Fishman's
Pulmonary Diseases and Disorders

Volume 1

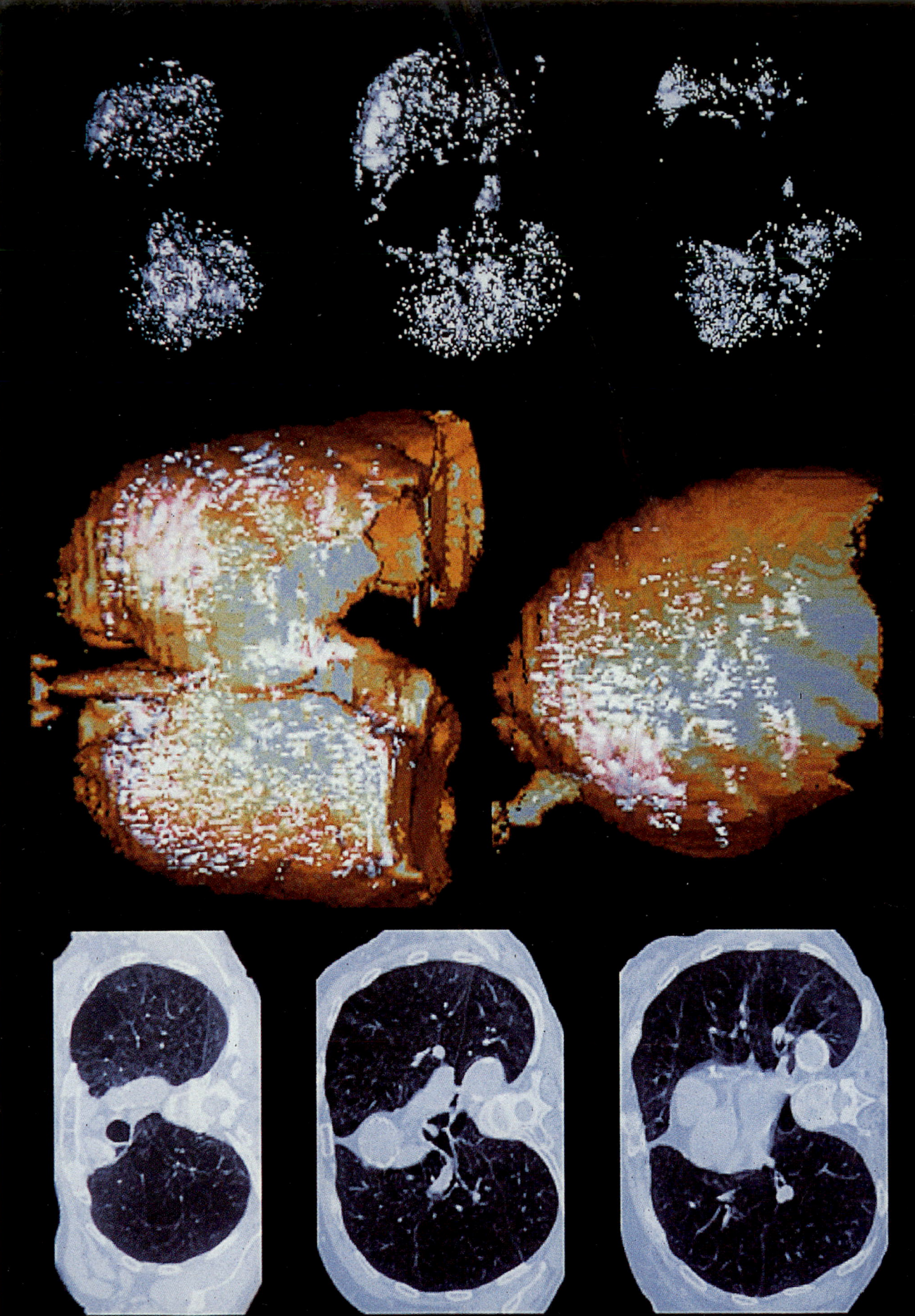

Frontispiece: Legend appears on page v.

Fishman's
Pulmonary Diseases
and Disorders
Third Edition

Volume 1

EDITOR-IN-CHIEF

Alfred P. Fishman, M.D.

William Maul Measey Professor of Medicine
University of Pennsylvania Medical Center
Philadelphia, Pennsylvania

SECTION EDITORS

Jack A. Elias, M.D.

Chief, Pulmonary and Critical Care Medicine
Yale University School of Medicine
New Haven, Connecticut

Jay A. Fishman, M.D.

Infectious Diseases Unit
Massachusetts General Hospital-East
Charlestown, Massachusetts

Michael A. Grippi, M.D.

Vice Chairman, Clinical Affairs
University of Pennsylvania Medical Center
Philadelphia, Pennsylvania

Larry R. Kaiser, M.D.

Director, Lung Transplant
Division of Cardiothoracic Surgery
University of Pennsylvania Medical Center
Philadelphia, Pennsylvania

Robert M. Senior, M.D.

Professor, Jewish Hospital
Washington University Medical Center
St. Louis, Missouri

McGraw-Hill
Health Professions Division

New York St. Louis San Francisco Auckland Bogotá Caracas Lisbon London Madrid
Mexico City Milan Montreal New Delhi San Juan Singapore Sydney Tokyo Toronto

McGraw-Hill

A Division of The McGraw-Hill Companies

Fishman's
Pulmonary Diseases and Disorders

1234567890 DOWDOW 9987

ISBN 0-07-911167-X (set)
ISBN 0-07-021179-5 (volume 1)
ISBN 0-07-021180-9 (volume 2)

This book was set in Times Roman by York Graphic Services, Inc.
The editors were J. Dereck Jeffers and Lester A. Sheinis;
the production supervisors were Robert R. Laffler and Helene G. Landers;
the text designer was Marsha Cohen / Parallelogram;
the cover designer was Edward R. Schultheis;
the indexer was Irving Condé Tullar.
R. R. Donnelley & Sons Company was printer and binder.
This book is printed on acid-free paper.

Library of Congress Cataloging-in-Publication Data

Fishman's pulmonary diseases and disorders / editor-in-chief, Alfred P. Fishman; section
editors, Jack A. Elias . . . [et al.].—3rd ed.
    p. cm.
  Rev. ed. of: Pulmonary diseases and disorders. 2nd ed. c1988.
  Includes bibliographical references and index.
  ISBN 0-07-911167-X (set).—ISBN 0-07-021179-5 (v. 1).—ISBN 0-07-021180-9 (v. 2)
  1. Lungs—Diseases. I. Fishman, Alfred P. II. Elias, Jack A. III. Pulmonary diseases and
disorders. IV. Title: Pulmonary diseases and disorders.
  [DNLM: 1. Lung Diseases. WF 600 F537 1997]
RC756.P826 1997
616.2′4—DC20
DNLM/DLC
for Library of Congress   96-26303

Front cover: Lateral view of resin-cast of left human lung, with airways (yellow), pulmonary
arteries (red), and pulmonary veins (blue) filled out to fine lobular branches. *(Courtesy of
Dr. H. C. Walter Weber, Department of Anatomy, University of Bern, Switzerland.)*

Alfred P. Fishman, M.D.

To Linda, Hannah; Mark, Martha, Eric; Sarah; Jay, Gayle, Aaron, and Brian

Jack A. Elias, M.D.

To Sandy, Lauren, Alma, and Gabby

Jay A. Fishman, M.D.

To Aaron, Brian, and Gayle

Michael A. Grippi, M.D.

To Barbara, Kristen, and Amy

Larry R. Kaiser, M.D.

To Ruthy, Jeffrey, and Jonathan

Robert Senior, M.D.

To Jerry Flance, Jack Pierce, and Martha

FRONTISPIECE: Quantification of regional emphysema by three-dimensional maps of the lungs using newer CT techniques. *Left column:* High-resolution CT (HRCT) scans through upper, middle, and lower lobes. Areas of emphysema characterized by hypoattenuation and diminished pulmonary vasculature. *Center column:* Single breath-holding spiral CT scan. Three-dimensional shaded-surface displays. Areas of emphysema appear in white. *Top.* Both lungs, frontal projection. *Bottom.* Left lung, lateral projection. Distribution of emphysema is heterogeneous affecting predominantly the upper and middle zones. *Right column:* High-resolution CT (HRCT). Regional, three-dimensional axial projections of the upper, middle, and lower thirds of the lungs. The brightest areas correspond to the regions with highest concentrations of emphysema. *Right lung.* Emphysema occupies 23% of the total lung volume. *From top-to-bottom:* Emphysema occupies 43% of top third, 20% of middle third, and 17% of lower third. *Left lung.* Emphysema occupies 15% of the total lung volume. *From top-to-bottom:* 25%, 17%, and 7%, respectively. *(Courtesy of Krishanu B. Gupta, M.D., Ph.D., and Warren B. Gefter, M.D., Department of Radiology, University of Pennsylvania Medical Center.)*

Notice

Contents

Section 3
The Lungs in Different Physiological States

Section 4
Lung Immunology

Section 5
Lung Injury and Repair

Part Three

SYMPTOMS AND SIGNS OF RESPIRATORY DISEASE / 359

Section 6
Clinical Approach to the Patient

Section 7
Diagnostic Procedures

Part Four
OBSTRUCTIVE LUNG DISEASES / 643

Section 8
Chronic Obstructive Pulmonary Disease

Section 9
Asthma

Section 10
Other Obstructive Disorders

Part Seven

INTERSTITIAL AND INFLAMMATORY LUNG DISEASES / 1035

Section 13
Immunologic and Interstitial Diseases

Section 14
Depositional and Infiltrative Disorders

Part Eight

ALVEOLAR DISEASES / 1191

Part Nine

DISORDERS OF THE PULMONARY CIRCULATION / 1231

Part Ten

DISORDERS OF THE PLEURAL SPACE / 1387

APPENDIXES

Part Fifteen
NEOPLASMS OF THE LUNGS / 1693

Section 15
Cancer of the Lungs

Section 16
Lymphoproliferative Disorders

Section 19
Special Hosts and Opportunistic Infections

Section 20
Specific Microorganisms

Section 21
Mycobacterial Infections

Part Seventeen

ACUTE RESPIRATORY FAILURE / 2523

Section 22
Lung Failure

Section 23
Respiratory Pump Failure

Section 24
Management and Therapeutic Interventions

APPENDIXES

Contributors

MASAZUMI ADACHI, M.D., SC.D.
Director of Laboratories,
Isaac Albert Research Institute,
Kingsbrook Jewish Medical Center,
Brooklyn, New York
(Chapter 78)

ABASS ALAVI, M.D.
Professor of Radiology,
Chief, Nuclear Medicine,
Department of Radiology,
University of Pennsylvania,
Philadelphia, Pennsylvania
(Chapter 35)

STEVEN ALBELDA, M.D.
Associate Professor of Medicine,
Pulmonary and Critical Care Division,
University of Pennsylvania Medical Center,
Philadelphia, Pennsylvania
(Chapter 92)

MURRAY D. ALTOSE, M.D.
Professor of Medicine,
Chief of Staff,
Case Western Reserve University,
VA Medical Center,
Cleveland, Ohio
(Chapter 10)

MICHEL AOUN, M.D.
Attending Physician,
Department of Medicine,
Institut Jules Bordet,
Brussels, Belgium
(Chapter 123)

CARLOS A. ARES, M.D.
Pulmonary and Critical Care Medicine,
Winthrop Pulmonary Associates, PC,
Mineola, New York
(Chapter 110)

DONALD ARMSTRONG, M.D.
Chief, Infectious Disease Service,
Memorial Sloan-Kettering Cancer Center,
New York, New York
(Chapter 146)

JOHN R. BACH, M.D.
Professor and Chair,
Department of Pulmonary Medicine and Rehabilitation,
UMD-New Jersey Medical School,
University Hospital,
Newark, New Jersey
(Chapter 99)

ANN SULLIVAN BAKER, M.D.[†]
Associate Professor of Medicine, HMS,
Infectious Disease Unit,
Massachusetts General Hospital,
Boston, Massachusetts
(Chapter 126)

JOHN G. BARTLETT, M.D.
Professor of Medicine and Chief,
Division of Infectious Disease,
Johns Hopkins University School of Medicine,
Baltimore, Maryland
(Chapter 129)

† Deceased.

MICHAEL F. BEERS, M.D.
Assistant Professor of Medicine,
Institute for Environmental Medicine,
University of Pennsylvania School of Medicine,
Philadelphia, Pennsylvania
(Chapter 172)

JEFFREY S. BERMAN, M.D.
Associate Professor of Medicine
Chief, Pulmonary and Critical Care Medicine,
Pulmonary Center,
Boston University School of Medicine,
Boston, Massachusetts
(Chapter 21)

ALAN L. BISNO, M.D.
Chief, Medical Service,
Miami VA Medical Center,
Miami, Florida
(Chapter 142)

PETER D. BITTERMAN, M.D.
Professor of Medicine,
Division of Pulmonary and Critical Care Medicine,
University of Minnesota,
Minneapolis, Minnesota
(Chapter 27)

CHARLES D. BLANKE, M.D.
Assistant Professor of Medicine,
Division of Medical Oncology,
Vanderbilt University School of Medicine,
The Vanderbilt Clinic,
Nashville, Tennessee
(Chapter 114)

CHRISTINE A. BLASKI, M.D.
Division of Pulmonary, Critical Care, and Occupational Medicine,
University of Iowa Hospitals and Clinics,
Iowa City, Iowa
(Chapter 61)

ALAN B. BLOCH, M.D., M.P.H.
Medical Epidemiologist,
Division of Tuberculosis Elimination,
National Center for HIV, STD, TB Prevention,
Centers for Disease Control and Prevention,
Atlanta, Georgia
(Chapter 161)

SIDNEY S. BRAMAN, M.D.
Professor of Medicine,
Brown University School of Medicine,
Rhode Island Hospital,
Providence, Rhode Island
(Chapter 52)

PETER H. BURRI, M.D.
Professor and Chairman
Institute of Anatomy
University of Bern
Bern, Switzerland
(Chapter 5)

MICHAEL E. BURT, M.D., PH.D.
Attending Surgeon,
Thoracic Surgery Department,
Memorial Sloan-Kettering Cancer Center,
New York, New York
(Chapter 117)

WILLIAM W. BUSSE, M.D.
Professor, Department of Medicine,
Head, Allergy and Clinical Immunology,
Clinical Science Center,
University of Wisconsin Hospital and Clinics,
Madison, Wisconsin
(Chapter 47)

JAY C. BUTLER, M.D.
Assistant Chief, Respiratory Diseases,
Division of Bacterial and Mycotic Diseases,
National Center for Infectious Disease, Centers for
Disease Control and Prevention,
Atlanta, Georgia
(Chapter 153)

EDWARD J. CAMPBELL, M.D.
Associate Professor of Medicine,
Division of Respiratory, Critical Care, and Occupational Pulmonary Medicine,
University of Utah,
Salt Lake City, Utah
(Chapter 19)

DAVID M. CENTER, M.D.
Professor of Medicine
Chief, Pulmonary and Critical Care Medicine,
Boston University School of Medicine,
The Pulmonary Center,
Boston, Massachusetts
(Chapter 21)

RICHARD E. CHAISSON, M.D.
Director, AIDS Service,
Division of Infectious Diseases,
Johns Hopkins University,
Baltimore, Maryland
(Chapter 163)

NEIL S. CHERNIACK, M.D.
Director, Clinical Affairs,
Dean's Office,
Case Western Reserve University,
Cleveland, Ohio
(Chapter 11)

JOHN W. CHRISTMAN, M.D.
Assistant Professor of Medicine,
Division of Pulmonary Medicine,
Vanderbilt University School of Medicine,
Nashville, Tennessee
(Chapter 166)

JOHN P. CHUTE, M.D.
National Cancer Institute–Navy Medical Oncology Branch,
National Naval Medical Center,
Bethesda, Maryland
(Chapter 116)

JAMES M. CLARK, M.D., PH.D.
Clinical Associate Professor of Environmental Medicine in Pharmacology,
Institute for Environmental Medicine,
University of Pennsylvania,
Philadelphia, Pennsylvania
(Chapter 64)

J. ALLEN D. COOPER, JR., M.D.
Associate Professor of Medicine,
Chief, Pulmonary Section,
University of Alabama at Birmingham,
Birmingham, Alabama
(Chapter 60)

ANTHONY CORBET, M.B.B.S.
Clinical Professor of Pediatrics,
University of Texas Health Science Center,
San Antonio, Texas
(Chapter 169)

ROBERT O. CRAPO, M.D.
Medical Director, Pulmonary Laboratory,
LDS Hospital,
Salt Lake City, Utah
(Chapter 19)

ROBERT S. CRAUSMAN, M.D.
Director, Internal Medicine Residency Program,
Memorial Hospital of Rhode Island,
Pawtucket, Rhode Island
(Chapters 76, 77)

STEPHEN W. CRAWFORD, M.D.
Associate Professor of Medicine,
Critical Care Director,
University of Washington,
Fred Hutchinson Cancer Research Center,
Seattle, Washington
(Chapter 137)

GERARD JOSEPH CRINER, M.D.
Associate Professor of Medicine,
Director, Pulmonary and Critical Care Medicine,
Temple University Hospital,
Philadelphia, Pennsylvania
(Chapters 98, 171)

ARTHUR M. DANNENBERG, JR., M.D., PH.D.
Professor, Environmental Health Sciences, Molecular Microbiology and
Immunology, and Epidemiology
Johns Hopkins School of Hygiene and Public Health,
Baltimore, Maryland
(Chapter 160)

DAVID M. DAUGHTON, M.S.
Behavioral Researcher,
Pulmonary and Critical Care Division,
University of Nebraska Medical Center,
Omaha, Nebraska
(Chapter 45)

PAUL T. DAVIDSON, M.D.
Director, Tuberculosis Control,
Public Health Programs and Services,
Los Angeles County Department of Health Services,
Los Angeles, California
(Chapter 164)

RICHARD O. DAVIES, D.V.M., PH.D.
Professor of Physiology,
Animal Biology,
University of Pennsylvania,
Philadelphia, Pennsylvania
(Chapter 101)

MALCOLM M. DECAMP, JR., M.D.
Assistant Professor of Surgery,
Division of Thoracic Surgery,
Brigham and Women's Hospital,
Boston, Massachusetts
(Chapter 95)

MARC DECRAMER, M.D., PH.D.
Professor of Medicine,
Respiratory Division,
University Hospitals,
Leuven, Belgium
(Chapter 3)

HORACE M. DELISSER, M.D.
Assistant Professor of Medicine,
Pulmonary and Critical Care Division,
University of Pennsylvania Medical Center,
Philadelphia, Pennsylvania
(Chapter 40)

RICHARD A. DEREMEE, M.D.
Professor of Medicine,
Mayo Medical School, Mayo Clinic,
Rochester, Minnesota
(Chapter 86)

CLIFFORD S. DEUTSCHMAN, M.D.
Associate Professor of Anesthesia,
University of Pennsylvania Medical Center,
Philadelphia, Pennsylvania
(Chapter 168)

LISA L. DEVER, M.D.
Assistant Professor,
Department of Medicine, VAMC,
Division of Infectious Diseases,
UMD-New Jersey Medical School,
East Orange, New Jersey
(Chapter 119)

GORDON M. DICKINSON, M.D.
Professor of Medicine,
Division of Infectious Diseases,
University of Miami School of Medicine,
Miami, Florida
(Chapter 142)

FRANCIS W. DIPIERRO, M.D.
Instructor, Department of Surgery,
University of Pennsylvania School of Medicine,
Philadelphia, Pennsylvania
(Chapter 105)

ROBERT J. DOWNEY, M.D.
Attending Thoracic Surgeon,
Director, Surgical Critical Care,
Memorial Sloan-Kettering Cancer Center,
New York, New York
(Chapter 104)

MARLENE DURAND, M.D.
Assistant in Medicine,
Infectious Disease Unit,
Massachusetts General Hospital,
Boston, Massachusetts
(Chapter 126)

JEFFREY D. EDELMAN, M.D.
Pulmonary and Critical Care Division,
University of Pennsylvania Medical Center,
Philadelphia, Pennsylvania
(Chapter 58)

JACK A. ELIAS, M.D.
Professor and Chief,
Pulmonary and Critical Care Medicine,
Department of Internal Medicine,
Yale University School of Medicine,
New Haven, Connecticut
(Chapter 20)

PAUL E. EPSTEIN, M.D.
Chief, Pulmonary Division,
Graduate Hospital,
Philadelphia, Pennsylvania
(Chapter 41)

ALAN M. FEIN, M.D.
Director, Pulmonary and Critical Care Medicine,
Winthrop Pulmonary Associates, PC,
Mineola, New York
(Chapter 110)

STEVEN H. FEINSILVER, M.D.
Director, Pulmonary and Critical Care Medicine, Training Program,
Winthrop Pulmonary Associates, PC,
Mineola, New York
(Chapter 110)

GREGORY A. FILICE, M.D.
Chief, Infectious Disease Section,
VA Medical Center,
Associate Professor of Medicine,
University of Minnesota Medical School,
Minneapolis, Minnesota
(Chapter 146)

SYDNEY M. FINEGOLD, M.D.
Staff Physician, Medical Services,
Department of Veterans Affairs Medical Center,
Los Angeles, California
(Chapter 130)

JAMES E. FISH, M.D.
Director, Pulmonary and Critical Care Medicine,
Jefferson Medical College,
Philadelphia, Pennsylvania
(Chapter 50)

ALFRED P. FISHMAN, M.D.
William Maul Measey Professor of Medicine,
Department of Rehabilitation Medicine,
University of Pennsylvania Medical Center,
Philadelphia, Pennsylvania
(Chapters 1, 16, 28, 30, 36, 42, 55, 75, 82, 83, 84, 109)

JAY ALAN FISHMAN, M.D., F.A.C.P.
Associate Physician,
Infectious Diseases Unit,
Massachusetts General Hospital-East,
Charlestown, Massachusetts
(Chapters 130, 133, 134, 135, 136, 138, 150)

HENNING A. GAISSERT, M.D.
Assistant Professor of Surgery,
Brown University School of Medicine,
Rhode Island Hospital,
Providence, Rhode Island
(Chapter 52)

GREGORY P. GEBA, M.D.
Assistant Professor of Medicine,
Pulmonary and Critical Care Medicine,
Yale University School of Medicine,
New Haven, Connecticut
(Chapter 49)

CHARLES F. P. GEORGE, M.D.
Associate Professor of Medicine,
University of Western Ontario,
Director of Sleep Laboratory,
London Health Sciences Centre–Victoria Campus,
London, Ontario, Canada
(Chapter 103)

RONALD B. GEORGE, M.D.
Professor and Chairman, Department of Medicine,
Louisiana State University,
Shreveport, Louisiana
(Chapter 44)

ANDREW N. GOLDBERG, M.D.
Assistant Professor,
Department of Otorhinolaryngology,
Hospital of the University of Pennsylvania,
Philadelphia, Pennsylvania
(Chapter 102)

STANLEY GOLDFARB, M.D.
Vice Chairman, Network Development,
Department of Medicine,
University of Pennsylvania Medical Center,
Philadelphia, Pennsylvania
(Chapter 15)

MITCHELL GOLDMAN, M.D.
Assistant Professor of Medicine,
Department of Medicine,
Wishard Memorial Hospital,
Indianapolis, Indiana
(Chapter 149)

DANIEL M. GOODENBERGER, M.D.
Associate Professor of Medicine,
Washington University School of Medicine,
St. Louis, Missouri
(Chapter 87)

JONATHAN GOTTLIEB, M.D.
Pulmonary and Critical Care Medicine
Thomas Jefferson University Hospital
Philadelphia, Pennsylvania
(Chapter 175)

STEPHEN B. GREENBERG, M.D.
Professor and Vice Chairman,
Department of Medicine,
Baylor College of Medicine,
Houston, Texas
(Chapter 151)

JEFFREY K. GRIFFITHS, M.D., M.P.H., T.M.
Assistant Professor of Medicine,
Tufts University School of Medicine,
Director, Microbiology,
St. Elizabeth's Medical Center,
Brighton, Massachusetts
(Chapter 155)

MICHAEL A. GRIPPI, M.D.
Associate Professor of Medicine,
Vice Chairman, Clinical Affairs,
University of Pennsylvania Medical Center,
Philadelphia, Pennsylvania
(Chapters 36, 40, 165)

PRABODH K. GUPTA, M.D.
Director, Cytopathology and Cytometry,
Pathology and Laboratory Medicine,
University of Pennsylvania Medical Center
Philadelphia, Pennsylvania
(Chapter 33)

IMAD Y. HADDAD, M.D.
Assistant Professor of Pediatrics,
University of Alabama at Birmingham,
Birmingham, Alabama
(Chapter 26)

JOHN HANSEN-FLASCHEN, M.D.
Associate Professor and Chief,
Pulmonary and Critical Care Division,
University of Pennsylvania Medical Center,
Philadelphia, Pennsylvania
(Chapter 179)

C. WILLIAM HANSON III, M.D.
Assistant Professor of Anesthesia, Surgery, and Internal Medicine,
University of Pennsylvania Medical Center,
Philadelphia, Pennsylvania
(Chapter 174)

WILLIAM D. HARDIN, JR., M.D.
Associate Professor of Surgery and Pediatrics,
The Children's Hospital of Alabama,
Birmingham, Alabama
(Chapter 140)

HOWARD M. HELLER, M.D.
Instructor in Medicine,
Harvard Medical School,
Massachusetts Institute of Technology,
Medical Department,
Cambridge, Massachusetts
(Chapter 157)

HARRY R. HILL, M.D.
Professor, Departments of Pathology and Pediatrics,
Head, Division of Clinical Immunology and Allergy,
University of Utah School of Medicine,
Salt Lake City, Utah
(Chapter 139)

MICHAEL P. HLASTALA, PH.D.
Professor, Physiology and Biophysics,
Pulmonary and Critical Care Medicine,
University of Washington,
Seattle, Washington
(Chapter 14)

ANN D. HOROWITZ, PH.D.
Instructor of Pediatrics,
Children's Hospital Medical Center,
Division of Pulmonary Biology,
Cincinnati, Ohio
(Chapter 7)

LEONARD D. HUDSON, M.D.
Head, Pulmonary and Critical Care Medicine,
University of Washington,
Harborview Medical Center,
Seattle, Washington
(Chapter 167)

SUZANNE S. HURD, PH.D.
Director, Division of Lung Diseases,
National Heart, Lung, and Blood Institute, National Institutes of Health,
Bethesda, Maryland
(Chapter 182)

BRIAN V. JEGASOTHY, M.D.
Professor and Chairman,
Department of Dermatology,
University of Pittsburgh,
Pittsburgh, Pennsylvania
(Chapter 29)

WALDEMAR G. JOHANSON, JR., M.D.
Professor and Chairman,
Department of Medicine,
UMD-New Jersey Medical School,
Newark, New Jersey
(Chapter 119)

BRUCE E. JOHNSON, M.D.
National Cancer Institute,
Navy Medical Oncology Branch,
National Naval Medical Center,
Bethesda, Maryland
(Chapter 116)

DAVID H. JOHNSON, M.D.
Director,
Vanderbilt University School of Medicine,
Division of Medical Oncology,
The Vanderbilt Clinic,
Nashville, Tennessee
(Chapter 114)

LARRY R. KAISER, M.D.
Associate Professor of Surgery,
Department of Surgery,
University of Pennsylvania Medical Center,
Philadelphia, Pennsylvania
[Chapters 39, 96, 105, 113 (Part I)]

KUSHAGRA KATARIYA, M.D.
Chief Resident,
Department of Surgery,
Beth Israel Medical Center,
New York, New York
(Chapter 115)

STEVEN M. KELLER, M.D.
Chief, Division of Thoracic Surgery,
Director, David B. Kriser Lung Cancer Center,
Department of Surgery,
Beth Israel Medical Center,
New York, New York
(Chapter 115)

MARK A. KELLEY, M.D.
Professor of Medicine,
Vice Dean for Clinical Affairs,
University of Pennsylvania Medical Center,
Philadelphia, Pennsylvania
(Chapters 84, 180)

STEVEN G. KELSEN, M.D.
Professor of Medicine and Physiology,
Temple University Hospital,
Philadelphia, Pennsylvania
(Chapters 98, 171)

DAVID KENT, M.D.
Chief Medical Resident,
The Cambridge Hospital,
Cambridge, Massachusetts
(Chapter 141)

JEFFREY A. KERN, M.D.
Associate Professor of Medicine,
Department of Internal Medicine,
University of Iowa Hospitals and Clinics,
Iowa City, Iowa
(Chapter 107)

GARY T. KINASEWITZ, M.D.
Professor of Medicine, Physiology, and Biophysics,
University of Oklahoma,
Oklahoma City, Oklahoma
(Chapter 88)

TALMADGE E. KING, JR., M.D.
Senior Faculty Member,
Vice Chairman for Clinical Affairs,
Department of Medicine,
National Jewish Center for Immunology and Respiratory Medicine,
Denver, Colorado
(Chapters 54, 76, 77)

JEAN A. KLASTERSKY, M.D.
Professor and Chief of Medicine,
Department of Medicine,
Institut Jules Bordet,
Brussels, Belgium
(Chapter 123)

ROBERT A. KLOCKE, M.D.
Professor and Chairman,
Department of Medicine,
State University of New York at Buffalo,
Buffalo, New York
(Chapter 13)

MICHAEL I. KOTLIKOFF, PH.D., D.V.M.
Professor and Chairman, Animal Biology,
School of Veterinary Medicine,
University of Pennsylvania,
Philadelphia, Pennsylvania
(Chapter 6)

ROBERT M. KOTLOFF, M.D.
Assistant Professor of Medicine,
Pulmonary and Critical Care Medicine,
University of Pennsylvania Medical Center,
Philadelphia, Pennsylvania
(Chapter 170)

MEIR H. KRYGER, M.D.
Professor of Medicine,
Director, Sleep Research,
St. Boniface Hospital Research Center,
Winnipeg, Manitoba, Canada
(Chapter 103)

LESZEK KUBIN, PH.D.
Research Associate Professor,
Department of Animal Biology,
School of Veterinary Medicine,
Philadelphia, Pennsylvania
(Chapter 101)

STEVEN L. KUNKEL, PH.D.
Professor, Department of Pathology,
University of Michigan Medical School,
Ann Arbor, Michigan
(Chapter 24)

SUKHAMAY LAHIRI, PH.D.
Professor, Department of Physiology,
University of Pennsylvania School of Medicine,
Philadelphia, Pennsylvania
(Chapter 63)

KENNETH S. LANDRETH, PH.D.
Professor, Department of Microbiology and Immunology,
West Virginia University,
Mary Barb Randolph Cancer Center,
Morgantown, West Virginia
(Chapter 23)

PAUL N. LANKEN, M.D.
Associate Professor of Medicine,
Medical Intensive Care Unit,
University of Pennsylvania Medical Center,
Philadelphia, Pennsylvania
(Chapter 181)

JAMES W. LEATHERMAN, M.D.
Associate Professor of Medicine,
Pulmonary and Critical Care Medicine,
University of Minnesota,
Hennepin County Medical Center,
Minneapolis, Minnesota
(Chapter 79)

CLAUDE LENFANT, M.D.
Director, National Heart, Lung, and Blood Institute,
National Institutes of Health,
Bethesda, Maryland
(Chapter 182)

LESLIE A. LITZKY, M.D.
Assistant Professor of Medicine,
Department of Pathology and Laboratory Medicine,
University of Pennsylvania,
Philadelphia, Pennsylvania
(Chapters 92, 111)

JACOB S. LOKE, M.D.
Clinical Professor of Medicine,
Pulmonary Medicine,
Yale University School of Medicine,
New Haven, Connecticut
(Chapter 65)

WALKER A. LONG, M.D.
Associate Professor of Pediatrics,
Pediatric Cardiology Division,
University of North Carolina,
Chapel Hill, North Carolina
(Chapter 169)

JOSEPH P. LYNCH III, M.D.
Professor of Internal Medicine,
The University of Michigan Medical Center,
Ann Arbor, Michigan
(Chapters 70, 79)

MITCHELL MACHTAY, M.D.
Assistant Professor,
Department of Radiation Oncology,
University of Pennsylvania Medical Center,
Philadelphia, Pennsylvania
[Chapter 113 (Part III)]

ADEL A. F. MAHMOUD, M.D., PH.D.
The John H. Hord Professor and Chairman,
Department of Medicine,
University Hospitals of Cleveland,
Cleveland, Ohio
(Chapter 156)

SAVVAS C. MAKRIDES, PH.D.
Director of Molecular Biology,
T Cell Sciences, Inc.,
Needham, Massachusetts
(Chapter 9)

SCOTT MANAKER, M.D., PH.D.
Assistant Professor of Medicine and Pharmacology,
Pulmonary and Critical Care Division,
University of Pennsylvania,
Philadelphia, Pennsylvania
(Chapter 173)

MITCHELL L. MARGOLIS, M.D.
Chief, Pulmonary Division,
Philadelphia VA Medical Center,
Philadelphia, Pennsylvania
(Chapter 112)

JOHN J. MARINI, M.D.
Professor of Medicine,
University of Minnesota,
St. Paul Ramsey Medical Center,
St. Paul, Minnesota
(Chapter 177)

THOMAS J. MARRIE, M.D.
Professor of Medicine,
Victoria General Hospital,
Department of Medicine, Infectious Diseases,
Halifax, Nova Scotia, Canada
(Chapter 127)

SADIS MATALON, PH.D.
Professor, Department of Anesthesiology,
University of Alabama at Birmingham,
Birmingham, Alabama
(Chapter 26)

C. GLEN MAYHALL, M.D.
Department of Internal Medicine,
University of Texas Medical Branch at Galveston,
Galveston, Texas
(Chapter 143)

F. DENNIS McCOOL, M.D.
Associate Professor of Medicine,
Pulmonary Division,
Memorial Hospital of Rhode Island,
Pawtucket, Rhode Island
(Chapter 97)

PAUL B. McCRAY, JR., M.D.
Associate Professor,
Department of Pediatrics,
University of Iowa College of Medicine,
Iowa City, Iowa
(Chapter 8)

VINCENT G. McDERMOTT, M.B., M.R.C.P.I., F.R.C.R.
Assistant Professor of Radiology,
Department of Diagnostic Radiology,
Duke University Medical Center,
Durham, North Carolina
(Chapter 34)

DAVID S. McKINSEY, M.D.
Clinical Associate Professor of Medicine,
University of Kansas School of Medicine,
Research Medical Center,
Kansas City, Missouri
(Chapter 142)

GEOFFREY McLENNAN, M.B.B.S., F.R.A.C.P.
Associate Professor of Medicine,
Pulmonary and Critical Care Medicine,
University of Iowa Hospitals and Clinics,
Iowa City, Iowa
(Chapter 107)

JOSEPH L. MELNICK, M.D., PH.D.
Distinguished Service Professor of Virology,
Division of Molecular Virology,
Baylor College of Medicine,
Houston, Texas
(Chapter 154)

SAUMIL N. MERCHANT, M.D.
Assistant Professor, Otology and Laryngology,
Assistant Surgeon in Otolaryngology,
Massachusetts Eye and Ear Infirmary,
Boston, Massachusetts
(Chapter 126)

LOUIS F. METZGER, R.P.F.T.
Administrative Director,
Center for Sleep and Respiratory Neurobiology,
University of Pennsylvania Medical Center,
Philadelphia, Pennsylvania
(Chapter 36)

JAMES L. MICHEL, M.D., PH.D.
Assistant Professor of Medicine,
Microbiology and Molecular Genetics,
Channing Laboratory,
Harvard Medical School,
Boston, Massachusetts
(Chapter 125)

JAMES S. MILLEDGE, M.D.
Emeritus,
Clinical Research Centre,
Northwick Park Hospital,
Harrow, Middlesex, England
(Chapter 63)

WALLACE T. MILLER, M.D.
Professor of Radiology,
University of Pennsylvania,
Philadelphia, Pennsylvania
(Chapter 32)

DAVID R. MOLLER, M.D.
Assistant Professor of Medicine,
Director, Sarcoid Clinic,
Johns Hopkins School of Medicine,
Baltimore, Maryland
(Chapter 69)

ADRIAN R. MORRISON, D.V.M., PH.D.
Professor of Behavioral Neuroscience,
School of Veterinary Medicine,
University of Pennsylvania,
Philadelphia, Pennsylvania
(Chapter 100)

MAURICE A. MUFSON, M.D.
Professor and Chairman,
Department of Medicine,
Marshall University School of Medicine,
Huntington, West Virginia
(Chapter 145)

DAVID M. MURPHY, M.D.
Clinical Associate Professor of Medicine
Chief, Pulmonary Medicine Department,
Deborah Heart and Lung Center,
Browns Mills, New Jersey
(Chapter 55)

EDWARD A. NARDELL, M.D.
Chief, Pulmonary Medicine,
Assistant Professor of Medicine, HMS,
The Cambridge Hospital,
Cambridge, Massachusetts
(Chapter 141)

RONALD LEE NICHOLS, M.D.
William Henderson Professor of Surgery,
Department of Surgery,
Tulane University Medical Center,
New Orleans, Louisiana
(Chapter 140)

JERRY A. NICK, M.D.
Instructor, Division of Pulmonary Sciences and Critical Care Medicine,
Worthen Lab,
National Jewish Center,
Denver, Colorado
(Chapter 25)

MICHAEL S. NIEDERMAN, M.D.
Associate Professor of Medicine,
Director, Critical Care Subsection,
Pulmonary and Critical Care Unit,
Winthrop-University Hospital,
Mineola, New York
(Chapter 122)

RICHARD H. OCHS, M.D.
Adjunct Clinical Professor and Director,
Department of Pathology and Laboratory Medicine,
Bryn Mawr Hospital,
Bryn Mawr, Pennsylvania
(Chapter 75)

ELIZABETH A. OLEK, D.O.
Instructor in Medicine,
Infectious Diseases Section,
Boston University Medical Center Hospital,
Boston, Massachusetts
(Chapter 147)

A. FUSON ONER-EYUBOGLU, M.D.
Instructor in Medicine,
Pulmonary and Critical Care Medicine,
University of Pennsylvania Medical Center,
Philadelphia, Pennsylvania
(Chapter 162)

IDA M. ONORATO, M.D.
Chief, Surveillance and Epidemiologic Investigations Branch,
Division of TB Elimination, Centers for Disease Control and Prevention,
Atlanta, Georgia
(Chapter 158)

ALLAN I. PACK, M.D., PH.D.
Professor of Medicine,
Center for Sleep and Respiratory Neurobiology,
University of Pennsylvania Medical Center,
Philadelphia, Pennsylvania
(Chapters 11, 101, 102)

HAROLD I. PALEVSKY, M.D.
Associate Professor of Medicine,
Pulmonary and Critical Care Division,
University of Pennsylvania Medical Center,
Philadelphia, Pennsylvania
(Chapter 84)

REYNOLD A. PANETTIERI, JR., M.D.
Assistant Professor of Medicine,
Pulmonary and Critical Care Division,
University of Pennsylvania Medical Center,
Philadelphia, Pennsylvania
(Chapter 6)

JOHN E. PARKER, M.D.
Division of Respiratory Disease Studies,
National Institute for Occupational Safety and Health,
Morgantown, West Virginia
(Chapter 59)

DAVID E. PARRY, M.D.
Instructor, Allergy and Clinical Immunology,
University of Wisconsin Hospital and Clinics,
Madison, Wisconsin
(Chapter 47)

MARK S. PASTERNACK, M.D.
Chief, Pediatric Infectious Disease Unit,
Massachusetts General Hospital,
Charlestown, Massachusetts
(Chapter 128)

ROY PATTERSON, M.D.
Chief of Allergy and Immunology,
Northwestern University Medical School,
Chicago, Illinois
(Chapter 51)

CYNTHIA S. PAYNE, M.D.
Assistant Professor of Radiology,
Department of Diagnostic Radiology,
Duke University Medical Center,
Durham, North Carolina
(Chapter 34)

ANDERS PERSSON, M.D., PH.D.
Assistant Professor of Medicine,
Respiratory and Critical Care Division,
Barnes-Jewish Hospital (North Campus),
St. Louis, Missouri
(Chapter 81)

JAY I. PETERS, M.D.
Associate Professor of Medicine,
Department of Medicine,
University of Texas Health Sciences Center,
Audie Murphy VA,
San Antonio, Texas
(Chapter 91)

STEPHEN P. PETERS, M.D., PH.D.
Professor of Medicine,
Jefferson Medical College,
Philadelphia, Pennsylvania
(Chapter 50)

EDWARD L. PETSONK, M.D.
Chief of Clinical Section,
Division of Respiratory Disease Studies,
National Institute for Occupational Safety and Health,
Morgantown, West Virginia
(Chapter 59)

KATHLEEN D. PFEFFER, M.D.
Assistant Professor of Medicine,
Division of Pulmonary Medicine,
Department of Pediatrics,
University of Utah School of Medicine,
Salt Lake City, Utah
(Chapter 139)

GERALD B. PIER, PH.D.
Associate Professor of Medicine,
Microbiology and Molecular Genetics,
Harvard Medical School,
Channing Laboratory,
Boston, Massachusetts
(Chapter 125)

GIUSEPPE G. PIETRA, M.D.
Professor, Pathology and Laboratory Medicine,
Division of Anatomic Pathology,
University of Pennsylvania Medical Center,
Philadelphia, Pennsylvania
(Chapter 118)

SUSAN K. PINGLETON, M.D.
Professor of Medicine,
Pulmonary and Critical Care Medicine,
University of Kansas Medical Center,
Kansas City, Kansas
(Chapter 178)

BRUCE R. PITT, PH.D.
Professor of Pharmacology,
University of Pittsburgh School of Medicine,
Pittsburgh, Pennsylvania
(Chapter 26)

JOHN POPOVICH, JR., M.D.
Division Head,
Division of Pulmonary and Critical Care Medicine,
Henry Ford Hospital,
Detroit, Michigan
(Chapter 18)

PIETER E. POSTMUS, M.D.
Department of Pulmonology,
Free University Hospital,
Amsterdam, The Netherlands
(Chapter 108)

JOE B. PUTNAM, JR., M.D.
Associate Professor of Surgery,
Thoracic and Cardiovascular Surgery,
The University of Texas,
M.D. Anderson Cancer Center
Houston, Texas
(Chapter 93)

GANESH RAGHU, M.D.
Associate Professor of Medicine,
Pulmonary and Critical Care Medicine,
University of Washington Medical Center,
Seattle, Washington
(Chapter 68)

DONALD G. RAIBLE, M.D.
Associate Professor of Medicine,
Medical College of Pennsylvania and Hahnemann University,
Philadelphia, Pennsylvania
(Chapter 22)

CARRIE A. REDLICH, M.D.
Associate Professor of Medicine,
Pulmonary and Critical Care Medicine,
Yale University School of Medicine,
New Haven, Connecticut
(Chapter 56)

STEPHEN I. RENNARD, M.D.
Chief, Pulmonary and Critical Care Medicine,
University of Nebraska Medical Center,
Omaha, Nebraska
(Chapter 45)

HERBERT Y. REYNOLDS, M.D.
J. Lloyd Huck Professor of Medicine,
Department of Medicine,
Milton S. Hershey Medical Center,
The Pennsylvania State University,
Hershey, Pennsylvania
(Chapter 20)

ELIZABETH A. RICH, M.D.
Associate Professor of Medicine,
Division of Pulmonary and Critical Care Medicine,
Case Western Reserve University,
Cleveland, Ohio
(Chapter 152)

RENÉE RIDZON, M.D.
Medical Epidemiologist,
Division of TB Elimination,
Centers for Disease Control,
Atlanta, Georgia
(Chapter 158)

ANDREW L. RIES, M.D.
Professor of Medicine,
Associate Director, Pulmonary Rehabilitation,
University of California Medical Center,
San Diego, California
(Chapter 46)

JEAN E. RINALDO, M.D.
Professor of Medicine,
Division of Pulmonary Medicine,
Vanderbilt University School of Medicine,
Nashville, Tennessee
(Chapter 166)

JOHN R. ROBERTS, M.D.
Assistant Professor of Surgery,
University of Pennsylvania Medical Center,
Philadelphia, Pennsylvania
(Chapter 96)

KENNETH B. ROBERTS, M.D.
Assistant Professor,
Department of Therapeutic Radiology,
Yale University School of Medicine,
New Haven, Connecticut
(Chapter 72)

CYNTHIA ROBINSON, M.D.
Assistant Professor, Pulmonary and Critical Care,
University of Pennsylvania,
Philadelphia, Pennsylvania
(Chapter 53)

KEITH M. ROBINSON, M.D.
Vice Chairman for Clinical Services,
Department of Rehabilitation Medicine,
University of Pennsylvania Medical Center,
Philadelphia, Pennsylvania
(Chapter 80)

CAROLYN L. ROCHESTER, M.D.
Assistant Professor of Medicine,
Section of Pulmonary and Critical Care,
Yale University School of Medicine,
New Haven, Connecticut
(Chapter 74)

DUDLEY F. ROCHESTER, M.D.
Professor Emeritus,
Department of Medicine,
University of Virginia,
Charlottesville, Virginia
(Chapter 97)

SARA ROCKWELL, PH.D.
Professor, Department of Therapeutic Radiology and Cancer Center,
Yale University School of Medicine,
New Haven, Connecticut
(Chapter 72)

WILLIAM N. ROM, M.D.
Professor of Medicine and Environmental Medicine,
Pulmonary and Critical Care Medicine,
Bellevue,
New York University Medical Center,
New York, New York
(Chapter 57)

JESSE ROMAN, M.D.
Chief, Pulmonary and Critical Care Section,
Department of Medicine,
Atlanta VA Medical Center,
Decatur, Georgia
(Chapter 4)

MILTON D. ROSSMAN, M.D.
Professor, Pulmonary and Critical Care,
University of Pennsylvania Medical Center,
Philadelphia, Pennsylvania
(Chapters 58, 162)

ROBERT H. RUBIN, M.D., F.A.C.P., F.C.C.P.
Chief, Transplantation Infectious Disease,
Massachusetts General Hospital,
Boston, Massachusetts
(Chapter 138)

MARK E. RUPP, M.D.
Assistant Professor of Medicine,
Department of Internal Medicine,
University of Nebraska Medical Center,
Omaha, Nebraska
(Chapter 131)

WILLIAM A. RUTALA, PH.D., M.P.H.
Professor of Medicine,
University of North Carolina,
Chapel Hill, North Carolina
(Chapter 143)

UNA S. RYAN, PH.D.
Vice President of Research,
T Cell Services, Inc.,
Needham, Massachusetts
(Chapter 9)

ANN V. SACKS, B.S., R.P.F.T.
Associate Director,
Pulmonary and Critical Care Medicine,
University of Pennsylvania Medical Center,
Philadelphia, Pennsylvania
(Chapter 36)

STEVEN A. SAHN, M.D.
Professor, Pulmonary and Critical Care Medicine,
Medical University of South Carolina,
Charleston, South Carolina
(Chapter 90)

EDWARD Y. SAKO, M.D., PH.D.
Assistant Professor,
Department of Surgery,
Division of Cardiothoracic Surgery,
The University of Texas Health Sciences Center at San Antonio,
San Antonio, Texas
(Chapter 91)

KEVIN E. SALHANY, M.D.
Assistant Professor,
Division of Anatomic Pathology,
University of Pennsylvania Medical Center,
Philadelphia, Pennsylvania
(Chapter 118)

JONATHAN M. SAMET, M.D.
Professor and Chairman,
Department of Epidemiology,
Johns Hopkins School of Hygiene and Public Health,
Baltimore, Maryland
(Chapter 62)

GERARDO S. SAN PEDRO, M.D.
Associate Professor of Clinical Medicine,
Pulmonary and Critical Care Medicine,
Louisiana State University Medical Center,
Shreveport, Louisiana
(Chapter 44)

WILLIAM T. SAUSE, M.D., F.A.C.R.
Associate Professor of Radiology,
University of Utah,
LDS Hospital,
Salt Lake City, Utah
[Chapter 113 (Part III)]

THOMAS F. SCANLIN, M.D.
Professor, Pediatrics,
Abramson Pediatric Center,
Children's Hospital of Philadelphia,
Philadelphia, Pennsylvania
(Chapter 53)

EDWARD S. SCHULMAN, M.D.
Professor of Medicine,
Allegheny University Hospital, Hahnemann Division,
Pulmonary and Critical Care Medicine,
Philadelphia, Pennsylvania
(Chapter 22)

DANIEL P. SCHUSTER, M.D.
Associate Professor of Medicine and Radiology,
Department of Internal Medicine,
Washington University School of Medicine,
St. Louis, Missouri
(Chapter 85)

MARK R. SCHUYLER, M.D.
Professor of Medicine,
Chief, Medical Service,
VA Medical Center,
Albuquerque, New Mexico
(Chapter 71)

RICHARD J. SCHWAB, M.D.
Assistant Professor of Medicine,
Medical Director, Penn Center for Sleep Disorders,
Hospital of the University of Pennsylvania,
Philadelphia, Pennsylvania
(Chapter 102)

DAVID A. SCHWARTZ, M.D.
Associate Professor,
Director, Occupational Medicine,
University of Iowa College of Medicine,
Iowa City, Iowa
(Chapter 61)

MARVIN I. SCHWARZ, M.D.
Professor of Medicine,
Head, Division of Pulmonary Sciences and Critical Care Medicine,
University of Colorado Health Services Center,
Denver, Colorado
(Chapter 73)

ROBERT M. SENIOR, M.D.
Dorothy R. and Hubert C. Moog Professor of Pulmonary Diseases in Medicine,
Washington University Medical Center,
Barnes-Jewish Hospital (North Campus),
St. Louis, Missouri
(Chapter 43)

STEVEN D. SHAPIRO, M.D.
Associate Professor of Medicine,
Barnes-Jewish Hospital (North Campus),
St. Louis, Missouri
(Chapter 43)

KUMAR SHARMA, PH.D.
Assistant Professor of Medicine,
Thomas Jefferson University,
Philadelphia, Pennsylvania
(Chapter 15)

MICHAEL S. SIMBERKOFF, M.D.
Chief, Infectious Diseases Section,
Veteran Affairs Medical Center,
New York, New York
(Chapter 124)

TONY P. SMITH, M.D.
Professor of Radiology,
Department of Diagnostic Radiology,
Duke University Medical Center,
Durham, North Carolina
(Chapter 34)

KENNETH P. STEINBERG, M.D.
Assistant Professor of Medicine,
University of Washington,
Harborview Medical Center,
Seattle, Washington
(Chapter 167)

DANIEL H. STERMAN, M.D.
Instructor of Medicine,
University of Pennsylvania Medical Center,
Philadelphia, Pennsylvania
(Chapters 38, 92)

ROBERT M. STRIETER, M.D.
Professor of Internal Medicine,
Division of Pulmonary and Critical Care Medicine,
University of Michigan,
Ann Arbor, Michigan
(Chapter 24)

ALAN M. SUGAR, M.D.
Associate Professor of Medicine,
Boston University Medical Center Hospital,
Boston, Massachusetts
(Chapter 147)

MORTON N. SWARTZ, M.D.
Professor of Medicine,
Infectious Diseases Unit,
Massachusetts General Hospital,
Boston, Massachusetts
(Chapters 121, 132)

ERIK R. SWENSON, M.D.
Associate Professor of Medicine,
Pulmonary Section,
University of Washington,
VA Medical Center,
Seattle, Washington
(Chapter 14)

LYNN T. TANOUE, M.D.
Assistant Professor of Medicine,
Yale School of Medicine,
Pulmonary and Critical Care Medicine,
New Haven, Connecticut
(Chapter 66)

C. RICHARD TAYLOR, PH.D.†
Charles P. Lyman Professor of Biology,
Museum of Comparative Zoology,
Harvard University,
Cambridge, Massachusetts
(Chapter 2)
†Deceased.

RICHARD TEPLICK, M.D.
Associate Professor of Anesthesia,
Department of Anesthesia,
Massachusetts General Hospital,
Boston, Massachusetts
(Chapter 133)

KAREN J. TIETZE, PHARM.D.
Associate Professor of Clinical Pharmacy,
Philadelphia College of Pharmacy and Science,
Philadelphia, Pennsylvania
(Chapter 173)

MARTIN J. TOBIN, M.D.
Professor and Chief,
Pulmonary and Critical Care Division,
Loyola University of Chicago,
Maywood, Illinois
(Chapter 176)

GALEN B. TOEWS, M.D.
Professor of Internal Medicine,
Chief, Pulmonary Medicine,
The University of Michigan Medical Center,
Ann Arbor, Michigan
(Chapters 70, 120)

JOSEPH F. TOMASHEFSKI, JR., M.D.
Associate Professor of Pathology,
Case Western Reserve University,
Metro Health Medical Center,
Cleveland, Ohio
(Chapter 160)

JOSEPH TREAT, M.D.
Division of Hematology-Oncology,
Department of Medicine,
University of Pennsylvania,
Philadelphia, Pennsylvania
[Chapter 113 (Part II)]

PETER G. TUTEUR, M.D.
Associate Professor of Medicine,
Pulmonary and Critical Care Division,
Washington University School of Medicine,
St. Louis, Missouri
(Chapter 31)

MICHAEL UNGER, M.D.
Clinical Professor of Medicine,
Thomas Jefferson University,
Philadelphia, Pennsylvania
(Chapter 38)

MARK J. UTELL, M.D.
Professor, Medicine and Environmental Medicine,
Director, Pulmonary and Occupational Medical Units,
Strong Memorial Hospital,
University of Rochester School of Medicine,
Rochester, New York
(Chapter 62)

FRITS VAN DER KUYP, M.D., M.P.H.
Controller,
Tuberculosis for Cuyahoa County,
Metrohealth Medical Center,
Cleveland, Ohio
(Chapter 159)

EMANUEL N. VERGIS, M.D.
Instructor in Medicine,
University of Pittsburgh,
Infectious Disease Section,
VA Medical Center,
Pittsburgh, Pennsylvania
(Chapter 144)

PETER D. WAGNER, M.D.
Professor of Medicine,
Department of Medicine,
University of California / San Diego,
La Jolla, California
(Chapter 12)

JOHN C. WAIN, M.D.
Associate Visiting Surgeon,
Thoracic Surgery Unit,
Massachusetts General Hospital,
Boston, Massachusetts
(Chapter 106)

DAVID J. WEBER, M.D., M.P.H.
Associate Professor of Medicine,
Infectious Disease Division,
University of North Carolina,
Chapel Hill, North Carolina
(Chapter 143)

KARL T. WEBER, M.D.
Professor and Chairman, Internal Medicine,
Division of Cardiology,
University of Missouri at Columbia,
Columbia, Missouri
(Chapter 37)

EWALD R. WEIBEL, M.D.
Professor Emeritus of Anatomy,
University of Berne,
Fondation Maurice E. Müller,
Berne, Switzerland
(Chapter 2)

ARNOLD N. WEINBERG, M.D.
Professor of Medicine, H.M.S.,
Medical Director
Massachusetts Institute of Technology,
Health Services,
Cambridge, Massachusetts
(Chapter 157)

SCOTT T. WEISS, M.D.
Professor of Medicine,
Director, Respiratory and Environmental Epidemiology,
Channing Laboratory, Brigham and Women's Hospital,
Harvard Medical School,
Boston, Massachusetts
(Chapter 48)

DAVID N. WEISSMAN, M.D.
Associate Professor of Medicine,
Pulmonary and Critical Care Medicine,
West Virginia Health Sciences Center,
Robert C. Byrd Center,
Morgantown, West Virginia
(Chapter 23)

MICHAEL J. WELSH, M.D.
Professor of Medicine and Physiology and Biophysics
Howard Hughes Medical Institute
Department of Internal Medicine
University of Iowa College of Medicine,
Iowa City, Iowa
(Chapter 8)

CHRISTINE H. WENDT, M.D.
Assistant Professor of Medicine,
University of Minnesota,
Minneapolis, Minnesota
(Chapter 27)

L. JOSEPH WHEAT, M.D.
Professor of Medicine,
Division of Infectious Diseases,
Wishard Memorial Hospital,
Indianapolis, Indiana
(Chapters 148, 149)

BRIAN J. WHIPP, PH.D., D.SC.
Professor of Physiology,
University of London,
St. George's Hospital Medical School,
London, England
(Chapter 17)

JEFFREY A. WHITSETT, M.D.
Professor of Pediatrics,
Division of Pulmonary Biology,
Children's Hospital Medical Center,
Cincinnati, Ohio
(Chapter 7)

NEVIN W. WILSON, M.D.
Associate Professor of Pediatrics,
Department of Pediatrics,
West Virginia University,
Health Science Center,
Morgantown, West Virginia
(Chapter 23)

RICHARD H. WINTERBAUER, M.D.
Head, Pulmonary and Critical Care Medicine,
Virginia Mason Medical Center,
Seattle, Washington
(Chapter 89)

ERIC T. WITTBRODT, PHARM.D.
Assistant Professor of Clinical Pharmacy,
Philadelphia College of Pharmacy and Science,
Philadelphia, Pennsylvania
(Chapter 173)

DANIEL WORSLEY, M.D.
Assistant Professor of Radiology,
Division of Nuclear Medicine,
Department of Radiology,
Vancouver General Hospital,
Vancouver, Canada
(Chapter 35)

G. SCOTT WORTHEN, M.D.
Department of Medicine,
National Jewish Center for Immunology and Respiratory Medicine,
Denver, Colorado
(Chapter 25)

CAMERON D. WRIGHT, M.D.
Assistant Professor of Surgery,
Howard Medical School,
Massachusetts General Hospital,
Boston, Massachusetts
(Chapter 94)

DAVID J. WYLER, M.D.
Professor of Medicine,
Tufts University School of Medicine,
Division of Geographic and Infectious Diseases,
New England Medical Center,
Boston, Massachusetts
(Chapter 155)

VICTOR L. YU, M.D.
Professor of Medicine,
University of Pittsburgh,
Chief, Infectious Disease Section,
Veterans Affairs Medical Center,
Pittsburgh, Pennsylvania
(Chapter 144)

SHERIF R. ZAKI, M.D., PH.D.
Chief, Molecular Pathology and Ultrastructure Activity,
Division of Viral and Rickettsial Diseases,
Centers for Diseases Control and Prevention,
Atlanta, Georgia
(Chapter 153)

RALPH J. ZITNIK, M.D.
Assistant Professor of Medicine,
Pulmonary and Critical Care Medicine,
Department of Internal Medicine,
Yale University School of Medicine,
New Haven, Connecticut
(Chapter 67)

RICHARD D. ZOROWITZ, M.D.
Director, Stroke Rehabilitation,
Department of Rehabilitation Medicine,
University of Pennsylvania Medical Center,
Philadelphia, Pennsylvania
(Chapter 80)

Preface

This edition deserves a special word of explanation since it marks a radical departure from the two previous editions, not so much in format as in editorial lineup and, as an inevitable result, in content. Instead of a single editor, there is now an editor-in-chief abetted by five associate editors, each one of whom is expert in at least one domain of chest medicine.

Looking back, we may find it rewarding for the sake of perspective to recapitulate the changing scene in pulmonary medicine that the two previous editions had addressed. In 1980, when the first edition appeared after several years of preparation, pulmonary medicine was reveling in its solid substrates of anatomy and pathology buttressed by physiology. Quantification was in the air and science was providing fresh insights into the mechanisms of disease. Previous preoccupation with infectious disease had given way to a pervasive interest in pulmonary function testing and derangements in pulmonary mechanics; new therapeutic modalities were evolving based on the improved understanding of the mechanisms of disease. Chronic obstructive pulmonary disease (COPD) and diffuse interstitial diseases were recognized by epidemiologic and clinical studies to be widespread and formidable problems that needed to be addressed. Prevention focused on smoking as a prime cause of both COPD and of lung cancer. The scientific meetings and journals took on new life, and all concerned in the science or clinical aspects of pulmonary medicine were proud of the distinguished leaders: Wallace Fenn, Hermann Rahn, Cournand and Richards, Julius Comroe. The first edition reflected the solid base in structure-function and the promising vistas opened by respiratory physiology.

The second edition eight years later moved into higher gear. By then, structure-function was solidly in place as a foundation for new advances in related fields. Immunology had found its feet in pulmonary medicine aided by hypersensitivity diseases, chemotherapy, and the spread of AIDS. Biochemistry had paved the way for studies of vital substances, such as pulmonary surfactant. Genetic diseases, such as cystic fibrosis and alpha-1-antitrypsin deficiency, were attracting attention in molecular terms. Clinical medicine received an enormous boost from the newer technologies: bronchoscopy, imaging, mechanical ventilation. Sleep disorders were incorporated into the purview of pulmonary medicine. Critical care medicine became a burgeoning subset of pulmonary medicine that took advantage of virtually all advances in both the understanding of pulmonary diseases and its management.

This glimpse from the rearview mirror brings us back to a look at this edition, which, in dealing with the present state of pulmonary medicine, also looks ahead toward leading edges, where advances in understanding, knowledge, and their applications are to be anticipated. This goal is in keeping with the recent report by the American Thoracic Society which sets forth "the major problems in lung disease and possible pathways to their solution." The report, entitled "Future Directions for Research on Diseases of the Lung," is reassuring to the editors of the third edition in that each target listed in this report is dealt with substantively and expertly in this book. As expected, the third edition envisages even larger and brighter horizons in the years ahead because of the clear and discerning visions of the individual contributors who write in their chapters about their special fields of interest.

The experience and knowledge of each of the editors have been directed at ensuring that the specialized, as well as the general, aspects of pulmonary medicine have been expertly covered and well presented. Although the book is now a collective arbeit, discussion and debate among the editors and authors have led to a work integrated by a meeting of the minds. By the process of peer review, the book aspires to provide a readable and balanced coverage of what is latest and most meaningful in pulmonary diseases and disorders.

I have already indicated how much this book owes to the experts who comprise the editorial board. Clearly, they would have little to work with were it not for the splendid chapters contributed by the individual authors. Nor would the book be as well orchestrated were it not for the leadership (and prodding) of J. Dereck Jeffers, editor-in-chief at McGraw-Hill, who has been the shepherd for all three editions, latterly promoting camaraderie and productivity among the editors while ensuring that deadlines were met.

I owe a great deal to those close to home. Alice K. Glover handled the preparation of the book with great skill and speed, moving its pages along from manuscript to page proof. Betsy Ann Bozzarello freed time for me to devote to the book while catalyzing the efforts of others. Roger Webb continued to infiltrate the text with his telltale drawings, and Daniel Barrett was once again on continuing standby alert, ready and available to pitch in as needed.

My family provided the encouragement and peace of mind that such an effort inevitably calls for. My wife, Linda, was unwavering in her tolerance and support. My daughter, Hannah, who is trying her own hand at writing, was both impressed by the enormity of the undertaking and indulgent about anyone who would embark on such a venture. My sons, Mark and Jay, shared my conviction that this book is in keeping with our shared academic convictions. Their spouses, Gayle and Martha, helped to create the setting and frame of mind in which this book was put together.

Alfred P. Fishman, M.D.

Fishman's
Pulmonary Diseases and Disorders
Volume 1

PART ONE

PERSPECTIVES

CHAPTER 1

MILESTONES IN THE HISTORY OF PULMONARY MEDICINE

Alfred P. Fishman

It has taken medicine more than 2000 years to reach its present level of clinical, scientific, and technologic sophistication. From the beginning, pulmonary medicine has been an integral part of this growth and development. About three hundred years ago, progress toward scientific medicine accelerated markedly, and it has continued to gain speed ever since: In the seventeenth century, research and experimentation began to tilt clinical medicine toward the exact sciences; by the eighteenth century, pathology had become an integral part of clinical medicine, and clinical-pathologic correlations began to succeed empiricism, dogmatism, and metaphysics in medicine. The age of the great clinicians dawned in Europe early in the nineteenth century, when autopsies became legally permissible and socially acceptable, and when physicians who cared for the patients ultimately performed the autopsy.[5]

The road to current understanding and practice has been convoluted. Progress has been punctuated by delays, detours, and reversals. But it is possible to retrace the scientific trail by using certain figures and discoveries to draw the map. Chapter 1 uses these milestones to trace the course of scientific pulmonary medicine up to the early twentieth century. The chapter goes no further, since more recent advances are more a matter of report-

ing than of history. These advances are left to subsequent chapters in this book. This chapter deals only with certain of the key components of modern pulmonary medicine: alveolar-capillary gas exchange, lung volumes, mechanics of breathing, control of breathing, ventilation-perfusion relationships, and scientific clinical medicine.

ALVEOLAR-CAPILLARY GAS EXCHANGE

Ancient Greek Medicine

The beginnings of scientific medicine can be traced to ancient Greece in the sixth century B.C. Natural philosophers then speculated that air or some essential ingredient in air was inspired to generate a vital essence for distribution throughout the body.[7]

Hippocrates, the "father of medicine," is as much a symbol of the Greek physician of the fifth and fourth centuries B.C., as the name of a real figure (Fig. 1-1). As an individual, he exemplified the caring physician who kept accurate records, made cautious inferences, and relied more on nature, rest, and diet than on drugs for therapy. His name has been immortalized by affixing it to three major components of Greek medicine even though none of these seems to be the work of a single individual. The first is the *Hippocratic corpus,* a collection of about 70 works that includes case reports, textbooks, lectures, and notebooks. The collection contains a description of Cheyne-Stokes breathing and the use of *Hippocratic succession* for the diagnosis of fluid and air in the pleural cavity. The second item is a collection of aphorisms, a compilation of brief generalizations relating to medicine. The third, which seems more attributable to Pythagoras (c. 530 B.C.) than to Hippocrates, who lived about a century later (Table 1-1), is the *Hippocratic oath,* which not only represents the spirit of the physician of ancient Greece but has endured to modern times as a reflection of the ethical code of the physician.[46]

Aristotle needs mention at this juncture because of his permanent influence on the intellect of humankind in his own time and for two millennia thereafter. Not until the seventeenth century were his doctrine of the four elements (earth, air, fire, water) and that of Hippocrates (blood, phlegm, yellow bile, and black bile) laid to rest, thereby clearing the way for modern scientific medicine. Soon after Aristotle, about 300 B.C., an extraordinary medical school was founded at Alexandria in Egypt. One of the

TABLE 1-1

Landmark Figures in the Evolution of Modern Pulmonary Medicine

Alveolar-Capillary Gas Exchange

Ancient Greek Medicine

Hippocrates of CoS (c. 460–359 B.C.)
Aristotle (384–322 B.C.)
Erasistratus of Chios (c. 300–250 B.C.)
Galen of Pergamon (A.D. 129–99)
Ibn An Nafis (c. 1210–1288)
Leonardo da Vinci (1452–1519)
Miguel Servetus (1511–1553)
Andreas Vesalius of Brussels (1514–1564)
Realdus Columbus of Cremona (1516–1559)
Andreas Caesalpinus of Pisa (1519–1603)

William Harvey and the Oxford Physiologists

Galileo Galilei (1564–1642)
William Harvey (1578–1657)
Giovanni Alfonso Borelli (1608–1679)
Marcello Malpighi (1628–1694)
Robert Boyle (1627–1691)
Richard Lower (1631–1691)
Robert Hooke (1635–1703)
John Mayow (1640–1679)

Phlogiston: The Rise and Fall

Georg Erst Stahl (1660–1734)
John Black (1728–1799)
Joseph Priestley (1733–1804)
Carl Wilhelm Scheele (1742–1782)

Respiration and Metabolism

Antoine Laurent Lavoisier (1743–1794)
John Dalton (1766–1844)

Julius Robert von Mayer (1814–1878)
Carl von Voit (1831–1908)
Nathan Zuntz (1847–1920)

The Blood Gases

Joseph Black (1728–1799)
John Dalton (1766–1844)
Heinrich Gustav Magnus (1802–1870)
Felix Hoppe-Seyler (1825–1895)
Paul Bert (1833–1886)
Christian Bohr (1855–1911)
John Scott Haldane (1860–1936)
August Krogh (1874–1949)

Diffusion or Secretion of Oxygen

Joseph Barcroft (1872–1947)
Marie Krogh (1874–1943)

The Physical-Chemical Synthesis

Lawrence J. Henderson (1878–1942)

Mechanics of Breathing

John Hutchinson (1811–1861)
Karl Ludwig (1816–1895)
Franciscus Cornelius Donders (1818–1889)
Fritz Rohrer (1888–1926)
Wallace Osgood Fenn (1893–1971)

Control of Breathing

The Central Respiratory Centers

Thomas Lunsden (1874–1953)
Hans Winterstein (1878–1963)
Merkel Henry Jacobs (1884–1970)

The Peripheral Chemoreceptors

Ewald Hering (1834–1918)
Joseph Breuer (1842–1925)
Cornelius Heymans (1892–1968)

Scientific Clinical Medicine

Pathologic Anatomy

Gioranni Battista Morgagni (1682–1771)
Leopold Auenbrugger (1727–1809)
Jean Nicolas Corvisart (1755–1821)
René Theophile Hyacinthe Laënnec (1781–1826)

Microbiology

Robert Koch (1843–1910)

Physiology of the Pulmonary Circulation

Claude Bernard (1813–1878)
Auguste Chauveau (1827–1917)
Étienne Jules Marey (1830–1904)
Dickinson W. Richards (1895–1973)
André Frederic Cournand (1895–1988)
Werner Forssmann (1904–1979)

first teachers at this school, Erasistratus, postulated that the pneuma or spirit essential for life is somehow generated from an interplay between air and blood.[7] About four centuries after Erasistratus, Galen (Fig. 1-2) drew upon the medical, philosophic, and anatomic knowledge of his day to fashion a remarkable physiologic schema. His construct was largely teleological. Unfortunately, it was so convincing that even though it was ultimately proved fanciful, it sufficed to retard scientific progress for a millennium and a half.[5,17,46] Galen was a talented individual, well-educated, well-read, and well-positioned in society to popularize his beliefs. Moreover, his concepts fit well into the tenets of Christianity which was then beginning its ascendency; to contravert his authority was tantamount to blasphemy. Among his enduring, albeit erroneous, postulates, were the following: invisible pores in the ventricular septum that enabled the bulk of the blood flow from the right ventricle to bypass the lungs, a diminutive pulmonary circulation that served only to nourish the lungs, and two-way traffic of inspired air and effluent waste vapors going their respective ways in the pulmonary vein (Fig. 1-3).[15,18]

Every now and then, a voice did rise in protest—but without lasting effect. In the thirteenth century, Ibn An Nafis, writing in his *Canon of Avicenna,* objected that blood does not traverse the ventricular septum from right to left as Galen had proposed. However, this insight attracted little attention, as did similar misgivings voiced by Vesalius 300 years later. In the sixteenth century, Michael Servetus, a theologian trained in anatomy with Vesalius, included two important anatomical points in his theological treatise *Christianismi Restitutio:* Blood could not traverse the septum between the right and left ventricles, and the lumen of the pulmonary artery was too large for a nutrient vessel. Calvin had him burned at the stake for the heretical views expressed in the book. In 1559, Realdus Columbus of Cremona, pupil of Vesalius, came to similar conclusions as did Andreas Caesalpinus in 1571. Despite these challenging observations, Galen's schema was to last for more than another half century, i.e., until the physiologic experiments of William Harvey.[7]

William Harvey and the Oxford Physiologists

William Harvey (Fig. 1-4) was led to the discovery of the circulation of the blood by the anatomic observations of his mentor, Fabricus ab Aquapedente, on the disposition of the venous valves. Harvey's small book, *De Motu Cordis,* published in 1628, marked the birth of modern physiology.[22] However, the book shed no light on the physiology of breathing. To his dying day, Harvey clung to the theory that the main function of breathing is to

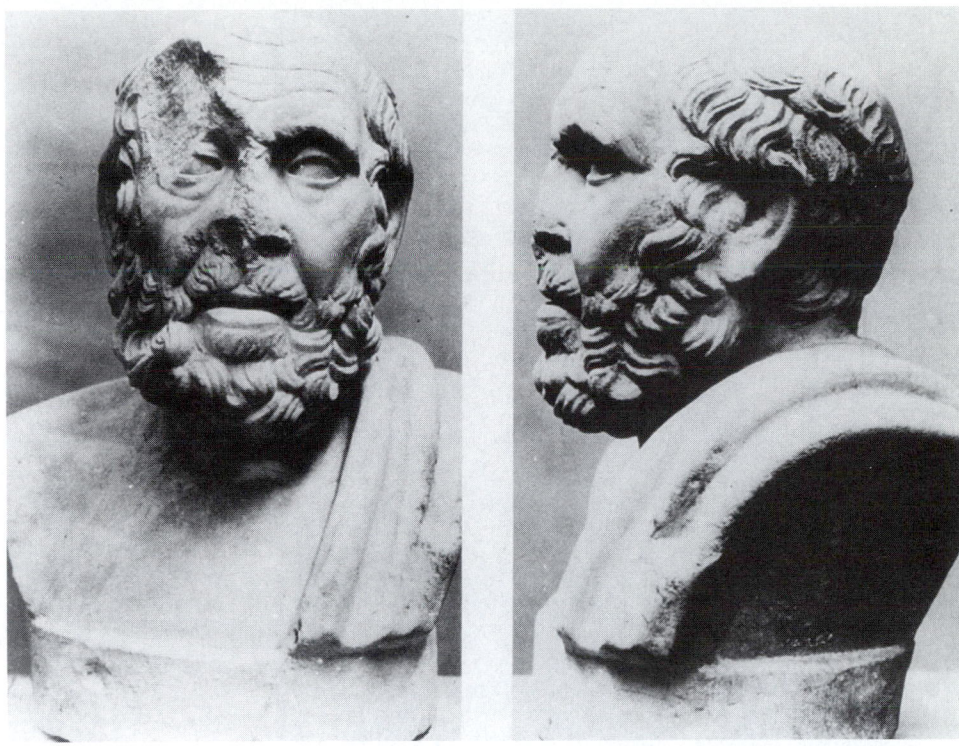

FIGURE 1-1   The Hippocrates of Ostia. This damaged bust is believed to represent Hippocrates as perceived in antiquity. It was found in a family tomb in excavations near Ostia. (*Courtesy of Dr. Dickinson W. Richards.*)

cool the heart. Moreover, since he made no use of the microscope, he could not picture how the pulmonary arteries made connection with the pulmonary veins. The connections were subsequently seen by Marcello Malpighi, using the compound microscope invented by Galileo; in 1661, Malpighi reported that alveoli were covered by capillaries and that blood and air were kept separate by the continuous alveolar-capillary barrier.[5,46]

Harvey's description in 1628 of the circulation of the blood had three major consequences for pulmonary medicine: (1) it oriented pulmonary medicine toward the basic sciences and away from philosophy and empiricism; (2) it demolished the Galenic concept of circulation; and (3) it set the stage for an upcoming generation of physiologists at Oxford University to explore breathing in terms of chemistry and physics.[17]

Harvey's disciplined approach to scientific inquiry made a deep impression on the physiologists working at Oxford in the 1660s. Many of these were medical practitioners who did research as a sideline ("the Oxford physiologists"). Four in particular began the systematic study of air and its constituents, thereby laying the foundations for contemporary respiratory physiology and medicine: Robert Boyle (Fig. 1-5), Robert Hooke, Richard Lower, and John Mayow.[16] In 1660, Robert Boyle proved by means of his air pump that air is necessary for life. In 1667, Robert Hooke showed that insufflation of the lungs with air while breathing movements were arrested, could keep alive an open-chest animal, i.e., that movement of the lungs was not essential for life. Richard Lower, the first to practice blood transfusion, took advantage of Hooke's continuously inflated lung preparation in the dog to observe that the dark venous blood becomes bright red as it traverses lungs insufflated with air.[33] In 1674,

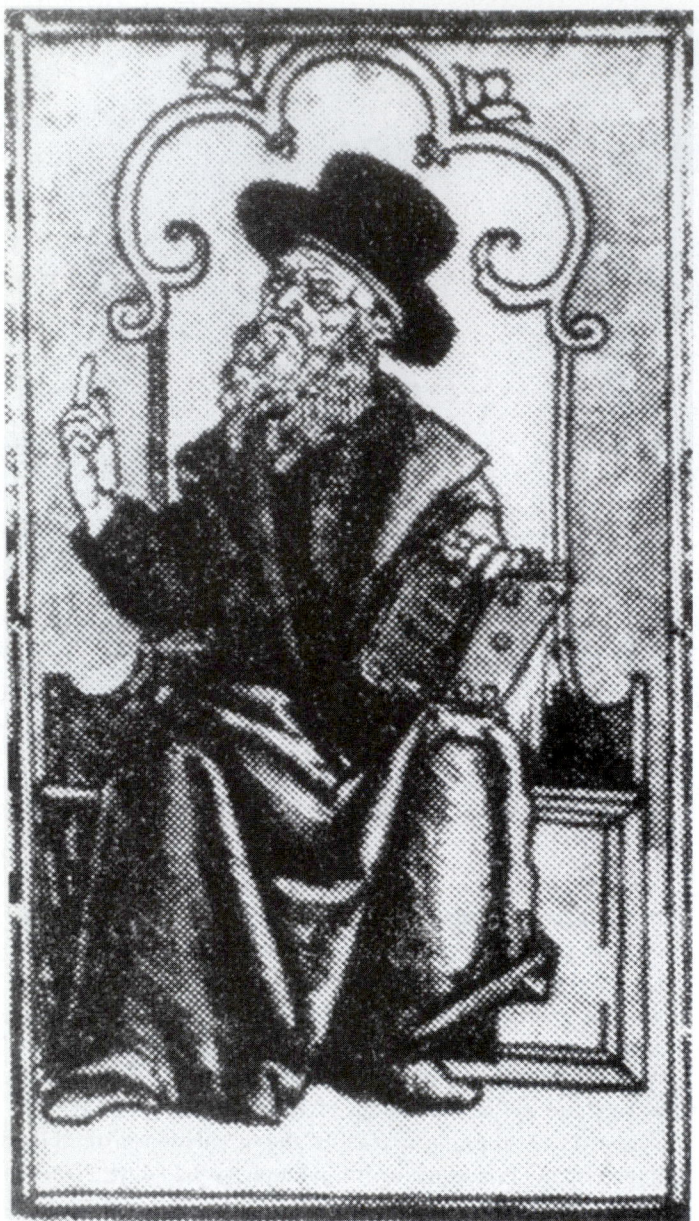

FIGURE 1-2 Galen of Pergamon as depicted in medieval times. No authentic reproduction exists of Galen in ancient times. *(From Galen's Therapeutica, published in Venice in 1500.)*

Mayow interpreted the change in the color of blood from venous to arterial as due to the uptake of "nitro-aerial particles" (later to be called "oxygen") from the air.[34]

Phlogiston: The Rise and Fall

Unfortunately, the discoveries and insights of the Oxford physiologists went largely unnoticed during the century that followed, overshadowed by the phlogiston theory of combustion.[39] This theory, advanced by Stahl, postulated that all combustible materials were composed of two ingredients: phlogiston, a principle which transformed into fire when heated, and an ash which was left behind after the fiery phlogiston escaped.[17] The phlogiston theory was sufficiently malleable to accommodate almost every

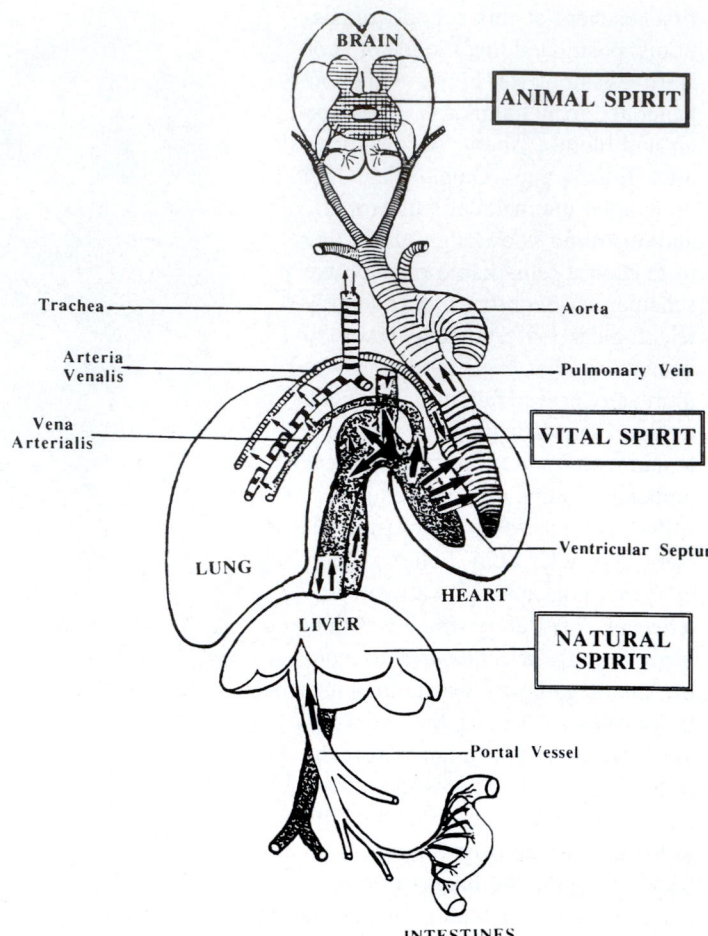

FIGURE 1-3 Galen's scheme of the circulation. The diagram shows the source and distribution of the three types of spirits. The validity of this scheme depended on invisible pores in the ventricular septum, two-way traffic in the pulmonary vein, and selective permeability of the mitral valve for sooty wastes but not for spirit-containing blood. Vena arterialis = pulmonary vein; arteria venalis = pulmonary artery. *(Modified after Singer.[46])*

new discovery that could have overthrown it, including the rediscovery of carbon dioxide in 1754 by John Black and the independent discoveries of oxygen by Priestley and Scheele. Although the respiratory gases had been discovered by the end of the eighteenth century and many of their properties characterized, the discoveries were misapplied to support, rather than destroy, the phlogiston theory.[17] The phlogiston theory was finally demolished by the experiments of Lavoisier.

Respiration and Metabolism

From the time of Hippocrates until early in the twentieth century, debate had continued about the site of heat production in the body. In 1777, Lavoisier suggested that air was composed of one respirable gas (which he later named "oxygine") and another (nitrogen) which remained unchanged in the course of respiration. Between 1782 and 1784, Lavoisier and Laplace concluded, on the basis of experiments using guinea pigs and involving calorimetry, that "respiration is therefore a combustion, admit-

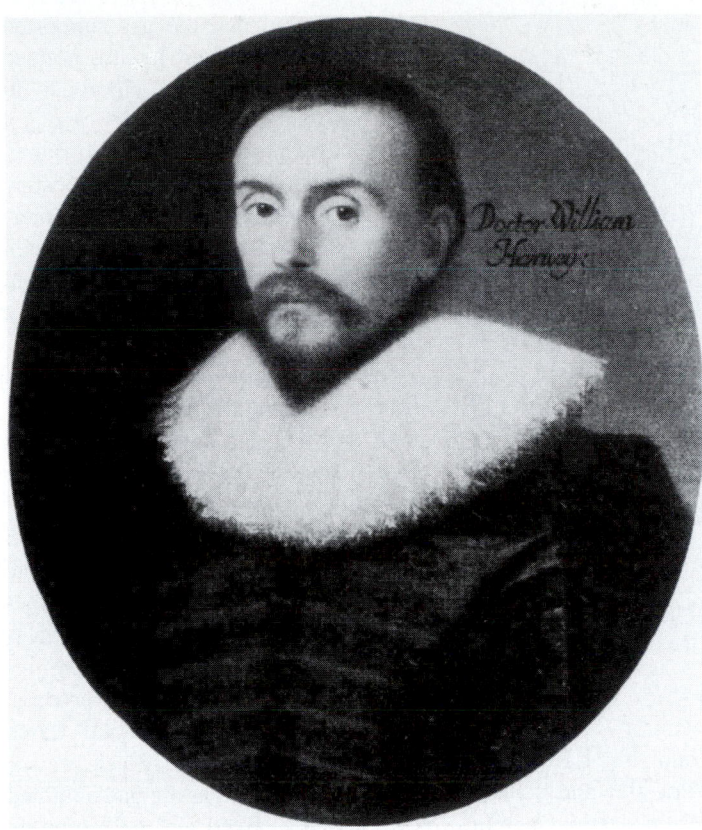

FIGURE 1-4   William Harvey (1578–1657). This portrait of William Harvey is part of a family group in which William Harvey and his five brothers are gathered around their father, William Harvey.

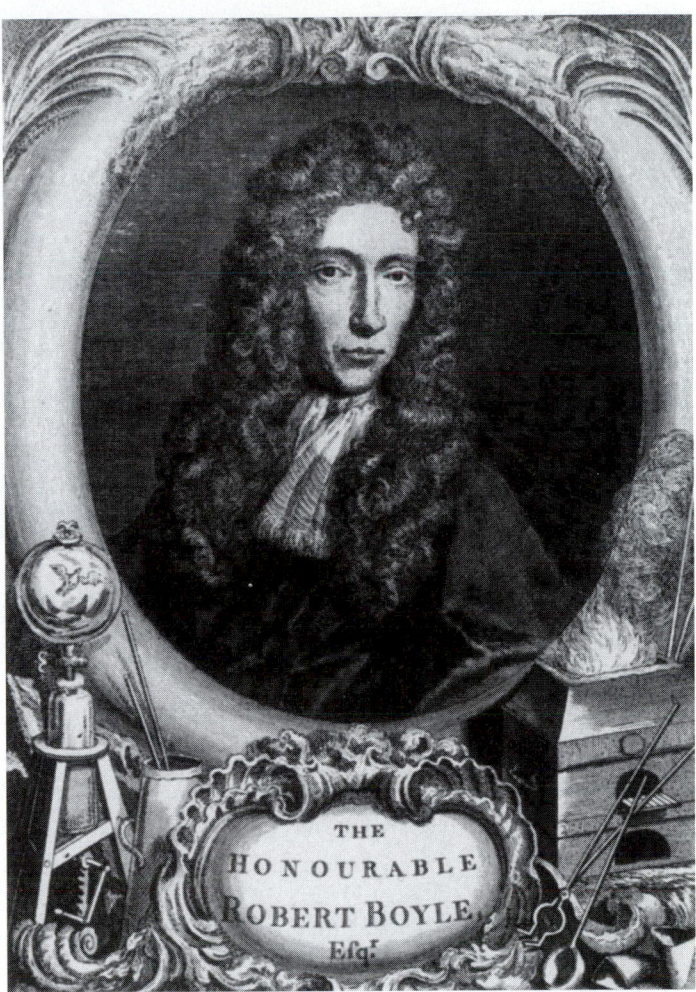

FIGURE 1-5   Robert Boyle (1627–1691). This engraving, from an original painting by Johann Kerseboom, hangs in the Royal Society, London. Boyle's invention of a pneumatic air pump and his publications concerning "the spring of air and its effect" stimulated considerable research on the physical properties of air and its role in respiration and combustion. He strongly influenced Hooke, Lower, and Mayow at Oxford.

tedly very slow, but otherwise exactly similar to that of charcoal" (Fig. 1-6). The similarity between respiration and combustion had previously been recognized by the Oxford physiologists, especially Mayow. By 1783, Lavoisier was accumulating evidence against the phlogiston theory and began to substitute for it an entirely new system of chemistry.[35]

As noted above, the ancients pictured the heart as the heat generator. Lavoisier favored the lungs. Others held that combustion occurred in the blood. Although Spallanzani had shown in the eighteenth century that isolated tissues take up oxygen and give off carbon dioxide,[39] the idea that combustion occurred in the tissues was slow in gaining acceptance. Strength was infused into this hypothesis by Pflüger in 1878. He measured oxygen consumption and carbon dioxide production in dogs and calculated respiratory quotients: The latter substantiated a concept that had been enunciated, but not named, by Lavoisier.

Once the idea that oxidation occurred in the tissues became generally accepted, investigators began to delve into the tissue utilization of foodstuffs, energetics, growth, and repair. Carl von Voit and Max von Pettenkofer, using a respiration chamber, drew upon chemical balances and respiratory quotients in humans to distinguish the nature of the foodstuffs being burned and to show that the amounts of fat protein and carbohydrate burned varied with the mechanical work done by the subject. The law of conservation of energy was formulated by Julius Robert von Mayer between 1842 and 1845. Subsequently, Max Rubner showed that

the law applied to the living body, and Herman von Helmholtz showed how its relevance to metabolism could be demonstrated experimentally. Application of these principles at the bedside were greatly facilitated by the development of portable metabolic apparatus by Nathan Zuntz. Pioneering bedside studies of diverse metabolic states were conducted by a succession of distinguished investigators, including Magnus-Levy, Graham Lusk, F. G. Benedict, and Eugene F. DuBois.[39]

The Blood Gases

The Oxford physiologists set the stage for the discovery of the blood gases. Using his vacuum pump, Robert Boyle extracted "air" from blood. John Mayow came close to discovering oxygen by showing that only part of air was necessary for life and that this part, his "nitro-aerial spirits," was removed both by respiration and fire (combustion).[34] One of his famous experiments

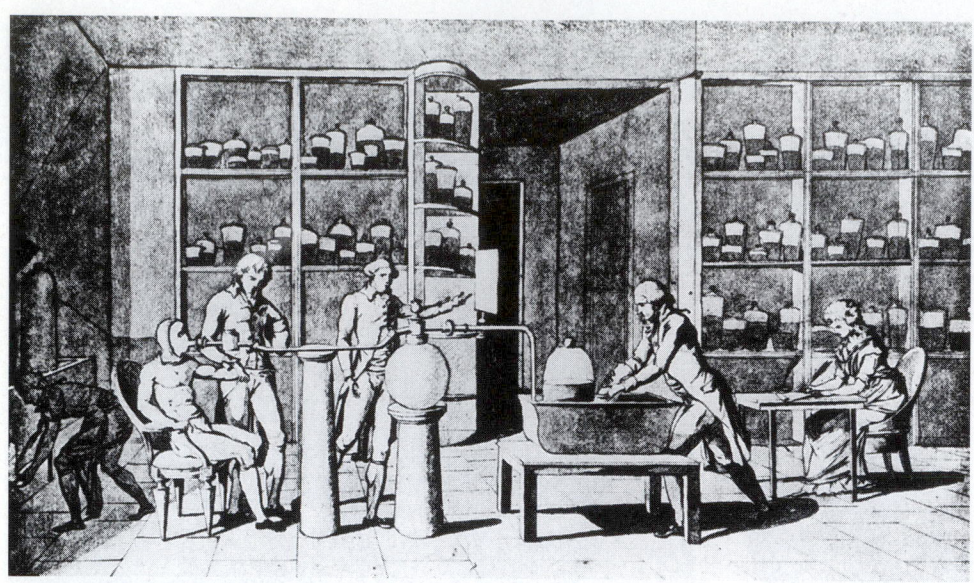

FIGURE 1-6 Scene from the laboratory of Antoine Laurent Lavoisier (1743–1794). His wife is acting as his assistant, and Sequin is the subject. Studies such as this led to the conclusion that respiration and circulation are similar processes.

ide and found that the gas supported life better than did air; he also noticed that a flame burned more vigorously in this gas than in air. Priestley was not alone in his preoccupation with flame. In 1773, about a year before Priestley had obtained oxygen by heating mercuric oxide, Scheele discovered oxygen independently because of his interest in fire, and he designated oxygen as "fire air."[17]

In 1662, Van Helmont, a Capuchin friar and talented chemist—a mystic with a drive to quantify—discovered carbon dioxide, coined the word *gas,* and called carbon dioxide "wild gas" ("gas sylvestre").[5] In 1755, Joseph Black rediscovered carbon dioxide. He showed that calcium carbonate (limestone) and magnesium carbonate (magnesia alba) lost weight on heating, releasing "fixed air" (CO_2) in the process. This fixed air extinguished both flame and life. Lavoisier knew of the observations of Black and of Priestley and Scheele. He decided in 1778 that the gas obtained from heating mercuric oxide was not "fixed air" or "common air," but "highly respirable air" (oxygen).[7]

entailed enclosing an animal and a lighted lamp in an air-tight container; the lamp went out first and then the mouse died.[6] However, Mayow did not realize that the "nitro-aerial spirits" could be isolated as a gas.

One hundred years after Mayow, Joseph Priestley (Fig. 1-7) exposed a mouse to the gas released from heated mercuric ox-

The story of hemoglobin, the essential element in the transport of the respiratory gases by the blood, begins with Hoppe-Seyler, who, between 1866 and 1871, crystallized hemoglobin, explored its chemical properties, and assigned it a proper role in the transport of oxygen by the blood.[6] At the turn of the nineteenth century, Dalton reported his experiments with the respiratory gases which led to the development of his atomic theory. In 1872, taking advantage of Dalton's law, Paul Bert published the first oxygen dissociation curve, i.e., oxygen content at different barometric pressures; he pictured the curve as hyperbolic. Christian Bohr subsequently identified its *s*-shaped contour (Fig. 1-8) and in 1904, together with Hasselbach and August Krogh, showed that increasing carbon dioxide tensions in blood drives out oxygen, i.e., the "Bohr effect."[7] Shortly thereafter, the various influences, e.g., temperature and electrolytes, on the affinity of oxygen for hemoglobin—and consequently the position of the oxygen dissociation curve—began to be explored in detail by Barcroft and his associates.[1] In 1914, Christiansen, Douglas, and Haldane reported that an increase in the oxygen tension of the blood drives out carbon dioxide, i.e., the "Haldane effect."[6,21] In 1967, a new dimension was added to the understanding of the position and configuration of the oxygen dissociation curve by the demonstration that diphosphoglycerate, a chemical constituent of red cells, regulates the release of oxygen from oxyhemoglobin.[6]

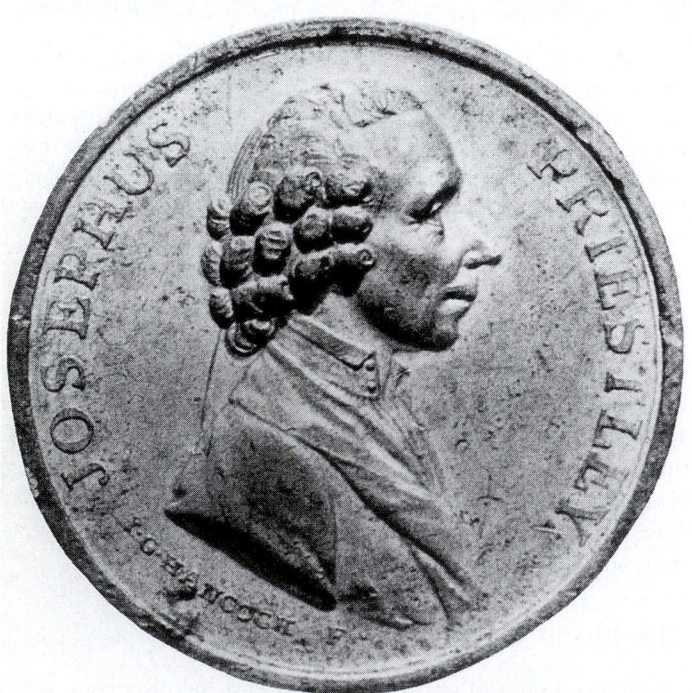

FIGURE 1-7 Joseph Priestley (1733–1804). A silver medal struck in his honor in 1783. The discoverer of oxygen. A Presbyterian minister, he was radical in his religious and political beliefs, inventive in science, and conservative in the interpretation of his findings. *(From Fishman AP, Richards DW: Circulation of the Blood: Men and Ideas, New York, Oxford University Press, 1964, with permission.)*

Diffusion or Secretion of Oxygen

Bohr is a central figure as an investigator and mentor in respiratory physiology. In 1904, he raised a troublesome issue that was not easily resolved, primarily because of limitations in

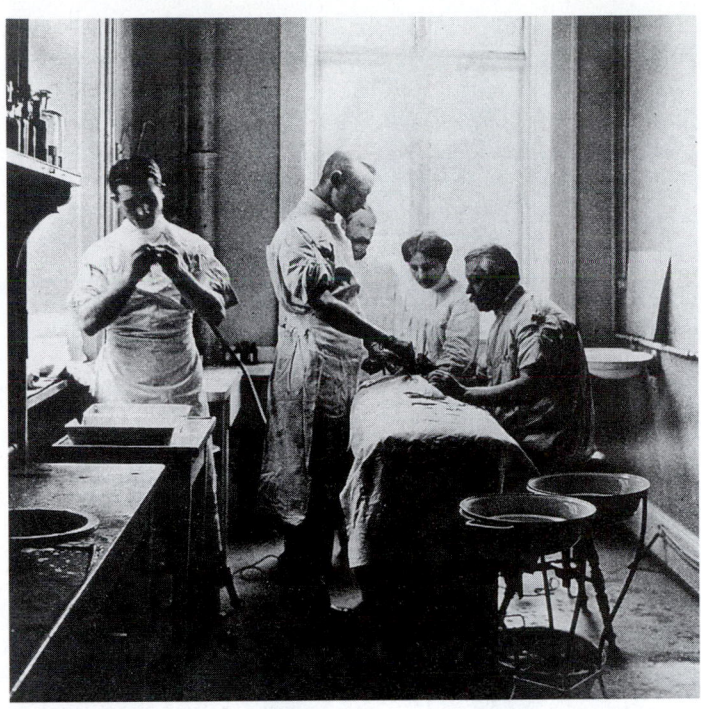

FIGURE 1-8 Christian Bohr (1855–1911). At work in his laboratory, Bohr (far right) and his associates systematically explored the interplay between the respiratory gases and hemoglobin which led to the discovery of the "Bohr effect." *(From Fishman AP, Richards DW: Circulation of the Blood: Men and Ideas, New York, Oxford University Press, 1964, with permission.)*

methodology. He postulated that even though diffusion could account for the oxygen uptake at rest,[2] it could not suffice during strenuous exercise, particularly at altitude. He held to this conviction for his lifetime supported by two major lines of evidence. The first was indirect, i.e., oxygen secretion by the swim bladder of fish which showed that, in principle, active transport of oxygen in the lungs was possible. The second was based on observations made during his expedition to Pike's Peak in 1912 which showed (erroneously), that during exercise at altitude, arterial oxygen tension exceeded alveolar oxygen tension.[1,2]

But, even before the report from high altitude, Bohr's former assistant August Krogh and his wife, Marie Krogh (Fig. 1-9), had marshaled new evidence to show that "the absorption of oxygen and the elimination of carbon dioxide in the lungs takes place by diffusion and diffusion alone."[29] The final blow to the secretion theory was delivered by Marie Krogh.[31] Based on the single-breath carbon monoxide method for determining diffusing capacity that she and her husband had developed in 1910, the Kroghs were able to account

for oxygen uptake in the lung by diffusion alone, even under strenuous exercise under conditions of low oxygen tension.[31] Refinements in the carbon monoxide method by Roughton and others extended its clinical applicability and provided further evidence against the secretion theory.[43] But Haldane would not let go. Throughout his life, despite mounting evidence to the contrary, he adhered to the idea of secretion of oxygen by the alveolar membrane.[21]

Finally, the issue was settled by Joseph Barcroft (Fig. 1-10). Using a chamber to reproduce the hypoxic-strenuous exercise circumstances of the Pike's Peak expedition, he found that under all conditions, the arterial oxygen saturation of arterial blood was less than that of blood exposed to a sample of alveolar gas obtained at the same time.[1,17] He subsequently confirmed these results by experiments done at high altitude, i.e., at Cerro de Pasco (1921–1922).[36]

The Physical-Chemical Synthesis

Lawrence J. Henderson undertook the herculean task of depicting the reactions of oxygen and carbon dioxide in blood not as cause and effect but as an interplay among physiochemical variables and functions (Fig. 1-10). In his theoretical considerations and practical applications via the Fatigue Laboratory at Harvard, he was greatly abetted by close collaboration with Van Slyke, Wu, and McLean at the Rockefeller Institute in New York, who were exploring the exchanges of blood constituents between red cells and plasma.[42a] In 1828, Henderson presented his synthesis in the form of a D'Ocagne nomogram which displayed the changes in the various elements that entered into the exchange of the respiratory gases between alveolar gas and blood: plasma; the red cell; hemoglobin; chloride, bicarbonate and hydrogen

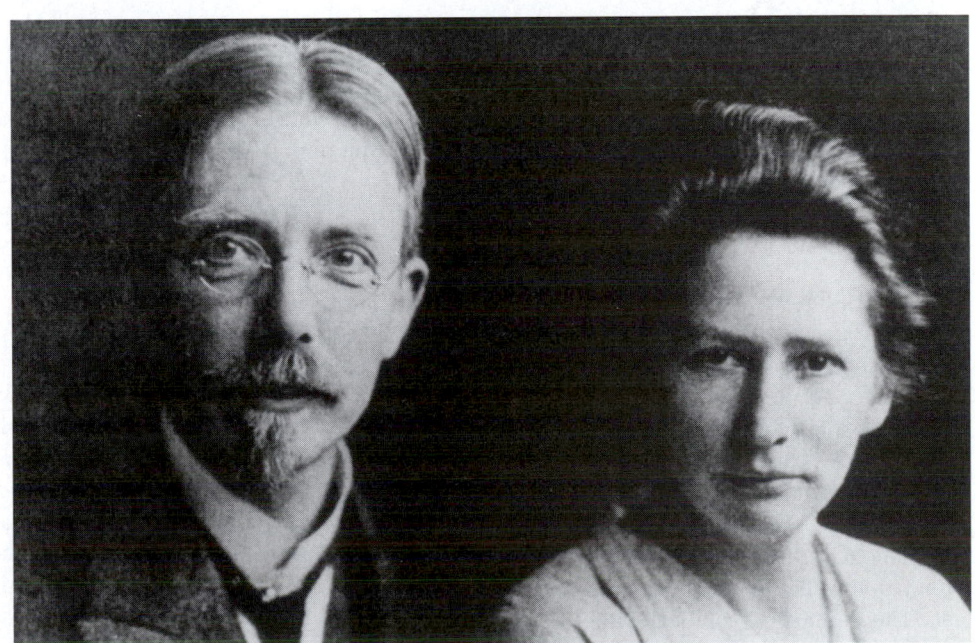

FIGURE 1-9 August and Marie Krogh in 1922 at the time of their first visit to the United States so that August Krogh could deliver the Silliman Lecture at Yale. They demonstrated that diffusion, without secretion, could account for the transfer of O_2 and CO_2 across the alveolar-capillary membranes of the lungs. *(Courtesy of their daughter, Dr. Bodil Schmidt-Nielsen.)*

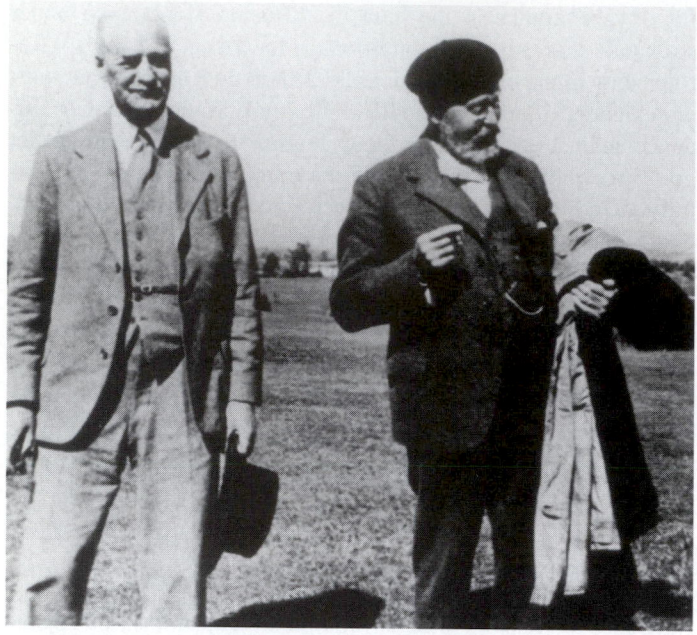

FIGURE 1-10 Two founders of contemporary respiratory physiology, in 1936. Sir Joseph Barcroft (1872–1947) *(left)* proved, in experiments on himself, that diffusion was the mechanism for gas exchange in the lungs and pioneered current understanding of the respiratory functions of the blood. Lawrence J. Henderson (1878–1942) *(right)* provided a mathematical analysis of blood as a physiochemical system and stimulated research on the complex interplay involved in respiratory gas exchange during exercise. *(From Fishman AP, Richards DW: Circulation of the Blood: Men and Ideas, New York, Oxford University Press, 1964, with permission.)*

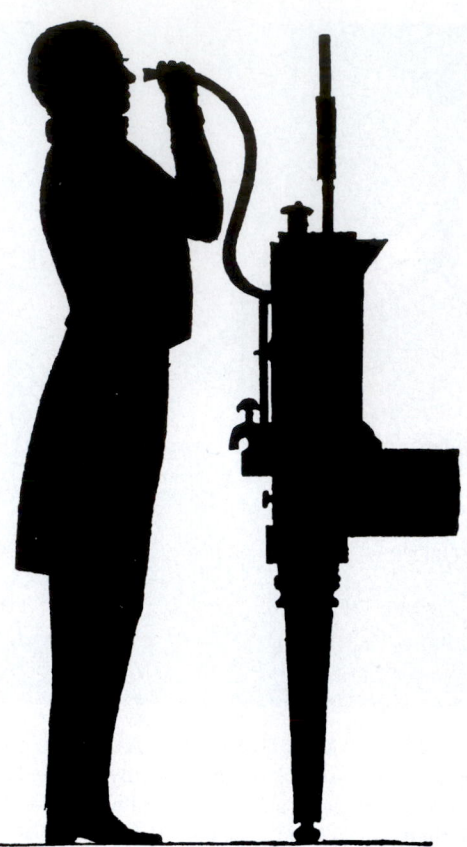

FIGURE 1-11 John Hutchinson's illustration of a subject about to undergo measurements of lung volumes. *[From Hutchinson J: Med Chir Soc (Lond) trans 29:137, 1846.]*

ions.[24] He presented nomograms not only for the normal subject at rest and during exercises but also for individuals with anemia, nephritis, diabetic coma, and other major clinical entities. Henderson dealt with steady-state observations. Roughton and associates enlarged the physiochemical horizons further by discovering carbonic anhydrase in the red cell and by dealing with transient phenomena relating to the transport of the respiratory gases and carbon monoxide in blood.[43a]

LUNG VOLUMES

Although Humphrey Davy had determined his own lung volume using hydrogen as test gas in 1800, it was not until the 1840s that John Hutchinson laid the groundwork for modern pulmonary function testing: He devised a spirometer and used it to determine the subdivisions of the lung in a large number of healthy subjects, relating the measurements to height and age (Fig. 1-11).[6,39] The many refinements since then are too numerous for mention in this chapter. A big step forward was the invention of the body plethysmograph many years later which made possible the determination of the thoracic gas volume along with airway resistance and pulmonary capillary blood flow.[6]

MECHANICS OF BREATHING

The ancients wondered about how air moved into and out of the lungs, and as far back as Erasistratus, the diaphragm was recognized to be involved in breathing.[17] Galen was aware that the

lungs fill the chest cavity, that they are moved by the actions of the thorax, and that the large airways enlarge and lengthen during inspiration.[19] He marveled at the long course of the nerves to the diaphragm and the innervation of the intercostal muscles. After Galen, interest in the mechanics of breathing waned except for sporadic observations and experiments by anatomists, notably, Leonardo da Vinci and Andreas Vesalius. Interest resumed in the sixteenth century largely as a result of progress in physics and mathematics exemplified by the works of Borelli and Galileo.

THE RESPIRATORY MUSCLES

Mayow, one of the Oxford physiologists (Fig. 1-5), drew heavily on the work of colleagues, such as Boyle and Hooke, to develop considerable insight into the mechanics of breathing. He also built the first model on record of the chest as a bellows, which contained a bladder within it (Fig. 1-12). He understood that air moved into the lungs as the chest expanded because of the pressure and elasticity of ambient air, that the chest expands because of the action of the intercostal muscles (internal and external), that the diaphragm is the primary muscle of inspiration, and that normal expiration is passive. After Mayow, little research was done on the role of the respiratory muscles in breathing until the mid-nineteenth century when Donders distinguished between the respective roles played by the inspiratory muscles, and elastic forces.[14,38]

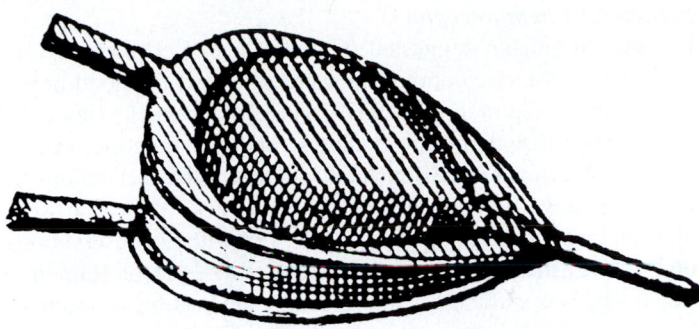

FIGURE 1-12 Mayow's model of the chest and lungs. The bellows encloses a bladder, the neck of which opens to the outside. A glass window on the upper side makes it possible to observe the bladder during inflation and deflation. *(From Mayow J.[34])*

ELASTIC PROPERTIES OF LUNGS AND CHEST

Until the twentieth century, observations on the elastic properties of the lungs and chest cage in humans were fragmentary. Access to the pleural space was the major limiting factor. With few exceptions, notably Neergaard and Wirz, who used pleural pressures to determine elastic recoil in normal human subjects, and Christie, who recorded pleural pressures to demonstrate loss of pulmonary elasticity in emphysematous patients, measurements in humans were largely confined either to therapeutic interventions, e.g., induction of a pneumothorax or aspiration of pleural fluid, or to experiments done at autopsy.[14,38] The number of observations on the mechanical properties of the lungs increased dramatically when it was shown by Buytendijk, in 1949, and again by Dornhurst and Leathart, in 1952, that esophageal pressures provided an accurate measure of pleural pressures.[6]

The role of alveolar surface tension in determining the elastic forces in the lungs began to be widely appreciated in the late 1950s. The stage had been set long before then. In 1812, Laplace had published the law of surface tension.[6] The implications of this law for the lungs began to be appreciated in 1929 when Neergaard compared pressure-volume curves of lungs filled with air with those filled with fluid. He concluded that unopposed surface tensions would favor alveolar collapse. Then, between 1954 and 1960, a remarkable outpouring of papers from different laboratories showed that a unique surfactant lined the alveoli, that this material was absent in premature infants with hyaline membrane disease (and alveolar collapse); these papers prompted extensive research, which continues to this day, on the chemical and physical properties of surfactant and on its sites of formation and removal.[14,38,39]

AIRWAY RESISTANCE

A giant step forward began in 1916 when Rohrer, as part of his doctoral dissertation, presented a conceptual framework for determining flow/resistance in airways.[44] His equations were based on precise anatomical measurements of airway dimensions in a human cadaver coupled with aerodynamic principles. During the following decade, he and his coworkers, Neergaard and Wirz, applied Poiseuille's law for laminar flow and his equations to the determination of airway resistance. Fleisch's pneumotachygraph with periodic interruptions of airflow was used as a strategy for

measuring alveolar pressure. Measurements of alveolar pressure that were more useful clinically became available in 1956 with the introduction by DuBois and associates of the whole-body plethysmograph which they coupled with the application of Boyle's law.[6]

SYNTHESIS OF MECHANICS

During the decade between 1915 and 1926, Rohrer and his colleagues provided a remarkably comprehensive synthesis of respiratory mechanics that included a description of the static pressure-volume characteristics of the respiratory system, the work of breathing, and they developed the principle of optimal frequencies of breathing to minimize respiratory work. Together with von Neergaard and Wirz, Rohrer developed and tested experimentally concepts involving pressures, flows, and volumes.[44] The full significance of Rohrer's work was not appreciated until the publications by Fenn and his group at the University of Rochester starting in the 1940s. Although it is still premature to evaluate the contributions of W. O. Fenn, H. Rahn, and A. B. Otis to our present understanding of the mechanics of breathing, there is little doubt that this group shaped much of the contemporary thinking of respiratory physiologists and pulmonary physicians along this line.[14,42]

CONTROL OF BREATHING

The control of breathing is a complex process which depends on the integrity of the entire respiratory system—lungs, airways, circulation, and control systems. Two dominant control systems exist: One is in the central nervous system, and the other is outside the brain. Control mechanisms in the central nervous system are influenced by the state of wakefulness or alertness and are subject to voluntary control. These mechanisms are also influenced reflexively by peripheral receptors of different kinds.

LOCALIZATION OF THE CENTRAL RESPIRATORY CENTERS

In 1812, Legallois, apparently intrigued by the gasp movements of the head after decapitation, identified an area in the medulla that was essential for life. In 1923, Lumsden systematically explored the effects of serial sections of the brain stem on respiration. This report marks the beginning of current lines of research on rhythmic breathing.[9] He designated an area in the caudal pons responsible for a sustained inspired drive as the "apneustic center" and an area in the rostral and lateral portions of the pons which presumably inhibited the apneustic drive as the "pneumotaxic center"; section of the vagi exaggerated the inhibition of the apneustic drive by the pneumotaxic center. Sixteen years later, Pitts and coworkers, using stereotactic stimulation of the cat medulla, identified inspiratory and expiratory centers and proposed a theory that could account for both rhythmic breathing and apneusis.[40]

CHEMICAL STIMULATION OF THE RESPIRATORY CENTERS

The chemical stimuli to breathing have been known for more than a century.[9,28] In 1885, Miescher-Ruesch showed in humans that ventilation at rest is primarily regulated by carbon dioxide.

Between 1887 and 1901, cross-perfusion experiments by Leon Fredericq underscored the role of carbon dioxide. But, it was not until 1905 to 1909 that Haldane, Priestley, and Douglas paved the way to the modern understanding of the role of carbon dioxide under a variety of experimental conditions.[21] In their experiments on humans, they relied heavily on the Haldane gas analyzer and an alveolar gas sampler of their own invention. However, their experiments did not distinguish clearly between CO_2 or H^+ in the stimulation of the respiratory centers. Winterstein[49] and later Gesell[20] advanced the idea that the chemical regulation of respiration is by the concentration of hydrogen ions within the respiratory centers.

The Winterstein theories provide a good example of the evolution of ideas prompted by new discoveries and inventions. The original theory in 1911 attributed increments in ventilation caused by hypoxic or hypercapnic inspired mixtures to a single mechanism, i.e., acidification of arterial blood by either carbonic acid or lactic acid. In 1921, largely because of chemoreceptors, Jacob's demonstration of the rapid diffusion of carbon dioxide into starfish eggs[27] implicated acidity within the respiratory centers as well as arterial blood acidity, as the sites of stimulation. In order to account for the stimulation of breathing by hypoxia (the peripheral chemoreceptors had not yet been discovered), he invoked the release of asphyxiating substances ("*Erstickungsstoffen*") within the respiratory centers themselves. A third theory in 1949, which attempted to incorporate the discovery of the peripheral chemoreceptors, finally gave way in 1955 to his fourth theory, which explained the effects of acid or hypoxia on both the central and peripheral chemoreceptors.

A major consequence of Winterstein's research was the impetus it gave to subsequent explorations of the chemical control of breathing. These explorations led to the identification of central chemoreceptors, distinct from mechanoreceptors, on the ventral surface of the medulla and clarification of the role of hydrogen ion activity as the central stimulus to breathing. It also prompted a search, which continues to this day, not only for the drives to ventilation arising from respiratory and metabolic acidosis but also for a unifying theory for the chemical control of breathing.[39]

THE REFLEX REGULATION OF BREATHING

A considerable and diverse number of peripheral receptors can influence breathing reflexively by supplying information to respiratory centers located in the brain. These include pain receptors, stretch receptors in the muscles and distensible structures, and organs and chemoreceptors in major systemic arteries.

Mechanoreceptors

Until the work of Hering and his student, J. Breuer, little was known about the role of afferent impulses to the central control mechanisms in the control of breathing except that electrical stimulation of the vagus nerves influenced respiration. In 1868, Hering and Breuer reported that inflation of the lungs stopped respiration in expiration and promoted expiration and that, conversely, a decrease in lung volume ended expiration and promoted inspiration. They inferred that inflation had mechanically stimulated nerve endings in the lungs and that the resulting impulses ascending the vagi were inhibitory to inspiration.[47]

Peripheral Chemoreceptors

In 1841, Volkmann suggested the existence of chemoreceptors in the systemic circulation that were sensitive to blood-borne stimulants to respiration. In 1927, J.F. Heymans and C. Heymans first showed that the aortic bodies served this function, and in 1930, C. Heymans and Bouckaert demonstrated the peripheral chemoreceptive function of the carotid bodies.[25,45] These were physiological observations that tallied well with the observations of F. De Castro, a student and later a colleague of Ramón y Cajal, who was sufficiently impressed by the histologic structure, location, and rich innervation of the carotid body to propose that it might be stimulated by blood-borne substances (Fig. 1-13).[10,26]

VENTILATION-PERFUSION RELATIONSHIPS

In 1946, William Dock attributed the apical localization of tuberculosis to hypoperfusion of well-ventilated alveoli in the lung apices in the upright position.[11] Shortly thereafter, ventilation–blood flow relationships were described in quantitative terms in papers by two separate groups: Rahn and Fenn[41] and Riley and Cournand.[43]

SCIENTIFIC CLINICAL MEDICINE

Four remarkable figures may serve to illustrate different stages in the evolution of scientific pulmonary medicine: Morgagni, Laënnec, Koch, Cournand, and Richards. They represent pathologic anatomy, microbiology, and physiology.

Pathologic Anatomy

Two figures, almost a century apart, stand out in the contributions of pathologic anatomy to pulmonary medicine.

MORGAGNI

In the eighteenth century, a major contribution to scientific clinical medicine was made by Morgagni, student of Valsalva (Fig. 1-14). Morgagni veered away from the undisciplined case reports of his predecessors. Instead, he adopted a logical system for relating findings at autopsy to their clinical manifestations. At age 79, he published a compilation of his lifelong experience in his famous work, *De Sedibus et Causis Morborum per Anatomen Indagatis*. *De Sedibus* includes about 700 cases. The clinical-pathologic correlations in this work benefited greatly from the fact that Morgagni was both a seasoned clinician and a pathologist. One of the compilation's five books is devoted to diseases of the thorax. Among his descriptions were those of a tubercle undergoing liquefaction and the hepatization stage of pneumonia.[37]

LAËNNEC

René Théophile Laënnec invented the stethoscope in 1816. At that time, clinical medicine in Europe, especially in France, was turning from metaphysic concepts and doctrinal systems to pathology as its scientific foundation. Eminent physicians, such as Bichat, Bayle, and Corvisart in France, and William and John

Hunter and Baillie in England, were turning to the anatomic findings at autopsy to understand the signs and symptoms of their patients. Percussion had been rediscovered by Corvisart: Although Auenbrugger had reported his "new invention" in 1761 in Latin, the idea had not caught on until Corvisart—eminent clinician and teacher and personal physician to Napoleon—published a translation in French in 1808. Corvisart's approach to medicine strongly influenced Laënnec. Laënnec applied the stethoscope and Corvisart's "sounding of the chest" to study individual patients with diseases of the lungs and heart throughout their clinical course to anatomical examination at autopsy. This was no simple matter. Since there were no pathologists in those days, the physician not only had to provide continuous care during the patient's lifetime but also had to arrange for, and perform, the autopsy and then to gather all that he had seen and learned and prepare it for publication.

In 1819, two years after the invention of the stethoscope, Laënnec published his famous monograph, *De l'Auscultation médiate,* which drew lessons from carefully documented cases that were studied throughout their clinical course and at autopsy. In this work, Laënnec built upon the monumental tome of Morgagni, who had, a generation before, related the clinical features of the diseases that he described to the morbid anatomy but had not been able to take the next step of relating the clinical course of individual patients to the anatomical findings after death.

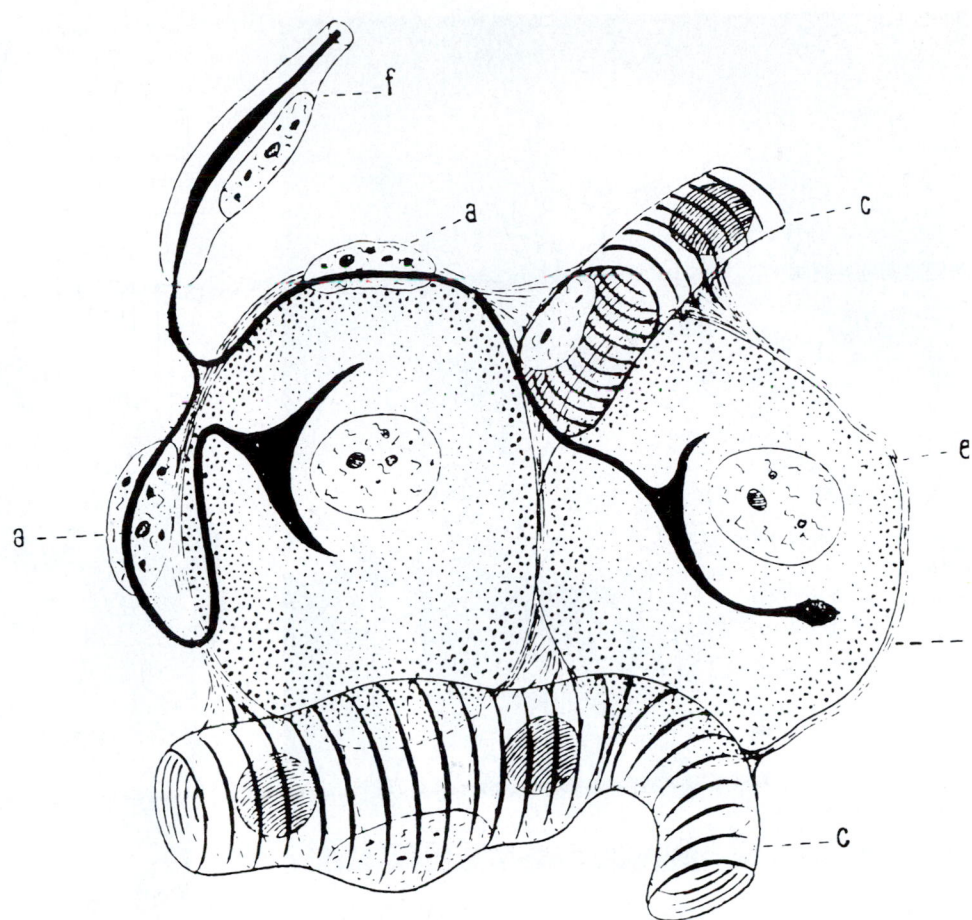

FIGURE 1-13   Drawing by De Castro showing the structure of the chemoreceptor. The glomus cells (*e*) present an ample cytoplasmic surface for contact with the perfusing blood delivered by the capillary (*c*); sensory nerve fiber (*f*) with sheath of myelin; Schwann cells (*a*) surrounded the unmyelinated fibers which form the terminal menisci; cell membrane (*b*). *(From De Castro F: Sur la structure de la synapse dans les chemocepteurs: leur mécanisme d'Excitation et Rôle dans la circulation sanguine locale. Acta Physiol Scand 22:14, 1951.)*

Laënnec's monograph contains descriptions of physical signs, clinical-pathologic correlations for tuberculosis, pneumonia, bronchiectasis, emphysema, and cancer of the lung, and instructions for the treatment of these conditions.[32] The descriptions of tuberculosis were outstanding in the history of tuberculosis before Koch discovered the causative agent of the disease.

Microbiology

Tuberculosis provides a remarkably illuminating example of the impact of a novel basic science on clinical medicine. The disease can be traced back to the ancients, who were familiar with the diverse clinical syndromes that we now take for granted as due to tuberculosis but had no way to relate them to a common etiologic agent. A synthesis by Morton in 1685 of all that was then known about tuberculosis focused on cavitory lesions, emaciation ("consumption") and the tubercle but was shrouded in Galenic humors. Understanding of the disease accelerated in the

eighteenth century when clinicians, such as William Cullen, began to sort out the various syndromes relating to phthisis, recognizing hemoptysis, empyema, catarrh, and asthma.[4]

The tempo of discovery increased dramatically in the nineteenth century, after the French Revolution. During the Napoleonic era, distinguished Parisian clinicians, including Bichat, Bayle, Louis, Broussais, and Laënnec, reported clinical-pathologic correlations of tuberculosis. Both Bayle and Laënnec died of tuberculosis. However, little advance was made in understanding the pathogenesis of tuberculosis until Villemin,[50] impressed by the analogy between glanders and syphilis on the one hand and tuberculosis on the other and by the fact that two of the three diseases had been shown to be infectious in origin, undertook experiments that showed that tuberculosis was an infectious disease that could be transmitted from humans to animals and from animals to animals.

KOCH

In 1876, Koch was a general practitioner in the German township of Wollestein in the province of Posen, where he was re-

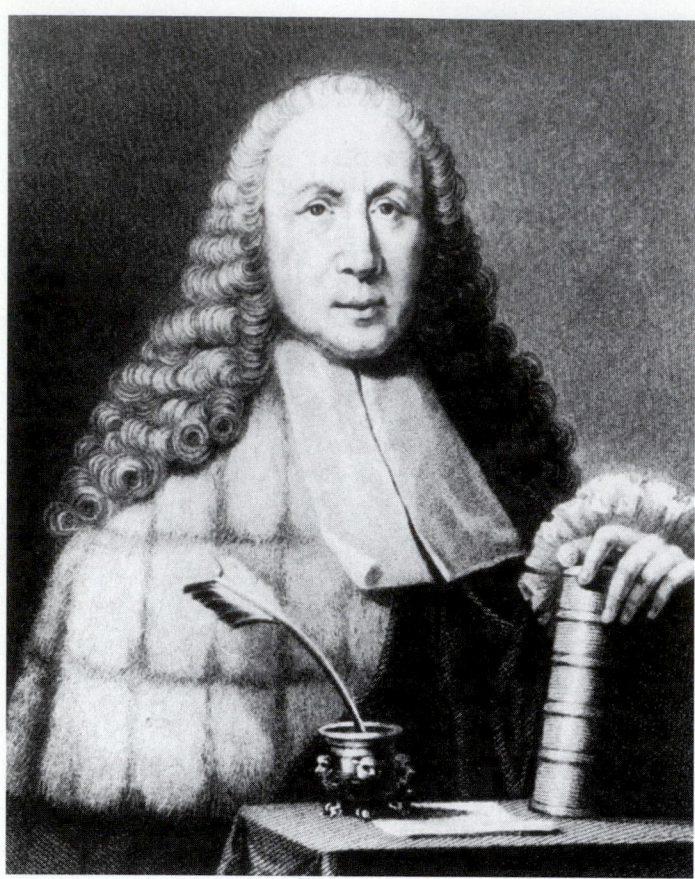

FIGURE 1-14 Giovanni Battista Morgagni (1682–1771). The five volumes of his *De Sedibus* contain the clinical and pathologic descriptions of approximately 700 cases. *(Courtesy of the Library of the College of Physicians of Philadelphia.)*

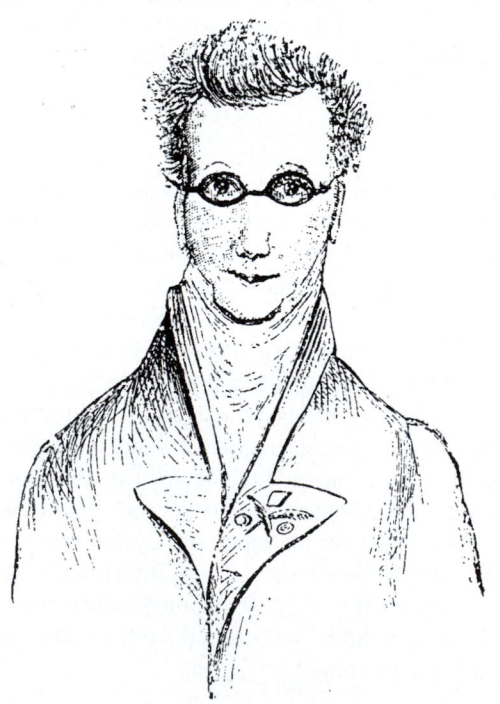

FIGURE 1-15 Rene T.H. Laënnec (1781–1826). *[Drawn from life in 1825 by Charles James Blasius Williams (1805–1889) and reproduced in his autobiography,* Memoirs of Life and Work, *London, Smith, Elder & Co, 1884.]*

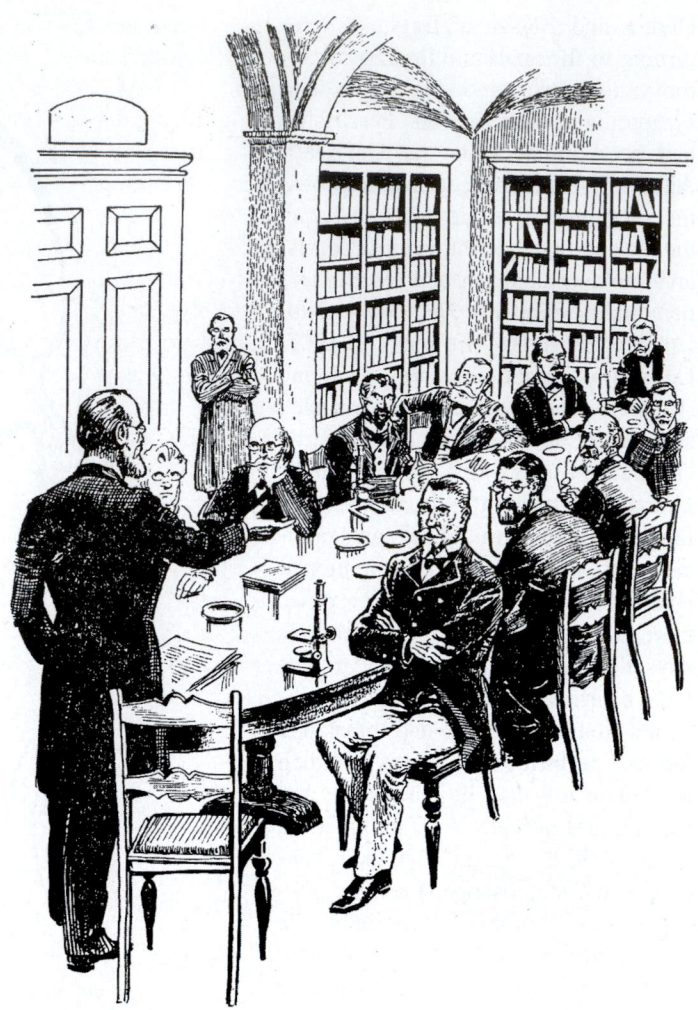

FIGURE 1-16 Robert Koch (1843–1910), announcing his discovery of the tubercle bacillus as the cause of tuberculosis. Berlin, March 28, 1882. *(Reproduced with permission from Knight D: Robert Koch: Founder of Bacteriology. New York: Franklin Watts, Inc., 1961, p 10.)*

sponsible for the health care of 4000 inhabitants (Fig. 1-16). Between obstetrical deliveries and satisfying the medical and surgical needs of patients of all ages, he managed to conduct research on the microbial causes of communicable diseases. His laboratory was homemade, either the barn or living room; his major instrument was a microscope to examine bacteriologic and tissue specimens. In pursuing his research, he kept in mind the dictum of Jacob Henle, one of his teachers in medical school, who counseled that: "Before microscopic organisms can be regarded as the cause of contagion in man, they must be found constantly in the contagious material, they must be isolated from it and their strength tested." This lesson was to be the keynote of the future Koch postulates.

In 1876, Koch, the busy medical practitioner, sent a letter to professor Ferdinand Cohn, director of the Botanical Institute in Breslau, indicating that he had discovered "the process of development of bacillus anthracis" and requesting permission to present his findings to Professor Cohn, "the foremost authority on bacteria." Koch had discovered the spores of anthrax bacilli. Cohn arranged for him to present his results before a formidable room full of distinguished scientists, i.e., Julius Cohnheim,

Carl Weigert, Moritz Traube, Ludwig Lichtheim, and Leopold Auerbach. Koch's demonstration of the complete life history of the anthrax bacillus, including sporulation, was entirely convincing to these scientists. After the meeting, Cohnheim, upon his return home, announced to his colleagues, "This man has made a splendid discovery which is all the more astonishing because Koch has had no scientific connections and has worked entirely on his own initiative and has produced something absolutely complete. There is nothing more to be done. I consider this the greatest discovery in the field of bacteriology. . . ."

During the next two years, Koch described novel procedures for the examination, preservation, and photography of bacteria and demonstrated the role of microorganisms in traumatic infections while continuing his dual existence as a country doctor and an independent investigator. In 1880, Cohn and Cohnheim arranged for him to move to Berlin as a member of the Imperial Sanitary Commission. This move freed more time for research. By 1881, he made another breakthrough. This was the pour-plate method for isolating pure cultures. The ability that this technique afforded of producing transparent solid media coupled with his invention of new staining methods paved the way for him to tackle the microbial cause of tuberculosis.

His scientific approach, which has become immortalized as the "Koch postulates," consisted of four essential steps:

1. To prove that a microbe is the cause of a disease, it must be present in all cases of the disease. (He showed this for the tubercle bacillus using methylene blue and a counter stain.)
2. The microbe must be grown outside of the body in pure culture. (He devised blood-serum jelly as a culture medium for the slow-growing tubercle bacillus.)
3. The pure culture must be capable of causing the disease in healthy animals. (He proved this initially by inoculation and subsequently by allowing animals to breathe contaminated air.)
4. The same microbe must then be isolated from the inoculated (infected) animal and grown outside of the body in pure culture.

Koch's discovery of the tubercle bacillus and its modes of transmission revolutionized the treatment of tuberculosis. Before the discovery, tubercular patients were treated in sanitaria which offered fresh air and altitude. Those who ran the sanitaria did not know that tuberculosis was a contagious disease: Sanitation was unregulated; neither sterilization nor fumigation were practiced; there were no laws about spitting; diagnostic capabilities were limited. Koch's discovery of the tubercle bacillus revolutionized therapy. For the rest of his life, while pursuing the causes of other diseases around the world—rinderpest in South Africa, Texas fever, tropical malaria, blackwater fever, bubonic plague in

Bombay—he maintained his interest in tuberculosis. His interest led him into a major mistake, i.e., advocacy of tuberculin as a vaccine instead of its present use as a diagnostic test. In 1905, he was awarded the Nobel prize. On April 7, 1910, the year of his death, he delivered a final address on the epidemiology of tuberculosis before the Berlin Academy of Sciences.

Physiology of the Pulmonary Circulation

Starting with William Harvey, studies of the pulmonary circulation have gone hand in hand with advances in pulmonary physiology and medicine. For many years, research on the pulmonary circulation was confined to animal experimentation. A giant step forward was made by the introduction of cardiac catheterization in humans.

Accurate measurement of pulmonary blood flow is a sine qua non for assessing pulmonary and cardiac performance in health and disease. The use of nitrous oxide in humans by Krogh and Lindhard[47] was an important beginning in this direction, but not until mixed venous blood could be sampled for application of the Fick principle could reliable determinations of pulmonary blood flow be made.

Claude Bernard in 1846, and Chauveau and Marey in 1861, had catheterized the right side of the heart in animal experiments.[6] Whether this technique could be safely used in humans was not known until 1929, when Werner Forssmann, a young surgeon in Germany, introduced a ureteral catheter into his own right atrium. In the 1940s, Cournand, Richards and their colleagues, resorted to right heart catheterization in order to obtain mixed venous blood for the determination of cardiac output by the Fick principle (Fig. 1-17). As everyone knows, the technique opened the way not only to the accurate determination of cardiac output but

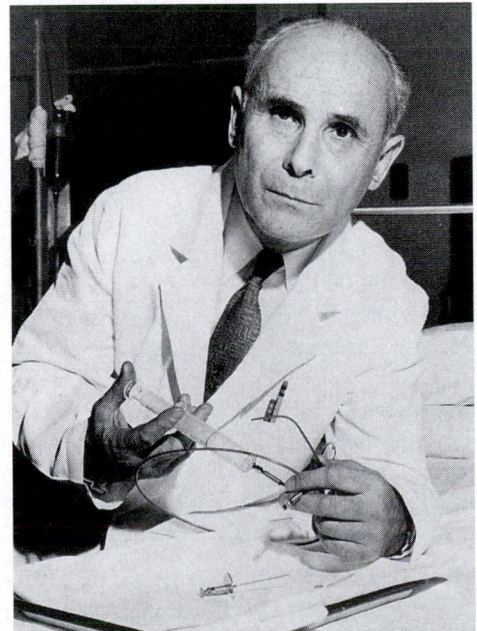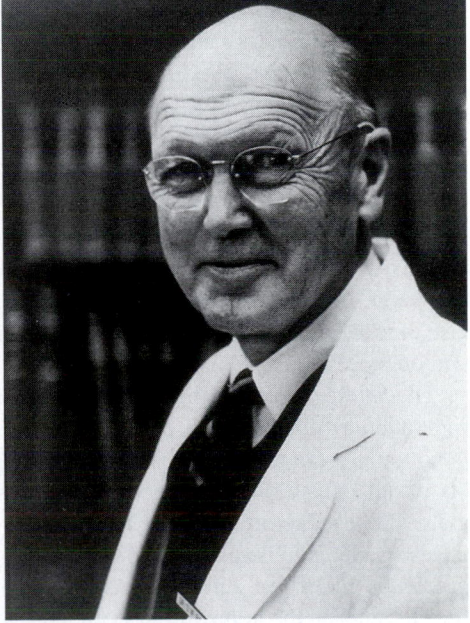

FIGURE 1-17 André Frederic Cournand (1895–1988) and Dickinson W. Richards (1895–1973). After Forssman's report of the uneventful catheterization of his own right heart, Cournand and Richards pioneered the use of cardiac catheterization for the study of the normal and abnormal pulmonary circulation and the standardization of pulmonary function tests.

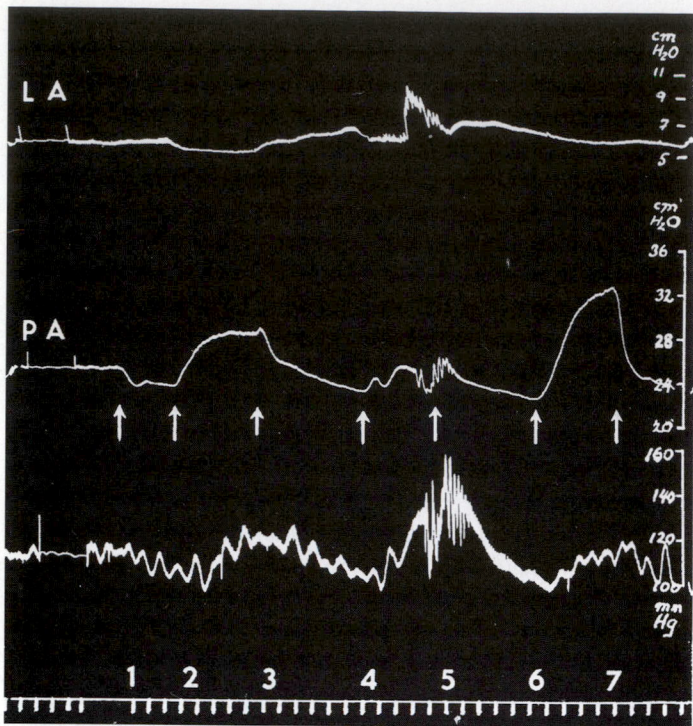

FIGURE 1-18 Effects of the blood gases on pulmonary arterial pressure in the open-chest cat, artificial respiration. LA = left atrial pressure; PA = pulmonary arterial pressure; lower trace = systemic arterial blood pressure. Numbers along the baseline represent the administration of test gases: 1 = O_2 (from air); 2 = 6.5% CO_2 in O_2; 3 = O_2; 4 = 18.7% CO_2 in CO_2; 5 = O_2; 6 = 10.5% O_2 in N_2; 7 = O_2. *(From Von Euler, US and Liljestrand, G: Observations on the pulmonary arterial blood pressure in the cat. Acta Physiol Scand 12:310, 1946.)*

also to exploring the heart and lungs in a wide variety of clinical cardiac and pulmonary disorders.[8]

Until 1946, when von Euler and Liljestrand reported the effects of hypoxia and hypercapnia on the pulmonary circulation of the open chest of an anesthetized cat (Fig. 1-18), there was little understanding of the regulation of the pulmonary circulation.[13] However, these studies, and the proposition of local control of the pulmonary circulation by local concentrations of the respiratory gases, paved the way to understanding pulmonary hypertension and the behavior of the pulmonary circulation on the one hand, in normal individuals at rest, after birth, during exercise, and at altitude, and on the other, in individuals with heart and/or lung disease.

The interposition of the pulmonary circulation between the right and left sides of the heart, an eventual step for life on earth, is not only prerequisite for gas exchange, but also serves a variety of other functions, e.g., mechanical, as a filter for particulate matter in blood returning to the heart, and metabolic, for the synthesis uptake, and breakdown for vital biologic functions and ingredients. Extensive studies have been conducted over the last few decades on the nonrespiratory functions of the lungs.[23] From these studies has emerged considerable understanding of the diverse functions served by the branching pulmonary circulation and by its components, i.e., endothelium and smooth muscle and their interplay in the pulmonary circulation.

TECHNOLOGICAL INVENTIONS AND IMPROVEMENTS

The road to contemporary pulmonary medicine could be just as easily traced by using technological advances as landmarks instead of people and discoveries. For example, the introduction of the manometer for pressure recording, the use of chambers to simulate high altitude, the development of accurate blood-gas analyzers, the application of sophisticated optical systems for viewing the lumens of the airways and the inside of the chest cavity are all notable milestones. However, probably no better example exists than the discovery of radiographs and the application of this discovery to the diagnosis, prevention, and management of pulmonary tuberculosis.

Wilhelm Conrad Roentgen (1845–1923) discovered radiographs in 1895 while experimenting with cathode ray tubes in his physics laboratory at the University of Wurzburg.[3] Although others before him had seen radiographs as early as 1890, Roentgen was apparently the first to grasp the full significance of the discovery, and his publication, quite unpretentious, immediately attracted worldwide attention because of its prospects for the study of anatomic structures and pathologic changes.

Within 2 years after Roentgen's discovery, fluoroscopy of the chest had been introduced into clinical practice, and its value in the early detection of tuberculosis and in the diagnosis of pleural effusions was appreciated. In 1901, an atlas of chest radiographs was published, and the use of chest radiography increased greatly with each subsequent improvement in hot-cathode radiograph tubes and intensifying screens. The radiographic evaluation of tuberculosis was superior to physical examination per se for the diagnosis and characterization of pulmonary tuberculosis. By 1910, all patients admitted to sanatoriums were undergoing chest radiographic examination, and by 1917 tuberculosis was being classified according to radiograph findings.[12]

REFERENCES

1. Barcroft J: *Features in the Architecture of Physiological Function.* New York, Hafner, 1972.
2. Bohr C: Ueber die spezifische Tätigkeit der Lungen bei der respiratorischen Gasaufnahme und irh Verhalten zu der durch die Alveolarwand staffindenden Gasdiffusion. *Skand Arch Physiol* 16:402–412, 1904.
3. Castiglione A: History of tuberculosis, Recht E (trans) *Medical Life,* 40:148–159, New York, Froben Press, 1933, pp 1–95.
4. Castiglione A: History of tuberculosis. *Medical Life* 40:5–96, 1933.
5. Castiglione A: *A History of Medicine.* New York, Alfred A. Knopf, 1947.
6. Comroe JH Jr: *Pulmonary and Respiratory Physiology.* Stroudsburg, PA, Dowden, Hutchinson and Ross, 1976.
7. Cournand A: Air and blood, in Fishman AP, Richards DW (eds), *Circulation of the Blood. Men and Ideas.* Bethesda, MD, American Physiological Society, 1982, pp 3–70.
8. Cournand A, Ranges HA: Catheterization of the right auricle in man. *Proc Soc Exp Biol Med* 46(3):462–466, 1941.
9. Cunningham DJC, Robbins PA, Wolff CB: Integration of respiratory responses to changes in alveolar partial pressures of CO_2 and O_2 and in arterial pH, in *Handbook of Physiology,* Section 3: *The Respiratory System,* vol 2, *Control of Breathing;* NS Cherniack, JG Widdicombe (eds). Bethesda, MD, American Physiological Society, 1986, pp 475–476.

10. De Castro F: Sur la structure et l'innervation de la glande inter-carotidienne (glomus caroticum) de l'homme et des mammifères et sur un nouveau système d'innervation autonome du nerf glossopharyngien. *Trav Lab Recherches Biol Univ Madrid* 24:365–432, 1926.

11. Dock W: Apical localization of phthisis. *Am Rev Tuber* 53:297–305, 1946.

12. Eisenberg RL: *Radiology. An Illustrated History.* St. Louis, Mosby Year Book, 1995.

13. Euler US von, Liljestrand G: Observations on the pulmonary arterial blood pressure in the cat. *Acta Physiol Scand* 12:301–320, 1946.

14. Fenn WO: Introduction to the mechanics of breathing, in Fenn WO, Rahn H (eds): *Handbook of Physiology,* Section 3: *Respiration,* vol 1. Bethesda, MD, American Physiological Society, 1964, pp 357–362.

15. Foster M: *Lectures on the History of Physiology.* London, Cambridge University Press, 1901.

16. Frank RG Jr: *Harvey and the Oxford Physiologists.* Berkeley, CA, University of California Press, 1980.

17. Franklin KJ: *A Short History of Physiology,* 2d ed. London, Staples, 1949.

18. Furley DJ, Wilkie JS: *Galen on Respiration and the Arteries.* Princeton, NJ, Princeton University Press, 1984.

19. Galen: *On the Usefulness of the Parts of the Body,* May MT (trans). Ithaca, NY, Cornell University Press, 1968, pp 279, 599–600.

20. Gesell R: On the chemical regulation of respiration: I. The regulation of respiration with special reference to the metabolism of the respiratory center and the coordination of the dual function of hemoglobin. *Am J Physiol* 66:40–47, 1923.

21. Haldane JS, Priestley JG: *Respiration.* Oxford, Clarendon Press, 1935.

22. Harvey W: *Movement of the Heart and Blood in Animals, an Anatomical Essay,* Franklin, KJ (trans). Oxford, Blackwell Scientific Publications, 1957.

23. Heinemann HO, Fishman AP: Non-respiration functions of mammalian lung. *Physiol Rev* 49:1–47, 1969.

24. Henderson LJ: *Blood. A Study in General Physiology.* New Haven, CT, Yale University Press, 1982.

25. Heymans C, Bouckaert JJ, Regniers P: *Le Sinus carotidien, et la zone homologue cardioaortique.* Paris, Doin, 1933.

26. Heymans C, Neil E: *Reflexogenic Areas of the Cardiovascular System.* London, Churchill, 1958.

27. Jacobs MH: The production of intracellular acidity by neutral and alkaline solutions containing carbon dioxide. *Am J Physiol* 53:457–463, 1920.

28. Kellogg RH: Central chemical regulation of respiration, in Fenn WO, Rahn H (eds), *Handbook of Physiology.* Section 3: *Respiration,* vol 1, Bethesda, MD, American Physiological Society, 1964, pp 507–534.

29. Krogh A, Krogh M: On the tensions of gases in the arterial blood. *Skand Arch Physiol* 23:179–192, 1910.

30. Krogh A, Lindhard J: Measurements of the blood flow through the lungs of man. *Skand Arch Physiol* 27:100–105, 106–109, 118–121, 124–125, 1912.

31. Krogh M: The diffusion of gases through the lungs of man. *J Physiol (Lond)* 49:271–300, 1915.

32. Laënnec R: On the diagnosis of diseases of the chest. *A Treatise on the Diseases of the Chest,* Forbes J (trans). London, 1821, Hafner Publishing Co, 1962.

33. Lower R: *Tractatus de Corde: Item De Motu & Colore Sanguinis et Chyli in cum Transitu.* Elzevir edition, 1669, p 176. English excerpt: On the color of the blood, Franklin KJ (trans), in *Early Science in Oxford,* vol 9, Oxford, Clarendon Press, 1932.

34. Mayow J: *Medico-Physical Works,* Crum A, Brown, Dobbin L (trans). Edinburgh, Alembic Club, Reprints, no 17, 1957. (Translated from *Tractatus quinque medico-physics,* 1674.)

35. McKie D: *Antoine Lavoissier: Scientist, Economist, Social Reformer.* New York, Schuman, 1952.

36. Milledge JS: The great oxygen secretion controversy. *Lancet* 2:1408–1411, 1985.

37. Morgagni GB: *The Seats and Causes of Diseases Investigated by Anatomy,* Alexander B (trans). London, A Miller, T Cadell, 1769.

38. Otis AB: History of respiratory mechanics, in Fishman AP (ed), *Handbook of Physiology.* Section 3: *The Respiratory System,* vol 3, *Mechanics of Breathing;* PT Macklem, J Mead (part 1 eds). Bethesda, MD, American Physiological Society, 1986, pp 1–12.

39. Perkins JF Jr: Historical development of respiratory physiology, in Fenn WO, Rahn H (eds), *Handbook of Physiology.* Section 3: *Respiration,* vol 1, Bethesda, MD, American Physiological Society, 1964, pp 1–62.

40. Pitts RF, Magoun HW, Ranson SW: Localization of the medullary respiratory centers in the cat. *Am J Physiol* 126:673–688, 1939.

41. Rahn H: A concept of mean alveolar air and the ventilation-blood flow relationships during pulmonary gas exchange. *Am J Physiol* 158:21–30, 1949.

42. Rahn H, Otis AB, Chadwick LE, Fenn WO: The pressure-volume diagram of the thorax and lung. *Am J Physiol* 146:161–178, 1946.

42a. Richards DW, Henderson LJ: Remarks made at Respiration Dinner, American Physiological Society, Chicago, April 17, 1957.

43. Riley RL, Cournand A: "Ideal" alveolar air and the analysis of ventilation-perfusion relationships in the lungs. *J Appl Physiol* 1(12):825–843, 846–847, 1949.

43a. Roughton FJW: The average time spent by the blood in the human lung capillary and *its* relation to the rates of CO uptake and elimination in man. *Am J Physiol* 143: 621–633, 1945.

44. Rohrer F: Der Zusammenhand der Atemkräfte und ihre Abhängigkeit vom Dehrungszustand der Atmungsorgame. *Pfügers Arch Gesamte Physiol Menschen Tiere* 165:419–444, 1916.

45. Schmidt CF, Comroe JH: Functions of the carotid and aortic bodies. *Physiol Rev* 20:115–157, 1940.

46. Singer C: *A Short History of Scientific Ideas to 1900.* London, Oxford University Press, 1959.

47. Ullmann E: About Hering and Breuer, in Porter R (ed), *Breathing: Hering-Breuer Centenary Symposium.* London, J & A Churchill, 1970, pp 3–15.

48. Underwood EA: The training of the greatest of chest physicians: Laënnec. *Brit J Dis Chest* 53:109–127, 1959.

49. Winterstein H: Die Reactionstheorie der Atmungsregulation. *Arch Ges Physiol* 187:293–298, 1921.

50. Villemin JA: *Études sur la tuberculose.* Paris, J-B Bailliere (ed) fils, 1868.

PART TWO

SCIENTIFIC BASIS OF LUNG FUNCTION IN HEALTH AND DISEASE

CHAPTER 2

FUNCTIONAL DESIGN OF THE HUMAN LUNG FOR GAS EXCHANGE

Ewald R. Weibel / C. Richard Taylor

At the end of a deep breath, about 80 percent of the lung volume is air, 10 percent is blood, and only the remaining 10 percent is tissue. Because this small mass of tissue is spread over an enormous area—nearly the size of a tennis court—the tissue framework of the lung must be extraordinarily delicate. It is indeed remarkable that the substance of the lung manages to maintain its integrity in the face of the multitude of insults that inevitably accompany a lifetime of exposure to ambient air and the complex necessity of keeping air and blood in intimate contact, but separate, for the sake of gas exchange.

Part of this success is undoubtedly attributable to the unique design of the lung, which ensures mechanical stability as well as nearly optimal conditions for the performance of the lung's primary function: to supply the blood with an adequate amount of oxygen even when the body's demands for oxygen are particularly high, as during heavy work. There are, however, some problems that limit this performance, such as inhomogeneities in the relations between perfusion and ventilation of the gas exchange units, basic functions that are, again, related to design properties of the lung, at least in part.

THE LUNG AS AN ORGAN

At total lung capacity, the lung fills the entire chest cavity and can reach a volume, in the adult human, of some 5 to 6 L, largely depending on body size. Upon expiration, the lung retracts, most conspicuously from the lower parts of the pleural cavity, the posterior bottom edge of the lung moving upward by some 4 to 6 cm. This preferential lifting of the bottom edge is caused by retraction of the tissue throughout the entire lung, the surfaces of which are freely movable within the thoracic cavity.

The structural background for this mobility of a healthy lung is the formation, during morphogenesis, of a serosal space that is lined on the interior of the chest wall and on the lung surface by a serosa, the parietal and visceral pleurae, respectively (Fig. 2-1). However, this serosal space is minimal, since the visceral pleura is closely apposed to the parietal pleura, with only a thin film of serous fluid intercalated as a lubricant between the two surfaces.[1] Both pleural surfaces are lined by a squamous epithelial layer, often called *mesothelium,* whose surface is richly endowed with long microvilli. It is unknown how the pleural fluid is secreted or how it is maintained as a minimal film. Whether lymphatics in the parietal pleura play an important role in rapidly draining excess fluid is unsettled.

The connective tissue of the visceral pleura consists of three layers. A superficial layer of predominantly elastic fibers follows the mesothelium, thereby forming an elastic "bag" that enwraps each lobe. A deep sheet of fine fibers follows the outline of alveoli and extends into the depth of the lung. Between these sheets lies a bed of loose connective tissue, containing free cells (histiocytes, plasma cells, and mast cells), that is often close to lymphatics and to systemic arterial branches from the bronchial arteries.

The lung is maintained in a stable position within the chest by the hilus, where airways and blood vessels enter from the mediastinum, and by the pulmonary ligament, a long, narrow band of attachment between visceral and mediastinal pleura which extends downward from the hilus. Because of these attachments, a pneumothorax causes the lung to retract and to form a lump of tissue that is attached to the mediastinal wall of the thoracic cavity.

The shape of the lung is congruent with that of the fully expanded pleural cavity. This shape is preformed in lung tissue and is hence also evident if an excised lung is inflated, revealing its three faces: the convex thoracic face apposed to the rib cage, the concave diaphragmatic face modeled by the diaphragmatic dome, and the mediastinal face, on which the contours of the heart are impressed beneath the hilus.

As the lung retracts during deflation, the acute edges between the thoracic face and the diaphragmatic and (anterior) mediastinal faces of the lung withdraw; the thoracic and diaphragmatic leaflets of the parietal pleura become apposed, thereby forming a costodiaphragmatic recess on each side (Fig. 2-1); similarly, as the ventral edge of the lung retracts, the costal and mediastinal pleurae form a recess on each side, corresponding topographically to the borders of the sternum.

The port through which airways and blood vessels enter the lung is the hilus, i.e., the attachment of lung tissue to the mediastinum (Fig. 2-1). The airways reach the two hili by the mainstem, or principal, bronchi (Figs. 2-1 and 2-2); the left main-

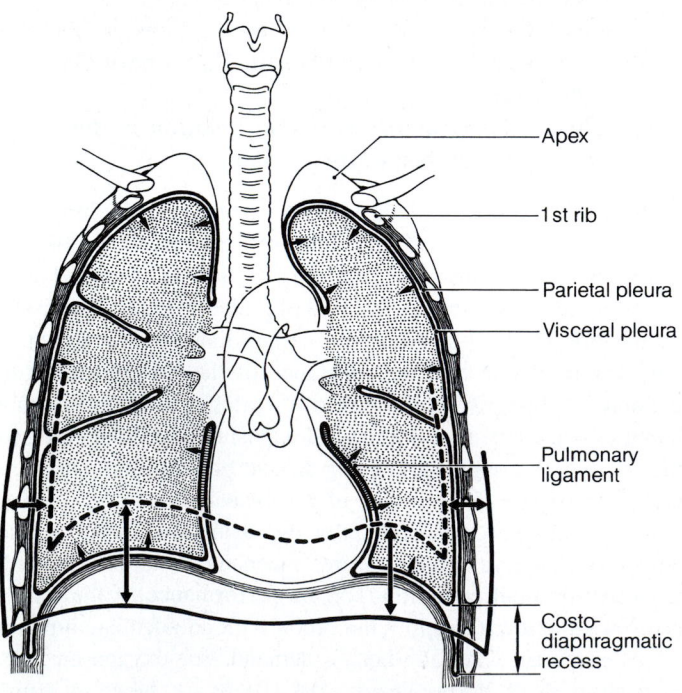

FIGURE 2-1 Frontal section of chest and lung showing pleural space. Single arrows indicate retractive force, double arrows show the excursion of the lung bases and periphery between deep inspiration and expiration.

Labels: Apex; 1st rib; Parietal pleura; Visceral pleura; Pulmonary ligament; Costo-diaphragmatic recess.

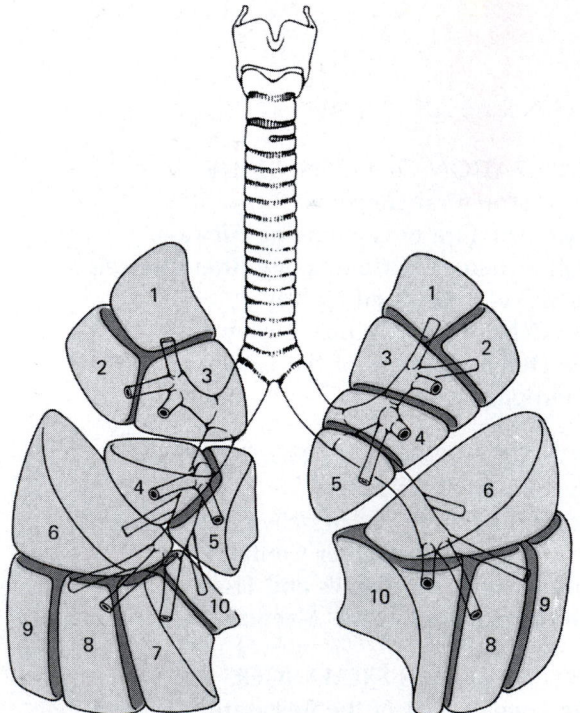

FIGURE 2-2 Bronchopulmonary segments of human lung. Left and right upper lobes: (1) apical, (2) posterior, (3) anterior, (4) superior lingular, and (5) inferior lingular segments. Right middle lobe: (4) lateral and (5) medial segments. Lower lobes: (6) superior (apical), (7) medial-basal, (8) anterior-basal, (9) lateral-basal, and (10) posterior-basal segments. The medial-basal segment (7) is absent in the left lung. (Note: The lungs are represented as turned inward slightly in order to display part of the lateral face.)

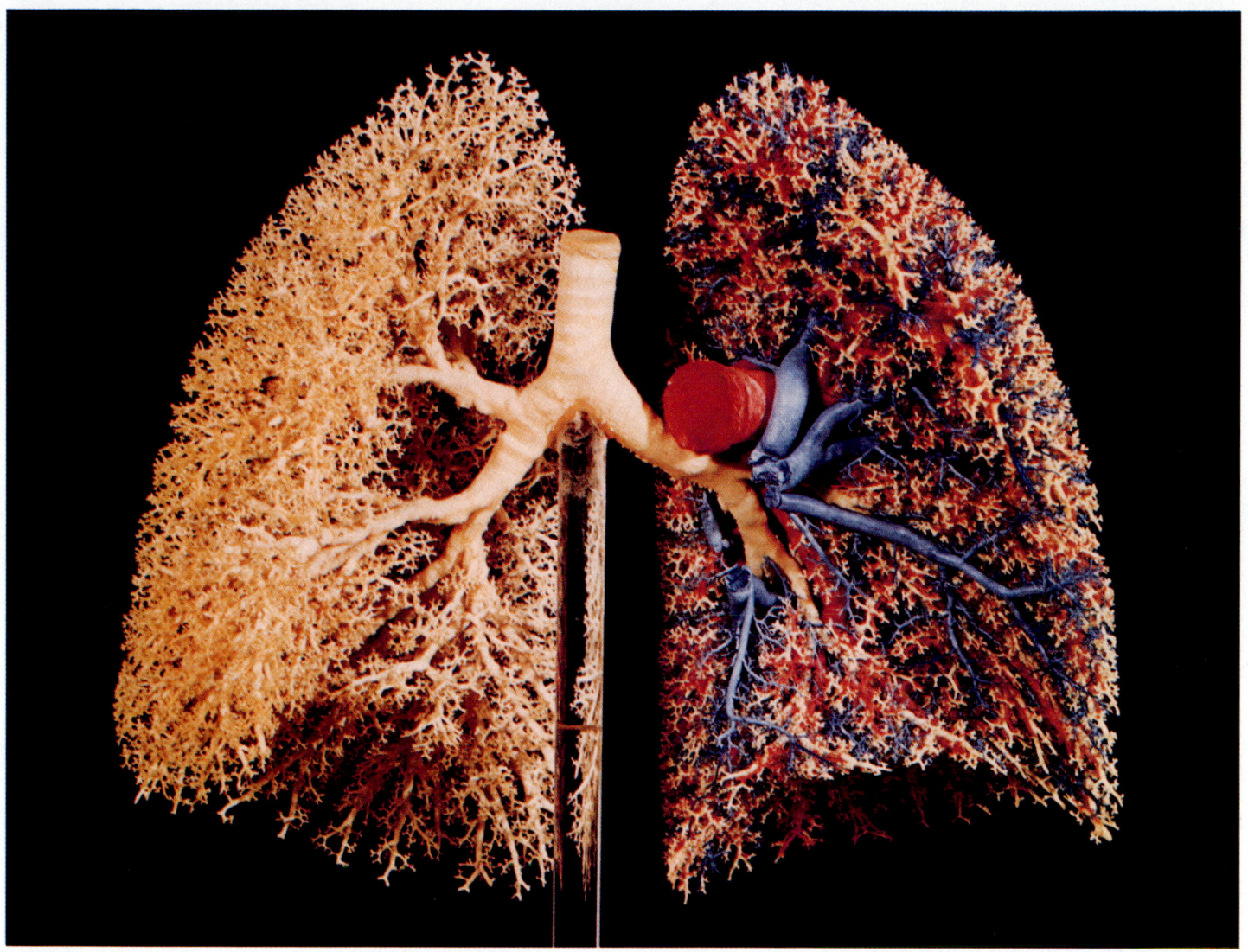

FIGURE 2-3   A resin cast of the human airway tree shows the dichotomous branching of the bronchi from the trachea and the systematic reduction of airway diameter and length with progressive branch-ing. In the left lung the pulmonary arteries (*red*) and veins (*blue*) are also shown.

stem bronchus is longer than the right because it must pass under the aortic arch before it reaches the lung. The two principal bronchi course downward and begin to divide sequentially shortly after entering the lung, first releasing the lobar bronchus to the upper lobe (Fig. 2-2). Since a middle lobe is formed only on the right side, there is no middle lobe bronchus on the left; instead, the corresponding parts form the lingula, which receives its airways from the superior bronchus of the upper lobe (Fig. 2-2). The last branch of the stem bronchus goes to the lower lobe.

The branching pattern of the human bronchial tree and of the pulmonary artery and veins are shown in a resin cast in Fig. 2-3. The pulmonary artery joins the bronchi while still in the mediastinum (Fig. 2-4A); its trunk lies to the left of the ascending aorta, and the right pulmonary artery turns dorsally to course between ascending aorta and right principal bronchus. In the hilus, the right pulmonary artery lies anterior to the right principal bronchus; the left pulmonary artery, however, "rides" on the principal bronchus and crosses over the superior lobar bronchus to the posterior side. From there on, the pulmonary artery branches

in parallel with the bronchi; characteristically, each bronchus is associated with one closely apposed pulmonary artery branch, and this relationship is strictly maintained to the periphery, i.e., to the respiratory bronchioles.

In contrast, the pulmonary veins (Fig. 2-4B) follow a course independent of the bronchial tree; rather, they lie about midway between two pairs of bronchi and arteries; this position is maintained to the periphery of the airway system. In the hilus, these veins are collected into at least two main veins on either side, which lead into the left atrium located at the back of the heart.

The airways systematically branch over an average of 23 generations of dichotomous branching,[45,50] ending eventually in a blind sac (Fig. 2-5). The last six to seven generations of these airways are connected to tightly packed alveoli, airway chambers in which gas exchange takes place, whereas the central airways serve the function of conducting the air to the gas-exchange parenchyma. In such a system of sequential branching, the unit of lung parenchyma could be defined according to the portion of parenchyma that is supplied by a particular branch of the

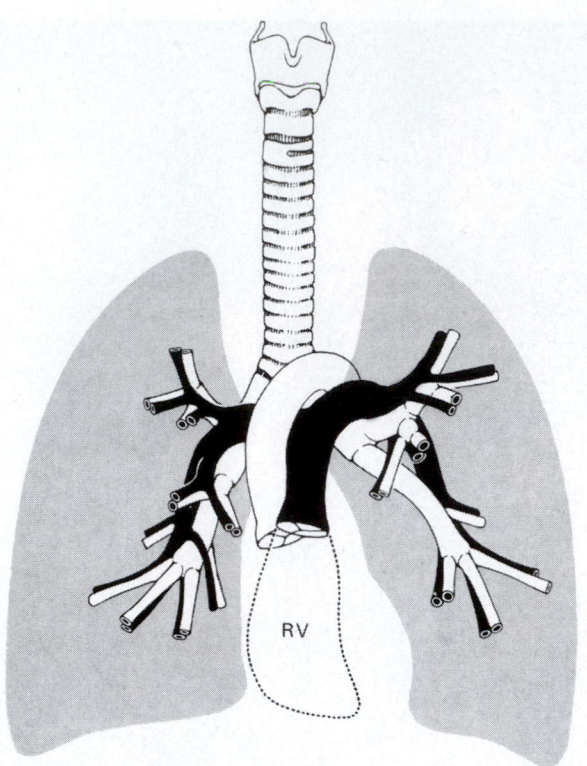

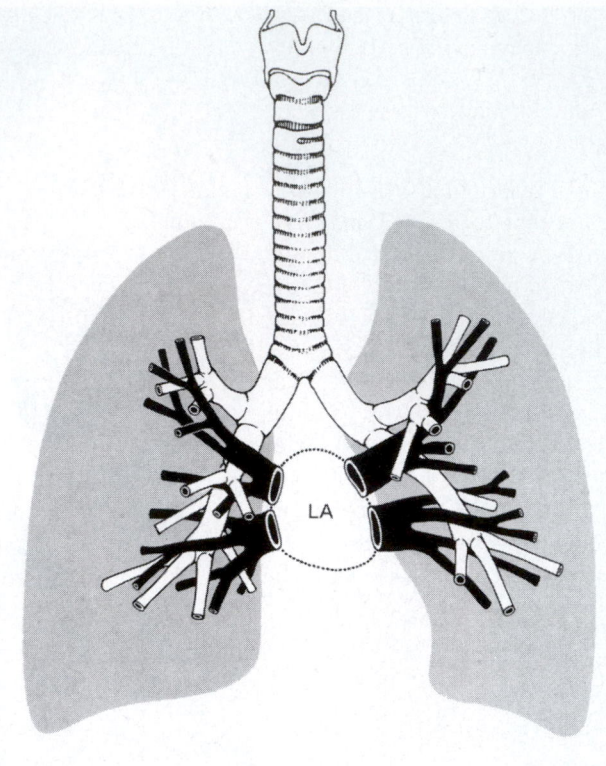

FIGURE 2-4 Schematic diagrams of the relation of the main branches of pulmonary arteries *(A)* and pulmonary veins *(B)* to the bronchial tree. The arteries follow the airways. Two main stems of pulmonary vein pen-

etrate independently into the lung on each side. RV = right ventricle, LA = left atrium.

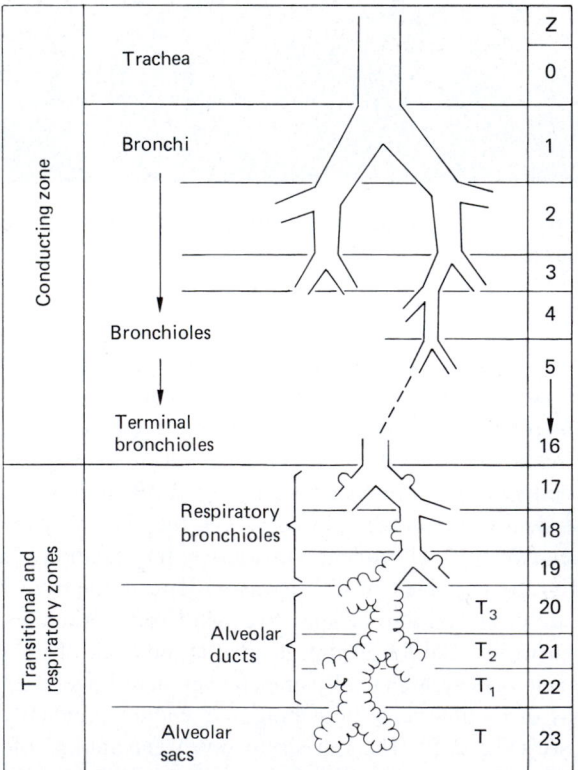

FIGURE 2-5 Airway branching in human lung by regularized dichotomy from trachea (generation z = 0) to alveolar ducts and sacs (generations 20 to 23). The first 16 generations are purely conducting; transitional airways lead into the respiratory zone made of alveoli. *(Adapted from Weibel,[45] with permission.)*

bronchial tree, and it is possible to conceive of as many types of units as there are generations unless clear definitions for such units are proposed. However, two units appear to be natural:

1. The *lobes,* which are demarcated by a more or less complete lining of pleura. There are three lobes on the right (superior, middle, and inferior lobes), and two on the left (superior and inferior lobes).
2. The *acinus,* which is defined as that portion of lung parenchyma that is supplied by a first-order respiratory bronchiole—i.e., a parenchymal unit in which all airways participate in gas exchange.[15]

Since all other units are somewhat arbitrarily defined, it is not surprising that some ambiguity exists in the literature about their meanings. Nonetheless, a certain convention has been adopted with respect to the following:

1. *The lung segments,* which are considered as the first subdivisions of lobes. Figure 2-2 shows the location and distribution of the segments to the various lobes. The symmetry is imperfect because on the left the two segments corresponding to the right middle lobe are incorporated into the superior lobe as the lingula and because the medial-basal segment of the lower lobe is generally missing on the left.
2. *The secondary lobule,* an old anatomic unit. It was introduced in the nineteenth century because "lobules" of about 1 cm³ are visible on the surface of the lung. These lobules are delineated by connective tissue septa that are connected to the pleura. The secondary lobule is difficult to define in terms of the bronchial tree, but it does seem to comprise

about a dozen acini and most often is said to include the parenchyma, which is supplied by about five terminal bronchioles. With reference to bronchograms, secondary lobules are supplied by airway branches that are about 1 mm in diameter.

The pulmonary blood vessels show a characteristic relationship to these units (Figs. 2-3 and 2-4). The pulmonary arteries, following the airways, course through the centers of the units and finally fan out into the capillaries located in the delicate alveolar septa of lung parenchyma. In contrast, the veins lie in the boundary between units and collect the blood from at least two or three adjacent units. This arrangement applies to acini and secondary lobules as well as to lung segments.

Therefore, it is evident that the units of lung parenchyma are bronchoarterial units, which share their venous drainage with neighboring units. This architecture has important functional and practical consequences. Except for the lobes, none of the units are separated from each other by complete connective tissue septa.

ORGANIZATION OF LUNG TISSUE

Basic Structural Elements

In looking at the tissue organization of the lung, we must first consider that the airways and the blood vessels each have their own lining by an uninterrupted cell layer. These layers extend all the way out to the gas-exchange region, but they show different properties in conducting as compared to respiratory structures. Likewise, the connective tissue forms a continuum throughout the lung all the way out to the pleura, but it, too, will be differently organized in the different functional zones: whereas it is reduced to a minimum in the alveolar walls, it contributes a number of different ancillary structures to the wall of conducting airways and blood vessels, such as smooth muscle sheaths or cartilage. This connective tissue space also houses the nutritive vessels and nerves as well as the elaborate defense system related to lymphatic vessels. In the gas-exchange region, however, very few of these accessory structures are found.

Wall Structure of Conducting Airways

The wall of conducting airways consists of three major components (Figs. 2-6 and 2-7): (1) a mucosa composed of an epithelial and a connective tissue lamina, (2) a smooth-muscle sleeve, and (3) an enveloping connective tissue tube partly provided with cartilage.[10]

Though derived from one and the same anlage,[46] the airway epithelium modifies its differentiation characteris-

tics as we proceed from large bronchi over bronchioles to the alveolar region (Fig. 2-6). A simple epithelium exists as a lining of smaller bronchioles: as we move upward toward larger bronchi, the epithelium becomes higher and some basal cells appear, making the epithelium pseudostratified; at the point of transition into the gas-exchange region—that is, at the entrance into the complex of alveoli—the epithelium abruptly becomes extremely thin.

Figure 2-6 also shows that the epithelium is not made of a uniform cell population but that it is, at each level, rather a mosaic of at least two cell types, in that secretory cells are interspersed into the complex of lining cells.[10] There are also some additional rarer cells, such as neuroendocrine cells that are capable of secreting some mediators into the blood, or so-called brush cells whose precise function is not yet understood.

If we now first have a closer look at the epithelium of larger conducting airways, we see that the lining cells are provided with a tuft of kinocilia at their apical cell face, whereas the secretory cells are goblet cells that produce and discharge to the surface a sticky mucus (Figs. 2-8 and 2-9). This mucus spreads out as a thin blanket on top of the cilia and is capable of trapping dust particles that are still contained in the air entering the lung. Kinocilia (Fig. 2-10) are organelles of movement that are known to beat rhythmically in a given direction and at a frequency of about 20 Hz.[36] In the airway epithelium, the cilia are oriented in such a fashion that their beat is directed outward. It is interesting that the cilia of airway epithelia develop at their tip fine claws with which they can grasp the mucus blanket in the phase of their forward beat, whereas on their return to the upright position they glide past the mucus blanket. The result of this is that the mucus blanket, together with trapped foreign material, moves

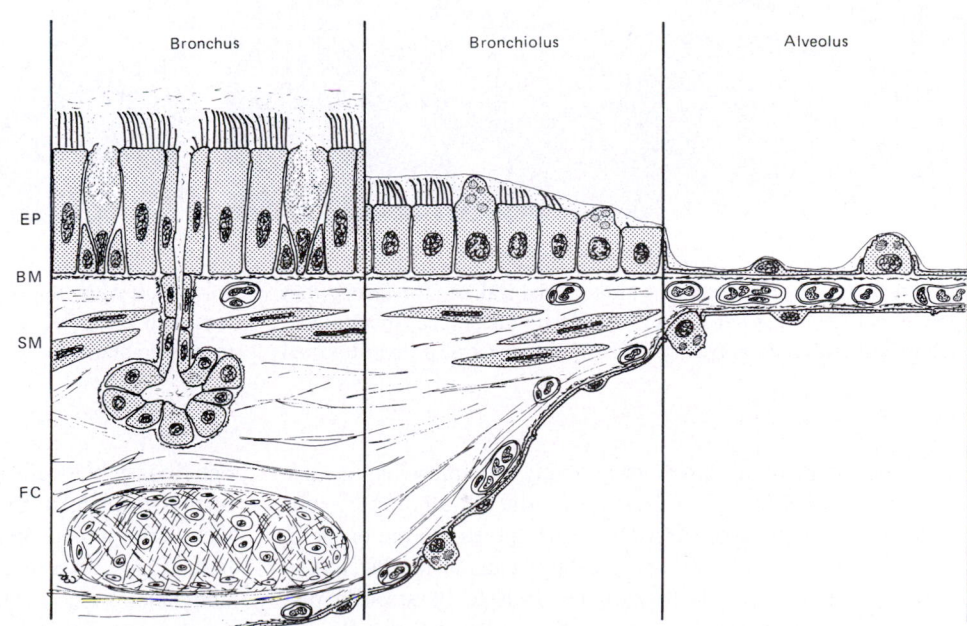

FIGURE 2-6   Airway wall structure at the three principal levels. The epithelial layer (EP) gradually becomes reduced from pseudostratified to cuboidal and then to squamous but retains its organization as a mosaic of lining and secretory cells. The smooth muscle layer (SM) disappears in the alveoli. The fibrous coat (FC) contains cartilage only in bronchi and gradually becomes thinner as the alveolus is approached. BM = basement membrane.

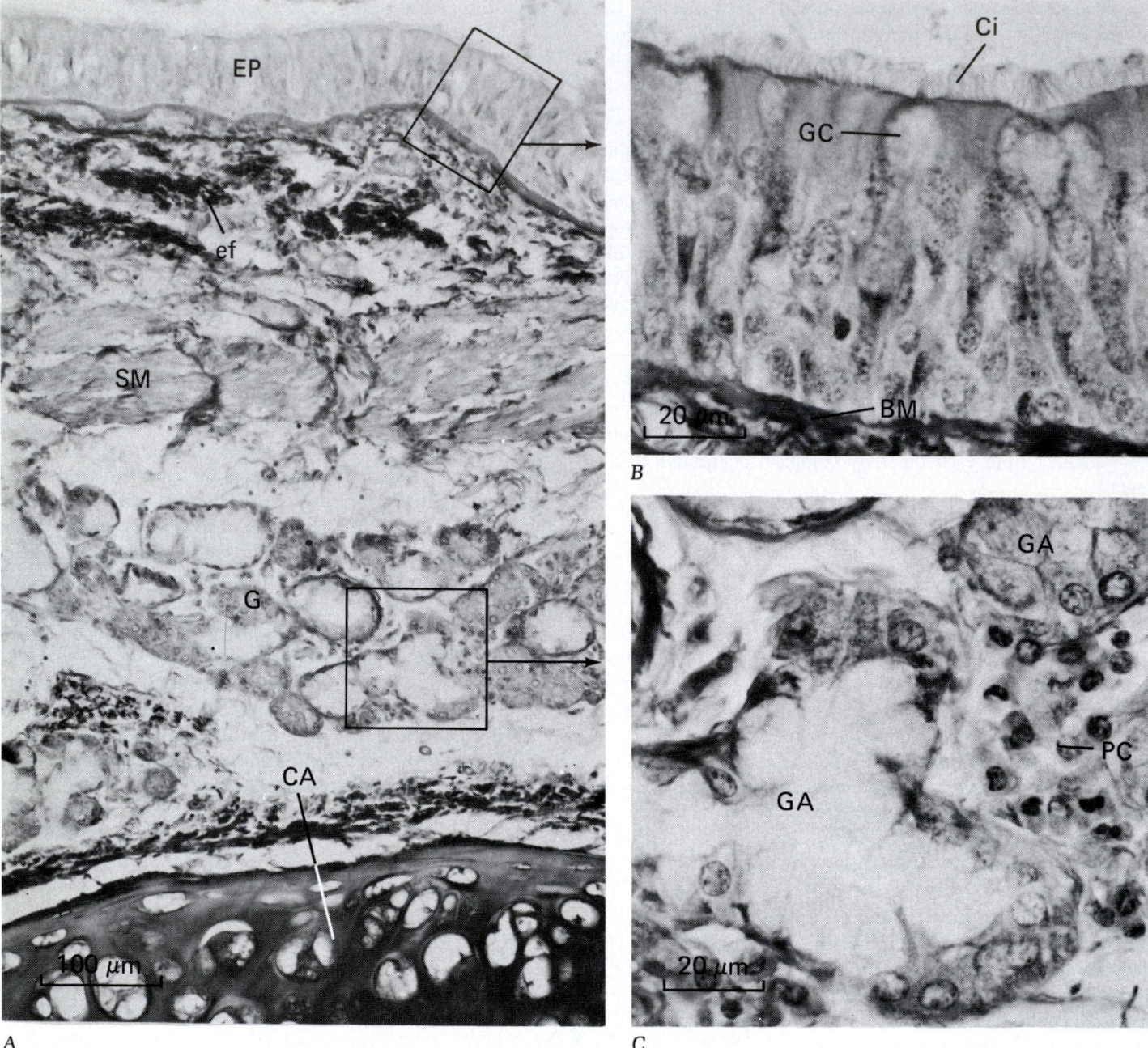

FIGURE 2-7   Light micrographs of bronchial wall. *A.* The layers from epithelium (EP) to cartilage (CA) with elastic fibers (ef), smooth-muscle bundles (SM), and glands (G). *B.* Higher power of pseudostratified epithelium with cilia (Ci). *C.* Details of gland with acini (GA) associated with groups of plasma cells (PC). GC = goblet cell; BM = basement membrane.

outward or "up the airways" in a steady stream, a feature appropriately called the *ciliary escalator.* Since the lining by ciliated cells is uninterrupted from the bronchioles, up the bronchi, to the trachea, this mucociliary escalator ends at the larynx, so that the normal fate of bronchial mucus is to be steadily discharged into the pharynx, whence it is swallowed, usually unnoticed. Only when an excessive amount of mucus accumulates in the trachea or in larger bronchi do we have to assist the system by coughing.

The secretory cell population shows a number of specialized features.[10] In the bronchi of all sizes and in larger bronchioles

one finds goblet cells interspersed between the ciliated cells; they form the mucus in their endoplasmic reticulum and Golgi complex, store it as droplets in their apical part, and discharge it in bulk (Figs. 2-8 and 2-9). In larger bronchi, one finds, in addition, small mucous glands located in the connective tissue; they are connected to the bronchial surface by long and narrow ducts (Figs. 2-6 and 2-7). In the normal bronchus the glandular acini are relatively small and composed of serous and mucous cells; enlargement of the acini and a relative increase of mucous cells are characteristics of chronic bronchitis. Finally, a special secretory cell appears in the smaller bronchioles—the Clara cell

(Fig. 2-11), whose secretory product is still unknown; this cell is rich in smooth endoplasmic reticulum and contains mixed-function oxidases that are involved in detoxification of foreign compounds.

The layer of connective tissue in the bronchial mucosa consists predominantly of elastic fibers that are oriented longitudinally; these fibers serve to maintain a smooth outline of the longitudinal profile of the bronchial lumen no matter how much the bronchi are stretched as the lungs are inflated. In this connective tissue lamina there are foci of lymphoid cells; often they form small lymphoid follicles.[29]

Smooth-muscle bundles form a continuous sleeve in the connective tissue underlying the epithelial tube that extends from the major bronchi to the respiratory bronchioles; beyond the respiratory bronchioles, the bundles extend into the wall of alveolar ducts where the muscle fibers lie in the alveolar entrance rings. The bundles have an oblique course and encircle the mucosal tube in a criss-cross pattern; hence, their contraction results primarily in a narrowing of the lumen.

In the small bronchioles there is little else to the airway wall; the smooth-muscle layer is ensheathed by a layer of delicate connective tissue that is in direct contact with adjacent alveoli (Fig. 2-6). In the larger bronchioles and even more in the bronchi, the outer connective tissue sheath forms a strong layer of fibers; in the bronchi, rings or plates of cartilage are incorporated into this layer.

The wall structure in the respiratory bronchioles is identical to that of terminal bronchioles except that in some regions the cuboidal epithelium is replaced by an alveolar epithelium of squamous cells (type I cells) closely apposed to capillaries. Very often, these single alveoli constitute outpouchings in these regions; sometimes simple "respiratory patches" form in the bronchiolar wall.

Wall Structure of Conducting Blood Vessels

The endothelial lining of pulmonary arteries and veins is basically similar to

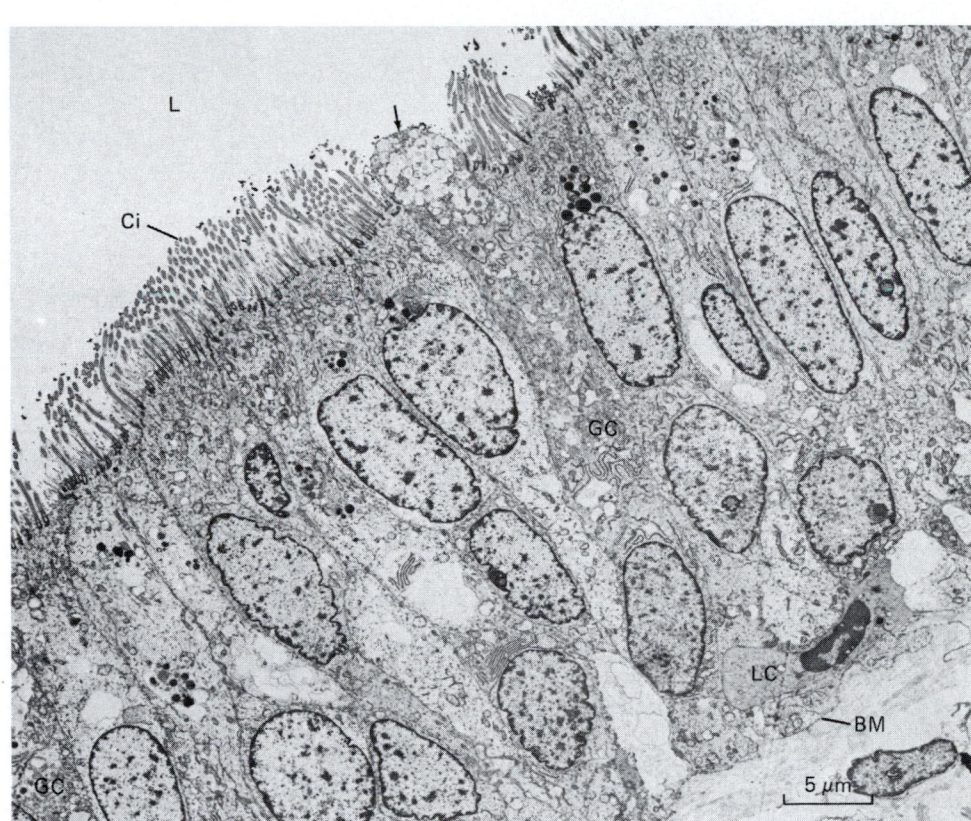

FIGURE 2-8 Electron micrograph of section across human bronchial epithelium made of high-columnar cells, most of which are ciliated (Ci). A goblet cell (GC) is cut lengthwise; note mucous droplets in process of accumulating at cell apex (*arrow*) and leukocyte (LC) caught in epithelium in process of diapedesis. L = lumen; BM = basement membrane.

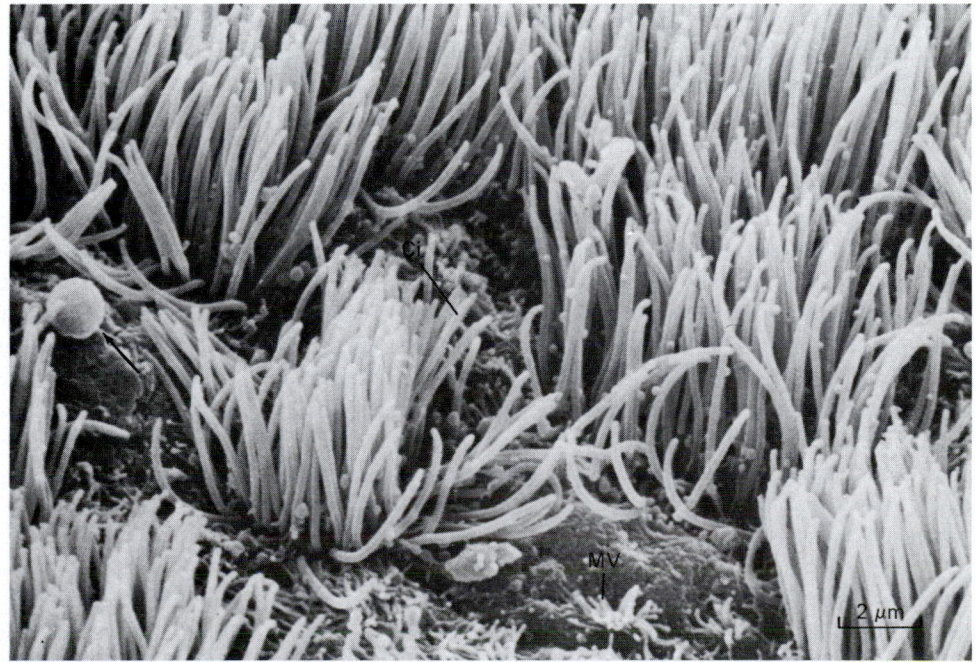

FIGURE 2-9 Surface view of bronchiolar epithelium shows tufts of cilia (Ci) forming on individual ciliated cells and microvilli (MV) on other cells. Note secretion droplet in process of release from goblet cell (*arrow*).

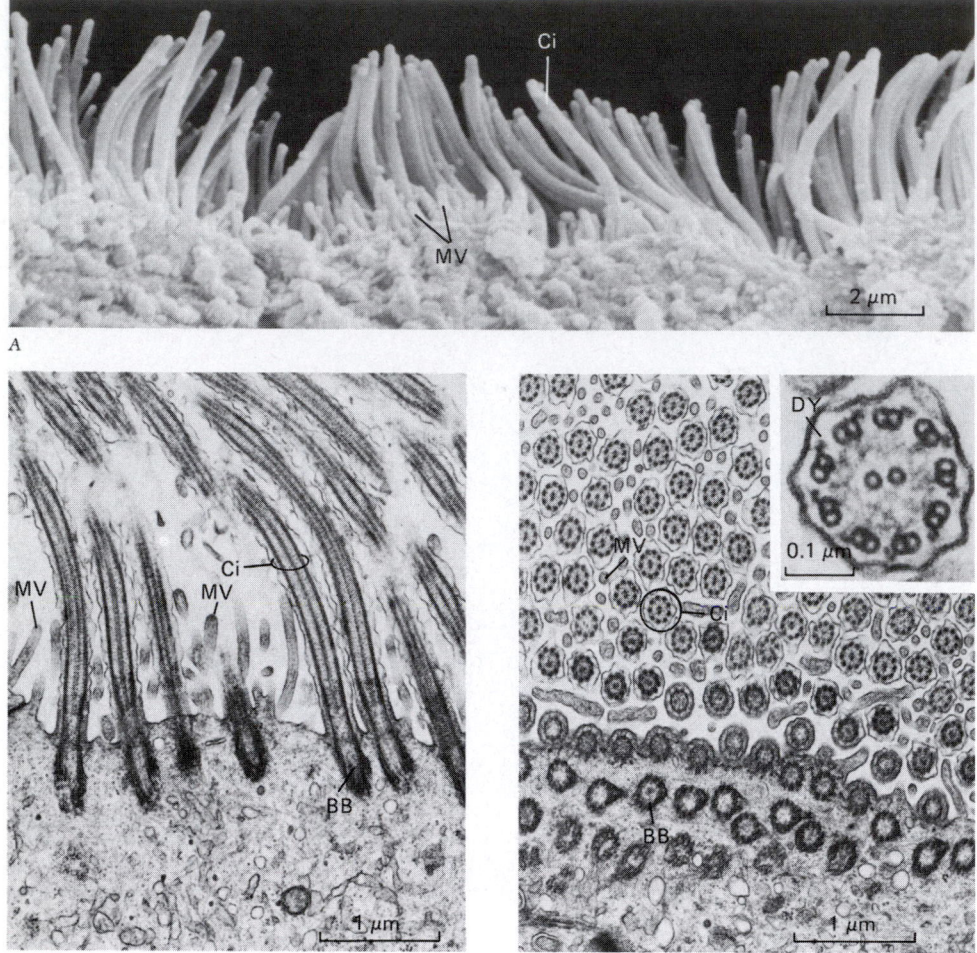

FIGURE 2-10   Cilia (Ci) from human bronchial epithelium seen on sections of epithelial cells in scanning electron micrograph (*A*), and on thin sections in longitudinal (*B*) and oblique cross section (*C*). They are implanted in the epithelial cell by a basal body (BB). Cross-sectioned cilium at high power (*inset, C*) reveals its membrane, which is enveloping a typical set of two axial tubules and nine peripheral duplex tubules with dynein arm (DY) attached. Note abundant short microvilli (MV) interspersed between cilia.

exposed to the pressure oscillations of large amplitude prevailing in the outflow tract of the right ventricle, are of the elastic type, i.e., layers of elastic lamellae are interconnected with smooth-muscle fibers as in the aorta; the tone of the smooth muscle regulates the elastic modulus of the vessel wall, thereby controlling the shape of the pulse wave. In the pulmonary arterial tree, this pattern prevails out to branches of about 1 mm diameter.

In contrast, branches less than l mm in diameter are of the muscular type, i.e., the smooth-muscle fibers encircle the vessel lumen; they can modify the vessel's cross section and can thus regulate blood flow through this vessel. Compared to systemic arteries, the thickness of the pulmonary arterial wall is reduced about in proportion to systolic pressure, i.e., by about a factor of 1:5; in pulmonary hypertension, the wall becomes thicker. Although arterioles are a well-defined entity in the systemic vascular bed, where they constitute the major site of arterial resistance, pulmonary arterioles are more difficult to locate and to define. A single muscle layer—the histologic definition of an arteriole—does occur in branches about 100 μm in diameter, but the arterial bed continues out to the precapillaries, which consist of vessels 20 to 40 μm in diameter that lack a complete smooth-muscle sheath. This poverty of smooth muscle contributes importantly to the low resistance to blood flow that is normally afforded by the pulmonary arterial tree.

that of capillaries. It is, however, thicker, and parts of its cytoplasm are richly endowed with organelles of various kinds (Fig. 2-12). Clearly, these cells are metabolically more active than those of the capillary endothelium. They are particularly rich in a rod-shaped granule,[51] specific for endothelial cells, the function of which is to store factors regulating clotting, such as von Willebrand protein,[39] as well as selectins, which regulate cell adhesion.

It is said that many of the nonrespiratory metabolic functions of the lung—particularly the transformation of certain bioactive substances, such as angiotensin and prostaglandins—are performed in endothelial cells; the exact site of execution of these functions is not yet known, but caveolae (i.e., invaginations of the surface plasma membrane) have been implicated.[35]

Accessory structures develop in the wall in accord with the functional properties of the vessels. Thus, the walls of the major pulmonary arteries that are close to the heart, and therefore

The pulmonary veins are similar to systemic veins of the upper half of the organism. Their walls are rich in connective tissue and contain irregular bundles of smooth muscle. Larger veins contain a large amount of elastic tissue. In some mammals—e.g., rodents but not humans—the larger branches of pulmonary veins have a sleeve of heart muscle fibers that is formed by extensions of left atrial muscle.

Nutritive Vessels and Nerves

The tissue of lung parenchyma is very well supplied with blood; the fact that it is venous is of no disadvantage, because O_2 is easily obtained from the air. Thus, nutrient supply from pulmonary arteries combined with O_2 supply from air appears to suffice not only for the parenchyma but also for bronchioles and for the smaller pulmonary vessels, whose outer surface is almost directly exposed to air. The thicker-walled bronchi, with their glands and

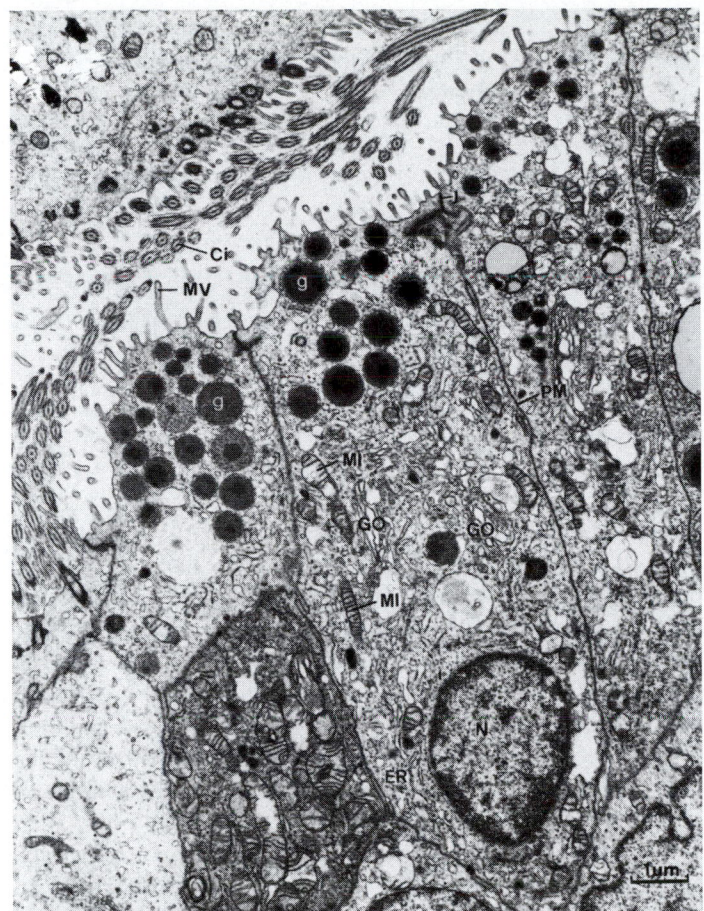

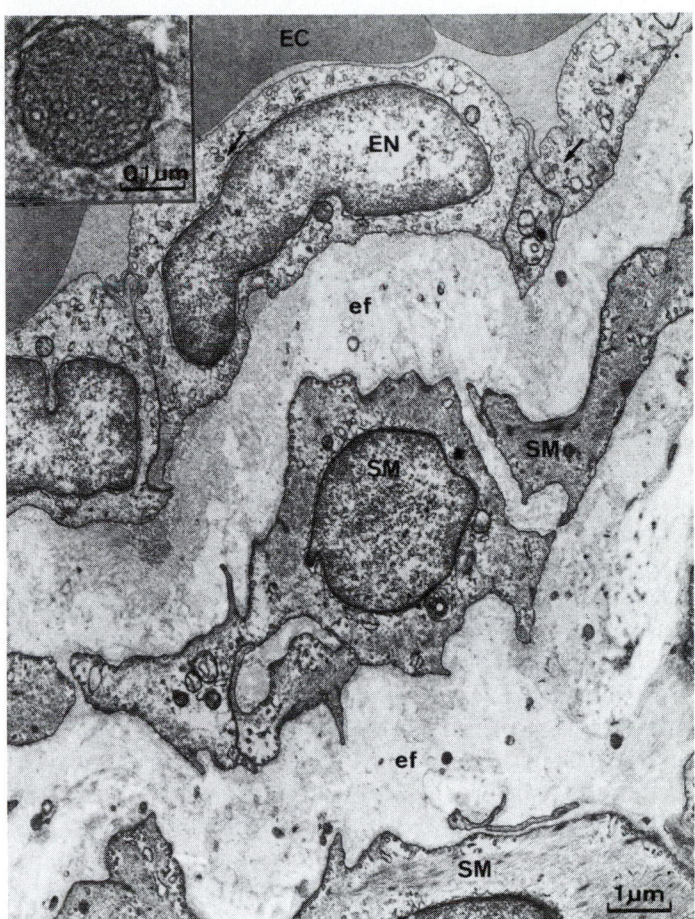

FIGURE 2-11   Clara cells from human bronchiolar epithelium contain dense secretion granules (g) at apex. Note abundant cytoplasmic organelles such as mitochondria (MI), Golgi complex (GO), or endoplasmic reticulum (ER) as well as microvilli (MV) at surface. Cell membranes are closely apposed and form tight junctions (J) at apical edge. Ci = cilia; N = nucleus; PM = plasma membrane.

FIGURE 2-12   Part of wall of pulmonary artery from human lung. Endothelial cells (EN) form thick layer; their cytoplasm is rich in organelles. Specific granules of endothelium *(arrows)*, a cross section of one of which is shown at high power in the inset, are enveloped by a membrane and contain tubules. The arterial wall is of the elastic type, formed of alternating layers of smooth muscle (SM) and elastic fibers (ef). EC = erythrocyte.

cartilage, require a nutrient blood supply from bronchial arteries.[10] These derive in part directly from anterior branches of the aorta and partly from the upper intercostal arteries. They course alongside the esophagus and penetrate on both sides into the hilus. The bronchial arteries extend to the most peripheral bronchi but not into the walls of bronchioles. On the other hand, some branches supply large pulmonary vessels, whereas others course along larger septa to reach the pleura. Some bronchial arteries form anastomoses with peripheral branches of the pulmonary arteries. There have been long discussions about the role that such anastomoses may play. It seems that in the normal lung their importance has been overrated. However, in certain pathological conditions, such as bronchiectasis and tumors, the bronchial arteries and perhaps the bronchopulmonary anastomoses appear to play an important role. They also enlarge to form a collateral circulation when branches of the pulmonary artery are obliterated.

Except for a few bronchial veins in the hilar region, the bronchial system does not have its own venous drainage into the systemic veins. Instead, the bronchial veins, which begin as a peribronchial venous plexus, drain into pulmonary veins; this drainage seems to constitute one source of normal venous admixture to arterial blood.

The lung is innervated by the autonomic nervous system. The parasympathetic fibers are derived from the vagal nerves and the sympathetic fibers from the upper thoracic and cervical ganglia; together they form the pulmonary nervous plexus in the region of the hilus before entering the lung. The fiber bundles follow the major bronchi and blood vessels, finally penetrating into the acini; some nerves also supply the pleura. In addition, motor nerves influence the smooth-muscle tone of airways and blood vessels, and sensory nerves are involved in reflex functions (e.g., cough reflex, Hering-Breuer reflex). Moreover, the secretory function of glands as well as of type II alveolar epithelial cells is at least partly under control of this nervous system. Nerve fibers are easily found in the wall of bronchioles and bronchi, where they often follow the course of bronchial arteries. However, fibers in alveolar septa are small and scarce.

The Cells of the Alveolar Region

BASIC DESIGN OF A GAS-EXCHANGE BARRIER

Efficient gas exchange in the lung depends on a very thin barrier of very large surface between air and blood.[46] Nevertheless, this barrier must be built of the three minimal tissue layers: an endothelium lining the capillaries, an epithelium lining the airspaces, and an interstitial layer to house the connective tissue fibers. The guiding principle in designing these cells must evidently be to minimize thickness and maximize extent. However, there is definitely a limit to this, set by the need to make the barrier and its constituent cells strong enough to resist the various forces that act on it—capillary blood pressure, tissue tension, and surface tension, in particular. Furthermore, the barrier must remain intact for a lifetime, and this requires continuous repair and turnover of the cells and their components.

In spite of this delicacy of tissue structure, we find that three-quarters of all the lung cells by volume or weight are contained in the lung parenchyma (Table 2-1). We also note that epithelium and endothelium make up about one-quarter each of the tissue barrier in the alveolar walls, whereas interstitial cells amount to 35 percent; the interstitial space with the connective tissue fibers makes up no more than 15 percent of the barrier.[42]

THE CELLS LINING THE BARRIER

If we now first look at the cell layers bounding the barrier, we note that by far the major part of the barrier surface is lined, on both the air and blood sides, by simple layers of squamous cells. This histologic description is sufficient for the endothelium, whose cell population is uniform. The epithelium, however, is a

TABLE 2-1

Estimated Cell Volumes in the Human Lung

Cell or Tissue	Volume, ml	Percent Septal Tissue
Tissue (excl. blood)	284	—
Nonparenchyma	99	—
Alveolar septa	185	—
Cells	213	—
Nonparenchyma	50	—
Alveolar septa	163	—
Parenchymal cells	163	—
Alveolar epithelium type I	23	12.6
Alveolar epithelium type II	18	9.7
Capillary endothelium	49	26.4
Interstitial cells	66	35.8
Alveolar macrophages	7	3.9

SOURCE: Weibel, 1984.[46]

TABLE 2-2

Morphometric Characteristics of Cell Population in Human Pulmonary Parenchyma

Cell Population	Percent of Total Cell Number*	Average Cell Volume, μm^3	Average Apical Cell Surface, μm^2
Alveolar epithelium			
Type I	8	1764	5098
Type II	16	889	183
Endothelium	30	632	1353
Interstitial cells	36	637	—
Alveolar macrophages	10	2492	—

*Total cell number in human lung 230×10^9.
SOURCE: Data from Crapo et al.[8]

mosaic of different cell types; one therefore finds a small fraction of the total surface—only a few percent (Table 2-2)—to be occupied by secretory cells; one usually calls the squamous lining cells type I and the secretory cells type II alveolar cells or pneumocytes. A rare third cell, the brush cell, is also found in some specific regions near the terminal bronchiole; its function is as yet unknown.

The squamous lining cells (the capillary endothelium and the type I epithelial cells) show very similar design features (Fig. 2-13). In terms of cell biology, they are rather simple cells. Their small, compact nucleus is surrounded by a slim rim of cytoplasm, where one finds a modest basic set of organelles, a few small mitochondria, and some cisternae of endoplasmic reticulum—the picture of a quiescent cell with no great metabolic activity.[34,35,42]

At the edge of the perinuclear region, a very attenuated cytoplasmic leaflet emerges (Fig. 2-13) and spreads out broadly over the basal lamina. This leaflet is made essentially of the two plasma membranes of the apical and basal cell face, respectively, with a very small amount of cytoplasmic ground substance interposed (Fig. 2-14). Here one rarely finds any organelles except for the numerous microvesicles implied in the transcellular transport of macromolecules.

Terminal bars are formed where the cytoplasmic leaflets of epithelial or endothelial cells meet (Fig. 2-15). Here there is a notable difference between these two linings in that the tight junction between epithelial cells constitutes a powerful seal of the intercellular cleft, whereas that in the endothelium is rather leaky, allowing a nearly uninhibited exchange of water, solutes, and even some smaller macromolecules between the blood plasma and the interstitial space.

There is another notable and important difference between these two basically similar lining cells: their size. Although the capillary surface is some 10 to 20 percent smaller than the alveolar surface, the capillary endothelial cells are about four times more numerous than type I cells;[8] this means that the surface covered by one type I epithelial cell must be about four times larger, namely 4000 to 5000 μm^2, as compared to about 1000 μm^2 in endothelial cells (Table 2-2). In some texts one may find the type I cell called the "small alveolar cell" because of its small nucleus; clearly this is a misnomer, as the type I cell is a rather large cell indeed, with respect to both surface and cell volume (Table 2-2).

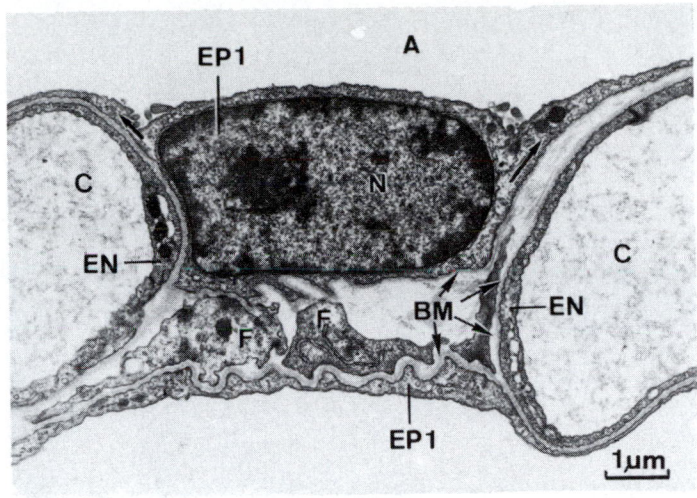

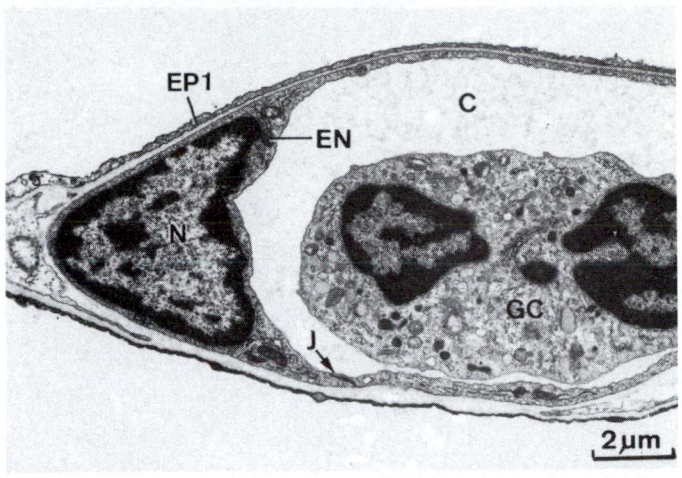

FIGURE 2-13 *A.* A type I alveolar epithelial cell (EP1) from human lung. The nucleus (N) is surrounded by very little cytoplasm, which extends as thin leaflets (*arrows*) to cover the capillaries 'C). Note the basement membranes (BM) of the epithelium and endothelium (EN), which become fused in a minimal barrier. Interstitial space contains fibroblast processes (F). *B.* An endothelial cell (EN) of capillary (C) is similar in basic structure to a type I epithelial cell (EP1). The nucleus is enwrapped by little cytoplasm but thin leaflets extend as capillary lining (*arrow*). Note the intercellular junction (J) and a white blood cell/granulocyte, (GC) in the capillary. *(From Weibel,[46] with permission.)*

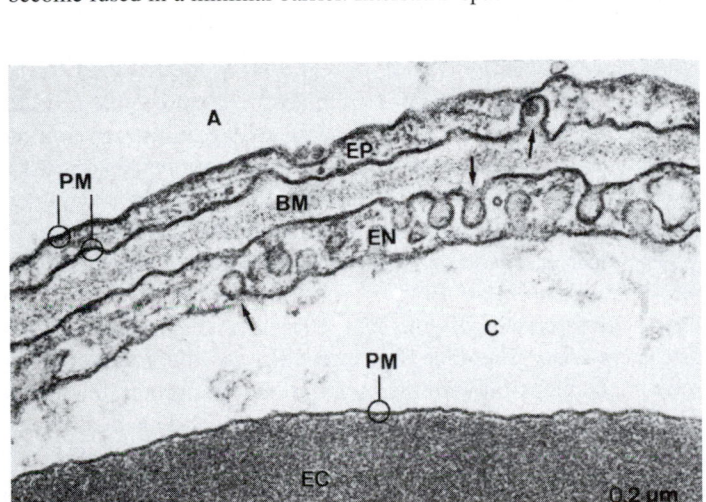

FIGURE 2-14 Thin, minimal tissue barrier between alveolar air (A) and capillary blood (C) is made of cytoplasmic leaflets of epithelium (EP) and endothelium (EN), joined by fused basement membranes (BM). Note that the epithelial and endothelial leaflets are bounded by plasma membranes (PM), as is the erythrocyte (EC). Arrows point to pinocytotic vesicles. *(From Weibel,[46] with permission.)*

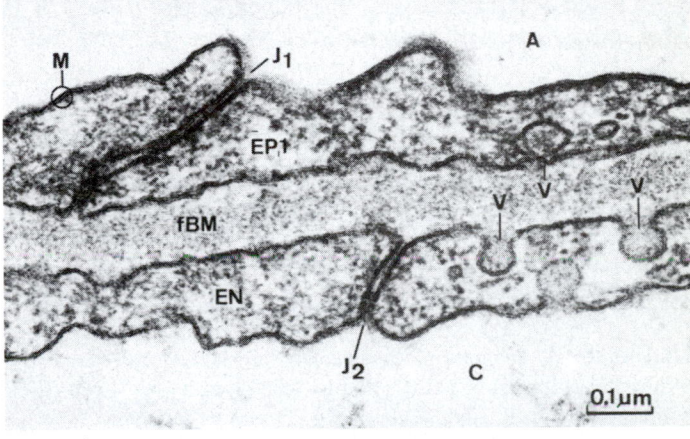

FIGURE 2-15 Minimal barrier part showing intercellular junctions. Between type I epithelial cells, a "tight" junction (J_1) is formed by close apposition of the cell membranes over a comparatively wide band; the junction between endothelial cells (J_2) is "leaky" because membranes become apposed over a narrow strip only. Note trilaminar structure of cell membranes (M), the occurrence of pinocytotic vesicles (V) in both epithelium and endothelium (EN), and the fused basement membranes (fBM). EC = erythrocyte; C = capillary; A = alveolus; EP1 = type I epithelial cell; M = membrane.

If one looks at the surface of the alveolar epithelium in scanning electron micrographs (Fig. 2-16), one notes that the patches covered by single type I cells are variable in size and that even the largest are much smaller than the 4000 to 5000 μm^2 given above, a number derived by dividing the total alveolar surface by the total number of type I cell nuclei; the one large type I cell seen in Fig. 2-16 has an area of only about 1400 μm^2, and there are not many that are larger. Why is this? There seem to be three to four times as many type I cell domains encircled by terminal bars as there are nuclei. Indeed, this observation was already made some hundred years ago by Albert Kölliker, German pio-

neer of histology; his interpretation was that part of the alveolar surface was lined by "nonnuclear" cytoplasmic plates rather than by complete cells. A modern cell biologist cannot accept this interpretation without scrutiny, and it turns out that an alternative explanation is possible. One finds that type I cells are not simple squamous cells but rather branched cells with multiple apical faces, as shown diagrammatically in Fig. 2-17. Thus, what appears as nonnucleated plates are cytoplasmic domains connected to the perinuclear region by a stalk, spreading out on one side of the alveolar wall or the other; it is evident that several such domains may share a nucleus.

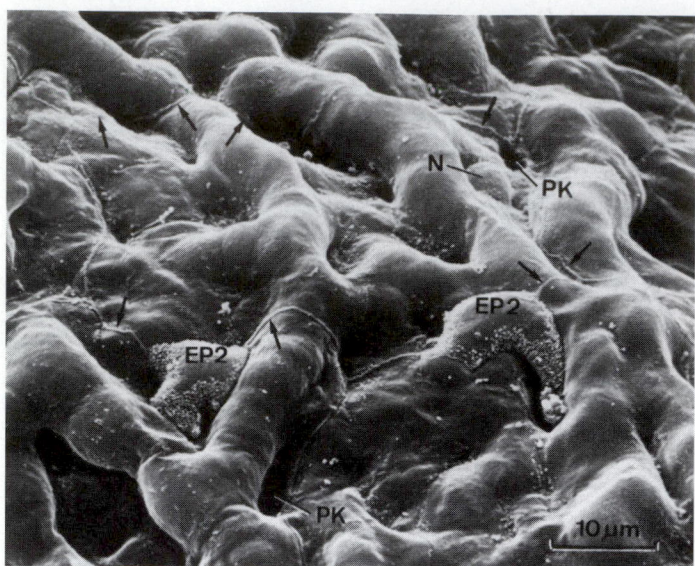

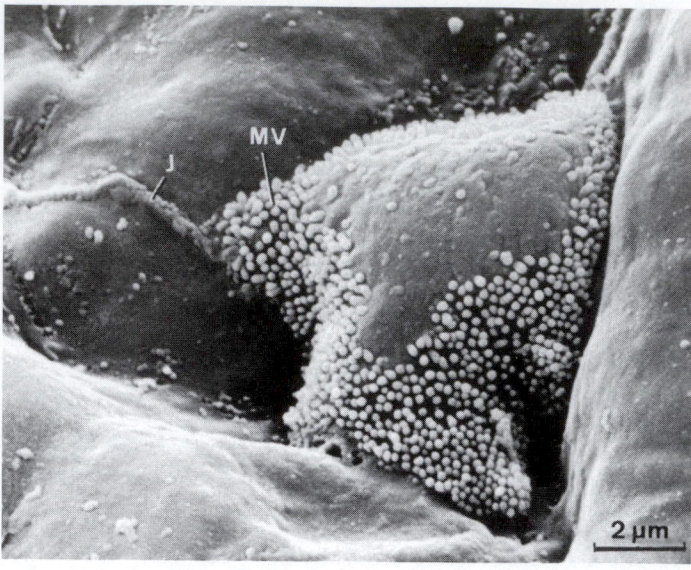

FIGURE 2-16   Surface of the alveolar wall in the human lung seen by scanning electron microscopy reveals a mosaic of alveolar epithelium made of type I and type II (EP2) cells. Arrows indicate boundary of the cytoplasmic leaflet of the type I cell which extends over many capillaries (C). Note the two interalveolar pores of Kohn (PK).

FIGURE 2-18   Higher magnification of a type II cell reveals a "crown" of short microvilli (MV) and a central "bald patch." Note junction lines of type I cells (J) meeting with the type II cell.

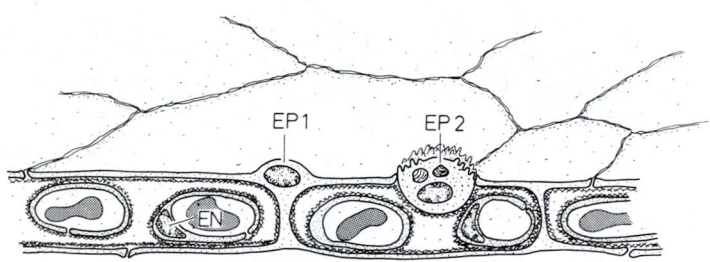

FIGURE 2-17   Diagram of the alveolar wall showing the complexity of a type I epithelial cell (EP1) and its relation to a type II cell (EP2) and endothelial cell (EN). *(From Weibel,[46] with permission.)*

THE ALVEOLAR SECRETORY CELL: SYNTHESIS OF SURFACTANT

The type II alveolar cell is a conspicuous but in fact relatively small cell whose mean volume is less than half that of the type I cell (Table 2-2), although it is often called the "large alveolar cell."[42] Its shape is cuboidal and it has no cytoplasmic extensions (Figs. 2-18 and 2-19). The apical cell surface bulges toward the lumen and is provided, mostly around its periphery, with a tuft of microvilli.

The most conspicuous feature of the type II cell is its wealth in cytoplasmic organelles of all kinds (Fig. 2-19): mitochondria, a lot of endoplasmic reticulum with ribosomes, and a well-developed Golgi complex surrounded by a set of small lysosomal granules among which so-called multivesicular bodies—membrane-bounded organelles containing a group of small vesicles—stand out (Fig. 2-20). In addition, one finds the characteristic lamellar bodies, larger membrane-bounded organelles that contain a dense stack of phospholipid lamellae, which stain black with osmium.

These structural properties are directly related to the type II cell's principal function: the synthesis, storage, and secretion of surfactant, a complex of phospholipids and proteins that spreads in a thin film on the alveolar surface and drastically lowers the surface tension at the air-tissue interface.[16,49]

The main surfactant phospholipid of the lung, dipalmitoyl-phosphatidylcholine (DPPC), is a lecithin whose two fatty acid chains are saturated palmitic acid;[16] it lowers the surface tension at an air-water interface by spreading on the surface as a monomolecular film with the hydrophilic polar group immersed in the water and the two hydrophobic palmitic acid residues sticking out. It is well established that the type II cells synthesize DPPC, store it in the lamellar bodies, and secrete it into the thin fluid layer that covers the alveolar epithelium.[16,42]

In spite of a large number of biochemical studies, it is less certain how the type II cells synthesize DPPC.[16] The problem is that the most common biochemical pathway for the synthesis of lecithins or phosphatidylcholines, the so-called Kennedy pathway, results in phosphatidylcholine where at least one of the two fatty acids is unsaturated; DPPC, where both fatty acid chains are fully saturated palmitic acids, therefore appears like an "unnatural" product which must be made by a two-step procedure, involving remodeling by reacylation.

The site of DPPC synthesis within the type II cells is not yet precisely localized; possible candidates are the endoplasmic reticulum, parts of the Golgi membranes, the multivesicular bodies, or the lamellar bodies themselves (Fig. 2-20); these organelles are arranged in a kind of complex (Fig. 2-21) and could thus establish a spatial sequence for the intracellular processing of phospholipids.[16,42] It is possible that all sites are involved at one step or another of the complex pathway leading to DPPC. One point is beyond doubt, however: the lamellar bodies are the storage sites for "mature," fully saturated DPPC, which becomes "crystallized" into a regular layered stack.

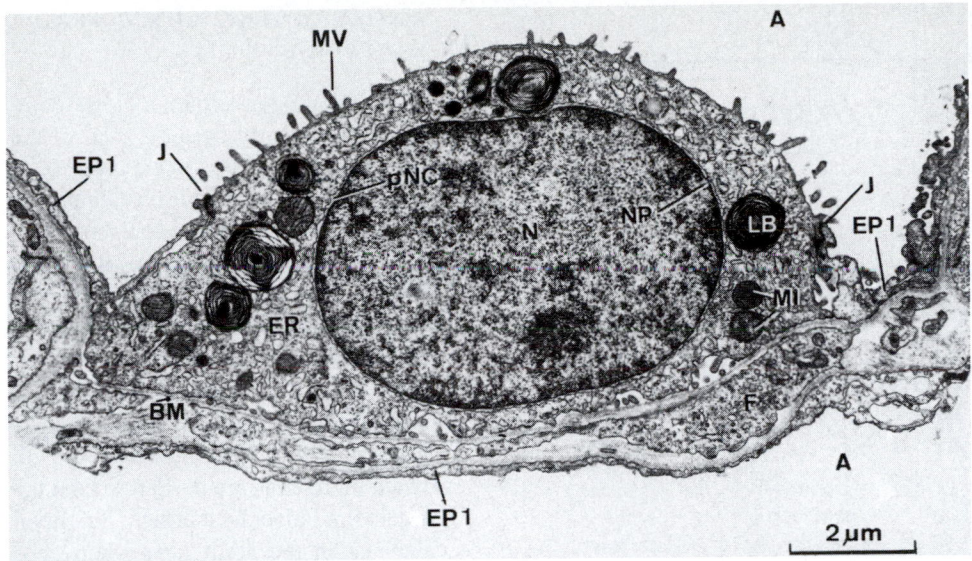

FIGURE 2-19   A type II epithelial cell from the human lung forms junction (J) with type I epithelial cells (EP1). Its cytoplasm contains osmiophilic lamellar bodies (LB) and a rich complement of organelles: mitochondria (M), endoplasmic reticulum (ER), and so on. The nucleus (N) is surrounded by a perinuclear cisterna (pNC) which is perforated by nuclear pores (NP). BM = basement membrane; F = fibroblast; MV = microvilli; A = alveolus.

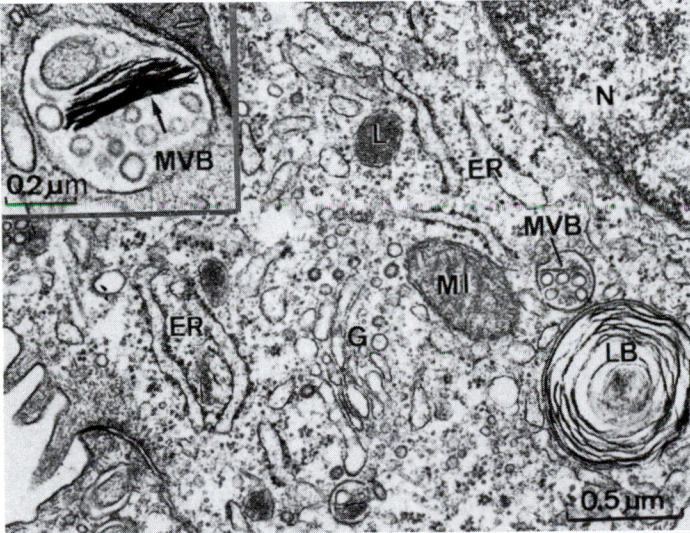

FIGURE 2-20   Cytoplasmic organelles of the type II cell implicated in the synthesis of surfactant are the endoplasmic reticulum (ER), Golgi complex (G), lysosomes (L), multivesicular bodies (MV), and finally lamellar bodies (LB). The inset shows a large multivesicular body with a stack of phospholipid lamellae (*arrow*). Scale markers: 0.5 μm; (*inset*) 0.2 μm. (*From Weibel,[46] with permission.*)

The content of lamellar bodies is eventually secreted onto the alveolar surface by exocytosis: the granule membrane fuses with the apical plasma membrane and the content is discharged (Fig. 2-22). In the alveolar lining layer, the once densely packed phospholipid lamellae unravel and become associated with an apoprotein, which is probably also synthesized by the type II cells by the usual pathway of protein synthesis in the endoplasmic reticulum (Fig. 2-21). Within the lining layer, this lipoprotein

complex now forms a new pattern of regular array (Figs. 2-21 and 2-22), so-called tubular myelin, and it can spread on its free surface as a monomolecular film.

Pulmonary surfactant is turned over rather rapidly. Continuous synthesis must therefore be coupled with regulated removal, for which two pathways are known; some of the surfactant leaves the alveolar region over the surface of terminal bronchioles; from there, it is removed by the mucociliary escalator; some is engulfed by alveolar macrophages (Fig. 2-21) and broken up in their lysosomes, which are known to contain, besides their usual complement of acid hydrolases, phospholipase A₂, the enzyme that cleaves fatty acids from phosphatidylcholine. It is not known whether there are other mechanisms for removing surfactant that has become inactivated, but some recent evidence suggests that part of it may be recycled through the type II cells.[16]

A difficult topic is the regulation of surfactant synthesis and turnover. One postulates "neurohumoral" pathways, but nothing very precise is as yet known. On the one hand, local regulatory effects must be postulated because one knows that surfactant production becomes stimulated by increased ventilation. However, it is possible that this increased surfactant production is the result of neural effects, since it can also be brought about by stimulation of the vagus nerve and by some neurotransmitters, mainly β-adrenergic agonists. The problem with respect to neural control is that the lung parenchyma contains very few nerve fibers, and they have not been shown to be related to type II cells.

There is reasonably good evidence that the potential for surfactant synthesis develops under the effect of some hormones, particularly corticosteroids.[16] This plays a major role during fetal lung development, when, between the 18th and 25th gestational weeks in humans, surfactant begins to be secreted into the lung fluid. This is evidently most crucial in view of the fact that, upon the first breath, the newborn baby must be able to instantaneously open up all its alveoli and keep them open. Sufficient quantities of surfactant have usually been produced by the 28th gestational week, although birth normally takes place at only about the 40th week. For this reason premature babies are capable of surviving in a protected environment after the 26th or 28th week. However, in some prematurely born infants, this is not the case, because the onset of surfactant production shows some variation. Such babies rapidly develop a severe, life-threatening disease called the respiratory distress syndrome of the newborn, because they cannot take up enough O₂ in their ever-collapsing lungs. It is noteworthy that the surfactant content of the lung can be monitored because the lung fluid communicates freely with amniotic fluid, which can be tapped by amniocentesis; when surfactant production has become adequate, one finds the DPPC concentration in amniotic fluid to have risen to a certain level.

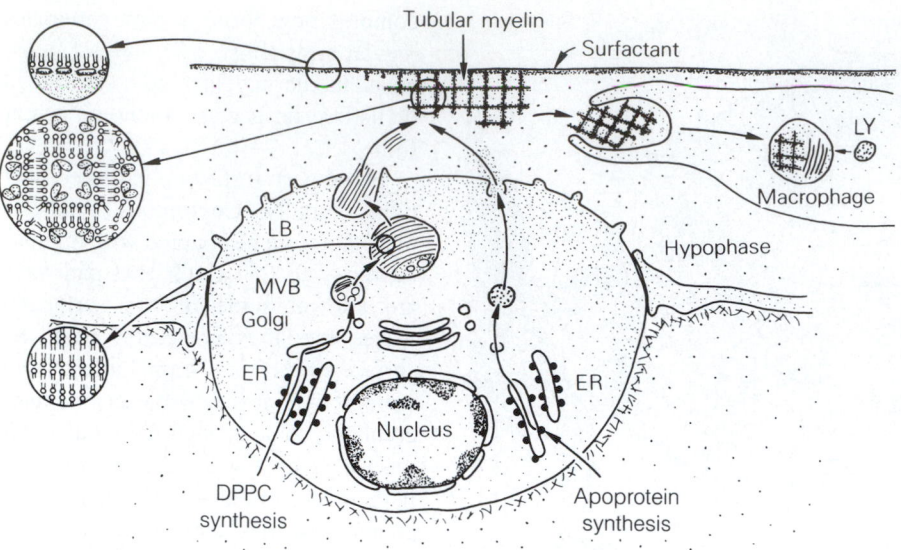

FIGURE 2-21   Schematic diagram of pathways for synthesis and secretion of surfactant DPPC and apoproteins by a type II cell, and for their removal by macrophages. Note the arrangement of phospholipids and apoproteins in the lamellar bodies, in tubular myelin, and in the surface film. *(From Weibel,[46] with permission.)*

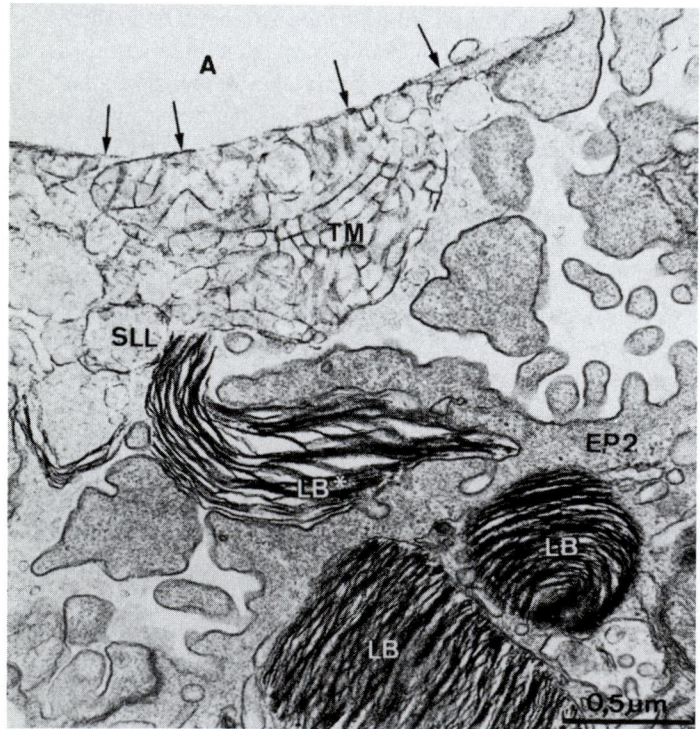

FIGURE 2-22   Apical part of type II cell (EP2) with lamellar bodies (LB); one of these (LB) is seen in the process of being secreted into the surface lining layer (SLL). The free surface of the lining layer is covered by a thin black film of DPPC *(arrows)*, which is connected with tubular myelin (TM) in the hypophase. *(From Weibel and Gil,[49] with permission.)*

KINETICS OF LUNG CELLS: COPING WITH VULNERABILITY

The alveolar epithelium is easily damaged, particularly because each of the very thin type I cells is exposed to air over a much larger surface than any other cell. It is, in fact, astonishing how little seems to happen to this cell, which, as we have seen, has only a limited potential for repairing membrane defects, for example. But there is an additional problem: one finds that type I cells are not capable of multiplying by mitosis, neither during lung growth when more cells are needed to coat the expanding alveolar surface nor upon damage in the adult lung when cells need to be replaced. In both instances new type I cells are made by mitotic division and transformation of type II cells which form squamous extensions and lose their potential for surfactant synthesis, a process which takes about 2 to 5 days.

This seems to work under normal circumstances. There are, however, conditions where this repair mechanism is too slow to cope with excessive damage, so that a syndrome of severe catastrophic respiratory failure develops, which requires intensive care, mechanical ventilation, and supplemental O_2 just to allow the patient to survive. This can happen when the lung becomes diffusely damaged by toxic fumes. Here it is noteworthy that breathing pure O_2 over a prolonged period is highly toxic to lung cells as well; but such damage also occurs in shock—for example, upon severe blood loss or as a consequence of multiple bone fractures. In such patients one finds large parts of the type I cell lining of the alveolar surface to be destroyed. As a consequence, the barrier has become leaky and the alveoli fill with alveolar edema, so that they can no longer take part in gas exchange.[2,5]

With proper medical care, this alveolar edema can often be resolved within a few days. The alveoli become again filled with air, but in spite of this, gas exchange does not improve. What has happened is that the repair of the severely damaged alveolar epithelium requires a lot of new cells to be made by division of type II cells.[5,6] These form a rather thick cuboidal lining of the barrier surface, and this thick barrier offers a high resistance to O_2 flow. It takes several weeks until a thin barrier is restored by transformation of the cuboidal cell lining into delicate type I cells.

The Defense System of the Lung

At the alveolar level, the lung appears to rely heavily on macrophages as primary defense cells;[42] they physically remove from direct contact with lung tissue all sorts of particulate matter that enters the peripheral airways, particularly bacteria and organic or inorganic dust particles. These cells are right at the forefront of the defense line, in the alveolar surface lining layer, as we shall discuss below.

Another set of these cells forms a second defense line just beneath the alveolar epithelium—i.e., in the interstitial space of the lung parenchyma. In the normal lung, these interstitial histiocytes are not found in alveolar septa; instead, they occur only in the connective tissue sleeves at the periphery and in the center of acini. Thus, they are found in regions where lymphatics begin their course toward the major airways in the hilar region, where lymph nodes are found.[28] In these juxta-alveolar regions of connective tissue, we usually find the common elements of the defense system (Fig. 2-23). These are as follows:

1. Lymphatic vessels.
2. Histiocytes, which may sometimes become permanent residents in the form of storage cells for "indigestible" foreign matter, such as carbon particles and silicates.
3. Plasma cells and lymphocytes, indicating that humoral defense factors (specific antibodies) may come into play.
4. Leukocytes, which are occasionally seen but are rare in the healthy lung.
5. Mast cells, which are also found, suggesting that effectors of bioactive substances can come into play, particularly in regulating vascular permeability and inflammatory responses.

Similar patches of defense cells are also found beneath the ciliated epithelium in bronchi and bronchioles;[29] here diapedesis is seen—i.e., lymphocytes and other leukocytes in the process of penetrating the epithelium to reach the mucous blanket. Plasma cells occur in relatively high numbers around the acini of the seromucous glands of bronchi (Fig. 2-7); hence, it is likely that antibodies are being secreted into the mucous blanket by these glands by a process similar to that occurring in the salivary glands or in the glands of the nasal mucosa.

The third defense line is constituted by the lymph nodes, which are arranged along the major bronchi and extend to subsegmental bronchi about 5 mm in diameter (Fig. 2-24). The most peripheral lymph nodes are tiny, a mere 1 to 2 mm in diameter; but closer to the hilus they become larger, reaching 5 to 10 mm in diameter in the region of the tracheal bifurcation and along the trachea. The lymph nodes from adult human lungs often appear gray or even black because of deposition in the medullary cords of large numbers of macrophages loaded with carbon pigment. This material entered the lung via the airways, primarily as smoke, soot, or coal dust; depending on the size of the particles, they were either deposited on the surface of conducting airways or reached the alveoli. The further down the deposition, the greater the likelihood that this material cannot be eliminated while in the airways, i.e., within the mucous blanket. The only

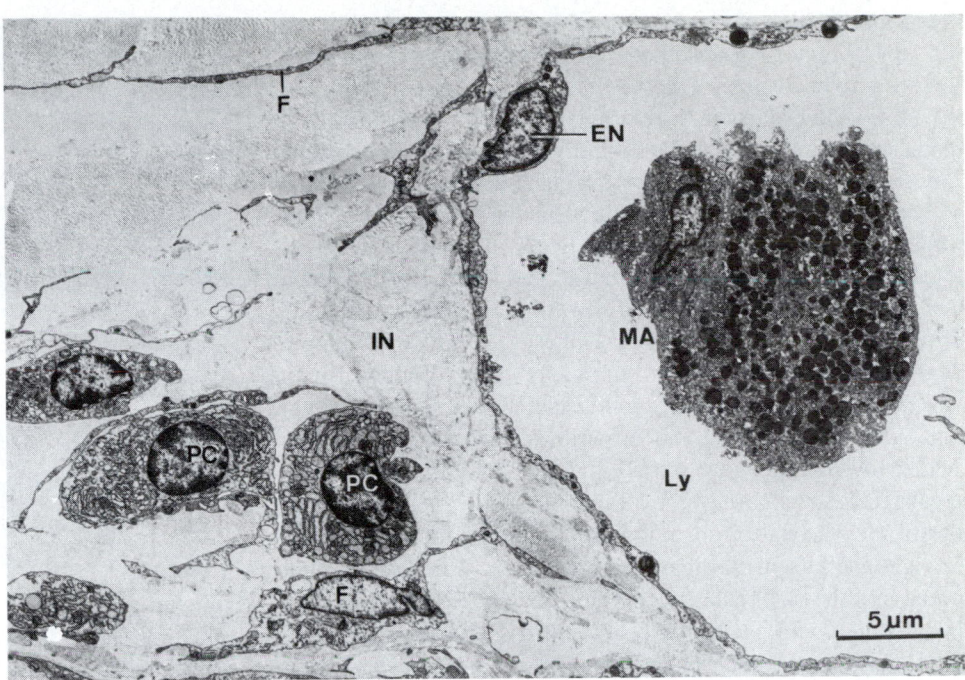

FIGURE 2-23 Perivascular connective tissue with lymphatic (Ly) containing a macrophage (MA) with heterogeneous population of "lysosomal" granules. Interstitium (IN) contains fibroblasts (F) and plasma cells (PC). EN = endothelium.

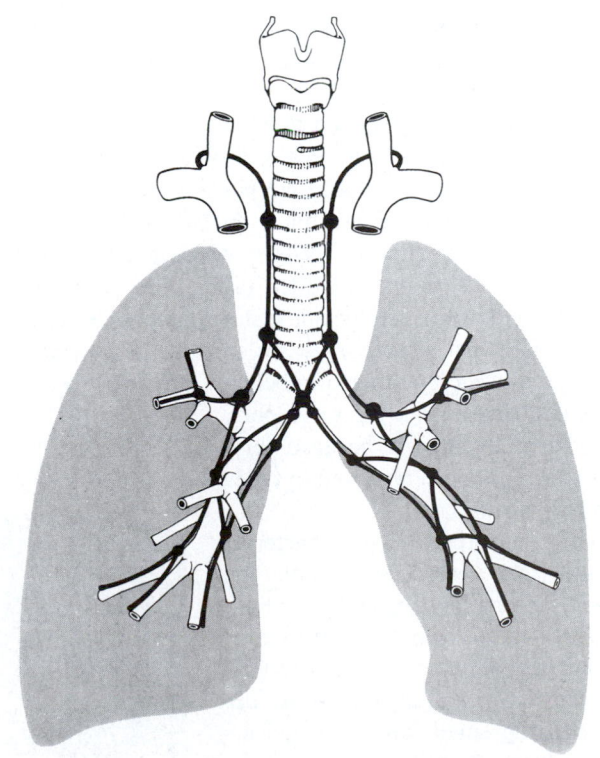

FIGURE 2-24 Schematic diagram of distribution of lymph nodes and main lymphatic channels along bronchial tree.

exit from the lung parenchyma then is via the lymphatics, but this exit ultimately leads to the blood, a circumstance that is obviously to be avoided. Filtering the lymph in lymph nodes and providing a depository in the medullary cords protects the blood and hence the entire organism from dissemination of indigestible foreign matter and also, in most instances, of infective agents.

Thus, the lymphatic "circulation" in the lung plays an important defense role.[29] It is unidirectional: it begins as interstitial fluid that seeps from the capillaries and is efficiently drained along the connective tissue fibers toward those connective tissue sleeves in the center and at the periphery of acini where lymph capillaries begin. From there, lymphatic vessels, endowed with valves and an irregular smooth-muscle wall, course in septal structures, in the pleura, and in peribronchial and perivascular sheaths toward the hilar region (Fig. 2-24). Lymph nodes are intercalated in the course of the lymphatics, which lead the lymph toward the tracheal bifurcation and then along the trachea into the right and left mediastinal lymph channels. The right channel drains into the right subclavian vein; the left, together with the thoracic duct, into the left subclavian vein. Because of the many anastomoses connecting parallel lymphatics, a particular lymph node receives lymph from various lung regions, but the closest regions tend to predominate.

Macrophages

Alveolar macrophages are the cell population of the surface lining layer.[42] They are free cells, endowed with a high phagocytic capacity, which are transiently attached to the surface of the alveolar epithelium by pseudopodia and can crawl over this surface by ameboid movement (Fig. 2-25). However, they are submerged beneath the surface film of phospholipids (Fig. 2-26) and are, therefore, part of the surface lining layer of alveoli, more specifically of its hypophase.

Alveolar macrophages exert their phagocytic activity within the surface lining layer (Fig. 2-21). Hence, it is not surprising that their vacuoles contain large amounts of phospholipid material, in part even tubular myelin; a considerable part of these phospholipids is dipalmitoyl-lecithin. Although it seems likely that this material has been ingested in the process of removing and breaking down the surfactant system, the possibility has not been excluded that macrophages are engaged in surfactant synthesis as well. The presence of tubular myelin in phagosomes tends to support the removal hypothesis because this material has not been observed in type II epithelial cells.

Foreign materials, such as bacteria or dust, that reach the alveoli in aerosols are first intercepted by the lining layer and are then ingested by the alveolar macrophages. Type I alveolar epithelial cells are also capable of phagocytizing small foreign particles, whereas type II cells are not. The acutely diseased lung shows pictures that are reminiscent of phagocytosis by type I cells.

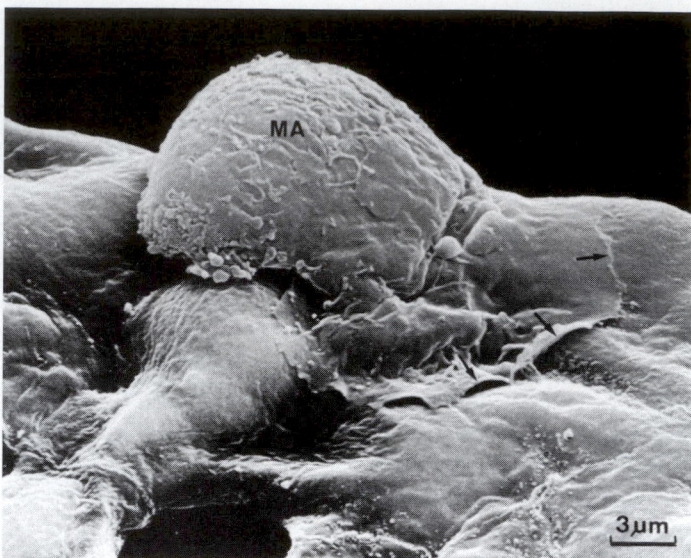

FIGURE 2-25 Alveolar macrophage (MA) seen sitting on epithelial surface of human lung. Note cytoplasmic lamella *(arrows)* which represents the advancing edge of the cell.

The kinetics of these macrophages is as yet unclear. They seem to be derived from monocytes—indirectly, therefore, from bone marrow cells—and probably reach the alveoli in two steps: first, by settling in the pulmonary interstitial tissue, and second, by migration from the interstitial tissue into the alveoli where they constitute a partly self-reproducing cell population. Their removal seems to involve two different pathways: (1) some of the macrophages undoubtedly move up the bronchial tree in the mucous blanket and eventually appear in the sputum (heart failure cells, dust cells) and (2) others possibly return into the interstitial space. In the normal lung, however, the second path seems to occur exclusively in those alveoli that abut on the connective tissue sleeves around larger vessels and conducting airways or on interacinar septa—i.e., where the lymphatic capillaries are located. A preferred location appears to be in the respiratory bronchioles at the entrance into the acinus or in the center of the acinus, where one often finds congregations of dust-laden macrophages; this may be at the origin of centroacinar damages observed in smokers, which lead to progressive emphysema. In these places, macrophages either settle as carbon

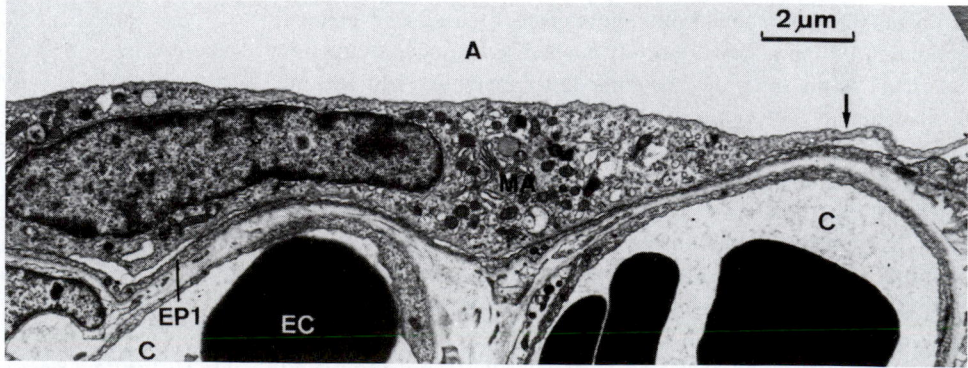

FIGURE 2-26 Alveolar macrophage (MA) fixed in its natural position of "flat" attachment to the alveolar epithelium. Arrow points to advancing cytoplasmic leaflet.

pigment–loaded histiocytes, or they leave the lung parenchyma via lymphatics (Fig. 2-23) to settle in the lymph nodes. The way in which macrophages and/or their ingested material are transferred from the alveolar surface to the interstitial space is still entirely unknown.

DESIGN OF PULMONARY PARENCHYMA

Alveoli and Capillaries

The airspaces and blood vessels of lung parenchyma are designed to facilitate gas exchange between air and blood.[46] To this end a very large area of contact between air and blood must be established; for the human lung it is sometimes compared to the area of a tennis court in size. Furthermore, the tissue barrier separating air and blood must be kept as thin as possible—it is found to be about fifty times thinner than a sheet of airmail stationery. This is important, because less than 1 s is available for loading O_2 onto the erythrocytes as they flow through the lung's gas exchange region.

The first design feature to this end is the formation of alveoli in the walls of all airways within the acinus—i.e. in the gas-exchange units derived from the first order respiratory bronchiole (Fig. 2-27). In the human lung, one estimates that there are about 30,000 acini and 300 million alveoli, so that each of the gas-exchange units contains some 10,000 alveoli, on average, connected to about seven to nine generations of acinar airways, respiratory bronchioles, and alveolar ducts.[15]

The alveoli are so densely packed that they occupy the entire surface of alveolar ducts; they are separated from each other by delicate alveolar septa that contain a single capillary network (Fig. 2-28). About half the space of the septum is taken up by blood, which is thus exposed to the air in two adjacent alveoli (Fig. 2-29A). Although the barrier separating air and blood is extremely thin, we find the capillaries to be provided with a complete endothelial lining, as the alveolar surface of the septum is lined by an epithelium. We have seen above that these two cell linings are very much attenuated over the greatest part of the surface.

To make the barrier very thin, the interstitial structures must also be reduced

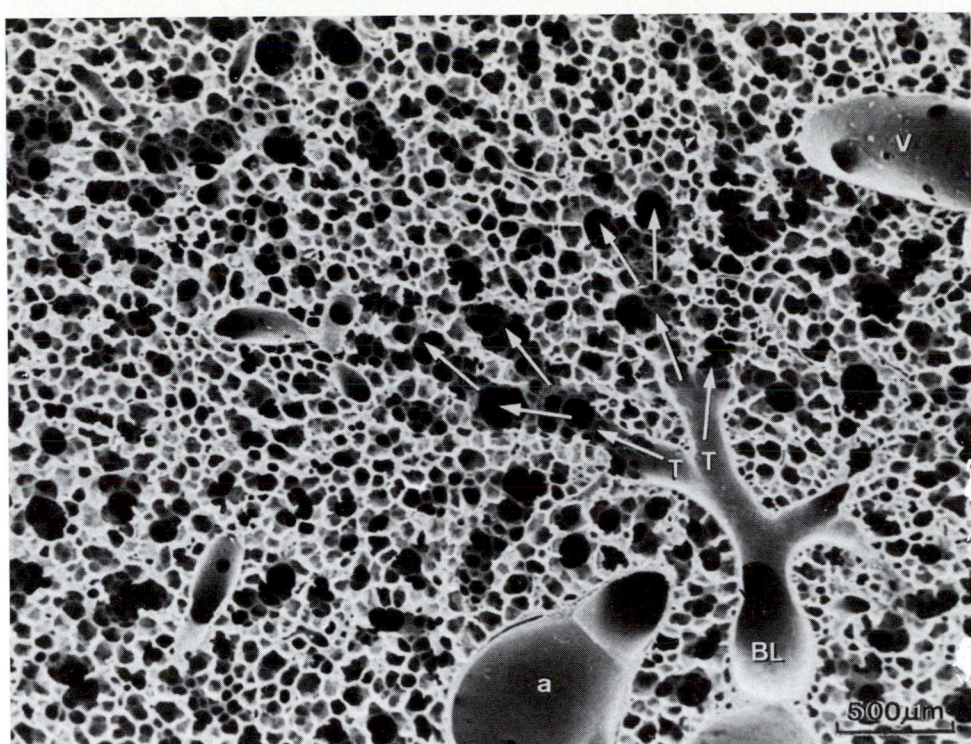

FIGURE 2-27 Scanning electron micrograph of lung shows branching of small peripheral bronchiole (BL) into terminal bronchioles (T), from where the airways continue into respiratory bronchioles and alveolar ducts (arrows). Note the location of the pulmonary artery (a) and vein (V). *(From Weibel,[46] with permission.)*

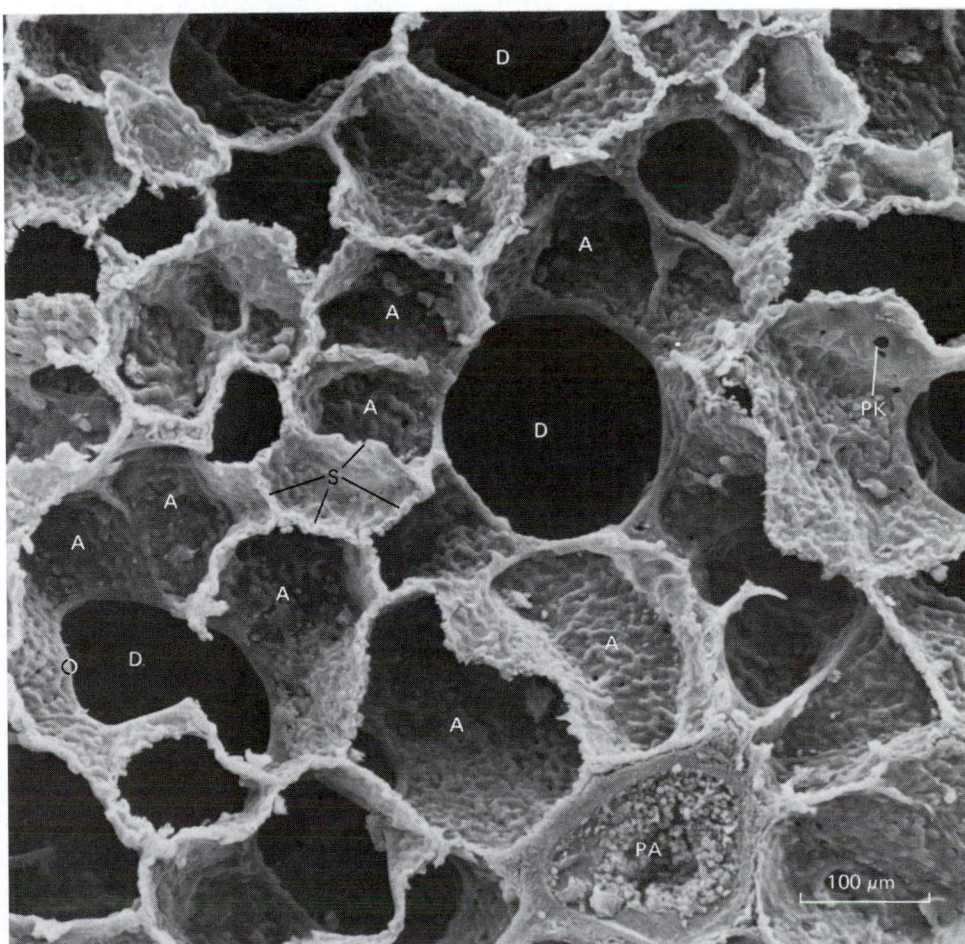

FIGURE 2-28 Scanning electron micrograph of human lung parenchyma. Alveolar ducts (D) are surrounded by alveoli (A), which are separated by thin septa (S). Note small branch of pulmonary artery (PA). PK = interalveolar pore of Kohn.

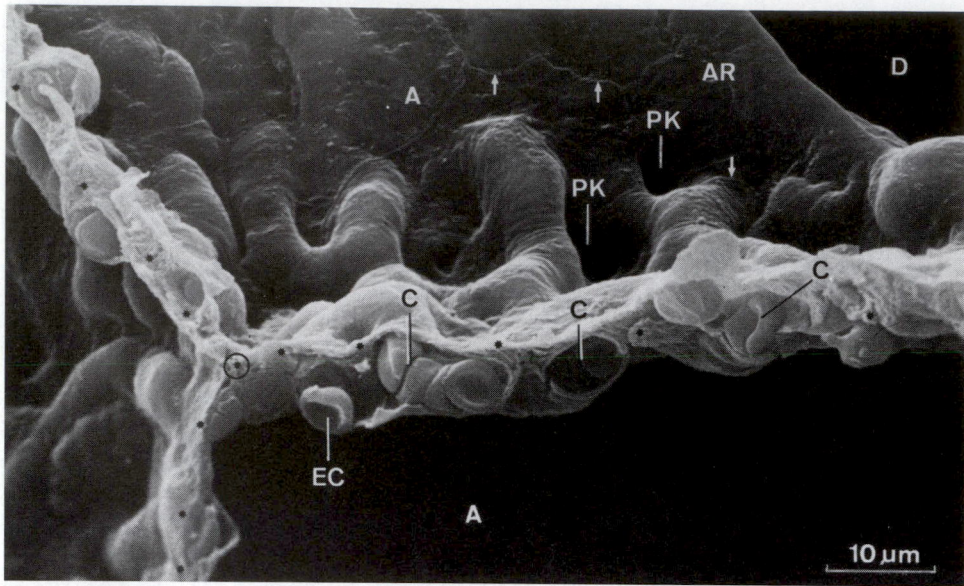

A

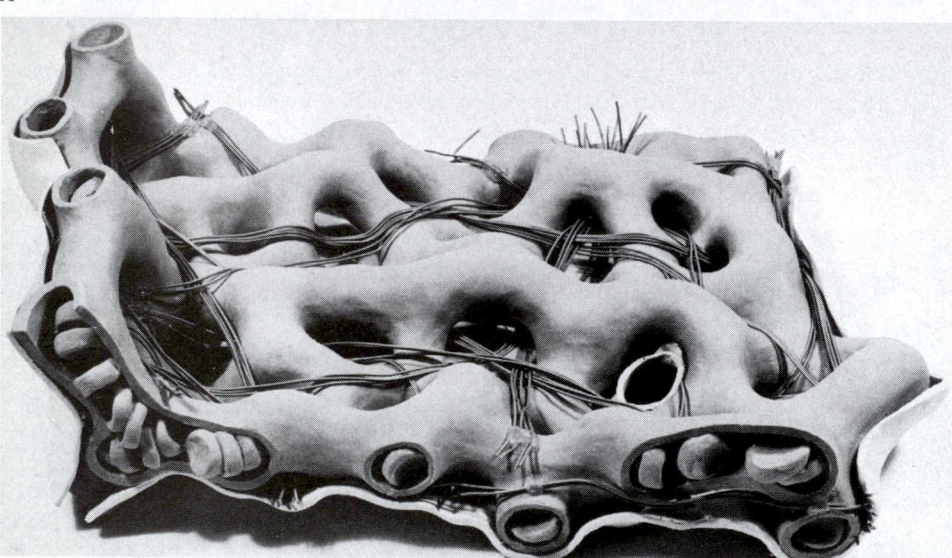

B

FIGURE 2-29 In the alveolar wall, shown in (a) in a scanning electron micrograph from a human lung, the capillary blood (C) is separated from the air by a very thin tissue barrier. Short arrows mark intercellular junctions of alveolar epithelium. The model (b) shows the capillary network to be interwoven with the meshwork of septal fibers, the course of which is marked by asterisks in (a). *(From Weibel,[46] with permission.)*

dency to disrupt it? The thin barrier must not only withstand the distending pressure of the capillary blood due both to hemodynamic forces and to gravity, particularly in the lower lung zones, but must also keep the capillary bed expanded over a very large surface—a task that is made difficult because surface forces that act on the complex alveolar surface would tend to collapse alveoli and capillaries. This requires a very subtle, economical design of the fibrous support system.[41,46,49]

The problem of supporting the capillaries on connective tissue fibers with as little tissue as possible has been solved ingeniously: we find that the fiber network is interlaced with the capillary network; Fig. 2-29B shows that, when the fibers are taut, the capillaries weave from one side of the septum to the other. This arrangement has a threefold advantage: (1) it allows the capillaries to be supported unit by unit directly on the fiber strands without the need of additional "binders," (2) it causes the capillaries to become spread out on the alveolar surface when the fibers are stretched, and (3) it optimizes the gas-exchange conditions by limiting the presence of fibers—which must interfere with O_2 flow—to half the capillary surface. The thin section of a capillary shown in Fig. 2-30 reveals that an interstitial space with fibers and fibroblasts exists on only one side of the capillary, whereas on the other the two lining cells, endothelium and epithelium, become closely joined with only a single common basement membrane interposed. Over half the surface the capillary blood is therefore separated from the air merely by a minimal tissue barrier made of epithelial and en-

to the minimum required (Fig. 2-30). The septal interstitium contains very few cells, mostly slim fibroblast with long extensions; these contain fine bundles of contractile filaments that serve an as yet unknown mechanical function.[26] The septal interstitium usually does not contain cells of the defense system or lymphatics.

dothelial cytoplasmic sheets with their basement membranes fused (Fig. 2-14).

The principal structural "backbone" of the lung is a continuous system of fibers anchored at the hilum and put under tension by the negative intrapleural pressure that tugs on the visceral pleura.[41,49] The general construction principle follows from the formation of the mesenchymal sheath of the airway units in the developing lung; as the airway tree grows, its branches remain separated by layers of mesenchyme within which blood vessels form. When fiber networks develop within this mesenchyme, they will enwrap all airway units and extend from the hilum right to the visceral pleura. The pulmonary fiber system hence forms a three-dimensional fibrous continuum that is structured by the airway system and is closely related to the blood ves-

Internal Support of Parenchymal Structures: the Pulmonary Fiber Continuum

This extraordinary reduction of the tissue mass in the alveolar septa inevitably introduces a number of major problems. How is it possible to secure the mechanical integrity of the system if we consider that several forces act on the septal tissue with a ten-

sels. By virtue of the design of this fibrous continuum, the lung becomes, in
fact, subdivided into millions of little
bellows that are connected to the airway tree, as represented schematically
in Fig. 2-31; these structures expand
with expansion of the chest because the
tension exerted on the visceral pleura
by the negative intrapleural pressure
becomes transmitted to the bellows'
walls through that fiber system.[41,49]

To try to put some order into this
fiber system, we can first single out two
major components that can easily be
identified (Fig. 2-31). First we find that
all airways, from the main-stem
bronchus that enters the lung at the
hilum out to the terminal bronchioles
and beyond, are enwrapped by a strong
sheath of fibers. These fibers constitute
the axial fiber system; they form the
"bark" of the tree whose roots are at
the hilum and whose branches pene-

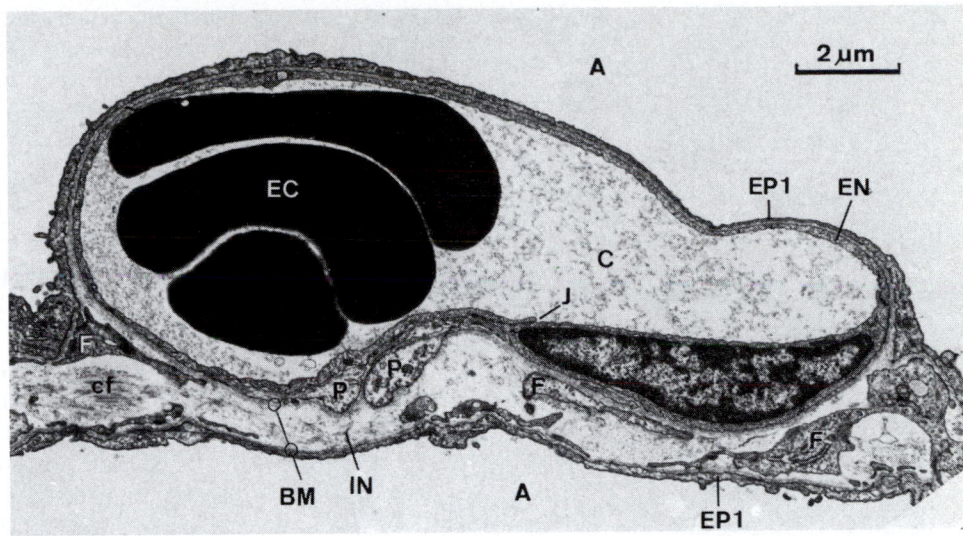

FIGURE 2-30   Alveolar capillary from human lung lined by endothelial cell (EN) which is associated with processes of pericytes (P). Substantial interstitial space with fibers (cf) and fibroblasts
(F) occurs on one side only, whereas minimal air-blood barrier is formed on other side by fusion
of basement membranes (BM).

trate deep into lung parenchyma, following the course of the airways. A second major fiber system is related to the visceral
pleura, which is made of strong fiber bags enwrapping all lobes.
We then find connective tissue septa penetrating from the visceral
pleura into lung parenchyma, separating units of the airway tree.
We call these fibers the *peripheral fiber system* because they
mark the boundaries between the units of respiratory lung tissue.

The peripheral fiber system subdivides the lung into a number of units that are not simple to define because they form a
continuous hierarchy in accordance with the pattern of airway
tree branching. As we have seen above, however, two such units
appear to be natural: the lobes, which are demarcated by a more
or less complete lining by visceral pleura with a serosal cleft interposed (Fig. 2-1); and the acinus, the parenchymal unit in which
all airways participate in gas exchange.

The acinus is the functional unit of the pulmonary parenchyma.
The airway that leads into the acinus, the first-order respiratory
bronchiole, continues branching within the acinus for about 6 to
10 additional generations (Figs. 2-5 and 2-27).[15] These intra-
acinar airways, called respiratory bronchioles and alveolar ducts,
also carry in their wall relatively strong fibers of the axial fiber
system, which extend to the end of the duct system. But since
the walls of intra-acinar air ducts are densely settled with alveoli, these fibers form a kind of network whose meshes encircle
the alveolar mouths (Figs. 2-28 and 2-32). These fiber rings serve
as a scaffold for a network of finer fibers that spread within the
alveolar septa (Fig. 2-32). But now we must note that in a fiber
system there may be no loose ends; accordingly the septal fiber
system must be anchored at both ends—on the network of axial
fibers around the alveolar ducts, and on extensions of the peripheral fibers that penetrate into the acinus from interlobular
septa. Thus the fiber system of the lung becomes a continuum
that spans the entire space of the lung, from the hilus to the visceral pleura (Fig. 2-31). It is put under varying tension as the
pleura is expanded by the chest wall and diaphragm.

The continuous nature of a well-ordered fiber system is an essential design feature of the lung.[41] This becomes evident in emphysema: when some fibers are disrupted they cannot be kept
under tension; they will retract, and larger airspaces will form as

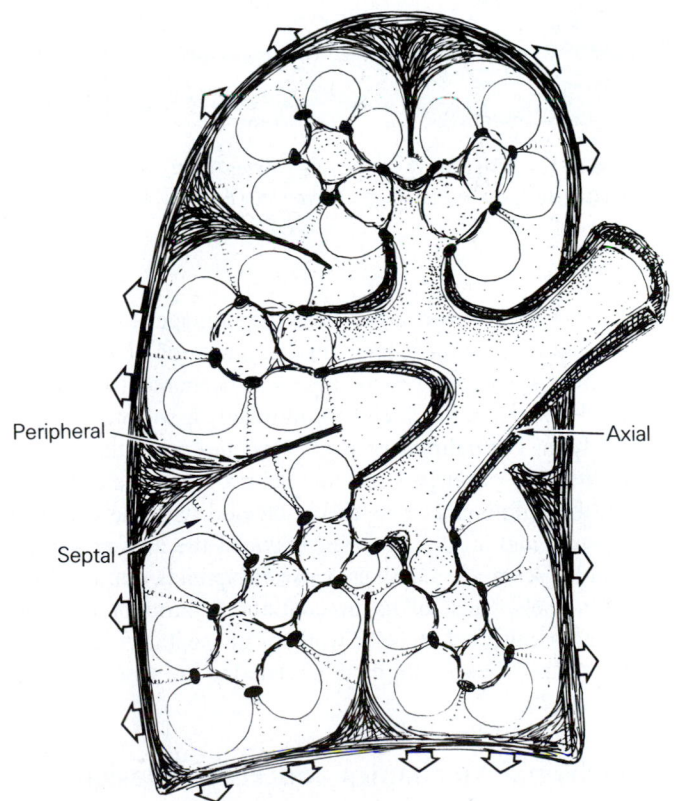

FIGURE 2-31   The major connective fiber tracts of the lung are divided into axial fibers along the airways and peripheral fibers connected
to the pleura. They are connected by fibers in the alveolar septa. *(From
Weibel and Gil,[49] with permission.)*

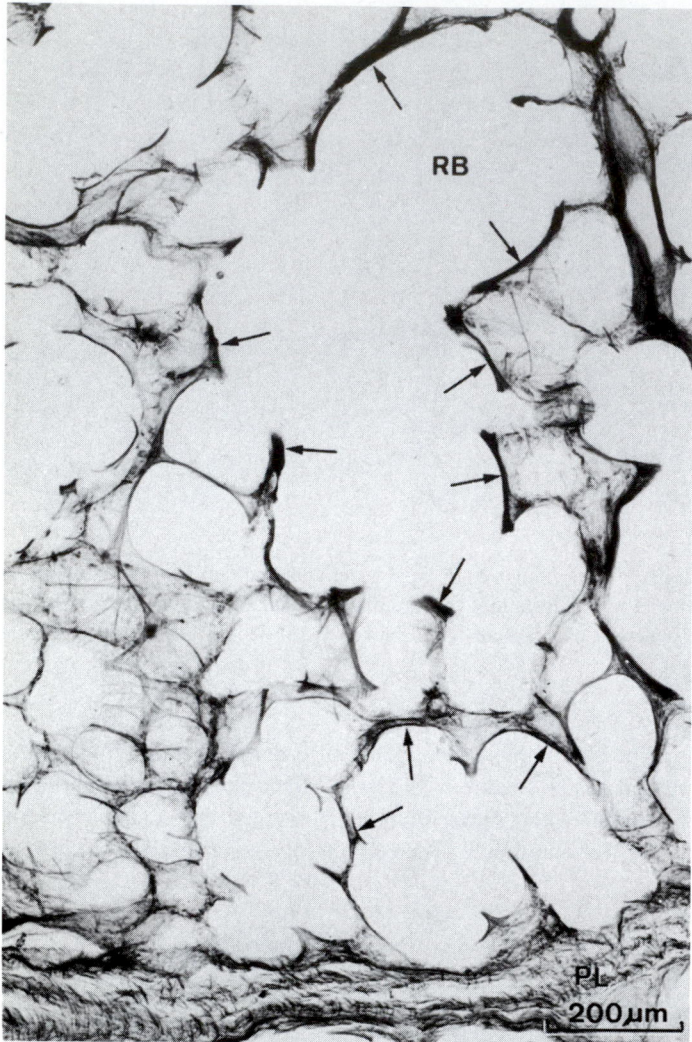

FIGURE 2-32 Connective tissue stain reveals the strong fiber rings that demarcate the alveolar ducts *(arrows). (From Weibel,*[46] *with permission.)*

the fiber system is rearranged near the damage. Small foci of emphysema form in most lungs in the course of time.

The fiber system serves mainly as a mechanical support for the blood vessels, with which it is intimately associated in an orderly fashion. The pulmonary artery branches in parallel with the airway tree and penetrates into the acinus along the axial fiber system; the pulmonary veins are associated with the peripheral fiber system and are thus located between the airway units. In the alveolar septa, the capillary network spreads out as a broad sheet of vessels whose paths are continuous throughout the system of interconnected alveolar walls of the septa. We have seen that these capillaries are intimately related to the septal fiber system (Fig. 2-29).

Parenchymal Mechanics and Tissue Design

As in all connective tissue, the fibers of the lung are composed of collagen and elastic fibers.[41] The collagen fibers are bundles of fibrils bound together by proteoglycans; they are practically inextensible (less than 2 percent) and have a very high tensile

strength, so that they rupture at loads of only 50 to 70 dyn/cm^{-2}, which means that a collagen fiber of 1 mm diameter can support a weight of over 500 g. In contrast, elastic fibers have a much lower tensile strength but a high extensibility: they can be stretched to about 130 percent of their relaxed length before rupturing.

In the fiber system of lung parenchyma, collagen and elastic fibers occur in a volume ratio of about 2.5:1, whereas this ratio is 10:1 for the visceral pleura. In a relaxed state, one will find the collagen fibers to be longer than the accompanying elastic fibers, so that they appear wavy. Because of the association between "rubberlike" elastic and "twinelike" collagen fibers, the connective tissue strands behave like an elastic band: they are easy to stretch up to the point where the collagen fibers are taut, but from there on they resist stretching very strongly.

The elastic properties of the lung's fiber system can be studied by filling the airways with fluid so as to eliminate the effects of surface tension. This reveals that the lung's fiber system has a high compliance until high levels of inflation are reached, and that the retractive or recoil force generated by the fiber system amounts to no more than a few millibars at physiological inflation levels. The actual recoil force in the air-filled lung, reflected by the negative pressure in the pleural space, is appreciably higher, but this is due to surface tension rather than to the retractive force of the fibers.[3,7,13,49]

Surface tension arises at any gas-liquid interface because the forces between the molecules of the liquid are much stronger than those between the liquid and the gas. As a result, the liquid surface will tend to become as small as possible. A curved surface, such as that of a bubble, generates a pressure that is proportional to the curvature and to the surface tension coefficient γ. The general formula of Gibbs relates this pressure, P_S, to the mean curvature $\bar{K}$:

$$P_S = 2\gamma \cdot \bar{K} \qquad (1)$$

In a sphere, the curvature is simply the reciprocal of the radius r:

$$P_S = \frac{2\gamma}{r} \qquad (2)$$

The most critical effect of surface tension is that it endangers stability of the air space, because a set of connected "bubbles," the alveoli, is inherently unstable: the small ones should contract and the large ones expand. Since the 300 million alveoli are all connected with each other through the airways, the lung is inherently unstable: why do the alveoli not all collapse and empty into one large bubble? There are two principal reasons.

The first reason is one of tissue structure. The alveoli are not simply soap bubbles in a froth; rather, their walls contain an intricate fiber system, as we have seen. Thus, when an alveolus tends to shrink, the fibers in the walls of adjoining alveoli are stretched, and this will prevent the alveolus from collapsing. It is said that alveoli are mechanically interdependent and that this stabilizes them.[56]

The second reason is related to the fact that the alveolar surface is not simply water exposed to air but is lined by surfactant (Fig. 2-33), which has peculiar properties in that its surface tension coefficient γ is variable:[7,13] from a large volume of evidence, it is now established that surface tension falls as the alveolar surface becomes smaller, and that it rises when the surface

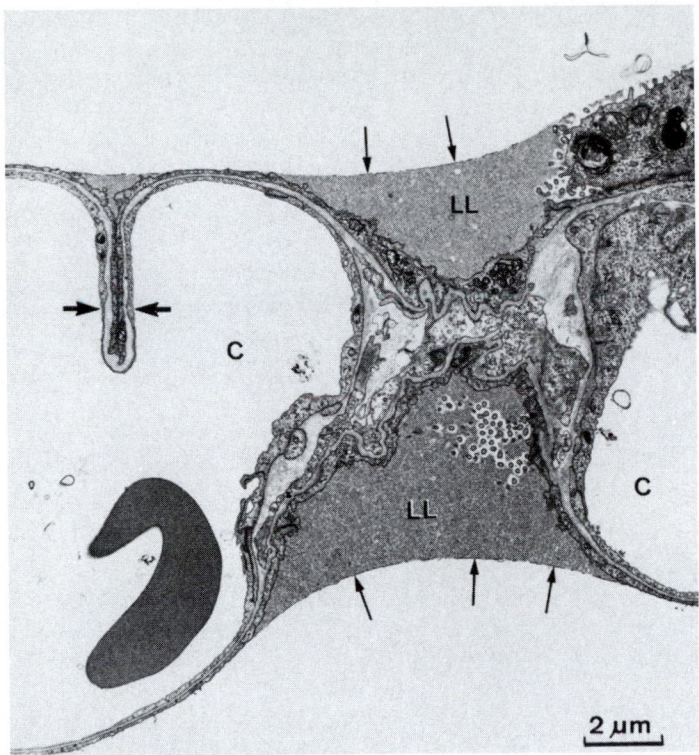

FIGURE 2-33 Alveolar septum of human lung fixed by perfusion through blood vessels shows alveolar lining layer (LL) in crevices between capillaries (C) topped by surfactant film which appears as a fine black line (*arrows*). Note the type II cell with lamellar bodies and the fold in thin tissue barrier (*bold arrows*). (*From Weibel, Am J Roentgenol 133:1021–1031, 1979, with permission.*)

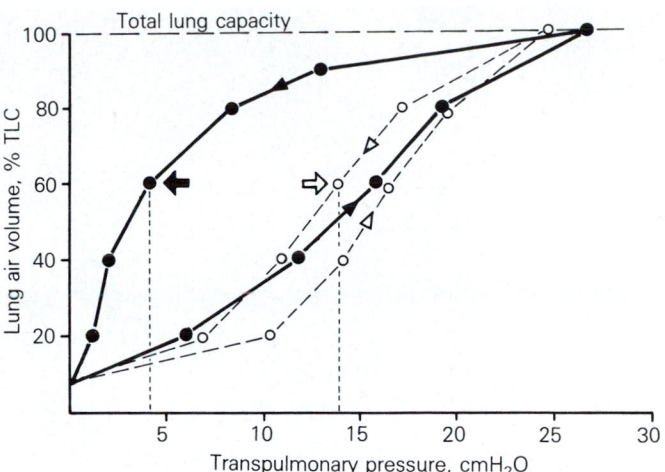

FIGURE 2-34 Comparison of pressure-volume curve of a normal air-filled rabbit lung with that of a surfactant depleted lung (*broken line*). The arrows indicate the points at which the lungs shown in Fig. 2-35 have been fixed by vascular perfusion. (*From Weibel,[46] with permission.*)

expands. Because of this feature, which is due to the phospholipid nature of alveolar surfactant, alveoli do not behave like soap bubbles whose surface tension remains constant. When an alveolus begins to shrink, the surface tension of its lining layer falls and the retractive force generated at the surface is reduced or even abolished. Combined with interdependence, this property of surfactant allows the complex of alveoli to remain stable.

Which of the two factors for stabilizing lung structure is now the most important: interdependence or surfactant properties? It turns out that both are essential. If one depletes the lung of its surfactant lining by washing with a detergent, the pressure-volume curve changes dramatically (Fig. 2-34): on deflation, lung volume falls rapidly.[3] If we look at samples from lungs fixed at the same volume (60 percent total lung capacity) but derived from either normal or detergent-rinsed lungs, we find that surfactant depletion causes the alveoli to collapse (Fig. 2-35). This, however, causes the alveolar ducts to enlarge, stretching the strong fiber nets at the mouths of the collapsed alveoli. The ducts do not collapse because of interdependence between adjacent units.[3]

In the normal air-filled lung, surfactant properties and interdependence due to fiber tension both contribute to stabilizing the complex of alveoli and alveolar ducts.[56] To understand this, let us examine Fig. 2-36, which shows a highly simplified diagram of a parenchymal unit. Interdependence is established by the continuum of axial, septal, and peripheral fibers. Surface tension

exerts an inward pull in the hollow alveoli, where curvature is negative. However, over the free edge of the alveolar septa, along the outline of the duct, the surface tension must pull outward because there the curvature is positive. The latter force must be rather strong, because the radius of curvature is very small on the septal edge; but this force is counteracted by the strong fiber strands, usually provided with some smooth muscle cells, that we find in the free edge of the alveolar septum (Figs. 2-27 and 2-32). Thus interdependence is an important factor in preventing the complex hollow of the lung, where negative and positive curvatures coexist, from collapsing. But its capacity to do so is limited and requires low surface tensions, particularly on deflation when the fibers tend to slack. If surface tension becomes too high, the lung's foamlike structure will partly collapse in spite of fiber interdependence (Fig. 2-35).

Micromechanics of the Alveolar Septum

We must finally consider the mechanical factors that shape the alveolar septum in the air-filled lung. As we have seen, the alveolar septum is made of a single capillary network that is interlaced with fibers (Fig. 2-29). When the fibers are stretched, the capillaries bulge alternatingly to one side or the other, and this will cause pits and crevices to occur in the meshes of the capillary network.

This irregular surface is to some extent evened out by the presence of an extracellular layer of lining fluid, which is rather thin over the capillaries but forms little pools in the intercapillary pits (Fig. 2-33). This lining consists of an aqueous layer of variable thickness, called the *hypophase,* and surfactant, which forms a film on the surface of the hypophase.[13,49] The hypophase seems to contain considerable amounts of reserve surfactant material, which occurs in a characteristic configuration called *tubular myelin* (Fig. 2-22).

In the alveolar septum, the tissue structures are extremely delicate, as we have seen; its configuration is therefore not exclusively determined by structural features but results from the

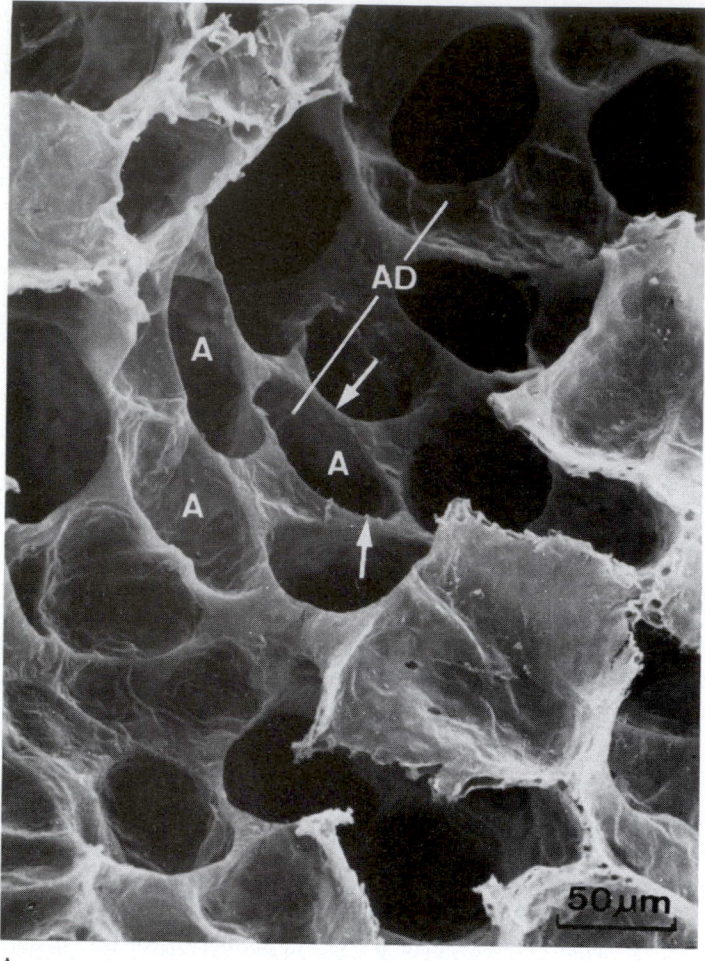

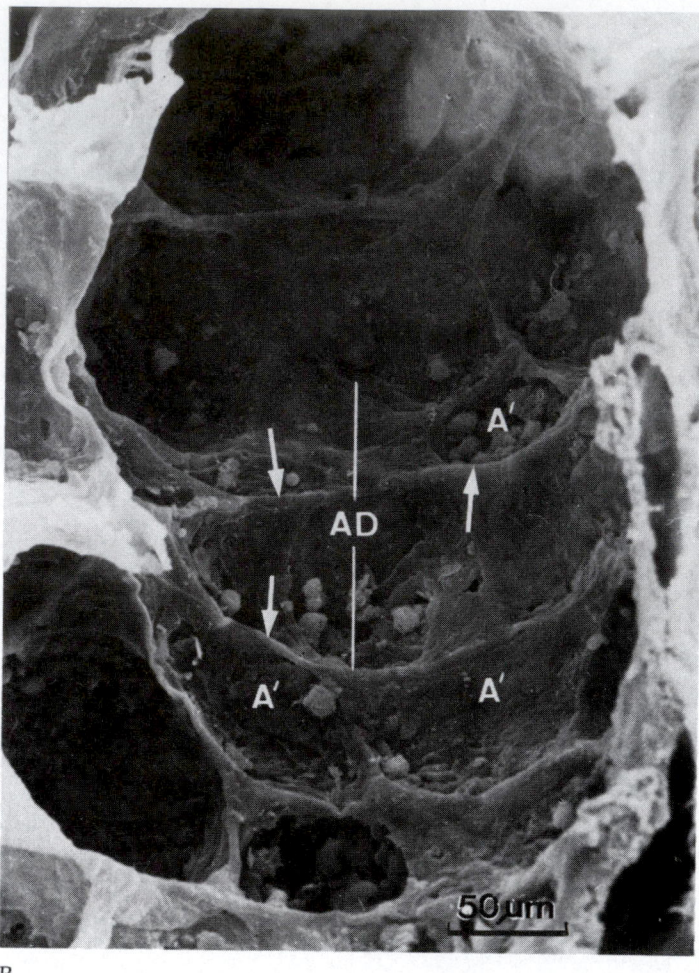

A

B

FIGURE 2-35   Scanning electron micrographs of normal air-filled (*A*) and surfactant-depleted (*B*) rabbit lungs fixed at 60 percent TLC on the deflation curve (Fig. 2-34) show alveoli to be open (A) in (*A*), collapsed (A′) in (*B*). The alveolar duct (AD) is widened in the surfactant-depleted lung, resulting in a stretching of the fiber strands around the alveolar mouths (*arrows*). (*From Wilson and Bachofen,[56] with permission.*)

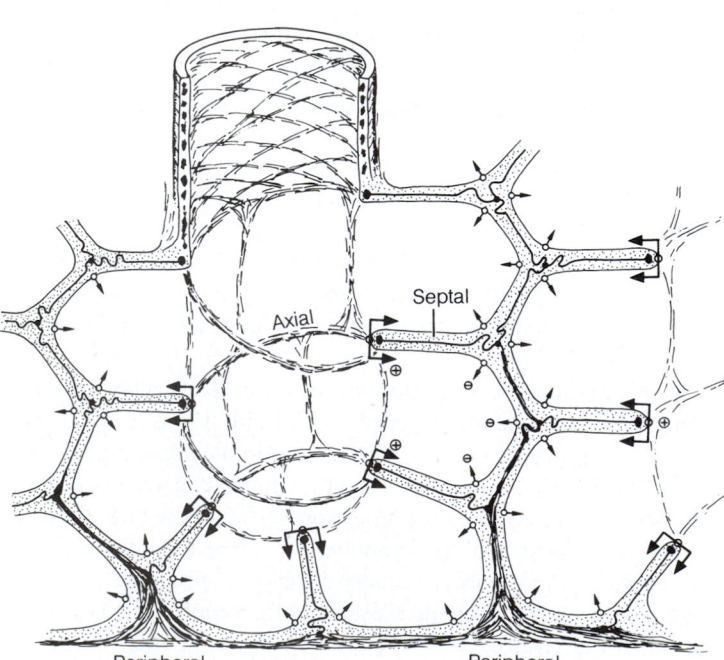

FIGURE 2-36   Model of the disposition of axial, septal, and peripheral fibers in an acinus showing the effect of surface forces (*arrows*). (*From Weibel,[46] with permission.*)

molding effect of various forces that must be kept in balance.[41,46,49] Figure 2-37 shows how the three principal mechanical forces—tissue tension, surface tension, and capillary distending pressure—interact in the septum. The fibers of the alveolar septum are under a tension whose magnitude depends on the level of lung inflation. This tends to straighten out the fibers, so that a force (pressure) normal to the fiber axis results, which is responsible for shifting the capillaries to one side of the septum or the other (Figs. 2-29*B* and 2-37). The walls of the capillaries are exposed to the luminal pressure, which is the result of blood pressure in pulmonary arteries and veins but also depends on gravity, for one finds wider capillaries at the bottom of the lung than at the top. If this distending pressure acts homogeneously over the circumference of the capillary, it will push against the fibers on one side but will cause the thin barrier on the opposite side to bulge outward. This effect is to some extent counteracted by surface tension, which exerts a force normal to the surface (Fig. 2-37). This force depends on two factors: its direction depends on the orientation of curvature, acting toward the alveolar space over concave regions (negative curvature) and toward the tissue over convexities (positive curvature); its magnitude depends on the degree of curvature and on the value of the surface tension coefficient γ.

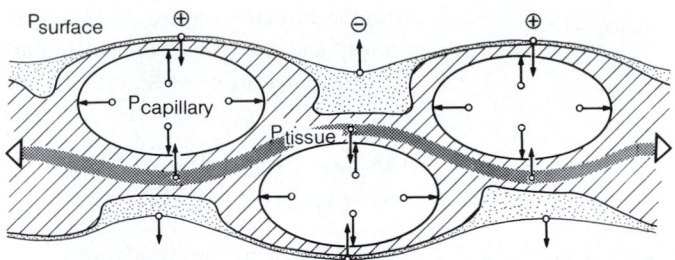

FIGURE 2-37 Model showing the micromechanical forces of surface tension, tissue tension, and capillary distending pressure that shape the alveolar septum. *(From Weibel,[46] with permission.)*

The alveolar septum achieves a stable configuration when all these interacting forces are in balance. Combined forces tend to squash the capillary flat; this happens at high levels of lung inflation when the fibers are under high tension and the surface tension coefficient of surfactant reaches its highest value due to expansion of the surface. On deflation, the fibers are relaxed and surface tension falls drastically; the capillary distending pressure now exceeds both the tissue and the surface forces, with the result that the slack fibers are bent, weaving through the capillary network, whereas the capillaries bulge slightly toward the airspace. Surface tension is apparently so low as to permit a considerable degree of surface "crumpling" to persist (Fig. 2-38).[3]

The importance of the balance between the forces that act on the septum is also shown in Fig. 2-39. The specimen of Fig. 2-39B was fixed under zone 3 perfusion conditions[4] and all the capillaries are wide, partly bulging toward the airspace, as in Fig. 2-38. This is different in Fig. 2-39A, which was fixed under zone 2 conditions: in the flat part of the septum, the capillaries are squashed flat, because the surface and tissue forces now exceed the vascular distending pressure. It is interesting, however, that the capillaries remain wide in the corners where three septa come together. The distribution of surface forces causes the internal pressure to be lower in the region of these corners, as we can see intuitively from Fig. 2-36.

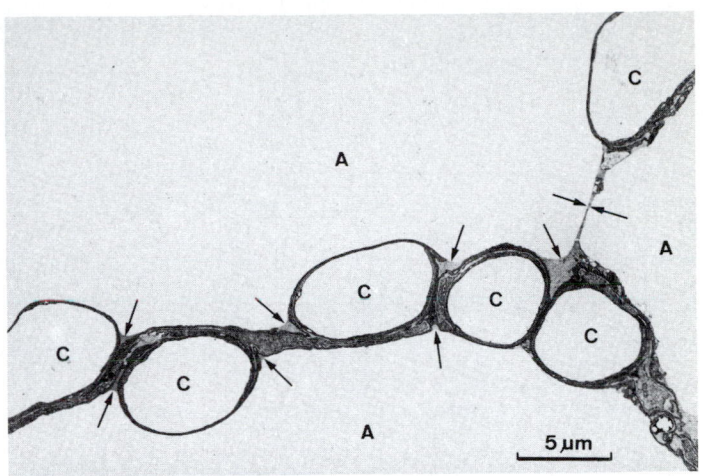

FIGURE 2-38 Alveolar septum of air-filled rabbit lung perfusion-fixed at 60 percent TLC shows empty capillaries (C) which bulge toward the alveolar air space (A). Note pools of surface lining layer in the crevices between capillaries (*arrows*) and film spanning across alveolar pore (*double arrows*). *(From Gil et al. J Appl Physiol 52:990–1001, 1979, with permission.)*

THE LUNG AS GAS EXCHANGER

Up to this juncture the principal design features of the lung have been considered with respect to the lung as an organ in its own right. When now discussing the implications of these design features on the lung's main function, gas exchange between air and blood, we must modify our approach in two ways: (1) we must consider the lung as a servant of the body, i.e. as one link in the chain of events that provide O_2 for energy production in the cells of the organism, and (2) we must adopt a quantitative approach, asking, in a way, how much lung is enough to serve the body's needs.

The Lung as Part of the Respiratory System

The O_2 needs of the body are set by the energetic demands of the cells and their mitochondria when these produce ATP by

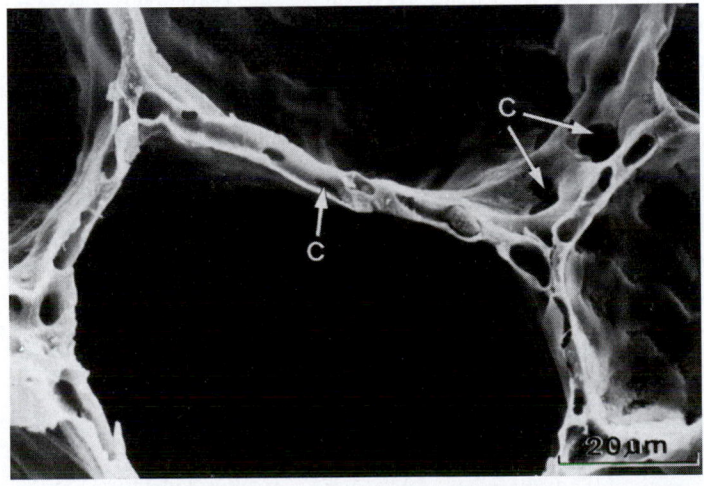

A

FIGURE 2-39 Scanning electron micrographs of alveolar walls of rabbit lungs fixed under (a) zone 2 and (b) zone 3 conditions of perfusion. Note that capillaries (C) are wide in zone 3 and slit-like in zone 2, ex-

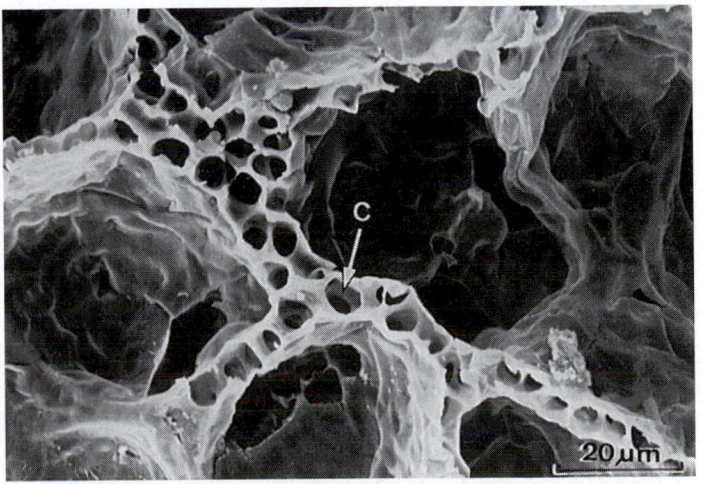

B

cept for "corner capillaries," which are wide in either case. *(From Bachofen, et al. Respir Physiol 52:41–52, 1983, with permission.)*

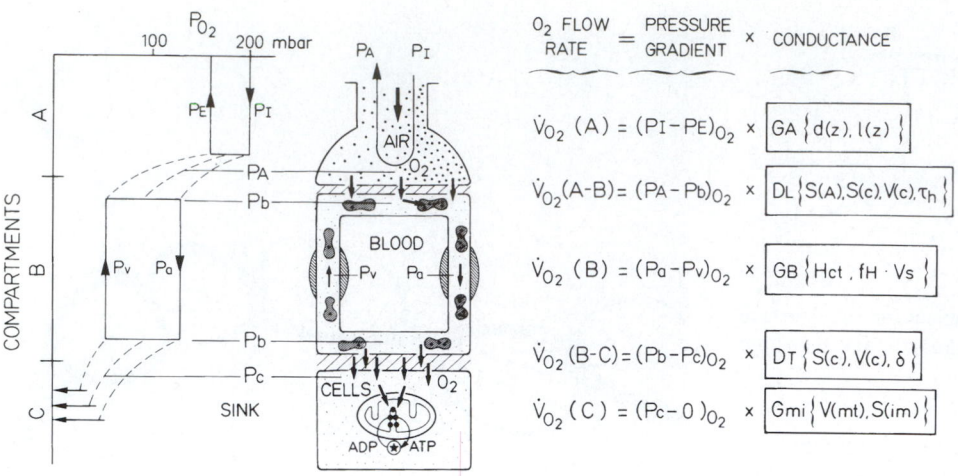

FIGURE 2-40   Model of the respiratory system from lung to cells. (*Modified from Weibel and Taylor,[52] with permission.*)

may be affected by the design of the airway and vascular trees, particularly by their quantitative properties.

Design of the Branching Airway Tree

The entrance to the lung's airways is the trachea, a single tube; the gas-exchange elements where air and blood are brought into close contact are contained in several million units. Between entrance and periphery lies a meticulously designed system of branching airways that serve to conduct the inspired air into those peripheral channels that carry alveoli in their walls and can thus contribute to the exchange of gases between air and blood (Fig. 2-5).

The pattern of airway branching can be studied on resin casts such as that illustrated in Fig. 2-3. Consistently each branch is seen to divide into two smaller branches—i.e., to undergo dichotomous branching.[32,45,50] The two daughter branches from the same parent often differ in diameter and/or in length (Fig. 2-42): dichotomy is hence irregular. Nonetheless, morphometric analysis of the casts reveals that the progression of airway dimensions from the trachea to the periphery follows strict laws.

oxidative phosphorylation to allow the cells to do work.[46] This process requires a flow of O_2 to be maintained from the lung to the cells. It proceeds along the respiratory system through various steps (Fig. 2-40): into the lung by ventilation, to the blood by diffusion, through the circulation by blood flow, from the blood capillaries by diffusion to the cells and mitochondria, where it disappears in the process of oxidative phosphorylation. A number of basic features characterize this system: (1) under steady-state conditions the O_2 flow rate, $\dot{V}_{O_2}$, is the same at all levels, i.e., O_2 uptake in the lung is equal to O_2 consumption in the tissues; (2) the basic driving force for O_2 flow through the system is a cascade of O_2 partial pressure which falls from inspired P_{O_2} down to near zero in the mitochondria; (3) the O_2 flow rate at each step is the product of a partial pressure difference and a conductance which is related to structural and functional properties of the organs participating in O_2 transfer. It can, for example, be shown that the O_2 flow rate into the O_2-consuming step in the cells is directly related to the amount of mitochondria that perform oxidative phosphorylation.

With respect to gas exchange in the lung (Fig. 2-41), the O_2 flow rate is determined by the Bohr equation:

$$\dot{V}_{O_2} = P_{AO_2} - \overline{P}_{cO_2}) \cdot DL_{O_2} \tag{3}$$

where

P_{AO_2} = the P_{O_2} in alveoli,
$\overline{P}_{cO_2}$ = the mean P_{O_2} in pulmonary capillaries, and

DL_{O_2} = the pulmonary diffusing capacity or the lung's O_2 conductance.

The important point is now that all parameters to the right of this equation may be significantly affected by design features. We have already pointed out that O_2 uptake may be affected by the surface available for gas exchange and by the thickness of the barrier between air and blood; we now need to find an appropriate formulation of how these features may be related to DL_{O_2}. The O_2 partial pressure difference is established by ventilation and perfusion of the gas exchange units, and this

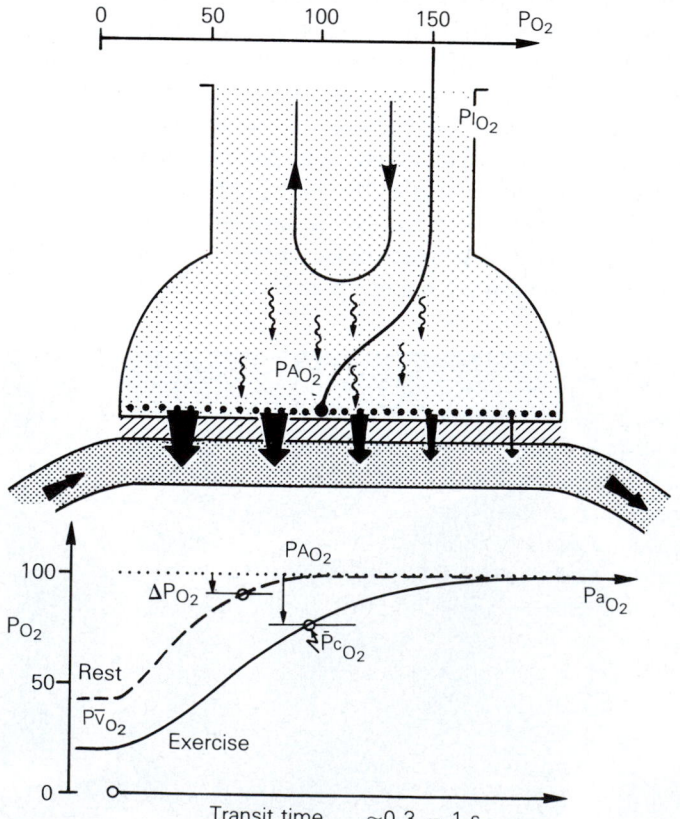

FIGURE 2-41   Model of gas exchange showing gradual rise of capillary P_{O_2} (P_{cO_2}) as blood flows through capillary until it approaches alveolar P_{O_2} (P_{AO_2}). (*From Weibel,[46] with permission.*)

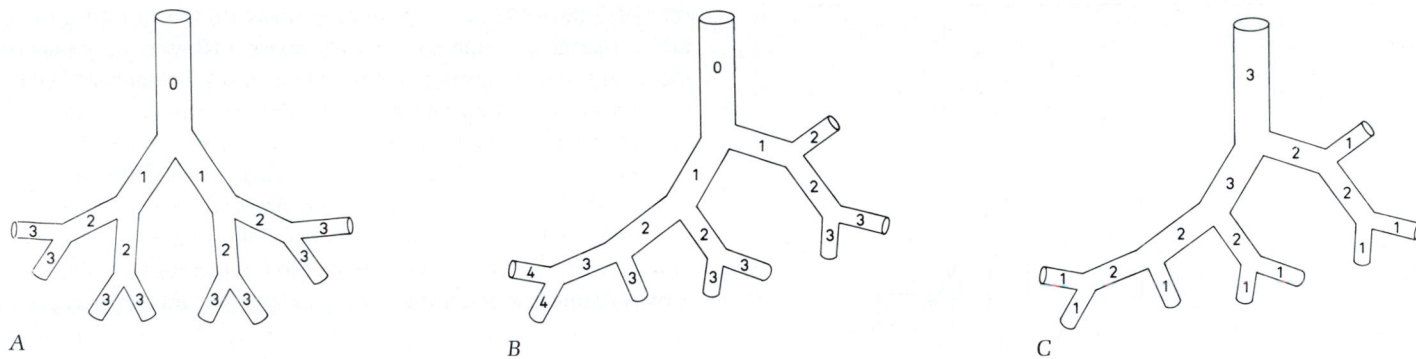

FIGURE 2-42   Patterns of airway branching: *A.* Regular dichotomy. *B.* Irregular dichotomy numbered by "generations down." *C.* Irregular dichotomy numbered by "orders up."

There are two ways of approaching such an analysis. In the first place, the pattern of branching is followed from trachea to the periphery: each bifurcation gives rise to a new generation of airways.[45] The number of branches in each new generation is twice that in the parent generation; the branching ratio of dichotomy is 2. Accordingly, the number (N) of branches in each generation (z) is

$$N(z) = 2^z \qquad (4)$$

Within each generation, the lengths and diameters of the branches have a characteristic range of sizes;[21] but the mean diameter of the conducting airways (to about the 16th generation) decreases systematically, following a simple law (Fig. 2-43):

$$d(z) = d_0 \cdot 2^{-z/3} \qquad (5)$$

where

$d(z)$ = the mean diameter of airways in generation z
d_0 = the diameter of the trachea

This equation shows that with each generation, the airway diameter is reduced by the cube root of the branching ratio 2, a law that is well known in hydrodynamics, as it defines an optimal design of a branched system of tubes, also called Murray's law.

Using this approach, it is possible to construct a model that takes into account irregularities in branching by considering the number of airways of a given diameter, d_μ, that exist in each generation, and the number of lengths of bronchial pathway that intervene between the larynx and the particular airways (Fig. 2-44).

The alternative is to regard the airways as a system of tubes converging from the periphery, the acinus, toward the center, the trachea.[22,23] By using an ordering system that is employed in analyzing rivers (Strahler system), branches are grouped into orders by size, beginning with the smallest designated as order 1 (Fig. 2-42C). This ordering pattern is particularly well adapted to a system of irregular dichotomy because the size of branches in one order varies less than with the other approach. A branching ratio is determined as the ratio of the number of branches in order μ to that in order $\mu + 1$. Remarkably, the progression of diameters through the various orders is again roughly proportional to the cube root of the branching ratio.[12] Hence, both models yield basically the same result.

The general conclusion drawn from this type of analysis is that the diameters of the conducting airways are such as to assure optimal conditions for airflow:[23,45,50] from an engineering point of view, the airways of the lung are well designed. The total volume of the conducting airways down to generation 16 (the

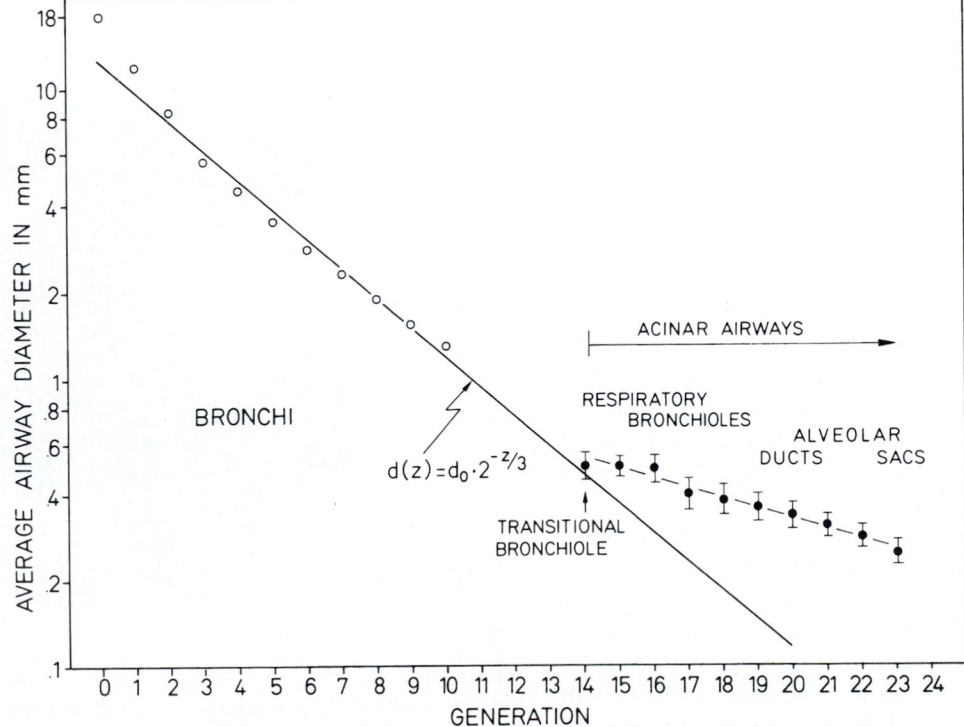

FIGURE 2-43   Average diameter of airways in human lung plotted by generations of regularized dichotomous branching. (*From Haefeli-Bleuer and Weibel,*[15] *with permission.*)

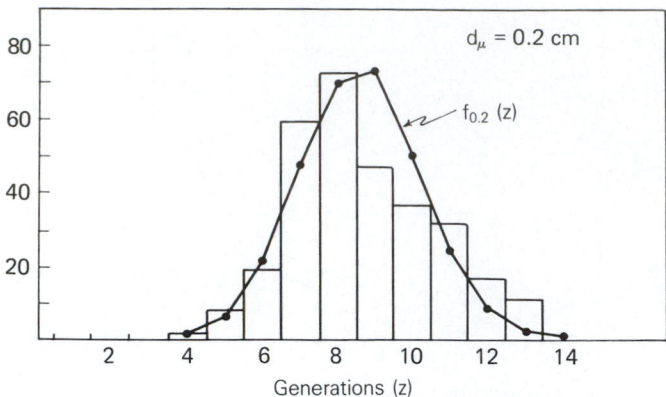

A

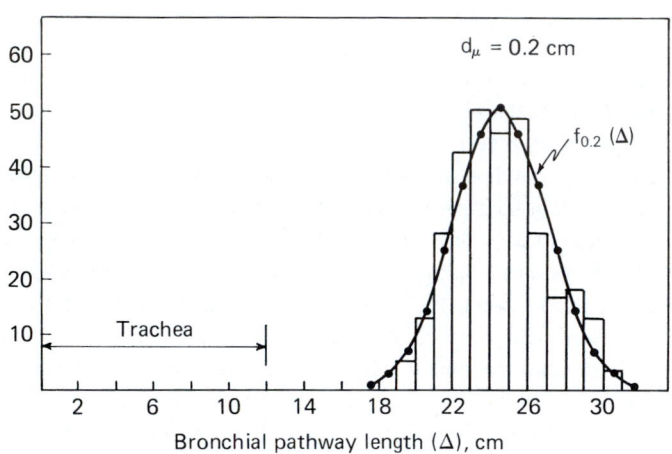

B

FIGURE 32-44 Distribution of airways of diameter $d_\mu = 2$ mm with respect to (*A*) generations of branching and (*B*) bronchial pathway lengths. (*From Weibel,*[45] *with permission.*)

root-of-2 law relates to optimizing mass flow of a liquid or of air. In the most peripheral airways, mass airflow is only part of the means of transporting O_2 toward the air-blood barrier:[43] since the airways are blind-ending tubes and since a sizable amount of residual air remains in the lung periphery after expiration, O_2 molecules must move into the residual air by diffusion (Fig. 2-46). But diffusion of O_2 in the gas phase is best served by establishing as large an interface as possible between residual air and the fresh air that flows in from the trachea. In fact, since the airway diameter remains nearly unchanged, the total airway cross section nearly doubles with each generation beyond generation 16 (Fig. 2-47).

The dimensions of the airway tree influence the ventilatory flow of air in a number of ways. First of all, airflow velocity falls along the airway tree because the total cross-sectional area of the airways increases with every generation (Fig. 2-47); whereas the cross-sectional area of the trachea is about 2.5 cm², that of the 1024 airways in the 10th generation taken together is 13 cm², and as we approach the acinar airways, the total cross section reaches 300 cm². But since the same air volume flows through all generations, the flow velocity falls by more than 100-fold from the trachea to the acini: at rest, the mean flow velocity on inspiration is about 1 m/s⁻¹ in the trachea and less than 1 cm/s⁻¹ in the first-order respiratory bronchioles. This shows that in the small airways the transport of O_2 by mass airflow is slower than that by diffusion, since O_2 molecules move through air at a velocity of about 5 cm/s⁻¹. In exercise, the flow velocities are up to 10 times greater, in proportion to the increased ventilation; accordingly, mass flow velocity is somewhat greater than molecular velocity at the entrance into the acini.

anatomic dead space) is about 150 ml; it is rapidly flushed by simple gas flow in the course of inhaling 500 ml of fresh air during quiet inspiration. For the larger airways, optimization for flow and its distribution to peripheral units is, therefore, the essential condition for good design.

Figure 2-45 shows the transition of peripheral airways from terminal bronchioles, which serve only as conducting tubes, to respiratory bronchioles, which contain alveoli in their walls. The terminal airways also branch by dichotomy (Fig. 2-27).

Figure 2-43 shows that the diameters of the most peripheral airways (generations 15 to 23) do not follow the law of reduction by the cube root of 2; the diameters of respiratory bronchioles and alveolar ducts change very little with each generation.[15] Does this arrangement imply less than an optimal design? No, on the contrary, the cube-

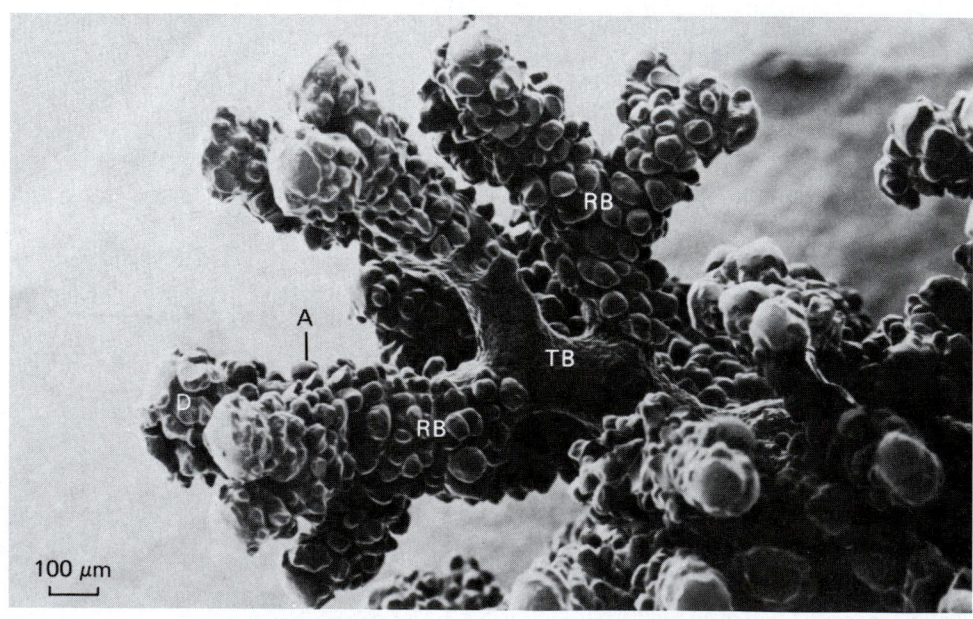

A

FIGURE 2-45 Scanning electron micrographs of airway branches peripheral to terminal bronchiole. *A.* In silicon-rubber cast of cat lung. *B.* In whole tissue preparation of air-filled, perfusion-fixed rabbit lung. Note that branching can be followed from terminal bronchiole to alveolar ducts. A = alveolus; D = alveolar duct; RB = respiratory bronchiole; TB = terminal bronchiole; S = alveolar septum.

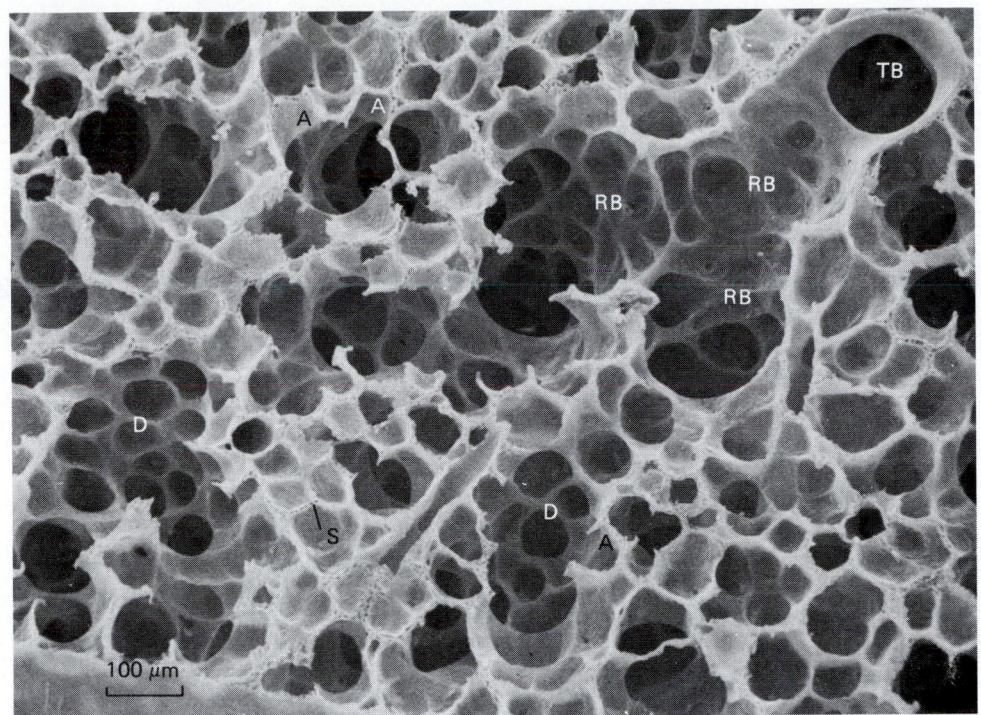

B

FIGURE 2-45   *(Cont.)*

The size of airways also determines the resistance to airflow. The overall resistance is, however, rather small; it is given by the reciprocal of the ratio of ventilatory airflow to the pressure difference between the mouth and alveoli, which is normally no greater than about 1 cmH$_2$O (mbar) or less than 1 mmHg. It is large enough, however, to potentially affect the distribution of ventilation to the many gas-exchange units.

Since the diameter of airways decreases as they branch (Fig. 2-43), one would suspect that their resistance increases toward the periphery. Apparently this is not the case, as the major pressure drop along the airways occurs in medium-sized bronchi;[31] mainly because the flow velocity falls so rapidly as airways branch, the small airways have a low resistance (Fig. 2-48). This is further accentuated by the fact that the thin-walled bronchioles become widened as the lung expands on inspiration because they are subject to the tissue tensions in the coarse fiber system of the lung. Airway resistance is therefore seen to fall as lung volume increases. When this effect of tissue tension is disturbed, as in emphysema, some small bronchioles may collapse. This causes ventilation of the peripheral lung units to become highly uneven.

This biophysical way of looking at the significance of the progression of airway dimensions has recently been complemented by the alternative notion that the airway and vascular trees could be determined by the laws of fractal geometry,[40,55] which appears to lie at the basis of the design of such hierarchical structures.

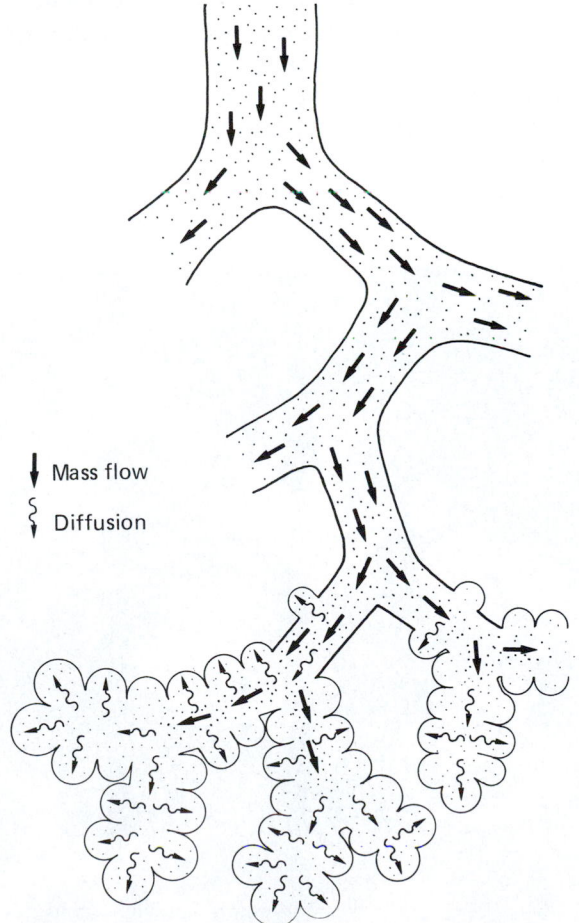

FIGURE 2-46   Oxygen molecules reach alveoli by combined mass airflow and molecular diffusion, the importance of diffusion increasing toward the periphery.

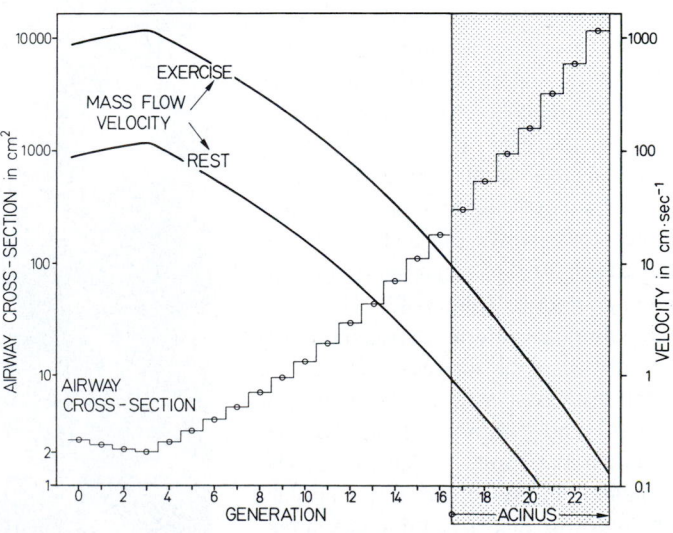

FIGURE 2-47   As total airway cross section increases with the generations of airway branching, the mass flow velocity of inspired air decreases rapidly, falling below the molecular velocity of O$_2$ diffusion in air as we enter the acinus. *(From Weibel,[46] with permission.)*

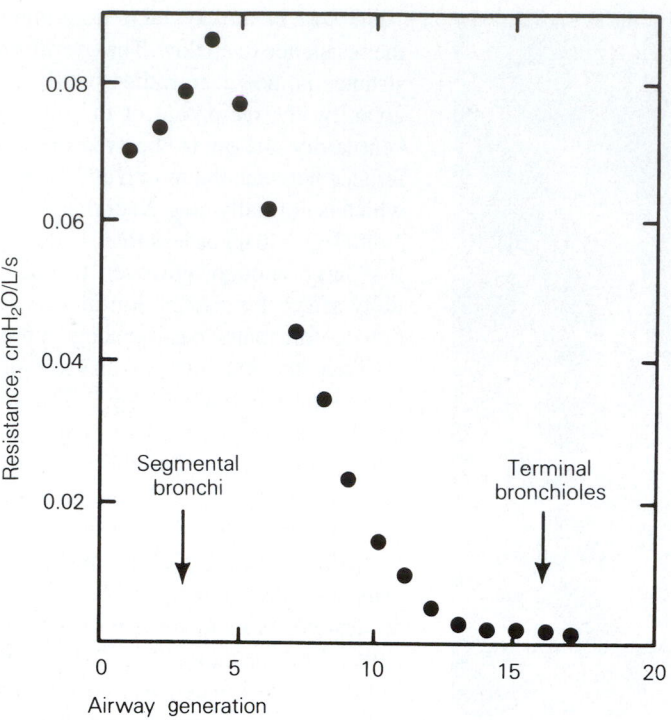

FIGURE 2-48 Airway resistance to mass air flow is located mostly in the conducting airways and falls rapidly toward the periphery. (*Redrawn after Pedley et al.,*[31] *with permission.*)

Design of the Vascular Trees

In many ways, the course and pattern of dimensional changes in the pulmonary blood vessels resemble those of the airways. Figure 2-3 shows that the pulmonary arteries follow the airways closely, out to the smallest branches; together they form the axis of lung parenchymal units of varying order: acinus, lobule, segment lobe. As indicated previously, the veins are differently disposed, lying in the boundary between two or three adjacent units.

The diameter of each pulmonary artery branch also approximates closely that of the accompanying bronchus (Fig. 2-49). Therefore it is evident that the diameter law presented above for airways must also hold for the first 10 to 16 generations of pulmonary arteries (Fig. 2-43). However, the pulmonary arteries divide more frequently than the airways; very often, small branches leave the artery at right angles and supply blood to the parenchymal units adjacent to the bronchus. From a count of precapillaries, it seems that the pulmonary arteries divide, on the average, over 28 generations, as compared to 23 for the airways.[50] The diameter of these terminal vessels is about 20 to 50 μm; if

this range is plotted onto an extension of the graph of Fig. 2-43 to generation 28, it falls on the curve that is obtained by extrapolation from the major branches, $d(z) = d_0 \cdot 2^{-z/3}$. Although no information exists about the entire sequence of dimensional changes throughout the pulmonary arterial tree, this finding suggests that the pulmonary arteries abide to the cube-root-of-2 law from beginning to end. Evidently, the blood is transported to the capillary bed by mass flow only. Therefore there is no reason to deviate from this fundamental law of design, which minimizes the loss of energy due to blood flow. By the way, this design principle seems to hold also for the systemic arteries.

Not much is known yet about the design of the venous tree. The cast shown in Fig. 2-3 suggests, however, that it is similar to that of the arterial tree.

The alveolar capillary network of the lung is very different from that of the systemic circulation. Whereas in muscle, for example, long capillaries are found to be joined in a loose network, the capillaries of the alveolar walls form dense meshworks made of very short segments[14,27] (Fig. 2-50). The meshes are so dense that some people believe blood flows through the alveolar walls like a sheet rather than through a system of interconnected tubes.[11] In this sheet-flow concept, the sheet is bounded by two flat membranes, the air-blood barrier, connected by numerous "posts." When blood flows through this sheet, it is not channeled in a given direction but has freedom to move in a tortuous way between the posts. Although this concept oversimplifies the actual structural conditions, it does provide a useful description of the pattern of blood flow through the alveolar walls and explains why blood flow is not interrupted when some parts of the capillary bed become squashed flat at high inflation levels, as discussed above (Fig. 2-39); the capillaries that remain open in the corners are simply some channels of this broad sheet. It is fur-

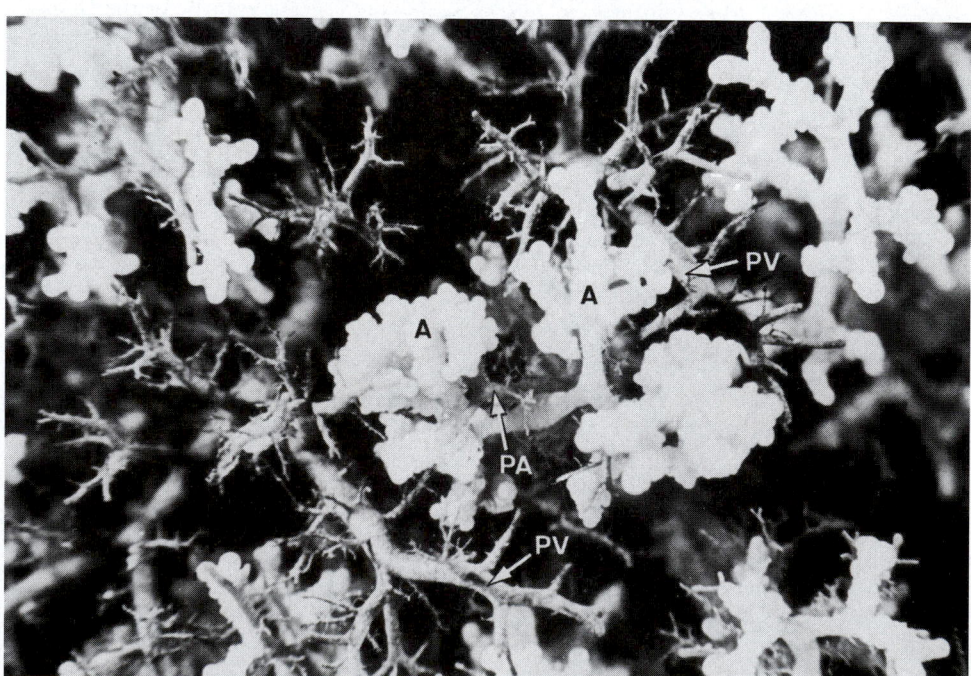

FIGURE 2-49 Detail of cast of airways and blood vessels of human lung shows how pulmonary artery (PA) closely follows the airways (A) to the periphery, whereas the pulmonary vein branches (PV) lie between the units. (*From Weibel,*[46] *with permission.*)

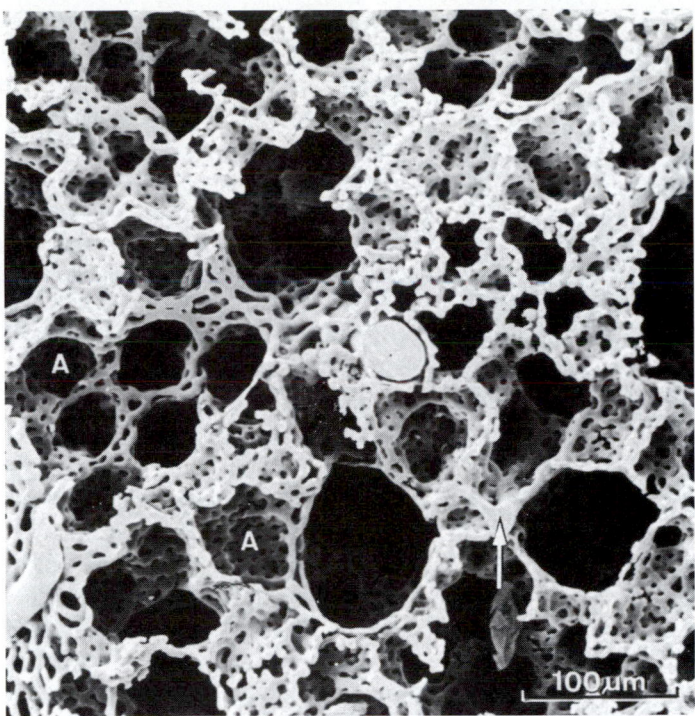

FIGURE 2-50   Alveolar capillary network in walls of alveoli (A) demonstrated by a casting technique. Note larger vessel which leads into network (*arrow*). (*Scanning electron micrograph courtesy Drs. L. Fischer and P. Burri; from Weibel,[46] with permission.*)

thermore important to note that the capillary network or sheet is continuous through many alveolar walls, probably at least throughout the entire acinus, if not for greater distances.[27] It is hence not possible to isolate microvascular units. One finds, rather, that arterial end branches simply feed into this broad sheet at more or less even distances and that the veins drain these sheets in a similar pattern (Fig. 2-51). But now we must remember that the arteries reach the acinus along the airways, whereas the veins are in a peripheral location (Fig. 2-49). In principle, therefore,

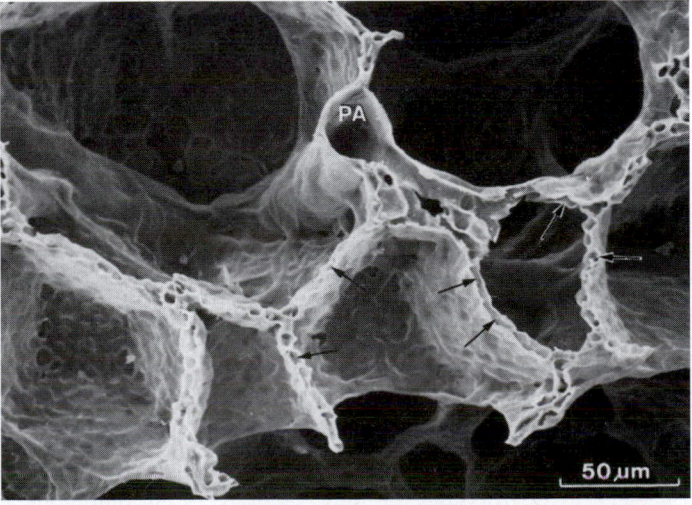

FIGURE 2-51   Scanning electron micrograph of perfusion-fixed rabbit lung shows small pulmonary arteriole (PA) connecting to (empty) capillaries in alveolar walls (*arrows*). (*From Weibel,[46] with permission.*)

blood flows through the acinar capillary sheet from the center to the periphery.

The Pulmonary Diffusing Capacity

In discussing the lung as part of the respiratory system we had noted that the flow of O_2 from air to blood is determined, according to the equation derived by Bohr in 1909,[46] by the product of the P_{O_2} difference between alveolar air and capillary blood with the lung's diffusion conductance or "diffusing capacity"—Eq. (3). Whereas alveolar and capillary P_{O_2} is, to some extent, determined by the design of airways and blood vessels, we must expect $D_{L_{O_2}}$ to be determined in part by the design properties of the gas exchanger established in lung parenchyma.[44]

It is well known that the conductance of any conductor—for example, of an electrical wire—can be calculated from its dimensions and its material properties. Accordingly, $D_{L_{O_2}}$ should be proportional to the barrier surface S and inversely proportional to the barrier thickness τ (Fig. 2-41). This ratio multiplied by the permeability coefficient of the lung for oxygen, K_{O_2}, provides a first approximation of $D_{L_{O_2}}$ based on structural parameters, i.e.:

$$D_{L_{O_2}} = K_{O_2} \cdot \frac{S}{\tau} \qquad (6)$$

We will see that this relationship is oversimplified as we develop a morphometric model for $D_{L_{O_2}}$, because oxygen passes through a series of barriers before binding to the hemoglobin in the red cell, but it still provides a good starting point.

There is also a functional approach, which physiologists utilize for measuring $D_{L_{O_2}}$. Rearranging Eq. (3), we see that:

$$D_{L_{O_2}} = \frac{\dot{V}_{O_2}}{(P_{A_{O_2}} - P_{C_{O_2}})} \qquad (7)$$

Thus, if one can measure O_2 consumption, $\dot{V}_{O_2}$, and the P_{O_2} in alveolar air and capillary blood, one can calculate $D_{L_{O_2}}$ from these functional parameters. In principle, therefore, if we can measure $\dot{V}_{O_2}$ and the P_{O_2} gradient as well as S and τ, we have two approaches in hand with which to estimate $D_{L_{O_2}}$, one based on function, the other on structure. This gives us one means of examining the question of how lung structure affects gas exchange in a quantitative way.

MORPHOMETRIC MODEL FOR PULMONARY DIFFUSION CAPACITY

Oxygen crosses a series of barriers as it diffuses from the air in an alveolus to the hemoglobin in a red blood cell.[44] Each barrier presents its own resistance to oxygen flow (Fig. 2-52): (1) the air-blood tissue barrier (R_t), consisting of alveolar and capillary endothelial cells and interstitial tissue; (2) the plasma barrier (R_p), consisting of the plasma separating the capillary endothelium from the red blood cell; and (3) the erythrocyte barrier (R_e). The total resistance of the lung (R_L) is the sum of all three resistances:

$$R_L = R_t + R_p + R_e \qquad (8)$$

or, expressed in terms of reciprocals of their conductances,

$$\frac{1}{DL} = \frac{1}{Dt} + \frac{1}{Dp} + \frac{1}{De} \qquad (9)$$

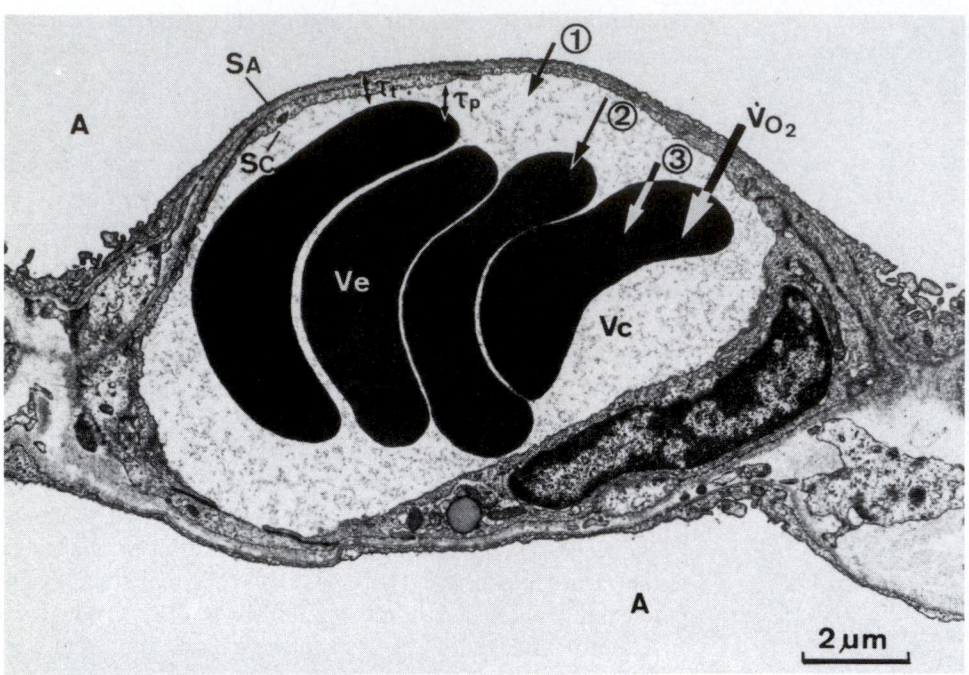

FIGURE 2-52 Morphometric model for calculating diffusion capacity, D. Flow of O_2 ($\dot{V}_{O_2}$) has to traverse in sequence three resistances: (1) tissue barrier, (2) plasma barrier, and (3) erythrocyte interior. (See text.)

It should be noted that the "membrane" diffusing capacity D_M derives from the sum of the resistances in tissue and plasma:

$$\frac{1}{D_M} = \frac{1}{D_t} + \frac{1}{D_p} \tag{10}$$

Each of these conductances is composed of a physical coefficient and some structural parameters that can be quantified morphometrically,[43] as shown in Fig. 2-52.

Conductance of Tissue Barrier (Dt)

The tissue barrier is a sheet of thickness τ which separates two compartments, alveolar air and plasma, over an area S; thus Fick's law determines O_2 flow across this barrier:

$$\dot{V}_{O_2}(t) = Kt \cdot \tau^{-1} \cdot (\Delta Pt_{O_2}) = Dt\,(\Delta Pt_{O_2}) \tag{11}$$

where

 Kt = Krogh's permeation coefficient of the tissue for oxygen (3.3×10^{-8} cm$^2 \cdot$ min$^{-1} \cdot$ mmHg^{-1})

and

 ΔPt_{O_2} = the pressure head for diffusion across the tissue barrier.

Rearranging this equation we find:

$$Dt = Kt \cdot \frac{S}{\tau} \tag{12}$$

As we discussed earlier in this chapter, the tissue barrier is a complex structure. Its two bounding surfaces are formed by independent cell layers, epithelium and endothelium, and they are related to two independent functional spaces, alveoli and capil-

laries. The two surfaces are not perfectly matched and the thickness of the barrier varies considerably. How can we take this into account when calculating S and τ? O_2 enters the barrier on its alveolar and leaves it through its capillary surface, so that it is reasonable to use the mean of these two surface areas, $(S_A + S_C)/2$, as an estimate of the effective area of the tissue barrier. The effect of varying barrier thickness is that the conductance for O_2 will be variable from point to point, in fact, about inversely proportional to the local thickness. If we imagine the barrier built of a set of units of equal area but varying thickness τ, we find the overall conductance of the barrier as the mean of the unit conductances, because they are all in parallel. The only variable being the thickness—whose reciprocal determines the conductance, as we saw—we find that the relevant estimate of barrier thickness is its harmonic mean, t_{ht}, that is, the mean of the reciprocal local thicknesses. This turns out to be quite important for we find that the value of the harmonic mean thickness of the pulmonary air-blood barrier is consistently about three times smaller than the arithmetic mean thickness $\bar{\tau}_t$; in humans, for example, t_{ht} is about 0.6 μm, as compared to 2.2 μm for $\bar{\tau}_t$; whereas in the rat, we find 0.5 μm versus 1.5 μm. This difference is the result of design features that must optimize various functional requirements. Thus we need fibers to support the capillaries; but it suffices to have them in only half of the barrier, keeping the other half very thin, as we saw above (Fig. 2-30). Or, the barrier needs cell bodies with bulky nuclei to maintain the cell linings alive; but these can be tucked away into the meshes of the capillary network (Fig. 2-13) where the tissue is already relatively thick because this is where the fiber tracts cross the capillary sheet from one side to the other. Thus the barrier must maintain a certain minimal mass to ensure its integrity, and this is reflected in the arithmetic mean barrier thickness; but it disposes of it in such a fashion as to interfere as little as possible with gas exchange. Barrier thickness becomes highly irregular, but this turns out to be an advantage in that it allows the diffusion-effective mean thickness to be three times smaller than if a barrier of the same total mass were made of even thickness—a remarkable finding!

On the basis of these arguments we find the conductance of the tissue barrier to be

$$Dt = Kt \cdot \frac{(S_A + S_C)}{(2t_{ht})} \tag{13}$$

The morphometric variables, S_A, S_C, and t_{ht}, can all be measured on electron micrographs of lung sections using stereological methods provided the micrographs are obtained by proper statistical random sampling.[43]

Conductance of the Plasma Barrier (Dp)

The plasma barrier consists of a sheet highly variable in thickness. Much of the surface of the red blood cells is "hidden" from the capillary surface by neighboring red cells (Fig. 2-52), so the red cell surface "accessible" for diffusion of oxygen is found to be similar to the capillary surface. Thus, the conductance of the plasma barrier is

$$Dp = Kp \cdot \frac{S_c}{t_{ht}} \qquad (14)$$

The permeation constants for plasma (Kp) and tissue (Kt) are approximately the same.

A number of arguments can be advanced in favor of combining tissue and plasma barriers into a single barrier of diffusion conductance D_{MO_2}.[48] One is that the permeability coefficients are about the same for tissue and plasma; another one that the plasma barrier thickness cannot be reliably estimated because some parts are so very thin. If the harmonic mean thickness of the total barrier τ_{hb} is estimated as the harmonic mean distance between the alveolar surface and the erythrocyte membrane, we can estimate D_{MO_2} directly as

$$D_{MO_2} = K_{O_2} \cdot \left\{ \frac{S_A}{\tau_{hb}} \right\} \qquad (15)$$

Erythrocyte Conductance (De)

The erythrocyte conductance is of a different nature in that it involves two coupled events: diffusion of molecular oxygen and oxyhemoglobin within the red blood cell as well as the chemical reaction of O_2 with hemoglobin. Roughton and Forster[33] developed a simplified expression based on an empirical measure of the rate at which O_2 is bound to whole blood, θ_{O_2},

$$De_{O_2} = \theta_{O_2} \cdot Vc \qquad (16)$$

where

Vc = the total capillary blood volume, which can again be estimated on sections by stereologic methods.

The estimation of the coefficient θ_{O_2} in vitro is difficult mainly because of the effect of variable unstirred layers around the red cells on the measurements of the initial reaction velocity of red cells when exposed to O_2 in solution;[18] from recent experiments, it was concluded that previously accepted estimates of θ_{O_2} are too small by about a factor of 2 due to this effect.[17,19,57] In addition, θ_{O_2} depends on the hematocrit or hemoglobin concentration, and it is not a constant as it falls with increasing O_2-hemoglobin saturation; recent studies have shown that, as blood moves through alveolar capillar-

ies, θ_{O_2} falls gradually from about 4 to 1 mL $O_2 \cdot min^{-1} \cdot torr^{-1} \cdot mL^{-1}$, so that the correct value can only be found after Bohr integration of capillary P_{O_2}. In Table 2-3, three different estimates of θ_{O_2} have been used to estimate D_{LO_2}.

MORPHOMETRY AND DIFFUSING CAPACITY OF THE HUMAN LUNG

With this model in hand, we can now attempt to estimate the diffusing capacity of the human lung on the basis of morphometric data, as listed in Table 2-3. These data, obtained by electron microscopic morphometry on seven young adults, reveal the alveolar surface area to amount to 130 m[2] and the capillary surface to be about 10 percent smaller.[12,43] These values are higher than those most commonly quoted in textbooks derived from light microscopic studies, which did not adequately resolve the alveolar surface texture. The harmonic mean thickness of the tissue barrier is 0.6 μm, whereas the total barrier, from alveolar to red cell surface (Fig. 2-52) measures 1.11 μm.[48] The capillary volume is estimated at about 200 mL. With these data we calculate D_{LO_2} for the adult human lung to be about 150 to 200 mL $O_2/min^{-1}/mmHg^{-1}$, the variation depending on the choice of θ_{O_2}.

These data also allow us to ask the question how the resistance to O_2 diffusion is distributed between the diffusion barrier and the red cells. Table 2-2 shows that the diffusion conductance of the "membrane" is some 20 percent larger than that of the red cells, which means that the resistance to O_2 uptake is nearly equally divided between membrane and red cell, perhaps being somewhat higher in the erythrocytes.

These morphometric estimates of the diffusing capacity are based on model assumptions that are considered reasonable. The test of their validity must be to compare them to physiological

---

TABLE 2-3

Morphometric Estimate of D_{LO_2} for Young, Healthy Adults of 70-kg Body Weight, Measuring 175 cm in Height[a]

Morphometric data (mean ± 1 SE)				
Total lung volume (60 % TLC)	4340		±285	ml
Alveolar surface area	130		±12	m[2]
Capillary surface area	115		±12	m[2]
Capillary volume	194		±30	ml
Air–blood tissue barrier thickness				
Arithmetic mean	2.2		± 0.2	μm
Harmonic mean	0.62		± 0.04	μm
Total barrier harmonic mean thickness	1.11		± 0.1	μm

Conductances (ml/min/mmHg)		θ_{O_2} (ml/ml/min/minHg)		
		1.5[b]	3.0[c]	1.8[d]
Membrane	D_{MO_2}	332	332	332
Erythrocytes	De_{O_2}	319	639	383
Total	D_{LO_2}	163	219	178

[a]From Gehr et al.[12] and Weibel et al.[13]
[b]Holland et al.[17]
[c]Introducing "slowing factor" of Holland et al.[19]
[d]"Effective" mean θ_{O_2} considering fall along capillaries.

estimates. The standard physiological value of $D_{L_{O_2}}$ of a healthy adult at rest is about 30 ml O_2/min^{-1}/mmHg^{-1}, thus considerably less than what we find on the basis of morphometric estimates. However, this is not a valid comparison, because, under resting conditions, we take up only one-tenth the amount of O_2 that our lungs are capable of absorbing under conditions of heavy work. There have been a number of estimates of $D_{L_{O_2}}$ in exercising humans, and these have yielded values of the order of 100 ml O_2/min^{-1}/mmHg^{-1}. This estimate should come closer to the "true capacity" of the lung for O_2 transfer to the blood than the value obtained at rest. The fact that this is only about 50 percent lower than the morphometric estimate is not disturbing, for we do not know whether the "true diffusing capacity" is completely exploited even in heavy exercise. Inhomogeneities in the distribution of ventilation and perfusion would, for example, limit the degree to which "true" $D_{L_{O_2}}$ can be exploited.

The apparent discrepancy between the morphometric and physiological estimates of $D_{L_{O_2}}$ in humans could obviously be due to the fact that morphometric and physiological estimates were obtained in separate studies. In order to test whether the two estimates measure the same thing, we performed, some years ago, a combined physiological and morphometric estimation of pulmonary diffusing capacity on four species of canids ranging from 4 to 30 kg in body mass.[54]

Because it is difficult to estimate mean capillary P_{O_2} reliably, most physiological measurements of the diffusing capacity use carbon monoxide (CO) as a tracer gas; CO binds to hemoglobin so avidly that, for practical purposes, the Pb_{CO} is zero, so that it suffices to measure CO uptake and alveolar CO concentration. It is also possible to revise the morphometric model of diffusing capacity to estimate the conductance for CO instead of O_2 by appropriately changing the permeability coefficients and the rate of CO binding to erythrocytes, θ_{CO}, whereas the morphometric parameters are not changed. In a study on dogs and on other canids, the calculated morphometric value of $D_{L_{CO}}$ was found to be larger than the physiological estimate by less than a factor of 1.5, thus confirming the observation made with respect to human lungs.[54]

We therefore conclude that the pulmonary gas exchanger is designed with a certain amount of redundancy or excess capacity, but this is by no means unreasonable from an engineering point of view. Indeed, to design the pulmonary gas exchanger with a certain degree of redundancy may make a lot of sense. The lung forms the interface to the environment and its functional performance will thus depend on environmental conditions, such as the prevailing O_2 partial pressure, which falls as we go from sea level to higher altitudes. It has been shown that goats, whose $D_{L_{O_2}}$ is about twice as large as seemingly required, can maintain their maximal level of exercise-induced $\dot{V}_{O_2}$ even under moderate hypoxia, and that the redundancy apparent under sea-level conditions then disappears. It has also been suggested that human athletes exercising at high altitude may fully exploit their $D_{L_{O_2}}$. This suggests that the apparent redundancy in $D_{L_{O_2}}$ may be a safety factor to protect the good functioning of the pulmonary gas exchanger even when environmental conditions are not optimal. Recent studies with partial pneumonectomy in dogs have shown that the lung can achieve 85 percent of its maximal O_2 uptake even when 40 percent of lung tissue is removed after left pneumonectomy, making use of some of this reserve capacity; but when right pneumonectomy removes 60 percent of lung tissue, adequate function can be achieved only after compensatory growth of the residual lung tissue to restore diffusing capacity.[24,25]

DESIGN OF THE LUNG FOR GAS EXCHANGE: IS THERE A MATCH BETWEEN STRUCTURES AND FUNCTIONS?

Concept and Approach

The principal design features of the lung that we have considered up to this point are (1) the walls between alveoli, which are densely populated with blood; (2) the tissue barrier separating air and blood, which is exceedingly thin—50 times thinner than a sheet of airmail stationery—and is yet tightly organized into three basic layers; (3) the surface of contact between air and blood, which is very large, approaching in humans the square footage of a tennis court; and (4) the airways and blood vessels, which are designed in such a way as to allow efficient ventilation and perfusion of the gas exchange units that number some 300 million in humans.

Intuitively, these structural design features, which determine essentially the pulmonary diffusing capacity, appear related to establishing efficient gas exchange within the lung, and it seems reasonable to expect them to be well matched to functional requirements. Now we must note that the requirements for O_2 flow through the lung are established by the O_2 needs of the cells that perform work, in exercise primarily by the muscle cells, where 98 percent of the O_2 taken up is consumed in oxidative ATP production.[46,53] In a first approximation, we could therefore propose the hypothesis that the lung is designed according to functional needs if $D_{L_{O_2}}$ is matched to $\dot{V}_{O_2}$ under conditions of maximal work (i.e., when the limit of O_2 supply to the working muscles is reached).[9,46,53] We have seen above (Fig. 2-40) that O_2 must flow through several steps from the lung to the mitochondria. Clearly, each step could be limiting $\dot{V}_{O_2}$, but in a well-designed system we should expect all steps to reach their functional limit at the same level; in other words, no step should have an excess capacity for O_2 flow.

To test whether this "perfect match" between functional needs and an economic design at all levels—which we have called *symmorphosis*[52]—is realized in the organism is a rather demanding task. The complexity of the system and the interdependence of the various steps make it impossible to approach it directly. We have therefore chosen a comparative approach, exploiting the fact that O_2 needs show a large degree of variation as we look at different species of the animal kingdom.[53]

It should be noted that, compared to mammals, the bird lung and the fish gills are very differently designed gas exchangers, particularly with respect to the relation between perfusion and ventilation patterns in the gas-exchange units.[46] The principal advantage of these designs is that the O_2 contained in the ventilating media—air or water, respectively—can be better extracted by blood flow, which is important for birds flying at high altitude or for fishes swimming in deep waters with a low O_2 content. This is not essential for mammals, because O_2 is plentiful in their normal environments. We therefore limit the following discussion to mammals which share the basic design of the respiratory system, particularly of the lung and the circulation.

The basic strategy in the approach followed here is to estimate maximal O_2 consumption ($\dot{V}_{O_2max}$) and to set it into relation with the parameters that determine design properties, such as the diffusing capacity of the lung. We focus here on the lung, but it is evident that all steps of the respiratory system must enter our considerations.

Maximal Oxygen Consumption

The procedure for measuring $\dot{V}_{O_2max}$ of humans under steady-state conditions consists of measuring O_2 consumption of a subject, running on a treadmill or bicycling on an ergometer, as a function of exercise intensity—i.e., speed or work rate (Fig. 2-53). Oxygen consumption increases linearly with exercise intensity up to a maximal rate ($\dot{V}_{O_2max}$); it does not increase with further increases in exercise intensity but rather stays constant, and the additional energy required to sustain these higher intensities is supplied by anaerobic glycolysis. Lactate, an end product of anaerobic glycolysis, accumulates, limiting the duration of exercise. This procedure for determining $\dot{V}_{O_2max}$ can be applied to animals as well as humans, and it provides very reproducible values.[37,38,52]

Large differences in $\dot{V}_{O_2max}$ occur between individuals of the same species (e.g., 1.5- to 2-fold between trained athletes and sedentary individuals[21]), between species of the same size (e.g., 2- to 3-fold between dogs and goats or horses and cows[37] and

5-fold from goat to pronghorn antelope[30]), and between species of different body size (e.g., 6-fold between mice and cows[52]). These large differences in $\dot{V}_{O_2max}$ provide us with the tools for testing the principle of symmorphosis, which predicts a quantitative match in $\dot{V}_{O_2max}$ and structure, determining the conductances for O_2 flow at each step in the flow of O_2 through the respiratory system, as diagrammed in Fig. 2-40.

Differences in $\dot{V}_{O_2max}$ occur particularly as a result of exercise training. This is evidenced in Fig. 2-53: at low energy requirements, $\dot{V}_{O_2}$ is the same for untrained and trained persons; in the athletes trained for endurance running, $\dot{V}_{O_2}$ reaches the plateau at a markedly higher level, and accordingly lactic acid production takes off at higher energy requirements. This indicates one important feature that has now been demonstrated for both humans and animals—namely, that the respiratory system is adaptable to functional needs in that the limit for O_2 supply to the working muscles can be pushed to higher values of $\dot{V}_{O_2max}$ when the energetic demands imposed on the muscles are increased. And it takes only a few weeks of relatively intense training—running at 70 percent of $\dot{V}_{O_2max}$ for 20 min every day—to achieve this.

The performance of the respiratory system as measured by the limit to O_2 flow, $\dot{V}_{O_2max}$, thus shows considerable variation, and we can now ask to what extent the structures that support O_2 flow at the various levels of the system are adapted to the functional needs—in other words, to what extent they can be considered to be limiting factors for O_2 flow.[53]

Structure-Function Relations at the Level of the Muscle: Mitochondria and Capillaries

During heavy physical exercise, over 90 percent of oxygen is consumed in the mitochondria of the active muscles as they produce ATP to power the exercise.[21] The process of oxidative phosphorylation occurs in a well-controlled manner within the mitochondria: the production of 6 mol ATP requires 1 mol O_2. The fact that $\dot{V}_{O_2}$ reaches a limit $\dot{V}_{O_2max}$ and that additional ATP required by higher workloads is produced anaerobically suggests that the mitochondria themselves may set the limit to aerobic metabolism.

In humans this can be tested by comparing untrained individuals with well-trained athletes whose $\dot{V}_{O_2max}$ differs by up to twofold. Mitochondrial content of their muscle cells (Fig. 2-54) can be measured using small muscle biopsies. Several such studies have demonstrated an almost direct proportionality between mitochondrial volume and $\dot{V}_{O_2max}$, as demonstrated in Fig. 2-55. Thus, at the level of the muscle's metabolic machinery, there appears to be a good match between structure and function.[21]

This proportionality can be demonstrated more quantitatively by comparing different species from the animal kingdom where the differences in $\dot{V}_{O_2max}$ are larger and where the total volume of mitochondria in the muscles can be measured instead of relying on biopsy samples of a few muscles. If we compare animals of different size, we find that the total volume of mitochondria scales in direct proportion to $\dot{V}_{O_2max}$ in a group of animals ranging in size from 20-g mice to 500-kg horses and steers (Fig. 2-56).[52] This same strict proportionality between $\dot{V}_{O_2max}$ and mitochondrial volume is also observed in compar-

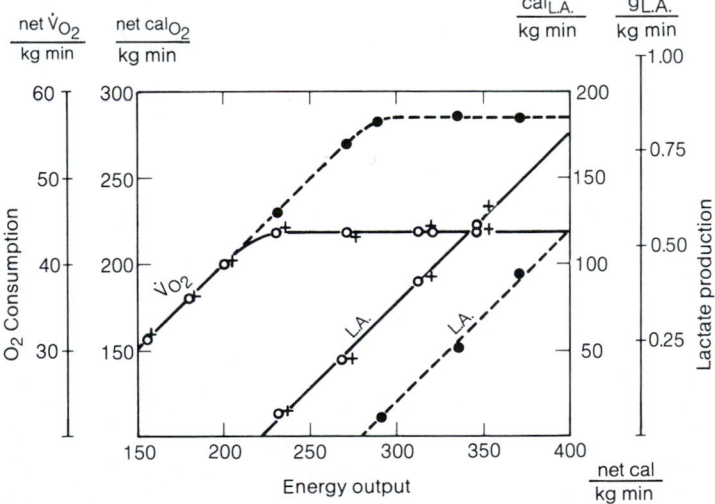

FIGURE 2-53 Rate of lactic acid production (g·min⁻¹) as an effect of exercise (ordinate at right) are plotted as a function of the work intensity and, therefore, of the energy requirement (abscissa). A straight line is obtained that cuts the abscissa at an energy requirement corresponding to 220 cal/kg min⁻¹; below this value no production of lactic acid takes place and the energy requirement is met solely by oxygen consumption (shown on the ordinate at left). The broken lines refer to athletes (middle- and long-distance runners) whose maximum oxygen consumption is higher; the line of the lactic acid for these subjects is correspondingly shifted to the right. *(From Margaria et al., J Appl Physiol 18:371–377, 1963, with permission.)*

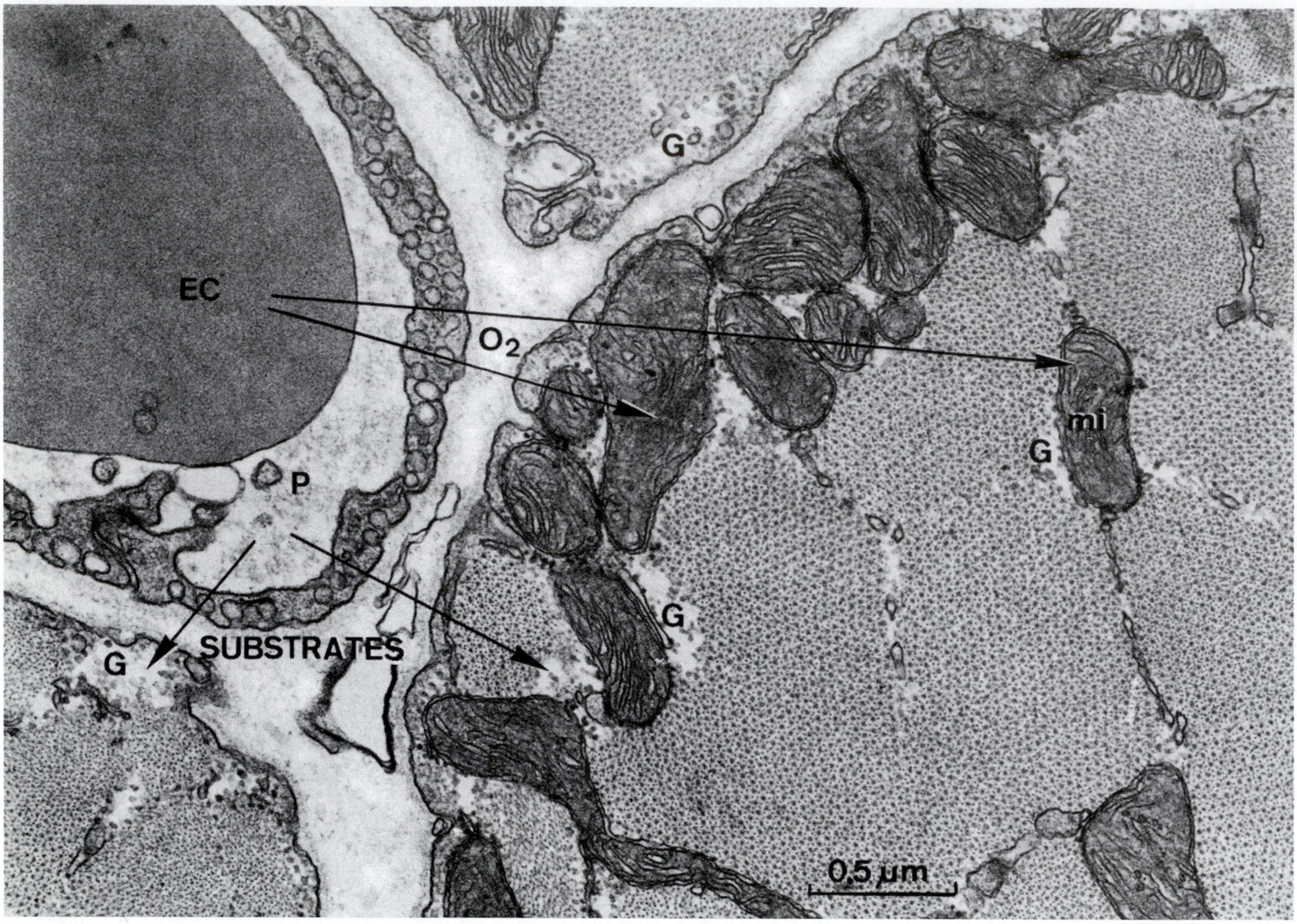

FIGURE 2-54   This electron micrograph of a capillary with its adjacent muscle fibers shows the pathways for O_2 supply from the erythrocyte (EC) to the mitochondria (mi) and for substrates from the plasma (P) to intracellular glycogen deposits (G). *(From Weibel,[46] with permission.)*

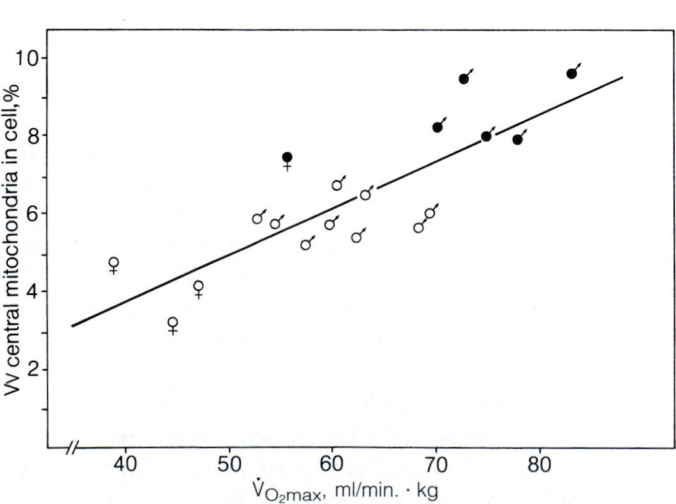

FIGURE 2-55   The volume density of mitochondria in leg muscle cells is proportional to $\dot{V}_{O_2}$ max in a population of untrained *(open circles)* and trained *(full circles)* humans. *(From Hoppeler, et al., Pflügers Arch 344:217–232, 1973, with permission.)*

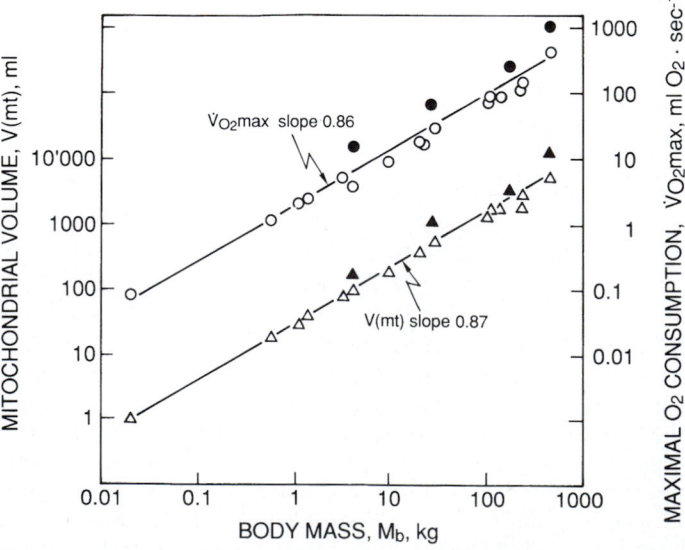

FIGURE 2-56 $\dot{V}_{O_2}$ max and whole body mitochondrial volume V(mt) plotted as function of body mass M_b on logarithmic coordinates. Open symbols are sedentary and full symbols athletic species. *(Data from Weibel et al.,[53] with permission.)*

TABLE 2-4

Differences in Morphometric and Physiologic Parameters of Muscle Mitochondria and Capillaries, and of Heart, Blood and Lung with Variation of $\dot{V}_{O_2}$ max in Three Pairs of Athletic and Sedentary Species

Design: Function:	$\dot{V}_{O_2}max/M_b$ ml/min^{-1}/kg^{-1}	Mitochondria V(mt)/M_b ml/kg^{-1}	Blood V_V(ec)	Capillaries V(c)/M_b ml/kg^{-1}	Heart f_H min^{-1}	Heart Vs/M_b ml/kg^{-1}	Lung D_{LO_2}/M_b ml·s^{-1}·mmHg^{-1}/kg^{-1}
25–30 kg							
Dog	137.4	40.6	0.50	8.2	274	3.17	7.08
Goat	57.0	13.8	0.30	4.5	268	2.07	4.80
D/G	2.4	2.9	1.68[a]	1.8[a]	1.02[a]	1.53[a]	1.48[a]
150 kg							
Pony	88.8	19.5	0.42	5.1	215	2.50	4.74
Calf	36.6	9.2	0.31	3.2	213	1.78	3.00
P/C	2.4	2.13	1.35[a]	1.6[a]	1.02[a]	1.40[a]	1.57[a]
450 kg							
Horse	133.8	30.0	0.55	8.3	202	3.11	6.48
Steer	51.0	11.6	0.40	5.3	216	1.52	3.24
H/S	2.6	2.6	1.4[a]	1.6[a]	0.94[a]	2.1[a]	2.0[a]
Ath/Sed[b]	2.5	2.5	1.5[a]	1.7[a]	1.0[a]	1.7[a]	1.7[a]

[a]These ratios are significantly different from that for $\dot{V}_{O_2}$max.
[b]This line presents overall ratios for athletic/sedentary species.
SOURCE: After Weibel et al: *Proc Natl Acad Sci USA* 88:10357, 1991, with permission.

ing pairs of mammals of the same body mass but with widely differing energy requirements, such as dog and goat or horse and cow (Table 2-4). When the animals exercise at $\dot{V}_{O_2}$max, each milliliter of mitochondria consumes about 4 to 5 ml O_2/min irrespective of size or adaptation.[21,53]

If the same calculation is done on humans, they appear as an exception to the general rule; they possess twice an many mitochondria as quadrupeds relative to their $\dot{V}_{O_2}$max. It seems likely that this is a result of their bipedal gait:[20] they use only about half of their muscles to reach $\dot{V}_{O_2}$max when running or bicycling, and the mitochondria in these muscles appear to operate at the same maximum rate of 4 to 5 mL O_2/ml per min, as in other animals. The difference appears to be that humans can reach $\dot{V}_{O_2}$max with only a fraction of their total musculature.

At the level of the mitochondria, the results are simple and consistent with the hypothesis: the limit to O_2 consumption is directly related to the quantity of mitochondria that can perform oxidative phosphorylation. If a muscle needs more oxidative capacity, it builds more mitochondria.

The capillary network is the second structural factor which determines O_2 flow in the muscles, as it must maintain an adequate supply of O_2 to the muscle cells (Fig. 2-54). The capillaries form more or less dense networks between the muscle cells (Fig. 2-57); the O_2 flow rate will depend on the distance from the capillary to the mitochondria and on the volume of blood available for unloading O_2. The hypothesis of symmorphosis predicts that capillary

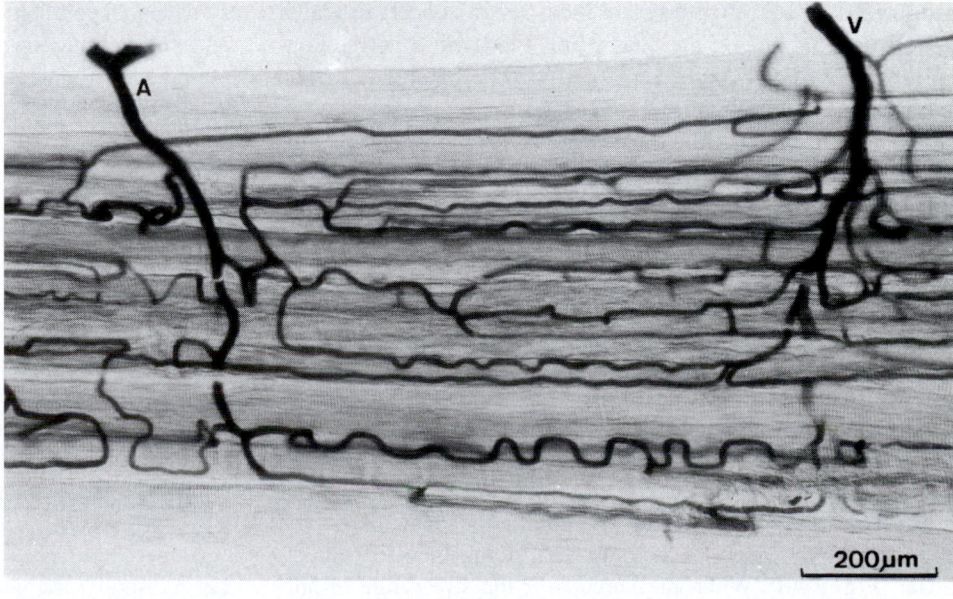

FIGURE 2-57 Capillary network in muscle shows a preferentially longitudinal orientation, parallel to muscle fibers. *(From Weibel,[46] with permission.)*

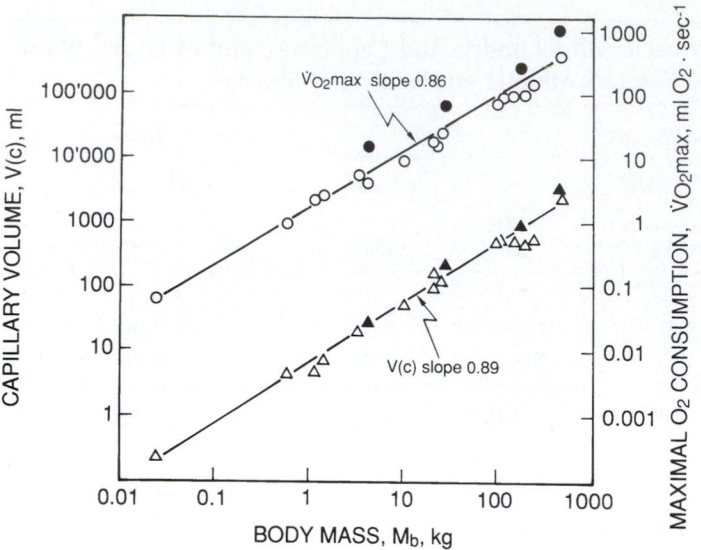

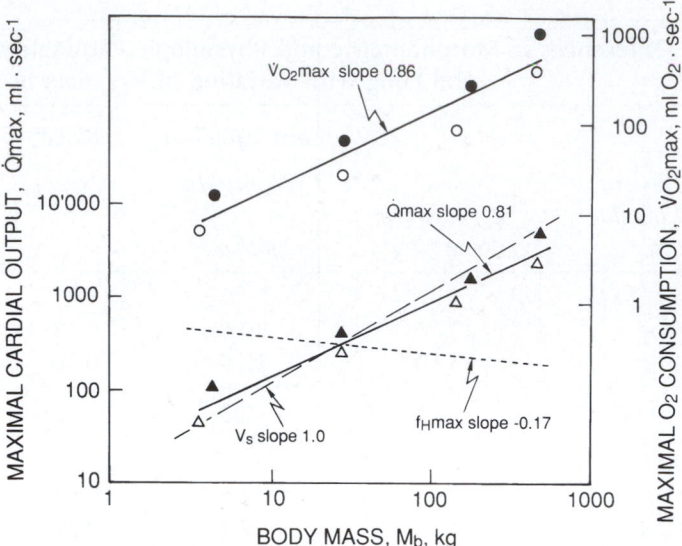

FIGURE 2-58 $\dot{V}_{O_2}$ max and whole-body muscle capillary volume V(c) plotted as function of body mass M_b on logarithmic coordinates. Open symbols are sedentary and full symbols athletic species. *(Data from Weibel et al.,[53] with permission.)*

FIGURE 2-59 $\dot{V}_{O_2}$ and cardiac output $\dot{Q}$ plotted as function of body mass M_b on logarithmic coordinates. Open symbols are sedentary and full symbols athletic species. The dotted lines show the allometric regressions for the two factors of cardiac output: heart frequency f_H and stroke volume V_s, which is proportional to heart mass. *(Data from Weibel et al.,[53] with permission.)*

volume, like mitochondrial volume, should vary directly with $\dot{V}_{O_2max}$. This is exactly what we find when we compare animals of different size.[52]

The length of capillaries in the muscle is directly related to $\dot{V}_{O_2max}$ (and to the volume of mitochondria they supply with O_2) over a range of body size from mice to horses (Fig. 2-58). From this relation we can calculate that there are about 3 μm^3 of mitochondria for every 1 μm^3 of capillary blood! Surprisingly, however, athletic species have a relatively smaller capillary volume than sedentary animals of the same size (Table 2-4);[37] on closer examination, however, the athletic species are found to have a higher hematocrit, so that the volume of oxygen-carrying red cells per volume of mitochondria remains constant. In this case, therefore, two structures are modified in concert to match O_2 delivery to demand: the quantity of capillaries and the concentration of red cells in the capillary blood. By shared effort the match becomes nearly perfect.

Thus it appears that, in the muscle, the O_2 consumer—the mitochondria—and the O_2 supply structures—the capillaries and their red blood cells—are directly related to $\dot{V}_{O_2max}$, and that both can therefore be considered to contribute equally to the limitation of O_2 flow.[38,53]

Structure-Function Relations at the Level of the Heart

The circulation of blood transports O_2 from the capillaries in the lung to those in the muscle. This convective transport is often considered the limiting step in O_2 transport during strenuous exercise. The transport of O_2 by the circulation depends on the properties of the heart as a pump and of the blood as an O_2 carrier (Fig. 2-40). When measured over the size range of animals where data are available, cardiac output increases directly

with maximal O_2 uptake (Fig. 2-59). This suggests a structure-function match as predicted by symmorphosis.[53] However, in this instance, the match does not appear to be achieved by adjusting a structural variable, as we found to be the case with mitochondria and capillaries. Cardiac output is the product of heart frequency and stroke volume, which are directly related to the size of the heart. On average, the heart makes up the same fraction of body mass over the size range of animals from mice to cows, about 0.58 percent. Furthermore, it pumps the same volume per gram of heart (about 43 percent) under rate-limiting conditions. Hemoglobin concentration and oxygen capacity of the blood are also about the same over the entire size range of mammals, namely 13 g hemoglobin and 17.5 mL O_2/100 mL of blood. This evidence taken together suggests that the two structural parameters determining O_2 delivery at this step, stroke volume/body mass and O_2 content of the blood, are invariant with body size. A functional variable, heart frequency, accounts entirely for the adjustment.[53]

It is interesting that maximal heart frequency appears to be tightly linked to body size. Our athletic and sedentary animals of the same size, dogs versus goats, ponies versus calves, and horses versus steers, have the same heart rate despite the two- to threefold difference in maximal oxygen uptake (Table 2-4). In this case, a match is achieved entirely by building more structure. Two structures are involved, just as we observed with the capillaries—namely, red cell volume and size of the heart. Both structures contribute nearly equally to the match (Table 2-4).

Structure-Function Relations in the Pulmonary Gas Exchanger

Let us finally ask whether the lung's gas-exchange capacity is adjusted to the body's O_2 needs.[9] A number of early compara-

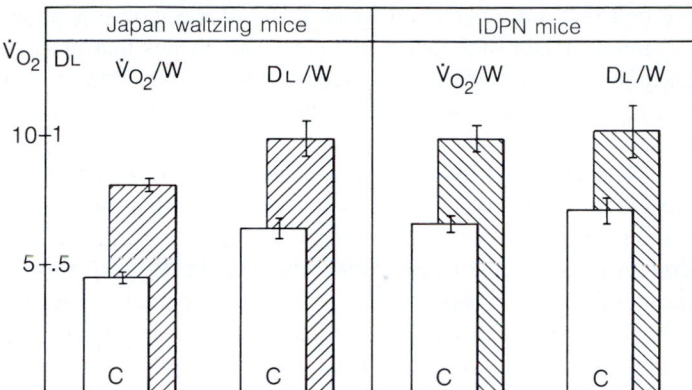

FIGURE 2-60   Increase of O_2 consumption and morphometric D_L in Japanese waltzing mice and in mice rendered waltzers artificially by treatment with β-iminodipropionitrile (IDPN). (*From Burri and Weibel, in Hudson WA (ed): Development of the Lung. New York, Marcel Dekker, 1977, pp 215–268, with permission.*)

tive and experimental studies had suggested this.[46] A particularly striking case was that of the Japanese waltzing mice (Fig. 2-60): their well-known hyperactivity results in rates of O_2 consumption that were about 60 percent higher than those of normal laboratory mice (Fig. 2-60). The morphometric study of their lungs revealed that their alveolar surface area and the diffusing capacity were also larger, about in proportion to their elevated O_2 needs. Some of this difference may have been genetic, but a subsequent experiment showed the same proportionality between $\dot{V}_{O_2 max}$ and $D_{L_{O_2}}$ to occur in mice in which a waltzing syndrome was induced by drug treatment during early growth (Fig. 2-60). This, then, suggested that $D_{L_{O_2}}$ is adapted to $\dot{V}_{O_2 max}$. In several experiments, it was subsequently attempted to induce a chronic increase in O_2 needs of the body, either by exercise training or by cold environment, in view of testing the hypothesis that the lung's gas exchanger will increase its diffusing capacity in response to elevated demand; the results of these studies were not consistent, however, perhaps because the degree of experimental $\dot{V}_{O_2 max}$ increase achieved was insufficient to trigger a response. On the other hand, some studies have shown convincingly that the lung may adapt to changes in the O_2 partial pressure: animals raised at high altitude develop a larger gas exchange surface than those raised at sea level; in contrast, chronic hyperoxia leads to a reduction in $D_{L_{O_2}}$.

An important type of experiment asks whether the lung can compensate for gas-exchange capacity lost as a consequence of partial pneumonectomy—a question of evident clinical signifi-

cance. Experiments done on growing rats revealed that the remaining lung expands in volume and alveolar surface area so as to fully compensate the lost diffusing capacity. This is achieved by proliferation of cells and tissue. When pneumonectomy was performed in adult dogs, the result was different.[24,25] Upon removal of the left lung, or 42 percent of the gas exchanger, the remaining right lung expanded to fill the available space in the chest cavity; in the process, the alveolar surface became stretched, but this was accompanied by only a very modest proliferation of capillaries and tissue, so that the diffusing capacity was not fully compensated. As a consequence, the pneumonectomized dogs did not regain their normal $\dot{V}_{O_2 max}$. On the other hand, removing the right lung, or 58 percent of the gas exchanger, appears to trigger proliferative processes, and the diffusing capacity becomes compensated to a higher degree.[25] We conclude from these experimental studies that the lung cannot easily make new gas-exchanger tissue so that its possibility to respond by adjustment of its diffusing capacity to elevated O_2 needs is very limited or nonexistent.

Another line of study that had suggested adjustment of the lung's gas-exchange capacity to the body's O_2 needs was the observation that very small mammals that have a high metabolic rate also have very small alveoli, which should give them a relatively large diffusing capacity. The Etruscan shrew, for instance, weighs only 2 g and has the highest metabolic rate of all mammals; its alveoli have a diameter of only about 20 μm (Fig. 2-61), so that several hundred shrew alveoli would fit into one human alveolus! This suggested that the allometric variation of metabolic rate could be matched by a similar allometric regression of $D_{L_{O_2}}$.[46]

The studies that had suggested a more or less close relationship between $D_{L_{O_2}}$ and the rate of O_2 consumption suffered from

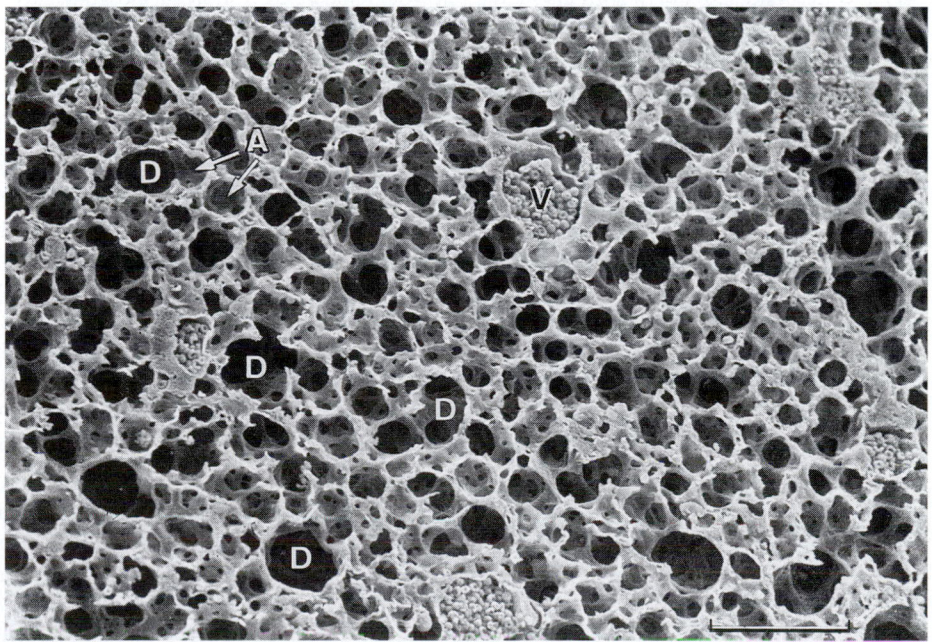

FIGURE 2-61   Scanning electron micrograph of lung parenchyma of the Etruscan shrew (*Suncus etruscus*) shows very small alveoli. D = alveolar duct; V = larger vessel. Compare with Fig. 2-28, which represents a similar picture for human lung. Scale marker 50 μm. (*From Weibel,[46] with permission.*)

two shortcomings: (1) they were more anecdotal case studies rather than systematic tests of a hypothesis and (2) they were mostly based on some ill-defined level of $\dot{V}_{O_2}$ rather than on a measure of the limit to oxidative metabolism, $\dot{V}_{O_2max}$. We have therefore undertaken a systematic study of the variation of the pulmonary diffusing capacity and its morphometric parameters using our comparative approach to obtain large differences in $\dot{V}_{O_2max}$.[53] The specific hypothesis, derived from the general hypothesis of symmorphosis, predicts that $D_{L_{O_2}}$ estimated by morphometry varies in parallel with $\dot{V}_{O_2max}$ both across animal size and between athletic and sedentary species, or that the ratio $D_{L_{O_2}}/\dot{V}_{O_2max}$ is invariant under both modes of variation.

We find that this hypothesis is not supported.[53] When we compare athletic and sedentary species of about the same body mass, we find that the athletic species have a $D_{L_{O_2}}$ that is about 1.7 times larger than in the sedentary species, but this is clearly not matched to the 2.5 times greater $\dot{V}_{O_2max}$ (Table 2-4). The higher $D_{L_{O_2}}$ is the result of both an enlargement of gas exchange surface and the increased hematocrit that we have already noted in the muscle capillaries. But it is evident that these adjustments fall short in comparison to the maximal needs for O_2 uptake.

In extensive studies on species ranging from shrews and mice to horses and cows, we found that $D_{L_{O_2}}$ increases more rapidly with body mass than $\dot{V}_{O_2max}$ (Fig. 2-62). The consequence of these different slopes is that, on average, a 30-g animal, like a mouse, has the same amount of diffusing capacity per unit body mass as one weighing 300 kg, like a cow, but it has to accommodate an O_2 flow rate which is six times greater.[38,52] As a consequence, the driving force for O_2 uptake, the alveolar-capillary P_{O_2} difference, must be much larger in the smaller animal. A recent reevaluation of these data suggests that the regressions in Fig. 2-62 may be somewhat distorted by the fact that athletic species occur only in the larger size classes. If we exclude the athletes and take the sedentary animals as the "normal" species,

we find that, on a per gram basis, $D_{L_{O_2}}$ of the mouse is about 2.5 times greater than that of the cow. This means that $D_{L_{O_2}}$ is partially—about halfway—adjusted to the sixfold difference in $\dot{V}_{O_2max}$—a result similar to that observed between athletic and sedentary species.[53]

The mismatch between $D_{L_{O_2}}$ and $\dot{V}_{O_2max}$ observed in the studies reviewed above leads to the conclusion that the driving force for O_2 diffusion from air to erythrocytes is variable. This driving force has two components: the alveolar P_{O_2} as pressure head and the mean capillary P_{O_2}. The latter parameter crucially depends on gas exchange itself, because the mean capillary P_{O_2} is the integrated mean of the instantaneous P_{O_2} along the capillary, which ranges from the mixed venous to the end-capillary or arterial P_{O_2}. The gradual increase of P_{O_2} along the capillary depends on the membrane diffusing capacity and on the rate of O_2 binding by hemoglobin; it can be calculated by combining the physiological and morphometric data we have obtained. Two examples are shown in Fig. 2-63, comparing the profiles of P_{O_2} change along the capillary path at rest and at $\dot{V}_{O_2max}$.[38] We first note that the transit time becomes shorter as $\dot{V}_{O_2}$ increases; from 1.5 s at rest it falls to about 0.3 s in the dog and 0.47 s in the goat, at $\dot{V}_{O_2max}$. Accordingly, loading O_2 onto the blood is completed at rest well before the blood leaves the capillary, both in dogs and in goats. At $\dot{V}_{O_2max}$, however, the dog uses most of its capillary length for oxygen uptake, with its blood reaching the P_{O_2} of arterial blood shortly before it exits from the lung (Fig. 2-63). In contrast, the goat arterial P_{O_2} utilizes less than half the capillary path for oxygen uptake even at $\dot{V}_{O_2max}$ (Fig. 2-63).

We conclude from this comparison that the athletic dog has very little if any redundancy at $\dot{V}_{O_2max}$. It is interesting, however, that the most athletic mammal, the pronghorn antelope of the Rocky Mountains, whose $\dot{V}_{O_2max}$ is five times greater than that of the goat, has a $D_{L_{O_2}}$ that is also five times greater.[30] Accordingly, this top athlete has an excess $D_{L_{O_2}}$ similar to that of the goat; this may well be the result of a survival strategy of this animal, which is capable of maintaining extraordinary running speeds for long periods at 2000- to 3000-m altitude—i.e., under severely hypoxic conditions, where high levels of gas exchange must be maintained with a reduced pressure head.

Since the goat lung appears to have a diffusing capacity vastly in excess of what is needed, it should be possible to decrease the pressure head for diffusion of O_2 drastically without reducing O_2 flow across the lung. In fact, using the morphometric value for $D_{L_{O_2}}$, one predicts that there will be excess diffusing capacity for O_2 across the lung until alveolar P_{O_2} is reduced to approximately 40 mmHg. When this prediction was tested, it was found that $\dot{V}_{O_2max}$ was not decreased until alveolar and arterial P_{O_2} dropped to approximately 40 mmHg (Fig. 2-64); at this P_{O_2}, capillary blood equilibrated with alveolar air just prior to leaving the lung.[38] The redundancy built into the pulmonary gas exchanger was hence fully exploited to allow the goats to maintain their maximal work capacity even in severe hypoxia. It can be predicted that this would not be possible in dogs or horses, which use most of their $D_{L_{O_2}}$ at $\dot{V}_{O_2max}$; indeed, it appears from several studies that in hypoxia, these species must reduce their level of aerobic exercise, since their O_2 consumption is nearly limited by pulmonary diffusing capacity, even under normoxic condi-

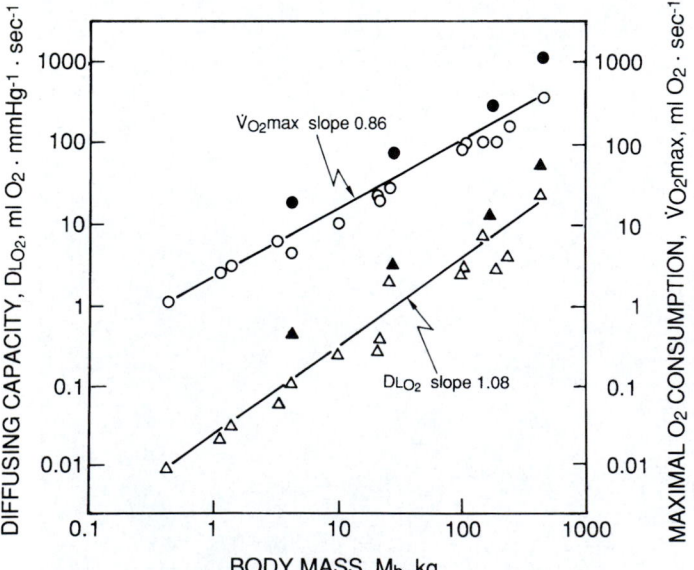

FIGURE 2-62 $\dot{V}_{O_2}$ max and morphometric pulmonary diffusing capacity $D_{L_{O_2}}$ plotted as function of body mass M_b on logarithmic coordinates. Open symbols are sedentary and full symbols athletic species. *(Data from Weibel et al.,[53] with permission.)*

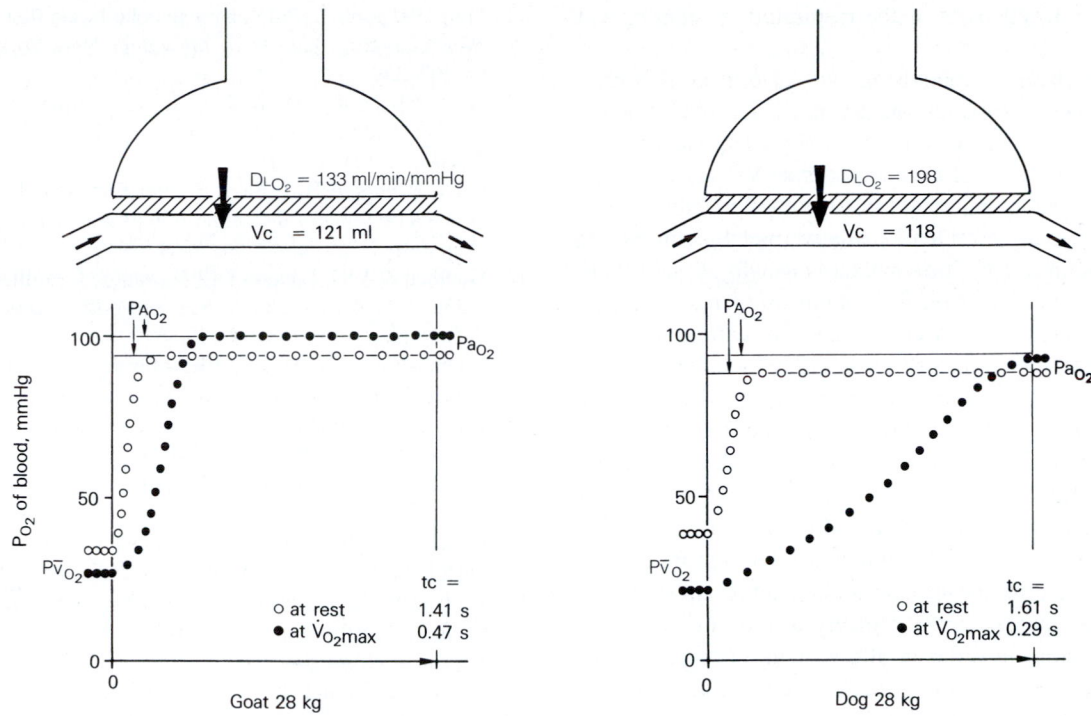

FIGURE 2-63   Bohr integrals of P_{O_2} for blood passing through lung capillaries in goat and dog, at rest and at exercise, respectively. In maximal exercise, the shorter transit times t_c cause a larger fraction of the capillary length to be required for equilibration of blood with alveolar air. Note that equilibration is reached later in the dog.

tions. This is apparently also the case in the highly trained human athlete.

This leads to the conclusion that the design of the pulmonary gas exchanger is not quantitatively matched to the body's O_2 needs at the limit of aerobic metabolism measured by $\dot{V}_{O_2max}$. In most species we find a certain redundancy to be maintained, but this redundancy is variable. The lung therefore deviates from the pattern of coadjustment of structure and function noted in the other steps of the respiratory system. What could the reasons be? We do not know, but several arguments can be advanced.

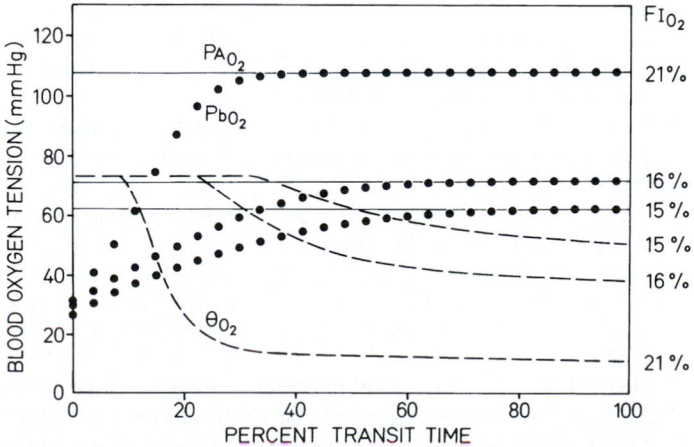

FIGURE 2-64   Bohr integrals for P_{O_2} in goats breathing air of different inspired O_2 concentrations $F_{I_{O_2}}$. At low concentrations a longer stretch of the capillary transit time is required for equilibration. *(From Taylor et al.[37])*

First, lung structure and size could be genetically determined and the target reached during development and growth—that is, long before the lung can "feel" the O_2 needs of the body. This is important in the light of the observation that the lung is nearly unable to upregulate its diffusing capacity by making new gas-exchange structure in later life. This limited malleability of lung structure may be related to mechanical design constraints of the parenchyma: it may be difficult to add new alveolar septa without disrupting the continuity essential to maintaining integrity of the alveolar complex. Second, the ideal gas-exchange conditions that we have supposed to exist when setting up the model for $D_{L_{O_2}}$ may not exist in vivo; functional heterogeneity in ventilation-perfusion matching may allow the design-determined $D_{L_{O_2}}$ to be exploited only to a certain degree, and there may well be species differences in this factor. Finally, the lung forms the interface to the environment, so that its structure must not only be adjusted to internal requirements but must also be capable of accounting for possible variations in the external boundary conditions of gas exchange, one of these being the prevailing ambient P_{O_2}.

Conclusions on Structure-Function Relations in the Lung as Part of the Respiratory System

The question whether the lung's design is commensurate to its main functional task, the uptake of O_2 from the air at the rate required by the body, has been asked for a long time, and it has usually been answered in the positive. Some of our own findings seemed to lead to the same conclusion, but it did not stand up to a more refined test. It now appears that the hypothesis of symmorphosis applies to all parts of the respiratory system except the lung.

In order to reach these conclusions we have used as overall functional reference parameter the animal's aerobic capacity, measured by $\dot{V}_{O_2max}$. This may not be totally adequate, because an animal will very rarely if ever experience $\dot{V}_{O_2max}$. A more suitable reference parameter might be sustained metabolic rate, $\dot{V}_{O_2sus}$—the time averaged rate of oxidative metabolism that an animal can maintain in free life—which is usually about two to five times basal metabolic rate, thus about up to half $\dot{V}_{O_2max}$. When measuring $\dot{V}_{O_2max}$ we were, in fact, estimating the break point of the system when all reserves or safety factors have been called upon. We found that this break point is reached at the same level of $\dot{V}_{O_2}$ in all steps of the respiratory system from the heart to the mitochondria, so that these structures can be considered coadjusted to the function they serve with about the same safety factors. The lung is designed with an additional safety margin. This may indeed be regarded as a sign of good design for at least two reasons. First, its limited structural malleability upon altered functional stress requires excess capacity at this initial step of the respiratory system in order to allow for the malleability of the subsequent steps to become effective. Second, as explained above, the lung is at the interface to the environment; it must ensure high levels of O_2 uptake even if ambient P_{O_2} is low. In addition, it may well be designed with additional safety margins to cope with external stresses of various kinds, because most pathological effects on lung structure will tend to reduce its gas-exchange capacity either by loss of functional surface area or by thickening of the exceptionally delicate tissue barrier.

REFERENCES

1. Agostoni E: Mechanics of the pleural space. *Physiol Rev* 52:5–128, 1972.
2. Bachofen H, Bachofen M, Weibel ER: Ultrastructural aspects of pulmonary edema. *J Thorac Imag* 3:1–7, 1988.
3. Bachofen M, Bachofen H: Parenchymal changes, in Crystal RG, West JB, Barnes PB, Weibel ER (eds): *The Lung: Scientific Foundations,* 2d ed. New York, Lippincott-Raven, 1997, pp 2499–2508.
4. Bachofen H, Gehr P, Weibel ER: Alterations of mechanical properties and morphology in excised rabbit lungs rinsed with a detergent. *J Appl Physiol* 47:1002–1010, 1979.
5. Bachofen H, Weber J, Wangensteen D, Weibel ER: Morphometric estimates of diffusing capacity in lungs fixed under zone II and zone III conditions. *Respir Physiol* 52:41–52, 1983.
6. Bachofen M, Weibel ER: Alterations of the gas exchange apparatus in adult respiratory insufficiency associated with septicemia. *Am Rev Respir Dis* 116:589–615, 1977.
7. Clements JA, Hustead RF, Johnson RB, Bribetz I: Pulmonary surface tension and alveolar stability. *J Appl Physiol* 16:444–450, 1961.
8. Crapo J, Barry BE, Gehr P, Bachofen M, Weibel ER: Cell number and cell characteristics of the normal human lung. *Am Rev Respir Dis* 125:332–337, 1982.
9. Dempsey JA: Is the lung built for exercise? *Med Sci Sports Exerc* 18:143–155, 1986.
10. Forrest JB, Lee MKW: The bronchial wall: integrated form and function, in Crystal RG, West JB, Barnes PB, Weibel ER (eds): *The Lung: Scientific Foundations,* 2d ed. New York, Lippincott-Raven, 1997, pp 1081–1092.
11. Fung YB, Sobin S: Pulmonary alveolar blood flow, in West JB (ed): *Bioengineering Aspects of the Lung.* New York, Dekker, 1977, pp 267–359.
12. Gehr P, Bachofen M, Weibel ER: The normal human lung: Ultrastructure and morphometric estimation of diffusion capacity. *Respir Physiol* 32:121–140, 1978.
13. Gil J, Bachofen H, Gehr P, Weibel ER: Alveolar volume–surface area relation in air- and saline-filled lungs fixed by vascular perfusion. *J Appl Physiol* 47:990–1001, 1979.
14. Guntherodt WG, Luchtel DL, Kawabori I: Pulmonary microcirculation: Tubules rather than sheet and post. *J Appl Physiol* 53:510–515, 1982.
15. Haefeli-Bleuer B, Weibel ER: Morphometry of the human pulmonary acinus. *Anat Rec* 220:401–414, 1988.
16. Hawgood S: Surfactant: Composition, structure, metabolism, in Crystal RG, West JB, Barnes PB, Weibel ER (eds): *The Lung: Scientific Foundations,* 2d ed. New York, Lippincott-Raven, 1997, pp 557–572.
17. Heidelberger E, Reeves RB: O_2 transfer kinetics in a whole blood unicellular thin layer. *J Appl Physiol* 68:1854–1864, 1990.
18. Holland RAB, van Hezewijk W, Zubazanda J: Velocity of oxygen uptake by partly saturated adult and fetal human red cells. *Respir Physiol* 29:303–364, 1977.
19. Holland RAB, Shibata H, Scheid P, Piiper J: Kinetics of O_2 uptake and release by red cells in stopped-flow apparatus: Effects of unstirred layer. *Respir Physiol* 59:71–91, 1985.
20. Hoppeler, H: The different relationship of $\dot{V}_{O_2max}$ to muscle mitochondria in humans and quadrupedal animals. *Respir Physiol* 80:137–146, 1990.
21. Hoppeler H, Lindstedt SL: Malleability of skeletal muscle tissue in overcoming limitations: Structural elements. *J Exp Biol* 115:355–364, 1985.
22. Horsfield K, Cumming G: Morphology of the bronchial tree in man. *J Appl Physiol* 24:373–383, 1968.
23. Horsfield K, Dart G, Olson DE, et al: Models of the human bronchial tree. *J Appl Physiol* 31:207–217, 1971.
24. Hsia, CCW, Carlin JI, Ramathan M, et al: Estimation of diffusion limitation after pneumonectomy from carbon monoxide diffusing capacity. *Respir Physiol* 83:11–22, 1991.
25. Hsia CCW, Johnson RL: Physiology and morphology of postpneumonectomy compensation, in Crystal RG, West JB, Barnes PB, Weibel ER (eds): *The Lung: Scientific Foundations,* 2d ed. New York, Lippincott-Raven, 1997, pp 1047–1060.
26. Kapanci Y, Assimacopoulos A, Irle C, et al: "Contractile interstitial cells" in pulmonary alveolar septa: A possible regulator of ventilation-perfusion ratio? Ultrastructural, immunofluorescence, and in vitro studies. *J Cell Biol* 375–392, 1974.
27. König MF, Lucocq JM, Weibel ER: Demonstration of pulmonary vascular perfusion by electron and light microscopy. *J Appl Physiol* 75:1877–1883, 1993.
28. Lauweryns JM: Alveolar clearance and the role of pulmonary lymphatics. *Am Rev Respir Dis* 115:625–683, 1977.
29. Leak LV, Ferrans VJ : Lymphatics and lymphoid tissue, in Crystal RG, West JB, Barnes PB, Weibel ER (eds): *The Lung: Scientific Foundations,* 2d ed. New York, Lippincott-Raven, 1997, pp 1129–1138.
30. Lindstedt SL, Hokanson JF, Wells DJ, et al: Running energetics in the most remarkable aerobic athlete, the pronghorn antelope. *Nature* 353:748–750, 1991.
31. Pedley TJ, Schroter RC, Sudlow MF: The prediction of pressure drop and variation of resistance within the human bronchial airways. *Respir Physiol* 9:387–405, 1970.

32. Phalen RF, Yeh HC, Schum GM, Raabe OG: Application of an idealized model to morphometry of the mammalian tracheobronchial tree. *Anat Rec* 190:167–176, 1978.

33. Roughton FJW, Forster RE: Relative importance of diffusion and chemical reaction rates in determining rate of exchange of gases in the human lung, with special reference to true diffusing capacity of pulmonary membrane and volume of blood in capillaries. *J Appl Physiol* 11:290–302, 1957.

34. Schneeberger EE: Alveolar type I cells, in Crystal RG, West JB, Barnes PB, Weibel ER (eds): *The Lung: Scientific Foundations,* 2d ed. New York, Lippincott-Raven, 1997, pp 535–542.

35. Simionescu M: Lung endothelium: Structure and function correlates, in Crystal RG, West JB, Barnes PB, Weibel ER (eds): *The Lung: Scientific Foundations,* 2d ed. New York, Lippincott-Raven, 1997, pp 615–628.

36. Sleigh MA: Mucus propulsion, in Crystal RG, West JB, Barnes PB, Weibel ER (eds): *The Lung: Scientific Foundations.* New York, Raven Press, 1991, vol I, pp 189–196.

37. Taylor CR, Karas RH, Weibel ER, Hoppeler H: Adaptive variation in the mammalian respiratory system in relation to energetic demand: I–VIII. *Respir Physiol* 69:1–127, 1987.

38. Taylor CR, Karas RH, Weibel ER, Hoppeler H: Matching structures and functions in the respiratory system, in Wood SC (ed): *Comparative Pulmonary Physiology: Current Contents.* New York, Marcel Dekker, 1989, pp 27–65.

39. Wagner DD, Olmsted JB, Marder VJ: Immunolocalization of von Willebrand protein in Weibel-Palade bodies of human endothelial cells. *J Cell Biol* 95:355–360, 1982.

40. Weibel ER: Design of biological organisms and fractal geometry, in Nonnenmacher TF, Losa GA, Weibel ER (eds): *Fractals in Biology and Medicine.* Basel, Birkhäuser, 1994, pp 68–85.

41. Weibel ER: Functional morphology of lung parenchyma, in Macklem PT, Mead J (eds): *Handbook of Physiology:* Section 3: *The Respiratory System.* Bethesda, MD, American Physiological Society, 1986, vol 3, pp 89–111.

42. Weibel ER: Lung cell biology, in Fishman A, Fisher AB (eds): *Handbook of Physiology.* Section 3: *The Respiratory System.* Bethesda, MD: American Physiological Society, 1985, vol 1, pp 47–91.

43. Weibel ER: Lung morphometry and models in respiratory physiology, in Chang HK, Paiva M (eds): *Respiratory Physiology: An Analytical Approach.* New York, Marcel Dekker, 1989, pp 1–56.

44. Weibel ER: Morphometric estimation of pulmonary diffusion capacity: I. Model and method. *Respir Physiol* 11:54–75, 1970/71.

45. Weibel ER: *Morphometry of the Human Lung.* Heidelberg, Springer-Verlag, 1963.

46. Weibel ER: *The Pathway for Oxygen.* Cambridge, MA, Harvard University Press, 1984.

47. Weibel ER, Bachofen H: Structural design of the alveolar septum and fluid exchange, in Fishman AP, Renkin EM (eds): *Pulmonary Edema.* Bethesda, MD: American Physiological Society, 1979, pp 1–20.

48. Weibel ER, Federspiel WJ, Fryder-Doffey F, et al: Morphometric model for pulmonary diffusing capacity: I. Membrane diffusing capacity. *Respir Physiol* 93:125–149, 1993.

49. Weibel ER, Gil J: Structure-function relationships at the alveolar level, in West JB (ed): *Bioengineering Aspects of the Lung.* New York, Marcel Dekker, 1977, pp 1–81.

50. Weibel ER, Gomez DM: Architecture of the human lung. *Science* 137:577–585, 1962.

51. Weibel ER, Palade GE: New cytoplasmic components in arterial endothelia. *J Cell Biol* 23:101–112, 1964.

52. Weibel ER, Taylor CR: Design of the mammalian respiratory system: I–IX. *Respir Physiol* 44:1–164, 1981.

53. Weibel ER, Taylor CR, Hoppeler H: Variations in function and design: Testing symmorphosis in the respiratory system. *Resp Physiol* 87:325–348, 1992.

54. Weibel ER, Taylor CR, O'Neil JJ, et al: Maximal oxygen consumption and pulmonary diffusing capacity: A direct comparison of physiologic and morphometric measurements in canids. *Respir Physiol* 54:173–188, 1983.

55. West BJ, Barghava V, Goldberger AL: Beyond the principle of similitude: Renormalization in the bronchial tree. *J Appl Physiol* 60:1089–1097, 1986.

56. Wilson TA, Bachofen H: A model for mechanical structure of the alveolar duct. *J Appl Physiol* 52:1064–1070, 1982.

57. Yamaguchi K, Nguyen-Phu D, Scheid P, Piiper J: Kinetics of O_2 uptake and release by human erythrocytes studied by a stopped-flow technique. *J Appl Physiol* 58:1215–1224, 1985.

CHAPTER 3

THE RESPIRATORY MUSCLES

Marc Decramer

The respiratory muscles constitute a complex pump system. Several muscles comprise this system, represented schematically in Fig. 3-1. Breathing under all circumstances requires a coordinated contraction of different respiratory muscles.[4] The most important inspiratory muscle is the diaphragm.[46] The conditions under which this respiratory muscle system weakens and eventually will fail are addressed in other chapters (see Chapters 98, 99, and 170). This chapter focuses on structural and functional properties of the respiratory muscles, respiratory muscle action, and respiration muscle interaction.

STRUCTURAL AND FUNCTIONAL PROPERTIES OF RESPIRATORY MUSCLES

The respiratory muscles are skeletal muscles, and, in essence, their structural and functional properties are within the range of other skeletal muscles located in the limbs. Adaptations to their specific function, however, make them distinctly different from other skeletal muscles in a number of respects. First, limb muscles are essentially designed to produce movements, and hence, primarily work against inertial loads. Respiratory muscles mainly have to overcome resistive and elastic loads. Second, peripheral muscles contract rhythmically during movements, while respiratory muscles contract rhythmically and continuously, and they are the only skeletal muscles on which life depends. These vital muscles thus have to be well equipped to sustain continuous

rhythmic contraction.[24] These adaptations include high fatigue resistance, high oxidative capacity, greater capillary density, and greater maximal blood flow, and they depend upon structural and functional properties of the muscles.

Structural Properties

Structural properties of muscles in general and respiratory muscles in particular depend upon fiber types present in the muscle, morphological characteristics of the fibers, and motor unit organization.

FIBER TYPES

Skeletal muscles are composed of several motor units, each with hundreds of muscle fibers. Three types of muscle fibers are usually present. They are distinguished on the basis of the myofibrillar myosin adenosine triphosphatase (ATPase) activity and its pH dependence.[2] Alternatively, the muscle fibers may be distinguished through myosin heavy chain gene expression. Type I fibers, or slow oxidative fibers, have a slow contraction profile but are high in endurance and rich in oxidative enzymes. Type II fibers are fast-twitch fibers which develop tension rapidly. They either are fatigue-resistant or glycolytic-oxidative (IIa), or fatigable or glycolytic (IIb). Type II fibers develop greater forces than do type I fibers.[23] Muscles primarily composed of type I fibers have high endurance, whereas those primarily composed of type IIb fibers are designed to develop high forces but have low endurance capacity. Type IIa fibers are intermediate and combine relatively high force development with relatively long endurance. In general, type I fibers have the smallest cross-sectional area, and type IIb fibers tend to have the largest.

Type IIb fibers were recently distinguished from the histochemically different type IIx fibers by means of myosin electrophoresis and histochemistry.[35] The respiratory muscles are mixed muscles containing both fast-twitch and slow-twitch fibers. The human diaphragm contains about 55 ± 5 percent type I fibers, 21 ± 6 percent type IIa fibers, and 23 ± 3 percent type IIb fibers. All respiratory muscles (i.e., intercostal muscles, abdominal muscles, sternomastoids, and diaphragm) contain at least 60 percent highly oxidative fibers.[24] No data are available on the scalenes. The respiratory muscles thus seem to be generally well equipped to sustain continuous rhythmic contraction.

MORPHOLOGICAL CHARACTERISTICS OF THE FIBERS

The respiratory muscles consist of muscle bundles oriented in a parallel fashion. These bundles consist of hundreds of muscle fibers, each of which in turn consists of hundreds of myofibrils.

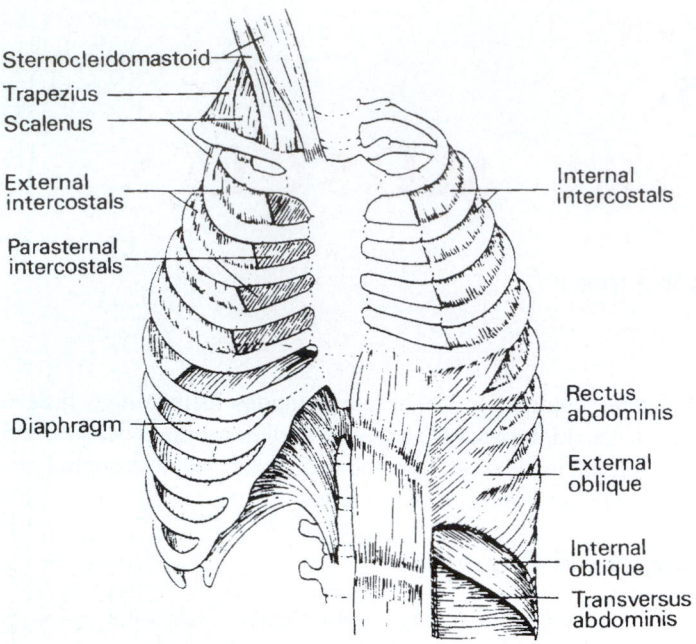

FIGURE 3-1   Idealized diaphragm of the respiratory muscles.

These myofibrils are made up of hundreds of sarcomeres arranged in series, each sarcomere consisting of a number of myosin (thick filaments) and twice the number of actin (thin) filaments. The capacity of the muscle to produce forces depends upon the number of myofibrils in parallel, since the forces developed by all these myofibrils are additive, whereas the displacement and velocity of shortening depend upon the number of sarcomeres in series. Indeed, the displacements of these sarcomeres arranged in series are additive.

The density of mitochondria in each of the three fiber types tends to be greater than in the same fiber types in limb muscles. In addition, in humans, the diaphragm is composed of about 80 percent oxidative fibers compared to 36 to 46 percent in the limb muscles of untrained men.[24] As a consequence, the volume density of mitochondria in the diaphragm is twofold greater than in limb muscles. Therefore, the oxygen uptake capacity of the diaphragm is considerably greater than that of limb muscles because of the high oxidative fiber content and the greater mitochondrial density. Moreover, the maximal blood flow also considerably exceeds that of limb muscles because of the greater capillary density, which is about twice the capillary density in limb muscle.[1] The diaphragm is thus well equipped to sustain rhythmic contraction at rest through its type I and IIa fibers: The type IIa fibers permit additional recruitment in power and rate during exercise, and the few type IIb fibers permit high power outputs necessary for sneezing and coughing.[24]

MOTOR UNIT ORGANIZATION

Muscle fibers are organized in motor units. The muscle fibers within a given motor unit are broadly dispersed throughout a region of the diaphragm. Dispersion occurs both horizontally across the surface of the diaphragm and vertically with fibers at different depths. There are three types of motor units in the respiratory muscles: fast-fatiguable (FF), fast-fatigue resistant (FR),

and slow (S). Motor units composed of fast fibers are large and develop forces in the range of 110 mN. These, however, are considerably smaller than in limb muscles.[47] Motor units composed of slow fibers are smaller and develop forces in the range of 30 to 60 mN. The recruitment pattern of the diaphragm follows the size principle, the smallest motor units being recruited first.

Functional Properties

Functional properties of muscles are generally described in terms of force-length relationships, time-dependent characteristics of the twitch, force-frequency, force-velocity, and power-frequency relationships.

The force-length characteristics of the diaphragm are in essence similar to other muscles.[40] Maximal tension is generated at the optimal length. Three aspects of the force-length curve of the diaphragm are potentially relevant to clinical medicine. First, with hyperinflation, the diaphragm shortens and its capacity to generate force is concomitantly reduced.[18,44] Second, when hyperinflation occurs chronically, adaptation occurs in the muscle. This adaptation consists of drop out of sarcomeres such that muscle shortening is then accommodated by a reduced number of sarcomeres rather than by alterations in filament overlap within the sarcomeres.[27,31] As a consequence, the force-generating capacity is restored, at least in part, at foreshortened length. This adaptation is summarized in Fig. 3-2. The consequences of this adaptation to patients with hyperinflation are discussed below. Third, although less-than-optimal filament overlap is the primary reason for a reduction in force with muscle shortening, calcium deactivation due to T-tubular failure also plays a role.[48] This is potentially significant for treatment, since inotropic agents restore T-tubular function in foreshortened muscle. Accordingly, inotropic agents exert much greater effects on foreshortened diaphragm than on diaphragm placed at its optimal length.[33] This concept opens up new perspectives for respiratory muscle pharmacotherapy in patients with severe hyperinflation. The length-tension curves of other respiratory muscles and their adaptation to hyperinflation have not been systematically studied.

A particularly interesting question, is the relationship between the in situ operational length of the respiratory muscles and the optimal length in vitro. For the diaphragm the length at functional residual capacity (FRC) comes close to the optimal length.[30] The length changes undergone by the diaphragm over the vital capacity range are large, 30 to 40 percent.[18,44] These length changes are considerably smaller for the parasternal intercostals, the scalenes, and the sternocleidomastoids.[17,28,29] For the parasternal intercostals, the length at FRC is clearly longer than optimal in supine dogs, so that with hyperinflation, the parasternal intercostals move toward their optimal length.[29,37] The scalenes and the sternocleidomastoids appear to operate on the ascending limbs of their length-tension curves in supine dogs.[28] How hyperinflation in patients affects the force-generating capacity of these muscles remains unclear. According to a recent analysis, the changes in length during passive inflation are proportional to the mechanical advantage of a particular respiratory muscle. In keeping with this analysis, the mechanical advantage of the diaphragm would be considerably greater than the mechanical advantage of the other inspiratory muscles[50] (see below).

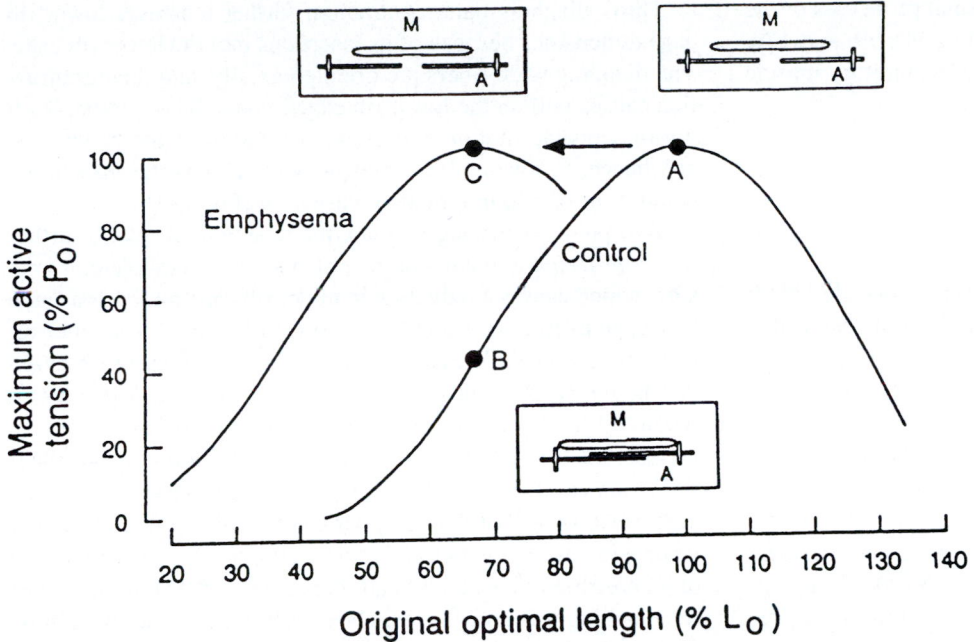

FIGURE 3-2 Diaphragmatic length–tension curve in normal hamsters and hamsters with elastase–induced emphysema. Tension is expressed as a percentage of maximum tetanic tension, P_O, and length is expressed as a percentage of original optimal length, L_O. The degree of filament overlap between actin, A, and myosin, M, filaments, in control, A, acute, B, and chronic hyperinflation C, is shown. Note that due to sarcomere adaptation in chronic hyperinflation, the degree of filament overlap is the same at a considerably shorter length. *(After Farkas,[27] with permission.)*

traction occurs. Particularly interesting is the effect of acute shortening on the force-frequency curve.[24] Since acute shortening is associated with a downward shift of the force-frequency curve, the detrimental effect of acute shortening on the force-generating capacity of the diaphragm appears to be twofold. With muscle shortening there is a clear reduction in maximal tetanic force. However, the decrease in force at submaximal stimulation frequencies is disproportionately greater (Fig. 3-3).

The force-velocity curve of the diaphragm is shown in Fig. 3-4. With increasing loads, the velocity of contraction is reduced. The velocity of contraction is a direct function of myosin ATPase activity, and, hence, the force-velocity curve is primarily determined by the muscle fiber composition. The diaphragm is intermediate between the force-velocity curve of a fast and a slow muscle (Fig. 3-4).[24] The production of airflow into the lungs requires power output by the respiratory muscles. Power may be calculated as the product of the values of velocity and force according to the force-velocity relationship (Fig. 3-4). Instantaneous peak power occurs at 30 percent of maximal force and at 30 percent of maximal velocity. The frequency–isometric force relationship, the frequency-shortening force and the frequency-power relationships show a similar dependency of force and power upon frequency of stimulation.[24]

Fatigue also affects profoundly the force-length, force-frequency, force-velocity and power-frequency characteristics of the

The force developed by a muscle increases with increasing frequency of stimulation (Fig. 3-3). The increase in force is considerably steeper for a slow muscle in which fusion occurs at lower frequency because of the longer relaxation time than for a fast muscle. The diaphragm is intermediate, so that at the in vivo stimulation frequencies (10 to 30 Hz), a fused tetanic con-

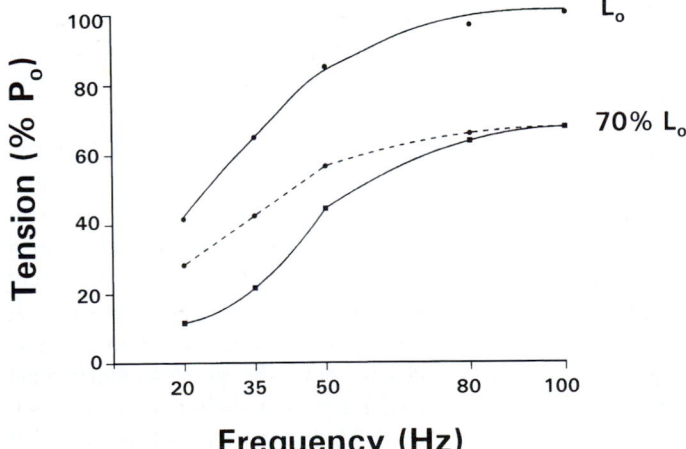

FIGURE 3-3 Force–frequency curve of human diaphragm at L_O and 70 percent L_O. Force is expressed as a percentage of maximal tetanic tension, P_O, and frequency is expressed in Hz. Dashed line is the predicted line at 70 percent L_O, whereas the solid line is the observed line. The predicted line is based on the assumption that a 30 percent change in length produces a 35 percent drop in force at all stimulation frequencies, as is observed for maximal tetanic force. Note that the decrease in force at lower stimulation frequencies is considerably greater than theoretically predicted. *(Modified after Farkas,[27] with permission.)*

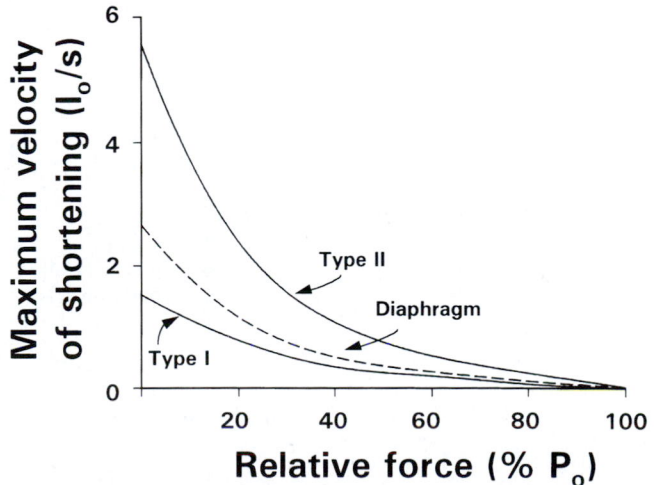

FIGURE 3-4 Force–velocity curve of human diaphragm (dashed line), which is intermediate between the force–velocity curve of a typical slow muscle (type I) and a typical fast muscle (type II). Maximum velocity is expressed in optimal length, l_O, per second and relative force is expressed as a percentage of maximum tetanic force, P_O.

diaphragm. The effects of fatigue on functional properties of the respiratory muscles are discussed in Chapters 98, 99, and 170. The factors determining the development of respiratory muscle fatigue are also discussed in these chapters.

ACTIONS OF RESPIRATORY MUSCLES

The Diaphragm

The diaphragm is the most important inspiratory muscle.[10,46] It consists of two distinct parts, the costal and crural parts, that have separate actions on the rib cage, separate segmental motor innervations, and a different embryological origin.[15] In respiratory activities, however, the diaphragm frequently operates as a functional unit, and in the following its action is described as such. Diaphragmatic action is schematically represented in Fig. 3-5. Diaphragmatic contraction increases chest wall dimensions because of three distinct reasons.[10] First, diaphragmatic descent increases the craniocaudal dimensions of the thorax. Diaphragmatic descent is tightly coupled to outward motion of the free abdominal wall.[20,42]

Second, diaphragmatic contraction increases the dimensions of the lower rib cage because of the increase in abdominal pressure that it causes. This increase in abdominal pressure acts through the zone of apposition (i.e., the zone in which the diaphragm is immediately apposed to the rib cage) to expand the lower rib cage. This action is the *appositional component* of diaphragmatic action (Fig. 3-5). The magnitude of the appositional component is determined by the magnitude of the zone of apposition, about 25 to 30 percent of the total internal surface area of the rib cage at FRC in standing humans, and by the magnitude of the increase in abdominal pressure caused by diaphragmatic contraction.[42]

Third, diaphragmatic contraction further increases lower rib cage dimensions because of its insertions into the lower rib cage. The diaphragmatic fibers are oriented axially, and their contraction causes pull on the lower rib cage in an axial direction, leading to cephalad motion and outward rotation of the lower ribs, and hence, to lower rib cage expansion. This is the *insertional component* of diaphragmatic contraction (Fig. 3-5).

Two points regarding diaphragmatic action are worth further mention. Diaphragmatic contraction also decreases pleural pressure, which causes a reduction in upper rib cage dimensions and, hence, an expiratory effect on the lower rib cage.[10] The latter reduction in upper rib cage dimensions is also clearly observed during diaphragm contraction or pacing in high quadriplegics, in whom all inspiratory muscles, except for sternocleidomastoids, are paralyzed.[25] The pattern of chest wall motion in quadriplegics is shown in Fig. 3-6. The displacement observed in quadriplegics suggests that diaphragmatic contraction alone cannot be responsible for the pattern of chest wall motion observed during quiet breathing (see below) and, hence, that other muscles assist the diaphragm in moving the chest wall during quiet breathing.

The Intercostal Muscles

The functional anatomy of intercostal muscles is schematically represented in Fig. 3-7. Between the chondral portions of the ribs only one layer of intercostal muscles, the parasternal intercostals, is present. Between the osseous portions of the ribs, two layers are present. The outermost layer runs obliquely downward and forward and is called the *external intercostal*. The innermost layer runs obliquely downward and backward and is called the *internal intercostal* (Fig. 3-7, left panel). Note that the internal intercostals and the parasternal intercostals have the same fiber orientation. Dorsally only an external intercostal is present. At its outside runs a fusiform muscle between the transverse processus of the vertebra and the angle of the lower rib. This muscle is called the *levator costae* (Fig. 3-7, right panel).[6,10]

The parasternal portion of the intercostal musculature, the "parasternals," is consistently active during quiet breathing both in animals and in human subjects,[14,17] and is the most important inspiratory portion of the intercostal musculature. The parasternal intercostals have the greatest mechanical advantage, and their contraction produces about 60 percent of the cephalad motion of the rib, during inspiration.[7,50] Within the parasternal intercostal, the medial fibers have a greater mechanical advantage and are activated more consistently and before the middle and the lateral fibers.[9]

The action and the respiratory role of the interosseus intercostals remain

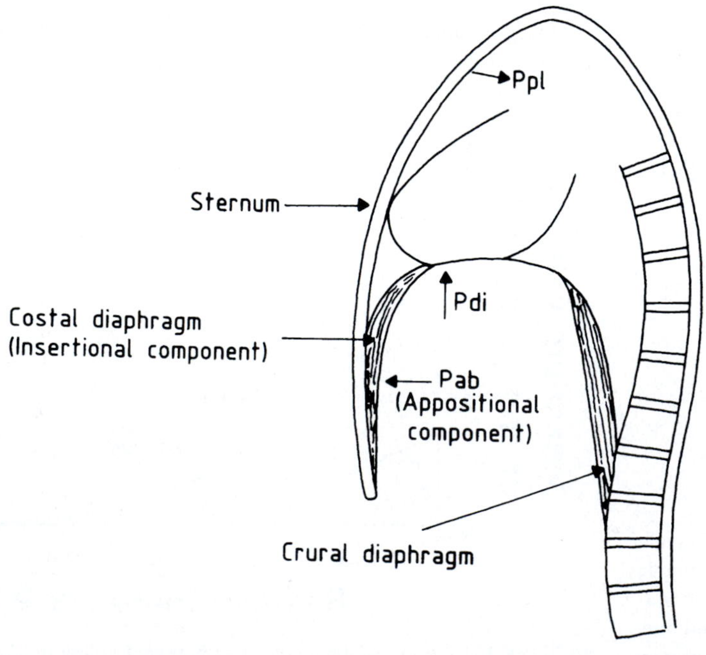

FIGURE 3-5 Diagram illustrating diaphragmatic action. Lateral view of the thorax. Ppl = pleural pressure, Pab = abdominal pressure. Costal and crural diaphragm are shown. See text for further explanation.

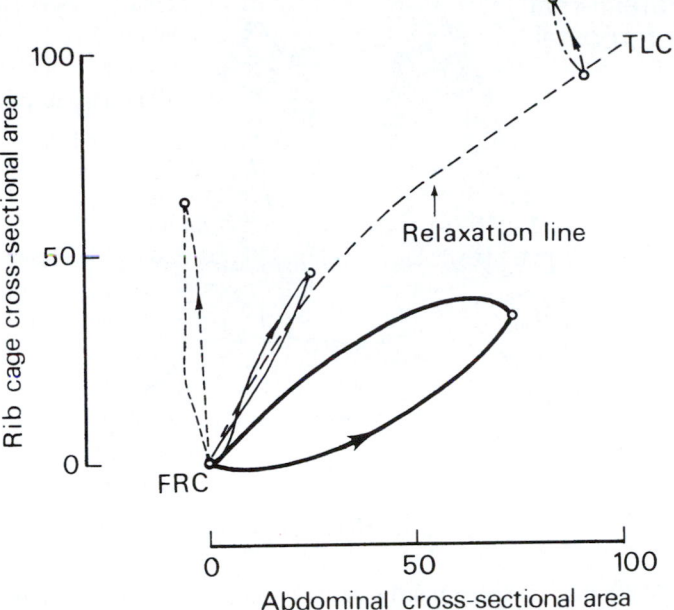

FIGURE 3-6 Konno–Mead diagram illustrating chest wall motion during quiet breathing (thin loop), diaphragmatic pacing or quiet breathing in tetraplegic patient (thick loop), breathing with diaphragm paralysis (dash loop), and breathing at severely elevated end–expiratory volume (dash–dot loop). Rib cage and abdominal cross-sectional areas are expressed as a percentage of inspiratory capacity. Dashed line is the relaxation line.

the subject of longstanding debate.[8,10] The most commonly accepted view on intercostal muscle action is based on a theory of intercostal muscle fiber orientation and rib geometry.[36] This theory states that the external intercostals are inspiratory in action, and the external intercostals are expiratory in action. Numerous experiments do not fit with this theory, although a recent finite

element analysis largely confirmed these actions.[38] It is commonly believed that the interosseus intercostals constitute a reserve system that may be recruited with increased ventilatory load. The external intercostals are recruited predominantly during inspiration, primarily in the upper interspaces, whereas the internal intercostals are recruited predominantly during expiration primarily in the lower interspaces.[11] In addition, they also may serve postural functions,[21] such as in rotation of the trunk. In the latter respect they appear as the continuation of the abdominal external and internal oblique (see below) in the thorax. Separate activation of the external and internal intercostals in humans during rotation of the trunk was demonstrated.[49]

Without question, the levator costae has an inspiratory action on the rib. It is frequently activated even during quiet inspiration in supine dogs.[6] The levator costae's contribution to inspiratory motion of the ribs during quiet breathing, however, appears substantially smaller than that of the parasternal intercostals. This contribution may further increase when the inspiratory motion of the ribs is appreciably increased.

The Scalenes

The scalenes run between the transverse processi of the five lower cervical vertebrae and the upper margin of the first (scalenus anterior) and the second (scalenus medius and posterior) ribs. The action of these muscles is to raise the first two ribs. The orientation of their axis in the neck[10] causes upward motion of these ribs ("pump handle" motion). Moreover, the scalenes are consistently active during quiet breathing in normal individuals and contribute to chest wall expansion.[4] They may be very important in the case of spinal cord injury. When the injury is below C_4-C_8, the scalenes' function is entirely or partially preserved, and they contribute importantly to upper rib cage motion in these patients.[25]

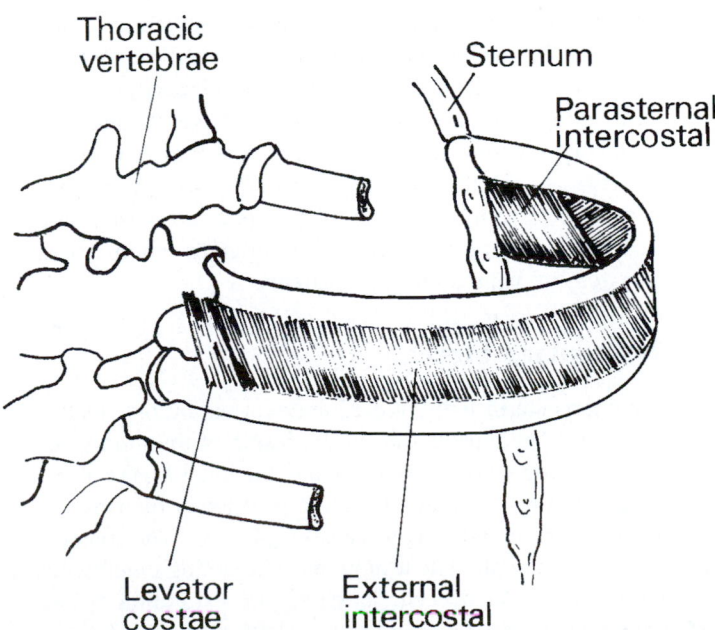

FIGURE 3-7 Diagram of the functional anatomy of the intercostal muscles, at their anterior (left) and posterior aspects (right). Notice the parasternal intercostals, the internal intercostals, the external intercostals, and the levator costae.

The Sternocleidomastoids

The sternocleidomastoids run between the mastoid processes of the temporal bone and the manubrium sterni and medial portion of the clavicle. In humans, these muscles are electrically silent during quiet breathing, but they may be recruited with increased ventilatory load. These muscles are particularly important in high quadriplegics in whom they preserve their function because they are innervated by the eleventh cranial nerve and spinal nerves C_1-C_2.[43] Through training the sternocleidomastoids may develop severe hypertrophy and contribute to several hours of ventilator independence in these patients.[10] They also may be recruited in patients with poliomyelitis and diaphragmatic dysfunction. These muscles are thought to be important in moving the upper rib cage in chronic obstructive pulmonary disease (COPD) patients even though a recent study failed to demonstrate consistent activity in these muscles in these patients.[13]

The Shoulder Girdle and Neck Muscles

Several shoulder girdle and neck muscles may contribute to inspiration under particular circumstances. Most of these muscles run from the rib cage to an extrathoracic extension. When the rib cage is fixed in the lean-forward position—a position commonly employed by COPD patients—these muscles contribute to expansion of the rib cage during inspiration. Muscles that may contribute to inspiration include: trapezius, latissimus dorsi, pectoralis major and minor, erector spinae, teres major, serratus anterior, platysma, mylohyoid, sternohyoid. Since these muscles commonly contribute to inspiration in patients with severe airflow obstruction, using these muscles for other activities, such as hair combing, may considerably increase dyspnea in these patients.[3]

The Clavicular Head of Pectoralis Major

The clavicular head of the pectoralis major runs laterally and caudally from the medial half of the clavicle and manubrium sterni to the humerus. If the arms are fixed and braced, contraction causes downward motion of the ribs and the sternum, increase in pleural pressure and, hence, expiration. Simultaneously, the lower rib cage and the abdomen move outward. Tetraplegics use this expiratory action when all other expiratory muscles are paralyzed.[26] Training increases pectoralis strength and increases expiratory reserve volume in these patients.

The Triangularis Sterni

The triangularis sterni is the most important expiratory muscle of the rib cage. The muscle runs at the inside of the thorax between the inner aspect of the sternum and the inner aspect of the five lower ribs (Fig. 3-8), and its action is to lower the ribs relative to the sternum and thus to cause expiration. The triangularis sterni is electrically silent in humans breathing quietly, but it is recruited during speech, laughing, or expiration below FRC.[12] Its recruitment threshold is low, lower than the recruitment threshold of most other expiratory muscles.

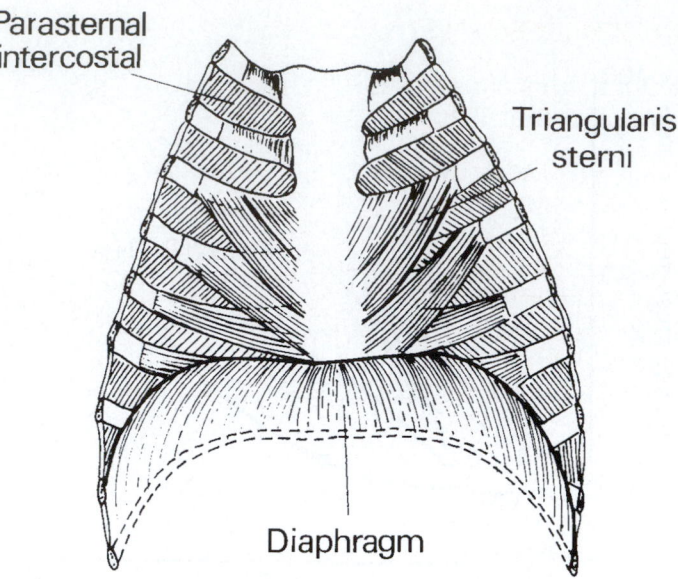

FIGURE 3-8 Diagram illustrating the functional anatomy of the triangularis sterni. View from the inside of the thorax.

The Abdominal Muscles

The abdominal muscles are composed of four different muscle layers (Fig. 3-1). Ventrally, a muscular sheet runs between the lower costal cartilages and the sternum and the pubis, the rectus abdominis. This muscle is enclosed in a sheath formed by the aponeuroses of the other three muscles. Laterally, an oblique muscle runs obliquely downward and forward between the lower eight ribs and the iliac crest, inguinal ligament, and the linea alba medially, the external oblique. At the inner surface of this muscle lies the internal oblique with a fiber orientation which is 90° perpendicular to the external oblique. These muscles are homologous to the external and internal intercostals. The innermost layer is the transversus abdominis, a circular muscular sheet surrounding the abdomen, with a fiber orientation that is parallel to the ribs. The transversus abdominis originates from the inner surface of the lower six ribs, where it interdigitates with the costal insertions of the diaphragm. It runs from this origin and from the lumbar fascia, iliac crest, and inguinal ligament, circumferentially around the abdominal visceral mass to terminate ventrally in the rectus sheet. These muscles all have an expiratory action, by virtue of the inward pull of the abdomen they cause and by virtue of the insertions they have in the rib cage. In addition, however, rib cage expansion may occur with contraction of some of these muscles through the increase in abdominal pressure accompanying their contraction.

The abdominal muscles are electrically silent during quiet breathing. Usually, however, tonic activity is present in the abdominal muscles in upright position, particularly in the upper segments.[5] During inspiratory loading, CO_2-induced hyperventilation, exercise, and forced expiration, these muscles are recruited. The transversus abdominis appears to have the lowest recruitment threshold.[10]

RESPIRATORY MUSCLE INTERACTION

Respiratory Muscle Interaction during Quiet Breathing

Respiratory muscle interaction is traditionally studied by means of a Konno-Mead diagram, relating rib cage diameter or cross-sectional area to abdominal diameter or cross-sectional area (Fig. 3-6). First, this relationship is determined in the absence of muscle contraction, during a relaxed expiration, yielding a relaxation line. During quiet breathing in the upright position, the chest wall moves along this relaxation line, which means that proportional expansion of rib cage and abdomen is occurring. In the supine position, abdominal movement is proportionally greater than rib cage movement. Since isolated diaphragmatic contraction in quadriplegics causes abdominal movement without rib cage motion or even inward movement of the upper rib cage (upper rib cage paradox), diaphragmatic contraction alone cannot be responsible for the pattern of motion occurring during quiet breathing (Fig. 3-6). Therefore, this motion requires concomitant contraction of other muscles (i.e., the parasternal intercostals and the scalenes). These muscles actively contribute to chest wall motion and cause upper rib cage expansion, whereas diaphragmatic contraction alone would cause upper rib cage paradox. During quiet breathing, the diaphragm probably contributes about 60 to 70 percent of the tidal volume, and the parasternal intercostals and the scalenes contribute the rest.[46]

Physiological Conditions Affecting Respiratory Muscle Interaction

Respiratory muscle interaction present during quiet breathing, and the chest wall motion resulting from it, may be altered in a number of circumstances in which ventilatory load is increased. During speech, laughing, and forced expiration, expiratory muscles are recruited. The expiratory muscles with the lowest recruitment threshold appear to be the triangularis sterni,[12] running between the sternum and the lower ribs at the inside of the thorax and the transversus abdominis, the innermost layer of the abdominal muscles.[10] Recruitment of these expiratory muscles may add significantly to inspiratory work; relaxation of these muscles just prior to the onset of inspiration contributes substantially to inspiration. Major recruitment of expiratory muscles occurs during exercise, inspiratory resistive loading, CO_2-induced hyperventilation, and anesthesia.[10]

Pathologic Conditions Affecting Respiratory Muscle Interaction

Respiratory muscle interaction is further profoundly affected by a number of pathologic conditions. Hyperinflation is a functional abnormality of lung diseases in which airflow obstruction or loss of elastic recoil are features. Hyperinflation may be particularly severe in COPD patients, in whom the FRC often exceeds predicted total lung capacity (TLC) (see below).

An overwhelming amount of evidence shows that hyperinflation reduces the diaphragmatic effectiveness as a pressure gen-erator and reduces diaphragm contribution to chest wall motion.[19,34,39] The contribution of the intercostal muscles and the scalenes is likely to be increased, such that chest wall motion becomes exclusively or predominantly rib cage motion (Fig. 3-6).

The ineffectiveness of the diaphragm may result from diaphragmatic shortening, geometrical alterations, alterations in diaphragm–rib cage interaction, alterations in mechanical arrangements among the costal and crural parts of the diaphragm, reduction in the zone of apposition, and so on. Among these, diaphragmatic shortening appears to be the most important. Indeed, with inflation from FRC to TLC, the diaphragm shortens about 30 to 40 percent,[18,44] which is expected to reduce significantly its pressure-generating capacity. Several studies indicate that diaphragmatic geometry is not affected significantly by hyperinflation.[32] The appositional component of diaphragmatic action is reduced substantially due to a reduction in the zone of apposition. The insertional component is affected so that diaphragmatic contraction causes inward retraction of the lower rib cage. This may be noticed clinically in patients with severe hyperinflation. The mechanical arrangement between the costal and crural parts of the diaphragm changes from a parallel arrangement at FRC to a series arrangement at TLC.[18] This is likely to further compromise the pressure-generating capacity of the diaphragm independently of its force-length characteristics.

It should be emphasized, however, that the above pertains to acute hyperinflation. In chronic hyperinflation, the diaphragm adapts to the chronically foreshortened state by dropping out sarcomeres. As a consequence, the filament overlap within each sarcomere is restored toward optimal overlap. This adaptation is shown in Fig. 3-2. It should be noticed, however, that this adaptation only partially restores diaphragmatic function. First, because part of the reduction in force with shortening is due to compression of the T-tubular system, blocking exit-electrolyte flow and impeding excitation-contraction coupling.[48] Whether adaptations in T-tubular function also occur with chronic foreshortening remains to be investigated. Second, sarcomere adaptation adapts only to the loss in diaphragmatic function associated with diaphragmatic shortening and not to the loss in function due to geometrical alterations, alterations in diaphragm-rib cage interaction, changes in mechanical arrangement among different parts of the diaphragm, or loss of zone of apposition. Third, although sarcomere adaptation restores the force-generating capacity of a foreshortened diaphragm, it reduces the number of sarcomere in series. Consequently, sarcomere adaptation compromises the capacity of the diaphragm to undergo changes in length and, hence, its capacity to produce volume changes, presumably its most important function.

The action of the parasternal intercostals, the scalenes, and the sternocleidomastoids is likely to be less disturbed by hyperinflation because the changes in length that these muscles undergo with hyperinflation are considerably smaller.[17,28] Moreover, the optimal length for the parasternal intercostals may be close to TLC rather than at FRC.[29,37] The role of the sternocleidomastoids in COPD patients remains unclear, since activity is usually absent even in severe airflow obstruction.[13] Expiratory muscle recruitment is frequently observed in COPD patients with severe airflow obstruction.[45] The transversus abdominis appears to be frequently recruited. Expiratory muscle recruitment may contribute to the intrinsic positive end-expiratory pressure (PEEP$_i$) that is frequently observed in these patients. PEEP$_i$ is primarily caused by impaired pulmonary mechanics and consequent dynamic hyperinflation. The functional significance of this expiratory muscle activation is poorly understood. Indeed, in severe airflow obstruction, expiratory flow limitation is frequently present. In the presence of expiratory flow limitation, recruitment of expiratory muscles no longer contributes to expiratory flow.

In patients with pulmonary disease in general and COPD in particular, several factors may contribute to generalized muscle weakness, in which the respiratory muscles partake. These include hypoxemia and hypercapnia, malnutrition, cardiac failure,[41] corticosteroid treatment,[16,22] infection, electrolyte disturbances, and inactivity with consequent disuse atrophy. Of particular importance appears to be treatment with corticosteroids in repetitive bursts,[16] which is often inadvertently administered to COPD patients. Typically this myopathy causes a myopathic pattern on muscle biopsy instead of selective type IIb fiber atrophy as is commonly believed.[16]

ACKNOWLEDGMENTS

The writer thanks Mr. Jean Sente for making excellent drawings. He further thanks the Nationaal Fonds voor Wetenschappelijk Onderzoek grant #3.0167.95, Actie Levenslijn grant #7.0002.94, Nationale Vereniging tot Steun aan de Gehandicapte Personen, and Astra Pharmaceuticals for their support of the research mentioned in this chapter.

REFERENCES

1. Boczkowski J, Vicaut E, Aubier M: A model for in vivo study of the diaphragmatic microcirculation in the rat. *Microvasc Res* 40:157–167, 1990.
2. Brooke MH, Kaiser KK: Muscle fiber types: how many and what kind. *Arch Neurol* 23:369–379, 1970.
3. Celli BR, Rassulo J, Make BJ: Dyssynchronous breathing during arm but not leg exercise in patients with chronic airflow obstruction. *New Engl J Med* 314:1485–1490, 1986.
4. De Troyer A, Estenne M: Coordination between rib cage muscles and diaphragm during quiet breathing in humans. *J Appl Physiol* 57:899–906, 1984.
5. De Troyer A, Estenne M: Functional anatomy of the respiratory muscles. *Clin Chest Med* 9:175–193, 1988.
6. De Troyer A, Farkas GA: Inspiratory function of the levator costae and external intercostal muscles in the dog. *J Appl Physiol* 67:2614–2621, 1989.
7. De Troyer A, Farkas GA: Linkage between parasternals and external intercostals during resting breathing. *J Appl Physiol* 69:509–516, 1990.
8. De Troyer A, Kelly S, Macklem PT, Zin WA: Mechanics of intercostal space and actions of external and internal intercostal muscles. *J Clin Invest* 75:850–857, 1985.
9. De Troyer A, Legrand A: Inhomogeneous activation of the parasternal intercostals during breathing. *J Appl Physiol* 79:55–62, 1995.
10. De Troyer A, Loring SH: Actions of the respiratory muscles, in Roussos C (ed): *The Thorax,* part A, *Physiology.* New York, Marcel Dekker, 1995, pp 535–563.
11. De Troyer A, Ninane V: Respiratory function of intercostal muscles in supine dog: an electromyographic study. *J Appl Physiol* 60:1692–1699, 1986.
12. De Troyer A, Ninane V, Gilmartin JJ, et al: Triangularis sterni use in supine humans. *J Appl Physiol* 62:919–925, 1987.
13. De Troyer A, Peche R, Yernault JC, Estenne M: Neck muscle activity in patients with severe chronic obstructive pulmonary disease. *Am J Respir Crit Care Med* 150:41–47, 1994.
14. De Troyer A, Sampson M: Activation of the parasternal intercostals during breathing efforts in human subjects. *J Appl Physiol* 52:524–529, 1982.
15. De Troyer A, Sampson M, Sigrist S, Macklem PT: The diaphragm: two muscles. *Science* 213:199–202, 1981.
16. Decramer M, de Bock V, Dom R: Functional and histologic picture of steroid-induced myopathy in COPD. *Am J Respir Crit Care Med* in press: 1996.
17. Decramer M, De Troyer A: Respiratory changes in parasternal intercostal length. *J Appl Physiol* 57:1254–1260, 1984.
18. Decramer M, De Troyer A, Kelly S, Macklem PT: Mechanical arrangement of costal and crural diaphragms in dogs. *J Appl Physiol* 56:1484–1490, 1984.
19. Decramer M, Jiang TX, Demedts M: Effects of acute hyperinflation on chest wall mechanics in dogs. *J Appl Physiol* 63:1493–1498, 1987.
20. Decramer M, Jiang TX, Reid MB, et al: Relationship between diaphragm length and abdominal dimensions. *J Appl Physiol* 61:1815–1820, 1986.
21. Decramer M, Kelly S, De Troyer A: Respiratory and postural changes in intercostal muscle length in supine dogs. *J Appl Physiol* 60:1686–1691, 1986.
22. Decramer M, Lacquet LM, Fagard R, Rogiers P: Corticosteroids contribute to muscle weakness in chronic airflow obstruction. *Am J Respir Crit Care Med* 150:11–16, 1994.
23. Eddinger TJ, Moss RL: Mechanical properties of skinned single fibers of identified types from rat diaphragm. *Am J Physiol* 253:C210–C218, 1987.
24. Edwards RHT, Faulkner JA: Structure and function of the respiratory muscles, in Roussos C (ed): *The Thorax,* part A, *Physiology.* New York, Marcel Dekker, 1995, pp 185–217.
25. Estenne M, De Troyer A: Relationship between respiratory muscle electromyogram and rib cage motion in tetraplegia. *Am Rev Respir Dis* 132:53–59, 1985.
26. Estenne M, De Troyer A: Cough in tetraplegic subjects: an active process. *Ann Intern Med* 112:22–28, 1990.
27. Farkas G: Functional characteristics of the respiratory muscles. *Sem Respir Med* 12:247–257, 1991.
28. Farkas G, Rochester DF: Contractile characteristics and operating lengths of canine neck inspiratory muscles. *J Appl Physiol* 65:2427–2433, 1988.
29. Farkas GA, Decramer M, Rochester DF, De Troyer A: Contractile properties of intercostal muscles and their functional significance. *J Appl Physiol* 59:528–535, 1985.
30. Farkas GA, Rochester DF: Functional characteristics of canine costal and crural diaphragm. *J Appl Physiol* 65:2253–2260, 1988.
31. Farkas GA, Roussos C: Diaphragm in emphysematous hamsters: sarcomere adaptability. *J Appl Physiol* 54:1635–1640, 1983.
32. Gauthier AP, Verbanck S, Estenne M, et al: Three-dimensional reconstruction of the in vivo human diaphragm shape at different lung volumes. *J Appl Physiol* 76:495–506, 1994.

33. Gayan-Ramirez G, Decramer M: Inotropic effects of theophylline on foreshortened canine diaphragm. *Am J Respir Crit Care Med* 149:920–924, 1994.

34. Gilmartin JJ, Gibson GJ: Abnormalities of chest wall motion in patients with chronic airflow obstruction. *Thorax* 39:264–271, 1984.

35. Gorza L: Identification of a novel type 2 fiber population in mammalian skeletal muscle by combined use of histochemical myosin ATPase and anti-myosin monoclonal antibodies. *J Histochem Cytochem* 38:257–265, 1990.

36. Hamberger GE: *De Respirationis Mechanismo et usu Genuino.* Jena, Germany, 1749.

37. Jiang TX, Deschepper K, Demedts M, Decramer M: Effects of acute hyperinflation on the mechanical effectiveness of the parasternal intercostals. *Am Rev Respir Dis* 139:522–528, 1989.

38. Loring SH, Woodbridge JA: Intercostal muscle action inferred from finite-element analysis. *J Appl Physiol* 70:2712–2718, 1991.

39. Martinez FJ, Couser JI, Celli BR: Factors influencing ventilatory muscle recruitment in patients with chronic airflow obstruction. *Am Rev Respir Dis* 142:276–282, 1990.

40. McCully KK, Faulkner JA: Length–tension relationship of mammalian diaphragm muscles. *J Appl Physiol* 54:1681–1686, 1983.

41. McParland C, Resch EF, Krishnan B, et al: Inspiratory muscle weakness in chronic heart failure: role of nutrition and electrolyte status and systemic myopathy. *Am J Respir Crit Care Med* 151:1101–1107, 1995.

42. Mead J, Loring SH: Analysis of volume displacement and length changes of the diaphragm during breathing. *J Appl Physiol* 53:750–755, 1982.

43. Mortola JP, Sant'Ambrogio G: Motion of the rib cage and the abdomen in tetraplegic patients. *Clin Sci Mol Med* 54:25–32, 1978.

44. Newman SL, Road J, Bellemare F, et al: Respiratory muscle length measured by sonomicrometry. *J Appl Physiol* 56:753–764, 1984.

45. Ninane V, Rypens F, Yernault JC, De Troyer A: Abdominal muscle use during breathing in patients with chronic airflow obstruction. *Am Rev Respir Dis* 146:16–21, 1992.

46. Rochester DF, Farkas GA: Performance of respiratory muscles in situ, in Roussos C (ed): *The Thorax,* part B, *Applied Physiology.* New York, Marcel Dekker, 1995, pp 1127–1159.

47. Sieck GC: Diaphragmatic muscle: structural and functional organization. *Clin Chest Med* 9:195–210, 1988.

48. Taylor SR, Rüdel R: Striated muscle fibers: inactivation of contraction induced by shortening. *Science* 167:882–884, 1970.

49. Whitelaw WA, Ford GT, Rimmer KP, De Troyer A: Intercostal muscles are used during rotation of the thorax in humans. *J Appl Physiol* 72:1940–1944, 1992.

50. Wilson TA, De Troyer A: Respiratory effect of the intercostal muscles in the dog. *J Appl Physiol* 75:2636–2645, 1993.

CHAPTER 4

CELLULAR MECHANISMS OF LUNG DEVELOPMENT

Jesse Roman

During embryogenesis, the lung develops from a single avascular epithelial bud into a specialized structure with a complex airway design, two complete circulatory systems, and millions of alveoli. The exact mechanisms responsible for this dramatic transformation remain undefined. However, several concepts are beginning to arise. During morphogenesis, the pulmonary structures (airways and vessels) organize into a single unit that accommodates a large surface area in a relatively small space. By enhancing surface area, the lung can efficiently accomplish its most important function, gas exchange. This chapter discusses the mechanisms considered important for the organization of embryonic cells into the functional multicellular structure characteristic of the lung.

Rather than providing a comprehensive review of the information available on this subject, the discussion will focus on the extracellular signals implicated in regulation of lung pattern formation during the early stages of development. In particular, the potential role of cell-matrix interactions and polypeptide growth factors in airways formation and lung vascularization will be discussed. Much less will be said about the intracellular signals or genetic codes (e.g., homeobox genes, proto-oncogenes) responsible for lung pattern formation, reflecting the limited information available on this subject. The speculative nature of the discussion is intended not to provide definitive answers but to stimulate research in this field, begin to close the gap between biologists and theoretical scientists, and provide a framework for the creation of physiological and mathematical models that adequately incorporate cellular and molecular mechanisms influencing lung development.

PATTERN FORMATION DURING LUNG DEVELOPMENT

To better understand its embryology, mammalian lung development has been divided into various overlapping stages characterized by the appearance of specific pulmonary structures (Table 4-1) (see Chapter 5). These structures are the epithelial lung bud (embryonic stage), airways (pseudoglandular stage), vessels (canalicular or vascular stage), and alveoli (saccular and alveolar stages).[55] At the end of the first or embryonic stage of lung development, the lung bud is essentially a hollow mass of proliferating epithelium surrounded by mesenchyme. The basic pattern of the lung is established afterward, during the pseudoglandular stage, by repetitive branching of the epithelial bud. This process, termed *lung-branching morphogenesis,* is responsible for development of the basic pattern characteristic of the bronchial tree. This rudimentary lung serves as the basis for the assembly of vascular structures and subsequent formation of gas exchange units or alveoli.

Using data obtained from anatomic studies, various models have been proposed to describe the airway branching pattern. Some of these models are useful in predicting the number of generations developed and pathway lengths between branches, while other models are more suitable for studying the function of an airway tree in relation to its structure (see Chapter 2). Unfortunately, in general, these models provide little insight into the processes responsible for the branching process itself. Furthermore, most are based on the notion that dichotomous branching is the only mode of branching, while others have suggested that monochotomous branching occurs as well.[55] Because of this, these models will not be discussed further. Instead, we shall explore the cellular mechanisms believed to regulate lung branching during pattern formation and how they may come together in a simple mechanistic model.

TABLE 4-1

Stages of Lung Development

Stage	Period			
	Human (weeks)	Mouse (days)	Rat (days)	Rabbit (days)
Embryonic	0–6	9–10	0–13	0–18
Pseudoglandular	5–16	11–16	13–18	18–24
Canalicular	16–26	15–17	18–20	24–27
Saccular and alveolar	26–postnatal period	17–term	20–term	27–term

LUNG-BRANCHING MORPHOGENESIS

Epithelial-Mesenchymal Interactions

Unlike other aspects of biology, pattern formation is less amenable to study using isolated cells in culture. Instead, organ culture models that display organogenesis and can be manipulated with reagents that affect specific molecules or functions are necessary. With the aid of such models, it has been found that pattern formation cannot take place in the absence of organ growth. On the other hand, uncontrolled proliferation of cells leads to an amorphous mass. To prevent this, cell differentiation is required. By expressing or suppressing cellular genetic or phenotypic markers that distinguish them from their progenitors (or by alterations in cell function), differentiated cells trigger morphologic changes that drive pattern formation. The result is the expression of a set of signals that alter the morphologic state of an organ and drive it into another. Thus, pattern formation during organogenesis depends on organ growth (cell proliferation) and maturation (cell differentiation). Intense efforts are directed at identifying the factors that control cell proliferation, differentiation, and organization during embryogenesis and how they interact during lung formation.

As described above, the lung obtains its characteristic pattern during the process of lung-branching morphogenesis. Much insight into the molecules implicated in and the mechanisms responsible for lung-branching morphogenesis has been obtained in experiments performed in cultured lung explants. Under these conditions, lung explants (usually of mammalian origin) grow and branch similarly to lung in the in vivo situation, albeit much more slowly (Fig. 4-1). Studies performed in this and similar models (i.e., salivary glands) have suggested a role for epithelial-mesenchymal interactions in control of both cleft formation and growth. This is best depicted in experiments showing that dissection of the mesenchyme away from the developing lung epithelium prevents branching (Fig. 4-2A and 2B).[58] It is interesting to note that mesenchyme obtained from a variety of tissues elicits budding of the primitive gut endoderm (from which the lung originates), but only lung mesenchyme induces branching. Furthermore, attachment of mesenchymal tissue from distal branching areas of the lung (bronchial mesenchyme) to a more proximal nonbranching tubule (trachea) leads to the formation of new buds, whereas mesenchyme from proximal nonbranching areas prevents cleft formation when transplanted to the distal part of a growing lung branch (Fig. 4-2C).[4] Together, these and other studies suggest that signals provided by the mesenchyme induce epithelial branching in an organ- and species-specific fashion. Additionally, they reveal that the signals are not distributed uniformly within the mesenchyme, with inductive signals being more abundant distally. A consequence of these signals is the activation of mechanisms at work in lung growth and branching. These two processes (cell proliferation and cleft formation) act in concert to determine the final pattern of the lung.

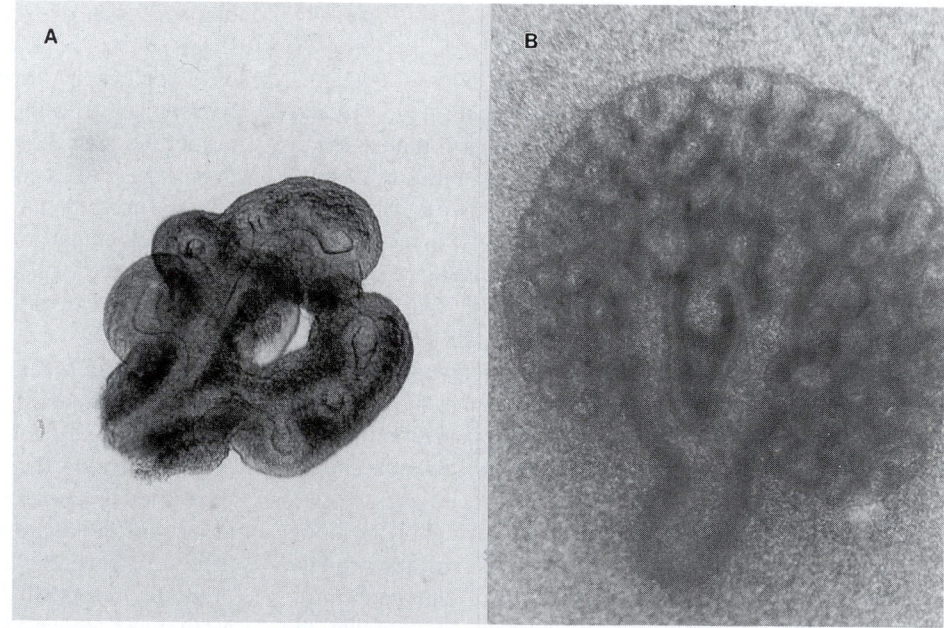

FIGURE 4-1 Lung-branching morphogenesis of cultured lung explants. Lungs from CD-1 murine embryos were obtained by microdissection at 11 days of gestation and maintained in the upper level of a culture chamber at the air-medium interface for 96 h. A lung was photographed at 11 days of gestation (*A*) and again after 3 days in culture (*B*). Note how the morphology has changed with growth of the organ and development of new branches. The dense background in *B* is due to the culture membrane on which the lung is resting.

Cell Proliferation

A critical role for cell proliferation in lung pattern formation is supported by studies showing that treatment of lung explants with reagents that block DNA synthesis (e.g., aphidicolin) results in aberrant lung branching. Epithelial-mesenchymal interactions are implicated in control of cell proliferation in lung.[16] This is demonstrated by studies showing that bronchial mesenchyme can maintain proliferation of epithelial cells. Furthermore, the rate of epithelial mitosis has been found to correlate well with the mass of lung mesenchyme present.[4,25]

Even though the aforementioned studies indicate that cell proliferation is necessary for branching, its exact role in this process remains unclear. Two hypotheses have been proposed that explain the role of cell proliferation in lung-branching morphogenesis. One hypothesis suggests that cell proliferation is supportive of this process in that, by providing an adequate cell mass, cleft formation can continue until further branching is prevented by spatial limitations imposed by thoracic size and contents. In other words, cell proliferation is important but not necessary for cleft formation. This concept is supported by in vitro studies showing that inhibition of DNA synthesis diminishes lung branching but does not abolish it completely.[44] In mammals, congenital diaphragmatic hernias cause lung agenesis or hypoplasia by impingement of the developing lung by the extravasated gastrointestinal tract. When present, the hypoplastic lungs show a decrease in number of airway generations, but the basic pattern of the bronchial tree is not lost.

A second hypothesis suggests a more active role for cell proliferation in lung pattern formation and is based on the observation that epithelial growth during lung development is not a uniform process. With use of autoradiography of lung explants, high rates of mitosis are found in epithelial cells present at the tips of developing airways, whereas low rates of mitosis are observed at the cleft site (Fig. 4-2D). Others have shown that the induction

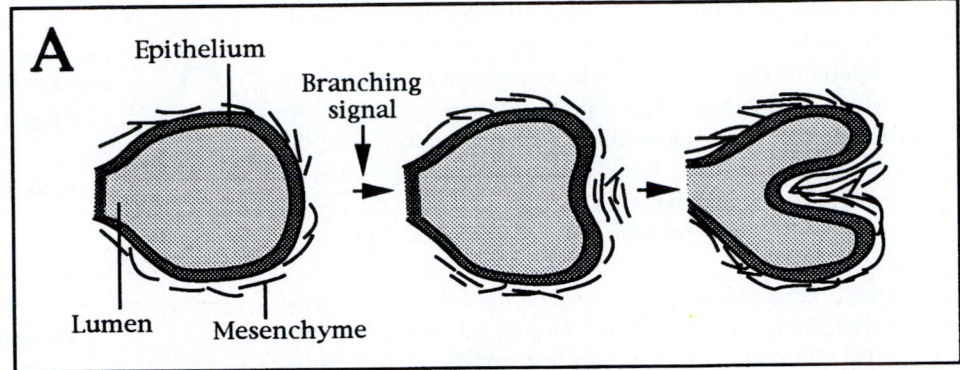

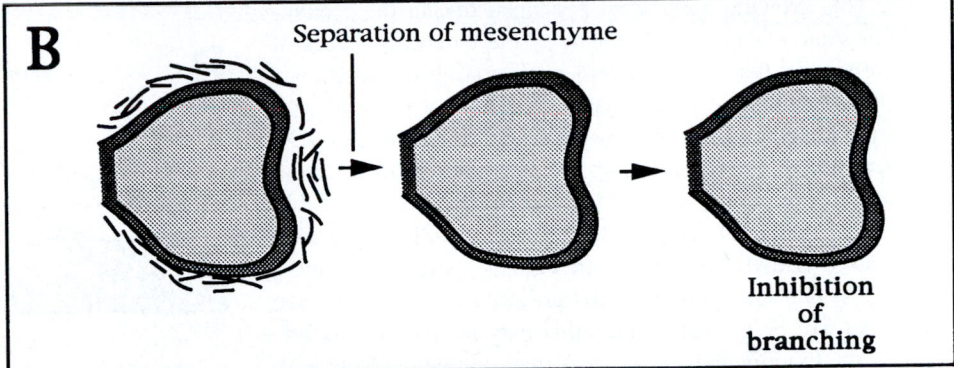

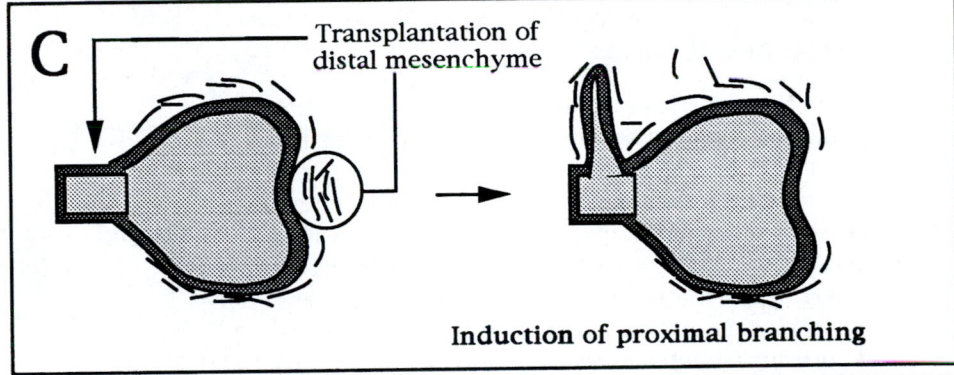

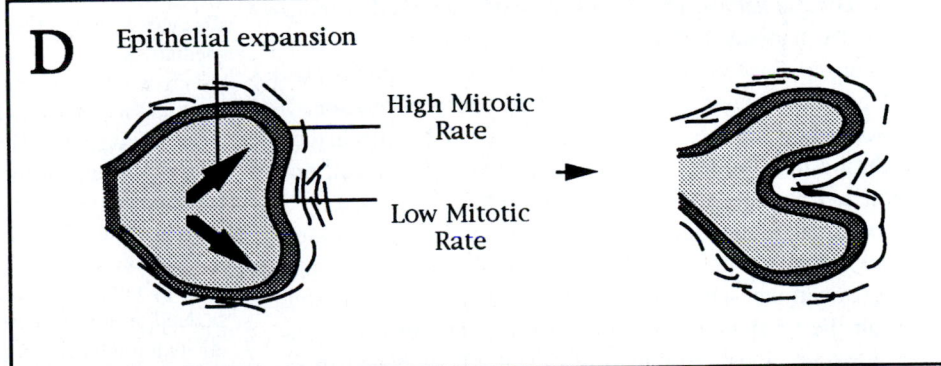

FIGURE 4-2   Epithelial-mesenchymal interactions in lung-branching morphogenesis. Experiments performed in cultured lung explants suggest epithelial-mesenchymal interactions are necessary for lung-branching morphogenesis. *A.* Schematic representation of cleft formation. Note that the airway bud is lined by epithelium and surrounded by mesenchyme. After several hours in culture, a cleft begins to appear, followed by branching of the airway. *B.* Removal of mesenchyme away from the epithelium prevents cleft formation. *C.* Transplantation of distal airway mesenchyme to the proximal portion of the airway results in budding of the proximal epithelium. On the contrary, transplantation of mesenchyme from proximal airways prevents branching of the distal epithelium (not shown). *D.* Epithelial cell proliferation in developing lungs is not uniform. High mitotic rates are found at the tips of the developing airways, whereas low mitotic rates are found at the cleft site.

of tracheal buds by bronchial mesenchyme correlates with the age of the trachea where the mesenchyme is implanted. For example, supernumerary budding can be induced in 11-day-old tracheas, which demonstrate high mitotic rates as determined by ^{3}H-thymidine uptake and autoradiography, but not in 13-day-old tracheas with lower mitotic rates. These studies suggest that by differentially affecting epithelial expansion, temporal and spatial control of epithelial cell proliferation is an integral part of the branching process.

Together, these and other data suggest the following scheme for lung-branching morphogenesis. During the late embryonic stage, cells within the primitive lung bud undergo active proliferation. This growing epithelium is shaped during the pseudoglandular stage of lung development by the balancing forces of inductive signals that maintain cells proliferating in specific areas of the growing bud, and negative signals that diminish cell proliferation in other areas, thereby creating the clefts (Fig. 4-2D). In general, it is believed that soluble polypeptide growth factors produced by both epithelium and mesenchyme are responsible for inducing epithelial cell growth, whereas insoluble extracellular matrix (ECM) deposited strategically within the mesenchyme around the epithelial mass prevents its expansion (see below). As will be discussed later, this may be an oversimplification of the function these molecules play in lung development.

Role of Mechanical Forces

Although the role of mechanical forces on lung development remains undefined, observations in humans with congenital anomalies and experimental animals suggest they are important. For example, conditions associated with impingement of developing lungs (e.g., congenital diaphragmatic hernias, chest wall deformities) are generally associated with pulmonary hypoplasia. Similarly, lung hypoplasia is observed in congenital disorders leading to abnormalities in fetal breathing movements or in animals with interruption of fetal breathing movements by severing of the phrenic nerves. These congenital and acquired disorders prevent cellular distention. This may have profound effects on organogenesis, since cellular distention has been demonstrated to be a potent stimulant for induction of cell proliferation. In other words, alterations in cell shape induced by mechanical forces during distention may result in abnormalities in cell proliferation and perhaps affect many other cellular processes.

The concept that alterations in cell shape may affect cell function is supported by many studies showing that rearrangements in the organizational state of the cell cytoskeleton cause profound effects on the expression of many genes.[30] The exact mechanisms by which cytoskeletal rearrangement affects gene expression are unknown. The cell cytoskeleton (actin microfilaments and microtubules) can be viewed as a network of cords that span from the internal surface of the plasma membrane to the surface of various organelles, including the nucleus. Some investigators have proposed that tension (developed at the plasma membrane) applies stress to certain membrane proteins linked to cytoskeletal structures. In turn, this results in "stiffening" of the cytoskeleton. The tension is transmitted to the nucleus, inducing, by unknown mechanisms, alterations in gene expression. This concept is known as *tensegrity* (Fig. 4-3).

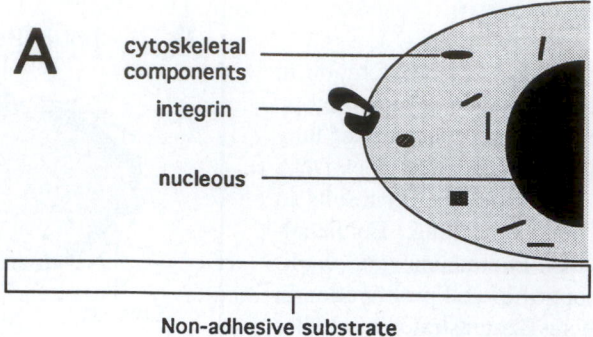

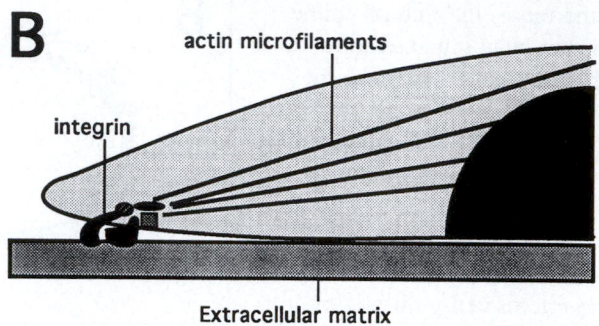

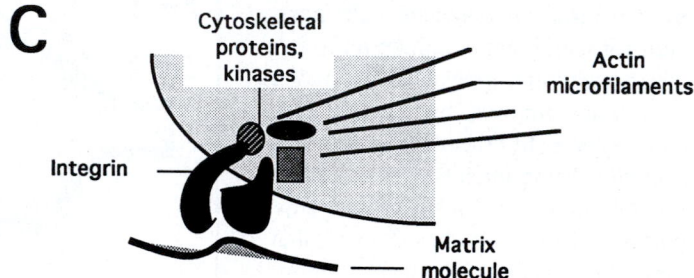

FIGURE 4-3 Interactions among extracellular matrices, integrins, and the cytoskeleton. Integrins are transmembrane cell surface receptors that mediate cell-matrix and cell-cell interactions. In the absence of adhesion to a substrate, integrins are diffusely distributed on the surface of cells and the cytoskeleton is disorganized (A). However, cell adhesion to a substrate induces the organization of integrins and cytoskeletal components (including the ends of actin microfilaments) into membrane structures termed focal adhesion complexes (B). Localization of integrins at focal adhesion complexes appears dependent on the β subunit cytoplasmic domain. This domain interacts with cytoskeletal proteins such as talin and α-actinin, which, in turn, interact with other cytoskeletal proteins, including vinculin and actin. In this manner, tension elicited at the cell surface by ligand binding to integrins is transmitted intracellularly. In addition to cytoskeletal components, focal adhesion complexes (C) contain many members of diverse signal transduction pathways, including protein kinases.

Tensegrity may explain why inhibition of cytoskeletal organization by reagents that affect actin polymerization (cytochalasins) prevents budding of mouse tracheal epithelium in a reversible manner. They may also explain the effects of fetal breathing movements on lung growth. However, it is difficult to envision how fetal breathing movements may affect lung pattern formation during branching morphogenesis, since they appear during the late stages of development, long after the bronchial tree is formed. Recently, attention has been directed to spontaneous airway contractions observed in embryonic mammalian and chick lung airways during the pseudoglandular stage of lung development, overlapping with the period of branching morphogenesis (Fig. 4-4).[44] The appearance of spontaneous contractile activity in developing airways coincides with the organization of smooth-muscle cells around the airways. In murine lung explants obtained at 11 days of gestation (corresponding to the first trimester in humans), proximal airway contractions are observed only after 48 h in culture. They occur every 20 to 60 s, are temperature dependent, and can be blocked by calcium channel blockers but not by tetrodotoxin or atropine, and can be enhanced by increased concentration of calcium, suggesting a myogenic rather than a neurogenic origin.[29] The airway contractions are associated with intraluminal fluid movement distally. This is probably due to contraction of the airway smooth muscle in the presence of a closed proximal portion of the trachea that is common in culture. With closing of the proximal airway, fluid is forced to move distally.

In vivo, airway contractions in the presence of proximal airway occlusion by the fetal glottis may increase intraluminal pressure and force the movement of intratubule fluid distally, causing distention of distal portions of the lung. As discussed before, distention may have profound effects on cell function. For example, it has been demonstrated that distention of cultured alveolar type II cells induces surfactant production. Cyclic mechanical deformation of cultured human lung fibroblasts results in increased cell proliferation.[6] This last observation correlates with the production of mitogenic factors secreted into the culture medium. Moreover, inhibition of airway contractions in embryonic murine lung explants by calcium channel blockade results in striking decreases in total lung DNA content.[44] Although definitive conclusions cannot be derived, these observations suggest that the airway contractions observed in embryonic lungs may increase the intraluminal pressure and promote distal cell distention, inducing cell proliferation and differentiation. If so, one would predict that manipulations leading to increased intraluminal pressure during contractions would enhance growth. This is indeed observed in lungs with laryngeal atresia and in experimental animals after tracheal ligation in which the fluid is forced to move distally.

Fetal lungs are known to generate mechanical forces that are likely to contribute to the process of lung-branching morpho-

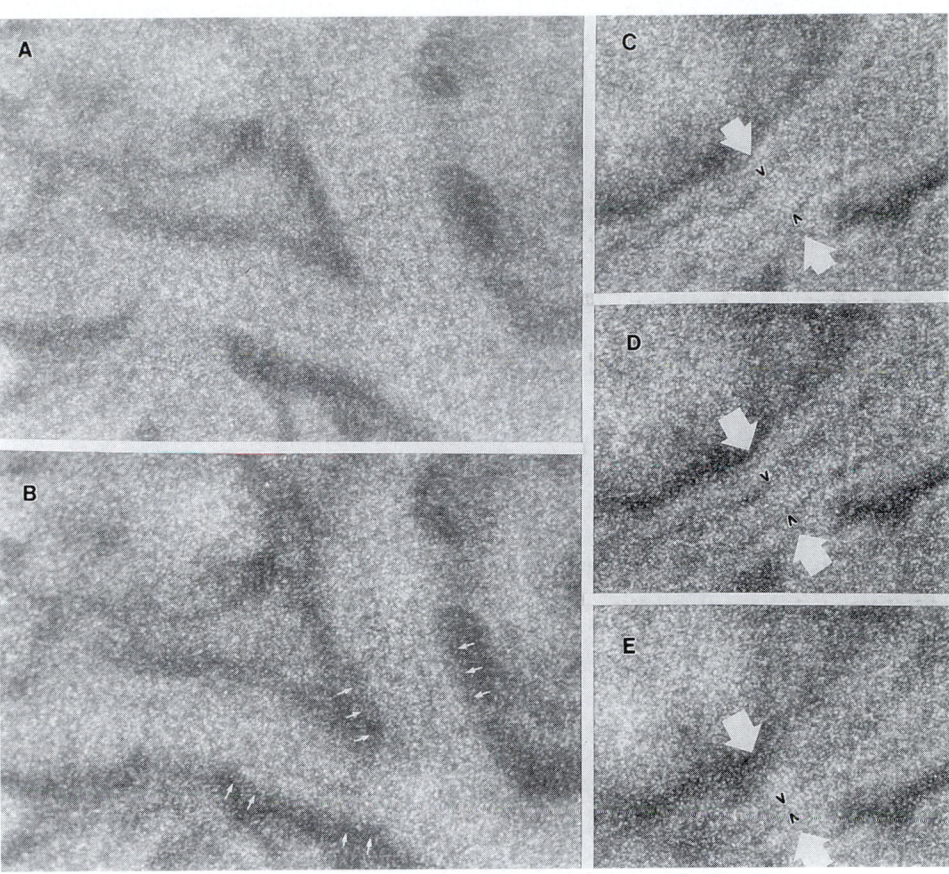

FIGURE 4-4   Airway contractions in cultured murine lungs. *A.* View of an early 13-day-old lung rudiment during relaxation phase (×200). *B.* Same lung rudiment during contraction of the proximal airways (small arrows). Note that at this stage, contractions of the proximal airways are weak. Fourteen-day-old lung rudiment during relaxation phase (*C*), midcontraction (*D*), and full contraction (*E*) (×400). White arrows show the location of the external diameter of the airways; small arrowheads show the location of the internal diameter. Note that the lumen becomes completely obliterated during a contraction.

genesis. Episodic contraction and relaxation of the fetal airways may increase the airway intraluminal pressure, cause fluid displacement, and induce alterations in tensile strength that are distributed across the entire primitive bronchial tree. This tension applied at the surface of cells may alter cell shape and elicit profound changes in cell proliferation, differentiation, and other functions.

Potential Role of Extracellular Matrices

It has already been mentioned that poorly defined epithelium- and mesenchyme-derived signals are likely to be important for induction of lung-branching morphogenesis. Of all the potential candidates, strong evidence favoring a role in lung-branching morphogenesis is available for ECM proteins. Embryogenesis is characterized by complex structural and compositional changes in the ECM of developing organs.[17,31] In lung, the ECM molecules laminin and collagen are present early on in development, and their amount increases steadily during embryogenesis. In rabbit, chick, and murine lungs, fibronectin concentration increases during the midpseudoglandular stage of lung development coinciding with branching morphogenesis; it decreases thereafter, coinciding with vessel formation during the canalicular stage.[47] In contrast, some thrombospondin variants increase during the late stages of lung development. As with thrombospondin, very little elastin content is found in lungs during the pseudoglandular stage, but it increases markedly during the saccular and alveolar stages. The types and amounts of glycosaminoglycans also change dramatically during lung development. In chick lung, hyaluronic acid is the predominant species in mesenchyme, and the content of sulfated glycosaminoglycans increases as development progresses.

These and other alterations in composition of the ECM in embryonic lungs are likely to influence lung-branching morphogenesis, since treatment of lung explants with various inhibitors of ECM deposition or degradation results in aberrant lung branching. This was found to be the case for reagents that affect collagen deposition. Incubation of lung explants with bacterial collagenases results in aberrant branching.[15,58] Similar results are obtained with reagents that affect collagen hydroxylation and secretion (e.g., α_1-dipyridyl, L-azetidine-2-carboxylic acid).[3] The importance of collagen in branching morphogenesis suggested by these studies is lessened by experiments performed with lungs obtained from Mov 3 mice, which are deficient in type I collagen.[24] In these mice, branching of the lung is observed as well as an increase in its content of type III collagen. The relevance of this last observation is unknown, but it is conceivable that although type I collagen may be important for branching, in its absence, other interstitial collagens (e.g., type III collagen) may replace it functionally. A redundancy in function of various related molecules may have the theoretical advantage to prevent abnormalities in pattern formation during such a critical embryonic stage.

Polyclonal antibodies to the basement membrane matrix molecule laminin also diminish lung branching, perhaps by affecting lung growth in vitro.[49] Synthetic peptides with sequences corresponding to SPARC, an ECM molecule with antiadhesive properties expressed in developing lungs, prevent normal lung branching morphogenesis. Inhibitors of synthesis of glycosaminoglycans (e.g., 6-diazo-5-oxo-L-norleucine, azaserine), which are also present in basal lamina, prevent branching morphogenesis of lungs. Similar observations were made in salivary glands with the inhibitor of proteoglycan synthesis β-xyloside.[56] Antiserum to tenascin-C, a matrix molecule also found in fetal lungs, inhibited branching of rat lung explants.[59] Finally, reagents that affect fibronectin matrix assembly in cultured lung fibroblasts diminish branching in murine lungs.[45]

Thus, the characteristic distribution of ECMs around developing airways, together with the aberrant branching observed in lung explants exposed to inhibitors of ECM expression and deposition, suggests a central role for ECMs in lung-branching morphogenesis. How can ECMs affect this process? One way in which ECMs can affect lung branching is by limiting or controlling epithelial expansion during lung-branching morphogenesis. Fibronectin, laminin, and collagens have been shown to induce the in vitro proliferation of epithelial cells, fibroblasts, and other cell types.[13] Of note, ECMs can enhance or diminish cell proliferation, depending on the cell type and culture conditions. Furthermore, ECMs may serve as a reservoir for growth-promoting factors, such as epidermal growth factor and fibroblast

growth factor, and may act synergistically with them to promote cell proliferation. Thus, ECMs can affect the proliferation of epithelial cells, and this effect could be enhanced or suppressed depending on the composition of the ECM. It should be noted that this concept implies a direct contact between epithelial cells and ECMs within the mesenchyme. Indeed, epithelial cells are in direct contact with ECMs present in their basement membrane. In addition, electron microscopic studies reveal that epithelial cells can directly contact other cells and matrix proteins present within the mesenchyme by extending foot processes through gaps present in the developing basement membrane.[7]

Another mechanism by which ECMs could affect cleft formation in the expanding lung epithelium is by mechanical obstruction to growth. Electron microscopy studies performed in salivary glands, which also undergo branching morphogenesis, revealed deposition of collagen in long cables at sites of cleft formation.[35] This is reminiscent of our own observations showing that fibronectin deposition is greatest at cleft sites in the developing lung, whereas little fibronectin is detected at the tips of growing airways (Fig. 4-5).[47] These observations suggest that ECM deposition is directed by unknown mechanisms to sites of future cleft formation, where they may limit epithelial expansion. This physical barrier may drive epithelial cells to migrate around the obstruction and, thus, bifurcate, forming a cleft. The more matrix "roadblocks" are deposited, more clefts are formed and, therefore, more airway branching occurs. This concept is consistent with the observation that reagents that inhibit matrix deposition or enhance matrix degradation can prevent normal branching. On the other hand, one would predict that an excessive number of matrix "roadblocks" could prevent normal branching from occurring.

For ECMs to serve as "roadblocks," they must be fixed in place to be able to transfer tension to the surface of cells. This is a complex process, since tension cannot be developed in the absence of contractile and expandable elements. Furthermore, for tension to be transmitted at a distance, a fulcrum is required for the stabilization of these contractile and expandable elements. The molecules and mechanisms described in the previous sections identify candidates for these elements. We propose that ECMs themselves provide the fulcrum by virtue of their singular distribution, which forms a continuous circular array around developing airways. This arrangement allows tension forces developed at any point along the airway to be distributed to all ECM molecules deposited around this structure. Thus, the tensile strength developed by contraction and relaxation of proximal airways would be transmitted distally to the ECM deposited at the tips of the growing airways, thereby inducing tension at the cell surface of distal epithelial cells. Ultimately, transmission of the force intracellularly may affect cytoskeletal organization—which, in turn, can affect gene expression, protein synthesis, and overall cell function, including mitosis, adhesion, migration, and differentiation, all necessary for normal lung development.

Differential regulation of epithelial expansion appears important for lung branching and pattern formation. ECMs may affect this process by localizing to specific sites, preventing mechanical expansion of the epithelium in some areas but not in others. In addition, ECMs may directly stimulate cells to proliferate at distinct points of the developing airway. Many processes other than cell proliferation can be affected by ECMs, including cell adhesion and migration, differentiation, and growth factor expression.[23,32] The molecules that mediate cell-matrix interactions (termed *integrins*) and the mechanisms entailed in the interpretation of matrix-induced messages by cells will be discussed next.

MATRIX-BINDING RECEPTORS OF THE INTEGRIN FAMILY

Integrins are cell surface glycoproteins that function in cell-cell and cell-matrix interactions.[10,23] These $\alpha\beta$ heterodimers are classified according to their β subunits into various subfamilies (i.e., β_1, β_2, β_3, etc.) (Fig. 4-6). The best-characterized matrix-binding integrins are members of the β_1 subfamily (also termed *VLAs,* for very late activation antigens) and include receptors for laminin, collagen, and fibronectin. Integrins in the β_2 (CD18) subfamily (*leucams*) are mainly concerned in cell-cell interactions. However, some β_2 integrins have been found to bind fibrin (i.e., CD11b/CD18 and CD11c/CD18). Integrins in the β_3 subfamily, or *cytoadhesins,* are expressed by endothelial cells and platelets and include receptors for vitronectin, fibrinogen, fibronectin, von Willebrand's factor, and thrombospondin.

In lung, integrins, particularly β_1 and β_3 integrins, are detected at very early stages of gestation. The α_5 subunit present in the fibronectin-binding $\alpha_5\beta_1$ complex is detected in mesenchymal cells of murine lungs as early as 11 to 12 days of gestation and is expressed in vascular structures as soon as they appear.[47] The appearance of $\alpha_5\beta_1$ in the mesenchyme coincides with the expression of α–smooth-muscle actin in spindle-shaped cells localized around the developing airways. This, and other data implicating fibronectin-$\alpha_5\beta_1$ binding in the differentiation of cultured muscle cells, suggests a role in airway smooth-muscle differentiation.[32] The α_4 subunit of the $\alpha_4\beta_1$ receptor is also detected in airway and vascular structures predominating in smooth-muscle cells. This receptor and one of its ligands, vascular cell adhesion molecule–1, or VCAM-1 ($\alpha_4\beta_1$

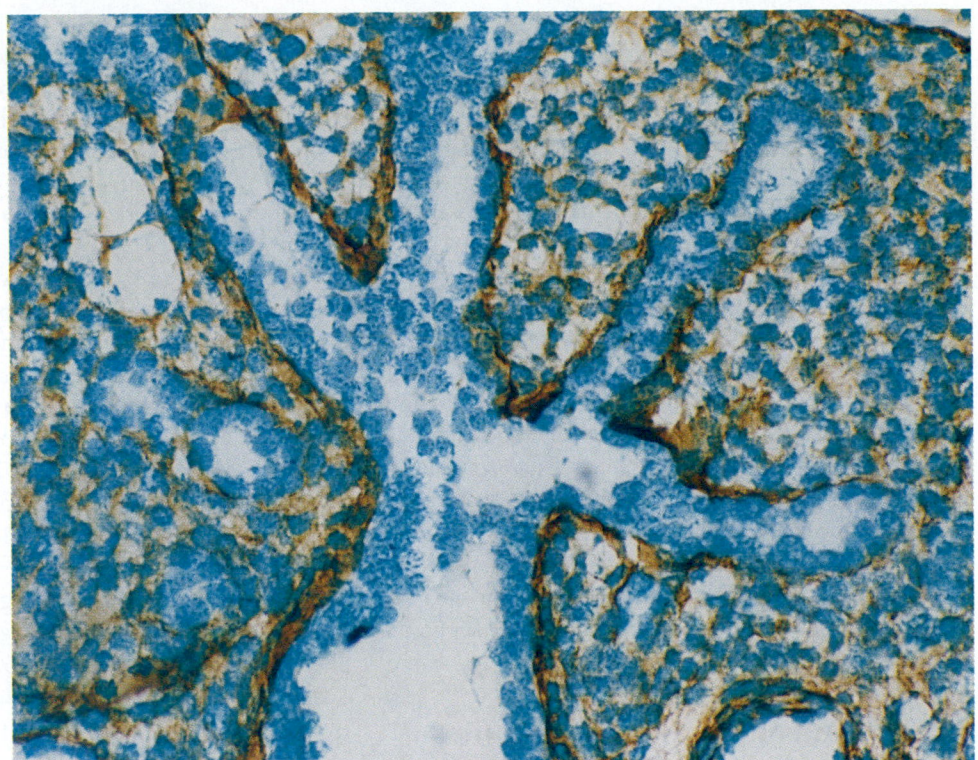

FIGURE 4-5   Distribution of fibronectin in developing lung. Murine lungs were obtained at 16 days of gestation, frozen, and processed for immunostaining with polyclonal antibodies to fibronectin. At this stage, fibronectin was detected with mesenchymal cells—in particular, cells localized around the developing airways and vessels. Note the intensity of the staining for fibronectin at the cleft sites, whereas little staining is found at the tips. (*Based on data of Roman and McDonald,*[47] *with permission.*)

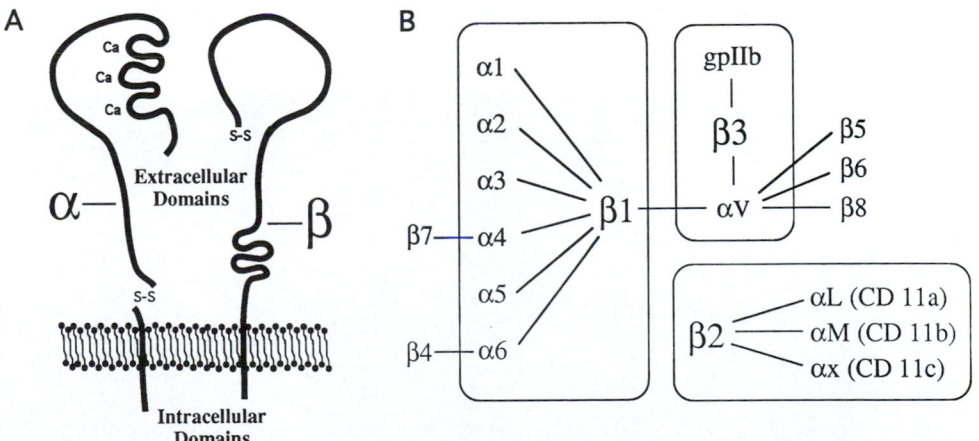

FIGURE 4-6   The integrin receptor family. *A.* Schematic representation of an integrin receptor. Integrins are heterodimeric glycoproteins expressed by diverse cell types, including fibroblasts, epithelial and endothelial cells, and leukocytes. Integrins consist of transmembrane α and β subunits. The α subunits contain several divalent cation binding sites considered important for ligand binding. In general, the β subunits contain various conserved cysteines, which are arranged in four repeating units. *B.* Integrin subunit associations. Integrin α subunits are known to associate with different β subunits. The identity of each subunit in any given heterodimer determines ligand-binding specificity. Initially, integrins were divided into 3 subfamilies according to their β subunit (e.g., β_1, β_2, and β_3). However, newly discovered integrin subunits and associations have limited the usefulness of this classification scheme.

also binds fibronectin), are also considered important in myogenic differentiation. The α_3 subunit is expressed in epithelial cells of developing airways, and $\alpha_v\beta_3$ receptors are present in epithelial and mesenchymal cells, including vessels.[46] It has recently been reported in preliminary form that integrin subunits α_1, α_2, α_6, and α_9 are present in developing lungs as well.

Extracellularly, many integrins, particularly some members of the β_1 and β_3 subfamilies, bind an RGD (Arg-Gly-Asp) amino acid sequence present in their ligands. The RGD sequence is found in various matrix proteins, including fibronectin, thrombospondin, fibrinogen, vitronectin, laminin, and type I collagen. This observation has been extremely important, as synthetic peptides containing this sequence inhibit ligand binding to integrin receptors and have been used to study the role of integrins in various biologic systems. Strong evidence for the role of integrins in lung development is derived from studies showing that incubation of murine lung explants with RGD peptides prevents lung branching, whereas control peptides had no effect (Fig. 4-7).[46] This information not only suggests a role for integrin receptors in lung development but also provides further support for the role of ECMs in this process.

Role of Growth Factors and Growth Factor Receptors

Polypeptide growth factors are also likely to play key roles in lung-branching morphogenesis. By binding to specific membrane-bound receptors, epithelial- and mesenchyme-derived polypeptide growth factors can affect cellular functions in autocrine and paracrine fashions. Many growth factors are detected in developing lungs, and their role in lung-branching morphogenesis has been tested in lung explant models. One potential player in lung-branching morphogenesis is *epidermal growth factor* (EGF). EGF is a polypeptide detected in many murine and human tissues, where it can bind to specific transmembrane receptors (EGFR). An important feature of these receptors is their intrinsic tyrosine kinase activity and their ability for autophosphorylation, an important step required for signal transduction and induction of mitogenesis. *Transforming growth factor–α* (TGF-α) is homologous to EGF and binds to the same receptor. EGF, TGF-α, and EGFR are found in embryonic tissues, including the lung—in particular, pseudoglandular-stage lungs—and EGF and TGF-α can induce proliferation of embryonic cells in culture.[57] When added exogenously, EGF stimulates branching morphogenesis of tracheal epithelium in embryonic chick lung explants. In embryonic murine lung explants, exogenous addition of EGF results in increased DNA, RNA, and protein content and enhances branching.[57] Antisense oligonucleotides against EGF can block murine lung branching and growth as well.[52] Like EGF, TNF-α is considered to have a stimulatory role in branching, since addition of exogenous TNF-α to murine lung explants results in increased lung branching and expression of surfactant protein A.[22] However, these results contrast with another report, showing that EGF- and TGF-α–treated lungs displayed fewer branches along with dilated end buds that lacked clefts.[15]

Transforming growth factor–β (TGF-β) has also been implicated in lung-branching morphogenesis. The mammalian TGF-β family consists of three related proteins—TGF-β_1, TGF-β_2, and TGF-β_3. TGF-βs are capable of varied effects that may be relevant during embryogenesis. For example, TGF-βs are known to stimulate the expression of various genes encoding for ECM molecules, including collagen and fibronectin. In addition, they stimulate cell surface expression of matrix-binding integrin receptors. Not only do TGF-βs enhance ECM expression, but they also decrease the expression of genes encoding proteases that degrade ECMs and enhance the expression of protease inhibitors. TGF-β may also enhance cell proliferation by inducing the expression of certain oncogenes (e.g., c-*sis*) and growth factors that regulate the cell cycle. The varied effects of TGF-β may be

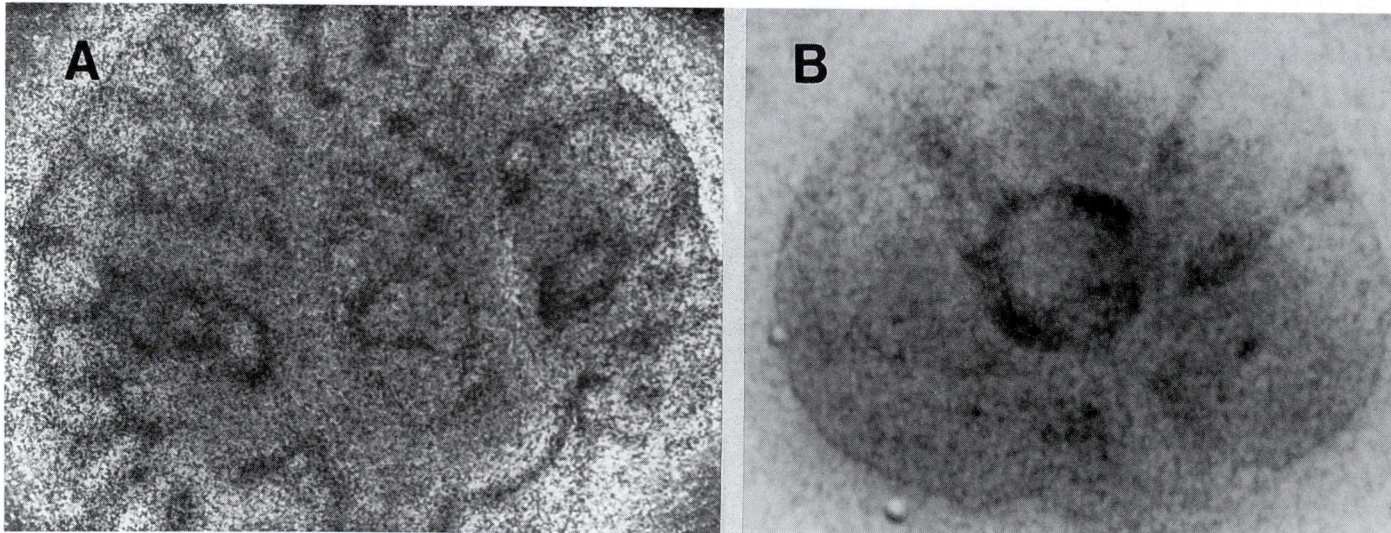

FIGURE 4-7 RGD peptides diminish branching of 11-day-old embryonic lung rudiments. *A.* Control murine lung rudiment obtained at 11 days of gestation and cultured for 37 h. Note the extensive amount of branches. *B.* Experimental 11-day-old lung rudiment cultured for 72 h in the presence of 1 mg/ml of peptide GRGDSP. There is asymmetry and enlargement of airways when compared to the control, as well as marked reduction in the number of branches. *(Based on data of Roman et al,[46] with permission.)*

explained by the fact that it binds not one but three receptors (termed TGFβR 1 through 3). With in situ hybridization, TGF-βs 1–3 have been detected in the lung and in regions of active morphogenesis involving epithelial-mesenchymal interactions.[33] Because, in general, TGF-β opposes the actions of other growth factors (e.g., EGF) when examined in cultured cells, one might predict that TGF-β would inhibit lung-branching morphogenesis. This is exactly what has been reported from examination in cultured lung explants.[51] Of interest, the ability of TGF-β to inhibit lung branching is associated with inhibition of expression of the proto-oncogene N-myc. Since lungs obtained from homozygous N-myc–deficient transgenic mice show failure to undergo branching morphogenesis, it has been speculated that N-myc is important for branching and that TGF-β inhibits lung branching by inhibiting N-myc expression. However, recent studies performed in transgenic animals with homozygous null mutation for the retinoblastoma gene (Rb), which is necessary for N-myc expression, suggest that the inhibitory effects of TGF-β on lung branching are independent of its ability to suppress N-myc expression.

The *platelet-derived growth factors* (PDGFs) were first identified in platelets. However, like other growth factors, they are now known to be produced by many cell types, including macrophages, smooth-muscle cells, and fibroblasts. PDGFs are dimers formed by A and B chains of 15-kD molecular weight. These dimers bind to PDGF receptors, which are related structurally to members of the immunoglobulin receptor family and, like the EGFR, possess intrinsic tyrosine kinase activity. PDGF receptors are expressed by mesenchymal cells; that explains the potent mitogenic and chemotactic effects of PDGFs on cells of mesenchymal origin. In lungs, PDGF-AA and PDGF-BB have been localized to airway epithelial cells as early as day 12 of gestation in rats. They are expressed in mesenchymal cells somewhat later. Rat lung explants exposed to PDGF-A antisense oligonucleotides or anti–PDGF-AA antibodies showed diminished DNA content, reduced size, and diminished number of terminal buds.[53] In contrast, PDGF-B chain-specific antisense oligonucleotides inhibited DNA synthesis in cultured lungs but did not have a significant effect on number of terminal buds.[54]

Among the heparin-binding growth factors is the *fibroblast growth factor* (FGF) family, which includes two highly homologous forms: acidic FGF (aFGF) and basic FGF (bFGF). By binding to specific FGF receptors, FGFs exert potent mitogenic effects on cells of mesodermal and neuroectodermal origin. In embryonic lungs, the FGF receptor gene FGFR2 is expressed in the epithelium of lung buds. Using the human surfactant protein C promoter to target expression of a dominant negative FGFR2 in lung epithelium in transgenic mice, investigators were able to study the potential role of FGFs in lung development.[41] Experimental animals expressed a striking phenotype showing that a dominant negative FGF receptor prevented lung branching, resulting in two undifferentiated epithelial tubes extending from the bifurcation of the trachea to the diaphragm.

The *somatomedins, or insulinlike growth factors* (IGFs), are expressed in early embryogenesis. These peptide hormones are well known for their growth-promoting activities in many tissues. The IGF receptor–1 (IGFR-1) is a transmembrane glycoprotein similar to the insulin receptor and, like the EGFR and

PDGFR, contains an insulin-dependent protein tyrosine kinase domain with intrinsic enzymatic activity. This contrasts with the IGFR-2, which does not possess intrinsic enzymatic activity. Members of the IGF system are present in lungs throughout development, including IGF-I and -II, IGF receptors, and the IGF-binding protein, which binds to IGFs.[34] Expression of IGF receptors appears to be developmentally regulated as assessed by PCR and in situ hybridization. For example, IGFR-1 and IGFR-2 are present in the epithelium of 14-day-old lungs but not in 18-day-old lungs, followed by reexpression in the postnatal period.[26]

Recently, the role of another class of growth factors in lung development has been investigated. *Bombesin-like peptides* (BLPs), derived from neuroendocrine cells, are transiently up-regulated during lung development. Expression of BLP receptors has also been demonstrated in pseudoglandular-stage lungs using reverse transcriptase polymerase chain reaction. Exogenous addition of bombesin to lung explants resulted in a modest increase in lung branching without significant changes in DNA content.[1] These effects were blocked by bombesin analogs and enhanced by phosphoramidon, an inhibitor of neutral endopeptidases capable of degrading neuropeptides (Fig. 4-8). Another neuropeptide, *endothelin,* has also been implicated in lung development, but its role in this process is less well defined. Together, these results suggest a prominent role for neuroendocrine cells and neuropeptides in lung development.

Polypeptide growth factors can affect many cellular processes directly or by inducing the expression of other factors with distinct effects. Although they were originally identified because of their mitogenic activity, these growth factors are known to affect many other aspects of cellular function. After secretion into the

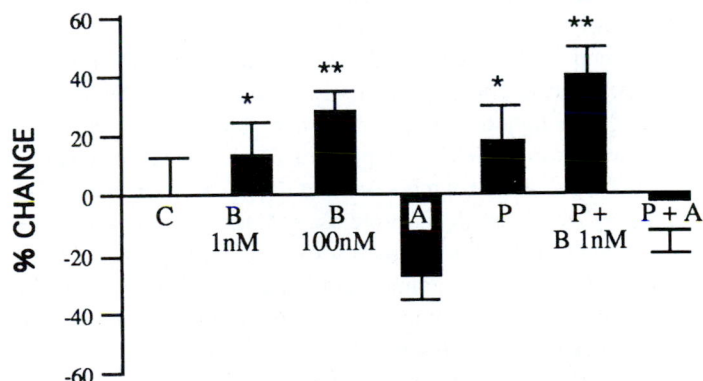

FIGURE 4-8 Effects of bombesin, bombesin-like peptide antagonist, and phosphoramidon on airways branching in vitro. Embryonic murine lungs were obtained at 11 days of gestation and cultured in the presence of bombesin (B), bombesin-like peptide (BLP) receptor antagonist (A), and phosphoramidon (P) for 96 h. Note that bombesin (B) and phosphoramidon (P) had a stimulatory effect. The receptor antagonist (A), the BLP analog (Leu13-psi[Ch2Nh]-Leu114)-bombesin, had an inhibitory effect. *p <0.05 in comparison with the embryonic lungs that were treated with the BLP receptor antagonist. **p <0.05 in comparison with the group that received both phosphoramidon and BLP receptor antagonist (P + A). Differences in fold increase in branching were examined with the Kruskal-Wallis test for multiple comparisons between the various experimental groups, and with the Mann-Whitney rank-sum test for comparisons between any two treatment groups. *(Based on data from Aguayo et al,[1] with permission.)*

extracellular space, they may bind to receptors present on epithelial and mesenchymal cells or may be sequestered in the extracellular matrix, where they remain until released by matrix-degrading enzymes activated during tissue remodeling. In general, their role in morphogenesis is considered to be inductive by promoting epithelial cell proliferation and/or differentiation; however, some polypeptide growth factors are negative inducers. Growth factors cannot sustain lung-branching morphogenesis, which requires the presence of ECM. The need for both ECMs and growth factors for lung-branching morphogenesis is best exemplified by recent studies showing that embryonic mouse lung epithelium separated from its mesenchyme and cultured in mesenchyme-free conditions can be induced to undergo branching morphogenesis by addition of basement membrane matrix and a growth factor (aFGF).[40]

SIGNAL TRANSDUCTION VIA INTEGRINS AND GROWTH FACTOR RECEPTORS

The mechanisms by which ECMs and growth factors affect cell function are not entirely understood. When bound,

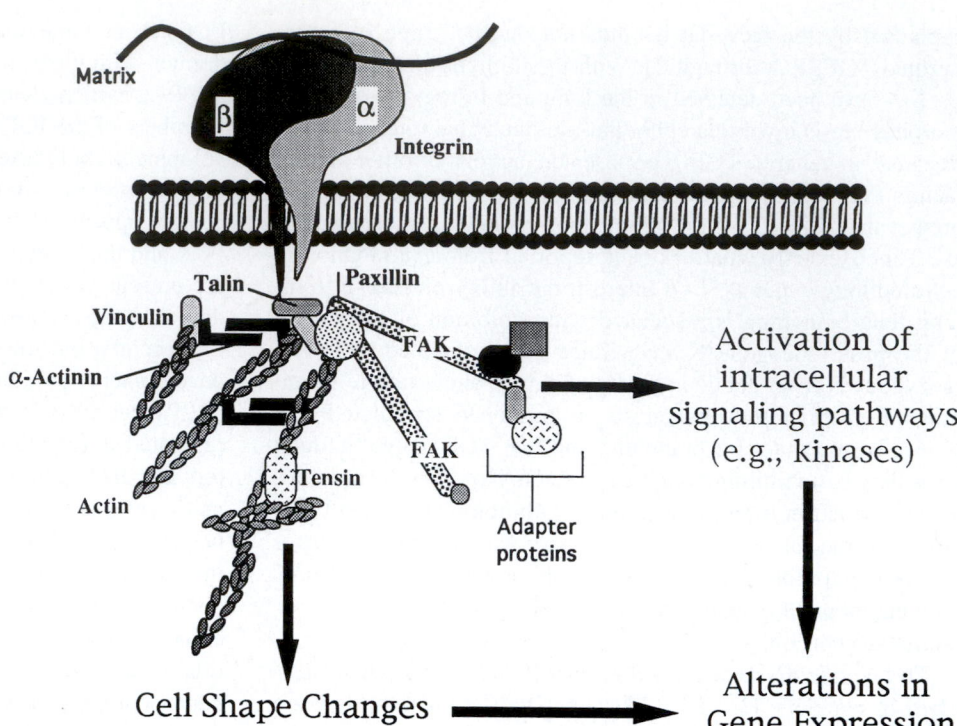

FIGURE 4-9 Signal transduction via matrix-binding integrins. Ligand binding to integrins induces their clustering at focal adhesion complexes (FACs), where they codistribute with cytoskeletal proteins. In addition to cytoskeletal proteins, proteins with kinase activity interact with integrins intracellularly. One example is pp120 kD focal adhesion kinase, or pp125^{FAK}. By interacting with "adapter" proteins (e.g., Grb2, Crk), FAK links integrins with other kinases (e.g., mitogen-activated protein) and components of the membrane phospholipid metabolism responsible for induction of protein kinase C, both regulators of gene transcription. Thus, by interactions with cytoplasmic proteins, integrins can induce signals that not only affect cell shape but also activate intracellular signal transduction pathways that result in altered gene expression.

these receptors induce the activation of various intracellular signal transduction pathways believed critical for the biologic effects of their ligands. Integrins, for example, interact intracellularly with cytoskeletal components such as talin, vinculin, α-actinin, and actin (Figures 4-3 and 4-9). The interaction of integrins with cytoskeletal proteins and the interaction of cytoskeletal proteins between themselves and other proteins appear dependent on specific amino acid sequences (termed SH_2 and SH_3 domains) that mediate these protein-protein interactions. This allows for ligand binding to integrins to alter the organizational state of the cytoskeleton, thereby affecting various cellular functions. It must be emphasized, however, that not all integrin-mediated signals are dependent on alterations in cytoskeletal organization and cell shape, at least as assessed by currently available techniques. Ligand binding to integrins elicits the activation of many intracellular signals implicated in signal transduction, including Na^+/H^+ antiporters, calcium fluxes, protein phosphorylations, and protein kinase C (Fig. 4-9).[10,23]

Similar to integrins, ligand binding to growth factor receptors elicits many cellular responses in signal transduction.[48] These include Na/H exchange, calcium fluxes, stimulation of glucose and amino acid transport, and phosphorylation of serine and threonine residues on many proteins. Another effect is activation of phospholipase C–γ, which leads to generation of phosphoinositol metabolites such as 1,4,5-triphosphate, which causes release

of calcium from intracellular compartments and generation of diacylglycerol. In turn, diacylglycerol induces activation of the serine/threonine kinase protein kinase C. In addition to the above, several peptide growth factor receptors contain intrinsic tyrosine kinase activity (e.g., PDGFR, EGFR, IGFR-1). Although the steps following tyrosine kinase phosphorylation of intracellular substrates have not been entirely defined, it is clear that this process is linked to various signaling pathways, since substrates for tyrosine kinases include phospholipase C–γ, phosphatidylinositol 3-kinase, the ras GTPase-activating protein, and the c-*raf* proto-oncogene.

From the discussion, it is evident that signal transduction elicited by ligand binding to growth factor receptors triggers the induction of molecules common to signaling pathways triggered by ligand binding to integrin receptors. This may explain how ECMs enhance the mitogenic effects of certain growth factors and vice versa. The mechanisms that link integrins and growth factor receptors are subject to intense investigation. Recently, the kinase pp125^{FAK} has been shown to exhibit both growth factor– and ECM-dependent phosphorylation on tyrosine. This tyrosine kinase codistributes with integrins at focal adhesion contacts or complexes (FACs), where it appears to bind to their β-cytoplasmic domain. FACs are membrane structures whose formation is elicited by ligand binding to integrins and which contain cytoskeletal and noncytoskeletal proteins (Fig. 4-10). Because

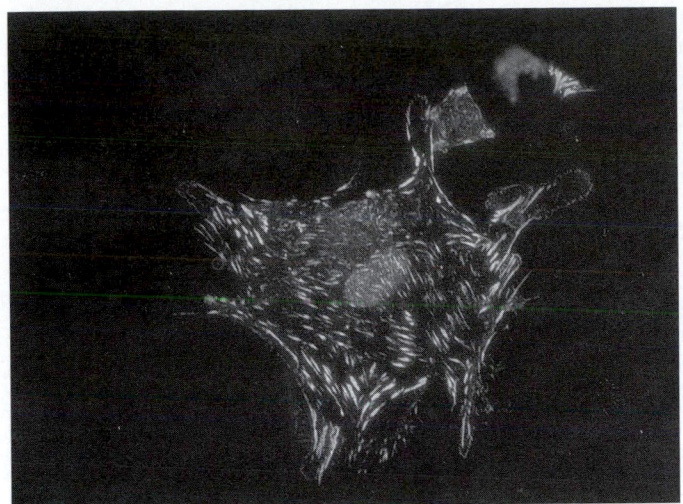

FIGURE 4-10   Distribution of focal adhesion complexes (FACs) on cultured human fetal lung fibroblasts. IMR-90 fetal lung fibroblasts were cultured overnight in the presence of serum on surfaces coated with fibronectin, fixed, permeabilized, and immunostained with an antibody to the fibronectin receptor $\alpha_5\beta_1$. Note that the receptor is concentrated in needle eye–shaped structures termed focal adhesion complexes that mediate cell-substrate adhesion and are typically found at the cell periphery.

pp125[FAK] and other kinases (e.g., *src,* protein kinase C) and signaling molecules have been found to codistribute with integrins at FACs when examined with immunofluorescence, it has been postulated that integrins "integrate" a variety of different signaling pathways (including those induced by growth factor receptors) by promoting the formation of a specialized cytoskeletal scaffold that serves to orient various receptors and chemical signaling molecules such as intracellular kinases. Evidence supporting this concept has been recently obtained.[42] Examination of endothelial cell FACs isolated using magnetic microbeads coated with fibronectin or RGD peptides revealed the presence of tyrosine kinases pp60c-*scr* and pp125[FAK], phospholipase C–γ, the Na/H antiporter, and high-affinity fibroblast growth factor receptors. Thus, cell adhesion to ECMs induces the formation of FACs that provide a substratum for the convergence of integrin and growth factor signaling pathways.

ECMs and growth factors can transmit key signals to embryonic lung cells that can drive their organization into a branching multicellular structure. By acting as positive and negative inducers, these molecules can induce differential cell proliferation and cleft formation, thereby leading to lung pattern formation.

Retinoic Acid and Retinoic Acid Receptors

Retinoids are considered *morphogens,* very small molecules known to influence pattern formation during organogenesis. Their effects on morphogenesis may be explained by effects on genes directly implicated in pattern formation such as matrix molecules and growth factors. Another group of genes targeted by retinoids are homeobox (Hox) genes. Hox genes are DNA transcription factors considered important for the expression of site- and time-specific signals needed for pattern formation. To date, at least 16 different Hox genes have been identified in newborn mouse lung.[8]

The role of retinoids in organogenesis has been extensively studied in limb formation. However, several reports suggest they play important roles in lung development as well. This is not surprising, since receptors for retinoic acid have been detected in developing lungs. Treatment with retinoic acid results in significant alterations in the expression of Hox genes in rat lung explants.[8] It also induces proliferation of isolated embryonic lung mesenchymal cells and increased branching of mouse lung explants.[50] It has been demonstrated that retinoic acid interferes with the transcription of epithelial genes typically expressed by distal segments of developing lungs (e.g., surfactant proteins) and that high concentrations of retinoic acid favor growth of proximal airway structures (Fig. 4-11).[11] This was interpreted as a

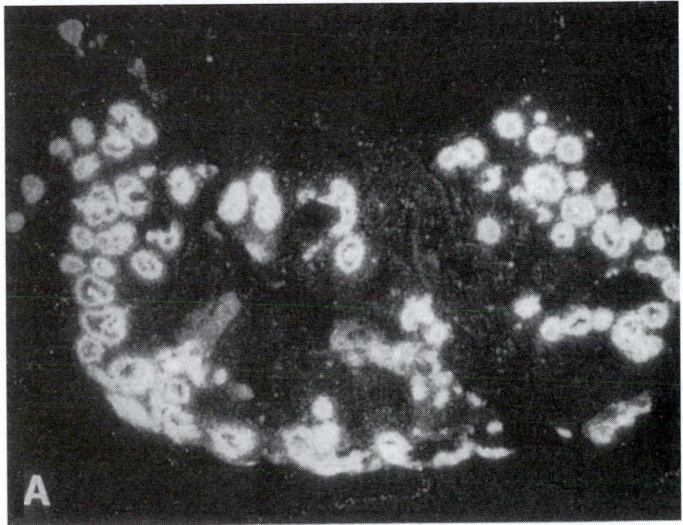

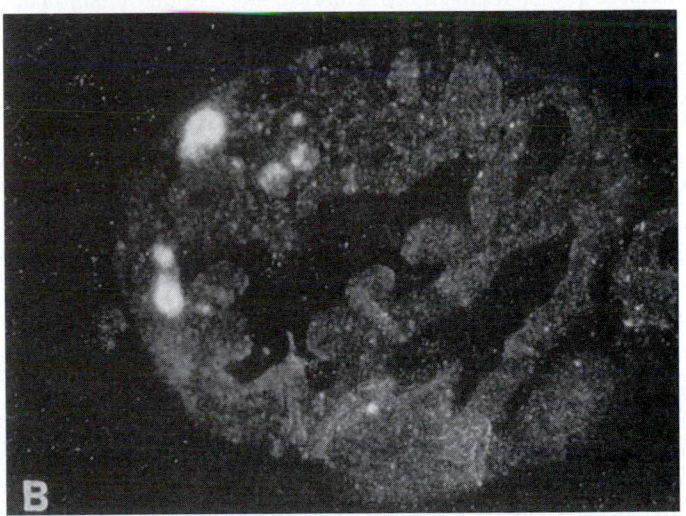

FIGURE 4-11   In situ hybridization of SP-C mRNA expression in control and retinoic acid (RA)–treated embryonic lungs. Rat lungs were cultured in the absence (*A*) or presence (*B*) of RA 10^{-5} M for 5 days. Note that the surfactant protein C (SP-C) mRNA is expressed in the epithelium of the most distal tubules of control lungs. In RA-treated explants, very few of these distal structures are still present in restricted areas and they express SP-C mRNA, while the great majority of the large tubules extending to the distal portions of the explant do not express SP-C mRNA. (*Based on data from Cardoso et al,*[11] *with permission.*)

"proximalizing" effect; in other words, retinoic acid altered the pattern of the lung to one dominated by proximal airway structures rather than distal differentiation into alveolar sacs. The aforementioned studies performed in lung explants revealed findings similar to those in animals with alterations in retinoic acid responsiveness. For example, compound null mutations of retinoic acid receptor genes are lethal in utero. When examined, these embryos show abnormalities in many organs, including the lung. In general, these abnormalities are similar to those described above and those described in the fetal vitamin A deficient syndrome. The above-mentioned studies suggest that retinoids may influence lung-branching morphogenesis by regulating the expression of specific genes affecting the differentiation of proximal/distal and medial/lateral structures necessary for pattern formation.

Role of Cell-Cell Interactions

In addition to receiving extracellular signals from ECMs and polypeptide growth factors, cells can communicate with each other. Cells interact physically with each other via specific surface receptors. Similar to the cell-matrix receptors, cell-cell adhesion molecules interact with cytoplasmic proteins, including the cytoskeleton. Unlike the cell-matrix receptors, some receptors that mediate cell-cell interactions are implicated in homophilic interactions (cadherins); in other words, they bind to similar molecules on other cells. In general, cell-cell adhesion molecules are members of the *cadherin, integrin,* and *immunoglobulin* families.

Although little is known about the expression and potential function of cell-cell adhesion molecules in developing lungs, studies of cadherins are tantalizing. Cadherins are surface receptors composed of a single transmembrane polypeptide chain. They are classified in four subgroups: the epithelial or E-cadherins (found mainly in epithelial cells), the neural or N-cadherins (found in adult neural tissues and muscle), the placental or P-cadherins (found in placenta and epithelial cells), and the vascular or V-cadherins (expressed mainly in endothelial cells). In lung, P- and E-cadherins have been detected in the epithelial cells of developing airways. Incubation of lung explants with monoclonal antibodies to both P- and E-cadherins partly suppressed branching and distorted the arrangement of epithelial cells showing flat epithelial lobules devoid of luminal space.[18]

LUNG VASCULARIZATION

Once the basic pattern of the lung is established, the rudimentary lung provides the scaffold on which endothelial cells organize into vascular structures. The mechanisms at work in vascular formation during lung development remain largely unknown. This is due in part to the absence of an appropriate experimental model for the study of lung vascularization, and to the fact that isolated congenital abnormalities (e.g., unilateral absence of a pulmonary artery) are very rare. Most abnormalities in pulmonary circulation are associated with major alterations in lung structure related to lung hypoplasia, dysplasia, and hyperplasia.[12] This suggests that the factors controlling vessel formation in lung are linked to the formation of the airways, and indicates that per-

haps a good understanding of vessel formation can be attained only after a better appreciation of the regulatory factors entailed in the formation of airways and the interdependence among the various processes responsible for their development.

Vascular structures appear within the mesenchyme of embryonic lungs during the late stages of development, when two separate vascular systems are formed and become connected before birth. One vascular system is composed of the central pulmonary and bronchial arteries and veins, which originate outside the lung, invade the lung parenchyma, and connect with the distal pulmonary circulation or microvasculature. This distal pulmonary circulation develops within the lung mesenchyme and is formed by endothelial cells (ECs) of nonpulmonary origin that have invaded the lung mesenchyme, and ECs of pulmonary origin that result from the in situ differentiation of mesodermal cells. ECs of both origins cluster into discrete areas around the developing airways, where they organize into elongated cords around a central lumen surrounded by cells that develop into smooth muscle. The idea that the pulmonary circulation develops as two separate systems is supported by reports of neonates' showing isolated absence of pulmonary artery capillaries or no connection between capillaries and the central pulmonary arteries.

BASIC MECHANISMS OF VESSEL FORMATION

By 16 weeks of human gestation, airway branching is almost complete and the *canalicular stage* (also termed *vascular stage*) of lung development begins (16 to 28 weeks). Formation of the acinus, differentiation of the acinar epithelium, and development of the distal pulmonary circulation take place during this stage. Capillary networks derived from EC precursors (also termed *angioblasts*) extend from and around distal airspaces and connect with the developing pulmonary arteries and veins. Two distinct processes are considered important for formation of these vascular networks: *vasculogenesis* and *angiogenesis*.[43] In this review, vasculogenesis is defined as the process by which randomly distributed mesodermal cells differentiate into ECs, proliferate, and organize into multicellular structures singularly arranged around a central lumen (Fig. 4-12). Angiogenesis is defined as the process by which differentiated ECs proliferate and sprout from previously formed vessels to form new vascular structures. The relative contribution of vasculogenesis and angiogenesis to development of the pulmonary vasculature has been studied in transplantation experiments performed in developing chick, quail, and, more recently, mouse tissues. These studies suggest that although some organs, such as the brain and kidney, are vascularized by sprouting of ECs from vessels that invade the rudiments (angiogenesis), vasculogenesis is the predominant method of vascularization in lung.[39]

Much of our knowledge related to vessel formation is derived from studies using EC lines (not from lung origin) in migration and proliferation assays, as well as in vitro assays of vasculogenesis and angiogenesis. In the vasculogenesis assay, ECs are cultured on two- or three-dimensional substrates containing one or more ECM components in the presence of serum or well-defined growth factors (Fig. 4-13). Studies using this system have shown that in vitro capillary tube or "cord" formation is characterized by a series of morphologic changes that include EC migration, invasion of the ECM, and development of cell-cell connections. Once the cords are formed, cellular retraction and elevation above the surface of the rigid substrate are followed by involution of cells around a lumen.[19] Other assays examine angiogenesis by culturing previously formed vascular structures, such as aortic vessel wall or rat corneal explants, on three-dimensional ECM substrates.[9]

As expected, experiments performed in such assays reveal that EC adhesion to the substrate, migration, and proliferation are necessary for the initiation and progression of both vasculogenesis and angiogenesis. As observed for lung-branching morphogenesis, these processes are regulated by growth factors and ECMs.[19] Although both signals are critical, studies directed at examining in vitro EC cord formation suggest that the influence of ECMs predominates.

Role of Cell-Matrix Interactions in Vessel Formation

In vitro, ECMs stimulate directional and nondirectional migration of cultured human umbilical ECs and bovine aortic ECs, among others. ECMs also influence the growth and differentiation of ECs in culture.[20] In addition, insoluble ECMs provide an adhesive scaffold for building elongated vascular structures in vitro. For example, fibronectin, a major component of the ECM of developing microvessels, promotes vessel elongation during angiogenesis.[37] Collagen matrices promote EC organization into capillary networks. Matrigel, a reconstituted basement membrane product of Engelbreth-Holm Swarm tumor—which is composed mainly of laminin, collagen type IV, and entactin—is a potent inducer of cord formation in vitro. Thrombospondin, a matrix component with antiadhesive properties, does not affect EC proliferation but promotes angiogenesis of explants of rat aorta, particularly when incorporated into fibrin and collagen gels.[38] In rabbit cornea, induction of angiogenesis by fibroblast growth factors is enhanced by thrombospondin. Conversely, others have demonstrated that thrombospondin-1 inhibits neovascularization and EC migration. SPARC stimulates angiogene-

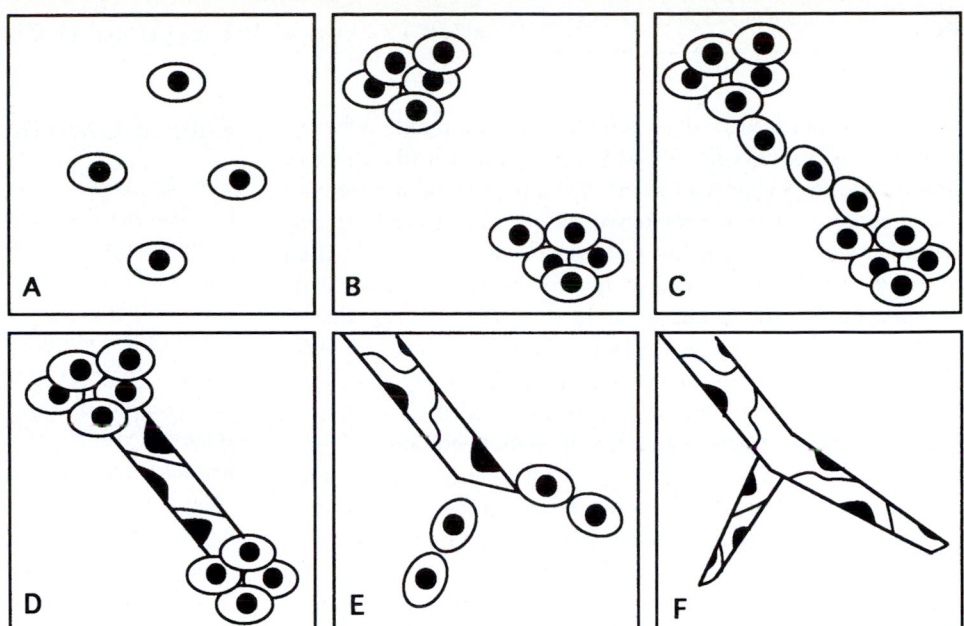

FIGURE 4-12 Scheme of vasculogenesis and angiogenesis. Vasculogenesis is the process by which vessels are formed from undifferentiated mesodermal cells. Once mesodermal cells differentiate into endothelial cells (ECs) (A), they proliferate and organize into clusters or islands (B). These islands send out ECs that will connect them with adjacent islands (C). Cells present between islands develop tight cell-cell interactions and organize around a central lumen forming a vessel (D). In angiogenesis, vascular structures are derived from existent vessels. These vessels send sprouts of ECs (E) that connect each other via cell-cell adhesion molecules and organize around a lumen extending the length of the vessel (F). Although both vasculogenesis and angiogenesis occur during embryogenesis, angiogenesis is considered to predominate in adult tissues, particularly during revascularization of injured tissues.

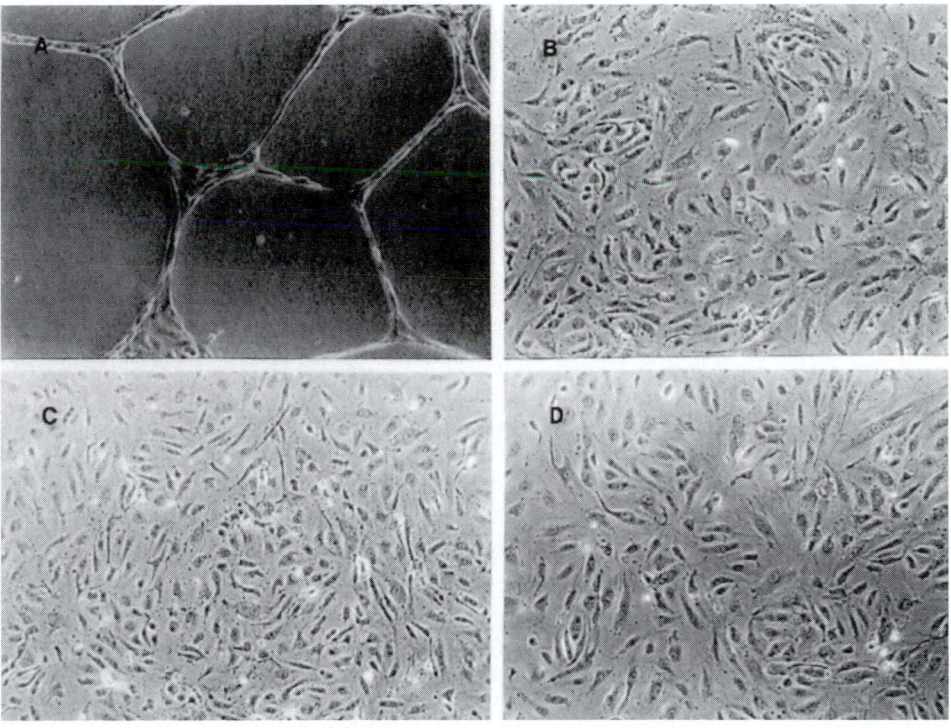

FIGURE 4-13 In vitro cord formation of human umbilical endothelial cells (HUVECs) cultured on various substrates. HUVECs were cultured on Matrigel (A), type I collagen (B), fibrin (C), or plastic for 12 h in the presence of 10 percent bovine calf serum. Note that on Matrigel, HUVECs organized into capillary-like structures or cords. Reorientation of cells into polygones was noticed as early as 3 h after culture, suggesting that although proliferation is important, the matrix can drive the organization of cells into cords in the absence of significant proliferation. In contrast to cells cultured on Matrigel, HUVECs cultured on other surfaces (B, C, and D) did not organize into cords and remained as a monolayer.

sis of bovine aortic ECs. Two peptides, containing the adhesive sequence YIGSR (Tyr-Ile-Gly-Ser-Arg), present in B1 chain of laminin, and PA 21, present in the A chain, prevent in vitro cord formation on Matrigel. Proteoglycans are also considered important in substrate adhesion and transmission of signals from the ECM. Hyaluronidase-sensitive proteoglycans predominate in migrating ECs of sprouting capillaries, whereas heparinase-sensitive proteoglycans predominate in quiescent ECs.[5] This difference in expression of various groups of proteoglycans in proliferating and migrating ECs compared with ECs present in quiescent capillaries suggests a role in vessel formation.

The ability to stimulate in vitro cord formation is not limited to the aforementioned matrix components. In fact, many matrix proteins tested to date are capable of inducing or sustaining this process if enough time is allowed (from hours to weeks). The effect of ECMs on EC phenotype is dependent on time of exposure, cell type, and configuration and composition of the matrix, as well as EC density and the presence or absence of growth factors. These studies suggest that switching of ECs between differentiation, growth, and spatial organization during vascular formation in developing lungs may be influenced by alterations in the adhesive or mechanical integrity of their ECM.

As described earlier, the effects of ECMs on EC function are mediated via integrins.[2] Through inhibition of EC integrin adhesion to matrices, RGD-containing peptides prevent the formation of microvessels from aortic explants placed on collagen gels, as well as cord formation of ECs placed on a reconstituted basement membrane.[36] Antibodies to various integrin subunits have also been used successfully to prevent vascular formation in vitro. Anti-$\alpha_v\beta_3$ antibodies have recently been shown to block growth factor–induced angiogenesis in the chick chorioallantoic membrane model.[9] In contrast, antibodies to $\alpha_2\beta_1$ and $\alpha_v\beta_3$ integrin receptors enhance capillary tube formation in vitro.[14] This seemingly paradoxical observation suggests that although EC adhesion to the matrix is important for vessel formation, antiadhesive events are also necessary because they allow detachment of the EC from their substrate and presumably facilitate mitosis and migration.

ECMs AND PROTEINASES IN VASCULAR FORMATION

Although in situ differentiation of mesodermal cells into ECs appears to be a major mechanism for vascularization of developing organs, invasion of avascular tissues by well-differentiated ECs, which may then become incorporated into developing vessels, is considered important as well. Tissue invasion by ECs requires the production of proteolytic enzymes necessary for traversing basement membranes and reorganizing ECM components.[28] The expression of interstitial collagenases and plasminogen activator (u-PA) in cultured capillary ECs is enhanced by growth factors such as bFGF. Type IV collagenase is another enzyme expressed by ECs with ECM-degrading activity. Some of these enzymes reside in the ECM and are released during tissue remodeling. In addition, ECMs may themselves stimulate the production of proteinases by lung fibroblasts. Thus, ECMs may affect regional expression of proteolytic enzymes by stimulating their production in mesenchymal cells other than ECs.

Role of Growth Factors in Vessel Formation

The angiogenic activity of multifunctional peptide growth factors has been studied extensively. Particular attention has been given to heparin-binding growth factors such as aFGF and bFGF. A recently discovered heparin-binding growth factor with mitogenic and angiogenic activity is *vascular endothelial growth factor* (VEGF). Unlike other angiogenic factors, this polypeptide is specific for ECs. Expression of VEGF and VEGF binding sites is regulated during lung development, increasing during late stages of gestation in blood vessels.[21] In addition to its ability to increase vascular permeability (for which it is also known as vascular permeability factor, or VPF), VEGF has been shown to promote angiogenesis in rat cornea and chicken chorioallantoic membrane assays. The effects of VEGF are mediated via at least two tyrosine kinase receptors: flt-1 and flk-1/kdr. The limited expression of these receptors to ECs has led to their consideration as good markers of EC precursors.

PDGF-A and -B chain mRNAs are present in microvascular ECs. While PDGF-AA has no mitogenic activity on microvascular ECs, PDGF-AB has a small but significant effect, and PDGF-BB has the strongest effect. The expression of PDGF receptors in these cells is down-regulated during induction of cord formation in 3D collagen gels, whereas they are up-regulated in 2D cultures—suggesting that differentiation of cells during in vitro vessel formation is associated with a reduction in proliferation, which may be due to down-regulation of PDGF receptors.[27]

Other growth factors implicated in vasculogenesis include *platelet-derived EC growth factor* (PD-ECGF), which is present in human placenta and stimulates EC proliferation and chemotaxis in vitro as well as angiogenesis in vivo. TGF-β inhibits the proliferation of ECs but induces a potent angiogenic response, depending on the cell substrate composition and organization. Both TGF-α and EGF stimulate microvascular EC proliferation. TGF-α has been shown to have angiogenic activity in rat airways. Other growth factors with angiogenic activity are the *granulocyte/monocyte colony–stimulating factor* and *angiogenin*.

SUMMARY AND RESEARCH NEEDS

The studies described above are part of the growing literature that is shaping our understanding of lung development. This literature reveals that lung pattern formation occurs during the pseudoglandular stage of lung development through the process of lung-branching morphogenesis. Lung-branching morphogenesis is responsible for the formation of the primitive bronchial tree and involves mechanisms responsible for control of cell proliferation and cleft formation, among other processes. Experimental data indicate that for normal lung-branching morphogenesis to occur, an exquisite balance needs to be maintained between inductive forces that maintain epithelial proliferation and restrictive forces that prevent the expansion of the epithelium in specific areas to form clefts. Although the molecules and mechanisms exerting these forces have not been entirely defined, there is much evidence suggesting a role for polypeptide growth factors and ECMs. In general, polypeptide growth factors expressed at both sides of the epithelial-mesenchymal interface induce the differentiation and proliferation of cells and are responsible for the continuous expansion of the epithelium. ECMs deposited strategically within the mesenchyme may prevent expansion of the epithelial sheet in specific areas, thereby creating clefts. In other words, expansion of the growing epithelial bud is not uniform, with clefts created in certain areas in response to signals provided by the mesenchyme. These balancing forces are elicited by direct binding of growth factors and ECMs to specific membrane receptors that are capable of converting extracellular messages into intracellular signals. In addition, ECMs can affect cell function by providing a mechanical obstruction to the expansion of the epithelial sheet. Extracellular signals can also be obtained from other cells. However, the role of cell-cell interactions in lung pattern formation is less well understood. Independent of the types of signaling mechanisms involved, the main consequence of these activities is to affect the proliferation (and differentiation) of cells and to drive their organization into a treelike functional structure. Differentiation of proximal versus distal and lateral versus medial structures may be driven by retinoids and other morphogens.

Once the rudimentary bronchial airway is formed, lung vascularization takes place during the canalicular phase of lung development. Formation of the pulmonary circulation appears to depend on invasion of the lung parenchyma by central extrapulmonary vessels formed by angiogenesis, and linkage of these vessels with distal capillary networks formed via vasculogenesis by EC precursors present within the lung mesenchyme. Both angiogenesis and vasculogenesis in lung can be driven by growth factors and cell-matrix and cell-cell interactions. However, as seen for lung-branching morphogenesis, the exact identity of the players and their specific actions on developing lung tissue remain to be elucidated.

It can be surmised that our understanding of the mechanisms responsible for lung pattern formation and vascularization is vague. Much still needs to be learned. The search for epithelial and mesenchymal factors important for lung development needs to continue. Recently, monoclonal antibodies to a novel mesenchymal cell protein termed *epimorphin* were shown to prevent epithelial lung-branching morphogenesis. However, the identity and exact role of this molecule await definition. Little is known about innervation of the lung during development and how this can affect cell function during pattern formation and vascularization. Thus, research is needed to ascertain the role of many poorly understood factors, such as nerve-derived factors and how they act in concert with ECMs and growth factors to drive pattern formation and vascularization.

Another important aspect that is poorly understood is smooth-muscle differentiation and epithelial cell– and endothelial cell–smooth-muscle interactions. Both ECMs and growth factors appear necessary for muscle differentiation, but it is not known whether airway or vascular smooth-muscle differentiation is tied to epithelial and endothelial cell differentiation. It is also not known whether vascular and airway smooth-muscle cells follow similar pathways of differentiation and organization around endothelial and epithelial structures, respectively.

Once the airspaces and vessels are formed, apposition of these structures needs to occur. This process takes place during the late stages of lung development and is crucial for developing functional gas-exchanging units. A major part of this process is the clearing of mesenchymal cells and connective tissue present between the developing airways and vessels. Activation of mechanisms leading to programmed cell death (also termed *apoptosis*) and expression of matrix-degrading enzymes during the late stages of development may be crucial for the formation of functional alveoli-capillaries barriers by allowing for the clearance of cells and connective tissue.

A key question that remains unanswered relates to the factors that control overall lung development. For example, how does the embryonic clock trigger the sequential expression of genes that leads to morphogenetic movements of cells during pattern formation? What induces the formation of the lung bud? What master genes (e.g., homeobox genes) control lung pattern formation? Appropriate answers to these questions cannot be obtained without appropriate models of lung formation and vascularization. We anticipate that these models will become available within the next decade. Technologic advances in this and other areas will accelerate our understanding of lung development— which, in turn, may affect the way we approach congenital lung malformations and other processes, such as lung inflammation and repair after injury, with common mechanisms of action with embryogenesis.

Finally, it must be mentioned that branching patterns such as those seen in the lung are characteristic of many other organs, including the salivary glands, pancreatic duct system, liver biliary tree, urinary collecting duct, and the His-Purkinje nerve fiber network in the heart. Branching patterns are also seen elsewhere in nature (e.g., snowflakes, crystals, lightning-like paths of electricity, tree branches). In general, these branching structures appear to adhere to the principles of fractal geometry as applied to nonequilibrium growth processes. Fractal trees such as the lung exhibit heterogeneity, lack a characteristic scale, and demonstrate self-similarity; in other words, their small-scale structure resembles their large-scale form. The universality of branching systems suggests there are functional advantages for this type of structure and, more important, that similar mechanisms are responsible for their development. Like physicists and mathematicians searching for clues to understand the geometry of nature, developmental and theoretical biologists are interested in learning the mechanisms responsible for organogenesis and the emergence of branching patterns during this process. We envision that sophisticated mathematical and physiological models that adequately incorporate observations made in biologic systems (e.g., lung explants) may greatly accelerate progress in this area.

REFERENCES

1. Aguayo SM, Schuyler WE, Murtagh JJ, Roman J: Regulation of lung branching morphogenesis by bombesin-like peptides and neutral endopeptidase. *Am J Respir Cell Mol Biol* 10:635–642, 1994.
2. Albelda SM: Endothelial and epithelial cell adhesion molecules. *Am J Respir Cell Mol Biol* 4:195–203, 1991.
3. Alescio T: Effect of a proline analogue, azetidine-2-carboxylic acid, on the morphogenesis in vitro of mouse embryonic lung. *J Embryol Exp Morphol* 29:439–451, 1973.
4. Alescio T, Di Michele M: Relationship of epithelial growth to mitotic rate in mouse embryonic lung developing in vitro. *J Embryol Exp Morphol* 19:227–237, 1968.

5. Ausprunk DH, Boudreau CL, Nelson DA: Proteoglycans in the microvasculature: II. Histochemical localization in proliferating capillaries of the rabbit cornea. *Am J Pathol* 103:367–375, 1981.

6. Bishop JE, Mitchell JJ, Absher PM, et al: Cyclic mechanical deformation stimulates human lung fibroblast proliferation and autocrine factor activity. *Am J Respir Cell Mol Biol* 9:126–133, 1993.

7. Bluemink JG, Van Maurik P, Lawson KA: Intimate cell contacts at the epithelial/mesenchymal interface in embryonic mouse lung. *J Ultrastruct Res* 55:257–270, 1976.

8. Bogue CW, Gross I, Vasavada H, et al: Identification of Hox genes in newborn lung and effects of gestational age and retinoic acid on their expression. *Am J Physiol* 266:L448–454, 1994.

9. Brooks PC, Clark RAF, Cheresh DA: Requirement of vascular integrin $\alpha v \beta 3$ for angiogenesis. *Science* 264:569–571, 1994.

10. Clark EA, Brugge JS: Integrins and signal transduction: The road taken. *Science* 268:233–239, 1995.

11. Cardoso WV, Williams MC, Mitsialis SA, et al: Retinoic acid induces changes in the pattern of airway branching and alters epithelial cell differentiation in the developing lung in vitro. *Am J Respir Cell Mol Biol* 12:464–476, 1995.

12. deMello DE, Reid LM: Pre- and postnatal development of the pulmonary circulation, in Chernick V, Mellins RB (eds), *Basic Mechanisms of Pediatric Respiratory Disease: Cellular and Integrative.* Philadelphia, BC Decker, 1991, pp 36–54.

13. End P, Engel J: Multidomain proteins of the extracellular matrix and cellular growth, in McDonald JA, Mecham RP (eds), *Receptors for Extracellular Matrices.* San Diego, Academic, 1991, pp 79–129.

14. Gamble JR, Matthias LJ, Meyer G, et al: Regulation of in vitro capillary tube formation by anti-integrin antibodies. *J Cell Biol* 121:931–943, 1993.

15. Ganser GL, Stricklin GP, Matrisian LM: EGF and TGF alpha influence in vitro lung development by the induction of matrix-degrading metalloproteinases. *Int J Dev Biol* 35:453–461, 1991.

16. Goldin GV, Hindman HM, Wessells NK: The role of cell proliferation and cellular shape change in branching morphogenesis of the embryonic mouse lung: Analysis using aphidicolin and cytochalasins. *J Exp Zool* 232:287–296, 1984.

17. Guzowski DE, Blau H, Bienkowski RS: *Extracellular Matrix in Developing Lung.* Philadelphia, Lea & Febiger, 1990.

18. Hirai Y, Nose A, Kobayashi S, Takeichi M: Expression and role of E- and P-cadherin adhesion molecules in embryonic histogenesis: I. Lung epithelial morphogenesis. *Development* 105:263–270, 1989.

19. Ingber DE, Folkman J: Mechanochemical switching between growth and differentiation during fibroblast growth factor–stimulated angiogenesis in vitro: Role of extracellular matrix. *J Cell Biol* 109:317–330, 1989.

20. Ingber DE, Madri JA, Folkman J: Endothelial growth factors and extracellular matrix regulate DNA synthesis through modulation of cell and nuclear expansion. *In Vitro Cell Dev Biol* 23:387–394, 1987.

21. Jakeman LB, Armanini M, Phillips HS, Ferrara N: Developmental expression of binding sites and messenger ribonucleic acid for vascular endothelial growth factor suggests a role for this protein in vasculogenesis and angiogenesis. *Endocrinology* 133:848–858, 1993.

22. Jaskoll T, Boyer PD, Melnick M: Tumor necrosis factor-alpha and embryonic mouse lung morphogenesis. *Dev Dynamics* 201:137–150, 1994.

23. Juliano RL, Haskill S: Signal transduction from the extracellular matrix. *J Cell Biol* 120:577–585, 1993.

24. Kratochwil K, Dziadek M, Löhler J, et al: Normal epithelial branching morphogenesis in the absence of collagen I. *Dev Biol* 117:596–606, 1986.

25. Lawson KA: Stage specificity in the mesenchyme requirement of rodent lung epithelium in vitro: A matter of growth control? *J Embryol Exp Morphol* 74:183–206, 1983.

26. Maitre B, Clement A, Williams MC, Brody JS: Expression of insulin-like growth factor receptors 1 and 2 in developing lung and their relation to epithelial cell differentiation. *Am J Respir Cell Mol Biol* 13:262–270, 1995.

27. Marx M, Perlmutter RA, Madri JA: Modulation of platelet-derived growth factor receptor expression in microvascular endothelial cells during in vitro angiogenesis. *J Clin Invest* 93:131–139, 1994.

28. Matrisian LM, Hogan BLM: Growth factor–regulated proteases and extracellular matrix remodeling during mammalian development, in Nilsen-Hamilton M (ed), *Growth Factors and Development.* San Diego, Academic, 1990, pp 219–259.

29. McCray PB, Joseph T: Spontaneous contractility of human airway smooth muscle. *Am J Respir Cell Mol Biol* 8:573–580, 1993.

30. McDonald JA: Extracellular matrix effects on cell shape and gene expression. *Curr Opin Cell Biol* 1:995–999, 1989.

31. McGowan SE: Extracellular matrix and the regulation of lung development and repair. *FASEB J* 6:2895–2904, 1992.

32. Menko AS, Boettiger D: Occupation of the extracellular matrix receptor, integrin, is a control point for myogenic differentiation. *Cell* 51:51–57, 1987.

33. Millan FA, Denhez F, Kondaiah P, Akhurst RJ: Embryonic gene expression patterns of TGF beta 1, beta 2 and beta 3 suggest different developmental functions in vivo. *Development* 111:131–143, 1991.

34. Moats-Staats BM, Price WA, Xu L, et al: Regulation of the insulin-like growth factor system during normal rat lung development. *Am J Respir Cell Mol Biol* 12:56–64, 1995.

35. Nakanishi Y, Sugiura F, Kishi J, Hayakawa T: Scanning electron microscopic observations of mouse embryonic submandibular glands during initial branching: Preferential localization of fibrillar structures at the mesenchymal ridges participating in cleft formation. *J Embryol Exp Morphol* 96:65–77, 1986.

36. Nicosia RF, Bonanno E: Inhibition of angiogenesis *in vitro* by Arg-Gly-Asp–containing synthetic peptide. *Am J Pathol* 138:829–833, 1991.

37. Nicosia RF, Bonanno E, Smith M: Fibronectin promotes the elongation of microvessels during angiogenesis in vitro. *J Cell Physiol* 154:654–661, 1993.

38. Nicosia RF, Tuszynski GP: Matrix-bound thrombospondin promotes angiogenesis *in vitro. J Cell Biol* 124:183–193, 1994.

39. Noden DM: Embryonic origins and assembly of blood vessels. *Am Rev Respir Dis* 140:1097–1103, 1989.

40. Nogawa H, Ito T: Branching morphogenesis of embryonic mouse lung epithelium in mesenchyme-free culture. *Development* 121:1015–1022, 1995.

41. Peter K, Werner S, Liao X, et al: Targeted expression of a dominant negative FGF receptor blocks branching morphogenesis and epithelial differentiation of the mouse lung. *EMBO J* 13:3296–3301, 1994.

42. Plopper GE, McNamee HP, Dike LE, et al: Convergence of integrin and growth factor receptor signaling pathways within the focal adhesion complex. *Mol Biol Cell* 6:1349–1365, 1995.

43. Poole TJ, Coffin JD: Vasculogenesis and angiogenesis: Two distinct morphogenetic mechanisms establish embryonic vascular pattern. *J Exp Zool* 251:224–231, 1989.

44. Roman J: Effects of calcium channel blockade on mammalian lung branching morphogenesis. *Exp Lung Res* 21:489–502, 1995.

45. Roman J, Crouch EC, McDonald JA: Reagents that inhibit fibronectin matrix assembly of cultured cells also inhibit lung branching morphogenesis *in vitro:* Implications for lung development, injury, and repair. *Chest* 99:20S–21S, 1991.

46. Roman J, Little CW, McDonald JA: Potential role of RGD-binding integrins in mammalian lung branching morphogenesis. *Development* 112:551–558, 1991.

47. Roman J, McDonald JA: Expression of fibronectin, the integrin VLA-5 and α–smooth muscle actin in lung and heart development. *Am J Respir Cell Mol Biol* 6:472–480, 1992.

48. Schlessinger J, Ullrich A: Growth factor signaling by receptor tyrosine kinases. *Neuron* 9:383–391, 1992.

49. Schuger L, O'Shea S, Rheinheimer J, Varani J: Laminin in lung development: Effects of anti-laminin antibody in murine lung morphogenesis. *Dev Biol* 137:26–32, 1990.

50. Schuger L, Varani J, Mitra R Jr, et al: Retinoic acid stimulates mouse lung development by a mechanism involving epithelial-mesenchymal interaction and regulation of epidermal growth factor receptors. *Dev Biol* 159:462–473, 1993.

51. Serra R, Pelton RW, Moses HL: TGF beta 1 inhibits branching morphogenesis and N-myc expression in lung bud organ cultures. *Development* 120:2153–2161, 1994.

52. Seth R, Shum L, Wu F, et al: Role of epidermal growth factor expression in early mouse embryo lung branching morphogenesis in culture: Antisense oligodeoxynucleotide inhibitory strategy. *Dev Biol* 158:555–559, 1993.

53. Souza P, Kuliszewski M, Wang J, et al: PDGF-AA and its receptor influence early lung branching via an epithelial-mesenchymal interaction. *Development* 121:2559–2567, 1995.

54. Souza P, Sedlackova L, Kuliszewski M, et al: Antisense oligonucleotides targeting PDGF B mRNA inhibit cell proliferation during embryonic rat lung development. *Development* 120:2163–2173, 1994.

55. Ten-Have-Opbroek AAW: The development of the lung in mammals: An analysis of concepts and findings. *Am J Anat* 162:201–219, 1981.

56. Thompson HA, Spooner BS: Proteoglycan and glycosaminoglycan synthesis in embryonic mouse salivary glands: Effects of beta-D-xyloside, an inhibitor of branching morphogenesis. *J Cell Biol* 96:1443–1450, 1983.

57. Warburton D, Seth R, Shum L, et al: Epigenetic role of epidermal growth factor expression and signaling in embryonic mouse lung morphogenesis. *Dev Biol* 149:123–133, 1992.

58. Wessels NK, Cohen JH: Effects of collagenase on developing epithelia in vitro: Lung, ureteric bud, and pancreas. *Dev Biol* 18:294–309, 1968.

59. Young SL, Chang LY, Erickson HP: Tenascin-C in rat lung: Distribution ontogeny and role in branching morphogenesis. *Dev Biol* 161:615–625, 1994.

DEVELOPMENT AND GROWTH OF THE LUNG

P e t e r   H .   B u r r i

With the replacement of lung liquid by air and the onset of respiration, birth represents a major caesura in pulmonary development.[21] The change from the amniotic into the atmospheric environment is, however, more a functionally than a structurally relevant step: lung development is continuous and proceeds from early fetal into postnatal life (Fig. 5-1). The staging of lung development is highly descriptive; it is based on the light microscopic morphologic changes that the prospective lung undergoes. Because maturation proceeds metachronically from the proximal to the peripheral portions of the airway tree, there can be some overlap between the stages. Whereas the beginning of pulmonary development is relatively clearly defined by the first appearance of the future trachea in the region of the foregut, there is no such clear limit to when it ends during childhood. Indeed, as will be discussed, the end of alveolar formation and of microvascular maturation cannot be precisely determined. This is partly due to methodologic limitations, but even more to the fact that development will slowly blend into growth.

PRENATAL LUNG DEVELOPMENT

Organogenesis

Following fertilization, the germ cells soon segregate into a cluster of trophoblastic cells to which a few embryoblastic cells adhere. The trophoblastic cells may be viewed as the future placenta, whereas the embryoblastic cells, after differentiation into the three germ layers, will form the human embryo.

The organs of the body are laid down by differentiation from the germ layers during the so-called embryonic period, which encompasses the first 8 weeks after fertilization. The lung appears around the 26th day of gestation as a ventral diverticulum of the foregut. In the region of the future esophagus, two lateral grooves appear, the "laryngotracheal sulci"; they deepen, join each other, and separate the lung bud from the gut except in its most proximal part, the site of the prospective hypopharynx. In the following days, the bud rapidly divides dichotomously, and both branches grow into the surrounding mesenchyme. The process of dichotomous division is repeated many times, and the future airways, covered by mesenchyme, push into the primitive pleuroperitoneal cavity. It is interesting to note that the tubular branching pattern already reflects the hierarchy of the future conducting airways: the lobar bronchi are formed by the 37th day, and 4 days later all the segmental bronchi are present.

As is evident from the above description, the high columnar epithelium of the tubular sprouts is of endodermal origin, whereas the mesenchyme is derived from the third germ layer, the mesoderm. This double origin of the lung tissues is important: many processes of lung development are dependent on the interaction between epithelium and mesenchyme. Indeed, as could be demonstrated in very elegant experiments,[47] removal of mesenchyme from the tip of a bud in these early phases of development and transplanting it to the side of a higher-ordered segment abolished further branching at the tip and induced a new branch at the site of transplantation. During later stages of pre- and postnatal lung development, and even in the adult lung, the interplay between differentiating pneumocytes, mesodermally derived interstitial cells, and extracellular matrix continues to be decisive for cell maturation and cell function regulation.

During the fourth week of gestation, the heart starts to beat, being the first organ to take up its function in the embryo. The development of the pulmonary vessels takes advantage of the early development of the systemic circulatory system. The pulmonary arteries develop as buds from the sixth pair of aortic arches and connect to the vascular plexus forming in the pulmonary mesenchyme. The sixth left and right aortic branches will follow different pathways of development (Fig. 5-2). Whereas the proximal (ventral) parts of the arches will be integrated into the pulmonary arterial tree to form permanent parts of the pulmonary vasculature, the distal (dorsal) parts will disappear completely on the right-hand side and form the ductus arteriosus on the left side. By connecting the pulmonary artery to the aortic arch, the ductus arteriosus enables the right ven-

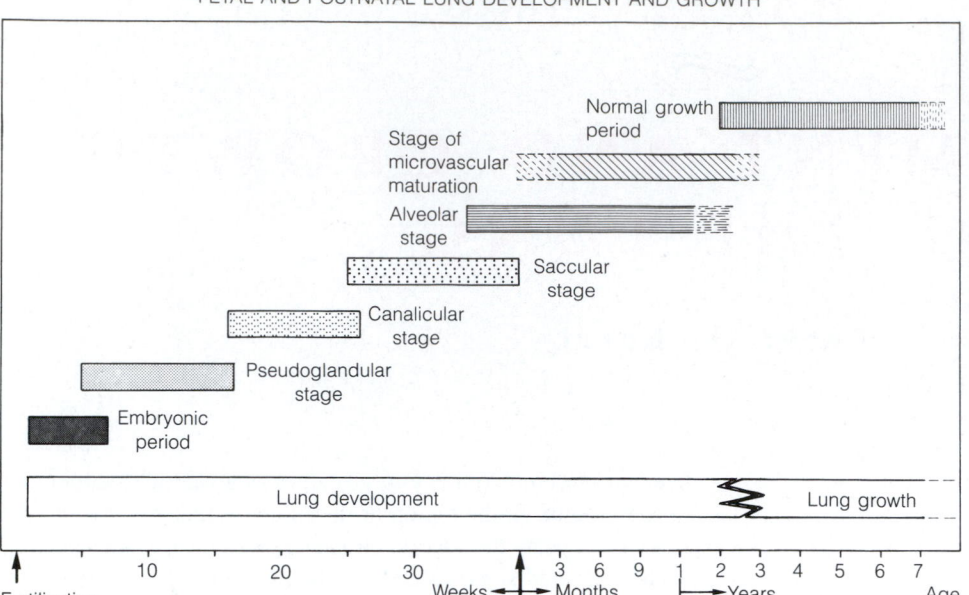

FIGURE 5-1 Stages of human lung development and their timing. Note overlapping between stages, particularly between the alveolar stage and the stage of microvascular maturation. Open-ended bars indicate uncertainty as to exact timing. The embryonic period is not a specific period for lung development. *(From Zeltner and Burri,[56] with permission.)*

veloping lung), the amount of future gas exchange tissue present during and at the end of the pseudoglandular stage has been severely underestimated. Already in the early 1980s, Ten Have–Opbroek had demonstrated by immunohistochemical techniques that epithelial cells at the periphery of the airway tree in the pseudoglandular stage had to be considered precursors of the later alveolar epithelium.[48,49] In morphologic and morphometric studies of fetal rat lungs, we found that half of the parenchymal epithelial cell mass in the saccular stage before birth was already present in the late pseudoglandular stage.[13,36] Furthermore, Kitaoka and coworkers[30] concluded from counts of the number of end segments in human lungs in the pseudoglandular and canalicular stages that all the airway divisions down to the level of alveolar ducts were present toward the end of the pseudoglandular stage. For these reasons, the view that the pseudoglandular stage is almost exclusively the stage of conducting airway development can no longer be maintained.

Although the appearance of the acinar structures apparently provides a well-defined morphologic characteristic for the transition to the next stage of development, a precise estimate of

tricular output to bypass the pulmonary vascular bed during fetal life. Shortly after birth the duct closes, redirecting the entire cardiac output to the lung. The pulmonary veins are derived from a single evagination of the left atrium, which divides several times and connects to the pulmonary vascular bed. Subsequently, the original bud and its first- and second-order branches are fully reintegrated into the left atrium, so that finally, from each lung side, a pair of veins delivers the oxygenated blood into the left heart.

At around 7 weeks, the period of organogenesis can be considered to merge imperceptibly with the period proper of lung development.

Fetal Lung Development

This period lasts till birth and comprises three phases of development, the names of which are derived from the changing morphology of the prospective gas exchange tissue: pseudoglandular, canalicular, and terminal sac (or saccular).

PSEUDOGLANDULAR STAGE

From the fifth week to the 17th week, the developing lung shows the characteristics of a tubular gland, giving rise to the name for this stage (Fig. 5-3*A, B*). Until the end of this stage, the tubular tree preforms, through growth and branching, all the conductive airways down to their last generations—i.e., the future terminal bronchioles. This stage has therefore often been referred to as the stage of conductive airway formation. Although Boyden[4] claimed that the transition to the next stage was marked by the first appearance of the pulmonary acinus (which means that the prospective lung parenchyma appears at the periphery of the de-

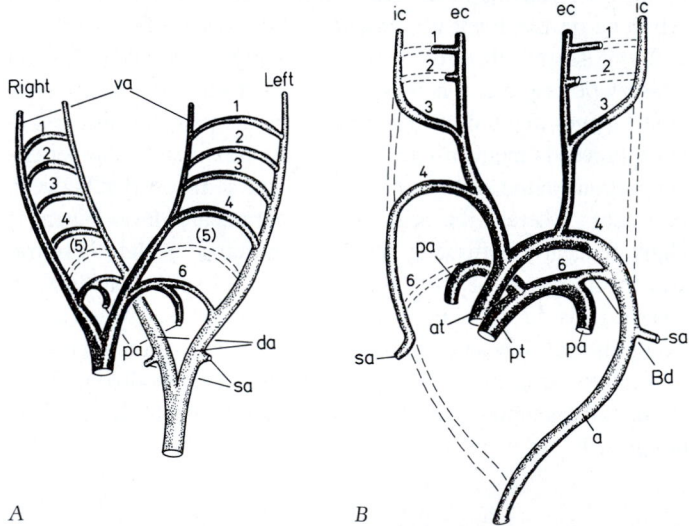

A   *B*

FIGURE 5-2 Development of pulmonary arteries. *A.* Ventral arteries (va) and dorsal arteries (da) are interconnected by six pairs of aortic arches numbered 1 to 6. Pulmonary arteries (pa) bud off from sixth pair of aortic arches and grow into the nearby pulmonary mesenchyme. Notice that formation of the aortic arches is sequential; they are never present simultaneously. Furthermore, the fifth pair is never formed. sa = subclavian artery. *B.* Fate of developing arterial vessels. Some segments regress and disappear (white); others develop and grow preferentially. a = aorta; at = aortic trunk; pa = pulmonary artery; pt = pulmonary trunk; Bd = Botallo's ductus arteriosus; ec = external carotid artery; ic = internal carotid artery; sa = subclavian artery.

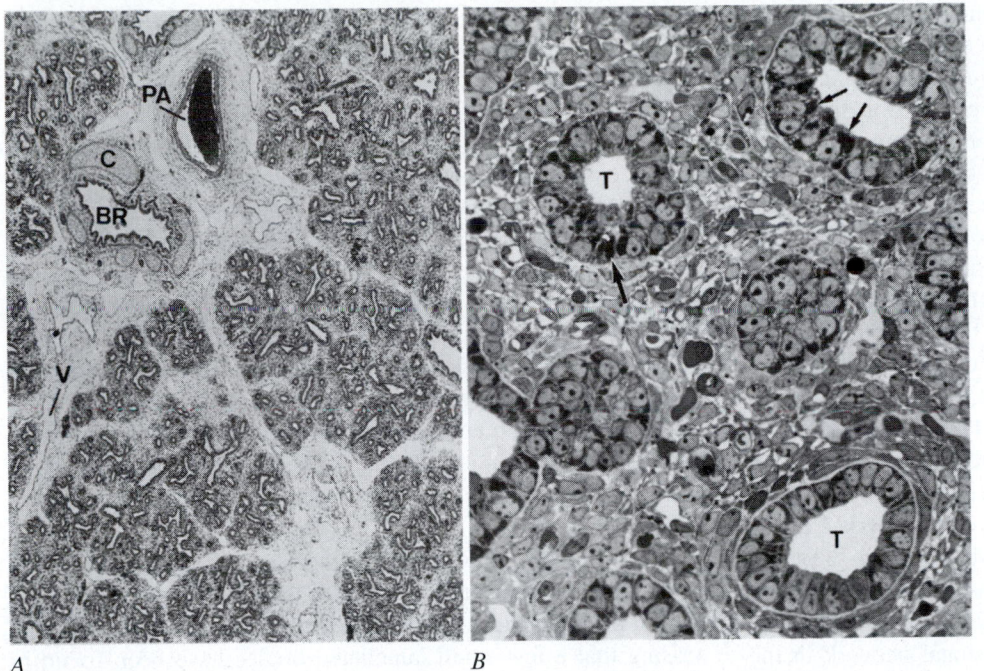

A   *B*

FIGURE 5-3   Pseudoglandular stage of human lung. *A.* Gestational age 15 weeks. Clear bands of loose mesenchyme containing veins (V) indicate septation of lung into segments and lobules. Denser mesenchyme surrounds the tubular sprouts. PA = pulmonary artery; BR = bronchus with embryonal cartilage (C). Light micrograph, ×25. *B.* Higher magnification of pseudoglandular stage in rat lung. Tubules (T) are lined by high columnar epithelium with large amounts of glycogen (dark spots, arrows). The mesenchyme is highly cellular and contains a loose capillary meshwork. Light micrograph. ×450.

first in the trachea in condensed areas of the mesenchyme. From the trachea, differentiation spreads toward the periphery, so that cartilage is commonly found in main bronchi around week 10 and in segmental bronchi in week 12 of gestation. However, cartilage formation continues almost until the end of the canalicular stage.

Mucous glands and goblet cells appear almost simultaneously in the airway epithelium. They develop from solid epithelial sprouts that invade the mesenchyme underneath the epithelium. At around weeks 12 to 13, mucous glands are found in bronchi; at week 14, mucus formation can be detected in the trachea.

During the pseudoglandular stage, the vascular system develops along with the bronchial tree, so that by the end of this stage, all the preacinar vessels, arteries and veins, are laid down in the characteristic pattern of the adult lung. In principle, arteries follow airway branching rather closely, whereas the veins run interaxially within the mesenchyme,[52] where they demarcate future segments and subsegments (Fig. 5-3*A*). However, the number of generations in the arterial tree is greater than in the airway system: on average, there are more than 28 generations in the arterial tree versus 23 in the airways. In addition to the conventional arteries that follow the bronchi and bronchioles, there are other branches (i.e., "supernumerary" arteries), which split off at right angles. Usually these branches are smaller vessels that irrigate the "recurrent" gas exchange tissue adjacent to the conducting airways.

gestational age cannot be made from it. Differentiation usually proceeds centrifugally, and the speed of growth varies during a developmental period, with an acceleration toward the end of a stage. Furthermore, animal studies have demonstrated that upper lobes develop faster than lower lobes. If the time differences in development observed between lobes in rabbits are transposed to the human lung, the differences in lobar development could amount to 2 weeks in view of the much longer gestation period. Such differences, however, have never been assessed. Recently it was postulated that human lung development proceeded homogeneously.[30]

During the pseudoglandular stage, the airway tubes are proximally lined by a very high columnar epithelium. The height of the cells decreases continuously toward the periphery, to reach a cuboidal shape in the terminal branches (Fig. 5-3*B*). Mitotic figures are frequent. The cytoplasmic organellar machinery looks relatively simple: mitochondria, many free ribosomes and a little rough endoplasmic reticulum, some lipid droplets, and large patches of glycogen. Remarkably, the epithelial barrier appears to be tight from the early stages of development. In freeze-fracture preparations, the morphology of the junctional complexes does not differ during development to full term; conversely, gap junctions are present early in gestation and disappear during the canalicular stage as the epithelial cells differentiate. Therefore, it may be that electrical coupling between cells plays a role in cellular differentiation.

The first ciliated, goblet, and basal cells appear in the central airways. Similarly, cartilage and smooth-muscle cells are found

CANALICULAR STAGE

The canalicular stage lasts from week 16 to 26 and comprises important steps in the development of the fetal lung. During this stage, lung morphology changes dramatically, owing primarily to the differentiation of the pulmonary epithelium, resulting in the formation of the typical air-blood barrier, to the beginning of surfactant synthesis and secretion, and to the "canalization" of the lung parenchyma by capillaries. The latter process gave this stage its name. These alterations have most important functional consequences: at the end of the canalicular stage, the lung has reached a state of development that, in principle, enables it to exchange gas. Before these developmental steps, a prematurely born infant has no chance to survive. However, as clinical experience unfortunately shows, at the end of the canalicular stage survival is by no means assured.

At the beginning of this stage, the future gas exchange region of the lung can be distinguished from the conductive tubules of the airway tree. Boyden[4] has characterized this step as "birth of the acinus," marking the transition from the pseudoglandular to the canalicular stage. The early acini are composed of several very short generations of tubules arranged in clusters and taking origin from the actual last segment of the conducting airways, a prospective terminal bronchiole. The acinar borders can be recognized because of rarefaction of the mesenchyme (Fig. 5-3A).

In subsequent weeks, the distal segments of the airways grow in length and widen at the expense of the mesenchymal mass. The cuboidal, glycogen-rich epithelium lining the tubules starts to flatten out. In some cells the junctional complexes localized around the cell apex are shifted to the lower half of the intercellular clefts. Where this happens, the cell develops cytoplasmic attenuations, which soon become so thin that they are invisible in the light microscope (Fig. 5-4). No wonder a controversy went on for years about whether the airspaces of mature lungs were lined by a continuous epithelium. This problem was rapidly solved by the first electron microscopic investigations of the lung of various species by Low in the early 1950s.[32] Important changes in the microvasculature accompany, or even precede, the attenuation of the epithelium. The capillaries, which originally form a three-dimensional network in the mesenchyme, rearrange around the tubules, and it seems that, where capillaries come into close contact with epithelium, the cuboidal cells differentiate into type I cells. In this way, the first thin portions of the future air-blood barrier are formed. The mechanisms responsible for this process are unknown. Whether the capillary contact initiates the differentiation of the epithe-

lium, or vice versa, is an open question. Nonetheless, it seems very likely that the two events are linked, since they coincide so closely in time.

The epithelial cells that remain cuboidal develop to type II cells, the secretory cells of the peripheral airspaces that will produce the pulmonary surfactant. Within their cytoplasm, these cells accumulate groups of lamellated bodies that, in turn, are often associated with multivesicular bodies. Lamellar bodies correspond to the intracellular storage form of the surface-active material present in the alveolar surfactant. Therefore, in all species, the appearance of lamellated bodies in type II cells precedes the presence of surfactant material in the airspaces. In most mammals, lamellated bodies appear at about 80 to 85 percent of total pregnancy duration, whereas in humans, the bodies are already present at about 60 percent of total gestation time; i.e., they appear during the sixth month of development.

Type II cells are also the progenitor cells of the type I cell population in adult lungs, as could be demonstrated during repair of the damaged alveolar epithelium.[2] Therefore, it is not surprising that a few small lamellated bodies have been found in the cytoplasm of immature epithelial cells *before* they started to differentiate into type I and type II cells.[35] In cytokinetic experiments using tritiated thymidine, it has been shown that during lung development, early type II cells (or, more precisely, cells resembling type II cells) also represented the stem cells of the type I and type II pulmonary epithelium.

At the uttermost periphery of the airspaces, the cuboidal cells of the epithelium remain undifferentiated until after birth (Fig. 5-5). Throughout this stage, the blood vessels grow in length and diameter, and new branches follow the developing peripheral airway tree.

SACCULAR (OR TERMINAL SAC) STAGE

This stage lasts from about week 24 almost to term. At the beginning of this stage, the peripheral airways form typical clusters of widened airspaces termed saccules or terminal sacs. By widening and lengthening of all airspace generations distal to the terminal bronchioles, and probably also by the addition of the last generations of airspaces, the future gas exchange region expands massively. According to Boyden,[4] until birth the terminal airspaces are thought to produce, on average, three generations of prospective alveolar ducts and one generation of alveolar sacs. In the light of more recent investigations, however, the increase in generation number in the saccular stage could be more limited, because more generations than assumed so far are already present at the end of the pseudoglandular stage.[30]

Each new generation of this pathway is originally formed as a blind-ending saccule. As soon as it divides distally, however, it is no longer a saccule, but an open-ended channel. As is discussed in the section on postnatal development, the morphology of all these channels and saccules undergoes change until the formation of the alveoli is completed in the postnatal period. Therefore, these structures have been designated as transitory ducts and transitory saccules[8] or, more generally, as transitory airways or airspaces, because their morphology changes further until alveoli are formed.

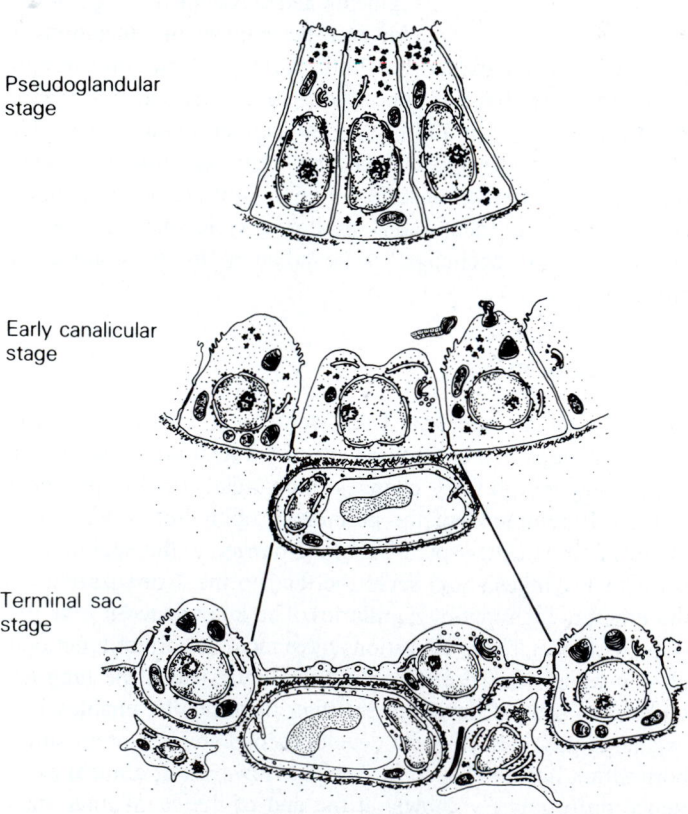

Pseudoglandular stage

Early canalicular stage

Terminal sac stage

FIGURE 5-4 Epithelial transformation during development. In the pseudoglandular phase the columnar epithelium is tall. During the canalicular phase two cell types appear: the prospective secretory and lining cells.

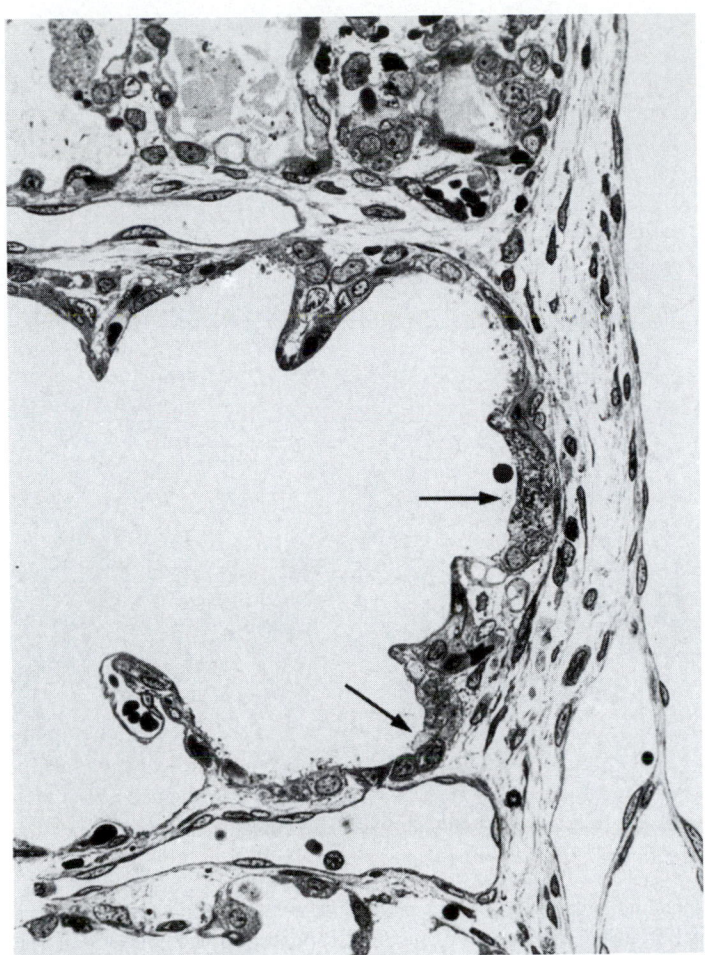

FIGURE 5-5   Periphery of gas-exchange region in human lung aged 26 days. The cuboidal epithelium persists at the uttermost periphery (arrows). Light micrograph, ×425.

Also at this stage, within the mesenchyme, one or two populations of fibroblastic cells have differentiated. Not only are these cells responsible for the deposition of extracellular matrix and fibers but also, by way of interactions with the epithelial cover, they presumably play a role in epithelial differentiation and in the control of surfactant secretion. Owing to the expansion of the lumina of the peripheral airspaces in the foregoing and in the present stage, the proportion of interstitial tissue within the interairspace septa has decreased. Nevertheless, the intersaccular and interductular septa are still relatively thick and contain two layers of capillaries. The interstitium is highly cellular; because its content in collagen is low, the fetal lung is delicate and fragile: under mechanical stress, it ruptures much more rapidly than the adult organ.

Finally, in anticipation of the next stage, during which the alveoli will be formed, the interstitial cells start to produce elastic fibers along the interductular and intersaccular walls. Elastin is found first in extracellular bays of large fibroblastic cells rich in organelles. The deposits later extend throughout the septal walls of the parenchyma, from the peribronchial and perivascular sheaths to the pleural sac.

Keeping pace with the intense growth of the gas exchange region during this stage, the vascular tree grows in length and diameter and by adding new generations. Measurements on ar-

teriograms by Hislop and Reid have shown that arterial diameter is practically constant at a given distance from the end of the arterial pathway.[24] This is true irrespective of age, either fetal or postnatal. Therefore, a vessel of a given size will, for example, supply a large portion of a lobe in an early fetal lung, but only an acinus in a child's lung. In late fetal life, the wall structure of arteries is similar to that of adult lungs. Proximal arteries are elastic, with many elastic lamellae strutted to each other by smooth-muscle cells that are arranged obliquely between the elastic sheets. Smaller arterial vessels show a transitional structure, the muscular component becoming increasingly prominent at the expense of the elastic component. Finally, the muscle layer of the media becomes irregular and assumes a spiral configuration. This configuration explains the "partly muscular" arteries seen in histologic sections. Unfortunately, there are no strict relationships between vessel diameter, size of the region supplied, and character of the wall structure; these relationships may differ from one pathway to the other. Intrapulmonary veins are practically devoid of smooth-muscle cells until the end of the canalicular period. In the following weeks, however, a thin muscle layer is formed that, at birth, extends down to vessels of about 100 μm diameter.[26]

POSTNATAL LUNG DEVELOPMENT

Around the time of birth, the complete set of airway generations seems to be present; the most peripheral ones, however, are still relatively short. The pulmonary parenchyma consists of several generations of transitory ducts and, as the last generation on each pathway, the transitory saccules. At birth, these structures are on the way to being transformed into alveolar ducts and sacs, respectively, by the process of alveolization. Although reports indicate that in humans the formation of alveoli starts during late intrauterine life,[31] the alveolar stage of lung development is discussed in this section because most alveoli (more than 85 percent) are formed after birth.

Alveolar Stage

Many of the general laws and principles that govern the development of the alveoli have been derived from animal studies, with the rat lung having proved to be a particularly useful model. The following description of the postnatal processes at work in the appearance of the alveoli and in the maturation of the alveolar walls will therefore be based on experimental findings obtained in the rat lung. Subsequent morphologic and morphometric investigations of human lungs have confirmed that the developmental processes leading to alveolization and maturation of the child's lung do not differ in structural essentials. Evidently, however, as expected, the timing of the events is different between species.

At birth, the parenchyma of the rat lung consists of smooth-walled channels and saccules corresponding to transitory ducts and definitive terminal saccules, respectively. The interductular or intersaccular septa are straight and relatively thick. Three weeks later, the parenchymal structures are much more complex, the septa are slender, and the airspaces are irregularly delineated

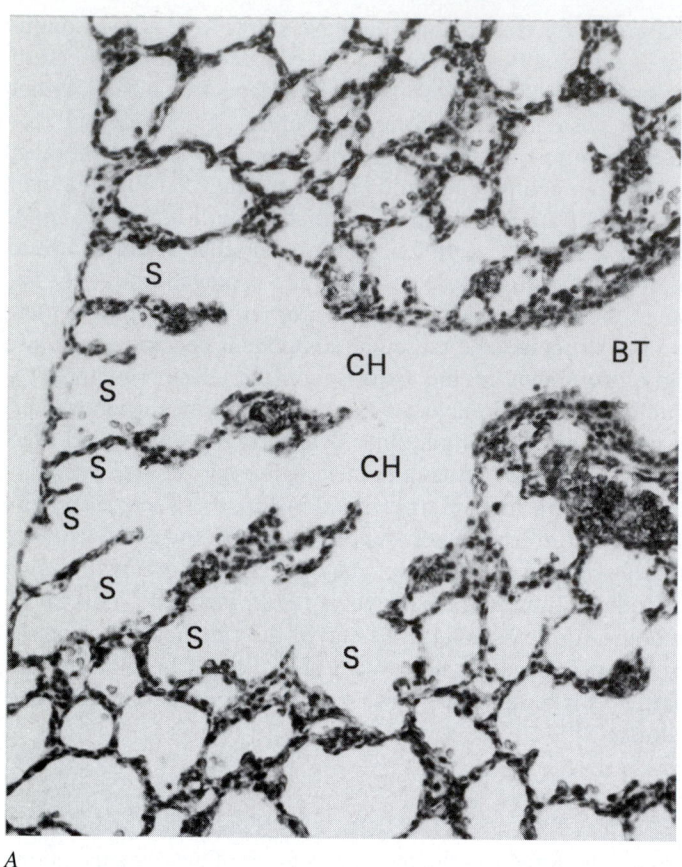

A

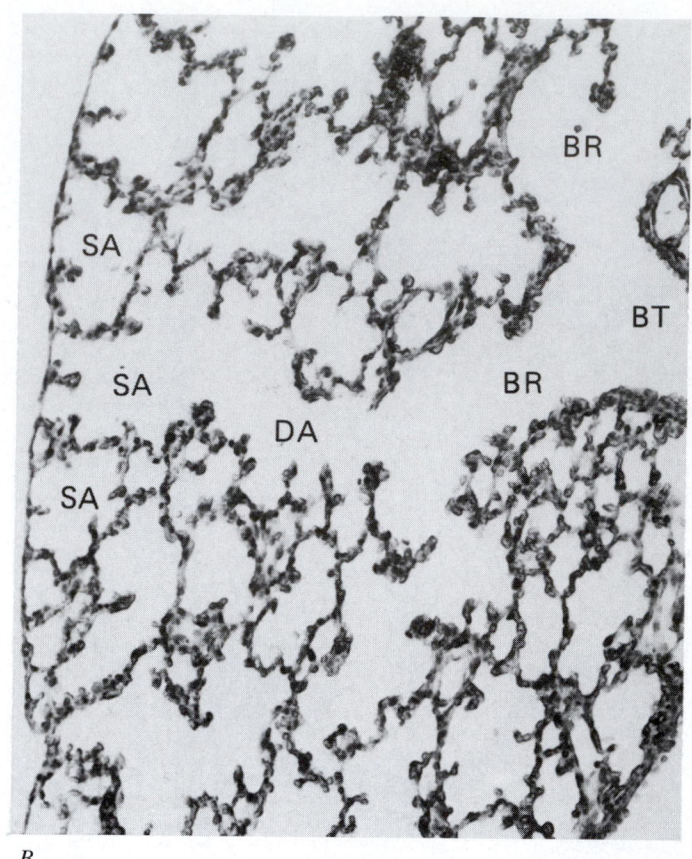

B

FIGURE 5-6   Termination portion of the airways of the rat lung. *A.* One day after birth. A terminal bronchiole (BT) divides into smooth-walled channels (CH) that terminate into small airspaces called saccules (S). No true alveoli are present. ×200. This figure can be directly compared with *B,* taken at the same magnification and showing the corre-sponding structures on postnatal day 17. *B.* Seventeen days. The terminal bronchiole (BT) now opens into respiratory bronchioles (BR). The originally smooth-walled channels have elongated and have transformed into alveolar ducts (DA). The saccules of *A* have been partitioned into alveolar sacs (SA) surrounded by alveoli.

(Fig. 5-6). This transformation is due to a honeycomblike partitioning of the airspaces into smaller units by a septation process. The newly formed units are the alveoli and the walls delineating them, the interalveolar septa. The process is nicely visualized with scanning electron microscopy (Fig. 5-7).

Besides alveolization, there is another marked difference between the newborn and the adult rat lung. The relatively thick septa present at birth and after alveolization contain two capillary networks, one on each side of a central layer of connective tissue. In contrast, not only are the septa of the adult lung thinner but also their central axis of connective tissue has disappeared; a single capillary meshwork makes up almost the entire width of the septum. This means, as is to be discussed below, that the pulmonary capillary system has to be completely restructured after birth.

Morphologic investigations supported by quantitative stereologic analyses have led to the following picture of alveolar formation. To begin with, as described above, the newborn rat lung is practically devoid of alveoli. The airspaces correspond to transitory ducts and sacs. The septa between ducts and sacs are called *primary septa* to distinguish them from the *secondary septa* that appear later to form the interalveolar walls. Within the first few days, the lung increases in volume by simple expansion of its airspaces. In the second half of the first postnatal week, a multitude of small ridges and crests appear along the primary septa.

These secondary septa[7] subdivide the airspaces into smaller units, the alveoli. As a consequence, the transitory ducts become alveolar ducts, and the terminal saccules become alveolar sacs (Fig. 5-8). The new partitions greatly increase airspace complexity and hence also alveolar surface area (Sa). With simple isotropic growth (expansion of airspaces in proportion to the increase in lung volume), Sa would be expected to increase to the two-thirds power of lung volume (V_L). As Fig. 5-9 shows, Sa, plotted double logarithmically against lung volume, increases with V_L to the power of 1.6.[12] This high rate of increase in internal surface area is explained by the very conspicuous changes in airspace morphology. In the rat, the septation process is so rapid that most of the alveoli are formed within approximately 10 days. However, this does not preclude the formation of additional alveoli later on. Of interest is that the rapid increase in alveolar surface area is paralleled by changes at the subcellular level in type II cells. The total mass of lamellated bodies is augmented in proportion to the increase in gas exchange surface area, so that lamellar body volume divided by total surface area remains almost unchanged.[53] This means that, if secreted, the lamellar bodies could cover the entire respiratory surface with a film of surfactant that is constant in thickness. Age-dependent changes in surfactant components in rats have been described by Ohashi and coworkers.[38]

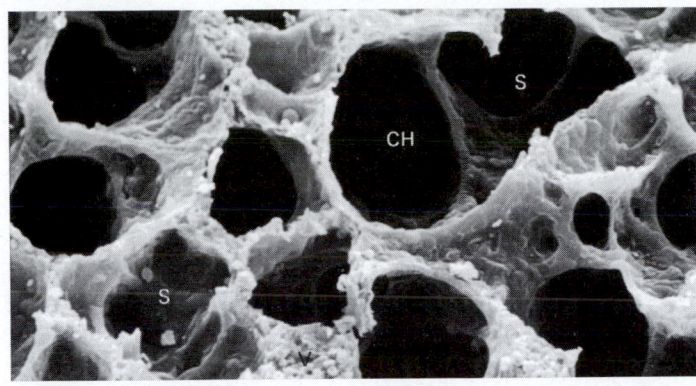

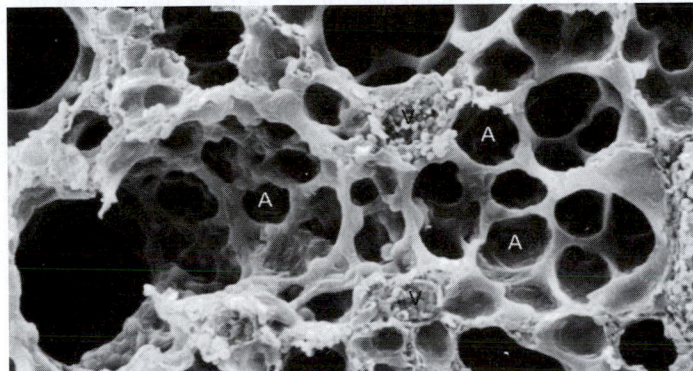

B

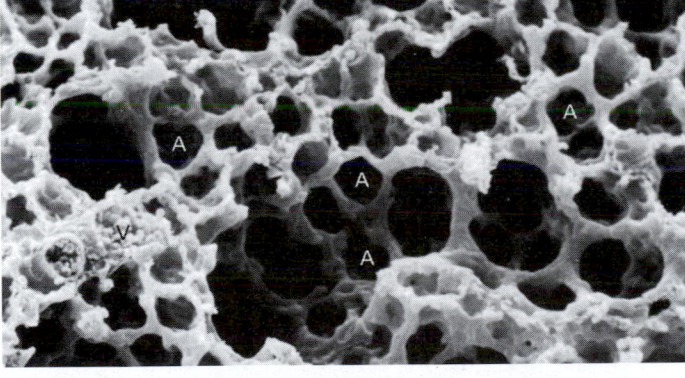

C

FIGURE 5-7 Series of scanning electron micrographs taken at the same magnification (×260) showing formation of alveoli. V = blood vessels containing erythrocytes. *A.* Lung parenchyma at day 4. Relatively large holes correspond to smooth-walled channels (CH) or saccules (S). No alveoli are present. *B.* Lung parenchyma at day 8. Within 4 days, numerous small, rounded outpocketings have formed that can now be called alveoli (A). *C.* Lung parenchyma at day 18. Alveoli (A) appear to be deeper and polygonal in shape. More mature aspect of lung parenchyma.

It seems that the formation of the secondary septa is closely linked to the deposition of elastic fibers in the primary septa. Indeed, in cross sections of forming septa, elastic tissue can regularly be found in the tip of the septum.[7] This strongly suggests that the secondary septa are formed by an up-folding of tissue from the primary septum, pulling up one of the two capillary layers, as is illustrated by the diagram of Fig. 5-10. Therefore,

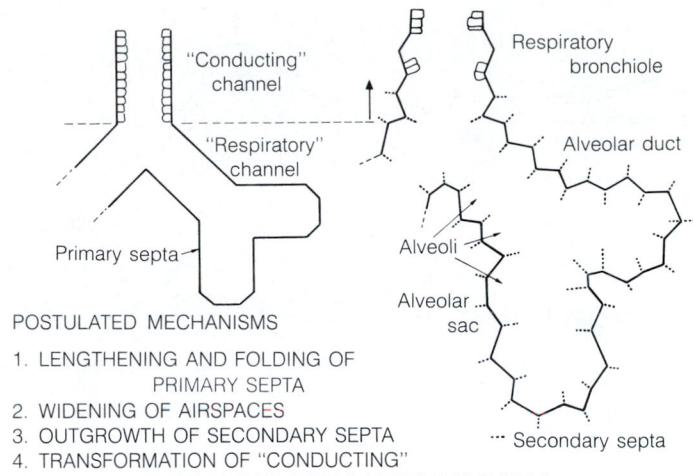

POSTULATED MECHANISMS

1. LENGTHENING AND FOLDING OF
      PRIMARY SEPTA
2. WIDENING OF AIRSPACES
3. OUTGROWTH OF SECONDARY SEPTA
4. TRANSFORMATION OF "CONDUCTING"
      INTO "RESPIRATORY" AIRWAYS [BOYDEN]

FIGURE 5-8 The formation of alveoli.

secondary septa invariably contain, as do primary ones, a double capillary network and a central layer of connective tissue.

Shortly before and also during the onset of septal formation, DNA synthesis is increased in cells located preferentially in the region of the forming crests. Autoradiographic studies with H_3-thymidine showed that DNA synthesis was high first in the mesodermally derived cells, like the interstitial and endothelial cells. A few days later (at the age of 1 week), type II cells exhibited the highest activity in DNA synthesis.[29] Within 1 h after the thymidine injection, not a single type I cell could be labeled, indicating clearly that type I cells are unable to divide. If, in some experiments, type I cell labeling could be detected, it was always with some delay, which allowed for the differentiation of labeled type II cells into type I cells. At the age of 2 weeks, all labeling indices were back to low levels. Nonetheless, alveolar surface

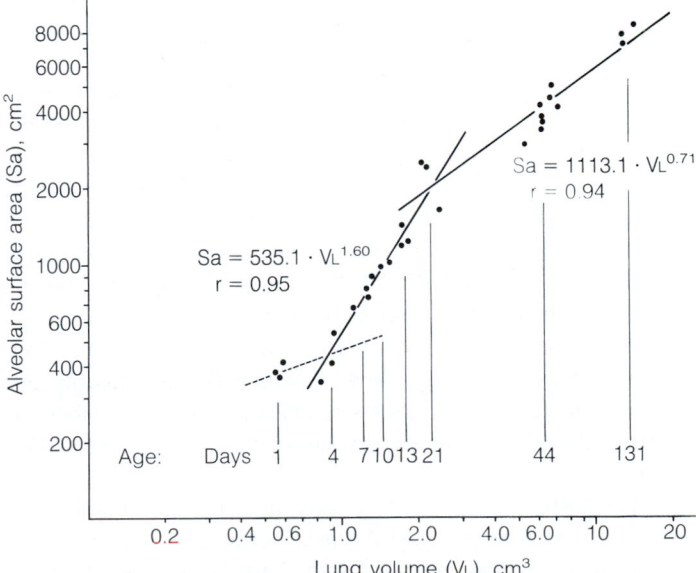

FIGURE 5-9 Postnatal increase in "alveolar" surface area. The alveolar surface area (Sa) is plotted double-logarithmically against lung volume (VL). Steep increase in alveolar surface area between days 4 and 21 corresponds to phase of alveolar formation and septal remodeling. r = correlation coefficient. (*After Burri et al,[12] with permission.*)

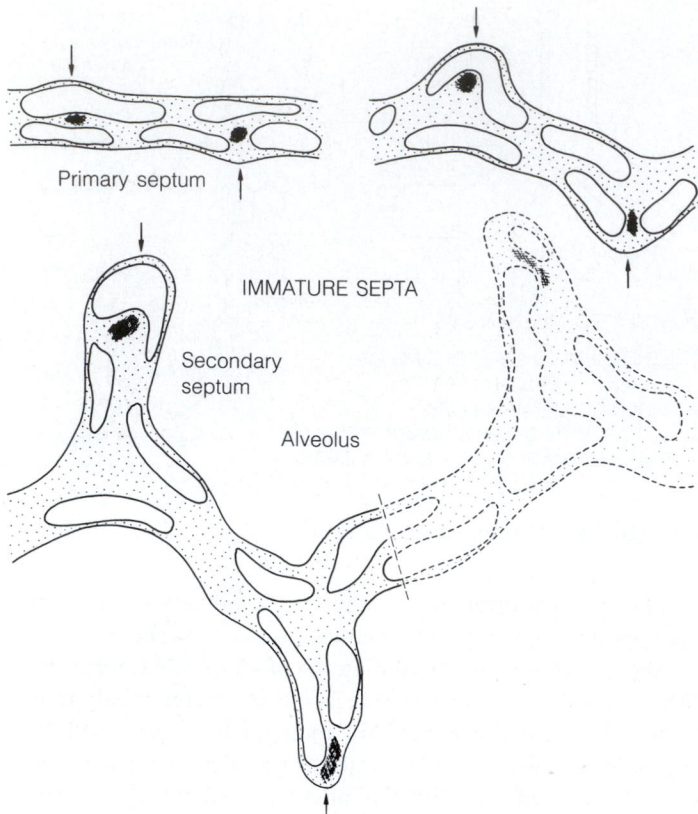

FIGURE 5-10 Formation of secondary septa. Secondary septa are formed by lifting off one of the two capillary layers of the primary septum (arrows). Deposition of elastin (dark spots) is closely linked with alveolar formation. Notice that secondary septa also contain a double capillary network.

area continued to increase at a high rate during the third week. The morphometric data indicate that this further gain in surface area was obtained by restructuring of the available tissue mass rather than by further proliferative activity.

Boyden has postulated an additional mechanism for formation of alveoli: the centripetal transformation of terminal bronchioles (purely conductive airways) into respiratory bronchioles. He described a flattening of the cuboidal epithelium in terminal bronchioles, followed by local outpocketings of the new air-blood barrier;[5] these first shallow depressions subsequently deepen to form true alveoli. Whether this is a completely different mechanism of alveolization or whether formation of secondary septa also occurs is not yet settled. A consequence of this putative process (the importance of which Boyden has played down in his later publications[4]) is that the average number of purely conducting airway generations would slightly decrease after birth.

In the postnatal rat lung, the interstitial tissue contains two clearly defined fibroblastic cell types:[6] a cell type with lipid inclusions (LIC), which is located at the base of the newly formed crests and has little signs of secretory activity, and a fibroblastic type, which has no lipid inclusions (NLICs) but does contain a well-developed machinery for protein synthesis and secretion. Whereas the LICs contain lipoprotein lipase and may be the

source of this chylomicron-degrading enzyme in the endothelial cells,[33] the NLICs seem to be responsible for the formation of collagen and elastin. In adult lungs, lipid droplets in fibroblasts are usually absent or sparse, so that the fate of the LICs is unknown. It has been suggested that because LICs contain microfilaments, they could be the source of the contractile fibroblasts (or myofibroblasts) of the lung parenchyma described by Kapanci and coworkers.[28]

According to the concept of alveolization described above, it is evident that interairspace walls with a double capillary layer represent a prerequisite for the formation of alveoli. It is, however, well established that the mature lung possesses slender interalveolar walls, where a single-layered capillary network occupies practically the whole width of the septum. Lung development therefore must undergo a last step: the stage of microvascular maturation.

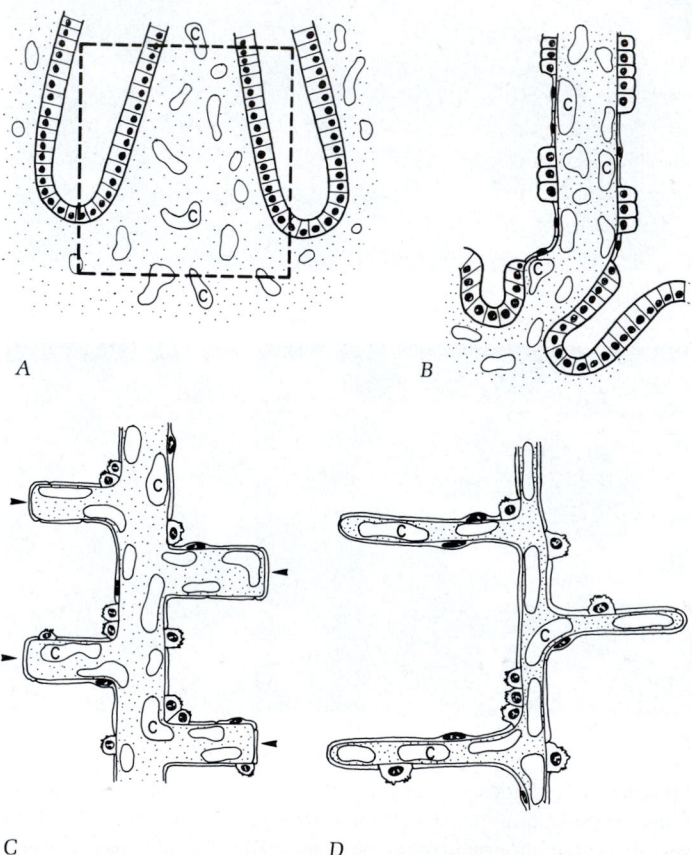

FIGURE 5-11 Fetal and postnatal development of the pulmonary capillary bed. *A.* Pseudoglandular stage with capillary network (c). Development of structures within frame is shown in *B* to *D. B.* Canalicular stage. Mesenchyme with capillaries is sandwiched between widening canaliculi. Capillaries begin to arrange around canaliculi. At sites of epithelio-capillary contact, thin air-blood barriers develop through differentiation of the epithelium. At the tip of the still-growing canaliculi the cuboidal epithelium is maintained for further branching and growth. *C.* Perinatally, the secondary septa develop from the primary septa (arrowheads). All septa are of the primitive type, i.e., contain a double capillary network (c) and a central layer of connective tissue. *D.* Mature lung with mostly a single capillary network meandering along the interalveolar septa. The interstitial layer is very thin.

Stage of Microvascular Maturation

This stage completely transforms the structure of the interalveolar walls. During the third week, low and thick septa change to high and slender ones, the double capillary layer disappears in most places, and, despite a size increase of the lung, the total mass of interstitium decreases.[12] The reduction of interstitial tissue mass is likely to be functionally linked to capillary restructuring.

A diagram of the capillary development during the fetal and postnatal periods may help to clarify the changes in the pulmonary microvasculature. Figure 5-11 illustrates schematically how the loose, three-dimensional capillary network formed in early stages of lung development is rearranged around the peripheral airspaces of the canalicular stage. The intervening mesenchyme thins out, bringing the pericanalicular capillary networks of adjacent tubules close together, which leads to the formation of the capillary bilayer in the intersaccular septa (Fig. 5-11). Since the secondary septa that form later also contain a double network, shortly after alveolar formation practically all septa are of the primitive or immature type. We have hypothesized that the further thinning of the central interstitial tissue layer could lead to intercapillary contacts and to capillary fusions. By electron microscopic examination of serial sections of interalveolar walls, we have recently been able to detect sites of capillary fusions (Burri, unpublished observations).

Local fusion of capillary segments, combined with subsequent preferential growth of the fused areas, finally leads to the classic adult septal morphology (Fig. 5-12).[15] The decrease in interstitial tissue mass and the ensuing thinning of the interalveolar wall have other consequences, too: the formation of the interalveolar pores of Kohn. In a recent study,[54] we demonstrated that, owing to the reduction of the interstitial tissue layer, there were sites of transseptal interepithelial cell contact; i.e., the epithelial covers of both sides of an interalveolar septum were meet-ing transseptally and fusioning in small spots. Subsequently, the epithelium thinned out and gave way to form an interalveolar opening. This process can occur as well between two type I cells as between a type I and a type II cell (Figs. 5-13 and 5-14). Because of their greater thickness, however, type II cells were more frequently involved in pore formation.

Based on animal experiments, postnatal lung development comprises two stages: alveolar formation, which is initiated by a phase of lung expansion that prepares for a phase of tissue proliferation and formation of the interalveolar septa, and the stage of microvascular maturation, during which the double-layered capillary system of the interalveolar septa is completely restructured into a single intraseptal network. The decrease in interstitial tissue mass related to these alterations also induces the formation of interalveolar pores, whose frequency differs greatly from one species to another. Concurrently with these alterations, the interalveolar walls increase in height in conjunction with deepening of the alveolar cups. It is well known that these processes and the postnatal growth of the lung are influenced by various external factors, such as hormones, malnutrition, and alterations in O_2 partial pressure of inspired air.[3,9,19,34,44,45,50] Glucocorticoids in particular, when injected at a very low dose into newborn rats during the period of alveolization, were found to prevent the formation of secondary septa almost completely. At the age of young adults, the lungs of treated rats showed much wider airspaces than controls, and their gas exchange surface area was decreased.

In view of our concept that interalveolar walls arise by folding up one of the two capillary layers, we hypothesized that glucocorticoids could prevent septum formation by acting on the interstitial tissue and inducing a premature maturation of the microvascular network. We recently obtained evidence for this theory: In rats treated with 0.1 μg of dexamethasone phosphate on postnatal days 2 to 15, alveolization was markedly impeded; more important, the stage of microvascular maturation, normally occuring in the third week, was already advanced at the age of 10 to 13 days.[51] Further

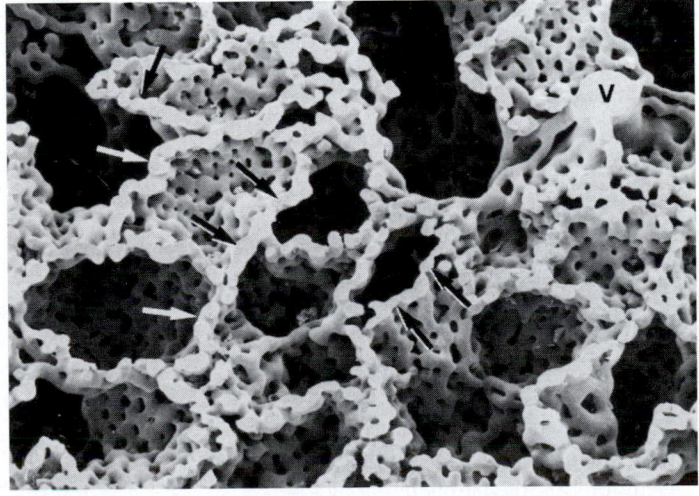

A   *B*

FIGURE 5-12   Mercox cast of pulmonary capillary bed of rat. *A*. Lung aged 7 days. Tissues are digested away; the vascular structures outline the saccular airspaces. The intersaccular walls contain two well-defined capillary networks (arrows). Secondary septa are low (arrowheads). Scanning electron micrograph, $\times250$. *B*. Lung aged 139 days. Same technique as above. Interalveolar septa contain a single and dense capillary network (arrows). V = collecting venule. Scanning electron micrograph, $\times270$.

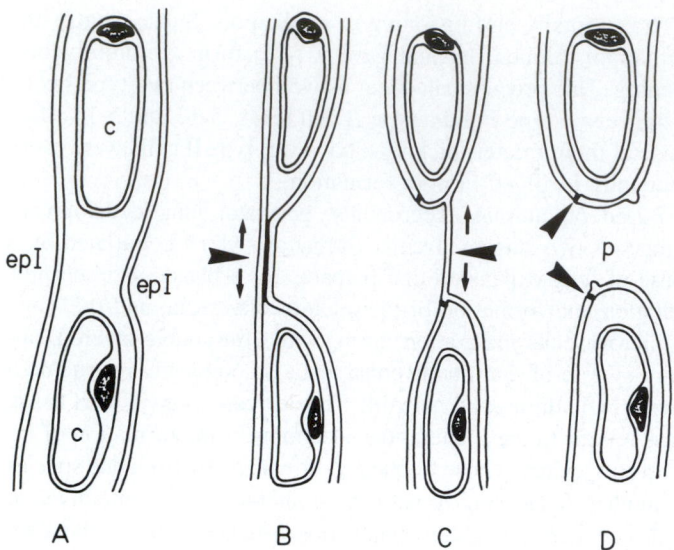

FIGURE 5-13 Diagrammatic sequence based on serial sections illustrating interalveolar pore formation by involvement of type I epithelial cells only. *A*. Normal interalveolar septum before pore formation. *B.* Thinning of interstitial layer permits interepithelial cell contact. Arrowhead points to spot of future thinning and opening of left epithelial leaflet. Notice formation of interepithelial cell junctions. *C.* Only a single type I cytoplasmic extension covers future pore. Membrane undergoes same process as in *B. D.* Pore of Kohn with intercellular junctions running all around it (arrowheads). *(From Weiss and Burri,[54] with permission.)*

passed its climax and that capillary remodeling is already taking place over wide areas by 6 months of age. These observations, however, do not preclude the addition of further alveoli at a much slower pace later in childhood. Some parenchymal regions with double capillary networks, prerequisite structures for alveolar formation, can still be found in the adult lung.

In summary, the stage of rapid alveolar formation in the human lung starts in late fetal life and is probably completed within the first 12 to 18 postnatal months. As in the rat, the human alveolar stage of lung development is followed and partly overlapped by a stage of microvascular maturation, which, in humans, is supposed to end somewhere between 2 and 5 years of age (Fig. 5-1). In this phase, the double capillary network present in the parenchymal septa during the first months of life is reduced to a single-layered system by a complex process combining capillary fusion with capillary network growth.

GROWTH OF THE LUNG

Transition from Development to Growth

In theory, normal lung growth starts when lung development is complete. The transition from the developmental phase into simple organ growth is, however, blurred—as is the transition from growth into aging, where further structural alterations are expected.[18] The difficulty in setting clear limits is both technical and biologic. Alveolar counting procedures are problematic,

experiments are needed, however, to clarify the mode of action of this potent hormone.

In humans, alveolization starts during the late fetal period, but the bulk alveolar formation occurs postnatally. The newborn human lung contains about 50 million alveoli, the adult lung about 300 million; individual variations are large.[31] The age up to which alveoli are formed is a much discussed issue. Before the 1980s, it was generally assumed that alveolization extended to the age of 8 years. Then the figure of 2 years was advanced,[31,56,57] and when lung morphology is considered, with most interalveolar walls already appearing mature in the first year of life, the figure is likely to be even lower. Although at 1 month the human lung looks very immature (Figs. 5-15*A* and 5-16*A*) and, except for airspace size, compares well with the lung of a 1-week-old rat, the parenchyma of a 6-month-old lung already has large regions in which interalveolar septa are slender (Figs. 5-15*B* and 5-16*B*). This finding strongly suggests that the stage of *intense* alveolar formation (which we call bulk alveolar formation) has

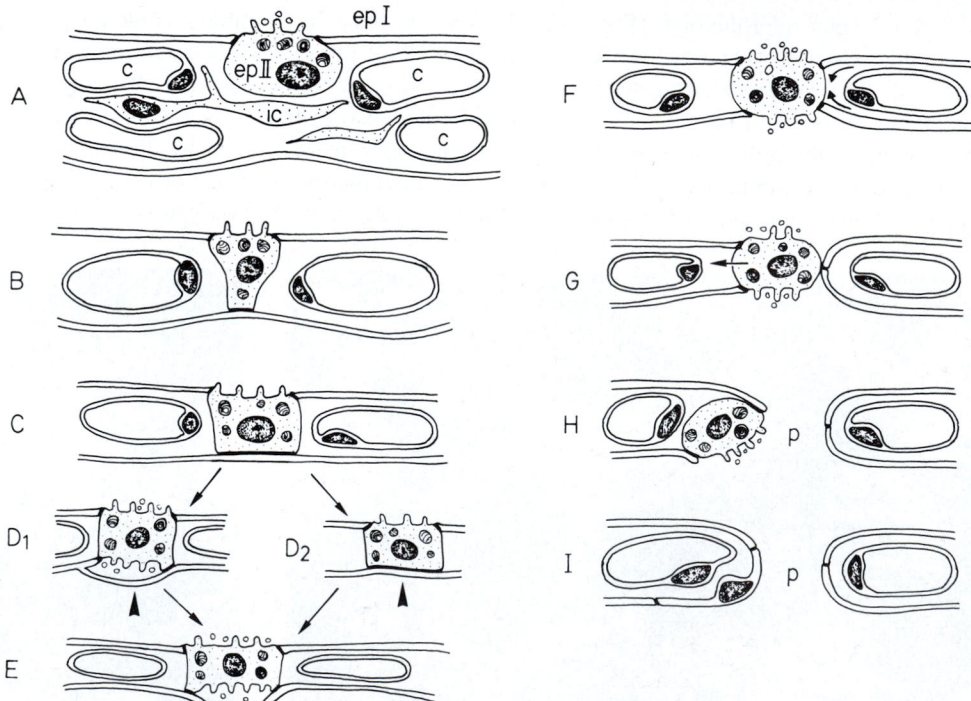

FIGURE 5-14 Diagrammatic illustration based on serial sections illustrating interalveolar pore formation involving a type II epithelial cell. *A.* Immature primary or secondary septum with double capillary layer. *B.* Same septum following microvascular maturation. Septum is slender, interstitial tissue mass has decreased, and type II cell has established transseptal contact to type I cell. *C–E.* Zone of contact enlarges and overlying extension of type I cell opens up by same process as in Fig. 5-13. *F.* Type II cell sits in future pore and abuts to two adjacent alveoli. *G–H.* Type II cell detaches from one side and forms a pore of Kohn. *I.* Type II cell may differentiate into type I cell. *(From Weiss and Burri,[54] with permission.)*

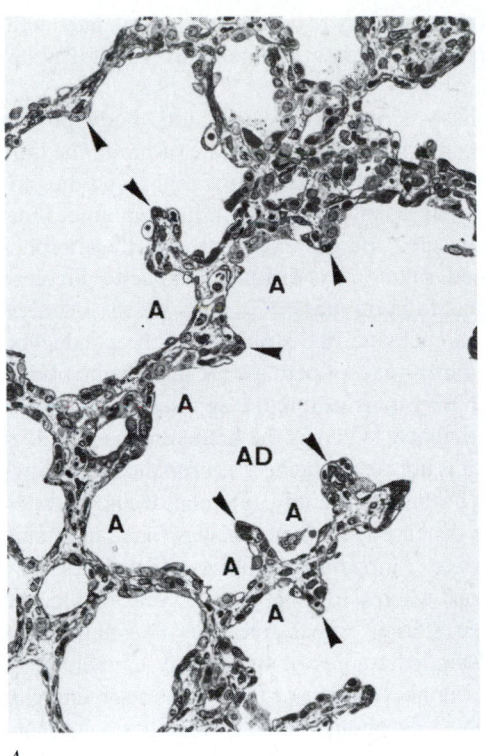

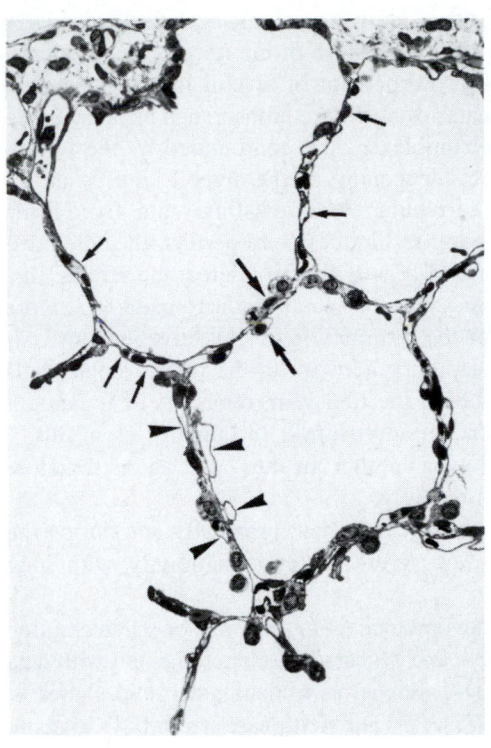

A   *B*

FIGURE 5-15 Development of pulmonary parenchyma in human lung. *A*. Alveolar formation in human lung aged $3\frac{1}{2}$ weeks. Thick and short secondary septa (arrowheads) bulge from the broad primary septa and subdivide the saccular airspaces into alveolar ducts (AD) with small alveoli (A). Light micrograph, ×250. *B*. Pulmonary parenchyma of a child aged 5.8 months. The interalveolar walls are already slender: they show mostly a single capillary network (short arrows) that appears alternately on either side of the septum (long arrows). In places, a double capillary network seems to be present (arrowheads). Light micrograph, ×360.

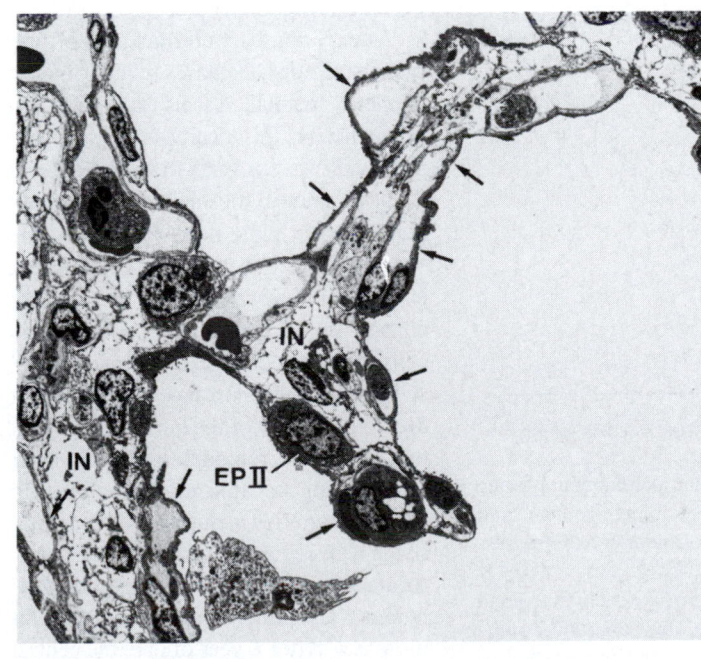

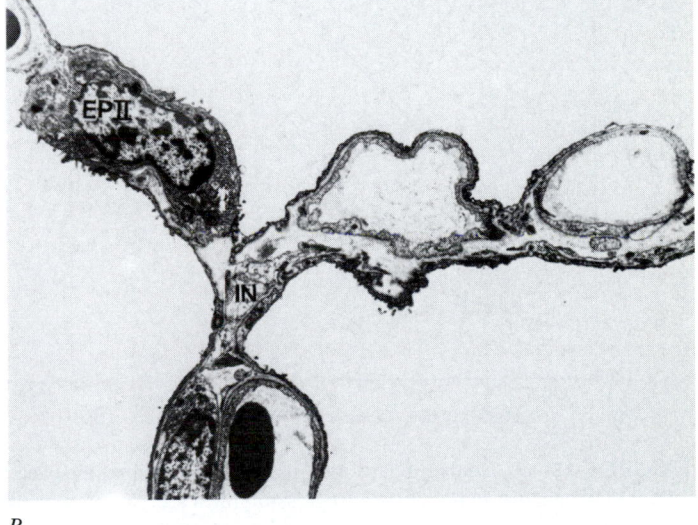

A   *B*

FIGURE 5-16 Transmission electron micrographs comparing parenchymal septa in the lung of a child. *A*. Human lung, 32 days. The septa are broad and primitive in type (arrows pointing to double capillary layer). *B*. Human lung, $6\frac{1}{2}$ months. The septa are now slender, the interstitial tissue mass being markedly reduced. IN = interstitium; EP = epithelial cell of type II. Magnification: *A* = ×960, *B* = ×2580.

even if they rely on the modern stereologic counting procedures introduced in the 1980s,[17] because of the uncertainty in identifying more than 70 to 80 percent of alveoli in histologic sections. Indirect estimates of alveolar number, such as those based on alveolar surface complexity, are confounded by the formation of new septa, by deepening of the alveoli, and by an increase in the surface irregularities of existing septa. Even if the counting and measuring techniques were perfect, the sole presence of biologic variability would partly defeat the efforts. In a similar way, the assessment of septal maturity cannot be more than an indicator for the termination of bulk alveolization. Although the double capillary network in the interalveolar walls disappears mostly within the first year, remnants of it can still be sporadically found in adult lungs. In humans, as in rats, a slow increase in alveolar number far into adult age is therefore conceivable, though unlikely.

From the above, it is evident that, prenatally and during the first years of life, lung growth occurs conjointly with lung development.

Morphometric data obtained from the lungs of seven children aged between 26 days and 5 years and complemented with data from eight adult lungs, allowed us to distinguish two phases of lung growth (Fig. 5-17).[56,57] The first phase (from birth to about 18 months) corresponds to the period of ongoing lung development (alveolization and microvascular maturation) and is therefore characterized by major shifts in the quantitative parameters of the parenchymal compartments. The parameters in close relationship with O_2 transport, the airspace and capillary volumes, grow faster than lung volume, mainly at the expense of the parenchymal tissue mass. The fact that capillary blood volume increases massively during the phase of microvascular matura-

tion is an indication that capillary restructuring is associated with intense capillary growth—a further argument in favor of the concept of preferential growth.

In the second phase (from 1 1/2 years until body growth stops), the lung grows in a highly proportionate fashion. The lung volume increases to the power of 1 to body weight, and the pulmonary compartments augment linearly with lung volume. Most important, the surface area for gas exchange and the morphometrically determined pulmonary diffusion capacity increase both to the power of 1 to body mass.[57]

Unlike the lung parenchyma, the structure of the conducting airways is mature at birth—except perhaps for the terminal bronchioles, part of which may transform into respiratory bronchioles, as has been described above. Whereas the branching pattern does not change with age, it is not clear whether the bronchial tree grows proportionately after birth. In one study, the relationship between diameter and relative distance from the hilus was found to remain almost constant with age.[23] In another analysis, this was true only after the age of 1 year, whereas during the first year of life, the larger bronchi showed a faster growth rate than the smaller conducting airways.[27] Detailed studies of the airway epithelium of hamsters and rhesus monkeys indicate that the airway lining is largely mature at birth.[39,43] Although there is some postnatal functional maturation, most developmental changes occur before birth.

During fetal life, blood flow through the lung is limited to between 10 and 15 percent of the cardiac output. Clearly, the most important vascular event accompanying the onset of air breathing is the closure of the ductus arteriosus and the shunting of the entire cardiac output through the lung. The ductus arteriosus, first obstructed by muscular contraction, is anatomically closed within a few weeks by the fibrotic organization of an intravascular clot. The ligamentum arteriosum represents the tombstone of this important prenatal structure.

After birth, the wall thickness of pulmonary arteries decreases relative to their diameter. In small vessels (up to 200 μm in diameter), this decrease occurs very rapidly. It was assumed that it was due to a fall in smooth-muscle tone.[25] A study performed in pigs, however, related the vascular dilatation more to a concurrent extensive rearrangement and shape change of the vascular smooth-muscle cells than to a change in muscle tone.[22] A similar adaptation has been noted in the small arteries of the human lung, with the structural remodeling being most rapid during the first month of life.[1] In the larger arteries in humans, the thinning of the wall occurs less abruptly: the transformation is achieved by structural adaptations and therefore takes several months.[25] After 1 year of age, the central pulmonary arteries no longer change their relative wall thickness appreciably; instead, they grow more or less proportionally.

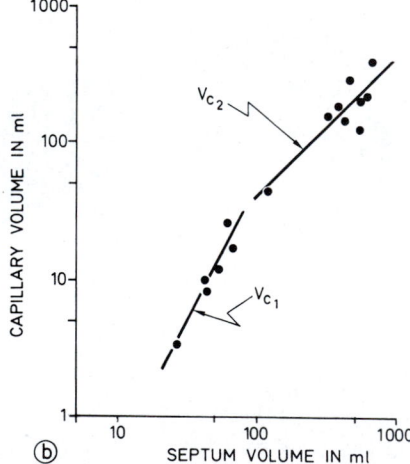

FIGURE 5-17 *A.* Double logarithmic plot of parenchymal airspace (Va) and parenchymal tissue volume (Vt) against lung volume. Regression lines are plotted separately for subjects younger and those older than 18 months of age (subscripts 1 and 2, respectively). The formulas for the regression lines are $Va_1 = 0.275 \times V_L^{1.155}$; $Va_2 = 0.476 \times V_L^{1.059}$; $Vt_1 = 5.60 \times V_L^{0.317}$; $Vt_2 = 0.08 \times V_L^{0.978}$. *B.* Double logarithmic plot of capillary volume (Vc) versus volume of parenchymal septa (Vs). Regression lines are plotted separately for subjects younger and those older than 18 months of age (subscripts 1 and 2, respectively). The formulas describing the regressions are $Vc_1 = 0.003 \times Vs^{2.114}$; $Vc_2 = 0.405 \times Vs^{0.997}$. Calculation of regression lines represents a mean to evaluate the growth rate of a parameter with respect to another one. An exponent of 1 means that growth is proportionate, smaller than 1 signals that growth is slower and larger than 1 that growth is faster than that of the structure referred to. (*From Zeltner et al,*[57] *with permission.*)

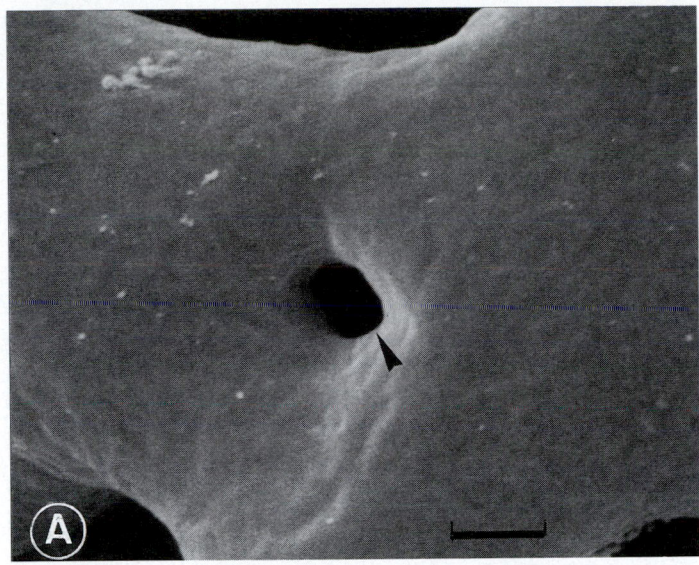

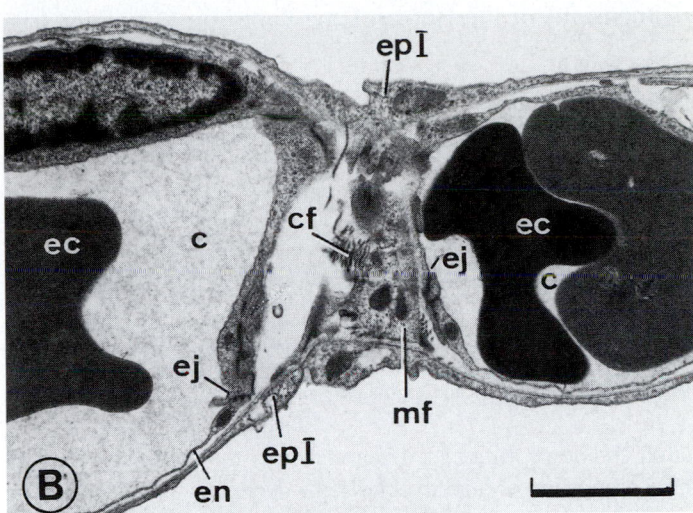

FIGURE 5-18 Transcapillary tissue pillars responsible for intussusceptive microvascular growth as observed in rat lung preparations. *A.* Mercox cast of lung microvascular bed. Pillars appear as tiny holes, often in the range of 1.5 μm in diameter. Scanning electron micrograph, ×5850, bar 2 μm. *B.* Longitudinal sections of transcapillary tissue pillar. The pillar structure exhibits a central axis formed by the cytoplasmic extension of a myofibroblast (mf) with actin filaments, and some collagen fibrils (cf); c = capillary; ec = erythrocyte; epI = type I cell; en = endothelial cell; ej = endothelial cell junctions. Electron micrograph, ×9400, bar 2 μm.

Although the central vessels that accompany the conductive airways do not multiply after birth, the situation is completely different for the peripheral vessels. During the first 1 or 2 years of life, intra-acinar arteries undergo intense development and growth as they follow the extension of the peripheral airspaces. The number of small vessels therefore increases both absolutely and relatively. The relative increase implies that their number augments per unit area of lung section. From the age of 5 years on, the relative number decreases again, reflecting the enlargement of the alveoli. The newly formed vessels are thin walled and are partly muscular or nonmuscular, because muscle formation lags behind the increase in diameter. Gradually, muscularization then proceeds toward the periphery—a process that continues into adulthood.

Veins have a smaller amount of smooth muscle than do arteries. But, in principle, the same observations apply to veins as well as to arterial development and growth.

Growth of the Pulmonary Capillary Bed

Between birth and adulthood, lung volume increases about 23 times both in rats and in humans.[57] The pulmonary capillary network grows even more: its surface area more than 20 times and its volume more than 35 times. Evidently this means that if the gas exchange system continues to function satisfactorily, the capillary network has to extend by addition of new capillary segments. Until about 10 years ago, general vascular network growth in organs was assumed to occur exclusively by capillary sprouting. This means that capillary network complexity—i.e., an increase in number of capillary segments—is achieved by the outgrowth of either solid buds or hollow protrusions from the side of capillaries. The proliferating endothelial cells would then contact a neighboring capillary and merge with its wall. With the formation of a lumen, the sprout becomes a new segment of the network and opens up to the blood circulation.

In 1950, Short,[46] investigating thick sections of rabbit lungs and studying en face views of interalveolar walls, suggested that the capillary network of septa would grow by the addition of new meshes; this was an idea, however, that went unnoticed. The investigation of the capillary maturation of the capillary bed by study of casts in the scanning electron microscope[15] revealed the presence in the capillary network of numerous holes of less than 1.5 μm in diameter (Fig. 5-18A). We considered these holes to represent newly formed intercapillary meshes, which would subsequently grow in diameter. By the continuous addition of such holes, the capillary network would increase its number of segments and hence gain in complexity. We termed this new process of capillary growth *intussusceptional* or *intussuceptive* microvascular growth (IMG).[10] The term is commonly used to describe the growth of cartilage, and means that a structure is able to grow within itself by the addition of new but similar elements of formative material among those already present. It is evident that the holes in the cast must correspond to some form of tissue pillars traversing the capillary lumina. By electron microscopic investigation of serial sections through the interalveolar walls, we demonstrated the presence of tissue pillars of corresponding diameters (Fig. 5-18B). From the analysis of their varying ultrastructure, we derived a mechanism for their formation.[14]

IMG has since been documented in various species and organ systems,[11,40,41,55] and even in tumor growth.[37] Also, further mechanisms of pillar formation have been described.[42] Today, IMG seems to represent a fundamental mechanism of angiogenesis and capillary network growth not only in the lung but in growing organisms in general.

Dimensions of the Adult Lung

Table 5-1 summarizes the dimensions of a "standard" adult human lung.[16,20] In a direct comparison of the quantitative data of

TABLE 5-1

Dimensions of the Human Lung Based on Morphometry*

Body weight, kg	74 ± 4
Lung volume, L	4.3 ± 0.3
Volume of compartments	
Parenchyma, L	3.9 ± 0.3
Parenchymal tissue, ml	298 ± 36
Parenchymal capillaries, ml	213 ± 31
Surface areas	
Airspace, m^2	143 ± 12
Capillary, m^2	126 ± 12

*Values represent mean values $\pm$ standard errors. Eight human lungs were used.
SOURCE: Based on data from Crapo et al[16] and Gehr et al.[20]

adult and newborn lungs, it is noteworthy that, with age, the volume proportion of interalveolar septa decreases, the airspace volume increases, and, within the interalveolar walls, the volume proportion of the blood compartment increases at the expense of tissue mass. It is interesting to note that the arithmetic mean thickness of the air-blood tissue interface (calculated by dividing total tissue mass by the alveolar surface area) falls from around 5 μm at birth to 2.5 μm in the adult, while the harmonic mean thickness of the air-blood tissue barrier, a measure of the average effective diffusion distance, remains largely unaffected by all the structural alterations of postnatal development.

It is most important that the gas exchange surface areas of airspaces and capillaries increase linearly with body weight.[57] These data indicate that lung development and growth represent a structural process that is well balanced to continuously meet the O_2 needs of the growing organism.

REFERENCES

1. Allen K, Haworth SG: Human postnatal pulmonary arterial remodeling: Ultrastructural studies of smooth muscle cell and connective tissue maturation. *Lab Invest* 59:702–709, 1988.
2. Bachofen M, Weibel ER: Alterations of the gas exchange apparatus in adult respiratory insufficiency associated with septicemia. *Am Rev Respir Dis* 116:589–615, 1977.
3. Blanco LN, Massaro D, Massaro GD: Alveolar size, number, and surface area: Developmentally dependent response to 13% O_2. *Am J Physiol* 261:L370–L377, 1991.
4. Boyden EA: Development and growth of the airways, in Hodson WA (ed), *Development of the Lung*. New York, Dekker, 1977, pp 3–35.
5. Boyden EA, Tompsett DH: The postnatal growth of the lung in the dog. *Acta Anat (Basel)* 47:185–215, 1961.
6. Brody JS, Vaccaro C: Postnatal formation of alveoli: Interstitial events and physiologic consequences. *Fed Proc* 38:215–223, 1979.
7. Burri PH: The postnatal growth of the rat lung: III. Morphology. *Anat Rec* 180:77–98, 1974.
8. Burri PH: Development and growth of the human lung, in Fishman AP, Fisher AB (eds), *Handbook of Physiology,* sec. 3: *The Respiratory System: Circulation and Nonrespiratory Functions*. Bethesda, MD, American Physiological Society, 1985, pp 1–46.
9. Burri PH: Postnatal lung development and modulation of lung growth, in Walters DV, Strang LB, Geubelle F (eds), *Physiology of the Fetal and Neonatal Lung*. Norwell, MA, Kluwer, 1987, pp 39–59.
10. Burri PH: Intussusceptive microvascular growth, a new mechanism of capillary network formation, in Steiner R, Weisz PB, Langer R (eds), *Angiogenesis*. Basel, Birkhäuser, 1992, pp 32–39.
11. Burri PH: Postnatal development and growth of the pulmonary microvasculature, in Motta PM, Murakami T, Fujita H (eds), *Scanning Electron Microscopy of Vascular Casts: Methods and Applications*. Norwell, MA, Kluwer, 1992, pp 139–156.
12. Burri PH, Dbaly J, Weibel ER: The postnatal growth of the rat lung: I. Morphometry. *Anat Rec* 178:711–730, 1974.
13. Burri PH, Moschopulos M: Structural analysis of fetal rat lung development. *Anat Rec* 234:399–418, 1992.
14. Burri PH, Tarek MR: A novel mechanism of capillary growth in the rat pulmonary microcirculation. *Anat Rec* 228:35–45, 1990.
15. Caduff JH, Fischer LC, Burri PH: Scanning electron microscopic study of the developing microvasculature in the postnatal rat lung. *Anat Rec* 216:154–164, 1986.
16. Crapo JD, Barry BE, Gehr P, Bachofen M: Cell numbers and cell characteristics of the normal human lung. *Am Rev Respir Dis* 126:332–337, 1982.
17. Cruz-Orive LM: Particle number can be estimated using a disector of unknown thickness: The selector. *J Microsc* 145:121–142, 1987.
18. Escolar JD, Gallego B, Tejero C, Escolar MA: Changes occurring with increasing age in the rat lung: Morphometrical study. *Anat Rec* 239:287–296, 1994.
19. Gaultier C: Malnutrition and lung growth. *Pediatr Pulmonol* 10:278–286, 1991.
20. Gehr P, Bachofen M, Weibel ER: The normal human lung: Ultrastructure and morphometric estimation of diffusion capacity. *Respir Physiol* 32:121–140, 1978.
21. Harding R, Hooper SB: Regulation of lung expansion and lung growth before birth. *J Appl Physiol* 81:209–224, 1996.
22. Haworth SG, Hall SM, Chew M, Allen K: Thinning of fetal pulmonary arterial wall and postnatal remodelling: Ultrastructural studies on the respiratory unit arteries of the pig. *Virchows Arch [A]* 411:161–171, 1987.
23. Hislop A, Muir DCF, Jacobsen M, et al: Postnatal growth and function of the pre-acinar airways. *Thorax* 27:265–274, 1972.
24. Hislop A, Reid L: Intra-pulmonary arterial development during fetal life: Branching pattern and structure. *J Anat* 113:35–48, 1972.
25. Hislop A, Reid L: Pulmonary arterial development during childhood: Branching pattern and structure. *Thorax* 28:129–135, 1973.
26. Hislop A, Reid L: Fetal and childhood development of the intrapulmonary veins in man: Branching pattern and structure. *Thorax* 28:313–319, 1973.
27. Horsfield K, Gordon WI, Kemp W, Phillips S: Growth of the bronchial tree in man. *Thorax* 42:383–388, 1987.
28. Kapanci Y, Assimacopoulos A, Irle C, et al: "Contractile interstitial cells" in pulmonary alveolar septa: A possible regulator of ventilation/perfusion ratio? *J Cell Biol* 60:375–392, 1974.
29. Kauffman SL, Burri PH, Weibel ER: The postnatal growth of the rat lung: II. Autoradiography. *Anat Rec* 180:63–76, 1974.
30. Kitaoka H, Burri PH, Weibel ER: Development of the human fetal airway tree—Analysis of the numerical density of airway endtips. *Anat Rec* 244:207–213, 1996.
31. Langston C, Kida K, Reed M, Thurlbeck WM: Human lung growth in late gestation and in the neonate. *Am Rev Respir Dis* 129:607–613, 1984.
32. Low FN: The pulmonary alveolar epithelium of laboratory mammals and man. *Anat Rec* 117:241–246, 1953.
33. Maksvytis HJ, Niles RM, Simanovsky L, et al: In vitro characteristics of the lipid-filled interstitial cell associated with postnatal lung growth: Evidence for fibroblast heterogeneity. *J Cell Physiol* 118:113–123, 1984.

34. Massaro D, Teich N, Maxwell S, et al: Postnatal development of alveoli: Regulation and evidence for a critical period in rats. *J Clin Invest* 76:1297–1305, 1985.

35. Mercurio AR, Rhodin JAG: An electron microscopic study on the type I pneumocyte in the cat: Differentiation. *Am J Anat* 146:255–272, 1976.

36. Moschopulos M, Burri PH: Morphometric analysis of fetal rat lung development. *Anat Rec* 237:38–48, 1993.

37. Nagy JA, Morgan ES, Herzberg KT, et al: Pathogenesis of ascites tumor growth: Angiogenesis, vascular remodeling, and stroma formation in the peritoneal lining. *Cancer Res* 55:376–385, 1995.

38. Ohashi T, Pinkerton K, Ikegami M, Jobe AH: Changes in alveolar surface area, surfactant protein A, and saturated phosphatidylcholine with postnatal rat lung growth. *Pediatr Res* 35:685–689, 1994.

39. Otani EM, Newkirk C, McDowell EM: Development of hamster tracheal epithelium: IV. Cell proliferation and cytodifferentiation in the neonate. *Anat Rec* 214:183–192, 1986.

40. Patan S, Alvarez MJ, Schittny JC, Burri PH: Intussusceptive microvascular growth: A common alternative to capillary sprouting. *Arch Histol Cytol* 55:65–75, 1992.

41. Patan S, Haenni B, Burri PH: Evidence for intussusceptive capillary growth in the chicken chorio-allantoic membrane (CAM). *Anat Embryol* 187:121–130, 1993.

42. Patan S, Haenni B, Burri PH: Implementation of intussusceptive capillary growth in the chicken chorio-allantoic membrane (CAM): 1. Pillar formation by folding of the capillary wall. *Microvasc Res* 51:80–98, 1996.

43. Plopper CG, Alley JL, Weir AJ: Differentiation of tracheal epithelium during fetal lung maturation in the rhesus monkey *Macaca mulatta*. *Am J Anat* 175:59–71, 1986.

44. Randell SH, Mercer RR, Young SL: Postnatal growth of pulmonary acini and alveoli in normal and oxygen-exposed rats studied by serial section reconstructions. *Am J Anat* 186:55–68, 1989.

45. Sahebjami H, Domino M: Effects of postnatal dexamethasone treatment on development of alveoli in adult rats. *Exp Lung Res* 15:961–973, 1989.

46. Short RHD: Alveolar epithelium in relation to growth of the lung. *Philos Trans R Soc Lond [Biol]* 235:35–87, 1950.

47. Spooner BS, Wessells NK: Mammalian lung development: Interactions in primordium formation and bronchial morphogenesis. *J Exp Zool* 175:445–454, 1970.

48. Ten Have–Opbroek AAW: Immunological study of lung development in the mouse embryo: II. First appearance of the great alveolar cell, as shown by immunofluorescence microscopy. *Dev Biol* 69:408–423, 1979.

49. Ten Have–Opbroek AAW: The development of the lung in mammals: An analysis of concepts and findings. *Am J Anat* 162:201–219, 1981.

50. Thibeault DW, Heimes B, Rezaiekhaligh M, Mabry S: Chronic modifications of lung and heart development in glucocorticoid-treated newborn rats exposed to hyperoxia or room air. *Pediatr Pulmonol* 16:81–88, 1993.

51. Tschanz SA, Damke BM, Burri PH: Influence of postnatally administered glucocorticoids on rat lung growth. *Biol Neonate* 68:229–245, 1995.

52. Verbeken EK, Cauberghs M, Van de Woestijne KP: Membranous bronchioles and connective tissue network of normal and emphysematous lungs. *J Appl Physiol* 81:2468–2480, 1996.

53. Vidic B, Burri PH: Quantitative cellular and subcellular changes in the rat type II pneumocyte during early postnatal development. *Am Rev Respir Dis* 124:174–178, 1981.

54. Weiss MJ, Burri PH: Formation of interalveolar pores in the rat lung. *Anat Rec* 244:481–489, 1996.

55. Wilting J, Christ B, Bokeloh M, Weich HA: In vivo effects of vascular endothelial growth factor on the chicken chorioallantoic membrane. *Cell Tissue Res* 274:163–172, 1993.

56. Zeltner TB, Burri PH: The postnatal development and growth of the human lung: II. Morphology. *Respir Physiol* 67:269–282, 1987.

57. Zeltner TB, Caduff JH, Gehr P, et al: The postnatal development and growth of the human lung: I. Morphometry. *Respir Physiol* 67:247–267, 1987.

CHAPTER 6

CELLULAR AND MOLECULAR MECHANISMS REGULATING AIRWAY SMOOTH MUSCLE CELL PHYSIOLOGY AND PHARMACOLOGY

Reynold A. Panettieri, Jr. / Michael I. Kotlikoff

Airway smooth muscle represents an important end-effector cell responsible for modulating bronchomotor tone in health and disease. In recent years, advances in the techniques and concepts of cell and molecular biology have provided fresh insights into the cellular and subcellular physiological processes that regulate smooth muscle cell contraction. Progress has also occurred in the study of the biochemistry and regulation of contractile proteins, transduction properties of the sarcolemma, and the pharmacology of neuropeptides, inflammatory agents, and other intracellular messenger sources. Together these advances have markedly improved our understanding of excitation-contraction coupling mechanisms and the pharmacology related to those processes that regulate force generation.

The role of airway smooth muscle in disease, however, may extend beyond the processes that regulate force generation in individual myocytes. Increased airway smooth muscle mass, which may be induced by myocyte hypertrophy or hyperplasia, has been a well-recognized pathologic finding in the bronchi of patients with chronic severe asthma. Increased smooth muscle cell mass profoundly affects the force generation of the muscle. In addition, the newly recognized immunomodulatory function of airway myocytes and the capacity of these cells to secrete extracellular matrix may implicate airway myocytes as an important effector cell that promotes the airway remodeling seen in patients with asthma, chronic bronchitis, or bronchiolitis obliterans.

This chapter will summarize several of the important molecular mechanisms of excitation-contraction coupling in airway smooth muscle and indicate how these processes are modulated by bronchoactive substances. The cellular and molecular mechanisms regulating airway smooth muscle cell proliferation will also be reviewed, as well as potential pharmacologic approaches to prevent airway smooth muscle cell growth.

EXCITATION-CONTRACTION COUPLING

Airway smooth muscle in vivo either is electrically quiescent or generates slow waves and some active tone, but it does not generate action potentials under resting conditions or when stimulated by neurotransmitters or autocoids. Excitatory stimulation—whether neural, hormonal, or due to the release of autocoids—results in a graded depolarization and increase in tone in the muscle. Since excitatory and inhibitory stimuli are imposed on a tissue with little intrinsic contractile tone, the degree of muscle stimulation (and bronchodilation) will be the summated effect of bronchoconstrictor and bronchodilator stimuli. This feature (electrical quiescence) almost certainly relates to the substantial expression and diversity of potassium channels in airway smooth muscle. A second general feature of airway smooth muscle is its relative resistance to dihydropyridines. Whereas some types of smooth muscle are quite sensitive to inhibitors of voltage-dependent calcium channels, their effects are variable in the airways. Although dihydropyridines are effective at antagonizing contractions associated with a low degree of stimulation, a high level of excitatory input results in the recruitment of different calcium-mobilizing mechanisms.

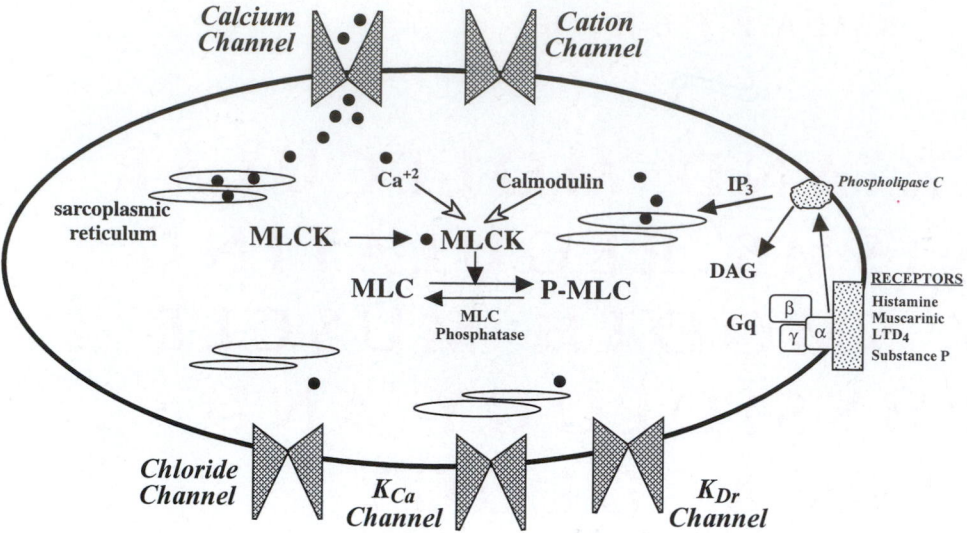

FIGURE 6-1 Major signaling molecules associated with contraction and relaxation of airway smooth muscle cells. Transmembrane proteins shown are G protein–coupled receptors with associated G protein subunits (α, β, and γ) and plasmalemmal ion channels. A Gq-coupled receptor is ligand bound, and the associated G protein has undergone nucleotide exchange. The next step will be dissociation of the α and $\beta\gamma$ subunits, activation of phospholipase C, and release of intracellular calcium stores. Sources of calcium for contraction are also shown. Calcium permeates voltage-dependent calcium channels and nonselective cation channels and is released by the sarcoplasmic reticulum (intracellular structures). Calcium molecules will bind calmodulin and activate myosin light-chain kinase (MLCK), which will phosphorylate myosin light chain (MLC). Dephosphorylation occurs by myosin light-chain phosphatase, which may be regulated during excitation-contraction coupling. DAG = diacylglycerol; IP_3 = inositol triphosphate; LTD_4 = leukotriene D_4; K_{Ca} = calcium-activated potassium channel; K_{DR} = delayed rectifying potassium channel. [*Data based on Kotlikoff MI, Barnes PJ: Pharmacology of airway smooth muscle, in Crystal RG et al (eds), The Lung: Scientific Foundations, 2d ed, Vol I. Philadelphia, Lippincott-Raven, 1996, pp 1345–1354, with permission.*]

Activation of an airway smooth muscle cell by a bronchoconstrictor results in a rapid rise in $[Ca^{2+}]_i$, associated with the release of intracellular calcium stores, to a peak level roughly 10 times higher than the resting level (100 nm to greater than 1 μm at maximum agonist concentration). Following this peak, calcium falls but remains elevated as long as the contractile stimulus is present. The elevation of $[Ca^{2+}]_i$ results in the activation of the calcium-calmodulin–sensitive myosin light-chain kinase, and the subsequent phosphorylation of the regulatory myosin light-chain (MLC_{20}) at Ser 19. Phosphorylation of this residue by myosin ATPase activity initiates cross-bridge cycling between myosin and actin. ATP binding, hydrolysis, and ADP release continue as long as MLC_{20} is phosphorylated; dephosphorylation terminates cross-bridge cycling and relaxes smooth muscle. In addition to the regulation of tension by $[Ca^{2+}]_i$, several mechanisms have been advanced to explain a lack of correlation between $[Ca^{2+}]_i$ and tension between different modes of stimulation. The G protein–coupled regulation of myosin phosphatase may be an important mechanism by which "sensitization" of myosin phosphorylation occurs.[54] Figure 6-1 illustrates several key signaling processes in smooth muscle cells that will be described in more detail below.

Ion Channels

CALCIUM CHANNELS

Studies with calcium indicators in single myocytes show that agonist exposure results in a rapid elevation of $[Ca^{2+}]_i$, followed by a return to an elevated level that is sustained as long as the myocyte is exposed to the agonist.[32] The source of calcium for contraction may derive from extracellular calcium ions that enter the cell through calcium-permeant channels or from intracellular stores. Two types of calcium-permeant channels have been definitively described in patch-clamp studies in airway myocytes: voltage-dependent calcium channels (VDCCs) and nonselective, calcium-permeant cation channels, which are opened by activation of certain surface receptors without depolarization.[54]

VOLTAGE-DEPENDENT CALCIUM CHANNELS

Depolarization of airway smooth muscle with potassium chloride (KCl) solutions results in a contraction that is due to influx of Ca^{2+} through VDCCs.[60] This contraction is blocked by the calcium antagonists verapamil and dihydropyridine (e.g., nifedipine). Furthermore, the Ca^{2+} agonist BAY K8644 augments KCl-induced contractions of airway smooth muscle.[1] Patch-clamp studies have shown that the calcium current is due to the opening of dihydropyridine-sensitive, L-type calcium channels.[18,32] The VDCC current in airway smooth muscle is relatively small (peak current is usually less than 100 pA under physiological conditions) and inactivates rapidly.[18] Although little measurable current is obtained at –50 mV in a smooth muscle cell, recordings of single-channel currents indicate that isolated channel openings can be resolved at potentials as negative as –70 mV.[18] Simultaneous measurements of VDCC currents and $[Ca^{2+}]_i$ in single airway myocytes indicate that these low-probability events substantially regulate $[Ca^{2+}]_i$ in airway smooth muscle cells, and this "low-activity mode" of VDCC function is probably the major mechanism by which VDCCs regulate $[Ca^{2+}]_i$ in nonspiking cells such as airway myocytes.[18] A major factor in this process is the absence of a rapid calcium extrusion mechanism analogous to that found in cardiac and neuronal cells.

Functional studies suggest that VDCCs are important in mediating the contractile response to depolarization in airway smooth muscle and constitute a substantial source of calcium at low doses of contractile agonists.[56] Calcium antagonists, however, have only weak effects against the contraction of human airway smooth muscle induced by higher concentrations of histamine or methacholine.[15] It also appears that differences exist between tracheal and bronchial smooth muscle, with bronchial contractions being more resistant to dihydropyridine block.[12] The pattern of muscle activation may also be a factor in the functional actions of VDCC, since blockade of VDCC effectively limits the refilling of calcium stores following agonist exposure,[9] and when contraction is first induced by a spasmogen, calcium antagonists may effectively reverse the contraction. Calcium antagonists have generally been found to be only weakly effective in human airways in vivo. They do not cause bronchodilation in normal or asthmatic subjects, and they give only weak protection against histamine-, methacholine-, allergen-, and exercise-induced bronchoconstriction.[4]

OTHER CALCIUM-PERMEANT CHANNELS

Numerous studies at the organ or single cell level[40] have indicated that dihydropyridine-resistant calcium influx occurs in airway smooth muscle. With the recent cloning and expression of the P_2 purinergic receptor channel from smooth muscle[59] and the measurement of nonselective cation channels with patch-clamp methods in several smooth muscle cell types,[5] definitive evidence for additional calcium influx mechanisms has been obtained. In airway smooth muscle cells, a nonselective cation current evoked by cholinergic agonists was first reported by Janssen and Sims.[29] Simultaneous measurements of current and calcium in single-airway myocytes show that this current satisfies the principal criteria identified for dihydropyridine-resistant calcium influx in human airway smooth muscle cells. That is, the current is dihydropyridine resistant, maintained as long as the cell is exposed to the muscarinic agonist, blocked by divalent cations such as Ni^{2+}, augmented by hyperpolarization, and permeant to Ca^{2+} ions. The cation current is preceded by a large calcium-activated chloride current following exposure to a contractile agonist. Of interest is that, unlike the chloride current, the calcium-permeant nonselective current is not activated by the release of intracellular calcium. Thus, caffeine activates the chloride current but not the calcium-permeant current. It now appears that substantial diversity exists in non–voltage-gated, calcium-permeant channels. Nonselective cation channels appear to be either calcium or G protein activated.[35] Unlike in airway myocytes, in some cells strong evidence exists for a calcium-selective channel activated following the release of intracellular calcium stores.[27]

Since the development and clinical use of dihydropyridines, it has been recognized that calcium channel antagonists were needed that more effectively dilate airways.[4] In the next few years, we should begin to learn about the structure of important calcium-permeant channels in airway myocytes and about the molecular coupling mechanisms associated with their activation. It is likely that this information will have a substantial impact on the development of bronchodilators.

POTASSIUM CHANNELS

Potassium (K^+) channels are associated with recovery of excitable cells after depolarization. Drugs that block these channels, such as tetraethylammonium (TEA) and 4-aminopyridine (4-AP), cause an increase in excitability. In airway smooth muscle, these agents result in spontaneous action potentials and a reduced threshold of excitation. Conversely, activation of K^+ channels results in depolarization or hyperpolarization of the cell.

There is great diversity of K^+ channels. Several selective blockers, many of which are insect venoms, have been useful tools in identifying these channels. K^+ channels may be activated by depolarization, by a rise in intracellular Ca^{2+}, by activation of certain receptors, or by changes in intracellular concentrations of ATP. With the development of new pharmacologic agents, an increasing number of K^+ channels have been recognized, providing an opportunity for the development of highly selective drugs in the future. The use of selective potassium channel agonists may be of particular use in the airways, since they could serve to inhibit the release of neurotransmitters as well as directly relax smooth muscle. Several drugs, which open K^+ channels in smooth muscle, have recently been developed; the most potent of these drugs is cromakalim (BRL 34915), which has been shown to hyperpolarize various smooth muscles, including guinea pig trachea.[2]

Potassium Channels in Airway Smooth Muscle

Electrophysiological studies of airway smooth muscle cells have indicated the existence of several types of potassium channels. A family of delayed-rectifier, calcium-insensitive channels has been identified by patch-clamp methods and the molecular identity of these channels determined. In airway myocytes from a variety of species, these channels appear to be responsible for the resting membrane potential and electrical stability of airway myocytes.[19] Recent experiments confirmed these findings in acutely dissociated human tracheal and bronchial myocytes. On the basis of subtype-specific toxin experiments, the functionally important channel in airway smooth muscle is likely to be Kv1.5. This channel is relatively insensitive to blockade by TEA and is not blocked by dendrotoxin or charybdotoxin. The release of acetylcholine from parasympathetic nerve endings in the airway appears to be controlled by the same channel subtype.[19]

High-conductance, Ca^{2+}-activated K^+ (K_{Ca}) channels (maxi-K channels)[34] have been recorded in airway smooth muscle. These K^+ channels are potentially of great importance in airway smooth muscle, since they are expressed in high abundance and are actively modulated during excitation-contraction coupling.[33] Thus, during cholinergic contraction K_{Ca} channels are inhibited, and disruption of this inhibitory linkage has predictable consequences on contraction. That is, if the inhibitory linkage between the muscarinic (presumably M_2) receptor is disrupted with pertussis toxin, substantially less force is produced at any given concentration of cholinergic agonist; the normal agonist/force relationship is restored if K_{Ca} channels are blocked by charybdotoxin. It thus appears that an important inhibitory system acts to prevent K_{Ca} channels from opening as calcium rises during cholinergic contractions. These channels are also likely to be key targets associated with cyclase-linked bronchodilation.

The K^+ channel activator cromakalim is effective in relaxing airway smooth muscle in vitro. Substantial evidence indicates that this action results from the opening of ATP-sensitive K^+ channels. These drugs induce hyperpolarization and cause an increase in the efflux of labeled rubidium ions.[6] The relaxant effect of cromakalim in airway smooth muscle is competitively inhibited by K^+ channel blocker glibenclamide.[39] This indicates that the channel involved belongs to the ATP-sensitive K^+ channel class, although the low sensitivity to glibenclamide distinguishes it from the high-affinity ATP-sensitive K^+ channel typical of pancreatic islets. Glibenclamide itself has no effect on airway smooth muscle tone, which suggests that K_{ATP} channels do not contribute substantially to the maintenance of the resting potential.

Adenylyl Cyclase

Adenylyl cyclase (AC) is a membrane-associated enzyme that consists of six membrane-spanning segments with a large cytoplasmic loop and a smaller extracellular section. Some receptors, such as β-adrenoreceptors, vasoactive intestinal peptide receptors, and prostaglandin E receptors, activate AC via a stimulatory G protein, Gs, resulting in an increase in intracellular cyclic AMP, which leads (through a sequence of events) to relaxation of airway smooth muscle. In contrast, other receptors, such as muscarinic M_2 receptors, inhibit AC via the coupling protein G_i. The balance between activation and inhibition of AC determines the intracellular concentration of cyclic AMP, which is an important determinant of bronchial tone. A terpine derivative from plants, forskolin, directly activates AC by binding to its catalytic subunit. Forskolin stimulates a very marked increase in cyclic AMP concentration via airway smooth muscle, yet it is less effective than a beta agonist as a bronchodilator, suggesting that β-receptor–linked activation of AC may involve certain parts of AC that are preferentially linked to relaxation.

Future Sites for Pharmacologic Therapy

Through a greater understanding of the fundamental mechanisms regulating excitation-contraction coupling, new therapeutic approaches may be developed. In the near future, there is promise in the development of specific calcium-permeant channel blockers of airway smooth muscle. In addition, the development of new K^+ channel activators may offer even greater potential as a new class of bronchodilators. As our understanding improves with regard to the critical signaling molecules that regulate excitation-contraction coupling, gene therapy to enhance K^+ channel activation or block calcium-permeant channel activity may become a reality.

AIRWAY SMOOTH MUSCLE CELL PROLIFERATION

The principal features of asthmatic airways include exaggerated narrowing to bronchoconstrictor agonists and attenuated relaxation to β-adrenoreceptor stimulation. These functional alterations are associated with inflammation and remodeling of the airways, which include an increase in airway smooth muscle cell mass, disruption of the airway epithelium, and changes in the airway tissue extracellular matrix. The complex interplay between these altered functional and structural features of the asthmatic airway remains to be identified. In recent years, many studies have provided compelling evidence to support two basic concepts: (1) the actions of infiltrating inflammatory cells, which release proinflammatory mediators and growth factors, significantly contribute to modulating airway structure and function; and (2) the structural remodeling of the airways, which includes an increase in airway smooth muscle cell mass, contributes to the enhanced airway constrictor responsiveness and airflow limitation in asthma. This section of the chapter will address the extracellular stimuli and receptors coupled to airway smooth muscle cell hyperplasia, and review the cellular and molecular signaling mechanisms implicated in regulating smooth muscle cell growth.

Pathophysiology

Evidence suggests that the structural changes of the airways in asthma contribute to their altered function in this disease. Recent theoretical models based on morphometric analyses of asthmatic airways[37] demonstrate that the mechanism of excessive airway narrowing may be attributed to intrinsic changes in the airway smooth muscle, a reduction in the load acting against the contracting myocytes, and/or altered airway wall geometry. The increase in airway smooth muscle cell mass, coupled with inflammation-induced changes in the surrounding extracellular matrix, may reduce the load acting on the muscle due to peribronchial inflammation and give rise to enhanced airway smooth muscle contractility.[28,37] This process may result in disruption of normal airway/parenchymal interdependence. As the latter phenomenon serves to maintain the integrity of volume dependency of airway caliber and patency, disruption of this interdependence may contribute to the fixed airway obstruction and gas trapping observed in asthmatic subjects in response to bronchoconstrictor agonists.[37]

An increase in smooth muscle cell mass may be intrinsically related to altered contractility of the airway smooth muscle, as evidenced by the finding of a positive correlation between the volume of airway smooth muscle and its degree of isometric force of contraction to in vitro administration of constrictor agonists. In considering the mechanics of airway narrowing in asthma, there exists evidence that airway wall thickening determines the enhanced magnitude of airway constrictor responsiveness seen in asthmatics. Calculations based on morphologic data indicate that the increased airway wall area in asthmatic bronchi, which is due to an increase in airway smooth muscle cell mass, allows for a relatively greater increase in airway resistance in response to a given degree of airway smooth muscle shortening. Other computational analyses demonstrate that among the morphologic changes seen in asthmatic airway, including adventitial and submucosal thickening and smooth muscle hyperplasia, the latter significantly contributes to the increase in airway resistance in response to bronchoconstrictor agonists.[37]

Signaling via Extracellular Stimuli

The binding of mitogens to their receptors promotes the generation of early signals in the membrane cytosol and the nucleus that lead to cell growth. Since the initiation of DNA synthesis occurs 10 to 15 h after the addition of mitogens, it is expected that knowledge of these early events will provide clues regarding the primary regulatory mechanisms.

Smooth muscle cell proliferation is stimulated by mitogens that fall into two broad categories: those that activate receptors with intrinsic tyrosine kinase activity and those that mediate their effects through receptors coupled to heterotrimeric GTP-binding proteins (G proteins) and activate non–receptor-linked tyrosine kinases found in the cytoplasm (Fig. 6-2). Although both pathways increase cytosolic calcium through activation of phospholipase C (PLC), different PLC isoenzymes appear to be operative. Activated PLC hydrolyzes phosphatidylinositol bisphosphate (PIP$_2$) to phosphatidylinositol trisphosphate (IP$_3$) and diacylglycerol. These second messengers activate other cytosolic tyrosine kinases as well as serine and threonine kinases (protein kinase C and G) that have pleotrophic effects, including the activation of proto-oncogenes. Proto-oncogenes, which are a family of cellular genes (c-onc) that control normal cellular growth and differentiation, were characterized initially from viral genes (v-onc) that induced cellular transformation in eukaryotic cells. The protein products of proto-oncogenes play a critical role in transducing growth signals from the cell surface to the nucleus and in regulating gene transcription.

Growth Factors and Receptors

Growth factors are defined as polypeptides that stimulate cell proliferation through binding to specific high-affinity cell membrane receptors.[43] Growth factor receptors with intrinsic tyrosine kinase activity (RTK) play a central role in the regulatory mechanisms controlling cell growth and proliferation. In smooth muscle, epidermal growth factor (EGF), basic fibroblast growth factor (FGF), platelet-derived growth factor (PDGF), insulinlike growth factor–1 (IGF-1), and colony-stimulating factor–1 (CSF-1) induce cell proliferation by binding to receptors with RTK activity.[10,43] These growth factors are among the most potent smooth muscle mitogens.

Receptor tyrosine kinases share molecular topology and possess a large extracellular ligand-binding region, a single hydrophobic transmembrane segment, a cytoplasmic portion that contains the tyrosine kinase catalytic domain, and a carboxy-terminal regulatory region.[10] Structural similarities among growth factor receptors have led to their classification into seven broad groups. First, the EGF receptor, the hepatocyte growth factor receptor (c-met) as well as the tetrameric containing insulin and IGF-1 receptors contain cysteine-rich segments in their extracellular domain. Second, PDGF, CSF-1, and FGF mediate their effects through receptors that contain regulatory regions that are inserted in the cytoplasmic kinase portion and contain extracellular immunoglobulinlike domains.[10] The third group is represented by the nerve growth factor receptor, which has also been identified as the oncoprotein trk, and contains neither cysteine-rich nor immunoglobulinlike regions. Finally, a variety of hematopoietic growth factor receptors as well as glycoprotein cytokine receptors belong to another group that transduce their signals by recruiting tyrosine kinases from the cytosol and by creating a signaling complex. The interleukin 2 receptor as well

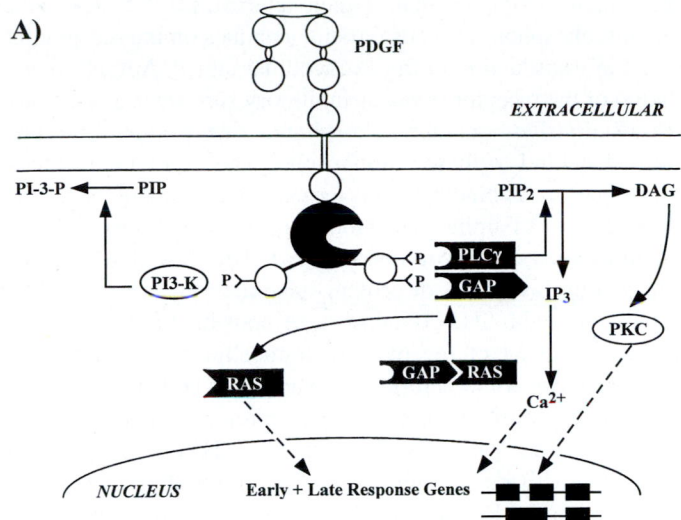

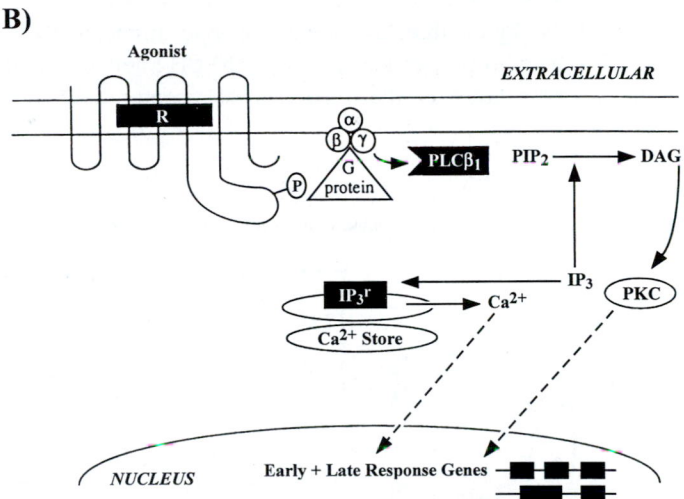

FIGURE 6-2 Characterization of smooth muscle cell mitogens: An overview. *A.* Some growth factors such as platelet-derived growth factor (PDGF) stimulate cell surface receptors with intrinsic tyrosine kinase activity (RTK). *B.* Other agonists activate receptors coupled to heterotrimeric G proteins. Activation of either receptor increases cytosolic calcium through activation of specific phospholipase C isozymes (PLC) that hydrolyze phosphatidylinositol 3,4-biphosphate (PIP$_2$) to phosphatidylinositol 3,4,5-triphosphate (IP$_3$) and diacylglycerol (DAG). These second messengers then activate other cytosolic tyrosine kinases as well as serine and threonine kinases such as protein kinase C (PKC). Stimulation of RTK-dependent receptors also activates phosphatidylinositol 3-phosphate kinase (PI 3-kinase); however, the role of 3'-inositol phosphates in signaling smooth muscle cell growth remains unknown. *(Based on data of Panettieri[43] with permission.)*

as interleukin 3 receptor are included in this group and appear to induce cell proliferation by coupling the ligand-activated receptor to nonreceptor kinases p56lck and Lyn kinase of the src family, respectively.[49]

Activation of the receptor tyrosine kinase is necessary for transduction of the growth factor–mediated responses. Although the precise mechanism by which the ligand activates the RTK is unknown, studies suggest that ligand binding to the receptor may induce oligomerization of receptor monomers or may form a receptor–ligand complex that is then internalized.[10,49] The next step, autophosphorylation of tyrosine residues on the receptor, is critical in transduction of the extracellular signal. Autophosphorylation of the receptor removes inhibitory substrates and creates high-affinity sites containing phosphotyrosine residues. The substrates that bind to these autophosphorylated tyrosine residues contain particular binding sites, termed SH2 domains. SH2 domains refer to an amino acid motif that is homologous with the protein product of the *Src* oncogene (p60*src*), the first member identified in this family of protein substrates.[10,11]

Substrates with SH2 domains are responsible for coupling activated growth factor receptors to intracellular signaling pathways operative in the control of a variety of cell functions, including cell proliferation, cytoskeletal protein remodeling, and gene expression. Proteins with one or more SH2 domains include the GTPase-activating protein of p21ras, phospholipase-γ_1, phosphatidylinositol 3-kinase (PI 3-kinase), Ras, and other cytoplasmic kinases (Fig. 6-3). Specificity of the growth factor response is determined not only by the SH2 recognition sites of the substrates but also by the three amino acid residues immediately C-terminal to the phosphotyrosine to which the SH2 domains bind. Studies suggest, however, that formation of receptor–SH2 complexes is important in some, but not all, responses of cells to growth factors.

Many proteins that possess SH2 domains also contain a distinct sequence of approximately 50 amino acid residues termed the SH3 domain. SH3 domains may modulate protein–protein interactions through the recognition of short peptide sequences that do not require phosphorylation. SH3 domains appear to regulate the interaction of the growth factor receptors with small Ras-like guanine nucleotide–binding proteins. Ultimately, the physical association of these proteins having SH2 and SH3 domains with that of RTK may require their translocation from the cytosol to the membrane. This translocation may result in an increased affinity of the receptor to become tyrosine phosphorylated.

Signaling complexes based on the formation of SH2/SH3 interactions are then followed by activation of downstream effector proteins, which involve, for example, Src nonreceptor tyrosine kinases, small GTP-binding proteins of the Ras family, serine/threonine kinases of Raf, and mitogen-activated protein kinase families (Fig. 6-3).[11,16] These intracellular enzymes are the products of oncogenes and proto-oncogenes whose function is to regulate expression of a large and diverse group of proteins active in complex cellular functions such as cell proliferation and growth.[16,36] Proto-oncogenes encode proteins in virtually every step of the growth factor–signaling cascade. Current challenges are directed at identifying proto-oncogenes that are both necessary and sufficient to induce cell proliferation so that new therapeutic approaches can be developed to alter expression of these genes and inhibit smooth muscle cell growth.

TYROSINE KINASE ACTIVITY

Airway inflammation, which is a hallmark of asthma, is represented by recruitment of various inflammatory cells to the airways, including macrophages, mast cells, basophils, platelets, eosinophils, and T lymphocytes. These cells have been suggested as important immune effector cells in modulating airway responsiveness (see Chapter 47). Many of these cells secrete a variety of smooth muscle cell mitogens, which may mediate their effects in an RTK-dependent manner and potentially induce airway smooth muscle cell growth.[43] In addition to direct stimulation of myocyte proliferation, these mitogens can stimulate myocyte growth in an autocrine manner. In vascular smooth muscle, stimulation of cells with PDGF or interleukin 1 induces myocytes to secrete PDGF and interleukin 1 that may further enhance the proliferative response.[22] Smooth

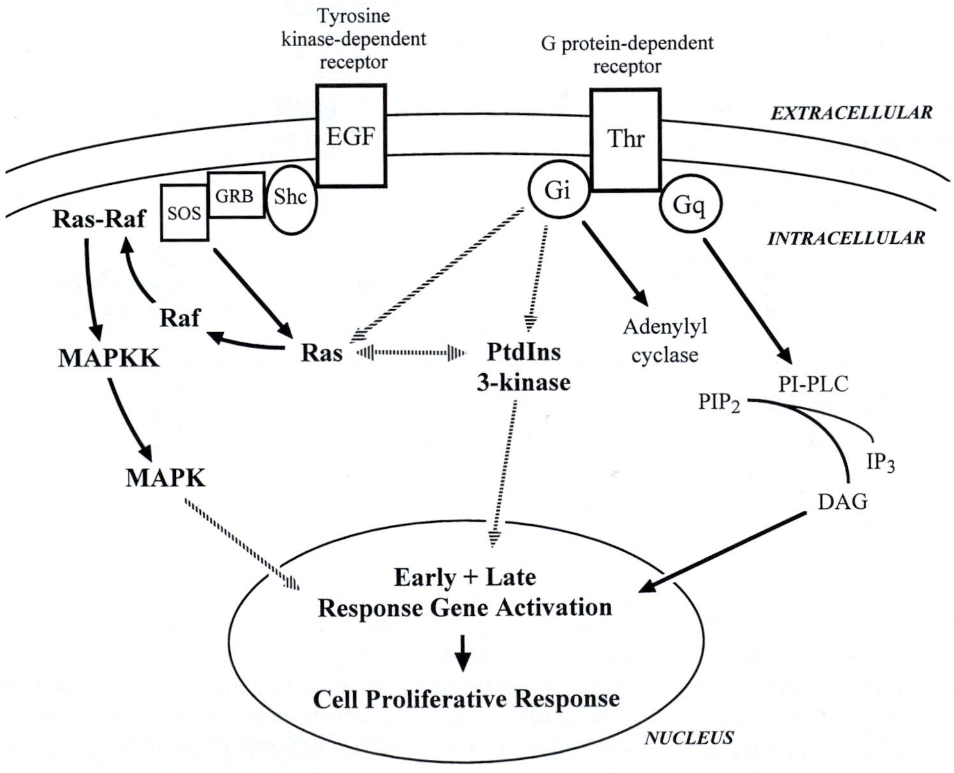

FIGURE 6-3   Possible mechanisms that regulate airway smooth muscle cell proliferation induced by contractile agonists and growth factors. Receptor tyrosine kinase–coupled receptors and those coupled to G proteins activate similar downstream signaling pathways. On the basis of recent data,[43,44] activation of PI-PLC is not essential for mediating airway smooth muscle cell proliferation. G proteins = guanine nucleotide–binding regulatory proteins; PIP_2 = phosphatidylinositol 4,5 biphosphate; DAG = 1,2-diacylglycerol; IP_3 = inositol 1,4,5-triphosphate; PI-PLC = phosphoinositol-specific phospholipase C; PtdIns 3-kinase = phosphotidylinositol 3-kinase; SOS, GRB, and Shc are growth factor receptor–binding proteins; MAPKK = mitogen-activated kinase kinase; MAPK = mitogen-activated kinase. The hatched lines represent possible signaling pathways that stimulate myocyte growth.

muscle cell hyperplasia is probably a consequence of the chronic stimulation of myocytes with a variety of cytokines and mitogens rather than a single growth factor. To date, however, there are no in vivo studies that have conclusively identified specific growth factors or mitogens that induce airway smooth muscle cell hyperplasia.

Since few studies have characterized airway smooth muscle cell hyperplasia or hypertrophy in animal models of asthma, investigators have used models of cultured human airway smooth muscle cells to study myocyte proliferation.[45,55] As a model, airway smooth muscle in culture has several advantages over wholeorgan or strip studies. The availability of large populations of pure airway myocytes without contamination from neuronal or epithelial cells allows for the precise control of extracellular conditions and provides the ability to reversibly synchronize the cells in G_0 (resting phase) of the cell cycle. Monolayers of cells eliminate variability in diffusion of agonists through tissue that may alter cellular concentrations. In addition, a human model eliminates interpretative difficulties from possible interspecies variations. Although extrapolation from cultured models to in vivo conditions may be problematic, human airway smooth muscle models demonstrate morphologic and functional compatibility with in vivo conditions.[43,45]

Recently, EGF in human cells[44] and PDGF in guinea pig,[55] human,[24] and bovine cells[31] have been characterized as airway smooth muscle cell mitogens. These growth factors probably mediate their effects through intrinsic RTK activity. In comparison to contractile agonists, which mediate their effects through G proteins, EGF and PDGF are more potent, with half-maximal concentrations in the nanomolar range.[43,44] In addition, EGF induces mRNA expression of c-*fos*, a proto-oncogene whose induction is one of the earliest markers of proliferation and differentiation in mesenchymal-derived cells.[46]

Other growth factors found to stimulate airway smooth muscle cell proliferation are the insulinlike growth factors IGF-I and IGF-II,[41] which are ubiquitous peptides that mediate cell proliferation and differentiation by acting via RTK-dependent type 1 and type 2 IGF receptors. Of interest is that cultured rabbit airway smooth muscle cells were found to release IGF-II, as well as the IGF-binding protein (IGFBP) IGFBP-2, which largely acts to inhibit the promitogenic action of IGFs by limiting their bioavailability to cell surface IGF receptors.[41] These findings suggest that, apart from any direct action of a growth factor on cell proliferation, the airway smooth muscle cell growth response may be significantly modulated by activation of an autocrine network involving the IGF axis (i.e., IGFs, IGFBPs, and proteases), which may up- or down-regulate the net proliferative response to the mitogen.

The downstream signaling events that modulate RTK-dependent proliferation of airway smooth muscle cells have not been well characterized. In a recent study of protein kinase C activation in modulating PDGF-induced airway smooth muscle cell growth, cell proliferation induced by PDGF was markedly attenuated by pretreating the cells with protein kinase C inhibitors.[25] Others have determined that pretreatment of rabbit airway smooth muscle cells with genistein and lavendustin A, which are tyrosine kinase inhibitors, inhibited serum-, EGF-, and PDGF-induced cell growth. Since these inhibitors lack specificity and block a variety of serine, threonine, or tyrosine kinases, further study is needed to identify specific kinases that regulate RTK-dependent airway myocyte growth.

RECEPTORS COUPLED TO GTP-BINDING PROTEINS

The recent observations that agonists that induce smooth muscle cell contraction can also induce myocyte proliferation may have important pathophysiological implications in diseases characterized by smooth muscle hyperplasia. A variety of contractile agonists have been identified as vascular and airway smooth muscle cell mitogens.[23,43]

Most contractile agonist receptors share a common topography that consists of a seven-membrane–spanning region and a site that couples the receptor to a heterotrimeric G protein (Fig. 6-2). In a similar manner to RTK-dependent growth factor receptors, those coupled to G proteins activate phosphoinositide (PI)-specific phospholipase C (PLC), which then hydrolyzes PIs to generate inositol triphosphate (IP$_3$) and diacylglycerol (DAG). In the case of G protein–coupled receptors, a specific PI-PLC isotype, PLC-β_1, is activated rather than PLC-γ, which is activated by RTK-dependent receptors.

Activation of protein kinase C by DAG is considered a pivotal event in regulating G protein–dependent cell proliferation. Activated protein kinase C, in conjunction with increased cytosolic calcium, induces intracellular alkalinization by promoting Na^+/H^+ exchange and by phosphorylating specific substrates that have been associated with cell proliferation. In addition, specific agonists induce expression of the proto-oncogenes c-*fos* and c-*myc*, whose activation regulates myriad cellular functions that include gene transcription and cell proliferation.[46,52]

Despite certain similarities in stimulatory signal transduction pathways between RTK-dependent growth factors and contractile agonists, important disparities exist. First, cell proliferation stimulated by most growth factors is mediated by receptor-linked tyrosine kinase activation; to date, no such activity has been noted in cell proliferation induced by agonists. Second, contractile agonists that both induce cell proliferation and contraction appear to do so by receptors coupled to different G proteins.[30,44] Finally, RTK-dependent cell proliferation is both protein kinase C dependent and independent,[7] whereas agonist-induced mitogenesis is thought to be protein kinase C dependent.

In addition to differences between the proliferative mechanisms of these mitogens, there exists substantial variability in the mitogenic capacity among contractile agonists. First, some contractile agonists stimulate smooth muscle cell proliferation, although most of these agonists induce comparable levels of polyphosphoinositide hydrolysis, cytosolic calcium transients, protein kinase C activation, and c-*fos* mRNA expression.[44] Second, the mitogenic effects of endothelin and serotonin[30] on vascular smooth muscle appear to be coupled to pertussis toxin–sensitive G proteins that differ from the pertussis toxin–insensitive G proteins that mediate agonist-induced PI hydrolysis, cytosolic calcium release, or smooth muscle contraction. The differences in proliferative responses induced by growth factors and contractile agonists, and differential contractile agonist effects, imply that other regulatory components are involved.

Intracellular Calcium as a Modulator

To a large extent, cellular processes regulated by alterations in the cytoplasmic concentration of ionized calcium are initiated by the release of this ion from sequestered intracellular stores. The best-studied example is the release mediated by IP_3 gating of its receptor/ion channel. Compelling evidence, however, suggests that there are more calcium storage pools and release mechanisms than can be explained by the action of IP_3 alone. The exact nature of these pools and how they interact are an intensely investigated topic.[58]

Numerous studies have postulated the participation of intracellular calcium signals in growth. Studies using the Ca^{2+} ionophore A23187 have determined that increases in cytosolic calcium induce proto-oncogene expression and cell proliferation,[17] but the interpretation of these experiments remains difficult because A23187 has pleiotrophic effects.[53] Despite these drawbacks, much evidence supports the role of growth factor–induced cytosolic Ca^{2+} signals as being necessary for activation of G_0 to G_1 transition and mitogenesis in some cell types.[49]

The levels of Ca^{2+} remaining in Ca^{2+}-accumulating organelles may also have important consequences for signaling and growth regulation.[51] Depletion of calcium stores within the endoplasmic reticulum by thapsigargin markedly inhibits growth factor–induced mitogenesis in a transformed smooth muscle cell line. Such effects may result from either an altered ability of the endoplasmic reticulum to generate specific Ca^{2+} signals necessary for cell growth or modulation of key endoplasmic reticulum functions that are dependent on intraluminal Ca^{2+} to induce mitogenesis. Current evidence suggests that cytosolic Ca^{2+} mobilization or depletion of Ca^{2+} stores in response to growth factors may be critical to modulate cell proliferation in some cells.

Although both growth factors and contractile agonists evoke calcium transients by stimulation of phospholipase C in smooth muscle cells, the role of Ca^{2+} in regulating smooth muscle cell growth remains controversial. Contractile agonists that induce both cell proliferation and contraction appear to do so by receptors coupled to different G proteins.[30,44] Some contractile agonists stimulate airway smooth muscle cell proliferation, although most of these agonists induce comparable levels of polyphosphoinositide hydrolysis, cytosolic calcium transients, and c-*fos* mRNA expression.[43] These studies and others[44,55] suggest that regulatory processes apart from calcium mobilization are important in mediating smooth muscle cell proliferation.

Cyclic Nucleotides

Recognition that vascular smooth muscle proliferation is important in the pathogenesis of atherosclerosis has focused attention on identifying cellular and molecular mechanisms that inhibit smooth muscle cell growth. An understanding of these mechanisms is critical not only in preventing cell growth but also in addressing whether the loss of inhibitory signals may induce myocyte proliferation. Activation of cAMP- or cGMP-dependent kinases and alterations in extracellular matrix proteins have been reported to inhibit myocyte proliferation. Several studies indicate that similar mechanisms inhibit airway smooth muscle cell growth.[42,43,46]

CYCLIC AMP

New insights into the mechanisms by which cAMP-dependent pathways inhibit cell growth have been described. The activation of A kinase results in the inhibition of Raf-1 activation in mammalian cells.[61] Raf-1, a serine–threonine protein kinase, is an effector for Ras-GTP, and the interaction of Raf-1 with Ras-GTP induces Raf activation (Fig. 6-3). Activation of Raf-1 phosphorylates and activates other serine–threonine protein kinases, ultimately activating the mitogen-activated protein kinase pathway. This pathway is thought to be important in modulating mitogen-induced cell proliferation of some cell types. Despite these advances in our knowledge concerning A kinase effects on cell growth, mitogenesis of some cell types appears to be independent of Raf-1 inhibition, suggesting substantial redundancy in signal transduction pathways that induce cell proliferation.[61]

In vascular as well as in airway smooth muscle cells, activation of receptors coupled to G_s, which increases cytosolic cAMP levels and activates A kinase, inhibits cell growth induced by growth factors.[42,43,57] A-kinase activation, however, appears to selectively inhibit mitogens that induce airway smooth muscle cell growth through PI-PLC– and protein kinase C–dependent pathways.[43] Alternatively, mitogens that stimulate cell proliferation through activation of receptor-linked tyrosine kinases are less sensitive to this inhibition.[43] These mitogens stimulate growth, in part, through protein kinase C–independent mechanisms. In smooth muscle, "cross talk" between intracellular kinases appears crucial in coordinating cell proliferation.

Identifying cellular mechanisms that inhibit cell growth may be relevant not only with regard to preventing airway smooth muscle cell proliferation but also in terms of understanding the full spectrum of pathways that regulate cell growth. For example, further studies may clarify whether myocyte proliferation results from a loss of tonic inhibitory effects of A kinase. Such studies may have important implications concerning the chronic use of therapeutic agents that manipulate these signal transduction pathways.

CYCLIC GMP

Atrial naturetic factor, sodium nitroprusside, and nitric oxide are potent vasodilators that mediate their effects by increasing cytosolic cGMP levels and activating cyclic GMP–dependent kinase (G kinase). Investigators have reported that vascular smooth muscle cell proliferation induced by serum or by serotonin is inhibited by pretreating the cells with atrial naturetic peptide or with permeant cGMP analogs.[3] In guinea pig airway smooth muscle cells, nitroprusside and dibutyryl cGMP, a permeable cGMP analog, also inhibited serum-induced cell proliferation.[13] However, the downstream signaling events that mediate G-kinase inhibition of cell growth remain unknown.

ACTIVATION OF DOWNSTREAM EFFECTORS

The above discussion focused on the second messenger systems that modulate airway smooth muscle cell proliferation. Although an exhaustive review of the sequential protein kinase cascades activated by mitogens extends beyond the scope of this chapter, it is important to review some recent advances in our understanding of downstream effector molecules that are activated by second messengers and may play critical roles in transducing growth signals in smooth muscle cells.

Ras   The proteins encoded by *ras* genes serve as essential transducers of diverse physiological signals, and Ras proteins, which are mutationally altered, can induce cell transformation. Although the *ras* gene was first identified in transforming retroviruses, the identification that retroviral oncogenes (v-*ras*) derived from normal cellular genes (c-*ras*) has led to the recognition that Ras activation is critical in mediating normal cell growth and differentiation.[16,36]

Ras, which migrates as a 21-kDa protein (p21ras), has served as a prototype for the superfamily of Ras-related proteins, a group of guanine nucleotide–binding proteins that share structural homology.[16,36] The discovery that Ras proteins bind guanine nucleotides (GTP and GDP) with high affinity and possess intrinsic GTPase activity suggested a mechanism by which Ras activity is regulated. Ras proteins are deactivated by interaction with GTPase-activating proteins that promote GTP hydrolysis by Ras. In some cell types, active Ras promotes cell proliferation; in others, it arrests cell division and induces the expression of differentiated phenotypes.[36] The role of Ras activation in mediating mitogen-induced smooth muscle cell proliferation remains unknown.

Recent studies have determined that activated Ras interacts with both Raf kinase and PtdIns 3-kinase, two important Ras effector proteins that modulate growth factor–induced proliferation of 3T3 and Rat-1 fibroblasts.[16,48] Ras binding alone does not activate the intrinsic kinase activity of Raf; rather, it localizes Raf to the plasma membrane, where it is activated. Activated Raf then stimulates a cascade of other kinases—including mitogen-activated protein kinase, whose activation in some cells is necessary to induce cell proliferation. A parallel pathway by which activated Ras may induce cell growth involves PtdIns 3-kinase activation.[48] To date, studies on airway smooth muscle have not addressed the role that Ras activation may play in regulating mitogen-induced airway smooth muscle proliferation.

Protein Kinase C   Activation of protein kinase C (PKC), either directly by phorbol esters or indirectly by mitogens, is an important signaling event for the proliferation of many cells,[50] including smooth muscle. PKC represents a family of protein kinases, activated by calcium and diacylglycerol, that induce protein phosphorylation of serine and threonine residues of many proteins. One such protein, with a molecular weight of 76,000 (p76), has been well characterized and its phosphorylation associated with mitogenesis.[7] Cloning and molecular biology studies have revealed the existence of multiple isotypes of PKC. To date, at least four calcium- and phosphatidyl serine–dependent PKC isotypes (α-, βI-, βII-, γ-PKC) and four calcium-independent isotypes (δ-, ϵ-, ζ-, and η-PKC) have been identified.[38] A recent study has determined that most of the above-mentioned PKC isotypes are found in canine airway smooth muscle—except for η-PKC, which was not present.[14] Currently, there is little evidence to designate specific functions for each PKC isotype; however, their distribution appears to be tissue specific.

The role of PKC activation in fibroblast and smooth muscle cell proliferation induced by contractile agonists has been demonstrated by down-regulation of PKC following prolonged pretreatment with phorbol esters. In these cells, pretreatment diminished phorbol ester–induced p76 phosphorylation by 80 to 90 percent, abolished phorbol ester stimulation of cell proliferation in 3T3 cells[21] and vascular smooth muscle cells, as well as markedly attenuated phorbol ester–induced c-*fos* expression. However, the mitogenic responses of PKC-deficient 3T3 cells to PDGF, EGF, and FGF were not attenuated. Other studies have demonstrated that rabbit airway smooth muscle cell proliferation induced by serum was inhibited by the selective PKC inhibitors RO-318220 and RO-317549.[26] These findings suggest that PKC activation is necessary in transducing growth signals from receptors coupled to G proteins and from receptors with intrinsic tyrosine kinases in some cell types.

The dependence of receptor-activated mitogenesis on PKC appears to be growth factor and cell specific. Some, but not all, contractile agonists that activate PKC induce vascular smooth muscle cell proliferation. Accordingly, PKC activation may be necessary but not sufficient to induce G protein–dependent cell growth, and other signaling pathways must modulate the proliferative response.

Mitogen-Activated Protein Kinases   MAP kinases, which are a family of 40-kD to 46-kD serine-threonine kinases activated early in response to extracellular signals, appear to play an integral role in the signaling cascade initiated by diverse stimuli. A variety of mitogens activate MAP kinase in vivo, including PDGF, EGF, and nerve growth factor—all of which induce autophosphorylation of their receptors on tyrosine residues.[20] Evidence also suggests that MAP kinase activation occurs in response to stimulation of receptors coupled to heterotrimeric G proteins. Although the precise signaling events that modulate MAP kinase activation remain unknown, a major pathway requires the sequential activation of Ras, Raf, and MAP kinase/Erk-activating kinase, also known as MAP kinase kinase (MAPKK). MAPKK has been shown to directly phosphorylate MAP kinase on both tyrosine and threonine residues.[8] The phosphorylation of both these residues is required for maximal enzymatic activation of MAP kinase.[8] Subsequently, the activated MAP kinase, which translocates from the cytoplasm to the nucleus,[8] induces expression of the proto-oncogenes c-*jun* and c-*myc*, which are necessary for cell proliferation.[47] The integration of signal events activated by tyrosine and serine–threonine phosphorylation at the level of MAP kinase suggests that MAP kinase plays a central role in the downstream regulation of cell proliferation.

Recent studies have revealed that growth factors that stimulate receptors with intrinsic tyrosine kinases and those that stimulate receptors coupled to G proteins activate MAP kinases in bovine airway smooth muscle cells.[31] Sustained activation of MAP kinase correlated with the proliferative response of bovine airway smooth muscle cells to the putative mitogen. Other data have also suggested that prolonged activation of MAP kinase is necessary to induce cell proliferation of CCL 39 cells stimulated with thrombin.[8] Despite these studies, the role of MAP kinase in regulating cell proliferation remains controversial. It is likely that the role of MAP kinase activation as a requirement for growth factor–stimulated DNA synthesis will vary among different cell types. More studies are needed to determine whether MAP kinase activation is necessary and sufficient to induce airway smooth muscle cell growth.

SUMMARY

Asthma, bronchiolitis obliterans, and chronic bronchitis are chronic lung diseases characterized by airflow obstruction. Despite considerable research effort, primary defects that underlie airway obstruction remain unknown, although an intrinsic abnormality of airway smooth muscle has been postulated.

Although asthma typically induces reversible airway obstruction, in some asthmatics, airflow obstruction can become irreversible. Such obstruction may be a consequence of persistent structural changes in the airway wall due to the frequent stimulation of airway smooth muscle by contractile agonists, inflammatory mediators, and growth factors. Increased smooth muscle mass, which has been attributed to increases in myocyte number, is a well-documented pathologic finding in the airways of patients with chronic severe asthma.

Although the mechanisms by which agonists induce cell proliferation are unknown, similarities exist between signal transduction processes activated by these agents and those of known growth factors. Diverse extracellular stimuli induce cell growth, in part, by activating common intracellular signal transduction pathways. The identification of critical regulatory sites in these pathways may provide new therapeutic approaches to alter the airway remodeling seen in patients with chronic airflow obstruction.

REFERENCES

1. Advenier C, Naline E, Rennier A: Effects of BAY K 8644 on contraction of the human isolated bronchus and guinea pig isolated trachea. *Br J Pharmacol* 88:33–39, 1986.

2. Allen SL, Boyle JP, Cortijo J, et al: Electrical and mechanical effects of BRL34915 in guinea-pig isolated trachealis. *Br J Pharmacol* 89:395–405, 1986.

3. Assender JW, Southgate KM, Hallet MB, Newby AC: Inhibition of proliferation, but not of Ca^{2+} mobilization, by cyclic AMP and GMP in rabbit aortic smooth muscle cells. *Biochem J* 288:527–532, 1992.

4. Barnes PJ: Clinical studies with calcium antagonists in asthma. *Br J Clin Pharmacol* 20 (Suppl 2):S289–S298, 1985.

5. Benham CD, Tsien RW: A novel receptor-operated Ca^{2+}-permeable channel activated by ATP in smooth muscle. *Nature* 328:275–278, 1987.

6. Black JL, Armour CL, Johnson PRA, et al: The action of potassium channel activator, BRL 38227 (lemakalim), on human airway smooth muscle. *Am Rev Respir Dis* 142:1384–1389, 1990.

7. Blackshear PJ, Witters LA, Girard PR, et al: Growth factor–stimulated protein phosphorylation in 3T3-L1 cells: Evidence for protein kinase C-dependent and -independent pathways. *J Biol Chem* 260:13304–13315, 1985.

8. Blenis J: Signal transduction via the MAP kinases: Proceed at your own RSK. *Proc Natl Acad Sci USA* 90:5889–5892, 1993.

9. Bourreau J-P, Abela AP, Kwan CY, Daniel EE: Acetylcholine Ca^{2+} stores refilling directly involves a dihydropyridine-sensitive channel in dog trachea. *Am J Physiol* 261:C497–C505, 1991.

10. Cadena DL, Gill GN: Receptor tyrosine kinases. *FASEB J* 6:2332–2337, 1992.

11. Carpenter G: Receptor tyrosine kinase substrates: *src* homology domains and signal transduction. *FASEB J* 6:3283–3289, 1992.

12. Croxton TL, Fleming C, Hirshman CA: Expression of dihydropyridine resistance differs in porcine bronchial and tracheal smooth muscle. *Am J Physiol* 267:L106–L112, 1994.

13. De S, Zelazny E, Souhrada JF, Souhrada M: Nitric oxide has an inhibitory effect on growth of airway smooth muscle (ASM) cells (abstract). *Am J Respir Crit Care Med* 151:A49, 1995.

14. Donnelly R, Yang K, Omary MB, et al: Expression of multiple isoenzymes of protein kinase C in airway smooth muscle. *Am J Respir Cell Mol Biol* 13:253–256, 1995.

15. Drazen JM, Fanta CH, Lacoutre PG: Effect of nifedipine on constriction of human tracheal strips in vitro. *Br J Pharmacol* 78:687–691, 1983.

16. Feig LA, Schaffhausen B: The hunt for Ras targets. *Nature* 370:508–509, 1994.

17. Fisch TM, Prywes R, Roeder RG: c-*fos* sequence necessary for basal expression and induction by epidermal growth factor, 12-O-tetradecanoyl phorbol-13-acetate and the calcium ionophore. *Mol Cell Biol* 7:3490–3502, 1987.

18. Fleischmann BK, Murray RK, Kotlikoff MI: A voltage window for sustained elevation of cytosolic calcium in smooth muscle cells. *Proc Natl Acad Sci USA* 91:11914–11918, 1994.

19. Fleischmann BK, Washabau RJ, Kotlikoff MI: Control of resting membrane potential by delayed rectifier potassium currents in ferret airway smooth muscle cells. *J Physiol (Lond)* 468:625–638, 1993.

20. Gotoh Y, Nishida E, Yamashita T, et al: Microtubule-associated-protein (MAP) kinase activated by nerve growth factor and epidermal growth factor in PC12 cells: Identity with mitogen-activated MAP kinase of fibroblastic cells. *Eur J Biochem* 193:661–669, 1990.

21. Greenberg ME, Hermanowski AL, Ziff EB: Effect of protein synthesis inhibitors on growth factor activation of c-*fos* and c-*myc* and actin gene transcription. *Mol Cell Biol* 6:1050–1057, 1986.

22. Hajjar DP, Pomerantz KB: Signal transduction in atherosclerosis: Integration of cytokines and the ekosanoid network. *FASEB J* 6:2933–2941, 1992.

23. Hepler JR, Gilman AG: G proteins. *Trends Biochem Sci* 17:383–387, 1992.

24. Hirst SJ, Barnes PJ, Twort CHC: Quantifying proliferation of cultured human and rabbit airway smooth muscle cells in response to serum and platelet-derived growth factor. *Am J Respir Cell Mol Biol* 7:574–581, 1992.

25. Hirst SJ, Barnes BJ, Twort CHC: Protein kinase inhibitors (PKC and PKA) and phorbol ester inhibit proliferation induced by serum in cultured rabbit airway smooth muscle cells (abstract). *Am Rev Respir Dis* 147:A252, 1993.

26. Hirst SJ, Webb BLJ, Giembycz MA, et al: Inhibition of fetal calf serum-stimulated proliferation of rabbit cultured tracheal smooth muscle cells by selective inhibitors of protein kinase C and protein tyrosine kinase. *Am J Respir Cell Mol Biol* 12:149–161, 1995.

27. Hoth M, Penner R: Depletion of intracellular calcium stores activates a calcium current in mast cells. *Nature* 355:353–356, 1992.

28. Ishida K, Paré PD, Blogg T, Schellenberg RR: Effects of elastic loading on porcine trachealis muscle mechanics. *J Appl Physiol* 69:1033–1039, 1990.

29. Janssen LJ, Sims SM: Acetylcholine activates non-selective cation and chloride conductances in canine and guinea-pig tracheal smooth muscle cells. *J Physiol (Lond)* 453:197–218, 1992.

30. Kavanaugh WM, Williams LT, Ives HE, Coughlin SR: Serotonin-induced deoxyribonucleic acid synthesis in vascular smooth mus-

cle cells involves a novel, pertussis toxin–sensitive pathway. *Mol Endocrinol* 123:599–605, 1988.

31. Kelleher MD, Abe MK, Chao TS, et al: Role of MAP kinase activation in bovine tracheal smooth muscle mitogenesis. *Am J Physiol* 268:L894–L901, 1995.

32. Kotlikoff MI: Calcium currents in isolated canine airway smooth muscle cells. *Am J Physiol* 254:C793–C801, 1988.

33. Kume H, Hall IP, Washabau RJ, et al: β-Adrenergic agonists regulate K_{Ca} channels in airway smooth muscle by cAMP-dependent and -independent mechanisms. *J Clin Invest* 93:371–379, 1994.

34. Kume H, Takai A, Tokuno H, Tomita T: Regulation of Ca^{2+}-dependent K^+-channel activity in tracheal myocytes by phosphorylation. *Nature* 341:152–154, 1989.

35. Loirand G, Pacaud P, Baron A, et al: Large conductance calcium-activated non-selective cation channel in smooth muscle cells isolated from rat portal vein. *J Physiol (Lond)* 437:461–475, 1991.

36. Lowy DR, Willumsen BM: Function and regulation of Ras. *Annu Rev Biochem* 62:851–891, 1993.

37. Macklem PT: A theoretical analysis of the effect of airway smooth muscle load on airway narrowing. *Am J Respir Crit Care Med* 153:83–89, 1996.

38. Majumdar S, Kane LH, Rossi MW, et al: Protein kinase C isotypes and signal-transduction in human neutrophils: Selective substrate specificity of calcium-dependent β PKC and novel calcium-independent η PKC. *Biochim Biophys Acta* 1176:276–286, 1993.

39. Miura M, Belvisi MG, Ward JK, et al: Bronchodilating effects of the novel potassium channel opener HOE 234 in human airways in vitro. *Br J Clin Pharmacol* 35:318–320, 1993.

40. Murray RK, Kotlikoff MI: Receptor-activated calcium influx in human airway smooth muscle cells. *J Physiol (Lond)* 435:123–144, 1991.

41. Noveral JP, Bhala A, Hintz RL, et al: The insulin-like growth factor axis in airway smooth muscle cells. *Am J Physiol* 267:L761–L765, 1994.

42. Noveral JP, Grunstein, MM: Adrenergic receptor-mediated regulation of cultured rabbit airway smooth muscle cell proliferation. *Am J Physiol* 267:L291–L299, 1994.

43. Panettieri RA: Airways smooth muscle cell growth and proliferation, in Raeburn D, Giembycz MA (eds), *Airways Smooth Muscle: Development and Regulation of Contractility.* Basel, Switzerland, Birkhauser, 1994, pp 41–68.

44. Panettieri RA, Hall IP, Maki CS, Murray RK: α-Thrombin increases cytosolic calcium and induces human airway smooth muscle cell proliferation. *Am J Respir Cell Mol Biol* 13:205–216, 1995.

45. Panettieri RA, Murray RK, DePalo LR, et al: A human airway smooth muscle cell line that retains physiological responsiveness. *Am J Physiol* 256:C329–C335, 1989.

46. Panettieri RA, Yadvish PA, Kelly AM, et al: Histamine stimulates proliferation of airway smooth muscle and induces c-*fos* expression. *Am J Physiol* 259:L365–L371, 1990.

47. Pulverer BJ, Kyriakis JM, Avruch J, et al: Phosphorylation of c-*jun* mediated by MAP kinases. *Nature* 353:670–674, 1991.

48. Rodriguez-Viciana P, Warne PH, Dhand R, et al: Phosphatidylinositol-3-OH kinase as a direct target of Ras. *Nature* 370:527–532, 1994.

49. Rozengurt E: Growth factors and cell proliferation. *Curr Opin Cell Biol* 4:161–165, 1992.

50. Rozengurt E, Rodriguez-Pena A, Coombs M, Sinnett-Smith J: Diacylglycerol stimulates DNA synthesis and cell division in mouse 3T3 cells: Role of Ca^{2+}-sensitive phospholipid-dependent protein kinase. *Proc Natl Acad Sci USA* 81:5748–5752, 1984.

51. Schönthal A, Sugarman J, Brown JH, et al: Regulation of c-*fos* and c-*jun* protooncogene expression by the Ca^{2+}-ATPase inhibitor thapsigargin. *Proc Natl Acad Sci USA* 88:7096–7100, 1991.

52. Sheng M, Dougan ST, McFadden G, Greenberg ME: Calcium and growth factor pathways of c-*fos* transcriptional activation require distinct upstream regulatory sequences. *Mol Cell Biol* 8:2787–2796, 1988.

53. Smith PL, McCabe RD: A23187-induced changes in colonic K and Cl transport are mediated by separate mechanisms. *Am J Physiol* 247:G695–G702, 1984.

54. Somlyo AP, Somlyo AV: Signal transduction and regulation in smooth muscle. *Nature* 372:231–236, 1994.

55. Stewart AG, Grigoriadis G, Harris T: Mitogenic actions of endothelin-1 and epidermal growth factor in cultured airway smooth muscle. *Clin Exp Pharmacol Physiol* 21:277–285, 1994.

56. Tomasic M, Boyle JP, Worley JI, Kotlikoff MI: Contractile agonists activate voltage-dependent channels in airway smooth muscle cells. *Am J Physiol* 263:C106–C113, 1994.

57. Tomlinson PR, Wilson JW, Stewart AG: Inhibition by salbutamol of the proliferation of human airway smooth muscle cells grown in culture. *Br J Pharmacol* 111:641–647, 1994.

58. Tsien RW, Tsien RY: Calcium channels, stores and oscillations. *Annu Rev Cell Biol* 6:715–760, 1990.

59. Valera S, Hussy N, Evans RJ, et al: A new class of ligand-gated ion channel defined by P_{2X} receptor for extracellular ATP. *Nature* 371:516–519, 1994.

60. Weiss GB, Pang I-H, Goodman FR: Relationship between ^{45}Ca movements, different calcium components and responses to acetylcholine and potassium in airway smooth muscle. *J Pharmacol Exp Ther* 233:389–394, 1985.

61. Wu J, Dent P, Jelinek T, et al: Inhibition of the EGF-activated MAP kinase signaling pathway by adenosine 3′, 5′-monophosphate. *Science* 262:1065–1069, 1993.

SURFACTANT AND ASSOCIATED PROTEINS

Jeffrey A. Whitsett / Ann D. Horowitz

Pulmonary surfactant, a complex mixture of phospholipids and proteins, creates a unique interface, separating alveolar gas and liquids at the alveolar cell surface, reducing surface tension, and maintaining lung volumes at end expiration. Reduction of the surface tension at the air-liquid interface is a requirement for respiratory function following birth. Deficiency of pulmonary surfactant causes respiratory failure in premature infants, or infantile respiratory distress syndrome (IRDS). The adequacy of pulmonary surfactant is maintained by unique and highly regulated systems mediating the synthesis, secretion, reuptake, re-utilization, and catabolism of surfactant. Loss of pulmonary surfactant later in life occurs in the adult respiratory distress syndrome (ARDS), a significant cause of morbidity and mortality following infection, shock, or trauma. This chapter reviews the biology of the surfactant system and its implications for the pathogenesis and treatment of respiratory distress syndromes in both premature infants and adults.

PHYSICAL FORCES AT THE AIR-LIQUID INTERFACE

In 1929, Van Neergard recognized the critical role of surface tension as a "retractile force" in the lung, observing the marked difference in inflation pressures required to inflate the air- versus water-filled lung.[40] Avery and Mead associated the lack of a lipid-rich material in the lungs of infants dying from IRDS with alveolar collapse and respiratory failure.[1] In the absence of pulmonary surfactant, molecular forces at the air-liquid interface create a region of high surface tension because intermolecular forces between water molecules are unopposed at the air-liquid interface, and an area of high retractile force at the surface is created. Forces of 70 dynes/cm^2 are generated at the air-water interface at 37°C; if unopposed in the alveolus, such forces lead to alveolar collapse and respiratory failure. A surface film composed of sheets of phospholipids creates a distinct phase separating air and liquid, reducing surface tension to nearly zero and maintaining residual lung volume at end expiration.[44] Complex interactions between surfactant phospholipids and proteins are required to maintain surfactant activity throughout life.

COMPOSITION OF PULMONARY SURFACTANT

Pulmonary surfactant isolated by lung lavage consists of highly heterogeneous forms of phospholipid-protein aggregates of distinct sizes, structural characteristics, and composition.[22] Tubular myelin is the most abundant form of alveolar phospholipid and consists of large, relatively dense aggregates composed of phospholipids and surfactant proteins. Tubular myelin is a highly organized form of surfactant phospholipid, forming square tubular arrays, as in Fig. 7-1. Tubular myelin is surface-active and likely represents an extracellular pool of surfactant lipids that move to the air-liquid interface to form the monolayer or multilayered sheets that reduce surface tension in the alveolus. Large lamellated structures, of composition similar to that of tubular myelin, are also seen within the alveolus and likely represent newly secreted lamellar bodies that unravel and form tubular myelin in the airspace. The phospholipid composition of lamellar bodies, the intracellular storage form of surfactant, tubular myelin, and lamellated forms present in the alveolus are virtually identical.

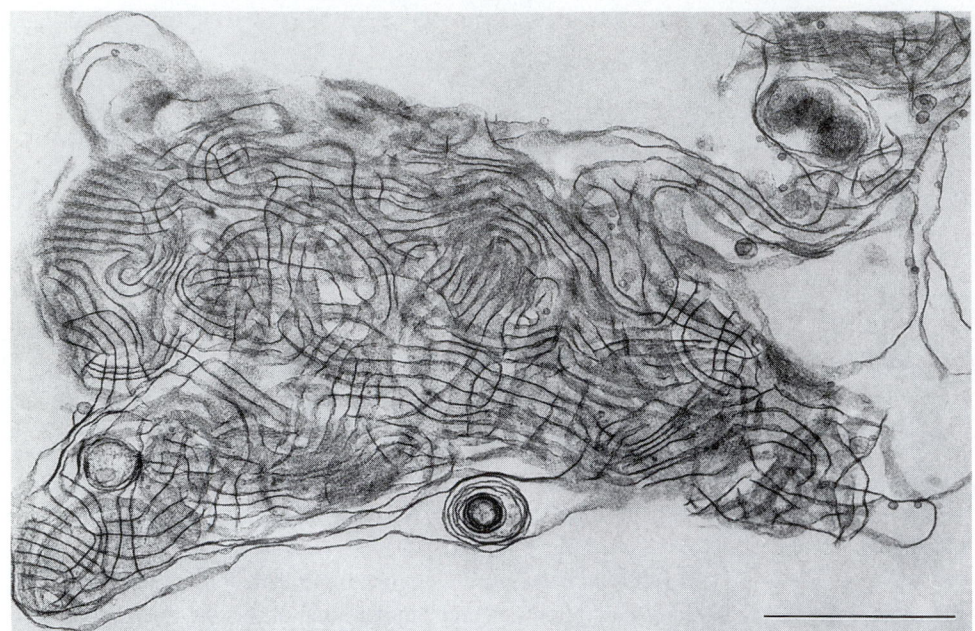

FIGURE 7-1   Tubular myelin. Tubular myelin is produced after secretion of lamellar bodies into the airspace by a process dependent upon surfactant proteins A, B, phospholipids and extracellular calcium. Tubular myelin is a relatively dense, highly organized form of phospholipid present in the alveolar subphase. Phospholipid molecules move from the tubular myelin to monolayer and multilayer sheets, reducing surface tension at the air-liquid interface. Bar = 1 μm.

Smaller, less dense particles (small aggregates) are also present within the alveolar space, representing remnants or catabolic forms of surfactant that are destined for uptake, reutilization, or catabolism by type II epithelial cells and alveolar macrophages.

Surfactant Phospholipids and Proteins

The composition of surfactant phospholipids is similar in all of the structural forms of surfactant isolated from mammalian lung, generally representing 80 to 90 percent of the mass of pulmonary surfactant.[43] In the adult lung, phosphatidylcholine (70 to 80 percent) and phosphatidylglycerol (10 percent) are the most abundant phospholipid constituents. Lesser amounts of phosphatidylserine, phosphatidylethanolamine, sphingomyelin, neutral lipids, and glycolipids are also detected in surfactant. The lung content of surfactant phospholipids increases markedly with advancing gestation. Surfactant is secreted into the amniotic fluid, and total phospholipid, dipalmitoylphosphatidylcholine (DPPC), or increased lecithin to sphingomyelin (L/S) ratio correlate with postnatal respiratory function. These tests are widely used to predict pulmonary maturity prior to the birth of preterm infants. Proteins represent approximately 5 to 15 percent of the mass of pulmonary surfactant and include serum proteins and proteins that are produced by respiratory epithelial cells. Four surfactant proteins—SP-A, SP-B, SP-C, and SP-D—named in the order of discovery, are produced primarily by respiratory epithelial cells, each playing specific roles in surfactant homeostasis or host defense.

Surfactant is uniquely enriched in disaturated DPPC. The saturated C16 acyl chains pack densely at an air-liquid interface, reducing tension at the surface. However, such dense and stable packing of DPPC occurs at a phase transition of 41°C, far above

physiological temperatures. Thus, at 37°C, pure DPPC maintains a semicrystalline or gel phase that is incapable of moving rapidly with the expansion and contraction of the alveolus during the respiratory cycle. The capability of DPPC pulmonary surfactant to move rapidly to the alveolar interface at 37°C and to maintain low surface tension during dynamic compression is conferred by the surfactant-associated proteins SP-B and SP-C.

Structure and Function of Surfactant Proteins

Four distinct proteins have been isolated from surfactant obtained by lung lavage (Fig. 7-2). Their cDNAs, genes, and structures have been identified and are relatively well characterized.[26] These surfactant proteins are expressed in a lung epithelial cell–selective manner and are secreted into the airspace, where they influence the structure, metabolism, and function of surfactant. Two classes of proteins have been distinguished on the basis of their structures. SP-A and SP-D are relatively abundant, hydrophilic, structurally related proteins that are members of the calcium-dependent lectin family of proteins. These molecules have relatively weak "surfactant"-like qualities but are able to bind complex carbohydrates, including those on the surface of bacteria, viruses, and other lung pathogens. They act as opsonins, activate alveolar macrophages, and therefore are likely to play important roles in host defense in the lung. In contrast, SP-B and SP-C are small, hydrophobic proteins that play critical roles in enhancing the rate of spreading and stability of surfactant phospholipids. SP-B and SP-C are the protein components of the animal-derived surfactant replacement preparations used for the treatment of IRDS.

SP-C

SP-C is encoded by a single gene on chromosome 8 in the human. SP-C mRNA is expressed exclusively in type II epithelial cells in the lung and is translated to produce a 22-kDa precursor that is proteolytically processed to form the active, hydrophobic peptide of 33 to 35 amino acids.[13] SP-C enhances the surface-active properties of lipid mixtures by lowering surface tension and enhancing adsorption rate of a lipid film at the air-water interface,[42] although to a smaller extent than SP-B. SP-C and SP-B together reduce surface tension of a lipid film to near zero, and they increase lung compliance in premature animals.[11] SP-C is palmitoylated on cysteine residues near the NH_2 terminus.[10] The surface activity of depalmitoylated SP-C is somewhat less than that of palmitoylated SP-C,[9] and the palmitoyl groups may be required for a posttranslational modification of the SP-C precursor. The carboxy-terminal two-thirds of SP-C is generally in an α-helical conformation, but depalmitoylation reduces

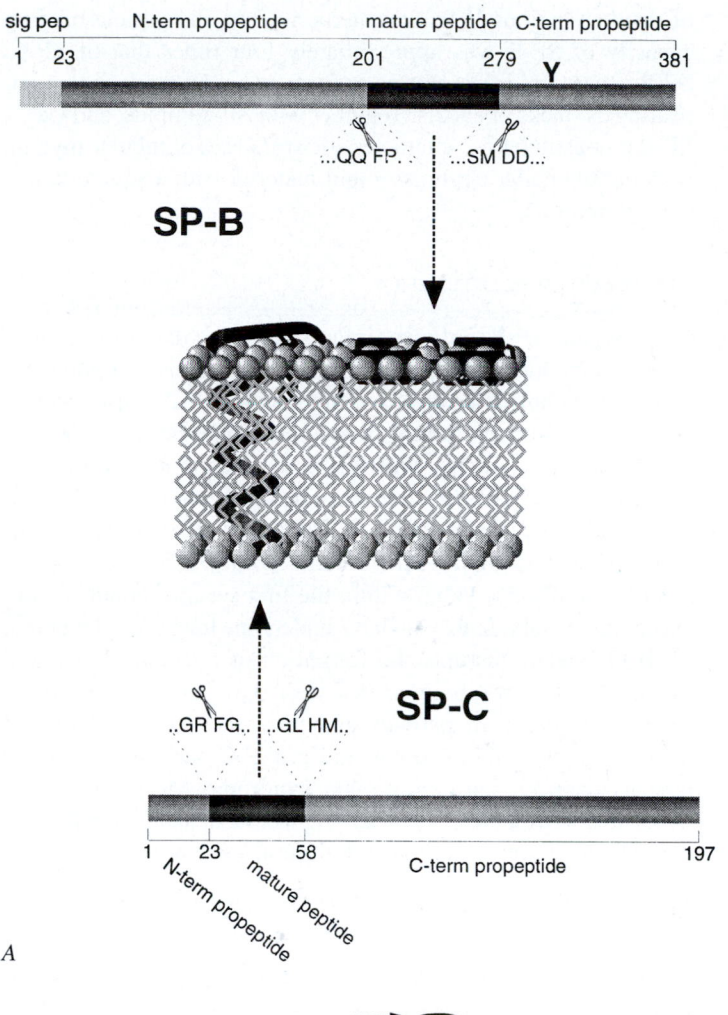

A

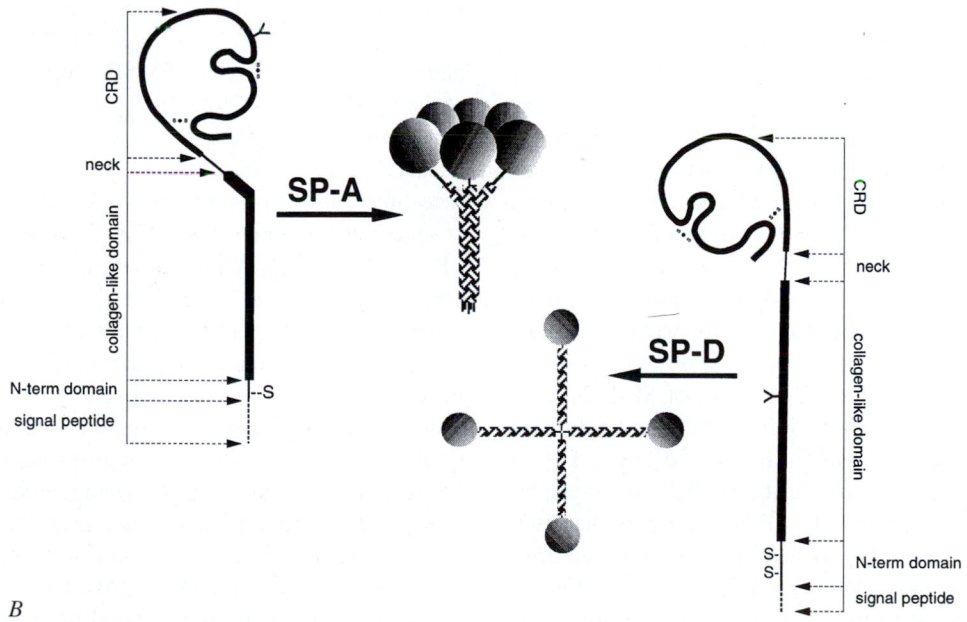

B

FIGURE 7-2 *A.* Hydrophobic surfactant proteins SP-B and SP-C. The active SP-B peptide is produced by proteolytic processing of pre-proSP-B protein consisting of 381 amino acids. The active 79–amino acid, SP-B peptide interacts with phospholipid head groups, altering the stability of phospholipid films and enhancing their rate of spreading at the air-liquid interface. SP-C is generated by proteolytic processing of a 197–amino acid preproprotein to form the 32– to 34–amino acid active hydrophobic peptide that inserts deeply into the acyl chains of lipid bilayers, disrupting acyl group packing and enhancing mobility of phospholipids at the membrane surface. *B.* Surfactant proteins A and D. Surfactant protein A is produced from a preproprotein that is proteolytically processed by the removal of the signal peptide and glycoslated (Y). SP-A consists of a carboxy-terminal globular, lectinlike domain (CRD) (*thin line*) and a more rigid, collagen-like domain (*dark line*) comprising the amino terminal region. Sulfhydryl-dependent interactions between SP-A monomers result in the organization of SP-A into hexamers that further associate to form the larger oligomers present in the alveolar space. SP-D is closely related to SP-A and is also a member of the calcium-dependent family of lectins. SP-D contains a C-terminal globular lectin domain (*thin line*) that is linked to a larger, NH_2-terminal, collagenlike domain. SP-D forms quatramers in the airspace that are relatively weakly associated with surfactant lipids. Human SP-A (two genes) and SP-D are located together on human chromosome 10 and are likely derived from duplications of an ancestral molecule.

the α-helical content of native SP-C. A form of depalmitoylated SP-C that forms a very stable dimer with a high β-sheet content has also been identified. Although the orientation of the palmitoyl groups in a lipid environment is not currently known, they are likely, due to their hydrophobicity, to hold the amino-terminal region of SP-C in close contact with lipids.

In a lipid bilayer, the orientation of the α-helical segment of SP-C is closely parallel with the lipid acyl chains, implying a transbilayer orientation (Fig. 7-2A). In a surface monolayer, SP-C has a preferential orientation parallel to the interface, as observed by circular dichroism of monolayer films.[9] The positive charges near the NH_2 terminus of SP-C may promote in the binding of phospholipid vesicles to the monolayer—a step required for insertion of phospholipids into the monolayer. Blocking of the positively charged residues arginine and lysine with phenylglyoxal produced a modified SP-C, which had lost the ability to enhance binding of lipid vesicles to the monolayer and did not catalyze insertion of lipids into the monolayer.[8] SP-C forms aggregates in DPPC/DPPG (dipalmitoylphosphatidylglycerol) mixtures below the phase transition temperature of the bulk lipid, as observed by fluorescence energy transfer among SP-C molecules labeled with fluorescent probes.[20] SP-C also affects the size and shape of lipid vesicles. It disrupts vesicular structure, causing the formation of larger vesicles and discoid particles.

In summary, SP-C is likely to be present in both phospholipid monolayers and bilayers. Insertion of SP-C into the phospholipid membranes disrupts acyl group packing; positive charges near the NH_2 terminus and located near the surface of the phospholipids may enhance insertion of phospholipid molecules into surfactant films.

SP-B

Surfactant protein SP-B is a hydrophobic 8.8-kDa protein produced from a single gene located on human chromosome 2.[46] The SP-B mRNA is expressed in bronchioles and type II alveolar cells and is translated to produce a 40- to 42-kDa precursor that is proteolytically processed to form the active 79–amino acid peptide found in surfactant. In combination with lipids, SP-B reconstitutes most of the surface activity of natural lung surfactant.[11] In combination with SP-C and SP-A, SP-B is even more effective. SP-B contains two regions, (Trp_9-Pro_{23}) and (Ile_{56}-Pro_{67}), predicted to form amphipathic α-helices.[20] Almost 50 percent of the protein is in an α-helical conformation, with approximately 20 percent β-sheet and 16 percent turns, as determined by Fourier transform infrared spectroscopy (FTIR). SP-B contains three intramolecular disulfide bonds, linking cysteines 8 with 77, 11 with 71, and 35 with 46. These disulfide bonds confine the amphipathic helices of SP-B in an antiparallel configuration. A seventh cysteine (Cys 48) is free to form an intermolecular disulfide bond, stabilizing the SP-B dimer. Dimers and higher multimers of SP-B, which are probably stabilized by noncovalent interactions, are also found in organic extracts of pulmonary surfactant.

The positively charged amino acid residues of SP-B interact with the negatively charged phospholipid DPPG, as determined by a variety of physical techniques.[46] In a mixed DPPC/DPPG monolayer, SP-B is believed to purify the DPPC monolayer by removal of DPPG in a complex with SP-B, a process that may require interaction with SP-C. SP-B increases order in the lipid head group region with little effect on order in the membrane interior.[13] The ability to order the lipid head group region is located in the amino- and carboxy-terminal regions of SP-B (1-20) and (53-78), which contain the predicted amphipathic helices.[14] Synthetic peptides that contain these two regions have surface-tension lowering activity similar to that of native SP-B.[14]

SP-B enhances the insertion of phospholipid vesicles into a preformed DPPC/DPPG monolayer, particularly in the presence of divalent cations.[33] In these experiments, the vesicle-binding capacity of SP-B was approximately four times that of SP-C. SP-B causes lipids in solution to form discoid particles often appearing as stacks or sheets. Together with SP-A, lipids, and Ca^{2+}, SP-B reconstitutes the characteristic structures of tubular myelin, both multilamellar aggregates and material with a square lattice configuration.[38]

HEREDITARY SP-B DEFICIENCY

Homozygous SP-B–deficient infants and mice die of respiratory failure immediately following birth.[14] While lung morphogenesis proceeds normally in utero, the lack of SP-B causes atelectasis and respiratory failure in the immediate postnatal period. More than forty infants with SP-B deficiency have now been identified since Nogee et al. first described the disorder in 1993.[30] SP-B deficiency is inherited as an autosomal recessive gene, generally presenting in full-term infants with IRDS. The disorder has been uniformly lethal within the first several months of life except in several infants who have undergone lung transplantation. SP-B deficiency disrupts the formation of lamellar bodies and tubular myelin, and it interferes with the routing of proSP-C. Thus SP-B–deficient patients and mice lack active SP-B and SP-C proteins in the alveolus and proSP-C accumulates in the airspace, causing a proteinosis-like syndrome. Most of these patients do not respond to surfactant replacement and generally succumb from chronic respiratory failure in spite of intensive care.

SP-A

SP-A is an abundant hydrophilic 26-kDa (monomer) glycoprotein that functions in the maintenance of tubular myelin structure,[38] host defense,[39] and regulation of surfactant lipid uptake and secretion,[36,47] (Fig. 7-2B). SP-A mRNA is expressed in bronchiolar and alveolar type II cells in the lung, being translated from two genes located on chromosome 10 in the human. In the absence of SP-C and SP-B, SP-A enhances formation of a surface lipid film in the presence of divalent ions, although SP-A is much less effective than the hydrophobic surfactant proteins SP-B and SP-C. SP-A also enhances surface activity of lipid films containing SP-C and SP-B. The amino-terminal third of SP-A is arranged in a collagenlike triple helix,[18] while a carboxy-terminal region bears homology to mammalian lectins and serum mannose-binding proteins. The hydrophobic domain, Gly 81 through Val 117, and the amino-terminal collagenlike domain, are required for lipid binding. Protein-protein interactions among SP-A molecules requiring the collagenlike domain and an intermolecular disulfide bond at Cys 9 are necessary for the aggregation of lipids by SP-A. When added to type II cells in vitro, SP-A decreases surfactant secretion.[35] Binding and uptake of SP-A by type II epithelial cells is mediated by a specific, saturable cell-surface receptor.[25,36] The noncollagenous C-terminal domain of SP-A binds to isolated type II cells and inhibits phospholipid secretion, suggesting that the receptor-binding site is in the C-terminal region of SP-A. SP-A increases the association of lipids with type II cells[39] but does not appear to increase internalization of lipid, as monitored by uptake of fluorescent lipid probes.[21]

SP-D

Surfactant protein D is a collagenous Ca^{2+}-dependent carbohydrate-binding protein that is structurally related to SP-A and other C-type lectins,[34] (Fig. 2B). SP-D is encoded by a single gene located near the SP-A gene on human chromosome 10. SP-D is synthesized by alveolar type II epithelial cells and is found in the endoplasmic reticulum and Golgi of Clara cells, but it is also expressed in the gastric mucosa. The interaction of SP-D with surfactant is Ca^{2+}- and carbohydrate-dependent. SP-D can be eluted from surfactant with glucose, maltose, and other saccharides. Thus, SP-D does not bind lipids hydrophobically, in contrast to the other surfactant-associated proteins. Like SP-A, SP-D plays a role in lung immune defense as an opsonin.

RECYCLING AND CATABOLISM OF SURFACTANT LIPIDS AND PROTEINS

Pulmonary surfactant is taken up rapidly in the lung, and much of the lipid is reutilized (Fig. 7-3). Measurements of the efficiency of recycling of phosphatidylcholine (PC) in adult rabbit lungs range between 23 and 85 percent, with approximately 10 percent of the alveolar pool of 10 to 15 mg/kg total body weight being recycled every hour.[23] In 3-day-old rabbits, 94 percent of the PC is reutilized, with a turnover time of the alveolar PC of 10 h. Some 30 to 50 percent of intratracheally injected ^{3}H-PC is sequestered from the alveolar space within a few minutes after instillation and cannot be removed by lavage. Since the initial uptake is immediate, it likely represents binding to lung surfaces rather than endocytosis by epithelial cells. Administered lipid appears in type II cells and alveolar macrophages, but little label appears in type I cells.

Isolated pulmonary epithelial type II cells internalize ^{3}H-PC and resecrete the internalized material or degrade it with reincorporation into other lipids. Isolated type II cells also endocytose SP-C. Association of labeled SP-C with isolated type II cells is nonsaturating up to 150 μg/ml, consistent with a non-receptor-mediated mechanism. SP-B is also endocytosed by isolated type II cells.[6] SP-A binds to type II cells and is endocytosed by a receptor-mediated mechanism.[25,36] In vivo, the rates of clearance of saturated PC, SP-B, and SP-A from the airspace are distinct.

Pulmonary surfactant as isolated from lavage fluid exists in several forms that can be fractionated based on density.[28] In vivo labeling indicates that phospholipid is initially secreted in the heaviest forms, followed by conversion into distinct heavy and light forms.[28] The most dense or ultraheavy form contains lamellar bodies and tubular myelin. The dense form contains tubular myelin and large vesicles. The heavy forms of tubular myelin are also referred to as large aggregates (LA). A light form, or small aggregates, is comprised of small unilamellar vesicles. Unlike the other two forms, the light form has little surface activity in vitro and is ineffective in enhancing lung compliance in preterm animals. Small aggregates are depleted of SP-A, SP-B, and SP-C,[5] and their lipid composition is similar to that of large aggregates except for an increase in lysoPC content. Cycling surfactant by expansion and contraction of surface film in vitro produces a conversion from large to small aggregates.[16] This conversion is blocked by serine protease inhibitors; however, the mechanism involved remains unclear at present.

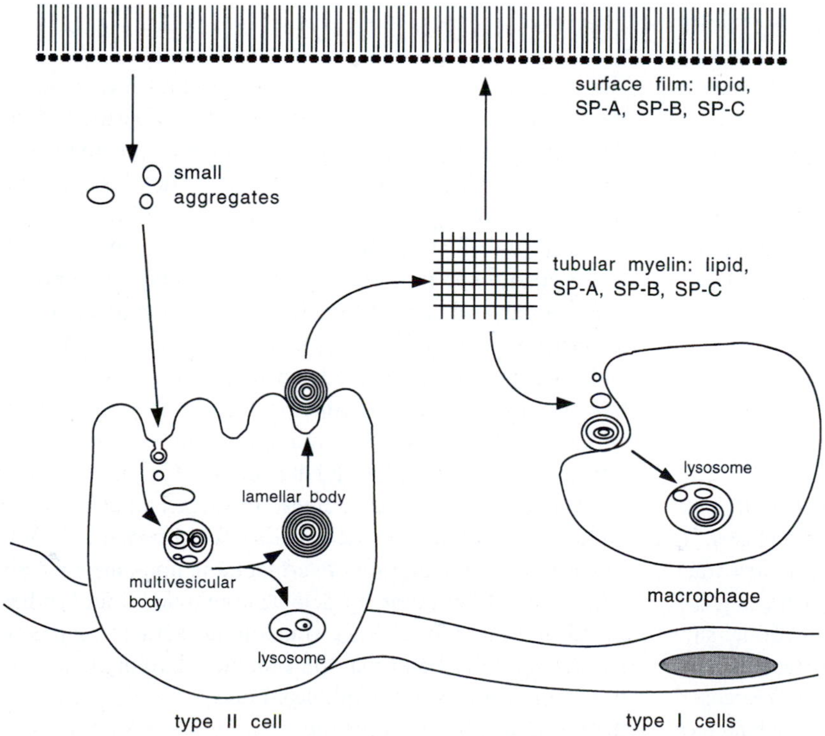

REGULATION OF SURFACTANT PRODUCTION

The synthesis of pulmonary surfactant is subject to precise regulatory controls both during development and postnatally.[29] Surfactant phospholipid synthesis increases markedly in late gestation and is enhanced by a variety of hormones, including glucocorticoids. Lung phospholipid content increases in the latter two-thirds of gestation in preparation for respiratory adaptation at birth. Prenatal glucocorticoids are routinely used to induce lung maturation and surfactant synthesis in infants at risk for preterm delivery. Glucocorticoids reduce the risk of IRDS and

FIGURE 7-3 Life cycle of pulmonary surfactant. SP-A, SP-B, SP-C and lipids are packaged in lamellar bodies and secreted by type II alveolar epithelial cells into the airspace. Lamellar bodies unfold into tubular myelin, which gives rise to the lipid/protein film at the air-liquid interface. Used surfactant lipids are released from the film as small vesicles, which are taken up and recycled or degraded by type II cells. Alveolar macrophages also take up surfactant and degrade it.

enhance the efficacy of surfactant replacement therapy after birth. Like surfactant phospholipids, the surfactant proteins are highly regulated, increasing in the latter two-thirds of gestation in the mammalian species studied. Expression of surfactant proteins is regulated in complex ways by a variety of hormonal agents. The levels of surfactant protein mRNA increase in the perinatal period in association with increased surfactant synthesis and secretion required for postnatal respiratory adaptation. Expression of the surfactant proteins is regulated at both transcriptional and posttranscriptional levels, maintaining steady-state protein concentrations within tight constraints in the adult lung. Surfactant production is, in general, enhanced by glucocorticoids, epidermal growth factor (EGF), and cyclic adenosine monophosphate (cAMP) but inhibited by tumor necrosis factor-alpha (TNF-α), transforming growth factor-beta (TGF-β) and insulin, depending on experimental conditions. Transcriptional control of the surfactant genes is modulated by interactions with nuclear transcription proteins including thyroid transcription factor-1 (TTF-1), and a variety of more ubiquitously expressed transcription factors including members of the HNF-3 family and AP-1.[45] Surfactant proteins A, B, and D are expressed in bronchiolar and alveolar type II cells, while SP-C is expressed exclusively in type II epithelial cells. Thus a variety of transcriptional and posttranscriptional controls influence the synthesis of surfactant proteins and lipids maintaining surfactant content, in part contributing to the maintenance of surfactant concentrations in the airspace.

While less than 10 to 15 percent of surfactant lipids are cleared by catabolism by alveolar macrophages, this pathway may be significant in the control of steady-state surfactant concentrations. Recent studies in granulocyte macrophage colony-stimulating factor (GM-CSF) knockout transgenic mice demonstrate the important role of GM-CSF in clearance of surfactant proteins and lipids. GM-CSF knockout mice develop severe alveolar proteinosis associated with failure to clear surfactant protein-A or phospholipids, implicating GM-CSF signaling in the clearance or catabolism by alveolar macrophages or respiratory epithelial cells.[12] As such, this regulation may be involved in the pathogenesis of idiopathic pulmonary alveolar proteinosis (PAP) (see Chapter 81).

SURFACTANT HOMEOSTASIS AND REPLACEMENT IN INFANTILE RESPIRATORY DISTRESS SYNDROME

Infantile respiratory distress syndrome is associated with prematurity, the risk increasing as the gestational age decreases. In addition to the morphologic immaturity of the respiratory tract seen in the lungs, lung phospholipid content and surfactant secretion are decreased in the preterm infant. While functional surfactant can be isolated from infants with IRDS, surfactant pool size is markedly decreased in the preterm infant.[23] Decreased alveolar surfactant concentrations following birth cause atelectasis, alveolar collapse, and hypoxemia, all characteristic of IRDS in the preterm infant.

Supplemental oxygen and ventilatory therapy are used to treat IRDS. However, during the last decade, widespread use of exogenous surfactant has markedly ameliorated the morbidity and mortality associated with this common disease of preterm in-

fants. Exogenous surfactants—in the form of synthetic mixtures of phospholipids and various extracts of lung or surfactant containing surfactant proteins B, C, and phospholipids—have been used extensively for prevention and therapy of RDS in newborn infants.[2] Surfactant replacement with preparations containing surfactant proteins B and C acts rapidly, increasing lung volumes, and compliance and decreasing the requirements for positive-pressure ventilation and oxygen. Morbidity and mortality have been markedly reduced since the application of surfactant replacement to preterm neonates, decreasing barotrauma, pneumothorax, and mortality from the disorder. Surfactant is given intratracheally, in several doses, in the first days of life, and this is generally associated with marked improvement in pulmonary function. Synthetic surfactants lacking surfactant proteins generally function in a somewhat delayed manner, but treatment with synthetic and protein-containing surfactant has been highly effective in decreasing morbidity and mortality from IRDS in clinical studies. The effectiveness of surfactant is likely related both to the immediate surface tension–reducing properties and to the reuptake and reutilization of the exogenous surfactant particles by the respiratory epithelium. Surfactant replacement is generally given for several days postnatally. Thereafter, production of endogenous surfactant lipids and proteins is maintained by the respiratory epithelium. Surfactant replacement preparations are presently being studied for treatment of meconium aspiration, pneumonia, and ARDS.

SURFACTANT IN ADULT RESPIRATORY DISTRESS SYNDROME

Adult respiratory distress syndrome occurs in association with trauma, sepsis, long bone fractures, thermal burns, and injury to the lung from aspiration of gastric contents, pneumonia, and inhalation of toxic gases (see Chapter 61). The prognosis in ARDS patients remains poor, with approximately 50 percent mortality in most studies. In ARDS, increased permeability of the microvasculature permits leakage of protein and fluid into the lung, inactivating surfactant. Epithelial cell injury may also contribute to surfactant deficiency in ARDS. Various nonsurfactant proteins and lipids present in elevated concentrations in the lung in ARDS have been implicated in reducing surface activity of pulmonary surfactant; these include immunoglobulins, albumin, fibrinogen, fatty acids, lyso-phosphatidylcholine, and C-reactive protein. The mechanisms causing the decrease in surfactant activity in ARDS include competition of the proteins for the air-liquid interface, sequestration and dilution of surfactant in non-surface-active particles, and inhibition of surfactant protein and lipid synthesis and secretion (Table 7-1). Alterations in surfactant composition occur during ARDS and may precede the development of respiratory failure. Lavage phospholipid and SP-A are decreased, and the minimum surface tension of surfactant tested in vitro is increased in patients at risk for ARDS.[15] In ARDS, total phospholipid, phosphatidylcholine, phosphatidylglycerol, and surfactant proteins SP-A and SP-B are decreased[15,41] and the ratio of small to large aggregates is significantly increased compared to that in non-ARDS patients.[41] Thus, ARDS leads to both a deficiency in pulmonary surfactant constituents and inhibition of the

TABLE 7-1

TABLE 7-1

Pathogenesis of ARDS

Agent	Effect on Pulmonary Surfactant
cell injury, TNF-α, TGF-β	↓ synthesis
oxidation, phospholipases, lysolipids	↑ inactivation
plasma proteins	↓ accessibility of air/liquid interface
edema fluid	↑ dilution
proteases	↑ conversion from large to small aggregates

activity of the remaining surfactant. Adult respiratory distress syndrome and related syndromes are associated with protein leak into alveolar space and inactivation of surfactant function.

INHIBITION OF SURFACTANT ACTIVITY

Phospholipases A_2 and C and their products, fatty acids, lysoPC, and dipalmitin inhibit surface activity in vitro. These molecules may be released or produced during lung injury. Inhibitory effects of oleic acid may be related to its miscibility with phospholipids, disrupting the interfacial surfactant film, rather than by competition for the interface. The inhibition by PAF, lysoPC, and oleic acid is not reversible, suggesting that their direct interaction with surfactant lipids disrupts lipid organization at the interface. However, not all fatty acids are inhibitory. Palmitic acid has been reported to improve surfactant function of an organic extract of surfactant. The surface activity of pulmonary surfactant is readily destroyed by phospholipase A_2 or phospholipase C. In injured lungs, inhibition of surface activity by fatty acids and proteins may be additive, since they appear to inhibit surfactant activity by different mechanisms.

Oxidant Injury

Oxygen therapy, used routinely for ARDS and IRDS, may influence surfactant homeostasis and function in the alveolus. The rate of synthesis of surfactant lipids and clearance of radiolabeled surfactant extracts decreased in rabbits exposed to 100% O_2 for 64 h.[32] In contrast, exposure of adult rats to 85% O_2 increased surfactant proteins SP-A, SP-B, and SP-C and phospholipids. The increase occurred at the pretranslational level, with mRNA levels of the various proteins increasing two- to five-fold after 5 days in 85% O_2.[31] Oxidants are also released locally in the lung by activated immune cells. Activated alveolar macrophages secrete NO and superoxide, which can then react to form peroxynitrite. Peroxynitrite in combination with Fe^{3+} EDTA inhibited the surface activity of surfactant[17] by damaging the lipid, SP-A, SP-B, and SP-C. The ability of the surfactant proteins to decrease surface tension when recombined with lipids is decreased by treatment with peroxynitrite.

Edema Fluid

Leakage of edema fluid into the airspace occurs in both ARDS and IRDS. Edema fluid obtained from hyperoxia-exposed rab-

bits contains various serum proteins capable of inhibiting the surface activity of surfactant extracts, as evaluated in the pulsating bubble apparatus.[24] Thus edema fluid may interfere with surfactant therapy, although the concentration dependence of the inhibition suggests that increased doses of surfactant may aid in overcoming the inhibitory effects of edema fluid. The mechanism of inhibition by edema fluid is consistent with the mechanisms reported for its plasma protein constituents; edema fluid also dilutes surfactant, thereby making it more susceptible to inhibition by proteins.

Plasma Proteins

Serum albumin, globulin, and fibrinogen reduce the rate of adsorption, increase the minimum surface tension of the surfactant film, and reduce the hysteresis area between compression and expansion curves in vitro. The mechanism by which plasma proteins inhibit the activity of pulmonary surfactant is likely to be one of competition for the interface,[19] because higher surfactant lipid concentrations overcome albumin inhibition even at high albumin concentrations. Inhibition by C-reactive protein, fibrinogen and other plasma proteins is reversible. Addition of SP-A and organic surfactant extracts reverses inhibition caused by soluble proteins but not by lysoPC.[7]

Both SP-C and SP-B increase the ability of a phospholipid mixture to resist inhibition of surface activity by plasma proteins. SP-B is more effective than SP-C at resisting inhibition by fibrinogen.[37] Addition of SP-B to SP-C/PL mix decreases its sensitivity to fibrinogen. In addition, incubation of an organic surfactant extract (CLSE) with anti-SP-B antibody produced little effect on surface tension alone, but markedly increased the sensitivity of CLSE to inhibition by fibrinogen.[37] The best resistance to inhibition was observed when both SP-C and SP-B were present.

REDUCTION OF SURFACTANT SYNTHESIS

In addition to the inactivation of pulmonary surfactant by proteins and lipids in edema fluid, a reduction of synthesis of surfactant may contribute to the decreased surfactant activity in ARDS. In an in vitro organotypic culture system, the effect of *Escherichia coli* endotoxin on lung cell surfactant synthesis was studied as a model system for pulmonary complications of postburn sepsis.[27] In those studies, endotoxin at 1 to 10 μg/ml suppressed the incorporation of ^{3}H-choline and ^{3}H-palmitate into de novo synthesized lamellar bodies and common myelin figures by 50 to 64 percent. Synthesis of surfactant proteins may be influenced by inflammatory response following lung injury infection. In vitro, TNF-α decreases de novo synthesis of SP-A, SP-B, and SP-C mRNA. When administered intratracheally in mice, TNF-α causes respiratory distress and decreases SP-C mRNA. Likewise, TGF-β1, a polypeptide produced by the injured lung, decreases the expression of SP-A and SP-C in vitro. Thus, sepsis or lung injury may reduce both the synthesis and functions of surfactant lipids and proteins.

SUMMARY

Decreased production or inactivation of pulmonary surfactant has been associated with both IRDS and ARDS (Table 7-1). Surfactant production and activity are inhibited following injury and alveolar capillary leak. Surfactant function may be further impaired by dilution caused by pulmonary edema and by the action of phospholipases, producing lysolipids and free fatty acids which disrupt the surfactant monolayer. Conversion of active large aggregate forms of surfactant, to inactive small aggregate forms, depleted of the surfactant proteins, may also be accelerated in the injured lung. Surface activity of the remaining surfactant is reduced further by competition with plasma proteins for the air-water interface. Surfactant deficiency and inactivation accompanying respiratory distress syndrome can be overcome by treatment with exogenous surfactant. Surfactant therapy for IRDS in premature infants has been highly successful, reducing morbidity and mortality from pulmonary disease. While in early phases of study, therapy with exogenous surfactant preparations containing the surfactant proteins SP-C and SP-B may also be useful in treatment of ARDS and other lung disorders associated with disruption of surfactant homeostasis.

REFERENCES

1. Avery ME, Mead J: Surface properties in relation to atelectasis and hyaline membrane disease. *Am J Dis Child* 97:517–523, 1959.
2. Avery ME, Merritt TA: Surfactant-replacement therapy. *New Engl J Med* 324:910–912, 1991.
3. Baatz JE, Elledge B, Whitsett JA: Surfactant protein SP-B induces ordering at the surface of model membrane bilayers. *Biochemistry* 29:6714–6720, 1990.
4. Baatz JE, Sarin V, Absolom DR, et al: Effects of surfactant-associated protein SP-B synthetic analogs on the structure and surface activity of model membrane bilayers. *Chem Phys Lipids* 60:163–178, 1991.
5. Baritussio A, Alberti A, Quaglino D, et al: SP-A, SP-B, and SP-C in surfactant subtypes around birth: Reexamination of the alveolar life cycle of surfactant. *Am J Physiol* 266 (*Lung Cell Mol Physiol* 10): L436–L447, 1994.
6. Breslin JS, Weaver TE: Binding, uptake, and localization of surfactant protein B in isolated rat alveolar type II cells. *Am J Physiol* (*Lung Cell Mol Physiol* 6) 262:L699–L707, 1992.
7. Cockshutt AM, Weitz J, Possmayer F: Pulmonary surfactant-associated protein A enhances the surface activity of lipid extract surfactant and reverses inhibition by blood proteins in vitro. *Biochemistry* 29:8424–8429, 1990.
8. Creuwels LAJM, Boer EJ, Demel RA, et al: Neutralization of the positive charges of surfactant protein C. *J Biol Chem* 270:16225–16229, 1995.
9. Creuwels LAJM, Demel RA, van Golde LMG, et al: Effect of acylation on structure and function of surfactant protein C at the air-liquid interface. *J Biol Chem* 268:26752–26758, 1993.
10. Curstedt T, Johansson J, Persson P, et al: Hydrophobic surfactant-associated peptides: SP-C is a lipopeptide with two palmitoylated cysteine residues, whereas SP-B lacks covalently linked fatty acyl groups. *Proc Natl Acad Sci USA* 87:2985–2989, 1990.
11. Curstedt T, Jornvall H, Robertson B, et al: Two hydrophobic low-molecular mass protein fractions of pulmonary surfactant: Characterization and biophysical activity. *Eur J Biochem* 168:255–262, 1987.
12. Dranoff G, Crawford AD, Sadelain M, et al: Involvement of granulocyte-macrophage colony-stimulating factor in pulmonary homeostasis. *Science* 264:713–716, 1994.
13. Glasser SW, Korfhagen TR, Weaver TE, et al: cDNA, deduced polypeptide structure and chromosomal assignment of human pulmonary surfactant proteolipid, SPL(pVal). *J Biol Chem* 263:9–12, 1988.
14. Glasser S, Korfhagen TR, Weaver TE, et al: cDNA and deduced amino acid sequence of human pulmonary surfactant-associated proteolipid SPL(Phe). *Proc Natl Acad Sci USA* 84:4007–4011, 1987.
15. Gregory TJ, Longmore WJ, Moxley MA, et al: Surfactant chemical composition and biophysical activity in acute respiratory distress syndrome. *J Clin Invest* 88:1976–1981, 1991.
16. Gross NJ, Narine KR: Surfactant subtypes in mice: Characteristics and quantitation. *J Appl Physiol* 66:342–349, 1989.
17. Haddad IY, Ischiropoulos H, Holm BA, et al: Mechanisms of peroxynitrite-induced injury to pulmonary surfactants. *Am J Physiol* 265:L555–L564, 1993.
18. Hawgood S: Pulmonary surfactant: A review of protein and genomic structure. *Am J Physiol* 257(*Lung Cell Mol Physiol*): L13–L22, 1989.
19. Holm BA, Notter RH, Finkelstein JN: Surface property changes from interactions of albumin with natural lung surfactant and extracted lung lipids. *Chem Phys Lipids* 38:287–298, 1985.
20. Horowitz AD, Baatz JE, Whitsett JA: Lipid effects on aggregation of pulmonary surfactant protein SP-C studied by fluorescence energy transfer. *Biochemistry* 32:9513–9523, 1993.
21. Horowitz AD, Moussavian B, Whitsett JA: Roles of SP-A, SP-B and SP-C in modulation of lipid uptake by pulmonary epithelial cells in vitro. *Am J Physiol* (*Lung Cell Mol Physiol* 14) 270: L69–L79, 1996.
22. Jobe A, Ikegami M: Surfactant metabolism. *Clin Perinatol* 20:683–686, 1993.
23. Jobe AH, Rider EO: Catabolism and recycling of surfactant, in Robertson B, van Golde LMG, Batenburg JJ (eds): *Pulmonary Surfactant: From Molecular Biology to Clinical Practice.* Amsterdam, Elsevier, 1992, pp 313–332.
24. Kobayashi T, Nitta K, Ganzuka M, et al: Inactivation of exogenous surfactant by pulmonary edema fluid. *Pediatr Res* 29:353–356, 1991.
25. Kuroki Y, Mason RJ, Voelker DR: Alveolar type II cells express a high affinity receptor for pulmonary surfactant protein A. *Proc Natl Acad Sci USA* 85:5566–5570, 1988.
26. Kuroki Y, Voelker DR: Pulmonary surfactant proteins. *J Biol Chem* 42:25943–25946, 1994.
27. Li JJ, Sanders RL, McAdam KPWJ, et al: Endotoxin suppresses surfactant synthesis in cultured rat lung cells. *J Trauma* 29:180–188, 1989.
28. Magoon MW, Wright JR, Baritussio A, et al: Subfractionation of lung surfactant: Implications for metabolism and specific activity. *Biochim Biophys Acta* 750:18–31, 1983.
29. Mendelson CR, Boggaram V: Hormonal control of the surfactant system in fetal lung. *Annu Rev Physiol* 53:415–440, 1991.
30. Nogee LM, deMello DE, Dehner LP, Colten HR: Brief report: Deficiency of pulmonary surfactant protein B in congenital alveolar proteinosis. *New Engl J Med* 328:406–410, 1993.
31. Nogee LM, Wispé JR, Clark JC, et al: Increased expression of pulmonary surfactant proteins in oxygen-exposed rats. *Am J Respir Cell Mol Biol* 4:102–107, 1991.

32. Novotny WE, Hudak BB, Matalon S, Holm BA: Hyperoxic lung injury reduces exogenous surfactant clearance in vivo. *Am J Respir Crit Care Med* 151:1843–1847, 1995.

33. Oosterlaken-Dijksterhuis MA, Haagsman HP, et al: Interaction of lipid vesicles with monomolecular layers containing lung surfactant proteins SP-B or SP-C. *Biochemistry* 30:8276–8281, 1991.

34. Persson A, Chang D, Crouch E: Surfactant protein D is a divalent cation-dependent carbohydrate-binding protein. *J Biol Chem* 265:5755–5760, 1990.

35. Rice WR, Ross GF, Singleton FM, et al: Surfactant-associated protein inhibits phospholipid secretion from type II cells. *J Appl Physiol* 63:692–698, 1987.

36. Ryan RM, Morris RE, Rice WR, et al: Binding and uptake of pulmonary surfactant protein (SP-A) by pulmonary type II cells. *J Histochem Cytochem* 37:429–440, 1989.

37. Seeger W, Günther A, Thede C: Differential sensitivity to fibrinogen inhibition of SP-C- vs. SP-B-based surfactants. *Am J Physiol (Lung Cell Mol Physiol 5)* 261:L286–L291, 1992.

38. Suzuki Y, Fujita Y, Kogishi K: Reconstitution of tubular myelin from synthetic lipids and proteins associated with pig pulmonary surfactant. *Am Rev Respir Dis* 140:75–81, 1989.

39. Van Iwaarden F, Welmers B, Verhoef J, et al: Pulmonary surfactant protein A enhances the host-defence mechanism of rat alveolar macrophages. *Am J Respir Cell Mol Biol* 2:91–98, 1990.

40. VanNeergaard K: Neue Auffassunder über einen Grundbegriff der Atemmechanik: Die Retraktionskraft der Lunge abhangig von der Oberflaschens Pannung in der Alveolar, 2. *Gesamte Exp Med* 66:373–394, 1929.

41. Veldhuizen RAW, McCaig LA, Akino T, Lewis JF: Pulmonary surfactant subfractions in patients with the acute respiratory distress syndrome. *Am J Respir Crit Care Med* 152:1867–1871, 1995.

42. Warr RG, Hawgood S, Buckley DI, et al: Low molecular weight human pulmonary surfactant protein (SP5): Isolation, characterization and cDNA and amino acid sequences. *Proc Natl Acad Sci USA* 84:7915–7919, 1987.

43. Whitsett JA: Composition of pulmonary surfactant lipids and proteins, in Polin RA, Fox WW (eds): *Fetal and Neonatal Physiology.* Philadelphia, Saunders, 1991, vol 2, pp 941–949.

44. Whitsett JA: Composition and structure of pulmonary surfactant, in, Boynton BR, Carlo WA, Jobe AH (eds): *New Therapies for Neonatal Respiratory Failure—A Physiological Approach.* New York, Cambridge University Press, 1994, pp 3–15.

45. Whitsett JA, Korfhagen TR: Regulation of gene transcription in respiratory epithelial cells. *Am J Respir Cell Mol Biol* 14:118–120, 1996.

46. Whitsett JA, Nogee LM, Weaver TE, Horowitz AD: Human surfactant protein B: Structure, function, regulation and genetic disease. *Physiol Rev* 75:749–757, 1995.

47. Wright JR, Wager RE, Hawgood S, et al: Surfactant apoprotein Mr = 26,000–36,000 enhances uptake of liposomes by type II cells. *J Biol Chem* 262:2888–2894, 1987.

CHAPTER 8

TRANSPORT FUNCTION OF AIRWAY EPITHELIA AND SUBMUCOSAL GLANDS

Paul B. McCray, Jr. / Michael J. Welsh

Secretion and solute transport by epithelial cells that are lining the conducting airways and comprising the submucosal glands play key roles in the biology of the normal lung. In addition, abnormalities in airway epithelial and submucosal gland function contribute to the pathogenesis and pathophysiology of several inherited and acquired diseases. Two major functions of these cells are the production and modification of airway surface fluid and the secretion of a number of factors that contribute to host defenses. The active transport of electrolytes by surface cells regulates the volume and composition of airway fluid. The specialized cells of submucosal glands also contribute to the secretion of airway surface fluid and are the major producer of macromolecules including mucins. Together the products and function of these epithelia generate a local host defense

mechanism that protects the lungs from inhaled organisms and particulate material.

Knowledge about the biology of the respiratory tract solute transport and secretion has increased dramatically in recent years. This chapter describes the function of the surface epithelia and the submucosal glands and their roles in host defense. Despite progress, significant gaps in knowledge persist; these are also noted.

BIOLOGY OF EPITHELIA COVERING THE AIRWAY SURFACE

Morphologic Features Related to Function

Although morphologic aspects of airway epithelia are covered in another chapter, two morphologic features required for transepithelial transport of solute and water are worth considering. First, the epithelial cells are joined at their apical surface by tight junctions. The tight junctions and sheet of epithelial cells form a continuous barrier to solute and water movement. Yet, despite their name, tight junctions do not constitute an impermeable barrier; they have selective permeabilities to ions, other solutes, and water. Thus, solutes and water can move across the epithelium through two pathways: between the cells through the tight junctions (the paracellular pathway) or through the epithelial cells (the cellular pathway). Second, epithelial cells are polar; the apical membrane, which faces the mucosal or lumenal surface, is different from the basolateral membrane, which faces the submucosal or interstitial space. The morphologic differences between the two membranes are paralleled by biochemical and functional differences. Hormone receptors and ion transporters are segregated to one or the other of the two cell membranes. These morphologic features allow the epithelium to serve as a barrier separating the lumenal compartment from the interstitial compartment and to modify the composition of those compartments by net vectoral transport of electrolytes and macromolecules.

Proximal airway epithelium is a pseudostratified, columnar epithelium composed predominantly of ciliated cells, goblet cells, nonciliated cells, and basal cells.[7] The distal airway epithelia contain mostly ciliated and nonciliated bronchiolar (Clara) cells. In the proximal airway epithelium, studies with intracellular microelectrodes suggest that the ciliated surface cells play an important role in both sodium (Na^+) and chloride (Cl^-) transport. Transepithelial electrical resistance (a measure of the ionic permeability of the epithelium) ranges from 150 to 1000 $\Omega \cdot cm^2$ in proximal airways and decreases in more distal airways.

In Vivo Studies of Electrolyte Transport

Electrolyte transport by human airway epithelia has been studied in vivo by measuring the voltage across the epithelium (Vt, mucosal surface referenced to interstitial surface).[21] Most frequently this has been done across the nasal epithelium, but qualitatively similar measurements have been made in the large intrapulmonary airways. As shown by the example in Fig. 8-1, Vt across normal human airway epithelia in vivo is in the range of −5 to −20 mV.

Knowledge obtained from in vivo studies is limited in scope because such studies do not accurately evaluate the quantitative aspects of transport, they provide only minimal insight into the cellular and molecular mechanisms involved, and they do not measure electrically silent transport. Nevertheless, important clues have been obtained from measurements of Vt in the presence of various agents perfused onto the epithelial surface. Figure 8-1 shows that when the apical surface is perfused with a solution containing amiloride, which blocks Na^+ channels, Vt decreases. This finding demonstrates the presence of electrogenic Na^+ transport. If the apical surface is then perfused with a solution containing a low Cl^- concentration and an agonist such as terbutaline, which increases cellular levels of adenosine 3′,5′-cyclic phosphate (cAMP), Vt hyperpolarizes. This result, plus the finding that Vt does not hyperpolarize in people with cystic fibrosis (Fig. 8-1*B*), indicates that the apical membrane contains Cl^- channels, which as described below are cystic fibrosis transmembrane conductance regulator (CFTR) Cl^- channels. Finally, if the apical surface is perfused with adenosine 5′-triphosphate (ATP) or another nucleotide in the presence of low Cl^- concentration, Vt transiently hyperpolarizes, indicating the presence of another type of Cl^- channel in the apical membrane. This is particularly prominent in cystic fibrosis epithelia that lack CFTR Cl^- channels (Fig. 8-1*B*).

Thus, measurements of Vt in vivo provide valuable qualitative information about the airways. As a result, they are being used increasingly as a measure of the function of airways in disease states and as an assay to test the effect of potential therapeutic agents.

In Vitro Studies of Airway Epithelia

In vitro studies have confirmed in vivo studies and greatly increased the understanding of the mechanisms of electrolyte transport. Studies of airway epithelia from many species have contributed to knowledge of airway biology, but here we focus on human airway epithelia. The ability to culture human airway epithelial cells was an important advance for many studies of the airways. Primary cultures of human airway epithelia can be grown on permeable filter supports, often at the air-liquid interface, so that they differentiate, develop tight junctions, form distinct apical and basolateral membranes, and generate a ciliated surface.[38] To study electrolyte transport, the cultured epithelia or native epithelia can be mounted in Ussing chambers where the apical and basolateral compartments are separated. Vt can be measured and controlled (clamped) to desired values. The transepithelial electrical resistance can be determined by measuring the change in Vt that results from an applied current pulse. The short-circuit current (Isc) is measured when Vt is clamped at 0 mV and both sides of the epithelium are bathed with identical solutions. Under these conditions, the Isc is equal to the sum of all active, electrogenic, transepithelial transport.

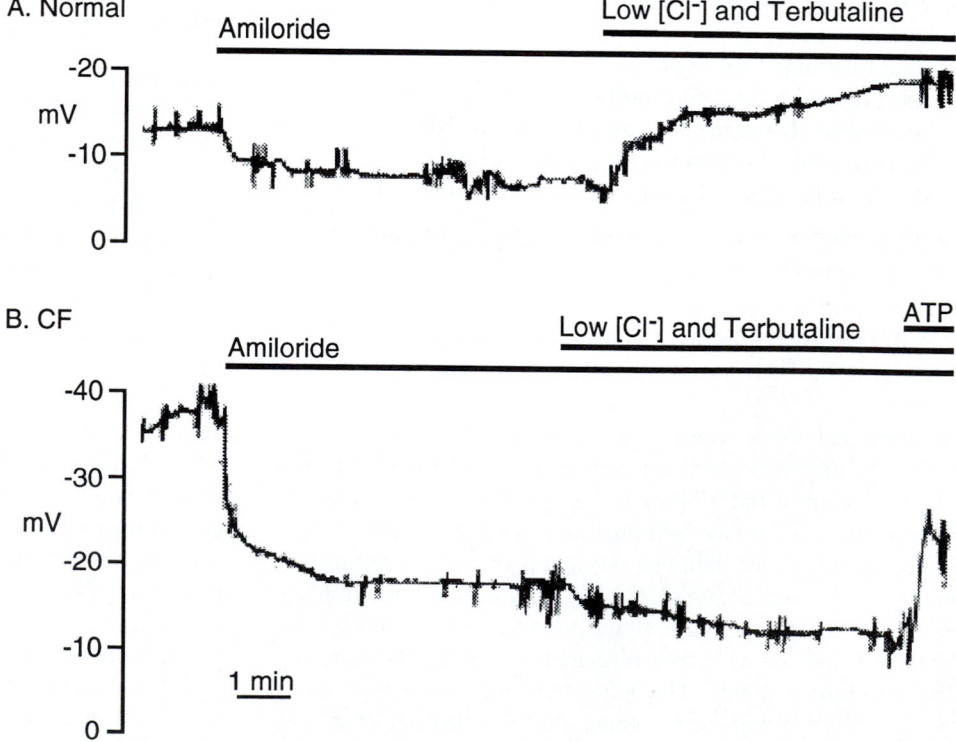

FIGURE 8-1   Examples of transepithelial voltage (Vt) measured in vivo across the airway epithelium of the nasal mucosa. Amiloride, a solution containing a low Cl^- concentration, terbutaline, and ATP were present during the times indicated by the bars. Top trace *(A)* was from a normal person and bottom trace *(B)* was from a person with cystic fibrosis. *(Provided by Dr. Joseph Zabner and Jan Launspach.)*

Cellular and Molecular Mechanisms of Electrolyte Transport

The cellular and molecular mechanisms of transepithelial transport are depicted graphically in Fig. 8-2 (for review, see references 6, 34, 40). Although the magnitude and contribution of specific processes to net transport vary depending on the airway region and experimental conditions, the cellular mechanisms appear similar throughout the airways. As described below, several aspects also apply to the function of submucosal gland epithelia. When the epithelium is studied in vitro, the Isc is accounted for by the absorption of Na^+ from the mucosal to the submucosal surface and by secretion of Cl^- from the submucosal to the mucosal surface. In humans, electrogenic absorption of Na^+ makes a much greater contribution to the short-circuit current than does secretion of Cl^-. In fact, definite identification of Cl^- secretion in human airway epithelia often requires inhibition of Na^+ absorption and stimulation of Cl^- secretion.

The main features of the model for Na^+ transport (Fig. 8-2) include: (1) Na^+ enters the cell through apical membrane *epithelial Na^+ channels* (ENaC). ENaC channels are inhibited by apical amiloride. Entry is a passive process, with Na^+ flowing down favorable concentration (the intracellular Na^+ concentration is lower than the extracellular concentration) and electrical (intracellular voltage is negative relative to the apical side of the membrane) gradients. (2) Na^+ then exits across the basolateral membrane via the Na^+-K^+-ATPase. This enzyme powers transepithelial transport by using energy from ATP hydrolysis to pump Na^+ out of the cell thereby maintaining a low intracellular Na^+ concentration. The Na^+-K^+-ATPase also accumulates K^+ inside the cell. (3) K^+ exits passively through a basolateral membrane K^+ channel. The basolateral K^+ conductance and the K^+ concentration gradient (high intracellular and low extracellular K^+ concentrations) hyperpolarize the cell, providing part of the driving force for Na^+ entry at the apical membrane.

Under short-circuit conditions in the presence of amiloride the mechanisms for Cl^- secretion (Fig. 8-2) are: (1) Cl^- enters the cell across the basolateral membrane via an electrically neutral cotransport process, coupled to Na^+ and K^+. The entry of Na^+ down its electrochemical gradient provides the driving force for accumulation of Cl^- at a concentration above electrochemical equilibrium. (2) Cl^- exits passively through apical membrane Cl^- channels, moving down a favorable electrochemical gradient. The regulation of the apical Cl^- permeability controls, in part, the rate of transepithelial Cl^- transport. There are at least two types of apical Cl^- channels[1]: CFTR Cl^- channels, which are regulated by phosphorylation by cAMP-dependent protein kinase, and Cl^- channels that are activated by an increase in the cytosolic concentration of free Ca^{2+}, $[Ca^{2+}]_c$. The molecular identity of the Cl^- channels controlled by $[Ca^{2+}]_c$ are not yet known. (3) Na^+ which enters the cell at the basolateral membrane coupled to Cl^- exits across the basolateral membrane via the Na^+-K^+-ATPase. (4) K^+ which enters coupled to Cl^- and on the Na^+-K^+-ATPase exits passively through basolateral membrane K^+ channels. When the epithelium is studied in an Ussing chamber under open-circuit conditions (i.e., when Vt is not clamped), often little net Cl^- transport is measured, and Cl^- absorption can occur.

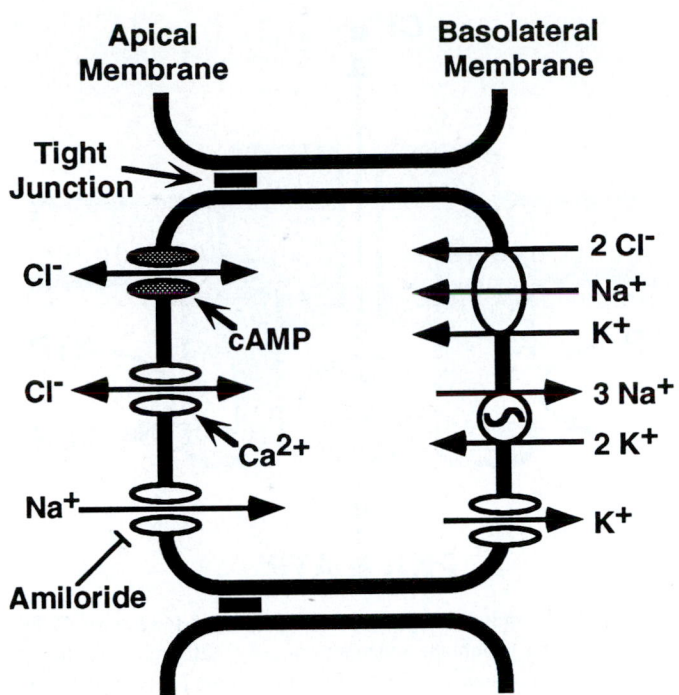

FIGURE 8-2   Cellular mechanism of electrolyte transport by airway epithelia. Note that cAMP-dependent and Ca^{2+}-dependent Cl^- secretion and amiloride-sensitive Na^+ absorption appear to occur in the same cell type. The CFTR Cl^- channel which is defective in CF is indicated by shading; all other channels, transporters, and pumps are indicated by open symbols.

The CFTR Cl^- Channel

Because the gene for CFTR is mutated in patients with cystic fibrosis,[36] the CFTR Cl^- channel has been studied extensively (for reviews see references 24, 35). CFTR is a member of a family of proteins named *ATP-binding cassette* (ABC) transporters. CFTR is located in the apical membrane and within intracellular vesicles beneath the apical membrane. Note that the epithelia lining the pulmonary airways express little CFTR, yet the Cl^- channel function (and its absence in CF) is easily measured. This is so because ion channels are very efficient, with an ability to transport 10^6 to 10^7 ions per second. Thus only a relatively few molecules of CFTR are sufficient to support transepithelial Cl^- transport.

As shown in Fig. 8-3, CFTR contains at least five domains: two membrane-spanning domains (MSDs), each composed of six transmembrane segments; an R domain, which contains several consensus phosphorylation sequences; and two nucleotide-binding domains (NBDs), which interact with ATP. Each of the different domains contributes to the protein's function. The MSDs combine to form the Cl^- channel pore. Several studies have shown that when specific residues in the MSDs are altered by site-directed mutagenesis, movement of ions through the pore is altered in specific ways. The R domain plays an important role in controlling the activity of the channel. The balance of kinase (especially cAMP-dependent protein kinase) and phosphatase activity in the cell determines the state of phosphorylation of the R domain. When the R domain is phosphorylated, the channel can open. Regulation by phosphorylation is complex because the R domain contains several sites that are phosphorylated, and we

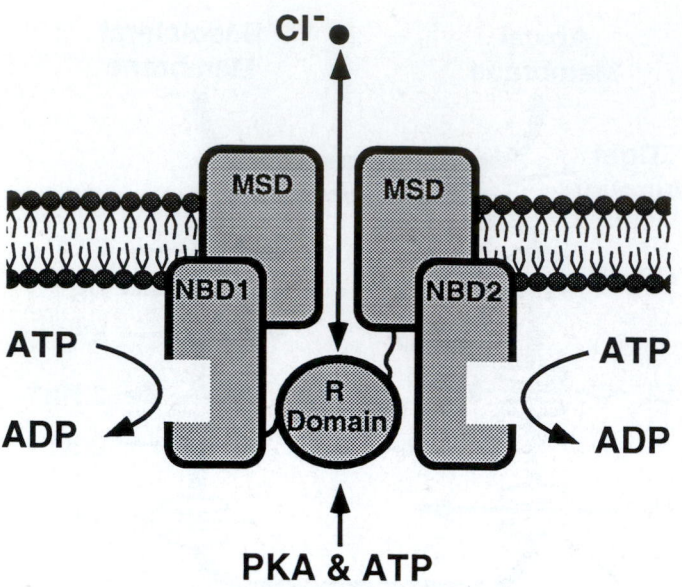

FIGURE 8-3 Model showing the proposed domain structure of CFTR. *MSD* refers to the membrane spanning domains, *NBD* refers to the nucleotide-binding domains, and *PKA* refers to cAMP-dependent protein kinase. The NBDs and R domain are on the cytosolic side of the membrane.

do not yet understand how individual phosphorylation sites interact to determine overall activity. The NBDs also determine channel activity. Current models suggest that hydrolysis of ATP by NBD1 opens the channel and hydrolysis of ATP by NBD2 closes the channel. But how hydrolysis changes the conformation of the molecule to cause it to open and close is not yet known. Much work will be required to understand the complex regulation of this interesting molecule and to understand better how mutations found in patients with cystic fibrosis disrupt its function.

Regulation of Electrolyte Transport

A variety of neurohumoral and pharmacologic agents regulate the rate of transepithelial electrolyte transport by the airway epithelia.[6,34,39] Extracellular signals regulate two main second messengers: cAMP and $[Ca^{2+}]_c$. An increase in levels of cAMP activates cAMP-dependent protein kinase, which phosphorylates and thereby activates CFTR Cl^- channels, basolateral $Na^+/K^+/Cl^-$ cotransporters, and probably some basolateral K^+ channels. An increase in $[Ca^{2+}]_c$ appears to activate a population of apical Cl^- channels and some basolateral K^+ channels. An increase in $[Ca^{2+}]_c$ and diacylglycerol may also activate protein kinase C which can modulate the activity of several transporters. Most agents that regulate transport tend to stimulate transepithelial Cl^- transport; much less is known about how Na^+ transport is regulated. Under some conditions cAMP may stimulate Na^+ absorption, and an increase in $[Ca^{2+}]_c$ may inhibit transport. As in a variety of other Na^+-absorbing epithelia, aldosterone may also regulate Na^+ absorption, although the effect appears to be variable. More work is required to understand better the control of Na^+ transport in airway epithelia.

A number of hormones, neurotransmitters, and autocoids regulate the intracellular levels of cAMP. The epithelia contain re-

ceptors for and respond to β-adrenergic agonists, prostaglandins, adenosine, and vasoactive intestinal peptide. In addition, pharmacologic agents such as methylxanthines increase cellular levels of cAMP. The level of $[Ca^{2+}]_c$ is controlled by bradykinin, substance P, leukotrienes, and nucleotides, such as ATP. Extracellular nucleotides are of particular interest, because they interact with receptors on the apical surface of the epithelium and, by activating Ca^{2+}-activated Cl^- channels, they stimulate transepithelial Cl^- transport through a pathway other than the CFTR Cl^- channel.

Effect of Electrolyte Transport on Fluid Transport and Ion Concentrations

Although much has been learned about the specific molecules involved in electrolyte transport and the function of the epithelium, there is a persistent lack of knowledge about the integrated physiology of the airways. Here we describe some aspects related to the biology of the airways, but we also note deficiencies in current knowledge.

Fluid transport has been studied in cultured human airway epithelial cells.[19,29] As predicted from measurements of electrolyte transport described above, active Na^+ absorption appears to be responsible for fluid absorption under baseline conditions. When the epithelium is treated with amiloride and agonists that increase cellular levels of cAMP, fluid secretion ensues. The measured rate of fluid transport suggests that fluid transport could easily modify the respiratory tract fluid. If it is estimated that the aqueous layer of surface fluid in vivo is approximately 5 μm in depth, one would predict a volume of 500 nl of fluid over each square centimeter of epithelium. Measurements of the rate of fluid transport under basal conditions correspond to the absorption of several times this volume over a 24-h period. In contrast, when epithelia are stimulated to secrete, the rate of fluid secretion is at least ten times this volume in a 24-h period. One major limitation of studies of fluid transport is that of necessity they have been performed with the mucosal surface bathed by a comparatively large volume of fluid. Yet as noted above, the amount of fluid covering the apical surface in vivo is very small. As a result, fluid transport might be influenced by surface forces or by the composition of the airway surface fluid (ion transport might change the composition of the fluid in vivo, but it would not change when a large volume of fluid is on the apical surface and measurements are made over short periods).

Current knowledge of the composition of the respiratory tract fluid and how electrolyte transport affects composition is inadequate. The paucity of knowledge results, in large part, from the small volumes and inaccessibility of the respiratory tract fluid. Sputum has been collected and analyzed, but sputum also contains mucus and may be modified by cellular debris, bacteria, and saliva, especially in subjects with increased respiratory secretions. Studies using bronchoscopy to obtain airway surface fluid from the trachea and main stem bronchi of normal and CF subjects[13,20] have reported that normally the fluid has a low salt concentration, with Cl^- concentrations of 80 to 90 mM. Of note, CF surface fluid had higher Cl^- concentrations in the range of 130 to 170 mM. These observations suggest that Na^+ absorption through ENaC accompanied by Cl^- absorption through CFTR tends to lower the salt concentration in the mucosal solution. More work is needed to learn how fluid composition varies in different airway regions, how it is modified by specific electrolyte transport processes, and how evaporation might change composition.

BIOLOGY OF AIRWAY SUBMUCOSAL GLANDS

Development

Human submucosal gland development is a prenatal event, beginning at 10 to 12 weeks of gestation. From then until about 25 weeks of gestation, glands appear first in the trachea, then outward to the cartilaginous bronchi. Gland formation is completed before birth and involves budding morphogenesis and migration of surface epithelial cells into the submucosa and formation of a progressively more complex system of branching ducts and tubules.[23,30–32] The area and complexity of glands continues to increase postnatally.[18] Recent evidence suggests that more than one surface epithelial cell type serves as a progenitor in the formation of submucosal glands.[10] Whereas gland hyperplasia may occur with disease states such as chronic bronchitis and cystic fibrosis, the total number of glands appears to be established before birth with little change in number postnatally. It is estimated that there are 4000 glands present in the adult human trachea.[32]

Structure and Cell Types

Submucosal glands are complex tubuloacinar structures reflecting the diverse functions of the gland.[17] The cell volume of submucosal glands is approximately forty times greater than that of the secretory (goblet) cells of the surface epithelium.[16] The glands are predominantly located in the submucosal tissue between cartilage plates in trachea and bronchi and are normally absent from the bronchiolar region. In the adult trachea, submucosal glands occur at a frequency of about one per square millimeter.[31] As shown in Fig. 8-4, each gland has four anatomic regions. A narrow ciliated duct is lined by ciliated epithelia in continuity with the surface epithelium. The ciliated duct epithelia are morphologically similar to ciliated cells of the surface epithelium. A wider collecting duct is lined by cells containing numerous mitochondria that stain positive with eosin and by

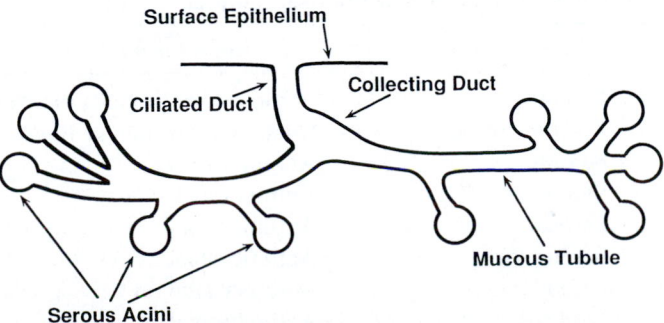

FIGURE 8-4 Model of submucosal gland from human trachea. The anatomic regions shown include ciliated duct, collecting duct, mucous tubules, and serous acini. See text for details.

other poorly characterized cells.[17] Mucous tubules and acini consist of cells rich in acidic glycoconjugates and stain positive with PAS and Alcian blue. Serous tubules and acini are composed of serous cells containing neutral glycoconjugates and are located distal to mucous tubules. Serous cells are also PAS positive but do not stain with Alcian blue. Mucous and serous cells can also be differentiated by specific patterns of staining with several lectins. Multiple branches of mucous and serous tubules occur from each collecting duct, terminating in a variable number of acini. The mucous and serous cells are the main epithelial components of the submucosal gland. In addition to these cells, contractile myoepithelial cells surround the acini and secretory tubules of glands and may be important in the short-term responses of glands, causing the ejection of secreted mucus and fluid from ducts and tubules.[26]

Submucosal Gland Physiology

The functions of submucosal glands appear to be twofold: (1) the secretion of fluid and electrolytes, which contributes to the periciliary fluid layer and hydration of mucus and (2) the secretion of macromolecules, including mucins and proteins that contribute to host defenses in the airways. The viscous secretions of mucous cells are rich in high-molecular-weight glycoconjugates. In contrast, the secretions of serous cells are less viscous. The thinner secretions of the distally oriented serous cells probably serve to hydrate and mobilize the thicker secretory products of mucous cells.[12] Submucosal glands are richly innervated by postganglionic fibers from both the sympathetic and parasympathetic nervous systems. These fibers release norepinephrine and acetylcholine and produce neuropeptides such as substance P, calcitonin gene-related peptide (CGRP), and vasoactive intestinal peptide (VIP).[2]

Electrolyte Transport in Submucosal Glands

The cellular mechanisms of ion transport in human submucosal glands is under investigation, and some data come from animal studies. Similar to the surface epithelium, the movement of water across submucosal gland epithelia is osmotically coupled to the net direction of active electrolyte transport. Both secretory and absorptive pathways for electrolyte movement are distributed in a polarized fashion in gland epithelia (see Fig. 8-2 above). Serous cells express CFTR at the apical membrane, and the level of expression is greater than the surface epithelium.[11,12] Submucosal glands also express ENaC in both ductal and acinar epithelia.[8] The Isc of mixed seromucous cell cultures is inhibited by ouabain on the basolateral membrane, indicating the presence of Na^+/K^+-ATPase.[41] Thus the pathways for ion movement across gland epithelia bear great similarity to those of the surface cells.

Recent advances in the isolation and culture of human serous and mucous cells from submucosal glands have brought new insights into submucosal gland physiology.[12,41] The serous cells of the submucosal gland contribute greatly to the secretion of electrolytes and airway surface fluid. Unlike the surface epithelia, which exhibit absorptive transport properties in the resting state, the serous cells are predominantly Cl^- secretory.[27,41] Serous gland epithelia exhibit cAMP-activated Cl^- secretion consistent with CFTR function.[4,12,41] The Cl^- secretory capacity and CFTR protein expression of serous cells is greater than the mucous cells, and thus the serous cell is probably the predominant source of fluid secreted by submucosal glands.[12,37] Cl^- secretion is induced by agents that increase $[Ca^{2+}]_c$, indicating that, like the surface epithelium, submucosal glands express Ca^{2+}-activated Cl^- channels.[27,41] When applied to the apical membrane of isolated human submucosal glands cell preparations amiloride inhibits the Isc, suggesting that in addition to secreting Cl^-, the cells of the gland can modify the volume and composition of secretions by absorbing Na^+.[41]

Electrolyte transport across submucosal gland epithelia is regulated by several secretagogues including cholinergic agonists, adrenergic agents, bradykinin, and neuropeptides. In contrast to the surface epithelium, cholinergic pathways and agents that increase intracellular Ca^{2+}, rather than β-adrenergic pathways, are the major stimuli for Cl^- secretion in gland epithelia. This information comes from several sources including receptor autoradiography, receptor binding assays and in vitro physiology studies.[27] A list of neurohumoral agents regulating Cl^- secretion in submucosal glands is listed in Table 8-1.

Secretion of Macromolecules and Proteins

In addition to the transport of fluid and electrolytes, submucosal glands are the major source of airway mucins and secrete several protein products listed in Table 8-2. Histochemical stains demonstrate that both the serous and mucous cells of the glands produce glycoproteins. Mucous cells contain predominantly acidic glycoconjugates, identified as large, electron neutral granules, whereas serous cells contain neutral, more heavily sulphated glycoconjugates in smaller, electron-dense granules. Although both mucous and serous cells express mRNAs for mucin genes, mucin production is restricted to the mucous cells.[9,15] The control of secretion by mucous cells is complex. Cholinergic stimuli cause degranulation of both mucous and serous cells.[3,27,41] Neuropeptides including substance P and VIP also regulate the secretion of macromolecules. In addition to cholinergic, adrenergic, and neuropeptide mediated secretion, several neural reflexes are associated with mucus secretion. These include cough due to irritation of the airways, hypoxia, and gastric distention.[2] Inflammatory mediators such as those associated with infections or allergic reactions can stimulate mucus secretion. These include histamine from mast cells, prostaglandins A_2, D_2 and $F_{2\alpha}$, and leukotrienes C_4 and D_4.

Macromolecular Products of Submucosal Glands

Submucosal glands play an important part in lung host defenses by contributing to mucociliary function and secreting products with antimicrobial activity. The fluid and electrolyte secretions produced predominantly by

TABLE 8-1

Neurohumoral Regulation of Submucosal Gland Cl^- Secretion

| | Target Cell Type | | |
Agent	Mucous	Serous	Reference
Methacholine	–	++	41,12
Histamine	–	+	41, 12
α adrenergic	+	+	41, 12
β adrenergic	+	++	12
Bradykinin	+	++	41, 12
Substance P	+	+	27

NOTE: Neurohumoral agents that have been shown to regulate Cl^- secretion in mucous and serous gland epithelia are listed with the associated references. A negative sign (–) indicates no demonstrated effect, and a plus sign (+) indicates stimulation of Cl^- secretion.

the serous cells of glands are in part responsible for the maintenance of the periciliary fluid layer on airway surface cells. These secretions also hydrate mucins secreted by mucous cells and thus are important for the production of the gel layer. Thus, submucosal gland products are key components of the mucociliary clearance system in the airways and support this first line of defense for handling inhaled infectious and noninfectious particulate matter.

The serous cells of glands elaborate a number of products which constitute additional host defense mechanisms in the airways. These factors act in a broad-spectrum fashion, in some cases exerting antimicrobial effects against bacteria, fungi, and viruses. The cationic, bacteriolytic protein lysozyme is a specific product of the serous cell and is found in measurable quantities in airway secretions.[9] Lactoferrin is found in airway secretions and is distributed in submucosal glands in a pattern similar to lysozyme. It is a cationic, iron-binding protein which may act by inhibiting growth of iron-requiring bacteria. The serous cells also produce the secretory component of IgA which is required for the translocation of IgA from the basolateral to apical membrane where it is released. A low-molecular-weight cationic proteinase inhibitor termed *antileukoprotease* or *secretory leukocyte proteinase inhibitor* (SLPI) is also produced by serous cells and

TABLE 8-2

Macromolecular Products of Submucosal Glands

Product	Cell of Origin	Proposed Function
Mucins	Mucous	Component of mucus blanket
Glycoconjugates	Mucous, serous	Component of mucus blanket
Lysozyme	Serous	Antimicrobial
Lactoferrin	Serous	Antimicrobial
Secretory component	Serous	Antimicrobial
Antileukoproteinase	Serous	Antimicrobial
Peroxidase	Serous	Antimicrobial
Proline-rich proteins	Serous	Antimicrobial

NOTE: The macromolecular products of submusal glands, the cell of origin (mucous, serous or both) and proposed function are listed. Note that glycoconjugates are a product of both cell types. Many of the products exhibit antimicrobial properties. See text for details.

comprises most of the antineutrophil proteinase activity produced in the airways. Additional products of serous cells with antimicrobial properties include peroxidase and proline-rich proteins. It is unknown whether any defensin-like molecules are secreted by human submucosal gland cells. It is likely that these multiple components of the nonspecific mucosal immune system act synergistically to prevent infection of the lung from a variety of inhaled or aspirated pathogens.

INTEGRATED PHYSIOLOGY AND HOST DEFENSE FUNCTIONS

Although much has been learned about the specific molecules involved in electrolyte transport and the function of the epithelium on the airway surface and submucosal glands, there is a continuing lack of knowledge about the integrated physiology of the airways. An important function of the airway epithelium is in local host defense, protecting the lung from inhaled microorganisms, particulate material, and toxins. Here we describe some aspects of the integrated physiology of the airways, but we also note deficiencies in current knowledge.

Mucociliary Clearance

An important function of airway secretions is in mucociliary clearance. Mucociliary clearance is a pulmonary defense mechanism that serves to remove inhaled particulate material from the lung. Effective clearance requires both ciliary activity and respiratory tract fluid. Cilia cover much of the airway surface, and their coordinated beating provides the mechanical force that propels particulate material toward the larynx. The cilia are immersed in a periciliary fluid layer, or sol phase of the fluid, that is about 5 μm thick. The periciliary fluid is covered by a mucous or gel layer, 5 to 10 μm thick, that exists as a discontinuous blanket, i.e., as islands of mucus. The viscoelastic mucus traps and carries inhaled material, whereas the watery periciliary fluid allows the cilia to move freely, with only the tops of the cilia contacting the overlying mucus and propelling it toward the mouth. The quantity and composition of the periciliary fluid, and perhaps hydration of the mucus, are controlled by the electrolyte transport properties of the cells of the surface and submucosal gland epithelia. The quantity and composition of macromolecules in the mucus are controlled by secretory cells in the surface epithelium and submucosal glands.

Antibacterial Activity at the Airway Surface

Recent work has shown that bacteria were killed when they were applied to the apical surface of normal human airway epithelia grown on permeable supports at the air-liquid interface.[28] The antibacterial activity was contained in the airway surface fluid because fluid removed from the epithelium killed bacteria in vitro and, after the apical surface was washed, the epithelium was no longer able to kill applied bacteria. It was discovered that bactericidal activity required low salt concentrations. Bactericidal activity in the airway surface fluid may be a first line of defense that protects the lung. Bacteria deposited on the airway surface after inhalation and aspiration may be killed by bactericidal ac-

tivity in airway surface fluid. This process could explain, in part, the ability of the airways to maintain a sterile intrapulmonary environment. Future studies will be required to reproduce these results and to identify the bactericidal factor (which may be a defensin-like molecule). Submucosal gland secretory products such as lysozyme, lactoferrin, and antileukoproteinase also exhibit antimicrobial activity and probably contribute to this important pulmonary defense mechanism.

In addition to mucociliary clearance and antibacterial activity in the airway surface fluid and products of submucosal glands, a second line of defense involves the recruitment of phagocytic cells such as neutrophils and macrophages to the airway surface. By releasing a variety of cytokines and inflammatory molecules, the epithelium mediates the inflammatory response to inhaled bacteria and other pathogens.[22]

Insights into Airway Biology from Disease States

Clues about the integrated function and biology of the airways have come from study of several disease states and the development of animal models in which specific genes have been disrupted. We discuss these only briefly here; they are discussed in greater depth in subsequent chapters.

In immotile cilia syndrome (ciliary dyskinesia), ciliary activity is disrupted. As a result, mucociliary activity is impaired. Patients often develop chronic infections of the middle ear, sinuses, and airways, which may advance to bronchiectasis. This observation underscores the important role of mucociliary clearance as a defense mechanism in humans.

In cystic fibrosis the gene encoding CFTR is mutated.[36] The resulting loss of CFTR Cl^- channels leads to chronic respiratory tract infections. This supports a central role for electrolyte transport in the normal biology and host defense of the airways. The mechanism by which loss of CFTR predisposes to infection is just beginning to be understood. It has been speculated that abnormal amounts or composition of the respiratory tract fluid might make mucociliary clearance less efficient. Disruption of CFTR function in submucosal gland epithelia may also contribute the pathogenesis of CF. Recent data suggest that the loss of CFTR Cl^- channels may impair the ability of the epithelium to absorb salt, much as occurs in the CF sweat gland duct. As a result, high salt concentrations in CF airway surface fluid would prevent bacterial killing by antibacterial factors produced by the epithelium.[28] Loss of this local host defense mechanism might then lead to airway infections. Alterations in the composition of airway surface fluid may also affect the normal hydration of mucus.

Diseases that alter Na^+ absorption can also provide clues about the role of this process in airway biology. In Liddle's syndrome,[5] gain-of-function mutations in the ENaC Na^+ channel increase the rate of amiloride-sensitive Na^+ absorption. In contrast, in pseudohypoaldosteronism, loss-of-function mutations in the ENaC Na^+ channel decrease the rate of Na^+ absorption. Patients with Liddle's syndrome are not reported to have evidence of airway disease, whereas patients with pseudohypoaldosteronism develop airway disease that shows some similarity to CF.[14] If, as expected, the gain or loss of ENaC function in the airways is similar to what has been reported in the kidney of patients with these diseases, then these observations would suggest that a reduced capacity for salt absorption would impair airway host defense mechanisms much as was suggested for the loss of CFTR Cl^- channels in CF.

The genes for the CFTR Cl^- channel and the ENaC Na^+ channel have also been disrupted in mice. Unfortunately these models have not faithfully reproduced the human disease. Mice lacking CFTR do not develop chronic airway disease; it has been speculated that this may be because mice have quantitatively more Ca^{2+}-activated Cl^- current in the airways than humans. Mice lacking the α subunit of the ENaC Na^+ channel die of respiratory distress because of a failure to clear fluid from the lungs after birth. While this establishes the important role of electrolyte transport in airway function, it did not produce an animal with disease that accurately mimics human disease. Future interventions may be of greater value, and a comparison of disease in mice and humans may yield additional clues as to the biology of the airways.

The appreciation that abnormalities in airway and submucosal gland function play central roles in the pathogenesis and pathophysiology of some inherited and acquired diseases has increased interest and focused research in this area. Future studies in this field should continue to increase our understanding of how airway surface fluid and its secretory products contribute to lung health and are altered in disease states.

REFERENCES

1. Anderson MP, Sheppard DN, Berger HA, Welsh MJ: Chloride channels in the apical membrane of normal and cystic fibrosis airway and intestinal epithelia. *Am J Physiol* 263:L1–L14, 1992.

2. Basbaum CB, Finkbeiner WE: Mucus-producing cells of the airways, in Massaro D (ed), *Lung Cell Biology.* New York, Dekker, 1989, pp 37–79.

3. Basbaum CB, Ueki I, Brezina L, Nadel JA: Tracheal submucosal gland serous cells stimulated in vitro with adrenergic and cholinergic agonists. A morphometric study. *Cell Tissue Res* 220:481–498, 1981.

4. Becq F, Merten MD, Voelckel MA, et al: Characterization of cAMP dependent CFTR-chloride channels in human tracheal gland cells. *FEBS Lett* 321:73–78, 1993.

5. Botero-Velez M, Curtis JJ, Warnock DG: Liddle's syndrome revisited—a disorder of sodium reabsorption in the distal tubule. *New Engl J Med* 330:178–181, 1994.

6. Boucher RC: Human airway ion transport. *Am J Respir Crit Care Med* 150:271–281, 1994.

7. Breeze RG, Wheeldon RB: The cells of the pulmonary airways. *Am Rev Respir Dis* 116:705–777, 1977.

8. Burch LH, Talbot CR, Knowles MR, et al: Relative expression of the human epithelial Na^+ channel subunits in normal and cystic fibrosis airways. *Am J Physiol* 269:C511–C518, 1995.

9. Dohrman A, Tsuda T, Escudier E, et al: Distribution of lysozyme and mucin (MUC2 and MUC3) mRNA in human bronchus. *Exp Lung Res* 20:367–380, 1994.

10. Engelhardt JF, Schlossberg H, Yankaskas JR, Dudus L: Progenitor cells of the adult human airway involved in submucosal gland development. *Development* 121:2031–2046, 1995.

11. Engelhardt JF, Yankaskas JR, Ernst SA, et al: Submucosal glands are the predominant site of CFTR expression in the human bronchus. *Nat Genet* 2:240–248, 1992.

12. Finkbeiner WE, Shen BQ, Widdicombe JH: Chloride secretion and function of serous and mucous cells of human airway glands. *Am J Physiol* 267:L206–L210, 1994.

13. Gilljam H, Ellin A, Strandvik B: Increased bronchial chloride concentration in cystic fibrosis. *Scand J Clin Lab Invest* 49:121–124, 1989.

14. Hanukoglu A, Bistritzer T, Rakover V, Mandelber A: Pseudohypoaldosteronism with increased sweat and saliva electrolyte values and frequent lower respiratory tract infections mimicking cystic fibrosis. *J Pediatr* 125:752–755, 1994.

15. Jany BH, Gallup MW, Yan P, et al: Human bronchus and intestine express the same mucin gene. *J Clin Invest* 87:77–82, 1991.

16. Jeffery, PK: Structure and function of adult tracheobronchial epithelium, in McDowell EM (ed), *Lung Carcinomas.* New York, Churchill Livingstone, 1987, pp 42–73.

17. Jeffery, PK: Microscopic structure of airway secretory cells: variation in hypersecretory disease and effects of drugs, in Takishima T, Shimura S (eds), *Airway Secretion—Physiological Bases for the Control of Mucous Hypersecretion.* New York, Dekker, 1994, pp 149–215.

18. Jeffery PK, Gaillard D, Moret S: Human airway secretory cells during development and in mature airway epithelium. *Eur Respir J* 5:93–104, 1992.

19. Jiang C, Finkbeiner WE, Widdicombe JH, et al: Altered fluid transport across airway epithelium in cystic fibrosis. *Science* 262:424–427, 1993.

20. Joris L, Dab I, Quinton PM: Elemental composition of human airway surface fluid in healthy and diseased airways. *Am Rev Respir Dis* 148:1633–1637, 1993.

21. Knowles M, Gatzy J, Boucher R: Increased bioelectric potential difference across respiratory epithelia in cystic fibrosis. *New Engl J Med* 305:1489–1495, 1981.

22. Konstan MW, Berger M: Infection and inflammation of the lung in cystic fibrosis, in Davis PB (ed), *Cystic Fibrosis.* New York, Dekker, 1993, pp 219–276.

23. Plopper CG, Weir AJ, Nishio SJ, et al: Tracheal submucosal gland development in the rhesus monkey, *Macaca mulatta:* ultrastructure and histochemistry. *Anat Embryol* 174:167–178, 1986.

24. Riordan JR: The cystic fibrosis transmembrane conductance regulator. *Annu Rev Physiol* 55:609–630, 1993.

25. Riordan JR, Alon N, Grzelczak Z, et al: The CF gene product as a member of a membrane transporter (TM6-NBF) super family. *Adv Exp Med Biol* 290:19–29, 1991.

26. Shimura S, Sasaki T, Sasaki H, Takishima T: Contractility of isolated single submucosal gland from trachea. *J Appl Physiol* 60:1237–1247, 1986.

27. Shimura S, Takishima T: Airway submucosal gland secretion, in Takishima T, Shimura S (eds), *Airway Secretion—Physiological Bases for the Control of Mucous Hypersecretion.* New York, Dekker, 1994, pp 325–398.

28. Smith JJ, Travis SM, Greenberg EP, Welsh MJ: Cystic fibrosis airway epithelia fail to kill bacteria because of abnormal airway surface fluid. *Cell* 85:229–236, 1996.

29. Smith JJ, Welsh MJ: Fluid and electrolyte transport by cultured human airway epithelia. *J Clin Invest* 91:1590–1597, 1993.

30. Thurlbeck WM, Benjamin B, Reid L: Development and distribution of mucous glands in the foetal human trachea. *Br J Dis Chest* 55:54–64, 1961.

31. Tos M: Development of the tracheal glands in man. *Acta Pathol Microbiol Scand* 68(supp. 185):3–128, 1966.

32. Tos M: Development of the mucous glands in the human main bronchus. *Anat Anz Bd* 123:S.376–S.389, 1968.

33. Warnock DG, Bubien JK: Liddle syndrome: clinical and cellular abnormalities. *Hosp Pract* 29:65–75, 1994.

34. Welsh MJ: Electrolyte transport by airway epithelia. *Physiol Rev* 67:1143–1184, 1987.

35. Welsh MJ, Anderson MP, Rich DP, et al: The CFTR chloride channel, in Guggino WB (ed), *The Current Topics in Membranes and Transport: Chloride Channels from Plants to Human Disease.* San Diego, Academic Press, 1994, pp 155–171.

36. Welsh MJ, Tsui L-C, Boat TF, Beaudet AL: Cystic fibrosis, in Scriver CR, Beaudet AL, Sly WS, Valle D (eds), *The Metabolic and Molecular Basis of Inherited Disease.* New York, McGraw-Hill, 1995, pp 3799–3876.

37. Widdicombe JH, Miller SS, Finkbeiner WE: Altered regulation of airway fluid content in cystic fibrosis, in Dodge JA, Brock DJH, Widdicombe JH: *Cystic Fibrosis: Current Topics,* Chichester, John Wiley & Sons, 1994, pp 109–129.

38. Widdicombe JH: Use of cultured airway epithelial cells in studies of ion transport. *Am J Physiol* 258:L13–L18, 1990.

39. Widdicombe JH: Ion and fluid transport by airway epithelium, in Takishima T, Shimura S (eds), *Airway Secretion: Physiological Bases for the Control of Mucous Hypersecretion.* New York, Dekker, 1994, pp 399–431.

40. Wine JJ, Brayden DJ, Hagiwara G, et al: Cystic fibrosis, the CFTR, and rectifying Cl⁻ channels, in Tsui L-C (ed), *The Identification of the CF Gene.* New York, Plenum Press, 1991, pp 253–272.

41. Yamaya M, Finkbeiner WE, Widdicombe JH: Altered ion transport by tracheal glands in cystic fibrosis. *Am J Physiol* 261:L491–L494, 1991.

CHAPTER 9

NONRESPIRATORY FUNCTIONS OF THE LUNGS

Una S. Ryan / Savvas C. Makrides

BIOLOGICALLY ACTIVE MOLECULES
  Vasoactive Polypeptides
  Vasoactive Amines
  Neuropeptides
  Hormones
  Lipoprotein Complexes
  Eicosanoids

HEMOSTATIC FUNCTIONS

LUNG DEFENSE
  Complement Activation
  Leukocyte Recruitment
  Cytokines and Growth Factors

CONCLUSION

The lungs constitute a major site of synthesis, activation, and inactivation of a host of vasoactive substances.[40–43] The extensive surface of the pulmonary vascular bed (Fig. 9-1) plays an essential role in regulating circulating levels of biologically active substances. The concentration of many bioactive molecules in the systemic circulation is determined in large part by their metabolic fate in the lungs, since it is there that the entire cardiac output is processed and its composition modified.[41,42] Pulmonary endothelial cells (Fig. 9-2) influence such important functions as blood pressure, hemostasis, and inflammatory and immunologic reactions. In addition to its diverse constitutive functions, the pulmonary endothelium is capable of responding to stimuli to express a broad spectrum of inducible functions.[42] These inducible functions can alter the properties of the endothelial layer and contribute to pulmonary disease. The wide range of chemical compounds processed by the lungs belies the specificity with which the lungs metabolize biologically active substances. This selectivity is in part achieved by the structural organization of the lung.[41,42]

Specific aspects of the nonventilatory functions of lungs have been covered in several excellent reviews, and the reader is referred to these for greater detail. Topics previously covered include host defense,[46,48] leukocyte traffic,[18] the metabolism of arachidonic acid,[19] and neuropeptides.[3,4] The uptake of environmental particulates and the biologic effects of nitric oxide on the lungs are beyond the scope of this chapter. Fishman[14] has provided a comprehensive review of nonrespiratory functions, as have others.[40–43] Our goal here is not to provide an exhaustive coverage of the published literature but, rather, to review recent progress in understanding of the processing of biologic substances by the lungs, as well as the effects of specific compounds and their metabolites on lung function.

BIOLOGICALLY ACTIVE MOLECULES

Vasoactive Polypeptides

The pulmonary vascular bed exhibits high selectivity in its processing of biologically active materials (Fig. 9-3). Although the lungs contain all the enzymes necessary to inactivate many bioactive peptides, the complex anatomic structure of the lungs effectively sequesters specific enzymes (Fig. 9-4) and their potential substrates.[41] Thus, early in vitro studies utilizing lung homogenates do not accurately reflect the metabolic processing of peptides in vivo.

Bradykinin (BK), so called for its slow onset of biologic activity, as contrasted to the faster-acting tachykinins, is a member of the kinin family of regulatory peptides, exerting numerous biologic effects in different tissues and organs. It causes vasodilatation and enhances vascular permeability, lowers systemic blood pressure, stimulates phospholipase A_2 to release prosta-

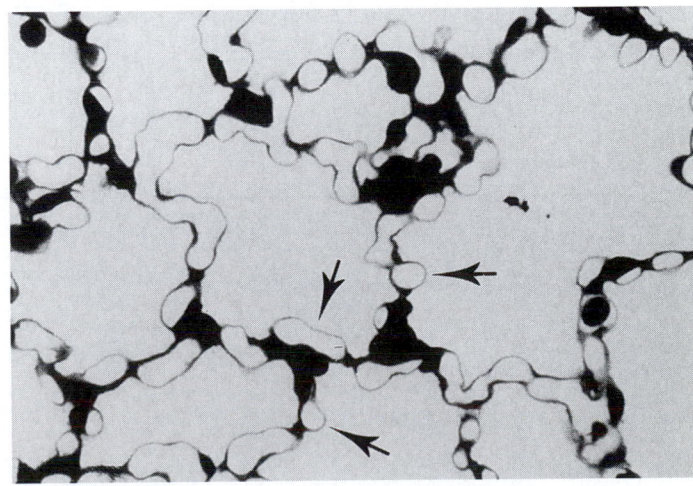

FIGURE 9-1 Light micrograph of a rat pulmonary capillary bed. The alveolar capillary unit (arrows) is extremely thin, representing a vast surface area for interaction with blood-borne and airborne molecules (×350). (*Based on data of Ryan,[42] with permission.*)

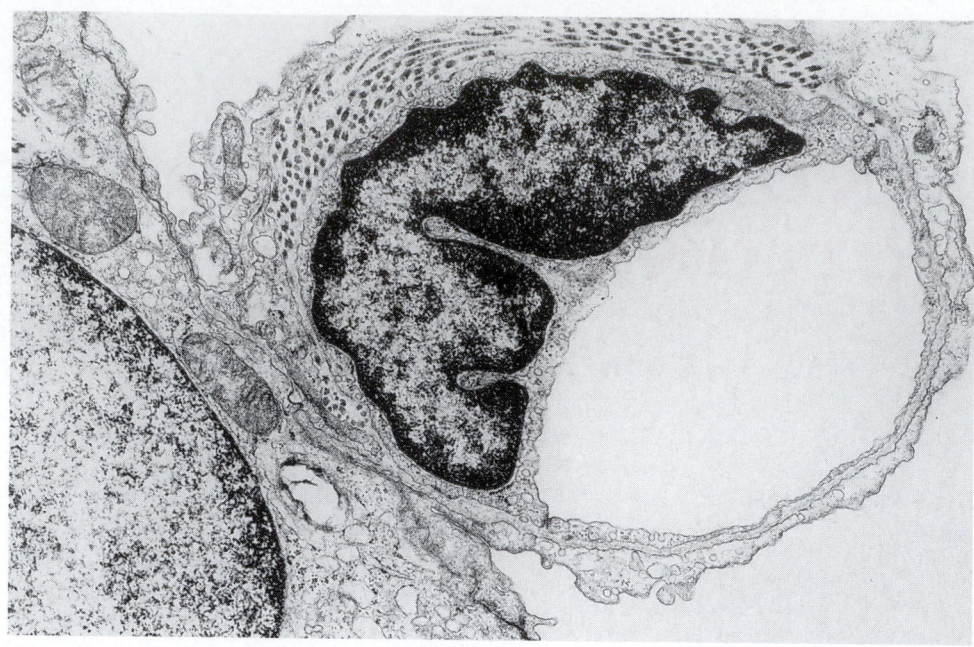

FIGURE 9-2 Pulmonary capillary loop from a rat lung showing the endothelial nucleus and narrow cytoplasmic extensions of the endothelial cell ($\times 21{,}000$). *(Based on data of Ryan,[40] with permission.)*

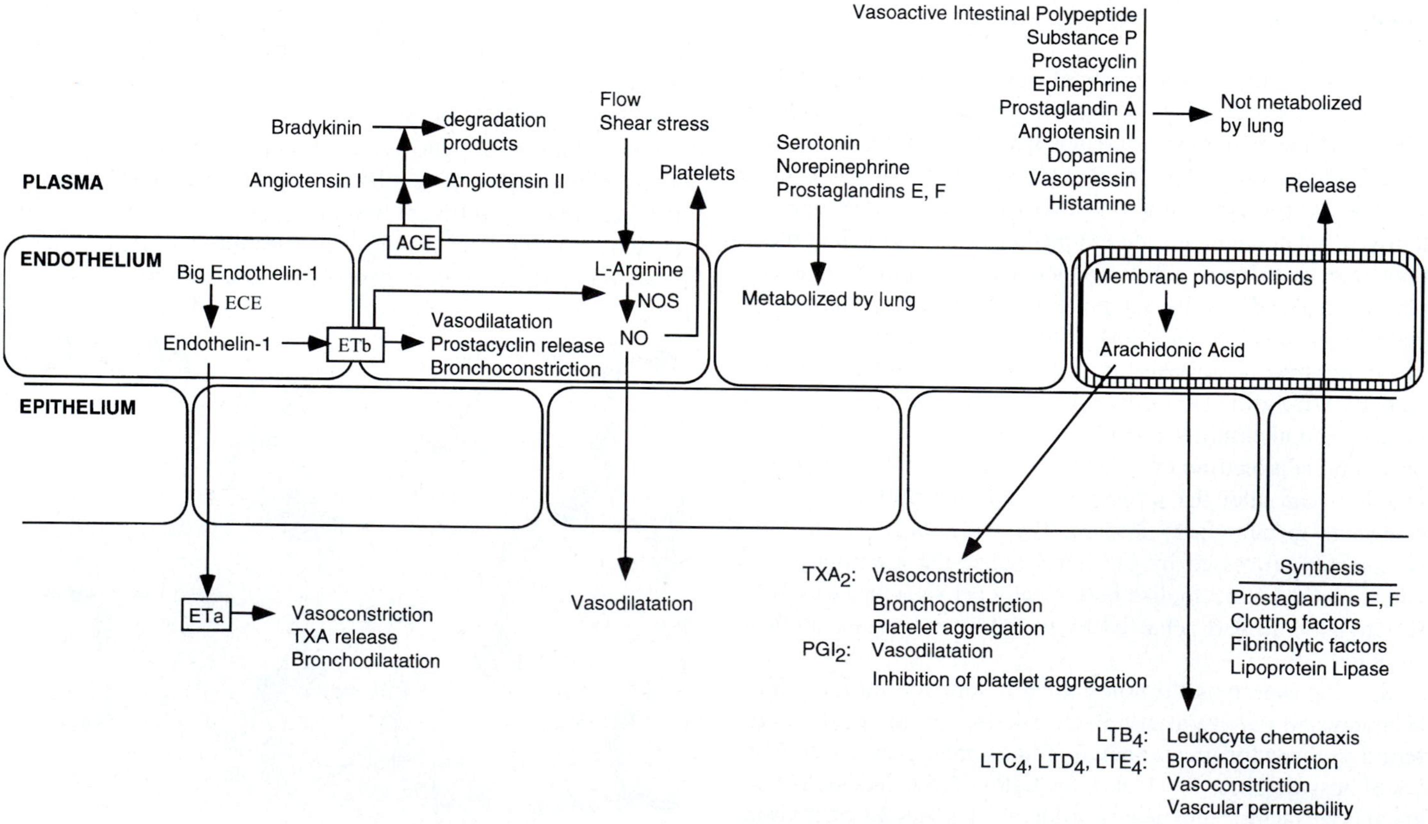

PLASMA

Vasoactive Intestinal Polypeptide
Substance P
Prostacyclin
Epinephrine
Prostaglandin A
Angiotensin II
Dopamine
Vasopressin
Histamine → Not metabolized by lung

Bradykinin → degradation products

Angiotensin I → Angiotensin II

Flow
Shear stress

Platelets

Serotonin
Norepinephrine
Prostaglandins E, F

Release

ACE

ENDOTHELIUM

Big Endothelin-1
↓ ECE
Endothelin-1 → ETb

L-Arginine
↓ NOS
NO

Metabolized by lung

Membrane phospholipids

Vasodilatation
Prostacyclin release
Bronchoconstriction

Arachidonic Acid

EPITHELIUM

ETa → Vasoconstriction
TXA release
Bronchodilatation

Vasodilatation

TXA$_2$: Vasoconstriction
           Bronchoconstriction
           Platelet aggregation
PGI$_2$: Vasodilatation
           Inhibition of platelet aggregation

Synthesis

Prostaglandins E, F
Clotting factors
Fibrinolytic factors
Lipoprotein Lipase

LTB$_4$: Leukocyte chemotaxis
LTC$_4$, LTD$_4$, LTE$_4$: Bronchoconstriction
           Vasoconstriction
           Vascular permeability

FIGURE 9-3 Schematic presentation of the processing of biologically active substances in the lung and diverse interactions with pulmonary endothelial and epithelial cells. ACE = angiotensin-converting enzyme; ECE = endothelin-converting enzyme; LT = leukotriene; NO = nitric oxide; NOS = nitric oxide synthase; PGI$_2$ = prostacyclin; TXA = thromboxane.

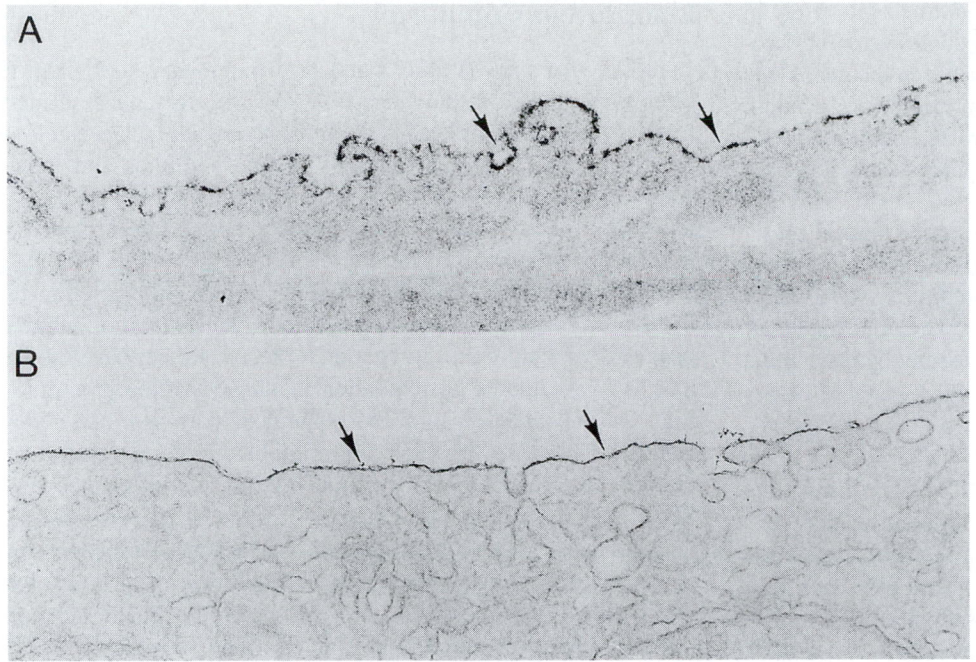

FIGURE 9-4   Immunocytochemical localization of sites of angiotensin-converting enzyme activity on the luminal plasma membrane, including caveolae, of an endothelial cell in a rat lung (*A*), and on a pulmonary endothelial cell in culture (*B*) (×75,000). *(Based on data of Ryan et al,[43] with permission.)*

three distinct endothelin receptors, designated ET_A, ET_B, and ET_C. Both ET_A and ET_B receptors exist in the lung. Stimulation of ET_A receptors effects vasoconstriction, release of thromboxane, and bronchodilatation, whereas stimulation of ET_B receptors results in vasodilatation, release of prostacyclin, and bronchoconstriction. ET-1 may play a role in the pathogenesis of asthma, and the proinflammatory action of ET-1 by activation mainly of the ET_A receptor might be a target for therapeutic intervention.

Li and colleagues[26] reported that chronic hypoxia in rats results in concomitant increases in mRNA levels for ET-1 and the ET_A and ET_B receptors in lung homogenates, but not in other organs. These findings are believed to support the hypothesis that increased synthesis of ET-1 in the lung participates in pulmonary vascular remodeling and the maintenance of chronic hypoxic pulmonary hypertension.[26] The source of the increased ET-1 production in the lung is currently unknown. Recently it was shown that ET-1 is produced in rat alveolar epithelial cells, where it binds to ET_A receptors concomitant with the accumulation of prostaglandin E_2 (PGE_2) and adenosine 3′,5′-cyclic monophosphate (cAMP).[29]

Adrenomedullin (ADM) is a recently discovered hypotensive peptide isolated from pheochromocytoma tissue of human adrenal medulla and subsequently cloned. The lung contains the largest amount of ADM, and the ADM gene is regulated by glucocorticoid and possibly by thyroid hormone.[21] The intact human ADM (amino acid residues 1-52) has marked vasodilator activity in the isolated perfused rat lung by a mechanism that is poorly understood. Only a fragment (residues 13-52) of the intact human ADM peptide appears to be necessary to dilate the vascular pulmonary bed, although the physiologically active form of ADM in vivo is unknown. Much remains to be learned about this novel peptide, which appears to control vascular tone as an autocrine/paracrine factor.

Heat shock proteins, also referred to as molecular chaperones, are up-regulated under conditions of stress, presumably to protect the cell from injury. The exposure of rats to hyperthermia resulted in the accumulation of calreticulin mRNA and protein in the lungs.[12] Hyperthermia and heat shock proteins have also been demonstrated to be protective in sepsis-induced lung injury in rats. It is possible that heat shock proteins have a protective function in the lungs during fever or other stresses.[12]

Vasoactive Amines

Serotonin (5-hydroxytryptamine, or 5-HT) inhibits or stimulates a variety of smooth muscles and nerves. In the respiratory sys-

glandins and leukotrienes, causes smooth-muscle contraction in the respiratory and gastrointestinal tracts and the uterus, and mediates immune cell stimulation and activation of sensory and sympathetic neurons.[5] Recent progress in the pharmacology and molecular biology of BK receptors, including the development of improved receptor antagonists, and the cloning of BK receptors provide powerful new tools for the study of BK metabolism.

BK is synthesized by the action of plasma and tissue kallikreins on kininogen precursors, and is cleaved by the membrane-bound kininase II (also known as angiotensin I–converting enzyme or dipeptidyl carboxypeptidase) localized on pulmonary endothelial cells[43] and other proteases in the lungs.[5] The quantitative removal of a hypotensive substance, BK, together with the conversion of angiotensin I to angiotensin II, established a role for the lungs in the control of blood pressure and provided the first evidence of metabolic or nonrespiratory functions of the lungs.[41,42] BK exerts its effects through at least two types of receptors, B_1 and B_2. The existence of additional kinin receptors—for example, B_3, B_4, and B_5—has been proposed; these studies, however, have been critically reviewed[39] and await confirmation. BK is thought to mediate most of its physiological activity through the B_2 receptor, whereas B_1 receptors may be involved in inflammation and other pathophysiological conditions.[5]

Endothelins are produced by a wide variety of cells and organs in the body; they are especially abundant in the lungs, where they act as vasoconstrictors and regulators of pulmonary vascular tone and permeability. The biologic properties of endothelins and their receptors have been reviewed.[31] Endothelin has been shown to be a member of a family of isopeptides—referred to as ET-1, ET-2, and ET-3—which bind with different affinity to

tem it causes bronchoconstriction in many animals but rarely in humans, except in asthmatic patients. The contribution of serotonin to allergic bronchoconstriction may be mediated by the direct activation of serotoninergic receptors present on smooth muscle as well as through indirect mechanisms, such as modulation of neurotransmission, increase in microvascular leakage, or other means.[51]

Histamine, a constrictor of bronchial smooth muscle and a vasodilator, is released from airway mast cells in response to stimulation by tachykinins by a mechanism that is mediated by activation of neurokinin-1 and -2 receptors.[27] Under normal conditions, the pulmonary vasculature does not metabolize histamine in vivo, although disrupted lung tissue is fully capable of degrading histamine. Recent work has shown that human pulmonary artery endothelial cells can express the enzymatic components necessary for histamine degradation, underlining the ability of the lungs to regulate histamine degradation in a cell- and tissue-specific manner.[2] Thus, injuries that elicit systemic inflammatory responses have the capacity to modify the clearance properties of the lung and augment the pulmonary uptake and degradation of histamine. This complex series of reactions underscores the ability of the lung to up-regulate a protective mechanism in dealing with inflammatory events at distant loci.

Neuropeptides

The respiratory tract contains a large number of neuropeptides that are localized in neurons, epithelium, and inflammatory cells, such as mast cells, eosinophils, and neutrophils. These chemical messengers play important roles in lung physiology and disease, and their diverse functions include neurotransmission, modulation of vascular permeability and airway tone, mucus secretion, chemotactic responses, and modulation of the functions of T and B cells of the immune system (Table 9-1). Neuropeptides reach their target cells by a variety of mechanisms, including transport in the general circulation, release from nerve endings to act locally, and secretion as paracrine and autocrine substances. The pathophysiology and metabolism of neuropeptides in the respiratory tract have been examined in detail, and the reader is referred to these reviews.[3,4]

Hormones

Using immunohistochemical techniques, Hastings and coworkers[16] showed that parathyroid hormone–related protein (PTHrP) is expressed in the adult rat lung and in cultured rat alveolar type II epithelial cells. The secretion of PTHrP by cultured cells is regulated by a protein kinase C–dependent pathway. The function of PTHrP in the adult lung is unknown, although it is speculated that it may have to do with control of cell growth and differentiation or control of surfactant lipid secretion.[16]

Glucocorticoids are active in the transcriptional regulation of the gene encoding the β_2-adrenergic receptor in human lung. This effect is mediated by glucocorticoid response elements located in the promoter region of the β_2-receptor gene. Glucocorticoids also prevent down-regulation of β_2-receptor number without affecting β_1-receptor levels.[28] This selective effect may be clinically important in preventing tolerance to β_2-agonists in asthmatic patients treated with β-agonist bronchodilators.[28]

Lipoprotein Complexes

Lung alveolar type II cells synthesize pulmonary surfactant, a lipoprotein complex that functions primarily to reduce surface tension at the alveolar lining and prevent alveolar collapse at low lung volumes. Surfactant consists of phospholipids and lung-specific proteins, which are known as surfactant-associated proteins SP-A, -B, -C, and -D. SP-A is the major surfactant-specific protein, with many nonrespiratory functions related to lung metabolism and host defense, including receptor binding, facilitated uptake of phospholipid by type II cells, enhancement of antigen phagocytosis, and lipid aggregation.[46] Recent studies have shown that SP-A facilitates up-regulation of phagocyte receptor function. During infection with the respiratory pathogen *Mycobacterium tuberculosis,* bacteria that are inhaled into the alveoli of the lung are phagocytosed by and multiply within phagocytes. SP-A appears to enhance phagocytosis of *M. tuberculosis* by macrophages.[15] Thus, although this surfactant-specific protein enhances the killing of extracellular microbes in the lung, for host-adapted pathogens such as *M. tuberculosis,* SP-A may facilitate uptake of these pathogens into their host niche.[15]

Platelet-activating factor (PAF), a potent lipid mediator of inflammation, is secreted within the airways from neutrophils, eosinophils, platelets, and resident cells of the lungs, including endothelial cells. It has various effects on the lungs, including activation of neutrophils, increased adherence of inflammatory cells to the endothelium, vascular leakage, bronchoconstriction, and pulmonary artery vasoconstriction.[9] The increase in PAF-induced vasopermeability appears to be mediated by products of arachidonic acid metabolism.

Eicosanoids

Eicosanoids, a family of compounds with wide-ranging biologic effects in the lungs and other organs, are metabolites of arachidonic acid (AA), a 20-carbon unsaturated fatty acid. AA is released from membrane phospholipids by the action of phospholipase, and is in turn metabolized by three pathways: 1. Cyclooxygenase produces prostaglandin endoperoxide (PGH_2), which is the precursor of prostaglandins, thromboxane, and prostacyclin. The cyclooxygenase pathway may be regulated by growth factors, cytokines, and oxygen radicals. 2. Lipoxygenases catalyze the formation of 5-, 12-, and 15-hydroperoxyeicosatetraenoic acids (HPETE), which participate in the synthesis of leukotrienes. 3. Cytochrome P-450 monooxygenase forms epoxyeicosatrienoic acid (EET).[19] The lungs have the capacity to synthesize as well as to inactivate AA metabolites. This has important implications for extrapulmonary pathophysiology, as the lungs receive the total cardiac output. Thus, the concentration of eicosanoids in the systemic circulation is dependent to a large extent on AA metabolism in the lungs.

Although phospholipids are thought to be the major pool of AA-containing lipid molecules, recent studies have identified a pool of AA associated with triglycerides (TGs) in human lung macrophages and other inflammatory cells.[52] The TG pool, the largest AA-containing pool of the mast cells, supplies AA to the phospholipids during cell activation. It appears that as inflammatory cells mature in the lungs, they compartmentalize AA into

TABLE 9-1

Functions of Selected Neuropeptides in the Lungs

Neuropeptide	Function	Reference
VIP-related peptides		
Vasoactive intestinal peptide	Vasodilatation, bronchodilatation, modulation of mucus secretion, modulation of cholinergic neurotransmission, anti-inflammatory activity	3
Peptide histidine isoleucine	Vasodilatation, bronchodilatation	3
Peptide histidine methionine	Vasodilatation, bronchodilatation	3
Peptide histidine valine	Bronchodilatation in guinea pig airways in vitro	3
Helodermin	Relaxation of airway smooth muscle in vitro	3
Pituitary adenylate cyclase–activating peptide	Similar to VIP?	3
Tachykinins		
Substance P	Vasodilatation, bronchoconstriction, increase in vascular permeability, up-regulation of the production of inflammatory cytokines, chemotactic for neutrophils, histamine release	27
Neurokinin A (substance K)	Vasodilatation, bronchoconstriction, increase in vascular permeability	3
Neurokinin B (neuromedin K)	Increase in vascular permeability	3
Bombesinlike peptides		
Bombesin	Vasoconstriction, bronchoconstriction, stimulation of airway mucus secretion, trophic effect on some cell types	4
Gastrin-releasing peptide	Vasoconstriction, bronchoconstriction, stimulation of airway mucus secretion, active in lung maturation?	4
Phyllolitorins	Bronchoconstriction, stimulation of branching morphogenesis in lung	24
Calcitonin gene-related peptide	Vasodilatation, bronchoconstriction?, amplification of SP-induced vascular permeability, proteolytic fragments of CGRP are chemotactic for eosinophils, inhibition of macrophage-induced activation of T lymphocytes, inhibition of SP degradation	4
Neuropeptide Y	Vasoconstriction, bronchoconstriction?, modulation of cholinergic transmission, increase in mucus secretion, reduction of microvascular leakage	4
Cholecystokinin octapeptide	Bronchoconstriction	4
Somatostatin	Potentiation of cholinergic neurotransmission	4
Galanin	Unknown physiological role in airways	4
Enkephalins	Unknown physiological role in airways	4

distinct subcellular locations.[52] These findings indicate that TGs may be important regulators of eicosanoid metabolism in inflammatory cells in the lungs.

Prostaglandins (PGs) are multifunctional mediators of cell homeostasis, including pulmonary vasoconstriction, peripheral vasodilation, platelet aggregation, inflammation, potentiation of the effects of histamine and bradykinin on vascular permeabil-ity, inhibition of gastric acid secretion, neuromodulation, and other biologic effects.[19] The recent demonstration of transcriptional induction of the hepatocyte growth factor (HGF) gene by PG analogues[30] adds a novel function to these eicosanoids. The modification of the PG metabolic pathway by overexpression of the prostaglandin G/H (PGH) synthase gene has been explored for the potential gene therapy of acute lung injury.[11] In vivo transfection of rabbits with a plasmid encoding the PGH synthase gene increased lung generation of PGE_2 and prostacyclin, and reduced endotoxin-stimulated pulmonary hypertension, edema, and thromboxane B_2 release.[11]

Leukotrienes (LTs), thromboxane, and PAF act in concert to enhance vascular permeability and contribute to pulmonary dysfunction and the pathogenesis of lung disease. LTs are synthesized via the 5-lipoxygenase pathway of AA metabolism, and promote neutrophil aggregation, chemotaxis, and adhesion to vascular endothelium.[25] Studies have employed selective inhibitors to LTs and their receptors in order to elucidate the role of these eicosanoids in lung injury. Leukotriene B_4 (LTB_4) was shown to mediate alveolitis and pulmonary edema formation in endotoxemic pigs, probably by facilitating transendothelial migration of neutrophils.[53] The intravenous administration of LTD_4 elicited vascular permeability in the trachea, main bronchi, and small airways of the guinea pig, as measured by dye extravasation.[6] The increase in microvascular leakage appears to be mediated through the formation of cyclooxygenase products, which act on the PG/TXA_2 receptors.[6]

HEMOSTATIC FUNCTIONS

The initiation of blood coagulation is effected predominantly by the extrinsic pathway.[38] Lung endothelial cells, as elsewhere in the vasculature, possess both procoagulant and anticoagulant properties. Under normal conditions, several substances are expressed by the endothelium that maintains its antithrombotic properties. For example, prostacyclin inhibits platelet aggregation, and heparan sulfate, thrombomodulin, and tissue factor pathway inhibitor (TFPI) interfere with thrombin activity. In addition, tissue plasminogen activator (t-PA) promotes fibrinolysis. On the other hand, perturbation of the endothelium by inflammatory molecules—such as endotoxin, interleukin-1 (IL-1), and tumor necrosis factor–α (TNF-α)—provokes its procoagulant properties, concomitant with the release or enhanced production of tissue factor, von Willebrand factor, the fibrinolytic inhibitor plasminogen activator inhibitor–1 (PAI-1), PAF, and extracellular matrix components.[38] Thus, the anticoagulant characteristics of the endothelial surface are maintained by the complex interactions of these counterbalancing substances. A key regulator of the extrinsic pathway of coagulation is TFPI. Recent work has demonstrated the presence of TFPI mRNA in rabbit and bovine lung endothelium.[1] This, and the observation that of all the organs the lung expresses the largest amount of TFPI, indicates that the lung endothelium is a primary physiological site of TFPI synthesis. It is interesting to note that, unlike thrombomodulin and fibrinolytic enzymes synthesized by the endothelium, TFPI synthesis is not down-regulated and may be slightly increased during inflammation.[1]

LUNG DEFENSE

The lungs possess many mechanisms for prevention of injury and infection from inhaled pathogens. These include upper-airway respiratory filters, secretions, airway reflexes, specialized cell-mediated defenses, and the microbicidal fatty acids of the alveolar lining fluid.[46] In addition, type II pneumocytes may function as immune accessory cells for major histocompatibility complex class II–restricted presentation of antigens to T cells; the same cells secrete opsonic and other proteins that participate in alveolar host defense.[46] Here we consider three topics—the complement system, cytokines, and leukocyte migration and adhesion.

Complement Activation

The complement system consists of approximately 30 different proteins, some of them membrane bound and others in plasma.[20] Two different pathways are involved in the activation of the complement cascade. The classic pathway is initiated by the binding of immune complexes to the C1q subunit of the C1 protein. The alternative pathway is initiated by the deposition of C3b on nucleophilic groups on target molecules—e.g. bacteria, lipopolysaccharides, fungi, yeast cell walls, viruses, and parasites—as well as injured host cells. Complement participates in antigen processing through the binding of bound components, such as C3b and C4b, to complement receptors on leukocytes and erythrocytes. Other complement components, C5a and C3a, known as anaphylatoxins, are potent mediators of the inflammatory response, and stimulate cells to release a wide variety of proinflammatory molecules, including histamine, LTs, and PGs.[17] The net effect at the site of inflammation is the accumulation of complement proteins, antibodies, and clotting factors, neutrophils, and phagocytes that ingest foreign antigens. Activation of the complement system is thought to be involved in the development of disease-associated pulmonary hypertension. This effect is likely mediated by C3a, which causes thromboxane-dependent pulmonary vascular constriction in lungs.[33] The C5a anaphylatoxin receptor has recently been shown to be expressed in bronchial and alveolar epithelial cells, as well as vascular smooth muscle and endothelial cells in the lungs.[17]

In rat models, intrapulmonary deposition of IgG immune complex causes inflammatory lung injury, which can be reduced with agents that interfere with neutrophil recruitment in the lungs. Thus, neutralization of ICAM-1, IL-1, or TNF-α using blocking Ab or the use of PAF receptor antagonists minimized injury.[54] Vaporciyan and colleagues found that after IgG immune complex deposition or airway instillation of TNF-α, there was a relationship between pulmonary vascular expression of ICAM-1 and a requirement for complement activation.[54]

A large number of studies have established convincingly that activation of complement is a key initial step in tissue injury in animal models of autoimmune disease.[55] Moreover, complement plays an essential role in the pathobiology of acute lung injury in animal models.[54] Complement-mediated damage to the host tissue is prevented by soluble and membrane-bound regulatory proteins of the complement system. Central among these is the complement receptor type 1 (CR1), a potent inhibitor of both the classic and alternative pathways and a cofactor in the factor I–dependent degradation of C3b and C4b.[55] A truncated soluble form of human CR1 (sCR1) has been produced,[55] and shown to effectively reduce the severity of acute lung injury in animal models.[34,35] sCR1 has the potential to become an important therapeutic agent in the wide variety of diseases where complement activation plays a role.

Leukocyte Recruitment

The migration of leukocytes throughout the vasculature provides the body with the ability to maintain immune surveillance and to protect tissues from injury caused by foreign antigens.[48] In addition to participating in host defense, leukocytes may be active in the mounting of pathologic inflammation in pulmonary disease. The recruitment of leukocytes is the result of a complex interplay of activated adhesion molecules[49] and the release of chemotactic molecules (Table 9-2).

The cell adhesion molecules that orchestrate the complex interactions between leukocytes and endothelium are classified into three families—the selectins, integrins, and immunoglobulin superfamily.[49] The precise mechanism of the binding of leukocytes to inflamed endothelium is complex and incompletely under-

stood. In the current consensus model, leukocytes interact with endothelium through a series of events: Initial attachment and "rolling" of leukocytes on endothelium is mediated by selectin molecules. Tethering leads to activation of integrins, which cause strong adhesion of leukocytes to the vessel wall. Migration of leukocytes into tissues is mediated by chemokines and possibly other cytokines that are secreted by subendothelial tissues or by the endothelium itself.

Our understanding of the regulation of leukocyte-endothelial interactions is derived mainly from studies of systemic vessels. The unique anatomic features of the lung, however, suggest that the series of steps worked out for systemic microvessels are not applicable to adhesion events in the pulmonary capillaries. Thus, space constraints (Fig. 9-5) in pulmonary capillaries preclude leukocyte rolling; furthermore, neutrophil adherence in the pul-

TABLE 9-2

Chemotactic Mediators in the Lungs

Substance	Source	Target	Potency	Reference
f-met Peptides	Bacteria	PMN, monocyte	+	46
MCP-1	Monocyte, macrophage	Monocyte, T cell	++	46
MIP-1	Macrophage	PMN, monocyte, T cell	++	50
TNFα	PMN, endothelial cells	PMN, monocyte	++	48
PAF		PMN, eosinophil	+	13
LTB4	PMN	PMN, monocyte	+	46
C5a	Serum	PMN, monocyte	++	46
IL-1	Monocyte, macrophage	PMN	++	45
IL-5	T cell, mast cell	Eosinophil	++	36
IL-8	PMN, monocyte, T cell	PMN, T cell	++	37
Lymphotactin	T cell	Lymphocyte	++	23
Immune complexes		PMN	+	48

NOTE: + = weak activity; ++ = strong activity.

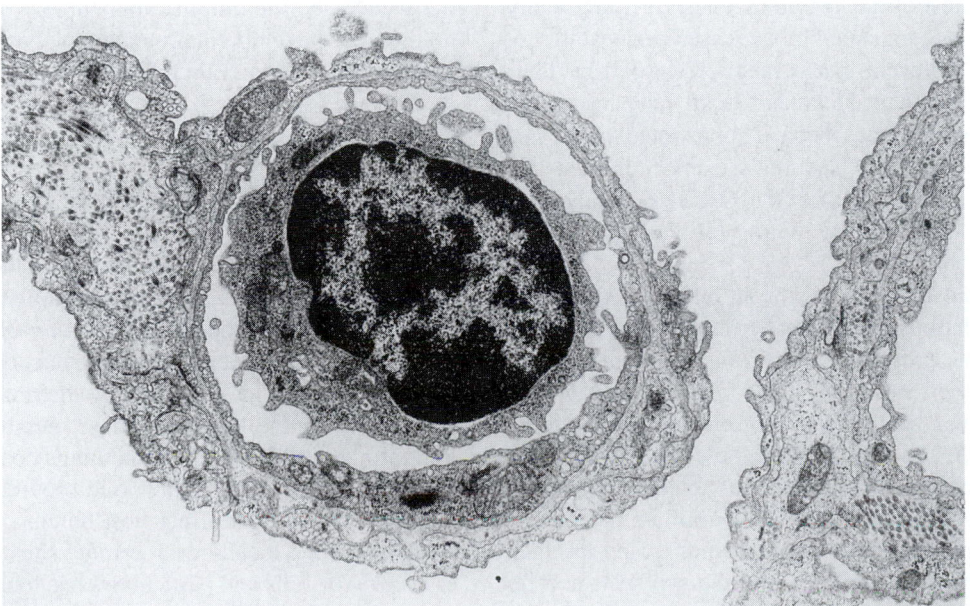

FIGURE 9-5   Transverse section of pulmonary alveolar capillary containing a leukocyte. The tight fit and opportunities for interaction between the leukocyte and endothelial cell can be appreciated (×15,000).

monary circulation may occur by either CD11/CD18-dependent or -independent mechanisms, whereas all neutrophil migration in the systemic circulation requires the CD11/CD18 complex.[18] In addition to neutrophils, pulmonary macrophages are engaged in the clearance of blood-borne pathogens, particulates, and damaged cells. These cells secrete eicosanoids, which affect airway smooth muscle. Eosinophils also secrete inflammatory substances, which can be toxic to endothelial cells.

The chemokines make up a family of chemoattractant cytokines that are classified into two subfamilies based on sequence homology and the sequence around two cysteine residues.[37] The C-X-C or α chemokine family acts predominantly on neutrophils and nonhematopoietic cells, and the C-C or β chemokine family acts mainly on monocytes as well as on eosinophils and lymphocytes. The recently discovered lymphotactin cytokine has been proposed to belong to a new group of chemokines designated the C family.[23] Chemokines are thought to play an important role in lung inflammatory cell recruitment and subsequent lung injury. The TNF-induced expression of the macrophage inflammatory protein–1α (MIP-1α), a member of the C-C chemokine family, has been shown to mediate neutrophil and macrophage influx into the lungs, probably by regulating the expression of ICAM-1 within the lung.[50]

Cytokines and Growth Factors

Cytokines modulate cellular communication and phenotype in response to pathophysiological stimuli. Numerous biologic events are orchestrated by these molecules, including modification of the anticoagulant properties of endothelium, leukocyte migration and adhesiveness, induction of cyclooxygenase and prostaglandin production, up-regulation of immune system components, induction of synthesis, and release of cytokines.[22] In addition to the secretion of cytokines in the pulmonary circulation by activated macrophages, the lungs themselves have the biosynthetic capacity to produce most of the known cytokines.[22] Lung injury and inflammation are accompanied by increased permeability of the endothelial layer, an event that is mediated in part by TNF. Two distinct TNF receptors, of 55 kd and 75 kd, have been identified, and their expression has been demonstrated in normal human lung tissue.[47] Recently Sakuma's team[44] reported that granulocyte colony–stimulating factor (G-CSF), synthesized in the human lung, increases the permeability of pulmonary endothelium.

The capacity of the lungs to mount an allergic response to IgE-dependent stimulation is mediated by mast cells that release eisosanoids, histamine, proteases, and various cytokines. Proinflammatory granulocytes, especially eosinophils, are recruited to the site of tissue damage by a variety of chemoattractants, including LTB$_4$, and PAF, as well as bacterial peptide fragments, which exhibit different eosinophilotactic potency profiles.[13] Eosinophils themselves secrete several proinflammatory cytokines. Okayama and coworkers[36] have demonstrated the IgE-dependent expression of IL-5 mRNA and the synthesis and release of immunoreactive IL-5 in human lung mast cells. IL-5 is known to regulate the recruitment and activation of eosinophils, which play an important role in allergy and inflammation. These

data support the hypothesis that mast cell activation releases cytokines that initiate and perhaps maintain allergic reactions in the lungs.[36]

IL-10 is known to be an anti-inflammatory cytokine, as it suppresses the release of the proinflammatory cytokines IL-1 and TNF-α from macrophages, slows down the accumulation of neutrophils, and inhibits antigen presentation.[32] Recent work showed that IL-10 is constitutively produced by bronchial epithelial cells from healthy persons, but it is down-regulated in patients with cystic fibrosis.[7] This finding suggests an important role for the bronchial epithelium in secreting IL-10 to attenuate lung inflammation.

The insulinlike growth factor (IGF) molecules regulate airway smooth-muscle cell proliferation. The IGF network includes IGF-1 and IGF-II, their receptors, a number of IGF-binding proteins (IGFBPs), and several IGFBP proteases that degrade IGFBP, regulating the biologic effects of IGF.[10] LTD$_4$ induces an IGFBP-2 protease that decreases the extracellular levels of IGFBP-2, allowing more free IGF to bind to its receptor and stimulate airway smooth-muscle cell proliferation.[10] The precise roles of the components of the IGF system in the lungs remain to be defined.

Clearly, an effective regulatory system must exist in order to maintain the appropriate levels of the numerous cytokines and growth factors in homeostasis of the healthy lung. The aberrant synthesis of these chemical signal transducers can accelerate pulmonary disease. Steady-state levels of cytokines are achieved by a variety of mechanisms, including transcriptional and translational controls, as well as by the intrinsic stability of each peptide. An additional level of control is provided by cytokine-binding proteins, defined as "extracellular proteins that do not transduce a cytokine signal as would be the case for a 'cytokine receptor.'"[8] These proteins are thought to provide a mechanism to clear, sequester, or inactivate cytokines following the successful resolution of an inflammatory event in the lungs. Additional functions could be the amplification of the biologic effects of cytokines and the temporal protection of cytokines from proteolytic degradation, followed by release and binding of the cytokine to its receptor.[8]

CONCLUSION

On account of their strategic position in the circulation, their extensive vascular bed, and the multiplicity of component cell types, the lungs are ideally suited to process circulating vasoactive substances, whether naturally occurring or xenobiotic. In addition, they are ideally suited to distribute both the molecules synthesized by the lungs and those metabolized during circulation through the lungs. Thus the lungs control which substances enter the systemic circulation, and provide an important regulatory function in controlling host defense and inflammatory responses elicited locally or at remote sites. The role of the lungs as a sieve for cells and particulates has long been known. Recognition of the nonrespiratory functions of the lungs[14,41] and progress in that understanding in recent years now allow acknowledgment of the role of the lungs as a molecular sieve.

REFERENCES

1. Ameri A, Kuppuswamy MN, Basu S, Bajaj SP: Expression of tissue factor pathway inhibitor by cultured endothelial cells in response to inflammatory mediators. *Blood* 79:3219–3226, 1992.

2. Baenziger NL, Dalemar LR, Mack P, Haddock RC: Histamine degradative uptake by cultured human pulmonary vascular endothelial cells utilizes an inflammatory cell diamine oxidase. *J Biol Chem* 269:32858–32864, 1994.

3. Barnes PJ, Baraniuk JN, Belvisi MG: Neuropeptides in the respiratory tract: Part I. *Am Rev Respir Dis* 144:1187–1198, 1991.

4. Barnes PJ, Baraniuk JN, Belvisi MG: Neuropeptides in the respiratory tract: Part II. *Am Rev Respir Dis* 144:1391–1399, 1991.

5. Bhoola KD, Figueroa CD, Worthy K: Bioregulation of kinins: Kallikreins, kininogens, and kininases. *Pharmacol Rev* 44:1–80, 1992.

6. Bochnowicz S, Underwood DC: Dose-dependent mediation of leukotriene D_4–induced airway microvascular leakage and bronchoconstriction in the guinea pig. *Prostaglandins Leukot Essent Fatty Acids* 52:403–411, 1995.

7. Bonfield TL, Konstan MW, Burfeind P, et al: Normal bronchial epithelial cells constitutively produce the anti-inflammatory cytokine interleukin-10, which is downregulated in cystic fibrosis. *Am J Respir Cell Mol Biol* 13:257–261, 1995.

8. Bonner JC, Brody AR: Cytokine-binding proteins in the lung. *Am J Physiol* 268:L869–L878, 1995.

9. Chung KF: Platelet-activating factor in inflammation and pulmonary disorders. *Clin Sci* 83:127–138, 1992.

10. Cohen P, Noveral JP, Bhala A, et al: Leukotriene D_4 facilitates airway smooth muscle cell proliferation via modulation of the IGF axis. *Am J Physiol* 269:L151–L157, 1995.

11. Conary JT, Parker RE, Christman BW, et al: Protection of rabbit lungs from endotoxin injury by in vivo hyperexpression of the prostaglandin G/H synthase gene. *J Clin Invest* 93:1834–1840, 1994.

12. Conway EM, Liu L, Nowakowski B, et al: Heat shock–sensitive expression of calreticulin: *In vitro* and *in vivo* up-regulation. *J Biol Chem* 270:17011–17016, 1995.

13. Erger RA, Casale TB: Comparative studies indicate that platelet-activating factor is a relatively weak eosinophilotactic mediator. *Am J Respir Cell Mol Biol* 12:65–70, 1995.

14. Fishman AP: The nonrespiratory functions of the lungs, in Fishman AP (ed), *Pulmonary Diseases and Disorders*, 2d ed. New York, McGraw-Hill, 1988, pp 205–219.

15. Gaynor CD, McCormack FX, Voelker DR, et al: Pulmonary surfactant protein A mediates enhanced phagocytosis of *Mycobacterium tuberculosis* by a direct interaction with human macrophages. *J Immunol* 155:5343–5351, 1995.

16. Hastings RH, Duong H, Burton DW, Deftos LJ: Alveolar epithelial cells express and secrete parathyroid hormone-related protein. *Am J Respir Cell Mol Biol* 11:701–706, 1994.

17. Haviland DL, McCoy RL, Whitehead WT, et al: Cellular expression of the C5a anaphylatoxin receptor (C5aR): Demonstration of C5aR on nonmyeloid cells of the liver and lung. *J Immunol* 154:1861–1869, 1995.

18. Hogg JC, Doerschuk CM: Leukocyte traffic in the lung. *Annu Rev Physiol* 57:97–114, 1995.

19. Holtzman MJ: Arachidonic acid metabolism in airway epithelial cells. *Annu Rev Physiol* 54:303–329, 1992.

20. Homeister JW, Lucchesi BR: Complement activation and inhibition in myocardial ischemia and reperfusion injury. *Annu Rev Pharmacol Toxicol* 34:17–40, 1994.

21. Imai T, Hirata Y, Iwashina M, Marumo F: Hormonal regulation of rat adrenomedullin gene in vasculature. *Endocrinology* 136:1544–1548, 1995.

22. Kelley J: Cytokines of the lung. *Am Rev Respir Dis* 141:765–788, 1990.

23. Kelner GS, Kennedy J, Bacon KB, et al: Lymphotactin: A cytokine that represents a new class of chemokine. *Science* 266:1395–1399, 1994.

24. King KA, Torday JS, Sunday ME: Bombesin and [Leu^8]phyllolitorin promote fetal mouse lung branching morphogenesis via a receptor-mediated mechanism. *Proc Natl Acad Sci USA* 92:4357–4361, 1995.

25. Lewis RA, Austen KF, Soberman RJ: Leukotrienes and other products of the 15-lipoxygenase pathway: Biochemistry and relation to pathobiology in human disease. *New Engl J Med* 323:645–655, 1990.

26. Li H, Chen SJ, Chen YF, et al: Enhanced endothelin-1 and endothelin receptor gene expression in chronic hypoxia. *J Appl Physiol* 77:1451–1459, 1994.

27. Lilly CM, Hall AE, Rodger IW, et al: Substance P–induced histamine release in tracheally perfused guinea pig lungs. *J Appl Physiol* 78:1234–1241, 1995.

28. Mak JCW, Nishikawa M, Shirasaki H, et al: Protective effects of a glucocorticoid on downregulation of pulmonary β_2-adrenergic receptors in vivo. *J Clin Invest* 96:99–106, 1995.

29. Markewitz BA, Kohan DE, Michael JR: Hypoxia decreases endothelin-1 synthesis by rat lung endothelial cells. *Am J Physiol* 269:L215–L220, 1995.

30. Matsumoto K, Okazaki H, Nakamura T: Novel function of prostaglandins as inducers of gene expression of HGF and putative mediators of tissue regeneration. *J Biochem* 117:458–464, 1995.

31. McMillen MA, Sumpio BE: Endothelins: Polyfunctional cytokines. *J Am Coll Surg* 180:621–637, 1995.

32. Moore KW, O'Garra A, Malefyt RW, et al: Interleukin 10. *Annu Rev Immunol* 11:165–190, 1993.

33. Morganroth ML, Schoeneich SO, Till GO, et al: C3a$_{57-77}$, a C-terminal peptide, causes thromboxane-dependent pulmonary vascular constriction in isolated perfused rat lungs. *Am Rev Respir Dis* 141:296–300, 1990.

34. Mulligan MS, Warren JS, Smith CW, et al: Lung injury after deposition of IgA immune complexes: Requirements for CD18 and L-arginine. *J Immunol* 148:3086–3092, 1992.

35. Mulligan MS, Yeh CG, Rudolph AR, Ward PA: Protective effects of soluble CR1 in complement- and neutrophil-mediated tissue injury. *J Immunol* 148:1479–1485, 1992.

36. Okayama Y, Petit-Frére C, Kassel O, et al: IgE-dependent expression of mRNA for IL-4 and IL-5 in human lung mast cells. *J Immunol* 155:1796–1808, 1995.

37. Oppenheim JJ, Zachariae COC, Mukaida N, Matsushima K: Properties of the novel proinflammatory supergene "intercrine" cytokine family. *Annu Rev Immunol* 9:617–648, 1991.

38. Rapaport SI: The extrinsic pathway inhibitor: A regulator of tissue factor-dependent blood coagulation. *Thromb Haemost* 66:6–15, 1991.

39. Regoli D, Jukic D, Gobeil F, Rhaleb N-E: Receptors for bradykinin and related kinins: A critical analysis. *Can J Physiol Pharmacol* 71:556–567, 1993.

40. Ryan US: Endothelial cell activation responses, in Ryan US (ed), *Pulmonary Endothelium in Health and Disease*, vol. 32. New York, Dekker, 1987, pp 3–33.

41. Ryan US: Metabolic activity of pulmonary endothelium: Modulations of structure and function. *Annu Rev Physiol* 48:263–277, 1986.

42. Ryan US: Structural bases for metabolic activity. *Annu Rev Physiol* 44:223–229, 1982.

43. Ryan US, Ryan JW, Whitaker C, Chiu A: Localization of angiotensin converting enzyme (kininase II): II. Immunocytochemistry and immunofluorescence. *Tissue Cell* 8:125–145, 1976.

44. Sakuma T, Nakada T, Nishimura T, et al: The granulocyte colony–stimulating factor produced in the human lung and its effect on liquid movement in the rabbit lung. *Surg Today* 24:1050–1055, 1994.

45. Sayers TJ, Wiltrout TA, Bull CA, et al: Effect of cytokines on polymorphonuclear neutrophil infiltration in the mouse: Prostaglandin- and leukotriene-independent induction of infiltration by IL-1 and tumor necrosis factor. *J Immunol* 141:1670–1677, 1988.

46. Sherman MP, Ganz T: Host defense in pulmonary alveoli. *Annu Rev Physiol* 54:331–350, 1992.

47. Shimomoto H, Hasegawa Y, Nozaki Y, et al: Expression of tumor necrosis factor receptors in human lung cancer cells and normal lung tissues. *Am J Respir Cell Mol Biol* 13:271–278, 1995.

48. Sibille Y, Reynolds HY: Macrophages and polymorphonuclear neutrophils in lung defense and injury. *Am Rev Respir Dis* 141:471–501, 1990.

49. Springer TA: Traffic signals for lymphocyte recirculation and leukocyte emigration: The multistep paradigm. *Cell* 76:301–314, 1994.

50. Standiford TJ, Kunkel SL, Lukacs NW, et al: Macrophage inflammatory protein–1a mediates lung leukocyte recruitment, lung capillary leak, and early mortality in murine endotoxemia. *J Immunol* 155:1515–1524, 1995.

51. Tolloczko B, Jia YL, Martin JG: Serotonin-evoked calcium transients in airway smooth muscle cells. *Am J Physiol* 269:L234–L240, 1995.

52. Triggiani M, Oriente A, Seeds MC, et al: Migration of human inflammatory cells into the lung results in the remodeling of arachidonic acid into a triglyceride pool. *J Exp Med* 182:1181–1190, 1995.

53. VanderMeer TJ, Menconi MJ, O'Sullivan BP, et al: Acute lung injury in endotoxemic pigs: Role of leukotriene B_4. *J Appl Physiol* 78:1121–1131, 1995.

54. Vaporciyan AA, Mulligan MS, Warren JS, et al: Up-regulation of lung vascular ICAM-1 in rats is complement dependent. *J Immunol* 155:1442–1449, 1995.

55. Weisman HF, Bartow T, Leppo MK, et al: Soluble human complement receptor type 1: In vivo inhibitor of complement suppressing post-ischemic myocardial inflammation and necrosis. *Science* 249:146–151, 1990.

CHAPTER 10

PULMONARY MECHANICS

Murray D. Altose

LUNG VOLUMES

**STATIC MECHANICAL PROPERTIES OF THE
RESPIRATORY SYSTEM**
    Elastic Properties of the Lungs (Pulmonary
      Compliance)
    Elastic Properties of the Thorax
    Elastic Properties of the Respiratory System as a Whole

**DYNAMIC MECHANICAL PROPERTIES OF THE
RESPIRATORY SYSTEM**
    Airway Resistance
    Isovolume Pressure-Flow Curves
    Equal Pressure Point Theory: Dynamic Compression of
      Airways
    Wave Speed Limitation Theory

**MECHANICAL DETERMINANTS OF REGIONAL
VENTILATION**
    Dynamic Compliance of the Lungs
    Interdependence and Collateral Ventilation

WORK AND ENERGY COST OF BREATHING
    Work of Breathing
    Oxygen Cost of Breathing

For venous blood to be properly arterialized, the distribution of air and blood within the lung is automatically matched in order to ensure effective gas exchange across alveolar-capillary membranes. Arterialization comprises a series of interrelated processes that begin with the mechanical performance of the ventilatory apparatus—i.e., the lungs and chest wall, including the rib cage, diaphragm, and abdominal wall. Although the function of each component of the lung and of the chest bellows can be deranged by injury or disease, the design of the ventilatory apparatus provides for considerable reserve. As a result, mechanical derangements are usually quite severe by the time clinical symptoms appear or arterial blood-gas levels become abnormal.

Depending on the nature of the underlying disorder, assessment of the mechanical properties of the ventilatory apparatus provides several different types of information. In some instances, characterization of the mechanical abnormality provides insight into pathogenesis and affords a quantitative measure of severity. In others, once the nature of the mechanical disorder is understood, the mystery surrounding a life-threatening disorder in gas exchange may be dispelled. Finally, certain breathing patterns make sense only if the mechanical performance of the chest bellows is taken into account.

During breathing, the lungs and chest wall operate in unison. The lungs fill the chest cavity so that the visceral pleura is in contact with the parietal pleura of the chest wall. The two pleural surfaces are separated by only a thin liquid film, which provides the bond holding the lungs and chest wall together.

At the end of a normal exhalation, the respiratory muscles are at rest. The pressure along the entire tracheobronchial tree from the airway opening to the alveoli is equal to atmospheric pressure. The tendency of the lung is to deflate, however, and lung elastic recoil is directed centripetally. This is counterbalanced by the elastic recoil of the chest wall, which is directed centrifugally to favor an increase in volume. These opposing forces generate a subatmospheric pleural pressure of about -5 cmH$_2$O (Fig. 10-1A). The tendency for the lung to recoil inward and for the chest wall to recoil outward is illustrated by the observation that when the chest is opened at autopsy, the lungs collapse and the thorax expands.

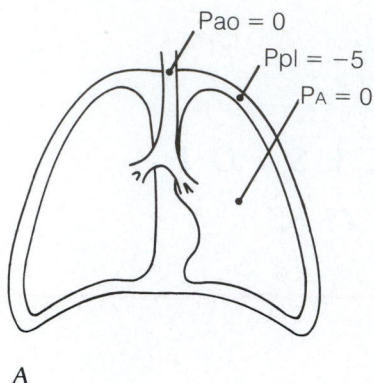
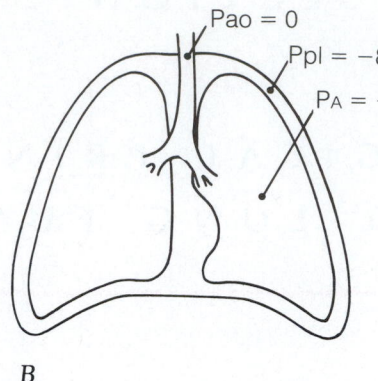
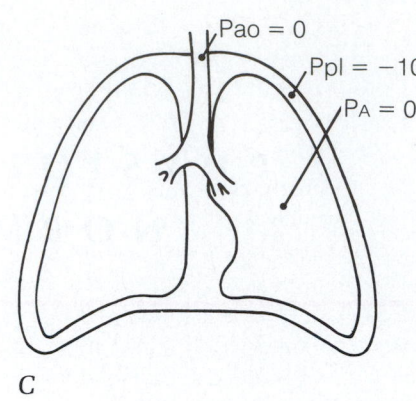

A   B   C

FIGURE 10-1 Respiratory pressures during a breathing cycle. Ppl = pleural pressure; PA = pressure in the alveoli; Pao = pressure at the air-way opening. *A*. End expiration. *B*. During inspiration. *C*. End inspiration.

Although it is conventional to consider pleural pressure as a single, mean value that reflects mechanical events within the entire ventilatory apparatus, this is clearly an oversimplification on several accounts: (1) pleural pressure is not directly determinable because normally there is only a potential space between the visceral and parietal pleura; (2) on conceptual grounds, distinctions exist between surface and liquid pleural pressures; (3) pleural pressures are not uniform over the surface of the lungs, being strongly affected by gravity; and (4) transmission of pleural pressures at the surface to alveoli located at different depths and loci with the lungs depends on the structural interplay among supporting structures in the alveolar walls (interdependence), which resists any inclination of individual alveoli or even a lobule to collapse. Nonetheless, the concept of mean pleural pressure, as generally used in considerations of respiratory system mechanics, has proved to be of great practical value.[31]

The contraction of the muscles of inspiration produces the forces that permit the flow of gas along the tracheobronchial tree and the expansion of the lungs and chest. The movement of air into the lungs requires a pressure difference between the airway opening and the alveoli sufficient to overcome the resistance to airflow of the tracheobronchial tree. During spontaneous breathing, the action of the inspiratory muscles causes an increase in the outward recoil of the chest wall. As a result, the pleural pressure becomes more subatmospheric. This pressure change is transmitted to the interior of the lungs, so alveolar pressure also becomes subatmospheric (Fig. 10-1*B*). In contrast, during artificial ventilation with a positive-pressure breathing machine, a supra-atmospheric pressure applied at the inlet to the airways creates the proper pressure gradient between the airway opening and alveoli for airflow.

Expansion of alveoli depends on the achievement of an appropriate distending pressure across alveolar walls. This distending pressure or transpulmonary pressure is the difference between alveolar (PA) and pleural (Ppl) pressures. As shown in Fig. 10-1*A,* the transpulmonary pressure at end-expiration (PA – Ppl) is 5 cmH$_2$O. At the end of inspiration (Fig. 10-1*C*), the transpulmonary distending pressure is higher and the lungs contain more air.

The energy used during inspiration to overcome the elastic resistance of the lungs is stored. Expiration occurs when these forces are released. When the inspiratory muscles relax, the recoil of the lungs causes the alveolar pressure to exceed the pressure at the mouth, and air flows out of the lungs. Although expiration during quiet breathing is passive, the expiratory muscles are engaged at high levels of ventilation to assist the movement of air out of the lungs.

LUNG VOLUMES

The lung volumes and capacities (Table 10-1) are also considered elsewhere in this book (see Appendix C). The end-expira-

---

TABLE 10-1

Lung Volumes and Subdivisions

The *functional residual capacity* (FRC) is the volume of air that remains in the lungs at the end of a normal expiration.

The *tidal volume* (TV) is the volume of air that is drawn into the lungs during inspiration from the end-expiratory position (and also leaves the lungs passively during expiration in the course of quiet breathing).

The *expiratory reserve volume* (ERV) is the maximum volume of air that can be forcibly exhaled after a quiet expiration has been completed (i.e., from the end-expiratory position).

The *residual volume* (RV) is the volume of air that remains in the lungs after a maximal expiratory effort.

The *inspiratory capacity* (IC) is the maximum volume of air that can be inhaled from the end-expiratory position. It consists of two subdivisions: tidal volume and the *inspiratory reserve volume* (IRV).

The *total lung capacity* (TLC) is the total volume of air contained in the lungs at the end of a maximum inspiration.

The *vital capacity* (VC) is the volume of air that is exhaled by a maximum expiration after a maximum inspiration.

tory position of the lungs, functional residual capacity (FRC), is the major reference point for the volume subdivisions of the lung. This position is set by the opposing recoil forces of the lung and chest wall when the respiratory muscles are at rest.

Total lung capacity (TLC) is determined by the balance between the force-generating capacity of the inspiratory muscles and the opposing elastic recoil forces of the lung and chest wall.[1] Weakness of the muscles of inspiration or increased stiffness of the lung reduces TLC. Loss of retractive forces exerted by the lung, as in emphysema, enlarges TLC.

Residual volume (RV) is set by the balance between the actions of the expiratory muscle and the recoil forces of the lung, which act to decrease lung volume, and the outward recoil forces of the chest wall, which favor lung expansion. In middle-aged and older people, closure of airways at low lung volumes, with air trapping in the lung, is an important determinant of residual volume.[21]

STATIC MECHANICAL PROPERTIES OF THE RESPIRATORY SYSTEM

To assess the elastic properties of the ventilatory apparatus, it is expedient to evaluate the elastic properties of the lungs and chest separately.

Elastic Properties of the Lungs (Pulmonary Compliance)

The change in transpulmonary pressure required to effect a given change in the volume of air in the lungs is a measure of the distensibility, or compliance, of the lungs.[13] Pulmonary compliance is calculated as the ratio of the change in lung volume to the change in transpulmonary pressure—i.e.,

$$C = \frac{\Delta V_L}{\Delta (P_A - Ppl)}$$

where

$$C = \text{lung compliance}$$
$$\Delta(P_A - Ppl) = \text{change in transpulmonary pressure}$$
$$\Delta V_L = \text{change in lung volume}$$

Compliance denotes the ease of stretch or inflation. The inverse of compliance (i.e., elastance) refers to the tendency to resist distortion and to return to the original configuration when the distorting force is removed.

In practice, pulmonary compliance is determined by relating the changes in transpulmonary pressures to the changes in lung volume in the course of an expiration after a maximal inspiration—i.e., starting from total lung capacity.

The pressure-volume characteristics of the lung are nonlinear.[35] As lung volume increases, the elastic elements approach their limits of distensibility, and a given change in transpulmonary pressure produces smaller and smaller increases in lung volume. Thus, the compliance of the lung is least at high lung volumes and greatest as the residual volume is approached (Fig. 10-2). Elastic recoil forces favoring collapse of the lung can be demonstrated throughout the range of the vital capacity, even at

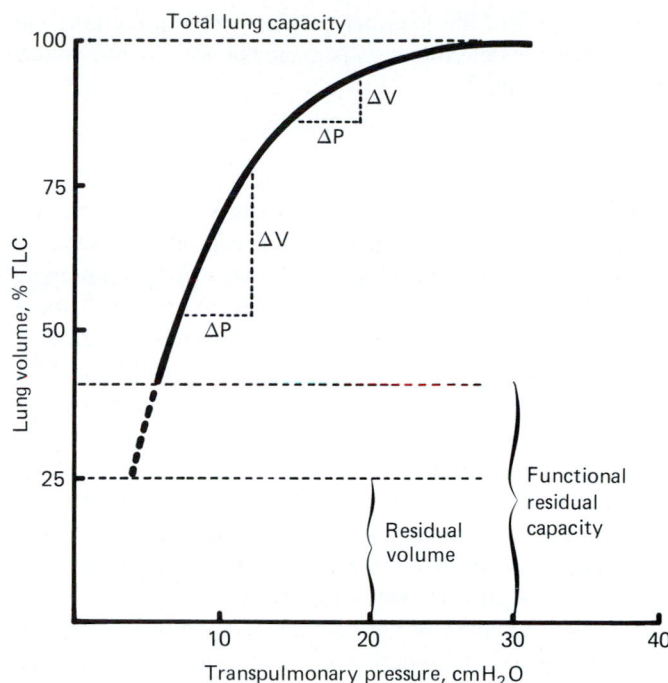

FIGURE 10-2 Pressure-volume curve of the lung. The static elastic recoil pressure of the lung is approximately 5 cmH$_2$O at FRC and 30 cmH$_2$O at TLC. The compliance of the lung ($\Delta V/\Delta P$) is greater at low lung volumes than at high lung volumes.

low lung volumes approaching the residual volume. If the opposing forces of the chest wall on the lungs are eliminated—for instance, by removing the lungs from the thorax or by opening the chest—the lung collapses to a virtually airless state.

If static measurements of transpulmonary pressure are made during lung inflation rather than deflation, the pressure-volume curve has a different configuration (Fig. 10-3). This indicates that

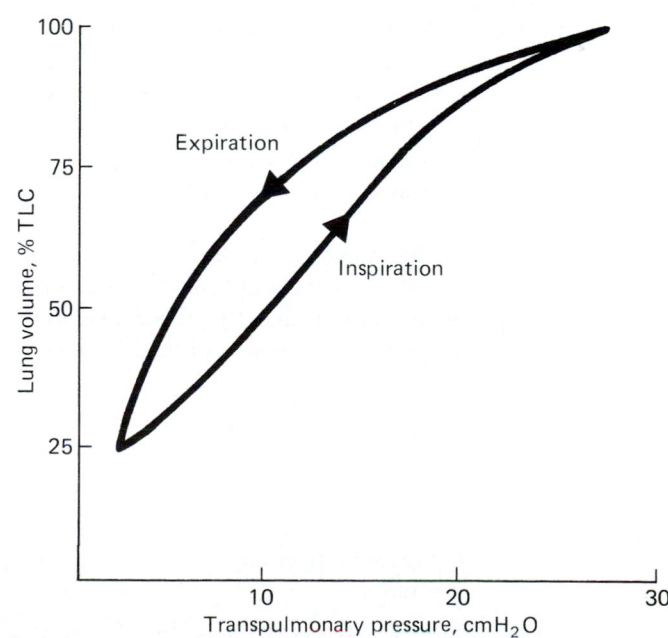

FIGURE 10-3 Pressure-volume curves of the lung during inspiration and expiration.

the elastic recoil of the lung depends not only on the lung volume at which the determination is made but also on the "volume history" of the lung.[15]

HYSTERESIS

Differences in the pathways of the pressure-volume curve during inspiration (when force is applied) and expiration (when force is withdrawn) are designated as hysteresis, which is a property of all elastic structures. In the lungs, it is due to the surface forces and the properties of the surface material lining the alveolar walls and also to the elastic properties of the tissues. An additional factor relates to the closure of small airways at low lung volumes. Once these airways close, the lung units that they serve will not expand during inspiration until a critical opening pressure has been exceeded; only then will the closed units inflate. Recruitment of additional lung units as increasing transpulmonary pressure expands the lungs from low lung volume contributes to the hysteresis of the pressure-volume curve.

The elastic behavior of the lung depends on two factors: the physical properties of the lung tissue, per se, and the surface tension of the film lining of the alveolar walls.[4]

SURFACE FORCES

In addition to the elastic properties of the parenchyma, the surface tension at the air-liquid interface of the alveoli contributes importantly to the elastic recoil of the lungs and acts to decrease lung compliance.[39] The cohesive forces between the molecules of the liquid lining of the alveoli are stronger than those between the film and alveolar gas, thereby causing the film to shrink to its smallest surface area. The behavior of this surface film has been examined in experimental animals by comparison of pressure-volume relationships of air-filled lungs with those of saline-filled lungs; saline eliminates the liquid-air interface without affecting elastic properties of the tissue. A lung distended with saline requires a lower transpulmonary pressure to maintain a given lung volume than a lung that is inflated with air.[2] Also, hysteresis is less in the saline-filled lung. The greater hysteresis in the air-filled lung is explained by the surface tension of the film lining the alveoli, which is higher during inflation as the film expands than it is during deflation as the film is compressed (Fig. 10-4).

By considering the alveolus to be a sphere, Laplace's law can be applied. Laplace's law states that the pressure inside a spherical structure—e.g., the alveolus—is directly proportional to the tension in the wall and inversely proportional to the radius of curvature:

$$\text{Alveolar pressure} = \frac{2T}{r}$$

where

$$T = \text{tension (dyn/cm)}$$
$$r = \text{radius}$$

Abolition of the liquid-air interface by the instillation of saline into the alveolar spaces eliminates surface forces, thereby reducing the transpulmonary pressure required to maintain a given lung volume.

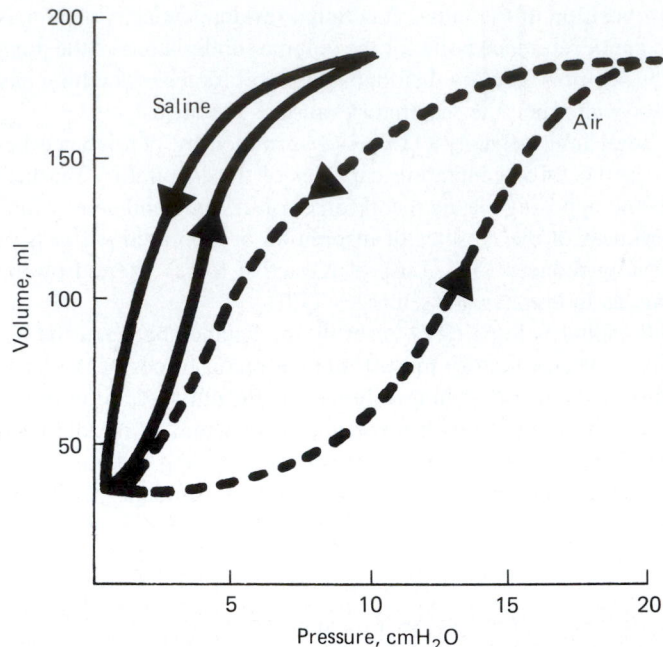

FIGURE 10-4   Comparison of pressure-volume relationships of air-filled and saline-filled excised lungs. Arrows directed upward indicate inflation; those directed downward indicate deflation. Since saline eliminates surface forces at the liquid-air interface without affecting tissue elasticity, the difference in pressure between the two curves, at any lung volume, is that required to overcome surface forces. To maintain a small lung volume, a large proportion of the pressure is used to overcome surface forces. In contrast, at high lung volumes a greater fraction of the pressure is used to overcome tissue elasticity.

The surface tension of the alveolar walls depends on the lung volume: surface tension is higher at large lung volumes and lower at small lung volumes. These variations in surface tension with lung volume are due to the surface film, which contains a special type of surface-active material: surfactant. This substance contains different phospholipids, notably dipalmitoyl lecithin, and special proteins. It is generated by type II alveolar cells and undergoes a continuous cycle of formation, removal, and replenishment.

Surfactant serves several important functions. The surface tension of surfactant is inherently low and decreases even further at low lung volumes when the surface area of the film is reduced. The minimization of surface forces, particularly at low lung volumes, increases the compliance of the lung and decreases the work required to inflate the lungs during the next breath. The automatic adjustment of surface tension as lung volume changes also promotes stability of alveoli at low lung volumes; if the surface tension were to remain constant instead of changing with lung volume, the transpulmonary pressure required to keep an alveolus open would increase as the radius of curvature diminished with decreasing lung volume. Therefore, small alveoli would empty into the larger ones with which they communicate, and atelectasis would be a regular occurrence (Fig. 10-5).

PHYSICAL PROPERTIES OF LUNG TISSUE

A number of different tissue components contribute to lung elasticity. The pleura, the intralobular septa, peripheral airway

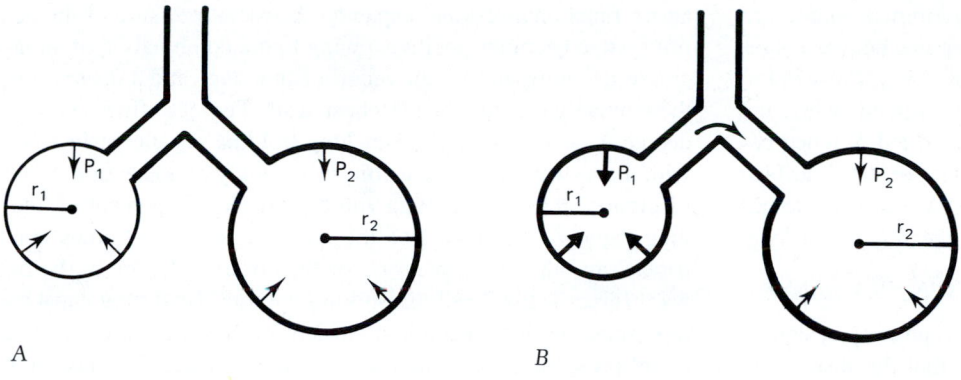

FIGURE 10-5 The effects of surfactant in maintaining alveolar stability. *A.* Surfactant lowers the tension (T) of the alveolar walls at low lung volumes. Consequently, the transpulmonary pressure (P) of large and small communicating airspaces is the same. $r_1 < r_2$, $T_1 < T_2$, $P_1 = P_2$. *B.* Without surfactant, the surface tension remains constant as lung volume changes, and the recoil pressure of small airspaces exceeds that of larger ones. As a result, small alveoli tend to empty into larger ones. $r_1 < r_2$, $T_1 = T_2$, $P_1 > P_2$.

smooth-muscle tone, and pulmonary vasomotor tone, as well as the tissues of the alveolar walls, play a role in shaping lung elastic recoil.

The major connective-tissue elements of the alveolar walls are the collagen and elastin fibers.[40] Elastin fibers in the alveolar walls and surrounding the bronchioles and pulmonary capillaries have a low tensile strength but can be stretched to over twice their resting length. Elastin fibers are thought to bear most of the stress in the lung at low volumes. Collagen fibers have high tensile strength but are poorly extensible and probably act to limit expansion at high lung volumes.[19] Like a stretched nylon stocking, expansion of the lungs appears to entail an unfolding and geometric rearrangement of the fibers and only slight elongation of individual fibers.

As a result of alterations in the elastin and collagen fibers in the lung, the distensibility of the lungs (measured as compliance) increases with age.[38] This is part of the normal aging process. Pulmonary compliance is also increased by the destruction of alveolar walls and the enlargement of alveolar spaces that characterize pulmonary emphysema. In contrast, the distensibility of the lungs is reduced by pulmonary fibrosis, which stiffens its interstitial tissues.[13]

Elastic Properties of the Thorax

The elastic recoil of the chest wall is such that if it were unopposed by the lungs, the chest would enlarge to approximately 70 percent of total lung capacity. This position represents its equilibrium or resting position.[6] In this position (when the respiratory muscles are completely relaxed), the pressure difference across the chest wall—i.e., the difference between pleural pressure and the pressure at the surface of the chest—is zero. If the chest were forced to enlarge further by an increasingly positive pleural pressure or by the application of subatmospheric pressure at the body surface, it would, like the lung, recoil inward, resisting expansion and favoring return to its equilibrium position. Conversely, at volumes less than 70 percent of total lung capacity, the recoil of the chest is opposite that of the lung and is directed outward (Fig. 10-6). The chest wall can also be represented as a two-compartment system consisting of the rib cage

and the abdomen, and volume changes can be partitioned between the two compartments.[20] Changing from the upright to the supine position at a constant overall lung volume produces a shift in volume from the abdominal to the rib cage compartment. The compliance of the rib cage is similar in the supine and upright positions, but the compliance of the abdominal compartment—particularly at high volumes—is greater in the supine position.

The elastic recoil properties of the chest wall play an important role in determining the subdivisions of lung volume. They may be seriously deranged by disorders affecting the chest wall, such as marked obesity, kyphoscoliosis, and ankylosing spondylitis.

Elastic Properties of the Respiratory System as a Whole

If we consider the lung and the chest wall to operate mechanically in series, the elastic recoil pressure of the total respiratory system (Prs) can be calculated as the algebraic sum of the pressures exerted by the elastic recoil of the lung (transpulmonary pressure) and the elastic recoil of the chest wall.[33]

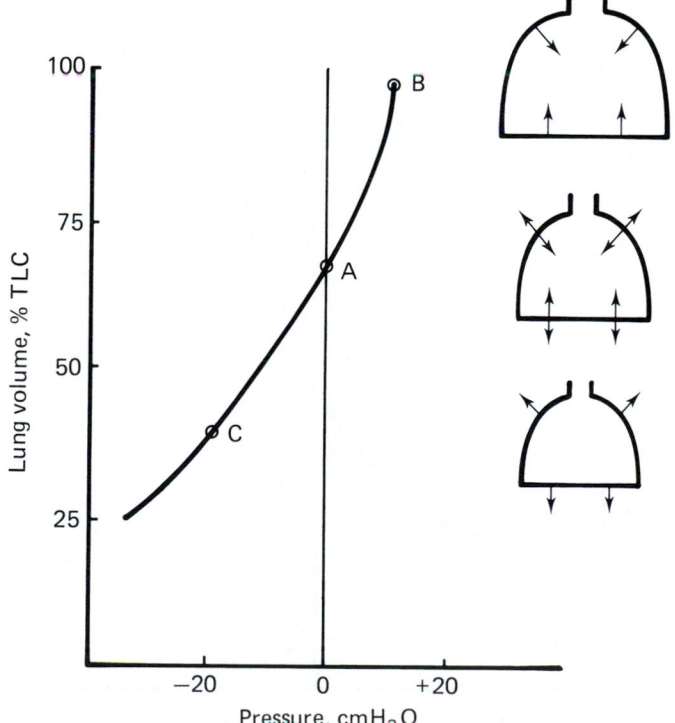

FIGURE 10-6 Pressure-volume relationships of the isolated chest wall. The equilibrium position of the chest wall *(A),* unopposed by the lungs, is approximately 70 percent of the total lung capacity. In this position, the pressure difference across the chest wall is zero. At larger volumes *(B),* there is inward recoil of the chest wall; at volumes below the equilibrium position *(C),* the recoil of the chest wall is directed outward, favoring expansion.

Since the elastic recoil of the lung is determined (under static conditions of arrested airflow) as the difference between alveolar pressure (Pa) and pleural pressure (Ppl)—i.e., Pa – Ppl—and the elastic recoil of the chest wall is determined (while the respiratory muscles are completely at rest) as the difference between pleural pressure and the pressure at the external surface of the chest (Pbs)—i.e., Ppl – Pbs, the elastic recoil of the entire respiratory system can be expressed as the sum of the two:

$$Prs = (Pa – Ppl) + (Ppl – Pbs) = Pa – Pbs$$

Thus, a measure of the elastic recoil of the respiratory system is supplied by the alveolar pressure, provided that the respiratory muscles are completely at rest and the pressure of the body surface is at atmospheric levels. In the absence of airflow into or out of the lung and when the glottis is open, alveolar pressure corresponds to the pressure at the mouth.

RELAXATION PRESSURE-VOLUME CURVE

The elastic properties of the entire respiratory system can be determined from the relaxation pressure-volume curve (Fig. 10-7). Functional residual capacity represents the equilibrium position of the lung-chest wall system while the respiratory muscles are relaxed. At this point, the opposing recoils of the lung and chest wall are of equal magnitude, and the recoil pressure of the entire respiratory system is zero. With increases in lung volume

above functional residual capacity, the recoil pressure of the entire system becomes positive, owing to the combination of an increase in centripetal elastic recoil of the lungs and a decrease in the centrifugal recoil of the chest wall. The net effect favors a decrease in lung volume, and lung volume can be maintained with the airway open to the atmosphere only by the action of the inspiratory muscles. As lung volume exceeds 75 percent of total lung capacity, the recoil of the chest wall also becomes centripetal and the recoil pressure of the chest wall adds to the inward forces acting to diminish lung volume. Total lung capacity represents the lung volume at which the inward passive elastic recoil pressure of the respiratory system reaches the maximum force that can be generated by the inspiratory muscles.

At lung volumes below functional residual capacity, when the centrifugal recoil of the chest wall exceeds the reduced centripetal recoil of the lungs, the relaxation pressure is negative and this net effect favors an increase in lung volume. Lung volumes below functional residual capacity are achieved and maintained by the muscles of expiration.

A switch from the sitting to the supine position decreases functional residual capacity because of the effects of gravity. In the upright position, gravity pulls the abdominal contents away from the chest wall. In contrast, in the supine position, the push of the abdominal contents against the diaphragm decreases the centrifugal recoil of the chest wall. The chest wall pressure-volume curve—and, consequently, the pressure-volume curve of the entire respiratory system—is displaced to the right.

DYNAMIC MECHANICAL PROPERTIES OF THE RESPIRATORY SYSTEM

The total nonelastic resistance of the lungs consists of the resistance of the airways to airflow (airway resistance), defined in terms of the driving pressure and the resulting rate of airflow, and the frictional resistance of the lung tissues to displacement during breathing (tissue resistance). Normally, tissue resistance makes up only 10 to 20 percent of the total pulmonary nonelastic resistance, but in diseases of the pulmonary parenchyma, it may increase considerably.

Airway Resistance

A large fraction of the resistance to airflow is in the upper respiratory tract, including the nose, mouth, pharynx, larynx, and trachea. During nasal breathing, the nose constitutes up to 50 percent of total airway resistance. During quiet mouth breathing, the mouth, pharynx, larynx, and trachea constitute 20 to 30 percent of the airway resistance; but they account for up to 50 percent of the total airway resistance when minute ventilation increases—during vigorous exercise, for example. Most of the remainder of airway resistance is in medium-sized lobar, segmental, and subsegmental bronchi up to about the seventh generation of airways.[9,10] Additional branching distally causes a progressive increase both in the number of airways in any generation and in the total cross-sectional area of the tracheobronchial tree. Consequently, in the normal lung, the small peripheral airways, particularly those less than 2 mm in diameter, constitute only about 10 to 20 percent of the total airway resistance.[22]

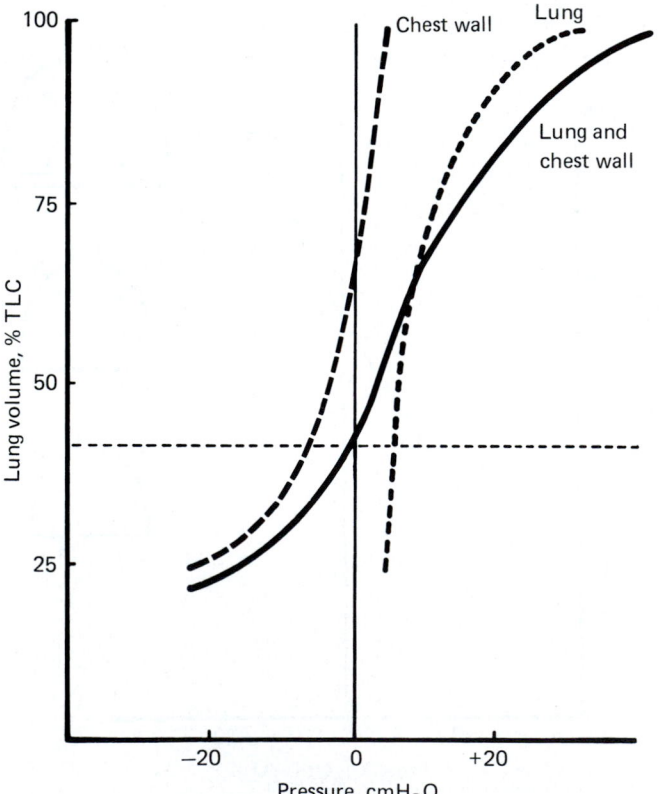

FIGURE 10-7 Relaxation pressure-volume curves. The elastic recoil pressures of the total respiratory system in the algebraic sum of the recoil pressures of the lung and chest wall are equal but opposite. Since the net recoil pressure is zero, the respiratory system is in a position of equilibrium.

AIRWAY CALIBER

The airways, like the pulmonary parenchyma, exhibit elasticity and can be compressed or distended. Therefore, the diameter of an airway varies with the transmural pressure applied to that airway—i.e., the difference between the pressure within the airway and the pressure surrounding the airway. The pressure surrounding intrathoracic airways approximates pleural pressure, since these airways are tethered to the parenchymal tissue and are exposed to the expansive forces that are active in overcoming the elastic recoil of the lung.[27]

As the lung volume increases, the elastic recoil forces of the lung increase; the traction applied to the walls of the intrathoracic airways also increases, widening the airways and decreasing their resistance to airflow. Conversely, at low lung volumes, the transmural airway pressure is lower and airway resistance increases.[16,37] If the elastic recoil of the lung is reduced—by destruction of alveolar walls in pulmonary emphysema, for instance—the transmural airway pressure at any given lung volume decreases correspondingly; the airways are narrower and airway resistance is greater even though there is no disease of the airways per se.

The effects of a change in transmural pressure on airway caliber depend on the compliance of the airways—which, in turn, is determined by their structural support. The trachea, for example, is almost completely surrounded by cartilaginous rings, which tend to prevent complete collapse even when the transmural pressure is negative. The bronchi are less well supported by incomplete cartilaginous rings and plates, whereas the bronchioles lack cartilaginous support. All airways can be stiffened, albeit to different degrees, by contraction of smooth muscle in their walls.

In patients with airway disease, mucosal edema, hypertrophy and hyperplasia of mucous glands, increased elaboration of mucus, and hypertrophy of smooth muscle further compromise airway caliber and increase airway resistance.

PRESSURE-FLOW RELATIONSHIPS:
THEORETICAL CONSIDERATIONS

In the lungs, pressure-flow relationships are extremely complicated because the airways consist of a system of irregular branching tubes that are neither rigid nor perfectly circular. For purposes of simplification, pressure-flow relationships in rigid tubes are generally regarded as a model for those in the airways.

The driving pressure that produces flow of air into and out of the lung must suffice to overcome friction and to accelerate the air. Acceleration in the lungs is of two types: local (i.e., changes in the rate of airflow with time when flow is initiated) and convective (i.e., acceleration of molecules of air over distance while flow is constant). The driving pressure required for convective acceleration is proportional to the gas density and to the square of the flow rate. It is important during expiration because, as air moves downstream from the alveoli toward the airway opening, the total cross-sectional airway diameter decreases; therefore, molecules of air must accelerate through the converging channels even though the overall flow rate remains unchanged. Also,

the driving pressure that produces high expiratory flow rates at large lung volume serves for convective acceleration rather than for overcoming friction.[18,36]

The driving pressure required to overcome friction depends on the rate and the pattern of airflow. Two major patterns of airflow warrant special consideration: laminar and turbulent. Laminar flow is characterized by streamlines that parallel the sides of the tube and are capable of sliding over one another. Also, because the streamlines at the center of the tube move faster than those closest to the walls, the flow profile is parabolic (Fig. 10-8). The pressure-flow characteristics of laminar flow depend on the length (l) and the radius (r) of the tube and the viscosity of the gas (n) according to Poiseuille's equation:

$$\Delta P = \frac{\dot{V}8nl}{\pi r^4}$$

where

ΔP = the driving pressure (pressure drop between the beginning and the end of the tube)

$\dot{V}$ = the flow rate that the driving pressure produces

r = the radius of the tube

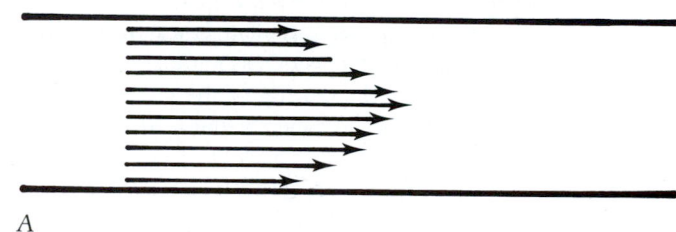

A

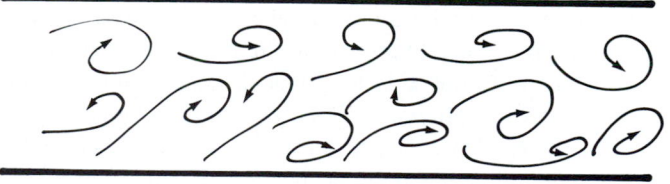

B

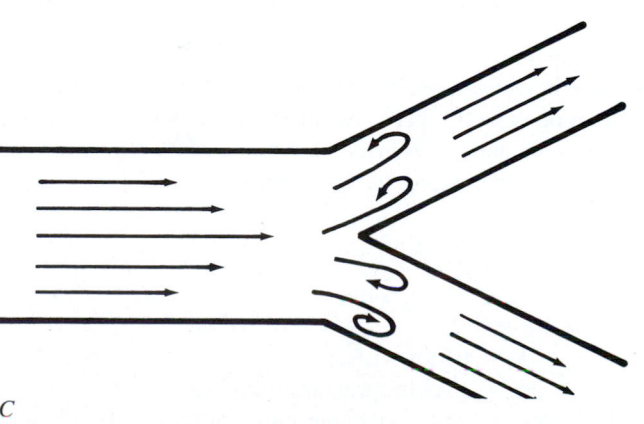

C

FIGURE 10-8   Patterns of airflow. A. Laminar flow. B. Turbulent flow. C. Transition flow.

The critical importance of tube radius in determining the driving pressure for a given flow is apparent in the above equation. If the radius of the tube is halved, the pressure that is required to maintain a given flow rate must be increased 16-fold. Laminar flow patterns occur only in small peripheral airways, where, because of the enormous overall cross-sectional area, flow through the individual airways is exceedingly slow.

Turbulent flow occurs at high flow rates and is characterized by a complete disorganization of streamlines, so that the molecules of gas move laterally, collide with each other, and change velocities. Under these circumstances, pressure-flow relationships change. In contrast to laminar flow, the rate of turbulent airflow is no longer proportional to the driving pressure. Instead, the driving pressure to produce a given rate of airflow is proportional to the square of flow and is dependent on gas density. Turbulent flow occurs regularly in the trachea.

At lower flow rates during expiration—particularly at branches in the tracheobronchial tree, where flow in two separate tubes comes together into a single channel—the parabolic profile of laminar flow becomes blunted, the streamlines separate from the walls of the tube, and minor eddy formation develops. This is referred to as a mixed, or transitional, flow pattern. In a mixed pattern of airflow, the driving pressure for a given flow depends on both the viscosity and the density of the gas.

Whether airflow is laminar or turbulent is predictable from the Reynolds number (Re), a dimensionless number that depends on the average velocity ($\overline{v}$), the density of the gas (ρ), the viscosity of the gas (η), and the diameter of the tube (D), so that

$$Re = \frac{\overline{v} \, D\rho}{\eta}$$

In straight, smooth, rigid tubes, turbulence occurs when the Reynolds number exceeds 2000. Therefore, turbulence is most apt to occur when the average velocity is high, gas density is high, gas viscosity is low, and the tube diameter is large. Since most of the resistance to airflow in the normal lung is in large airways, where resistance is density dependent, breathing a mixture of 80 percent helium and 20 percent oxygen (a mixture that is 64 percent less dense than air) increases airflow at a given driving pressure and substantially decreases airway resistance.[9]

CALCULATION OF AIRFLOW RESISTANCE

The driving pressure along the tracheobronchial tree—i.e., the difference between alveolar pressure and the pressure at the airway opening (mouth) that is required to produce a given rate of airflow into the lungs—provides a measure of the flow resistance of the airways, according to the equation

$$Raw = \frac{P_A - Pao}{\dot{V}}$$

where

$\dot{V}$ = airflow (L/s)
P_A = alveolar pressure (cmH_2O)
Pao = airway-opening pressure (cmH_2O)
Raw = airway resistance (cmH_2O/L/s)

FLOW-VOLUME RELATIONSHIPS

Considerable insight into the flow-resistive properties of the airways can be obtained from the relationship between airflow and lung volume during maximal expiratory and inspiratory maneuvers.[17] In practice, a person inhales maximally to total lung capacity; then exhales as forcefully, rapidly, and completely as possible to residual volume; and then returns to total lung capacity by a rapid, forceful inhalation (Fig. 10-9). During the maximal expiration, the rate of airflow peaks at a lung volume that is close to the total lung capacity; as the lung volume decreases and intrathoracic airways narrow, airway resistance increases, and the rate of airflow decreases progressively.

During the maximal inspiration, the pattern of airflow is different: because of the markedly negative pleural pressure and large transmural airway pressure, the bronchi are wide, and their calibers increase further as lung volume increases. Consequently, inspiratory flow becomes high while the lung volume is still low and remains high over much of the vital capacity even though the force generated by the inspiratory muscles decreases as they shorten.

A family of flow-volume loops is produced by repeating full expiratory and inspiratory maneuvers over the entire range of the vital capacity using different levels of effort (Fig. 10-10). The greater the effort exerted during inspiration, the greater is the rate of airflow over the entire range—i.e., from residual volume to total lung capacity. Similarly, during expiration, the rate of airflow increases progressively with increasing effort at large lung

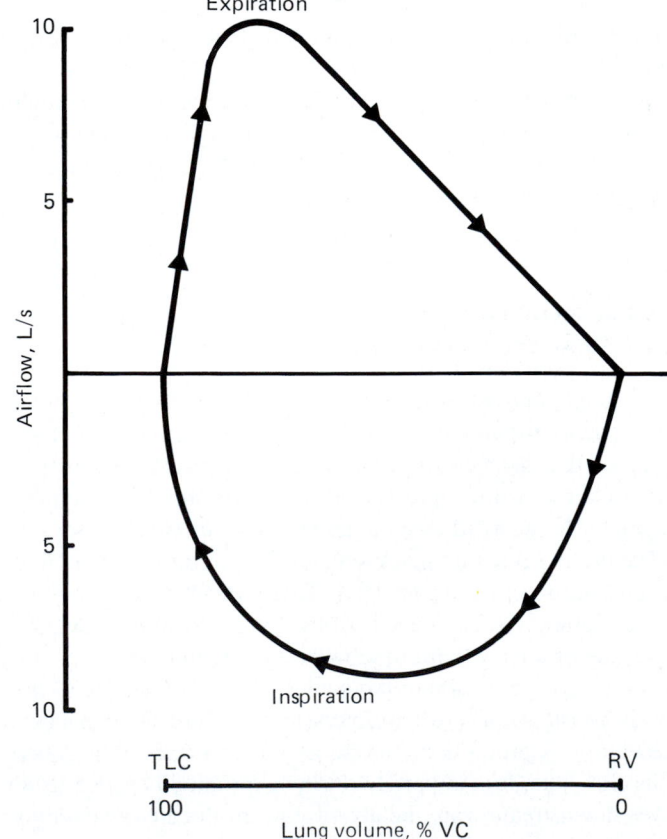

FIGURE 10-9   Maximal expiratory and inspiratory flow-volume loop.

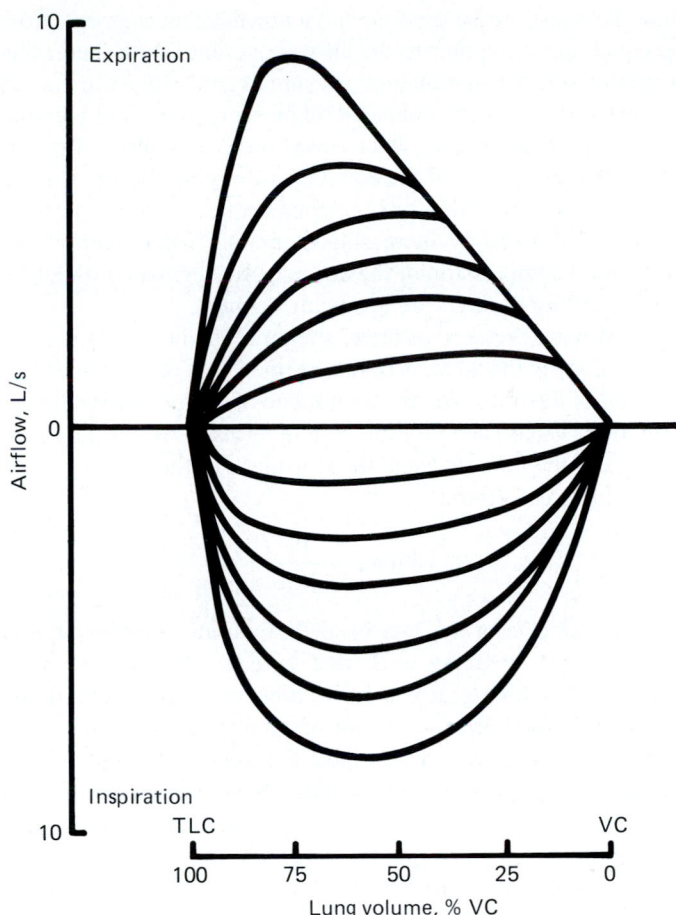

FIGURE 10-10   Series of flow-volume loops constructed from complete inspiratory and expiratory maneuvers repeated at different levels of effort.

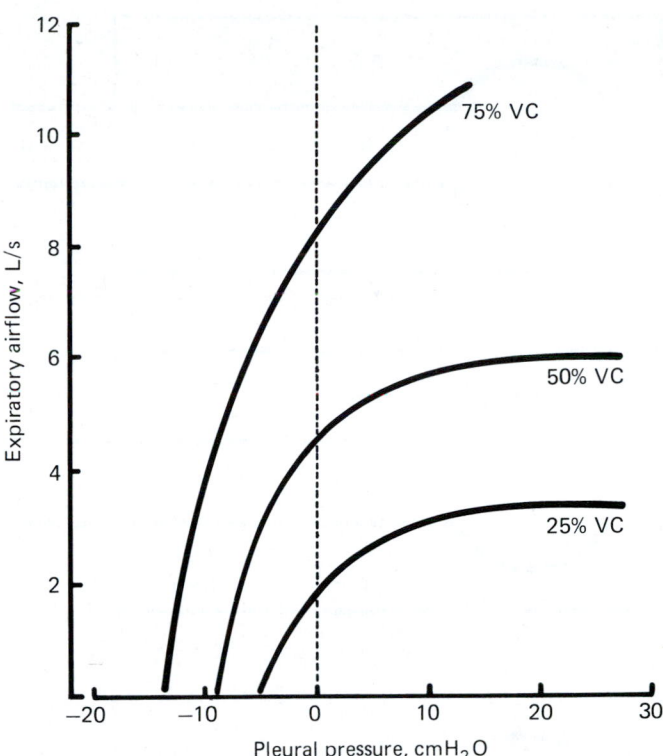

FIGURE 10-11   Isovolumetric pressure-flow curves. At lung volumes greater than 75 percent of the vital capacity, airflow is effort dependent; i.e., airflow increases progressively with increasing effort. At lower lung volumes, airflow is effort independent; i.e., airflow becomes fixed at a maximum level and does not increase despite further increases in effort.

volumes close to total lung capacity. At intermediate and low lung volumes, the rate of expiratory airflow reaches a maximum while the effort expended is only moderate; thereafter, airflow does not increase further despite increasing expiratory efforts.

Isovolume Pressure-Flow Curves

Separation of the effects of increasing effort from those of changes in lung volume on the rate of airflow during expiration can be accomplished by using isovolume pressure-flow curves (Fig. 10-11). During repeated expiratory maneuvers performed with varying degrees of effort, simultaneous measurements are made of airflow rate, lung volumes, and pleural pressure. For each lung volume the rate of airflow is plotted against the pleural pressure, an index of the degree of effort.[12]

As expiratory effort is increased at any given lung volume, the pleural pressure increases toward, and then exceeds, atmospheric pressure; correspondingly, the rate of airflow increases. At lung volumes greater than 75 percent of the vital capacity, airflow increases progressively as pleural pressure increases; it is considered to be effort dependent. In contrast, at lung volumes below 75 percent of the vital capacity, the rate of airflow levels off as the pleural pressure exceeds atmospheric pressure and becomes fixed at a maximum level. Thereafter, further increases in

effort, and in pleural pressure, effect no further increase in the rate of airflow; at these lower lung volumes, airflow is considered to be effort independent. Since the rate of airflow remains constant despite increasing driving pressure, it follows that the resistance to airflow must be increasing in direct proportion to the increase in driving pressure. This increase in resistance is attributed to compression and narrowing of large intrathoracic airways.

Equal Pressure Point Theory: Dynamic Compression of Airways

To illustrate the mechanisms that normally limit airflow during a maximal expiratory maneuver, it is useful to consider a model of the lung where the alveoli are represented by an elastic sac and the intrathoracic airways by a compressible tube, both enclosed within a pleural space (Fig. 10-12).[28]

At a given lung volume, when there is no airflow (as during breath holding with the glottis open), pleural pressure is subatmospheric, counterbalancing the elastic recoil pressure of the lung. The alveolar pressure (PA), which is the sum of the recoil pressure of the lung and pleural pressure (Ppl), is zero (Fig. 10-12A). Since airflow has ceased, the pressure along the entire airway is also atmospheric.

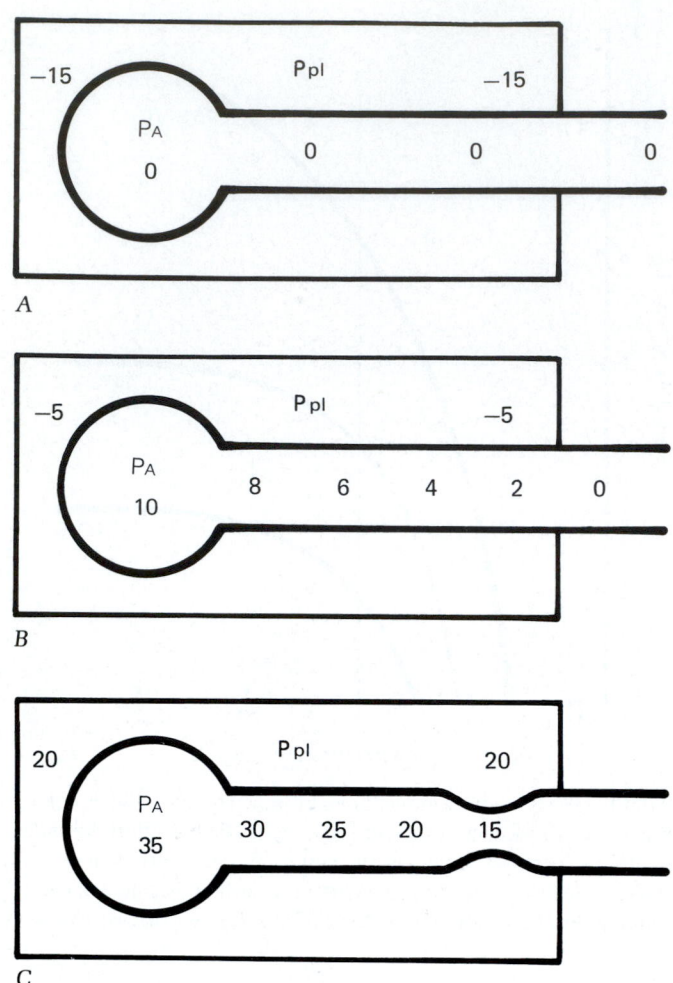

FIGURE 10-12 Schema of the distribution of pleural, alveolar, and airway pressures at rest and during expiration, illustrating the equal pressure point concept. *A.* End-expiration. *B.* Quiet expiration. *C.* Forced expiration.

At the same lung volume during a quiet expiration, pleural pressure is less subatmospheric. Since lung volume and the elastic recoil pressure of the lung are unchanged, alveolar pressure is now positive with respect to atmospheric pressure; airflow occurs. The alveolar pressure is gradually dissipated along the airway in overcoming resistance so that the pressure at the airway opening (Pao) is zero. All along the airway, however, the airway pressure exceeds pleural pressure and the transmural pressure is positive; the airways remain open, and flow continues (Fig. 10-12*B*).

A forceful expiration raises pleural pressure above atmospheric pressure and further increases alveolar pressure (Fig. 10-12*C*). Airway pressure again falls progressively from the alveolus toward the airway opening. But at some point along the airway—the equal pressure point—the drop in airway pressure is equal to the recoil pressure of the lung; intraluminal pressure and the pressure surrounding the airways are equal and the same as pleural pressure. Downstream (i.e., toward the airway opening) the transmural pressure is negative, because the intraluminal airway pressure is less than pleural pressure; the airways are subjected to dynamic compression.

The equal pressure point divides the airways into two components arranged in series: an upstream segment, from the alve-

oli to the equal pressure point, and a downstream segment, from the equal pressure point to the airway opening. With increasing expiratory effort as the pleural pressure becomes more and more positive with respect to atmospheric pressure, the equal pressure point moves upstream. Once maximum expiratory flow is achieved, the position of the equal pressure point becomes fixed in the region of the lobar or segmental bronchi. Further increase in pleural pressure by increasing expiratory force simply produces more compression of the downstream segment without affecting airflow through the upstream segment.

The driving pressure of the upstream segment—i.e., the pressure drop along the airways of that segment—is equal to the elastic recoil of the lung. The maximum rate of airflow during forced expiration ($\dot{V}max$) can be expressed in terms of the elastic recoil pressure of the lung (P_L) and the resistance of the upstream segment (Rus), as follows:

$$\dot{V}max = \frac{P_L}{Rus}$$

Measurements of the rate of airflow during force expiration form the basis of many tests used to assess the flow-resistive properties of the lung. It is evident, however, that the maximum rate of expiratory airflow depends on many factors: the lung volume at which airflow is determined, the force of expiration (particularly at high lung volumes—i.e., above 75 percent of vital capacity), the elastic recoil pressure of the lung, the cross-sectional area of large airways, the collapsibility of large intrathoracic airways, and the resistance of small peripheral airways.

Wave Speed Limitation Theory

An alternative explanation for airflow limitation during forced expiration is based on principles of wave speed theory.[8] The wave speed theory proposes that flow is limited by the velocity of propagation of pressure waves along the wall of the tube. The velocity of propagation (v) varies proportionally with the cross-sectional area of the tube (A) and the elastance of the tube walls (dP/dA). At a site where the linear velocity of gas molecules equals the velocity of propagation of pressure waves, a choke point develops, preventing further increases in flow rate. Where choke points occur in the tracheobronchial tree depends on the lung volume: at large lung volumes, a choke point is situated in the vicinity of the lower trachea; at lower lung volumes, choke points develop more upstream along the bronchial tree. Extension of the neck exerts longitudinal tension and stiffens the trachea, increases wave velocity, and increases maximum expiratory flow rates at large lung volumes.[26]

MECHANICAL DETERMINANTS OF REGIONAL VENTILATION

The lung is not homogeneous, and the mechanical properties of all airways in a given generation and of all alveoli are not the same. This results in important nonuniformities of regional ventilation.

Pleural pressure in the upright person is more subatmospheric at the apex than at the base of the lung, because of the effects of gravity and the weight of the lung.[14] Pleural pressure topography

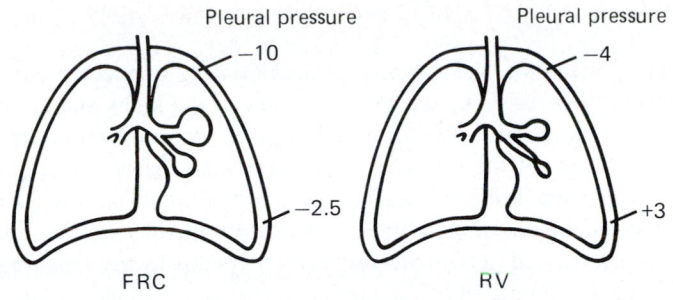

FIGURE 10-13 Pleural pressure gradients in the upright lung at FRC *(left)* and at RV *(right)*. The effect of the gradient on alveolar volumes is shown for each case.

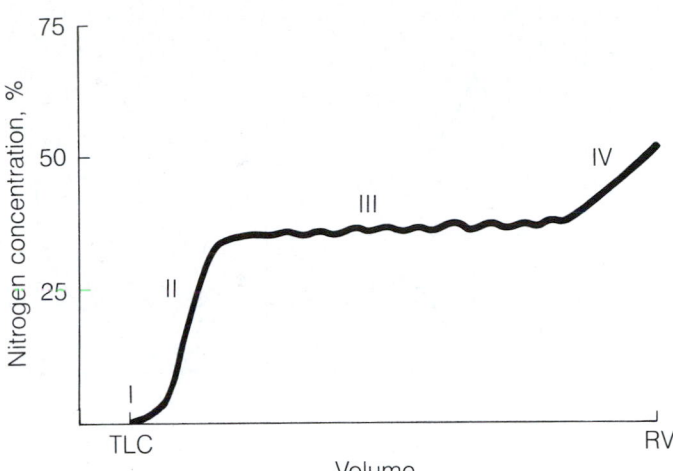

FIGURE 10-14 Tracing of expired nitrogen concentration during a slow expiration from TLC to RV after a full inspiration of pure O_2. The four phases are indicated.

and regional lung expansion are also determined by the shape of the chest wall and by the forces required for the lung to conform to the thoracic gravity shape.[7] The rate of increase in pleural pressure from top to bottom is approximately 0.25 cmH_2O per centimeter of vertical distance. Consequently, the transpulmonary pressure—i.e., alveolar pressure minus pleural pressure—is greater at the top than at the bottom of the lung. Therefore, at most lung volumes, the alveoli at the lung apexes are larger (more expanded) than those at the lung bases (Fig. 10-13).

Because of regional variations in lung compliance, ventilation is not uniform, even in the normal lung. With the use of external scanners after the inhalation of a radioactive gas, such as ^{133}Xe, it has been demonstrated that within the range of normal tidal volume, lung units are better ventilated, and ventilation per alveolus is greater, at the bottom than at the top of the lung.[30]

At low lung volumes (i.e., near the residual volume), pleural pressure at the bottom of the lung actually exceeds airway pressure and leads to closure of peripheral airways (Fig. 10-13). During a breath taken from residual volume, air that enters the lungs first is preferentially distributed to the lung apexes.

The distribution of ventilation within the lungs and the volume at which airways at the lung bases begin to close can be assessed by the single-breath N_2 washout test.[11] This test requires a maximum expiration into an N_2 meter after a maximal inspiration of pure O_2 from residual volume; the changing concentration of nitrogen is plotted against expired lung volume (Fig. 10-14). Because the inspiration starts at the residual volume, the initial portion of the breath containing dead-space gas, rich in nitrogen, is distributed to alveoli in the upper lung zones. The rest of the breath, which contains only O_2, goes preferentially to lower lung zones. Consequently, the concentration of nitrogen is lower in the alveoli at the lung bases than in the alveoli at the apexes of the lungs.

During expiration, the initial portion of the breath consists of O_2 remaining in the large airways; it contains no N_2 (phase I). As alveolar gas containing N_2 begins to be washed out, the concentration of N_2 in the expired air rises to reach a plateau. The portion of the curve where the concentration of N_2 rises steeply is phase II. The plateau is phase III. Phase III depends on the uniformity of the distribution of ventilation in the lung. If gas enters and leaves alveoli throughout the lung synchronously and equally, phase III is flat. But when the distribution of ventilation is nonuniform, so that gases coming from different alveoli have different N_2 concentration, phase III slopes upward.

At low lung volumes, airways at the lung bases close; only alveoli at the top of the lung continue to empty. Since the concentration of N_2 in the alveoli of upper lung zones is higher than in the alveoli at the lung bases, the slope of the N_2-volume curve increases abruptly, marking the start of phase IV. The volume, above residual volume, at which phase IV begins is the closing volume.[24]

Dynamic Compliance of the Lungs

The relationship between changes in volume and changes in pleural pressure during a normal breathing cycle is shown in Fig. 10-15. Airflow momentarily ceases at the end of expiration (A) and at the end of inspiration (C); the change in pleural pressure between these two points reflects the increasing elastic recoil of the lung as the volume of air in the lungs increases. The slope of the line connecting the end-expiratory and end-inspiratory points (AEC in the figure) on a pressure-volume loop provides a measure of the dynamic compliance of the lungs.

In normal persons, dynamic compliance closely approximates inspiratory static lung compliance and remains essentially unchanged even when breathing frequency is increased up to 60 breaths per min. This indicates that lung units that are parallel with each other normally fill and empty uniformly and synchronously, even when airflow is high and the change in lung volume is rapid. The rate of filling and emptying of a lung unit depends on its time constant—i.e., the product of its resistance and compliance. In order for the distribution of ventilation in parallel lung units to be independent of the rate of airflow, the resistance and compliance of these units must be matched so that the time constants of individual units throughout the lungs are approximately the same. The time constants of lung units distal to airways 2 mm in diameter are approximately 0.01 s, and fourfold differences in time constants are necessary to cause dynamic compliance to become frequency dependent.[23]

Patchy narrowing of small peripheral airways produces regional differences in time constants. At low breathing frequencies, when the rate of airflow is low, ventilation is fairly evenly

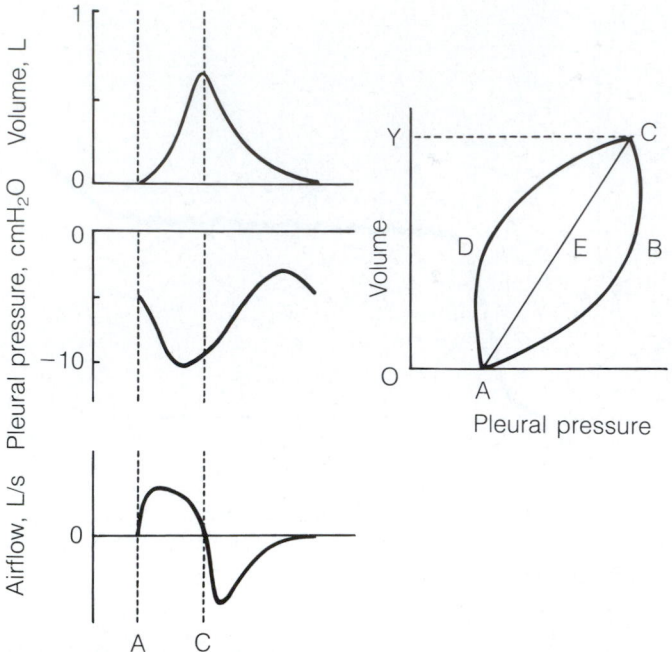

FIGURE 10-15 Individual tracings of tidal volume, pleural pressure, and airflow, taken simultaneously during a single complete breath, are shown on the left. The relationship between volume and pleural pressure is illustrated by the dynamic pressure-volume loop on the right. Dynamic compliance is determined as the slope of the line AEC. The work of breathing during inspiration to overcome the elastic forces of the lung is represented by the area of the trapezoid OAECY, and the work required to overcome nonelastic forces is represented by the area of the loop ABCEA.

distributed. As the breathing frequency increases, however, ventilation tends to be distributed to areas that offer the least resistance to airflow. Therefore, lung units fed by narrowed airways receive proportionally less ventilation than do areas of the lung where the airways remain normal; the change in pleural pressure required to effect the same change in overall lung volume increases. As a result, the dynamic compliance falls.

Measurements of frequency dependence of dynamic compliance are time-consuming and technically difficult, but this test has proved useful in the diagnosis of obstruction in small peripheral airways when results of other conventional tests of lung mechanics are still within normal limits.[41]

Interdependence and Collateral Ventilation

Important mechanisms in the lung promote a more even distribution of ventilation. For example, contiguous lung units attached by their connective-tissue framework are not free to move independently. This mechanical interdependence of adjacent lung units serves as a stabilizing influence and ensures uniform inflation.[42] Also, collateral channels of ventilation between alveoli (pores of Kohn) and from bronchioles to alveoli (canals of Lambert) enhance the uniformity of ventilation, particularly in patients with lung disease.[29]

WORK AND ENERGY COST OF BREATHING

During breathing, the respiratory muscles work to overcome the elastic, flow-resistive, and inertial forces of the lungs and chest wall.[32] The elastic work of breathing is done to overcome the elastic recoil of the lungs and chest wall; the resistive work is done in overcoming the resistance of airways and tissues. The mechanical work of breathing can be determined by relating the pressure exerted across the respiratory system to the resulting change in volume, since the product of pressure (P) and volume (V) has the dimension of work, according to the equation

$$\text{work} = \int P \, dV$$

Records of pleural pressure and lung volume changes during spontaneous breathing can be used to measure the work of breathing; the work of breathing performed on the lungs can be determined from the area of dynamic pressure-volume loop (Fig. 10-15) and fractionated into its elastic and resistive components. During inspiration, the work done to overcome the elastic forces of the lung is determined from the area of the trapezoid OAECY (Fig. 10-15). The area of the loop ABCEA is the work in overcoming nonelastic forces during inspiration, and the area of the loop OABCY is the total work of breathing during inspiration.

Expiration during quiet breathing is passive, since the elastic recoil of the lung suffices to overcome the expiratory airflow resistance. Some of the stored elastic energy is also used to overcome inspiratory muscle activity that persists into the expiratory phase of breathing. At high levels of ventilation and when airway resistance is increased, additional mechanical work during expiration is required to overcome nonelastic forces. Under these circumstances, the pleural pressure exceeds atmospheric pressure, and the loop AECDA extends beyond the confines of the trapezoid OAECY.

Work of Breathing

The work of breathing at any given level of ventilation depends on the pattern of breathing. Large tidal volumes increase the elastic work of breathing, whereas rapid breathing frequencies increase the work against flow-resistive forces. During quiet breathing and during exercise, people tend to adjust tidal volume and breathing frequency at values that minimize the force and the work of breathing.[25] Similar adjustments are also seen in patients with pulmonary disorders: patients with pulmonary fibrosis, which is characterized by an increased elastic work of breathing, tend to breathe shallowly and rapidly; those with airway obstruction and increased nonelastic work of breathing usually breathe more deeply and slowly.

The work done on the chest wall during breathing is calculated by subtracting the work performed on the lung from the total mechanical work of breathing. The total mechanical work of breathing cannot be readily measured during spontaneous breathing because the respiratory muscles that perform the work also make up part of the resistance offered by the chest wall. But the total mechanical work can be determined during artificial ventilation by using either intermittent positive airway pressure or negative pressure applied to the chest, provided that the respiratory muscles are completely at rest. For this determination, the change in lung volume is related to the pressure difference across the respiratory system—i.e., differential pressure between the mouth and the body surface. Disturbances of the chest wall, such as kyphoscoliosis and obesity, usually increase the work of breathing severalfold.

Oxygen Cost of Breathing

In order to perform their work, the respiratory muscles require O_2. The O_2 cost of breathing, which reflects the energy requirements of the respiratory muscles, provides an indirect measure of the work of breathing.[3,5] The O_2 cost of breathing is assessed by determining the total O_2 consumption of the body at rest and at an increased level of ventilation produced by voluntary hyperventilation or CO_2 breathing. Provided there are no other factors acting to increase O_2 consumption, the added O_2 uptake is attributed to the metabolism of the respiratory muscles.

The O_2 cost of breathing in normal subjects is approximately 1 ml/L of ventilation and constitutes less than 5 percent of the total O_2 consumption. At high levels of ventilation, however, the O_2 cost of breathing becomes progressively greater. There is a dramatic increase in the O_2 cost of breathing at high levels of ventilation in some diseases of the lung, such as pneumonia, pulmonary fibrosis, and emphysema, and in disorders of the chest wall, such as obesity and kyphoscoliosis. The increase in the energy requirement of the respiratory muscles during increased ventilation, concomitant with a decrease in O_2 supply secondary to arterial hypoxemia, probably produces muscle fatigue, thereby limiting the amount of exertion that these patients can sustain.[34]

REFERENCES

1. Altose MD, Crapo RO, Wanner A: Statement on the determination of static lung volumes. *Chest* 86:471–474, 1984.
2. Bachofen H, Hildebrandt J, Bachofen M: Pressure-volume curves of air- and liquid-filled excised lungs: Surface tension in situ. *J Appl Physiol* 29:422–431, 1970.
3. Campbell EJM, Westlake EK, Cherniack RM: Simple methods of estimating oxygen consumption and efficiency of the muscles of breathing. *J Appl Physiol* 11:303–308, 1957.
4. Clements JA: Surface phenomena in relation to pulmonary function. *Physiologist* 5:11–28, 1962.
5. Cournand A, Richards DW, Bader RA, et al: The oxygen cost of breathing. *Trans Assoc Am Phys* 67:162–173, 1954.
6. D'Angelo E, Agostoni E: Statics of the chest wall, in Roussos C (ed), *The Thorax,* 2d ed, Part A. New York, Dekker, 1995, pp 457–493.
7. D'Angelo E, Michelini S, Agostoni E: Partition of factors contributing to the vertical gradient of transpulmonary pressure. *Respir Physiol* 12:90–101, 1971.
8. Dawson SV, Elliott EA: Wave-speed limitation on expiratory flow—a unifying concept. *J Appl Physiol* 43:498–515, 1977.
9. Drazen JM, Loring SH, Ingram RH Jr: Distribution of pulmonary resistance: Effects of gas density, viscosity and flow rate. *J Appl Physiol* 41:388–395, 1976.
10. Ferris BJ Jr, Mead J, Opie LH: Partitioning of respiratory flow resistance in man. *J Appl Physiol* 19:653–658, 1964.

11. Fowler WS: Intrapulmonary distribution of inspired gas. *Physiol Rev* 32:1–20, 1952.
12. Fry DL, Hyatt RE: Pulmonary mechanics: A unified analysis of the relationship between pressure, volume and gas flow in the lungs of normal and diseased human subjects. *Am J Med* 29:672–689, 1960.
13. Gibson GJ, Pride NB: Lung distensibility: The static pressure-volume curve of the lungs and its use in clinical assessment. *Br J Dis Chest* 70:143–184, 1976.
14. Hoffman EA, Behrenbeck T, Chevalier PA, Wood EH: Estimation of regional pleural pressure surface espansile forces in intact dogs. *J Appl Physiol* 55:935–948, 1983.
15. Hoppin FG Jr, Stothert JC Jr, Greaves IA, et al: Lung recoil: Elastic and rheological properties, in Macklem PT, Mead J (eds), *Handbook of Physiology,* Sec 3, *The Respiratory System,* vol 3, Part I. Bethesda, MD, American Physiological Society, 1986, pp 195–216.
16. Hughes JMB, Hoppin FG Jr, Mead J: Effect of lung inflation on bronchial length and diameter in exercise lungs. *J Appl Physiol* 32:25–35, 1972.
17. Hyatt RE, Black LF: The flow-volume curve: A current perspective. *Am Rev Respir Dis* 107:191–199, 1973.
18. Hyatt RE, Wilson TA, Bar-Yishay E: Prediction of maximum expiratory flow in excised human lungs. *J Appl Physiol* 48:991–998, 1980.
19. Karlinsky JB, Snyder GL, Fanzblau C, et al: In vitro effects of elastase and collagenase on mechanical properties of hamster lungs. *Am Rev Respir Dis* 113:769–777, 1976.
20. Konno K, Mead J: Measurement of separate volume changes of rib cage and abdomen. *J Appl Physiol* 22:407–422, 1967.
21. Leith DE, Mead J: Mechanisms determining residual volume of the lungs in normal subjects. *J Appl Physiol* 23:221–227, 1967.
22. Macklem PT, Mead J: Resistance of central and peripheral airways measured by a retrograde catheter. *J Appl Physiol* 22:395–401, 1967.
23. Macklem PT, Mead J: Factors determining maximum expiratory flow in dogs. *J Appl Physiol* 25:159–169, 1968.
24. McCarthy DS, Spencer R, Greene R, Milic-Emili J: Measurement of "closing volume" as a simple and sensitive test for early detection of small airway disease. *Am J Med* 52:747–753, 1972.
25. Mead J: Control of respiratory frequency. *J Appl Physiol* 15:325–336, 1960.
26. Mead J: Respiratory flow limitation: A physiologist's point of view. *Fed Proc* 39:2771–2775, 1980.
27. Mead J, Takishima T, Leith D: Stress distribution in lungs: A model of pulmonary elasticity. *J Appl Physiol* 28:596–608, 1970.
28. Mead J, Turner JM, Macklem PT, Little JB: Significance of the relationship between lung recoil and maximum expiratory flow. *J Appl Physiol* 22:95–108, 1967.
29. Menkes HA, Traystman RJ: Collateral ventilation. *Am Rev Respir Dis* 116:287–309, 1977.
30. Milic-Emili J, Henderson JAM, Dolovich MB, et al: Regional distribution of inspired gas in the lung. *J Appl Physiol* 21:749–759, 1966.
31. Milic-Emili J, Mead J, Turner JM, Glauser EM: Improved technique for estimating pleural pressure from esophageal balloons. *J Appl Physiol* 19:207–211, 1964.
32. Otis AB: The work of breathing. *Physiol Rev* 34:449–458, 1954.
33. Rahn H, Otis AB, Chadwick LE, Fenn WO: The pressure-volume relationship of the thorax and lung. *Am J Physiol* 146:161–178, 1946.
34. Roussos C, Zakynthinos S: Respiratory muscle energetics, in Roussos C (ed), *Thorax,* 2d ed, Part A. New York, Dekker, 1995, pp 681–749.
35. Salazar E, Knowles JH: An analysis of pressure volume characteristics of the lungs. *J Appl Physiol* 19:97–104, 1964.

36. Schilder DP, Roberts A, Fry DL: Effect of gas density and viscosity on the maximal expiratory flow-volume relationships. *J Clin Invest* 42:1705–1713, 1963.

37. Stubbs SE, Hyatt RE: Effect of increased lung recoil pressure on maximal expiratory flow in normal subjects. *J Appl Physiol* 32:325–331, 1972.

38. Turner JM, Mead J, Wohl ME: Elasticity of human lungs in relation to age. *J Appl Physiol* 25:664–671, 1968.

39. Van Golde IMG, Tatenberg JJ, Robertson B: The pulmonary surfactant system: Biochemical aspects and functional significance. *Physiol Rev* 68:374–455, 1988.

40. Weibel ER: Functional morphology of lung parenchyma, in Macklem PT, Mead J (eds), *Handbook of Physiology,* sec 3, *The Respiratory System,* vol 3, Part I. Bethesda, MD, American Physiological Society, 1986, pp 80–112.

41. Woolcock AJ, Vincent NJ, Macklem PT: Frequency of dependence of compliance as a test for obstruction on the small airways. *J Clin Invest* 48:1097–1106, 1969.

42. Zidulka A, Sylvester JT, Nadler S, Anthonisen NR: Lung interdependence and lung–chest wall interaction of sublobar units in pigs. *J Appl Physiol* 46:8–13, 1979.

CHAPTER 11

CONTROL OF VENTILATION

Neil S. Cherniack / Allan I. Pack

Breathing is produced by the coordinated action of a relatively large number of muscles.[2] Principal among these is the diaphragm, which generates negative pressure in the thorax, thereby causing inflation of the lung. The diaphragm's action is complemented by that of other inspiratory muscles. Expiration, in turn, involves the coordinated action of muscles, which brakes the rate of air flow from the lung, and of the abdominal and other expiratory muscles, which can act to supplement the expulsive force provided by the recoil of the respiratory system. Since the action of each of these muscles has to be controlled, the control system for breathing has a number of distinct neural outputs (Fig. 11-1).

The action of these muscles is regulated to match the level of ventilation to metabolic demand.[5] Since the latter undergoes wide variations during normal behavior, there is a need for feedback systems (Fig. 11-1). Principal among these are the peripheral and central chemoreceptors monitoring the chemical status of the organism. Not only, however, does ventilation have to be set but so, too, does its pattern (e.g., the durations of inspiration and expiration and the magnitude of tidal volume).[4,8] One might anticipate that ventilatory pattern should be set to minimize the work of breathing, and certain evidence suggests that this is so. Control of pattern requires a different set of afferent information

that is provided principally by receptors in the lung monitoring its deformation. Finally, there is a need for more local feedback loops for each of the respiratory muscles to ensure that the central command to the muscle is executed. Such local feedback loops involve segmental reflexes in the spinal cord and are based on information provided by muscle spindles and tendon organs about the mechanical state of the muscle.

Thus, the respiratory control system is hierarchical.[1,8,10] Neural circuits must match efferent outflow to the need for ventilation (drive component) and generate appropriate oscillatory signals to the inspiratory muscles (control of ventilatory pattern). These descending signals can be modulated at the spinal cord by segmental afferent inputs (local control). To accomplish this, the central neuronal circuits produce a variety of efferent outflow signals (multi-output) and receive a large variety of afferent information (multi-input) (for schematic of system, see Fig. 11-1). In this chapter we discuss briefly the functioning of each of the major afferent systems, current knowledge as to the central pattern generator, and the role of the different respiratory muscles. The chapter concludes with consideration of certain of the integrated responses of the total system.

MAJOR AFFERENT SYSTEMS

Peripheral Chemoreceptors

The peripheral chemoreceptors affecting ventilation consist of the carotid and aortic bodies. Quantitatively, the carotid bodies are considerably more important. Indeed in humans (but not in all species) ventilation does not increase when subjects with denervated carotid bodies are exposed to hypoxia. During normal quiet breathing of ambient air (eupnea), the carotid bodies contribute about 15 percent of the ventilatory drive. They also account for about 30 percent of the ventilatory response to hypercapnia.[2,6,7]

The carotid bodies are situated in the neck at the bifurcations of the common carotid arteries (Fig. 11-2). The carotid bodies are supplied by blood from a branch of the external carotid artery, and their venous drainage is to the internal jugular. They have an enormous blood flow when one considers their small mass (of the order of 10 mg in humans); their blood flow is equivalent to 2 L/100 g per minute. Because of the large blood flow, the arteriovenous difference for oxygen is extremely small (0.2 to 0.5 ml per 100 ml). This large blood flow, coupled with the low extraction of oxygen, makes the carotid body relatively insensitive to variations in oxygen delivery (O_2 content $\times$ blood flow). Instead, carotid bodies respond primarily to changes in oxygen tension.[2]

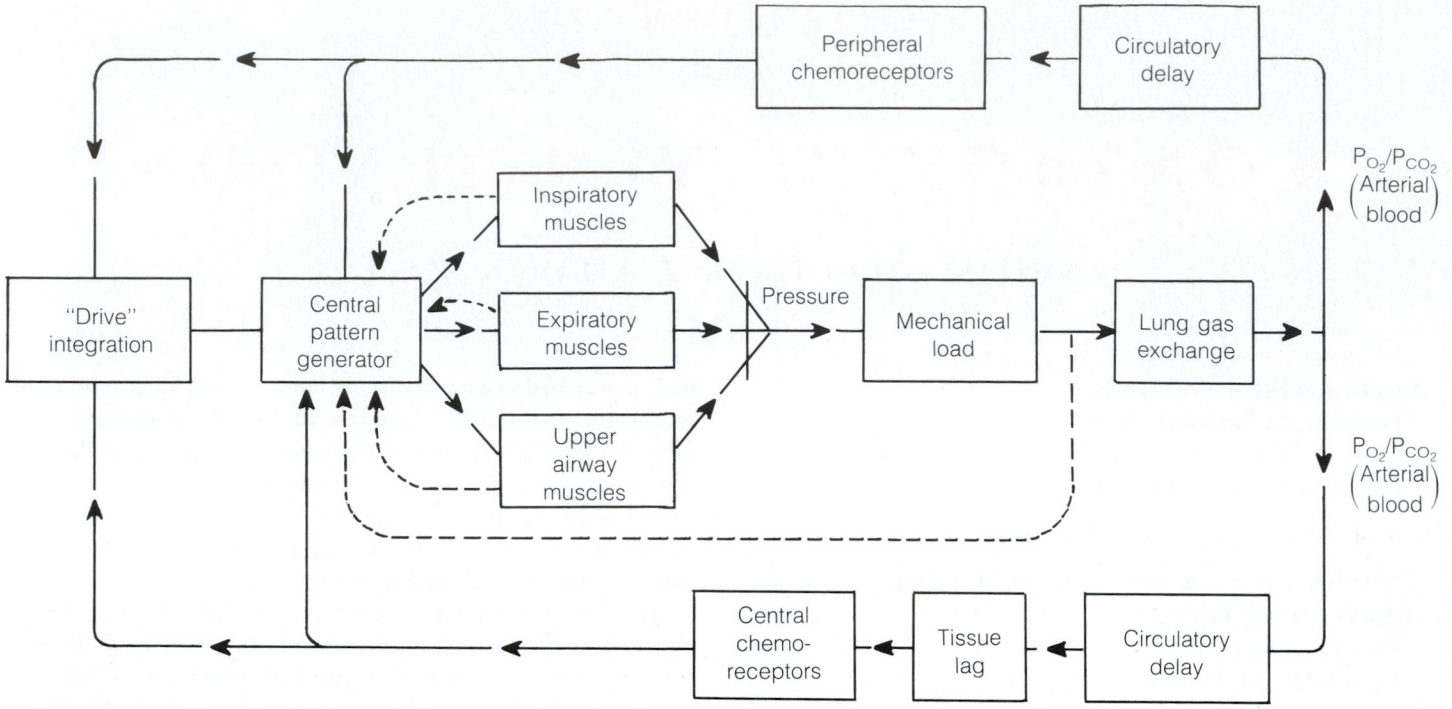

FIGURE 11-1   Block diagram of multi-input, multioutput system that controls ventilation. For further details see text.

The carotid bodies respond not only to hypoxia but also to increasing P_{CO_2}. At a constant P_{CO_2}, a hyperbolic relationship exists between receptor discharge and P_{O_2} (Fig. 11-3A), whereas at a constant P_{O_2}, the relationship between activity and P_{CO_2} is linear (Fig. 11-3B). The interaction is such that the receptors become more sensitive to P_{CO_2}, with increasing degrees of hypoxia (Fig. 11-3B). In addition to these characteristics, most, but not all, studies indicate that the receptors are sensitive to the rate of change of P_{CO_2}. This rate sensitivity involves carbonic anhydrase in some way, since it is abolished by acetazolamide.[2,5,7]

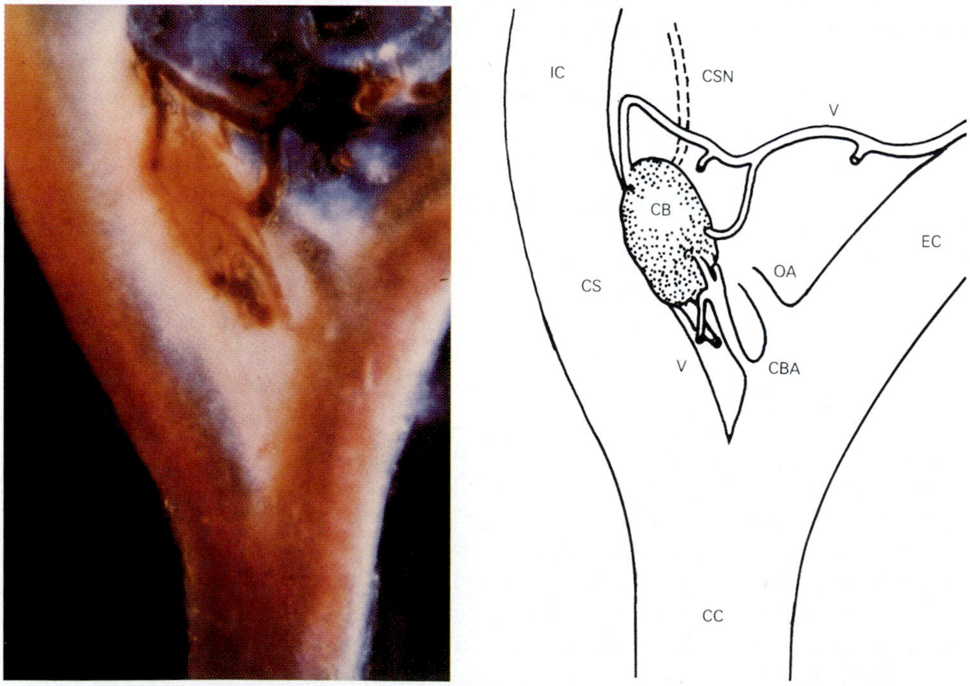

The rate sensitivity of the receptors, and their rapid response to changes in P_{CO_2} and P_{O_2}, enable the carotid body to follow respiratory-related oscillations in arterial blood-gas tensions. Since the magnitude of oscillations in arterial P_{CO_2} is directly related to metabolic CO_2 production, it has been proposed that this oscillatory signal contains the necessary information to produce the coupling between metabolic production of CO_2 and ventilation that occurs during exercise. This postulate has been the subject of much study, but experimental results have been conflicting.

The afferent signals from the carotid body are relayed in fibers in the glossopharyngeal nerve to the nucleus tractus solitarius. The chemoreceptor fibers are both myelinated and unmyelinated. In addition to the afferent fibers, there is both a sympathetic innervation of the carotid body and an afferent pathway in the glossopharyngeal nerve. Stimu-

FIGURE 11-2   *A.* Photograph (×40) of the carotid body in the rat situated at the bifurcation of the common carotid artery. The organ is highly vascular. *B.* Schematic representation of the various structures: CB = carotid body; CBA = carotid body artery; CS = carotid sinus; CSN = carotid sinus nerve; CC = common carotid artery; EC = external carotid artery; IC = internal carotid body; OA = occipital artery; V = vein from carotid body. *(Reprinted with permission from DM McDonald: Peripheral Chemoreceptors in Regulation of Breathing. New York, Dekker, 1981.)*

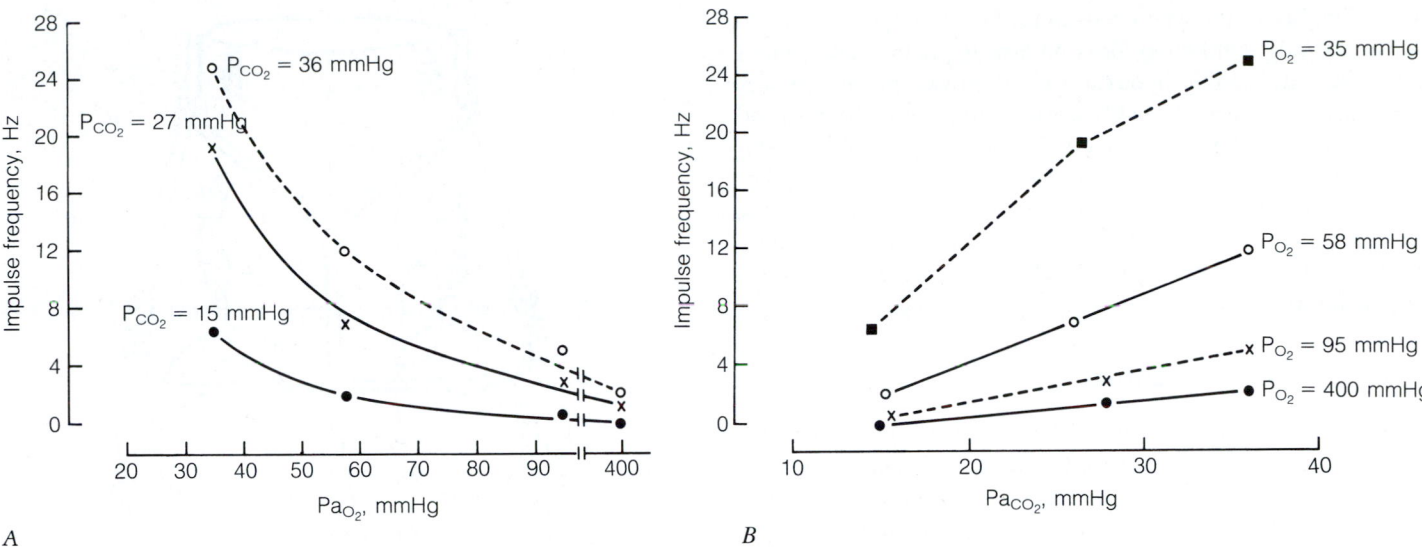

FIGURE 11-3 *A.* Relationship between carotid body afferent activity (single fiber) and P_{O_2} (at different levels of P_{CO_2}). *B.* Relationship between single-fiber carotid body afferent activity and P_{CO_2} at different levels of P_{O_2}. *(These data are redrawn from S Lahiri, RG deLaney: Respir Physiol 24:249–266, 1975.)*

lation of the sympathetic nervous system leads to an increase in carotid body discharge, an effect that is probably due to local changes in blood flow within the organ. In contrast, increased activity of the efferent glossopharyngeal pathway inhibits chemoreceptor discharge. Thus, the system makes possible direct control of the sensitivity (gain) of the carotid body.[2,6]

The majority of the afferent fibers terminate on glomus cells (i.e., the type I cells which constitute most of the specific cell types of the carotid body) (60 to 80 percent in different species). The type I cells appear to be secretory in nature, since they contain rough endoplasmic reticulum, aggregates of ribosomes, a well-developed Golgi apparatus, and dense core vesicles. The glomus cells are arranged in groups (glomerules), and each group is surrounded by the second main cell type of the carotid body (i.e., the sheath, or type II cell). These cells do not appear to be innervated, nor do they contain the dense core vesicles of the type I glomus cell.[6]

The type I cells contain catecholamines (dopamine, norepinephrine, and epinephrine) in their dense core vesicles. Of these, dopamine is the principal catecholamine (60 to 90 percent of the total catecholamine present), and its concentration is about the same as that in the adrenal medulla. The carotid bodies can take up circulating catecholamines and their precursors and can synthesize catecholamines from tyrosine. Enzymes responsible for each of the synthetic steps are present in the carotid body, the rate-limiting enzyme being tyrosine hydroxylase, which catalyzes the conversion of tyrosine to dopamine. Hypoxia affects the levels of dopamine in two ways: (1) by increasing secretion from glomus cells, thereby depleting their content of catecholamine; and (2) over a long time, by increasing production of tyrosine hydroxylase and, hence, of dopamine. The role of dopamine in chemoreception remains uncertain: we do not know if dopamine is an essential neurotransmitter or, as seems more likely, if it modulates the chemoreceptor process. What is known is that exogenously administered dopamine depresses chemoreceptor discharge.[2]

Catecholamines are not the only potential neurotransmitter in the carotid body. Also present are 5-hydroxy-tryptamine (serotonin), acetylcholine, and some of the neuropeptides—substance P, vasoactive intestinal polypeptide (VIP), met- and leuenkephalin. The role of these substances in the transduction process is also unknown. Acetylcholine has been proposed as an essential transmitter, since it is present in glomus cells, and exogenously administered acetylcholine stimulates afferent discharge. A plausible idea is that hypoxia stimulates glomus cells to release acetylcholine which in turn stimulates sensory endings. However, although plausible, this theory is probably incorrect, since pharmacologic blockade of acetylcholine's actions causes no change in the carotid body responses to hypoxia.[2,6]

Recent data indicate that both carbon monoxide (CO) and nitric oxide (NO) inhibit carotid body activity, although there is more compelling evidence for the more extensively studied NO. Mammals can synthesize NO and CO, and both act as chemical messengers in the body. NO formation from arginine is catalyzed by the enzyme nitric oxide synthase which is found in the carotid body, mainly in nerve fibers. Inhibition of NO synthase by a variety of I-arginine derivatives increases carotid body activity both in vivo and in vitro. Since NO is a vasodilator, its inhibitory action in vivo may be due to an increase in carotid body blood flow. But in addition, its effect in vitro and in vivo seems to be caused by an increase in NO produced by guanylate cyclase activity. Since NO synthase is itself inhibited by hypoxia, a decrease in NO formation in the carotid body may contribute to hypoxic stimulation of the carotid body.

Heme-oxygenase 2 (HO-2), which catalyzes CO production, is also found in type I cells. Metalloprotoporphyrins which inhibit HO-2 enhance carotid body discharge. CO like NO increases CPMP by activating guanylate cyclase.[7]

There is currently no agreement as to which component of the carotid body senses the change in oxygen tension. Some favor the sensory nerve terminals as the site of the sensing mechanism or even the sheath (type II) cell. The predominance of evidence implicates the type I cells as the O_2 sensor. There are two not necessarily conflicting ideas on how hypoxia excites type I cells: One idea is that hypoxia acts at the cell membrane, decreasing the conductance in O_2 sensitive potassium channels and thus leading to cell depolarization. The other, the so-called metabolic hypothesis, is that hypoxia interferes with respiratory energy production in type I cells, and this in turn triggers the increase in chemoreceptor discharge; cytochrome A_3 according to this idea is the biochemical substance responsible for O_2 responsibility.

Central Chemoreceptors

Knowledge of the functioning of the so-called central chemoreceptors is less complete than for the peripheral chemoreceptors. Indeed, whether the term *central chemoreceptors* should be used is debatable. What is known is that after denervation of the peripheral chemoreceptors, most of the response to hypercapnia is retained. Also, this central sensitivity to CO_2 is not mediated by the respiratory neurons themselves, since, if anything, they are inhibited (hyperpolarized) by the direct effects of increasing CO_2.[2,4,11]

That this central chemosensitivity is located in the ventral medulla was originally suggested by experiments involving infusion of acidic cerebrospinal fluid (CSF). More precise localization was achieved by applying pledgets saturated with solutions of low pH directly to different regions of the ventral medulla. Two chemosensitive regions were identified by these experiments. The first (rostral or Mitchell's) area extends caudally from the pontomedullary junction; it is bordered laterally by the roots of the seventh to tenth cranial nerve (Fig. 11-4). The second, smaller (caudal or Loeschcke's) area is situated at the origin of the twelfth nerve (Fig. 11-4). Since ventilation was increased by changes in H+ ion at the surface and decreased by local application of procaine, it was hypothesized that the chemosensitive elements were close to the surface of the medulla where they were influenced by the pH of the CSF.[2,11]

Between the two chemosensitive areas lies an interesting region, i.e., the intermediate area (IA) or "Schläfke's area" (Fig. 11-4). Cooling this small area, or applying procaine to it, markedly depresses ventilation and abolishes the response to inhaled CO_2. These observations have been interpreted to mean that the intermediate area is a site of convergence of fibers from the two adjacent chemosensitive areas as they pass to the respiratory complex in the dorsal medulla. But other evidence suggests that the intermediate area has a more general role in the regulation of ventilation and that its function is not just related to that of the central chemoreceptors.[11]

Although it is clear that experimental manipulations in regions near the ventral surface of the medulla (particularly near its rostral borders) can dramatically alter respiratory responsiveness to CO_2; it is not established whether these regions are integrating centers in a chemoreceptive pathway, the exclusive central chemoreceptors or one of many chemosensitive regions in the brain. Microinjections in the dorsal and the ventral medulla of acetazolamide, which inhibits the enzyme carbonic anhydrase and increases pH locally, can substantially increase phrenic nerve activity. This suggests that there are at least potential chemosen-

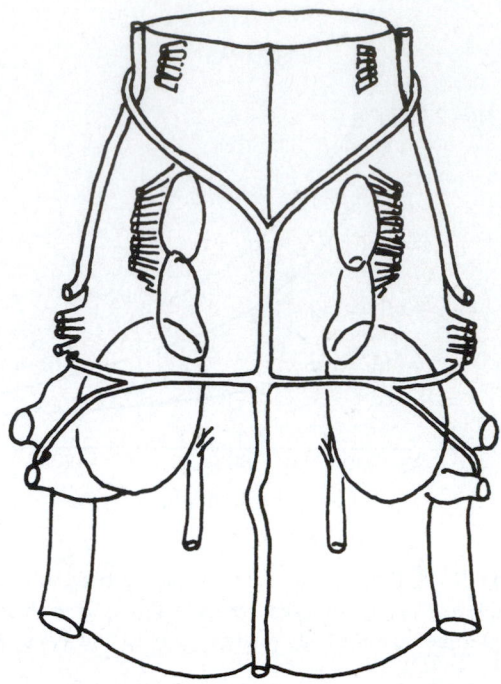

FIGURE 11-4 Outline of various regions on the ventral aspect of the medulla that are associated with the central chemoreceptor mechanism. The largest most rostral area is the chemosensitive area described by Mitchell. The smaller most caudal area is the chemosensitive area of Loeschcke. Between these areas is the region that is known as the *intermediate area*. (*This schematic is reproduced with permission from ME Schläfke, M Pokorski, WR See, RK Prill, HH Loeschcke: Bull Physiopath Respir 11:277–284, 1975.*)

sitive regions which are not located at the ventral surface. How important these areas are in mediating CO_2 response under more physiologic circumstances remains to be determined.[2,11]

The specific stimulus for the central chemoreceptors also continues to be a subject of debate. The prevailing theory is that the stimulus is uniquely related to hydrogen ion concentration at the receptor site. However, much of the evidence is indirect, based on mathematical predictions of extracellular pH. Most recent experiments, using techniques for measuring extracellular pH directly in this region of the brain, have cast doubt on the role of H+ ion as the unique stimulus, since different relationships between stimulation of respiration and H+ ion concentration are obtained depending on whether the changes in the H+ ion concentration are produced by respiratory or metabolic perturbations. A given decrease in pH produced by CO_2 inhalation has more marked effects on respiration than does the same decrease produced by metabolic acidosis, suggesting that CO_2 may, per se, have an additional stimulatory action. However, such experiments are somewhat problematic, since the precise location of the receptors is unknown and quantification of the pH "stimulus" can only be approximate.

Pulmonary Vagal Afferents

Complementing the information from the chemoreceptors are afferent systems that provide information about the state of the lungs and of the respiratory muscles; the latter are provided by muscle spindles and tendon organs. The intercostal and abdominal muscles are relatively richly innervated with both muscle spindles and tendon organs, whereas the diaphragm is relatively poor in muscle spindles.[2,4,8,10]

Within the lung there are thought to be four major receptor types: stretch receptors, rapidly adapting ("irritant") receptors, and two receptors that are innervated by nonmyelinated afferents. The last group of receptors is classified according to the receptors' different locations [i.e., either in the pulmonary interstitium (*juxtacapillary,* or *J, receptors*) or in the bronchi (*bronchial C receptors*)].[3] Although this separation for nonmyelinated afferents may seem somewhat artificial, the responses of the receptors in the two locations to different chemical stimuli are different. Moreover, certain theories center around the role of J receptors in the genesis of the increase in ventilation during exercise and during interstitial edema.

STRETCH RECEPTORS

The *pulmonary stretch receptor* shows a slowly adapting response to inflation of the lung that is maintained (Fig. 11-5A). This receptor is situated within the smooth muscle of the airway, and the highest density of receptors is in the more proximal airways.

The firing of the stretch receptors increases as the lung is inflated, and the receptors continue to fire even when the lung is static (Fig. 11-5A). However, their firing also depends on the rate of inflation (dynamic response).[2] At higher lung volumes, the receptor shows more marked sensitivity to changes in flow rate than to changes in lung volume (i.e., stretch receptors act increasingly as rate receptors at higher lung volumes).

RAPIDLY ADAPTING RECEPTORS

The *rapidly adapting receptors* (also called *irritant receptors* and *deflation* or *collapse receptors*) are also mainly in the larger airways; indirect evidence indicates that they are situated in the epithelium and submucosa.[3] Originally identified by their rapidly adapting response to lung inflation (Fig. 11-5B), the receptors quickly became known as irritant receptors. This change in nomenclature was based on observations that the receptors respond to a variety of chemical irritants (e.g., ammonia, cigarette smoke, ether vapor, and inert dust particles). Their response to inhaled irritants was thought to produce a defense reflex (i.e., coughing, bronchoconstriction, laryngeal constriction, and increased production of respiratory tract mucus). However, only a minority of receptors that respond to lung inflation by a rapidly adapting discharge show any response to inhaled irritants, and the firing of the rapidly adapting receptors, although somewhat erratic (compared to carotid chemoreceptors), shows a definite deterministic relationship between the rate and magnitude of inflation on the one hand and receptor activity on the other.

The irritant receptor fires predominantly during the inflation part of the respiratory cycle, and its firing depends strongly on the rate of air flow; also, decreases in compliance during inflation lead to increased firing of the receptor. The rapidly adapting receptor may be responsible for the generation of intermittent sighs without which pulmonary compliance decreases progressively.[2,3]

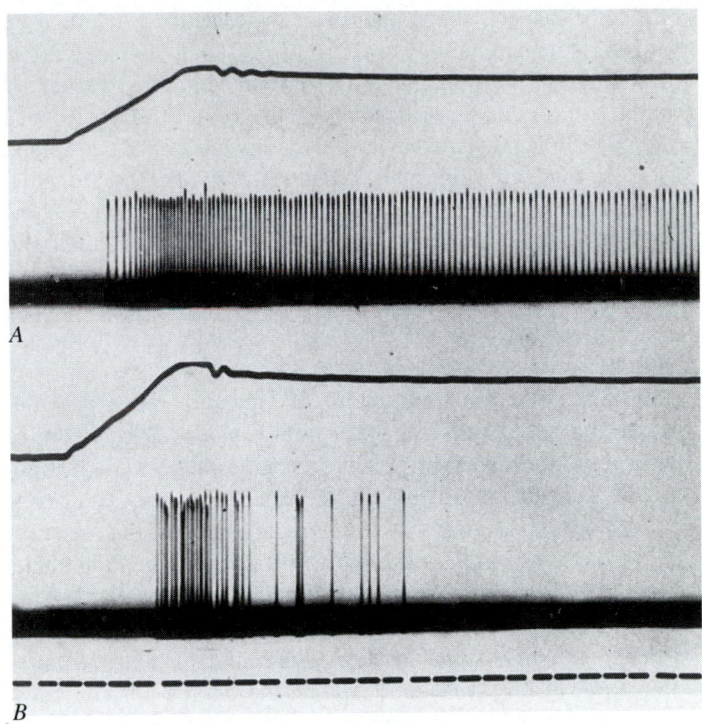

FIGURE 11-5   Response characteristics of the two major mechanoreceptors in the airways. *A.* A response of pulmonary stretch receptor. This shows the slowly adapting nature of the response and the continued discharge of the receptor during maintained inflation of the lung. *B.* Response of rapidly adapting ("irritant") receptor which fires largely during the period while the lung is being inflated and then adapts. (*Reproduced with permission from GC Knowlton, MG Larabee: Am J Physiol 147:100–114, 1946.*)

The rapidly adapting receptors have also been implicated in reflex bronchoconstriction. Chemicals released in asthma, such as histamine, cause bronchoconstriction not only by a direct action on smooth muscle but also by a reflex pathway. That rapidly adapting receptors might be an afferent component of such a reflex is largely based on demonstrations of their marked sensitivity to histamine.

BRONCHIAL C AND J RECEPTORS

A "new" group of nonmyelinated afferent endings appears to be mediators of reflex bronchoconstriction in asthma. These endings, identified by Coleridge and Coleridge, innervate receptors in the bronchi.[2,3] The bronchial C receptors are stimulated by phenyldiguanide and capsaicin, chemicals that are known to increase the firing of nonmyelinated endings. The receptors also respond to a variety of pulmonary autocoids released in asthma and inflammatory disease [i.e., bradykinin, serotonin, prostaglandins (PGF_{2a}, PGE_2, PGI_2), prostacyclin] as well as to inhaled irritants such as sulfur dioxide. The sensitivity of the receptors to bradykinin is marked, particularly when bradykinin is infused into the bronchial circulation. Activation of the receptors produces reflex tachypnea, increased tracheobronchial secretion, and bronchoconstriction. The low baseline firing of the receptors may contribute to baseline bronchomotor tone.

In some respects the responses of the receptors identified by the Coleridges are similar to those of the nonmyelinated afferent endings in the pulmonary interstitium described earlier by Paintal (i.e., the juxtacapillary or J receptors).[3] J receptors also respond to chemicals such as phenyldiguanide and capsaicin. However, there are important differences between the bronchial C receptors and the J receptors. In particular, J receptors show only weak stimulation in response to histamine and virtually no response to bradykinin. Whether this represents differences in the receptors themselves or in the metabolic properties of the different endothelia—since the chemicals are injected into the circulation in these experiments—is unknown.

The reflex effects of stimulation of J receptors are also somewhat different from those of bronchial C fibers. Stimulation of J receptors produces the pulmonary chemoreflex, a triad of apnea, bradycardia, and hypotension. Apnea may not be an integral part of this response but simply a reflection of intense stimulation, since less intense but more sustained stimulation elicits tachypnea rather than apnea. The cardiac depressor effects are due to both cardiac slowing and a fall in right ventricular stroke volume. Although some cardiac depression also occurs after stimulation of bronchial C receptors, the depression is modest compared to that for J receptors.

Stimulation of J receptors also inhibits motoneurons of the spinal cord by a central reflex mechanism; affected by this inhibition are the motoneurons that innervate the respiratory muscles and those involved in monosynaptic and polysynaptic, spinal reflexes. This component of the reflex response, which has been called the *J reflex,* led Paintal to propose that the receptors function to limit exercise by inhibiting motoneuron discharge whenever alveolar-capillary interstitial pressure increases as the result of interstitial deformation (e.g., by an increase in interstitial water). At present, the role of the J receptors can only be regarded as unsettled.

CENTRAL NEURAL MECHANISMS

Since respiration is a rhythmic motor act, the central neural circuits for respiration have to produce a rhythmic efferent outflow.[2,4,6,8,10] Of the various neural mechanisms that are capable of producing such rhythmic behavior, the prevailing view is that rhythmicity is a property of the synaptic interactions between the various types of respiratory neurons in the network. The rhythm which is generated consists of three parts: inspiration, postinspiration (phase 1, expiration), and late expiration (phase 2, expiration). Identification of these phases is based not only on the different mechanical functions of each (lung inflation, passive expira-

tion with braking of expiratory air flow, and active expiration, respectively) but also, perhaps more important, on the fact that each is controlled by different components of the neural network. These different components of the cycle are shown on a recording of phrenic nerve activity (Fig. 11-6).

During inspiration, inspiratory neurons in the medulla which are premotor to the phrenic and intercostal motor nuclei display an augmenting discharge. Intracellular recording from such neurons reveals that they receive increasing excitatory postsynaptic activity throughout inspiration. This activity is due, in part, to these neurons reexciting each other but, more than that, to an excitatory input, central inspiratory activity, that they receive from an unidentified source. Thus, these premotor neurons are driven by an "upstream" pattern generator.[2,6,8,10]

At the end of inspiration, discharge from these inspiratory neurons is extinguished by an "off switch." This seemingly simple concept, introduced by von Euler and colleagues, was based on examination of relationships between various afferent stimuli (e.g., lung volume and the duration of inspiration). The concept has since been supported in toto by neurophysiological studies. Inspiratory neurons receive a strong transient inhibition at the end of inspiration (off switch) that terminates the ramp increase of inspiratory neural activity (Fig. 11-6). The source of this inhibition is unknown, although activity has been recorded in certain neurons which fire just at the time of the inspiratory off switch (late inspiratory neurons).

However, the off switch is not totally abrupt as originally conceived. Instead, a period of graded inhibition, when the off switch is reversible, precedes the final off switch. Certain afferent in-

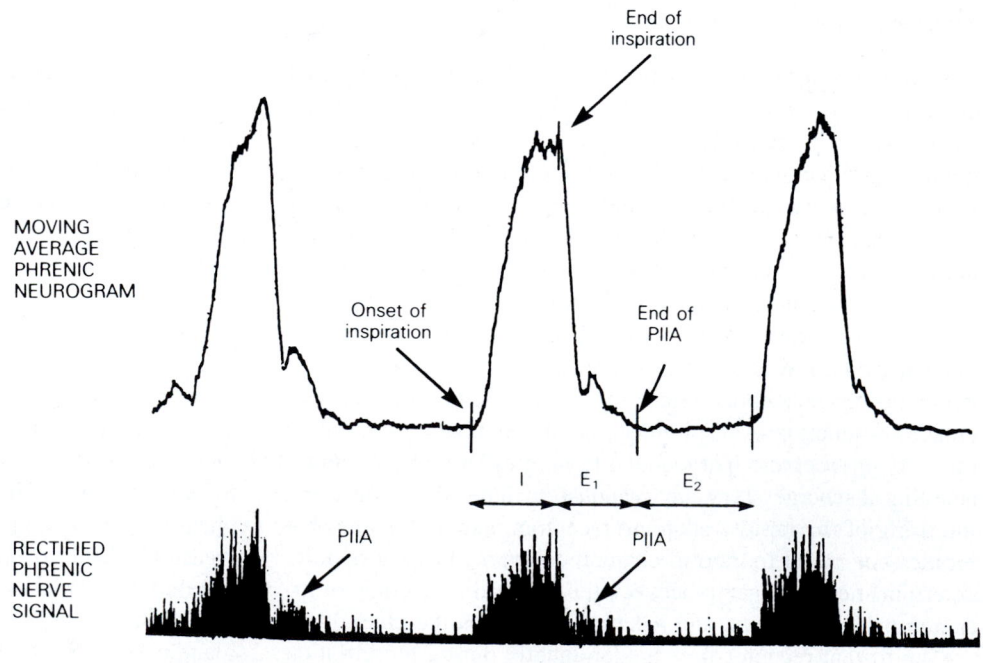

FIGURE 11-6   Different phases of the respiratory cycle shown by a recording of phrenic nerve activity (below) together with its moving average (above). The three phases are inspiration, postinspiratory activity (expiration, phase 1), and late expiration (expiration, phase 2). For further details, see text.

puts like the pulmonary stretch receptor affect the operation of the switching circuits. Increased activity of pulmonary stretch receptors shortens inspiratory duration. As a result, the larger the tidal volume, the shorter the duration of inspiration.[4]

The end of inspiration is followed by a period of postinspiratory activity on the part of certain inspiratory neurons. During this period of declining activity, the inspiratory neurons receive both excitatory and inhibitory postsynaptic potentials. This neural activity is associated with active braking of air flow at the beginning of expiration. The duration of this postinspiratory phase of the respiratory cycle seems to be an important determinant of total duration of expiration.[6,8]

After the postinspiratory phase of the respiratory cycle, there is a period during which the expiratory muscles may undergo active contraction. In this phase of the cycle, inspiratory bulbospinal neurons receive inhibitory postsynaptic potentials in an augmenting pattern. A particular group of expiratory neurons in the retrofacial nucleus (Botzinger complex) has been shown to be capable of generating this inhibition.[8,10]

Although the duration of expiration, like inspiration, can be set by intrinsic brainstem mechanisms, normally it is modulated by afferent inputs. Throughout expiration, there is a decreasing inhibition of the following inspiration. Thus, early in expiration larger stimuli (e.g., pulmonary deflations) are needed to trigger the onset of inspiration than later in expiration. In addition to this intrinsic process, there are various afferent inputs. As in the case of inspiration, afferents from pulmonary stretch receptors are particularly important. Activity of these stretch receptors prolongs expiration (i.e., the Hering-Breuer expiratory promoting reflex). Central processing of this afferent activity is complex and involves a process akin to leaky integration. The time constants of this processing are now known.

Some investigations consider the breathing pattern to be produced by the interaction of a rhythm-generating circuitry and a central pattern-forming network.

The site of the rhythm-generating circuitry is unknown. Several sites in the ventral medulla have been implicated, including the pre-Bötzinger complex and the retrotrapezoid nucleus. The rhythm generator is believed to consist of conditional pacemaker neurons embedded within an oscillating network. Although pacemaker neurons seem to be involved in breathing in immature animals, their importance in the adult is questionable. The rhythm generated, produced or not by pacemaker neurons, is formed and shaped through the interactions of groups of premotor, motor, and sensory neurons.[6,10]

Recent studies have focused on the cellular mechanisms that shape the respiratory burst. These include levels of membrane polarization, concentrations of calcium and potassium channels and the level of their currents, and actions of excitation and inhibitory neurotransmitters.

COORDINATION OF THE ACTIVITY OF THE RESPIRATORY MUSCLES

The chest wall itself is flexible and, although the ribs and the spine act as a framework to preserve its shape, the coordinated activity of the muscles which insert upon the thoracic cage not only brings air to the alveoli but also prevents the waste of energy that could be caused by chest wall distortion during breathing.[2]

The pharyngeal channels, which air must traverse before arriving at the lungs, also have flexible walls and contain valve-like mobile structures that can be displaced to obstruct the airways by the negative and positive swings in pressure that occur during normal breathing. The rigidity and configuration of these channels and their patency again depend on the skeletal muscles, and the activity of this group of muscles has a respiratory modulation that increases as breathing is stimulated.

Thoracic Muscles

During quiet breathing the diaphragm is the muscle mainly responsible for the tidal excursions of air. As the diaphragm contracts, it presses on the abdominal contents, which are primarily fluid, to push the abdominal wall outward. At the same time, through its insertions on the lower ribs, the diaphragm elevates the costal margins and expands the chest cavity.

Even the small transthoracic pressure changes that occur during breathing are sufficient to distort the chest wall. Acting alone, the diaphragm would use energy not only to overcome the resistance of the airways and the stiffness of the chest wall but also to distort the ribs. Contraction of the parasternal intercostal muscles, and perhaps the scalene muscles, prevents this distortion.[2]

Expiration is largely passively determined by the elastic recoil of the chest wall. But usually the inspiratory muscles continue to contract, albeit at a steadily decreasing rate, during early expiration to retard the egress of air from the lungs. This postinspiratory activity may help to improve the efficiency of gas exchange and, in infants (in whom the chest wall is extremely pliable), may help to preserve the functional residual capacity by preventing too much air from leaving the lungs during the expiratory period.

The diaphragm itself does not behave as if it were a single muscle. The costal portion of the diaphragm is supplied mainly by the upper cervical roots which make up the phrenic nerve, whereas the crural portion of the diaphragm receives its innervation mainly through the lower phrenic roots. Isolated contraction of the crural diaphragm causes primarily expansion of the abdomen, whereas contraction of the costal portion, in addition to causing movement of the abdominal wall, enlarges the rib cage. The crural diaphragm may also act as a part of the sphincter mechanism for the lower esophagus; its contraction compresses the sphincter. For this role the action of the crural diaphragm is coordinated with motor events for the gastrointestinal system. As an example, the activity of the crural diaphragm is inhibited during swallowing and vomiting.

The phrenic motor neurons themselves have been divided into early firing units, the activity of which begins at the very onset of inspiration, and late firing units, which commence their activity much later in inspiration. It is interesting that the early units are the ones that are responsible for postinspiratory activity. The crural diaphragm may contain more of these early units, since electrical activity of that part of the diaphragm generally precedes activity in the costal portion.

As respiration increases, the frequency of firing of both the early and late units increases; in addition, more and larger motor units are recruited according to a "size principle." Phrenic neurons supplying larger motor units (which contain more fibers) are recruited later than are neurons that innervate smaller units (Fig. 11-7). Also, as ventilation increases, the intercostal muscles come into play, the upper intercostals becoming active first and then the lower intercostals. The expiratory muscles begin to contract at higher levels of ventilation, and the duration of the postinspiratory inspiratory activity decreases. At high levels of ventilation, the "accessory" muscles of respiration, such as the sternocleidomastoid, the hyoid muscle, and muscles attaching to the spine, also contribute to breathing.[2,5,9]

The diaphragm, like other skeletal muscles, has less ability to produce force as the velocity of contraction and the degree of shortening increase. The ability of the respiratory system to increase tidal volume is preserved by at least three compensatory mechanisms: (1) Motor output to the diaphragm grows greater; (2) as air flow accelerates, reflex mechanisms (possibly from rapidly adapting receptors) further increase motor output; and (3) the recruitment of more muscles helps curtail the load on the diaphragm.[2]

When skeletal muscles are made to contract forcibly over long periods, they tire (i.e., are unable to generate as much pressure). The diaphragm can also become fatigued when it is obliged to develop large pressure changes because of either sustained respiratory stimulation or chronic mechanical impairment of the lungs. Fatigue leads to decreasing tidal volume and, ultimately, to CO_2 retention. Diaphragm fatigue can result from interference with cellular contractile mechanisms but can also be central in origin. Afferent signals from the diaphragm, originating from unspecified receptors that project to the brain via the phrenic nerves, may signal impending fatigue and enable motor output to diminish, thereby preventing irreversible damage to the muscle itself.[2]

Upper Airway Muscles

The muscles of the upper airways also serve an important respiratory function. Contraction of the posterior cricoarytenoid muscle during inspiration to open the laryngeal aperture, an important site of airway resistance, increases the efficiency of energy used by the thoracic muscles during breathing. Changes in the laryngeal aperture are thus synchronized with breathing. When respiratory drive is increased, as during exercise or acute hypercapnia, the magnitude of this modulation increases.[9]

In addition to the larynx, activity of the cranial nerves that innervate muscles of the upper airways, such as the alae nasi (the nasal dilator), the genioglossus (the protrussor muscle of the tongue), and the muscles inserting on the hyoid, varies with the breathing cycle. During inspiration these muscles contract, dilating the upper airway passages and overcoming the negative intraluminal pressures produced by shortening of the thoracic muscles. This inspiratory activity may be of particular importance during sleep when the alignment of gravitational forces favors occlusion of the upper airways. Inspiratory activity of the

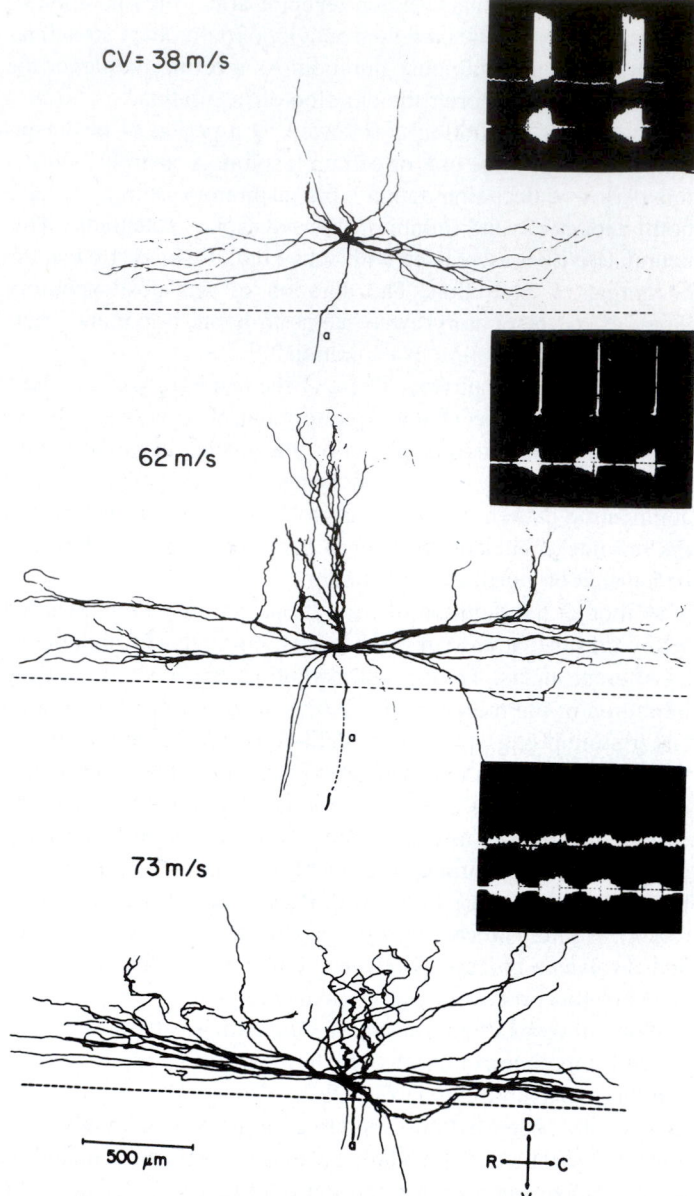

FIGURE 11-7   Examples of structure of these phrenic motor neurons which fire at different times during inspiration. The cellular structures were obtained by reconstruction of structure of neurons labeled by intracellular horseradish peroxidase. The inserts show the intracellular recording from the neuron above and recording of mass phrenic nerve activity (below). CV is the conduction velocity of the axon. The cell in the top panel is the smallest with lowest conduction velocity. It fires throughout inspiration. The cell in the bottom panel is the largest with highest conduction velocity. Its membrane potential is modulated with respiration, but it does not fire during eupnea. The cell in the middle is between these extremes and fires only at the end of the inspiratory burst. These data conform to the size principle. The broken line indicates the ventral margin of the gray matter and *A* indicates the axon. D = dorsal; V = ventral; R = rostral; C = caudal. (*From WE Cameron, DB Averill, AJ Berger: Neurogenesis of Central Respiratory Rhythm, London, MTP Press, 1985.*)

upper airways also begins slightly before the onset of activity of the chest wall muscles. This difference in time of onset within a breath may also help to prevent airway obstruction.

The upper airway muscles seem to be far more susceptible to the inspiratory inhibiting action of pulmonary stretch receptor input than are the muscles of the chest wall. The reduction in stretch receptor stimulation that occurs during airway occlusion increases the inspiratory activity of the upper airway muscles far more than that of either diaphragm or intercostal muscles. This heightening of discharge helps to dilate the upper airways and to prevent obstruction during breathing.

DISTURBANCES OF RESPIRATORY RHYTHM

Regularity of Breathing

The normal range of variability of breathing has been studied by only a few investigators. Tidal volume and inspiratory and expiratory times tend to fluctuate more than ventilation because breath duration in general is longer with larger tidal volumes and is shorter when tidal volume is smaller. Variability tends to be less with exercise and hypercapnia, but hypoxia has a less consistent effect, sometimes improving the constancy of breathing but at times causing cyclic fluctuations in ventilation level. Individuals with absent or poor ventilatory responses to hypercapnia and hypoxia frequently have irregular breathing patterns at rest.[2,9]

Whereas these random variations can be considered an unwanted feature of breathing, these fluctuations in breathing patterns may serve a useful purpose in allowing the controller to better detect changes in the mechanical characteristics of the respiratory muscles and lungs.

Irregularities in breathing depth may also help improve lung function. When patients are artificially ventilated at constant rates for prolonged periods, areas of atelectasis form, and lung compliance decreases. This reduction in compliance can be reversed by intermittently causing the patient to sigh (allowing the ventilator to produce large tidal volumes). Sighs also occur during normal spontaneous breathing and seem to have the same purpose of reopening atelectatic lung regions. Sighs occur more frequently when breathing is stimulated, particularly when the stimulus is hypoxia.

In addition to random disturbances and sighs, regularly recurring short-period oscillations in ventilation, gas exchange, and blood-gas tensions have been reported, but variations in arterial P_{O_2} rarely exceed 3 to 4 mmHg and in P_{CO_2} are even less. Techniques such as autocorrelation, power spectral density analysis, and, more recently, comb filtering have been used to uncover periodicities in ventilation and in blood pressure and heart rate that are not immediately obvious because of the masking effect of noise.[2]

In addition to these short ultradian oscillations, circadian oscillations in ventilation and circulation have been described. Circadian oscillations are found in many biologic systems and seem to depend on the presence of internal clocks. In higher animals it is believed that there is a multiplicity of such clocks arranged in an hierarchical order. Circadian changes seem to be under the control of at least two master clocks. One master clock seems to be located in the suprachiasmatic nucleus (SCN) of the hypothalamus and is responsible for the circadian variation in calcium secretion in the urine, growth hormone release, recurrence of nonrapid eye movement (NREM) sleep, and skin temperature. Destruction of the SCN produces sleep fragmentation. A retinohypothalamic projection between the SCN and the eye apparently accounts for the entrainment of the circadian activity cycle to the light-dark variation.

However, even when the SCN is destroyed, the circadian oscillation in core temperature persists. Hence there seems to be still another master clock with as yet undetermined location. In addition to temperature this clock also appears to control the circadian secretion of cortisols, the REM sleep pattern, and urinary excretion of potassium.

It is known that the amplitude of circadian oscillations in activity temperature shows considerable interindividual differences. It is possible that similar variability occurs in circadian respiratory oscillations, depending on the relative sensitivity of ventilation to temperature and metabolic changes.

Feedback Control

Instability in feedback control can affect the regularity of breathing. Ventilation is adjusted to meet changes in external conditions and internal demands by regulating systems which limit variations in arterial P_{CO_2} and P_{O_2} using feedback control. Although biologic control systems are much more complex than physical ones, design principles seem similar, and some abnormalities in breathing resemble disturbances occurring in systems used to control machines. Ideally, biologic control systems minimize the effects of disturbances and rapidly restore steady-state conditions to prevent wide swings in the internal conditions and to operate with minimal use of energy. It may not be possible for the control system to meet all these objectives simultaneously. Fluctuations in arterial blood-gas tensions can arise if the system is excessively stressed or from destruction of key components in the control system which render it insensitive; less obviously, they may also occur if control is too rigorous.[2,5,9]

Like physical control systems, the feedback system that regulates P_{O_2} and P_{CO_2} can be considered to consist of a controller and controller elements linked by feedback loops. In this system the controller consists of the central and peripheral chemoreceptor neurons in the brain. The peripheral chemoreceptors which monitor arterial P_{CO_2} and P_{O_2} and the central chemoreceptors which monitor hydrogen ion concentration in the interstitial fluid communicate with groups of neurons in the brain (most heavily concentrated in the bulbopontine areas) which govern the activity of the muscles of breathing, allowing the lungs to be ventilated. The controlled system consists of these respiratory muscles and the O_2 and CO_2 chemically bound and physically dissolved in the body (the gas stores). Hypoxia and hypercapnia may affect the electrical activity and the forces generated by the upper airway and chest wall muscles dissimilarly so that coordination of the activity of these different muscles is crucial. Changes in ventilation alter the amount of CO_2 and O_2 stored in the lung, blood, and tissues and so adjust the level of P_{CO_2} and O_2. Information on gas tension is transmitted to the sensors by the circulation. The bulbopontine neurons sense the difference between the input from the chemosensors and desired reference value levels and readjust the output to the respiratory muscles to reduce the discrepancy. State of alertness and sleep alter reference values.

Although the function of feedback control systems is to maintain oxygen and acid-base homeostasis and not to regularize ventilation, in steady states they have this effect. In feedback control systems, cyclic changes in both the rate of breathing and tidal volume can result from rhythmic changes in input or instability in control system operation. Common mechanisms that produce instability include transport delays and increased loop gain (caused by greater controller sensitivity or changes in operating point which allow the controller to exert a larger effect of the controlled system). In linear control systems, the occurrence of instability and the characteristics of the cyclic changes can be predicted by graphic techniques, for example, by the Bode and Nyquist diagrams. However, the respiratory control system behaves alinearly, and the prediction of the effects of specific alterations in system components usually requires the use of mathematical models. Although they differ somewhat in details, models of the respiratory system show that unstable operations can occur with alterations in the activity of the components of the system or can be triggered by disturbances that are well within the range of physiological possibility.

Because the respiratory control system interacts with other systems that regulate circulation and body temperature, the stability of respiratory control can be affected by operation of these systems.

Apneas

Apnea is probably the most frequent and striking abnormality in respiratory rhythm. Apneas are observed most often in premature infants but can occur in healthy adults, especially during sleep, and can be isolated events or can be recurrent. Because apneas sometimes produce severe hypoxia and hypercapnia, they may cause clinically significant cardiac arrhythmias or have long-lasting effects such as pulmonary hypertension.

Several different mechanisms can potentially produce random apneas. These include (1) loss of nonspecific respiratory excitatory stimulation (noise, light, tactile stimuli) and (2) active suppression of breathing by respiratory inhibitory reflexes arising from the cardiovascular system, the lung and chest wall, or via somatic and visceral afferents. For example, excitation of receptors located in the upper airway can, via the superior laryngeal nerve, trigger an apnea. Stimulation of J receptors in the lungs by inhaled irritants may produce a temporary apnea. Apnea may also occur as a result of a stimulus which produces hypocapnia but represses mechanisms which normally help maintain breathing even when chemical stimulation is minimal, such as posthyperventilation hyperpnea.[2]

Recurrent apneas may appear as part of a pattern of grossly irregular ataxic breathing. Patients with this kind of breathing usually have functional or actual structural medullary damage. The breathing disturbance results from a kind of sputtering of

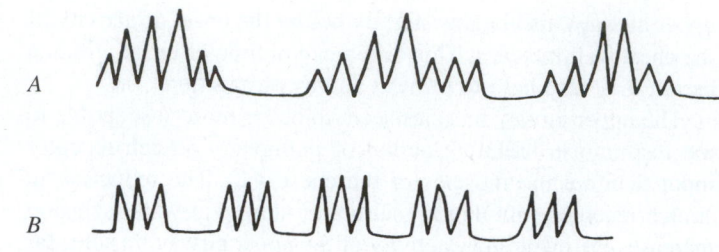

FIGURE 11-8 *A.* Cheyne-Stokes breathing. Regularly recurring swings in ventilation separated by periods of apnea. *B.* Biot's breathing. Unlike Cheyne-Stokes breathing, the tidal volumes between periods of apnea are uniform. It is unclear whether Cheyne-Stokes breathing and Biot's breathing are produced by the same mechanism.

damaged respiratory neuronal circuits. Breathing responds poorly to stimulants, and the patients with this disorder tend to hypoventilate.

In other types of abnormalities, such as Cheyne-Stokes breathing and Biot's breathing, apneas occur more predictably (Fig. 11-8). Apneas may be separated by periods of gradually increasing and decreasing breathing, as in Cheyne-Stokes breathing, and often in sleep apnea, or as in Biot's breathing, by breaths with a fixed tidal volume. Recurrent apneas may be associated with either hypoventilation or hyperventilation.

Different mechanisms may be involved in producing recurrent apneas: an instability in the feedback control of respiration which produces periodic breathing by the same mechanisms that produce oscillatory output in the physical control systems when they become unstable; an exaggeration of the mechanisms which may normally produce oscillations in ventilation; and recurrent apnea producing disturbances.[2]

SLEEP APNEA

On the basis of EEG criteria, sleep has been divided into rapid eye movement (REM) and NREM sleep.[9] Sleep usually begins in the NREM stage, which has been divided into two substages on the basis of a progressive slowing in EEG frequencies. REM sleep (the stage in which dreaming tends to occur) usually follows NREM states. It is characterized by the occurrence of a desynchronized EEG and periods of abrupt eye movements. REM sleep is also accompanied by inhibition of motor neurons, which leads to a profound loss of muscle tone that affects the diaphragm less than other respiratory muscles.

In both REM and NREM sleep, ventilatory responses to hypoxia and hypercapnia are reduced. Changes in lung mechanisms occurring during sleep (increased upper airway resistance and decreased compliance) may also contribute to depressed ventilatory responses.

Responses to stimulation of mechanoreceptors are also altered by sleep. For example, the compensatory response in motor activity which occurs during wakefulness when the airway is obstructed is reduced or eliminated during sleep.[2,9]

Apneas occur occasionally during sleep in considerable numbers of healthy individuals. But in those who have the sleep apnea syndrome, apneas are frequent and prolonged so that much of the night is spent hypoxemic. These same individuals are frequently sleepy during the day and may have elevated levels of arterial P_{CO_2} and pulmonary artery pressure. Sleep apnea occurs most frequently in premature infants, adult males, and postmenopausal women. Apneas are often, but not always associated with obesity, anatomic narrowing of the upper airway passages, and snoring. Sleep apneas generally occur in clusters, each of the apneas separated by a gradual increase and decrease in ventilation. Arousal terminates some of the periods of apnea. Apneas are most frequent in the lighter forms of NREM sleep and in REM sleep.

The interruptions in breathing that occur during the night have been divided into two types, central apneas and obstructive apneas. In central apneas there is no detectable respiratory activity, whereas in obstructive apneas respiratory efforts continue but there is no flow of air at either the nose or mouth. It is believed that a block in the upper airway occurs during obstructive apnea which prevents the movement of air into the lungs.

The distinction between obstructive and central apnea is not always clear. Frequently apneas are mixed in type, beginning with a central component followed by an obstructive period of ineffectual respiratory efforts.[9] Many patients have both kinds of apnea even within the same night. Also, theraputic interventions that are designed to prevent the occurrence of one or the other forms of apnea sometimes just substitute one type for the other.

Differences in the response of upper airway and chest wall muscles to chemical and mechanical stimuli could cause obstructive apnea. When the diaphragm contracts, a negative intrapharyngeal pressure is produced which tends to displace mobile upper airway structure and block airflow. Contraction of the upper airway muscles counterbalances this force to prevent obstruction during inspiration. According to this idea, maintenance of upper airway patency depends on fine coordination of the movements of upper airway and chest wall muscles. This coordination is more crucial when the airway is anatomically narrow.

The decrease in drive occurring during sleep may silence upper airway muscles before it stops the diaphragm, creating an imbalance of forces that promotes the collapse of the upper airway. Also, altered alignment of the respiratory muscles in the upper airway caused by changes in posture and the effects in gravity tend to increase the forces needed to maintain airway patency during sleep. Both mechanisms tend to produce an obstructive apnea.

CHEYNE-STOKES BREATHING

Cheyne-Stokes breathing is characterized by a cyclic rise and fall in ventilation with recurrent periods of apnea.[2] It was initially observed in patients with cardiac or neurologic disease, but it has since been reported in seemingly normal humans. The appearance of Cheyne-Stokes breathing can be triggered by the administration of sedatives and opiates and is more common during sleep. The period of the oscillations in ventilation in Cheyne-Stokes breathing is related to the circulation time measured from the lung to a systemic artery. Cycle length increases when circulation time is prolonged. Arterial blood P_{CO_2} is highest during the phase of hyperpnea and arterial P_{O_2} is then at its minimum, but alveolar gas tensions cycle in the opposite way.

Changes in the level of alertness occur coincidentally with the respiratory oscillations. Arousal tends to occur during the hyperpneic phase along with an increase in cerebral blood flow. The EEG shows greater fast-wave activity. The pupils dilate, and muscle tone is increased. The sensorium seems more depressed during apnea, the pupils are constricted, and muscle tone is diminished. Cerebral blood flow is often less during apnea, and there is a higher percentage of slow-wave activity in the EEG. Interestingly, arousal also frequently seems to terminate an episode of apnea during sleep.

Although the apneas occurring in Cheyne-Stokes breathing are more commonly central in type, recurrent obstructive apneas may resemble Cheyne-Stokes breathing.[2]

Cheyne-Stokes breathing has not been consistently produced in animals by lesions in the central nervous system, but it has been shown to follow manipulations that are likely to produce unstable feedback control of breathing. For example, the steadiness of the output in a feedback control system depends on the ability of the control system to be adequately informed of the consequences of its actions. If delays in information transfer are sufficiently great, the controller action to correct the effects of a disturbance may result in cyclic output changes. Delays can occur in the respiratory system when circulation time is prolonged between the lungs and the respiratory chemoreceptors. Experiments have shown that artificial prolongation of the circulation time causes Cheyne-Stokes breathing in anesthetized dogs.

Increased controller gains also enhance tendencies for instability in physical control systems. One way to increase the gain of the respiratory controller is to produce hypoxia. Posthyperventilation apnea can be used as a device to produce hypoxia at subnormal levels of CO_2 drive. In anesthetized dogs with normal circulation times, periodic breathing can occur following a period of artificial hyperventilation.[2]

Recent studies in humans have demonstrated that artificial hyperventilation during NREM sleep is frequently followed by a period of apnea and then Cheyne-Stokes-type breathing. Also, although Cheyne-Stokes breathing is common at high altitude, it occurs mainly in lowlanders who have much greater ventilatory responses to hypoxia than the natives of high altitude who have much lower hypoxic sensitivity.

Periodic breathing has also been produced in anesthetized cats ventilated with a respirator governed by phrenic nerve output so that feedback loops remained intact. Periodic breathing could be elicited sometimes just by increasing the gain of the servorespirator but at other times also required respiring the cat with hypoxic gas mixtures. Cooling the ventral medullary surface of the cat, which increased controller set point (the P_{CO_2} during resting breathing), also led to periodic breathing.

INTEGRATED RESPONSES OF THE CONTROL SYSTEM

The afferent and efferent systems described above, coordinated by the central neural circuits, respond to a variety of challenges of different severity that face both normal individuals and patients with pulmonary disease.[2,9] These challenges can disturb the respiratory rhythm and the level of ventilation or both.

Respiratory Adaptation to Altitude

Acute exposure to decreased barometric pressure produces an immediate increase in ventilation mediated through the peripheral chemoreceptors which is caused by the reduced partial pressure of oxygen. With continued exposure, ventilation in humans continues to increase for several days resulting in a gradual decrease in arterial P_{CO_2}. This process, called *acclimatization,* is poorly understood, as is the slow return of ventilation (deacclimatization) when the acclimatized individual returns to sea level pressures. It has been proposed that these ventilatory transients are caused by changes in blood and cerebrospinal fluid bicarbonate concentrations, which return pH from the alkalotic levels produced by acute hypoxic hyperventilation toward more normal levels. But recent studies have failed to find a reasonable correspondence between ventilation and pH. Rather than accounting for the gradual rises and falls in breathing, H+ concentrations in the blood and cerebrospinal fluid seem to follow the ventilatory changes. Recent animal studies show that these slow processes probably depend on the presence of intact peripheral chemoreceptors.[2,7]

At least three different possibilities may account for ventilatory changes during acclimatization and deacclimatization: (1) slow pH changes may occur at central chemoreceptors that as yet have been undetected by experimental measurements— these changes could take place either in brain interstitial fluid or even within the receptors themselves; (2) over time, hypoxia may produce specific chemical mediators, such as glutamate, which stimulate breathing and appear and disappear slowly; and (3) the gradual breathing changes may not be peculiar to hypoxia; any mechanism that causes active hyperventilation may produce long-lasting stimulation regardless of the initiating mechanism, for example, long-lasting stimulation of the central ends of the carotid sinus nerves.

Hypoxic Depression of Ventilation

In conscious animals with intact peripheral chemoreceptors exposed to sustained hypoxia at constant levels of arterial P_{CO_2}, ventilation after an initial increase will after 5 min or so decline. The initial rise is produced by peripheral chemoreceptor stimulation, but the subsequent reduction in ventilation may involve decreased sensitivity of the chemoreceptors as well as central depressive mechanisms.[2,7]

If the peripheral chemoreceptors are removed, respiration tends to be depressed by hypoxia. Several different factors seem to contribute to this ventilatory depression: (1) hypoxia, which may be quite severe in some regions of the brain, may interfere with the metabolic function of some neurons in the brain; (2) by dilating cerebral vessels and increasing cerebral blood flow, brain H+ concentration is decreased, thereby reducing stimulation of the central chemoreceptors; and (3) hypoxia seems to release mediators, such as γ-aminobutyric acid (GABA) and adenosine, that reduce breathing. These may overpower the effect of excitatory neurotransmitters that may also be released by hypoxia.

Since the brain is heterogeneous both in its cellular organization and with respect to blood flow rates, the effects of prolonged hypoxia in animals without peripheral chemoreceptors are complex depending on the susceptibility of different brain regions to low oxygen; for example, prolonged hypoxia produces an inhibitory action on ventilation but an overall excitatory effect on the hypothalamic regions.

Adaptation to Metabolic Acid-Base Disturbances

Chronic changes in blood bicarbonate levels which reduce arterial pH increase ventilation and cause hypocapnia. For example, hyperventilation is a feature of diabetic ketoacidosis and renal failure. Conversely, diseases which elevate blood bicarbonate levels and raise arterial pH, such as aldosteronism or hypercalcemia, frequently cause hypoventilation and hypercapnia. As a rule, the arterial P_{CO_2} increases by about 1 mmHg for each milliequivalent per liter change in bicarbonate. The changes in P_{CO_2} help restore pH toward normal.

Although reductions in P_{CO_2} invariably accompany metabolic acidosis, P_{CO_2} does not always rise in response to metabolic alkalosis. For example, it is widely held that blood alkalosis produced by K depletion does not elicit hypoventilation, presumably as a result of the intracellular acidosis that seems to accompany K loss. Also, in hypoxic, hypercapnic patients, complete compensation for metabolic alkalosis is limited by the hypoxia that accompanies hypoventilation.[2]

Like the ventilatory response to altitude, the compensatory responses to chronic metabolic disturbance occur over hours and days rather than immediately. Because of this time course, it seems likely that central, as well as peripheral, chemoreceptors contribute to the ventilatory compensation.

Acidosis either leaves ventilatory responses to inhaled CO_2 unaltered or causes them to increase; ventilatory responses tend to decrease with metabolic alkalosis. In chronic metabolic acidosis, the ventilatory response to exercise remains nearly isocapnic. Because of lower resting levels of arterial P_{CO_2} in the chronically acidotic individual than in the normal individual, ventilation increases more for the same rise in V_{CO_2} in the chronically acidotic individual.

Although both peripheral and central chemoreceptors participate in the ventilatory compensations that occur in response to acid-base derangements, the relative role of each is still unclear.

Response to Mechanical Loading

The control system for respiration can also readjust to maintain homeostasis in the face of mechanical impediments to breathing. Both resistive loads, mimicking obstructive lung disease, and elastic loads, mimicking interstitial disease, have been used experimentally. But, whether externally applied loads correspond to the mechanical impairments of pulmonary disease is questionable. In particular, the pattern of afferent activity from the lungs and the resulting pattern of ventilation differ in patients with pulmonary disease from those of normal subjects breathing with mechanical loads in place.[2,5]

Several factors act to maintain ventilation during mechanical loading. First are the factors intrinsic to the respiratory muscles. The force that the muscle develops for a fixed electrical input depends on the length of the muscle (the force-length relationship). As the muscle shortens, less force is developed. The force also depends on the velocity of shortening (force-velocity relationship), with less force being developed as the velocity of shortening increases. During loading, both the magnitude and the velocity of shortening tend to decrease. These intrinsic properties of the respiratory muscles help to compensate for the effects of mechanical loads.

In addition to intrinsic muscular effects, there are reflex effects. At the spinal level, less shortening of the inspiratory muscles increases the signal from muscle spindles that, in turn, augments contraction of these muscles. Because the number of spindles in the diaphragm is small, this phenomenon is most marked for the intercostal muscles. During loading, afferent information from pulmonary mechanoreceptors also changes. Since tidal volume is depressed, inspiratory duration tends to be prolonged because of the inspiratory off switch mechanism (Hering-Breuer inspiratory terminating reflex). This reflex has the characteristics of a negative feedback mechanism, since impeding inspiration causes its duration to be prolonged, thereby maintaining tidal volume. However, in humans this mechanism is of little importance in compensating for mechanical loads.

In conscious humans both resistive and elastic loads elicit an increase in neuromuscular output as reflected in the occlusion pressure. This increase in occlusion pressure occurs in the face of a constant chemical drive; the magnitude of the increase in occlusion pressure is related to the severity of the mechanical load. The intensity of this load-compensating mechanism is variable: In patients with chronic obstructive disease of the airways, no increase in occlusion pressure occurs during flow-resistive loading. When present, the mechanism seems to depend on higher, possibly cortical, influences; this aspect of load compensation is abolished by anesthesia.

The final compensation for mechanical loads is provided by the chemoreceptors, peripheral and central. When loads are so severe that hypoventilation ensues, the resulting changes in arterial blood-gas tensions (increase in P_{CO_2}, reduction in P_{O_2}) act to sustain ventilation. The magnitude of this component of the response depends on the gain of the peripheral and central chemoreflexes.

Response to Bronchoconstriction

Major differences exist between the neural responses to bronchoconstriction and the neural responses to loading. In particular, inspiratory muscle activity increases during bronchoconstriction even in anesthetized animals, even though this component of the compensation to external loads is, as noted above, abolished by anesthesia. These differences can be attributed to the different pattern of afferent activity in the two states. During bronchoconstriction, many of the pulmonary receptor systems described above undergo stimulation: Both stretch receptors and, more particularly, rapidly adapting receptors can be stimulated by the mechanical changes in the airway walls during bronchoconstriction. In addition, both rapidly adapting receptors and nonmyelinated afferents in the bronchi can be stimulated chemically by a number of autocoids (e.g., histamine and bradykinin) that are released in the lungs in asthma.

During asthma, or induced bronchoconstriction, changes in these afferent systems in the lung cause reflex changes in respiratory timing. The durations of all phases of the respiratory cycle are reduced so that respiratory frequency increases. This shortening of duration is unequally distributed across the different phases of respiration: Expiratory duration shortens more than inspiratory duration; within expiration, larger changes take place in the second phase of the expiratory part of the cycle. Indeed, during bronchoconstriction, the duration of the postinspiratory phase of the cycle changes least. Since the work of breathing during airway obstruction is minimized by using slow, deep breaths (lower air flows and, hence, resistive work), these changes in timing during bronchoconstriction are opposite from those produced by afferent stimulation. Thus, part of the reason for the increased work of respiration in asthma is that the respirator pattern adopted is nonoptimal.

The changes in afferent activity in the lungs described above also change reflexly the magnitude of the inspiratory neural output. For example, vagal blockade abolishes the increase in neuromuscular output. Thus, the increase in inspiratory neural output that occurs during bronchoconstriction is vagally mediated.

Changes in the activity of the inspiratory muscles are not confined to the inspiratory phase of the cycle. During expiration, tonic activity of the inspiratory muscles increases. This neural phenomenon leads to an increase in functional residual capacity. Thus, the increase in functional residual capacity in asthma is due not just to mechanical changes within the airways that lead to air trapping but also to altered neural control of the respiratory muscles. This alteration in the activity of the inspiratory muscles during expiration also seems to be vagally mediated, probably by way of stimulation of the rapidly adapting receptors.

Muscles other than the inpiratory muscles undergo changes in activity. For example, inhalation of histamine narrows the larynx, an effect that is most marked in expiration, thereby contributing reflexly to the increased airway resistance in asthma. This component of the response can be ameliorated by continuous positive airway pressure.[2]

VOLUNTARY CONTROL OF BREATHING AND DYSPNEA

Normally breathing does not reach the level of awareness except during exposure to severe hypoxia or intense exercise. But patients with lung disease may complain of shortness of breath or dyspnea even at rest. Since dyspnea itself can become an incapacitating symptom, considerable attention has been given to its etiology.[1,2,9]

Earlier experiments used breath holding as a model for the investigation of dyspnea. These studies showed that hypercapnia and hypoxia decreased breath-holding times, supporting the idea that increased levels of input promote dyspnea; conversely, increased lung volume lengthened breath-holding time. Since combined blockade of the phrenic nerves and of the vagi extend the time apnea could be voluntarily maintained, these studies led to the idea that contraction of muscles was an important contributor to the sense of dyspnea.

More recent studies have used standard psychophysical tests to evaluate respiratory sensations and relate these sensations to dyspnea. These tests have had several goals: (1) to determine the ability of subjects to detect loads applied to the mouth, (2) to scale the respiratory sensations produced either by breathing with a load in place or by changing respiratory pressures and tidal volumes, and (3) to scale the respiratory sensations evoked by increasing ventilation using a variety of maneuvers. Although these approaches have not settled the mechanisms responsible for dyspnea, they have provided fresh insights.

With respect to load detection, the ability to sense added loads depends on background mechanical conditions. Resistive loads, for example, are more difficult to detect by patients with increased airway resistance.

The scaling of easily detectable loads depends mainly on the pressure developed while breathing with the load in place and far less on inspiratory duration and the frequency of breathing. The relationship between respiratory pressure and sensory intensity follows a power law. The sensations produced by pressure changes (produced, for example, by breathing with different efforts against an occluded valve), like the sensations produced by changes in tidal volume, grow disproportionately greater as the magnitude of the stimulus (i.e., change in pressure or tidal volume) increases.

Respiratory effort as well as pressure or tidal volume changes can be scaled, suggesting that subjects can sense intent (i.e., the motor command to the respiratory muscles directly), even if there is little afferent input from the respiratory muscles. Finally, dyspnea seems to be related to the effort (motor command), expressed as a percentage of its maximum. Thus, dyspnea increases as the pressures used for tidal breathing grow greater or the maximal inspiratory pressure decreases (e.g., as by paresis, disease, or respiratory muscle fatigue).

Although these observations seem to equate dyspnea with the intensity of the sense of effort and, thus, only indirectly to input, this is probably not the complete story. New observations indicate that dyspnea is less when ventilations are voluntarily increased than when they are produced by chemical stimulation. This suggests that cognitive factors, and probably affective factors which determine the relative pleasantness of a sensation as well as sensory intensity, affect the level of dyspnea.

Some data show that responses to chemical stimuli can be affected by voluntary control. The respiratory response to hypoxia can be conditioned in animals, and brainstem mechanisms may modulate the ventilatory response to CO_2. For example, a respiratory-related discharge is present in CO_2-responsive neurons in the thalmus. Also, stimulation or ablation of different regions of the cortex modify the magnitude of the respiratory CO_2 response. Positron emission tomography (PET) scans show activation of the limbic system during CO_2 inhalation in humans. The dyspnea experienced during CO_2 breathing may be mediated through the limbic system.

Another important, unresolved issue is whether the sense of dyspnea can induce patients to alter their breathing patterns or to deliberately hypoventilate in order to avoid discomfort. This seems possible, since breathing can be controlled voluntarily as well as automatically. Separate pathways to respiratory motoneurons have been described by which the cortex can influence respiratory activity. Moreover, it has been demonstrated that the automatic and behavioral pathways for breathing can be independently altered by disease. Ondine's curse (primary alveolar hypoventilation) is probably mainly caused by an abnormality in the automatic control of breathing. However, patients have been described who have respiratory apraxia, that is, they breathe normally at rest and respond appropriately during exercise but are unable to voluntarily change their breathing. Thus, through voluntary action, patients who are short of breath may be able to alter the way they breathe.[1,2,5]

It is also likely that the response of some respiratory sensors (e.g., the carotid body) can be modified by pathways which project from the brain to the receptor.[2]

Some studies suggest that by the judicious use of analgesics the sense of dyspnea can be relieved without causing dangerous hypoventilation. However, much better success in alleviating dyspnea in lung disease patients has occurred through interventions which strengthen or augment the endurance of the respiratory muscles.

REFERENCES

1. Carfield DR, Fink GR, Ramsay SC, et al: Evidence for limbic system activation during CO_2-stimulated breathing in man. *J Physiol* (*Lond*) 488:77–84, 1995.
2. Cherniack NS, Widdicombe JG (eds): *Handbook of Physiology.* Section 3: *The Respiratory System,* vol 3, *Control of Breathing.* Bethesda, Md, American Physiological Society, 1986.
3. Coleridge JCG, Coleridge HM: Afferent vagal C fibre innervation of the lungs and airways and its functional significance. *Rev Physiol Biochem Pharmacol* 99:2–110, 1984.
4. Von Euler C: On the central pattern generator for the basic breathing rhythmicity. *J Appl Physiol* 55:1647–1659, 1983.
5. Von Euler C, Lagercrantz H: *Neurobiology of Control of Breathing.* New York, Raven, 1987.
6. Feldman JL, Ellenberger HH: Central coordination of respiratory and cardiovascular control in mammals. *Ann Rev Physiol* 50:593–606, 1988.
7. Lahiri S, Iturrigia R, Mokashi A, et al: CO reveals dual mechanisms of O_2 chemoreception in the cat carotid body. *Resp Physiol* 94:227–240, 1993.
8. Long S, Duffin J: The neuronal determinants of respiratory rhythm. *Prog Neurobiol* 27:101–182, 1986.
9. Pack AI, Millma RP: Changes in control of ventilation, awake and asleep, in the elderly. *J Am Geriatr Soc* 34:533–544, 1986.
10. Richter DW: Generation and maintenance of the respiratory rhythm. *J Exp Biol* 100:93–107, 1982.
11. Severinghaus JW: Widespread sites of brainstem ventilatory chemoreceptors. *J Appl Physiol* 75:3–4, 1993.

CHAPTER 12

VENTILATION, PULMONARY BLOOD FLOW, AND VENTILATION-PERFUSION RELATIONSHIPS

Peter D. Wagner

BASIC OUTLINE OF THE GAS EXCHANGE PATHWAY

POTENTIAL DISRUPTION OF THE GAS TRANSPORT PATHWAY
   Hypoventilation
   Diffusion Limitation
   Shunt
   Ventilation/Perfusion ($\dot{V}_A/\dot{Q}$) Inequality
   Assessment of Ventilation/Perfusion Inequality

This chapter and that succeeding it together share responsibility for presenting the physiological basis of normal pulmonary gas exchange. Gas exchange occurs by an integrated series of gas transport steps between the environmental air we breathe and the hemoglobin (Hb) molecule of the red cells passing through the pulmonary capillaries. These transport steps are of two types—diffusive and convective, and a number of conceptually separate diffusive as well as convective processes interact to accomplish the gas exchange mission. This is true both for gases that are taken up from the environment into the blood (i.e., O_2 and occasional toxic gases or volatile anesthetics) and for gases that are eliminated from the body (i.e., CO_2 and volatile anesthetic agents).

This chapter deals principally with the convective processes and the following chapter with those involving diffusion. However, since the two types of process occur simultaneously, they are closely linked.

BASIC OUTLINE OF THE GAS EXCHANGE PATHWAY

This section dwells on O_2, the gas of principal physiological interest, although the pathway components are of course identical for all gases and furthermore do not depend on whether the gas is being taken up (O_2) or eliminated (CO_2). However, distinct quantitative differences in the uptake or elimination patterns of different gases exist, but those are readily explained by differences in their fundamental physical or chemical properties and not by transport pathway differences.

To understand the gas transport pathway one must first appreciate the anatomy of the lungs, laid out in detail in Chapter 2. The salient functional features are presented in Fig. 12-1.

The chest wall (rib cage and diaphragm) contain muscles that on contraction expand the volume of the chest cavity and thus reduce the intrathoracic pressure of the pleural space, expanding the lungs with air drawn in via the mouth and nose. Although there is but a single air passage in the neck (i.e., the trachea), this soon branches into right and left main bronchi. These also divide many times, essentially dichotomously. There are some 16 such orders of branching of these bronchi,[33] resulting in a structure that resembles an inverted deciduous tree without its leaves in winter. With each successive branch the airways become shorter and narrower but ever greater in number, usually doubling at each branching. Thus although the cross-sectional area of any one airway becomes smaller with each branching, the greater number of airways more than makes up for loss of individual cross-sectional area such that the sum of cross-sectional areas of all airways of a given generation rises essentially exponentially with each branching (Fig. 12-2). The total volume of gas in these 16 conducting airway generations is called the *anatomic* or *conducting airway dead space*, and approximates 1 ml per pound of body weight. After these 16 or so successive branches, the tubular, purely conducting airways begin to show alveolar units in their wall (generation 17 to 19 or so), and these finally give way to fully alveolated structures (in succession: alveolar ducts, alveolar sacs, and alveoli). There are some 300 million alveoli, each about 300 μm in diameter. They are blind structures so that ventilation has to be accomplished by a tidal, in-and-out process (rather than a flow-through process as for pulmonary blood flow). The alveoli can be seen in Fig. 12-1, from a different perspective. For gas exchange to occur, O_2 must be moved from the mouth all the way to the alveoli—it is only within alveoli that gas exchange occurs.

Each alveolus is densely covered in a capillary network, seen from various perspectives in Fig. 12-1. This network is closely applied to the alveolar gas space as Fig. 12-1 shows, with on average only about 1/2 μm of cellular and interstitial tissue be-

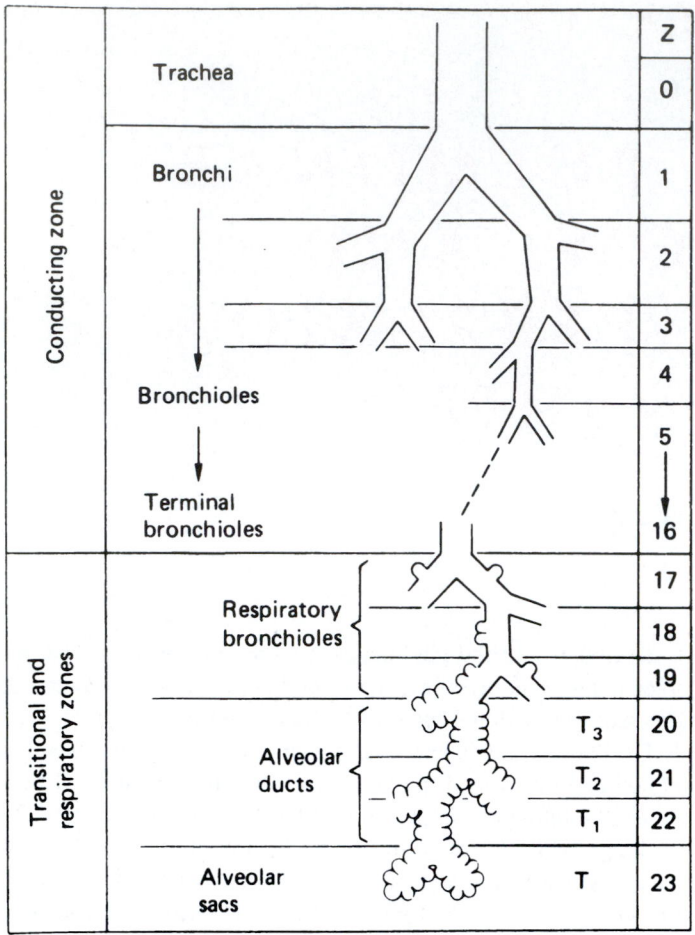

A

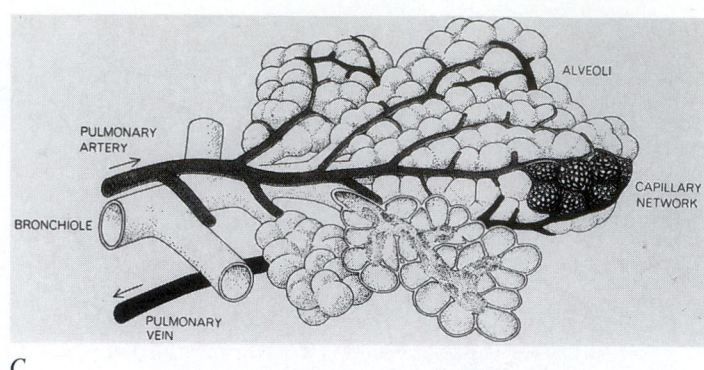

C

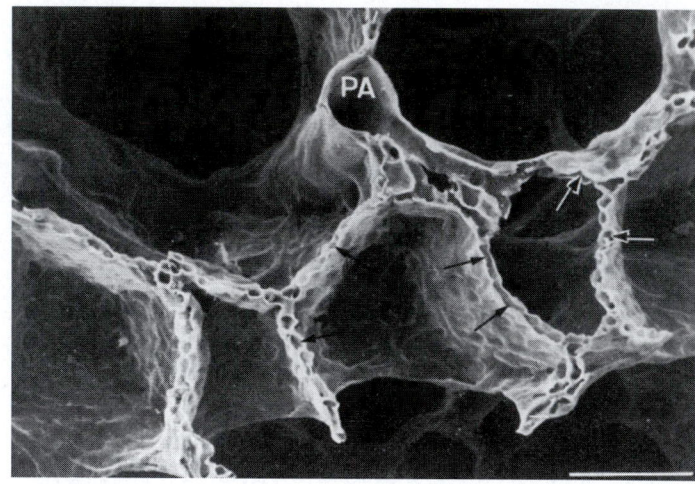

D

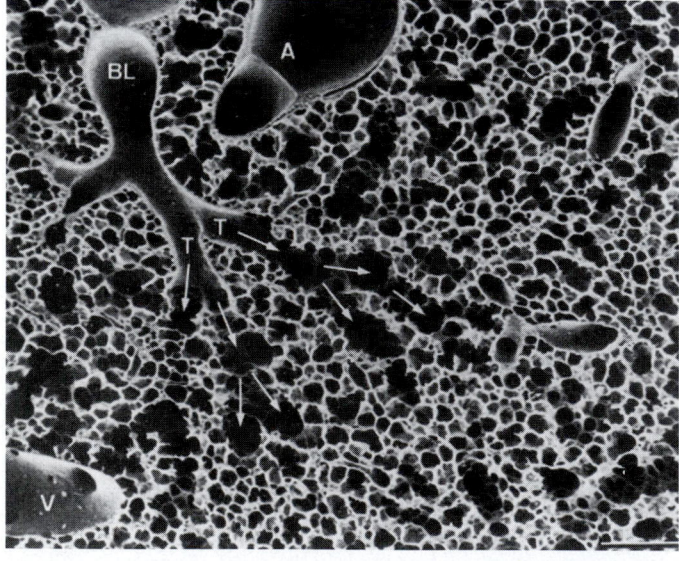

B

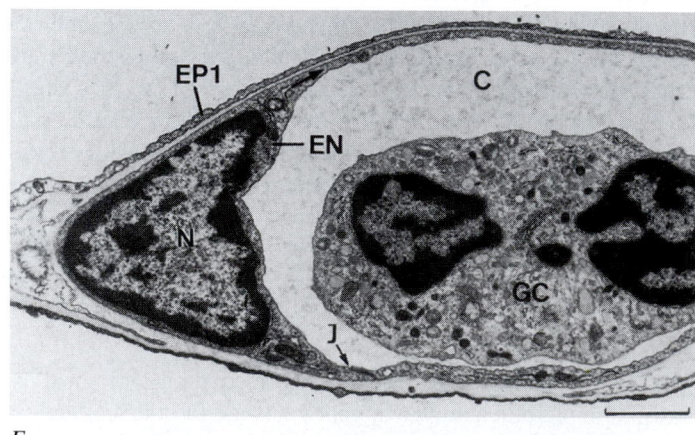

E

FIGURE 12-1   Principal anatomical features of the lung related to gas exchange. *A* shows the organization of branching airways, mirrored by a photograph of a lung slice showing terminal and respiratory bronchioles and the alveolar parenchyma in B. *C* shows how the capillaries are wrapped around alveoli, and *D* is a scanning electron micrograph indicating the rich capillary networks in the alveolar walls. *E* is a transmission electron micrograph showing the capillaries (C) and the three layers of the blood-gas barrier (endothelium, EN, basement membrane, and epithelium, EP1). *(Panels A,B,D, and E reproduced from Weibel,[34] with permission.)*

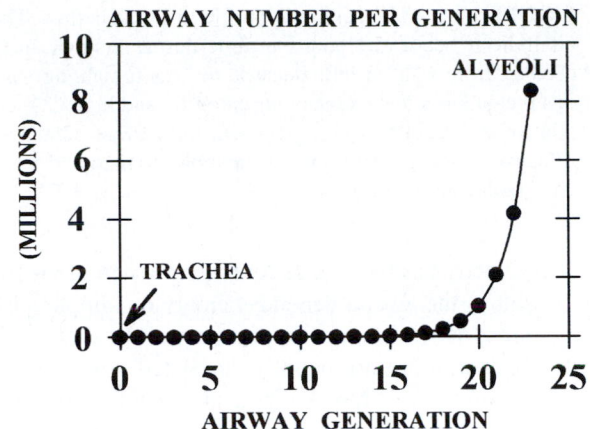

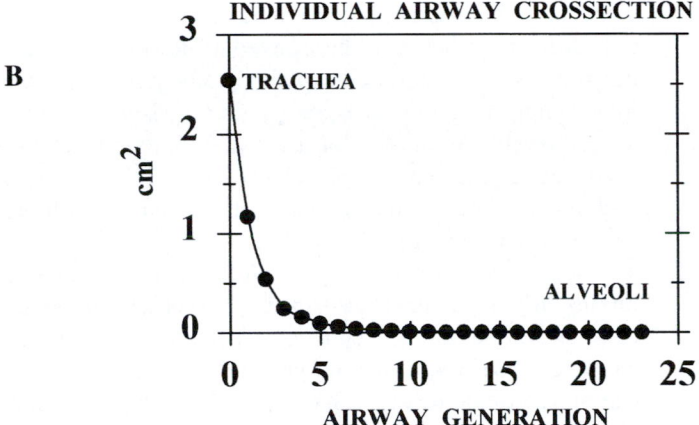

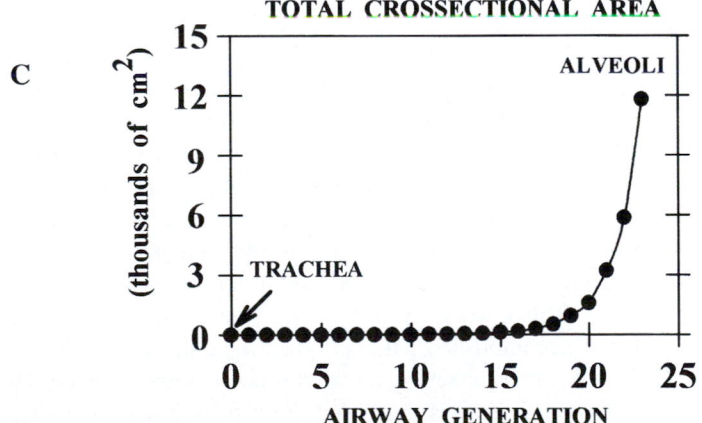

FIGURE 12-2   Relationship between number (*A*) and cross-sectional area (*B*) of the airways at a given generation. Note that total airway cross-sectional area (*C*) increases extremely rapidly beyond airway generation 15 or so, the beginning of the respiratory zone for gas exchange.

tween the blood inside the capillary and the alveolar gas outside. The capillary network is fed by the pulmonary arterial tree which branches alongside the airways in a very similar pattern as the airways. The capillaries then drain into venules that join to form larger and larger vessels, eventually becoming the pulmonary veins that drain oxygenated blood into the left atrium. This coalescence of venous vessels forms a similar branching tree to the

pulmonary arteries and airways, but in reverse. The right ventricle is responsible for unidirectional pumping of blood through this vascular system.

The gas exchange pathway from the lips to the left atrium is therefore highly complex structurally, and understanding how gases pass along the pathway requires following the events an O_2 molecule must participate in between the lips and the left atrium:

1. The first step is inspiration of air into the trachea via mouth and nose. Accomplished by inspiratory chest wall muscle contraction, which reduces intrathoracic pressure, this step is convective (like water flowing from a region of high to low pressure along a garden hose). All the respired air must pass the trachea, but at the first branch point some air goes to the right lung, the rest to the left. At each successive branch point, similar mass-conserving distribution of air must occur between the daughter branches of each parent pathway. Remembering that there are some 23 total branchings from the mouth to the 300 million alveoli, there is a very real risk of quite uneven distribution of that inspired air amongst those alveoli. The principal determinants of how air is distributed at branch points (i.e., between daughter branches) are the mechanical properties of the respiratory system: the compliance (elastic properties), the resistance, and the inertial properties. These concepts are more fully treated in Chapter 10.

2. During normal resting inspiration, flow is laminar in most of the airways. Thus inspired gas develops a parabolic profile due to higher molecular velocities in the center than periphery of the airway (Fig. 12-3). The parabolic "tongue" of inspired gas in Fig. 12-3 moves down an airway, while around the tongue is gas remaining from the previous expiration. The tongue therefore has O_2 at a concentration of 21 percent and essentially no CO_2. The gas around the tongue, having undergone gas exchange during the preceding breath, has about 14 percent O_2 and 5 percent CO_2. Consequently, during forward motion of this tongue toward the alveoli, O_2 will diffuse from the tongue to its surrounding gas, and CO_2 will diffuse in the opposite direction. This is called Taylor dispersion,[26] and it reduces the forward transport of O_2 produced by the onward convective movement of the tongue. This effect however is considered quite small and is generally not of significance to overall gas exchange. Note that if inspiration occurs at high rates as in exercise, such laminar flow may not occur in the larger airways—it may be turbulent, and then Taylor dispersion is essentially noncontributory, as the turbulent mixing evens gas concentrations across the airway lumen.

3. Figure 12-2 shows the exponential increase in airway cross-sectional surface area as one proceeds deeper and deeper into the lungs.[33] The significance of this curve is that since the mass flow rate of inspired gas is the same at every generation (because the airways are simply a conducting system), the forward velocity of O_2 molecules falls (since its flow rate is the product of velocity and cross-sectional surface area). As it happens, by about generations 17 to 19, where the alveoli are just beginning to appear, this forward

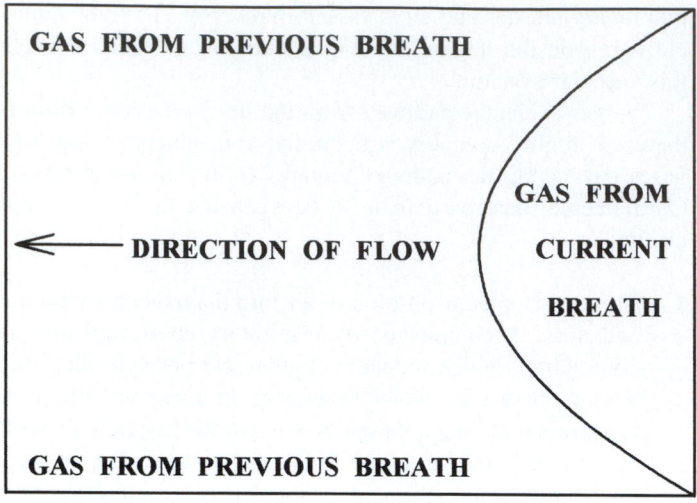

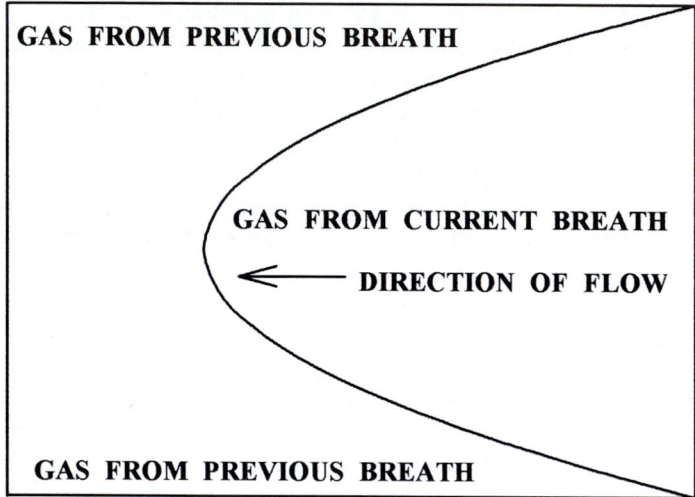

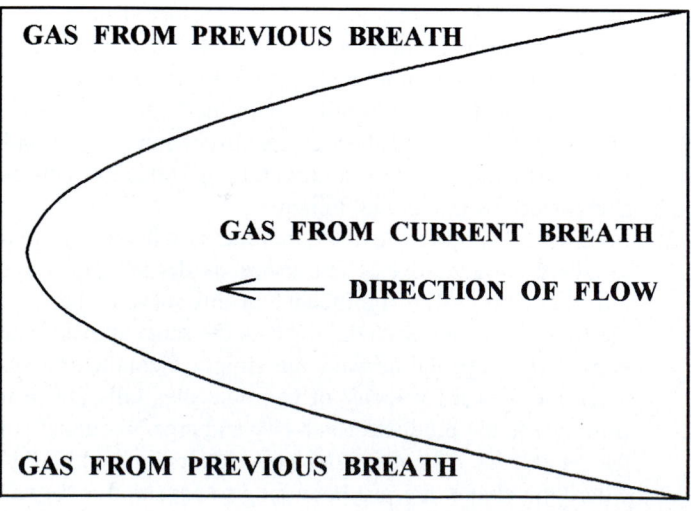

FIGURE 12-3 The parabolic profile of laminar flow. The three panels indicate sequential points in time during a single inspiration proceeding from right to left. Because the gas remaining from the previous breath has a low oxygen concentration and high CO_2 concentration relative to that of the inspired gas in the current breath, there will be diffusive exchange between the parabolic tongue and the surrounding gas (Taylor dispersion).

velocity has become so low that passage of O_2 from here on out to the alveoli depends heavily on simple gaseous diffusion, not just on continuing convective flow.

4. If alveoli are not equally ventilated with gas (and equally perfused with blood), their alveolar O_2 concentration will differ, as explained later in this chapter. Because adjacent alveoli are so physically close, there can be considerable diffusion of O_2 between such alveoli when their O_2 levels are different.[5] This passive process tends to reduce concentration differences between these alveoli. However, although this process can be detected experimentally, it is of probably minor clinical significance. Step 3 (and to some extent 4) are responsible for most of the alveolar gas mixing that must occur for gas exchange to take place—that is, the mixing of each breath of newly inspired gas with alveolar gas still present from prior breaths.

5. The heart acts as a massaging pump to further enhance gas mixing into the alveolar gas spaces.[37] Alternate filling and emptying of the cardiac chambers respectively facilitates exhaling and inhaling of airway gas into those alveoli physically close to the heart but has little effect on more distant alveoli. Although a well-known and easily demonstrated phenomenon, this so-called cardiogenic mixing is probably also of minimal physiological impact for gas exchange.

6. Once the dominant convective and diffusive gas transport steps have brought O_2 from the lips to the alveolar gas spaces, O_2 physically dissolves in the tissues separating alveolar gas from capillary blood, the blood-gas barrier (Fig. 12-1). O_2 then moves by diffusion through the blood-gas barrier and into the plasma. Over 98 percent of these O_2 molecules diffuse further, (i.e., into the red cell interior) and then bind rapidly to hemoglobin. The remaining 2 percent or so remain physically dissolved in the plasma and red cell water. This transport process from alveolar gas to hemoglobin is accomplished passively by simple diffusion: No convective forces or active transport processes are involved. The diffusion process is discussed more fully in the next chapter. In normal lungs at rest, this process is very rapid and causes no O_2 transport limitation.

7. Finally, the red cells are transported convectively by cardiac pumping action out of the pulmonary capillaries and into the pulmonary veins and then to the left atrium, and left ventricle, finally reaching the various body tissues.

POTENTIAL DISRUPTION OF THE GAS TRANSPORT PATHWAY

If all the above elements of the transport pathway were functionally perfect, the partial pressure of O_2 (and other gases) would be identical in the gas of all 300 million alveoli and equal to that in systemic arterial blood. The system comes close to perfection in health, but there is never complete equivalence of alveolar and arterial pressures, even in healthy young, normal people. Aging further leads to a progressive impairment of the pathway with arterial P_{O_2} falling from 95 to 100 mmHg at age 20 to 75 to 80 mmHg at age 80 or thereabouts.[22] However, alveolar P_{O_2} tends to be invariant with age. Thus, the difference between alveolar and arterial P_{O_2} steadily increases from about 5 to 10 mmHg to about 20 to 25 mmHg over this age range. Pulmonary diseases such as asthma, emphysema and bronchitis, fibrosis, pneumonia, and many others can greatly disrupt gas transport to the point of causing death from insufficient tissue O_2 supply. Consequently, it is essential to have a good understanding of the O_2 transport pathway and what may affect it even in health, in order to appreciate the problems seen in pulmonary diseases.

A traditional view of how to consider abnormalities of the transport pathway has evolved over the years and is very useful as a framework for discussion. This view is based upon the end result of gas exchange—the arterial P_{O_2}—and listing the reasons why this variable can fall below normal values.

Four principal potential mechanisms of failure of the O_2 transport pathway can lead to a reduced arterial P_{O_2} (i.e., to arterial hypoxemia):

1. Hypoventilation
2. Diffusion limitation
3. Shunt
4. Ventilation-perfusion ($\dot{V}_A/\dot{Q}$) inequality.

These are the so-called intrapulmonary factors that directly cause hypoxemia. Modulating extrapulmonary factors are also important. These include changes in inspired O_2 concentration, in total cardiac output, in overall metabolic rate, and in Hb concentration. The four intrapulmonary factors are now defined and discussed.

Hypoventilation

Normal levels of ventilation produce a tightly regulated arterial P_{CO_2} at 40 ± 2 mmHg in normal subjects with several control systems in place to ensure this.[3] However, if overall ventilation is reduced for any reason, alveolar P_{CO_2} ($P_{A_{CO_2}}$), and therefore arterial P_{CO_2}, must rise to maintain constant the elimination of metabolically produced CO_2. Reciprocally, alveolar P_{O_2} ($P_{A_{O_2}}$), and hence arterial P_{O_2}, will fall (and by relatively similar amounts as P_{CO_2} will rise). The alveolar gas equation[21] quantitatively relates $P_{A_{O_2}}$ and $P_{A_{CO_2}}$ and is used to calculate how much $P_{A_{O_2}}$ will change for a change in $P_{A_{CO_2}}$:

$$P_{A_{O_2}} = P_{I_{O_2}} - \frac{P_{A_{CO_2}}}{R} + P_{A_{CO_2}} \cdot F_{I_{O_2}} \cdot \frac{1 - R}{R} \qquad (1)$$

$P_{I_{O_2}}$ and $F_{I_{O_2}}$ are inspired O_2 partial pressure and fractional concentration, respectively, and R is the respiratory exchange ratio.

Hypoventilation represents a failure of step 1 of the gas transport pathway (see above) and can occur for several reasons: (1) The control centers in the nervous system that regulate ventilation could malfunction due to diseases, drugs, or anesthetics; (2) there could be neuronal or neuromuscular dysfunction of the nerves supplying the chest wall muscles of respiration; (3) the

chest wall muscles could be fatigued, damaged, or paralyzed; or (4) the airways or chest wall could be disrupted from trauma or other mechanical derangement such as compression, or, in the case of airways, obstruction.

Conceptually this type of problem is usually thought of as a whole-lung issue, usually with obvious causes, and can be reversed by recognizing the cause and taking appropriate reparative or ventilatory supportive steps.

Diffusion Limitation

Whereas diffusive transport plays a recognizable if small role within the airways and alveolar gas (see above), the concept of diffusive limitation affecting arterial P_{O_2} is more usually associated with transport step 6 above—diffusion of O_2 from alveolar gas into the capillary and red cell.

This topic is specifically the focus of the following chapter and will not be dealt with here. Indeed, the ensuing discussion of other factors will set aside diffusion limitation of O_2 transport for the sake of simplicity and assume that the diffusive exchange of O_2 (and CO_2) between alveolar gas and capillary blood proceeds to completion within a single red cell's passage through the pulmonary microcirculation. Under most conditions this is reasonable.[29]

Shunt

A shunt is a blood pathway that does not allow any contact between alveolar gas and red cells, so that no gas exchange occurs in the affected region. Consequently, blood passes through a shunt maintaining a mixed venous blood composition. When this blood reaches pulmonary veins, the left atrium, and eventually arterial blood, it mixes with other blood that has undergone alveolar gas exchange. The result is a fall in arterial P_{O_2} and potentially an increase in arterial P_{CO_2} (arterial P_{CO_2} may not increase if the patient raises his or her level of ventilation, but hypoxemia will persist).[35]

Classical pathophysiological scenarios giving rise to shunts are: (1) pulmonary edema, which fills alveoli with fluid, thereby abolishing their ventilation and any gas exchange; (2) alveolar filling with cellular and microorganismal debris as in pneumonia, with the same result as in edema; (3) collapse of a region of lung due to pneumothorax, gas absorption distal to a fully obstructed airway, or to external compression; (4) rarely, the presence of abnormal arteriovenous vascular channels in the lungs, that can occur in, for example, hepatic cirrhosis; and (5) direct right-to-left vascular communications at the level of the heart or great (extrapulmonary) blood vessels.

Ventilation-Perfusion ($\dot{V}_A/\dot{Q}$) Inequality

The exquisite and complex branching architecture of the airways and of the blood vessels makes the lungs very susceptible to the potential problem of nonuniform distribution of alveolar ventilation and of pulmonary blood flow. Whenever alveoli are ventilated at less than average rates, for example if their feeding airways become partially obstructed for any reason, the ratio of ventilation to blood flow ($\dot{V}_A/\dot{Q}$ ratio) will fall. In certain other conditions, lung regions may suffer a reduction in local blood flow rather than ventilation, so that the $\dot{V}_A/\dot{Q}$ ratio rises above the average value in those areas.

Whenever there is a range of $\dot{V}_A/\dot{Q}$ ratios in a lung such that the $\dot{V}_A/\dot{Q}$ ratio is not everywhere identical, it is said that $\dot{V}_A/\dot{Q}$ inequality exists. It matters not what the pathologic cause of $\dot{V}_A/\dot{Q}$ inequality is, nor whether the problem originates in the airways or blood vessels. The principal concept is that, compared to a lung having the same total alveolar ventilation and blood flow, a lung that has $\dot{V}_A/\dot{Q}$ inequality will exchange (all) gases in an inefficient manner. The result will be hypoxemia and, potentially, hypercapnia (raised arterial P_{CO_2}). A large section of this chapter presents the physiological reasons for this effect of $\dot{V}_A/\dot{Q}$ inequality.

Understanding of $\dot{V}_A/\dot{Q}$ inequality can be demanding, but no matter what its pathologic origins, the concepts are similar. $\dot{V}_A/\dot{Q}$ inequality can occur at many different scales. Not uncommonly, it can be manifest on a large scale as differences between the right and left lungs. Classical examples of this include unilateral atelectasis, pneumothorax, pulmonary embolus, or pneumonia. All these are relatively common phenomena that can lead to severe gas exchange disturbances. At the other end of the scale, there can be $\dot{V}_A/\dot{Q}$ ratio differences between essentially adjacent alveoli. However, research has shown that small groups of contiguous alveoli can maintain functional homogeneity of $\dot{V}_A/\dot{Q}$ ratios via rapid gas diffusion rates, possibly augmented by collateral ventilation and blood flow.[39] It is likely that all alveoli distal to individual respiratory (or perhaps terminal) bronchioles can retain functional homogeneity for gas exchange through these mechanisms.

In between these two extremes of scale, vascular or airway obstruction at all levels will produce $\dot{V}_A/\dot{Q}$ inequality that, depending on how widespread it is, causes hypoxemia and potentially hypercapnia.

Even the young normal lung is usually subject to $\dot{V}_A/\dot{Q}$ inequality,[28] which explains the 5- to 10-mmHg P_{O_2} difference between alveolar gas and arterial blood generally observed in healthy young subjects. There are several mechanisms for the existence of such $\dot{V}_A/\dot{Q}$ inequality.

GRAVITY-BASED INEQUALITY

Ventilation, and, even more so, blood flow are unevenly distributed in a manner systematically influenced by gravity.[36] This is due respectively to the weight of the lungs and of the blood in the blood vessels. Thus, dependent lung regions receive far more blood flow than nondependent regions, a finding that is in concept independent of body position. It turns out that the gravitational gradient in blood flow considerably exceeds that of ventilation. As a result, the nondependent lung regions are of *higher* than average $\dot{V}_A/\dot{Q}$ ratio, and the dependent regions are of *lower* than average $\dot{V}_A/\dot{Q}$ ratio.[36] Average $\dot{V}_A/\dot{Q}$ ratio is about 1.0, because total alveolar ventilation and blood flow are similar. At the apex of the upright human lung, the $\dot{V}_A/\dot{Q}$ ratio is about 3; at the base it is about 0.6, 5-fold lower. There is a smooth gradation between the two extremes depicted in Fig. 12-4. This large-scale apex-to-base gradient in $\dot{V}_A/\dot{Q}$ ratios does not produce more than about a 4-mmHg drop in arterial P_{O_2} (compared to expectations

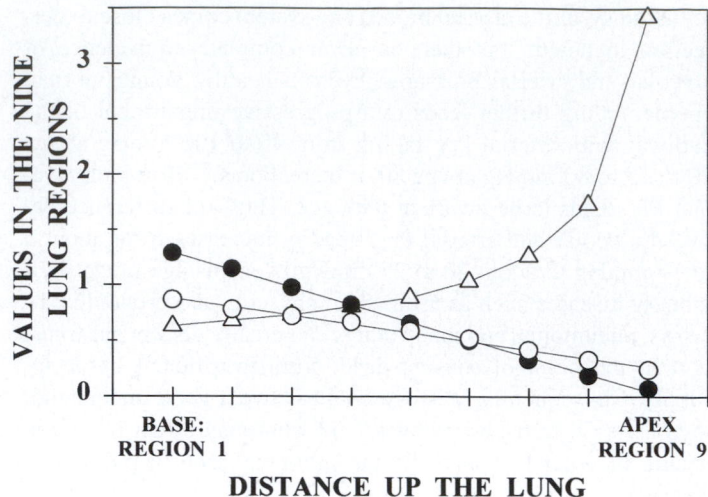

FIGURE 12-4   Topographical relationships between ventilation and blood flow as a function of distance up and down the upright lung (divided into nine contiguous regions). Although both ventilation and blood flow are higher at the base than at the apex, the ventilation-perfusion ratio ($\dot{V}_A/\dot{Q}$) rises exponentially from the bottom to the top of the lung. *(Adapted from West.[36])*

in the absence of this phenomenon), and thus a 4-mmHg alveolar-arterial P_{O_2} difference.

FRACTALLY BASED $\dot{V}_A/\dot{Q}$ INEQUALITY

The branching airway and blood vessel structure of the lung constitutes a fractal system that is innately susceptible to $\dot{V}_A/\dot{Q}$ inequality independently of gravity.[8] With some 23 sequential orders of branching, very small random inequalities in gas or blood flow distribution repeated at each branch point of the system can rapidly escalate into very significant degrees of nonuniform ventilation or blood flow. To illustrate, consider a branching system of just 16 dichotomous sequences—at each of the 16 branch points, air is *not* precisely split 50/50 between each daughter pair. Rather, suppose a 49 to 51 percent split—a nonuniform effect of trivial proportions at any one airway branch. The most poorly ventilated regions (receiving 49 percent of the split at every one of the 16 branchings) end up with only about half as much ventilation as the best ventilated regions that receive 51 percent of the split at each branch.

Unless the fractal structure somehow distributes both ventilation and blood flow in a correlated manner to preserve $\dot{V}_A/\dot{Q}$ ratios (even as $\dot{V}_A$ or $\dot{Q}$ individually vary), significant hypoxemia could result. Understanding the consequences of the fractal nature of the lung is a topic of much current interest. It would appear that there must be correlation of $\dot{V}_A$ with $\dot{Q}$, since the large potential for fractally based hypoxemia does not generally get realized.

LONGITUDINALLY BASED INEQUALITY

As airways and blood vessels progressively narrow with each branch point, resistance to gas and blood flow increases. Not all alveoli receive gas or blood from airways that have gone through the same number of branchings. Hence, some alveoli will be more and some will be less distant from the mouth. Such simple principles suggest the possibility of reduced $\dot{V}_A$ and/or $\dot{Q}$ of those alveoli further from the mouth compared to more proximal alveoli and therefore the chance of a central to peripheral, or longitudinal, gradient in ventilation and blood flow. Although not universally observed, there is a fair amount of evidence that such inequality exists, but its contribution to gas exchange is hard to establish.[9] To the extent that similar physical principles apply to both gas and blood flow in the present context, one can theorize that more distant alveoli have both less ventilation and less blood flow, so that again there is a natural tendency to preserve the $\dot{V}_A/\dot{Q}$ *ratio* between central and peripheral regions.

ANATOMICALLY BASED INEQUALITY

Another potential reason for nonuniform gas or blood flow distribution is intrinsic anatomical differences between lung regions. Perhaps the best example is in the dog[1] and horse[10] where, independent of body position in relation to gravity, the dorsal regions of the lower lobes often can be shown to have an unduly high share of total pulmonary perfusion. This tendency, presumably based on the overall branching architectural differences between lobes or within lobes, becomes important in concept when patients are moved from one body position to another, in order to best understand consequent changes in gas exchange.

COLLATERAL VENTILATION AND BLOOD FLOW

To this point, a picture has been painted of a branching architecture that has no lateral connections between either adjacent airways or blood vessels at any level of branching. Such lateral connections can exist at several airway levels[15,16] from large airways down to alveoli. This is a species-dependent phenomenon,[17] so that while the pig has few or no such collateral pathway structures, the dog has extensive collateral ventilatory channels. Humans are somewhere between these extremes.

Whatever the evolutionary pressure for collateral channel development, the ability to move gas around obstructions in airways by the use of collateral channels appears to be a useful property of human lungs. This is because total airway obstruction in the absence of collateral channels often leads to rapid alveolar gas absorption into the blood from the alveoli distal to the obstructed airway, and this in turn leads to atelectasis and therefore vascular shunts and hypoxemia. Remarkably, chronic human lung diseases typified by airway obstruction—chronic obstructive pulmonary disease (COPD), asthma—produce $\dot{V}_A/\dot{Q}$ inequality due to presence of poorly ventilated areas but only uncommonly lead to true shunts.[31,30] The likely explanation for the paucity of shunts in COPD and asthma is the existence of collateral ventilation. Collateral ventilation in humans therefore appears to be a naturally occurring structural phenomenon that can to some extent counteract the gas exchange consequences of diseases.

Collateral perfusion must also occur in the alveolar capillary network. This is deduced simply from the richly interconnecting microvascular network that has the potential to allow blood to flow easily around microvascular obstructions into adjacent vessels. Just how much collateral blood flow potential exists at a larger scale is not clear, because it is difficult to study. However, well-documented connections occur between the bronchial and pulmonary circulations, creating a different kind of collateral circulatory network.[4] The importance of this connection is evident when the pulmonary artery is either absent or embolized. Then, the bronchial circulation expands considerably and can support function of the affected lung regions long term.

REACTIVE VASOCONSTRICTION AND BRONCHOCONSTRICTION

The distribution of ventilation or blood flow in the lung can be modified by vasoreactive or bronchoreactive functional changes that appear triggered by changes in alveolar gas composition. The most well-documented phenomenon is that of hypoxic pulmonary vasoconstriction.[2,27] Here, in response to local alveolar hypoxia produced by locally reduced ventilation, local pulmonary arterial constriction reduces blood flow in the hypoxic region. Whether this system developed to counteract disease or to cope with intrauterine life and the abrupt transition to air-breathing is arguable, although most people favor the latter explanation.

Irrespective of the reasons, the effect of hypoxic vasoconstriction is to help to return the local ratio of ventilation to blood flow toward normal. This automatic effect (whose basic biochemical basis remains controversial) is rarely able to fully restore $\dot{V}_A/\dot{Q}$ ratios to normal, but even partial improvements in $\dot{V}_A/\dot{Q}$ ratio facilitate gas exchange significantly. The negative aspect of hypoxic vasoconstriction is a rise in pulmonary vascular resistance. If this is substantial and protracted over time, pulmonary hypertension can develop, eventually leading to right heart failure. However, factors other than hypoxic vasoconstriction are then also generally present—microvascular destruction and alveolar distortion—and these may be more important to heart failure than hypoxia per se. However, hypoxic vasoconstriction has provided a rationale for enriched O_2 therapy in patients with chronic disease to reduce the severity, or to delay the progression, of pulmonary hypertension.

To a much less obvious extent, a counterpart to hypoxic vasoconstriction occurs in the airways: hypocapnic bronchoconstriction.[11,18] Here, especially when pulmonary embolism occurs, the $\dot{V}_A/\dot{Q}$ ratio in the embolized area rises due to loss of blood flow from vascular obstruction. This increase in $\dot{V}_A/\dot{Q}$ ratio leads to a lower local P_{CO_2} (see below), which causes bronchoconstriction in the local area. This reduces local ventilation and thus tends to normalize the local $\dot{V}_A/\dot{Q}$ ratio. Radioactive tracer ventilation scans routinely show evidence of this as a modest reduction in the ventilation of embolized regions.

THE $\dot{V}_A/\dot{Q}$ RATIO AND GAS EXCHANGE

To this point, much space has been given to the concepts underlying the distribution of ventilation ($\dot{V}_A$), blood flow ($\dot{Q}$), and hence their ratio, $\dot{V}_A/\dot{Q}$. The reason for this lies in the importance of $\dot{V}A/\dot{Q}$ ratios to the basic function of the lung—to exchange O_2 and CO_2 between the blood and the air. $\dot{V}A/\dot{Q}$ inequality, no matter what its physiological basis or pathologic cause, interferes with gas exchange and causes hypoxemia and sometimes hypercapnia.[35]

The following section will explain the relationship of $\dot{V}A/\dot{Q}$ inequality to gas exchange. The subject is complex and must be considered at several "concentric" levels. To start, we will consider how the $\dot{V}A/\dot{Q}$ ratio in a small local lung region controls local P_{O_2}, P_{CO_2}, and, therefore, how much O_2 and CO_2 are exchanged in that region. This isolated approach requires at first some key assumptions. Removing the restrictions of these assumptions is the next "concentric" step in understanding $\dot{V}A/\dot{Q}$ relationships. A final outer shell of modifying factors that can further affect gas exchange forms a third level of the analysis.

The $\dot{V}A/\dot{Q}$ Ratio of a Small Homogeneous Unit of Lung, and Gas Exchange

How the $\dot{V}A/\dot{Q}$ ratio determines gas exchange is best explained by considering the flux of O_2 from the environment into and out of the alveolus with each breath as well as from the alveolar gas into the capillary blood. Equations that describe these processes and follow the fundamental principle of mass conservation must be used. Original descriptions of these appeared some 50 years ago.[7,23–25] Figure 12-5 provides a model of a homogeneous lung and specifies the ventilation ($\dot{V}A$) and blood flow ($\dot{Q}$) together with the key locations of the relevant O_2 levels, also appropriate to consideration of a small homogeneous unit of lung.

Convention has long considered ventilation over a period of time as a constant in spite of the tidal nature of breathing. This is in fact a very reasonable approximation that has stood the test of time. Similarly, blood flow is considered constant, and this too has proved reasonable. If $\dot{V}A$ and $\dot{Q}$ are therefore considered as alveolar minute ventilation and blood flow of the small ho-

mogeneous unit respectively, the following simple mass conservation equations can be written for O_2:

$$\dot{V}_{O_2} = \dot{V}I \cdot F_{I_{O_2}} - \dot{V}A \cdot F_{A_{O_2}} \quad (2)$$

and

$$\dot{V}_{O_2} = \dot{Q} \cdot Cc'_{O_2} - \dot{Q} \cdot C\bar{v}_{O_2} \quad (3)$$

In these equations, $\dot{V}_{O_2}$ is amount of O_2 transferred from the environment into the blood per unit time and, given the assumption of steady-state conditions, this, when summed over all such units in the lungs, equals metabolic rate. $\dot{V}I$ and $\dot{V}A$ are, respectively, the inspired and expired volumes of gas respired per minute, less that amount remaining in the conducting airways. As anticipated, $\dot{V}I$ and $\dot{V}A$ are close to identical, otherwise the lungs would blow up or collapse in a short period. However, $\dot{V}I$ does not generally equal $\dot{V}A$ because slightly more O_2 is consumed per minute than is CO_2 produced (i.e., the respiratory quotient is in general not 1.0). Thus, $\dot{V}A = \dot{V}I - \dot{V}_{O_2} + \dot{V}_{CO_2}$. Mostly, the inequality of $\dot{V}I$ and $\dot{V}A$ can be ignored because the difference is only about 1 percent—if $\dot{V}I$ is 6 L/min and $\dot{V}_{O_2}$ is 300 ml/min with $\dot{V}_{CO_2}$ at 240 ml/min, $\dot{V}A = 5.94$ L/min. Although this small difference is not ignored in research applications, it can be for the present purposes, so that $\dot{V}I$ is replaced by $\dot{V}A$ in Eq. (1), simplifying the analysis below. In Eq. (1), $F_{I_{O_2}}$ and $F_{A_{O_2}}$ are the fractional concentrations (F) of O_2 in inspired (I) and exhaled alveolar (A) gas, respectively, from the small unit of Fig. 12-5. In Eq. (2), Cc'_{O_2} and $C\bar{v}_{O_2}$ are the O_2 concentrations (C) in the oxygenated blood leaving (c') and the deoxygenated blood entering ($\bar{v}$) the vasculature respectively. The abbreviation c' stands for end capillary blood; $\bar{v}$ for mixed venous (pulmonary arterial) blood.

Since Eqs. (2) and (3) both describe the same O_2 flux rate ($\dot{V}_{O_2}$) they may be set equal to each other

$$\dot{V}A [F_{I_{O_2}} - F_{A_{O_2}}] = \dot{Q} [Cc'_{O_2} - C\bar{v}_{O_2}] \quad (4)$$

and rearranged so that

$$\frac{\dot{V}A}{\dot{Q}} = \frac{[Cc'_{O_2} - C\bar{v}_{O_2}]}{[F_{I_{O_2}} - F_{A_{O_2}}]} \quad (5)$$

It should further be noted that because diffusion equilibration of O_2 transfer across the alveolar-capillary membrane is assumed to be complete, alveolar P_{O_2} and end capillary P_{O_2} are identical. Hence, the relationship between $F_{A_{O_2}}$ and Cc'_{O_2} is uniquely dictated by the O_2-Hb dissociation curve such that knowing $F_{A_{O_2}}$ allows us to determine directly Cc'_{O_2} (or vice versa).

Equation (5) is very revealing and explains directly the role of the $\dot{V}A/\dot{Q}$ ratio in governing alveolar gas exchange. This equation states that for a *given* set of what may be called boundary conditions (i.e., composition of inspired gas and mixed venous blood, represented here by $F_{I_{O_2}}$ and $C\bar{v}_{O_2}$, respectively, and for a known O_2-Hb dissociation curve), alveolar (and thus end capillary) P_{O_2} is *uniquely* determined by the ratio of alveolar ventilation ($\dot{V}A$) to blood flow ($\dot{Q}$).

Under the given assumptions, summarized as (1) continuous and constant ventilation and blood flow; (2) steady-state conditions; (3) diffusion equilibration of alveolar-capillary exchange; and (4) equality of inspired and expired ventilation, equations

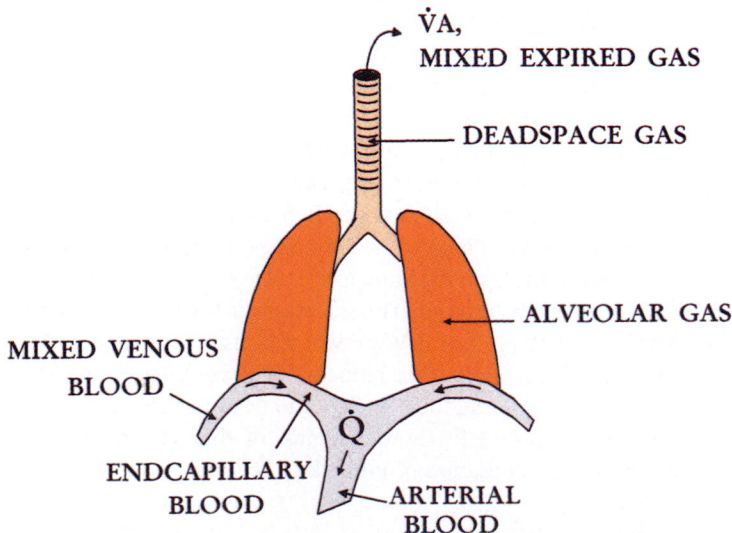

FIGURE 12-5 Conceptual model of the lungs indicating main sites in which oxygen and carbon dioxide partial pressures are different, together with the principal convective processes accomplishing gas exchange, ventilation ($\dot{V}A$) and blood flow ($\dot{Q}$).

The figure is labeled: $\dot{V}A$, MIXED EXPIRED GAS; DEADSPACE GAS; ALVEOLAR GAS; MIXED VENOUS BLOOD; ENDCAPILLARY BLOOD; $\dot{Q}$; ARTERIAL BLOOD.

identical in construct to Eq. (5) can be written for any gas being exchanged by the lung.

For CO_2, this produces Eq. (6):

$$\frac{\dot{V}_A}{\dot{Q}} = \frac{[C\bar{v}_{CO_2} - Cc'_{CO_2}]}{[F_{ACO_2} - F_{ICO_2}]} \quad (6)$$

The order of bracketed terms on the right is reversed to maintain positive numbers, since CO_2 is being eliminated from the blood. Of course, F_{ICO_2} is almost always zero and thus drops out of the equation.

Unfortunately, neither equation (5 or 6) is amenable to simple quantitative solutions, because of the complexity of the O_2 and CO_2 dissociation curves. The equations are however readily explored by appropriate computerized numerical analyses.[12–14,19,20,38] Using such programs, one can explore the relationship between $\dot{V}_A/\dot{Q}$ ratio and alveolar P_{O_2} and P_{CO_2}, and this is done in Fig. 12-6. These relationships are important because they indicate what degrees of $\dot{V}_A/\dot{Q}$ abnormality are required to affect gas exchange for both O_2 and CO_2. The four panels of Fig. 12-6 show alveolar P_{O_2} and P_{CO_2} as well as end capillary O_2 and CO_2 concentrations. The latter better reflect total gas exchange as a function of $\dot{V}_A/\dot{Q}$ ratio.

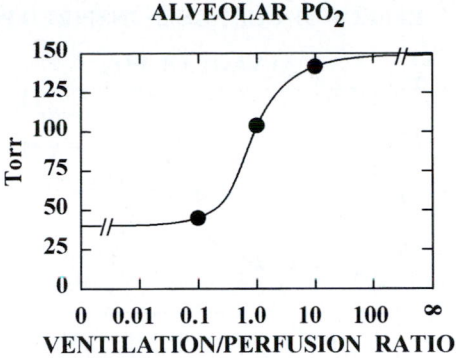

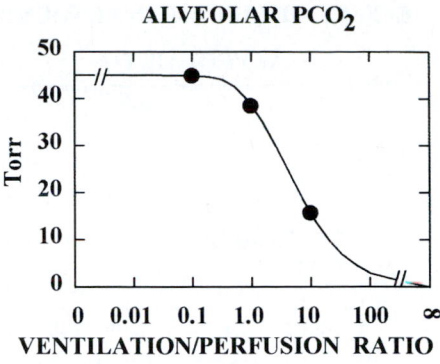

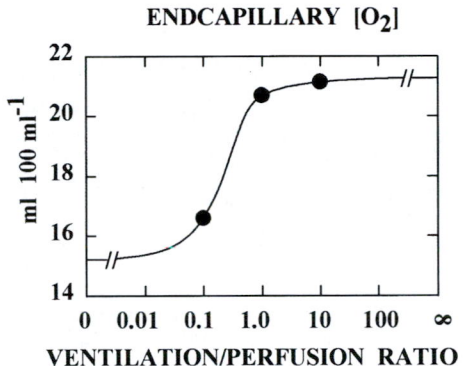

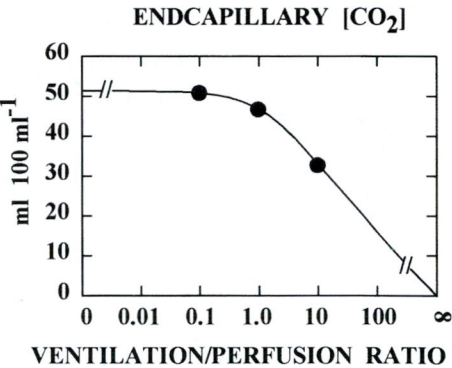

FIGURE 12-6 Calculated relationships between alveolar P_{O_2} and P_{CO_2} and the ventilation-perfusion ratio (top panels) and their corresponding end capillary blood concentrations (lower panels). The three solid circles in each case represent values for ventilation-perfusion ratios of 0.1, 1.0, and 10. (See text for further details.)

Specific conditions for Fig. 12-6 are that mixed venous blood P_{O_2} is 40 mmHg and P_{CO_2} 45 mmHg, normal resting values. Also, inspired gas is room air, and [Hb] is 15 gm dl⁻¹. In each panel, the three solid circles are positioned at the normal $\dot{V}_A/\dot{Q}$ ratio (of about 1.0) and at $\dot{V}_A/\dot{Q}$ ratios 10 times greater and less. All four relationships are highly nonlinear. Focusing on the two lower panels, it is evident for O_2 that a 10-fold reduction in $\dot{V}_A/\dot{Q}$ greatly reduces local O_2 transport, whereas a 10-fold increase barely improves it. Furthermore, as $\dot{V}_A/\dot{Q}$ falls even lower than 0.1, there is little further loss in O_2 transport. There is however little protection against a fall in $\dot{V}_A/\dot{Q}$ below 1.0—the curve is very steep below a $\dot{V}_A/\dot{Q}$ of 1.0, as the lower left panel shows. For CO_2, the curves are opposite in slope (P_{CO_2} falls as $\dot{V}_A/\dot{Q}$ increases). However, unlike the case for O_2, there is little difference between a $\dot{V}_A/\dot{Q}$ of 1.0 and a 10-fold reduction, whereas an increase in $\dot{V}_A/\dot{Q}$ considerably reduces alveolar P_{CO_2} and end capillary CO_2 concentration. The reason for the differences between O_2 and CO_2 lies mainly in the slopes of their dissociation curves: that for CO_2 is about 10-fold greater than that for O_2. It has been shown that the higher the slope of the dissociation curve (or equivalently for an anesthetic gas, its solubility) the more it is sensitive to areas of high $\dot{V}_A/\dot{Q}$. The lower the slope or solubility, the more the gas is affected by areas of low $\dot{V}_A/\dot{Q}$. Consequently, areas of low $\dot{V}_A/\dot{Q}$ predictably cause more reduction in arterial P_{O_2} than increase in arterial P_{CO_2}.[35] Although Fig. 12-6 is true strictly only for the stated "boundary" conditions

(i.e., mixed venous blood and inspired gas composition), the principles hold even for different conditions, as shown in Fig. 12-7 for O_2. The left panels illustrate how changes in mixed venous P_{O_2} alone will affect alveolar P_{O_2} and end capillary $[O_2]$ via Eq. (4). The right panels correspondingly show how change in inspired P_{O_2} affects O_2. Venous P_{O_2} is selected at 30, 40, and 50 mmHg, and inspired P_{O_2} is chosen to be 120, 150, and 180 mmHg. Changes in venous P_{O_2} dramatically affect P_{O_2} and $[O_2]$ in unventilated and poorly ventilated regions as well as regions approaching normal but have no real effect on high $\dot{V}_A/\dot{Q}$ alveoli. Altering inspired P_{O_2} (but not venous) has the converse effect if P_{O_2} is examined (top right panel), but, due to the nonlinear shape of the O_2-Hb dissociation curve, effects on $[O_2]$ are minimal in high $\dot{V}_A/\dot{Q}$ areas, small in very low $\dot{V}_A/\dot{Q}$ areas, and more significant between $\dot{V}_A/\dot{Q}$ ratios of 0.1 and 1.0 (bottom right panel). This figure shows how the inspired and mixed venous "boundary conditions" alter the magnitude (but not basic patterns) of alveolar gas exchange.

If one returns to the normal boundary conditions ($P\bar{v}_{O_2} = 40$ mmHg, $P_{IO_2} = 150$ mmHg), one can explore the consequences of $\dot{V}_A/\dot{Q}$ inequality on gas exchange. In reality, the complex structure of the lungs defies a simple analysis but conceptually even a two-compartment model is an invaluable aid to understanding this difficult area.

Figure 12-8 shows such a simple two-compartment model in three configurations: (1) each compartment equally ventilated

EFFECT OF CHANGE IN VENOUS P$_{O_2}$

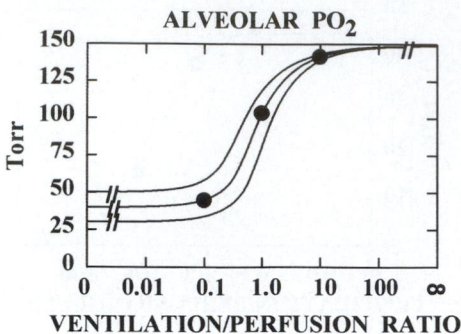

EFFECT OF CHANGE IN INSPIRED P$_{O_2}$

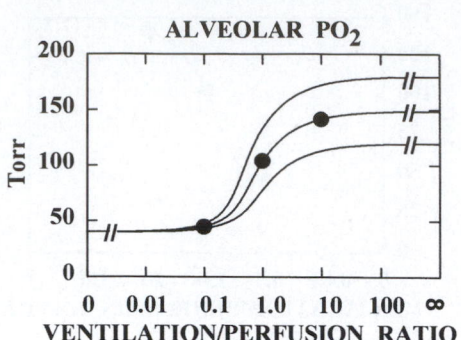

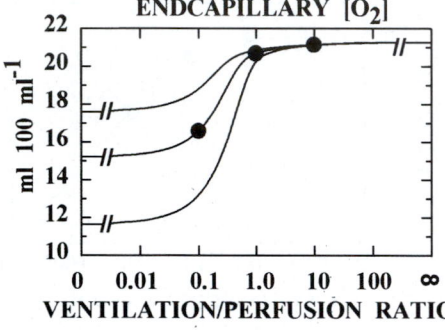

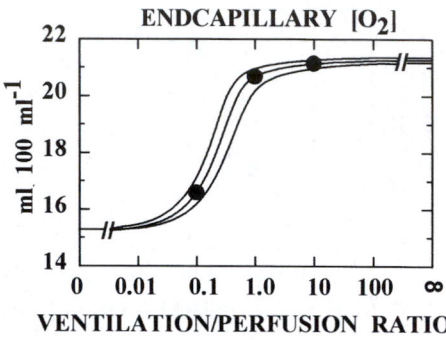

FIGURE 12-7 Effects of changes in mixed venous P$_{O_2}$ (left panels) or inspired P$_{O_2}$ (right panels) on alveolar P$_{O_2}$ and associated end capillary oxygen concentrations. Note that changes in venous P$_{O_2}$ mostly affect values associated with low ventilation-perfusion ratios, whereas changes in inspired P$_{O_2}$ affect units throughout the $\dot{V}_A/\dot{Q}$ range, especially those with medium to high $\dot{V}_A/\dot{Q}$ ratios.

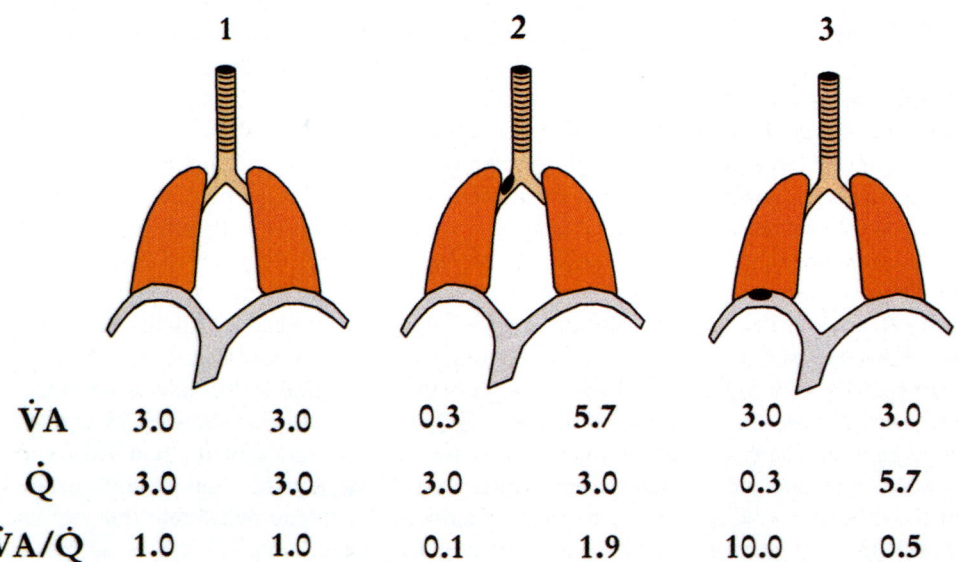

FIGURE 12-8 Three two-compartment models of ventilation-perfusion relationships. Model 1 represents an ideal lung without ventilation-perfusion mismatch. Model 2 represents a lung in which one compartment has a 90 percent reduction in its alveolar ventilation due to airway obstruction, and model 3 is a lung in which one compartment has a 90 percent reduction in capillary blood flow due to vascular obstruction. Ventilation, blood flow, and ventilation-perfusion ratio of each compartment are indicated. Total ventilation and total blood flow remain the same among the three models. (See text for further details.)

and perfused such that there is no $\dot{V}_A/\dot{Q}$ inequality; (2) the left compartment hypoventilated due to airway obstruction, causing $\dot{V}_A/\dot{Q}$ inequality; and (3) the left compartment hypoperfused from vascular obstruction. Table 12-1 shows the corresponding O_2 and CO_2 calculations for each compartment. Specific assumptions common to all three models are (1) the mixed venous P$_{O_2}$ remains at 40 mmHg; inspired P$_{O_2}$ is constant at 150 mmHg; total alveolar ventilation summed over both compartments is constant as is total blood flow, both taken to be 6 L · min^{-1}; [Hb] is constant at 15 gm dl^{-1}. Further, airways obstruction reduces L-hand compartmental ventilation from 3.0 to 0.3 L · min^{-1}, redistributing the balance to the R-hand compartment. Vascular obstruction is of the same order as the right panel of the figure shows. Note that for *both* obstructive models, one compartment has developed a $\dot{V}_A/\dot{Q}$ ratio less than average and the other a $\dot{V}_A/\dot{Q}$ ratio greater than average, irrespective of the location of the obstruction.

Using the curves of Fig. 12-6, for $P\bar{v}_{O_2} = 40$ mmHg and $P_{I_{O_2}} = 150$ mmHg, $P\bar{v}_{CO_2} = 45$ mmHg, and $P_{I_{CO_2}} = 0$ mmHg, alveolar P$_{O_2}$ and P$_{CO_2}$ are listed for each compartment of Fig. 12-8 in Table 12-1.

In Table 12-1, alveolar diffusion equilibration is assumed to be complete such that alveolar P$_{O_2}$ (P$_{A_{O_2}}$) equals end capillary P$_{O_2}$ (Pc'$_{O_2}$); the same holds for P$_{CO_2}$. In each obstructive model, the low $\dot{V}_A/\dot{Q}$ compartment has a lower-than-average P$_{O_2}$ and higher-than-average P$_{CO_2}$ as Fig. 12-6 dictates. The converse is seen for the compartment of high $\dot{V}_A/\dot{Q}$ ratio. Corresponding end capillary O_2 and CO_2 concentrations are also listed in Table 12-1.

The question is what will the mixed arterial blood and mixed expired gas O_2 and CO_2 levels change to as a result of obstruction of one compartment, and how will this affect the ability of the total system to exchange O_2 and CO_2? To answer these questions one applies simple mixing equations to the two individual compartments [left (L) and right (R)]. For O_2:

TABLE 12-1

O_2 and CO_2 Calculations for the Models of Fig. 12-8

	Normal		Airways Obstruction Model		Vascular Obstruction Model	
	Left	Right	Left	Right	Left	Right
P_{AO_2}, Pc'_{O_2}, mmHg	103.0	103.0	45.0	120.0	142.0	77.0
P_{ACO_2}, Pc'_{CO_2}, mmHg	38.8	38.8	44.9	32.5	15.5	42.7
Cc'_{O_2}, ml $\cdot$ dl^{-1}	20.7	20.7	16.7	20.9	21.1	20.1
Cc'_{O_2}, ml $\cdot$ dl^{-1}	46.9	46.9	50.8	43.9	32.5	48.8
Ca_{O_2}, ml $\cdot$ dl^{-1}	20.7		18.8		20.1	
Ca_{CO_2}, ml $\cdot$ dl^{-1}	46.9		47.5		48.0	
Pa_{O_2}, mmHg	103.0		55.0		77.0	
Pa_{CO_2}, mmHg	38.8		39.0		40.9	
$P\overline{A}_{O_2}$, mmHg	103.0		118.0		110.0	
$P\overline{A}_{CO_2}$, mmHg	38.8		33.7		29.2	
Total O_2 exchange, ml $\cdot$ min^{-1}	328.0		212 (65%)		294 (90%)	
Total CO_2 exchange, ml $\cdot$ min^{-1}	270.0		234 (87%)		203 (75%)	
$P\overline{A}_{CO_2}$, $-$ Pa_{O_2}, mmHg	0.0		63.0		33.0	
Pa_{CO_2} $-$ $P\overline{A}_{CO_2}$, mmHg	0.0		5.3		11.7	

$$P\overline{A}_{O_2} = \frac{P_{AO_{2L}} \cdot \dot{V}_{AL} + P_{AO_{2R}} \cdot \dot{V}_{AR}}{\dot{V}_{AL} + \dot{V}_{AR}}$$

$$Ca_{O_2} = \frac{Cc'_{O_{2L}} \cdot \dot{Q}_L + Cc'_{O_{2R}} \cdot \dot{Q}_R}{\dot{Q}_L + \dot{Q}_R} \quad (7)$$

For CO_2, identical equations apply. These mixing equations conserve mass and use the principle that the two gas or blood streams combine in a manner proportional to their relative ventilation and blood flow, respectively. Table 12-1 lists the results of these calculations, giving mixed alveolar partial pressure ($P\overline{A}_{O_2}$, $P\overline{A}_{CO_2}$) and mixed arterial concentrations (Ca_{O_2}, Ca_{CO_2}). From the blood gas concentration, corresponding arterial partial pressures (Pa_{O_2}, Pa_{CO_2}) are read directly off the O_2 and CO_2 dissociation curves. Finally, whole-lung computations of O_2 and CO_2 exchange rates (ml $\cdot$ min^{-1}) are determined using either equations 1 or 2 and the mixed alveolar or arterial data respectively, and the mixed alveolar to arterial partial pressure differences expressed for each gas.

The results are very instructive. Both obstructive models result in hypoxemia and slight hypercapnia, but the effects on arterial P_{O_2} and on the alveolar-arterial P_{O_2} difference greatly exceed those for CO_2 due to both shape and slope differences between the dissociation curves of the two gases. Airways obstruction produces more hypoxemia but *less* hypercapnia than the identical degree of vascular obstruction. This reflects the 10-fold greater dissociation curve slope of CO_2 compared to O_2, rendering O_2 relatively more susceptible to the lower $\dot{V}_A/\dot{Q}$ areas seen in the airway obstruction model (0.1 versus 0.5) (Fig. 12-8) and CO_2 relatively more susceptible to the higher $\dot{V}_A/\dot{Q}$ areas of vascular obstruction (10.0 vs. 1.9) (Fig. 12-8) as Fig. 12-6 would predict.

Both models have impaired overall O_2 and CO_2 exchange (recall that venous blood, inspired gas, total ventilation, and blood flow were all considered fixed and identical for all three models)

as a result of the development of $\dot{V}_A/\dot{Q}$ mixmatch. In keeping with the differential sensitivity of O_2 and CO_2 to regions of low and high $\dot{V}_A/\dot{Q}$ discussed above, total O_2 transport is diminished to a greater extent in the airway obstruction model than in the vascular obstruction model (Table 12-1). The converse is true for CO_2, also shown in Table 12-1.

The principal effects of $\dot{V}_A/\dot{Q}$ inequality as they apply to O_2 and CO_2 exchange may thus be listed. $\dot{V}_A/\dot{Q}$ inequality

1. Affects both gases, no matter what the pathological basis of the inequality.
2. Causes arterial hypoxemia and hypercapnia.
3. Causes usually more severe hypoxemia than hypercapnia.
4. Affects O_2 more than CO_2 when very low $\dot{V}_A/\dot{Q}$ regions develop.
5. Affects CO_2 more than O_2 when very high $\dot{V}_A/\dot{Q}$ regions develop.
6. Impairs total O_2 and CO_2 exchange by the lung.
7. Creates alveolar-arterial differences for both gases.

Compensation for Effects of $\dot{V}_A/\dot{Q}$ Mismatch

The preceding analysis shows that if no changes in total ventilation, blood flow, mixed venous blood or inspired gas composition occur, O_2 and CO_2 transfer across the lung is compromised. This is not viable in the steady state: the lungs must find a way to restore total O_2 and CO_2 transfer to levels equal to metabolic use of O_2 and production of CO_2. This leads to the next concentric level of consideration of $\dot{V}_A/\dot{Q}$ inequality referred to at the start of this section.

Here we ask what compensatory mechanisms exist to achieve restoration of O_2 and CO_2 transfer assuming that the initial pathophysiologic insults have persisted unchanged. The same models as in Fig. 12-8 and Table 12-1 will be used.

Changes in Mixed Venous Blood   The only possible short-term compensatory changes are in mixed venous blood, total ventilation, and cardiac output. (Hb change in response to tissue hypoxia requires days to weeks to develop and then is by no means always observed; changing inspired P_{O_2} is not usually an option until the patient seeks medical attention.) To reduce complexity, changes in venous blood alone are first addressed.

If it is assumed that there is no limit to how much O_2 can be extracted from the arterial blood by the peripheral tissues, it is evident that $\dot{V}_A/\dot{Q}$ inequality will passively lead to a reduced venous P_{O_2} and increased venous P_{CO_2}. This is deduced simply from the hypoxemia and hypercapnia initially produced by the $\dot{V}_A/\dot{Q}$ insult, together with the need to extract the same amount of O_2 (and add CO_2) to each ml of blood perfusing the tissues as before the $\dot{V}_A/\dot{Q}$ insult developed.

If venous P_{O_2} falls (and P_{CO_2} rises), Fig. 12-7 indicates that alveolar P_{O_2} will fall in each $\dot{V}_A/\dot{Q}$ compartment (as will P_{CO_2} rise). Thus a circle of events is set up such that if a single red cell were followed around the circulation, at each passage through the lungs and then tissues, P_{O_2} would fall progressively with each circuit of the body.

Although not intuitively obvious, this reduction in both arterial and venous P_{O_2} will not "bottom out" at zero (or in the case of CO_2 rise toward infinity) unless the $\dot{V}_A/\dot{Q}$ insult was fatally overwhelming in the first place: Both arterial and venous P_{O_2} will restabilize at new lower values (P_{CO_2} values will be higher) than were present immediately after the $\dot{V}_A/\dot{Q}$ insult developed. In so doing, $\dot{V}_{O_2}$ and $\dot{V}_{CO_2}$ will have been restored to normal values.

To explore this quantitatively, we will continue on with the models of Fig. 12-8 and Table 12-1 to show just what changes in venous and arterial P_{O_2} and P_{CO_2} must occur as a result of this process to restore pulmonary O_2 and CO_2 exchange to normal. The values are shown in Table 12-2. For the airways obstruction model, the passive blood gas changes are greater for O_2 than CO_2, consonant with the greater initial decrement in O_2 exchange caused by airways obstruction in the first place. For the vascular obstruction model, the effects are more marked for CO_2, for corresponding reasons. To restore $\dot{V}_{O_2}$ and $\dot{V}_{CO_2}$ in the airways obstruction model, hypoxemia is now more severe, but hypercapnia is mild. However, with vascular obstruction, hypoxemia remains mild but hypercapnia is severe. In both cases, the lung is meeting the original healthy requirement of transferring 328 and 270 ml/min of O_2 and CO_2, respectively.

The speed of passive venous blood composition changes is very rapid, taking place in seconds to minutes as the blood moves

continuously around the vascular system between lungs and tissues. The principal effects of the changes can be summarized as follows:

1. Following development of $\dot{V}_A/\dot{Q}$ mismatch, and a fall in $\dot{V}_{O_2}$ and $\dot{V}_{CO_2}$ at the lungs, mixed venous P_{O_2} will fall and mixed venous P_{CO_2} will rise to restore pulmonary $\dot{V}_{O_2}$ and $\dot{V}_{CO_2}$ to equal the original metabolic requirements for O_2 and CO_2 transport.
2. As a result, there will always be a further fall in arterial P_{O_2} and rise in arterial P_{CO_2}, compared to conditions prior to mixed venous blood changes.
3. When the $\dot{V}_A/\dot{Q}$ insult primarily involves development of extremely low $\dot{V}_A/\dot{Q}$ areas, those effects are more marked for O_2 than for CO_2.
4. When the $\dot{V}_A/\dot{Q}$ insult primarily consists of high $\dot{V}_A/\dot{Q}$ areas, CO_2 is affected more than O_2.

Changes in Total Ventilation   When either low or high $\dot{V}_A/\dot{Q}$ areas develop and the mixed venous and arterial adjustments occur as described above, there is hypoxemia and hypercapnia. Either or both may well stimulate an immediate increase in total ventilation, which will alleviate to some extent both the hypoxemia and hypercapnia. Figure 12-9 shows for the same two examples used above how increases in alveolar ventilation (distributed in the same proportions as in each of the two $\dot{V}_A/\dot{Q}$ models of Fig. 12-8) variably improve arterial P_{O_2} and P_{CO_2}. In the low $\dot{V}_A/\dot{Q}$ (airways obstruction) model, a 50 percent increase in total alveolar ventilation from the normal value of $6\ L \cdot min^{-1}$ to $9\ L \cdot min^{-1}$ drops arterial P_{CO_2} to almost 30 mmHg, well below the normal standard value of 40 mmHg. Arterial P_{O_2}, however, is not affected at all. This is because even a 50 percent increase in ventilation of the very poorly ventilated unit fails to significantly increase end capillary P_{O_2} of that unit (Fig. 12-6), whereas in the better ventilated unit of that model, Hb in the end capillary blood was already virtually fully saturated before the increase in ventilation.

For the model with vascular obstruction, a 50 percent increase in alveolar ventilation returns both P_{O_2} and P_{CO_2} to near-normal values (Fig. 12-9, lower panel). The difference in the two model responses to ventilation reflects the original $\dot{V}_A/\dot{Q}$ ratios of the two compartments—that is, where they lie on the curves of Fig. 12-6.

Changes in Cardiac Output   One final compensatory adjustment is possible—an increase in cardiac output. Adrenergic stimulation by arterial hypoxemia can raise cardiac output by 50 percent or more, and this will also tend to improve arterial blood gases by raising mixed venous P_{O_2} (and lowering mixed venous P_{CO_2}). Figure 12-10 shows the effects on arterial P_{O_2} and P_{CO_2} of such increases, as done for ventilation in Fig. 12-9, again assuming that the relative distribution of blood flow remains unaltered between the two compartments as total blood

TABLE 12-2

Gas Exchange Effects of Passive Changes in Mixed Venous Blood-Gas Values Required to Restore $\dot{V}_{O_2}$ and $\dot{V}_{CO_2}$ to Normal in the Models of Fig. 12-8

	Airways Obstruction Model		Vascular Obstruction Model	
	Before Change	*After Change*	*Before Change*	*After Change*
$P\bar{v}_{O_2}$, mmHg	40.0	30.4	40.0	39.5
$P\bar{v}_{CO_2}$, mmHg	45.0	50.7	45.0	62.4
Pa_{O_2}, mmHg	55.0	46.0	77.0	67.0
Pa_{CO_2}, ml $\cdot$ min^{-1}	39.0	44.5	40.9	55.6
$\dot{V}_{O_2}$, ml $\cdot$ min^{-1}	212.0	328 (normal)	294.0	328.0
$\dot{V}_{CO_2}$, ml $\cdot$ min^{-1}	234.0	270 (normal)	203.0	270.0

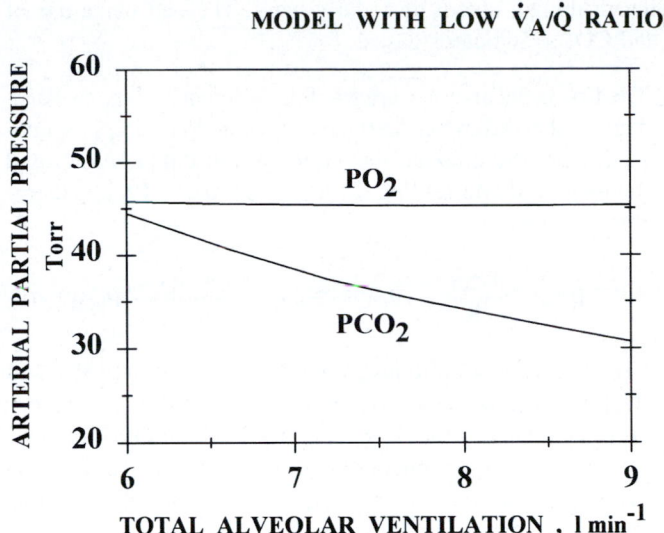

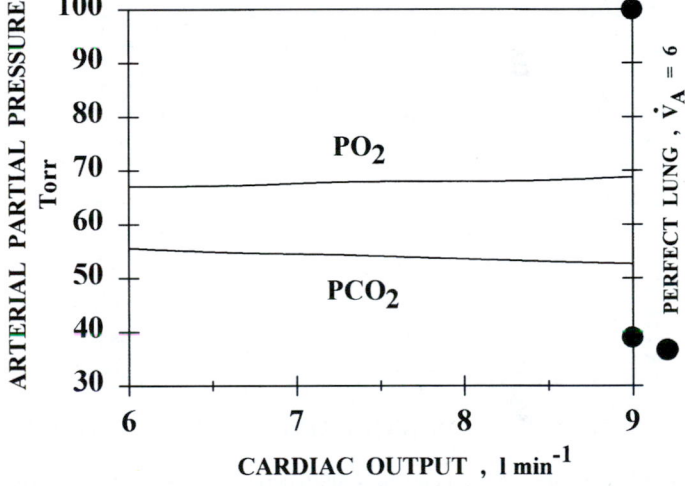

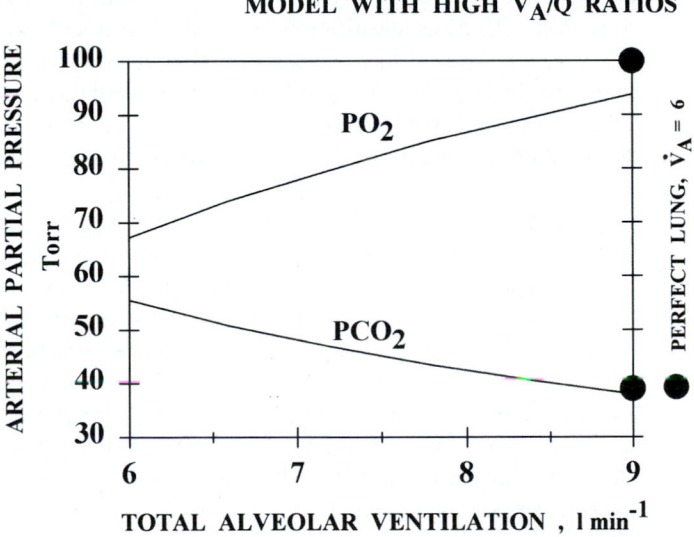

FIGURE 12-9   Effect of increasing alveolar ventilation on arterial P_{O_2} and P_{CO_2} in the two models with ventilation-perfusion inequalities in Fig. 12-8. Top panel is that for model 2, and bottom panel is that for model 3. Increasing ventilation is ineffective in restoring arterial P_{O_2} in the low $\dot{V}A/\dot{Q}$ model 2, but much more effective in the high $\dot{V}A/\dot{Q}$ model 3. Both models respond in terms of P_{CO_2}.

FIGURE 12-10   Effects of increases in cardiac output on arterial P_{O_2} and P_{CO_2} in models 2 and 3 of Fig. 12-8. Cardiac output produces a significant rise in P_{O_2} in the presence of regions of very low ventilation-perfusion ratio (top panel) but has little influence in the presence of higher ventilation-perfusion ratios (bottom panel). P_{CO_2} is affected only minimally in either case.

flow is increased. For a lung with airways obstruction causing very low $\dot{V}A/\dot{Q}$ regions (upper panel), an increase in cardiac output significantly improves arterial oxygenation—more so than does the same relative increase in ventilation. However, arterial P_{CO_2} is only slightly improved. In stark contrast, increases in cardiac output barely alter arterial P_{O_2} and P_{CO_2} in the high $\dot{V}A/\dot{Q}$ ratio model, especially when one recalls (Fig. 12-9) how effective an increase in ventilation is in restoring arterial P_{O_2} and P_{CO_2}.

When both ventilation and cardiac output are simultaneously increased, there is no real synergistic effect (Fig. 12-11): P_{O_2} and P_{CO_2} are improved as predicted from the individual changes (i.e., as shown above in Figs. 12-9 and 12-10).

In all the calculations depicted in figures 12-9, 12-10, and 12-11, the two-compartment models are exchanging the necessary amounts of O_2 and CO_2 to sustain normal metabolism. Depending on (1) the ventilatory and cardiovascular responses to the original insult causing $\dot{V}A/\dot{Q}$ mismatch and (2) the fundamental pattern of $\dot{V}A/\dot{Q}$ mismatch (i.e., the preponderance of low and/or high $\dot{V}A/\dot{Q}$ areas), it is possible to observe hypercapnia, normocapnia, or hypocapnia. However, it is very uncommon for arterial P_{O_2} to be fully normalized by the compensatory mechanisms, and the observed degree of hypoxemia can be extremely variable. As an important clinical corollary, it becomes difficult to establish the severity of the $\dot{V}A/\dot{Q}$ insult per se when the extent of compensating mechanisms cannot be easily established, since

MODEL WITH LOW $\dot{V}_A/\dot{Q}$ RATIOS

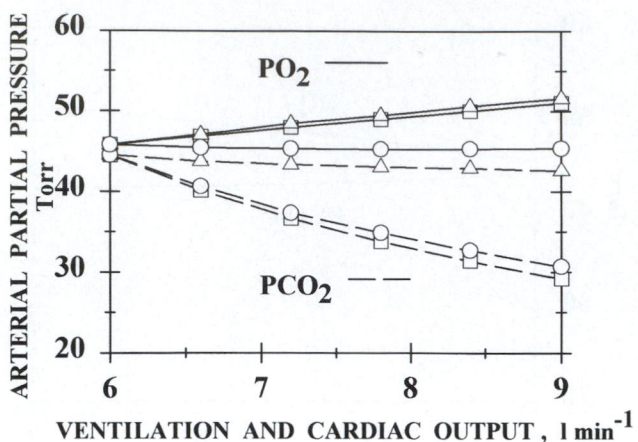

VENTILATION AND CARDIAC OUTPUT , $l\ min^{-1}$

MODEL WITH HIGH $\dot{V}_A/\dot{Q}$ RATIOS

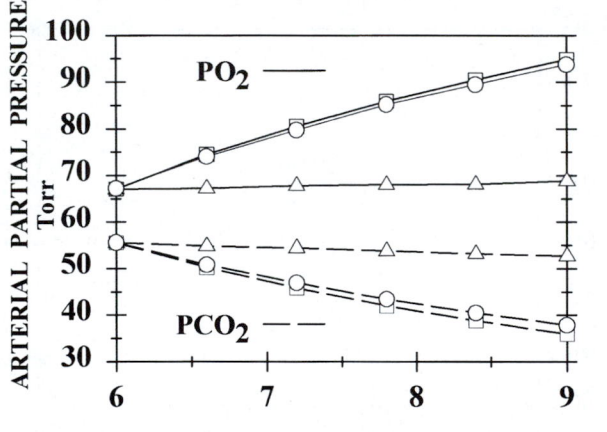

VENTILATION AND CARDIAC OUTPUT , $l\ min^{-1}$

FIGURE 12-11 Responses to simultaneous increases in ventilation and cardiac output (compared to responses to individual increases as shown in Fig. 12-9 and 12-10). Simultaneous increases do not provide for significantly more improvement than with either alone. ○–○ = response to increased ventilation only; △–△ = response to increased cardiac output only; □–□ = response to increased ventilation cardiac output.

these two aspects are so intertwined in their resulting effect on gas exchange.

Assessment of Ventilation-Perfusion Inequality

Whereas the preceding discussion highlights the complexity of how $\dot{V}_A/\dot{Q}$ inequality impairs gas exchange, there is a need for methods to assess the extent of such mismatch in the clinical setting. The *multiple inert gas elimination technique* was developed expressly for this purpose.[32] Although the technique provides the necessary descriptions of the extent and pattern of inequality, it remains a complex technique that is not well-suited to routine clinical use. Several traditional quantifying indexes of $\dot{V}_A/\dot{Q}$

mismatch remain useful on a daily basis. They all make use of O_2 and CO_2 as indicator gases:

1. The first is the alveolar-arterial P_{O_2} difference, $P_{A_{O_2}} - P_{a_{O_2}}$. This is the difference between alveolar P_{O_2} ($P_{A_{O_2}}$, calculated from the alveolar gas equation presented below) and the measured arterial P_{O_2} ($P_{a_{O_2}}$). The $P_{A_{O_2}} - P_{a_{O_2}}$ is therefore given by

$$P_{I_{O_2}} - \frac{P_{CO_2}}{R} + P_{CO_2} \cdot F_{I_{O_2}} \cdot \frac{(1-R)}{R} - P_{a_{O_2}} \quad (8)$$

Use of this equation requires knowledge of inspired P_{O_2} and $[O_2]$, the respiratory exchange ratio R, and the ideal alveolar P_{CO_2}, which is that P_{CO_2} that would be observed in alveolar gas of a homogeneous lung having the R value of the patient's actual lung at the time.[23–25] Three problems arise with the application of this equation: First, the result is very dependent on $P_{I_{O_2}}$ even when the amount of $\dot{V}_A/\dot{Q}$ inequality does not change as $P_{I_{O_2}}$ is varied. Second, the value of R is generally not known and must be assumed. Third, in some cases, the usual substitution for the ideal alveolar P_{CO_2}, the measured arterial P_{CO_2}, leads to a systematic error because arterial P_{CO_2} can be significantly higher than the ideal alveolar value. However, $P_{A_{O_2}} - P_{a_{O_2}}$ remains a useful index of $\dot{V}_A/\dot{Q}$ inequality providing these limitations are kept in mind.

2. The second index is simply the ratio of arterial P_{O_2} to $F_{I_{O_2}}$ which in a perfectly normal lung is virtually insensitive to $P_{I_{O_2}}$, a major advantage. However, even that is an oversimplification, because this ratio may not be as constant as hoped for depending on the pattern of $\dot{V}_A/\dot{Q}$ inequality present.

A third index is venous admixture (QSQT) or, equivalently, physiological shunt. This is a parameter that expresses what magnitude shunt would have to be present in a particular case to explain a patient's arterial P_{O_2} if that shunt were the sole cause of hypoxemia. The formula is:

$$\% QSQT = 100 \cdot \frac{[Cc'_{O_2} - Ca_{O_2}]}{[Cc'_{O_2} - C\overline{v}_{O_2}]} \quad (9)$$

where Cc'_{O_2} is the calculated end capillary $[O_2]$ of blood perfusing a hypothetical alveolus exchanging gas at the overall respiratory exchange ratio of the patient's actual lungs. Ca_{O_2} is arterial and $C\overline{v}_{O_2}$ mixed venous $[O_2]$, respectively. This parameter, working in the O_2 concentration domain (rather than the partial pressure domain of the $P_{A_{O_2}} - P_{a_{O_2}}$), better reflects the degree of gas exchange defect but requires knowledge of the ideal alveolar conditions to calculate Cc'_{O_2}, as well as [Hb]. This parameter also is sensitive to $P_{I_{O_2}}$ in that when $\dot{V}_A/\dot{Q}$ inequality is present, its contribution to QSQT diminishes progressively as $P_{I_{O_2}}$ is raised. The most limiting aspect of this parameter however is the need to know the value of $C\overline{v}_{O_2}$, reflecting mixed venous blood. If this must be assumed rather than measured, the value of QSQT will be only as good as the assumption, which may be extremely misleading if changes in $C\overline{v}_{O_2}$ in fact occur but are not accounted for in the QSQT calculation.

4. Finally, using the arterial and mixed expired partial pressures of CO_2 (Pa_{CO_2}, $P\bar{E}_{CO_2}$, respectively), a very similar calculation to QSQT can be performed to compute the percentage of total ventilation that is wasted on non-gas-exchanging ("dead space") areas of the lungs. As for QSQT, the calculation determines the magnitude of the dead space that would have to be present to dilute the arterial P_{CO_2} down to the mixed expired level if that dead space were the only abnormality in ventilation. Expressed as deadspace (VD) over tidal volume (VT) percentage,

$$\% \, VDVT = \frac{100 \cdot [Pa_{CO_2} - P\bar{E}_{CO_2}]}{[Pa_{CO_2}]} \qquad (10)$$

This parameter is independent of P_{IO_2} but is weakened by the fact that the normal airway conducting volume is included in the computed result. Thus it may be difficult to separate how much the VDVT value represents this normal anatomic dead space as opposed to reflecting $\dot{V}A/\dot{Q}$ inequality amongst the alveoli. This problem is amplified because even normally VDVT is very dependent on the size of the tidal volume even if the dead space volume itself is essentially constant. Thus, for a dead space volume of 150 ml and a tidal volume of 500 ml, VDVT is 30 percent, but if tidal volume were to drop to 400 ml, VDVT now becomes 38 percent—not because $\dot{V}A/\dot{Q}$ inequality has developed, but simply because smaller breaths are being taken.

In summary, no index of $\dot{V}A/\dot{Q}$ inequality is without potentially significant limitations both quantitative and qualitative. However, if these limitations are recognized and the data interpreted accordingly, they still remain very useful indexes of clinical gas exchange function.

REFERENCES

1. Albert RK, Lease D, Sanderson M, et al: The prone position improves arterial oxygenation and reduces shunt in oleic-acid-induced acute lung injury. *Am Rev Respir Dis* 135:628–633, 1987.
2. Barer GR, Howard P, Shaw JW: Stimulus-response curves for the pulmonary vascular bed to hypoxia and hypercapnia. *J Physiol (Lond)* 211:139–155, 1970.
3. Cunningham DJC, Robbins PA, Wolff CB: Integration of respiratory responses to changes in alveolar partial pressures of CO_2 and O_2 and in arterial pH, in Fishman AP, Charniack NS, Widdicombe JG, Greiger SR (eds), *Handbook of Physiology*, Section 3: *The Respiratory System,* vol 2. Bethesda, MD, American Physiological Society, 1986, pp 475–528.
4. Deffebach ME, Widdicombe J: The bronchial circulation, in Crystal RG, West JB, Barnes PJ, et al (eds), *The Lung: Scientific Foundations,* vol 1. New York, Raven Press, 1991, pp 741–757.
5. Engel LA: Dynamic distribution of gas flow, in Fishman AP, Macklem PT, Mead J, Geiger SR (eds), *Handbook of Physiology. Section 3: The Respiratory System,* vol 3. Bethesda, MD, American Physiological Society, 1986, pp 575–593.
6. Evans JW, Wagner PD: Limits on $\dot{V}A/\dot{Q}$ distributions from analysis of experimental inert gas elimination. *J Appl Physiol* 42:889–898, 1977.
7. Fenn WO, Rahn H, Otis AB: A theoretical study of composition of alveolar air at altitude. *Am J Physiol* 146:637–653, 1946.
8. Glenny RW, Lamm WJ, Albert RK, Robertson HT: Gravity is a minor determinant of pulmonary blood flow distribution. *J Appl Physiol* 71:620–629, 1991.
9. Hakim TS, Dean GW, Lisbona R: Effect of body posture on spatial distribution of pulmonary blood flow. *J Appl Physiol* 64:1160–1170, 1988.
10. Hlastala MP, Bernard SL, Erickson HH, et al: Pulmonary blood flow distribution in standing horses is not dominated by gravity. *J Appl Physiol,* in press.
11. Ingram Jr RH: Effects of airway versus arterial CO_2 changes on lung mechanics in dogs. *J Appl Physiol* 38:603–607, 1975.
12. Kelman GR: Digital computer subroutine for the conversion of oxygen tension into saturation. *J Appl Physiol* 1:1375–1376, 1966.
13. Kelman GR: Digital computer procedure for the conversion of P_{CO_2} into blood CO_2 content. *Respir Physiol* 3:111–115, 1967.
14. Kelman GR: Computer programs for the production of O_2-CO_2 diagrams. *Respir Physiol* 4:260–269, 1968.
15. Macklem PT: Airway obstruction and collateral ventilation. *Physiol Rev* 51:368–436, 1971.
16. Menkes HA, Traystman RJ: State of the art—collateral ventilation. *Am Rev Respir Dis* 116:287–309, 1977.
17. Mitzner W: Collateral ventilation, in Crystal RG, West JB, Barnes PJ, et al (eds), *The Lung: Scientific Foundations,* vol 1. New York, Raven Press, 1991, pp 1053–1063.
18. Newhouse MT, Becklake MR, Macklem PT, MacGregor M: Effect of alterations in end-tidal CO_2 tension on flow resistance. *J Appl Physiol* 19:745–749, 1964.
19. Olszowka AJ, Farhi LE: A system of digital computer subroutines for blood gas calculations. *Respir Physiol* 4:270–280, 1968.
20. Olszowka AJ, Farhi LE: A digital computer program for constructing ventilation/perfusion lines. *J Appl Physiol* 26:141–146, 1969.
21. Rahn H, Fenn WO: *A Graphical Analysis of the Respiratory Gas Exchange.* Washington, DC, American Physiological Society, 1955.
22. Raine JM, Bishop JM: A-a difference in O_2 tension and physiological dead space in normal man. *J Appl Physiol* 18:284–288, 1963.
23. Riley RL, Cournand A: "Ideal" alveolar air and the analysis of ventilation/perfusion relationships in the lung. *J Appl Physiol* 1:825–847, 1949.
24. Riley RL, Cournand A: Analysis of factors affecting partial pressures of oxygen and carbon dioxide in gas and blood of lungs: Theory. *J Appl Physiol* 4:77–101, 1951.
25. Riley RL, Cournand A, Donald KW: Analysis of factors affecting partial pressures of oxygen and carbon dioxide in gas and blood of lungs: Methods. *J Appl Physiol* 4:102–120, 1951.
26. Taylor GI: Dispersion of soluble matter in solvent flowing slowly through a tube. *Proc R Soc Lond* Ser A 219:186–203, 1953.
27. Von Euler US, Liejestrand G: Observations on the pulmonary arterial blood pressure in the cat. *Acta Physical Scand* 12:301–320, 1947.
28. Wagner PD, Laravuso RB, Uhl RR, West JB: Continuous distributions of ventilation-perfusion ratios in normal subjects breathing air and 100% O_2. *J Clin Invest* 54:54–68, 1974.
29. Wagner PD: Diffusion and chemical reaction in pulmonary gas exchange. *Physiol Rev* 57:257–312, 1977.
30. Wagner PD, Dantzker DR, Dueck R, et al: Ventilation-perfusion inequality in chronic obstructive pulmonary disease. *J Clin Invest* 59:203–216, 1977.
31. Wagner PD, Hedenstierna G, Bylin G: Ventilation-perfusion inequality in chronic asthma. *Am Rev Respir Dis* 136:605–612, 1987.
32. Wagner PD, West JB: Ventilation-perfusion relationships, in West JB (ed), *Ventilation, Blood Flow and Diffusion, Pulmonary Gas Exchange,* vol 1. New York, Academic Press, 1980, pp 219–262.

33. Weibel ER: *Morphometry of the Human Lung.* Berlin, Springer-Verlag, 1963.
34. Weibel ER: *The Pathway for Oxygen.* Cambridge, MA, Harvard University Press, 1984.
35. West JB: Ventilation/perfusion inequality and overall gas exchange in computer models of the lung. *Respir Physiol* 7:88–110, 1969.
36. West JB: *Ventilation/Blood Flow and Gas Exchange.* Oxford and Philadelphia, Blackwell Scientific Publications and Lippincott, 1990.
37. West JB, Hugh-Jones P: Pulsatile gas flow in bronchi caused by the heart beat. *J Appl Physiol* 16:697–702, 1961.
38. West JB, Wagner PD: Pulmonary gas exchange, in West JB (ed), *Bioengineering Aspects of the Lung,* vol 3. New York, Dekker, 1977, pp 361–458.
39. Young IH, Mazzone RW, Wagner PD: Identification of functional lung unit in the dog by graded vascular embolization. *J Appl Physiol* 49:132–141, 1980.

CHAPTER 13

DIFFUSION, CHEMICAL REACTIONS INVOLVING RESPIRATORY GASES, AND DIFFUSING CAPACITY

Robert A. Klocke

Uptake of oxygen, the principal substrate of metabolism, and excretion of carbon dioxide, the primary metabolic product, require rapid, efficient exchange of respiratory gases in the lung. The quantities of exchanged gases are staggering. For example, an 1800-calorie diet requires exchange of 375 L of oxygen per day, as well as an almost equal volume of carbon dioxide. Because of the limited time that blood remains in the pulmonary capillary bed, the process of exchange is accomplished in less than 1 s at rest and one-half that time during exercise.[24] This rapid, high-volume exchange occurs efficiently despite numerous interacting processes of diffusion and chemical reaction that occur in the lung. The rates of these processes not only are affected by intrinsic characteristics of blood but also are determined by a host of other factors, including inspired oxygen fraction, alveolar gas tensions, cardiac output, and metabolic activity. The ease of exchange of respiratory gases belies the complexity of the overall process.

DIFFUSION

Normally, diffusion is treated as movement of material in a medium from a higher to a lower concentration. It is more ex-

act to consider diffusion down an electrochemical gradient. This is especially important when a substance is moving between two phases, as occurs when O_2 and CO_2 are exchanged between alveolar gas and blood. The most accurate and practical measures of the electrochemical activities of the respiratory gases are their partial pressures. Movement of O_2 and CO_2 proceeds between the gas and liquid phases by diffusion down electrochemical, not concentration, gradients. For example, dissolved CO_2 diffuses down a partial pressure gradient from blood (46 mmHg) into the alveolus (40 mmHg) even though its actual concentration (millimoles of molecular CO_2 per liter of gas or blood) is greater in alveolar gas (2.5) than it is in venous blood (1.3).

Influence of Physical Properties

The concentration (C) of gas x dissolved in fluid depends upon its partial pressure (P) and solubility (α)

$$C_X = \alpha_X P_X \qquad (1)$$

Gas diffusion occurs down a partial pressure gradient, but the quantity of gas transported is critically dependent on its solubility in the medium in which diffusion occurs. Hence, the rate ($\dot{V}_X$) of gas x crossing the alveolar-capillary membrane at any instant in time (t) is

$$\dot{V}_X(t) = \frac{A\,k_X\,\alpha_X[P_{A_X}(t) - P_{C_X}(t)]}{h} \qquad (2)$$

where A and h are properties of the membrane barrier (the surface area and thickness), k_X and α_X are physical properties of the gas in the membrane (diffusion coefficient and solubility), and $[P_{A_X}(t) - P_{C_X}(t)]$ is the instantaneous partial-pressure gradient between alveolar and capillary blood.

The diffusion coefficient (k_X) of a gas in the alveolar-capillary membrane is largely a function of the size of the gas molecule, which is approximately proportional to the reciprocal of the square root of its molecular weight. Oxygen ($1/\sqrt{32}$) has a slightly larger diffusion coefficient than carbon dioxide ($1/\sqrt{44}$) in the alveolar membrane. However, the solubility of CO_2 in water, the major component of the tissue composing the membrane, is more than 20-fold greater than the solubility of O_2. This difference far outweighs the effect of the slightly smaller size of the oxygen molecule. Thus, CO_2 transfer across the alveolar membrane is 20 times greater than O_2 transfer when both gases diffuse under the same partial-pressure gradient. A much greater alveolar-capillary P_{O_2} gradient is required to maintain O_2 transfer approximately equal to that of CO_2.

Diffusion is affected by the viscosity of the medium in which diffusion occurs. As a result, diffusion of a gas in air occurs at a rate that is four orders of magnitude greater than diffusion in water. Gaseous diffusion coefficients in tissues are only moderately less than those in water, since most tissues are composed primarily of water. The interior of the erythrocyte is an exception to this general rule in that the viscosity of the red cell contents is substantially greater than that of water, resulting in a diffusion coefficient for oxygen that is only one-third of the aqueous coefficient.[33] The combination of the viscosity inside the erythrocyte and the large size of the hemoglobin molecules lowers the diffusion coefficient of hemoglobin in the red cell to 4 to 9 percent of hemoglobin in dilute aqueous solution. As a result, significant diffusion gradients are thought to exist within the red cell even though the distance of the cell membrane to the innermost portion of the cell is only a few microns.[30]

Capacitance and Diffusion Exchange

The alveolar-capillary membrane provides the barrier to diffusion between the alveoli and the interior of the capillaries. The rate of exchange and attainment of diffusion equilibrium for a gas such as oxygen is dependent on the capacitance of the gas in its reservoir (i.e., the alveoli) and the diffusion sink (i.e., blood) relative to its capacitance in the membrane. The reservoir of a gas provides a pressure head to drive the diffusive process. In the case of oxygen, the alveolar reservoir provides a larger capacitance than the capacitance of the alveolar-capillary membrane because O_2 is poorly soluble in the membrane. Hence, alveolar P_{O_2} decreases relatively slowly as O_2 traverses the membrane. If the alveolus receives a normal quantity of ventilation relative to its blood flow, sufficient oxygen is brought into the alveolus to maintain a pressure head for O_2 diffusion across the membrane as mixed venous blood enters the capillary bed. The presence of hemoglobin in blood increases its capacity for O_2 two orders of magnitude compared to the solubility of O_2 in the alveolar-capillary membrane. The large sink for oxygen provided by hemoglobin tends to maintain the difference between alveolar and capillary P_{O_2}, facilitating transfer of O_2 across the alveolar-capillary membrane. In normal circumstances, oxygen exchange across the membrane does not take place instantaneously but does reach completion in approximately 0.3 s[44]—well below the average time of 0.5 to 0.8 s that blood remains in the capillary bed.[24] The lesser membrane capacitance compared to the capacitances of alveolar gas and blood is responsible for this delay in completion of exchange. If the membrane were not extremely thin (less than 1 μm),[45] the process of O_2 exchange would not be completed during capillary transit time.

In contrast to oxygen, the capacitance of carbon dioxide in the membrane is sufficiently great compared to the capacitances

in blood and alveoli to permit rapid equilibration of CO_2 across the alveolar-capillary membrane.[42] As discussed below, CO_2 exchange requires a finite time for completion, but this delay is the result of time needed to complete processes in blood, not diffusion across the alveolar-capillary membrane.

Inert gases (i.e., gases that are carried in physical solution and not bound or transported in different forms in blood) are exchanged almost instantaneously between the alveolus and the capillary.[44] Inert gases have similar solubilities in the alveolar-capillary membrane and blood. If an inert gas is poorly soluble, such as nitrogen, small quantities of gas dissolve in the membrane and blood, maintaining alveolar pressure essentially constant to support the diffusive process. Even though the quantity of gas traversing the membrane is small, the low capacity of blood for the gas is saturated quickly and diffusive transfer is completed rapidly. In the case of extremely soluble gases, such as ether, the great solubility of the gas in membrane and blood leads to rapid depletion of ether in the alveoli, stopping the diffusive process. Equilibrium is reached quickly because of the rapid decrease in gas tension in the alveoli. Uptake of poorly soluble gases is limited by the quantity of blood perfusing an alveolus because the sink is smaller than the reservoir.[29] In the case of highly soluble gases, uptake is limited by ventilation because the reservoir is smaller than the sink. With gases of intermediate solubility, the combination of matched capacitances in the reservoir, membrane and sink also produces rapid diffusion equilibrium. Only gases such as O_2 or CO, which have capacitances in the reservoir and sink that are substantially greater than that in the alveolar-capillary membrane, will require finite time to reach diffusive equilibrium.

CHEMICAL REACTIONS INVOLVING RESPIRATORY GASES

Transport of respiratory gases not only requires diffusion across the alveolar capillary membrane but also entails numerous chemical reactions with components of the blood. Like diffusive transport of oxygen, these chemical reactions are not instantaneous and require finite periods for completion. It is commonly thought that diffusion provides the greatest time-dependent impediment to gas exchange, but in actuality, chemical processes, especially those occurring in combination with diffusion or other chemical reactions, are more likely to slow rates of exchange.

Oxygen and Carbon Monoxide

From a stoichiometric viewpoint, the binding of O_2 to each of the four heme moieties of the hemoglobin tetramer is described by four successive step

$$Hb_i + O_2 \underset{k_i}{\overset{k'_i}{\rightleftharpoons}} Hb_iO_2 \qquad (3)$$

where i = 1 to 4, k'_i and k_i are the association and dissociation kinetic constants. If the four heme rings were similar and acted independently, k'_i and k would be the same for each heme ring and the resulting dissociation curve would have a hyperbolic shape. However, binding of oxygen to one of the heme rings affects the affinity for O_2 of the remaining heme moieties of the tetrameric molecule, leading to the familiar sigmoid shape of the oxygen dissociation curve (see Chapter 14). Attempts to determine the values of each of the four association constants and the four dissociation constants have been only partly successful. The exact values for these constants are not important, however, because the rate of uptake of O_2 by hemoglobin contained within the erythrocyte is not determined only by the rate of chemical reaction.

The binding and release of oxygen occur quite rapidly in dilute solutions of hemoglobin but proceed more slowly in red cell suspensions.[13,30] The high concentration of hemoglobin within the erythrocyte is responsible for this slower rate of reaction. Because of the large size of the hemoglobin molecule and increased viscosity of the red cell contents, hemoglobin remains relatively immobile.[33] As the red cell enters the capillary, oxygen molecules bind to reduced hemoglobin molecules just inside the erythrocyte membrane. As these hemoglobin molecules become saturated, however, subsequent oxygen molecules entering the red cell must diffuse more deeply into the interior of the cell to reach reduced hemoglobin molecules.

This combination of diffusion and chemical reaction causes oxygen uptake to occur as an "advancing front," which proceeds at a rate that is an order of magnitude slower than O_2 uptake in well-mixed, dilute hemoglobin solution.[39] This combined process is complex and is not easily described from a theoretical standpoint. As a result, the rate of oxygen uptake by hemoglobin contained in red cells is described by a single overall descriptive rate constant, k_c', which incorporates all the processes into a single phenomenologic value. Similarly, the release of oxygen from erythrocytes is described by k_c, also a descriptive constant. In reality, k_c' and k_c are not true constants and vary with oxygen saturation, pH, and hemoglobin type.[19,30] The same is true regarding constants used to describe carbon monoxide uptake in blood, as well as description of the replacement of O_2 in blood by CO. The rate at which CO replaces bound O_2 in blood with a normal hemoglobin concentration is described by the constant θ, which appears in the familiar equation used to describe the CO diffusing capacity.[40]

The rate of O_2 and CO uptake by erythrocyte suspensions is determined in vitro and assumed to be representative of the rates of gas exchange in vivo.[13] However, classic in vitro measurements of these rate constants in red cell suspensions have been affected adversely by methodologic artifacts.[4] Rate constants measured in thin layers of erythrocytes indicate that gas exchange can occur twice as rapidly as previously thought.[18]

Carbon Dioxide

CO_2 is transported in blood as dissolved molecular CO_2, bicarbonate ion, and carbamate. The latter is a salt of carbamic acid formed by reaction of CO_2 with certain amino groups on the hemoglobin molecule. The relation between the partial pressure of CO_2 and the total content of CO_2 in all forms is described by the CO_2 dissociation curve of blood (see Chapter 14). Because CO_2 is more soluble than O_2 in the alveolar-capillary membrane, it has been assumed that CO_2 exchange occurs much more rapidly than O_2 exchange. However, only dissolved CO_2 can cross the alveolar capillary membrane, and conversion of bicar-

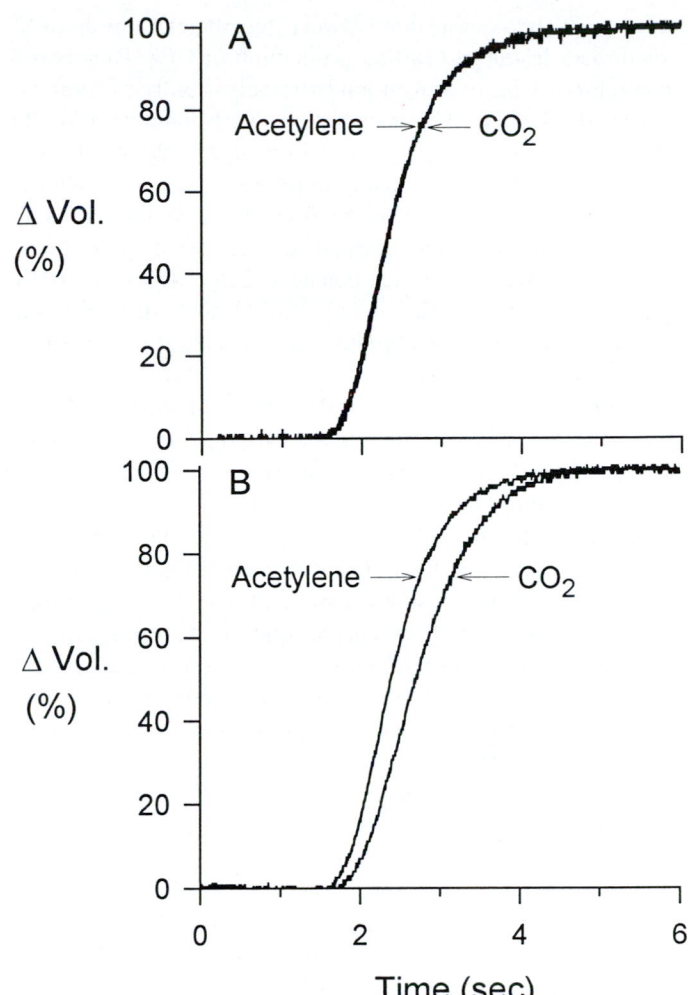

FIGURE 13-1   Rate of acetylene and CO_2 excretion after bolus injections into the pulmonary artery of isolated lungs perfused with buffer. Volume changes are normalized to facilitate comparison. *A.* The excretion of both acetylene and CO_2 proceed at the same rate after injections of buffer containing either dissolved CO_2 or acetylene. *B.* The excretion of CO_2 lags behind that of acetylene after injections of buffer containing either bicarbonate ion or acetylene. In this example, the mean time of CO_2 excretion lags 0.312 s behind that of acetylene. This slower excretion of CO_2 is caused by the time required to convert bicarbonate to CO_2 with catalysis in this experiment provided by carbonic anhydrase localized to the capillary endothelium. *(Based on data of Schünemann and Klocke[42]; reproduced from Klocke,[27] with permission.)*

bonate and carbamate to dissolved CO_2 limits the rate of CO_2 exchange. As indicated in Fig. 13-1*A,* when a bolus of CO_2 is injected into an isolated lung perfused with saline buffer, CO_2 is rapidly exchanged at the same rate as the inert gas acetylene. In contrast, when a bicarbonate bolus is injected into the same preparation (Fig. 13-1*B*), CO_2 exchange lags behind acetylene excretion because a finite period is required to process bicarbonate to dissolved CO_2.

Dissolved CO_2 is excreted almost instantaneously as blood enters the pulmonary capillary bed,[42] but it constitutes only 8 percent of the total quantity of CO_2 exchanged during capillary transit.[31] The majority (79 percent) of excreted CO_2 enters the capillary bed as bicarbonate ion. As dissolved CO_2 leaves capillary blood, the equilibrium between bicarbonate ion and CO_2 is disturbed, leading to further production of CO_2. Bicarbonate ion combines with hydrogen ion extremely rapidly to form carbonic acid (H_2CO_3). The dehydration of carbonic acid to CO_2 and water is a slow process, but it is catalyzed about 10,000 to 16,000 times by the large concentration of carbonic anhydrase inside the erythrocyte.[31] This rapid catalysis depletes the concentration of intracellular bicarbonate after a short time (0.1 s), slowing the conversion of bicarbonate to CO_2.[20] Depletion of hydrogen ions in this reaction is not a factor, since the substantial buffering provided by hemoglobin maintains intracellular pH relatively constant.

As intracellular stores of bicarbonate are depleted, extracellular bicarbonate enters the cell in exchange for intracellular chloride (Fig. 13-2). Bicarbonate-chloride movement across the erythrocyte membrane occurs in an electrically neutral one-for-one exchange that is facilitated by a carrier, termed band 3 protein, present in the erythrocyte membrane.[27] Despite the presence of approximately 1 million carrier sites with extremely rapid turnover number (50,000 ions per second) on the surface of each erythrocyte,[32] bicarbonate-chloride exchange has a half-time of 0.1 s and requires 0.4 to 0.5 s to reach completion.[28] Drugs such as aspirin can inhibit this transmembrane exchange to some extent in vitro,[5] but it is not clear whether these agents have a major effect on CO_2 excretion in vivo. In some circumstances the time required for the combined processes of dehydration of carbonic acid and transmembrane ionic exchange is sufficiently long that CO_2 exchange is not completed prior to blood leaving the pulmonary capillary.[1] The degree of disequilibrium is small, however, and a minimal increase in ventilation can easily compensate for the slight impairment of CO_2 exchange.[1]

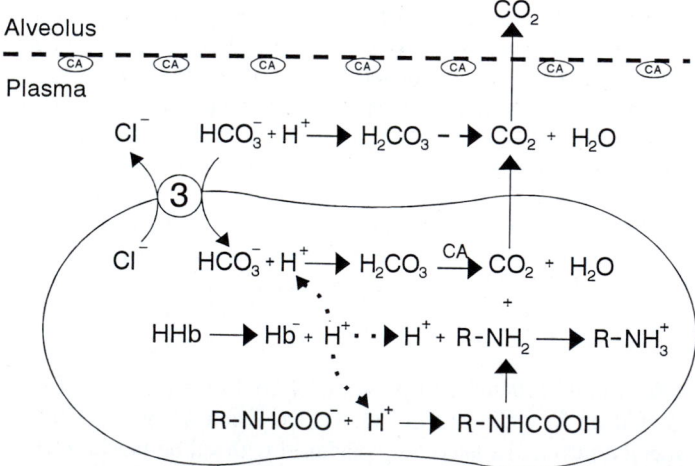

FIGURE 13-2 Pathways of CO_2 transport and exchange in the lung. CA=carbonic anhydrase within the erythrocyte or localized to the capillary endothelium; dashed arrow indicates that the production of CO_2 from plasma bicarbonate proceeds more slowly than the same reaction inside the erythrocyte; dotted arrows indicate that hemoglobin provides protons that partake in these reactions; R-NH_2=amino groups of hemoglobin molecule that bind CO_2 to form carbamate compounds, R-NHCOOH; 3=band 3 anion exchange protein in the cell membrane, which facilitates exchange of bicarbonate and chloride ions across the membrane. (*Reproduced from Klocke,[27] with permission.*)

In the past, it was assumed that plasma bicarbonate ion could participate in CO_2 exchange only after entering the erythrocyte.[39] However, carbonic anhydrase is present on the interior surface of the pulmonary capillary in sufficient concentration to catalyze the dehydration reaction by a factor of 100 to 150.[27] Mathematical models of CO_2 exchange indicate that this lesser catalytic activity, together with a plasma buffering power substantially less than that present within the red cell, results in relatively little production of CO_2 from bicarbonate outside the confines of the erythrocyte.[1] Experiments have not yet been performed in vivo to confirm these computations.

Besides exchange of dissolved CO_2 and bicarbonate, a modest amount of CO_2 excretion (13 percent) results from release of CO_2 bound to hemoglobin as carbamate (Fig. 13-2).[27] This exchange depends on change in the molecular conformation of hemoglobin that accompanies oxygenation. This pathway accounts for a portion of the Haldane effect, the change in the CO_2 dissociation curve that results from oxygenation of blood (see Chapter 14).

DIFFUSING CAPACITY

The pulmonary diffusing capacity (D_L) for a gas provides an estimate of the rate of transfer of that gas from the alveoli into capillary blood. Initially it was thought that only diffusion across the membrane limited gas exchange and this process could be described by equation 1 above. This is the case for inert gases, and equilibrium is achieved rapidly even in the case of severe reduction of the diffusing capacity.[44] However, transfer of gases that combine with elements of blood or are transported in different chemical forms can be limited both by diffusion across the alveolar membrane and by the rate of chemical reactions in blood. As noted previously, CO_2 equilibrium may not be reached in the pulmonary capillary bed because of the time required to complete chemical reactions. However, CO_2 itself crosses the alveolar-capillary membrane as rapidly as an inert gas,[42] and D_L for CO_2 is so great that it cannot be measured accurately.[22] The only gases that have measurable diffusing capacities are those with low solubility in the pulmonary membrane and high capacitance in blood secondary to liganding with intracellular hemoglobin. These gases include oxygen, carbon monoxide, and nitric oxide.

Diffusing Capacity for Oxygen

The diffusing capacity is calculated as the volume of gas absorbed by pulmonary blood per unit time ($\dot{V}$) divided by the pressure gradient between alveolar gas (P_A) and capillary blood (P_C). For oxygen

$$D_{L_{O_2}} = \frac{\dot{V}_{O_2}}{P_{A_{O_2}} - P_{C_{O_2}}} \tag{4}$$

Measurement of $D_{L_{O_2}}$ is difficult because, in addition to diffusion, O_2 transfer is limited by other mechanisms, such as ventilation-perfusion mismatching and shunting (see Chapter 12). Therefore, $D_{L_{O_2}}$ must be measured under conditions in which these other pathophysiological mechanisms are absent. With deliberate reduction of alveolar P_{O_2} produced by inhaling hypoxic

O_2 gases (~about 10 percent), O_2 exchange is predominantly limited by diffusion,[12] so $D_{L_{O_2}}$ can be measured. However, this reduction in alveolar, and hence arterial P_{O_2} precludes measurement of $D_{L_{O_2}}$ in many patients. The measurement is further complicated by a changing alveolar-capillary P_{O_2} gradient during capillary transit, and calculation of the time course of capillary P_{O_2} requires the complex Bohr integration procedure.[26] These difficulties have led clinicians and investigators to abandon attempts to measure $D_{L_{O_2}}$.

Diffusing Capacity for Carbon Monoxide

Carbon monoxide provides an excellent alternative to measure the diffusing capacity because CO is present in minimal amount in venous blood and binds to hemoglobin in the same manner as O_2. $D_{L_{CO}}$ is calculated by dividing CO uptake by mean alveolar CO tension. CO uptake originally was presumed to be limited by diffusion alone and CO thought to bind rapidly to hemoglobin. Thus, capillary P_{CO} should remain essentially zero and could be ignored in the calculation. However, in their pioneering work, Roughton and Forster,[40] demonstrated that CO uptake was limited both by diffusion across the alveolar-capillary membrane and by chemical reaction of CO with intracellular hemoglobin. $D_{L_{CO}}$ is influenced by both processes and is described mathematically by the well-known equation

$$\frac{1}{D_{L_{CO}}} = \frac{1}{Dm_{CO}} + \frac{1}{\Theta V_c} \tag{5}$$

where Dm_{CO} is the diffusing capacity of the alveolar-capillary membrane for CO, θ the rate of displacement of O_2 from intracellular hemoglobin by CO, and V_c the volume of blood in the pulmonary capillary bed. As pointed out in the original report,[40] there are certain assumptions implicit in the derivation. For example, at elevated $P_{A_{O_2}}$ the limiting rate of chemical reaction is the displacement of O_2 from hemoglobin by CO, since O_2 binds before CO. At lower $F_{I_{O_2}}$ (e.g., as provided in room air), this is not exactly the case, and to some extent the two gases compete for binding sites. However, the assumption is sufficiently accurate to allow calculation of Dm and Vc from measurements of $D_{L_{CO}}$ at two different $F_{I_{O_2}}$ if the value of θ at each $F_{I_{O_2}}$ is known. Equation 5 has been used to describe pulmonary exchange of other gases, but the mathematical basis for the equation is valid only for CO exchange. Extrapolation of this theoretical framework to exchange of other gases may lead to inaccuracies. Finally, estimates of the diffusing capacity measured with any gas are based on the assumptions that the lung is homogeneous, that all portions of the lung have the same ventilation-perfusion ratio, and that gas exchange units have the same relative volume and ability to exchange the test gas.

Diffusing Capacity for Nitric Oxide

Nitric oxide binds to hemoglobin in the same manner as O_2 and CO, but the rate of NO binding is more rapid than that of the other two gases. Thus, the chemical reaction term $1/\theta V_c$ in equation 5 should contribute little to the overall diffusing capacity when NO is used to measure D_L. Measurements of D_L with CO and NO in the same subjects have indicated that $D_{L_{NO}}$ is ap-

proximately three to five times greater than $D_{L_{CO}}$.[15,34] Since the physical characteristics of NO and CO are similar except for the differing kinetics of their reactions with hemoglobin, this has allowed calculation of Dm and Vc in a single measurement at normal alveolar P_{O_2}. These experiments support previous work that indicates that diffusion and chemical reaction provide approximately equal resistance to the uptake of CO and O_2.[24,40]

Interpretation of these observations should be confirmed with different experimental approaches to avoid potential artifacts of $D_{L_{NO}}$ measurements. A key assumption in the measurement of $D_{L_{NO}}$ is that NO binds negligibly to receptors other than hemoglobin. Binding to ligands other than hemoglobin would lead to overestimates of the true $D_{L_{NO}}$. NO is especially prone to this type of artifact, since it must be administered in very low concentrations during the measurement to avoid its cardiovascular effects. In addition, recent work indicates that the lung and nasal sinuses can produce NO, further confusing interpretation of measurements of NO exchange.[25] Because of these effects and the uncertainty of the interpretation of $D_{L_{NO}}$, it has no clinical role at present.

Methods for Measuring Diffusing Capacity

SINGLE-BREATH TECHNIQUE

The single-breath technique to measure the diffusing capacity is the method used almost exclusively in clinical practice. The subject exhales to residual volume, inhales a maximal breath of dilute CO in air, holds the breath for approximately 10 s, and then exhales maximally. A gas sample obtained after sufficient expiration to clear the dead space is used to estimate final alveolar CO fraction. After inhalation of a single breath of a gas mixture containing CO, the alveolar partial pressure of CO falls exponentially as CO enters the capillary blood. The volume of CO taken up in the lungs can be calculated from the volume of inspired gas and the initial and final concentrations of CO in alveolar gas. The rate of CO uptake during the breath-hold varies as a function of the alveolar $P_{A_{CO}}$, which falls throughout the breath-hold. Capillary CO pressure is assumed to be equal to zero. The diffusing capacity is calculated by

$$D_{L_{CO}} = \frac{60\,V_A}{t_{bh}\,(P_B - 47)} \ln \frac{F_{A_{CO}}\,\text{initial}}{F_{A_{CO}}\,\text{final}} \tag{6}$$

where V_A is the volume of gas present in the lung (ml_{STPD}) at the start of the breath-hold, P_B the barometric pressure (mmHg), t_{bh} the duration of the breath-hold (seconds), 60 the number of seconds per minute, and $F_{A_{CO}}$ the alveolar fraction of carbon monoxide at the beginning and end of the breath-holding period.[36] An insoluble inert gas such as helium or neon is included in the inspirate. Then V_A can be calculated from the dilution of the inert gas (in this case, helium) and the inspired volume (V_I)

$$V_A = V_I \frac{F_{I_{He}}}{F_{A_{He}}} \tag{7}$$

where $F_{I_{He}}$ and $F_{A_{He}}$ are the inspired and alveolar helium concentrations. As originally described,[36] V_A was calculated from the inspired volume and a separate determination of the residual volume. However, automated instruments that are now used to measure $D_{L_{CO}}$ calculate V_A from the inspired and alveolar concentrations of the inert gas. The final alveolar CO fraction is obtained by measuring CO in the alveolar gas sample. The initial alveolar CO fraction is calculated from the dilution of the CO in the inspired volume in the volume of gas present in the lung during the breathhold,

$$F_{A_{CO}} \text{ initial} = F_{I_{CO}} \frac{V_I}{V_A} \qquad (8)$$

where $F_{I_{CO}}$ is the inspired CO fraction.

The single-breath method requires some degree of patient cooperation to perform the required respiratory maneuvers. A patient with reduced lung volume may not have a sufficiently large vital capacity to clear the dead space and provide a large enough sample to analyze for alveolar gas concentration. This is now less of a problem with automated equipment and current gas analyzers which can utilize small samples for measurements. The ability to hold the breath for 10 s also limits applicability to some patients. Finally, this method can be employed only in the resting state, since few patients can hold the breath for 10 s during strenuous exercise. Despite these limitations, the single-breath $D_{L_{CO}}$ is the most practical of all available methods.

STEADY-STATE TECHNIQUE

With this method, the patient inhales a low concentration of CO for a prolonged time (usually 6 min), until a steady state of CO uptake is reached. $D_{L_{CO}}$ is calculated from the rate of CO uptake in the final minute of the test and the alveolar pressure of CO. CO uptake is calculated from minute ventilation and the difference between inspired and expired CO fraction. Alveolar P_{CO} is calculated from inspired P_{CO} and alveolar dead space. This method requires either an arterial blood gas sample to measure dead space, a necessity that makes the test impractical, or the assumption of a value for dead space. $D_{L_{CO}}$ measured with the steady-state technique is usually performed during exercise, since the smaller dead space/tidal volume ratio present during exercise decreases errors associated with the assumption of a dead space.[11]

The requirement of measuring D_L during exercise sharply limits the practicality of steady-state measurements in patients with extensive lung disease. Furthermore, the prolonged inhalation of a CO mixture leads to elevated blood CO levels, violating the assumption of zero P_{CO} in blood and leading to possible underestimates of the true $D_{L_{CO}}$. In contrast, substantially less CO is absorbed by blood with the single-breath method, and the measurement is completed before absorbed CO recirculates into the pulmonary capillary bed. Finally, the prolonged steady-state procedure is less convenient to perform than the single-breath method.

REBREATHING METHOD

Sackner and colleagues[41] developed a means of assessing $D_{L_{CO}}$ by measuring the breath-by-breath decrease in alveolar CO as the subject repeatedly rebreathes into an anesthesia bag containing CO. $D_{L_{CO}}$ is calculated from the exponential decline in alveolar CO in a manner similar to that of the single-breath method. An insoluble inert gas is included in the rebreathed gas mixture to estimate lung volume. Addition of a relatively soluble inert gas (e.g., acetylene) permits simultaneous estimation of cardiac output and lung water. The additional information obtained from the measurement is attractive, and the rebreathing maneuver tends to reduce artifactual reduction of the true $D_{L_{CO}}$ caused by maldistribution of inspired gas in relation to lung volume and blood flow. Unfortunately, technical problems restrict this method to the research laboratory. The requirement of quasi-instantaneous measurement of CO during the rebreathing maneuver cannot be accomplished with the infrared equipment used to measure CO in most clinical laboratories. Measurement of rapid changes in CO concentration requires mass spectrometry, a much more expensive technique. In addition, the mass spectrometer cannot distinguish between N_2 and CO because both have the same mass, so ^{13}CO must be utilized for the measurement.

MEASUREMENT OF Dm, Vc

If $D_{L_{CO}}$ is measured, the remaining variables in equation 5 are Dm, θ, and Vc. The process of diffusion across the alveolar-capillary membrane is described by equation 2, and the diffusing capacity of the membrane (Dm) is the combination of the characteristics of membrane surface area (A), diffusion coefficient (k) and gas solubility (α) in the membrane, and the thickness of the membrane (h). Dm cannot be measured directly. θ, the rate of replacement of O_2 bound to hemoglobin by CO, can be measured in vitro. A variety of techniques have been used to measure θ,[30] and values of this constant are available over a wide spectrum of O_2 tension.[38] Because O_2 and CO compete for the same sites on hemoglobin, the rate of CO binding is inhibited by increasing P_{O_2} and θ varies inversely with P_{O_2}. Thus, measured $D_{L_{CO}}$ decreases as θ is reduced with increasing P_{O_2}. Vc, the volume of blood present in the pulmonary capillaries, also cannot be measured directly. Since the relation between θ and P_{O_2} is established, only Dm and Vc in equation 5 are unknown. If these two variables are unaffected by P_{O_2}, measurement of $D_{L_{CO}}$ at two different oxygen tensions permits solution for Dm and Vc by mathematical or graphic procedures (Fig. 13-3). This approach, developed by Roughton and Forster,[40] indicates that uptake of CO—and, by analogy, uptake of O_2—is limited equally by the processes of diffusion across the alveolar-capillary membrane and chemical reaction within capillary blood. This method has been used extensively to determine the effects on Dm and Vc in a variety of normal physiological conditions and differing diseases.

Factors Influencing Diffusing Capacity

The CO diffusing capacity was thought to reflect the resistance of the alveolar-capillary membrane to transfer of CO from the alveoli to capillary blood. The classic work of Roughton and Forster[40] further elucidated the influence of chemical reactions on transfer of CO. In this work, the authors clearly indicated the assumptions underlying the measurements of these processes, but these cautionary warnings have frequently gone unheeded. An abnormal value of the diffusing capacity does not necessarily in-

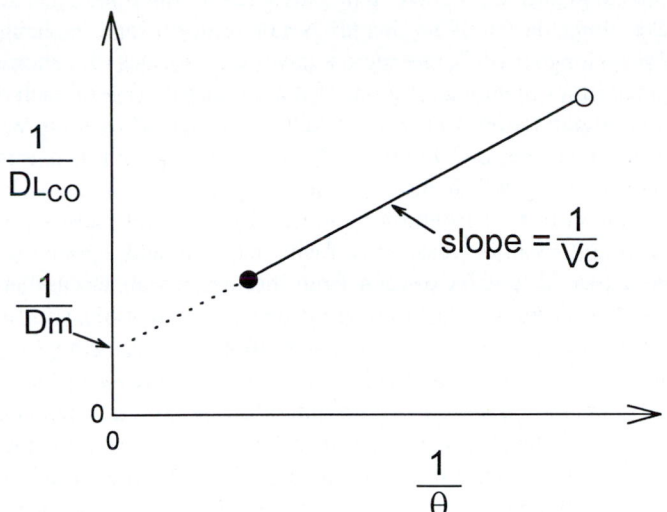

FIGURE 13-3 Graphic solution for Dm and Vc from measurements of $D_{L_{CO}}$ at normal (●) and elevated (○) alveolar P_{O_2}. θ varies inversely with alveolar P_{O_2}, and $D_{L_{CO}}$ decreases with increasing alveolar P_{O_2}. The reciprocal of $D_{L_{CO}}$ is plotted as a function of the reciprocal of θ. The line joining two measurements at differing alveolar P_{O_2} is extrapolated to the ordinate to obtain the reciprocal of Dm. The slope of this line is the reciprocal of Vc.

dicate abnormal diffusive transfer of CO or O_2 in the lung. $D_{L_{CO}}$ reflects an abnormality in gas transfer that may be indicative of abnormal diffusion, but it also can reflect abnormalities in the gas-carrying capacity of blood, the nonuniformity of distribution of physiological properties throughout the lung, the loss of lung tissue, or artifacts in measurement. For these reasons, in Europe this test is termed the CO transfer factor, rather than the CO diffusing capacity. Perhaps the specificity of the diffusing capacity is best compared to the specificity of the serum creatinine. An abnormal value of serum creatinine can reflect primary renal disease, but it can also be affected by extrarenal factors (muscle mass, state of hydration, cardiac output, obstruction to outflow, etc.). These limitations do not negate the usefulness of the serum creatinine in clinical medicine, but they require careful thought in interpretation of the test results. Similar caution is required in interpreting determinations of the CO diffusing capacity.

HEMOGLOBIN CONCENTRATION

Capillary blood volume (Vc) is a prime variable in the diffusing capacity; its importance is due to the quantity of hemoglobin present within the capillary bed. This quantity can be reduced directly through disease, which decreases the capillary blood volume, but it also can vary with the concentration of hemoglobin within the capillary. Hence, in the absence of lung disease, $D_{L_{CO}}$ is affected by the hemoglobin concentration in blood.[10] To compensate for alteration in hemoglobin concentration, $D_{L_{CO}}$ can be corrected to a standard hemoglobin concentration of 14.4 gm/dl by

$$D_{L_{CO}} \text{ corrected } = \frac{D_{L_{CO}} \text{ uncorrected}}{0.06965 \, [\text{Hb}]} \quad (9)$$

where [Hb] is hemoglobin concentration (in grams per deciliter).[10]

ALVEOLAR PARTIAL PRESSURE OF OXYGEN

As indicated previously, θ depends on P_{O_2}, and increased alveolar P_{O_2} will reduce measured $D_{L_{CO}}$. Therefore, patients cannot be given supplemental oxygen when the measurement is made. Conversely, reduced alveolar P_{O_2} will lead to an increment in measured $D_{L_{CO}}$. This has led some investigators to advocate using slight increases in inspired O_2 fraction in measuring $D_{L_{CO}}$ at altitude, to facilitate comparison to values measured at sea level.[6] Even when alveolar P_{O_2} is kept constant, lifelong residents of a community located 10,000 feet above sea level have slightly greater diffusing capacities than sea-level residents.[8] Short-term residence (6 weeks) at altitude does not cause an increase in $D_{L_{CO}}$. Beagles raised at altitude have slightly greater diffusing capacities even when reacclimated to sea level than similar animals raised at sea level.[23] However, dogs taken to altitude for 3 years after reaching adulthood do not exhibit an increased $D_{L_{CO}}$, suggesting that residence at altitude during growth is the basis for the increased $D_{L_{CO}}$. It is not clear at this point whether these data can be extrapolated to humans.

BODY POSITION

$D_{L_{CO}}$ is 5 to 15 percent greater in the supine position than in the erect position.[3] This difference is within the usual variability of the determination, but it leads to a slight systematic increase that can be detected by comparisons in the same subjects. With assumption of the supine position, there is a shift in blood volume from the lower trunk and limbs to the lungs. Most of the increase appears to be due to a 13 to 27 percent increase in Vc accompanying the fluid shift. However, there is also a minimal increase in Dm in the supine position. The effect of posture on $D_{L_{CO}}$ decreases with age, but the reasons underlying this observation remain unknown.[3]

EXERCISE

$D_{L_{CO}}$ can increase approximately twofold during exercise. The increase is attributed to increases in both Dm and Vc as alveolar-capillary surface area and capillary volume increase with recruitment of previously nonperfused capillary segments.[24] The transit time through the capillary bed decreases, but not as much as would be predicted in a fixed vascular bed. The potential reduction in transit time is offset to some degree by recruitment of capillaries that previously were not perfused.

Theoretically, $D_{L_{CO}}$ must have a maximum that cannot be exceeded when the entire pulmonary capillary bed and alveolar surface have been recruited. This should lead to a plateau in measured $D_{L_{CO}}$ even though the level of exercise continues to increase. This has never been observed in humans. Using a unique animal preparation of conscious greyhounds exercising on a treadmill, Carlin and coworkers[2] could not demonstrate a plateau in $D_{L_{CO}}$ with increasing exercise even though oxygen uptake reached a level of approximately 120 ml/kg/min. This level of O_2 uptake is almost twice that seen in highly trained humans.[9] It seems unlikely that the diffusing capacity in humans reaches a plateau during maximal exercise, but this does not rule out the possibility that gas exchange is limited by diffusion. Disequilibrium may occur before maximum recruitment of the diffusing capacity, because capillary transit time may be less than the time required for O_2 exchange to be completed. Indirect evidence in humans suggests that blood leaves the capillary bed without attaining complete equilibrium between alveolar P_{O_2} and capillary P_{O_2} during heavy exercise at sea level.[9,16]

The determination of $D_{L_{CO}}$ after exercise has led to the interesting observation that $D_{L_{CO}}$ decreases by approximately 10 to 15 percent after strenuous exercise of any type.[17,37] This decrement persists for at least 6 h and returns to its preexercise level by 20 h.[17] A second bout of exercise 2 h after the first period does not produce a further decrement in $D_{L_{CO}}$.[17] Arterial P_{O_2} falls similarly during both exercise periods. Furthermore, there is no response to diuretic administration, suggesting that the decrease in $D_{L_{CO}}$ is not the result of interstitial pulmonary edema.[17] The cause of the decrease in $D_{L_{CO}}$ associated with strenuous exercise remains uncertain.

LUNG VOLUME

The measured value of $D_{L_{CO}}$ decreases with reduction in lung volume. This can be seen with an inadequate inspiration to total lung capacity in a person with normal lungs, or with a maximal inspiration in a patient whose total lung capacity has been reduced by disease. In an effort to correct for alterations in lung volume rather than a true loss of diffusing capacity, clinicians and investigators have attempted to correct $D_{L_{CO}}$ measurements by dividing by lung volume. This ratio of $D_{L_{CO}}/V_A$, also termed the Krogh coefficient, will be a useful index only if two assumptions are valid. First, there must be an approximately linear relation between $D_{L_{CO}}$ and V_A. This appears to be the case. Second, the relation between $D_{L_{CO}}$ and V_A must be directly proportional (i.e., a graph of $D_{L_{CO}}$ versus V_A must pass through the origin of the graph). This clearly is not the case. Stam and colleagues[43] have shown that $D_{L_{CO}}/V_A$ is not a constant in normal persons and varies as lung volume changes. There is no point in using the $D_{L_{CO}}/V_A$ ratio unless normal values are provided for the lung volume present during the breath-hold. Furthermore, this approach embodies the implicit assumption that the mechanism of reduction of $D_{L_{CO}}$ associated with lower lung volumes in normal persons is the same as that caused by disease in patients. This caveat is tenuous in view of the lack of data supporting it.

MALDISTRIBUTION OF PHYSIOLOGICAL PROPERTIES

Calculations of $D_{L_{CO}}$, regardless of the method used to make the measurement, employ a theoretical framework that assumes that the lung is completely uniform with regard to its ventilation, volume, perfusion, and diffusive properties. This requires that each alveolus has the same relationship between all these physiological properties—a conclusion known to be invalid even in normal, healthy persons. For example, if two alveoli are exactly the same except for the surface area of the alveolar-capillary membrane, CO uptake will be greater in the alveolus with increased surface area. Similarly, if one alveolus receives more ventilation than another alveolus, the resulting increased P_{CO}

leads to greater CO uptake in that alveolus. Furthermore, gas uptake along the capillary length is not uniform, and exchange along a longer path in one region may not compensate for shorter transit times in another region. Disparate distribution of each of these important physiological variables throughout the lung will result in decreased CO uptake. O_2 uptake, because of its similar characteristics, will behave in a similar fashion.

Nonuniform distribution of these physiological factors produces an overall decrease in diffusing capacity and, by analogy, the ability to transfer oxygen from the inspired air to capillary blood. This transfer is further impeded by the nonlinear nature of the processes involved. The dissociation curve of hemoglobin and either O_2 or CO is highly nonlinear. An increase in P_{O_2} or P_{CO} may have a large or a minimal effect on gas exchange, depending on the absolute value of the P_{O_2} or P_{CO}. The complex relationship among important physiological variables results in increased impediment to gas transfer beyond the fractional decrement of each physiological variable. The cumulative effect of a combination of abnormalities is large, and the contributions of individual pathophysiological deviations cannot be assessed by a global measurement such as the diffusing capacity. Thus, $D_{L_{CO}}$ provides a means of assessing overall gas transport but does not indicate the specific problems in gas transfer that influence the overall measurement.

TECHNICAL PROBLEMS

The diffusing capacity measurement has greater intrinsic variation than spirometric observations. The coefficient of variation (100 × standard deviation/mean) of $D_{L_{CO}}$ measurements is 5 percent,[6] which indicates that a change in $D_{L_{CO}}$ must be at least 10 percent to be considered significant. Besides the usual technical problems of measurement of volumes and gas concentrations, other factors influence the variability of $D_{L_{CO}}$. Although the time of the breath-holding maneuver in the single-breath method is better controlled with newer electronic equipment, patient cooperation is still necessary. Because of nonuniform distribution of physiological variables, CO uptake does not occur in a strictly exponential fashion even in healthy persons. As a result, the magnitude of CO uptake and measured $D_{L_{CO}}$ decreases slightly with breath-holding time.[36] The empirical breath-holding time of 10 s was chosen as a practical compromise to permit measurable CO uptake but still be feasible for the patient to perform. The size of the alveolar sample obtained during expiration with automated equipment is an order of magnitude less than that of the sample utilized in the original description of the single-breath measurement. This could lead to a less representative alveolar sample in patients with significant lung disease. Thus the technique of measurement has changed subtly with automation, but current normal values have been obtained with the newer automated procedures.[6,35]

With repeated measurements of $D_{L_{CO}}$, blood CO levels increase. If venous P_{CO} rises substantially, CO uptake will decrease because of the lower gradient, and the calculated $D_{L_{CO}}$ will be lowered as a result of this artifact. Because CO uptake is minimal with the single-breath method, this is usually not a problem. However, markedly elevated blood CO levels due to heavy smoking can produce an artifactually low $D_{L_{CO}}$.

Finally, patients with lung disease, especially of the obstructive variety, cannot rapidly perform the respiratory maneuvers required by the single-breath D_{LCO} measurement. Slower maximal flow rates prolong the time required for inspiration and expiration. As a result, the assumed conditions for calculation of D_{LCO} are not achieved. However, using a series of three equations, rather than a single equation, to accurately describe conditions during CO uptake can help to avoid this difficulty.[14] Further experience is required to determine the practicality of this new method in improving the accuracy of D_{LCO} estimations.

Controversies in Interpretation

As estimated by equation 5, resistance to O_2 and CO uptake is evenly divided between the transfer of gas across the alveolar-capillary membrane and the chemical processes of binding O_2 or CO to intracellular hemoglobin.[40] Recent data have provided conflicting evidence regarding the partitioning of these two processes to overall gas exchange. Recent morphometric measurements indicate that the alveolar-capillary membrane is more permeable to O_2 than predicted by physiological estimations of Dm, although the estimates are lower than the initial morphometric measurements.[47] Earlier morphometric measurements of Dm are 2 to 10 times greater than physiological measurements of Dm in the same lungs.[7,46] If these estimates are accurate, Dm is very large and the term 1/Dm in equation 5 should vanish. This would indicate that gas uptake is dependent only on chemical reactions (i.e., the $1/\theta Vc$ term in equation 5).

The measurements of θ in vitro are affected by artifacts produced by stagnant layers that impede gas diffusion, leading to significant underestimates of the rate of gas uptake by erythrocytes.[4] The rate of O_2 and CO uptake[18,38] in thin layers (17 μm) of erythrocyte suspensions are more rapid than previous estimates of these processes made in dilute cell suspensions. These observations suggest that gas uptake by blood is very rapid and that the term $1/\theta Vc$ in equation 5 contributes little resistance to overall O_2 or CO exchange. However, if both the 1/Dm and $1/\theta Vc$ terms in equation 5 become insignificant, the diffusing capacity itself becomes nonexistent.

These observations that Dm and θ could be much greater than previously appreciated underlie conflicts in interpreting and understanding D_{LCO}. If these data can be extrapolated to the in vivo situation, the time-honored construct of gas exchange embodied in equation 5 may be erroneous. A recent mathematical model of CO exchange and the diffusing capacity provides evidence that morphometric measurements seriously overestimate Dm. Hsia and coworkers[21] concluded that resistance to gas diffusion across the alveolar-capillary membrane to the erythrocyte surface is underestimated because (1) diffusion pathways are longer than measured by morphometry, (2) pathways are curvilinear rather than straight, and (3) not all of the alveolar surface area participates in diffusion at a physiological level of hematocrit. Using this mathematical model, the classic Roughton-Forster approach[40] appeared to provide a more realistic estimate of Dm, especially at normal levels of hematocrit.

In addition, in vitro measurements of θ may not accurately reflect events that occur in vivo. Early estimates of θ underestimated the speed of cellular gas exchange because of artifacts resulting from stagnant layers of fluid surrounding red cells in experiments conducted in vitro.[4] Removal of these stagnant layers results in substantially greater measured values of θ.[19,38] However, conditions in the pulmonary capillary bed may impair the speed of gas exchange. For example, the velocity of flow in the capillary is quite low, and stagnant layers of plasma may surround erythrocytes in vivo, analogous to earlier in vitro experiments. Furthermore, erythrocytes are substantially deformed as they pass through the capillary bed and the entire cell membrane may not be exposed directly to the alveolar-capillary membrane. It is challenging to duplicate in vivo conditions with in vitro experiments.

These uncertainties in our understanding of gas exchange underscore the need for review of previous theoretical constructs and new experimental approaches to investigate the factors that limit O_2 and CO exchange.

REFERENCES

1. Bidani A: Analysis of abnormalities of capillary CO_2 exchange in vivo. *J Appl Physiol* 70:1686–1699, 1991.
2. Carlin JI, Hsia CCW, Cassidy SS, et al: Recruitment of lung diffusing capacity with exercise before and after pneumonectomy in dogs. *J Appl Physiol* 70:135–142, 1991.
3. Chang S-C, Chang H-I, Liu S-Y, et al: Effects of body position and age on membrane diffusing capacity and pulmonary capillary blood volume. *Chest* 102:139–142, 1992.
4. Coin JT, Olson JS: The rate of oxygen uptake by human red blood cells. *J Biol Chem* 254:1178–1190, 1979.
5. Crandall ED, Winter HI, Schaeffer JD, Bidani A: Effects of salicylate on HCO_3/Cl exchange across the human erythrocyte membrane. *J Membrane Biol* 65:139–145, 1982.
6. Crapo RO, Morris AH: Standardized single breath normal values for carbon monoxide diffusing capacity. *Am Rev Respir Dis* 123:185–189, 1981.
7. Crapo JD, Crapo RO, Jensen RL, et al: Evaluation of lung diffusing capacity by physiological and morphometric techniques. *J Appl Physiol* 64:2083–2091, 1988.
8. DeGraff AC Jr, Grover RF, Johnson RL Jr, et al: Diffusing capacity of the lung in Caucasians native to 3,100 m. *J Appl Physiol* 29:71–76, 1970.
9. Dempsey JA, Hanson PG, Henderson KS: Exercise-induced arterial hypoxaemia in healthy human subjects at sea level. *J Physiol (Lond)* 355:161–175, 1984.
10. Dinakara P, Solnick PB, Kaufmann LA, et al: The effect of anemia on pulmonary diffusing capacity with derivation of a correction equation. *Am Rev Respir Dis* 102:965–969, 1970.
11. Donevan RE, Palmer WH, Varvis CJ, Bates DV: Influence of age on pulmonary diffusing capacity. *J Appl Physiol* 14:483–492, 1959.
12. Farhi LE, Rahn H: A theoretical analysis of the alveolar-arterial O_2 difference with special reference to the distribution effect. *J Appl Physiol* 7:699–703, 1955.
13. Forster RE: Rate of gas uptake by red cells, in Fenn WO, Rahn H (eds), *Handbook of Physiology,* section 3, *Respiration,* vol I. Washington, DC, American Physiological Society, 1964, pp 827–837.
14. Graham BL, Mink JT, Cotton DJ: Improved accuracy and precision of single-breath CO diffusing capacity measurements. *J Appl Physiol: Respirat Environ Exercise Physiol* 51:1306–1313, 1981.
15. Guenard H, Varene N, Vaida P: Determination of lung capillary blood volume and membrane diffusing capacity in man by the measurements of NO and CO transfer. *Respir Physiol* 70:113–120, 1987.

16. Hammond MD, Gale GE, Kapitan KS, et al: Pulmonary gas exchange in humans during exercise at sea level. *J Appl Physiol* 60:1590–1598, 1986.

17. Hanel B, Clifford PS, Secher NH: Restricted postexercise pulmonary diffusion capacity does not impair maximal transport for O_2. *J Appl Physiol* 77:2408–2412, 1994.

18. Heidelberger E, Reeves RB: O_2 transfer kinetics in a whole blood unicellular thin layer. *J Appl Physiol* 68:1854–1864, 1990.

19. Heidelberger E, Reeves RB: Factors affecting whole blood O_2 transfer kinetics: implications for $\theta(O_2)$. *J Appl Physiol* 68:1865–1874, 1990.

20. Holland RAB, Forster RE: Effect of temperature on rate of CO_2 uptake by human red cell suspensions. *Am J Physiol* 228:1589–1596, 1975.

21. Hsia CCW, Chuong CJC, Johnson RL Jr: Critique of conceptual basis of diffusing capacity estimates: A finite element analysis. *J Appl Physiol* 79:1039–1047, 1995.

22. Hyde RW, Puy RJM, Raub WF, Forster RE: Rate of disappearance of labeled carbon dioxide from the lungs of humans during breath holding: A method for studying the dynamics of pulmonary CO_2 exchange. *J Clin Invest* 47:1535–1552, 1968.

23. Johnson RL Jr, Cassidy SS, Grover RF, et al: Functional capacities of lungs and thorax in beagles after prolonged residence at 3,100 m. *J Appl Physiol* 59:1773–1782, 1985.

24. Johnson RL Jr, Spicer WS, Bishop JM, Forster RE: Pulmonary capillary blood volume, flow and diffusing capacity during exercise. *J Appl Physiol* 15:893–902, 1960.

25. Kimberly B, Nejadnik B, Giraud G, Holden WE: Nasal contribution to exhaled nitric oxide at rest and during breathholding in humans. *Am J Respir Crit Care Med* 153:829–836, 1996.

26. King TKC, Briscoe WA: Bohr integral isopleths in the study of blood gas exchange in the lung. *J Appl Physiol* 22:659–674, 1967.

27. Klocke RA: CO_2 transport, in Crystal RG, West JB (eds), *The Lung: Scientific Foundation.* New York, Lippincott-Raven, 1997, pp 1633–1642.

28. Klocke RA: The rate of bicarbonate-chloride exchange in human red cells at 37°C. *J Appl Physiol* 40:707–714, 1976.

29. Klocke RA: Pulmonary excretion of absorbed gases, in Lee DHK, Falk GL, Murphy SD (eds), *Handbook of Physiology,* section 9, *Reactions to Environmental Agents.* Bethesda, MD, American Physiological Society, 1977, pp 555–562.

30. Klocke RA: Kinetics of pulmonary gas exchange, in West JB (ed), *Pulmonary Gas Exchange.* New York, Academic, 1980, pp 173–218.

31. Klocke RA: Carbon dioxide transport, in Farhi LE, Tenney SM (eds), *Handbook of Physiology.* section 3, *The Respiratory System,* vol IV. Bethesda, MD, American Physiological Society, 1987, pp 173–197.

32. Knauf P: Erythrocyte anion exchange and the band 3 protein: Transport kinetics and molecular structure, in Bronner F, Kleinzeller A (eds), *Current Topics in Membranes and Transport,* vol 12. New York, Academic, 1979, pp 249–363.

33. Kreuzer F: Facilitated diffusion of oxygen and its possible significance: A review. *Respir Physiol* 9:1–30, 1970.

34. Meyer M, Schuster K-D, Schulz H, et al: Pulmonary diffusing capacities for nitric oxide and carbon monoxide determined by rebreathing in dogs. *J Appl Physiol* 68:2344–2357, 1990.

35. Miller A, Thornton JC, Warshaw R, et al: Single breath diffusing capacity in a representative sample of the population of Michigan, a large industrial state. *Am Rev Respir Dis* 127:270–277, 1983.

36. Ogilvie CM, Forster RE, Blakemore WS, Morton JW: A standardized breath holding technique for the clinical measurement of the diffusing capacity of the lung for carbon monoxide. *J Clin Invest* 36:1–17, 1957.

37. Rasmussen JR, Hanel B, Saunamaki K, Secher NH: Recovery of pulmonary diffusing capacity after maximal exercise. *J Sports Sci* 10:525–531, 1992.

38. Reeves RB, Park HK: CO uptake kinetics of red cells and CO diffusing capacity. *Respir Physiol* 88:1–21, 1992.

39. Roughton FJW: Transport of oxygen and carbon dioxide, in Fenn WO, Rahn H (eds), *Handbook of Physiology,* section 3, *Respiration,* vol I. Washington, DC, American Physiological Society, 1964, pp 767–825.

40. Roughton FJW, Forster RE: Relative importance of diffusion and chemical reaction rates in determining rate of exchange of gases in the human lung, with special reference to true diffusing capacity of pulmonary membrane and volume of blood in lung capillaries. *J Appl Physiol* 11:290–302, 1957.

41. Sackner MA, Greeneltch G, Heiman MS, et al: Diffusing capacity, membrane diffusing capacity, capillary blood volume, pulmonary tissue volume and cardiac output measured by a rebreathing technique. *Am Rev Respir Dis* 111:157–165, 1975.

42. Schünemann HJ, Klocke RA: Influence of CO_2 kinetics on pulmonary carbon dioxide exchange. *J Appl Physiol* 74:715–721, 1993.

43. Stam H, Hrachovina V, Stijnen T, Versprille A: Diffusing capacity dependent on lung volume and age in normal subjects. *J Appl Physiol* 76:2356–2363, 1994.

44. Wagner PD: Diffusion and chemical reaction in pulmonary gas exchange. *Physiol Rev* 57:257–312, 1977.

45. Weibel ER: Morphometric estimation of pulmonary diffusion capacity: I. Model and method. *Respir Physiol* 14:26–43, 1972.

46. Weibel ER, Taylor CR, O'Neil JJ, et al: Maximal oxygen consumption and pulmonary diffusing capacity: A direct comparison of physiologic and morphometric measurements in canids. *Respir Physiol* 54:173–188, 1983.

47. Weibel ER, Federspiel WJ, Fryder-Doffey F, et al: Morphometric model for pulmonary diffusing capacity: I. Membrane diffusing capacity. *Respir Physiol* 93:125–149, 1993.

CHAPTER 14

BLOOD-GAS TRANSPORT

Michael P. Hlastala / Erik R. Swenson

OXYGEN TRANSPORT

The circulatory system provides special mechanisms in order to deliver the large quantities of oxygen required by the peripheral tissues. The major factor is the presence of hemoglobin in blood. Reversible binding of O_2 greatly enhances the effective solubility of O_2 in blood compared to that in other body fluids. In addition to quantitative transport requirements, O_2 must be delivered at a pressure sufficient to allow for its diffusion to the intracellular mitochondria, where it is utilized.

Oxygen Equilibrium Curve

The relationship between content and pressure for gases dissolved in blood is linear (Henry's law). Inert gases (such as nitrogen and argon) are carried only in the dissolved form in blood. Oxygen differs from inert gases because of its binding with hemoglobin. Four O_2 molecules can bind with each hemoglobin molecule through a complex interaction that occurs between the four heme components. Binding of an O_2 molecule to one heme site affects the affinity for ligands at other heme sites on the molecule.[1] The resulting S-shaped content-pressure relationship, the *O_2 equilibrium curve* (also called the *O_2 dissociation curve*) of blood, is shown in Fig. 14-1. The physiological portion of the curve includes the partial pressures and contents normally seen in arterial blood and in the venous effluent of various organs under both resting and exercising conditions. The flatness of the curve in the arterial range is an advantage because decrements in arterial P_{O_2} (as might be caused by lung disease or excursions to altitude) will still allow for a relatively normal arterial O_2 content. Because of the steepness of the equilibrium curve below

50 mmHg, large quantities of O_2 can be released and the partial pressure of O_2 remains relatively high. Increased O_2 extraction can be achieved with only a relatively small decrease in partial pressure.[2] Although the O_2 content of mixed venous blood is approximately 15 ml per 100 ml of blood (15 volume percent) at rest, and may fall to 10 ml per 100 ml during exercise, the O_2 contents of venous blood leaving some organs, such as the heart, are even less. Under pathologic circumstances, venous O_2 content may decrease even further. Adequacy of blood oxygenation can be expressed in a variety of ways. The most common, the arterial P_{O_2}, indicates the partial pressure but not the content of O_2 in blood.

Oxygen Affinity

The relative affinity of hemoglobin for oxygen, and the position of the O_2 equilibrium curve, can change under a variety of different physiological conditions.[5] However, the sigmoid shape of the curve remains unchanged. A change in O_2 affinity of hemoglobin results in a shift in the position of the equilibrium curve. The magnitude of change in O_2 affinity is indicated by the change in P_{50}, i.e., the oxygen partial pressure needed to achieve 50 percent saturation of hemoglobin. The curve to the left of the normal curve in Fig. 14-1 has a P_{50} of 22 mmHg, indicating that the O_2 affinity is high, since the P_{O_2} required to half-saturate blood is less than normal (27 mmHg). Shifts of the equilibrium curve can be physiologically important—a left shift permits greater O_2 binding, an important factor in O_2 uptake in the fetus in utero or in normal lungs at altitude. However, an increased affinity (lower P_{50}) may impair tissue O_2 delivery, since greater binding can limit O_2 release in the periphery. A shift of the curve to the right may enhance O_2 delivery to tissues because oxygen can be delivered while maintaining a higher-than-normal P_{O_2}, thereby promoting diffusion from the capillary to the cells. Shifts in the curve in either direction are mediated by several factors, all additive in their effect on the position of the O_2 equilibrium curve.[5]

Bohr Effect

An increase in plasma and, therefore, in the intracellular hydrogen ion concentration [H^+] displaces the equilibrium curve to the right. Originally, the shift in the curve was attributed entirely to a change in pH, whether mediated by the addition of fixed acid or a change in P_{CO_2}. However, CO_2 does have a direct effect on O_2 affinity in addition to that associated with a change in pH. This direct effect results from binding of CO_2 to the

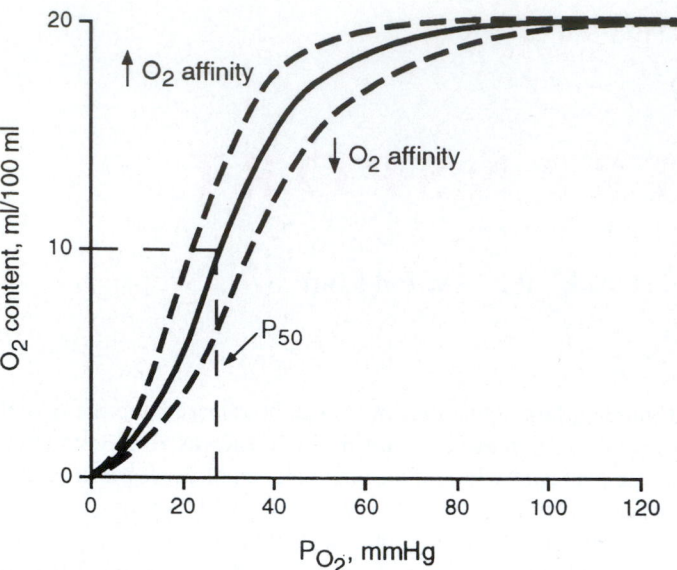

FIGURE 14-1 The oxygen equilibrium curve of human blood. The normal curve (solid line) has a P_{50} (PO_2 at 50 percent saturation) of 27 mmHg. Two other curves, one with increased oxygen affinity (decreased P_{50}) and one with decreased oxygen affinity (increased P_{50}), are also shown.

hemoglobin molecule. But it is small compared to the H^+ effect. A shift of the curve caused by a fixed acid, such as lactic acid, is less than a shift to a comparable pH caused by CO_2.

The Bohr effect assists O_2 exchange to a small extent.[4] In the tissues, addition of CO_2 to blood shifts the O_2 equilibrium curve to the right, releasing O_2 bound to hemoglobin. In the lungs, as the equilibrium curve returns to its normal position with excretion of CO_2, O_2 binding is enhanced. It has been calculated that the Bohr effect accounts for only a small percent of total O_2 uptake, less than assumed previously, because of the small pH changes that occur between arterial and venous blood.

2,3-Diphosphoglycerate

The human erythrocyte contains large quantities of 2,3-diphosphoglycerate (DPG), an organic phosphate that binds to hemoglobin and affects the O_2 affinty.[2] Two mechanisms are involved: (1) DPG binds more readily to reduced hemoglobin than to oxyhemoglobin, tending to "hold" the molecule in the reduced configuration, and (2) at body pH, the organic phosphate has four negative charges and reduces intraerythrocytic pH by the Donnan effect, since the large DPG molecule does not cross the cell membrane; the reduction in intracellular pH causes a decrease in affinity through the Bohr mechanism.

An increased concentration of DPG is a compensatory mechanism in pathologic states characterized by reduced O_2 transport. The shift of the O_2 dissociation curve to the right facilitates O_2 delivery, maintaining tissue oxygenation despite a reduction in the absolute quantity of O_2 delivered to peripheral tissues.

Blood stored in acid solution is deficient in DPG, leading to questions concerning its efficacy after transfusion in O_2 delivery. Fortunately, normal levels of DPG are regenerated in transfused cells within a day after transfusion. In the intervening period, O_2 exchange continues to take place even though efficiency may be somewhat reduced.

Abnormal Hemoglobins

Most hemoglobins have normal equilibrium curves despite differences in amino acid sequence. However, a few hemoglobins are exceptions to the rule and exhibit altered O_2 affinity.[3] Although shifts of the equilibrium curve to the right are common in hemoglobinopathies, this alteration is usually due to other factors, such as increased DPG concentration or mean corpuscular hemoglobin concentration.

Carbon Monoxide

Carbon monoxide (CO) has an affinity for hemoglobin nearly 250 times that of oxygen. Although small quantities are produced in the body by the breakdown of heme proteins, CO is important clinically only when it contaminates inspired air (as caused by cigarette smoke or automobile exhaust). Competition between CO and O_2 for ligand-binding sites on hemoglobin reduces the number of sites available for O_2 binding and causes the O_2 equilibrium curve to shift to the left. This combined effect produces a greater deficit in the ability to exchange O_2 than the loss of comparable O_2-carrying capacity in anemia.[1]

The half-time of CO clearance from the body is 4 h. Breathing 100 percent O_2 reduces the half-time to less than 1 h because of the competition between CO and O_2. Inhalation of 5 percent CO_2 in O_2 has been used to treat CO poisoning. Although it was once postulated that CO_2 has a specific effect on CO release from hemoglobin, it has now been demonstrated that the faster elimination of CO while breathing CO_2-O_2 mixtures is the result of the hyperventilation produced by CO_2 inhalation. If patients treated with CO_2-O_2 mixtures cannot increase ventilation sufficiently to avoid respiratory acidosis during CO_2 inhalation, this treatment can be dangerous. For this reason, the treatment of choice for CO poisoning is O_2 inhalation, either at ambient pressure or, when available, in a hyperbaric chamber.

CARBON DIOXIDE TRANSPORT

Carbon dioxide (CO_2) is produced within cells of the body principally by aerobic metabolism but also from the generation of CO_2 when intra- and extracellular bicarbonate stores are utilized to buffer organic acids such as lactic and ketoacids generated by anaerobic metabolism, starvation, and uncontrolled diabetes. CO_2 diffuses from tissue cells into the capillary blood and is carried in chemical combination and physical solution in the venous blood to the lungs, where a portion of it diffuses into alveolar gas and is eliminated in the expired breath. As is the case with the transport of O_2 by blood, most CO_2 is not carried as the gas itself but rather in several chemical forms directly or indirectly dependent on hemoglobin. CO_2 itself is not an acid but forms carbonic acid in combination with water and needs to be eliminated continuously by the lungs to avoid acidosis. Body acid-base status is maintained by a balance in the ventilatory excretion of CO_2 and renal regulation of body HCO_3^- stores.

Carbon Dioxide Equilibrium Curve

The relationship between blood content and partial pressure is considerably different for CO_2 than for O_2.[6] The total quantity of CO_2 contained in arterial blood is more than twice that of O_2

despite the generally lower CO_2 partial pressures that are involved. Because the slope of the CO_2 equilibrium curve is quite steep, CO_2 partial pressures in venous and arterial blood normally range between 40 and 50 mmHg in contrast to large arterial-venous differences in blood P_{O_2}. The entire CO_2 curve is curvilinear, but over the range encountered under normal conditions the content-pressure relationship is nearly linear (Fig. 14-2). This characteristic helps to maintain efficiency of CO_2 exchange when maldistribution of ventilation to blood flow occurs in the lungs.[7] Despite the 20-fold greater solubility of CO_2 over that of oxygen, there still must be a form of storage of CO_2 in blood other than simple physical solution if CO_2 transport is to be maintained without an obligatory high cardiac output or venous P_{CO_2}. The content of CO_2, i.e., the vertical axis of the CO_2 equilibrium curve, is the sum of these forms: dissolved CO_2, bicarbonate, and carbamates.

Dissolved Carbon Dioxide

Approximately 5 percent of total CO_2 content is transported in physical solution in plasma and red cell water. This dissolved form is critical for CO_2 transport because molecular CO_2 can rapidly cross cell membranes and be excreted in the lungs. The partial pressure of carbon dioxide, P_{CO_2}, is directly proportional to the quantity of dissolved CO_2. It is indirectly related to CO_2 content through the equilibrium curve.

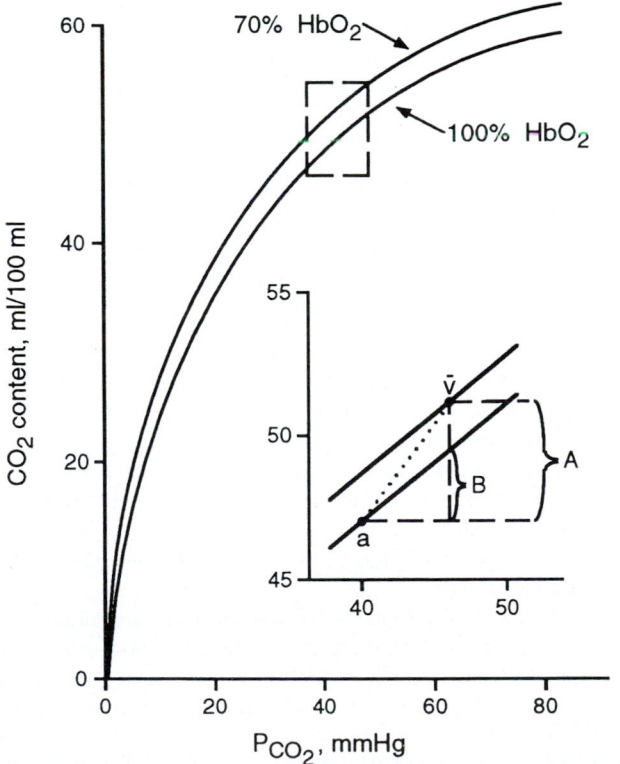

Bicarbonate

Under the influence of the enzyme carbonic anhydrase (CA) which is contained largely within the cytosol of the erythrocyte, approximately 85 percent of CO_2 entering blood from the tissues is rapidly converted into bicarbonate ion (HCO_3^-):

$$CO_2 + H_2O \leftrightarrow H_2CO_3 \leftrightarrow H^+ + HCO_3^-$$

Catalysis of this otherwise very slow reaction permits rapid interconversion between CO_2 and HCO_3 so that large quantities of CO_2 can be absorbed by the blood in the periphery and excreted in the lungs.[8] The H^+ generated by the conversion of CO_2 into HCO_3^- must be buffered to prevent large changes in pH and limitation on CO_2 uptake. In blood, this is accomplished by proton binding to hemoglobin, enhanced to a significant degree by the simultaneous off-loading of oxygen (the Haldane effect—see below). A rate-limiting buildup of bicarbonate is slowed by one-for-one electroneutral exchange of red cell bicarbonate for plasma chloride across the red cell membrane (Hamburger shift) mediated by band 3 protein, an integral membrane glycoprotein.

Carbamates

Another 10 percent of the CO_2 binds directly to terminal amino groups of hemoglobin. Because reduced hemoglobin binds more CO_2 than the oxygenated protein, more CO_2 can be carried in venous blood at any given P_{CO_2} than in oxygenated arterial blood. The physiological importance of this process is diminished somewhat by the binding of DPG to hemoglobin (Hb) at a portion of the sites involved in carbamate formation. However, due to the Haldane effect, changes in carbamate concentration account for one-sixth of the difference between arterial and venous CO_2 contents during normal gas exchange.

Haldane Effect

Oxygenated blood at any P_{CO_2} has a lower CO_2 content than reduced blood at the same partial pressure. This difference, illustrated in Fig. 14-2, is known as the *Haldane effect*.[6] The effect of oxygenation on CO_2 transport is analogous to the Bohr effect but has far greater physiological importance. Deoxygenation of hemoglobin permits greater binding of H^+, since reduced hemoglobin is a weaker acid (stronger base) than oxyhemoglobin. In peripheral blood, H^+ formed by the conversion of CO_2 into HCO_3^- is bound to hemoglobin. As a result of this proton binding, at any P_{CO_2}, more HCO_3^- is present in blood, and hence its CO_2 content is greater when hemoglobin is reduced. As mentioned previously, direct CO_2 binding to hemoglobin is also facilitated in deoxygenated blood, increasing the total CO_2 content in deoxygenated as compared to oxygenated blood. Under normal circumstances, approximately one-third of the Haldane effect is the result of direct binding of CO_2; the remainder is the result of H^+-binding hemoglobin.

The physiological importance of the Haldane effect is illustrated in the inset in Fig. 14-2. The change in CO_2 content between normal arterial and mixed venous CO_2 partial pressure in partially oxygenated blood is indicated by bracket B on the right side of the inset. However, under physiological circumstances, the CO_2 equilibrium curve shifts from the position of the partially oxygenated curve to that of fully oxygenated blood. Thus, as is

FIGURE 14-2 The carbon dioxide equilibrium curves of completely oxygenated (100 percent HbO_2) and partially oxygenated (70 percent HbO_2) human blood. The inset shows the enhancement of pulmonary CO_2 exchange by the Haldane effect. Mixed venous ($\overline{v}$) and arterial (a) points are shown. The CO_2 exchange resulting from the Haldane effect is the difference between the total ($\overline{v}$-a) difference (A) and the exchange that would occur without the Haldane effect (B).

shown by bracket A on the right side of the inset, the shift from one curve to the other produces a greater change in blood CO_2 content between arterial and mixed venous partial pressures. As a result, the changes in venous pH and P_{CO_2} are minimized despite transport of large amounts of CO_2.

Quantitatively, the Haldane effect has a much larger effect on gas transport under physiological circumstances than does the Bohr effect. Under resting normoxic conditions, the Bohr effect is responsible for less than 5 percent of O_2 uptake in the lung and 10 to 15 percent in the systemic capillaries. The binding of oxygen to hemoglobin alters both its binding of CO_2 directly as carbamino-CO_2 and its overall pK (its buffering capacity). The first effect accounts for virtually all the contribution of carbamino-CO_2 to CO_2 transfer between blood and tissues or lungs, i.e., all carbamino-CO_2 contribution is linked. It probably accounts for about one-third of the Haldane effect. The other two-thirds derives from the reduced buffering capacity of hemoglobin as it is fully oxygenated. Model calculations and in vitro data suggest that the Haldane effect accounts for 35 to 40 percent of CO_2 exchange under normal conditions.[4]

Kinetic Aspects of CO_2 Exchange

It is conventionally taught that there is early CO_2 equilibration during capillary gas exchange, because CO_2 is some 20 times more diffusible than O_2. If CO_2 transport by blood were solely by its carriage as dissolved CO_2, this would be correct. However, like oxygen, the transport of CO_2 is critically dependent on its interactions directly and indirectly with hemoglobin. Whereas rates of oxygen binding to and release from hemoglobin are essentially instantaneous, several of the chemical reaction and exchange rates of CO_2 are much slower. Although controversy persists about the true magnitude and physiological significance of end-capillary CO_2 disequilibrium, it is becoming increasingly clear that CO_2 exchange cannot be considered fully complete in the duration of normal capillary transit times. Table 14-1 lists the times for 90 percent completion of all the diffusion and reaction steps in CO_2 exchange. The critical value to be considered is the average transit time of blood through capillaries, which, depending on the tissue and its metabolic rate, blood flow, and capillary density, ranges between 0.4 and 1.0 seconds. It is immediately apparent that the uncatalyzed rates of CO_2 hydration and HCO_3 dehydration are exceedingly slow but are accelerated sufficiently by carbonic anhydrase. The degree of catalysis by carbonic anhydrase is so extraordinarily in excess that more than 99 percent inhibition is necessary before CO_2 hydration becomes a limiting factor in CO_2 exchange.[8]

However, the rate of red cell anion exchange, on which 15 to 20 percent of CO_2 exchange depends, may be rate-limiting even at rest.[6] As capillary transit times fall with increased cardiac output, especially if capillary reserve is limited, as may occur in many diseases, the potential exists for significant CO_2 disequilibrium between arterial blood and alveolar gas and between tissue and venous blood. To further compound the problem, end-capillary CO_2 equilibration may not occur under these conditions. Since the Haldane effect plays a large role in CO_2 exchange, any end-capillary O_2 disequilibrium magnifies further

the CO_2 disequilibrium. The physiological consequences of any in vivo CO_2 end-capillary disequilibrium at rest in a healthy person are minimal. This is because CO_2 is such a soluble gas that P_{CO_2} gradients across tissues and the lungs are fairly small (about 4 to 8 mmHg). Lack of equilibration that would cause CO_2 retention and therefore raise P_{CO_2} can be countered easily by slight increases in ventilation and cardiac output. At rest, lung CO_2 equilibration is roughly 97 percent complete, which would lead to less than a 1 mmHg difference between arterial and alveolar P_{CO_2}. With maximal exercise, comparable values would be 87 percent equilibration and a 6-mmHg arterial-alveolar P_{CO_2} difference. However, if normal ventilatory and cardiac responses are limited, and/or parenchymal lung disease exists, significant CO_2 retention and respiratory acidosis could develop. It should also be noted that with severe $\dot{V}_A/\dot{Q}$ mismatching and reduction in diffusing capacity, large arterial-alveolar P_{CO_2} differences can develop, which have been ascribed to these factors alone and not end-capillary CO_2 disequilibrium. Probably all three factors are important. Drugs interfering with either carbonic anhydrase (acetazolamide, methazolamide) or red cell anion exchange (high-dose salicylate or loop diuretic therapy) will clearly cause end-capillary CO_2 disequilibrium. In healthy individuals this can be tolerated with minimal problems, but these agents may be harmful in patients with cardiopulmonary insufficiency.

REFERENCES

1. Bauer C: On the respiratory function of hemoglobin. *Rev Physiol Biochem Pharmacol* 70:1–31, 1974.
2. Baumann R, Bartels H, Bauer C: Blood oxygen transport, in Farhi LE, Tenney SM (eds), *Handbook of Physiology*. Section 3: *The Respiratory System,* vol 4. Bethesda, Md, American Physiological Society, 1987, pp 147–172.
3. Bunn HF, Iorget BG, Ranney HM: *Human Hemoglobins.* Philadelphia, Saunders, 1977.
4. Hill EP, Power GG, Longo LD: Mathematical simulation of pulmonary O_2 and CO_2 exchange. *Am J Physiol* 24:904–917, 1973.
5. Hlastala MP, Woodson RD: Saturation dependency of the Bohr effect interactions among H^+, CO_2, and DPG. *J Appl Physiol* 38:1126–1131, 1975.
6. Klocke RA. Carbon dioxide transport, in Farhi LE, Tenney SM (eds), *Handbook of Physiology*. Section 3: *The Respiratory System,* vol 4. Bethesda, Md, American Physiological Society, 1987, pp 173–197.
7. Piiper J. Gas exchange and acid-base status, in Heisler N (ed), *Acid Base Regulation in Animals.* New York, Elsevier, 1986, pp 49–89.
8. Swenson ER, Grønlund J, Ohlsson J, Hlastala MP: In vivo quantitation of carbonic anhydrase and band 3 protein contributions to pulmonary gas exchange. *J Appl Physiol* 74:838–848, 1993.

TABLE 14-1

Rates of CO_2 and O_2 Exchange Processes

Reaction	Time to 90% Completion, msec
Diffusion of CO_2	1–3
Carbamino-CO_2 binding/release*	250–300
Chloride-bicarbonate exchange	400–500
Bohr/Haldane effects	250
CO_2 hydration/HCO_3^- dehydration	
Uncatalyzed	$>4 \times 10^4$
Catalyzed by carbonic anhydrase	5
Diffusion of O_2	50–100
Hemoglobin-O_2 binding	5–10

*This value reflects the predominant rate-limiting effect of O_2 diffusion, because all the carbamino-CO_2 contribution is O_2-exchange dependent.

CHAPTER 15

ACID-BASE BALANCE

Stanley Goldfarb / Kumar Sharma

Regulation of [H$^+$] is of crucial importance for maintenance of normal cellular functions. The normal [H$^+$] is maintained at about 40 neq/L. When there is even a small change in the [H$^+$], intracellular proteins gain or lose H$^+$ ions resulting in alterations in charge distribution which may affect molecular structure and protein function. The hydrogen ion concentration in bodily fluids is largely regulated by the ratio of the concentrations of carbon dioxide and bicarbonate. This is predicated upon the relationship demonstrated in the Henderson-Hasselbalch equation:

$$pH = pKa + \log \frac{[HCO_3^-]}{0.03\ P_{CO_2}} \qquad (1)$$

where pH $= -\log[H^+]$ (the H$^+$ concentration measured in moles per liter) and pK$_a$ = 6.10. Whereas the lungs are responsible for modulating arterial P$_{CO_2}$, the kidneys are primarily responsible for modulating the concentration of bicarbonate in plasma. In concert these organs maintain a stable extracellular acid-base milieu that is readily assessed by measuring arterial pH.

The normal internal environment is maintained within narrow limits: The arterial blood pH is kept remarkably close to 7.40, the bicarbonate concentration is maintained around 24.5 meq/L, and the P$_{CO_2}$ is maintained at about 40 mmHg. Deviations of the pH with accompanying changes in the P$_{CO_2}$ and [HCO$_3^-$] result in the four major categories denoted in Table 15-1. Metabolic acidosis is characterized by acidemia (pH < 7.35) that is due to a reduced plasma [HCO$_3^-$]. Metabolic alkalosis is characterized by an alkalemia (pH > 7.45) that results from an elevation in the plasma [HCO$_3^-$]. Respiratory acidosis is due to hypoventilation resulting in a net increase in P$_{CO_2}$ (hypercapnia) and a concomitant fall in pH. Respiratory alkalosis is due to primary hyperventilation leading to a fall in P$_{CO_2}$ (hypocapnia) and a rise in pH.

In this chapter, we first review the basic physiological roles that the kidneys and lungs play in maintaining acid-base balance and then discuss their adaptation in primary acid-base disorders. The following section then focuses on clinical application of physiological concepts in analyzing acid-base problems as encountered by the clinician.

BASIC PHYSIOLOGY OF THE ROLE OF THE KIDNEY IN ACID-BASE BALANCE

Normal metabolism generates large quantities of volatile acid (CO$_2$) and nonvolatile acid daily. The complete metabolism of carbohydrates and fats generates 15,000 mmol of CO$_2$ daily. This leads to acid generation as the CO$_2$ combines with H$_2$O to form carbonic acid (H$_2$CO$_3$). As the volatile fraction is excreted by the lungs during respiration, acid accumulation does not occur. The nonvolatile or "fixed" fraction is produced at a rate of 1 meq/kg per day. The major source of the nonvolatile acid fraction is the oxidation of sulfur-containing proteins from the diet to sulfuric acid. If this amount of nonvolatile acid is not excreted, life-threatening metabolic acidosis ensues. Therefore, for a normal individual to maintain acid-base balance, 50 to 100 meq of nonvolatile acid must be excreted daily by the kidneys.

The addition of 50 to 100 meq of acid requires initial buffering before it can be excreted. Whole-body buffering capacity is composed of interacting buffer systems: the bicarbonate and nonbicarbonate buffers (Buf$^-$), consisting primarily of hemoglobin, proteins and phosphates. The sum of the buffer anions [HCO$_3^-$] and [Buf$^-$] is the total buffer base and defines total-body buffering capacity. Since all body buffer systems are in equilibrium, a

TABLE 15-1

Patterns of P_{CO_2} and HCO_3 Changes in Acid-Base Disorders

Primary Disturbance	Initial Abnormality	Compensatory Response	Expected Compensation
Metabolic acidosis	Decreased pH, decreased $[HCO_3^-]$	Decreased P_{CO_2}	$P_{CO_2} = 1.5 \times [HCO_3^-] + 8 \pm 2$ (Winter's formula)
Metabolic alkalosis	Increased pH, increased $[HCO_3^-]$	Increased P_{CO_2}	P_{CO_2} increases 0.6 mmHg per meq/L rise in $[HCO_3^-]$
Respiratory acidosis	Decreased pH, increased P_{CO_2}	Increased $[HCO_3^-]$	Acute: $[HCO_3^-]$ increases 1 meq/L per 10 mmHg rise in P_{CO_2} Chronic: $[HCO_3^-]$ increases 3.5 meq/L per 10 mmHg rise in P_{CO_2}
Respiratory alkalosis	Increased pH, increased P_{CO_2}	Decreased $[HCO_3^-]$	Acute: $[HCO_3^-]$ falls 2 meq/L per 10 mmHg fall in P_{CO_2} Chronic: $[HCO_3^-]$ falls 5 meq/L per 10 mmHg fall in P_{CO_2}

change in the serum $[HCO_3^-]$ reflects concurrent changes in the other body buffer systems. The importance of bicarbonate in buffering is due to its relationship with CO_2. As H^+ are buffered by HCO_3^-, there is a decrease in the $[HCO_3^-]$ and a concurrent increase in the dissolved $[CO_2]$. As the $[CO_2]$ can be excreted by the lungs to maintain a constant $[CO_2]$, this substantially increases the buffering capacity of bicarbonate. Since the kidney plays a major role in controlling the $[HCO_3^-]$ and $[HCO_3^-]$ is easily measured in serum, the HCO_3^- anion is a useful parameter to evaluate the renal response to an acid load.

The H^+ ions released from the dissociation of sulfuric acid are titrated by blood bicarbonate and nonbicarbonate buffers.

$$H_2SO_4 + 2NaHCO_3 \rightarrow Na_2SO_4 + 2H_2CO_3 \rightarrow$$
$$2H_2O + CO_2 \quad (2)$$

Although the added H^+ is excreted via CO_2 elimination by the lungs, this occurs at the cost of depletion of $[HCO_3^-]$. In order to *replenish* the consumed base, bicarbonate is reabsorbed by the kidneys and returned to the blood. This process does not accomplish the replacement of consumed base, since continuous metabolic production of acid will ultimately decrease the available base present. The process of renal *regeneration* of base requires the urinary excretion of acid or H^+ ions in the absence of any urinary bicarbonate. For every H^+ ion excreted, a bicarbonate is returned to the body. If there is any bicarbonate in the urine, there will be a net gain of H^+. Therefore the kidney has two major functions in this context: (1) reabsorption of all the filtered bicarbonate—this takes place primarily in the proximal tubule—and (2) the base consumed by metabolism must be generated in the process of urinary acid excretion. This takes place in the distal portions of the nephron, the distal collecting tubule, and the collecting ducts.

BICARBONATE RECLAMATION

The proximal tubule is responsible for reclaiming 70 to 90 percent of the filtered bicarbonate. This may occur either by direct bicarbonate absorption at the proximal tubule or via proton secretion into the lumen of the tubule. The latter mechanism appears to be the predominant pathway.[22] Protons generated from intracellular water are secreted into the tubular lumen via a Na^+/H^+ antiporter, where they can then combine with filtered bicarbonate to form carbonic acid. The carbonic acid is dehydrated by carbonic anhydrase in the brush border of the proximal tubular epithelium to form CO_2 and H_2O. The CO_2 diffuses into the cell and combines with hydronium ion (OH^-) to form bicarbonate (via intracellular carbonic anhydrase). The bicarbonate is transported in the basolateral direction back into the blood via a Na^+/HCO_3^- cotransporter. (See Fig. 15-1.) It is important to understand that this process reclaims filtered bicarbonate but does not result in a net gain of bicarbonate. At the end of the proximal tubule there is a lowering of the luminal pH from 7.26 to 6.70, and the bicarbonate concentration is lowered from 24 meq/L to 8 meq/L.[22] The fluid delivered to the distal tubule is essentially the same with respect to pH and bicarbonate concentration as that which leaves the proximal tubule. The reclamation of the remaining bicarbonate occurs in the thick ascending limb and in the outer medullary collecting tubule. At the collecting tubule, H^+ secretion occurs primarily by an H^+-ATPase pump at the luminal membrane and bicarbonate entry to the blood is via a Cl^-/HCO_3^- exchanger at the basolateral membrane.[26]

The crucial role of carbonic anhydrase is demonstrated by the fact that carbonic anhydrase inhibitors, i.e., acetazolamide, result in bicarbonate wasting and the generation and maintenance of metabolic acidosis. The most physiologically important regulators of reclamation of bicarbonate are the pH, the P_{CO_2} and the extracellular volume status of the patient. In states of acidosis, there is enhanced luminal Na^+/H^+ exchange that may be mediated by an increase in intracellular H^+ ions and by increasing the number of new exchangers and increased activity of the Na^+/HCO_3^- cotransporter at the basolateral membrane. Elevation of the P_{CO_2} will promote higher proximal tubular concentration of CO_2 and lead to intracellular acidosis, giving rise to further secretion of H^+ ions and reclamation of bicarbonate. If there is volume depletion, there will be avid Na^+ reabsorption

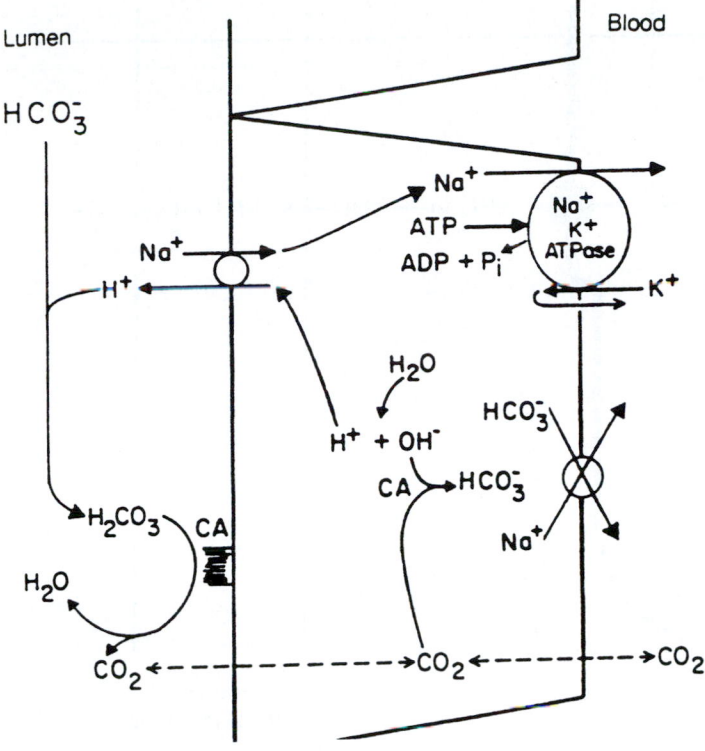

Lumen   Blood

HCO_3^-

FIGURE 15-1   Schematic representation of proximal tubular reclamation of filtered bicarbonate. In the lumen, filtered bicarbonate reacts with secreted H^+, generating carbonic acid, which is dehydrated by carbonic anhydrase, CA, located on the brush border. The cell secretes H^+ by a process that exchanges H^+ for filtered Na^+. The source of secreted H^+ is water, which in turn generates OH^- and subsequently bicarbonate because of the presence of intracellular CA. Bicarbonate exits the basolateral side of the cell linked in some fashion with Na^+; sodium is also actively pumped out of the cell.

at the proximal tubule in exchange for H^+ and thus greater reabsorption of bicarbonate. Other factors that are important include the luminal bicarbonate concentration, the tubular flow rate, and the serum potassium.

NET RENAL ACID EXCRETION

Net excretion of acid occurs primarily in the distal nephron and is largely mediated by the active secretory pumps, H^+-K^+ ATPase and H^+-ATPase. The latter appears to be linked in some way to Cl^- reabsorption to preserve electroneutrality. By definition, to produce net H^+ excretion the secreted H^+ will have to be excreted in processes that do not consume bicarbonate.

To achieve net secretion of protons in the luminal fluid of the distal nephron requires association of the protons with urinary buffers other than bicarbonate. Although secreted protons lower the urinary pH to 4.5 resulting in a 3 pH unit differential from arterial pH (a thousandfold increase in H^+ concentration), the quantity of acid excreted as free H^+ is trivial. For example, daily excretion of 2 L of urine with a pH of 5 would result in excretion of only 0.02 meq of dissociated H^+ ions in contrast to the 50 to 100 meq of H^+ generated each day from dietary sources. The nonbicarbonate buffers present in the urine that carry out the role of net acid excretion are the titratable buffers, primarily

phosphate, which accounts for 40 percent of net acid excretion, and ammonia, which accounts for the remainder.

The ability of phosphate to act as proton acceptor in the urine is based on its pK_a of 6.8. As the urine pH is lowered below the pK_a of 6.8, there is conversion of HPO_4^- to H_2PO_4. This transfer continues until the urine pH reaches 5.5, at which point almost all the phosphate present is in the associated form, H_2PO_4. Other components of this system are uric acid ($pK_a = 5.75$) and creatinine ($pK_a = 4.97$). Although the titratable buffers account for a sizable fraction of net basal acid excretion, they cannot increase in amount to enhance acid excretion in settings of acid loading.

The rate of ammonium (NH_4^+) production and excretion can, however, be varied according to physiological needs. Ammonia (NH_3) combines with H^+ to form ammonium, which is trapped in the collecting tubule lumen and excreted in the urine. The pK_a for this reaction is 9.0. The majority of ammonia is synthesized in the proximal tubular cell by the enzymatic breakdown of glutamine. Glutamine is actively taken up by the proximal tubule at the apical and basolateral membranes and transported to mitochondria.[22] Deamidation by glutaminase forms ammonium and glutamate. The latter is further metabolized by glutamate dehydrogenase to form ammonium and α-ketoglutarate. Metabolism of α-ketoglutarate to bicarbonate in the liver leads to return of bicarbonate to the systemic circulation (Fig. 15-2).

The ammonium that is formed is transported into the proximal tubular lumen via the Na^+-H^+ antiporter, working in this case as a Na^+-NH_4^+ antiporter. The ammonium is then reabsorbed in the thick ascending limb by substitution of NH_4^+ for K^+ on the Na^+-K^+-$2Cl^-$ carrier. The intracellular ammonium in the thick ascending limb cell is then dissociated into ammonia and H^+. The ammonia accumulates in the medullary interstitium and is finally secreted into the lumen of the medullary collecting tubule. At this site, due to the low lumen pH (4.5 to 5), the ammonia accepts a H^+ and is trapped in the lumen and excreted in the urine as NH_4Cl.

The importance of the ammonia system is that it can be regulated by the systemic acid-base state. An acid load initially leads to an increase in ammonium excretion within 2 h due to formation of a more acid urine which enhances ammonia diffusion into the lumen at the collecting duct. After 5 to 6 days there is maximal NH_4^+ excretion due to increased glutamine uptake and enhanced activity of phosphate dependent glutaminase and glutamate dehydrogenase to produce more ammonium in the proximal tubule.[26] This is presumably mediated by intracellular acidosis of the proximal tubular cell. The net effect is that NH_4^+ excretion can increase from about 30 meq per day to as much as 300 meq per day in severe metabolic acidosis. The plasma potassium is an important regulator of ammonia synthesis as hyperkalemia will result in a transcellular influx of K^+ in exchange for H^+ resulting in lowering of the intracellular H^+ concentration, thus causing an intracellular alkalosis with consequent inhibition of ammonia synthesis. Hypokalemia would have the opposite effect. Urinary acidification is also very important, since an inability to lower urinary pH will result in a reduction in NH_3 trapping in the collecting duct lumen and a subsequent inhibition of the degree of ammonium formation. Inadequate acidification of the urine will also inhibit H_2PO_4 formation.

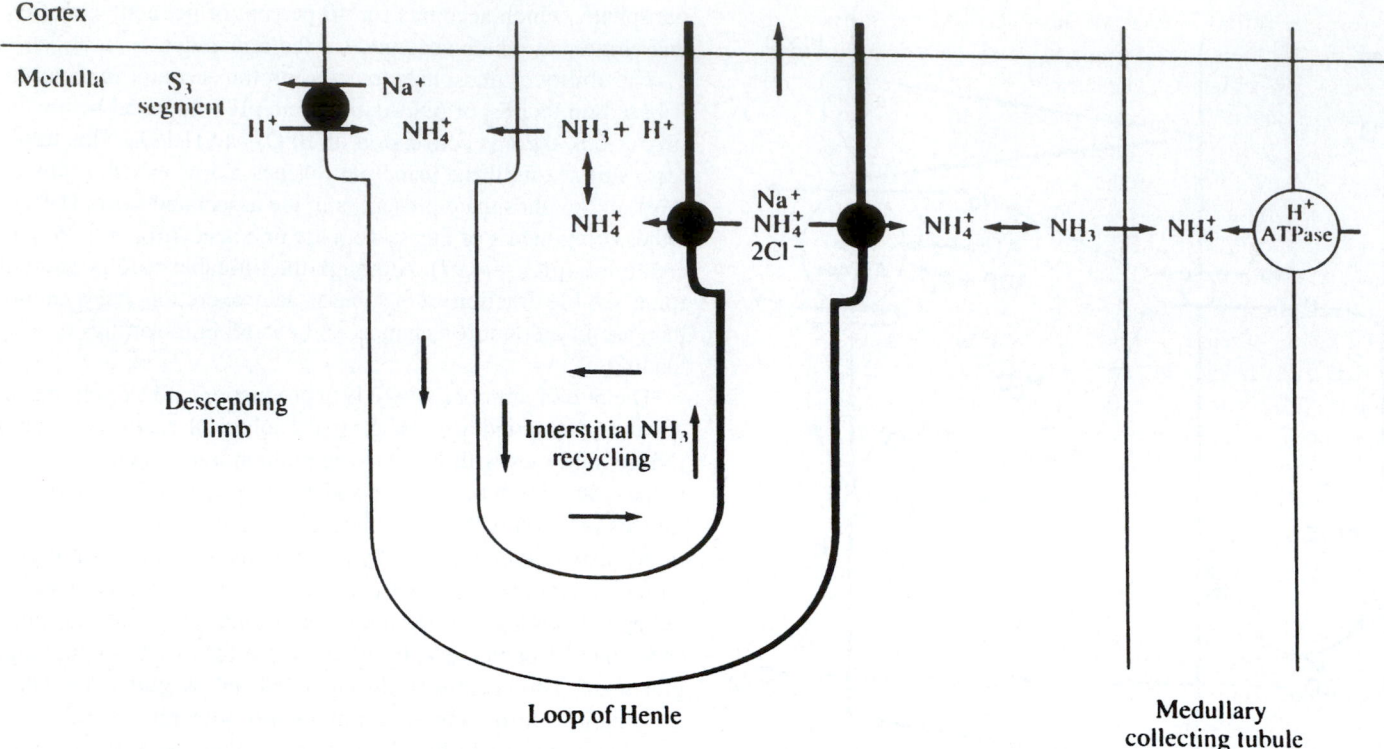

FIGURE 15-2 Schematic representation of ammonia recycling within the renal medulla. Although NH_4^+ production occurs predominantly in the proximal tubule, most of the NH_4^+ is then reabsorbed in the thick ascending limb, apparently by substitution for K^+ on the Na^+-K^+-$2Cl^-$ carrier in the luminal membrane. Partial dissociation into NH_3 and H^+ then occurs in the less acid tubular cell. The NH_3 diffuses into the medullary interstitium, where it reaches relatively high concentrations; it then diffuses back into those segments that have the lowest pH and therefore have the most favorable gradient: the S_3 segment of the late proximal tubule and, more important, the medullary collecting tubule, where the secreted NH_3 is trapped as NH_4^+ and then excreted. *(From Rose,[26] with permission.)*

RESPIRATORY CONTRIBUTION TO ACID-BASE BALANCE

The major roles of the lungs in acid-base balance are to excrete the CO_2 produced daily by aerobic metabolism and to compensate for primary metabolic acid-base disturbances by altering the rate and depth of ventilation. The CO_2 generated by the tissues diffuses into the plasma, at the peripheral capillaries, and is present in the blood in three compartments. Part of the CO_2 remains in the gas phase, but the amount is limited by the solubility coefficient of CO_2 (0.03 mM/mmHg). CO_2 may also react with amino groups of proteins and form carbamino compounds. The majority of the CO_2 is carried within red blood cells.[19] The red cells contain carbonic anhydrase which hydrates the CO_2 and thus forms carbonic acid which dissociates to H^+ and HCO_3^-. The protons are buffered by hemoglobin which has an increased affinity for H^+ at the low oxygen tension present in the peripheral capillaries and venous blood. The bicarbonate produced in the red cell leaves the cell in exchange for chloride. This chloride shift is a characteristic response to elevation of CO_2 in the blood resulting in an acute elevation of bicarbonate in exchange for a drop in serum chloride. When the blood enters the pulmonary circulation, the enhanced oxygenation of hemoglobin promotes release of bound H^+. The H^+ and HCO_3^-, via carbonic anhydrase, combine to reform CO_2, which passively diffuses from the blood into the pulmonary interstitium where the CO_2 tension is very low. Subsequently CO_2 is lost into the alveolar space.

The rate of minute ventilation is controlled by two sets of chemoreceptors: those in the respiratory center in the brainstem and those in the carotid and aortic bodies located at the bifurcation of the carotid arteries and in the aortic arch, respectively. The central chemoreceptors are stimulated by an increase in the P_{CO_2} or by metabolic acidosis, both of which appear to be sensed by a fall in the pH of the surrounding cerebral interstitial fluid. The peripheral chemoreceptors are primarily stimulated by hypoxemia, although they may also respond to acidemia. The level of alveolar or effective ventilation varies in accord with the total minute ventilation. Level of total ventilation changes as a function of metabolic demand. Under normal circumstances, P_{CO_2} is well controlled between 38 and 42 mmHg according to the relationship

$$P_{CO_2} = \frac{\dot{V}_{CO_2}}{\dot{V}_A} \qquad (3)$$

where $\dot{V}_{CO_2}$ is CO_2 production (reflecting metabolic rate) and $\dot{V}_A$ is alveolar ventilation (reflecting CO_2 clearance).

Under basal conditions the volatile acid production or CO_2 that is metabolically generated is completely eliminated by the lungs. The mechanism of the central stimulation of respiration in response to an elevated CO_2 is a topic of intense debate and will not be focused upon in this section. However, intracranial adjustments to pH have been consistently observed and have interesting parallels to the effects of acidosis on the proximal tubular cell in the kidney. Increased concentrations of CO_2 in the cerebrospinal fluid (CSF) result in intracellular acidosis, an increase in CSF bicarbonate concentration, and an equimolar reduction in CSF chloride concentration.[19] As brain cells increase their bicarbonate concentration, there is increased buffering, and intracellular brain pH is returned toward normal. The major group of cells within the central nervous system (CNS) responsible for acid-base regulation are the glial cells and the cells of the choroid plexus.[19,32] These cells contain carbonic anhydrase[14] which converts intracellular $CO_2 + H_2O$ to H^+ and HCO_3^-. The H^+ is exchanged for Na^+ on the blood side, allowing the intracellular pH to increase. The administration of acetazolamide into the cerebral ventricles blocks the expected increase in CSF bicarbonate in response to hypercapnia.[32] In addition to changes in bicarbonate concentration in the CSF in response to hypercapnia, there are also changes in the levels of ammonia.[19] Brain and CSF ammonia increase in hypercapnia; ammonia acts to enhance H^+ buffering thereby preventing a fall in the bicarbonate concentration.

ACUTE AND CHRONIC ADAPTATION TO RESPIRATORY ACIDOSIS

Figure 15-3 depicts the acute steady-state relationships among P_{CO_2} plasma bicarbonate concentration, and plasma hydrogen concentration during graded degrees of acute hypercapnia.[7] These observations were obtained by sequentially exposing

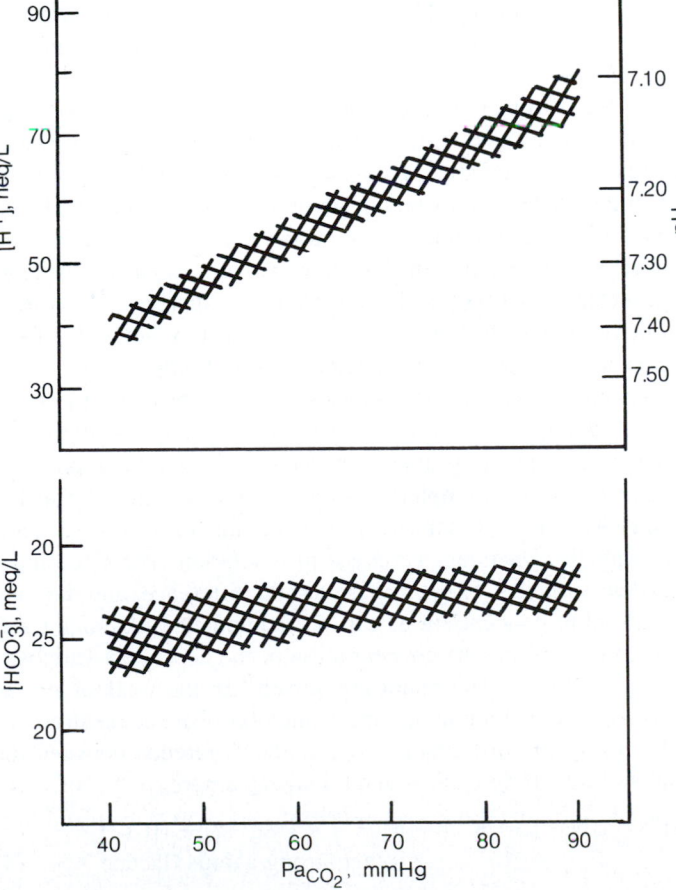

FIGURE 15-3 Ninety-five percent confidence bands for plasma hydrogen ion and bicarbonate concentrations during acute hypercapnia in normal humans. *(From Brackett et al,[7] with permission.)*

unanesthetized normal human volunteers to increasing concentrations of inspired carbon dioxide in a large environmental chamber. Increasing degrees of hypercapnia are associated with a curvilinear rise in plasma bicarbonate concentration, with higher levels of P_{CO_2} resulting in lesser incremental changes in bicarbonate concentration. This acute rise in bicarbonate is largely due to the chloride shift as described above. As a result of the modest increment in bicarbonate, the average rise in plasma $[H^+]$ is limited to 0.75 neq/L per mmHg rise in P_{CO_2} rather than the 1 neq/mmHg rise that would have occurred if the plasma bicarbonate concentration did not change.[7]

The quantitative aspects of the adaptive response to acute hypercapnia are influenced markedly by the baseline acid-base status. Acute hypercapnia induces a larger increment in both plasma bicarbonate and H^+ ion concentrations in animals with preexisting hypobicarbonatemia (whether from metabolic acidosis or from chronic respiratory alkalosis) than in animals with preexisting hyperbicarbonatemia (whether from metabolic alkalosis or from chronic respiratory acidosis).[1] This points out that the factor controlling the amount of bicarbonate generated from an acute rise in P_{CO_2} is not only the initial pH but also the initial bicarbonate concentration. Although the rise in bicarbonate in response to hypercapnia limits the fall in pH acutely, to excrete the gain of H^+ produced from the rise in P_{CO_2} requires renal compensatory mechanisms.

During the initial period of respiratory acidosis, renal compensation takes about three to five days, during which time there is enhanced reabsorption of proximal tubular bicarbonate, enhanced secretion of H^+, and increased ammonia production.[31] These processes will lead to an increase of the serum bicarbonate concentration and a rise in the systemic pH toward normal. However, when steady state is achieved and a stable P_{CO_2} is present, there is no longer an increase in ammonia production: As filtered bicarbonate is increased, there is enhanced proximal secretion of H^+ and a normalization of intracellular pH removing the stimulus for ammonia synthesis.[31]

RENAL ADAPTATION TO RESPIRATORY ALKALOSIS

The adaptive responses to respiratory alkalosis occurs in two distinct steps, in close analogy with respiratory acidosis. Hypocapnia reduces the carbonic acid concentration and causes a prompt fall in H^+. Acutely this alkalemia is ameliorated by a secondary, adaptive reduction in plasma bicarbonate concentration that stems principally from titration of nonbicarbonate body buffers.[12] During protracted hypocapnia, renal adaptive mechanisms yield a further and larger secondary reduction in plasma bicarbonate that results in still greater amelioration of the alkalemia.[12]

In acute uncomplicated respiratory alkalosis the plasma bicarbonate concentration falls by approximately 0.2 meq/L for each mmHg reduction in P_{CO_2}[4]; thus a reduction in plasma bicarbonate of 3 to 4 meq/L occurs within minutes after P_{CO_2} is lowered to 20 to 25 mmHg. The resulting change in plasma H^+ concentration is approximately 0.75 meq/L for each mmHg fall in P_{CO_2}, similar to the relationship between P_{CO_2} and H^+ in acute hypercapnia.

When hypocapnia persists beyond the acute phase, the additional decrement in plasma bicarbonate concentration is a consequence of renal adaptive responses and reflects a dampening of hydrogen ion secretion by the renal tubule.[22] As a result, a transient suppression of net acid excretion occurs, largely manifested by a fall in ammonium excretion and by an increase in net bicarbonate excretion. These changes lead, in turn, to a positive hydrogen ion balance and a reduction in the body's bicarbonate stores. Persistence of the resulting hypobicarbonatemia is explained by the continued inhibition of tubular hydrogen ion secretion and suppression of bicarbonate reabsorption.

The adaptive retention of acid during chronic hypocapnia is normally accompanied by a loss of sodium into the urine; the resultant decrease in the extracellular volume promotes chloride retention and the typical hyperchloremia of chronic respiratory alkalosis.[20] Upon reaching a new steady state, the net excretion of acid returns to control levels, and the altered anionic concentration of the extracellular fluid (ECF), namely hypobicarbonatemia and hyperchloremia, is maintained by a reduced bicarbonate reabsorption and enhanced chloride reabsorption. On average, the combined effect of cell buffers and renal compensation results in a new steady state in which the plasma HCO_3^- concentration falls approximately 4 meq/L for each 10 mmHg reduction in the P_{CO_2}.[13] The renal adaptation to persistent hypocapnia appears to be mediated by some direct effect of P_{CO_2} itself, not the systemic pH. In animals in which plasma bicarbonate was reduced by HCl loading prior to adaptation to sustained hypocapnia, the renal response to a primary reduction in P_{CO_2} was the same as in normal individuals, even though the net effect of this adaptation was an overt fall in pH.

RESPIRATORY ADJUSTMENT TO METABOLIC ACIDOSIS

Metabolic acidosis stimulates both central and peripheral chemoreceptors to increase alveolar ventilation and decrease P_{CO_2} to limit the fall in pH. Although peripheral chemoreceptors appear to play a role, in animal experiments the same degree of respiratory compensation occurs with intact and with ablated peripheral chemoreceptors. The increase in ventilation begins within 1 to 2 h and reaches its maximal level at 12 to 24 h. The stereotype is Kussmaul's breathing in acute diabetic ketoacidosis, in which tidal volume is characteristically large with minute ventilation increasing by as much as 35 L. On average, studies in otherwise normal patients with metabolic acidosis reveal that the P_{CO_2} will fall 1.2 mmHg for every 1.0 meq/L reduction in plasma HCO_3^- down to a minimum P_{CO_2} of 10 to 15 mmHg.[2]

RESPIRATORY ADJUSTMENT TO METABOLIC ALKALOSIS

The development of metabolic alkalosis is sensed by the respiratory chemoreceptors resulting in a decline in alveolar ventilation and an elevation of the P_{CO_2}. On average, the P_{CO_2} rises 0.7 mmHg for every 1.0 meq/L increment in the plasma HCO_3^- concentration.[16] Values significantly different from the predicted value represent superimposed respiratory acidosis or alkalosis. However, it is unclear whether this response significantly pro-

tects the pH from rising. In experimental animals, the rise in P_{CO_2} in metabolic alkalosis increases net H^+ excretion leading to an increase in the HCO_3^- concentration. The effect after several days is that the arterial pH is the same as it would have been if there had been no respiratory compensation.[20,26]

Ventilation may be strongly affected by influences other than acid-base balance. Among these influences are body temperature, increases in circulating catecholamines, changes in cerebral blood flow, changes in systemic blood pressure, and changes in metabolic activities of different organs (e.g., liver), as well as the physiological state of the lung itself. Perhaps for teleological reasons, the defense of chronic metabolic acid-base imbalances by ventilatory compensation is not of major importance.

ALTERNATIVE CONCEPTS OF ACID-BASE BALANCE

The preceding discussion has tacitly assumed that the systemic pH is the final control that affects the renal and respiratory response to an acid-base disorder; however, this issue is certainly not settled. The proximal tubular cell of the kidney can often have effects that are more predictably based on the P_{CO_2} rather than the arterial pH. If P_{CO_2} is elevated, the proximal tubular cells acts to secrete protons and reabsorb bicarbonate whether or not there is systemic alkalosis or acidosis. This may be explained if an elevation in P_{CO_2} results in intracellular acidosis and the cell is responding appropriately to its internal milieu.[20,26] Similarly, in the central control of respiration, it is controversial as to whether it is CSF pH, interstitial pH, P_{CO_2}, or the bicarbonate concentration that stimulates compensatory changes in ventilation.[19]

In addition to the above observations, it is also known that changes in salt and water balance may affect acid-base status. For example, Schwartz's group[20] found that a low dietary sodium chloride intake in dogs with a stable amount of water intake results in hypoventilation, increased P_{CO_2}, and increased HCO_3^- concentration. Studies in dogs have demonstrated that increasing dietary NaCl with a fixed water intake increases the acidity of body fluids, whereas decreasing the NaCl in diet with a fixed water intake decreases the acidity of body fluids.[17]

An alternative view to understanding acid-base disorders and the regulatory response of the lungs and kidneys is offered by the theories initially proposed by Stewart.[9,30] Based on physicochemistry, Stewart emphasized the important principle that H^+ and HCO_3^- as well as the acidic and anionic forms of weak acids are actually dependent variables in a solution. The three independent variables, P_{CO_2}, the strong ion difference, and the total weak anion concentration, can be manipulated externally and serve to determine the concentration of the dependent variables, H^+ and HCO_3^-. The major components of the weak anions in plasma are the albumin and inorganic phosphate concentrations. The strong ion difference (SID) is the difference between the sums of all strong cations and all strong anions:

$$SID = ([Na^+] + [K^+] + [Ca^{2+}] + [Mg^{2+}]) - ([Cl^-] + [\text{other strong anions (lactate}^-)]) \quad (4)$$

This equation is based on the principles of (1) electroneutrality, (2) dissociation equilibria of all incompletely dissociated substances, and (3) conservation of mass. This concept appears to better explain the basis for renal and ventilatory response in a variety of states which also affect acid-base balance. Practically, it is observed that the plasma SID is primarily regulated by the kidneys, whereas the P_{CO_2} is regulated by alveolar ventilation. The weak anion concentration is generally not regulated and may often be assumed to be stable.

This concept has primarily been used by investigators in relation to the study of central regulation of ventilation.[19] As albumin and other proteins are not present in the CSF, it is the SID and P_{CO_2} that determine the concentration of weakly dissociating electrolytes, H^+, OH^-, and HCO_3^-. In analyzing various acid-base disturbances, it appears that the change in CSF SID can predict the concentration of CSF bicarbonate.[19]

In evaluating acid-base balance in many species, note that there is a consistent inverse relationship between the pH and body temperature, whereas the CO_2 content remains stable.[8,25] To explain this relationship Reeves and his coworkers provided evidence that the imidazole ring structure of histidine is responsible for the pH-temperature relationship.[24] This is because imidazole has a pK_a in the physiologic range (7.00), is relatively ubiquitous, and has enthalpy of ionization (7 kcal/mol). To integrate acid-base regulation with receptor function and control of respiration, Reeves and Rahn[25] have proposed the hypothesis that it is not the arterial or intracellular pH that is being regulated per se but rather the constancy of the fractional dissociation of the imidazole moiety of histidine contained in proteins throughout the body. α-imidazole is defined as the ratio of the absolute amount of unprotonated imidazole (Im) to total imidazole (HIm + Im):

$$\alpha\text{-imidazole} = \frac{Im}{HIm + Im} \quad (5)$$

α-Imidazole regulation (alphastat regulation) would have the effect of maintaining cellular protein charge states and enzymatic functions constant. It would also maintain the OH^-/H^+ ratio constant in all compartments. There is also evidence that alphastat regulation directly influences ventilatory status. For example, application of an imidazole blocker to the chemosensitive area of the medulla in cats blocked increases in ventilation caused by local application of acid.[23] Thus, changes in P_{CO_2}, reflecting alveolar ventilation, may be determined by alphastat regulation, which maintains the OH^-/H^+ ratio constant in membranes of the cells in the chemosensitive areas of the medulla.

The difficulty with using these concepts lies in the practical measurement of the relevant molecules. For example, although the imidazole moiety of histidine is considered the most important of the intracellular buffers,[24] its pK_a and enthalpy of ionization may vary widely due to the influence of the local configuration of molecules into which they are incorporated. Thus, even in lower animals such as fish under different temperatures, calculations based on the alphastat model do not accurately predict the acid-base disturbance, since the pK_a and enthalpy of ionization vary with temperature and are difficult to measure.

Similarly, measurement of the plasma SID is problematic and is often replaced by the "SID effective," which is roughly equal to the bicarbonate concentration plus albumin and inorganic phosphate.[9] Calculation of the anion gap—$[Na^+] - [Cl^-] +$

$[HCO_3^-]$—accounts for the roles of the strong ions Na^+ and Cl^- as well as bicarbonate but does not account for the role of inorganic phosphate or plasma proteins. Although the bicarbonate concentration may not be strictly speaking an independent variable, the anion gap calculation does indicate the quantity of unmeasured anions and hence is an indirect measure of the strong ion difference. If one considers the impact of serum proteins and inorganic phosphate in the unmeasured anion pool, the anion gap gives a very useful parameter in evaluating acid-base disturbances. As will be described in more detail in the following section, the use of the anion gap is still the most clinically useful tool to determine the contribution of different metabolic etiologies of metabolic acidosis.

APPROACH TO THE PATIENT WITH AN ACID-BASE DISTURBANCE

In this section, we examine the diagnostic approach to disorders of acid-base balance with a particular emphasis on the ventilatory response and its role in mitigating or exacerbating acid-base disorders. We will also review the approach to the patient with complex acid base disorders.

Analysis of Clinical Information

Table 15-1 summarizes the pattern of abnormality of arterial blood acid-base parameters in the four classic acid-base disorders. It also indicates the physiological or compensatory response induced in pulmonary or renal function in response to the initial disturbance.

BASE EXCESS AND BASE DEFICIT NOTATIONS

Base excess and *base deficit* are terms applied to an analytic method for determination of the appropriateness of responses to disorders of acid-base metabolism.[29] The base excess or deficit is determined by measuring blood pH against ambient P_{CO_2} and against a P_{CO_2} of 40 mmHg. If the calculated HCO_3^- is below 25 when the P_{CO_2} is 40 mmHg and the original pH is low, a base deficit is indicated. The magnitude of the deficit is expressed as the number of meq of bicarbonate needed to restore the serum bicarbonate to 25 meq/L at a P_{CO_2} of 40 mmHg compared to that at the ambient P_{CO_2}. The use of notations for base excess and deficit has been debated in the medical literature. This notation is favored in the evaluation of acid-base status in the operating room because acute changes in P_{CO_2} and in HCO_3^- can be simply evaluated by this approach. However this notation can be misleading in chronic respiratory alkalosis or acidosis, since the patient with chronic respiratory alkalosis will be categorized as suffering from a base deficit because of the low serum bicarbonate induced as compensation for the reduced P_{CO_2}. In fact, a "base deficit" is a normal physiological response to the chronic reduction in P_{CO_2}. Unfortunately, lack of familiarity with the complete analytical paradigm used for this analysis of acid-base disorders has led some to focus on the designations "base deficit" and "base excess" as guides to bicarbonate or acid therapy in chronic respiratory disorders. In addition, discrepancies between the buffering characteristics of plasma, blood, and whole body have also been cited as potential weaknesses in a system for assessing acid-base disorders which relies on in vitro CO_2 titration methods. We therefore recommend that the physiological evaluation of the patient be the mode of analysis of acid-base disorders rather than an emphasis on derived formulae.

USE OF NOMOGRAMS

As indicated above, the body buffers and the kidneys respond in a predictable fashion to a change in P_{CO_2} whereas ventilatory response to changes in $[HCO_3^-]$ is also predictable. Also, the resulting changes in bicarbonate and pH are time dependent so that a larger change occurs in several days than in the first hours. The confidence bands for changes in P_{CO_2} or HCO_3^- in response to primary disturbances are shown in Fig. 15-4.[15] Any deviation can be interpreted as a reflection of processes other than a compensatory response. For example, in a patient with chronic obstructive airways disease, other factors affecting the acid-base status are the concentration of potassium in the plasma, the size of extracellular fluid volume, chloride depletion, diuretics, renal hypoperfusion, and co-existing renal disease. The special case of posthypercapneic alkalosis is discussed in the next section.

In evaluating an acid-base disorder, the history and physical examination are invaluable in focusing attention on potential pathologic processes.[21] The composition of blood, with respect to serum electrolytes and blood gases, is then examined for consistency with the clinical impressions. However, in using the acid-base map (Fig. 15-4), remember that the map is based on data from individuals who had a single disorder. Therefore, the map does not take into account the possibility of multiple disorders. For example, in a patient with chronic obstructive airways disease whose sputum has turned purulent and who develops nausea and vomiting, the possibility arises of coexistent metabolic alkalosis and acute respiratory acidosis. However, ill-advised application of the arterial blood-gas values from this patient (e.g., pH = 7.25 and P_{CO_2} = 75 mmHg) to the acid-base map would lead to the erroneous conclusion that a chronic respiratory acidosis is present. Thus the clinician needs to integrate laboratory data with clinical assessments to properly analyze clinical disorders of acid-base balance.

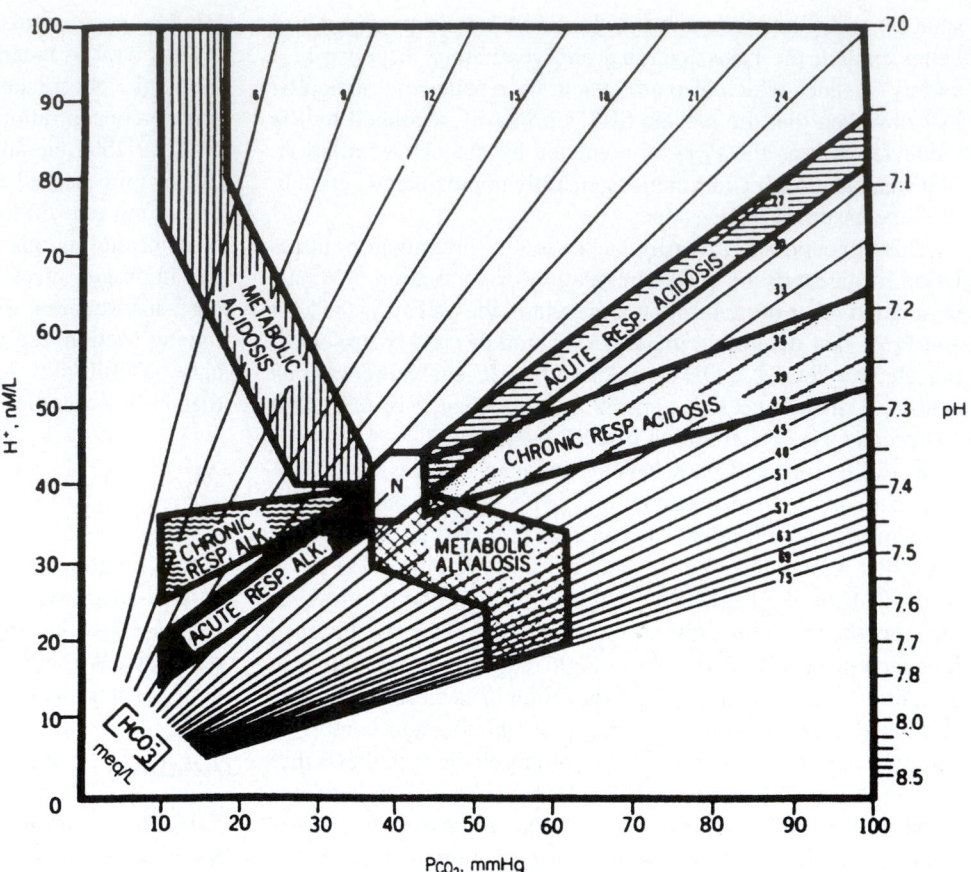

FIGURE 15-4   Acid-base map showing the normal range (N) and the confidence bands for acute or chronic respiratory and metabolic acid-base disturbances. The ordinates are the partial pressure of CO_2 and the hydrogen-ion activity given in nmol/L and pH units. Isopleths for bicarbonate concentration, in milliequivalents per liter, are also shown. *(From Goldberg et al,*[15] *with permission.)*

clinician to ascertain the appropriateness of organized homeostatic responses to the perturbation.[2] The pathophysiological basis for the initiation of metabolic acidosis and homeostatic responses in the defense of systemic pH have been defined above in descriptions of the buffering of newly introduced acid [see Eq. (1)] and in the demonstration of the normal confidence band for the ventilatory response to metabolic acidosis as detailed in the acid-base nomogram (Fig. 15-4).

A key clinical distinction in the pathogenesis of metabolic acidosis is whether the production of the acidosis is rapid or slow. If the etiology of the metabolic acidosis is merely the continued ingestion of a diet which generates a variety of fixed acids such as H_2SO_4 [see Eq. (2)] from the metabolism of methionine residues, then the serum HCO_3^- will fall slowly as only that fraction of the 50 to 100 meq of H^+ generated from diet that is not excreted would be added to the body fluids each day. However, if the addition occurs because of an acute increase in the acid load such as may occur with lactic acidosis, the kidney capacity can be rapidly overwhelmed, and serum bicarbonate may fall precipitously. See Table 15-2 for the common causes of metabolic acidosis.

Approach to the Patient with Metabolic Acidosis

An increase in the H^+ concentration of the extracellular fluid will result in a series of predictable responses which allow the

UTILITY OF THE ANION GAP

As seen in Eq. (6), the buffering of mineral acids will result in the production of the salt of the acid, NaA.

TABLE 15-2

Causes of Metabolic Acidosis (Common)

Failure to generate new bicarbonate to replace that consumed in buffering dietary acid load

    Diminished NH_4^+ production and excretion
        Reduced renal mass
        Chronic hyperkalemia
        Chronic aldosterone deficiency

    Decreased H^+ ion secretion (primary)
        Distal renal tubular acidosis

    Increased H^+ ion production
        Lactic acidosis
        Ketoacidosis
        Toxic ingestion

    Bicarbonate or equivalent losses from body fluids
        Renal-proximal RTA, carbonic anhydrase inhibitors
        GI-diarrhea, villous adenoma, fistula

$$NaHCO_3 + HA \rightleftarrows NaA + H_2CO_3 \rightleftarrows HCO_3^- + H^+ \rightleftarrows$$
$$CO_2 + H_2O + NaA \quad (6)$$

If the kidney is able to excrete this salt or, in the case of the production of the salts of organic acids such as lactic acid, if the liver can metabolize the anion to HCO_3^-, then there will be no accumulation of the anion in the extracellular fluid. Typically, anions associated with strong organic acids are not measured with routine electrolyte determinations and contribute to the so-called anion gap. Determination of the plasma anion gap is primarily used in the differential diagnosis of metabolic acidosis. However, the anion gap also changes in other conditions, a finding that may be of diagnostic importance.

The plasma anion gap (AG) is calculated from the following formula based on routine laboratory determination:[10]

$$AG = (cations) - (anions)$$

Since Na^+ is the primary measured cation and Cl^- and HCO_3^- are the primary measured anions,

$$AG = [Na^+] - ([Cl^-] + [HCO_3^-]) \quad (7)$$

and normal $= 12 \pm 2$ meq/L.

An increase in the anion gap can be produced by an increase in unmeasured anions or by a reduction in unmeasured cations. Hypokalemia, hypocalcemia, or hypomagnesemia can only raise the anion gap by a few meq/L, since these ions can only deviate from normal by a meq/L or less and maintain a physiological condition. The predominant extracellular unmeasured anion is actually albumin with many negative charge sites per molecule. Hence, a mild elevation in the anion gap can occur in conditions in which the albumin concentration or the charge characteristics of albumin are altered, for example in metabolic alkalosis. In that instance, a number of factors may contribute to the increment, including a rise in the plasma albumin concentration due to extracellular volume depletion and contraction of plasma constituents, an increase in the number of negative charges per albumin molecule induced by the rise in extracellular pH titrating

protons off the albumin molecule, and a tendency for systemic alkalemia to induce an increase in lactate production. This latter response serves a homeostatically beneficial function.

In forms of metabolic acidosis in which there is buffering of excess hydrochloric acid by extracellular bicarbonate, then

$$HCl + NaHCO_3 \rightleftarrows NaCl + H_2CO_3 \rightleftarrows CO_2 + H_2O \quad (8)$$

Bicarbonate is replaced on an equimolar basis by chloride, and there is no change in the anion gap; this disorder is also called a *hyperchloremic acidosis* because of the rise in the plasma chloride concentration. Both diarrhea and type 2 (proximal) renal tubular acidosis can lead to the loss of $NaHCO_3$. The kidneys compensate by retaining NaCl in an attempt to preserve volume, with the net effect being a meq-for-meq exchange of chloride for bicarbonate.

If the retained acid is not HCl but an organic acid whose anion is not routinely measured such as lactic acid, then the increase in the unmeasured lactate anion will raise the anion gap. It is important to emphasize that the acidosis is due to the retained proton; the anion is irrelevant to the change in acid-base status or systemic pH but is important as a diagnostic tool. The major causes of a high anion gap metabolic acidosis include those listed in Table 15-2 under disorders of increased H^+ production. Although renal failure produces an acidosis because of failure of H^+ excretion and bicarbonate production, most patients with severe renal failure retain both hydrogen and anions, such as sulfate, phosphate, and urate, and hence demonstrate a high anion gap.

The diagnostic utility of a high anion gap is greatest when the anion gap is above 20 meq/L; in this setting, renal failure, lactic acidosis, or evidence of a toxic ingestion will almost always be present. When the anion gap is less than 20 meq/L, identifying the anions which contribute to the mild elevation[10] often is impossible.

URINE ANION GAP

Estimation of the urinary ammonia content may be a useful clue to the etiology of metabolic acidosis as the value will increase in diseases in which kidney function affecting acid-base balance is completely intact but in which bicarbonate is lost from the body fluids.[6] The calculation of the urinary anion gap is shown in Eq. (9):

$$\text{Urine anion gap} = (\text{Urine } [Na^+] + \text{Urine } [K^+]) - \text{Urine } [Cl^-] \quad (9)$$

The usual value will be negative, between -25 and -50 meq/L, as the ammonium content of the urine is typically in this range, and ammonium accounts for the apparent discrepancy between the level of cations and anions in the urine. In states of metabolic acidosis due to diarrhea or to chronic acid ingestion, the value will be greater than -50 meq/L as ammonium production is stimulated.

In three conditions, the urine anion gap will be very low or even positive in the face of metabolic acidosis. In all forms of renal insufficiency, ammonia production by the kidney will be deficient and significantly contribute to a reduced urinary anion gap and to metabolic acidosis. In type I distal RTA, inability to maintain a steep gradient for protons in the distal tubular lumen and in the collecting duct results in a deficiency in ammonia trapping in the luminal fluid and therefore a decreased excretory rate for ammonia. This in turn leads to metabolic acidosis, a low ammonia excretion, and an abnormally low urinary anion gap. Type IV RTA, a condition in which hyperkalemia and mild renal insufficiency are found, hyperkalemia suppresses renal ammonia production, and a low urinary anion gap is found.

In any condition associated with hypokalemia, increased intracellular proton accumulation (which results from the exchange of cellular potassium for extracellular protons) will lead to an exaggerated ammonia production in the kidney. Hence, the use of the anion gap in the urine will be particularly useful to differentiate classic type I RTA from hypokalemia and acidosis due to diarrhea. The former will show a very low urine anion gap. Typically, a careful history will elicit the crucial information, and measurement of the urine anion gap will be confirmatory.

CLINICAL ASSESSMENT OF METABOLIC ACIDOSIS

In approaching a patient with metabolic acidosis, the clinician should first assess the history and clinical circumstances. For example, patients with renal failure or with uncontrolled diabetes may be presumed to have a metabolic acidosis until disproved by laboratory analysis. The next step is to evaluate the serum electrolytes to determine the level of the serum HCO_3^- and the presence of a anion gap of greater than 12 ± 2 meq/L. If both are present, then one must consider the possibility of a metabolic acidosis secondary to increased acid production as listed in Table 15-2. If the HCO_3^- is reduced but the serum anion gap is normal, then one is dealing with either a respiratory alkalosis or a metabolic acidosis due to reduced renal capacity to generate replacement HCO_3^- to compensate for that lost as a result of decreased acid excretion or increased HCO_3^- loss.

At this point arterial blood gases should be assessed to determine the pH and the ventilatory response. Finding a low pH establishes the diagnosis of metabolic acidosis. Reference to the acid-base nomogram (Fig. 15-4) will verify whether the clinical response is consistent with a simple metabolic acidosis with a normal ventilatory response or whether some other disturbance in ventilation is present.

Metabolic Alkalosis

Two separate processes are involved in metabolic alkalosis: an excess load of base that is generated either endogenously or exogenously (see Table 15-3) and maintenance of an abnormally high concentration of bicarbonate in the plasma.[18] During hypercapnia, the load of base is the result of renal compensation and de novo bicarbonate generation; in posthypercapneic alkalosis, the key abnormality is maintaining the bicarbonate level in plasma at inordinately high levels, as will be discussed below.

GENERATION OF METABOLIC ALKALOSIS

Causes of metabolic alkalosis are predominantly events that remove H^+ ions from the body but also include circumstances in which excess base is added to the body fluids. Hydrogen loss can occur from the gastrointestinal tract or in the urine. Each

TABLE 15-3

Causes of Metabolic Alkalosis

Gastrointestinal hydrogen loss
  Removal of gastric secretions
Renal hydrogen loss
  Primary mineralocorticoid excess
  Loop or thiazide diuretics
  Posthypercapneic alkalosis
Intracellular shift of hydrogen
  Hypokalemia
Alkali administration
Contraction alkalosis

meq of hydrogen lost generates 1 meq of bicarbonate, as the source of hydrogen ions in cells which produce and secrete protons is

$$H_2O \rightleftarrows H^+ + OH^- \rightleftarrows OH^- + CO_2 \rightleftarrows HCO_3^- \quad (10)$$

When vomiting or tube drainage prevents stomach acid from reaching the duodenum and combining with HCO_3^- released from pancreatic secretions, the net balance of bicarbonate in body fluids becomes positive, and serum HCO_3^- begins to rise.

Increased renal acid losses may result from enhanced distal hydrogen secretion. Aldosterone acts both by directly stimulating the secretory H^+-ATPase pump and, via the stimulation of sodium reabsorption, by making the lumen more electronegative, thereby favoring hydrogen ion secretion. Increased distal nephron delivery and reabsorption of sodium further stimulates hydrogen ion secretion as the accompanying anion is less avidly reabsorbed than is sodium, and the lumen of the distal nephron becomes more negatively charged. Excess secretion of mineralocorticoids can lead to metabolic alkalosis by this pathway. In patients treated with loop-active or thiazide diuretics, enhanced distal delivery of sodium and increased secretion of aldosterone are usually present, thereby enhancing renal bicarbonate production as a result of enhanced hydrogen ion secretion. This pattern commonly leads to the development of metabolic alkalosis.

Chronic respiratory acidosis leads to a secondary increase in renal hydrogen secretion, as the subsequent rise in the plasma bicarbonate concentration will restore the pH toward normal as a compensatory response. If the patient undergoes a therapeutic maneuver such as rapid lowering of the P_{CO_2} by mechanical ventilation, a posthypercapneic form of metabolic alkalosis will ensue as the patient is left with an elevated plasma bicarbonate concentration.

Hypokalemia is a frequent finding in patients with metabolic alkalosis and may not only be the consequence of some of the disorders which lead to the initiation of metabolic alkalosis but may also actually induce an alkalotic tendency. Gastric drainage, diuretics, and mineralocorticoid excess all induce potassium as well as hydrogen losses through the GI tract and kidney, respectively. Hypokalemia also induces a transcellular shift in which potassium is exchanged in an electroneutral fashion for hydrogen ions in the extracellular fluid. This exchange directly raises the extracellular pH, lowers the intracellular pH, and mitigates the hypokalemia. Intracellular acidosis in renal tubular cells promotes hydrogen secretion and therefore bicarbonate reabsorption (see above).

Administering large amounts of alkali does not maintain metabolic alkalosis in normal individuals because of rapid urinary excretion, but it may induce the initiation stage of metabolic alkalosis if factors are active to sustain a high rate of renal HCO_3^- reabsorption. A form of metabolic alkalosis termed *contraction alkalosis* occurs when there is loss of relatively large volumes of bicarbonate-free fluid. Administration of a loop diuretic to induce rapid fluid removal in a markedly edematous patient is the most common cause of a contraction alkalosis. The plasma bicarbonate concentration rises in this setting because there is contraction of the extracellular volume around a relatively constant quantity of extracellular bicarbonate. The degree to which this occurs is in part minimized by intracellular buffering, as the release of hydrogen ions from cells buffers lowers the plasma bicarbonate concentration toward the baseline value. Even this form of alkalosis is probably critically dependent on increases in renal bicarbonate production for its manifestation, since the diuretics promote excess renal hydrogen ion secretion as noted above.

MAINTENANCE PHASE OF METABOLIC ALKALOSIS

Maintenance of metabolic alkalosis requires an increase in the reabsorption of bicarbonate by the renal tubule.[27] Four factors are known to be important in the maintenance phase of metabolic alkalosis: extracellular volume depletion, chloride depletion, hypokalemia, and mineralocorticoid excess.

A reduction in extracellular fluid volume and possibly a fall in the glomerular filtration rate secondary to extracellular volume depletion are major stimuli for increasing the proximal reabsorption of bicarbonate. The enhanced proximal tubular bicarbonate reabsorption is likely the most important factor. This reabsorption is stimulated by extracellular volume depletion which is a frequent accompaniment of metabolic alkalosis. Enhanced proximal tubular reabsorption of sodium ions is a major factor in the enhanced rate of proton secretion, a key factor in the proximal tubular reabsorptive pathway for bicarbonate. Enhanced activity of the sodium-proton exchanger in the luminal membrane of the proximal tubule is an important component of the transport system.

In addition, an important role is played by the distal nephron in maintaining metabolic alkalosis by way of the secondary phenomena of chloride depletion, extracellular volume depletion, and hypokalemia.[11] Cells of the cortical collecting tubule can either reabsorb or secrete bicarbonate depending on homeostatic requirements. For example, during excess bicarbonate ingestion, the secretory process predominates, and excess bicarbonate is lost into the urine. Chloride depletion enhances the bicarbonate reabsorptive pathway by reducing chloride availability at an anion exchange site on the luminal membrane of the type A intercalated cell. This exchange process normally allows bicarbonate entry into the urine in exchange for chloride absorption. Chloride depletion thus blocks bicarbonate loss.

Hypokalemia acts to stimulate bicarbonate reabsorption through several mechanisms. First, loss of potassium from the extracellular fluid leads to a shift of protons into the cell as potassium leaves the cell. Hence, intracellular pH falls, driving enhanced tubular bicarbonate reabsorption. Also, severe potassium depletion produces a defect in tubular fluid chloride reabsorption thus mimicking a chloride depletion state. Finally, excess mineralocorticoid hormone, either as a result of primary overproduction or due to a variety of secondary hyperreninemic states, stimulates H^+ secretion in the cortical collecting tubule and thereby stimulates increased renal tubular bicarbonate production and helps maintain metabolic alkalosis.

Typically, all four components coexist in patients with metabolic alkalosis secondary to vomiting or gastric drainage following gastric intubation. If any of the factors is present in a patient with metabolic alkalosis, therapy will be only partially successful until all the factors have been eliminated.

Depression of ventilation in metabolic alkalosis is a normal physiological response to the elevation in serum bicarbonate but is difficult to assess clinically and may not be found in many patients as detailed above.[16]

POSTHYPERCAPNEIC METABOLIC ALKALOSIS

In response to sustained hypercapnia, the increased excretion of hydrogen ion in the urine and the increased bicarbonate generated by the acid secretory process increase the concentration of bicarbonate in the plasma as described above. During this process, the total sodium content of the body remains stable as does the extracellular fluid volume (unless there is a separate reason for a volume abnormality, e.g., right ventricular failure and the use of diuretics). If correction of hypercapnia occurs, for example through the use of mechanical ventilation without simultaneous replacement of sodium chloride, the urinary loss of sodium bicarbonate may lag for several hours or days. This is particularly true if there is concomitant depletion of the extracellular fluid volume. This leads to an increase in the reabsorption of solute, including sodium bicarbonate, by the proximal tubule, sustaining the high bicarbonate concentration in blood. This process is similar to the maintenance phase of metabolic alkalosis described above; the other processes outlined also could pertain to this posthypercapneic state and produce a persistent metabolic alkalosis following correction of hypercapnia.[28]

Approach to the Patient with a Mixed Acid-Base Disorder

The approach to patients with mixed acid-base disorders, that is, more than one disturbance in acid-base metabolism, is particularly challenging because no nomogram, calculation of base excess or deficit, or other formula can allow the clinician to parse the pathophysiological disorders and allow a rational therapeutic plan.[20] Rather, it is the combination of clinical assessment, application of expected compensatory responses, assessment of the anion gap, and application of principles of physiology that together allow a successful analysis.

In order to determine the presence of a mixed or complex acid-base disorder, the clinician must follow a rigorous approach that integrates clinical observation with assessment of a variety of laboratory parameters. No single nomogram or other shortcut device will suffice. The initial step is to perform a history and physical examination to seek processes which could contribute to acid-base disorders. For example, any patient who has vomited has the potential for developing a metabolic alkalosis, and any patient with chronic renal failure surely has metabolic acidosis as an ongoing process for which compensation will be necessary. Moreover, many clinical conditions are typically characterized by the presence of more than one concurrent disorder. Patients with severe liver failure will usually experience respiratory alkalosis as a consequence of hepatic encephalopathy so that any other conditions associated with abnormalities of acid-base balance which may develop in these patients will result in mixed acid-base disorders. Septic shock is associated with the mixed disorders of respiratory alkalosis and metabolic acidosis due to lactic acid production. Immediately following cardiac arrest, patients will have both a respiratory and a metabolic acidosis. Patients with renal failure who undergo gastric drainage will manifest both metabolic alkalosis and metabolic acidosis as a result of the underlying conditions. The clinician must consider these expected abnormalities in acid-base balance when addressing laboratory results.

The second step in the process is to evaluate a venous blood sample for determination of the electrolytes, blood urea nitrogen (BUN), creatinine, and other parameters indicative of liver function. Here, the evaluation of the $[HCO_3^-]$ and analysis of the anion gap is invaluable. Decrements or elevations of $[HCO_3^-]$ will point toward a disturbance in the body's buffering system. The anion gap measurement, if elevated, will clarify whether a metabolic acidosis is present, as described above. Also, analyzing the anion gap together with the venous $[HCO_3^-]$ can provide important information. Because the anions which accumulate in most forms of organic acidosis (lactic acidosis, ketoacidosis, many toxic ingestions) can be metabolized in the liver to bicarbonate through the Kreb's cycle, adding the unmeasured anion concentration to the current plasma HCO_3^- concentration indicates the level of $[HCO_3^-]$ prior to the onset of the metabolic acidosis.

APPENDIX

The following cases illustrate the clinical approach to the patient with acid-base disturbances.

Metabolic Acidosis

A 75-year-old patient presented with a 7-day history of intermittent diarrhea and a 5-lb weight loss. The rest of the history was unrevealing. Physical examination only revealed signs of volume depletion. Laboratory values were as follows:

$[BUN] = 18$ mg/dl
$[Na^+] = 138$ meq/L
$[K^+] = 3.0$ meq/L
$[Cl^-] = 110$ meq/L
$[HCO_3^-] = 13$ meq/L

At this point, the lack of an elevated anion gap (12 meq/L) and the reduced bicarbonate concentration together suggest the pos-

sibility of either respiratory alkalosis or metabolic acidosis of the non-anion-gap variety, i.e., in which the chloride concentration has risen as bicarbonate has been utilized in buffering reactions or has been lost from body fluids. The history of diarrhea strongly suggests that a metabolic acidosis is the culprit in the disorder. The relatively low BUN supports the theory that diarrhea and not renal insufficiency is the main etiologic factor.

Arterial blood gases are then obtained:

$pH = 7.24$
$P_{CO_2} = 27$ mmHg
$P_{CO_2} = 100$ mmHg
$[HCO_3^-] = 13$ meq/L

The low serum bicarbonate in association with a low arterial blood pH indicates that the patient has a metabolic acidosis. Finding that the rate of ventilation produces a P_{CO_2} of 27 is consistent with the expected P_{CO_2} of 27.5 ± 2 mmHg calculated from Winters's formula (see Table 15-1). Reference to the acid-base nomogram (see Fig. 15-4) reveals the graphical equivalent of this calculation as the values for pH, P_{CO_2}, and $[HCO_3^-]$ fall in the confidence band for metabolic acidosis. Other possible etiologies for this form of non-anion-gap metabolic acidosis would include mild renal insufficiency, wherein the decline of GFR has not reached a level where the unmeasured anions such as SO_4^{2-} would begin to accumulate in plasma, and the ingestion of salts such as ammonium chloride which are metabolized in the liver to urea and hydrochloric acid. Urinary electrolyte analysis confirms the diagnosis:

$[Na^+] = 50$ meq/L
$[K^+] = 20$ meq/L
$[Cl^-] = 140$ meq/L
Urine volume $= 2$ L
Urinary anion gap $= -70$ meq/L

The discrepancy between the sum of urine cations and anions in the negative range indicates that an unmeasured cation, in this case ammonium, is being excreted into the urine. It is the excretion of protons in association with ammonia that allows the renal excretion of the accumulated acid load and the attempted regeneration of body HCO_3^- stores. If this value were not greater than -20 to -50 meq/L, a defect in ammonia production or excretion such as could be found in renal insufficiency or in renal tubular acidosis could be present. In this case, diarrhea is the culprit.

Metabolic Alkalosis

A 65-year-old patient experienced severe and unremitting vomiting for 4 days. He has had a history of peptic ulcer disease, but he decided to medicate himself with an antacid, which he could not keep from vomiting. There was no other significant past medical history. Physical examination showed a moderate degree of orthostatic hypotension as blood pressure fell from 100/70 mmHg supine to 90/60 mmHg when seated. The rest of the examination was not remarkable except for some abdominal tenderness.

Laboratory results revealed the following:

[BUN] = 28 mg/dl

[Na$^+$] = 43 meq/L

[K$^+$] = 3.0 meq/L

[Cl$^-$] = 85 meq/L

[HCO$_3^-$] = 39 meq/L

The elevation in HCO$_3^-$ content is consistent with either metabolic alkalosis or with chronic respiratory acidosis with renal compensation. The clinical circumstances strongly imply that metabolic alkalosis will be found, since the patient has been vomiting and has therefore been generating new alkali in the body fluids as gastric hydrochloric acid is lost. Also, the vomiting-induced deficit in extracellular fluid volume and in body fluid chloride content will likely act to help sustain the metabolic alkalosis by stimulating a high rate of renal bicarbonate transport by the proximal tubule and inhibiting distal nephron bicarbonate secretion.

Arterial blood gases are then obtained:

pH = 7.52

P$_{CO_2}$ = 46 mmHg

[HCO$_3^-$] = 36 meq/L

These confirm the diagnosis. Note that the hypoventilatory response is modest, probably because of the degree of hypokalemia which tends to acidify the intracellular fluid and stimulate ventilation. Correction of this abnormality will require both replacement of fluid with sodium and chloride and adequate intake of potassium to fully restore acid-base balance to normal.

Mixed Acid-Base Disturbance

An insulin-dependent diabetic patient with several days of vomiting developed diabetic ketoacidosis. The following set of electrolytes is obtained:

[Na$^+$] = 140 meq/L

[K$^+$] = 5 meq/L

[Cl$^-$] = 90 meq/L

[HCO$_3^-$] = 15 meq/L

Anion gap = 35 meq/L

Since the normal anion gap is 12 ± 2 meq/L, this individual has utilized 23 meq/L of HCO$_3^-$ to buffer the ketoacids. If the production of ketoacids ceases and hepatic metabolism is restored through insulin administration, then 23 meq/L of HCO$_3^-$ could be added to body fluids. The new set of electrolytes would be

[Na$^+$] = 140 meq/L

[K$^+$] = 5 meq/L

[Cl$^-$] = 90 meq/L

[HCO$_3^-$] = 38 meq/L

Anion gap = 12 meq/L

By assessing the value—(anion gap increment above 12 meq/L) + (serum [HCO$_3^-$])—and finding a value greater than 30, one can infer that some process has previously raised the bicarbonate content above normal even if the ambient total CO$_2$ level is subnormal at the current moment. Hence either metabolic alkalosis or respiratory acidosis is a component process of the acid-base

disorder. Conversely, finding a value less than 20 suggests that the patient had a preexistent metabolic acidosis or a respiratory alkalosis prior to the onset of the organic acidosis. Finally, the clinician may assess the alveolar-arteriolar O$_2$ gradient to determine the effectiveness of oxygenation as an initial assessment of respiratory intactness.

At this point the clinician is able to ascertain a tentative diagnosis and perform an arterial blood gas determination to conclude the process. Measurement of the blood gas will show whether the respiratory response to a metabolic disturbance (metabolic alkalosis or metabolic acidosis) or the metabolic (renal) response to a respiratory disturbance is as expected. The acid-base disorder could still be labeled a simple disturbance if the initial assessment of the clinical condition and the anion gap support that conclusion. Consulting the acid-base map (see Fig. 15-4) will provide the expected compensatory response to each disturbance. In the case above of a patient with diabetic ketoacidosis and an initially increased [anion gap + total CO$_2$] concentration, the following arterial blood gases were obtained:

pH = 7.18

P$_{CO_2}$ = 38 mmHg

[HCO$_3^-$] = 15 meq/L

In pure metabolic acidosis the ventilatory response to a [HCO$_3^-$] lowered to 15 meq/L would be a P$_{CO_2}$ of 25 mmHg (see Table 15-1 and Fig. 15-4). In this example, the patient shows a P$_{CO_2}$ that is higher than the expected value of 25 for a patient with pure metabolic acidosis and a depressed HCO$_3^-$ value of 15 meq/L. Hence this patient demonstrates a so-called triple disturbance, metabolic acidosis (low HCO$_3^-$, high anion gap), a metabolic alkalosis [(HCO$_3^-$ + anion gap increment above 12) > 30 meq/L] and a respiratory acidosis (P$_{CO_2}$ higher than expected value given the lowering of HCO$_3^-$ level as determined from the acid-base nomogram or the formula for expected compensation). Therapy for this patient will require awareness of these various processes, since removal of a counter disturbance can induce a more severe expression of the still-present abnormality.

REFERENCES

1. Adrogué HJ, Madias NE: Influence of chronic respiratory acid-base disorders on acute CO$_2$ titration curve. *J Appl Physiol* 58:1231–1238, 1985.
2. Albert MS, Dell RB, Winters RW: Quantitative displacement of acid-base equilibrium in metabolic acidosis. *Ann Intern Med* 66:312–319, 1967.
3. Alpern RJ, Moe OW, Preisig PA: Chronic regulation of the proximal tubular Na/H antiporter: from HCO$_3$ to SRC. *Kidney Int* 48:1386–1396, 1995.
4. Arbus GS, Hebert LA, Levesque PR, et al: Characteristics and clinical application of the "significance band" for acute respiratory alkalosis. *New Engl J Med* 280:117–123, 1969.
5. Aronson PS, Nee J, Suhm MA: Modifier role of internal H$^+$ in activating the Na$^+$-H$^+$ exchanger in renal microvillus membrane vesicles. *Nature* 299:161–163, 1982.
6. Batlle DC, Hizon M, Cohen E, et al: The use of the urine anion gap in the diagnosis of hyperchloremic metabolic acidosis. *New Engl J Med* 318:594–599, 1988.

7. Brackett NC Jr, Cohen JJ, Schwartz WB: Carbon dioxide titration curve of normal man: Effect of increasing degrees of acute hypercapnia on acid-base equilibrium. *New Engl J Med* 272:6–12, 1965.

8. Cameron JN: Acid-base status of fish at different temperatures. *Am J Physiol* 246:R452–R459, 1984.

9. Fencl V, Leith DE: Stewart's quantitative acid-base chemistry: applications in biology and medicine. *Respir Physiol* 91:1–16, 1993.

10. Gabow PA: Disorders associated with an altered anion gap. *Kidney Int* 27:472–484, 1985.

11. Galla JH, Bonduris DN, Luke RG: Effects of chloride and extracellular fluid volume on bicarbonate reabsorption along the nephron in metabolic alkalosis in the rat. Reassessment of the classic hypothesis on the pathogenesis of metabolic alkalosis. *J Clin Invest* 80:41–52, 1987.

12. Gennari FJ, Goldstein MB, Schwartz WB: The nature of the renal adaptation to chronic hypocapnia. *J Clin Invest* 51:1722–1730, 1972.

13. Gennari FJ, Kassirer JP: Respiratory alkalosis, in Cohen JJ, Kassirer JP (eds), *Acid-Base.* Boston, Little, Brown, 1982, pp 349–376.

14. Giacobini E: Cytochemical study of the localization of carbonic anhydrase in the nervous system. *J Neurochem* 9:169–176, 1962.

15. Goldberg M, Green SB, Moss ML, et al: Computer-based instruction and diagnosis of acid-base disorders. A systematic approach. *JAMA* 223:269–278, 1973.

16. Javaheri S, Kazemi H: Metabolic alkalosis and hypoventilation in humans. *Am Rev Respir Dis* 136:1011–1020, 1987.

17. Jennings DB: The physicochemistry of [H$^+$] and respiratory control: roles of P_{CO_2}, strong ions, and their hormonal regulators. *Can J Physiol Pharmacol* 72:1499–1512, 1994.

18. Kassirer JP, Schwartz WB: The response of normal man to selective depletion of hydrochloric acid. Factors in the genesis of persistent gastric alkalosis. *Am J Med* 40:10–21, 1966.

19. Kazemi H, Hitzig B: Control of ventilation: Central chemical drive, in Narins RG (ed), *Maxwell & Kleeman's Clinical Disorders of Fluid and Electrolyte Metabolism,* 5th ed. New York, McGraw-Hill, 1994, pp 175–186.

20. Madias NE, Adrogue HJ, Cohen JJ, Schwartz WB: Effect of natural variations in P_{CO_2} on plasma [HCO$_3^-$] in dogs: A redefinition of normal. *Am J Physiol* 236:F30–F35, 1979.

21. McCurdy DK: Mixed metabolic and respiratory acid-base disturbances: Diagnosis and treatment. *Chest* 62:35S–44S, 1972.

22. Moe OW, Rector FC, Alpern RJ: Renal regulation of acid-base metabolism, in Narins RG (ed), *Maxwell & Kleeman's Clinical Disorders of Fluid and Electrolyte Metabolism,* 5th ed. New York, McGraw-Hill, 1994, pp 203–242.

23. Nattie EE: Intracisternal diethylpyrocarbonate inhibits central chemosensitivity in conscious rabbits. *Respir Physiol* 64:161–176, 1986.

24. Reeves RB: The interaction of body temperature and acid-base balance in ectothermic vertebrates. *Ann Rev Physiol* 39:559–586, 1977.

25. Reeves RB, Rahn H: Patterns in vertebrate acid-base regulation, in Wood S, Lenfant C (eds), *Evolution of the Respiratory Process: A Comparative Approach.* New York, Dekker, 1979, pp 225–252.

26. Rose B: *Clinical Physiology of Acid-Base and Electrolyte Disorders,* 4th ed. New York, McGraw-Hill, 1994.

27. Sabatini S, Kurtzman NA: The maintenance of metabolic alkalosis: Factors which decrease bicarbonate excretion. *Kidney Int* 25:357–364, 1984.

28. Schwartz WB, Hays RM, Polak A, Haynie GD: Effects of chronic hypercapnia on electrolyte and acid-base equilibrium: Recovery, with special reference to the influence of chloride intake. *J Clin Invest* 40:1238–1249, 1961.

29. Severinghaus JW: Acid-base balance nomogram: A Boston-Copenhagen detente. *Anesthesiology* 45:539–541, 1976.

30. Stewart PA: How to understand acid-base balance, in *A Quantitative Acid-Base Primer for Biology and Medicine.* New York, Elsevier, 1981.

31. Trivedi B, Tannen RL: Effect of respiratory acidosis on intracellular pH of the proximal tubule. *Am J Physiol* 250:F1039–F1045, 1986.

32. Wichser J, Kazemi H: CSF bicarbonate regulation in respiratory acidosis and alkalosis. *J Appl Physiol* 44:504–511, 1975.

SECTION 3

THE LUNGS IN DIFFERENT PHYSIOLOGICAL STATES

CHAPTER 16

EXERCISE, INTEGRATION, AND ADAPTATION

Alfred P. Fishman

Muscular exercise is such a regular feature of daily life that little heed is apt to be paid to the complexity of the underlying physiological processes. The range of daily activity and its limits vary greatly from person to person. The range is shorter in persons who lead a sedentary existence than in those who engage in competitive sports, walk briskly, jog, or perform calisthenics. In the athlete who regularly engages in competitive sports, the physiological adjustments are of a degree and type different from those in people who engage in less demanding activities.[18] Moreover, these functional changes are generally accompanied by structural changes in the heart and lungs (see "Adaptation" below).

In recent years, participation in moderate exercise has been advocated as healthful and personally gratifying. However, the rewards of exercise are not confined to normal subjects. More than a few days' bed rest, such as a weeklong convalescence from an acute illness, is accompanied by a decrease in strength and physical capacity. Physical inactivity also imposes a continuing threat to persons for whom freedom of motion is limited, such as those who get about in motorized wheelchairs. In these people, physical deconditioning is inevitable unless physical exercise is deliberately incorporated into their way of life.

Over the years, studies of physiological adjustments during exercise invoked such concepts as "fixity of the internal environment,"[15] "homeostasis,"[3] and adaptation.[1] Recently, increasing attention has been paid to structural changes such as hypertrophy and hyperplasia.[19] This introductory chapter deals with some of these traditional concepts as they apply to the physiological processes of normal subjects during exercise. Against this background, diseases of the cardiorespiratory apparatus emerge as failures in one or more components of the integrative and compensatory responses.

THE INTEGRATED RESPONSE

Principles of the Integrated Response

Barcroft's classic monograph of 60 years ago, titled *Features in the Architecture of Physiological Function*, includes three chapters under the heading "Every Adaptation Is an Integration."[1] One chapter deals with exercise; the other two deal with pregnancy and anoxia (i.e., hypoxia), respectively. All three are concerned with the physiological changes that make possible the successful transition from one biologic state to another (e.g., rest to exercise) (Fig. 16-1).

His considerations of the three states led Barcroft to several generalizations about cardiorespiratory adjustments that can be paraphrased as follows: (1) after a person adjusts to a new environment or to a changed demand for oxygen, the blood gases undergo measurable changes instead of remaining constant; (2) the changes in blood gases occur in an orderly way and reverse upon return to the person's original condition or environment; and (3) the physiological adjustment is usually due to a summation or multiplication of several small changes rather than to a single major change (e.g., the cardiac output can undergo a 9-fold change because of 3-fold variations in stroke volume and heart rate).[1]

The Integrated Response for O_2 Uptake

The increase in energy called for by the exercising muscles has to be delivered by the heart, lungs, and blood, working as a coordinated system for the delivery of oxygen and removal of car-bon dioxide.[21] The amount of oxygen required can be quite large and impose large demands on the heart as a pump, the transport system between the alveolar capillaries and the mitochondria, and the ventilatory apparatus. Traditionally, the capacity to respond has been tested by progressive, steady-state exercise calibrated according to successive levels of oxygen uptake. For each level of exercise, the normal response of the cardiorespiratory apparatus has been quantified. For example, to satisfy the need for a 10-fold increase in oxygen uptake, the ventilation is expected to increase to about 20 times the resting minute volume and the cardiac output (predominantly by an increase in heart rate) to about three times the resting minute volume. These changes operate in concert with a striking redistribution of blood flow to the exercising muscles.

In 1925, Morgan and Murray, close collaborators of Barcroft and Henderson (see below), used a four-quadrant diagram to graphically demonstrate the complex interplay in oxygen uptake by the lungs at rest (Fig. 16-2).[1,17] Since then, the same type of representation has been used to depict related aspects of oxygen uptake by the lungs during steady-state exercise (Fig. 16-3). It can also be used to illustrate oxygen delivery to the exercising muscles and carbon dioxide elimination by the lungs in health and disease (Fig. 16-4).[14]

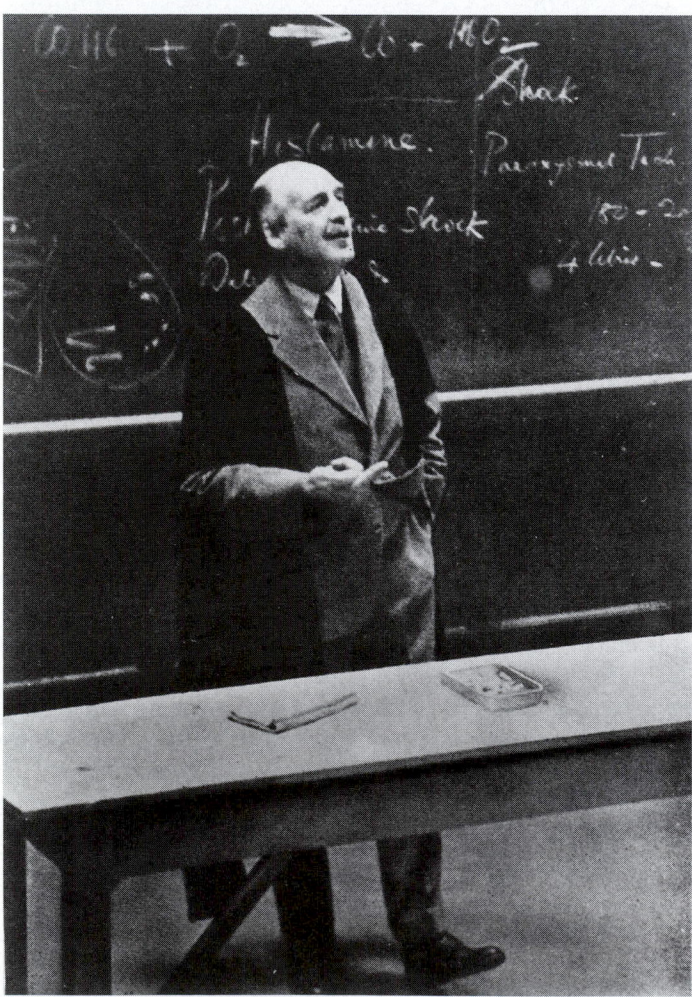

FIGURE 16-1 Joseph Barcroft (1872–1947) explored the integrating functions responsible for adjustments to diverse external environments, such as high altitude and fetal life. He maintained a lifelong interest in the properties of the oxygen dissociation curve and proved that oxygen entered pulmonary capillary blood by diffusion rather than by secretion.

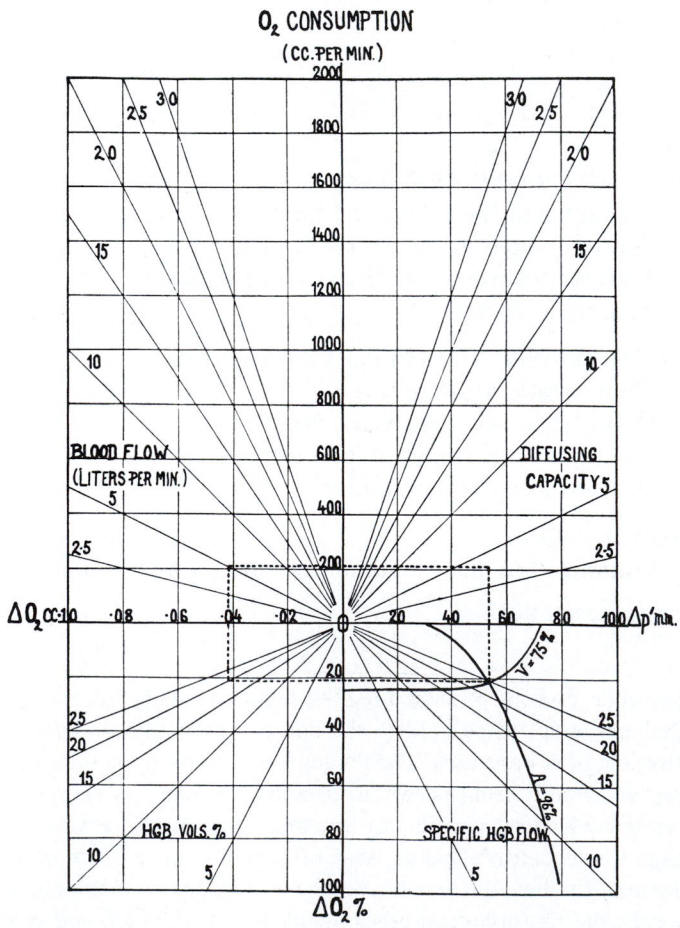

FIGURE 16-2 The original Morgan-Murray diagram. This diagram illustrates the linkages between physiological mechanisms at work in achieving adequate O_2 uptake by the lungs. (*From Richards DW Jr: Lawrence Joseph Henderson, in Medical Priesthoods and Other Essays, 1970, p 81.*)

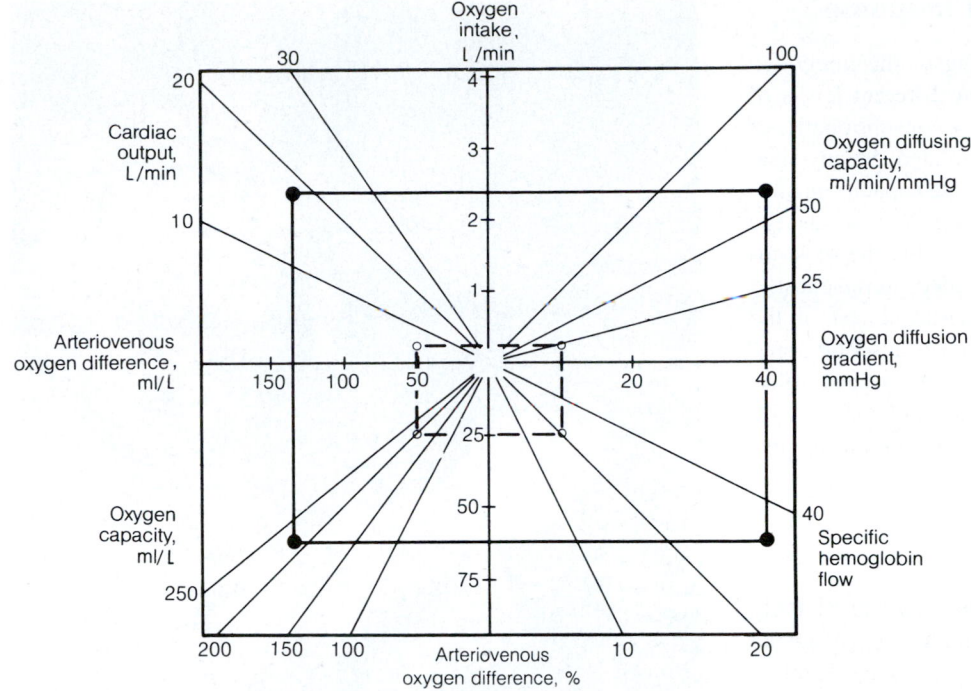

FIGURE 16-3 A more recent edition of the Morgan-Murray diagram, modified to show mechanisms of oxygen uptake by the lungs at rest (inner dashed rectangle) and during moderate exercise (solid rectangle). The oxygen uptake increased from 240 ml/min at rest to 2400 ml/min during exercise.

right of the O_2 dissociation curve due to increased release of CO_2 by the exercising muscle, and an increase in temperature of blood.[22]

The circulatory component of the cardiorespiratory system imposes more of a limit on the O_2 delivery system than does the ventilation. Thus, at $\dot{V}_{O_2max}$, the cardiac output reaches almost 90 percent of the capability of the heart, whereas the ventilation is only at 65 percent of the capability of the ventilatory apparatus.[6]

Not illustrated in graphic representations are the underlying automatic adjustments in both the autonomic nervous system and local mechanisms. For example, even though muscle arteries are compressed during exercise, resulting in increased resistance to blood flow, the dramatic increase in blood flow and O_2 delivery to the exercising muscles suffices to keep pace with the increase in energy requirement. Helping to increase blood flow and O_2 delivery are vasodilation induced by the metabolic products of the exercising muscles and the modest increase in blood pressure that accompanies exercise.

During recent decades, the physiological parameters that make up the individual quadrants of the Morgan-Murray diagram have been extensively studied at rest and during graded exercise.[1] For example, at consecutive levels of exercise, the cardiac output increases by a combination of an increase in heart rate and stroke volume. However, the increase in cardiac output is proportionally less than the increase in oxygen consumption. The difference between the two is made up by redistribution of the cardiac output. Thus, at the maximum rate of oxygen uptake ($\dot{V}_{O_2max}$)—i.e., when oxygen uptake levels off despite further increases in work rate—blood flow to skeletal muscle increases from about 20 percent of the cardiac output at rest to almost 90 percent during exercise; concomitantly, the splanchnic blood flow decreases from about 25 percent of the cardiac output to about 1 percent.[19] In addition to redistribution of the cardiac output in favor of the exercising muscles, the arteriovenous O_2 difference increases greatly; i.e., the O_2 extraction from each unit volume of perfusing blood increases. This increase in O_2 extraction is, in turn, a consequence of several physiological adjustments: an increase in the hemoglobin concentration of blood, a shift to the

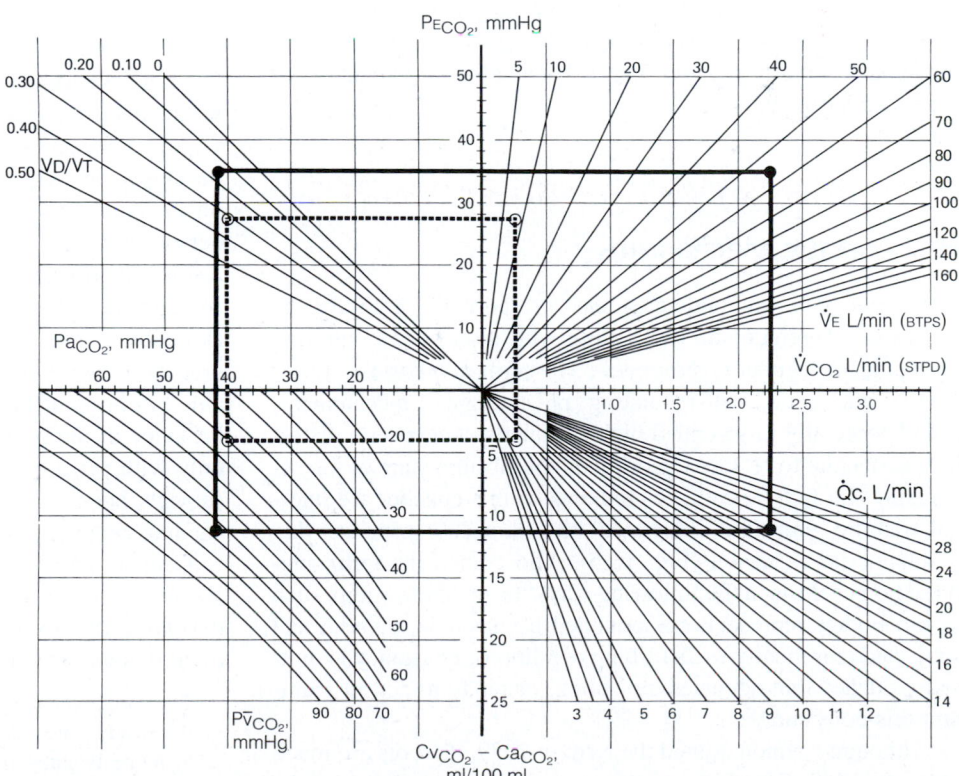

FIGURE 16-4 Application of the Morgan-Murray diagram to CO_2 elimination in the lungs. The inner (dashed) rectangle represents CO_2 output at a $\dot{V}_{O_2}$ of 200 ml/min; the outer rectangle (solid line) is for a $\dot{V}_{O_2}$ of 2250 ml/min. *(From Jones.[14])*

Exercise Testing of the Integrated Response

Steady-state, graded exercise enables testing of the integrated response of the cardiorespiratory system, at different levels of work, in terms of power output ($\dot{W}$) or, more conventionally, of oxygen uptake ($\dot{V}_{O_2}$). The two are closely related. Steady state is also useful in defining the ceiling of exercise capacity in similar terms ($\dot{W}max$, $\dot{V}_{O_2max}$).[24] The peak power ($\dot{W}max$) and the maximum O_2 consumption ($\dot{V}_{O_2max}$) are probably the most informative measurements obtained from a graded exercise test.[14]

For clinical purposes, however, a standardized test of the global aerobic capacity of the cardiorespiratory-muscular apparatus (e.g., the 6-min walk) is often substituted for tests utilizing graded exercise.[2,9] When global testing is supplemental with specific pulmonary function tests, precise localization of the impaired structure or function can be achieved.

Anaerobic Threshold

During exercise, the rate of oxygen uptake increases predictably until a plateau is reached—i.e., the maximum oxygen uptake ($\dot{V}_{O_2max}$). In the course of increasing exercise to the level of $\dot{V}_{O_2max}$, as oxygen delivery to the muscles cannot keep pace with oxygen requirements, anaerobic metabolism becomes evident. As indicated in Chapter 17, at the "anaerobic threshold," serum lactate levels begin to increase when the energy requirements of exercise exceed the ability of the combined respiratory and circulatory systems to supply oxygen at a sufficiently high rate. At this juncture, ventilation increases inordinately, accompanied by decreases in blood pH and bicarbonate levels. In normal nonathletic subjects, this anaerobic threshold is reached at about 50 to 60 percent of predicted $\dot{V}_{O_2max}$.[21] In persons with impaired ability to transport oxygen (e.g., heart failure), this threshold occurs at a lower $\dot{V}_{O_2}$ (expressed as a percentage of predicted $\dot{V}_{O_2max}$).

HOMEOSTASIS AND ITS PERTURBATIONS

Homeostatic Mechanisms

For clinicians, an understanding of normal physiological processes is prerequisite for dealing with disease and with disturbances in regulatory processes. The term *homeostasis* refers to the automatic, self-regulating physiological mechanisms, found especially in so-called higher animals, that, after a disturbance, operate to restore the original equilibrium state of the organism. The two essential ingredients of this concept are internal stability and the integrated (coordinated) response that maintains it.[15] Cannon (Fig. 16-5), who coined the term, pictured homeostasis in the following way: "In an open system, such as our bodies represent, compounded by unstable material and subjected continually to disturbing conditions, constancy is in itself evidence that agencies are acting, or ready to act, to maintain this constancy."

Although Cannon coined the term in 1939, its roots are much older. In 1859, Claude Bernard, concerned with stability of the internal environment of the body as a prerequisite for a free and independent life in the face of a changing external environment,

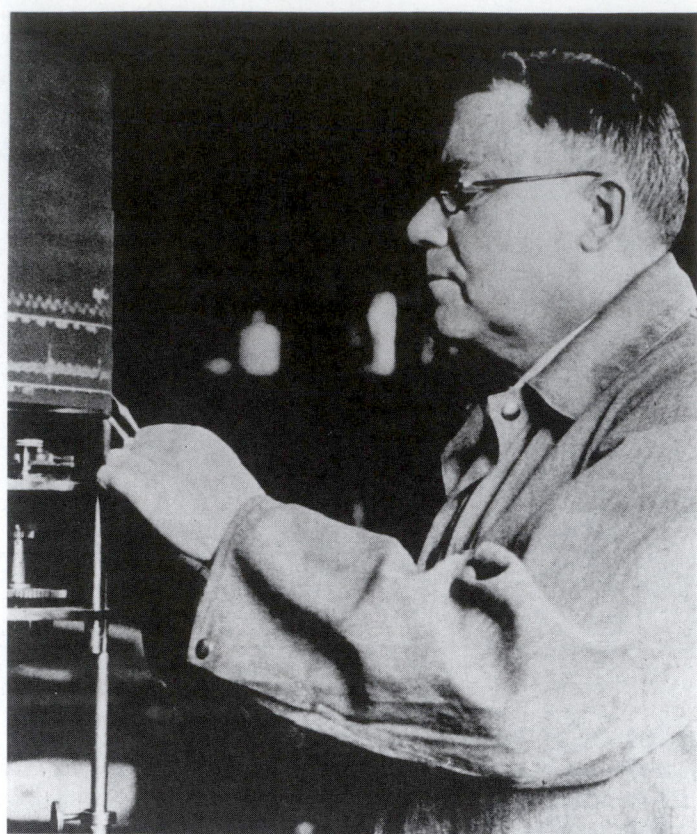

FIGURE 16-5 Walter B. Cannon (1871–1945) incorporated the idea of stability of the internal environment into the larger concept of *homeostasis*. He appreciated the role of the autonomic nervous system in maintaining the stability of the internal environment.

identified blood and lymph, the circulating body fluids, as the internal environment (Fig. 16-6). His experiments dealt with the mechanisms for ensuring this stability. The concept of blood as a critical element in the internal environment was subsequently developed by other physiologists and reached its peak of sophistication early in the 20th century when Lawrence J. Henderson (Fig. 16-7) described the physicochemical properties and respiratory function of blood. For these classic works, Henderson drew heavily on collaborative efforts with Van Slyke's group at the Rockefeller Institute and his own group in the Fatigue Laboratory at Harvard. Henderson's monograph affords a remarkable synthesis of the composition of the blood and its biologic behavior in the transport of the respiratory gases. It deals not only with perturbations in the composition of blood in normal subjects but also with abnormalities induced by disease (e.g., anemia, nephritis, and diabetic coma).[12]

Cannon envisaged homeostatic mechanisms as part of *The Wisdom of the Body*. His concept of homeostasis extended far beyond Bernard's ideas about the internal environment. He pictured homeostasis in the following way:

> The coordinated physiological processes which maintain most of the steady states in the organism are so complex and so peculiar to living beings—involving, as they may, the brain and nerves, the heart, lungs, kidneys, and spleen, all working cooperatively—that I have suggested a special designation for these states, *homeostasis*. The word does not imply something set and immobile, a

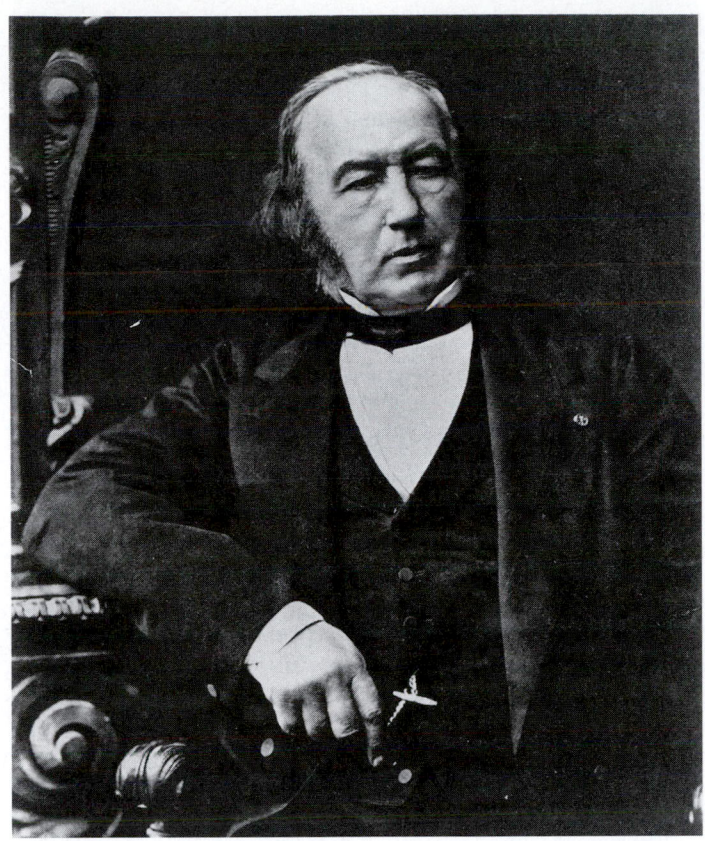

FIGURE 16-6 Claude Bernard (1813–1878) enunciated the principle that the ability of humans and animals to function in the external environment (i.e., to maintain a "free life") is due to the stability of its internal environment (i.e., the circulating body fluids that bathe organs and tissues). *(From Fishman and Richards.[8])*

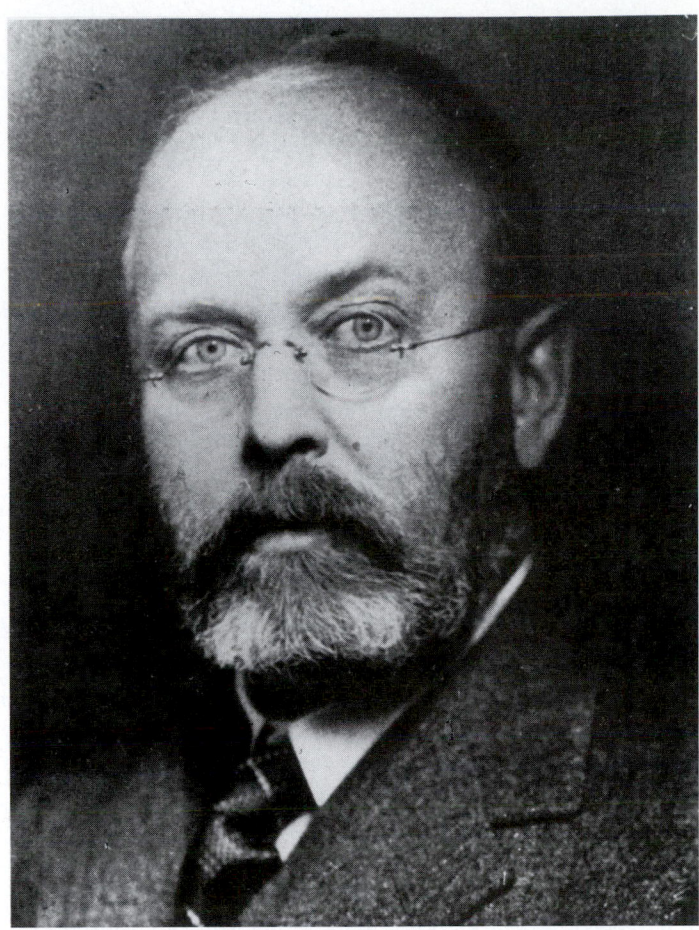

FIGURE 16-7 Lawrence J. Henderson (1878–1942) developed seminal concepts of acid-base balance and the regulation of the neutrality of the blood based on his explorations of blood as a physicochemical system. Founder of the Fatigue Laboratory at Harvard, he created nomograms to illustrate graphically the interrelations of the major chemical constituents of the blood in normal humans and in various pathologic states (e.g., anemia, nephritis, diabetic acidosis).

stagnation. It means a condition—a condition which may vary, but which is relatively constant.[3]

Restorative mechanisms per se, without intervening mechanisms to tide the body over abrupt and marked disturbances (e.g., temperature, body water, blood pressure), could not suffice to sustain the stability of the internal environment. Henderson appreciated that "the body seems to contain what may be likened to marshes or swamps into which substances may disappear and be lost to view." Aerobic metabolism illustrates the need for such "marshes." Faced with abrupt changes in ambient air or with pulmonary function sufficient to elicit disease that compromises arterial hypoxemia, the body draws upon oxygen-containing "swamps" to satisfy its need for oxygen. Thus, between ambient air and the mitochondrion are several distinct stores—the alveolar air, the blood, and the metabolizing cells. These are interposed seriatim between the processes of respiration, circulation, and metabolism (Fig. 16-8).

Disease can affect the "marshes" (stores) or the processes. With respect to the "marshes," pulmonary edema compromises oxygen uptake by replacing alveolar air with liquid; anemia limits the oxygen transport function of the blood; occlusive arterial disease can compromise oxygen delivery to the metabolizing cells. Considerations such as these prompt the idea that disease and regulatory disorders can be viewed as failure or insufficiency of normal processes and stores, components of the homeostatic

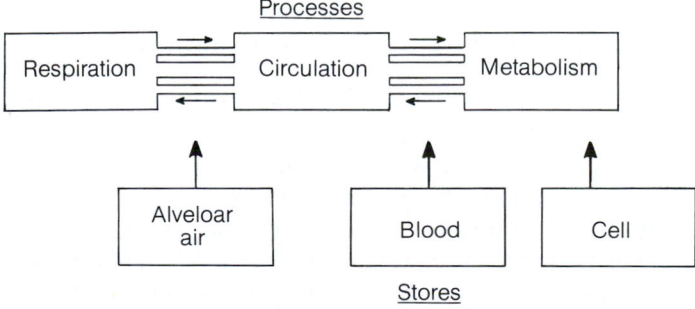

FIGURE 16-8 Processes and stores that maintain stable levels of P_{O_2} within cells. The alveolar air acts as a store for O_2 between ambient air and blood, serving as a tonometer of fairly stable composition. The blood, interposed between alveolar air and metabolizing tissues, has hemoglobin as the store. Within the cells are stores in the form of high-energy phosphates, dissolved O_2, myoglobin, and substrates for metabolic processes. Rearrangements in the distribution of blood by vasomotor activity determine the rate of delivery of O_2 to the different tissues. *(Modified from Weibel.[22])*

system originally designed to sustain stability of the internal environment.[8] Arterial hypotension or abnormal hemoglobins can interfere with oxygen transport. Various toxic substances, by accelerating cellular metabolism, can deplete oxygen stored in myoglobin.

Homeostasis as a Feedback Process

The principles that govern man-made control systems apply equally well to the self-regulatory mechanisms of living organisms.[5,10] The paradigm of a man-made control system is the control of temperature by means of a thermostat, which, in turn, is an example of a closed-loop (negative feedback) control system—one in which any deviation of the controlled output (room temperature) from the desired value automatically signals a change in input (fuel supply that generates heat) to the system in order to minimize the discrepancy between controlled output and desired output. There are two types of feedback: *negative*, which operates to the advantage of the system to minimize the original deviation in the controlled output, and *positive*, which perpetuates the deprivation, promotes instability, and runs the risk of destroying the organism unless turned off by the calling of another mechanism into play. Clearly, in a biologic system, failure of a negative-feedback system or unbridled positive feedback is capable of causing disorder or disease.

Although it is instructive to draw an analogy between man-made and living systems, it should be noted that a living system is infinitely more complex, entailing endless interplay (information transfer) among all levels in the biologic hierarchy, from cell to organ. Also, the sensory part of the regulatory apparatus is almost invariably more intricate than the effectors. Finally, the desired value ("set point") of a biologic parameter often depends on the physiological state (e.g., as dictated by the diurnal rhythm or the level of physical activity): during sleep, arterial P_{CO_2} is kept higher than during waking hours; while the subject is upright, the set point of the arterial P_{CO_2} is lower than it is while the subject is supine. Larger biologic rhythms, such as the monthly cycles in females, also are associated with different set points for the arterial P_{CO_2}.

The Bounds of Homeostatic Mechanisms

Before we consider the limitations imposed by disease, it is important to recall that the concept of homeostasis was conceived by physiologists to deal with adjustments of normal subjects to changing environments and circumstances. As a rule, considerations of homeostatic mechanisms in normal persons deal with acute or subacute adjustments. As noted above, even in normal subjects, the capacity of the cardiorespiratory-muscular system to transport, deliver, and utilize oxygen in aerobic metabolism is limited.[20] Although compensatory mechanisms such as widening of the arteriovenous difference for oxygen can raise the ceiling, the limit, as defined by the $\dot{V}_{O_2max}$, remains and is measurable.

A flaw or malfunction at any point in the uptake, transport, and delivery system for oxygen can lower the limit. In normal persons breathing ambient air at sea level, the weak link in the O_2 delivery system is the heart, which has only a modest ca-

pacity for increasing stroke volume. When this limitation coexists with hypoxia, as may occur at altitude, oxygen delivery (cardiac output multiplied by O_2 content) can be seriously impaired.

One special case of limitation in the aerobic capacity of the human organism under stress in a hypoxic environment has been seen in mountain climbers who have ascended to the summit of Mount Everest without supplementary oxygen. At this peak (altitude 8848 m), where the inspired P_{O_2} is about 42 mmHg, the $\dot{V}_{O_2max}$ is at a level that barely suffices for basal metabolism. The oxygen consumption is then limited, in part, by a marked alveolar-arterial P_{O_2} gradient (attributable to diffusion limitation of O_2 uptake across the alveolar-capillary barriers) and the dependence of O_2 uptake and delivery on O_2 exchanges conducted on the steep part of the O_2 dissociation curve.[23]

Homeostatic Malfunctioning

D. W. Richards analyzed the applicability of concepts about homeostatic mechanism to disease.[16,17] He took into account that integrative mechanisms designed to restore the internal environment to normal levels operate within constraints imposed by the structures and functions of the coordinating system. He recognized that diseases of the cardiorespiratory-muscular system often impose additional limits and generate distortions that may cause physiological mechanisms to undershoot or overshoot their mark, or to display instabilities (Fig. 16-9).[16]

Undershooting of homeostatic mechanisms is commonplace in cardiac diseases such as acute myocardial infarction, in which a low cardiac output may compromise oxygen delivery to the tissues despite other compensatory mechanisms, such as widening of the arteriovenous oxygen difference. *Overshooting* can be illustrated by renal failure in the course of the adult respiratory distress syndrome: ischemic necrosis of the kidney can follow intense systemic homeostatic vasoconstriction to counteract systemic hypotension. *Instabilities* are exemplified by Cheyne-Stokes breathing, in which rhythmic changes in ventilation are accompanied by swings in arterial blood gas composition. These examples represent instances in which homeostatic mechanisms can miss the mark, to the detriment of the organism. In the clinical setting, well-intentioned therapeutic interventions can contribute to homeostatic malfunction. Such iatrogenic disturbances pose continuing threats in emergency or intensive care settings, where urgency often dictates or dominates therapeutic interventions.

ADAPTATION

Adaptation signifies changes in both physiological and biochemical function and in structure that enhance performance or facilitate survival.[13] It signifies the adjustment of an organism to its environment. In a setting in which O_2 is chronically in short supply, it entails enhancement of the O_2 delivery system coupled with redirection of metabolic activities toward sustaining oxidative functions. In doing so, it spares undue reliance on the anaerobic machinery. As a rule, adaptation is a gradual process in which anatomic changes flow prominently.[11]

Homeostatic (physiological and biochemical) mechanisms are the first line of defense upon exposure to a threatening environment. Subsequently, structural changes come into play (e.g., mus-

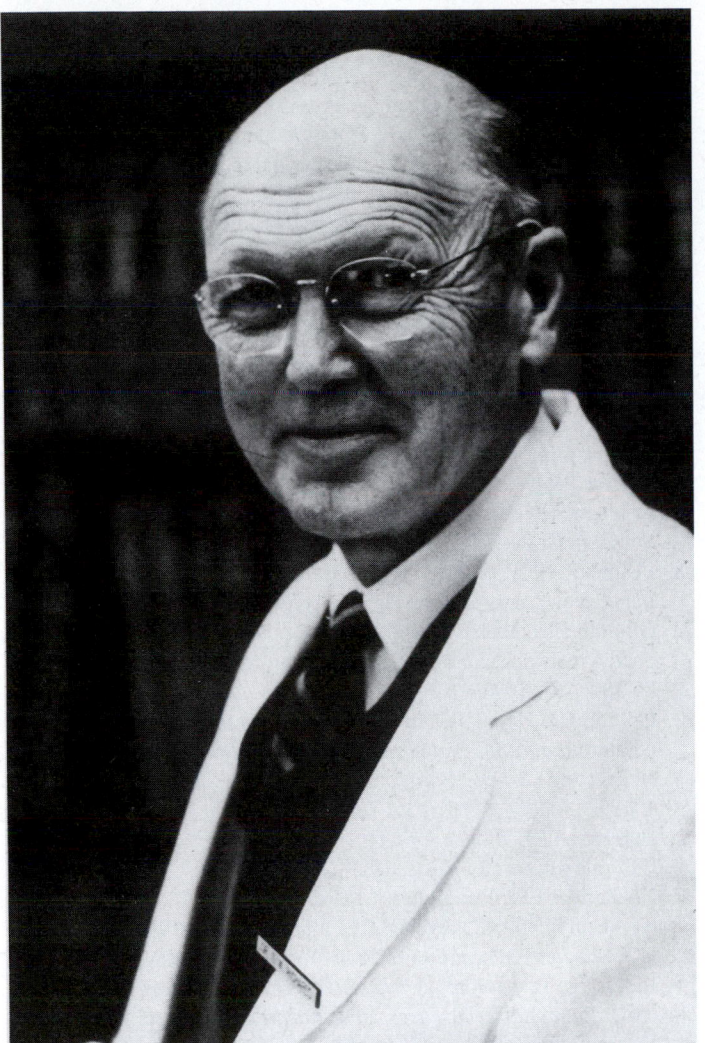

FIGURE 16-9   Dickinson W. Richards (1895–1973), a physician-scientist, related disturbances in homeostatic mechanisms to clinical disorders. Strongly influenced by L. J. Henderson, he shared the Nobel Prize with André Cournand and Werner Forssmann for contributing to the development of cardiac catheterization and to standardization of measurements of pulmonary function.

cularization of the pulmonary arteries and arterioles at altitude and right ventricular hypertrophy). When the new steady state has been achieved (i.e., when adaptation has occurred), the person at altitude can carry on the activities of daily life, including moderate exercise, about as effectively as at sea level. However, should control mechanisms, such as the sensitivity of the carotid bodies to hypoxia, fail to reset properly, maladaptation ensues. (For example, Monge's disease is caused by failure to increase alveolar ventilation due to inadequate responsiveness of the carotid bodies to the hypoxic stimulus.) The approach to disease in terms of malfunctioning of homeostatic and adaptive mechanisms is not confined to the cardiorespiratory-muscular system. In a similar fashion, many diseases, such as those due to hypersecretion by endocrine glands or tumors (e.g., thyrotoxicosis, Addison's disease), can be considered in terms of failure of homeostatic and adaptive mechanisms.

Adaptation may be *inherited*, as in native residents at high altitude in whom the process of natural selection, operating over

the ages, has yielded a population that can exist, thrive, and reproduce in a hypoxic environment. On the other hand, adaptation may be *nonhereditary*, as in the case of the sea-level native who becomes a permanent dweller at high altitude.

Adaptation is commonly studied in people who relocate to different environments (e.g., from sea level to altitude). Upon arrival at altitude, the newcomer is tachycardic (to sustain cardiac output) and breathes rapidly. In time, these changes are succeeded by adjustments that favor O_2 uptake by the lungs and O_2 delivery to the tissues (e.g., a left shift of the O_2 dissociation curve and increased capillary density in the muscles). Another common approach to the study of adaptation is to compare populations of animals and humans, born and raised in different environments, not only with respect to adaptive mechanisms but also with respect to genetic influences in adaptation.

Adaptation has also been studied in people exposed to a wide variety of other chronically stressful circumstances. One large group is made up of endurance athletes who, over time, undergo biologic changes that enable them to perform optimally in competitive sports that require maximum oxygen delivery to the exercising muscles. These changes are evident both in the cardiorespiratory system and in the exercising muscles. The changes in the components of the cardiorespiratory system proceed at different rates: the plasma volume increases (in weeks), the pump capacity of the heart increases (in months to years), the red cell mass increases the O_2-carrying capacity of the blood (in months), the number of capillaries in skeletal muscles increases (in weeks to months), and the mitochondrial enzymes in skeletal muscle increase (in weeks).

During endurance athletic training, not only do the muscles employed in exercise undergo hypertrophy but also the heart enlarges by combined hypertrophy and dilation, thereby raising the capacity for increasing the cardiac output. Finally, at the maximum level and intensity of the exercise, the $\dot{V}_{O_2}$ reaches a plateau ($\dot{V}_{O_2}max$). Whether the heart or the peripheral muscles (i.e., the mitochondria and capillaries) set the limit for maximal O_2 uptake in the endurance-trained athlete continues to be debated. However, the bulk of the evidence currently assigns the limitation to the heart rather than to the number of capillaries and mitochondrial enzymes in the peripheral muscles.[19,22]

Chronic respiratory disease often calls forth adaptive mechanisms that sometimes overshoot their mark. For example, polycythemia, which originates as a homeostatic response to hypoxia and serves to increase the oxygen-carrying capacity of the blood, if continued, increases the circulating blood volume. Cardiac volume and mass then increase to handle the increased circulatory load; i.e., a homeostatic mechanism has been succeeded by adaptive change in the heart. If carried to excess (the so-called hyperexis of Richards), venous thrombosis, on the one hand, or cardiac failure, on the other, may ensue.[17]

Optimization and Limitation of Human Adaptation

The cardiorespiratory-muscular system operates within limits imposed by the structure and the integrated functioning of its components. The maximum oxygen uptake ($\dot{V}_{O_2max}$) provides a measure of the limit of the capacity of this system to transport and utilize oxygen. The activities of daily life are generally conducted well below this limit. In sports, however, this ceiling is apt to be approached, usually in spurts but occasionally in sustained effort.

The capability of the cardiorespiratory-muscular system to satisfy the energy needs of the cells depends on its ability to match oxygen delivery to their aerobic needs. The system is vulnerable at many sites, particularly where respiration and circulation cross paths—i.e., in the lungs, where O_2 is taken up from the environment and transferred across alveolar-capillary barriers into flowing blood; in the blood, which transports the oxygen to the tissues; in the tissues, where the blood releases oxygen for diffusion into cells; within cells, where oxygen moves to mitochondria for oxidative phosphorylation, which generates the high-energy organic phosphates for biologic work. Each of these sites operates within its own limits, which, if exceeded, could set the limit of O_2 uptake and delivery for the entire organization (i.e., the $\dot{V}_{O_2max}$). At each site, buffer mechanisms exist: between ambient air and the blood is the large volume of alveolar air; in the blood is the large reservoir of hemoglobin; in the muscle cells is the bank of myoglobin; and within the muscle cells are stores of high-energy phosphates.[4] In addition to these stores, which neutralize abrupt changes in oxygen supply, compensatory mechanisms, such as an increase in heart rate to sustain oxygen delivery by increasing cardiac output, are on standby alert. The autonomic nerve system plays a critical role in orchestrating the response to the call for oxygen as the energy needs increase.

In disease, adaptation to a chronic impairment may favor realignment of physiological process to compensate for a deficiency in either a component or process of the system. For example, in patients with severe kyphoscoliosis and dwarfing, a breathing pattern is adopted that minimizes the energy cost of breathing; this pattern consists of rapid frequency and small tidal volumes. However, as indicated above for homeostatic overshoot, this pattern may pay the penalty of alveolar hypoventilation, which, in turn, results in respiratory acidosis and arterial hypoxemia and their consequences, respiratory and cardiac failure. Thus, by adopting a respiratory pattern that minimizes the work, energy cost, and discomfort of breathing, the individual may be put at risk of losing life because of the consequences of alveolar hypoventilation.

Limitation of the adaptive potential can also vary with the disease or circumstance. For example, after lung transplantation, limitation to maximal exercise is imposed not by the heart or lungs but by abnormalities in the peripheral muscles, probably secondary to preoperative muscle disuse and atrophy.[9]

CONCLUSIONS

Exercise is a remarkable example of the integrative and adaptive capacities of the body. Disease may impose limitations on the capacity of the body to acquire, transport, and utilize oxygen. This limitation in aerobic capacity can be tested by calibrated exercise, either graded or global, and the malfunctioning component uncovered by a combination of clinical evaluation and pulmonary function testing.

REFERENCES

1. Barcroft J: *Features in the Architecture of Physiological Function.* London, Cambridge University Press, 1934.
2. Cahalin LP, Mathier MA, Semigran MJ, et al: The six-minute walk predicts peak oxygen uptake and survival in patients with advanced heart failure. *Chest* 110:325–332, 1996.
3. Cannon WB: *The Wisdom of the Body*, 2d ed. New York, Norton, 1932.
4. Cherniack NS, Longobardo GS: Oxygen and carbon dioxide gas stores of the body. *Physiol Rev* 70:196–243, 1970.
5. DeFares JG: Principles of feedback control and their application to the respiratory control system, in Fenn WO, Rahn H (eds), *Handbook of Physiology*, Sec 3: *Respiration.* Washington, DC, American Physiological Society, 1964, pp 649–680.
6. Dempsey JA, Pack AI: *Regulation of Breathing*, 2d ed. New York, Dekker, 1995.
7. Fishman AP (ed): *Pulmonary Diseases and Disorders,* 2d ed. New York, McGraw-Hill, 1988.
8. Fishman AP, Richards DW: *Circulation of the Blood: Men and Ideas.* New York, Oxford University Press, 1964.
9. Gilbreth EM, Weisman IM: Role of exercise stress testing in preoperative evaluation of patients for lung resection. *Clin Chest Med* 15:389–403, 1994.
10. Gordon CJ, Heath JE: Integration and central processing in temperature regulation. *Annu Rev Physiol* 48:595–612, 1986.
11. Henderson LJ: *The Fitness of the Environment.* Boston, Beacon, 1913.
12. Henderson LJ: *Blood: A Study in General Physiology.* New Haven, CT, Yale University Press, 1928.
13. Hochachka PW: Principles of physiological and biochemical adaptation, in Wood SC, Weber RE, Hargens AR, Millard RW (eds), *Physiological Adaptation in Vertebrates.* New York, Dekker, 1992.
14. Jones NL: Physiological basis of exercise testing, in Fishman AP (ed), *Pulmonary Diseases and Disorders,* 2d ed. New York, McGraw-Hill, 1988, pp 235–249.
15. Langley LL: *Homeostasis: Origins of the Concept.* Stroudsburg, PA, Dowden, Hutchinson and Ross, 1973.
16. Richards DW: Homeostasis versus hyperexis, or Saint George and the Dragon. *Sci Mon* 77:289–294, 1953.
17. Richards DW: Homeostasis: Its dislocations and perturbations. *Perspec Biol Med* 3:238–251, 1960.
18. Rowell LB, Shepherd JT (eds): *Exercise: Regulation and Integration of Multiple Systems, Handbook of Physiology*, Sec 12. New York, Oxford University Press, 1996.
19. Saltin B: Maximal oxygen uptake: Limitation and malleability, in Nazar K, Terjung RL, Kaciuba-Ûscilko H, Budohoski L (eds), *International Perspectives in Exercise Physiology.* Champaign, Ill., Human Kinetics Books, 1990, pp 26–40.
20. Stern N, Tuck ML: Homeostatic fragility in the elderly. *Cardiol Clin* 4:201–211, 1986.
21. Wasserman K, Hansen JE, Sue DY, Whipp BJ: *Principles of Exercise Testing and Interpretation.* Philadelphia, Lea & Febiger, 1987.
22. Weibel ER: *The Pathway for Oxygen.* Cambridge, MA, Harvard University Press, 1984.
23. West JB, Lahiri S: *High Altitude and Man.* Washington, DC, American Physiological Society, 1984.
24. Whipp BJ: The bioenergetic and gas exchange basis of exercise testing. *Clin Chest Med* 15:173–192, 1994.

CHAPTER 17

BREATHING DURING EXERCISE

Brian J. Whipp

Although many of the integrative aspects of the control of exercise hyperpnea remain to be elucidated, the general patterns of ventilatory response are not topics of serious dispute. These response profiles, especially their dynamics, provide the clues to the elements of the control processes. Too often, however, authoritative reviews on this topic fail to address this fundamental issue: a congeries of mechanisms capable of stimulating ventilation under some circumstances during exercise is not sufficient. The challenge is to establish the integrative aspects of the control which accounts for the actual dynamic features of the ventilatory responses in humans.

VENTILATORY REQUIREMENTS

The ventilatory demands of muscular exercise depend not only on the work rate being performed but also on its intensity. The range of work rates within which there is no sustained metabolic acidemia may be considered to be of moderate intensity.

Alveolar, and hence arterial, P$_{O_2}$ and P$_{CO_2}$ can be regulated at—or close to—resting levels only if alveolar ventilation ($\dot{V}$A) increases in proportion to metabolic rate. And, indeed, this is normally the case (i.e., arterial P$_{CO_2}$ is well regulated at or close

to resting values in the steady state of moderate exercise). With respect to CO$_2$ exchange:

$$F_{ACO_2} = \frac{\dot{V}_{CO_2(STPD)}}{\dot{V}_{A(STPD)}} \qquad (1)$$

where F is the fractional concentration of alveolar (A) gas and $\dot{V}$ is the volume per unit time or flow. Note that in this equation both gas volumes are determined under the same conditions, i.e., standard temperature (0°C) and pressure (one atmosphere) dry (STPD).

But as convention has reasonably dictated that ventilatory volumes are expressed under the conditions at which they actually operate (i.e., at body temperature and pressure, saturated with water vapor), and as the partial pressure P of the gas is of more interest physiologically than the concentration, then:

$$P_{ACO_2} = \frac{863 \times \dot{V}_{CO_2(STPD)}}{\dot{V}_{A(BTPS)}} \qquad (2)$$

Similarly, for oxygen exchange:

$$P_{AO_2} = P_{IO_2} - \frac{863 \times \dot{V}_{O_2(STPD)}}{\dot{V}_{A(BTPS)}} \qquad (3)$$

where 863 is the constant that corrects for these different conditions of reporting the gas volumes (at a body temperature of 37°C) and the transformation of the fractional concentration to the partial pressure.

However, neither the alveolar ventilation nor the alveolar gas partial pressures in Eqs. (1) and (2) are conceptually straightforward. Establishing a single average value for the alveolar gas tensions is difficult in a structure as complex as the lung which has significant regional differences of alveolar ventilation-to-perfusion ratios. The expedient of assigning P$_{ACO_2}$ to be exactly equal to the arterial CO$_2$ (P$_{aCO_2}$) dispenses with this difficulty and allows alveolar ventilation to be computed readily from Eq. (1). This alveolar ventilation, however, is figmentary. Similarly, the alveolar P$_{O_2}$ in Eq. (2) is also that of the ideal lung. The "real" alveolar P$_{CO_2}$ would be lower, and the "real" alveolar P$_{O_2}$ would be higher than the "ideal" alveolar values calculated from Eqs. (1) and (2).

Accepting these definitions, and ignoring the slight effect on P$_{O_2}$ of the small difference in $\dot{V}$I and $\dot{V}$E that occurs when the respiratory exchange ratio R does not equal 1, it becomes apparent from Eqs. (1) and (2) that alveolar P_{CO_2} and P_{O_2} can only be maintained at constant levels during exercise if $\dot{V}_A$ changes in precise proportion to $\dot{V}_{CO_2}$ and $\dot{V}_{O_2}$, respectively. Note, however, that $\dot{V}_A$ is common to both equations, that is,

$$\frac{863 \times \dot{V}_{CO_2}}{P_{A_{CO_2}}} \longleftarrow \dot{V}_A \longrightarrow \frac{863 \times \dot{V}_{O_2}}{P_{I_{O_2}} - P_{A_{O_2}}} \qquad (4)$$

Alveolar ventilation cannot therefore meet the demands of both O_2 and CO_2 exchange under conditions in which the pulmonary exchange rates for O_2 and CO_2 differ. These conditions can occur during exercise, either because of differences in substrate utilization (e.g., Fig. 17-1) or because of transient variations in the body gas stores (e.g. Fig. 17-2). Under such conditions, ventilation has been consistently demonstrated to change in closer proportion to CO_2 output than to O_2 uptake.[22,55] $P_{A_{CO_2}}$ is therefore the more closely regulated variable, with alveolar P_{O_2} changing as a consequence. In normal subjects at sea level these P_{O_2} changes normally vary only over the relatively flat region of the oxyhemoglobin dissociation curve, with little consequent effect on the O_2 content or saturation of arterial blood.

It is more appropriate, therefore, to consider the ventilatory demands of exercise using CO_2 exchange rather than O_2 exchange as the frame of reference. It follows from Eq. (2) that the demands for alveolar ventilation increase as a linear function of $\dot{V}_{CO_2}$ at any "set point" level of $P_{A_{CO_2}}$. Consequently, the greater the CO_2 output is, the greater the ventilatory requirement. But if $P_{A_{CO_2}}$ is regulated at a lower level, the alveolar ventilation must be appropriately higher for any given level of CO_2 output. However, ventilating the alveoli requires simultaneous ventilation of the dead space. That is, the ventilatory demand is expressed through the total or minute ventilation ($\dot{V}_E$), rather than alveolar ventilation. But as

$$\dot{V}_A = \dot{V}_E - \dot{V}_{DS} \qquad (5)$$

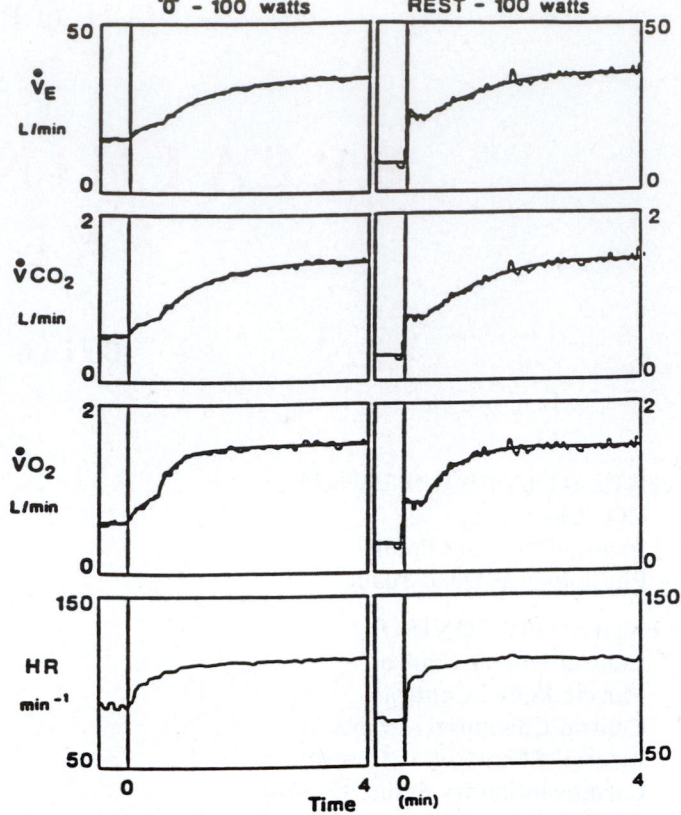

FIGURE 17-2   Ventilatory and pulmonary gas exchange responses to a constant-load work rate of 100 watts on a cycle ergometer beginning either at rest or from unloaded pedalling ("0" watts). Note the more abrupt changes at the transition from rest and, in both cases, the slower time course for $\dot{V}_E$ and $\dot{V}_{CO_2}$ toward the steady state than for $\dot{V}_{O_2}$. *(Reprinted from Whipp and Ward,[55] by courtesy of Marcel Dekker, Inc.)*

or

$$\dot{V}_A = \dot{V}_E \left(1 - \frac{V_{DS}}{V_T}\right) \qquad (6)$$

then

$$\dot{V}_E = \frac{863 \times \dot{V}_{CO_2}}{P_{A_{CO_2}}(1 - V_{DS}/V_T)} \qquad (7)$$

where V_{DS}/V_T is the physiological dead space fraction of the breath.

The ventilatory demands of exercise (Fig. 17-3) should therefore be considered with respect to the three defining variables of Eq. (7):

1. The rate of pulmonary CO_2 clearance
2. The set point at which $P_{A_{CO_2}}$ is regulated
3. The physiological dead space fraction of the breath which represents an index of the inefficiency of pulmonary gas exchange

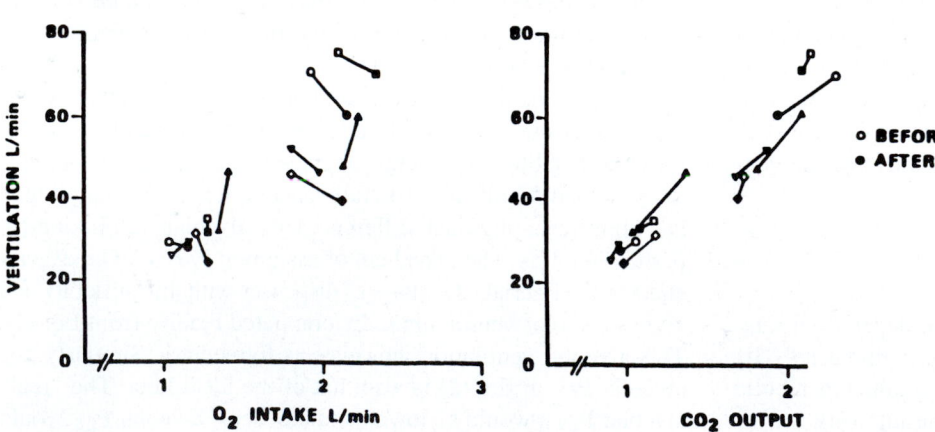

FIGURE 17-1   Steady-state relationship among ventilation, O_2 uptake, and CO_2 output before and after endurance training in normal subjects. Note that the training-induced reduction in CO_2 output is matched by a proportional reduction in ventilation. The relation between ventilation and O_2 uptake, however, is highly variable. *(By permission of R Taylor and NL Jones, Eur J Cardiol 9:53–62, 1979.)*

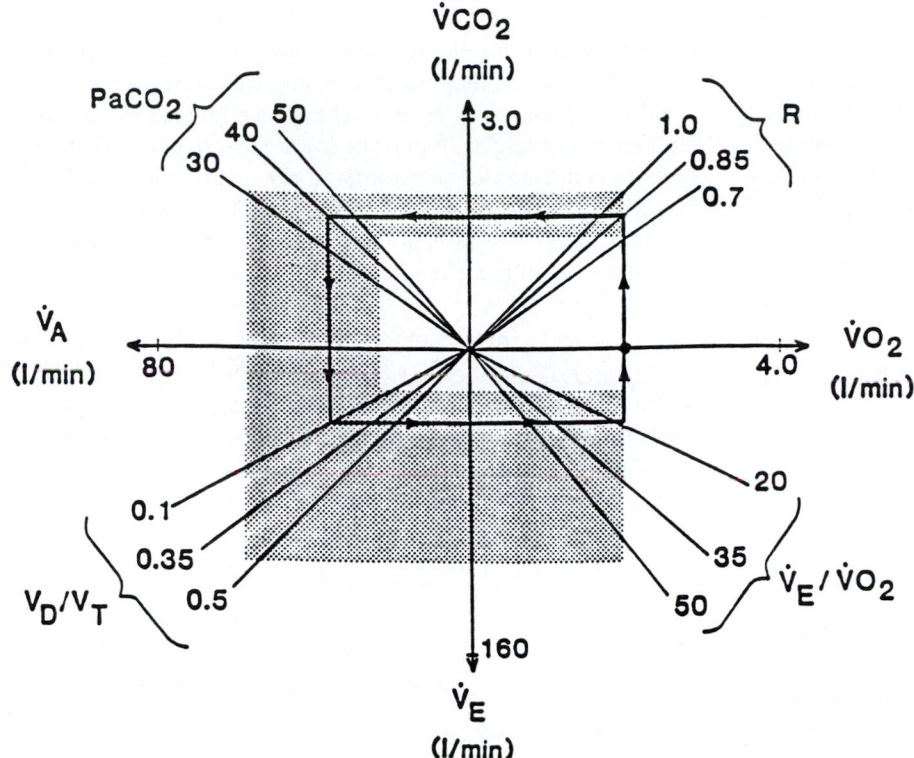

FIGURE 17-3   Influence of the respiratory exchange ratio (R), the regulated level of arterial P_{CO_2} (Pa_{CO_2}), the physiological dead space fraction of the tidal volume (V_D/V_T) on the ventilatory response to a given O_2 uptake (V_{O_2}). Beginning in the first quadrant with a $\dot{V}_{O_2}$ requirement of 2 L/min and proceeding counter-clockwise through the quadrants, the resulting range of values are represented by the stippled area. *(Reprinted from Whipp and Ward,[55] by courtesy of Marcel Dekker, Inc.)*

CO₂ Clearance

CO_2 measured at the lung ($\dot{V}_{CO_2}$) only equals the CO_2 production rate in the tissues ($\dot{Q}_{CO_2}$) in the steady state of exercise. Under these conditions the respiratory exchange ratio R equals the metabolic RQ. The substrates being catabolized, and therefore contributing to the RQ, place fundamental demands upon the pulmonary system. For example, a given rate of high-energy phosphate formation requires some 6 percent less O_2 when carbohydrate is metabolized than when fatty acids serve as the substrate (Table 17-1).

The carbohydrate metabolism, however, yields some 40 percent more CO_2 than for a typical fatty acid, leading to a greater demand for CO_2 clearance and, by extension, ventilation. To minimize the ventilatory demands for CO_2 clearance, fatty acids may therefore be considered a more suitable substrate. The conse-

quence, however, is that alveolar and arterial P_{O_2} will necessarily be reduced as $\dot{V}_E$ is now low for the O_2 requirement of the task. Conversely, alveolar and arterial P_{O_2} will be higher in subjects metabolizing carbohydrate.

Under non-steady-state conditions, $\dot{V}_{CO_2}$ is disassociated from $\dot{Q}_{CO_2}$ as a result of transient changes in the body CO_2 stores. During the on-transient of constant-load exercise, some of the metabolically produced CO_2 never reaches the lung for exchange as a result of the capacitative storage of CO_2 in the muscle and the venous blood. $\dot{V}_{CO_2}$ is therefore less than $\dot{Q}_{CO_2}$ during this phase. And as the changes in the muscle O_2 stores are trivially small with respect to those of CO_2, R therefore *falls* transiently to reach a minimum at the point of the maximum *rate* of CO_2 storage. R subsequently rises again to equal the new metabolic steady-state RQ as the muscle P_{CO_2} stabilizes at its new, and higher, exercise value. Whereas the ventilatory change during the transient is closely coupled to that of $\dot{V}_{CO_2}$, it changes slowly with respect to $\dot{V}_{O_2}$ (Fig. 16-2) which, of course, has a more rapid time constant of response. Consequently, alveolar and arterial P_{O_2} are reduced in the transient. At the off-transient, the increased levels of the CO_2 stores now discharge, leading the pulmonary R to increase to levels *above* that of the metabolic RQ.

At work rates associated with a metabolic (chiefly lactate) acidosis, pulmonary CO_2 exchange is increased further. Additional CO_2 is produced as a result of the bicarbonate (HCO_3^-) component of the proton buffering which is formed in concert with the increased lactate at these work rates; thus

$$CH_3 \cdot CHOH \cdot COO^- + H^+ + NaHCO_3 \longrightarrow$$
$$CH_3 \cdot CHOH \cdot COONa + H_2CO_3$$
$$\swarrow \qquad \searrow$$
$$CO_2 + H_2O$$

It is important to recognize here, however, that the extra CO_2 which is formed in these reactions is quantitatively large. For example, although the complete aerobic catabolism of one gluco-

TABLE 17-1

Energetics of Substrate Catabolism

	RQ	$\dot{V}_{O_2}$ (L/min)	$\dot{V}_{CO_2}$ (L/min)	~P:O₂	~P:CO₂	O₂:~P	CO₂:~P
Glycogen	1.0	1.0	1.0	6.00	6.00	0.17	0.17
Palmitate	0.7	1.0	0.7	5.65	8.13	0.18	0.12
Glycogen/palmitate	1.43	1.0	1.43	1.06	0.74	0.94	1.42

Values are expressed at a particular $\dot{V}_{O_2}$.

syl unit of glycogen to CO_2 and H_2O yields 37 adenosine triphosphate (ATP) molecules, its breakdown to two lactates and associated protons yields only three ATP molecules. Glycolytic flux must therefore increase by 12.3-fold (i.e., 37/3) in order to sustain the required ATP production rate. This leads to 24.6 meq of lactate (i.e., 2×12.3 meq) being formed. The accompanying proton production will therefore decrease $[HCO_3^-]$ by ~22 meq (i.e., HCO_3^- only accounts for some 90 percent of this buffering, with phosphate and protein buffers accounting for the remainder). Of this *additional* yield of ~22 mmol of CO_2 production, however, 6 mmol replace the CO_2 that would have been produced aerobically for this rate of ATP formation:

$$22 \text{ m}M \text{ anaerobic } CO_2 - 6 \text{ m}M \text{ aerobic } CO_2 =$$
$$16 \text{ m}M \text{ net } CO_2 \text{ yield}$$

This represents a ~2.5-fold increase in $\dot{V}_{CO_2}$ for these "anaerobic" reactions.

The extra *amount* of CO_2 produced under these conditions is a direct function of the *amount* of $[HCO_3^-]$ decrease in the blood and muscle compartments. Any contribution from nonbicarbonate buffering mechanisms (such as phosphate and protein), although important for $[H^+]$ regulation, does not produce extra CO_2. The *rate* at which extra CO_2 is produced from these reactions will consequently be directly related to the *rate* at which the HCO_3^- levels fall—not, it should be recognized, the amount of the decrease.

Consequently, the more rapid the rate of rise of [lactate], the greater is the increase in the pulmonary CO_2 exchange rate, $\dot{V}_{CO_2}$. This accounts for both $\dot{V}_{CO_2}$ and R being appreciably higher in the period of increasing blood lactate during rapid-increment exercise, compared to tests where the increment rate is relatively slow.

Arterial P_{CO_2} Set Point

Arterial P_{CO_2} is normally regulated at, or near, resting levels in the steady state of moderate-intensity exercise. Hyperventilation can occur transiently, however, at the onset of exercise, especially in "excitable" subjects; this is more common in treadmill than in cycle ergometry. But as the time constant for $\dot{V}_E$ ($T\dot{V}_E$) during the subsequent increase to the steady state is slightly longer than that of $\dot{V}_{CO_2}$ ($T\dot{V}_{CO_2}$), a small and transient increase in $P_{A_{CO_2}}$ and Pa_{CO_2} is both predictable and has been measured. The ratio $T\dot{V}_E/T\dot{V}_{CO_2}$ seems to depend, in large part, on the sensitivity of the subject's peripheral chemoreceptors (Fig. 17-4), in humans predominantly the carotid bodies. $T\dot{V}_E$ is short when carotid body sensitivity is high (e.g., with hypoxia or metabolic acidemia),

whereas $T\dot{V}_E$ is long when carotid body sensitivity is low (e.g., hyperoxia, pharmacologic suppression with drugs such as dopamine or when they have been surgically resected.[55]

Although arterial P_{CO_2} appears to be a regulated variable during moderate exercise, it must be lowered by hyperventilation in order to constrain the fall of arterial pH (pHa) at levels of exercise which induce a metabolic acidemia. This compensatory decrease in Pa_{CO_2} washes CO_2 out of the body stores and provides an additional source of extra CO_2 at high work rates:

$$pHa = pK' + \log \frac{[HCO_3^-]a}{\alpha \cdot Pa_{CO_2}} \qquad (8)$$

where α is the CO_2 solubility coefficient which relates Pa_{CO_2} (in mmHg) to CO_2 content (in mM/L). The interrelationship among the ventilatory-related variables, in this regard, is apparent in an alternative way of considering this equation:

$$pHa = pK' + \log \left[\left(\frac{[HCO_3^-]a}{25.8} \right) \cdot \left(\frac{\dot{V}_E}{\dot{V}_{CO_2}} \right) \cdot \left(1 - \frac{V_{DS}}{V_T} \right) \right] \qquad (9)$$

$$\downarrow \qquad\qquad \downarrow \qquad\qquad \downarrow$$
$$\text{set point} \qquad \text{control} \qquad \text{efficiency}$$

where the bracketed terms may be considered to represent the metabolic set point, the control component, and the ventilatory efficiency terms, respectively.

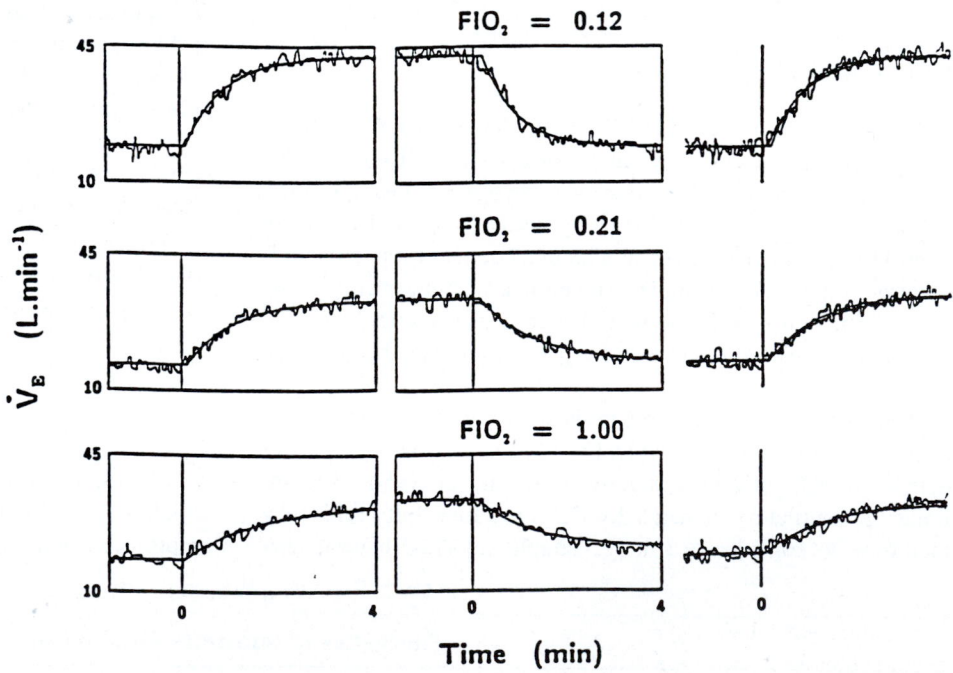

FIGURE 17-4   Influence of inhaled O_2 fraction ($F_{I_{O_2}} = 0.12$, 0.21, and 1.00) on the time course of the phase 2 $\dot{V}_E$ response to moderate constant-load cycling (90 watts) from unloaded pedalling, for a single subject. *Left panel:* On-transient responses, with the best-fit monoexponential superimposed. *Center panel:* Off-transient responses, with the best-fit monoexponential superimposed. *Right panel:* Off-transient responses (reversed) superimposed on the corresponding on-transient responses; note that these superimposed responses are effectively indistinguishable. (*Reprinted from Whipp and Ward,[55] by courtesy of Marcel Dekker, Inc.*)

Physiological Dead Space

The total requirement for dead space ventilation must, of course, consider both the anatomical and the alveolar dead space volumes. In healthy subjects at rest, the alveolar dead space is small and reflects, in large part, the relative underperfusion of apical alveoli. However, during exercise, the increased pulmonary artery pressure leads to a more even perfusion throughout the lung, thus reducing the alveolar dead space. Furthermore, as the end-inspiratory expansion of the conducting airways during exercise is small compared to the total volume increase, the physiological dead space fraction of the breath (V_{DS}/V_T) falls, despite absolute value of the dead space increasing.

VENTILATORY CONTROL

Although the postulated mechanisms of ventilatory control during exercise continue to foment considerable debate, neurogenic, chemoreflex and circulatory-coupled processes are considered to contribute to the control. The challenge is to establish a justifiable control model which integrates these processes and which accounts for both the dynamic and steady-state ventilatory responses. Such a model is not yet available.

Central Neural Control

As the ventilatory and cardiovascular responses to dynamic muscular exercise are initiated with little or no discernible delay, they are considered to result from *neurogenic* mechanisms, of central and peripheral origin.

CENTRAL COMMAND

The cortical somatomotor command that triggers locomotion also may influence brain-stem respiratory (and cardiovascular) control "centers." This has been termed the *central command.* The consequent ventilatory responses are proportional to the magnitude of the central command. Proponents of a central command argue that feedback control need only be modest via humoral mediation (or related to muscle contraction) to provide a ventilatory response which is appropriate for the metabolic demands of the exercise.

The descending motor influences on the medullary ventilatory integrating regions[14] include:

- Direct "irradiation" of the cortical somatomotor drive
- Subcortical projections from regions such as the paraventricular locomotor region of the hypothalamus and the fields of Forel

Evidence which supports central neurogenesis has been derived from animal studies in which discrete focal central nervous system (CNS) stimulation is utilized to activate descending central command pathways to ventilatory control regions and from experiments in humans which attempt to dissociate the magnitude of central command from its subsequent motor outcome.

Fink and coworkers[15] have recently provided evidence of motor cortical involvement in the exercise hyperpnea in humans. Using positron emission tomography to estimate regional cerebral blood flow (indicative of regional neuronal activation), they demonstrated significant increases in the superomedial primary motor cortical activity (i.e., spatially consistent with the motor cortical leg region) during leg exercise but not during recovery. In contrast, although the activity of the superolateral primary cortical areas also increased during exercise, the activity remained during recovery. As these superolateral regions have been associated with volitional activation of the respiratory muscles, the researchers concluded that this provided evidence for a feed-forward component of the exercise hyperpnea in humans, of motor cortical origin.

There is, however, evidence from experiments on animals which suggests that the cerebral cortex is not the sole origin of this control component. Spontaneous locomotion can be elicited in decorticate animals that is associated with prompt respiratory and cardiovascular responses.[14]

Focal stimulation (either electrical or chemical) of the paraventricular locomotor region of the posterior hypothalamus or the H_2 field of Forel leads to locomotor activity accompanied by rapid hyperpnea, tachycardia, and arterial hypertension.[14,49] Furthermore, efferent neural connections have been demonstrated from these hypothalamic sites to medullary sites of cardiovascular and respiratory control, such as the nucleus of the solitary tract (NTS), the nucleus ambiguus (NA), and the dorsal vagal nucleus (DVN).[45]

These evoked responses are essentially unaffected by muscle paralysis[14] and hence appear not to depend upon actual muscular contraction and increased metabolic rate. Although neural projections from the NTS to hypothalamic "locomotor" regions have been demonstrated (i.e., consistent with central command modulation by respiratory-related neuronal feedback),[30] to what *extent* the hypothalamus is involved in the normal ventilatory responses to exercise is unclear. For example, the normal exercise response profile has been reported to be abolished by hypothalamic lesioning,[19] as was also the case for the "fictive" locomotory model reported by Eldridge and colleagues.[14] However, in other studies,[35] removal of hypothalamic influences had no clear effect. Furthermore, Fink and coworkers[15] could find no evidence of increased neuronal activity in these hypothalamic motor regions during exercise in conscious humans using positron emission tomography, despite evidence of increased cortical respiratory motor activity.

These hypothalamically induced ventilatory responses are also typically accompanied by a rapid and usually marked hypocapnia.[14] This is not characteristic of the normal response to moderate exercise in humans—although it does appear to be the case for many,[16] but not all, experimental animals.[20]

Procedures designed to augment or diminish the central command for a task have also been used to characterize its role in the exercise hyperpnea. For example, selective stimulation of muscle spindles by means of the high-frequency vibration applied to the contracting muscle in humans has been shown to reduce the central command required to maintain a given force of muscle contraction. In this case, the reflex facilitation of motor neurons to the exercised muscle takes over a component of force generation from central command sources. The $\dot{V}_E$ response was less than under control conditions. Furthermore, when an antagonist muscle was stimulated in this way, the respiratory response was exaggerated. This was thought to be a consequence of the greater effort now being required to sustain the force.

Other evidence seems inconsistent with the view that central command subserves the dominant component controlling the respiratory responses during exercise. At the onset of exercise, there is an initial short period in which pulmonary gas exchange is effectively isolated from the demands of increased muscle metabolic rate (phase 1). The subsequent phase of pulmonary gas exchange in which mixed venous composition is changing may be termed phase 2, with the new steady state being phase 3. The magnitude of the initial (or phase 1)[2] ventilatory response to exercise is not a simple function either of the number of motor units recruited to generate the muscle force or of the magnitude of the central command for their recruitment. The magnitude of the $\phi 1$ $\dot{V}E$ responses is relatively constant over a wide range of imposed work loads.

Furthermore, when the work-rate increment is imposed from a background of light exercise (Fig. 16-2), the initial hyperpneic response develops more slowly and is of a smaller magnitude.[55] The initial hyperpnea is also slow when subjects initiate rest-to-work transitions in the supine position. We are not told by supporters of the central command hypothesis how body position *per se* would so markedly reduce this component of control. And so, while neurogenesis as the mechanism mediating the $\phi 1$ ventilatory response seems beyond serious challenge, the nature and functional organization of the signals themselves remain to be elucidated.

The results of sinusoidal exercise are also instructive in this regard. When the work rate is "forced" sinusoidally over a range of increasing input frequencies, the $\dot{V}E$ response amplitude decreases as a close linear function of the decrease in $\dot{V}_{CO_2}$ amplitude (Fig. 17-5). The relationship extrapolates at, or close to, the origin at high frequencies.[8] The control system therefore cannot "keep up" with the amplitude demands of the task at high forcing frequencies: a rapid neurogenic mechanism should! Consequently, the central command, which continues to drive the force-generating muscle units over the same amplitude range, either subserves a trivially small role in the exercise hyperpnea under the non-steady-state condition, or these mechanisms themselves exhibit slow neural dynamics.

A servo-assisted positive-pressure ventilator has been used as a means of dissociating a subject's intrinsic ventilatory drive from the motor task. That is, the applied pressure is synchronized with the respiratory cycle to "take over" a proportion of the normal inspiratory flow.[29,38] Were the $\dot{V}E$ dictated wholly by the the central command, then the subject's intrinsic ventilatory drive would be expected to remain unchanged despite the external assistance to ventilation imposed by the ventilator. Consequently, overall ventilation would be expected to increase—with a

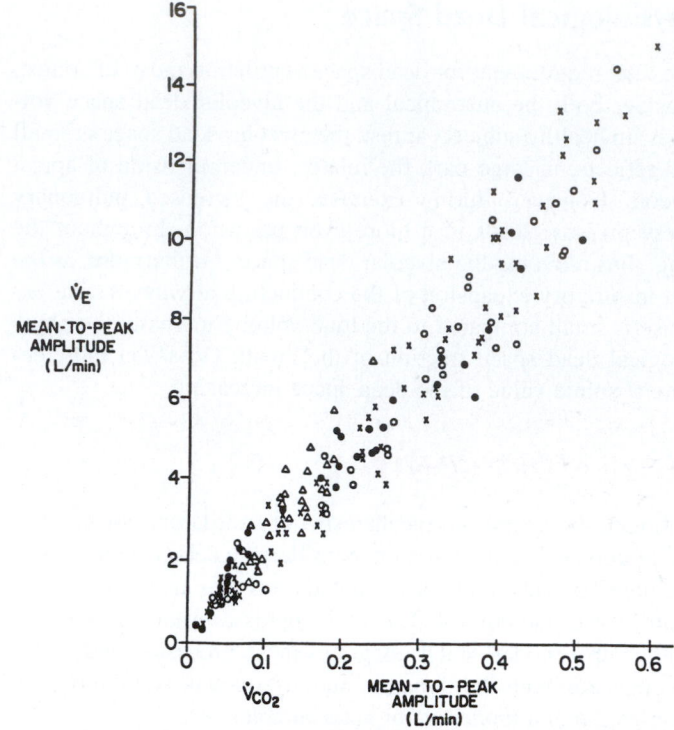

FIGURE 17-5   Relationship between the amplitude of $\dot{V}E$ and $\dot{V}_{CO_2}$ in response to exercise of sinusoidally varying work rate. Note that the reduction in $\dot{V}_{CO_2}$ amplitude is matched by a proportional reduction in $\dot{V}E$ amplitude as the forcing frequency of the work-rate sinusoid is increased. The relationship extrapolates to the origin. (*Reprinted from Casaburi et al,*[8] *with permission.*)

sustained hypocapnia resulting. This is *not* the case, however (Fig. 17-6). Rather, a proportional compensatory reduction in the intrinsic ventilatory drive results.

Finally, were central command a major and obligatory component of the exercise hyperpnea, then one would expect an attenuated response when exercise is performed in the absence of

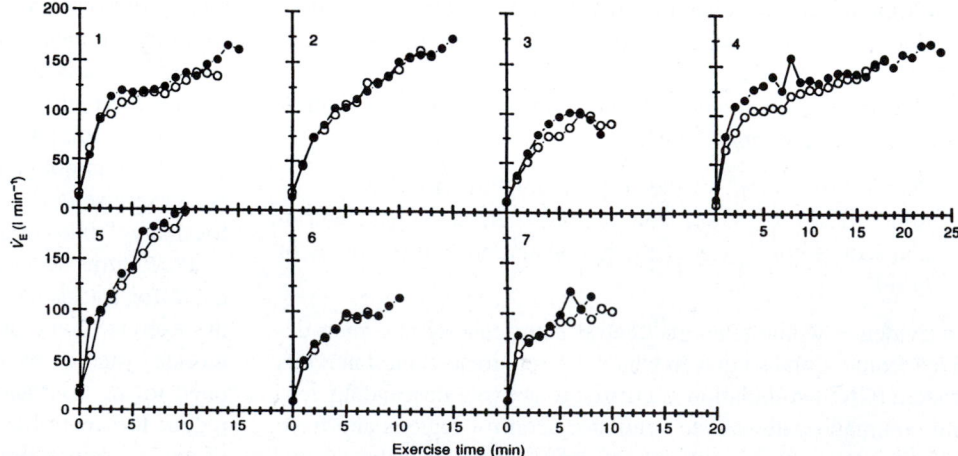

FIGURE 17-6   Profile of ventilatory response to high-intensity exercise in normal subjects under control conditions (○) and when the respiratory muscular demands for pressure generation were reduced by approximately one-third by means of a proportional ventilatory assist (●). (*Reprinted from Krishnan et al,*[29] *with permission.*)

central command. However, in subjects with clinically complete spinal cord transection, in whom exercise has been induced by direct electrical stimulation of the quadriceps muscles,[1,5,55] both the magnitude and time course of the ventilatory response have been shown to be essentially normal with respect to $\dot{V}_{CO_2}$—albeit over a restricted range of metabolic response. These observations argue against a major obligatory involvement of central command in ventilatory control during moderate exercise. Rather, they reinforce the notion of redundancy of ventilatory control system drives during exercise.

SHORT-TERM POTENTIATION

Eldridge and his associates have demonstrated that exercise activates a slowly developing neurogenic drive to ventilation in the cat—*short-term potentiation* or *reverberation*.[13,14] The hyperpneic response to the abrupt cessation of afferent activity from sources such as limb muscle afferents, the carotid bodies, and the ventral medullary surface results in a slowly decaying exponential decrement of ventilation.

A similarly slow decrement of $\dot{V}_E$ can also be demonstrated in humans following the abrupt cessation of volitional isocapnic "hyperventilation."[46] However, the onset of the $\dot{V}_E$ response in the cat is much more rapid when the stimulus is imposed, i.e., the mechanism exhibits dynamic *asymmetry*. The reverberatory component itself, however, is symmetrical, as evidenced by Eldridge and Gill-Kumar's cleverly designed "alternate-breath" stimulation study.[14] That is, the intrinsic symmetry of the reverberatory component appears to be masked by a direct component at the on-transient that renders the overall response asymmetrical. The exercise hyperpnea in humans, however, exhibits symmetry of the mono-exponential $\phi 2$ $\dot{V}_E$ responses at the onset and cessation of moderate exercise.[55] This symmetry of the on- and off-transient kinetics is maintained even when the response time constants are varied by up to fourfold (Fig. 16-4) by altered levels of inspired O_2 and peripheral chemoreceptor gain. Studies addressing this issue have not, to date, been performed in the cat.

LONG-TERM POTENTIATION

Martin and Mitchell[31] have proposed that a component of the exercise hyperpnea may be the result of long-term modulation or potentiation resulting from repeated exposure to activity, akin to associative motor learning. They demonstrated that goats consistently overbreathed during a standard treadmill task after they had been trained to exercise repeatedly for 2 days at that level, with an additional stimulus to breathing in the form of added dead space (0.8 L). This resulted in appreciable hypercapnia ($\Delta Pa_{CO_2} \simeq 10$ mmHg) during the exercise, in contrast to the 0.5-mmHg average decrease in Pa_{CO_2} during the initial pretraining trial and the $\simeq 3$-mmHg decrease during the posttraining trial without the added dead space. This augmented hyperpnea during exercise as a result of the hyperpneic "history" resolved over a period of 6 h or so. As the training had no effect on the ventilatory response to inhaled CO_2, they concluded that the neural mechanisms controlling the exercise hyperpnea evidences adaptability, plasticity, or "learning." This would be consistent with the postulate of Somjen[44] that functionally error-free physiological control systems may operate through central nervous system control that "anticipates present and future needs on the basis of past experience."

Muscle Reflex Control

There is a wide range of receptors and free nerve endings in skeletal muscles, the afferent projections of which have been proposed to contribute to the control of the exercise hyperpnea. For example, $\dot{V}_E$, heart rate, and arterial blood pressure all increase[48] when the muscle contraction is induced in experimental animals by stimulation of (1) ventral spinal roots, (2) motor nerves, or (3) the muscles themselves. These responses are abolished by section of the dorsal spinal roots, suggesting that they originate in the exercising muscles.

More specifically, electrical stimulation of small-diameter group III and IV afferents (but not of the larger group I and II afferents) leads to an increase in $\dot{V}_E$, heart rate, and arterial blood pressure (see references 14 and 33 for example) which can be abolished by differential blockade of these small-diameter fibers. Other stimuli such as local mechanical "distortion" and increased intramuscular pressure[26,33] have also been demonstrated to activate a subpopulation of the small-diameter afferents. A second subpopulation of small-diameter afferents are responsive to humoral mediators such as intramuscular levels of H^+, K^+, bradykinin, and possibly arachidonic acid derivatives.[26,33,41,42]

However, a simple interpretation of the role of skeletal muscle metabo- or chemoreception in the exercise hyperpnea is confounded by the consistent demonstration that when pneumatic thigh cuffs are inflated to suprasystolic pressures at the end of exercise, the $\dot{V}_E$ response decreases more rapidly than normal and not more slowly, despite the local accumulation of exercise-induced metabolites[17] and presumably the sustained activation of chemosensitive muscle afferents *after* the cessation of the work (Fig. 17-7). Consequently, although there appears to be little doubt that respiratory drives originate within contracting muscles, whether these represent an obligatory or necessary control component during normal volitional exercise is by no means certain.

Removing the influence of somatic limb afferents does not seem to impair the ventilatory response to dynamic exercise to any appreciable extent in humans—at least over the usual range of metabolic rates achieved. The respiratory response to dynamic exercise has been shown to be essentially normal, both in normal subjects with muscle sensory blockade induced by epidural anesthesia and in patients with sensory neuropathies (i.e., despite the absence of functioning afferent projections from the exercising limbs).

And finally, the results of the "assisted" inspiration experiments[29,38] described above are relevant in this regard. That is, the subjects' ventilation was not significantly affected by the "assist" as a result of the intrinsic ventilatory drive being proportionally reduced, i.e., despite neither central command nor mechanical feedback from the exercising muscles presumably being altered.

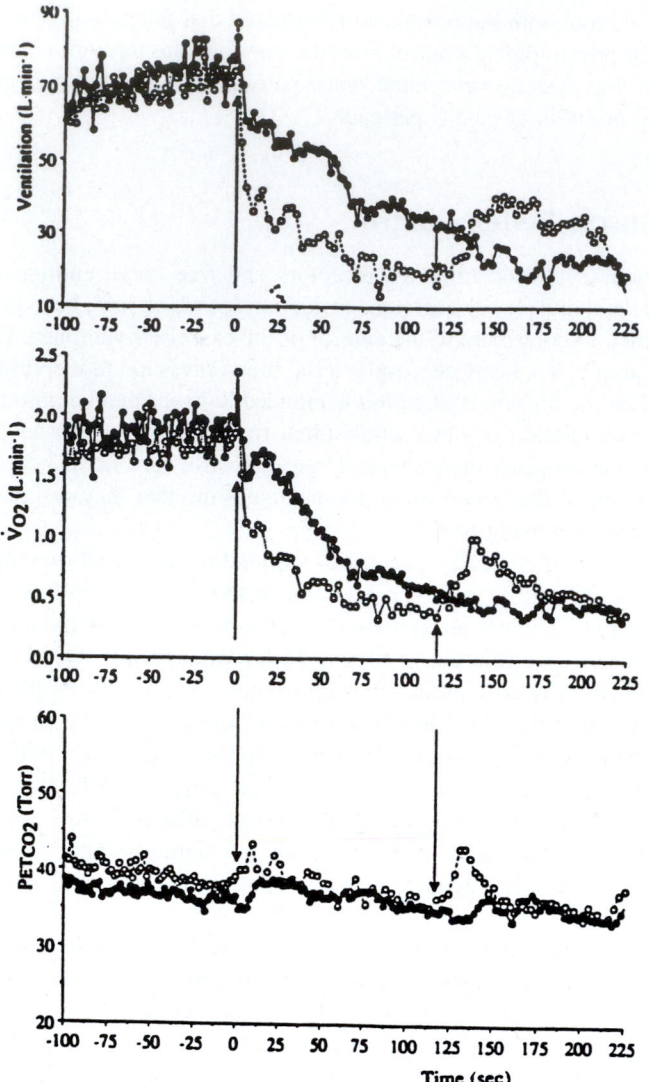

FIGURE 17-7 Dynamics of the ventilatory response during recovery from heavy-cycle ergometer exercise in normal human individuals under control conditions (●) and when thigh cuffs were inflated to suprasystolic pressures at the cessation of exercise (○). Note ventilation decreases appreciably more rapidly with the thigh cuffs inflated. The subsequent release of the cuff pressure is marked by the right arrow. *(Reprinted from Haouzi et al,[17] with permission.)*

Central Chemoreflex Control

Studying central chemoreflex function in humans is difficult owing to the inaccessibility of the receptors themselves. Hyperoxic hypercapnia is commonly used to assess the "sensitivity," and in some studies, the dynamics, of the central chemoreflex: The hyperoxia is necessary to suppress peripheral chemosensitivity. There is no consistent evidence, however, that central chemosensitivity is increased significantly with exercise. Patients with *congenital central hypoventilation syndromes* (CCHS)[37,43] have impaired central chemosensitivity, with little or no ventilatory response in inhaled CO_2. Important in this regard, their response to exercise is often remarkably normal.

The onset of the slower $\phi2$ component of the exercise hyperpnea has a time delay consistent with the limb-to-lung transit time,[55] suggestive of "downstream" chemoreceptor mediation.

Although the $\phi1$-$\phi2$ transition is prolonged with hyperoxic inspirates, any significant involvement of the central chemoreceptors in this response is unlikely, as CCHS patients demonstrate essentially normal $\phi2$ $\dot{V}E$ kinetics despite the absence of central CO_2 chemosensitivity.[43]

The central chemoreceptors also appear not to play an essential role in $\dot{V}E$ control for $\phi3$ of moderate exercise. First, there is the issue of a discernible chemical stimulus: The pH of cerebrospinal fluid (csf) remains relatively stable during the steady state of moderate exercise.[4] And, despite significant increases in arterial [K^+], csf [K^+] does not increase.[11] The demonstration that the normal ventilatory responses to exercise in CCHS patients regulate P_{CO_2} close to their resting levels (although these are often elevated in these patients)[37,43] appears decisive in this regard.

Above the lactate threshold (θL), the ventilatory compensation for the lactic acidosis results in a respiratory alkalosis in the cerebrospinal fluid.[4] Under these conditions, the central chemoreceptors are likely to provide *constraint* on the hyperpnea. The alkalotic csf would not only reduce ongoing central chemoreceptor activity but also stimulate efferent projections to the carotid chemoreceptors which have been demonstrated to inhibit afferent chemosensory discharge from the carotid bodies.

During prolonged exercise, designed to produce a high constant level of arterial blood lactate, there was a slow, but systematic, restoration of arterial pH back toward normal after the transient fall even with hyperoxic suppression of peripheral chemosensitivity.[39] This slow compensatory response might reflect a slow "leak" of H^+ ions into the csf from the blood or, possibly, slow central chemoreflex response to the transiently elevated Pa_{CO_2} that was a consistent finding of the study.

Arterial Chemoreflex Control

It seems unlikely that the carotid bodies mediate the $\phi1$ $\dot{V}E$ response to exercise. This response is typically unaffected when hypoxic or hyperoxic gas mixtures are breathed[10,12] or in subjects whose carotid bodies have been surgically resected (CBR)[52]: procedures which respectively increase, decrease, and, of course, abolish carotid chemosensitivity.

In contrast, the carotid bodies do appear to play a prominent role in $\phi2$ ventilatory control.[55] For example, increasing carotid body sensitivity by hypoxia or ammonium chloride ingestion results in a faster time course of response for $\dot{V}E$, both in absolute terms and relative to CO_2 output. Procedures which reduce or abolish carotid chemosensitivity such as hyperoxia, sodium bicarbonate ingestion, intravenous infusion of dopamine, and, perhaps most specifically, CBR all lead to an appreciable slowing of the $\phi2$ $\dot{V}E$ kinetics.

The carotid bodies therefore appear to modulate the dynamics of the $\dot{V}E$ response relative to those of $\dot{V}_{O_2}$ and $\dot{V}_{CO_2}$. Consequently they play an important role in the "tightness" with which Pa_{O_2}, Pa_{CO_2} and pHa are regulated throughout the nonsteady-state phase of muscular exercise.

There seems to be no dispute that the carotid bodies provide a component of the $\phi3$ $\dot{V}E$ control.[12,53–55] Some have termed this a "fine-tuning" component of the control system. The proportional contribution of the carotid bodies to the φ3 hyperpnea has been estimated using the *Dejours test*[12] in which high inspired O_2 fractions are used surreptitiously to abolish abruptly any carotid body contribution to the hyperpnea. These tests have demonstrated that the carotid bodies normally appear to account for approximately 20 percent of the steady-state hyperpnea[54]—although there is some concern that the Dejours test may underestimate the carotid body component of the exercise hyperpnea.[50,54] CBR subjects have no ventilatory decrease during the Dejours test.[54]

The proportional role of the various stimuli in the arterial blood during exercise, however, is unclear. Components of the oscillating CO_2-H^+ pattern, such as the amplitude and rate of change of the oscillation, have been proposed to provide a CO_2-linked drive to $\dot{V}E$ in φ3. The carotid bodies in animals have been shown to be capable of transducing such signals into respiratory stimulation.[9] However, whether such oscillating signals provide any significant humoral feedback for ventilatory control in exercising humans remains to be demonstrated.

The increased arterial K^+ that is released from contracting muscle cells during exercise has been demonstrated to stimulate $\dot{V}E$ through an action on the carotid bodies.[2,6] As K^+ does not cross the blood-brain barrier,[11] the increased arterial $[K^+]$ apparently does not influence sites of central chemosensitivity. Consequently, the increased arterial K^+ may account for or contribute a component of the 20 percent or so of the steady-state exercise hyperpnea that is mediated by the carotid bodies. However, other known carotid body stimuli, such as increases in the plasma levels of H^+, adenosine, osmolarity, catechol-amines, temperature, and rate of change of the P_{CO_2}-H^+ oscillations, also increase during exercise. These presumably also contribute to this ~20 percent of the exercise hyperpnea.

It has been argued that the carotid bodies normally appear to be largely responsible for mediating the respiratory compensation for the lactic acidosis above θL in humans,[52] responding to stimuli such as $[H^+]$, $[K^+]$, and catecholamines. Evidence against this view has been presented, however. Individuals deficient in the glycogenolytic enzyme myophosphorylase b (McArdle's syndrome) are constrained to exercise only at relatively low work rates as they are unable to catabolize glycogen anaerobically. These subjects have been reported to hyperventilate despite there being no metabolic acidemia at these low work rates. This suggests, to some investigators, that the compensatory hyperventilation seen in normal subjects above θL therefore does not require a lowered pHa for its mediation. Other mechanisms, however, such as apprehension, discomfort, increased intramuscular pressure, or pain, can induce acute hyperventilatory *alkalosis* under some circumstances[40,54]—and indeed, muscle pain is a cardinal symptom of McArdle's syndrome. Another important distinction is that respiratory alkalemia is *not* normally seen in humans performing high-intensity isotonic exercise.

In response to constant-load exercise above θL, the compensatory hyperventilation has been reported to be nonexistent in CBR subjects—not only did pHa fall more for a given decrease in $[HCO_3^-]a$ in these subjects, but P_{aCO_2} was actually higher than the corresponding control values.[52] It has been proposed, however, that this marked reduction in the compensatory hyperventilation for the metabolic acidemia in these subjects may be

a consequence of their asthmatic history rather than of the absence of carotid bodies.[16]

In studies designed to induce a standard, and more prolonged, degree of metabolic acidemia during constant-load exercise (Δ standard $[HCO_3^-]$ of 5 meq/l) in normal subjects, there was a significant O_2-labile (and presumably a carotid-body-mediated) component of the hyperpnea.[39] This constrained the magnitude of the transient decrease in pHa (Fig. 17-8). When carotid-body chemosensitivity was suppressed by inhalation of 80 percent O_2, a *slower* compensatory component was still evident. The carotid bodies in humans may therefore be considered to play a significant and even dominant role in constraining variations of pHa in response to the acute metabolic acidemia of exercise in humans. However, there are secondary—presumably central chemosensory—mechanisms which subserve a slower compensatory role. An alternative interpretation of these findings, consistent with the demonstration that ventilation evidences an upward concavity at high work rates during hyperoxic incremental

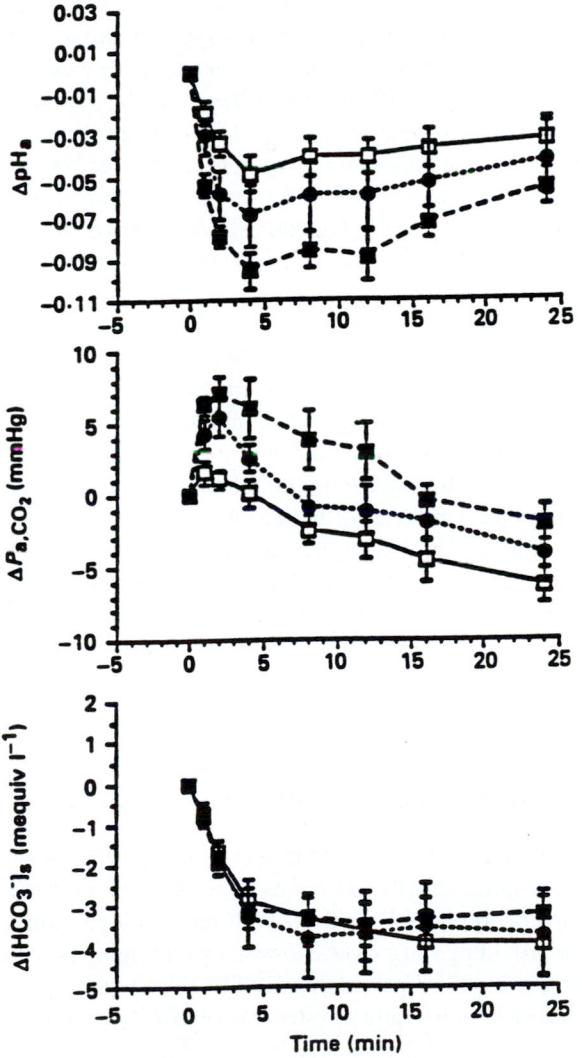

FIGURE 17-8 Responses of arterial pH, P_{CO_2} and standard $[HCO_3^-]$ to a suprathreshold square-wave exercise for three inspired oxygen fractions (□ = 12% O_2; ● = 21% O_2; ■ = 80% O_2), expressed as changes (Δ) from unloaded cycling. Values are means ± SEM (n = 7). (*Reprinted from Rausch et al,*[39] *with permission.*)

exercise, is that hyperoxia does not abolish peripheral chemosensitivity. However, the absence of an early ventilatory response to altered inspired CO_2 fraction in hyperoxia, either at rest or during exercise,[50] suggests that this is not the case.

Cardioventilatory Reflex Control

Some investigators have proposed that a component of ventilatory control during exercise may be of cardiac or circulatory origin.[18] Vascular distension of the heart and adjacent vasculature, for example, can elicit tachycardia and hyperpnea.[24,28] Might the increased venous return of exercise therefore contribute to the ventilatory control during exercise in humans?

The relative stability of the end-tidal gas tensions and R, as a result of the close proportionality of the $\phi 1$ cardiovascular and ventilatory responses,[55] has suggested to some investigators that there may be a component of *cardiodynamic* ventilatory control in this early phase of exercise. However, recent evidence from several sources has questioned the role of such cardiodynamic mechanisms in exercise hyperpnea. When the resting heart rate (and therefore cardiac output) was abruptly increased in patients with permanent, demand-type pacemakers, there was no immediate $\dot{V}E$ response—although both $\dot{V}_{CO_2}$ and $\dot{V}_{O_2}$ started to increase.[23] It is also clear that cardiac afferents do not subserve an obligatory role in the exercise hyperpnea, although they can, under some circumstances, stimulate ventilation. Humans who have undergone cardiac transplantation[3,47] and calves with an implanted pneumatically driven artificial heart (Jarvik type),[20] have no reduction in either the magnitude or the rapidity of onset of the exercise hyperpnea.

Recent studies have suggested that ventilation may respond to a signal mediated by altered vascular conductance and/or tissue pressure in the exercising muscles themselves.[17,18] This proposal therefore changes the focus of a cardiorespiratory linkage during exercise from a central circulatory site of control to one more intimately related to the peripheral microvasculature and its innervation.[18,32] Although a control link between the peripheral gas exchange surface and breathing is intuitively attractive, the extent to which such a mechanism actually contributes to the exercise hyperpnea in humans, if at all, remains to be determined.

VENTILATORY COSTS

Mechanical Costs to Respiratory Muscles

The intrapleural pressure changes resulting from respiratory muscle contraction (Pmus) serves to expand the lung and generate tracheobronchial air flow, with an additional small component providing lung-tissue flow and overcoming inertia.

The pressure, or power, required to overcome the total impedance of the respiratory system is therefore given by:

$$Pmus = E \cdot V + R \cdot \dot{V} + I \cdot \ddot{V} \qquad (10)$$

where E, R, and I are the respiratory system elastance, resistance, and inertance respectively.

The relationship between ventilation and respiratory muscle power during exercise is not linear.[21,27] At high work rates a given increment in $\dot{V}E$ requires a larger increase in Pmus than at low work rates. People who are moderately fit, however, utilize only some 30 to 40 percent of their maximum available respiratory power at maximal work rates and have a considerable "breathing reserve," i.e., the difference between the maximum exercise $\dot{V}E$ and that achieved volitionally during a maximal voluntary ventilation (MVV) maneuver. Very fit individuals, however, typically have a low breathing reserve at maximum exercise as a result of the higher maximum exercise $\dot{V}E$. The MVV is essentially unaffected by training status and fitness.

The mechanical costs of ventilation are appreciably greater at high work rates[27] because of (1) increased contributions from turbulence (and even inertia) when air flow is high; (2) increased elastic work of breathing, owing both to decreased lung compliance even in the tidal range, during exercise (an effect ascribed to increased pulmonary blood volume) and end-inspiratory lung volume approaching the poorly compliant upper region of the compliance curve at high tidal volumes, although the decrease in end-expiratory lung volume tends to ameliorate this effect; and (3) the recruitment of respiratory muscles with low mechanical efficiencies at high levels of ventilation.

Metabolic Costs to Respiratory Muscles

These increased mechanical costs of the exercise hyperpnea require both an increased respiratory muscle work rate and respiratory muscle O_2 consumption ($\dot{V}rm_{O_2}$). The relationship between $\dot{V}rm_{O_2}$ and $\dot{V}E$ during exercise is not linear; rather it is concave upward, i.e., greater increments in $\dot{V}rm_{O_2}$ are required as work rate increases.[21] Estimation of $\dot{V}rm_{O_2}$, however, is technically difficult in humans, as it represents such a small fraction of the whole-body $\dot{V}_{O_2}$ during exercise.

A further complication results from the fact that whole-body $\dot{V}_{O_2}$ can change not solely as a consequence of the increased respiratory muscle work rate (in tests that attempt to reproduce the exercise hyperpnea in a resting subject) but also as a result of the altered pH if Pa_{CO_2} is not maintained precisely. Acute respiratory alkalosis has been shown to increase whole-body $\dot{V}_{O_2}$ by ~10 percent per 10-mmHg reduction in Pa_{CO_2}.[25]

Although $\dot{V}rm_{O_2}$ is small at resting levels of $\dot{V}E$, it can be appreciable at high levels of exercise, especially in highly fit athletes. In moderately fit individuals a $\dot{V}rm_{O_2}$ of ~0.5 L/min, ~15 percent of the current total $\dot{V}_{O_2}$, has been reported[27] for a $\dot{V}E$ in excess of 120 L/min. This is presumably even greater in athletes, who are capable of attaining appeciably higher levels of $\dot{V}E$ at maximum exercise.

Might the O_2 demands of the respiratory muscles therefore actually outstrip the vascular O_2 supply mechanisms during exercise? That is, do the respiratory muscles exercise beyond their "lactate threshold"?

Although this relationship for spontaneous breathing during exercise may be expected to be qualitatively similar to that of volitional hyperpnea at rest, there may be significant quantitative differences. For example, the respiratory muscle recruitment pattern, the muscles' mechanical efficiencies, their operating length, and the metabolic cost of the $\dot{V}E$ which is attained are all likely to be different.

SYSTEM CONSTRAINTS AND LIMITATIONS

The mechanical and metabolic costs of ventilation during muscular exercise are themselves sources of *constraint* and potential *limitation* of exercise tolerance. Constraint, in this context, reflects a condition in which the ventilatory response is less than that of its regulatory requirement as a result of the influence of an opposing mechanism, e.g., an added resistive load. Ventilation in this case is not actually limited, as higher work rates lead to greater hyperpnea.

Limitation occurs when the variable cannot increase, despite further increases in ventilatory drive. Maximum expiratory airflow during exercise (at a particular lung volume) becomes limited during exercise in subjects with reduced lung recoil and/or increased airways resistance, despite further increases in ventilatory drive; similarly, the achievable tidal volume is limited during exercise in patients with diffuse interstitial fibrosis as a result of the increased elastance (Fig. 17-9).

Ventilatory Constraints

The tidal volume (V_T) limit theoretically extends from zero to vital capacity, whereas the breathing frequency extends from zero to ~5 to 7 Hz. Normally, however, the ventilatory system "only" operates at a V_T of only ~50 to 60 percent of the vital capacity and a frequency of ≤ 1 Hz even during maximum exercise. The maximum airflow that can be attained, at a given lung volume, during exercise in normal individuals, is that generated by a maximal forced volitional effort, i.e., the maximum expiratory flow volume (MEFV) relationship. During maximum exercise the spontaneously generated expiratory flow profiles fall well below the maxima of the MEFV curve[27] in people of poor or moderate fitness. However, in highly fit athletes, who are capable of generating high instantaneous airflows at the high levels of $\dot{V}_E$, these maxima may be encroached upon.

The postulate that respiratory work would be minimized, at a particular level of $\dot{V}_E$, with a particular breathing frequency, is largely based upon the recognition that when $\dot{V}_E$ is achieved with a high frequency and a low V_T, the flow-resistive component of the respiratory work increases; when this is accomplished with a large V_T and a low breathing frequency, there would be an increased contribution from the elastic component of the respiratory work, as the lung volume encroaches on the flatter portion of the lung compliance curve. Exercising individuals normally seem to "choose" a breathing pattern at, or near, the optimum for minimum respiratory muscle work rate—unless, of course, this is prevented by the breathing demands of the event (e.g., swimming).

There is likely to be turbulent constraint of airflow during exercise even in moderately fit subjects. When the inspired nitrogen is replaced by the lower-density gas helium (care being taken to mask the sudden sensation of cold in the airways), no effect on $\dot{V}_E$ is discernible at low levels of ventilation. But at higher levels of work rate and hence of ventilation, replacing the nitrogen with helium induces a prompt and sustained hyperventilation.[34,51] This is consistent with the removal of a constraint on $\dot{V}_E$ imposed by the turbulent component of airflow.

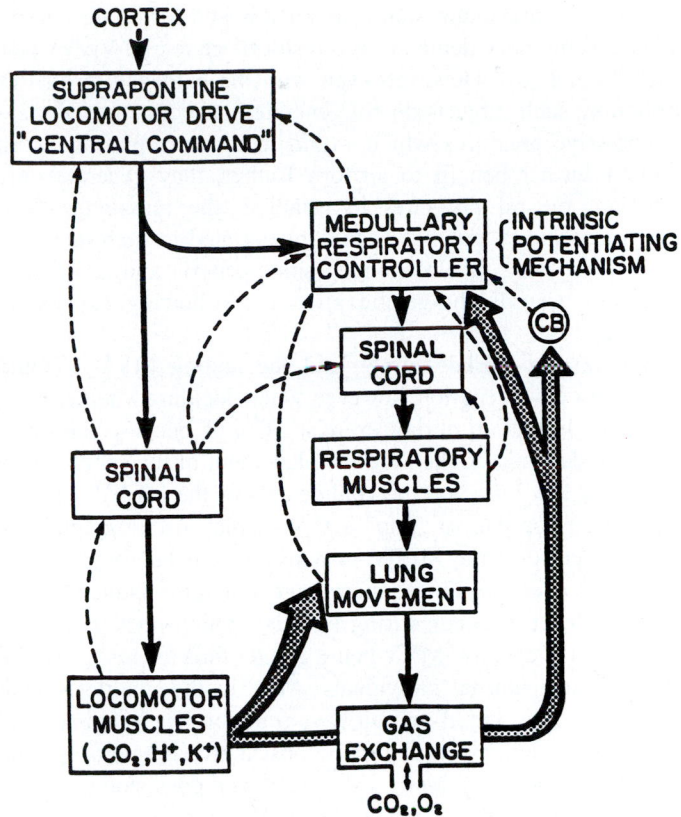

FIGURE 17-9 Schematic representation of neural mechanisms involved in the hyperpnea of exercise. *(Reprinted from Eldridge and Waldrop,[14] by courtesy of Marcel Dekker, Inc.)*

However, the extent to which such turbulent constraint impairs the respiratory compensation for the metabolic acidemia in athletes is not clear at present.

Ventilatory Limitations

MECHANICAL LIMITATIONS

In moderately fit young individuals, ventilation appears not to be mechanically limited during maximal exercise: (1) They can volitionally increase $\dot{V}_E$ to appreciably greater levels than those attained spontaneously at maximum exercise; (2) the ratio of maximum exercise $\dot{V}_E$ to MVV ($\dot{V}_E$/MVV) is relatively low (i.e., ~60 to 70 percent); (3) the spontaneously generated expiratory F-V curve does not encroach on the boundaries of the MEFV curve even at maximum exercise, and (4) there is also no evidence of significant respiratory muscle fatigue.

There is evidence of both ventilatory-mechanical limitation and inspiratory muscle fatigue, however, in people who are more fit. For example, the spontaneous expiratory F-V curve commonly impacts on the envelope of the MEFV curve during maximal exercise in individuals with a $\mu\dot{V}_{O_2}$ of ~5 to 6 L/min and a maximum exercise $\dot{V}_E$ of ~110 to 160 L/min (i.e., some 80 percent of MVV). In older individuals who have developed or maintained high levels of fitness, such airflow limitation has been demonstrated at lower levels of $\dot{V}_E$ during exercise.[21] This is predominantly caused by the aging-related reduction in lung recoil reducing the maximum attainable airflow and MVV, despite increased ventilatory demands as a result of increased V_D/V_T [see Eqs. (7) and (8)]. However, even with the evidence of airflow limitation, such subjects do not generate nonproductive, airway-compressive pressures which would increase respiratory work without further benefit to airflow. Rather, they generate only sufficient pleural pressures to establish the maximum flow. Diaphragmatic fatigue has been demonstrated in such individuals both in terms of electromyographic criteria and as reduced maximum transdiaphragmatic pressures following exhausting exercise.

The resting MEFV curve—and the resting MVV—should only be used with caution, however, when deciding whether there is airflow limitation during exercise. This is because the interpretation depends on the accurate placement of the spontaneous expiratory F-V curve on the volume axis of the MEFV curve. It is more appropriate to "trap" a F-V display oscillographically and then perform the MEFV maneuver immediately afterward during the exercise. Furthermore, catecholamine-induced bronchodilatation can occur during exercise which presumably accounts for the exercise MVV being greater than the resting MVV even in some normal individuals. Also, in older athletes with diminished lung recoil and airways function, for example, and especially in patients with chronic obstructive lung disease, the maximum expiratory *effort* F-V maneuver does not yield the optimum maximum expiratory *flow* F-V curve.

And finally, there have been reports of reduction of vital capacity, respiratory muscle strength, and endurance following exercise, but this reduction has been consistently observed only following prolonged exercise in athletes.[7]

CONCLUSIONS

Our understanding of the control of the exercise hyperpnea since Dejours's seminal review in 1964[12] has advanced both in detail and in perspective. The details encompass both humoral sources of ventilatory stimulation, such as potassium and adenosine, and neural pathways of information transmission, such as the type III and type IV afferents from skeletal muscle. The change of perspective has resulted from the studies which have challenged the notion that the terms *rapid* and *slow* are necessarily synonymous with neural and humoral control mechanisms respectively. It is difficult, however, to incorporate many of the recently proposed mechanisms into a justifiable control scheme, the most satisfying at present being that of Eldridge and Waldrop.[14] This is because the proponents often neglect to suggest what proportion of the control might be attributable to the specific mechanisms. But, perhaps more challenging is the fact that in many cases the absence of what is normally a demonstrably stimulatory mechanism has little or no effect on the overall control. The adage that "anyone not confused by this doesn't understand the problem" is one that is currently apposite to the control of the exercise hyperpnea. Much of the confusion could be clarified if the "what" of the proposed stimulus and the "so what" of its integrative role were viewed as cooperative control concerns.

REFERENCES

1. Adams L, Frankel H, Garlick J, et al: The role of spinal cord transmission in the ventilatory response to exercise in man. *J Physiol* (Lond) 355:85–97, 1984.
2. Band DM, Linton RAF, Kent R, Kurer FL: The effect of peripheral chemodenervation on the ventilatory response to potassium. *Respir Physiol* 60:217–225, 1985.
3. Banner N, Guz A, Heaton R, et al: Ventilatory and circulatory responses at the onset of exercise in man following heart or heart-lung transplantation. *J Physiol* (Lond) 399:437–449, 1988.
4. Bisgard GE, Forster HV, Byrnes B, et al: Cerebrospinal fluid acid-base balance during muscular exercise. *J Appl Physiol* 45:94–101, 1978.
5. Brice AG, Forster HV, Pan LG, et al: Is the hyperpnea of muscular contractions critically dependent on spinal afferents? *J Appl Physiol* 64:226–233, 1988.
6. Burger RE, Estavillo JA, Kumar P, et al: Effects of potassium, oxygen and carbon dioxide on the steady-state discharge of cat carotid body chemoreceptors. *J Physiol* (Lond) 401:519–531, 1988.
7. Bye PTP, Farkas GA, Roussos C: Respiratory factors limiting exercise. *Ann Rev Physiol* 45:439–451, 1983.
8. Casaburi R, Whipp BJ, Wasserman K, Stremel RW: Ventilatory control characteristics of the exercise hyperpnea as discerned from dynamic forcing techniques. *Chest* 73S:280S–283S, 1978.
9. Cross BA, Davey A, Guz A, et al: The pH oscillations in arterial blood during exercise; a potential signal for the ventilatory response in the dog. *J Physiol* (Lond) 329:57–73, 1982.
10. Cunningham DJC: Integrative aspects of the regulation of breathing: a personal view, in Guyton AC, Widdicombe JG (eds), *MTP International Review of Science,* series 1, vol 2, *Physiology.* Baltimore, University Park Press, 1974, pp 303–369.
11. Davson H: *Physiology of the Cerebrospinal Fluid.* London, Churchill, 1970.
12. Dejours P: Control of respiration in muscular exercise, in Fenn WO, Rahn H (eds), *Handbook of Physiology,* vol 1, *Respiration.* Washington DC, American Physiology Society, 1964, pp 631–648.
13. Eldridge FL: Maintenance of respiration by central neural feedback mechanisms. *Fed Proc* 36:2400–2404, 1977.
14. Eldridge FL, Waldrop TG: Neural control of breathing, in Whipp BJ, Wasserman K (eds), *Pulmonary Physiology and Pathophysiology of Exercise.* New York, Dekker, 1991, pp 309–370.
15. Fink GR, Adams L, Watson JDG, et al: Hyperpnoea during and immediately after exercise in man: Evidence of motor cortical involvement. *J Physiol* (Lond) 489:663–675, 1995.
16. Forster HV, Pan LG: Exercise hyperpnea, in Crystal RG, West JB (eds), *The Lung: Scientific Foundations.* New York, Raven, 1991, pp 1553–1564.
17. Haouzi P, Huszczuk A, Porszasz J, et al: Femoral vascular occlusion and ventilation during recovery from heavy exercise. *Respir Physiol* 94:137–150, 1993.
18. Haouzi P, Marchal F, Huszczuk A: Muscle perfusion and control of breathing: Is there a neural link? in Semple SJG, Adams L, Whipp BJ (eds), *Modelling and Control of Ventilation.* New York, Plenum, 1995, pp 363–368.
19. Hobbs SF: Central command during exercise: Parallel activation of the cardiovascular and motor systems by descending command signals, in Smith OA, Galosy RA, Weiss SM (eds), *Circulation, Neurobiology and Behavior.* New York, Elsevier, 1982, pp 217–232.
20. Huszczuk A, Whipp BJ, Adams TD, et al: Ventilatory control during exercise in calves with artificial hearts. *J Appl Physiol* 68:2604–2611, 1990.

21. Johnson BD, Dempsey JA: Demand vs. capacity in the aging pulmonary system. *Ex Sports Sci Rev* 19:171–210, 1991.

22. Jones NL: Exercise testing in pulmonary evaluation: Rationale, methods, and the normal respiratory response to exercise. *New Engl J Med* 293:541–544, 1975.

23. Jones PW, French W, Weissman ML, Wasserman K: Ventilatory responses to cardiac output changes in patients with pacemakers. *J Appl Physiol* 51:1103–1107, 1981.

24. Jones PW, Huszczuk A, Wasserman K: Cardiac output as a controller of ventilation through changes in right ventricular load. *J Appl Physiol* 53:218–244, 1982.

25. Karetsky MS, Cain SM: Factors controlling O_2 uptake. *Chest* 61(suppl):48S–49S, 1972.

26. Kaufman MP, Rybicki KJ: Discharge properties of group III and IV muscle afferents: Their responses to mechanical and metabolic stimuli. *Circ Res* 61(suppl I):60–65, 1987.

27. Klas JV, Dempsey JA: Voluntary versus reflex regulation of maximal exercise flow: volume loops. *Am Rev Respir Dis* 139:150–156, 1989.

28. Kostreva DR, Zuperku EJ, Purtock RV, et al: Sympathetic afferent nerve activity of right heart origin. *Am J Physiol* 229:911–915, 1975.

29. Krishnan B, Zintel T, McParland C, Gallagher CG: Lack of importance of respiratory muscle load in ventilatory regulation during heavy exercise. *J Physiol* (Lond) 490:537–550, 1996.

30. Loewy AD: Central autonomic pathways, in Loewy AD, Spyer KM (eds), *Central Regulation of Autonomic Functions*. New York, Oxford University, 1990, pp 88–103.

31. Martin PA, Mitchell GS: Long-term modulation of the exercise ventilatory response in goats. *J Physiol* (Lond), 470:601–617, 1993.

32. Mense S, Stanke M: Responses in muscle afferent fibers of slow conduction velocity to contractions and ischaemia in the cat. *J Physiol* (Lond) 342:383–397, 1983.

33. Mitchell JH, Schmidt RF: Cardiovascular reflex control by afferent fibers from skeletal muscle receptors, in Shepherd JT, Abboud FM, Geiger SR (eds), *Handbook of Physiology*, sec 2, vol 3, *The Cardiovascular System: Peripheral Circulation and Organ Blood Flow*. Bethesda, MD, American Physiology Society, 1983, pp 623–658.

34. Nattie EE, Tenney SM: The ventilatory response to resistance unloading during muscular exercise. *Respir Physiol* 10:249–262, 1970.

35. Ordway GA, Waldrop TG, Iwamoto GA, Gentile BJ: Hypothalamic influences on cardiovascular response of beagles to dynamic exercise. *Am J Physiol* 257:H1247–H1253, 1989.

36. Paterson DJ: Potassium and ventilation in exercise. *J Appl Physiol* 72:811–820, 1992.

37. Paton JY, Swaminathan S, Sargent CW, et al: Ventilatory response to exercise in children with congenital central hypoventilation syndrome. *Am Rev Respir Dis* 147:1185–1191, 1993.

38. Poon CS, Ward SA, Whipp BJ: Influence of inspiratory assistance on ventilatory control during moderate exercise. *J Appl Physiol* 62:551–560, 1987.

39. Rausch SM, Whipp BJ, Wasserman K, Huszczuk A: Role of the carotid bodies in the respiratory compensation for the metabolic acidosis of exercise in humans. *J Physiol* (Lond) 444:567–578, 1991.

40. Riley M, Nicholls DP, Nugent A-M, et al: Respiratory gas exchange and metabolic responses during exercise in McArdle's disease. *J Appl Physiol* 75:745–754, 1993.

41. Rotto DM, Schultz HD, Longhurst JC, Kaufman MP: Sensitization of group III muscle afferents to static contraction by arachidonic acid. *J Appl Physiol* 68:861–867, 1990.

42. Rybicki KJ, Waldrop TG, Kaufman MP: Increasing gracilis muscle interstitial potassium concentrations stimulate group III and IV afferents. *J Appl Physiol* 58:936–941, 1985.

43. Shea SA, Andrews LP, Shannon DC, Banzett RB: Ventilatory responses to exercise in humans lacking ventilatory chemosensitivity. *J Physiol* (Lond) 469:623–640, 1993.

44. Somjen GG: The missing error signal—regulation beyond negative feedback. *News Physiol Sci* 7:184–185, 1992.

45. Spyer KM: Central nervous mechanisms contributing to cardiovascular control. *J Physiol* (Lond) 474:1–19, 1994.

46. Swanson GD, Bellville JW, Ward DS: Posthyperventilation isocapnic hyperpnea. *J Appl Physiol* 40:592–596, 1974.

47. Theodore J, Morris AJ, Burker CM, et al: Cardiopulmonary function at maximum tolerable constant work rate exercise following human heart-lung transplantation. *Chest* 92:433–439, 1987.

48. Tibes U: Reflex inputs to the cardiovascular and respiratory centers from dynamically working canine muscles. *Circ Res* 42:332–341, 1977.

49. Waldrop TG, Henderson MC, Iwamoto GA, Mitchell JH: Regional blood flow responses to stimulation of the subthalamic locomotor region. *Respir Physiol* 64:93–102, 1986.

50. Ward SA: Assessment of peripheral chemoreflex contributions to ventilation during exercise. *Med Sci Sports Ex* 26:303–310, 1994.

51. Ward SA, Whipp BJ, Poon CS: Density-dependent air flow and ventilatory control in exercise. *Respir Physiol* 49:267–277, 1982.

52. Wasserman K, Whipp BJ, Koyal SN, Cleary MG: Effect of carotid body resection on ventilatory and acid-base control during exercise. *J Appl Physiol* 39:354–358, 1975.

53. Weil JV, Swanson GD: Peripheral chemoreceptors and the control of breathing, in Whipp BJ, Wasserman K (eds), *Pulmonary Physiology and Pathophysiology of Exercise*. New York, Dekker, 1991, pp 371–403.

54. Whipp BJ: Peripheral chemoreceptor control of the exercise hyperpnea in humans. *Med Sci Sports Ex* 26:337–347, 1994.

55. Whipp BJ, Ward SA: The coupling of ventilation to pulmonary gas exchange during exercise, in Whipp BJ, Wasserman K (eds), *Pulmonary Physiology and Pathophysiology of Exercise*. New York, Dekker, 1991, pp 271–307.

CHAPTER 18

THE LUNGS IN PREGNANCY

John Popovich, Jr.

ANATOMICAL CHANGES OF NORMAL PREGNANCY
    Airways
    Respiratory Muscles and the Thoracic Cage
PHYSIOLOGICAL CHANGES OF NORMAL PREGNANCY
    Respiratory Physiology
    Sleep Disturbances
    Cardiovascular Physiology
    Dyspnea of Pregnancy
ACUTE RESPIRATORY DISTRESS IN PREGNANCY

Pregnancy induces a number of alterations in anatomy and physiology which have major pulmonary and cardiovascular consequences occurring throughout the gravid period. Physiological values and requirements, as well as normal laboratory assessment parameters, dynamically change in preparation for fetal support and parturition. The understanding of the clinical cardiopulmonary manifestations of disease states occurring during pregnancy requires a thorough comprehension of these transformations and the interplay of the various factors leading to these conditions.

ANATOMICAL CHANGES OF NORMAL PREGNANCY

Components of respiratory and cardiac anatomy change as a process of normal pregnancy. Basic structural changes occur in the upper and lower airways, thoracic cage, and the respiratory muscles, most notably the diaphragm.

Airways

Mucosal changes of the airways, consisting of hyperemia, friability, mucosal edema, and hypersecretion, occur throughout pregnancy. These changes are most pronounced in the upper airways, especially during the third trimester.[41] Associated medical conditions, such as preeclampsia, upper respiratory tract infection, or allergic rhinitis, may aggravate these changes. Nasal obstruction, epistaxis, sneezing episodes, and vocal changes may occur and may worsen when the individual lies down. Nasal and sinusoidal polyposis is often seen and tends to recur in women with each pregnancy. Common complaints in these individuals are recurrent or chronic "head colds" which are often treated with over-the-counter medications for relief.[13] Nasal obstruction may contribute to upper airway obstruction during sleep, leading to snoring and even obstructive sleep apnea.[14]

Anatomical changes in the upper airway may have important ramifications in complicated clinical conditions associated with delivery. Patients with such changes may significantly prefer mouth breathing and may not tolerate nasal cannula delivery of oxygen, if required. Nasopharyngeal obstruction may make the pregnant parturient poorly tolerant of the introduction of nasogastric tubes, nasal airways, or nasotracheal tubes. The placement of such devices requires significant lubrication and careful insertion technique to avoid local trauma and epistaxis. Smaller endotracheal tubes, such as 6.0 mm or less, may be advised for nasotracheal intubations.[25]

The anatomical changes that occur in the lower airways during pregnancy have not been characterized, but some of the mucosal changes that affect the upper airways may also occur in the central portion of the airway, such as the larynx and trachea. Nonspecific complaints of airway irritation, such as irritant cough or sputum production, may be intensified during pregnancy, often in association with functional changes in airway reactivity and/or coexistent pulmonary conditions. Other more tangible symptoms and signs of lower-airway irritation, such as hemoptysis and wheezing, should not be considered the result of normal anatomic changes associated with pregnancy, and other etiologies for these findings should be sought.

The physiological causes of nasal mucosal changes appear to be predominantly mediated by estrogens. Estrogens increase tissue hydration and edema through an increase in the hyaluronic acid component of ground substance. They also cause capillary congestion and hyperplastic and hypersecretory mucous glands.[31]

Respiratory Muscles and the Thoracic Cage

Upward displacement of the diaphragm is produced by the enlarging uterus. Although the diaphragm may be elevated up to 4 cm cephalad, diaphragmatic function is not impaired.[7,17] The anatomical effects of the elevation of the diaphragm are offset by an increase in the anteroposterior and transverse diameter of the thoracic cage.[7] Diminished tone and activity of the abdominal muscles serve to also counterbalance this effect of the gravid uterus. Diaphragmatic excursion during breathing may be greater in pregnancy than during the puerperium, suggesting that breathing may tend to be more diaphragmatic than costal during pregnancy. Progressive relaxation of the ligamentous attachments of the ribs broadens the subcostal angle by approximately 50 percent (68 to 103 degrees). Consequently, there is a 5- to 7-cm increase in chest circumference. These parameters, with the exception of subcostal angle, return to prepregnancy values after delivery.[7]

The anatomic changes of pregnancy cause shortening and widening of the lungs, with upward, lateral displacement of the cardiac apex on chest radiography.[7] Except for the appearance of smaller lung volumes and/or positional effects, such as lordotic or rotational views, no other radiographic change should be attributed to the anatomic changes of normal pregnancy.[13]

PHYSIOLOGICAL CHANGES OF NORMAL PREGNANCY

Profound physiological changes coincide with the structural preparation for fetal growth and childbirth. Both respiratory and cardiovascular changes ensure the delivery of necessary oxygenated blood and other nutrient factors required for this process.

Respiratory Physiology

The anatomical changes induced by the enlarging uterus cause serial changes in lung volumes (Fig. 18-1).[1,8,9,13,15,25] During pregnancy, the expiratory reserve volume decreases by 8 to 40 percent and the residual volume by 7 to 22 percent.[12] As a result, there is a 10 to 25 percent decrease in functional residual capacity after the fifth or sixth month of pregnancy. Functional residual capacity decreases due to a reduction in both expiratory reserve volume and residual volume.[9] This decline in functional residual capacity is more pronounced in the supine position. Due to the counterbalancing effects of widening of the lower rib cage, attenuation of the abdominal musculature, and unimpaired diaphragmatic movement, inspiratory capacity increases. Vital capacity and total lung capacity are not substantially changed in normal healthy gravidas, although total lung capacity does minimally decrease in the third trimester. Residual volume to total lung capacity ratio is low in the third trimester.

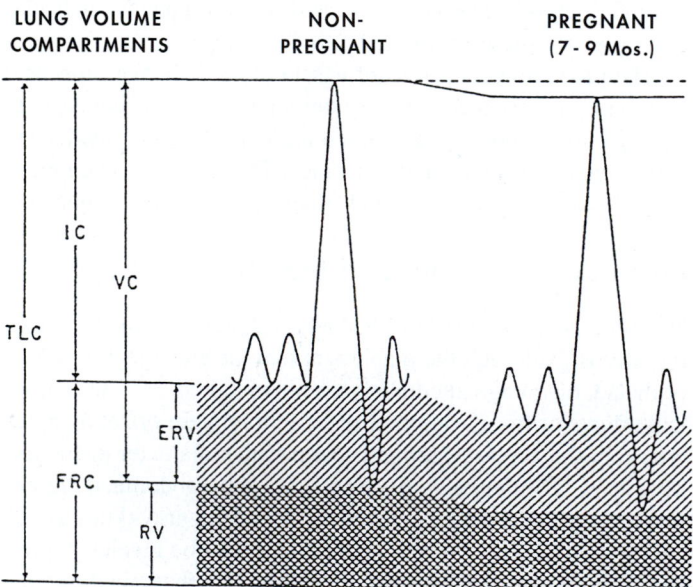

FIGURE 18-1 Lung volume changes associated with pregnancy. Although total lung capacity, residual volume, and expiratory reserve volume diminish, vital capacity is preserved in values similar to non-pregnant women.[9] TLC = total lung capacity, IC = inspiratory capacity, FRC = functional residual capacity, VC = vital capacity, RV = residual volume, ERV = expiratory reserve volume.

In late pregnancy, airway closure may occur at a lung volume close to or greater than functional residual capacity.[8] This phenomenon is more significant in the supine position. It is unclear if this is due entirely to a decreasing functional residual capacity while closing volume remains unchanged or if an absolute decrease in closing capacity is also involved. Increased gastric and esophageal pressure occurring in late pregnancy have been considered major factors that produce a decrease in transpulmonary pressure leading to peripheral airway collapse.[7] An increase in lung water, resulting in a change in the elastic properties of the lungs and in the tethering small airways, may also play a role.

Tidal volume increases considerably, i.e., from 450 ml to 600 ml (30 to 35%), as a result of increased ventilatory drive and excursions of the thoracic cage.[1,17,35] The increase in tidal volume is the predominant mechanism for the increase in minute ventilation during pregnancy, since respiratory rate either does not change appreciably or increases slightly, especially after the middle of the second trimester (Fig. 18-2A).[1,9,13,35] This observation suggests that the occurrence of tachypnea during pregnancy is an important abnormal finding that must be investigated. Maximum voluntary ventilation does not change greatly during pregnancy.[9,13]

Values of forced expiratory volume (FEV$_1$) measured throughout pregnancy are not significantly different from the nonpregnant condition.[1,15,30] Nevertheless, it is not clear how pregnancy affects lower airway function. In theory, changes in maternal prostaglandin and cyclic nucleotide concentrations may affect bronchomotor tone, but their respiratory effects are unclear.[50] Progressive increases of airway conductance have been reported to occur between 6 months of pregnancy and term along with a decrease in airway resistance.[13,15] Other reports have failed to document significant changes in the function of the lower airways during pregnancy.[13,24] In a study of serial specific conductance involving 30 pregnant women, no significant changes were found throughout pregnancy compared with the postpartum period.[30] Few studies have been directed at categorizing airway reactivity of airways during pregnancy, but one study involving few subjects did demonstrate an improvement in airway responsiveness and a decrease in the severity of asthma during pregnancy.[20]

Lung compliance does not change significantly during pregnancy.[15] Total pulmonary resistance, consisting of both airway and tissue resistance, is reduced by approximately 50 percent in pregnancy, most of the decrease attributable to a reduction in airways resistance.[13,15] Compliance of the thoracic cage decreases, although the anatomical changes in chest wall and the decrease in tone and activity of the abdominal musculature counterbalance the uterine enlargement.[7]

In early pregnancy, the diffusing capacity is either unchanged or slightly increased.[24] Throughout the rest of pregnancy, the diffusing capacity decreases, returning to normal or slightly lower than normal values. The relative contributions of the specific factors that affect diffusion, such as membrane diffusing capacity and pulmonary capillary blood volume, are not known.[50]

Minute ventilation significantly increases by 20 to 50 percent before the end of the first trimester (Fig. 18-2B).[1,9,35] Two factors appear to explain this increase in minute ventilation: (1) an

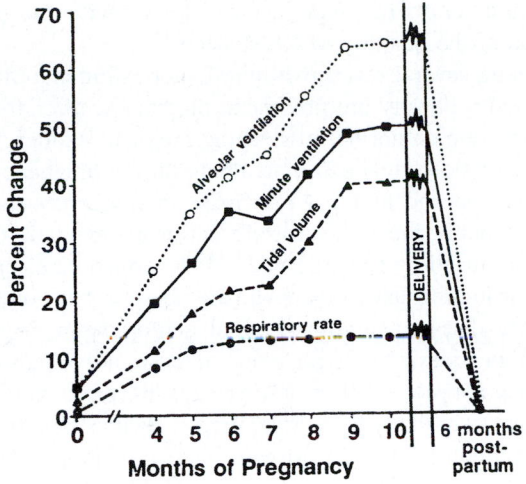

A

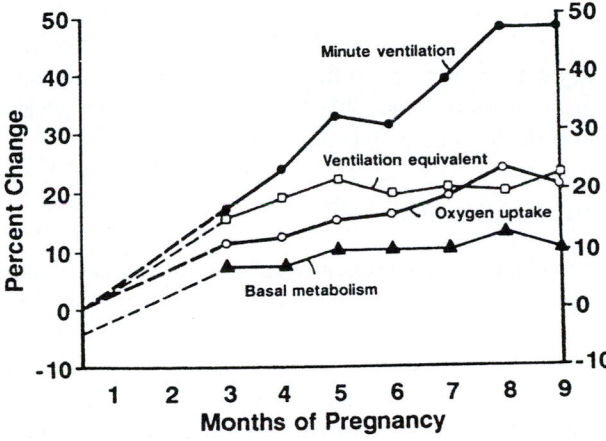

B

FIGURE 18-2 Ventilatory changes during pregnancy. *A.* The increase in minute ventilation is produced primarily by augmentation of tidal volume. This produces the significant increase in alveolar ventilation of approximately 70 percent noted at term. *(From Bonica*[3]*and Cugell et al.*[9]*) B.* Minute ventilation increases out of proportion to the increase in oxygen consumption, basal metabolism, and ventilatory equivalent. This demonstrates the physiological hyperventilation associated with pregnancy. *(From Prowse and Gaensler.*[34]*)*

increase in respiratory drive, presumably due to the effect of increased serum progesterone acting either as a direct respiratory stimulant or by increasing chemosensitivity of the respiratory center to P_{CO_2},[7,9,44] and (2) an increase in the production of carbon dioxide. Carbon dioxide production and oxygen consumption increase as a result of the increase in basal metabolic rate, coupled with growth in the mass of fetal and maternal tissue and a small increase in cardiac and respiratory work.[2,33,35] Since the increase in minute ventilation is approximately two times greater than the increase in oxygen consumption, without significant change in respiratory exchange ratio, an increase in respiratory drive with resultant physiological hyperventilation of pregnancy appears to be the principal physiological factor.[34] The physiological hyperventilation induced by altitude has been reported to

be greater in pregnant women than in nongravid control subjects, again suggesting a predominant increase in respiratory drive.[18]

Increasing progesterone levels play the major role in the increase in respiratory center activity and, subsequent, ventilatory response to pregnancy. Progesterone levels increase gradually during pregnancy from 25 ng/ml at 6 weeks to 150 ng/ml at 37 weeks. This hormone has been shown in normal nonpregnant women to increase both the resting minute ventilation and the slope of the ventilatory response curve to changes in alveolar P_{CO_2}.[44] Mouth occlusion pressures have been found to increase progressively during pregnancy in keeping with increasing progesterone levels.[7] Estrogen may have an additional effect by causing an increased responsivity of the respiratory center.[50]

The greater increase in minute ventilation than in carbon dioxide production produces a respiratory alkalosis with compensatory renal excretion of bicarbonate.[25,45] As a rule, arterial P_{CO_2} falls to levels of 28 to 32 mmHg. Arterial pH is maintained in the range of 7.40 to 7.45, and plasma bicarbonate decreases to 18 to 21 meq/L.[45] In contrast, the acute hyperventilation superimposed on the chronic hyperventilation during active labor and delivery is not easily compensated and may produce dangerous levels of pH, such as 7.6 or greater.[25,36] Blunting of the increase in ventilatory drive evoked by pain and/or anxiety control can minimize this abnormality. The increase in ventilatory drive and the decrease in functional residual capacity accelerate induction and recovery from inhalational anesthesia.

Values for arterial P_{O_2} are generally greater than 100 mmHg during pregnancy.[25,45] In the upright position, values for the alveolar-arterial oxygen gradient, physiological shunt, and VD/VT ratios remain similar to nonpregnant values.[45] With the supine position, the alveolar-arterial gradient may widen, and mild hypoxemia may develop, due to decrease in functional residual capacity and to increase in closure of small airways. The decrease in functional residual capacity, the increase in closing volumes, and the increase in oxygen consumption leads to a more precipitous decline in arterial P_{O_2} in pregnant patients who are apneic or hypoventilating.[2,25] Arterial P_{O_2} has been reported to decrease to 50 to 60 mmHg after 30 s of apnea during endotracheal intubation.[13]

Exercise poses certain physiological challenges to the pregnant patient which may adversely affect the fetus. The oxygen reserve, which is diminished by the reduction in the functional residual capacity and the increase in oxygen consumption, may be further depleted during exercise.[2] Minute ventilation is approximately 40 percent higher during exercise in pregnancy than in nonpregnant control subjects.[2,32,33] In addition, the initial response to exercise, as characterized by alveolar ventilation and the rate of change of minute ventilation during the first 90 s of exercise, is greater during pregnancy than at 3 months postpartum.[12,32] Absolute oxygen consumption during exercise is primarily affected by the increase in body mass and weight that occurs with pregnancy rather than to a change in basal aerobic metabolism. During pregnancy, there is neither a significant change in the absolute oxygen cost of non-weight-bearing (e.g., cycling) exercise nor in the oxygen cost per kilogram during weight-bearing exercise. Because of the increase in minute ventilation during pregnancy, the ventilatory equivalent ($\dot{V}_E/\dot{V}_{O_2}$) is higher during prepartum exercise than during postpartum exercise.

Respiratory responses during parturition are greatly affected by stage of labor and the response to pain and anxiety. During labor, tidal volume ranging from 350 to 2250 ml and minute ventilation from 7 to 90 L/min have been recorded.[13] The higher values were close to the maximum voluntary ventilation and were associated with the second stage of labor, whereas the lower values were obtained in the first stage of labor while the patient was sedated. Mean alveolar P_{CO_2} measured during the contractions of uncomplicated labor in patients medicated with meperidine, nitrous oxide, and oxygen is of the order of 32 mmHg during early labor, 24 mmHg at the end of the first stage, and 26 mmHg during the second stage.[36] This supports the observation that the physiological hyperventilation of pregnancy that occurs during labor and delivery is independent of appreciable pain. Along with the physiological hyperventilation, oxygen consumption during labor doubles and can even triple (e.g., to 750 ml/min) during uterine contractions.[13] The possibility of relative hypoventilation between contractions coupled with the grave implications of fetal hypoxemia makes it reasonable to be liberal in the use of oxygen in order to keep maternal oxygen saturation at 95 percent or greater.

Sleep Disturbances

Several alterations in maternal physiology can affect respiration in pregnant women during sleep. Sleep quality is often poor. Sleep disruption can be due to leg cramps, low back pain, urinary frequency, or responsibilities relating to child care.[14] Total sleep time and daytime sleepiness increase during the first trimester, whereas sleep time decreases and complaints of an increase in the number of nocturnal arousals increase in the third trimester.[14] Polysomnographic studies have shown an increase in sleep latency, an increase in the amount of stage I sleep and a decrease in REM sleep and delta sleep, as well as an increase in the number of wakenings.[14] Most sleep difficulties during pregnancy appear to relate to maintaining, rather than to initiating, sleep. After childbirth, most parameters of sleep quality and architecture return to prepregnancy values, with the possible exception of the quantity of REM sleep.[14]

Although several restrictive lung factors similar to those associated with obesity are present in pregnancy, arterial oxygen saturations remain normal in sleeping pregnant women.[4,14] The incidence of sleep-disordered breathing during pregnancy is unknown. Apnea and hypopnea decrease in frequency and duration, presumably due to the centrally acting augmentation of ventilation produced by progesterone.[4,14] Nevertheless, sleep apnea may occur in pregnant women who are obese or have underlying respiratory disease, significant nasal and/or upper airway obstruction, or preexistent hypoxemia. In these individuals progesterone may not prove sufficient to provide this protection.[5] These disturbances are likely to be magnified particularly in the supine position, although pregnant women frequently adopt a preferential left tilt position, possibly to reduce the likelihood of the aortocaval compression syndrome.[29] Women who manifest severe snoring, who are observed to develop irregular breathing during sleep, or who manifest excessive daytime somnolence should be referred for clinical polysomnography. Therapeutic intervention, generally with continuous nasal positive airway pressure, should be initiated as soon as possible because of the potential danger of hypoxemia to both mother and fetus.[5]

Cardiovascular Physiology

Profound changes in cardiovascular physiology occur during pregnancy (Table 18-1). Beginning around the fifth week of pregnancy and continuing into the postpartum period, cardiac output increases and peaks near term at 30 to 50 percent above normal.[6,48] Multiple gestations are accompanied by greater change in cardiac output.[6,39] The principal mechanisms of this change in cardiac output are increases in heart rate (maximum of 10 to 30 percent above prepartum values by week 12) and stroke volume and a decrease (20 to 30 percent in pulmonary and peripheral vascular resistances.[6,25,27,40] Cardiac output is increased further by 10 to 15 percent (1 to 2 L) to meet the challenges of

TABLE 18-1

Central Hemodynamic Changes of Normal Pregnancy

Parameter	Nonpregnant	Pregnant*	Significance
Cardiac output, L/min	4.3 +/− 0.9	6.2 +/− 1.0	p < 0.05
Heart rate, beats/min	71 +/− 10.0	83.0 +/− 10.0	p < 0.05
Systemic vascular resistance, (dyne/cm/s^{-5})	1,530 +/− 520	1,210 +/− 266	p < 0.05
Pulmonary vascular resistance, (dyne/cm/s^{-5})	119 +/− 47.0	78 +/− 22	p < 0.05
Colloid oncotic pressure	20.8 +/− 1.0	18.0 +/− 1.5	p < 0.05
Colloid oncotic pressure − pulmonary capillary wedge pressure (mmHg)	14.5 +/− 2.5	10.5 +/− 2.7	n.s.
Mean arterial pressure (mmHg)	86.4 +/− 7.5	90.3 +/− 5.8	n.s.
Pulmonary capillary wedge pressure, mmHg	6.3 +/− 2.1	7.5 +/− 1.8	n.s.
Central venous pressure, mmHg	3.7 +/− 2.6	3.6 +/− 2.5	n.s.
Left ventricular stroke work index, g/m/m^{-2}	41 +/− 8	48 +/− 6	n.s.

*36–38 weeks' gestation
SOURCE: Data from Clark et al,[6] with permission.

labor and delivery.[26,28,37,40] This response is principally a result of an increase in endogenous catecholamines and an increase in venous return of up to 300 to 500 ml of blood that occurs during uterine contractions.[26,37] Immediately after delivery, cardiac output increases further to levels as high as 40 to 50 percent greater than values during labor; this is probably due to an increase in venous return and autotransfusion resulting from the contracted uterus, as well as a release of the aortocaval compression (see below) caused by the enlarged uterus.[25] Although cardiac output remains high for the first few days after delivery, cardiac output returns to prepregnancy values over the ensuing 2 weeks.[19]

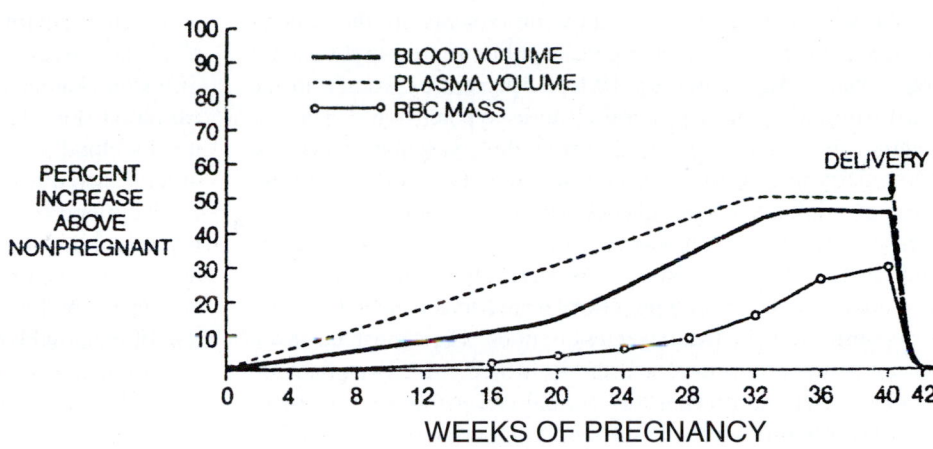

FIGURE 18-3   Blood volume changes during pregnancy. Plasma volume more significantly increases than red blood cell mass, especially during the first two terms. This produces the relative anemia and the hypervolemia state of pregnancy. *(From Scott.[43])*

Maternal blood volume increases progressively throughout pregnancy, beginning as early as 4 to 6 weeks of gestation and plateauing at approximately 32 to 34 weeks of gestation (Fig. 18-3). Total blood volume increases up to 35 to 50 percent above baseline (approximately 1.6 L), peaking by the third trimester.[47] The magnitude of the increases is greater in multiparous pregnancies or in multigravida mothers. The increase in blood volume provides some protection against peripartum blood loss, which averages approximately 0.6 L following uncomplicated vaginal delivery and 1.0 L following cesarean section.[25] Plasma volume increases to a greater degree than red blood cell mass, which increases less, and more gradually, to an average increase of about 25 percent. These changes result in a decrease of hemoglobin and hematocrit (absolute value decreased by 0.05), producing the "physiological anemia of pregnancy."[43] The increase in blood volume is probably determined by multiple primarily endocrinological factors, such as estrogen stimulation of aldosterone, nonrenal renin, and atrial natriuretic factor. Chorionic somatomammotropin (a growth-hormone-like substance produced by the placenta), progesterone, and possibly prolactin probably stimulate the increase in red blood cell mass. Extracellular water increases by 1 to 2 L, which, in addition to inferior vena caval compression by the enlarging uterus and fetus, results in the peripheral edema that occurs in 50 to 80 percent of normal pregnancies.[13]

Cardiac morphology changes progressively during pregnancy. Left ventricular wall thickness increases by 28 percent, and left ventricular mass by 52 percent above baseline, resulting in a decrease in left ventricular compliance.[21,27,40] Nevertheless, left atrial and left ventricular diastolic dimensions increase due to significant increases in filling volumes. Central venous pressure, pulmonary capillary wedge pressure, and left ventricular stroke work do not change significantly when compared to prepregnancy values.[6] Although left ventricular end-diastolic and left atrial dimensions return to normal during the 2 weeks after delivery, left ventricular wall thickness does not return to normal for approximately 24 weeks.[38]

The changes in cardiovascular physiology during pregnancy affect maternal tolerance to preexistent cardiac disease in different ways. Thus, the increased blood volume and decreased afterload of pregnancy may cause overt heart failure in patients with stenotic lesions of heart valves or worsen right-to-left shunts in uncorrected congenital heart defects. In contrast, pregnant women with regurgitant valvular heart disease often tolerate pregnancy well.[25] A decrease in the colloid oncotic pressure-pulmonary capillary wedge pressure gradient has been found and the suggestion made that the pregnant woman is predisposed to hydrostatic pulmonary edema. However, the clinical significance of the observation is unclear.[6]

Two theories have been proffered to account for the expansion of the blood volume in pregnancy: The "overfill" hypothesis proposes a primary mineralocorticoid excess in pregnancy, stimulating sodium and water retention and, subsequently, increasing blood volume; more likely is the "underfill" hypothesis which implicates a secondary response of volume-restoring mechanisms and cardiac output in response to a primary fall in systemic vascular resistance.[11] This primary fall in systemic vascular resistance is produced both by hormonally mediated vasodilation (due to vasodilating prostaglandins E2 and I2) and by the utero-placental unit acting as a functional low-resistance shunt.[42] Secondary hormonal responses include a 10-fold increase in plasma aldosterone levels by the third trimester, without a significant increase in levels of plasma arginine vasopressin.[10,25] Water intake is stimulated during pregnancy, as manifested in a decrease of 10 mosmol/kg in the plasma osmolarity level, provoking thirst.[10] Plasma osmolarity is significantly lowered to about 280 mosmol/kg.[10]

Systemic blood pressure, especially the diastolic component, is slightly lower during pregnancy.[13,42] Diastolic blood pressure reaches its nadir in the middle of the third trimester, falling by 10 to 20 percent of prepregnancy values.[23] Subsequently, blood pressure increases to near prepregnancy levels. The mechanism for this reduction in blood pressure appears to be hormonally mediated decreases in systemic vascular resistance. Although the resultant blood pressures in the third trimester appear to be distinctly hypotensive when compared to nonpregnant patients, prenatal blood pressure records should be reviewed to ascertain the extent and the significance of the blood pressure changes associated with pregnancy, especially in patients in the second trimester. Pregnant women are susceptible to profound postural hypotension. Approximately 10 to 30 percent of women in the third trimester exhibit postural systolic hypotension.[25] The enlarging uterus may compress surrounding vascular structures, particularly the inferior vena cava and the distal aorta. The principal physiological consequence of this compression is a decrease in venous return leading to a decrease in stroke volume and cardiac output.[22,49] Reflex vasovagal effects may also occur. The normal maternal compensatory response is tachycardia with vasoconstriction in the lower extremities. Care must be taken during spinal or epidural anesthesia, which causes sympathetic blockade that can prevent this normal compensatory phenomenon. Hypotension from aortocaval compression can be minimized by adequate restoration of intravascular volume and by displacement of the uterus, which is achieved by right or left lateral tilt of the pelvis. Although not found consistently, cardiac output in late pregnancy may be increased by about 20 percent when the patient is turned from supine to the lateral decubitus position.[25]

Reductions in maternal cardiac output may have profound fetal implications. Uterine blood flow is estimated to be 10 percent of maternal cardiac output, or, approximately, 500 ml/min.[25] Reductions in maternal cardiac output occurring during positional changes or due to underlying heart disease may significantly impair uterine blood flow, leading to fetal distress and potential fetal loss.[25] The low resistance nature of the uteroplacental unit makes this region highly dependent on global flow rates, and compensation by increasing vasodilation is poor when flow is impaired.

The umbilical vein supplies fetal blood, which has a P_{O_2} of 26 to 32 mmHg, an oxyhemoglobin saturation of 80 to 90 percent, a P_{CO_2} of 38 to 42 mmHg, and a pH of 7.30 to 7.35.[13] Several factors determine the rate of transfer of oxygen across the placenta: the higher affinity of fetal hemoglobin for oxygen, the diffusion characteristics of the placenta, and the rate of umbilical blood flow. Transfer of gas across the placenta is more limited by blood flow than by diffusion. Consequently, clinical conditions that diminish maternal cardiac output and/or regional uterine blood flow, such as shock, vasoconstricting agents (epinephrine, norepinephrine, phenylephrine, or high-dose dopamine), and severe respiratory alkalosis, could have serious detrimental effects on the fetus. Likewise, any decrease in the oxygen content of maternal blood resulting from profound hypoxemia, anemia, or alterations in oxyhemoglobin saturation (carbon monoxide, cyanide toxicity, severe alkalosis) could also compromise fetal health.[25]

Dyspnea of Pregnancy

Sixty to 70 percent of normal healthy pregnant women complain of dyspnea during pregnancy even though they have no prior history of cardiopulmonary disease.[34,46] These complaints commonly occur during the first and second trimester and remain stable or improve near term, suggesting that the etiology is not the mechanical burden of the enlarging uterus. Pulmonary function tests do not appear to correlate with symptomatology in this group, although one study suggested a reduction in diffusing capacity as a factor in dyspneic pregnant women.[9,13]

Several investigations have suggested a relationship between the physiological hyperventilation of pregnancy and the complaint of dyspnea in this population. Lower values for arterial P_{CO_2} at rest, substantial decrements in the values of arterial P_{CO_2} from prepregnancy, and a heightened response to hypercapnic ventilatory stimulation have been implicated.[16] It seems most likely that the awareness of overbreathing may be caused by

TABLE 18-2

Differential Diagnosis of Acute Respiratory Distress in Pregnancy

Disorder	Distinguishing Features	Chest Radiograph
Venous thromboembolism	Evidence of DVT, pleuritic chest pain, positive $\dot{V}/Q$ scan, leg dopplers, angiogram	Normal/atelectasis/effusion
Amniotic fluid embolism	Hemodynamic collapse, seizures, DIC	Normal/pulmonary edema
Pulmonary edema secondary to preeclampsia	Hypertension, proteinuria	Pulmonary edema
Tocolytic pulmonary edema	Tocolytic administration, rapid improvement	Pulmonary edema
Aspiration pneumonitis	Vomiting, reflux, fever	Focal infiltrate/pulmonary edema
Peripartum cardiomyopathy	Gradual onset, cardiac gallop	Cardiomegaly, pulmonary edema
Pneumomediastinum	Occurs during delivery, subcutaneous emphysema	Pneumomediastinum, subcutaneous air
Air embolism	Profound hypotension, cardiac murmur	Normal/pulmonary edema
Other: asthma pneumonia cardiac disease ARDS	As for nonpregnant patient	As for nonpregnant patient

DVT = deep venous thrombosis; $\dot{V}/Q$ = ventilation-perfusion; DIC = disseminated intravascular coagulopathy; ARDS = adult respiratory distress syndrome.
SOURCE: Data from Lapinsky et al,[25] with permission.

altered chest wall muscle proprioception due to increased muscle activity in response to progesterone-induced respiratory stimulation.[13]

ACUTE RESPIRATORY DISTRESS IN PREGNANCY

Although a number of preexistent cardiac and pulmonary disorders may be aggravated by pregnancy, several conditions that develop during or are specific for pregnancy need to be considered in evaluating acute onset of respiratory distress during pregnancy.[25] Most of these conditions, with the exception of pulmonary thromboembolic disease, pneumonia, or delivery-related pneumothorax, are attributable to the development of pulmonary edema (Table 18-2). Critical to the clinical evaluation of acute respiratory distress in pregnancy is the careful search for preexistent heart and/or lung disease, a detailed history to characterize precipitating and associated events (e.g., tocolytic therapy, aspiration, obstetrical complications), and the meticulous examination of the patient and chest radiograph to determine the presence of cardiogenic failure. As a rule, causes of respiratory distress due to conditions specific to pregnancy (e.g., amniotic fluid embolism, pulmonary edema secondary to preeclampsia) pose little problem in clinical diagnosis. However, more complicated presentations often require invasive hemodynamic monitoring to differentiate between cardiogenic and noncardiogenic pulmonary edema. Pulmonary thromboembolism should always be strongly considered in the absence of other explanatory conditions or as a complicating process.

REFERENCES

1. Alaily AB, Carrol KB: Pulmonary ventilation in pregnancy. *Br J Obstet Gynaecol* 85:518–524, 1978.
2. Artal R, Wiswell R, Romem Y, Dorey F: Pulmonary responses to exercise in pregnancy. *Am J Obstet Gynecol* 154:378–383, 1986.
3. Bonica JJ: *Principles and Practice of Obstetric Analgesia and Anesthesia.* Philadelphia, FA Davis, 1967.
4. Brownell LG, West P, Kryger MH: Breathing during sleep in normal pregnant women. *Am Rev Respir Dis* 133:38–41, 1986.
5. Charbonneau M, Falcone T, Cosio MG, Levy RD: Obstructive sleep apnea during pregnancy. Therapy and implications for fetal health. *Am Rev Respir Dis* 144:461–463, 1991.
6. Clark SL, Cotton DB, Lee W, et al: Central hemodynamic assessment of normal term pregnancy. *Am J Obstet Gynecol* 161:1439–1442, 1989.
7. Contreras G, Gutierrez M, Beroiza T, et al: Ventilatory drive and respiratory muscle function in pregnancy. *Am Rev Respir Dis* 144:837–841, 1991.
8. Craig DB, Toole MA: Airway closure in pregnancy. *Can Anaesth Soc J* 22:665–672, 1975.
9. Cugell DW, Frank NR, Gaensler EA, Badger TL: Pulmonary function in pregnancy: I. Serial observations in normal women. *Am Rev Tuberc Pulm Dis* 67:568–589, 1953.
10. Davison JM, Shiells EA, Philips PR, Lindheimer MD: Serial evaluation of vasopressin release and thirst in human pregnancy: Role of human chorionic gonadotropin in the osmoregulatory changes of gestation. *J Clin Invest* 81:798–806, 1988.
11. Duvekot JJ, Cheriex EC, Pieters FAA, et al: Early pregnancy changes in hemodynamics and volume homeostasis are consecutive adjustments triggered by a primary fall in systemic vascular tone. *Am J Obstet Gynecol* 169:1382–1392, 1993.
12. Edwards MJ, Metcalfe J, Dunham MJ, Paul MS: Accelerated respiratory response to moderate exercise in late pregnancy. *Respir Physiol* 45:229–241, 1981.
13. Elkus R, Popovich J: Respiratory physiology in pregnancy. *Clin Chest Med* 13:555–565, 1992.
14. Feinsilver SH, Hertz G: Respiration during sleep in pregnancy. *Clin Chest Med* 13:637–44, 1992.
15. Gee JBL, Packer BS, Millen JE, Robin ED: Pulmonary mechanics during pregnancy. *J Clin Invest* 46:945–952, 1967.
16. Gilbert R, Auchincloss JH Jr: Dyspnea of pregnancy: Clinical and physiological observations. *Am J Med Sci* 252:270–276, 1966.
17. Gilroy RJ, Mangura BT, Lavietes MH: Rib cage and abdominal volume displacements during breathing in pregnancy. *Am Rev Respir Dis* 137:668–672, 1988.
18. Hellegers A, Metcalfe J, Huckabee W, et al: The alveolar P_{CO_2} in pregnant and nonpregnant women at altitude. *J Clin Invest* 38:1010, 1959.
19. Hunter S, Robson SC: Adaptation of the maternal heart in pregnancy. *Br Heart J* 68:540–543, 1992.
20. Juniper EF, Daniel EE, Roberts RS, et al: Improvement in airway responsiveness and asthma severity during pregnancy: A prospective study. *Am Rev Respir Dis* 140:924–931, 1989.
21. Katz R, Karliner JS, Resnick R: Effects of a natural volume overload state (pregnancy) on left ventricular performance in normal human subjects. *Circulation* 58:434–441, 1978.
22. Kinsella SM, Lohmann G: Supine hypotensive syndrome. *Obstet Gynecol* 83:774–788, 1994.
23. Kirshon B, Hinkley CM, Cotton DB, Miller J: Maternal mortality in a maternal-fetal medicine intensive care unit. *J Reprod Med* 35:25–28, 1990.
24. Krumholz RA: Pulmonary diffusing capacity, capillary blood volume, lung volumes, and mechanics of ventilation in early and late pregnancy. *J Lab Clin Med* 63:648–655, 1964.
25. Lapinsky SE, Kruczynski K, Slutsky AS: Critical care in the pregnant patient. *Am J Respir Crit Care Med* 152:427–455, 1995.
26. Lee W, Rokey R, Miller J, Cotton DB: Maternal hemodynamic effects of uterine contractions by M-mode and pulsed-Doppler echocardiography. *Am J Obstet Gynecol* 161:974–977, 1989.
27. Mabie WC, DiSessa TG, Crocker LG, et al: A longitudinal study of cardiac output in normal human pregnancy. *Am J Obstet Gynecol* 170:849–856, 1994.
28. Mashini IS, Albazzaz SJ, Fadel HE, et al: Serial noninvasive evaluation of cardiovascular hemodynamics during pregnancy. *Am J Obstet Gynecol* 156:1208–1213, 1987.
29. Mills GH, Chafe AG: Sleeping positions adopted by pregnant women of more than 30 weeks gestation. *Anaesthesia* 49:249–250, 1994.
30. Milne JA, Mills RJ, Howie AD, Pack AI: Large airways function during normal pregnancy. *Br J Obstet Gynaecol* 84:448–451, 1977.
31. Paparella MM, Shumrick BA, Gluckman JL, Meyhoff WL: *Otolaryngology,* 3d ed. Philadelphia, WB Saunders, 1991, pp 1892–1893.
32. Pernoll ML, Metcalfe J, Kovach PA, et al: Ventilation during rest and exercise in pregnancy and postpartum. *Respir Physiol* 25:295–310, 1975.
33. Pernoll ML, Metcalfe J, Schlenker TL, et al: Oxygen consumption at rest and during exercise in pregnancy. *Respir Physiol* 25:285–293, 1975.
34. Prowse CM, Gaensler EA: Respiratory and acid-base changes during pregnancy. *Anesthesiology* 26:381–392, 1965.

35. Rees GB, Pipkin FB, Symonds EM, Patrick JM: A longitudinal study of respiratory changes in normal human pregnancy with cross-sectional data on subjects with pregnancy-induced hypertension. *Am J Obstet Gynecol* 162:826–830, 1990.

36. Reid DHS: Respiratory changes in labour. *Lancet* 1:784–785, 1966.

37. Robson SC, Dunlop W, Boys RJ, Hunter S: Cardiac output during labour. *Br Med J* 295:1169–1171, 1987.

38. Robson SC, Hunter S, Moore M, Dunlop W: Haemodynamic changes during the puerperium: A Doppler and M-mode echocardiographic study. *Br J Obstet Gynaecol* 94:1028–1039, 1987.

39. Robson SC, Hunter S, Boys RJ, Dunlop W: Hemodynamic changes during twin pregnancy: A doppler and M-mode echocardiographic study. *Am J Obstet Gynecol* 161:1273–1278, 1989.

40. Robson SC, Hunter S, Boys RJ, Dunlop W: Serial study of factors influencing changes in cardiac output during human pregnancy. *Am J Physiol* 256(H):1060–1065, 1989.

41. Schofman MA: The nose and pregnancy. *J Fla Med Assoc* 48:160–161, 1961.

42. Schrier FW: Pathogenesis of sodium and water retention in high-output and low-output cardiac failure, nephrotic syndrome, cirrhosis, and pregnancy. *New Eng J Med* 319:1127–1134, 1988.

43. Scott AE: Anemia in pregnancy. *Obstet Gynecol* 1:219, 1972.

44. Skatrud JB, Dempsey JA, Kaiser DG: Ventilatory response to medroxyprogesterone acetate in normal subjects: Time course and mechanism. *J Appl Physiol* 44:393–344, 1978.

45. Templeton A, Kelman GR: Maternal blood-gases ($P_{A_{O_2}} - Pa_{O_2}$), physiological shunt, and VD/VT in normal pregnancy. *Br J Anaesth* 48:1001–1003, 1976.

46. Tenholder MF, South-Paul J: Dyspnea in pregnancy. *Chest* 196:381–388, 1989.

47. Ueland K: Maternal cardiovascular dynamics, VII: Intrapartum blood volume changes. *Am J Obstet Gynecol* 126:671–677, 1976.

48. Ueland K, Novy MJ, Metcalfe J: Cardiorespiratory responses to pregnancy and exercise in normal women and patients with heart disease. *Am J Obstet Gynecol* 115:4–10, 1973.

49. Ueland K, Novey MJ, Peterson EN, Metcalfe J: Maternal cardiovascular dynamics, IV: The influence of gestational age on the maternal cardiovascular response to posture and exercise. *Am J Obstet Gynecol* 104:856–864, 1969.

50. Weinberger ST, Weiss ST, Cohen WR, et al: Pregnancy and the lung. *Am Rev Respir Dis* 121:559–581, 1980.

CHAPTER 19

AGING OF THE RESPIRATORY SYSTEM

Robert O. Crapo / Edward J. Campbell

Even in individuals who enjoy apparently good health, there are measurable decrements in function of the respiratory system with age. These changes occur progressively as a healthy individual grows older and are most marked beyond 60 years of age. Cross-sectional studies show clear differences between elderly and young persons with regard to the structure and function of the components of the respiratory system (Table 19-1). However, caution must be exercised in ascribing observed changes to age alone, since the lungs are exposed to a lifetime of environmental stresses, including tobacco smoke, respiratory infections, air pollutants, and occupational exposures to dusts and fumes. Increasingly sedentary life-styles and decreasing fitness with age have marked effects, especially upon cardiovascular function. Longitudinal studies of "healthy" individuals followed to old age are essentially not available. Despite these caveats, age-related changes in the respiratory system clearly exist, although the magnitude of the changes attributable to aging alone may be somewhat uncertain. Where appropriate, methodological problems in the available cross-sectional studies are described.

Although age-associated changes can easily be measured by objective testing, it is important to note that the routine activities of healthy elderly persons are not limited by decreasing respiratory system function. However, whereas youthful persons have a marked excess of functional capacity over the amount required to meet metabolic needs at rest or with stress (physiological reserve), the respiratory system draws on this reserve as its function declines with age. Thus, the physiological reserve, especially for alveolar gas exchange, is reduced with aging. This leaves elderly individuals vulnerable to stresses, diseases, and injuries that are weathered much more easily in the young.

STRUCTURAL CHANGES IN THE LUNG

Studies of the aging lung have shown changes in shape, with increases in anteroposterior diameter that lead to a "rounding" of the shape of the lung. These changes are presumably secondary to changes in the shape of the surrounding thoracic cage and are not thought to have functional consequences.

Conducting Airways

The conducting airways consist of the air passages from the mouth to the level of the respiratory bronchioles. Their volume comprises the anatomic dead space, and their geometry is a primary determinant of airway resistance. The larger cartilaginous airways show a modest increase in size with age, resulting in slight but probably functionally insignificant increases in anatomic dead space.[13] Although calcification of cartilage in the walls of the central airways and hypertrophy of bronchial mucous glands is seen in advanced age, these and other changes in the extraparenchymal conducting airways appear to have little or no physiological significance.

Lung Parenchyma

After age 30 or 40, the respiratory bronchioles and alveolar ducts undergo progressive enlargement (Fig. 19-1). This change has

TABLE 19-1

Respiratory System: Functional Divisions and Changes with Aging

Functional Division	Components	Function	Change(s) with Aging
Conducting airways	All airways not involved in gas exchange (mouth to terminal bronchioles)	Gas movement between environment and alveolar space	Slight changes in size; calcification; glandular hypertrophy
Lung parenchyma	Gas-exchanging airways and vessels; connective tissue framework	Gas exchange between alveolar space and capillary blood	Enlarged terminal airspaces; ventilation/perfusion mismatching
Bellows apparatus	Chest wall and muscles of respiration	Provide mechanical forces for ventilation	Increased rigidity of chest wall; decreased respiratory muscle strength
Ventilatory control	Respiratory control center (pons and medulla); carotid and aortic bodies	Maintaining homeostasis by altering ventilation to match metabolic needs	Markedly decreased responses to hypercapnia and hypoxemia
Cardiovascular system	Heart and systemic vasculature	Blood transport and tissue exchange of respiratory gases	Decreased maximal heart rate and cardiac output; decreased responsiveness to hypoxemia

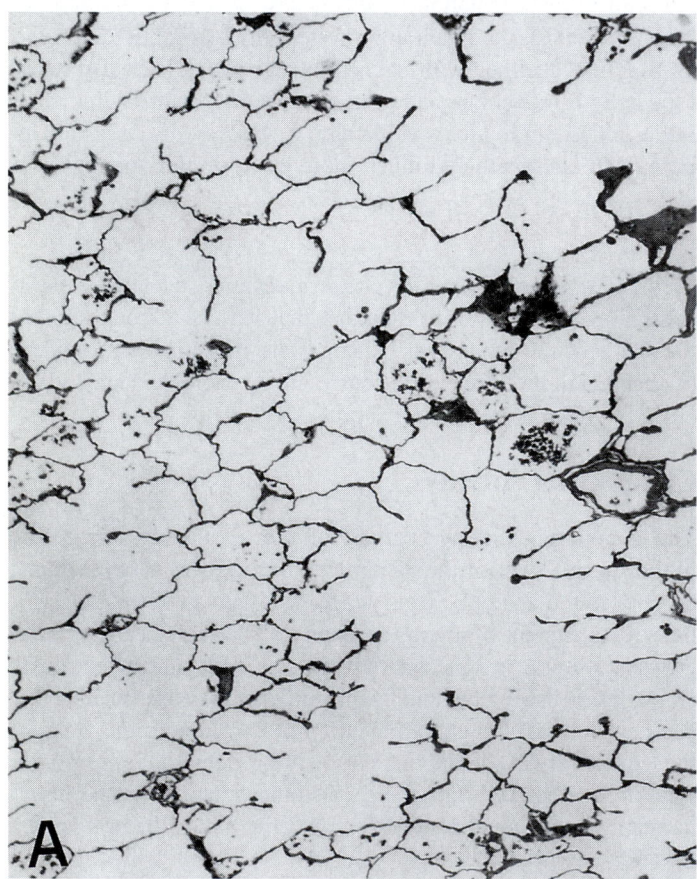 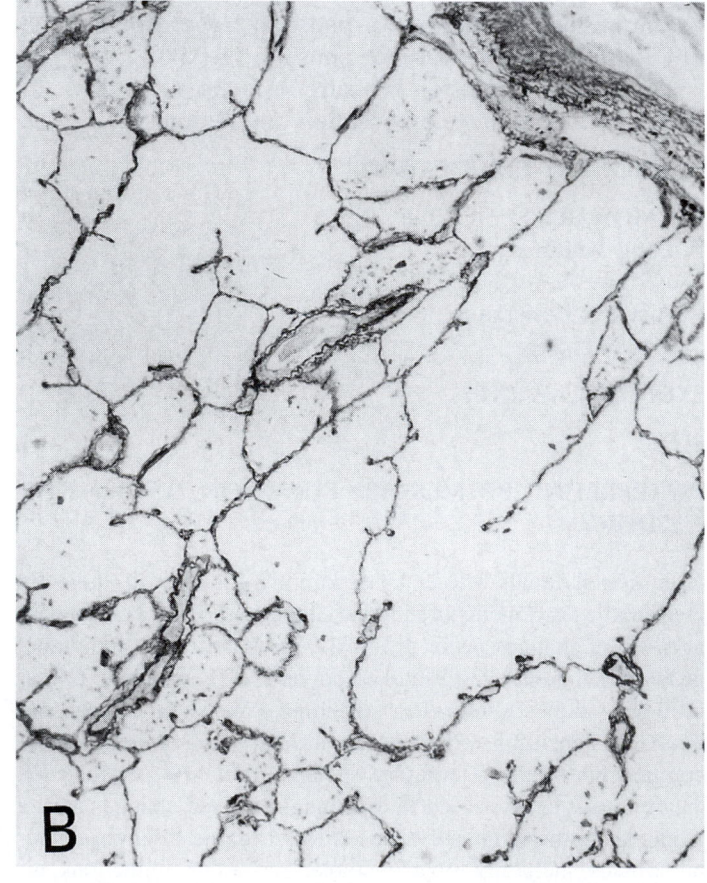

FIGURE 19-1   Histologic changes in the aging lung. *A.* Normal lung of a 36-year-old woman. *B.* Lung of a 93-year-old woman. In (*B*), the alveolar ducts are dilated, and shortening of interalveolar septa is ob-served. (*By permission of the Mayo Foundation; photomicrographs courtesy of Charles Kuhn III, M.D.*)

been termed "ductectasia" because of the prominent finding of enlargement of alveolar ducts. The proportion of the lung made up of alveolar ducts increases, and alveolar septa become shortened, leading to a "flattened" appearance of the alveoli. With the change in geometry, the distance between alveolar walls (known to morphologists as the mean linear intercept, or MLI) increases, while the surface-to-volume ratio of the lung decreases. The age-related enlargement of the terminal respiratory units also produces a decrease in the percentage of parenchymal air contained within alveoli. The net result of these structural changes is that the alveolar surface area decreases by approximately 15 percent by age 70.

Pulmonary emphysema is also characterized by an increase in the size of terminal airspaces, an increase in MLI, and a decrease in surface area; however, destruction of alveolar septa with fusion of terminal airspaces is a defining characteristic of emphysema. There have been some reports of emphysematous lesions in aged lungs, but it is not certain that smokers were excluded from these studies. Since the fate of individual alveolar septa during the aging process has been somewhat controversial, some have referred to the histological changes in aged lungs as "senile emphysema." A National Heart, Lung, and Blood Institute Workshop on the definition of emphysema weighed the available evidence and decided not to include age-related changes in the lung parenchyma under the definition of *emphysema*.[8] To simplify terms and avoid confusion, they recommended use of the term *aging lung* to apply to the uniform airspace enlargement that develops with increasing age.

CHANGES IN MECHANICAL PROPERTIES OF THE LUNGS

The lungs and chest wall are both elastic. The resting volume of excised lungs is smaller than that of the lungs contained within an intact thoracic cage, because the lungs are held at an increased volume by the outward recoil forces of the chest wall. Thus, in the intact thoracic cage, the lungs exert an inward recoil force. The retractile force of the lungs, or "elastic recoil," can be measured during life by estimating the pleural pressure with an esophageal balloon at progressively decreasing lung volumes from total lung capacity to functional residual capacity, when the airways are open and there is no air flow. The negative pleural pressure is generated by the lungs' elastic recoil forces.

The pressure measurements may be displayed on a pressure-volume diagram (Fig. 19-2). Figure 19-2 compares, at the same volume, the elastic recoil pressures of a young man, a normal elderly adult, and a patient with emphysema. The normal elderly individual and the patient with emphysema both have a greater decrease in elastic recoil pressure than does a young person. This is reflected in the leftward shift of their pressure-volume curves.[16,21,34] This loss of elastic recoil is the physiological hallmark of emphysema. However, emphysema is characterized by a much greater loss of elastic recoil than is caused by aging alone.

There has been some disagreement regarding the effects of aging on lung compliance (Δ volume/Δ pressure; i.e., the slope of the pressure-volume relationship, Fig. 19-2). The question is

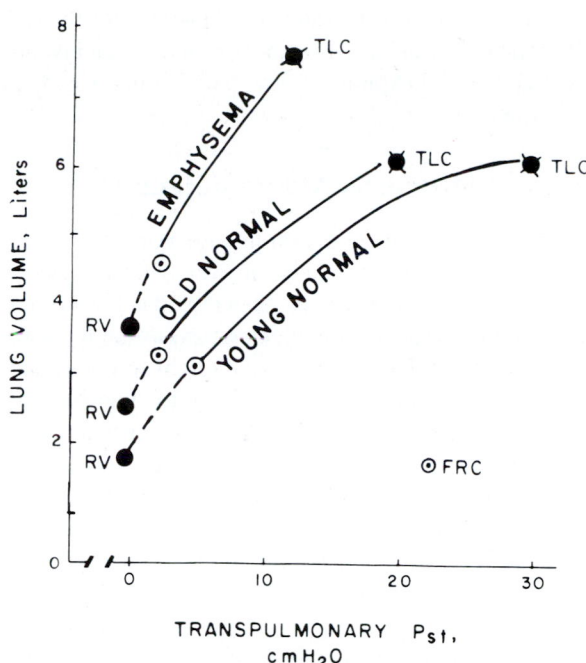

FIGURE 19-2   Static pressure-volume curves of the lungs. Static recoil pressure, expressed as transpulmonary pressure measured at various lung volumes, is plotted against lung volume on the ordinate. Note that at any lung volume, the recoil pressure is less in the aged individual than in the young, normal control, resulting in a pressure-volume curve that is shifted upward and to the left. For comparison, a curve for a patient with emphysema is shown. In emphysema, recoil pressures are reduced much more, and lung compliance (the slope of the pressure-volume relationship) is clearly abnormal. *(From Pride,[29] with permission.)*

whether there is a parallel leftward shift of the pressure-volume curve with aging (no change in compliance), or, instead, a steeper slope in addition to a shift (indicating an increase in compliance), as seen in emphysema. In aged individuals, the static pressure-volume curve is slightly steeper and is more concave in relation to the pressure axis. However, there is general agreement that changes in lung compliance with aging are not physiologically significant.

Two forces in the lung parenchyma are responsible for producing the elastic recoil of the lungs. The greatest part of the elastic recoil forces is provided by the surface tension at the curved air-fluid interface of the small airways and alveoli. The second retractive force is that produced when the fibrous skeleton of the lung (primarily the elastic fibers) is stretched.

Changes in Surface Forces

Most of the loss in lung recoil with age is likely to be related to the decrease in lung surface area with age. The loss of surface area that accompanies aging can be expected to reduce the area of gas-liquid interface, resulting in a decrease in the surface tension forces and, ultimately, a decrease in the total elastic recoil of the lung. Whether it is due to loss of air-liquid interface or to changes in lung structural macromolecules (see below), the reduced elastic recoil has important consequences for the function of the intraparenchymal airways and, ultimately, on alveolar gas exchange and forced expiratory flow (see "Pulmonary Function Tests," below).

Changes in Structural Macromolecules

Elastic fibers, which are composed in large part of an extremely hydrophobic, highly cross-linked, and very elastic macromolecule (elastin), form a continuous skeleton that follows the airways and pulmonary vessels and extends to a fine meshwork in the alveolar septa.[28] These fibers are thought to contribute substantially to lung elasticity. Analysis of whole lungs has revealed that the elastin content actually increases (rather than decreases) with age. More recent evidence indicates that the increase in lung elastin with age is accounted for by an increase in pleural elastin; parenchymal elastin does not change.

Careful studies of the elastic fibers in the lung parenchyma have shown that they are remarkably stable following postnatal lung growth. Certain biochemical changes in very long-lived proteins (change of amino acids into their mirror-image structures, or racemization) provide a type of "biological clock" that permits an estimate of the time that has elapsed since the proteins were synthesized.[32] Because of the constraints of the protein synthetic mechanisms, only L-amino acids are incorporated into newly synthesized proteins. With the passage of years at body temperature, however, there is a readily measurable accumulation of D-aspartic acid. When all of the lung proteins are examined together, minimal D-aspartic acid is found. In purified lung elastin, however, there is an age-related accumulation of D-aspartic acid, indicating that lung elastin is turning over very slowly if at all (Fig. 19-3). It has also been possible to estimate lung elastin turnover by measurement of the incorporation into elastic fibers of carbon 14 (^{14}C) from atmospheric nuclear weapons testing.[32] For example, individuals who completed their postnatal lung growth prior to the nuclear age show no excess ^{14}C in their lung elastin, indicating absence of new elastin synthesis. In contrast, an appropriate excess of ^{14}C is found in the lung elastin of individuals whose lungs were growing in the post–weapons testing era. Modeling of the radiocarbon data indicates that the "mean carbon residence time" in elastin is 74 years.

Taken together, the amino acid racemization and radiocarbon data indicate that lung parenchymal elastin is stable over the human life span, and it appears that the elastin content of the lung parenchyma not only does not change with age but that the individual fibers persist for at least many decades. The remarkable longevity of lung elastic fibers raises the strong possibility that these connective tissue structures provide a metabolically inert scaffold for the structure of the lung. This may explain the appearance of structural abnormalities in the lung parenchyma (such as pulmonary emphysema) when the elastic fibers are injured.

Other studies of lung elastic fibers have shown changes in the location and orientation of individual fibers with age as well as changes in the cross-linking of elastin. Thus, some authors have suggested that remodeling of the lung architecture may occur without replacement of elastic fibers. In any case, at the present

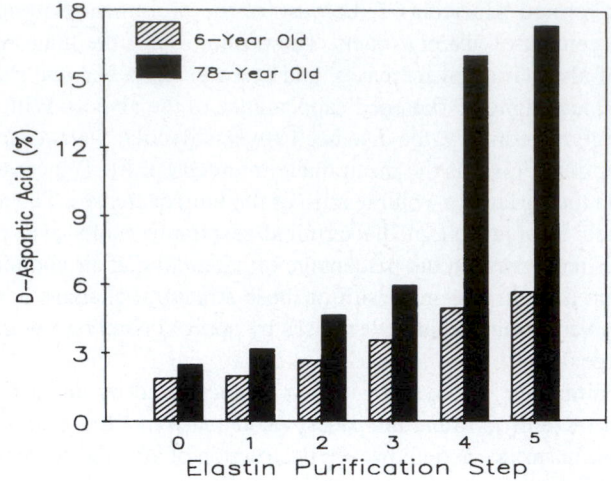

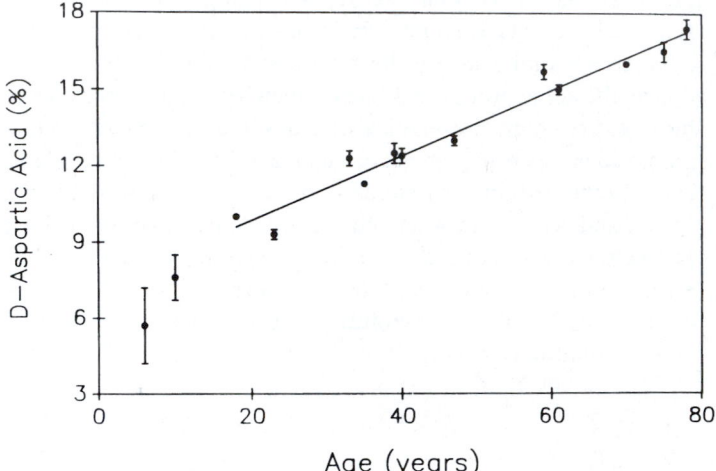

FIGURE 19-3 Longevity of human lung parenchymal elastin, as evidenced by in vivo racemization of aspartic acid. *Top panel.* Each pair of bars shows results from two individuals with greatly differing ages at time of death. Step 0 of elastin purification represents whole lung parenchyma, while step 5 is purified elastin. D-aspartic acid detected in the 6-year-old specimen can be attributed to racemization that occurs during the analytical procedures, whereas the difference in prevalence of D-aspartic acid between the young and old individual has resulted from racemization in vivo. Note that results from whole-lung hydrolysates (step 0) are similar for both specimens, reflecting their composition of proteins, having predominantly rapid turnover. However, purified elastin from the oldest specimen has racemized extensively in vivo, indicating that it was synthesized many decades before death. *Bottom panel.* D-aspartate in elastic fibers is shown as correlated with age at death. The relationship of D-aspartic acid to the age of the subject indicates that parenchymal elastin is markedly persistent after its synthesis. The data for elastin agree well with results for other very long lived proteins. *(From Shapiro et al,[32] with permission.)*

time, the age-related changes in connective tissue do not provide a sufficient explanation for the decrease in elastic recoil forces observed in the elderly.

Studies of lung collagen have failed to show a consistent change in its quantity during aging. Although human studies have not been done, studies in rodents and birds suggest that lung collagen fibers, like elastic fibers, are very long-lived. Finally, although some qualitative changes in collagen during aging have been described (decreases in solubility and increases in inter-molecular cross-links), these appear to have no relationship to changes in lung elastic recoil.

CHANGES IN CHEST WALL

There is good evidence that the chest wall becomes more rigid with advancing age. As may be seen in Fig. 19-4, the static pressure-volume curve of the chest wall is shifted to the right and is less steep with increasing age.[10,18,24] The articulations of the ribs with the sternum and the spinal column may become calcified, and the compliance of the rib articulations decreases. The changes in rib articulations may be compounded by the development of kyphosis due to osteoporosis. The decreasing compliance of the chest wall demands greater work from the respiratory muscles.[10] For example, in a 70-year-old person, approximately 70 percent of the total elastic work of breathing is expended on the chest wall, whereas this value is 40 percent in a 20-year-old.

Fig. 19-4 also demonstrates that the compliance of the total respiratory system decreases with age because the decrease in lung elastic recoil is outweighed by the changes in the mechanical properties of the chest wall.[21,34]

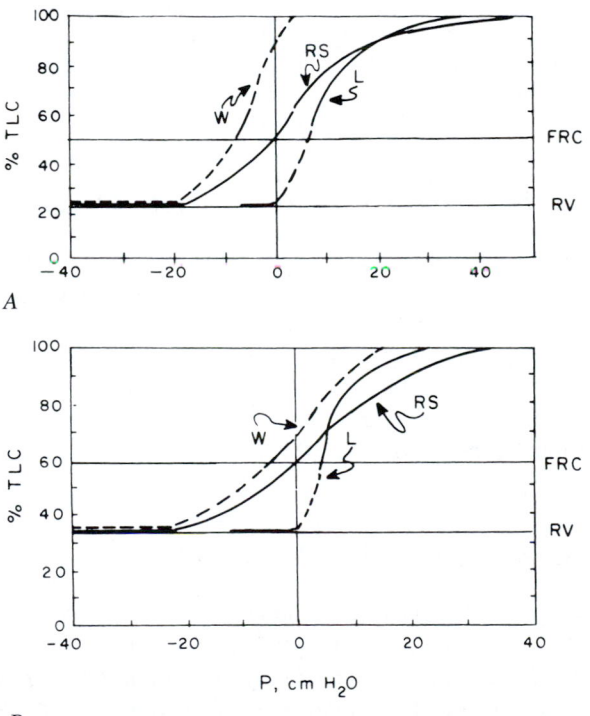

FIGURE 19-4 Static compliance relationships of the components of the respiratory system. (L = lungs; W = chest wall; RS = total respiratory system.) *A.* A 20-year-old man. *B.* A 60-year-old man. Note that the static compliance of the chest wall is substantially decreased (reduced slope) in the older individual, while functional residual capacity (the resting volume of the respiratory system, or the point at which the pressure gradient across the respiratory system is zero) increases. As in Fig. 19-2, it is also apparent that the static recoil pressure of the lungs is reduced in the older subject. (*Based on data from Mittman et al,[21] and Turner et al,[34] with permission.*)

CHANGES IN MUSCLES OF RESPIRATION

Age-related changes in nonrespiratory skeletal muscle include decreased work capacity due to alterations in the efficiency of muscle energy metabolism, atrophy of motor units, and electromyographic abnormalities. Based upon lessons learned with other skeletal muscles, it appeared likely that age-related abnormalities in respiratory muscles would also be found.

An early study by Black and Hyatt[3] appeared to confirm age-related decrements in respiratory muscle function by measuring maximal inspiratory pressure (P_{Imax}) and maximal expiratory pressures (P_{Emax}) in 120 normal individuals (both smokers and nonsmokers) between the ages of 20 and 70. Maximal respiratory pressures in females were 65 to 70 percent of those in males. No significant age-related changes were observed in individuals under the age of 55. Trends toward reduced maximal respiratory pressures with age were seen in both genders and with both P_{Imax} and P_{Emax}. With the numbers of males studied, the change with age in P_{Imax} was not statistically significant for male gender.

More recently, McElvaney and coworkers[20] came to a different conclusion in a similar study of 104 healthy individuals over the age of 55. They found large variation in maximal respiratory pressures from individual to individual (as had Black and Hyatt) but no significant correlation with age. In contrast, in a third population of 160 healthy individuals who ranged in age from 16 to 75 years, Chen and Kuo found significant gender differences in maximal respiratory pressures as well as trends toward decrements with age for both P_{Imax} and P_{Emax} in both genders.[7] The age-related change in P_{Emax} in males was not statistically significant with the sample size studied. When the 40 individuals of both genders in the youngest age group (16 to 30 years) were compared with the 40 individuals in the oldest group (61 to 75 years), the decrement in P_{Imax} was 32 to 36 percent, while the decrement in P_{Emax} was 13 to 23 percent. Representative findings for maximal respiratory pressures in women are illustrated in Fig. 19-5.

Chen and Kuo also measured inspiratory muscle endurance against a resistive load, and found significant decrements with age.[7] Physically active men had greater inspiratory muscle endurance than sedentary men.

In summary, it appears that when populations of healthy individuals of widely differing ages are studied, moderate age-related decrements in respiratory muscle strength and endurance can be found. These studies usually define *healthy* only by the absence of disease and do not control for physical activity. They are complicated by marked interindividual variability, and longitudinal studies have not been reported. Continuous respiratory muscle activity may have a training effect that leads to better preservation of respiratory muscle function when compared with other skeletal muscles. Finally, physical activity may have an additional training effect that enhances inspiratory muscle endurance in all age groups.

CONTROL OF BREATHING

In young individuals, minute ventilation is matched to metabolic demands. As a result, arterial blood gas values remain stable

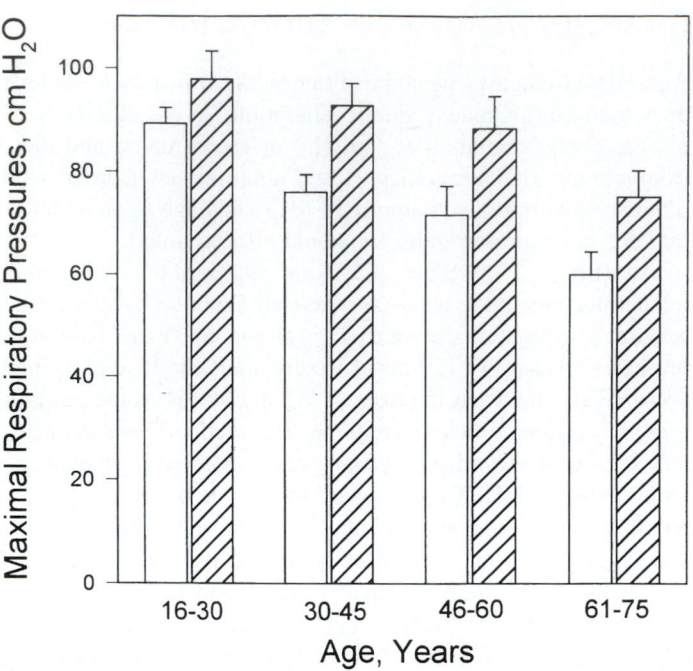

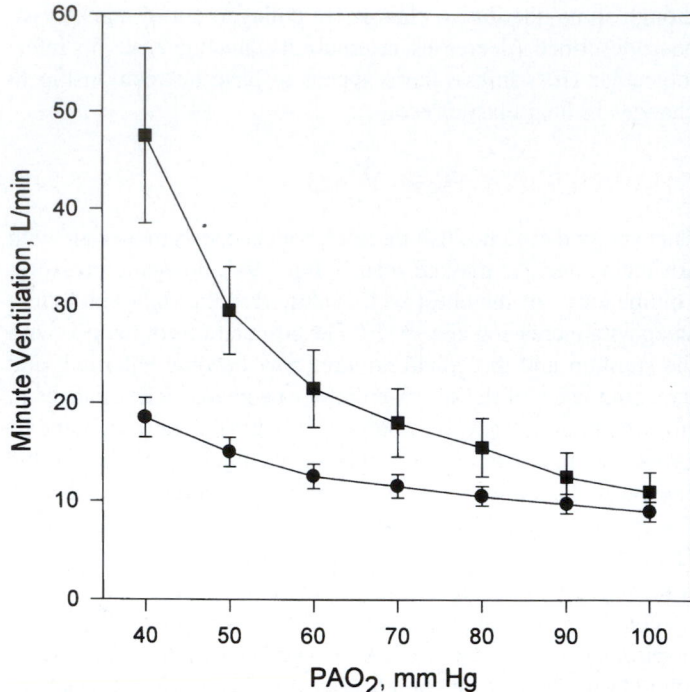

FIGURE 19-5 Representative variations in maximal respiratory pressures with age among women. Inspiratory and expiratory measurements were made at residual volume and total lung capacity, respectively. Maximal inspiratory pressure (*open bars*) and maximal expiratory pressure (*hatched bars*). Error bars are standard errors of the mean. Although quantitatively moderate, variations with age were statistically significant for both measurements. *(From Chen and Kuo,[7] with permission.)*

FIGURE 19-6 Variations with age in ventilatory responses to hypoxia. Eight normal men aged 64 to 73 (*squares*) and eight controls aged 22 to 30 (*circles*) were subjected to isocapnic progressive hypoxia by a rebreathing method. Data values are means, with standard errors of the mean shown by the error bars. Note that the ventilatory responses differ strikingly between the elderly individuals and the controls. *(From Kronenberg and Drage,[17] with permission.)*

throughout a wide range of activities from rest to strenuous exertion, while oxygen consumption and carbon dioxide production are varying widely. Similarly, when the efficiency of gas exchange is diminished by lung disease or congestive heart failure, appropriate increases in minute ventilation minimize the resulting hypercapnia and/or hypoxemia in healthy young individuals. The ventilatory control system is described in detail in Chapter 11.

Ventilatory control mechanisms are typically tested by stressing the respiratory system, by inducing either hypoxemia or hypercapnia while monitoring ventilatory parameters (and often cardiac parameters as well). Such tests have shown striking differences between young and elderly individuals in both ventilatory and cardiac responses.[5,6,17,27]

Diminished Ventilatory Response to Hypercapnia

Kronenberg and Drage[17] compared the ventilatory responses to hypercapnia in 8 young (mean age, 25.6 years) and 8 elderly (mean age, 69.6 years) individuals. During the tests, the subjects were asked to rebreathe 5% CO_2 while their $P_{A_{O_2}}$ was held above 200 mmHg by supplemental oxygen to eliminate hypoxic ventilatory drive. Measurements were made while $P_{A_{CO_2}}$ was allowed to rise to 65 mmHg. Although there was considerable individual variation and some overlap between the groups, the elderly individuals had a significantly diminished ventilatory response to hypercapnia, measured as the slope of the relationship between ventilation and $P_{A_{CO_2}}$.

Diminished Ventilatory Response to Hypoxia

When Kronenberg and Drage[17] measured the ventilatory response to hypoxia at constant CO_2, they found even more striking differences between the young and elderly subjects (Fig. 19-6). For example, the ventilatory response to a $P_{A_{O_2}}$ of 40 mmHg was uniformly smaller in the older subjects, and there was no overlap between the groups. The mean minute ventilation at a $P_{A_{O_2}}$ of 40 mmHg was 40.1 and 10.2 L/min in the young and old groups respectively.

Diminished Occlusion Pressure Responses

Peterson and colleagues[26] confirmed the above observations and have shown that the differences in responses of elderly subjects to both hypercapnia and hypoxia are due to a lesser increase in tidal volume while the ventilatory rate increases normally. Since this observation could be caused by differences in respiratory muscle strength or by increases in chest wall stiffness, the authors also measured airway occlusion pressures, which are valuable indices of respiratory drive that are not affected by respiratory muscle strength or respiratory mechanics. The measurement (P_{100}) is the negative pressure at the mouth, measured 100 ms after the start of inspiration against an occluded airway. The occlusion pressure responses to both hypoxia and hypercapnia (Fig. 19-7) were significantly reduced in the 10 elderly subjects studied by Peterson (mean age, 73.3 years) when compared to 9 young control subjects (mean age, 24.4 years).[27] Although the

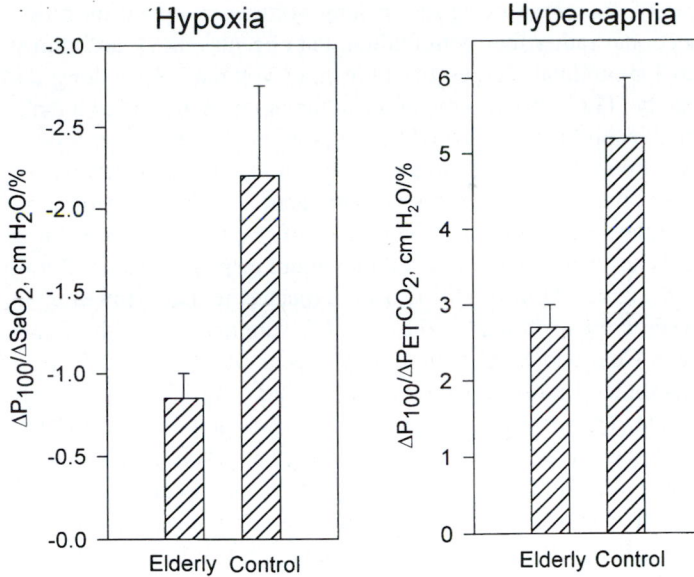

FIGURE 19-7   Variations with age in occlusion pressure responses to hypoxia and hypercapnia. Data shown are slopes of relationships between occlusion pressure responses and either SaO_2 or end-tidal P_{CO_2}; error bars are standard errors of the mean. Elderly individuals had significantly diminished occlusion pressures in response to both hypoxia and hypercapnia. Both differences were significant, with $p < 0.01$. *(From Peterson et al,*[27] *with permission.)*

elderly individuals had reduced respiratory muscle strength (mean, 24 percent lower maximal static inspiratory pressure), the differences in occlusion pressure persisted when normalized for these differences.

In summary, the reduced responsiveness in tidal volume to either hypoxemia or hypercapnia with age is apparently due to a reduced responsiveness of ventilatory drive or neural output from the respiratory center. It has not been determined whether the diminished ventilatory drive results from altered chemoreceptor function or from altered function of the respiratory center. Kronenberg and Drage favor altered receptor function based on their observation that elderly subjects responded to an alveolar oxygen tension of 40 torr with only an 11 percent increase in heart rate, whereas the young subjects responded with a 34 percent increase.

Respiratory Load Compensation and Dyspnea

Reflex compensation for a change in respiratory mechanical load (as in lung disease, changes in posture, and mouth versus nose breathing) normally serves to maintain ventilation constant during the change. Akiyama and colleagues[1] measured responses to inspiratory flow-resistive loading in young and elderly individuals and found significant differences. In the young control group, inspiratory loading resulted in an increase in P_{100} at each level of induced hypercapnia, such that inspiratory loading did not change the ventilatory response to hypercapnia when compared with unloaded responses. In marked contrast, the P_{100} in the elderly group did not change when an inspiratory load was applied. In the absence of a compensatory change in ventilatory

drive, ventilatory responses to hypercapnia were reduced during inspiratory loading in the elderly group.

At each level of P_{CO_2}, the intensity of perceived dyspnea in response to inspiratory loading was greater in the elderly than in the control group. Thus, the sensation of dyspnea was intact or enhanced in the elderly subjects while their compensatory responses were reduced. This suggests the possibility that elderly individuals may complain of greater dyspnea than younger individuals with similar pathophysiological deterioration.

PULMONARY CIRCULATION

Invasive physiological studies of pulmonary artery catheterization have typically been biased by including only subsets of patients whose signs and symptoms led to referral for heart catheterization and who, therefore, may not be representative of a "healthy" cohort. Further, age-related changes in the pulmonary circulation are difficult or impossible to separate from changes due to heart disease or age-related changes in cardiac function.

Ehrsam and colleagues[12] reported a retrospective analysis of right heart catheterization studies performed in 125 asymptomatic subjects who ranged from 14 to 68 years of age. Small increases in right atrial, pulmonary artery, and pulmonary artery wedge pressures observed in the highest age group disappeared when values were adjusted for sex, weight, and height. No significant age-related changes were found in cardiac output, stroke volume, or oxygen uptake. Age explained 10 percent or less of the total variation in the hemodynamic and pressure variables when assessed by multiple regression. During supine exercise with a bicycle ergometer, however, pulmonary artery and wedge pressures increased with age, particularly in subjects over age 45. The changes were highly significant, with age accounting for 12 to 30 percent of the total variation when assessed by multiple regression. Finally, pulmonary artery resistance showed a highly significant increase with age, whether measured at rest or during exercise, with age contributing 12 to 27 percent to the total variation in pulmonary artery resistance. Although the cohort studied were all asymptomatic and ambulatory, it is possible that silent coronary artery disease was present in some of the subjects, and the prevalence of coronary artery disease can be expected to increase with age. Moreover, younger patients tended to be referred for evaluation of a heart murmur, whereas the older patients were referred for "pulmonary investigation" that included coin lesions, hilar lymphadenopathy, "previous pulmonary infiltrates," and smoke inhalation. Cigarette smoking history was not discussed. Thus, it is not certain that the younger and older patients were strictly comparable.

More recently, Davidson and Fee[11] reported the results of right-heart catheterization at rest in 47 normal subjects who were free of coronary disease and had normal left ventricular systolic function. Smokers were included. The investigators found highly significant but quantitatively modest age-related increases in mean pulmonary artery pressure, pulmonary vascular resistance, and pulmonary/systemic vascular resistance ratio, but they found no age-related differences in pulmonary artery wedge pressure. The authors felt that the most likely explanation for the age-related changes in pulmonary artery pressure and pulmonary vascular resistance was a primary abnormality of the pulmonary vascular bed, but they could not exclude effects of subtle abnormalities in left ventricular function.

In summary, studies of pulmonary hemodynamics with aging are limited by retrospective design, bias in patient selection, and potential effects of smoking. Minor increases in pulmonary vascular resistance and age-related increases in pulmonary artery wedge pressure during exercise have been reported. These age-related changes may not be physiologically significant.

PULMONARY FUNCTION TESTS

Lung function and exercise capacity decline with age in concert with numerous other physiological, morphological, and biochemical changes. Descriptions of "normal" age-related changes are confounded by an increasing prevalence of disease, chronic illness, medication use, and an increasingly sedentary life-style. Further, chronological age only approximates physiological age; the two often differ significantly. Chronological age is, therefore an imperfect measure for indexing changes with senescence. While it would be desirable to isolate the effects of "normal aging" (aging in the absence of disease), it is essentially impossible to do so. The best studies to do so are longitudinal, tracing change with time, because they avoid the obvious biases of cross-sectional studies. Longitudinal studies, however, have methodologic problems and biases of their own, the most obvious being that the healthy elderly represent a healthy survival population. If, as a group, they have better than average lung function, they would not represent the general population of elderly people well.

Lung Volumes

Figure 19-8 illustrates typical lung volume changes with aging based on cross-sectional studies. With the exception of vital ca-

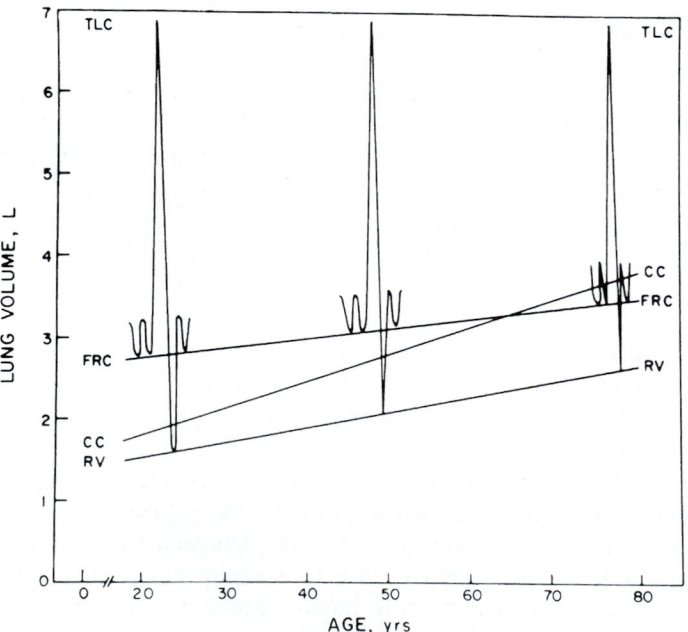

FIGURE 19-8   Schematic illustration of lung volume changes with age based on cross-sectional studies in seated individuals. (TLC = total lung capacity; FRC = functional residual capacity; RV = residual volume; CC = closing capacity.) Although not labeled, vital capacity (VC) is TLC minus RV. The most consistent changes are an increase in RV and a decrease in VC. *(From Peterson and Fishman,[26] with permission.)*

pacity, the effect of aging on lung volumes is based on cross-sectional rather than longitudinal data because there are almost no longitudinal studies of static lung volumes. Total lung capacity (TLC), the volume of air in the lungs at the end of a maximal inspiration, is marked by the point at which the recoil pressure exerted by the respiratory system is exactly counterbalanced by the maximal inspiratory pressure generated by the respiratory muscles. Since both the compliance of respiratory system (lung and chest wall combined) and maximum inspiratory pressure fall with aging, TLC might also be expected to fall. However, in seven cross-sectional studies of TLC summarized by the European Coal and Steel Community,[30] four of the studies in men and three of those in women did not find a significant age coefficient. The remaining studies found only small declines in TLC with age, on the order of -8 to -19 ml/year. When these study results were combined into average equations, no significant age coefficients were reported for either men or women.[20] McClaran and colleagues[19] measured lung volumes twice in 18 healthy, fit men. The first measurement was at a mean age of 67 and the second was 6 years later. Though average TLC fell 25 ml/year, the change was not statistically significant. The study was small and the interval was short.

In summary, current cross-sectional studies suggest that TLC either does not decline with age or declines very slowly. It is interesting to speculate on the possibility that cross-sectional studies of TLC might be confounded because they typically index TLC to both age and height. Height declines with aging, and maximum height during a life span appears to increase with successive generations. The authors believe that longitudinal studies of TLC with age are likely to show small but significant declines with age.

Both slow and forced vital capacity (FVC) decline with age, more rapidly in men than women. Average decrements in vital capacity per year vary considerably; in cross-sectional studies, declines range from 21 to 33 ml/year in men and 18 to 29 ml/year in women. Theoretically, longitudinal studies should provide better estimates of the effect of aging on lung function. Ware and colleagues,[22] in a study containing both longitudinal and cross-sectional computations, found cross-sectional falls in FVC for men and women to be -34 and -27.8 ml/year respectively. The longitudinal estimates were -40 ml and -31.3 ml/year respectively. This study contradicts the generally held concept that longitudinal studies show smaller declines in FVC than cross-sectional studies. Currently, it is not certain whether longitudinal studies are all that much different from cross-sectional studies in describing declines in FVC and forced expiratory volume in 1 s (FEV$_1$).[35] Longitudinal studies tend to show an acceleration in the rate of loss of in FVC and FEV$_1$ as age advances.

Cross-sectional studies of residual volume (RV) and the RV/TLC ratio consistently show increases with age. In the young, RV, the volume of air in the lungs at the end of a maximal expiration, is the volume at which the outward static recoil pressure of the respiratory system is counterbalanced by the maximal pressure exerted by the expiratory muscles. In older subjects, expiratory flow never completely reaches zero and the determination of RV is made partly by the length of time an individual can maintain expiratory effort. Other factors leading to an increased residual volume with aging include loss of lung recoil, decreased chest wall compliance, decreased expiratory muscle force, and increased small airway closure (air trapping) in dependent lung zones.[16] Time of exhalation and increase in air trapping are probably more important than changes in lung and chest wall compliance in explaining the increase in RV with aging.

Functional residual capacity (FRC) is also determined by the balance of the elastic recoil forces of the lung and chest wall, but, in this instance, the equilibrium occurs at the end of a quiet (unforced) exhalation. Since lung recoil falls and the chest wall stiffens with age, one would expect FRC to increase. Cross-sectional studies, however, show inconsistent results, with most showing no change in FRC with aging. Studies that do find an increase in FRC with aging show a small positive age coefficient on the order of 7 to 16 ml/year. McClaran's longitudinal study found FRC to increase 40 ml/year, but, again, the change was not significant.[19] Despite the conflicting data, it is generally believed that FRC increases with aging.

Loss of lung recoil also changes the volume at which airway closure occurs. When adults exhale fully, small airways close in the region of the terminal bronchioles in dependent lung zones. The lung volume at which this closure begins is measured as closing volume or, if it is added to residual volume, closing capacity. Closing volume increases linearly with age from about 5 to 10 percent of TLC at age 20 to about 30 percent of TLC at age 70. The loss of lung elastic recoil, a possible decrease in the recoil of the intrapulmonic airways, and decreases in small airway diameter probably explain most of the change in CV.

Closing volume encroaches on tidal volume by about age 44 when subjects are supine and about age 65 when they are seated (Fig. 19-8). Airway closure during tidal breathing explains part of the decrease in arterial oxygen tension (P_{AO_2}) observed with aging and may contribute to an aging-related increased frequency dependency of compliance.

Airflow

While essentially all expiratory flows measured during a maximum expiratory maneuver decrease with age, the declines are most evident at lower lung volumes (Fig. 19-9). Nunn and colleagues,[23] in a study of 225 male and 228 healthy female nonsmokers, reported a modest, nonlinear decrease in peak expiratory flow (PEF) with aging (Fig. 19-10), which reached a high point at age 30 to 35; decline became evident at about age 45. After age 50, the average decline in men was about 4 L/min per year, about 2.5 L/min per year for women.

Figure 19-11, from Paoletti et al.,[25] illustrates changes in FEV_1 during growth, maturation, and senescence. Changes in FVC are similar. In one model of aging, FVC and FEV_1 increase progressively during the growth phase until about age 12. In the

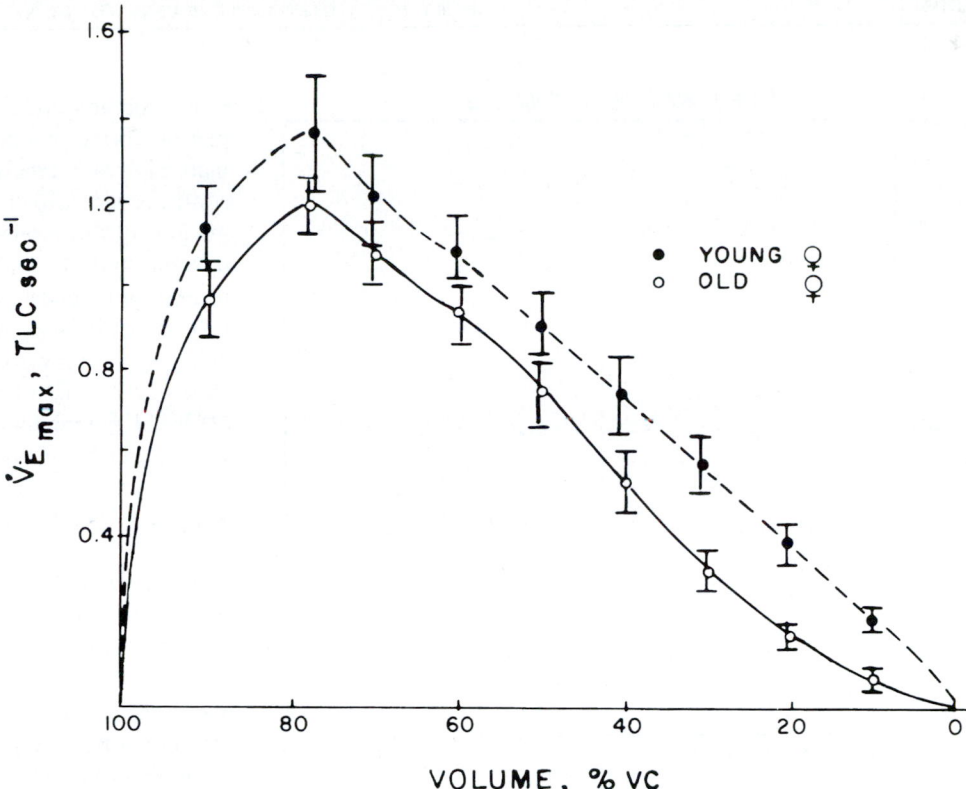

FIGURE 19-9 Illustrative maximal flow-volume curves for healthy "elderly" women (mean age, 63 years) and healthy young women (mean age, 25 years). Although all flows tend to be reduced with aging, the reduction in flow is most evident at lower lung volumes, where the flow-volume curve is clearly concave to the volume axis. *(From Peterson and Fishman,[27] with permission.)*

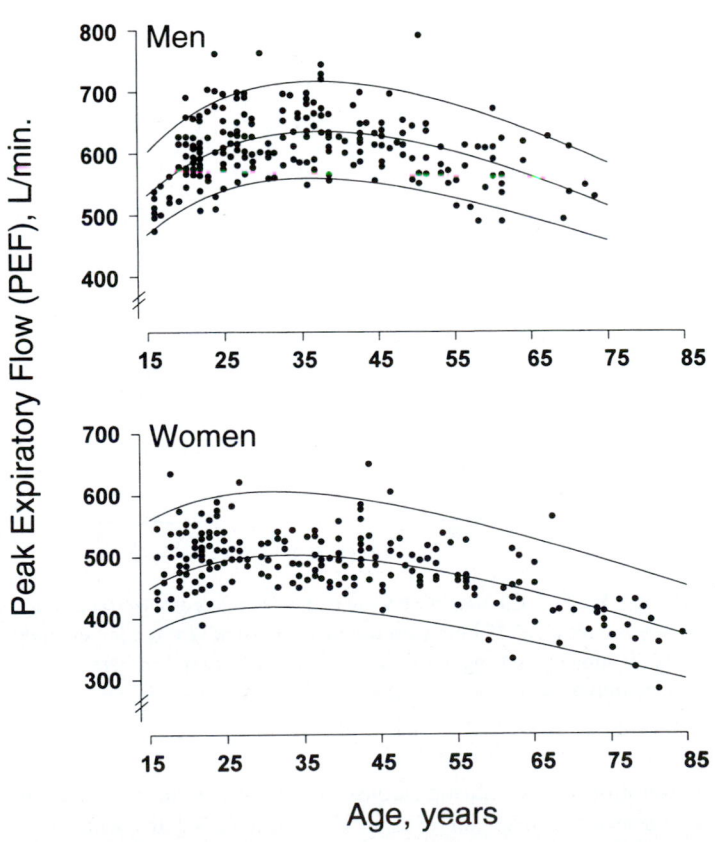

FIGURE 19-10 Changes in peak expiratory flow (PEF) in 225 males and 228 females who were healthy nonsmokers. The center line is a regression curve representing mean data and the boundaries are 90 percent confidence intervals. *(From Nunn and Gregg,[23] with permission.)*

FEV₁ BY AGE IN FEMALES

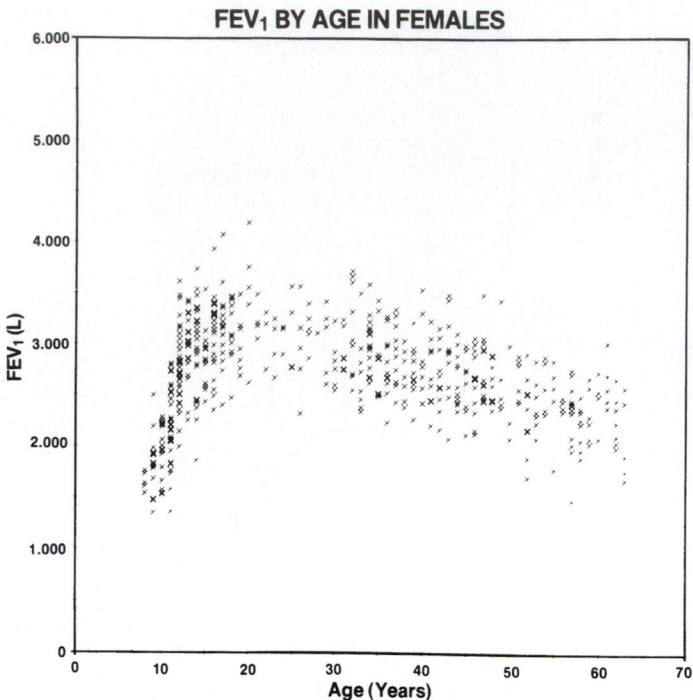

FEV₁ BY AGE IN MALES

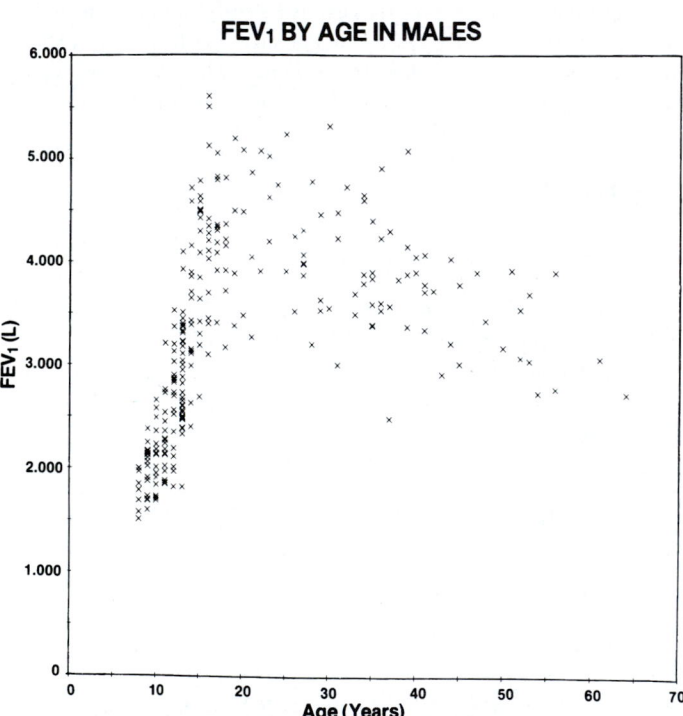

FIGURE 19-11 Change in FEV_1 with age from a cross-sectional study of 538 females and 263 males selected as "normal" from a larger study of 3289 subjects. Changes in FVC are similar. *(From Paoletti et al,[25] with permission.)*

maturation phase (during adolescence) there is an acceleration of these increases. Increases in FVC and FEV_1 are seen up to about age 20 years in women and about 25 years in men; increases in lung volumes occur even after somatic growth ceases. There appears to be a plateau phase where there is little or no change in FVC or FEV_1 prior to the onset of a decline. How-

ever, Robbins and colleagues[31] demonstrated that, while the plateau correctly represents average data, lung function is often increasing or decreasing in individuals (Fig. 19-12). Their study confirms the suspicion that the "plateau" phase represents the merging of slower maturation-related increases in FVC and FEV_1 in some subjects, with subtle decreases in others. In the decline phase, there appears to be an acceleration in the rate of loss of FVC and FEV_1 as age progresses. An accelerated rate loss at older ages is, however, not found in all studies. The rate of decline in FVC and FEV_1 with age tends to be greater (1) in men, (2) in taller individuals, (3) in individuals with larger baseline values, and (4) in individuals with increased airway reactivity.

Airways Resistance

Total airway resistance measured at FRC does not change with aging. Since upper airways increase and smaller airways decrease in size with aging, it is likely that peripheral airway resistance increases and central airway resistance decreases. That total airway resistance does not change with aging may be a function of the counterbalancing of these two opposite changes. However, since about 90 percent of total airway resistance resides in the upper airways, significant changes in peripheral airway resistance might not be readily reflected in total airway resistance. Significant increases in peripheral airway resistance with age would also be consistent with the more dramatic decreases in maximum flow observed at low lung volumes.

Gas Exchange

The carbon monoxide diffusing capacity ($D_{L_{CO}}$), also known as transfer factor ($T_{L_{CO}}$), declines with age. Earlier cross-sectional studies report a linear decline in $D_{L_{CO}}$ of about -0.2 ml CO/min per mmHg per year for men and -0.15 mL CO/min per mmHg per year for women.[9,33] These declines are roughly 0.5 percent per year. In a large representative sample of U.S. adult men, Neas and Schwartz[29] found an almost identical linear fall in $D_{L_{CO}}$. In women, however, they found a nonlinear, quadratic decline in $D_{L_{CO}}$ with age. After age 47, the nonlinear component was not significant and the decline in $D_{L_{CO}}$ was identical to that in earlier studies. The decline in $D_{L_{CO}}$ with age did not vary with race.

The decline in $D_{L_{CO}}$ with age is not explained by increased nonhomogeneity of gas distribution. Measured $D_{L_{CO}}$ falls as alveolar P_{O_2} increases and venous hemoglobin concentration falls. Neither alveolar P_{O_2} nor hemoglobin concentration varies enough with age to explain the aging decline in $D_{L_{CO}}$. The magnitude of the decline in $D_{L_{CO}}$ corresponds fairly well to the magnitude of the known aging-related decrease in the internal surface area of the lung.

The components of $D_{L_{CO}}$ are membrane diffusing capacity (Dm) and pulmonary capillary blood volume (Vc). Both Dm and Vc decrease with age. In a cross-sectional reference value study of 54 male and 36 female healthy nonsmokers, the declines in Dm and Vc with age were found to be linear.[10] Membrane diffusing capacity fell at about 0.6 percent per year in both men and women. Pulmonary capillary blood volume fell at about 0.3 percent per year.

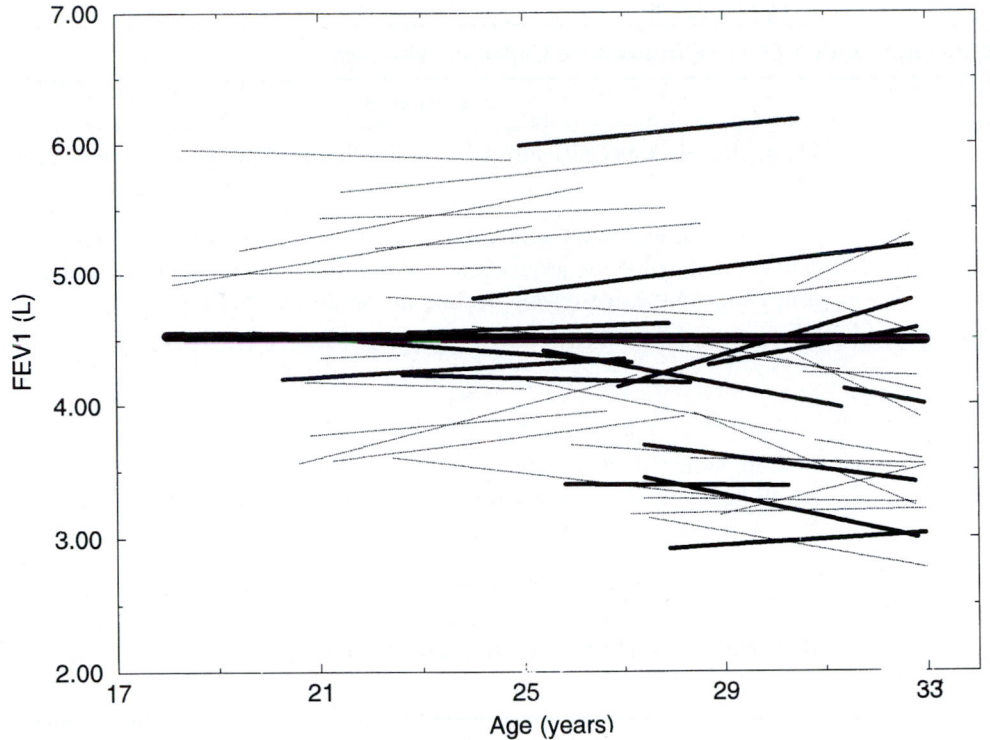

FIGURE 19-12   Predicted FEV_1 trajectories from 44 men based on linear regressions of longitudinal data. Nonsmokers (*fine lines*) and smokers (*dashed lines*). The heavy line is based on the entire group's data. While the group's data show no change with age, data for individuals show both increases and declines with age during this time period, when a plateau in lung function was theorized to occur. (*From Robbins et al,[26] with permission.*)

aging is increased mismatching of ventilation to blood flow ($\dot{V}/\dot{Q}$) as airway closure begins to occur during tidal breathing. Increased $\dot{V}/\dot{Q}$ mismatching with aging is also associated with an increase in physiological dead space. Hypoventilation does not contribute to the age-related fall in Pa_{O_2}, since Pa_{CO_2} and pH do not change with age (Fig. 19-13).

EXERCISE CAPACITY

Peak $\dot{V}_{O_2}$ ($\dot{V}_{O_2peak}$) and maximum work capacity decrease with aging in both sedentary and active individuals.[14,15,38] $\dot{V}_{O_2peak}$ (L/min) increases until about age 20. Declines are evident at about age 25 in both men and women and continue at about 1 percent per year (Fig. 19-14). If one expresses $\dot{V}_{O_2peak}$ as a function of body weight (L/kg per min), the decline is evident much earlier, perhaps in the first decade of life. The magnitude of the decline in $\dot{V}_{O_2peak}$ tends to be greater in longitudinal than in cross-sectional studies and occurs roughly twice as fast in sedentary than in physically active persons. Most but not all studies report linear declines in $\dot{V}_{O_2peak}$ with age, even though a nonlinear decline would be expected based on the number and type of variables that affect exercise capacity.[15,38]

Although alveolar oxygen pressure (Pa_{O_2}) remains constant with age, arterial P_{O_2} (Pa_{O_2}) decreases and the alveolar-arterial oxygen tension gradient ($P_A - a_{O_2}$) increases with aging (Fig. 19-13). The decline in Pa_{O_2} with aging is more pronounced when subjects are studied in a recumbent as contrasted with an upright position. The most likely explanation for the decline in Pa_{O_2} with

The decline in exercise capacity with age occurs as a result of normal aging but is accelerated by life-style issues. Aging is associated with significant changes in body configuration.

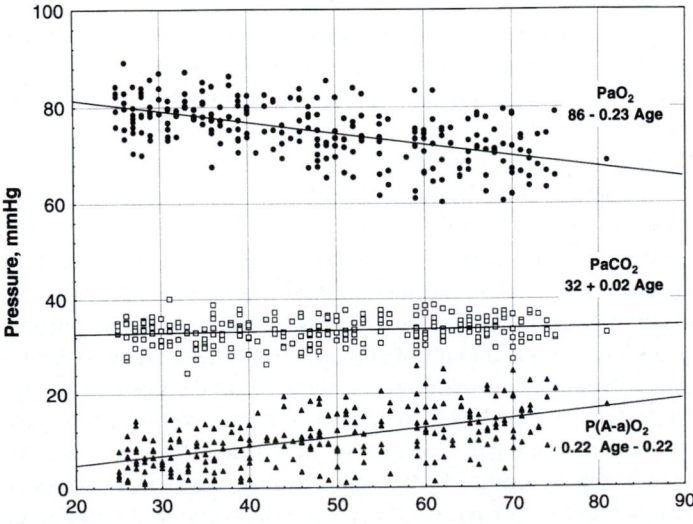

FIGURE 19-13   Change in Pa_{O_2}, Pa_{CO_2} and A − a gradient [$P(A − a)_{O_2}$] with age. Data were obtained from 200 healthy men and women living in Salt Lake City, UT (altitude = 1400 m). Sea level data would be similar, with a small upward shift in Pa_{O_2} and Pa_{CO_2}.

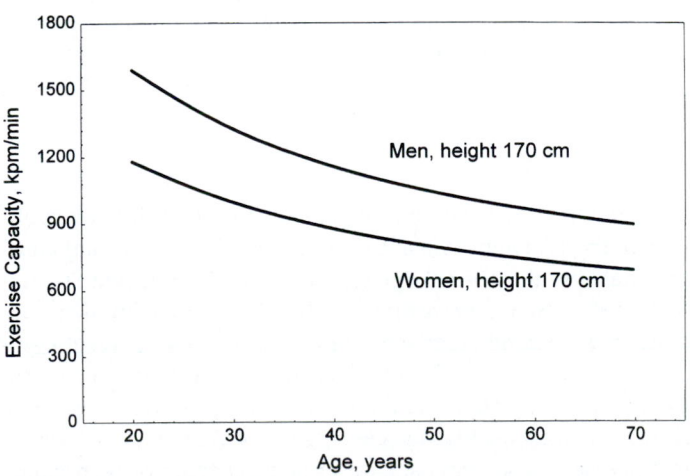

FIGURE 19-14   Decline in maximum exercise capacity with age. Exercise capacity declines nonlinearly with age. Maximum work capacity correlates strongly with peak oxygen uptake. (*From Jones et al,[15] with permission.*)

TABLE 19-2

Variables Associated with a Decline in Exercise Capacity with Age

Variable	Comment
Decreased muscle mass Increased fat mass	These changes especially affect $\dot{V}_{O_2peak}$ calculated per kg of body weight

Decreased cardiac output
oxygen
  Decreased maximal stroke volume
  Decreased maximal heart rate
Decreased maximal $C(a - \bar{v})O_2$ difference
Decreased maximum voluntary ventilation
	As a result of the decreased cardiac output and maximal $C(a - \bar{v})O_2$, delivery and extraction are reduced; decreased cardiac output is a major contributor to the age-related decline in exercise capacity

Increased ventilation at each workload Increased oxygen cost of breathing	At each workload, older individuals breathe more and work harder for each breath than younger persons; however, the effect is small and contributes little to the decline in exercise capacity with aging
Sedentary life-style Decreased training intensity in active persons Decreased willingness to work to maximal level during tests	Life-style issues play a large role in the rate at which exercise capacity is lost with age; the good news is that, like other deconditioned groups, the elderly respond very well to exercise training

Specifically, there is an increase in total body weight, primarily representing an increase in fat mass, since fat-free mass (mostly muscle mass) decreases with aging. The changes are most pronounced in sedentary persons. Muscle mass decreases, with a preferential atrophy of type II muscle fibers, and is associated with a decrease in muscle capillarization and oxidative activity. Muscle strength decreases on the order of 2 percent/year from ages 20 to 70. Variables associated with loss of exercise capacity with aging are listed in Table 19-2.

While exercise capacity declines with aging, it is also clear that the ability to respond to exercise conditioning is well maintained even at very advanced ages. Elderly individuals respond to both endurance and resistive training with improvements similar in magnitude to those seen in the young. There are equivalent increases in $\dot{V}_{O_2peak}$, muscle mass, capillarization of muscle tissue, muscle oxidative activity, and general muscle strength.

SLEEP

Sleep complaints from elderly patients present a difficult problem for the clinician, who must determine whether the complaints are related to the normal aging process, to sleep hygiene issues, or to the presence of pathology.[33,34] Problems with sleep are widespread among elderly persons, with 25 to 40 percent complaining about sleep difficulties. There is no evidence to confirm the widely held belief that the need for sleep declines with age. However, sleep quality decreases, and the frequency of various primary sleep disorders increases. The most common age-related change in sleep pattern is a striking increase in the number of nocturnal awakenings, resulting in lower total sleep time and lower sleep efficiency (total sleep time/time in bed). Whether or not sleep latency changes with aging is equivocal. The amount of

time spent in stage 1 non–rapid eye movement (NREM or light) sleep tends to increase with age. The decrease in total sleep time at night is associated with an increase in unwanted daytime naps. Disrupted sleep in the elderly is, in large part, explained by medical and psychological issues and the lack of structured physical and social activity during the day. Chronic illnesses, nocturia, medication and alcohol use, periodic leg movements, bereavement, and depression also play a role. Not surprisingly, the elderly are more likely to be using sedatives or hypnotics; their use is more frequent in elderly women than in elderly men. While hypnotics and sedatives are occasionally necessary, their chronic use may contribute to sleep disruption and aggravate certain sleep disturbances, such as sleep apnea. Increased autonomic activity, increased sensitivity to external stimuli (which may increase arousals as a result of environmental factors), decreased exposure to outdoor light, inactivity, and daytime napping also play a role in sleep disruptions in the elderly. Alterations in endogenous circadian rhythms for variables like temperature and cortisol or thyroid-stimulating hormone (TSH) levels may also contribute to sleep disruption in the elderly.

However, the neural system that regulates sleep is, like most other systems, subject to the "normal" aging process, and sleep disruption occurs in the elderly in the absence of any pathological process. The amount of stages 3 and 4 sleep (slow- or delta-wave sleep) declines with aging, though some argue that the aging decline is mostly a technical issue related to how delta-wave amplitude is defined. Changes in slow-wave sleep appear to be evident early, perhaps by 20 years of age. Arguments have been made both for and against declines in the amount of REM sleep with age. The persistent controversy about REM sleep and aging suggests that if REM sleep does change with aging, the magnitude of decline is so small that it does not overwhelm the confounding factors in studies.

Sleep disorders such as sleep apnea and restless legs syndrome, with periodic limb movements, appear to be more prevalent in older persons, and they are also more marked among nursing home residents than the independent elderly. For example, using an apnea index of five per hour as a threshold, one study found evidence of sleep apnea in 42 percent of elderly nursing home residents, in contrast to 24 percent of the independent elderly. Some argue that sleep disorders are associated with less morbidity and mortality in the elderly, but the data are inconsistent and remain inconclusive.

INTERPRETING PULMONARY FUNCTION TESTS IN THE ELDERLY

Several issues complicate the interpretation of lung function tests in the elderly.[2] The elderly are not well represented in most reference value reports; the number of subjects usually falls off significantly after age 60. The number of subjects over age 80 is usually so small that mean values calculated from regression equations are essentially an extrapolation of the data for younger persons. This means that the average or "predicted" value may not be as representative for the elderly as it is for middle-aged persons. The fall in sample size with aging likely reflects the reduced total number of candidates for participation and the larger number of individuals who fail screening criteria. In reference value studies, individuals are screened so as to be free of symptoms and illnesses that alter lung function. These selection criteria may eliminate more older than younger candidates because of their increased prevalence of illness. Also, test quality is carefully standardized. Cognitive impairment may compromise test quality. As a result, older individuals may have more difficulty meeting test quality criteria, increasing their likelihood of exclusion and potentially increasing the variability of reference data for the elderly. In summary, the selection processes may make the older individuals who participate in reference studies less representative of the individuals who present for clinical lung function testing.

These same issues also affect the limits applied to determine whether a tested individual is within the "normal" range. Limits are often defined assuming that the distribution of data is gaussian. Although tests of this assumption are sparse, there is reason to suspect that it is more likely to fail in the elderly. Even when the "normal" range is defined using methods that avoid assumptions about data distribution, data from the elderly are often lumped with those of younger subjects. The result may be an erroneous "normal" range. These reference value issues all suggest that increased caution should be used in interpreting lung function tests in the elderly. This caution is especially important for those over age 80 and in any elderly person whose data lie near the limits of a "normal" range.

REFERENCES

1. Akiyama Y, Nishimure M, Kobayaski S, et al: Effects of aging on respiratory load compensation and dyspnea sensation. *Am Rev Respir Dis* 148:1586–1591, 1993.

2. Becklake MR, Crapo RO (co-chairs): Lung function testing: Selection of reference values and interpretative strategies—Official Statement of the American Thoracic Society. *Am Rev Respir Dis* 144:1202–1218, 1991.

3. Black LF, Hyatt, RE: Maximal respiratory pressures: Normal values and relationship to age and sex. *Am Rev Respir Dis* 99:696–702, 1969.

4. Bliwise DL: Normal aging, in Kryger MH, Roth T, Dement WC (eds): *Principles and Practice of Sleep Medicine,* 2d ed. Philadelphia, Saunders, 1994, pp 26–37.

5. Brischetto MJ, Millman RP, Peterson DD, et al: Effect of aging on ventilatory response to exercise and CO_2. *J Appl Physiol* 56:1143–1150, 1984.

6. Chapman KR, Cherniack NS: Aging effects on the interaction of hypercapnia and hypoxia as ventilatory stimuli. *J Gerontol* 42:202–209, 1987.

7. Chen H-S, Kuo C-S: Relationship between respiratory muscle function and age, sex, and other factors. *J Appl Physiol* 66:943–948, 1989.

8. Crapo RO: The aging lung, in Mahler DA (ed): *Pulmonary Disease in the Elderly Patient.* Vol 63: Lenfant C (ed): *Lung Biology in Health and Disease.* New York: Marcel Dekker, 1993, pp 1–25.

9. Crapo RO, Gardner RM (co-chairs): Single breath carbon monoxide diffusing capacity (transfer factor): Recommendations for a standard technique. *Am Rev Respir Dis* 136:1299–1307, 1987.

10. Crapo RO, Morris AH, Gardner RM: Reference values for pulmonary tissue volume, membrane diffusing capacity, and pulmonary capillary blood volume. *Bull Eur Physiopathol Respir* 18:893–899, 1982.

11. Davidson WR, Fee EC: Influence of aging on pulmonary hemodynamics in a population free of coronary artery disease. *Am J Cardiol* 65:1454–1458, 1990.

12. Ehrsam RE, Perruchaud A, Oberholzer M, et al: Influence of age on pulmonary hemodynamics at rest and during supine exercise. *Clin Sci* 65:653–660, 1983.

13. Gibellino F, Osmanliev DP, Watson A, Pride NB: Increase in tracheal size with age: Implications for maximal expiratory flow. *Am Rev Respir Dis* 132:784–787, 1985.

14. Johnson BD, Dempsey JA: Demand vs capacity in the aging pulmonary systems. *Exec Sport Sci Rev* 19:171–210, 1991.

15. Jones NL, Summers E, Killian KG: Influence of age and stature on exercise capacity during incremental cycle ergometry in men and women. *Am Rev Respir Dis* 140:1373–1380, 1969.

16. Knudson RJ, Clark DF, Kennedy TC, Knudson DE: Effect of aging alone on mechanical properties of the normal adult human lung. *J Appl Physiol: Respir Environ Exerc Physiol* 43:1054–1062, 1977.

17. Kronenberg RS, Drage CW: Attenuation of the ventilatory and heart rate responses to hypoxia and hypercapnia with aging in normal men. *J Clin Invest* 53:1812–1819, 1973.

18. Mahler DA, Rosiello RA, Loke J: The aging lung. *Geriatr Clin North Am* 2:215–225, 1986.

19. McClaran SR, Babcock MA, Pegelow DF, et al: Longitudinal effects of aging on lung function at rest and exercise in healthy active fit elderly adults. *J Appl Physiol* 78:1957–1958, 1995.

20. McElvaney GL, Blackie S, Morrison NJ, et al: Maximal static respiratory pressures in the normal elderly. *Am Rev Respir Dis* 139:277–281, 1989.

21. Mittman C, Edelman NH, Norris AH, Shock NW: Relationship between chest wall and pulmonary compliance and age. *J Appl Physiol* 20:1211–1216, 1965.

22. Neas LM, Schwartz J. The determinants of pulmonary diffusing capacity in a national sample of U.S. adults. *Am J Respir Crit Care Med* 153:656–664, 1996.

23. Nunn AJ, Gregg I: New regression equations for predicting peak expiratory flow in adults. *Br Med J* 298:1068–1070, 1989.

24. Pack AI, Millman RP: The lungs in later life, in Fishman AP (ed): *Pulmonary Diseases and Disorders.* New York, McGraw Hill, 1988, pp 79–90.

25. Paoletti P, Pistelli G, Fazzi P, et al: Reference values for vital capacity and flow-volume curves from a general population study. *Bull Eur Physiopathol Respir* 22:451–459, 1986.

26. Peterson DD, Fishman AP: Aging of the respiratory system, in Fishman AP (ed): *Update: Pulmonary Diseases and Disorders.* New York: McGraw-Hill, 1992, pp 1–17.

27. Peterson DD, Pack AI, Silage DA, Fishman AP: Effects of aging on the ventilatory and occlusion pressure responses to hypoxia and hypercapnia. *Am Rev Respir Dis* 124:387–391, 1981.

28. Pierce JA, Ebert RV: Fibrous network of the lung and its change with age. *Thorax* 20:469–476, 1965.

29. Pride NB: *Bull Eur Physiopathol Respir* 10:103–108, 1974.

30. Quanjer PH, (ed): Standardized lung function. *Bull Eur Physiopathol Res* 19:45–51, 66–92, 1983.

31. Robbins DR, Enright PL, Sherrill DL: Lung function development in young adults: Is there a plateau phase? *Eur Respir J* 8:768–772, 1995.

32. Shapiro SD, Endicott SK, Province MA, et al: Marked longevity of human lung parenchymal elastic fibers deduced from prevalence of D-aspartate and nuclear weapons–related radiocarbon. *J Clin Invest* 87:1828–1834, 1990.

33. Stam H, Hrachovina V, Stijnen T, Versprille A: Diffusing capacity dependent on lung volume and age in normal subjects. *J Appl Physiol* 76:2356–2363, 1994.

34. Turner JM, Mead J, Wohl ME: Elasticity of human lungs in relation to age. *J Appl Physiol* 25:664–671, 1968.

35. Van Pelt W, Borsboom GJJM, Rijcken B, et al: Discrepancies between longitudinal and cross-sectional change in ventilatory function in 12 years of follow-up. *Am J Respir Crit Care Med* 149:1218–1226, 1994.

36. Vitiello MV, Prinz PN: Sleep and sleep disorders in normal aging in Thorpy MJ (ed): *Handbook of Sleep Disorders.* New York, Marcel Dekker, 1990, pp 139–151.

37. Ware JH, Dockery DW, Louis TA, et al: Longitudinal and cross-sectional estimates of pulmonary function decline in never-smoking adults. *Am J Epidemiol* 132:685–700, 1990.

38. Wasserman K, Hansen JE, Sue DY, et al: *Principles of Exercise Testing and Interpretation,* 2d ed. Philadelphia, Lea & Febiger, 1994.

CHAPTER 20

PULMONARY DEFENSE MECHANISMS AGAINST INFECTIONS

Herbert Y. Reynolds / Jack A. Elias

SPECIALIZED REGIONAL DEFENSES
    Nose and Oropharynx
    Conducting Airways
    The Alveolar Spaces
    Lymphocytes in the Alveolar Space

DEFECTS IN HOST DEFENSES THAT CAN BE ASSOCIATED WITH RESPIRATORY INFECTIONS

HOST DEFENSES IN THE APPROACH TO PATIENTS WITH PULMONARY DISEASE

The atmosphere that we breathe is more than just "air." In reality, it is a complex mixture of gases and particulates to which virus- and bacteria-containing droplets can be added when respiratory secretions are coughed or sneezed out by others. Moreover, humans frequently aspirate secretions from the upper respiratory tract, particularly during sleep. The respiratory system must recognize and eliminate these unwanted elements in inspired air to keep pulmonary structures free of infection. This is accomplished by the complex and multifaceted defenses that protect the respiratory tract. The fact that the normal respiratory tract is infection-free despite its constant exposure to foreign antigens and infectious agents is testimony to the efficiency of these defense mechanisms. The evolving appreciation of direct associations between breakdowns of these defenses and pulmonary diseases and disorders emphasizes the need for all physicians to be familiar with these critical protective processes.

Elements of the defense system are spaced along the entire respiratory tract, from the point of air intake at the nose and mouth to the level of oxygen uptake at the alveolar surface. The conducting airways functionally include the segments from the nares down to the respiratory bronchioles. In these segments the nasal turbinates, epiglottis, larynx, and other anatomic barriers are prominent. The dichotomous branching of the respiratory tree in this region also causes the airstream to deflect the particles it contains onto the mucosal surface, trapping them in airway mucus. In this location, inhaled particulates and infectious agents also interact with other locally produced proteins, such as secretory IgA. As a result of these interactions, ciliary clearance, and coughing, these particulates are efficiently removed from the respiratory tree. Beyond the respiratory bronchioles, other host defenses are important in protecting the alveolar units (Fig. 20-1). These defenses are in the lining material of the alveoli, which contains surfactant and glycoproteins such as fibronectin, immunoglobulins such as IgG opsonins, and complement (properdin factor B), which are active against aerosolized, inhaled particles or microorganisms.

Alveolar macrophages are the principal phagocytic and scavenger cells on alveolar surfaces. Materials that evade other host defense mechanisms and arrive on the alveolar surface are efficiently removed by these roaming cells. When further assistance is required, an inflammatory reaction can be initiated,[35,44] which attracts polymorphonuclear neutrophils (PMNs) and other vasomediators and humoral immune elements from systemic sources.

At all levels of the respiratory tract, specific and nonspecific defense mechanisms exist to protect respiratory structures. The nonspecific mechanisms, as noted above, include the mechanical barriers, mucociliary elevator, and macrophage phagocytosis,

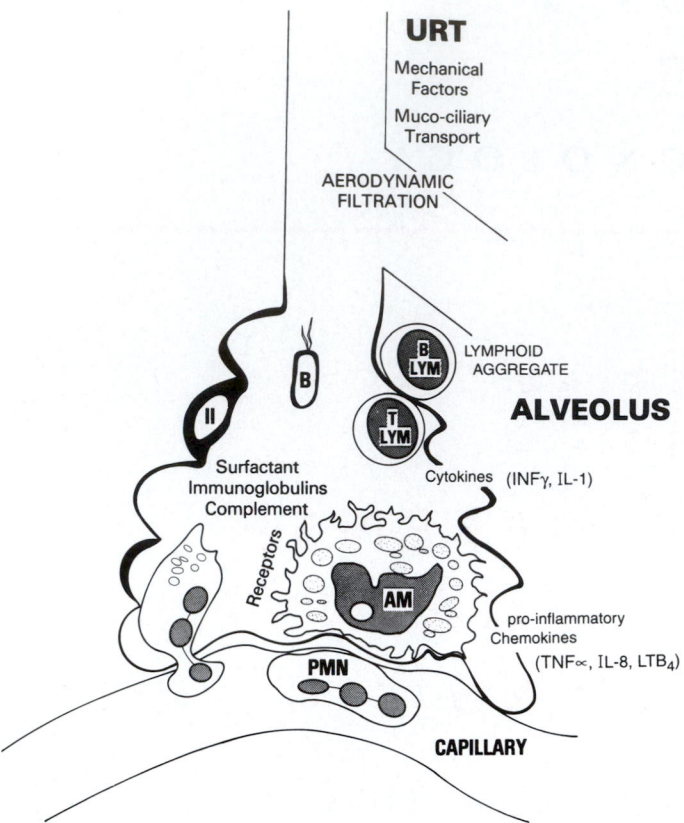

FIGURE 20-1 Defenses mechanisms in the alveolar spaces. If a bacterium (B) should elude the filtration mechanisms in the upper respiratory tract (URT) and enter the alveolus, several host mechanisms can defend against it: various opsonins, phagocytes such as an alveolar macrophage (AM), or PMNs attracted from an adjacent capillary site. T-lymphocytes (T-lym) can stimulate AM by cytokines and in turn AM can initiate an inflammatory response with chemokines. *(Modified from Reynolds,[33] with permission.)*

which behave similarly regardless of the inhaled particulate. In contrast, prior contact with a microbial agent or a sensitizing substance can induce antigen-specific cellular or humoral immune responses. The latter includes the production of secretory IgA in the airway, which prevents mucosal adherence, and IgG opsonins that facilitate phagocytosis. Such responses help the lung deal more efficiently with these agents and substances on rechallenge in the future.

In summary, the integrated action of diverse pulmonary defense mechanisms along the respiratory tract acts to remove or neutralize microorganisms, particulates, and noxious gases that are inhaled or aspirated into respiratory structures. Many are mechanical barriers and reflex actions that are concentrated in the nasooropharynx and along the conducting airways. There is also phagocytosis, which occurs in the alveoli and airways. These are surveillance mechanisms that function mechanically and can be activated by nonspecific (nonimmunologic) or immunogenic stimuli. In addition, several augmenting mechanisms exist that enhance the responsiveness of this defense system and make it flexible and adaptable. Crucial in this regard is the ability of the lung to mount antigen-specific immune responses (humoral and cellular) and to mount a local inflammatory reaction. This allows components in plasma and blood cells to bolster local resources

in the airways and alveoli. A more in-depth review of these defense mechanisms is detailed below.

SPECIALIZED REGIONAL DEFENSES

Nose and Oropharynx

Inhaled air passes through the glottis and into the extrathoracic portion of the trachea before it enters the thorax. With nasal breathing, air is filtered and conditioned for humidity and body temperature as it flows over the nasal turbinates and mucosa of the posterior pharynx. With nasal obstruction or ventilatory requirements for exertion that exceed about 20 to 30 L/min, mouth breathing occurs. Inhaled air then passes into the trachea without optimal filtering and climatic conditioning.

The nose provides formidable barriers to inhaled particulates. The nasal hairs help to exclude large particles, and materials greater than 10 μm in diameter that bypass the hairs impact upon the nasal mucosa. Sneezing (or blowing) then has the effect of coughing and provides high-velocity ejection from the mucosal surface. For substances that attach to the nasal mucosa, production of large quantities of watery secretions helps to wash off the surface (rhinorrhea). Mucociliary clearance is also operant in the nasal cavity. "Downspouts" leading from the ears, lacrimal glands, and sinus cavities provide numerous points for the addition of fluid to the nasal secretions. However, these drainage systems also contain vulnerable points that are prone to blockage.[33] The complex plumbing found in the nose works well if there is good gravitational flow and orifices stay open. If not, sinusitis, otitis media, and occluded tear ducts result.

Several substances in nasal secretions help control bacteria or viruses. Prominent in this regard are lysozyme and immunoglobulins, especially secretory IgA (SIgA). The nose has been studied extensively (see review[33]). Nasal secretions, like those from other external or mucosal surfaces, are rich in IgA,[51] which is synthesized locally by submucosal plasma cells. Free secretory component (SC) can also be detected in nasal wash fluid. Of the nasal immunoglobulins, SIgA is the major source of antibody, accounting for approximately 10 percent of the total protein content of nasal washings. IgG is present in smaller amounts. IgE probably is not secreted by normal, nonatopic people. Only in people with allergic rhinitis will IgE antibody be substantial. The usual specificity of IgA antibody is antiviral. After nasal immunization of normal subjects with various viral or mycoplasmal vaccines, many experimental studies have shown that appropriate neutralizing IgA antibody can be elicited.[33] Although these antibodies are protective against homologous and live microbial challenge, the duration of protection is often brief, and the antibody titers diminish rapidly unless repeated exposure occurs.

In the oral cavity, the tongue sweeps against many surfaces during chewing and swallowing. This should make it difficult for bacteria to persist in these locations. However, bacteria adhere to buccal squamous cells,[25] and many accumulate in crevices around teeth and gums. Many kinds of bacteria are present: aerobes and anaerobes, spirochetes, gram-positive and gram-negative species, and some that specialize in making dental plaque and causing tooth decay. A common feature of host defense in the mouth and nose is the plentiful amount of SIgA in secretions that bathe each area. The parotid glands and probably the submandibular salivary glands secrete IgA as their principal humoral immune substance; this immunoglobulin accounts for 12 to 15 percent of the total protein in their secretions.[50] In this fluid, albumin represents about 10 percent of the protein, but IgG is barely detectable (under 1 percent). In parotid fluid, IgA is found in monomeric and dimeric forms, and free secretory component can be detected as well. Thus, normal nasal and parotid (or salivary) secretions have about the same composition of immunoglobulins. As with the nasal immune system, it has been possible to manipulate SIgA in the mouth to produce antibodies against certain cariogenic strains of streptococci that will subsequently prevent bacterial adherence to teeth. The importance of this approach for augmenting dental defenses has yet to be determined.

Host defenses in the nose and mouth serve as a reminder that the upper portion of the respiratory tract has features in common with the lower part, particularly at the mucosal surfaces. They also demonstrate that infections in the nose, sinuses, ears, teeth, and gums may have ramifications for the diagnosis or successful treatment of illness in the lower respiratory tract. As examples, aspiration of anaerobic bacteria in oral secretions contributes to lung abscess formation; chronic sinusitis can be present with cystic fibrosis, dyskinetic ciliary syndromes, and dysgammaglobulinemia; atopic diseases can manifest with rhinitis, sinusitis, and asthma; and control of asthma symptoms often requires vigorous treatment of concomitant sinus infection.

Conducting Airways

Bridging the upper airway (nose, oropharynx, and larynx) and the alveolar air-exchange area distal to the terminal bronchioles are the conducting airways. Mucociliary clearance and coughing are the principal means of cleansing the mucosal surfaces of these airways. SIgA antibodies also prevent epithelial attachment of certain bacteria and viruses to the ciliated and nonciliated airway epithelial cells. The branching structure of the airways also causes airborne particulates to impact against the mucosa, enhancing the efficiency of mucociliary clearance. This segment is susceptible to many diseases—e.g., epithelial cell infection with viruses or bacteria such as *Bordetella pertussis, Chlamydia pneumoniae,* or *Mycoplasma pneumoniae;* inflammation, edema, and bronchoconstriction in asthmatic syndromes; chronic infection in bronchiectasis; irritation from noxious gases; and lung cancer.

The airway mucosa is coated with viscous fluid, which has a low pH (6.8 to 6.9)[28] and is secreted by bronchial glands, globlet cells, and probably Clara cells (nonciliated bronchiolar secretory cells found in the terminal bronchioles). Fluid is also derived from the intravascular space by diffusion through the blood-air barrier. Special proteins, such as SIgA and SC, can be added locally along airways by immunoglobulin-secreting plasma cells and epithelial cells.

The mucosal epithelial cells have beating cilia that propel secretions up the respiratory tree. Periodic coughing can assist the process. An intact mucosal lining and overlying mucous layer provide a protective barrier that prevents inhaled particulates

from penetrating or sticking to the respiratory surface. This seems to be an important component of host defense. Bacteria and other infectious agents may transiently colonize the airways, but mucociliary clearance effectively removes them.[34] Tight junctions between epithelial cells also prevent the passage of macromolecules into the submucosa. A number of circumstances can alter these protective barriers, making this portion of the respiratory tract susceptible to disease. They include (1) malnutrition, which affects the integrity of mucosal epithelial cells and enhances bacterial adherence;[24] (2) cigarette smoke and noxious fumes which disrupt the anatomy of epithelial junctions and enhance the passage of airway substances into areas that are usually inaccessible; and (3) some bacteria, which elaborate proteolytic enzymes that may break down IgA, promoting selective colonization.

Lymphoid tissue is present along the entire respiratory tract, but the level of organization of the lymphoid tissue varies greatly. Lymphoid nodules may occur in the mucosal surface of large and medium-sized bronchi and are particularly numerous at points of airway branching.[4] On the airway side, these submucosal follicles are covered by a layer of flattened, nonciliated surface epithelium, which is often observed to be infiltrated with lymphocytes.[31] These bronchial-associated lymphoid tissues (BALT) bear some resemblance to gut-associated lymphoid tissues (Peyer's patches).[4] Whereas BALT is easily demonstrated in some rodents and rabbits, subhuman primates and humans have decidedly less obvious amounts of this lymphoid tissue, and it may not be as relevant to airway defenses as initially thought, especially in adults.[27]

Loosely organized collections of lymphocytes (lymphoid aggregates) are concentrated in the distal airways, especially at the bronchoalveolar junctions at the interface between the ciliated epithelial cells of the terminal bronchioles and the alveolar lining cells. These aggregates provide an opportunity for close interaction between lymphoid cells and inhaled antigens that have been deposited in the lower respiratory tract. Also, in the vicinity of the respiratory bronchioles, lymphatic channels begin that might provide these lymphocytes with a route to draining lymph nodes (hilar nodes) where immunologic responses develop.

The Alveolar Spaces

Defenses in the airways (Fig. 20-1) eliminate most particles and microbes inspired into the lungs. As a result, the airways distal to the major bronchi are probably sterile in normal subjects.[10] However, some particles of small size and special geometry can elude the above-named mechanisms and reach the air-exchange surface of the alveolar spaces. When this occurs, another set of host defense mechanisms must take over. Anatomically, lung structure changes at the level of respiratory bronchioles so that in the acinar units (alveolar ducts and alveoli) ciliated epithelium and mucus-secreting cells (goblet cells and mucous glands) are no longer present. Mucociliary clearance is not operant, nor does coughing effectively clear material from the alveoli. Microbial clearance and the removal of other antigenic material from alveoli depend on cellular and humoral factors such as the lipoproteins, immunoglobulins, and complement factors in the alveolar lining material and phagocytic cells such as alveolar macrophages and PMNs.[44]

Inhaled microbes are an appropriate example. If a bacterium of critical size (0.5 to 3 μm in diameter) is deposited in an alveolus, it is likely to make contact with the alveolar wall and roll along in the alveolar lining fluid. In the process, it encounters several substances that can inactivate it and assist in its eventual phagocytosis. These substances include a variety of soluble lipoprotein substances, IgG, complement factor (C3b), and nonimmune opsonins, such as high-molecular-weight fibronectin fragments. The lipoproteins, in the form of surfactant, are secreted by type II pneumocytes and may have opsonic effects and antibacterial activity against staphylococci and rough colony strains of some gram-negative rod bacteria.[7,29] The immunoglobulins[17] are principally of the IgG class. They account for 5 percent of the total protein in alveolar fluid, with subclasses IgG1 and IgG3 being the most important and lesser concentrations of monomeric and secretory forms of IgA being noted. These immunoglobulins have specific opsonic antibody activity for the bacterium. The complement components, especially properdin factor B, interact with the bacterium and can trigger the alternative complement pathway, thereby lysing the microbe directly.[38] One or all of these interactions can prepare the bacterium for ingestion by an alveolar macrophage. Although alveolar macrophages avidly phagocytose some inert particles, they ingest viable bacteria with considerably less enthusiasm. Coating or opsonizing the organisms will enhance phagocytosis appreciably in an in vitro culture system. The nonimmune opsonins nonspecifically enhance this process. The immunoglobulins are capable of enhancing alveolar macrophage phagocytosis in an antigen-specific fashion, and the C3b complement fragment can function in concert with IgG to enhance or amplify this process.[37]

Phagocytosis, the ingestion of particulate matter by cells, is divided into two phases: attachment of the particle to the cell surface and internalization. Attachment of the particle to the surface of the phagocytic cell is essential before ingestion occurs. Although binding occurs randomly, it is greatly enhanced by opsonization of the particle by antibody (especially IgG) or a component of the complement system, C3b.[37] Opsonin-dependent phagocytosis is mediated by receptors on the cell surface for the Fc component of the opsonizing immunoglobulin or complement. Receptors for the Fc portion of IgG (Fcγ) (IgG3 and IgG1 primarily) and for the third component of complement (C3b) are present on human monocytes and alveolar macrophages.[37] Receptors for IgA are also found on alveolar macrophages.[43] There is evidence that the number and function of these receptors can be modulated by lymphocyte-derived cytokines such as γ-interferon.[22] Ingestion of membrane-bound particles occurs via a process that is energy-dependent as the plasma membrane of the ingesting cell surrounds the bound particle, enclosing it in an endocytic vesicle. This is followed by the activation of a number of well-developed mechanisms that operate to kill internalized pathogens.[44]

Following internalization of bacteria, the fate of alveolar macrophages is not certain. They are long-lived tissue cells that can survive at least for several months and presumably are capable of handling repeated bacterial and other microbial challenges (reusable phagocytes). Because they are mobile cells, they can migrate quickly to other alveoli through the pores of Kohn, or move to more proximal areas of the respiratory tract (to the region of the respiratory bronchioles) for elimination from the lungs by the mucociliary escalator. In addition, macrophages may gain entry into lung lymphatics at the same place and be carried to regional lymph nodes. This exit gives them access to systemic lymphoid tissue and is important in initiating cellular immune responses. Undoubtedly, macrophages are also instrumental in degrading antigenic material and presenting it in an appropriate manner to local T lymphocytes.

Increasingly, attention is being given to the immune effector role of macrophages. The alveolar macrophage has a dual role in the respiratory tract—one as a phagocyte to dispose of debris, process foreign antigens, and kill ingested microorganisms and a second as an effector cell to initiate immune and inflammatory responses. Alveolar macrophages are usually successful in inactivating inhaled microorganisms. As a result, clinical disease and pneumonitis rarely develop after day-to-day exposures. However, if a sufficiently large bacterial inoculum reaches the lower respiratory tract, or if particularly virulent microorganisms are inhaled, the macrophage system can be overwhelmed. By the secretion of proinflammatory chemotactic factors such as the chemokine family cytokines, alveolar macrophages then recruit PMNs and other cells to the lung,[32,44,49] and pneumonitis develops.

Gram-negative rod bacteria provide an interesting example. Some complement components, particularly factor B, are present in small amounts in bronchoalveolar fluids.[38] The bacterial endotoxin in the gram-negative rod bacteria can directly activate the alternative complement pathway—leading to the formation of C5a, which is a potent stimulus for PMN chemotaxis. Also, the inflammatory response may activate the kinin system; this results in generation of kallikrein, which has chemotactic activity, and bradykinin, which is capable of increasing vascular permeability. The latter allows for the seepage of fluid and other humoral and bioactive substances from the intravascular compartment into the alveoli.[35] Another mechanism of inflammation emanates from the alveolar macrophage itself. Following phagocytosis of opsonized bacteria or other forms of activation, proinflammatory chemokines are synthesized and secreted by macrophages that will attract PMNs and other cells.[32,44,49] Several substances with chemotactic activity have been found to be produced by human alveolar macrophages. These include interleukin-8 (IL-8),[14,32,49] macrophage-inflammatory protein-1α (MIP-1α),[49] monocyte chemotactic protein–1 (MCP-1),[49] tumor necrosis factor (TNF),[3] and lipoxygenase pathway metabolites of arachidonic acid, namely leukotrienes.[16,32] Leukotriene B$_4$ is one of the most important of these.[16,32]

Inflammation is the ultimate host response to contain common bacteria that reach the alveolar space. This response can be activated in several ways: (1) directly by microbes or substances such as lipopolysaccharide (endotoxin) that can activate the complement cascade, probably via the alternate complement pathway;[38] (2) through the generation of phlogistic factors from the kallikrein and bradykinin pathways; and (3) from the effector cell function of macrophages.[3,14,16,32,44,49] It is also known that other airway cells, such as epithelial cells,[23] elsewhere in the respiratory tract, can produce chemokines like IL-8 and that this can stimulate inflammation in other sites (bronchitis).

Special interest has focused on the macrophage-secreted proinflammatory chemokines,[44,49] a family of cytokines that can stimulate cellular motion (chemokinesis) and promote directed migration of different populations of responder cells (chemotaxis). These populations are primarily PMNs in the acute inflammatory responses. Lymphocytes, monocytes, and eosinophils are also recruited in the chronic phase of pneumonia, chronic inflammatory disorders such as hypersensitivity pneumonitis and sarcoidosis, and atopic and eosinophilic syndromes.[35,49] Recently, investigation has elucidated the cellular mechanisms whereby chemokines activate and initiate the migratory process of PMNs. This now extensive literature cannot be fully reviewed here.[15,46,49] Suffice it to say that this process involves a number of cell surface adhesion molecules, found on endothelial cells and granulocytes, that bind to one another.[15,35,46,49] At sites of inflammation mediators such as IL-1, tumor necrosis factor and γ-interferon induce or augment the expression of these adhesion molecules. As a result, intravascular PMNs slow down, roll along, and then anchor[15] on the endothelium. They then enter the interstitium via poorly understood processes.

Eventually, all pneumonic responses run their course. If the host is successful in containing the infective microbes or particles that initially incited the host response, resolution usually occurs. Resolution can be passive, resulting from the removal of the initiating agent. Resolution can have an active phase as well.[35] In this active phase, signals must go out to begin the healing and resorption phases that will restore the lung to normal respiratory function and architecture. Less is known about active resolution of inflammation. However, cytokines such as transforming growth factor-β, IL-6, IL-10, and the IL-1 receptor antagonist released by macrophages and possibly other cells are believed to be important mediators of this process.[1,8,20,52] As such, they provide a view of potential anti-inflammatory therapies of the future.

Lymphocytes in the Alveolar Space

When cells are retrieved from the alveolar surface by bronchoalveolar lavage (BAL), approximately 7 to 10 percent of the respiratory cells are lymphocytes. The characteristics of these cells are given in Table 20-1.[12] Two major populations of lymphoid cells are recognized, those that depend on the thymus gland for differentiation (T cells) and those that differentiate independently of the thymus in the bone marrow (B cells). The T and B lymphocytes are indistinguishable by usual morphologic criteria but can be differentiated by membrane surface markers. They are also functionally distinct, with T cells playing an important role in cell-mediated immunity and cell-mediated cytotoxicity while the B cells serve as precursors for cells that synthesize immunoglobulins and, hence, antibody molecules that are the basis of the humoral immune response.

As shown in Table 20-1, approximately 70 percent of the lymphocytes in lavage fluid are T cells and approx-imately 5 percent are B cells. The ratio of T to B cells in lavage fluid is roughly that of peripheral blood, although in blood more circulating B cells are usually identified (approximately 15 percent). Approximately 1 to 5 percent of lung lymphocytes seem to be able to release or secrete class-specific immunoglobulin. Enumeration of these cells has found that IgG- and IgA-secreting cells are much more numerous than IgM-producing cells. Natural killer lymphocytes make up about 5 to 8 percent of lung lymphocytes, but they are not especially active in the normal lung.[39]

With phenotypic markers, T cells can be divided into two principal groups. The CD8 cells usually have a suppressor-cytotoxic phenotype. The CD4 cells usually have a helper-inducer phenotype and thus are also called T helper (TH) cells. In the BAL fluid from normal subjects there is a greater percentage of CD4 cells, with approximately 45 percent of the total T cells expressing this surface marker. In contrast, approximately 25 percent of lung T cells express the CD8 phenotype. In lung lavage fluid, the ratio of these subtypes of T cells is approximately 1.5 to 2:1, which is approximately the same ratio found among peripheral blood lymphocytes.

As noted, most of the T lymphocytes in the alveoli are CD4-positive. When activated, these T-helper cells are capable of producing regulatory cytokines that in turn modulate the function of other immune and structural cells. Recent studies suggest that there are at least two subsets of CD4 TH cells, T helper–1 (TH1) and T helper–2 (TH2) cells. These cell populations have different functions based on the different array of cytokines that they produce.[19,21] The TH1 cells secrete inteferon-γ and IL-2, which activate macrophages and play a major role in cell-mediated immunity. The TH2 cells produce IL-4, IL-5, and IL-6, which stimulate B lymphocytes to produce immunoglobulins and, by their production of IL-10 and IL-13, suppress monocyte/macrophage activity and cell-mediated immune responses.[18,21,30] Thus, TH2 cells play a particularly important role in generating tissue eosinophilia and stimulating IgE production, processes that are extremely important in atopy, allergic asthma, and other inflammatory pulmonary disorders. Interleukin-2 (IL-2), formerly called T-cell growth factor (TCGF), is among the most important T-cell–regulating cytokines. It is produced by activated T cells[42] and acts in an autocrine or paracrine fashion to stimulate TH1 cells and TH2 cell precursors. IL-2 can also activate killer T cells. A few killer lymphocytes can be identified among alveolar T cells, but these cells seem to be dormant in normal subjects until stim-

TABLE 20-1

T-Lymphocyte Subgroups in Lung Lavage Fluid from Normal Subjects

Fluid	Cell Count ×10⁶	Lymphocytes (%)	T Cells (%)	CD4 (T Helper) (%)	CD8 (T Suppressor) (%)
Lung lavage*	10±4†	7±1	73±5	46 (35–55)	25 (18–32)
Blood				48 (40–60)	28 (22–40)

*Cells from 300-ml lavages of six normal nonsmokers.
†Mean ± SEM; range observed in parentheses.
SOURCE: From Hunninghake and Crystal.[12]

ulated.[39] Lastly, IL-2 can stimulate B lymphocytes to differentiate into plasma cells that synthesize various classes of immunoglobulins. This is a mechanism by which local production of immunoglobulin in the lung can occur. In all cases, the effects of IL-2 are mediated by the multimeric IL-2 receptor, a component of which is the Tac surface ligand. The expression of the IL-2 receptor is highly regulatable, and the expression of the Tac antigen can be used as a marker of T-cell activation.

Most T cells have T-cell receptors with alpha and beta subunits (α/β T-cell receptors). In the normal lung, a lesser number of T cells have gamma and delta T-cell receptors. The function of these cells is poorly understood. They may, however, play an important role in mucosal immunity, since they are increased in atopic allergic subsets.[47]

Alveolar macrophages and lymphocytes have the capacity to produce many cellular mediators (cytokines) that in turn affect each other as well as other inflammatory, structural, and immune effector cells.[13,36,48] This dynamic and complex interaction is illustrated in Fig. 20-2, which reviews alveolar macrophage/lymphocyte interactions in the alveolar milieu. Monocyte precursors from the blood differentiate into mature macrophages under the influence of vitamin D metabolites and undoubtedly other stimuli and become long-lived, aerobically metabolizing alveolar phagocytes. Their principal activity is to cleanse the alveolar surface and ingest debris that accumulates or microbes aerosolized into the lungs. In the process, the macrophages may become "activated" and are then are capable of secreting an enormous array of enzymes and cytokines. These moieties can affect the function of resident cells of the lung such as lymphocytes or epithelial cells. In addition, the release of proinflammatory chemokines attracts PMNs, lymphocytes, monocytes, and other cells into the alveoli. Of particular note are LTB4, IL-8, TNFα, MIP-1α, MCP-1, and IL-1. The last, when secreted by activated macrophages (especially in active lung forms of sarcoidosis), may attract T lymphocytes to the lungs.[11]

In the other direction, activated TH cells can produce several monokines that affect macrophage function. Such a substance is migration inhibition factor, which immobilizes macrophages engaged in phagocytosis. Of special interest is γ-interferon, which activates macrophages, increasing their expression of membrane receptors, which in turn enhances macrophage phagocytic uptake. γ-Interferon also has other functions that promote cellular immunity.[22] The scheme shown in Fig. 20-2 may help to explain certain derangements found in a number of lung diseases that have excessive or deficient secretion of cytokines and feature changes in the relative proportions of macrophages and lymphocytes. Examples of such cellular imbalances include sarcoidosis, hypersensitivity pneumonitis, and the acquired immunodeficiency syndrome (reviewed elsewhere[36]).

DEFECTS IN HOST DEFENSES THAT CAN BE ASSOCIATED WITH RESPIRATORY INFECTIONS

Infection can occur everywhere along the respiratory tract—upper airways (nose, sinuses, and oropharynx), conducting airways (trachea and bronchi down to the respiratory bronchioles), or the alveolar area. Although exposure to a virulent microorganism or to a large inoculum, if inhaled or aspirated into the lungs, may cause illness in a normal person, recurrent or chronic infections may point to deficiency or malfunction of a particular component of the host defense system (Table 20-2).[33] A number of situations associated with frequent respiratory infections serve as examples. Endotracheal tubes give direct access to the lung but, in so doing, bypass the larynx and the other upper-airway protective structures. Patients with depressed consciousness or with postoperative chest or abdominal pain become infected because of their inability to cough and clear airway secretions. In addition, patients with viral infections have an increased incidence of bacterial superinfection. The cause of this association appears to be multifactorial, including the ability of these infectious agents to damage ciliated epithelial cells and diminish the clearance of airway secretions and to infect alveolar macrophages, diminishing their bactericidal activity. In

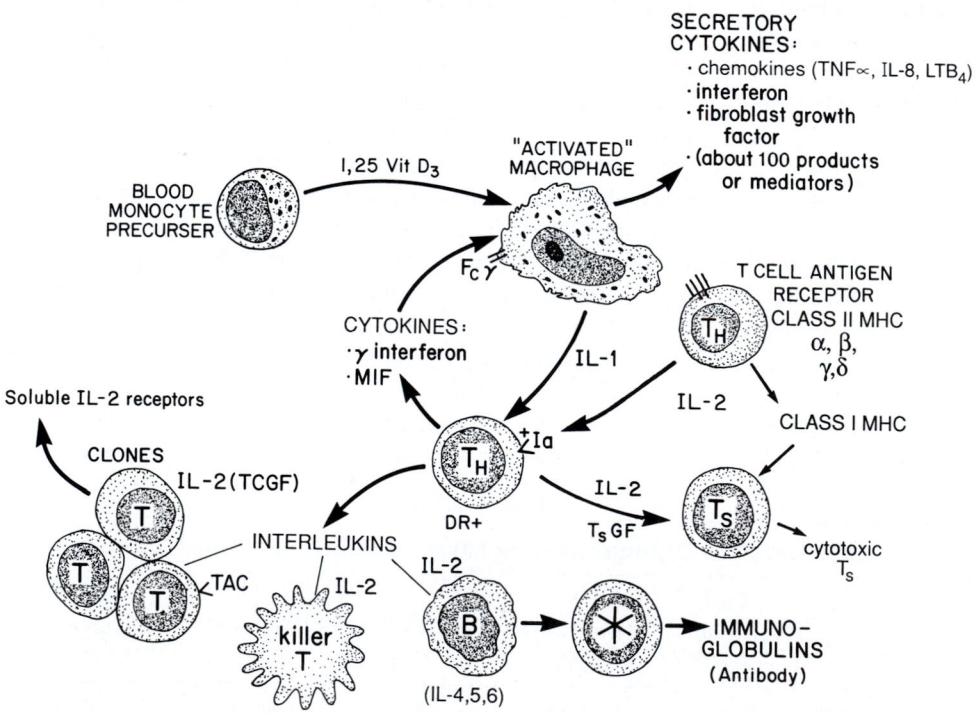

FIGURE 20-2   Some immunologic interactions on the alveolar surface involving macrophages and lymphocytes. Focusing on helper T-lymphocyte subtypes (T_H), these can produce cytokines that activate the alveolar macrophage, which in turn can secrete many cytokines itself with autocrine or paracrine functions. T_H through interleukins can promote cell function of the clonal expansion other T cells; also, B-lymphocytes or plasma cells can be stimulated to produce immunoglobulins. See text for further details. *(Modified from Reynolds HY: J Allergy Clin Immunol 78:833, 1986, with permission.)*

TABLE 20-2

Pulmonary Host Defenses

Component	Possible Impairment Defect	Related Impact or Infection
Conducting airways		
Mechanical barriers (larynx, etc.)	Bypassing barriers with an endo-tracheal tube or tracheostomy	Aspiration, direct aerosol of microbes into airway
Mucociliary clearance (cough)	Intrinsic structural defect in cilia; ciliotoxic infections	Stagnant secretions, coughing, bronchiectasis, sinusitis, pneumonitis
Bronchoconstriction and mucosal edema	Hyperactive airways; asthma	Poor removal of secretions; excessive secretions
Local immunoglobulin coating—secretory IgA	IgA deficiency or functional deficiency from breakdown by bacterial IgA1 proteases	Sinopulmonary infections; abnormal colonization with bacteria
Iron-containing proteins (transferrin, lactoferrin)	Iron deficiency	May not inhibit certain bacteria (*Pseudomonas, Legionella*)
Alveolar space		
Other immunoglobulin classes (opsonic IgG)	Acquired hypogammaglobulinemia; selective IgG2 and IgG4 deficiency	Sinopulmonary infections; pneumonia with encapsulated bacteria
Alternative complement pathway activation	C3 and C5 deficiency	Recurrent infection possible
Surfactant (protein)	Decreased synthesis; acute lung injury	Loss of opsonization activity; alveolar collapse (atelectasis)
Alveolar macrophages	Subtle effects from immunosuppression; cannot kill intracellular microbes	Propensity for intracellular microbes and *Legionella* infections; poor containment of *Mycobacterium* spp
Polymorphonuclear granulocytes	Absent because of immunosuppression; intrinsic defects of motility; lack of chemokine stimulus	Poor inflammatory response, associated with gram-negative bacillary infection and fungi (*Aspergillus*)
Augmenting mechanisms		
Initiation of immune responses (humoral antibody and cellular immunity)	Immunosuppression	Inadequate SIgA or IgG antibody available (more susceptible to viral, mycoplasmal, and bacterial infections)
Generation of an inflammatory response (influx of PMN granulocytes, eosinophils, lymphocytes, and fluid components)	Generally reflects status and supply of PMN granulocytes; impaired adherence to endothelium	Inadequate inflammatory response, recurrent infection

SOURCE: Modified from Reynolds,[33] with permission.

combination, these host defense defects are believed to contribute to the frequent association of influenza infection and staphylococcal superinfection.

Ultrastructural defects in the cilia[40,41] located on the apical edge of the airway epithelial lining cells cause mucociliary dysfunction. As a result, the removal of mucus and respiratory secretions is depressed, and recurrent infections and bronchiectasis occur. The constellation of multiple upper and lower respiratory infections and bronchiectasis should raise the possibility of a ciliary dyskinesis syndrome.[33] Infertility, especially in males, may be associated, and the evaluation of this problem may bring the respiratory symptoms to the physician's attention.

A variety of γ-globulin abnormalities are associated with recurrent infection. In patients with hypogammaglobulinemia, the lack of opsonic antibody can promote infections with encapsulated bacteria. Several common bacteria that colonize the airways of patients with chronic bronchitis and chronic obstructive pulmonary disease (*Streptococcus pneumoniae, Hemophilus influenzae,* and *Neisseria*) can also produce a specific IgA protease that cleaves the IgA heavy chain in its hinge region adjacent to the Fc portion.[34] By this mechanism, these bacteria could inactivate a substantial portion of the secretory IgA coating the conducting airways and gain better access to the ciliated epithelial cells for attachment. While this mechanism is somewhat theoretical, associations between deficiencies in IgG and recurrent infection are well documented. Particularly important are the associations between deficiencies of IgG subclasses IgG2 and IgG4, alone and in combination with IgA deficiencies and chronic inflammation and bronchiectasis.[2,26] Presumably, an absence of these subclasses denies phagocytic cells potential opsonic antibody, thereby diminishing membrane receptor attachment of opsonized particles or bacteria and subsequent phagocyte ingestion. Clinically, establishing the diagnosis of an IgG deficiency is quite important because, in contrast to many other immunodeficiencies, replacement preparations of IgG are often available for these patients.

Cytotoxic antineoplastic chemotherapy and other forms of immunosuppression also compromise host defenses in a major way. A major side effect of these therapies is granulocytopenia, which prevents the mobilization of PMNs and creates a poor inflammatory reaction.

HOST DEFENSES IN THE APPROACH TO PATIENTS WITH PULMONARY DISEASE

As noted above, normal hosts can develop respiratory infections or inflammation as a result of exposure to particularly virulent agents or a large inoculum of aerosolized particulates. In others, respiratory infections are associated with obvious clinical features that compromise pulmonary defenses (Table 20-2). Occasionally, however, the physician is confronted with a relatively young person who has an unexpected number of respiratory problems that seem inappropriate.[33] The illness can manifest as recurrent infection or poorly controlled allergic rhinitis, asthma, frequent sinusitis, recurrent nasal polyps, and/or bouts of otitis media. Because the severity of these respiratory problems may not seem great, the physician may not initially suspect that something unusual is present. The propensity for infection may not have been obvious in childhood but became apparent as the patient reached adolescence or adulthood. Although genetic defects usually are manifested in infancy, minor forms of host deficiency may not be recognized until later in life. Cystic fibrosis (adult onset), selective absence of IgG subclass immunoglobulins, structural ciliary defects, and IgA deficiency are the principal diseases that should be considered in this differential diagnosis. Recurrent sinopulmonary infections are an important clue to all these syndromes.

The physician should be prepared to examine such a patient thoroughly. A detailed history will immediately provide important information about affected siblings, infertility, or a striking change in respiratory health that makes an acquired abnormality likely. Preliminary screening tests are also indicated and may include microbial cultures of respiratory secretions and analysis of the electrolytes contained in a sample of sweat. Mucoid strains of *Pseudomonas aeruginosa* and elevated sweat chloride values can be noted in cystic fibrosis. Other useful screening tests are evaluations of quantitative serum immunoglobulins, including subclasses of IgG; secretory IgA as sampled in parotid fluid or nasal wash samples; subtyping of blood lymphocytes; assessment of ciliary clearance with an aerosolized, isotopic tracer; nasal mucosal biopsy for electron-microscopic ultrastructural analysis of cilia; sperm motility in males of appropriate age; and documentation of bronchiectasis by high-resolution chest computed tomographic scans. A thorough evaluation by an otolaryngologist is also often helpful because of the recurrent sinusitis, otitis media, and nasal polyps that might be present.

Alternatively, certain forms of pneumonia point to possible deficiencies in lung cells such as alveolar macrophages, lymphocytes, or PMNs. As opsonization of certain encapsulated bacteria is necessary for optimal phagocytosis by macrophages and PMNs, the lack of appropriate IgG antibodies against pneumococci, *Hemophilus* species, *Klebsiella pneumoniae,* and staphylococci may contribute to infections with these common bacteria. However, other causes of pneumonia may reflect abnormal lymphocyte function and cell-mediated immunity. Infection with *Legionella* bacteria is an example. After an infection with *L. pneumophila,* the host develops specific IgM and IgG serum antibodies. These antibodies, in the presence of complement, do not create a lytic state that is sufficient to kill the bacteria. However, they do behave as opsonins to ensure that the *Legionella* organisms can attach and be ingested by various phagocytic cells, including PMNs, blood monocytes, and alveolar macrophages. Once inside the phagocytes, *Legionella* multiply and eventually can kill and disrupt the host cells. When alveolar macrophages are activated with interferon-γ these stimulated phagocytes will inhibit the growth of the bacteria. This may be the result of the ability of interferon-γ to downregulate the transferrin receptors on these cells—limiting the accumulation of intracellular iron, which is an essential metabolite for *Legionella*.[6] Support for this concept comes from experiments with an experimental *Legionella* pulmonary infection rat model,[45] in which administration of intratracheal interferon-γ reduced intrapulmonary replication of the bacteria, improving host defenses. It is anticipated that this kind of immunomodulatory treatment may prove useful in human infection.[36]

Another example of defects at the level of the lymphocyte is the acquired immunodeficiency syndrome (AIDS), in which the human host is infected with HIV virus that destroys CD4 T-helper lymphocytes.[9] These patients experience recurrent respiratory infections with diverse organisms, including viruses (cytomegalovirus or herpes simplex), *Pneumocystis carinii, Mycobacterium tuberculosis, M. avium-intracellulare,* fungi such as *Cryptococcus* species, and *Toxoplasma gondii* and *Legionella.* These infectious agents have a common feature of residing in macrophages or similar cells as facultative intracellular organisms. One reason why an AIDS patient has trouble with this group of infections relates to the relative imbalance of lymphocytes found in the alveoli, as sampled by BAL of the lung. Normal values for T lymphocytes have been given in Table 20-1. From subjects with AIDS, the recoverable alveolar lymphocytes reflect a decrease in the CD4 T-helper cells from HIV infection, offset by an increase in the suppresser-cytotoxic species of T lymphocytes.[5,53] Although alveolar macrophages normally exist in an environment where they can be activated sufficiently to kill or control microbes of this sort, the CD4 deficiency in lungs of AIDS patients compromises this activation process.[5] This causes an impressive defect in cell-mediated immunity and the ability of macrophages to contain or kill organisms such as *Pneumocystis* or Mycobacterial species.

REFERENCES

1. Arend WP: Interleukin-1 receptor antagonist. *Adv Immunol* 54:167–227, 1993.

2. Beck CS, Heiner DC: Selective immunoglobulin G4 deficiency and recurrent infections of the respiratory tract. *Am Rev Respir Dis* 124:94–96, 1981.

3. Beutler B: TNF, immunity and inflammatory disease: Lessons of the past decade. *J Invest Med* 43:227–235, 1995.

4. Bienenstock J: Bronchus-associated lymphoid tissue, in Bienenstock J (ed), *Immunology of Lung and Upper Respiratory Tract.* New York, McGraw-Hill, 1984, pp 96–118.

5. Buhl R, Jaffe HA, Holroyd, KJ et al: Activation of alveolar macrophages in asymptomatic HIV-infected individuals. *J Immunol* 150:1019–1028, 1993.

6. Byrd TF, Horwitz, MA: Interferon gamma-activated human monocytes downregulate transferrin receptors and inhibit the intracellular multiplication of *Legionella pneumophila* by limiting the availability of iron. *J Clin Invest* 83:1457–1465, 1989.

7. Coonrod JD: The role of extracellular bactericidal factors in pulmonary host defense. *Semin Respir Infect* 1:118–129, 1986.

8. Denis M: Interleukin-6 in mouse hypersensitivity pneumonitis: Changes in lung free cells following depletion of endogenous IL–6 or direct administration of IL-6. *J Leukoc Biol* 52:197–201, 1992.

9. Fauci AS, Pantaleo G, Stanley S, Weissman D: Immunopathogenic mechanisms of HIV infection. *Ann Intern Med* 124:654–663, 1996.

10. Halperin SA, Suratt PM, Gwaltney JM, et al: Bacterial cultures from the lower respiratory tract in normal volunteers with and without experimental rhinovirus infection using a plugged double catheter system. *Am Rev Respir Dis* 125:678–680, 1982.

11. Hunninghake GW: Release of interleukin-1 by alveolar macrophages of patients with active pulmonary sarcoidosis. *Am Rev Respir Dis* 129:569–572, 1984.

12. Hunninghake GW, Crystal RG: Pulmonary sarcoidosis: A disorder mediated by excess helper T-lymphocyte activity at sites of disease activity. *New Engl J Med* 305:429–434, 1981.

13. Kelley J: Cytokines of the lung—State of the art. *Am Rev Respir Dis* 141:765–788, 1990.

14. Leonard EJ, Yoshimura T: Neutrophil attractant/activation protein–1 (NAP-1 [interleukin-8]). *Am J Respir Cell Mol Biol* 2:479–486, 1990.

15. Ley K, Tedder TF: Leukocyte interactions with vascular endothelium—New insights into selection-mediated attachment and rolling. *J Immunol* 155:525–528, 1995.

16. Martin TR, Raghu G, Merritt TL, Henderson WR Jr: Relative contribution of leukotriene B4 to the neutrophil chemotactic activity produced by the resident human alveolar macrophage. *J Clin Invest* 80:1114–1124, 1987.

17. Merrill WW, Naegel GP, Olchowski JJ, Reynolds HY: Immunoglobulin G subclass proteins in serum and lavage fluid of normal subjects: Quantitation and comparison with immunoglobulins A and E. *Am Rev Respir Dis* 131:584–591, 1985.

18. Minty A, Chalon P, Derocq JM, et al: Interleukin-13 is a new human lymphokine regulating inflammatory and immune responses. *Nature* 362:248–250, 1993.

19. Mosmann TR, Cherwinski H, Bond MW, et al: Two types of murine helper T cell clone: I. Definition according to profiles of lymphokine activities and secreted proteins. *J Immunol* 136:2348–2357, 1986.

20. Mosmann TR: Properties and functions of interleukin-10. *Adv Immunol* 56:1–26, 1994.

21. Mosmann TR, Sad S: The expanding universe of T-cell subsets: Th1, Th2 and more. *Immunol Today* 17:138–146, 1996.

22. Murray HW: Interferon-gamma and host antimicrobial defense: Current and future clinical applications. *Am J Med* 97:459–467, 1994.

23. Nakamura H, Yoshimura K, McElvaney NG, et al: Neutrophil elastase in respiratory epithelial lining fluid of individuals with cystic fibrosis induces interleukin-8 gene expression in a human bronchial epithelial cell line. *J Clin Invest* 89:1478–1484, 1992.

24. Niederman MS, Merrill WW, Ferranti RD, et al: Nutritional status and bacterial binding in the lower respiratory tract in patients with chronic tracheostomy. *Ann Intern Med* 100:795–800, 1984.

25. Niederman MS, Rafferty TD, Sasaki CT, et al: Comparison of bacterial adherence to ciliated and squamous epithelial cells obtained from the human respiratory tract. *Am Rev Respir Dis* 127:85–90. 1983.

26. Oxelius VA, Laurell A-B, Lindquist B, et al: IgG subclasses in selective IgA deficiency—Importance of IgG2-IgA deficiency. *New Engl J Med* 304:1476–1477, 1981.

27. Pabst R, Gehrke I: Is the bronchus-associated lymphoid tissue (BALT) an integral structure of the lung in normal mammals, including humans? *Am J Respir Cell Mol Biol* 3:131–135, 1990.

28. Palmer LP, Ferranti RD, Merrill WW, et al: Bacterial adherence to respiratory tract cells: Relationships between in vivo and in vitro pH and bacterial attachment. *Am Rev Respir Dis* 133:784–788, 1986.

29. Pikaar JC, Voorhout WF, van Golde LMG, et al: Opsonic activities of surfactant proteins A and D in phagocytosis of gram-negative bacteria by alveolar macrophages. *J Infect Dis* 172:481–489, 1995.

30. Punnonen J, de Waal Malefyt R, van Vlasselaer P, et al: IL-10 and viral IL-10 prevent IL-4–induced IgE synthesis by inhibiting the accessory cell function of monocytes. *J Immunol* 151:1280–1289, 1993.

31. Racz PK, Tenner-Racz Q, Myrvik N, Fainter LK: Functional architecture of bronchial associated lymphoid tissue and lymphoepithelium in pulmonary cell-mediated reactions in the rabbit. *J Reticuloendothel Soc* 22:59–83, 1977.

32. Rankin JA, Sylvester I, Smith S, et al: Macrophages cultured in vitro release leukotriene B4 and neutrophil attractant/activation protein (interleukin 8) sequentially in response to stimulation with lipopolysaccharide and zymosan. *J Clin Invest* 86:1556–1564, 1990.

33. Reynolds HY: Respiratory infections may reflect deficiencies in host defense mechanisms. *Dis Mon* 31:1–98, 1985.

34. Reynolds HY: Bacterial adherence to respiratory tract mucosa—A dynamic interaction leading to colonization. *Semin Respir Med* 2:8–19, 1987.

35. Reynolds HY: Lung inflammation: Normal host defense or a complication of some diseases. *Annu Rev Med* 38:295–323, 1987.

36. Reynolds HY: Cytokines: Role in respiratory illnesses and potential control with immunomodulatory therapy. *Focus Opinion Intern Med* 1:1–10, 1994.

37. Reynolds HY, Atkinson JP, Newball HH, Frank MM: Receptors for immunoglobulin and complement on human alveolar macrophages. *J Immunol* 114:1813–1819, 1975.

38. Robertson J, Caldwell JR, Castle JR, Waldman RH: Evidence for the presence of components of the alternate (properdin) pathway of complement activation in respiratory secretions. *J Immunol* 117:900–903, 1976.

39. Robinson BWS, Pinkston P, Crystal RG: Natural killer cells are present in the normal human lung but are functionally impotent. *J Clin Invest* 74:942–950, 1984.

40. Rossman CM, Lee RMKW, Forrest JB, Newhouse MT: Nasal ciliary ultrastructure and function in patients with primary ciliary dyskinesia compared with that in normal subjects and in subjects with various respiratory diseases. *Am Rev Respir Dis* 129:161–167, 1984.

41. Rutland J, de Iongh RU: Random ciliary orientation—A cause of respiratory tract disease. *New Engl J Med* 323:1681–1684, 1990.

42. Saltini C, Spurzem JR, Lee JJ, et al: Spontaneous release of inter-leukin 2 by lung T lymphocytes in active pulmonary sarcoidosis is primarily from the Leu + DR + T cell subset. *J Clin Invest* 77:1962–1970, 1986.

43. Sibille Y, Chatelain B, Staquet P, et al: Surface IgA and Fc-alpha receptors on human alveolar macrophages from normal subjects and from patients with sarcoidosis. *Am Rev Respir Dis* 139:740–747, 1986.

44. Sibille Y, Reynolds HY: Macrophages and polymorphonuclear neutrophils in lung defense and injury—State of the art. *Am Rev Respir Dis* 141:471–501, 1990.

45. Skerrett SJ, Martin TR: Intratracheal interferon–γ augments pulmonary defenses in experimental legionellosis. *Am J Respir Crit Care Med* 149:50–58, 1994.

46. Smith CW: Molecular determinants of neutrophil adhesion. *Am J Respir Cell Mol Biol* 2:487–489, 1990.

47. Spinozzi F, Agea E, Bistoni O, et al: Increased allergen-specific, steroid-sensitive gamma/delta T cells in bronchoalveolar lavage fluid from patients with asthma. *Ann Intern Med* 124:223–227, 1996.

48. Strieter RM, Kunkel SL: Acute lung injury: The role of cytokines in the elicitation of neutrophils. *J Invest Med* 42:640–651, 1994.

49. Strieter RM, Standiford TJ, Huffnagle GB, et al: The good, the bad, and the ugly: The role of chemokines in models of human disease. *J Immunol* 156:3583–3586, 1996.

50. Strober W, Krakauer R, Klaeveman HL, et al: Secretory component deficiency: A unique disorder of the IgA immune system. *New Engl J Med* 294:351–366, 1976.

51. Tomasi TB, Zigelbaum S: The selective occurrence of gamma A globulins in certain body fluids. *J Clin Invest* 42:1551–1560, 1963.

52. Ulich TR, Yin S, Guo K, et al: Intratracheal injection of endotoxin and cytokines: II. Interleukin-6 and transforming growth factor-β inhibit acute inflammation. *Am J Pathol* 138:1097–1101, 1991.

53. Young KR, Rankin JA, Naegel GP, et al: Bronchoalveolar lavage cells and proteins in patients with the acquired immunodeficiency syndrome: An immunologic analysis. *Ann Intern Med* 103:522–533, 1985.

CHAPTER 21

LYMPHOCYTE- AND MACROPHAGE-MEDIATED INFLAMMATION IN THE LUNG

Jeffrey S. Berman / David M. Center

LYMPHOCYTES IN THE LUNG
    Lymphocytes at the Epithelial Surface
    Bronchus-Associated Lymphoid Tissue
    Interstitial Lymphocytes
    Intravascular Lymphocytes
    Lymphocyte Recruitment to the Lung
    Lymphocyte Function in the Lung
    Lymphocyte Activation in the Lung
    Lymphocyte Clearance and Death in the Lung

MACROPHAGES IN THE LUNG
    Alveolar Macrophages
    Dendritic Cells and Langerhans' Cells
    Monocytes
    Intravascular Macrophages
    Recruitment of Monocytes and Macrophages
    Activation of Lung Macrophages

LYMPHOCYTE-MACROPHAGE INTERACTIONS IN THE LUNG

The lung constantly receives a flow of foreign infectious and noninfectious antigens on the tide of airflow. Like the gut, genitourinary tract, and skin, it is one of the interfaces of the sterile body sanctuary with the environment. The defense systems of the respiratory tract are designed to deal with this particulate and antigen load. The structural and mechanical features of these defenses trap and clear many of these particulates before they reach respiratory structures. Those that avoid these defenses interact with inflammatory and immune processes that work to sterilize or clear lung tissues. Two cells of hematopoietic origin, the lung lymphocyte and lung macrophage, play key roles in these responses. In many ways, they represent two very different sides of this inflammatory response. The macrophage, as a phagocytic cell, is of ancient phylogenetic lineage, is not antigen specific, and may be triggered by many inflammatory stimuli. The lymphocyte is present only in vertebrates and represents a significant refinement in the inflammatory response: antigen specificity and discrimination of self and nonself.

To understand the importance of lymphocytes and macrophages in respiratory inflammation, one must become familiar with the biologic properties and functions of each cell population. It is incorrect, however, to think solely of lymphocytes and macrophages as independent effector cells. In reality, they interact extensively and in many ways are codependent. Macrophages or macrophage-like cells are required for optimal presentation of antigens to lymphocytes, and for optimal lymphocyte activation and cytokine production. Conversely, macrophage microbicidal function and release of arachidonate and oxygen metabolites are influenced by cytokines produced by activated T lymphocytes, and phagocytosis is markedly enhanced by opsonic antibodies produced by B lymphocytes. The cooperation between these two cell types represents a cornerstone of lung defense against antigenic challenge or microbial infection. In this chapter, we will present an overview of the macrophage and lymphocyte populations in the human lung, their function and interactions, and a synthesis of their role in lung inflammation and disease. To assist in this review, we have defined, in Table 21-1, the cell surface markers that will be referred to in this chapter using the now standardized "clusters of differentiation" (CD) nomenclature.

LYMPHOCYTES IN THE LUNG

In the normal lung, lymphocytes are distributed in one of four compartments (Fig. 21-1). The compartments include lymphocytes at the epithelial surface, including those in the bronchoalveolar space; lymphocytes associated with the epithelium in lymphoid aggregates (also known as bronchus-associated lymphoid tissue, or BALT); interstitial and intraepithelial lymphocytes; and an intravascular pool. Each compartment has a distinct phenotypic and functional repertoire. It is not yet clear whether there is a sequential influx of lymphocytes from the blood/intravascular pool to the interstitium or BALT and finally to the epithelial surface. Alternatively, lymphocytes may be destined to reside in one or another of these pools from the time of maturation or activation in primary or secondary lymphoid organs. Finally, while the lung has a large blood volume and receives the entire cardiac output, the exact nature of influx and turnover of these lung lymphocyte populations is not clear.

TABLE 21-1

Cluster of Differentiation Antigens and Surface Molecules Discussed in This Chapter

Name/CD Designation	Function
CD1	Accessory molecule for antigen presentation on APCs
Sheep RBC receptor / CD2	Accesory molecule for T-lymphocyte activation, adhesion receptor (ligand for LFA-3)
T3 / CD3	Signaling subunit of TCR
$\alpha\beta$ TCR	T-cell receptor for antigen containing α and β chains
$\gamma\delta$ TCR	Alternative form of the T-cell receptor for antigen containing γ and δ chains
CD4	T-cell coreceptor (ligand for MHC class II); marker for helper/inducer cells
CD8	T-cell coreceptor (ligand for MHC class I); marker for cytotoxic cells
CD11a,b,c	α chains of the β_2 integrin; CD11a (also called LFA-1); CD11b (also called Mac-1/CR3); CD11c (also called CR4)
CD14	Macrophage receptor for lipopolysaccharide
CD18	β_2 integrin chain
CD25	p55 IL-2 receptor; T-cell activation antigen (also called Tac antigen)
CD31 / PECAM-1	Platelet-endothelial cell-adhesion molecule-1
HLA-DR	Class II MHC; expressed on APCs; activation antigen for T cells
CD28	Accessory molecule for T-lymphocyte activation (ligands for B7-1, B7-2, and CTLA-4)
CD29	Common beta chain of the β_1 integrins
VLA-1 - 6 / CD49a-f	Adhesion molecules; α chains of the β_1 integrins (ligands for ECM proteins)
VLA-4 / $\alpha_4\beta_1$ integrin	Adhesion molecule (ligand for VCAM expressed on endothelium, fibronectin)
$\alpha_4\beta_7$ integrin	Adhesion molecule (ligand for VCAM, fibronectin)
HML-1 / $\alpha_E\beta_7$ integrin / CD130	Adhesion molecule (ligand for epithelial cell carbohydrate antigen)
ICAM-1 / CD54	Cell adhesion molecule for cell-cell interaction (ligand for LFA-1 / CD11a/ CD18)
B7-1, B7-2/CD80	Accessory molecule for T-cell activation; ligand for CD28
CD95/Fas	Receptor for Fas ligand, induction of apoptosis
VCAM / CD106	Adhesion molecule expressed on activated endothelium (ligand α_4 integrins)

NOTE: Abbreviations: CD = cluster of differentiation; RBC = red blood cell; TCR = T-cell receptor; VLA = very late activation antigen; LFA = lymphocyte function–associated antigen; APC = antigen-presenting cells; MHC = major histocompatibility complex; CR = complement receptor; ECM = extracellular matrix; ICAM = intercellular adhesion molecule; VCAM = vascular cell adhesion molecule.

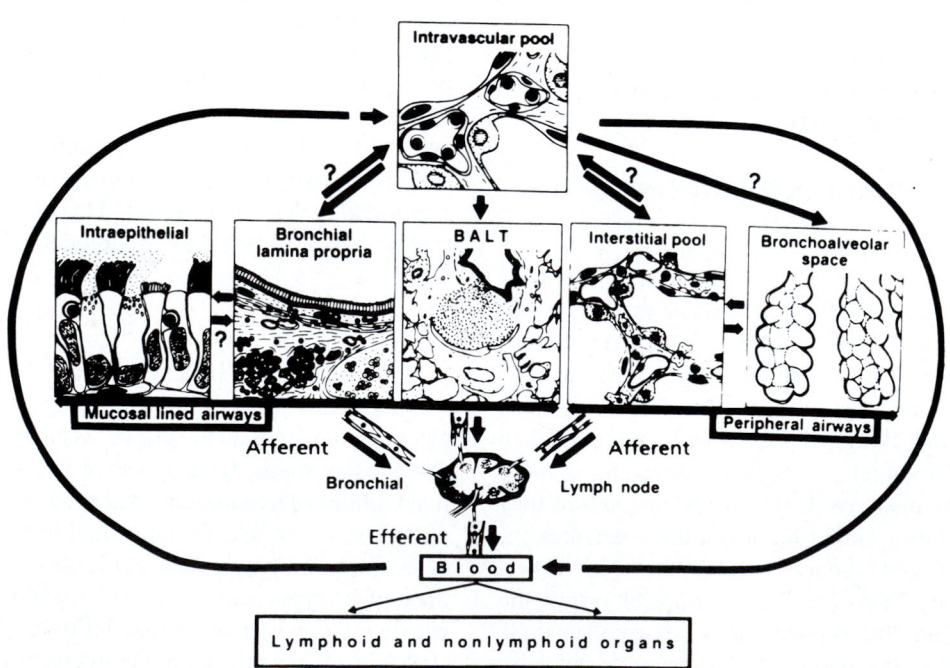

FIGURE 21-1 Lymphocytes are found in the lung in distinct sites. These include lymphocytes in the bronchoalveolar space (on the epithelial surface); the interstitial, lamina propria, and intraepithelial lymphocytes; BALT lymphocytes; and an intravascular pool. Lymphocytes travel from lymph nodes to blood and into the lung via interaction with lung endothelial cells. Hypothesized trafficking from one pulmonary compartment to another is indicated by arrows. Some lymphocytes from these various compartments may be able to leave the lung and travel to lymph nodes. Others become effete and die. (*Based on data of Pabst,*[31] *with permission.*)

Lymphocytes at the Epithelial Surface

This population is best studied as lymphocytes from the bronchoalveolar space, which are easily recovered from the lung using bronchoalveolar lavage (BAL). In normal nonsmoking subjects, lymphocytes make up only about 5 to 15 percent of the 10^5 cells recovered per milliliter of returned BAL fluid. The numbers of lymphocytes, however, increase dramatically during a variety of inflammatory responses.[2,3,4] Lymphocytes at the epithelial surface (LES) differ markedly from blood lymphocytes suggesting a selection or maturation process between blood and lung (Table 21-2).[2,4] Approximately 70 percent of LES are T cells. The CD4:CD8 ratio of these T cells is approximately the same as in the blood, though with a larger scatter from one person to another. More than 90 percent of BAL T cells are of the previously activated memory type, as determined by expression of a low-molecular-weight form of the leukocyte common antigen CD45 (CD45RO). Many have been chronically activated, as shown by the expression of the $\alpha_1\beta_1$ integrin. LES are more likely than blood T cells to express the activation antigen HLA-DR, and CD8$^+$ (cytotoxic/suppressor) LES are more likely to express markers associated with cytotoxic cell function.[2] An unusual population of memory cytotoxic cells that lack the accessory molecule CD28 have also been found in normal LES.[38] In the rodent lung, most T cells express the γ/δ T-cell receptor. In humans there is a small population of γ/δ T cells at the epithelial surface, though the vast majority express the α/β T-cell receptor. As might be expected in an area of microbial and antigen assault, there are a variable number of natural killer (NK) cells in this compartment. However, the bulk of NK activity in the lung is found in the interstitial population.[2] B cells are also present in the LES population derived by BAL. They have been documented to produce antibodies of all types.[2] It is unknown whether there are selected B-cell subpopulations among LES.

The source and fate of these T and B cells are unknown. It seems reasonable to hypothesize that epithelial surface T cells (and other lung T cells) emerge from the circulation, perhaps proliferate locally and differentiate further while in the lung, and then die or exit. The appearance of labeled blood T cells in LES has been documented in animals. The uniform memory phenotype of epithelial surface and interstitial T cells strongly suggests that such differentiation occurs before entry into the lung.

Many LES adhere to and interact with airway epithelial cells through the expression of a unique adhesion molecule, Human Mucosal Lymphocyte ([HML]-1/$\alpha\epsilon\beta_7$ integrin).[1] This integrin is expressed on 40 percent of LES (60 percent of CD8$^+$ cells are HML-1$^+$, while fewer CD4$^+$ cells express it) and on intestinal lymphocytes, but only rarely on blood or lung interstitial lymphocytes. It is likely that local influences, such as epithelial-derived cytokines like transforming growth factor–β_1 (TGF-β_1), induce the expression of this molecule on LES.[11,35] This suggests that LES are not necessarily effete or dying cells that are present in the airway only to be cleared by the mucociliary escalator and expectorated. Rather, they include a specialized lymphocyte population involved in the surveillance of the airway and interaction with epithelial cells. Among these interactions might be modulation of the normal turnover of epithelium-expressing Fas (CD95), by LES-expressing Fas ligand (A. Fine, personal communication). The possibility that LES reenter the interstitium and lymphoid tissue has recently been confirmed experimentally in the rat.[32]

LES can be stimulated to proliferate, produce cytokines and antibodies, and perform cytolytic functions. However, they are in general hyporeactive in proliferative or antibody responses to

---

TABLE 21-2

Characteristics of Lung Lymphocytes

Location	Number	Cell Type	Comments
Epithelial surface	10^4/ml BAL Approximately 10^8 total	CD4/CD8 ratio = blood 70% T cells >90% memory cells 40% express $\alpha_\epsilon\beta_7$ integrin (70% of CD8$^+$) Memory CTL NK phenotype present, decreased function	Specialized for interaction with epithelial cells; first line of defense?
BALT	? If present in normal human lung	B cells in center T cells scattered in center and surrounding follicle	Local antigen sampling and antibody production
Interstitium	10^7/gm lung tissue Approximately 6×10^9 total	CD4:CD8 ratio < blood >90% memory T cells Bulk of NK activity	With intravascular, equal to total blood lymphocyte pool
Intravascular	?Characteristics in human	?	Possible mobilizable cells poised for lung entry

NOTE: ELF = epithelial lining fluid; BAL = bronchoalveolar lavage; CD = cluster of differentiation; CTL = cytotoxic T lymphocyte; BALT = bronchus-associated lymphoid tissue. For a review, see reference 2.

antigen or mitogens when compared to blood T cells or even when compared to memory T cells from the lung interstitium. The reason for this is not known, but may relate to immuno-suppressive influences in the airways mediated by alveolar macrophages (AM),[16,43] locally produced TGF-β_1,[48] and pulmonary surfactant lipids or proteins.[22]

Bronchus-Associated Lymphoid Tissue

BALT is the term applied to localized subepithelial collections of lymphocytes in the airways.[6] These lymphoid aggregates are similar to gut-associated lymphoid tissue (GALT; e.g. Peyer's patches) in appearance and association with epithelium and a blood vessel, presence of specialized cuboidal or "high" venular endothelium (HEV) characteristic of lymphoid tissues, and a specialized thinned overlying epithelium facilitating antigen entry from the bronchial lumen and exit of lymphocytes and lymphocyte products. The resemblance of BALT to GALT, as well as the similarity of lymphocyte recirculation patterns from lung- and gut-associated lymphoid tissue, has suggested to some authors that these structures represent a common mucosal immune system. In this paradigm, recirculating blood lymphocytes exit into these structures, which provide an efficient exposure to antigens sampled from the environment. Activated memory cells are then a source of local antibody production, and disperse through the circulation to other mucosal sites to disseminate immunologic memory.

Immunohistochemistry has revealed a preponderance of B cells staining with IgM, IgG, and IgA, with a scattering (approximately 20 percent) of T cells, especially CD4$^+$ helper cells, within and surrounding the BALT aggregate. BALT lacks the organized germinal centers found in other secondary lymphoid tissue. It seems likely that BALT is a center for local antibody production in the airway in response to antigen challenge or immunization.

BALT is present in the normal rodent airway and increases in amount with age. BALT is reduced or absent in germ-free animals. Current evidence suggests that these structures are uncommon or absent in normal humans but may appear and proliferate in response to infection or inflammation.[31,33] Hyperplastic BALT has been reported in the setting of chronic airway infection. These data suggest that antigen, infection-induced cytokine production, or some other stimulus is required for the development of these lymphoid aggregates. The formation of these structures could be mediated through the development of HEV structures, which facilitate lymphocyte exit from the postcapillary venule.

Interstitial Lymphocytes

Lymphocytes are rarely seen in histologic sections of normal human lung. However, several investigators have prepared lymphocytes from human lungs extensively washed to remove airway cells using minced tissue and enzymatic digestion. The resulting population of interstitial lymphocytes in normal subjects appears to be distinct from lymphocytes recovered from normal BAL.[17,24] Specifically, approximately 20 × 10^6 mononuclear cells were found per gram of wet lung tissue. Of these, 70

percent were lymphocytes, of which 90 percent were CD2$^+$ T lymphocytes. There was enrichment for memory T cells similar to that seen in LES, but the CD4:CD8 ratio among IL T cells was lower than that seen in blood or LES. Memory T lymphocytes from the interstitial compartment can be stimulated to produce cytokines, and to proliferate in response to interleukin-2 despite a decreased proliferative response to mitogens.[2] Most, if not all, NK activity in the lung has been localized to the cells in the interstitial compartment.[2]

It is unknown to what extent the existing characterization of human IL are based on preparations that were contaminated with intravascular lymphocytes. In studies using human tissue, this is not unlikely. However, studies in rodents using extensively perfused and lavaged lungs have demonstrated a distinct IL population. This is an important point, since the estimate of the number of total lung IL extrapolated from the number per gram of tissue (6 × 10^9) is large, even exceeding the estimated blood lymphocyte pool. These estimates no doubt reflect the intravascular pool to some extent. The exact origin, fate, and function of IL are not known.

Intravascular Lymphocytes

The presence of this lymphocyte pool has been convincingly shown in animals, especially the pig.[31,34] Experimental data include lung perfusion studies showing the continued slow elution of lymphocytes from lung after elimination of red blood cells. The presence of an intravascular lymphocyte pool in humans has not been directly confirmed. However, labeled lymphocytes injected into humans are "held up" in the lung whether injected intravenously or intra-arterially.[4] These data suggest that lung lymphocyte trapping in the human is not an artifact of capillary flow and may be lung specific. Whether this phenomenon represents margination of lymphocytes in capillaries due to adhesion molecule interactions, entrapment due to slow capillary laminar flow, or physical forces (as has been shown for activated neutrophils) is unclear. The phenotypic characteristics of this pool in the human are unknown. The size and role of this pool in populating the interstitial and epithelial lymphocyte compartments are also poorly understood.

Lymphocyte Recruitment to the Lung

Lymphocytes are recruited to extravascular sites through a complex process involving adhesion to endothelial cells (EC), release from adhesion, transendothelial migration, interaction with cellular matrix, and response to locally produced chemoattractants.[4,35,39] The interaction of adhesion molecules expressed on blood T cells with complementary adhesion molecules on EC is a critical first step to T-cell emigration from the blood. This step is closely regulated at the level of adhesion molecule expression by T cells at different stages of development, and by transiently increased adhesion molecule function after T-cell activation. Similarly, expression of adhesion molecules by EC may be increased markedly by proinflammatory cytokines, especially tumor necrosis factor–α (TNF-α), IL-1, and γ-interferon.[5,45] Treatment of EC with these cytokines markedly alters the adhesiveness of EC for leukocytes, including certain subsets of T cells. The result of such EC activation by locally produced cytokines or other factors is that the exit of T cells from the blood is not random, but rather is restricted to lymphoid tissues, mucosal structures, or sites of tissue inflammation.[5]

The specific events in T-cell transendothelial migration have been dissected at the molecular level. T lymphocytes first appear to "roll" along the endothelium—an interaction requires loose adhesion via T-cell $\alpha_4\beta_1$ integrin and endothelial vascular cell adhesion molecule–1 (VCAM-1). As the result of a signaling event, this rolling is replaced with firm adhesion, which requires other integrin molecules, particularly an interaction between lymphocyte function–associated antigen–1 (LFA-1) ($\alpha L\beta_2$ integrin) and intracellular adhesion molecule–1 (ICAM-1) or other ligands on endothelium. This signal, often a chemokine or another chemotactic factor, strengthens adhesion by enhancing the avidity of integrins for their ligands. Other interactions—including decay of integrin affinity, homotypic interaction of T cell and endothelial PECAM (CD31) at endothelial cell junctions, and release of matrix degrading enzymes—permit release of this firm adhesion and T-cell migration into matrix.[39]

T cells are constantly recirculating from blood to tissue and back, with an average half-life in the blood of only about 18 h.[4] In addition, the sites of migration in vivo appear to be quite different for naïve or virgin cells, as opposed to previously activated memory cells. Naïve cells preferentially traffic to lymphoid tissue, where they are likely to encounter antigen, while memory cells traffic to nonlymphoid tissues such as skin or lung.[35]

The normal lung vasculature may have unique properties that facilitate the retention of circulating lymphocytes. Whether injected intravenously or intra-arterially, labeled lymphocytes are held up in the lung disproportionately in comparison to other organs. Thus, this is not just a "first pass" clearance effect from capillary passage.[4] Lymphocyte–endothelial cell adhesion may mediate this retention, since several investigators have found that antibodies to adhesion molecules, particularly LFA-1, decrease lymphocyte retention in the lung. Capillary size may also mediate this retention by mechanically trapping activated cells. This has been shown to be a significant process in the retention of activated neutrophils and monocytes in the lung. Lymphocytes also become larger, and lose deformability with activation. The role of this process in the retention of lung lymphocytes, however, has yet to be defined.

Lymphocyte chemoattractants represent another step in the regulation of the exit of adherent or trapped T cells from the capillary circulation. Multiple T-cell chemoattractants have been described that are relevant to the lung, many of which also alter the growth and activation of T cells.[4,25,47,42] A partial listing of known chemoattractants

may be found in Table 21-3. Most recently described is the chemokine family of cytokines. These low-molecular-weight peptides share a cysteine repeat motif (either C-C or C-X-C), a strong cationic charge, and the property of heparin binding.[25] Chemokine chemoattractants alter leukocyte function through binding to seven transmembrane-spanning receptors. The chemokines may bind to heparinlike regions of endothelial cell membrane receptors, preventing dilution of locally produced chemoattractant signal by blood flow. The chemokines have been shown to enhance both adhesion to endothelial cells and endothelial transmigration of many leukocyte types, including T-cell subsets and monocytes. The chemokines have also been found to act as accessory growth factors for T lymphocytes.[42] In lung diseases, multiple T-cell chemoattractants have been found in BAL or in tissue specimens, including the chemotactic growth factors IL-2,[18,21] IL-16,[9] insulinlike growth factor–1 (IGF-1),[4] the C-X-C chemokine IL-8, and the C-C chemokines macrophage chemoattractant protein–1 (MCP-1), RANTES, and macrophage inflammatory protein–1α (MIP-1α).[8,9,40] IL-2 is presumed to be of lymphocyte origin, while IGF-1 and IL-16 have many potential cellular sources, including T cells, eosinophils, and epithelial cells. The chemokines likewise have numerous cellular origins, including macrophages, endothelial cells, and epithelial cells.

IL-16 is a chemoattractant for CD4$^+$ cells, including T cells, monocytes, and eosinophils. The chemokines and IL-16 share a strong cationic charge at physiological pH, and enhance both adhesion and migration of target T cells[25] (J. Berman, unpublished data). Of importance to the lung, IL-16 and the chemokines MIP-1α and RANTES are rapidly released (within 4 h) after antigen challenge in atopic asthmatics.[9]

TABLE 21-3

Lymphocyte Chemoattractants*

Interleukins	Activation stimuli
IL-1	Antibody to T-cell receptor (T cells)
IL-2	Antisurface immunoglobulin (B cells)
IL-6	Phorbol esters
IL-10	
IL-15	
IL-16	

Chemokine chemoattractants	Growth factors
IL-8	Insulin
RANTES	IGF-1
MIP-1-α,β	TGF-β_1
MCP-1, -2, -3	
IP-10	

Matrix proteins	Miscellaneous chemoattractants
Laminin	Lysophosphatidylcholine
Fibronectin	fMLP, mycobacterial lipoarabinomannan
Amyloid protein AA	Casein/denatured protein

NOTE: IL = interleukin; RANTES = regulated activated normal T cells expressed, secreted; MIP = macrophage inflammatory protein; MCP = monocyte chemotactic peptide; IGF = insulinlike growth factor; TGF = transforming growth factor.
*Not a complete listing. For reviews, see references 4, 25, 42.

Lymphocyte Function in the Lung

Lymphocytes in the lung subserve three major functions: (1) antibody production; (2) cytotoxic activity, including lysis of virally infected cells, which have bound antibody, and tumor cells; and (3) cytokine production (Table 21-4).[3,32]

Antibody production in the lung by B lymphocytes serves to bind antigen and facilitate the inactivation of bioactive materials and phagocytosis by macrophages. Mucosal IgA is of particular interest in its active transepithelial transport to the bronchial lumen. Antibody production by lung B cells has been extensively studied in mouse lung. After challenge, antigen is removed to regional lymph nodes by motile phagocytic cells (macrophages and dendritic cells), where optimal activation of T and B cells occurs. Activated cells relocate into the circulation and migrate into the lung at areas of inflammation, and local antibody production results. Rechallenge with antigen results in a more rapid local response derived from resident memory cells.[2,4,10] While it has long been assumed that memory B and T cells are long-lived, such memory requires persistence of antigen in many systems. Thus, the true longevity of pulmonary memory lymphocytes is not known.

The lung contains many types of cytotoxic cells, including NK cells (not antigen-restricted), antigen restricted cytotoxic cells, and cells exhibiting antibody-dependent cytotoxicity. One unusual aspect of lung cytotoxic cells is the preeminence of $CD3^+$ cytotoxic T cells with NK activity (non–antigen receptor–mediated killing of tumor cell targets). This is in contradistinction to the blood, where most cells expressing NK activity are CD3 negative.[2] NK activity is found in the interstitial compartment of lung T cells. NK cells are phenotypically present among LES, but these cells have been found to be functionally impotent.[2]

In contrast to B cells, whose major products are immunoglobulins, T cells produce a broad range of cytokines under a variety of circumstances (Table 21-4). In many situations, the complexion of the inflammatory response correlates with the cytokines produced by local T cells, suggesting that T cells orchestrate many important tissue reactions. As a result, the pattern of cytokine production by T-cell populations has emerged as a major focus of investigation in lung inflammation.

Activated T-helper (TH) cells produce a distinct spectrum of lymphokines.[26,37] The repertoire of a single T cell to produce lymphokines appears to be limited and stereotyped, depending on the circumstances of activation. According to data accumulated in mice, virgin T cells produce mainly IL-2 in response to activation. After proliferation and switch to memory cell phenotype, T cells produce one of two major clusters of cytokines, either TH1 (IFN-γ, IL-2) or TH2 (IL-4, IL-5, IL-10). In humans this distinction between phenotypes has not been as predictable as in the mouse, and IL-10 may be produced by either TH1 or TH2 cells.[26] These two phenotypes roughly conform to polarized expressions of cell-mediated immune responses: granuloma formation with activation of mononuclear phagocytes and production of opsonizing IgG2 antibody (TH1) or optimal antibody response including reaginic antibody (IgE) formation, often with associated eosinophilia (TH2).

Certain immune responses are dominated by either a TH1 or TH2 response, while others are mixed. In human asthma, for example, T cells producing IL-4 or IL-5 predominate,[36] but IFN-γ–producing cells are found in the airways, suggesting a mixed response. In contrast, granulomas at sites of tuberculin reactions in skin show evidence for production of IFN-γ and IL-2 but not IL-4.[37] In leprosy or leishmaniasis, an ineffective host reaction is associated with a TH2 response, and an effective granulomatous response is associated with a TH1 response. In accord with this finding, treatment of ineffective responses to leishmania with IFN-γ has been reported to increase the efficacy of chemotherapy.[37] In sarcoidosis, airway and granuloma cells, particularly activated $CD4^+$ (HLA-DR$^+$) T cells, have been found to produce both IL-2 and IFN-γ, suggesting the predominance of a TH1 response.

There is considerable cross-regulation of TH1 and TH2 subsets, even after commitment to the production of these cytokines. This has led to the general concept that the character of an immune response as well as its termination may depend on the sequential predominance of TH1 or TH2 responses. The appropriate termination of inflammation is an important event in a normal healing response. Chronic inflammation or an aberrant repair process after inflammation may underlie lung fibrosis. While the cellular events that terminate inflammation, dictate normal repair, and generate tissue fibrosis remain to be elucidated, it is likely that transforming growth factor–β_1 (TGF-β_1) plays an important role in these processes. In addition to its complex actions on the regulation of

TABLE 21-4

Function of Lung Lymphocyte Subpopulations*

Cell Type	Function	Secreted Products
TH1 cell	Antiviral and antifungal defense, granuloma formation, CMI, graft rejection	IL-2, IFN-γ, IL-3, IL-6, IL-12, IL-16, GM-CSF, TGF-β_1
TH2 cell	Allergic inflammation, antiparasite defense	IL-2, IL-4, IL-5, IL-9, IL-10, IL-3, IL-13, IL-16, GM-CSF, TGF-β1
TCTL	Antigen-restricted lysis of viral- or mycobacteria-infected macrophages or epithelia; lysis of fungi, tumor cells	TH1 cytokines, perforin, IL-4
NK cell	Non–antigen-restricted lysis of tumor cells	IL-2
B cell	Antibody production	IgM, IgG subtypes, IgE, IgA, IL-10

NOTE: TH1 = T helper type 1; TH2 = T helper type 2; TCTL = cytotoxic T lymphocyte; NK = natural killer cell; IL = interleukin; CMI = cell-mediated immunity; GM-CSF = granulocyte-macrophage colony–stimulating factor; TGF-β_1 = transforming growth factor–beta$_1$.
*Not a complete listing. Listed are cytokines or other products produced under in vitro conditions or documented in lung disease. See references 2, 26.

growth and matrix production by mesenchymal cells, TGF-β_1 is a potent immunosuppressant and has been implicated as an immunomodulator in immunoregulatory mucosal-derived TH2-like suppressor cells.[26]

Lymphocyte Activation in the Lung

T and B lymphocytes are designed to require specific (antigenic) signals for activation, restricting their involvement in inflammation to situations where antigen overwhelms the mucociliary escalator and macrophage and neutrophil defenses. Lymphocytes are activated after engagement of an antigen receptor of remarkably fine specificity. This receptor is unique to a given lymphocyte clone, and is generated by recombination of gene segments in the antibody (for B cells) or T-cell receptor genes. B-cell receptors consist of single membrane-spanning antibody molecules of the same specificity as the B cell. T-cell receptors are heterodimeric structures made up of dimers of α/β or γ/δ chains. Like the antibody molecule, the T-cell receptor is highly antigen specific and has structural homology to the immunoglobulin molecule. B lymphocytes are activated by the cross-linking of membrane antibody by antigen. T cells are activated by engagement of their antigen receptor by antigen bound to major histocompatibility complex (MHC) molecules on the surface of so-called antigen-presenting cells (APC), also known as accessory cells. APC provide many "accessories" for T-cell activation, including (1) a source of MHC molecules to which antigen can bind; (2) the internalization and "processing" of antigen, including protease digestion into antigenic fragments; (3) multiple cell adhesion molecules, which bind to complementary adhesion molecules on T cells and serve to strengthen T cell–accessory cell interactions and transduce activation signals required for optimal lymphocyte activation; and (4) production of cytokines that amplify activation, including IL-1.[16]

APC in the lung include pulmonary macrophages of all varieties. However, dendritic cells and Langerhans cells are most efficient in this function (see below). These cells express "accessory" cell adhesion molecules important to accessory cell function, including ICAM-1, LFA-2, LFA-3, and the CD28 ligands B7-1, B7-2, and CTLA-4.[13,29] Other cells that may be induced to express class II MHC molecules may also act as weak accessory cells. Such cells include local B cells, epithelial cells, smooth-muscle cells, and fibroblasts. Uncommitted naïve T cells require intense accessory cell interaction in order to be activated by antigen. In contrast, previously activated (memory) T cells re-

quire less accessory cell input and might be influenced by interaction with such weak accessory cells. Since most lung T cells are memory cells, even the relatively weak lung accessory cells may play a role in T-cell activation in the pulmonary inflammatory response (Table 21-5).

Despite the need for T-cell responses after antigen or microbial challenge, the lung has also proved to contain major immunosuppressive elements that may serve to prevent inappropriate or excessive T-cell activation in an area of the body characterized by constant antigen bombardment. These influences include surfactant lipids, which have been shown to inhibit T-cell activation, proliferation, and cytokine production;[22] basal production (perhaps by epithelial cells) of the potent immunosupressive cytokine TGF-β_1;[48] and an inhibitory effect of AM.[43] These inhibitory effects may be moderated, reduced, or increased in various disease states. The weak accessory cell function and inhibitory effects of AM on T-cell activation, transmembrane signaling, and proliferation have always been considered paradoxic or perhaps laboratory artifacts. Two lines of evidence suggest, however, that these findings are real. First, some of the inability of AM to provide an adequate accessory signal lies in the observation that most of these cells lack the essential complementary ligand B7 for the T-cell accessory molecule CD28.[16] Second, it has become clear that subpopulations of pulmonary macrophages with potent accessory cell activity are present in the epithelium and interstitium, providing a mechanism for local antigen presentation and T-cell activation in the lung.

Lymphocyte Clearance and Death in the Lung

The means by which lymphocytes leave the lung or are cleared during homeostasis or after an inflammatory response are largely unknown. It is not known how long memory T or B cells reside in any of the compartments of the lung. In addition, the extent to which lymphocytes leave the lung utilizing lymph channels to enter nodes or the circulation has not been well characterized. It is clear from studies in the mouse, however, that programmed cell death, or apoptosis, is involved in the termination of antigen-induced inflammatory responses. In lymphocytes, this energy-requiring form of cell death may result from one of three events: (1) "neglect" or absence of stimulation; (2) stimulation out of context or without the appropriate second signals (such as CD28 or matrix interactions); or (3) signaling via Fas (CD95) engagement with Fas ligand. Fas is an apoptosis-signaling cell surface receptor that is a member of the tumor necrosis fac-

TABLE 21-5

Function of Lung Macrophage Populations*

Cell Type	Phagocytosis	Microbial Killing	Ag Presentation	Cytokine Production
Alveolar macrophage	++++	++++	± (suppression)	++++
Interstitial macrophage	++	++	++	++
Dendritic cell	+	+	++++	++
Langerhans' cell	++	+	++++	++
Blood monocyte	++	++	+++	+++

SOURCE: Condensed from Hance,[13] Holt,[16] and Lohmann-Matthes et al.[23]

tor/nerve growth factor receptor family. Fas ligand is expressed largely on T cells and is a member of the TNF family. This regulation of cell death appears to be critically important for the termination of an immune response once antigen has been cleared, preventing the accumulation of activated lymphocytes.[47]

MACROPHAGES IN THE LUNG

Macrophages are large phagocytic cells that reside in various compartments of many organs. They are especially prominent in the lung, where they serve a number of functions. They ingest inhaled particles or antigens, augmenting their removal on the mucociliary escalator, transporting them to regional lymph, and allowing the generation of sensitized T and B cells. In this last capacity, these cells serve as "professional" accessory cells for optimal T-cell antigen presentation. Lung macrophages also release a variety of cytokines and biologically active arachidonate metabolites that influence the function of nearby cells, including T cells, B cells, endothelial cells, and fibroblasts. Finally, macrophages have the capacity to ingest microorganisms and, when appropriately stimulated, kill them using a variety of means, including toxic oxygen metabolites and nitric oxide.

Macrophages or macrophage-like cells are found in several lung compartments, including the epithelial fluid lining the alveolus and large and small airways, the epithelium and interstitium, and the intravascular compartment. Several types of macrophage lineage cells with varying functional repertoires are found in the lung, including blood monocytes, interstitial and alveolar macrophages, dendritic cells, and Langerhans' cells. Each of these sites and cell types will be discussed.

Alveolar Macrophages

Because of their accessibility via BAL, alveolar macrophages (AM) have been the most intensively studied of human macrophage populations. They are large cells that make up more than 90 percent of the 10^7 cells harvested from the usual BAL in a normal nonsmoker. BAL in normal smokers yields a fourfold greater number of cells, approximately 90 percent of which are also AM (3). The difference in the number of AM in the BAL of smokers and nonsmokers may represent an increase in the lavageable pool without an increase in the total number of pulmonary macrophages. Alternatively, it may reflect the recruitment of more cells to the airway compartment in response to cigarette smoke–induced locally secreted cytokines. Based on the recovery from lavage of a subsegmental bronchus, the total lung AM population has been estimated at between 10^9 and 10^{10} cells. This may, however, be an underestimate. It is also estimated that macrophages make up 10 to 15 percent of all cells in the alveolar interstitium.[23] In the lung, macrophages are situated throughout the airway from large bronchi to the alveolus. They appear to be the first line for the clearance of inhaled antigens and pathogens. As such, they have well-developed phagocytic functions, and are able to turn over their cell membranes several times each hour. This capacity may be markedly increased by opsonization of the antigen and by secreted inflammatory signals that act directly on the macrophage, exemplified by the T-cell–derived cytokine IFN-γ.[1,12,28]

AM appear to derive from a bone marrow cell, possibly the blood monocyte.[12,19,23,27] Their numbers in the lung appear to be regulated, at least in part, by local cell influx, since, after bone marrow ablation in animals, AM numbers begin to decline at 20 to 30 days. There is also convincing evidence that in situ proliferation of AM occurs and that AM populations may be self-sustaining.[7] In addition, the level of in situ proliferation of AM may be markedly increased in some inflammatory states. The relative contribution of recruitment of bone marrow–derived cells versus in situ proliferation to the maintenance of AM in normal human lungs has not been firmly delineated. It is likely, however, that local production of hematopoietic growth factors such as granulocyte-macrophage colony–stimulating factor (GM-CSF) and monocyte-specific chemotactic cytokines such as the chemokine MCP-1 play a role in normal development and trafficking of monocytes into the lung in addition to their roles in the inflammatory states.[27] There is also a population of macrophages distinct from dendritic cells (see below) that are found in the interstitium of the lung as opposed to the airway lumen. These cells have been studied in animals and, to a lesser extent, in humans. They appear to have less phagocytic and cytokine production capacity than AM. One hypothesis is that they are direct precursors of AM in transit to the airways.[23]

As the sentinel of the immune system in the lung, AM are equipped with various functional capacities, including phagocytosis, migratory capability, production of a variety of enzymes and toxic oxygen and nitrogen metabolites, secretion of bioactive substances (including lipid mediators and cytokines), and expression of receptors facilitating cell-cell interaction with many cells, particularly lymphocytes.[12,13,16,23] To facilitate these diverse functions, AM express a large variety of receptors (Table 21-6).[12,23] These include receptors for bacterial endotoxin (CD14), receptors for opsonizing antibodies and complement fragments, a mannose receptor that mediates binding to *Pneumocystis carinii* and *Mycobacterium tuberculosis,* lectin receptors that bind carbohydrate antigens, and cytokine receptors. Efforts to characterize subpopulations of AM based on the differential expression of membrane receptors have been hampered by intense autofluorescence. However, the use of immunohistochemistry and, more recently, novel techniques using fluorescent dyes have facilitated the characterization of AM receptors. It is worth noting that while AM and other macrophages lack antigen receptors, they are able to take advantage of the antigen specificity of immunoglobulins. Most phagocytosis of microorganisms occurs after opsonization with antibody or complement. These processes utilize receptors for the Fc portion of the Ig molecule and complement, respectively.

AM release a variety of inflammatory mediators, including arachidonate products, peptide cytokines, and enzymes such as acid hydrolases, elastase, and plasminogen activator inhibitor (Table 21-7). Release of these mediators is increased with macrophage activation. These mediators interact to alter the function of a broad range of leukocytes and lung cells, and may alter extracellular matrix and fibrin deposition at sites of immune injury.[12,23,28]

In general, and with few exceptions, AM activation enhances mediator release, phagocytic function, and microbial killing.[1,23,28] Macrophages can also be "primed" by activation stimuli to release increased amounts of arachidonic acid metabolites. It is impossible to accurately assess the relative phagocytic, microbicidal, inflammation-generating, and other capabilities of

AM compared to other lung macrophage populations because it is likely that a large majority of the accessible AM are those that have previously "seen action." As a result, many may already be "preactivated" or depleted of a portion of their functional capacities. There is considerable heterogeneity in size of AM, ranging from small cells similar to blood monocytes to multinucleated cells 40 μm in size. In general, the smaller monocytelike cells are more efficient at phagocytosis and microbial killing than the large cells. The smaller cells probably represent younger, recently emigrated phagocytes.[23]

Under certain circumstances, it is likely that AM function as antigen-presenting cells for memory T-lymphocyte activation—a function that may be enhanced in such disorders as HIV infection, graft rejection, and sarcoidosis. In general, however, interstitial macrophages and blood monocytes are more efficient at antigen presentation than AM. In fact, the major function of AM in this regard may be suppression of T-lymphocyte activation at the level of antigen receptor signal transduction. This supposition is corroborated by one animal model in which depletion of AM enhanced lymphocyte activation, suggesting that AM function to suppress T-lymphocyte activation in normal lung homeostasis.[43]

Dendritic Cells and Langerhans' Cells

Seminal studies showing the immunosuppressive effects of AM led to the search for antigen-presenting cells in the lung. Like the spleen and skin, the lung is a residence site for dendritic cells (DC). DC are phagocytelike cells, presumably of hematopoetic origin, that have impressive antigen-presenting capabilities.[13] They are 10- 100-fold more potent than monocytes as antigen-presenting cells for naïve T lymphocytes (Table 21-5). They also account for a significant proportion of the MHC expression in the lung and thus probably make a significant contribution to T-cell activation in response to antigen challenge. Furthermore, they express the adhesion molecules and "accessory functions" essential for T-cell activation, including MHC molecules, antigen-processing capability, ICAM/CD54, LFA-3/CD58, β_1 and β_2 integrins, and possibly the CD28 lig-

TABLE 21-6

Receptors Expressed and Ligands Recognized by Alveolar Macrophages*

Immunoglobulins (Fc receptors):	Complement receptors for:
IgG1, IgG2a (murine)	C3b, iC3b, C4b, C3d, C5a
IgG2b, IgG3 (murine)	
IgG1, IgG3 monomers (human)	
IgE, IgA (murine, human)	
Protein, cytokine and matrix receptors:	Lipoprotein receptors for:
Fibronectin	Low-density lipoprotein
Fibrin	β–very-low-density lipoprotein
Lactoferrin, transferrin	
GM-CSF	
IFN-γ, IL-2, IL-4, IL-1, IL-1RA	
Insulin	
Chemotactic factor receptors	
Other receptors and adhesion molecules:	Lectin receptors for:
Class II MHC (HLA-DR, -DP, -DQ)	α-linked galactose residues
CD4	N-acetylgalactosamine residues
β_2 integrins (CD18; CD11a, b, c)	α-linked fucose residues
β_1 integrins (CD29; CD49a, b, c, e, f)	N-acetylneuraminic acid residues
CD54 (ICAM-1)	Mannose residues (mannose receptor)
CD14 (lipopolysaccharide receptor)	

NOTE: Ig = immunoglobulin; Fc = complement-binding fragment of immunoglobulin; IL = interleukin; IFN = interferon; GM-CSF = granulocyte-macrophage colony–stimulating factor; MHC = major histocompatibility complex antigen; R = receptor; RA = receptor antagonist; CD = cluster of differentiation.
*Not a complete listing.
SOURCE: Adapted from Fels and Cohn,[12] and Lohmann-Matthes et al.[23]

TABLE 21-7

Cytokines and Other Bioactive Substances Released from Lung Macrophages*

Arachidonate metabolites	Cytokines	Chemokine chemotactic factors
Thromboxane A$_2$	IL-1	IL-10
PGE$_2$, D$_2$, F$_{2a}$	IL-1RA	IL-12
LTB$_4$,	IL-6	IL-15
5-HETE	TNF-α	MIF
	IFN-α/β	
Reactive oxygen metabolites	Nitric oxide	
Superoxide anion (O2$^-$)	Constitutive	
H$_2$O$_2$	Inducible ?	
Hydroxyl radical (OH$\cdot$)		
Enzymes		
Metalloproteases		
Elastase		
Procoagulant activity		

NOTE: Tx = thromboxane; PG = prostaglandin; LT = leukotriene; HETE = hydroxyeicosatetraenoic acid; MIF = macrophage inhibitory factor; IL = interleukin; TNF = tumor necrosis factor; IFN = interferon.
*Not a complete listing. See references 12, 23, 28.

ands.[13,29] DC are found in the epithelium of the large airways in high density and decrease in number as airway size decreases.[13] Histologic sections along the long axis of airways have revealed a meshwork of DC processes that provide a mechanism for airway antigen sampling and interaction with epithelial T cells. Such a meshwork is also found in BALT.[13]

DC are found in the blood (0.5 percent of blood mononuclear cells), and are highly motile. It is assumed that pulmonary DC have translocated from the blood, though the stimuli for this translocation are not known and the role of in situ proliferation is not well understood.[13] Recent studies documented the translocation of dendritic cells, but not AM from the rodent airway to regional lymph nodes, suggesting that DC play a role in initiating a lymph node memory response to antigen challenge.[15] Specialized dendritic cells with distinctive infoldings of the plasma membrane seen only on electron microscopy (Langerhans' cells) are also found in lungs, especially those of smokers. Like DC, these cells are less efficient at phagocytosis, microbial killing, and generation of cytokines, but they are potent APC.[13]

Monocytes

Monocytes are a blood leukocyte type, and are presumed to be precursors of lung macrophages. The average monocyte spends 1 to 3 days in the circulation, leaves the circulation, and differentiates into a tissue macrophage. There is probably some baseline monocyte traffic into the lung that can be markedly increased in inflammation.[30] As mentioned above, monocytes can be induced under in vitro culture conditions to express receptors characteristic of AM over a period of days.

Intravascular Macrophages

A population of intravacular macrophages is found in the lung vasculature of many species. While they are most prominent in pigs and ruminants, a small intravascular population is present in humans.[46] They are characteristically located in postcapillary venules, strongly adherent, and positioned facing the flow of blood. These cells have been difficult to isolate in pure form and study in isolation. They are presumed to act as intravascular inflammatory sentinels, ingesting antigens and releasing mediators in response to inflammatory stimuli that reach the lung vasculature from the blood.[46]

Recruitment of Monocytes and Macrophages

There is evidence in both humans and animal models that lung macrophages are derived from bone marrow precursors, presumably monocytes.[44] There is also extensive evidence for the enhanced recruitment of circulating monocytes during acute lung inflammation.[23,30] Support for the concept that AM are derived from blood monocytes also comes from studies from a number of investigators demonstrating that monocytes develop phenotypic and functional characteristics of tissue macrophages when cultured *ex vivo* on various adhesion substrata. The present paradigm suggests that a blood-borne cell, likely the monocyte, adheres to pulmonary capillaries, with subsequent migration into the interstitium of lung.[27] Migration into the airway and further differentiation into a tissue macrophage are influenced by local tissue-specific factors, including chemotactic cytokines, matrix components, complement fragments, antigens released in the local environment, cell-cell interactions with fibroblasts and epithelial cells, and perhaps surfactant itself.[23,27]

Monocytes are motile cells that adhere to endothelial cells and transmigrate in vitro with extraordinary efficiency. Adhesion of monocytes to endothelial cells is mediated by a set of adhesion molecules similar to that of lymphocytes.[5,20,39] Like lymphocytes, monocytes "roll" along vascular walls in order to facilitate interaction with endothelial adhesion molecules. This rolling is mediated by adhesion molecules of the selectin family. The dominant adhesive function in monocytes appears to be mediated by the β_2 integrins $\alpha_L\beta_2$ and $\alpha_M\beta_2$, as well as $\alpha_4\beta_1$ integrin interaction with VCAM. Finally, alterations in monocyte deformability that occur with activation may enhance retention in lung capillaries. Blood monocytes adherent to endothelium respond to a variety of chemotactic influences, ranging from the complement fragments (C5a), the bacterial peptide f-MLP, leukotriene B4, and the chemokine chemoattractant cytokines—particularly MCP-1 and MIP-1α and $-\beta$.[23] Of interest is that IL-8 and MCP-1 are released by monocytes or by endothelial cells interacting with adherent monocytes. In extracellular matrix, monocytes and macrophages interact with extracellular matrix components via a variety of β_1 integrins.

The motility of AM and dendritic cells (DC) has also been studied. DC are present in blood and are presumed to be highly motile cells.[13,15] DC introduced into the airways have been found to efficiently translocate to regional lymph nodes, while AM were less efficient.[15] However, AM have been documented to transport phagocytosed antigen (e.g., fluorescent beads) from airway to regional lymph nodes in the dog.[14]

Activation of Lung Macrophages

A major feature of tissue macrophages is their ability to be "activated" by interacting with their environment via the many receptors they express at various stages of their development.[1,12,23] Classic examples of activation stimuli include interaction with antigen-antibody complexes via Fc receptors, with complement via complement receptors, or with cytokines such as γ-interferon. Activation causes an increase in cell size, augments the extrusion of pseudopodia, and increases membrane ruffling and cell membrane turnover. It also commonly upregulates one or all of the multifarious functions of macrophages, with enhanced phagocytosis being prominently noted. Metabolic activation is evidenced by an increase in oxygen and glucose metabolism, including the production of toxic oxygen metabolites. The presence of an inducible nitric oxide synthase has been documented in murine alveolar macrophages, but the human equivalent has proved controversial. As a result of activation, the expression and function of adhesion and chemotactic receptors, particularly the $\alpha_M\beta_2$ integrin, are increased. Secretory function is also increased, and the release of cytokines, toxic oxygen metabolites, and enzymes is augmented.[1] Arachidonate metabolism is more complex, and the release of AA metabolites may be either increased or decreased by various activation stimuli. Some activation signals, particularly IFN-γ, also potently increase the expression of class II MHC, enhancing interaction with T cells and antigen presentation. Macrophage activation after interaction with environmental stimuli is a key event in the inflammatory cascade in the lung.

LYMPHOCYTE-MACROPHAGE INTERACTIONS IN THE LUNG

The interactions between lymphocytes and macrophages, and their effects on lung inflammation and healing, are summarized in Fig. 21-2. AM and lymphocytes each perform important functions and influence the differentiation and function of a large variety of cells. The phenotype of the inflammatory and healing response that occurs also depends on interactions between AM and lymphocytes. These interactions include direct cell-cell contact during antigen presentation and mutual coactivation.

AM and related cells are the initial sentinels of the inflammatory response, phagocytosing and eliminating invading anti-gens and microbes. After interaction with microbial invaders, especially in conditions of overwhelming invasion, AM activation results in the release of inflammatory mediators, which activate adhesion molecule expression on endothelial cells and promote the migration and activation of blood leukocytes, including polymorphonuclear leukocytes (PMN), monocytes, lymphocytes, and eosinophils (Fig. 21-2). The rapid induction of selectin molecules stored in the Weibel-Palade bodies of the endothelium results in the rolling adhesion of neutrophils and monocytes. Migration of these leukocytes may be rapidly modulated by the release of arachidonate products such as LTB4, bacterial peptide f-MLP, and complement fragments. More time is required for the optimal expression of adhesion molecules such as VCAM,

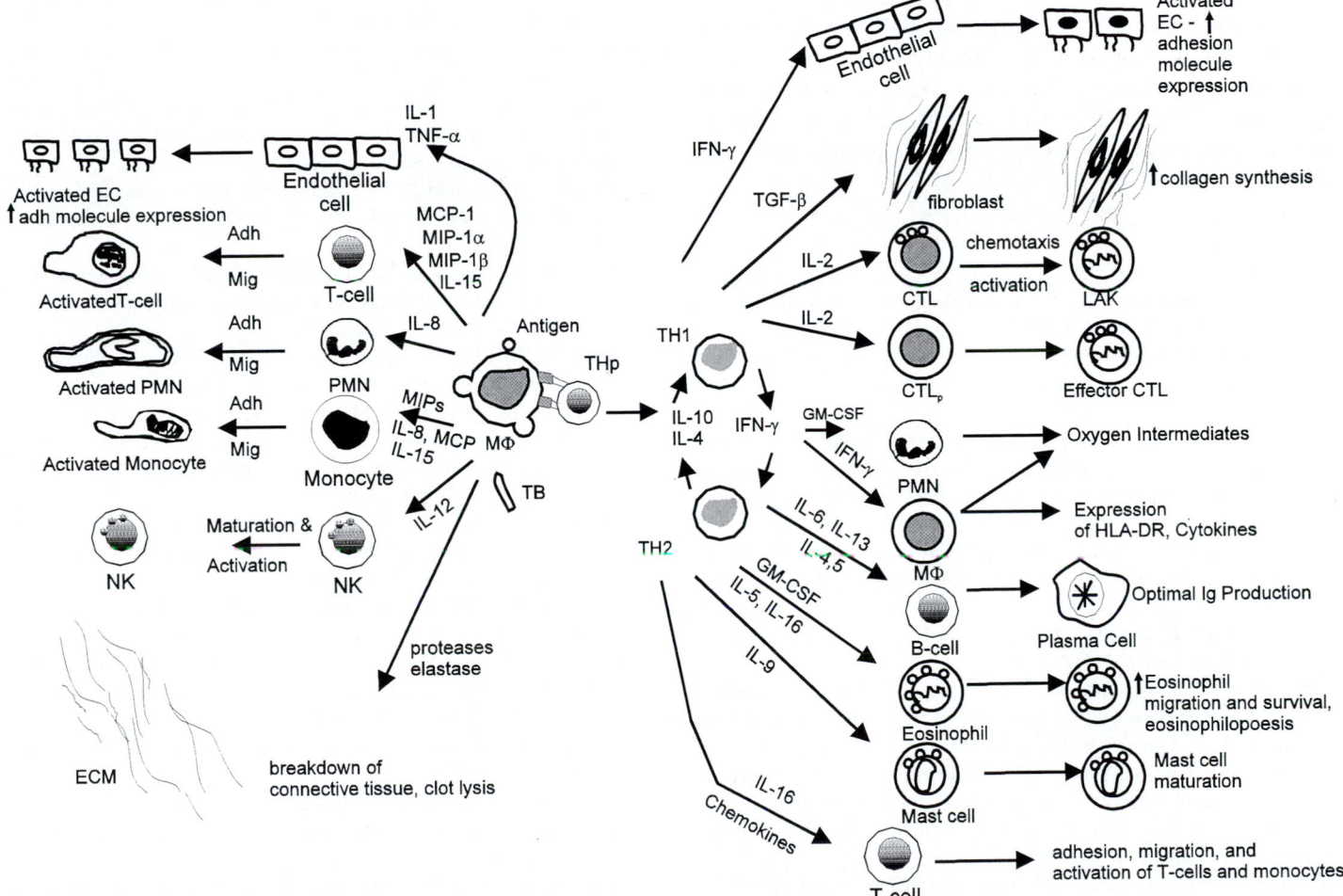

FIGURE 21-2 Lymphocyte and macrophage interactions in lung inflammation. Lymphocytes and macrophages interact directly and indirectly to influence lung inflammation. These interactions are complex—as illustrated by this diagram, which contains a necessarily incomplete sampling of these processes. Lymphocytes and macrophages interact directly in the process of lymphocyte activation. Activated T lymphocytes express a broad range of cytokines, which have far-reaching effects. They stimulate B cells to become plasma cells and make antibodies, regulate fibroblast proliferation and matrix molecule production, activate PMN and macrophages, stimulate eosinophil chemotaxis and activation, induce mast cell maturation, and augment the migration and activation of other lymphocytes. Macrophages similarly produce a large number of cytokines, which alter the functions of a variety of cells. Prominent effects include the elaboration of IL-1 and TNF, whose pro-tein effects include EC activation; chemotactic chemokines, which play a major role in the recruitment and activation of PMN, lymphocytes, monocytes, and eosinophils; and IL-12, which induces the activation and maturation of NK cells. Macrophages also release arachidonate metabolites and reactive oxygen species, nitric oxides, and a large number of proteases, which alter the function of surrounding cells, kill invading microorganisms, and degrade matrix proteins. See text for further explanation. NOTE: EC = endothelial cell; Adh = adhere; Mig = migratrion; IL = interleukin; TNF = tumor necrosis factor; MCP = monocyte chemotactic peptide; MIP = macrophage inflammatory protein; ECM = extracellular matrix; NK = natural killer cells; CTL = cytotoxic T lymphocyte; MØ = macrophage; Ig = immunoglobulin; IFN = interferon; THp = precursor T helper cell; TH1 = T helper–1; TH2 = T helper–2. (*Based on data of Agostini et al,*[12] *with permission.*)

which enhance lymphocyte entry, and the expression of the chemokine chemoattractant cytokines. One exception is the release within hours of IL-16 from the epithelium or resident T cells in response to mast cell–derived histamine.

Interaction of resident or infiltrating T cells with APC (mainly DC, Langerhans' cells, and monocytes) results in optimal T-cell activation, with resultant production of cytokines that act on a variety of cytokine receptor–bearing cells (Fig. 21-2). This results in the activation of endothelium, optimal B-cell production of antibody, generation of cytotoxic effector T cells, and, depending on the nature of the cytokines produced, a delayed-type hypersensitivity or granulomatous response (TH1 cytokines) or an allergic or eosinophilic response (TH2 cytokines). Fibrosis or repair may also be influenced by the production of proteases[28] and protease inhibitors by AM, or by the elaboration of the fibrogenic cytokines such as TGF-β_1 and IGF-1 by T lymphocytes, macrophages, or other cells. Remodeling of the resulting scar also occurs, mediated in part by enzymes that accelerate the degradation of fibrin and other matrix components, including laminin, fibronectin, hyaluronen, glycosaminoglycans, and elastin.

REFERENCES

1. Adams DO, Hamilton TA: The cell biology of macrophage activation. *Annu Rev Immunol* 2:283–318, 1984.
2. Agostini C, Chilosi M, Zambello R, et al: Pulmonary immune cells in health and disease: Lymphocytes. *Eur Respir J* 6:1378–1401, 1993.
3. BAL Cooperative Steering Committee: Bronchoalveolar lavage constituents in healthy individuals, idiopathic pulmonary fibrosis, and selected comparison groups. *Am Rev Respir Dis* 141:S169–S201, 1990.
4. Berman JS, Beer DJ, Theodore AC, et al: State of the art: Lymphocyte recruitment to the lung. *Am Rev Respir Dis* 142:238–257, 1990.
5. Bevilacqua MP: Endothelial-leukocyte adhesion molecules. *Annu Rev Immunol* 11:767–804, 1993.
6. Bienenstock J: Bronchus-associated lymphoid tissue, in Bienenstock J (ed), *Immunology of the Lung and Upper Respiratory Tract*. New York, McGraw-Hill, 1984, pp 157–173.
7. Bitterman RB, Saltzman LE, Adelberg S, et al: Alveolar macrophage replication: One mechanism for the expansion of the mononuclear phagocyte population in the chronically inflamed lung. *J Clin Invest* 74:460–469, 1984.
8. Car BD, Meloni F, Luisetti M, et al: Elevated IL-8 and MCP-1 in the bronchoalveolar lavage fluid of patients with idiopathic pulmonary fibrosis and pulmonary sarcoidosis. *Am J Respir Crit Care Med* 149:655–659, 1994.
9. Cruikshank WW, Long A, Tarpy RE, et al: Early identification of IL-16 (lymphocyte chemoattractant factor) and macrophage inflammatory protein 1a in BAL of antigen challenged asthmatics. *Am J Resp Cell Mol Biol* 13:738–747, 1995.
10. Curtis JL, Kaltreider HB: Characterization of bronchoalveolar lymphocytes during a specific antibody-forming cell response in the lungs of mice. *Am Rev Respir Dis* 139:393–400, 1989.
11. Erle DJ, Brown T, Cristian D, Aris R: Lung epithelial lining fluid T cell subsets defined by distinct patterns of beta 7 and beta 1 integrin expression. *Am J Respir Cell Mol Biol* 10:237–244, 1994.
12. Fels AOS, Cohn ZA: The alveolar macrophage. *J Appl Physiol* 60:353–369, 1986.
13. Hance AJ: Pulmonary immune cells in health and disease: Dendritic cells and Langerhans' cells. *Eur Respir J* 6:1213–1220, 1993.
14. Harmsen AG, Muggenburg BA, Snipes MB, Bice DE: The role of macrophages in particle transfer from lungs to lymph nodes. *Science* 230:1277–1280, 1985.
15. Havenith CE, van Miert PP, Breedijk AJ, et al: Migration of dendritic cells into the draining lymph nodes of the lung after intratracheal instillation. *Am J Resp Cell Mol Biol* 9:484–488, 1993.
16. Holt PG: Regulation of antigen-presenting cell function(s) in lung and airway tissues. *Eur Respir J* 6:120–129, 1993.
17. Holt PG, Robinson BWS, Reid M, et al: Extraction of immune and inflammatory cells from human lung parenchyma: Evaluation of an enzymatic digestion procedure. *Clin Exp Immunol* 66:188–200, 1986.
18. Hunninghake GW, Bedell GN, Zavala DC, Brady M: Role of interleukin-2 release by lung T cells in active pulmonary sarcoidosis. *Am Rev Respir Dis* 128:634–638, 1983.
19. Johnston RB: Monocytes and macrophages. *New Engl J Med* 318:747–752, 1988.
20. Jonjic N, Jilek P, Bernasconi S, et al: Molecules involved in the adhesion and cytotoxicity of activated monocytes on endothelial cells. *J Immunol* 148:2080–2083, 1992.
21. Kornfeld H, Berman JS, Beer DJ, Center DM: Chemotactic activity of interleukin-2 for human T-lymphocytes. *J Immunol* 134:3887–3890, 1985.
22. Kremlev SG, Umstead TM, Phelps DS: Effects of surfactant protein A and surfactant lipids on lymphocyte proliferation in vitro. *Am J Physiol* 267:L357–L364, 1994.
23. Lohmann-Matthes M, Steinmuller C, Franke-Ullman G: Pulmonary macrophages. *Eur Respir J* 7:1678–1689, 1994.
24. Marathias KP, Preffer FI, Pinto C, Kradin RL: Most human pulmonary infiltrating lymphocytes display the surface immune phenotype and functional responses of sensitized T cells. *Am J Respir Cell Mol Biol* 5:470–476, 1991.
25. Miller MD, Krangel MS: Biology and biochemistry of the chemokines: A family of chemotactic and inflammatory cytokines. *Crit Rev Immunol* 12:17–46, 1992.
26. Mossman TR, Sad S: The expanding universe of T cell subsets: Th1, Th2, and more. *Immunol Today* 17:138–146, 1996.
27. Naito M, Umeda S, Yamamoto T, et al: Development, differentiation and phenotypic heterogeneity of murine tissue macrophages. *J Leukocyte Biol* 59:133–138, 1996.
28. Nathan CF: Secretory products of macrophages. *J Clin Invest* 79:319–326, 1987.
29. Nicod LP, el Habre F: Adhesion molecules on human lung dendritic cells and their role for T-cell activation. *Am J Respir Cell Mol Biol* 7:207–13, 1992.
30. Ohgami M, Doerschuk CM, Gie RP, et al: Monocyte kinetics in rabbits. *J Appl Physiol* 70:152–157, 1991.
31. Pabst R: The immune system of the respiratory tract in the pig, in Busse W, Holgate ST (eds), *Asthma and Rhinitis*. Cambridge, MA, Blackwell, pp 415–425.
32. Pabst R, Binns RM: Lymphocytes migrate from the bronchoalveolar space to regional bronchial lymph nodes. *Am J Respir Crit Care Med* 151:495–499, 1995.
33. Pabst RM, Gehourke I: Is the bronchus-associated lymphoid tissue an integral structure of the lung in normal animals, including humans? *Am J Respir Cell Mol Biol* 3:131–135, 1990.
34. Pabst R, Binns RM, Licence ST, Peter M: Evidence of a selective major vascular marginal pool of lymphocytes in the lung. *Am Rev Respir Dis* 136:1213–1218, 1987.
35. Picker LJ: Control of lymphocyte homing. *Curr Opin Immunol* 6:394–406, 1994.

36. Robinson DS, Hamid Q, Ying S, et al: Predominant TH2-like bronchoalveolar T-lymphocyte population in atopic asthma. *New Engl J Med* 326:298–304, 1992.

37. Romagnani S: Lymphokine production by human T cells in disease states. *Ann Rev Immunol* 12:227–257, 1994.

38. Saukkonen JJ, Kornfeld H, Berman JS: Expansion of a CD8+ CD28– cell population in the blood and lung of HIV-positive patients. *J Acquir Immune Defic Syndr* 6:1194–1204, 1993.

39. Springer TA: Traffic signals on endothelium for lymphocyte recirculation and leukocyte emigration. *Annu Rev Physiol* 57:827–872, 1995.

40. Standiford TJ, Rolfe MW, Kunkel SL, et al: Macrophage inflammatory protein–1 alpha expression in intersitial lung disease. *J Immunol* 151:2852–2863, 1993.

41. Taub DD, Turcovski-Corrales, Key ML, et al: Chemokines and T lymphocyte activation: I. Beta chemokines costimulate human T lymphocyte activation in vitro. *J Immunol* 156:2095–2103, 1996.

42. Taub DD, Proost P, Murphy WJ, et al: Monocyte chemotactic proteins-1, 2, and 3 are chemotactic for human T lymphocytes. *J Clin Invest* 95:1370–1376, 1995.

43. Thepen T, Kraal G, Holt PG: The role of alveolar macrophages in regulation of lung inflammation. *Ann NY Acad Sci* 725:200–206, 1994.

44. Thomas ED, Ramberg RE, Sale GE, et al: Direct evidence for a bone marrow origin of the alveolar macrophage in man. *Science* 192:1016–1018, 1976.

45. van Dinther-Janssen AC, van Maarsseveen TC, Eckert H, et al: Identical expression of ELAM-1, VCAM-1, and ICAM-1 in sarcoidosis and usual interstitial pneumonitis. *J Pathol* 170:157–164, 1993.

46. Warner AE, Brain JD: The cell biology and pathogenic role of pulmonary intravascular macrophages. *Am J Physiol* 258:L1–L12, 1990.

47. Williams GT: Apoptosis in the immune system. *J Pathol* 173:1–4, 1994.

48. Yamauchi K, Martinet Y, Basset P, et al: High levels of transforming growth factor-β are present in the epithelial lining fluid of the normal lower respiratory tract. *Am Rev Respir Dis* 137:1360–1363, 1988.

CHAPTER 22

MAST CELLS AND EOSINOPHILS

Edward S. Schulman / Donald G. Raible

MAST CELLS
 Anatomic Localization
 Origins of Mast Cells
 Mast Cell Heterogeneity
 Morphology
 Biochemical Analysis of HLMC Activation
 Chemical Mediators
 Preformed Mediators
 Nonpreformed Mediators
 Pharmacologic Modulation of Mast Cell Function
 Mast Cells in Pulmonary Disease

EOSINOPHILS
 Eosinophil Development
 Morphology and Structure
 Granule Proteins
 Eosinophil Recruitment
 Eosinophil Receptors and Mechanisms of Activation
 Chemical Mediators
 Pharmacologic Modulation of Eosinophil Function
 Mast Cell–Eosinophil Interactions
 Eosinophil–Disease Associations

For more than a century physicians have noted a clear connection between mast cell activation and the subsequent appearance of eosinophils both within the circulation and in tissues. Only recently, however, have basic insights been gained into the mechanisms of this cellular collusion. In keeping with this association, human mast cells and eosinophils will be considered together in this chapter.

Mast cells and eosinophils were discovered in the 1870s by the same observer, Paul Ehrlich. He noted that some cells stained in a peculiar fashion when incubated with standard aniline dyes such as toluidine blue and alcian blue. He used the term *metachromasie* or *metachromasia* to describe the peculiar color modifications that occurred and the term *Mastzellen,* meaning "well fed" or "fattened" in German, to describe what we now call mast cells. Interestingly, this latter term is now known to be a misnomer, since mast cell cytoplasmic granules are not phagocytosized but rather synthesized during cell growth and again during regranulation. Ehrlich also noted that some cells stained intensely when incubated with the acidic dye eosin. As a result, these cells were called *eosinophils*. Studies of these two cell types, over the ensuing years, have provided great insight into

their roles in biology. They have also highlighted the differences that exist in these cells among different species and their heterogeneity in a single species in different organs.

MAST CELLS

The capacity of strategically localized human mast cells to release rapidly a panoply of powerful chemical mediators makes this cell a unique member of the body's immune response network.[38] Although most frequently discussed in the context of hypersensitivity responses, mast cells are also known to participate in normal physiological processes including gastric acid secretion and lipid clearance. Mast cells also participate in nonallergic pathophysiological processes such as inflammatory bowel disease, arthritis, scleroderma, tumors, interstitial pulmonary fibrosis, and atherosclerosis. Over the years, basophils have been confused with mast cells in a number of contexts. This confusion is due, in part, to a number of similarities between the cells, including the shared expression of FcεRI (high-affinity receptor for Fc fragment of IgE), release of preformed histamine, and metachromatic staining. However, mast cells are mononuclear cells and are almost exclusively localized to tissues. In contrast, basophils are circulating polymorphonuclear cells that are less commonly found in tissue reactions. In addition, significant differences in the two cell populations exist in cell lineage, ultrastructure, mediator release biochemistry, mediator profiles, pharmacology, and surface antigenicity.

Anatomic Localization

Mast cells are present in all organs but are in particular abundance in the nose, skin, GI tract, and lung. They reside primarily near blood vessels, within the adventitia of arteries, and also near lymph vessels and nerves. Estimated concentrations of human lung mast cells (HLMC) range from 500 to 4000 mm^{-3}. Mediator release from the small numbers of HLMC within the epithelium may subserve initial antigen recognition. The resulting airway permeabilization enhances antigen exposure to deeper mast-cell-rich regions. Within bronchial walls, these deeper sites include the areas near airway smooth muscle and beneath airway mucous gland capsules. In these locations the released mediators can effect bronchoconstriction and mucous secretion, respectively. In the lung periphery, abundant mast cells[39] reside within small airways and in the alveolar septa, within a few microns of the alveolar lumen. The small numbers of mast cells in bronchoalveolar lavage (BAL) fluid (≤0.1 percent of all cells) may result from epithelial shedding.

Origins of Mast Cells

Mast cells are derived from the multipotential hematopoietic stem cell. Tryptase-negative mast cell–colony-forming cells leave the marrow and circulate with a surface phenotype that is CD (cluster of differentiation) 34+, c-kit(CD117)+, LY-, CD14-, and CD17-.[2] After homing to either connective tissue or mucosal areas, the cells undergo differentiation and maturation and synthesize granule proteases in response to microenvironmental factors from fibroblasts and possibly T cells. One important microenvironmental factor is stem cell factor (c-kit ligand or SCF), the ligand for the c-kit tyrosine kinase receptor.

Mast Cell Heterogeneity

Mast cell heterogeneity was first appreciated in rats when it was found that mast cells in intestines and other tissues that were undetectable following formalin fixation were readily observed after basic lead acetate fixation.[13] Mast cells were thus designated as "mucosal" or "formalin-sensitive" if they were undetectable after formalin fixation, and "connective tissue" or "formalin-resistant" if they retained their metachromatic staining after formalin exposure.[13] Using these tinctorial properties to define mast cell subtypes, many investigators have reported striking differences in the morphology, T-cell dependence, resident proteoglycans, and responsiveness to secretagogues and drugs of these cell populations. Multiple types of human mast cells have been described.[38] The ontogeny of this heterogeneity, as well as the differing roles these mast cells play, in physiology and disease remain speculative. The nature of this heterogeneity is summarized below.

Proteases   The most commonly recognized system for classifying human mast cells is based on the expression of protease profiles as determined by immunohistochemical staining using monoclonal antibodies.[17] According to this system, the serine proteinase tryptase (T) is expressed in all human mast cells, and a subset, predominantly in the submucosa of the gut and in the skin, also express chymase (C) and multiple other proteases.[8] Those that express tryptase alone are classified as the MC_T type, and those with additional proteases as the MC_{TC} type. Based largely on their similar anatomic distribution in rodents, mast cells of the T and TC type have also been likened to the mucosal and connective tissue subtypes, respectively. However, the precision of this analogy in humans has not been firmly established. Because significant numbers of both types can be found in the same organ (e.g., lung), tissue location alone cannot dictate the protease type. Recently, cells positive for chymase alone (MC_C) have been described and shown to constitute up to 17 percent of mast cells in bowel submucosa. In the connective-tissue-rich environment of lung, only 8 to 35 percent of mast cells are MC_{TC}, 1 percent are MC_C, and the remainder are MC_T.

Airway versus Parenchyma   Anatomic location dictates disparate releasility.

Morphology: Diameter and Density   This heterogeneity was discovered following the development of techniques to dissociate lungs into single-cell suspensions. HLMC diameters vary between 8 and 18 μm with the majority being 12 to 15 μm. Histamine content is 2.5 to 10.0 pg per cell and varies directly with cell diameter. HLMC densities vary from 1.053 g/ml to 1.123 g/ml with the majority (67 percent) between 1.077 g/ml and 1.088 g/ml. These morphology-based subtypes also are distinct with respect to mediator content and function.

Morphology: Ultrastructure   These differences are most profound following anaphylactic release and recovery. The morphologies include small, large, immature, and poorly versus fully granulated mast cells.[28]

Formalin Sensitivity versus Resistance   Mast cells with staining properties analogous to those described in rodents are present in human lung and other organs.[40]

Proteoglycans   At least two types of proteoglycans are present in HLMC: chondroitin sulfates, predominantly chondroitin sulfate E, and heparin.[47] HLMC both positive and negative for the heparin-sensitive dye berberine sulfate have been described. Interestingly, human stomach mucosal mast cells are reported to synthesize exclusively chondroitin sulfate E ("E"-mast cells) and not heparin.

Cytokines   The MC_{TC} subtype preferentially expresses interleukin (IL)-4 (85 percent MC_{TC} versus 15 percent MC_T) as detected by immunohistochemical staining. IL-5 and IL-6 are almost exclusively restricted to the MC_T subtype.[7]

Morphology

"RESTING" MORPHOLOGY

HLMC ultrastructure at rest, during degranulation, and during recovery from stimulation, has been detailed.[28] All mast cells are mononuclear cells with heterogeneous cytoplasmic granules (Fig. 22-1). A variety of granule-filling patterns occur within individual cells: scrolls, crystals, particles (the least seen in pure form), and combinations (mixed). The appearance of individual patterns can be influenced by cross section. Granules are outlined by a perigranular membrane. Cell membranes are outlined by short, narrow surface folds.

MORPHOLOGY OF DEGRANULATION AND REGRANULATION

Following IgE-mediated (anaphylactic) activation, granules swell and then granule membranes fuse to form canaliculi that open through multiple pores to the cell exterior. Within 20 min of activation, granular matrix materials solubilize within these intracytoplasmic channels and empty. In HLMC, only rarely is extrusion of nonsolubilized granules observed. Lipid bodies, which are electron-dense nonmembrane-bound organelles, remain adjacent to these channels. Similar bodies are found in multiple cell types. They appear to serve as repositories of arachidonic acid and occasionally release lipid into the degranulation channels.

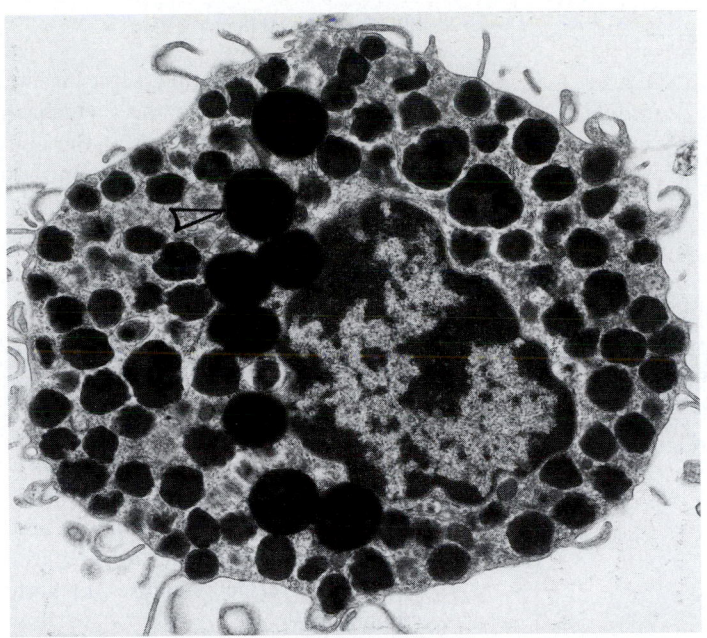

FIGURE 22-1 Ultrastructure of the human lung mast cell after purification. The mast cell is a mononuclear cell packed with multiple dense cytoplasmic granules that vary in size and shape. Eight electron-dense lipid bodies (open arrow) are bunched near the nucleus ($\times 15,000$). *(Reproduced with permission from Dvorak AM, Recovery of human lung mast cells from anaphylactic degranulation utilizes a mixture of conservation and synthetic mechanisms, in Galli SJ, Austen KF (eds), Mast Cell and Basophil Differentiation and Function in Health and Disease. New York, Raven, 1989, p 124.)*

In vivo, a process termed "piecemeal degranulation" is more frequently observed than the anaphylactic degranulation response described above. Though not well characterized in lung, this process involves the budding of small vesicles from granule membranes and their movement to the cell surface.

Depending on the extent to which an individual cell has degranulated, one of two predominant types of regranulation are observed individually or in combination. In cells that have only partially degranulated, the channel (formerly perigranular) membranes are reutilized, and regranulation events resemble degranulation in reverse. In cells that have experienced nearly complete degranulation, the channel membranes are placed in continuity with the plasma membrane and externalized. This results in the appearance of elongated, activated cell surface folds. These excessive folds can be internalized or shed. Shedding results in cells that are initially small (7 μm), but then these cells enter a rapidly expanding recovery cycle to produce a fully mature cell.

ACTIVATION

Immunologic activation of mast cells results from antigen cross-linking of antigen-specific cell surface IgE molecules and subsequent aggregation of the high-affinity receptors termed FcɛRI to which they are attached. Receptor dimerization is the minimum cross-linkage requirement for IgE-mediated activation. In vitro, immunologic activation can be achieved using antibodies directed against human IgE or the FcɛRI-receptor itself.

Non-IgE-mediated release triggers of mast cells are also well characterized. In general, the profile of agents that degranulate human gastrointestinal and synovial mast cells is similar to that of lung parenchymal cells but differs from that of skin cells. These agents include ionophores, hyperosmolar stimuli, "histamine-releasing activities" derived from human alveolar macrophages, and adenosine 5'-monophosphate. The purified anaphylatoxin C5a, an active trigger of human basophils and dermal mast cells, is inactive in HLMC. Degranulators of dermal but not HLMC include substance P, morphine, polyamines such as 48/80, and SCF. Even within lung compartments, responsiveness to triggers may vary. Compound 48/80 is reported to degranulate BAL mast cells, whereas those from lung parenchyma are minimally responsive. To date, neuropeptides have been inactive on HLMC.

Mast cells appear to possess receptors for multiple cytokines including IL-4 and IL-13. The modulatory effects of these cytokines on mast cell expression of leukocyte adhesion molecules [e.g., intercellular adhesion molecule-1(ICAM-1)] and response to other perturbations is poorly understood. Fibronectin and possibly other components of the connective tissue matrix also modulate mast cell reactivity.

Biochemical Analysis of HLMC Activation

Studies of the biochemical events following FcɛRI aggregation of authentic human mast cells have been few. The studies that have been performed, however, have provided evidence for the following sequence of events. IgE-mediated HLMC activation is followed at 15 s by phospholipid methylation. At 30 s a monophasic rise in cyclic AMP has been shown by some but not all investigators. Calcium influx occurs at 2 min and is followed by histamine release, which maximizes at 5 to 20 min.[18] Other "early phase" granule-associated and lipid mediators (e.g., arachidonate metabolites) are also released over 20 min. Over the ensuing 1 to 24 h, mRNAs for select cytokines are generated followed by their synthesis and release.[14,20] Other release events inferred from studies examining FcɛRI-bearing cells usually relate to exocytosis rather than lipid or cytokine synthesis. However, many pathways may be used in common by these mechanistic processes.

Chemical Mediators

The clinical expression of mast cell–mediated responses may reflect the individual mediators or in certain instances, the interplay of the multiple mediators these cells release (Table 22-1). The temporal sequence of their release appears critical to the development of both the early and late phase responses after antigen challenge (Figs. 22-2 and 22-3). Certain mediators are virtually unique to mast cells, (e.g., tryptase, chymase, heparin), and others are shared with one or more other cells [e.g., histamine, leukotriene (LT)C$_4$, and IL-5].

Classically, mediators released within minutes after activation are divided into preformed, or secretory, granule-associated mediators (e.g., histamine) and nonpreformed, or newly synthe-

TABLE 22-1

Human Mast Cell and Eosinophil Mediators

	Mast Cells	Eosinophils
Granule-associated (preformed) mediators	Histamine Heparin Chondroitin-sulfate E TNFα	MBP ECP EDN
Enzymes	Tryptase Chymase Cathepsin-G Elastase Carboxypeptidase-A	Eosinophil peroxidase (EPO) Lysophospholipase (CLC) Collagenase 92 kD gelatinase β-glucuronidase
Acid hydrolases	β-hexosaminidase β-glucuronidase Arylsulfatase	
Lipid mediators (nonpreformed)	PGD_2 LTC_4 LTB_4 PAF Thromboxane-A_2	LTC_4 Thromboxane-A_2 15-HETE PAF
Cytokines	IL-4, IL-5, IL-13 IL-6, IL-8 TNFα TGFβ bFGF	GM-CSF IL-3, IL-4, IL-5, IL-8 IL-6 TNFα TGF α/β PDGF
Reactive oxygen products	None detected	O_2^-, H_2O_2, OH· HOBr, HOCl

sized, mediators (e.g., lipids). It is now known that mast cell cytokines may be both preformed and newly synthesized over time (tumor necrosis factor alpha, TNFα). Other cytokine mediators, including IL-5 and IL-13, are only detected over time and may be critical to the evolution of the "late phase" response.

Preformed Mediators

HISTAMINE

Histamine measurements have served as an unequivocal marker of mast cell–mediated events. The actual role of histamine in asthma, however, remains less clear. Plasma histamine levels increase two- to fivefold following airway antigen challenge. Most histamine-induced allergic reactions are mediated via the H1 histamine receptor subclass producing enhancement of vascular permeability, initiation of neurogenic reflexes, and smooth muscle contraction. The reasons for the marginal value of H1 receptor blocking drugs in asthma may be due to high local tissue concentrations of histamine that exceed the inhibitory capacity of these agents and/or the redundancy of histamine actions with the multiple other mediators that are released. Histamine also induces the release of the CD4+ cell-specific cytokine, lymphocyte chemoattractant factor (IL-16) from CD8+ cells.[22] This effect is H2 receptor mediated.

PROTEOGLYCANS

Mast cell proteoglycans serve as the major determinant for the metachromatic tinctorial properties of the cell and form the granule backbone to which other preformed mediators, including histamine and neutral proteases, are bound. HLMC synthesize heparin and chondroitin sulfate E proteoglycans in roughly a 2:1 ratio.[47] In humans, heparin appears to be unique to mast cells. The role that heparin plays in HLMC-mediated reactions remains subject to conjecture. In addition to anticoagulant activity, heparin possesses both anti-inflammatory and immunoregulatory properties. Heparin may limit allergic responses in both skin and lung.[12]

CHEMOTACTIC FACTORS

Within hours of mast cell activation, airway inflammation at the tissue level is characterized by the infiltration of leukocytes. This response is principally eosinophilic but also contains neutrophils and, over time, lymphocytes. A variety of mast cell–derived mediators have been implicated in the generation of this response. These chemotactic mediators may be derived directly from mast cells and/or other cells through secondary stimulation. Known early-phase mast cell–derived eosinophilic chemotactic activities include leukotriene B_4 (LTB_4), platelet activating factor, histamine, and eosinophil chemotactic factor of anaphylaxis (ECF-A). The latter two factors are only weak perpetrators of this activity. A high-molecular-weight (750 kDa) chemotactic factor for neutrophils (NCF-A) can be measured in the blood of cold urticaria patients following cold challenge, and in sensitive asthmatics following antigen, aspirin, and exercise challenge. This factor may actually represent a small mast cell–derived lipid [e.g., LTB_4 and 8(S),15(s)-diHETE] bound to a high-molecular-weight carrier. Recently, over thirty highly active eosinophil, mononuclear, and neutrophil-derived chemotactic cytokines (chemokines) have been discovered. They can be classified into two distinct supergene families, the C-X-C and C-C families. At least seven C-X-C family members are known. They share receptors and, as typified by IL-8, are primarily chemotactic for neutrophils. In contrast, C-C chemokines are active on lymphocytes, monocytes, basophils, and eosinophils. Chemokines probably are released at sites of mast cell activation, and these cytokines may play a role in the late-phase allergic-hypersensitivity response. In accord with this belief, IL-8 has been appreciated in tissue mast cells using immunolocalization techniques. However, the ability of authentic human mast cells to produce diverse chemokines remains poorly defined.

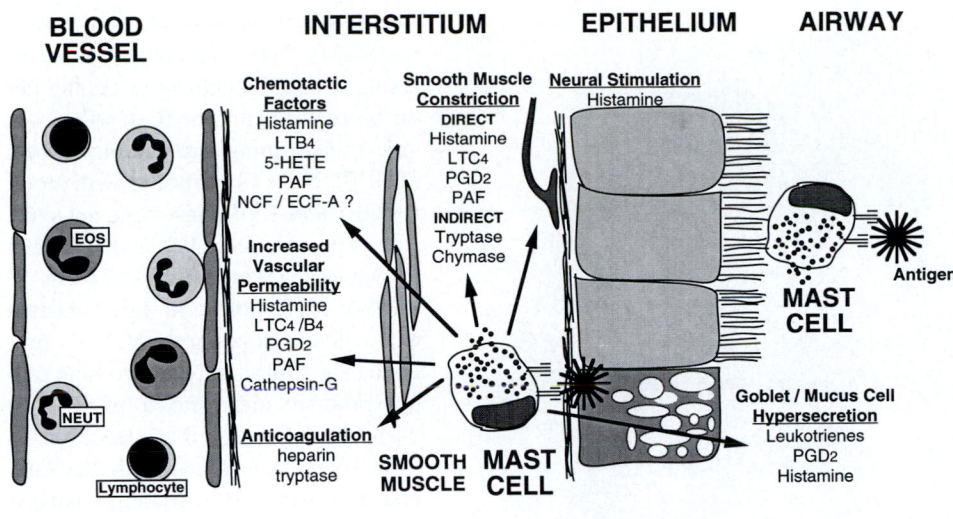

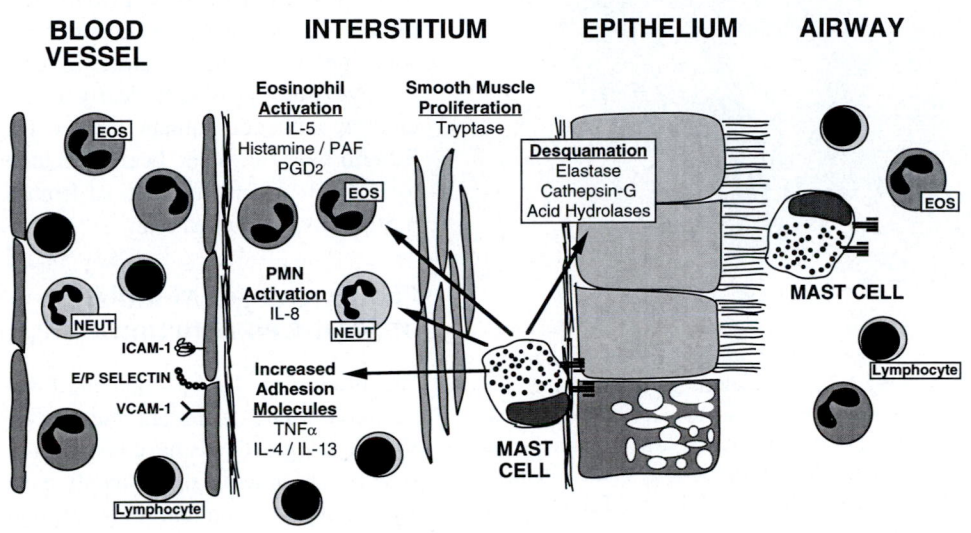

FIGURE 22-2   Effects of mast cell mediators in the early- and late-phase responses following airway allergen challenge. *A*. Early phase: Mediators are released within minutes following antigen cross-linking of allergen-specific IgE on the cell surface. Mechanisms of the initial airflow obstruction that persists for 30 to 60 min include smooth muscle constriction, edema formation due to increased vascular permeability, nerve stimulation, and mucus hypersecretion from both goblet cells and submucosal glands. *B*. Late phase. Within hours, the effects of newly synthesized and released cytokine mediators along with delayed effects of early-phase mediators produce recurrent airway obstruction. Mast cell mediators and cytokines can increase the expression of adhesion molecules on endothelial cells, both recruit and activate leukocytes, particularly eosinophils, contribute to epithelial desquamation, and stimulate smooth muscle proliferation.

PROTEASES

Large quantities of neutral proteases are contained within mast cells and constitute the predominant protein component of the secretory granule. The proteases include tryptase, chymase, cathepsin-G, elastase, and carboxypeptidase A.[8]

Tryptase

The first mast cell protease to be recognized was tryptase. Tryptase is the predominant neutral protease of the mast cell granule. The concentration of tryptase in pulmonary mast cells is 11 pg per mast cell. Since the concentration of tryptase in cir-

culating basophils (α tryptase, see below) is negligible at 0.05 pg per cell, responses characterized by the presence of histamine but not tryptase at the reaction site or in the circulation have been taken to be mediated by basophils and not mast cells. Recently, two forms of tryptase (α and β) have been identified.[42] The α form is constitutively secreted in an inactive form and reflects systemic mast cell burden. The active β form is packaged in the secretory granule and undergoes acute elevation in anaphylactic reactions.

Postulated roles for tryptase in pathophysiology remain to be established. Described actions include the degradation of the neuropeptide bronchodilator vasoactive intestinal peptide (VIP), mitogenic effects on smooth muscle and epithelial cells, inactivation of procoagulant proteins, and activation of urokinase. These latter activities may help inhibit clot formation and allow rapid resolution of edema reactions.

Chymase

Chymase received its name based on a similarity to chymotrypsin. It is associated with heparin in a manner similar to tryptase. Chymase substrates include angiotensin I, converting it to the vasoconstrictor angiotensin II, VIP (inactivates), substance P, bradykinin, and kallidin (inactivates).

Other Enzymes

Cathepsin-G is a neutral protease with chymotryptic specificities. The concentration of cathepsin-G in HLMC is roughly 100 to 700 ng/10[6] cells. The *elastase* in HLMC appears to be identical to human neutrophil elastase. The elastase measurement of 40 to 170 ng/10[6] cells assumes all HLMC contain this enzyme. This may not be the case, since elastase may be localized to an HLMC subset. *Carboxypeptidase A* is a metalloexopeptidase with a neutral-to-basic pH optimum. Among carboxypeptidases, the mast cell enzyme is unique. *Acid hydrolases* are granule-associated and include β-hexosaminidase, β-glucuronidase, and arylsulfatase. Their presence indicates that the granule organelle is a modified primary lysosome.

Nonpreformed Mediators

Arachidonic acid metabolites are generated within minutes of mast cell activation and play a crucial role in the early phases of

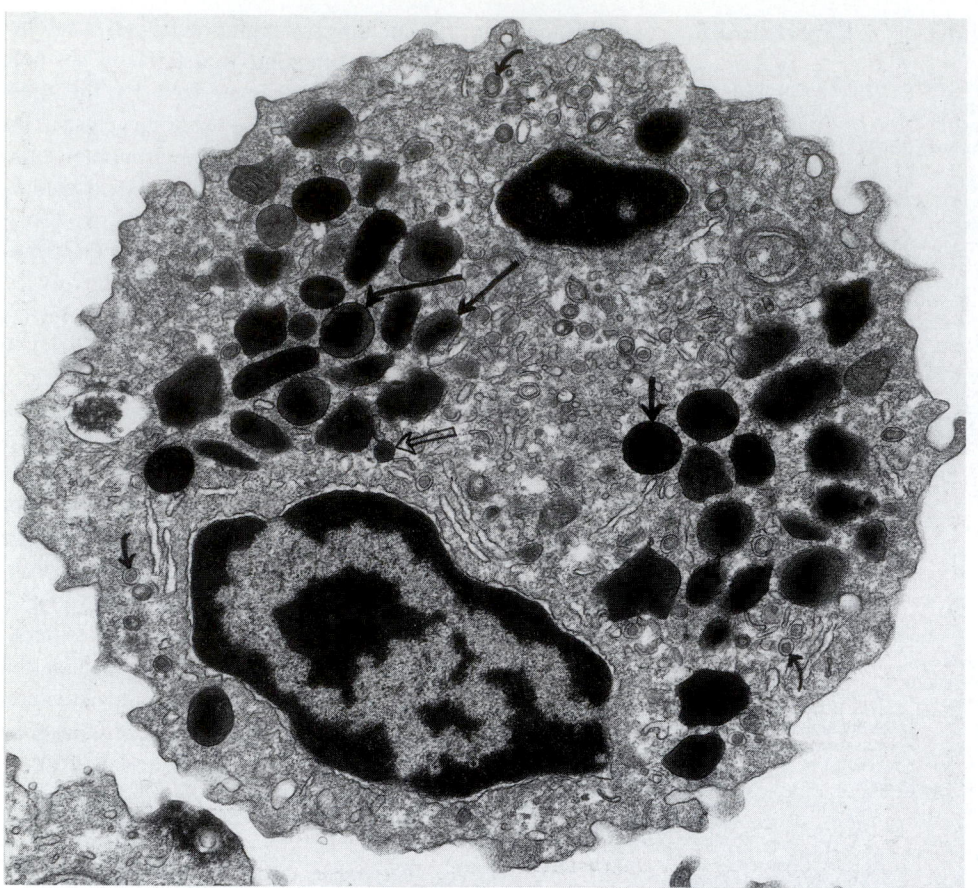

FIGURE 22-3 Ultrastructure of the human blood eosinophil. The primary granules are homogeneously dense and core-free (short closed arrow). The secondary or specific granules have a characteristic electron-dense core containing MBP (long closed arrows). Also shown are round, dense, small granules (open arrow) and curved, elongated, and round vesiculotubular structures (curved arrows) ($\times 13,650$). *(Reproduced with permission from Dvorak AM, Ultrastructural studies on mechanisms of human eosinophil activation and secretion, in Gleich GJ, Kay AB (eds), Eosinophils in Allergy and Inflammation. New York, Dekker, 1994, p 160.)*

man tissue mast cells are now known to generate "TH2" and other cytokines. Using immunolocalization techniques on biopsy specimens, IL-4, -5, -6, -8, -13, transforming growth factor beta (TGFβ), basic fibroblast growth factor (bFGF), and TNFα have been detected. Recently, purified HLMC have been shown to generate both IL-5 and IL-13 mRNA in response to IgE-mediated and calcium ionophore A23187–provoked signaling.[14,20] The cytokine protein products are released over a 4- to 24-h period following activation, a time course consistent with the late-phase response. IL-4 protein has been immunolocalized to HLMC. In addition, generation of IL-4 mRNA and protein release have been reported by some, but not all, investigators. To date, few cytokines have been clearly attributed to authentic human mast cells. Several have, however, been attributed to HMC-1, a cell line derived from a mast cell leukemia patient.

Pharmacologic Modulation of Mast Cell Function

The effects on HLMC activation-secretion of only a limited number of pharmacologic agents have been tested in vitro. In general, these agents have been tested on human parenchymal mast cells rather than those in bronchi or resident in BAL. The common classes of antiallergic and/or antiasthmatic drugs used in clinical practice have received most of the attention. To date, the beta-agonist pharmacologic agents, as typified by fenoterol, are reported to be among the most potent global inhibitors of HLMC mediator release.[30] In the chopped human lung model, the concentration of fenoterol that inhibits histamine release by 50 percent (IC_{50}) is less than $10^{-8}M$. Less effective inhibitors include the theophyllinelike phosphodiesterase inhibitor isobutylmethylxanthine ($IC_{50} = 0.5$ mM) and PGE_2 ($IC_{50} = 10^{-5}M$). Though widely touted as "mast cell stabilizers," disodium cromoglycate and nedocromil sodium poorly inhibit purified HLMC histamine release. Inhibition of BAL mast cell activation is reportedly more striking.

GLUCOCORTICOSTEROIDS

The effects of glucocorticosteroids are diverse including both stimulatory and inhibitory effects on the transcription of select genes. Release of early-phase mediators (e.g., histamine, LTC_4) in vitro and acute airway responses in vivo is unaffected by short pretreatment (up to 24 h) with corticosteroids. In contrast, IgE-

the asthmatic response.[29] Following mast cell activation, arachidonic acid is liberated from both electron-dense cytoplasmic lipid bodies and membrane phospholipids. Cyclooxygenase metabolism generates large quantities of prostaglandin (PG) D_2 and a small quantity of thromboxane A_2. PGD_2 is the most potent of the cyclooxygenase bronchoconstrictors, produces increased capillary permeability, and acts as a vasodilator. Metabolism along the 5-lipoxygenase pathway results in formation of LTC_4, LTB_4, and small quantities of 5-HETE. Mast cells appear to be the predominant source of LTC_4 immediately following IgE-mediated human lung reactions.

Platelet activating factor (PAF) is a phospholipid mediator that consists of a family of molecules. Generation is complete within 5 to 10 min following an anti-IgE stimulus. In contrast to the other lipid mediators, mast cells appear to retain PAF intracellularly or demonstrate rapid reuptake of any that may be released. PAF induces bronchoconstriction and may produce sustained increases in nonspecific bronchial hyperresponsiveness.

Cytokines attributable to the TH2 subtype of CD4+ T lymphocytes, notably IL-4, -5, -10, and -13, are felt to be central in directing the late-phase allergic-hypersensitivity response.[35] Hu-mediated generation of late-phase cytokine mRNA and protein (e.g., IL-5) is suppressed ($IC_{50} = 10^{-8}$ to 10^{-9}M).[37,43] Long-term (days to weeks) corticosteroid treatment in vivo has been shown to decrease mast cell numbers in both skin and lung.

IMMUNOSUPPRESSANT AGENTS

FK-506, a macrolide that binds to a specific binding protein, inhibits HLMC mediator release at low concentrations (0.1 to 300nM). Cyclosporin A, presumably by binding to cyclophilin, and auranofin, an orally absorbable gold compound, both inhibit HLMC mediator release.

ARACHIDONATE PATHWAY INHIBITORS

Agents that selectively inhibit arachidonic acid metabolic pathways are of considerable importance, although they may leave the release of other allergic mediators (e.g., histamine, proteases) unaffected.

Inhibitors of 5-Lipoxygenase

Specific inhibitors of leukotriene generation include direct 5-lipoxygenase enzyme inhibitors such as A-60477 (Zileuton) or indirect inhibitors such as MK-886 that bind to an 18 kD protein termed *5-lipoxygenase activating protein* (FLAP). Mast cell release of LTC_4 is virtually abolished by MK-886 at 10^{-8}M ($IC_{50} = 3.5 \times 10^{-9}$M) without affecting histamine release. Interestingly, PGD_2 release is markedly enhanced by FLAP inhibiton. This phenomenon has been termed a *reverse shunt effect*.

Inhibitors of Cyclooxygenase

Cyclooxygenase inhibition plays a critical role in a certain subset of "aspirin-sensitive" asthmatic patients (see below). Agents such as indomethacin potently inhibit HLMC PGD_2 generation ($IC_{50} = 5.5 \times 10^{-10}$M) while producing significant enhancement of LTC_4 release.

"ENDOGENOUS" REGULATORS OF RELEASE

Adenosine can induce bronchospasm in asthmatic subjects. It also has concentration-dependent effects on HLMC mediator release. When added alone to purified HLMC, it has no effect. However, at low concentrations (μM) it enhances IgE-mediated histamine and LTC_4 release and at high concentrations (1 mM), it inhibits histamine release.[30] Low-density lipoproteins (LDL), but not other classes of lipoproteins, also inhibit anti-IgE-induced histamine release by purified HLMC in a dose-dependent manner ($IC_{50} = 50$ to 80 μg/ml).[41]

Mast Cells in Pulmonary Disease

Mast cells have been implicated in a variety of pulmonary disorders based, to a great extent, on their presence in increased numbers and/or percentages in diseased tissues and the recovery of increased concentrations of mast cell–derived mediators (particularly histamine) in BAL fluid. Implicated pulmonary disorders include asthma, idiopathic pulmonary fibrosis, sarcoidosis, extrinsic allergic alveolitis, and chronic bronchitis.

ASTHMA

At baseline, even very mild asthmatics show evidence of mast cell degranulation in bronchial mucosa and increased histamine content in BAL.[24,44] Analysis of BAL in allergen-challenged atopic subjects and asthmatics demonstrates increased release of the HLMC mediators histamine, tryptase, and PGD_2. Increased numbers of lumenal mast cells are also noted and correlate with mediator content, airflow obstruction, and bronchial hyperresponsiveness. Even though some studies utilizing endobronchial biopsy have been unable to show increased mast cell numbers in individual asthmatic subjects, in general, asthmatic mast cells exhibited ultrastructural evidence of degranulation. Following chronic corticosteroid treatment, allergic reactions are diminished in association with depletion of mucosal mast cells in both the epithelium and submucosa.

Though much attention has been given to IgE-mediated mechanisms of asthmatic airway activation, it is likely that multiple other mast cell–triggering mechanisms operate under a variety of immunologic and environmental conditions. One mechanism proposed for exercise-induced asthma (EIA) relates to airway cooling and the generation of hyperosmolarity on the airway surface leading to mast cell degranulation. Evidence against a direct role of mast cells is the failure to detect increases in histamine, tryptase, PGD_2, or LTC_4 in BAL during EIA. In contrast, evidence in support of mast cell involvement comes from pharmacologic studies. The antihistamine cetirizine inhibited EIA by the inhaled (though not by the oral) route, suggesting the critical requirement for high drug concentrations at the airway surface.

Up to 10 to 20 percent of asthmatics are intolerant of aspirin and other non chemically related nonsteroidal anti-inflammatory drugs (NSAIDs). The potential role for mast cells in this disorder remains controversial. Support for mast cell involvement in aspirin-induced asthma includes the demonstration of a neutrophil chemotactic activity following challenge and the finding that indomethacin pretreatment of sensitized human airway tissues results in increased LTC_4 generation following IgE-mediated stimulation.

FIBROSIS

The cellular composition of diffuse fibrotic reactions includes striking increases in mast cell numbers.[27] The hypothesis that mast cells and their mediators are critical to the development of fibrotic reactions is supported by animal models where mast cell hyperplasia has been a constant finding in pulmonary fibrosis induced by bleomycin, ionizing radiation, and asbestos. Bronchial remodeling with subepithelial fibrosis is also a prominent feature of the asthmatic airway. The culpable mast cell mediators (histamine, tryptase, TGFβ, TNFα, and bFGF) in asthmatic or other forms of fibrosis are subject to conjecture. In addition, it is not clear whether mast cell proliferation and activation drive and/or are secondary to the fibrotic process. The latter mechanism could be effected through fibroblast generation of SCF, producing mast cell proliferation, chemotaxis, and inhibition of apoptosis.

EOSINOPHILS

Even though eosinophils are often thought of as circulating blood cells, they are actually more prevalent in tissues than the circulation. It has been estimated that for every circulating eosinophil, there are 100 to 300 tissue eosinophils. They have a tissue distribution similar to that of mast cells, being located below the epithelium in the lung, gut, and skin. Whereas mast cells and eosinophils are anatomically and often pathologically associated, eosinophil development and function differ significantly from those of the mast cell.

Eosinophil Development

Eosinophils develop into fully differentiated granulocytes from stem cells in the bone marrow.[11,15] Using cultures of bone marrow cells, eosinophils and basophils may be derived from a common progenitor cell. These eosinophil–basophil progenitors can also be found in the circulation, though the function of these circulating progenitors is not known. It has been known for years that eosinophil development is T-lymphocyte dependent. Several T-cell-derived hematopoietic growth factors are responsible for this effect. In in vitro culture experiments, IL-3 and granulocyte-macrophage colony stimulating factor (GM-CSF) stimulate eosinophil differentiation and the growth of other hematopoietic cells. In contrast, IL-5 supports the selective differentiation of progenitor cells into mature eosinophils. Transgenic mice that constitutively express IL-5 develop profound eosinophilia, whereas IL-5 gene-deficient knockout mice have markedly reduced numbers of circulating and tissue eosinophils. In an animal model, a pool of mature eosinophils in the bone marrow can be mobilized within hours in response to IL-5.[9] These findings have made IL-5 an important target for pharmacologic intervention in eosinophil-associated diseases. All the cytokines that participate in eosinophil differentiation are produced by cells resident in the lung. However, the actual contribution of lung-produced cytokines compared to bone marrow–derived factors in eosinophil growth and differentiation is not known.

Morphology and Structure

When viewed with standard blood stains, eosinophils are 10 to 15 μm in diameter, have a bilobed nucleus, and contain characteristic yellow-pink granules when stained with acidic aniline dyes (eosin or chromotrope-2R). Three eosinophil granules have been described based on ultrastructural studies.[15] The *primary* granules appear during the promyelocytic stage of eosinophil development. Later, the *secondary* or eosinophil-*specific* granules appear and have a characteristic electron-dense core when viewed by electron microscopy (Fig. 22-3). This core contains eosinophil major basic protein (MBP), the predominant granule protein of eosinophils (see below). Eosinophils also have smaller granules that contain enzymes with unknown physiological roles including acid phosphatase and arylsulfatase. Clear cytoplasmic vacuoles are often seen in eosinophils and have been shown to contain arachidonic acid–rich lipids.

Granule Proteins

Eosinophils contain several unique cationic granule proteins that have toxic effects on invading helminths and on normal lung cells. MBP is synthesized as a preproprotein, then cleaved to a 14,000-MW highly cationic molecule. The pro-sequence is anionic and is thought to protect the eosinophil from the toxic effects of the cationic mature MBP molecule.[4] MBP is localized to the core of the eosinophil-specific granule. Small amounts of MBP have also been found in basophils, consistent with their derivation from a common progenitor cell. MBP is known to be toxic to numerous parasites, including the larvae of *Schistosoma mansoni*. The role of MBP in the pathophysiology of lung disease has received increasing attention. When airway epithelial cells are exposed to MBP, ciliary function is inhibited. At higher MBP concentrations, equivalent to those commonly found in sputum of asthmatics, epithelial damage occurs. In addition, MBP administration to primates results in airway hyperresponsiveness. An interesting recent observation is that MBP binds to inhibitory muscarinic M2 receptors on airway nerve endings.[19] These M2 receptors function to decrease acetylcholine release from muscarinic nerves in the lung. By blocking the M2 receptors, MBP may enhance vagally mediated bronchoconstriction. Another unexpected effect of MBP is its procoagulant properties. MBP binds to thrombomodulin on the surface of endothelial cells and interferes with its anticoagulant activity.[45] This may account for the thromboembolic problems seen in the hypereosinophilic syndrome.

Eosinophil cationic protein (ECP) is localized to the matrix of the specific granule and is also synthesized as a preproprotein. ECP has significant structural homology with a third specific granule protein, eosinophil-derived neurotoxin (EDN), and with human pancreatic ribonuclease. Thus, the gene sequence for ECP and EDN shows that they are part of the mammalian ribonuclease gene family. ECP is more toxic to parasites than is MBP and may cause tissue damage. There are two forms of ECP, a storage form and a secreted form. Antibodies directed against the secreted form (the EG2 antibody) serve as markers of activated airway eosinophils and are used to assay circulating levels of ECP. Even though commercial assays for serum ECP are available, the clinical utility of these determinations has not yet been established. EDN has effects similar to ECP and has ribonuclease activity.

Eosinophil-specific granules also contain a unique peroxidase, eosinophil peroxidase (EPO), which differs structurally and functionally from neutrophil myeloperoxidase. EPO, in the presence of chloride, catalyzes the conversion of H_2O_2 to the toxic hypochlorous acid (HOCl). Bromide is the preferred substrate for EPO, however, forming hypobromous acid (HOBr), a very potent oxidant.[25] Another protein, found in both eosinophils and basophils, is the Charcot-Leyden crystal protein (CLC), now known to possess lysophospholipase activity. This exact role of CLC is unknown. It is thought, however, to degrade potentially toxic lysophospholipids and may degrade lysophospholipid components of lung surfactant. The protein structure of CLC is similar to several IgE-binding proteins that are members of a β-galactoside binding S-type animal lectin superfamily of proteins.[1] Eosinophils contain numerous other enzymes, including β-glucuronidase, histaminase, arylsulfatase, and collagenases that cleave types I and III collagen. Recently, a 92-kD gelatinase, also called *matrix metalloproteinase-9,* with proteolytic activity toward collagen-IV and other extracellular matrix proteins, has been found in skin eosinophils associated with bullous pemphigoid lesions. It is not known, however, whether this enzyme is expressed by lung eosinophils.

Eosinophil Recruitment

The observation that certain pathologic conditions are associated with predominant eosinophilic infiltrates has stimulated intense investigation into the mechanisms of their selective recruitment.[34] Early research efforts focused on identification of factors that selectively stimulated eosinophil chemotaxis. One such putative factor was felt to be mast cell–derived and called *eosinophil chemotactic factor of anaphylaxis* (ECF-A). Histamine was also shown to be chemotactic for eosinophils. However, both ECF-A and histamine have proved weak in this regard. The list of eosinophil chemotactic mediators active in vitro has grown significantly and now includes lipid mediators (PAF, LTB_4), complement proteins (C3a, C5a), and cytokines (Table 22-2). However, few of these mediators are thought to be selective for eosinophils. Moreover, some of these agents are chemotactic only for eosinophils from eosinophilic donors, or eosinophils primed by prior exposure to another mediator.

Recent advances have been made in our understanding of the leukocyte–endothelial cell interactions involved in eosinophil recruitment to sites of inflammation.[5] Eosinophils express adhesion molecules common to many leukocytes, including LFA-1 (CD11a/CD18), MAC-1/CR3 (CD11b/CD18), and p150,95 (CD11c/CD18), L-selectin, and the sialylated Lewis-x antigen. These eosinophil surface receptors mediate adhesion through counter-receptors on the endothelium, such as ICAM-1, E-selectin, and P-selectin. Eosinophils also express VLA-4 (CD49d/CD29), which binds to VCAM-1 on activated endothelium. Since neutrophils do not express VLA-4, this VLA-4/VCAM-1 pairing appears to be one mechanism that mediates selective eosinophil recruitment into tissues. Evidence for this comes from animal models that have shown that antibodies to VLA-4 block antigen-induced airway eosinophilia and the associated antigen-induced bronchial hyperreactivity. Expression of adhesion molecules on endothelial cells occurs in response to cytokines such as IL-1 and TNF. Note that VCAM-1 is expressed on vascular endothelium in response to the TH2 cytokines IL-4 and IL-13, which would lead to selective eosinophil recruitment. Eosinophils also express the adhesion receptors VLA-6 (CD49f/CD29) and Act-1 ($\alpha 4\beta 7$).

As noted above, an array of chemokines has been described, several of which have activity for eosinophils. Although the C-C class of chemokines is more active toward eosinophils than the C-X-C chemokines, primed eosinophils can respond to the C-X-C chemokine IL-8. The C-C chemokines and other moieties that attract eosinophils include RANTES, MIP-1α, MCP-3, and LCF (IL-16). These chemokines also attract basophils and lymphocytes. A recently described chemokine, eotaxin, appears to recruit only eosinophils and is homologous to MCP-3 and RANTES.[31] What remains unknown is how the various chemotactic agents and cytokines interact to produce eosinophil recruitment in vivo.

The fate of eosinophils once they are recruited to tissues is poorly understood. Similar to neutrophils, eosinophils rapidly undergo apoptotic cell death when cultured without critical anti-apoptotic cytokines.[46] In the lung, it is hypothesized that certain cytokines, specifically GM-CSF, IL-3, and IL-5, prolong eosinophil survival. Other cytokines such as TGF-β may trigger apoptosis. It is assumed that apoptotic eosinophils are removed by macrophages and other cells, limiting the unstimulated release of the toxic granule constituents. One proposed mechanism of eosinophil-mediated tissue damage is necrotic, versus apoptotic, cell death, which leads to the uncontrolled release of toxic eosinophil granule products.

Eosinophil Receptors and Mechanisms of Activation

Resident pulmonary and newly recruited eosinophils function along with mast cells as a first defense against invading organisms. Eosinophils participate in lung defense through specific immunoglobulin and complement re-

TABLE 22-2

Mediators Implicated in Eosinophil Chemotaxis

Lipid	PAF*
	LTB_4*
Cytokines	IL-2
	IL-5*†
	IL-3
	Lymphocyte chemotactic factor (LCF/IL-16)
	IL-4 *
	GM-CSF
Chemokines	RANTES
	MCP-3
	MIP-1α
	Eotaxin†
	IL-8*
	Platelet Factor 4
Complement factors	C3a†
	C5a
Miscellaneous	Histamine†‡
	ECF-A†‡

*Mast cell– and other-cell-derived
†Selectively attracts eosinophils
‡Mast cell derived

ceptors on their membrane surface. Immunoglobulin receptors permit eosinophils to respond specifically to opsonized organisms and lead to antibody-dependent cell cytotoxicity. Blood eosinophils have only one of the three receptors for the Fc portion of IgG, the low-affinity IgG receptor, FcγRII (CD32). They do not express FcγRI (CD64) or FcγRIII (CD16). Airway secretions contain large quantities of secretory IgA. Eosinophils express a highly glycosylated form of the IgA receptor and, in vitro, activation using secretory IgA is one of the most potent stimuli for eosinophil degranulation. The circulating eosinophils from hypereosinophilic subjects express the high-affinity IgE receptor, FcϵRI. Normal subjects and tissue eosinophils do not express significant amounts of this receptor. Eosinophils bind myeloma IgE through a low-affinity receptor that is similar if not identical to FcϵRII (CD23). Eosinophils also have complement receptors (CR1, CR3) that mediate responses to complement-opsonized organisms.

Activation through immunoglobulin and complement receptors by "particulate" stimuli (e.g., parasite) occurs predominantly through cross-linking of two or more receptors and produces degranulation along with LTC$_4$ and superoxide release. In general, "soluble" eosinophil activators (e.g., PAF) that do not cross-link receptors are relatively weak direct-release stimuli. However, these activators can produce a "priming" effect causing an enhanced response to cross-linking agents. This priming response has been observed with a large number of soluble factors, including PAF, PGD$_2$, LTB$_4$, the eosinophil chemotactic agents noted above, IL-5, and GM-CSF. In atopic individuals, circulating eosinophils are primed, presumably by the action of eosinophil-active mediators. These primed eosinophils adhere better, release larger quantities of mediators following stimulation, and survive better in culture. The molecular events that mediate these priming responses are incompletely understood.

Not all mediator and cytokine effects on eosinophils are stimulatory. For example, IFNγ has been shown to directly inhibit eosinophil activation in vitro. In addition, long-term exposure of eosinophils to IL-4 decreases the degranulation response.

One manifestation of priming is the generation of eosinophils with a "hypodense" phenotype. When evaluated with density gradient techniques, eosinophils are normally more dense than neutrophils or lymphocytes. In hypereosinophilic states, most eosinophils are less dense than normal. These hypodense eosinophils are metabolically activated, express increased quantities of immunoglobulin receptors, release more LTC$_4$, and have enhanced cytotoxic capabilities when compared to normodense cells.

Recently, it has been shown that eosinophils have many membrane receptors in common with lymphocytes including the VLA-4 ($\alpha4\beta1$) and $\alpha4\beta7$ adhesion molecules. HLA-DR and ICAM-1, although absent on blood eosinophils, are expressed on eosinophils isolated from asthmatic sputum and BAL. Also, expression can be induced by coculture of blood eosinophils with combinations of proinflammatory cytokines. Cytokine coculture can also induce the expression of CD4, functional IL-2 receptors, and CD69 (a marker for activated T cells). How these receptors influence eosinophil function is unknown.

Chemical Mediators

LIPID MEDIATORS

Eosinophils, along with mast cells and basophils, synthesize large quantities of the sulfidopeptide LTC$_4$ upon activation. LTC$_4$ diffuses from the cell and is subsequently metabolized in the lung to LTD$_4$ and LTE$_4$. Eosinophils are also a major source of 15-lipoxygenase products, such as 15-HETE and synthesized PAF, which is thought to act only locally, since it is rapidly reacylated into phospholipids. Eosinophils produce a variety of mediators listed in Table 22-1.

REACTIVE OXYGEN METABOLITES

Superoxide and hydrogen peroxide are synthesized and released from activated eosinophils in larger quantities than from neutrophils under in vitro conditions. In addition, eosinophils can produce the highly reactive hydroxyl radical OH$\cdot$ by a reaction of EPO with HOCl and superoxide anion (O$_2^-$).[26] As noted above, EPO preferentially uses bromide instead of chloride to form the potent oxidant HOBr from hydrogen peroxide (H$_2$O$_2$).

CYTOKINES

It has been appreciated relatively recently that eosinophils can produce immunologically active cytokines. Circulating normal eosinophils rarely express cytokines. However, blood eosinophils from asthmatic subjects do contain IL-8, and eosinophils from hypereosinophilic subjects have been shown to contain IL-5, IL-6, TNFα, MIP-1α, and TGF-β1. Tissue-infiltrating eosinophils in nasal polyps and bronchial walls have been shown to produce these cytokines and to synthesize GM-CSF, IL-3, IL-4, and platelet-derived growth factor (PDGF). Tumor-infiltrating eosinophils also produce TGFα. These observations suggest that the local tissue microenvironment plays a crucial role in the induction of eosinophil cytokine production. Tissue eosinophil–derived GM-CSF, IL-3, and IL-5 are thought to have autocoid effects, inhibiting eosinophil apoptosis and prolonging survival. Similar to mast cell cytokines, these eosinophil cytokines are thought to participate in the complex inflammatory processes in the lung, especially in asthma, host defense, and pulmonary fibrosis.

Only a few years ago, it was thought that eosinophils were present in pathologic states to dampen the inflammatory response. As our understanding of the biology of eosinophils has increased, their pathogenic potential has become more evident. The current belief is that eosinophils play an important role in the generation and/or amplification of inflammatory and tissue-damaging visceral events and that they do so, in great extent, via the release of the granule proteins, lipid mediators, cytokines, and oxidant moieties noted above. One important caveat is that it is difficult to establish the in vivo significance of many in vitro measures of eosinophil activation. Validation of these in vitro observations will require pharmacologic intervention or gene manipulation in animal models of various diseases.

In summary, eosinophils have many unique properties that distinguish them from other inflammatory cells. As discussed below, eosinophils are associated with a number of important clinical entities. Because of their strong association with allergic diseases and asthma, they have become a target for pharmacologic intervention.

Pharmacologic Modulation of Eosinophil Function

The realization that eosinophil activation can be an important event in tissue injury and disease pathogenesis has led to studies of the pharmacologic regulation of this process. One long-standing observation is that the administration of glucocorticoids frequently results in a rapid decrease in circulating and tissue eosinophil numbers. A number of mechanisms are felt to mediate this inhibition.[36] Glucocorticoids induce eosinophil apoptosis. They also inhibit the synthesis of IL-5 and other cytokines that are growth and survival factors for eosinophils. Lastly, they suppress the production of the cytokines responsible for inducing the endothelial adhesion molecules that eosinophils use to enter tissue structures. Steroids do not, however, inhibit eosinophil degranulation.

Eosinophils express surface β2-adrenergic receptors. Although receptor stimulation results in an increase in cAMP levels,[48] treatment with isoproterenol does not inhibit eosinophil superoxide release or degranulation. Other agents that increase cAMP such as theophylline or isobutylmethyl xanthine do inhibit IgG- and IgA-induced eosinophil degranulation.

Mast Cell–Eosinophil Interaction

As noted above, eosinophils and mast cells have been associated since their discovery by Ehrlich in the late 1800s. Early work on the interactions between these cells emphasized the roles of eosinophil-derived histaminase and arylsulfatase-B in the degradation of mast cell–derived histamine and slow-reacting substance of anaphylaxis (SRS-A), respectively. Later, when SRS-A was shown to be composed of the sulfidopeptide leukotrienes, it was thought that eosinophil-derived oxidants contributed to leukotriene degradation.

More recent evidence has highlighted the potential proinflammatory interaction of these two cell types. Eosinophil products may trigger mast cell degranulation, since both MBP and EPO stimulate histamine release from mast cells. Many mast cell mediators also activate eosinophils. Eosinophils have H1 and H2 histamine receptors. They also appear to have a novel histamine receptor, similar to the H3 receptor, which mediates histamine-induced calcium mobilization.[32] LCF (IL-16), a potent chemotactic agent for eosinophils, is released from CD8$^+$ lymphocytes by histamine.[22] Mast cell–derived PGD$_2$ increases intracellular calcium in eosinophils and primes eosinophils for enhanced LTC$_4$ release.[33] Mast cell–derived IL-5 may play an important role in recruiting and activating eosinophils.[14,20]

Eosinophil–Disease Associations

Blood eosinophilia is a commonly encountered clinical problem. Clinical conditions associated with eosinophilia include allergic conditions such as rhinitis, asthma, eczema, and drug reactions. Eosinophilia is also observed in certain malignancies, helminthic

infections, infectious and noninfectious granulomatous disorders, Churg-Strauss syndrome (allergic angiitis and granulomatosis), and a variety of eosinophilic pneumonias (see Chapter 74). In the absence of these diseases, extreme persistent elevations of blood eosinophils ($\geqq 1500$ eosinophils/mm^3) associated with neurologic, cardiac, lung, skin, and/or other organ involvement can occur as a result of the hypereosinophilic syndrome. A syndrome distinct from the hypereosinophilic syndrome, characterized by eosinophilia, fever, angioedema, and urticaria, but without vital organ involvement, has been described.[16]

Pulmonary eosinophilia is a less commonly recognized condition[3] (Table 22-3). Eosinophilic infiltration of the lung can result in mild, indolent symptoms (as seen in simple pulmonary eosinophilia) or the acute onset of a syndrome similar to adult respiratory distress (ARDS) (as seen in acute eosinophilic pneumonia). Airway eosinophilia and sputum Charcot-Leyden crystals have been recognized for years in asthma. These eosinophils have been implicated in the pathogenesis of the asthmatic diathesis, since they can generate airway hyperresponsiveness,[23] and the degree of eosinophilia correlates with the severity of the disorder.[6] Unremitting asthma associated with eosinophilia and IgE antibodies to Aspergillus is characteristic of allergic bronchopulmonary aspergillosis. Chronic asthma with eosinophilia that progresses to a systemic vasculitis is seen in allergic angiitis and granulomatosis or the Churg-Strauss syndrome. Pulmonary eosinophilia can be seen in idiosyncratic reactions to numerous drugs.

The presence of pulmonary eosinophilia may have prognostic value in other lung diseases, such as idiopathic pulmonary fibrosis and cystic fibrosis. In cystic fibrosis, clinical severity correlates with levels of ECP in sputum. This correlation exists even though the numbers of eosinophils in the lungs of these patients are not elevated. This suggests that there is an increased propensity for eosinophils to degranulate in these patients.[21] In idiopathic pulmonary fibrosis, an elevated number of eosinophils in BAL fluid is considered to be a poor prognostic sign. BAL eosinophilia is occasionally found in other interstitial lung diseases as well.[10] The biologic and prognostic significance of this finding is unknown.

Although the focus of the previous discussion has been on the role of eosinophils in disease pathogenesis, it should be noted that eosinophils also play an important role in host defenses against parasitic infections. Many helminthic infections have a tissue phase of their life cycle. Examples of helminthic infections that have an associated lung phase are schistosomiasis,

TABLE 22-3

Eosinophilic Lung Diseases

Asthma
Allergic bronchopulmonary aspergillosis/mycosis
Allergic angiitis and granulomatosis (Churg-Strauss syndrome)
Simple pulmonary eosinophilia
Chronic eosinophilic pneumonia
Acute eosinophilic pneumonia
Helminthic infections
Drug hypersensitivity reactions

paragonimiasis, strongyloidiasis, ascariasis, filariasis, and echino-coccosis. This tissue phase of infection results in an intense eosinophilia and eosinophilic infiltration. This occurs, at least in part, in response to signals from IgE-activated mast cells. The eosinophils are known to bind to the parasites through eosinophil surface immunoglobulin (IgG and IgE) and complement receptors. The eosinophils then degranulate onto the surface of the parasite. The eosinophil granule proteins are toxic to the parasite, and eosinophil-derived oxidants may also play a role in parasite killing.

REFERENCES

1. Ackerman SJ, Corrette SE, Rosenberg HF, et al: Molecular cloning and characterization of human eosinophil Charcot-Leyden crystal protein (lysophospholipase). Similarities to IgE binding-proteins and the S-type animal lectin superfamily. *J Immunol* 150(2):456–468, 1993.
2. Agis H, Willheim M, Sperr WR, et al: Monocytes do not make mast cells when cultured in the presence of SCF. Characterization of the circulating mast cell progenitor as a c-kit+, CD34+, Ly-, CD14-, CD17-, colony-forming cell. *J Immunol* 151:4221–4227, 1993.
3. Allen JN, Davis WB: Eosinophilic lung diseases. *Am J Respir Crit Care Med* 150(5, pt 1):1423–1438, 1994.
4. Barker RL, Gundel RH, Gleich GJ, et al: Acidic polyamino acids inhibit human eosinophil granule major basic protein toxicity. Evidence of a functional role for ProMBP. *J Clin Invest* 88(3):798–805, 1991.
5. Bochner BS, Schleimer RP: The role of adhesion molecules in human eosinophil and basophil recruitment. *J Allergy Clin Immunol* 94(3, pt 1):427–438, 1994.
6. Bousquet J, Chanez P, Lacoste JY, et al: Eosinophilic inflammation in asthma. *New Engl J Med* 323(15):1033–1039, 1990.
7. Bradding P, Okayama Y, Howarth PH, et al: Heterogeneity of human mast cells based on cytokine content. *J Immunol* 155:297–307, 1995.
8. Caughey GH: Serine proteinases of mast cell and leukocyte granules. A league of their own. *Am J Respir Crit Care Med* 150:S138–S142, 1994.
9. Collins PD, Marleau S, Griffiths-Johnson DA, et al: Cooperation between interleukin-5 and the chemokine eotaxin to induce eosinophil accumulation *in vivo*. *J Exp Med* 182(4):1169–1174, 1995.
10. Davis WB, Fells GA, Sun XH, et al: Eosinophil-mediated injury to lung parenchymal cells and interstitial matrix. A possible role for eosinophils in chronic inflammatory disorders of the lower respiratory tract. *J Clin Invest* 74(1):269–278, 1984.
11. Denburg JA, Woolley M, Leber B, et al: Basophil and eosinophil differentiation in allergic reactions. *J Allergy Clin Immunol* 94(6, pt 2):1135–1141, 1994.
12. Diamant Z, Timmers MC, van der Veen H, et al: Effect of inhaled heparin on allergen-induced early and late asthmatic responses in patients with atopic asthma. *Am J Respir Crit Care Med* 153:1790–1795, 1996.
13. Enerback L: Mast cells in rat gastrointestinal mucosa. I: Effects of fixation. *Acta Pathol Microbiol Scand* 66:289–302, 1966.
14. Glaum MC, Jaffe JS, Gillespie DH, et al: IgE-dependent expression of interleukin-5 mRNA and protein in human lung: Modulation by dexamethasone. *Clin Immunol Immunopathol* 75:171–178, 1995.
15. Gleich GJ, Adolphson CR, Leiferman KM: The biology of the eosinophilic leukocyte. *Ann Rev Med* 44:85–101, 1993.
16. Gleich GJ, Schroeter AL, Marcoux JP, et al: Episodic angioedema associated with eosinophilia. *New Engl J Med* 310(25):1621–1626, 1984.
17. Irani AA, Schechter NM, Craig SS, et al: Two types of human mast cells that have distinct neutral protease compositions. *Proc Natl Acad Sci USA* 83:4464–4468, 1986.
18. Ishizaka T, Conrad DH, Schulman ES, et al: Biochemical analysis of initial triggering events of IgE-mediated histamine release from human lung mast cells. *J Immunol* 130:2357–2362, 1983.
19. Jacoby DB, Gleich GJ, Fryer AD: Human eosinophil major basic protein is an endogenous allosteric antagonist at the inhibitory muscarinic M2 receptor. *J Clin Invest* 91(4):1314–1318, 1993.
20. Jaffe JS, Glaum MC, Raible DG, et al: Human lung mast cell IL-5 gene and protein expression: Temporal analysis of upregulation following IgE-mediated activation. *Am J Respir Cell Mol Biol* 13:665–675, 1995.
21. Koller DY, Urbanek R, Gotz M: Increased degranulation of eosinophil and neutrophil granulocytes in cystic fibrosis. *Am J Respir Crit Care Med* 152(2):629–633, 1995.
22. Laberge S, Cruikshank WW, Kornfeld H, Center DM: Histamine-induced secretion of lymphocyte chemoattractant factor from CD8+ T cells is independent of transcription and translation. Evidence for constitutive protein synthesis and storage. *J Immunol* 155(6):2902–2910, 1995.
23. Leff AR, Hamann KJ, Wegner CD: Inflammation and cell-cell interactions in airway hyperresponsiveness. *Am J Physiol* 260:L189–L206, 1991.
24. Liu MC, Hubbard WC, Proud D, et al: Immediate and late inflammatory responses to ragweed antigen challenge of the peripheral airways in allergic asthmatics. Cellular, mediator, and permeability changes. *Am Rev Respir Dis* 144:51–58, 1991.
25. Mayeno AN, Curran AJ, Roberts RL, Foote CS: Eosinophils preferentially use bromide to generate halogenating agents. *J Biol Chem* 264(10):5660–5668, 1989.
26. McCormick ML, Roeder TL, Railsback MA, Britigan BE: Eosinophil peroxidase-dependent hydroxyl radical generation by human eosinophils. *J Biol Chem* 269(45):27914–27919, 1994.
27. Pesci A, Bertorelli G, Gabrielli M, Olivieri D: Mast cells in fibrotic lung disorders. *Chest* 103:989–996, 1993.
28. Peters SP, Dvorak AM, Schulman ES: Mast cells in lung biology, in Massaro D (ed), *Vol 41: Lung Biology in Health and Disease.* New York, Decker, 1989, pp 345–399.
29. Peters SP, MacGlashan DW Jr, Schulman ES, et al: Arachidonic acid metabolism in purified human lung mast cells. *J Immunol* 132:1972–1979, 1984.
30. Peters SP, Schulman ES, Schleimer RP, et al: Dispersed human lung mast cells. Pharmacologic aspects and comparison with human lung tissue fragments. *Am Rev Respir Dis* 126:1034–1039, 1982.
31. Ponath PD, Qin S, Ringler DJ, et al: Cloning of the human eosinophil chemoattractant, eotaxin. Expression, receptor binding and functional properties provide a mechanism for the selective recruitment of eosinophils. *J Clin Invest* 97(3):604–612, 1996.
32. Raible DG, Lenahan T, Fayvilevich Y, et al: Pharmacologic characterization of a novel histamine receptor on human eosinophils. *Am J Respir Crit Care Med* 149(6):1506–1511, 1994.
33. Raible DG, Schulman ES, DiMuzio J, et al: Mast cell mediators prostaglandin-D$_2$ and histamine activate human eosinophils. *J Immunol* 148(11):3536–3542, 1992.
34. Resnick MB, Weller PF: Mechanisms of eosinophil recruitment. *Am J Respir Cell Molec Biol* 8(4):349–355, 1993.
35. Robinson DS, Hamid Q, Ying S, et al: Predominant TH2-like bronchoalveolar T-lymphocyte population in atopic asthma. *New Engl J Med* 326:298–304, 1992.

36. Schleimer RP, Bochner BS: The effects of glucocorticoids on human eosinophils. *J Allergy Clin Immunol* 94(6, pt 2):1202–1213, 1994.

37. Schleimer RP, Schulman ES, MacGlashan DW Jr, et al: Effects of dexamethasone on mediator release from human lung fragments and purified human lung mast cells. *J Clin Invest* 71:1830–1835, 1983.

38. Schulman ES: The role of mast cells in inflammatory responses in the lung. *Clin Rev Immunol* 13:35–70, 1993.

39. Schulman ES, MacGlashan DW Jr, Peters SP, et al: Human lung mast cells: purification and characterization. *J Immunol* 129:2662–2667, 1982.

40. Schulman ES, Pollack RB, Post TJ, Peters SP: Histochemical heterogeneity of dispersed human lung mast cells. *J Immunol* 144:4195–4201, 1990.

41. Schulman ES, Quinn TJ, Post TJ, et al: Low density lipoprotein (LDL) inhibits histamine release from human mast cells. *Biochem Biophys Res Commun* 148:553–559, 1987.

42. Schwartz LB, Sakai K, Bradford TR, et al: The alpha form of human tryptase is the predominant type present in the blood at baseline in normal subjects and is elevated in those with systemic mastocytosis. *J Clin Invest* 96:2702–2710, 1995.

43. Schwiebert LA, Beck LA, Stellato C, et al: Glucocorticosteroid inhibition of cytokine production: Relevance to antiallergic actions. *J Allergy Clin Immunol* 97(1, pt 2):143–152, 1996.

44. Sedgwick JB, Calhoun WJ, Gleich GJ, et al: Immediate and late airway response of allergic rhinitis patients to segmental antigen challenge. Characterization of eosinophil and mast cell mediators. *Am Rev Respir Dis* 144:1274–1281, 1991.

45. Slungaard A, Vercellotti GM, Tran T, et al: Eosinophil cationic granule proteins impair thrombomodulin function. A potential mechanism for thromboembolism in hypereosinophilic heart disease. *J Clin Invest* 91(4):1721–1730, 1993.

46. Stern M, Meagher L, Savill J, Haslett C: Apoptosis in human eosinophils. Programmed cell death in the eosinophil leads to phagocytosis by macrophages and is modulated by IL-5. *J Immunol* 148(11):3543–3549, 1992.

47. Thompson HL, Schulman ES, Metcalfe DD: Identification of chondroitin sulfate E in human lung mast cells. *J Immunol* 140:2708–2713, 1988.

48. Yukawa T, Ukena D, Kroegel C, et al: Beta 2-adrenergic receptors on eosinophils. Binding and functional studies. *Am Rev Respir Dis* 141(6):1446–1452, 1990.

CHAPTER 23

ANTIBODY-MEDIATED LUNG DEFENSES AND HUMORAL IMMUNODEFICIENCY

David N. Weissman / Kenneth S. Landreth / Nevin W. Wilson

Immunoglobulins (Ig) are proteins with the ability to recognize and bind a broad diversity of antigens as well as to modulate subsequent effector responses to bound antigens. As a result, Ig plays a key role in both normal respiratory tract homeostasis and in pathology of the lung. Appropriate Ig responses promote clearance of antigens from the lung and minimize injury responses. In contrast, inadequate or inappropriate Ig responses can allow or actually induce lung injury. In this chapter, we briefly review mechanisms underlying antibody synthesis and secretion by B cells, physical and functional characteristics of Ig, and features specific to pulmonary antibody immunity. Humoral immunodeficiency syndromes relevant to the lung are also discussed.

OVERVIEW OF B-LYMPHOCYTE BIOLOGY

Immunoglobulins are members of the immunoglobulin superfamily of adhesive proteins.[7] Production of immunoglobulin by B cells is the hallmark of a humoral immune response.[23] B lymphocytes express immunoglobulins both as integral cell membrane receptors and as secreted protein. Serum immunoglobulins produced in response to antigen exposure that bind specifically to the stimulating antigen are defined as antibody. In vivo antibody production normally results from the combined activation of a number of B-lymphocyte clones that respond to different antigenic determinants, or epitopes, on the same antigen. This discussion first focuses on the development of systemic humoral immunity before turning to antibody-mediated immunity of the lung.

Development of B Lymphocytes

B-lymphocyte progenitor cells are first detectable at 9 weeks of gestation in the developing liver of prenatal humans, subsequently appearing in the developing spleen and bone marrow.[23] The anatomic migration of primary B lymphocytes from the liver embryonically to the marrow during postnatal life is thought to result from developmental relocation of relevant hemopoietic stem cells. In postnatal mammals, B lymphocytes are continuously generated in the bone marrow throughout life. Although other sites of B lymphocyte production have been proposed,[15,21] these reports remain controversial. In the marrow, B lymphopoiesis and myelopoiesis anatomically cohabit, their development is regulated by the same hemopoietic stromal cells, and both cell types derive from common hemopoietic stem cells.

The steps involved in the differentiation and commitment of stem cells to the B lymphoid lineage are best characterized by the progressive rearrangement of immunoglobulin genes and surface expression of immunoglobulin molecules that occur as stem cells evolve into B cells and eventually plasma cells (Fig. 23-1).[19,26,40]

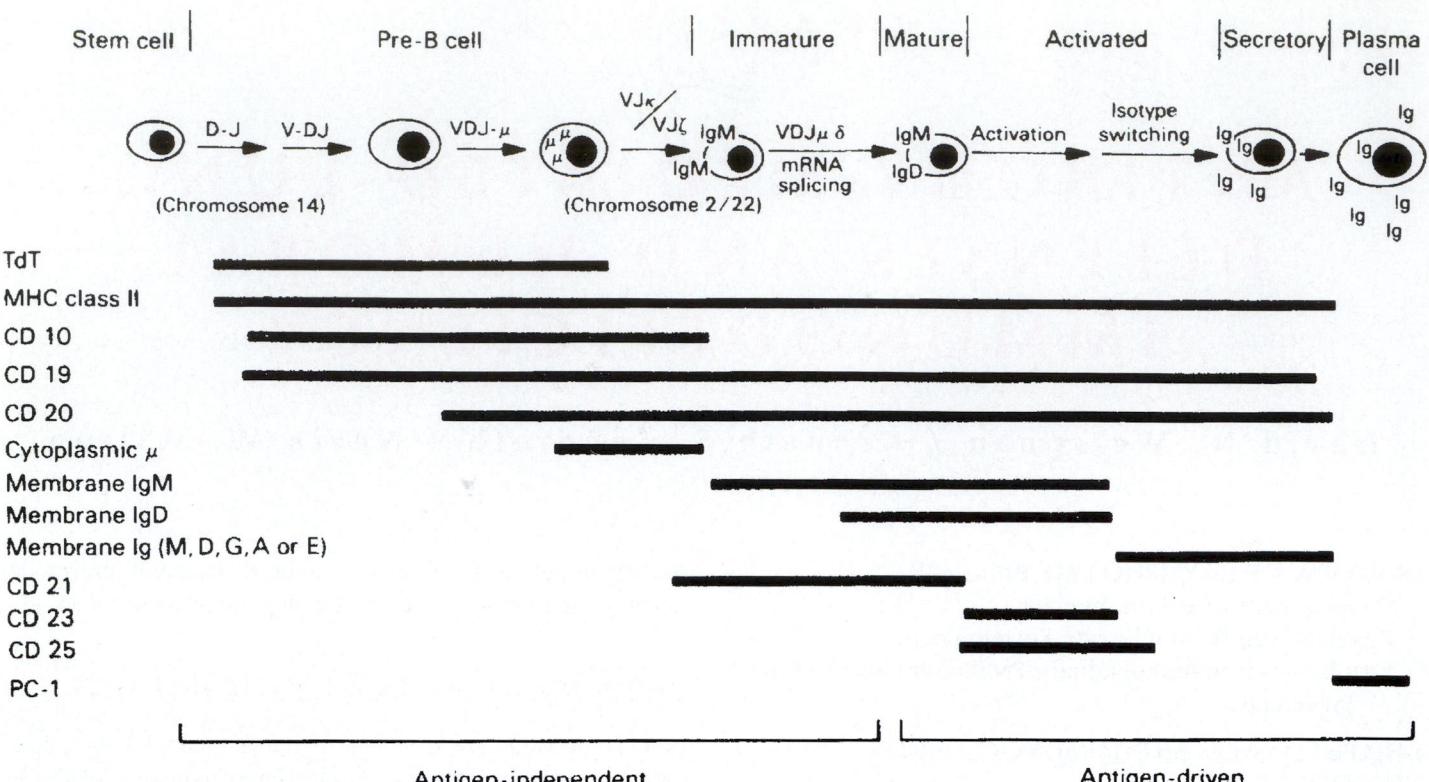

FIGURE 23-1 B-cell differentiation from bone marrow stem cell to Ig-secreting plasma cell. Stages of B-cell development are as demarcated at the top of the figure. Just below, the Ig gene rearrangements leading to Ig secretion are depicted (see text and Fig. 23-2). Briefly, initial rearrangements are between diversity (D) and joining (J) segments of the Ig heavy-chain gene located on chromosome 14. Subsequent gene rearrangement joins a variable (V) segment with the DJ segment, producing a pre-B cell expressing high levels of cytoplasmic μ heavy chain. Next, VJ recombination occurs in either κ or λ light chain genes located on chromosomes 2 or 22, respectively. After light-chain gene rearrangement, the immature B cell expresses surface IgM. Mature B cells coexpress IgM and IgD on the cell surface. Activation of mature B cells by factors such as antigen, T cells, and cytokines leads to proliferation, isotype switching, and production of cells capable of secreting the various Ig isotypes. Fully differentiated plasma cells are the most efficient secretors of Ig. Timing of expression of several antigenic markers of B-cell differentiation are shown in the lower portion of the figure. These include the enzyme terminal deoxynucleotidyl transferase (TdT), cytoplasmic μ heavy chain, the various Ig (M, D, G, A, and E), and several clusters of differentiation (CD) antigens, including CD10, CD19, CD20, CD21, CD23, and CD25. Terminally differentiated plasma cells do not express a number of surface antigens present earlier in development but do express the plasma cell marker PC-1. *(From Huston et al.,[18] with permission.)*

In humans, B lymphocytes express membrane immunoglobulin molecules made up of two identical protein heavy chains and two identical protein light chains. The immunoglobulin heavy-chain gene complex resides on chromosome 14. Immunoglobulin light chain can be either derived from the Igκ-locus on chromosome 2 or the Igλ locus on chromosome 22. The unique expression of either κ or λ gene products by an individual B lymphocyte is known as light chain isotype exclusion. Both immunoglobulin heavy-(Ig$_H$) and light-chain (Ig$_\kappa$ or Ig$_\lambda$) molecules contain constant and variable regions, the latter of which confer the antigen specificity of the mature Ig molecule. The variable component of the heavy chain contains variable (V), diversity (D), and junctional (J) regions, while that of the light chain contains V and J regions only. The many possible VDJ segments that can be used to produce an Ig molecule are encoded by different exons in the immunoglobulin genes. These exons are upstream of the exons encoding the constant regions employed in the generation of the different classes of Ig. This can be best appreciated in Fig. 23-2, which shows representative exons encoding the V, D, and J segments of the heavy chain and the tandemly arranged constant regions (μ through α_2). The production of immunoglobulin heavy and light chains initially involves a series of DNA rearrangements that join specific VDJ heavy chain exons and V and J light chain exons while eliminating intervening V, D, and J sequences and intervening introns. The constant regions remain separated from the VDJ and VJ segments by residual DNA including residual introns and J exons. At this stage newly formed B cells express IgM predominantly by termination of transcription immediately 3' to the μ constant region. The primary mRNA heavy chain transcript is processed to remove unused J sequences and introns and splice VDJ and μ constant regions. Within 24 h, coexpression of IgD occurs by transcription of long mRNA transcripts containing VDJ regions, μ constant regions, and δ constant regions, followed by splicing out of μ constant regions. Coexpression of IgD occurs as B cells exit the marrow and populate peripheral lymphoid tissues (spleen and lymph nodes). Thus, most newly formed naive mature B cells in peripheral lymphoid tissues are IgM$^+$, IgD$^+$.

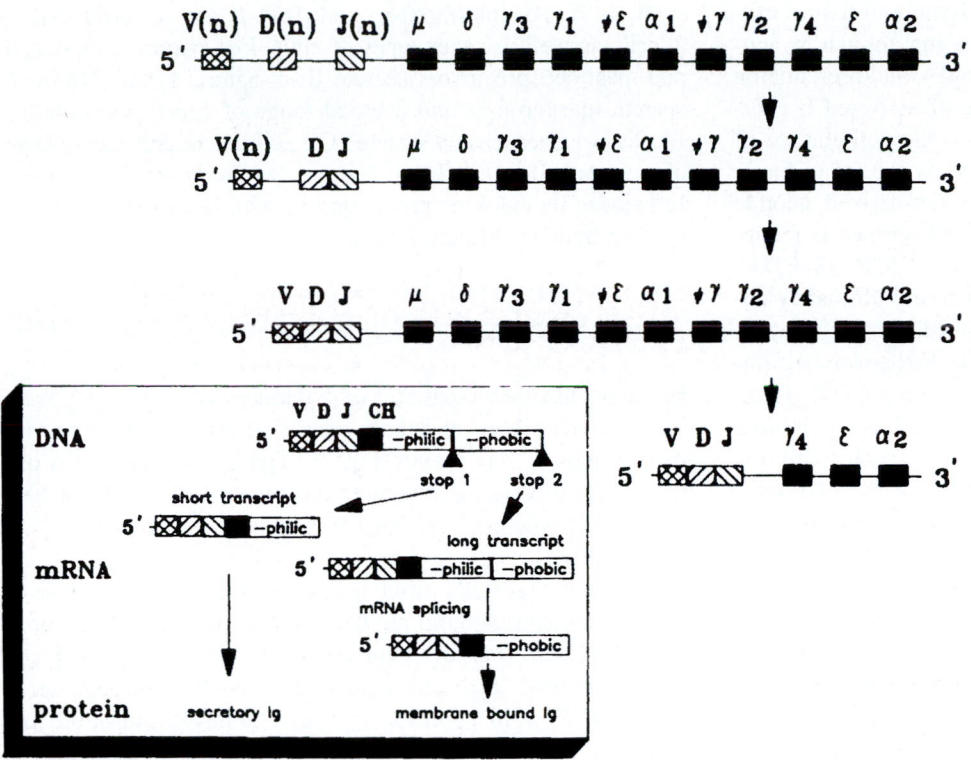

FIGURE 23-2 Progressive rearrangement of the heavy-chain gene exons (see text). Heavy-chain germ-line DNA on chromosome 14 is depicted in the upper gene sequence. Exons are shown as rectangles and introns as connecting lines. A full complement of exonic gene segments coding for multiple variable (V), diversity (D), and joining (J) regions is present in germ-line DNA. Exonic DNA segments coding for each of the constant heavy-chain (CH) regions are also present in germ-line DNA, including the various subclasses for IgG ($\lambda 1$–4), IgA ($\alpha 1$–2), IgM (μ), IgD (δ), and IgE (ϵ). Rearrangement between gene segments encoding a single D and a single J exon is shown in the next gene sequence, with elimination of intervening D segments, J segments, and introns. Rearrangement next occurs between the DJ segment and a single variable segment, with further elimination from the gene of intervening D segments, V segments, and introns. This VDJ recombination allows for the transcription of mRNA complementary to the specific VDJ segment along with the μ CH region exon producing IgM heavy chain. Isotype switching requires further rearrangement to juxtapose the same VDJ segment with a more 3' CH region, as is demonstrated for switching from μ to $\lambda 4$. As is the case in VDJ recombination, isotype switching results in elimination of intervening intronic and exonic DNA segments from the heavy-chain gene. The inset illustrates how membrane-bound or secretory immunoglobulin can be produced from the same genes. This is done by using different stop codons at the 3' end of the gene, leading to the production of proteins with either a hydrophilic carboxy terminus that is secreted or with a hydrophobic carboxy terminus that remains membrane bound. *(From Huston et al.,[18] with permission.)*

Regulation of B-Lymphocyte Development

Development of B lymphocytes is largely regulated by the stromal cells of the hemopoietic microenvironment.[13] Marrow stromal cells produce at least three cytokines that regulate the tempo of B lymphocyte production, interleukin-7 (IL-7), *ckit*- ligand (or stem-cell factor), and insulinlike growth factor-1 (IGF-1).[5,14] IL-7 is the primary proliferative cytokine for developing lymphocyte precursors, and both *ckit*- ligand and IGF-1 potentiate the effect of IL-7 on these cells. Failure of stem-cell differentiation into the B-lymphocyte pathway, or failure to appropriately produce (or respond to) either IL-7, *ckit*- ligand, or IGF-1 may result in humoral immunodeficiency.

The process of Ig gene rearrangement is random and generates B cells producing immunoprotective antibodies as well as

potentially harmful self-reactive cells and cells without protective value.[40] Self-reactive cells are largely removed by clonal deletion. Following expression of IgM on newly formed B lymphocytes, these cells are characterized by a transient period during which exposure to cognate antigen results in disappearance of stimulated B cells and tolerance to that specific antigen. This period of tolerability persists for approximately 12 to 24 h. After this period, exposure to antigen results in B-cell activation, renewal of cell proliferation, and secretion of specific immunoglobulin or antibody. B lymphocytes without protective value that are not stimulated by cognate antigen within 1 week die by programmed cell death, or apoptosis.

Selection of immunoprotective-protective B lymphocytes is accomplished by clonal selection. B lymphocytes that bind cognate antigen in peripheral lymphoid tissues within the first week following expression of IgM are activated. Activated cells enlarge and prepare to enter the cell cycle. Activated B cells require additional signals for continued response and cell division. These additional signals can be provided by T lymphocytes and include secretion of IL-2, IL-4, IL-5, and IL-6 as well as expression of stimulatory molecules on the T-cell surface such as CD40 ligand (CD40-L).[2,33] With appropriate stimulation, activated B cells undergo 6 to 10 rounds of cell division and produce up to 1000 plasma cells. Plasma cells are the most efficient producers of immunoprotective-protective antibody, secreting 3000 to 30,000 molecules of immunoglobulin per minute. In addition, activation and differentiation of immunocompetent B lymphocytes leads to the production of a set of memory B cells, which are long-lived and confer enhanced protective immunity to subsequent antigen exposures.

Regulation of Immunoglobulin Production and Isotype Switching

Activation of B lymphocytes results from Ig binding to cognate antigen.[24] Thymus-independent antigens such as bacterial polysaccharides can directly activate B cells and induce antibody production without T-cell cooperation.[41] Most antigens, including proteins, are thymus-dependent and require T-cell help by antigen-specific T cells to generate an antibody response. Activation of appropriate T-helper cells in peripheral lymphoid tissues usually results by internalization of the stimulating antigen by activated B cells, intracellular digestion of antigen, and presentation of antigen-derived peptides on the surface of activated B cells. Antigen-derived peptides are transported to the cell surface of activated B cells bound to proteins encoded by the major histocompatibility gene complex (MHC). Antigen-derived peptide bound to MHC class II protein on the B-cell surface is recognized by the antigen-specific T-cell receptor (TCR) of $CD4^+$ T cells. This process of antigen presentation and ultimately antibody production is therefore MHC restricted.

The specific interactions between peptide:MHC class II complexes on a B cell and antigen-specific TCRs on a $CD4^+$ T cell trigger the T cell to make membrane and secreted molecules that drive B cell proliferation and differentiation. One such T-cell surface molecule is CD40-L, which is a member of the TNF family. CD40-L binding to CD40 on the B cell surface results in intracellular signaling necessary for B cells to enter the cell cycle. This interaction is essential for B-cell responses to thymus dependent antigens, as demonstrated by the effect of absent CD40L function in the X-linked hyper-IgM syndrome.[2] Interactions between B and T cells also stimulate T cells to secrete a variety of B-cell stimulatory cytokines, such as IL-4, IL-5, and IL-6.

During an antibody-mediated immune response, individual B cells switch immunoglobulin isotype expression; e.g., cells producing IgM and/or IgD switch to producing IgE or one of the IgG or IgA subclasses (Fig. 23-2).[19,26,41] Isotype switching involves translocation of the V_HDJ_H gene to a position immediately 5′ to one of the constant gene regions. Although the mechanism of isotype switching has not been fully elucidated, sequence studies have demonstrated that 5′ to each heavy chain constant region gene (except the δ gene) lie repetitive DNA sequences called *switch regions*. Switching occurs by recombination between the switch regions, with deletion of intervening DNA. Switching occurs during B-cell proliferation and does not occur in nondividing plasma cells. Ability of the same heavy-chain variable gene segment to become associated with different heavy-chain constant gene segments provides a mechanism for dissemination of a given antigen-binding specificity to different Ig heavy-chain classes. No isotype switching occurs in light chains.

Isotype switching is regulated by T lymphocytes and cytokines. T cells affect isotype switching in B cells both through cell surface interactions, such as those between CD40-L on T cells and CD40 on B cells, and by secreting cytokines. Cytokines alone are not sufficient to induce isotype switching in resting B cells but must act in concert with B cell activators such as LPS, antigen-receptor cross-linkers, or activated T cells.[41] Cytokines appear to act by selectively inducing transcriptional activation of the constant heavy (C_H) genes that encode the Ig class that is subsequently induced. C_H gene activation, in turn, makes switch regions accessible to switch recombinases. Different cytokines can preferentially induce switching to certain isotypes. For example, in humans, IL-4 is able to promote isotype switching and production of IgE and IgG4;[41] IL-10 may act as switch factor for IgG1 and IgG3 production;[2] gamma-interferon (IFN-γ) supports IgG2 production;[51] and transforming growth factor-beta (TGF-β) induces IgA production.[41]

IL-4, IL-10, interferon-γ, and TGF-β are all produced by T cells as well as other types of cells. For example, mast cells and mast cell precursors secrete IL-4, natural killer (NK) cells secrete interferon-γ, and a broad range of cell types including B cells and macrophages secrete TGF-β.[41] B cells and macrophages also secrete IL-10.[36] Thus, isotype switching in vivo is likely influenced by cytokine production by a variety of cell types, including both T and non-T cells.

T-HELPER SUBSETS AND IMMUNOGLOBULIN PRODUCTION

Based on differential patterns of cytokine secretion, two types of T-helper cell subsets have been identified in both murine and human systems—"T_H1" and "T_H2."[36] T_H1 but not T_H2 cells produce IL-2, IFN-γ, and lymphotoxin (tumor necrosis factor-beta, or TNF-β), whereas T_H2 but not T_H1 cells produce IL-4, IL-5, IL-6, and IL-10.

T_H1 and T_H2 cells differ markedly with respect to their effects on immunoglobulin production. Due to their production of IL-4, T_H2 cells strongly support isotype switching to IgE and IgG_4 in humans. T_H1 cells antagonize this effect through secretion of IFN-γ. In addition, in vitro studies demonstrate that T_H2 clones are much more efficient providers of B-cell help than T_H1 clones. This is also the case in vivo, where T_H2-cell–like responses are associated with strong antibody production and T_H1-cell–like responses are associated with delayed-type hypersensitivity.[36]

SUBCLASSES OF B LYMPHOCYTES

Several lines of evidence suggest that functional subclasses of B lymphocytes arise in distinct anatomic sites and express unique cell surface proteins.[21] Most of our understanding of B-cell subpopulations comes from studies of the immune system of mice. Whereas conventional B cells are generated in the bone marrow and express both IgM and IgD as cell surface receptors, a subset of cells termed CD5 B cells fail to express IgD, but express a unique cell surface protein, CD5. CD5 B cells appear to be produced during embryonic development in the liver and are maintained throughout life as replicating cells primarily in the peritoneal and pleural cavities. Importantly, they do not appear to be produced in the hemopoietic bone marrow along with conventional B cells, as described above. CD5 B cells appear to be functionally unique in responding primarily to bacterial polysaccharides and may have evolved as a primary antibacterial defense mechanism predating the dramatic diversification of antibody responses that takes place in the marrow. The extent to which CD5 B cells contribute to antibody responses in the lung is not known.

IMMUNOGLOBULIN STRUCTURE AND FUNCTION

Immunoglobulins are expressed with five unique heavy-chain isotypes encoded in the immunoglobulin heavy-chain gene complex. Each heavy chain isotype or class has unique structure and properties (Table 23-1).[19,26] The basic structure of immuno-

TABLE 23-1

Structural and Functional Characteristics of Human Immunoglobulin Classes

	IgM	IgD	IgG1	IgG2	IgG3	IgG4	IgA1	IgA2	IgE
Heavy chain	μ	δ	γ_1	γ_2	γ_3	γ_4	α_1	α_2	ε
Molecular weight, kDa	970+	184	146	146	165	146	160*	160*	188
Serum level, mg/mL	0.5–1.5	0–0.4	5–12	2–6	0.5–1.0	0.2–1.0	0.5–2.0	0–0.2	0–0.002
Half-life days	10	3	21	20	7	21	6	6	2
Complement fixation++	+++	−	++	+	+++	−	+/−	+/−	−
FcR binding++	−	−	+++	+/−	+++	+/−	+	+	+++
Relevant Fc receptor	−	−	FcγRI, FcγRII FcγRIII	FcγRI, FcγRII FcγRIII	FcγRI, FcγRII, FcγRIII	FcγRI, FcγRII FcγRIII	FcαR	FcαR	FcεRI, FcεRII

+Pentameric form.
*Monomeric form.
++Relative importance.
SOURCE: Data from Janeway and Travers[19] and Li.[26]

globulin is a protein complex composed of two identical immunoglobulin heavy chains and two identical immunoglobulin light chains held together by intrachain disulfide bonds. An immunoglobulin monomer has an approximate molecular weight of 160,000 Da. This immunoglobulin monomer has two antibody binding sites, composed of the amino terminal ends of both heavy and light chains, and a single carboxy-terminal Fc region (the name deriving from the historical observation that it could be crystallized), which binds to specific Fc receptors on other cells. Fc-receptor binding of specific immunoglobulin classes confers the specificity of antibody passively to cells that do not synthesize immunoglobulin.

IgM

Immunoglobulin M is the first immunoglobulin isotype expressed on newly formed B cells and is expressed as both a cell surface protein and a circulating immunoglobulin making up approximately 10 percent of total plasma Ig. Circulating IgM is a pentamer of IgM molecules, polymerized by a unique B-cell–derived J-chain protein. The approximate molecular weight of pentameric IgM is 960,000.

IgM is the most effective complement-fixing immunoglobulin class and the 10 antigen binding sites on the pentameric form make it a good agglutinating antibody.[9] It is the first antibody to be detected in the blood during primary and secondary antibody responses. Its main role is thought to be neutralization of pathogens, especially viruses, in the intravascular compartment.

IgD

Immunoglobulin D is expressed primarily as a cell surface receptor, making up less than 1 percent of total plasma immunoglobulin. Although IgD is thought to function in B cell signaling and activation, its unique function remains unknown.

IgG

Immunoglobulin G is the major circulating plasma immunoglobulin class, making up some 70 to 75 percent of total detectable circulating antibody. IgG is also expressed as a cell membrane immunoglobulin, primarily on memory cells. Circulating IgG is found as a monomer of approximately 150,000 molecular weight and in humans can be subdivided into four subclasses each with a unique heavy-chain structure (serum concentrations of IgG1 > IgG2 > IgG3 and IgG4).

Considerable functional differences exist between the four subclasses. For example, differing antigenic stimuli induce differing IgG subclass responses.[9,17,18,31,37] In general, polysaccharide antigens evoke a predominantly IgG2 response systemically, whereas protein antigens induce IgG1 and IgG3 responses. IgG4 responses appear to evolve with chronic antigen exposure. The subclasses also differ in their ability to fix complement with IgG1 and IgG3 > IgG2 in this respect. IgG4 does not fix complement.

IgG subclasses also differ with regard to ability to bind Fcγ-receptors (FcγRs). Three subclasses of FcγRs have been identified: FcγRI, FcγRII, and FcγRIII.[11] These receptors are found on a number of cell types, including neutrophils, monocytes, macrophages (including alveolar macrophages), eosinophils, platelets, NK cells, and other lymphocytes. FcγRI is the only FcγR capable of binding monomeric IgG with high affinity. FcγRIII can also bind monomeric IgG but with moderate affinity. FcγRII receptors do not bind monomeric IgG but only IgG in aggregates or immune complexes. In general, IgG3 binds best to the various FcγRs, followed closely by IgG1, with IgG2 and IgG4 binding to a far lesser degree.

IgA

Humans produce more IgA than any other immunoglobulin class.[26] The major role of IgA is mucosal immunity. Although

IgA is a major constituent of external secretions, it constitutes only about 20 percent of plasma immunoglobulin. In humans, 80 percent of circulating IgA is in monomeric form and 20 percent is in polymeric form. Dimeric IgA polymerized by J chain is the predominant IgA polymer.[22,46] As compared to circulating IgA, which is mostly monomeric and derived from bone marrow B cells, most IgA in secretions is dimeric, associated with J chain, and derived from mucosal B cells. Two subclasses of IgA exist— IgA1 and IgA2. Circulating IgA and IgA in secretions differ in IgA subclass composition, with the IgA2 subclass constituting a lesser proportion (10 to 20 percent) of circulating IgA and a greater proportion (25 to 50 percent) of IgA in secretions.[22,46] Thus, IgA2 may be particularly important for mucosal immunity, especially in view of its resistance to bacterial proteases specific to the hinge region of IgA1 produced by certain pathologic strains of *Streptococcus pneumoniae, Haemophilus influenzae, Neisseria gonorrheae,* and *Neisseria meningitides.*

Polymeric IgA is actively secreted onto mucosal surfaces by epithelial cells, which express a polymeric immunoglobulin receptor (pIg-R) on their basolateral surfaces (Fig. 23-3).[22,29,46]

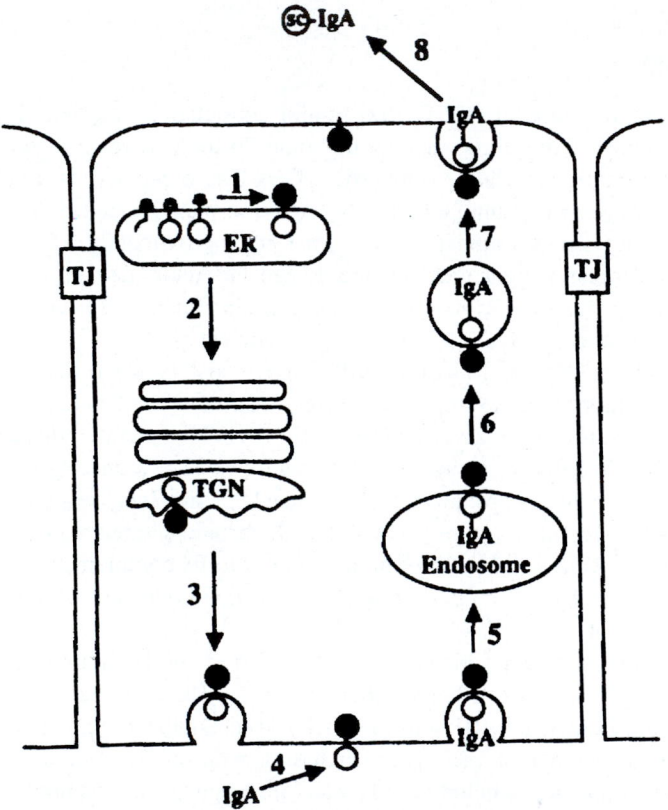

FIGURE 23-3 The general intracellular pathway taken by the PIg-R. An epithelial cell is depicted with the apical surface at the top and the basolateral surface at the bottom. The receptor is synthesized in the endoplasmic reticulum (step 1) and is then transported to the Golgi apparatus (step 2). From the *trans*-Golgi network, the pIg-R is delivered to the basolateral surface (step 3), where it can bind IgA (step 4) and can be subsequently endocytosed (step 5). The receptor is packaged into transcytotic vesicles (step 6) and transported to the apical cell surface (step 7), where the extracellular, ligand-binding portion of the PIg-R is cleaved off and released (step 8). This cleaved fragment is known as secretory component (SC) and remains associated with IgA in the extracellular secretions. *(From Mostov,[29] with permission.)*

After binding of polymeric IgA to the pIg-R, the IgA-pIg-R complex is endocytosed into intracellular vesicles that transport the complex to the apical (luminal) surface of the epithelial cell. The complex is cleaved with release of the polymeric IgA onto the mucosal surface by exocytosis, still bound to a cleavage fragment of the pIg-R known as secretory component (SC). Polymeric IgA bound to secretory component is termed secretory IgA (sIgA). Binding of secretory component probably prolongs IgA half-life by increasing resistance to proteolysis. Of note is that sIgA on the mucosal surface is mostly derived from locally produced, not plasma-derived, IgA.[26]

In many mucosal tissues, the primary site for induction of IgA responses is in mucosa-associated lymphoepithelial tissue (MALT), where precursors of IgA-producing cells are generated in response to antigen and T-cell regulation.[6,46] These lymphoid tissues—which include Peyer's patches and other gut-associated lymphoid tissue (GALT), bronchus-associated lymphoid tissue (BALT), and nasal-associated lymphoid tissues like the palatine and nasophyaryngeal tonsils (NALT)—are covered by specialized epithelium facilitating uptake and processing of antigen from the mucosal lumen. They are also supplied with high endothelial venules (HEV) facilitating entry of circulating lymphocytes from the vasculature.

Immunoregulation in MALT is incompletely understood. However, it is clear that factors such as T cells and cytokines promote development of antigen-specific B cells committed to IgA production. These cells leave MALT and recirculate to mucosal surfaces, where they are subjected to further immunoregulatory signals, causing both local proliferation and terminal differentiation to IgA plasma cells. MALT is a key component of the common mucosal immune system, as immunocytes generated in MALT are capable of migrating to distant mucosal surfaces and producing IgA at these sites. For example, immunocytes generated in GALT can migrate to breast and secrete IgA into breast milk.

From a functional standpoint, sIgA has four binding sites, making it an effective agglutinating antibody, yet it is less able to induce inflammation via Fc interactions than IgM or IgG. Thus, IgA's primary function is felt to be immune exclusion and/or neutralization of bound antigens.[6,9,22,46] More controversial is IgA's ability to orchestrate effector responses via its Fc portion. Under appropriate conditions, IgA can activate complement by either the alternative or classic pathway, but the clinical significance is unclear. Similarly, an FcαR has been identified on macrophages, including alveolar macrophages, and neutrophils of human beings, but the importance of this receptor in vivo remains unclear.[39]

IgE

Immunoglobulin E (IgE) constitutes only a minuscule fraction of the total antibody in human serum.[45] However, the biological effects of IgE are not mediated by free antibody but rather by IgE bound to cell surface receptors. The high-affinity receptor for IgE (FcεRI) binds IgE via its Fc portion and is found on mast cells and basophils. IgE bound to FcεRI is responsible for immediate hypersensitivity reactions such as occur in asthma and allergic rhinitis. Cross-linking of cell surface IgE by multivalent antigen triggers degranulation of mast cells and basophils, with rapid release of stored mediators such as histamine. IgE cross-linking also leads to synthesis and secretion of cytokines that subsequently attract and activate inflammatory cells, leading to the "late-phase response." FcεRI has also been demonstrated on eosinophils, Langerhans' cells, and activated monocytes. On eosinophils, it can mediate IgE dependent killing of parasites. Its biological role in other cell types such as Langerhans' cells and monocytes is unclear.

IgE also binds to a low-affinity receptor, FcεRII (CD23). FcεRII is the only known antibody receptor that is not a member of the immunoglobulin superfamily and has been identified on a broad range of cell types, including B cells, T cells, follicular dendritic cells, Langerhans' cells, epithelial cells of bone marrow and thymus, and various inflammatory cells such as macrophages (including alveolar macrophages), eosinophils, platelets, and NK cells. IgE bound to FcεRII has been thought capable of mediating cytotoxic activities of inflammatory cells, although coexpression of FcεRI on many of these cell types is a confounding factor.

FcεRII also has important immunoregulatory functions both with and without IgE binding. For example, binding of IgE to FcεRII on the B-cell surface downregulates IgE synthesis. Complement receptor 2 (CR2; CD21) also binds to B-cell surface FcεRII at a different binding site than IgE. Interestingly, CR2 binding of FcεRII on the B-cell surface upregulates IgE synthesis and prevents elimination of B cells by apoptosis. FcεRII is also secreted in soluble form and stimulates growth and differentiation of precursors of plasma cells, T cells, and basophils. Thus, IgE and its receptors mediate a broad range of biological activities.

ORIGINS AND FATE OF RESPIRATORY TRACT IMMUNOGLOBULINS

There are two major sources for respiratory tract Ig.[9] The first is passive transudation (diffusion) from the vascular compartment across lung tissue. The rate of transudation is dependent on several factors, including plasma Ig concentration, "resistance" to diffusion, and effective Ig size. Transudation rate may be elevated during increased permeability states such as inflammation.

The second source of respiratory tract Ig is local production by B cells within lung tissue. By far the most active site for Ig production is the bronchial mucosa, although, under certain conditions, Ig production can also be demonstrated in other compartments of the lung, such as the parenchymal interstitium and within the airways. After synthesis, Ig reach airways lumina by either passive diffusion across epithelial barriers or, in the case of polymeric IgA and IgM, by active transport through epithelial cells via the pIg-R.

Determination whether Ig in respiratory secretions are serum-derived or locally produced is often accomplished by standardizing Ig concentrations to proteins which are purely serum-derived, such as albumin.[9,43] By this approach, similar Ig/albumin ratios at both sites are interpreted as evidence for passive transudation of Ig from blood to lung. Increased Ig/albumin ratio in respiratory secretion relative to blood is interpreted as evidence for lo-

cal antibody production. A limitation to this approach is that Ig are larger than albumin, so the lung is less permeable to Ig. For this reason, use of Ig/albumin ratios to standardize data may lead to overestimation of Ig proportion derived from serum.[43]

Relative to production, far less is known about the fate of respiratory tract Ig. It is likely that inflammatory conditions associated with increased epithelial permeability and the presence of endogenous and bacterial proteases increase Ig clearance and contribute to pathology.[6]

ANTIGEN-SPECIFIC PULMONARY ANTIBODY RESPONSES

Pulmonary antibody responses have been evaluated in a number of animal species using models based on instillation of antigen into the lower respiratory tract (Fig. 23-4).[3,4] In general, exposure of the lung to low doses of antigen is not sufficient to induce a primary antibody response, even after repeated antigen exposures. These low doses of antigen appear to be cleared by nonspecific defense mechanisms, such as mucociliary clearance and nonspecific phagocytosis. Induction of an antibody response requires a dose of antigen sufficient to overwhelm nonspecific clearance mechanisms and induce pulmonary inflammation, leading to translocation of antigen from the lung to the draining lung-associated lymph node (LALN). This is the primary site for induction of an antibody response to intralobar antigen. Antibody-forming cells (AFC) generated in LALN are then released

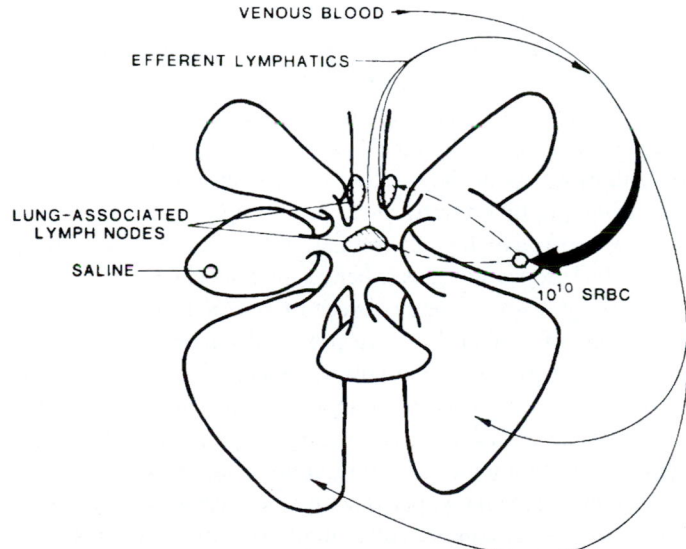

FIGURE 23-4   Summary of events leading to the development of antibody-mediated immunity in the lower respiratory tracts of dogs and nonhuman primates after primary immunization by intralobar instillation of sheep red blood cells (SRBC). The SRBC are cleared to draining lung-associated lymph nodes, which are the primary sites for induction of a B-cell response. Specific antibody and antibody-forming cells are released from the lung-associated lymph nodes into the blood. Antibody and antibody-forming cells enter predominantly into inflamed immunized lung, as indicated by the heavy arrow. Antibody and antibody-forming cells also enter uninflamed saline control and unexposed lung lobes, but at a significantly lower level than occurs in inflamed immunized lung. *(From Bice,[4a] with permission.)*

into efferent lymphatics and blood. AFC reach the lung parenchyma from blood. Nonspecific pulmonary inflammation promotes recruitment of AFC from blood to lung, regardless of antigen specificity or lymph node of origin. Findings in humans are consistent with this sequence of events.[50]

In addition to recruiting AFC to the lung, localized antigen exposure leads to recruitment and/or production of immune memory cells only in the immunized lung lobe.[3,4] These cells are able to function locally and manifest their presence in several ways. First, they confer the ability on immunized and challenged lung to mount AFC and antibody responses to far lower doses of antigen than can induce these responses in previously unimmunized lung lobes. Second, after local challenge with a given dose of antigen, they allow previously immunized and challenged lung lobes to mount AFC responses of markedly greater magnitude than occur after antigen instillation in previously unimmunized lobes. Finally, in the dog model, B cells recruited to and/or produced in the lung interstitium are able to produce antibody for years after localized immunization and challenge. Thus, primary antibody responses induced in the lung by intrapulmonary deposition of antigen are mediated by B cells recruited from regional lymph nodes via the circulation. Subsequent local antigen exposure can result in antibody responses that are compartmentalized within the lung and mediated by memory cells recruited to and/or produced in the pulmonary interstitium.

IMMUNOGLOBULIN MEASUREMENT IN THE HUMAN LUNG

Immunoglobulins are prominent protein constituents of normal respiratory secretions, with IgG, IgM, and IgA accounting for approximately 20 percent of total protein in bronchoalveolar lavage (BAL) fluids.[1] IgG and IgA are the Ig present in greatest concentrations, with the relative content of IgA progressively decreasing and IgG progressively increasing as one moves from oral cavity to alveolus. In canines, saliva IgA concentrations exceed IgG concentrations whereas in tracheal and bronchial washings IgG concentrations exceed those of IgA (with higher proportions of IgA in the more proximal tracheal washings).[20] Similarly, in humans the ratio (by weight) of IgG to IgA in nasal washings has been reported at about 1:3 as compared to 2.5:1 in lung lavage obtained via a bronchography catheter.[48] Thus, the relative contribution of IgA to respiratory tract host defense appears greater proximally than distally; the reverse is true for IgG.

Due to ease of sample collection, most measurements of Ig levels in the human respiratory tract have been performed using BAL fluid.[1,37] Bronchoalveolar lavage samples both conducting airways and the alveolar surface. Levels of IgG, IgM, and IgA have been reported in a large multicenter study using a standardized BAL technique.[1] In 76 never-smokers, mean BAL IgG, IgA, and IgM concentrations were 5.9, 6.2, and 0.2 μg/ml respectively. Current smoking significantly increased mean BAL IgG and IgM concentrations to 10.2 and 0.23 μg/ml respectively (62 subjects studied). Mean BAL IgA concentrations were unaffected by smoking (5.9 μg/ml).

Data were also presented for serum and BAL Ig/albumin ratios for all 184 subjects studied (including an ex-smoker group).

Mean IgG/albumin and IgM/albumin ratios were significantly lower in BAL than in serum, suggesting that these Ig were largely serum-derived. In contrast, mean IgA/albumin ratios documented were significantly greater in BAL than in serum, suggesting that a significant proportion of BAL IgA was locally produced.

Respiratory Tract IgA

As noted above, BAL data support local production and active secretion of total IgA into the human respiratory tract. The various forms of IgA have also been evaluated in human BAL. With regard to relative proportions of monomeric and polymeric forms, approximately 84 percent of BAL IgA is polymeric sIgA.[34] With regard to IgA subclass levels, IgA2 constitutes 10 to 20 percent of total IgA in blood and about 30 percent of total IgA in BAL.[12] Free secretory component can also be recovered by BAL.[27] SC recovery ranges from < 25 to 500 μg per BAL. Of interest is that SC recovery is markedly decreased in about 20 percent of smokers, perhaps as a result of epithelial dysfunction.

Immunohistologic studies have documented sites of IgA production and secretion in the human lung. IgA-producing plasma cells are most abundant in the glands and lamina propria of the major bronchi but are also found in small bronchi, bronchioles, and alveolar septa.[9] The proportion of IgA plasma cells producing IgA2 is somewhat greater in bronchial mucosa (26 to 33 percent) than in bone marrow or peripheral lymph node (10 to 20 percent) but less than in large bowel mucosa (about 60 percent).[6,9] As staining for SC is also most intense in the bronchial glands (in glandular epithelial cells), bronchial glands appear to be particularly important sites for production and transepithelial secretion of IgA. SC and IgA associated with J chain have also been demonstrated in bronchiolar nonciliated epithelium and type II alveolar cells, so IgA production and secretion also appears to occur at other sites, including the lower respiratory tract.

The extent to which human pulmonary IgA responses fit the model of common mucosal immunity is controversial.[6,32] A typical MALT-like structure, BALT, is a prominent feature in the lungs of laboratory animals such as rabbits and rats and is variably present in other species. In rabbits and rats, BALT has functional properties similar to other types of MALT. However, the role of BALT is unclear in humans, as very little or no BALT can be identified in the healthy human lung. Furthermore, it is unknown if some other structure in the human lung is capable of assuming MALT-like functions after exposure to antigen. For these reasons, it has been proposed that nasal associated lymphoid tissue (NALT) may be an important site of origin for pulmonary IgA-producing immunocytes. In any event, it is unclear how closely generation of IgA-producing immunocytes by the human lung conforms to patterns seen in other mucosal tissues, such as the gut.

Respiratory Tract IgG

As previously noted, respiratory tract IgG is to a far greater extent serum-derived than is IgA. However, some variation in the level of local production has been noted amongst the IgG subclasses. All IgG subclasses have been identified in human

BAL.[28,37] In healthy nonsmokers, the various subclasses constitute the following percentages of BAL IgG: IgG1, 65 percent; IgG2, 28 percent; IgG3, 1.8 percent; and IgG4, 1.3 percent. Based on albumin ratios, IgG1 and IgG2 appear to reach the airways lumen primarily by passive transudation, IgG4 originates to a significant degree from local antibody production, and demonstrable local IgG3 production occurs only in some individuals. Smoking is associated with increased levels of IgG1 in both serum and lavage and evidence for increased local production of IgG3 (based on BAL and serum IgG3/albumin ratios).

Using immunostaining techniques, IgG-producing cells have been identified in human bronchial mucosa and are present in relatively greater proportions than at other mucosal surfaces, such as the intestine.[6,9] Unlike IgA-producing cells, IgG-producing cells in bronchial mucosa do not localize to glandular areas.

In contrast to IgA, whose main role is immune exclusion, the main role of respiratory tract IgG appears to be immune elimination of foreign antigens penetrating the respiratory mucosal barrier.[6] Immune elimination is facilitated by interactions with Fc receptors on inflammatory cells such as neutrophils, monocytes, macrophages, and NK cells as well as interactions with soluble factors such as the complement system.

Respiratory Tract IgE

IgE appears to be locally produced in the human respiratory tract. In healthy nonsmokers, mean BAL IgE concentrations have been reported to be 9.1 ng/mL with mean IgE/albumin ratios significantly greater in BAL than in serum, suggesting local IgE production.[28] Healthy smokers' mean BAL IgE concentrations appeared elevated at 14.0 ng/mL, but the study lacked sufficient power to document statistical significance. Based on albumin ratios, IgE production also appeared to be occurring in the lungs of smokers.

IgE bound to histamine-containing cells can also be identified in the human lung by BAL.[16] Over 95 percent of such cells obtained during the late-phase response to segmental challenge with antigen are basophils.

PATHOLOGY INDUCED BY RESPIRATORY TRACT IMMUNOGLOBULIN

The Gell and Coombs classification system classifies immune-mediated tissue injury into four types. Types I to III are antibody-mediated and type IV is cell-mediated. Type I, or allergic, responses are mediated by IgE. Type II and III responses are usually mediated by IgG or IgM, with activation of either complement-mediated or phagocytic effector mechanisms. Type II responses are the result of antibodies directed against cell surface– or matrix-associated antigen. Type III responses are directed against soluble antigens with tissue damage caused by responses to immune complexes. All three types of tissue injury can occur in the lungs and respiratory tract.

A common pulmonary disease associated with type I injury is atopic asthma.[16] An example of a disease causing type II injury is Goodpasture's syndrome. Type III injury may contribute to the pathogenesis of hypersensitivity pneumonitis, but to what degree is controversial.[42]

In a rat model system, type III injury to the lung can be mediated by either IgG or IgA immune complexes.[30] In this system, IgG immune complex injury involves products from both neutrophils and macrophages. IgA immune complex injury is mediated by pulmonary macrophages, which release toxic products from oxygen and L-arginine in a manner leading to intrapulmonary injury.

Elevated BAL Ig levels are noted in a variety of pulmonary diseases, including interstitial diseases such as hypersensitivity pneumonitis, idiopathic pulmonary fibrosis, and sarcoidosis as well as in acquired immunodeficiency syndrome (AIDS).[9,37] It is often unclear whether increased Ig levels are of pathogenic importance or simply a marker of some other underlying disease process. For example, BAL IgG1/IgG2 ratios have been proposed as a biomarker to assess for underlying T_H1-mediated lung allograft rejection after lung transplantation.[51]

HUMORAL IMMUNODEFICIENCY AND THE LUNG

The respiratory tract is profoundly affected by systemic humoral immunodeficiency. Patients with defects in the B-lymphocyte (humoral) system have a tendency to develop sinopulmonary infections such as otitis media, sinusitis, bronchitis, and pneumonia as well as complications of recurrent bacteremia such as sepsis or meningitis. Encapsulated bacteria such as *S. pneumoniae, H. influenzae,* and *N. meningitides* or, less commonly, gram-negative bacteria are often the etiologic organisms. Recurrent infection often leads to chronic disease such as bronchiectasis as well as respiratory dysfunction.[18,49]

Humoral immune deficiencies can vary from a complete failure of B-cell development, such as Bruton's agammaglobulinemia, to relatively mild conditions, such as selective IgG subclass deficiency. These B-cell deficiencies are characterized by either a decreased ability to produce all or some immunoglobulin classes or a diminished ability to make an antigen-specific antibody response. Failure of antibody function results in recurrent infection and is the primary indication for antibody replacement with intravenous immunoglobulin.[8,18]

Bruton's Agammaglobulinemia

Bruton's agammaglobulinemia or X-linked hypogammagobulinemia was the first immunodeficiency to be described. It is an X-linked disorder caused by a mutation in the gene of the B-cell-specific tyrosine kinase *Btk*.[47] In this disorder, affected infants are relatively infection free for the first 6 to 9 months of life as a result of transplacental IgG. They then develop recurrent chronic middle ear, sinus, and pulmonary infections. Sepsis, meningitis, septic arthritis, osteomyelitis, pyoderma, and encephalitis may also occur. Gastrointestinal infections and malabsorption may develop. Occasionally, viruses such as echoviruses have caused a progressive, fatal neurological infection in these patients. Prior to antibiotics and immunoglobulin replacement, few patients survived past infancy.

IgG levels are usually below 200 mg/dl, and IgM, IgA, IgD, and IgE levels are extremely low or absent. There is a complete inability to make antigen-specific antibody to either protein and polysaccharide antigens after stimulation. Pre-B cells are present in the bone marrow, but B lymphocytes bearing surface immunoglobulin are almost completely absent from the circulation. Lymph nodes without germinal centers and hypoplastic adenoids and tonsils are found due to the lack of B cells. Immunity involving T lymphocytes is completely intact.

Prior to diagnosis, multiple or recurrent pulmonary infections may occur due to *S. pneumoniae, H. influenzae, N. meningitidis* and *Staphylococcus aureus.* This leads to the development of bronchiectasis. Even after diagnosis and the institution of antibody replacement with intravenous immunoglobulin (IVIG), chronic sinopulmonary disease may continue and worsen due to the inability to replace mucosal IgA. Delay in diagnosis and treatment with IVIG results in severe chronic pulmonary disease. In one study, approximately 75 percent of patients over 20 years of age had chronic lung disease, either obstructive disease or mixed obstructive and restrictive disease.[25] Most of these older patients had received intramuscular immunoglobulin, which results in lower serum IgG levels. High doses of IVIG in the range of 400 mg/kg given every 3 weeks, leading to serum trough IgG levels of around 500 mg/dl, are associated with decreased infections, especially pneumonias. With early diagnosis and appropriate treatment, many of these patients now reach adulthood.

Common Variable Immune Deficiency

Common variable immune deficiency (CVID) presents with hypogammaglobulinemia, decreased antigen-specific antibody function and increased recurrent infections.[18] It is likely that there is more than one underlying etiology for this disorder. Unlike X-linked agammaglobulinemia, some ability to develop a functional antibody response is present. In addition, tonsils, adenoids, and lymph nodes are usually enlarged and splenomegaly is generally present. Cellular immune defects, such as a decrease CD4/CD8 ratio may be present. CVID generally has a later onset than Bruton's agammaglobulinemia and occurs in either sex. There is a marked predisposition to autoimmune disease, malignancy, and gastrointestinal malabsorption.

Patients with CVID tend to develop chronic and recurrent otitis media, sinusitis, and pneumonia due to *S. pneumoniae, H. influenzae,* and *S. aureus.* Recurrent pulmonary infections with *Mycoplasma pneumoniae* are frequently seen. Due to the cellular immunologic abnormalities observed in these patients, infections with fungi, mycobacteria, and *Pneumocystis carinii* are possible. Bronchiectasis and pulmonary compromise are common sequelae in these patients.[49] Many of them are followed for chronic lung disease for years before the underlying immune abnormalities are discovered.

Patients with common variable immune deficiency exhibit a variety of immune abnormalities; IgG levels are generally below 300 mg/dl. IgA and IgM levels are usually low. Antibody responses to specific antigens such as tetanus toxoid, pneumococcal vaccine, or the neoantigen bacteriophage ØX 174 are diminished or absent. Peripheral B-cell numbers are usually normal but may be decreased. Lymphocytes do not differentiate into immunoglobulin-producing plasma cells in vivo and in vitro. B-cell activators such as pokeweed mitogen are also incapable of stimulating immunoglobulin production. Standard in vitro proliferation assays for mitogens and antigens are abnormal in about 50 percent of patients with CVID. Thus the most likely explanation for CVID is an arrest of terminal differentiation of B cells, probably due to the absence of some outside stimuli, possibly from the T-helper cell.

The most important aspect of therapy for patients with CVID is antibody replacement with intravenous immunoglobulin. Most patients are started on a dose of 400 mg/kg given once per month and will show considerable improvement on these doses. Those patients with increased frequency of infection will usually have the dose increased or the interval between doses decreased. There is evidence that patients with CVID and chronic lung disease will respond to considerably higher doses of IVIG, in the range of 600 to 800 mg/kg.[38] Chronic pulmonary infections may require long-term treatment with oral broad-spectrum antibiotics in addition to IVIG. Those patients with evidence of T-cell dysfunction are at risk of developing a wider variety of pulmonary infections, and appropriate investigations for *P. carinii,* mycobacteria, viruses, and fungi should be instituted in those patients when appropriate.

IgA Deficiency

IgA deficiency is a relatively common disorder, with a prevalence estimated to be between 1/300 to 1/2000.[18,44] It is usually defined as an IgA level of less than 5 mg/dl, which is 1 to 3 percent of the normal age-adjusted levels. There is an increased incidence of IgA deficiency in first-degree relatives as well as evidence that it occurs more commonly in relatives of patients with common variable immune deficiency.

The ability to produce Ig isotypes other than IgA is usually intact, as is the ability to produce antigen-specific antibody. Occasionally, IgA deficiency is associated with a deficiency of one or more IgG subclasses. When this happens, inability to make antigen-specific antibody may occur.

Infections of the sinopulmonary tract and gastrointestinal tract are usually due to encapsulated bacterial organisms rather than opportunistic infections. These infections are similar to CVID but with a greatly decreased frequency and severity. Patients with extremely low IgA levels combined with IgG subclass deficiencies tend to have more severe infections. While recurrent pneumonias, bronchiectasis, chronic obstructive lung disease, and chronic bronchitis have all been described in patients with IgA deficiency, these clearly do not occur as often as with disorders associated with antigen-specific antibody deficiencies. IgE mediated allergy is strongly associated with IgA deficiency, and allergic asthma occurs frequently in these patients.[35] The asthma in these patients can be quite severe and difficult to manage. Gastrointestinal problems are also similar to CVID, with an increased risk of giardiasis, nodular lymphoid hyperplasia, and celiac disease. Malignancies, especially B-cell lymphoma, occur at a higher rate in IgA deficient patients.

For patients with selective IgA deficiency, there is no specific therapy. Rapid identification of bacterial infections and prompt antibiotic therapy is usually all that is required. Prophylactic antibiotics may be of value in those patients with recurrent bronchitis or sinusitis. Asthma in these patients can be treated in the usual manner, although they are often resistant to therapy, and aggressive use of inhaled steroids and oral corticosteroids may be required. Those patients with both an IgA deficiency and a IgG subclass deficiency with a functional antibody defect can be cautiously treated with IVIG. Immunoglobulin replacement is complicated in these patients because of the possibility of IgA deficient patients making anti-IgA antibodies capable of causing an anaphylactic reaction. Use of an IgA-depleted IVIG in these patients may be helpful in decreasing these reactions.[10] For the same reasons, anaphylactic reactions to blood transfusions may occur, and anti-IgA antibody titers should be checked prior to the administration of any blood product. If anti-IgA antibody is detected, the red blood cells should be washed with saline to remove IgA.

IgG Subclass Deficiency

Clinical presentation of the IgG subclass deficiencies depends upon the subclass or subclasses involved.[17,18,31] Deficiency of IgG1 is associated with lifelong increased susceptibility to pyogenic infection and progressive deteriorating lung disease. It is commonly linked with deficiency of IgG2 and IgG3 and many consider it to be a form of CVID, particularly if the total IgG level is low. Most patients with IgG2 deficiency have normal total IgG levels and even elevated IgG1 and IgG3 levels. These patients tend to have difficulty making antibody to polysaccharide antigens. They tend to have infections with encapsulated organisms and will develop sinusitis, otitis media, and pneumonias leading to chronic lung disease or recurrent meningitis. IgG2 subclass deficiency may be associated with IgA deficiency, and these patients tend to have more severe lung disease than those with either deficiency alone. Patients with IgG3 deficiency tend to develop recurrent respiratory infections, and some have been reported with chronic lung disease. Defining IgG4 deficiency is problematic since 20 to 30 percent of the general population have levels that are undetectable using standard techniques.[31] Patients defined as absolutely IgG4-deficient using the most sensitive techniques (<0.005 mg/dl) have been reported with recurrent pulmonary infections and bronchiectasis.

It is important to realize that individuals exist who are completely healthy yet have one or more IgG subclasses missing. Before a diagnosis of IgG subclass deficiency is made, a thorough evaluation of the patient's ability to make a specific antibody response to tetanus toxoid and the pneumococcal vaccine must be pursued.[8] Response to IVIG is good in those patients with a defect in specific antibody production.

REFERENCES

1. BAL Cooperative Group Steering Committee: Bronchoalveolar lavage constituents in healthy individuals, idiopathic pulmonary fibrosis, and selected comparison groups. *Am Rev Respir Dis* 141: S169–S202, 1990.
2. Banchereau J, Bazan F, Blanchard D, et al: The CD40 antigen and its ligand. *Annu Rev Immunol* 12:881–922, 1994.
3. Bice DE, Shopp GM: Antibody responses after lung immunization. *Exp Lung Res* 14:133–155, 1988.
4. Bice DE: Pulmonary responses to antigen. *Chest* 103:95S–98S, 1993.
4a. Bice DE, Muggenburg BA: Lung response to antigen. *Semin Respir Med* 5:217–228, 1984.
5. Billips LG, Petitte D, Dorshkind K, et al: Differential roles of stromal cells, interleukin 7, and *kit*-ligand in regulation of B lymphopoiesis. *Blood* 79:1185–1192, 1992.
6. Brandtzaeg P: The role of humoral mucosal immunity in the induction and maintenance of chronic airway infections. *Am J Respir Crit Care Med* 151:2081–2086, 1995.
7. Buck, CA: Immunoglobulin superfamily: Structure, function and relationship to other receptor molecules. *Semin Cell Biol* 3:179–188, 1992.
8. Buckley RH, Schiff RI: The use of intravenous immune globulin in immunodeficiency diseases. *New Engl J Med* 325:110–117, 1991.
9. Burnett D: Immunoglobulins in the lung. *Thorax* 41:337–344, 1986.
10. Cunningham-Rundles C, Zhou Z, Mankarious S, Courter S: Long-term use of IgA depleted intravenous immunoglobulin in immunodeficient subjects with anti-IgA antibodies. *J Clin Immunol* 13: 272–278, 1993.
11. de Haas M, Vossebeld PJM, von dem Borne AEGK, Roos D: Fc receptors of phagocytes. *J Lab Clin Med* 126:330–341, 1995.
12. Delacroix DL, Dive C, Rambaud JC, Vaerman JP: IgA subclasses in various secretions and serum. *Immunology* 47:383–385, 1982.
13. Dorshkind K, Landreth KS: Regulation of B cell differentiation by bone marrow stromal cells. *Int J Cell Cloning* 10:12–17, 1992.
14. Gibson LF, Piktel D, Landreth KS: Insulin-like growth factor-1 potentiates expansion of interleukin-7 dependent pro-B cells. *Blood:* 82:3005–3011, 1993.
15. Griebel PJ, Hein WR: Expanding the role of Peyer's patches in B-cell ontogeny. *Immunol Today* 17:30–39, 1996.
16. Guo CB, Liu MC, Galli SJ, et al: Identification of IgE-bearing cells in the late-phase response to antigen in the lung as basophils. *Am J Respir Cell Mol Biol* 10:384–390, 1994.
17. Hanson LA, Soderstrom R, Avanzini A, et al: Immunoglobulin subclass deficiency. *Pediatr Infect Dis J* 7:S17–S21, 1988.
18. Huston DP, Kavanaugh AF, Rohane PW, Huston MM: Immunoglobulin deficiency syndromes and therapy. *J Allergy Clin Immunol* 87:1–17, 1991.
19. Janeway CA, Travers P: *Immunobiology—the Immune System in Health and Disease.* New York, Garland Publishing, 1994, pp 3: 1–3:46.
20. Kaltreider HB, Chan MKL: The class-specific immunoglobulin composition of fluids obtained from various levels of the canine respiratory tract. *J Immunol* 116:423–429, 1976.
21. Kantor AB, Herzenberg LA: Origin of B cell lineages. *Annu Rev Immunol* 11:501–538, 1993.
22. Kerr MA: The structure and function of human IgA. *Biochem J* 271:285–296, 1990.
23. Landreth KS: B lymphocyte generation as a developmental process, in Cooper EL, Nesbit-Brown E (eds.): *Developmental Immunology.* New York, Oxford University Press, 1993, pp 238–273.
24. Lanzavecchia A: Receptor-mediated antigen uptake and its effect on antigen presentation to class-II restricted T lymphocytes. *Annu Rev Immunol* 8:773–793, 1990.
25. Lederman HM, Winkelstein JA: X-linked agammaglobulinemia: An analysis of 96 patients. *Medicine* 64:145–156, 1985.
26. Li JTC: Immunoglobulin structure and function, in Middleton E, Reed CE, Ellis EF, et al (eds.): *Allergy Principles and Practice,* 4th ed. St. Louis, Mosby-Year Book, 1993, pp 73–92.
27. Merrill WW, Goodenberger D, Strober W, et al: Free secretory component and other proteins in human lung lavage. *Am Rev Respir Dis* 122:156–161, 1980.
28. Merrill WW, Naegel GP, Olchowski JJ, Reynolds HY: Immunoglobulin G subclass proteins in serum and lavage fluid of normal subjects—Quantitation and comparison with immunoglobulins A and E. *Am Rev Respir Dis* 131:584–587, 1985.

29. Mostov KE: Transepithelial transport of immunoglobulins. *Annu Rev Immunol* 12:63–84, 1994.

30. Mulligan MS, Wilson GP, Todd RF, et al: Role of β_1, β_2 integrins and ICAM-1 in lung injury after deposition of IgG and IgA immune complexes. *J Immunol* 150:2407–2417, 1993.

31. Ochs HD, Wedgwood RJ: IgG subclass deficiencies. *Annu Rev Med* 38:325–340, 1987.

32. Pabst R: Is BALT a major component of the human lung immune system? *Immunol Today* 13:119–122, 1992.

33. Parker DC: T cell dependent B cell activation. *Annu Rev Immunol* 11:331–360, 1993.

34. Peebles RS, Liu MC, Lichtenstein LM, Hamilton RG: IgA, IgG, and IgM quantification in bronchoalveolar lavage fluids from allergic rhinitics, allergic asthmatics, and normal subjects by monoclonal antibody-based immunoenzymetric assays. *J Immunol Methods* 179:77–86, 1995.

35. Plebani A, Monafo V, Ugazio AG, et al: Comparison of the frequency of atopic disease in children with severe and partial IgA deficiency. *Int Arch Allergy Appl Immunol* 82:485–486, 1987.

36. Rennick D, Davidson N, Berg D: Interleukin-10 gene knock-out mice: A model of chronic inflammation. *Clin Immunol Immunopathol* 76:S174–S178, 1995.

37. Reynolds, HY: Immunoglobulin G and its function in the human respiratory tract. *Mayo Clin Proc* 63:161–174, 1988.

38. Roifman CM, Levison H, Gelfand EW: High-dose vs. low dose intravenous immunoglobulin in hypogammaglobulinemia and chronic lung disease. *Lancet* 1:1075–1077, 1987.

39. Saito K, Suzuki K, Matsuda H, et al: Physical association of Fc receptor chain homodimer with IgA receptor. *J Allergy Clin Immunol* 96:1152–1160, 1995.

40. Shatz GG, Oettinger MA, Schlissel MS: V(D)J recombination: Molecular biology and regulation. *Annu Rev Immunol* 10:359–384, 1992.

41. Snapper CM, Mond JJ: Towards a comprehensive view of immunoglobulin class switching. *Immunol Today* 14:15–17, 1993.

42. Soda K, Ando M, Sakata T, et al: C1q and C3 in bronchoalveolar lavage fluid from patients with summer-type hypersensitivity pneumonitis. *Chest* 93:76–80, 1988.

43. Stockley RA, Burnett D: Local IgA production in patients with chronic bronchitis: Effect of acute respiratory infection. *Thorax* 35: 202–206, 1980.

44. Strober W, Sneller MC: IgA deficiency. *Ann Allergy* 66:363–379, 1991.

45. Sutton BJ, Gould HJ: The human IgE network. *Nature* 366:421–428, 1993.

46. Tomasi TB: Regulation of the mucosal IgA response—An overview. *Immunol Invest* 18:1–15, 1989.

47. Vetrie D, Vorchovsky I, Sideras P, et al: The gene involved in X-linked agammaglobulinemia is a member of the src family of protein-tyrosine kinases. *Nature* 361:226–233, 1993.

48. Waldman RH, Jurgensen PF, Olsen GN, et al: Immune response of the human respiratory tract: I. Immunoglobulin levels and influenza virus vaccine antibody response. *J Immunol* 111:38–41, 1973.

49. Watts WJ, Watts MB, Dai W, et al: Respiratory dysfunction in patients with common variable hypogammaglobulinemia. *Am Rev Respir Dis* 134:699–703, 1986.

50. Weissman DN, Bice DE, Crowell RE, Schuyler MR: Intrapulmonary antigen deposition in the human lung: Local responses. *Am J Respir Cell Mol Biol* 11:607–614, 1994.

51. Wilkes DS, Heidler KM, Niemeier M, et al: Increased bronchoalveolar IgG2/IgG1 ratio is a marker for human lung allograft rejection. *J Inves Med* 42:652–659, 1994.

CHAPTER 24

CYTOKINES AND CHEMOKINES IN LUNG INFLAMMATION AND INJURY

Steven L. Kunkel / Robert M. Strieter

CYTOKINES IN ACUTE PULMONARY INFLAMMATION

EARLY-RESPONSE CYTOKINES AND INITIATION OF PULMONARY INFLAMMATION

CHEMOTACTIC CYTOKINES AND THE INFLAMMATORY RESPONSE

CHEMOKINE-INDUCED PATHOLOGY AND TISSUE INJURY

CHEMOKINES IN MODELS OF ACUTE LUNG INJURY

CHEMOKINES IN EXPERIMENTAL LUNG INJURY DUE TO ENDOTOXEMIA

CHEMOKINES IN EXPERIMENTAL ALLERGIC AIRWAY INFLAMMATION

CYTOKINES IN CHRONIC LUNG INFLAMMATION

CYTOKINES IN INTERSTITIAL FIBROSIS

CONCLUSIONS

The cascade of events which dictate the initiation, maintenance, and resolution of pulmonary inflammation are usually the consequence of the host responding to direct and indirect insults. Infection, trauma, ischemia/reperfusion injury, and autoimmune disease are examples of clinically important insults which produce lung injury associated with inflammatory cell infiltration. These inflammatory responses involve coordinated interactions of specific signals which dictate the evolution of the inflammatory process. The signals which are generated as the inflammatory

response evolves serve as important communication networks between the different cellular components of the local response. A variety of mediators are involved in the coordination of these networks. These include nucleotides, reactive oxygen and nitrogen intermediates, lipids, peptides, and polypeptides (Table 24-1). This latter group of inflammatory agents comprise a large number of mediators collectively identified as *cytokines*. Research into the mechanisms of cytokine action in various diseases is currently being conducted in both clinical and basic research settings, as these polypeptide mediators are known to play key roles in a spectrum of pulmonary diseases.

TABLE 24-1
Inflammatory Mediators

Polypeptides	*Lipids*
Cytokines	Thromboxane
Complement activation products	Leukotrienes
Clotting cascade products	Prostaglandins
Reactive Oxygen Intermediates	*Vasoactive Amines*
Superoxide	Histamine
Hydrogen peroxide	Serotonin
Metabolites of Arginine	*Nucleotides*
Nitric oxide	ADP

Note: The diversity of inflammatory mediators is demonstrated by the wide range of chemically distinct, biologically active compounds.

A basic definition for most cytokines would classify these mediators as soluble, hormonelike proteins produced by a variety of cells. Historically, cytokines were referred to as monokines or lymphokines depending upon whether their source of synthesis was a monocyte/macrophage or lymphocyte, respectively. However, recent evidence has demonstrated that the cellular source and biological targets of these polypeptides are not restricted to cells of the immune system, since endothelial cells, stromal cells, and epithelial cells are all capable of both producing and responding to a number of different cytokines.[36,44,48] An area of increasing importance in cytokine biology is the ability of non-immune cells to participate as effector cells in the perpetuation of an inflammatory response by producing cytokines (Table 24-2). This is particularly true in the lung, as pulmonary epithelial cells and stromal cells produce both proinflammatory and immuno-regulatory cytokines under specific conditions.

The interest promoted by the biotechnology industry during the last decade has focused on the role of cytokines as mediators of immune/inflammatory function. However, the function of cytokines extends beyond orchestrating immune responses, as these signals are clearly operative during normal physiological responses. Normal circadian body temperature fluctuations, appetite regulation, and lethargy/sleep patterns appear to be controlled, at least in part, by cytokines. Thus, it is not too surprising that both professional immune/inflammatory cells and stromal cells contribute to the overall biology of cytokines during health and disease.

Cytokines appear to have a wide range of concentration-dependent physiological activities, but they are most distinguished

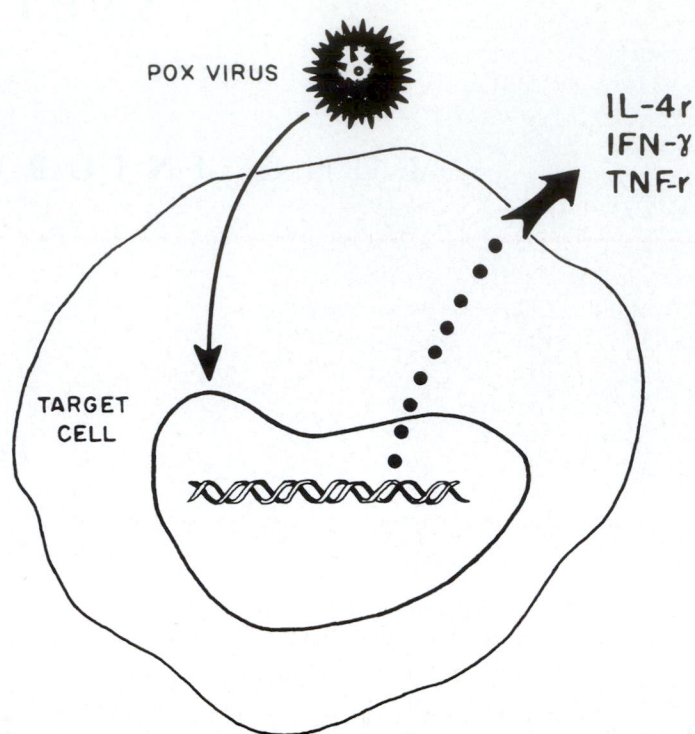

FIGURE 24-1   Certain viruses (pox virus) encode polypeptides which are versions of key cytokine receptors secreted from infected cells. These secreted soluble receptors block the biologic activity of cognate cytokines.

for their activities associated with inflammation, immune reactivity, tissue injury, and potential loss of organ function. The broad scope of biologic activities of cytokines is fundamental to their ability to participate in various aspects of inflammation. For example, specific cytokines are known to initiate inflammation via the activities of early response cytokines, such as interleukin-1 (IL-1) and tumor necrosis factor (TNF), regulate inflammation through the effects of interleukin-10, and repair tissue injury through the activities of transforming growth factor beta.[20,23,46] These mediators are only representative of the many redundant polypeptides which participate in different facets of the evolving pulmonary response. Evidence for the importance of cytokines during the evolution of an inflammatory response is derived from recent studies demonstrating that certain viruses encode soluble receptors for different cytokines (Fig. 24-1). Upon expression of these genes, the infected cells release an immunoregulatory protein or polypeptide which possesses immunoregulating activity via their ability to bind and inactivate the reciprocal ligand cytokine.[1,42,43,54]

CYTOKINES IN ACUTE PULMONARY INFLAMMATION

The evolution of an acute pulmonary inflammatory response is usually the consequence of the host responding to a set of mediators initiated by a known or unknown etiologic agent. The acute response in the lung can cover a wide gamut of diseases, including bronchitis, pneumonia, and adult respiratory distress syndrome (ARDS). The histopathology of acute bronchitis and bacterial pneumonia is usually characterized by the presence of

TABLE 24-2

Cytokine Source and Function

Cytokine	Cell Source	Function
IL-1	Macrophages, stromal cells	Cell activation and proliferation
IL-2	Lymphocytes	Lymphocyte proliferation
IL-6	Immune and nonimmune cells	Acute phase response
IL-8	Immune cells, fibroblasts, lung epithelial cells	Chemotaxis and angiogensis
IL-10	Immune cells, lung epithelial cells	Immunoregulatory
IL-12	Macrophages	Immunoregulatory
IL-16	Mononuclear cells	Immunoregulatory
MCP-1	Endothelial cells, fibroblasts, epithelial cells	Chemotaxis
TNF	Macrophages, lymphocytes	Immunoregulatory

Note: The diverse repertoire of cells that express cytokines include a number of immune/inflammatory cells and nonprofessional immune cells. This latter category includes stromal cells and lung epithelial cells.

proteinaceous exudate and polymorphonuclear leukocytes. In pneumonia the extravasation of neutrophils and exudate may be significant and lead to consolidation of the lung. Interestingly, once the inciting agent is removed, the inflammatory response usually resolves, lung architecture is restored, and normal lung function is reestablished without the sequela of pulmonary fibrosis. In contrast, certain types of acute lung inflammation, such as ARDS, may culminate in severe tissue injury and threaten host survival. The pathology of this syndrome also includes the participation of neutrophils and heightened vascular permeability, leading to exudate in the lungs. However, the resolution phase of ARDS is quite different than that observed during pneumonia, as abnormal lung function is frequently observed with fibrotic changes after recovery. Although many of the basic mechanisms that mediate the progression of the acute inflammatory response in the lung are not clear, it is known that neutrophil-mediated lung inflammation involves the interplay of early-response cytokines, adhesion molecules, and chemokines.

EARLY-RESPONSE CYTOKINES AND THE INITIATION OF PULMONARY INFLAMMATION

The importance of inflammatory mediators to the evolution of acute lung injury has been investigated intensely for a number of years. These studies originally focused on the participation of serum-derived mediators, such as split products of the complement and coagulation cascades. However, research conducted during the past decade has underscored the important role of cytokines in orchestrating lung inflammation. A number of seminal observations have established cytokines as important communication links to initiate, maintain, and resolve the inflammatory response.[8,21,22,39] These polypeptide mediators function as communication links via their ability to establish cytokine networks, whereby one cytokine can bind to an appropriate receptor on a specific cell and induce the expression of an additional cytokine, which may then interact with other cells and cause the expression of still another cytokine in a cascadelike manner (Fig. 24-2). An exogenous challenge can induce the expression of cytokines by alveolar or interstitial macrophages which can subsequently activate resident tissue cells, such as lung fibroblasts or epithelial cells, resulting in the production of additional cytokines. The importance of this cytokine network lies in the facts that (1) a relatively small group of mediators may initiate diverse inflammatory/immune responses, (2) a variety of immune and nonimmune cells can fully participate in the evolution of the inflammatory response, and (3) control of the evolving response is under the direction of many transcriptional and posttranscriptional regulatory steps. This latter aspect of cytokine networking is of great interest in immune regulation, since suppression of polypeptide mediators which function early in the response may control the subsequent steps of inflammation. Furthermore, the regulation of protein synthesis at the transcriptional and posttranscriptional levels inherently allows for additional cellular and molecular targets to develop novel therapies.

Although structurally unrelated, IL-1 and TNF possess similar functional activities during the evolution of an inflammatory response and have been classified as *early-response cytokines*.

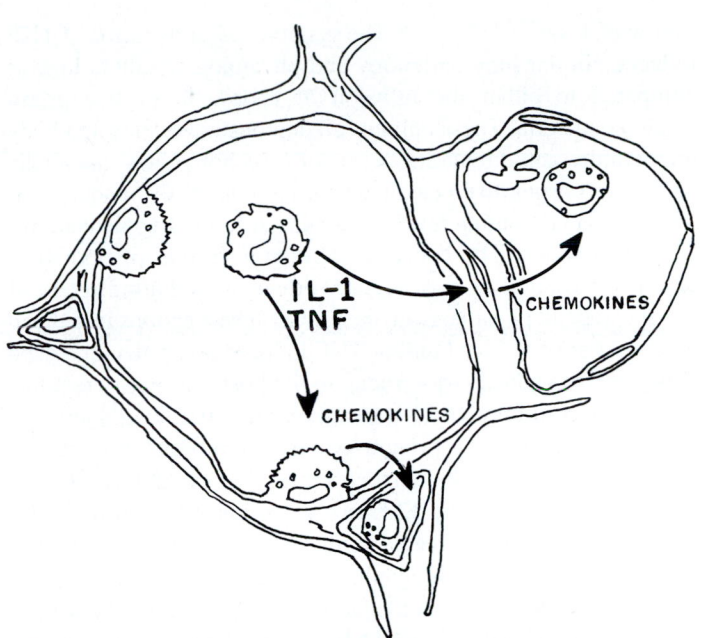

FIGURE 24-2 The production of early-response cytokines, such as IL-1 and/or TNF, by resident macrophages can initiate a cytokine cascade via activating stromal or epithelial cells in the lung and inducing the expression of additional cytokines. These more distal cytokines can in turn activate other cells and promote their participation in the inflammatory response.

This designation stems from the fact that TNF and IL-1 are among the first polypeptide mediators synthesized at a site of inflammation. These cytokines are primarily produced by monocytes and fixed macrophages after cell stimulation and, depending upon the levels released, can induce autocrine, paracrine, and endocrine effects.[39] Thus, TNF and IL-1 possess a wide-range of overlapping activities on most cells in the body. Interestingly, almost all cells in the body possess a functional receptor for IL-1 and TNF, suggesting that these cytokines are important in local and systemic cell communication.

IL-1 and TNF have been associated with a variety of cell activation events, and circumstantial evidence suggests that these mediators are involved in the initiation of specific human lung diseases. For example, both experimental and clinical studies indicate that IL-1 and TNF appear to play a significant role in the pathogenesis of septic shock and the development of acute lung injury. Investigations of TNF levels in serum samples from patients with meningococcal septicemia with associated acute lung injury demonstrated a significant correlation between serum TNF levels and mortality.[55] Subsequent investigations have correlated TNF and IL-1 levels with mortality in patients with sepsis and purpura fulminans due to meningococcemia.[15] In a prospective study, serum of 33 percent of patients with clinical correlates of septic shock possessed elevated levels of TNF.[27] The TNF levels correlated with the incidence and severity of ARDS, lung injury, and subsequent mortality. Interestingly, TNF levels were elevated with equal frequency in shock patients due to gram-negative or gram-positive bacteria.

The role of TNF in the pathogenesis of sepsis has been examined through the use of established animal models of endotoxemia, cecal ligation and puncture, or by the direct administration of TNF.[17,35,38,46,51,53] The systemic administration of TNF induced similar lung pathology and physiological alterations as compared to either the infusion of endotoxin or live gram-negative bacteria. These animals all demonstrated: elevated body temperature and circulating levels of catecholamines, metabolic acidosis, consumptive coagulopathy, pulmonary dysfunction, alterations in circulating levels of leukocytes, and hypotension resulting in shock. The concomitant administration of both IL-1 and TNF resulted in a synergistic effect in mediating many of the above pathophysiological alterations. Investigations into the in vivo mechanism of IL-1 and/or TNF-induced injury demonstrated that protein synthesis was crucial to the host's ability to regulate the pathophysiology. In vivo treatment of experimental animals with actinomycin D, a protein synthesis inhibitor, in combination with a sublethal challenge of either IL-1 or TNF resulted in 100 percent mortality by 12 hours, as compared to no mortality in non-actinomycin-D-treated animals.[38] These experiments suggest that de novo protein synthesis is necessary in vivo to protect against TNF or IL-1-induced tissue injury and lethality.

Inhibition of endogenous TNF activity during gram-negative bacteria-induced sepsis significantly attenuates lung pathology and mortality.[51] The administration of neutralizing antibodies against TNF prior to challenging baboons with an LD_{100} (lethal dose) of E. coli resulted in a significant reduction in mortality. However, delaying antibody therapy until after E. coli challenge did not salvage the experimental animals, suggesting that the production of TNF occurred early and set into motion a cascade of events which ultimately ended in the death of the challenged animal. Among the interesting pathologic findings in these animals were histologic alterations of leukocyte infiltration associated with permeability changes in the lung. Similar studies in rodents have demonstrated that TNF is expressed very rapidly after endotoxin challenge. After an LD_{100} administration of endotoxin, TNF levels peaked in vivo at 1 h and then rapidly declined to undetectable levels.[35] Human volunteers challenged with low concentrations of endotoxin also have a rapid rise and abrupt fall in the circulating levels of TNF.[29] These studies support previous findings that the expression of TNF is under strict regulation in vivo.

Intratracheal delivery of IL-1 or TNF into experimental animals induces an intraalveolar inflammatory response.[52] The response is characterized by a neutrophilic infiltrate that peaks by 12 h, followed by a monocytic and lymphocytic infiltrate that peaks at 24 and 48 h, respectively. Intratracheal administration of endotoxin increases the presence of both IL-1 and TNF in the lung and mimics the leukocyte trafficking induced by either exogenous IL-1 or TNF.

Whereas endotoxin clearly induces the expression of early response cytokines such as IL-1 and TNF, this same exogenous activating agent can also cause the expression of certain antagonists of IL-1 and TNF.[2,12,14,19,24,31] For example, endotoxin can induce the production of the IL-1 receptor antagonist (IRAP) and soluble TNF receptors (sTNFr) from monocytes and macrophages. The inhibitory activity of IRAP appears to be at the level of competitive occupancy of the IL-1 receptor without any inherent agonist activity, and while the activity of the sTNFr occurs via binding TNF and rendering it inactive. IRAP inhibits the in vitro activity of IL-1 by blocking the ability of IL-1-stimulated fi-

broblasts to increase PGE production and decrease neutrophil adherence to IL-1-challenged endothelial cells. In vivo, IRAP inhibits E.-coli-induced septic shock and lung injury in experimental animals. Subsequent studies demonstrated that IRAP could protect the lungs of endotoxin challenged animals from tissue injury found in untreated animals.

CHEMOTACTIC CYTOKINES AND THE INFLAMMATORY RESPONSE

An important aspect of cytokine networks is the interactive cascade of early-response cytokines and distal cytokines, which result in the recruitment of specific leukocyte subpopulations to an area of immune reactivity. One of the primary features of IL-1 and TNF-induced lung injury is the sequestration of leukocytes to the pulmonary tissue. Although TNF and IL-1 were originally thought of as chemotactic factors, evidence has now demonstrated that these cytokines lack chemotactic activity.[59] Chemotactic activity associated with in vivo expression of either IL-1 or TNF is likely to have occurred via networks involving IL-1- or TNF-induced chemokines.[28]

Chemokines, defined as *chemotactic cytokines,* belong to two groups of related polypeptides, identified by the location of two of the four cysteine amino acids comprising their primary amino acid structure.[4,5,32] Accumulating evidence supports the concept that members of these chemokine families have proinflammatory and reparative activities. In their monomeric form chemokines are fewer than 10,000 daltons and are basic heparin-binding proteins. One of the chemokine families displays a conserved amino acid motif characterized by the location of two amino terminal cysteines separated by one nonconserved amino acid residue. This chemokine family is designated the C-X-C chemokines and appears to have specificity for the elicitation of mainly neutrophils. The C-X-C chemokines are all clustered on human chromosome 4 and possess approximately 20 to 55 percent homology in their primary structure. Interest in this field is exemplified by investigations which have identified several different C-X-C chemokines (Table 24-3). Interestingly, connective-tissue-activating protein 3, beta thromboglobulin, and neutrophil-activating protein 2 are all N-terminal truncations of platelet basic protein. These cleavage products are formed when platelet basic protein is released from platelet alpha granules and is proteolytically digested by leukocyte-derived proteases.

Recent investigations have demonstrated that an important feature in the primary structure of C-X-C chemokines may account for the neutrophil chemotactic and activating properties of these mediators (Table 24-4). These studies identified three critical amino acid residues immediately preceding the first N-terminal cysteine residue, which are important in binding to a neutrophil receptor and activating neutrophils. These amino acids are Glu-Leu-Arg or the *ELR motif,* which is absent in certain members of the C-X-C chemokine family. In particular, IP-10, platelet factor 4, and monokine induced by gamma interferon (MIG) all lack the ELR motif and are not potent in neutrophil activation. Interestingly, when the ELR motif was synthetically introduced into platelet factor 4, this polypeptide gained chemotactic activity. Therefore, certain members of the C-X-C supergene family may have different biological activities. Platelet factor 4 (a non-

TABLE 24-3

Selected Chemotactic Cytokines

TABLE 24-3

Selected Chemotactic Cytokines

C-X-C Chemokines	*C-C Chemokines*
Interleukin-8	Monocyte chemoattractant protein
Growth-related oncogene α, β, γ	RANTES
Neutrophil-activating factor 2	Macrophage inflammatory protein
Platelet basic protein	Eotaxin
β thromboglobulin	
ENA-78	
Platelet factor 4	
γ interferon-inducible protein	

Note: These representative members of chemotactic cytokines belong to either the C-X-C chemokine or C-C chemokine supergene family.

ELR-containing C-X-C chemokine) was one of the first members of this family to be described. This factor was originally identified for its ability to bind heparin, leading to the inactivation of the anticoagulation function of heparin. All members of the chemokine supergene family appear to possess heparin-binding domains in their primary amino acid structure. Interleukin-8 has been the most studied C-X-C chemokine and is produced by an array of cells, including monocytes, alveolar macrophages, neutrophils, keratinocytes, mesangial cells, alveolar epithelial cells, hepatocytes, fibroblasts, and endothelial cells.[34,36,47,48,49,50] In addition, IL-8 is expressed by a number of neoplastic cell lines.

An additional related supergene family of polypeptide chemokines is the C-C chemokine family. This group is defined by the juxaposition of the first two N-terminal cysteines (Table 24-3). In general terms, the C-C chemokine family has relative specificity for the elicitation of mononuclear cells. Certain members of the C-C chemokine family also appear to be potent chemotactic factors for eosinophils. Like the C-X-C family, certain of the C-C members are produced by a number of cell types, including lymphocytes, monocytes, neutrophils, and a variety of noninflammatory cells and tumor cell lines.

TABLE 24-4

C-X-C Chemokines

ELR-C-X-C Chemokines with Neutrophil Chemotactic Activity

Interleukin-8 (IL-8)
Granulocyte chemotactic protein 2 (GCP-2)
Growth-regulated oncogene alpha (GRO-alpha)
Growth-regulated oncogene beta (GRO-beta)
Growth-regulated oncogene gamma (GRO-gamma)
Epithelial neutrophil-activating protein (ENA-78)
Neutrophil-activating protein 2 (NAP-2)

Non-ELR-C-X-C Chemokines That Lack Neutrophil Chemotactic Activity

Monokine induced by gamma interferon (MIG)
Platelet factor 4 (PF4)
gamma-interferon inducible protein-10 (IP-10)

Note: The ELR amino acid motif comprises the primary structure of specific C-X-C chemokine family members. The ELR containing chemokines possess activity for the directed movement of neutrophils, whereas non-ELR-containing C-X-C chemokines are not potent inducers of neutrophil chemotaxis.

CHEMOKINE-INDUCED PATHOLOGY AND TISSUE INJURY

Initial experimental animal studies assessing the in vivo activity of human IL-8 demonstrated that a single 100 μg intravenous injection into rats or rabbits caused a marked neutrophilia 15 minutes after administration, which peaked by 1 to 2 h.[11,60] Histological examination revealed both leukostasis and aggregration mainly in the microvasculature of the lung. Interestingly, repeated intravenous administration of IL-8 resulted in significant pathology, which was restricted only to the lungs.[60] These pathologic features included neutrophil aggregates in the small to medium-size pulmonary vessels, diffuse septal and intraalveolar edema, and foci of hemorrhage. Animals that received injections over 5 consecutive days (5 nmol each) showed a substantial broadening of the alveolar septa, which contained fibroblasts and a mixed leukocytic infiltrate. This information supported earlier studies demonstrating that the intradermal administration of IL-8 in experimental animals induces cutaneous leukocyte accumulation.[34] Furthermore it provided interesting information concerning the lung as an especially sensitive target for the pathologic effects of IL-8 and other C-X-C chemokines.

Although the exact rodent homologue of human IL-8 has not been identified,[58] murine macrophage inflammatory protein 2 (MIP-2), a murine chemokine functionally equivalent to human IL-8, is a major LPS-inducible chemokine.[40,56] This was first demonstrated during the original isolation studies, as murine MIP-2 was purified from the conditioned media of lipopolysaccharide (LPS)-stimulated mouse RAW 264.7 cells, a macrophage cell line, hence the name macrophage inflammatory protein 2. Although murine MIP-2 does have functional and some structural homology to human IL-8, including an E-L-R-C-X-C motif near the amino terminus, this murine chemokine also has structural homology to human growth-regulated oncogene (GRO) beta and GRO gamma (also known as human MIP-2 alpha and MIP-2 beta, respectively).[40]

Investigations have shown murine MIP-2 is highly chemotactic for neutrophils and elicits a localized neutrophil infiltrate when administered in vivo. Initial in vitro studies demonstrated that MIP-2 was significantly chemotactic for human neutrophils at 10 ng/ml and was more chemotactic for neutrophils than formyl methionyl leucyl phenylalanine (fMLP) on an nM basis. In vivo investigations demonstrated that an intratracheal, subcutaneous, or intracisternal challenge of MIP-2 to mice or rabbits induced a significant and rapid neutrophilic accumulation.[13,18,57] Further analyses of alveolar macrophages challenged in vitro with LPS demonstrated a marked increase in steady-state MIP-2 mRNA levels within 30 min after challenge. The levels of MIP-2 mRNA peaked at 1 h and remained elevated for the next 4 to 6 h. Similar MIP-2 mRNA kinetic data were obtained from alveolar macrophages recovered from animals intratracheally challenged with LPS. Thus, MIP-2 is probably an important chemokine involved in the elicitation of leukocytes to the lung during infectious processes.

CHEMOKINES IN MODELS OF ACUTE LUNG INJURY

In a rabbit model of lung reperfusion injury, antigenic IL-8 was observed both in the bronchoalveolar lavage (BAL) fluid and in lung tissue homogenates after 2 h of ischemia followed by 2 h of reperfusion.[37] The levels of IL-8 correlated with neutrophil infiltration and injury of the pulmonary parenchyma. The administration of neutralizing IL-8 antibodies prevented neutrophil infiltration and lung injury, suggesting a causal role for IL-8 in this model. Furthermore, the initiation of endotoxin-induced pleural inflammation in the rabbit was associated with a significant increase in IL-8 expression in the pleural space, associated with a profound influx of neutrophils.[7] Passive immunization of rabbits with neutralizing antibodies to rabbit IL-8 resulted in a marked reduction in neutrophil influx into the pleural space. This study was important in that species-specific reagents confirmed the role of IL-8 in an experimental model of acute inflammation, in contrast to previous reports which had demonstrated some efficacy of antibodies to human IL-8 in a rodent model of acute lung injury.[30] In addition, these findings support previous studies that the mesothelium is a likely source of IL-8 in human diseases.

CHEMOKINES IN EXPERIMENTAL LUNG INJURY DUE TO ENDOTOXEMIA

During sepsis bacteria or bacterial products, such as LPS, probably result in the early generation of TNF and IL-1. Subsequently, TNF and IL-1 can lead to the systemic activation and accumulation of neutrophils in several organs. One well-characterized model of systemic inflammation with accompanying lung injury is the mouse endotoxemia model, which is usually induced by a bolus intraperitoneal injection of LPS. This model has been used to outline many basic mechanisms of cytokine activation pathways which affect multiple organ systems, including lung, liver, kidney, heart, and intestinal tract. During endotoxemia there appears to be an early peak in TNF and IL-1 production, followed by the accumulation of neutrophils in multiple organs. The examination of neutrophil-specific chemokines has identified MIP-2, a functional homologue of IL-8, as a potential mediator of neutrophil accumulation leading to the lung injury. The induction of MIP-2 occurs very quickly after LPS injection, with detectable protein in the serum by 30 min post LPS challenge. MIP-2 does not appear to be induced by TNF, but directly activated by LPS, as in vivo neutralization of TNF does not significantly inhibit the early MIP-2 production. The primary source of MIP-2 during endotoxemia appears to be monocytes and macrophages, as indicated by immunohistochemical localization.

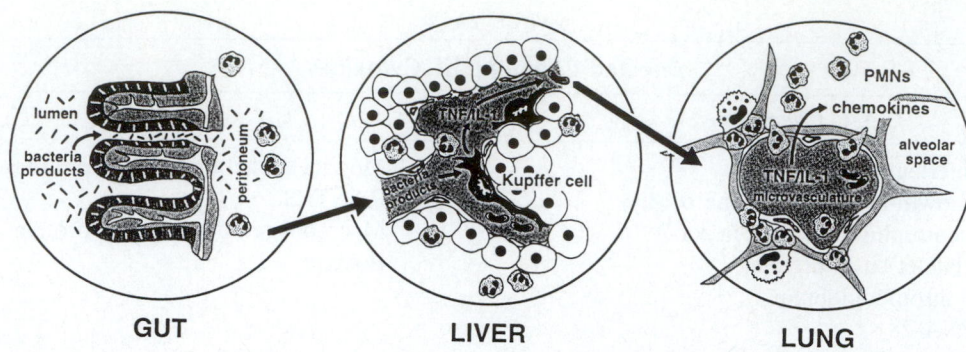

FIGURE 24-3 Although cytokine cascades are important in localizing inflammation to specific tissue, systemic inflammation is directed, in part, by organ-to-organ communication. The translocation of material from the gut can impact on the fixed macrophages found in the liver, which can affect the vasculature of the lung and cause pulmonary injury.

Interestingly, epithelial cell populations within the lung have also been identified as cellular sources of MIP-2 by in situ hybridization, indicating that several cellular sources likely contribute to the MIP-2 levels. Neutralization of MIP-2 by passive immunization with anti–mouse-MIP-2 polyclonal serum during LPS-mediated sepsis decreased neutrophil accumulation within the lung but had a minimal effect on LPS-induced mortality. However, combined neutralization of MIP-2 and TNF synergistically decreased mortality in this model, suggesting that multiple mechanisms of injury were responsible for mortality.

This injury pattern involving specific cytokines appears to depend upon organ-to-organ communication that is established during acute, systemic inflammation (Fig. 24-3). In this scenario, the gut-liver-lungs are involved in a network whereby an insult to the intestinal epithelium may translocate bacteria or bacteria products to the vasculature and impact on the liver. The fixed macrophages in the liver can become activated and release mediators which activate both leukocytes and resident cells in the lungs. The strategic anatomical location of the lungs increases their vulnerability to "downstream" mediators and may explain why they are often injured.

C-C chemokines are also expressed in models of endotoxemia. For example, MIP-1α and regulated on activation normal T-cell expressed and secreted (RANTES) appear to be generated in significant levels within the lung after LPS challenge. These members of the C-C chemokine family have chemotactic activity for monocytes, lymphocytes, and eosinophils. During endotoxemia, both RANTES and MIP-1α appear to mediate mononuclear phagocytic cell recruitment into the lungs. Passive immunization of mice with anti-MIP-1α antibodies significantly reduced inflammation, monocyte accumulation, and mortality associated with the host's response to LPS. Interestingly, passive neutralization of RANTES significantly inhibited macrophage, but not lymphocyte or neutrophil, influx during LPS challenge. In addition, neutralization of TNF in the endotoxin model significantly reduced RANTES mRNA expression and protein production within the lung. Taken together, it appears that multiple chemokines are operative during endotoxemia, leading to both neutrophil and monocyte infiltration.

The results from these studies may give significant insight into the development of pharmacologic agents to inhibit the production, release, or activity of chemokines during acute lung inflammation. This may be especially pertinent in endotoxemia or sepsis-related disorders, as it appears that targeting early response cytokines, such as IL-1 and TNF, has not been effective in altering lung injury in these patient populations.

CHEMOKINES IN EXPERIMENTAL ALLERGIC AIRWAY INFLAMMATION

The production of chemokines during asthmatic responses may specifically contribute to the influx of eosinophils, a major effector cell inducing airway injury and subsequent late-phase reactivity. A number of C-C chemokines appear to preferentially recruit human eosinophils in vitro, including RANTES, MIP-1α, and MCP-3. To determine the relative contribution of eosinophil-specific chemokines, a murine model of allergic airway inflammation utilizing schistosome parasite soluble egg antigen (SEA) has been developed. The ability of SEA to induce a Th2-type (IL-4, IL-5) response, with high serum IgE ($\sim 10^5$ titer) and hypereosinophilia, appeared to be instrumental for the development of this model. Localization of the soluble SEA antigen to the airway, 21 days after primary challenge, induces an airway localized Th2-type response characterized by intense peribronchial leukocyte accumulation, airway eosinophilia, antigen-specific histamine release, and airway hyperreactivity. These responses appear to be similar to those observed in patient populations with allergic asthma.

In this model the eosinophilic influx appears to be regulated by both IL-4 and TNF, as neutralization of these cytokines in vivo significantly attenuates the eosinophil recruitment into the lung and airway. Although IL-4 and TNF are not directly chemotactic for leukocytes, they have been reported to induce various C-C and C-X-C chemokines. Of particular interest has been the induction of C-C chemokines by these cytokines which promote eosinophil chemotaxis. During the development of the eosinophilic response, MIP-1α and RANTES levels are elevated in the lung homogenates and BAL, peaking between 8 and 48 h after airway allergen challenge. MIP-1α appears to be produced by macrophages and airway epithelial cells, whereas RANTES appears to be produced primarily by epithelial cells within the lung. In addition, the production of both MIP-1α and RANTES was significantly decreased in lung homogenates when either IL-4 or TNF were neutralized in vivo. Furthermore, the neutralization of either chemokine resulted in a significant reduction in airway eosinophilia, indicating that multiple chemokines may contribute to the recruitment of eosinophils. Interestingly, passive immunization with anti-MCP-1 did not reduce the influx of eosinophils into the airway, thus demonstrating chemokine specificity for the response. This animal model, which has many of the histopathologic and physiological attributes of human asthma, is useful in defining the specific role that cytokines play in allergic airway inflammation.

CYTOKINES IN CHRONIC LUNG INFLAMMATION

Chronic pulmonary inflammation is associated with a wide variety of disease states ranging from infectious etiologies, such as tuberculosis, to idiopathic process, such as idiopathic pulmonary fibrosis. Often these disease states are accompanied by significant lung injury caused by active and progressive inflammation, leading to end-stage fibrosis. At present, treatment of idiopathic chronic lung diseases is difficult, reflecting, in part, the limited understanding of the mechanisms that orchestrate and maintain the inflammatory lesion. The progression of chronic pulmonary inflammation is usually characterized by an intense mononuclear leukocyte recruitment phase followed by a fibroproliferative response and deposition of extracellular matrix. Research into chronic lung diseases has underscored the idea that efficacious therapeutic interventions must be directed at the active inflammatory cell or fibroproliferative stage of the disease, as end-stage fibrosis is not responsive to treatment. Although there is heterogeneity in the various types of interstitial lung lesions, the presence of mononuclear leukocytes is clearly one unifying feature of chronic lung inflammation. Distinct cytokine-directed mechanisms appear to be important to ensure the appropriate host response to a particular etiologic agent.

Historically, research directed at understanding the inflammatory processes accompanying chronic lung inflammation has identified lymphocytes, monocytes, and macrophages and their derivatives (giant cells and epitheloid cells) as important participants of the developing lesion. However, many of the mechanisms involved in the elicitation and subsequent chronic activation of these leukocytes have remained an enigma. This latter aspect of leukocyte activation is especially interesting, as the continued response appears to be directed by ill-defined mechanisms which influence the chronicity, composition, and intensity of the lesion.

A variety of cytokines are associated with chronic pulmonary inflammation, including IL-1,[9] IL-6,[41] IL-8,[26] MIP-1α,[45] MCP-1,[10] TNF,[3] transforming growth factors,[20] and growth factor.[6] Although this list is not all-inclusive, it does contain representative cytokines which possess early activation, chemotactic growth and differentiation, and remodeling activity (Table 24-5). During the evolution of chronic lung disease, early activation events are likely initiated by IL-1 and TNF. These early-response cytokines,

---

TABLE 24-5

Sequential Expression of Specific Cytokines

I. Early Activation
   Tumor necrosis factor α, β
   Interleukin-1 α, β

II. Chemotactic
   Monocyte chemoattractant protein 1
   Macrophage inflammatory protein 1 α, β

III. Growth and Differentiation
   Interferons
   Colony-stimulating factors
   Fibroblast growth factor
   Transforming growth factors

IV. Remodeling
   Platelet-derived growth factor
   Transforming growth factor

Note: The sequential expression of specific cytokines during the evolution and resolution of chronic inflammation involves cytokines with various activities.

which are involved in acute lung injury, are also important in triggering a number of events that perpetuate and maintain the chronic response. These events include the initiation of cascades that result in the production of more distal cytokines, such as chemokines, which elicit leukocyte subpopulations. Activated leukocytes in turn serve as important sources for a number of cytokines, including those with growth, differentiation, and remodeling activity. For example, the expression of leukocyte-derived TGF-beta may increase the production of extracellular matrix molecules by stromal cells, inhibit collagenase production, and influence fibroblast proliferation via the induction of fibroblast growth factors.[20] These cytokine-induced events are all important to the growth and remodeling phases of chronic lung disease.

CYTOKINES IN INTERSTITIAL FIBROSIS

The identification of different cytokines from patients with sarcoidosis or idiopathic pulmonary fibrosis or animal models that mimic human pulmonary fibrosis has provided clues that specific immune mediators are involved in the evolution of interstitial lung disease. However, a causal role of these cytokines in the initiation and maintenance of lung lesions has not been established. Thus, the biomedical community is still far from understanding the mechanisms which dictate either the restoration of normal lung tissue or the progression to irreversible fibrotic derangements of the pulmonary interstitium following chronic lung disorders. Evidence suggests that the cytokine profile of the natural immune/inflammatory response likely determines the disease phenotype responsible for either resolution of the pulmonary response or progression to end-stage fibrosis. Much of the supporting evidence is derived from studies demonstrating that interferons, especially gamma interferon (IFN-γ), have profound suppressive effects on the production of extracellular matrix proteins such as collagen and fibronectin.[16] Interferons can inhibit fibroblast collagen production in vitro as well as decrease the expression of steady-state type I and III procollagen mRNA levels in this cell population. In addition, the administration of IFN-γ in vivo can cause a reduction of extracellular matrix in animal models of pulmonary fibrosis. This information supports the concept that IFN-γ, one of the major Th1-type cytokines, possesses profound regulatory activity for collagen deposition during chronic inflammation.

Interleukin-4 (IL-4), one of the major Th2-type cytokines, is a potent stimulus for the production of fibroblast-derived extracellular matrix, including type I and III collagen and fibronectin.[33] These studies have demonstrated that IL-4 treatment of fibroblasts can increase steady state levels of extracellular matrix mRNA and subsequent production of extracellular matrix protein. In addition, IL-4 has been identified as a chemotactic factor for directed movement of fibroblasts.[33] These studies lend support to the theory that the disease phenotype characterized by either Th1 or Th2 like cytokines may be paramount in determining the course of chronic pulmonary inflammation, leading to interstitial fibrosis.

A model of granulomatous inflammation induced via the embolization of S. mansoni parasite egg or egg antigen (SEA) into the lungs of naive and sensitized mice has provided a convenient

model to study chronic lung inflammation characterized as a delayed-type hypersensitivity response. The primary granulomatous response induced in naive mice is a Th1 immune reaction that is IFN-γ-mediated. The cellular response in this model peaks at 16 days after challenge. A secondary granuloma can be initiated in SEA-sensitized mice, and this lung granuloma is mediated by a Th2 immune reaction and IL-4-dependent responses. The Th2 response represents an accelerated granulomatous reaction, peaking at 4 days and resolving by 16 days after challenge. The primary granuloma is characterized by mainly mononuclear cell accumulation, whereas the secondary granuloma formation is characterized by macrophages, eosinophils, and fibroblasts. These two distinct phases of granuloma formation provide the unique opportunity to examine the differential role of chemokines during the progression of inflammation in lesions with distinct cytokine profiles.

There is also a significant induction of MIP-1α mRNA in the primary lung granulomas in this model.[25] The production of MIP-1α protein from isolated granulomas demonstrated a progressive increase during primary lesion development. In vivo neutralization of MIP-1α during primary and secondary granuloma formation demonstrated different results. During primary granuloma formation the size of the lesion was reduced by approximately 60 percent, whereas secondary granuloma formation was reduced by only 15 to 20 percent. Immunohistochemical localization of MIP-1α identified mononuclear phagocytes as the primary source of this C-C chemokine. These results suggest that MIP-1α plays a greater role in leukocyte recruitment during primary, Th1-mediated, than in secondary, Th2-mediated granuloma formation.

An additional C-C chemokine, monocyte chemotactic protein 1 (MCP-1), was also assessed for its production pattern during lung granuloma development. MCP-1 is chemotactic for mononuclear cells and can be induced in a number of cell populations by specific cytokines. Interestingly, IL-4 has been shown to induce MCP-1 from endothelial cells, as well as smooth-muscle cell populations. The expression of MCP-1 mRNA in granulomatous lungs was much stronger in Th2-type inflammatory lung lesions than in Th1-type lung granulomas. The production of MCP-1 in isolated granulomas demonstrated high constitutive levels of MCP-1 in Th2 lesions, which correlated with the size of the Th2-mediated response. When MCP-1 was neutralized in vivo, there was no evidence of diminished formation of Th-1 lesions, but a significant decrease was observed in Th2-type granulomas. The predominant cellular expression of MCP-1 appeared to be associated with vascular cell populations within the Th2-type lesions. These data contrast with MIP-1α neutralization and suggest that specific chemokines operate at certain stages of the granulomatous processes, possibly dependent upon the local expression of supporting cytokine profiles (Th1-versus Th2-type cytokines).

CONCLUSIONS

Cytokine and chemokine expression often occurs via an amplified cascade or network that involves cellular activation by an early-response cytokine which triggers the expression of more distal cytokines. The generation of cytokine networks is necessary for both the pathogenesis and resolution of a variety of acute and chronic lung diseases, as these mediators are fundamental to the initiation, maintenance, and final resolution of the inflammatory response. Studies that illuminate the mechanistic role of cytokines and chemokines in mediating lung inflammation are likely to lead to novel cytokine-based forms of therapies, which will significantly aid in treating enigmatic lung disease.

REFERENCES

1. Alcami A, Smith GL: Cytokine receptors encoded by poxviruses: a lession in cytokine biology. *Immunol Today* 16:474–478, 1995.

2. Arend WP: Interleukin-1 receptor antagonist a new member of the interleukin-1 family. *J Clin Invest* 88:1445–1451, 1991.

3. Bachwich PR, Lynch JP, Larrick J, et al: Tumor necrosis factor production by human sarcoid alveolar macrophages. *Am J Pathol* 125: 421–425, 1986.

4. Baggiolini M, DeWald B, Moser B: Interleukin 8 and related chemotactic cytokines-CXC and CC chemokines. *Adv Immunol* 555:97–179, 1994.

5. Baggiolini M, Walz A, Kunkel SL: Neutrophil-activating peptide-1/IL-8, a novel cytokine that activates neutrophils. *J Clin Invest* 84: 1045–1049, 1989.

6. Bonner JC, Osornio-Vargas AR, Badgett A, Brody AR: Differential proliferation of rat lung fibroblasts induced by the platelet-derived growth factor-AA, AB, and BB isoforms secreted by alveolar macrophages. *Am J Respir Cell Mol Biol* 5:539–547, 1991.

7. Broaddus VC, Boylan AM, Hoeffel JM, et al: Neutralization of IL-8 inhibits neutrophil influx in a rabbit model of endotoxin-induced pleurisy. *J Immunol* 152:2960–2967, 1994.

8. Cerami A: Inflammatory cytokines. *Clin Immunol Immunopathol* 62:S3–S10, 1992.

9. Chensue SW, Ottrness IG, Higashi GI, et al: Monokine production by hypersensitivity (Schistosoma mansoni egg) and foreign body (Sephadex bead)-type granuloma macrophages. Evidence for sequential production of IL-1 and TNF. *J Immunol* 142:1281–1286, 1989.

10. Chensue SW, Warmington KS, Lukacs N, et al: Monocyte chemotactic protein (MCP-1) expression during schistosome egg granuloma formation: sequence of production, localization, contribution, and regulation. *Am J Pathol* 146:130–138, 1995.

11. Coldtiz I, Zwahlen R, Dewald B, Baggiolini M: In vivo inflammatory activity of neutrophil-activating factor, a novel chemotactic peptide derived from monocytes. *Am J Pathol* 134:755–764, 1989.

12. Dinarello CA: Interleukin-1 and interleukin-1 antagonism. *Blood.* 77:1627–1652, 1991.

13. Driscoll KE, Hassenbein DG, Carter J, et al: Macrophage inflammatory proteins 1 and 2: expression by rat alveolar macrophages, fibroblasts, and epithelial cells and in rat lungs after mineral dust exposure. *Am J Respir Cell Mol Biol* 8:311–318, 1993.

14. Gershenwald JE, Fong Y, Fahey TJ, et al: Interleukin-1 receptor blockade attenuates the host inflammatory response. *Proc Natl Acad Sci USA* 87:4966–4973, 1990.

15. Girardin E, Grau GE, Dayer JM, Roux-Lombard P: Tumor necrosis factor and interleukin-1 in the serum of children with severe infectious purpura. *New Engl J Med* 319:397–400, 1988.

16. Goldring MB, Sandell LJ, Stephenson ML: Immune interferon suppresses levels of procollagen mRNA and type II collagen synthesis in cultured human articular and costal chondrocytes. *J Immunol* 261:9049–9056, 1986.

17. Hinshaw LB, Tekamp-Olson P, Chang ACK, et al: Survival of primates in LD100 septic shock following therapy with antibody to tumor necrosis factor (TNF alpha). *Cir Shock* 30:279–292, 1990.

18. Huang S, Paulauskis JD, Godleski JJ, Kobzik L: Expression of macrophage inflammatory protein 2 and KC mRNA in pulmonary inflammation. *Am J Pathol* 141:981–988, 1992.

19. Jansen J, van der Poll T, Levi M, et al: Inhibition of the release of soluble tumor necrosis factor receptors in experimental endotoxemia by an antitumor necrosis factor antibody. *J Clin Invest* 15:45–54, 1995.

20. Khalil N, Bereznay O, Sporin M, Greenberg AH: Macrophage production of TGF-beta and fibroblast collagen synthesis in chronic pulmonary fibrosis. *J Exp Med* 170:727–737, 1989.

21. Kunkel SL, Remick DG, Strieter RM, Larrick JW: Mechanisms that regulate the production and effects of tumor necrosis factor. *Crit Rev Immunol* 9:93–117, 1988.

22. Larrick JW, Kunkel SL: The role of tumor necrosis factor and interleukin-1 in the immunoinflammatory response. *Pharm Res* 5: 129–139, 1988.

23. Le J, Vilcek J: TNF and IL-1: cytokines with multiple overlapping biological activities. *Lab Invest* 56:234–282, 1987.

24. Leeuwenberg JFM, Jeunhomme TMAA, Buurman WA: Slow release of soluble TNF receptors by monocytes in vitro. *J Immunol* 152:4036–4042, 1994.

25. Lukacs NW, Kunkel SL, Strieter RM, et al: The role of macrophage inflammatory protein 1 alpha in *Schistosoma mansoni* egg-induced granulomatous inflammation. *J Exp Med* 177:1551–1559, 1993.

26. Lynch JP, Standiford TJ, Rolfe MW, et al: Neutrophilic alveolitis in idiopathic pulmonary fibrosis. The role of interleukin-8. *Am Rev Res Dis* 145:1433–1439, 1992.

27. Marks JD, Marks CB, Luce JM, et al: Plasma tumor necrosis factor in patients with septic shock: mortality rate, incidence of adult respiratory distress syndrome. *Am Rev Respir Dis* 141:94–97, 1990.

28. Matsushima K, Oppenheim JJ: Interleukin-8 and MCAF: novel inflammatory cytokines inducible by IL-1 and TNF. *Cytokine* 1:2–13, 1989.

29. Michie HR, Mangue KR, Spriggs DR, et al: Detection of circulating tumor necrosis factor after endotoxin administration. *New Engl J Med* 318:1481–1486, 1988.

30. Mulligan MS, Jones ML, Bolanowski MA, et al: Inhibition of lung inflammatory reactions in rats by an anti-human IL-8 antibody. *J Immunol* 150:5585–5592, 1993.

31. Ohlsson K, Bjork P, Bergenfeldt M, et al: IL-1ra reduces mortality from endotoxin shock. *Nature* 348:550–552, 1990.

32. Oppenheim JJ, Zachariae OC, Mukaida N, Matsushima K: Properties of the novel proinflammatory supergene intercrine cytokine family. *Ann Rev Immunol* 9:617–648, 1991.

33. Postlewaite AE, Holness MA, Katai H, Raghow R: Human fibroblasts synthesize elevated levels of extracellular matrix proteins in response to interleukin-4. *J Clin Invest* 90:1479–1485, 1992.

34. Rampart M, Van Damme J, Zonnekeyn L, Herman AG: Granulocyte chemotactic protein-interleukin-8 induces plasma leakage and neutrophil accumulation in rabbit skin. *Am J Pathol* 345:21–30, 1989.

35. Remick DG, Strieter RM, Lynch JP, et al: In vivo dynamics of murine tumor necrosis factor gene expression: kinetics of dexamethasone-induced supression. *Lab Invest* 60:766–771, 1989.

36. Rolfe MW, Kunkel SL, Standiford TJ, et al: Expression and regulation of human pulmonary fibroblast-derived monocyte chemotactic peptide-1. *Am J Physiol* 7:536–545, 1992.

37. Sekido N, Mukaida N, Harada A, et al: Prevention of lung reperfusion injury in rabbits by a monoclonal antibody against interleukin-8. *Nature* 365:654–657, 1994.

38. Shalaby MR, Halgunset J, Haugen OA, et al: Cytokine associated tissue injury and lethality in mice: a comparative study. *Clin Immunol Immunopath* 61:69–82, 1991.

39. Sherry B, Cerami A: Cachectin/tumor necrosis factor exert endocrine, paracrine, and autocrine control of the inflammatory response. *J Cell Biol* 107:1269–1277, 1988.

40. Sherry B, Horii Y, Manogue KR, et al: Macrophage inflammatory proteins 1 and 2: an overview. *Cytokine* 4:127–130, 1992.

41. Sibille Y, Houssiau F, Pochet JM, et al: Alpha 2 macroglobulin and Interleukin-6 release by human alveolar macrophages from normal and sarcoidosis patients. *Am Rev Resp Dis* 141:A8712, 1990.

42. Smith CA, Davis T, Wignall JM, et al: T2 open reading frame from the shope fibroma virus encodes a soluble form of the TNF receptor. *Biochem Biophys Res Comm* 176:35–340, 1991.

43. Spriggs CA, Hruby DE, Maliszewski CR, et al: Vaccina and cowpox viruses encode a novel secreted IL-1 binding protein. *Cell* 71:145–153, 1992.

44. Standiford TJ, Kunkel SL, Chensue SW, et al: Interleukin-8 gene expression by a pulmonary epithelial cell line; a model for cytokine networks in the lung. *J Biol Chem* 266:9912–9918, 1991.

45. Standiford TJ, Rolfe MW, Kunkel SL, et al: Macrophage inflammatory protein-1 alpha expression in interstitial lung disease. *J Immunol* 151:2852–2863, 1993.

46. Standiford TJ, Strieter RM, Lukacs NW, Kunkel SL: Neutralization of IL-10 increases lethality in endotoxemia. *J Immunol* 155:2222–2229, 1995.

47. Strieter RM, Chensue SW, Basha MA, et al: Human alveolar macrophage gene expression of interleukin-8 by TNF-α, LPS and IL-1β. *Am J Respir Cell Mol Biol* 2:321–326, 1990.

48. Strieter RM, Kunkel SL, Showell HJ, et al: Endothelial cell gene expression of a neutrophil chemotactic factor by TNF, LPS, and IL-1. *Science* 243:1467–1469, 1989.

49. Strieter RM, Phan SH, Showell HJ, et al: Monokine-induced neutrophil chemotactic factor gene expression in human fibroblasts. *J Biol Chem* 264:10621–10626, 1989.

50. Thornton AJ, Strieter RM, Lindley I, et al: Cytokine-induced gene expression of a neutrophil chemotactic factor/interleukin-8 by human hepatocytes. *J Immunol* 144:2609–2613, 1990.

51. Tracey KJ, Fong Y, Hesse DG, et al: Anti-cachectin/TNF monoclonal antibodies prevent septic shock during lethal bacteremia. *Nature* 330:662–664, 1987.

52. Ulich TR, Watson LR, Songmei Y, et al: The intratracheal administration of endotoxin and cytokines. *Am J Pathol* 138:1485–1496.

53. Van der Poll T, Mardfhant A, Buurman WA, et al: Endogenous IL-10 protects mice from death during septic peritonitis. *J Immunol* 155:5397–5401, 1995.

54. Vieira P, Waal-Malefyt RD, Dang MN, et al: Isolation and expression of human cytokine synthesis inhibitory factor cDNA clones: homology to Epstein-Barr virus open reading frame BCRFI. *Proc Natl Acad Sci USA* 88:1172–1176, 1991.

55. Waage A, Halstensen A, Espevik T: Association between tumor necrosis factor in serum and fatal outcome in patients with meningococcal disease. *Lancet* 1:255–357, 1987.

56. Wolpe SD, Sherry B, Juers D, et al: Identification and characterization of macrophage inflammatory protein-2. *Proc Natl Acad Sci USA* 272:911–927, 1990.

57. Xing Z, Jordana M, Kirpalani H, et al: Cytokine expression by neutrophils and macrophages in vivo: endotoxin induces TNF, MIP-2, IL-1, IL-6, but not RANTES or TGF mRNA expression in acute lung inflammation. *Am J Respir Cell Mol Biol* 10:148–153, 1994.

58. Yoshimura T: The gene for neutrophil attractant protein-1 (NAP-1) is highly conserved in guinea pig but not in rat or mouse. *J Immunol* 151:6225–6236, 1993.

59. Yoshimura T, Matsushima K, Oppenheim JJ, Leonard EJ: Neutrophil chemotactic factor produced by LPS-stimulated human blood mononuclear leukocytes: partial characterization and separation from interleukin-1. *J Immunol* 139:788–794, 1987.

60. Zwahlen R, Walz A, Rot A: In vitro and in vivo activity and pathophysiology of human interleukin-8 and related peptides. *Int Rev Exp Pathol* 34B:27–42, 1993.

LEUKOCYTE ACCUMULATION IN THE LUNG

G. Scott Worthen / Jerry A. Nick

The ability of the lung to regulate the accumulation of leukocytes is one of the central issues of pulmonary homeostasis, the importance of which is highlighted by lung diseases associated with an overexuburant inflammatory response. In health, the airspaces and interstitium maintain a sparse population of leukocytes, primarily macrophages. In the face of continuous exposure to the external environment, pulmonary defense mechanisms are capable of recognizing and disposing of a vast array of antigenic and noxious stimuli by recruitment of inflammatory cells without injury to the lung. When it is fully mobilized, however, the intensity of the pulmonary inflammatory response is overwhelming. Through the presence of the so-called marginating pool of leukocytes within the pulmonary circulation, the lung appears to harbor at any given time an extraordinary number of neutrophils, monocytes, and (to a lesser extent) lymphocytes and other leukocytes. Indeed, it is estimated that the lung contains approximately half of the neutrophils that are present in the circulating blood volume, a number much greater than can be accounted for by the relatively small blood volume within the pulmonary vascular bed.

Thus the presence of this marginating pool provides a reservoir of leukocytes already positioned within the lung. These cells are predominantly located within the lung capillaries. In contrast, the marginating pool of neutrophils in other organs and systemic tissue occurs in the postcapillary venules. Teleologically, it would appear to be an advantage to have host defense mechanisms located precisely at the site where external agents are likely to come in contact with the delicate alveolar capillary membrane. Were neutrophils to localize in postcapillary venules, the length of their journey to the actual site at which environmental agents are most likely to come in contact with lung structures would be greatly extended. The high-volume, low-perfusion pressure circuit that is necessary for the lung to perform gas exchange may thus also be critical for host defense purposes.

As this chapter will explain, the normal physiological balance between leukocytes and the lung is characterized by large numbers of leukocytes in the capillary, just microns away from the external environment. This arrangement is ideally suited to a rapid initial response. In addition, however, the leukocytes in the circulation may be quickly mobilized (within seconds) to further increase the number of leukocytes within the lung capillary, dramatically increasing the ability of the lung to respond acutely to initial offense. It is now widely believed that the intensity of this rapid response of the lungs to external agents is central to the pathogenesis of lung injury during the acute inflammatory response in vivo, but perhaps it represents an almost inevitable result of the measures taken to ensure that the lung is adequately protected. We will discuss in some detail the mechanisms responsible for the stimulated sequestration of leukocytes within the lung, as the leukocyte migrates from the vascular space into the alveolar space under a diverse range of conditions. This migration is rapid and associated with alterations in the behavior of the leukocyte. Remarkably enough, however, migration of leukocytes into the lung may have diverse consequences, ranging from almost no derangement of lung function to the nearly complete loss of gas-exchanging surface, as is seen in the adult respiratory distress syndrome (ARDS). Under many circumstances, the lung appears to tolerate the accumulation of a large number of leukocytes within the airspace without a dramatic decrease in its gas exchange function. This is essential if host defenses of the lung are to be focused on invading microorganisms and not hinder life-sustaining functions of the lung. Lung injury, as a result of an excessive inflammatory response, can thus be viewed as a direct consequence of the processes developed to protect the lung from microorganisms.

Much of what is known about leukocyte accumulation in the lung is a result of studies of the neutrophil. It has long been known that neutrophil accumulation is one of the first recognizable events in the pathogenesis of lung inflammation. As neutrophils can rapidly accumulate in the airspaces as a result of a focal pulmonary inflammatory event (for example, bacterial pneumonia) or of an insult distant from the lungs (for example, ARDS secondary to endotoxemia), the neutrophil must respond to a wide range of inflammatory mediators. It has been recognized that the functional response of the neutrophil does vary according to the type of external stimuli. These observations have led to the concept that individualized response to stimuli is initiated by the activation of stimuli-specific cell surface receptors and preserved by distinct intracellular signaling pathways.

As certain inflammatory processes progress, selective recruitment of monocytes, eosinophils, and lymphocytes can occur. Elucidation of the mechanisms by which specific cell types accumulate in response to a select group of pulmonary insults is a field of intense investigation. The importance of an ever-expanding array of chemokines as well as the less specific chemoattractants is now recognized in the selective accumulation of monocytes and eosinophils to the lung. Although less well studied than the neutrophil, other types of leukocytes share some common mechanisms of accumulation as well as possessing unique cell-type specific responses. Attention has recently focused on the mechanisms by which lymphocytes are recruited to the lung. To a greater extent than that of other leukocytes, the accumulation of lymphocytes appears to depend on cell-cell interactions that are fundamentally different from other described mechanisms. The focus of this chapter will be the mechanisms by which neutrophil, eosinophil, and monocyte accumulation occurs.

REGULATION OF LEUKOCYTE RETENTION IN THE LUNG

It is well known that exercise, β-agonists, and other maneuvers result in the release of large numbers of neutrophils into the

bloodstream, and that a primary site from which these cells are released is the pulmonary microcirculation.[19] The mechanisms that account for the formation, maintenance, and release of this pool remain the subject of some controversy, but a great deal has been learned over the past 10 years.

Neutrophil Margination in the Lung Occurs in the Pulmonary Capillary

An important clue to the mechanisms of margination was the recognition that, in contrast to neutrophil behavior in most circulatory beds, in the lung, retention occurs almost exclusively within the pulmonary capillaries. Normal unstimulated neutrophils entering the lung microvascular bed form the marginating pool through retention within the lung capillary bed.[24] Furthermore, the cells sequestered do not pass in a continuous fashion through the capillary but, rather, are retained at discrete sites within the lung vasculature,[25] resulting in a stuttering movement. This suggests that preferred sites exist within the lung for leukocyte sequestration (Fig. 25-1). Even neutrophils that eventually transit the lung capillary may remain stationary for short periods, ranging from 1 to 2 s to as long as a few minutes. The distribution of transit times for unstimulated neutrophils is affected by a number of factors, including pulmonary circulation.[25] Increases in pulmonary artery pressure or local flow rates diminish transit time. Hence, the low-pressure nature of the pulmonary circulation appears to contribute significantly to capillary localization.

A simple calculation will suffice to consider the formation of the marginating pool in the lung. If the mean transit time across the pulmonary capillary of a dog[24] is 30 s, and the circulation time (i.e., the time for neutrophils in blood to travel from the left ventricle to the right atrium) is also 30 s, at equilibrium there will be similar numbers of neutrophils in the marginated (lung) pool and the circulating systemic pool. Under conditions of severe stress, reproduced by the infusion of epinephrine, the transit time across the pulmonary capillary bed can fall from 30 s to 2 s, and neutrophils are released out of the marginating pool into the circulating pool. This release of neutrophils into the circulatory pool can thus be explained, at least in part, by the dynamic reduction in time of transit across the lung and the resulting increase in size of the circulating systemic pool relative to the marginating pool.

Retention of Leukocytes in the Pulmonary Capillary Occurs Through Mechanisms Different from Those in the Systemic Circulation

While it is likely that several processes are at work in neutrophil retention in the capillary, adhesive properties and mechanical/structural properties of the neutrophil have received the most attention to date. The neutrophil has an average diameter of 8 μ, compared with a mean diameter of the pulmonary capillary of 5.5 μ. Thus, the neutrophil must deform in order to transit the pulmonary capillary. We have suggested that neutrophils are fairly deformable at rest and respond to chemoattractants by increasing size and stiffness.[53] In addition, we have suggested that the size and stiffness properties of the other circulating leukocytes, monocytes, and lymphocytes may also regulate the circu-

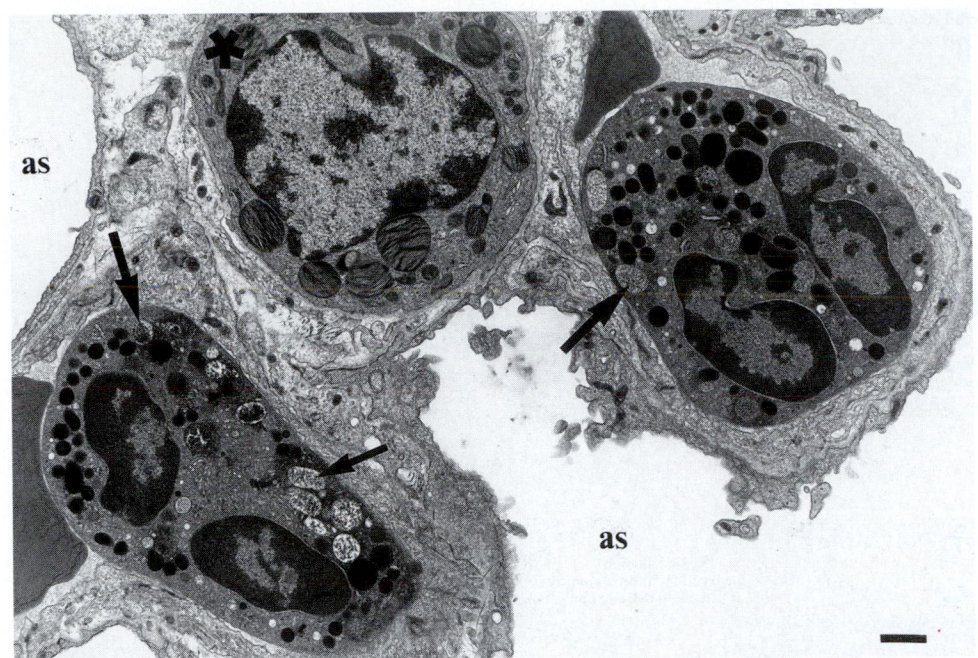

FIGURE 25-1   Electron micrograph of rabbit lung 4 h after intravenous infusion of lipopolysaccharide (LPS) and the chemoattractant formyl-methionyl-leucyl-phenylalanine (fMLP). Neutrophils (arrows) are seen in pulmonary capillaries within the alveolar walls, the typical site of retention of these leukocytes both during the normal formation of the marginating pool and in pathologic states of inflammation, as shown here. Of interest is that the neutrophils appear to be beginning to degranulate, as shown by the different density within a few peripheral granules at the arrows. The capillaries involved appear at a corner of an alveolus, further indicated by the appearance of an alveolar type II cell (*). The close approximation of the retained neutrophils to the alveolar space (as) is readily apparent ($\times 8100$; bar = 1 μm). *(Photograph prepared by Jan Henson.)*

latory behavior of unstimulated cells.[13] Exposure to chemoattractants dramatically prolongs the mean transit time.[26] However, the pulmonary capillary remains the site of neutrophil transit (Fig. 25-1), and the mode of transit (stuttering or hopping) remains similar, although the magnitude of these effects is much greater than in unstimulated cells.

These data highlight an important difference between the pulmonary circulation and other circulatory beds (Fig. 25-2). Even though neutrophils travel more slowly than erythrocytes in both pulmonary and systemic beds, neutrophils spend considerable time in stationary contact with the pulmonary endothelium—a condition that may greatly predispose to adhesive and other interactions between the neutrophil and the subjacent endothelium. Although pulmonary and systemic capillaries are of equivalent size, the much greater pressure head of the systemic circulation does not allow neutrophils prolonged contact with the systemic capillary endothelium. Instead, the initial event of neutrophil slowing in the systemic vascular beds is postponed to the postcapillary venules. Thus, neutrophils are slowed relative to erythrocytes by rolling along the walls of postcapillary venules of the systemic vacular beds—in contrast to the pulmonary circulation, where neutrophil slowing occurs in the capillaries.

Resistance to Deformation (Stiffness) Underlies Initial Retention in Pulmonary Capillaries

The increase in stiffness consequent to chemoattractant stimulation of neutrophils is accounted for largely by induction of cy-

toskeletal assembly and is accompanied by a redistribution of actin. At the same time, however, the cells express increased numbers of adhesion-related glycoproteins, which may also contribute to the retention of these cells within the pulmonary microvasculature. Increased neutrophil adhesivity has been demonstrated in response to complement fragment C5a, tumor necrosis factor (TNF), interleukin-1 (IL-1), and lipopolysaccharide (LPS).[6,51] Neutrophils from patients with a deficiency of β_2 integrins do not adhere to the endothelium. Only a few studies have directly assessed the role of adhesion molecules in neutrophil sequestration in vivo. These studies suggest that antibodies directed against the common beta chain of the MAC-1 (CD11b/CD18), LFA-1 (CD11a/CD18), P150,95 (CD11c/18) family can materially diminish neutrophil retention in skin[10] and gut[44] but appear to have less effect on neutrophil retention within the pulmonary microvasculature. Whether these data reflect (as we believe) an important role for the mechanical properties of the leukocyte or, rather, a different set of adhesion-related molecules or a fundamentally different endothelial surface in the lung than in systemic vascular beds remains unclear, but attempts to resolve this issue promise to yield a vigorous and constructive debate for several years.

MECHANISMS OF LEUKOCYTE ADHESION: CLUES TO SPECIFICITY OF ACCUMULATION

A number of other features may modify neutrophil retention within the lung microcirculation—in particular, the expression of endothelial cell-derived adhesion molecules. Treatment of endothelial cells with LPS, TNF, or IL-1[6] results in enhanced adhesion due to up-regulation of endothelial-derived adhesion molecules. The relative importance of increased neutrophil adherence compared with endothelial adherence is not yet known with clarity in any in vivo system. It is known that the adherence of neutrophils to the endothelium occurs quickly, and the neutrophil response is very rapid,[18] whereas the maximal endothelial response can take as long as 4 to 6 hours (see below). The endothelium is, however, capable of rapid responses due to generation of chemoattractants[57] and through up-regulation of already formed adhesion molecules such as P-selectin.[6] Thus, the resulting adhesive interaction is regulated with respect to time, intensity, and cell specificity by both the endothelium and the leukocyte.

Several families of adhesion molecules have been identified, including the CAM members of the immunoglobulin superfamily; intercellular cell adhesion molecule (ICAM-1, -2, and -3; the last two have not been implicated in neutrophil adherence); vas-

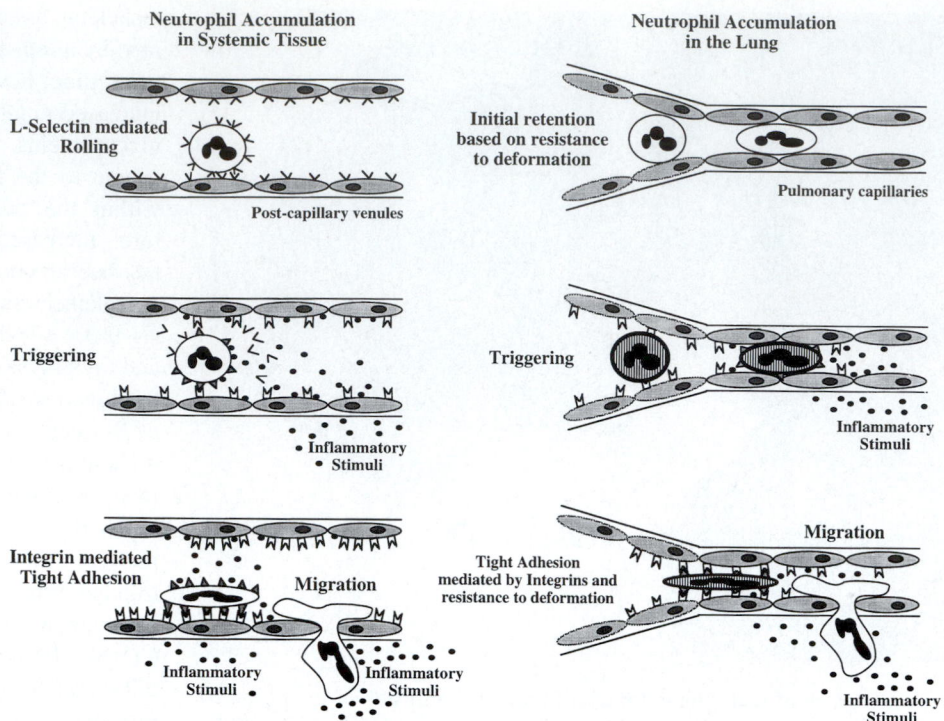

FIGURE 25-2 Mechanisms of retention of neutrophils in the lung compared to vascular beds supplied by the systemic circulation. Retention is shown in response to the local generation of stimuli such as chemoattractants in the tissue. In the systemic circulation *(left panel)*, retention proceeds through a three-step process that has been fairly well defined (see text for full details). Leukocytes are slowed by rolling through selectin-based mechanisms (depicted by V) that are essential for subsequent steps. The slowed leukocytes are then triggered by stimuli (typically chemoattractants; depicted by ●) to activate and up-regulate integrins (depicted by ▲), which interact with their cognate ligands to induce tight adhesion that seems essential for subsequent migratory

events. In the pulmonary microcirculation *(right panel)*, the initial slowing of leukocytes occurs in capillaries, and is accomplished by quite different mechanisms. Neutrophils are normally slowed in their passage through capillaries as a result of their resistance to deformation as the 8-μm-diameter neutrophil passes through the 5.5-μm-diameter capillary. Selectins do not appear to be engaged in this process. The triggering step (discussed in text) induces cytoskeletal assembly, shown by a striped pattern, resulting in a further increase in resistance to deformation (stiffness). In addition, triggering results in activation and up-regulation of integrins, which lead to tight, long-lasting adhesion and contribute to migratory events.

cular cell adhesion molecule (VCAM-1) and platelet-endothelial cell adhesion molecule (PECAM-1); and the members of the selectin family (E-, P-, and L-selectin). It is likely that more will be forthcoming.[6] The identity of the cognate ligands on the neutrophil identified by these molecules is the subject of considerable controversy. ICAM-1 appears to interact with CD11a/CD18 (LFA-1) and CD11b/CD18 (Mac-1) on the surface of the neutrophil,[43] while at least some selectins interact with sialated Lewis x (sialyl-le^x),[45] displayed on surface molecules. Recent studies indicate that ligand function may be more complex than was initially appreciated. The specificity of accumulation of distinct leukocyte populations (e.g., neutrophils in ARDS, eosinophils in asthma, and T cells in sarcoidosis), each with distinct timing (and persistence), has led to consideration of leukocyte interaction with the endothelium as a form of information transfer. Signals from the underlying tissue elicit unique and specific responses from circulating leukocytes.[14]

Retention of Leukocytes Modeled as a Three-Step Process

Adhesion to endothelium has been conceptualized as a three-step process.[5] The first step is typically depicted as rolling of neu-

trophils along the endothelial surface under the influence of selectins.[6] This step has been considered the most important, as it is necessary in positioning the neutrophil where subsequent information can then be transferred. This paradigm, however, probably does not hold in the pulmonary microcirculation (although it is likely to be important in the bronchial microcirculation), where cessation of movement and close association of the leukocyte to the endothelium occur because of fundamental mechanical properties rather than selectin-mediated events. Support for this notion comes from experiments in which inhibition of neither L-selectin on the neutrophil nor P- or E-selectin on the endothelium significantly prevents retention of neutrophils in the lung. Likewise, genetically modified mice lacking both P-selectin and ICAM-1 demonstrated normal neutrophil accumulation in the lung in response to *Streptococcus pneumoniae*–induced pneumonia, but absence of neutrophil accumulation into the peritoneum in response to *S. pneumoniae*–induced peritonitis.[4] The tethering step thought to be crucial in other vascular beds is thus effectively bypassed in the lung. Alternatively, the lung may be considered to be promiscuous in its tethering. Thinking teleologically again, it is possible that defense of the lung has encouraged the development of "shortcuts" to accumulation of leukocytes.

Triggers (Stimuli) Are Presented to the Leukocyte Within the Vascular Environment

The next step is conceptualized as "triggering," in which stimulation of the leukocyte leads to activation and up-regulation of integrin-class adhesion molecules, as well as activation of cytoskeletal assembly. This is particularly important in the case of the neutrophil β_2 integrins. Triggering not only dramatically stiffens the cell to assist in capillary retention but also allows integrins to establish "tight adhesion." In a section below, we will consider some of the intracellular cascades by which these triggering stimuli act to modify cellular behavior.

In this section, we will consider how the triggers (stimuli) might be presented to the leukocyte. First, it is clear that some type of leukocyte stimulus must be present for retention in systemic vascular beds to occur. For instance, blocking interleukin-8 (IL-8)[37] or platelet-activating factor (PAF)[23] in models of ischemia-reperfusion injury prevents tight adhesion but not rolling. The same is likely to be the case in the lung, although the effect of the trigger (adherence versus alteration of stiffness) may well be different. In the lung a variety of processes result in delivery of leukocyte stimuli to the capillary, including release by alveolar macrophages, epithelium, fibroblasts, local mast cells, and the endothelium itself. The recognition of the C-C (typically monocyte, T-cell, and eosinophil chemoattractants) and C-X-C chemokines (largely neutrophil chemoattractants) (see Chapter 24) has allowed for a dramatic shift in our understanding of the mechanisms accounting for the specificity of leukocyte accumulation in different pathologic processes. Chemokines are basic polypeptides that share a four-cysteine motif, and are divided into two groups based on the position of the first two of the conserved cysteines. In the C-X-C subfamily the cysteines are divided by an amino acid, while in the C-C family the cysteines are adjacent.

Endothelial cells are capable of several mechanisms that allow for presentation of chemokines to cells circulating in close approximation to the endothelium cells. First, almost all the chemokines have heparin-binding domains that permit binding and retention of these molecules on the endothelial glycocalyx.[49] This may not only allow presentation in high local concentration but also provide a "trail" of surface-bound chemokine for leukocytes to follow. Second, the endothelial cell expresses the Duffy antigen receptor for chemokines,[34] a promiscuous receptor that, although expressed typically in postcapillary venules, has not been studied fully in the lung. Both of these mechanisms allow the triggers to be presented at the site where leukocytes come into contact with the endothelial cells.

Furthermore, as indicated above, the endothelial cell is capable of synthesizing and releasing (thus expressing on its surface) a variety of both C-C and C-X-C chemokines. In response to LPS, IL-1, or TNF, human endothelial cells in culture transcribe IL-8, Gro-α, monocyte chemotactic protein-1 (MCP-1), and RANTES (though probably not MIP1-α). How, then, is specificity encoded in such a system? While the answer eludes us at present, there are several points worth considering. The concentrations of stimuli used in vitro are typically high, approximating those seen in only the most severely ill patients, in whom selectivity may have been lost. Few studies have yet addressed the relative concentration dependence in detail. Similarly, most studies have addressed the stimulation using single defined agents. In contrast, pathologic settings typically involve a complex mixture of stimuli. Accordingly, the combination of IL-1, TNF-α, and interferon-γ (IFN-γ) stimulates the endothelial cell to produce much larger amounts of RANTES than does any single agent.[29] Whether mixtures such as this confer selectivity is unknown, but other components of acute inflammatory responses, such as interleukin-4 (IL-4), can inhibit the effect of combining TNF-α and IFN-γ. Because IL-4 can enhance IL-1–induced production of MCP-1 and IL-8,[9] inhibitory effects attributed to IL-4 may in fact be a result of locally increased MCP-1 and/or IL-8 concentrations. These studies support the conclusion that the complex milieu of stimuli present at a site of inflammation contributes significantly to the specific chemokines produced, and hence to the inflammatory response that develops.

Although patterns of expression of adhesion molecules are complex, it is clear that adhesion molecules may have significant effects on neutrophil sequestration, particularly after the initial deformability events. Studies have begun to dissect the relative roles of these molecules in pulmonary inflammatory responses. In inflammation induced in rat lungs by immune complexes, CD11a (but not CD11b), L-selectin, and ICAM-1 appear important in regulating the accumulation of neutrophils from the vascular compartment. In contrast, CD11b and ICAM-1 appear important in regulation of neutrophil appearance in the airway compartment, and in manifestations of lung injury, linked perhaps to induction of TNF expression.[31]

It would appear that neutrophil sequestration per se in the pulmonary capillary bed is not necessarily associated with lung injury. For example, in a rabbit model of complement fragment–induced lung injury, there was no change in pulmonary permeability or apparent tissue injury associated with neutrophil sequestration.[47] In addition, intratracheal instillation of CD11b blocks injurious consequences of immune complexes while exerting no effect on neutrophil sequestration.[31] Likewise, instillation of leukotriene B4 (LTB4) into human lungs resulted in recruitment of neutrophils into the alveolar space without evidence of lung injury.[30] However, if, as we have suggested, initial retention may occur by mechanisms other than adherence, it remains possible that adherence is a critical prelude to injury. From in vitro studies it is known that activated neutrophils can cause endothelial damage even in the absence of adherence through the release of toxic mediators, including oxidants and elastase. However, in patients with leukocyte glycoprotein deficiency whose neutrophils neither adhere nor migrate, localized inflammation and injury are not seen, suggesting that adherence is necessary for development of injury.

REGULATION OF NEUTROPHIL MIGRATION

To reach the alveolus from the vascular space, neutrophils must migrate through the vascular endothelium, basement membrane, and alveolar epithelium. The route across the capillary endothelium appears to be almost exclusively along the thick segment of the alveolar capillary membrane rather than the thin one, but the mechanisms responsible remain unclear. In vitro it has been shown that neutrophils will migrate through endothelial monolayers without the addition of exogenous stimuli. This phenomenon is not seen with fibroblast, smooth muscle, or epithelial monolayers and suggests that endothelium may actually facilitate neutrophil migration, which is believed (based on ultrastructural examination) to occur between the endothelial cells. The early notion that the endothelium participated in the migratory process has been given a molecular basis. The demonstration that ICAM-1 up-regulation[6] on the endothelial cell, particularly in the context of coexpression of E-selectin,[28] actively facilitates neutrophil migration across the endothelial cell and into the subendothelial spaces may underlie certain migratory events in vivo and suggests new ways in which migration may be regulated.

The Neutrophil Increases Cell Volume as It Migrates

In the interstitium, neutrophil migration may be regulated by external factors, such as the intensity of the chemoattractant gradient, and by the motility of the cell. In the course of quantifying the inflammatory response to C5a in the lung, we measured the volume of neutrophils in the lung using serial 0.5-μm sections and three-dimensional reconstruction.[52] We found that neutrophils reconstructed within the vascular space, in arterioles (158 μm^3), capillaries (128 μm^3), or venules (128 μm^3), were of similar volume, while those in the airspace were markedly larger (266 μm^3). Neutrophils that had migrated into the abdominal wall (150 μm^3) were also significantly larger than those in the abdominal wall vasculature (100 μm^3). These increases in volume are much greater than the increase in volume (about 15 percent) that neutrophils undergo when stimulated in suspension. The much larger increase observed in vivo suggested to us that the process might have significance to the biology of the leukocyte and to the inflammatory process.

A major component of the volume response of neutrophils in suspension appears to be due to activation of the Na^+/H^+ antiport (NHE), a ubiquitous family of molecules that migrate as 110-kd glycoproteins on SDS gels.[39] These transporters catalyze the electroneutral exchange of one Na^+ for one H^+. Under resting conditions, Na^+/H^+ exchange is nearly inactive. The induction of exchange requires activation. A major role of the exchanger appears to be in response to imposed shrinking. Activation of exchange leads to a one-for-one exchange of H^+ for Na^+, which increases cell volume because the proton disequilibrium is converted into a bicarbonate disequilibrium through action of Cl^-/HCO_3^- exchange. The net result is entry of osmotically active NaCl, followed by water entry. Inhibitors of the antiport, such as amiloride and its analogs, bind without being transported, resulting in inhibition of ion exchange and therefore blocking both volume change and alkalinization.

Cellular Swelling Improves Migration

Migrating neutrophils undergo substantial shape changes from the round, resting state to a complex polarized phenotype, making assessment of volume difficult. We measured cell volume changes in neutrophils migrating toward formyl-methionyl-leucyl-phenylalanine (fMLP) in collagen gels, using optical sec-

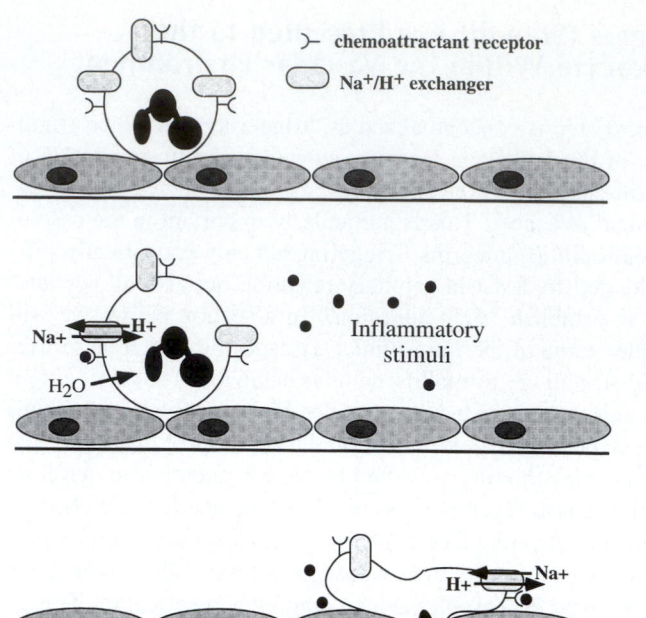

FIGURE 25-3   Cartoon depicting the increase in cell volumes of stimulated neutrophils that accompanies migration. The linkage between chemoattractant receptors and activation of the Na^+/H^+ exchange (NHE) is not depicted, as the mechanism remains unknown. The top panel depicts the unstimulated neutrophil. In the middle panel, binding of chemoattractants (inflammatory stimuli) to receptors activates the NHE, and Na^+ entry coupled to Cl^- entry (not shown) leads to net water accumulation. Under certain conditions of stimulation in suspensions or on surfaces, this net volume increase is on the order of 10 to 15 percent. In contrast, during directed migration (*bottom panel*) there is much greater apparent activation of NHE, leading to an increase in volume of approximately 50 percent and enhancing migratory efficiency. (*From Worthen et al,*[52] *with permission.*)

tioning on a confocal microscope and three-dimensional reconstruction. Migrating neutrophils displayed a significant volume increase of 35 to 60 percent, as depicted in Fig. 25-3. Cell swelling depended on sodium/proton antiport activity, since it was abrogated by amiloride and dimethyl-amiloride and by substitution of choline for sodium in the buffers, which is not transported by the antiport. The volume increase appeared to facilitate neutrophil migration, as indicated by two lines of evidence. First, hypotonic swelling enhanced, and hypertonic shrinking decreased, neutrophil migration toward fMLP in Boyden chambers. Second, sodium/proton antiport inhibitors lessened the extent of neutrophil migration in a fashion that was overcome in hypotonic buffers, which induced a volume increase similar to that seen in normal migrating cells. Hence, the volume increase associated with migration may be essential for optimal migration, suggesting that activation of the antiport is an important step in the signaling pathways used to initiate migration.

SELECTIVE RECRUITMENT OF EOSINOPHILS OCCURS THROUGH CELL-SPECIFIC MECHANISMS

Over the past decade, a tremendous amount of attention has been focused on the eosinophil and its role in a wide range of pulmonary and systemic diseases. Eosinophils are produced in the bone marrow and, when mature, are slightly larger than the neutrophil.[16] In healthy subjects, eosinophils account for less than 5 percent of leukocytes in blood, with an estimated half-life of 13 to 18 h in the circulation. The cell typically migrates from the peripheral circulation into tissues, where its life span is estimated to last up to 6 days. Like mast cells, eosinophil concentrations are highest in tissues that have epithelial surfaces in contact with the external environment, as in the lung.[48]

The role of eosinophils in human lung disease is complex. While in a few specific infections eosinophils are probably beneficial, for the most part they have been implicated as the effector of inflammatory responses resulting in tissue damage. Eosinophilia (along with significantly increased numbers of lung eosinophils) occurs in certain helminthic parasite infections, and has long been recognized to represent a specific host defense response.[16,48] The presence of increased circulating and pulmonary eosinophils in many other conditions—including several non-parasitic respiratory infections, drug reactions, certain autoimmune disorders, and some of the interstitial lung diseases—has been noted with varying degrees of predictability. The pulmonary eosinophilia in many of these conditions seems to account for much of the pathology.[22,48]

Asthma as a Model of Eosinophil Accumulation in the Bronchial Microcirculation

A variety of studies have provided evidence for the role of eosinophils in asthma. Bronchial biopsies, bronchoalveolar lavage (BAL), and peripheral blood samples have correlated the numbers of eosinophils present with the severity of the disease.[3] Bronchial hyperresponsiveness following allergen inhalation correlates with a marked increase of eosinophils in BAL samples. The preferential accumulation of eosinophils in the airways of asthmatics serves as a framework for studying the recruitment mechanism of eosinophils from the circulation to a site of inflammation. A stepwise process has been described, starting with the fairly nonspecific random contact of the cell to the vascular endothelium of the bronchial microvasculature. Since this circulation is systemic in origin, the mechanisms to be discussed will be similar to those described for the neutrophil in the systemic circulation. In the vicinity of an inflammatory foci, L-selectin on the nonactivated eosinophil bind reversibly to the locally activated endothelial surface, probably in the postcapillary venule. This early "rolling" interaction between the eosinophil and the endothelium appears similar to that of the neutrophil in the post-capillary venules; it results in a slowing of eosinophils, which may allow time for cellular activation by locally released mediators. Activation of the eosinophils, so-called triggering, results in an increased expression and affinity of adhesion molecules on the eosinophil surface, allowing more specific binding to an array of adhesion molecules on the endothelium surface. Impor-

tant endothelial ligands include ICAM-1 and ICAM-2, which can bind to LFA-1 or Mac-1 on the eosinophil cell surface. In asthma the cytokine-stimulated vascular endothelium has been shown to express the VCAM-1; the same cytokines result in the activation of the adherent eosinophils, resulting in the expression and increase in affinity of adhesion molecules on the cell surface.[21] Among the best studied of these adhesion molecules is the very late antigen–4 (VLA-4), which binds to VCAM-1 on endothelial cells and results in the most specific eosinophil-endothelial adhesion. The relatively selective transmigration ("diapedesis") across the endothelium by the eosinophil is induced by chemoattractants diffusing from the vicinity of the inflammatory focus.[2,16] The eosinophil thus migrates between endothelial cells and enters the extracellular space, facilitated in part by an ability of the eosinophil to loosen initial adhesive interactions by down-regulation or shedding of adhesion receptors at the time of activation,[20] as is also seen in the neutrophil. Whether the eosinophil also activates ion exchange mechanisms to modify its structural properties during migration is unknown.

Eotaxin, a Prototypic Chemokine That Leads to Eosinophil Accumulation

The selective accumulation of eosinophils in certain inflammatory diseases suggests that differences exist between the mechanisms of recruitment and accumulation of eosinophils and neutrophils in the lung. Following the discovery of chemokines with biologic activity for distinct subsets of leukocytes, intensive investigation has been directed toward the isolation and characterization of a cytokine with selective activity toward eosinophils. The first described C-X-C chemokine, IL-8, can induce the accumulation of eosinophils pretreated with IL-3 or granulocyte-macrophage colony–stimulating factor (GM-CSF),[46] but like all C-X-C chemokines, it is predominantly a neutrophil chemoattractant. Members of the C-C chemokine family, which include MCP-3 and RANTES, are more effective chemoattractants of unprimed eosinophils, with little activity toward neutrophils. Over the past several years, another C-C chemokine, referred to as "eotaxin," has been described that appears to be the most highly selective for eosinophils.[17] Originally purified from BAL fluid from guinea pigs after aerosol antigen challenge, the murine and human eotaxin genes[35] have now been cloned. It appears that eotaxin, MCP-3, and RANTES are all capable of binding to a single receptor on the eosinophil, but eotaxin binds with the strongest affinity.[35] Other mediators that can serve as relatively nonspecific eosinophil chemoattractants are PAF, GM-CSF, IL-2, IL-3, IL-5, IL-16, LTB4, TNF-α, LCF, MCP-3, and C5a.[21]

The coordinated role of a number of cell types in the recruitment of eosinophils into lung tissue remains an area of active investigation. Epithelial cells in the airways produce GM-CSF, PAF, PGE$_2$, PGF$_{2\alpha}$, and 15-lipoxygenase pathway–derived eicosanoids, which no doubt modify eosinophil function in diseases such as asthma when eosinophils are in the bronchoalveolar space. Platelets have the ability to produce two potent eosinophil chemoattractants, PAF and RANTES, implicating a role for platelets in eosinophil recruitment in certain inflammatory states.[21] RANTES, which is also produced by T lymphocytes, can serve as a potent chemoattractant for T lymphocytes as well as eosinophils (but not for neutrophils), and thus may be important in the pathogenesis of asthma. The cytokine IL-4, which is also released from T cells, is known to induce VCAM-1 expression on the vascular endothelium. These findings support the idea that eosinophil recruitment into the airways occurs via a T cell–dependent mechanism.[41]

Eotaxin has been found to be expressed in a number of human tissues, including the respiratory epithelium, endothelial cells, leukocytes, and fibroblasts of inflamed nasal mucosal tissue.[35] Lymphocytes are also the source of lymphocyte chemoattractant factor (LCF) and IL-2, both of which can act as potent eosinophil chemoattractants. Other cytokines—including IL-3, IL-5, and GM-CSF—are produced by lymphocytes and appear to promote eosinophilopoiesis, eosinophil recruitment, prolonged eosinophil survival, and enhanced function. Human lung-derived fibroblasts can promote eosinophil survival in vitro, and eosinophils can in turn produce factors that induce and maintain fibrogenesis.[21]

Defining the chain of events that must occur for activated eosinophils to accumulate in the lung will provide a number of possible strategies for pharmacologic intervention. Specifically, the application of antiadhesion molecules and anticytokines, as well as drugs with potentially direct antieosinophil properties, may have significant therapeutic benefit in eosinophil-dominated diseases, as well as providing further information on their respective role in eosinophil accumulation in the lung.[22]

MONOCYTE AND MACROPHAGE ACCUMULATION IN THE LUNG FOLLOWS NEUTROPHIL INFLUX

The mechanisms of monocyte and macrophage accumulation in the lung have been only partly elucidated. Several aspects of monocyte accumulation have been described, and they are of particular interest because strategies employed by the neutrophil and the eosinophil have now been observed in the monocyte as well. Progression of an acute inflammatory response in the lung typically features initial recruitment of neutrophils, followed by a subsequent accumulation of monocytes. In the rabbit model of C5 fragment–induced lung inflammation, neutrophil accumulation in the airspaces preceded monocyte accumulation by 2 to 3 hours. In animals rendered neutropenic, the C5 fragment–induced accumulation of monocytes in the airspaces did not occur.[12] This argues that in certain settings of acute inflammation, the accumulation of monocytes in the lung is neutrophil dependent.

Monocytes Respond to Selective Chemoattractants

The requirement of neutrophil accumulation before monocytes supports a model in which inflammatory mediators contribute to relatively selective recruitment of a cell type, as seen with the accumulation of eosinophils. In the initial inflammatory state, activation of alveolar macrophages and neutrophils, as well as interactions between inflammatory cells and lung fibroblasts and epithelia, produces a wide variety of chemotactic factors. Although not monocyte specific, such factors as the complement

fragment C5a, fibronectin fragments, platelet-derived growth factor (PDGF), transforming growth factor–B (TGF-B), and GM-CSF have been reported to induce monocyte migration.[42] Recently, a subfamily of C-C chemokines named the monocyte chemotactic proteins (MCP-1, -2, -3) have been found to be produced by a wide range of cell types upon induction with a variety of inflammatory stimuli.[36] The MCPs are capable of inducing chemotactic responses in monocytes (and lymphocytes) at very low concentrations, but at higher concentrations they are active on a broad range of cells. MCP-1 has been found in association with a number of inflammatory lung diseases, including idiopathic pulmonary fibrosis, asthma, tuberculosis effusions, pleural infections, sepsis, and pulmonary *Cryptococcus neoformans* infections.[36] Monocytes have a greater ability to adhere to and migrate across the endothelium than do neutrophils.[33]

A second mechanism by which monocytes accumulate in the lung is through morphologic changes, as seen with neutrophils. Administration of LPS to human monocytes results in a rapid increase in cell stiffness, net filamentous actin assembly, and retention in a filtration model of pulmonary capillaries.[11] This decreased ability to deform and cross the pulmonary capillary network is accompanied by increased CD18-dependent and -independent human monocyte adhesion to unstimulated human endothelial cell monolayers.

Prolonged Survival of Monocytes and Their Differentiation into Macrophages

A third mechanism by which human monocytes accumulate in the lung is through increased time of survival induced by inflammatory cytokines. In the circulation, peripheral blood monocytes have a half-life ranging from several hours to 2 days. Following accumulation in tissue surrounding an inflammatory focus, monocytes differentiate into macrophages, with a much longer life span. Upper-airway epithelium and lung fibroblasts have been shown to produce a number of differentiating and growth-promoting cytokines that allow for prolonged monocyte survival and differentiation into macrophages.[56] The cytokines most closely associated with this process are GM-CSF and M-CSF.

The accumulation of macrophages in the lung is closely linked to the accumulation of monocytes. It is currently believed that two mechanisms contribute to the recruitment of alveolar and interstitial macrophages. The first is chemotactic migration of monocytes from the lung blood pool into the alveoli, with concurrent differentiation into macrophages. Second, a relatively low rate of local proliferation of macrophages occurs within the lung. In the presence of inflammatory conditions, both monocyte influx and local macrophage proliferation increase.[27]

DISTINCT INTRACELLULAR SIGNALING PATHWAYS ALLOW FOR DIFFERENCES IN LEUKOCYTE ACCUMULATION IN THE LUNG

As outlined above, many processes contribute to leukocyte recruitment, including the structural design of the pulmonary vascular bed and complex interactions with the vascular endothelium. However, the accumulation of leukocytes in the lung depends on the ability of the cell to respond specifically to proinflammatory mediators. The vast array of potential cellular responses elicited in leukocytes by chemoattractants and proinflammatory stimuli has been broadly termed "activation." Neutrophil activation can include specific functional response such as adhesion, actin assembly, superoxide production, and granule enzyme release, as well as more complex and coordinated events, including increasing size, stiffness, and migration. The abilities of particular stimuli to induce a specific functional response differ significantly, and therefore "activation" must be considered in the context of the stimuli to which the leukocyte is exposed. Clearly, not every stimulus has an equal ability to induce leukocyte accumulation in the lung. This ability of leukocytes to respond in a selective fashion to a wide range of chemotactic and inflammatory stimuli is due in part to the presence of stimulus-specific cell surface receptors. Following receptor activation, intracellular signaling mechanisms must be present to link external stimuli to cellular responses.

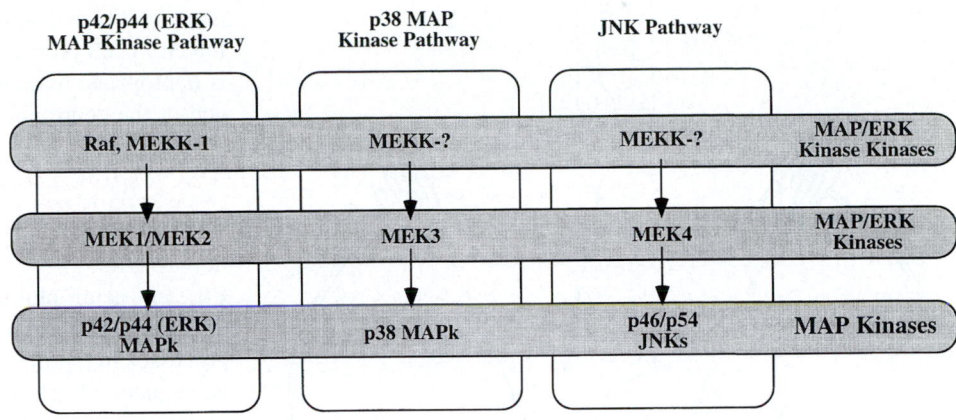

FIGURE 25-4 MAP kinase modules in human leukocytes. Three distinct MAP kinase cascades have been identified to date in human leukocytes and a variety of other mammalian cell types. Each consists of an MEKK family member (or Raf) that serves to phosphorylate and activate an MEK family member, which in turn phosphorylates and activates an MAP kinase.

Intracellular Signaling Occurs Through Phosphorylation of Protein Kinases

A fundamental theme in signal transduction is the sequential phosphorylation (resulting in the activation) of distinct families of intracellular proteins (protein kinases). Identical amino acid sequences provide sites of phosphorylation within each family in highly conserved regions of the proteins. Hundreds of protein kinases have been identified, but definition of the functional roles of these signaling proteins is, for the most part, lacking.

Among the most common components of signal transduction pathways are members of the mitogen-activated protein (MAP) kinase family. Activation of MAP kinases affects processes in the cytoplasm, the nucleus, the cytoskeleton, and the membrane. The MAP kinases are activated through the phosphorylation of a specific Thr and Tyr residue by members of the MAP/ERK kinase (MEK) family. MEK is activated through phosphorylation of two serine residues by MEK kinase (MEKK) or by Raf. The consistent appearance of these 3-kinase cascades has fostered the concept of distinct MAP kinase modules[7] acting sequentially within a pathway: a MEKK (a MEK activator), a MEK (a MAP kinase activator), and a MAP kinase (Fig. 25-4). In yeast, at least five parallel intracellular signaling pathways exist, each with a distinct MAP kinase module. For each pathway a unique cellular response occurs as a result of the interaction of a receptor-like molecule with a specific environmental stimuli.[15] In mammalian cells, at least three MAP kinase modules have been noted. Compelling evidence now exists that selectivity in neutrophil and monocyte response to specific stimuli occurs through divergence in the intracellular signaling pathways initiated by binding of various cell surface receptors.

Neutrophils Respond to Stimuli with a Distinct Repertoire of Functions and Discrete Signaling Pathways

One of the best-described signaling pathways in a primary human cell is the pathway utilized by neutrophils in response to the chemoattractant fMLP, a formylated tripeptide derived from bacterial cell walls. The binding of fMLP to a seven transmembrane-spanning G-protein–linked receptor on the surface of human neutrophils initiates a sequence of protein phosphorylation. The activation of G_i, in turn, activates a number of downstream protein kinases through the activation of the Ras-dependent kinases (Raf and MEKK-1),[1] which then phosphorylate and activate the MAP/ERK kinases (MEK-1 and MEK-2). These, in turn, activate the p42/p44 (ERK) MAP kinase.[50] In addition, exposure of human neutrophils to fMLP results in the activation of a second MAP kinase module, in which p38 MAPk is activated, apparently through the activation of MKK3.[32] The activation of both p42/p44 (ERK) and p38 MAP kinases in this pathway is maximal within 1 to 2 min after exposure to fMLP. Activation of the human neutrophil by fMLP results in a broad range of rapid functional responses, including actin assembly, adherence, calcium influx, migration, superoxide production, and granule enzyme release.[38]

In contrast, PAF, a distinctly different chemoattractant, appears capable of significant activation of only one branch of the MAP kinase cascade. As with fMLP, external stimulation of the human neutrophil with PAF results in binding of a seven transmembrane-spanning G-protein–linked receptor. Although early signaling events are less well characterized than those initiated in response to fMLP, we have shown that PAF selectively activates p38 MAP kinase (via MKK3), with only slight activation of the p42/p44 (ERK) MAP kinases. Activation of the human neutrophil by PAF results in rapid actin assembly and adherence, but fails to evoke the functional responses (such as superoxide production and granule enzyme release) that are seen after stimulation with fMLP. Migration of neutrophils stimulated with PAF is reduced in comparison to cells exposed to fMLP, and supports

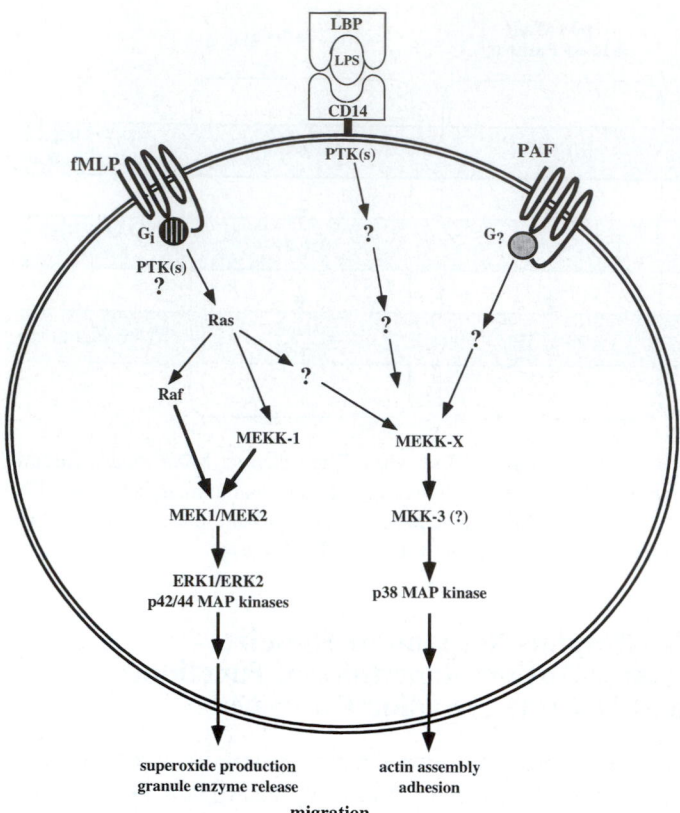

FIGURE 25-5 Proposed intracellular signaling pathways in the human neutrophil in response to LPS, fMLP, and PAF. Following binding of the cell surface receptor, intracellular signaling occurs through the sequential phosphorylation and activation of protein kinases. Although important early regulatory events have yet to be defined, the divergence in activation of MAP kinase modules allows for distinct (yet partly overlapping) sets of functional responses to various external stimuli. Neutrophil migration, which requires a complex spatial and temporal coordination of adhesion, actin assembly, and granule release, appears to require the activation of more than one MAP kinase module.

the conclusion that activation of p42/p44 (ERK) MAP kinases—or perhaps a yet unidentified MAP kinase family member—is more closely associated with this function (Fig. 25-5).

Purified LPS, following binding to CD14,[54] a glycosylphosphatidylinositol-anchored cell-surface glycoprotein in complex with LPS-binding protein,[51] results in the activation of p38 MAP kinase. However, LPS stimulation does not result in the activation of Raf, MEKK1, MEK1/MEK2, or p42/p44 (ERK) MAP kinase. As with PAF, the functional response of the neutrophil to LPS includes adherence and actin assembly. Both the maximal activation of p38 MAP kinase and the functional responses following exposure to LPS are 10- to 20-fold slower than those of neutrophils stimulated with fMLP or PAF.[32] This implies that a different "upstream" signaling mechanism is employed in response to LPS binding of CD14 (Fig. 25-5).

Thus, an outline is forming of different intracellular signaling pathways that allow distinct (but overlapping) functional response by the cell to a variety of different stimuli. As additional branches of the MAP kinase cascade are described, it is likely that further divergence in signaling patterns will be evident. In

many cell types, activation of p42/p44 and p38 MAP kinases is linked to cell proliferation, survival, and death.[55] Accordingly, it is appropriate to conclude this chapter with a discussion of the end of the neutrophil lifespan.

ACCUMULATION OF NEUTROPHILS IN THE LUNG REPRESENTS THE BALANCE BETWEEN INFLUX AND DISPOSAL

Efficient neutrophil disposal from lung tissue is apparent from the rapid disappearance of neutrophils from acute inflammatory processes in the lung.[12] To date, the mechanisms of disposal remain incompletely understood, but at least two processes have been described. Inflammatory cells are rapidly transported in exudate up the mucociliary escalator in a functional airway. Disorders of this process in cystic fibrosis or primary ciliary dysmotility syndromes are associated with prolonged and severe inflammation in the distal airway. The neutrophil in inflammatory lesions rapidly becomes apoptotic if removed from the inflamed site,[8] consistent with the known short life span of these cells in vivo. Of interest is that, apoptotic neutrophils are rapidly phagocytosed by macrophages isolated from the same site. Neutrophils engulfed by macrophages have been seen in inflammatory settings,[8] but the relative proportion of neutrophils disposed by this mechanism compared to movement up the mucociliary escalator has not been determined with certainty in any inflammatory lesion. The recognition of apoptotic neutrophils by macrophages is remarkably specific, involving a macrophage surface molecule, CD36, and the macrophage $\alpha_v\beta_3$ integrin that recognizes either vitronectin[40] or a mechanism that recognizes phosphatidylserine on the surface of the apoptotic cell.[8] The existence of several strategies for removal of senescent neutrophils suggests the importance of this process in regulation of inflammation. Thus, the potential for modulation of the inflammatory response through manipulation of disposal mechanisms seems as great as that for manipulating the initiating mechanisms that have been the predominant subject of this chapter.

REFERENCES

1. Avdi N, Winston BW, Russel M, et al: Activation of MEKK by fMLP in human neutrophils: Mapping pathways for MAP kinase activation. Unpublished manuscript.
2. Bentley AM, Durham SR, Robinson DS, et al: Allergens, IgE, mediators, inflammatory mechanisms: Expression of endothelial and leukocyte adhesion molecules intercellular adhesion molecule–1, E-selectin, and vascular cell adhesion molecule–1 in the bronchial mucosa in steady-state and allergen-induced asthma. *J Allergy Clin Immunol* 92:857–868, 1993.
3. Bousquet J, Chanez P, Lacoste JY, et al: Eosinophilic inflammation in asthma. *New Engl J Med* 323:1033–1039, 1990.
4. Bullard DC, Qin L, Lorenzo I, et al: P-selectin/ICAM-1 double mutant mice: Acute emigration of neutrophils into the peritoneum is completely absent but is normal into pulmonary alveoli. *J Clin Invest* 95:1782–1788, 1995.
5. Butcher EC: Leukocyte-endothelial cell recognition: Three (or more) steps to specificity and diversity. *Cell* 67:1033–1036, 1991.
6. Carlos TM, Harlan JM: Leukocyte-endothelial adhesion molecules. *Blood* 84:2068–2101, 1994.

7. Cobb MH, Goldsmith EJ: How MAP kinases are regulated. *J Biol Chem* 270:14843–14846, 1995.

8. Cohen JJ, Duke RC, Fadok VA, Sellins KS: Apoptosis and programmed cell death in immunity. *Annu Rev Immunol* 10:267–293, 1992.

9. Colotta F, Sironi M, Borrè A, et al: Interleukin 4 amplifies monocyte chemotactic protein and interleukin 6 production by endothelial cells. *Cytokine* 4:24–28, 1992.

10. Doerschuk CM, Winn RK, Coxson HO, Harlan JM: CD18-dependent and independent mechanisms of neutrophil emigration in the pulmonary and systemic microcirculation of rabbits. *J Immunol* 144:2327–2333, 1990.

11. Doherty DE, Downey GP, Schwab BI, et al: Lipopolysaccharide-induced monocyte retention in the lung: Role of monocyte stiffness, actin assembly, and CD18-dependent adherence. *J Immunol* 153:241–255, 1994.

12. Doherty DE, Haslett C, Downey GP, et al: Monocyte retention and migration in pulmonary inflammation: Requirement for neutrophils. *Lab Invest* 59:200–213, 1988.

13. Downey GP, Doherty DE, Schwab B III, et al: Retention of leukocytes in capillaries: Role of cell size and deformability. *J Appl Physiol* 69:1767–1778, 1990.

14. Ebnet K, Kaldjian EP, Anderson AO, Shaw S: Orchestrated information transfer underlying leukocyte endothelial interactions. *Annu Rev Immunol* 14:155–177, 1996.

15. Galcheva-Gargova Z, Dérijard B, Wu I-H, Davis RJ: An osmosensing signal transduction pathway in mammalian cells. *Science* 265:806–808, 1994.

16. Gleich GJ, Adolphson CR, Leiferman KM: The biology of the eosinophilic leukocyte. *Annu Rev Med* 44:85–101, 1993.

17. Griffiths-Johnson DA, Collins PD, Rossi AG, et al: The chemokine, eotaxin, activates guinea-pig eosinophils *in vitro* and causes their accumulation into the lung *in vivo*. *Biochem Biophys Res Commun* 197:1167–1172, 1993.

18. Harlan JM, Killen PD, Senecal FM, et al: The role of neutrophil membrane glycoprotein GP-150 in neutrophil adherence to endothelium *in vitro*. *Blood* 66:167–178, 1985.

19. Hogg JC: Neutrophil kinetics and lung injury. *Physiol Rev* 67:1249–1295, 1987.

20. Kishimoto T, Kei, Jutila MA, Butcher EC: Identification of a human peripheral lymph node homing receptor: A rapidly down-regulated adhesion molecule. *Proc Natl Acad Sci USA* 87:2244–2248, 1990.

21. Kroegel C, Virchow J-C Jr, Luttman W, et al: Pulmonary immune cells in health and disease: The eosinophil leucocyte (Part I). *Eur Respir J* 7:519–543, 1994.

22. Kroegel C, Warner JA, Virchow J-C Jr, Matthys H: Pulmonary immune cells in health and disease: The eosinophil leucocyte (Part II). *Eur Respir J* 7:743–760, 1994.

23. Kubes P, Ibbotson G, Russell J, et al: Role of platelet-activating factor in ischemia/reperfusion–induced leukocyte adherence. *Am J Physiol* 259:G300–G305, 1990.

24. Lien DC, Wagner WW, Capen RL, et al: Physiologic neutrophil sequestration in the canine pulmonary circulation: Evidence for localization in capillaries. *J Appl Physiol* 62:1236–1243, 1987.

25. Lien DC, Worthen GS, Capen RL, et al: Neutrophil kinetics in the pulmonary microcirculation: Effects of pressure and flow in the dependent lung. *Am Rev Respir Dis* 141:953–959, 1990.

26. Lien DC, Worthen GS, Henson PM, Bethel RA: Platelet-activating factor causes neutrophil accumulation and neutrophil-mediated increased vascular permeability in canine trachea. *Am Rev Respir Dis* 145:693–700, 1992.

27. Lohmann-Matthes M-L, Steinmüller C, Franke-Ullmann G: Pulmonary macrophages. *Eur Respir J* 7:1678–1689, 1994.

28. Luscinskas FW, Cybulsky MI, Kiely JM, et al: Cytokine-activated human endothelial monolayers support enhanced neutrophil transmigration via a mechanism involving both endothelial-leukocyte adhesion molecule–1 and intercellular adhesion molecule–1. *J Immunol* 146:1617–1625, 1991.

29. Marfaing-Koka A, Devergne O, Gorgone G, et al: Regulation of the production of the RANTES chemokine by endothelial cells. *J Immunol* 154:1870–1878, 1995.

30. Martin TR, Pistorese BP, Chi EY, et al: Effects of leukotriene B$_4$ in the human lung: Recruitment of neutrophils into the alveolar spaces without a change in protein permeability. *J Clin Invest* 84:1609–1619, 1989.

31. Mulligan MS, Vaporciyan AA, Warner RL, et al: Compartmentalized roles for leukocytic adhesion molecules in lung inflammatory injury. *J Immunol* 154:1350–1363, 1995.

32. Nick JA, Avdi NJ, Gerwins P, et al: Activation of a p38 mitogen-activated protein kinase in human neutrophils by lipopolysaccharide. *J Immunol* 156:4867–4875, 1996.

33. Pawlowski NA, Kaplan G, Abraham E, Cohn ZA: The selective binding and transmigration of monocytes through the junctional complexes of human endothelium. *J Exp Med* 168:1865–1882, 1988.

34. Peiper SC, Wang Z-X, Neote K, et al: The Duffy antigen/receptor for chemokines (DARC) is expressed in endothelial cells of Duffy negative individuals who lack the erythrocyte receptor. *J Exp Med* 181:1311–1317, 1995.

35. Ponath PD, Qin S, Ringler DJ, et al: Cloning of the human eosinophil chemoattractant, eotaxin: Expression, receptor binding, and functional properties suggest a mechanism for the selective recruitment of eosinophils. *J Clin Invest* 97:604–612, 1995.

36. Proost P, Wuyts A, Van Damme J: Human monocyte chemotactic proteins–2 and –3: Structural and functional comparison with MCP-1. *J Leukoc Biol* 59:67–74, 1996.

37. Rainger GE, Fisher A, Shearman C, Nash GB. Adhesion of flowing neutrophils to cultured endothelial cells after hypoxia and reoxygenation in vitro. *Am J Physiol* 269:H1398–H1406, 1995.

38. Sandborg RR, Smolen JE: Biology of disease: Early biochemical events in leukocyte activation. *Lab Invest* 59:300–320, 1988.

39. Sardet C, Counillon O, Franchi A, Pouysségur J: Growth factors induce phosphorylation of the Na$^+$/H$^+$ antiporter, a glycoprotein of 110 kD. *Science* 247:723–726, 1990.

40. Savill J, Hogg N, Ren Y, Haslett C: Thrombospondin cooperates with CD36 and the vitronectin receptor in macrophage recognition of neutrophils undergoing apoptosis. *J Clin Invest* 90:1513–1522, 1992.

41. Seminario M-C, Gleich GJ: The role of eosinophils in the pathogenesis of asthma. *Curr Opin Immunol* 6:860–864, 1994.

42. Sibille Y, Marchandise F-XP, Massion PP: Humoral and cellular mediators in the lung, in Bone RC, Dantzker DR, George RB (eds), *Pulmonary and Critical Care Medicine*, vol 1. St. Louis, Mosby–Year Book, 1996, pp 1–14.

43. Smith CW, Marlin SD, Rothlein R, et al: Cooperative interactions of LFA-1 and Mac-1 with intercellular adhesion molecule-1 in facilitating adherence and transendothelial migration of human neutrophils in vitro. *J Clin Invest* 83:2008–2017, 1989.

44. Vedder NB, Winn RK, Rice CL, et al: A monoclonal antibody to the adherence-promoting leukocyte glycoprotein, CD18, reduces organ injury and improves surivival from hemorrhagic shock and resuscitation in rabbits. *J Clin Invest* 81:939–944, 1988.

45. Walz G, Aruffo A, Kolanus W, et al: Recognition by ELAM-1 of the sialyl-le^x determinant on myeloid and tumor cells. *Science* 250:1132–1135, 1990.

46. Warringa RAJ, Koenderman L, Kok PTM, et al: Modulation and induction of eosinophil chemotaxis by granulocyte-macrophage colony–stimulating factor and interleukin-3. *Blood* 77:2694–2700, 1991.

47. Webster RO, Larsen GL, Mitchell BC, et al: Absence of inflammatory injury in rabbits challenged intravascularly with complement-derived chemotactic factors. *Am Rev Respir Dis* 125:335–340, 1982.

48. Weller PF: The immunobiology of eosinophils. *New Engl J Med* 324:1110–1118, 1991.

49. Witt DP, Lander AD: Differential binding of chemokines to glycosamino-glycan subpopulations. *Curr Biol* 4:394–400, 1994.

50. Worthen GS, Avdi N, Buhl AM, et al: FMLP activates Ras and Raf in human neutrophils: Potential role in activation of MAP kinase. *J Clin Invest* 94:815–823, 1994.

51. Worthen GS, Avdi N, Vukajlovich S, Tobias PS: Neutrophil adherence induced by lipopolysaccharide *in vitro:* Role of plasma component interaction with lipopolysaccharide. *J Clin Invest* 90:2526–2535, 1993.

52. Worthen GS, Henson PM, Rosengren S, et al: Neutrophils increase volume during migration *in vivo* and *in vitro. Am J Respir Cell Mol Biol* 10:1–7, 1994.

53. Worthen GS, Schwab B, Elson EL, Downey GP: Mechanics of stimulated neutrophils: Cell stiffening induces retention in capillaries. *Science* 245:183–185, 1989.

54. Wright SD, Ramos RA, Tobias PS, et al: CD14, a receptor for complexes of lipopolysaccharide (LPS) and LPS-binding protein. *Science* 249:1431–1433, 1990.

55. Xia Z, Dickens M, Raingeaud J, et al: Opposing effects of ERK and JNK-p38 MAP kinases on apoptosis. *Science* 270:1326–1331, 1995.

56. Xing Z, Ohtoshi T, Ralph P, et al: Human upper airway structural cell–derived cytokines support human peripheral blood monocyte survival: A potential mechanism for monocyte/macrophage accumulation in the tissue. *Am J Respir Cell Mol Biol* 6:212–218, 1992.

57. Zimmerman GA, McIntyre TM, Prescott SM, Otsuka K: Brief review: Molecular mechanisms of neutrophil binding to endothelium involving platelet-activating factor and cytokines. *J Lipid Mediat* 2(Suppl):S31–S43, 1990.

CHAPTER 26

NITRIC OXIDE AND LUNG INJURY

Imad Y. Haddad / Bruce R. Pitt / Sadis Matalon

MOLECULAR BIOLOGY OF ·NO
    Nitric Oxide Synthases
    Regulation of Constitutive (I and III) NOS Genes
    Regulation of Inducible NOS-II Gene

PHYSIOLOGICAL EFFECTS OF ·NO
    Biologic Targets
    Effect of ·NO on Gene Expression
    Cytotoxic Potential of ·NO/ONOO⁻
    Protective Effects of ·NO

SUMMARY AND CONCLUSIONS

The major function of the lung is gas exchange. The movement of both oxygen and carbon dioxide across the blood-gas barrier is by simple diffusion. This process is optimized by the large alveolar surface area, the close proximity of the alveolar and pulmonary capillary membranes, and the lack of any significant amount of fluid in the alveolar space. The relative dryness of the alveolar space is thought to be due to the low permeability of the alveolar epithelium to the presence of plasma proteins, surfactant (which lowers the surface tension of the blood-gas barrier), and the ability of alveolar epithelial cells to actively transport sodium ions from the alveolar to the basolateral spaces.

Prolonged exposure of animals to high concentrations of various oxidant gases damages the pulmonary surfactant system and alveolar epithelium, resulting in increased amounts of protein in the alveolar space, pulmonary atelectasis, arterial hypoxemia, and eventually death from respiratory failure. These injuries have been attributed mainly to increased intracellular and extracellular production of reactive oxygen species, including superoxide anion ($O_2^{·-}$), hydrogen peroxide (H_2O_2), and hydroxyl radical (·OH). Indeed, in vitro exposure of alveolar type II cells to various oxidants resulted in decreased incorporation of palmitate and choline into disaturated phosphatidylcholine and reduced activity of glycerol-3-phosphate acyltransferase, a sulfhydryl-containing enzyme catalyzing one of the early reactions of phospholipid biosynthesis.[23]

However, the precise contribution of various reactive oxygen species in vivo in the development of alveolar epithelial injury is poorly understood and debatable. While $O_2^{·-}$ can be directly toxic to biologic targets, its limited reactivity with many biologic molecules raises questions about its toxicity per se. Instead, it has been proposed that $O_2^{·-}$ toxicity in vivo may be due to its participation as a reducing agent in the production of the very reactive ·OH by the iron-catalyzed Haber-Weiss reaction. Generation of significant amounts of ·OH by this reaction in the epithelial-lining fluid (ELF) is unlikely for the following reasons: (1) $O_2^{·-}$ and H_2O_2 are kept in low concentrations by superoxide dismutase (SOD), catalase, and reduced glutathione;[8,33] (2) the rate of Fe^{+3} reaction with $O_2^{·-}$ is slow, and the rate of Fe^{+2} reaction with H_2O_2 is even slower; and (3) most iron is chelated in a noncatalytic form by ELF transferrin and ceruloplasmin.[43] These observations suggest that alternative reactions are important in $O_2^{·-}$ toxicity to the pulmonary surfactant system in vivo.

The free radical nitric oxide (·NO) is the major form of the endothelial-derived relaxing factor that is enzymatically synthesized from arginine oxidation by NADPH-dependent nitric oxide synthases. ·NO causes smooth-muscle relaxation by activating soluble guanylate cyclase, and inhibits platelet aggregation and adhesion to endothelium by increasing cGMP. Because of the vasorelaxant properties of ·NO and its rapid inactivation in the blood by its reaction with hemoglobin, ·NO inhalation has been advocated as a means of selectively reducing pulmonary hypertension and improving ventilation/perfusion mismatching in a variety of clinical situations.

In spite of its therapeutic value, there is evidence that in pathologic conditions where there is increased production of oxygen free radicals by lung cells, inhalation or overproduction of ·NO may damage alveolar cells and pulmonary surfactant. Because ·NO is a free radical, it can undergo a radical-radical reaction with $O_2^{·-}$ at near–diffusion-limited rates to yield peroxynitrite (ONOO⁻), a potent oxidizing agent known to initiate lipid peroxidation of biologic membranes, hydroxylation, and nitration of aromatic amino acid residues and sulfhydryl oxidation of proteins. Furthermore, ONOO⁻ may decompose to yield nitrogen dioxide (·NO₂) and species with hydroxyl radical–like reactivity without the need for metal catalysis.

Following stimulation by cytokines and lipopolysaccharide, alveolar macrophages and epithelial cells produce large amounts of ·NO and $O_2^{·-}$ for prolonged periods, and can act as foci for intense and localized production of ONOO⁻ and its toxic intermediates, in close proximity to pulmonary surfactant. On the other hand, some studies suggest that ·NO may actually decrease oxidant lung injury by reducing lung inflammation, inducing antioxidant enzymes, and decreasing lipid peroxidation of biologic membranes. This chapter summarizes the cellular and molecular mechanisms responsible for the regulation of ·NO synthesis, and reviews the beneficial and detrimental functions of ·NO during oxidant stress in the lung.

MOLECULAR BIOLOGY OF ·NO

Nitric Oxide Synthases

·NO is synthesized from the five-electron oxidation of either of the two equivalent guanidine nitrogens of L-arginine. The reaction is catalyzed by one of three isozymes of nitric oxide synthase (NOS), using reduced NADPH as the source of electrons and cofactors, including tetrahydrobiopterin (H_4B) and flavin nucleotides (FMN, FAD). Molecular oxygen is a cosubstrate, guanidino (N^G)-hydroxy-L-arginine is formed as a short-lived intermediate, and L-citrulline is a byproduct. All isoforms of NOS bind calmodulin and contain heme. Electrons are supplied by NADPH, transferred along the flavins and calmodulin, and presented to the catalytic heme.[40,59a]

Understanding of how the simple, small, diffusible, lipophilic short-lived molecule ·NO performs an extraordinarily diverse array of physiological and pathophysiological functions remains quite rudimentary. Nonetheless, it appears that regulation of ·NO biosynthesis explains, in part, its diverse functions, and thus significant advances have been made from the study of unique characteristics of NOS isoforms. Collectively, NOS are homodimeric cytochrome P450–like hemoproteins that have oxygenase and reductase domains in the NH_2 and COOH termini, respectively. The active dimeric form is hypothesized to depend on H_4B. The domains are separated by a Ca^{2+}/calmodulin–binding region. The reductase domain is homologous to NADPH-cytochrome P450, including binding sites for FMN, FAD, and NADPH. The constitutive forms have similar phosphorylation sites and one of them (NOS-III) has a unique NH_2 terminal myristoylation site.

Differences between the isozymes, however, underscore the function of ·NO in various biologic systems. The nomenclature evolved from descriptions of cellular source of the enzyme (e.g., neuronal, macrophage, or endothelial) or its expression (constitutive versus inducible), and by many conventions it is now relegated to the chronology in which the enzyme was purified and cloned (Table 26-1). NOS-I and -III are constitutively expressed, and their activity is regulated by intracellular calcium; prototypical sources are neuronal and endothelial cell, respectively. NOS-II is induced by cytokines, its activity is largely independent of calcium, and it is regulated at a transcriptional level. The prototypical source is the macrophage. Although the human genes are present on discrete chromosomes, considerable homology exists between the three isoforms, suggesting common ancestral origin with subsequent gene duplication and transposition. NOS-I and NOS-III derived ·NO is produced in small quantities for brief periods and underscores intra- and intercellular signaling events such as neurotransmission or vascular homeostasis. In contrast, NOS-II produces large amounts of ·NO for prolonged periods (assuming availability of substrate and cofactors) and contributes to more diffuse physiological roles associated with inflammation or infection.

Regulation of Constitutive (I and III) NOS Genes

Both isoforms of constitutive NOS have been identified in human lung. As shown in Table 26-2, NOS-I is localized to nerve terminals that probably contribute to nonadrenergic, noncholinergic innervation of the airways, and NOS-III is localized to pulmonary endothelium. In addition, NOS-I has a prominent location in human and rat airway epithelium. As in other tissues, their activities are closely regulated by changes in intracellular calcium.

TABLE 26-1

Characterizations of Nitric Oxide Synthase (NOS) Genes*

NOS isoform	nNOS	iNOS	ecNOS
Human Genome Nomenclature Committee	NOS-I	NOS-II	NOS-III
Calcium dependence	+	−	+
Calmodulin dependence	+	+	+
Size of the human gene (kb)	>200	~37	~23
Number of exons	29	26	26
Size of the mRNA (kb)	8.5–9.5	4.2–4.5	4.3–4.8
Size of the protein/number of amino acids	160 kDa/1434	130 kDa/1153	135 kDa/1203
Human chromosomal localization	12q24.2	17q11.2-q12	7q35-q36
Cell prototype	Neurons	Hepatocytes, macrophages	Endothelial cells
Subcellular localization	Cytosolic/membrane	Cytosolic	Membrane
Expression	Constitutive but regulated	Inducible	Constitutive but regulated

NOTE: n = neuronal; i = inducible; ec = endothelial constitutive.
SOURCE: Reprinted from Wang and Marsden,[59a] with permission.

TABLE 26-2

Intrapulmonary Localization of NOS in Humans and Rats

	NOS-I	NOS-II	NOS-III
Human	A549, BEAS 2B, HBE[4]	Alveolar macrophages[29,56] Endothelium[29] Airway epithelium[15,29] A549, BEAS 2B[4]	Endothelium[29] Nerve endings[29]
Rat	Bronchial epithelium[41,51]	Alveolar macrophage[29,60] Bronchial epithelium[65] Alveolar type II[16,49,60] Vascular smooth muscle[27,39] Mesothelial cell[42]	Endothelium[64,65] Nerve endings[29]

NOTE: A549 = human alveolar type II epithelium-like cell line; BEAS 2B = transformed human bronchial epithelial cell line; HBE = primary culture human bronchial epithelial cells.

REGULATION OF NOS-I

Human NOS-I is the largest and most complex of the three isoforms (Table 26-1). Although considered a constitutive enzyme, the 5′ flanking region contains multiple transcriptional factor binding sites. Human NOS-I mRNA contains significant structural and allelic diversity, including variations at the 3′ noncoding region that may affect mRNA stability and processing. Some of the tissue and cell diversity of NOS-I expression resides in alternative promoter usage. Despite this wealth of mRNA variants, little is known of the function of such regulation within the central nervous system, skeletal muscle, or lung. For instance, it is unclear what accounts for developmental changes in NOS-I within rat lung.[41]

REGULATION OF NOS-III

Although NOS-III expression is clearly associated with vascular endothelium, it does exist in extraendothelial locations, including human bronchial epithelial cells (Table 26-2). Its 5′ flanking region contains multiple putative transcriptional factor binding sites, including shear stress, sterol regulatory, acute-phase response, and activating protein-1 (AP-1) and AP-2 cis-acting DNA elements. These regions may account for increases in NOS-III mRNA in response to shear stress in vitro and in vivo. GATA and serum protein-1 (SP-1) regions contribute to the relative endothelial cell specific expression of NOS-III. TNF-α and oxidized low-density lipoproteins decrease stability of NOS-III mRNA, suggesting important posttranscriptional regulation. Hypoxia decreases NOS-III expression in cultured human umbilical vein endothelial cells[35] but appears to up-regulate NOS-III expression in chronic hypoxia in rats. Implications of regulation by shear stress, hypoxia, and perhaps oxidized low-density lipoproteins may have profound implications in the transition from the fetal to adultlike circulation at birth, as well as congenital or acquired cardiorespiratory disorders of the newborn and primary pulmonary hypertension in the adult.

Posttranslational modification of NOS-III is an important regulatory mechanism. Various roles are emerging for acylation, palmitoylation, myristoylation, and membrane phospholipid interactions in modifying the activity of this enzyme.

Regulation of Inducible NOS-II Gene

In general, resting cells do not express detectable NOS-II (at mRNA or protein level). After appropriate simulation, however, virtually every mammalian cell studied in culture has the capacity to express NOS-II. Originally cloned from murine macrophages, NOS-II was subsequently cloned from human hepatocytes, chondrocytes, and a colorectal adenocarcinoma cell line. The human NOS-II gene appears to be a single isoenzyme (Table 26-1). In situ expression of NOS-II has not been extensively characterized. Nonetheless, exposure of rats to lipopolysaccharide (LPS) (with or without various immunomodulating preexposure conditioning) results in widespread expression of NOS-II. Considerably less is known regarding NOS-II localization in human tissue in situ, with significant controversy regarding macrophage distribution. It is interesting that in lung, NOS-II appears to be constitutively expressed in human airway epithelium.[15]

Originally, factors that enhance NOS-II expression were limited to microbial products and inflammatory cytokines. More recently, it has been shown that stress and oxidative injury can also enhance NOS-II expression. Important general observations regarding regulation are that critical differences exist between cells and species regarding contributions of various regulatory stimuli and synergy is usually noted between various stimuli in a cell- and species-specific fashion. Several important hormones (glucocorticoids), cytokines (IL-4, -8, and -10), and growth factors (TGF-β) have been shown to inhibit NOS-II gene expression at several different steps. There is considerable controversy regarding the capacity of human monocytes and macrophages to express NOS-II.

TRANSCRIPTIONAL AND POSTTRANSCRIPTIONAL REGULATION OF NOS-II

Extraordinarily complex regulation of the high output ·NO system is consistent with its multifunctional physiological roles. Thus, it is not surprising that several levels of regulation have been identified. Almost all of the information about regulation of NOS-II mRNA is from work in murine macrophages, although recent data pertain to a variety of other cells, including those of the respiratory system. In particular, critical roles are apparent for sentinel cytokines, including IFN-γ, TNF-α, and IL-1β, in affecting NOS-II expression in cultured rat pulmonary artery smooth muscle cells (RPASMC)[39] and type II cells.[49] In murine macrophages, NF-κB and IRF-1 binding sites in the NOS-II 5′ flanking promoter region are important. The former binding site is intimately involved in redox gene regulation and has been associated with NOS-II regulation in RPASMC; the latter links

NOS-II expression to intracellular iron, further coupling NO biosynthesis with free radical–mediated pathology and redox gene regulation.[40]

Posttranscriptional regulation of NOS-II has been shown primarily in murine macrophages, in which IFN-γ increases ·NO formation by stabilizing NOS-II mRNA (without affecting basal transcriptional rates). Other factors—including TGF-β, IL-4, IL-8, and IL-10—decrease stability of NOS-II mRNA and thereby account for down-regulation of NOS-II expression.[59] Such effects presumably account for similar observations in cultured lung cells.[13] An interesting observation is that induction of heat shock protein 70 in RPASMC results in inhibition of cytokine-mediated induction of NOS-II in RPASMC, suggesting that NOS-II expression may be analogous to acute-phase genes and other proinflammatory genes whose expression is silenced during prioritization via HSP-70 induction.[63a]

POSTTRANSLATIONAL REGULATION OF NOS-II SYNTHESIS

Again, much of the potential posttranslational target of NOS-II regulation is derived from murine macrophages; thus, the lung-specific and human-specific aspects await confirmation. Nonetheless, substrate availability is modified by many of the same stimuli noted to affect NOS-II induction; thus, arginine transport and synthesis are affected as well as components of the partial urea cycle. Induction of arginosuccinate synthetase at mRNA levels supports the NO-citrulline cycle and may be important in conditions of substrate limitation. GTP cyclohydrolase I, the enzyme catalyzing the rate-limiting step in H_4B synthesis, is coinduced with NOS-II, supporting activation of newly synthesized enzyme with the critical biopterin cofactors.[38]

PHYSIOLOGICAL EFFECTS OF ·NO

Biologic Targets

The biologic actions of ·NO are dictated by the reactions it undergoes with different target molecules in cells, membranes, and in the extracellular milieu. For each target, depending on the amount and duration of induction, ·NO can exert beneficial or detrimental effects. Known targets for ·NO include:

1. Guanylate cyclase ·NO binds the heme group of soluble guanylate cyclase, leading to an increase in cyclic guanosine-3'-5'-monophosphate (cGMP) levels. Many effects of cGMP are mediated by a group of enzymes, known as cGMP-associated protein kinases (PKGs). These PKGs act to reduce intracellular calcium, relax smooth-muscle and increase activity of calcium ATPases. ·NO-mediated increased cGMP levels also prevent platelet aggregation and decrease adhesion of neutrophils. However, excessive ·NO-mediated cGMP production has been implicated in sepsis-induced refractory hypotension and shock.[61]

2. Hemoglobin The major route for the removal of ·NO in vivo is the fast and irreversible reaction with *oxy*-hemoglobin (Hb-Fe^{2+}–O_2) or *oxy*-myoglobin to produce nitrate and methemoglobin, according to the following reactions:

$$Hb-Fe^{2+}-O_2 + \cdot NO \rightarrow Hb-Fe^{2+}ONOO \rightarrow$$
$$Hb-Fe^{+3} + NO_3^- \quad (1)$$

Because of its vasorelaxant properties and rapid inactivation in the blood by its reaction with hemoglobin, ·NO inhalation has been advocated as a means of selectively reducing pulmonary hypertension and improving systemic oxygenation in a variety of clinical situations, including bronchopulmonary dysplasia and the adult respiratory distress syndrome (ARDS).[53] However, patients with diminished methemoglobin reductase activity, such as neonates, are unable to efficiently convert methemoglobin to ferrous hemoglobin and could therefore be at greater risk for developing methemoglobinemia and decreased oxygen transport.

3. Iron/sulfur (4Fe/4S) centers of enzymes Production of ·NO by activated macrophages defends the host against infectious agents, including bacteria, parasites, and viruses, and destroys tumor cells. The proposed mechanism responsible for these effects is the reaction of ·NO with the nonheme iron of iron-sulfur complexes, resulting in the inactivation of iron-sulfur–containing enzymes, including mitochondrial aconitase, cytochrome *c* oxidase,[9] and the DNA synthesis rate-limiting enzyme, ribonucleotide reductase. Inhibition of these critical enzymes leads to suppression of mitochondrial respiration, energy metabolism, and cell replication. ·NO effects are nonspecific, however, and its overproduction may be cytotoxic not only for microbes but also for the cells and tissues that produce it.[22]

4. Other free radicals ·NO has an unpaired electron, and thus can readily react with other free radicals, as specified below:

a. Reaction with oxygen If a tank of ·NO is allowed to leak into air, a cloud of lethal and highly reactive orange-brown nitrogen dioxide (·NO_2) is formed, according to the following reactions:

$$2 \cdot NO + O_2 \rightarrow 2 \cdot NO_2 \quad (2)$$

At low ·NO concentrations (under 5 μM), observed in vivo at physiological and most pathologic conditions, the low probability of any two ·NO molecules encountering each other makes the formation of ·NO_2 extremely slow. Instead, ·NO may react with a single molecule of oxygen in a second-order reaction to form a nitrosyldioxyl radical (ONOO·).

b. Reaction with $O_2^{·-}$ ·NO reacts with $O_2^{·-}$ at a near–diffusion-limited rate constant of about 7×10^9 M^{-1} s^{-1} to form $ONOO^-$. This reaction was mistakenly thought to be protective, since it decreased the amount of $O_2^{·-}$ detected. $ONOO^-$ has a pK_a of 6.8 at 37°C and thus may remain stable for months in alkaline solutions. The protonated form of peroxynitrous acid (ONOOH) forms ·NO_2 and an intermediate with a reactivity equivalent to the hydroxyl radical (·OH), derived from the transisomerization of ONOOH, as shown in Eq. 3:

$$O_2^{·-} + \cdot NO \rightarrow ONOO^- + H^+ \rightleftharpoons ONOOH \rightarrow {''} \cdot OH \cdots \cdot NO_2{''} \quad (3)$$

Under physiological conditions, a minimum of 25 percent of $ONOO^-$ decomposes to form the "·OH ··· ·NO_2," with the remainder recombining to form nitrate. Thus, peroxynitrite may serve as a source for ·OH-type species without the requirement of metal catalysis.

Although it is highly reactive, its modest rate of decomposition under physiological conditions allows $ONOO^-$ to diffuse for up to several cell diameters to critical cellular targets before becoming protonated and decomposing. $ONOO^-$ initiates iron-

independent lipid peroxidation and ox-
idizes thiols, damages the mitochondria electron transport chain,[50] and
causes lipid peroxidation of human
low-density lipoproteins. In addition,
metal ions, such as Fe^{3+} EDTA and
copper in the active site of SOD, catalyze the heterolytic cleavage of
$ONOO^-$ to form a nitronium ion–like
species (NO_2^+), which nitrates phenolics, including tyrosine, in proteins.[5]

Under normal conditions, intracellular $O_2^{·-}$ concentrations are kept at remarkably low levels (10 pM) because
eukaryotic cells contain large amounts
of SOD (4 to 10 μM). Under these conditions, $ONOO^-$ formation is prevented. However, pathologic conditions can greatly increase the synthesis
of both $·NO$ and $O_2^{·-}$. When the concentration of $·NO$ increases to the micromolar range, it can effectively compete with SOD for $O_2^{·-}$ to form
$ONOO^-$ (the rate constant of the reaction of $O_2^{·-}$ with $·NO$ is three times
faster than that with SOD). Indeed, ac-
tivated rat alveolar macrophages, human neutrophils, and ago-
nist-stimulated bovine endothelial cells have been shown to produce $ONOO^-$.

5. Thiols.   It has been suggested that various forms of $·NO$ (such
as N_2O_3, NO^+, and $ONOO^-$) may react with thiols to yield
S-nitrosothiols (RS-NO) and that $·NO$ circulates in plasma
mainly as an S-nitroso adduct of serum albumin. Micromolar
concentrations of S-nitrosoglutathione have been detected in the
airway fluid of normal subjects, and significantly higher levels
were observed in the lungs of patients with pneumonia or during inhalation of 80 ppm $·NO$.[14] It has been suggested that formation of RS-NO adducts stabilizes $·NO$, decreasing its cytotoxic potential while maintaining its bioactive properties. $·NO$
can also be transported on cysteine residues of hemoglobin,
which may facilitate efficient delivery of oxygen to tissues.[26]

Effect of $·NO$ on Gene Expression

$·NO$ is modulator of gene expression (Table 26-3). $·NO$ decreases
cytokine-induced endothelial cell activation by inhibiting NF-κB
expression and subsequently either VCAM transcription[11] or
NOS-II expression itself.[10] $·NO$ affects not only NF-κB function
(in part by altering IκBα expression)[45] but also other redox-
sensitive transcription factors, including AP-1 components
(Table 26-4).[47] $·NO$ modulates inflammation by altering the production of soluble cytokines[12,46] and chemoattractant factors
(MCP-1)[67] and by inhibiting adhesion molecules expression in
various cells (Table 26-3).

It is well known that iron is an important target and signaling molecule for $·NO$. The iron sulfur clusters of many proteins
are affected by $·NO$; in particular, *cis-* aconitase serves as a
bifunctional protein, depending on its iron sulfur status. In its

TABLE 26-3

Effect of $·NO$ on Cytokines

Gene	Cell Type	mRNA/protein level	Reference
Chemoattractant protein 1 (MCP-1)	Human umbilical vein endothelial cells	Decreased	67
TNF-α, IL-1α	Macrophages	Increased	31
IL-1α, IL-6	Macrophages	Decreased	46
IFN-γ	Splenocytes	Decreased	57
IL-8	Melanocytes	Increased	3

TABLE 26-4

Effect of $·NO$ on Expression and/or Activity of Transcription Factors

Transcription Factor	Cell Type	Observation	Reference
c-fos/c-jun B	Pheochromocytoma PC12	Increased	17
AP-1	Cerebellar granule	Decreased	55
IκBα	Endothelial	Increased	45

3Fe-4S complex, aconitase functions as the iron-regulatory protein (IRP). In this apo-IRP form (after $·NO$ attack), it can bind
to iron-responsive elements (IRE) and lead to inhibition of translation of ferritin and aminolevulinate synthase mRNA by forming an IRE/IRP complex in their 5' untranslated regions (UTR)
and stabilizing transcription of transferrin receptor mRNA
against targeted endonucleolytic degradation by interacting with
5 IREs in the 3' UTR. Accordingly, iron acts as both a sensory
and regulatory molecule in $·NO$ signaling, and IRP is the switch
in affecting gene expression. Although less is known regarding
similar mechanisms in lung, exposure of pulmonary artery endothelial cells in culture to S-nitrosoacetylpenicillamine (SNAP)
resulted in induction of heme oxygenase, transient increase in
iron, and a repression in the binding activity of IRP.[66]

Cytotoxic Potential of $·NO/ONOO^-$

The neutrality of $·NO$ and its low Stokes' radius permit facile
transmembrane diffusion, and its relatively long biologic half-
life allows it to react with targets distant from the point of its
origin. Thus, smooth-muscle cell– and endothelial cell–derived
$·NO$ may combine with epithelial cell–derived $O_2^{·-}$ to form
$ONOO^-$ in the epithelial lining fluid. The following observations establish the potential involvement of $·NO$, $ONOO^-$ and
various reactive nitrogen species in the generation and propagation of pulmonary epithelial injury in a variety of pathologic situations: 1. Induction of immune complex alveolitis in rat lungs
results in significant elevation of $·NO$ decomposition products
and albumin levels in bronchoalveolar lavage (BAL), indicating
the presence of increased alveolar permeability to solute. Alveolar instillation of N^G–monomethyl-L-arginine (L-NMMA)
mitigates $·NO$ production and alveolar epithelial injury.[37]

2. Paraquat-induced injury to the lung results in stimulation of ·NO synthesis. All signs of injury, including increased airway resistance and alveolar permeability to solute, are mitigated by administration of selective and competitive inhibitors of nitric oxide synthase.[7] 3. Ischemia-reperfusion injury to isolated rat lungs is associated with an increase in protein nitrotyrosine in lung homogenates, increased nitrate and nitrite levels in perfusate fluid, and formation of tissue oxidized protein and lipid products. Administration of N^G–nitro-L-argine-methyl ester (L-NAME) (NOS inhibitor) 30 min before induction of ischemia abolishes the increases in both nitrotyrosine and nitrate and nitrite and significantly reduces the formation of lung thiobarbituric acid reactive substances and protein carbonyl levels.[24] 4. Infecting hamster tracheal rings with *Bordetella pertussis* in vitro produces epithelial cytopathology. Destruction of ciliated cells and inhibition of DNA synthesis are associated with induction of ·NO synthesis by the tracheal epithelial cells. The cytopathology is dramatically attenuated by the NOS inhibitors L-NMMA and aminoguanidine. These results indicate that pertussis toxins elicit ·NO production in the same cells that suffer the subsequent dele-

terious effects.[22] 5. Pneumonia due to influenza virus results in increased production of both ·NO and $O_2^{\cdot-}$.[2] Increased expression and activity of NOS-II are observed in lungs infected with the influenza virus. L-NMMA, administered intraperitoneally daily to mice from day 3 after virus inoculation, improves survival.

EVIDENCE FOR THE PRODUCTION OF ONOO⁻ IN HUMAN LUNGS

One way to demonstrate ONOO⁻ formation in vivo is to detect the presence of stable byproducts of its reaction with various biologic compounds. 3-Nitrotyrosine, the product of the addition of a nitro group (NO_2) to the *ortho* position of the hydroxyl group of tyrosine, is such a stable compound. Nitrotyrosine has been demonstrated by indirect immunofluorescence and ELISA in lung sections obtained from rats exposed to hyperoxia, ozone,[44] endotoxin, and influenza virus.[2] Lung sections of children who died of pulmonary complications of ARDS[20] and cystic fibrosis (Fig. 26-1) stain positive for nitrotyrosine. No staining was ob-

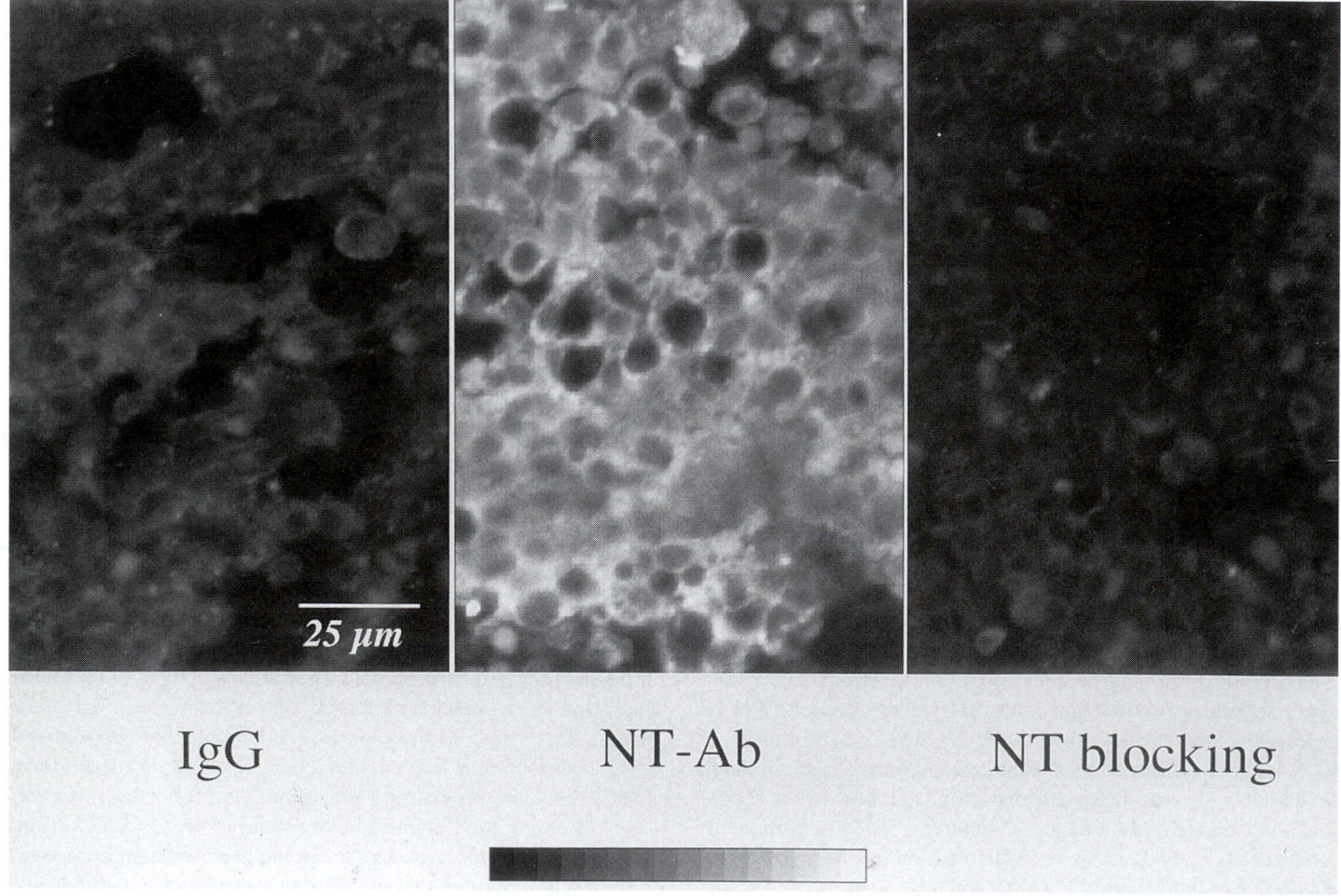

IgG   NT-Ab   NT blocking

FIGURE 26-1 Detection of nitrotyrosine in lungs of a patient who died from pulmonary complications of cystic fibrosis. Epifluorescence images of paraffin-embedded, semithin lung sections were incubated with nonspecific IgG, nitrotyrosine antibody (NT-Ab), or NT-Ab in the presence of 10 mm nitrotyrosine (NT blocking). All sections were then incubated with a secondary antibody coupled to rhodamine. All pictures were obtained with identical camera and computer settings. Significantly higher specific immunostaining (white areas) was noted with lung sections incubated with NT-Ab. The staining was completely blocked by excess amounts of nitrotyrosine, which can compete for the reaction with the antibody. Increased nitrotyrosine levels were observed in three of six cystic fibrosis patients, but none of controls.

served in the lungs of patients who died from nonpulmonary causes.[20] In additional experiments, we demonstrated nitrotyrosine formation in rat lung sections incubated in vitro with $ONOO^-$ (Fig. 26-2), but not with reactive oxygen species generated by xanthine oxidase plus Fe^{3+} EDTA or with $\cdot NO$ generated by SNAP (100 μM plus 100 μM L-cysteine). This amount of SNAP has been shown to generate $\cdot NO$ at a mean concentration of 1 μM over the 2-h exposure time.[18] With the use of HPLC, Nitrotyrosine has also been detected in homogenates of ischemic rat lungs[24] and in $ONOO^-$-treated surfactant protein A.[21]

However, $ONOO^-$ may not be the only species capable of tyrosine nitration. $\cdot NO_2$ can also nitrate tyrosine, although it is much less efficient than $ONOO^-$ because two molecules of $\cdot NO_2$ are required to nitrate one of tyrosine. Another possible nitration pathway is the reaction of $\cdot NO$-derived nitrite, under acidic conditions with oxidants such as H_2O_2 and hypochlorous acid, to form the nitrating species nitrosyl chloride.[58]

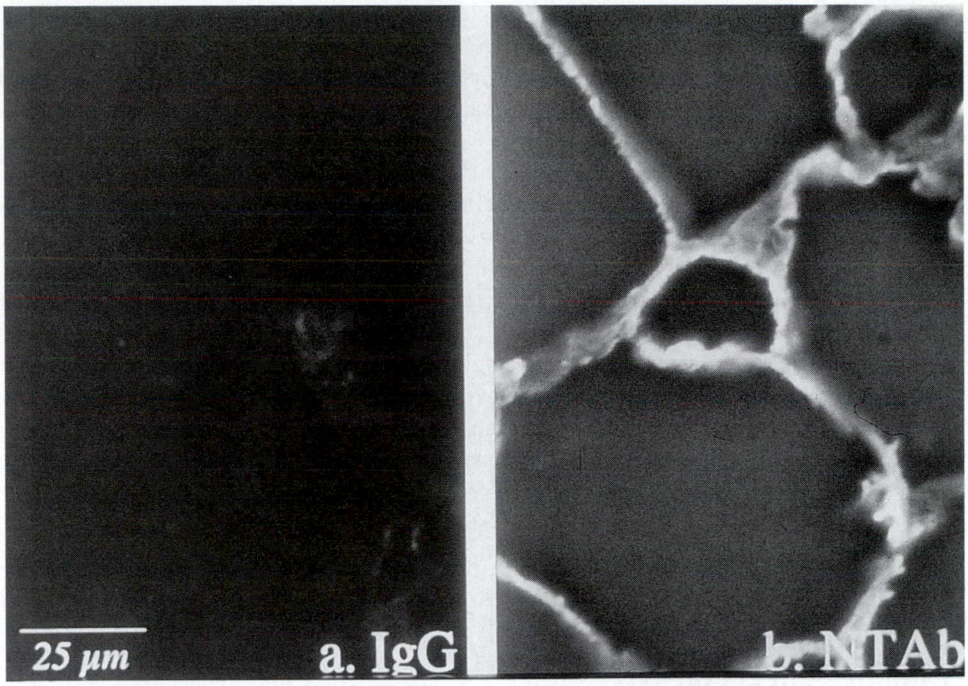

FIGURE 26-2   Detection of nitrotyrosine in rat lung section exposed to $ONOO^-$ in vitro. Epifluorescence images of semithin (4 to 6 μm) frozen rat lung sections immunostained with polyclonal antibody to nitrotyrosine (NTAb, right panel) or an equivalent amount of nonspecific IgG (IgG, left panel), followed by the secondary antibody. Exposures were taken under identical conditions. (*Based on data of Haddad et al,[20] with permission.*)

CONSEQUENCES OF NITRATION

Tyrosine nitration may be associated with important alterations in both the structure and function of proteins. Nitration of tyrosine residues of human IgG, but not rabbit IgG, abrogated their C1q-binding activity.[34] This was consistent with the presence of a tyrosine residue at the C1q receptor site of human but not rabbit IgG. Nitration of tyrosine residues of α_1-antitrypsin resulted in selective loss of elastase inhibitory activity, but not chymotrypsin or trypsin-inhibitory activity. Tyrosine nitration has also been shown to inhibit protein phosphorylation, which may interfere with intracellular signal transduction.

Nitration-Induced Injury to Surfactant Protein A
Pulmonary surfactant is a lipoprotein complex synthesized by alveolar type II cells and secreted into the epithelial lining fluid in close proximity to sites of production of reactive oxygen-nitrogen species. Surfactant consists mainly of phospholipids and at least four different associated proteins, labeled SP-A, SP-B, SP-C, and SP-D (see Chapter 7).

Nitration of human SP-A, isolated from the BAL of patients with alveolar proteinosis, by $ONOO^-$,[19] 3-morpholinosydnonimine, which simultaneously generates $\cdot NO$ and $O_2^{\cdot-}$ and forms $ONOO^-$,[18] and tetranitromethane, a specific nitrating agent at pH 7.4 and 8,[21] significantly inhibited the ability of the protein to enhance the aggregation of lipids and bind mannose in the presence of calcium. SP-A isolated from the BAL of dogs treated with oleic acid exhibited increased levels of nitration, as demon-

strated by ELISA, indicating the production of sufficient levels of reactive nitrogen species in animals with acute lung injury to nitrate SP-A in vivo.

The final translational product of human SP-A monomer contains eight tyrosine residues in the globular carboxy-terminal region of the protein, the region of SP-A responsible for enhancement of lipid aggregation. Nitration of tyrosine decreases the pK_a of tyrosine from 10 to 7.5, rendering nitrotyrosine more hydrophilic and thus potentially inducing conformational change of the tertiary structure of the carboxy-terminal region of SP-A secondary to alterations in the ionic charge.

INJURY TO PULMONARY SURFACTANT AND ALVEOLAR EPITHELIUM IN VIVO

Because of its vasorelaxant properties and its rapid inactivation in the blood by its reaction with hemoglobin, $\cdot NO$ inhalation has been advocated as a means of selectively reducing pulmonary hypertension and improving systemic oxygenation in a variety of clinical situations, including bronchopulmonary dysplasia and ARDS. However, there is concern that inhalation of $\cdot NO$ in the presence of acute inflammation may lead to the formation of reactive oxygen-nitrogen species that may damage the alveolar epithelium and pulmonary surfactant system.

A number of recent reports seem to indicate that $\cdot NO$ inhalation may indeed damage the lungs. Exposure of newborn piglets to 100 ppm $\cdot NO$ and 95 percent O_2 for 48 h resulted in significant injury to pulmonary surfactant, manifested by inhibition of surface activity, and worsened pulmonary inflammation.[52]

Pulmonary surfactant samples isolated from newborn lambs exposed to ·NO gas (200 ppm) for 6 h exhibited abnormal surface properties. SP-A, isolated from the lungs of lambs that breathed 200 ppm ·NO, exhibited a small but significant decrease in the ability to aggregate lipids in vitro.[32]

It may be argued that the concentrations of inhaled ·NO in these studies were outside the range used clinically. However, owing to the short exposure period utilized in these experiments, the value of the product of *concentration x time* of inhaled ·NO is comparable to the corresponding value in a patient who breathes 20 ppm ·NO for 3 days. Exposure of rats to 0.5 ppm ·NO for 9 weeks resulted in significantly higher injury to lung interstitial cells and matrix than an equivalent exposure to ·NO$_2$, implicating ·NO as an agent more toxic than ·NO$_2$.[36] None of the animals showed overt evidence of pulmonary injury, such as arterial hypoxemia, increased albumin content in the BAL, or respiratory failure. Accordingly, prolonged inhalation of ·NO in ARDS may lead to subacute lung injury, which may compound the existing pathology.

Protective Effects of ·NO

·NO, produced in the lung during inflammation or exposure to invading microorganisms, may initially represent an adaptive response of the host to defend against injurious stimuli. ·NO-mediated protective physiological responses include antimicrobial activity, increased mucin secretion,[1] and increased ciliary motility.[25] However, prolonged exposure to large concentrations of ·NO may lead to tissue injury by the formation of ·NO-derived species as detailed above.

INHIBITION OF OXIDANT-MEDIATED INJURY

·NO reaction with O$_2$$^{·-}$ will reduce the [O$_2$$^{·-}$] and thus decrease O$_2$$^{·-}$ injury. Also, it will limit the accumulation of H$_2$O$_2$ and decrease the formation of secondary reactive species with transition metals. ·NO donors inhibited reactive oxygen species-mediated cellular damage and cytotoxicity.[63] ·NO can also react with other free radicals, such as lipid alkoxyl (LO·) and peroxyl (LOO·) radicals, decreasing their steady-state concentration and terminating free radical chain reactions. When the molar concentration exceeds that of O$_2$$^{·-}$, ·NO protects against O$_2$$^{·-}$- and ONOO$^-$-dependent lipid peroxidation.[54] These reactions are especially important to consider, inasmuch as ·NO significantly concentrates in lipid-containing cell compartments, having a lipid-water partition coefficient of about 6.5. ·NO may also alleviate tissue injury by activating guanylate cyclase with subsequent induction of cGMP-dependent effects, such as reducing platelet and neutrophil adhesion to endothelium[30] and reacting with iron to form iron-nitrosyl compounds. By binding free coordination sites of iron, ·NO can limit iron-dependent electron transfer reactions. Also, ·NO has been shown to increase cellular reduced glutathione, an important antioxidant, in a variety of cell lines.[62]

Several observations suggest that ·NO can protect the lungs from oxidant stress. In buffer-perfused isolated rabbit lungs, inhaled ·NO (24 ppm) alleviated the increase in pulmonary vascular permeability produced by the intravascular generation of H$_2$O$_2$,[48] while inhibition of endogenous ·NO exacerbated the oxidant-mediated increase in capillary filtration coefficient (K$_{f,c}$).[28] In patients with acute lung injury, inhaled ·NO decreased permeability pulmonary edema[6] and suppressed proinflammatory cytokine production in the lung. Rats given aminoguanidine during exposure to hyperoxia had significantly increased lung injury as assessed by total protein concentrations in the BAL (unpublished observations). Although these data suggest that upregulation of ·NO production may serve a protective role, this conclusion is complicated by the fact that inhibitors of NOS-II activity also affect NOS-III, to varying degrees, and aminoguanidine interferes with glucose metabolism and thus may have diverse biologic functions in addition to blocking NOS-II.

SUMMARY AND CONCLUSIONS

Oxidant stress affects virtually all aspects of biologic existence by reaction with, and modification of, structural, metabolic, and genetic material. Protective mechanisms have evolved to defend cell components, but disease states and other environmental stresses can overwhelm defense mechanisms and cause cytotoxicity. The discovery of the L-arginine-·NO pathway has modified our understanding of the nature of the injurious species and the role ·NO plays in oxidant stress in the lung. Studies aimed at identifying regulation of the NOS genes will help us understand the wide range of functional manifestations of NOS-derived ·NO from modulating perfusion to mediating cytotoxicity. The reaction of ·NO with O$_2$$^{·-}$ is critical to understanding of the role of ·NO in oxidant stress and inflammation.

·NO plays a dual role in the modification of oxidant-mediated injury. It acts as a chain reaction–breaking antioxidant to inhibit O$_2$$^{·-}$-mediated lipid peroxidation by scavenging alkoxyl and peroxyl radicals. However, it may also promote oxidant injury to proteins by rapidly reacting with O$_2$$^{·-}$ to form a potent oxidizing and nitrating agent, ONOO$^-$. These results clarify, in part, the often confusing literature describing ·NO reactivity during oxidant stress, and provide evidence that the target molecule is an important determinant of the final outcome.

Finally, there is controversy as to whether ·NO is produced by human cells. Evidence presented herein is consistent with the presence of nitrotyrosine, the product of interaction of ONOO$^-$ with protein tyrosine residues, in the lungs of infants with various inflammatory lung diseases. These observations confirm that both ·NO and ONOO$^-$ are produced by human lung cells in vivo during inflammation.

REFERENCES

1. Adler KB, Fischer BM, Li H, et al: Hypersecretion of mucin in response to inflammatory mediators by guinea pig tracheal epithelial cells in vitro is blocked by inhibition of nitric oxide synthase. *Am J Respir Cell Mol Biol* 13:526–530, 1995.
2. Akaike T, Noguchi Y, Ijiri S, et al: Pathogenesis of influenza virus-induced pneumonia: Involvement of both nitric oxide and oxygen radicals. *Proc Natl Acad Sci USA* 93:2448–2453, 1996.

3. Andrew PJ, Harant H, Lindley IJ: Nitric oxide regulates IL-8 expression in melanoma cells at the transcriptional level. *Biochem Biophys Res Commun* 214:949–956, 1995.

4. Asano K, Chee CB, Gaston B, et al: Constitutive and inducible nitric oxide synthase gene expression, regulation, and activity in human lung epithelial cells. *Proc Natl Acad Sci USA* 91:10089–10093, 1994.

5. Beckman JS, Ischiropoulos H, Zhu L, et al: Kinetics of superoxide dismutase- and iron-catalyzed nitration of phenolics by peroxynitrite. *Arch Biochem Biophys* 298:438–445, 1992.

6. Benzing A, Brautigam P, Geiger K, et al: Inhaled nitric oxide reduces pulmonary transvascular albumin flux in patients with acute lung injury. *Anesthesiology* 83:1153–1161, 1995.

7. Berisha HI, Pakbaz H, Absood A, Said SI: Nitric oxide as a mediator of oxidant lung injury due to paraquat. *Proc Natl Acad Sci USA* 91:7445–7449, 1994.

8. Cantin AM, Fells GA, Hubbard RC, Crystal RG: Crystal: Antioxidant macromolecules in the epithelial lining fluid of the normal human lower respiratory tract. *J Clin Invest* 86:962–971, 1990.

9. Cleeter MW, Cooper JM, Darley-Usmar VM, et al: Reversible inhibition of cytochrome c oxidase, the terminal enzyme of the mitochondrial respiratory chain, by nitric oxide: Implications for neurodegenerative diseases. *FEBS Lett* 345:50–54, 1994.

10. Colasanti M, Persichini T, Menegazzi M, et al: Induction of nitric oxide synthase mRNA expression: Suppression by exogenous nitric oxide. *J Biol Chem* 270:26731–26733, 1995.

11. De Caterina R, Libby P, Peng H-B, et al: Nitric oxide decreases cytokine-induced endothelial activation: Nitric oxide selectively reduces endothelial expression of adhesion molecules and proinflammatory cytokines. *J Clin Invest* 96:60–68, 1995.

12. Eigler A, Moeller J, Endres S. Exogenous and endogenous nitric oxide attenuates tumor necrosis factor synthesis in the murine macrophage cell line RAW 264.7. *J Immunol* 154:4048–4054, 1995.

13. Finder J, Stark WW Jr, Nakayama DK, et al: TGF-beta regulates production of NO in pulmonary artery smooth muscle cells by inhibiting expression of NOS. *Am J Physiol* 268:L862-L867, 1995.

14. Gaston B, Reilly J, Drazen JM, et al: Endogenous nitrogen oxides and bronchodilator S-nitrosothiols in human airways. *Proc Natl Acad Sci USA* 90:10957–10961, 1993.

15. Guo FH, De Raeve HR, Rice TW, et al: Continuous nitric oxide synthesis by inducible nitric oxide synthase in normal human airway epithelium in vivo. *Proc Natl Acad Sci USA* 92:7809–7813, 1995.

16. Gutierrez HH, Pitt BR, Schwarz M, et al: Pulmonary alveolar epithelial inducible NO synthase gene expression: Regulation by inflammatory mediators. *Am J Physiol* 268:L501–L508, 1995.

17. Haby C, Lisovoski F, Aunis D, Zwiller J: Stimulation of the cyclic GMP pathway by NO induces expression of the immediate early genes c-fos and junB in PC12 cells. *J Neurochem* 62:496–501, 1994.

18. Haddad IY, Crow JP, Hu P, et al: Concurrent generation of nitric oxide and superoxide damages surfactant protein A. *Am J Physiol* 267:L242–L249, 1994.

19. Haddad IY, Ischiropoulos H, Holm BA, et al: Mechanisms of peroxynitrite-induced injury to pulmonary surfactants. *Am J Physiol* 265:L555–L564, 1993.

20. Haddad IY, Pataki G, Hu P, et al: Quantitation of nitrotyrosine levels in lung sections of patients and animals with acute lung injury. *J Clin Invest* 94:2407–2413, 1994.

21. Haddad IY, Zhu S, Ischiropoulos H, Matalon S: Nitration of surfactant protein A results in decreased ability to aggregate lipids. *Am J Physiol* 270:L281–L288, 1996.

22. Heiss LN, Lancaster JR Jr, Corbett JA, Goldman WE: Epithelial autotoxicity of nitric oxide: Role in the respiratory cytopathology of pertussis. *Proc Natl Acad Sci USA* 91:267–270, 1994.

23. Holm BA, Hudak BB, Keicher L, et al: Mechanisms of H_2O_2-mediated injury to type II cell surfactant metabolism and protection with PEG-catalase. *Am J Physiol* 261:C751–C757, 1991.

24. Ischiropoulos H, al-Mehdi AB, Fisher AB: Reactive species in ischemic rat lung injury: Contribution of peroxynitrite. *Am J Physiol* 269:L158–L164, 1995.

25. Jain B, Rubinstein I, Robbins RA, Sisson JH: TNF-alpha and IL-1 beta upregulate nitric oxide–dependent ciliary motility in bovine airway epithelium. *Am J Physiol* 268:L911–L917, 1995.

26. Jia L, Bonaventura C, Bonaventura J, Stamler JS: S-nitrosohaemoglobin: A dynamic activity of blood involved in vascular control. *Nature* 380:221–226, 1996.

27. Johnson BA, Lowenstein CJ, Schwarz MA, et al: Culture of pulmonary microvascular smooth muscle cells from intraacinar arteries of the rat: Characterization and inducible production of nitric oxide. *Am J Respir Cell Mol Biol* 10:604–612, 1994.

28. Kavanagh BP, Mouchawar A, Goldsmith J, Pearl RG: Effects of inhaled NO and inhibition of endogenous NO synthesis in oxidant-induced acute lung injury. *J Appl Physiol* 76:1324–1329, 1994.

29. Kobzik L, Bredt DS, Lowenstein CJ, et al: Nitric oxide synthase in human and rat lung: Immunocytochemical and histochemical localization. *Am J Respir Cell Mol Biol* 9:371–377, 1993.

30. Kubes P, Suzuki M, Granger DN: Nitric oxide: An endogenous modulator of leukocyte adhesion. *Proc Natl Acad Sci USA* 88:4651–4655, 1991.

31. Marcinkiewicz J, Grabowska A, Chain B: Nitric oxide up-regulates the release of inflammatory mediators by mouse macrophages. *Eur J Immunol* 25:947–951, 1995.

32. Matalon S, DeMarco V, Haddad IY, et al: Inhaled nitric oxide injures the pulmonary surfactant system of lambs in vivo. *Am J Physiol Lung Cell Mol Physiol* 270:L273–L280, 1996.

33. Matalon S, Holm BA, Baker RR, et al: Characterization of antioxidant activities of pulmonary surfactant mixtures. *Biochim Biophys Acta* 1035:121–127, 1990.

34. McCall MN, Easterbrook-Smith SB: Comparison of the role of tyrosine residues in human IgG and rabbit IgG in binding of complement subcomponent C1q. *Biochem J* 257:845–851, 1989.

35. McQuillan LP, Leung GK, Marsden PA, et al: Hypoxia inhibits expression of eNOS via transcriptional and posttranscriptional mechanisms. *Am J Physiol* 267:H1921–H1927, 1994.

36. Mercer RR, Costa DL, Crapo JD: Effects of prolonged exposure to low doses of nitric oxide or nitrogen dioxide on the alveolar septa of the adult rat lung. *Lab Invest* 73:20–28, 1995.

37. Mulligan MS, Hevel JM, Marletta MA, Ward PA: Tissue injury caused by deposition of immune complexes is L-arginine dependent. *Proc Natl Acad Sci USA* 88:6338–6342, 1991.

38. Nakayama DK, Geller DA, Di Silvio M, et al: Tetrahydrobiopterin synthesis and inducible nitric oxide production in pulmonary artery smooth muscle. *Am J Physiol* 266:L455–L460, 1994.

39. Nakayama DK, Geller DA, Lowenstein CJ, et al: Cytokines and lipopolysaccharide induce nitric oxide synthase in cultured rat pulmonary artery smooth muscle. *Am J Respir Cell Mol Biol* 7:471–476, 1992.

40. Nathan C, Xie QW: Nitric oxide synthases: Roles, tolls, and controls. *Cell* 78:915–918, 1994.

41. North AJ, Star RA, Brannon TS, et al: Nitric oxide synthase type I and type III gene expression are developmentally regulated in rat lung. *Am J Physiol* 266:L635–L641, 1994.

42. Owens MW, Grisham MB: Nitric oxide synthesis by rat pleural mesothelial cells: Induction by cytokines and lipopolysaccharide. *Am J Physiol* 265:L110–L116, 1993.

43. Pacht ER, Davis WB: Role of transferrin and ceruloplasmin in antioxidant activity of lung epithelial lining fluid. *J Appl Physiol* 64:2092–2099, 1988.

44. Pendino KJ, Laskin JD, Shuler RL, et al: Enhanced production of nitric oxide by rat alveolar macrophages after inhalation of a pulmonary irritant is associated with increased expression of nitric oxide synthase. *J Immunol* 151:7196–7205, 1993.

45. Peng HB, Libby P, Liao JK: Induction and stabilization of I kappa B alpha by nitric oxide mediates inhibition of NF-kappa B. *J Biol Chem* 270:14214–14219, 1995.

46. Persson AHJ, Schornagel K, Tilders HFF, et al: Alveolar macrophages autoregulate IL-1 and IL-6 production by endogenous nitric oxide. *Am J Respir Cell Mol Biol* 14:272–278, 1996.

47. Pilz RB, Suhasini M, Idriss S, et al: Nitric oxide and cGMP analogs activate transcription from AP-1-responsive promoters in mammalian cells. *FASEB J* 9:552–558, 1995.

48. Poss WB, Timmons OD, Farrukh IS, et al: Inhaled nitric oxide prevents the increase in pulmonary vascular permeability caused by hydrogen peroxide. *J Appl Physiol* 79:886–891, 1995.

49. Punjabi CJ, Laskin JD, Pendino KJ, et al: Production of nitric oxide by rat type II pneumocytes: Increased expression of inducible nitric oxide synthase following inhalation of a pulmonary irritant. *Am J Respir Cell Mol Biol* 11:165–172, 1994.

50. Radi R, Rodriguez M, Castro L, Telleri R: Inhibition of mitochondrial electron transport by peroxynitrite. *Arch Biochem Biophys* 308:89–95, 1994.

51. Rengasamy A, Xue C, Johns RA: Immunohistochemical demonstration of a paracrine role of nitric oxide in bronchial function. *Am J Physiol* 267:L704–L711, 1994.

52. Robbins CG, Davis JM, Merritt TA, et al: Combined effects of nitric oxide and hyperoxia on surfactant function and pulmonary inflammation. *Am J Physiol* 269:L545–L550, 1995.

53. Rossaint R, Falke KJ, Lopez F, et al: Inhaled nitric oxide for the adult respiratory distress syndrome. *New Engl J Med* 328:399–405, 1993.

54. Rubbo H, Radi R, Trujillo M, et al: Nitric oxide regulation of superoxide and peroxynitrite-dependent lipid peroxidation: Formation of novel nitrogen-containing oxidized lipid derivatives. *J Biol Chem* 269:26066–26075, 1994.

55. Tabuchi A, Sano K, Oh E, et al: Modulation of AP-1 activity by nitric oxide (NO) in vitro: NO-mediated modulations of AP-1. *FEBS Lett* 351:123–127, 1994.

56. Tracey WR, Xue C, Klinghofer V, et al: Immunochemical detection of inducible NO synthase in human lung. *Am J Physiol Lung Cell Mol Physiol* 266:L722–L727, 1994.

57. van der Meide PH, de Labie MC, Botman CA, et al: Nitric oxide suppresses IFN-gamma production in the spleen of mercuric chloride-exposed brown Norway rats. *Cell Immunol* 161:195–206, 1995.

58. van der Vliet A, Eiserich JP, O'Neill CA, et al: Tyrosine modification by reactive nitrogen species: A closer look. *Arch Biochem Biophys* 319:341–349, 1995.

59. Vodovotz Y, Kwon NS, Pospischil M, et al: Inactivation of nitric oxide synthase after prolonged incubation of mouse macrophages with IFN-gamma and bacterial lipopolysaccharide. *J Immunol* 152:4110–4118, 1994.

59a. Wang Y, Marsden PA. Nitric oxide synthases: Gene structure and regulation, in Ignarro L, Murad F (eds), *Nitric Oxide. Biochemistry, Molecular Biology, and Therapeutic Implications.* San Diego, CA: Academic Press, *Adv Pharmacol* 34:71–90, 1996.

60. Warner RL, Paine R 3rd, Christensen PJ, et al: Lung sources and cytokine requirements for in vivo expression of inducible nitric oxide synthase. *Am J Respir Cell Mol Biol* 12:649–661, 1995.

61. Wei XQ, Charles IG, Smith A, et al: Altered immune responses in mice lacking inducible nitric oxide synthase. *Nature* 375:408–411, 1995.

62. White AC, Maloney EK, Boustani MR, et al: Nitric oxide increases cellular glutathione levels in rat lung fibroblasts. *Am J Respir Cell Mol Biol* 13:442–448, 1995.

63. Wink DA, Hanbauer I, Krishna MC, et al: Nitric oxide protects against cellular damage and cytotoxicity from reactive oxygen species. *Proc Natl Acad Sci USA* 90:9813–9817, 1993.

63a. Wong HR, Finder JD, Wasserloos K, Pitt BR. Expression of iNOS in cultured rat pulmonary artery smooth muscle cells is inhibited by the heat shock response. *Am J Physiol: Lung Cell Mol Physiol* 13:L843–L848, 1995.

64. Xue C, Rengasamy A, Le Cras TD, et al: Distribution of NOS in normoxic vs. hypoxic rat lung: Upregulation of NOS by chronic hypoxia. *Am J Physiol* 267:L667–L678, 1994.

65. Xue C, Reynolds PR, Johns RA: Developmental expression of NOS isoforms in fetal rat lung: Implications for transitional circulation and pulmonary angiogenesis. *Am J Physiol Lung Cell Mol Physiol* 270:L88–L100, 1996.

66. Yee EL, Pitt BR, Billiar TR, Kim Y-M: Effect of nitric oxide on heme metabolism in pulmonary artery endothelial cells. *Am J Physiol: Lung Cell Mol Physiol* 15:L512–L518, 1996.

67. Zeiher AM, Fisslthaler B, Schray-Utz B, Busse R. Nitric oxide modulates the expression of monocyte chemoattractant protein 1 in cultured human endothelial cells. *Circ Res* 76:980–986, 1995.

CHAPTER 27

THE PATHOGENESIS OF PULMONARY FIBROSIS

Peter D. Bitterman / Christine H. Wendt

Morphologic studies in patients and model systems suggest that in fibrotic lung diseases of determined origin, the process begins with injury to the alveolar wall, resulting in activation of the coagulation cascade.[26] This leads to intra-alveolar deposition of a provisional matrix, along with an inflammatory response. Fibroproliferation follows, in which activated myofibroblasts migrate from the interstitium onto the luminal surface of the alveolus through gaps in the epithelial basement membrane. These cells attach to the intra-alveolar provisional matrix, where they proliferate. Alveolar walls fuse as collagen is deposited and myofibroblasts contract, eventually leading to remodeled, nonfunctional gas exchange units.

This pathologic sequence of injury, coagulation, inflammation, and fibrosis has been documented to occur following acute lung injury, and is supported by experimental evidence in the subacute and chronic fibrotic lung disorders of known cause, such as silicosis and asbestosis.[13] The experimental evidence for this sequence is so compelling that it has been accepted as axiomatic for all forms of pulmonary fibrosis. Moreover, it provides the rationale for therapeutic strategies in the fibrotic lung disorders of unknown cause. One tenet of therapy is that if inflammation can be suppressed, fibrosis can be prevented. However, available information does not fully support this possibility. In heavily (and immediately) immunosuppressed lung transplant patients, chronic rejection manifests as exuberant fibroproliferation in the bronchioles.[7] The same is true even for more profoundly immunosuppressed bone marrow transplant patients, in whom both infection and chronic graft-versus-host disease lead to fibroproliferation in the lung.[10]

The possibility has been raised that all pulmonary fibroproliferation that begins with alveolar injury follows the pathophysiological sequence that occurs after lung injury of defined cause. Instead, evidence has accumulated to indicate that the process may begin with changes in the differentiated state of interstitial fibroblasts induced by pathologic concentrations of profibrotic ligands. Data from two forms of genetic pulmonary fibrosis, familial idiopathic pulmonary fibrosis and the Hermansky-Pudlak syndrome, suggest that profibrotic ligands such as insulinlike growth factor–1 (IGF-1) and platelet-derived growth factor (PDGF) are present well before clinical imaging and physiological testing demonstrate fibroproliferative changes.[4,27] These studies do not, however, tell whether profibrotic ligands are present before or after alveolar injury. Until recently, the biologic plausibility of the profibrotic ligand–first hypothesis was low, and the intuitive appeal of the accepted sequence, beginning with injury and ending with fibrosis, was great. Studies indicating anatomic and biochemical identity between fibroproliferation in acute lung injury and the chronic fibrotic disorders further strengthened this position.[38] Nonetheless, in the idiopathic fibrotic disorders the cause of injury to the alveolar wall, presumably the first step in the process, remains elusive despite intensive search.

The pathophysiological basis for the profibrotic ligand–first hypothesis is suggested by several lines of evidence. For example, experimentally, profibrotic ligands have been shown to be capable of altering the state of differentiation of mesenchymal cells. Transforming growth factor–β (TGF-β) was identified from its ability to induce anchorage independent growth in fibroblasts, and has been demonstrated to modulate connective-tissue biosynthesis.[52] Fibroblast overexpression of *v-sis,* a close relative of the *PDGFB* gene, leads to frank sarcomatous transformation. In vivo, mesenchymal cells obtained from fibrotic lesions in numerous tissues—including blood vessels, skin, kidney, and lung—manifest an enhanced ability to proliferate and synthesize connective tissue. In theory, such phenotypic changes in mesenchymal cells could lead to a stromal microenvironment that is not hospitable to the overlying epithelium or the microvascular endothelium. This possibility has experimental support. Epithelial cells in culture remain viable when attached to the substratum by RGD-dependent integrins, but undergo apoptosis when this binding is interrupted.[23] If this formulation is correct, epithelial death would not be the initiating event in fibrosis; rather, it would be a consequence of ligand-induced mesenchymal cell phenotypic changes that result in alterations of the stromal microenvironment.

If the fibroproliferative process begins with ligand-induced changes in fibroblast phenotype that cause epithelial and endothelial cell injury or death, therapeutic efforts should logically focus on blocking the release or action of these profibrotic ligands. In contrast, if injury to the alveolar wall must occur before a fibroproliferative response ensues, identifying the injurious agent and preventing the injury along with promoting repair assume the highest therapeutic priority. This chapter will review information about the biology and pathophysiology of lung fibroproliferation with the goal of highlighting prospects for new therapeutic possibilities.

BIOLOGY OF LUNG INJURY

Both acute and chronic alveolar injury have been implicated in the initiation of the fibroproliferative response. Following an injury, the lung may respond with inflammation, tissue formation, and tissue remodeling, leading to a normal reparative process. Many of these processes may overlap temporally. However, if the injury is severe or chronic, the stages of inflammation and tissue formation may be prolonged and lead to fibrosis and physiological dysfunction of the lung.

In some fibrotic conditions, epithelial and endothelial cell damage and death may be obvious within areas of inflammation and fibroproliferation (Fig. 27-1). However, not all fibroproliferative disorders show widespread cellular damage, and cellular injury may be subtle histologically. Although the injury may appear slight, it may trigger cellular events that will lead to fibroproliferation. Identifying the cellular responses following injury may lead to a better understanding of the patterns that are protective in contrast to those that will ultimately lead to fibroproliferation.

Cellular Injury

The earliest discernible anatomic change in fibroproliferative lung diseases is the loss of alveolar epithelium, leaving denuded basement membrane at the air lung interface. The molecular mechanisms responsible for epithelial cell loss in the idiopathic fibroproliferative disorders remain unknown. Numerous candidate physiological and pathophysiological stressors have been identified, including oxidants and proteinases derived from resident and recruited leukocytes. However, the stimuli inducing these leukocytes have not been clearly identified, nor have the pathophysiological consequences of their presence been defined.

Excessive oxidant stress can clearly fall outside the boundary of an epithelial cell's antioxidant capacity and lead to necrotic death, with its well-defined inflammatory and fibrotic consequences. However, oxidant stress within the boundary of the epithelial cell's antioxidant capacity may trigger apoptosis, averting the proinflammatory consequences of necrotic death. There is also evidence that in addition to cellular loss, compensatory cellular proliferation may be inhibited by oxidant injury. Whether loss of epithelial integrity in idiopathic fibroproliferative lung disease results from necrosis, apoptosis, or failure of the progenitor function of type II epithelial cells in the course of physiological epithelial cell turnover is not definite. In addition, it is not clear what effect the loss of epithelial integrity has on the formation of fibrosis.

Injury of epithelial and endothelial cells result not only in cell death but also in the loss of tight junctions in areas where cells

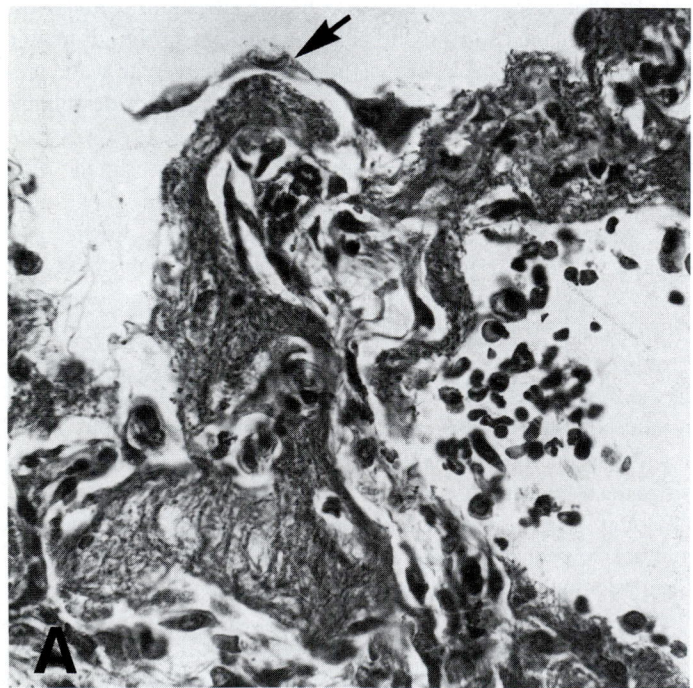

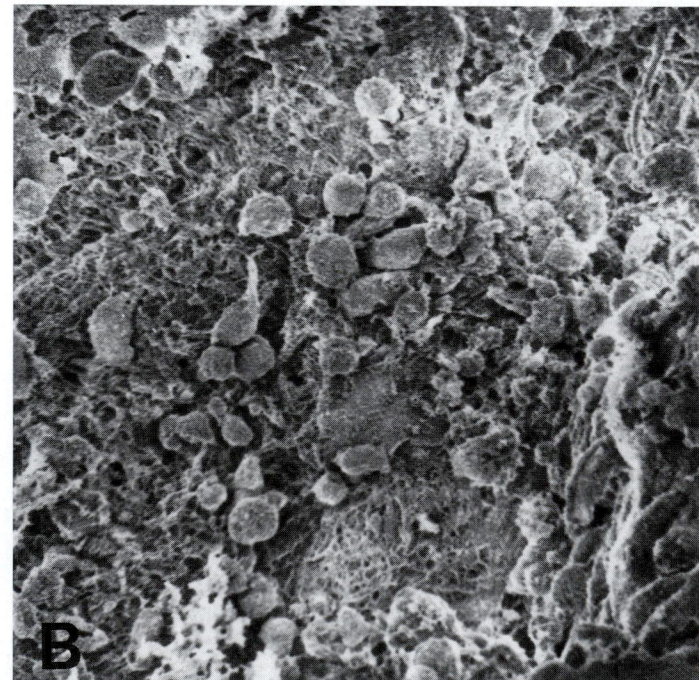

FIGURE 27-1 Alveolar epithelial cell injury. *A.* Early organization of hyaline membranes with extensions of proliferating alveolar pneumocytes after acute lung injury, ×810. *B.* Scanning electron micrograph of a similar area in the same lung showing proliferation of type II pneumocytes over hyaline membrane material, ×1170. (*From Anderson et al, Ultrastruct Pathol 16:615–628, 1992, with permission.*)

are still viable. Type I epithelial cells appear to be more susceptible to oxidant injury than are type II epithelial cells. Since type I cells cover a larger surface area than do type II cells, their susceptibility to oxidants can lead to an increase in cell permeability and edema fluid that is rich in proteins and neutrophils.[58] Independent of the biologic processes that denude the basement membrane, a predictable sequence of events ensues and follows the same pattern observed after any wound, either dermal or visceral. In the lung, plasma escapes into the airspace, leading to the activation of the coagulation cascade. This includes platelet degranulation with release of proinflammatory and profibrotic signals, as well as polymerization of fibrin within the wounded airspace.

INFLAMMATION

In the classic models of pulmonary fibrosis, in which injury precedes inflammation that leads to fibrosis, the injury and necrotic death of epithelial and endothelial cells incite the initial inflammatory response. Key to the recruitment of neutrophils into the lung is their initial adhesion to endothelial cells at sites of alveolar injury. This occurs through a number of adhesion molecules found on the surface of the leukocytes, such as members of the β_2 integrin adhesion molecule family, and on the surface of the injured endothelium, including members of the selectin family and intercellular adhesion molecule–1 (see Chapter 24).

Once adhesion to injured endothelium has occurred, neutrophils leave the circulation and move into the lung. The early response mediators released by activated macrophages, tumor necrosis factor (TNF) and interleuken 1 (IL-1), are important in the initial inflammatory response.[2,16] They lead to neutrophil sequestration and the initiation of cytokine networks necessary for neutrophil chemotaxis (see Chapter 25). In addition, TNF is a potent inducer of endothelial cell apoptosis. This can lead to the loss of capillary integrity and permit further neutrophil recruitment into the lung. Neither TNF nor IL-1 has chemotactic activity by itself. However, both can induce the expression of chemoattractants, such as IL-8, a member of the C-X-C chemokine supergene family, which has both neutrophil chemoattractant and activating activity. Recruited leukocytes can produce oxidants, which in turn can induce injury and expression of cytokines, such as IL-8.

PROTEINASES

Extracellular matrix turnover by carefully regulated proteolysis is essential for normal cell growth and function. This can be accomplished by proteinase members in the matrix metalloproteinase (MMP) and serine proteinase families. In the lung, the alveolar macrophage is the source of several MMPs, including interstitial collagenase and stromelysin, while other cells produce gelatinases and neutrophil collagenases. These enzymes are released as zymogens—in contrast to the serine proteinases, which are released in active form. Serine proteinases (e.g., plasminogen activators, neutrophil elastase, cathepsin G, and proteinase 3) and MMPs can further influence matrix turnover by augmentation of their activity through inactivation of proteinase inhibitors.

In addition to cellular injury, the extracellular matrix composition is altered during oxidant injury. This may be due to an alteration in the synthesis of matrix material by injured cells or by direct oxidation of matrix. Oxidant injury increases the expression of proteinases and plasminogen activator, which are important in the degradation and remodeling of the extracellular matrix components.[31,48] The activation of collagenases by oxidants can result in the direct loss of collagen within the extracellular matrix. In addition to a loss of collagen content, collagen fragmentation also occurs during oxidant injury.[35]

Epithelial cells have an absolute substratum requirement to remain viable. Loss of appropriate input from cell surface receptors, including integrins and possibly proteoglycans, can trigger programmed death. Therefore, it is possible that enzymatic alterations of the epithelial basement membrane by inflammatory or parenchymal cell—derived matrix active enzymes could create an environment no longer capable of supporting the viability of the epithelial cells. Proteolytic enzymes have been detected within the lungs of patients with idiopathic fibroproliferative disorders; they include collagenases, elastases, and gelatinases. What is unclear is whether these enzymes operate in the pathogenesis of the disease or whether they are mainly engaged in subsequent tissue remodeling and, therefore, play their principal role in disease progression.

OXIDANTS

Oxidants appear to play an important role in the injury that leads to the fibroproliferative response.[5,43] In idiopathic pulmonary fibrosis (IPF), the inflammatory process is marked by an increase in macrophages and neutrophils. These cells, found in the bronchoalveolar lavage (BAL) fluid of patients with IPF, release larger amounts of oxidants, such as O_2–radicals and H_2O_2, compared to healthy controls.[8] In addition, many of the animal models for pulmonary fibrosis are produced by exposure to oxidants. The classic model of bleomycin-induced pulmonary fibrosis results in oxidant production,[39] and antioxidants, such as liposome-entrapped catalase or N-acetylcysteine, can abrogate the effects of this injury.[39,54] These oxidants represent a mechanism of injury and may influence the repair process.

Although oxygen is essential for all aerobic life forms, excessive oxygen or its conversion to reactive oxidant species can be toxic to cells and tissues (see Chapter 26). Oxidant species can be derived from any cell by the formation of cellular adenosine triphosphate via the four-electron reduction of oxygen to form hydrogen peroxide (H_2O_2) in the mitochondrial electron transport system. In addition, stimulated macrophages and neutrophils generate oxidants that are helpful in host defenses against infection; however, oxidants can be harmful if produced in excess of normal host defenses.[36]

One oxidant produced in the lung is the superoxide anion radical of oxygen ($O_2°$). It is commonly generated by electrons leaking from the respiratory chain onto oxygen. Superoxide is a weak oxidant and is relatively unstable at neutral pH, with a half-life of milliseconds. It can oxidize a few compounds, including ascorbate, sulfhydryl groups, and certain catecholamines. Superoxide exerts cytotoxicity by inactivating essential cellular enzymes, such as tRNase, RNase, and glyceraldehyde-3-phosphate dehydrogenase. Although these reactions may occur, superoxide seems to exert most of its toxicity by acting as a precursor to more reactive oxidants, via superoxide dismutase (SOD).[36]

H_2O_2, a second oxidant, is produced in mitochondria by the reduction of O_2 or the dismutation of superoxide. From there, it can diffuse across the cytoplasm and out of the cell. H_2O_2 is a slow oxidant; however, in the presence of trace metals, it can form hydroxyl radicals (e.g., in the iron-catalyzed Fenton reaction). In areas of lung injury where heme and therefore iron have accumulated owing to endothelial cell damage and the extravasation of erythrocytes, the Fenton reaction may play a significant role in the formation of oxidants. Although high concentrations of H_2O_2 are required to damage cells, low concentrations can damage cellular DNA and alter molecular events. H_2O_2 is broken down to water by catalase or the glutathione peroxidase system.[36]

The hydroxyl radical (OH^-) is the most potent of the three oxidants. It is produced from superoxide-reducing H_2O_2 to produce hydroxyl radical in the Haber-Weiss reaction. This reaction can be accelerated by iron released from such compounds as ferritin, hemoglobin, and transferrin during inflammatory processes. The rate of reaction is fast, approaching diffusion-limited rates, making this oxidant very reactive, although short-lived.[36]

Oxidants can damage cellular lipids and proteins.[3] These reactive species lead to the oxidation of alveolar epithelial lining fluid proteins, specifically through the oxidation of methionine residues. When cellular plasma membranes are exposed to oxidants, such as hydroxyl radicals, the membrane lipids undergo peroxidation. This reaction is self-perpetuating and results in a decrease in membrane fluidity. In addition, oxidation can inactivate membrane proteins by the cross linkage of aldehyde groups to lipids. Other proteins, including enzymes, can be inactivated by the oxidation of sulfhydryl groups. These changes can affect all aspects of cellular homeostasis, such as ion transport, the uptake of essential nutrients, and cellular metabolism.[12]

Oxidant damage can affect cellular functions that will affect the entire organ. Oxidation of membrane proteins, such as the Na,K-ATPase, can decrease cellular ion transport. This can disrupt cellular and organ homeostasis, since ion and fluid transport is necessary to keep alveoli free of excess fluid and to maintain normal gas exchange. The oxidation of surfactant and inhibition of surfactant metabolism by oxidants can lead to abnormalities in both oxygen and fluid transport.[1] Therefore, the loss of specific epithelial cellular functions by oxidants can lead to organ dysfunction and loss of normal gas exchange.

Before loss of cell membrane integrity, oxidants perturb cellular energy stores and damage DNA. The presence of oxidants, such as H_2O_2, can lead to the depression of ATP and the inhibition of adenosine diphosphate phosphorylation.[56] Cellular energy stores can be affected by the inhibition of glucose uptake and the inhibition of glycolysis. Cellular DNA damage from nicking by hydroxyl radicals results in abnormal cross linking, mutations, and even, in extreme cases, cellular death.[55]

Cellular Defense

The mechanism of injury in pulmonary fibrosis is thought to be due to the excess production of oxygen radicals from recruited leukocytes and the activation of proteinases that damage stromal structures. This results in cell death and dysfunction, loss of normal architecture, and organ dysfunction. In many fibroproliferative disorders, however, extensive cellular injury and death are not always evident. Alternatively, oxidants and injury may induce certain cellular responses that may lead to the fibroproliferative response. This may be especially true during chronic or repeated exposure to oxidant injury, when molecular events necessary for the reparative process are persistent. The normal reparative process may entail an orchestration of molecular and cellular events that turn on and off at appropriate times. The loss of this control may result in a maladaptive reparative process and a resultant fibroproliferative state.

Injury can result in epithelial cell death by either necrosis or apoptosis, leaving areas of denuded basement membrane requiring repopulation. Oxidants, such as hyperoxia, have been shown to have both positive and negative effects on cellular proliferation in the lung. In animal models in vivo, cellular proliferation can be induced by acute exposures to oxidants.[20] This may require the induction of cell cycle genes, causing quiescent cells to enter the cell cycle. Cellular proliferation may have a beneficial effect if it results in the proliferation of type II cells and the reepithelialization of the denuded basement membrane. On the other hand, exposure of alveolar epithelial cells to repeated or sustained injury has been shown to result in decreased proliferation and continued loss of epithelium. Exacerbating this loss of epithelium is the stimulation of fibroblasts. Therefore, in the absence of the reepithelialization of the alveolus, proliferation of fibroblasts can lead to invasion of the alveolus and fibrosis.

During lung injury, genes are up-regulated that may be protective. These include the induction of type II epithelial cell surfactant apoproteins, sodium channel, and the Na,K-ATPase.[28,44,41] Oxidation of surfactant can result in regional atelectasis, which can decrease fluid and oxygen transport.[19] Therefore, maintaining appropriate surfactant levels by the up-regulation of surfactant gene expression can help preserve normal homeostasis in the lung.[41] The sodium pump and Na,K-ATPase are important proteins for the homeostasis of the cell and are especially important for ion and fluid transport in the lung. Oxidants injure cellular tight junctions and increase the amount of fluid in the alveoli. To counteract this, cells increase sodium transport via an increase in sodium channel and Na,K-ATPase expression and activity.[28] Active sodium transport may be an important determinant of physiological recovery from pulmonary edema and may influence survival.

ANTI-INFLAMMATORY DEFENSE

The events leading to the resolution of lung inflammation are not entirely clear. TNF and IL-1, which trigger cytokine networks and are necessary for neutrophil chemotaxis and activation, must be down-regulated, in order to prevent further recruitment and activation of leukocytes. One important step in the elimination of recruited leukocytes is apoptosis of neutrophils, followed by their phagocytosis by resident macrophages.[17] Apoptosis, as opposed to necrotic death, does not promote further cytokine release, which could continue the inflammatory response. In the absence of such counterregulation and orderly elimination of leukocytes, persistent inflammation with continued oxidant injury will occur. This, in turn, will sustain the cytokine network and result in continued injury.

ANTIPROTEINASES

Matrix degradation by proteinases is necessary for normal matrix turnover. This maintains a healthy substratum for lung epithelial and endothelial cells. Balancing proteinase activity is important in preventing excessive matrix degradation, which can result in cellular and organ dysfunction. Proteinase activity can be regulated by antiproteinases, such as alpha-1 proteinase inhibitor and the tissue inhibitors of metalloproteinases (TIMP). Antiproteinases appear to play a significant role in attenuating lung injury. In addition to the inhibition of protease activity, antiproteinases can have anti-inflammatory activity. These include suppression of neutrophil chemotaxis, antioxidant activity, inhibition of fibroblast proliferation, and reduced neutrophil adherence to epithelial cells. Injury to the lung, as by hyperoxia, increases expression of antiproteases such as TIMP.[31] This may have a protective effect, since experimental studies have shown that bleomycin-induced fibrosis can be attenuated by the administration of antiproteinases.[42]

ANTIOXIDANTS

There are several host defenses against oxidants. Metals can be sequestered by cellular and extracellular proteins, such as ferritin and metallothionin, to protect against the Fenton reaction. A variety of endogenous compounds—such as vitamins A, C, and E—can behave as weak antioxidants. More effective antioxidants include superoxide dismutase, catalase, and glutathione (GSH). Superoxide dismutase converts superoxide anion into H_2O_2, while catalase and glutathione peroxidase break H_2O_2 down to H_2O plus oxygen (Table 27-1). Small amounts of SOD and catalase are present in alveolar lining fluid, but these antioxidants are mainly intracellular. Glutathione is predominantly extracellular and is present in significant quantities in alveolar lining fluid; the origin of the intracellular glutathione remains unknown.[36]

There is increasing evidence that oxidants and injury regulate gene expression in mammalian cells, including the lung's epithelial and endothelial cells.[31] The redox state of regulatory proteins can influence both transcriptional and posttranscriptional events, such as increasing transcription or mRNA stability or affecting translation directly.[21] Many of the genes regulated by oxidants are at work in the anti-inflammatory response. Oxidants or injury can result in a 10- to 40-fold increase in gene expression of certain acute-phase reactant proteins, such as heat shock proteins.[21] Other genes regulated by oxidants or injury, such as certain housekeeping genes, may need only a three- to fivefold increase in gene expression to have a significant physiological effect.[31,44]

An initial response by many cells is to inhibit further oxidant damage by producing antioxidant enzymes. During lung injury, especially oxidant injury, many of the antioxidant enzymes undergo an increase in gene expression, with a concomitant increase in activity. Among these enzymes are catalase, MnSOD, and glutathione peroxidase.[11,21,30,31,37,50] These enzymes are directly involved in the elimination of oxidant species and can protect the epithelium and endothelium from injury. The mechanism by which these genes are up-regulated has been most clearly elucidated in the glutathione-S-transferase and NAD(P)H quinone reductase genes. In these genes, an "antioxidant response element" has been noted that up-regulates gene expression in the presence of oxidants.[53] Indirectly, oxidants also can modulate gene expression via signal transduction pathways, such as the activation of S6 kinase and protein kinase C by superoxide and hydrogen peroxide.[21]

Oxidant injury can both inhibit cellular function and induce the expression of genes needed in the anti-inflammatory and reparative response. However, the influx of inflammatory cells and loss of GSH may overwhelm the endogenous antioxidant activity, tipping the balance toward continued oxidant injury. This, in turn, may prevent the suppression of genes engaged in the reparative process and lead to the fibroproliferative response. The delivery of antioxidant enzymes to lungs exposed to oxidizing agents, such as bleomycin, has a protective effect against the injury and the fibroproliferative state. Therefore, if injury can be prevented or attenuated by the induction of antioxidant enzymes, processes in the generation of the fibroproliferative state may be aborted and the normal reparative process may proceed.

BIOLOGY OF LUNG FIBROPROLIFERATION

Fibroproliferation evolves in the setting of an injured alveolus. The anatomic alterations characterizing this injury involve cells and stroma constituting each of the three major anatomic compartments of the alveolus: the air-lung interface, the interstitum, and the microcirculation. Despite dramatic differences in clinical presentation among acute, subacute, and chronic fibroproliferative processes, the anatomic patterns of injury in gas exchange units are similar (Fig. 27-2). What appears to distinguish the pace of alveolar fibroproliferation in the acute respiratory distress syndrome from that observed in IPF is the number of alveolar units affected at any point in time. As a result, in biopsies from patients with chronic fibroproliferative disorders, it is common to see a combination of normal architecture, organizing pneumonitis, and alveolar collapse, whereas in acute lung injury with diffuse alveolar damage there is far more spatial synchrony of the anatomic perturbations.

In the wake of the tissue destruction inflicted on the alveolar wall by inflammatory processes, the fibroproliferative response is manifest. It consists of a series of structural and functional changes in the resident population of mesenchymal cells, resulting in partial or complete obliteration of the airspace. In the pro-

---

TABLE 27-1

Pathways of Reactive Oxygen Species

$$2O_2^\circ + 2H^- \xrightarrow{\text{SOD}} H_2O_2 + O_2$$
$$2H_2O_2 \xrightarrow{\text{catalase}} 2H_2O + O_2$$
$$ROOH + 2GSH \xrightarrow{\text{GSH-Px}} ROH + H_2O + GSSG$$

NOTE: SOD = superoxide dismutase; GSH-Px = glutathione peroxidase.

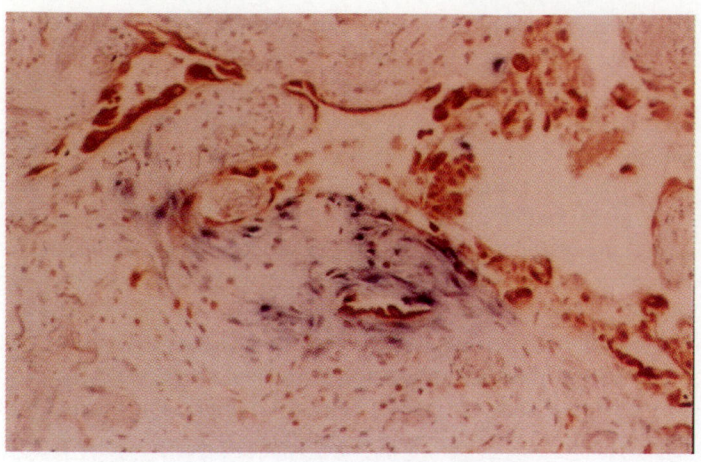
A

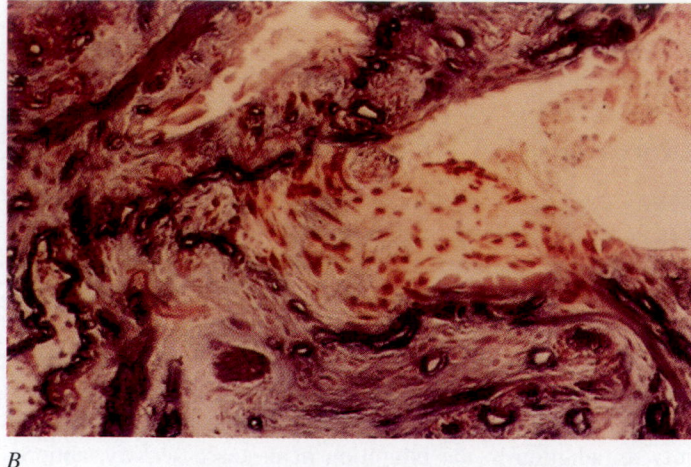
B

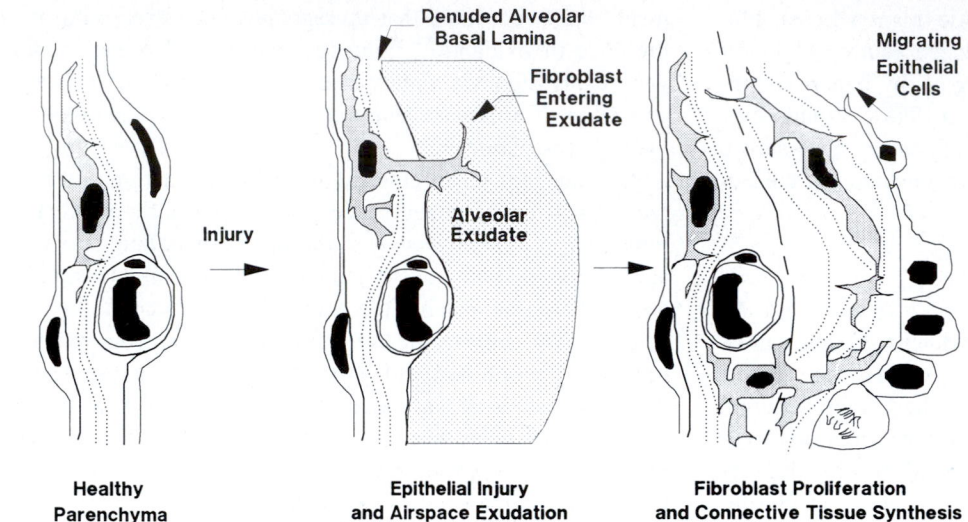
C

FIGURE 27-2 Morphologic evidence that in chronic pulmonary fibrosis interstitial fibroblasts are intraalveolar. *A.* Double stain for procollagen I (pCI) (blue) and cytokeratin (brown). There are blue-stained fibroblasts close to the epithelium. This staining combination gives the impression that the fibroblasts are interstitial. Note sloughed epithelium in the lumen identified by the cytokeratin reaction product. *B.* Serial section stained with anti-pCI (brown) and anti–type IV collagen (CIV) (dark blue). The underlying lung architecture is outlined by CIV, and the fibroblasts are now shown to be on the luminal side of the basal lamina. Original magnification ×160. *C.* Proposed pathogenetic sequence of events in chronic pulmonary fibrosis: formation of foci of intraluminal extracellular matrix. *(Based on data of Kuhn et al,[38] with permission.)*

gressive fibrotic disorders, this fibroproliferative response results in alveolar organization, including collagen deposition and myofibroblast contraction, leading to apposition of alveolar walls and loss of ventilatory function. Entrapped capillaries in such units contribute to the fixed venous shunting characteristic of fibroproliferative lung disease. Capillaries that course through stiff or partly collapsed alveoli contribute to the shunt when the minute ventilatory requirement increases with exercise or systemic stress, thereby creating a situation in which ventilation cannot increase to match the flow of blood.

In the next section, the mechanisms of lung fibroproliferation are considered with a focus on discrete functional and phenotypic changes in mesenchymal cells and epithelial cells. These changes include acquisition of a motile phenotype, migration, proliferation, apoptosis, and connective-tissue remodeling. This emphasis

is to direct attention to the cell populations effecting the structural derangements that make up pulmonary fibrosis.

Lung Parenchymal Cells Acquire a Motile Phenotype

FIBROBLASTS

Immunomorphologic and ultrastructural studies indicate that when regions of the alveolar epithelium are lost, the alveolar airspace is repopulated by mesenchymal cells containing smooth-muscle actin and vinculin (Fig. 27-3).[34,45] These cells, termed *myofibroblasts,* account for essentially all of the increased fibroblast population in the fibroproliferative lung disorders. They probably derive from resident interstitial mesenchymal cells that differentiate into myofibroblasts under the influence of peptide differentiation factors. One such peptide, TGF-β_1, is released from degranulated platelets, activated macrophages, and parenchymal cells. Although it is temporally and functionally associated with myofibroblast appearance in vivo, the molecular mechanism by which TGF-β_1 induces this change in differentiated state remains to be elucidated. Along with alterations in cytoskeletal anatomy, myofibroblasts display and utilize a repertoire of matrix receptors that provide them with the ability to migrate on provisional matrix components residing at the injured air-lung interface, including fibrin, fibronectin, and hyaluronic acid. These receptors include the fibronectin receptor $\alpha_5\beta_1$ integrin, CD_{44}, and receptor for hyaluronic acid–mediated motility (RHAMM).

EPITHELIAL CELLS

In IPF, alveolar epithelial cells manifest significant changes in cytoskeletal anatomy and matrix receptor expression. In areas where

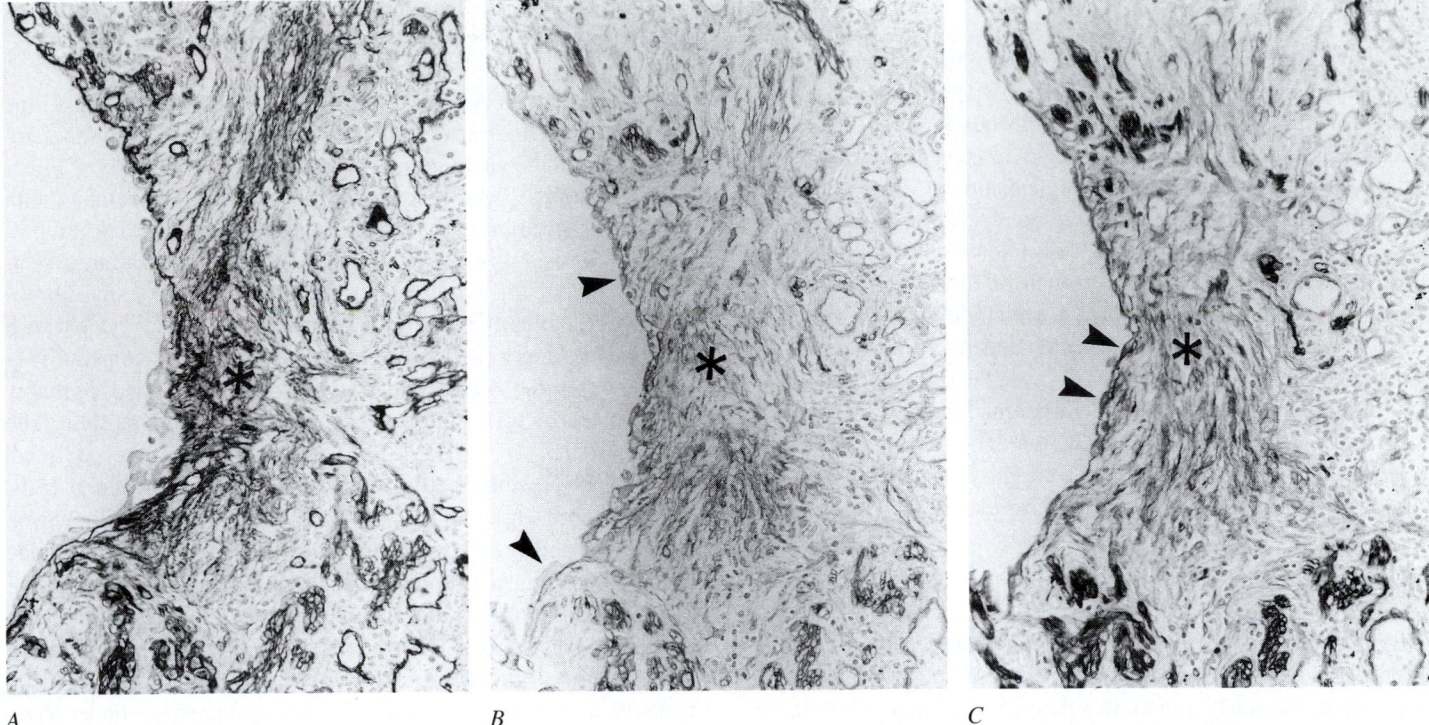

A   *B*   *C*

FIGURE 27-3   Views of three serially cut sections of an area of early fibrosis showing an intra-alveolar lesion. (Original magnification ×150.) *A*. Staining of epithelial basement membrane with anti–type IV collagen antibody shows the incorporated area of intra-alveolar fibrosis (asterisk). *B*. Integrin $\alpha_5\beta_1$ is found in smooth-muscle cells of the original alveo-lar walls and vessels, the basal layer of epithelial cells (arrows), and the mesenchymal cells in an area of intra-alveolar fibrosis (asterisk). *C*. Vin-culin is detected in smooth-muscle cells, epithelial cells (arrows), and mesenchymal cells in an area of intra-alveolar fibrosis (asterisk). (*Based on data of Fukuda et al,*[24] *with permission.*)

reepithelilization is occurring, expression of the fibronectin receptor $\alpha_5\beta_1$ is increased at the basal and lateral surfaces in association with increased vinculin expression and cytoskeletal organization.[24] This pattern is very similar to what occurs as the airways and airspaces form in development. Another fibronectin receptor, $\alpha_v\beta_6$, is induced in lung epithelium in vitro by TGF-β. Although data from patients with fibroproliferative lung disease are not yet available, TGF-β_1 induces several fibronectin-binding integrins in skin epithelial cells in vitro, including $\alpha_v\beta_6$ and $\alpha_5\beta_1$, in a pattern similar to that seen in healing wounds.[59] While the functional importance of these changes remains to be established, they provide a plausible mechanism to account for epithelial cell migration on the denuded basement membrane.

Migration on Provisional Matrix

FIBROBLASTS

Equipped with an enhanced cytoskeletal apparatus and cell surface receptors suited to the wound environment (see above), myofibroblasts depart from the interstitium and migrate into the provisional matrix. The precise identity of the haptotactic (crawling toward a solid-phase concentration gradient) stimuli that mediate this process in the fibrosing lung is not fully defined, but can be inferred from models of wound healing and in vitro studies. Platelet α granule release products, particularly PDGF family ligands, are potent stimuli for myofibroblast-directed migration

on a fibronectin substratum. In addition, both CD$_{44}$ and RHAMM have been closely associated with myofibroblast directed migration after injury.

EPITHELIAL CELLS

Information regarding the migration of lung epithelial cells on fibrin and fibronectin is limited. Nearly everything known about physiological reconstitution of the air-lung interface after injury is inferred from the profile of integrins expressed, the matrix macromolecules present to support their migration, and direct experimental evidence in models of wound healing. Together, these strongly implicate fibronectin- and fibrin-binding integrins such as $\alpha_v\beta_6$, $\alpha_5\beta_1$, and $\alpha_v\beta_3$ in the process. Functional data are available for bronchial epithelial cells in vitro, where TGF-β potently stimulates directed migration on a gelatin substrate.[57]

Experimental models indicate that proteinases with activity against basement membrane components, such as MMP-9, are rapidly expressed after wounding.[46] Fibrin- and fibronectin-binding integrins are increased in amount and redistributed to the advancing edge of the migrating epithelial cell. A concomitant early event is the co-localization of the surface receptor CD44, and one of its provisional matrix binding sites, hyaluronic acid. Even in these experimental models, however, the relative importance of the candidate enzymes and their substrates, receptors, cognate matrix ligands, and sequence of function remains to be precisely elucidated.

Proliferation

The transition from quiescence to a proliferative state and subsequent cell cycle transit is regulated by polypeptide growth factors. Each growth factor acts upon target cells bearing specific cell surface receptors. To respond to the signal received, each target cell must be in the appropriate physiological context. This includes its substratum and matrix receptor-binding repertoire. Growth factors act in a sequence, some signaling cells to emerge from quiescence and others acting to facilitate transit at therestriction point (R point) in G_1 phase of the cell cycle, which demarcates the events in cycle transit that are growth factor dependent from those that are autonomously programmed. Growth factors can derive from the processes of coagulation, inflammation, or autocrine or paracrine parenchymal cell production. The presence and functional state of the growth factors are tightly associated with both normal and pathologic fibroproliferative events.

FIBROBLASTS

Once they have moved into the injured alveolar airspace, lung myofibroblasts respond to a set of positive proliferative signals. Many of the same signals that modulate their directed migration, including fibronectin and PDGF, can also signal their emergence from quiescence. As a result, the myofibroblast population expands—leading to partial or, in some cases, complete effacement of the alveolar-capillary gas exchange apparatus. While a number of positive proliferative signals have the potential to participate in pathologic fibroproliferation, the focus here will be on three polypeptide growth factors for which an in vivo role has been established.

Platelet-Derived Growth Factors This family of dimeric ligands has been implicated in pathologic fibroproliferation of the lung and blood vessels, as well as in physiological wound healing.[22] Encoded by two genes, designated A and B, homodimeric or heterodimeric ligands bind to receptors on the surface of target cells to stimulate both directed migration and transit from the G_0 phase of the cell cycle to G_1.

The myofibroblast response to PDGF is determined by the receptor populations on its surface. In common with other growth factor receptors of the tyrosine kinase family, ligand binding leads to receptor dimerization, autophosphorylation, and signal transduction. Receptor monomers exist in two forms, α and β, with the α chain exhibiting affinity for both A and B chains of PDGF, whereas the β subunit binds only the β chain. β chains predominate on myofibroblasts, explaining its more robust response to dimers containing B chain.

There are several cellular sources of PDGF in fibroproliferative lung disease. Early on in the fibroproliferative response, PDGF probably derives from platelet α granules discharged when epithelial and endothelial cells are lost and denuded basement membrane collagen is exposed to the circulation. During later phases, macrophages and eventually parenchymal cells—including epithelial cells, endothelial cells, and myofibroblasts—may produce PDGF. The specific signals directing macrophage and parenchymal cell PDGF production, and those active in termination of ligand release, remain incompletely defined. One signal that may be involved in PDGF release is IL-1,

which is present in the fibrotic lung and can induce fibroblast production of PDGF B in vitro.[51]

Fibroblast Growth Factors This family consists of at least nine members.[40] FGF2 (basic FGF) has been identified immunohistochemically at the air-lung interface following lung injury.[29] Functional ligand has been recovered from the lungs of patients with active fibroproliferation, further strengthening its link to pulmonary fibrosis. Similar to PDGF, receptor dimerization is generally required for a cellular response to ligand. For myofibroblasts, FGF2 potently stimulates exit from G_0 and cell cycle transit in vitro. Lacking a classic leader sequence, FGF2 is constitutively secreted through alternative secretory pathways and probably binds to nearby glycosaminoglycans in the lung interstitium. The cellular sources of FGF2 in fibrosing lung are not well defined, but probably include both inflammatory and parenchymal cells.

Even more important than its proliferative function, however, may be the ability of growth factors of the FGF family to provide topographic information to mesenchymal cells. During development, FGF functions in the induction of ventral mesoderm and in the spatial patterning as limbs develop. A similar role in morphogenesis during fibroproliferation or physiological repair is consistent with its constitutive secretory pattern and presence under physiological conditions. This role, however, remains to be established.

Transforming Growth Factor–β TGF-β_1 participates in fibroproliferation as a potent modulator of mesenchymal cell differentiation. The TGF family of peptides includes more than 20 members that share structural similarities.[6] TGF-β_1 has been most closely associated with fibroproliferative processes, including atherosclerosis and pulmonary fibrosis. Produced as a large precursor protein, TGF-β_1 is cleaved into a mature C-terminal dimer and an N-terminal pro-region. Dissociation into an active ligand requires further enzymatic processing or an acidic microenvironment. There are three TGF-β_1 receptors, designated 1, 2, and 3. Ligand binding leads to heteromeric protein kinase complexes, which initiate the signal transduction cascade.

In the earliest stages of injury, TGF-β_1 derived from platelet α granules signals interstitial mesenchymal cells to differentiate into myofibroblasts. Later in the process, as the airspace fills with myofibroblasts, TGF-β_1 derived from macrophages and possibly parenchymal cells signals the transition from a motile, proliferative phenotype to a collagen synthetic phenotype. This critical transition in the course of physiological surface wound healing may in the lung lead to intra-alveolar deposition of collagens I and III, contraction of the airspace contents, and alveolar collapse.

TGF-β_1 may provide both positive and negative proliferative signals to mesenchymal cells. During the proliferative phase of alveolar fibrosis, TGF-β_1 can serve indirectly as a positive proliferative influence by stimulating production of autocrine myofibroblast PDGF B. As the airspace fills, TGF-β may directly lead to cycle arrest by down-regulation of cyclin-dependent kinases 2 and 4, which are both essential for the cell cycle transition from G_1 to S. Later, TGF-β_1 may function to stimulate fibroblast collagen synthesis.

Fibroproliferative Phenotype As important as proliferative and differentiation signals are in the initiation of fibroproliferation, their role in disease progression is less certain. A number of studies examining myofibroblasts recovered from a variety of fibroproliferative lesions indicate that they have an altered phenotype that is stably expressed in vitro. In atherosclerosis, pulmonary fibrosis, cirrhosis, scleroderma, and nephrosclerosis, myofibroblasts manifest an enhanced state of motility, increased collagen synthesis, and an enhanced proliferative state.[9,33] The biologic importance of this fibroproliferative phenotype in the evolution of pathologic fibroproliferation remains to be established.

EPITHELIAL CELLS

Repair after lung injury is dependent upon prompt and orderly reepithelialization at the alveolar surface. In acute injury of defined cause, the sequence of events and anatomic patterns are well defined. In idiopathic fibroproliferative disorders, this is not the case. It is generally agreed that epithelial repair depends on intact stromal scaffolding, which defines the correct pattern to be followed as reepithelialization occurs. As a result, when alveolar fibroproliferation supervenes, it may reflect loss of key stromal signals. There may be survival signals provided by ligation of integrin or proteoglycan receptors, or sites in the matrix itself that bind and make available peptide growth factors essential for epithelial cell proliferation. These stromal signals may also be important for immobilizing epithelial cells when they have correctly docked in the desired anatomic locus.

A number of ligands with tropism for alveolar epithelial cells have been identified. Among these, kerotinocyte growth factor (KGF), a protein released by fibroblasts, is active in vitro and in vivo to stimulate alveolar type II cell proliferation.[47] In addition, experiments in animal models of lung injury strongly suggest that KGF functions as a survival signal. Studies to directly evaluate whether defects in the KGF–epithelial cell axis are present in fibroproliferative lung disease are not yet available. Also undefined is the adequacy of epithelial cell progenitor function in patients with fibroproliferative lung disease.

Apoptosis

Apoptosis is a form of genetically regulated death characterized by a distinct sequence of anatomic rearrangements.[35] The nucleus and cytoplasm condense, followed by fragmentation into membrane-bound vesicles known as apoptotic bodies. In many systems, changes are accompanied by alterations of the plasma membrane, providing recognition signals to professional phagocytes and neighboring parenchymal cells. Recognition is followed by phagocytosis and degradation of the apoptotic cells without evoking a respiratory burst or overt inflammation. Apoptosis can be triggered by an intrinsic genetic program, lack of key survival signals, or interaction with specific death signals.

FIBROBLASTS

In surface wound healing, myofibroblast apoptosis is the principal process responsible for regression of granulation tissue as the wound space contracts (Fig. 27-4).[15] Apoptosis has also been implicated in the regression of intra-alveolar fibroproliferation in

lung repair, a process closely coordinated with reepithalization of the gas exchange surface.[49] In chronic fibroproliferative lung disease, dysregulation of myofibroblast survival seems to prevent restoration of physiological function. Some alveolar units behave as classic integumentary wound spaces, filling in with myofibroblasts, which deposit collagen. This durable matrix replaces the provisional matrix composed of polymerized fibrin, fibronectin, and proteoglycans. Myofibroblasts contract the airspace and undergo apoptosis as the alveolus is collapsed. In other alveolar units, myofibroblasts persist in the alveolar airspace and are eventually covered by a metaplastic epithelium, resulting in their being incorporated into a thick and remodeled alveolar wall.

Fibroblasts, in common with all eukaryotic cells, have specific requirements to remain viable. Among these are signals provided by the extracellular matrix through their cognate integrin and proteoglycan receptors. Fibroblasts also require survival signals from polypeptide growth factors such as PDGF and IGF-1. However, this requirement is dependent both on the proliferative and differentiated state of the cell and on whether the fibroblast resides on provisional or physiological matrix. For example, cycling cells are far more dependent on polypeptide growth factors for their survival than are quiescent cells. Fibroblasts also bear receptors for death signals, including TNF-α and Fas/Apo 1. While the functional importance of these receptors on myofibroblasts remains to be established, a dynamic interplay clearly exists between signals provided by matrix and polypeptide growth factors in regulating the fibroproliferative response, both physiological and pathologic. The molecular details of this interplay will undoubtedly come into sharper focus as more information becomes available about the intracellular signaling pathways involved.

EPITHELIAL CELLS

An invariant morphologic observation in fibroproliferative lung processes is the presence of a hyperplastic, cuboidal epithelium composed mainly of type II cells. Such an epithelium is found following acute lung injury when alveolar anatomy is to be restored. Type II cell hyperplasia is also found in subacute and chronic pulmonary fibrosis. This finding has two obvious implications. First, even after the most devastating injury, the progenitor function of type II cells is at least partly preserved. Second, if the alveolar structures are to be restored, a major geometric hurdle must be overcome.

In the normal alveolar epithelium, type II cells and type I cells are present in equal numbers, yet type I cells cover 95 percent of the air lung interface.[14] Thus, in a hyperplastic epithelium there is a 10-fold excess of type II cells. For restoration of a physiological epithelium, these excess cells must undergo programmed death to make room for the type I cells as they differentiate from parental type II cells. This problem is compounded by the need for maintenance of an edema-free functional airspace, suggesting that the elimination of a type II cell must be precisely coordinated with the differentiation of an adjacent type I cell. This geometric problem is reminiscent of that solved by the fetus as its lung differentiates from the bronchiolar stage into a mature lung. The molecular mechanisms regulating the programmed death of type II cells in ontogeny and during physio-

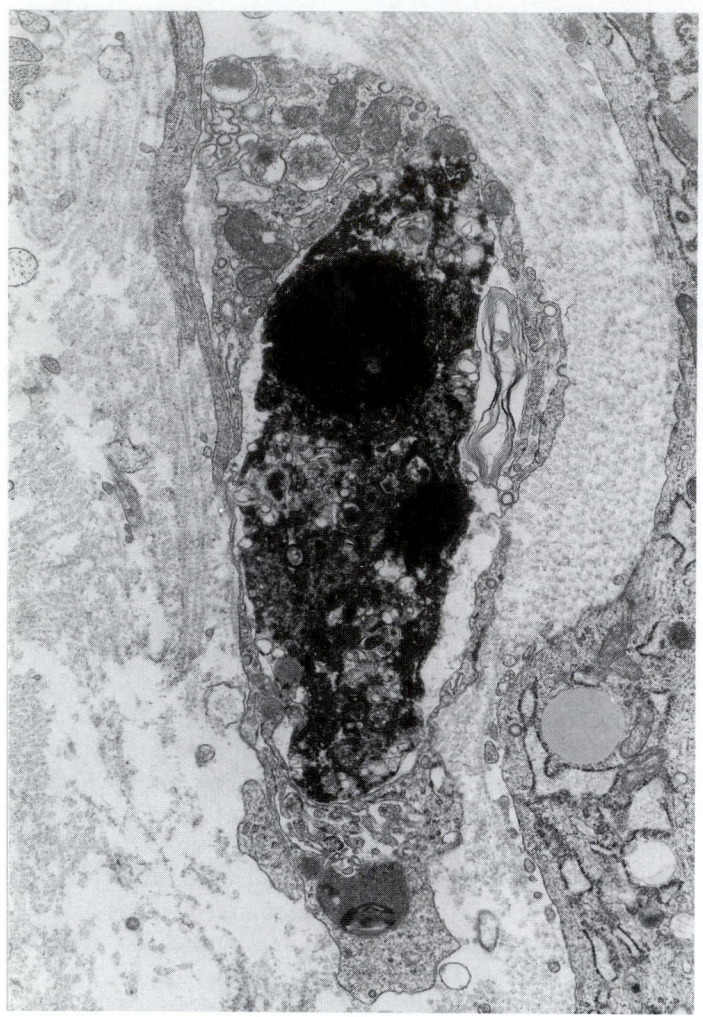

A

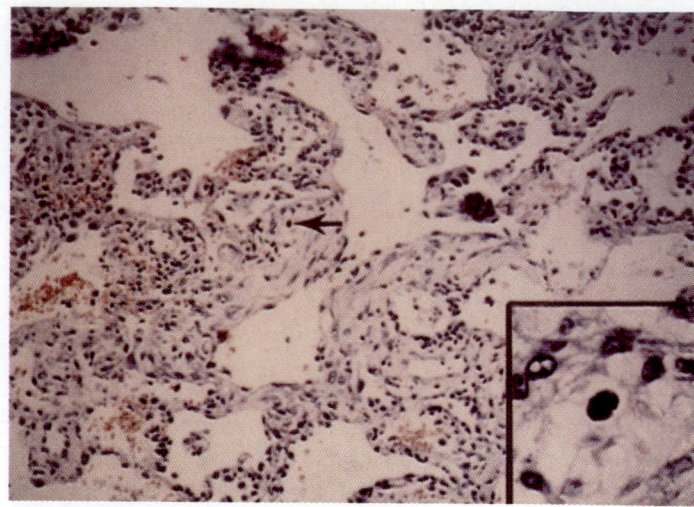

B

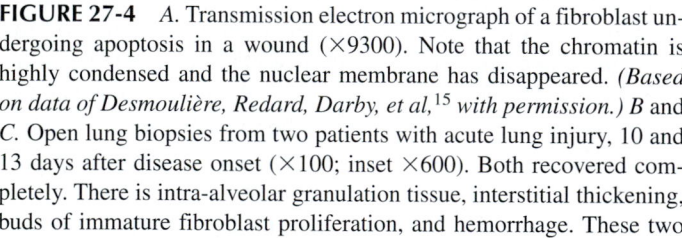

C

FIGURE 27-4 *A.* Transmission electron micrograph of a fibroblast undergoing apoptosis in a wound (×9300). Note that the chromatin is highly condensed and the nuclear membrane has disappeared. *(Based on data of Desmoulière, Redard, Darby, et al,*[15] *with permission.) B and C.* Open lung biopsies from two patients with acute lung injury, 10 and 13 days after disease onset (×100; inset ×600). Both recovered completely. There is intra-alveolar granulation tissue, interstitial thickening, buds of immature fibroblast proliferation, and hemorrhage. These two biopsies show, in addition, occasional cells (arrows) morphologically similar to human lung fibroblasts undergoing programmed death in vitro after culture with bronchoalveolar lavage fluid obtained from patients with acute lung injury (shown in the insets). Note that in *B* the cell appearing to undergo programmed death is present in an area where the fibroplastic plug has clearly reepithelialized. *(Based on data of Polunovsky et al,*[49] *with permission.)*

logical repair are not yet defined. Learning if and how the process of epithelial reconstitution fails in pathologic fibroproliferative processes awaits this critical information.

Connective-Tissue Remodeling

A fibroproliferative response is pathologic when it leads to a stable alteration of alveolar connective-tissue architecture that is incompatible with normal gas exchange. The process begins with activation of the coagulation cascade in regions where epithelial cells are lost. There is deposition of provisional matrix macromolecules, including fibrin, fibronectin, and hyaluronic acid. Of note, the pattern of fibrin deposition in experimental fibrosis correlates closely with the pattern of durable matrix deposition in fibrotic lesions.[25,26] Another product of the coagulation cascade, thrombospondin, which inhibits plasmin, also localizes to fibrotic lesions and forms part of the substratum for metaplastic epithelial cells in mature fibrotic lesions. Aberrant local regulation of coagulation occurs in the lungs of patients with IPF, where there is a net decrease in fibrinolytic activity.[32] Direct experimental manipulation of lung fibronolytic activity using transgenic mice that are either null or overexpressors of plasminogen activator inhibitor strongly links persistence of the provisional matrix with a pathologic outcome in fibroproliferation.[18]

Peptide signals may promote collagenous fibrosis in provisional matrix. In particular, TGF-β_1 has been localized by in situ hybridization and immunohistochemistry to regions where fibroblasts are actively synthetizing new type I collagen. TGF-β_1

is capable of directly stimulating fibroblast collagen synthesis, providing one mechanism driving fibroproliferation. Where TGF-β_1 and its receptors fit into normal repair, and whether dysregulation of the TGF-β_1 system leads to fibrosis, has not been clearly defined.

CONCLUSION

The pathologic sequence in pulmonary fibrosis may have several scenarios. Clearly, there is experimental evidence that pulmonary fibrosis can evolve from a series of events initiated by an oxidant injury leading to coagulation, inflammation, and eventually fibrosis. In most clinical cases of pulmonary fibrosis, however, no such orderly process can be identified. In these cases, injured cells may exist with inflammation and fibrosis, and it is not clear which are the initiating or sustaining events. When cells are exposed to a stress, such as oxidants, they have several choices. The stress may be mild, or the cell may be poised to adapt to this insult and manifest normal physiological function. In some instances, this stress may induce the molecular and cellular events leading to apoptosis. If the stress is severe enough or the cell is susceptible, necrosis may occur. Unlike apoptosis, this can lead to inflammation and further cellular stress through the release of oxidants. However, the inflammatory process does not always continue unchecked. Often, inflammation resolves and the normal reparative process proceeds.

Pulmonary fibroproliferation may occur following the orderly occurrence of stress or injury, inflammation, and fibrosis. There is clinical evidence, however, that inducers of fibroblast proliferation may be able to initiate pulmonary fibrosis. This change in fibroblast phenotype can alter the microenvironment, leading to cellular stress and the inflammatory response. Once initiated, the inciting event is difficult to differentiate, since injury, inflammation, and fibrosis can coincide. In these instances, treating with antioxidants and anti-inflammatory agents may minimize some of the injury and inflammation, but it will not eliminate the underlying fibroproliferative process. If pulmonary fibrosis is the result of an orderly sequence, early treatment with antioxidants and anti-inflammatory agents may have a therapeutic effect. However, if the phenotypic change of the fibroblast is the initial or even the final event that directly leads to cellular injury and inflammation, therapy should be aimed toward inhibiting the ligands or molecular events that induce these changes. While it is not clear how these processes interact, investigations into cellular injury, the inflammatory process, and fibroblast proliferation may elucidate the requisite cellular and molecular events necessary for the fibroproliferative state and may subsequently help us to focus our therapeutic efforts.

REFERENCES

1. Baker RR, Panus PC, Holm BA, et al: Endogenous xanthine oxidase–derived O_2 metabolites inhibit surfactant metabolism. *Am J Physiol* 259:L328–L334, 1990.
2. Bazzoni F, Beutler B: The tumor necrosis factor ligand and receptor families, in Flier JS, Underhill LH (eds), *Semin Med Beth Israel Hosp* 334:1717–1725, 1996.
3. Berger NA: Oxidant-induced cytoxicity: A challenge for metabolic modulation. *Am J Respir Cell Mol Biol* 4:1–3, 1991.
4. Bitterman PB, Rennard SI, Keogh BA, et al: Familial pulmonary fibrosis: Evidence of lung inflammation in unaffected family members. *New Engl J Med* 314:1343–1347, 1986.
5. Borzì RM, Grigolo B, Meliconi R, et al: Elevated serum superoxide dismutase levels correlate with disease severity and neutrophil degranulation in idiopathic pulmonary fibrosis. *Clin Sci* 85:353–359, 1993.
6. Brand T, Schneider MD: Transforming growth factor–β signal transduction. *Circulation Res* 78:173–179, 1996.
7. Burke CM, Theodore J, Dawkins KD, et al: Post-transplant obliterative bronchiolitis and other late lung sequelae in human heart-lung transplantation. *Chest* 86:824–829, 1984.
8. Cantin AM, North SL, Fells GA, et al: Oxidant-mediated epithelial cell injury in idiopathic pulmonary fibrosis. *J Clin Invest* 79:1665–1673, 1987.
9. Chen B, Polunovsky V, White J, et al: Mesenchymal cells isolated after acute lung injury manifest an enhanced proliferative phenotype. *J Clin Invest* 90:1778–1785, 1992.
10. Clark JG, Crawford SW, Madtes DK, et. al.: Obstructive Lung Disease after allogeneic marrow transplantation. *Ann Intern Med* 11:368–376, 1989.
11. Clerch LB, Massaro D: Oxidation-reduction-sensitive binding of lung protein to rat catalase mRNA. *J Biol Chem* 267:2853–2855, 1992.
12. Clerici C, Friedlander G, Amiel C: Impairment of sodium-coupled uptakes by hydrogen peroxide in alveolar type II cells: Protective effect of d-α-tocopherol. *Am J Physiol* 262:L542–L548, 1992.
13. Craighead JE, Abraham JL, Churg A, et al: The pathology of asbestos-associated diseases of the lung and pleural plaques: Diagnostic criteria and proposed grading system. *Arch Pathol Lab Med* 106:543–559, 1982.
14. Crapo JD, Barry BE, Gehr P, et al: Cell number and cell characteristics of the normal human lung. *Am Rev Respir Dis* 125:332–337, 1982.
15. Desmoulière A, Redard M, Darby I, Gabbiani G: Apoptosis mediates the decrease in cellularity during the transition between granulation tissue and scar. *Am J Pathol* 146:56–66, 1995.
16. Dinarello CA, Wolff SM: The role of interleukin-1 in disease. *New Engl J Med* 328:106–113, 1993.
17. Dransfield I, Stocks SC, Haslett C: Regulation of cell adhesion molecule expression and function associated with neutrophil apoptosis. *Blood* 85:3264–3273, 1995.
18. Eitzman DT, McCoy RD, Zheng X, et al: Bleomycin-induced pulmonary fibrosis in transgenic mice that either lack or overexpress the murine plasminogen activator–1 gene. *J Clin Invest* 97:232–237, 1996.
19. Engstrom PC, Holm BA, Matalon S: Surfactant replacement attenuates the increase in alveolar permeability in hyperoxia. *J Appl Physiol* 67:688–693, 1989.
20. Everett MM, King RJ, Jones MB, et al: Lung fibroblasts from animals breathing 100% oxygen produce growth factors for alveolar type II cells. *Am J Physiol* 259:L247–L254, 1990.
21. Fanburg BL, Massaro DJ, Cerutti PA, et al: Regulation of gene expression by O_2 tension. *Am J Physiol* 262:L235–L241, 1992.
22. Ferns GAA, Raines EW, Spruge KH, et al: Inhibition of neointimal smooth muscle accumulation after angioplasty by an antibody to PDGF. *Science* 253:1129–1132, 1991.
23. Frisch SM, Francis H: Disruption of epithelial cell-matrix interactions induces apoptosis. *J Cell Biol* 124:619–626, 1994.
24. Fukuda Y, Basset F, Ferrans VJ, Yamanaka N: Significance of early intra-alveolar fibrotic lesions and integrin expression in lung biopsy

specimens from patients with idiopathic pulmonary fibrosis. *Hum Pathol* 26:53–61, 1995.

25. Fukuda Y, Ferrans VJ, Schoenberger CI: Patterns of pulmonary structural remodeling after experimental paraquat toxicity. *Am J Pathol* 118:452–475, 1985.

26. Fukuda Y, Ishizaki M, Masuda Y, et al: The role of intraalveolar fibrosis in the process of pulmonary structural remodeling in patients with diffuse alveolar damage. *Am J Pathol* 126:171–182, 1987.

27. Harmon KR, Witkop CJ, White JG, et al: Pathogenesis of pulmonary fibrosis—PDGF precedes structural alterations in the Hermansky-Pudlak syndrome. *J Lab Clin Med* 123:617–627, 1994.

28. Haskell JF, Yue G, Benos DJ, Matalon S: Upregulation of sodium conductive pathways in alveolar type II cells in sublethal hyperoxia. *Am J Physiol* 266:L30–L37, 1994.

29. Henke C, Marinelli W, Jessurun J, et al: Macrophage production of basic fibroblast growth factor in the fibroproliferative disorder of alveolar fibrosis after lung injury. *Am J Pathol* 143:1189–1199, 1993.

30. Ho Y-S, Dey MS, Crapo JD: Antioxidant enzyme expression in rat lungs during hyperoxia. *Am J Physiol* 270:L810–L818, 1996.

31. Horowitz S, Dafni N, Shapiro DL, et al: Hyperoxic exposure alters gene expression in the lung. *J Biol Chem* 264:7092–7095, 1989.

32. Idell S, James KK, Levin EG, et al: Local abnormalities in coagulation and fibrinolytic pathways predispose to alveolar fibrin deposition in the adult respiratory distress syndrome. *J Clin Invest* 84:695–705, 1989.

33. Jordana M, Schulman J, McSharry C: Heterogeneous proliferative characteristics of human adult lung fibroblast lines and clonally derived fibroblasts from control and fibrotic tissue. *Am Rev Respir Dis* 137:579–584, 1988.

34. Kapanci Y, Desmouliere A, Pache JC, et al: Cytoskeletal protein modulation in pulmonary alveolar myofibroblasts during idiopathic pulmonary fibrosis: Possible role of transforming growth factor beta and tumor necrosis factor alpha. *Am J Respir Crit Care Med* 152:2163–2169, 1995.

35. Kerr JF, Wyllie AH, Currie AR: Apoptosis: A basic biological phenomenon with wide-ranging implications in tissue kinetics. *Br J Cancer* 26:239–257, 1972.

36. Kinnula VL, Crapo JD, Raivio KO: Biology of disease: Generation and disposal of reactive oxygen metabolites in the lung. *Lab Invest* 73:3–19, 1995.

37. Knickelbein RG, Ingbar DH, Seres T, et al: Hyperoxia enhances expression of γ-glutamyl transpeptidase and increases protein s-glutathiolation in rat lung. *Am J Physiol* 270:L115–L122, 1996.

38. Kuhn C III, Boldt J, King TE Jr, et al: An immunohistochemical study of architectural remodeling and connective tissue synthesis in pulmonary fibrosis. *Am Rev Respir Dis* 140:1693–1703, 1989.

39. Ledwozyw A: Protective effect of liposome-entrapped superoxide dismutase and catalase on bleomycin-induced lung injury in rats: II. Phospholipids of the lung surfactant. *Acta Physiol Hung* 78:157–162, 1991.

40. Mason IJ: The ins and outs of fibroblast growth factors. *Cell* 78:547–552, 1994.

41. Minoo P, King RJ, Coalson JJ: Surfactant proteins and lipids are regulated independently during hyperoxia. *Am J Physiol* 263:L291–L298, 1992.

42. Nagai A, Aoshiba K, Ishihara Y, et al: Administration of α_1-proteinase inhibitor ameliorates bleomycin-induced pulmonary fibrosis in hamsters. *Am Rev Respir Dis* 145:651–656, 1992.

43. Nakashima JM, Levin JR, Hyde DM, et al: Repeated exposures to enzyme-generated oxidants cause alveolitis, epithelial hyperplasia, and fibrosis in hamsters. *Am J Pathol* 139:1485–1499, 1991.

44. Nici L, Dowin R, Gilmore-Hebert M, et al: Upregulation of rat lung Na-K-ATPase during hyperoxic injury. *Am J Physiol* 261:L307–L314, 1991.

45. Ohta K, Mortenson RL, Clark RA, et al: Immunohistochemical identification and characterization of smooth muscle–like cells in idiopathic pulmonary fibrosis. *Am J Respir Crit Care Med* 152:1659–1665, 1995.

46. Oksala O, Salo T, Tammi R, et al: Expression of proteoglycans and hyaluronan during wound healing. *J Histochem Cytochem* 43:125–135, 1995.

47. Panos RJ, Bak PM, Simonet WS, et al: Intratracheal instillation of keratinocyte growth factor decreases hyperoxia-induced mortality in rats. *J Clin Invest* 96:2026–2033, 1995.

48. Phillips PG, Birnby L, Di Bernardo LA, et al: Hyperoxia increases plasminogen activator activity of cultured endothelial cells. *Am J Physiol* 262:L21–L31, 1992.

49. Polunovsky V, Chen B, Henke C, et al: Role of mesenchymal cell death in lung remodeling following injury. *J Clin Invest* 92:388–397, 1993.

50. Rahman I-U, Clerch LB, Massaro D: Rat lung antioxidant enzyme induction by ozone. *Am J Physiol* 260:L412–L418, 1991.

51. Raines EW, Dower SK, Ross R: Interleukin-1 mitogenic activity for fibroblasts and smooth muscle cells is due to PDGF-AA. *Science* 243:393–396, 1989.

52. Roberts AB, Anzano MA, Lamb LC, et al: New class of transforming growth factors potentiated by epidermal growth factor: Isolation from non-neoplastic tissues. *Proc Natl Acad Sci USA* 78:5339–5343, 1981.

53. Rushmore TH, Morton MR, Pickett CB: The antioxidant responsive element. *J Biol Chem* 266:11632–11639, 1991.

54. Shahzeidi S, Sarnstrand B, Jeffery PK, et al: Oral *N*-acetylcysteine reduces bleomycin-induced collagen deposition in the lungs of mice. *Eur Respir J* 4:845–852, 1991.

55. Spragg RG: DNA strand break formation following exposure of bovine pulmonary artery and aortic endothelial cells to reactivate oxygen products. *Am J Respir Cell Mol Biol* 4:4–10, 1991.

56. Spragg RG, Hinshaw DB, Hyslop PA, et al: Alterations in adenosine triphosphate and energy charge in cultured endothelial and P388D$_1$ cells after oxidant injury. *J Clin Invest* 76:1471–1476, 1985.

57. Spurzem JR, Sacco O, Rickard KA, et al: Transforming growth factor-β increases adhesion but not migration of bovine bronchial epithelial cells to matrix proteins. *J Lab Clin Med* 122:92–102, 1993.

58. Yamaya M, Sekizawa K, Masuda T, et al: Oxidants affect permeability and repair of the cultured human tracheal epithelium. *Am J Physiol* 268:L284–L293, 1995.

59. Zambruno G, Marchisio PC, Marconi A, et al: Transforming growth Factor-β_1 modulates β_1 and β_5 integrin receptors and induces the de novo expression of the $\alpha_V\beta_6$ heterodimer in normal human keratinocytes: Implications for wound healing. *J Cell Biol* 129:853–865, 1995.

PART THREE

SYMPTOMS AND SIGNS OF RESPIRATORY DISEASE

SECTION 6

CLINICAL APPROACH TO THE PATIENT

CHAPTER 28

APPROACH TO THE PATIENT WITH RESPIRATORY SYMPTOMS

Alfred P. Fishman

The most common respiratory complaint for which a person seeks medical help is either shortness of breath or cough. Less common are hemoptysis, thoracic pain, cyanosis, and an abnormal breathing pattern. As in the case of any medical evaluation, the paramount diagnostic mainstays are the history and physical examination. The use of chest radiography for routine screening, once popular in the hope of uncovering silent disease amenable to therapy, has fallen into disuse because it has not proved to be cost-effective or worth either the inconvenience to the patient or the exposure to radiation. Instead, chest radiography is now generally reserved for patients who have clinical manifestations of chest disease or are from families or populations known to be particularly vulnerable to chest disease. Serial chest radiographs are often invaluable in providing clues to the nature of chest lesions. More sophisticated diagnostic measures and interventions are described in subsequent chapters. Regardless of whether the analysis and diagnostic synthesis are accomplished in the clinician's mind or by computer-assisted mathematical modeling, the history, physical examination, and chest radiograph generally constitute the three-legged underpinning for diagnosis in chest medicine.[4,7,9,12]

HISTORY

Even though seasoned clinicians may be adept at spotting telltale diagnostic clues, there still is no substitute for a comprehensive, penetrating medical history. This should include a detailed inventory of substances in the air that can harm the lungs. One of the most common is cigarette smoking. An attempt should be made to quantify the exposure. When did it begin? When did

it stop? How many per day (expressed in number of pack-years)? The workplace is often the site where toxic air is breathed. An almost forgotten exposure to materials 20 years ago can explain certain types of pulmonary or pleural diseases. A newly installed home humidifier or an air-conditioning system that incorporates stagnant pools of water can point the way to resolving a mysterious illness. A brief residence in an area where either cryptococcosis (southwestern United States) or histoplasmosis (south and midwest United States) is endemic may help to clarify the nature of an illness that mimics tuberculosis. A recent visit to a Latin American country may bring into focus a more remote possibility (e.g., South American blastomycosis) (Fig. 28-1).[18,37,45,47]

Personal habits of the patient, such as intravenous drug abuse or unorthodox sexual practices, may also help to uncover the cause of an unusual pulmonary disorder. Recent treatment of a neoplastic disorder with immunosuppressive agents can raise suspicion of toxicity caused by the therapeutic agent or pulmonary infection by organisms that are usually noninvasive.

Certain pharmacologic agents have the propensity for inflicting lung damage. Among these are bleomycin, nitrofurantoin, and methotrexate (Fig. 28-2). Beta blockers, administered as part of a cardiac regimen, can evoke undesirable bronchoconstriction. Even a common agent like aspirin may, on rare occasions, cause a severe pulmonary disorder (e.g., pulmonary edema).[11]

The family history is an essential ingredient of the medical inventory. This history can be particularly helpful in uncovering heritable diseases of the lungs (e.g., cystic fibrosis, α_1-antitrypsin deficiency, alveolar microlithiasis, and hereditary telangiectasia). The unraveling of a familial history of asthma, a common disease, and of primary pulmonary hypertension, a rare disease, can be much more difficult.

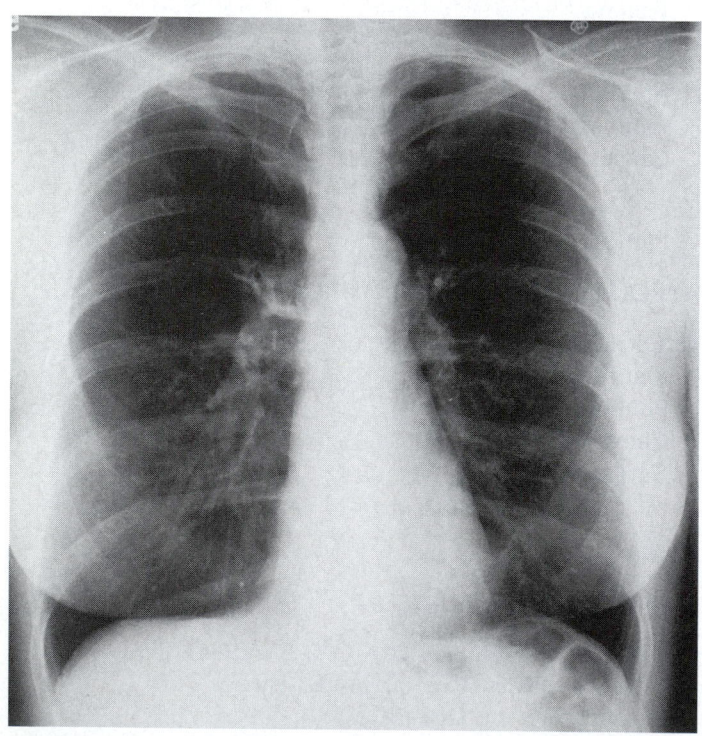

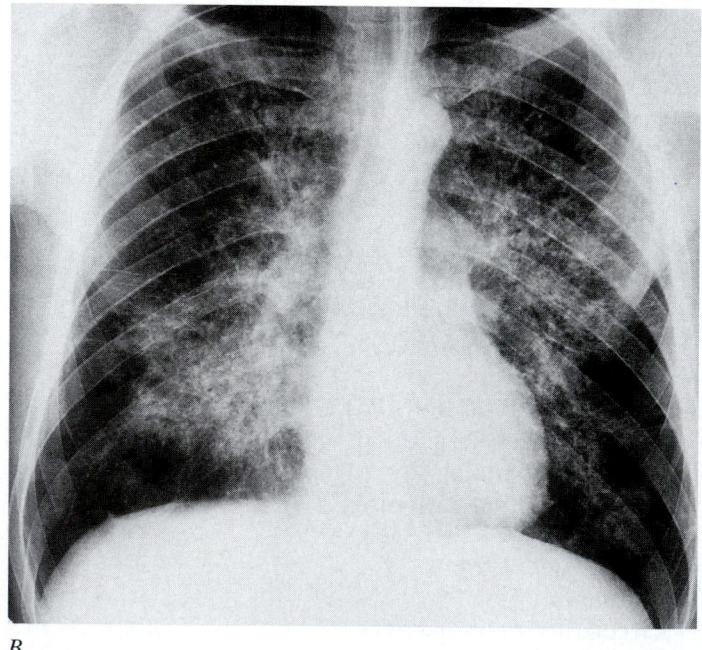

A

B

FIGURE 28-1   Exposure in an edemic area. *A.* Histoplasmosis. Nodule in right middle lobe.

B. South American blastomycosis. *(Courtesy of Dr. Nelson Porto.)*

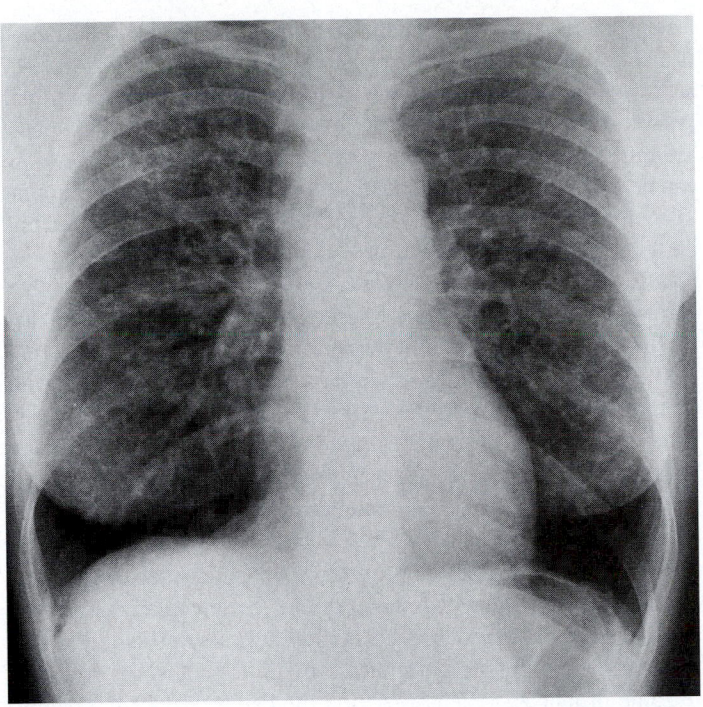

FIGURE 28-2 Nitrofurantoin hypersensitivity pneumonitis. The ingestion of nitrofurantoin, 50 mg qid, was accompanied by the appearance of patchy interstitial and alveolar changes throughout both lungs.

PHYSICAL EXAMINATION

Before the widespread use of chest radiography, the physical examination, along with the history, played a more pivotal role in the diagnosis of pulmonary disease. Although the advent of chest radiography and of more sophisticated methods of imaging has tended to deemphasize the value of the physical examination, recent emphasis on cost-effectiveness and efficiency in medical evaluations has underscored the proper role of physical examination in the diagnostic appraisal.

General Aspects   Important clues are often available before attention is directed to examination of the chest. Neglected pyorrheal teeth raise the prospect of a necrotizing aspiration pneumonia. A lacerated tongue suggests that a convulsive episode may have led to aspiration (Fig. 28-3). Subtle changes in consciousness or coordination may signal that metastasis has occurred to the brain from a primary carcinoma of the lung. In the patient with chronic obstructive pulmonary disease (COPD), a clouded sensorium or a disturbed personality can signify acute CO_2 retention.

Traditionally, evidence to support the diagnosis of pulmonary sarcoidosis is sought in the eyes and skin. Petechiae in the skin may reflect a systemic vasculitis that also affects the vessels of the lungs. The presence of a gallop rhythm alerts the examiner to a cardiac, rather than a pulmonary, origin of an asthmatic attack. The skin lesions of von Recklinghausen's disease may signify that a solitary pulmonary nodule in the paraspinal region may be a neurofibroma.

A variety of endocrine syndromes can accompany a carcinoma of the lung. Also, a number of clinical disorders can be associated with clubbing of the digits (Table 28-1). Among these

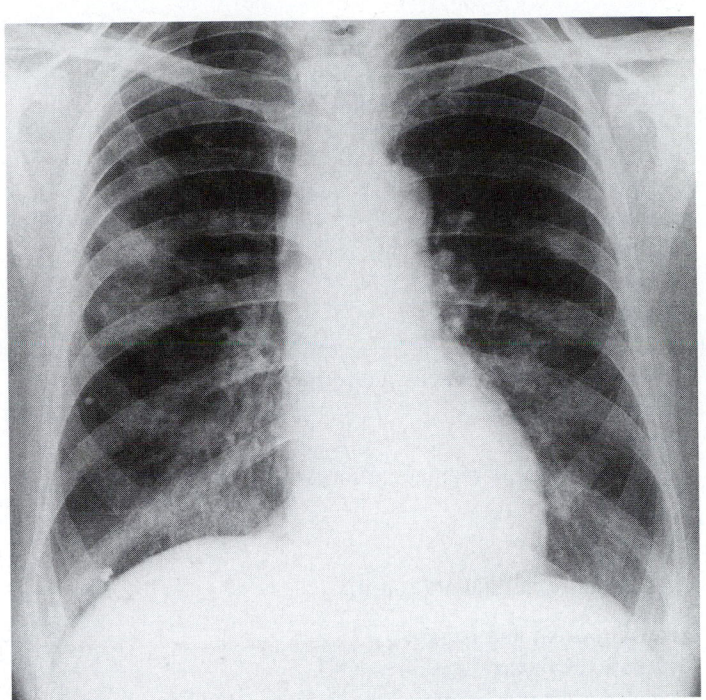

A

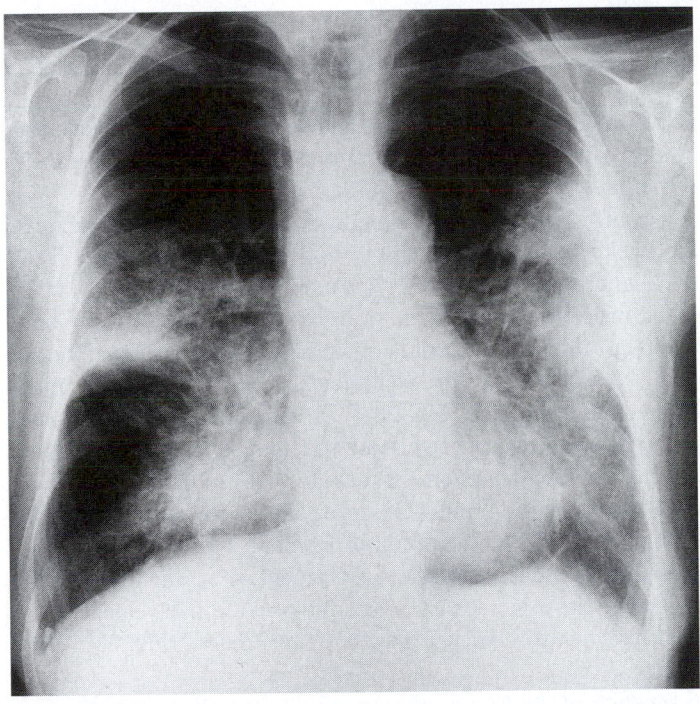

B

FIGURE 28-3 Chronic aspiration pneumonia. *A.* Chronic aspiration pneumonia in a 72-year-old man hospitalized for repair of hernia. Patchy infiltrates bilaterally. No pulmonary manifestations. Initiating cause was achalasia of esophagus. *B.* Eighteen months later. Persistent cough and breathlessness. Initiating cause was achalasia of the esophagus.

are idiopathic pulmonary fibrosis, bronchiectasis, and certain carcinomas of the lung. A minute skin abscess can turn out to be the source of multiple lung abscesses. Distinctive scars over the antecubital veins of a drug addict can help to clarify the etiology of old lesions in the lungs as well as of fresh abscesses. Erythema

TABLE 28-1

Clinical Disorders Commonly Associated with Clubbing of Digits

Pulmonary and thoracic
   Primary lung cancer
   Metastatic lung cancer
   Bronchiectasis
   Cystic fibrosis
   Lung abscess
   Pulmonary fibrosis
   Pulmonary arteriovenous malformations
   Empyema
   Mesothelioma
   Neurogenic diaphragmatic tumors

Cardiac
   Congenital
   Subacute bacterial endocarditis

Gastrointestinal and hepatic
   Hepatic cirrhosis
   Chronic ulcerative colitis
   Regional enteritis (Crohn's disease)

Miscellaneous
   Hemiplegia

nodosum and erythema multiforme occasionally complicate sarcoidosis, tuberculosis, histoplasmosis, and coccidioidomycosis; sometimes they are part of a drug reaction.

A puffy face, neck, and eyelids, coupled with dilated veins of the neck, shoulder, thorax, and upper arm (i.e., superior vena cava syndrome), occasionally constitute the first clinical evidence of extrinsic obstruction of the superior vena cava by a neoplasm of the lung. Although the causes of superior vena cava syndrome are many and diverse, at least 80 percent are attributable to a primary carcinoma of the lung (Fig. 28-4). In the patient in whom a neoplasm has evoked acute signs and symptoms of increased systemic venous pressure that progresses rapidly (e.g., to laryngeal edema), early diagnosis and prompt treatment of the neoplasm may be lifesaving. Similarly, the detection of Horner's syndrome—unilateral ptosis, miosis, and anhidrosis—in a patient with a carcinoma of the lung suggests a pulmonary sulcus tumor with involvement of the ipsilateral sympathetic pathway within the thorax (Fig. 28-5).

Inspection of the Chest   Observation of the chest from the foot of the bed can be informative: a visible lag of one side of the thorax localizes a pleural effusion, pulmonary infection, or paralyzed diaphragm. The position of the trachea with respect to the midline can be a useful clue to atelectasis of one lobe or to obstruction of a major bronchus. Inspection of the chest and abdomen during sleep may reveal the paradoxical inward movement of the abdomen that is characteristic of obstructive sleep apnea. Thoracoabdominal discoordination in the supine position raises the possibility of bilateral diaphragmatic paresis or paralysis.

Palpation of the Chest   Over the years, the role of palpation in the examination of the chest has been considerably devalued. Nonethe-

less, palpation can provide helpful diagnostic clues as well as confirmatory evidence for other physical signs. For example, the position of the trachea determined by palpation in the suprasternal notch can be helpful in detecting a lateral shift of the upper mediastinum. Displacement of the apical impulse and cardiac dullness can be useful as indices in detecting shift of the lower mediastinum. Tenderness over a rib may reflect a fracture, a metastasis, or an underlying pleuritis. Enlargement of the right ventricle can be more readily detected by palpation in the subxiphoid region than by other surface examination. Hoover's sign (elicited by comparing the displacement from the midline during a deep inspiration of the examinee's hands, each placed lightly over one hemithorax, with thumbs touching beneath the xiphoid at the start of the breath) can be useful in disclosing a unilateral lag in motion of one side of the chest due to pleuritis or a pleural effusion.

Consolidation of the lung, which causes increased transmission of sound, can be detected as femitus (i.e., as a palpable vibration) over the affected area while the patient repeats the traditional "one, two, three" as the examiner systematically moves the palms over the two hemithoraces. Conversely, impairment of sound transmission, as by a pleural effusion, diminishes vocal fremitus. In some instances, a pleural friction rub can be palpated. Overall, the more seasoned the chest physician, the more likely is palpation to get its full due in the physical examination of the chest.

Percussion of the Chest   Percussion for physical examination has followed Auenbrugger's sounding of beer barrels to determine their fluid levels. The response to percussion is impaired whenever something other than air-filled lung lies directly beneath the chest wall. Common causes are consolidation or atelectasis of the lung, fluid in the pleural space, pleural thickening, and a large mass at the surface of the lung. Distinction should be made between dullness and flatness: dullness is characteristic of pneumonic consolidation or atelectasis, whereas flatness is characteristic of a large pleural effusion or a high diaphragm. Widespread hyperresonance can often be elicited in emphysema and circumscribed hyperresonance over a pneumothorax or large bulla. As a rule, a decrease in breath sounds, as over a large bulla, is more characteristic than an increase in resonance.

Ausculation of Lungs   Ever since the time of Laennec, physicians have applied the stethoscope to the chest in search of sounds of disease. The intensity and transmission of breath sounds, as well as adventitious sounds, feature prominently in this search.[8,23,24,26,30]

Intensity and Duration of Lung Sounds   A global decrease in the intensity of breath sounds over the thorax or hemithorax can be due to a variety of abnormalities: impaired movement of air (e.g., in emphysema), paralysis of a diaphragm, complete obstruction of a bronchus, and impaired transmission of sounds to the chest wall (e.g., in pleural effusion, pleural thickening, pneumothorax). A bulla gives rise to a more circumscribed diminution in breath sounds. In a patient with COPD, regional variations in breath sounds correspond to the distribution of ventilation.

An abnormal increase in intensity of breath sounds is accompanied by a change in their character (the sounds become either harsh or bronchial). The abnormal sounds are heard over consolidated, atelectatic, or compressed lung as long as the air-

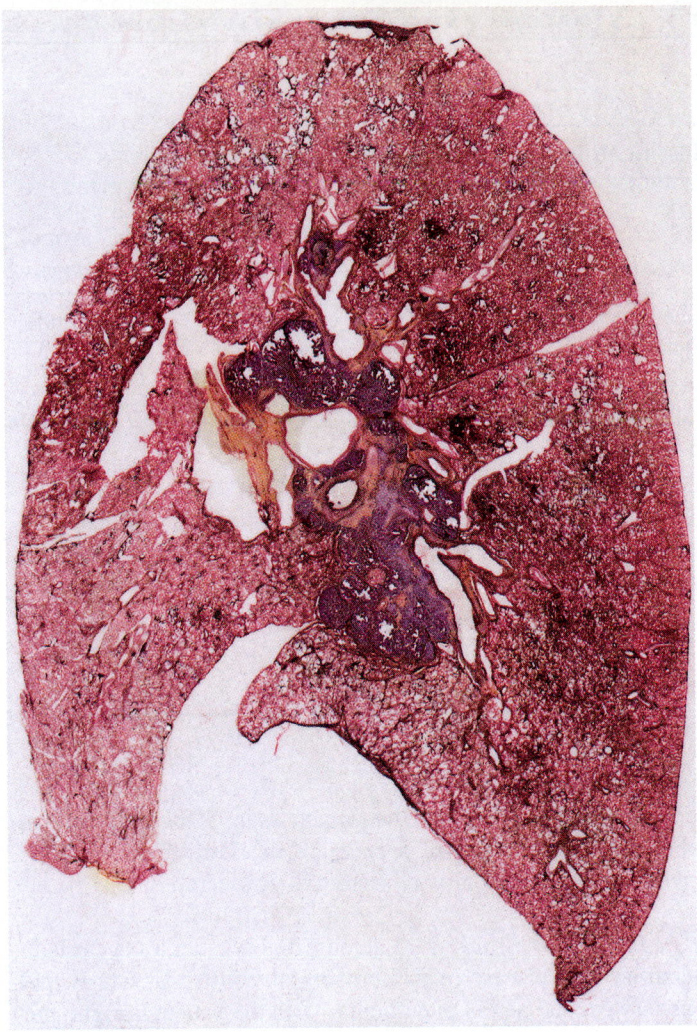

A

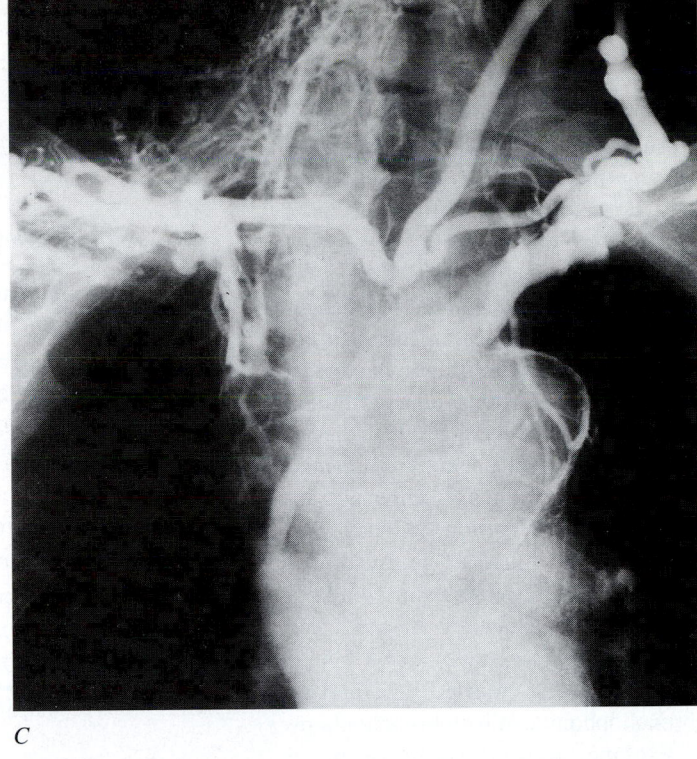

C

FIGURE 28-4 Local invasiveness of carcinoma of the lung. *A.* Sagittal section of the lung illustrating a carcinoma (blue) of the lung in the vicinity of the hilus. *B.* Chest radiograph showing right hilar mass. *C.* Angiogram showing site of obstruction (arrow) and extensive collateral circulation.

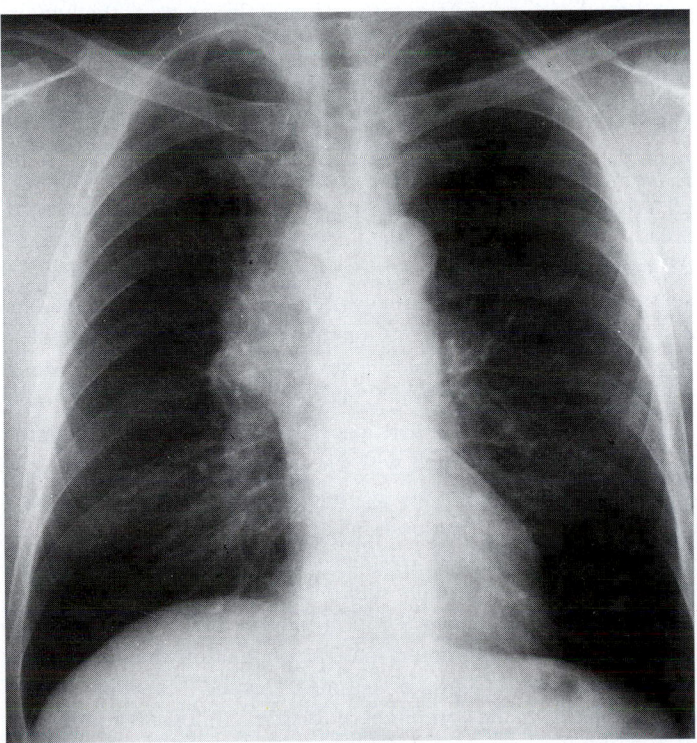

B

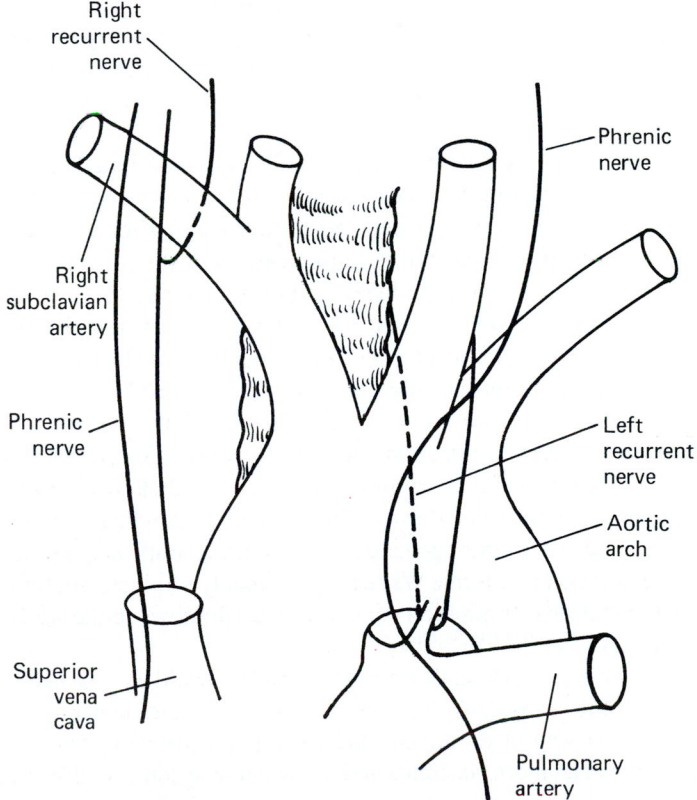

FIGURE 28-5 Courses of the recurrent laryngeal nerves. Invasion or compression of a nerve by a carcinoma of the lung causes ipselateral paralysis of the ipselateral vocal cord.

way to the affected portion of the lung remains patent. Consolidated lung is presumed to act as an acoustic conducting medium that, unlike normal lung, does not attenuate transmission of tracheal sounds to the periphery.

Transmission of Lung Sounds   Changes in voice sounds are often easier to appreciate than changes in breath sounds. Large pleural effusions, pneumothorax, and bronchial occlusion produce distant or inaudible breath sounds. Transmission of voice sounds is enhanced by consolidation, infarction, atelectasis, or compressions of lung tissue. Accompanying the increased transmission is a change in the character of the voice sounds that causes them to be higher pitched and less muffled than normal (bronchophony). When bronchophony is extreme, spoken words assume a nasal or bleating quality (egophony) and the sound "ee" is heard through the stethoscope as "ay." Egophony is most common when consolidated lung and pleural fluid coexist; sometimes it is heard over an uncomplicated lobar pneumonia or pulmonary infarction. Transmission of whispered voice sounds with abnormal clarity (whispered pectoriloquy) has the same significance as bronchophony.

A pleural friction rub is a coarse, grating, or leathery sound that is usually heard late in inspiration and early in expiration, most often low in the axilla or over the lung base posteriorly. It sounds close to the ear and usually is not altered by coughing.

Adventitious Lung Sounds   Lung sounds have traditionally been resistant to meaningful clinical classification. The American Thoracic Society attempted to develop a rational and clinically useful classification based on acoustic analysis of tape recordings and the nomenclature introduced by Forgacs (Table 28-2). With this approach, lung sounds are categorized as continuous (wheezes, rhonchi, or stridor) or discontinuous (crackles). Crackles (or rales) are further identified as fine or coarse.[8]

Wheezes, rhonchi, and stridor are musical adventitious sounds. Wheezes originate in airways narrowed by spasm, thickening of the mucosa, or luminal obstruction. Although wheezes are more apt to occur during forced expiration, which further narrows airways, they generally occur during both inspiration and expiration in asthma. Wheezes presumably originate through a combination of limitation to airflow and vibrations in the walls of the airways.[10,13,14,36,49]

Stridor is predominantly inspiratory and best heard over the neck. The common causes of stridor are a foreign body in the upper intrathoracic airway or esophagus and an acquired lesion of the airway (e.g., carcinoma in adults and a congenital lesion in children).

Early Inspiratory Crackles   Early inspiratory crackles are probably due to a rapid succession of explosive openings of small airways that closed prematurely during the previous expiration. Crackles that clear after a cough or two probably reflect secre-

TABLE 28-2

Classification of Common Lung Sounds

Acoustic Characteristics	American Thoracic Society Nomenclature	Common Synonyms
Discontinuous, interrupted explosive sounds; loud, low in pitch	Coarse crackle	Coarse rale
Discontinuous, interrupted explosive sounds; less loud than above and of shorter duration; higher in pitch than course crackles or rales	Fine crackle	Fine rale, crepitation
Continuous sounds longer than 250 ms, high-pitched; dominant frequency of 400 Hz or more, hissing sound	Wheeze	Sibilant rhonchus
Continuous sounds longer than 250 ms, low-pitched; dominant frequency about 200 Hz or less, snoring sound	Rhonchus	Sonorous rhonchus

SOURCE: Loudon R, Murphy RLH: Lung sounds: *Am Rev Respir Dis* 130:663–673, 1984.

tions in the airways; those that linger, as in COPD, are presumably the consequences of a decrease in elastic recoil (emphysema) or increase in airway secretions (bronchitis).[42]

Late Inspiratory Crackles   Late inspiratory crackles occur in interstitial lung disease (e.g., fibrosing alveolitis, asbestosis, pulmonary edema) and in pneumonia. With the patient upright, they are best heard at the lung bases; they shift toward the dependent parts of the lungs when the position changes. These crackles persist throughout the course of the disease. In contrast, the late inspiratory crackles that occur at the lung bases in the elderly or bedridden can be made to disappear with a few deep breaths.

DYSPNEA

Dyspnea is the medical term for breathlessness or shortness of breath. In the extensive medical, physiological, and psychological literature, this single term is used to designate a variety of sensations that range from an awareness of breathing, on the one hand, to respiratory distress, on the other. The wide range of meanings is understandable on several counts: (1) dyspnea is a subjective complaint without consistency in objective signs such as tachypnea; (2) few physicians have experienced the respiratory discomfort associated with chest disease, so most interpretations of the complaint are extrapolations from normal breathlessness (e.g., after strenuous exercise); (3) most experimental observations relating to dyspnea are based on the study of normal subjects or animals under artificial circumstances; and (4) most physicians apply the term loosely, based on their experience with the predominant patient population that they serve (e.g., patients with COPD or asthma). Despite this variability, in clinical medicine the complaint of dyspnea almost invariably implies respiratory discomfort.[1,19]

Because of its subjective nature, the sensation of dyspnea is an amalgam of two components.[15,33] The *first* is the sensory input to the cerebral cortex, which consists of information from specialized receptors, predominantly mechanoreceptors, at various sites in the respiratory apparatus (predominantly upper airways) and face (Fig. 28-6). The different sites of stimulation may contribute to the disparities in the sensation. No specific area in the central nervous system has been identified as the sensory site for dyspnea. The input—from airways, lungs (via the vagus nerves), respiratory muscles, chest wall, and chemoreceptors—is processed at consecutive levels of the nervous system (i.e., spinal cord and supraspinal regions en route to the sensorimotor cortex). The *second* component is the perception of the sensation, which rests heavily on the interpretation of information arriving at the sensorimotor cortex. The interpretation depends greatly on the psychological makeup of the person.[53]

A variety of influences can modify the psychological component of dyspnea.[29] During "Kussmaul breathing" (see page 376),

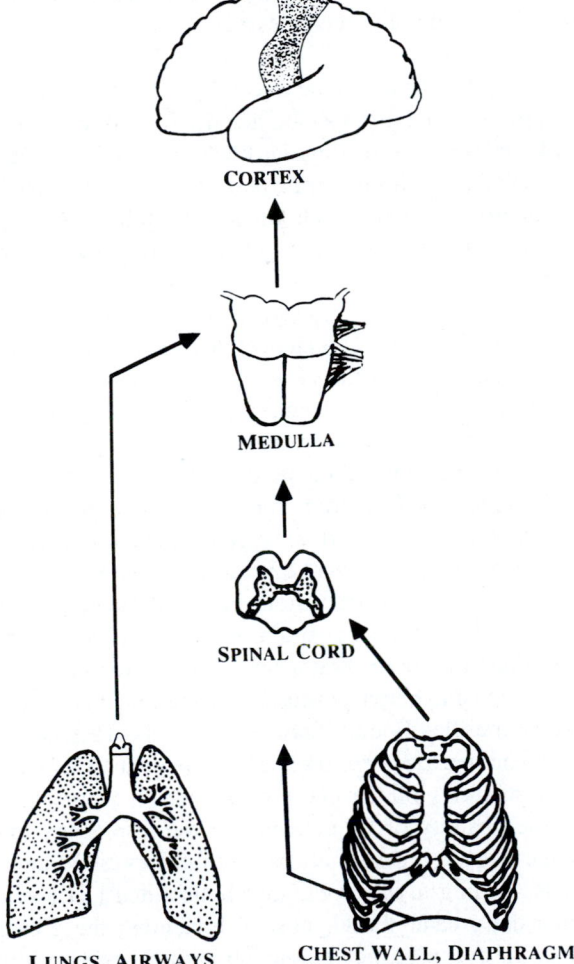

CORTEX

MEDULLA

SPINAL CORD

LUNGS, AIRWAYS

CHEST WALL, DIAPHRAGM

MECHANORECEPTORS
LARYNGEAL
AIRWAY SMOOTH MUSCLES
AIRWAY EPITHELIUM
INTERSTITIUM

MECHANORECEPTORS
INTERCOSTAL MUSCLES
DIAPHRAGM
TENDONS, JOINTS
CHEMORECEPTORS

FIGURE 28-6 Pathways to the sensation of breathlessness. Multiple sources of sensory information from mechanoreceptors in the upper airways, thorax, and muscles are integrated in the central nervous system and perceived according to the psychological makeup of the patient. The combination of sensory input and perception is responsible for the sensation of dyspnea. In turn, the output from the sensorimotor cortex provides the motor drive to the respiratory muscles.

"air hunger" may seem obvious to the observer, even though the patient does not feel short of breath. In contrast, patients with congestive heart failure or COPD frequently volunteer the complaint of "air hunger." Blunting of the sensorium, as by narcotics or by acute hypercapnia, can eliminate the sensation of breathlessness, even though the breathing pattern remains unchanged. Anxiety can heighten the sense of breathlessness. Indeed, anxiety can be responsible for the clinical syndrome of psychogenic dyspnea, in which the patient experiences "a sense of smothering" or "an inability to take a deep breath" without somatic cause. These ill-defined sensations may accompany a full-blown hyperventilation syndrome consisting of light-headedness, tingling of the hands and feet, tachycardia, inversion of T waves on the electrocardiogram, and even syncope. Usually, psychogenic dyspnea poses no diagnostic problem.

The quality of dyspnea can vary greatly. In normal persons, as well as in those with chest disease, dyspnea may simply signify the transition from an effortless process that is ordinarily conducted at a subconscious level to the awareness that muscular effort is being expended in breathing. The healthy athlete completing a dash experiences breathlessness that can be exhilarating rather than uncomfortable. The asthmatic often interprets breathlessness in terms of "tightness in the chest." The patient with COPD often complains of less-severe breathlessness than would be expected from the degree of airway obstruction, possibly reflecting adaptation either to the chronic obstructive airway disease or to CO_2 retention.

TABLE 28-3

Causes of Acute and Chronic Dyspnea*

Acute
  Pulmonary edema
  Asthma
  Injury to chest wall and intrathoracic structures
  Spontaneous pneumothorax
  Pulmonary embolism
  Pneumonia
  Adult respiratory distress syndrome
  Pleural effusion
  Pulmonary hemorrhage

Chronic, progressive
  Chronic obstructive pulmonary disease
  Left ventricular failure
  Diffuse interstitial fibrosis
  Asthma
  Pleural effusions
  Pulmonary thromboembolic disease
  Pulmonary vascular disease
  Psychogenic dyspnea
  Anemia, severe
  Postintubation tracheal stenosis
  Hypersensitivity disorders

*Asthma and acute left ventricular failure represent chronic causes with paroxysmal exacerbations.

Clinical Presentations

Dyspnea may be acute, chronic, or paroxysmal (Table 28-3).

Acute   The causes of acute dyspnea in children differ from those in adults. In children, upper-airway infection (epiglotitis, laryngitis, or acute laryngotracheobronchitis) is a common cause. In adults, the causes of acute dyspnea are much more varied (Table 28-2). Among the most common are an episode of acute left ventricular failure, a thromboembolic event, pneumonia, and spontaneous pneumothorax. Less common, but not unusual, is massive collapse of one lung due to inability to clear the airways of thick tenacious secretions (e.g., chronic bronchitis or asthma) or the first attack of asthma.

Chronic (and Progressive) Dyspnea   Chronic dyspnea is almost invariably progressive. As a rule, this type of dyspnea begins with breathlessness on exertion—which, in time, progresses to dyspnea at rest. Chest physicians commonly encounter dyspnea due to COPD; cardiologists are more often faced with patients in chronic congestive heart failure. Especially in older patients, distinction between the heart and lungs in the etiology of dyspnea, or the relative contributions of each, can be difficult to establish.

The most common cause of recurrent bouts of dyspnea is asthma. As a rule, in these patients breathlessness is accompanied by cough and wheezing. One special type of asthma, especially in middle-aged or elderly persons, is cardiac asthma, which is a manifestation of paroxysmal nocturnal dyspnea due to acute left ventricular failure and resultant pulmonary edema. Another, much less frequent cause of paroxysmal wheezing and breathlessness is bronchopulmonary aspergillosis. In parts of the world where schistosomiasis is endemic, an attack of asthma may signal the migratory stage of schistosomiasis (i.e., larvae traversing the lungs). An extraordinary cause of episodic asthma can be a carcinoid that has metastasized to the liver.

Physiological Correlates of Dyspnea

Historically, attempts to understand the physiological bases of dyspnea have evolved along four separate lines: ventilatory performance, mechanics of breathing, chemoreception, and exercise testing.[34,35,5,50]

Ventilatory Performance   The earliest investigations related dyspnea to minute ventilation. Dyspnea was found to correlate with an excessive minute ventilation for the level of oxygen uptake. Most of the increase in ventilation was accounted for by an increase in respiratory rate, especially in patients with stiff lungs. In patients who continued to ventilate excessively for the level of oxygen uptake (e.g., those with chronic left ventricular failure), the sensation of breathlessness gradually diminished, suggesting adaptation to the continued stimulus.

A second ventilatory measurement that proved to correlate well with dyspnea is the maximum voluntary ventilation (MVV). MVV is decreased by diseases of the lungs, airways, or chest cage. The smaller the maximum breathing capacity, the more apt is dyspnea to occur.

A third time-honored approach to measurement is the "breathing reserve." This value is determined as the difference between MVV and the actual minute ventilation. In principle, the sensation of breathlessness during the performance of any ventilatory task may be related to the fraction of the maximum capacity that is used for force generation by the respiratory apparatus. Thus, the closer the minute ventilation to the maximum breathing capacity, the more likely is the subject to complain of breathlessness. Indeed, when the actual level of ventilation reaches 30 to 40 percent of the maximum breathing capacity, dyspnea is inevitable. Unfortunately, the breathing reserve correlates better with the dyspnea of normal subjects during exertion than with the dyspnea of chronic bronchitis and COPD or of left ventricular failure. Thus, in COPD the minute ventilation may be a very large fraction of the MVV (greater than 50 percent) without eliciting dyspnea. In contrast, in acute left ventricular failure, a mild increase in ventilation and a nearly normal MVV may be associated with considerable breathlessness.

Mechanics of Breathing   One teleologic way to regard dyspnea is as a sensation that prompts an unconscious effort to minimize the work, energy cost, or force of breathing. In this light, dyspnea protects the respiratory apparatus from overwork and inefficient operation. This approach has led to exploration of the relationships between dyspnea and work or oxygen cost of breathing.

Work, Oxygen Cost, and Efficiency of Breathing   It has not been possible to identify a critical level for the work of breathing at which dyspnea will occur. However, a breakdown of the work of breathing into its elastic, resistive, and inertial components has helped to relate physiological disturbances to particular diseases. For example, in chronic mitral stenosis with pulmonary congestion, the elastic work is greatly increased (Fig. 28-7), whereas in obstructive airway disease, resistive work predominates. Moreover, such observations have reinforced the concept that patterns of breathing are automatically adjusted to minimize the work done by the respiratory muscles in breathing.

The relationship between ventilation and O_2 consumed by the respiratory muscles is curvilinear (Fig. 28-8). This O_2 cost of breathing can increase extraordinarily in patients with COPD or with abnormalities of the chest wall. Indeed, in patients with COPD, the quantity of O_2 delivered to the respiratory muscles during the large ventilatory effort may fail to satisfy their aerobic needs, leading to anaerobic metabolism and lactic acidosis. Although the greater the O_2 cost of breathing, the greater the likelihood of dyspnea, the determination of O_2 cost provides no more useful insight into the mechanism of dyspnea than does the work of breathing. Calculation of the efficiency of breathing (i.e., the work of breathing related to energy cost) provides no further clarification.

Length-Tension Inappropriateness   The concept of "length-tension inappropriateness" explains dyspnea as a mismatch between the central motor command to the respiratory muscles (i.e., the motor signal emitted from the brain) and the suboptimal ("inappropriate") shortening of the respiratory muscles that this command elicits (e.g., suboptimal thoracic expansion for any level of central motor command). In essence, this concept pictures a

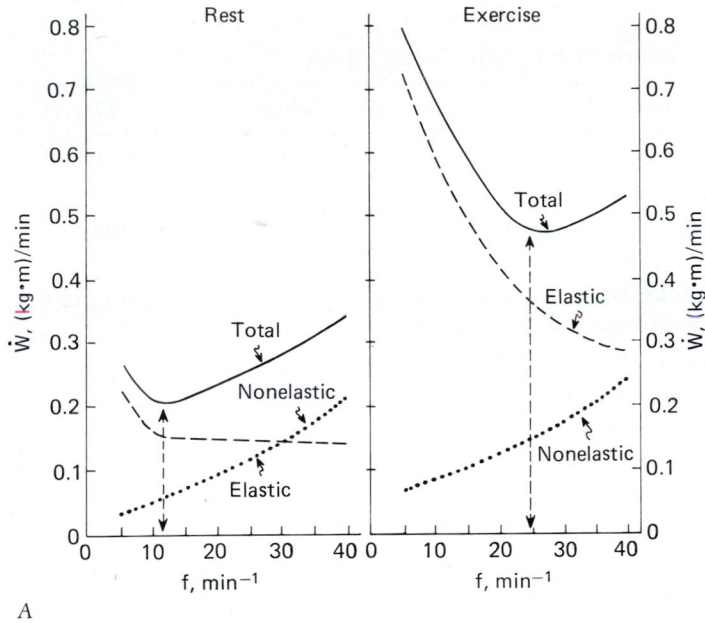

A

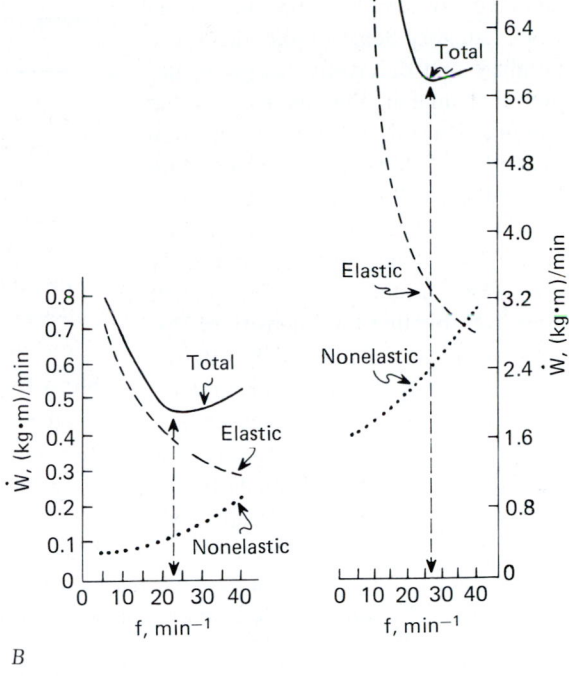

B

FIGURE 28-7 Partition of the work of breathing in pulmonary congestion and edema at rest and during exercise. *A.* Normal. The minimal work of breathing at rest was at a respiratory frequency of 12 breaths per min; during exercise, the minimal work was done at a higher frequency (25 breaths per min). *B.* Mitral stenosis. At rest, the frequency for least respiratory work was abnormally high (22 breaths per min);

during exercise it increased further (to 28 breaths per min). The dashed vertical line (capped by arrowheads) in each frame indicates the respiratory frequency at which respiratory work was minimal. *(From Christie RV: Dyspnea in relation to the visco-elastic properties of the lung. Proc R Soc Med 46:381–386, 1953, with permission.)*

decrease, instead of an increase, in the pressure-generating capacity of the respiratory muscles in the face of the increased need arising from the heightened respiratory drive.

Chemoreception   Acute hypoxia, hypercapnia, and acidosis are traditional stimuli for ventilation. For example, upon ascent to

altitude, acute hypoxia can stimulate ventilation to the level of awareness that may progress to discomfort during exertion. The effects of these stimuli on breathing decrease if they continue unabated. In addition, side effects, such as blunting of the sensorium during chronic CO_2 retention, diminish the likelihood of dyspnea, even though the level of ventilation is increased. In patients with abnormal pulmonary mechanics, the onset of abnormalities in blood gas composition, as during exercise, can aggravate or contribute to dyspnea.

Scaling   A variety of scaling methods have been devised in the attempt to quantify dyspnea during exercise and various experi-

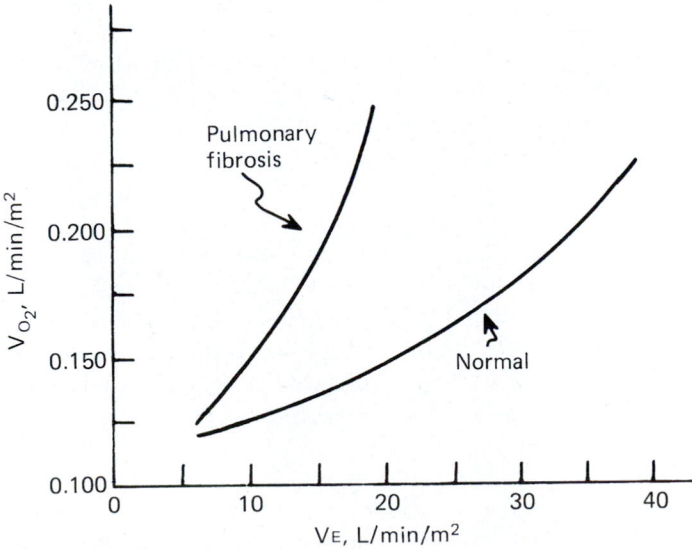

FIGURE 28-8   Oxygen cost of breathing in restrictive lung disease. Relationship between ventilation and O_2 consumption in pulmonary fibrosis. At each level of ventilation, the patient with pulmonary fibrosis does more work and expends more energy in breathing than does the normal subject.

TABLE 28-4

Modified Borg Category Scale

Rating	Intensity of Sensation
0	Nothing at all
0.5	Very, very slight (just noticeable)
1	Very slight
2	Slight
3	Moderate
4	Somewhat severe
5	Severe
6	
7	Very severe
8	
9	Very, very severe (almost maximal)
10	Maximal

mental conditions.[38] Some, such as the Borg Category Scale (Table 28-4), use numbers and descriptive terms to depict a change in the intensity of the stimulus ("threshold stimulus detection methods"). Others rely on visual analog scales, which are straight lines, usually 10 cm long, that extend from "not breathless" at one end to "extremely breathless" at the other. The patient marks on this line the intensity of respiratory discomfort elicited by external stimuli, such as resistive loads or exercise testing. The score is measured as the length of the line between "not breathless" and the mark made by the patient. The Shortness of Breath Scale issued by the American Thoracic Society (Table 28-5) has been used for years in one form or another, particularly in epidemiologic studies. No single scale is applicable to all subjects or patients.

TABLE 28-5

American Thoracic Society Scale

Descriptions	Grade	Degree
Not troubled by shortness of breath when hurrying on the level or walking up a slight hill	0	None
Troubled by shortness of breath when hurrying on the level or walking up a slight hill	1	Mild
Walks more slowly than people of the same age on the level because of breathlessness or has to stop for breath when walking at own pace on the level	2	Moderate
Stops for breath after walking about 100 yards or after a few minutes on the level	3	Severe
Too breathless to leave the house; breathless on dressing or undressing	4	Very severe

Dyspnea: Overview

In general, the sensation of dyspnea seems to be related to the intensity of afferent input from thoracic structures (especially the respiratory muscles) and from the chemoreceptors (central, peripheral, local). In patients with respiratory disease, dyspnea occurs most often when breathing is impeded, mechanics of breathing are abnormal, the lungs are stiffened, ventilatory musculature is weakened, and/or chemoreceptor input is increased.[32,46,54]

Dyspnea in Chronic Pulmonary Disease

Two common types of pulmonary disease in which dyspnea features prominently are considered here: chronic obstructive airway disease and restrictive lung disease.

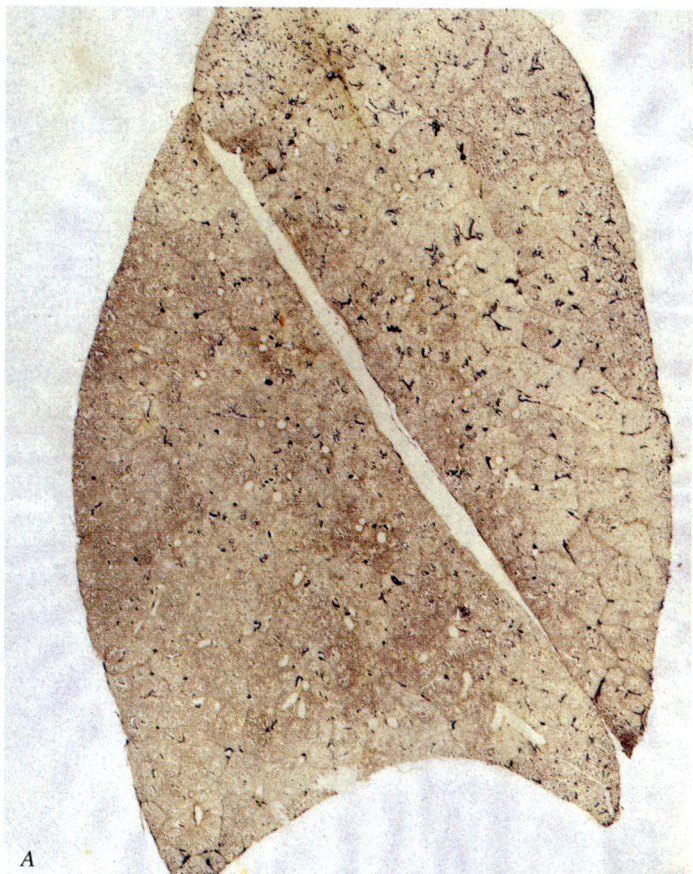

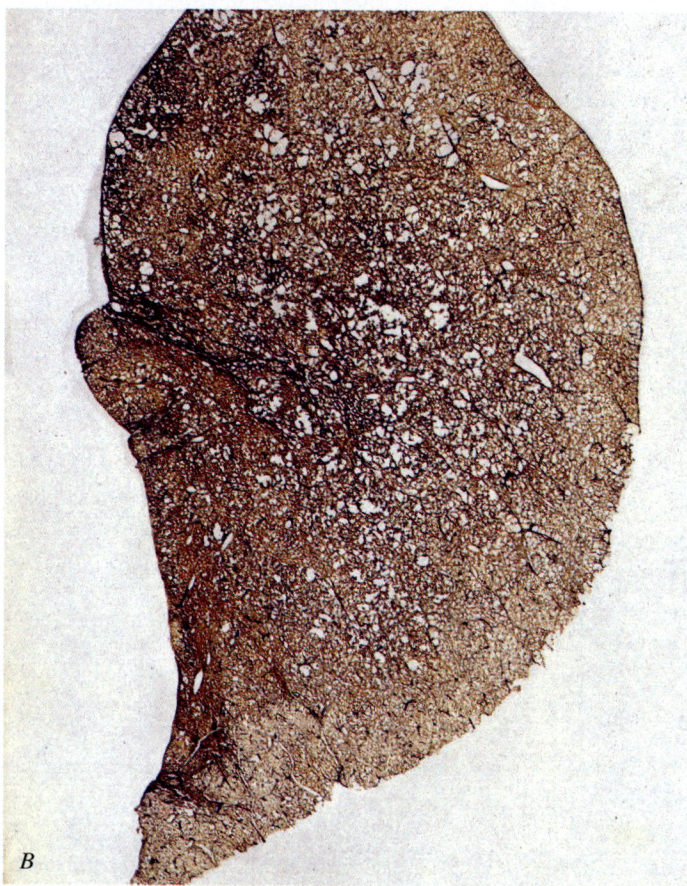

FIGURE 28-9   Chronic obstructive pulmonary disease (COPD). Sagittal sections showing patterns of emphysema. *A.* Normal lung from a patient who died of unrelated causes. *B.* Predominantly centrilobular emphysema in patient. *C.* Predominantly centrilobular and panlobular emphysema. *D.* Predominantly panlobular emphysema. Centrilobular emphysema is less marked. The three patients with emphysema also had clinical manifestations of chronic bronchitis confirmed by histologic sections.

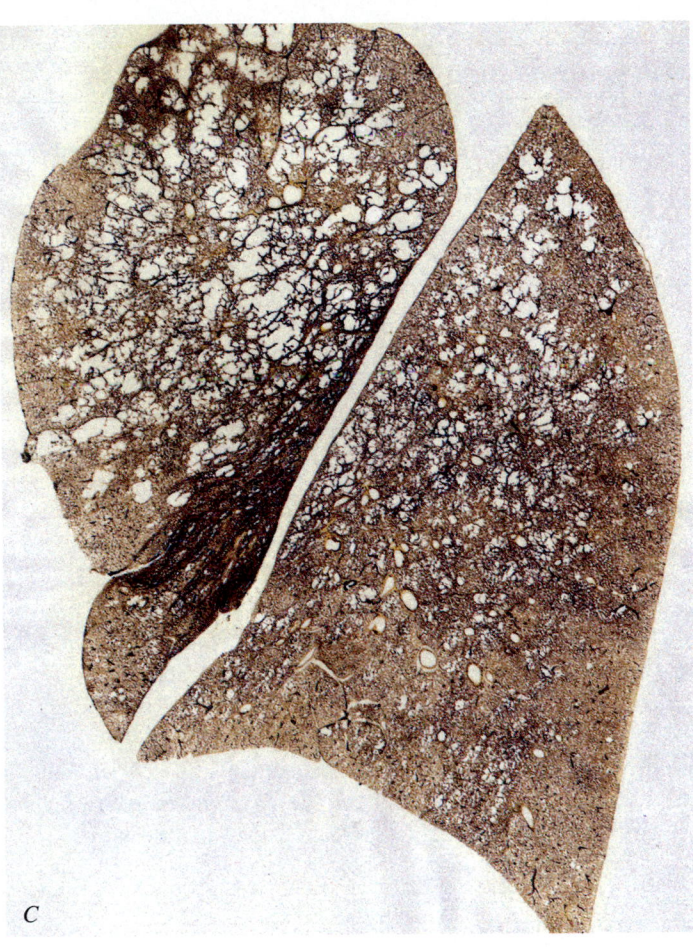

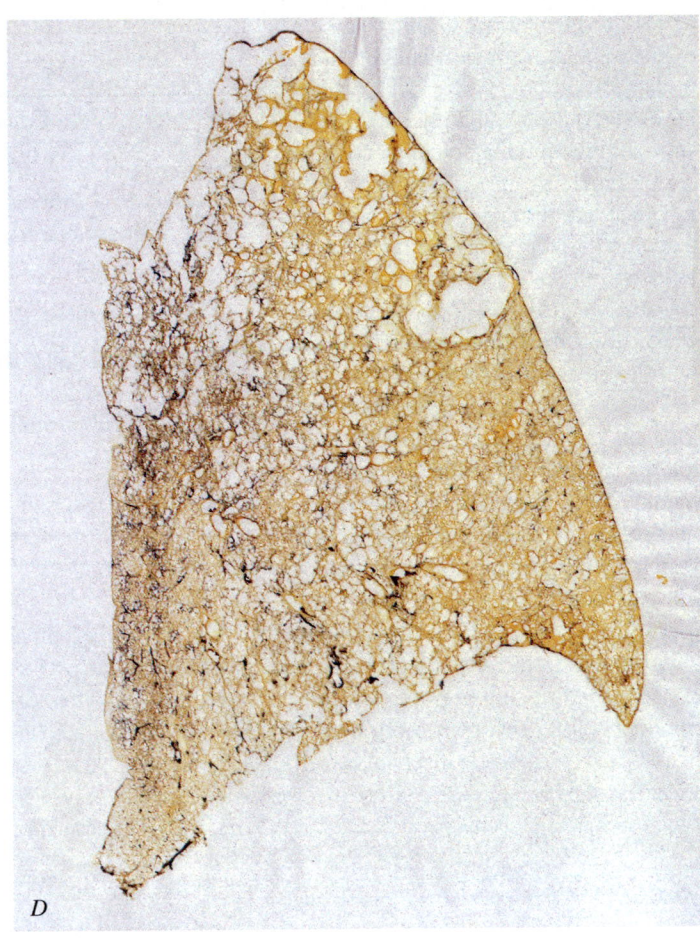

FIGURE 28-9   *(Cont.)*

Chronic Obstructive Pulmonary Disease (COPD)   COPD refers to a spectrum of airway diseases in which obstruction to airflow is the common denominator. Cigarette smoking is the leading cause of COPD. The outer limits of the spectrum are marked by chronic bronchitis at one end and emphysema at the other. Most patients with COPD fall into categories between those limits (i.e., they manifest mixtures of chronic bronchitis and emphysema that vary in degrees) (Fig. 28-9).

Asthma constitutes a different entity, not only in its clinical expressions but also because it is usually episodic, is unrelated to smoking, is often related to allergic manifestations, and generally affects younger people. Cystic fibrosis is another distinct entity because of its genetic basis, clinical and radiographic presentations, and nature of the airway obstruction (i.e., by inspissated mucus) and proclivity to superinfection.

Dyspnea is a regular feature of each of these subsets of chronic airways obstruction. Should CO_2 retention ensue, the sensation of dyspnea is apt to diminish, despite further progression in pulmonary function.

Patients with COPD suffer from disturbances in the mechanics of breathing, abnormal lung volumes, and derangements in gas exchange. The minute ventilation, which may be only slightly increased at rest, constitutes an abnormally large fraction of the maximum breathing capacity (i.e., the "breathing reserve" is low).

Abnormalities in the mechanics of breathing dominate the scene: resistance to airflow is high; the thorax assumes a hyperinflated position, placing the inspiratory muscles at mechanical disadvantage; the work of breathing is greatly increased. The O_2 cost of breathing is correspondingly high. Derangements in dead space ventilation and in alveolar-capillary gas exchange add to the afferent stimuli. As a result of the disturbances in mechanics and gas exchange, swings in pleural pressure (a measure of force applied to the lungs) are large, and a considerable muscular effort is expended in breathing; instead of the normal increase of about 1 ml of O_2 uptake per liter of ventilation per minute, the O_2 uptake increases enormously (up to 25 ml/min). Should O_2 delivery to the overworked respiratory muscles be insufficient, fatigue and exhaustion may send nervous and chemical signals of their own to the brain. Finally, should the patient accumulate excess water in the lungs, the juxtacapillary ("J") receptors provide additional sensory input to the central integrating mechanism. As noted above (see "Length-Tension Inappropriateness"), the convergence of these diverse stimuli upon the sensori-motor cortex may generate an inordinate motor command to the respiratory muscles, which cannot mobilize the thorax sufficiently to generate the pleural pressures needed for adequate ventilation.

One enigma is why some patients with COPD settle for a lower ventilation than others. For example, despite equal abnormalities in conventional pulmonary function tests, the "CO_2 retainer," with respiratory acidosis and arterial hypoxemia, often breathes less than does the non–CO_2 retainer in whom blood gas levels are near normal. One teleologic explanation is that the lower ventilation in the CO_2 retainer causes less dyspnea. However, this explanation affords no insight into the physiological mechanism.

Treatment of the patient with COPD is directed at diminishing airways resistance and restoring arterial blood gases toward normal. Unfortunately, bronchodilators and corticosteroids generally exert little effect, and the basic abnormalities in the mechanics of the lungs and airways remain. Consequently, the load on the respiratory muscles is not readily alleviated by medical management. Accordingly, therapeutic interest in these disorders has turned to ways by which the performance of the respiratory muscles can be improved. These have generally taken the form of training exercises to facilitate adaptive changes and to increase both muscle strength and endurance. Exercise reconditioning in patients with COPD has been shown to diminish breathlessness, possibly owing to three interactive mechanisms: (1) increased mechanical efficiency of the exercising muscles, which decrease ventilatory requirements; (2) improved function of the respiratory muscles; and (3) increased tolerance of the dyspneagenic sensory input to the brain.[40] Attempts to rest the respiratory muscles have no lasting effect on dyspnea.

Asthma   The mechanisms described above for COPD apply as well to asthma. However, these mechanisms do not account for the sensation of "tightness in the chest" or the inordinate sense of labored breathing that accompanies the breathlessness.

TABLE 28-6

Common Causes of Restrictive Lung Disease

Cause	Example
Interstitium	
Interstitial fibrosis and/or infiltration	Asbestosis
Pulmonary edema	Left ventricular failure
Pleura	
Pleural disease	Fibrothorax
Thoracic cage and abdomen	
Neuromuscular disease	Poliomyelitis
Skeletal abnormalities	Severe kyphoscoliosis
Marked obesity	Grossly overweight
Pulmonary vascular disease	
Pulmonary hypertensive disorders	Primary pulmonary hypertension

TABLE 28-7

Common Types of Diffuse Interstitial Disease

Etiology	Example	Common Features
Acute		
Infections	Miliary tuberculosis, histoplasmosis	Opportunity for exposure to organism
	Pneumocystis, cytomegalic inclusion virus, fungi	Immunosuppression
Radiation therapy	After mastectomy	Shortly after treatment
Pulmonary edema	Narcotic overdosage, nitrogen dioxide (silo-filler's disease), uremia	Distinctive history
Inhalation	Byssinosis	Monday morning asthma and fever
Aspiration	After loss of consciousness	History and alcoholism or epilepsy
Immunologic	Goodpasture's syndrome	Renal and pulmonary involvement
Carcinoma of lung	Alveolar cell carcinoma	
Idiopathic	Idiopathic pulmonary fibrosis	
Chronic		
Inhalation	Pneumoconioses	History of exposure
Radiation therapy	After mastectomy	Gradual evolution after treatment
Lymphangitic spread	Carcinoma of breast, lung, stomach, pancreas	Evidence of primary carcinoma
Medications	Hexamethonium, hydralazine, bleomycin, busulfan, nitrofurantoin	History, suggestive chest radiograph
Systemic disorders	Sarcoidosis, collagen disorders, histiocytosis X, amyloidosis, tuberous sclerosis	Multiorgan involvement; biopsy
Idiopathic	Diffuse interstitial fibrosis	Exclusion of known causes

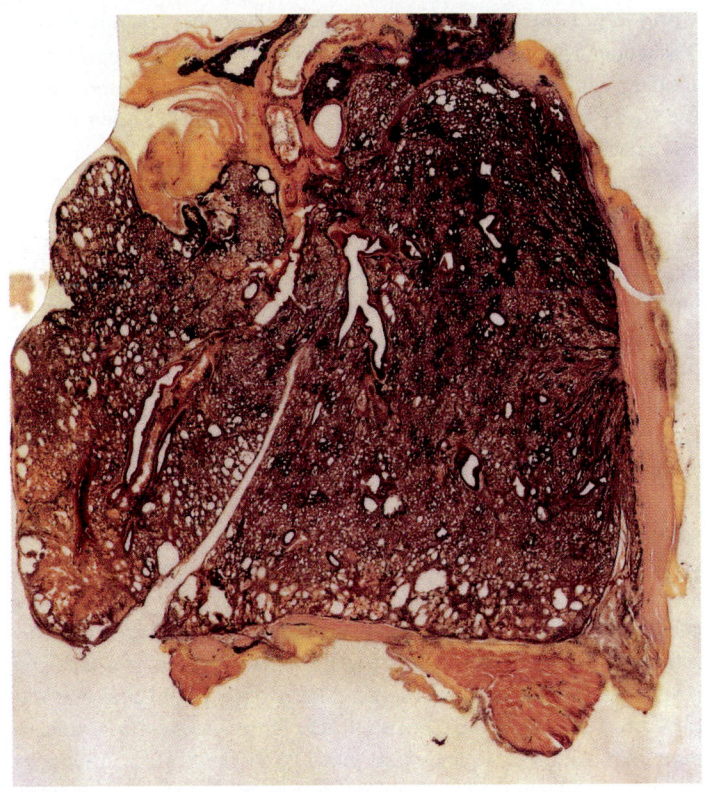

A

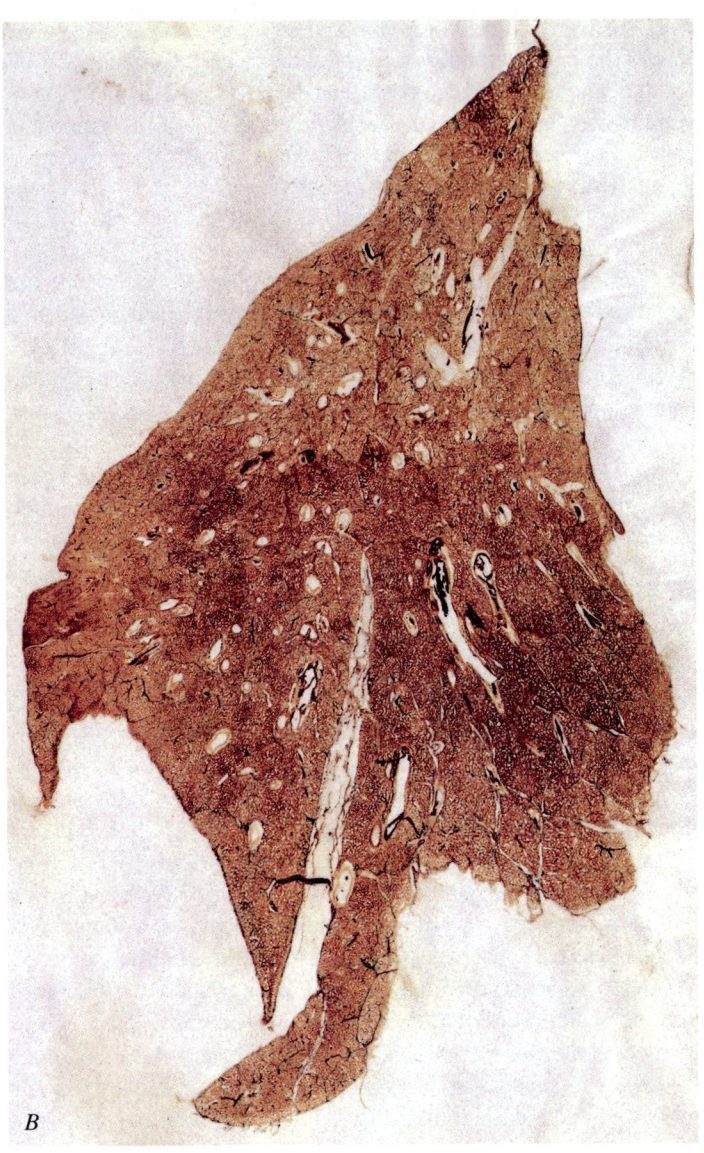

B

FIGURE 28-10   Restrictive lung disease. *A.* Asbestosis with markedly thickened pleura that encases and compresses the lungs. In addition, the lungs were afflicted with diffuse interstitial fibrosis. *B.* Compressed, distorted lung in patient with kyphoscoliosis. The lungs were otherwise normal, so that in this instance restriction was imposed by the chest wall rather than by intrapulmonary or pleural disease.

Restrictive Lung Disease   Restrictive lung diseases can be due to different causes, but usually they have in common a reduction in lung volumes and diffusing capacity (Table 28-6). One major category of restrictive lung disease is diffuse interstitial disease. Diffuse interstitial disease, in turn, has many different causes and may be either acute or chronic in onset (Table 28-7). Characteristically, in widespread interstitial disease, diffusing capacity is low and accompanied by a considerable decrease in total lung capacity and vital capacity in association with lesser decrements in functional residual capacity and residual volume. Similar findings occur in severe kyphoscoliosis or encasement of the lung by pleural thickening (Fig. 28-10). In contrast, in pulmonary vascular disease, such as primary pulmonary hypertension, a low diffusing capacity may be accompanied by normal lung volumes. Neuromuscular disease that affects the inspiratory muscles sufficiently to diminish maximum inspiratory pressures may only decrease the vital and total lung capacities, leaving the functional residual capacity and residual volume unaffected.

Patients with widespread pulmonary fibrosis breathe faster and maintain a higher minute ventilation than do normal subjects, both at rest and during exercise. The work and oxygen cost of ventilating the stiff lungs are increased. The maximum breathing capacity is well preserved. In these patients, dyspnea is at-tributable to the considerable effort by the respiratory muscles in ventilating the stiff lungs and in sustaining the high ventilatory rate. During exercise, dyspnea may become intolerable.[31]

Dyspnea in Chronic Cardiac Disease

The mechanisms responsible for dyspnea in cardiac disease vary with the extent to which the lungs are stiffened.

Without Stiff Lungs   Dyspnea occurs in many forms of heart disease that are not associated with congestion of the lungs. Uncomplicated pulmonic stenosis is an excellent example. Probably the symptom is related to an inadequate cardiac output during exercise. In tetralogy of Fallot, dyspnea is sometimes severe and often relieved by assuming a squatting position. In this and other forms of cyanotic heart disease, both dyspnea and fatigue appear during exertion when the arterial oxyhemoglobin saturation has fallen appreciably below the resting level.

With Stiff Lungs   Cardiac dyspnea is associated with expanded blood and water content of the lungs. It is a common occurrence in left ventricular failure and mitral stenosis, both of which are accompanied by increases in pulmonary venous and capillary pressures. The engorged pulmonary circulatory bed, coupled with interstitial and alveolar edema, stiffens the lungs (i.e., decreases their compliance) and stimulates the ventilation via "J" receptors. In chronic left ventricular failure, pulmonary fibrosis, consequent to long-standing interstitial edema, contributes to the stiff lungs. Edema of the tracheobronchial mucosa increases airway resistance.

As a result of the stiff lungs and increased airway resistance, the swings in pleural pressure during the respiratory cycle are large and the work and energy cost of breathing are increased. Arterial hypoxemia, generally mild, may add to the ventilatory drive. Exercise exaggerates the pulmonary congestion and edema, promotes arterial and mixed venous hypoxemia, and increases the dyspnea.

In patients with pulmonary congestion and edema, tachypnea is a regular feature at rest and increases during exercise. Although tachypnea is consistent, its degree is generally modest and probably not entirely responsible for the dyspnea. Fatigue is a common concomitant of low cardiac output and may stem from diminished O_2 delivery to the respiratory muscles, contributing to respiratory discomfort.

Orthopnea and Other Positional Forms of Breathlessness Orthopnea signifies dyspnea in the recumbent, but not in the upright or semivertical position; it is usually relieved by two or three pillows under the head and back. Oppositely, platypnea signifies dyspnea induced by assuming the upright position and relieved by assuming the recumbent position.[44] Orthopnea is a hallmark of pulmonary congestion that stiffens the lungs (i.e., decreases their compliance). The decrease in compliance on lying flat is attributable to the fact that more of the lung is located at or below the level of the heart. During recumbency, the swings in pleural pressure, the work of breathing, and the respiratory frequency increase. The increase in respiratory frequency appears to be optimal (i.e., automatically adjusted to minimize the work of ventilating the more rigid lungs).

Some patients with chronic lung disease or asthma are also intolerant of recumbency. In these people, the discomfort is attributed to the greater difficulty of performing vigorous movements of the chest bellows in the recumbent position.

Paroxysmal Nocturnal Dyspnea In an episode of paroxysmal nocturnal dyspnea, the patient is aroused from sleep gasping for air and must sit up or stand to catch his or her breath; sweating may be profuse. Sometimes the patient throws a window open wide in an attempt to relieve the oppressive sensation of suffocation. The chest tends to become fixed in the position of forced inspiration. Both inspiratory and expiratory wheezes, often simulating typical asthma, are heard. In some instances, overt pulmonary edema occurs, accompanied by many crackles at end-inspiration; the acute pulmonary edema rarely terminates fatally. Occasionally, the attacks recur several times a night, forcing the patient to sleep upright in a chair.

The episode represents precipitous failure of the left ventricle caused by the factors that produce orthopnea (see above), abetted by pulmonary hypervolemia caused by a surge in systemic venous return. Mobilization of peripheral edema from the periphery as the extremities are elevated from the dependent po-

sition may contribute to the increase in systemic venous return. The acute increase in pulmonary blood volume increases pulmonary capillary pressures, promoting pulmonary edema, while the surge in venous return imposes an additional burden on the left ventricle.

The acute episode is often triggered by coughing, abdominal distention, the hypercapnic phase of Cheyne-Stokes respiration, a startling noise, or anything that causes a rise in heart rate and further increases the pulmonary capillary and venous pressures. Usually the attack is terminated by assumption of the erect position and a few deep breaths. Cough, an important manifestation of pulmonary congestion, frequently occurs during the attack.

Cardiac Asthma The asthmatic wheezes often heard in patients with pulmonary congestion have given rise to the term *cardiac asthma*. The wheezes are a manifestation of tracheobronchial edema and often are accompanied by overt signs of pulmonary edema. In addition to the reduction in the lumen of the airways and thickening of bronchial walls by edema, high intrathoracic pressures are required to overcome the obstruction during expiration, and these tend to narrow the airways even further. The resistance to airflow is increased during both inspiration and expiration, and the compliance of the lungs is greatly reduced, reaching values as low as one-tenth of normal. Upon recovery from the acute episode of pulmonary edema, airway resistance and pulmonary compliance return toward normal unless previous episodes have left a residue of pulmonary fibrosis.

Dyspnea in Anemia

Shortness of breath during exercise or excitement is a common complaint in severe anemia (e.g., hemoglobin concentration under 6–7g/dl). It is more common in acute than in chronic anemia. Often the dyspnea is associated with dizziness or faintness, and invariably the patient manifests signs of a high cardiac output and low peripheral resistance (i.e., bounding pulse, warm skin, and systolic cardiac murmurs). Although the pathogenesis of the dyspnea is not entirely clear, inadequate O_2 delivery to the respiratory muscles has been proposed.

Miscellaneous Disorders

Breathlessness is not uncommon in patients with musculoskeletal disorders. The usual explanation is the heightened motor drive that is needed to activate the weakened respiratory muscles. In the intensive-care unit, inadequate ventilator settings for flow and tidal volume may fail to satisfy the intrinsic ventilatory drive of the patient, generating the sensation of breathlessness.

ABNORMAL BREATHING PATTERNS

An important clue to the nature of a clinical problem in pulmonary disease is sometimes provided by bedside observation of a patient's respiratory pattern. The pertinent features are the rate, regularity, depth, and apparent effort being expended in breathing. A normal person at rest breathes about 12 to 15 times per min, with a tidal volume of 400 to 800 ml. As a result, minute ventilation is normally greater than 5 L/min. The pattern is quite regular except for an occasional slow, deep breath, and the respiratory movements appear effortless. In the patient with lobar pneumonia, both the rate and depth of breathing increase along with the increase in body temperature.

Severe skeletal deformity, as well as massive obesity, can limit chest excursions to cause alveolar hypoventilation. Neuromuscular weakness, as in myasthenia gravis or Guillain-Barré syndrome, can do the same, not only by diminishing ventilatory excursions as a result of generalized weakness of the respiratory muscles but also by improving overloads of unaffected muscles (e.g., residual effects of poliomyelitis). Unilateral involvement of one pleural space by pneumothorax, effusion, or fibrothorax limits excursions on the affected side. Massive chest trauma can cause flail chest.

In COPD, a slow respiratory rate and large tidal volumes are characteristic. This pattern presumably serves to minimize the work of breathing in these patients. Pursed-lip breathing, a self-induced type of positive-pressure breathing, is often part of the picture, In contrast, persons with restrictive lung disease adopt a breathing pattern that is characterized by small tidal volumes and a rapid respiration rate, often with little apparent effort. It is seen in patients with a decrease in distensibility of the lung or chest wall or with reduction of the vital capacity from any other cause. During exercise, minute ventilation increases inordinately with respect to the level of O_2 uptake and frequency increases more than tidal volume.

Fatigue of the diaphragm and intercoastal muscles, sufficient to disturb their coordinated contractions, can give rise to paradoxical breathing that heralds the onset of respiratory failure.

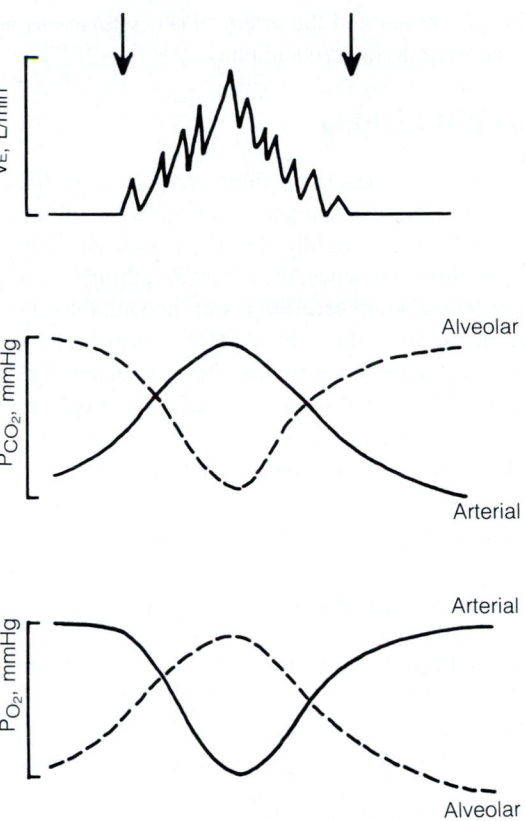

FIGURE 28-11   Cheyne-Stokes breathing, illustrating the relationship between the ventilation and the blood and alveolar gas tensions during the periods of apnea and hyperpnea. *(From Cherniack NS, Fishman AP: Abnormal breathing patterns. Dis Mon 3–45, 1975, with permission.)*

Cheyne-Stokes Respiration

In the fourth century B.C., in a preterminally ill person with fever, sweats, and black urine, Hippocrates described a pattern of breathing in which "the respiration throughout [was] like that of a man correcting himself, and rare and large." Presumably he had observed Cheyne-Stokes breathing, which was described more graphically by William Stokes two millennia later (in 1854) as follows:

> The symptom in question (previously described by Dr. Cheyne) consists in the occurrence of a series of inspirating, increasing to a maximum, and then declining in force and length, until a state of apparent apnoea is established. In this condition the patient may remain for such a length of time as to make his attendants believe that he is dead, when a low inspiration, followed by one more decided, marks the commencement of a new ascending and descending series of inspirations.[33]

Cheyne-Stokes breathing is characterized by alternating periods of hypoventilation and hyperventilation (Fig. 28-11). In its typical form, an apneic phase that lasts for 15 to 60 s is followed by a phase during which tidal volume increases with each breath to a peak level and then decreases in a progressive fashion to the apneic phase. At the onset of apnea, CO_2 tension in brachial or femoral arterial blood is at its lowest. As apnea persists, CO_2 tension gradually increases, and respiration is stimulated. CO_2 tension continues to increase until maximum hyperventilation is attained, after which ventilation decreases until apnea again occurs.

The arterial oxyhemoglobin saturation varies in an inverse manner, being highest at onset of apnea and lower during midhyperpnea. During the cycle, CO_2 tension varies by as much as 14 mmHg and oxyhemoglobin saturation by as much as 18 percent.

In patients with congestive heart failure, the respiratory oscillations are attributable to slowing of the circulation so that the blood gases reaching the respiratory centers in the brain are 180° out of phase with those in pulmonary capillary blood.

This mechanism has been verified experimentally by eliciting Cheyne-Stokes breathing in dogs by prolonging the circulation time from heart to brain by way of an extracorporeal circuit. Fluctuations in mental state and electroencephalographic patterns, and evidence of nervous system dysfunctioning, may occur during Cheyne-Stokes breathing because of swings in cerebral blood flow. In neurologic disorders, Cheyne-Stokes breathing can be due to supramedullary dysfunctions, particularly in patients who have destructive lesions in the tegmentum of the pons. Less common than in heart failure or neurologic disorders is the occurrence of Cheyne-Stokes respiration in normal infants, in healthy elderly persons, and in normal persons at high altitude. It is also seen occasionally after the administration of respiratory depressants (e.g., morphine) and often accompanies an increase in intracranial pressure, uremia, or coma. At one time, the respiratory center was believed to be depressed in Cheyne-Stokes respiration. This hypothesis was in error, since it has been shown that the respiratory response to inhalation of CO_2 is greater than normal. Respiratory alkalosis is common and the arterial P_{CO_2} remains subnormal in both the apneic and hyperpneic phases.

Kussmaul Breathing

In 1874, Kussmaul described three patients with diabetic ketosis who manifested "air hunger": they were breathing with large tidal volumes and so rapidly that there was virtually no pause between breaths. In essence, they were breathing at rest as though they were exercising; breathing was accomplished with little apparent effort. Since then, this pattern of breathing has been observed in other types of severe metabolic acidosis (e.g., alcoholic ketoacidosis). The usual sequence leading to this type of breathing is renal failure leading to a progressive decrease in plasma bicarbonate and acidosis. The "compensatory" increase in ventilation that Kussmaul described mitigates the fall in systemic pH caused by the fall in plasma bicarbonate.

Other Abnormal Patterns

Gasping respirations are characteristic of severe cerebral hypoxia. The pattern consists of irregular, quick inspirations associated with extensions of the neck and followed by a long expiratory pause. It is commonly seen in shock or in other conditions associated with severe reduction in cardiac output.

Hyperventilation is commonly seen in anxious patients without structural disease of the lungs. In some of these patients, striking deep sighs dominate the ventilatory pattern.

COUGH

A cough is an explosive expiration that protects the lungs against aspiration and promotes the movement of secretions and other airway constituents upward toward the mouth. It is a critical element in the self-cleansing and protective mechanisms of the lungs—a reflex act that usually, but not invariably, arises from stimulation of the bronchial mucosa somewhere between the larynx and the second-order bronchi. On rare occasions the cause is remote: impacted cerumen in an external ear or an inflammatory process of the pleura (see "Mechanism"). The stimuli that can elicit a cough are diverse: inhaled particles, mucus that has been elaborated by the lining of the airways, inflammatory exudate in airways or parenchyma, a new growth or foreign body in an airway, pressure on the external wall of the bronchus.

A cough may be voluntary, involuntary, or a combination of the two if the subject attempts to control an involuntary cough. Three categories of stimuli are commonly at work in producing an involuntary cough: mechanical, inflammatory, and psychogenic. Mechanical causes range from inhalation of irritants, such as smoke or dust, to distortions of the airways produced by pulmonary fibrosis or atelectasis. Most often, coughs are due to tracheobronchial inflammation. The cigarette smoker is particularly vulnerable to exacerbation of cough by inhaled particles and fumes because of underlying chronic pharyngitis, laryngitis, and tracheobronchitis. As a rule, cough represents organic disease. But on occasion, psychogenic influences are responsible for a dry cough that is related to anxiety. Psychogenic stress can aggravate cough due to organic causes.[6,22,25]

The site and significance of a cough can sometimes be localized from telltale signs and symptoms (Table 28-8). For example, the cough of acute tracheitis is often associated with retrosternal "burning." Acute laryngitis is usually associated with hoarseness and sore throat as well as cough. Tuberculosis of the larynx is associated not only with painful swallowing but also with unequivocal evidence of pulmonary tuberculosis. In asthma, cough is part of a constellation of airway obstruction. Body position can influence the persistence of a cough. When the pathologic process is changing, as in pneumonia or a neoplasm, the cough undergoes concomitant change, reflecting the evolution of the disorder.[16,20,28,39]

Interpretation of the significance of a cough depends on the clinical company that it keeps. It has to be viewed in context: Is it acute or chronic, productive, or nonproductive? How long has it lasted? What is the general condition of the patient, and what comorbidities are present? For example, the acute onset of a hacking, nonproductive cough accompanied by coryza, sore throat, malaise, sweating, and fever generally heralds a viral upper respiratory infection. An episode of asthma may begin with cough and wheezing. In contrast, a persistent cough, even if virtually ignored by the patient, may be a harbinger of serious disease (e.g., carcinoma of the lung). In a cigarette smoker, in whom bronchi are chronically irritated, a change in the nature of the cough from nonproductive to productive may signify the onset of a serious tracheobronchial infection or pneumonia. Alternatively, a lung neoplasm may present with a dry cough that not only persists and intensifies but also gradually becomes associated with systemic manifestations (e.g., loss of weight). As a rule, the endobronchial neoplasm responsible for the chronic cough is usually visible on the chest radiograph or on bronchoscopic examination. Occasionally, however, a cough due to extraluminal pressure on the trachea or bronchus by a tumor can be displayed only with more-sophisticated imaging techniques (e.g., CAT scan).

The implications of dry cough are different from those of productive cough. Before a cough can be regarded as nonproductive, the possibility should be weighed carefully that sputum has been produced but swallowed. Failure to probe deeply into this possibility once led to the notion that British and American patients suffered from different types of chronic bronchitis. Improved history-taking and interviews discounted this idea.[41]

A cough that is productive of purulent sputum is generally a reliable indication of infection in the tracheobronchial tree or lungs. When this symptom is associated with an acute illness, the characteristics of the sputum can be of considerable diagnostic help. Rust-colored sputum, which contains its distinctive coloration from the even dispersion of blood in yellow, purulent sputum, ocurs most often in pneumococcal pneumonia. The classic description of sputum in Friedländer's pneumonia is that it often resembles currant jelly; it also contains blood, but it is bright red and more translucent and viscid than the sputum of pneumococcal pneumonia. Purulent sputum with a foul odor usually indicates an anaerobic infection, commonly due to streptococci or *Bacteroides* in a lung abscess. A persistent cough that is productive of purulent sputum occurs in chronic bronchitis, bronchiectasis, and a variety of other suppurative disorders. Sputum that is mucoid can be a consequence of any long-standing bronchial irritant.

TABLE 28-8

Some Causes and Characteristics of Cough

Cause	Characteristics
Acute infections of lungs	
Tracheobronchitis	Cough associated with sore throat, running nose and eyes
Lobar pneumonia	Cough often preceded by symptoms of upper respiratory infection; cough dry, painful at first; later becomes productive
Bronchopneumonia	Cough dry or productive, usually begins as acute bronchitis
Mycoplasma and viral pneumonia	Paroxysmal cough, productive of mucoid or blood-stained sputum associated with flulike syndrome
Exacerbation of chronic bronchitis	Cough productive of mucoid sputum becomes purulent
Chronic infections of lungs	
Bronchitis	Cough productive of sputum on most days for more than 3 consecutive months and for more than 2 years
	Sputum mucoid until acute exacerbation, when it becomes mucopurulent
Bronchiectasis	Cough copious, foul, purulent, often since childhood; forms layers upon standing
Tuberculosis or fungus	Persistent cough for weeks to months, often with blood-tinged sputum
Parenchymal inflammatory processes	
Interstitial fibrosis and infiltrations	Cough nonproductive, persistent, depends on origin
Smoking	Cough usually associated with injected pharynx; persistent, most marked in morning, usually only slightly productive unless succeeded by chronic bronchitis
Tumors	
Bronchogenic carcinoma	Cough nonproductive to productive for weeks to months; recurrent small hemoptysis common
Alveolar cell carcinoma	Cough similar to that with bronchogenic carcinoma except in occasional instances, when large quantities of watery, mucoid sputum are produced
Benign tumors in airways	Cough nonproductive; occasionally hemoptysis
Mediastinal tumors	Cough, often with breathlessness, caused by compression of trachea and bronchi
Aortic aneurysm	Brassy cough
Foreign body	
Immediate, while still in upper airway	Cough associated with progressive evidence of asphyxiation
Later, when lodged in lower airway	Nonproductive cough, persistent, associated with localizing wheeze
Cardiovascular	
Left ventricular failure	Cough intensifies while supine, along with aggravation of dyspnea
Pulmonary infarction	Cough associated with hemoptysis, usually with pleural effusion

Mechanism

The cough begins with a rapid inspiration, followed, in rapid sequence, by closure of the glottis, contraction of the abdominal and thoracic expiratory muscles, abrupt increase in pleural and intrapulmonary pressures, sudden opening of the glottis, and expulsion of a burst of air from the mouth (Fig. 28-12). The high intrathoracic pressures, which often exceed 100 to 200 mmHg, increase the velocity of airflow through the airways, hastening the propulsion of the offending particles and producing the sound of a cough by setting into vibration airway secretions, the tracheobronchial walls, and the adjacent parenchyma (Fig. 28-13).

Afferent stimuli for a cough originate in irritant receptors and are conveyed centrally by the vagus, glossopharyngeal, trigeminal, and phrenic nerves. In subjects with an idiopathic, persistent, nonproductive cough, increased sensitivity of the afferent nerves of the airways due to neuropeptides stored in them has been proposed. The vagus nerve carries impulses not only from the larynx, trachea, and bronchi but also from the pleura and stomach. Receptors in the airways are most concentrated in the

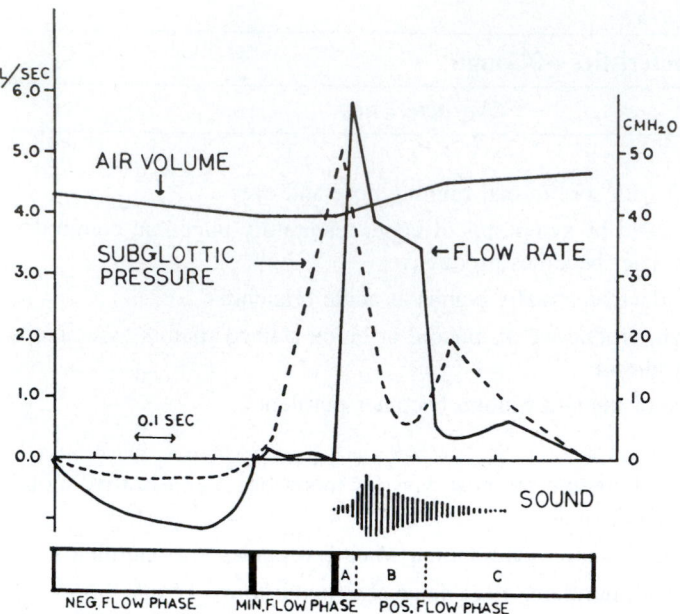

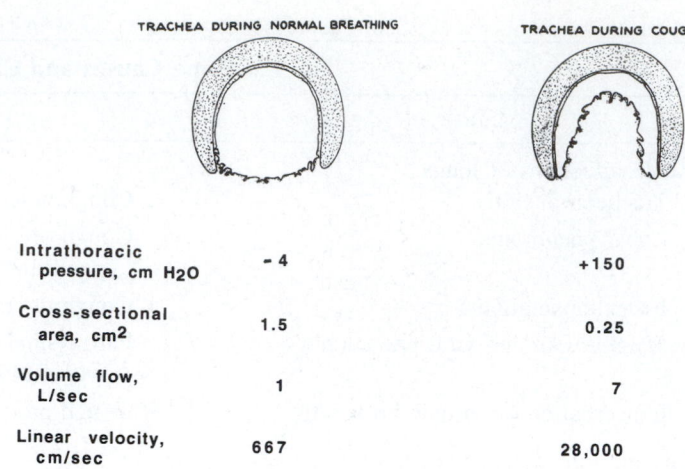

	TRACHEA DURING NORMAL BREATHING	TRACHEA DURING COUGH
Intrathoracic pressure, cm H_2O	– 4	+150
Cross-sectional area, cm^2	1.5	0.25
Volume flow, L/sec	1	7
Linear velocity, cm/sec	667	28,000

FIGURE 28-13 Effects of tracheal narrowing during a cough. The forced expiratory effort during coughing causes invagination of the non-cartilaginous part of the intrathoracic trachea by the high intrathoracic pressure. Air rushing with a high linear velocity through the exceedingly narrow trachea dislodges the material to be dispelled and propels it into the throat. *(From Comroe: Physiology of Respiration, Mosby–Year Book, 1965, p 122.)*

FIGURE 28-12 Sequence of events during a cough. Simultaneous recordings obtained during a single explosive cough by a normal subject. The three phases of a cough are identified by the boxes at the bottom of the figure. They correspond to (1) a deep initial inspiration, (2) compression of air in the lungs and airways by forceful contraction of the expiratory muscles coupled with tight closure of the glottis and opening of the larynx, and (3) sudden explosive expiration followed by narrowing of the glottis and return of the larynx to its normal inspiratory position. *(From Yanagihara, von Leiden, Werner-Kukuk: Acta Otolaryngol 61:495–510, 1965.)*

larynx, diminish in density in the conducting airways, and are absent from the distal airways, enabling the pooling of secretions in the periphery. The glossopharyngeal nerve carries stimuli from the pharynx; the trigeminal nerve, from the nose and paranasal sinuses; the phrenic nerve, from the pericardium and diaphragm. The motor pathways are even more extensive, comprising not only the cranial and phrenic nerves but also the nerves to the muscles of the rib cage and the accessory muscles.[52]

The effectiveness of a cough is strongly influenced by the lung volume at which it occurs. As indicated elsewhere in this volume, cough only removes particles toward the mouth ("downstream" from the "equal pressure points"). In healthy persons at high lung volumes, the equal pressure points are located in the larger airways; they move toward the alveoli ("upstream") as lung volume decreases. A series of coughs without any intervening inspiration moves the equal pressure points even closer to the small airways, helping to clear the depths of the lungs.

The cough reflex may be impaired by interrupting or blunting any step in the sequence. Irritant receptors can be damaged by a local destructive process (e.g., bronchiectasis), or their sensitivity can be diminished by narcotics or anesthetics.

The reflex pathways can be damaged as part of a neurologic disease. Tracheostomy, which eliminates glottic closure, decreases peak intrapulmonary pressures. Contraction of the respiratory muscles can be impaired by weakness due to illness, age, or neuromuscular disease. In general, as long as the patient can achieve maximum expiratory pressures greater than about

60 cm H_2O, the peak flow will suffice to produce effective coughs.

Circulatory Consequences

The increase in intrathoracic pressure that is part of the cough mechanism exerts considerable circulatory effects. However, because the increase in intrathoracic pressure is accompanied by an equal rise in vascular (and cerebrospinal fluid) pressures, distending pressures on the vessels of the heart, lungs, and other vital organs are unaltered, so they are spared the ill consequences of marked swings in transmural pressures.

The increase in intrathoracic pressure is accompanied by reflex vasodilation of systemic arteries and veins. Both of these effects contribute to a decrease in cardiac output. In patients with cor pulmonale and right heart failure, cough impedes systemic venous return, decreasing cardiac overload and improving stroke output.

Posttussive Syncope

Charcot recognized the syndrome of posttussive syncope 100 years ago. Originally conceived of as a form of epilepsy or a consequence of a laryngeal reflex, it is now attributed to the same circulatory consequences of raised intrathoracic pressures that coughing evokes in a normal person. However, the patient with cough syncope probably coughs more forcefully and longer than do normal persons.

The syncope usually develops within a few seconds after the onset of a paroxysm of coughing and ends quickly once the coughing has stopped. Return to consciousness is without sequelae unless the subject falls and is injured during the faint. Posttussive syncope nearly always occurs in men, probably because they generate a higher intrathoracic pressure and much more profound decrease in cardiac output than do women. It is not clear why this type of fainting occurs in the supine as well as the upright position; this occurrence suggests that the reduction in cerebral blood flow during posttussive syncope reflects more than interference with cardiac output. The extent to which intense reflex vasodilation contributes to posttussive syncope is unclear. In this regard, patients in severe heart failure who do not experience a posttussive drop in systemic arterial blood pressure also do not experience posttussive syncope. (Posttussive syncope is presumptive evidence of a good circulation with intact reflexes.)

HEMOPTYSIS

The coughing up of blood is termed *hemoptysis*. The material that is produced varies from blood-tinged sputum to virtually pure blood. The first decision faced by the physician who is told that blood has been coughed up is whether to conclude that the blood is coming from the respiratory tract. Although any portion of the respiratory tract can be the source, bleeding more often comes from a main bronchus or the lungs than from the nose or throat. On occasion, blood from the nose and throat is inhaled and then expectorated. As long as this possibility is kept in mind, bleeding that originates in the nose, throat, or larynx is not apt to be overlooked.[17,21]

There is usually no problem in distinguishing hemoptysis from hematemesis (vomited blood). Even if the blood is aspirated and then coughed up, the patient can usually tell if the blood originated in the respiratory or alimentary tract. The appearance of the bloody material also helps to distinguish between hemoptysis and hematemesis: blood that originates in the airways is usually bright red, is mixed with frothy sputum, has an alkaline pH, and contains alveolar macrophages that are laden with hemosiderin; in contrast, blood from the stomach usually is dark, has an acid pH, contains food particles, and occurs in patients with a long history of gastric complaints.

Mention was made earlier in this chapter of the need to rule out a systemic disorder, such as Goodpasture's syndrome or Wegener's granulomatosis, as the cause for hemoptysis (Fig. 28-14). Once it has been determined that the blood comes from the lungs, an earnest effort should be made to localize the intrapulmonary site of bleeding. The patient can be exceedingly helpful in this regard, particularly if the chest radiograph discloses any abnormality or shows bilateral pulmonary lesions. Occasionally, the detection of rales or rhonchi over one side or area of the lung directs the search. Sputum is zealously collected and examined: venous blood comes from the pulmonary arterial tree; bright-red blood stems either from a bronchial vein (as in mitral stenosis) or from a bronchial artery (as in bronchiectasis). Expectorated blood clots indicate that blood has been sitting in the lung for a while.

Because hunting for the cause and the source of bleeding is generally uncomfortable for the patient and expensive, the intensity of the search depends on the circumstances. For example, rarely is a search for the bleeding site needed in a patient with acute bronchitis, pneumonia, or bronchopulmonary suppuration. But as a rule, unless the cause is evident, a full-scale investigation is mandatory, particularly if this is not the first episode.

The list of causes of hemoptysis is long and diverse (Table 28-9). The clinical setting is usually helpful in identifying the cause. Hemoptysis before middle age usually brings to mind mitral stenosis, tuberculosis, pneumonia, or bronchiectasis; after 40 to 45 years of age, bronchogenic carcinoma and tuberculosis head the list. In patients left with a pulmonary cavity after pulmonary disease (e.g., tuberculosis) has healed, and in regions of the country where pulmonary fungal diseases are prevalent, a bout of hemoptysis is occasionally the first sign of the disease. In patients who have a predisposing cause, such as oral contraceptives or chronic heart failure, pulmonary embolism must be considered.

Neoplasms

Hemoptysis is so common in bronchogenic carcinoma that it should be regarded as the likeliest possibility in patients between 40 and 60 years of age. The likelihood is greatly increased if there is a long history of cigarette smoking. Usually a troublesome cough and vague chest pain precede and accompany the hemoptysis. For hemoptysis to occur, the lesion must communicate with the airways (Fig. 28-5). Most often the bleeding is a consequence of ulceration caused by the expanding tumor; sometimes it is due to a pneumonic process or an abscess in the lung behind the obstruction. Hemoptysis rarely complicates metastatic tumors of the lungs, since few (primarily renal and colon carcinomas) intrude on the airways until preterminal stages.

Not only malignant but also benign tumors of the lung cause bleeding. The classic example is bronchial carcinoid, which often causes bleeding that is generally difficult to arrest.

Infections

Hemoptysis can accompany a severe infection anywhere from the top to the bottom of the respiratory tract. It is uncommon in the usual viral or bacterial pneumonia. Conversely, it is not uncommon in the pneumonia that complicates bronchogenic carcinoma or in the pneumonia that is caused by staphylococci, influenzavirus, or *Klebsiella.*

The organism determines the appearance and composition of the material that is expectorated with the blood. As indicated above, in pneumococcal lobar pneumonia, the sputum at the onset is characteristically rusty-looking, but sometimes it is faintly or grossly bloody. In staphylococcal pneumonia, the blood is mixed with pus. In *Klebsiella* pneumonia, the bloody sputum often resembles currant jelly. Brisk bleeding is common in lung abscess; the blood is mixed with copious amounts of foulsmelling pus. In lung gangrene, blood is associated with necrotic lung tissue.

Bleeding is common in bronchiectasis. Because it usually originates in a bronchial artery, bleeding is often brisk. It is rarely life-threatening but tends to recur, and almost invariable each episode stops spontaneously.

Fungal infections of the lungs can cause hemoptysis (Fig. 28-14). As in tuberculosis, hemoptysis is generally a consequence of a continuing necrotizing and ulcerating inflammation process

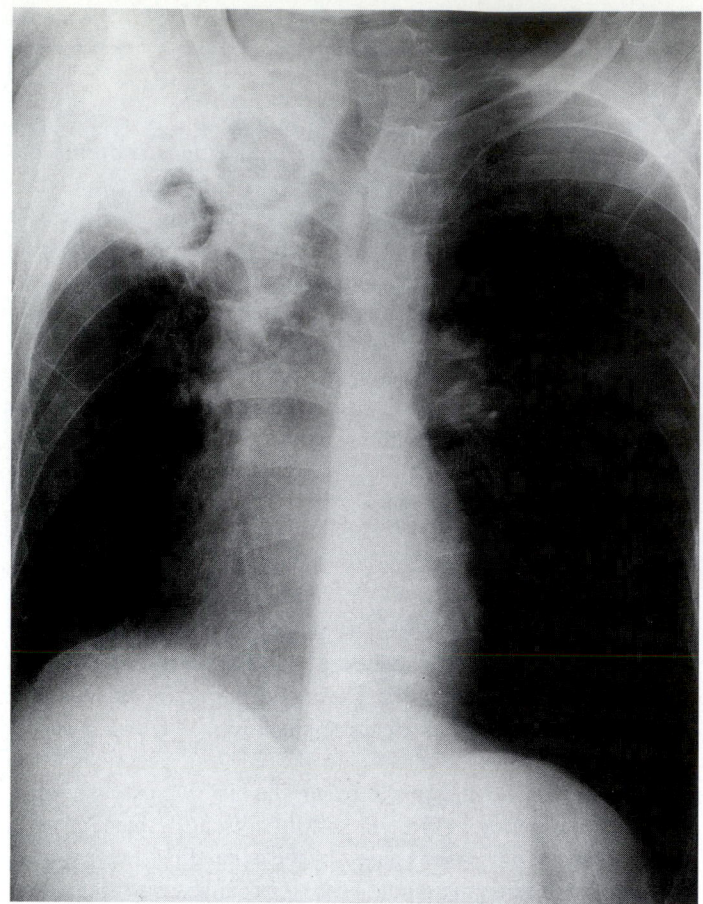

A

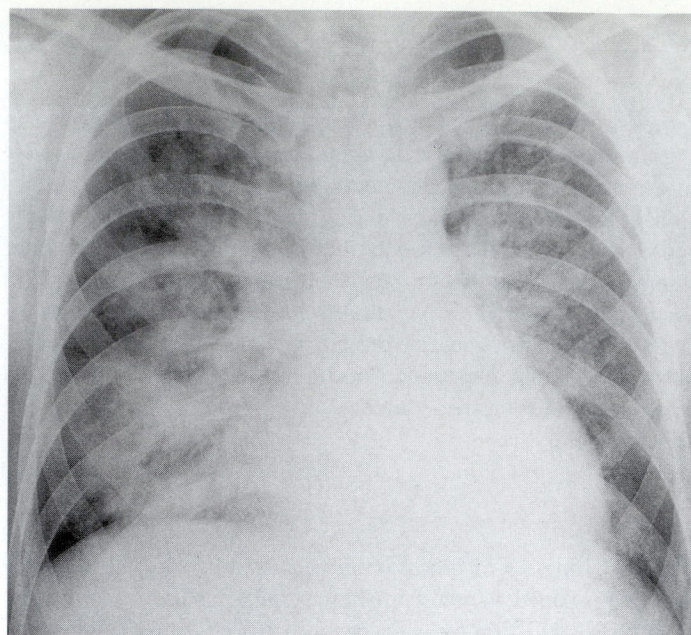

B

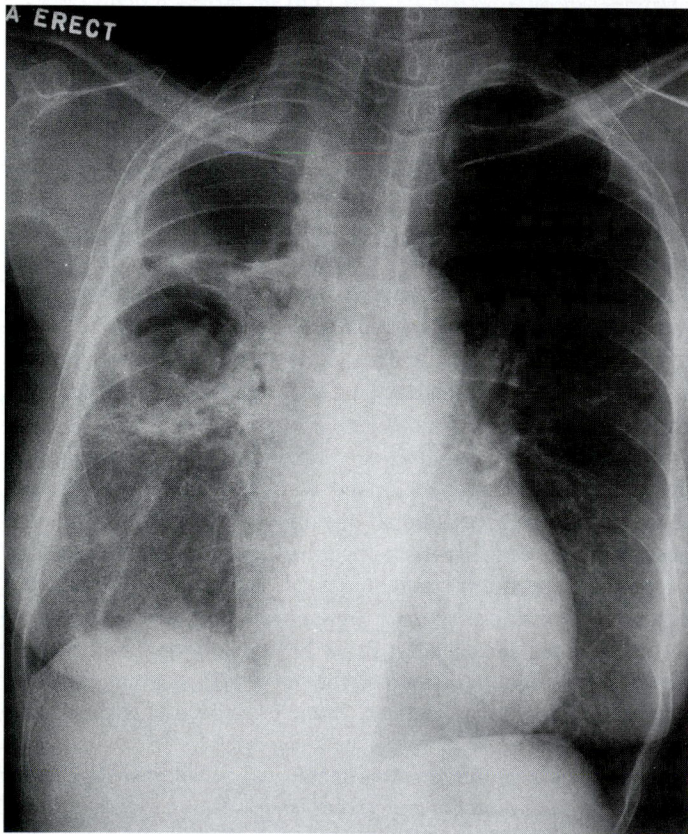

C

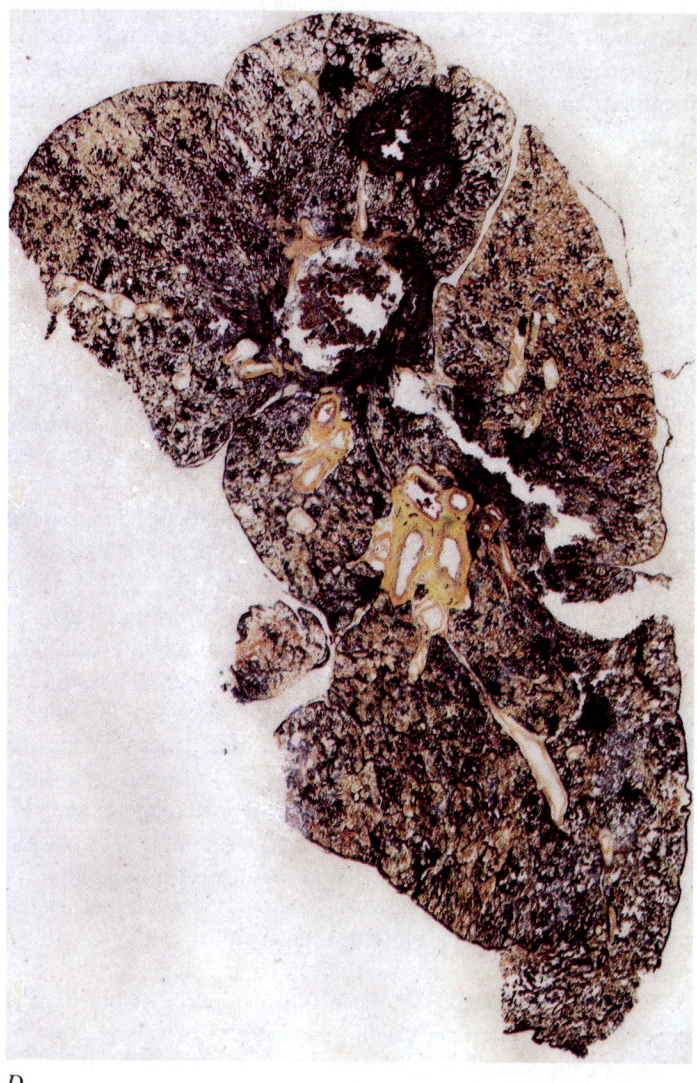

D

FIGURE 28-14 Causes of hemoptysis. *A.* Old tuberculosis cavities in right apex. They were removed surgically to control hemoptysis. *B.* Goodpasture's syndrome. *C.* Fungus ball in coal miner's pneumoco- niosis. Sagittal section of lung. *(Courtesy of J. Gough.) D.* Fungus ball due to aspergillosis in old tuberculosis cavity. Recurrent hemoptysis was arrested by surgical removal of right upper lobe.

TABLE 28-9

Some Common Causes of Hemoptysis

Infections
    Bronchitis
    Tuberculosis
    Fungal infections
    Pneumonia
    Lung abscess
    Bronchiectasis

Neoplasms
    Bronchogenic carcinoma
    Bronchial adenoma

Cardiovascular disorders
    Pulmonary infarction
    Mitral stenosis

Trauma
    Foreign body
    Blood dyscrasia
    Goodpasture's syndrome

or of bronchiectasis. The most common fungal disorder associated with hemoptysis is a "fungus ball" that resides either in a healed tuberculous or bronchiectatic area or in a cystic residue of sarcoidosis. Aspergillus is the usual fungal agent; less often another fungus is the cause.

The most common source of hemoptysis used to be an active tuberculous cavity. But now tuberculous pneumonia is a more common cause of hemoptysis than is active cavitation. Despite the growing incidence of tuberculosis, because of effective anti-tuberculous therapy, hemoptysis is uncommon. If tuberculosis is allowed to progress to the point of extensive fibrosis and caseation, or becomes complicated by bronchiectasis, hemoptysis can be troublesome and persistent.

The right middle lobe syndrome is frequently associated with hemoptysis. It is due to a partial or complete obstruction of the right middle lobe bronchus, resulting in atelectasis and/or pneumonitis in the right middle lobe. The obstruction is more often caused by scarring and/or inflammation than by physical compression of the lumen by an enlarged lymph node. The cause is usually infectious, and the infection can be tuberculous.

In parts of the world where amebiasis is endemic, hemoptysis follows perforation into the airways of a lung abscess that is continuous with hepatic abscess. The sputum resembles anchovy sauce.

Cardiovascular Disorders

Pulmonary congestion and alveolar edema (Fig. 28-7) sometimes produce blood-tinged sputum. In chronic pulmonary congestion secondary to left ventricular failure or to mitral valve disease, alveolar macrophages are often laden with hemosiderin ("heart failure cells"). In severe congestion and edema, the sputum is often pink and frothy. Usually there is no difficulty in recognizing that inadequate performance of the left ventricle is the cause of the bloody sputum.

Pulmonary embolism and, less often, pulmonary thrombosis produce hemoptysis only when associated with infarction (Fig. 28-15). The hemoptysis of pulmonary infarction is usually associated with pleuritic pain and often with a small pleural effusion because of the peripheral location of the infarct.

Tight mitral stenosis is sometimes first manifested by a bout of brisk, bright-red hemoptysis that is difficult to control. The source of the bleeding is the submucosal bronchial veins, which proliferate considerably in this disorder. Massive hemoptysis due to mitral stenosis is a medical emergency and is an indication for surgical intervention to relieve the obstruction at the mitral valve.

Hemoptysis from other circulatory disorders is much less common. Occasionally, an aortic aneurysm penetrates into the tracheobronchial tree, causing death by exsanguination and asphyxiation. An extraordinary event is the communication of an arteriovenous fistula with a small airway, causing bleeding that is exceedingly difficult to arrest.

Trauma

Hemoptysis follows a variety of chest injuries: puncture of a lung by a fractured rib, contusions of a lung by severe blunt trauma to the chest, and necrosis of the lining of the tracheobronchial

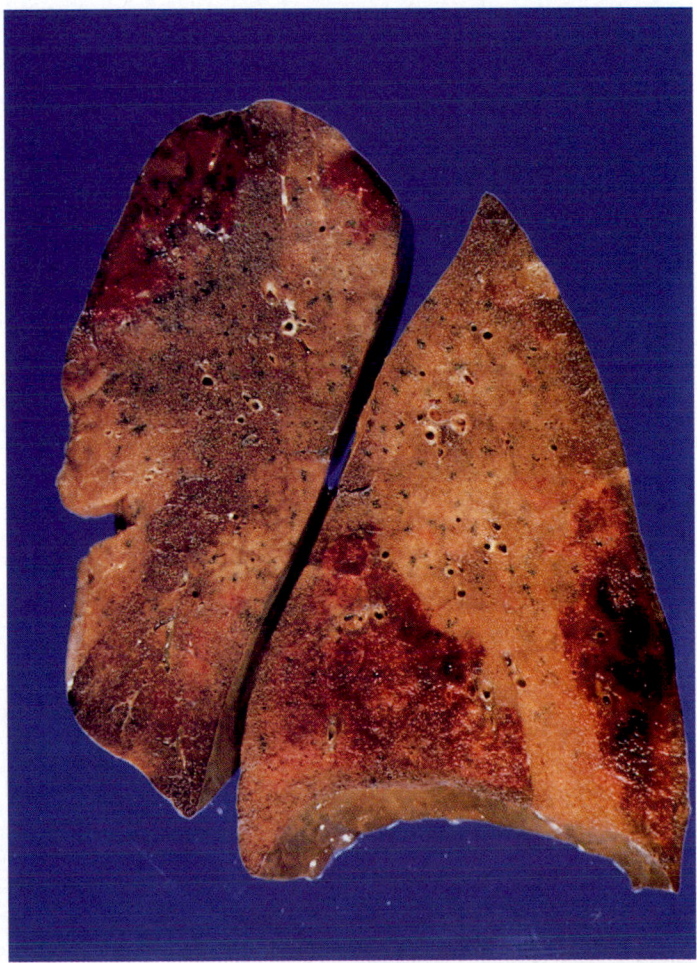

FIGURE 28-15 Hemorrhagic pulmonary infarcts. Several subpleural areas of infarction are clearly demarcated.

tree by inhaled fumes or smoke. Blunt trauma from the steering wheel during an automobile collision sometimes lacerates or fractures the tracheobronchial tree. Stab or gunshot wounds often tear the lungs or airways. On occasion, mucosal lacerations in the course of severe coughing evoke hemoptysis.

After pneumonectomy or lobectomy, a large hemothorax sometimes empties into the airways. This is an alarming and ominous event. Its imminent occurrence is often heralded by the expectoration of blood-stained sputum after a paroxysm of coughing. The hemothorax must be promptly evacuated and the bronchus surgically repaired. Hemoptysis within a few weeks to months after pneumonectomy has different implications: recurrence of tumor, granulation tissue, or bronchial sutures. Prompt bronchoscopy is necessary for accurate appraisal of the situation.

Miscellaneous

Other causes of hemoptysis are listed in Table 28-9. They vary enormously in severity, urgency, and prognosis. Sometimes the cause is obscure, as in the occasional instances of hemoptysis that accompany menstruation ("vicarious menstruation"). An aspirated foreign body produces bleeding by damaging the mucosa on impact; if allowed to remain in place, it sometimes causes bronchiectasis, which, in turn, may cause bleeding. Pulmonary calcific foci, either in the pulmonary parenchyma or in lymph nodes, sometimes cause hemoptysis by ulcerating into a bronchus.

Blood dyscrasias, notably thrombocytopenic purpura and hemophilia, and the therapeutic use of anticoagulants are occasional causes of hemoptysis. In areas where scurvy is endemic, vitamin C deficiency becomes a major cause.

Hemoptysis in Goodpasture's syndrome (Fig. 28-14) or in idiopathic hemosiderosis is life-threatening. This grim prospect has led to an aggressive therapeutic approach, including use of plasmapheresis and immunosuppressive agents.

CYANOSIS

A bluish discoloration of the skin that is caused by increased amounts of reduced hemoglobin in the subcapillary venous plexus is designated as *cyanosis*. The discoloration is most apparent in the lobes of the ears, the cutaneous surfaces of the lips, and the nail beds. In patients with dark skin, the mucous membranes and the retina are important sites to examine for cyanosis. Unless flow through the skin is slowed, as in heart failure, cyanosis implies arterial hypoxemia. Cyanosis does not appear in CO poisoning or in severe anemia in which arterial O_2 content is extremely low. The presence of abnormal pigments in blood, such as methemoglobin or bilirubin, complicates the detection of cyanosis.

Capillary O2 Content

An increase in the amount of reduced hemoglobin in the capillaries of the skin, as elsewhere, results from inadequate oxygenation of arterial blood, excessive removal of O_2 from capillary blood (as when the circulation through a region is slowed

by vasoconstriction), or a combination of the two. The concentration of reduced hemoglobin in the skin capillaries must reach about 5 g/dl before cyanosis becomes discernible. In severe pernicious anemia, in which hemoglobin concentrations are exceedingly low (on the order of 3 to 4 g/dl), virtually all the hemoglobin can be reduced in traversing the skin capillaries without causing cyanosis. Oppositely, the polycythemic patient develops cyanosis at a higher arterial O_2 saturation than does the normal subject.

The combination of intense vasoconstriction and excess reduced hemoglobin is responsible for the distinctive gray or heliotrope color that is frequently seen in patients with circulatory collapse and severe pulmonary edema.

Causes of Cyanosis

Several types of cyanosis are usually identified according to the underlying mechanism. They include peripheral cyanosis, cyanosis arising from pulmonary disease, cyanosis from venous admixture, and cyanosis due to abnormal pigments in the blood.

PERIPHERAL CYANOSIS

This type is secondary to abnormally large extraction of O_2 as blood flows through peripheral capillaries. The most common cause is diminished cardiac output associated with peripheral vasoconstriction. Not only the hands and feet but also the tip of the nose becomes blue in severe heart failure. Indeed, in patients with intractable heart failure, necrosis occasionally develops at the tip of the nose.

Peripheral vasoconstriction per se, as in Raynaud's disease, also produces cyanosis of the nail beds.

CYANOSIS IN PULMONARY DISEASE

Patients with chronic bronchitis and emphysema characteristically manifest derangements in ventilation-perfusion relationships. In some, arterial hypoxemia results. In patients with diffuse interstitial fibrosis, normal arterial oxygenation at rest is succeeded by arterial hypoxemia, and sometimes by cyanosis, during exercise. Another cause of arterial hypoxemia is the syndrome of alveolar hypoventilation in patients with normal lungs. In any of these situations, cyanosis is intensified by heart failure that slows blood flow through the skin (i.e., decreases O_2 delivery).

CYANOSIS DUE TO VENOUS ADMIXTURE

In patients with intracardiac right-to-left shunts, cyanosis arises from a mixture of venous and arterial blood. The effect of venous admixture is particularly striking if the O_2 content of mixed venous blood is inordinately low, as in some types of congenital heart disease and in severe heart failure. Often secondary polycythemia contributes to the cyanosis. On occasion, regional cyanosis is diagnostic. For example, in patent ductus arteriosus with reversal of blood flow, the lower extremities are deeply cyanotic, whereas the upper extremities are virtually normal in color.

CYANOSIS DUE TO ABNORMAL PIGMENTS IN BLOOD

Methemoglobinemia is an occasional cause of cyanosis. Methemoglobinemic blood is chocolate brown, and spectrophotometric examination of blood reveals the characteristic pigment. Arterial blood examination discloses a normal P_{O_2}.

The cause of methemoglobinemia may be hereditary (i.e., due to the presence of hemoglobin M or a deficiency in methemoglobin reductase) or, more often, acquired (e.g., by exposure to chemical agents such as analine dyes, chlorates, nitrates, and nitrites); or it may derive from use of drugs such as acetanilide, nitroglycerin, phenacetin, and primaquine. Nitrates are a common cause of methemoglobinemia. Nitrates are reduced to nitrites by bacteria in the intestinal tract. Excessive use of nitroglycerin, an organic nitrate, leads to methemoglobinemia.

In methemoglobinemia, the ferrous iron is oxidized to ferric iron, rendering the hemoglobin molecule incapable of binding O_2 or CO_2. Methemoglobin is formed continuously in the normal erythrocyte, but its level within the cell is kept low (less than 2 percent) by intracellular reductive mechanisms. High levels of methemoglobin result from hereditary abnormalities (e.g., a deficiency in methemoglobin reductase) or from exposure to drugs or chemicals that increase the rate of oxidation beyond the reductive capacity of the erythrocytes. Clinical manifestations of methemoglobinemia vary with the blood levels. Concentrations of methemoglobin between 10 and 25 percent usually cause asymptomatic cyanosis. When these levels are exceeded, dizziness, fatigue, and headache appear.

Because of the normal methemoglobin reductase and NADH generated during anaerobic glycosis, treatment is unnecessary unless serious manifestations occur (angina, stupor, or coma). Then methylene blue is given intravenously (1 to 2 mg/kg as a 1 percent solution) over 5 to 10 min. Cyanosis should disappear within 1 h; if not, the dose should be repeated. Larger doses of methylene blue engender the risk of aggravating the methemoglobinemia.

CLUBBING

Clubbing is a classic finding in medicine that dates back to Hippocrates' awareness of the association between characteristic changes in the fingertips and empyema. Occasionally it constitutes a valuable clue to clinically inapparent disease of the lungs and pleura. Clubbing of the fingers designates the selective bulbous enlargement of the distal segments of the digits due to an increase in soft tissue (Fig. 28-16). Most often it is painless.

When full-blown, clubbing is easy to recognize: (1) the nails, particularly the index finger, become abnormally curved in the longitudinal and coronal planes; (2) the hyponychial angle, viewed in profile, becomes blunted, often in conjunction with softening and sponginess of the base of the nail; and (3) the undersurface of the terminal digit becomes large and bulbous. Early stages of clubbing are subtle and generally difficult to diagnose. Clubbing often has to be distinguished from simple curvature of the nails and occasionally from chronic paronychia and Heberden's nodes. A variety of methods have been proposed for quantifying clubbing (e.g., measuring casts of the fingertips), but none has become popular.

Clubbing is generally acquired, but it may be hereditary. Acquired clubbing is seen in a wide variety of disorders, both extrathoracic and thoracic (Table 28-1). As a rule, clubbing is bilaterally symmetric, affecting hands and feet; on occasion, local factors, such as injury of a finger or of the median nerve, may cause clubbing that is confined to a single finger. On rare occasions, clubbing may be confined to the digits of one hand (e.g., in an ipsilateral pulmonary sulcus tumor that has invaded the brachial plexus or following hemiplegia). In certain types of congenital heart disease, a telltale distribution of clubbing is of considerable diagnostic value. For example, in patent ductus arteriosus associated with reversal of shunt through the ductus, clubbing affects only the toes.

Pathogenesis

The pathogenesis of clubbing is unknown, and no suitable animal model of clubbed fingers has yet been developed, largely because so few species other than primates have fingers. A common denominator in the pathogenesis of clubbing appears to be vasodilation of vessels in the fingertip, including formation of the arteriovenous connections. As a result, hydrostatic pressures increase in the capillaries and venules, promoting the transduction of fluid into the interstitium. The reason for this preferential vasodilation is unclear. A popular notion is that a humoral substance escapes normal deactivation by pulmonary capillaries. This theory could account for clubbing in cyanotic congenital heart disease, in various pulmonary diseases in which proliferation of the bronchial circulation occurs, and in hepatic cirrhosis in which pulmonary arteriovenous anastomoses and right-to-left shunts are common. However, it is difficult to relate this theory to the high incidence of clubbing in subacute bacterial endocarditis.

At present, a single hypothesis that would account for the clubbing that occurs in such diverse disorders as subacute bacterial endocarditis, carcinoma of the lung, hemiplegia, chronic mountain sickness, and purgative abuse is not possible. Indeed, it seems likely that clubbing of the digits is a stereotyped consequence of diverse influences that have in common the capacity to induce marked digital vasodilatation and soft-tissue interstitial edema.

HYPERTROPHIC OSTEOARTHROPATHY

Occasionally, clubbing of the digits is accompanied by hypertrophic osteoarthropathy, a separate entity both clinically and radiographically. Clinically, hypertrophic osteoarthropathy is manifested by pain and swelling of the soft tissues over the distal ends of the long and tubular bones. Radiographically, the distinctive feature of hypertrophic osteoarthropathy is the formation of new bone beneath the periosteum of the distal diaphyses of the long bones of the extremities (Fig. 28-16).

The most common disorder associated with hypertrophic osteoarthropathy is carcinoma of the lung. The incidence is about 5 percent and is unrelated to the cell type of the cancer, except that oat cell carcinoma is rarely implicated. A peripheral carci-

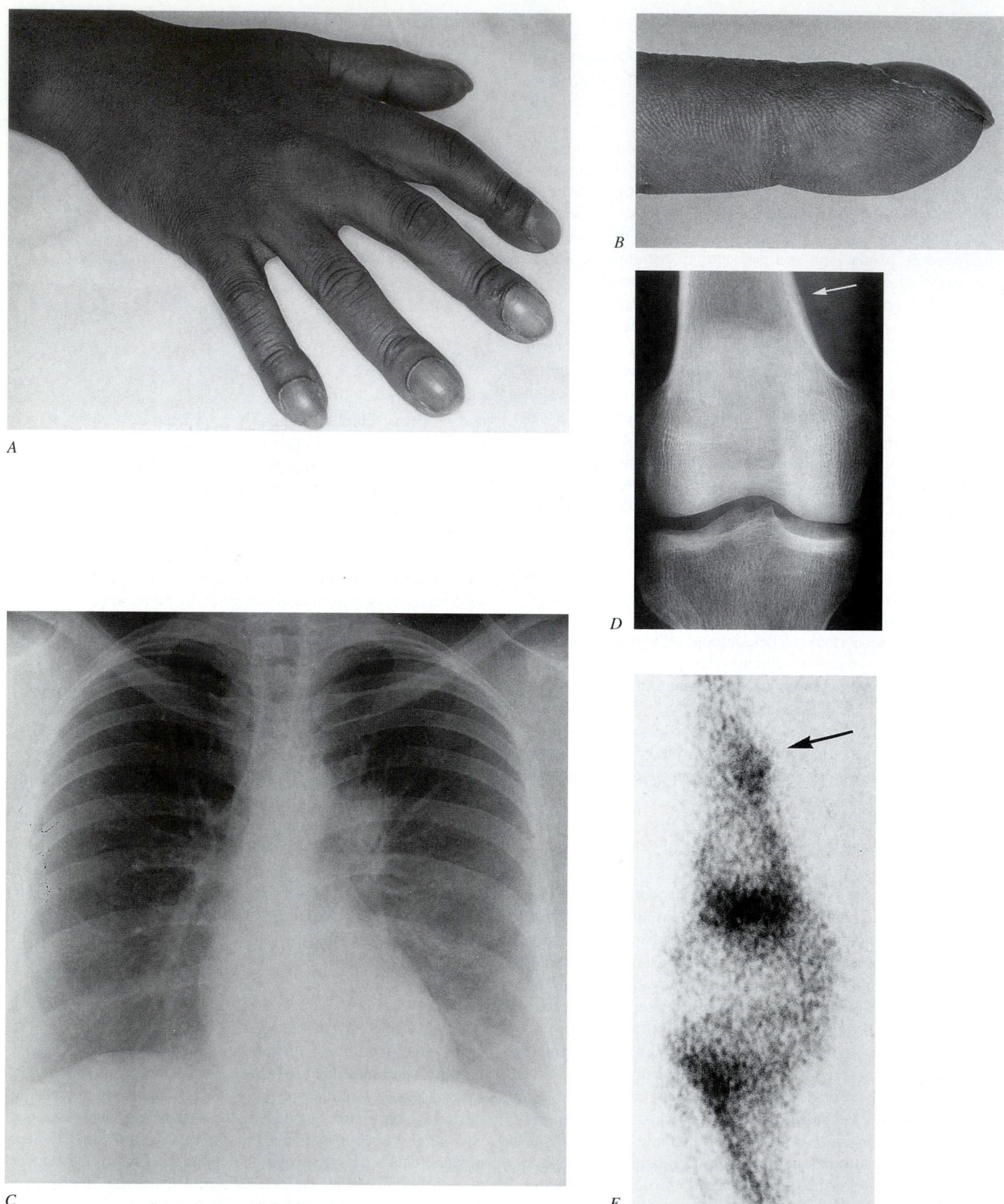

FIGURE 28-16 Clubbing and hypertrophic osteoartrophy. Clubbing of the digits and hypertrophic osteoarthropathy. A 40-year-old woman developed swelling and tingling of the fingertips in association with painful swelling of both knees. She was a heavy smoker (36 pack-years) and had an 8-month history of a dry cough. *A.* Clubbing of all fingers. *B.* Index finger. *C.* Left hilar mass that proved to be a primary adenocarcinoma of the lung. *D.* Subperiosteal formation of new bone on the medial aspect of the diaphysis of the femur. *E.* Bone scan, using ^{99m}Tc methylene diphosphonate. An abnormal accumulation of isotope is seen in the area of new bone (arrow).

noma of the lung is slightly more common than a central one. Joint symptoms precede the local signs of tumor in about one-third of the cases; the interval is sometimes as long as 2 years. Pulmonary metastases rarely cause hypertrophic osteoarthropathy. Pulmonary tuberculosis is seldom, if ever, associated with hypertrophic osteoarthropathy.

As in the case of clubbing of the digits, theories about pathogenesis tend to focus on humoral factors generated elsewhere. However, a neurogenic theory has also been advanced on the basis of two types of observations: (1) in a few patients, vagotomy relieves the symptoms of inoperable carcinoma of the lung and leads to regression of the bony lesions; and (2) in keeping with the observations on the few patients, in dogs, vagotomy is usually followed by a decrease in blood flow to the limbs. At present, neither theory has much convincing support, but both suggest future directions for exploration.

In contrast to clubbing of the digits, which is rarely painful, hypertrophic osteoarthritis associated with carcinoma of the lung often causes severe rheumatic symptoms. These symptoms vanish after resection of the carcinoma, even though clubbing usually remains. In patients who are treated with radiotherapy for unresectable carcinoma, pains in the vicinity of the joints usually decrease greatly and usually do not recur even if metastases develop to the lungs or elsewhere.

THORACIC PAIN

First thoughts about chest pain almost invariably turn to the pain of myocardial ischemia. However, cardiac pain is generally distinguishable from other types of chest pain because of its vice-like nature; its characteristic radiation to the left arm, shoulder, or neck; and its lack of relation to breathing. Extracardiac painful sensations can arise from various sites within the thorax, most often from the pleura, the lungs, and the chest wall.[2,51] Pain may also be referred to the thorax as a result of gastroesophageal reflux.[43]

Pleuritic Pain

The most characteristic pain associated with the respiratory apparatus is pleural pain. It originates in the parietal pleura and endothoracic fascia; the visceral pleura is insensitive to pain. In contrast to the deep, oppressive substernal pain of myocardial infarction, pleuritic pain is identified as being close to the thoracic cage. It is predominantly an inspiratory pain reflecting the stretching of inflamed parietal pleura during movement of the thorax; coughing or laughing is exceedingly distressing, and the patient often clutches the chest to minimize its excursion. The pain is usually local, but sometimes it spreads along the course of the intercostal nerves that supply the affected area.

As a rule, pleural pain is part of a syndrome of pleural infection that includes malaise and fever; an important exception to this generalization is the pleural pain of pulmonary infarction, which is often unassociated with any premonitory signs. Irritation of the diaphragmatic pleura by an inflammatory process either below or above the diaphragm often causes ipsilateral shoulder pain; sometimes the pain is referred to the abdomen.

Pulmonary Pain

A second distinctive type of respiratory chest pain accompanies a tracheitis or tracheobronchitis. The pain is searing and is most pronounced after cough. Invariably this central chest pain is associated with evidence of upper respiratory infection.

An uncommon type of respiratory pain is due to pulmonary hypertension. It is usually absent at rest and appears during exertion. The pain is substernal and is invariably associated with dyspnea; it subsides promptly when exercise stops. It is often mistaken for angina until the presence of pulmonary hypertension is uncovered.[55]

Chest Wall Pain

Pain in the chest is a common clinical problem. It may arise from within the thorax (the heart, pericardium, lungs, pleura, chest wall) or be referred from elsewhere (e.g., from below the diaphragm). Characteristic patterns and associations may help to clarify the source of the pain.

Pleural pain is generally associated with fever or dyspnea. Most often it is abrupt in onset, unilateral, and incapacitating. As a rule, it affects the lower part of the chest, but occasionally it is referred to the shoulder or abdomen. Almost invariably, pleural pain is aggravated by deep breathing or coughing. The patient tends to splint the chest on the affected side. Tachypnea and shallow tidal volumes are a consistent pattern.

Musculoskeletal pain arising in the chest that is also aggravated by breathing may be confused with pleuritic pain. It is rarely severe and incapacitating, is often bilateral, and generally is intensified by changes in body position or flexing the thorax. The affected muscles are often tender to gentle pressure. A fractured rib is usually identified as the source of pain by a history of a fall, injury, or trauma; point tenderness and crepitus of the affected area; reproduction of the pain upon manual compression of the chest; and radiographic evidence of the broken rib.

Pain arising from the large airways is usually burning in nature and retrosternal in location and is disturbing rather than incapacitating. It is aggravated by cough and is commonly accompanied by evidence of a bronchitis.

The pain of a pulmonary sulcus tumor (Fig. 28-17) is quite distinctive. This unusual location of a carcinoma of the lung was originally described in 1932 as characterized by pain along the distribution of the eighth cervical and the first and second thoracic nerves, Horner's syndrome, local destruction of bone by the tumor, and atrophy of hand muscles. The chest radiograph is distinctive in showing a small, sharply defined shadow at one apex. Destruction of one or more of the upper three ribs posteriorly and of their adjacent transverse processes may also be observed.

Cardiac Pain

Attention was called above to the pain of myocardial ischemia. Another type of cardiac pain is that of pericarditis. Pericardial pain is often aggravated by deep breathing and, almost invariably, is accompanied by a telltale rub that is synchronous with the heartbeat.

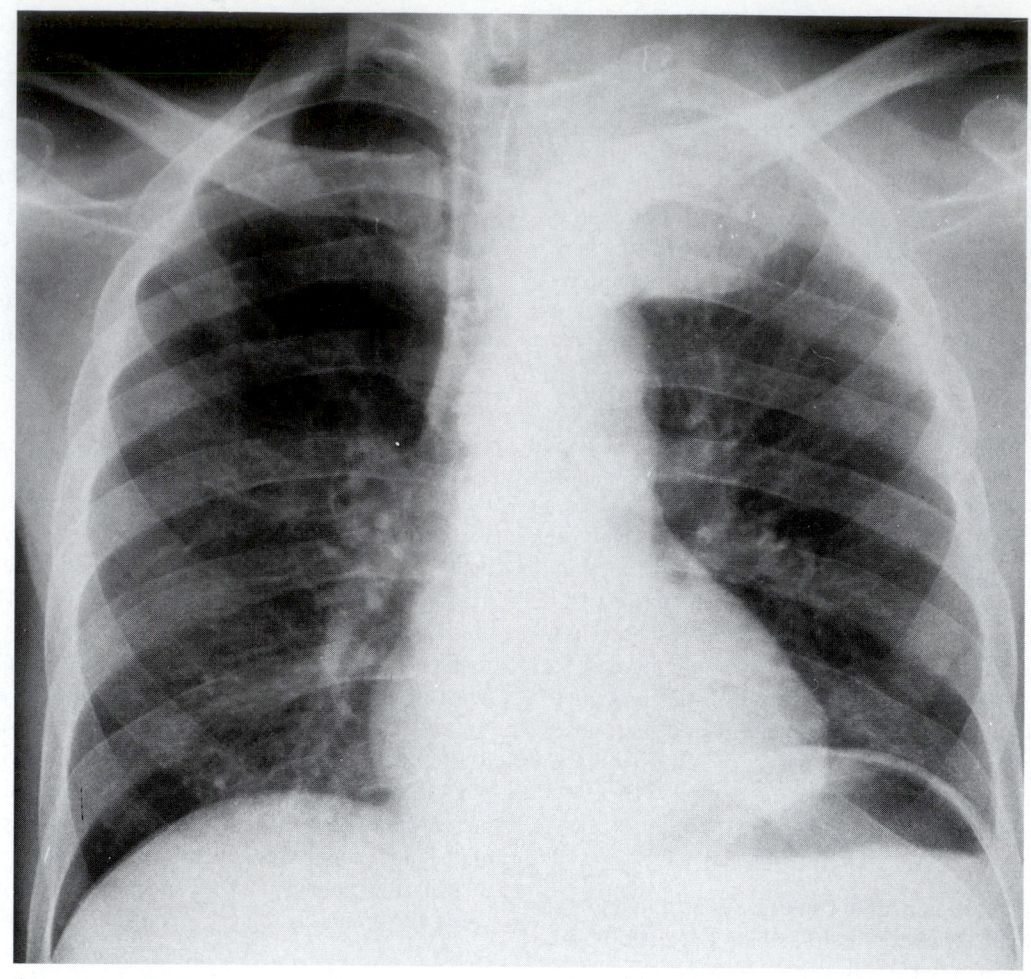

A

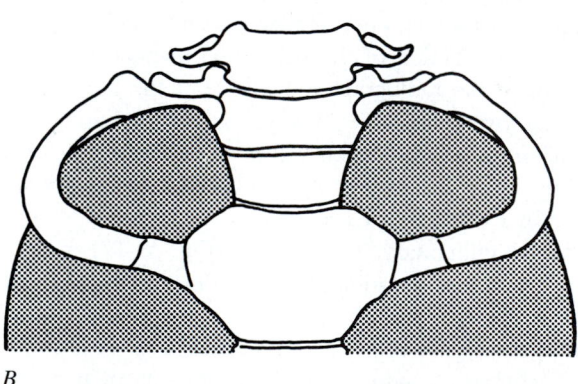

B

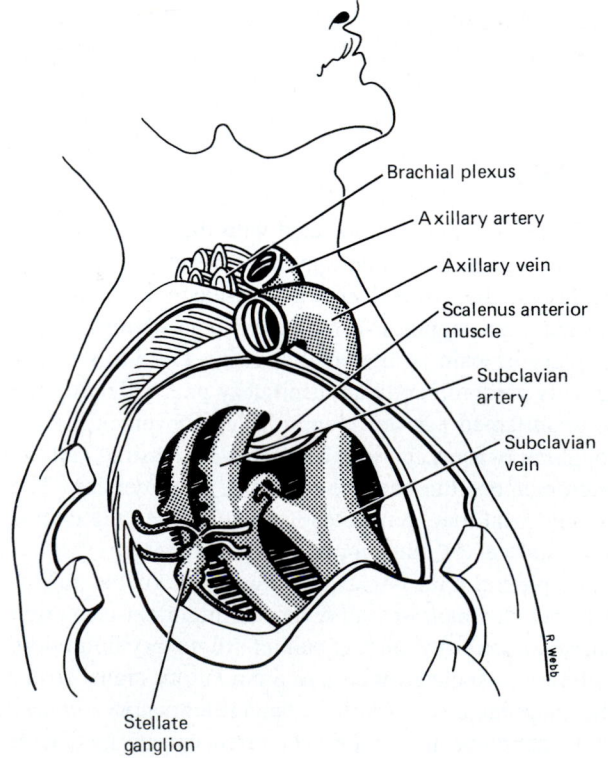

C

FIGURE 28-17   Pulmonary sulcus tumor. *A.* Chest radiograph. *B.* Relationships of apex of the lung to adjacent bony structures. *C.* Lateral view of area occupied by apex of lung, showing proximity not only to nerves of brachial plexus but also to sympathetic chain and to blood vessels. A mass that grows posteriorly and laterally can encounter sympathetic chain and bony structures; superiorly, the axillary vessels, brachial plexus, and bony structures; anteriorly, the subclavian vein and its tributaries. *(From Pernkopf: Atlas of Topographical and Applied Human Anatomy, WB Saunders, 1964, p 22.)*

The postcommissurotomy (postpericardiotomy) syndrome is characterized by chest pain that develops within a few days to weeks after cardiac surgery or pericardiotomy. The pain is usually sudden in onset and substernal, with radiation to the left side of the neck; often it is aggravated by deep breathing. Low-grade fever and a high sedimentation rate are regular concomitants. Chest pain can also be troublesome in patients who have undergone cardiac transplantation.[48] The diagnosis is usually self-evident when account is taken of the antecedent history of cardiac surgery. Indeed, confusion is more apt to arise with the pain of myocardial infarction than with respiratory causes of chest pain.

Miscellaneous Pain

Other structures in the mediastinum can be the source of chest pain. Noteworthy are the types of pain arising from the esophagus (peptic esophagitis) and dissection of the aorta. Their patterns and intensity serve to distinguish them from respiratory pain.

Arthritis of the cervical spine is a common cause of theoracic pain. Usually the cause is quite clear because of the characteristic distribution of the pain. Cervical spondylosis occasionally causes severe pain in the chest and arms, but it is more apt to mimic myocardial infarction than respiratory pain. A metastatic tumor to the thoracic spine often causes bilateral symmetric pain, whereas unilateral pain, along with distribution of an intercostal nerve, is characteristic of herpes zoster before the appearance of the skin eruption.

Anxiety can produce or intensify chest pain. Usually, pain related to anxiety is accompanied by dyspnea and hyperventilation. Manifestations of vasomotor instability, such as excessive palmar sweating, flushing, and tachycardia, may accompany the complaint of chest pain. Rarely does the pain conform to a characteristic or consistent pattern. Anxiety also interferes with the quantification of pain originating in a somatic lesion and with its management.

FEVER

In the patient with lung disease, fever usually, but not invariably, signifies infection. When the lung disease is chronic, as in bronchitis and emphysema, a bout of acute bronchitis usually elicits only a modest fever, even though the sputum turns purulent. In contrast, an acute pneumonia of lung abscess may be associated with high fever.

The possibility that fever is due to infection lends urgency to the situation. Elsewhere in this book, the patterns of acute pulmonary infection are considered with particular attention to systemic effects, chest radiography, white blood cell count, sedimentation rate, and sputum examination. Often overlooked at the outset is miliary tuberculosis, which occasionally escapes detection on the initial chest radiograph. Favoring this diagnosis is a history of recent contact with active tuberculosis, general malaise, easy fatigability, and anorexia during the previous few weeks. This insidious onset differs strikingly from the more sudden onset of acute pneumonia. A therapeutic trial of antituberculosis therapy is warranted while concrete evidence of disseminated tuberculosis is sought.

Neoplasms are also associated with fever. In certain neoplasms, such as carcinoma of the bronchus, the fever is generally a secondary effect attributable to infection distal to obstruction; necrosis within the tumor is a less common cause. In others, such as hypernephroma, fever and chills are striking, even though evidence of infection is absent. A mesothelioma of the pleura is often associated with fever; removal of the tumor is generally followed by defervescence. Presumably, in patients with neoplasms who have no evidence of infection, necrosis within the tumor leads to the elaboration of pyogenic substances within and around the tumor.

Extrinsic allergic alveolitis is sometimes followed by fever as well as by pulmonary disability after exposure to the offending antigen. Usually, the diagnosis poses no problem once the nature of the illness is suspected.

In contrast to the pulmonary disorders in which fever is a characteristic feature, pulmonary sarcoidosis is uncommonly associated with fever unless widespread extrapulmonary impairment, or erythema nodosum, coexists. Nor is pneumoconiosis associated with fever unless complicated by necrosis in the midst of conglomerate fibrosis or by superimposed tuberculosis. Among the other extensive disorders of the lungs that cause no fever (and few systemic complaints) are idiopathic pulmonary fibrosis, lymphangitic carcinomatosis, multiple pulmonary metastases, alveolar proteinosis, idiopathic pulmonary hemosiderosis, and alveolar microlithiasis.

RADIOLOGIC EVALUATION

The radiologic evaluation of the patient presenting with respiratory symptoms is dealt with in considerable detail elsewhere in this book (see Chapter 32). Over the years, the chest radiograph has become an invaluable tool, not only for diagnosis but also for following the result of treatment (Fig. 28-18) and for directing interventions. The value of routine screening films in asymptomatic subjects (e.g., as part of annual physicals or in chronic cigarette smokers to detect cancer) is still a matter of debate. The diagnostic yield of such studies has not been impressive. In contrast, the chest radiograph is an integral component of the initial evaluation of the patient with new respiratory symptoms.

In recent years, the conventional chest radiograph has been supplemented by a succession of imaging techniques, such as computed tomography, magnetic resonance imaging, and positron emission tomography. Although these powerful tools are generally used as complementary techniques, often they assume primary roles (e.g., examination of the mediastinum for lymphadenopathy or invasion of the chest wall in a patient with carcinoma of the lung). As successive improvements in these techniques continue to be made, the future seems to hold even brighter prospects for these noninvasive methods (e.g., delineation of pulmonary vessels for the diagnosis of pulmonary embolism or pulmonary hypertension).

COMMON CHRONIC PULMONARY DISEASES

The great majority of chronic pulmonary diseases that affect both lungs fall into four categories: chronic obstructive airway diseases, restrictive lung diseases, global alveolar hypoventilation, and obliterative pulmonary vascular diseases.

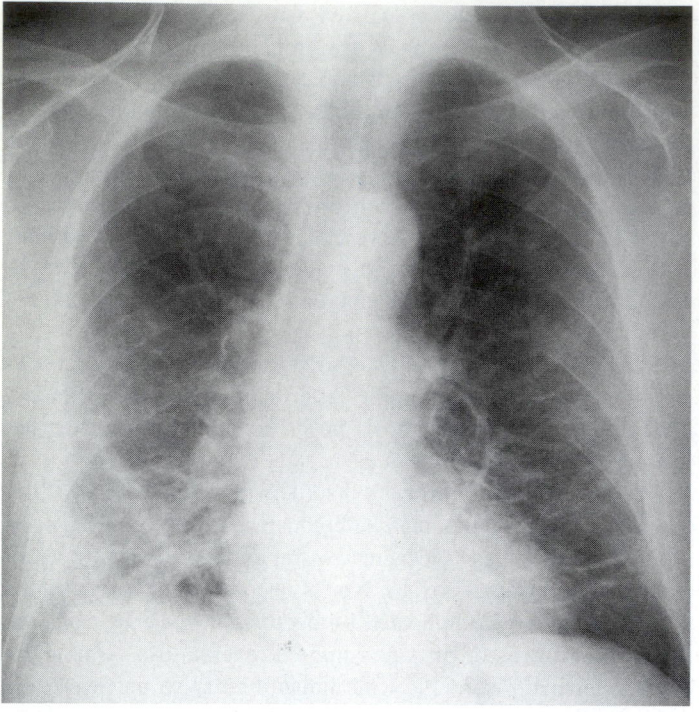

A

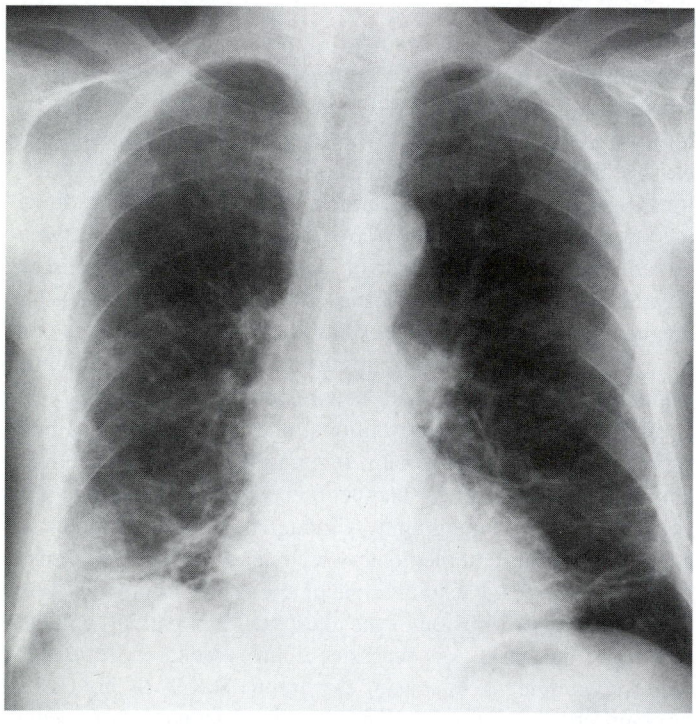

B

FIGURE 28-18 Response of interstitial lung disease to cortico-steroids. *A.* Interstitial lung disease ("usual interstitial pneumonitis") in a 67-year-old man before administration of corticosteroids. Widespread interstitial lung disease, more marked on the right. The lung function tests were characteristic of severe restrictive lung disease. *B.* After corticosteroids. Pulmonary function tests improved dramatically along with clearing of the pulmonary lesions on the chest radiograph.

Chronic Obstructive Airway Disease

Obstruction of the airways generally occurs during expiration. Based on expiratory maneuvers, airway obstruction has been categorized by a wide variety of tests (see Chapter 52). But it is remarkable how much information about the obstruction can be obtained from two traditional tests: (1) the FEV_1, determined serially, before and after administration of a bronchodilator; and (2) arterial blood gas analyses.

Preoccupation with expiration tended for a while to obscure disorders that were characterized primarily by inspiratory obstruction. These were commonly overlooked because of the failure to elicit stridor on the physical examination. But more and more instances of inspiratory obstruction are being uncovered, particularly in patients who have undergone prolonged tracheal intubation. Once the physician has been alerted to this prospect by detecting a wheeze over the trachea—usually, but not invariably, during inspiration—a comparison of maximum inspiratory and expiratory flow rates generally points to the upper airways as the site of obstruction. Other tests, particularly tomography, bronchography, and aortography, are often needed to complete the appraisal of the affected area.

In asthma, generalized wheezing occurs during both inspiration and expiration. Except for attacks precipitated by specific antigens, two common mechanisms often precipitate an episode: a respiratory infection, usually viral rather than bacterial, and an emotional event. Between episodes, most asthmatics, even those who are symptom-free, can be shown to have heightened bronchomotor tone (Fig. 28-19). In a latent asthmatic, a brief period of hyperventilation generally suffices to induce a bout of asthma. In patients with left ventricular failure, a paroxysm of wheezing ("cardiac asthma") occasionally heralds the onset of acute pulmonary congestion and edema. The new onset of asthma in an elderly person should be carefully assessed with respect to the state of the left ventricle before vigorous bronchodilator therapy is initiated; this often entails use of sympathomimetic drugs.

Restrictive Lung Disease

The diagnosis of restrictive lung disease usually begins with a complaint of dyspnea, reinforced by a telltale chest radiograph. Indeed, without abnormalities on the chest radiograph, detection of interstitial disease by pulmonary function testing is uncommon. The combination of tachypnea, the typical chest radiography, concentric reduction in lung volumes, and the appearance of arterial hypoxemia during exercise almost invariably clinches the diagnosis; a low value for the diffusing capacity of the lungs is final proof and is useful in following the course of the disease. Much more troublesome is the identification of the cause (Table 28-4).

An important distinction at the outset is whether the disease is acute or chronic (Table 28-3). Some types of interstitial disease, such as asbestosis, take years to become symptomatic. Others, such as idiopathic pulmonary fibrosis, run a fulminating course from start of symptoms to death within weeks.

Another help in categorization is the presence of systemic complaints. Sometimes, particularly in immunosuppressed patients, distinction between interstitial infection and interstitial

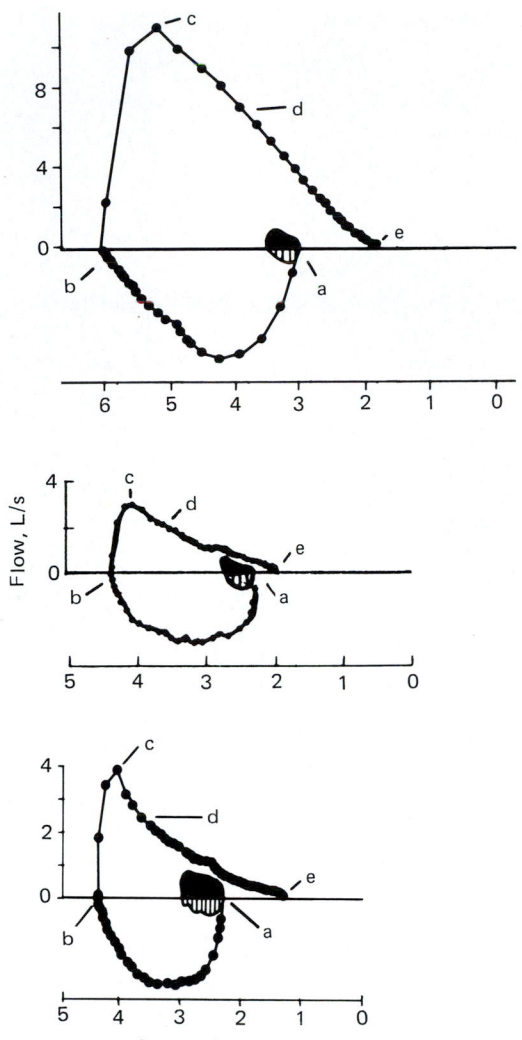

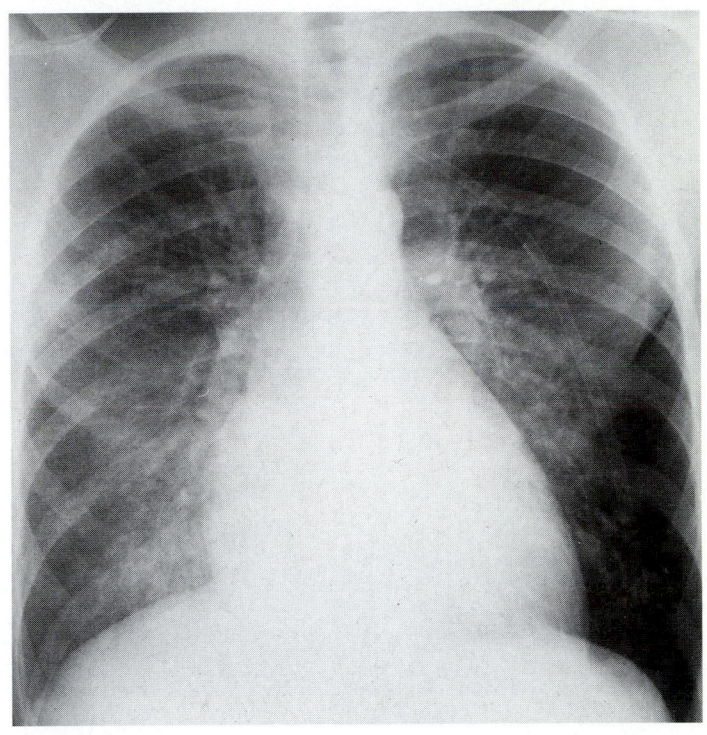

A

FIGURE 28-19 Simultaneous flow-volume curves in asthma. Top: Normal subject. Beginning at the end of a quiet expiration (a), the curves were recorded during a normal tidal breath (small, shaded loops) and during a forced expiration from peak lung inflation (b) to full expiration (e). Peak flow rates were reached at c. Expiration then continued along segment cde. In the record of the tidal breath, inspiration is hatched and expiration is solid black. The interval between each dot is 0.05 s. Center: Asthmatic subject. The vital capacity (be) is abnormally small, and flow rates along cde are diminished. Bottom: Same asthmatic subject 2 weeks after clinical recovery. Although flow rates are considerably higher than during the acute attack, the slope of segment de is still abnormally low, indicating that the resistance to airflow as lung volume decreases is still inordinately high. *(From Mellins et al,*[36] *with permission.)*

edema may be difficult to make (Fig. 28-20). Persistent fever suggests infection. Lung impairment by a systemic disease, such as scleroderma, is often suggested by telltale stigmas in extra-pulmonary sites (Fig. 28-21). In some instances, the cause is self-evident. This relationship is striking in some occupational disorders (e.g., silo-filler's disease that occurs after exposure to moldy hay). Also, the chest radiograph in sarcoidosis or silicosis is sometimes so characteristic as to be virtually diagnostic (Fig. 28-22). But sometimes the cause remains enigmatic or

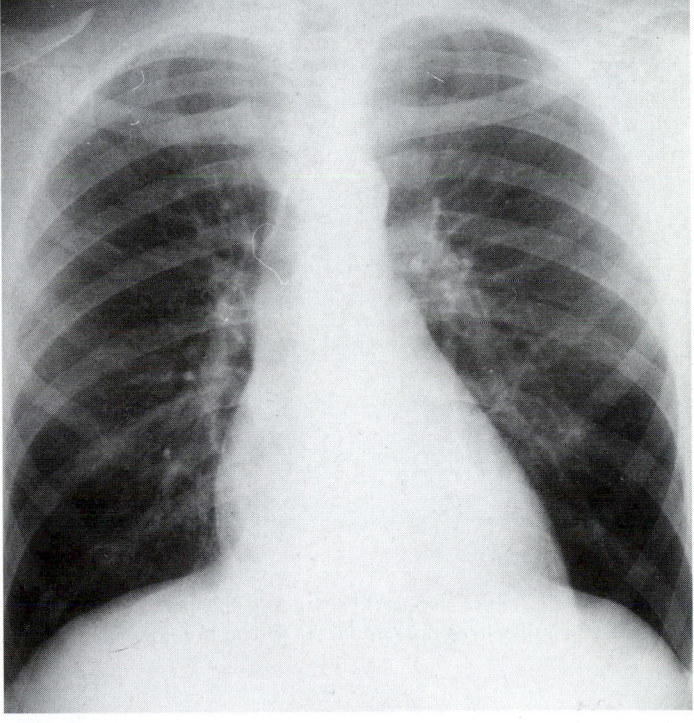

B

FIGURE 28-20 Interstitial edema and infection. Pneumocystis infection in an immunosuppressed patient in uremia. *A.* Bilateral interstitial and alveolar pattern and enlarged cardiac silhouette suggestive of pulmonary edema. *Pneumocystis carinii* was obtained by bronchial lavage. *B.* Three weeks later. Reduction in size of cardiac silhouette and clearing of infiltrates after marked diuresis and treatment with pentamidine isethionate.

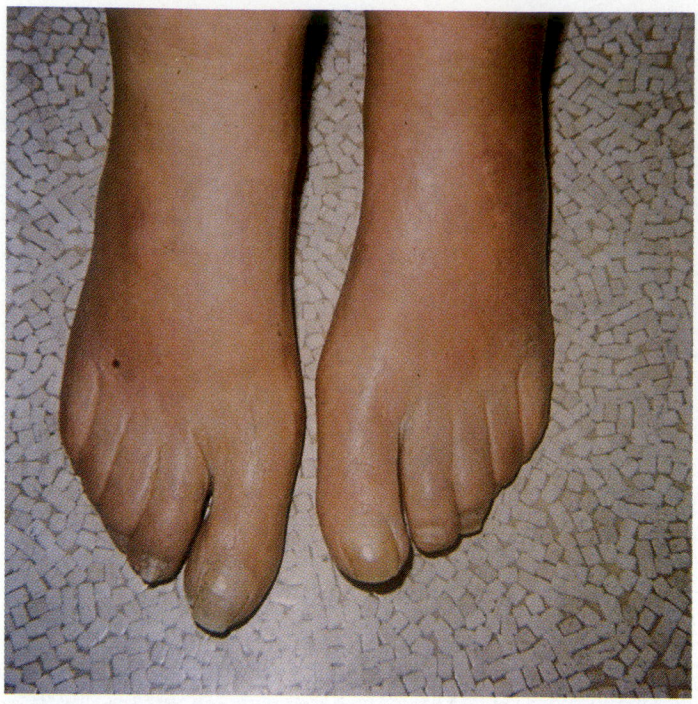

A

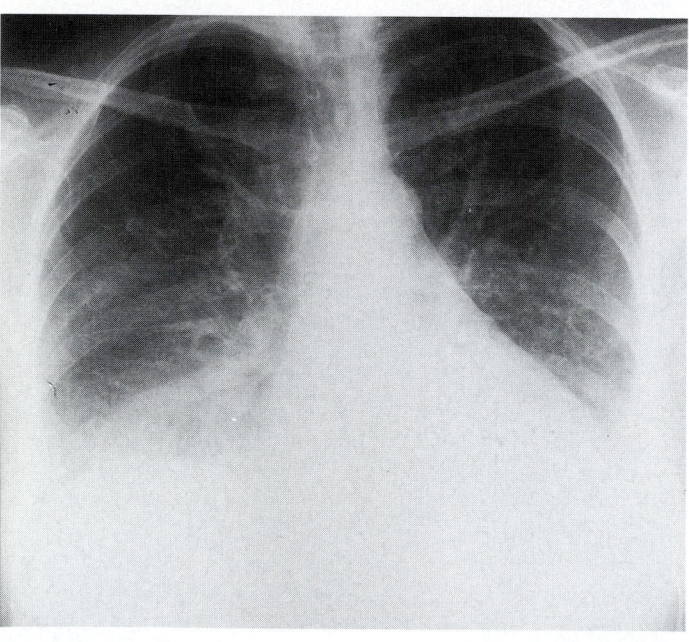

B

FIGURE 28-21   Scleroderma. *A.* Raynaud's phenomenon of the toes. *B.* Diffuse bibasilar interstitial infiltrates on chest radiograph.

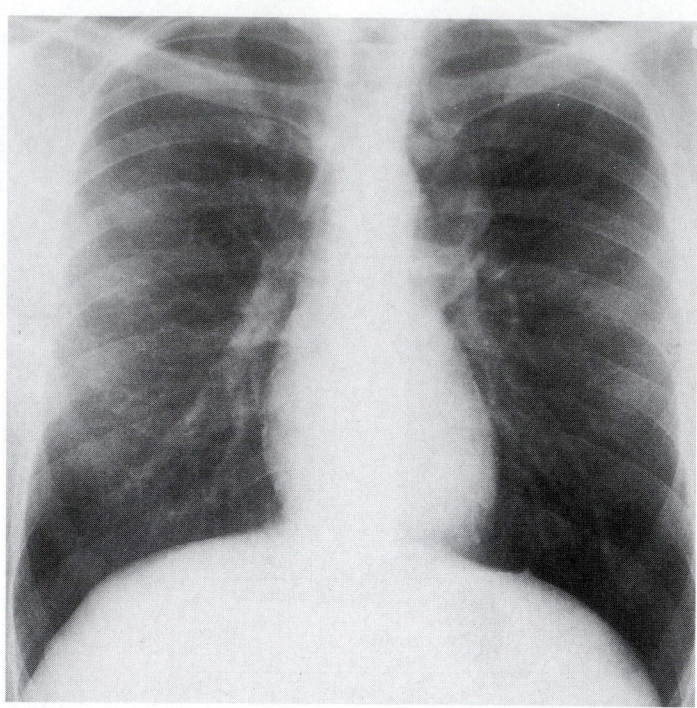

FIGURE 28-22   Sarcoidosis. Unilateral hilar adenopathy due to sarcoidosis. Twenty-seven-year-old asymptomatic man with left hilar adenopathy and interstitial lung disease of upper lobes. Bronchoscopic biopsy disclosed widespread noncaseating granulomas.

idiopathic despite elaborate laboratory investigations, including lung biopsy.

In essence, uncovering the cause of diffuse interstitial fibrosis is often a matter of painstaking and discriminating medical detection. The flash of brilliant insight, in the tradition of Sherlock Holmes or Lord Peter Wimsey, is apt to be less revealing about cause than is a meticulous, systematic account of lifestyle, habits, occupation, and background. The distribution and pattern of disease on the chest radiograph often provide clues to the next step in diagnosis. Sometimes the identification of abnormal constituents in sputum is diagnostically helpful (e.g., blood or blood products in the macrophages of the patient with Goodpasture's syndrome or eosinophils in the patient with a hypersensitivity disorder). In many instances, diagnosis rests on lung biopsy. Unfortunately, except in diseases such as sarcoidosis, biopsy is often deferred to the stage of nonspecific interstitial fibrosis when scarring is so indiscriminate that neither etiology nor pathogenic mechanisms are decipherable.

As pointed out above, the physiological hallmarks of diffuse interstitial disease are those of restrictive lung disease (i.e., stiffening of the lung [low compliance] and concentric reduction in lung volumes [decrease in vital capacity, residual volume, and total lung capacity]). Accompanying the decrease in compliance is an increase in the work of breathing and a breathing pattern of rapid, shallow tidal volumes. The chest radiograph demonstrates the inability of the patient to expand fully the stiffened lungs. Dyspnea is evoked at first by mild exercise and later persists at rest.

The once-popular picture of widespread disease confined to the alveolar-capillary interstitium has been modified by the recognition that alveoli are generally implicated in the underlying process. In interstitial pulmonary edema, groups of alveoli are often flooded. In inflammatory processes, such as sarcoidosis or desquamative interstitial pneumonia, alveoli, as well as the interstitial space, are commonly caught up in the process. In pneumonia caused by *Pneumocystis carinii,* the organisms are found in alveoli as well as in the interstitial spaces. Therefore, the designation of diffuse interstitial disease should not be mis-

TABLE 28-10

Practical Initial Approaches to Assessing Pulmonary Disorders*

Clinical State	First-Order Tests	Comments
Obstructive disease of airways		
Expiration		
Asthma	FEV_1; before and after bronchodilator	Detect bronchospasm
	Arterial blood-gas levels	Increasing P_{CO_2} requires assisted ventilation
Chronic bronchitis	FEV_1; before and after bronchodilator	Degree of obstruction; reversibility
	Arterial blood-gas levels	Magnitude of ventilation-perfusion abnormalities
Emphysema	FEV_1	Degree of obstruction; reversibility
	Arterial blood-gas levels	Extent of ventilation-perfusion abnormalities
	Elastic recoil pressure	Abnormally low if emphysema predominates over bronchitis
Inspiration	FEV_1	Normal
	Maximal inspiratory and expiratory flow curves	Characteristic configurations of curves (Fig. 28-19)
Restrictive lung disease		
Diffuse interstitial	Chest radiograph	Characteristic patterns
Inflammation, infiltration, fibrosis, thickened pleura	Lung volumes	Concentric reduction
	Arterial P_{O_2} at rest and exercise	Arterial hypoxemia during exercise
	Diffusing capacity	Conformity
Alveolar hypoventilation		
Secondary to obstructive disease of airways ("net")	Same as obstructive diseases of airways	Seriously abnormal lungs
	Arterial blood-gas levels	Hypoxemia, hypercapnia, respiratory acidosis
Primary mechanism lungs; respiratory centers, chest bellows; coordinating mechanisms	FEV_1; spirometry	Normal
	Arterial blood-gas levels	Hypoxemia, hypercapnia, respiratory acidosis
	Response to assisted ventilation	Normalization of blood-gas levels
	Maximum inspiratory and expiratory pressures	Assess muscle weakness
Obliterative pulmonary vascular disease	Chest radiograph	Characteristic
	Electrocardiogram	Right ventricular hypertrophy
	Spirometry; FEV_1	Normal
	Right-sided heart catheterization	Pulmonary hypertension
Complications or sources of ambiguity		
Respiratory failure	Arterial blood-gas levels; identify cause	Guide to therapy
Pulmonary congestion edema	Chest radiograph	Enlarged heart; vascular and interstitial pattern
	Viral capacity	Response to diuretics and cardiotonic agents
Cyanosis		
Polycythemia vera	Spirometry; FEV_1; arterial blood-gas levels	All near-normal
Anatomic right-to-left shunt	Same	Severe hypoxemia without hypercapnia
Abnormal pigment	Arterial P_{O_2}; spectrophotometry	Normal; identify pigments

*Emphasizing simplicity of tests as well as their specificity in substantiating clinical diagnosis. The more elaborate tests that are used for further discrimination are discussed elsewhere.

construed as being confined solely to the interstitium of the lungs, even though it generally does identify the predominant seat of disease.

Syndromes of Alveolar Hypoventilation

The common denominator in disorders characterized by alveolar hypoventilation is an abnormally high value for arterial (and alveolar) Pco_2. The most common cause is chronic bronchitis and emphysema, which produce hypercapnia by deranging ventilation-perfusion relationships. This "net" alveolar hypoventilation is conceptually different from the "generalized" alveolar hypoventilation that results from a disorder of respiratory control or of the chest bellows. The usual manifestation of generalized alveolar hypoventilation is the combination of normal lung volumes and FEV_1, normal chest radiograph in conjunction with arterial hypoxemia, hypercapnia, and respiratory acidosis.

Obliterative Vascular Disease

Pulmonary thromboemboli usually affect large as well as small vessels. Occlusive vascular diseases, such as primary pulmonary hypertension, which are confined to small ("resistance") pulmonary vessels, are uncommon. More often, the pulmonary resistance vessels are caught up in diffuse interstitial disease. In pulmonary vascular disease that compromises the area available for gas exchange, the diffusing capacity becomes subnormal. Occlusive vascular diseases of the lung are usually recognized when the extent of the disease is sufficient to cause considerable pulmonary hypertension. At that time, a characteristic constellation of findings usually prevails: (1) the chest radiograph shows central pulmonary arteries that are unduly large, in conjunction with pruning of the peripheral pulmonary vessels; (2) the electrocardiogram reveals right ventricular enlargement; and (3) pulmonary function tests show normal lung volumes and arterial blood-gas composition. Right-sided heart catheterization settles the diagnosis by revealing pulmonary arterial hypertension without evidence of pulmonary venous hypertension.

CHOOSING PULMONARY FUNCTION TESTS

In Chapter 36, pulmonary function testing is discussed in some detail. Often a combination of pulmonary function tests is needed to characterize a patient's abnormalities (Table 28-10). Pulmonary function tests can be particularly helpful in obstructive diseases of the airways, for which chest radiographs are often normal. Some of the tests are simple; others require special facilities and personnel. For example, closing volume and closing capacity, previously popular as "sensitive" tests for obstruction of small airways, have proved to be of little clinical value. There is certainly no value to these tests once the FEV_1 is abnormal. Nonetheless, the possibility exists that such sensitive tests may be useful in special conditions (e.g., in assessing obstruction of small airways in occupational disease).

The battery of tests that is used experimentally to portray the full length and breadth of the patient's pulmonary disorder is rarely needed for clinical purposes. However, only a few physi-

ological test patterns result from a wide variety of causes. Indeed, virtually all diffuse diseases of the lungs and airways that compromise pulmonary performance can be categorized into four distinctive patterns: (1) obstructive disease of the airways, (2) restrictive lung disease, (3) obliterative vascular disease, and (4) alveolar hypoventilation due to malfunctioning of the chest bellows or control mechanisms (Table 28-10).

REFERENCES

1. Adams L, Guz A: Dyspnea on exertion, in Whipp BJ, Wasserman K (eds), *Exercise: Pulmonary Physiology and Pathophysiology.* New York, Dekker, 1991, pp 449–494.
2. Bonica JJ: Painful disorders of the respiratory system, in Bonica JJ (ed), *The Management of Pain.* Philadelphia, Lea & Febiger 1990, pp 1043–1061.
3. Bonnet R, Jorres R, Downey R, et al: Intractable cough associated with the supine body position: Effective therapy with nasal CPAP. *Chest* 108:581–585, 1995.
4. Braman SS, Corrao WM: Cough: Differential diagnosis and treatment. *Clin Chest Med* 8:177–188, 1987.
5. Cherniack NS, Altose MD: Mechanisms of dyspnea. *Clin Chest Med* 8:207–214, 1987.
6. Coleridge HM, Coleridge JCG: Reflexes evoked from tracheobronchial tree and lungs, in Cherniack NS, Widdicombe JG (eds), *Handbook of Physiology,* Section 3: *Respiration,* vol 2, *Control of Breathing.* Bethesda, MD, American Physiological Society, 1986, pp 395–429.
7. Enelow AJ, Swisher SN: *Interviewing and Patient Care,* 3d ed. New York, Oxford University Press, 1986.
8. Forgacs P: The functional basis of pulmonary sounds. *Chest* 73:398–405, 1978.
9. Fraser RG, Paré JAP: *Diagnosis of Disease of the Chest,* 2d ed. Philadelphia, WB Saunders, 1978.
10. Gavriely N, Kelly KB, Grotberg JB, Loring SH: Forced expiratory wheezes are a manifestation of airway flow limitation. *J Appl Physiol* 62:2398–2403, 1987.
11. Goodwin SD, Glenny RW: Nonsteroidal anti-inflammatory drug–associated pulmonary infiltrates with eosinophilia: Review of the literature and Food and Drug Administration Adverse Drug Reaction reports. *Arch Intern Med* 152:1521–1524, 1992.
12. Gottlieb JE, Fanburg BL, Pauker SG: A decision analytic view of the diagnosis of sarcoidosis, in Fanburg BL (ed), *Sarcoidosis and Other Granulomatous Diseases of the Lung.* New York, Dekker, 1983, pp 349–380.
13. Hilman BC: Evaluation of the wheezing infant. *Allergy Proc* 15:1–5, 1994.
14. Holden DA, Mehta AC: Evaluation of wheezing in the nonasthmatic patient. *Cleve Clin J Med* 57:345–352, 1990.
15. Holt GA, Kelsen SG: Dyspnea, in Tierney DF (ed), *Current Pulmonology,* vol 14. St Louis, Mosby–Year Book, 1993, pp 293–320.
16. Irwin RS, Curley FJ, French CL: Chronic cough: The spectrum and frequency of causes, key components of the diagnostic evaluation, and outcome of specific therapy. *Am Rev Respir Dis* 141:640–647, 1990.
17. Israel RH, Poe RH: Hemoptysis. *Clin Chest Med* 8:197–205, 1987.
18. Jaakkola MS, Jaakkola JJK, Ernst P, Becklake MR: Respiratory symptoms should not be overlooked. *Am Rev Respir Dis* 147:359–366, 1993.
19. Johnson BD, Badr MS, Dempsey JA: Impact of the aging pulmonary system on the response to exercise. *Clin Chest Med* 15:229–246, 1994.

20. Johnson D, Osborn LM. Cough variant asthma: A review of the clinical literature. *J Asthma* 28:85–90, 1991.

21. Johnston H, Reisz G: Changing spectrum of hemoptysis: Underlying causes in 148 patients undergoing diagnostic flexible fiberoptic bronchoscopy. *Arch Intern Med* 149:1666–1668, 1989.

22. Karlsson JA, Sant'Ambrogio G, Widdicombe J: Afferent neural pathways in cough and reflex bronchoconstriction. *J Appl Physiol* 65:1007–1023, 1988.

23. Koster ME, Baughman RP, Loudon RG: Continuous adventitious lung sounds. *J Asthma* 27:237–249, 1990.

24. Kramin SS (ed): Lung sounds. *Semin Respir Med* 6:157–242, 1985.

25. Lacourcière Y, Lefebvre J: Modulation of the renin-angiotension-aldosterone system and cough. *Can J Cardiol* 11 (Suppl F):33F–39F, 1995.

26. Laennec RTH: *A Treatise on the Diseases of the Chest and Mediate Auscultation.* Translated by John Forbes. New York, Hafner, 1962.

27. Lanken PN, Fishman AP: Clubbing and hypertrophic osteoarthropathy, in Fishman AP (ed): *Pulmonary Diseases and Disorders.* New York, McGraw-Hill, 1980, pp 84–91.

28. Leith DE, Butler JP, Sneddon SL, Brain JD: Cough, in Cherniack NS, Widdicombe JG (eds): *Handbook of Physiology,* Section 3: *Respiration,* vol 3, *Mechanisms of Breathing.* Bethesda, MD, American Physiological Society, 1986, pp 315–336.

29. Light RW, Muro JR, Sato RI, et al: Effects of oral morphine on breathlessness and exercise tolerance in patients with chronic obstructive pulmonary disease. *Am Rev Respir Dis* 139:126–133, 1989.

30. Loudon RC: The lung exam. *Clin Chest Med* 8:265–272, 1987.

31. Lourenço RV, Turino GM, Davidson LAG, Fishman AP: The regulation of ventilation in diffuse fibrosis. *Am J Med* 38:199–216, 1965.

32. Mahler DA, Horowitz MB: Clinical evaluation of exertional dyspnea. *Clin Chest Med* 15:259–269, 1994.

33. Major RH: *Classic Descriptions of Disease,* 2d ed. Springfield, IL, Charles C Thomas, 1939, pp 596–603.

34. Manning HL, Schwartzstein RM: Pathophysiology of dyspnea. *New Engl J Med* 333:1547–1553, 1995.

35. Marshall R, Stone PW, Christie RV: The relationship of dyspnea to respiratory effort in normal subjects: Mitral stenosis and emphysema. *Clin Sci* 13:625–631, 1954.

36. Mellins RB, Lord GP, Fishman AP: Dynamic behavior of the lung in acute asthma. *Med Thorac* 24:81–98, 1967.

37. Murray JF: History and physical examination, in Murray JF, Nadel JA (eds), *Textbook of Respiratory Medicine,* 2d ed. Philadelphia, Saunders, pp 563–584.

38. Muza SR, Silverman MT, Gilmore GC, Hellerstein, HK, Kelsen SG: Comparison of scales used to quantitate the sense of effort to breathe in patients with chronic obstructive pulmonary disease. *Am Rev Respir Dis* 141:909–913, 1990.

39. O'Connell, Springall DR, Moradoghli-Faftvani A, et al: Abnormal intraepithelial airway nerves in persistent unexplained cough? *Am J Respir Crit Care Med* 152:2068–2075, 1995.

40. O'Donnell DE, McGuire M, Samis L, Webb KA: The impact of exercise reconditioning on breathlessness in severe chronic airflow limitation. *Am J Respir Crit Care Med* 152:2005–2013, 1995.

41. Patrick H, Patrick F: Chronic cough. *Med Clin North Am* 79:361–372, 1995.

42. Piirila P, Sovijärvi ARA, Kaisla T, Rajala HM, Katila T: Crackles in patients with fibrosing alveolitis, bronchiectasis, COPD, and heart failure. *Chest* 99:1076–1083, 1991.

43. Richter JE: Gastroesophageal reflux as a cause of chest pain. *Med Clin North Am* 75:1065–1080, 1991.

44. Schwenk NR, Schapira RM, Byrd JC: Laryngeal carcinoma presenting as platypnea. *Chest* 106:1609–1611, 1994.

45. Sharma OP: Symptoms and signs in pulmonary medicine: old observations and new interpretations. *Dis Mon* 41:577–638, 1995.

46. Simon PM, Schwartzstein RM, Weiss JW, et al: Distinguishable types of dyspnea in patients with shortness of breath. *Am Rev Respir Dis* 142:1009–1014, 1990.

47. Snider GL: History and physical examination, in Baum GL, Wolinsky E (eds), *Textbook of Pulmonary Diseases,* 5th ed. New York, Little, Brown, 1993, pp 243–272.

48. Stark RP, McGinn AL, Wilson RF: Chest pain in cardiac transplant recipients: Evidence of sensory reinervation after cardiac transplantation. *New Engl J Med* 324:1791–1794, 1991.

49. Tunkel DE, Zalzal GH: Stridor in infants and children: Ambulatory evaluation and operative diagnosis. *Clin Pediatr (Phila)* 31:48–55, 1992.

50. Wasserman K, Whipp BJ, Casaburi R: Respiratory control during exercise, in Fishman AP, et al (eds). *Handbook of Physiology,* Section 3: *The Respiratory System,* vol 2, *Control of Breathing,* Part II. Bethesda, MD, American Physiological Society, 1986, pp 595–619.

51. Weisenberg M: Cognitive aspects of pain, in Wall PD, Melzack R (eds), *Textbook of Pain.* Edinburgh, Churchill Livingstone, 1989, pp 231–241.

52. Widdicombe JG: Physiology of cough, in Braga PC, Allegra L (eds), *Cough.* New York, Raven, 1989, pp 3–25.

53. Wilson RC, Jones PW: Differentiation between the intensity of breathlessness and the distress it evokes in normal subjects during exercise. *Clin Sci* 80:65–70, 1991.

54. Zechman FW, Wiley RL: Afferent inputs to breathing: Respiratory sensation, in Cherniack NS, Widdicombe JG (eds), *Handbook of Physiology,* Section 3: *The Respiratory System,* vol. 2, *Control of Breathing.* Bethesda, MD, American Physiological Society, 1986, pp 449–474.

55. Zimmerman D, Parker B: The pain of pulmonary hypertension: Fact or fancy? *JAMA* 246:2345–2349, 1981.

CHAPTER 29

PULMONARY CUTANEOUS DISORDERS

Brian V. Jegasothy

Examination of the skin can provide important clues in the diagnosis and treatment of persons with pulmonary disease: some skin lesions either accompany pulmonary disease or complicate its treatment; occasionally, systemic diseases that affect both skin and lung first manifest themselves in the skin; certain primary diseases of the skin, such as mucosal erythema multiforme, are associated with important pulmonary complications. In addition, common skin lesions, many of which are unrelated to lung disease, have to be taken into account in patients being examined for pulmonary disease.[1]

TYPES OF SKIN LESIONS

The pattern of the skin lesion—i.e., macule, nodule, vesicle, and coloration—can be useful in clarifying the type of process that is occurring in the skin and its relevance to the pulmonary disease in question.

White Macules

Macules are areas of whitish or hypopigmented color change that are not palpable. For example, in young adults or in patients taking steroids, tinea versicolor is a common eruption of white or red-brown macules over the upper torso (Fig. 29-1A). In infants, nonscaling macules or ash-leaf spots concurrent with adenoma sebaceum (smooth pink papules over the central face) may be an early sign of tuberous sclerosis. Vitiligo occurs in patients with thyroid disease, Addison's disease, pernicious anemia, diabetes, and polyglandular failure. It is characterized by white macules that are usually symmetrically disposed over the extremities and around body orifices; occasionally, vitiligo is segmental over a dermatome.

Brown Macules

Brown macules occur as a consequence of sun exposure (freckles) or at the site of previously inflamed lesions, such as acne.

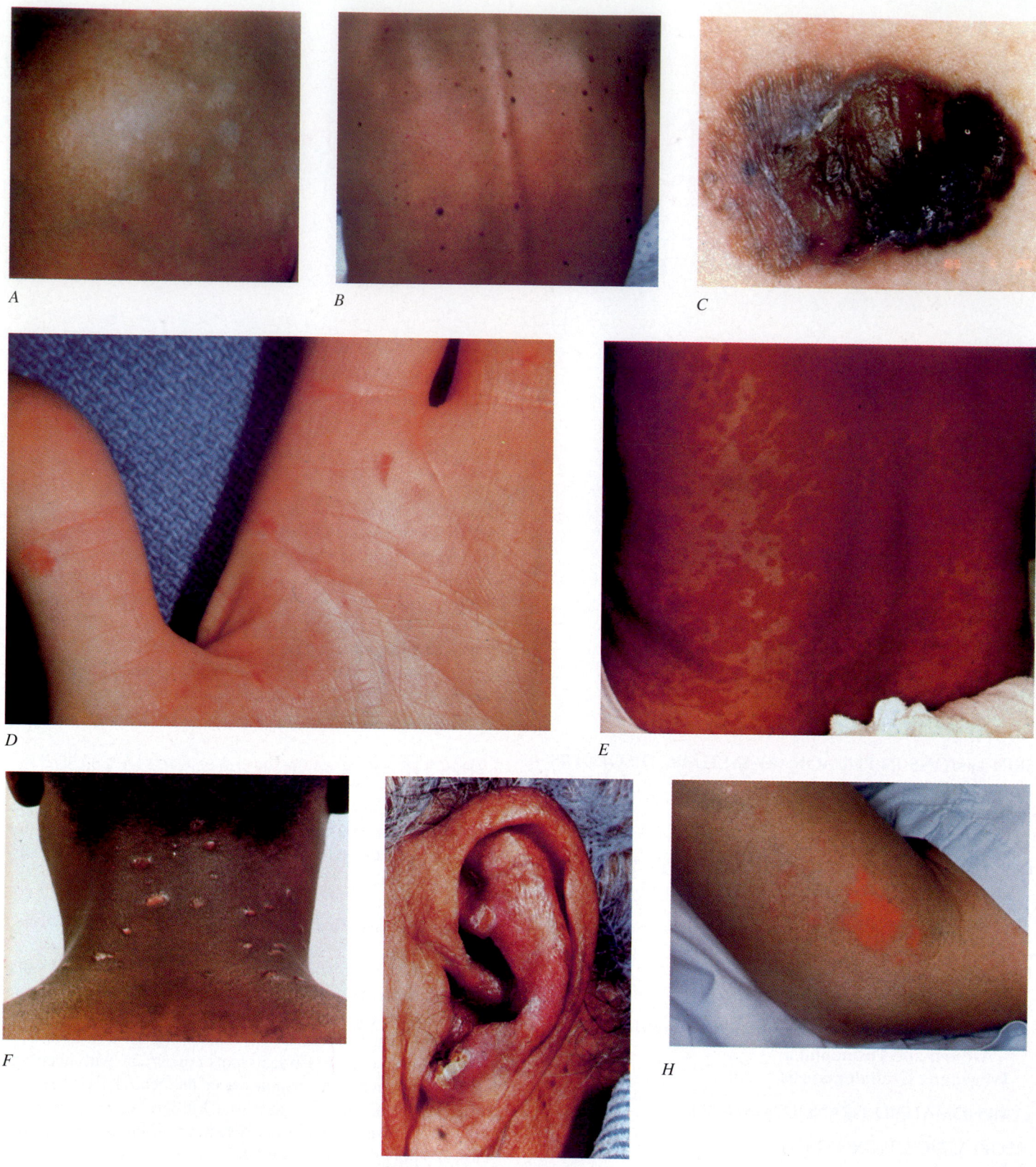

FIGURE 29-1 Prototypic skin lesions. *A.* Tinea versicolor. *B.* Melanocytic nevi. *C.* Malignant melanoma. *D.* "Mat" telangiectasia as seen in scleroderma, or Osler-Weber-Rendu disease. *E.* Exanthematous eruption. *F.* Sarcoid. Flesh-colored papules of upper eyelid and inner canthus. *G.* Metastatic nodule from primary lung carcinoma. *H.* Urticaria.

Pigment cell nevi are brown macules that usually develop in childhood or young adulthood; as a rule, they are symmetric and uniform in color (Fig. 29-1B); suspicion of melanoma should arise when the lesions are irregular in shape; blue, red, brown, or black in color (Fig. 29-1C); rapidly growing; or bleeding. In older people, seborrheic keratosis may first appear as oval brown macules before becoming papules.

Larger (2 to 20 cm) circumscribed brown macules—i.e., café-au-lait spots—occur in 10 percent of the population. The presence of six or more of such lesions larger than 1.5 cm raises the prospect of neurofibromatosis.

Diffuse flat hyperpigmentation occurs after sun exposure (tanning). The skin of patients with scleroderma occasionally develops a pattern of mottled "salt and pepper" hyperpigmentation. In obese persons, flexural pigmentation about the neck and under the axillae, at times associated with flesh-colored skin tags, suggest scaled pseudoacanthosis nigricans; in the nonobese adult, these lesions raise the possibility of acanthosis nigricans, a potential marker of internal malignancy. Although acanthosis nigricans is generally associated with adenocarcinoma of the gastrointestinal tract, it occasionally accompanies carcinoma of the lung.

Red Macules

Telangiectasias are red macules or papules that are usually vascular in appearance. Scattered telangiectasias are common in sun-exposed areas of the skin, such as the V of the anterior neck and the upper back. In patients with obstructive airway disease, linear telangiectasia is sometimes seen along the anterior costal margins; this pattern is known as *costal fringe*. Well-formed spider telangiectasias, common on the upper chest, occur in chronic liver disease or in states of hyperestrogenism. Spider telangiectasia of the trunk, mucosa, fingers, and hands is seen in Osler-Weber-Rendu disease, whereas larger, "mat" telangiectasias distributed in the same areas are seen in scleroderma (Fig. 29-1D). Telangiectasia and persistent edema of the face sometimes occur after repeated bouts of flushing in the carcinoid syndrome. On rare occasions, telangiectasia with mottled hyperpigmentation occurs in systemic mastocytosis.

Diffuse Erythema

This type of erythema may be acute or chronic in onset.

ACUTE

A maculopapular, or exanthematous, eruption is characterized by the acute appearance of many red macules that become confluent to form a diffuse erythema (Fig. 29-1E). The pattern is nonspecific and, in adults, is due either to a drug reaction or to an infectious, especially viral, process. The drugs most often responsible for this type of reaction are antibiotics, especially trimethoprim-sulfamethoxazole, the penicillins, phenytoin, allopurinol, blood products, isoniazid, and carbamazepine. Aminophylline sometimes elicits this type of eruption, especially in patients who have been previously sensitized to ethylenediamine, a common stabilizer in some topical products, such as Mycolog cream.

Viral and bacterial systemic infections can also cause an exanthematous eruption. In classic measles (rubeola) and rubella, fever and upper respiratory symptoms sometimes precede the exanthem, which usually starts on the face. In atypical measles, which occasionally occurs in adults who have developed partial immunity after receiving killed measles vaccine, the onset is generally more insidious and the skin eruption ranges from urticarial to petechial, favors the extremities, and is associated with pneumonia and high fever. Other respiratory viral infections are sometimes accompanied by nonspecific exanthems that are usually truncal; ordinarily the eruption lasts for only a few days and is followed by superficial scaling. In the immunocompromised host, an exanthem sometimes accompanies a fulminant cytomegaloviral infection; cytomegalic inclusions have been seen in skin biopsies from some of these patients.

Among the bacterial infections, streptococcal scarlet fever and the staphylococcal scaled skin syndrome are most often associated with a diffuse erythematous eruption. The toxic shock syndrome, a systemic illness induced by staphylococcal toxin, may be associated with bright-red truncal erythema and, subsequently, with desquamation of palmar and digital skin. Systemic bacterial sepsis due to a variety of organisms (e.g., the meningococci or *Pseudomonas*) occasionally elicits a generalized, nonspecific erythematous eruption; Legionnaires' disease can do the same. As a rule, biopsy or culture of the eruption is unrewarding.

CHRONIC

This category is characterized by the subacute or insidious development (over weeks to months) of a generalized or diffuse erythema (erythroderma). One example is atopic dermatitis, which, in adults, often represents an irritant or allergic reaction to a topical product such as soap or occupational exposure. Exposed areas show erythema, evidence of scratching, and secondary scaling and thickening of the skin. Usually there is a history of childhood eczema or sensitive skin and a personal or family history of asthma, hay fever, or environmental allergies. In some patients with atopic dermatitis, increased itching of the skin appears to be a prodrome to asthma attacks.

In dermatomyositis, a red violaceous hue commonly appears around the eyes (heliotrope), accompanied by fine scaling; the upper trunk and extensor surfaces of the extremities may be similarly affected. Gottron's papules—red, atrophic papules over the finger joints—are present in about one-third of patients. In lupus erythematosus, erythema, telangiectasia, and atrophy tend to affect the sun-exposed areas of the face and arms; sometimes the upper trunk is similarly involved.

A chronic insidious onset of generalized erythroderma may be secondary to drugs, to infiltrative skin disease (such as cutaneous lymphoma or leukemia), or to mastocytosis, or it may be a reaction to an internal malignancy, including carcinoma of the lung.

Flesh-Colored Papules and Nodules

In neurofibromatosis, flat, pigmented, café-au-lait patches that appear in childhood are often accompanied in adulthood by soft, flesh-colored papules and nodules. The lesions of basal cell carcinoma are flesh-colored or translucent papules with telangiectasia and erosion, and they occur particularly in sun-exposed areas of fair skinned people.

In sarcoidosis, distinctive lesions in the form of firm, flesh-colored papules of the face and upper trunk occur in 20 to 25 percent of affected subjects (Fig. 29-1F). Environmental exposure to beryllium can also reproduce the lesions clinically and histologically.

Neoplastic or metastatic lesions (Fig. 29-1G) are noninflamed, asymptomatic, firm to rock-hard flesh-colored or red nodules of the skin. Metastases from a carcinoma of the lung or breast or cutaneous infiltrates due to B-cell lymphomas are particularly likely to invade the anterior upper trunk. In men, carcinoma of the lung is a common cause of cutaneous metastases; the skin metastases usually involve the scalp, the anterior chest, and the abdomen.

Red Papules and Nodules

Cherry angiomas are typically persistent cherry-red papules, 1 to 8 mm in diameter; they commonly affect the trunk and proximal extremities in the elderly, in pregnant women, and in persons who are in a state of hyperestrogenism. They occur in Osler-Weber-Rendu disease, occasionally in association with pulmonary arteriovenous fistulas. Dermatomal hemangiomas are congenital vascular patches that may be associated with underlying spinal vascular malformations.

Urticarial lesions take the form of scattered, transient red papules, plaques, and wheals that may be annular or serpiginous in shape and edematous pink to dusky in color (Fig. 29-1H). The wheals may occur anywhere on the body. Pruritus is generally a prominent feature. The individual lesions usually last for only 24 to 48 h.

Urticaria is common and generally nonspecific; on the one hand, it may herald a life-threatening anaphylactic reaction; on the other, it may be a fleeting localized reaction of no great moment. Among the potential causes of urticaria are topical or systemic medications, food inhalant allergens, infections, and psychological factors.[16]

Dermatographism is a type of urticaria in which wheals develop in response to stroking of the skin; it occurs in up to 5 percent of normal persons but may also develop transiently after upper respiratory tract illness and from some medications. *White dermatographism* is a vasoconstrictive response to skin stroking that may be quite prominent in patients with atopic dermatitis. Cholinergic urticaria (Fig. 29-2A) is characterized by small (1 to 3 mm) pruritic wheals with surrounding red flare reactions; they occur in response to heat, cold, exercise, and emotional stress. Transient symptoms of wheezing or shortness of breath may accompany the onset of cholinergic urticaria, and pulmonary function tests may provide evidence of bronchospasm. The process seems to be mast cell mediated; treatment with antihistamines, such as hydroxyzine, is usually of benefit.[22]

In erythema multiforme, annular erythematous papules sometimes progress to target lesions with overlying blisters (Fig. 29-2B). The lesions can occur anywhere on the body but may be limited to the hands and feet. When erythema multiforme is accompanied by fever, skin lesions, and mucosal involvement of the mouth or eyes, it is called *Stevens-Johnson syndrome* (Fig. 29-2C). Erythema multiforme may occur as a reaction to drugs, including penicillin, sulfa derivatives, gold, and barbiturates. A long list of organisms and infections may also elicit erythema multiforme: herpes simplex I and II, influenza A, *Mycoplasia pneumoniae,* adenovirus, psittacosis, β-hemolytic streptococcus, *Pseudomonas,* tularemia, histoplasmosis, coccidioidomycosis, and tuberculosis.[21]

Several types of large (over 1 cm) erythematous nodules occur in patients with pulmonary disease. One type that has no bearing on the pulmonary process is a simple infected epidermal cyst that develops suddenly as a tender red nodule at the site of a preexisting lesion, commonly on the posterior neck and back. Oppositely, red nodules may represent vascular, inflammatory, or neoplastic processes that cannot be distinguished without excisional biopsy. The nodular vasculitides—including allergic, Wegener's, and lymphomatoid granulomatosis—are discussed later in this chapter.

The presence of many tender red nodules over the anterior surfaces of the lower extremities suggests erythema nodosum (Fig. 29-2D), a reactive inflammation of the subcutaneous fat that may be associated with a number of infections, drugs, and underlying inflammatory diseases. In the patient undergoing treatment for acute or subacute pulmonary disease, medications may be the cause—especially oral contraceptives, sulfonamides, other antibiotics, isodides, or bromides. In up to 16 percent of patients with erythema nodosum, sarcoidosis is the cause. Occasionally, sarcoidosis is first manifested as an acute febrile illness with erythema nodosum, hilar adenopathy, malaise, and arthritis (Lofgren's syndrome). As a rule, sarcoidosis that begins with erythema nodosum is a self-limited disease. Erythema nodosum also occurs in some people with tuberculosis, psittacosis, histoplasmosis, blastomycosis, and coccidioidomycosis.

A variety of pulmonary infections (blastomycosis, coccidioidomycosis, histoplasmosis, cryptococcosis, tuberculosis, actinomycosis, and nocardiosis) may be accompanied by skin lesions in the form of crusted, erythematous nodules and plaques (Figs. 29-2E and F). They may occur anywhere on the skin; as a rule, they are nonspecific in appearance and asymptomatic. The development of this type of crusted plaque or nodule in a patient with a chronic pulmonary infection calls for biopsy and histopathologic examination using special stains and cultures for suspected organisms.

Blue Papules and Nodules

Blue color is generally transmitted from vascular structures or melanin pigment deep in the dermis. Blue nevi are benign dermal melanocytic neoplasms that are uniform in shape; they may occur over the head or the paraspinal area of the trunk. A blue-black, irregular, or friable lesion raises the possibility of a melanoma. A vascular lesion is generally partly compressible or palpable. Venous angiomas occur over the lips, ears, and upper trunk of older people. Kaposi's sarcoma, particularly in patients with acquired immunodeficiency syndrome, may present as asymptomatic bluish papules or plaques on the mucosa, upper trunk, and extremities (Fig. 29-3A); these lesions may become quite extensive.

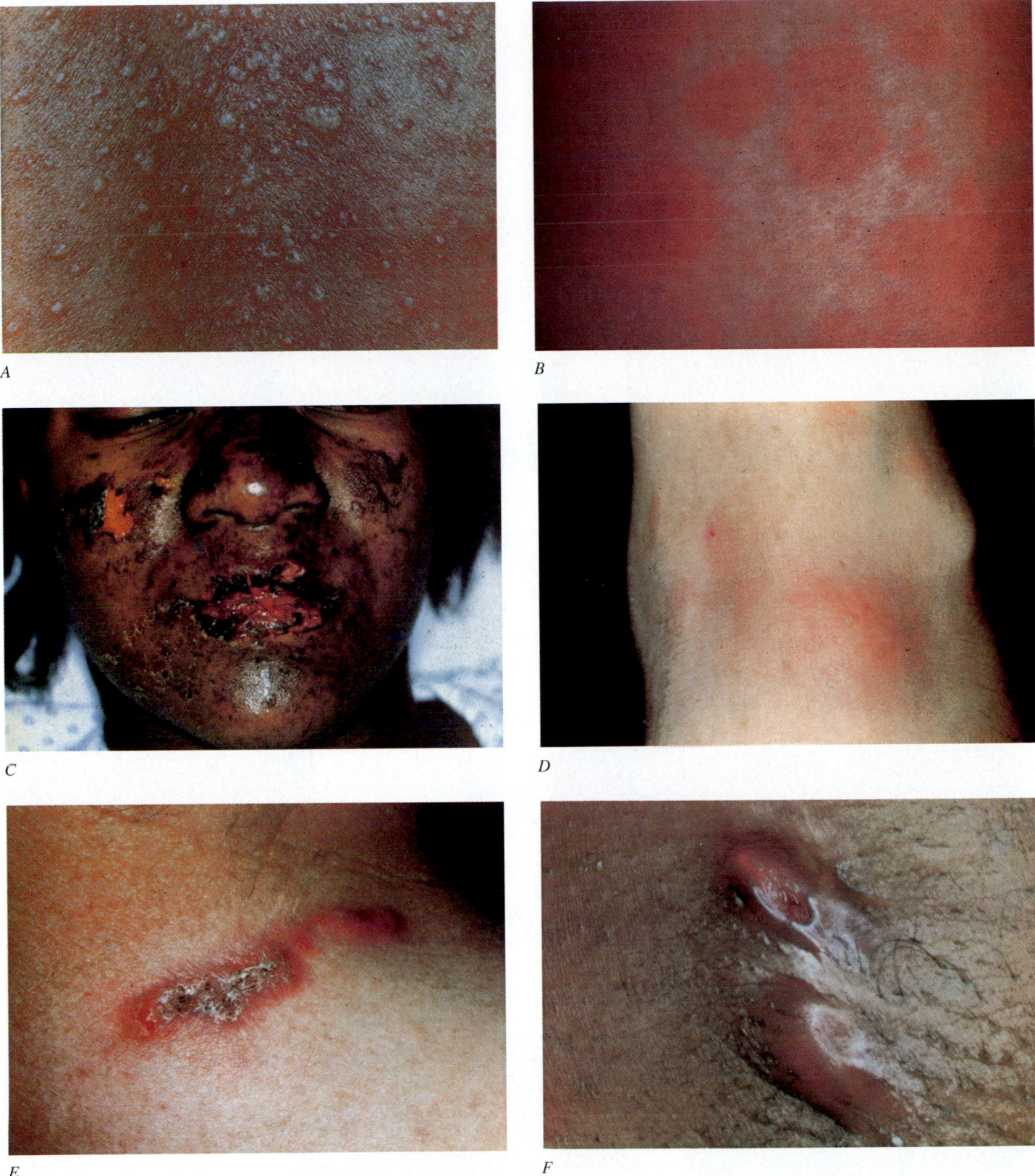

FIGURE 29-2 Skin lesions that may occur in pulmonary patients. *A*. Cholinergic urticaria. *B*. Erythema multiforme. *C*. Stevens-Johnson syndrome. *D*. Erythema nodosum. *E*. Blastomycosis. *F*. Tuberculous abscess.

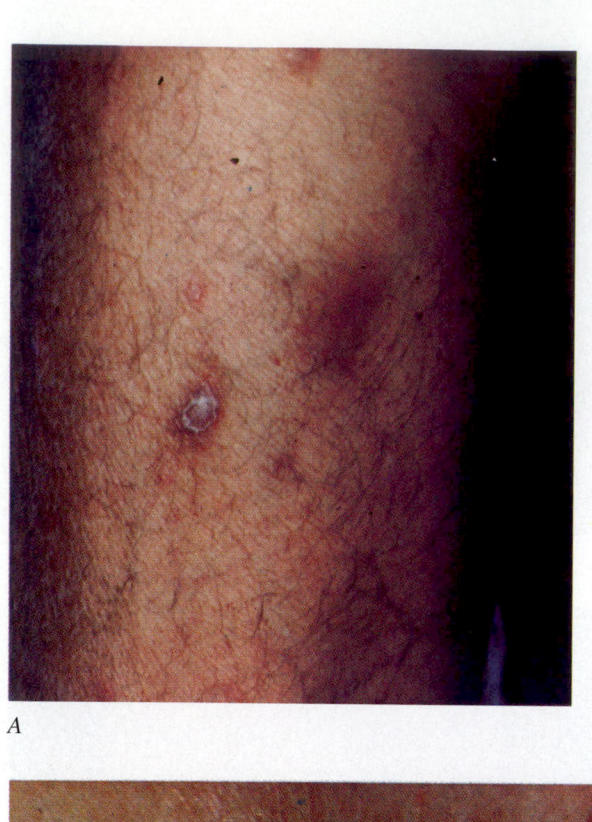

A

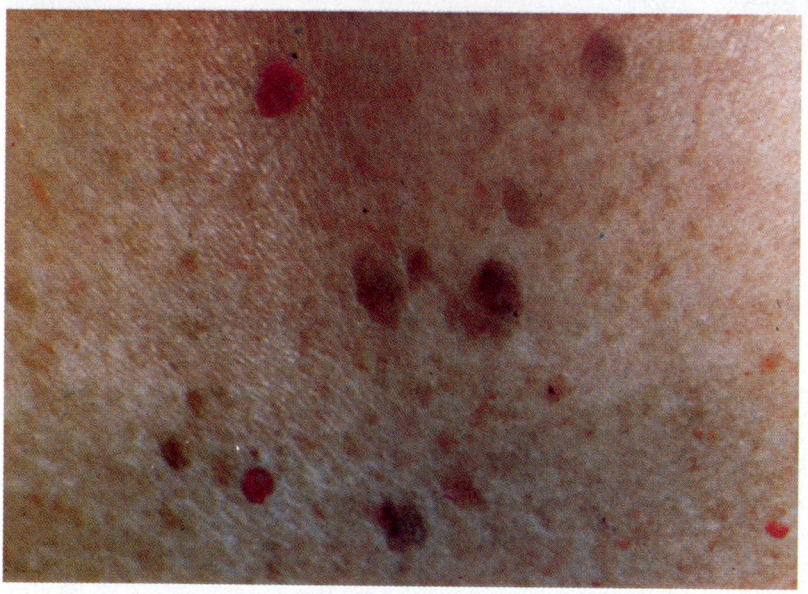

B

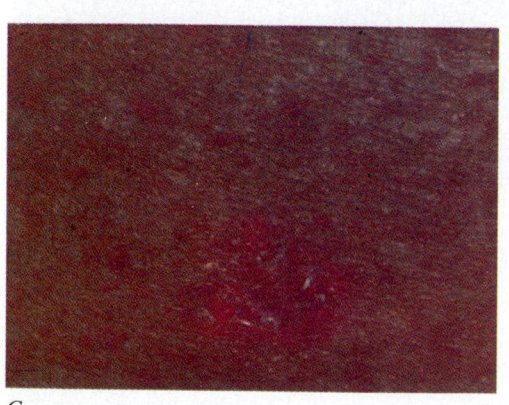

C

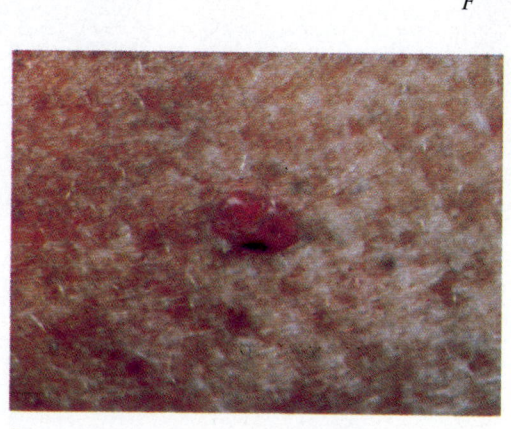

D

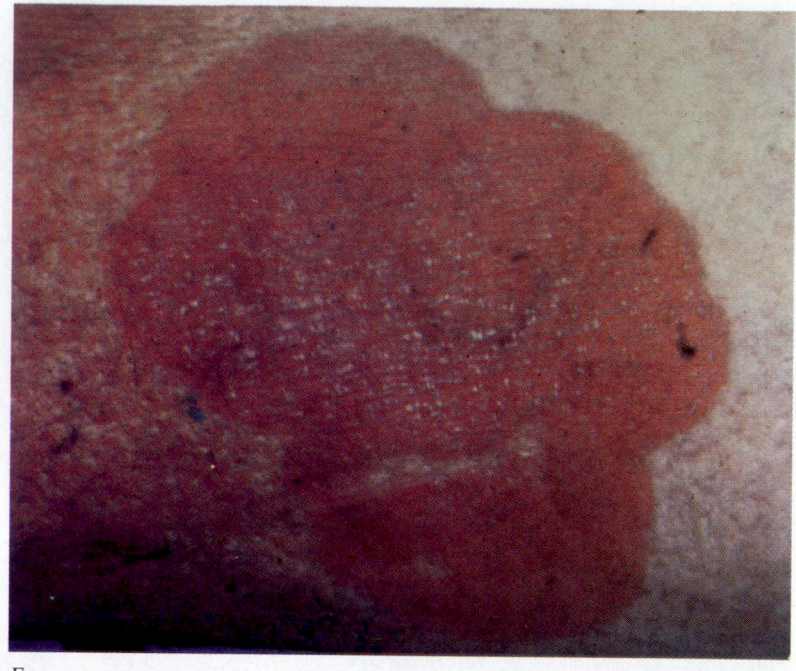

E

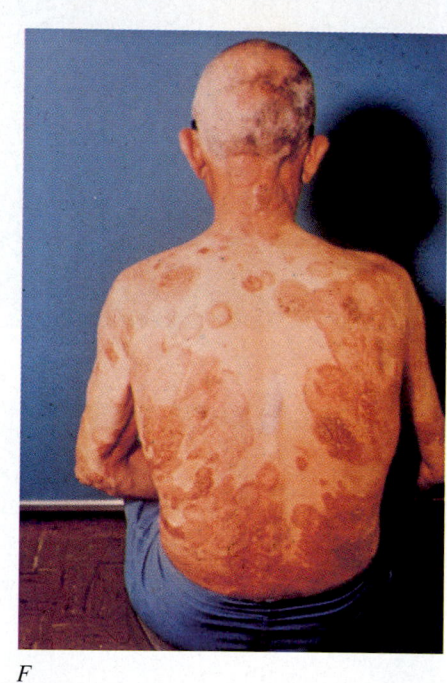

F

FIGURE 29-3

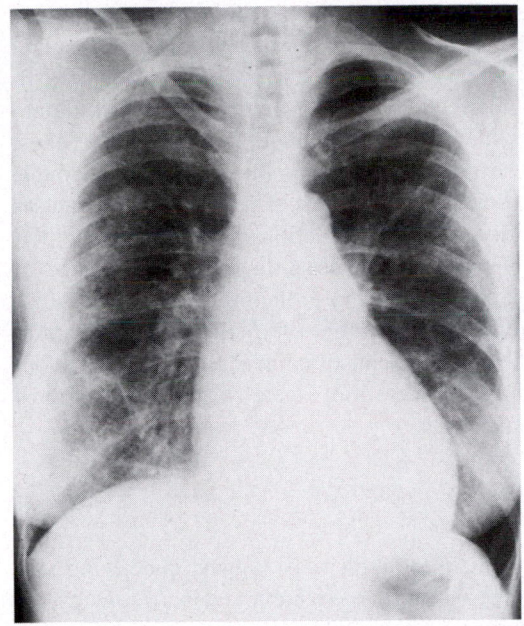

G

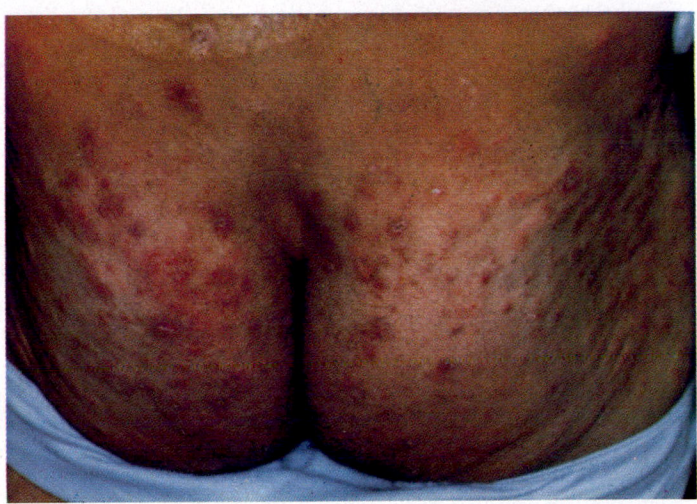

H

FIGURE 29-3 *(cont.)* Skin lesions that may be encountered in patients with pulmonary disease. *A.* Kaposi's sarcoma in a patient with acquired immunodeficiency syndrome. *B.* Seborrheic keratoses (brown) and cherry (red) angiomata. *C.* Basal cell carcinoma, superficial type. *D.* Basal cell carcinoma. *E.* Mycosis fungoides. *F.* Mycosis fungoides. Asymmetric diffuse, superficial, gyrate plaques of dermatitis. *G.* Chest radiograph shows diffuse reticular nodular density, proved by open lung biopsy to be mycosis fungoides. *H.* Larva migrans in a patient with Loeffler's syndrome. *(From Katz and Beerman.[11a])*

Brown Papules

Melanocytic nevi (Fig. 29-1*B*) and seborrheic keratoses (Fig. 29-3*B*) are the most common lesions of this type. Pigmented nevi are usually uniform, in both brown color and shape. Dysplastic nevi are atypical lesions that are irregular and reddish-brown; they may give rise to malignant melanoma. As indicated above, irregular borders or surface or blue-black or red color of the lesions should raise concern about malignant melanoma (Fig. 29-1*C*). Seborrheic keratoses are waxy or rough-shaped superficial brown papules usually found in the elderly, particularly over the back, neck, and face.

Scaling Papules

A number of skin disorders can present as multiple scaling red papules or plaques; among these are psoriasis, pityriasis rosea, secondary syphilis, and fungal infections. Sarcoid may also have scaling plaques and papules that resemble psoriasis.

Certain scaling lesions are common over the neck and back. Among these are actinic keratoses, which are small, rough lesions on sun-exposed areas of the face, neck, back, and arms. They are most prominent in fair-skinned persons with outdoor occupations. Bowen's disease (in situ squamous cell carcinoma) is usually a single scaling or eczematous plaque that may occur anywhere on the body; this type of persistent solitary lesion requires biopsy to establish the diagnosis. The occurrence of Bowen's disease in non–sun-exposed areas raises the possibility of an internal neoplasm, including a carcinoma of the respiratory tract; a latent period of 8 years may intervene between the onset of Bowen's disease and detection of the variant of this common sun-induced tumor; it presents as a single patch or as several scaling red patches, often on the trunk (Figs. 29-3*C* and *D*).

Mycosis fungoides,[2] also called cutaneous T-cell lymphoma, is a malignant lymphoma of the skin that progresses through three stages. The first, or *premycotic,* phase is characterized by lesions that resemble psoriasis, seborrheic dermatitis, or eczema; characteristically, the lesions are very pruritic (Fig. 29-3*E*). In the second phase, which may be long delayed, the lesions become infiltrative, forming indurated red-to-purple plaques in conjunction with exfoliative dermatitis and erythroderma (Fig. 29-3*F* and *G*). The final stage is characterized by the formation of tumors that usually become necrotic. This sequence may take 8 to 12 years to evolve. On occasion, however, mycosis fungoides blossoms de novo as a mushroomlike growth on normal skin (d'emblée form). The final stage is often accompanied by systemic manifestations, including Sézary syndrome.

The lungs are frequently affected in mycosis fungoides. Two-thirds of patients who die of disseminated mycosis fungoides have pulmonary involvement at autopsy; usually the lesions are in the form of multiple nodules; few have diffuse patchy or confluent infiltrates. Histologically, tumor cells are seen infiltrating alveolar walls. The neoplasm spreads via the bloodstream, leaving uninvolved contiguous or regional lymph nodes. Chest radiographs usually show mediastinal and hilar adenopathy, reticulonodular parenchymal lesions, and, occasionally, pleural effusions.

The extracutaneous sites that are most often affected by cutaneous T-cell lymphoma are blood, lymph nodes (in 75 percent of patients at autopsy), and lungs (in 66 percent at autopsy). This visceral involvement is often asymptomatic but is important in clinical staging and survival. When the lungs are affected, the chest radiograph may show hilar and mediastinal adenopathy (Fig. 29-3*G*) and a reticulonodular pattern of pulmonary infiltration. Lung biopsy shows the tumor lymphocytes infiltrating alveolar walls.

Vesiculobullous Lesions

Of the skin lesions that present as fluid-filled blisters, the herpesvirus group of diseases are the most relevant to pulmonary disease. These are discussed subsequently.

Primary blistering disorders may also affect the respiratory mucosa. Stevens-Johnson syndrome has already been mentioned. Pemphigus vulgaris, an immunologically mediated bullous disease in which IgG antibodies develop against the epidermal intracellular substance, presents as multiple flaccid bullous lesions. The mouth and oropharynx may be the initial and most prominent sites of invasion. Certain variants of a congenital bullous disorder, epidermolysis bullosa, may also afflict the pharyngeal and respiratory mucosa, leading to erosions, scarring and stricture.

Pustules

Skin lesions that present as pustules should raise the possibility of bacterial infection. The most common of these is probably a folliculitis, in which pustules develop around hair follicles. Most often a folliculitis is due to *Staphylococcus aureus* infection, and the lesions may progress to furuncles or to deep cutaneous abscesses. Manipulation of such lesions can lead to bacteremia and numerous septic pulmonary abscesses. Parenteral drug users are at risk for developing cutaneous abscesses at needle sites. Patients with underlying deep fungal disease, actinomycosis, or nocardiosis may develop indurated, pustular plaques or cutaneous abscesses. For identification of the causative organism, the lesions may have to be incised or biopsied for staining and culture.

Drug-induced acne presents as multiple small pustules, often over the upper chest. Steroids in high doses, bromides, or iodides are common causes. In areas and societies where larvae of nematodes can gain access to the skin, secondary pyoderma caused by scratching of the pruritic lesions is often superimposed on the linear tracts or papules produced by the entering larvae. The skin pattern is often a bizarre combination of lesions, and larva migrans should be considered in a patient who presents with a compatible history and skin lesions, especially over the buttocks and back (Fig. 29-3*H*). *Strongyloides stercoralis* and some other nematodes can cause these skin lesions (larva currens) in association with acute fever, asthma, and eosinophilia (Loeffler's syndrome).

Purpura

Purpura results from disruption or extravasation of blood from cutaneous vessels; it is a nonspecific finding. It occurs commonly over traumatized sites in older patients, particularly in sun-exposed areas. Patients receiving steroid or anticoagulant therapy, or with defects in collagen (e.g., Ehlers-Danlos syndrome or amyloidosis), are prone to traumatic purpura. Punctate petechiae may develop on the palate, face, and upper chest of patients with severe coughing spasms. Raised or palpable purpuric lesions should suggest a vasculitis. Because the causes of vasculitis are diverse (e.g., infections, medications, hypersensitivity reactions, and small-vessel disease), examination of the skin must be followed by more elaborate diagnostic studies, including biopsy. Involvement of medium or large cutaneous vessels with vasculitis causes painful red to purpuric nodules with secondary ulceration; once again, the clinical appearance is nonspecific.

NAILS

A number of changes in the nails may suggest underlying systemic disease. Clubbing and hypertrophic osteoarthropathy are discussed elsewhere (see Chapter 26). Yellow-brown staining of the nails where cigarettes are held is very common in persons with obstructive airway disease who have not stopped smoking. The designation *yellow nail syndrome* refers to thickening, yellowing, and curvature of all the nails in association with lymphedema; it may be associated with pleural effusions, chronic pulmonary infections, and bronchiectasis.[19]

Periungual telangiectasia and digital infarcts are seen in patients with lupus erythematosus, scleroderma, dermatomyositis, and overlap syndromes. Splinter hemorrhages are often due to trauma and are generally nonspecific despite their historical link to bacterial endocarditis. Sarcoidosis in the form of lupus pernio may affect the nails and underlying bones, leading to dystrophic, ridged nails and distal swelling.

SKIN TEXTURE CHANGES

Thickening or sclerosis of the skin is most often associated with scleroderma; this disorder may present as distal digital sclerosis or it may be diffuse, most prominently over the trunk, and cause the typical drawn facies of scleroderma. The pulmonary changes are discussed in Chapter 43. Scleredema adultorum is a rare cutaneous disorder with striking mucopolysaccharide infiltration of the face, neck, and trunk; it may be confused clinically with scleroderma.

Increased elasticity of the skin is associated with certain types of Ehlers-Danlos syndrome; it is associated with defects in collagen synthesis. Conversely, in cutis laxa, the skin loses its elasticity because of a defect in the formation of elastin. Both disorders are considered below (see "Disorders of Collagen and Elastin").

SKIN LESIONS IN PULMONARY-SYSTEMIC DISORDERS

A variety of cutaneous findings are sometimes evident in patients with systemic diseases. Some of the most common are highlighted below.

Atopic Dermatitis

Atopy refers to a group of disorders—including asthma, hay fever, and atopic dermatitis—in which immune and pharmacologic responses are characteristically abnormal.[8] The atopic person usually has a family history of one or more of these disorders. Atopic dermatitis is a common disorder, affecting 1 to 3 percent of the population in the United States. In 85 percent of affected subjects, the skin lesions appear before 5 years of age. The dermatitis generally resolves as the patient reaches adulthood; in the adult, either the skin lesions or respiratory systems may predominate.

In infants, the skin lesions often begin as dry, erythematous plaques on the cheeks; excoriations and scaling may be prominent. In older children, the lesions localize in flexures; lichenification and excoriated papules are prominent features (Fig. 29-4A). In adults, the lesions favor the hands and extremities (nummular dermatitis) (Fig. 29-4B). Atopic subjects also manifest prominent folds of the lower eyelids, periorbital hyperpigmentation with facial pallor, generalized dry skin, and white dermatographism. At any age, pruritus may be prominent and become secondarily infected, leading to bacterial impetigo within the lesions. In some patients, increased itching may be a prodrome to exacerbation of asthma.

The cause of atopic dermatitis is unknown. In all likelihood, the pathogenesis is multifactorial, probably including disordered immune regulation as a causative factor. In persons with atopic dermatitis, abnormalities in cell-mediated immunity and in lymphocyte function increase the risk of disseminated viral and fungal skin lesions. The role of food or environmental antigenic challenge in flares of atopic dermatitis is unsettled, but it is known that asthma can be precipitated by such challenges. Treatment of atopic dermatitis in adults is aimed at eliminating possible environmental irritants and allergens.

Infectious Disorders

The skin and lungs are sometimes affected simultaneously in infectious disorders, including viral, bacterial, mycoplasma, and fungal diseases.

VIRAL

Three types of viral infection are often responsible for pulmonary cutaneous syndromes: herpes simplex, herpes zoster-varicella, and measles.

Herpes Simplex

The lesions of herpes simplex appear as groups of small vesicles (1 to 5 mm) on an erythematous base; they may occur anywhere on the body surface, but the most common sites are around the lips or genital area. Recurrence of the lesions can be triggered by fever, upper respiratory infection, trauma, or exposure to sunlight. Patients with underlying skin diseases such as atopic dermatitis may be at risk for developing generalized herpes simplex (i.e., eczema herpeticum). In immunocompromised patients, the lesions may be atypical and take the form of persistent crusted ulcers or erosions. This should be kept in mind when one is do-

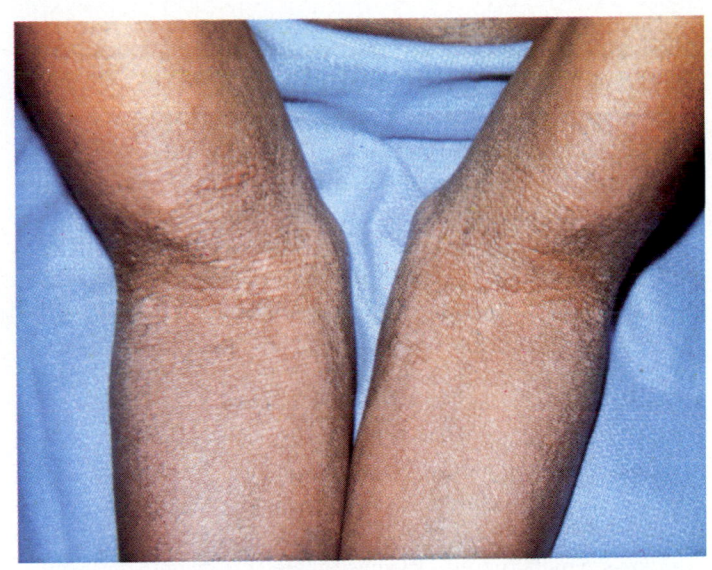

A

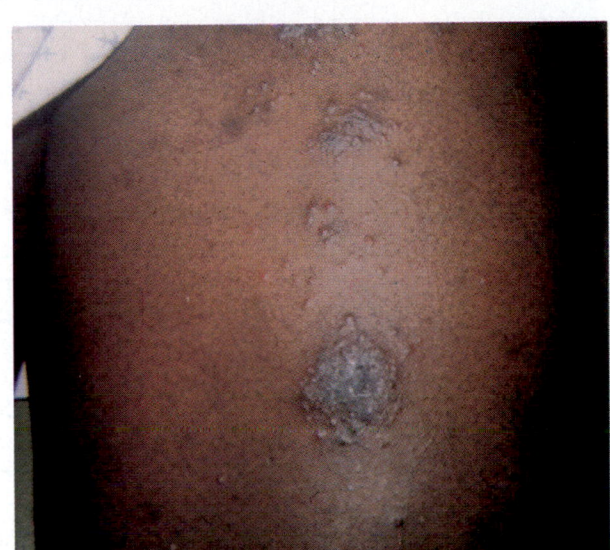

B

FIGURE 29-4 Skin lesions in pulmonary-systemic disorders. *A.* Atopic dermatitis—flexural lichenification. *B.* Atopic dermatitis—nummular lesions.

ing bronchoscopy, suctioning, or other procedures on patients with perioral ulcerations. Medical personnel are at risk for acquiring herpes simplex infection of the fingers—such as herpetic whitlow, a tender vesicular cellulitis of the digit.

Herpes Zoster and Varicella

Herpes zoster and varicella have potential pulmonary complications. Varicella often starts with a prodromal fever, malaise, headache, and sore throat, followed by onset of small (1 to 3 mm), distinct vesicles on a red base that rapidly progress to umbilicated and crusted lesions. Lesions appear in crops over the body and may also invade the mucous membranes. The major complication of adult varicella is pneumonia, and the extent of pulmonary impairment tends to correlate with the extent of the cutaneous eruption. Radiographic findings may be more prominent than symptoms; infiltrates are seen in up to 16 percent of adult patients with varicella, whereas respiratory symptoms occur in only about 5 percent of adults.

In more than two-thirds of patients with herpes zoster, the lesions affect the thoracic region. Prodromal symptoms of localized pain before the eruption may mimic pleuritic pain, angina, or an acute abdomen; local itching, tenderness, or hyperesthesia may be followed by erythematous papules or urticarial plaques over the distribution of one or two sensory ganglia. Within 12 to 24 h, the lesions develop into vesicles; crusting occurs within 7 to 10 days. Overlapping dermatomes may be affected, and a few isolated vesicles may lie outside these dermatomes. The associated pain is usually most severe early in the course and may lead to respiratory splinting. Affliction of the cervical roots may lead to diaphragmatic paralysis on the same side. The lesions cluster on the face, scalp, chest, and abdomen; the palms and soles are spared. The hard palate, tonsillar pillars, and larynx also develop vesicles—which rupture, leaving white ulcers with an erythematous halo. Histologically, zoster and varicella lesions contain interepidermal bullae. Infected cells contain eosinophilic, intranuclear inclusions surrounded by a clear halo and a circle of dark-staining chromatin. Multinucleated giant "balloon" cells are often present.

Pneumonia is the most common pulmonary complication of active infection with the varicella-zoster virus; pulmonary infarction has also been seen. Although the cutaneous form of the disease is common in children, 90 percent of people who develop pneumonia are more than 20 years old; most of them are in the third to fifth decade. The most frequent symptoms of varicella pneumonia develop 1 to 6 days after the onset of rash; they consist of cough, fever, cyanosis, dyspnea, and hemoptysis. Chest radiographs show a nodular or reticulonodular infiltrate throughout all lung fields, with a tendency toward coalescence at the base. Pleural effusions and hilar adenopathy have also been reported. Radiographic changes correlate well with cutaneous lesions; the chest radiograph clears rapidly as the skin manifestations resolve, leaving only minor abnormalities as residue; these often persist for months. Small calcifications in both lungs, especially at the bases, are common sequelae of varicella pneumonia.

Measles

Measles, a myxoviral infection, characteristically develops cutaneous manifestations after an incubation period of about 10 days. The initial phase of cutaneous manifestations, which lasts 4 to 7 days, consists of an erythematous or petechial eruption in the soft palate, followed by the appearance of blue-white lesions surrounded by a bright-red halo on the buccal mucosa (Koplik's spots). The buccal lesions proliferate, become confluent, and resolve within 72 h of their appearance. The characteristic macular eruption in the scalp then develops and rapidly spreads to the upper part of the neck, extremities, and trunk. This exanthema progresses to soft papules and becomes confluent over the face before beginning to scale. Systemic manifestations include high fever, chills, conjunctivitis, coryza, and a dry, hacking cough. This cough is a common symptom in the initial invasion phase, and it sometimes recurs as the disease progresses.

Segmental pneumonia and atelectasis are common in patients with measles. In most instances, these are complications of super-

infection with bacteria. However, the virus per se sometimes causes a giant-cell pneumonia, especially in children. Giant-cell pneumonia occurs before or coincident with the peak of the measles exanthema. In these children, the chest radiograph shows a diffuse reticular pattern, usually accompanied by hilar adenopathy.

MYCOPLASMA

Pneumonia caused by *M. pneumonia* is associated with a wide variety of mucocutaneous lesions. Approximately 25 percent of patients with pneumonia have dermatologic manifestations, including erythema nodosum, pityriasis rosea, scaly erythema, and urticaria, as well as petechiae and macular, papulovesicular, and morbilliform rashes. Occasionally, patients with *M. pneumonia* infection develop Stevens-Johnson syndrome. Erythema multiforme also occurs as vesicles or bullae in the oropharynx, which appear within 2 weeks of the onset of respiratory illness and frequently persist despite resolution of pulmonary signs and symptoms.

FUNGAL

Fungal infections of the lungs in people with normal immune mechanisms are not often accompanied by skin lesions. In the immunocompromised host, however, a disseminated fungemia often evokes striking and distinctive manifestations in the lungs and skin.

Blastomycosis

In blastomycosis, skin lesions are common as pulmonary lesions: Cutaneous, localized blastomycosis usually arises from a pulmonary focus that is often small and inapparent. Its typical presentation is as a solitary papule or nodule on the face, wrists, hands, or feet, which subsequently ulcerates and discharges pus. The lesions grow eccentrically at the periphery and atrophy centrally over a period of months, eventually forming an acriform or serpiginous contour with sharply elevated and verrucous borders. Miliary abscesses are seen along the borders of the lesions. In disseminated blastomycosis, multiple subcutaneous nodules are common, generally in association with osteolytic lesions: the skin lesions tend to ulcerate.

Actinomycosis

The thoracic form of this disease presents as a pulmonary parenchymal process that sometimes forms multiple draining sinus tracts. The draining exudate contains the characteristic sulfur granules.

Coccidioidomycosis

This fungal disease sometimes produces acute or chronic cutaneous manifestations. During the initial primary pulmonary infection, approximately one-fifth of patients develop an erythema nodosum, often accompanied by arthropathy and eosinophilia. As the pulmonary disease progresses, the skin is one of the organs most likely to be affected. Subcutaneous granulomatous eruptions form and undergo necrosis and ulceration. After several months, they tend to become verrucous. Disseminated disease has a poor prognosis.

Sporotrichosis

Almost invariably, this is strictly a dermatologic disorder. Following injury to the skin by an object contaminated with the spores of *Sporothrix schenckii,* the affected person develops the primary cutaneous eruption. These lesions, often mistaken for boils or luetic chancres, usually remain localized, but on rare occasions they disseminate via lymphatics to other organs, including the lungs.

Aspergillosis

The invasive form of this disease is occasionally associated with skin lesions. In most cases, the cutaneous eruptions are multiple and scattered, suggesting hematogenous spread from a primary pulmonary focus. It is uncertain whether direct cutaneous inoculation with *Aspergillus* can lead to disseminated disease. The dermatologic manifestations of systemic aspergillosis are nonspecific and include solitary necrotizing plaques, subcutaneous granulomas and abscesses, suppurative maculopapules, and a variety of other lesions. *A. fumigatus* is the species most frequently cultured from skin lesions in patients with systemic aspergillosis.

Candidiasis

Patients with disseminated candidiasis sometimes develop diffuse, macronodular, erythematous skin lesions. Biopsy of the skin lesions demonstrates pseudohyphae in the dermis and blood vessels, whereas the dermis is intact. Blood cultures are as often positive for *Candida* species, as are cultures of cutaneous lesions in this disseminated form of the disease.

TUBERCULOSIS

Cutaneous affliction results from direct inoculation with the tubercle bacillus, via either the skin or mucous membranes or as a consequence of widespread organ involvement that begins in the respiratory tract. The skin lesion occurs either as a primary infection or as a result of reactivation of infection with *Mycobacterium tuberculosis.*

When the tubercle is introduced via the skin or mucous membranes by a contaminated syringe or a wound in a previously unexposed host, a nodule usually develops at the site of injury. Within several weeks, the nodule evolves into a chancre, a well-circumscribed ulcer. Particularly if host defenses are impaired, these chancriform lesions, which are typically located on the extremities, develop associated regional lymphadenitis, followed by systemic dissemination of the organism.

A person who was previously infected with *M. tuberculosis* is apt to develop *tuberculosis verrucosa cutis* after receiving a cutaneous inoculation. The characteristic lesion in a sensitized person is a papule or a pustule, which becomes verrucous. On occasion, this disorder produces plaquelike lesions of the extremities consisting of verrucoid–indurated papules surrounded by an erythematous halo.

Lupus vulgaris is the most common form of cutaneous postprimary tuberculosis that follows inoculation or lymphatic or hematogenous spread of *M. tuberculosis.* Patients with this disorder typically present with reddish-brown plaques surrounded peripherally by yellowish nodules, especially on the neck or extremities. The skin lesions tend to spread centrifugally as the center of the cutaneous disorder atrophies. Papillary growths also occur in the nasal, buccal, and conjunctival mucosa. Histologically, lupus vulgaris generally shows epithelioid tubercles without caseation necrosis. Tubercle bacilli are rarely observed or cultured from skin biopsy specimens. Chronic cutaneous eruptions tend to involute, leaving considerable scarring. Chemotherapy with the usual antituberculosis drugs is effective in treating these skin manifestations.

Disseminated miliary tuberculosis can result in macules, papules, or vesicles. In children, especially those who are debilitated, subcutaneous nodules or gummas appear, ulcerate, and eventually develop draining sinus tracts, especially in the extremities and trunk. *Scrofuloderma,* which occurs following the necrosis of cervical nodules, is associated with fistula and sinus tract formation in the overlying cutaneous tissues.

Tuberculids are skin lesions that are considered to represent either a hypersensitivity reaction to *M. tuberculosis* or an embolic response to atypical *Mycobacteria.* Erythema nodosum also occurs in association with primary tuberculosis (Fig. 29-5).

Cutaneous Sarcoidosis

Sarcoidosis is a systemic disease with a number of cutaneous presentations. The clinical manifestations, course, and treatment of cutaneous sarcoidosis are discussed below. Systemic and pulmonary sarcoidoses are discussed in Chapter 69.

CLINICAL

Twenty to 35 percent of patients with systemic sarcoidosis develop cutaneous lesions at some time; in up to 10 percent, skin lesions are the initial complaint (Fig. 29-6).[9,24] Some of the skin lesions are specific microscopically (i.e., they show noncaseating granulomas on histologic examination), whereas others, notably erythema nodosum, are nonspecific (i.e., they do not show the characteristic—but not unique—granulomas of sarcoidosis). Erythema nodosum (Fig. 29-2D) occurs in 3 to 25 percent of patients with sarcoidosis and, as noted previously, is often associated with the acute onset of self-limited pulmonary disease. Other nonspecific skin lesions, such as generalized pruritus and erythema multiforme, are uncommon and may be coincidental.

The specific lesions of cutaneous sarcoid are commonly flesh-colored to violaceous papules that have a predilection for the face, neck, and upper trunk (Figs. 29-1F and 29-6 A–C) and are firm and sometimes annular or serpiginous; "angiolupoid" lesions are large violaceous plaques in which telangiectasia features prominently. Most papular and plaque forms of cutaneous sarcoid resolve without scarring.[18] However, the violaceous plaques of lupus pernio, which occur over the nose, ears, and digits and invade underlying bone, do scar and are both permanent and disfiguring (Fig. 29-6D). Lupus pernio accompanies invasion of various systems by sarcoidosis, including the upper respiratory tract.[17]

Other lesions that prove to be sarcoid on histologic examination may be nonspecific in appearance; among these are alopecia, ichthyosislike impairment of the lower legs, and psoriasiform, erythrodermic, follicular, and hypopigmented lesions. Deep subcuta-

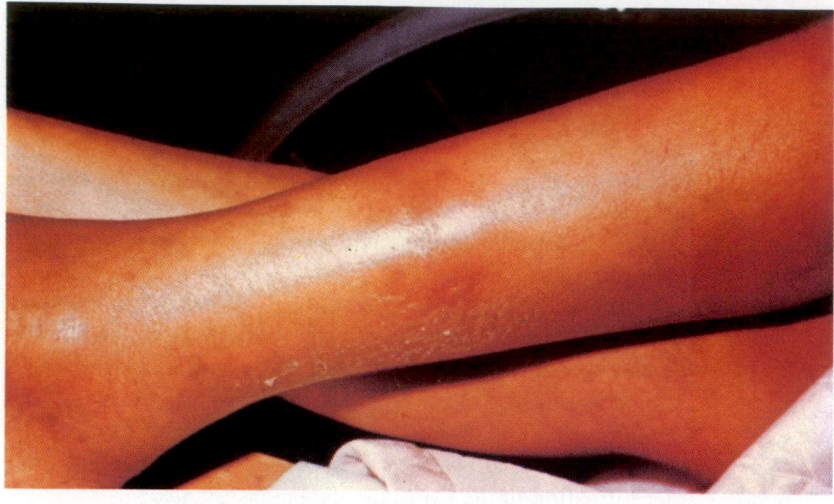

A

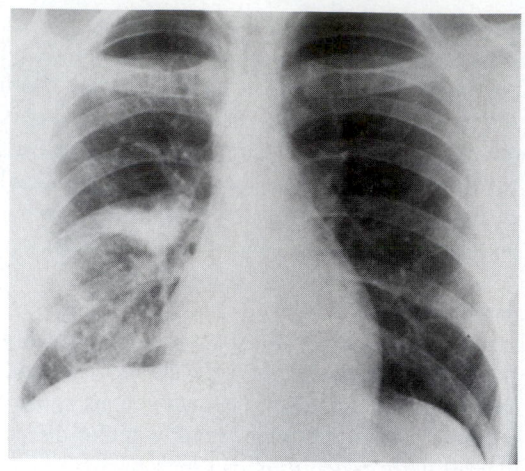

B

FIGURE 29-5 Erythema nodosum and primary tuberculosis. *A.* Discrete, tender, erythematous nodules over the pretibial region. *B.* and *C.* Infiltrates in the right middle lobe and the superior segment of the right lower lobe. Sputum smears and cultures were positive for *M. tuberculosis.* (From Katz and Beerman.[11a])

neous nodules also occur. Sarcoidal lesions sometimes develop at sites of previous trauma or surgical scars. Unless accompanied by systemic findings, however, skin biopsy of a scar cannot be used as the basis for a diagnosis of systemic sarcoidosis.

COURSE

Patients with systemic sarcoidosis who have specific cutaneous lesions tend to have a chronic course that often includes pulmonary fibrosis and uveitis.[15]

THERAPY

The management of cutaneous lesions depends on the type and extent of skin involvement as well as on the need to treat systemic lesions. In acute sarcoidosis, nonsteroidal anti-inflammatory drugs, such as indomethacin, may be adequate for the symptoms of erythema nodosum and the arthralgias. Lupus pernio is treated more aggressively—e.g., with systemic steroids, antimalarials such as hydroxychloroquine, weekly low-dose systemic methotrexate, or oral retinoids. In some patients with localized lesions (e.g., cutaneous papules or plaques) but in whom there is no evidence of systemic involvement, treatment of the local lesions with topical or intralesional steroids is often helpful.

CONGENITAL AND DEVELOPMENTAL DISORDERS

A wide variety of heredocongenital anomalies, as well as normal development itself, affect both the skin and the lung. Among these are disorders of collagen and elastin, vascular malformations, neurocutaneous syndromes, and miscellaneous processes.

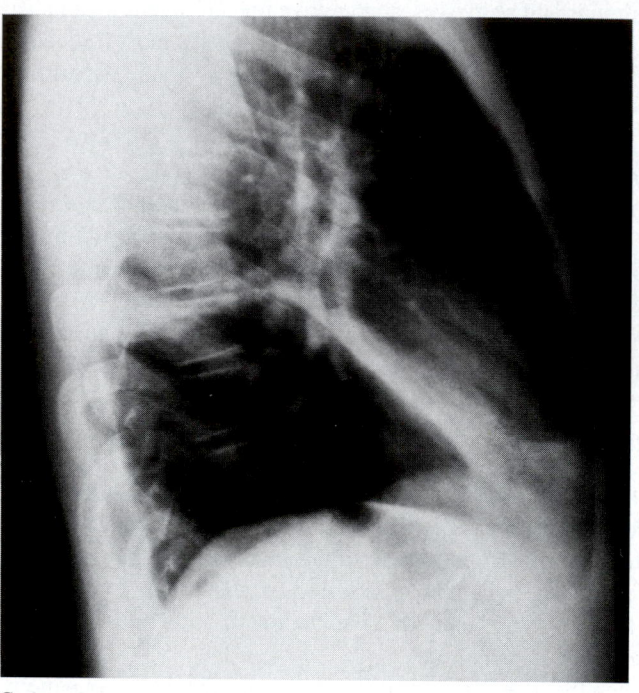

C

Disorders of Collagen and Elastin

The most important disorder of collagen affecting the skin and the lungs is Ehlers-Danlos syndrome (cutis hyperelastica), a hereditary disorder of collagen in which the skin and blood vessels are unduly elastic and fragile and the joints are hyperextensible. The skin is smooth, rubbery, and bruisable; the joints are hypermobile. Associated systemic abnormalities include megaesophagus, megacolon, dissecting aortic aneurysm, and diaphragmatic and inguinal hernias. Among the pulmonary disorders are spontaneous pneumothorax, arteriovenous fistulas, megatrachea, and bronchial ectasia.

   Cutis laxa is due to a disorder in the formation of elastin that is transmitted as a dominant hereditary trait. In children with this disorder, skinfolds of the abdomen and face are large and pendulous. The pulmonary manifestations of cutis laxa are emphysema and pulmonary artery stenosis.[10]

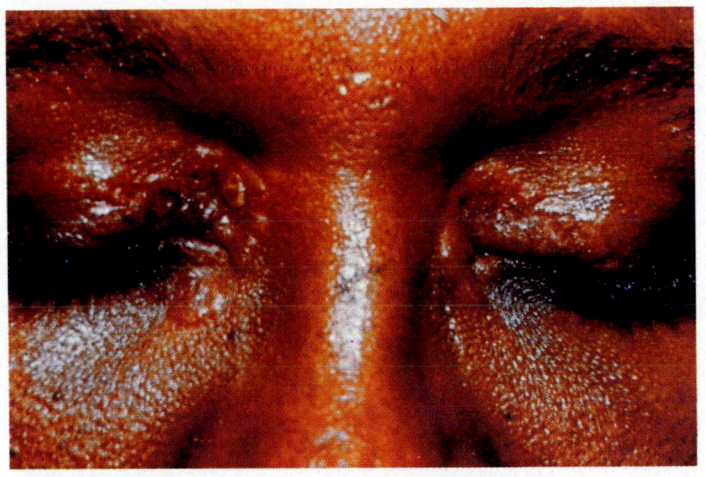

A

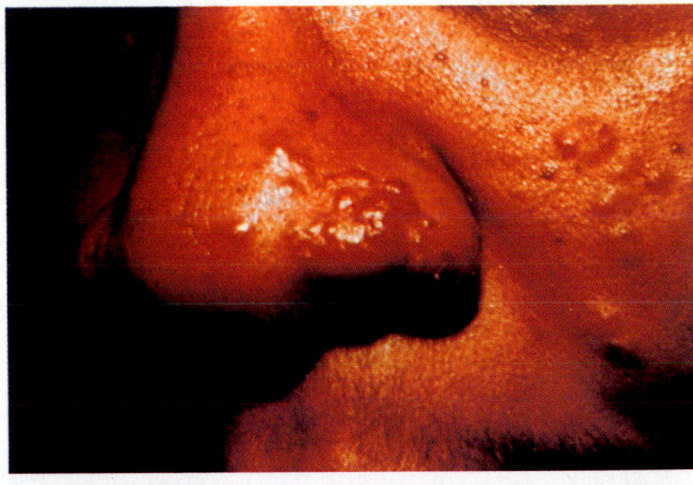

B

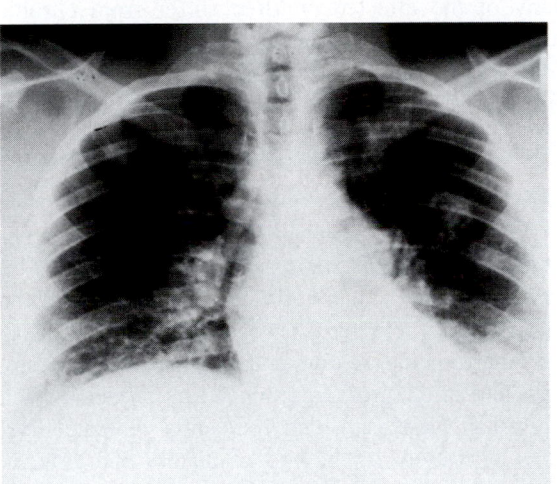

C

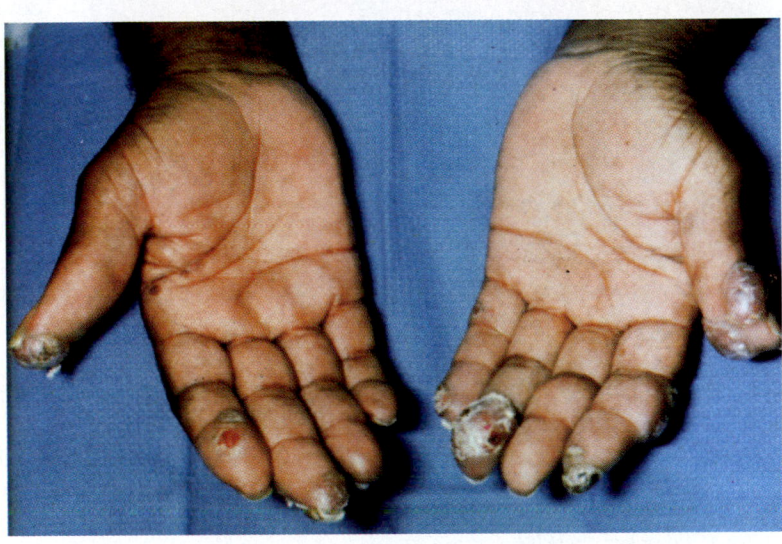

D

FIGURE 29-6   Sarcoidosis. *A.* and *B.* Grouped papular lesion on the medial aspects of the eyelids, alae nasi, and cheek. *C.* Bilateral hilar adenopathy and reticular nodular lung infiltrates. Skin and lung biop- sies demonstrated noncaseating granulomas consistent with sarcoidosis. *D.* Sarcoid lupus pernio involving fingers. *(A to C from Katz and Beerman.[11a])*

Vascular Malformations

The most common congenital vascular malformation of the skin and the lungs is hereditary hemorrhagic telangiectasia (Osler-Rendu-Weber syndrome). This is an autosomal dominant disorder that is manifested by hemangiomas in various organs, including the skin, and it may affect the lips, tongue, nasal mucosa, palate, and palms; on rare occasions, it is accompanied by arteriovenous fistulas in the lungs (Fig. 29-7). Epistaxis, melena, and hemoptysis are common in adults. The typical cutaneous lesion is slightly raised with an ill-defined border and one or more branching "legs" radiating from an eccentrically placed punctum; it is easily overlooked if it is located under the nails or on the soles of the feet. Large pulmonary arteriovenous communications are accompanied by clubbing, cyanosis, and polycythemia.

Neurocutaneous Syndromes

These disorders are characterized by dysplasia of ectodermally derived tissues, such as the skin and brain, as well as by disruption of organs formed from mesoderm, including the lungs. This group includes neurofibromatosis, tuberous sclerosis, and ataxia-telangiectasia. Pulmonary disease in patients with these disorders may be either a manifestation of the systemic involvement by the disease process or an indirect consequence of neuromuscular weakness that causes aspiration pneumonia and lung abscess.

Neurofibromatosis (von Recklinghausen's disease) (Fig. 29-8) is a hereditary disorder, transmitted as a dominant trait, that is characterized by cutaneous neurofibromas, café-au-lait spots, and axillary freckles. The cutaneous tumors derive from the nerve sheaths of the Schwann cells. A feature of these lesions that is virtually pathognomonic is the ability to invaginate small lesions by digital pressure. The café-au-lait spots represent giant pigmented granules in the melanocytes and epidermal cells; they are specific for neurofibromatosis only if they are larger than 1.5 cm and numerous (i.e., more than five spots). Approximately 15 percent of patients with cutaneous lesions have intrathoracic neurofibromas. In some patients with neurofibromatosis, the lungs are the seat of interstitial fibrosis, leiomyomas, and bullae.

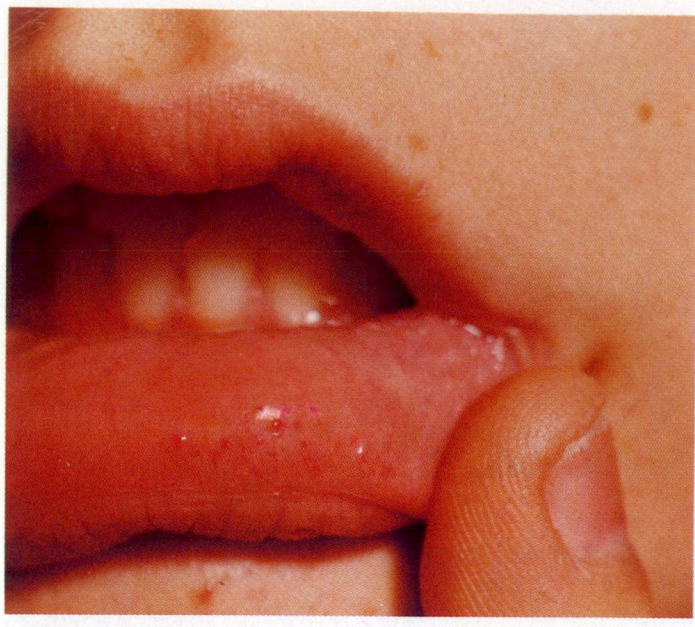

A

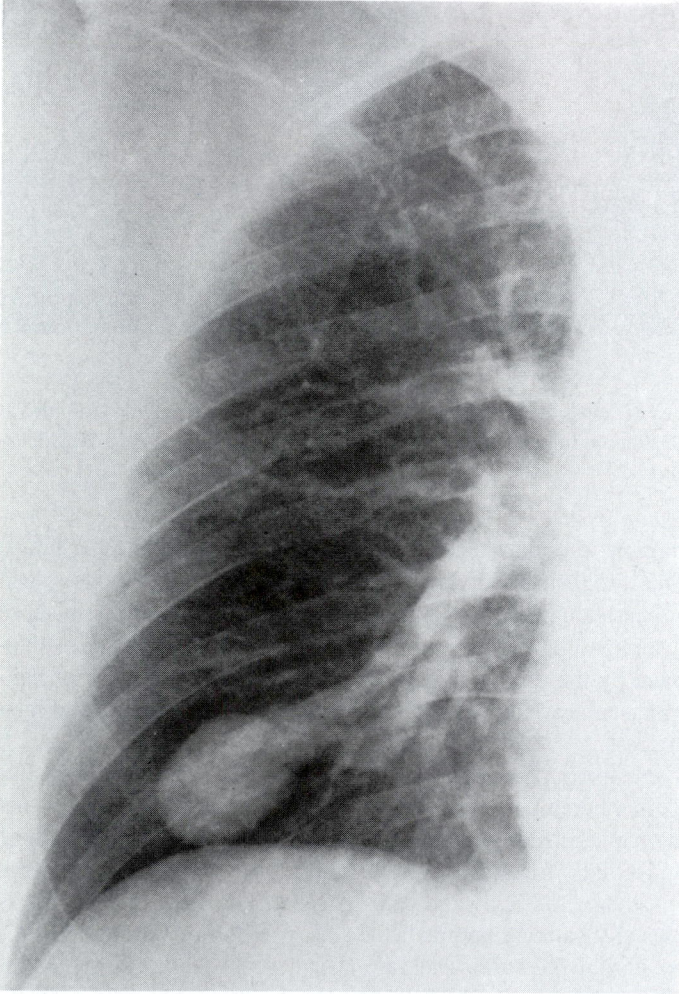

B

FIGURE 29-7   Osler-Rendu-Weber syndrome. *A.* Punctate hemangiomas of the lower lip. *B.* Arteriovenous fistulas of right lower lobe shown by angiography. *(From Katz and Beerman.[11a])*

Tuberous sclerosis is a hereditary disorder that is characterized by mental retardation, epilepsy, and, as indicated previously, adenoma sebaceum. Also seen as part of this disorder are retinal phakomas, calcification of basal ganglia, and ungual fibromas. Shagreen patches occur in approximately one-fifth of patients; they consist of soft plaques, with a pebbly appearance, in the lumbosacral region. Approximately 9 percent of patients with visceral tuberous sclerosis have pulmonary manifestations; some of the pulmonary lesions are cystic and may be associated with recurrent spontaneous pneumothorax and hamartomas. Certain poorly understood diseases, such as fibrocystic pulmonary dysplasia, may represent forme fruste of tuberous sclerosis.

Ataxia-telangiectasia is a recessively transmitted disorder that is characterized by choreoathetosis, ocular apraxia, and progressive cerebellar ataxia. These manifestations appear in early childhood; subsequently, telangiectasia of the conjunctiva and skin develops. Many of the affected children suffer from chronic sinopulmonary infections in association with an abnormality in delayed hypersensitivity and a decrease in the production of the immunoglobulin IgA.

EOSINOPHILIC GRANULOMA

Eosinophilic granuloma, also known as histiocytosis X, often begins with dermatologic manifestations. The characteristic lesions, most often seen in infants and young children with the Letterer-Siwe and Hand-Schüller-Christian forms of this disorder, consist of seborrheiclike scaling and erythema in the scalp, behind the ears, and in the groin, surrounded by reddish-brown and yellowish-brown papules, which frequently ulcerate. Purpura, as well as ulcerations of the buccal mucosa and gingiva, also occur. Eosinophilic granuloma rarely has cutaneous manifestations.

PULMONARY VASCULITIS

This category includes three entities: systemic vasculitis with asthma and eosinophilia, lymphomatoid granulomatosis, and Wegener's granulomatosis.[14,20] Here, only the skin manifestations of these disorders are considered.

Churg-Strauss Syndrome (Systemic Vasculitis with Asthma and Eosinophilia)

The clinical picture of allergic rhinitis, asthma, peripheral eosinophilia, and pulmonary infiltrates concomitant with systemic vasculitis has been designated the Churg-Strauss syndrome (see Chapter 69).[4] However, the histologic finding of necrotizing granulomas and tissue eosinophilia is not unique to this clinical syndrome.[7] Indeed, the same histologic appearance may be seen in a wide variety of systemic diseases, including allergic granulomatosis, Wegener's granulomatosis, rheumatoid arthritis, and lymphoproliferative disease.

One or more types of skin lesions develop in 70 percent of patients with Churg-Strauss syndrome.[13] Most common is palpable purpura of the extremities; histologically, these lesions show necrotizing vasculitis without granuloma formation. In one-third of the patients, the cutaneous lesions are nonspecific—i.e.,

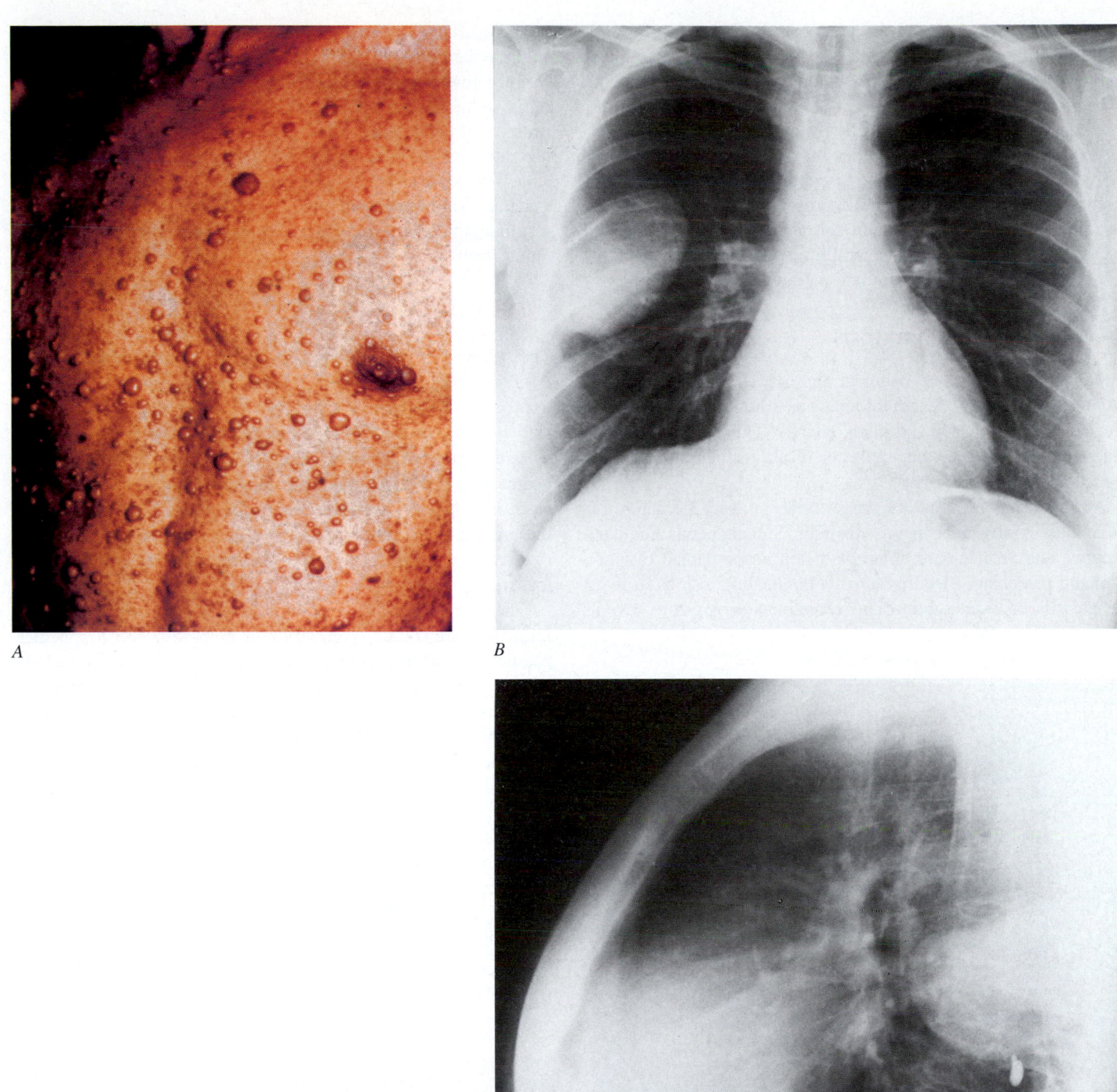

A

B

C

FIGURE 29-8   Von Recklinghausen's disease. *A.* Multiple soft, sub-cutaneous neurofibromas over the chest and abdomen. *B.* Chest radi-ograph shows an extrapleural soft-tissue mass eroding the right sixth rib as well as bilateral apical masses and a widened mediastinum. These lesions are caused by neurofibromas. *C.* Lateral film demonstrates scal-loping of the posterior bodies of the lower thoracic vertebrae as a con-sequence of dural ectasia. *(From Katz and Beerman.*[11a]*)*

erythematous and urticarial. In another third, however, the skin lesions are distinctive—i.e., tender red to violaceous, indurated nodules, measuring 0.5 to 2 cm, which develop central crusting or become infarcted (Fig. 29-9). These nodules occur most often over the scalp or symmetrically over the extensor surfaces of the extremities. It is these nodules that are most likely to have the histologic picture of necrotizing granulomatous vasculitis and eosinophilic infiltration; immunofluorescence staining may show vascular deposition of fibrin and complement. The skin lesions in Churg-Strauss syndrome generally respond to systemic corticosteroids or to adjuvant cytotoxic therapy.

Wegener's Granulomatosis

Although skin lesions do occur in approximately 45 percent of patients with Wegener's granulomatosis,[3] they are usually nonspecific, both clinically and histologically. Thus, biopsy of skin lesions is not apt to either make or refute a diagnosis of Wegener's granulomatosis.

Attention has been called above to the nonspecific nature of cutaneous involvement in this disorder. Subcutaneous nodules, papules, and vesicles are common, often accompanied by purpura and petechiae. Bleeding, crusty, nonhealing lesions form at the nostrils or nasal septum and sometimes progress to severe paranasal sinusitis and to nasopharyngeal ulceration; the end result may be perforation of the nasal septum and saddle-nose deformity. Involvement of the middle ear is signaled by a purulent otitis; in the mouth, the process leads to extensive gingivitis with necrosis of the alveolar ridge, palatal ulcers, and perforation and ulceration of the tongue. Except for infarcts or gangrenous lesions, the skin affliction generally resolves in response to the systemic administration of corticosteroids and cyclophosphamide; the recurrence of cutaneous lesions often presages systemic relapse.[6]

LYMPHOMATOID GRANULOMATOSIS

The skin is the most commonly affected extrapulmonary site in lymphomatoid granulomatosis, cutaneous lesions occurring in 40 to 50 percent of patients.[11,12] In 10 to 25 percent of patients, the skin lesions are the first clinical evidence of the disorder; the skin lesions precede involvement of the lungs by 2 weeks to 9 years. Because of the frequent occurrence of skin lesions, the ease of biopsying the skin, and the characteristic histology of these disease, careful dermatologic examination should be carried out in patients suspected of having lymphomatoid granulomatosis.

The characteristic cutaneous lesions in lymphomatoid granulomatosis are 1- to 4-cm erythematous-to-purplish macules, papules, or subcutaneous nodules that sometimes ulcerate; the lesions generally occur over the buttocks, thighs, and lower extremities (Fig. 29-10) but may occur anywhere. Healing is often accompanied by scarring and hyperpigmentation. Other cutaneous lesions are nonspecific—i.e., small vesicles, generalized ichthyosis, patchy alopecia, localized lack of sweating, and annular plaques.

This histopathology of the skin lesions is similar to that of the lesions in the lungs; a mild to deep dermal angiocentric and angiodestructive vasculitis with a mixed-cell granulomatous infiltrate; some atypical lymphoreticular cells are seen,[5] but eosinophils are sparse. Secondary inflammation and destruction of skin appendages, such as sweat glands and nerves, may occur; should deep vessels be affected, adjacent fat necrosis evokes

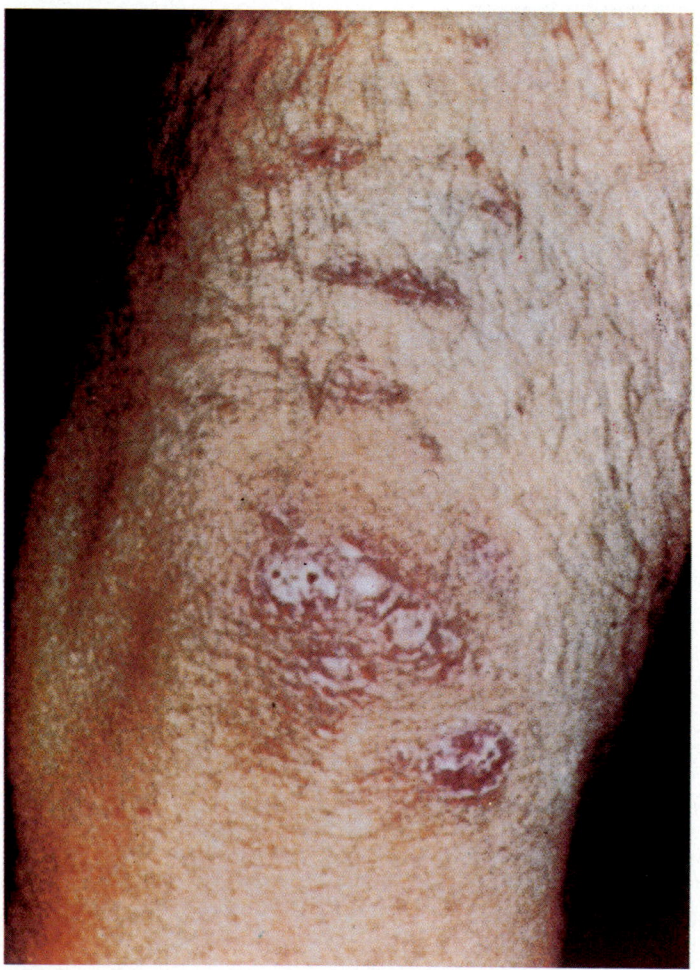

FIGURE 29-9   Churg-Strauss granulomatous vasculitis.

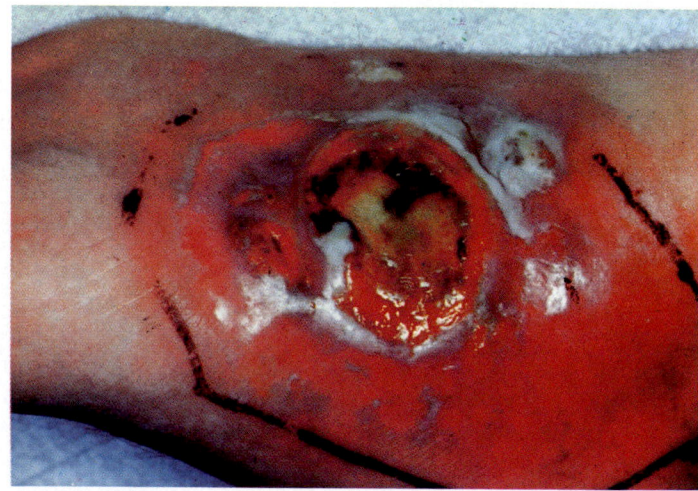

FIGURE 29-10   Lymphomatoid granulomatosis.

a panniculitis. Ultrastructurally, the histiocytosis shows certain distinctive features, including ruffling of the cell membrane, a well-developed Golgi apparatus, and collections of microfilaments and microtubules in the cytoplasm.

The papules or nodules in lymphomatoid granulomatosis sometimes clear spontaneously; more often, they recur. The skin lesions do seem to respond to therapy with systemic corticosteroids and cyclophosphamide. Localized radiation therapy has been used for some refractory skin lesions.

NEOPLASTIC DISORDERS

In some patients, carcinoma of the lung metastasizes to the skin; in others, nonspecific cutaneous lesions are part of the systemic effects of a pulmonary neoplasm. Neoplasms of the skin sometimes metastasize to the lung and pleura.

Although the skin is an uncommon site for metastases, carcinoma of the lung is the third most common source; the breast and the stomach are more common primary sites. Neoplastic lesions of the skin are rock-hard, subcutaneous, or intradermal nodules; in color, they range from fleshy to purple to brownish black; often they are localized to the chest wall. Occasionally, a cutaneous metastasis is first discovered in the scalp. Except for those in the scalp, skin lesions rarely ulcerate; sometimes the scalp lesions are associated with alopecia.

Ectopic Hormones

Various systemic syndromes that include cutaneous manifestations occur in conjunction with malignant neoplasms of the lungs. The most common systemic manifestations of a primary carcinoma of the lungs are due to ectopic production of hormones. Hyperpigmentation is part of the Cushing's syndrome produced by ACTH-like and/or melanin-stimulating hormone–like peptides arising in the pulmonary neoplasm; most often, the pulmonary neoplasm is a small-cell carcinoma. Cushing's syndrome is a harbinger of death in pulmonary neoplasm: most affected persons die within weeks of the appearance of the hyperpigmentation. Gynecomastia, often painful, complicates carcinoma of the lung, especially the undifferentiated variety that elaborates gonadotropins.

The carcinoid syndrome, usually secondary to appendiceal or intestinal tumors, is occasionally produced by bronchial adenomas. Occasionally, the repeated vasomotor episodes are followed by a lingering cyanotic flush of the face and telangiectasia.

Nonspecific Dermatologic Syndromes

Cutaneous abnormalities associated with carcinoma of the lungs (and with other visceral carcinomas as well) include dermatomyositis, scleroderma, pachydermoperiostosis, acanthosis nigricans, and pruritus.

In 15 to 34 percent of patients with dermatomyositis, a carcinoma of the lung is present. The dermatomyositis sometimes precedes, and at other times follows, the discovery of the internal malignancy. Moreover, about three-quarters of patients older than 50 years who present with late-onset myopathy prove to have an internal neoplasm.

Scleroderma occasionally accompanies a pulmonary neoplasm, particularly a bronchoalveolar carcinoma or an adenocarcinoma. Conversely, patients with the extensive pulmonary fibrosis of chronic scleroderma are at high risk of developing carcinoma of the lung.

Pachydermoperiostosis is a syndrome in which hypertrophic osteoarthropathy is associated with cutaneous changes of the face and extremities that are similar to those that occur in patients with acromegaly. Although this disorder is generally benign, occasionally it is associated with bronchogenic carcinoma.

Acanthosis nigricans is a frequent concomitant of internal neoplasia. Approximately 80 to 90 percent of malignant acanthosis is associated with abdominal cancer. But neoplasms of the lungs have also been associated with this skin disorder. The characteristic skin lesion is a brownish-black area of pigmentation that is extensively folded and appears dirty; later on, the lesion becomes papillomatous, verrucous, and shaggy. The skin lesions favor sites of flexion, including the neck, axillae, groin, and antecubital spaces; they also occur on the areolae and around the perineal and umbilical regions. The average survival time between the onset of acanthosis nigricans and death is 12 months.

Lymphomas and Leukemias

About half of all patients with lymphomas develop dermatologic manifestations during the course of the disease. Among the nonspecific markers of lymphomas and leukemias are pruritus exfoliative dermatitis, ichthyosis, mycosis fungoides, and bullous eruptions. The nonspecific dermatoses include nodules, papules, and skin tumors that originate from the epidermis or subcutaneous regions. These lesions vary in size and pigmentation and occur anywhere on the body surface. Dermatologic manifestations of malignant lymphomas often antedate systemic disease by months to years. Bluefarb has identified "11 p's" as characterizing the cutaneous lesions of Hodgkin's disease: pallor, pruritus, prurigolike papules, pigmentation, pyoderma, purpura, pemphigoid, post–spinal root ganglionitis (herpes zoster), pityriasis rubra, phlebitis, and poikilodermatomyositis. Pruritus is particularly common; the 11 manifestations are found in 25 to 35 percent of patients with this type of lymphoma.

Bowen's Disease

Epidermoid carcinoma in situ of the skin (Bowen's disease) is commonly associated with neoplasms of any organ, including the lungs. The lesions are asymptomatic, slow growing, psoriasiform, or eczematoid.

Arsenicals and Chromates

Inorganic arsenicals are carcinogens that cause neoplasms of both skin and viscera. The skin lesions may occur years after chronic exposure to inorganic arsenicals, as in drinking water. They are characterized by hyperpigmentation and palmar and plantar dermatoses; frequently, they are confused with Bowen's disease (squamous cell carcinoma of the skin in situ). Like Bowen's disease, arsenical toxicity is associated with a high incidence of visceral neoplasms—respiratory, gastrointestinal, and genitourinary.

Exposure to chromate dusts or vapors is associated with a frequency of pulmonary neoplasms that is about 30 times greater than that of the unexposed population. Chromate workers also develop perforations of the nasal septum, as well as ulcerations of the hands, forearms, and feet.

Primary Cutaneous Neoplasms

Certain primary neoplasms of the skin invade the lungs. Paramount in this group are malignant melanoma and mycosis fungoides. The latter has been noted above (see "Scaling Papules").

Malignant melanomas constitute approximately 1 to 2 percent of all neoplasms. They occur most often in the 5th to 7th decade, particularly in fair complexioned persons of North European descent. The typical lesion is a deeply pigmented nodule with irregular borders (Fig. 29-11). The usual course is progressive enlargement of the skin lesion, metastasis to regional lymph nodes, and hematogenous dissemination to the lungs and liver. Widespread metastasis is associated with diffuse hyperpigmentation of the skin and mucous membranes. Among the pulmonary manifestations of melanoma are nodules in the lungs (solitary, multiple, or miliary), hilar and mediastinal lymphadenopathy, and exudative pleural effusions caused by pleural metastases. Primary melanomas of the lungs are exceedingly rare. When they do occur, they usually masquerade as carcinoma, lymphoma, or sarcoma, often causing bronchial obstruction and distal atelectasis.

KAPOSI'S SARCOMA

Until the AIDS epidemic, Kaposi's sarcoma encountered in the United States was a rare disorder seen predominantly in middle-aged men. Its usual course was indolent and confined primarily to the lower extremities. At the outset, the lesions were dark-blue, purplish, or reddish papules, macules, and nodules; after months to years, plaques evolved in association with thickening of the skin from midtibia to ankle and lymphedema.

The AIDS epidemic brought to light an aggressive form of the disease that is widespread in its cutaneous manifestations. In AIDS patients, the respiratory tract is second only to the gastrointestinal tract in frequency of involvement. Tumors sometimes involve the larynx, trachea, bronchi, pulmonary parenchyma, and pleura. Accordingly, local manifestations of respiratory tract involvement range from hoarseness, signs of airway obstruction, cough, and hemoptysis to dyspnea. When the parenchyma of the lung is affected, chest radiographs usually show many small nodules; occasionally, parenchymal infiltration of the lung is massive. On bronchoscopic examination, bronchial and tracheal lesions appear as small bluish nodules. Bloody pleural effusions are rare.

COLLAGEN VASCULAR DISORDERS

Many of the collagen vascular diseases begin clinically with cutaneous lesions, or they develop in the course of the illness.

Systemic Lupus Erythematosus

Cutaneous lupus erythematosus usually takes the form of well-circumscribed discoid lesions that are raised, firm, and red to violaceous. Often the lesions are accompanied by telangiectasia, atrophy, and scarring. Silvery-white discolorations of the lips and of the mucosa of the mouth and lips are characteristic. A butterfly configuration over the bridge of the nose and on the cheeks is both less common and less specific. Subcutaneous nodules develop underneath the typical discoid lesions of lupus (lupus profundus). In addition to the discoid type of plaque and telangiectasia, patients sometimes exhibit urticarial plaques and alopecia. Discoid and systemic forms of lupus are believed to be different expressions of the same disorder. About 10 percent of patients who present only with cutaneous disease eventually develop generalized manifestations; on the other hand, 50 to 90 percent of those with systemic disease eventually develop some cutaneous abnormalities.

Rheumatoid Arthritis

A wide variety of dermatologic manifestations occur in rheumatoid arthritis, often together with pulmonary disease. Subcutaneous nodules occur in about 20 percent of patients with systemic rheumatoid disease. The lesions are generally located around the elbows, hands, ankles, and feet. Similar nodules also occur in the pulmonary parenchyma, heart, sclera, and dura mater and within the visceral pleura. Histologically, fibrinoid necrosis in vascular walls is surrounded by palisading. Other dermatologic manifestations of rheumatoid arthritides are secondary to widespread angiitis and include necrotic leg ulcers, gangrene of the extremities, and hemorrhagic infarcts along the finger pulp or nail. Involvement of the lungs is often associated with characteristic abnormalities of the hands (Fig. 29-12).

Dermatomyositis

The characteristic skin lesions of dermatomyositis are blotchy, purplish macules located on the extensor surfaces of the elbows, knuckles and knees, anterior chest, and malar area of the face. Periorbital and eyelid edema is common in association with a heliotrope discoloration of the affected skin. Raynaud's phenomenon occurs in about 10 to 20 percent of patients with this disorder. A fine, scaly erythema sometimes appears over the extensor surfaces of the large and interphalangeal joints as well as on the plantar and palmar surfaces of the hands. Periungual and linear telangiectasias occur at the cuticle. As the disease progresses, bullous lesions and poikiloderma—a speckled pattern of hypopigmented and hyperpigmented small macules—are sometimes interspersed with telangiectasia and cutaneous atrophy. Another late and specific manifestation of dermatomyositis is Gottron's papule, a purplish rash that appears on the dorsal interphalangeal joints.

The cutaneous manifestations of dermatomyositis usually precede muscle impairment by several months; on occasion, however, the skin is affected after muscle disease is extensive and quite evident. Biopsy of the skin lesions in dermatomyositis usually reveals a nonspecific inflammatory reaction. If the myositis is prolonged and severe, widespread calcification of the skin and muscle sometimes occurs, as early as 2 years after the onset of the disease.

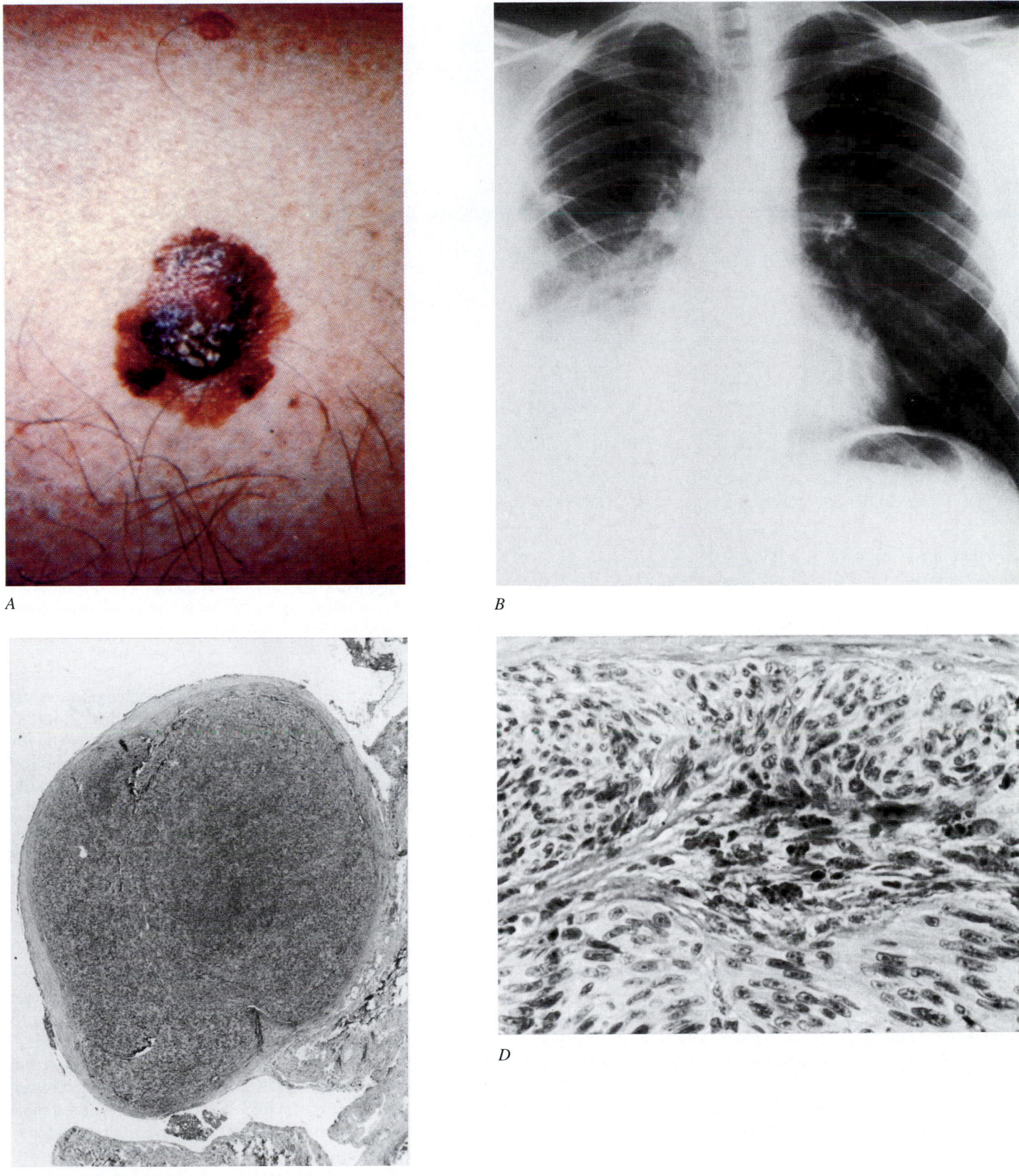

FIGURE 29-11   Metastatic melanoma. *A.* Deeply pigmented, raised facial lesion with irregular surface. *B.* Chest radiograph shows right pleural effusion with nodulation. *C.* Biopsy of the lung (× 27) reveals a large nodule on pleural surface. *D.* Spindle-shaped cells, some of which are filled with melanin pigment (× 400). *(From Katz and Beerman.*[11a]*)*

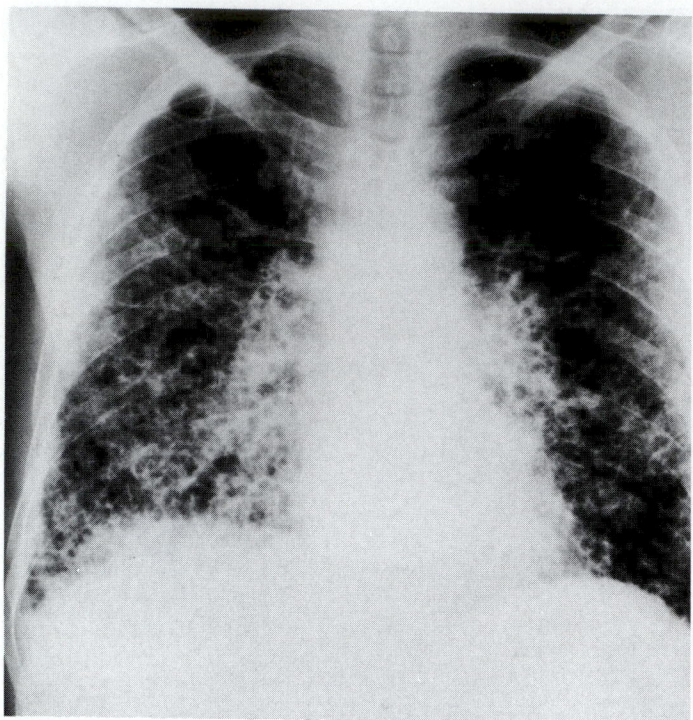

A

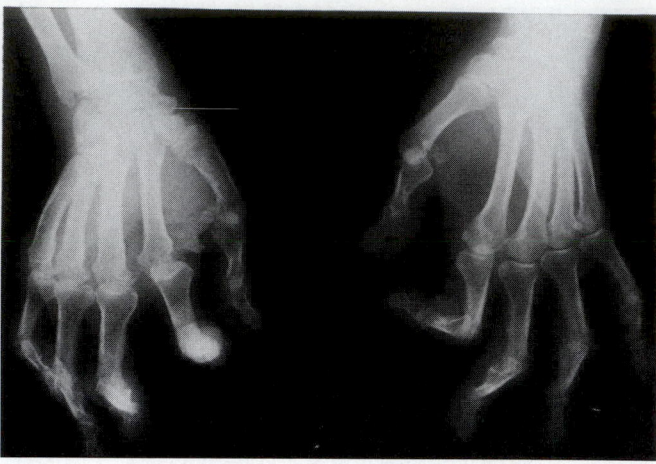

B

FIGURE 29-12 Rheumatoid arthritis. *A.* Chest radiograph shows a course, reticulonodular, honeycomb pattern, most prominent at the bases, consistent with rheumatoid arthritis. *B.* Hand radiographs show typical rheumatoid changes consisting of (1) synovitis, with erosions of the metacarpal heads; (2) soft-tissue swelling around several joints (intercarpal, metaphalangeal, proximal interphalangeal); (3) periarticular demineralization secondary to hyperemia; (4) fusion of carpal bones; and (5) early ulnar deviation. *(From Katz and Beerman.[11a])*

Scleroderma

The two principal forms of systemic scleroderma are acrosclerosis and diffuse scleroderma. Acrosclerosis, by far the more common of the two, is characterized by sclerosis of the skin of the fingers (sclerodactyly) and Raynaud's phenomenon. In contrast, diffuse scleroderma presents with tightening of the skin, especially over the chest, without Raynaud's phenomenon; the prognosis for diffuse scleroderma is much worse than for acrosclerosis. Acrosclerosis is often preceded by diffuse arthralgias or arthritis resembling rheumatoid arthritis. The skin manifestations begin with transient, recurrent swelling of the hands and progress to tapered fingers with shiny, hidebound skin (sclerodactyly). The feet, chest, face, and scalp are often involved in the sclerotic process. In time, the skin becomes taut, leading to contractures of the large and small joints that culminate in a claw-like deformity of the hand. A variety of pigmentary disturbances in scleroderma have been noted, including generalized hyperpigmentation that resembles adrenal insufficiency, focal hyperpigmentation and hypopigmentation, and areas of perifollicular pigmentation that resemble vitiligo (Fig. 29-13). Raynaud's phenomenon leads to small pitted scars at the fingertips or frank ulceration with or without gangrene of the fingertips, toes, knuckles, and ankles, especially the malleoli. Calcium is sometimes deposited in the major joints; fingers are affected late in the course of scleroderma (Thibierge-Weissenbach syndrome).

The face often undergoes distinctive changes, leading to a fixed stare, wrinkled forebrow, and inability to wrinkle the fore-head. As facial tissues shrink, the nose becomes pinched, the cheeks sunken, and the mouth small with thin lips. In diffuse scleroderma, cutaneous sclerosis, accompanied by a yellowish-brown hue, spreads from the chest to the head and extremities. Sharply delineated, broad telangiectatic macules appear on the face, buccal mucosa, lips, and hands. The constellation of calcinosis cutis, Raynaud's phenomenon, sclerodactyly, and telangiectasia is known as the CRST syndrome. This form of scleroderma is usually benign but is occasionally associated with pulmonary hypertension.

COMPLICATIONS OF MEDICATIONS

Medications used to treat respiratory disorders sometimes cause cutaneous reactions. Major offenders are antibiotics, particularly the penicillins, ampicillin, and trimethoprim-sulfamethoxazole—all of which can cause exanthematous, urticarial, or erythema multiforme–type reactions. The continued administration of corticosteroids systemically can elicit the cutaneous manifestations of Cushing's syndrome. In addition, chronic corticosteroid therapy may predispose to poor wound healing and to fungal infections of the skin, such as tinea versicolor and dermatophytes.

Aminophylline administered parenterally occasionally causes a generalized papulovesicular eruption.[23] The usual setting for this reaction is the patient who has been previously sensitized to ethylenediamine by using a topical preparation of Mycolog cream or certain antihistamines (promethazine or tripelennamine). Since the delayed hypersensitivity reactions to amino-

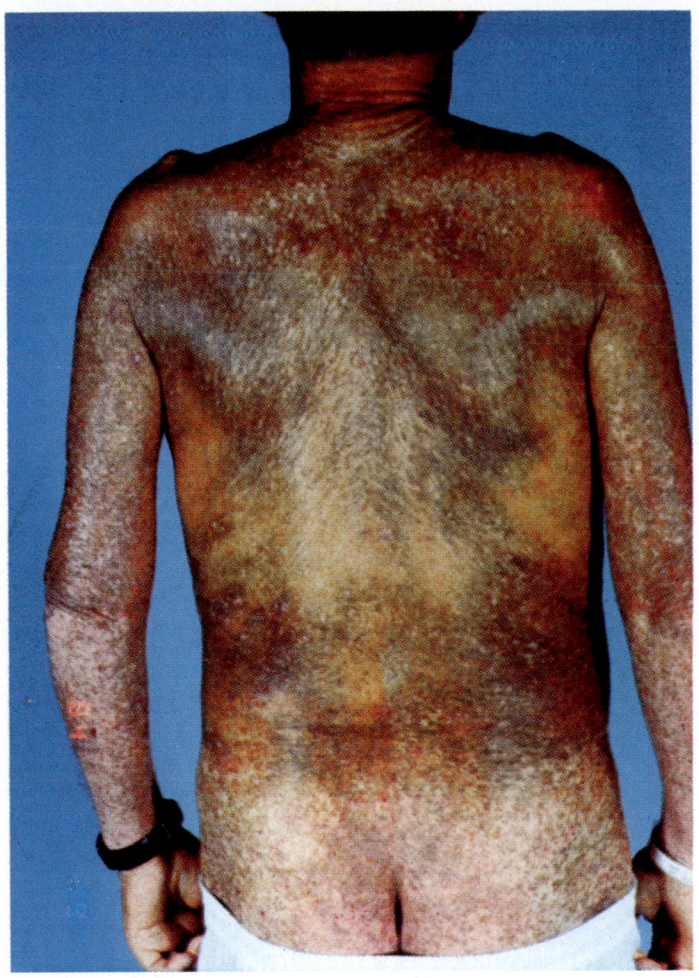

FIGURE 29-13   Scleroderma. Mottled hyperpigmentation.

phylline in this setting are due to the ethylenediamine component, theophylline preparations can be substituted. Immediate hypersensitivity reactions (urticarial) are uncommon for theophylline or aminophylline.

Codeine also can cause a number of cutaneous reactions, including generalized exanthematous eruptions, pruritus with or without skin lesions, and urticaria. The last may occur because of a nonimmunologic release of histamine owing to a direct effect of codeine on mast cells. Potassium iodide, once often used as an expectorant, may cause urticaria, an acneiform eruption, erythema nodosum, or iododerma. Heparin and warfarin anticoagulants can cause a temporary hair thinning; hair loss begins 6 weeks to 4 months after the start of therapy. Other medications used in pulmonary therapy have a fairly low incidence of cutaneous reactions, but drug eruption should be considered in the differential diagnosis of almost any cutaneous pattern.

REFERENCES

1. Callen JP: Cardiopulmonary disorders, in Callen JP (ed), *Cutaneous Aspects of Internal Disease*. Chicago, Year Book, 1981, pp 311–414.
2. Epstein EH, Levin DL, Croft JD Jr, Lutaner MA: Mycosis fungoides: Survival, prognostic features, response to therapy and autopsy findings. *Medicine* 51:61–72, 1982.
3. Fauci AS, Haynes BF, Katz P, Wolff SM: Wegener's granulomatosis: Prospective clinical and therapeutic experience with 85 patients for 21 years. *Ann Intern Med* 98:76–85, 1983.
4. Finan MC, Winkelmann RK: The cutaneous extravascular necrotizing granuloma (Churg-Strauss granuloma) and systemic disease: A review of 27 cases. *Medicine* 62:142–158, 1983.
5. Foley JF, Linder J, Koh J, et al: Cutaneous necrotizing granulomatous vasculitis with evolution to T-cell lymphoma. *Am J Med* 82:839–844, 1987.
6. Gibson LE, Winkelmann RK: Cutaneous granulomatous vasculitis: Its relationship to systemic disease. *J Am Acad Dermatol* 14:492–501, 1986.
7. Guillevin L, Guittard T, Bletry O, et al: Systemic necrotizing angiitis with asthma: Causes and precipitating factors in 43 cases. *Lung* 165:165–172, 1987.
8. Hanafin JM: Atopic dermatitis. *J Am Acad Dermatol* 6:1–13, 1982.
9. Hanno R, Needelman A, Eiferman RA, Callen JP: Cutaneous sarcoidal granulomas and the development of systemic sarcoidosis. *Arch Dermatol* 117:203–207, 1981.
10. Harris RB, Heaphy MR, Perry HO: Generalized elastolysis (cutis laxa). *Am J Med* 65:815–822, 1978.
11. James WD, Odom RB, Katzenstein A-LA: Cutaneous manifestations of lymphomatoid granulomatosis. *Arch Dermatol* 117:196–202, 1981.
11a. Katz AS, Beerman H: Pulmonary-cutaneous disorders, in Fishman AP (ed), *Pulmonary Diseases and Disorders*. New York, McGraw-Hill, 1980.
12. Katzenstein A-LA, Carrington CB, Liebow AA: Lymphomatoid granulomatosis: A clinicopathologic study of 152 cases. *Cancer* 43:360–373, 1979.
13. Lanham JG, Elkon KG, Pusey CD, Hughes GR: Systemic vasculitis with asthma and eosinophilia: A clinical approach to Churg-Strauss syndrome. *Medicine* 63:65–81, 1984.
14. Leavitt RY, Fauci AS: Pulmonary vasculitis. *Am Rev Respir Dis* 134:149–166, 1986.
15. Martin AG, Kleinhenz ME, Elmets CA: Immunohistologic identification of antigen-presenting cells in cutaneous sarcoidosis. *J Invest Dermatol* 86:625–629, 1986.
16. Mathews KP: Urticaria and angioedema. *J Allergy Clin Immunol* 72:1–14, 1983.
17. Neville E, Mills RGS, Jash DK, et al: Sarcoidosis of the upper respiratory tract and its association with lupus pernio. *Thorax* 31:660–664, 1976.
18. Olive KE, Kataria YP: Cutaneous manifestations of sarcoidosis: Relationships to other organ system involvement, abnormal laboratory measurements, and disease course. *Arch Intern Med* 145:1811–1814, 1985.
19. Pavlidakey GP, Hashimoto K, Blum D: Yellow nail syndrome. *J Am Acad Dermatol* 11:509–512, 1984.
20. Robin JB, Schanzlin DJ, Meisler DM, et al: Ocular involvement in the respiratory vasculitides. *Surv Ophthalmol* 30:127–140, 1985.
21. Sontheimer RD, Garibaldi RA, Krueger GC: Stevens-Johnson syndrome associated with *Mycoplasma pneumoniae* infections. *Arch Dermatol* 114:241–244, 1978.
22. Soter NA, Wasserman SI, Austen KF, McFadden ER: Release of mast cell mediators and alterations in lung function in patients with cholinergic urticaria. *New Engl J Med* 302:604–608, 1980.
23. Thompson PJ, Gibb WRG, Cole P, Citron KM: Generalized allergic reactions to aminophylline. *Thorax* 39:600–603, 1984.
24. Veien NK, Stahl D, Brodthagen H: Cutaneous sarcoidosis in caucasians. *J Am Acad Dermatol* 16:534–540, 1987.

PULMONARY-SYSTEMIC INTERACTIONS

Alfred P. Fishman

The lungs are incorporated into the body in such a way as to serve a variety of functions other than external gas exchange. These include hemodynamic, metabolic, endocrine, and immunologic activities. Inadequacy or failure on the part of any of these functions can have serious systemic repercussions. Moreover, as part of the total body fabric, the lungs share in diverse pathologic processes, such as collagen vascular diseases, and inherit susceptibility to others, such as cystic fibrosis, in which a generalized defect in ion transport across epithelial surfaces affects the liver, gastrointestinal tract, and pancreas, as well as the lungs.

Because of its strategic location between the two ventricles and as the recipient of the entire output of the right ventricle, the pulmonary circulation is uniquely situated to transmit the products of pulmonary metabolism and injury to systemic organs and tissues. Its position at the exit of the right ventricle also enables the pulmonary vascular bed to serve as a filter for particulate matter arising in the systemic venous circulation (e.g., thromboemboli). Finally, the arrangement in series of the gastrointestinal tract, liver, and lungs enables interdependence in the handling of biologically active materials that release in health (Fig. 30-1) and disease (e.g., hepatic cirrhosis, gastrointestinal disorders, and splenic dysfunctions).

The diversity of cells that constitute the pulmonary parenchyma, the vasculature, and the airways, coupled with the ready access of blood constituents to the structures in the lungs, affords great opportunity for the lungs to influence systemic organs and vice versa. For example, the endothelial cells that line the enormous expanse of pulmonary vessels can release vasodilator or vasoconstrictor substances, anticoagulants, and a wide variety of enzymes and cytokines into the circulation. Mast cells in the vicinity of the pulmonary vessels can release a variety of substances that can influence both intrapulmonary and extrapulmonary vessels and structures. Chloride-secreting cells, not only in the airways but also in other glandular structures (e.g., sweat glands, pancreas), can suffer inherited defects that disturb different kinds of bodily functions. Immunologically competent cells in the lungs that are part of natural body defenses can open the way for serious systemic infections if their guard is dropped or if environmental pollutants are overwhelming.

The large pulmonary blood flow and the brief pulmonary transit time ensure virtually instantaneous exposure to biologically active substances originating in the lungs. Among these substances are hormones (e.g., angiotensin II), mediators (e.g., nitric oxide), and neurotransmitters. Disease, such as pneumonia, can promote the release of inflammatory and immunologic mediators from both the resident cells and the migratory blood cells (e.g., leukocytes).

Another access route to the lungs is the bronchial circulation. This systemic blood supply can undergo remarkable proliferation in some diseases (e.g., bronchiectasis), but remain small in others (e.g., primary carcinoma of the lung). As is noted below, proliferation of the bronchial circulation often accompanies clubbing of the digits.

THE LUNG AS AN ENDOCRINE ORGAN

In addition to its roles in gas exchange and water exchange, the lung is active metabolically. The metabolic processes entail uptake, storage, and elaboration of substances, many of which (such as nitric oxide) function locally, whereas others, such as an-

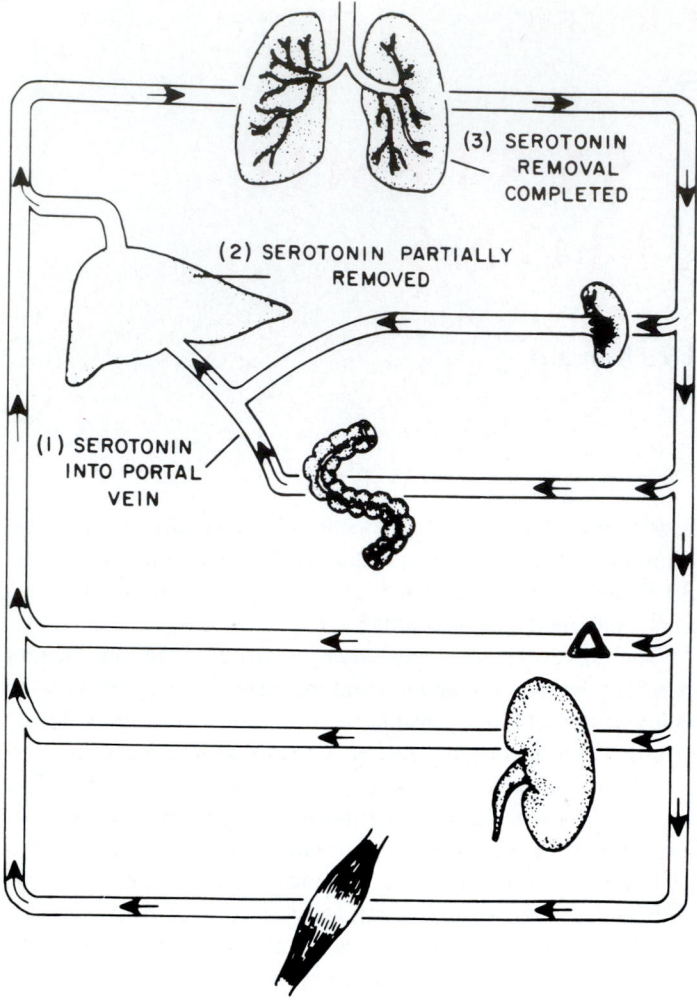

FIGURE 30-1   The sequential processing of serotonin.

giotensin II (Fig. 30-2), exert their effects on remote tissues and organs; i.e., they enter the bloodstream and influence systemic tissues and organs.

In addition to such chemical messengers, the lungs secrete amines and peptides, whose functions are far less well defined. These messengers are released by a system of epithelial cells—i.e., *pulmonary endocrine cells*—which are part of a widespread system that is contained within other organs as well as within the lungs. The so-called pulmonary endocrine cells have attracted the attention of clinicians more because of their potential for undergoing neoplastic transformation than because of recognizable biologic functions.

The Pulmonary Endocrine System

Pulmonary endocrine cells, or *pulmonary neuroendocrine cells*, have been found in a wide variety of species, ranging from the African lungfish to humans.[2,24] These cells can be found in the respiratory epithelium from trachea to alveolar walls, where they may appear as single cells, as clusters associated with nerve terminals (*neuroepithelial bodies*), or in mounds (*tumorlets*).[5] The typical pulmonary endocrine cell is usually argyrophilic and is characterized ultrastructurally by a dense-core vesicle surrounded

by clear scant cytoplasm; within the core are granular chromatin bodies and prominent nucleoli. Histochemistry and immunochemistry have displayed a large spectrum of biologically active mediators, including serotonin, calcitonin, substance P, cholecystokinin, somatostatin, calcitonin gene-related peptide, and bombesinlike peptides. Although these substances have been identified in cells and in serum, few have yet proved to be of clinical significance, although a variety of physiological functions—i.e., vasomotor, bronchomotor, secretomotor, and inflammatory—have been attributed to them. The basal aspect of these cells is often closely related to nerve endings or nerve varicosities. Acute hypoxia has been shown to cause exocytosis of the dense-core vesicles in neuroepithelial bodies,[35] presumably a reflection of a receptor or effector function.

Cells of the pulmonary endocrine system can give rise to neoplasms with endocrine characteristics. These endocrine tumors can be pictured as a continuum of neoplasms that range from benign to malignant (i.e., from carcinoid to small cell carcinoma). The carcinoids mark one end of the continuum: they are the more highly differentiated, and their endocrine features are the most marked. Toward the opposite end are the small cell carcinomas, which are poorly differentiated. Non–small cell carcinomas are less apt to show endocrine differentiation. In this continuum, carcinoids are generally indolent, whereas small cell carcinomas are very aggressive.

Paraneoplastic Syndromes

Pulmonary neoplasms are more commonly associated with paraneoplastic syndromes than are any other types of neoplasms. Three types of paraneoplastic syndromes illustrate the systemic effects of pulmonary neoplasms: the carcinoid syndrome, Cushing's syndrome, and inappropriate secretion of antidiuretic hormone.[28] Clubbing of the digits is considered below.

The carcinoid syndrome is attributed to the release of various mediators from the neoplasm, owing to either a carcinoid tumor or, less often, a small cell carcinoma. Various mediators have been implicated, including serotonin, histamine kinins, and prostaglandins. The systemic effects include flushing, diarrhea, bronchospasm, and heart disease.

Cushing's syndrome is due to excessive secretion of adrenocorticotropic hormone (ACTH) or ACTH-like peptides by the neoplasm, generally a small cell carcinoma. The systemic effects are hypokalemic alkalosis, systemic hypertension, impaired carbohydrate tolerance, muscle weakness and wasting, edema, and weight loss.

The syndrome of inappropriate antidiuretic hormone (SIADH) generally occurs in association with pulmonary tuberculosis or bronchial carcinoma. The clinical syndrome, caused by inappropriate secretion of arginine vasopressin and antidiuretic hormone, is manifested by hyponatremia (not attributable to drugs), water retention, hyperosmolar plasma accompanied by disproportionately high hyperosmolarity of the urine, persistent natriuresis without volume depletion, and hypouricemia. These disorders may lead to altered mental state, lethargy, confusion, psychosis, or coma.

Other familiar syndromes involving pulmonary neoplasms in association with systemic effects are clubbing of the digits, gy-

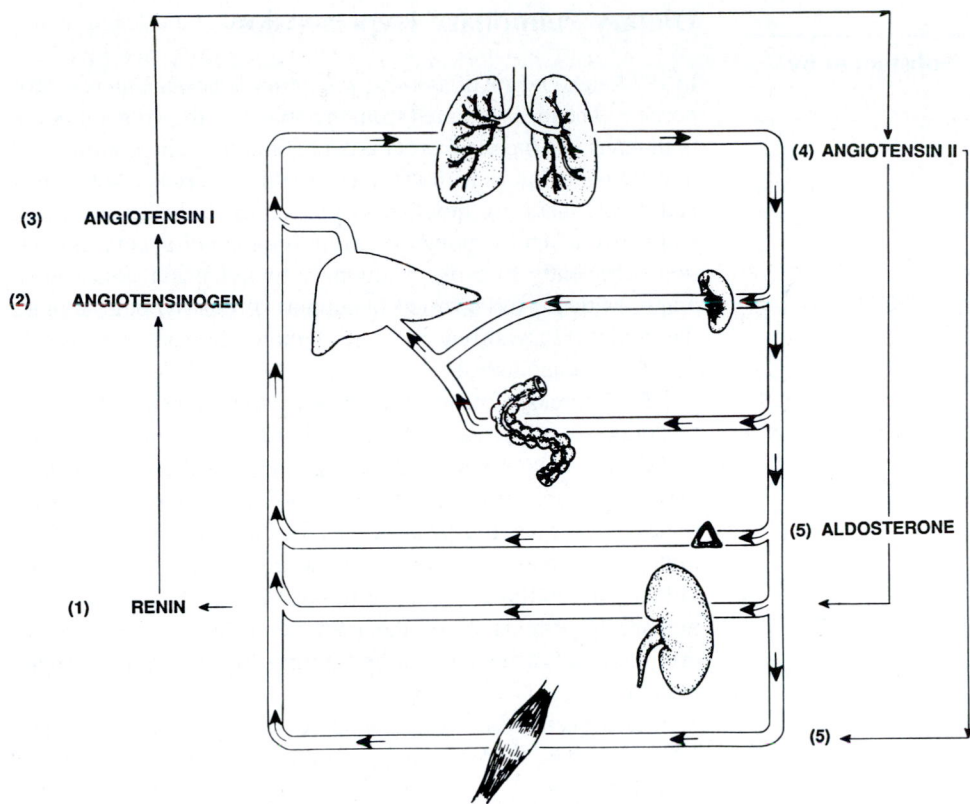

FIGURE 30-2   The renin-angiotensin system. The interplay among kidney, liver, and lungs results in the formation of angiotensin II. This hormone, generated in the lungs from precursors in the kidneys and blood, is active in the regulation of systemic blood pressure. It does so by way of its effects as a systemic vasoconstrictor and as a regulator of the circulating blood volume. The latter operates through the salt- and water-retaining effects of aldosterone.

necomastia, a variety of cutaneous disorders (e.g., acanthosis nigricans), neurologic disorders (e.g., cerebellar degeneration), and autonomic disturbances (e.g., orthostatic hypotension).

PULMONARY VASCULAR ENDOTHELIUM

The lungs contain the largest expanse of endothelium in the body. This lining of the pulmonary circulation is engaged in a variety of vital functions (Table 30-1). Some, such as pulmonary vasodilation, are served by local mediators, such as nitric oxide and prostacyclin. Countering these effects are local vasoconstrictors, such as the endothelins. As noted above, other products, such as angiotensin II, exert their effects on remote functions (e.g., in the regulation of systemic blood pressure).

The pulmonary circulation, like the systemic venous circulation, remains virtually free of atherosclerotic lesions unless pulmonary arterial blood pressures increase to hypertensive levels. Acute injury to endothelium can provide access of circulating proteins, such as fibrinogen, and blood cells to the pulmonary interstitium, thereby setting the stage for interstitial fibrosis. Aside from leakage, endothelial injury can stimulate a complex array of local reactions: circulating white blood cells and platelets are drawn to the injured site, undergo activation, and release factors that contribute to the response.

Interplay between endothelium and circulating cells and humors is exceedingly complex. Thrombin is one example of the many interactive substances. It plays a pivotal role in all coagulant processes: on the one hand, it is procoagulant (i.e., it activates platelets, stimulates monocyte and neutrophil chemotaxis, cleaves fibrinogen, stimulates the endothelial release of tissue factors, and releases von Willebrand factor from Weibel-Palade bodies); on the other, it can serve as an anticoagulant molecule that stimulates protein C activity, promotes prostacyclin secretion, and causes the liberation of tissue plasminogen activators.[3,10,19,25] Thrombin is also a potent growth factor that initiates proliferation of smooth-muscle cells at the site of injury. These diverse effects are due to the prevalence of thrombin receptors in many cell types. A variety of strategies to inhibit thrombin are being tested for therapeutic purposes: hirudin has been used to prevent the cleavage of fibrinogen and activation of thrombin receptors;[31] peptides that act as antagonists for thrombin receptors are being tested; monoclonal and polyclonal antibodies are being developed that prevent activation of thrombin receptors; antisense oligonucleotides are being tried to block expression of thrombin receptors.

Chronic injury to the pulmonary vascular endothelium can evoke proliferation of the intima, invasion of the endothelial lining by underlying smooth muscle and adventitial cells, and accumulation of blood cells at the blood-endothelial interface. The end result is replacement of the single endothelial lining layer by occlusive heaps of endothelial–smooth muscle–connective-tissue cells (Figs. 30-3 and 30-4). How well the heaped-up endothelium preserves the functions of normal endothelial function (e.g., anticoagulation) is not clear.[14]

THE GUT-LIVER-LUNG AXIS

Perhaps nowhere is the principle of effluent from one organ influencing the behavior of its neighbor better illustrated than in the gut-liver-lung axis (Fig. 30-5). Misbehavior by any one of the series can seriously derange the workings of the next in line and the entire organism.[13,17,47] For example, in liver failure, not only are noxious substances added to its effluent but also injurious substances from the gut, spleen, and other systemic organs, which are normally detoxified by the liver, gain access to the pulmonary circulation. The remote consequences of liver injury, such as clubbing of the digits in patients with liver cirrhosis, are considered below.

TABLE 30-1

The Processing of Certain Vasoactive Substances by the Lungs

Metabolized at the luminal surface
   Angiotensin I
   Bradykinin
   Adenine nucleotides
Uptake by endothelium and then metabolized
   Serotonin
   Norepinephrine
   Prostaglandins E and F
Released by endothelium
   Lipoprotein lipase
   Heparin
   Prostacyclin
   Kallikrein
   Leukotrienes
Unaffected in traversing the lungs
   Angiotensin II
   Epinephrine
   Dopamine
   Vasopressin
   Prostaglandin A
   Vasoactive intestinal polypeptide
   Oxytocin

The Generation of Vasoactive Substances by the Lungs
   Endothelins
   Nitric oxide
   Prostacyclin
   Hyperpolarizing factor

Dietary Pulmonary Hypertension

In 1974, the concept of *dietary pulmonary hypertension* was proposed.[22] The idea stemmed from the ability of the drug aminorex in humans and the plant crotalaria in animals to elicit pulmonary hypertension. The generalization from this experience with drugs and plants taken by mouth was that other medications, foods, and herbs, taken by mouth, might injure the pulmonary circulation sufficiently to evoke pulmonary hypertension. Since then, ample evidence has accrued in support of this hypothesis (e.g., the toxic oil syndrome;[23] fenfluramine derivatives;[1] female "crack-cocaine" users).

The outbreak of primary pulmonary hypertension attributed to aminorex occurred in Austria, Switzerland, and Germany, and came to a close after the sale of the over-the-counter drug was stopped.[29] Aminorex is a catechol derivative that acts by releasing norepinephrine at nerve terminals and synapses. One important lesson from the aminorex experience was that individual susceptibility was prerequisite for developing pulmonary hypertension: of the many thousands who used the drug, only a few developed the findings of primary pulmonary hypertension.

It now seems that history is about to repeat itself. In April 1996, another anorexigenic agent, dexfenfluramine, became available in drugstores throughout the United States, and its use is becoming widespread. In contrast to aminorex, dexfenfluramine exerts its pharmacologic effects by its enhancing effects on serotonin-mediated neurotransmission: it blocks serotonin reuptake, whereas its principal metabolite, dexnorfenfluramine, not only releases serotonin into synapses but also activates 5-HT_2 receptors.

The threat of an outbreak of pulmonary hypertension in people taking dexfenfluramine, the *d*-isomer of fenfluramine, or fenfluramine is serious. After sporadic case reports in the early 1980s of the association of pulmonary hypertension with the use of fenfluramine, Brenot and colleagues published a retrospective analysis that linked fenfluramine use with primary pulmonary hypertension.[11] A follow-up case-controlled study under the auspices of the Medical Research Council of Canada confirmed the higher incidence of primary pulmonary hypertension in people taking anorexigens, predominantly fenfluramine or dexfenfluramine.[1] Moreover, the use of the anorexigen for more than a few months was associated with increased risk of primary pulmonary hypertension. Because of the widespread use of anorexigens, an outbreak of primary pulmonary hypertension seems inevitable. Indeed, a registry set up to keep track of such cases has already received reports of people in whom the use of anorexigens is associated with primary pulmonary hypertension.

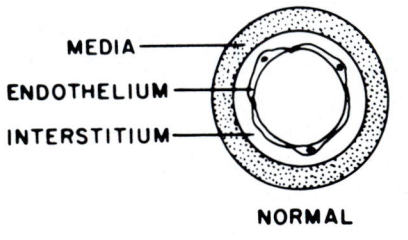
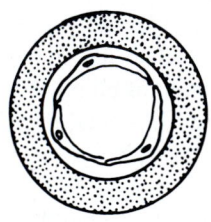
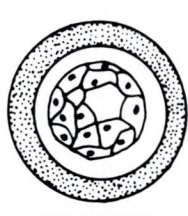
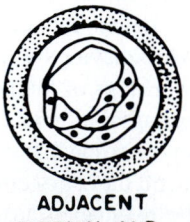
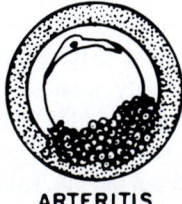
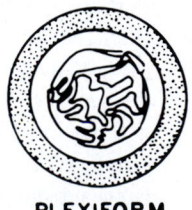
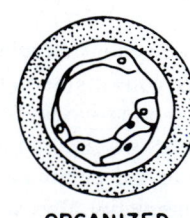

FIGURE 30-3   Normal and abnormal endothelium. Various endothelial abnormalities illustrating the different surfaces encountered by the perfusing blood.

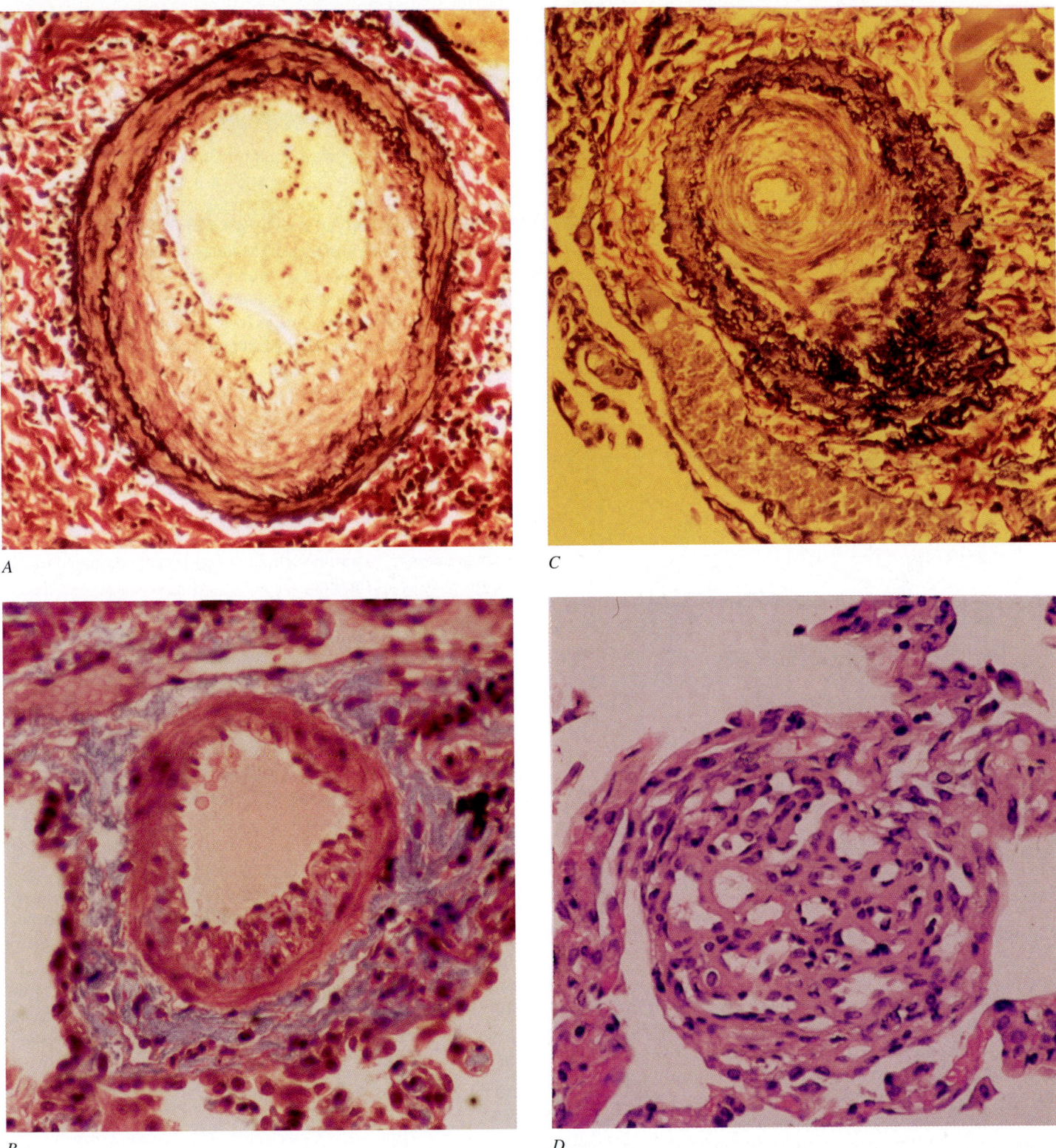

A

C

B

D

FIGURE 30-4 Microscopic appearance of small pulmonary muscular arteries, and arterioles, illustrating different degrees of intimal prolifer- ation and vascular occlusion. Plexiform lesion is at bottom right.

The Ventilation and Circulation in Liver Cirrhosis

Liver cirrhosis, and the accompanying portal hypertension, is of- ten associated with striking changes in the pulmonary circula-

tion.[40] Some of these changes appear to be diametrically oppo- site. Thus, on the one hand the minute vessels of the lungs of- ten show evidence of vasodilation in the pulmonary microcircu- lation (e.g., dilated arterioles and capillaries), whereas on the other hand the pulmonary microcirculation may be affected in

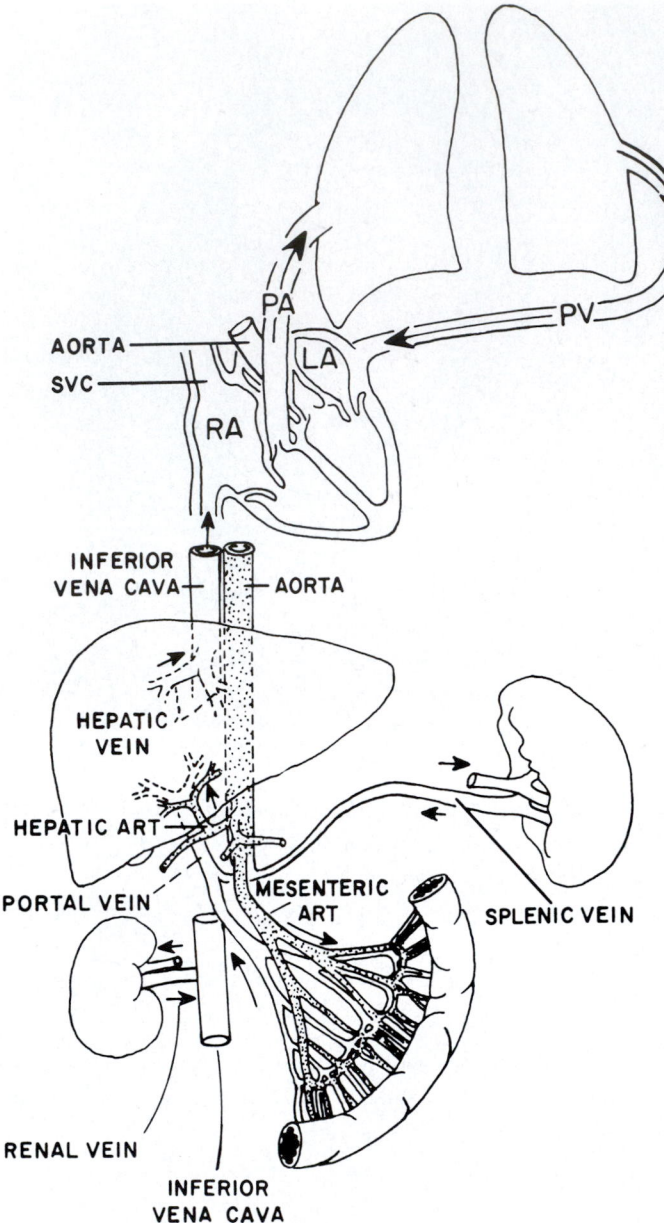

FIGURE 30-5   The gut-liver-lung axis.

obliterative vascular disease. The mechanisms at work are speculative. For example, the commonly held view that the obliterative pulmonary disease originates in pulmonary vasoconstriction, presumably because of some unknown vasoconstrictor mechanism, is unproven. Three aspects of the lung-liver relationship in liver cirrhosis have received special attention: pulmonary vasomotor control, pulmonary vasodilation, and pulmonary hypertension.

VENTILATORY RESPONSES TO HYPOXIA IN LIVER CIRRHOSIS

Hypoxic pulmonary vasoconstriction is blunted in patients with chronic liver disease,[17] indicating a defect in intrinsic autonomic control.[44] This blunting is in the face of the characteristic high-cardiac-output state that is a feature of patients with liver cirrhosis. The mechanism responsible for both the high-output state

and the blunted hypoxic pulmonary pressor response is unknown. Nitric oxide is the most recent candidate to explain the high output state associated with liver cirrhosis.

CIRCULATORY ADAPTATIONS IN LIVER CIRRHOSIS

Mild arterial hypoxemia is found in 30 to 70 percent of patients with hepatic cirrhosis.[47] This arterial hypoxemia is attributable to "anatomic" venous admixture—i.e., to anatomic shunts or to their equivalent: the rapid passage of unoxygenated blood past the gas-exchanging surfaces of the lungs.[44] This abbreviated transit time is, in turn, due to a combination of high cardiac output and dilation of the pulmonary precapillaries and capillaries.

Dilatation of microvessels in liver cirrhosis is not confined to the lungs. Instead, it occurs throughout the body, including the skin and kidneys. In the fingers, it contributes to the rare occurrence of clubbing in patients with liver cirrhosis.

Inexplicably, the blood vessels on the pleural surface are more affected by dilatation than are the intrapulmonary vessels.[7] The *spider naevi* on the pleural surface are fed by the pulmonary circulation. They are composed of short vessels, less than 1 mm in diameter, and are generally quite conspicuous. Although anatomic dilation of intrapulmonary microvessels has often been seen at autopsy, as a rule such dilatation is rare compared to that on the surface of the lung.[46]

PORTAL-PULMONARY HYPERTENSION

The association of pulmonary hypertension with liver cirrhosis has attracted considerable attention.[30] The pulmonary hypertension is due to obliterative pulmonary vascular disease.

In the 1960s, the obliterative pulmonary vascular disease in patients with liver cirrhosis was attributed to organized pulmonary emboli that originated in thrombi in the portal vein.[42] Since then, this possibility has largely been discounted, and it is now generally recognized that the pulmonary vascular lesions are identical with those of primary pulmonary hypertension.

The etiology of portal-pulmonary hypertension remains speculative. Among the possibilities being entertained is the prospect that vasoconstrictor substances or autoimmune substances,[27] or other injurious agents, might start the obliterative process by injuring pulmonary vascular endothelium. The arrangement of the gut, liver, and lungs in series nurtures this hypothesis. One intriguing aspect of this proposition is why the endothelium of pulmonary resistance vessels should be extensively affected by the injury while the more extensive endothelium of the pulmonary capillary bed is spared.

SEPSIS-INDUCED MULTIPLE ORGAN FAILURE

Probably the most striking impact of the lungs on the rest of the body is exemplified by multiple-organ failure that complicates the adult respiratory distress syndrome (ARDS). Indeed, most patients who die of ARDS do so because of multiple-organ failure rather than from the lung disease.[4,6,9,15] In recent years, the liver, as well as the kidneys, has been recognized to be a major determinant of the outcome of ARDS.[41]

In its systemic effects, ARDS behaves like sepsis elsewhere

in the body, overwhelming host defenses by the release into the circulation of inflammatiory cytokines, such as tumor necrosis factor (TNF) and interleukin 1 (IL-1).[8,12] TNF continues to be the major center of attention. Endotoxin is the most potent stimulus known for the production of TNF. Instead of acting directly to cause injury, endotoxin (or its lipopolysaccharide) prompts the formation of host factors that cause the damage. Macrophages are deeply implicated in generating these host factors. In addition to releasing injurious agents, sepsis interferes with the biologic inactivation of mediators of inflammation. Novel therapies have been directed at countering the role of TNF in the septic shock syndrome. These include anti-TNF monoclonal antibodies, soluble TNF receptors, and soluble TNF receptor–immunoglobulin G heavy-chain fusion proteins. These approaches are still under development.

Recently, attention has turned to attempts at blocking the production of nitric oxide, an endogenous vasodilator and immune modulator that may be active in inducing the systemic hypotension associated with sepsis. The target has been nitric oxide synthase (NOS), the enzyme that produces nitric oxide. Blocking NOS affords promise not only of relieving systemic hypotension but also of favorably influencing other harmful processes that may contribute to organ failure, including direct tissue injury, myocardial depression, derangement of cellular metabolism, and release of inflammatory cytokines (e.g., TNF) from macrophages.[49] However, the therapeutic role of inhibiting nitric oxide has not yet been settled because nitric oxide may have beneficial as well as harmful properties.

INJURY BY OXYGEN-DERIVED PRODUCTS

Mechanisms of Action

In recent years, mounting evidence has implicated oxidative injury in the pathogenesis of a wide array of biologic processes, ranging from the normal aging process to a variety of disease states, including atherosclerosis, carcinoma, and ischemia-perfusion injury.[32,45] Oxidative injury has also been increasingly held responsible for diverse diseases of the lungs and airways, such as emphysema, interstitial pulmonary fibrosis, asthma, and ARDS. The relationship between cigarette smoking and the development of emphysema illustrates one pathway: oxygen-derived products, either contained in cigarette smoke or generated by activated leukocytes attracted to the lungs by smoking, oxidize the methionine residue of α_1-antitrypsin, an antiprotease, thereby inactivating it and enabling the destruction by proteases of alveolar walls (see Chapter 43). The abnormal pulmonary function that ensues exerts systemic effects by way of abnormal blood gases and mechanics of breathing, stimulation of respiratory control mechanisms, and the sensation of dyspnea. The oxidant injury may be aggravated by administration of supplementary oxygen in the form of O_2-enriched inspired air mixtures.

Sensitized asthmatics respond to an allergen by degranulation of mast cells, which causes the release of TNFα. In turn, TNFα prompts the migration of neutrophils and eosinophils to the site of the allergic reaction. At this site, the leukocytes release toxic oxygen products, which contribute importantly to the inflammatory response.

Most of the molecular oxygen entering the body is reduced sequentially to water via the respiratory chain. However, in the course of the serial reductions that are part of normal intermediary metabolism, superoxide anion (O_2^-) and hydrogen peroxide (H_2O_2) are generated as undesirable by-products.

Generation of Toxic Reactive Oxygen Species

Cells that respire aerobically generate toxic reactive oxygen species. These reactive species are produced not only in the course of normal aerobic metabolism but also as by-products of inflammatory reactions. The toxic reactive species known as free radicals include the superoxide anion and hydroxyl radicals and hydrogen peroxide (Fig. 30-6). Cellular damage is inflicted by these species on proteins, nucleic acids carbohydrates, and lipids. Damage to the lungs inflicted by free radicals (e.g., ARDS) can exert disastrous effects on systemic organs (e.g., renal failure). In turn, the cell damage causes the induction of antioxidant genes that prompt the elaboration of enzymes directed at scavenging the reactive oxygen species. Among the clinical situations in which free radicals feature prominently are reperfusion injury and the adverse immunologic responses elicited by organ transplant action.[21]

In the lungs, reactive oxygen species from the environment can inflict damage. Oxygen toxicity, produced by breathing O_2-enriched inspired air, affords a traditional example of injury produced by O_2-derived products. Within 24 h of the start of oxygen breathing, the endothelium of the pulmonary microcirculation is damaged and becomes "leaky," enabling blood plasma to gain access to the interstitial spaces and alveoli. Along with excess fluid and serum proteins, inflammatory cells accumulate in the lungs. Should exposure to the O_2-rich inspired gas continue, the end-point can be ARDS. One experimental strategy for mimicking the pathologic and pathophysiological changes in the lungs induced by oxygen toxicity is the administration of endotoxin.

$$O_2 \xrightarrow{1e^-} O_2^{\cdot -} \underset{pK\ 4.7}{\rightleftharpoons} HO_2^{\cdot -}$$

$$O_2 \xrightarrow[2H^+]{2e^-} H_2O_2$$

$$2O_2^{\cdot -} + 2H^+ \xrightarrow{SOD} H_2O + O_2$$

$$2H_2O_2 \xrightarrow{Catalase} 2H_2O + O_2$$

$$H_2O_2 + O_2^{\cdot -} \xrightarrow{\underset{Fe^{2+}}{Fe^{3+}}} OH^- + \cdot OH + {}^1O_2$$

(Metal catalyzed Haber-Weiss)

$$H_2O_2 + Fe^{2+} \longrightarrow OH^\cdot + OH^- + Fe^{3+}$$

(Fenton reaction)

FIGURE 30-6 The generation of oxygen-free radicals by the addition of electrons.

Another mechanism for causing oxidant injury involves nitric oxide (see Chapter 26). Nitric oxide, a mediator of signal transduction with diverse physiological functions, is categorized as a free radical because of its unpaired electron. Because of this property, it has biologically important reactivities with certain kinds of proteins, carbohydrates, and other free radicals (e.g., superoxide radicals). In its reactions with other free radicals, it can yield even more potent oxidants (e.g., peroxynitrite).[45] Some toxic reactions, originally attributed to its chemical precursors, superoxide and nitric oxide, are now attributed to peroxynitrite. Oppositely, nitric oxide can also exert a protective action against free radicals, such as the superoxides. Thus, nitric oxide can either inflict damage or ward it off, depending on the oxidative environment in which the reactions are taking place. An intense research effort is currently directed at unraveling the nature of reactions involving nitric oxide and peroxynitrite with proteins, lipids, carbohydrates, and gene expression in a variety of pathologic processes.

The amino acid homocysteine is operative in another mechanism by which oxidative injury can damage endothelium.[36,39] This mechanism is mediated primarily by auto-oxidation, which generates the superoxide anion radical (O_2^-) and H_2O_2 and the hydroxyl radical ($OH\cdot$). Abnormally high levels of homocysteine in plasma blunt the responses of endothelium to endothelium-dependent vasodilators (e.g., nitric oxide) by way of the damage caused by products of homocysteine oxidation.[36] The antithrombotic function of endothelium and the migration and proliferation of vasocular smooth-muscle cells are also affected by high levels of homocysteine.

Two other clinical areas in which oxidant-produced injury features prominently are the inhalation or ingestion of oxidants (e.g., paraquat) and the chronic injury caused by smoking, which predisposes to low-level inflammation, pulmonary damage, and neoplasm.

GENERAL SYSTEMIC EFFECTS OF PULMONARY DISEASE

Pulmonary infections and neoplasms are notorious for the systemic effects that they can elicit (Table 30-2). Pneumonias caused by bacteria, mycoplasma, viruses, or fungi can cause a spectrum of disturbances, ranging from mild fever to bacteremia and circulatory collapse.[18,26,33,37] Viral infections are notorious for inducing leukopenia, anemia, and thrombocytopenia. Metabolic

TABLE 30-2

General Systemic Effects of Nonrespiratory Diseases of the Lung

Disturbances in the control of body temperature (fever, chills, sweating)

Central nervous system abnormalities (euphoria, irritability, confusion, delirium)

Faintness, reduced alertness, syncope (postural hypotension, arrhythmias, decreased blood flow to the brain)

Anorexia, asthenia, cachexia

Remote organ failure

derangements are also the rule in these acute disorders; abnormal hepatic and bone marrow functions are the bases for common abnormalities (e.g., high erythrocyte sedimentation rate and leukocytosis). The span of disturbances is just as great for neoplasms, not only because they encroach on adjacent structures and functions but also because of derangements in remote bodily functions that they cause by releasing biologically active materials (see Chapter 151). The impact of pulmonary disease on the rest of the body rises exponentially when infectious organisms or neoplastic cells escape the confines of the lungs to enter the bloodstream.

Bacteremia, viruses, fungi, and other microorganisms can invade the bloodstream from the lungs. Such infections gain in virulence with increasing numbers of organisms and their products; the elderly are particularly vulnerable to the systemic effects of pulmonary infections. Among the common consequences of diseases that begin in the lungs and affect the rest of the body are fever and body wasting.

Fever, Chills, Sweating

There are many causes of fever. Among the most common are infections, inflammation, injury to the central nervous system, thrombosis, hematoma, vasculitis, and necrosis. Fever is generally regarded as harmful. However, fever has enhancing functions. For example, in infections, it enhances neutrophil migration and the production of antibiotic substances by neutrophils.

The body is constructed to keep internal core temperature stable at about 37.1°C (corresponding to a rectal temperature of about 37.6°C) and equipped with automatic feedback devices that minimize fluctuations in the core temperature. Regulation of the core temperature is accomplished almost entirely by neural feedback mechanisms, virtually all of which are controlled by temperature-regulating mechanisms in the hypothalamus. Fever represents an upward shift in the thermostatic set point. The automatic attempt by the body to restore body temperature to normal includes cutaneous vasodilatation, sweating, decreased chemical thermogenesis, and a widespread decrease in muscle tone due to reflex inhibition of the *primary motor center for shivering.*

Chills are a response to an abrupt disparity between the set point of the thermostat in the hypothalamus and the temperature of the blood. Certain substances, notably pyrogens and products of tissue destruction (see next paragraph), can suddenly raise the hypothalamic set point without raising body temperature. Until the body temperature catches up, mechanisms to raise it are turned on, and the subject feels cold and experiences chills—even while the body temperature is increasing to match the hypothalamus set point: the cold sensation is a consequence of cutaneous vasoconstriction, whereas shivering causes the "shakes." When the body temperature reaches the higher set point, chills cease and the subject feels neither cold nor hot. Until the factor responsible for increasing the set point stops, the febrile state is maintained by the usual mechanisms. Precipitous discontinuance of the initiating factor results in widespread cutaneous dilatation and flushing and intense sweating—i.e., "the crisis."

Pyrogens feature prominently in causing clinical fevers. They do so, directly or indirectly, by raising the thermostatic set point in the hypothalamus. Particularly effective in this regard are en-

TABLE 30-3

Some Substances from Pulmonary Endocrine Neoplasms That Can Affect Systemic Organs and Tissues

Adrenocorticotropin
Calcitonin and calcitonin gene-related peptide
Arginine vasopressin
Growth hormone
Serotonin
Pituitary gonadotropins
Thyroid-stimulating hormone
Vasoactive intestinal polypeptide
Insulin
Parathyroid hormone
Somatostatin
Renin
Gastrin
Prolactin
Bombesinlike peptides

dotoxins produced by gram-negative bacteria. Leukocytes and macrophages act as intermediaries in this process: these phagocytic cells, after digesting the bacterial products, release leukocyte or endogenous pyrogen, which, in minute amounts, stimulates the hypothalamus to raise its set point; prostaglandin E_1 is presumably the intermediary within the cells of the hypothalamus that effects the febrile response. Blockage of prostaglandin formation, as by aspirin, can prevent or reduce the febrile response.

Chills, fever, and sweating are familiar manifestations of the syndrome of pneumococcal pneumonia and its complications. Some infecting organisms tend to be associated with distinctive diurnal fever patterns. Although these patterns were once regarded as diagnostic clues to the etiologic agent, not much clinical attention is now paid to patterns, although the peaks and valleys in the fever curves can suggest clues to origin, and undue persistence of fever may signal a complication.

Body Wasting

Progressive infection or the growth of a neoplasm often elicits anorexia, weight loss, and cachexia.[16] Cachexia is characterized by an inexorable loss of weight that is inordinate for the degree of anorexia and the decrease in food intake. Both adipose tissue and muscle mass are depleted; death usually is the end result of progressive depletion of lean body tissue.[38,43]

Anorexia and underlying metabolic abnormalities appear to be at work in the pathogenesis of cachexia. Anorexia regularly accompanies weight loss. Although the initiating mechanism for anorexia seems to relate to the infection or neoplasm, in time other mechanisms supervene. Among these are depression, continued immobilization, and co-morbid conditions. Appetite suppression is often aggravated further by medications. Attempts to reverse cachexia by nutritional supplements are rarely successful.[20]

Key factors in the production of cachexia fall into three categories: (1) metabolic products of the pathogen or neoplasm; (2) catabolic hormones and a lipid-mobilizing factor (LMF) produced by neoplasms that acts to cause breakdown of adipose tissue; and (3) cytokines, such as $TNF\alpha$ and interleukin 6 (IL-6), which seem to affect adipose tissue by inhibiting lipoprotein lipase. $TNF\alpha$ plays a pivotal role. It is produced by macrophages, monocytes, and T cells, and its toxic effects are exceedingly diverse: it is a pyrogen, directly damages endothelium, can suppress adipose-specific enzymes, and is a mediator of the inflammatory process.[50]

During the past 2 years, since the discovery of leptin, a hormone active in the control of body weight, interest in starvation has taken a new turn. Leptin is a hormone produced by the obesity gene (ob), manufactured by adipocytes, and delivered to receptors in the hypothalamus (arcuate nucleus and paraventricular nucleus). Leptin functions as a lipostat: when fat stores increase, adipocytes produce leptin, which tells the brain to decrease appetite and increase activity.

Leptin exerts its effects via a complex interplay that involves neuropeptide Y and the melanocortins, a family of peptides. Decreased leptin levels work through neuropeptide Y to deal with the stresses of starvation; high levels may work through melanocortins to resist overweight. One feature of starvation is altered endocrine activity (e.g., decreased production of thyroid and sex hormones and increased production of adrenal stress hormones). Low levels of leptin elicit starvation-induced changes in endocrine function. The components of the hormone-neuropeptide system and their interplay in the control of body weight are currently under intense investigation. Most studies have been conducted in the rat, however, and their implications for human disorders, such as starvation, are incompletely understood.

Some success in reversing cachexia has been accomplished by the use of two groups of agents: those that stimulate intake of food (e.g., megestrol acetate, which can also stimulate tumor growth) and those that inhibit LMF (e.g., eicosapentaenoic adic[48]).

SYSTEMIC EFFECTS OF PULMONARY DISEASE

Certain systemic manifestations, although not unique to pulmonary disease, occur often enough to warrant special mention. Among these is clubbing of the digits.

Clubbing of the Digits and Hypertrophic Osteoarthropathy

The characteristic and preferential bulbous enlargement of the distal segment of the digits (Fig. 30-7) and the distinctive bony lesions of secondary hypertrophic osteoarthropathy are generally explained in terms of humoral mediators that cause selective vasodilatation of the digital precapillary vessels. As is noted in Chapter 116, this explanation seems to suffice in certain disorders (e.g., the clubbing of the digits and the hypertrophic osteoarthropathy that accompany carcinoma of the lungs) but not in others (e.g., subacute bacterial endocarditis). One other intriguing aspect of clubbing is its association both with chronic bronchiectasis, in which the adjacent collateral circulation of the lungs undergoes remarkable proliferation, and with carcinoma of the lung, in which the collateral blood supply is modest.[34]

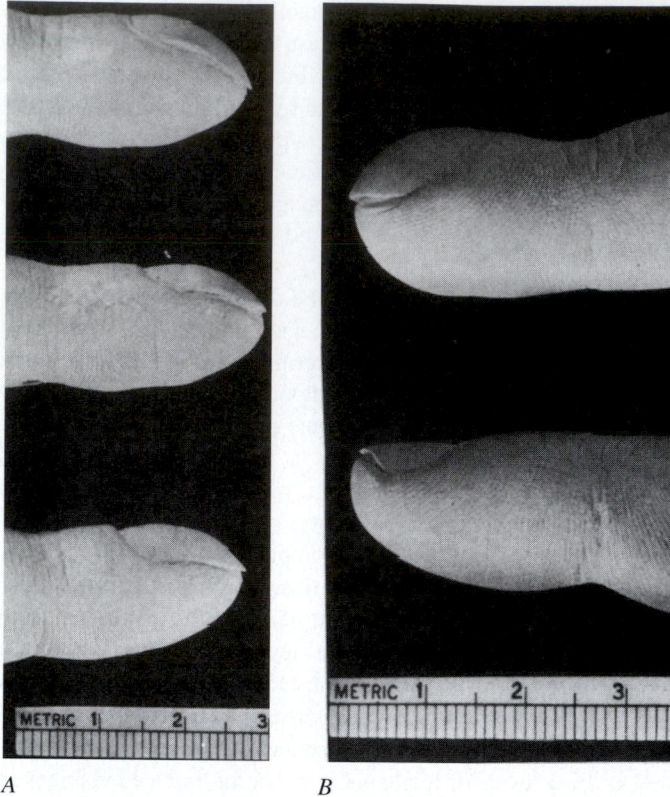

A   *B*

FIGURE 30-7 Casts of clubbed fingers. *A.* The second right finger of an 18-year-old woman with tetralogy of Fallot before and after surgery. *Upper:* Preoperatively, showing marked clubbing. *Middle:* Two months later, showing partial reversal of changes. *Lower:* Regression of the clubbing. *B.* The third right finger of a 40-year-old woman with digital clubbing *(above),* compared with that of a normal 36-year-old woman *(below). (From Mellins, Fishman: Circulation 33:143–145, 1966.)*

CONCLUDING COMMENT

Once the metabolic functions of the lungs were fully appreciated, it became evident that interplay between the lungs and systemic tissues and organs was part of normal body functioning and that more than nervous connections is operative. This interplay became even more evident in clinical syndromes that involved the transport by the circulation (and possibly lymph) of products of inflammation from one part of the body to the other. Syndromes such as the hepatorenal syndrome and organ failure in ARDS underscored the interplay. Others, such as coexistent portal and pulmonary hypertension, remain enigmas to be resolved. With these insights came the realization that understanding of the interplay between the lungs and other organs is still in its infancy.

REFERENCES

1. Abenheim L, Moride Y, Brenot F, et al: Appetite-suppressant drugs and the risk of primary pulmonary hypertension. *New Engl J Med* 335:609–616, 1996.
2. Adriaensen D, Scheuermann DW, Timmermans JP, DeGroodt-Lasseel MH: Neuroepithelial endocrine cells in the lung of the lungfish *Protopterus arthiopicus*: An electron- and fluorescence-microscopical investigation. *Acta Anat (Basel)* 139:70–77, 1990.
3. Badimon L, Meyer BJ, Badimon JS: Thrombin in arterial thrombosis. *Haemostasis* 24:69–80, 1994.
4. Barie PS: Organ-specific support in multiple organ failure: pulmonary support. *World J Surg* 19:581–591, 1995.
5. Becker KL, Gazdar AF: *The Endocrine Lung in Health and Disease.* New York: Saunders, 1984.
6. Bernard ER, Artigas A, Brigham KL, et al: The American-European Consensus Conference on ARDS. *Am J Respir Crit Care Med* 149:818–824, 1994.
7. Berthelot P, Walker JC, Sherlock S, et al: Arterial changes in the lungs in cirrhosis of the liver-lung spider nevi. *New Engl J Med* 274:291–298, 1966.
8. Blackwell TS, Christman JW: Sepsis and cytokines: current status. *Br J Anaesth* 77:110–117, 1996.
9. Bone RC: Toward a theory regarding the pathogenesis of the systemic inflammatory response syndrome. *Crit Care Med* 24:163–172, 1996.
10. Brass LF, Ahuja M, Belmonte E, et al: Thrombin receptors: Turning them off after turning them on. *Semin Hematol* 31:251–260, 1994.
11. Brenot F, Hervé P, Petipretz P, et al: Primary pulmonary hypertension and fenfluramine use. *Br Heart J* 70:537–541, 1993.
12. Casale TB, Costa JJ, Galli SJ: TNFα is important in human lung allergic reactions. *Am J Respir Cell Mol Biol* 15:35–44, 1996.
13. Castro M, Krowka MJ, Schroeder DR, et al: Frequency and clinical implications of increased pulmonary artery pressures in liver transplant patients. *Mayo Clin Proc* 71:543–551, 1996.
14. Chaouat A, Weitzenblum E, Higenbottam T: The role of thrombosis in severe pulmonary hypertension. *Eur Respir J* 9:356–363, 1996.
15. Cipolle MD, Pasquale MD, Cerra FB: Secondary organ dysfunction: From clinical perspectives to molecular mediators. *Crit Care Clin* 9:261–298, 1993.
16. Coodley GO, Loveless MO, Merrill TM: The HIV wasting syndrome: A review. *J Acquir Immune Defic Synd* 7:681–694, 1994.
17. Daoud FS, Reeves JT, Schaefer JW: Failure of hypoxic vasoconstriction in patients with liver cirrhosis. *J Clin Invest* 51:1076–1080, 1972.
18. Demling RH: The modern version of adult respiratory distress syndrome. *Annu Rev Med* 46:193–202, 1995.
19. Esmon CT: Cell mediated events that control blood coagulation and vascular injury. *Annu Rev Cell Biol* 9:1–26, 1993.
20. Espat NJ, Moldawer LL, Copeland EM 3rd, Copeland EM: Cytokine-mediated alterations in host metabolism prevent nutritional repletion in cachectic cancer patients. *J Surg Oncol* 58:77–82, 1995.
21. Fisher A, Forman HJ: Oxygen utilization and toxicity in the lungs, in Fishman AP, Fisher AB (eds), *Handbook of Physiology,* sec. 3: *The Respiratory System,* vol I: *Circulation and Nonrespiratory Functions.* Bethesda, MD, American Physiological Society, 1985, pp 231–254.
22. Fishman AP: Dietary pulmonary hypertension. *Circ Res* 35:657–660, 1974.
23. Garcia-Dorado D, Miller DD, Garcia EJ, et al: An epidemic of pulmonary hypertension after toxic rapeseed ingestion in Spain. *J Am Coll Cardiol* 1:1216–1222, 1983.
24. Gosney JR: *Pulmonary Endocrine Pathology.* Oxford, Butterworth-Heinemann, 1992.
25. Griffin JA: The thrombin paradox. *Nature* 378:337–338, 1995.
26. Grootendorst AF: Hemodynamic aspects of multiple organ failure. *Intensive Care Med* 16(Suppl):S165–S167, 1990.
27. Groves BM, Brundage BH, Elliot CG, et al: Pulmonary hypertension associated with hepatic cirrhosis, in Fishman AP (ed), *The Pulmonary Circulation: Normal and Abnormal.* Philadelphia, University of Pennsylvania, 1990, pp 359–369.

28. Grunwald GB: Autoimmune paraneoplastic syndromes: Manifestations and mechanisms, in Fishman AP (ed), *Update: Pulmonary Diseases and Disorders.* New York: McGraw-Hill, 1992, pp 137–146.

29. Gurtner HP: Aminorex pulmonary hypertension, in Fishman AP (ed), *The Pulmonary Circulation: Normal and Abnormal.* Philadelphia, University of Pennsylvania, 1990, pp 397–411.

30. Hadengue A, Benhavoun MK, Lebrec D, et al: Pulmonary hypertension complicating portal hypertension. *Gastroenterology* 100: 520–528, 1991.

31. Johnson PH. Hirudin: Clinical potential of a thrombin inhibitor. *Annu Rev Med* 45:165–177, 1994.

32. Kerr ME, Bender CM, Monti EJ: An introduction to oxygen free radicals. *Heart Lung* 25:200–209, 1996.

33. Knox JB: Oxygen consumption-oxygen delivery dependency in adult respiratory distress syndrome. *New Horiz* 1:381–387, 1993.

34. Lanken PN, Fishman AP: Clubbing and hypertrophic osteoarthropathy, in Fishman AP (ed), *Pulmonary Diseases and Disorders.* New York, McGraw-Hill, 1980, pp 84–91.

35. Lauweryns JM, Van Ranst L: Immunocytochemical localization of aromatic L–amino acid decarboxylase in human, rat, and mouse bronchopulmonary and gastrointestinal endocrine cells. *J Histochem Cytochem* 36:1181–1186, 1988.

36. Lentz SR, Sobey CG, Piegors DJ, et al: Vascular dysfunction in monkeys with diet-induced hyperhomocyst(e)inemia. *J Clin Invest* 98:24–29, 1996.

37. Livingston DH, Deitch EA: Multiple organ failure: A common problem in surgical intensive care unit patients. *Ann Med* 27:13–20, 1995.

38. Loprinzi CL: Management of cancer anorexia/cachexia. *Support Care Cancer* 3:120–122, 1995.

39. Loscalzo J: The oxidant stress of hyperhomocyst(e)inemia (editorial). *J Clin Invest* 98:5–7, 1996.

40. Mandelli MS, Groves BM: Pulmonary hypertension in chronic liver disease. *Clin Chest Med* 17:17–34, 1996.

41. Matuschak GM: Liver-lung interactions in sepsis and multiple organ failure syndrome. *Clin Chest Med* 17:83–98, 1996.

42. Naeye RL: "Primary" pulmonary hypertension with coexisting portal hypertension. *Circulation* 22:376–384, 1960.

43. Ottery FD: Supportive nutrition to prevent cachexia and improve quality of life. *Semin Oncol* 22:98–111, 1995.

44. Rodriguez-Roisin R, Roca J, Agust AG, et al: Gas exchange and pulmonary vascular reactivity in patients with liver cirrhosis. *Am Rev Respir Dis* 135:1085–1092, 1987.

45. Rubbo H, Radi R, Trujillo M, et al: Nitric oxide regulation of superoxide and peroxynitrite-dependent lipid peroxidation. *J Biol Chem* 269:26066–26075, 1994.

46. Schraufnagel DE, Kay JM: Structural and pathologic changes in the lung vasculature in chronic liver disease. *Clin Chest Med* 17:1–15, 1996.

47. Sherlock S: The liver-lung interface. *Semin Respir Med* 9:247–253, 1988.

48. Tinsdale MJ: Cancer cachexia. *Anticancer Drugs* 4:115–125, 1993.

49. Tracey KJ, Cerami A: Tumor necrosis factor: A pleiotropic cytokine and therapeutic agent. *Annu Rev Med* 45:491–503, 1994.

50. Wilmore DW: Catabolic illness. Strategies for enhancing recovery. *New Engl J Med* 325:695–702, 1991.

CHAPTER 31

PRINCIPLES OF EFFECTIVE CARE

Peter G. Tuteur

COST-EFFECTIVE ANALYSIS: THE DEVELOPMENTAL
  NEED

COST-EFFECTIVE ANALYSIS: THE DISCIPLINE

COST-EFFECTIVE ANALYSIS: THE DEVELOPMENTAL NEED

Since the beginning of the 20th century, physicians have been trained to view the health needs of their patients as paramount. To meet these needs, physicians are required to exemplify empathy, compassion, patience, scientific knowledge, objective reasoning, and expert decision-making. The physician must know the patient and his or her family and assess the meaning of what is said and the feelings behind the meanings. The doctor is to be professional and, thus, uninfluenced by personal gain, potential loss, or perverse incentives. Then, with one hand on the patient's shoulder and the other on the stethoscope, the physician must synthesize all information into an efficient plan, often despite inadequate data. This, collectively, is the art of medicine; when perfected, it is viewed as a good.[2]

By the 1930s, physician-patient encounters grew more likely to result in a positive outcome, and society attached increasing value to health-care services. After World War II, employers, unions, and governments facilitated access to care through payer systems that nurtured this perceived good. Subsequently, health-care expenditures grew rapidly. By the late 1970s, American health planners began to voice concern about limited, unequally distributed resources. To counter this dilemma, external systems that managed provider (hospital and doctor) behavior were proposed, promoting efficiency without adversely influencing ef-

fectiveness. The idea took hold, and today managed care often dramatically affects the practice of medicine, forcing physicians individually and organizationally to reassess the way clinical problems are approached.

Two decades ago, for no discernible or consistent reasons, wide variations in practice patterns were demonstrated among geographically adjacent communities of similar demographic composition. Moreover, in these communities, costs varied, but health outcomes differed little.[6] There were numerous responses to these observations. Initially, closed-panel health maintenance organizations (HMOs) claimed to provide efficient, high-quality health care at lower costs by stressing disease prevention, primary care evaluation and management, and outpatient surgical services. Also, savings were incurred with the use of home-based professional support. More recently, regulated and unregulated systems employing prescribing pattern control, care pathways, case managers, step-down units, and hospitalists have been introduced as organizational components designed to lead to more efficient and, at least, satisfactory care. These approaches are based largely on population studies and make use of techniques of *cost-effective analysis* (CEA). Overall, the rate of increase in American health-care costs has slowed; however, some payers profess that there is even more room for efficiency and more to be saved or, for some, earned.

This chapter creates a framework for guiding clinicians to effectively approach diagnostic problems and manage therapeutic issues encountered in pulmonary medicine. An understanding of the basic concepts, tools, and role of formal CEA is developed. In addition, the forces affecting clinicians are explored, including professional responsibility to the individual patient and the influence of those who view delivery of health care not from the examining table but from the fiscal perspective. To reach a compromise between these sometimes diametrically opposed positions, an assumption is made that although the fiscal "bottom line" is of critical programmatic import, it is not the ultimate goal. Furthermore, the end point of greatest value is assumed to be the provision of clinically sensitive, scientifically valid health care. This requires effective use of data collection methods and their proper application to problem-solving techniques. The potential consequences of actions on health, both short- and long-term, as well as monetary implications both to the individual and to the health-care system, must be kept in mind.

COST-EFFECTIVE ANALYSIS: THE DISCIPLINE

The formal discipline of cost-effective analysis was developed in response to a programmatic need to evaluate the relationship of health outcomes and resource costs of health interventions in defined populations. This quantitative approach often assumes that the target population is rather homogeneous, and that health benefits are distributed equally. Furthermore, it is assumed that both health services and expected outcomes are assigned similar values by individual members of the group. Unfortunately, these conditions may not hold universally. What is the value of a year of life or a year of life adjusted for quality? Costs, too, are difficult to define. Are they equal to charges—average, marginal, or discounted for future payment? Under such conditions, how can these evaluations aid the clinician in managing his or her patients' care?

Clearly, instruments designed to answer a question in one field of inquiry may not be as useful in addressing similar questions in another. An example is the International Labor Organization (ILO) system used to describe standard chest radiographs of patients with suspected pneumoconioses. The system employs a semiquantitative scale to depict the degree of profusion of an interstitial pulmonary process. The ILO system was designed for, and validated by, epidemiologists for population studies. For clinicians, it has less value, particularly when used to determine the presence or absence of coal worker's pneumoconiosis in an individual patient when a complete personal, environmental, and medical history is assembled and supplemented by a detailed and focused physical examination, laboratory studies, and imaging techniques. Extending this concept, one must question the applicability, accuracy, and appropriateness of broad-based cost-effective analysis in caring for an individual patient.

Over the past two decades, health-care costs in the United States have increased at a rate greater than the growth in the general economy. Among planners, this has stimulated two general concerns: recognition that resources are limited and heterogeneously distributed and dissatisfaction with measured national health outcomes. Additionally, the appreciation of behavioral variation among providers serves as a great stimulus for the development of tools to investigate the efficiency of differing strategies of health-care delivery, with a goal of defining "the right way of doing it." Cost-effective analysis has become a focus.

At an initial glance, the meaning of the terms *cost* and *effectiveness* appears to be intuitively obvious. The unit of cost is currency. However, one must think of the relationship of cost to charges, mean costs, marginal costs, and discounted costs. Nonmonetary costs pose a dilemma when one is attempting to assign value to factors such as stress, risk, time, suffering, and partial disability. Similarly, effectiveness in clinical terms might be thought of as "cure" or years of life prolongation; soon, however, discounts for suboptimal quality, pain, cognitive level, and other factors are required. In an attempt to quantify costs and effectiveness in population studies comparing alternative clinical strategies, a variety of terms have been used.

The incremental (marginal) cost-*effective* ratio is the number of dollars per life year gained. This term simply relates monetary cost of an intervention to a year of life gained by that intervention. Valid criticism that variation in the quality of an additional year of life determines its value has prompted development of a term that adjusts for a survival of lesser quality—incremental (marginal) cost-*utility* ratio, which is the number of dollars per quality-adjusted year of life gained. Finally, concern that not all persons attach similar value to given characteristics of life has led to a third term: incremental (marginal) cost-*benefit* ratio, which is the number of dollars in cost difference versus the dollar value attributed to the outcome anticipated by the patient.

TABLE 31-1

Cost and Effect Guidelines in Disease Diagnosis and Management

- Health-care activities conducted in the hospital are more costly than the same activities performed in an outpatient venue.
- An activity that influences neither care nor outcome reduces overall efficiency.
- Less costly activities positively influencing health care are more efficient than more expensive ones with similar influence.
- The higher the morbidity and mortality of an activity, the greater the adverse effect on efficiency, all other factors remaining constant.
- Unneeded therapy can produce only side effects, without benefit.
- Short-term advantages must be weighed against potential long-term disadvantages; however, this often is a difficult calculation.
- A test that definitely establishes a diagnosis does not require confirmation.
- A test without morbidity, with low to moderate sensitivity, and with generous specificity may be a valuable replacement for one of high morbidity and high specificity.
- Two procedures performed simultaneously are more efficient than the same two performed sequentially.
- A beneficial and desirable clinical outcome is more valuable than the efficiency of the route of attainment. The cost of the route determines value. The ratio of the two is the basis of the concept of cost-effectiveness.
- An activity done for "academic" interest may be associated with beneficence both to the individual patient and to the body of scientific knowledge. However, it must be initiated formally in a prospectively defined, independently supported manner.

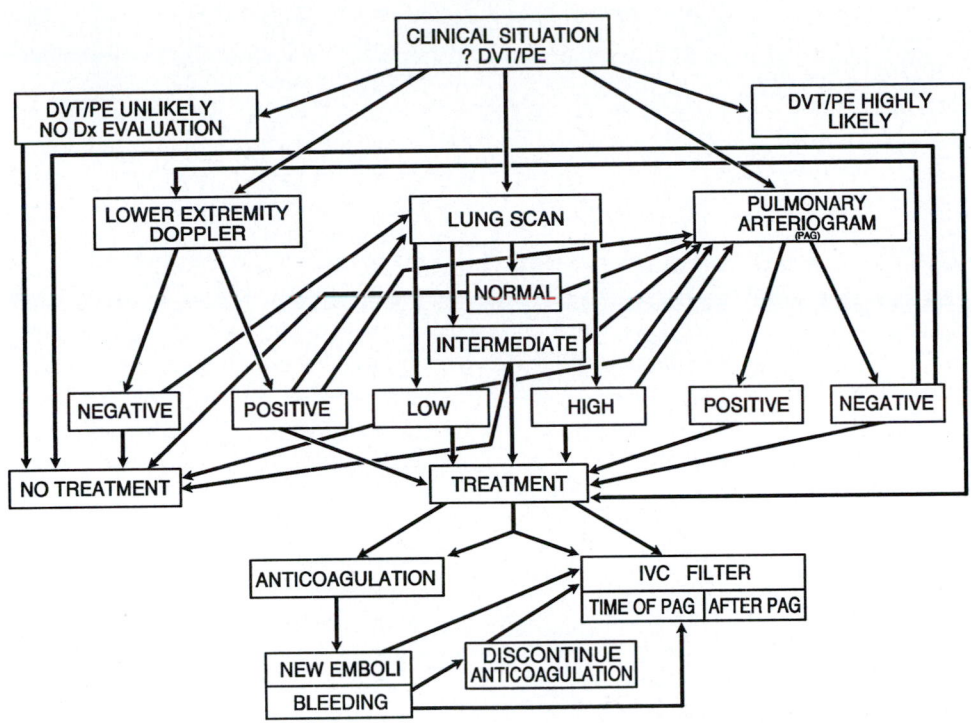

FIGURE 31-1   This figure represents only some of the possible decision pathways associated with the care of a patient suspected of having deep venous thrombosis (DVT) and/or pulmonary emboli (PE).

Using the tools that define relationships between cost and effect in population studies often helps the clinician explore ways to improve efficiency in the practice of medicine, without adversely affecting outcome. Applying general principles derived from global studies may guide the clinician in the care of individual patients. Since costs and prices neither are stable nor change in parallel in any market, including healthcare, the guidelines noted here are qualitative and expressed first as widely accepted truisms, often intuitively obvious yet supported by formal CEA. The guidelines are summarized in Table 31-1.

With this background in mind, one can view common clinical situations either as "routine" or as an opportunity to navigate through a complex decision network employing the concepts of efficiency and effectiveness. To this calculus one may also add consideration of cost. Participation in this exercise brings about the recognition that available data universally applicable to each task may be incomplete. One such often considered routine clinical problem is caring for the patient with suspected deep venous thrombosis (DVT) and/or pulmonary emboli (PE). Figure 31-1 illustrates some of the many potential decision pathways toward resolution. Each junction affords the clinician an opportunity to use the principles of clinical effectiveness and efficiency.

These terms and the meaning assigned to their components have been used and validated in population studies. In achieving standardization, however, interpretation of results is limited by definitions that are narrow, subject to significant inaccuracies when used more broadly, and applied in a rapidly changing clinical world after significant delay from the time of data collection. Also, various authors often use identical terms that differ in definition, making comparison among studies difficult. When different instruments are employed, global application becomes even less successful. However, these calculations, when properly applied, aid health planners in ranking different strategies in an attempt to provide improvements in health status to populations for which health resources are limited.[3–5]

As noted above, use of these terms is a tool for allocating funding priorities for populations.[1] In contrast, for most clinicians making decisions about resource allocation for individual patients, the effect of fiscal resource constraint is secondary—if it is considered at all. This contrasts with *facility limitation*. Physicians traditionally search for maximal effectiveness for individual patients—a philosophy that is in conflict with those who primarily wish to minimize costs. However, tradition must be modified, because society's agents have not only limited resources but also increased expectations. The goal of attempting to accomplish both poses a challenge that, if met, results in a productive outcome.

REFERENCES

1. Detsky, Allan S, Naglie IG: A clinician's guide to cost-effectiveness analysis. *Ann Intern Med* 113:147–154, 1990.
2. Ludmerer, KM: *The Development of American Medical Education: Learning to Heal.* New York, Basic Books, 1995.
3. Russell LB, Gold MR, Siegel JE, et al, for the Panel on Cost-Effectiveness in Health and Medicine: The role of cost-effectiveness analysis in health medicine. *JAMA* 276:1172–1177, 1996.
4. Siegel JE, Weinstein MC, Russell LB, Gold MR, for the Panel on Cost-Effectiveness in Health and Medicine: Recommendations for reporting cost-effectiveness analysis. *JAMA* 276:1339–1341, 1996.
5. Weinstein MC, Siegel JE, Gold MR, et al, for the Panel on Cost-Effectiveness in Health and Medicine: Recommendations of the Panel on Cost-Effectiveness in Health and Medicine. *JAMA* 276:1253–1258, 1996.
6. Wennberg JE: Dealing with medical practice variations: A proposal for action, in Iglehart JK (ed), *Health Affairs,* vol III. Milwood, Virginia, Project Hope, 1984, pp 6–32.

CHAPTER 32

RADIOGRAPHIC EVALUATION OF THE CHEST

Wallace T. Miller

Radiographic evaluation of the chest constitutes an important component in assessment of the patient with known or suspected pulmonary disease. In fact, the chest x-ray may provide the earliest or only clue to the presence of clinically significant respiratory disease. This chapter provides a brief overview of chest radiology. First, general aspects are covered; use of more specialized techniques, including computed tomography, nuclear

magnetic resonance, and arteriography, is highlighted. Subsequently, radiographic manifestations of diseases that affect the distribution of pulmonary blood flow, the airways, and the lung parenchyma are considered. Finally, disorders are reviewed that are predominantly or exclusively confined to anatomically distinct areas of the thorax, including the mediastinum, diaphragm and chest wall, and pleura. Throughout the presentation, examples of radiographs are provided to highlight the principles and disorders discussed.

GENERAL ASPECTS

In recent years, fresh concepts and new techniques have greatly expanded the diagnostic armamentarium of chest radiology. As a rule, the new approaches have strengthened the underpinnings of conventional methods and our diagnostic abilities. Evaluation invariably begins with routine chest radiographs, supplemented, as indicated, by more specialized techniques.

The Routine Examination

In asymptomatic patients, a posteroanterior (PA) chest radiograph is generally used as the sole screening procedure. This projection is easiest to interpret, since the anatomy is quite familiar, and most pathologic respiratory conditions are demonstrable in this view. Ideally, a lateral view should also be part of the routine examination. The lateral view adds valuable information about areas that are not well seen in the PA projection. This is particularly true of the anterior portion of the lung, adjacent to the mediastinum—an area that may be obscured by the overlying heart and aortic shadows (Fig. 32-1). The region of the vertebral column is also seen to better advantage on the lateral view. A small pleural effusion is best seen, and often only seen, as blunting of a costophrenic sulcus posteriorly (Fig. 32-2).

In determining which costophrenic angle is blunted, correct identification of each hemidiaphragm on the lateral view is helpful. If the lateral radiograph is taken in the left lateral position, as is usual, the magnified ribs are on the right side; the unmagnified ribs are on the left side and are associated with the corresponding left hemidiaphragm (Fig. 32-2). In addition, the outline of the left hemidiaphragm is often obscured anteriorly because it merges with the heart shadow. Finally, the left hemidiaphragm may be recognized from its proximity to the stomach bubble.

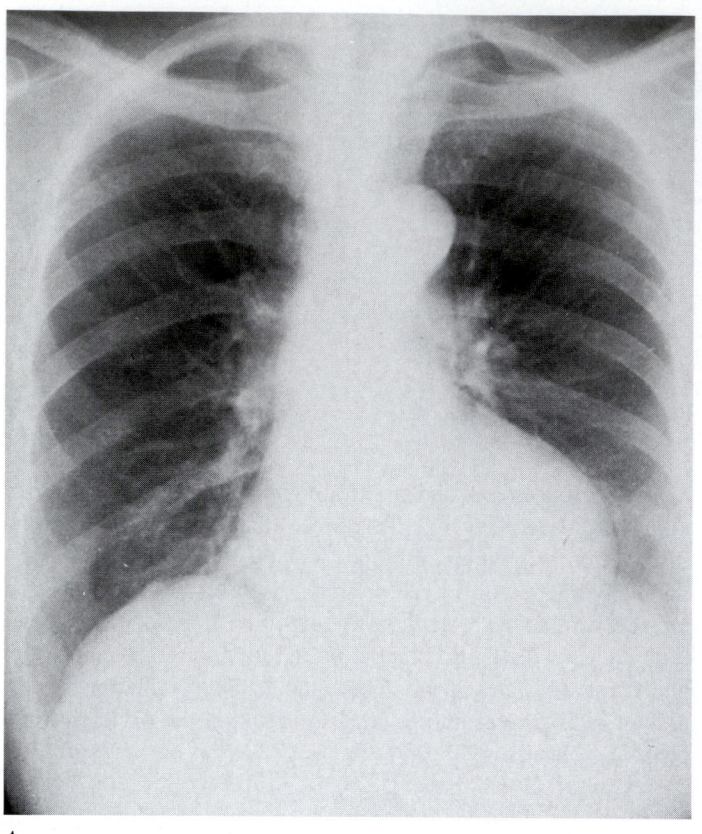

A

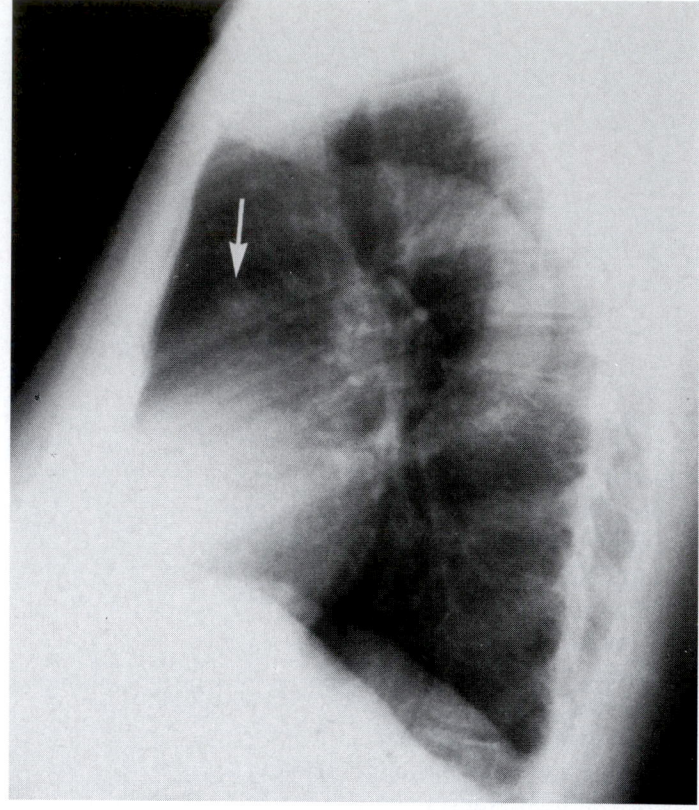

B

FIGURE 32-1   The lateral view in uncovering a solitary nodule. *A.* PA view. No nodule is discernible. *B.* Lateral view. A small nodule (arrow) overlies the left hilus. The nodule proved to be a granuloma.

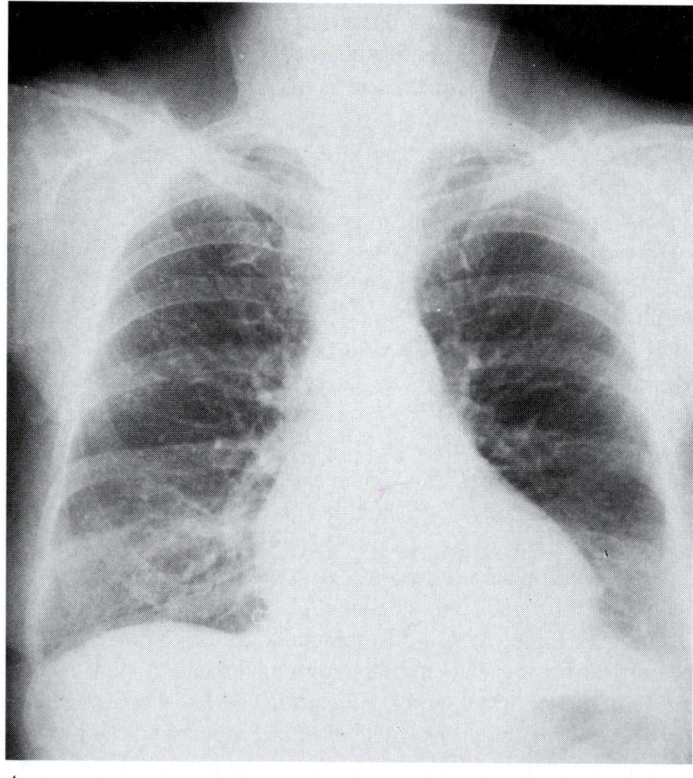

A

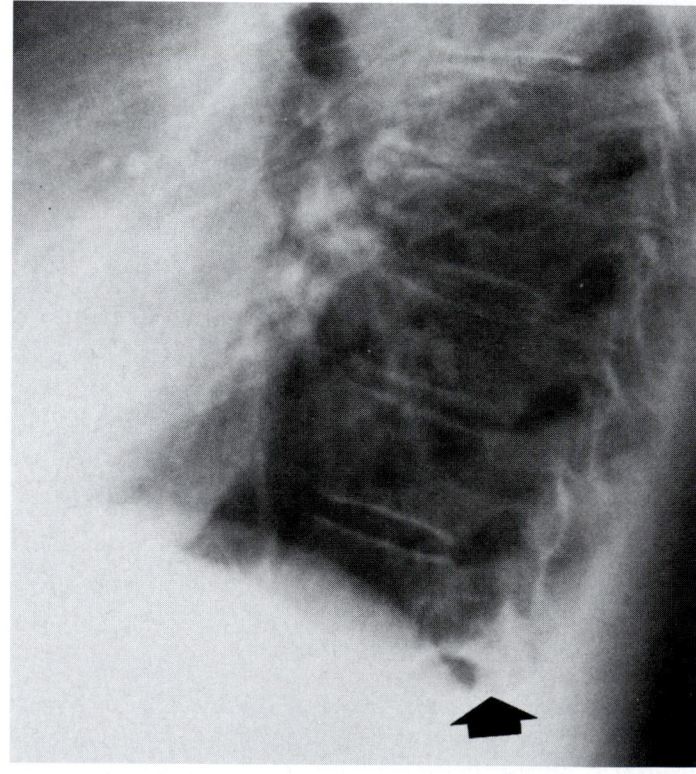

B

FIGURE 32-2   The lateral view in uncovering a small pleural effusion. *A.* PA view. No evidence of a pleural effusion. *B.* Lateral view. The right costophrenic sulcus in blunted (arrow). *C.* Lateral view. After treatment for heart failure, the effusion is gone. Note the magnification of the posterior (right) ribs.

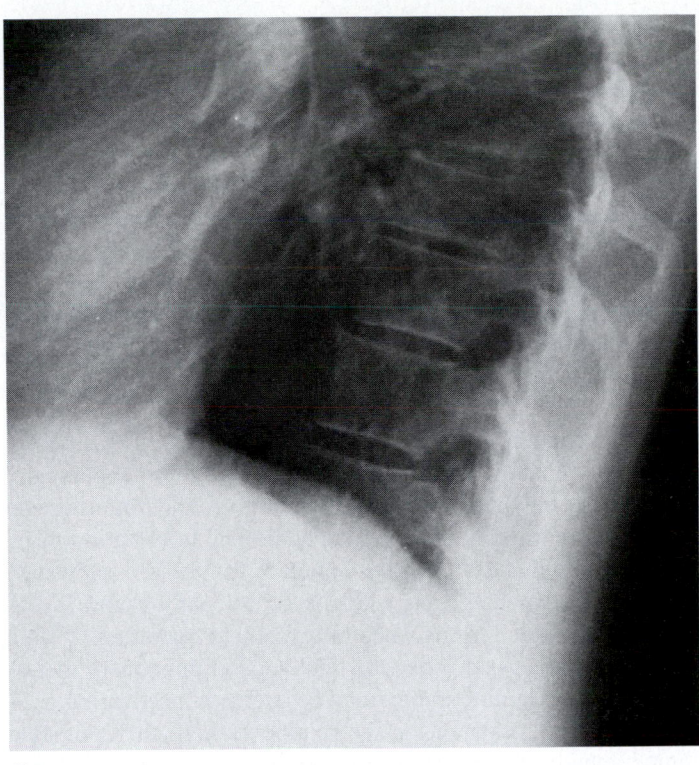

C

FIGURE 32-2 *(Cont.)*

Supplementary Plain Radiographs

In addition to the PA and lateral chest radiographs, other projections serve special purposes.

Oblique views are sometimes invaluable in delineating a pulmonary mass or infiltrate from structures that overlie it on the PA and lateral views. Barium in the esophagus serves as a useful adjunct in clarifying the location of mediastinal lesions on oblique films.

In interpreting oblique films, it is helpful to keep in mind that a pulmonary lesion that maintains a fairly constant relationship to the heart as the patient is rotated lies in the anterior portion of the chest; a lesion that maintains a constant relationship with respect to the spine is posterior.[4]

The *lateral decubitus* projection (Fig. 32-3C) is often used to identify the presence of a pleural effusion. As little as 25 to 50 ml of pleural fluid can be visualized, even though 300 ml may be required to blunt the costophrenic sulcus on the PA view. The decubitus view is particularly useful in determining if blunting of a costophrenic sulcus is due to a pleural effusion or pleural thickening. Although a pleural effusion may be an important finding, pleural thickening most often is a sequel to an exudate or blood in the pleural space and is usually unimportant.

On the PA film, shadows created by the first rib and clavicle may make interpretation of the lung apices difficult (Fig. 32-4A). The *lordotic* projection enables evaluation of the apices by displacing these overlying shadows (Fig. 32-4B). The lordotic view may also be useful in demonstrating collapse of the right middle lobe.

The *overpenetrated grid* radiograph (Fig. 32-5A) is useful for evaluating densities that lie behind the heart or diaphragm and are poorly seen on routine radiographs. *Expiratory* films often disclose air trapping or demonstrate a pneumothorax that is poorly shown on the inspiratory film. *Stereoscopic* views can be helpful in localizing any pulmonary lesion, but are particularly

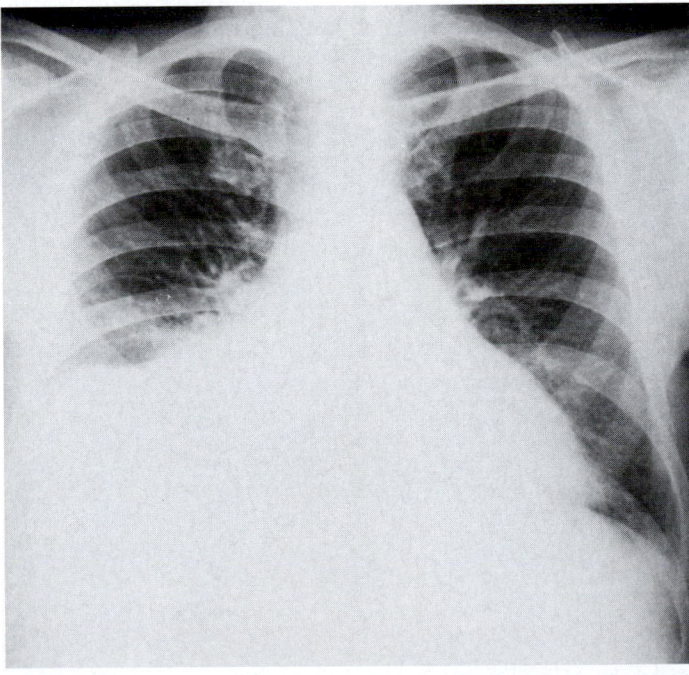

A

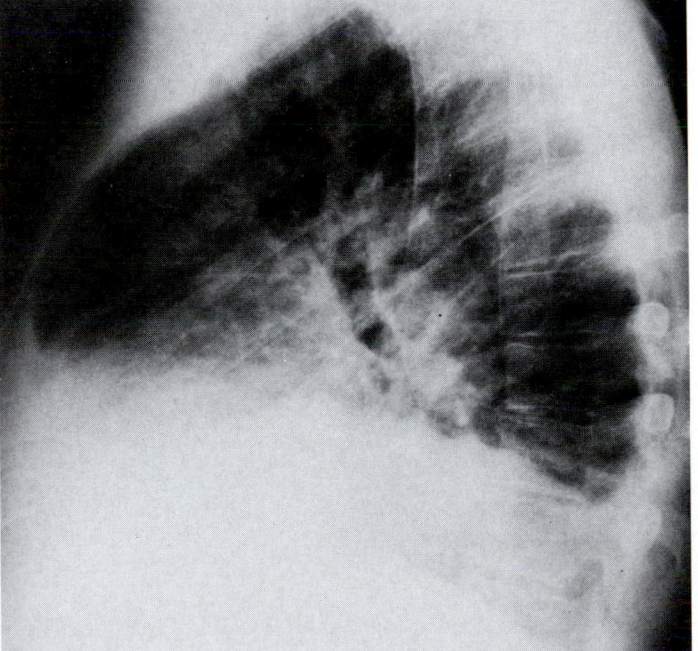

B

FIGURE 32-3 Infrapulmonary effusion. Neither the PA view (*A*) nor the lateral view (*B*) shows blunting of the costophrenic sulcus. However, elevation of the right hemidiaphragm suggests the presence of an infrapulmonary effusion. A right lateral decubitus film (*C*) shows the presence of a free pleural effusion on the right. The effusion was secondary to congestive heart failure.

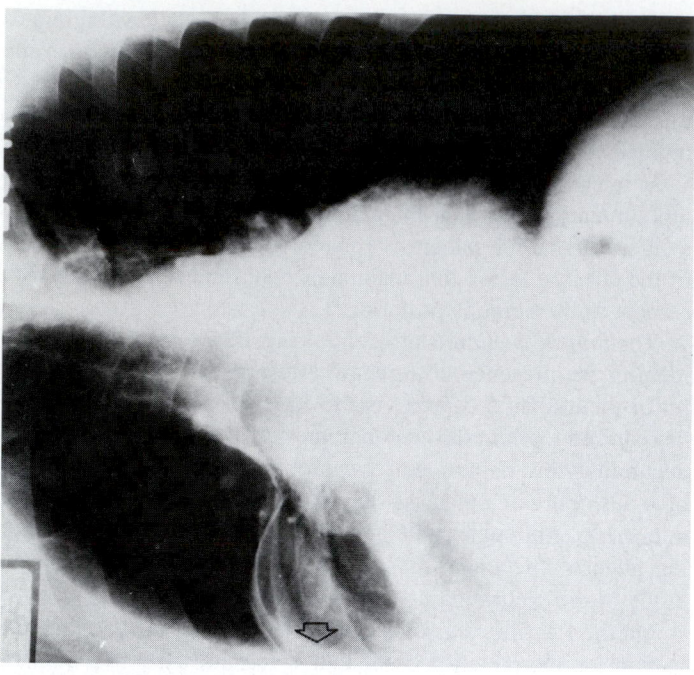

C

FIGURE 32-3   *(Cont.)*

useful for apical abnormalities because they permit separation of pulmonary lesions from the overlying clavicle and first rib.

Magnification radiographs are occasionally used in evaluating diffuse lung disease to clarify minute details of the pulmonary parenchyma. Supravoltage radiographs (1000 kV or more) are occasionally helpful in assessing pulmonary or mediastinal lesions.

Laminography

The technique of laminography (also known as tomography, body section radiography, or planigraphy) utilizes movement of

the radiography tube and film about a fixed point to generate a radiograph of a tissue plane that is several millimeters thick; the designated plane is in focus, while surrounding anatomic details are blurred. In effect, this technique provides a view of a thin slice of lung and affords a "close look" at a suspected abnormality. It is useful in demonstrating the presence of calcification within a pulmonary nodule (Fig. 32-6) and, occasionally, in providing insight into its cause. For example, the finding of scattered, "popcorn" calcifications indicates benign disease. The clinical implications of various types of calcifications seen in pulmonary radiographs are considered later in this chapter.

Laminography occasionally discloses cavitation within a pulmonary lesion, particularly in pulmonary tuberculosis—a finding that may not be evident on the routine radiograph.[3] Laminography is seldom useful in searching blindly for a clinically suspected lesion that cannot be seen on the routine film. It is also apt to be unrewarding in supplying additional information when a routine study has clearly depicted the lesion. However, laminography of both lung fields is occasionally useful in uncovering multiple lesions when only a solitary nodule is visible on routine films. Also, when the likelihood of pulmonary metastasis is strong, laminography may be useful in uncovering a lesion that is not apparent on the routine radiograph. Computed tomography is even more sensitive in this regard and has largely supplanted laminography.

Fluoroscopy

Fluoroscopy of the chest is useful for examining the movement of pulmonary and cardiac structures and for localizing a pulmonary lesion that is visible in only one of the two conventional radiographic projections.[4] It is particularly helpful for examining diaphragmatic motion. When one is searching for diaphragmatic paralysis, the patient is best fluoroscoped in the lateral projection so that the motion of both hemidiaphragms can be

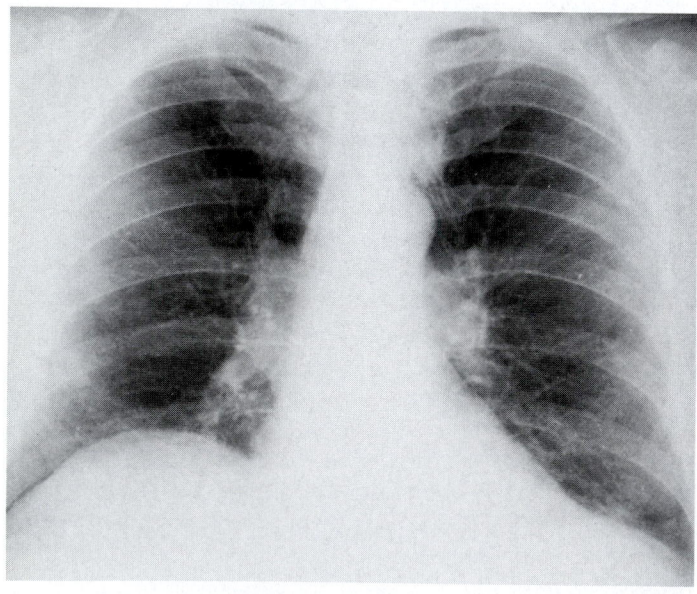

A

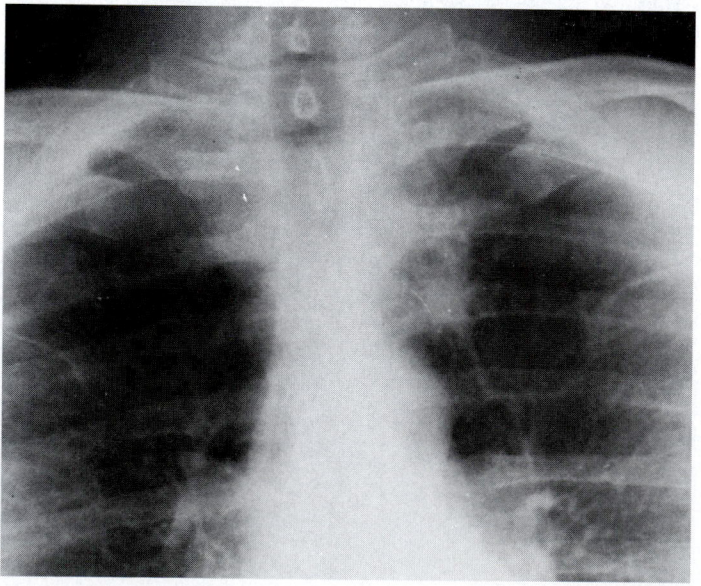

B

FIGURE 32-4   Carcinoma of the left upper lobe. *A*. PA view. A small nodule is present in the left upper lobe adjacent to the mediastinum, just above the aortic knob. *B*. Lordotic view. The nodule is much more apparent. It proved to be a primary adenocarcinoma of the lung.

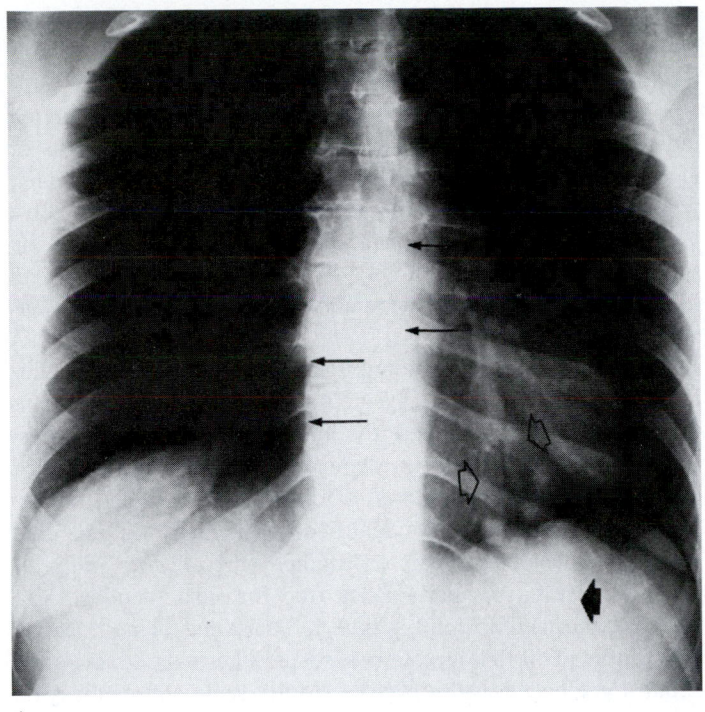

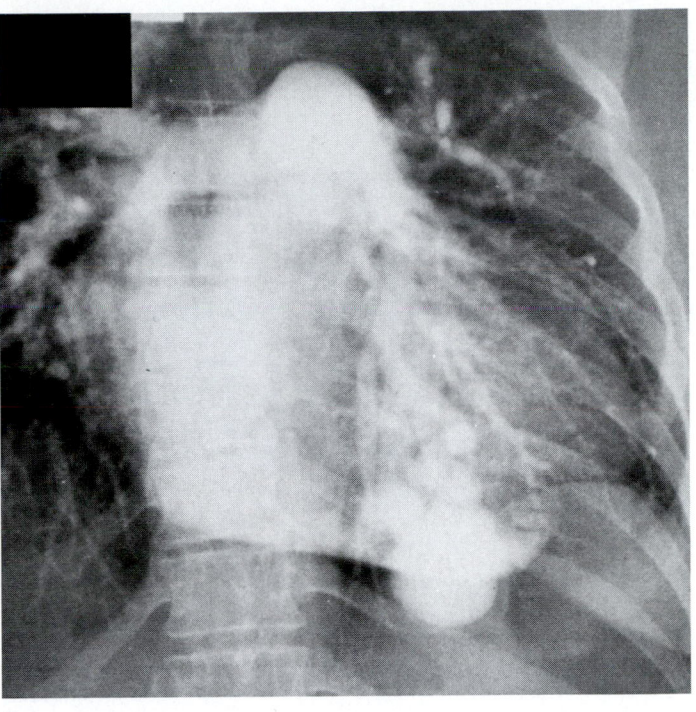

A

B

FIGURE 32-5 Pulmonary arteriovenous malformation, *A*. Overpenetrated grid (Bucky) radiograph shows a nodule behind the diaphragm (closed arrow). *B*. Pulmonary angiogram confirmed the diagnosis of arteriovenous malformation. Also visible bilaterally on the overpenetrated Bucky film are the posterior paraspinal lines (small arrows). The left posterior paraspinal line is medial to the aorta. The right paraspinal line is ordinarily not discernible; however, it can be seen in this patient because small osteophytes arising from the vertebral bodies displace the pleura laterally on the right.

observed simultaneously. A paralyzed hemidiaphragm moves paradoxically. This paradoxical motion may be difficult to see during quiet breathing, but it usually becomes readily apparent during a quick, short "sniff" (sniff test). Localized weakness in part of one hemidiaphragm—i.e., *diaphragmatic eventration*

(Fig. 32-7)—is often misinterpreted as diaphragmatic paralysis. This error can be avoided by performing fluoroscopy with the patient in the lateral projection; partial eventration is then manifested by paradoxical motion of one portion of the hemidiaphragm, while the remainder moves normally. Eventration of an entire hemidiaphragm is impossible to distinguish from paralysis, since in both instances the entire hemidiaphragm moves paradoxically.

Fluoroscopy is sometimes useful in determining whether a nodule is truly in the lung. In an upright subject, nodules that are in the lung move in the caudal direction with inspiration, while nodules in the chest wall or ribs move cephalad.

Fluoroscopy of the heart is useful in demonstrating calcifications in cardiac valves and in coronary arteries. It often suggests the presence of pericardial effusion much more convincingly than does the chest radiograph. However, fluoroscopy is rarely definitive for detecting a pericardial effusion, and other procedures, particularly ultrasound, computed tomography, and magnetic resonance imaging, are generally used to confirm a suspected pericardial effusion.

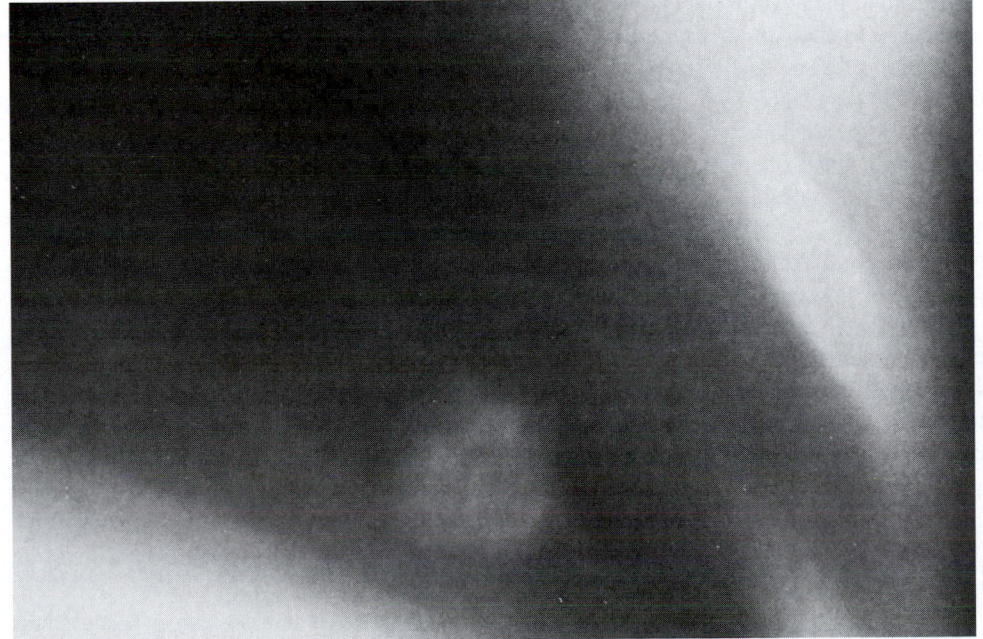

FIGURE 32-6 Hamartoma. A tomogram of a pulmonary nodule shows that the nodule contains several calcifications at its center. The nodule proved to be a hamartoma.

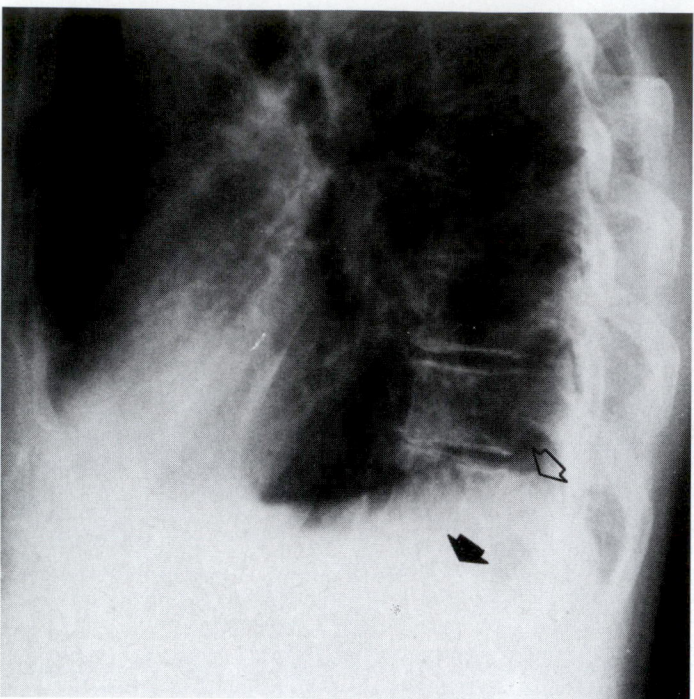

FIGURE 32-7 Partial eventration of the diaphragm. The lateral view shows elevation of the posterior portion of the right hemidiaphragm (open arrow). The normal contour of the left hemidiaphragm (closed arrow) appears immediately beneath. This partial eventration is due to a localized waekness in the posterior aspect of the right hemidiaphragm.

Fluoroscopy often helps to identify the nature of a mediastinal lesion. When it is coupled with a barium swallow, lesions within the esophagus can be demonstrated. Moreover, the pattern of displacement of the esophagus by a mass in the middle mediastinum often helps to determine the nature of the mass.[4] Respiratory maneuvers affect the size of large venous structures in the chest; they become smaller during the Valsalva maneuver and larger during the Hills-Müller maneuver. These maneuvers leave unchanged the size of solid masses. Pulsation of a mediastinal mass raises the prospect that it is vascular. However, pulsation has to be interpreted with care; masses that are adjacent to the aorta often transmit its pulsations and appear to pulsate themselves; conversely, large aortic aneurysms often pulsate poorly.

In the past, fluoroscopy was used as a screening procedure for routine examination of the chest. This is no longer acceptable for several reasons: (1) the patient's x-ray exposure is much greater during a short fluoroscopic examination than during the performance of standard chest radiographs; (2) small lesions in the lung fields are easily overlooked at fluoroscopy; and (3) no permanent record of the fluoroscopic examination is created. Indeed, unless specific information is being sought, fluoroscopy of the chest is not warranted.

Computed Tomography

Computed tomography (CT) is a radiologic technique for scanning cross sections of the entire body. The underlying principle

is the production of radiographic absorption profiles that are made at different angles in the same cross-sectional plane. A pencil-thin beam of x-rays passes through the body as the radiographic tube rotates around the patient, and the transmitted radiation is detected by a sodium iodide crystal. By means of electronic transformation, the signals are fed into a computer, which synthesizes them into a picture that displays the relative absorption coefficients of each small area in the plane of the scan.[17] The technique is highly accurate, and its sensitivity to differences in density is considerably greater than that of the standard radiograph.

While the plain chest radiograph remains the primary radiologic technique in evaluating the chest, CT has added tremendous insight into disorders of the lungs, mediastinum, and chest wall. Cross-sectional images depicted by CT provide an added dimension in the investigation of chest pathology, and the increased resolution permits identification of many findings that are not visible on the plain radiograph (Fig. 32-8).[17] This increased sensitivity is particularly true for small nodules.[11] In addition, the mediastinum, which is somewhat of an "occult" area on the plain radiograph, is seen in rather marked anatomic detail. Lymphadenopathy may be readily seen, and mediastinal lesions of uncertain nature may be elucidated (Fig. 32-9). The use of intravenous contrast material as part of the examination permits separation of vascular from nonvascular mediastinal lesions and identification of vascular invasion by neoplasm (Fig. 32-10).[11] The technique is also extremely useful in investigating chest wall lesions or the extension of pulmonary or pleural tumors into the chest wall (Fig. 32-11)[11]—an important consideration, since the chest wall is not readily studied with the plain radiograph unless bone destruction is present.

CT ANGIOGRAPHY

CT angiography is an exciting application of helical (spiral) CT technology. Axial, multiplanar, reformatted images and three-dimensional images of the vascular system are possible with this technique.

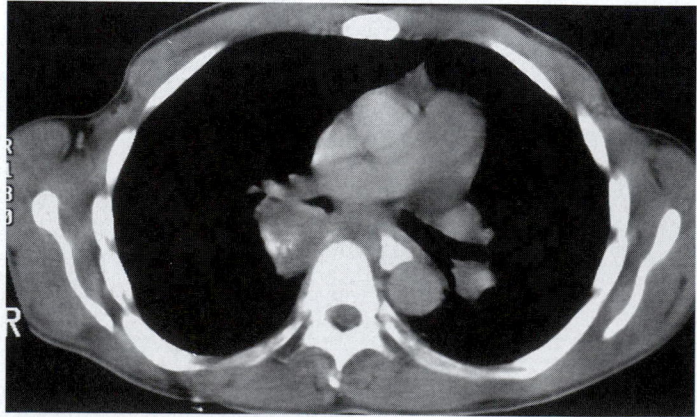

FIGURE 32-8 CT showing lung carcinoma not seen on routine chest radiograph. A large mass narrowing the right main stem bronchus can be seen in the right lower lobe. The mass contains some calcification.

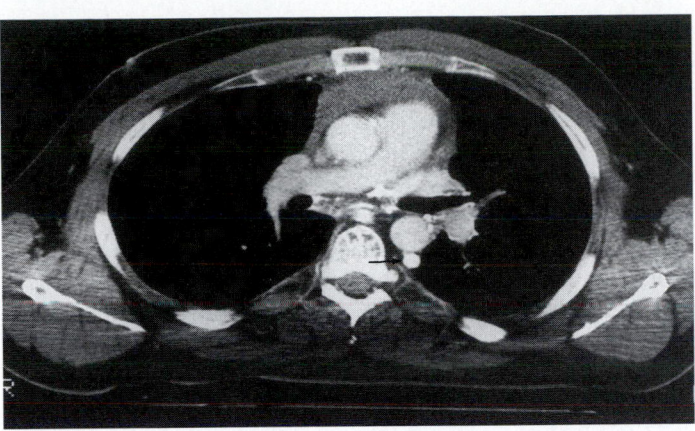

A

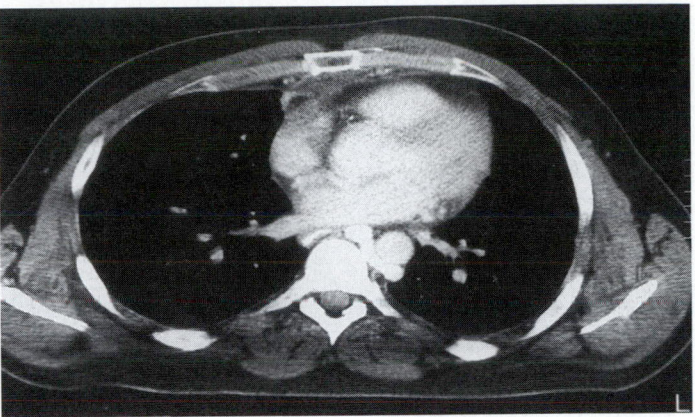

B

FIGURE 32-9 CT demonstrating Hodgkin's disease obstructing the superior vena cava. *A.* A mass is seen in the anterior mediastinum, just beneath the sternum. The mass completely obstructs the superior vena cava, which cannot be seen. However, the accessory azygos vein (ar- row) is unusually bright, since it is carrying blood that would ordinar- ily pass through the superior vena cava. *B.* A lower section shows con- trast material crossing into the azygos vein, where it then enters the su- perior vena cava, adjacent to the right atrium.

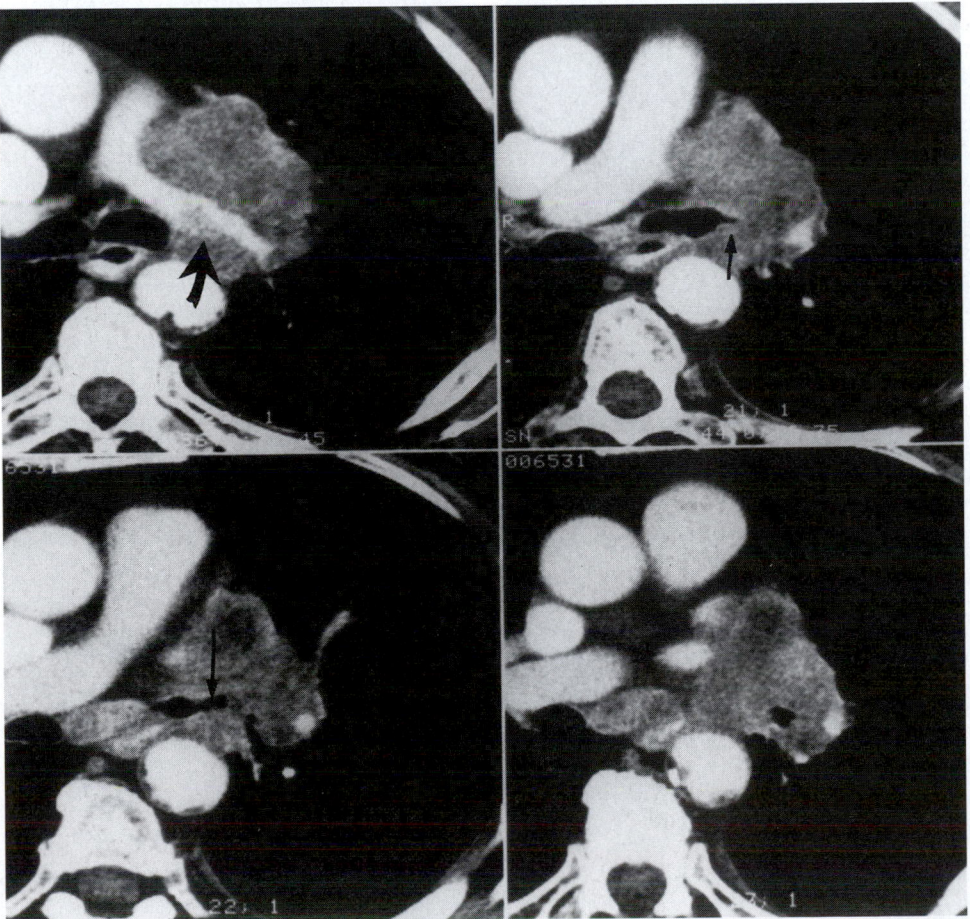

FIGURE 32-10 CT demonstration of extent of left-upper-lobe carcinoma. A mass is seen invad- ing the pulmonary artery (large arrow) and left main-stem bronchus (small arrows).

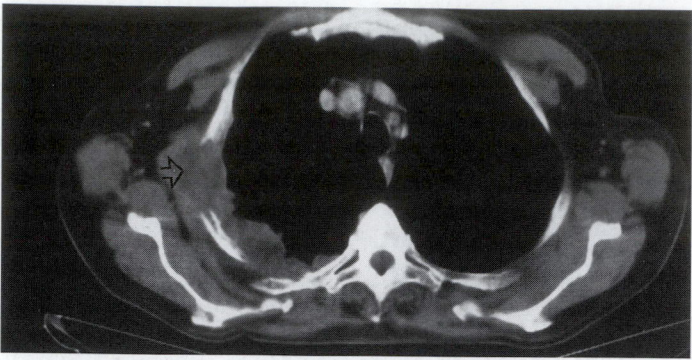

FIGURE 32-11   Mesothelioma extending into the chest wall. A pleural mesothelioma is seen on the right side; it directly invades the chest wall (arrow). The nodular character of the pleural involvement is characteristic of mesothelioma.

CT angiography is emerging as an excellent tool for identifying pulmonary embolism. Preliminary reports indicate that direct visualization of the pulmonary embolus by CT angiography provides a specificity similar to that of pulmonary angiography and a sensitivity similar to that of ventilation-perfusion scanning (Fig. 32-12).[23] It is also useful in pinpointing chronic thromboembolic disease. Various aortic lesions, such as aortic dissection, traumatic pseudoaneurysm, aortic aneurysms, and vascular anomalies of the aorta are well visualized with CT angiography.[23] Likewise, pulmonary venous malformations are readily recognized noninvasively.

HIGH-RESOLUTION CT

High-resolution CT is a special method for evaluating pulmonary pathology.[15] The technique is based on generation of images of

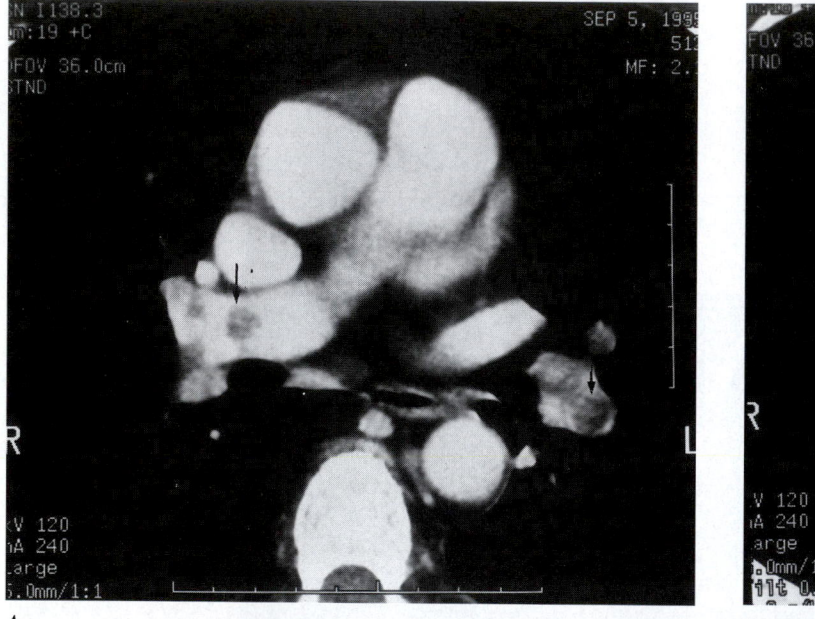

A

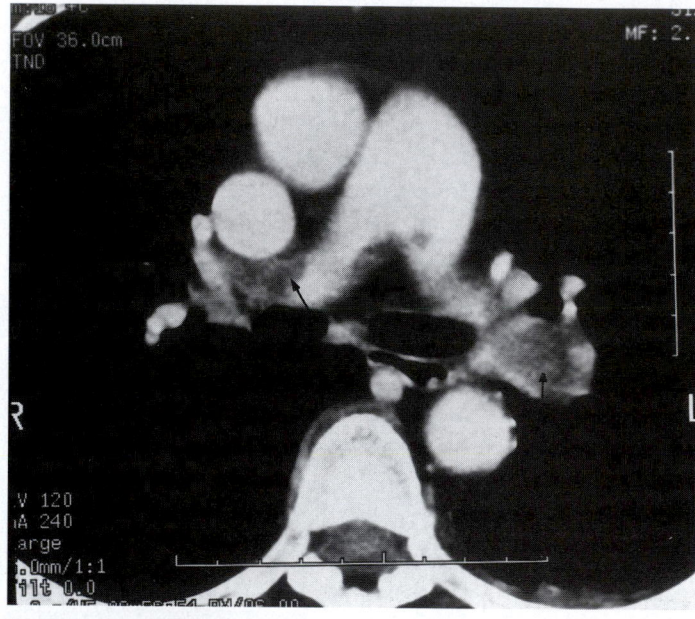

B

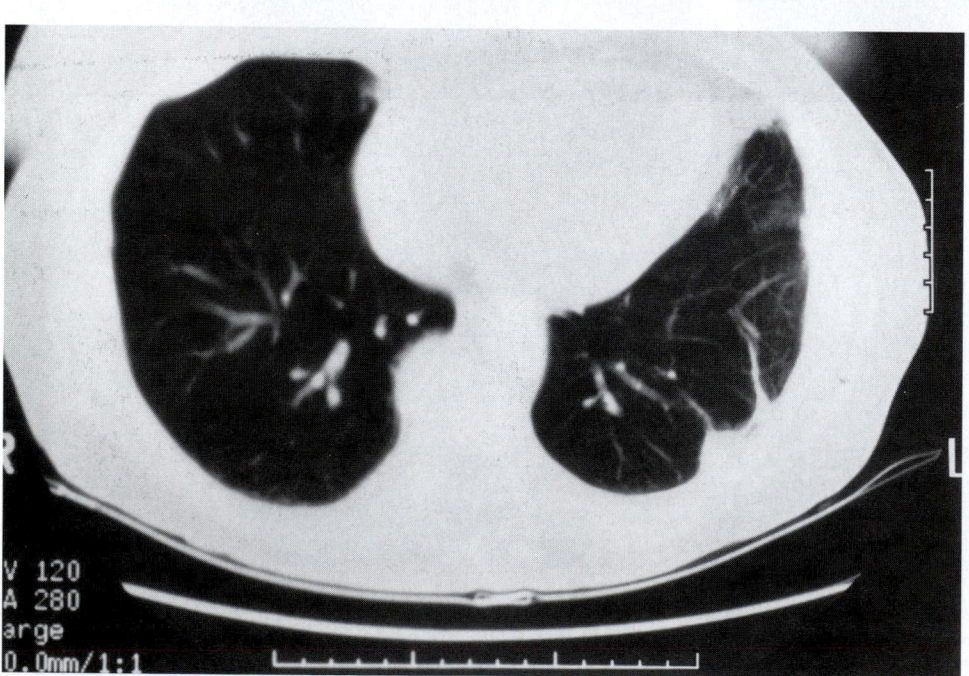

C

FIGURE 32-12   Spiral CT showing pulmonary embolus. *A* and *B*. Axial tomographic cuts at two levels show multiple central pulmonary emboli (arrows). *C*. Lung windows demonstrate a pulmonary infarct in the left lower lobe.

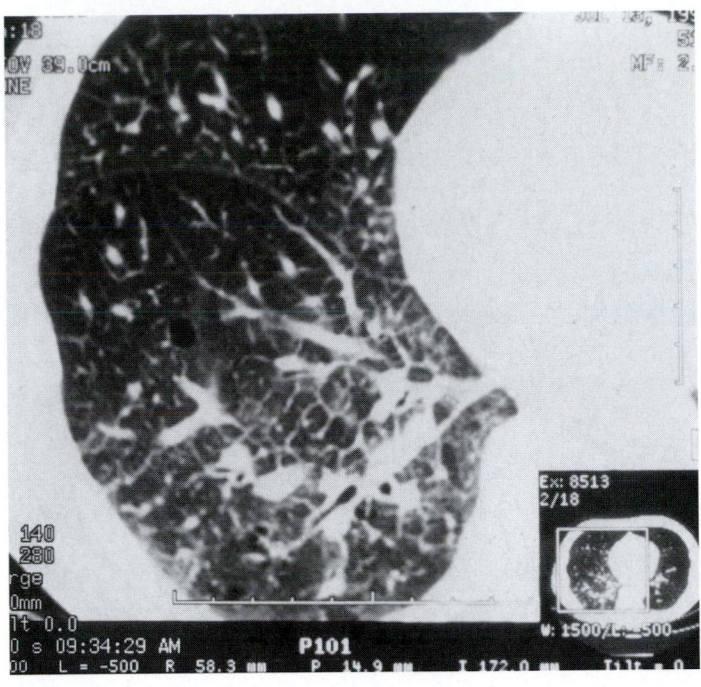

A

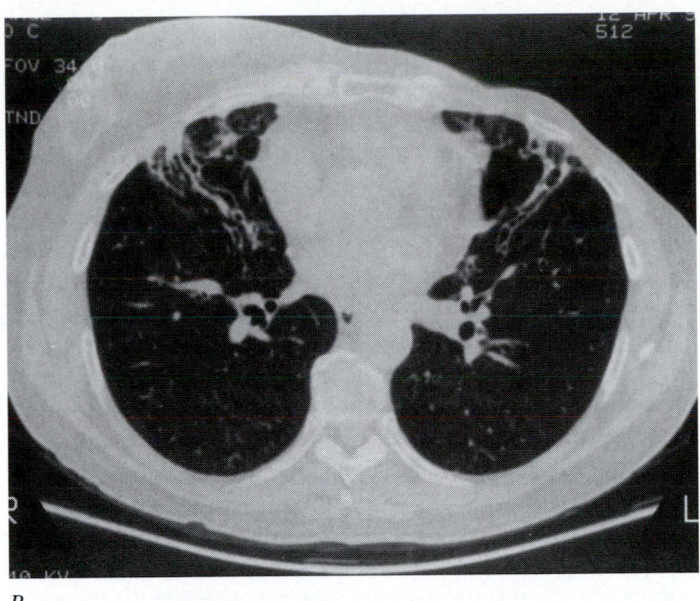

B

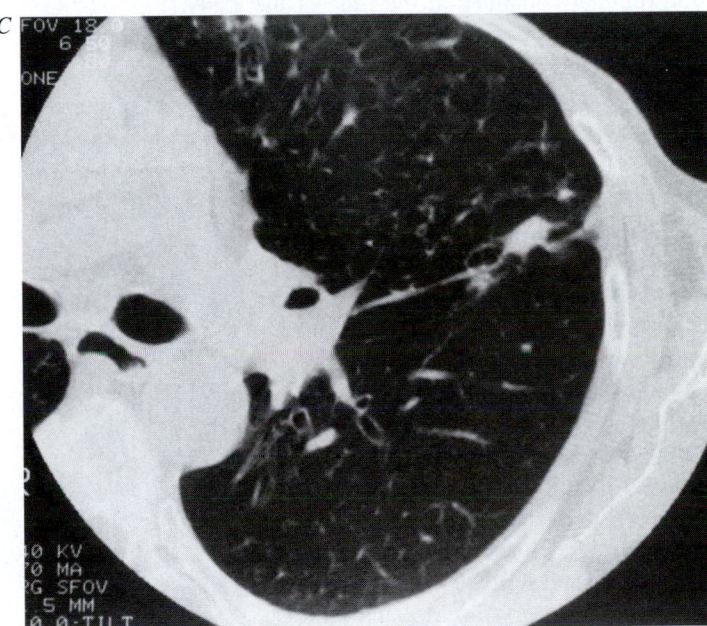

C

FIGURE 32-13 High-resolution CT. *A*. Interstitial lung disease. Pulmonary lobules are nicely outlined by an interstitial process that affects the interlobular septae. This pattern is characteristic of lymphangitic spread of carcinoma, which, in this patient, was due to pancreatic carcinoma. *B*. Bronchiectasis. Focal areas of tubular bronchiectasis are demonstrated in the middle lobe and lingula. *C*. High-resolution scan from another patient demonstrates more subtle bronchiectasis, with many small areas of invasion in the lingula.

very thin anatomic slices (1 to 2 mm, versus 8 to 10 mm for the usual CT slice) and a special "bone algorithm" for reconstruction of the information obtained in each slice. The result is a very high-contrast image that provides excellent insight into many pulmonary disorders.

High-resolution CT is especially useful in investigating interstitial lung disease and bronchiectasis (Fig. 32-13). This technique has supplanted bronchography in evaluation of bronchiectasis, as it is of comparable diagnostic accuracy.[15] In addition, high-resolution CT is helpful in identifying low-grade interstitial lung disease, which is not visible on the plain radiograph.[15] While useful in stratifying differential diagnostic considerations in interstitial lung disease, high-resolution CT will not supplant tissue biopsy in most instances; rather, the technique serves mainly as an adjunct diagnostic method. Finally, while not ideal

for studying mediastinal and chest wall lesions, high-resolution CT is adequate to investigate these areas if the main objective is delineation of the extent of the pulmonary process.

Nuclear Magnetic Resonance

Magnetic resonance (MR) or nuclear magnetic resonance (NMR) is a technique that uses radiowaves modified by a strong magnetic field to produce a diagnostic image. The images generated are somewhat similar to CT images, but they differ in that in the NMR images, vascular structures are usually well seen without use of contrast material. In addition, with NMR different images can be obtained by manipulation of the radiowave frequency and timing of the impulses delivered.

Although magnetic resonance imaging (MRI) has not had quite as great an impact as CT in the investigation of thoracic lesions, it has major promise in the study of various chest disorders, particularly those of the mediastinum and pulmonary vasculature.[11] In some institutions, MRI has become the primary technique used in the study of aortic dissection. MRI may also have a major role in the investigation of pulmonary embolism, either acute or chronic (Fig. 32-14).[23] Finally, MRI has become a major means of investigation of congenital heart disease, and it shows great promise in the evaluation of myocardial ischemia.[11]

New techniques have emerged in this rapidly developing area. Intravenous administration of gadolinium as a "contrast agent" allows better visualization of vascular structures, as do a variety of MRI scanning techniques ("time of flight" imaging, etc.) (Figs. 32-15 and 32-16). Scanning can now be done extremely quickly, almost rivaling CT in rapidity of image acquisition.

MRI provides a unique feature in investigating the thorax and other body parts: the images obtained can be reconstructed in any one of several anatomic planes. While the standard MR image is usually an axial view, similar to that obtained with CT, sagittal and coronal images can be easily created from the information routinely obtained at the time of the study (Fig. 32-14).[11] Although CT can create reformatted images in the coronal or sagittal planes—planes that often provide similar information—the images are usually better and more easily obtained with MRI.

Contrast Examinations

Air in the bronchi and alveoli is a superb contrast medium, outlining the pulmonary vasculature, heart, aorta and other mediastinal structures, diaphragm, and chest wall. In addition, pathologic processes in the lung often produce characteristic changes in the pattern of the pulmonary vessels or air-filled alveoli. Hence, the plain chest film is a very useful tool in the diagnosis of pulmonary disease, and more sophisticated radiographic techniques are usually not necessary. However, supplementary information may be gained by placement of extraneous contrast material into different components of the chest. Positive contrast material, such as barium sulfate suspension, is commonly introduced into the esophagus; other suitable media are used to visualize cardiac chambers, the trachea and bronchi, pulmonary vessels, vena cava and mediastinal veins, and mediastinal lymphatics. For negative contrast, air or other gases are introduced into the pleural cavity, the peritoneal cavity, or the mediastinum.

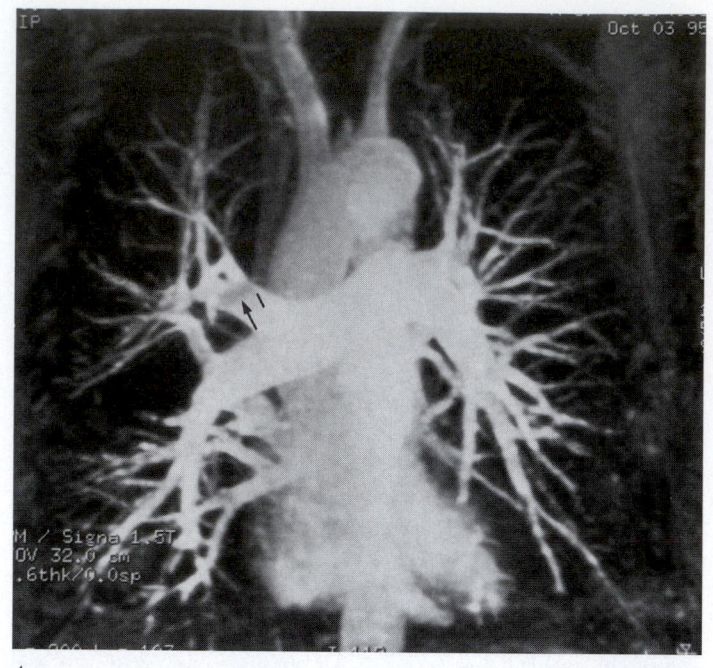

A

B

FIGURE 32-14 Pulmonary embolus demonstrated by "time of flight" MRI. This technique shows the blood vessels in detail, rivaling images obtained with pulmonary arteriography. *A.* A pulmonary embolus can be seen in the right upper lobe (arrow). *B.* Reproductions in various degrees of obliquity show that the defect of the pulmonary embolus remains constant.

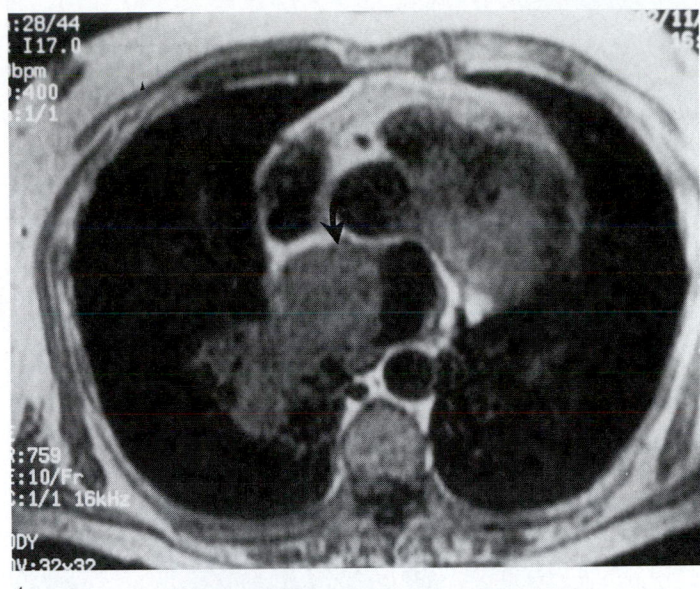

FIGURE 32-15 MRI demonstration of partial anomalous pulmonary venous return. Time of flight image shows the pulmonary arteries (straight arrow), pulmonary veins (curved arrow), and an anomalous pulmonary vein entering the superior vena cava (small arrow).

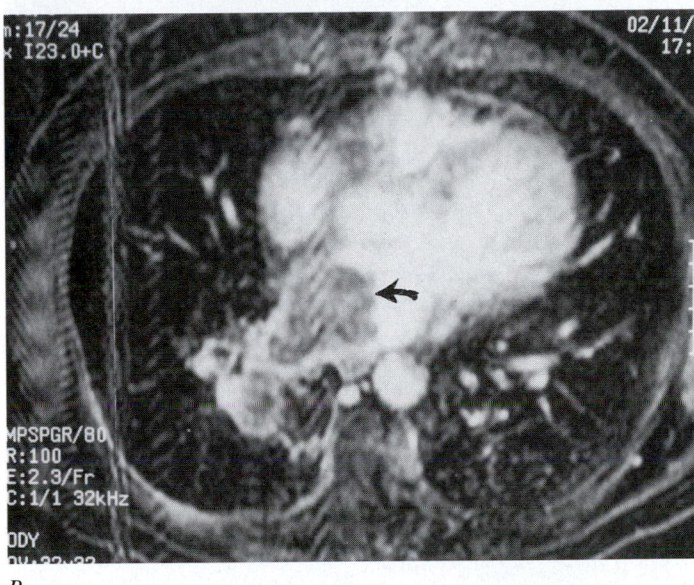

B

FIGURE 32-16 Metastatic renal cell carcinoma (arrows) to the right-lower-lobe pulmonary veins and right atrium. *A*. Tumor in the right atrium (T1 image). *B*. Tumor in the pulmonary veins (T2 image).

Carbon dioxide and nitrous oxide have been used to outline the right-sided cardiac chambers.

Intravenous contrast material is extremely useful in investigating mediastinal lesions. In many institutions, administration of intravenous contrast material is standard for the chest CT examination. Oral contrast agents (e.g., Gastrografin) may be used to outline the esophagus and the GI tract in the upper abdomen. Similarly, in MRI, intravenous gadolinium is frequently used to better depict vascular structures or highly vascular organs such as the liver.

Of all the contrast examinations available, the barium swallow, generally carried out under fluoroscopic guidance, is the simplest to perform. A thick mixture of swallowed barium sulfate outlines the esophageal contour, making it easy to detect displacement of the esophagus by adjacent mediastinal structures, such as tumor-containing lymph nodes or a large left atrium (Fig. 32-17). Abnormalities of the esophagus itself, such as achalasia or tumor, are also easily seen.

Although the trachea and major bronchi are readily visualized in the mediastinum and hili, bronchography or CT is necessary to demonstrate abnormalities in peripheral bronchi, whose thin walls are not sharply delineated from the alveolar portions of the lungs. Bronchography is performed with one of several contrast materials. Figure 32-18 is a bronchogram obtained by using oily Dionosil.

With the advent of fiberoptic bronchoscopy, bronchography fell into disuse as a technique for exploring the tracheobronchial tree for tumor. Bronchoscopy yields much more information without much additional patient discomfort. Furthermore, although bronchography has also been used to identify bronchiec-

tasis (Fig. 32-19), the advent of high-resolution CT has made the bronchogram a study of historical interest, since CT provides similar information using a much simpler and less invasive technique (Fig. 32-13*B* and 32-13*C*).[16]

Pulmonary Angiography

Pulmonary angiography entails the rapid injection of a radiopaque dye into the pulmonary circulation through a catheter introduced into the pulmonary arterial tree or into a large systemic vein leading into the right atrium. Angiography is the gold-standard test in the investigation of pulmonary thromboembolic disease (Figs. 32-20 and 32-21) (see Chapter 34). Ventilation and

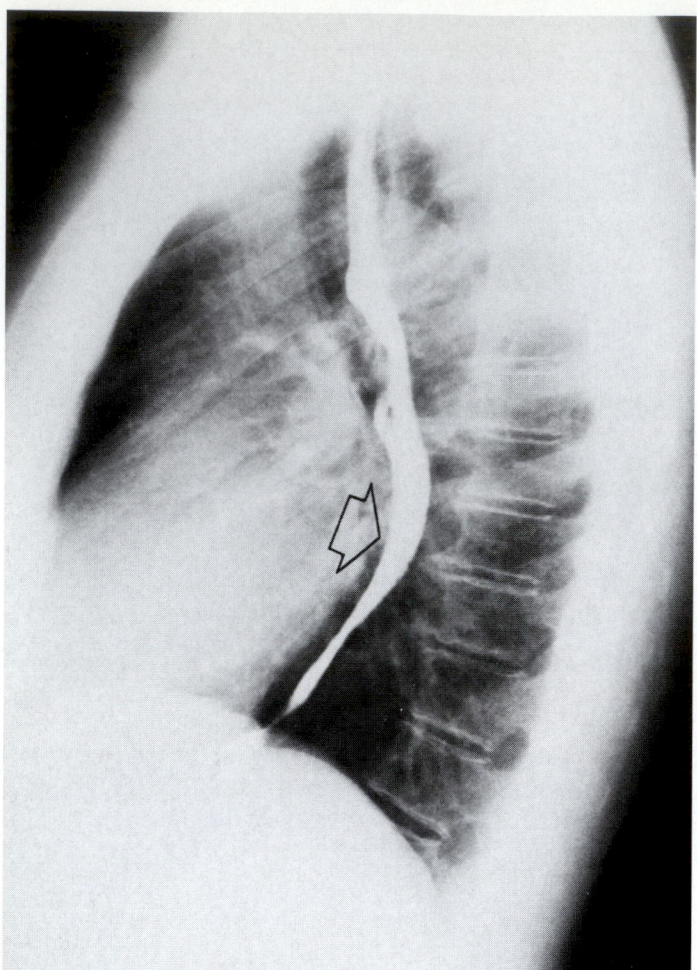

FIGURE 32-17 Enlarged left atrium. The esophagus is displaced posteriorly by an enlarged left atrium (arrow).

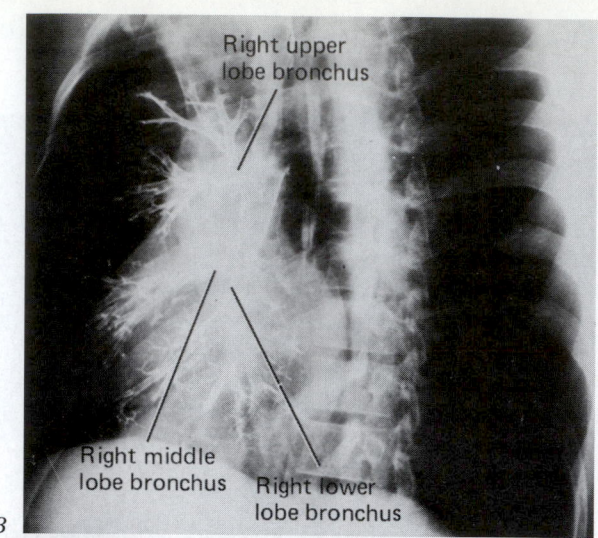

B

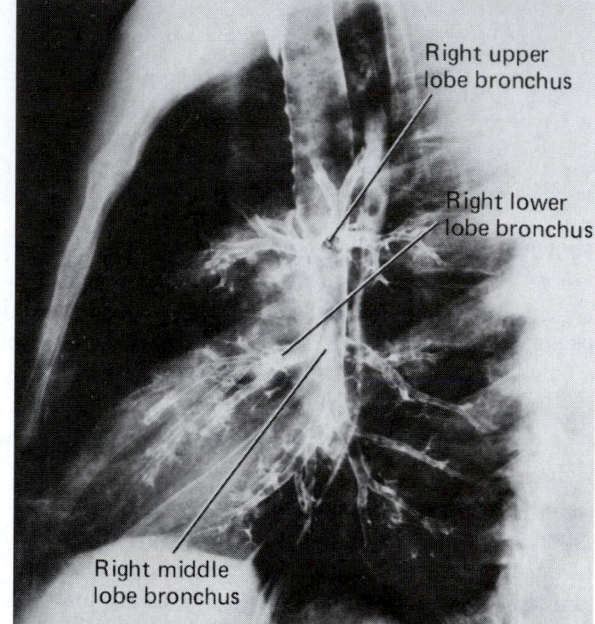

C

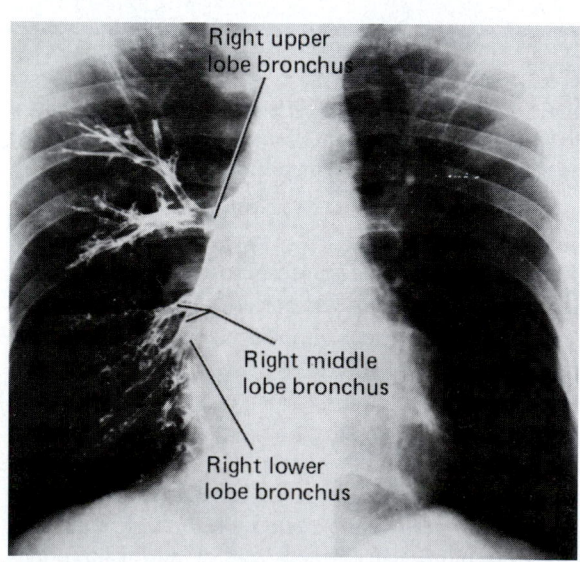

A

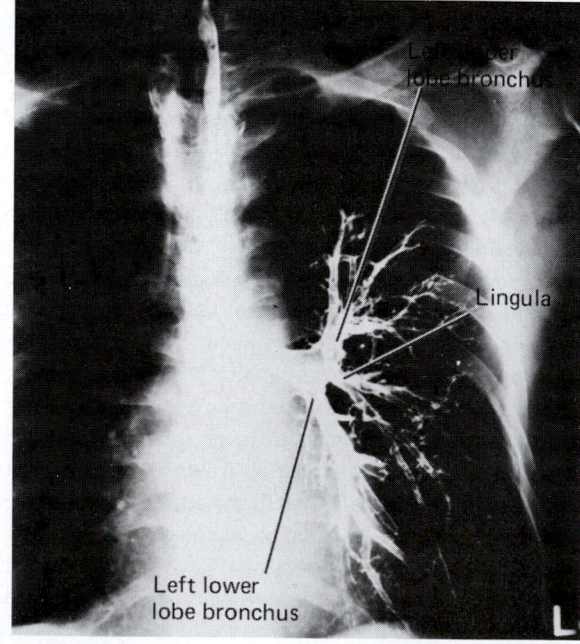

D

FIGURE 32-18 Normal bronchogram. The normal bronchial anatomy of the right lung is shown in the PA (*A*), oblique (*B*), and lateral (*C*) projections. The corresponding anatomy of the left lung is demonstrated in the PA (*D*) and oblique (*E*) projections. The lateral projection for the left lung appears in Figure 32-19, which also illustrates bronchiectasis. A schematic representation of the bronchial tree in the PA projection appears in Figure 32-38.

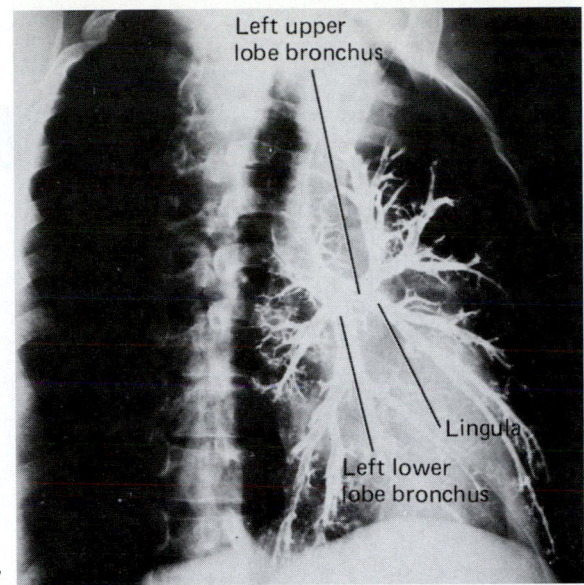

E

FIGURE 32-18 *(Cont.)*

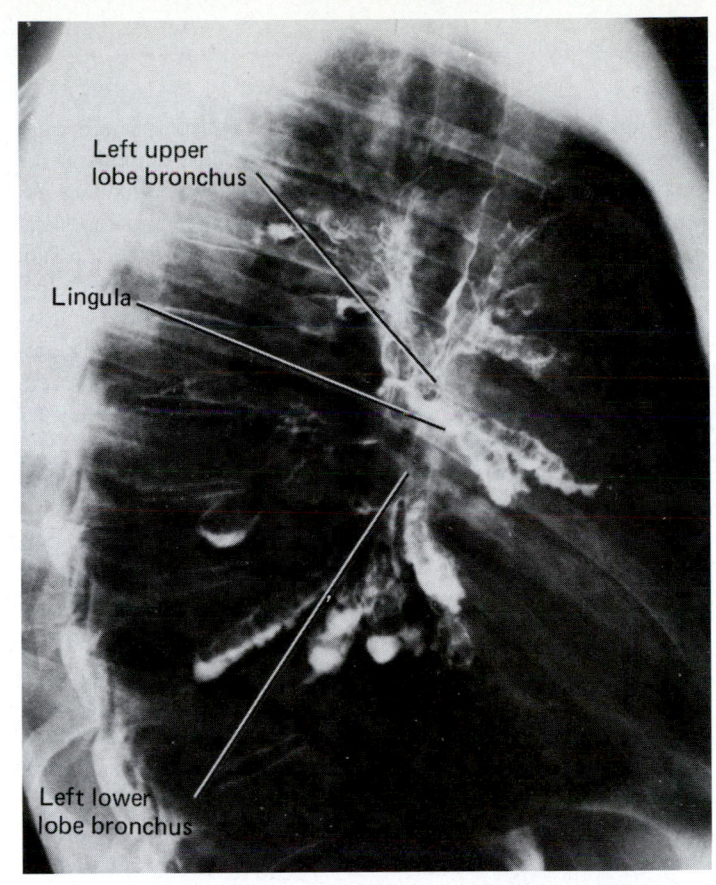

FIGURE 32-19 Bronchiectasis. The lateral view shows extensive bronchiectasis of the left lung. All the bronchi that contain contrast medium show saccular dilatation of their segments.

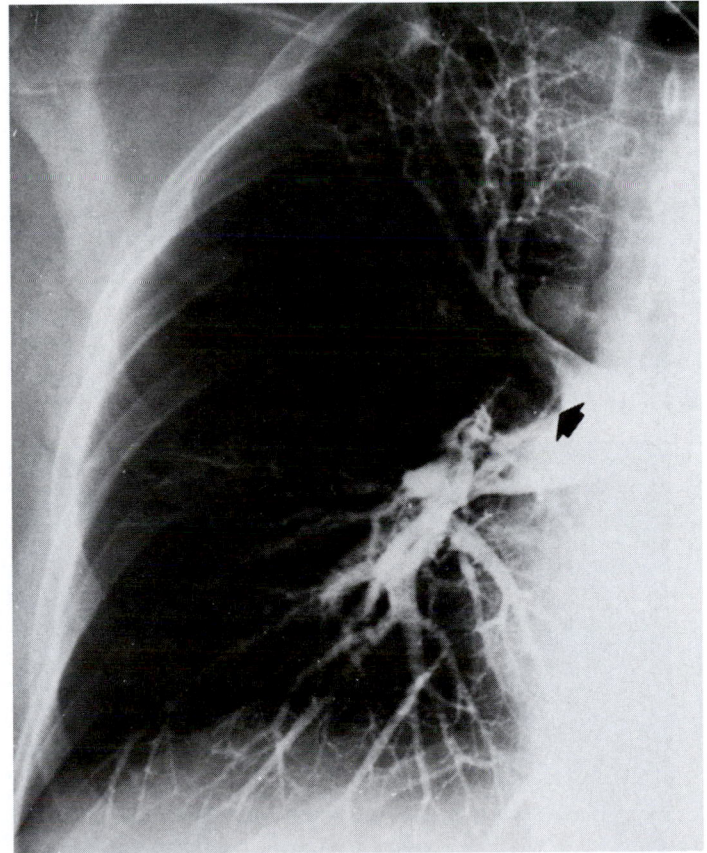

FIGURE 32-20 Large pulmonary embolus. A large pulmonary embolus is lodged in the right main pulmonary artery and has compromised blood flow primarily to the arteries of the right upper lobe (arrow). The peripheral vessels in the right midlung zone are not filled.

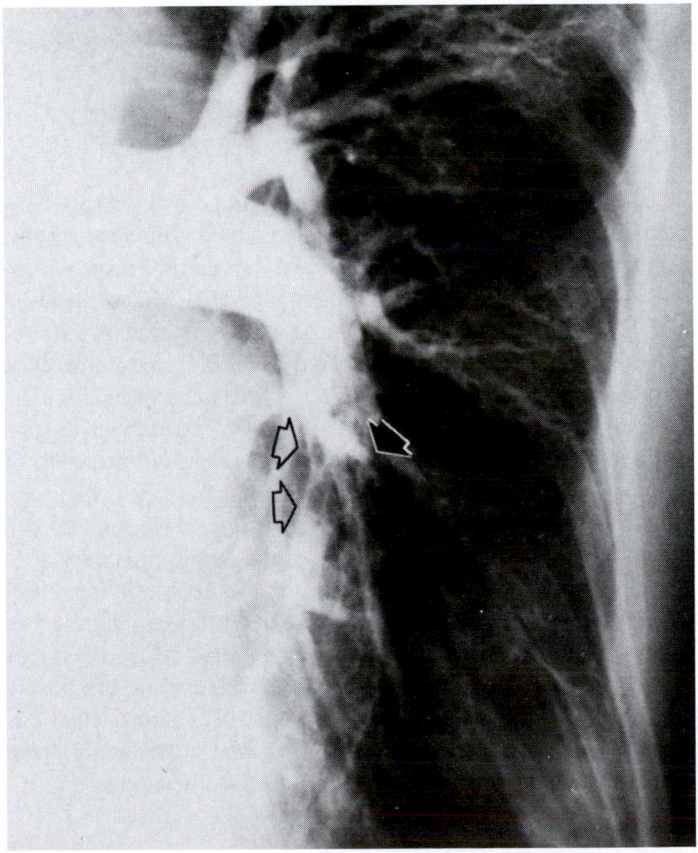

FIGURE 32-21 Small pulmonary emboli. Angiography shows small filling defects in the posterior basal artery (open arrows). Several of the other basal divisions are cut off (closed arrow). Blood flow to the left upper lobe is well preserved. Angiography was helpful diagnostically in this patient because the lung scan was equivocal.

perfusion scans of the lung using radioactive isotopes are valuable screening procedures in detecting pulmonary embolism (see Chapter 84), but if diagnostic uncertainty exists, pulmonary angiography is generally indicated. Both helical (spiral) CT and MRI are emerging as techniques that have the power to supplant more invasive pulmonary angiography (Figs. 32-12 and 32-14). Indeed, these techniques might even eventually replace ventilation-perfusion scanning as the preferred methods for investigating pulmonary embolism. A major practical problem at present is limited access to the heavily used scanners in emergency investigation of suspected pulmonary embolism.

Congenital abnormalities of the pulmonary vascular tree, such as hypoplasia or agenesis of the pulmonary artery, arteriovenous malformation, pulmonary varix, or anomalous pulmonary venous return, are also identified with pulmonary angiography (Fig. 32-5*B*). These abnormalities are often suspected on the basis of routine radiographs, but angiography may be necessary for confirmation. As with pulmonary embolism, both CT and MRI have the potential to supplant pulmonary angiography in investigating these lesions (Fig. 32-15).

Pulmonary angiographic procedures may also be used therapeutically (see Chapter 34). Arteriovenous malformations can be treated with pulmonary artery embolization using a variety of embolic materials, as can bleeding from the pulmonary or bronchial arteries. A strategically placed pulmonary artery catheter may be used to infuse streptokinase or other lytic agents to dissolve an acute pulmonary embolus. Similarly, techniques are available to fragment and extract pulmonary emboli through pulmonary artery catheters.

Aortography and Systemic Arteriography

Puzzling shadows in the vicinity of the middle (visceral) compartment of the mediastinum can be explored with aortography, a technique that takes advantage of the fact that the aorta is contained primarily within the middle mediastinal compartment.

Opacification of the aorta using contrast material usually requires retrograde catheterization of the aorta for direct injection. Middle mediastinal masses frequently prove to be vascular—e.g., dissecting aneurysms of the aorta, sacular or fusiform aneurysms of the aorta (Fig. 32-22), or anomalies or unusual tortuosity of the aorta or great vessels. In current practice, CT or MRI usually makes arteriography unnecessary (Figs. 32-23 and 32-24).

Owing to the dual blood supply of the lung, pulmonary arteriography may not be rewarding in the evaluation of some pulmonary lesions; in these cases, bronchial arteriography may be more useful. In patients with massive hemoptysis due to tumor or infection (e.g., tuberculosis, bronchiectasis, or aspergillosis), the major pulmonary blood supply is usually the bronchial circulation. Embolization of feeding bronchial arteries may yield temporary, or even permanent, control of the bleeding.

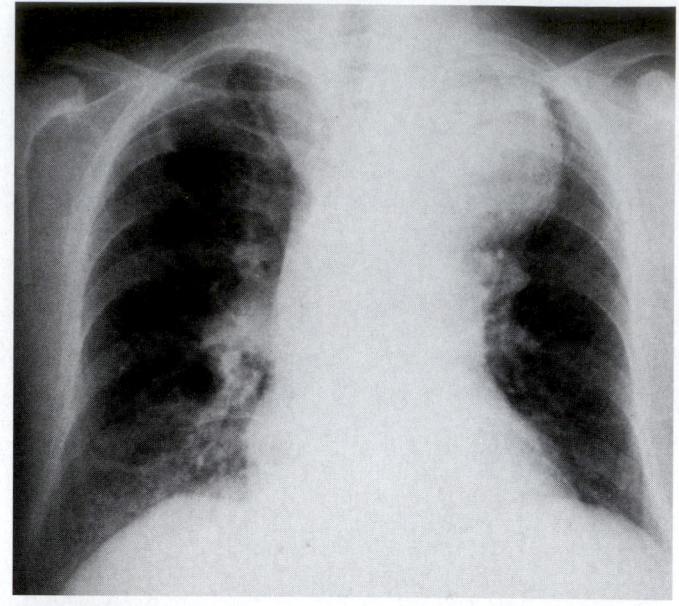

A

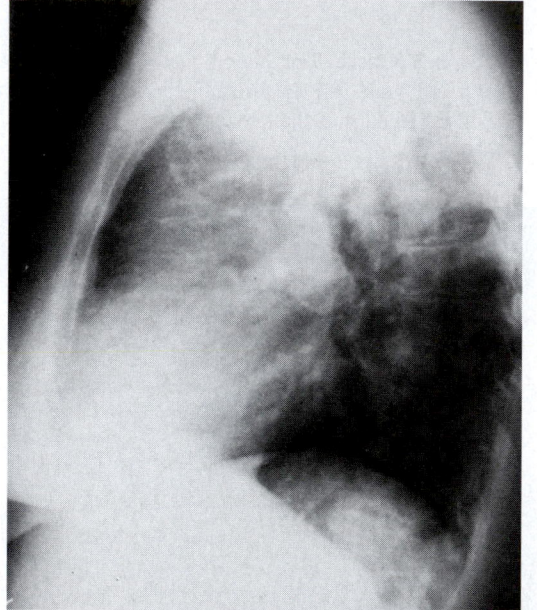

B

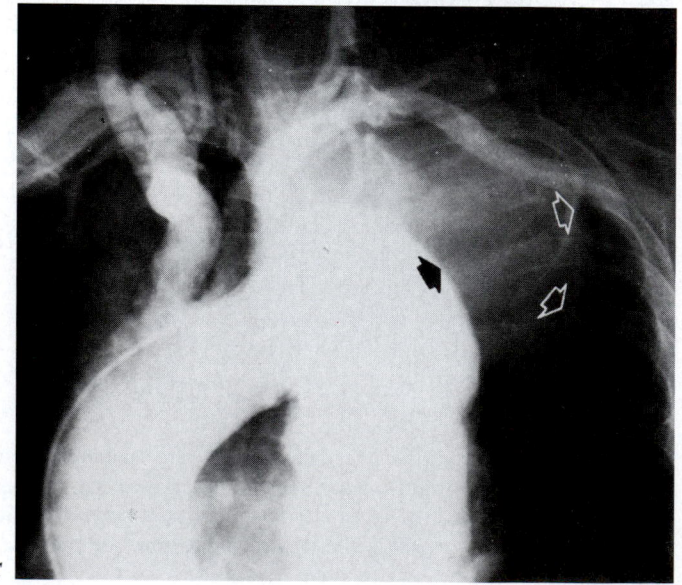

C

FIGURE 32-22   Aortic aneurysm. *A*. PA view. A large mass is in the left upper mediastinum. *B*. Lateral view. This mass appears to be within the middle mediastinal (visceral) compartment. *C*. Aortogram. The dye column is irregular at the site of the aortic aneurysm (closed arrow), most of which is filled with clot (open arrows).

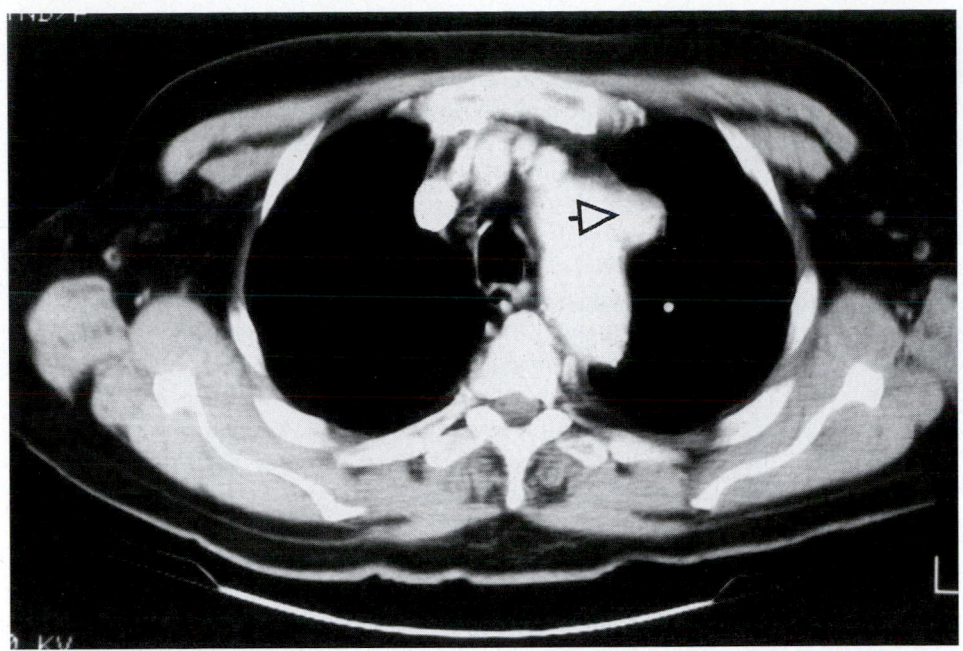

FIGURE 32-23   Aortic aneurysm shown by CT. A saccular aneurysm of the aortic arch (arrow) is readily demonstrated.

Bronchial arteries supply most lung tumors.[21] Infusion of various chemotherapeutic agents into these tumors via the bronchial circulation has been attempted for palliative control of nonresectable malignancies. So far, this has not been a very fruitful approach.

Venography can also be helpful in the diagnostic evaluation of pulmonary abnormalities. After injection of radiopaque material into a large vein of one or both upper extremities, displacement or obstruction of the superior vena cava by mediasti-

nal masses or scarring due to inflammatory processes can be identified (Fig. 32-25). The azygos vein can also be opacified, and visualization of this structure is occasionally helpful in evaluating mediastinal lesions or suspected bronchogenic carcinoma. Once again, these techniques have been largely supplanted by CT (Fig. 32-9) and MRI.

Air Contrast Studies

Occasionally, air has been introduced into various compartments of the chest for diagnostic purposes. For example, deliberate introduction of air into the pleural space (diagnostic pneumothorax) has been used to demonstrate pleural lesions. Diagnostic pneumothorax has fallen out of vogue because other methods, such as thoracoscopy, yield much more definitive and reliable information. Diagnostic pneumothorax and diagnostic pneumoperitoneum are still useful occasionally in investigating masses in the vicinity of the diaphragm. Air in the peritoneal cavity is particularly useful in demonstrating a subphrenic abscess.

PULMONARY ARTERIES AND VEINS

The pulmonary arteries are recognized as structures that accompany the bronchi and branch in a similar fashion (Fig. 32-26A).

In contrast, the pulmonary veins take a somewhat different course (Fig. 32-26B). In the lower lobes, the pulmonary veins are considerably more caudal than the corresponding arteries; the veins are situated at the level of the eighth to tenth ribs posteriorly, whereas the arteries are at the level of the seventh and eighth ribs. In the upper lobes, the pulmonary veins are lateral to the pulmonary arteries (Fig. 32-15).

The direction taken by a pulmonary vessel is the most useful basis for establishing its identity. Near the hili, particularly in the lower lobes, the pulmonary veins are more horizontal than the pulmonary arteries. At the hili, the pulmonary veins lie below and lateral to the arteries (Figs. 32-15 and 32-26). Although it is often possible to distinguish arteries from veins, this distinction is seldom useful and the generic terms *pulmonary vessels* and *pulmonary vasculature* are used. Laminography enhances distinctions between pulmonary

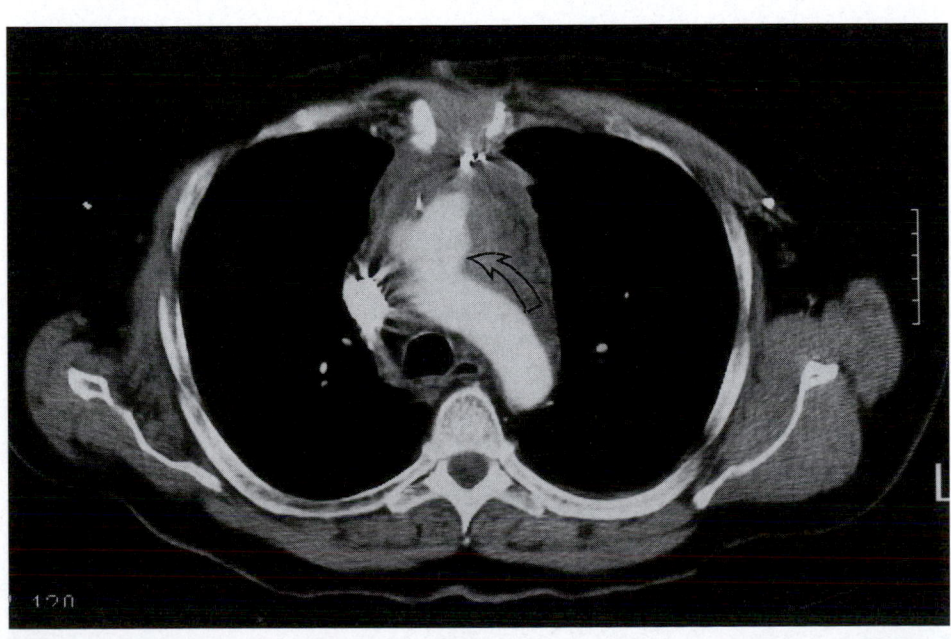

FIGURE 32-24   Aortic psuedoaneurysm demonstrated by CT. Anterior mediastinal infection led to development of a pseudoaneurysm at an aortotomy site. The CT not only demonstrates the pseudoaneurysm (arrow) but also shows masses caused by infection in the anterior mediastinum and chest wall.

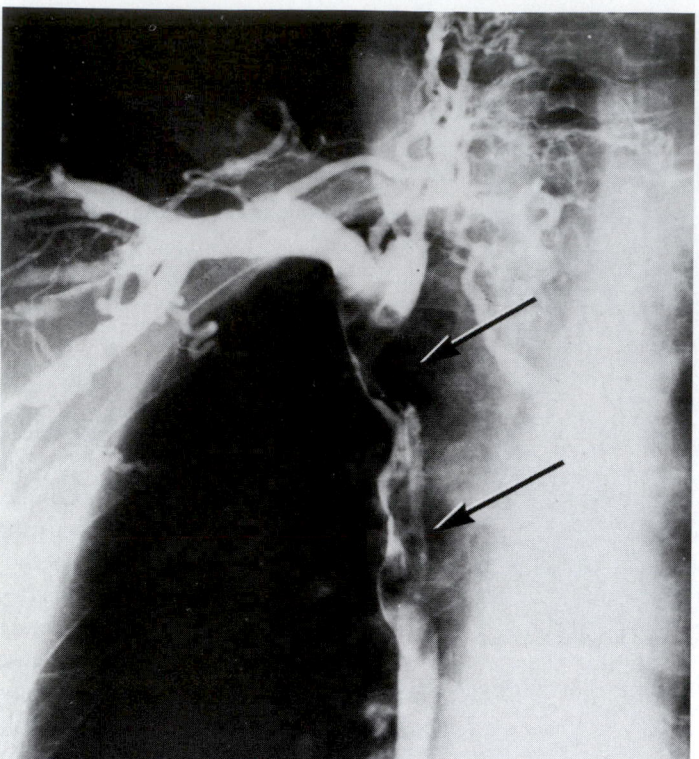

FIGURE 32-25 Superior vena caval invasion by metastatic tumor. A superior venacavogram shows invasion of the superior vena cava in several places (arrows) by metastic tumor involving the mediastinal lymph nodes.

arteries and veins; angiography is the most definitive procedure for making the distinction.

CT and MRI readily depict the pulmonary arteries and veins. The pulmonary arteries arise from the main pulmonary artery trunk, while the pulmonary veins enter the left atrium (Fig. 32-15).

Distribution of Pulmonary Blood Flow

Blood flow is not uniform in the normal, upright human lung. Moreover, the blood flow pattern shifts with changes in posture, during exercise, and in a variety of heart and lung diseases. In the normal pulmonary circulation, gravity is the predominant determinant of the pattern of blood flow (and blood volume). Under the influence of gravity, hydrostatic pressure in pulmonary arteries, capillaries, and veins decreases by approximately 1 cm H_2O per centimeter of distance from the bottom to the top of the lung. Accordingly, in the upright position, blood flow is minimal at the apex and maximal at the base. In the supine position, blood flow becomes much more uniform. If the lung is inverted, the normal pattern is reversed, so that flow to the apex, now dependent, increases considerably and exceeds blood flow to the base (Fig. 32-27). During walking or with any mild exercise in the upright position, total pulmonary flow increases, but flow to the lung apex increases proportionately more than flow to the base, resulting in a more uniform distribution.[22]

If pulmonary arterial pressure at the top of the lung fails to exceed alveolar pressure, capillaries in the apices collapse. In the normal lung, pulsatile pulmonary blood flow suffices to perfuse the apices; but when pulmonary arterial pressure falls, as in hemorrhagic hypotension, the normal marginal perfusion of the apices may give way to cessation of blood flow. Gravity plays less of a role once an increase in pulmonary vascular resistance has raised pulmonary arterial pressure to hypertensive levels.[22]

Lung disease often modifies the pattern of pulmonary blood flow by mechanical means and by development of pulmonary vasoconstriction (Fig. 32-28). Heart disease may also affect the pattern of flow.[10,14] For example, in left-to-right intracardiac shunts, pulmonary blood flow not only increases but also becomes more uniform than normal. The pattern is quite similar to that in exercise. In heart disease associated with high pulmonary

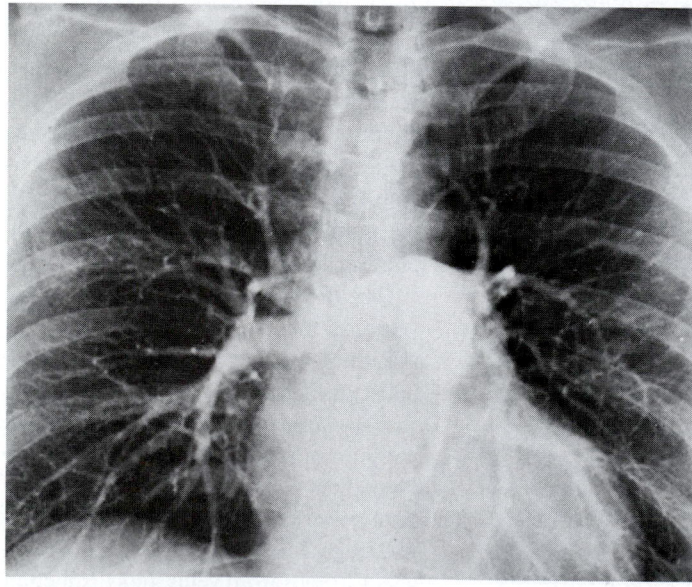

A

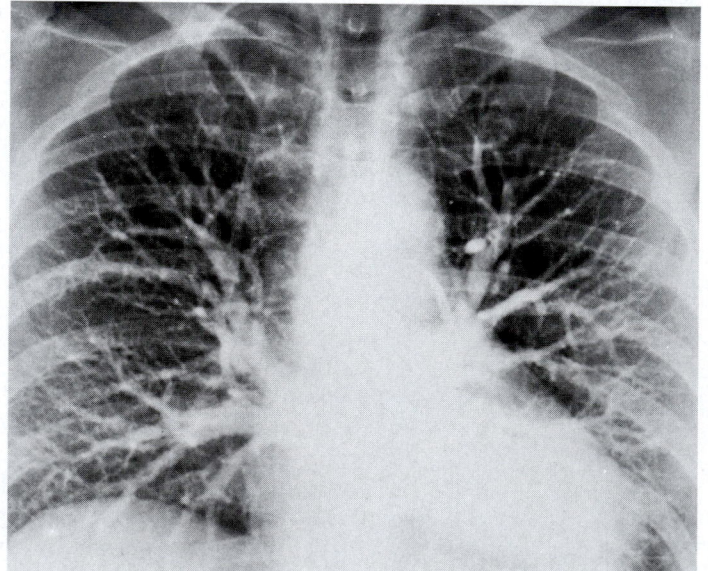

B

FIGURE 32-26 Pulmonary arteries and veings. *A.* The early phase of the pulmonary angiogram depicts the normal course of the pulmonary arteries. *B.* The late phase shows the normal course of the pulmonary veins. The veins have a more horizontal course than the arteries and enter the hilus below the arteries.

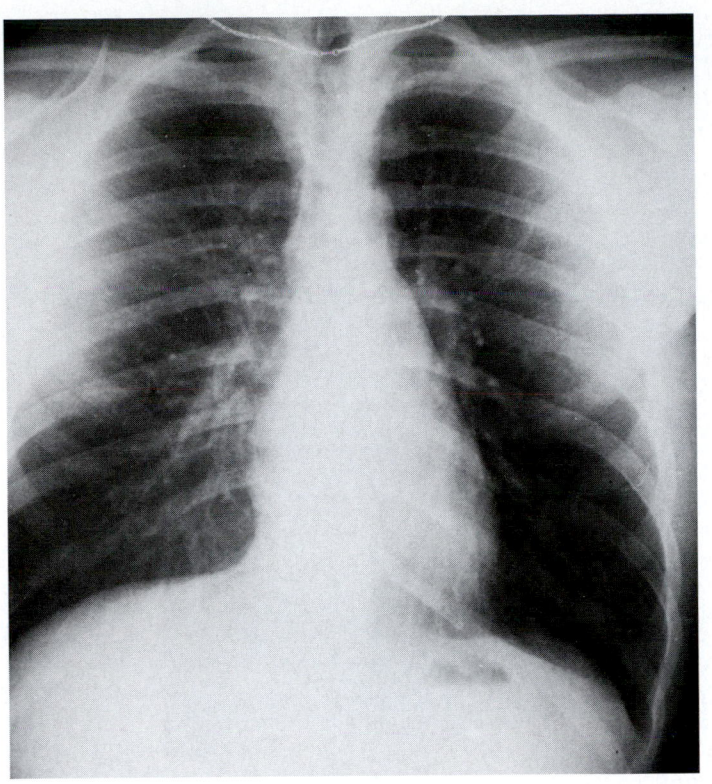

A

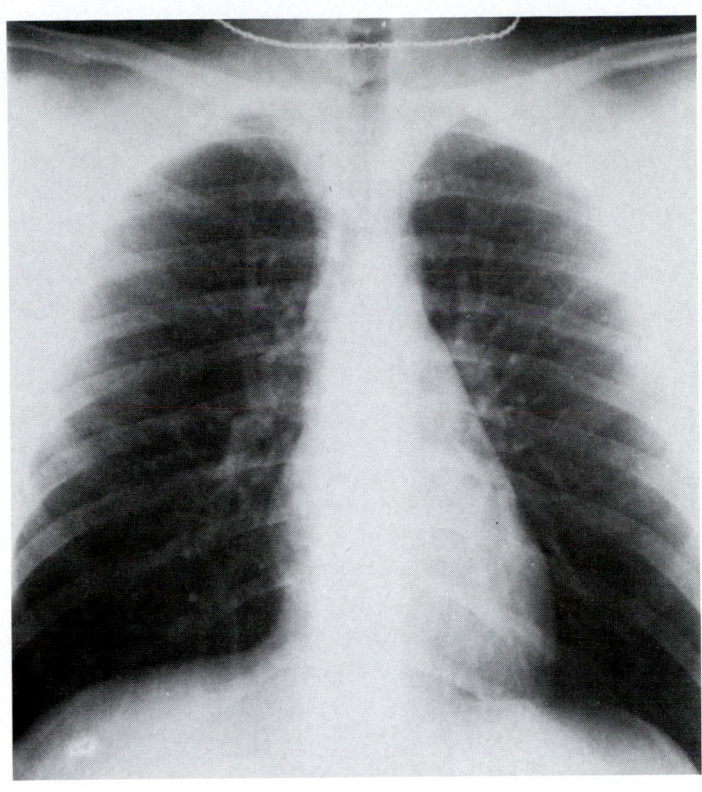

B

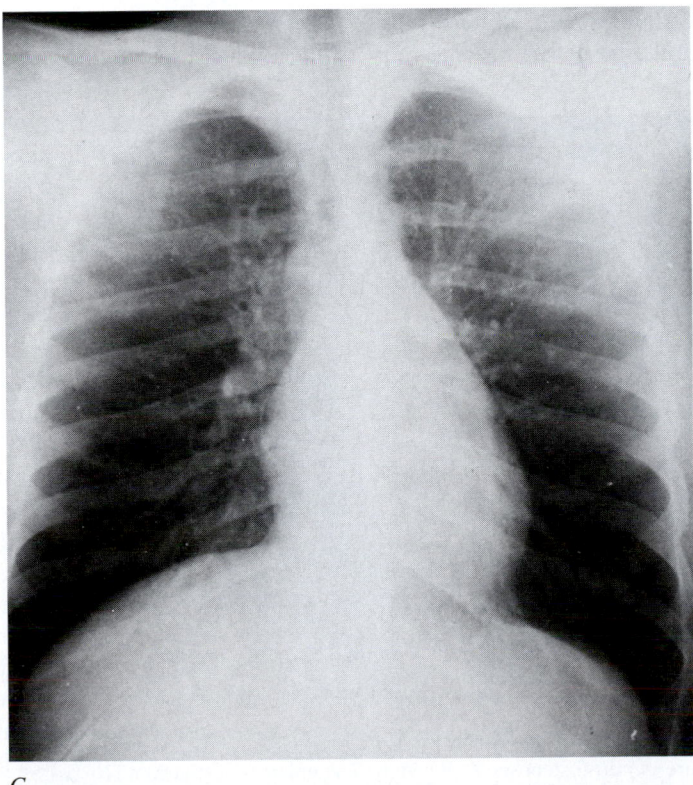

C

FIGURE 32-27   Effect of gravity on the pulmonary vasculature. Vascular patterns are compared in a normal subject in the erect, supine, and upside-down positions. *A*. Erect posture. The vascular pattern is more prominent at the bases. *B*. Supine position. The vascular pattern is more uniform. *C*. Upside-down position. The vascular pattern is more marked at the apices.

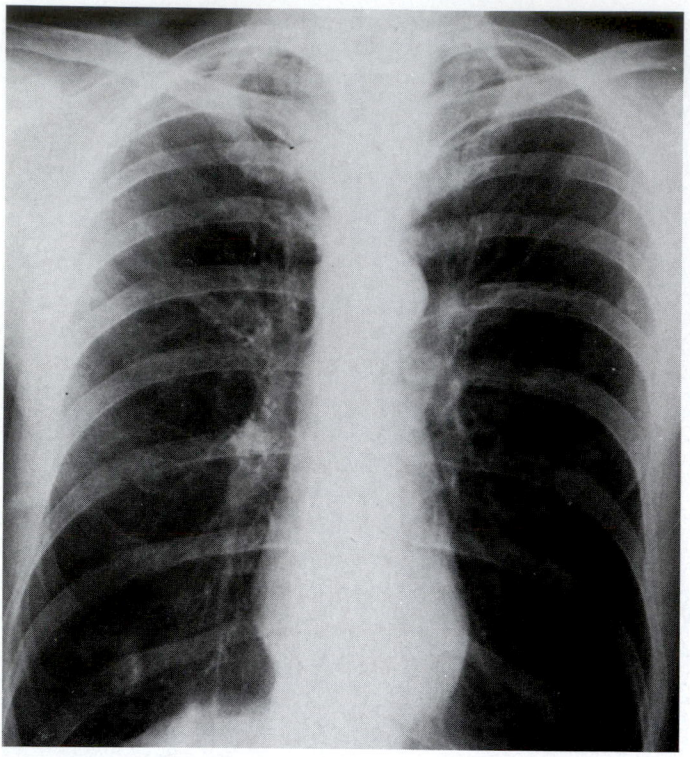

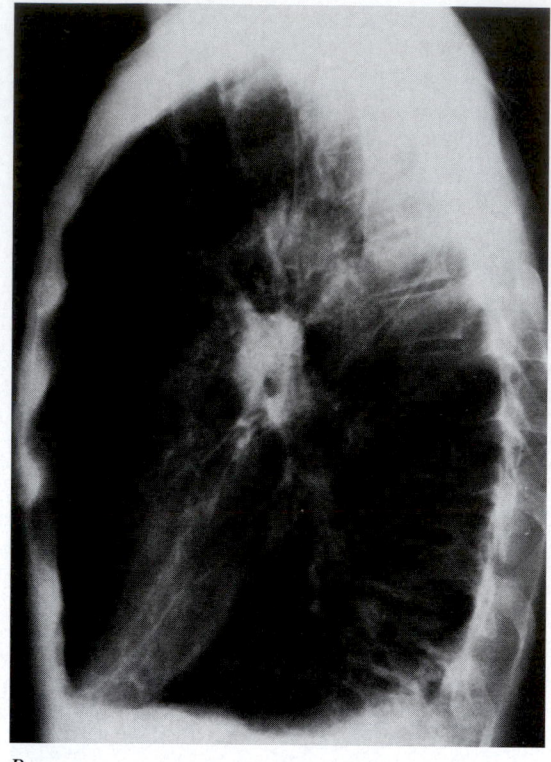

A

B

FIGURE 32-28 Pulmonary emphysema. *A.* PA view. Both lungs appear to be hyperradiolucent. Blood flow to the left lower lobe is particularly reduced. *B.* Lateral view. The marked hyperradiolucency is associated with a flat diaphragm, a wide anteroposterior diameter of the chest, and an increase in the retrosternal space.

venous pressure (e.g., chronic left ventricular failure or mitral stenosis), the distribution of blood flow tends to become more uniform early in the disease. In time, the apices become relatively hyperperfused as a result of interstitial edema, pulmonary fibrosis, and hypoxic vasoconstriction of the lung bases. As a consequence, pulmonary vascular resistance at the lung bases is increased in the setting of pulmonary venous hypertension, and blood flow is directed toward the apices (Fig. 32-29).[10] In prolonged, severe pulmonary venous hypertension, further constriction of the pulmonary vasculature occurs diffusely through the lungs, resulting in the "pruned tree" appearance of pulmonary arterial hypertension.[14] Chronic lung disease or idiopathic pulmonary hypertension (Fig. 32-30) may also result in the radiographic findings of pulmonary arterial hypertension. In general, the diagnostic accuracy of the radiologist is much greater for pulmonary venous hypertension than for pulmonary arterial hypertension.

The influence of gravity on the distribution of blood flow bears on the interpretation of the chest radiograph.[14] The mainstay of the concept, illustrated in Figure 32-31, is that in the normal upright lung, although gravity causes pulmonary arterial and venous pressures to increase from top to bottom of the lung, alveolar pressure remains

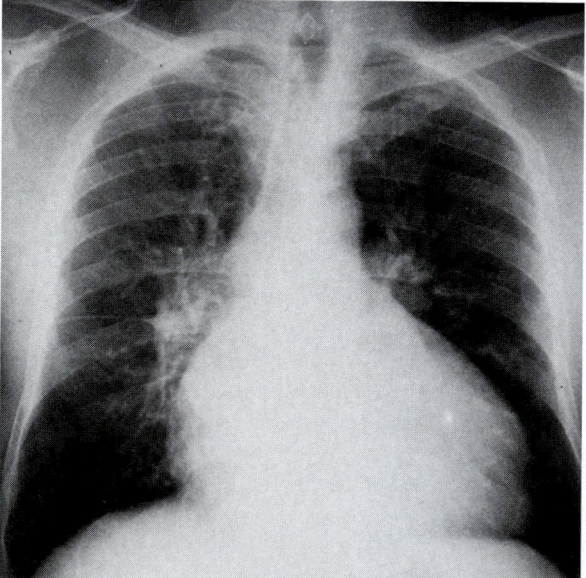

A

B

FIGURE 32-29 Pulmonary vasculature in mitral stenosis. *A.* PA view. The enlarged left atrium is seen as a double density within the cardiac shadow. Cephalization of the pulmonary blood vessels is also present as a result of an increase in blood flow to the apices, in conjunction with a decrease in flow to the lung bases. *B.* Close-up view. The increase in vascular markings at the apices is more striking.

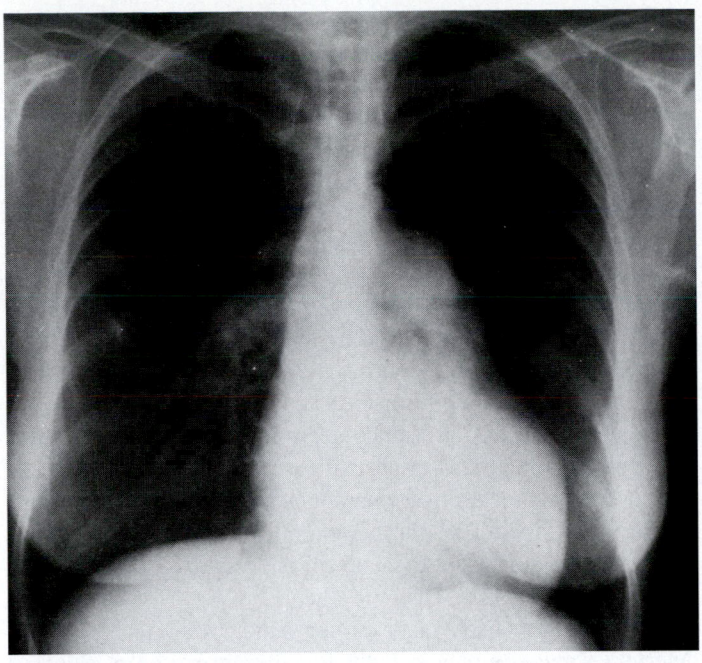

FIGURE 32-30 *Primary pulmonary hypertension. The pulmonary trunk and its right and left main bronchi are markedly enlarged. In contrast, the peripheral vasculature is sparse.*

Zone			Behavior of capillary	Flow depends on
I $P_A>Ppa>Ppv$	Ppa	Ppv	Collapsed	No flow*
II $Ppa>P_A>Ppv$	Ppa	Ppv	Starling resistor	$Ppa - P_A$
III $Ppa>Ppv>P_A$	Ppa	Ppv	Open or distended	$Ppa - Ppv$

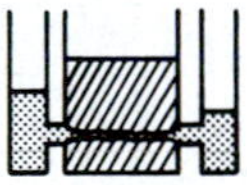

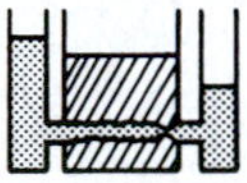

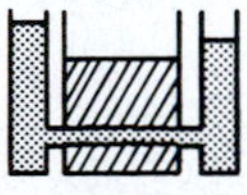

*Except for flow through corner vessels.

FIGURE 32-31 *Schematic representation of the behavior of small vessels in different parts of the lung. The lung is pictured as consisting of three vertical zones. In zone I, alveolar pressure is greater than arterial pressure, so collapsible vessels in the pulmonary microcirculation close; there is no flow. In zone II, arterial pressure exceeds alveolar pressure, which exceeds venous pressure. The pulmonary arterial-alveolar pressure difference determines the blood flow. Microvessels in this zone behave like Starling's resistors. The arterial-alveolar pressure difference increases linearly from top to bottom of the lung and produces corresponding changes in blood flow. In zone III, blood flow is determined by the difference between pulmonary arterial and venous pressures, since venous pressure exceeds alveolar. The collapsible vessels are open, and the pressure difference is constant throughout the zone (From West.[22])*

virtually constant (see Chapter 12). Alterations in the normal relationships among pulmonary arterial, pulmonary venous, and alveolar pressures from top to bottom of the upright lung cause derangements in the pattern of blood flow. For example, a regional increase in alveolar pressure may arise because of "ball-valve" physiology as a result of bronchoconstriction or bronchial obstruction by a foreign body or mucous plug. In chronic obstructive airway disease, this mechanism contributes to rearrangement of blood flow, adding a functional component to the anatomic effect of obliteration of parts of the pulmonary vascular bed by disease.[20]

Other disease processes also cause a characteristic redistribution of pulmonary blood flow.[14] For example, although uncommonly seen, the oligemic pattern distal to a large pulmonary embolus is of great diagnostic value (Fig. 32-32). In primary pulmonary hypertension, the peripheral vessels are small and the central vessels are quite large, resulting in the pruned-tree appearance of the pulmonary vasculature described earlier (Fig. 32-30). In emphysema, local destruction of pulmonary vasculature results in bizarre and unpredictable patterns of pulmonary blood flow (Fig. 32-28A).

DISTRIBUTION OF AIR WITHIN THE LUNGS

Just as is the case for pulmonary blood flow, the distribution of ventilation is affected by gravity. Normally, ventilation to the base is greater than to the apex because of the greater alveolar distention caused by gravity and a higher transpulmonary pressure at the apex (see Chapter 12).[22] Changes in ventilation from top to bottom of the upright lung are much more modest than are changes in blood flow. When the lung is supine, ventilation, as well as blood flow, is much more uniform. If the lung is turned upside down, the normal pattern is reversed, so the apex is better ventilated than the base.

Radiographic techniques can be of considerable value in providing information about the distribution of air within the lungs. For example, fluoroscopy of the chest and comparison of chest radiographs taken during inspiration and expiration are useful in detecting and localizing air trapping; blebs and bullae appear as avascular, excessively radiolucent areas. Extensive pleural encasement of one lung often is associated with a disproportionately small hemithorax and diminished ventilation of the affected side. Marked reduction in pulmonary vascular markings also occurs in unilateral hypoventilation or hypoplasia of the pulmonary artery (Swyer-James or Macleod's syndrome); the hemithorax on the affected

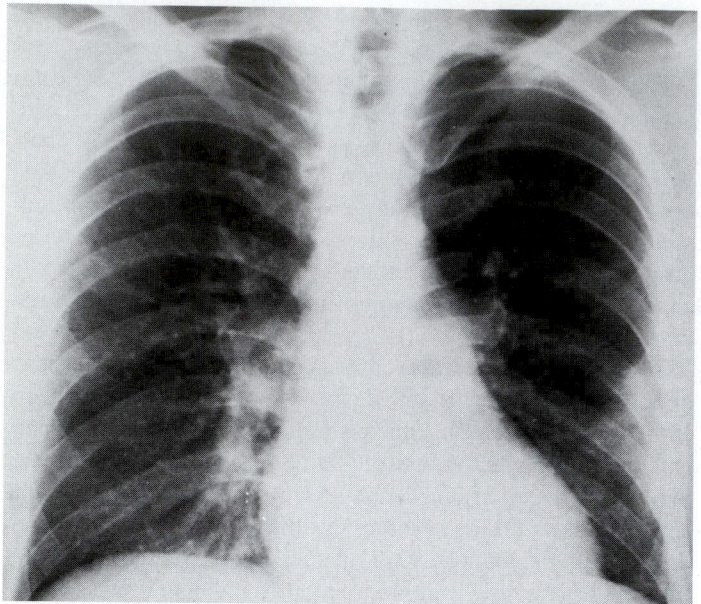

FIGURE 32-32 Massive pulmonary embolus. The PA view demonstrates marked diminution of the pulmonary vasculature to the left lung, secondary to a chronic massive pulmonary embolus in the left main pulmonary artery.

side is also usually small. Syndromes associated with unilateral hypoplasia often show air trapping on the affected side.[19]

Obstructive Airway Disease

The radiologist generally has little to offer in the early diagnosis of obstructive disease of the airways.[20] Chest radiographs are nearly always normal in patients in whom the airway obstruction is reversible. For example, in asthma, the chest radiograph is usually normal except during an acute episode, when the lungs often appear hyperinflated.

Similarly, the diagnosis of chronic bronchitis is a clinical one, based upon a history of chronic sputum production (see Chapter 42) and supplemented by characteristic abnormalities in pulmonary function tests (see Chapter 36). The radiograph rarely provides substantive help. Vascular markings throughout the lung fields are sometimes prominent, but this finding is nonspecific.

Even the practice of using the radiograph to assess the coexistence of emphysema and chronic bronchitis is generally unrewarding, unless emphysema is marked. The classic radiographic appearance of emphysema is hyperinflation and diminution of vascular markings (Fig. 32-28). Hyperinflation is manifested by increased radiolucency of the lungs; low, flat diaphragms; exaggerated verticality of the heart; increased anteroposterior diameter of the chest; and widening of the retrosternal space. Of all these criteria, diaphragmatic flattening is probably the most reliable in supporting a diagnosis of chronic obstructive airway disease.

Hyperinflation can be simulated radiographically when a normal, robust person exerts a maximal inspiratory effort. The lungs also appear hyperinflated in very slender persons. Therefore, it is unwise to make the diagnosis of emphysema on the sole basis of the radiographic finding of hyperinflation.

Supplemental radiographic evidence for the diagnosis of emphysema is afforded by examination of the pulmonary vessels. Two distinctly different vascular patterns have been identified in patients with chronic bronchitis and emphysema: arterial "deficiency" and increased lung markings.[20] Patients who show the arterial deficiency pattern (Fig. 32-28) often have panlobular emphysema and manifest the clinical syndrome of the "pink puffer." Those who have the pattern of increased lung markings (Fig. 32-33) often have centrilobular emphysema and manifest the "blue bloater" syndrome (see Chapter 42). It must be emphasized that these radiographic findings occur relatively late in the clinical course of emphysema.

Patients with chronic bronchitis and emphysema who develop pulmonary hypertension usually show the characteristic features of hyperinflation and an abnormal vascular pattern. In addition, they may show distinctive enlargement of the hilar pulmonary arteries and oligemia of the peripheral lung fields. These findings constitute important evidence of the existence of pulmonary hypertension.

Attempts have been made to use radiographic techniques to determine lung volumes in patients with chronic bronchitis and emphysema.[13] Numerous measurements made on PA and lateral chest radiographs have served as the basis for the calculations; results have compared favorably with those obtained directly with spirometric or body plethysmographic techniques. Recently, the radiographic approach has been reinforced by the availability of sophisticated computer techniques. These methods have not been widely adopted, however, because of the availability and accuracy of body plethysmography (see Chapter 10).

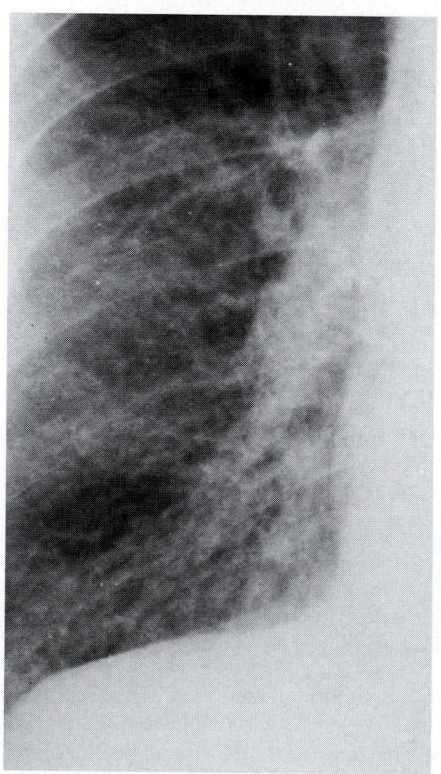

FIGURE 32-33 Increased markings pattern. The vascular markings are prominent throughout the lung fields. The patient has chronic bronchitis and emphysema. Hyperaeration is minimal.

CT is much more sensitive to the presence of emphysema than the plain chest radiograph. Centrilobular emphysema is readily demonstrated by CT; bullae, which may be difficult to see on the plain radiograph, are easily recognized. CT is especially useful in demonstrating the presence and location of bullae when bullectomy or lung reduction techniques are planned (see Chapter 55).

Heart Failure Complicating Chronic Bronchitis and Emphysema

Both right and left ventricular failure occur in the patient with chronic obstructive airway disease, but the underlying mechanisms and the radiographic appearances are different. Right ventricular failure in chronic obstructive airway disease is generally a consequence of pulmonary hypertension—which, in turn, is secondary to severe hypoxia and respiratory acidosis. As a consequence of the right ventricular failure, lung water increases, but rarely to the point of overt pulmonary edema. In contrast, left ventricular failure is generally caused by unrelated disease of the coronary circulation or left ventricular myocardium; as a result, pulmonary venous pressure is abnormally high, resulting in the formation of hemodynamic pulmonary edema.

Recognition of left ventricular failure in patients with chronic obstructive airway disease is difficult.[14] The low diaphragm and rarefield lungs obscure enlargement of the heart. Changes in pulmonary vasculature that are associated with left ventricular failure are difficult to recognize in the patient with a pattern of increased lung markings. Moreover, pulmonary edema often assumes unusual appearances in patients with underlying structural lung diseases. Most helpful is comparison of recent and old chest radiographs, with particular attention focused on changes in cardiac size and vascular pattern. Frequently the presence of left ventricular failure is recognized retrospectively, as heart size decreases and vascular markings become attenuated following diuretic therapy.

DISEASES AFFECTING THE PULMONARY PARENCHYMA

In sorting out the many diseases that can affect the lung parenchyma, it is useful to know if the process involves primarily the alveoli or the interstitium.[4] Frequently, but not invariably, this distinction can be made on the chest radiograph.

An alveolar radiographic pattern is created when alveolar airspaces are filled with material (e.g., blood, pus, or fluid). Characteristic radiographic features of alveolar filling diseases are exemplified in Figs. 32-34, 32-35, and

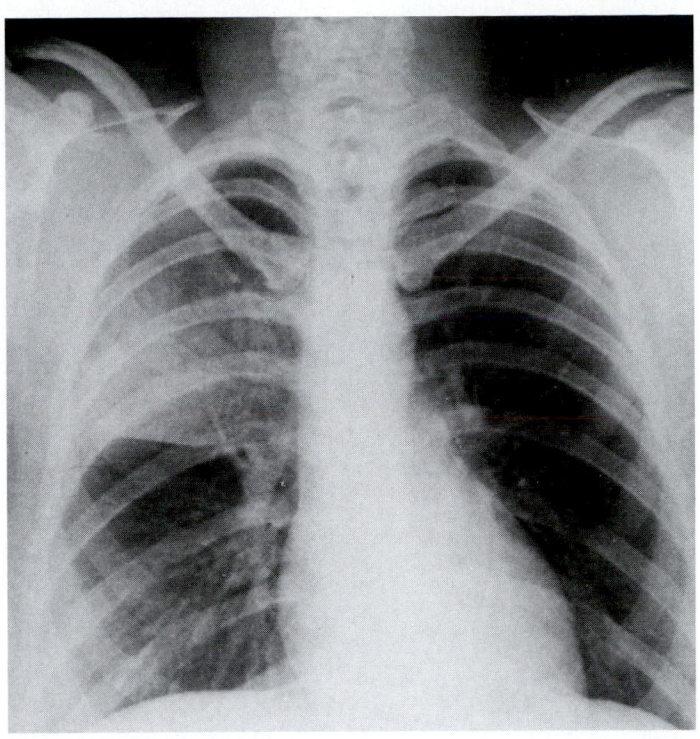

FIGURE 32-34 Right-upper-lobe pneumonia. The PA radiograph shows diffuse consolidation of the right upper lobe. The alveolar pattern is characteristic. The radiolucent streaks that run through the consolidation represent air in the bronchi (air bronchogram).

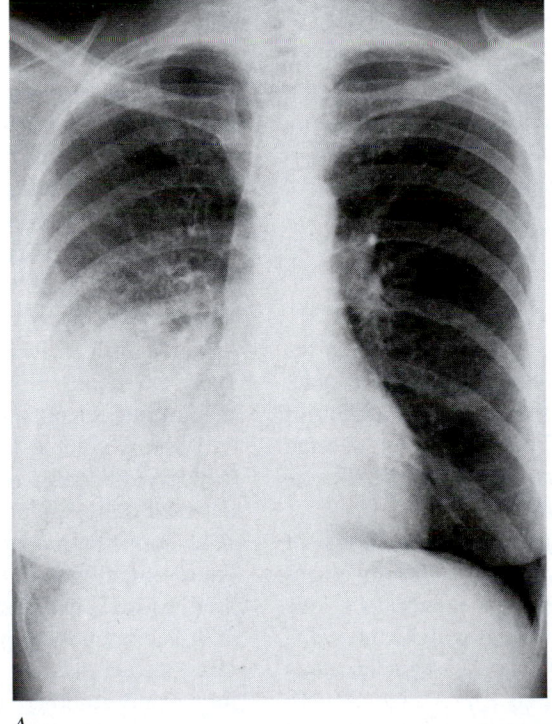
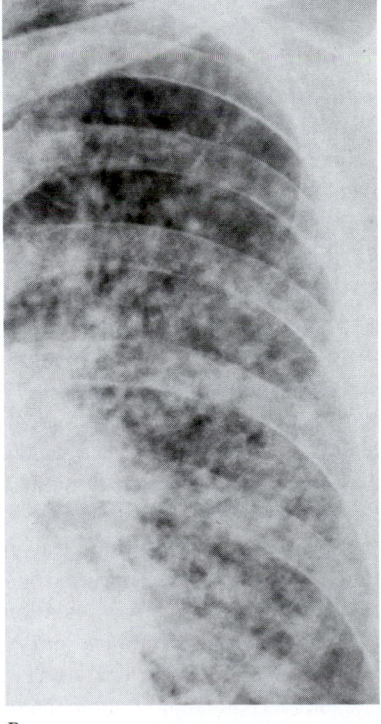

A   *B*

FIGURE 32-35 Patterns of alveolar cell carcinoma. *A.* A large area of consolidation in the right lower lobe. The alveolar pattern suggests pneumonia. *B.* The more distinctive pattern for alveolar cell carcinoma consists of multiple alveolar nodules. The nodules have irregular or fuzzy margins that are characteristic of alveolar, rather than interstitial, nodulation.

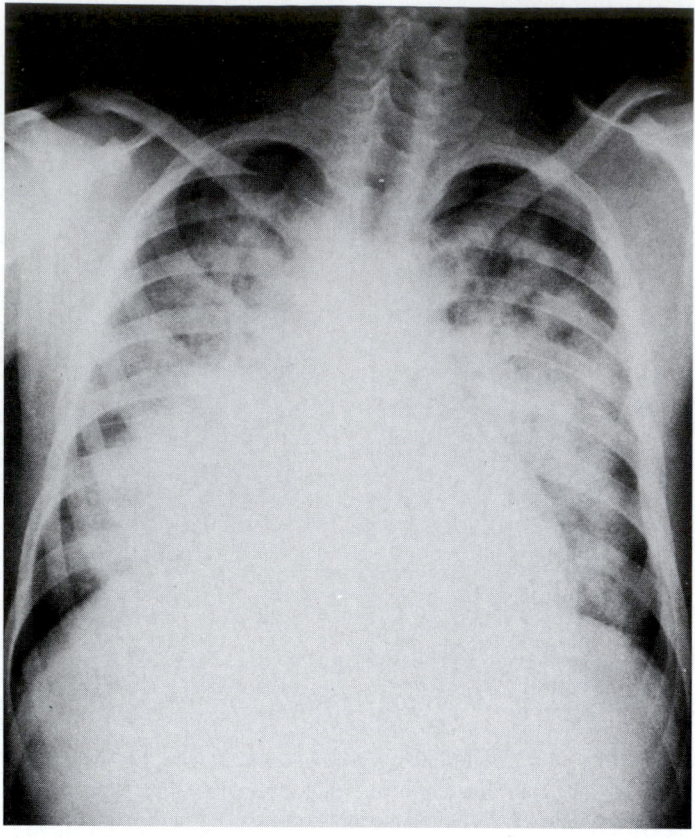

A

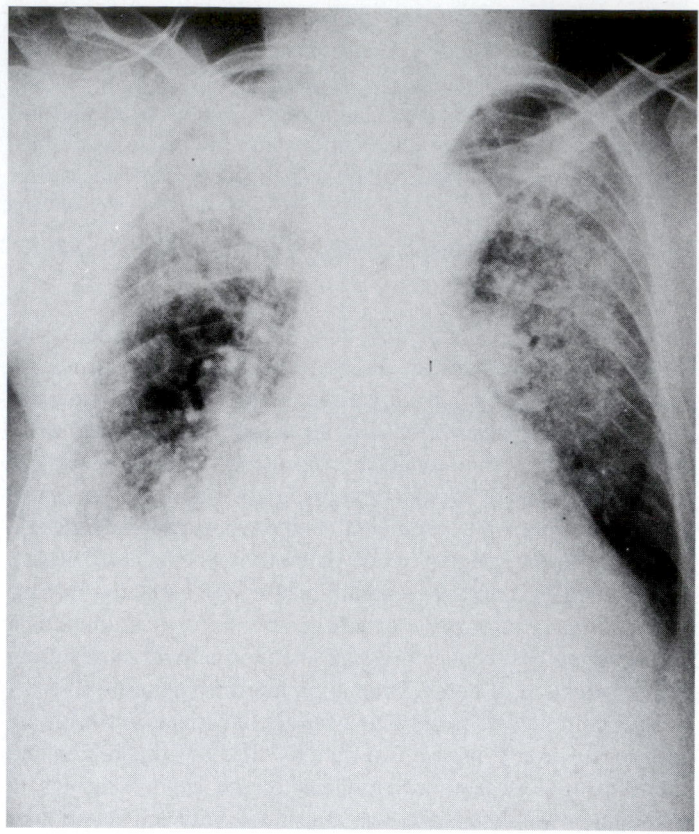

B

FIGURE 32-36 Pulmonary edema. Pulmonary edema may be either localized or diffuse. *A*. Most distinctive, but not most common, is a "bat wing" pattern of central alveolar consolidation. *B*. more often, pul-

monary edema affects one or more areas of the lung and appears as patchy alveolar consolidation.

32-36. These features include coalescence of densities and creation of large homogeneous shadows; presence of air bronchograms (i.e., visualization of peripheral bronchi due to consolidation of surrounding alveoli); fluffy, irregular margins of localized areas of consolidation; and rapid changes in areas of consolidation.[4]

Localized Alveolar Disease

Localized alveolar disease assumes two primary patterns on the chest radiograph: patchy consolidation of airspaces without a decrease in the volume of the affected area and consolidation of airspaces associated with a decrease in the volume of the affected area (atelectasis). The differential diagnosis depends heavily on the extent to which lung volume is decreased.

Localized consolidation of alveolar airspaces without loss of lung volume, or with minimal loss, is usually a sign of pneumonia (Fig. 32-34). Consolidation may be localized to a lobe (Fig. 32-35) or a pulmonary subsegment, or it may be more diffuse (Fig. 32-36). Consolidation of a pulmonary subsegment causes a characteristic radiographic pattern (Figs. 32-37 and 32-38). Among other causes of consolidation without loss of volume is pulmonary edema, which occasionally occurs as a local consolidation, even though more often it is diffuse, and pulmonary infarction (Fig. 32-12*C*).

In most instances, localized pulmonary consolidation without loss of lung volume indicates an acute inflammatory process. If

consolidation persists without change for several weeks, however, a less common pathologic process should be suspected: alveolar cell carcinoma (Figs. 35*A* and 32-39); lymphoma; metastatic carcinoma, particularly from a breast primary; fungal infection; eosinophilic lung disease; or granulomatous vasculitis, such as Wegener's disease.[6,7]

CT is not very useful in distinguishing between the various causes of localized alveolar disease. The technique can readily depict the extent of the process, but the underlying cause is usually not further elucidated (Fig. 32-39). CT is useful in identifying cavitation (Figs. 32-40 and 32-41) and in demonstrating mediastinal adenopathy, which may not have been suspected.[17]

Loss of volume (atelectasis) commonly accompanies localized consolidation of the lung. In most instances, atelectasis detected radiographically is lobar in distribution, since collapse of anatomic pulmonary units smaller than a lobe (e.g., segments) is prevented by collateral air drift. Lobar patterns of atelectasis are illustrated in Figures 32-42, 32-43, 32-44, 32-45, and 32-46.

It is extremely important to recognize the various patterns of lobar atelectasis, since this radiographic finding is a very common manifestation of carcinoma of the lung. In addition, its presence suggests an endobronchial neoplasm. Atelectasis is also common in the postoperative patient, presumably because of hypoventilation of dependent parts of the lungs and inadequate clearing of respiratory secretions. Finally, atelectasis may occur as a consequence of inflammatory disease of the airways or aspiration of a foreign body.[7]

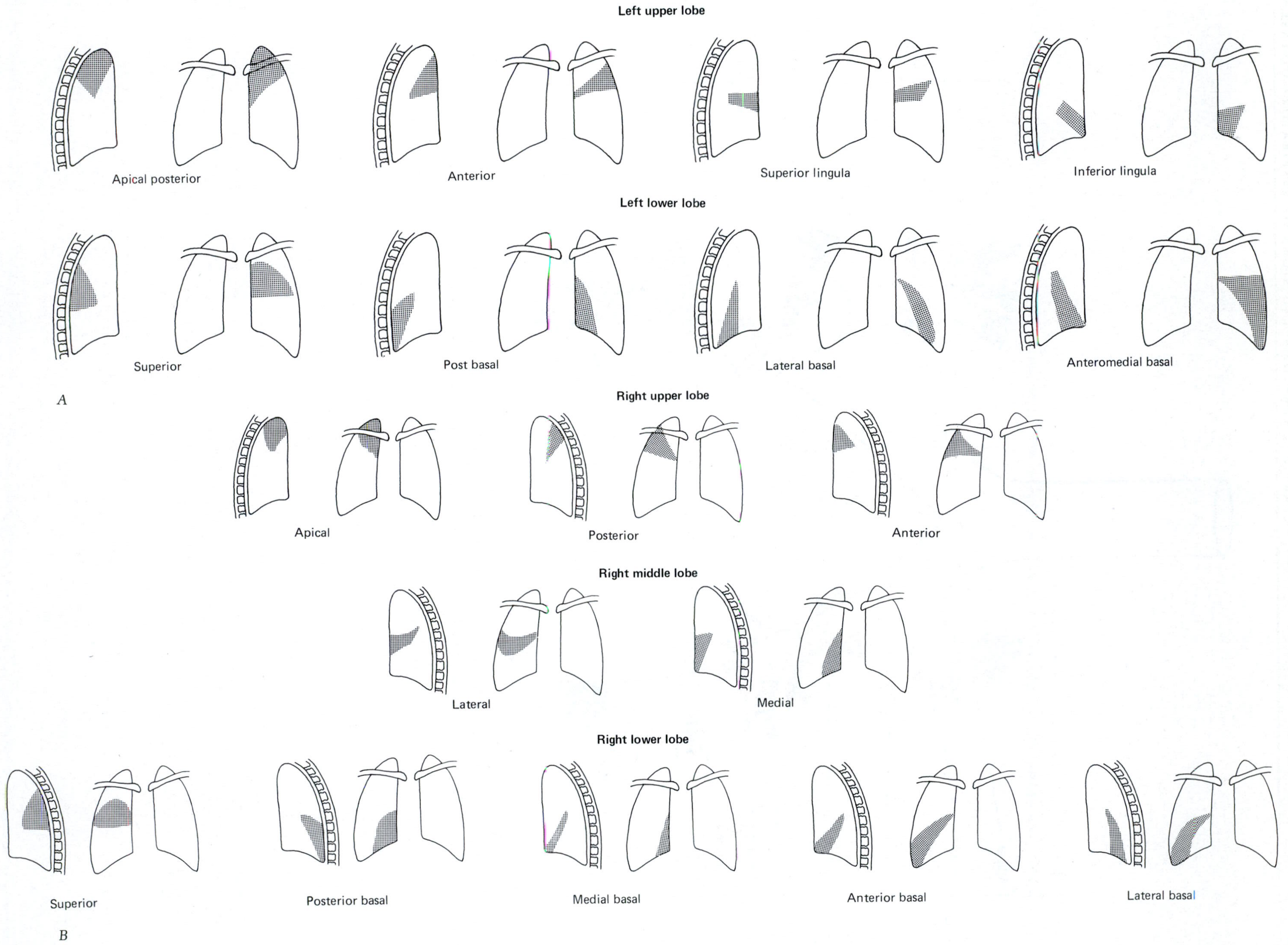

Left upper lobe

Apical posterior

Anterior

Superior lingula

Inferior lingula

Left lower lobe

Superior

Post basal

Lateral basal

Anteromedial basal

Right upper lobe

Apical

Posterior

Anterior

Right middle lobe

Lateral

Medial

Right lower lobe

Superior

Posterior basal

Medial basal

Anterior basal

Lateral basal

A

B

FIGURE 32-37 Radiographic anatomy of the pulmonary subsegments. Schematic representations of characteristic patterns of consolidation for each of the pulmonary subsegments are shown. *A.* Left lung. *B.* Right lung.

455

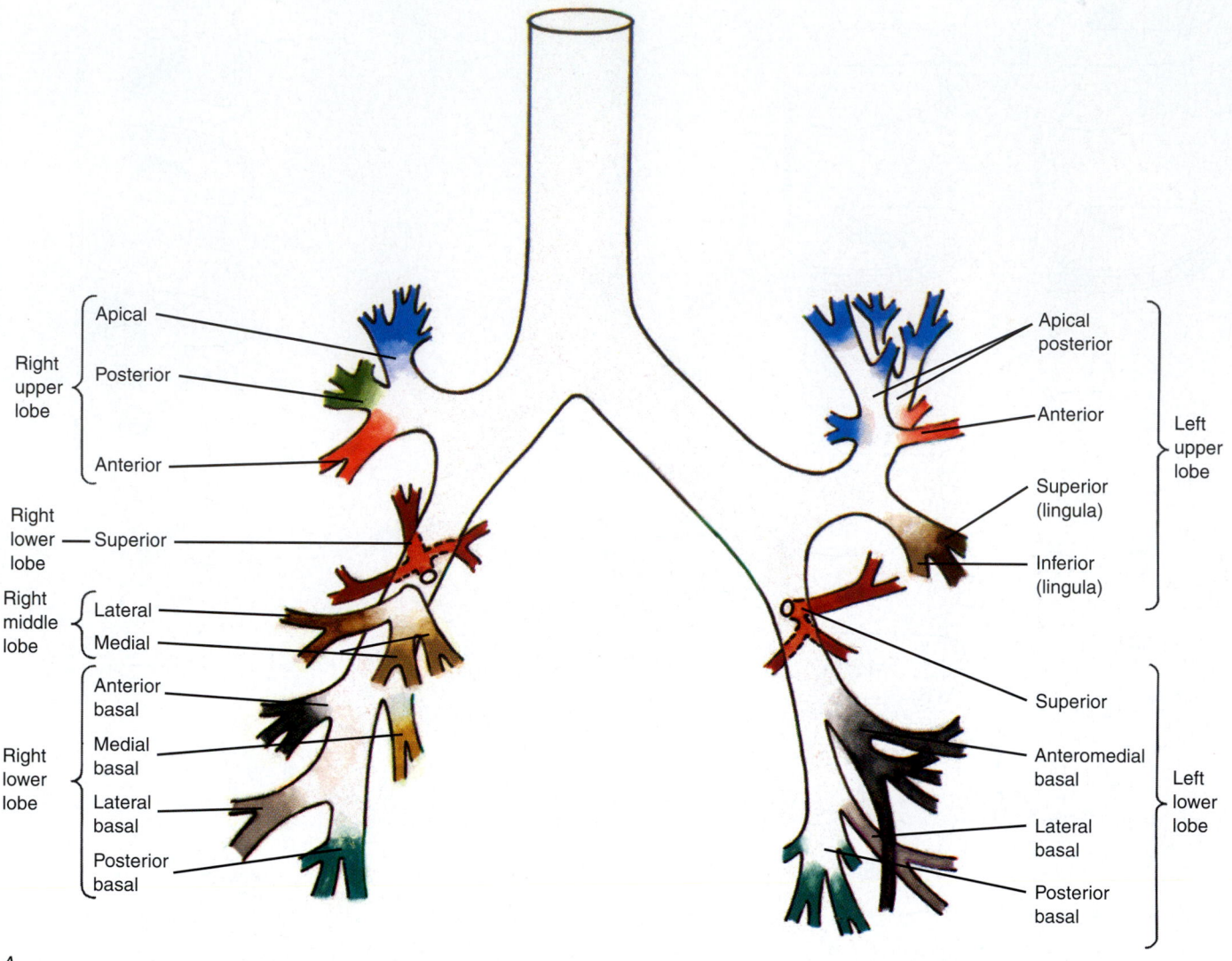

A

FIGURE 32-38 Topographic anatomy of the tracheobronchial tree and pulmonary subsegments. *A*. Tracheobronchial tree. *B*. Left anterior. *C*. Left lateral. *D*. Left cutaway. *E*. Left posterior. *F*. Right anterior. *G*. Right lateral. *H*. Right cutaway. *I*. Right posterior.

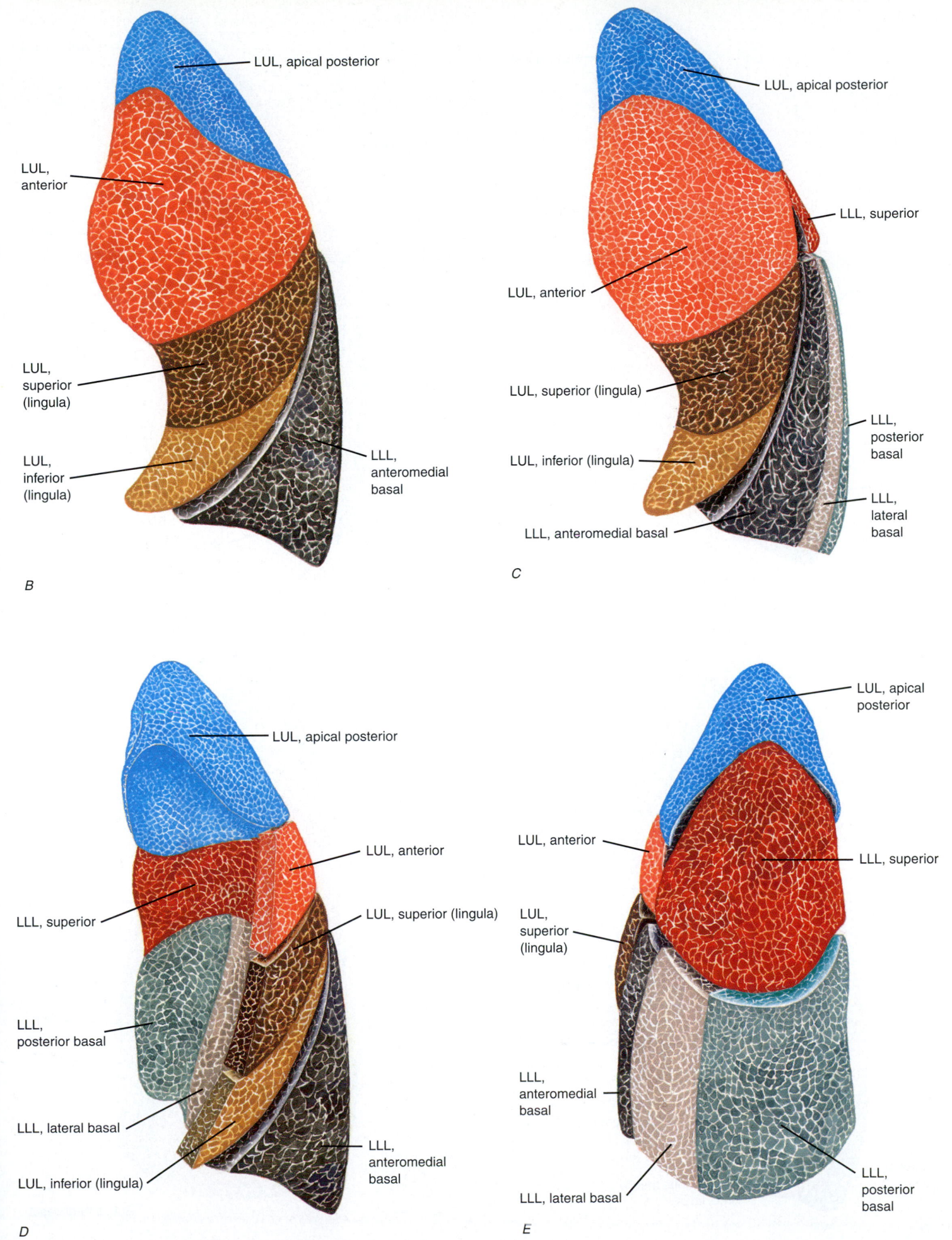

B

LUL, apical posterior

LUL, anterior

LUL, superior (lingula)

LUL, inferior (lingula)

LLL, anteromedial basal

C

LUL, apical posterior

LLL, superior

LUL, anterior

LUL, superior (lingula)

LUL, inferior (lingula)

LLL, anteromedial basal

LLL, posterior basal

LLL, lateral basal

D

LUL, apical posterior

LUL, anterior

LLL, superior

LUL, superior (lingula)

LLL, posterior basal

LLL, lateral basal

LUL, inferior (lingula)

LLL, anteromedial basal

E

LUL, apical posterior

LUL, anterior

LLL, superior

LUL, superior (lingula)

LLL, anteromedial basal

LLL, lateral basal

LLL, posterior basal

FIGURE 32-38 *(Cont.)*

457

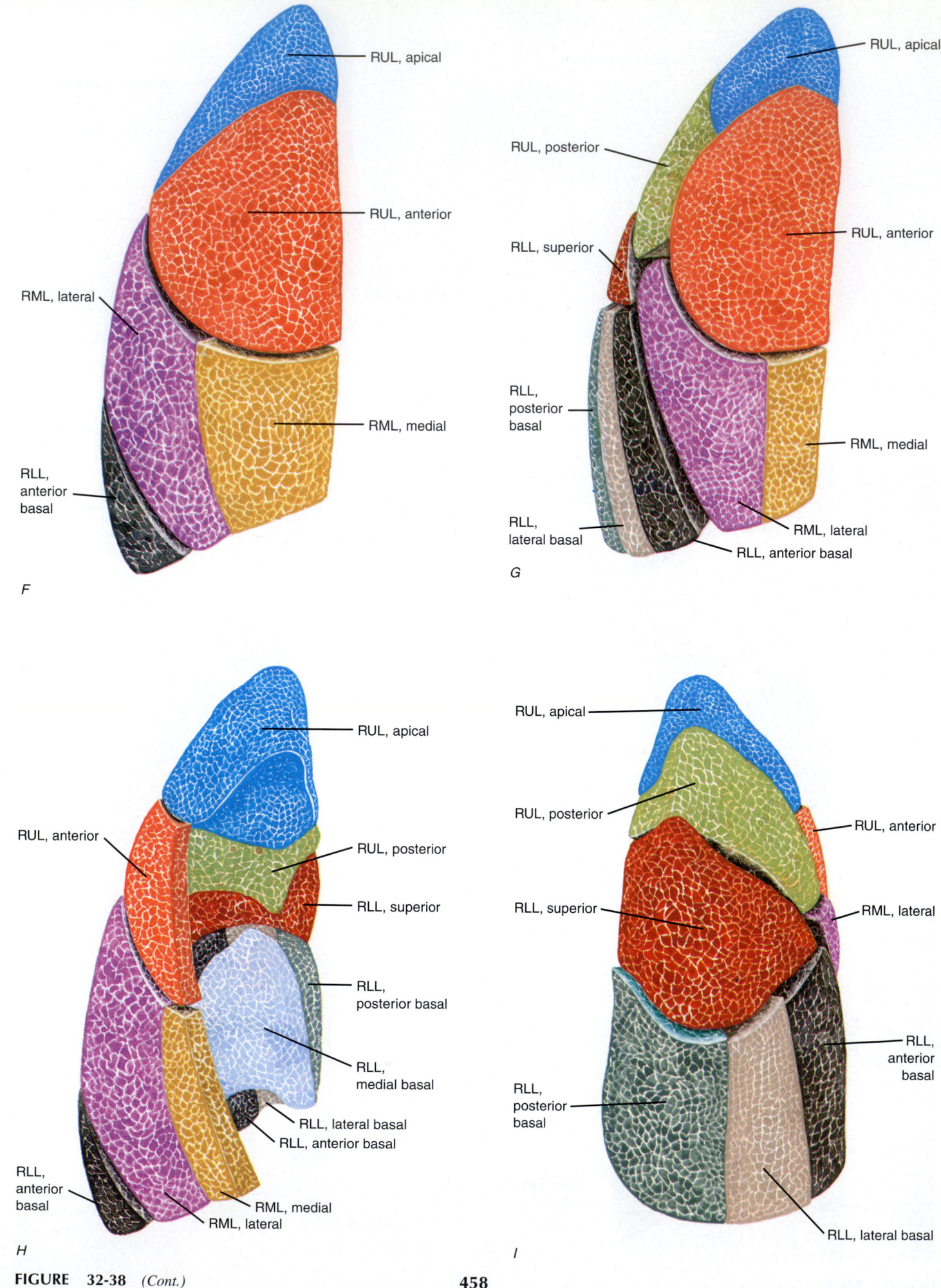

FIGURE   32-38   (Cont.)   **458**

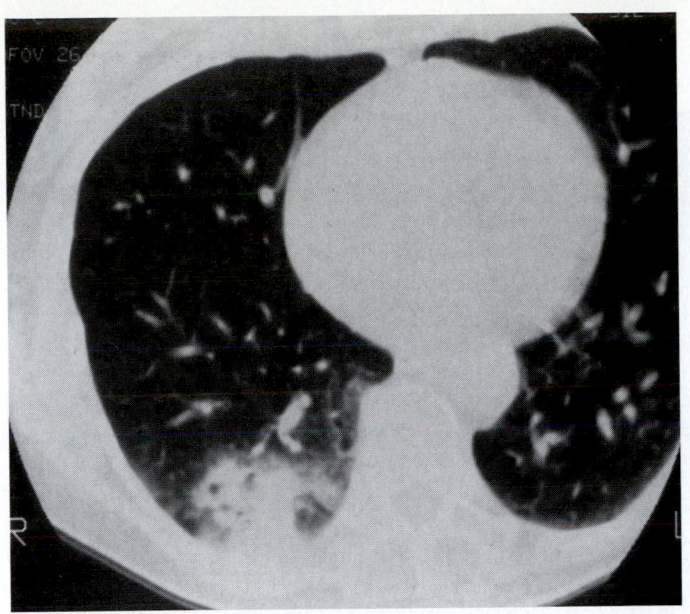

FIGURE 32-39 CT image of localized alveolar cell carcinoma. A patchy right-lower-lobe infiltrate is present. The characteristic alveolar infiltrate is consistent with lobar-type alveolar cell carcinoma. However, the findings are not specific. In this instance, CT adds little to the diagnosis.

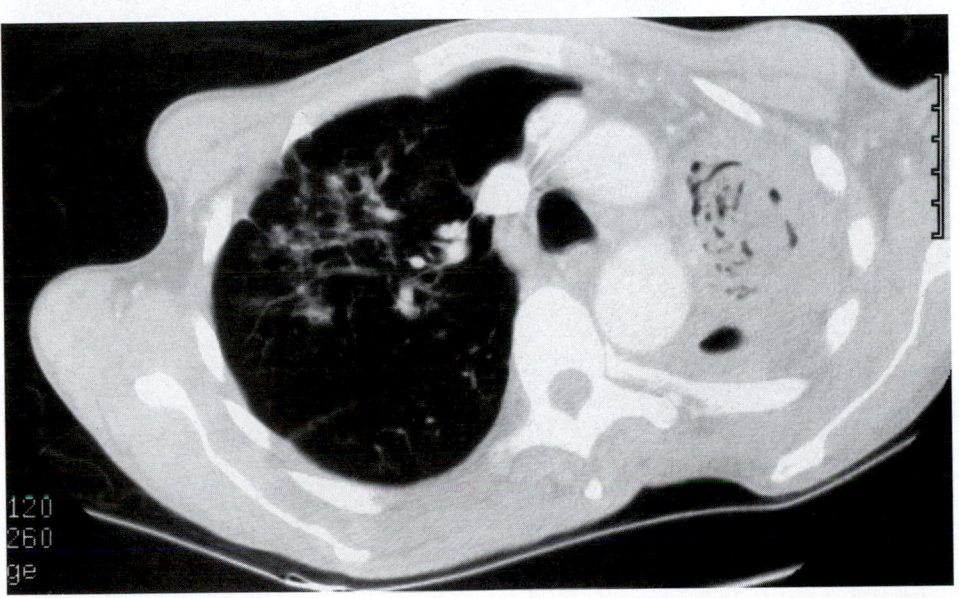

FIGURE 32-40 CT demonstrating characteristic crescent sign of aspergillosis. A right-upper-lobe infiltrate is seen that, in this case, was due to tuberculosis. In the left upper lobe, a crescent of air is seen within the matted mycelia of a fungus ball. The finding is characteristic of noninvasive aspergillosis, in which saprophytic aspergillus has invaded a tuberculous cavity.

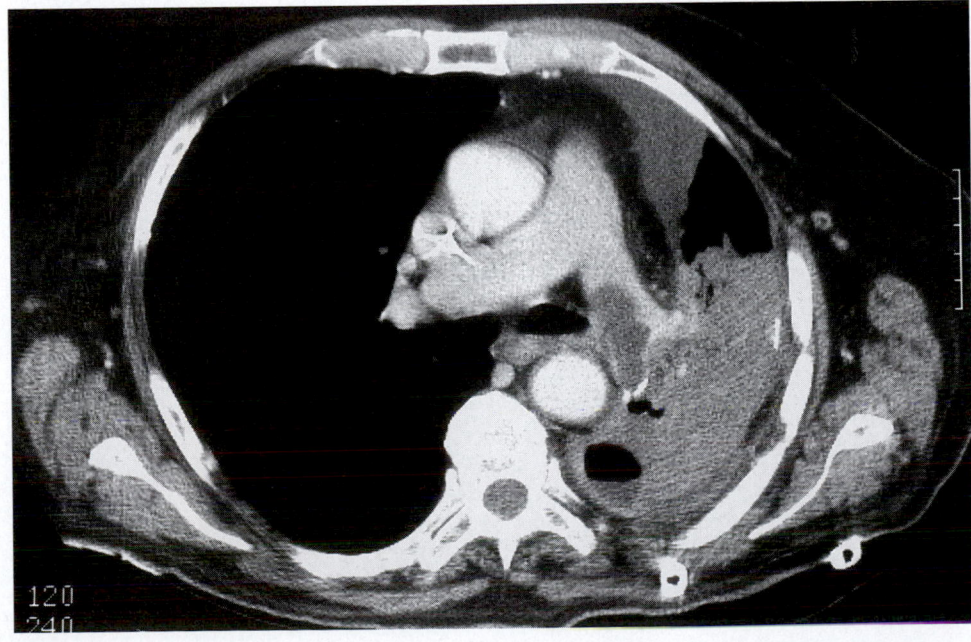

FIGURE 32-41 CT showing gangrene of the lung due to a pulmonary artery thrombus. The patient had a prior left upper lobectomy; in the postoperative period, consolidation of the remaining left lung developed. The scan shows a lung cavity that was not previously suspected, as well as a thrombus in the left pulmonary artery. The cavity represents a rapidly developing lung abscess due to lung infarction (gangrene).

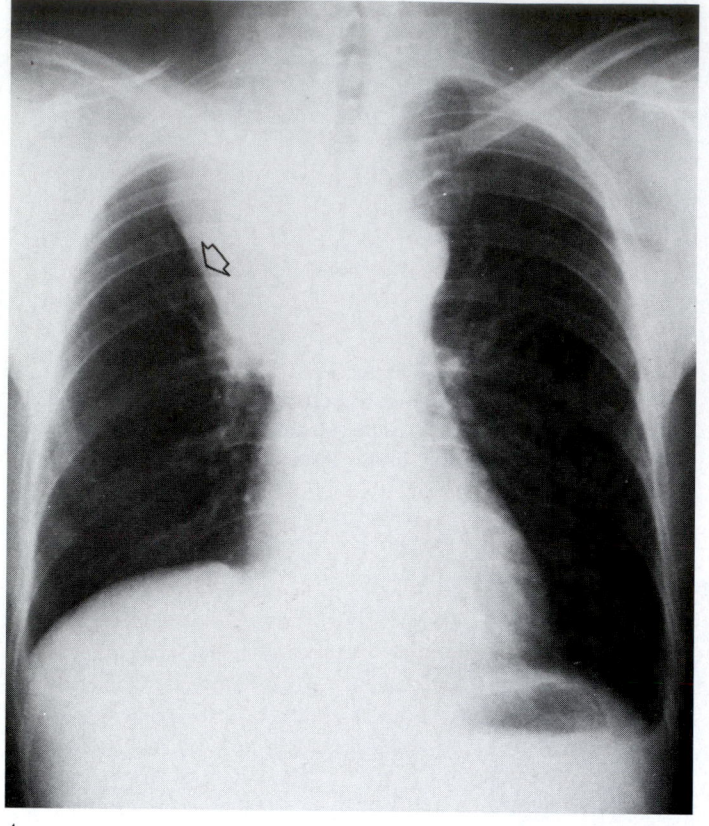

A

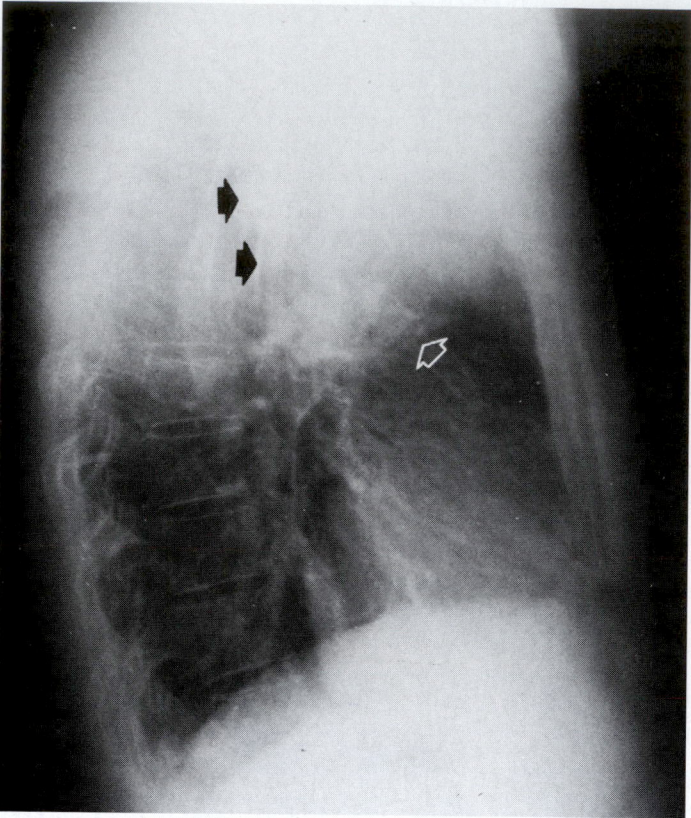

B

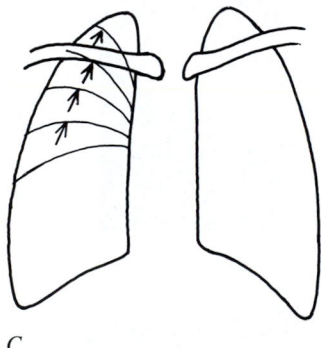

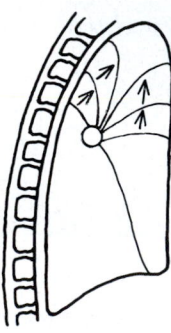

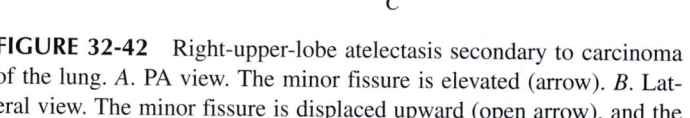

C

FIGURE 32-42   Right-upper-lobe atelectasis secondary to carcinoma of the lung. *A*. PA view. The minor fissure is elevated (arrow). *B*. Lateral view. The minor fissure is displaced upward (open arrow), and the major fissure is displaced anteriorly (closed arrows). *C*. Schematic representation of atelectasis of the right upper lobe.

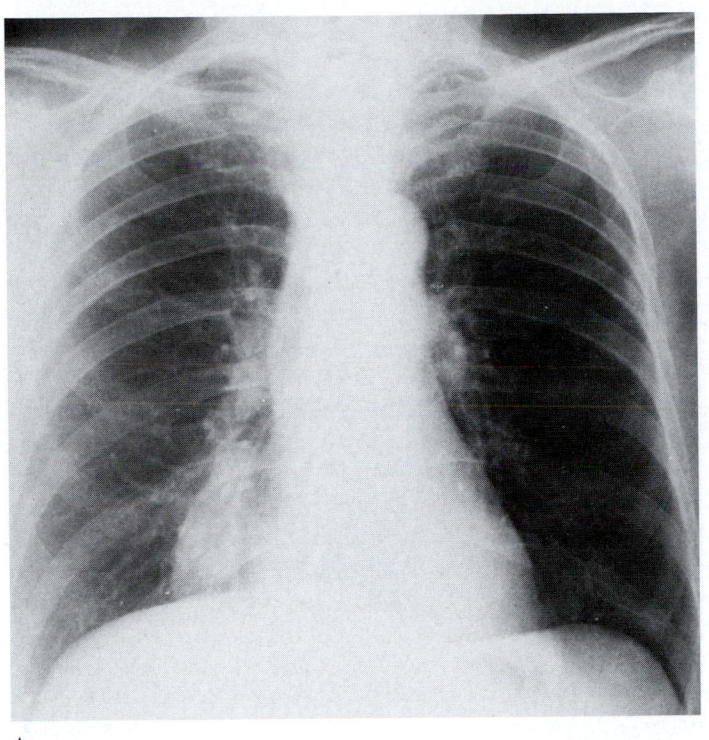

A

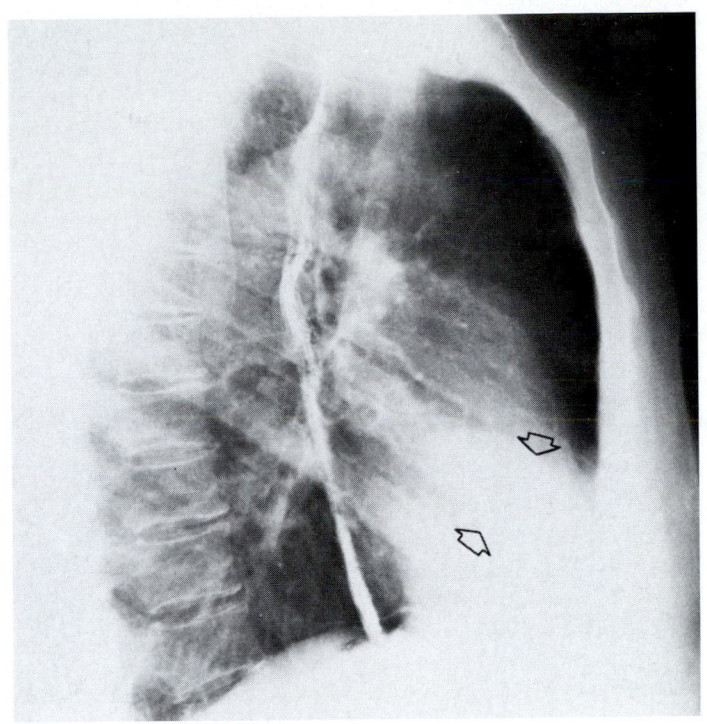

B

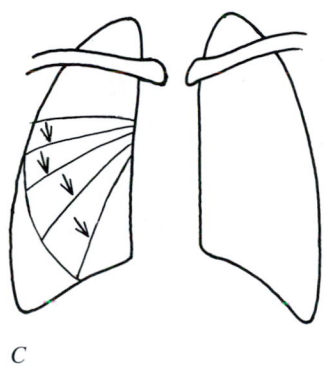
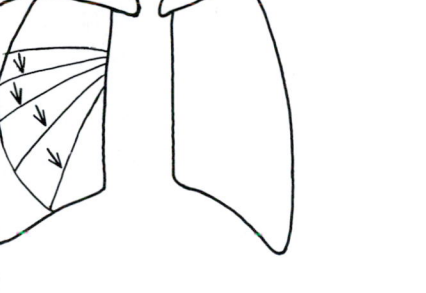
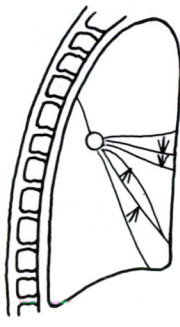

C

FIGURE 32-43   Right-middle-lobe atelectasis secondary to right-middle-lobe syndrome. *A*. PA view. The middle lobe is collapsed against the right side of the heart. *B*. Lateral view. The major and minor fissures are drawn together (arrows), creating a density that overlies the cardiac shadow. *C*. Schematic representation of right-middle-lobe atelectasis.

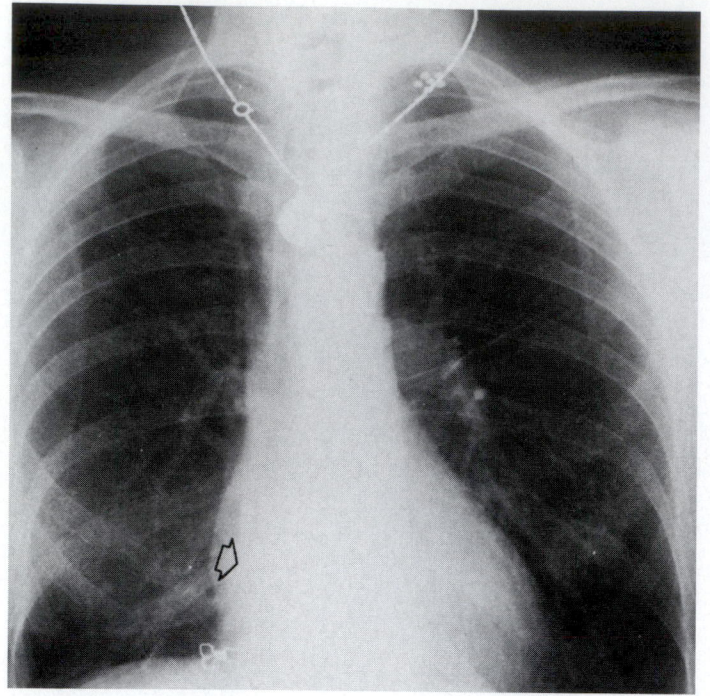

A

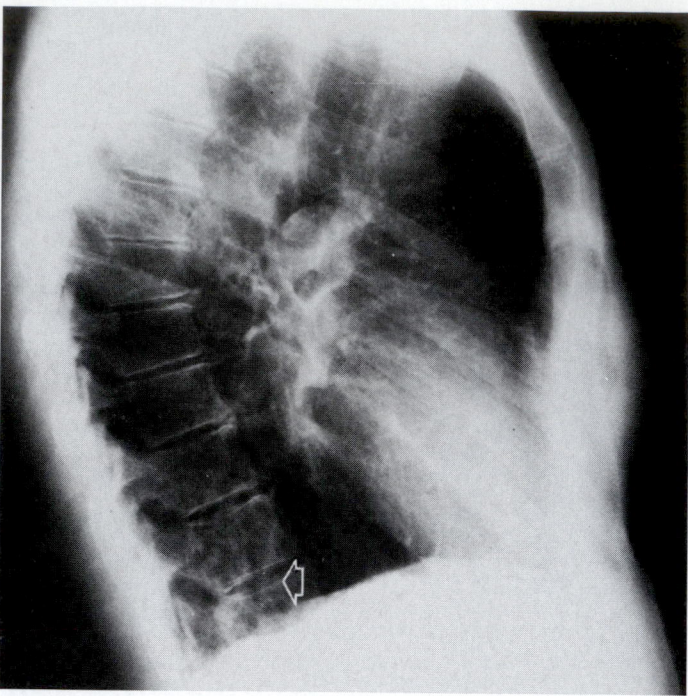

B

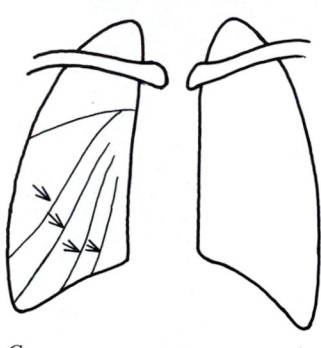

C

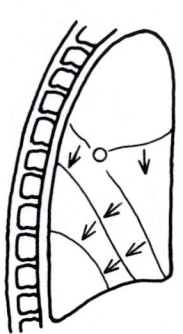

FIGURE 32-44   Atelectasis (severe) of the right lower lobe due to chronic inflammatory disease. *A*. PA view. Secondary signs of atelectasis are present in the right lung: small hemithorax, stretching of the pulmonary vessels, hyperlucent lung, and small hilus. In addition, there is downward displacement of the right hilus, and the collapsed lower lobe can be seen through the right heart border (arrow). *B*. Lateral view. The entire right lower lobe appears only as a diffuse density overlying the spine (arrow). The posterior portion of the right hemidiaphragm cannot be identified (silhouette sign). *C*. Schematic representation of right-lower-lobe collapse.

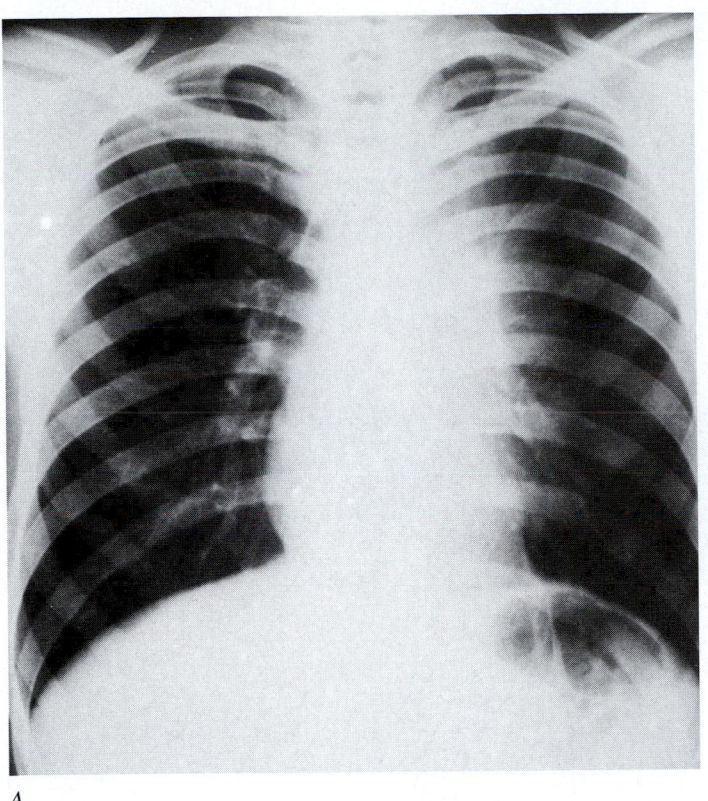

A

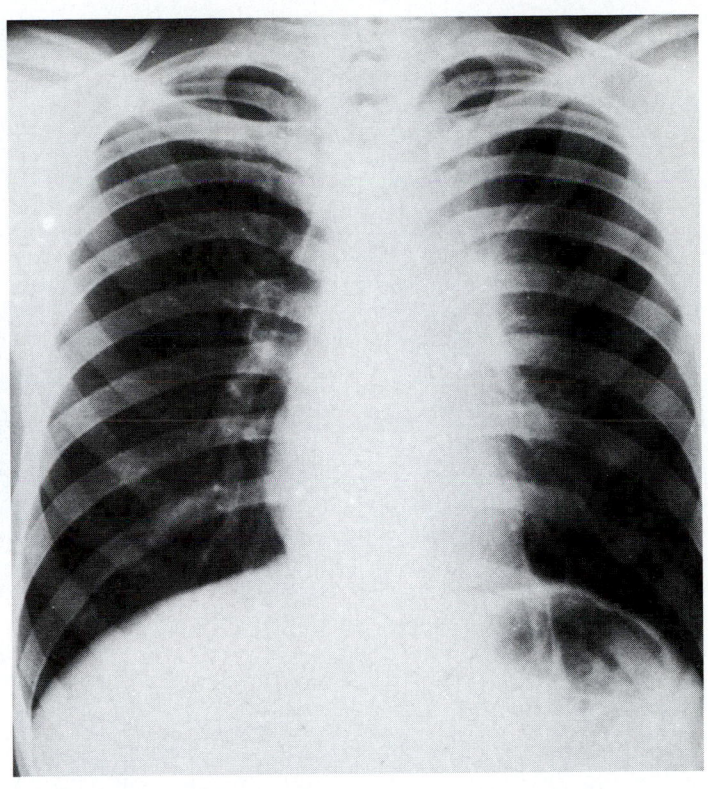

B

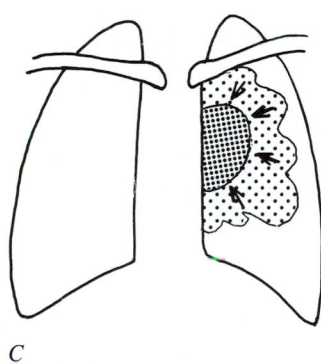
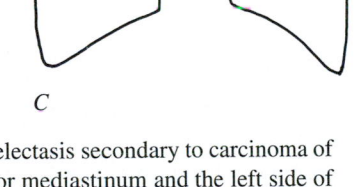

C

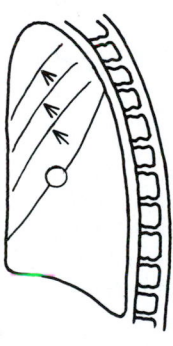

FIGURE 32-45   Left-upper-lobe atelectasis secondary to carcinoma of the lung. *A*. PA view. The left superior mediastinum and the left side of the heart are indistinct, owing to collapse of the left upper lobe medi- ally. *B*. Lateral view. The collapsed lung is seen as a density anterior to the major fissure (arrows), which is displaced far anteriorly. *C*. Schematic representation of left-upper-lobe collapse.

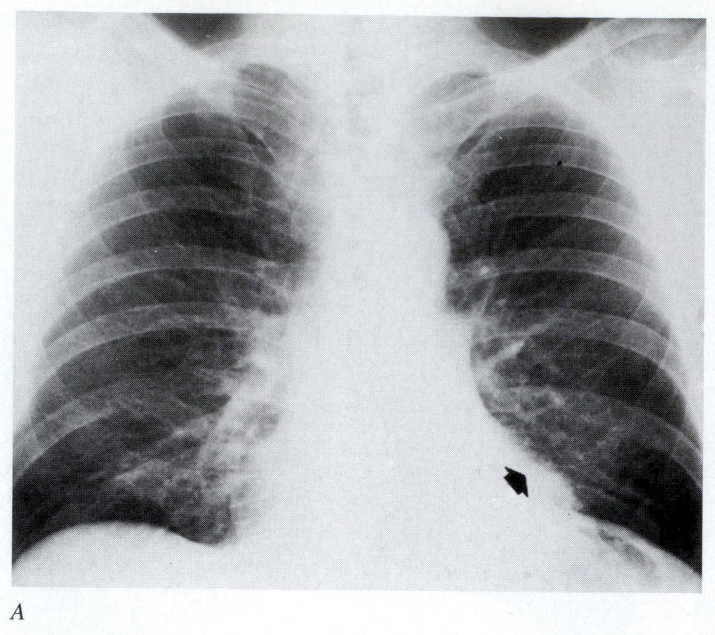
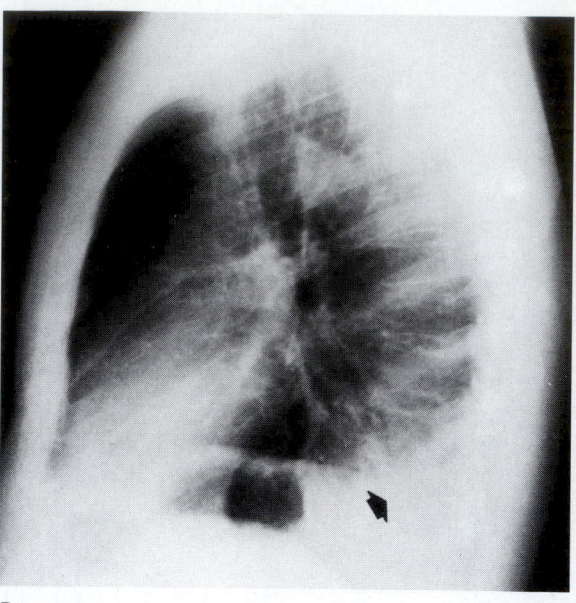

A

B

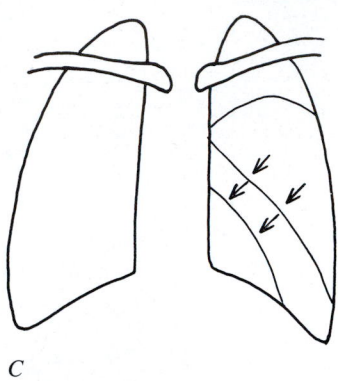
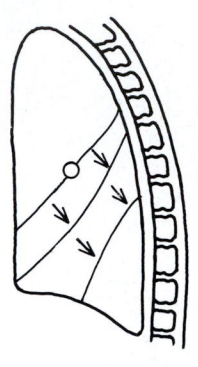

C

FIGURE 32-46 Left-lower-lobe atelectasis (postoperative). *A*. PA view. The collapsed left lower lobe is seen as a straight line (arrow) behind the left heart border. No vasculature can be seen through the heart shadow, and the medial border of the left hemidiaphragm is obscured by the collapsed left lower lobe (arrow). *B*. Lateral view. Density over spine and absence of left posterior diaphragm. *C*. Schematic representation of left-lower-lobe collapse.

CT is extremely useful in the evaluation of atelectasis, since the technique may clearly demonstrate the cause—for example, a primary carcinoma of the lung. Conversely, CT may demonstrate an open bronchus, strongly suggesting that the atelectasis is not due to an endobronchial tumor. In this regard, it is important to note that some tumors (e.g., alveolar cell carcinoma and lymphoma) may cause atelectasis with an open bronchus.

Finally, CT may suggest the diagnosis of rounded atelectasis (Fig. 32-47) or may be particularly useful in demonstrating mediastinal adenopathy or the extent of a tumor that invades the mediastinum or great vessels.

Diffuse Alveolar Disease

The prototype of a pathologic process that affects alveoli diffusely is pulmonary edema (Fig. 32-36). Most often, pulmonary edema is secondary to left ventricular failure. However, noncardiac pulmonary edema is common and may have several underlying causes, including hypersensitivity reactions to drugs or inhaled toxins, adult respiratory distress syndrome, uremia, drug overdose, oxygen toxicity, and near-drowning.[6,7] Cardiac pulmonary edema characteristically clears rapidly after appropriate therapy, whereas noncardiac pulmonary edema often requires days or weeks to clear (see Chapter 85).

If diffuse alveolar consolidation persists for weeks or months, chronic disorders, such as pulmonary alveolar proteinosis (Fig. 32-48), alveolar cell carcinoma (Figs. 32-35 and 32-39), sarcoidosis, metastatic carcinoma, desquamative interstitial pneumonitis, and lymphoma are among the disorders that should be considered as reasons for this rather unusual radiographic pattern.[6,7]

As with localized disease, CT is not particularly useful in distinguishing one type of diffuse alveolar disease from another. However, CT may show unsuspected cavitation or mediastinal adenopathy, which may be useful in differential diagnosis.

Interstitial Lung Disease

The radiographic features of interstitial lung disease differ from those of the alveolar disorders (Fig. 32-49). In interstitial disease, the pattern is discrete and sharp, rather than fluffy and ir-

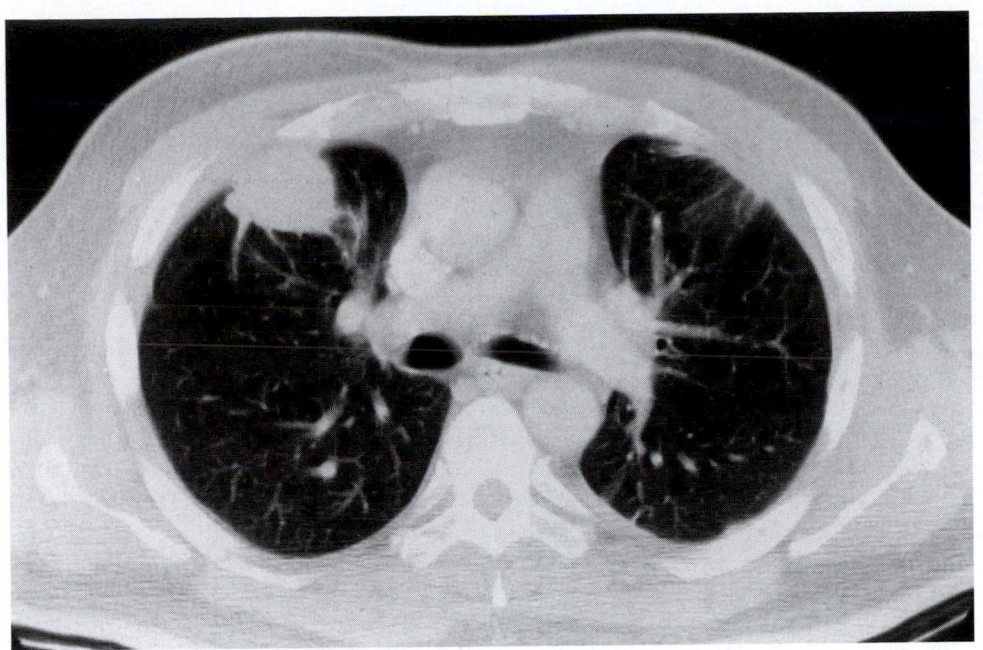

FIGURE 32-47   Rounded atelectasis. A mass with a "tail" can be seen in the anterior segment of the right upper lobe. Pleural thickening is seen on the left side, with transpulmonary bands extending into the left upper lobe. The mass on the right represents rounded atelectasis, a finding usually associated with asbestos exposure. The changes on the right probably represent an early stage in the development of rounded atelectasis.

regular, and the lesions tend to be diffuse, rather than localized. In addition, coalescence is not a feature, and the small densities are characteristically nodular, reticular, or linear.

Pathologic interstitial processes may be acute or chronic, although the chronic causes are more common. Within the acute category, a pattern changing over hours to days usually represents interstitial pulmonary edema. Occasionally, a rapidly changing interstitial pattern represents pneumonia due to *Pneumocystis carinii* or cytomegalovirus. The acute interstitial disorders typically cause a linear or reticular pattern, which is characterized by prominent Kerley's lines throughout the lung fields (Fig. 32-49A).

In his original description in 1951, Kerley associated thin, radiographic parenchymal opacities with left ventricular failure. At first, Kerley's lines were thought to represent swollen pulmonary lymphatics. It is now recognized that Kerley's lines usually represent edematous septa within the pulmonary interstitium. Three patterns exist. Kerley type B lines are the most familiar and are particularly prominent at the lung bases, where they appear as straight, thin lines approximately 1 cm long; they are oriented parallel to the diaphragm. Kerley type A lines represent septae deep within the substance of the lungs; they radiate from the hili. Kerley type C lines probably represent coalescence of A and B lines.

Chronic interstitial lung diseases may be caused by a wide variety of diseases (Figs. 32-49 and 32-50), including pneumoconioses; sarcoidosis; lymphangitic spread of tumors; infections, such as miliary tuberculosis, interstitial pneumonia, and fungal diseases; allergic lung disease; collagen vascular diseases; eosinophilic granuloma; and idiopathic interstitial fibrosis.[6,7]

Characterization of the pattern of interstitial disease as nodular, reticular, or linear may help in differential diagnosis, since many of the interstitial lung diseases assume, almost exclusively, one of these three patterns.

Interstitial nodules range in size from minute to massive. Large nodules generally represent metastatic tumor (Fig. 32-51). Smaller nodules are found in pneumoconiosis or silicosis, miliary tuberculosis, sarcoidosis (Fig. 32-49B), and allergic lung disease.

Linear densities, as noted previously, are more characteristic of acute lung disease [e.g., interstitial pulmonary edema (Fig. 32-49A) or interstitial pneumonia]. A similar, but chronic, pattern occurs in lymphangitic spread of metastatic tumor (Figs. 32-49C and 32-13A).

A reticular pattern suggests collagen vascular disease when the reticular or cystic changes are tiny and are confined primarily to the lung bases (Fig. 32-49D). Asbestosis, desquamative interstitial pneumonitis, and usual interstitial pneumonitis also cause a basilar reticular pattern (Fig. 32-52). Eosinophilic granuloma of the lung causes a similar pattern at the lung apices. A larger reticular pattern suggests idiopathic pulmonary fibrosis or the end-stage lung pattern that often represents the final common denominator of a variety of chronic interstitial lung diseases.

Most interstitial diseases cause loss of lung volume on the radiograph, since these disorders are truly restrictive in their pathophysiological effect. However, two interstitial diseases that produce diffuse, small bullous changes are characteristically associated with preserved lung volume: eosinophilic granuloma and lymphangioleiomyomatosis. These are relatively uncommon causes of interstitial lung disease.[7] It should be recognized that patients with interstitial lung disease may have concurrent chronic obstructive pulmonary disease, in which case lung volumes may be preserved.

High-resolution CT has emerged as a useful technique for evaluating interstitial lung disease.[2] CT may be useful in identifying interstitial disease that is not seen on the plain radiograph and in identifying the underlying cause.

CT patterns of interstitial lung disease follow, to some degree, the patterns seen on the plain radiograph. Collagen vascular disease and idiopathic pulmonary fibrosis typically have reticular or cystic changes in the periphery of the lung and at the lung bases (Fig. 32-52). Sarcoidosis and lymphangitic spread of tumor demonstrate a bronchovascular distribution; occasionally, densities may be seen outlining the pulmonary lobule (Fig. 32-13). Hypersensitivity disease frequently is associated with an alveolar or "ground glass" pattern. Finally, metastatic tumor (Fig. 32-51) and miliary tuberculosis usually are characterized by fine nodules.

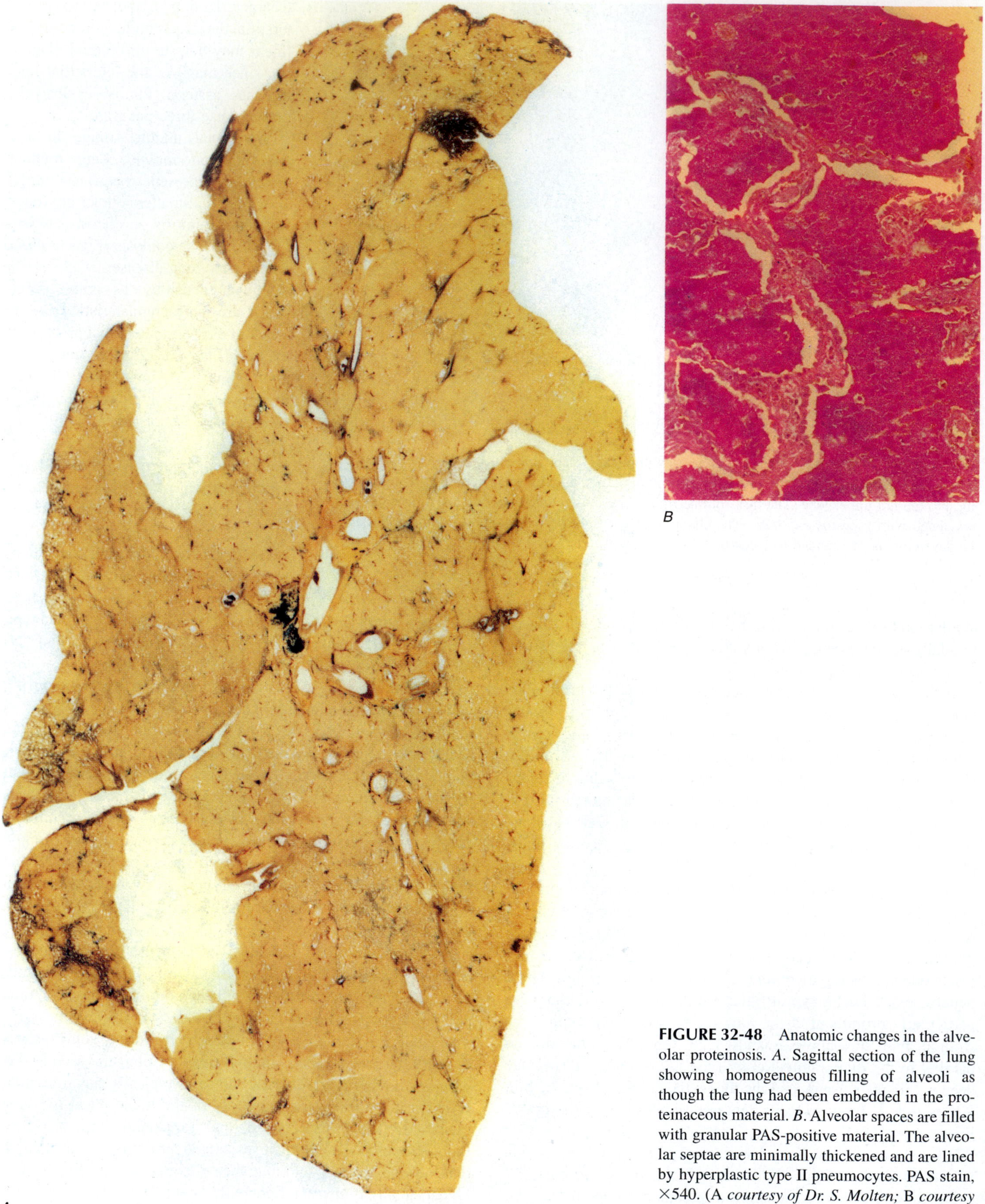

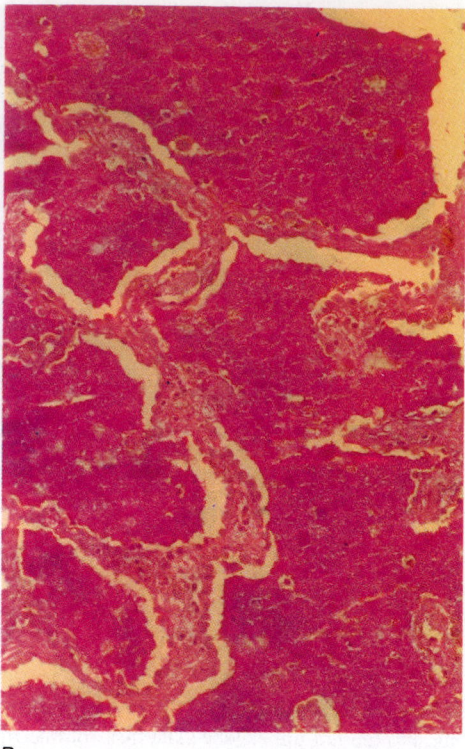

B

A

FIGURE 32-48   Anatomic changes in the alveolar proteinosis. *A.* Sagittal section of the lung showing homogeneous filling of alveoli as though the lung had been embedded in the proteinaceous material. *B.* Alveolar spaces are filled with granular PAS-positive material. The alveolar septae are minimally thickened and are lined by hyperplastic type II pneumocytes. PAS stain, ×540. (A *courtesy of Dr. S. Molten;* B *courtesy of Dr. G. G. Pietra.*)

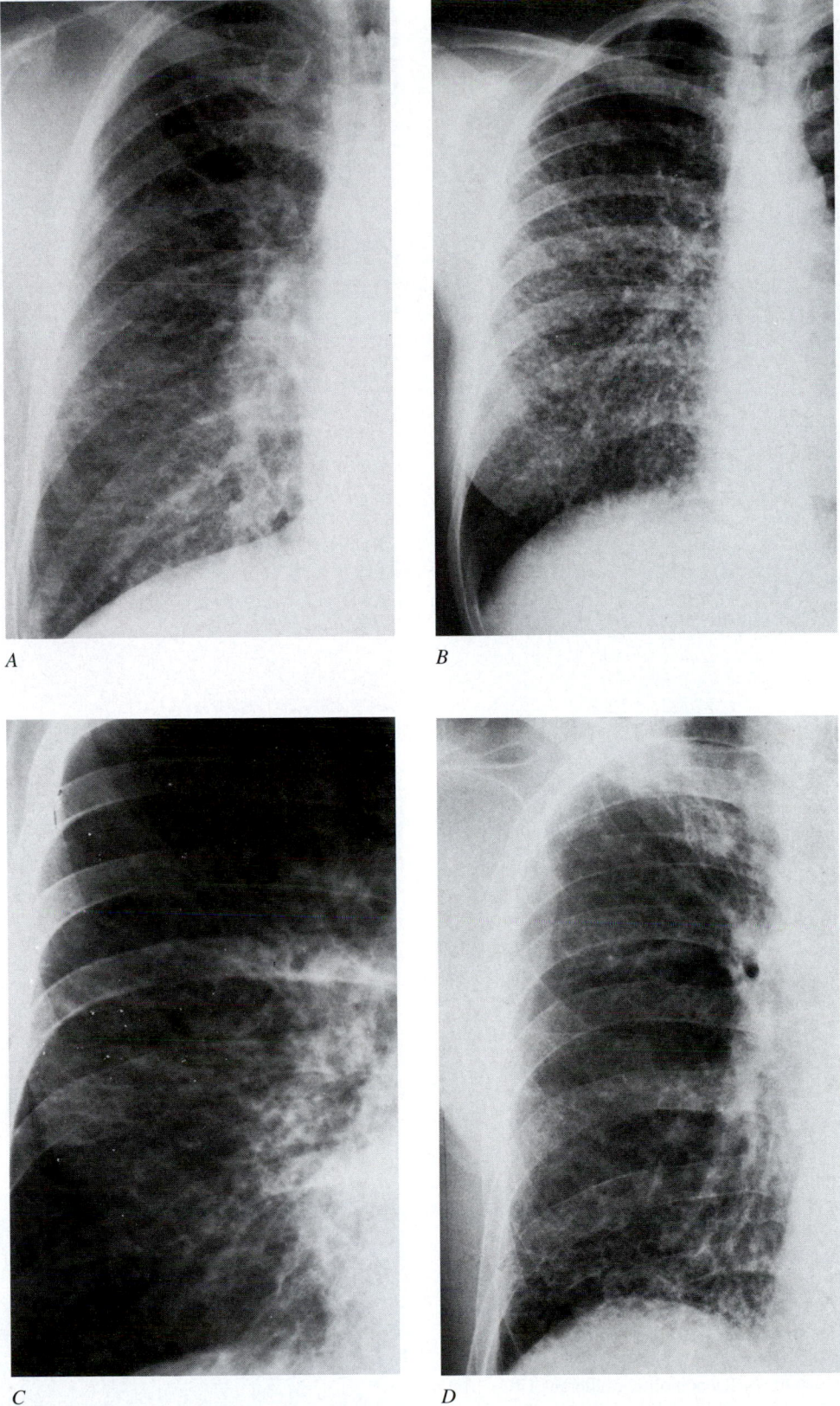

FIGURE 32-49   Diffuse interstitial disease. *A.* Linear interstitial pattern produced by interstitial pulmonary edema. The pattern is caused by fluid in the interstitial spaces of the lungs, particularly in interlobar septae. *B.* Nodular interstitial pattern produced by Boeck's sarcoid. Multiple small, discrete nodules involve both lung fields diffusely. Adenopathy is absent. *C.* Lymphagitic spread of tumore. The linear interstitial pattern was caused by metastatic carcinoma of the pancreas. *D.* Reticular or cystic interstitial lung pattern. The pattern is most marked at the bases and is characteristic of the collagen vascular disease, particularly scleroderma (as in this patient).

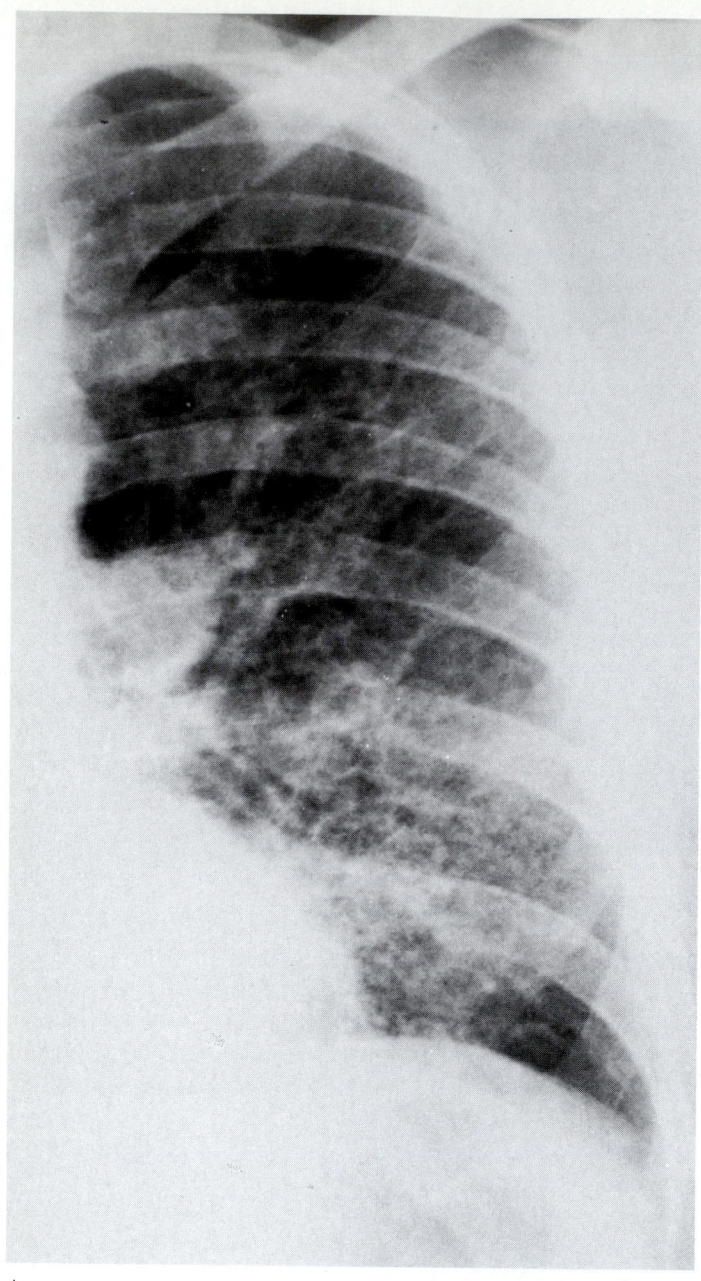

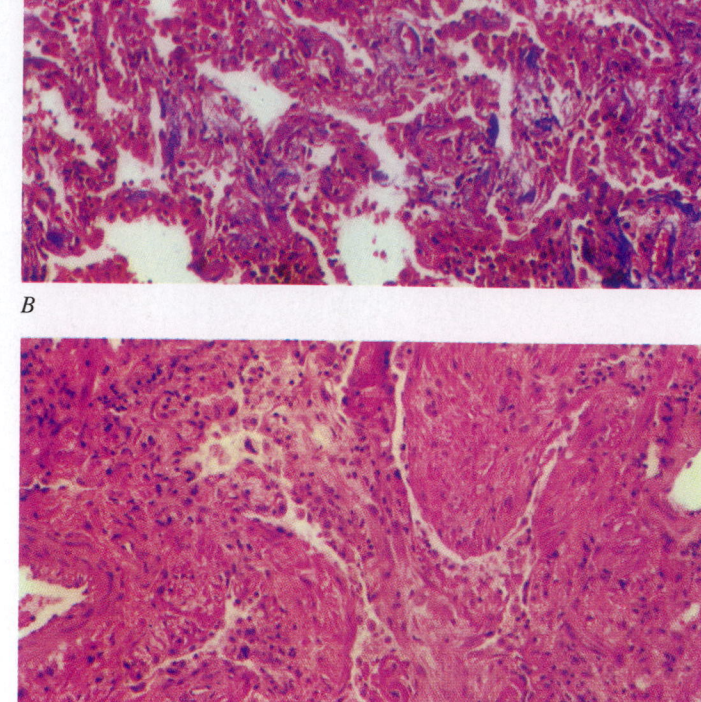

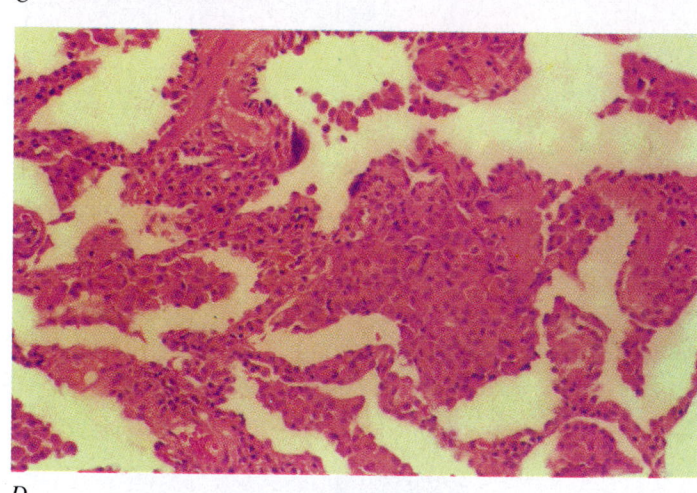

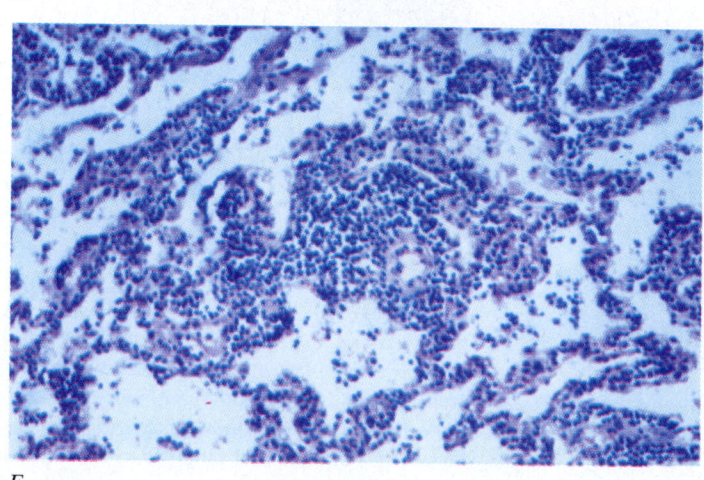

FIGURE 32-50 Different types of interstitial pneumonia. *A*. Chest radiograph of fibrosing alveolitis (usual interstitial pneumonia). *B*. Usual interstitial pneumonia (UIP). The alveolar septae are irregularly thickened by collagen (blue) and mononuclear cells. The airspaces contain desquamated epithelial cells, macrophages, and newly formed fibrous tissue. Masson trichrome, ×540. *C*. Bronchiolitis obliterans (BO). The luman of a small bronchus is obliterated by fibrin (bright red), collagenous tissue, and macrophages. H&E, ×540. *D*. Desquamative interstitial pneumonia (DIP). The airspaces are filled with desquamated epithelial cells and occasional eosinophils. The alveolar walls are lined by hyperplastic type II cells. Giant cells are also present. H&E, ×400. *E*. Lymphocytic interstitial pneumonia (LIP). The alveolar septae are infiltrated by monoculear cells, primarily mature lymphocytes and plasma cells. H&E, ×405. (B *to* E, *courtesy of Dr. G. G. Pietra.*)

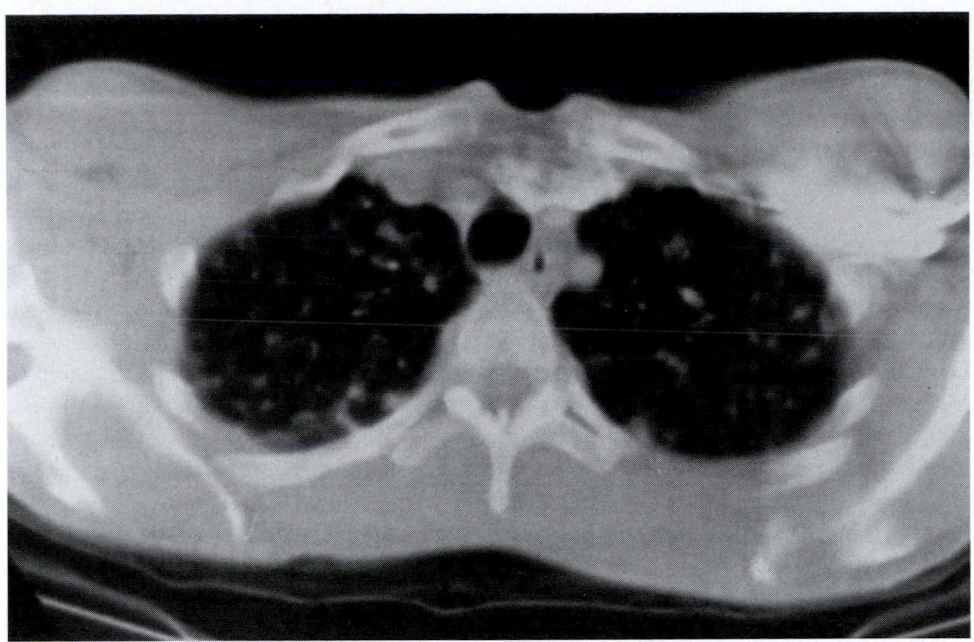

FIGURE 32-51 Metastic tumor causing a nodular interstitial pattern. Multiple fine nodules can be seen throughout the lung. The moderate-size nodules are characteristic of metastatic tumor. Finer nodules suggest miliary tuberculosis or other types of nodular interstitial disease.

The Solitary Nodule

A wide variety of pathologic processes appear on the chest radiograph as a solitary nodule (see Chapter 110).[5,12] Among the most common are primary carcinoma of the lung, granulomas due to tuberculosis or fungal infection, metastatic carcinoma, and organizing pneumonia. Less common are hamartoma, bron-

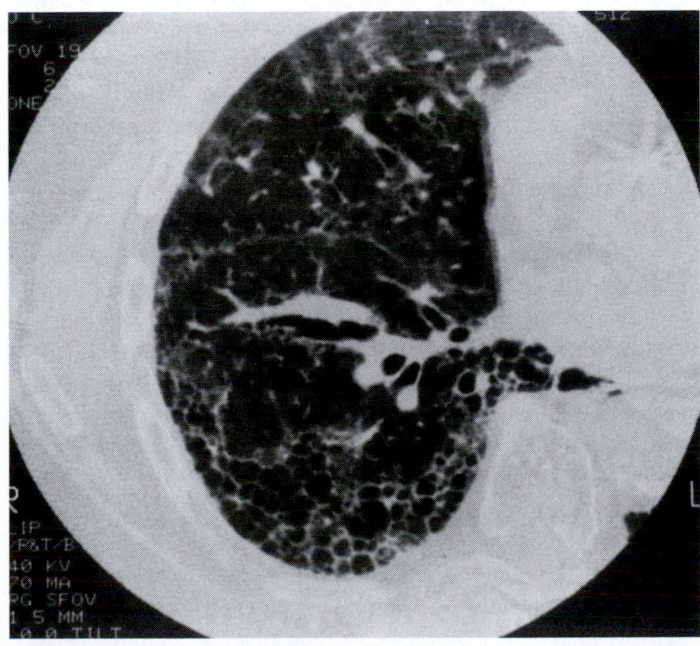

FIGURE 32-52 High-resolution CT of reticular interstitial lung disease. The characteristic peripheral reticular pattern is from a patient with idiopathic pulmonary fibrosis. Collagen vascular disease causes an indistinguishable pattern.

chogenic cyst, bronchial adenoma, arteriovenous malformation, pulmonary sequestration, necrobiotic nodule due to rheumatoid arthritis, or Wegener's granulomatosis, lymphoma, inflammatory pseudotumor, and lipoid granuloma.[2,7] Although the radiograph is invaluable for detection of a pulmonary nodule, it is usually of little help in elucidating the underlying cause. Although certain radiographic aspects of a nodule may suggest its benign or malignant nature, in most instances histologic or cytologic proof is required.[1]

One radiologic clue to the origin of a pulmonary nodule is the character of its border. Ill-defined margins suggest an inflammatory lesion (e.g., tuberculosis or pneumonia). On the other hand, a very sharply circumscribed pulmonary nodule with a regular contour is more likely to be a granuloma or hamartoma. However, metastatic tumor often presents with a sharply circumscribed edge, and primary lung neoplasms may present either as sharply circumscribed nodules or nodules with ill-defined margins.

The age of the patient is useful in the differential diagnosis of a solitary nodule. Primary carcinoma of the lung is extremely rare in patients less than 30 years old, whereas in patients older than 50 years, more than half of solitary nodules are primary carcinomas of the lung.

Occasionally, the radiograph may be sufficiently convincing of the benignity of a pulmonary nodule to preclude the need for diagnostic evaluation, including possible thoracoscopy or thoracotomy. Extensive calcification within the nodule suggests that the process is benign; laminography may be helpful in demonstrating the calcification. Benignity is also suggested by calcification that is central, concentric, diffuse, or punctate ("popcorn" calcification). On the other hand, eccentric calcification is of no diagnostic help, since it also occurs in malignant disease, presumably as a consequence of envelopment of a preexisting benign calcified focus within an expanding neoplastic process. In some centers, CT density numbers have been definitive in distinguishing benign from malignant pulmonary nodules; unfortunately, this experience has not been universal.

Prominent vascular shadows extending from a nodule suggest that the nodule is an arteriovenous malformation; the shadows actually represent veins. Arteriography is useful in confirming the vascular nature of the lesion (Fig. 32-5B). CT and MRI are also helpful in diagnosing arteriovenous malformations. A basal lung nodule that is suggestive of a pulmonary sequestration can be identified arteriographically. The study demonstrates that the mass is supplied by an anomalous artery arising from the abdominal aorta. The artery can usually be identified by either CT or MRI as well.

The lung is uniquely suited for serial radiographic estimates of the size of a solitary pulmonary nodule. This feature has led to the practical concept of *doubling time*—the time required for a tumor to double in volume (not diameter). A previous radiograph in which the nodule was present, even if unrecognized, serves as a useful baseline for estimating the rate of nodule growth. If a nodule does not change in size for 2 years, it is likely that the process is benign. Conversely, any growth of the nodule within 1 year should raise suspicion of malignancy.[18] Usually, malignant tumors grow quickly, with a doubling in volume between 1 and 15 months (Fig. 32-53). Not uncommonly, however, a slowly growing nodule proves to be a primary carcinoma of the lung—usually an adenocarcinoma or alveolar cell carcinoma.

The presence of cavitation within a pulmonary nodule is usually unhelpful in determining whether the nodule is benign or malignant.[7] Other radiographic features, including the presence of stranding, satellite lesions, or associated pleural disease, are seen in both benign and malignant processes and do not constitute bases for distinction.

Occasionally, CT is helpful in identifying calcification within a solitary nodule, or in suggesting that a nodule is probably benign by virtue of having a high CT density.[1,17] CT can also help distinguish an arteriovenous malformation (see above). However, perhaps the main use of CT is in determining whether a solitary nodule is indeed solitary. Many nodules that appear to be solitary on the plain radiograph are shown by CT to be multiple; many of the other nodules are much smaller than the nodule originally identified. The presence of multiple nodules strongly suggests the diagnosis of metastatic tumor.

It should be emphasized that a definitive diagnosis is rarely possible with radiographic techniques alone. Sputum cytology, bronchoscopy with bronchial washings, brushings, and biopsy, transthoracic lung aspiration or biopsy, thoracoscopic biopsy, or open lung biopsy is necessary (see Chapters 38 and 39).

Multiple Pulmonary Nodules

Although a solitary pulmonary nodule may be benign or malignant, multiple nodules strongly suggest metastatic tumor. Occasional exceptions to this rule include rheumatoid nodules (Fig. 32-54), fungal infections, alveolar sarcoidosis, and Wegener's granulomatosis.[6] CT is usually not very helpful when multiple pulmonary nodules have already been identified on the plain chest radiograph. Although CT may detect additional nodules, this information is generally not useful clinically.

Left Ventricular Failure

Failure of the left ventricle is generally easy to recognize on the chest radiograph. The heart is enlarged, and the pulmonary vasculature is prominent. Changes in the size of the heart and central vessels are most evident on consecutive radiographs.

In chronic left ventricular failure, chronic dependent edema and interstitial fibrosis at the lung bases result in redirection of pulmonary blood flow from the bases to the apices (see above); the vessels of the upper lobes become more prominent than those of the lower lobes, a finding referred to as *cephalization*. Interstitial edema often accompanies pulmonary venous congestion and is manifested by a diffuse increase in interstitial markings,

usually in a linear distribution (Fig. 32-49A); Kerley's lines are characteristic features of interstitial edema. Alveolar edema may follow the development of interstitial edema and is characterized by diffuse bilateral consolidation (Fig. 32-36).[14]

Pleural effusions often accompany biventricular heart failure. At first, the pleural effusions are associated with prominence of the pulmonary vascular markings, cephalization, or both. However, while the pulmonary congestion clears in response to therapy, the pleural effusions often remain after the pulmonary vessels have returned to normal size. Pleural effusions in congestive heart failure may be unilateral or bilateral. If unilateral, the effusion almost invariably occurs on the right side.[14] As noted previously, recognition of left ventricular failure is difficult in the patient with obstructive lung disease because hyperinflated lungs and an elongated heart make it difficult to recognize cardiomegaly and pulmonary vascular engorgement. Comparison with previous films is paramount in recognizing subtle changes in cardiac size and in pulmonary vascular engorgement.

THE MEDIASTINUM

As pointed out in Chapter 93, the anatomic delineations of "compartments" of the mediastinum are not defined consistently throughout the medical literature. For radiographic diagnosis, a simple classification has been employed (Fig. 32-55): 1. The *anterior* compartment, which extends from the sternum anteriorly to the heart, aorta, and brachiocephalic vessels posteriorly, comprises only the thymus and a few lymph nodes. 2. The *middle,* or *visceral,* compartment contains the heart, great vessels, trachea and its branches, esophagus, and descending aorta. It extends from the posterior border of the anterior compartment to the anterior border of the vertebral column. These boundaries differ from the anatomist's classification (Fig. 32-55A), which relegates portions of the esophagus and the descending aorta to the posterior mediastinum. 3. The *posterior* compartment contains the vertebrae and the paravertebral sulci. Applying this classification to the lateral chest radiograph, one may categorize mediastinal masses readily according to their position with the mediastinum.

Common findings in the anterior compartment include enlarged lymph nodes, substernal goiter, thymus and thymic tumors, and teratomas.[9] Distinction among these can be made on the basis of their position within the anterior mediastinum and their appearance. Thyroid masses almost invariably lie high in the anterior mediastinum and displace the trachea and esophagus (Fig. 32-56A and B); benign, or minimally invasive, thymomas and teratomas generally lie below the aortic arch and present as a single, well-demarcated mass (Fig. 32-56C and D). Lymph node enlargement is generally more diffuse and often nodular or lumpy in character (Figs. 32-57 and 32-58). Lymph node enlargement may be produced by metastatic tumor, particularly from a primary neoplasm of the lung, or by sarcoidosis, lymphoma, or primary tuberculosis. Less common causes of mediastinal lymphadenopathy include other inflammatory processes, such as fungal infection or infectious mononucleosis. Highly invasive thymoma and malignant teratoma may be diffuse and, therefore, indistinguishable from diffuse lymphadenopathy (Fig. 32-59).

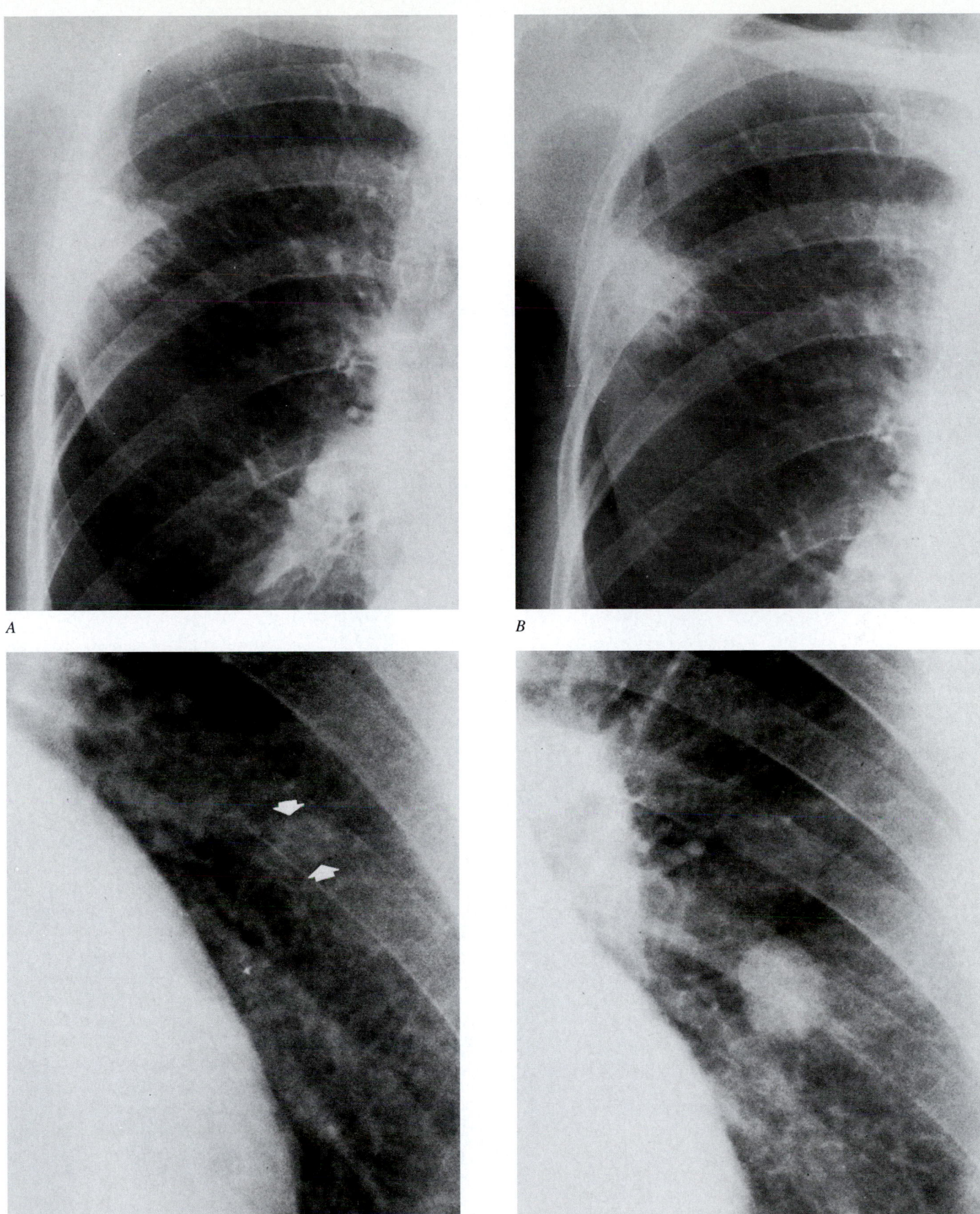

FIGURE 32-53 *Top,* carcinoma of the lung with a long doubling time. An interval of 18 months elapsed between *A* and *B*. The right-upper-lobe lesion, which enlarged minimally during that time, proved to be squamous cell carcinoma of the lung. *Bottom,* carcinoma of the lung with a short doubling time. An interval of 4 months elapsed between *C* and *D*. The nodule was not detected on the first radiograph (*C*). It proved to be an oat cell carcinoma of the lung.

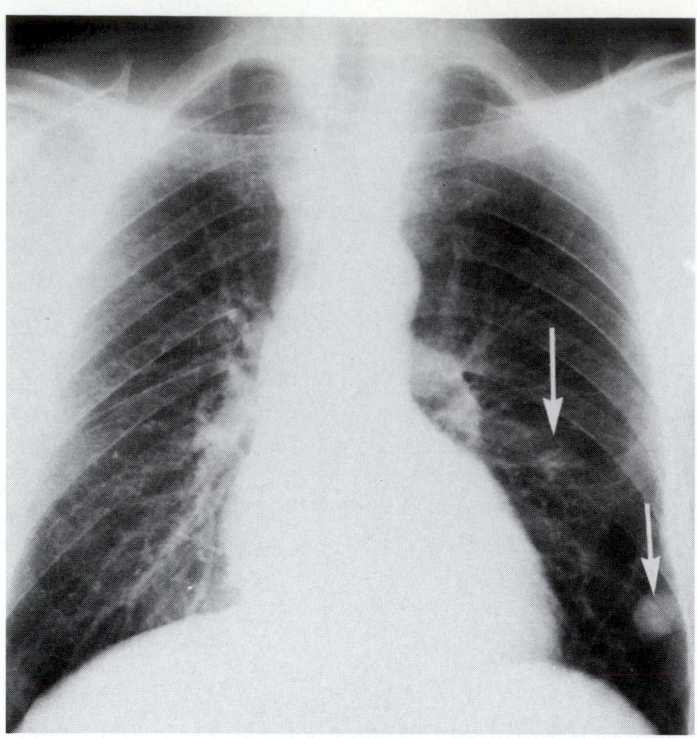

FIGURE 32-54 Rheumatoid nodules. the nodules in the left lung of this patient with rheumatoid arthritis regressed 4 months later.

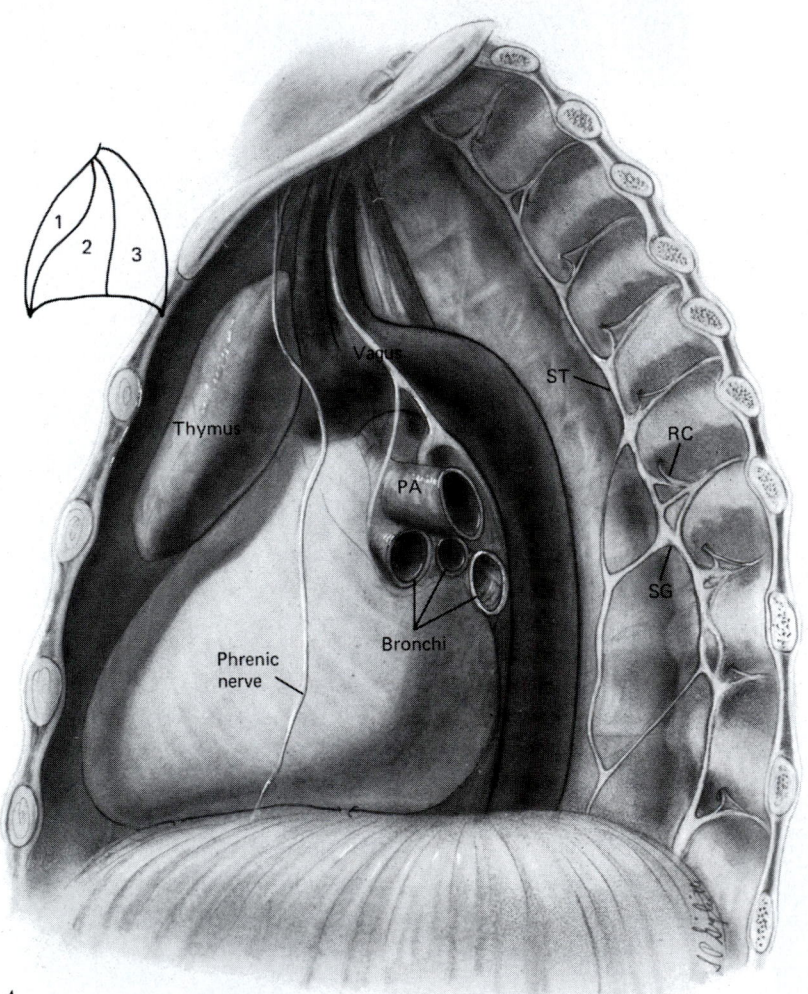

A

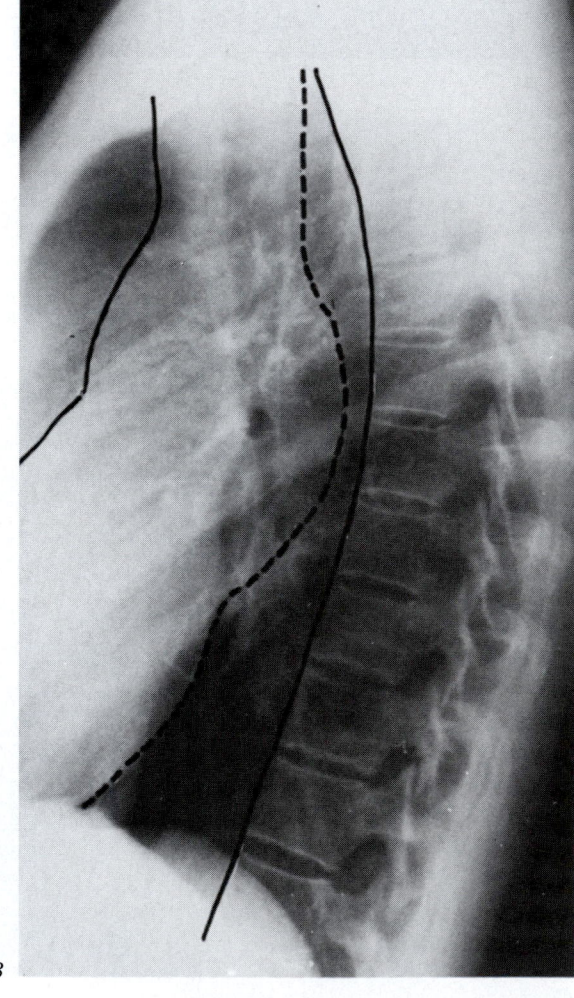

B

FIGURE 32-55 Compartments of the mediastinum. *A.* Anatomic view of the compartments of the mediastinum. The subdivisions in the small schematic (top left) correspond to those designated by the solid black lines in *B*. PA = pulmonary artery; ST = sympathetic trunk; SG = sympathetic ganglion; RC = ramus communicans. (*From Jones et al, 1980.*)

B. Radiographic division of the mediastinum. The closed lines delineate the anterior, middle, and posterior compartments. The dashed line represents the division of the middle and posterior mediastinum that is conventionally used by anatomists.

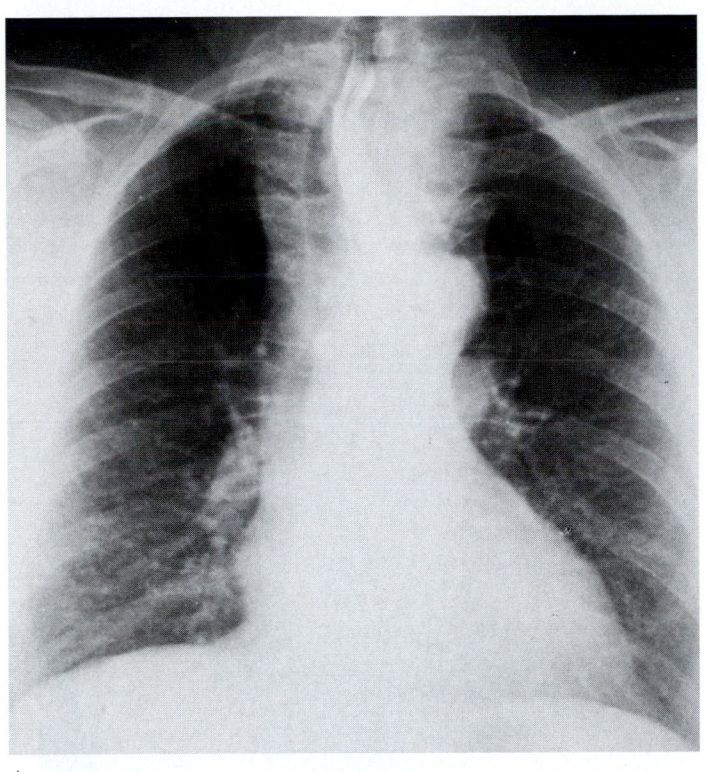

A

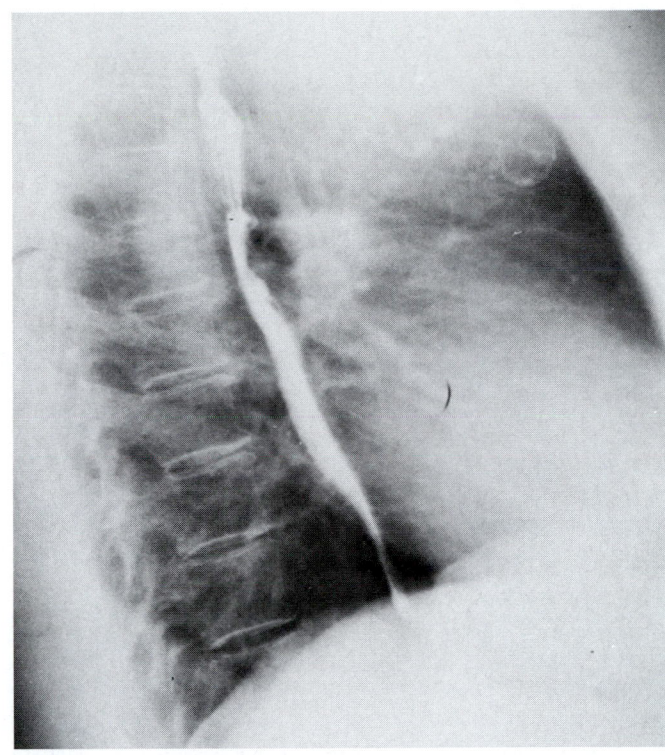

B

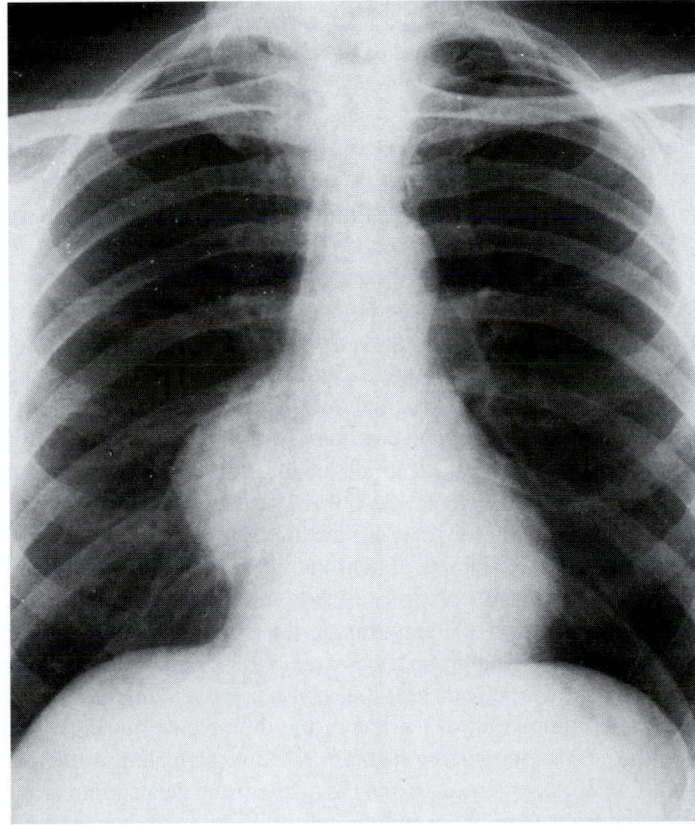

C

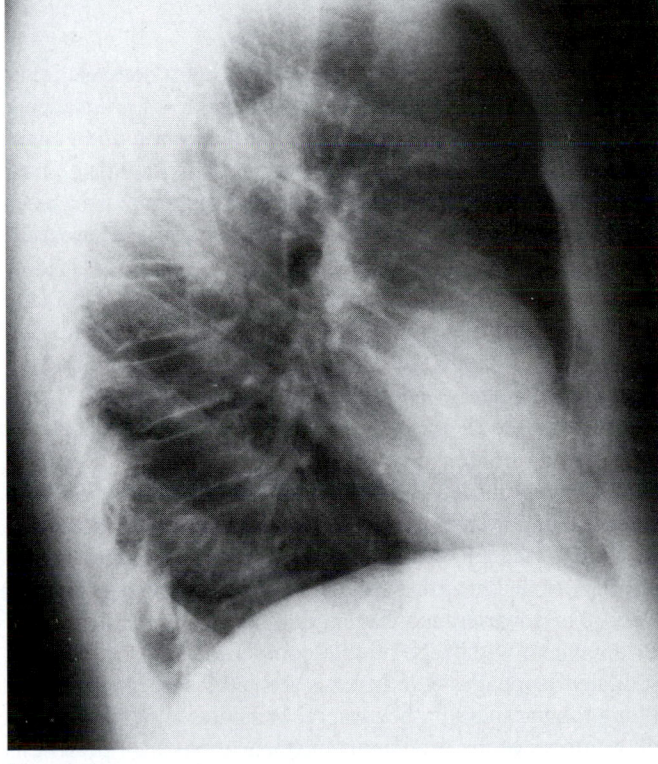

D

FIGURE 32-56 *Top,* substernal thyroid. *A.* PA view. A large mass in the neck extends below the clavicle. The trachea and esophagus are displaced to the right. *B.* Lateral view. The trachea and esophagus are also displaced posteriorly. Several calcifications are present within the mass. *Bottom,* thymoma. *C.* PA view. A discrete mass (thymoma) lies along the right heart border. *D.* Lateral view. The mass also overlies the anterior portion of the cardiac shadow.

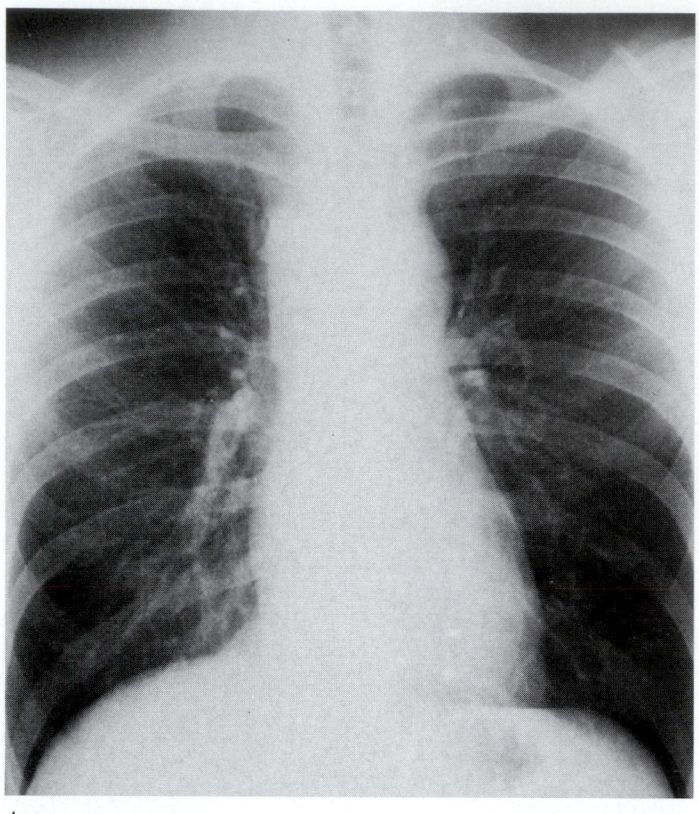

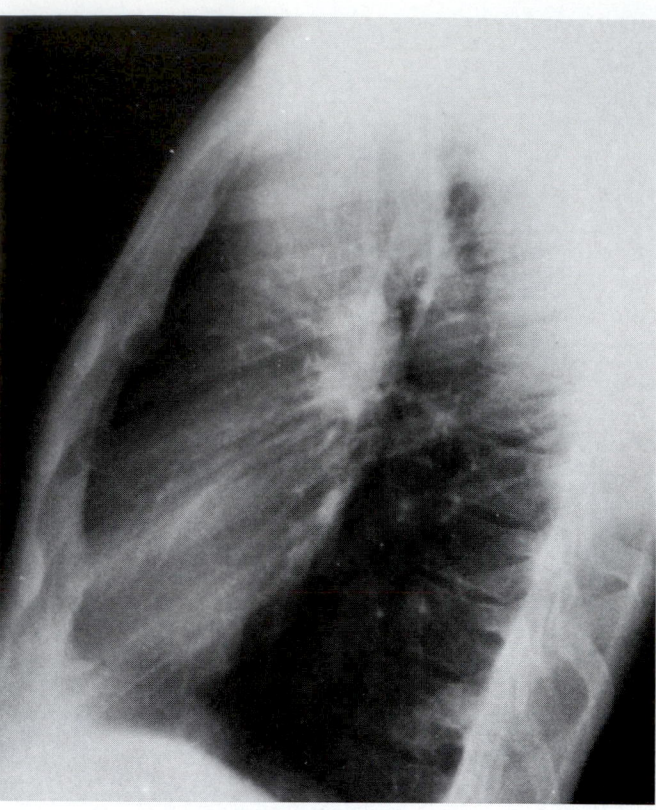

A

B

FIGURE 32-57 Hodgkin's disease. *A.* PA view. A lobulated mass widens the mediastinum on both sides of the trachea. *B.* Lateral view. The mass lies anterior to the trachea.

The middle compartment of the mediastinum contains all of the mediastinal viscera, as well as lymph nodes. Lymphadenopathy in the middle compartment is quite common and is generally seen as a diffuse mass, often associated with enlargement of one or both hili (Fig. 32-58). A localized mass may be caused by an aneurysm or other anomaly of the aorta or great vessels. Its vascular nature is suggested by proximity to the aortic shadow and is readily confirmed by aortography (Fig. 32-60). CT and MRI are also extremely well suited to evaluation of vascular lesions (Fig. 32-61); MRI is somewhat safer, since it does not require administration of intravenous contrast material. Duplication cysts of the esophagus and the tracheobronchial tree are also common in the visceral compartment. These localized masses are smooth and well circumscribed; generally, they do not contain air. Bronchogenic cysts commonly occur at the tracheal carina, whereas esophageal duplication cysts are characteristically located near the distal end of the esophagus (Fig. 32-62*A* and *B*). However, esophageal and bronchogenic cysts may occur anywhere within the middle compartment.[9]

A dilated esophagus is sometimes seen on the chest radiograph as a long tubular mass in the visceral compartment (Fig. 32-62*C* and *D*); tumors of the esophagus or trachea may also present as more localized mediastinal masses. Radiographs taken with barium in the esophagus are particularly helpful in characterizing masses in the visceral compartment.

In the posterior (paraspinal) compartment, the most common radiographic abnormalities are neurogenic tumors (Fig. 32-63).[9]

However, tumors or infections of the vertebral column may also present as masses in the posterior compartment (Fig. 32-64).

CT is ideally suited to the evaluation of mediastinal masses (Fig. 32-65). The technique clearly shows the compartment in which the mediastinal mass lies, and it readily permits distinction between adenopathy and other abnormalities.[11] Adenopathy tends to occur in several areas of the mediastinum, rather than remaining confined to a single compartment or area within the compartment. Other mediastinal masses can be distinguished following the same basic rules for plain film differentiation. Use of contrast material permits identification of vascular structures, which may appear masslike (Fig. 32-66). MRI is also very useful for identifying vascular lesions of the mediastinum (Fig. 32-61). Certain tumors (e.g., those of neurogenic origin) are readily characterized by MRI.[11]

Finally, a variety of radiographic lines or stripes seen in and around the mediastinum on the PA radiograph can be very useful diagnostically. Among these is the *posterior paraspinal line,* which is a pleural reflection to the left of the thoracic spine (Figs. 32-5 and 32-64). The posterior paraspinal line is related to the descending aorta; it is seen on the right side if the descending aorta is on the right. Tumors or inflammatory diseases in the vertebral bodies displace the posterior paraspinal line to the left, creating a posterior paraspinal line on the right, where one is not ordinarily present. Large spurs arising from the vertebral body on the right also push out the pleura, creating a paraspinal line on the right (Fig. 32-5*A*); this is not clinically important.

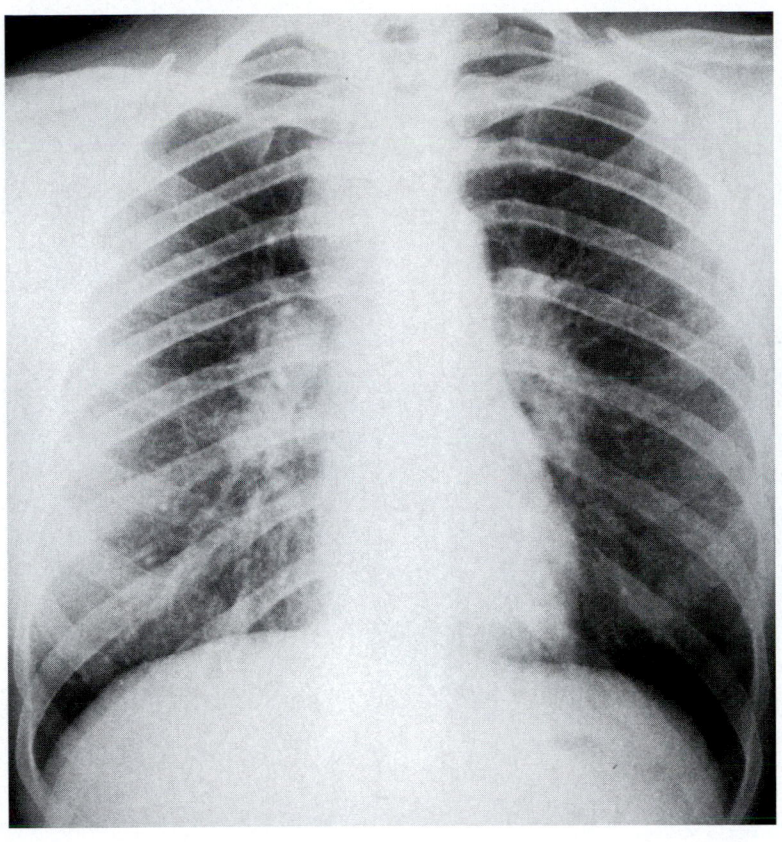

A

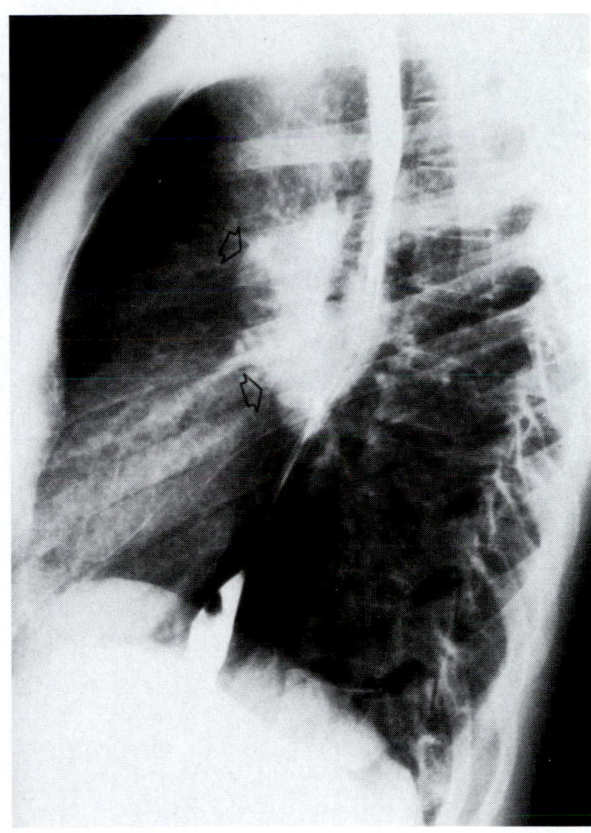

B

FIGURE 32-58 Sarcoidosis. *A*. PA view. A mass is present in the right paratracheal area, and both hili are enlarged. *B*. Lateral view. The hilar enlargement (arrows) is striking. Enlargement in these three node-bearing areas is characteristic of sarcoidosis.

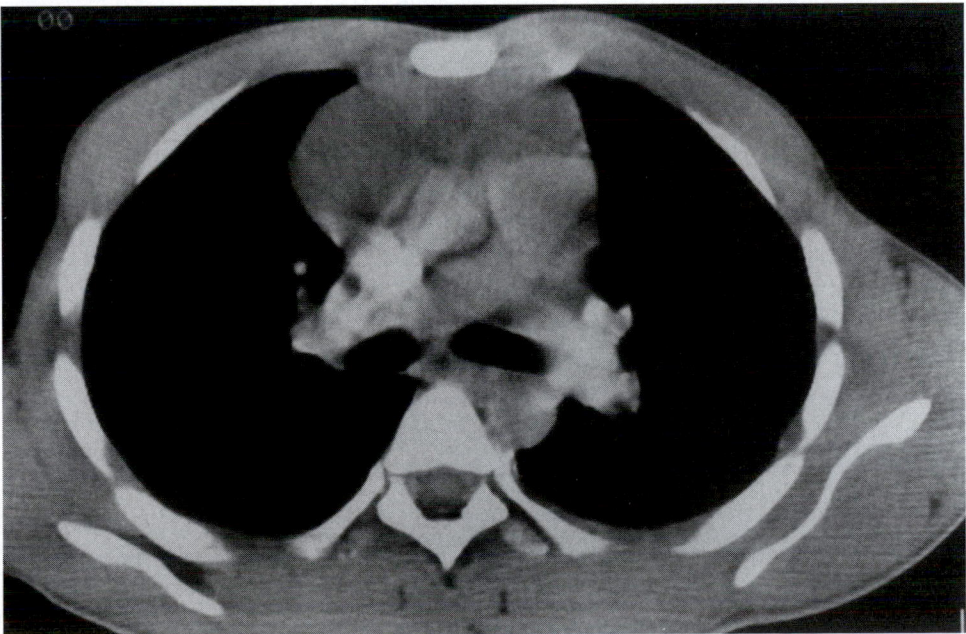

FIGURE 32-59 Malignant teratoma. A poorly circumscribed, diffuse mass can be seen anterior to the great vessels. Although the mass could represent lymphadenopathy from a number of causes, it is also consistent with malignant thymoma or teratoma. In this patient with AIDS, the mass was shown to be a teratoma.

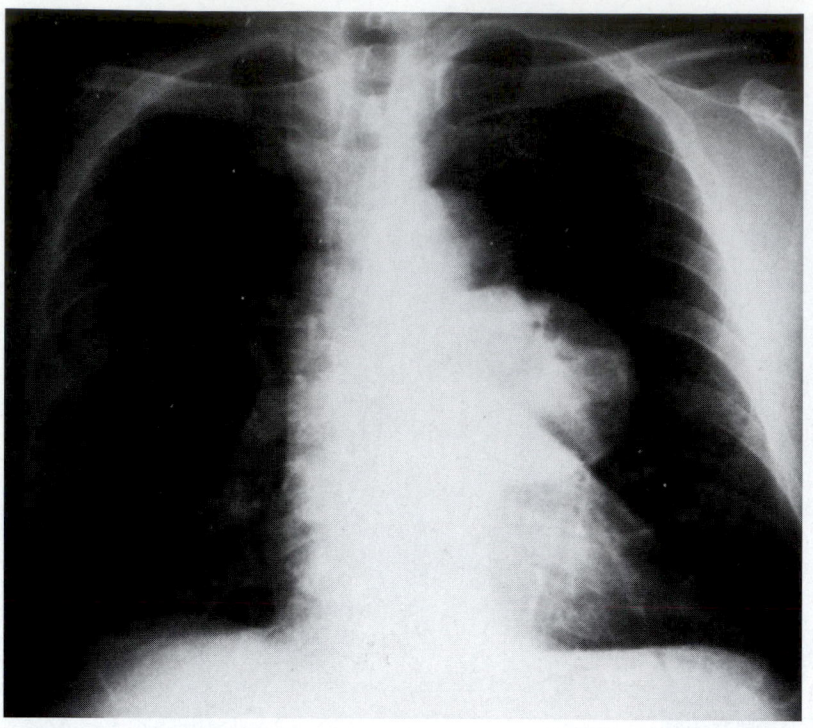

A

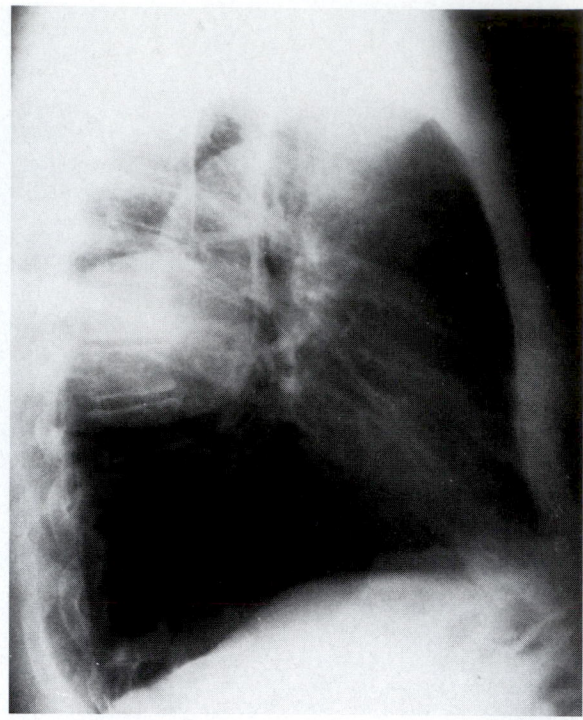

B

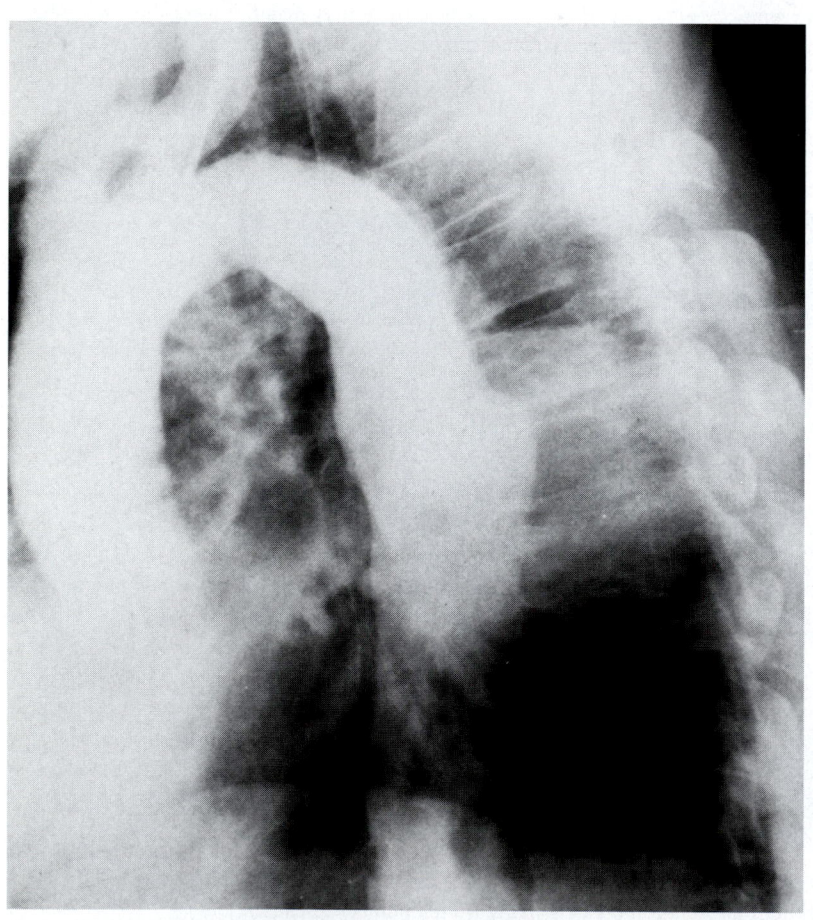

C

FIGURE 32-60 Mediastinal mass. *A.* Aortic aneurysm, PA view. A mass is seen to the left of the aorta. *B.* Aortic aneurysm, lateral view. The mass is also posterior to, and intimately associated with, the aorta. *C.* Aortic aneurysm, aortogram. An irregularity in the wall of the opacified aorta indicates the aneurysm. Most of the aneurysm is filled with clot. This type of mass is often mistaken for a neurogenic tumor in the posterior mediastinal compartment.

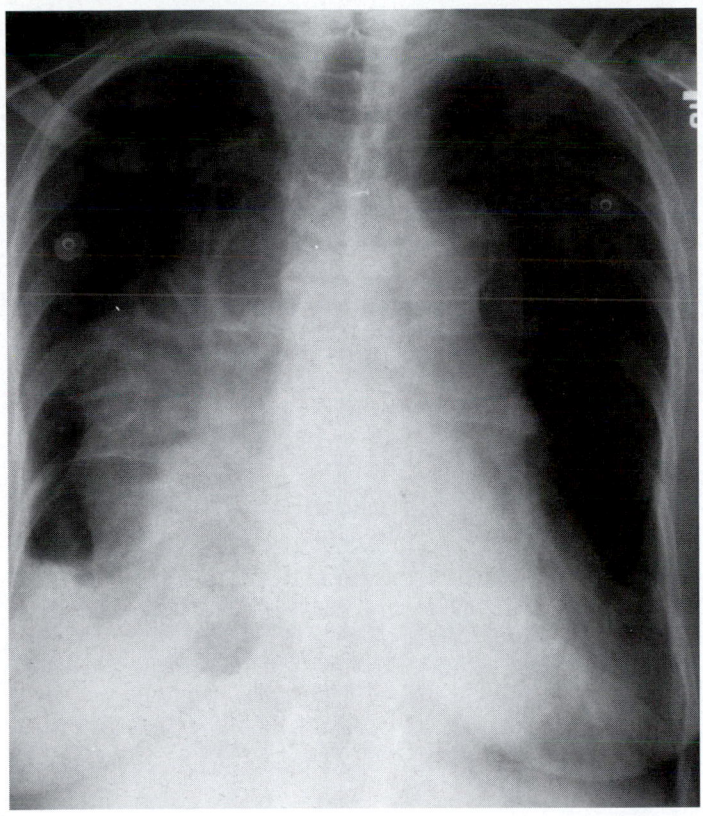

A

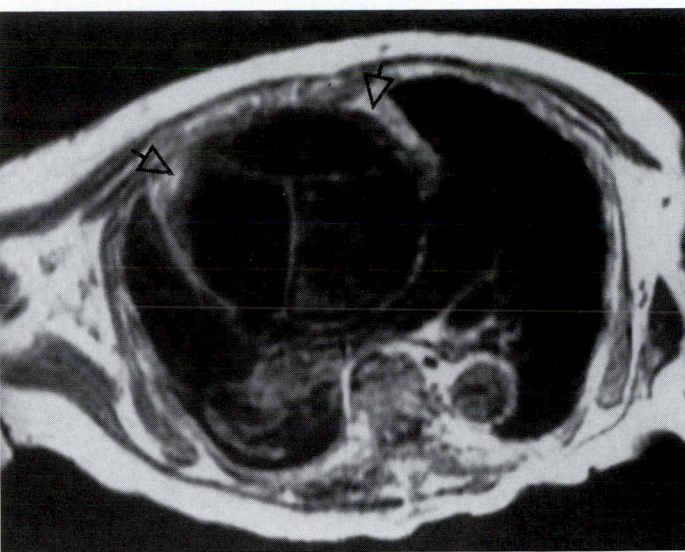

B

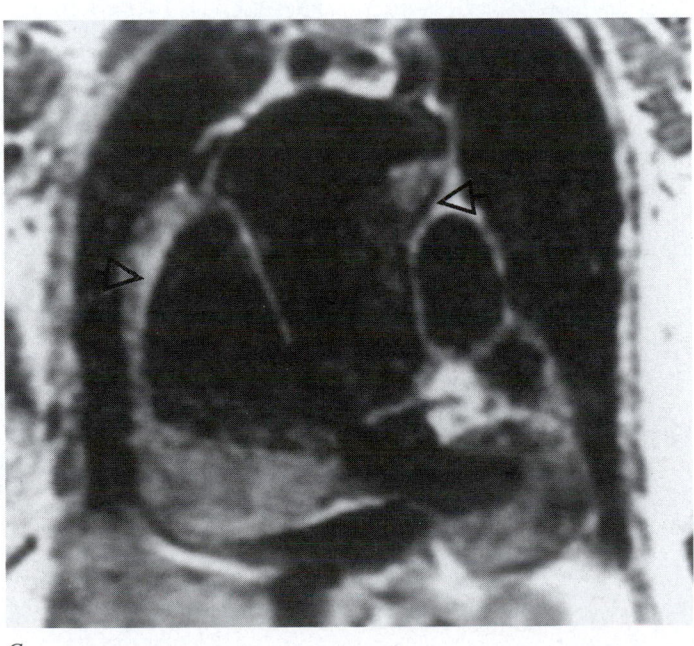

C

FIGURE 32-61   Ascending aortic aneurysm demonstrated by magnetic resonance imaging. *A.* A large anterior mediastinal mass was suspected in the plain chest film. *B.* An axial MRI shows a huge dissecting aneurysm of the ascending aorta (arrows) containing multiple septations (arrows). *C.* A saggital image is more graphic in its depiction of the huge ascending aortic aneurysm (arrows).

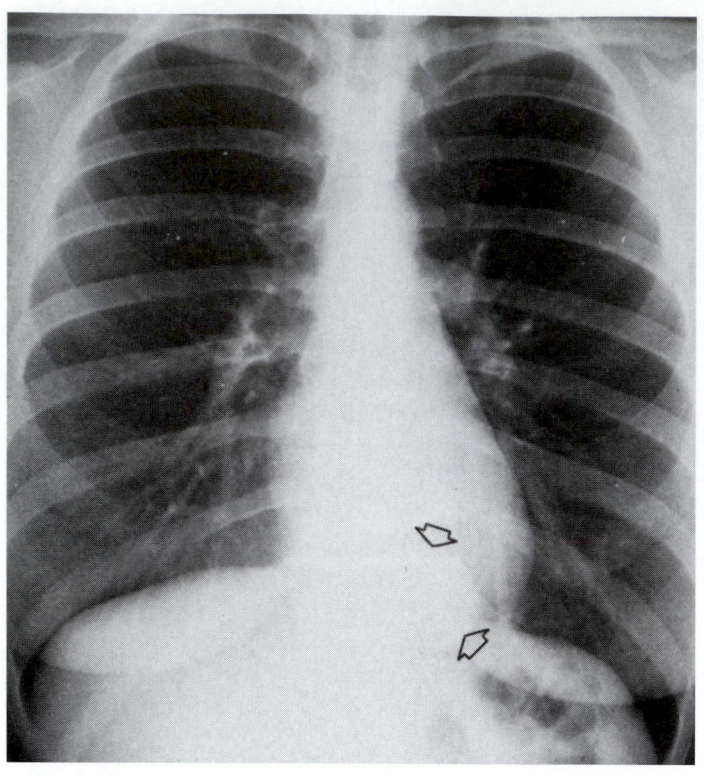

A

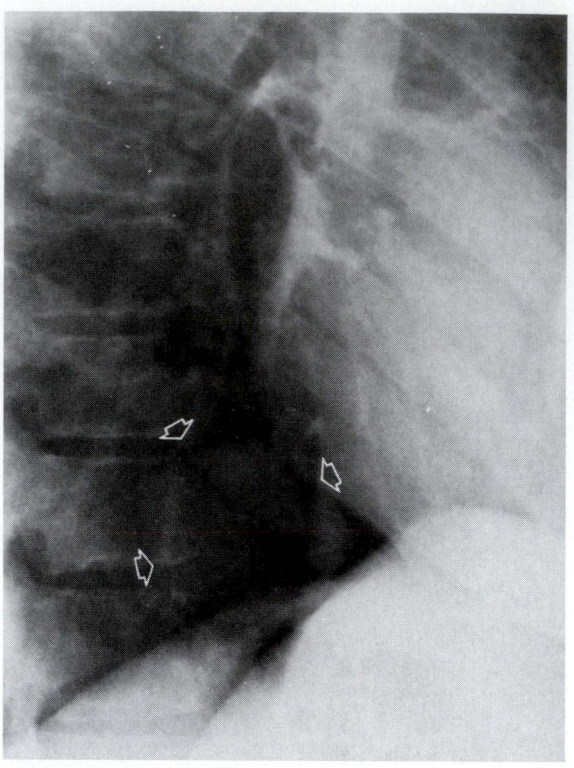

B

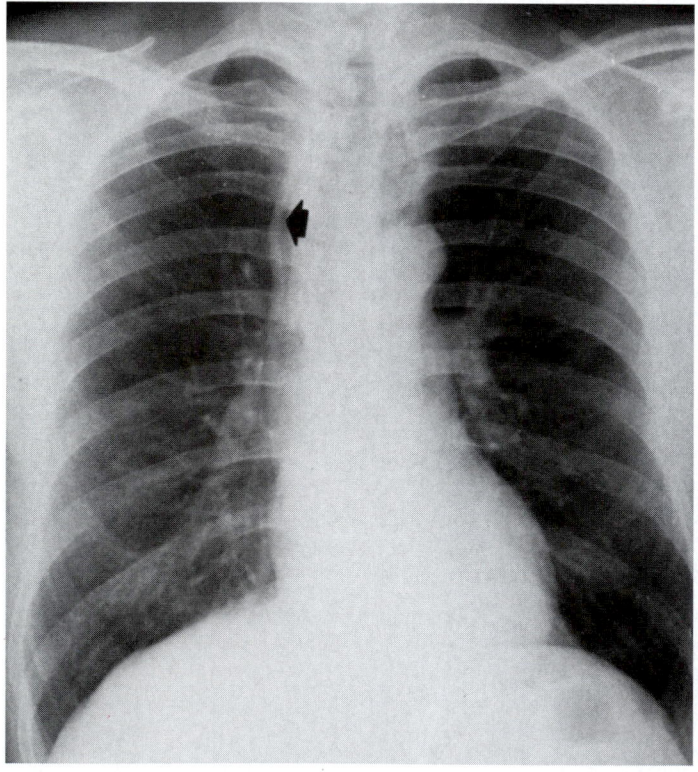

C

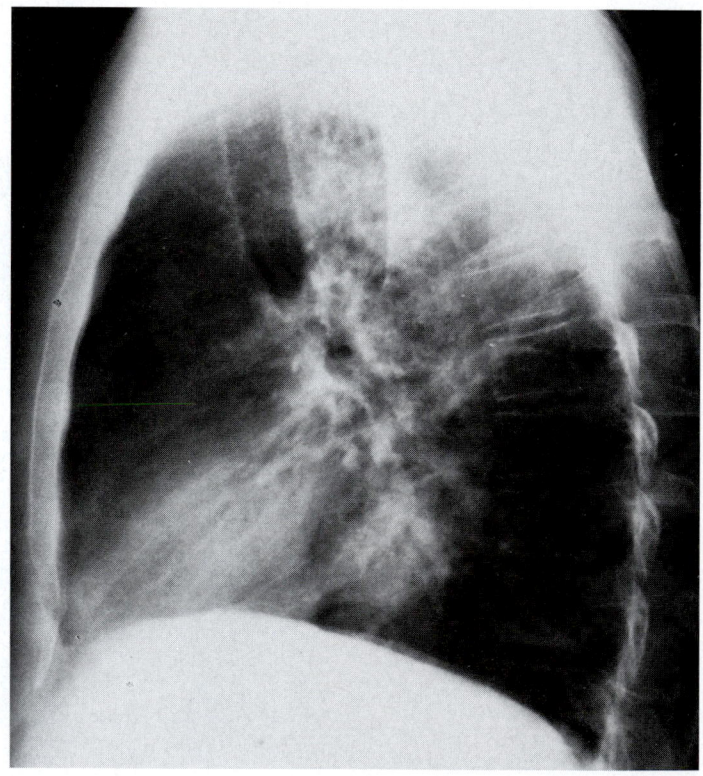

D

FIGURE 32-62 *Top,* esophageal duplication cyst. *A, B.* The small round mass behind the heart (arrows) has the characteristic location and appearance for an esophageal duplication cyst. *Bottom,* achalasia. *C.* PA view. The dilated esophagus is visible as a mass in the mediastinum. Air outlines the wall of the upper esophagus above the aortic arch (arrow). *D.* Lateral view. The mass appears to consist of an amorphous cluster of material lying posterior to the trachea and the heart.

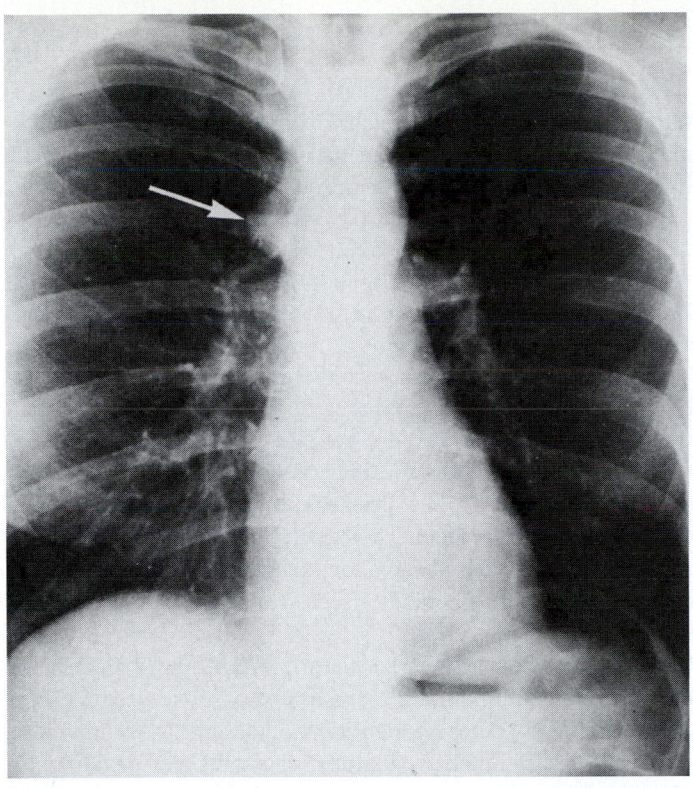

A

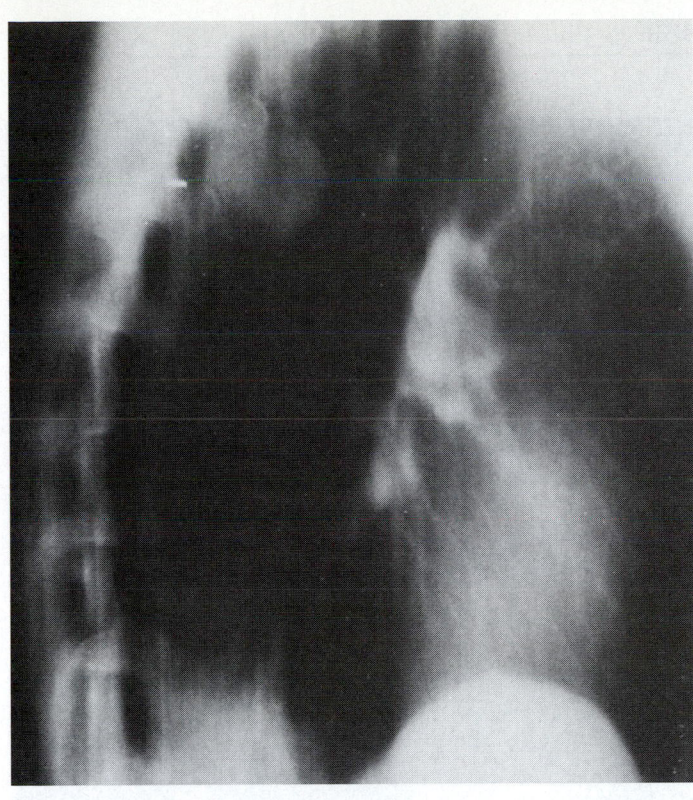

B

FIGURE 32-63 Neurogenic tumor (pheochromocytoma). *A*. PA view. A small mass (arrow) lies to the right side of the spine. *B*. Lateral view. The mass overlies the spine. The location is typical for a neurogenic tu-mor, usually a schwannoma or ganglioneuroma. This mass proved to be a thoracic pheochromocytoma.

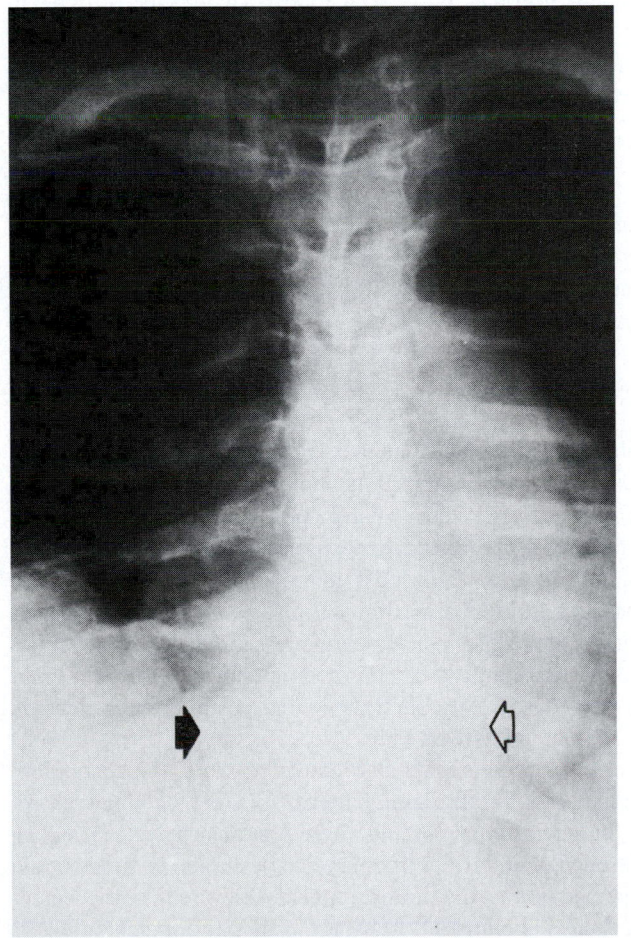

FIGURE 32-65 Mediastinal mass not seen on the routine chest radio-graph. A large lymph node (arrow) is well seen on the CT scan lying just anterior to the descending aorta. This could not be seen on the rou-tine chest radiograph. This node contained adenocarcinoma, and its pres-ence on the scan was an important finding in staging a primary carci-noma of the left lower lobe.

FIGURE 32-64 Tuberculosis. The normal left paraspinal line is displaced later-ally (open arrow) by a paraspinal mass; the right paraspinal line, which is usually not seen, is present and displaced laterally (closed arrow). These findings are char-acteristic of infection near the spine, in this case tuberculosis.

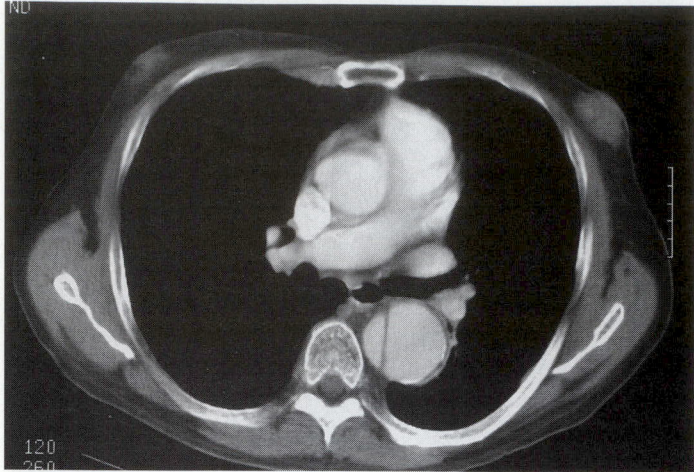

A

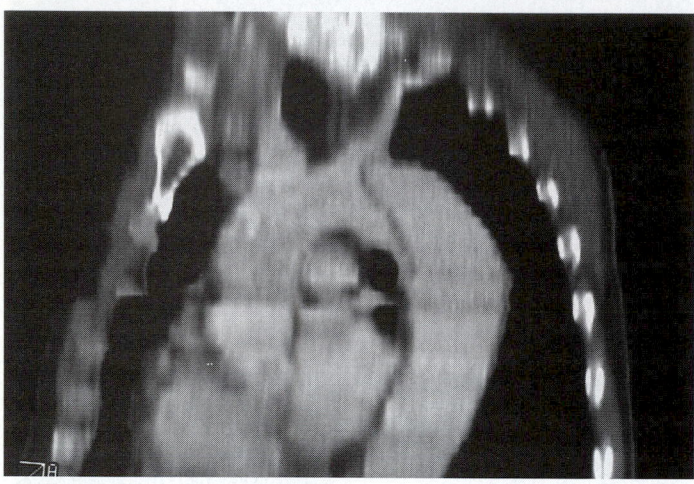

B

FIGURE 32-66 Dissecting arotic aneurysm shown by CT. *A*. A saggital image shows a dissecting aneurysm in the descending aorta; a prominent flap is seen medially, crossing the aortic lumen. *B*. An oblique saggital reconstruction of the image shows the flap in the proximal descending aorta.

THE DIAPHRAGM AND CHEST WALL

The left hemidiaphragm is generally lower than the right; in only about 9 percent of subjects is the left hemidiaphragm higher. Variations in diaphragmatic contour are common. Most common is a localized eventration of the diaphragm (Fig. 32-7), in which a segment of diaphragmatic muscle is replaced by a thin fibrous membrane. The use of fluoroscopy in identifying local eventration of the diaphragm has been described previously.

Foramina traverse the normal diaphragm to connect the thorax and abdomen. Sometimes the foramina enlarge sufficiently to allow herniation of abdominal viscera into the chest. The paired foramina of Morgagni lie anteriorly and medially; hernias through one of these foramina occur frequently on the right (Fig. 32-67*A* and *B*) but rarely on the left. Generally, diaphragmatic hernias contain only omentum or fat, but they may sometimes contain colon. Hernias through the centrally placed esophageal hiatus (Fig. 32-67*C, D,* and *E*) are much more common than

through the foramina of Morgagni. The stomach is the usual herniating viscus; less often, the hernia contains colon or small bowel. Traversing the diaphragm posteriorly and slightly laterally are the paired foramina of Bochdalek. The massive congenital hernias occasionally seen in newborns generally occur through a large foramen of Bochdalek, usually on the left side. Hernias through these foramina are unusual in adults; when present, they may contain a kidney.

On the plain film, masses of the chest wall generally cause bone destruction or erosion; if they do not, they may not be readily visualized. The masses also may be seen if they protrude into the lung as densities. Most lesions of the chest wall are metastatic tumors of the ribs, but primary tumors of the ribs and soft-tissue sarcomas also occur. Their encroachment into the lung tissue causes a characteristic shadow that has smooth margins and tapering edges and is generally seen well in only one of the two standard views of the chest (Fig. 32-68*A*); this characteristic configuration has been designated the *extrapleural sign.*[4] Since many pleural lesions mimic the extrapleural sign, bone destruction is the key finding in accurate identification of an extrapleural mass. CT is very useful in the evaluation of chest wall lesions (Fig. 32-11), which often are not well seen on routine radiographs. MRI also is an excellent technique for demonstrating chest wall masses.

In addition to hernias through the diaphragm, tumors of the diaphragm occasionally present as masses on the chest radiograph. MRI is ideally suited to demonstrating diaphragmatic lesions, since coronal sections are much better than transaxial ones for this anatomic region. This is also true for pleural lesions, such as a pleural fibroma. With axial images, it may be difficult to clearly show that a pleural lesion is in the chest, above the diaphragm, rather than in the abdomen. Coronal images will usually clearly demonstrate the location of the lesion.

THE PLEURA

The pleura and its disorders are considered in Chapters 88–92. Radiographic involvement of the pleura is generally manifested by pleural fluid, localized or diffuse pleural thickening, or pleural nodules.

Pleural Effusions

Fluid in the pleural cavity appears radiographically as a homogeneous opacity that generally occupies a dependent position. A small pleural effusion that is barely perceptible or is overlooked on the PA view is often readily apparent on the lateral radiograph as blunting of the posterior costophrenic sulcus (Fig. 32-2). The best radiographic technique for demonstrating small quantities of pleural fluid is the lateral decubitus film (Fig. 32-3*C*). With this technique, as little as 25 ml of fluid can be detected. Larger pleural effusions usually blunt the lateral costophrenic sulcus on the PA radiograph as well (Fig. 32-68*B*).

Occasionally, pleural fluid remains between the diaphragm and the lung (i.e., is infrapulmonary), displacing the lung upward, so that the lateral costophrenic angle remains sharp (Fig. 32-3). The presence of an infrapulmonary accumulation of fluid should be suspected if the diaphragm appears elevated, if the costophrenic sulcus is blunted posteriorly, or if the stomach bubble is

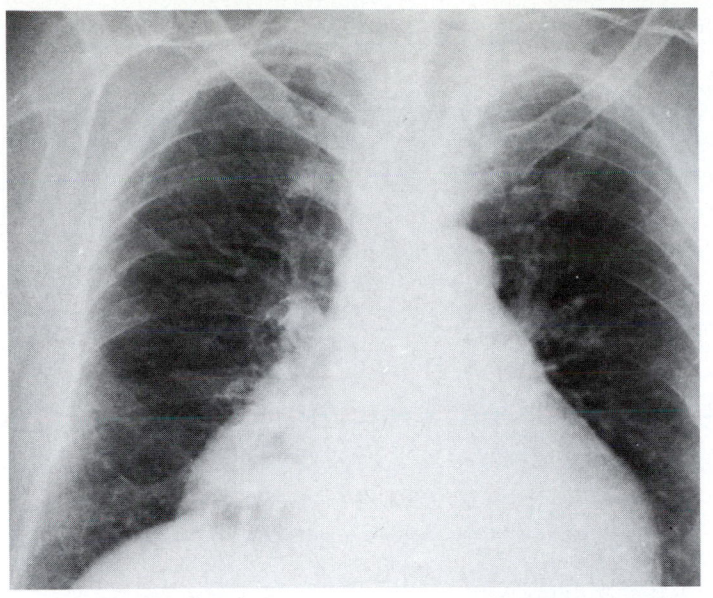

A

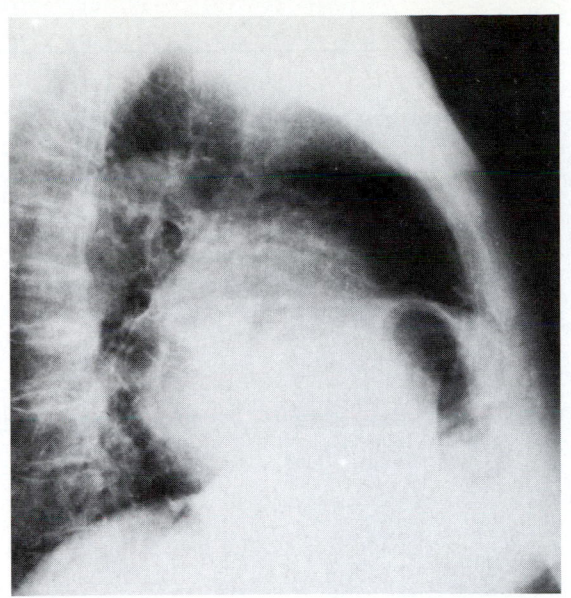

B

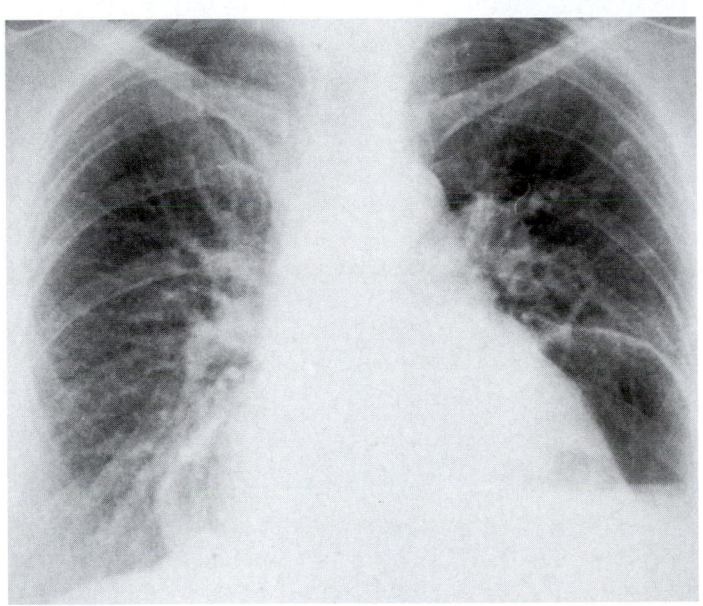

C

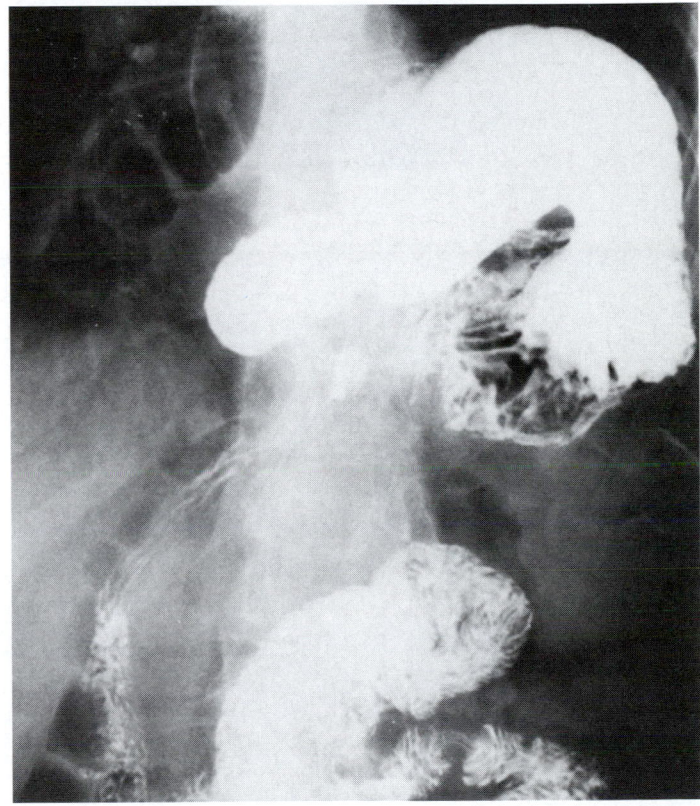

E

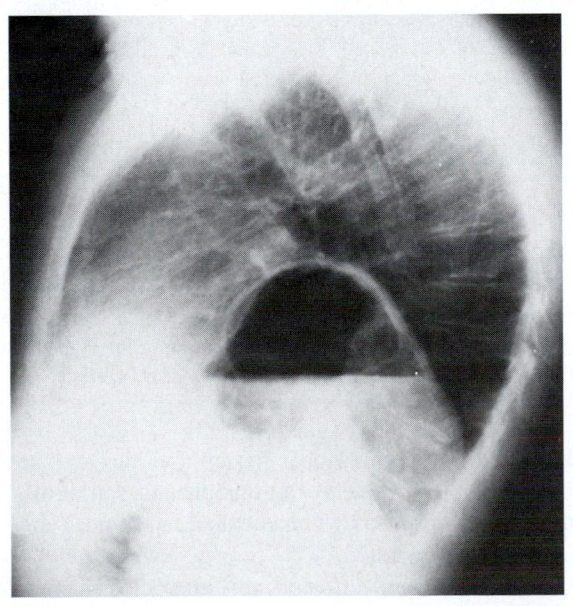

D

FIGURE 32-67 *Facing page,* foramen of Morgagni hernia. *A.* PA view. *A* mass containing a loop of bowel lies just to the right of the cardiac silhouette. *B.* Lateral view. The mass is also anterior to the cardiac silhouette. The location of the mass is characteristic for a foramen of Morgagni hernia. The hernia usually contains only omentum, but in this instance, it also contained a loop of colon. *Above,* hiatus hernia. *C.* PA view. An air-fluid level is present on the left. *D.* Lateral view. The mass is also posterior to the heart. *E.* An upper GI series demonstrates the air-fluid level to be within the stomach, which has herniated into the chest and lies in an upside-down position.

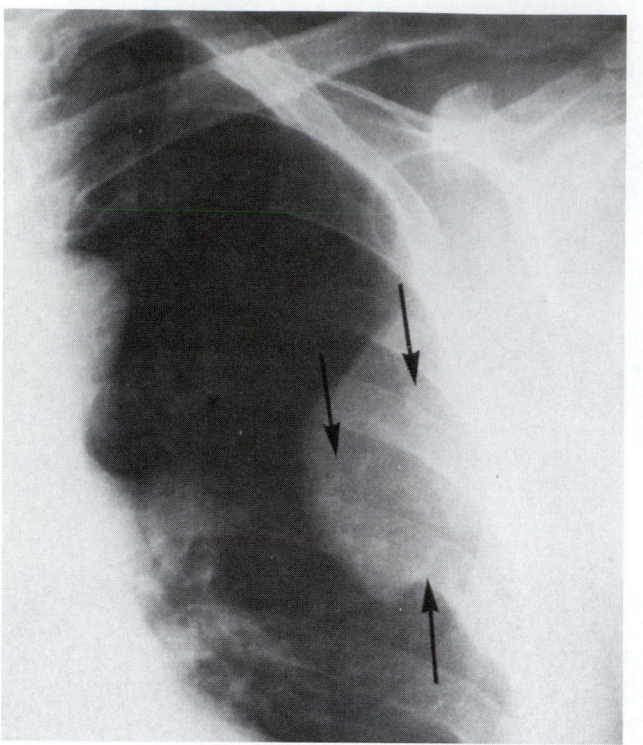

A

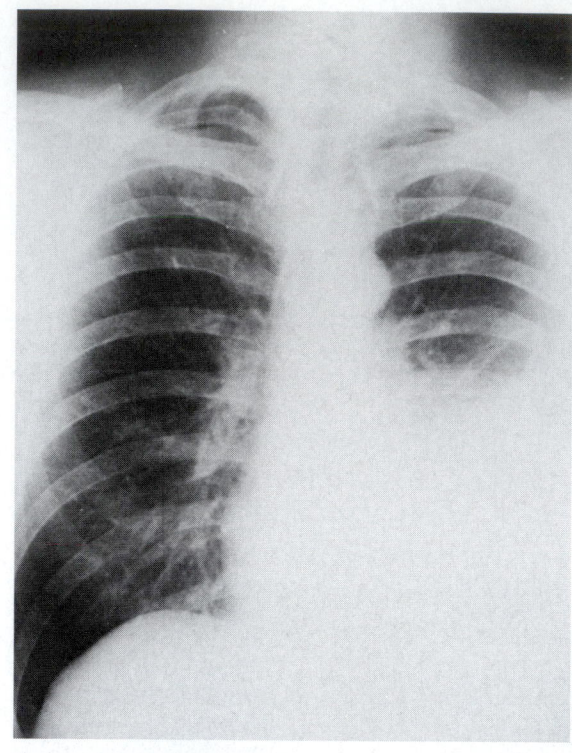

B

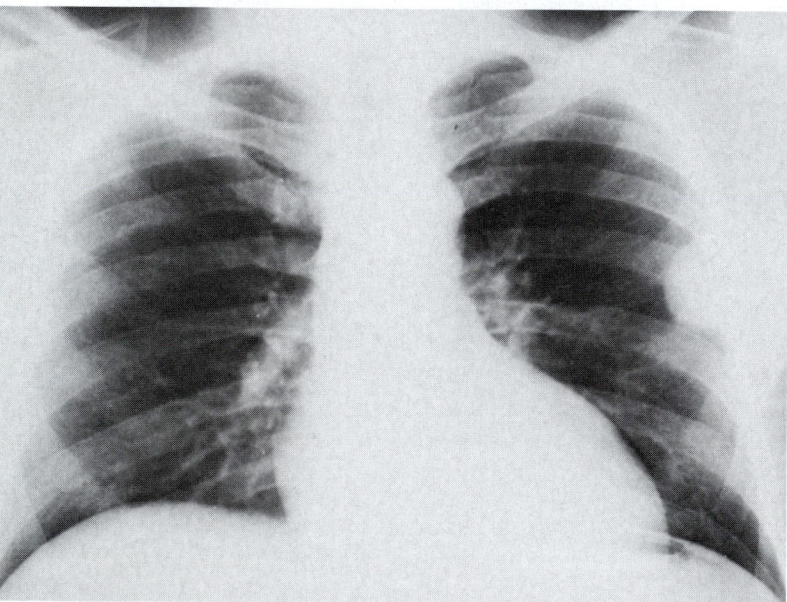

C

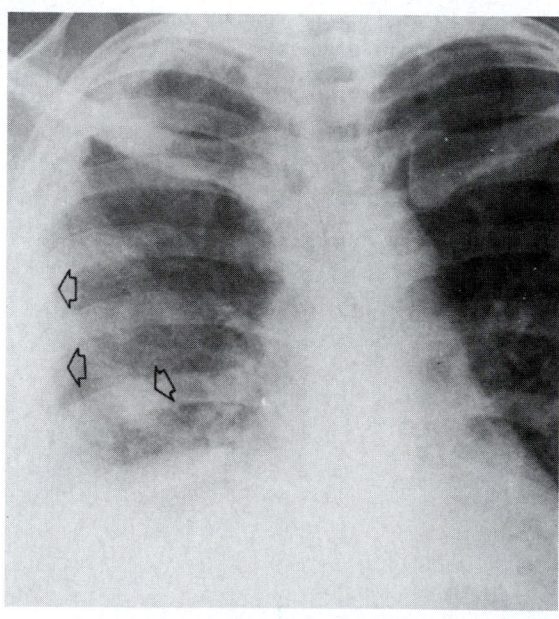

D

FIGURE 32-68 *A.* Rib metastases (extrapleural sign). A smooth mass protrudes into the lung. This mass has tapering edges, characteristic of an extrapleural lesion. The destroyed anterior rib (arrows) is secondary to a metastatic tumor that is invading the rib. *B.* Rheumatoid effusion. The characteristic meniscus of a free pleural effusion is seen in the left hemithorax. This patient had rheumatoid arthritis. *C.* Pleural lipoma. A smooth mass along the left lateral chest wall proved to be a lipoma. *D.* Pleural metastases. A right pleural effusion, showing a meniscus, blunts the right costophrenic sulcus. The lobulation along the right lateral chest wall is characteristic of tumor nodulation (arrows).

separated from the dome of the apparent hemidiaphragm by more than a few millimeters. CT is especially sensitive in identifying small pleural effusions (Fig. 32-69).

Pleural fluid sometimes is loculated and difficult to distinguish from localized pleural thickening. A pleural effusion generally has a convex border toward the hilus, whereas pleural thickening more often presents a concave border toward the hilus.

Loculated pleural fluid in an interlobar fissure assumes a cigar-shaped configuration on the lateral radiograph and sometimes simulates a mass. This mass, known as a "phantom tumor," disappears as the fluid is eliminated.

Common causes of pleural effusion are tuberculosis, pneumonia, pulmonary infarction, metastatic tumor, primary pleural tumor, lymphoma, collagen vascular disease, chest trauma, and

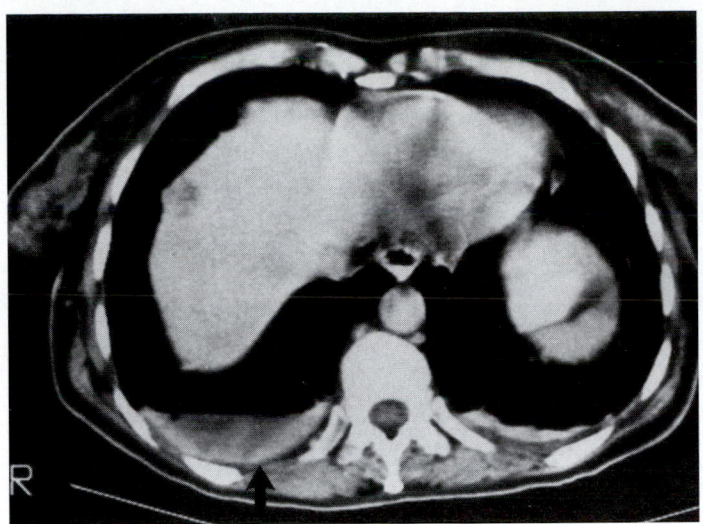

FIGURE 32-69   A right pleural effusion (arrow) is identified by CT. This was not seen on the routine chest radiograph. Pleural thickening is seen in a similar location of the left side.

intra-abdominal inflammatory processes, such as subphrenic abscess or pancreatitis.[8] Thoracentesis and pleural biopsy may be necessary to establish the nature of a pleural effusion that has been recognized radiographically. CT and MRI are generally not useful in determining the exact cause of a pleural effusion. The lumpy, masslike character of a mesothelioma can be nicely demonstrated by CT (Fig. 32-70), but findings are usually apparent on the plain chest radiograph. Many mesotheliomas demonstrate only a pleural effusion, without any specific findings to indicate the malignant nature of the process. CT or MRI may show associated mediastinal adenopathy that was not suspected on the plain radiograph.

Pleural Thickening

Fibrosis of the pleura may be localized or generalized. Localized pleural thickening is common at the lung apices and is suggestive of tuberculosis. Most often, however, apical scarring remains unexplained and is attributed to aging. Blunting of the costophrenic sulcus is occasionally the result of a previous pleural effusion. A costophrenic sulcus that appears to be blunted laterally on the PA radiograph, but not posteriorly on the lateral radiograph, usually represents pleural thickening, rather than pleural fluid.

Generalized pleural thickening confined to one hemithorax is usually secondary to previous tuberculosis, empyema, or hemothorax. Bilateral pleural thickening, either localized or generalized, is strongly suggestive of asbestos exposure.[11] Although such thickening is sometimes accompanied by pleural calcification or interstitial lung disease, it is important to recognize that pleural thickening may be the sole radiographic manifestation of asbestos exposure.

Pleural Nodules

A localized pleural nodule suggests a benign pleural tumor (Fig. 32-68C and D). The nodule may be difficult to distinguish

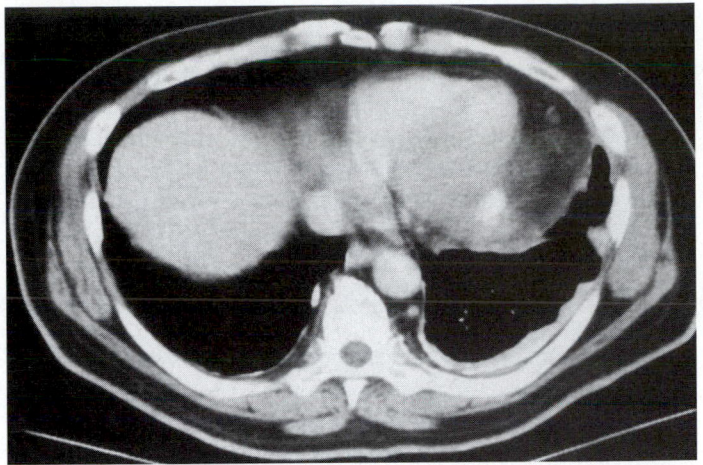

A

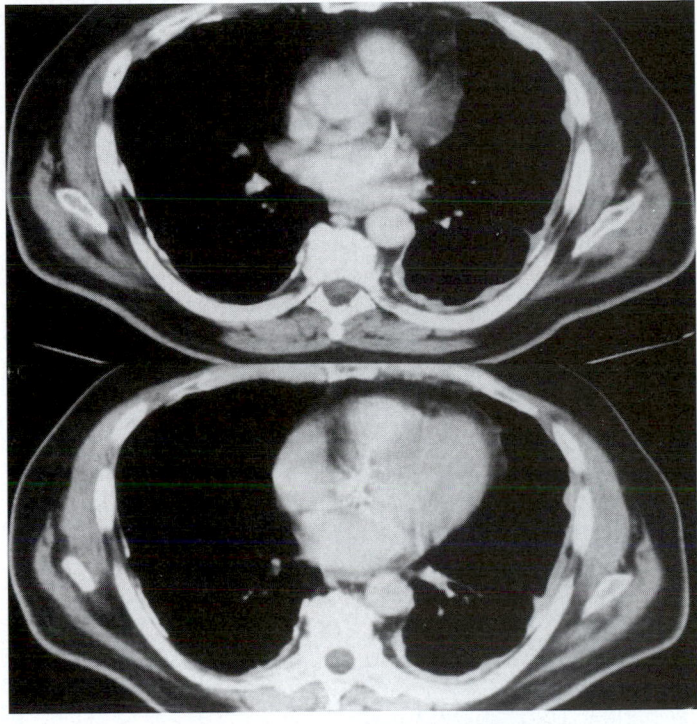

B

FIGURE 32-70   Pleural mesothelioma. Asbestos-related pleural plaques are seen in the right chest; pleural thickening and pleural calcification are present. On the left side, the pleura is thickened and quite lumpy. This is characteristic of mesothelioma, but the finding is not specific for this disorder.

from a localized area of pleural thickening, but generally it is larger and more symmetric in contour. Diffuse pleural nodulation (Fig. 32-68D) indicates diffuse mesothelioma or metastatic malignancy, although empyema can sometimes be quite nodular in appearance. Mesotheliomas and pleural metastatic tumor are impossible to distinguish radiographically; they also may be difficult to distinguish histologically. Both are commonly associated with pleural effusion. As with pleural effusions, CT is extremely useful in identifying localized or diffuse pleural abnormalities.[1]

Pneumothorax

In the conventional upright radiograph, air within the pleural cavity is best seen at the apices, where the thin line of visceral pleura surrounding the partly collapsed lung is easily identified. If doubt exists, a radiograph taken during expiration may make a pneumothorax more obvious. In supine patients or in patients with pleural adhesions, pneumothorax may be seen only at the bases, medially or laterally. CT is useful in demonstrating small pneumothoraces, which may not be appreciated on conventional radiographs.

Trauma, including that of iatrogenic origin, is the most common cause of pneumothorax. Spontaneous pneumothorax occurs in a variety of conditions. Most often the cause is unknown. On occasion, pneumothorax may be clearly attributed to a ruptured apical bleb. Diffuse lung disease, such as eosinophilic granuloma, is sometimes the cause of spontaneous pneumothorax.

Chronic pneumothoraces are almost invariably associated with pleural effusions. The interface of air and fluid causes the fluid to assume a flat-line configuration (Fig. 32-71), rather than the usual curved-line configuration (meniscus) seen when air is absent. A pneumothorax is ordinarily rapidly reabsorbed or replaced by fluid in the pleural space. A chronic pneumothorax strongly suggests a bronchopleural fistula.

PORTABLE CHEST EXAMINATION

Portable radiographic examination of seriously ill patients has become routine. Interpretation of the portable radiograph is often difficult because the film may be of poor technical quality.

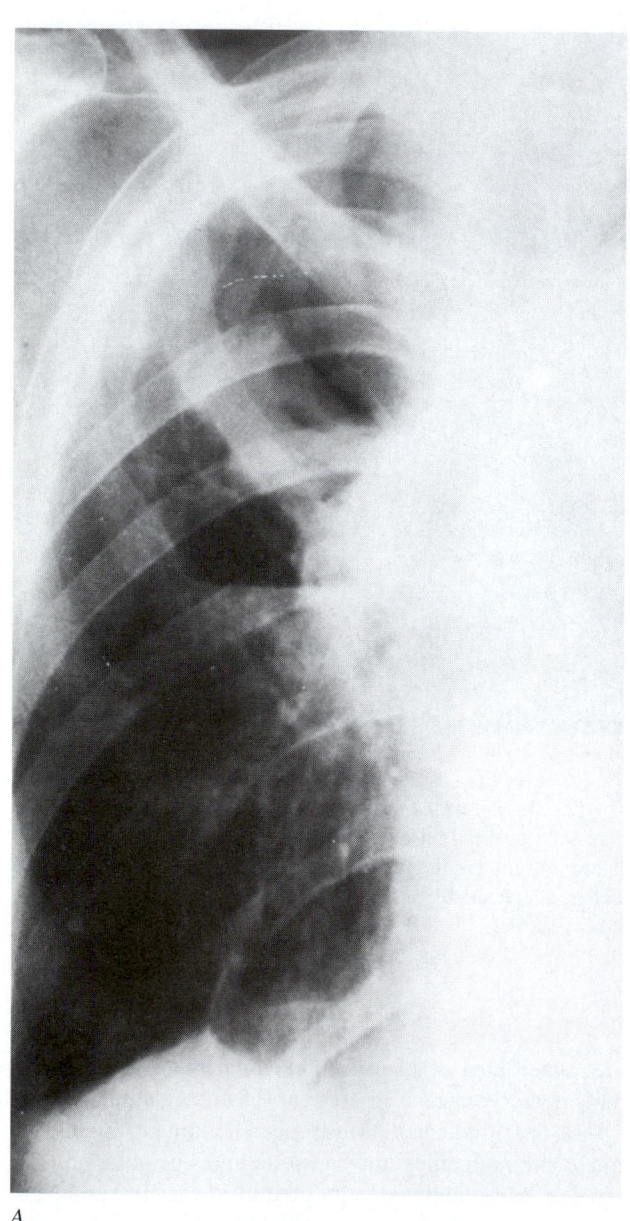

A

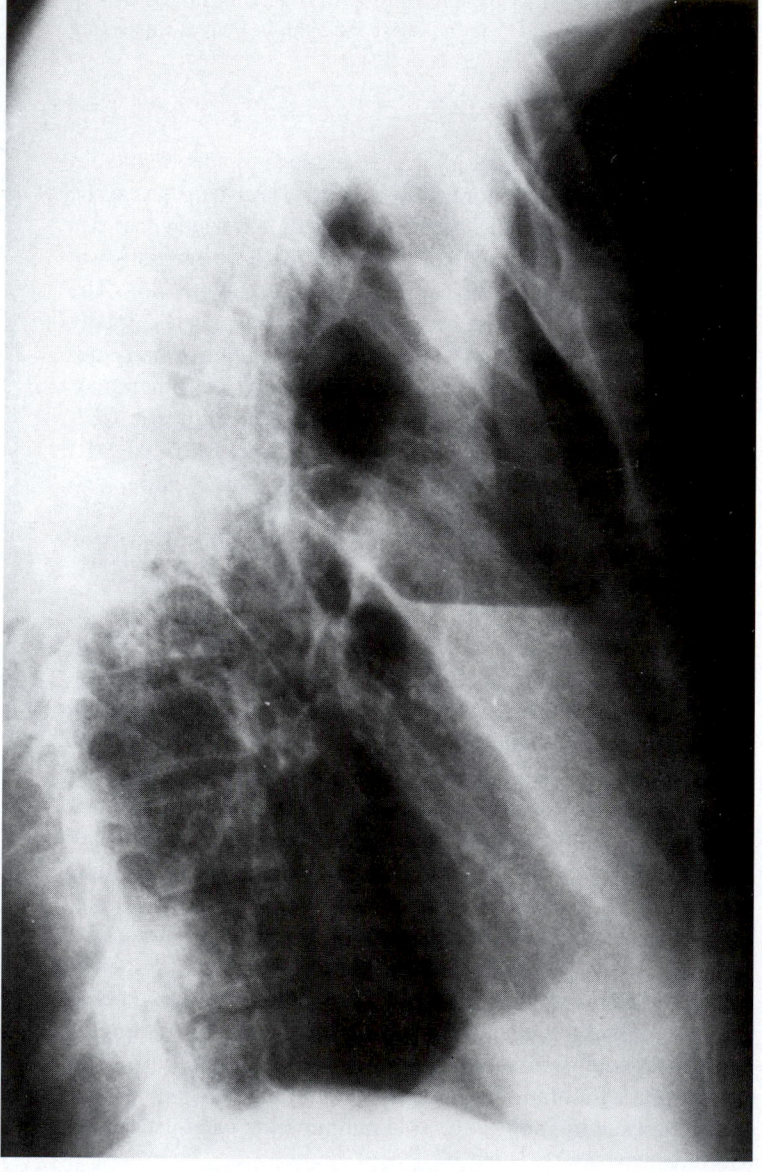

B

FIGURE 32-71 Hydropneumothorax. *A*. Posteroanterior view. A distinct air-fluid level is seen overlying the left hilus. *B*. Lateral view. The fluid and air are anterior to the hilus, indicating that they are in the pleural space. The hydropneumothorax was secondary to a postoperative bronchopleural fistula.

Despite its problems, the portable radiograph usually provides useful information in postoperative patients, who may be difficult to examine clinically, and in critically ill patients being mechanically ventilated.

Localized pulmonary consolidation seen in the postoperative radiograph generally indicates one of three possibilities: pulmonary contusion, pneumonia, or atelectasis (segmental or lobar). Pulmonary contusion is common after thoracic surgery. It is generally noted immediately after the surgery and gradually resolves. In contrast, pneumonia generally occurs after the second or third postoperative day; it may be diffuse or localized. If localized, it is often difficult to distinguish from atelectasis; if diffuse, it is sometimes difficult to distinguish from pulmonary edema.

Atelectasis is a frequent postoperative complication. It occurs most often in the lower lobes, more commonly on the left than on the right. An increased density behind the cardiac shadow or obliteration of the diaphragmatic shadow behind the cardiac silhouette constitutes presumptive evidence of left-lower-lobe atelectasis. It is frequently difficult to distinguish between atelectasis and pleural fluid on the portable radiograph.

Basilar atelectasis, also known as platelike atelectasis, Fleischner's lines, or discoid atelectasis, frequently occurs in very ill patients, particularly after abdominal surgery. It is manifested by linear densities at the bases that generally are oriented parallel to the diaphragmatic surface; the densities do not follow the usual patterns of lobar collapse. Basilar atelectasis is generally considered an indication of poor diaphragmatic motion and often occurs with abdominal pain. Basilar atelectasis may be seen in patients who are obese, who have poor diaphragm motion, or who have diaphragm eventration (Fig. 32-72).

Pleural effusions are often difficult to identify in a portable examination, since the patient is rarely upright in bed or optimally positioned; a lateral radiograph is generally not available. On occasion, a large pleural effusion mimics lower-lobe atelectasis. Although difficult to perform, portable decubitus radiographs can be useful in distinguishing a pleural effusion from atelectasis.

In patients who have recently undergone thoracic surgery, fluid may accumulate in the extrapleural space in the area of the incision and may simulate a loculated collection of pleural fluid. With mediastinal incisions, fluid that may be accumulating within the mediastinum is detected as diffuse widening of the mediastinal shadow. Once again, comparison with earlier films is particularly useful in evaluating the process.

Left ventricular failure is another common clinical problem that is often difficult to recognize on the portable radiograph. Distortions in heart size produced by inconsistent distances of the radiographic tube from the patient's chest complicate study interpretation. Enlargement of the pulmonary vessels is probably the most reliable sign of left-sided heart failure. The finding must be interpreted with care, however, since the portable radiograph is often made while the patient is supine, a position that results in redistribution of blood flow toward the apices (see above). Pulmonary interstitial edema and alveolar edema are additional signs of left-sided heart failure that are generally recognizable in the portable radiograph.

The presence of diffuse alveolar consolidation in the portable film generally signifies pulmonary edema, just as it does in the routine radiograph. In the critically ill patient, however, pul-

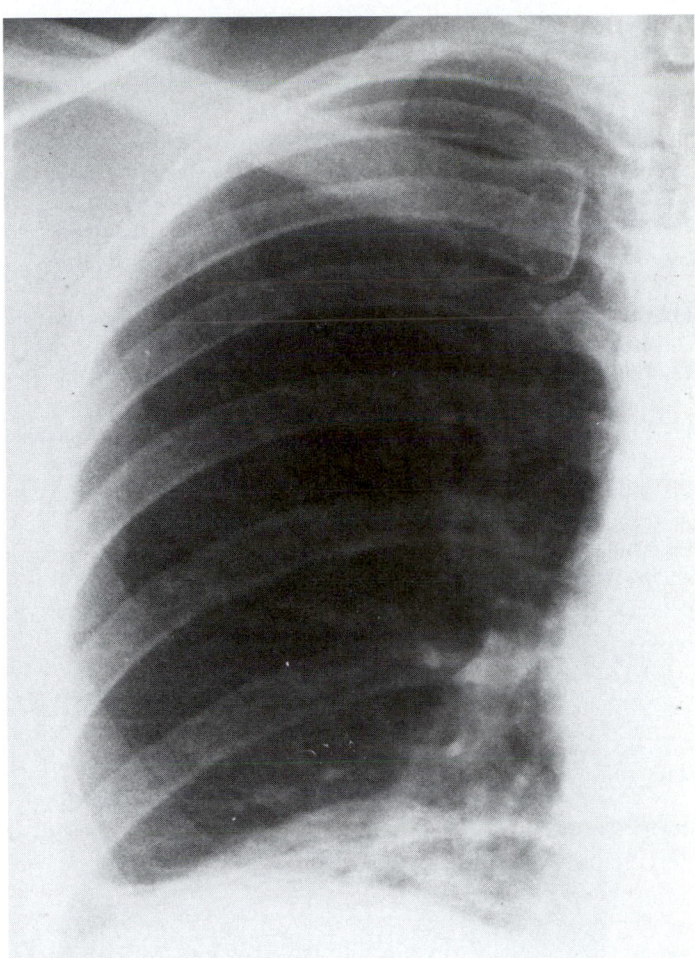

FIGURE 32-72   Platelike atelectasis. A linear density above the right hemidiaphragm in the postoperative patient represents platelike atelectasis. The configuration of this density does not correspond to that of an pulmonary subsegment, and it crosses segmental boundaries.

monary edema is often noncardiac in origin (see Chapter 85). Massive aspiration pneumonia and sepsis may also produce the radiographic picture of diffuse alveolar consolidation.

REFERENCES

1. Albelda SM, Epstein DM, Gefter WB, Miller WT: Pleural thickening: Its significance and relationship to asbestos dust exposure. *Am Rev Respir Dis* 116:621–624, 1982.
2. Colby TV, Swenson SJ: State of the art: Anatomic distribution and histopathologic patterns in diffuse lung disease: Correlation with HRCT. *J Thorac Imaging* 11:1–25, 1996.
3. Favis EA: Planigraphy (body section radiography) in detecting tuberculous pulmonary cavitation. *Dis Chest* 27:668–673, 1955.
4. Felson B: *Chest Roentgenology.* Philadelphia, WB Saunders, 1973.
5. Fraser RG, Pare JAP: *Diagnosis of Diseases of the Chest*, 3d ed. Philadelphia, WB Saunders, 1989.
6. Fraser RG, Pare JAP: *Synopsis of Diseases of the Chest*, 2d ed. Philadelphia, WB Saunders, 1994.
7. Freundlich IM, Bragg DG: *A Radiologic Approach to Diseases of the Chest.* Williams & Wilkins, 1995.

8. Hessen J: Roentgen examination of pleural fluid: A study of the localization of free effusions, the potentialities of diagnosing minimal quantities of fluid and its existence of physiological conditions. *Acta Radiol* 86 (Suppl):1–80, 1951.

9. Jones KW, Pietra GG, Sabiston DC: Primary neoplasms and cysts of the mediastinum, in Fishman AP (ed), *Pulmonary Diseases and Disorders*. New York, McGraw-Hill, 1980, pp 1490–1521.

10. Lavender JP, Doppman J, Shawdon HE, Steiner RE: Pulmonary veins in left ventricular failure and mitral stenosis. *Br J Radiol* 35:293–302, 1962.

11. Lee JKT, Sagel SS, Stanley RS: *Computed Body Tomography with MRI Correlation*. New York, Raven, 1989.

12. Lillington GA: The solitary pulmonary nodule–1974. *Am Rev Respir Dis* 110:699–707, 1974.

13. Lloyd HM, Strong ST, DuBois AB: Radiographic plethysmographic determination of total lung capacity. *Radiology* 86:7–14, 1966.

14. Milne EC: Correlation of physiologic findings with chest roentgenology. *Radiol Clin North Am* 11:17–44, 1973.

15. Muller N (ed): High resolution CT of the chest *Semin Roentgenol* 26:104–192, 1991.

16. Naidich DP, Harkins TJ: Airways and lungs: Correlation of CT with fiberoptic bronchoscopy. *Radiology* 197:1–12, 1995.

17. Naidich DP, Zerhouni E, Siegelman S: *Computed Tomography and Magnetic Resonance of the Thorax*, 2d ed. New York, Raven, 1991.

18. Nathan MH, Collins VP, Adams RA: Differentiation of benign and malignant pulmonary nodules by growth rate. *Radiology* 79:221–232, 1962.

19. Swyer PE, James GOW: A case of unilateral pulmonary emphysema. *Thorax* 8:133–136, 1953.

20. Thurlbeck WM: Chronic airflow obstruction in lung disease, in Bennington JL (ed), *Major Problems in Pathology*, vol 5: *Chronic Airflow Obstruction in Lung Disease*. Philadelphia, WB Saunders, 1976.

21. Viamonte M Jr: Angiographic evaluation of lung neoplasms. *Radiol Clin North Am* 3:529–542, 1965.

22. West JB: *Regional Differences in the Lung*. New York, Academic, 1977.

23. Zeman RK, Silverman JM, Vieco PT, Costello P: CT angiography. *AJR Am J Roentgenol* 165:1079–1088, 1995.

PULMONARY CYTOPATHOLOGY

Prabodh K. Gupta

In his *Atlas of Exfoliative Cytology,* George N. Papanicolaou described the success and utility of cytopathology in the detection and diagnosis of malignant lesions of the respiratory tract.[33] During the past 20 years, however, the advent of flexible fiberoptic bronchoscopy and transthoracic and transbronchial fine-needle aspiration and refinements in cytopreparation and immunocytochemical techniques have established pulmonary cytopathology as an accurate, economical, safe, and rapid diagnostic procedure. Frost and colleagues,[11–13] Woolner,[48] Koss,[27] and Wang,[46] among others, have contributed to our present understanding of pulmonary cytopathology.

THE CYTOPATHOLOGY REPORT

A number of neoplastic and nonneoplastic pulmonary lesions can be accurately diagnosed with cytologic techniques. For a valid and reliable diagnosis, the specimen must be satisfactory—that is, representative of the lesion(s) under investigation, adequate in quantity, well preserved, and prepared and examined with utmost care. In addition, the relevant clinical information must be reviewed by the cytopathologist. A cytopathology report should carry the same clinical and diagnostic significance as does a report from a representative and accurate histologic study. At times, cytologic findings may be neither specific nor diagnostic. The need for proper communication between the cytopathologist and pulmonologist cannot be overemphasized.

PULMONARY SAMPLES

A wide variety of pulmonary specimens may be examined cytologically. Those most commonly used are described below.

Spontaneously Produced Sputum

Spontaneously expectorated sputum is the most easily collected sample submitted to the laboratory; unfortunately, it is also the least valuable. A sputum sample contains mucus and mature and immature squamous cells exfoliated from the oral cavity. It may also contain lymphoid cells from the tonsils and adenoids. A satisfactory sputum specimen is one that is representative of the bronchial mucosa and pulmonary parenchyma. Besides squamous cells, the specimen should contain macrophages (generally carbon-bearing) derived from the alveolar spaces. Inspissated mucus from the terminal airways (Curschmann's spirals) and columnar cells from the bronchial tree and nasopharynx may also be observed (Fig. 33-1). The presence of only squamous cells is an indication of an unsatisfactory pulmonary sample.

The patient should be instructed in the proper technique to produce a satisfactory sputum specimen. After rinsing the mouth and cleaning the throat, the patient takes a deep breath, holds it for up to 20 s, and then coughs. With this method, material is forcefully expectorated from the airways. The procedure should be repeated for up to 30 min to produce a sufficient quantity of sputum.

Induced Sputum

Asymptomatic patients often are unable to spontaneously produce a satisfactory sputum specimen by deep coughing. Such patients may be successfully "induced" to produce a sample. After the patient is given appropriate instructions, a preheated (37°C) hypertonic saline solution or mucolytic agent (Mucomyst) is administered through the inhalational route for 10 to 15 min. The patient is asked to cough for up to an additional 20 min, and a pooled sputum sample is collected. The patient may be instructed to collect sputum specimens for an additional 2 to 3 days after the induction procedure. Such specimens are valuable diagnostically. Postinduction specimens should be pooled and preserved in a polyethylene glycol and alcohol mixture, using the technique described by Saccomanno,[37] as discussed below.

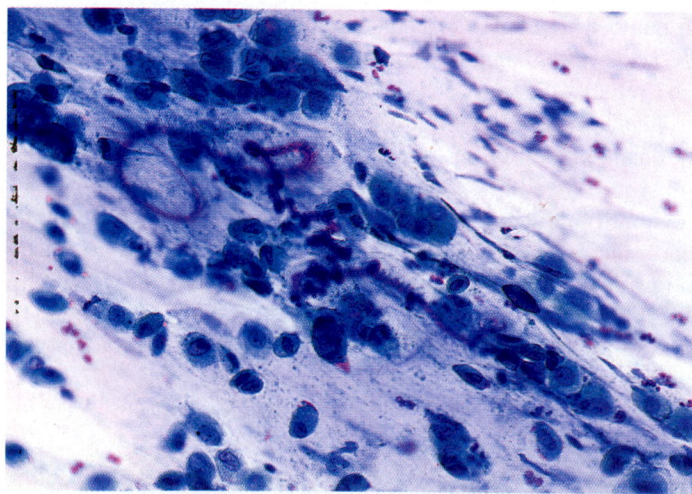

FIGURE 33-1 A satisfactory respiratory specimen (bronchial washing). Note the presence of macrophages, a Curschmann's spiral, and a few macrophages, indicative of a deep cough specimen. Squamous cells most often indicate oral material. (Papanicolaou stain, ×105.)

Sputum-induction techniques were investigated extensively as part of the Early Lung Cancer Detection Project, and standardized procedures were published by the National Cancer Institute (NCI) in 1979.[30] In the late 1960s, the NCI established the Cooperative Early Lung Cancer Group, which included the Johns Hopkins University School of Medicine, Memorial Sloan-Kettering Cancer Center, and the Mayo Clinic and Mayo Foundation. Based upon a large prospective study, this group concluded that although sputum cytology can detect "early" squamous cancers at a resectable stage, mortality does not seem to be affected by early detection. The observation may be related to the natural biologic behavior of malignant pulmonary tumors and the currently available treatment methods.

Bronchial Washings

Cytologic examination of bronchial washings has been in use for a number of years. Developments in its application have been summarized recently.[45] While normal saline may be used to obtain bronchial washings, use of a physiological solution such as Normosol or Plasmalyte may be preferable. The collected specimens should be submitted fresh to the laboratory. In certain circumstances, fresh smears may be made on site and fixed immediately in 95 percent ethyl alcohol for at least 20 min; alternatively, spray fixation (using Surgipath cytology fixative) may be employed. Such preparations are generally diagnostically inferior to specimens submitted fresh to the laboratory and processed utilizing cellulosic (Millipore) filters or other concentration techniques. On many occasions, sampling variability exists, and the most valuable material may not be smeared on the slides; hence, the diagnostic value of the procedure is compromised. A segmental sampling of the bronchial tree, taking adequate precautions against contamination of the specimen, can be useful in localization of the lesion.

Bronchoalveolar Lavage

Using bronchoalveolar lavage (BAL), a physiological solution under pressure is instilled in a specified area of the pulmonary parenchyma and, subsequently, aspirated (Chapter 38). A physiological solution like Normosol, or Plasmalyte, rather than normal saline, should be used. The samples obtained with this technique are representative of the alveolar compartment, rather than the tracheobronchial tree.

BAL samples are most useful in investigating diffuse alveolar processes such as *Pneumocystis carinii* pneumonia, viral infections, chemotherapy- or radiation-related changes, or lesions with transalveolar spread, such as alveolar proteinosis and bronchoalveolar cell carcinoma.[29] BAL specimens must be differentiated from bronchial washings, as the cellular contents and diagnostic yields of the two specimens are usually different.

Bronchial Brushings

Bronchial brushings are generally obtained under direct visualization or by employing imaging guidance techniques (e.g., fluoroscopy). When an epithelial abnormality is noted with the bronchoscope, diagnostic material can be obtained by gently scraping the lesion with a brush. Cytology samples tend to be extremely cellular, containing well-preserved fragments of the bronchial epithelium. Caution must be exercised in evaluating such samples, since the cells seen may be hyperchromatic and reactive and may display altered nucleocytoplasmic (N:C) ratios, mimicking undifferentiated tumors. Reserve cells can be obtained with ease during these procedures and may be mistaken for small-cell neoplasms. In hypersensitivity and inflammatory processes, proliferative goblet cells and columnar cells may be recovered.[24,32]

Postbronchoscopy Sputum

Analysis of postbronchoscopy sputum may be a valuable cytologic technique. The patient is directed to collect morning sputum specimens for 2 to 3 days after bronchoscopy. The samples tend to be clean, more cellular, and representative of the underlying pathology. Caution in interpretation is necessary, as extremely reactive and bizarre bronchial cells may be seen in the samples. An adequate clinical history and communication between the bronchoscopist and cytopathologist are necessary for proper collection and interpretation of postbronchoscopy specimens. The technique may be of particular value in patients who are unwilling or unable to undergo additional diagnostic procedures.

Transbronchial Aspiration

Transbronchial aspiration of pulmonary masses and thoracic lymph nodes is generally utilized to evaluate peritracheal, peribronchial, and, occasionally, anterior mediastinal lesions. An aspirating needle is introduced through the bronchoscope and directed to the area of interest.[46] Considerable experience is needed for specimen collection and interpretation to obtain diagnostic results consistently; samples should be examined on site.

Transthoracic Fine-Needle Aspiration

Fine-needle aspiration (FNA) is generally performed utilizing a thin needle (20 gauge or smaller) under imaging guidance. The technique is extremely accurate, rapid, and economical; results are comparable to those from tissue biopsies.[8,23] The yield is excellent, and the complication rate is minimal. While pneumothorax and hemorrhage may occur, they are rare. The incidence of tumor seeding along the needle track is negligible.

SPECIMEN PROCESSING

A variety of techniques may be employed in the cytopreparation of pulmonary specimens.

Direct Smears

Direct smears, analyzed by the "pick and choose" technique, are best prepared in the laboratory from fresh specimens. A biologic hood should be employed and adequate precautions taken by staff. Samples are transferred to a Petri dish and examined against a dark background in order to improve contrast and visualization. Any thick, pink, or dark suspicious areas are transferred to clear, prelabeled slides for preparation of smears. At least four

smears should be made from each sample; the remaining material is processed as described below.

Saccomanno's Fixative

Saccomanno's fixative is a popular technique in which a mixture of 50 percent ethyl alcohol and polyethylene glycol (Carbowax 1540) is added to the specimen. The specimen is either smeared directly on glass slides or used to prepare a slurry after mixing in a blender and subsequent centrifugation.[30,37] However, alcohol causes coagulation of proteinaceous material, making direct smearing of the specimen difficult. The cells are trapped in mucus, they stick together and appear hyperchromatic. In addition, blending may result in fraying of the delicate cell cytoplasm and cilia. Although the technique is useful in detection of squamous and other large-cell tumors and certain infections, it is less valuable for the diagnosis of small-cell neoplasms and related lesions.

Cytospin Preparations

Cytospin preparations are generally prepared from fixed and, sometimes, fresh specimens. Inadequate sampling and artifactual clumping of the cells occur commonly. At least four slides should be examined from each specimen when cytospins are used exclusively.

Thinprep Preparations

Thinprep preparations are popular as a cell-concentration technique and are superior to cytospin slides. The slide background is clean, and screening is easier. In addition, slides can be utilized for other special investigations, such as morphometry and immunocytochemistry. With this technique, however, cells tend to clump together, appearing hyperchromatic and often losing the delicate morphologic and background features necessary for correct evaluation and diagnosis.

Cellulosic (Millipore) Filters

Cellulosic or Millipore filters are used in the processing of fresh specimens. A 5-nm pore filter is employed in the collection of all cells; artifacts of fixation are minimal. Adequate sampling and maintenance of intercellular relationships and background features are facilitated with this technique. However, the procedure is expensive and time-consuming; it requires a special setup and experienced technicians.

Cell Block

Preparation of cytology specimens utilizing paraffin processing is not desirable for routine pulmonary specimens. Slides prepared with this technique may permit accurate diagnosis when specimens contain abundant abnormalities; however, when abnormalities are limited, they are of little value. On the other hand, cell blocks may be used for specimens obtained through fine-needle aspiration, when the available particulate material cannot be examined by other cytologic techniques, such as smears and filter preparations. Cell blocks are useful in evaluating specimens obtained by fine-needle aspiration, as they provide a representative, concentrated sample that can be utilized for a variety of histochemical and immunocytologic techniques.

Specialized Techniques

Specialized investigations, such as electron microscopy, may be undertaken in evaluating selected cytology specimens. Based upon the on-site evaluation of fine-needle aspirates, specimens for ultrastructural and immunocytochemical studies can be appropriately collected and processed. These techniques are especially useful in differentiation of adenocarcinoma from mesothelioma, diagnosis of bronchoalveolar carcinoma, and further characterization of poorly differentiated tumors. In addition, molecular diagnostic procedures may be applied in the diagnosis of pulmonary infections.[42]

NORMAL BRONCHOPULMONARY CYTOLOGY

A variety of cells are normally seen in a pulmonary specimen that has been obtained with a deep cough. These cells are representative of those within the airways and lung parenchyma.

Squamous Cells

The squamous cells seen in an expectorated specimen are flat squames, occurring singly. In general, they are uniform and have pyknotic nuclei. Sometimes the nuclei are vesicular. Most cells are large and keratinized and exhibit little variation in size. Nonuniform, small, hyperkeratinized cells with altered nucleocytoplasmic ratios and hyperchromasia may be observed in the presence of oropharyngeal and laryngeal squamous lesions. The presence of abnormally shaped keratinized cells, with or without necrosis, should prompt an examination of the upper airway (Fig. 33-2). Mechanical irritation in the oral cavity, generally by ill-fitting dentures or similar prosthetic devices, can cause exfoliation of bizarrely shaped keratinized cells that may occur in

small tissue fragments. Small, dense, keratinized metaplastic cells may be seen in patients who are endotracheally intubated or who have undergone tracheotomy. Other chronic pulmonary diseases can produce metaplasia and atypical cell morphology, causing concern about a possible underlying malignancy.

Ciliated Bronchial Columnar Cells

Ciliated bronchial columnar cells may occur singly and in small tissue fragments. The cells are tall and columnar and contain basal, vesicular nuclei and pale cytoplasm. The cells have cilia of uniform length; the cilia exhibit periodicity and attach at right angles to the terminal plates. The cilia must be accurately identified because, as a rule, true cilia, which are visible by light microscopy, do not occur on malignant cells. Cellular degeneration and trapped mucus can be a source of error in the proper identification of cilia.

Goblet Cells

Goblet cells are recognized less commonly in normal pulmonary specimens. When present, they appear as swollen, pale cells. In general, goblet cells possess a single large vacuole or multiple small vacuoles that may contain mucus. Hyperplastic columnar and goblet cells may be seen in chronic pulmonary diseases, such as bronchitis or bronchial asthma, and in allergic conditions. In bronchial asthma, Curschmann's spirals also may be observed in cytologic specimens. These are composed of a mucous shroud with numerous neutrophils and some eosinophils (Fig. 33-3). Occasionally, needle-shaped Charcot-Leyden crystals, which appear orangophilic with Papanicolaou staining, may be seen (Fig. 33-4).

Hyperplastic bronchial columnar cells may appear quite bizarre. They occur in tight tissue fragments with overlapping, reactive nuclei that are hyperchromatic and enlarged and contain prominent nucleoli. Such structures are known as creola bodies,[32] which, on careful examination, reveal cilia on the edge

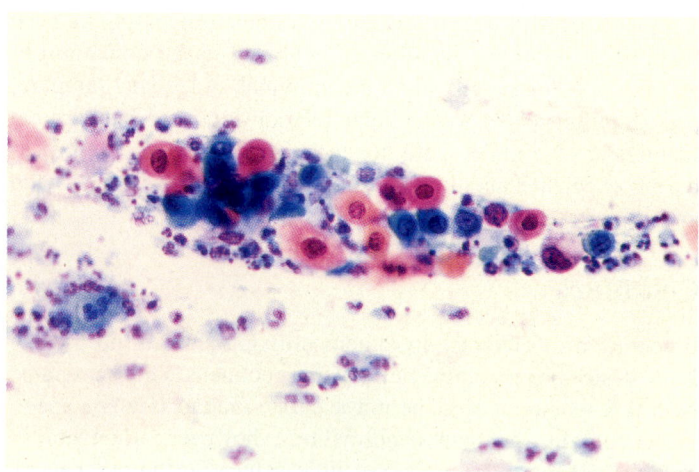

FIGURE 33-2 Brush specimen showing squamous cell carcinoma of the larynx. Note the group of small abnormal, keratinized cells occurring in a necrotic background. The patient had a normal chest radiograph. (Papanicolaou stain, ×166.)

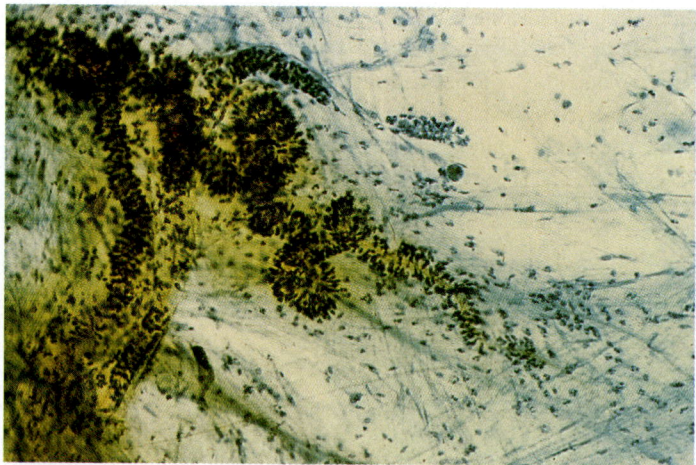

FIGURE 33-3 Bronchial washing showing Curschmann's spiral in bronchial asthma. In comparison to that shown in Fig. 33-1, this spiral has a mantle of acute inflammatory cells and occurs in a background that contains mucus strands. (Papanicolaou stain, ×83.)

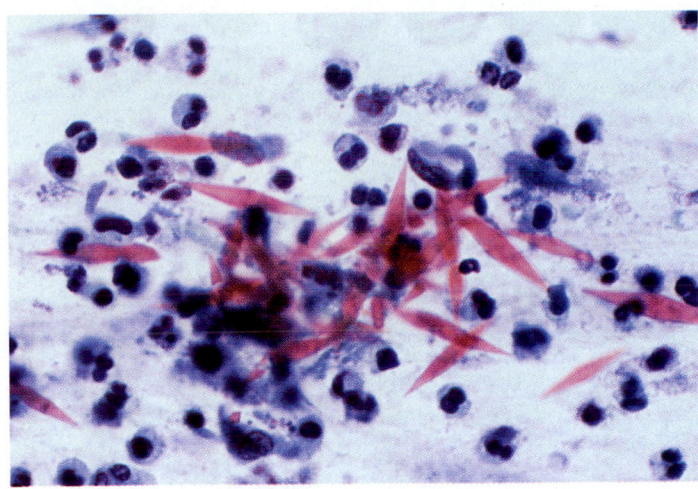

FIGURE 33-4   Bronchial washing showing Charcot-Leyden crystals. Note the numerous needle-shaped crystals occurring in an acute inflammatory background. The crystals are orangophilic with the Papanicolaou method. (Papanicolaou stain, ×166.)

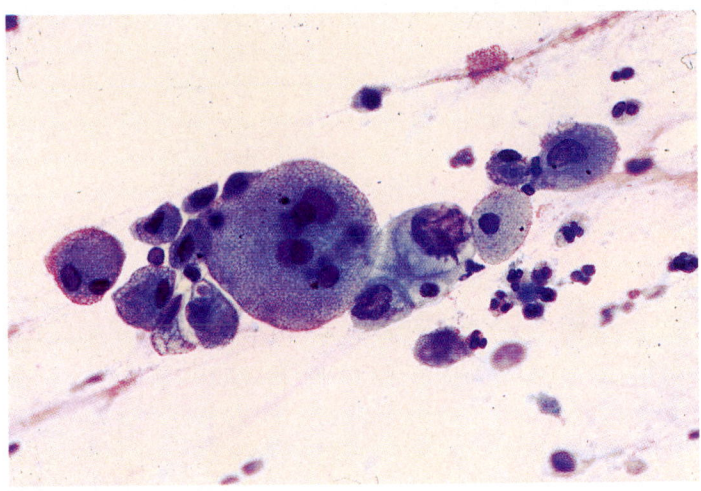

FIGURE 33-6   Bronchial washing showing multinucleated giant cell in pulmonary specimen from a cigarette smoker. Note the acute inflammatory background, mucus, and foreign body–type giant cell. (Papanicolaou stain, ×208.)

or cell surface (Fig. 33-5). Creola bodies are a common cause of false-positive diagnosis of adenocarcinoma. Similar hyperplastic structures can be seen in postbronchoscopy sputum specimens. The occurrence of large numbers of mucus-producing columnar cells in tissue fragments obtained by fine-needle aspiration may be indicative of a mucus-producing adenocarcinoma.

Alveolar Macrophages

The presence of alveolar macrophages or type II pneumocytes in a pulmonary specimen is an excellent criterion for the adequacy of the specimen. These cells occur singly. They are round or cuboidal and typically have a kidney-shaped, vesicular nucleus;

the nucleus may contain a single prominent nucleolus. The cytoplasm of these cells is pale and demonstrates fine vacuolation. Occasionally, ingested foreign material or blood products (e.g., hemosiderin) may be observed in the cytoplasm. Multinucleated forms may occur in bronchoalveolar specimens obtained from patients who have alveolar proteinosis or granulomatous diseases or have been exposed to pollutants[11,25] (Fig. 33-6).

Alveolar macrophages must be examined in the context of the specimen background. Whereas evidence of old hemorrhage and necrosis may suggest a neoplasm, acute inflammation may signify an inflammatory process. Pulmonary infarcts, organizing pneumonia, prior chemotherapy, and other factors produce atypical cellular changes in macrophages and epithelial cells. The cytopathologist must be provided proper clinical information in evaluating these specimens.

TOXIC ENVIRONMENTAL INHALATION EFFECTS

Respiratory squamous and columnar cells and alveolar macrophages react to various environmental pollutants.[11] As examples, the cytologic responses of these cells to exposure to cigarette smoke, asbestos, beryllium, and "crack" cocaine are described briefly below.

Cigarette Smoking

Exposure of the respiratory system to cigarette smoke produces the accumulation of a golden-brown refractile pigment within macrophages—so-called pink-tailed macrophages. Generally, these alveolar macrophages are ringed by material composed of α_1-antitrypsin, which stains orange-red with Papanicolaou stain. This material has been further investigated with appropriate immunocytochemical procedures.[11,17,44] α_1-Antitrypsin accumulation may be tapered at one or both ends of the macrophage, creating the "tailed" appearance (Fig. 33-7).

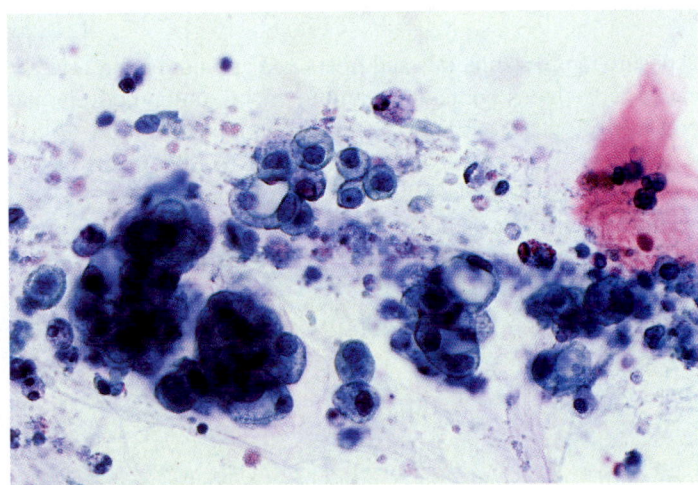

FIGURE 33-5   Bronchial washing showing creola bodies. Note the numerous glandular structures. Cells have prominent nucleoli, hyperchromasia, and evidence of mucus production. Some cells reveal terminal plates and cilia. Cilia may be few, poorly stained, and difficult to recognize. (Papanicolaou stain, ×208.)

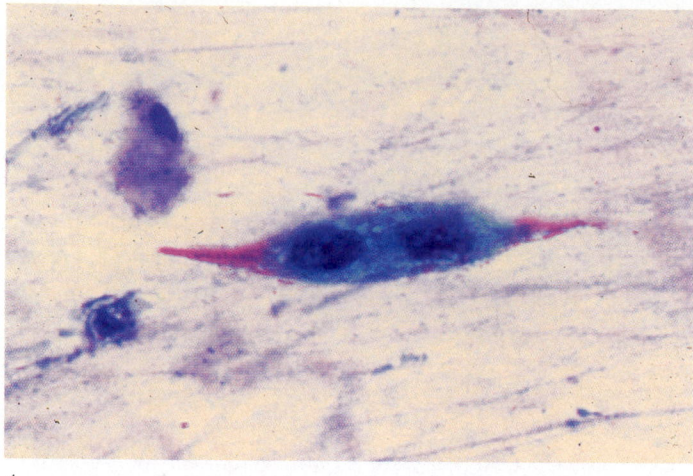

A

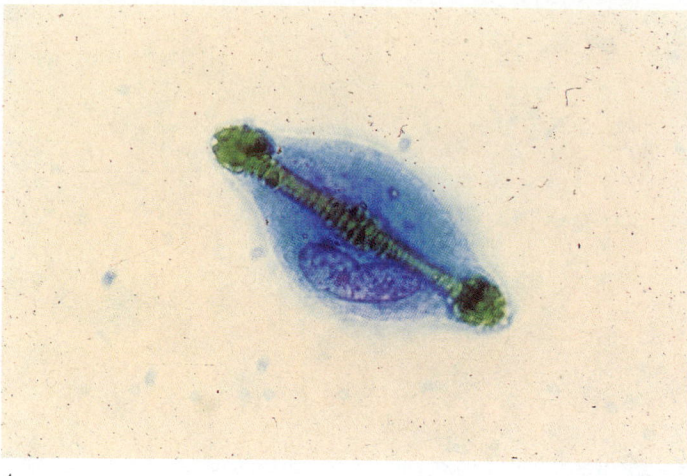

A

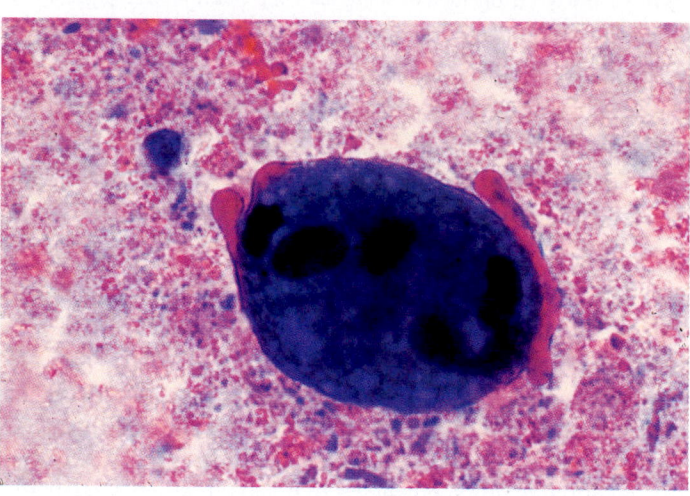

B

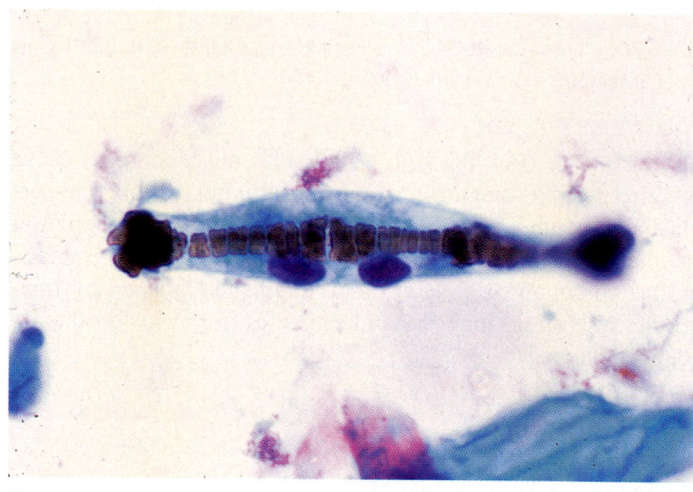

B

FIGURE 33-7 *A.* Bronchial washing showing "pink-tailed" macrophages in pulmonary specimen from a patient with a cigarette-smoking history of 15 pack-years. *B.* Even distribution of α_1-antitrypsin around macrophages. While α_1-antitrypsin is distributed in the "points" in *A,* it is seen in close apposition to the cell in *B.* (Papanicolaou stain, $\times 330$.)

FIGURE 33-8 Induced sputum showing ferruginous bodies in pulmonary specimens from a shipyard worker. *A.* Details of the central fiber core are visible. *B.* The surrounding core with segmented appearance is evident. (Papanicolaou stain, $\times 330$.)

Asbestosis

Asbestosis generally arises from exposure to dust containing mainly chrysolite and other forms of asbestos fibers. Elongated ferruginous bodies may be observed in pulmonary specimens from subjects exposed to asbestos.

Ferruginous bodies vary in size from 4 to 5 nm to over 200 nm. They are generally dumbbell-shaped; a central translucent fiber core is surrounded by layers of a material containing minerals (iron, calcium) and mucopolysaccharides. The color of ferruginous bodies is variable, from a pale golden yellow to dark brown or black. The outer coat tends to be segmented and to exist at right angles to the axis of the fiber.

Ferruginous bodies generally have a macrophage and giant-cell reaction surrounding them (Fig. 33-8). On rare occasions, needle-shaped asbestos fibers without any surrounding deposits are observed within the macrophages.[11,27] These structures were described originally in relation to asbestos inhalation and referred to as "asbestos bodies." However, they are also observed after exposure to other minerals and fibers and are more appropriately called ferruginous bodies. No definitive correlation between the presence of asbestos bodies and occupational exposure to asbestos fibers has been described. Although large numbers of ferruginous bodies may be seen after massive exposure to asbestos, occasional ferruginous bodies are observed as a nonspecific finding.[36] Prussian blue stain for iron compounds helps further identify ferruginous bodies.

Berylliosis

Chronic exposure to beryllium and certain other heavy metals may result in profound pneumocyte proliferation and giant-cell formation.[41] The giant cells tend to be syncytial and often occur as large tissue fragments (Fig. 33-9).

Crack Cocaine Inhalation

Repeated inhalation of recreational drugs may result in large quantities of black soot within the alveoli and pulmonary

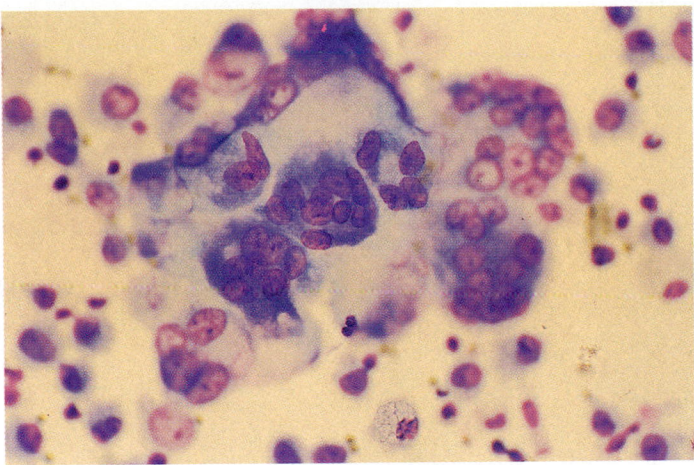

FIGURE 33-9 Bronchoalveolar lavage (BAL) specimen showing multinucleated giant cell in beryllium exposure. Note the extremely large foreign body–type giant cell and alveolar macrophages. (Diff-Quik stain, ×208.)

macrophages[14] (Fig. 33-10). The occurrence of large amounts of carbonaceous material within macrophages obtained by BAL appears to be unique to this patient population. The finding of similar pigmented macrophages within pleural fluid cells has been reported.

INFECTION

A variety of infections of the respiratory system result in cytopathologic changes seen in specimens obtained by the aforementioned methods. The following sections outline changes that may be observed in respiratory bacterial, fungal, and viral infections.

Bacterial Infections

Although bacterial infections of the respiratory tract are extremely common, cytopathology does not offer much help in their

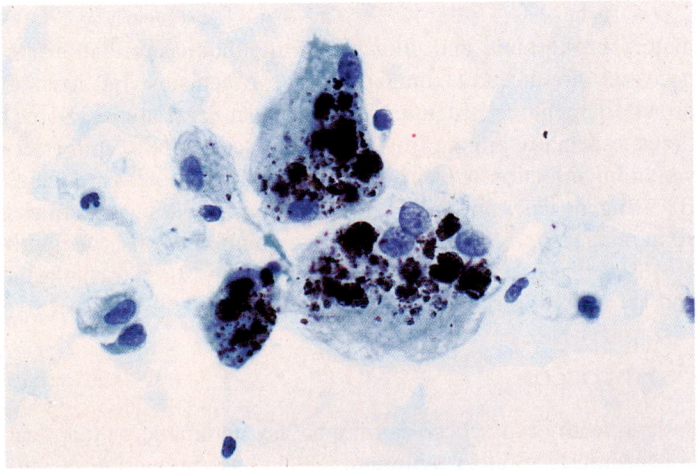

FIGURE 33-10 Bronchoalveolar lavage specimen showing pulmonary macrophages in crack cocaine user. Note the abundant pigmented material in the cytoplasm of the cells, some of which appear reactive. Occurrence of pigment, per se, is a nonspecific finding. (Papanicolaou stain, ×208.)

diagnosis or management. In selected cases, cytopathology may be useful.

ACTINOMYOSIS

In patients with infection caused by species of *Actinomycetes,* pulmonary specimens generally contain large aggregates of filamentous, branching, thin organisms seen as tight, "woolly" clumps. The organisms are easily recognized in routine preparations and are correctly identified with appropriate immunohistochemical techniques.[18] Concurrent findings of significant acute inflammation and pulmonary macrophages should be sought, and diagnostic interpretation made in view of the clinical and radiographic features. The *constellation* of findings is important, since occurrence of actinomycetes in the oral cavity is extremely common, and morphologic detection may not indicate pulmonary infection.

NOCARDIOSIS

Nocardia may be associated with pneumonia and cavitary pulmonary lesions. The organisms are visualized as delicate, filamentous, branching structures. The diagnosis can be made on specimens obtained from fine-needle aspiration or bronchoscopy. Generally, a histochemical (modified acid-fast) stain is used for further identification.

MYCOBACTERIOSIS

Acid-fast organisms may be detected in a variety of pulmonary specimens from patients with mycobacterial infections. Both tuberculous and nontuberculous mycobacterial infections are seen in immunocompetent and immunosuppressed patients. In immunosuppressed patients (e.g., those with HIV infection) the sample background is variable and may not be diagnostically helpful; only foamy macrophages, neutrophils, and a few lymphocytes may be seen (Fig. 33-11). While infection with *Mycobacterium tuberculosis* may yield only a few organisms in respiratory samples, specimens obtained from patients with atypical mycobacterial infections may yield abundant numbers of organisms that are recognized easily on histochemical staining.[22,35] Appropriate cultures should be performed in all such cases for a specific microbiologic diagnosis.

Fungal Infections

A number of fungal organisms can be easily recognized in pulmonary specimens with the use of the Papanicolaou stain. These include both true pathogens and a number of contaminants.

CANDIDIASIS

Candida albicans may be seen in many specimens that are not freshly prepared and were stored at room temperature before fixation; most of the fungal forms are budding yeasts. This finding is of little clinical significance and is generally not reported by the cytology laboratory. In contradistinction, the occurrence of filamentous *Candida* forms, especially in specimens obtained by fine-needle aspiration, may be clinically important and should

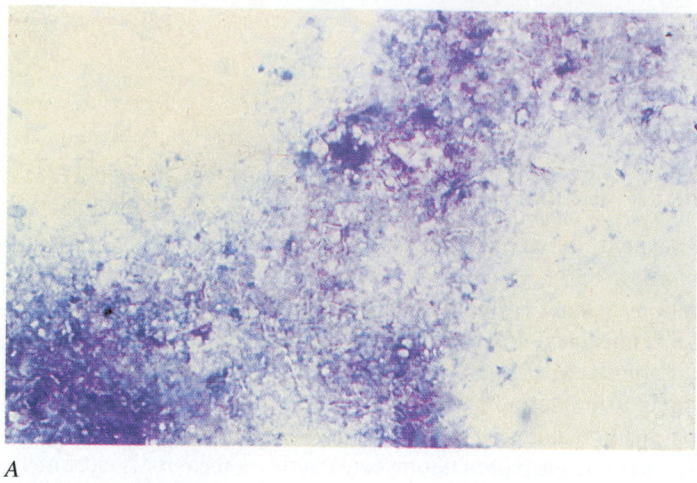

A

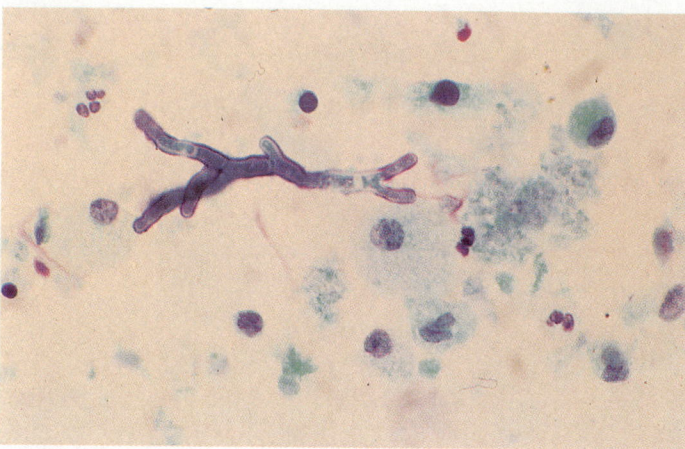

A

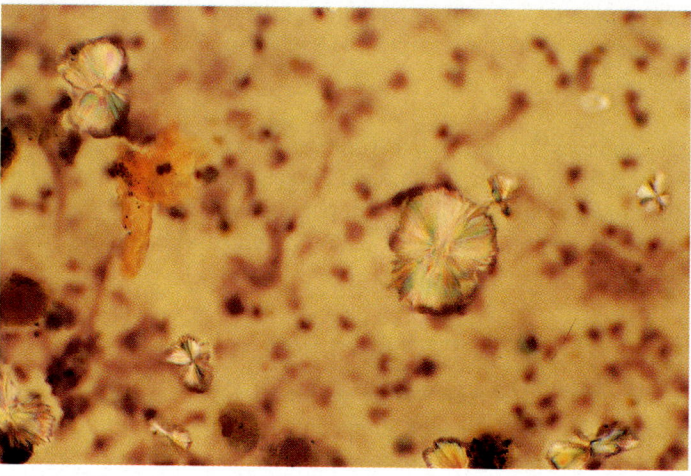

B

FIGURE 33-11 *A.* Fine-needle aspirate of the lung from a patient with atypical mycobacterial infection. Necrotic background, lack of inflammatory cells, and "ghost" forms of bacillary organisms are seen. These can be seen in air-dried smears using Ramonovsky's stain. (Diff-Quik stain, ×330.) *B.* Induced sputum showing acid-fast organisms in another case of atypical mycobacterial infection. (Ziehl-Neelsen stain, ×330.)

FIGURE 33-12 *A.* BAL specimen showing broad filamentous forms and acute angle branching of *Aspergillus. B.* Calcium oxalate crystals in association with aspergillus infection seen with partially polarized light. (Papanicolaou stain, ×208.)

be reported. Such findings are seen in patients who are immunocompromised or suffer from diabetes or other disabling conditions.

ASPERGILLOSIS

Aspergillus-related pulmonary disorders are quite varied in their clinical presentation, ranging from allergic-mediated airway disease to frank parenchymal infiltration. While the diagnosis of tissue invasion may be difficult, pneumonic and cavitary lesions can be accurately diagnosed cytologically. Most parenchymal infections are caused by *A. fumigatus,* although *A. niger* and *A. flavus* infections also occur. Sputum specimens, bronchial washings, bronchial brushings, and fine-needle aspirations can be diagnostic.

Aspergillus is an opportunistic airborne organism that sometimes contaminates pulmonary specimens. Care should be exercised in reporting infection with *Aspergillus* if it is seen only on one slide or one set of slides. The presence of an acute inflam-

matory background and clinical and radiologic correlation are necessary for accurate diagnosis. The organisms are seen as broad, filamentous structures that branch at acute angles. Sometimes, especially among immunosuppressed patients with overwhelming infections, "fruiting bodies" (conidiospores) are seen.[5] Birefringent calcium oxalate crystals may occur in specimens containing *Aspergillus;* they are more commonly observed with *A. niger*[9,28] (Fig. 33-12). Epithelial cells may show metaplastic and atypical morphologic features.[27]

CRYPTOCOCCOSIS

Patients with cryptococcosis may be asymptomatic or manifest nonspecific respiratory symptoms, including production of mucoid or blood-streaked sputum.[20] Organisms can be visualized in sputum, bronchial washings, bronchial brushings, or fine-needle aspirations. Most commonly, narrow-necked budding yeast forms are observed that show marked variation in size

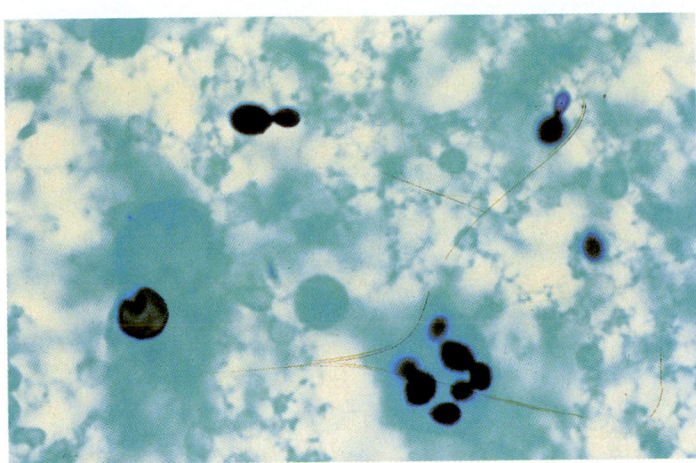

FIGURE 33-13 Bronchial washing showing *Cryptococcus*. Note the numerous budding organisms. Budding is narrow, and organisms show variation in size. (Silver stain, ×260.)

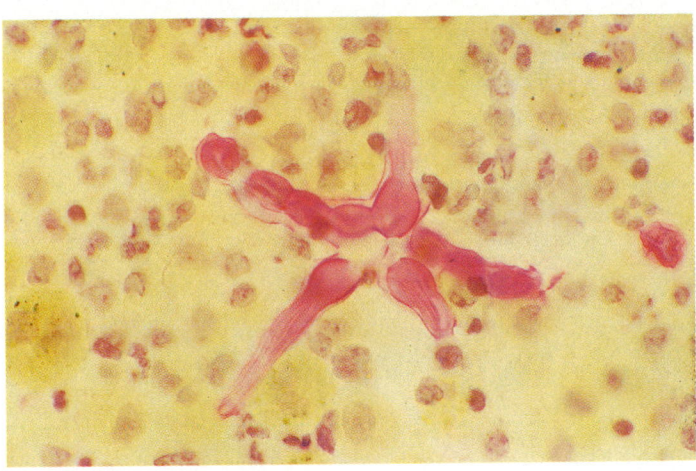

FIGURE 33-15 Bronchoalveolar lavage showing *Cryptococcus*. Note the broad, filamentous forms. Budding organisms are seen at the tips of the filaments. (Mucicarmine stain, ×330.)

(5 to 40 nm) (Fig. 33-13). The organism has a surrounding mucopolysaccharide-rich capsule that can be stained with mucicarmine or other histochemical agents (Fig. 33-14). In fresh, unfixed specimens, an India-ink preparation outlines the organisms quite well. Occasionally, broad filamentous forms are observed (Fig. 33-15).

HISTOPLASMOSIS

Pulmonary infection with *Histoplasma capsulatum* may be asymptomatic or associated with chronic signs and symptoms, mimicking tuberculosis. The organisms are small (2 to 4 nm) and are generally intracellular, occurring within pulmonary macrophages, bronchial epithelial cells, or neutrophils.[22] Organisms are best identified with a silver-methenamine technique.

BLASTOMYCOSIS

Patients with respiratory infection caused by *Blastomyces dermatidis* may be asymptomatic or have signs and symptoms of

chronic suppurative pulmonary disease. A clinical history demonstrating exposure in an endemic area (e.g., Ohio, the Mississippi River Valley, or southeastern United States) is usually helpful. The organism is seen as a budding yeast, generally with single, broad-based refractile walls. The budding form has a short neck, and the daughter bud is found in close apposition to the mother bud.

COCCIDIOIDOMYCOSIS

Patients with coccidioidomycosis generally present with features of a respiratory tract infection, including productive cough; alternatively, the principal clinical finding may be a solitary pulmonary mass. *Coccidioides immitis* is found in dry, sandy areas of the southwestern United States, including California, Arizona, New Mexico, and Texas. The organism is large (20 to 60 nm) and occurs as a nonbudding spherical structure. Spherules have a distinct thick wall and contain a variable number of endospores. The endospores are small (1 to 3 nm), round, and nonbudding. With most specimens, the background examination reveals a heavy acute inflammatory exudate that obscures the faintly stained organisms. Pulmonary fine-needle aspirates may be helpful in the diagnostic evaluation of solitary pulmonary nodules caused by coccidioidomycosis.

Other fungi, including *Paracoccidioides, Mucor,* and *Sporothrix,* are seen occasionally in pulmonary specimens.

Viral Infections

Influenza and parainfluenza viruses commonly infect the respiratory tract. Bronchial epithelial cells are affected and may demonstrate ciliocytophthoria (CCP), in which bronchial ciliated cells degenerate when the cytoplasmic tip and attached cilia are exfoliated. In CCP, the basal portion of the cell shows a pyknotic, degenerated nucleus (Fig. 33-16). Specimens generally have an acute inflammatory background and may contain numerous reactive bronchial cells that can be mistaken for neoplasm. In addition to CCP, which may be observed with other viral infections, influenza produces intracytoplasmic and intranuclear

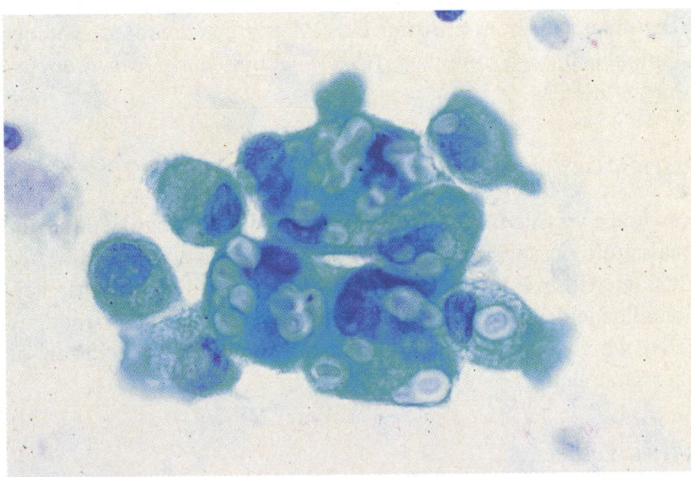

FIGURE 33-14 Bronchial washing showing *Cryptococcus*. Intracytoplasmic organisms show variation in size and a pale thick capsule. (Papanicolaou stain, ×330.)

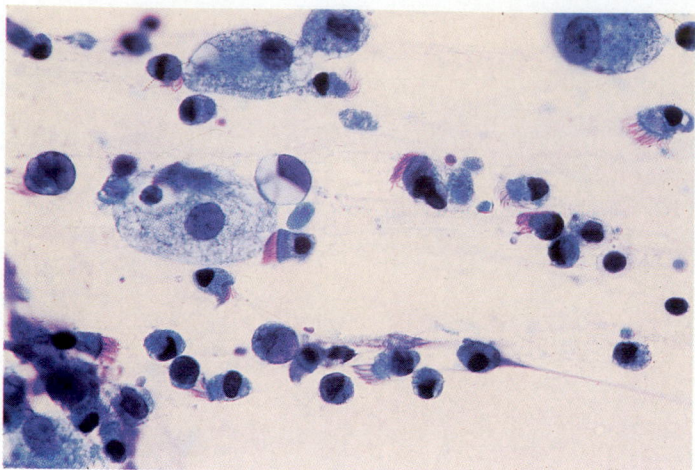

A

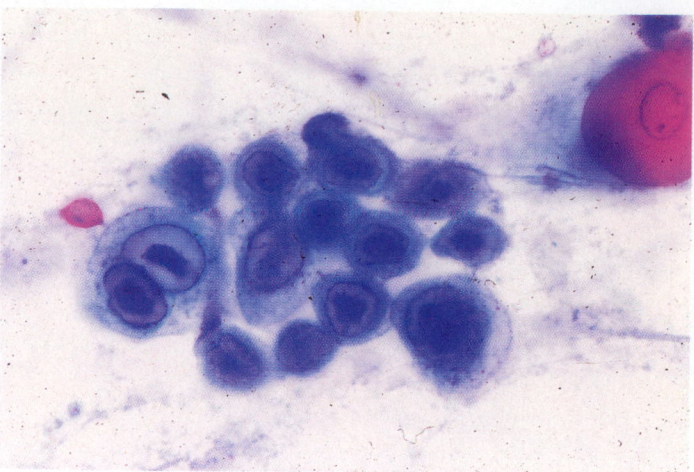

FIGURE 33-17 Bronchial washing showing herpes simplex virus (HSV). Note the large single cells with prominent intranuclear inclusions and gelatinous nuclear chromatin. (Papanicolaou stain, ×260.)

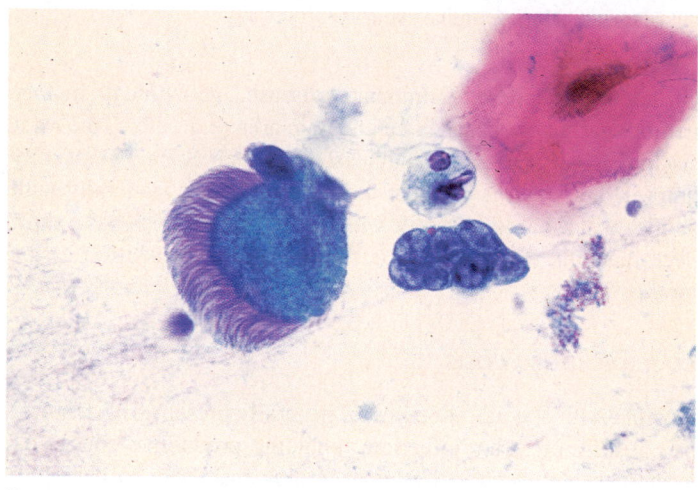

B

FIGURE 33-16 *A.* Bronchial washing showing ciliocytophthoria (CCP) in a pulmonary viral infection. Notice numerous fragmented, ciliated macrophages and columnar cells. (Papanicolaou stain, ×208.) *B.* Details of CCP. Note the cilia in a degenerated cell. (Papanicolaou stain, ×330.)

acidophilic, columnar cell inclusions. These inclusions may be single or multiple; cells are generally of normal size and are degenerate.[37]

HERPES SIMPLEX VIRUS

Herpes simplex virus (HSV) may infect the oral mucosa, the tracheobronchial tree, or the pulmonary parenchyma. The finding of HSV in a pulmonary cytologic specimen is useful only in localizing the infection to the lower respiratory tract when the specimen is "uncontaminated"—i.e., obtained from fine-needle aspiration, tracheal aspiration, bronchial washing, or BAL. Clinical and radiologic correlation is necessary in most cases. When pulmonary parenchymal infection is present, the specimen background generally is extremely inflammatory, showing numerous neutrophils, abundant mucus, and cellular degeneration. Unless adequate pulmonary material is carefully examined, pulmonary HSV infection can be easily overlooked.

The infected cells may be small (10 to 15 nm) and round and contain intranuclear evidence of the virus as a "ground glass" appearance. This pattern is commonly seen with tracheobronchial infection or in specimens obtained from aspiration of material through a tracheotomy tube. In cases of severe pulmonary infection, multinucleated giant cells demonstrating internuclear molding, intranuclear acidophilic inclusions, or a gelatin chromatin pattern may be seen (Fig. 33-17). Care should be exercised in distinguishing HSV inclusions and prominent nucleoli within bronchial cells.

CYTOMEGALOVIRUS

A member of the herpesvirus family, cytomegalovirus (CMV) may infect the bronchial epithelium and alveolar lining cells. Infection is common among immunocompromised patients. Infected cells show cytomegaly and large, generally distinct acidophilic intranuclear inclusions. Thin strips of nuclear chromatin bridge the space between the inclusion and the nuclear envelope (Fig. 33-18). Occasionally, the inclusions are basophilic and intracytoplasmic. In rare instances, CMV-infected cells may show multinucleation. Pulmonary HSV infection may occur concurrently with CMV.

RESPIRATORY SYNCYTIAL VIRUS

Respiratory syncytial virus (RSV) is often not recognized in routine cytologic specimens. The virus produces two types of inclusions within bronchial and alveolar living cells: (1) dense acidophilic inclusions with clear halos around them and (2) "smudge" cells, which contain a basophilic nucleus with obliteration of chromatic details.[51]

OTHER VIRUSES

Multinucleation and eosinophilic cellular inclusions may be observed in measles and adenovirus infections. Human papillomavirus (HPV) may cause tracheal papillomatosis and produce

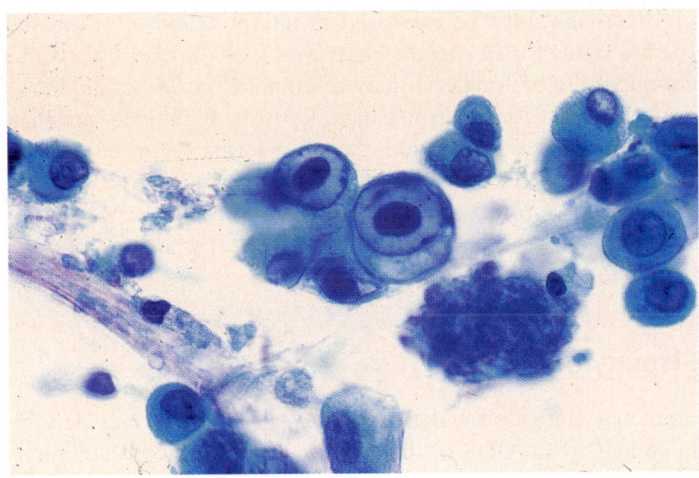

A

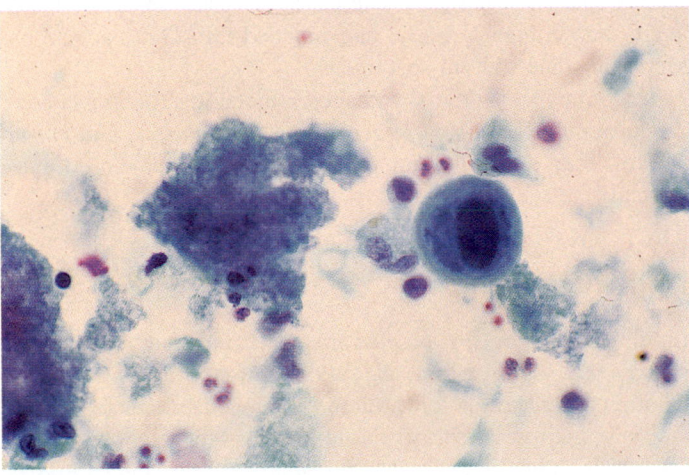

B

FIGURE 33-18 *A.* Bronchial brush showing cytomegalovirus (CMV). Note the large intranuclear acidophilic inclusions with radiating chromatin threads. *B.* Basophilic intranuclear and intracytoplasmic inclusions are seen. (Papanicolaou stain, ×330.)

fragments of squamous epithelium containing typical koilocytes. Koilocytes are squamous cells with eccentric, vesicular nuclei and a distinct cytoplasmic halo or cavity. These cells contain intranuclear HPV antigens, which can be demonstrated by use of various tissue and molecular techniques. Most HPV infections are caused by viral types 6 and 11.

OTHER NONNEOPLASTIC CONDITIONS

Cytopathologic findings may be observed in a number of other nonneoplastic conditions, several of which are described briefly below.

Pneumocystis carinii Pneumonia

Pneumocystis carinii infection was originally described by Chagas in 1909 and confirmed a year later by Carinii. It has been most commonly reported among patients with underlying neoplastic or immunodeficiency diseases. Initial reports of *P. carinii*

pneumonia (PCP) in homosexual men date back to 1981.[4] In current practice, pulmonary infection with *P. carinii* may be observed at some time in up to 60 percent of patients with acquired immunodeficiency syndrome (AIDS).[19,26] Systemic chemotherapy for neoplastic diseases and transplantation may result in immunosupression and subsequent infection.

Initially regarded as a fungus, *P. carinii* is now considered a protozoon, based on ribosomal RNA studies.[7] The precise life cycle is unknown, and attempts to culture the organism have been unsuccessful. *P. carinii* occurs in the trophozoite form, which is 1 to 5 nm in diameter and has a distinct nucleus. Up to eight organisms may be contained within the cyst, which measures 6 to 8 nm in diameter, roughly the size of a red blood cell. Parasites infect adjacent tissue after being liberated from the ruptured cysts. *P. carinii* infects alveolar macrophages; in rare instances, it may be seen in macrophages in pleural fluid, in lymph nodes, and in other reticuloendothelial cells.

Whereas, historically, PCP was often diagnosed from examination of lung tissue obtained by open lung biopsy, carefully collected pulmonary cytology specimens from fiberoptic bronchoscopy give comparable or better results with minimal risk to the patient. The technique is sensitive, rapid, and economical. While early reports on the diagnostic yield from examination of induced sputum specimens were encouraging, the data have not been uniformly confirmed. The best results are obtained with BAL. Table 33-1 summarizes the diagnostic value of various pulmonary specimens in the diagnosis of PCP.

Pneumocystis infection may be suspected from inspection of routine Papanicolaou stains, as well as hematoxylin-and-eosin–stained pulmonary preparations. For a definitive diagnosis, a variety of histochemical, immunologic, and recently introduced molecular techniques are utilized. Trophozoites can be visualized using selected stains (e.g., Romanovsky), basic dye (crystal violet, toluidine blue), periodic acid–Schiff (PAS), Papanicolaou, and Gram-Weigert. The most commonly used histochemical procedure, the silver-methenamine (Grocott) stain, outlines the cyst wall. Immunocytochemical and molecular techniques can be used to identify the organisms, as well as the cyst walls.

CYTOMORPHOLOGY

In air-dried specimens prepared using the Romanovsky, Papanicolaou, or hematoxylin-eosin method, *P. carinii* appears within the alveolar material or foamy "coagulum." The organism occurs

TABLE 33-1

Sensitivity of Pulmonary Cytopathology Specimens

Specimen	Sensitivity
Sputum (induced)	50–55%
Bronchial washings	70–80%
Bronchial brushings	55–75%
Bronchoalveolar lavage	90–95%
Lung biopsy (transbronchial)	85–90%

SOURCE: Modified from Gupta.[19]

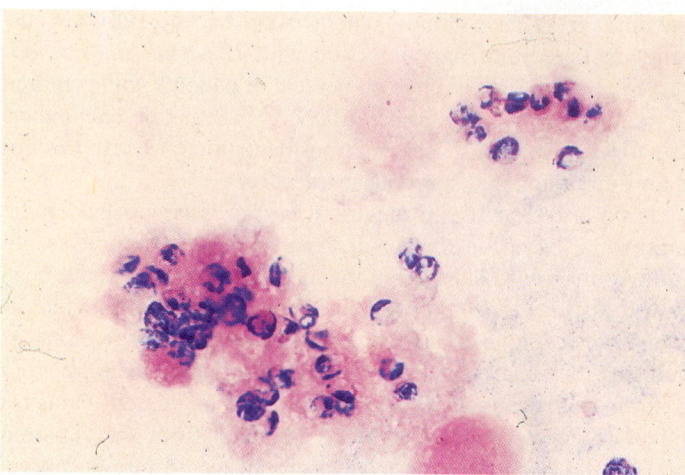

FIGURE 33-19 Bronchoalveolar lavage showing *Pneumocystis carinii.* Note the cluster of organisms with collapsed cyst walls and central clearing. These forms should be distinguished from the yeast form of Candida, which is commonly seen in pulmonary specimens. (Gram-Weigert's stain, ×260.)

in cyst forms that may contain trophozoites (see above). In silver- and Gram-Weigert–stained preparations, the cysts frequently collapse, giving a crescent or "poached egg" appearance (Fig. 33-19).

The sensitivity of the staining techniques varies according to the quality of preparation, content of pulmonary material, and duration of therapy, if any, before the diagnostic procedure. Silver stains and some of the immunologic techniques may give negative results in specimens collected from patients who have received prior therapy. After treatment, the cysts undergo lysis, with fragmentation of the walls, necrosis, and ingestion of the organisms by pulmonary macrophages[19,34] (Fig. 33-20). The sensitivity of commonly utilized special staining techniques for PCP has been discussed.[16] Based on our own experience and that of others,[16] among the commonly utilized histochemical stains, Gram-Weigert appears slightly more sensitive and specific than silver-methenamine; Giemsa's stain is the least sensitive technique.

Great care must be exercised in interpretation of silver and special stains for *P. carinii.* Yeast forms of *Candida* that occur commonly in oral material may resemble *P. carinii* cysts. However, the yeast forms do not have the soft, wrinkled, "poached egg" appearance. In addition, the yeast forms occur in oral mucoid material, not in the proteinaceous, granular alveolar contents. In situ hybridization and molecular techniques provide results similar to other diagnostic procedures; however, there appear to be quantitative differences.[34]

Strongyloidosis

Pulmonary infection with *Strongyloides stercoralis* may be seen in patients with AIDS or those who are iatrogenically immunosuppressed (e.g., by prolonged corticosteroid administration). Filariform larvae, which are easily identifiable, may be seen in bloody sputum specimens. The larvae measure up to 500 nm in length and contain a gullet and notched tail. Ova may be observed in some sputum specimens.

Uncommonly, other parasites, including *Echinococcus, Trichomonas, Entamoeba,* microfilaria, *Toxoplasma,* and *Paragonimus,* may infect pulmonary tissues and be diagnosed cytologically.

Lipid Pneumonia

Lipids may enter the respiratory system through exogenous sources (e.g., by ingestion, aspiration, or use of nasal sprays containing fatty materials) or through endogenous routes (e.g., from the bone marrow after soft-tissue injuries—fat embolism). Cytologically, large foamy cells with small vesicular nuclei may be seen, either singly or in small tissue fragments (Fig. 33-21). The presence of endogenous or exogenous fats can be confirmed by appropriate histochemical stains.[39] Such differentiation and diagnosis can be valuable for infants and children with pneumonia.[6]

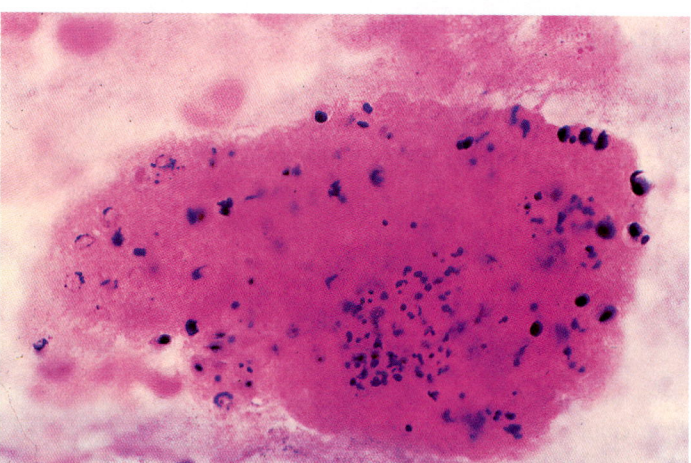

FIGURE 33-20 Bronchoalveolar lavage showing *P. carinii* after therapy. Note the degenerated and ghost forms of the organisms in the alveolar cast material. (Gram-Weigert's stain, ×330.)

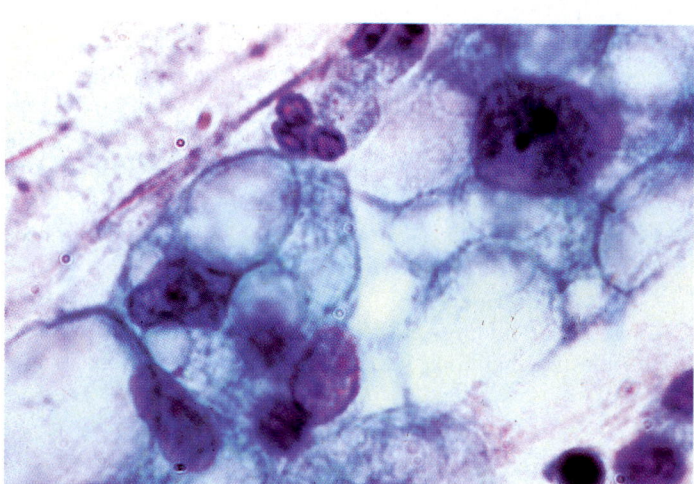

FIGURE 33-21 Bronchial wash specimen showing lipid pneumonia. Note the large vacuolated cells with hyperchromatic nuclei and prominent nucleoli. Such cells can be mistaken for adenocarcinoma cells. (Papanicolaou stain, ×260.)

Aspiration Pneumonia

Generally, both severe acute inflammation and foreign-body giant-cell reactions may be observed in pulmonary specimens obtained from patients with aspiration pneumonia. The latter reaction is related to the duration of the disease.

Sarcoidosis

In pulmonary parenchymal involvement with sarcoidosis, diagnostic cytologic changes may be observed.[1,49] BAL specimens are most useful in the evaluation. Typical findings include a clean background, a few lymphocytes, Langhan's multinucleated giant cells, and syncytial forms of histiocytic cells. Giant cells often have a clear cytoplasm and vesicular or pyknotic nucleus (Fig. 33-22). These giant cells should be distinguished from the multinucleated cells associated with cigarette smoking, bronchial irritation, or pneumonia. The multinucleated giant cells from cigarette smokers often contain golden-brown pigment; the irritative processes are characterized by numerous reactive columnar cells; the pneumonic processes commonly include an inflammatory background. Concentrically laminated Schaumann's bodies or spiderlike asteroid bodies may be observed in pulmonary specimens.[1] It must be appreciated that these findings are uncommon and not specific for sarcoidosis. Clinical and radiologic correlation is necessary for proper interpretation of such specimens.

Radiation and Chemotherapy Effects

Some of the most bizarre and atypical cytologic changes are seen in pulmonary specimens obtained after radiation therapy or chemotherapy. The value of obtaining a proper clinical history in this regard cannot be overemphasized. Radiation may affect both squamous and bronchial columnar cells; the effect is long-term and dose-dependent. General features include cytomegaly and karyomegaly; nucleocytoplasmic ratios are unaltered. Irradiated nuclei are generally pale and have a finely divided, evenly

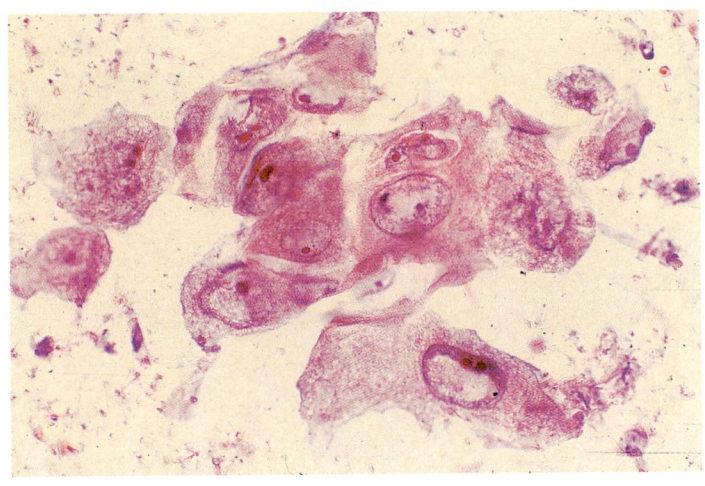

A

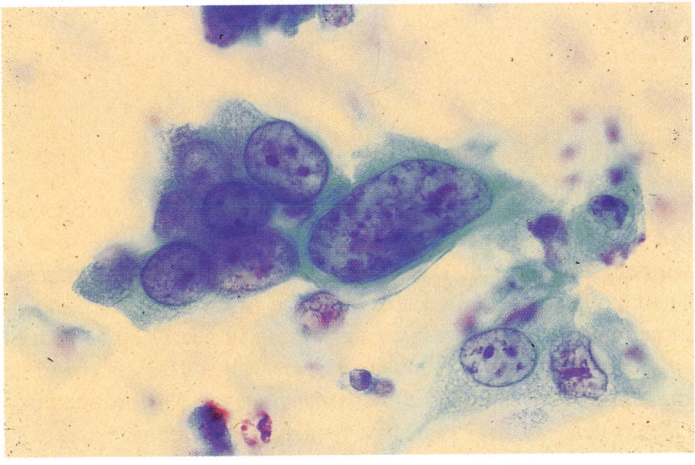

B

FIGURE 33-23 *A.* Bronchial washing showing radiation changes in bronchial epithelial cells. Notice the extremely bizarre cells with marked variation in size. *B.* Prominent nucleoli are evident. Cells have thin and uniform nuclear membranes and pale chromatin. (Papanicolaou stain, ×260.)

distributed chromatin (Fig. 33-23). These cells reveal minimum pleomorphism and contain prominent acidophilic inclusions. The cytoplasm may be variable, dense, or vacuolated.

As first reported by Weston and Guin,[47] chemotherapeutic agents, including alkylating drugs (e.g., busulfan and cyclophosphamide) and antimetabolites (e.g., methotrexate and azathioprine), generally produce changes that affect bronchial epithelial cells and type II pneumocytes. These cells enlarge and become hyperchromatic, although the chromatin remains uniform and generally does not show abnormal clumping and clearing. Nucleoli are single or multiple and appear prominent. The nuclei may appear smudged, with loss of chromatin granularity and nuclear detail (Fig. 33-24). Great care should be exercised in diagnosing neoplasm in such cases. A proper history, comparison of cells with the original tumor, and familiarity of cytomorphologic changes are useful adjuncts to correct diagnosis. Similar cellular changes may be associated with amiodarone therapy.[40]

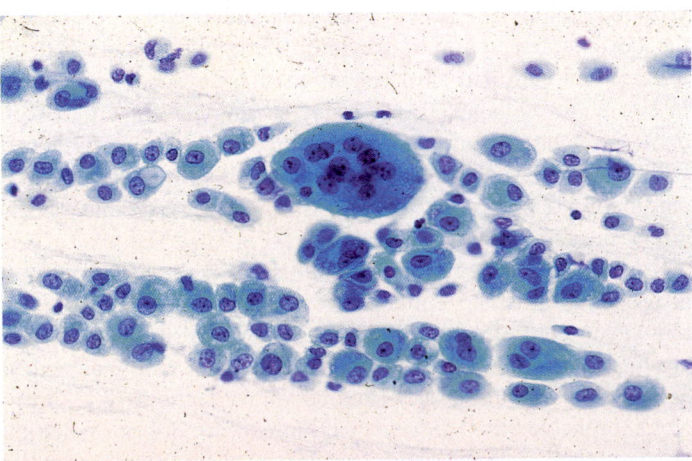

FIGURE 33-22 Bronchial washing showing pulmonary sarcoidosis. Note the numerous macrophages and a giant cell. Intermixed are a few lymphocytes. (Papanicolaou stain, ×166.)

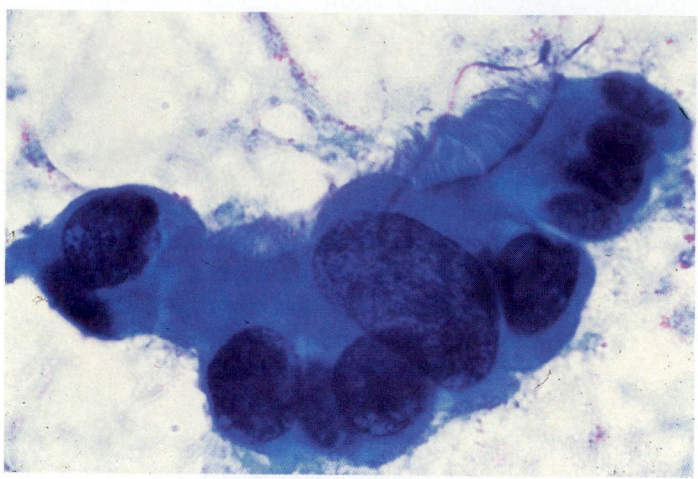

FIGURE 33-24 Bronchial washing showing chemotherapy effect on bronchial epithelial cells. Note the fragment of cells with cytomegaly, nuclear atypia, and large cilia. (Papanicolaou stain, ×330.)

PULMONARY NEOPLASMS

More than 100,000 new cases of lung cancer were reported in the United States in 1994; the majority (72,000) were seen in women, a statistic that continues to escalate.[3] Only 16 percent of lung cancers are detected when the disease is localized; regional and distant metastases are present in nearly 70 percent of cases at the time of diagnosis. The overall 5-year survival rate for lung cancer is under 20 percent; however, for localized disease, 5-year survival is nearly 60 percent. Death rates seem to have stabilized in the past decade.

The cytopathologic changes observed with several common pulmonary neoplasms are described below.

Early Lung Cancer

In some lung cancers (e.g., squamous cell carcinoma), precursor lesions, including squamous dysplasia and in situ changes, precede development of invasive cancer. The early detection of this type of tumor improves survival; however, the multicentric origin of the tumors, along with coexisting illnesses, contributes to the mortality. Furthermore, moderate, atypical squamous metaplasia of the bronchial epithelium represents a lesion that, in a significant number of cases, may develop into squamous carcinoma.[2,42] Application of antibody techniques to analysis of sputum specimens can detect moderately and markedly atypical metaplastic cells in patients at risk of subsequent lung cancer, a second primary, or recurrent tumor.[42] Attempts to identify the at-risk population using immunocytochemical techniques have been only partly successful. The labor and costs associated with sputum collection, sampling, and cell concentration have contributed to the limited use of these techniques. Molecular methods are currently being evaluated for early lung cancer detection; results have been encouraging.

Based on experience from an early Veterans Administration study, and using the evolution of cervical cancer as a model, a multi-institutional, early lung cancer detection project was launched by the National Cancer Institute in the early 1970s.[13] Guidelines were outlined for the early detection of lung cancer, using chest radiographs, sputum cytology, and, when indicated, fiberoptic bronchoscopy. In addition, treatment methods were delineated for "early" cancer, which was defined as an unsuspected, asymptomatic tumor detected by cytologic or imaging techniques.

Nearly 30,000 high-risk participants were screened using sputum cytology or chest radiographs (or both) at the three participating centers. Cases were followed for up to 15 years. While sputum cytology and chest radiography detected a number of presymptomatic, early-stage lung cancers (especially squamous cell carcinomas), higher resectability and survival rates among the study group did not result in a lower overall mortality. Accordingly, the American Cancer Society does not recommend an annual sputum examination or chest radiography in its guidelines for early lung cancer detection.[43]

Established Lung Cancer

Although pulmonary cytology in its present form has been used for detection and diagnosis of lung cancer for about 50 fifty years, the earliest description of the technique dates back to 1767, when exfoliated respiratory cells were first described. In patients with suspected pulmonary malignancies, examination of a single expectorated sputum has a diagnostic yield as low as 20 percent; when five early-morning, deep-cough specimens are examined, the yield is as high as 90 percent.[8] The type of pulmonary specimen (random, early-morning, induced, pooled, bronchial washing, bronchial brushing, transbronchial aspiration, or transthoracic needle aspiration), technique of collection (fresh or fixed), quantity of specimen examined, and technique of specimen preparation have bearing on the value of pulmonary cytology in cancer detection. Additionally, the location of the lesion, associated pathology, and sampling techniques may contribute to the number of diagnostic tumor cells present in a specimen.

EARLY SQUAMOUS CELL CARCINOMA

From a cytology perspective, early squamous cell carcinoma is the best-studied tumor of the lung; definitive precursor (dysplastic) and early (in situ) lesions have been documented.[2,8,48] In situ tumor cells are recognizable as single cells with a high nucleocytoplasmic ratio. The cells have hyperchromatic nuclei with no nucleoli; chromatin is uniformly distributed, with little chromatin clumping and clearing. Cytoplasm is variable, generally scant, and frequently keratinized (Fig. 33-25).

A few cells may be seen in small tissue fragments, especially in bronchial brush specimens. The smear background is generally clean; cells should be distinguished from similar cells that are mostly metaplastic and may be associated with mechanical irritation (e.g., from tracheal intubation), infections (e.g., bronchitis, bronchiectasis, abscess, viral infection), or prior radiation or chemotherapy. Successful resection of in situ lung cancer has resulted in a 5-year survival rate of 80 to 85 percent, but tumors frequently tend to be multicentric and difficult to successfully eradicate.

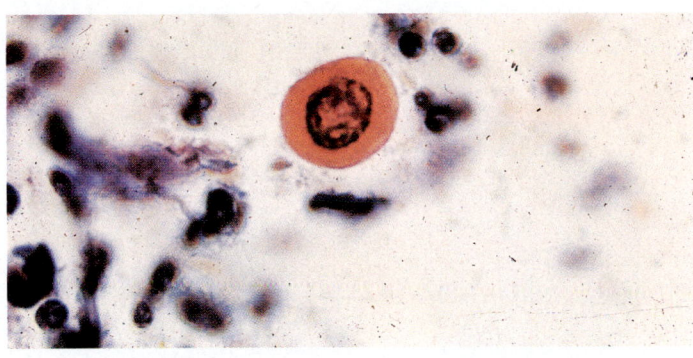

A

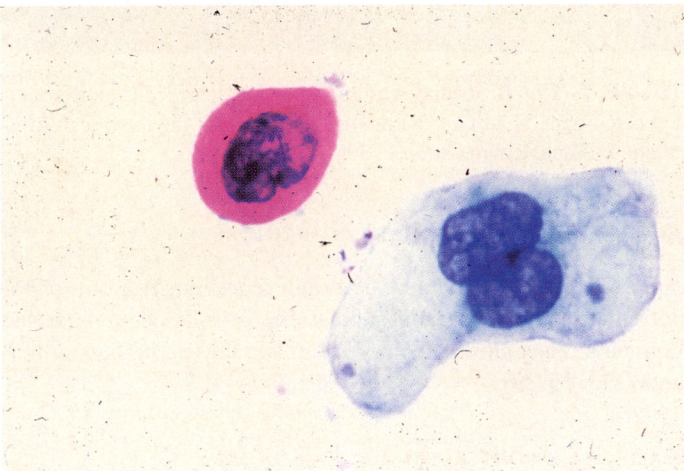

B

FIGURE 33-25   Bronchial washing showing "early" lung cancer. The cells in (*A*) and (*B*) represent nuclear and cytoplasmic features that are indicative of early squamous cell carcinoma. (Papanicolaou stain, A ×260, B ×330.)

INVASIVE SQUAMOUS CELL CARCINOMA

Invasive squamous cell carcinoma often results in a mass or cavitary lesion with tumor necrosis and secondary infection. The background of such specimens may be acutely inflammatory or necrotic, with numerous infarcted, necrotic cells, little nuclear detail, and malignant features. Typical cells reveal pleomorphism that may appear as "tadpole" or fiber forms. Bizarre, irregularly shaped cells with obvious malignant features, such as nuclear membrane irregularities, abnormal chromatin clearing and clumping, and prominent nucleoli, may occur. Cytoplasm is variable, but it reveals squamous differentiation (Fig. 33-26). Careful examination of cells for intercellular bridges or keratohyaline granules is necessary before a definitive diagnosis of squamous cell carcinoma can be established.

The cytomorphologic diagnosis of squamous cell cancer is highly accurate and approaches 100 percent.[8] Tumor cells detected in expectorated sputum or bronchial wash specimens generally are more keratinized and poorly preserved than those obtained using bronchial brush and fine-needle aspiration techniques. Reactive changes, especially after instrumentation, with therapy, or with viral infections and pulmonary infarction, can be extremely atypical and must be distinguished from tumor

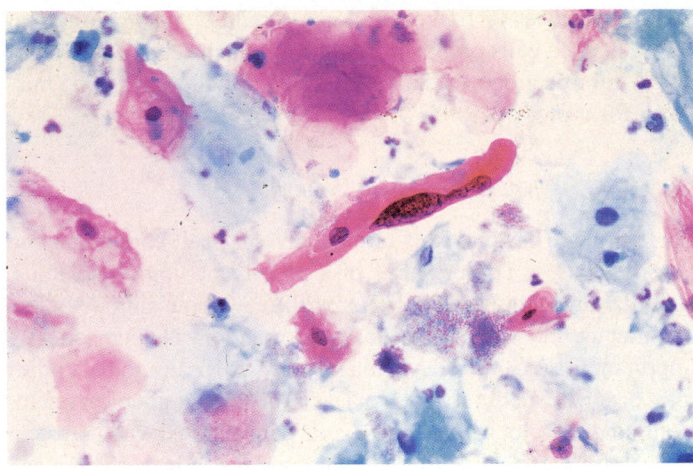

FIGURE 33-26   Induced sputum showing invasive squamous cell carcinoma. Note an obvious malignant cell with necrotic background and numerous squamous cells. (Papanicolaou stain, ×208.)

cells. Communication between the clinician and the laboratory is necessary for proper interpretation of pulmonary specimens.

ADENOCARCINOMA

Cytodiagnosis of adenocarcinoma is generally highly accurate (70 to 80 percent). Pulmonary adenocarcinoma can be diagnosed relatively easy when the tumor is located within central airways; however, diagnosis is extremely difficult with peripheral tumors or scar-associated malignancies. Tumor cells generally occur in tissue fragments, which may appear as acinar and papillary structures (Fig. 33-27). Cells have a soft, molding cytoplasm that may contain evidence of secretion. Tumor cells may exhibit bizarre, malignant nuclei with obvious nuclear membrane and chromatinic abnormalities and prominent nucleoli. Nucleoli can be large and abnormally shaped; they may be variable in number.

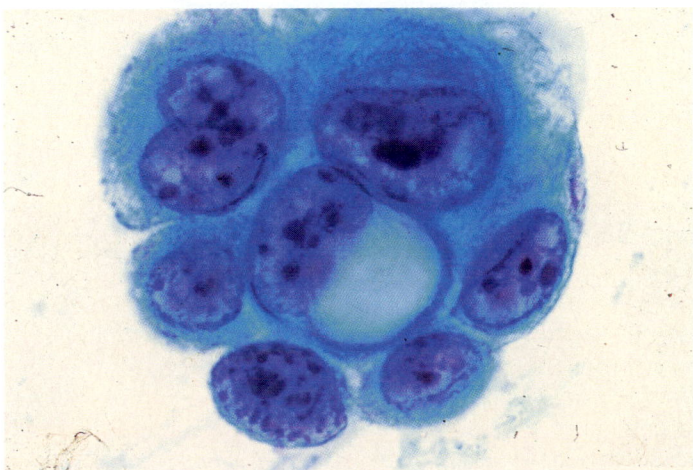

FIGURE 33-27   Bronchial washing showing adenocarcinoma of the lung. Note the glandular features with nuclear chromatin and nucleolar variability. There is evidence of mucus secretion in the cell in the center of the field. (Papanicolaou stain, ×330.)

The diagnosis of adenocarcinoma should be made with great care. Shedded cells obtained from postbronchoscopy specimens, after viral infections, or during pulmonary infarction can be mistaken for tumor cells.

BRONCHOALVEOLAR CELL CARCINOMA

The cytologic diagnosis of bronchoalveolar cell carcinoma can be problematic. The presence of a prominent single nucleolus, cuboidal or columnar cell forms with or without intracytoplasmic mucus, and papillary and acinar formations is diagnostically important (Fig. 33-28). At times, calcified psammoma bodies may occur in such tumors. Nuclear grooves, intranuclear inclusions, and tenacious intracytoplasmic connections, when present, are helpful diagnostically.[24,50] Cytologic diagnosis of cases can be extremely accurate (60 to 80 percent).

Bronchoalveolar tumor cells can often be confused with reactive bronchial cells, which may be seen with inflammation or after instrumentation or treatment.

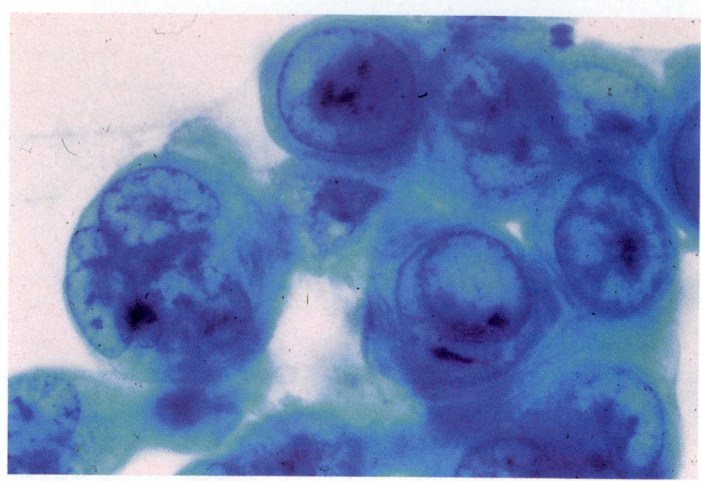

FIGURE 33-29   Bronchial washing showing large cell undifferentiated carcinoma. Note that the malignant cells lack any obvious differentiation. (Papanicolaou stain, ×330.)

LARGE-CELL UNDIFFERENTIATED CARCINOMA

Large-cell undifferentiated carcinoma represents a group of tumors that cannot be easily subclassified. Cells occur in tissue fragments. They show pleomorphism and classic malignant features (Fig. 33-29).

SMALL-CELL UNDIFFERENTIATED CARCINOMA

Small-cell undifferentiated carcinoma is relatively easy to diagnose when the specimen is of good technical quality and representative of the lesion. In fresh smears or filter preparations, tumor cells are seen in association with mucous strands. The cells have a high nucleocytoplasmic ratio and uniformly distributed chromatin. Nuclei are absent or inconspicuous, intercellular molding is prominent; and cytoplasm is distinct, delicate, and scant (Fig. 33-30). Well-preserved cells must be examined for a definitive diagnosis. Invariably, such tumor cells have tumor-type necrosis (diathesis) that appears to remain confined to adjacent

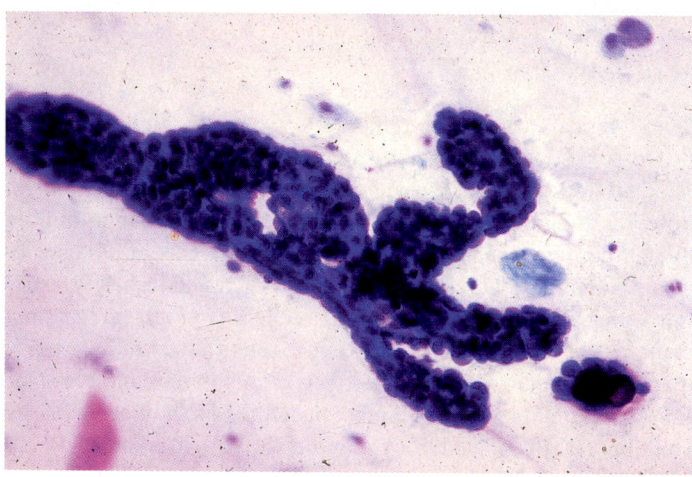

A

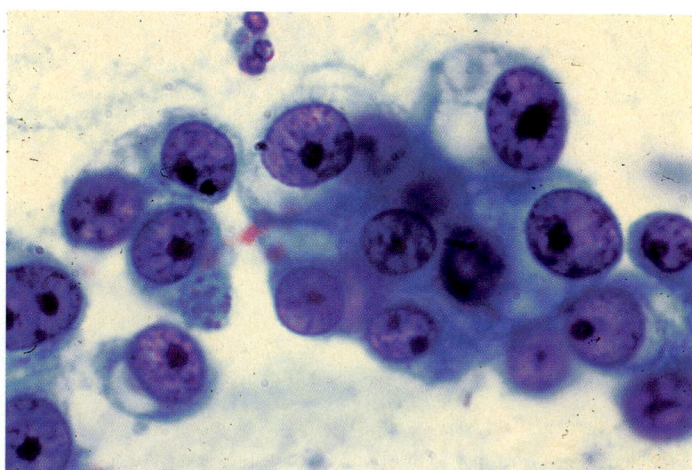

B

FIGURE 33-28   Bronchial washing showing bronchioloalveolar carcinoma. *A.* Papillary formation. *B.* Prominent nucleoli and tenacious intercytoplasmic connection (TIC). (Papanicolaou stain, *A* ×105, *B* ×330.)

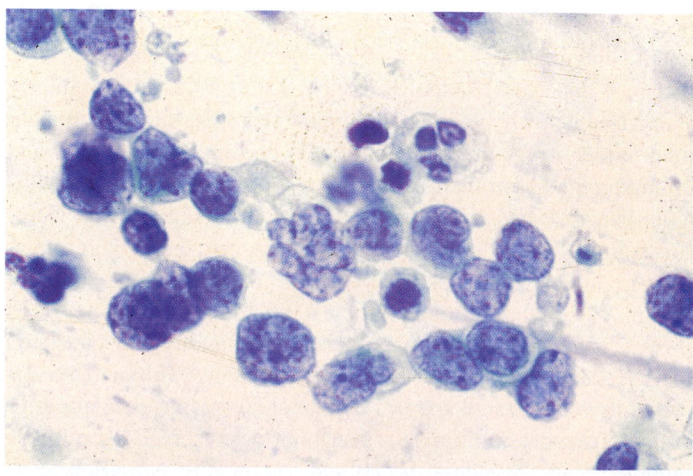

FIGURE 33-30   Bronchial washing showing small cell undifferentiated carcinoma. Note the soft cells with uniformly granular chromatin, intercellular molding, and scant cytoplasm. (Papanicolaou stain, ×330.)

areas. Bronchial brush specimens and fine-needle aspirations may provide better preservation of tumor cells, as well as larger tissue fragments. It may be possible to subclassify these tumors as oat cell or intermediate variety, but this distinction is generally not possible on the basis of cytologic preparations.

Great care needs to be exercised in the proper diagnosis of small-cell undifferentiated tumors. Vegetable cells, lymphoid cells from tonsils and adenoids, reserve cells, degenerated bronchial columnar cells, and lymphoma may all resemble small cell carcinoma of the lung. Diagnostic accuracy with this tumor type approaches 100 percent in certain laboratories; most centers report 70 to 80 percent predictability of cytologic diagnosis.[8]

At times, not all small cell tumors possess all the typical morphologic changes. They may contain a few nucleoli, coarser chromatin, and a variable amount of cytoplasm; they may occur in tissue fragments. Such tumors are best classified as "undifferentiated tumors with neuroendocrine features." Immunocytochemical stains for chromogranin and neuron-specific enolase and ultrastructural studies may be helpful in such cases.

Carcinoid

The vast majority of pulmonary carcinoid tumors occur submucosally and do not exfoliate diagnostic cells. Diagnostic cells can, however, be obtained by bronchial brush and fine-needle aspiration techniques. When present, the cells are small and round or oval; they possess scant, delicate cytoplasm and contain one or two nucleoli. The cell exists in microacinic formations or in trabecular and papillary structures. Little evidence of intercellular molding, pleomorphism, or necrosis is present in these specimens.

Atypical Carcinoid

Atypical carcinoid tumors are classified morphologically as midway along the pathologic spectrum between carcinoids and small cell undifferentiated carcinomas. Although the cells may not have the nuclear features typical of a small cell carcinoma or the microacinic and trabecular pattern of a carcinoid, they may reveal an occasional mitosis and focal necrosis.

Lymphoma

A diagnosis of lymphoma may be made from pulmonary specimens. A proper clinical history and use of marker studies are necessary for accurate diagnosis. Hodgkin's disease can be diagnosed by recognition of typical Reed-Sternberg cells in a variety of pulmonary specimens.

Metastatic Tumors

Malignant melanoma and breast, prostate, kidney, and gastrointestinal tumors commonly metastasize to the lungs. A knowledge of the patient's history, coupled with typical morphologic changes and immunohistochemical studies, is often helpful. Of course, patients with an extrapulmonary primary tumor may develop a primary pulmonary malignancy. Concurrent or sequential development of malignancies is common in cigarette smokers, particularly laryngeal and pulmonary squamous cell tumors.

SUMMARY

Cytology is an accurate, economical, and rapid technique that can be useful in diagnosing a large number of nonneoplastic and neoplastic pulmonary lesions. Proper sampling, procurement of high-quality specimens, adequate specimen preparation, careful examination of material, and correlation with clinical and radiographic features are essential for accurate diagnosis.

REFERENCES

1. Aisner S, Gupta PK, Frost JK: Sputum cytology in pulmonary sarcoidosis. *Acta Cytol* 21:394–398, 1977.
2. National Cancer Institute, National Institutes of Health, US Department of Health and Human Services: *Atlas of Early Lung Cancer.* New York, Igaku-Shoin, 1983.
3. Boring C, Squires TS, Tong T, Montgomery S: Cancer statistics, 1994. *CA* 44:7–42,1994.
4. Centers for Disease Control: *Pneumocystis* pneumonia—Los Angeles. *MMWR* 30:250–252, 1981.
5. Chandler FM, Watts JC: Fungal infections, in Dail DH, Hammer SP (eds), *Pulmonary Pathology.* New York, Springer-Verlag, 1987, pp 189–258.
6. Collins KA, Geisinger KR, Wagner PH, et al: The cytologic evaluation of lipid-laden alveolar macrophages as an indicator of aspiration pneumonia in young children. *Arch Pathol Lab Med* 119: 229–231,1995.
7. Edman JC, Kovacs JA, Masor H, et al: Ribosomal RNA sequence shows *Pneumocystis carinii* to be a member of the Fungi. *Nature* 334:519–522, 1988.
8. Erozan YS, Frost JK: Cytopathologic diagnosis of lung cancer, in Straus MJ (ed), *Lung Cancer: Clinical Diagnosis and Treatment,* 2d ed. New York, Grune & Stratton, 1983, pp 113–125.
9. Farley ML, Mabry L, Munoz LA, Diserens HW: Crystals occurring in pulmonary cytology specimens: Association with aspergillus infection. *Acta Cytol* 29:737–744, 1985.
10. Freedman SI, Ang EP, Haley RS: Identification of coccidiidomycosis of the lung by fine needle aspiration biopsy. *Acta Cytol* 30:420–424, 1986.
11. Frost JK, Gupta PK, Erozan YS, et al: Pulmonary cytologic alterations in toxic environmental inhalation. *Hum Pathol* 4:521–553, 1973.
12. Frost JK: *The Cell in Health and Disease,* 2d ed. New York, Karger, 1986.
13. Frost JK, Ball WC Jr, Levin ML, et al: The National Cancer Institute cooperative early lung cancer detection program results of initial screen (prevalence). Early lung cancer detection: Summary and conclusions. *Am Rev Respir Dis* 130:656–670, 1984.
14. Greenbaum E, Copeland A, Grewal R: Blackened bronchoalveolar lavage fluid in crack smokers: A preliminary study. *Am J Clin Pathol* 100:481–487, 1993.
15. Greenberg SD: Asbestos, in Dail DH, Hammer SP (eds), *Pulmonary Pathology.* New York, Springer, 1987, pp 619–636.
16. Guarner J, Robey SS, Gupta PK: Cytologic detection of *Pneumocystis carinii:* Comparison of Papanicolaou and other histochemical stains. *Diagn Cytopathol* 2:133–137, 1986.
17. Gupta PK, Frost JK, Geddes SS, et al: Morphologic identification of alpha-1 antitrypsin in pulmonary macrophages. *Hum Pathol* 10: 345–347, 1979.
18. Gupta PK: Intrauterine contraceptive device: Vaginal cytology, pathologic changes and their clinical implications. *Acta Cytol* 26: 571–613, 1982.

19. Gupta PK: Cytopathology of *Pneumocystis carinii,* in Wied GL, Keebler CM, Koss LG, et al (eds), *Compendium on Diagnostic Cytology,* 7th ed. Chicago, Tutorials of Cytology, 1992, pp 205–211.

20. Gupta RK: Identification of unsuspected pulmonary cryptococcosis in sputum cytology. *Acta Cytol* 39:154–156, 1985.

21. Johnston WW, Frable WJ: *Diagnostic Respiratory Cytopathology.* New York, Masson, 1979.

22. Johnston WW: Pulmonary cytopathology in the compromised host, in Greenberg SD (ed), *Lung Pathology for Clinicians.* New York, Thieme-Stratton, 1982.

23. Johnston WW: Percutaneous FNAB of the lung. *Acta Cytol* 28:218–224, 1984.

24. Johnston WW: Cytopatholgy of the lung, diagnostic applications of sputum, bronchial brushings and fine needle aspiration specimens, in Wied GL, Keebler CM, Koss LG, et al (eds), *Compendium on Diagnostic Cytology,* 7th ed. Chicago, Tutorials of Cytology, 1992, pp 225–238.

25. Johnston WW, Elson CE: Respiratory tract, in Bibbo M (ed), *Comprehensive Cytopatholgy.* Philadelphia, Saunders, 1992, pp 320–398.

26. Johnston WW: Role of cytopathology in the diagnosis of opportunistic infections of the respiratory tract and other nongynecologic sites, in Wied GL, Keebler CM, Koss LG, et al (eds), *Compendium on Diagnostic Cytology,* 7th ed. Chicago, Tutorials of Cytology, 1992, pp 194–204.

27. Koss LG: *Diagnostic Cytology and Its Histopathologic Bases,* 3d ed. Philadelphia, Lippincott, 1979.

28. Lee SH, Barnes WG, Scaetzel WP: Pulmonary aspergillosis and the importance of oxalte crystals recognition in cytology specimen. *Arch Pathol Lab Med* 110:1176–1179, 1986.

29. Linder J, Rennard S: *Bronchoalveolar Lavage.* Chicago, American Society of Clinical Pathologists, 1988.

30. National Cancer Institute Cooperative Early Lung Cancer Group: *Manual of Procedures,* 2d ed. Washington, DC, NIH# 79-1972, US Dept. of Health, Education, and Welfare, 1979.

31. Naib ZM, Stewart JA, Dowdle WR, et al: Cytological features of viral respiratory tract infections. *Acta Cytol* 12:162–171, 1968.

32. Naylor B, Railey C: A pitfall in the cytodiagnosis of sputum of asthmatics. *J Clin Pathol* 17:84–89, 1964.

33. Papanicolaou GN: *Atlas of Exfoliative Cytology.* Cambridge, MA, Commonwealth Fund, Harvard University Press, 1954.

34. Peraz L, Gupta PK, Montone K: Detection of *Pneumocystis carinii* in transbronchial biopsy and bronchoalveolar lavage specimens by in situ hybridization and immunohistochemical techniques. *Cell Vision* 2:462–467, 1996.

35. Rajwanshi A, Bhambhani S, Das DK: Fine-needle aspiration cytology diagnosis of tuberculosis. *Diagn Cytopathol* 3:13–16, 1987.

36. Roggli VL, Piantadosi CA, Bell DY: Asbestos bodies in bronchoalveolar lavage fluid: A study of 20 asbestos exposed individu-

als and comparison to patients with other chronic interstitial lung diseases. *Acta Cytol* 30:470–476, 1986.

37. Saccomanno G, Saunders RP, Ellis H, et al: Concentration of carcinoma or atypical cells in sputum. *Acta Cytol* 7:305–310, 1963.

38. Singh B, Greenbaum E, Cole R: Carbon-laden macrophages in pleural fluid of crack smoker. *Diagn Cytopathol* 13:316–319,1995.

39. Spencer H: *Pathology of the Lung,* 3d ed. Philadelphia, Saunders, 1978.

40. Stein B, Zaatari GS, Pine JR: Amiodarone pulmonary toxicity: Clinical, cytologic and ultrastructural findings. *Acta Cytol* 31:357–361, 1987.

41. Tabatowski K, Roggli VL, Fulkerson WJ, et al: Giant cell interstitial pneumonia in a hard-metal worker: Cytologic, histologic and analytical electron microscopic investigation. *Acta Cytol* 32:240–246, 1988.

42. Tochman MS, Gupta PK, Pressman NJ, Mulshine JL: Biomarkers of pulmonary disease, in Schulte PA, Perera EP (eds), *Molecular Epidemiology: Principles and Practices.* New York, Academic Press, 1993, pp 443–468.

43. Tochman MS, Erozan YS, Gupta P, et al: The early detection of second lung cancers by sputum immunostaining. *Chest* 106:385s–390s, 1994.

44. Walker KR, Fullmer CD: Observations of eosinophilic extracytoplasmic processes in pulmonary macrophages: Progress report. *Acta Cytol* 15:363–364, 1971.

45. Walloch J: Pulmonary cytopathology in historical perspective, in Gruhn JG, Rosen ST (eds), *Lung Cancer: The Evolution of Concepts.* New York, Field and Wood, 1989.

46. Wang KP, Terry PB: Transbronchial needle aspiration in the diagnosis and staging of bronchogenic carcinoma. *Am Rev Respir Dis* 127:344–347, 1983.

47. Weston JT, Guin GH: Epithelial atypias with chemotherapy in 100 acute childhood leukemias. *Cancer* 8:179–186, 1955.

48. Woolner LB: Recent advances in pulmonary cytology: Early detection and localization of occult lung cancer in symptomless males. In Koss LG, Colman D (eds), *Advances in Clinical Cytology,* vol 1. London, Butterworth, 1981, pp 95–135.

49. Zaman SS, Elshami A, Gupta PK: Bronchoalveolar lavage cytology in pulmonary sarcoidosis. *Acta Cytol* 39:1117–1123, 1995.

50. Zaman SS, vanHoeven KH, Slott S, Gupta PK: The distinction between bronchoalveolar carcinoma and hyperplastic pulmonary proliferation: A cytologic and morphologic analysis. *Acta Cytol* (in press).

51. Zaman SS, Seykora JT, Hodinka RL, et al: Cytologic manifestations of respiratory syncytial virus pneumonia in bronchoalveolar lavage: A case report. *Acta Cytol* (in press).

CHAPTER 34

ANGIOGRAPHIC TECHNIQUES IN THE EVALUATION AND MANAGEMENT OF SUSPECTED PULMONARY DISEASE

Vincent G. McDermott / Cynthia S. Payne / Tony P. Smith

In the past decade, many advances have been made in the field of radiology of the pulmonary vasculature. These advances include refinement of techniques and interpretation of isotope lung scanning, development of spiral computed tomography (CT), and introduction of magnetic resonance angiography, which creates the possibility of noninvasive confirmation of the diagnosis of such disorders as pulmonary embolism (PE) and pulmonary arteriovenous malformation. However, contrast angiography remains the best technique for reliably producing high-resolution images of the pulmonary vasculature. Furthermore, with the development of transcatheter interventional techniques, the angiographer continues to play a significant role in the diagnosis and management of patients with pulmonary disease. This chapter focuses on pulmonary angiography and bronchial angiography and embolization. In addition, since insertion of inferior venal caval filters constitutes an important aspect of management of venous thromboembolic disease, a discussion of the indications for the technique, methods, and results is provided.

PULMONARY ANGIOGRAPHY

Pulmonary angiography plays a valuable role in the diagnostic evaluation of patients with suspected pulmonary vascular disorders. Indications for the procedure, patient preparation, an overview of the technique and its complications, and specific diagnostic applications are described below.

Indications

The indications for pulmonary angiography are listed in Table 34-1. Lung scanning for ventilation-perfusion abnormalities using radioisotopes is the most widely applied imaging test for PE (see Chapter 35); the most common indication for pulmonary angiography remains the diagnosis of acute PE. Using the modified criteria of the Prospective Investigation of Pulmonary Embolism Diagnosis (PIOPED), 87 percent of patients with ventilation-perfusion scans that were interpreted as showing a high probability of PE had angiographic evidence of PE; 30 percent of those with intermediate-probability scans and 14 percent with low-probability scans had PE on angiography.[40] Thus, therapeutic decisions based solely on lung scans will be incorrect in a significant number of cases. Therefore, for any patient in whom the clinical picture and ventilation-perfusion scan result are not concordant, or in whom the lung scan is indeterminate, pulmonary angiography should be considered before anticoagulation is instituted.

Pulmonary angiography may be obviated by the finding of deep venous thrombosis (DVT) with use of a noninvasive technique (ultrasonography or impedance plethysmography). The presence of DVT in the proximal lower-extremity indicates that anticoagulation is required; its absence, in the appropriate clinical setting, may indicate that the likelihood of a PE is low or that clinically significant thromboembolism is not present. However, a significant number of patients in whom pulmonary embolism is suspected require pulmonary angiography; at our institution, one pulmonary angiogram is performed for every four or five ventilation-perfusion scans.

TABLE 34-1

Indications for Pulmonary Angiography

High-probability ventilation-perfusion study and a contraindication to anticoagulation

Low-probability ventilation-perfusion study and a high clinical suspicion of PE

Indeterminate-probability ventilation-perfusion study

Candidate for thrombolytic therapy

Candidate for inferior vena caval filter placement for documented PE

Suspicion of nonembolic process causing perfusion abnormality (e.g., extrinsic compression, vasculitis)

Suspicion of vascular abnormality (e.g., arteriovenous malformation)

Suspected congenital abnormality (e.g., pulmonary sequestration)

Pulmonary artery stenosis

Preangiographic Preparation

Informed consent is necessary to perform the procedure. The patient should be fasting from solids. Before iodinated contrast is administered intravascularly, renal function must be assessed and any history of allergy to contrast material must be elicited. Marked renal impairment in a patient who is not on hemodialysis or a history of life-threatening allergy to contrast material is a contraindication to angiography. Any significant history of allergy to contrast material calls for premedication with corticosteroids in order to avoid a serious reaction. One premedication regimen currently in use is prednisone, 20 mg every 6 h for four doses before the procedure. The electrocardiogram should be assessed for the presence of left bundle branch block (LBBB). Although the risk of clinically significant complete heart block from a right heart catheterization in the presence of LBBB is small, the angiographer must be prepared to treat complete heart block. If complete heart block does occur, it may revert to LBBB after the catheter is repositioned. If LBBB is present, however, it is preferable to apply an external or transvenous pacemaker before performing the study.

Because pulmonary angiography requires a venous rather than an arterial puncture, hemostasis at the groin is rarely a problem. Heparin that is being administered intravenously can be stopped immediately before the procedure as long as the partial thromboplastin time is not increased significantly above the therapeutic range. Conversely, heparin can be safely restarted about 1 h after the procedure.

A decision about whether an inferior vena caval filter (see below) will be required if pulmonary embolism is documented should be made before the procedure. Placement of a filter through the existing access site immediately after the arteriogram is performed saves time, reduces cost, and is more convenient for the patient.

Technique

Sedation is routinely administered for the comfort of the conscious patient during angiography. Continuous monitoring of the electrocardiogram, blood pressure, and oxygen saturation is standard. Most often, the catheter is introduced via the right common femoral vein. Alternative sites include the contralateral femoral vein, the jugular veins, and brachial veins. The choice of the site of access is influenced by information obtained before the procedure about whether any of these vessels is occluded.

In the past, pulmonary angiography was performed with straight end-hole catheters. These catheters ran the risk of cardiac perforation, however, and have been replaced universally by curved, pigtail-type catheters with many side holes. Among the catheters currently in use are the pigtail catheter, the Grollman catheter, and the Van Aman catheter.

The catheter is advanced over a guidewire into the proximal pulmonary artery on the side that is most suspect, according to the ventilation-perfusion scan, of containing an embolus. Ventricular ectopic beats commonly occur during manipulation of the catheter through the right ventricle. The ectopy ceases once the catheter is in the pulmonary artery and manipulation is stopped. If ventricular tachycardia does occur, the catheter is rapidly withdrawn into the right atrium—a maneuver that usually aborts the arrhythmia. Another attempt to manipulate the catheter is made after administration of an antiarrhythmic agent (e.g., lidocaine). Once the catheter is positioned in the appropriate pulmonary artery, pulmonary arterial pressures are measured before the contrast material is injected.

Digital filming is increasingly supplanting the use of cut film in angiography. Modern digital images provide adequate resolution for a high-quality diagnostic study (Fig. 34-1). The angiographic run may be viewed on a monitor, permitting the radiologist to watch the pulmonary tree fill with contrast in "real time." Thus, each run can be examined on the monitor without the need to wait for hard-copy images to be processed—significantly decreasing the time for the procedure and, in many instances, reducing the volume of contrast material. Regardless of whether digital or cut film technique is used, at least two views of each lung must be obtained before pulmonary embolism is excluded. When necessary, subselective injections may be performed by advancing the catheter into a lobar or segmental branch (Fig. 34-2). The total volume of contrast used is customarily in the range of 150 to 200 ml. Nonionic, low-osmolality agents are used routinely to increase the comfort and safety of the patient. Upon completion of the study, the catheter is removed over a guidewire and hemostasis is achieved by manual compression of the access site.

Pulmonary angiography at the patient's bedside through an indwelling Swan-Ganz catheter is a tempting alternative to transferring the critically ill patient to an angiography suite. However, the technique has been shown to be dangerously misleading, with an accuracy of 29 percent—considerably less than that for conventional angiography.[24]

Complications

Potential complications of pulmonary angiography include formation of a hematoma or arteriovenous fistula at the access site, infection of the groin, allergic reaction to contrast agent, contrast nephropathy, cardiac perforation, cardiac arrhythmias, and sudden death. Complications at the groin site are uncommon. The risk of an allergic reaction to contrast agent is no greater than that from intravenous urography or CT scanning. Contrast

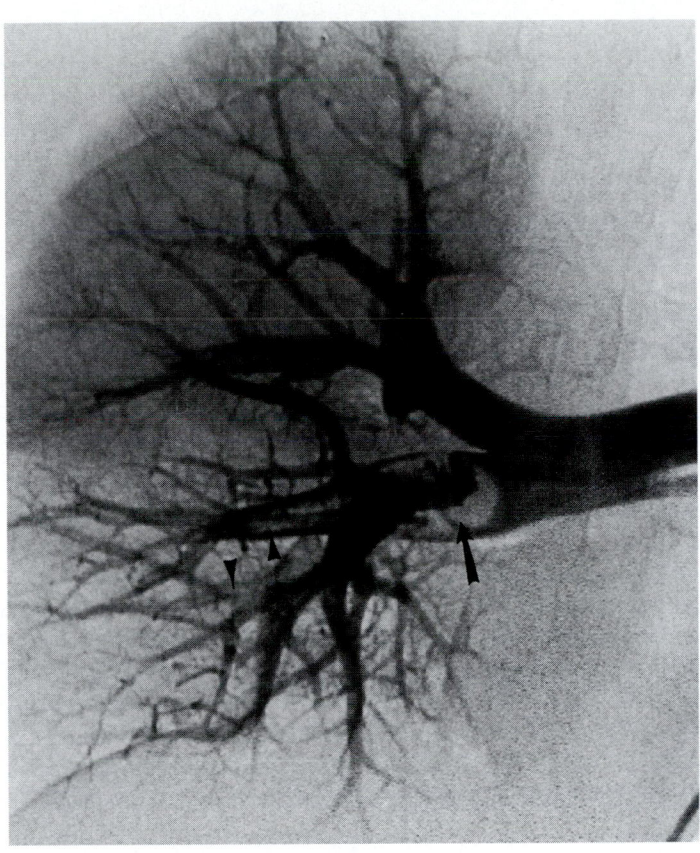

FIGURE 34-1 Acute pulmonary embolism. Digital subtraction right pulmonary arteriogram shows a radiolucent filling defect in the right lower-lobe pulmonary artery (arrow), with extensions of the thrombus into segmental branches (arrowheads).

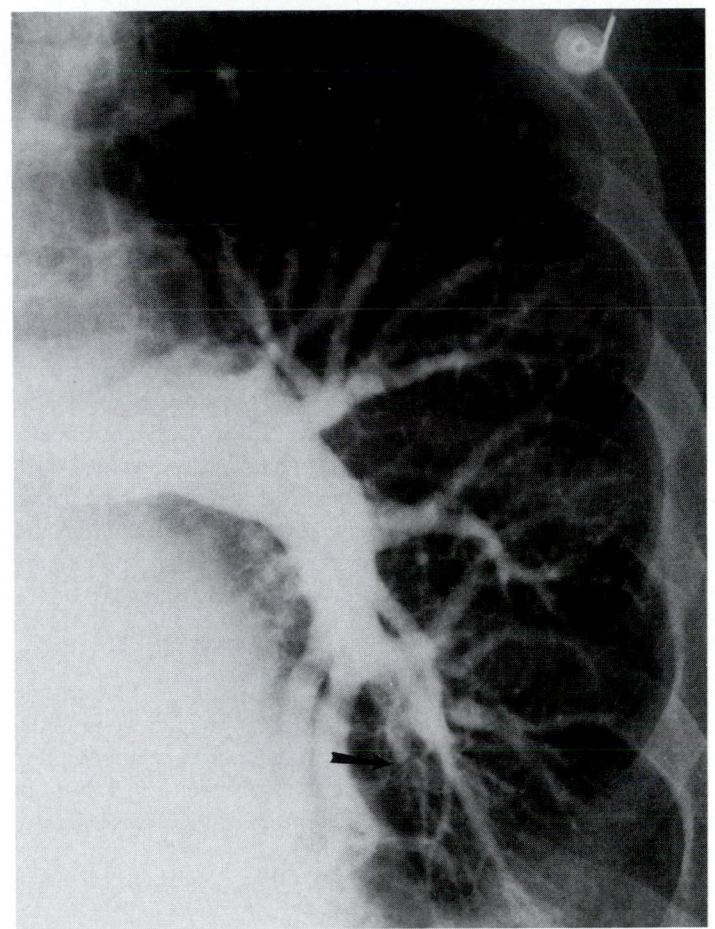

A

nephropathy is rare unless the patient has diabetes and the serum creatinine level is abnormally high. As mentioned previously, clinically significant cardiac perforation is very rare when modern pigtail catheters are used. The major concerns regarding pulmonary angiography have centered on the risk of sudden death in patients with cor pulmonale.

Four large studies on the complications of pulmonary angiography, each including more than 1000 patients, have been published. In a series of 1350 patients who underwent pulmonary angiography for PE,[27] three deaths (0.2 percent) and an overall complication rate of 5 percent, including 20 endocardial or myocardial injuries (none of them fatal), were reported. All three deaths were in patients with cor pulmonale. However, the data did not include the total number of patients with pulmonary hypertension. In a follow-up series, 27 percent of 1434 patients who underwent pulmonary angiography had pulmonary hypertension, defined as a pulmonary artery systolic pressure greater than 40 mmHg.[31] There were two deaths (mortality of 0.14 percent), both in patients with severe pulmonary hypertension. These death rates are similar to that reported in PIOPED (0.18 percent).[41]

Two major changes have occurred in the technique of pulmonary angiography since publication of these studies. One is that angiography is now performed almost exclusively with pigtail-type catheters. As a result, cardiac injuries have become rare. The second is that nonionic, low-osmolar contrast agents have almost completely replaced ionic contrast agents. In a review of 1432 patients who underwent pulmonary angiography at

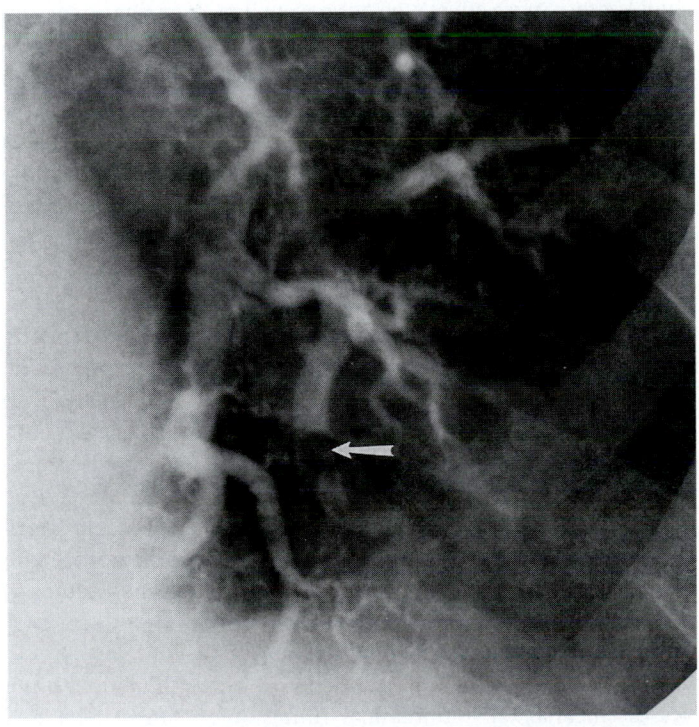

B

FIGURE 34-2 Acute pulmonary embolism. *A*. Cut-film left pulmonary angiogram shows occlusion of a left basal segmental pulmonary artery (arrow). *B*. Selective angiogram that confirms the presence of an embolus (arrow).

one institution after 1987, no cardiac injuries were reported and no deaths related to the procedure occurred. The overall major complication rate was only 0.3 percent.[18] The absence of procedure-related mortality is believed to be due to the use of nonionic, low-osmolar contrast media.

Recognition of the potential complications of pulmonary angiography, including sudden death, has engendered some reluctance to perform the procedure. In a survey of 126 hospitals in the United Kingdom, it was found that 47,000 ventilation-perfusion scans were performed over a 1-year period. Only 490 pulmonary angiograms were done, however, even though angiography was available in most centers.[8] Fear of sudden death may also affect technical success of the procedure. In one study, 37 percent of pulmonary angiograms either could not be successfully completed or were nondiagnostic.[19] Concern over procedure-related mortality may be well founded when ionic media are used for pulmonary angiography. However, the significantly greater safety margin of nonionic media has made pulmonary angiography a much safer procedure.

Specific Diagnostic Applications

Pulmonary angiography has found its greatest application in the diagnostic evaluation of acute and chronic thromboembolic disease (see Chapter 84) and pulmonary arteriovenous malformations (see Chapter 87).

ACUTE PULMONARY THROMBOEMBOLISM

Pulmonary angiography is most often performed to exclude the diagnosis of acute pulmonary embolism. Ventilation-perfusion studies are almost always performed before pulmonary angiography. Although a ventilation-perfusion scan provides only indirect evidence for PE and may not be diagnostic, the procedure is relatively inexpensive, noninvasive, and safe, obviating pulmonary angiography in most cases. When necessary, perfusion studies may be performed at the bedside of patients in clinically unstable condition. Even for patients in whom perfusion scanning is nondiagnostic, a unilateral abnormality directs the angiographer to the site of interest and may significantly reduce procedure time, contrast dose, and cost.

Pulmonary emboli usually do not lyse for 1 to 2 weeks after the acute event.[11] Thus, if a pulmonary angiogram is performed within 1 to 2 days of a suspected PE, it is unlikely that the diagnosis will be missed. Since most patients do not have a contraindication to anticoagulation, heparin can be started empirically when pulmonary embolism is considered, and diagnostic pulmonary angiography can be performed as a nonemergency procedure. Pulmonary angiography as an emergency procedure should be reserved for patients who have a contraindication to anticoagulation, who are in unstable condition, or who are possible candidates for thrombolytic therapy.

The primary angiographic finding of acute PE is an abrupt vessel cutoff or an intraluminal filling defect (Figs. 34-1 and 34-2).[30] Without these findings, the diagnosis cannot be definitively established. Secondary signs of PE include diminished perfusion, prolonged arterial phase, tortuous peripheral vessels, and delayed venous phase or absence of draining veins. Secondary

findings may be associated with chronic or previous pulmonary embolism, rather than acute PE. Potential diagnostic pitfalls include artifacts resulting from the mingling of contrast material with unopacified blood, overlapping vessels, hypoperfusion caused by hypoxic vasoconstriction, slowed flow due to pneumonia, and vascular crowding caused by atelectasis.[3]

These pitfalls can often be obviated by increasing the injection rate and obtaining several views. Interpretation of pulmonary angiograms can be difficult, however, and interobserver variation in interpretation does occur. In a study of 60 patients in which the interpretations of three blinded observers were compared, interobserver agreement was noted in 86 percent; the greatest disagreement occurred in the reading of subsegmental filling defects.[32] Nonetheless, negative pulmonary angiography is a very good indicator of a low risk for subsequent PE. In a retrospective review of 380 patients in PIOPED who had negative pulmonary angiograms and did not receive anticoagulation,[17] only six patients experienced documented pulmonary embolism in the following year: in four of these, PE occurred in the first month after the angiogram; five of the six patients had either thrombophlebitis or an objective test suggestive of deep venous thrombosis. Thus, the risk of subsequent PE following a negative pulmonary angiogram is less than 2 percent. In patients in whom clinical uncertainty continues, however, definitive studies of the lower extremities to exclude deep venous thrombosis are indicated.

If a patient experiences a massive, life-threatening PE, transcatheter therapy may be lifesaving. The methods that are available include suction embolectomy; clot fragmentation using catheters, guidewires, or mechanical thrombolytic devices; and stenting of narrowed pulmonary arteries in patients with acute severe cor pulmonale.[4,15,44] None of these methods has been validated in a large, prospective clinical trial. Direct thrombolysis has also been tried. This technique does not have an immediate effect, however, and it has not been shown to be any more efficacious than systemic thrombolysis instituted via a peripheral vein.[38]

CHRONIC PULMONARY THROMBOEMBOLISM

Pulmonary hypertension due to chronic thromboembolic obstruction of the pulmonary arteries usually presents insidiously with exertional dyspnea, right heart failure, and cyanosis. Although the diagnosis may be suggested by the clinical picture and noninvasive studies, it is frequently delayed, and confirmation requires pulmonary angiography. Ventilation-perfusion scans underestimate the degree of involvement of proximal vessels. Therefore, bilateral pulmonary angiography is recommended for any patient suspected of having chronic pulmonary thromboembolic disease, even if the ventilation-perfusion scan is unimpressive.

Recognition that pulmonary hypertension is due to thromboembolism of large pulmonary arteries is vital because it affords the prospect of surgical thromboendarterectomy to decrease pulmonary arterial pressures, thereby relieving right ventricular overload and cor pulmonale.[29] In a review of angiographic findings in 250 patients with surgically confirmed chronic thromboembolic pulmonary hypertension, five angiographic findings were noted: (1) a pouchlike appearance of a central pulmonary artery, characterized by a smooth, concave appearance to an organized obstructing or partly occlusive thrombus; (2) pulmonary arterial webs, which are lucent lines crossing the width of the vessel, which is usually stenotic, and associated with poststenotic dilatation (Fig. 34-3); (3) intimal irregularity due to organized thrombus lining the wall of the vessel; (4) hypertrophied main pulmonary arteries, with abrupt narrowing of the lumen of the main vessels and proximal lobar branches (Fig. 34-3); and (5) obstruction of lobar vessels at their point of origin from the main pulmonary artery.[1] At least one of these findings was present in every patient. Moreover, in almost all patients, both the right and left pulmonary arteries were affected.

The differential angiographic diagnosis of chronic thromboembolic pulmonary disease can be difficult if the angiogram shows only one or two of the typical findings. For example, multiple pulmonary webs can also be caused by congenital multiple pulmonary arterial stenoses or Takayasu's arteritis. Other clinical findings usually help to clarify the situation. For example, congenital multiple pulmonary stenoses are usually recognized at a younger age and are associated with other cardiovascular abnormalities, whereas Takayasu's arteritis is generally associated with systemic manifestations of the disease. Total obstruction or abrupt narrowing of the major pulmonary arteries may be caused by carcinoma, extrinsic compression, fibrosing mediastinitis, or pulmonary agenesis. Mass lesions can be excluded with a CT scan. Although chronic pulmonary thromboembolic occlusion has been misinterpreted on angiography as unilateral pulmonary artery agenesis, this misdiagnosis can be avoided by careful review of the patient's history, other radiologic examinations, and, in particular, examination of the contralateral pulmonary angiogram for evidence of thromboembolic disease.

PULMONARY ARTERIOVENOUS MALFORMATION

Pulmonary arteriovenous malformations (AVMs) are usually congenital, although they may be acquired as a consequence of trauma, infection, or schistosomiasis. In 50 percent of patients with this anomaly, the lesion is solitary; in the rest, it is part of the Rendu-Osler-Weber syndrome.[47] Pulmonary AVMs are present in only 15 percent of patients with the Rendu-Osler-Weber syndrome. Morphologically, 80 percent of the malformations are simple, direct arteriovenous fistulas; in the remaining 20 percent the lesions are complex, with two or more feeding or draining vessels.[47]

In about 50 percent of patients, the AVMs are less than 2 cm in diameter and are asymptomatic. Patients with larger AVMs often become hypoxemic because of right-to-left shunting. These patients may develop dyspnea, cyanosis, clubbing of digits, polycythemia, or hemoptysis. The most serious potential complications of the shunt are related to loss of the filtering function of the pulmonary capillary bed. Bacteria and particulate matter can pass through the AVM to the brain, causing cerebrovascular accidents or brain abscesses.[47] Thus, it is recommended that AVMs with a feeding vessel greater than 3 mm in diameter be occluded to avoid these complications (Fig. 34-4).[48]

On the chest radiograph or CT scan, AVMs are usually seen in the lower lobes as round or lobulated masses with a feeding artery and draining vein. The AVMs are multiple in 33 percent of patients. Contrast-enhanced CT has been shown to be the most sensitive method for the diagnosis of pulmonary AVM and has made angiography unnecessary, unless treatment is in prospect.[35] CT scanning has also been shown to be useful for the diagnosis of recurrence: in up to 10 percent of such patients, CT scanning has revealed an unembolized feeding vessel or blood flow through the embolic material.[37]

Before treatment, bilateral pulmonary angiography is performed in order to delineate the size and number of feeding arteries and draining veins for each AVM. Pulmonary AVMs are best occluded by use of detachable balloons or Gianturco coils (Fig. 34-4). In a follow-up study of 27 patients who underwent therapy using Gianturco coils over a period of 4 years, CT scanning revealed that 96 percent of the AVMs either became undetectable or decreased in size.[36]

Pulmonary angiodysplasia occurs occasionally in patients with hepatic cirrhosis but does not cause discrete AVMs.[25] In these patients, pulmonary angiography reveals subtle peripheral vascular dilatation with early venous filling. Pulmonary angiodysplasia is a diffuse process and is not amenable to endovascular therapy.

INFERIOR VENA CAVAL FILTERS

Insertion of filters into the inferior vena cava (IVC) has become an important element in the therapeutic armanentarium of venous thromboembolic disease. A clear understanding of the indications for the technique and its complications is important for proper clinical decision making.

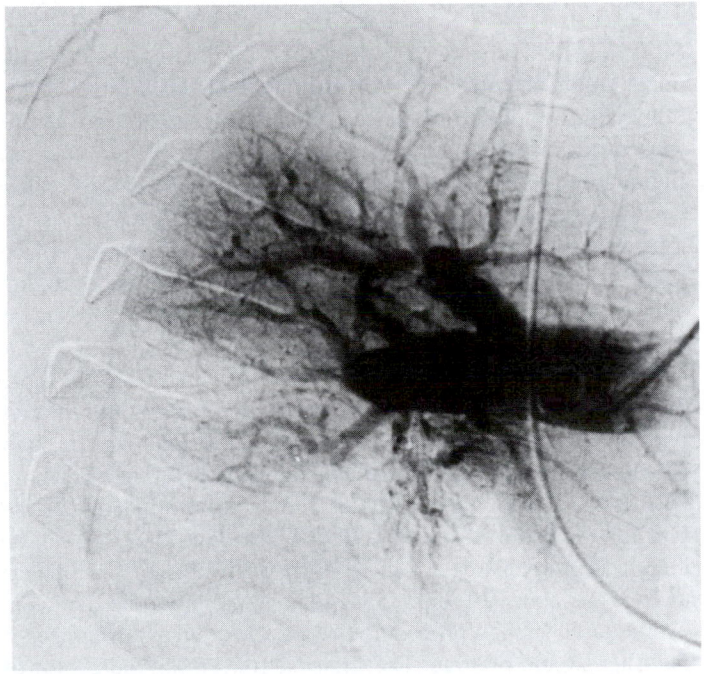

FIGURE 34-3 Chronic pulmonary embolism. Right anterior oblique view. Digital subtraction arteriogram of the right pulmonary artery shows that the artery is markedly enlarged, with irregularity and webbing of peripheral branches and relative oligemia of the upper and lower lobes.

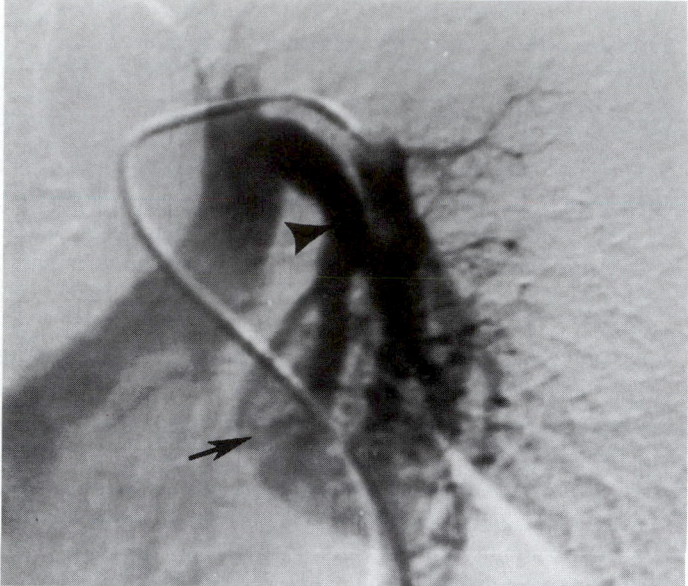

A

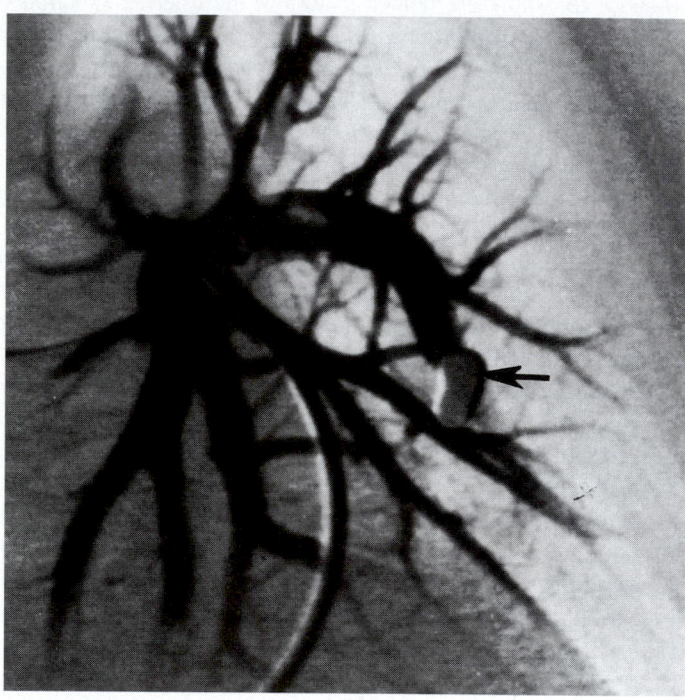

B

FIGURE 34-4 Pulmonary arteriovenous malformation (AVM). This middle-aged woman had an episode of transient hemiplegia. *A.* Left lower lobe. Selective digital subtraction pulmonary angiogram shows a large AVM (arrow) with early venous filling (arrowhead). *B.* The AVM was successfully treated with use of balloon occlusion (arrow) of the feeding segmental artery.

Indications

Percutaneous interruption of the IVC to avoid fatal pulmonary embolism has been possible since the introduction of the stainless-steel Greenfield (SSG) filter in 1973. Both the SSG and the subsequently introduced Mobin-Udin umbrella required venotomy for placement. In the past decade, however, various filters have been developed (Table 34-2) that can be safely placed

TABLE 34-2

FDA-Approved Inferior Vena Caval Filters in Current Use

Titanium Greenfield (Boston Scientific Corp., Watertown, MA)

24 Fr. Stainless-Steel Greenfield (Boston Scientific Corp.)

12 Fr. Stainless-Steel Greenfield (Boston Scientific Corp.)

Vena-Tech LGM (B. Braun VenaTech, Evanston, IL)

Simon-Nitinol (Nitinol Medical Technologies, Boston, MA)

Gianturco-Roehm Bird's Nest (Cook Co., Bloomington, IN)

through 9-15 French introducer sheaths, obviating a surgical "cutdown." Owing to decreased cost, increased ease of deployment, fewer complications, and ready availability, the insertion of IVC filters has steadily increased and indications for their use have broadened.

Accepted indications for placement of an IVC filter include (1) a contraindication to anticoagulation in a patient with documented DVT or PE; (2) a complication of current anticoagulation; (3) failure of anticoagulation, as reflected in recurrent DVT or PE; and (4) a high-risk patient (e.g., a patient who has a large residual DVT and limited pulmonary reserve). Not as widely accepted is the use of IVC filters in other situations— for example, in patients who have recently undergone surgery and develop DVT or PE postoperatively, are poorly compliant with anticoagulant medication, or are difficult to adequately anticoagulate or require prophylaxis because of high risk for DVT (e.g., a patient with paraplegia or hip replacement surgery).[22]

Types of Filters

Six IVC filters have been approved by the Food and Drug Administration and are currently available in the United States (Table 34-2). All can be placed percutaneously, and all permit subsequent magnetic resonance imaging (MRI). While titanium filters are not subject to migration during MRI, the SSG filter has displayed some mild torque in a magnetic field. Generally, a patient can undergo MRI once a steel filter has been in place for 6 weeks, since, by that time, fibrosis around the retaining struts in the caval wall is unlikely to allow significant movement of the device.

The currently available IVC filters that are listed in Table 34-2 have several distinguishing characteristics: (1) the Simon-Nitinol (SN) is malleable and, therefore, can be deployed through a 9-French sheath using a brachial approach in patients in whom both femoral and jugular access routes are occluded; (2) the Gianturco-Roehm Bird's Nest (BN) is the only filter that can be deployed in a vena cava that is larger than 28 mm in diameter; and (3) the new 12-French SSG filter is the only one deployed over a guidewire—a procedure that has theoretical advantages if the filter should migrate. The decision concerning the choice of filter is influenced by various factors, including the availability of venous access and the diameter of the vena cava. The most important practical factor, however, is familiarity of the surgeon or angiographer with the various types of filters and their personal preferences.

Technique of Insertion

The right femoral vein is the preferred site of access and permits convenient and rapid deployment following pulmonary angiography. Alternative sites include the left femoral vein, the internal jugular veins, and, in the case of the SN filter, the brachial vein. In cases of DVT, the radiologist should be informed about whether the thrombus extends proximally into the common femoral veins, since this situation dictates the site of venous puncture. Because of the tortuosity of the vessels, kinking of the introducer sheath may be a significant problem when left femoral or jugular venous access is used. In these cases, the more pliable BN or SN filter or the over-the-wire Greenfield filter may be easier to place.

An inferior vena cavagram is mandatory before the filter is placed in order to document the level of the renal veins and the absence of thrombus and to permit accurate measurement of IVC diameter. If the patient has a megacava (a cava greater than 28 mm diameter, corrected for magnification), a BN filter must be placed or, alternatively, one of the other filters can be deployed in each common iliac vein. IVC anomalies are not uncommon, and occasionally it is necessary to place two parallel filters in a duplicated IVC. The tip of the IVC filter is ideally deployed approximately 1 cm below the lowest renal vein. Placement at or above the renal veins may allow for propagation of clot into the renal veins, with subsequent renal vein thrombosis.[34] Placement above the renal veins is only rarely indicated and can be technically difficult because of the proximity of the hepatic veins and right atrium.

Complications

Complications of IVC filter placement include those at the puncture site, IVC penetration or thrombosis, and malposition, incomplete opening, tilting, migration or dislodgment of the filter.[34] The incidence of puncture site bleeding, malposition of the filter, injury to the cava, caval injury, and thrombosis are all greater with the surgically placed 24-French SSG. Placement in the angiography suite enables precise measurement of the cava, accurate placement, and visualization during advancement in the cava—all of which are associated with a reduced incidence of complications. The smaller delivery devices are also less traumatic at the access site.

Even with the newer filters, thrombosis at the access site occurs in 14 to 35 percent of patients, but it is occlusive in fewer than 10 percent and symptomatic in only 3 percent.[28,34] Significant bleeding requiring transfusion and surgical intervention is rare. Caval penetration occurs in up to 10 percent of patients and is usually asymptomatic, although duodenal perforation and arterial injury have been noted.[34] Thrombus may be imaged in the IVC following 15 to 25 percent of filter placements, but it is difficult to say whether this represents emboli trapped by the filter or thrombus formation on the filter.[13] Placement of a filter in the IVC leads to new, or worsening, edema of the lower extremity in 5 to 6 percent of patients.[2]

Malposition of the filter is uncommon when the procedure is performed by an experienced operator in a modern angiography suite. Placement above the renal veins increases the risk of renal vein thrombosis, and malposition in the iliac vein leaves the patient unprotected from clotting in the contralateral lower extremity.[34] The stainless-steel wires of a BN filter may prolapse, but this does not significantly impair the filter's effectiveness.[34] Once deployed, the filter may lie tilted or incompletely opened, thereby reducing its clot-trapping ability. Tilting is most common with the SN filter, occurring in up to 50 percent of patients, whereas incomplete opening, due to overlapping struts, is seen most often with the TG filter.[34] Postdeployment manipulation of these filters, using curved catheters and guidewires, is discouraged by the manufacturers of the devices because manipulation may lead to further complications. If the configuration of the filter is completely unsatisfactory, a second filter may be placed. Filter migration has been noted with most types of filters and may be caused by massive thromboembolism, incorrect sizing of the IVC, poor positioning of the filter in the IVC, or fracture of the struts. Migration usually occurs in a caudal direction into the wider infrarenal IVC; embolization to the heart is rare. If clinically significant migration does occur, the filter can often be retrieved percutaneously.[34]

Results

IVC filters are designed to trap large emboli, but they do permit small, clinically insignificant emboli to pass. Therefore, the efficiency of an IVC filter is measured by the rate of recurrent PE. The incidence varies from 0.5 to 4 percent in different series,[10,14,34,39] but, overall, there does not appear to be a significant difference among the various filters. Clinically overt recurrent PE in a patient with an IVC filter is a serious event and should be confirmed by ventilation-perfusion scan or angiography. Imaging studies should then be obtained to examine for migration of the filter, fracture of the filter, or thrombosis of the IVC with development of large collaterals.

BRONCHIAL ANGIOGRAPHY AND EMBOLIZATION

Visualization of the bronchial arteries and therapeutic embolization have assumed a useful role in the management of a variety of pulmonary disorders.

Indications

Clinical indications for bronchial angiography include preoperative investigation of patients in whom the pulmonary arteries have been obstructed by emboli; evaluation of types of congenital heart disease that involve interruption of the pulmonary artery; assessment of pulmonary malformations (e.g., sequestration); evaluation of the bronchial arterial system following lung transplantation; and assessment during complete spinal angiography. The most common indication for bronchial angiography, however, is investigation of the cause of uncontrollable hemoptysis. The procedure is then almost always performed in anticipation of transcatheter occlusion (embolization) of an abnormal bronchial arterial supply.

Anatomic Considerations

Successful bronchial angiography requires a complete understanding of the anatomy of the bronchial arterial system, which is very variable.[5,45] Bronchial arteries usually arise from the descending thoracic aorta between T3 and T8. The right bronchial arteries originate from the lateral or dorsolateral aorta, whereas the left bronchial arteries arise from the anterior thoracic aorta or concavity of the aortic arch. Based on findings at autopsy, the most common variations are two left and one right bronchial artery in 41 percent of patients, bilateral single bronchial arteries in 21 percent, two left and two right bronchial arteries arising separately or in combination in 21 percent, and a single left and two right bronchial arteries in 9 percent.[5] The remaining 8 percent consist of other variations, all including at least three bronchial arteries on one side. The right bronchial artery often arises from a common trunk with an intercostal artery, termed an *intercostobronchial trunk.*

The angiographic anatomy differs from the anatomy seen at autopsy, since angiographic visualization is usually only of abnormal (i.e., enlarged) bronchial arteries and depends on the ease of catheterization.[45] In addition to aortic and intercostobronchial origins, bronchial arteries have been reported to arise from other locations, including the phrenic arteries, the subclavian arteries, and their branches and, most notably, the thyrocervical and internal mammary arteries.[26]

The arterial supply to the bronchi may also originate from the systemic arterial system via transpleural collaterals that become enlarged because of chronic pulmonary inflammation, or after the native bronchial supply has been occluded by embolization.[23] Therefore, bronchial angiography that is performed for evaluation of hemoptysis must always take into account the anatomy and its variations, including the possibility of systemic collaterals.

Technique and Findings

Bronchial angiography is usually performed with a femoral arterial approach. A thoracic aortogram is often obtained at the outset in order to delineate the vascular anatomy, including the presence of any grossly enlarged bronchial arteries. This step may be omitted, however, to minimize the dose of contrast agent. Although the site of hemorrhage may have been previously localized by clinical, radiographic, and bronchoscopic findings, both lungs should be evaluated. Selective catheterization of the bronchial arterial supply can be performed with a number of different catheter types and shapes.

A number of angiographic findings may be seen in patients presenting with hemoptysis. Some depend on the underlying cause. For example, vascularity of the tumor may be visualized in patients with mass lesions. Extravasation of contrast material is rarely seen, because hemorrhage is usually intermittent and not sufficient to cause extravasation of the contrast agent.[43] Hemoptysis usually originates from bronchial arteries that are enlarged and angiographically abnormal. Focal hypervascularity is usual, and systemic-to-pulmonary arterial or venous shunting may be seen (Fig. 34-5). If an abnormal bronchial supply is not visualized, pulmonary angiography should be performed. In 26 of 28 patients who had no initial response to bronchial em-

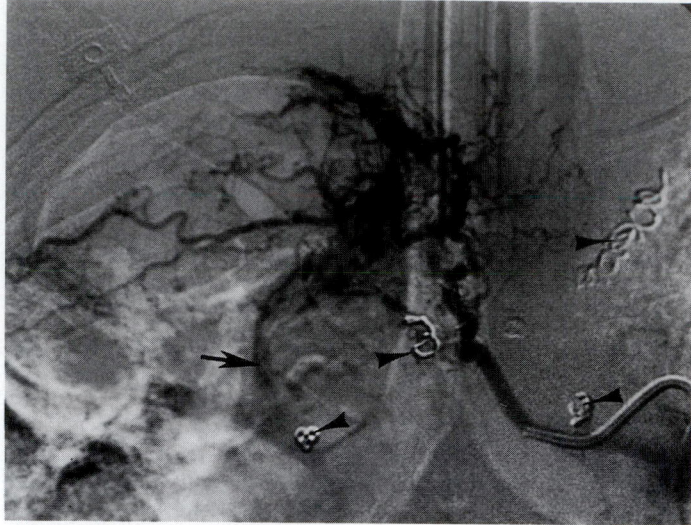

A

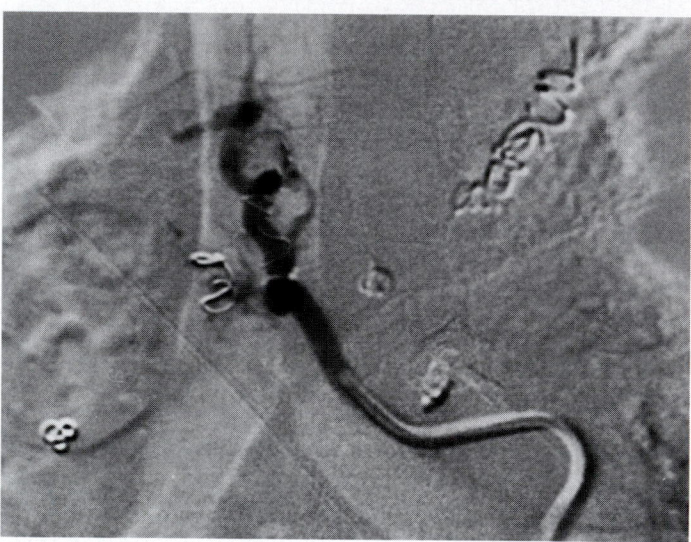

B

FIGURE 34-5 Bronchial arteriograms before and after embolization. The patient had sarcoidosis and developed massive recurrent hemoptysis. *A.* Digital subtraction arteriography of the right bronchial artery shows a hypertrophied bronchial artery supplying hyperemic pulmonary parenchyma, with fistulization to pulmonary vein (arrow). Coils from prior embolization can be identified (arrowheads). *B.* The bronchial artery was successfully embolized with polyvinyl alcohol.

bolization, the pulmonary artery proved to be the source of hemorrhage.[33]

In assessing a bronchial arteriogram, it is necessary to search carefully to determine whether the spinal cord arterial supply originates from the bronchial arteries. The reported rates of radicular supply to the cord from the bronchial arteries is variable (up to 55 percent in one report).[7] Bronchial angiography for hemoptysis is usually a precursor to transarterial embolization. Once an abnormal bronchial supply is visualized and lack of supply to the spinal cord verified, embolization may be performed.

Since bronchial embolization for hemoptysis was first reported in 1974, a number of changes in technique have been made. Bronchial angiography is usually performed with 5-French

TABLE 34-3

Results of Bronchial Artery Embolization for Hemoptysis

Study	Number of Patients	Initial Success	Maximum Follow-Up Interval (months)	Rehemorrhage		Complications	
				Patients	Mean Time (months)	Major	Minor
Cremaschi et al, 1993[9]	209	205/209 (98%)	168	29/209 (14%)	NA	0	0
Rabkin et al, 1987[33]	306	278/306 (91%)	60	36/158† (23%)	NA	0	0
Zhang et al, 1994[49]	35	32/35 (91%)	6	7/35 (20%)	4	0	0
Uflacker et al, 1985[45]	67	49/67 (73%)	47	18/59†† (31%)	25	0	5
Sweezey & Fellows, 1990[42]*	25	21/25 (84%)	101	8/25 (32%)	35	0	0
Cohen et al, 1990[7]*	20	19/20 (95%)	62	7/20 (35%)	34	0	1
Keller et al, 1987[23]	20	20/20 (100%)	NA	16/20 (80%)	NA	0	0
Cipolli, 1995[6]*	14	14/14 (100%)	38	8/14 (57%)	15	0	0
Hayakawa et al, 1992[16]	58	50/58 (86%)	120	25/58 (43%)	22	0	4
Katoh et al, 1990[21]	33	33/33 (100%)	48	7/33 (21%)	12	0	2
Totals	787	721/787 (92%)		161/631 (26%)		0	12 (1.5%)

*Series consisting of patients with cystic fibrosis only as their primary diagnosis.

†Only 158 patients did not have surgery as an initial plan in addition to embolization.

††Eight patients successfully embolized initially were lost to long-term follow-up; some patients had additional surgery or chemotherapy planned.

catheters (1 French caliber = 0.33 mm). If a catheter can be well seated in the bronchial artery, embolization can be performed effectively; if not, subselective catheterization may be necessary, using microcatheters that are 3-French or less in size and can be advanced farther into the artery through the 5-French catheter.

In early series, embolization entailed the use of embolic agents (e.g., absorbable gelatin sponge [Gelfoam; Upjohn, Kalamazoo MI] and stainless-steel coils), which lodged proximally in the bronchial artery. Although these agents were effective for acute hemoptysis, proximal embolization proved to have the disadvantage of allowing collaterals to form, supplying the distal bronchial artery beyond the area of therapeutic occlusion. In addition, the gelatin sponge is a temporary agent; recanalization of the vessel occurs after a few weeks.

Embolic agents that permit more distal occlusion, such as polyvinyl alcohol sponge particles, and liquid agents, such as cyanoacrylates and absolute ethanol, are now available. Bronchial necrosis, although very rare, has been reported with the two liquid agents.[33] Therefore, polyvinyl alcohol sponge has become the agent of choice in most centers. Polyvinyl alcohol particles are available in various sizes. Particles of 250 to 750 μm are suitable to produce distal occlusion of bronchial vessels, but they are large enough to occlude vessels at a precapillary level, reducing the chances of shunting into the pulmonary venous system. In addition, such particles preserve the capillary supply to critical organs supplied by the bronchial arteries, including the lungs, tracheobronchial tree, portions of the visceral pleura, esophagus, and other mediastinal tissues.

Results

The results of bronchial embolization for treatment of hemoptysis are variable (Table 34-3), owing to differences in patient population, etiology of the hemoptysis, techniques of embolization, and differing reporting standards in different series. The causes of hemoptysis in most series are heterogeneous and include bronchiectasis, tuberculosis, cystic fibrosis, lung carcinoma, aspergillosis, chronic pneumonia with or without pulmonary abscess, and idiopathic hemorrhage, as well as a host of more unusual conditions. In the two largest series published to date, bronchiectasis and infection, including tuberculosis, accounted for most of the cases.[9,33] Currently, in the United States, cystic fibrosis has become a common indication for embolization as the mean age of this patient population continues to increase.

Comparison of studies (Table 34-3) is difficult, owing to differing reporting standards and follow-up. Key issues include whether primary technical success has been achieved and rates of rehemorrhage and complications. The data compiled in Table 34-3 show an initial success rate of 92 percent in the combined series of 787 patients.[6,7,9,16,21,33,42,45,49] However, rehemorrhage occurs in 26 percent of patients, with a mean time to rehemorrhage of 4 to 35 months. In one of the two largest series,[33] 306 patients with acute pulmonary hemorrhage were evaluated by bronchial angiography and treated with the use of transcatheter embolization. Hemostasis was effective initially in 278 patients (90.8 percent). Early recurrent bleeding requiring surgery occurred in 39 patients (14 percent). Of 158 patients who were

treated without additional surgery, subsequent episodes of hemoptysis occurred in 36 (23 percent), including 24 (15 percent) within 1 year. In the other large series,[9] bronchial artery embolization was performed in 209 patients with hemoptysis. In 98 percent, hemoptysis was controlled in the first 24 h; a 16 percent relapse rate occurred within the first year.

In a review of hemoptysis following repeat arterial embolization,[21] recurrent bleeding was noted in three of five patients.[21] Hemoptysis recurred again in two patients after a third embolization, prompting the authors to conclude that embolization is a palliative procedure. This is not unexpected, since the underlying origin of hemorrhage is not cured by the embolization procedure.

Diseases causing life-threatening hemoptysis are usually difficult to treat, are prone to exacerbation, and often have a progressively worsening course. Few data exist to correlate rehemorrhage following embolization with the nature of the underlying disease. In a study of 58 patients who underwent therapeutic embolization, treatment was successful in 100 percent of cases in which the hemorrhage was idiopathic or due to bronchiectasis.[16] Ninety percent of patients in whom inflammation was the underlying cause were successfully treated, whereas hemoptysis of neoplastic origin was successfully treated in 58 percent.

Complications

Complications from bronchial angiography and embolization are infrequent, usually consisting of minor events, such as intimal dissections, which do not require therapy. The most feared complication is spinal cord injury. However, the only reported case of damage to the spinal cord from embolization was that of a patient in whom the bronchial artery arose from the seventh intercostal artery.[46] Cases of transverse myelitis following bronchial angiography using high-osmolar contrast agents[12,20] have been reported. The risk of spinal cord damage from bronchial angiography and embolization is low when the procedure is performed in a high-quality angiography suite with digital technology and nonionic, low-osmolar contrast agents.

REFERENCES

1. Auger WR, Fedullo PF, Moser KM, et al: Chronic major-vessel thromboembolic pulmonary artery obstruction: Appearance at angiography. *Radiology* 182:393–398, 1992.
2. Becker DM, Philbrick JT, Selby JB: Inferior vena caval filters: Indications, safety, effectiveness. *Arch Intern Med* 152:1985–1994, 1992.
3. Bookstein JJ, Silver TM: The angiographic differential diagnosis of acute pulmonary embolism. *Radiology* 110:25–33, 1974.
4. Brady AJB, Crake T, Oakley CM: Percutaneous catheter fragmentation and distal dispersion of proximal pulmonary embolus. *Lancet* 338:1186–1189, 1991.
5. Cauldwell EW, Siekert RG, Lininger RE, Anson BJ: The bronchial arteries. *Surg Gynecol Obstet* 86:395–412, 1948.
6. Cipolli M, Perini S, Valletta EA, Mastella G: Bronchial artery embolization in the management of hemoptysis in cystic fibrosis. *Pediatr Pulmonol* 19:344–347, 1995.
7. Cohen AM, Doershuk CF, Stern RC: Bronchial artery embolization to control hemoptysis in cystic fibrosis. *Radiology* 175:401–405, 1990.

8. Cooper TJ, Hayward MWJ, Hartog M: Survey on the use of pulmonary scintigraphy and angiography for suspected pulmonary thromboembolism in the UK. *Clin Radiol* 43:243–245, 1991.

9. Cremaschi P, Nascimbene C, Vitulo P, et al: Therapeutic embolization of bronchial artery: A successful treatment in 209 cases of relapse hemoptysis. *Angiology* 44:295–299, 1993.

10. Crochet DP, Stora O, Ferry D, et al: Vena Tech-LGM filter: Long-term results of a prospective study. *Radiology* 188:857–860, 1993.

11. Dalen JE, Banas JS Jr, Brooks HL, et al: Resolution rate of acute pulmonary embolism in man. *New Engl J Med* 280:1194–1199, 1969.

12. Feigelson HH, Ravin HA: Tranverse myelitis following selective bronchial arteriography. *Radiology* 85:663–665, 1965.

13. Ferris EF, McCowan TC, Carver DK, McFarland DR: Percutaneous inferior vena caval filters: Follow-up of seven designs in 320 patients. *Radiology* 188:851–856, 1993.

14. Greenfield L, Cho KJ, Proctor M, et al: Results of a multicenter study of the modified hook-titanium Greenfield filter. *J Vasc Surg* 14:253–257, 1991.

15. Haskal ZJ, Soulen MC, Huettl EA, et al: Life-threatening pulmonary emboli and cor pulmonale: Treatment with percutaneous pulmonary artery stent placement. *Radiology* 191:473–475, 1994.

16. Hayakawa K, Tanaka F, Torizuka T, et al: Bronchial artery embolization for hemoptysis: Immediate and long-term results. *Cardiovasc Intervent Radiol* 15:154–159, 1992.

17. Henry JW, Relyea B, Stein PD: Continuing risk of thromboemboli among patients with normal pulmonary angiograms. *Chest* 107:1375–1378, 1995.

18. Hudson ER, Smith TP, McDermott VG, et al: Pulmonary angiography using low osmolar nonionic contrast material: Complications in 1432 patients. *Radiology* 198:61–65, 1996.

19. Hull RD, Hirsh J, Carter CJ, et al: Diagnostic value of ventilation-perfusion lung scanning in patients with suspected pulmonary embolism. *Chest* 88:819–828, 1985.

20. Kardjiev V, Symeonov A, Chankov I: Etiology, pathogenesis, and prevention of spinal cord lesions in selective angiography of the bronchial and intercostal arteries. *Neuroradiology* 112:81–83, 1974.

21. Katoh O, Kishikawa T, Yamada H, et al: Recurrent bleeding after arterial embolization in patients with hemoptysis. *Chest* 97:541–546, 1990.

22. Kaufman JA, Geller SG: Indications for vena caval filters. *AJR Am J Roentgenol* 164:256–257, 1995.

23. Keller FS, Rosch J, Loflin TG, et al: Nonbronchial systemic collateral arteries: Significance in percutaneous embolotherapy for hemoptysis. *Radiology* 164:687–692, 1987.

24. Le Page JR, Gracia RM: The value of bedside wedge pulmonary angiography in the detection of pulmonary emboli: A predictive and prospective evaluation. *Radiology* 144:67–73, 1982.

25. McAdams HP, Erasmus J, Crockett R, et al: The hepatopulmonary syndrome: Radiologic findings in 10 patients. *AJR Am J Roentgenol* 166:1379–1385, 1996.

26. McPherson S, Routh WD, Nath H, Keller FS: Anomalous origin of bronchial arteries: potential pitfall of embolotherapy for hemoptysis. *J Intervent Radiol* 1:86–88, 1990.

27. Mills SR, Jackson DC, Older RA, et al: The incidence, etiologies, and avoidance of complications of pulmonary angiography in a large series. *Radiology* 136:295–299, 1980.

28. Molgaard CP, Yucel EK, Geller SC, et al: Access-site thrombosis after placement of inferior vena cava filters with 12–14-F delivery sheaths. *Radiology* 185:257–261, 1992.

29. Moser KM, Auger WR, Fedullo PF: Chronic major vessel thromboembolic pulmonary hypertension. *Circulation* 81:1735–1743, 1990.

30. Newman GE: Pulmonary angiography in pulmonary embolic disease. *J Thorac Imag* 4:28–39, 1989.

31. Perlmutt LM, Braun SD, Newman GE, et al: Pulmonary arteriography in the high-risk patient. *Radiology* 162:187–189, 1987.

32. Quinn MF, Lundell CJ, Klotz TA, et al: Reliability of selective pulmonary arteriography in the diagnosis of pulmonary embolism. *AJR Am J Roentgenol* 149:469–471, 1987.

33. Rabkin JE, Astafjev VI, Gothman LN, Grigorjev YG: Transcatheter embolization in the management of pulmonary hemorrhage. *Radiology* 163:361–365, 1987.

34. Ray CE Jr, Kaufman JA: Complications of inferior vena cava filters. *Abdom Imag* 21:368–374, 1996.

35. Remy J, Remy-Jardin M, Giraud F, Wattinne L: Angioarchitecture of pulmonary arteriovenous malformations: Clinical utility of three-dimensional helical CT. *Radiology* 191:657–664, 1994.

36. Remy J, Remy-Jardin M, Wattinne L, Deffontaines C: Pulmonary arteriovenous malformations: Evaluation with CT of the chest before and after treatment. *Radiology* 182:809–816, 1992.

37. Remy-Jardin M, Wattinne L, Remy J: Transcatheter occlusion of pulmonary arterial circulation and collateral supply: Failures, incidents, and complications. *Radiology* 180:699–705, 1991.

38. Rosenthal D, Evans RD, Borrero E, et al: Massive pulmonary embolism: Triple-armed therapy. *J Vasc Surg* 9:261–270, 1989.

39. Simon M, Athanasoulis CA, Kim D, et al: Simon nitinol inferior vena caval filter: Initial clinical experience. *Radiology* 172:99–103, 1989.

40. Sostman HD, Coleman RE, DeLong DM, et al: Evaluation of revised criteria for ventilation-perfusion scintigraphy in patients with suspected pulmonary embolism. *Radiology* 193:103–107, 1994.

41. Stein PD, Athanasoulis C, Alavi A, et al: Complications and validity of pulmonary angiography in acute pulmonary embolism. *Circulation* 85:462–468, 1992.

42. Sweezey NB, Fellows KE: Bronchial artery embolization for severe hemoptysis in cystic fibrosis. *Chest* 97:1322–1326, 1990.

43. Tan RT, McGahan JP, Link DP, Lantz BMT: Bronchial artery embolization in management of haemoptysis. *J Intervent Radiol* 6:67–76, 1991.

44. Timsit J-F, Reynaud P, Meyres G, Sors H: Pulmonary embolectomy by catheter suction device in massive pulmonary embolism. *Chest* 100:655–658, 1991.

45. Uflacker R, Kaemmerer A, Picon PD, et al: Bronchial artery embolization in the management of hemoptysis: Technical aspects and long-term results. *Radiology* 157:637–644, 1985.

46. Vujic I, Pyle R, Parker E, Mithoefer J: Control of massive hemoptysis by embolization of intercostal arteries. *Radiology* 137:617–620, 1980.

47. White RI Jr: Pulmonary arteriovenous malformations: How do we diagnose them and why is it important to do so? *Radiology* 182:633–635, 1992.

48. White RI, Lynch-Nyhan A, Terry P, et al: Pulmonary arteriovenous malformations: Techniques and long-term outcome of embolotherapy. *Radiology* 169:663–669, 1988.

49. Zhang J, Cui Z, Wang M, Yang L: Bronchial arteriography and transcatheter embolization in the management of hemoptysis. *Cardiovasc Intervent Radiol* 17:276–279, 1994.

SCINTIGRAPHIC EVALUATION OF PULMONARY DISEASE

Abass Alavi / Daniel Worsley

The use of radionuclide tracers has made it possible to assess regional pulmonary function in a variety of pulmonary disorders. In 1955, ^{133}Xe was introduced for the study of regional ventilation. Shortly thereafter, it became possible to evaluate regional pulmonary blood flow using $^{15}CO_2$ by inspiration or ^{135}Xe by injection. In 1964, intravenous injection of ^{133}I-macroaggregated albumin made it feasible to obtain perfusion scans of the lungs. Although these techniques soon gained wide acceptance as tests of regional abnormalities in ventilation and pulmonary blood flow, the major practical application of radionuclide tracers has been in the diagnosis of pulmonary embolism. Increasingly, the role of radiotracers has been expanded to include disorders such as inflammatory lung disease and lung cancer. With the intro-

duction of positron emission tomography as a powerful research and clinical tool, functional and metabolic imaging of the lungs is expected to be employed frequently in the future. These techniques are essential and complementary to routine anatomic studies for optimal management of patients with a variety of pulmonary disorders.

RADIOPHARMACEUTICALS AND TECHNIQUES IN VENTILATION-PERFUSION LUNG SCANNING

Clinical application of perfusion lung scanning was first described in 1964, when iodine 131–labeled macroaggregates of albumin were utilized in the evaluation of pulmonary perfusion.[38,42] Currently, the agents of choice for pulmonary perfusion imaging are technetium 99m–labeled human albumin microspheres (^{99m}Tc HAM) and macroaggregated albumin (^{99m}Tc MAA). ^{99m}Tc MAA particles range in size from 10 to 150 μm; however, more than 90 percent of injected particles measure between 10 and 90 μm. ^{99m}Tc HAM particles are relatively uniform in size and range between 35 and 60 μm. However, ^{99m}Tc MAA is considered the agent of choice for routine perfusion lung scanning because of its availability, short residence time in the lungs, and relatively low cost.

Radiolabeled particles are injected intravenously while the patient is in the supine position, thereby limiting the effect of gravity on regional pulmonary arterial blood flow. Following the administration of ^{99m}Tc MAA, particles are mixed uniformly with the blood that is traveling to the heart and then lodge in precapillary arterioles in the lungs. The usual administered dose of radioactivity is between 74 and 148 MBq (2 to 4 mCi).

The distribution of particles in the lungs is proportional to regional pulmonary blood flow at the time of injection. Approximately 200,000 to 500,000 particles are injected during a routine clinical perfusion lung scan. The normal adult human lung contains approximately 300 million precapillary arterioles and 300 billion capillaries. Therefore, only about 0.1 percent of precapillary arterioles are blocked following the procedure. In addition, the blockage of pulmonary precapillary arterioles by ^{99m}Tc MAA is transient; the biologic half-life in the lung ranges between 2 and 6 h. In pediatric patients and patients with suspected or known right-to-left shunts, pulmonary hypertension, prior pneumonectomy, or a single lung transplant, the number of particles injected should be reduced. Based on past experience, a minimum of 60,000 particles is necessary to obtain relatively uniform and statistically reliable distribution of particles in the pulmonary arterial circulation and to avoid suboptimal studies.

A routine perfusion scan should include at least six views of the lungs; anterior, posterior, right and left lateral, and right and left posterior oblique views (Fig. 35-1). Right and left anterior oblique views may be helpful in selected cases.

Perfusion lung scans are routinely utilized to examine patients with suspected pulmonary embolism. Unfortunately, perfusion imaging is sensitive, but not specific, for diagnosing pulmonary embolism. Virtually all lung diseases (including tumors, infections, asthma, and chronic obstructive pulmonary disease) may cause decreased pulmonary arterial blood flow in the affected lung zones. Therefore, combined use of perfusion ventilation studies can improve the diagnostic specificity of lung scanning for pulmonary embolism.[15] Pulmonary embolism almost always causes abnormal perfusion, while ventilation is preserved (*mismatched defects*) (Fig. 35-2). In contrast, in parenchymal pulmonary disorders, decreased ventilation and perfusion are noted in the same lung region (*matched defects*). Conditions in which the ventilation abnormality may appear larger than the perfusion abnormality (*reverse mismatch*) include airway obstruction, mucous plug, atelectasis, and pneumonia (Fig. 35-3). Patients with metabolic alkalosis or patients treated with inhaled albuterol fail to respond to hypoxic insults by vasoconstriction. Such inappropriate reaction can be demonstrated as reverse mismatch (perfusion of poorly ventilated sites) on ventilation-perfusion scans.

^{133}Xe has been widely used to determine regional ventila-tion in the lungs. However, other tracers, such as xenon 127, krypton 81m, and, recently, technetium 99m–labeled aerosols, Technegas and Pertechnegas, are utilized for this purpose. Studies that compare various ventilation agents are limited; however, based on the data available, there appear to be no major differences with regard to diagnostic yield among various radiotracers.[1,14]

Utilizing a closed breathing system and ^{133}Xe, the first inspiration image demonstrates regional ventilation in major airway systems (Fig. 35-4). Equilibrium images are obtained while the patient rebreathes the gas for several minutes. Regions of the lung that appear to ventilate poorly in the initial image may fill in the equilibrium phase of the study because of collateral air drift. During the washout phase, while the patient inspires room air, areas of poor ventilation are detected as focal spots of gas retention on the image. Diagnostic yield from the ventilation-perfusion scan is significantly higher if studies are performed in the erect, rather than supine, position. Generally, for technical reasons (lower energy of gamma radiation of ^{133}Xe compared to ^{99m}Tc), ventilation images with ^{133}Xe are obtained before perfusion imaging.

The imaging technique for ^{127}Xe is similar to that for ^{133}Xe. However, because ^{127}Xe has a higher energy than ^{99m}Tc, ventilation scanning with ^{127}Xe can be performed following perfusion imaging. The advantages of acquiring ventilation imaging following perfusion studies are that the patient can be positioned so ventilation to the areas of the lungs that reveal the greatest perfusion abnormality can be imaged with optimal detail and ventilation imaging may be avoided altogether in selected cases when the perfusion lung scan appears normal.

However, ^{127}Xe scanning has several disadvantages. It is more costly than ^{133}Xe and requires medium energy collimation, which degrades image resolution. With either ^{133}Xe or ^{127}Xe, images can be obtained only in a limited number of views—in contrast to perfusion images, which are obtained in multiple projections.

Krypton 81m is a noble gas that can be used to evaluate regional ventilation. This radioactive gas has a very short physical half-life (13 s), and images acquired with this agent reveal ventilation to major airway systems only. However, the short physical half-life of ^{81m}Kr allows generation of images of the lungs in multiple projections. ^{81m}Kr is produced from a rubidium 81 generator. The parent radionuclide has a physical half-life of 4.7 h, which limits the useful lifetime of the generator to only 1 day. As with ^{127}Xe ventilation studies, imaging with ^{81m}Kr is generally performed following the perfusion scan.

Technetium-labeled aerosol studies can be performed following the inhalation of several preparations, in-

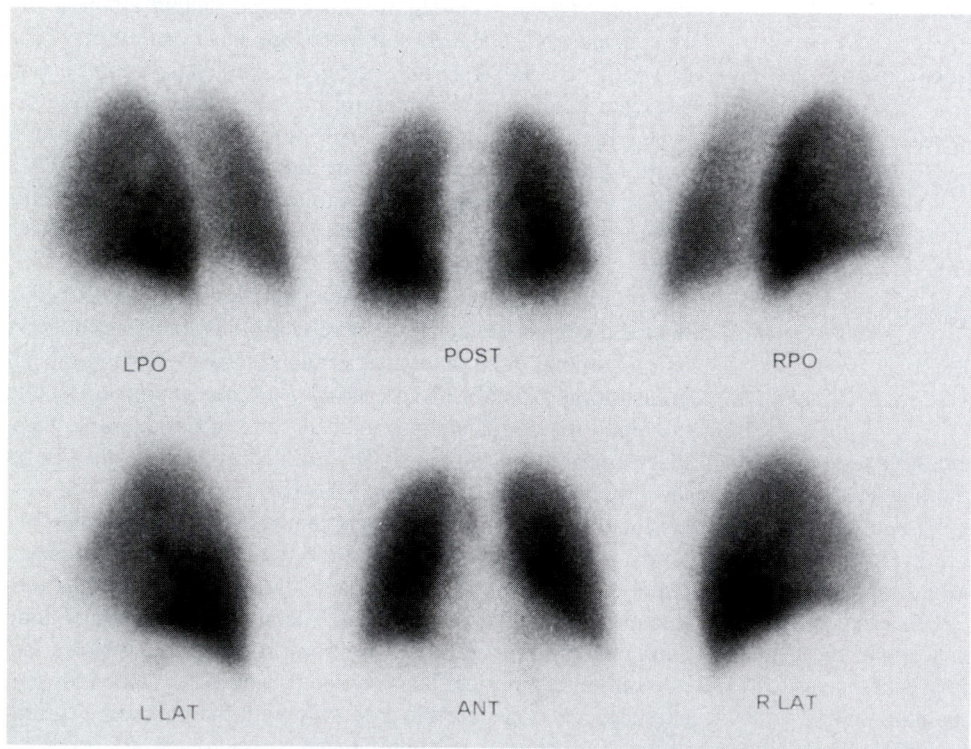

FIGURE 35-1   Normal lung scans. Normal perfusion scan using ^{99m}Tc MAA. The distribution of particles is uniform, with a minimum gradient of activity from the apex to the base of the lungs. The six views (left posterior oblique, posterior, right posterior oblique, right anterior oblique, anterior, left anterior oblique) shown here correspond to those shown in subsequent figures.

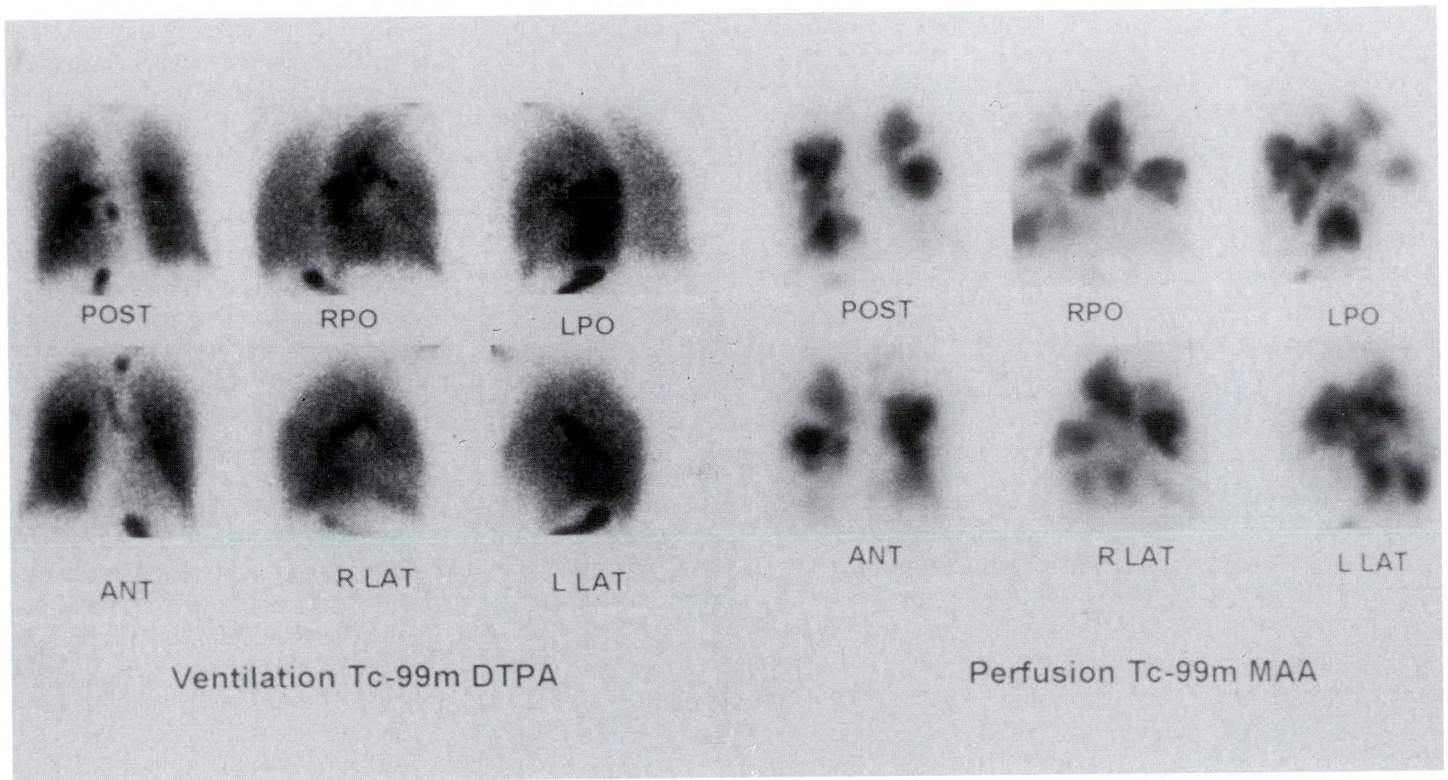

FIGURE 35-2 High-probability scan for pulmonary embolism. Ventilation scan utilizing ^{99m}Tc DTPA aerosol is within normal limits. Perfusion scan shows large segmental defects in both lungs. This combination of findings is most consistent with pulmonary embolism.

cluding ^{99m}Tc DTPA (diethylene triamine penta-acetic acid), ^{99m}Tc sulfur colloid, ^{99m}Tc pyrophosphate, ^{99m}Tc MDP (methylene diphosphate), and ^{99m}Tc glucoheptanate. The most popular is ^{99m}Tc DTPA. However, this agent has a relatively short residence time within the lung, especially in smokers. In such patients, use of ^{99m}Tc-labeled sulfur colloid or pyrophosphate may be more appropriate. ^{99m}Tc-labeled radioaerosols have particles between 0.5 and 3 μm in size and are produced by utilizing recently introduced commercially available nebulizers. For a routine ventilation study, 1.11 GBq (30 mCi) of ^{99m}Tc DTPA in 3 ml of saline is placed in the nebulizer. Oxygen is then forced through the nebulizer at high pressure to produce aerosolized droplets, which are inhaled by the patient through a mask or mouthpiece. The patient generally breathes from the nebulizer for 3 to 5 min or until 37 MBq (1 mCi) of radioactivity is deposited in the lungs. The regional distribution of radioactivity in the lungs is proportional to local ventilation. ^{99m}Tc-labeled radioaerosol studies are generally performed before perfusion imaging. The lungs are imaged in multiple projections, which correspond to those obtained during the subsequent perfusion study. Ventilation studies using ^{99m}Tc-labeled radioaerosols require minimal patient cooperation and can be performed at the bedside and on patients who are on ventilators. Disadvantages of ^{99m}Tc-labeled radioaerosols include the central deposition of radioactivity in patients with chronic obstructive pulmonary disease (COPD) or airway obstruction and the need to dispose of the substantial unused amount of radioactivity that is deposited in the nebulizer.

Central deposition of ^{99m}Tc-labeled radioaerosol in patients with COPD is a major drawback to the use of aerosol agents, and newer agents have been developed to overcome this defi-

ciency, including ^{99m}Tc Technegas and ^{99m}Tc Pertechnegas. These agents are generated by burning ^{99m}Tc pertechnetate in a carbon crucible at very high temperatures, which produces an ultrafine radiolabeled aerosol (particle size, 0.02 to 0.2 μm). Pertechnegas is purged with 5 percent oxygen and 95 percent argon; Technegas is purged with 100 percent argon. This rela-

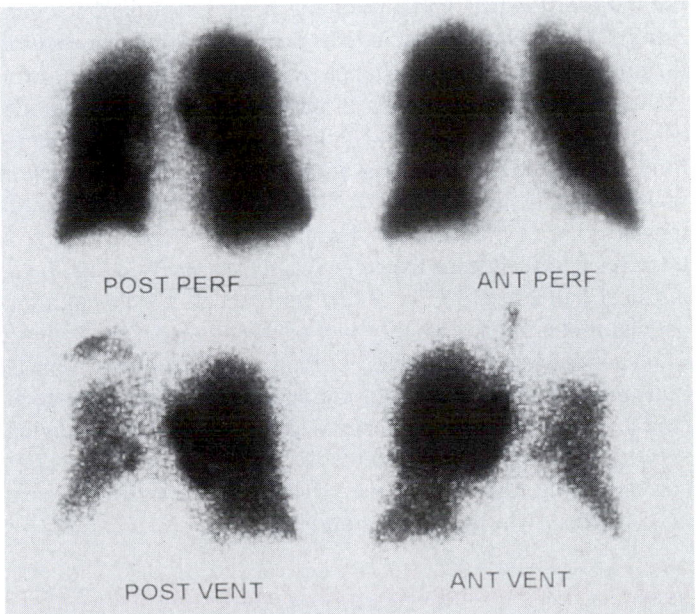

FIGURE 35-3 Reverse V/Q mismatch. Posterior and anterior perfusion scans appear within normal limits (upper row). Posterior and anterior aerosol ventilation scans show significantly reduced perfusion in the left lung.

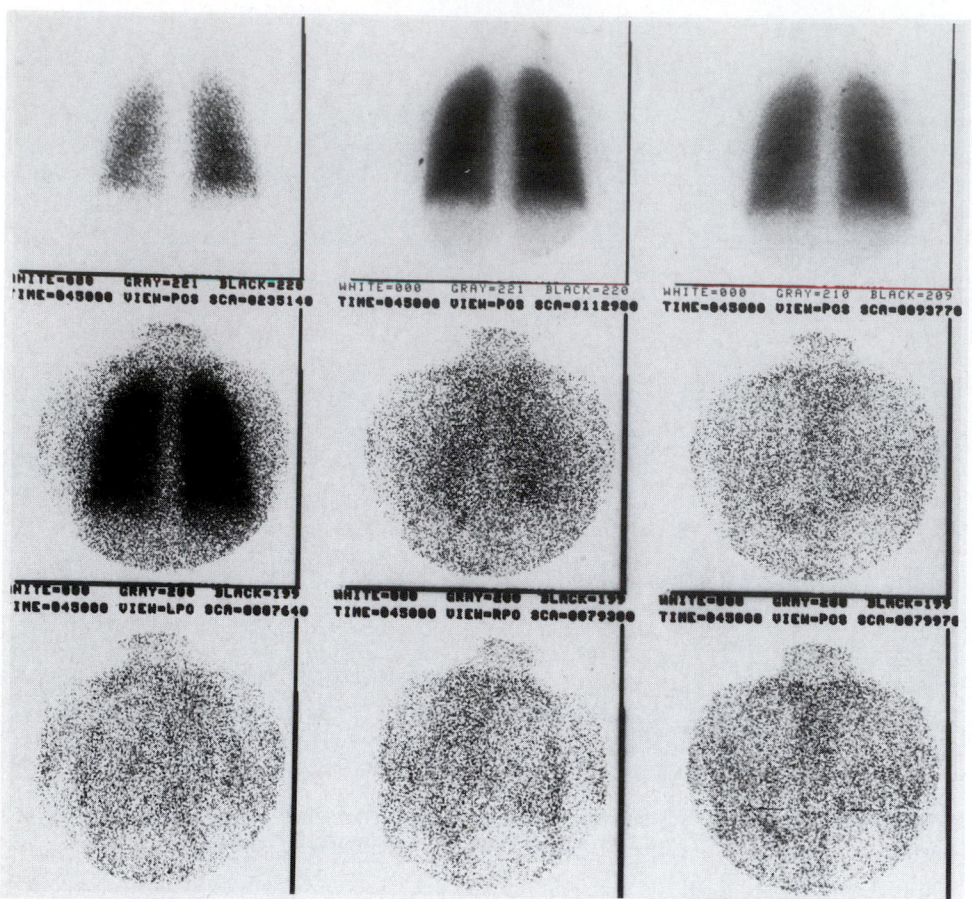

FIGURE 35-4 Normal ventilation scan using ^{133}Xe. The distribution of gas is uniform during the wash-in and equilibrium-phase images (left to right in upper row). During the washout phase, the radioisotope is rapidly cleared from both lungs (lower-row images). Ventilation images were obtained in the posterior projection.

tality and morbidity if initiated soon after the event. The accurate and expeditious diagnosis of acute PE can be difficult because of the nonspecificity of the clinical, laboratory, and radiographic findings.[24] Approximately 10 percent of patients with PE die within 1 h.[2] For patients who survive beyond the first hour, anticoagulation with heparin or thrombolysis with thrombolytic agents is effective therapy.[2] The mortality in patients with PE who are not treated is as high as 30 percent. In contrast, correct diagnosis and appropriate therapy significantly lower mortality to 2.5 to 8 percent.[2,4]

Although anticoagulant therapy is effective in treating PE and in reducing mortality, it is not without risks. The prevalence of major hemorrhagic complications has been reported to be as high as 10 to 15 percent among patients receiving anticoagulant therapy.[21] Therefore, the accurate diagnosis of PE is essential, not only to prevent death from recurrent embolism but also to avoid complications related to unnecessary anticoagulant therapy.

Ventilation-perfusion (V̇/Q̇) lung imaging has been shown to be a safe, noninvasive technique in evaluating regional pulmonary function for a variety of purposes. The technique has been widely used in the assessment of patients with suspected PE. In spite of its proven value in the management of patients with PE and studies suggesting the underdiagnosis of PE, critics have suggested that this powerful method has been overutilized and has minimal impact on patient outcome.[11,28]

The first major study that utilized perfusion lung scanning as a screening test for the diagnosis of PE was the Urokinase Pulmonary Embolism Trial (UPET). In more then 90 percent of patients enrolled in the trial, perfusion lung scanning was performed following intravenous administration of ^{131}I-labeled MAA. Since lung imaging was carried out using rectilinear scanners, ventilation studies were not performed during the study. Despite utilizing a suboptimal radiopharmaceutical and somewhat primitive instruments (as judged by today's standards), the UPET study established perfusion lung scanning as an effective technique in both screening for PE and assessing restoration of pulmonary blood flow following an embolic event.[40]

Most patients with acute PE either completely lyse the thrombi or partly recanalize the pulmonary artery clots. In UPET, approximately 75 to 80 percent of perfusion defects resolved by 3 months, and those that did not remained largely persistent when followed for 1 year. The degree of clot resolution observed in UPET may represent an underestimate, since ventilation scanning was not performed, and many of the unresolved perfusion defects might have been due to preexisting COPD. Therefore, al-

tively minor step in production of the final preparation causes profound differences in the biologic behavior of particles generated. When inhaled, both agents distribute homogeneously in the lung in proportion to regional ventilation and with very minimal central deposition, even in patients with COPD. Pertechnegas readily penetrates the alveolar epithelial membrane; therefore, its biologic half-life in the lungs is quite short (approximately 6 to 10 min). On the other hand, very little transalveolar or mucociliary clearance is seen with Technegas; thus, residence time in the lung is approximately equal to the physical half-life of ^{99m}Tc (6 h). Both agents require minimal patient cooperation, and only two or three breaths are required to obtain sufficient deposition in the lungs for optimal ventilation imaging. In general, ventilation imaging with both Technegas and Pertechnegas is performed before perfusion imaging. As with ^{99m}Tc-radiolabeled aerosols, multiple views of the lungs corresponding to those acquired during perfusion imaging can be generated with these preparations.

LUNG SCANNING IN THE DIAGNOSIS OF ACUTE PULMONARY EMBOLISM

Pulmonary embolism (PE) is a common and potentially fatal disorder for which treatment is highly effective and decreases mor-

though chronic pulmonary thromboembolism can be erroneously diagnosed as an acute event based on $\dot{V}/\dot{Q}$ images, the overall diagnostic performance of this method does not appear to be significantly altered by the history of PE. Based on the data from UPET, we recommend that a repeat perfusion lung scan be performed approximately 3 months after the initial diagnosis of PE; the scan can serve as a baseline for future comparisons and aids in evaluating clot resolution.

Data from three large studies using modern imaging agents and instruments have clearly revealed the efficacy of $\dot{V}/\dot{Q}$ scanning in the management of patients with acute PE.[12,13,26] In a prospective study of 874 patients, $\dot{V}/\dot{Q}$ scan interpretation was grouped into three diagnostic categories with regard to probability of PE: normal (no evidence of PE), non–high-probability, and high-probability patterns.[12] The purpose of the study was to determine whether anticoagulation could be withheld from patients who had either a normal or a non–high-probability scan pattern, adequate cardiorespiratory reserve, and absent proximal vein thrombosis, as determined by negative serial impedance plethysmography (IPG). The diagnostic approach was based on the pathophysiological concept that venous thromboembolism is a systemic disorder and that pulmonary embolism is merely the respiratory manifestation of this process. High-probability and normal $\dot{V}/\dot{Q}$ scan patterns were interpreted in 8 and 36 percent of patients, respectively. Nine percent of patients had non–high-probability scan interpretation and inadequate cardiorespiratory reserve as defined by the presence of pulmonary edema, right ventricular failure, systolic blood pressure less than 90 mmHg, syncope, acute tachyarrhythmias, or significantly abnormal spirometry values or arterial blood gases; 47 percent of patients had non–high-probability scan patterns and adequate cardiorespiratory reserve.

The outcome in each group in the study was assessed during a 3-month follow-up period. In patients with a non–high-probability lung scan interpretation, adequate cardiorespiratory reserve, and negative serial IPGs, anticoagulants were withheld. Only 2.7 percent of these patients had evidence of venous thromboembolism during the follow-up period. The conclusion from the study is that patients with a non–high-probability $\dot{V}/\dot{Q}$ scan pattern, adequate cardiorespiratory reserve, and negative serial IPGs can be managed safely without anticoagulation. In addition, the results confirm findings from previous studies suggesting that the incidence of recurrent PE is very low in the absence of proximal, lower-extremity venous thrombi. Unfortunately, the interpretation criteria used to categorize the probability of PE were, to some extent, unconventional (conventional categories include "normal," "low," "nondiagnostic," and "high" probability patterns). Consequently, the results of the study cannot be optimally compared with those of the PIOPED study (see below).

Recently, 1564 consecutive patients with suspected pulmonary embolism who underwent both $\dot{V}/\dot{Q}$ scanning and IPGs of the lower extremities were examined prospectively.[13] In 40 percent, $\dot{V}/\dot{Q}$ scans were interpreted as nondiagnostic, and serial IPGs were negative. All these patients had adequate cardiorespiratory reserve and were managed without anticoagulation. Using this algorithm, only 1.9 percent had evidence of either deep venous thrombosis or PE during follow-up.

Prospective Investigation of Pulmonary Embolism Diagnosis Study

To date, the most comprehensive prospective investigation addressing the role of $\dot{V}/\dot{Q}$ scanning in the diagnosis of PE has been the Prospective Investigation of Pulmonary Embolism Diagnosis (PIOPED) study.[26] This multi-institutional study was designed to evaluate the efficacy of various conventional methods for diagnosing acute PE. In particular, the PIOPED study was designed to determine the sensitivity and specificity of $\dot{V}/\dot{Q}$ lung scanning for the diagnosis of acute PE. In addition, the relative contribution of clinical assessment, the chest radiograph, and other routine studies were assessed. The PIOPED study also provided an opportunity to determine the validity of pulmonary angiography for establishing the diagnosis of acute PE and to measure the incidence of complications related to this procedure. Finally, the study design allowed monitoring of the clinical course and outcome of patients with PE.

In this study, risk factors and clinical signs and symptoms suggestive of PE in males and females were similar.[27] The clinical findings in patients with no preexisting cardiac or pulmonary disease were evaluated in a subgroup of patients.[36] A total of 117 patients with PE and 248 patients in whom PE was excluded were included in the analysis.

Immobilization (strict bed rest for more than 3 continuous days) and surgery (an incision under regional or general anesthesia) within 3 months before enrollment were more common in patients with PE than in those without this diagnosis.[36] The frequency of other risk factors recorded was approximately the same, regardless of the presence or absence of PE.

The most common symptoms in patients with PE and no preexisting cardiac or pulmonary disease were shortness of breath, pleuritic chest pain, and cough.[36] However, the prevalence of these symptoms was not significantly different between patients with and those without PE. Shortness of breath, tachypnea, and pleuritic chest pain alone, or in combination, were present in 97 percent of patients with PE.[35] Based on this observation, the investigators concluded that only a very small percentage of patients do not have at least one of the important clinical manifestations of PE.

Although this statement is valid for patients who were evaluated in the PIOPED study, selection bias, which was forced by the study design, could have affected study findings. Entry criteria into the PIOPED study required that only patients with risk factors, signs, symptoms, or laboratory findings suggestive of acute PE be enrolled in the study. Therefore, it is not surprising that very few patients had no important clinical manifestations of acute PE.

Although the clinical diagnosis of PE is not definitive in most instances, results from the PIOPED study emphasize the importance of incorporating the clinical assessment in the evaluation of patients suspected of having acute PE. As expected, combining clinical assessment with $\dot{V}/\dot{Q}$ scan interpretation improved diagnostic accuracy of the imaging technique.

In patients with low- or very-low-probability $\dot{V}/\dot{Q}$ scan patterns and no history of immobilization, recent surgery, trauma to the lower extremities, or central venous instrumentation, the prevalence of PE was only 4.5 percent.[45,47] In patients with low- or very-low-probability scan interpretation and one or more than one of the above-mentioned risk factors, the prevalence of PE was 12 and 21 percent, respectively (Table 35-1). In PIOPED, however, most of the patients had intermediate-probability $\dot{V}/\dot{Q}$ scan patterns and an intermediate clinical likelihood of PE. For these patients, the combination of clinical assessment and $\dot{V}/\dot{Q}$ scan interpretation does not appear to be adequate for optimal management; therefore, further investigation using peripheral venous studies or pulmonary angiography may be warranted in such circumstances.

Chest radiographs in the PIOPED study in patients with angiographically documented PE were interpreted as normal in only 12 percent.[44] Even among patients with no preexisting cardiac or pulmonary disease, only 16 percent of those with PE had normal chest radiographs.[36] The most common chest radiographic findings in patients with PE were atelectasis or parenchymal opacities in the affected lung zone.[36,44] However, the same abnormalities were noted with the same frequency in patients in whom PE was excluded. Although chest radiographic findings alone are not specific for PE, they are essential for diagnosing conditions that can clinically mimic PE. Also, chest radiographic findings heavily influence the criteria utilized for estimating the probability of PE based on $\dot{V}/\dot{Q}$ scan patterns.

The sensitivity and specificity of $\dot{V}/\dot{Q}$ lung scanning for detecting acute PE are presented in Table 35-2. The sensitivity and specificity, positive predictive value, and negative predictive value of $\dot{V}/\dot{Q}$ scanning in women and men are not significantly different.[27] Similarly, the overall diagnostic performance of the scan is similar among patients of varying ages.[34] The diagnostic utility of $\dot{V}/\dot{Q}$ scanning for detecting PE among patients with preexisting cardiac or pulmonary disease and in those with no such underlying disorders is similar.[33] In a subgroup of patients with COPD, the sensitivity of a high-probability $\dot{V}/\dot{Q}$ scan pattern was significantly lower than that in patients with no preexisting cardiopulmonary disease.[18] In the PIOPED study, however, the positive predictive value of a high-probability $\dot{V}/\dot{Q}$ scan interpretation was 100 percent, and the negative predictive value of a low- or very-low-probability scan pattern was 94 percent.

The most common cause of ventilation-perfusion mismatch in patients without proven PE is chronic or unresolved PE. Other causes of ventilation-perfusion mismatch are compression of the pulmonary vasculature (by mass lesions, adenopathy, or mediastinal fibrosis), blood vessel wall lesions (e.g., pulmonary artery sarcoma, vasculitis), intraluminal obstruction (tumor or foreign-body emboli), and congenital vascular abnormalities (e.g., pulmonary artery agenesis or hypoplasia).

Interpretation Criteria and Amendments to Original PIOPED Criteria

Several diagnostic schemes have been suggested for the interpretation of $\dot{V}/\dot{Q}$ lung scans. The original PIOPED criteria were developed to interpret the $\dot{V}/\dot{Q}$ scans generated from the study based on experience over the preceding decade. However, several revisions of the original PIOPED criteria have been made since it was introduced (Table 35-3). By utilizing a series of these revisions, it has become possible to decrease the number of intermediate $\dot{V}/\dot{Q}$ scan interpretations and to correctly interpret the scans as consistent with a low probability for acute PE. The use of revised PIOPED criteria has already been shown to provide a more accurate assessment of angiographically proven PE than the original criteria.[6]

Based on revised PIOPED criteria, the prevalence of PE in patients with extensive matched defects and no chest radiographic evidence of pleural effusion or parenchymal abnormalities is 14 percent.[8] Therefore, $\dot{V}/\dot{Q}$ scans in patients with COPD, regardless of the extent of the disease, can be categorized as representing low probability for acute PE.

With the revised PIOPED criteria, 36 percent of patients with a moderate-sized mismatch $\dot{V}/\dot{Q}$ scan abnormality were found to have PE; therefore, this finding represents an intermediate probability for acute PE.[8]

In the PIOPED study, the overall prevalence of PE in patients with matching ventilation-perfusion defects and chest radiographic opacities ("triple matches") was 26 percent.[46] However, when triple matches were present in the upper and middle lung zones, the prevalence of PE was 11 and 12 percent, respectively. In contrast, PE was present in 33 percent of lower lung zones that demonstrated triple matches.[46] Therefore, matching ventilation-perfusion defects and chest radi-

---

TABLE 35-2

Sensitivity, Specificity, and Positive Predictive Value of Lung Scans in Detecting Pulmonary Embolism in Patients Enrolled in PIOPED

Lung Scan Interpretation (Probability)	Sensitivity	Specificity	Positive Predictive Value
High	40%	98%	87%
High, intermediate	82%	64%	49%
High, intermediate, low	98%	12%	32%

TABLE 35-1

Risk Factors and Prevalence of Pulmonary Embolism in Patients with False-Negative and True-Negative Lung Scans Enrolled in PIOPED

	Patients with 0 Risk Factors (%)*	Patients with 1 Risk Factors (%)*	Patients with ≥ 2 Risk Factors (%)*	Total
PE positive	14 (2.2%)	19 (2.9%)	37 (5.7%)	70
PE negative	301 (46.4%)	136 (21.0%)	142 (21.9%)	579
Prevalence of PE	4.5%	12.2%	20.7%	10.8%

*Risk factors include immobilization, trauma to lower extremities, surgery, and central venous instrumentation within 3 months of enrollment.

TABLE 35-3

Revised PIOPED Criteria for Interpretation of Lung Scans*

High Probability

≥2 large segmental perfusion defects (>75% of a segment) without corresponding ventilation or radiographic abnormalities

1 large segmental perfusion defect and ≥2 moderate segmental perfusion defects (25–75% of a segment) without corresponding ventilation or radiographic abnormalities

≥4 moderate segmental perfusion defects without corresponding ventilation or radiographic abnormalities

Intermediate Probability

1 moderate to <2 large segmental perfusion defects without corresponding ventilation or radiographic abnormalities

Corresponding ventilation-perfusion defects and radiographic parenchymal opacity in lower lung zone

Single, moderate, matched ventilation-perfusion defects with normal radiographic findings

Corresponding ventilation-perfusion defects and small pleural effusion

Difficult to categorize as normal, low, or high probability

Low Probability

Multiple matched ventilation-perfusion defects, regardless of size, with normal radiographic findings

Corresponding ventilation-perfusion defects and radiographic parenchymal opacity in upper or middle lung zone

Corresponding ventilation-perfusion defects and large pleural effusion

Any perfusion defects with substantially larger radiographic abnormality

Defects surrounded by normally perfused lung (stripe sign)

>3 small segmental perfusion defects (<25% of a segment) with a normal radiograph

Nonsegmental perfusion defects (cardiomegaly, aortic impression, enlarged hila)

Very Low Probability

≤3 small segmental perfusion defects (<25% of a segment) with a normal radiograph

Normal Probability

No perfusion defects; perfusion outlines the shape of the lung seen on the radiograph

*Criteria generated after completion of prospective study.

ographic opacities isolated to the upper or middle lung zones represent a low probability for acute PE. Similar findings in the lower lung zones are evidence for an intermediate probability of acute PE.

An additional interesting finding from the PIOPED study was that among patients with no previous cardiopulmonary disease, no patient with PE had radiographic evidence of a pleural effusion that occupied more than one-third of the hemithorax.[36] Therefore, ventilation-perfusion defects with a large pleural effusion represent a low probability of acute PE. In contrast, most patients with PE and pleural effusions had small effusions that caused only blunting of the costophrenic angles. The prevalence of PE in the lower lung zones in patients with small pleural effusions was 32 percent in the right hemithorax and 25

percent in the left hemithorax.[44] Therefore, matching ventilation-perfusion defects with a small effusion represent an interme-diate probability for acute PE.

The *stripe sign* is defined as a rim of perfused lung tissue between the perfusion defect and the adjacent pleural surface (Fig. 35-5). In the PIOPED study, the presence of the sign excluded the diagnosis of PE within the affected zone in 93 percent of cases.[31] Therefore, perfusion defects that demonstrate a stripe sign are unlikely to be due to PE, and in the absence of perfusion defects elsewhere, such findings should be interpreted as representing a low probability of PE.

Finally, the nuclear medicine physician's subjective estimate of the likelihood of PE (without using specific interpretation criteria) correlated well with the fraction of patients with angiographic evidence of PE in the PIOPED study. Thus, experienced readers (such as the PIOPED investigators) can provide an accurate estimate of the probability of PE based on radiographic and scintigraphic findings.

Pulmonary Angiography in Pulmonary Embolism

In the PIOPED study, the angiographic diagnosis of acute PE was based strictly on the identification of an intraluminal filling defect or the trailing edge of a thrombus obstructing a vessel. All pulmonary angiograms were interpreted by two independent readers who were not from the institutions where the study was performed. The angiograms were interpreted with regard to the presence, absence, or uncertainty of acute PE. If the two readers agreed, the interpretation was considered final. If the first two readers disagreed, the interpretation was adjudicated by a third reader. If all three readers disagreed, the final interpretation was rendered by an angiography working group panel.

For patients who had angiographic evidence of PE, reader agreement among experts was 86 percent. For patients with angiograms interpreted as negative or uncertain for PE, reader agreement was 80 and 40 percent, respectively.

Pulmonary angiography was completed in 99 percent of patients who consented to undergo the procedure.[32] The frequency distribution of final angiographic interpretations is presented in Fig. 35-6. In most patients in whom angiography was not com-

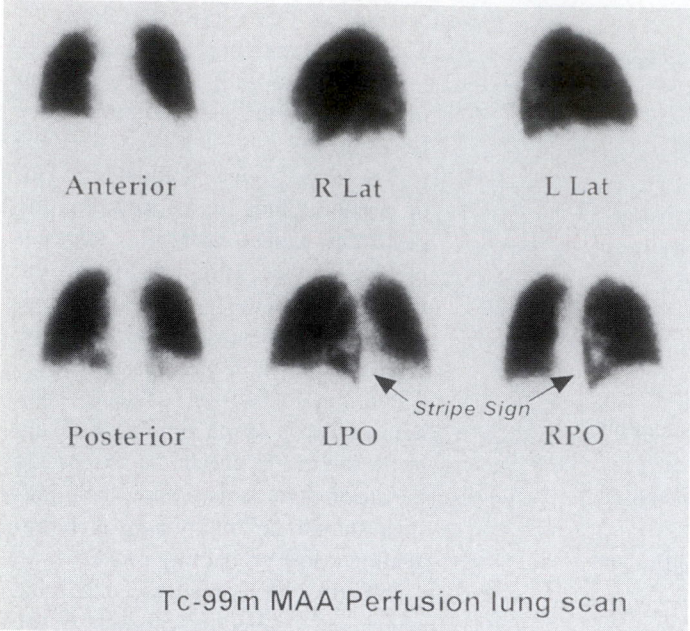

Tc-99m MAA Perfusion lung scan

FIGURE 35-5 Stripe sign. Both left posterior and right posterior oblique views (lower row) demonstrate a defect surrounded by perfused lung. This pattern is very rarely seen in pulmonary embolism.

An analysis of the regional distribution of PE on angiography demonstrated that PE occurred more frequently on the right than on the left and more frequently in the lower lung zones than in the middle or upper lung zones.

Complications related to pulmonary angiography in the PIOPED study have been well documented.[32] Death attributed to pulmonary angiography occurred in 0.5 percent of patients. Nonfatal major complications, including respiratory distress, severe renal failure, and hematoma requiring transfusion, occurred in 1 percent of patients. The frequency of major complications was higher in patients from medical intensive care units than in those from other inpatient settings. Minor complications, which were not life-threatening and responded promptly to pharmacologic intervention, occurred in 5 percent. The most common minor complications were urticaria or pruritus and mild renal dysfunction. The frequency of complications was not related to patient age, the presence of PE, or pulmonary artery pressure.

Outcome in Pulmonary Embolism

Of the 399 patients in the PIOPED study who had confirmed PE, treatment was initiated for 94 percent. Among the 24 patients who were not treated, in 19 patients, pulmonary angiograms were interpreted as negative for PE at the local hospital, which was in disagreement with the final angiographic interpretation. Death attributed to pulmonary embolism occurred in only 2.5 percent of patients with PE.[4] Patients were far more likely to die from co-morbid conditions than from PE. Among patients who died from PE, only one was untreated, and nine of the deaths were due to clinically suspected recurrent PE. Therefore, when the disorder was properly diagnosed and treated, death attributed to PE was relatively uncommon.

Based on the PIOPED study, the following conclusions regarding the role of radionuclide imaging in the diagnosis of PE can be reached:

1. A normal ventilation-perfusion scan excludes the diagnosis of clinically significant PE (Fig. 35-6).

pleted, a complication was encountered during the procedure. Nondiagnostic pulmonary angiograms were obtained in only 3 percent of patients.

The validity of pulmonary angiography was assessed by an outcome classification committee. Among 681 patients whose angiograms were interpreted as negative for PE, only in four patients was the diagnosis reversed by the outcome committee. Thus, a negative pulmonary angiogram excluded the diagnosis of acute PE in 99 percent of cases. Since angiography was considered the gold standard in the PIOPED study, the validity of a positive angiogram representing PE could not be verified. In one patient with an angiographic diagnosis of PE, however, the outcome classification committee failed to document PE at autopsy.

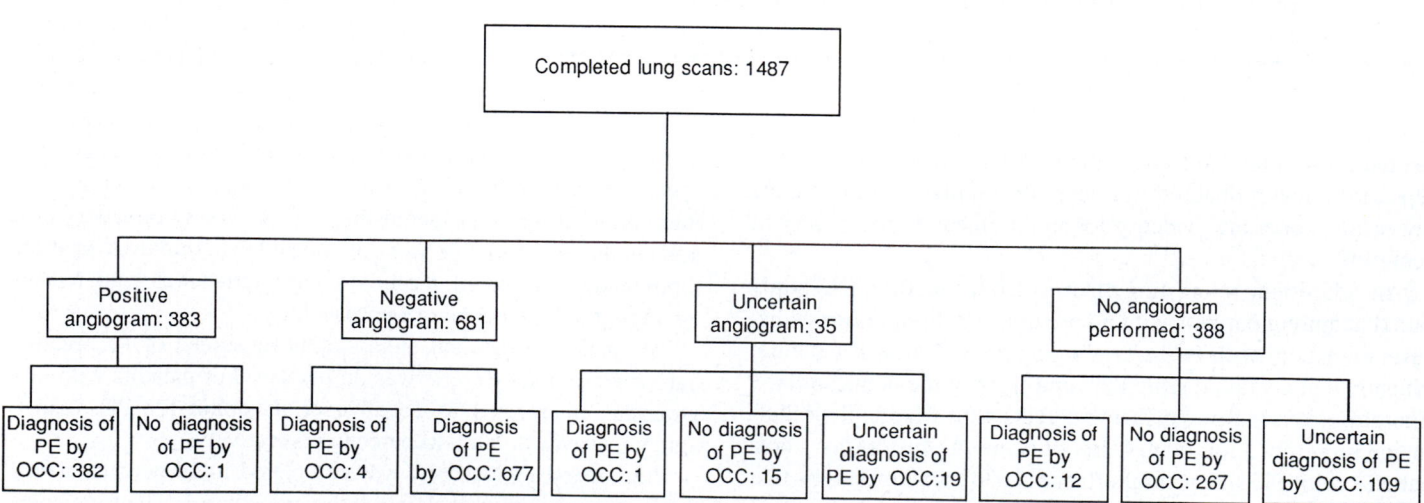

FIGURE 35-6 Outcome classification of patients enrolled in PIOPED. Data are from patients who completed ventilation-perfusion scans. See text for details. PE = pulmonary embolism; OCC = Outcome Classification Committee.

2. A patient with a very-low- or low-probability scan pattern and a low clinical likelihood of PE does not require angiography or anticoagulation.

3. A patient with very-low- or low-probability scan interpretation, intermediate or high clinical likelihood of PE, and negative serial noninvasive venous studies of the lower extremities does not require anticoagulation or angiography. If serial noninvasive venous studies of the lower extremities are positive, the patient should be treated.

4. A clinically stable patient with an intermediate-probability scan pattern requires a noninvasive venous study of the legs; if the study is negative, the patient may require pulmonary angiography or spiral computed tomography (CT).

5. A clinically stable patient with a high-probability scan interpretation and a high clinical likelihood of PE requires treatment, and no further diagnostic tests are required to confirm the diagnosis.

6. A clinically stable patient with a high-probability scan pattern and a low or intermediate clinical likelihood of PE requires a noninvasive venous study of the legs; if the study is negative, the patient may require pulmonary angiography or spiral CT.

One of the deficiencies of the PIOPED study was that non-invasive evaluation of the lower extremities was not included as a mandatory procedure. As has been demonstrated, the combination of ventilation-perfusion scan findings and impedance plethysmography can be very useful in selecting patients who have not had substantial PE and in whom there is no evidence of proximal lower-extremity venous thrombi. In these patients, the risk of recurrent embolic events is low, and anticoagulation may not be required.[10,12,13,17] Current clinical strategies for diagnosing PE appropriately include both $\dot{V}/\dot{Q}$ scanning and an evaluation of the deep venous system of the lower extremities.

EVALUATION OF PULMONARY HYPERTENSION

Pulmonary hypertension (PHT) as a consequence of chronic pulmonary thromboembolism is a serious and potentially surgically treatable disease. It has been estimated that between 0.5 and 4 percent of patients with acute pulmonary emboli eventually develop chronic thromboembolic PHT.[20] Unfortunately, the clinical features, laboratory studies, and other noninvasive assessments employed are often unreliable in distinguishing chronic thromboembolic PHT from primary and nonthromboembolic secondary PHT. Pulmonary angiography is usually required to confirm the diagnosis and to determine whether surgical intervention is indicated. Although some authors have reported that pulmonary angiography may be performed safely in patients with severe PHT, others have documented a high frequency of complications, including death.[22,32] Ventilation-perfusion lung scanning is a safe, noninvasive technique that facilitates selection of patients with PHT for pulmonary angiography to confirm the diagnosis of chronic PE. However, both ventilation-perfusion lung scanning and pulmonary angiography may produce underestimations of the magnitude of vascular occlusion by chronic emboli, as determined at thromboendarterectomy.[29]

When $\dot{V}/\dot{Q}$ lung scans are performed in patients with PHT, in order to prevent potential adverse hemodynamic effects, the number of ^{99m}Tc MAA particles to be administered should be reduced substantially. We recommend that patients with PHT be injected with approximately 100,000 particles of ^{99m}Tc MAA. Published studies have documented the safety of perfusion lung scanning in patients with PHT when the number of particles is reduced.[48]

In a recent study of patients with chronic thromboembolic PHT, 96 percent of $\dot{V}/\dot{Q}$ lung scans were interpreted as indicative of a high probability of pulmonary embolism.[48] In one patient (the remaining 4 percent), the lung scan suggested an intermediate probability of pulmonary embolism. Therefore, based on this retrospective study, pulmonary angiography appears justifiable in patients with intermediate or high-probability $\dot{V}/\dot{Q}$ lung scan interpretations to confirm the diagnosis of chronic PE. Most patients with primary PHT and nonthromboembolic secondary PHT have low-probability scan patterns, with diffuse, inhomogeneous distribution of ^{99m}Tc MAA particles within both lungs. Patients with PHT rarely, if ever, have normal or very-low-probability $\dot{V}/\dot{Q}$ lung scan patterns. Thus, a low-probability $\dot{V}/\dot{Q}$ lung scan effectively excludes chronic thromboembolism as the cause of PHT.

QUANTITATIVE VENTILATION-PERFUSION LUNG SCANNING

In patients undergoing pulmonary resection or lung transplantation, quantitative $\dot{V}/\dot{Q}$ lung scanning has been shown to be a useful method for determining regional lung function. The major use of the quantitative $\dot{V}/\dot{Q}$ lung scan is the prediction of postoperative pulmonary function following lung volume reduction for treatment of COPD or pneumonectomy for other reasons. Lung carcinomas located in the periphery of the lung reveal matched ventilation and perfusion defects that correspond to the abnormalities noted on the chest radiograph. In patients with central bronchogenic carcinomas, mismatches between ventilation and perfusion patterns may be noted. In these cases, either the primary lung tumor or adenopathy may compress the main pulmonary artery or vein—which, in turn, may result in decreased perfusion to the affected areas of the lungs. When the airway is partly or totally occluded by cancer, a matching $\dot{V}/\dot{Q}$ pattern is seen in affected zones of the lungs. In patients with central bronchogenic carcinomas, regional perfusion values correlate well with regional lung physiology and should be utilized to predict postoperative pulmonary function. The postoperative FEV_1 is calculated by multiplying the preoperative value by the ratio of the counts in the remaining lung to total lung activity (Fig. 35-7).

ASSESSMENT OF INFLAMMATORY AND GRANULOMATOUS LUNG DISEASE

Gallium 67 citrate and labeled white blood cells are the radiopharmaceuticals of choice for imaging pulmonary infection and inflammation. Gallium 67, which has a physical half-life of 78 h, is an iron analog. Following intravenous administration, approximately 90 percent of the dose injected is bound to transferrin. Only 25 percent of the administered preparation is ex-

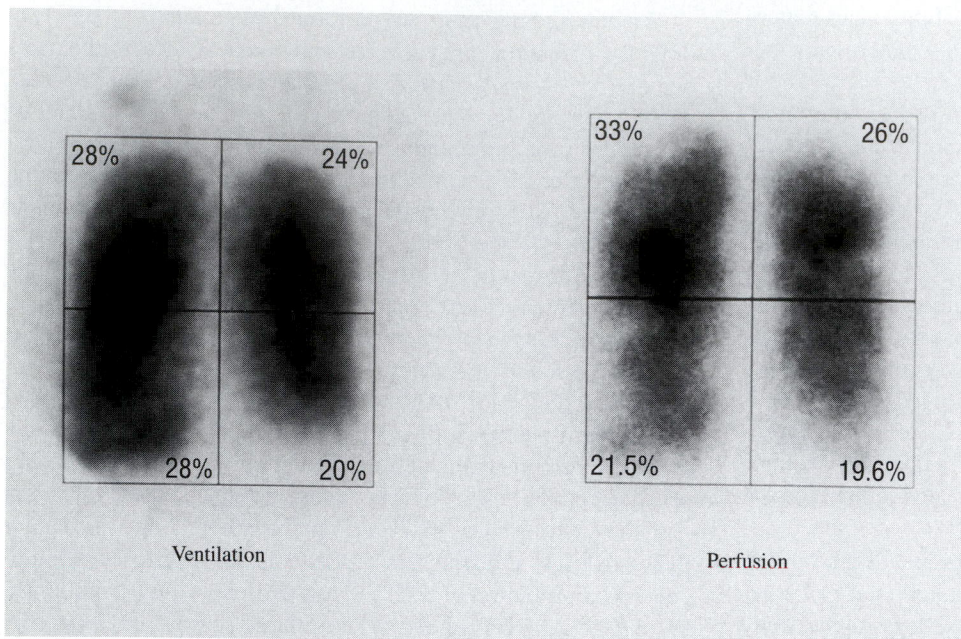

Ventilation

Perfusion

FIGURE 35-7 Quantitative ventilation-perfusion lung scan. Regional ventilation and perfusion can be quantified by outlining regular or irregular regions of interest and generating ratios that correspond to percent of total pulmonary function. Images shown were analyzed by dividing each lung into two equal rectangles.

creted by the kidneys during the first 24 h after injection. Another 10 percent of the injected activity is excreted in stool over the next several days. The remaining 65 percent is distributed within the body. Typically, gallium is taken up in the liver, skeleton, bone marrow, spleen, nasopharynx, lacrimal and salivary glands, and external genitalia. The precise mechanism of gallium localization at sites of inflammation or infection is not completely understood. Increased vascular permeability, direct bacterial uptake (binding to siderophores), binding to lactoferrin (which is secreted by activated leukocytes), and direct binding to circulating leukocytes have been postulated.

The optimal time for imaging the thorax is at least 48 to 72 h following the administration of gallium. Increased gallium activity in the lungs is a sensitive, but relatively nonspecific, indicator of pulmonary infection or inflammation. A variety of conditions, including acute (adult) respiratory distress syndrome, pneumonia, drug reactions (e.g., those due to busulfan, cyclophosphamide, amiodarone, or contrast agent following lymphangiography), pneumoconiosis, idiopathic pulmonary fibrosis, and sarcoidosis may cause increased radiogallium accumulation in the lungs. The intensity and distribution of radiogallium accu-

mulation in the lungs can be quantified to determine the degree of parenchymal inflammation. Malignant processes such as lymphoma, leukemia, mesothelioma, and lung metastases may also result in increased radiogallium uptake when disease activity generally appears focal.

Gallium 67 Citrate Imaging of the Thorax in the Immunocompromised Host

Gallium 67 scintigraphy of the chest is more sensitive than plain chest radiographs for detection of inflammatory processes in immunocompromised patients.[19] Diffuse gallium uptake in the lungs of HIV-infected patients with normal chest radiographs is highly suggestive of *Pneumocystis carinii* pneumonia (PCP) (Fig. 35-8). The sensitivity of gallium scanning for detecting PCP is approximately 95 percent, and when gallium uptake in the lungs is intense (greater than the liver), the specificity also approaches 95 percent.

Other conditions associated with diffuse lung uptake in immunocompromised patients are cytomegalovirus pneumonitis, cryptococcal infections, and lymphoma. Although localized lung

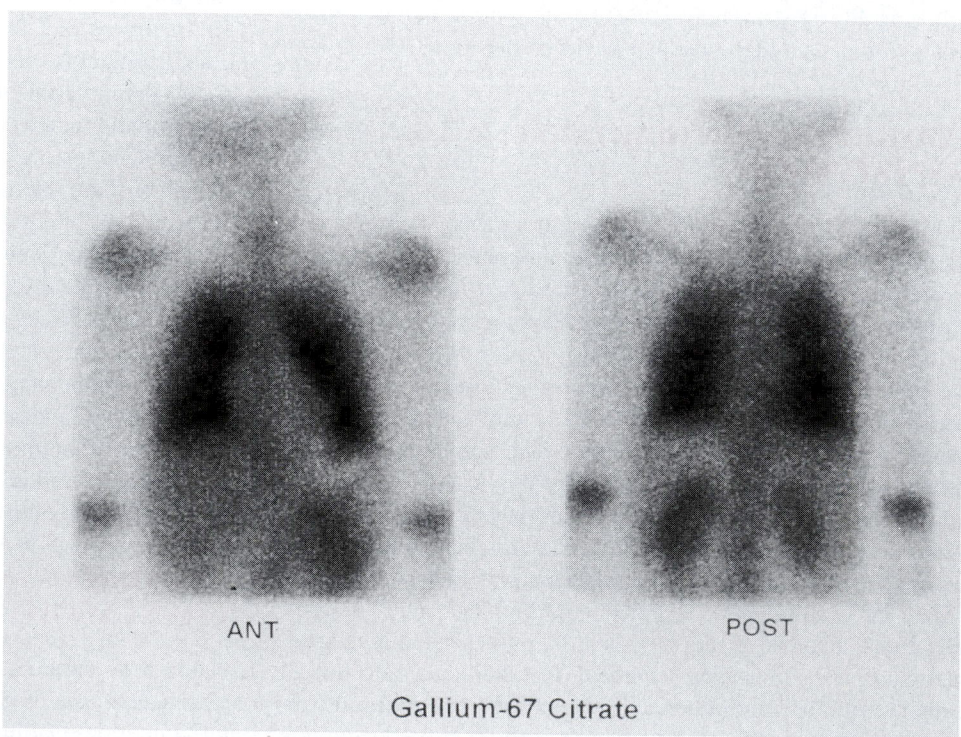

ANT

POST

Gallium-67 Citrate

FIGURE 35-8 *Pneumocystis carinii* pneumonia with diffuse parenchymal lung uptake. Anterior and posterior gallium scans of the chest and abdomen reveal intense uptake of radiogallium, indicating a diffuse inflammatory process in both lungs.

uptake may be associated with PCP, particularly in patients treated with prophylactic aerosolized pentamidine, often focal accumulation is secondary to bacterial pneumonia or immunoblastic lymphoma. Focal activity in the lung and corresponding regional lymph nodes is typical for infection with *Mycobacterium avium-intracellulare* or *M. tuberculosis.* Kaposi's sarcoma does not accumulate radiogallium, but the lesions are clearly visualized following the administration of thallium 201 chloride. Combined imaging with gallium 67 citrate and thallium 201 chloride has been suggested to distinguish Kaposi's sarcoma from PCP and lymphoma in HIV-infected patients.[17]

Noninfectious Inflammatory Lung Disease

Gallium 67 citrate lung imaging has been used to quantify the degree of alveolitis in various interstitial lung diseases, particularly sarcoidosis and idiopathic pulmonary fibrosis. In patients with idiopathic pulmonary fibrosis, the intensity of radiogallium uptake has been shown to correlate with the degree of alveolitis assessed by open lung biopsy and the percentage of neutrophils present in bronchoalveolar lavage fluid. However, pulmonary uptake of gallium 67 citrate may be normal in patients with low-grade alveolitis. Unfortunately, pulmonary accumulation of radiogallium in idopathic pulmonary fibrosis is not a reliable indication of the patient's response to treatment with cortico-steroids or prognosis. Patients who have normal thoracic gallium scans may eventually develop pulmonary fibrosis, whereas the condition of patients with marked increased uptake may remain stable or improve. Therefore, the routine use of gallium 67 scintigraphy in patients with idiopathic pulmonary fibrosis is not recommended.

Scintigraphy with gallium 67 citrate has been advocated for assessment of disease activity in pulmonary sarcoidosis. In patients with sarcoidosis, radiogallium activity in the lung correlates well with the presence of alveolitis detected by lung biopsy and the percentage of T lymphocytes detected by bronchoalveolar lavage. Although it is not specific for sarcoidosis, this disorder is characterized by bilateral, perihilar, or peritracheal uptake of gallium 67 citrate (Fig. 35-9). This appearance, combined with increased uptake in the parotid glands, is virtually pathognomonic for sarcoidosis. Parenchymal activity can also be seen, with or without hilar activity. Parenchymal uptake is usually in the midlung, with relative sparing of the upper and lower lung zones. Gallium 67 citrate imaging in sarcoidosis is useful in selecting the site for lung biopsy to confirm the diagnosis and in distinguishing fibrotic changes from active inflammatory disease. Several studies have also shown a correlation between the degree of uptake of radiogallium with the level of response to

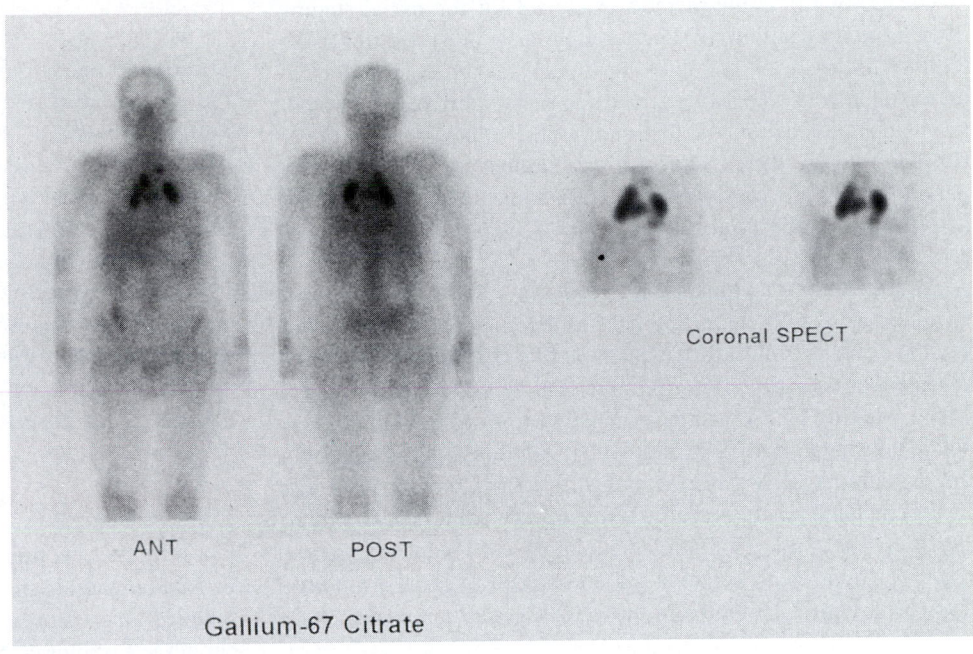

Coronal SPECT

ANT POST

Gallium-67 Citrate

FIGURE 35-9 Bilateral hilar lymphadenopathy in sarcoidosis. Anterior and posterior whole-body images demonstrate intense uptake of radiogallium in both hilar regions. These areas are clearly defined on tomographic (SPECT) images in coronal planes. Similar patterns are seen in patients with lymphoma.

therapy with corticosteroids. Gallium 67 citrate scintigraphy is also useful in assessing extrapulmonary manifestations of sarcoidosis.[3,16]

Radiogallium accumulation in the lungs compared to the soft tissues elsewhere may be graded as follows:

Grade	Radiogallium Uptake
0	lung less than soft tissue
1+	lung equal to soft tisses
2+	lung greater than soft tissues but less than liver
3+	lung equal to liver
4+	lung greater than liver

The grade of gallium uptake may then be multiplied by the area of the lung affected to yield the "gallium index." Semiquanitative indices, including the ratio of lung activity to liver activity, may also be calculated and followed serially in patients with interstitial lung disease.

GALLIUM 67 CITRATE IMAGING IN LYMPHOMA

Gallium 67 scanning has been shown to be useful in detecting mediastinal disease in both Hodgkin's and non-Hodgkin's lymphomas. Because of the frequent localization in the liver, spleen, and large bowel, gallium scintigraphy is insensitive for detecting intra-abdominal or para-aortic disease. There is also some variation in the accumulation in the various histologic subtypes of non-Hodgkin's lymphoma. Patients with moderate- or high-grade lymphoma usually show increased accumulation of gallium, whereas patients with low-grade lymphoma usually demonstrate minimal uptake.

Currently, CT is the method of choice for the initial staging of lymphoma. Gallium 67 citrate imaging is most useful for detecting disease activity following therapy, when anatomic evaluation of mediastinal nodes may not be conclusive.[7] Radiogallium accumulates in viable tumor, rather than in necrotic or fibrotic tissues. When radiogallium studies are performed in patients with previously treated lymphoma, it is important to determine that the tumor takes up this agent before therapy is initiated.

In one study of patients with Hodgkin's and non-Hodgkin's lymphomas, significant differences in disease-free survival were seen in patients with positive and negative gallium scan results.[7] Differences in survival do not appear to be significantly different in patients with positive or negative findings on CT. In this study, the mean period of survival in patients with Hodgkin's disease and negative gallium studies was 20.1 months, whereas in patients with positive scans, the mean survival was 9.4 months. In patients with non-Hodgkin's lymphoma, the mean survival period in patients with negative gallium studies was 18.3 months, compared with 8.4 months in those with positive results.

SCINTIGRAPHIC ASSESSMENT OF ALVEOLAR-CAPILLARY MEMBRANE PERMEABILITY

Assessment of alveolar-capillary membrane permeability requires the inhalation of ^{99m}Tc-labeled radioaerosols. The rate of aerosol clearance from the lung is measured with a counting probe or gamma camera. Several factors influence the rate at which inhaled aerosols "wash out" from the lungs. The most important determinant is the site of aerosol deposition. Aerosols of relatively small aerodynamic diameter (e.g., ^{99m}Tc DTPA) are deposited largely within the small airways and alveoli, whereas larger particles (e.g., ^{99m}Tc MAA or ^{99m}Tc sulfur colloid) are deposited within the proximal airways. The normal half-time of ^{99m}Tc DTPA washout from the lungs is 86 ± 26 min. In the presence of epithelial alveolar damage, the clearance of ^{99m}Tc DTPA is accelerated.

A variety of acute or chronic pulmonary conditions may cause increased clearance of ^{99m}Tc DTPA from the lungs, including pneumoconiosis, idiopathic pulmonary fibrosis, collagen vascular diseases, sarcoidosis, acute (adult) respiratory distress syndrome, and pneumocystis pneumonia. Cigarette smoking or physiological factors, such as posture and exercise, also influence epithelial lung clearance. Since increased alveolar-capillary membrane permeability is relatively nonspecific, ^{99m}Tc DTPA clearance studies have been utilized only to assess the effects of therapy in patients with known pulmonary diseases. Comparison of serial studies is of value only if a consistent pattern of distribution of radiotracer activity is demonstrated on repeated studies. Otherwise, results from such studies are of little help in determining the course of the disease.

EVALUATION OF MUCOCILIARY CLEARANCE

Determination of mucociliary clearance may be obtained after the inhalation of relatively large aerosolized particles, followed by measurement of the rate of clearance with a gamma camera. The rate of mucociliary clearance depends on several factors, including ciliary activity and mucus production. Inhaled particles, such as ^{99m}Tc MAA or ^{99m}Tc sulfur colloid, tend to be deposited within the proximal airways. The normal mucociliary clearance half-time is approximately 24 h. Delayed mucociliary clearance is seen in patients with airway inflammation (e.g., due to COPD, asthma, or viral respiratory tract infections), following bronchial surgery, or after irradiation. Physiological factors, such as aging and sleep, can also delay mucociliary clearance.

ASSESSMENT OF LUNG CANCER

Not infrequently, pulmonary nodules pose a diagnostic dilemma in routine radiologic studies of the lungs. Solitary pulmonary nodules may represent a potentially curable stage of bronchogenic carcinoma. Most solitary pulmonary nodules, however, represent benign processes, such as granulomas.

In the United States alone, approximately 130,000 solitary pulmonary nodules are diagnosed each year. The incidence of solitary pulmonary nodules in adult radiographic surveys varies from 0.1 to 0.2 percent.

Before the advent of CT, approximately 60 percent of resected lung nodules were shown by histologic examination to be benign. Studies utilizing CT have revealed a prevalence of about 20 to 40 percent[37,39] of such processes. Despite recent radiographic advances in the assessment of pulmonary nodules, however, a significant number of patients with benign lesions require further invasive testing. Such patients with "indeterminate" solitary pulmonary nodules usually undergo intensive examination, including bronchoscopy, percutaneous biopsy, and, eventually, surgical excision. Bronchoscopic and percutaneous biopsies have a sensitivity of 71 to 93 percent. The specificity is higher and varies from 91 to 96 percent. False-negative test results occur largely because of sampling error. These techniques are invasive and have been associated with pneumothorax in as many as 30 per-

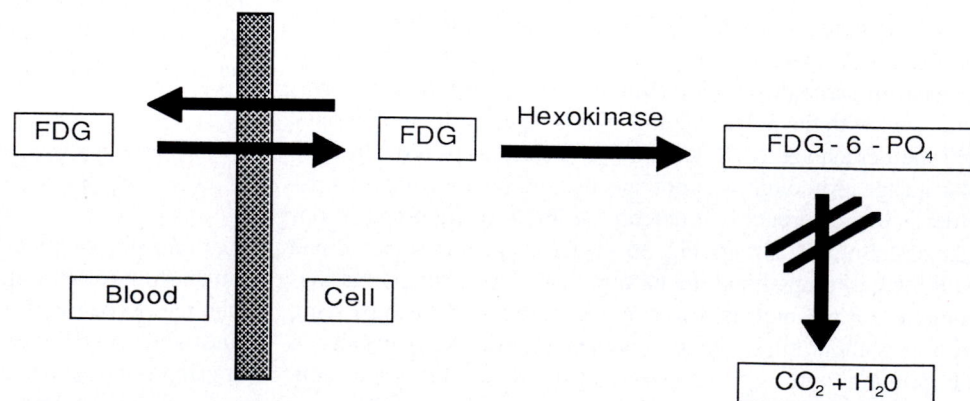

FIGURE 35-10 Schematic representation of FDG metabolism in metabolically active cell. FDG is preferentially transported through the cell membrane. Following phosphorylation to FDG-6-phosphate by the hexokinase system, FDG remains trapped in the cell for a while, facilitating imaging of the abnormal tissue with PET.

cent of cases. To determine whether a nodule is benign or malignant requires surgical excision, followed by histologic examination of resected tissue. Some authors have advocated immediate resection of all radiologically indeterminate solitary pulmonary nodules. However, such a drastic intervention exposes the patient to unnecessary complications, including death, for the diagnosis of a potentially benign disease. Thoracotomy for malignant lesions has an operative mortality of 3 to 7 percent.[39] Therefore, it is imperative to develop a noninvasive procedure to complement the radiographic studies in these patients.

Specific contrast enhancement patterns detected by spiral CT have been suggested as a means for differentiating benign from malignant pulmonary nodules. Enhancement greater than 20 Hounsfield units has a positive predictive value of 90 percent in detecting malignancy. Contrast enhancement is directly related to the vascularity of the nodule and not necessarily to the metabolism within the nodule.

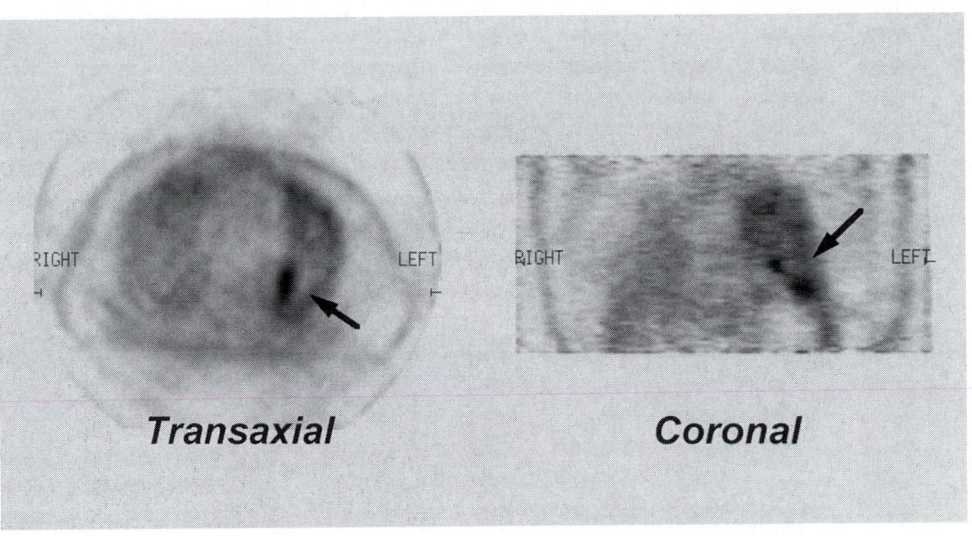

Transaxial   **Coronal**

FIGURE 35-12 FDG images of mesothelioma. Transaxial and coronal images of the lungs in a patient with proven mesothelioma show overall increased metabolic activity in the entire left pleural space, with intense focal accumulation in the area adjacent to the lateral wall of the left ventricle. FDG images of the lung can distinguish between benign and malignant pleural disease and may assist in choosing the appropriate sites for biopsy.

Positron Emission Tomography

Differences between benign and malignant tissues can be demonstrated by using noninvasive imaging techniques such as positive emission tomography (PET) with a radiotracer—e.g., F-18-fluorodeoxy-D-glucose (FDG). The mechanism of uptake and initial phosphorylation of this compound is similar to that of glucose. However, once FDG is phosphorylated (FDG-6-phosphate), it is trapped within the cell and can be imaged with PET (Fig. 35-10). The amount of FDG within the cell is proportional

to glucose uptake and, therefore, metabolic activity of the tissue examined. Relative to benign cells, malignant cells have increased glucose transport and metabolism due to accelerated cell proliferation and increased messenger RNA.

The sensitivity and specificity of PET with FDG for detecting benign and malignant (Fig. 35-11) lesions range from 94 to 97 percent and 80 to 100 percent, respectively.[25,41,43] False-positive studies have been reported with active inflammation due to aspergillosis, tuberculosis, or sarcoidosis.

An additional advantage of PET FDG in the evaluation of solitary pulmonary nodules is the ability to stage mediastinal nodes in non–small-cell lung cancer. In a preliminary study, PET FDG was shown to be more accurate than CT for staging the mediastinum in patients with non–small-cell lung cancer.[43] The accuracy of PET was 81 percent, compared with 52 percent for CT. The combination of PET and CT findings did not improve the accuracy of either technique. In a report on 53 patients with non–small-cell lung cancer who were staged with both CT and PET FDG, the sensitivity and specificity of the latter were significantly higher (sensitivity, 83 percent; specificity, 91 percent) than those of the former (sensitivity, 61 percent; specificity, 71 percent).[41] In addition, whole-body PET imaging detected unsuspected distant metastases in 11 percent (6 of 53) of patients.

Current indications for PET FDG imaging in patients with suspected lung cancer include distinction of benign from malignant pulmonary nodules, mediastinal staging of non–small-cell lung cancer, and differentiation between parenchymal scarring and recurrent tumor in patients who have had previous therapy for lung neoplasm.

In patients with residual parenchymal abnormalities following radiotherapy for lung cancer, PET FDG scanning can be used to distinguish between persistent or recurrent lung cancer and radiation fibrosis. In a study of 35 patients who had recurrent or persistent parenchymal abnormalities following radiotherapy, the sensitivity and specificity for detecting recurrent tumor were 97

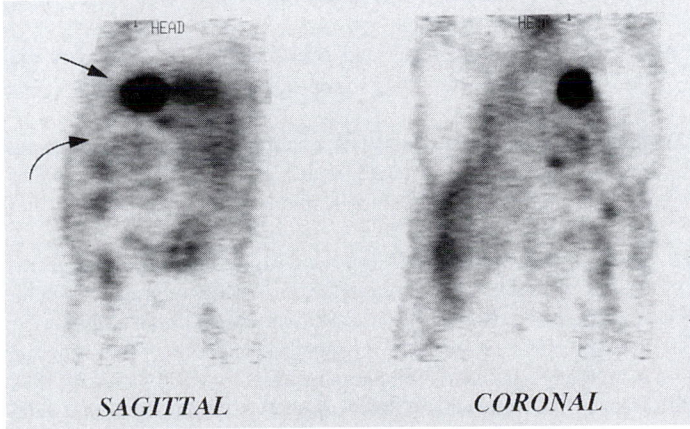

SAGITTAL   *CORONAL*

FIGURE 35-11 Abnormal accumulation of FDG in lung cancer. Sagittal and coronal images of the chest and abdomen reveal intense uptake of FDG in the left upper lung, corresponding to the site of known lung cancer. No evidence of metastases is seen in the mediastinum or other sites.

and 100 percent, respectively. Only one patient, who had a very thin pleural tumor rind, had a false-negative study.[25]

Study of patients with mesothelioma with PET FDG scans has revealed more accurate localization of the tumor activity sites than with anatomic imaging such as CT (Fig. 35-12). In these patients, PET may be of considerable value in establishing the diagnosis and the management plans. PET FDG imaging may play a major role in distinguishing benign peural disease from malignant mesothelioma in patients who have been exposed to asbestos fibers.

It is becoming increasingly clear that PET imaging can significantly influence the outcome of patients with a variety of pulmonary disorders. Even in patients with suspected inflammatory disorders such as sarcoidosis, PET may prove to be superior to conventional nuclear medicine techniques, such as gallium imaging. Unfortunately, PET is available in only a limited number of centers in the United States, and its impact on the day-to-day practice of medicine is very limited. The major impediment for its widespread and routine utilization is the complexity of the technology and the lack of standard reimbursement for the procedure. It is expected that these obstacles will be overcome in the near future, and this powerful technique will be available for routine management of patients.

REFERENCES

1. Alderson PO, Biello DR, Gottschalk A, et al: Tc-99m-DTPA aerosol and radioactive gases compared as adjuncts to perfusion scintigraphy in patients with suspected pulmonary embolism. *Radiology* 153:515–521, 1984.

2. Alpert JS, Smith R, Carlson J, et al: Mortality in patients treated for pulmonary embolism. *JAMA* 236:1477–1480, 1976.

3. Baughman RP, Fernandez M, Bosken CH, et al: Comparison of gallium-67 scanning, bronchoalveolar lavage, and serum angiotensin-converting enzyme levels in pulmonary sarcoidosis: Predicting response to therapy. *Am Rev Respir Dis* 129:676–681, 1984.

4. Carson JL, Kelley MA, Duff A, et al: The clinical course of pulmonary embolism. *New Engl J Med* 326:1240–1245, 1992.

5. DeNardo GL, Goodwin DA, Ravasini R, Dietrich PA: The ventilatory lung scan in the diagnosis of pulmonary embolism. *New Engl J Med* 282:1334–1336, 1970.

6. Freitas FE, Sarosi MG, Nagle CC, et al: Modified PIOPED criteria used in clinical practice. *J Nucl Med* 36:1573–1578, 1995.

7. Front D, Israel O: The role of Ga-67 scintigraphy in evaluating the results of therapy of lymphoma patients. *Semin Nucl Med* 25:60–71, 1995.

8. Gottschalk A, Sostman HD, Coleman RE, et al: Ventilation-perfusion scintigraphy in the PIOPED study: Part II. Evaluation of the scintigraphic criteria and interpretations. *J Nucl Med* 34:1119–1126, 1993.

9. Gupta NC, Frank AR, Dewan NA, et al: Solitary pulmonary nodules: Detection of malignancy with PET with 2-[F-18]-fluoro-2-deoxy-D-glucose. *Radiology* 184:441–444, 1992.

10. Hull RD, Feldstein W, Stein PD, Pineo GF: Cost-effectiveness of pulmonary embolism diagnosis. *Arch Intern Med* 156:68–72, 1996.

11. Hull RD, Raskob GE: Low-probability lung scan findings: A need for change. *Ann Intern Med* 114:142–143, 1991.

12. Hull RD, Raskob GE, Coates G, et al: A new noninvasive management strategy for patients with suspected pulmonary embolism. *Arch Intern Med* 149:2549–2555, 1989.

13. Hull RD, Raskob GE, Ginsberg JS, et al: A noninvasive strategy for the treatment of patients with suspected pulmonary embolism. *Arch Intern Med* 154:289–297, 1994.

14. James JM, Herman KJ, Lloyd JJ, et al: Evaluation of ^{99}Tcm Technegas ventilation scintigraphy in the diagnosis of pulmonary embolism. *Br J Radiol* 64:711–719, 1991.

15. Kelley MA, Carson JL, Palevsky HI, Schwatz JS: Diagnosing pulmonary embolism: New facts and strategies. *Ann Intern Med* 114:300–306, 1991.

16. Lawrence EC, Teague RB, Gottlieb MS, et al: Serial changes in markers of disease activity with corticosteroid treatment in sarcoidosis. *Am J Med* 74:747–756, 1983.

17. Lee VW, Fuller JD, O'Brien MJ, et al: Pulmonary Kaposi sarcoma in patients with AIDS: Scintigraphic diagnosis with sequential thallium and gallium scanning. *Radiology* 180:409–412, 1991.

18. Lesser BA, Leeper KV Jr, Stein PD, et al: The diagnosis of acute pulmonary embolism in patients with chronic obstructive pulmonary disease. *Chest* 102:17–22, 1992.

19. Miller RF: Nuclear medicine and AIDS. *Eur J Nucl Med* 16:103–118, 1990.

20. Moser KM, Auger WR, Fedullo PF, Jamieson SW: Chronic thromboembolic pulmonary hypertension: Clinical picture and surgical treatment. *Eur Respir J* 5:334–342, 1992.

21. Nelson PH, Moser KM, Stoner C, Moser KS: Risk of complications during intravenous heparin therapy. *West J Med* 136:189–197, 1982.

22. Nicod P, Peterson K, Levine M, et al: Pulmonary angiography in severe chronic pulmonary hypertension. *Ann Intern Med* 107:565–568, 1987.

23. Nolop KB, Rodes CG, Brudin LH, et al: Glucose utilization in vivo by human pulmonary neoplasms. *Cancer* 60:2682–2689, 1987.

24. Palevsky HI: The problems of the clinical and laboratory diagnosis of pulmonary embolism (Review). *Semin Nucl Med* 21:276–280, 1991.

25. Patz EF Jr, Lowe VJ, Hoffman JM, et al: Persistent or recurrent bronchogenic carcinoma: Detection with PET and 2-[F-18]-2-deoxy-D-glucose. *Radiology* 191:379–382, 1994.

26. PIOPED Investigators : Value of the ventilation/perfusion scan in acute pulmonary embolism: Results of the prospective investigation of pulmonary embolism diagnosis (PIOPED). *JAMA* 263:2753–2759, 1990.

27. Quinn DA, Thompson BT, Terrin ML, et al: A prospective investigation of pulmonary embolism in women and men. *JAMA* 268:1689–1696, 1992.

28. Robin ED: Overdiagnosis and overtreatment of pulmonary embolism: The emperor may have no clothes. *Ann Intern Med* 87:775–781, 1977.

29. Ryan KL, Fedullo PF, Davis GB, et al: Perfusion scan findings understate the severity of angiographic and hemodynamic compromise in chronic thromboembolic pulmonary hypertension. *Chest* 93:1180–1185, 1988.

30. Sostman HD, Coleman RE, Delong DM, Newman GE: Prospective trial of revised PIOPED criteria for lung scan interpretation in clinically selected patients (abstract). *J Nucl Med* 35:25P, 1994.

31. Sostman HD, Gottschalk A: Prospective validation of the stripe sign in ventilation-perfusion scintigraphy. *Radiology* 184:455–459, 1992.

32. Stein PD, Athanasoulis C, Alavi A, et al: Complications and validity of pulmonary angiography in acute pulmonary embolism. *Circulation* 85:462–468, 1992.

33. Stein PD, Coleman RE, Gottschalk A, et al: Diagnostic utility of ventilation/perfusion lung scans in acute pulmonart embolism is not diminished by pre-existing cardiac or pulmonary disease. *Chest* 100:604–606, 1991.

34. Stein PD, Gottschalk A, Saltzman HA, Terrin ML: Diagnosis of acute pulmonary embolism in the elderly. *J Am Coll Cardiol* 18:1452–1457, 1991.

35. Stein PD, Saltzman HA, Weg JG: Clinical characteristics of patients with acute pulmonary embolism. *Am J Cardiol* 68:1723–1724, 1991.

36. Stein PD: Clinical, laboratory, roentgenographic, and electrocardiographic findings in patients with acute pulmonary embolism and no pre-existing cardiac or pulmonary disease. *Chest* 100:598–603, 1991.

37. Stoller JK, Ahmad M, Rice TW: Solitary pulmonary nodule. *Cleve Clin J Med* 55:68–74, 1988.

38. Taplin GV, Johnson DE, Dore EK, et al: Suspensions of radioalbumin aggregates for photoscanning the liver, spleen, lung and other organs. *J Nucl Med* 5:259–275, 1964.

39. Toomes H, Delphendahl A, Manke H-G, Vogt-Moykopf I: The coin lesion of the lung: A review of 955 resected coin lesions. *Cancer* 51:534–537, 1983.

40. UPET Investigators: The urokinase pulmonary embolism trial: A national cooperative. *Circulation* 47:46–50, 1973.

41. Valk PE, Pounds TR, Hopkins DM, et al: Staging lung cancer by whole-body PET-FDG imaging (abstract). *J Nucl Med* 36:95P, 1995.

42. Wagner HN Jr, Lopez-Majano V, Langan JK, Joshi RC: Radioactive xenon in the differential diagnosis of pulmonary embolism. *Radiology* 91:1168–1174, 1968.

43. Wahl RL, Quint LE, Greenough RL, et al: Staging of mediastinal non–small cell lung cancer with FDG PET, CT, and fusion images: Preliminary prospective evaluation. *Radiology* 191:371–377, 1994.

44. Worsley DF, Alavi A, Aronchick JM, et al: Chest radiographic findings in patients with acute pulmonary embolism: Observations from the PIOPED study. *Radiology* 189:133–136, 1993.

45. Worsley DF, Alavi A, Palevsky HI: A detailed evaluation of patients with pulmonary embolism and low or very low probability lung scan interpretations (abstract). *J Nucl Med* 35:25P, 1994.

46. Worsley DF, Kim CK, Alavi A, Palevsky HI: Detailed analysis of patients with matched ventilation-perfusion defects and chest radiographic opacities. *J Nucl Med* 34:1851–1853, 1993.

47. Worsley DF, Palevsky HI, Alavi A: Clinical characteristic of patients with pulmonary embolism and low or very low probability lung scan interpretations. *Arch Intern Med* 154:2737–2741, 1994.

48. Worsley DF, Palevsky HI, Alavi A: Ventilation/perfusion lung scanning in the evaluation of pulmonary hypertension. *J Nucl Med* 35:793–796, 1994.

49. Yamashita K, Matsunobe S, Tsuda T, et al: Solitary pulmonary nodule: Preliminary study of evaluation with incremental dynamic CT. *Radiology* 194:399–405, 1995.

50. Zerhouni EA, Stitik FP, Siegelman SS, et al: CT of the pulmonary nodule: A cooperative study. *Radiology* 160:319–327, 1986.

PULMONARY FUNCTION TESTING

Michael A. Grippi / Louis F. Metzger
Ann V. Sacks / Alfred P. Fishman

The evaluation of human pulmonary function dates back to the seventeenth century. According to John Hutchinson, writing in 1846, "Borelli is the earliest physiologist [1679] who established an experimental inquiry into the quantity of air received by a single inspiration." In 1700, Humphrey Davy used his "mercurial air-holding machine" and a hydrogen dilution technique to measure his own residual volume. Subsequently, Hutchinson, in his treatise, *On the Capacity of the Lungs and on Respiratory Functions,* defined the functional subdivisions of lung volume. He reported the results of vital-capacity measurements performed in more than 1800 "healthy cases," relating these values to the height, age, and weight of his subjects and, thereby, establishing a basis for determining normal values.

For the next century, progress in developing techniques for pulmonary function testing was slow. In the 1950s, however, pulmonary physiologists took advantage of the opportunities afforded by the burgeoning fields of electronics, transducers, and computers. Currently, there are many techniques for assessing both the integrated performance of the cardiovascular and respiratory systems and their individual components.

LUNG VOLUMES AND SUBDIVISIONS

Important quantitative aspects of respiratory function are the changes in lung volume with inspiration and expiration and the absolute volume of air that the lungs hold at various times during the respiratory cycle. These volumes and changes in volume are described below.

Definitions and Assessment

For purposes of quantification and comparison, the total volume of gas in the lungs is conventionally subdivided into compartments (volumes) and combinations of two or more volumes (capacities). For many of these subdivisions, the end-expiratory volume—the volume of gas remaining in the lungs at the end of normal expiration—is the point of reference. Lung volumes and capacities are defined in Table 36-1 and are depicted schematically in the tracing shown in Fig. 36-1, which was obtained using a device called a spirometer. The relationships between the volumes recorded directly by the spirometer and the other lung volumes and capacities—including total lung capacity (TLC), functional residual capacity (FRC), residual volume (RV), and inspiratory capacity (IC)—are highlighted in the figure.

Spirometers are available in a variety of configurations. Some spirometers primarily sense volume and track time (volume type), while others primarily sense airflow at particular times (flow type). In either case, by using manual calculations or employing computers, one can define the relationships among volume, flow, and time to generate displays and numeric values to provide a measure of the respiratory system's ability to move air.

Two styles of volume-type spirometers are in common use: water-sealed and dry rolling-seal. In the water-sealed spirometer (Fig. 36-2A), a mouthpiece is attached to the tube through which air passes into a lightweight bell that is inverted over a water bath. Air movement through the mouthpiece into the bell during expiration causes the bell to rise; conversely, as air is withdrawn from the system during inspiration, the bell falls. The change in

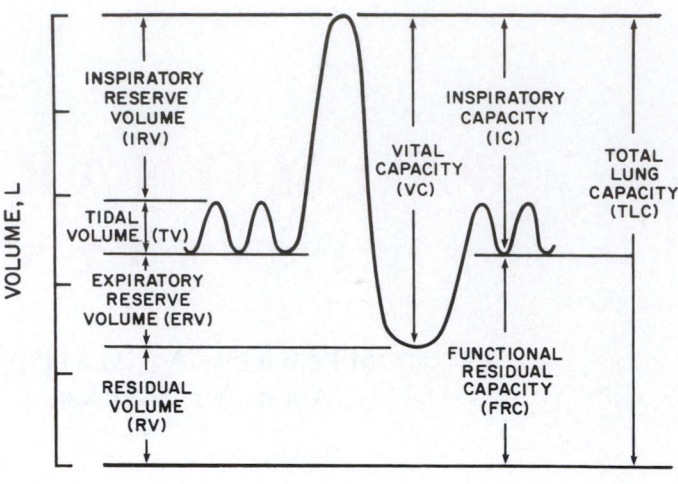

FIGURE 36-1   The subdivisions of lung volume as recorded by a spirometer. The record is generated on paper calibrated for volume in the vertical direction and time in the horizontal. The term *capacity* is applied to a subdivision composed of two or more *volumes*. The definitions of these subdivisions are found in Table 36-1.

volume with time can be recorded by an attached pen on a rotating, paper-covered drum or can be digitally noted by a computer and displayed on a screen in both graphic and numeric formats.

In dry, rolling-seal spirometers, a cylinder with a rolling plastic seal (Fig. 36-2B) is substituted for the spirometer bell and its water seal. Movement of air through the mouthpiece effects a change in the position of the piston, which is attached to a variable resistor. The resistor, in turn, generates voltage signals proportional to volume changes reflected in displacement of the pis-

---

TABLE 36-1

Glossary for Static Lung Volumes and Capacities

Term	Symbol	Definition
Volumes		
Residual volume	RV	Volume of air remaining in the lungs after maximal expiration
Expiratory reserve volume	ERV	Maximal volume of air expired from the resting end–expiratory level
Tidal volume	TV*	Volume of air inspired or expired with each breath during quiet breathing
Inspiratory reserve volume	IRV	Maximal volume of air inspired from the resting end-inspiratory level
Capacities		
Inspiratory capacity	IC	Maximal volume of air inspired from the end-expiratory level (the sum of IRV and TV)
Vital capacity	VC	Maximal volume of air expired form the maximal inspiratory level
Inspiratory vital capacity	IVC	Maximal volume of air inspired form the maximal expiratory level
Functional residual capacity	FRC	Volume of air remaining in the lungs at the end-expiratory level (the sum of RV and ERV)
Total lung capacity	TLC	Volume of air in the lungs after maximal inspiration (the sum of all volume compartments)

*The symbol TV is traditionally used for tidal volume to indicate a subdivision of static lung volumes. However, the symbol V_T is used for tidal volume in formulas for gas exchange.

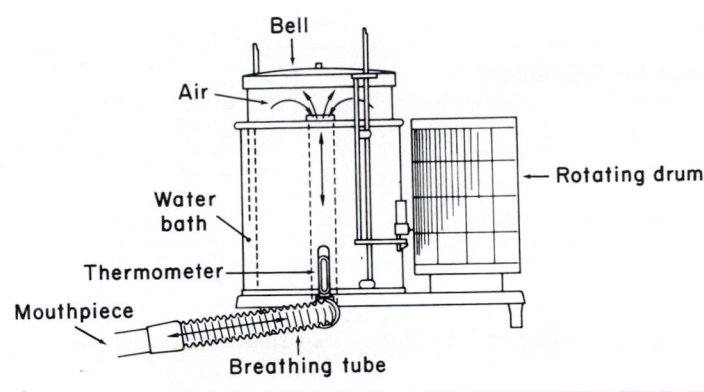

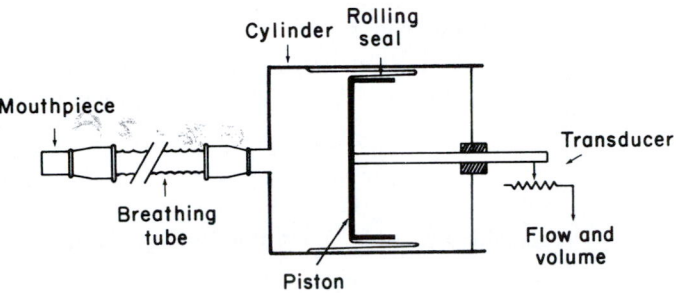

A

B

FIGURE 36-2   Two types of spirometers: water-sealed (*A*) and dry rolling-seal (*B*). Movement of air through the breathing tube results in movement of the bell (*A*) or piston (*B*). The output signal is either mechanical (pen on rotating drum) or electrical (flow and volume as voltage changes). The primary design criteria for these instruments are that inertia and resistance to airflow must be held to negligible levels, and the calibration must be accurate and stable.

ton. These signals are processed by a computer to generate graphic and numeric outputs similar to those of the water-sealed spirometer.

Flow-type spirometers use pneumotachographs or rotating turbines to determine airflow. Two types of pneumotachographs are in general use: hot-wire and flow-resistive. In the hot-wire type, air flowing past a heated wire cools the wire, thereby altering its resistance in proportion to changes in airflow. Flow-resistive pneumotachographs contain a resistive element composed of parallel tubes (Fig. 36-3), a wire mesh, or a fibrous, paperlike element. Airflow through the resistive element results in a pressure gradient across the device, which can be measured by a very sensitive differential pressure gauge. In the model depicted in Figure 36-3, the array of parallel small-bore tubes maintains a laminar gas flow pattern through the pneumotachograph. As a result, the pressure-flow characteristics of the system can be described by Poiseuille's law:

$$\Delta P = \dot{V}\frac{8\eta l}{\pi r^4}$$

where

ΔP = pressure drop across the resistive element, dyn/cm^2

$\dot{V}$ = gas flow, cm^3/s

η = viscosity of gas, dyn · s/cm^2

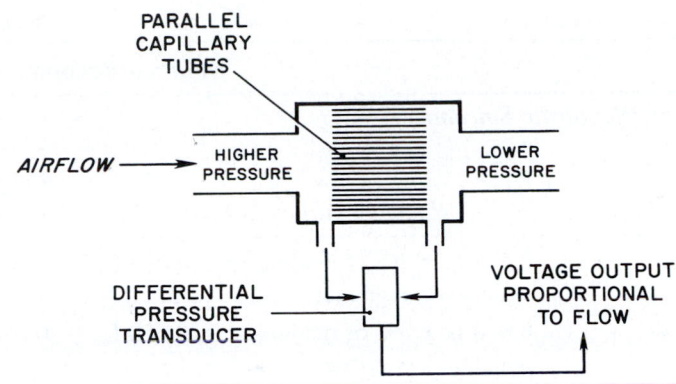

FIGURE 36-3   Principle of pneumotachography. During unidirectional airflow, a pressure drop is created across a resistive element made up of an array of parallel capillary tubes. The magnitude of the pressure drop is related to airflow, as described by Poiseuille's law for a laminar flow system. The pressure drop is transduced to a proportional voltage output, which can be recorded. A heating element (not shown) maintains the temperature of the expired gas near body temperature.

l = length of resistive element, cm

r = radius of resistive element, cm

Hence, under laminar flow conditions, the flow of gas in each tube is proportional to the pressure drop across the tube. The calculation for the overall pressure drop across the entire resistive element is based on the parallel arrangement of the array of tubes.

The pressure drop across the resistive element is sensed by a pressure transducer and converted to a voltage output that is proportional to flow. Moreover, the flow signal can be integrated electronically to yield volume. The output signals for flow and volume are displayed on a monitor and recorded.

Not all commercial spirometers are equally precise. Minimal standards have been established by the American Thoracic Society (Table 36-2) for spirometers used for diagnostic purposes and for patient monitoring.[1,2,19]

In a diagnostic setting, spirometers are used (1) to evaluate symptoms, signs, or abnormal laboratory tests; (2) to measure the effect of disease on pulmonary function; (3) to screen persons at risk of having pulmonary disease; (4) to assess preoperative risk; (5) to assess prognosis; and (6) to assess health status before enrollment in strenuous physical activity programs.

On the other hand, spirometers used for patient monitoring must meet less rigorous criteria and are used (1) to assess therapeutic interventions, including bronchodilator therapy, management of congestive heart failure, etc.; (2) to characterize the course of diseases affecting lung function (e.g., obstructive or interstitial lung diseases, congestive heart failure, or neuromuscular diseases); (3) to track pulmonary function in persons working in occupations or receiving medications known to affect the lung; (4) to evaluate large numbers of people in disability assessments; and (5) to provide data as part of epidemiologic surveys.[2]

In general, the diagnostic spirometer is used to assess a patient's lung function for purposes of comparison with values expected in a normal population. In contradistinction, the monitoring spirometer, which is less expensive and more portable, is used to study a patient's performance over time and to study large numbers of people for epidemiologic or other purposes.

TABLE 36-2

Minimal Recommendations for Spirometry

For Diagnostic Spirometry*

Test	Range/Accuracy (BTPS)	Flow Range (L/s)	Time(s)	Resistance and Back Pressure	Test Signal
VC	0.5–8 L ± 3% of reading or ± 0.050 L, whichever is greater	0–14	30		3-L cal syringe
FVC	0.5–8 L ± 3% of reading or ± 0.050 L, whichever is greater	0–14	15	<1.5 cm H_2O/L/s	24 standard waveforms 3-L cal syringe
FEV_1	0.5–8 L ± 3% of reading or ± 0.050 L, whichever is greater	0–14	1	<1.5 cm H_2O/L/s	24 standard waveforms
Time zero	The time point from which all FEV_t measurements are taken			Back extrapolation	
PEF	Accuracy: ± 10% of reading or ± 0.400 L/s, whichever is greater	0–14		Same as FEV_1	26 flow standard waveforms
	Precision: ± 5% of reading or ± 0.200 L/s, whichever is greater				
$FEF_{25-75\%}$	7.0 L/s ± 5% of reading or ± 0.200 L/s, whichever is even greater	±14	15	Same as FEV_1	24 standard waveforms
$\dot{V}$	±14 L/s ± 5% of reading or 0.200 L/s, whichever is greater	0–14	15	Same as FEV_1	Proof from manufacturer
MVV	250 L/min at TV of 2 L within ± 10% of reading or ± 15 L/min, whichever is greater	±14 ±3%	12–15	Pressure less than ±10 cm H_2O at 2 L TV at 2.0 Hz	Sine wave pump

For Monitoring Devices

Requirement	FVC & FEV_t (BTPS)	PEF (BTPS)
Range	High: 0.50–8 L Low: 0.5–6 L	High: 100 L/min to ≥700 L/min but ≤850 L/min Low: 60 L/min to ≥275 L/min but ≤400 L/min
Accuracy	±5% of reading or ±0.100 L, whichever is greater	± 10 percent of reading or ±20 L/min, whichever is greater
Precision	±3% of reading or ±0.050 L, whichever is greater	Intradevice: ≤5% of reading or ≤10 L/min, whichever is greater Interdevice: ≤10% of reading or ≤20 L/min, whichever is greater
Linearity	Within 3% over range	Within 5% over range
Graduations	Constant over entire range High: 0.100 L Low: 0.050 L	Constant over entire range High: 20 L/min Low: 10 L/min
Resolution	High: 0.050 L Low: 0.025 L	High: 10 L/min Low: 5 L/min
Resistance	Less than 2.5 cm H_2O/L/s, from 0 to 14 L/s	<2.5 cm H_2O/L/s, from 0 to 14 L/s
Minimal detectable volume	0.030 L	—
Test signal	24 standard volume-time waveforms	26 standard flow-time waveforms

*Unless specifically stated, precision requirements are the same as the accuracy requirements.
NOTE: High = high range devices; Low = low range devices.
SOURCE: Condensed from American Thoracic Society[2], with permission.

The Vital Capacity and Its Subdivisions

Two methods of performing a vital-capacity maneuver are in common use: closed-circuit and open-circuit methods. In the closed-circuit method, the seated patient, with nose clip in place, breathes quietly into the apparatus. After several breaths to establish the resting end-expiratory level, which serves as a point of reference for all subsequent measurements, the patient is urged to inspire fully and then, after reaching a plateau at maximal inspiration, to expire maximally. This expiration must be performed slowly and evenly; attempts by the patient with obstructive pulmonary disease to maximize flow often reduce expiratory volumes because of dynamic compression of the airways caused by high positive pleural pressures (see Chapter 10). Figure 36-1 illustrates schematically this slow or relaxed vital-capacity maneuver. From this record, tidal volume, inspiratory reserve volume, expiratory reserve volume, vital capacity, and inspiratory capacity are calculated. A similar maneuver in which the subject breathes out as rapidly and forcefully as possible after a maximal inspiration provides a measure of the forced vital capacity (FVC). Other timed measurements of expiratory airflow (e.g., the forced expiratory volume in one second, or FEV_1) are also determined from this type of record (see "Dynamic Mechanical Properties of the Respiratory System," below).

In the open-circuit method of determining vital capacity, the patient inspires maximally, inserts the mouthpiece, and then exhales with a slow, constant effort to the point of maximal expiration. With this technique, the resting end-expiratory position is not recorded. Thus, only the vital capacity, not its component volumes, can be measured. There are two advantages of the open-circuit technique: 1. Since the patient inspires from room air before expiring into the apparatus, concern over acquisition of infection from contaminated inspired air is minimized. 2. The open-circuit method is generally completed in a briefer time, providing a major advantage when epidemiologic studies are being performed on large numbers of subjects.

Functional Residual Capacity and Residual Volume

One compartment of the total lung capacity that cannot be measured by spirometry is residual volume (RV), the volume of air remaining in the lungs at the end of a maximal expiration. RV is determined indirectly in three steps: 1. Functional residual capacity (FRC) is typically measured using one of three techniques: closed-circuit helium, open-circuit nitrogen, or total-body plethysmograph. 2. Expiratory reserve volume (ERV) is determined spirometrically. 3. RV is calculated as the difference between FRC and ERV. In principle, it is possible to determine the RV using a dilution technique or body plethysmography after maximal expiration. In practice, however, the resting end-expiratory level is a more reproducible starting point for determining FRC than is the maximal end-expiratory level for determining RV.

CLOSED-CIRCUIT HELIUM METHOD

The closed-circuit helium dilution method for determining FRC is a variation of the hydrogen dilution method first used by Davy

in 1800. Both take advantage of the virtual insolubility of the test gas in body tissues and the law of conservation of mass. The development and simplification of this test were accomplished over a 20-year span, starting in 1941. Schematic depictions of the principle upon which the technique is based and the apparatus used are shown in Fig. 36-4.

When a fully manual device is used for measuring FRC, the system is readied by the addition of about 2 L of air and sufficient helium to achieve an initial helium concentration of approximately 10 percent in the apparatus. The patient, with nose clip in place, then breathes room air through the mouthpiece (Fig. 36-4A). After a preliminary period of quiet breathing to familiarize the patient with the mouthpiece, apparatus, and environment, and after the baseline resting end-expiratory level is established, the test begins.

At the end of a normal expiration, the valve at the mouthpiece is turned to connect the patient to the spirometer system (Fig. 36-4B). As the patient rebreathes from the closed circuit, the blower circulates the gas mixture. The CO_2 is absorbed by soda lime (CO_2 absorber), while O_2 is added through a valve and flowme-

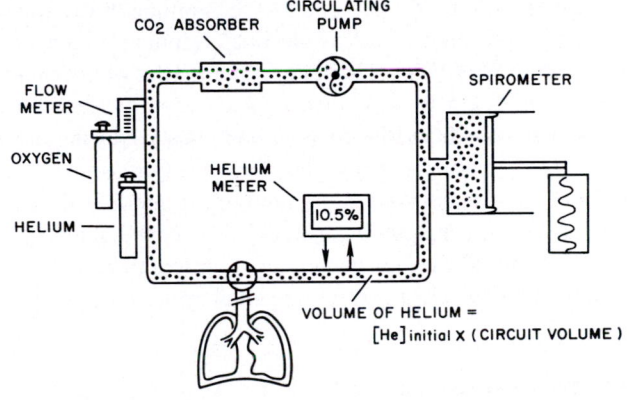

A

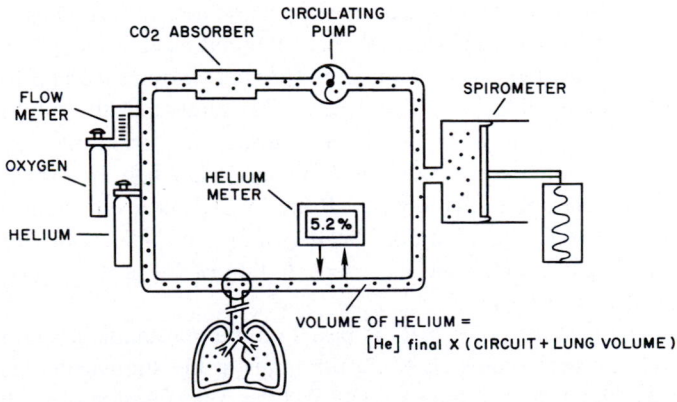

B

FIGURE 36-4 Closed-circuit helium dilution method for measurement of FRC. *A.* Spirometer and tubing system with helium before subject begins breathing through the circuit. At the end of an expiration, the mouthpiece valve is turned and the patient rebreathes through the circuit. Expired CO_2 is "scrubbed" out of the system, and O_2 is added to compensate for continued O_2 uptake in the lungs. *B.* During equilibration, the measured helium concentration falls, reflecting a dilutional effect of the additional volume (FRC) on the spirometer circuit.

ter at a rate corresponding to the subject's O_2 consumption. As the helium, which was at first contained entirely within the apparatus, mixes with air contained in the lungs, its concentration, as monitored by the helium analyzer, falls. Stabilization of the helium concentration, indicated by a rate of change in concentration of less than 0.02 percent over a 30-s interval, signals the point at which the helium concentration has equilibrated throughout the lung-breathing circuit system; equilibration, the end-point of the test, occurs within 7 min in normal persons. However, in patients in whom the distribution of ventilation is abnormal—e.g., those with chronic obstructive disease of the airways—equilibration may take much longer. Upon equilibration, the following equation, based on the law of conservation of mass, is applied:

$$F_{0He} \times V_0 = F_{FHe} \times V_F$$

where

F_{0He} = initial concentration of helium
V_0 = initial volume of system, L
F_{FHe} = final concentration of helium
V_F = final volume of system, L

The initial volume of the system is the volume of the spirometer and circuit tubing, whereas the final volume consists of the initial volume plus FRC. The latter value is the only unknown in the preceding equation. Corrections are usually made for the small amount of helium dissolved in body tissues during the test and for slight volume changes caused by a respiratory exchange ratio that is not equal to 1.0.[6] Although the method described here is based on a manually operated device, the same principles hold when all the mechanical and computational steps are accomplished with a computer-controlled system.

NITROGEN WASHOUT METHOD

Conceptually, the nitrogen washout method is similar to the helium dilution method described previously; however, it relies on an open circuit rather than the closed circuit used in the helium dilution method. The open-circuit nitrogen washout method for determining FRC, proposed in 1940,[9] requires that the subject breathe 100 percent O_2 for 7 min; during this period, the concentration of N_2 in expired gas is monitored. When the expired N_2 concentration falls to zero, all the N_2 present in the lungs at the start of O_2 breathing has been "washed out." The total volume of gas expired and the concentration of N_2 in the expired gas are measured.

The calculation of FRC is based on the reasonable assumption that the volume of N_2 in the lungs at the start of the test (i.e., the product of lung volume and the concentration of N_2 in the lungs) is the same as the total volume of N_2 expired and collected during the period of the test—i.e., the product of the total volume of gas expired and the concentration of N_2 in the expired gas:

$$F_{0N_2} \times V_0 = F_{EN_2} \times V_E$$

where

F_{0N_2} = concentration of N_2 in the lungs

V_0 = volume of gas in the lungs, L
F_{EN_2} = concentration of N_2 in the expired gas
V_E = volume of expired gas, L

Since the test is started at the end of a quiet expiration, the volume of gas in the lungs is FRC. This volume is calculated by substituting into the above equation the initial concentration of N_2 in the lungs, estimated at 0.81 in fasting and 0.79 to 0.80 in nonfasting subjects,[6] and the measured values for volume and N_2 concentration of expired gas.

BODY PLETHYSMOGRAPHY

The word *plethysmography* is derived form the Greek *plethysmos,* meaning "enlargement." Although the concept of measuring FRC by recording changes in the volume of the body during "enlargement" of the chest was described in 1882, not until 1956 did DuBois and coworkers introduce a practical plethysmographic technique, based on Boyle's law, for determining thoracic gas volume.[13]

Three types of body plethysmographs are currently used: (1) the *pressure plethysmograph,* in which pressure during breathing varies while volume remains constant; (2) the *volume plethysmograph,* in which volume varies during breathing while pressure remains constant; and (3) the *pressure-corrected flow plethysmograph,* which couples the pressure plethysmograph's fidelity of response to high-speed events with the volume plethysmograph's ability to follow large changes in volume. Since the conceptual basis for all three devices is about the same, only the most popular one—the pressure plethysmograph—will be described.

The pressure plethysmograph (Fig. 36-5) contains a pneumotachograph and transducer for measuring flow and volume and two strain-gauge transducers, one for sensing pressure at the mouth (Pm) and the other for sensing pressure in the box (Pbx). A solenoid-operated shutter mechanism is situated between the

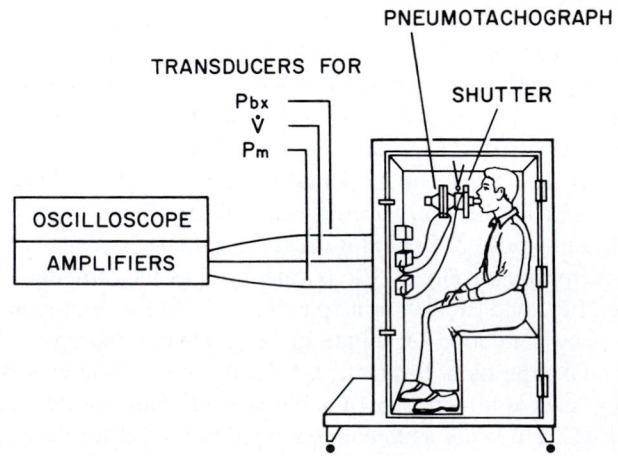

FIGURE 36-5 Constant-volume, variable-pressure plethysmograph used for measuring functional residual capacity and airway resistance. The device has a fixed volume. Thoracic gas volume changes associated with changes in alveolar pressure are reflected as changes in pressure within the plethysmograph.

mouthpiece and the pneumotachograph. The three transducers are connected to an amplifying and monitoring system so that box pressure (or lung volume) and mouth pressure are displayed simultaneously on the X and Y axes, respectively, of an oscilloscope (Fig. 36-6).

In order to determine FRC, the patient, seated comfortably within the box with nose clip in place, is asked to breathe quietly through the mouthpiece. At the end of a quiet expiration, the shutter is closed and the patient is instructed to pant gently against it. The panting movements cause both mouth pressure and box pressure to change. With each inspiratory effort, as mouth pressure falls and gas in the lungs is rarefied, lung volume increases. Because the plethysmograph is a closed box, the increase in lung volume produces a corresponding increase in box pressure. With each expiratory effort, as lung volume decreases, box pressure falls. Because the shutter is closed while the measurements are made, mouth pressure equals alveolar pressure (P_A). These oscillations in mouth pressure and box pressure or lung volume appear on the oscilloscope as a closed loop (Fig. 36-6). Measurement of the slope of this loop is used to determine the volume of gas in the lungs at the time of shutter closure (see below).

Applying Boyle's law to the plethysmographic determination of lung volume,

$$PV = (P + \Delta P)(V + \Delta V)$$

where

> P = pressure in the lungs at end-expiration (atmospheric pressure), cm H_2O
> ΔP = change in pulmonary pressure produced by respiratory efforts, cm H_2O
> V = volume of gas in the lungs at end-expiration (FRC), L
> ΔV = change in gas volume in the lungs produced by compression (during expiration) and rarefaction (during inspiration) secondary to respiratory efforts, L

In the pressure plethysmograph, ΔV is sensed as a change in pressure within the box, and ΔP is determined from the change in mouth pressure during breathing efforts against the closed shutter.

Rearranging the above equation and solving for V yield

$$V = \frac{\Delta V}{\Delta P}(P + \Delta P)$$

However, since ΔP is small compared to P (atmospheric pressure), it may be disregarded. The equation then becomes

$$V = P \times \frac{\Delta V}{\Delta P}$$

where

> V = functional residual capacity, L
> P = atmospheric pressure, cm H_2O
> $\Delta V/\Delta P$ = inverse of slope of the loop on the oscilloscope

Therefore, the only unknown in this equation is V, which can be calculated by incorporating values for barometric pressure and

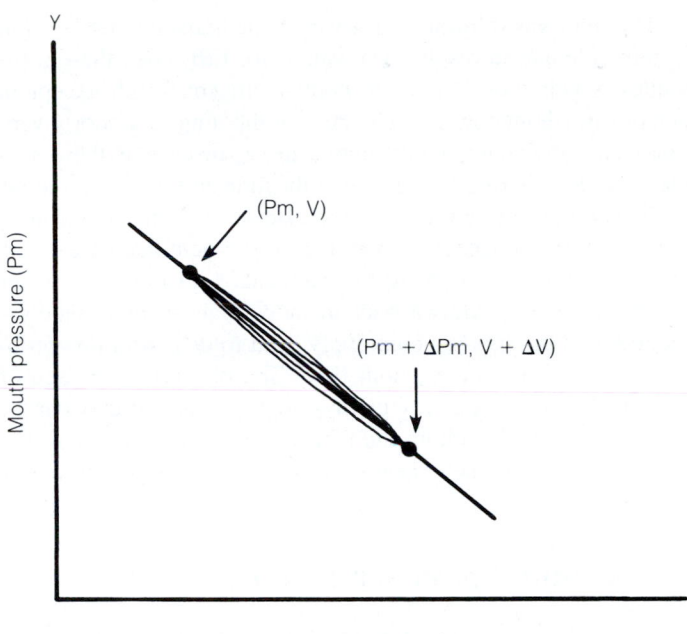

FIGURE 36-6   Pressure-volume loop obtained from a person seated in a body plethysmograph. Pressure at the mouth represents alveolar pressure; pressure in the box represents thoracic gas volume. After the shutter has closed at end-expiration (Pm, V), the subject attempts to inspire. Pm falls, and the pressure in the box increases. This increase in box pressure is calibrated in terms of an equivalent volume change. The new position of the trace at the end of the inspiratory effort is (Pm + ΔPm, V + ΔV). The slope of the loop depends on the volume of gas in the lungs when the shutter is closed (FRC).

the inverse of the slope of the plot of mouth pressure versus box pressure ($\Delta P/\Delta V$).

COMPARISON OF METHODS

Compared to the dilution and washout techniques, body plethysmography is, by far, the fastest method available for determining FRC. Indeed, it enables several determinations to be made per minute. Although the equipment required for body plethysmography is more expensive than that required for the other methods, in a busy laboratory this technique generally proves to be more economical because of the time saved and the additional uses to which the equipment can be put (e.g., measurement of airway resistance; see "Airway Resistance," below). Technically, the test is only slightly more difficult than the inert gas dilution method.

Sources of error inherent in the use of body plethysmography and discrepancies between results obtained by body plethysmography and the inert gas techniques have attracted considerable attention. For example, in patients with chronic obstructive airway disease[46] and asthma,[49] values for FRC obtained by body plethysmography may be artifactually high because of pressure differences between the mouth and alveoli generated during panting across narrowed airways. Consequently, pressures recorded at the mouth during shutter occlusion of the airway underestimate changes in alveolar pressure.

The inert gas dilution and washout methods are similar both in principle and in results. The values for FRC with these techniques match those from the body plethysmograph except in persons in whom considerable areas of the lungs are poorly ventilated, usually owing to obstructive airway disease. In these people, complete mixing or washout of the indicator gas is very slow, at times requiring 45 min or longer. Because of the slow equilibration of gas concentrations in the poorly ventilated areas, the usual time allotted for the test is inadequate, resulting in a lower value for FRC by the washout methods than by body plethysmography. One strategy commonly used to deal with this problem is to prolong the washout time. The primary advantage of these techniques over body plethysmography is that they can be used in persons for whom the plethysmograph is impractical—e.g., those with marked obesity, skeletal abnormalities, or claustrophobia.

Temperature Correction Factors

By convention, all lung volumes described above and airflows (see below) are expressed in terms of body temperature and pressure, saturated with water vapor (BTPS). This practice enables direct comparison of pulmonary function data from laboratories operating at different ambient temperatures and altitudes. To convert the volume of gas collected in a volume-type spirometer under ambient conditions (i.e., ambient temperature and pressure, saturated with water vapor, or ATPS) to BTPS, a conversion factor is applied (Table 36-3). Previously, it was presupposed that ambient air entering a spirometer was cooled *immediately* to ambient temperature and remained saturated with water vapor (ATPS). Under this assumption, only ambient temperature was considered in determining the appropriate correction factor. However, more recent studies have addressed the assumption that expired gas is immediately cooled,[20,41] as well as the practical consequences of temperature correction errors.[25] Currently, the American Thoracic Society recommends temperature correction of results from volume-type spirometers based on *measured* gas temperature at the time of testing. Similar corrections for flow-style spirometers are more problematic. They should be based

on the location of the flow sensor in the system and whether the airflow to be corrected is inspiratory or expiratory.

STATIC MECHANICAL PROPERTIES OF THE RESPIRATORY SYSTEM

Exploration of the elastic properties of the respiratory system and their effect on lung volumes and work of breathing began in earnest during the earlier part of this century. Although the groundwork had been laid long before then (by Robert Hooke's *The Theory of Springs* in 1678), between 1923 and 1956 investigators provided a wealth of information about the elastic properties of the respiratory system and its components and the work done in overcoming these elastic forces during breathing.

Static Compliance of the Lungs

The elastic properties of the lungs are determined by relating the change in the volume of air contained in the lungs to the corresponding change in the recoil force of the lungs. Change in lung volume is most easily measured by determining the volume of gas inspired or expired at the mouth. Although expedient, this approach to determining the elastic properties of the lungs can underestimate the change in lung volume when incorporated into techniques (see below) that require the subject to expire gently against a closed shutter, a maneuver that compresses thoracic gas. However, the problem can be circumvented by placing the subject in a volume plethysmograph that uses a spirometer attached to the plethysmograph to record changes in thoracic gas volume due to gas compression.

The recoil force of the lungs, measured as the transpulmonary pressure (Fig. 36-7), is the difference between the alveolar and pleural pressures (PA and Ppl, respectively). Alveolar pressure is determined as the pressure at the airway opening (Pao)—i.e., the mouth—when airflow is arrested and the glottis is open. The pleural pressure is determined indirectly by measuring the pressure in the esophagus using an esophageal balloon catheter. This technique, first introduced in 1949, has been improved over the years and provides accurate reflections of changes in pleural pressure at all lung volumes except those below FRC.[33]

The balloon, about 10 cm long and made of thin rubber, is placed over a small-diameter polyethylene catheter. Several holes

TABLE 36-3

Factors for Converting Volumes from *ATPS* to *BTPS* at Barometric Pressure of 760 mmHg*

Ambient Temperature, °C	*Multiplier to Convert Volumes to BTPS†*
20	1.101
21	1.096
22	1.091
23	1.085
24	1.080
25	1.074
26	1.069
27	1.062

*Based on Boyle's, Charles's, and Dalton's laws.
†Volume at ATPS × multiplier = volume at BTPS.

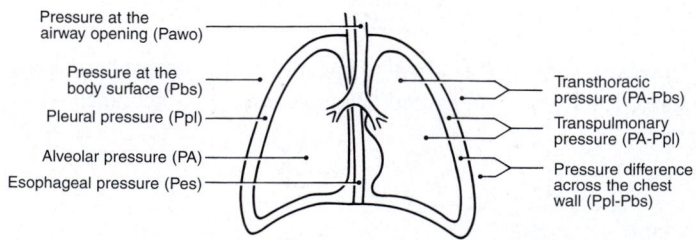

FIGURE 36-7   Schematic representation of the chest depicting pressure terms and gradients used in analysis of the mechanics of breathing. The expressions for individual pressure measurements on the left are relative to atmospheric pressure. Pleural pressure (Ppl) is not routinely measured directly but is approximated by esophageal pressure (Pes) measured with a balloon catheter.

in the terminal portion of the catheter allow pressure to be transmitted from the balloon, through the catheter, to a transducer. The balloon is positioned in the lower third of the esophagus, where esophageal pressure and, therefore, balloon pressure accurately reflect the pressure acting on the lung surface (pleural pressure). Use of an elongated balloon of low volume helps to minimize changes in pressure due to esophageal contractions. By conveying mouth pressure and esophageal pressure to opposite sides of a differential pressure transducer, an output signal is generated that is proportional to the difference between these two pressures—i.e., the transpulmonary pressure (PA–Ppl).

To determine the elastic properties of the lungs, the patient with esophageal balloon in place is seated in a closed body plethysmograph. The patient then breathes ambient air through a tube to the outside until the volume trace, inscribed by the plethysmograph spirometer, indicates that the end-expiratory level is stable. At this juncture, the patient is instructed to first inspire slowly to TLC and then to expire slowly to the resting end-expiratory level (FRC). This maneuver is then repeated; during the second expiration, the shutter is activated to occlude the airway intermittently. Since each closure of the shutter interrupts the expiration briefly, the recorded trace of expiratory volume versus time displays a staircase pattern (Fig. 36-8A). The plateau resulting from each closure of the shutter marks a finite period of zero change in lung volume as the lungs empty during expiration. Associated with each plateau is a corresponding plateau in transpulmonary pressure.

The relationship between the change in volume and the change in pressure is a measure of the *recoil force* of the lungs at each of the lung volumes that are registered (Fig. 36-8B). The resulting curve provides several useful indices of the elastic behavior of the lungs. The slope of the curve over the range corresponding to the tidal volume is the *static lung compliance*. The transpulmonary pressure attained at TLC is the *maximal static recoil pressure*. The ratio of the maximal static recoil pressure to the corresponding maximal lung volume is the *coefficient of retraction*. However, since these values are derived from only small segments of the curve, inspection of the total static pressure-volume curve remains the most comprehensive means of assessing the elastic properties of the lungs.

Static Compliance of the Chest Wall

Functionally, the chest wall includes the bony thorax, intercostal muscles, overlying soft tissue, pleura, and diaphragm. The chest wall is distensible and has its own distinctive elastic properties. In the normal, end-expiratory, resting position of the respiratory system (FRC), the inward recoil of the lung is balanced by the outward recoil of the chest wall (Fig. 36-9B). As the volume of the thoracic cavity enlarges progressively during inspiration from FRC to TLC, the outward recoil pressure of the chest wall lessens, becoming zero at approximately 70 percent of TLC; beyond this point, the chest wall begins to recoil inwardly (Fig. 36-9C). Conversely, as the chest wall is compressed below FRC by the action of the expiratory muscles, the natural outward recoil tendency is increased (Fig. 36-9A).

In practice, assessment of the elastic properties of the chest wall is accomplished by first determining the compliance curve

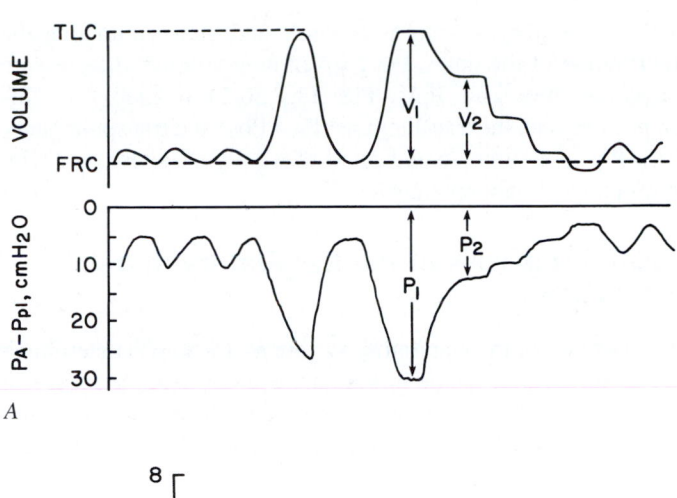

A

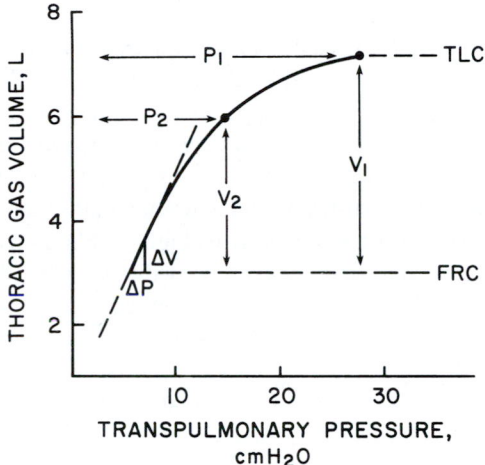

B

FIGURE 36-8 Measurement of the elastic properties of the lungs. *A.* Recordings of changes in lung volume and transpulmonary pressure (PA-Ppl) using the esophageal balloon technique described in the text. Simultaneous measurements of volume and pressure are obtained during periods of arrested airflow at lung volumes ranging from TLC to just below FRC. *B.* Thoracic gas volume is plotted on the ordinate and transpulmonary pressure on the abscissa. The curve formed by the plot using values from *A* describes the elastic properties of the lungs. The slope of the line, $\Delta V/\Delta P$, over the range of the tidal volume is the static compliance of the lungs.

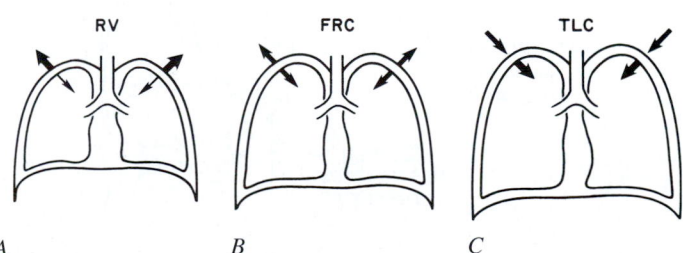

A   *B*   *C*

FIGURE 36-9 Schematic depiction of elastic recoil vectors across the lung and chest wall as determined by the level of inflation. *A.* At RV, the outwardly directed recoil pressure of the chest wall is large and the inwardly directed recoil pressure of the lung is small. *B.* At FRC, the recoil pressures of the lung and chest wall are equal and in opposite directions. *C.* At TLC, both recoil pressures are directed inward, and each contributes substantially to the overall recoil pressure of the respiratory system.

of the respiratory system as a whole and then subtracting the contribution of the lungs. For a given lung volume, the pressure across the chest wall, Ppl – Pbs (Fig. 36-7), is simply the difference between the transthoracic (PA – Pbs) and transpulmonary (PA – Ppl) pressures. As indicated above, Ppl is determined with an esophageal balloon catheter.

Elastic Properties of the Respiratory System as a Whole

The elasticity of the respiratory system as a whole is determined by measuring the change in volume resulting from a change in pressure applied to the system—i.e., the transthoracic pressure (PA – Pbs)—*while the respiratory muscles are completely relaxed.*

The first method used for this evaluation employed the relaxation technique described by Rahn and associates.[42] The subject breathes quietly into an apparatus consisting of a spirometer, a shutter, and a pressure transducer connected to the subject's side of the shutter (Fig. 36-10). After a period of quiet breathing, the subject is instructed to inspire maximally; the shutter is closed at peak inspiration, and the subject is then asked to relax the respiratory muscles completely while keeping the glottis open. Periodically, the shutter is opened, allowing a small volume of air to move from the subject into the spirometer; the shutter is then closed again. This maneuver is repeated until FRC is reached. During the periods of arrested airflow, pressure at the mouth (Pao) is equal to the pressure in the alveoli (PA). Provided the pressure at the body surface is atmospheric and the respiratory muscles are completely at rest, this value represents transthoracic pressure. In practice, however, full relaxation of the respiratory muscles is difficult, and a contribution by them to the pressure at the airway opening is frequently unavoidable.

A more practical technique entails the application of continuous positive pressure to the airways during spontaneous breathing. The subject breathes quietly into a water-sealed spirometer until a constant end-tidal level is achieved. A weight is then placed on the spirometer bell to increase the pressure in the respiratory system and, thereby, to raise the resting end-expiratory lung volume. This procedure is repeated using several different weights so that a pressure-volume curve of the total respiratory system can be constructed.

The individual pressure-volume curves for the lungs and chest wall and the composite curve for the intact respiratory system are shown in Fig. 36-11. As illustrated, the elastic recoil of the chest wall alone is determined by subtracting the recoil pressure of the lung from that of the total respiratory system. Chest wall elasticity is an important determinant of the subdivisions of lung volume and the overall compliance of the respiratory system; the latter is, in turn, an important determinant of the work of breathing.

Several features of the pressure-volume relationships shown in Fig. 36-11 are worth emphasizing. As lung volume approaches RV, the elastic recoil pressure of the respiratory system is largely due to the outwardly directed recoil pressure of the chest wall. At RV, the contribution of the lung to the recoil pressure of the respiratory system is minimal. At the other extreme of lung volume, TLC, elastic recoil pressure is high and directed inwardly, owing to the combined elastic recoils of the lung and chest wall. At FRC, the outwardly directed recoil of the chest wall balances the inwardly directed recoil of the lung, and the transthoracic pressure is zero (i.e., PA – Pbs = 0). Indeed, the system "comes to rest" at FRC because of the counterbalancing of these forces at that volume. Since alveolar pressure at FRC is zero, no pressure gradient exists for airflow. Therefore, the system remains stationary until acted upon by the muscles of inspiration or expiration.

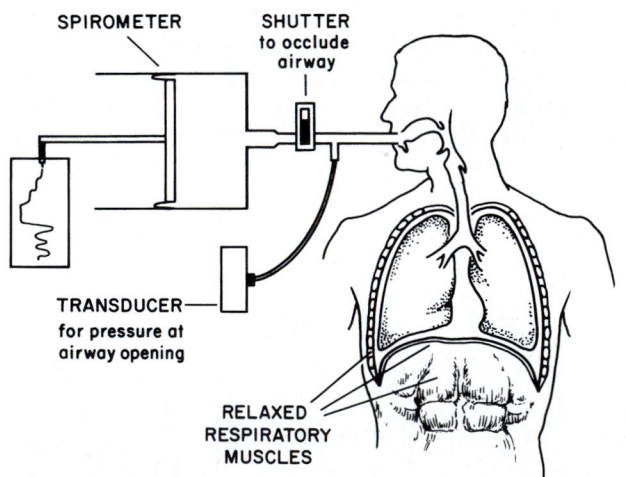

FIGURE 36-10 Relaxation technique for measurement of elastic recoil pressure of the respiratory system. After a period of normal tidal volume breathing, the subject inspires to TLC. A shutter in the airway is closed, and the subject relaxes his or her respiratory muscles. The shutter is periodically opened, permitting exhalation of a small volume of air measured by the spirometer. Airway pressures are recorded at times of shutter closure (i.e., during no airflow, when mouth pressure equals alveolar pressure). A pressure-volume curve is then constructed from the simultaneously recorded values for pressure and volume.

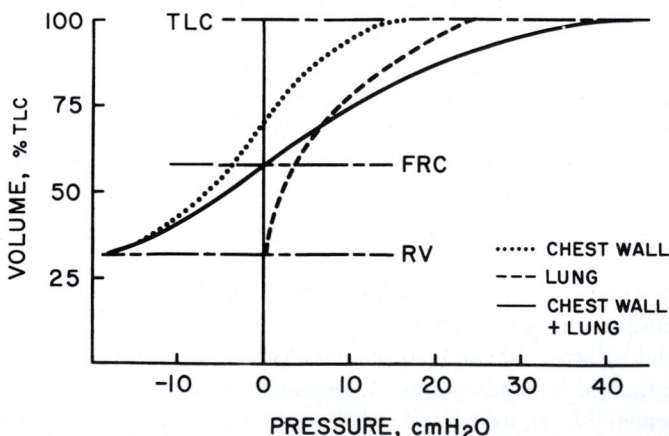

FIGURE 36-11 The pressure-volume curves of the respiratory system and its components. The elastic recoil pressures of the total respiratory system (solid line) over the vital capacity range are the sum of the recoil pressures of the lung (dashed line) and chest wall (dotted line). At FRC, the chest wall recoil pressure is counterbalanced by the lung recoil pressure. The net result is a total system recoil pressure of 0. The total system recoil pressure is obtained by relaxation pressure or continuous positive-pressure breathing techniques. The chest wall recoil pressure is calculated as the difference between the recoil pressure of the entire respiratory system and the recoil pressure of the lungs.

TABLE 36-4

Normal Maximal Static Recoil Pressures for Adults (cm H₂O)

	Male Age (Years)			Female Age (Years)		
	25–35	36–64	65–75	25–35	36–64	65–75
Mean ± SD	35.9 ± 8.5	33.0 ± 8.7	33.0 ± 2.9	36.4 ± 5.8	25.7 ± 4.0	23.7 ± 3.9
Range	24.0 − 48.0	21.5 − 48.0	17.0 − 42.2	21.0 − 48.0	20.0 − 30.0	18.0 − 31.6

SOURCE: Data from Knudson et al.[27]

Elastic Properties of the Respiratory System in Health and Disease

The elastic properties of the respiratory system are altered by a wide variety of diseases that can affect the lung parenchyma or chest wall, either selectively or in concert. Most instances of clinically significant reductions in static compliance are due to abnormalities in the lung. The two standard clinical measures of the elastic properties of the lung are static lung compliance and maximal static recoil pressure.

Static lung compliance, Cst,L, is determined over the linear portion of the pressure-volume curve, between FRC and a lung volume corresponding to FRC plus 0.5 L. Normal values vary from laboratory to laboratory, ranging from 0.147 to 0.375 L/cm H₂O, with a mean of 0.262 L/cm H₂O. Some variability is related to age and sex; Cst,L decreases with age and is higher in males than in females.

Maximal static recoil pressure is the recoil pressure at TLC. Once again, normal values vary. Data from one series of 51 normal subjects[27] are shown in Table 36-4.

In disease states characterized by an increased elastic recoil pressure, such as diffuse interstitial fibrosis, the pressure-volume curve is shifted to the right and the static lung compliance decreases (Fig. 36-12A and B). The increased elastic recoil pressure contributes to a decrease in FRC and TLC. By expressing the volume axis of the pressure-volume curve in terms of *percent predicted TLC* (Fig. 36-12B), instead of *absolute TLC* (Fig. 36-12A), the reduction in maximal lung volume is clearly evident; i.e., maximal recoil pressure is increased, despite the reduced TLC.

In contrast to the effects of fibrosis, emphysema, which destroys alveolar walls and enlarges alveolar spaces, reduces lung elastic recoil pressure (Pel). This change increases both TLC and FRC. The shift of the pressure-volume curve upward and to the left (Fig. 36-12A and B) indicates that lung compliance increases and that the maximal recoil pressure decreases. If the volume axis is expressed as percent predicted TLC (Fig. 36-12B), the increase in lung volume is more clearly demonstrated.

As noted previously, disorders affecting primarily the chest wall can also significantly alter the elastic properties of the respiratory system. Among these are obesity, kyphoscoliosis, and fibrothorax. These disorders limit chest wall excursion and lung expansion and reduce FRC. In addition, they produce decreases in static compliance of the lung and chest wall and maximal recoil pressure.

Respiratory Muscle Strength

Ventilatory performance depends not only on the mechanical properties of the lungs and chest wall but also on the strength of the respiratory muscles. Evaluation of respiratory muscle

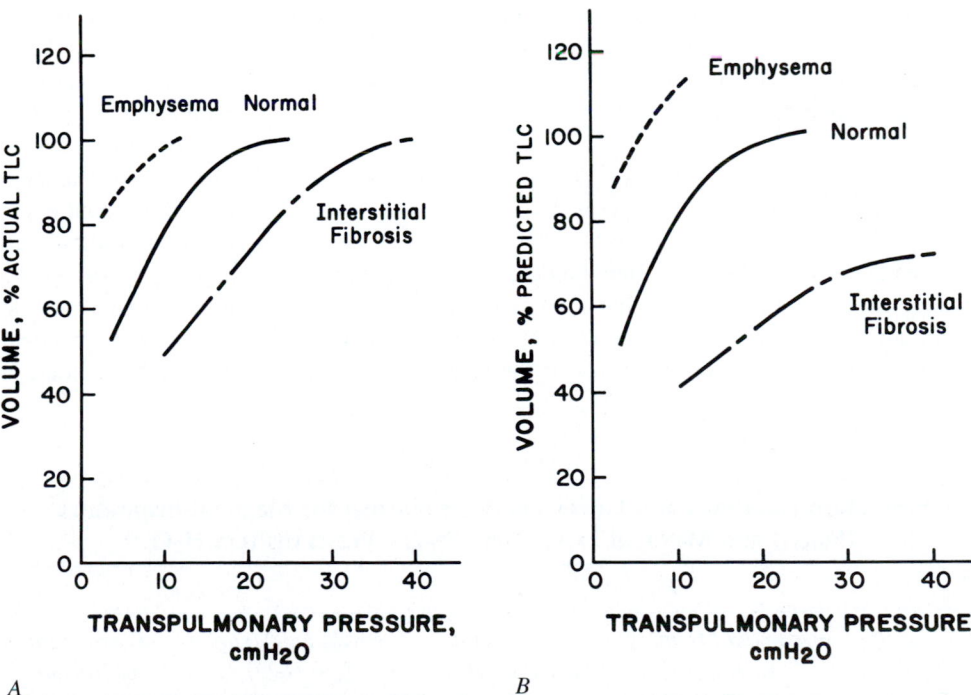

A   *B*

FIGURE 36-12 Pressure-volume curves of the lungs in health and disease. *A.* Volume expressed as percent of actual TLC. Differences in transpulmonary pressures in normal and diseases states are evident. Changes in lung volume that occur with disease are demonstrated on the plots. *B.* Volume expressed as percent of predicted TLC. In addition to the differences in transpulmonary pressures, alterations in lung volumes in the disease states are evident.

strength was made as early as 1846 by Hutchinson. Subsequently, using simplified methods of measurement, Black and Hyatt[3] established normal values (Table 36-5).

The maximal pressure generated by an isometric contraction varies directly with the resting length of the muscle. Consequently, values for maximal inspiratory and expiratory pressures depend on the lung volume at which the tests are performed (Fig. 36-13).[45] When TLC is less than 70 percent of the predicted value, the maximal expiratory pressure will be low. Similarly, when RV exceeds 40 percent of the predicted TLC, the maximal inspiratory pressure will be low.

The only equipment required for measurement of maximal inspiratory or expiratory pressure is an aneroid vacuum and pressure gauge. To determine maximal expiratory pressure, the patient is urged to inspire fully to TLC and then to expire as forcefully as possible into the gauge. The highest pressure attained and held for at least 1 s is the *maximal expiratory pressure* (PE_{max}). The *maximal inspiratory pressure* (PI_{max}) is determined by having the patient inspire maximally from the gauge after having expired completely to RV. The value recorded is the lowest pressure attained and held for at least one second.

Measurement of maximal static respiratory pressures is particularly important in evaluating respiratory muscle weakness in patients with neuromuscular disease, as described in Chapter 98. In these patients, spirometric tests are often normal, despite respiratory muscle weakness, because maximal pressures are not required to achieve maximal expiratory flow rates (see "Flow-Volume Curves," below).

Another useful function of these measurements is in examining patients whose coordination in performing spirometry or whose degree of motivation is suspect. In such patients, determination of maximal pressures is often helpful in determining whether optimal efforts are being expended during pulmonary function testing (see "Approach to Interpreting Commonly Performed Pulmonary Function Tests," below).

DYNAMIC MECHANICAL PROPERTIES OF THE RESPIRATORY SYSTEM

The static tests of pulmonary function described in the previous section are based on measurements of volume and pressure made while airflow is arrested. These static tests are particularly useful in defining the elastic properties of the respiratory system.

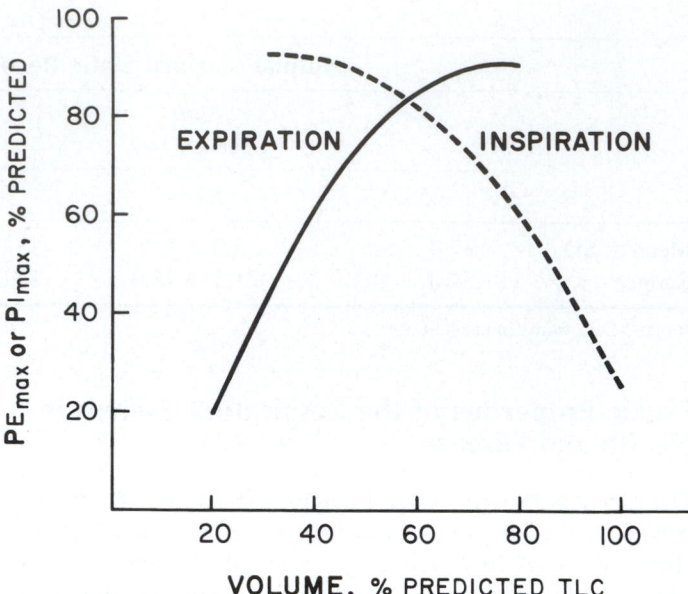

FIGURE 36-13 Effect of lung volume on maximal inspiratory (dashed line) and maximal expiratory (solid line) pressures. See text for discussion.

Considerable additional information can be gained from tests done during airflow—i.e., under "dynamic" conditions.

Although measurements of static lung volumes began about 300 years ago, the assessment of pulmonary function while air is flowing into or out of the lungs began in 1933, when the test now known as the *maximal voluntary ventilation* was first proposed. This test did not become popular until 1941, when Cournand and Richards developed regression equations to determine normal values. Subsequently, investigators proposed that the volume of air expired during specific time intervals be determined. In 1955, determination of the average airflow during the middle half of a forced expiratory vital capacity was described. Determination of these indices of dynamic lung function is now generally part of the battery of tests, both static and dynamic, included under the designation *spirometry*.

The more practical tests of dynamic function can, for convenience, be divided into four categories: forced vital capacity, flow-volume curves, maximal voluntary ventilation, and airway resistance. Other dynamic tests, including assessment of airway reactivity and the function of small airways, will be considered separately.

Forced Vital Capacity

Both expiratory and inspiratory measurements of the forced vital capacity are routinely made in pulmonary function laboratories. Unless otherwise specified, FVC refers to the forced *expiratory* maneuver.

TABLE 36-5

Prediction Equations and Lower Limits of Normal for Maximal Inspiratory (PI_{max}) and Maximal Expiratory (PE_{max}) Pressures (cm H_2O)*

	PI_{max}		PE_{max}	
	Predicted Mean, (cm H_2O)	Lower Limit of Normal[†]	Predicted Mean (cm H_2O)	Lower Limit of Normal[†]
Male	$143 - (0.55 \times age)$	71	$268 - (1.03 \times age)$	111
Female	$104 - (0.51 \times age)$	39	$170 - (0.53 \times age)$	88

*Age range = 20 to 86 years.
[†]Independent of age.
SOURCE: Equations and lower limits of normal from Black and Hyatt.[3]

FORCED EXPIRATORY VITAL CAPACITY

The forced expiratory vital capacity is measured during expiration. The maneuver entails two steps: a full inspiration to total lung capacity, followed by a rapid, forceful, maximal expiration (to RV) into a spirometer. The forced expiratory vital capacity (FVC) is normally equal to the slow vital capacity (VC), which requires a more relaxed expiration to RV. However, a discrepancy between FVC and VC appears in obstructive disease of the airways: the FVC is less than the VC. The relationship between expired volume and time during an FVC maneuver is used to determine airflow during expiration and the volume of air expired within designated intervals; these values provide an indirect measure of the flow-resistive properties of the lung. The FVC is displayed in one of two ways: expired volume plotted against time (Fig. 36-14) and airflow plotted against lung volume—i.e., an expiratory "flow-volume curve" (see below).

The normal volume-time display of the FVC consists of a smooth curve with a gradually and progressively decreasing slope. Irregularities in the curve suggest either a failure of coordination or a suboptimal effort. At times, the onset of the forced expiration is unclear (Fig. 36-15) because of hesitation on the part of the patient. When this occurs, the start of expiration ("zero time") is determined with the "back extrapolation" method (Fig. 36-15)[2]: a tangent taken through the part of the curve with the steepest slope is extrapolated back to the maximal inspiratory volume; the point of intersection is considered to be the time of onset of expiration. Several values are commonly determined from the volume-time plot of the forced vital capacity (Table 36-6, Fig. 36-14): (1) the *volume expired in the first second,* expressed either as an absolute volume (FEV_1) or as a percentage of the forced vital capacity ($FEV_1/FVC\%$); (2) *the volume expired in the first 3 s,* expressed either as an absolute volume (FEV_3) or as a percentage of the forced vital capacity ($FEV_3/FVC\%$); and (3) *the forced midexpiratory flow rate* ($FEF_{25-75\%}$). The $FEF_{25-75\%}$ is determined by locating the points on the volume-time curve corresponding to 25 and 75 percent of the FVC and then calculating the slope of a straight line passing through those two points. The slope of this line represents the average airflow over the midportion of the FVC.

Although the *slow* vital capacity (VC) may be normal or only modestly reduced in patients with obstructive disease of the airways, the volume-time relationship of the FVC maneuver is usually distinctly abnormal in such patients (Fig. 36-16A and B). Most obvious is a flattening of the slope of the curve at any given lung volume, reflecting the reduced airflow. In addition, the duration of the forced expiratory maneuver is prolonged. Normally, expiration is complete within 5 s; in obstructive airway disease, expiratory airflow may continue for 10 to 12 s. These changes in the expiratory airflow reduce the FEV_1 and FEV_3, the $FEV_1/FVC\%$, the $FEV_3/FVC\%$, and the $FEF_{25-75\%}$.

Restrictive lung disorders reduce the slow vital capacity. However, the *configuration* of the volume-time relation-

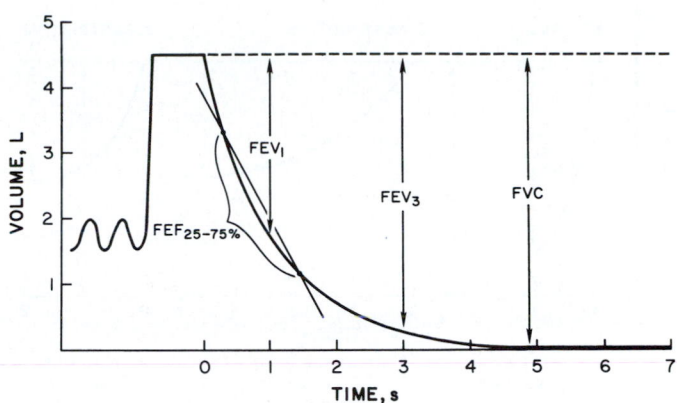

FIGURE 36-14 Forced expiratory vital capacity maneuver. After an initial period of tidal volume breathing, the patient inspires maximally to TLC and then exhales as rapidly and as forcefully as possible into a spirometer. Shown on the left of the tracing are a series of tidal volume breaths and the maximal inspiration to TLC. The forced expiration begins at time 0. Nearly all the volume is exhaled in the first 3 s of the maneuver. The values for FVC, FEV_1, and FEV_3 are measured from the maximal inspiratory level. The $FEF_{25-75\%}$ is the slope of the line connecting the points on the volume-time trace that correspond to 25% and 75% of the FVC.

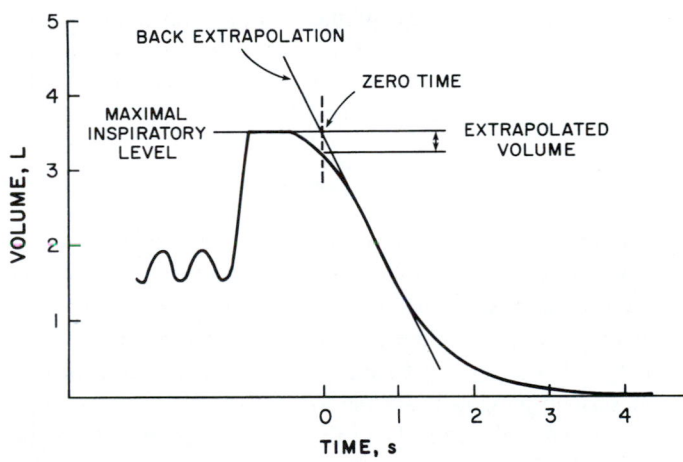

FIGURE 36-15 Technique of back extrapolation for determining the zero time in calculation of FEV_1. Zero time is determined as the point of intersection of a tangent drawn through the steepest portion of the spirogram and a line drawn horizontally through the maximal inspiratory level.

TABLE 36-6

Values Obtained from Forced Expiratory Volume-Time Curves

FVC (BTPS), L	Forced vital capacity; the total volume expired
FEV_1 (BTPS), L	Volume of air expired in the first second
$FEV_1/FVC\%$	Volume of air expired in the first second, expressed as percent of the FVC
$FEV_3/FVC\%$	Volume of air expired in the first 3 s, expressed as percent of the FVC
$FEF_{25-75\%}$ (BTPS), L/s	Forced midexpiratory airflow

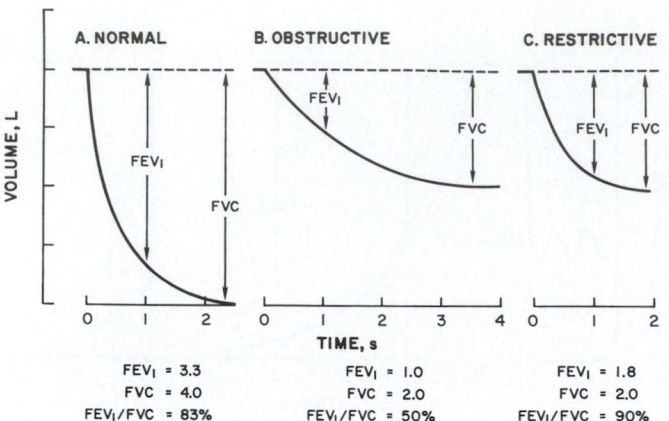

FIGURE 36-16 Representative spirograms from a normal subject (*A*), a patient with obstructive lung disease (*B*), and a patient with restrictive lung disease (*C*), obtained during a forced expiratory vital capacity maneuver. In the normal subject, expiration is completed within 3 s, and 83% of the volume is expired in the first second ($FEV_1/FVC\% = 83$). In the patient with obstructive disease, expiration is prolonged, and only half the volume is expired in the first second ($FEV_1/FVC\% = 50$). In the patient with restrictive disease, although the magnitude of the reduction in exhaled volume is the same as in the obstructed patient, most of the volume is exhaled within the first second ($FEV_1/FVC\% = 90$).

ship may not be abnormal (Fig. 36-16*C*). Although the FEV_1 and FEV_3 are reduced because of the reduced vital capacity, the $FEV_1/FVC\%$ and $FEV_3/FVC\%$ remain normal or even exceed normal values. Often, because of the reduced vital capacity, the $FEF_{25-75\%}$ is also less than predicted.

FORCED INSPIRATORY VITAL CAPACITY

Measurement of the forced inspiratory vital capacity (FIVC) consists of two steps: (1) full expiration to residual volume, followed by (2) a rapid maximal inspiratory effort (Fig. 36-17). The rate of airflow over the middle half of the forced inspiratory vital capacity ($FIF_{25-75\%}$) is determined using a procedure similar to that described previously for the $FEF_{25-75\%}$.

In normal subjects, the $FIF_{25-75\%}$ is greater than the $FEF_{25-75\%}$. Since inspiratory flow is more dependent on effort

than is expiratory flow, a fall in the $FIF_{25-75\%}$ is usually a more sensitive indicator of respiratory muscle dysfunction or a suboptimal effort than is the $FEF_{25-75\%}$. When airway resistance is high, a disproportionate fall in $FIF_{25-75\%}$ relative to $FEF_{25-75\%}$ suggests an extrathoracic site of airway obstruction (see "Approach to Interpreting Commonly Performed Pulmonary Function Tests," below).

Flow-Volume Relationships

In addition to analysis of the relationship between volume and time depicted on a spirogram, examination of the relationship between flow and volume provides useful information about lung function. A flow-volume curve, which shows the relationship between lung volume and maximal airflow as lung volume changes during a forced expiration, is shown in Fig. 36-18. The test comprises four phases of breathing into a spirometer: (1) tidal breathing for several breaths, (2) a maximal inspiratory effort to TLC, followed by (3) a maximal expiration to RV done as forcefully and quickly as possible, and (4) another maximal inspiratory effort to TLC. Volume is displayed on the horizontal axis and airflow on the vertical axis. Airflow is measured at the mouth with a pneumotachograph; volume is measured either by integrating the pneumotachographic record during expiration or as a change in thoracic gas volume, determined by a pressure-corrected flow plethysmograph. The records obtained by the two techniques for determining volume differ because the body plethysmograph senses compression of intrathoracic gas during

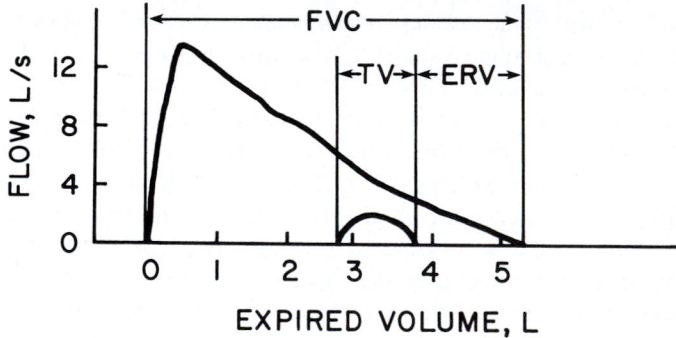

A

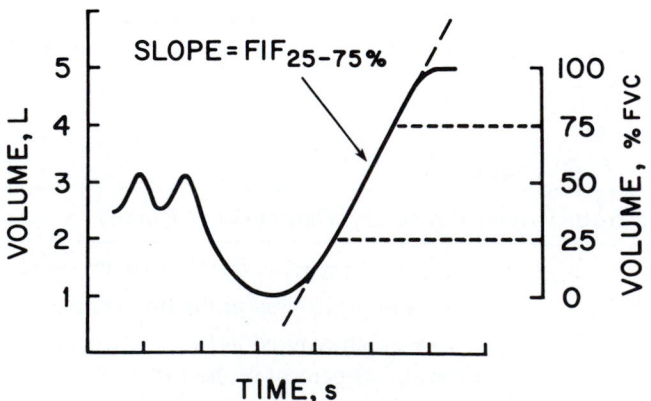

FIGURE 36-17 Forced inspiratory volume-time curve. The $FIF_{25-75\%}$ is the slope of a line between the points on the trace corresponding to 25% and 75% of the inspired volume.

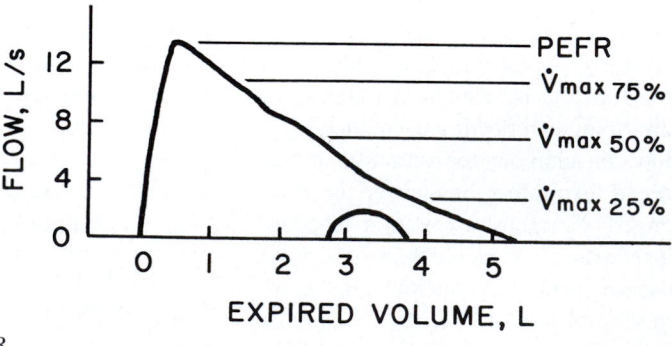

B

FIGURE 36-18 Flow-volume plots during forced expiration (outer trace) and quiet expiration (inner trace). *A.* The subdivisions of lung volume. *B.* The common flow measurements. PEFR = peak expiratory flow rate; $\dot{V}_{max75\%}$, $\dot{V}_{max50\%}$, and $\dot{V}_{max25\%}$ = flows at 75, 50, and 25 percent of the vital capacity, respectively.

a forced expiration, whereas measurements of volume made at the mouth do not (Fig. 36-19). Differences between curves obtained with the two techniques for measuring volume are most marked in patients with airway obstruction in whom considerable gas compression occurs during a forced expiration.

For the sake of comparison, tracings of flow vs. volume and volume vs. time, recorded during the same forced vital capacity maneuver and aligned by using a common volume axis as the abscissa, are shown in Fig. 36-20. Selected measurements are more evident in one tracing or the other—e.g., maximal expiratory flow in the flow-volume curve and volume expired in 1 s (FEV_1) in the volume-time curve.

Comparison of serial curves from a single person or curves from different subjects requires that the curves be aligned on the volume (horizontal) axis so that points of maximal inspiration or maximal expiration coincide. As may be seen in Fig. 36-21A, which illustrates typical curves from a normal subject and two patients, one with pulmonary fibrosis and the other with obstructive airway disease, the information provided by this form of representation is limited; i.e., the vital capacities and airflows from the patients are abnormally low. The limitation stems from the fact that the change in volume during expiration is shown relative to the *maximal inspiratory level* rather than to an *absolute volume* of gas in the lungs—i.e., RV or TLC. When RV or TLC is known so that absolute volumes can be plotted on the horizontal axis (Fig. 36-21B), additional insight is gained into the flow-volume relationship depicted in Figure 36-21A. The patient with obstructive disease of the airways manifests a reduction in expiratory airflow at elevated lung volumes, which should enhance airflow. In contrast, the reduced rate of airflow in the patient with pulmonary fibrosis is normal, or even supranormal, when the lung volume at which the airflow occurs is taken into account; i.e., the reduced airflow is primarily a function of the reduced lung volume, rather than of airway obstruction.

Maximal Voluntary Ventilation

The previous considerations of dynamic lung function focus on a single timed maximal expiratory or inspiratory maneuver. In contrast, the maximal voluntary ventilation (MVV) depends on the movement of air into and out of the lungs during continued

maximal effort throughout a preset interval (Fig. 36-22). The MVV is a simple, informative test that provides an overall assessment of effort, coordination, and the elastic and flow-resistive properties of the respiratory system.

In performing the test, the patient is urged to breathe as hard and as fast as possible. As a rule, the patient automatically adjusts frequency and tidal volume for optimal performance. However, extremes of frequency or tidal volume are to be avoided, since neither panting nor slow deep breathing leads to the highest possible values. The total volume that is expired during a 12-s interval, expressed in liters per minute (BTPS), is the maximal voluntary ventilation. In some patients the test cannot be done because of an inability to continue the necessary effort for 12 s.

A normal value for MVV indicates that the overall integrated performance of the respiratory system is intact, thereby excluding moderate to severe restrictive or obstructive disease. In addition, a normal value suggests that the elastic and flow-resistive properties of the respiratory system, respiratory muscle

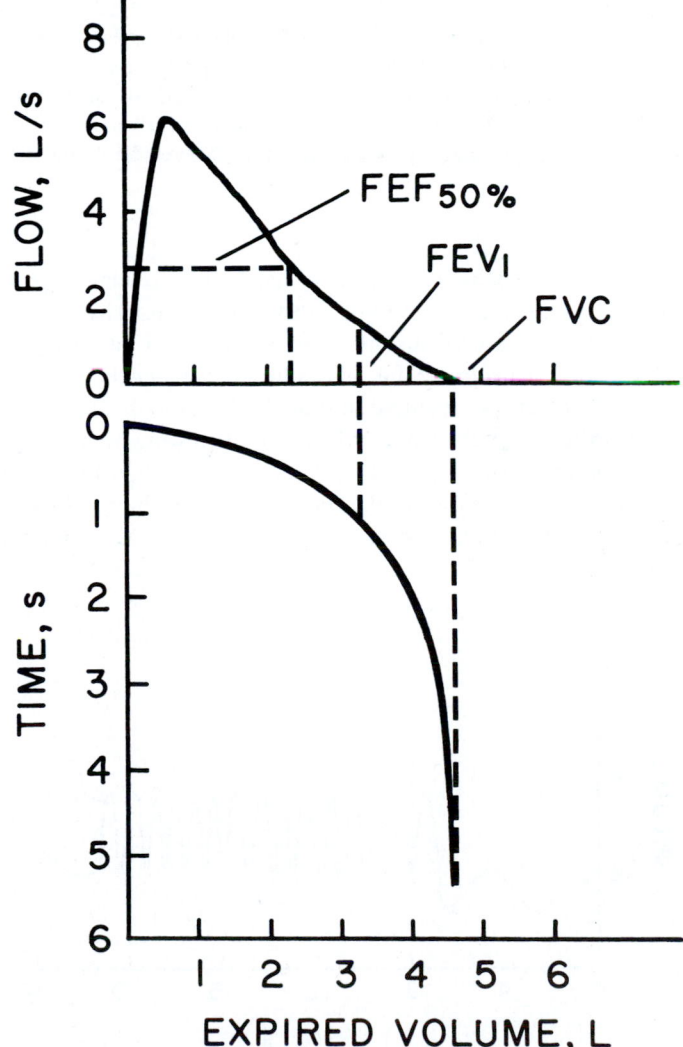

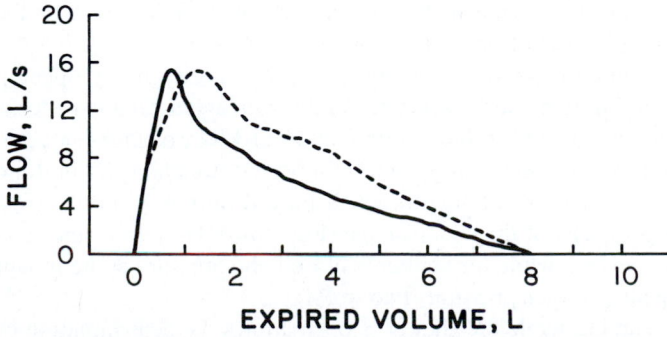

FIGURE 36-19 Comparison of the flow-expired volume curve (solid line) with a simultaneously recorded flow-thoracic gas volume curve (dashed line). The difference between the two curves results from the compression of gas in the lungs during a forced expiration.

FIGURE 36-20 Flow-volume and volume-time curves depicting the same forced expiration aligned along a common volume axis (abscissa). Points corresponding to the FEV_1, FVC, and $FEF_{50\%}$ obtained from the volume-time plot are shown on the flow-volume curve.

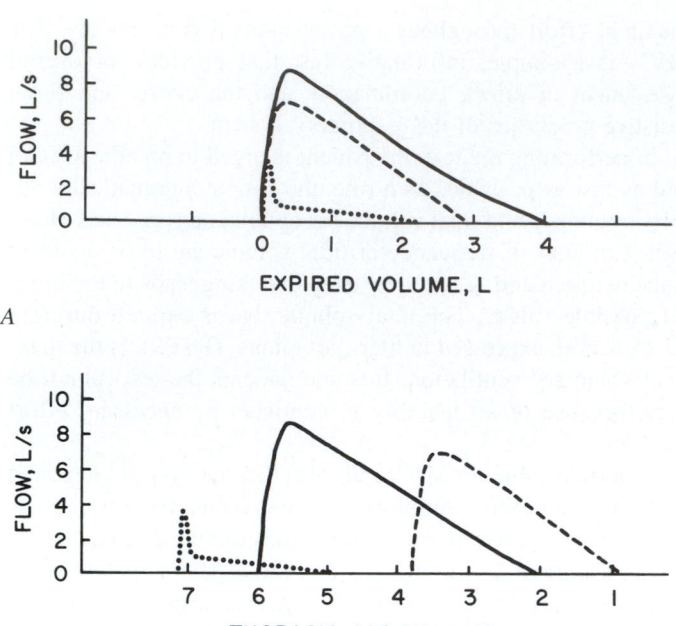

FIGURE 36-21   Airflow at different lung volumes. *A.* Flow-volume curves aligned at TLC. *B.* Flow-volume curves displayed relative to thoracic gas volume. Although the curves aligned at TLC (*A*) show striking differences in the pattern of airflow, they provide no insight into the relationship between lung volumes and airflow. See text for discussion.

strength, coordination of respiratory performance, and motivation of the patient are all normal. Although this test is very useful in detecting overall disturbances in integrated performance and diffuse tracheobronchial and pulmonary parenchymal diseases, other tests are required to pinpoint specific disorders.

The difference between the MVV and the resting minute ventilation is the *breathing reserve.* At one time, a low breathing reserve was correlated with the breathlessness in lung diseases. However, this determination is now primarily of historical interest.

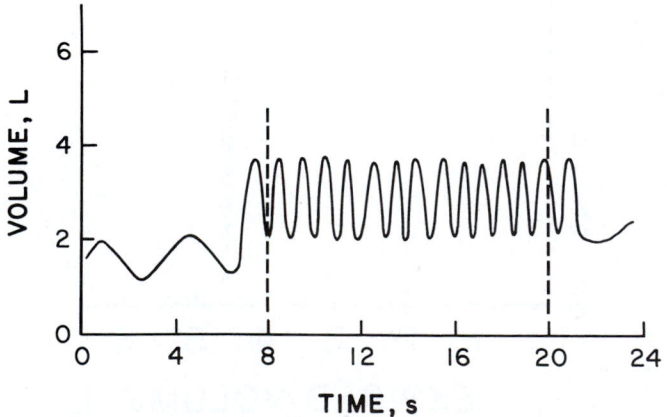

FIGURE 36-22   Maximal voluntary ventilation (MVV). After a period of relaxed breathing, the subject breathes rapidly and as forcefully as possible. The total volume of air inspired over 12 s and expressed in L/min is the MVV.

Respiratory Resistance

Total respiratory resistance (Rrs) is the resistance to airflow and chest expansion offered by the airways (Raw), chest wall (Rw), and lung tissue (Rti):

$$Rrs = Raw + Rw + Rti$$

Although the overall resistance of the respiratory system can be determined with a technique employing forced oscillation, this approach has, to date, exhibited limited practical usefulness. In addition, further methodologic refinements permitting determination of *pulmonary resistance*—the sum of airway and tissue resistances (Raw + Rti)—have not proved to be worthwhile clinically, particularly since measurement of transpulmonary pressure with an esophageal balloon is necessary. Other variations of the determination of resistance measurements have also been explored.[40] However, the only clinically useful measurement of resistance is airway resistance, which is now routinely determined in pulmonary function laboratories.

AIRWAY RESISTANCE

Airway resistance (Raw) is defined as the ratio of the driving pressure (P) required to produce a given airflow ($\dot{V}$) along the airways—i.e., the mouth, nasopharynx, larynx, and central and peripheral airways:

$$Raw = \frac{\Delta P}{\dot{V}}$$

where ΔP, the drop in pressure over the entire length of the airways, is determined as the difference between alveolar pressure (PA) and pressure at the mouth (Pm) or airway opening (Pao).

Although airflow and pressure at the airway opening are easily measured, the difficulty in measuring alveolar pressure prevented the routine determination of airway resistance until DuBois and colleagues introduced the plethysmographic technique in 1956.[14]

With this techique, the patient, seated in the body plethysmograph, pants at a rate of about two breaths per second while airflow is measured using a pneumotachograph. During inspiration and expiration, gas in the alveoli is alternately rarefied and compressed, causing changes in pressure within the sealed plethysmograph. The relationship between plethysmograph pressure and airflow during the panting maneuver is displayed on the X and Y axes of an oscilloscope (Fig. 36-23).

While the panting continues, a shutter at the airway opening is closed so that airflow is transiently interrupted. Using the technique employed in the determination of FRC, changes in pressure in the plethysmograph (equivalent to changes in lung volume) and at the mouth are displayed on the X and Y axes, respectively, of the oscilloscope (Fig. 36-6). However, since airflow is zero while the shutter is closed, the pressure at the mouth equals alveolar pressure (Pao = PA).

Panting while the shutter is open allows the determination of the relationship between airflow ($\dot{V}$) and plethysmograph pressure (Pbx)—i.e., $\dot{V}$/Pbx. Similarly, panting against a closed shutter enables the determination of the relationship between alveolar pressure (PA) and plethysmograph pressure—i.e., PA/Pbx.

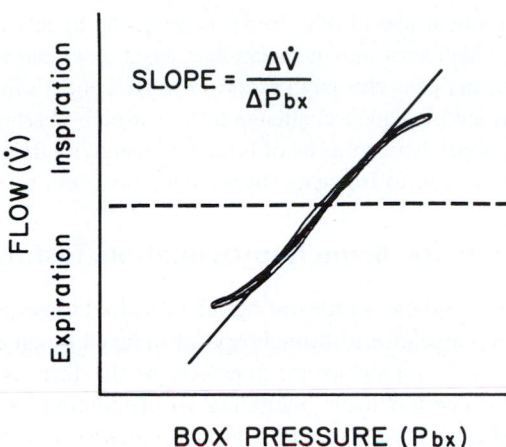

FIGURE 36-23   Plot of airflow ($\dot{V}$) versus body plethysmograph pressure (Pbx). The slope of this curve, in the range of 0 to 0.5 L/s of inspiratory flow, divided into the slope of the loop obtained when the shutter is closed (see Fig. 36-7) provides a measure of airway resistance (Raw).

Airway resistance is calculated by dividing the slope of the loop obtained by plotting PA versus Pbx while the shutter is closed by the slope obtained by plotting $\dot{V}$ versus Pbx while the shutter is open:

$$Raw = \frac{PA/Pbx}{\dot{V}/Pbx} = \frac{PA}{\dot{V}}$$

where

>   Raw = airway resistance, cm H_2O/L/s
>   PA = alveolar pressure, cm H_2O
> $\dot{V}$ = airflow, L/s

Raw is measured during a panting maneuver for several reasons[57]: 1. The rapid respiratory frequency in panting circumvents the poor low-frequency response characteristics of many plethysmographs. 2. The small inspired and expired volumes minimize temperature fluctuations in the plethysmograph that would otherwise occur as tidal breaths of air at body temperature are exchanged with breaths of air at room temperature. 3. During panting, the glottis remains open, thereby minimizing its contribution to overall airway resistance. Recently, plethysmographs linked to microprocessors that automatically correct for temperature-related volume differences have made possible the determination of airway resistance during quiet breathing instead of during panting.

Airway resistance varies inversely with lung volume: it is low at large lung volumes and increases curvilinearly as lung volume and, consequently, airway diameters are reduced (Fig. 36-24A).[4] In contrast, the inverse of airway resistance, airway *conductance,* is linearly related to lung volume (Fig. 36-24B). Interpretation of a given value for airway resistance or airway conductance requires that the lung volume at which the measurement is made be taken into account. *Specific conductance* (SGaw) is calculated by dividing airway conductance by the lung volume.

Defining the range of normal for Raw is difficult because of the lack of data obtained from populations sorted into smoking and nonsmoking groups and because of the inter- and intraindi-

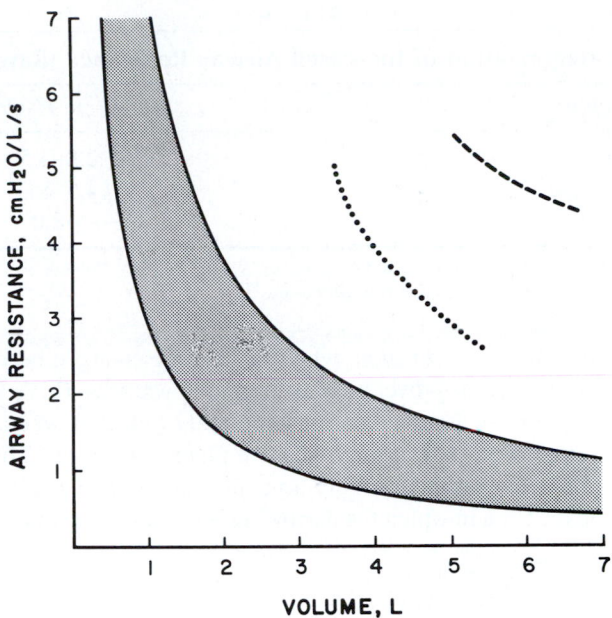

A

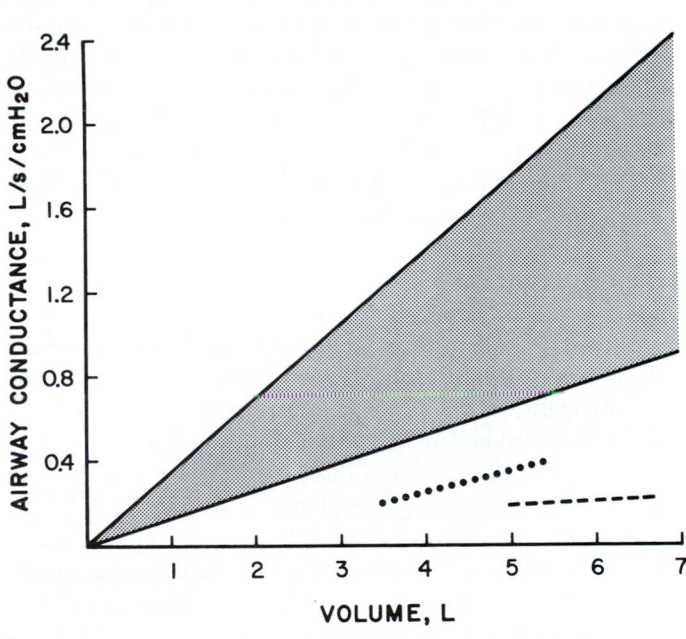

B

FIGURE 36-24   The relationship between airway resistance (*A*) and airway conductance (*B*). The shaded area represents the predicted normal range.[14] Values are shown for an asthmatic patient before (dashed line) and after (dotted line) bronchodilator therapy. Airway resistance increases as lung volume decreases. Conversely, airway conductance, the inverse of resistance, decreases as lung volume decreases.

vidual variations of Raw with lung volume. One classification scheme proposed for defining normal and abnormal Raw in adults in whom FRC exceeds 2 L is given in Table 36-7.

At times, an apparent discrepancy occurs between forced expiratory flow rates and values for airway resistance. For example, although the FEV_1 and $FEF_{25-75\%}$ may be abnormally low (suggesting some degree of airway obstruction), Raw may be within normal limits (mitigating against appreciable airway obstruction). This apparent contradiction arises because Raw is de-

Categorization of Increased Airway Resistance (Raw)

Category	Raw (cm $H_2O/L/s$)
Mild	2.8–4.5
Moderate	4.5–8.0
Severe	>8.0

SOURCE: Modified from Ries and Clausen, in Wilson AF (ed), *Pulmonary Function Testing: Indications and Interpretations.*[57]

termined during *inspiration,* when airways are enlarged because of surrounding negative pleural pressure, whereas FEV_1 and $FEF_{25-75\%}$ are determined during a forceful *expiration,* when airways are compressed by high positive pleural pressures. Therefore, the discrepancy is simply a manifestation of dynamic airway obstruction in which the narrowing is confined to expiration.

AIRWAY REACTIVITY

The dynamic tests of airway function described previously are designed to determine intrinsic properties of the airways in a subject breathing room air at rest. This section deals with reactivity of the airways to certain pharmacologic or environmental agents—i.e., *bronchoprovocation testing.*[50] One test of bronchial reactivity that has been incorporated into routine pulmonary function testing is determination of the effect on airflow of administration of a nebulized bronchodilator agent.

Background

Bronchoprovocation tests are designed to quantify the degree of bronchoconstriction that follows application of a particular stimulus. Originally, in the 1940s, the test stimulus was tailored to the patient's history of extrinsic influences that appeared to trigger respiratory symptoms. However, this approach was flawed by the fact that stimuli held responsible for evoking bronchoconstriction during daily life do not always work in the laboratory. Furthermore, it proved difficult in many instances to distinguish between normal reactivity and hyperreactivity. Consequently, a considerable effort has been expended in recent years to establish normal response characteristics of the airways and to standardize the setting and the test. For example, in inhalation testing with pharmacologic agents such as methacholine, the response depends not only on the dose but also on the maneuver used in testing. Also, during testing for exercise-induced asthma, the humidity and temperature of the inhaled gas profoundly influence the response. A number of tests of bronchial reactivity are cur-

rently in clinical use (Table 36-8). Among the agents used for inhalation challenges are methacholine, histamine, carbacholine, and specific antigens chosen in accord with the patient's history. In addition to the inhalation challenge tests in which pharmacologic agents are used, there are tests of bronchial reactivity to inhalation of cold or dry air, to isocapnic hyperventilation, and to exercise.

Indications for Bronchoprovocation Testing

The principal indication for testing for bronchial hyperreactivity is a history suggestive of bronchospasm induced by an environmental or occupational agent, generally in the face of normal pulmonary function tests (including determination of airflow before and after administering a bronchodilator). For example, comparison of FEV_1 before and after administration of a pharmacologic agent such as methacholine or histamine can be useful in establishing the diagnosis of asthma. Also, inhalation of a suspected specific antigen may be useful in uncovering asthma when skin tests are equivocal, or in proving that asthma in a particular patient is occupation related. In some instances, exercise testing may disclose airway hyperreactivity in persons who are free of bronchoconstriction while at rest. Airway hyperresponsiveness to methacholine may presage an accelerated decline in pulmonary function.[36] However, interpretation of this finding with regard to the need to treat (e.g., with inhaled bronchodilators or corticosteroids) to prevent progression is unclear.

Methods of Bronchoprovocation Testing

Several methods of bronchoprovocation testing are in general clinical use. These include methacholine challenge, exercise challenge, and antigen challenge, each of which is described briefly below.

Tests of Bronchial Reactivity

Test	Reference
Inhalational challenges	
Pharmacologic agents	
Methacholine	Chai et al: *J Allergy Clin Immunol* 56:323–327, 1975
Histamine	Chai et al: *J Allergy Clin Immunol* 56:323–327, 1975
Carbacholine	Orehek et al: *Br Med J* 1:123–125, 1975
Specific antigens	
Toluene diisocyanate	Salvaggio: *J Allergy Clin Immunol* 64:646–649, 1979
Bacillus subtilis	Salvaggio: *J Allergy Clin Immunol* 64:646–649, 1979
Pollen	Spector: *J Allergy Clin Immunol* 64:580–586, 1979
Molds	Spector: *J Allergy Clin Immunol* 64:580–586, 1979
House dust	Spector: *J Allergy Clin Immunol* 64:580–586, 1979
Exercise-induced asthma	
Cold-air challenge	Strauss et al: *N Engl J Med* 297:743–747, 1977
Dry-air challenge	Hahn et al: *Am Rev Respir Dis* 130:575–579, 1984
Isocapnic hyperventilation	Eschenbacher et al: *Am Rev Respir Dis* 131:894–901, 1985

INHALATION CHALLENGE: METHACHOLINE

Inhalation challenge using methacholine has become popular because of standardization of the technique, ease and safety of performing the test, and high sensitivity of the test in detecting asthma.[53] Methacholine is a cholinomimetic agent that evokes constriction of both the central and peripheral airways. Because baseline pulmonary function and breathing pattern influence the site of deposition of the inhaled methacholine particles and, thereby, the response, a standard method for aerosolizing the agent is used to ensure reproducible results.[53]

One method in common use is that of intermittent aerosol generation. Standardization entails the delivery of a 0.6-s pulse of airflow at 20 lb/in² to a nebulizer, which, in turn, discharges particles that range from 0.3 to 4 μm in diameter into the airways. Methacholine for delivery by aerosol is prepared in concentrations ranging from 0.1 to 25 mg/ml using bicarbonate-buffered isotonic saline (containing 0.4 percent phenol) as the diluent. The cumulative dose delivered is expressed in inhalation units. One inhalation unit is equivalent to the single inhalation of a solution containing 1 mg of methacholine per milliliter (Table 36-9).

At the outset, the patient is challenged with five inhalations containing only aerosolized diluent. If the FEV_1 falls below 90 percent of the baseline value (i.e., the prechallenge control FEV_1) the test is discontinued, since this result establishes that the airways are hyperreactive. However, if the FEV_1 does not fall below 90 percent of the control value, increasing concentrations of methacholine are given in stepwise increments, each by five-breath inhalations. The breaths are taken slowly from FRC to TLC. Then, 1 to 1.5 min after each dose, an FVC maneuver is performed. The interval between each increase in concentration is kept to a minimum because the response is judged in terms of the *cumulative* dose. However, the deep inspiration that immediately precedes the expiratory portion of the FVC maneuver may decrease bronchomotor tone in airways narrowed by methacholine. This effect lasts up to 6 min, thus limiting the shortest acceptable interval between dosage steps.[31] At any step, if the postchallenge FEV_1 falls below 80 percent of the control FEV_1, or if the patient experiences cough or chest tightness, the test is stopped. The magnitude of the bronchoconstrictor response to

inhalational challenge is related to the control FEV_1. A lower baseline FEV_1 (even in the normal range) correlates with increased bronchial reactivity.[5,22,38,54] Additional measurements of dynamic airway function (e.g., specific conductance) may provide supplemental data but also prolong the study.

The results are plotted on four-cycle semilog graph paper: the number of cumulative inhalation units, expressed logarithmically, against the FEV_1, as percent of control (Fig. 36-25). A curve is constructed through the points; the dose corresponding to the point at which the FEV_1 is 80 percent of the control FEV_1 is designated as the *provocation dose*, or PD_{20} FEV_1. If specific conductance (SGaw) is used as the index of bronchial reactivity, the dose that produces a 35 percent drop in the baseline SGaw is regarded as the "provocation dose" and is designated as PD_{35} SGaw.

EXERCISE CHALLENGE

Persons without a history of asthma who develop cough, wheezing, or dyspnea after exercise may have exercise-induced asthma (EIA). In these people, an exercise test may prove useful in establishing the diagnosis.

Several factors that may influence the outcome of the test should be kept in mind. The temperature and humidity of the laboratory should be tightly controlled. In addition, the duration of the test needs to be monitored. In particular, exercise testing for EIA should not continue for more than 6 to 8 min, in order to avoid "run-through" of the bronchospasm—i.e., reversal at the end of the test.

The type of exercise also influences the outcome. Free-range running provides the most potent stimulus for bronchoconstriction, followed by treadmill running, bicycle ergometry, swimming, and walking. An asthmatic may swim comfortably at a level of exercise that is incapacitating on the treadmill. Also, as a rule, the more intense the exercise, the more likely is bron-

---

TABLE 36-9

Concentrations and Cumulative Doses of Methacholine Employed in the Methacholine Challenge Test

Methacholine Concentration (mg/ml)	Cumulative Dose* (Inhalation Units)
0.1	0.5
0.5	3
1.0	8
2.0	18
5.0	43
10.0	93
25.0	218

*After five inhalations of a nebulized solution containing methacholine in a concentration of 1 mg/ml.

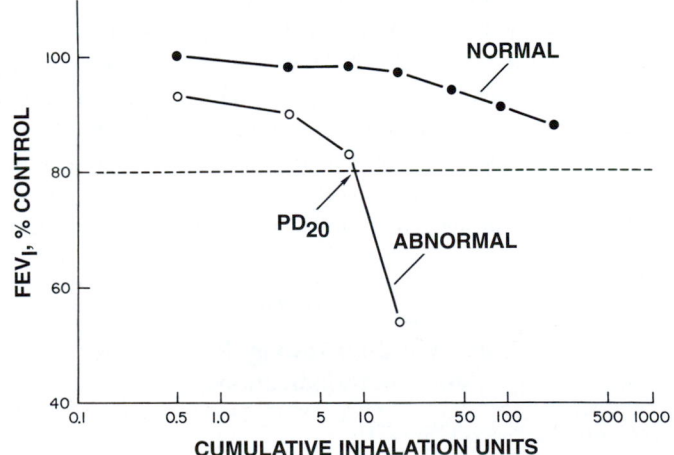

FIGURE 36-25 Plot of FEV_1, % control versus cumulative dose of methacholine administered by inhalation (logarithmic scale), to a normal subject and a subject with hyperreactive airways. The PD_{20} is the cumulative dose, which results in a 20% drop in the FEV_1 from the baseline measurement (after inhalation of diluent alone). In the subject with normal airway reactivity, the maximal cumulative dose of methacholine administered fails to elicit a 20% drop in FEV_1.

choconstriction to occur. Finally, despite elaborate controls and exercise typing, a person who may ultimately be shown to have exercise-induced asthma fails to develop bronchoconstriction under laboratory conditions.

The FEV_1 and peak expiratory flow are the most useful measurements made during testing for EIA. These measurements are made just before and immediately after the exercise and at 2- 5-min intervals for the following 30 min. A decrease in FEV_1 of 10 percent or more below the preexercise value constitutes a positive test.

INHALATION CHALLENGE: ANTIGEN

Compared with the relatively safe methacholine challenge test, bronchoprovocation testing with a specific antigen is unpredictable and potentially hazardous. Since establishing the minimum dose required to induce bronchoconstriction is difficult, too much of the antigen may be given. A late response, far more severe than the initial one, often develops about 6 h after the challenge. Despite these reservations about antigen challenge, testing is warranted under certain circumstances: to uncover a particular agent in the environment that causes bronchoconstriction, to establish the diagnosis of occupational asthma, to prove that bronchoconstriction is caused by a particular antigen after routine skin tests have failed to support the clinical suspicion, and to convince a skeptical patient about the cause of his or her asthma. Recommendations for preparing concentrations of antigens and the technique of antigen challenge testing are specific to the antigen in question and may be found in the literature.

Precautions and Contraindications

For certain patients in whom bronchial hyperreactivity is suspected, bronchoprovocation tests may be unnecessary, invalid, or even dangerous (Table 36-10). For example, the patient who manifests appreciable airway obstruction by conventional testing (e.g., FEV_1/FVC percent under 70) may undergo life-threatening airway narrowing during a bronchoprovocation test. In such a patient, a bronchodilator study would be more appropriate. If bronchodilators fail to reverse the increase in airway resistance, and if it is important to prove that bronchial hyperreactivity does exist, bronchoprovocation testing is sometimes done, with extreme caution, on another day, as antigen dosages are titrated carefully and details of the procedure monitored closely.

TABLE 36-10

Bronchoprovocation Testing: Precautions and Contraindications

- Baseline $FEV_1/FVC\%$ <70
- Recent upper respiratory tract infection
- Recent influenza vaccination
- Recent administration of bronchodilator
- Ingestion of caffeine within 6 h before testing
- Cold-air breathing, hyperventilation, exercise within 6 h before testing

A recent viral upper respiratory tract infection can cause airway hyperreactivity for up to 6 weeks in normal subjects. Similarly, influenza vaccination increases responsiveness to inhalation challenges in asthmatics for a few days to a week. In these conditions, bronchoprovocation testing should not be undertaken until the sensitization effects of the infection or vaccination have worn off. Also, bronchodilators, including caffeine, should be withheld for at least 6 h before a bronchoprovocation test, if possible, in order to prevent blunting of the bronchoconstrictor response. Finally, cold air, hyperventilation, and exercise should be avoided for at least 6 h before testing in order to prevent the induction of a refractory period or late response that would overlap the test results.

SMALL-AIRWAY FUNCTION

Up to this point, discussion of tests of dynamic lung function has addressed the tracheobronchial tree as a unit. Sometimes, however, particularly in cigarette smokers, obstructive disease is confined to the peripheral airways—i.e., those 2 mm or smaller in diameter. Consequently, tests to detect small-airway disease have been devised in the hope of early intervention for the sake of reversing and arresting further progression of the inflammatory process.[7] In otherwise normal persons, obstructive disease of the peripheral airways, generally entailing local edema and, ultimately, fibrosis in the small airways, contributes little to total resistance of the airways, particularly at moderate to large lung volumes.[21] Because of their small contribution to airway resistance, estimated to be about 10 to 38 percent (at a lung volume equivalent to 50 percent of VC), the small airways can undergo considerable damage before the usual tests of either static or dynamic lung function become abnormal.

In obstructive disease of the peripheral airways, however, the small airways' contribution to overall resistance increases, and abnormalities in their function may be detected from the expiratory VC maneuver. In particular, abnormal values for $FEF_{25-75\%}$, in conjunction with normal values for FVC and FEV_1, are often useful in identifying small-airway disease. The basis for this approach is that $FEF_{25-75\%}$ measures airflow during the effort-independent part of the FVC, when the small airways contribute substantially to the limitation of airflow (see Chapter 10).

In addition to limiting airflow during expiration, obstruction of small airways results in abnormal distribution of ventilation to peripheral lung units. This abnormality forms the basis for two tests that merit additional comment: frequency dependence of dynamic compliance and closing volume.

Dynamic Compliance

Dynamic compliance, the change in lung volume during airflow produced by a given change in transpulmonary pressure, is normally independent of breathing frequency. However, under conditions of nonuniformity of ventilation throughout the lung (see Chapter 10), increases in breathing frequency are associated with a fall in dynamic compliance. This frequency dependence of compliance was first noted in a patient with emphysema.[32] The finding was attributed to the asynchronous filling and emptying of alveoli throughout the emphysematous lung. Subsequent work led to the idea that frequency-related changes in dynamic compliance, in the presence of normal values for airway resistance and static lung compliance, indicated obstruction of small peripheral airways.[58] Since then the test for frequency dependence of dynamic compliance has become the "gold standard" against which newer tests of small-airway function are compared. Unfortunately, the standard is not pure gold, since results are far from reproducible, in large measure because of technical difficulties in performing the test.

The same equipment is used to determine dynamic and static compliance. However, the demands on the equipment with respect to frequency response are more stringent for the dynamic measurements. The pneumotachograph, esophageal balloon, transducers, and recording device must be capable of detecting and recording faithfully the rapidly changing volumes and pressures. Artifacts in amplitude and in phase relationships of these volume and pressure signals introduce errors into the determinations.

During the test, the patient, with esophageal balloon in place, first inspires maximally to TLC and then expires to the resting end-expiratory position (FRC); the patient then breathes at a normal tidal volume and respiratory rate (15 breaths per minute). In order to enable the patient to monitor these parameters, tidal volume and the resting end-expiratory level are displayed on an oscilloscope within sight of the patient. At the same time, changes in tidal volume and transpulmonary pressure are displayed on another oscilloscope (Fig. 36-26). The slope of the line connecting the end-inspiratory and end-expiratory points on the pressure-volume loop—i.e., the points of zero airflow—is the dynamic compliance. This procedure is repeated with breathing frequencies of 30 and 60 breaths per minute. Values for dynamic compliance ($C_{dyn,L}$) at the various frequencies are expressed as a ratio of the dynamic compliance to the static inspiratory compliance ($C_{st,L}$) or as a percentage of $C_{st,L}$ (Fig. 36-27) for the same range of tidal volumes.

In normal subjects, $C_{dyn,L}/C_{st,L}$ remains above 0.8, even at frequencies greater than 60 breaths per min. However, in the presence of obstructive disease of the small airways, $C_{dyn,L}/C_{st,L}$ falls progressively to values below 0.8 as breathing frequency increases. It is worth emphasizing that interpretation of frequency dependence of compliance with regard to small-airway disease is valid only if the static compliance and overall airway resistance are normal. Abnormalities in these other measurements indicate disease that is not likely to be confined to the small airways and whose frequency dependence of dynamic compliance is another manifestation. The physiological basis for the fall in $C_{dyn,L}/C_{st,L}$ as respiratory frequency increases is the presence of unequal time constants throughout the lung (see Chapter 10).

The value of this test lies in its sensitivity to increased resistance to airflow in small airways, while other measurements, such as lung volumes and expiratory airflow, are still normal. For example, it has been shown that smoking and upper respiratory tract infections, which produce isolated small-airway disease, elicit frequency-related changes in compliance, even though results of other tests, including FEV_1, $FEF_{25-75\%}$, and lung volumes, are normal.

Closing Volume

In 1949, Fowler described the single-breath nitrogen washout test for assessing the uniformity of ventilation throughout the lungs.[17] In performing this test, the patient first expires maximally to RV, then fills his or her lungs by taking a maximal breath of 100 percent O_2. During the subsequent expiration, the concentration of nitrogen at the mouth is continuously recorded and plotted against the volume of expired gas. Originally, interest focused on the initial part of the tracing that depicts the changing concentration in expired nitrogen as the first 750 to 1200 ml of gas is exhaled. Over this range, the change in nitrogen concentration

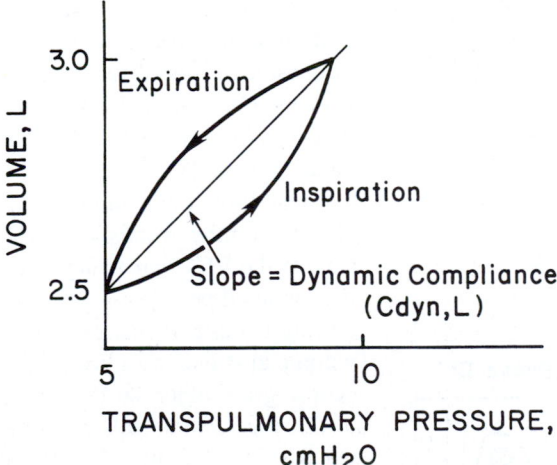

FIGURE 36-26 Measurement of dynamic lung compliance ($C_{dyn,L}$). During the inspiratory and expiratory phases of the respiratory cycle, a loop relating volume to transpulmonary pressure is generated. The slope of a line drawn through the points of zero airflow (at end-inspiration and end-expiration) is the dynamic compliance. Determination of $C_{dyn,L}$ can be done at a variety of respiratory frequencies to assess the frequency dependence of compliance (Fig. 36-27).

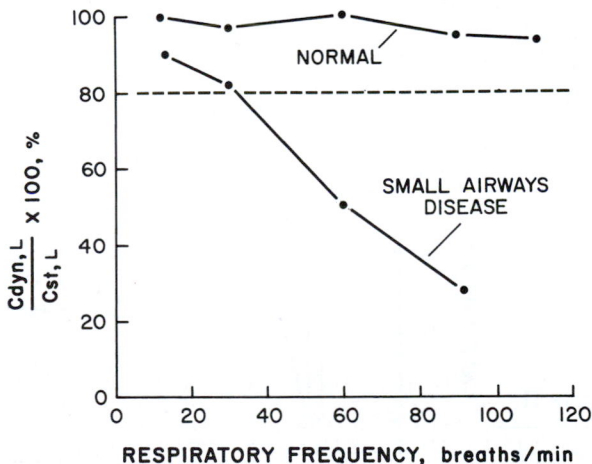

FIGURE 36-27 Determination of frequency dependence of dynamic compliance. Dynamic compliance is determined as shown in Fig. 36-26 and is expressed as a percentage of static lung compliance ($C_{dyn,L}/C_{st,L} \times 100$, %) at a variety of respiratory frequencies. Normally, $C_{dyn,L}$ is $\geq 80\%$ of $C_{st,L}$ and is independent of respiratory frequency. In patients with obstructive airway disease, including those with disease limited to the small airways, $C_{dyn,L}$ falls relative to $C_{st,L}$ as respiratory frequency increases.

in persons with normal lungs is less than 2.5 percent. In contrast, when abnormal lungs or disease of the tracheobronchial tree result in abnormal intrapulmonary distribution of inspired gas, the change in nitrogen concentration exceeds 2.5 percent.

Almost 20 years later, Fowler's test was modified to include a bolus of xenon at the beginning of inspiration and to record the concentration of xenon during the following expiration.[11] Abrupt changes in the concentration of expired xenon as RV was approached suggested that important information about the small airways could be obtained from the terminal portion of the curve.

These observations with xenon rekindled interest in Fowler's original technique but also directed attention to the terminal portion of expiration. The procedure currently in use is shown in Fig. 36-28. To perform the maneuver for this measurement, the seated patient takes two deep breaths of air and then expires to RV. At the end of this maximal expiration, a valve is opened so that the patient can take a full breath of 100 percent O_2 to TLC. The patient then expires slowly to RV while N_2 concentration and expired volume are recorded continuously.

Four distinct phases can be identified in the continuous record relating N_2 concentration to expired volume. Phase I, the initial expirate, contains virtually no N_2, since it derives from the O_2-containing dead space (Fig. 36-28). Phase II represents a mixture of gases from the dead space and the alveoli. Phase III is due to a mixture of gases from alveoli located at the apices, mid-lung fields, and bases. Phase IV, characterized by an upward shift in N_2 concentration, is caused by closure of alveoli in the dependent parts of the lungs at low lung volumes. This final expirate derives from alveoli in the middle and upper regions of the lungs, where N_2 concentrations are higher than at the bases.

The explanation for these phases resides in the intrapulmonary distribution of gases during the respiratory maneuvers used in performing the test. In the normal upright person, a gradient of pleural pressures exists from apex to base, so that pleural pressure is more negative at the apices than at the bases. Because the alveoli at the bases operate on a lower portion of their pressure-volume curve (Fig. 36-11), they expand more than do apical alveoli per unit change in pleural pressure. However, the less negative pleural pressures and decrease in elastic recoil pressure at the bases also cause small airways to close during expiration as lung volume approaches RV. Thus, the pleural pressure gradient from top to bottom of the chest causes nonuniform distribution of gas within the normal upright lungs.

In the single-breath nitrogen washout test, a breath of 100% O_2 is taken, starting from RV. At RV, small basal airways are closed. Therefore, at the start of the O_2 breath, the N_2-containing air remaining in the dead space is preferentially drawn into the middle and apical lung zones as 100% O_2 gradually replaces air in the dead space. As the inspiration continues, the small airways at the bases open. Since their compliances are greater than those in the middle or at the top of the upright lungs, the inspired O_2 is then preferentially distributed to the bases.

During the expiration from TLC, the four phases then represent, as indicated above, the sequential emptying of dead-space gas and a mixture of dead-space and alveolar gas, followed by mixtures of alveolar gases from different parts of the lungs, as determined by the preceding intrapulmonary distribution of inspired O_2.

The volume from the onset of phase IV to the completion of the full expiratory maneuver is termed the *closing volume* (CV). It is generally expressed as a percentage of the VC: (CV/VC) × 100%. The *closing capacity* (CC), expressed as a percentage of TLC, is calculated by adding RV to the closing volume—i.e., CC = CV + RV—and dividing the sum by TLC: (CC/TLC) × 100%.

Although not a test of small airway function, the slope of phase III, expressed as change in the percentage of N_2 per liter, is a useful index of the uniformity of the distribution of ventilation. In normal young people, the slope of phase III is less than 5% per liter. In persons more than 50 years of age, however, the upper limit of normal may be as high as 9%.[47]

In healthy young adults, the normal closing volume averages about 10 percent of the VC. Narrowing or obstruction of small peripheral airways causes closing volume to enlarge. The closing volume also increases progressively as people grow older, so that by the age of 50, the closing volume sometimes reaches 25% of the VC (Fig. 36-29). Cigarette smokers consistently experience an increase in closing volume. In both aging normal persons and cigarette smokers at any age, a decrease in pulmonary elasticity seems to be responsible for the increase in closing volume.

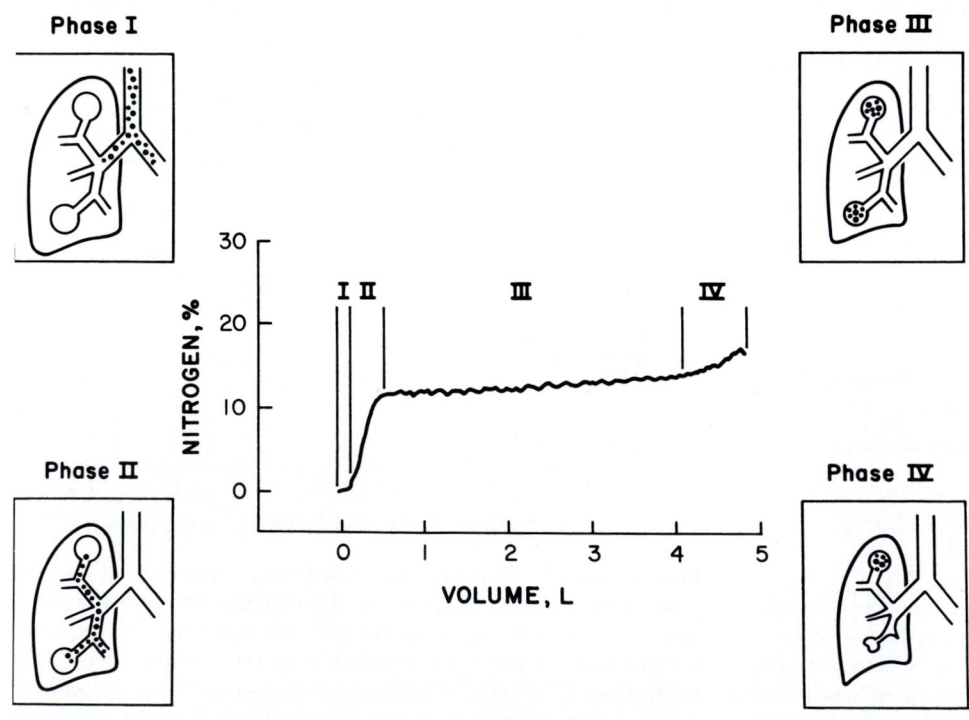

FIGURE 36-28 Contributions of different lung regions to the nitrogen concentration-volume curve obtained during the single-breath nitrogen washout test. See text for discussion.

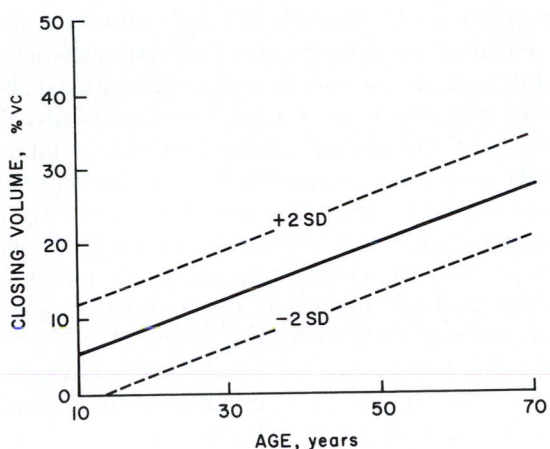

FIGURE 36-29 Relationship between closing volume, expressed as percent of vital capacity, and age. *(From McCarthy et al: Am J Med 52:747–753, 1972.)*

Helium-Oxygen Flow-Volume Curves

In 1963, the effects of changes in gas density and viscosity on maximal expiratory flow throughout the vital capacity range were described.[48] Almost 10 years later, gas density and viscosity-related concepts were applied to determine the site of airway obstruction in asthma.[10] These principles were then applied for the specific purpose of detecting obstruction of small airways when other tests of pulmonary function were within normal limits.[24]

The use of a helium-oxygen mixture to detect small-airway disease requires comparison of two maximal expiratory flow-volume curves, one that is generated while the patient breathes air and the other while the patient breathes helium and oxygen (Fig. 36-30). At least three maximal expiratory flow curves are obtained with room air and three with helium-oxygen.[57]

In normal subjects, at lung volumes greater than 10% of the VC, the primary site of resistance to airflow is in the larger airways, where flow is turbulent and, therefore, density dependent. At these lung volumes, the flow attained with the helium-oxygen mixture will be higher than that attained with air. At lung volumes less than 10% of the VC, the primary site of resistance is in the smaller airways, where flow is laminar and, therefore, not density dependent. In this circumstance, the less dense helium mixture has no effect on flow (Fig. 36-30). In disease of the small airways, the primary site of resistance shifts at large volumes from the larger to the smaller airways. As a result, the flow-enhancing effect of the less dense gas disappears at volumes well above 10% of the VC.

In practice, two sets of maximal expiratory flow-volume curves are obtained, one while the subject is breathing air and the other after three VC breaths of the helium-oxygen mixture to replace at least 95% of the alveolar N_2. Comparisons are then made of the superimposed curves (Fig. 36-30). One comparison is made at 50% of the VC in order to compare maximal expiratory flows (i.e., the $\Delta\dot{V}_{max,50\%}$); the other is at the volume at which the flows become identical—i.e., the *volume of isoflow* ($V_{iso}\dot{V}$).[12] The curves are superimposed at RV or TLC, as long as the vital capacities of each curve are within 2.5 to 5.0% of the largest VC recorded.[57]

The percentage change in expiratory flow while breathing helium-oxygen compared to air at 50% of the VC, $\Delta\dot{V}_{Emax,50\%}$, is calculated as

$$\Delta\dot{V}_{Emax,50\%} =$$

$$\frac{\dot{V}_{Emax,50\%}\ (\text{helium-oxygen}) - \dot{V}_{Emax,50\%}\ (\text{air})}{\dot{V}_{max,50\%}\ (\text{air})} \times 100$$

where $\dot{V}_{Emax,50\%}$ (helium-oxygen) and $\dot{V}_{Emax,50\%}$ (air) are the expiratory flows at 50% of the VC during helium-oxygen and air breathing, respectively. As noted previously, the volume of isoflow is normally less than 10% of the VC; when it is increased, it indicates small-airway obstruction. The $\Delta\dot{V}_{Emax,50\%}$ is also specific for small-airway disease, and unlike the closing volume, it is considered to be unaffected by changes in the elastic properties of the lung. Questions remain, however, about the validity and sensitivity of tests of density dependence of flow in assessing small-airway disease. Although they are conceptually attractive, the practical value of helium-oxygen flow-volume curves in detecting small-airway disease is debatable.

GAS EXCHANGE FUNCTIONS

Traditional measurements of the gas exchange functions of the lung include oxygen uptake ($\dot{V}_{O_2}$), carbon dioxide elimination ($\dot{V}_{CO_2}$), respiratory dead space (V_D), alveolar gas composition ($P_{A_{O_2}}$ and $P_{A_{CO_2}}$), diffusing capacity for carbon monoxide ($D_{L_{CO}}$), and arterial blood gas tensions (Pa_{O_2} and Pa_{CO_2}). These determinations require a steady state of the ventilation and circulation and constant body stores of O_2 and CO_2. A steady state with respect to O_2 implies that O_2 uptake measured at the mouth equals the rate of O_2 transport across the alveolar membrane, and that, in turn, both rates are equal to O_2 consumption by the tissues. The same type of definition applies to CO_2 exchange in the tissues, in the alveolar capillaries, and at the mouth.

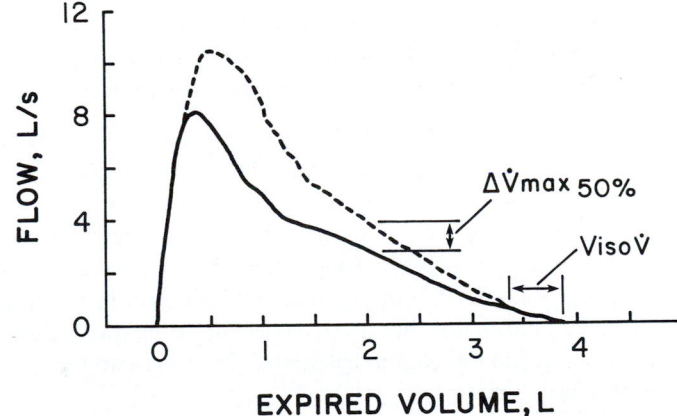

FIGURE 36-30 Maximal expiratory flow-volume curves generated in breathing room air (solid line) and breathing a helium-oxygen mixture (dashed line). The airflows achieved with the less dense helium mixture are higher than those with air at all but the lowest lung volumes. The point of first intersection of these two curves demarcates the volume of isoflow ($V_{iso\ \dot{v}}$). The difference between the flows achieved when 50% of the vital capacity has been expired is the $\Delta V_{max,\%}$. The use of these measurements as indicators of small-airway disease is described in the text.

Ventilation, Oxygen Uptake, and Carbon Dioxide Elimination

The total volume of air breathed per minute ($\dot{V}_E$) is the *minute ventilation*. It is equal to the product of the tidal volume (V_T) and the breathing frequency (f). As a rule, minute ventilation is determined by measuring the volume of expired gas relative to time. When the measurement is performed manually, the necessary equipment includes gas-collecting bags, low-resistance directional valves, a stopwatch, and a device for measuring gas volume. In practice, the patient, with nose clip in place, breathes through a mouthpiece for at least 3 to 5 min while expired gas is vented to the atmosphere. This preliminary period is intended to put the patient at ease and to achieve a steady state of respiration and circulation. When a steady heart rate and breathing pattern are achieved, a valve is turned without the patient's knowledge, and expired gas is collected for 3 min.

The minute ventilation is determined by dividing the total volume of expired gas collected in the spirometer by the time of collection (3 min). The average tidal volume is obtained by dividing $\dot{V}_E$ by the number of breaths per minute. Values for minute ventilation and tidal volume are expressed in terms of body conditions (BTPS). In the resting adult, the minute ventilation is typically 6 to 8 L/min; the corresponding tidal volume is 0.4 to 0.6 L.

The quantity of CO_2 in inspired air is negligible. Consequently, the amount of CO_2 produced per minute ($\dot{V}_{CO_2}$) can be calculated as the product of the expired volume of ventilation ($\dot{V}_E$) and the concentration of CO_2 in the expired air ($F_{E_{CO_2}}$):

$$\dot{V}_{CO_2} = \dot{V}_E \times F_{E_{CO_2}}$$

Oxygen uptake ($\dot{V}_{O_2}$) is calculated as the difference between the amounts of O_2 in inspired and expired air:

$$\dot{V}_{O_2} = (\dot{V}_I \times F_{I_{O_2}}) - (\dot{V}_E \times F_{E_{O_2}})$$

where

$\dot{V}_I$ = inspired volume of ventilation, L/min
$F_{I_{O_2}}$ = concentration of O_2 in the inspired air
$F_{E_{O_2}}$ = concentration of O_2 in the expired air

In the steady state, O_2 uptake by alveolar capillary blood exceeds CO_2 output from alveolar capillary blood. As a result, the expired volume of gas is less than the corresponding inspired volume. Since N_2 does not undergo exchange in the lungs, the difference between CO_2 output and O_2 uptake results in a higher concentration of N_2 in expired air than in inspired air. Based on the change in nitrogen concentration, the inspired volume of ventilation can be calculated from the expired volume of ventilation:

$$\dot{V}_I = \dot{V}_E \frac{F_{E_{N_2}}}{F_{I_{N_2}}}$$

where

$F_{E_{N_2}}$ = concentration of N_2 in expired air
$F_{I_{N_2}}$ = concentration of N_2 in inspired air

In the normal, resting subject who is tested after several hours of fasting, the ratio of CO_2 output to O_2 uptake, the *respiratory exchange ratio* (R), is about 0.8. The respiratory exchange ratio at any instant is calculated by simultaneously determining the P_{O_2} and P_{CO_2} in an alveolar gas sample. As indicated above, in the steady state, the R determined by sampling alveolar gas equals the R of alveolar capillary blood, which, in turn, equals the R of the tissues. The steady-state R, when alveolar gas, blood, and tissue are all in dynamic equilibrium, is the *respiratory quotient* (RQ). Hence, in the steady state, when the O_2 and CO_2 stores of the body are not changing, the RQ, reflecting cellular metabolism, can be determined by analyzing alveolar gas for O_2 and CO_2.

Unlike tidal volume and ventilation, which are expressed in terms of BTPS, $\dot{V}_{O_2}$ and $\dot{V}_{CO_2}$ are given in terms of standard temperature and pressure, dry (STPD).

Dead Space

Not all of the air breathed participates in gas exchange. Part of each breath remains in the mouth, nose, pharynx, larynx, trachea, bronchi, and bronchioles. This volume, the *anatomic dead space,* is about equal, in milliliters, to the subject's ideal body weight, in pounds (e.g., about 150 ml in a typical adult male). Inspired air reaching alveoli that are not exposed to pulmonary capillary blood also does not participate in gas exchange. This volume plus the anatomic dead space equals the *physiological dead space.* In a normal person, the anatomic and physiological dead spaces are virtually identical and constitute about one-third of the tidal volume.

Determination of the physiological dead space has proved to be of practical importance in a variety of clinical conditions. It is calculated by considering each breath (V_T) to consist of dead space (V_D) and an alveolar volume that participates in gas exchange (V_A):

$$V_T = V_D + V_A$$

Physiological dead space can be calculated using a modification of the *Bohr equation,* which recognizes that all of the test gas expired derives from two sources: the physiological dead space and the alveolar gas-exchanging volume. If we use CO_2 as the marker gas, the total amount of CO_2 eliminated per minute equals the sum of the CO_2 coming from the dead space per minute and from the alveolar compartment per minute:

$$\dot{V}_E \times F_{E_{CO_2}} = (\dot{V}_D \times F_{I_{CO_2}}) + (\dot{V}_A \times F_{A_{CO_2}})$$

where

$\dot{V}_E$ = minute ventilation, L/min
$F_{E_{CO_2}}$ = fractional concentration of CO_2 in expired gas
$\dot{V}_D$ = minute dead space ventilation, L/min
$F_{I_{CO_2}}$ = fractional concentration of CO_2 in inspired gas
$\dot{V}_A$ = alveolar ventilation, L/min
$F_{A_{CO_2}}$ = fractional concentration of CO_2 in alveolar gas

Since, in a subject breathing room air, $F_{I_{CO_2}}$ is practically zero, the last equation is generally simplified as follows.

$$V_E \times F_{E_{CO_2}} = V_A \times F_{A_{CO_2}}$$

where V_E and V_A represent volumes of ventilation, rather than rates.

If we recall that $V_A = V_T - V_D$ and substitute partial pressures for the fractional concentration terms, the relationship becomes

$$V_E \times P_{ECO_2} = (V_T - V_D)\, P_{ACO_2}$$

where P_{ECO_2} and P_{ACO_2} are the partial pressures of CO_2 in mixed expired gas and alveolar gas, respectively.

Assuming that arterial blood and alveolar gas are in equilibrium with respect to CO_2, when P_{ACO_2} is substituted for P_{ACO_2} and the equation rearranged, it becomes

$$V_D = V_T \frac{P_{ACO_2} - P_{ECO_2}}{P_{ACO_2}}$$

Thus, if arterial blood is sampled during collection of expired gas, and if the partial pressures of CO_2 in expired gas and arterial blood are determined, the physiological dead space can be calculated. In order for the physiological dead space to be separated from the total dead space determined by the above equation, the dead space of the apparatus is subtracted from the value for total dead space.

Alveolar Gas Composition

In normal subjects, values for P_{O_2} and P_{CO_2} in an end-tidal sample approximate mean alveolar values. However, when imbalances exist in alveolar ventilation and blood flow because of lung disease, inhomogeneity in alveolar gas composition often invalidates the use of end-tidal gas tensions as a measure of mean alveolar gas composition.

In practice, mean alveolar P_{O_2} ($\bar{P}_{AO_2}$) and mean alveolar P_{CO_2} ($\bar{P}_{ACO_2}$) are often determined indirectly. Arterial P_{CO_2} is assumed to equal mean alveolar P_{CO_2} on the grounds of the narrow arteriovenous difference for P_{CO_2} across the lungs, the high solubility of CO_2, and the presumed role of pulmonary capillary blood as a tonometer. Mean alveolar P_{O_2} is calculated with the alveolar gas equation:

$$\bar{P}_{AO_2} = P_{IO_2} - \bar{P}_{ACO_2}\left(F_{IO_2} + \frac{1 - F_{IO_2}}{R}\right)$$

The alveolar gas equation takes advantage of the fact that the total pressure of gases in the alveoli is equal to the sum of the partial pressures of the individual gases. This equation simply states that the mean alveolar P_{O_2} is the difference between inspired P_{O_2} and mean alveolar P_{CO_2}, allowing for a correction factor when the respiratory exchange ratio differs from 1.0.

Diffusing Capacity

The diffusing capacity of the lung for carbon monoxide (D_{LCO}), known in Europe as the transfer factor, can be determined by steady-state, rebreathing, and single-breath methods. The most frequently used method is a modification of the single-breath method first described in 1915 and subsequently modified in 1957.[37] Although the single-breath test has been shown to exhibit a large interlaboratory variation, it has proved to be a valuable measure of lung function in a wide variety of disease states. In fact, with continuing refinement of the standards,[1,23,35] the variability, which may be as much as 12 percent or greater, is

likely to decrease; however, the variability will probably not be reduced to the range for vital capacity measurements (about 4 percent).

The diffusing capacity is intended to provide an estimate of the rate at which test molecules—usually either O_2 or CO—move by diffusion from alveolar gas to combine with hemoglobin in the red blood cells. Factors that influence the measurement are the physicochemical properties of the test gas, the extent and thickness of the alveolar-capillary barrier, the resistance to diffusion offered by the red blood cell membrane, and the reaction rates of the test gas and hemoglobin. As a rule, the diffusing capacity is interpreted as an index of the surface area engaged in alveolar-capillary diffusion.

Carbon monoxide has emerged as the most practical test gas. It is usually administered by a single-breath method. The diffusing capacity for CO is defined as the amount of CO transferred per minute per mm Hg of driving pressure:

$$D_{LCO} = \frac{\dot{V}_{CO}}{\bar{P}_{ACO} - \bar{P}_{CCO}}$$

where

$$D_{LCO} = \text{the diffusing capacity of the lung for CO,}$$
$$\text{ml/min/mm Hg (STPD)}$$
$$\dot{V}_{CO} = \text{the amount of CO transferred, ml/min}$$
$$\bar{P}_{ACO} = \text{the mean alveolar } P_{CO}, \text{ mm Hg}$$
$$\bar{P}_{CCO} = \text{the mean capillary } P_{CO}, \text{ mm Hg}$$

Since the blood P_{CO} in nonsmokers is essentially zero, the term $\bar{P}_{CCO}$ is customarily neglected. In practice, D_{LCO} is determined by calculating $\dot{V}_{CO}$ as the difference between inspired and expired samples and estimating the mean alveolar P_{CO}. Generally, one of two techniques is used to determine D_{LCO}: the single-breath or the steady-state technique.

THE SINGLE-BREATH METHOD

The breathing maneuvers required for the single-breath method consist of quiet breathing for a few breaths, expiration to residual volume, and then a single full, rapid inspiration of a gas mixture containing approximately 0.3% CO and 10% helium. The breath is held for 10 s and then rapidly expired. The initial portion of the expirate containing dead-space gas is discarded; the remainder is collected, and the concentrations of CO and helium are measured.[37] A variety of systems are commercially available for performing the single-breath diffusing capacity. However, the essential components in all systems are a source of the special inspired gas mixture, a device for measuring the volume of gas inspired and expired, analyzers to measure the concentration of gases (see below), a timer, and appropriate valving and collection devices to trap the desired portion of the expirate.

The diffusing capacity of the lung for CO is calculated according to the following equation.

$$D_{LCO} = \frac{V_A \times 60}{(\text{barometric pressure} - 47)} \times \text{time}$$
$$\times \ln \frac{F_{ACO}, \text{ initial}}{F_{ACO}, \text{ final}}$$

where

$$V_A = \text{alveolar volume}$$
$$F_{A_{CO}}, \text{initial} = \text{alveolar concentration of CO at start of breath hold}$$
$$F_{A_{CO}}, \text{final} = \text{alveolar concentration of CO at end of breath hold}$$

The concentration of CO in the alveoli at the start of the period of breath holding ($F_{A_{CO}}$, initial) is calculated from the inspired concentration of CO, the inspired concentration of helium, and the expired concentration of helium according to the equation

$$F_{A_{CO}}, \text{initial} = \frac{F_{E_{He}}}{F_{I_{He}}} \times F_{I_{CO}}$$

where

$$F_{E_{He}} = \text{expired concentration of helium}$$
$$F_{I_{He}} = \text{inspired concentration of helium}$$
$$F_{I_{CO}} = \text{inspired concentration of CO}$$

The concentration of CO in the alveoli at the end of the breath-holding period ($F_{A_{CO}}$, final) is equal to the concentration of CO in the expired gas. The alveolar volume (V_A) is determined in one of two ways. Originally, V_A was calculated as the sum of the residual volume, determined by the closed-circuit helium or body plethysmograph techniques described previously, and the volume of inspired gas, as recorded on the spirometer. Later, V_A came to be calculated from the single-breath dilution of helium that occurs during the determination of $D_{L_{CO}}$. Finally, the time of breath holding is measured (in seconds) from the spirometer recording of the maneuver.

Although the single-breath method is relatively simple and has the advantage of requiring no blood samples, breath holding is clearly artificial, and the maneuver is difficult for dyspneic patients. Therefore, a steady-state method is sometimes used.

THE STEADY-STATE METHOD

In the steady-state method, a gas mixture containing 0.1% carbon monoxide is breathed until the rate of CO uptake from the lung is constant.[16] CO uptake ($\dot{V}_{CO}$) is determined from the difference between the amount of CO in the inspired and expired gas using an equation similar to that presented previously for calculation of O_2 consumption.

COMPARISON OF SINGLE-BREATH AND STEADY-STATE METHODS

Certain differences between the single-breath and steady-state techniques merit special mention.[57] The single-breath method is more popular because it is relatively easy to perform; it is well standardized, and it is less affected by nonuniformity of ventilation in comparison to the steady-state method. However, one drawback is that the patient is required to perform an inspiratory vital capacity maneuver of at least 90% of the VC and to hold his or her breath for 10 s. Another is that the test is extremely difficult to perform during exercise. The steady-state method is more attractive intrinsically than the single-breath method, since it requires no respiratory maneuvers and can be done during exercise. However, it does require an arterial blood sample (for determination of P_{CO_2}), and it is technically more difficult to perform.

The steady-state method for determining diffusing capacity tends to give lower values for the resting subject than does the single-breath method. The discrepancy is generally attributed to the fact that the surface area for diffusion is smaller during the quiet tidal breathing employed in the steady-state method than during the full inspiration to TLC, as required in the single-breath method. Also, during quiet breathing, some areas of the lung receive considerably less ventilation than during a breath hold at TLC.

FACTORS OTHER THAN DIFFUSION THAT INFLUENCE TEST RESULTS

A low $D_{L_{CO}}$ need not indicate a diffusion defect. A number of additional respiratory and nonrespiratory factors may reduce or increase the $D_{L_{CO}}$. A reduction in the lung volume alone can reduce the $D_{L_{CO}}$. Therefore, some laboratories "normalize" the diffusing capacity for lung volume by dividing $D_{L_{CO}}$ by alveolar volume—a manipulation that assumes a linear relationship between $D_{L_{CO}}$ and V_A, which is not the case.

Ventilation-perfusion inequalities may affect the $D_{L_{CO}}$, but they exert a greater influence on results obtained by the steady-state method. Since current techniques provide only a mean value for $D_{L_{CO}}$, inhomogeneities in diffusing capacity throughout the lung are obscured.

Anemia artificially decreases the $D_{L_{CO}}$ as determined by either method, but the effect of low hemoglobin concentration can be adjusted by application of a correction factor.[8] Conversely, polycythemia and intrapulmonary hemorrhage tend to increase the value for $D_{L_{CO}}$. In fact, an unexpectedly high value for $D_{L_{CO}}$ may be a helpful clinical clue in detecting radiographically occult pulmonary hemorrhage.

Although the equation for $D_{L_{CO}}$ assumes that the CO back pressure in blood is negligible, the blood of a heavy smoker sometimes contains as much as 10 percent CO Hb. Such levels of CO Hb will be accompanied by appreciable concentrations of dissolved CO in the plasma. The resulting back pressure of CO will reduce the $D_{L_{CO}}$. A correction equation may be applied to adjust the $D_{L_{CO}}$ for this effect.

Altitude also affects the $D_{L_{CO}}$. Pa_{O_2} falls with increasing altitude above sea level. The reduction in Pa_{O_2} allows CO to diffuse more rapidly into the blood. The American Thoracic Society has adopted the position that an adjustment for altitude is permitted, but it is not required.[1]

Arterial Blood Gas Composition

The determination of arterial P_{O_2} and P_{CO_2} provides useful information about the overall efficiency of external gas exchange. Heavy reliance is placed upon them for this purpose in managing acute respiratory failure, particularly in intensive care units. Less dramatic, but important, is their use in a variety of other settings (e.g., exercise testing) and for assorted calculations (e.g., the alveolar-arterial O_2 gradient and respiratory dead space).

TECHNIQUE FOR SAMPLING ARTERIAL BLOOD

Arterial blood is sampled either through an indwelling arterial catheter or by percutaneous arterial puncture. Sampling through an indwelling catheter avoids the acute changes in ventilation that sometimes result from apprehension and pain associated with percutaneous puncture.

Three anatomic sites are generally used for obtaining arterial blood samples: the radial, brachial, and femoral arteries. For several reasons, the radial artery is the preferred sampling site. Because of its superficial location at the wrist, the radial artery is easy to palpate and easy to compress by direct pressure, facilitating hemostasis when sampling is complete. In addition, no large veins lie in its immediate vicinity. Furthermore, the ulnar artery usually provides an adequate collateral circulation to the hand in the rare instance of postsampling thrombosis of the radial artery.

Adequacy of the ulnar collateral system is easily assessed with a modified Allen's test (Fig. 36-31). This test comprises several steps. 1. By tightly clenching the fist, the patient's hand is drained of much of its blood. 2. While the fist is kept clenched, blood flow to the hand is arrested by compression of the radial and ulnar arteries at the wrist (Fig. 36-31A). 3. Relaxation of the fist while arterial compressions are maintained causes the hand to blanch (Fig. 36-31B). 4. The ulnar artery is then released while the radial artery is still compressed. When the ulnar collateral circulation is normal, the hand flushes within 15 s (Fig. 36-31C), suggesting that if radial artery occlusion were to occur after radial arterial puncture, ulnar blood flow would suffice to avoid ischemic damage to the hand.

Arterial blood samples are drawn anaerobically into plastic or glass syringes coated with heparin. Because room air at sea level has a P_{O_2} of approximately 150 mmHg and a P_{CO_2} of approximately zero mmHg, air bubbles in the syringe will artificially increase the arterial P_{O_2} and reduce the arterial P_{CO_2}. The sample either is immediately analyzed or is placed on ice in order to minimize the metabolism of blood cells, particularly the white cells. If the icing precaution is neglected and the analysis is delayed, the Pa_{CO_2} of the sample will increase and the Pa_{O_2} and pH will decrease; the rate of change depends on the temperature of the sample and the elapsed time before analysis (Table 36-11).[26]

INTERPRETATIONS

Analysis of arterial blood gases as part of pulmonary function testing is based primarily on determination of Pa_{O_2}, Pa_{CO_2}, and pH. As a rule, these parameters are measured directly. Other val-

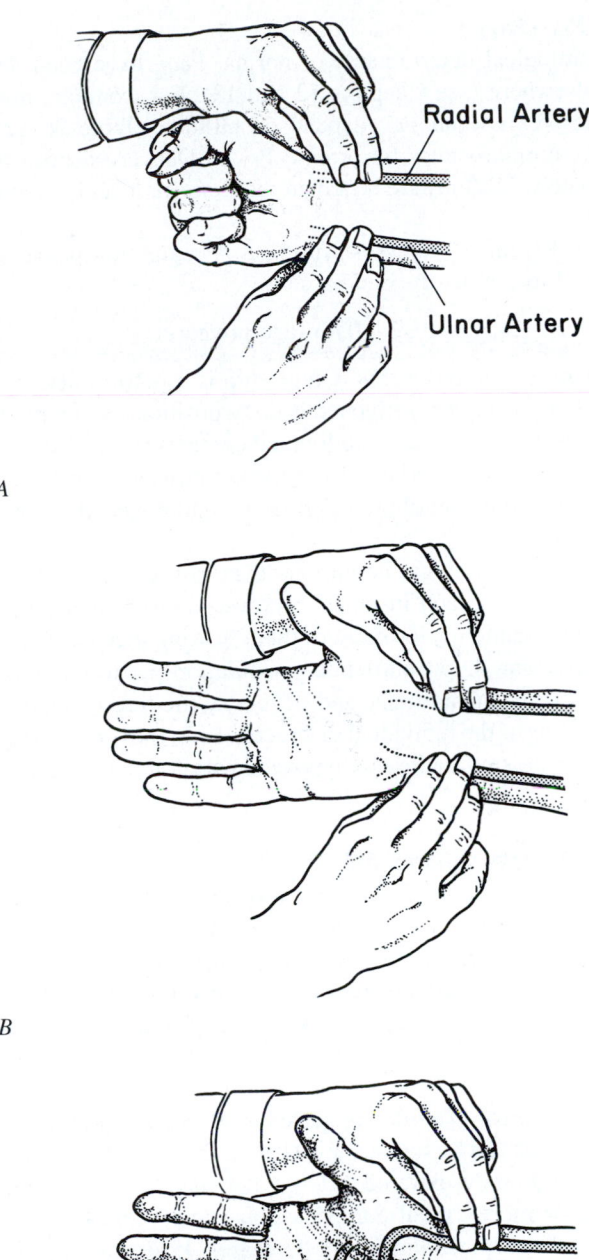

FIGURE 36-31   Modified Allen's test for assessing ulnar arterial flow to the hand. *A.* The subject is instructed to make a fist as the examiner firmly compresses the radial and ulnar arteries at the wrist. *B.* As the fist is released and radial and ulnar arterial compressions are maintained, the hand appears blanched. *C.* An adequate ulnar collateral flow is indicated by reperfusion of the hand within 15 s of release of ulnar compression as radial compression is maintained. *(From Shapiro et al: Clinical Application of Blood Gases, 3d ed. Chicago, Year Book Medical Publishers, 1982.)*

ues, including O_2 saturation, bicarbonate concentration, and base excess (or deficit), are usually calculated. This section deals with the interpretation of Pa_{O_2}, Pa_{CO_2}, and pH. Additional consideration of arterial blood gases, with particular reference to acid-base balance, is found in Chapter 15.

TABLE 36-11

In Vitro Changes in Arterial Blood Gas Values at 37°C

Measurement	Change over 10 Min
pH (units)	−0.01
P_{CO_2} (mmHg)	+1
O_2 content (vol %)	−0.001

SOURCE: Data from Kelman and Nunn.[26]

Arterial P_{O_2} (Pa_{O_2})

The physiological determinants of normal Pa_{O_2} have been described elsewhere (see Chapters 12 and 13). For example, normal values for arterial P_{O_2} depend on altitude (Table 36-12). Therefore, normal values for arterial P_{O_2} in Denver (altitude of approximately 1500 m) are less than those at sea level by about 20 mmHg.

Arterial P_{O_2} also decreases with age. A regression equation can be used to predict the decrease.[51]

$$Pa_{O_2} = 109 - 0.43 \text{ (age in years)}$$

The standard deviation of this relationship is ± 4.10 mmHg.

A third physiological influence is body position. Assumption of the supine position causes abdominal contents to displace the diaphragm cephalad, thereby closing small airways at the lung bases and creating ventilation-perfusion inhomogeneities that decrease Pa_{O_2}.

Many more pathologic conditions than physiological states can lower Pa_{O_2}. In each instance, however, arterial hypoxemia may be attributed to one or more of the following generic mechanisms: alveolar hypoventilation, ventilation-perfusion mismatch, diffusion impairment, and venous admixture ("shunt"). Considerations of the individual disorders within these categories and the mechanisms leading to hypoxemia are found throughout this book.

Arterial P_{CO_2} (Pa_{CO_2}) and pH

In a steady state, the level of Pa_{CO_2} reflects the level of alveolar ventilation. In the absence of a disorder in metabolic acid-base balance, an increase or decrease in Pa_{CO_2} beyond normal limits indicates a primary disorder in alveolar ventilation. A summary of these disorders and useful criteria for distinguishing among them, based on arterial blood gas composition, are given in Table 36-13.

Acute *respiratory alkalosis,* produced by alveolar hyperventilation, is characterized by hypocapnia (Pa_{CO_2} less than 33 mmHg) and an appropriately elevated pH (greater than 7.45). In time (e.g., 24 h or more), renal compensation occurs, and the concentration of bicarbonate in serum decreases. If alveolar hyperventilation continues, a chronic respiratory alkalosis, partly or completely "compensated," ensues.

A low Pa_{CO_2} is not necessarily indicative of a primary disturbance in alveolar ventilation. Instead, it may be a consequence of respiratory compensation (partial or complete) for metabolic acidosis; this possibility is signaled by the coexistence of hypocapnia and a low pH (under 7.35). Since the kidney and respiratory system do not overcompensate for acid-base derangements, the coexistence of hypocapnia and acidemia is inconsistent with renal compensation for a chronic respiratory alkalosis.

Acute respiratory acidosis, caused by alveolar hypoventilation, is characterized by an abnormally high Pa_{CO_2} (over 47 mmHg) and a subnormal pH (under 7.35). Again, in time (24 h or more), renal compensation for the primary respiratory disorder restores the serum bicarbonate concentration and blood pH toward normal. A high value for Pa_{CO_2} may also reflect respiratory compensation for a primary metabolic alkalosis ([HCO_3^-] greater than 30 mEq/L). In this circumstance, however, blood pH will be abnormally high (pH over 7.45), rather than low. In general, the elevation in Pa_{CO_2} in compensation for metabolic alkalosis does not exceed about 55 mmHg. A Pa_{CO_2} exceeding this value in the setting of a metabolic alkalosis suggests the likely coexistence of a primary respiratory acidosis.

This discussion has been limited primarily to alterations in arterial blood gas values in primary respiratory acidosis or alkalosis. Metabolic derangements often complicate the picture. These disorders are considered elsewhere (Chapter 15).

CONTROL OF BREATHING

The rate, depth, and pattern of breathing reflect a complex interplay of neurohumoral and chemical regulatory mechanisms that drive the respiratory apparatus. Tests that are sometimes used clinically to evaluate the control of breathing are based on assessment of the ventilatory response to controlled hypercapnia or hypoxia.

Ventilatory Response to CO_2

The ventilatory response to changes in Pa_{CO_2} is linear over a broad range (Fig. 36-32). Determination of the ventilatory response to controlled hypercapnia generally is based on one of two methods: the steady-state method[30] or the rebreathing method.[43]

TABLE 36-12

Effect of Altitude on Mean Alveolar and Arterial O_2 Pressures

Altitude (Feet)	Barometric Pressure (mmHg)	Ambient P_{O_2} (mmHg)	Alveolar P_{O_2} (mmHg)
0	760	159	103
1000	733	154	98
2000	707	148	94
3000	681	143	90
4000	656	138	85
5000	632	133	81
6000	609	128	77
8000	565	118	69
10,000	523	110	61
12,000	484	101	54

SOURCE: Modified from Wasserman: *Clin Notes Respir Dis* 12:3–10, 1973.

Classification of Primary Respiratory Disorders of Acid-Base Balance

Disorder	*Definition*
Acute respiratory alkalosis (acute alveolar hyperventilation)	Pa_{CO_2} below lower limit of normal (<33 mmHg), with accompanying alkalemia (pH >7.45)
Chronic respiratory alkalosis (chronic alveolar hyperventilation)	Pa_{CO_2} below lower limit of normal, with pH normal (or near normal) due to renal compensation and lowered serum bicarbonate concentration (<19 mEq/L)
Acute respiratory acidosis (acute alveolar hypoventilation)	Pa_{CO_2} above upper limit of normal (>47 mmHg), with accompanying acidemia (pH <7.35)
Chronic respiratory acidosis (chronic alveolar hypoventilation)	Pa_{CO_2} above upper limit of normal, with pH normal (or near normal) due to renal compensation and elevated serum bicarbonate concentration (>30 mEq/L)

STEADY-STATE METHOD

After a control period in which CO_2-free air is breathed to establish a baseline, the patient is subjected to two or more periods of breathing CO_2-enriched air. Care is taken to achieve a steady state of ventilation and circulation during each exposure. Especially at the higher concentrations of inspired CO_2, at least 10 to 20 min is required for a steady state to be reached in alveoli, arterial blood, cerebrospinal fluid, and the chemosensitive areas of the brain. The ventilatory response to CO_2 is then determined from a plot of $\dot{V}E$ versus Pa_{CO_2}. In patients without underlying lung disease, end-tidal CO_2 concentration is often substituted for Pa_{CO_2}. In addition, in order to eliminate the influence of variations in arterial PO_2 on the ventilatory response to CO_2, the inspired gas is enriched with O_2 during the control and test periods.

REBREATHING METHOD

Because the steady-state method is tedious and time-consuming, it has largely been replaced by the rebreathing method. The procedure entails rebreathing a CO_2-enriched gas mixture from a

bag for approximately 4 min. The validity of this approach requires rapid equilibration of CO_2 among alveolar gas, arterial and mixed venous blood, and the chemosensitive areas of the brain. In order to promote equilibration, the volume of the bag is adjusted to about 1 L greater than the patient's vital capacity. It is filled at the outset with a mixture of 7% CO_2 in O_2; O_2 is substituted for air in this mixture to avoid the ambiguity of a hypoxic stimulus to ventilatory drive. The use of a small bag and the gas mixture generally enables equilibration within 30 to 40 s (Fig. 36-33).

During the test, the fasting patient rests quietly while seated or semirecumbent. The procedure is conducted in a quiet room to minimize environmental effects on the ventilatory response. The rebreathing test is stopped after 4 min if the patient complains of dyspnea or if the end-tidal CO_2 concentration exceeds 9%.

The result of the CO_2 rebreathing test is described by use of two terms: (1) the *slope* of the line relating change in ventilation response to change in end-tidal P_{CO_2} ($\Delta\dot{V}E/P_{CO_2}$), determined by using the method of least squares linear regression analysis,

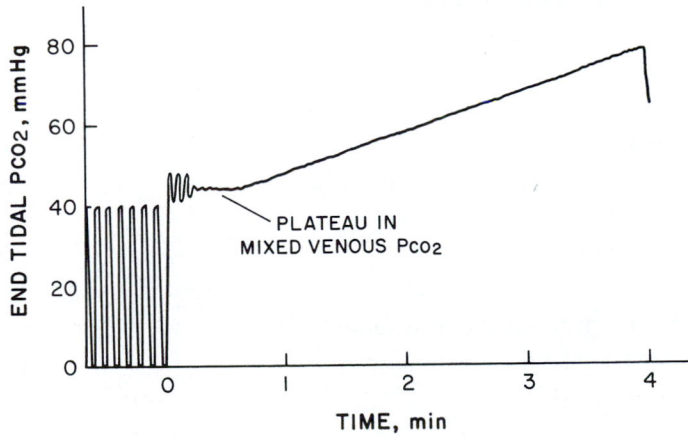

FIGURE 36-33   Rebreathing techniques for assessing the ventilatory response to CO_2. As a gas mixture containing 7% CO_2 is rebreathed, rapid equilibration of P_{CO_2} in alveoli, mixed venous and arterial blood, and the brain chemosensitive areas occurs. Changes in P_{CO_2} at the chemosenors are then reflected in changes in the concentration of CO_2 in the end-tidal gas.

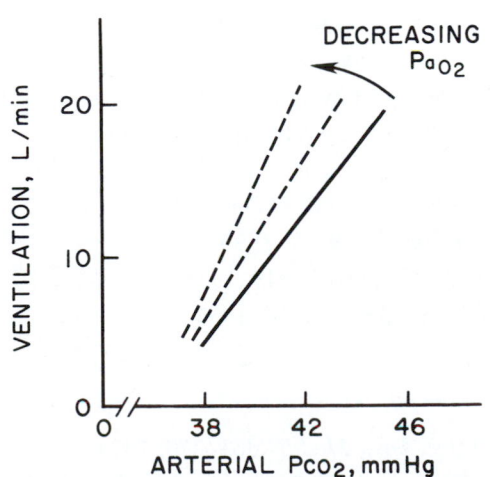

FIGURE 36-32   Linear relationship between minute ventilation ($\dot{V}E$) and arterial P_{CO_2}. The dashed lines show the increased slope of the relationship of $\dot{V}E$ versus P_{CO_2} as Pa_{O_2} decreases.

and (2) the *x-intercept* of the relationship between $\dot{V}_E$ and end-tidal P_{CO_2}. The slope is regarded as the sensitivity or "gain" of the control system, and the x-intercept as the threshold or "set point."

Even though the slope of the ventilatory response to P_{CO_2} may be the same by the steady-state and rebreathing methods, the P_{CO_2} thresholds determined by the methods are different (Fig. 36-34). The higher threshold measured by the rebreathing method may reflect discrepancies between end-tidal P_{CO_2} (and, hence, alveolar and arterial P_{CO_2}) and values of P_{CO_2} in the chemosensitive areas of the brain. Because of this likelihood, the steady-state method is generally considered to be a more meaningful test for determining CO_2 threshold. Nevertheless, the rebreathing test is more popular because of its relative simplicity and the close correspondence between end-tidal (alveolar) P_{CO_2} and arterial P_{CO_2}, even in the presence of lung disease.

NORMAL RESPONSE TO CO2 AND MODIFYING INFLUENCES

As indicated above, the normal increase in ventilatory response to increasing concentrations of inspired CO_2 is linear (Fig. 36-32). Although a subject's ventilatory response determined in the course of a single testing session is usually reproducible, reproducibility often falls off when tests are repeated on different days. In addition, responses differ from person to person. In order to take this variability into account, "normal" responses are categorized as low (under 1.5 L/min/mmHg), intermediate (1.5 to 5.0 L/min/mmHg), and high (more than 5.0 L/min/mmHg). Most normal persons (about 80 percent) have an intermediate ventilatory response.

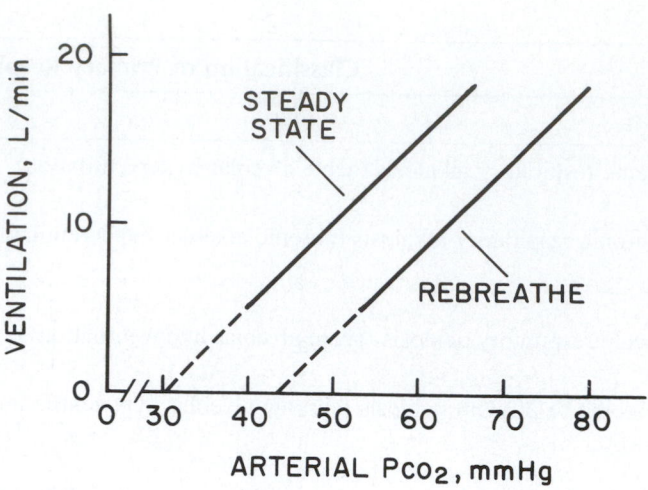

FIGURE 36-34   The relationship between ventilation and arterial P_{CO_2} as determined by the steady-state and rebreathing techniques. Each technique demonstrates the linear relationship between ventilation and P_{CO_2}, and each generates the same slope. However, the thresholds determined by the two methods are different, as discussed in the text.

A variety of factors, both genetic and environmental, seem to influence the ventilatory response to CO_2 (Table 36-14). Also, tidal volume and respiratory frequency are often influenced differently. For example, the tidal volume response appears to be genetically determined, whereas the frequency response appears to depend heavily on environmental or psychological factors.

TABLE 36-14

Factors Associated with an Altered Ventilatory Response to CO₂

Factor	Reference
Depressed Response	
Endurance training	Byrne-Quinn et al: *J Appl Physiol* 30:91–98, 1971
Aging	Peterson et al: *Am Rev Respir Dis* 124:387–391, 1981
Genetic/racial predilection	Beral et al: *Lancet* 2:1290–1294, 1971
Metabolic alkalosis	Koboyashi et al: *Am Rev Respir Dis* 147:1192–1198, 1993
	Heinemann, Goldring: *Am J Med* 57:361–370, 1974
Narcotics, barbiturates, and other CNS depressants	Lambertsen: *Handbook of Physiology,* section 3, *Respiration,* vol I. Washington DC, American Physiological Society, 1964, pp 545–555
Neurologic disorders (encephalitis, brainstem disease)	Plum, Brown: *Ann NY Acad Sci* 109:915–931, 1963
Myxedema	Zwillich et al: *N Engl J Med* 292:662–665, 1975
	Duranti et al: *Am J Med* 95:29–37, 1993
Obesity-hypoventilation syndrome	Zwillich et al: *Am J Med* 59:343–348, 1975
Chronic obstructive pulmonary disease (COPD)	Flenley, Millar: *Clin Sci* 33:319–334, 1967
Accentuated Response	
Metabolic acidosis	Heinemann, Goldring: *Am J Med* 57:361–370, 1974
Drugs (e.g., aminophylline, salicylates, thyroxine, progesterone)	Lambertsen: *Handbook of Physiology,* section 3: *Respiration,* vol I. Washington, DC, American Physiological Society, 1964, pp 545–555

A decreased ventilatory response to CO_2 occurs in endurance athletes, with aging, and in certain racial groups (e.g., the Enges of New Guinea). Acid-base imbalances modify the ventilatory response to CO_2. Low concentrations of bicarbonate in serum and in the brain enhance the response to CO_2 (i.e., increase the slope and decrease the threshold of the $\dot{V}E$ versus-P_{CO_2} curve); high concentrations of bicarbonate have the opposite effect. Drugs and hormones may also alter the CO_2 response. Aminophylline, salicylates, thyroxine, and progesterone increase responsiveness to CO_2, whereas narcotics, barbiturates, and other CNS depressants decrease it. Finally, the ventilatory response to CO_2 is sometimes reduced in certain neurologic diseases (e.g., encephalitis and brain-stem disease), metabolic disorders (e.g., myxedema), the obesity-hypoventilation syndrome, and chronic obstructive disease of the airways.

Ventilatory Response to Hypoxia

The response to acute hypoxia in normal persons is largely shaped by the peripheral arterial chemoreceptors, as long as the level of hypoxia is mild to moderate. Even at sea level, the level of arterial P_{O_2} in normal persons provides an appreciable chemoreceptor drive, accounting for about 10% of the minute ventilation. Unlike the linear response of $\dot{V}E$ to progressive hypercapnia, the response to hypoxemia is curvilinear (Fig. 36-35). The magnitude of the ventilatory response to a decrease in arterial P_{O_2} depends on the Pa_{CO_2}, increasing as the concentration of CO_2 in arterial blood is increased.

As may be seen from the hyperbolic curves in Fig. 36-35, the rate of change in ventilation is greater over the lower range of oxygenation (when Pa_{O_2} falls below 60 mmHg). Not shown in Fig. 36-35 is the depression of ventilation brought about by severe hypoxemia, presumably because of the central depressing effect of severe hypoxia on respiratory neurons.

Although tests for assessing the ventilatory response to hypoxia are less well standardized than those for measuring the hypercapnic response, they, too, may be conveniently categorized into steady-state and non–steady-state methods.

STEADY-STATE METHODS

Because steady-state methods require prolonged exposure to potentially hazardous levels of hypoxemia, clinical testing relies predominantly on non–steady-state methods. However, research laboratories have used two approaches, based on different principles. In one method,[30] successive ventilatory responses are determined to a series of increasingly severe hypoxic gas mixtures, each administered for at least 10 min; Pa_{CO_2} is kept constant by the addition of CO_2 to the inspired gas mixture as hypoxia-induced hyperventilation develops. Another steady-state method tests the effect of hypoxia on the slope of the plot of $\dot{V}E$ versus P_{CO_2} as P_{O_2} is lowered from hyperoxic (at least 200 mmHg) to hypoxic (40 mmHg) levels (Fig. 36-36). As in the previous method, each hypoxic inspired gas mixture is breathed for at least 10 min. The normal response to diminished inspired oxygen concentrations is characterized by an increase in sensitivity (slope) without a change in the CO_2 threshold. The magnitude of the increase is designated as $\Delta\dot{V}_{40}$ (the difference between the minute ventilation in breathing gas with a P_{O_2} of at least 200 mmHg and in breathing gas with a P_{O_2} of 40 mmHg at a P_{CO_2} of 40 mmHg).

NON–STEADY-STATE METHODS

Three non–steady-state techniques are currently in use. Two are rebreathing tests; the other is a "few breaths" test.

In the hypoxic rebreathing test,[44] the subject rebreathes a hypoxic gas mixture containing 7% CO_2. As arterial hypoxemia intensifies, causing an increase in ventilation and in CO_2 elimination into the closed circuit, the P_{CO_2} in the system is held constant at a predetermined level by the diversion of a fraction of the expired gas through a CO_2 absorber. The ventilatory response is determined at two or more levels of P_{CO_2}, since the hypoxic response is influenced by P_{CO_2} (Fig. 36-35). $\dot{V}E$ is plotted against

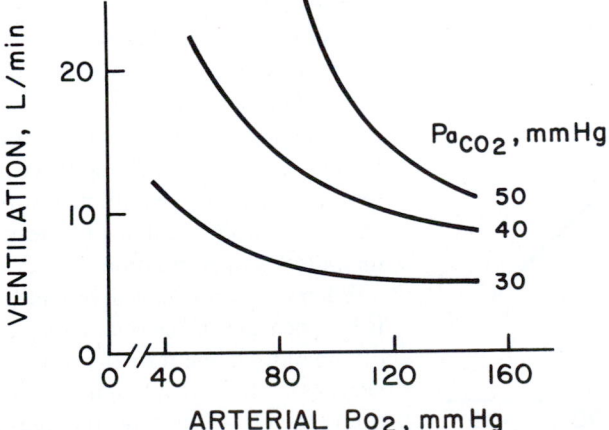

FIGURE 36-35 The curvilinear relationship between ventilation and arterial P_{O_2} at various levels of arterial P_{CO_2}. The rate of change of ventilation as P_{O_2} falls (slope) increases precipitously at a P_{O_2} of approximately 60 mmHg when P_{CO_2} is 40 mmHg. The abrupt increase in ventilation occurs at a higher P_{O_2} when the level of P_{CO_2} is elevated, and at a lower P_{O_2} when the prevailing P_{CO_2} is lower.

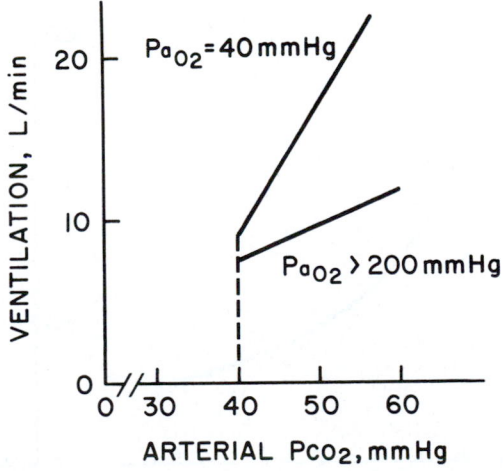

FIGURE 36-36 Method proposed for expressing the ventilatory response to hypoxia. The change in ventilation as a function of the change in arterial P_{CO_2} is determined under hyperoxic (P_{O_2} >200 mmHg) and hypoxic (P_{O_2} = 40 mmHg) conditions. The hypoxic response is measured as the difference in ventilation between the hyperoxic and hypoxic determination at a P_{CO_2} of 40 mmHg. *(From Severinghaus, Chest 70(Suppl):129–131, 1976.)*

arterial P_{O_2} (Fig. 36-37A) or arterial O_2 saturation (Fig. 36-37B). The advantage of using O_2 saturation instead of arterial P_{O_2} is that the $\dot{V}_E$–O_2 saturation relationship is linear (Fig. 36-37B).

An alternative rebreathing test[55] induces progressive hypoxemia by adding N_2 to the inspired gas mixture over a 20-min period. Ventilation is plotted as a function of the term $1/(P_{O_2} - 32)$, to produce a linear relationship that is described by the slope "A," also known as the "shape parameter" (Fig. 36-38). The greater the sensitivity to hypoxia, the greater is the slope and the larger is the shape parameter. When $\dot{V}_E$ is plotted as a function of Pa_{O_2}, the shape parameter provides a measure of the degree of curvature of the plot.

Finally, in a relatively simple test,[15] the patient induces a transient drop in arterial P_{O_2} by inhaling pure N_2 for a few breaths. The relationship between $\dot{V}_E$ and Pa_{O_2} is plotted; the slope of the relationship is the sensitivity to hypoxia. Because the duration of the hypoxia is brief, presumably only the peripheral chemoreceptors are stimulated. No adjustment is made for the drop in P_{CO_2} that occurs during the hypoxia-stimulated increase in ventilation.

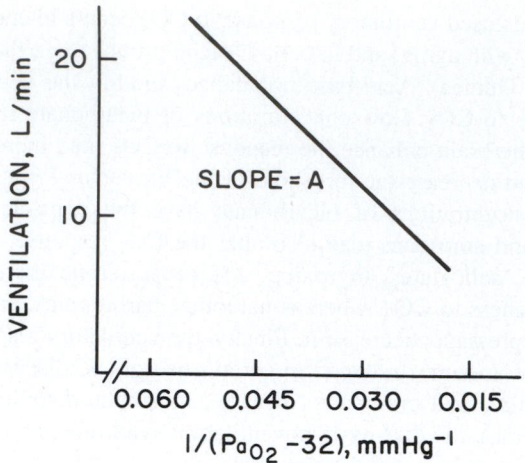

FIGURE 36-38 Measurement of the ventilatory response to hypoxia using the method of Weil et al.[55] The relationship between ventilation and the term, $1/(Pa_{O_2}-32)$, is linear. The slope of the line, A, is known as the "shape parameter" and is an expression of hypoxic chemosensitivity.

NORMAL RESPONSES TO HYPOXIA AND MODIFYING INFLUENCES

The normal ventilatory response to acute hypoxia varies from person to person. Several factors may influence the relationship (Table 36-15): 1. A high ventilatory response to CO_2 may be associated with a high sensitivity to hypoxia. 2. The level of arterial P_{CO_2} influences the magnitude of the hypoxic response (Fig. 36-35): at higher levels of arterial P_{CO_2}, the ventilatory response to hypoxia increases. 3. The duration of hypoxia before the test period is important: native residents at high altitude and persons with cyanotic congenital heart disease manifest a diminished sensitivity ("blunted response") to acute hypoxia. In cardiac patients, hypoxic insensitivity is reversed after successful surgery. 4. The normal aging process is associated with a

depressed response. 5. A variety of other clinical disorders, including myxedema and hypothyroidism, autonomic nervous system dysfunction, chronic narcotic addiction, and the chronic use of methadone, are characterized by a reduced hypoxic response. 6. Carotid endarterectomy diminishes the ventilatory response to acute hypoxia.

Nonventilatory Measures of Ventilatory Drive

Measurement of ventilation in response to acute hypoxia or hypercapnia provides a useful index of respiratory output when the ventilatory apparatus (thorax, diaphragm, abdominal muscles, lung, and airways) is normal. This situation obviously does not apply in certain neuromuscular disorders in which the thorax and diaphragm behave abnormally. In addition, it does not apply in some instances of pulmonary disease, notably obstructive airway disease, in which the respiratory apparatus may not be capable of responding normally, even though it is intact and chemosensitivity is normal. In this instance, a decrease in ventilatory response may be attributable to the excessive mechanical load placed on the muscles of respiration.

When ventilation fails to provide a reliable measure of the ventilatory drive (efferent discharge from the respiratory neurons), the diaphragmatic electromyograph (EMG) or the pressure generated by the inspiratory muscles during the first 0.1 s of an occluded inspiration (the $P_{0.1}$)[56] has been used for the clinical assessment of the control of breathing.

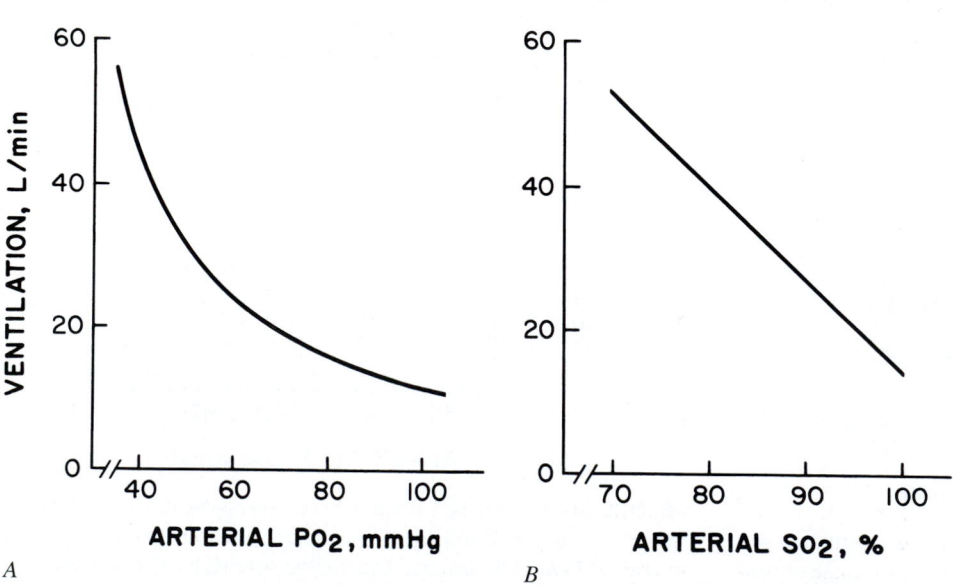

FIGURE 36-37 The ventilatory response to hypoxia. The relationship between ventilation and arterial P_{O_2} (A) is curvilinear, while that between ventilation and arterial saturation (B) is linear.

TABLE 36-15

Factors Associated With an Altered Ventilatory Response to Hypoxia

Factor	Reference
Depressed Response	
Long-standing hypoxia	
High-altitude dwelling	Severinghaus et al: *Respir Physiol* 1:308–334, 1966
Congenital cyanotic heart disease	Blesa et al: *N Engl J Med* 296:237–241, 1977 Blesa et al: *N Engl J Med* 296:237–241, 1977
Aging	Kronenberg et al: *J Clin Invest* 52:1812–1819, 1973
Hypothyroidism	Zwillich et al: *N Engl J Med* 292:662–665, 1975
Riley-Day syndrome	Edelman et al: *J Clin Invest* 49:1153–1165, 1970
Chronic use of methadone	Marks: *Am Rev Respir Dis* 108:1088–1093, 1970
Following carotid endarterectomy	Wade et al: *N Engl J Med* 282:823–829, 1970
Accentuated Response	
Heightened CO_2 response	Rebuck et al: *J Appl Physiol* 35:173–177, 1973
Hypercapnia	Rebuck, Woodley: *J Appl Physiol* 38:16–19, 1975

The electrical activity of the diaphragm is directly related to neural activity of the phrenic nerve. Therefore, it provides a measure of efferent neural traffic to the diaphragm. The diaphragmatic EMG may be recorded in patients by placing the tip of an esophageal catheter, containing bipolar electrodes, at the level of the diaphragm.

The second approach to obtaining a nonventilatory measure of ventilatory drive is the determination of $P_{0.1}$, which is the negative pressure generated by the inspiratory muscles during the first 100 ms of an inspiratory effort made against an occluded airway. During this brief period, contraction of the respiratory muscles is virtually isometric, and the force generated correlates with activity recorded by the diaphragmatic EMG.

In performing the test, airflow in the inspiratory line of the breathing circuit is randomly interrupted during the preceding expiration. The 100-ms period has proved to be so brief as to be imperceptible, thereby obviating any corrective action by the subject during the breath against the occlusion. However, the $P_{0.1}$ is far from foolproof. A major concern is that $P_{0.1}$ is affected by resting lung volume: $P_{0.1}$ is reduced when FRC is abnormally high, a common occurrence in obstructive disease of the airways.

QUALITY CONTROL IN THE PULMONARY FUNCTION LABORATORY

Meaningful interpretation of pulmonary function tests requires confidence in the accuracy and reproducibility of results provided by the pulmonary function laboratory. Until recently, it was tacitly assumed that all data from all laboratories, especially when reported as "percent predicted," were equally reliable. In recent years, the fallacy of this assumption has been explicitly recognized, and steps have been taken to standardize equipment and procedures and to ensure accuracy, reproducibility, and uniformity in testing and reporting.[1,2] To accomplish this goal, both analytical and nonanalytical factors must be taken into account.

Nonanalytical Factors in Quality Control

A familiar example of a confounding influence that may distort test results is the anxious patient who pauses outside the laboratory door to "calm the nerves" by smoking one or more cigarettes before undergoing pulmonary function testing. Cigarette smoking before the diffusing capacity of the lungs is determined can generate enough carboxyhemoglobin to reduce a normal value to subnormal levels.

Another example of a nonanalytical factor is the failure to achieve patient understanding and comfort for tests that usually require patient cooperation. Unfortunately, preliminary explanations before the patient arrives at the laboratory or prior exposure of the patient to the laboratory and its personnel is usually impractical. Use of explanatory sheets or descriptive brochures may prove helpful. If such materials are not available, laboratory personnel are obligated to make the patient comfortable and even perform "practice runs" before undertaking final testing.

When the patient arrives at the pulmonary function laboratory, an assessment should be made of his or her prior experiences. Did the patient undergo other tests or procedures that could alter the outcome of the pulmonary function tests in question? Is the patient fatigued or in pain? Should a period of rest precede the tests in order to ensure optimal performance? If delay is impractical, the test report should include the fact that the patient was fatigued or in pain.

Medication use before pulmonary function testing can seriously affect the results. For example, self-administration of bronchodilators before testing can artificially enhance tests of airflow. If medications have been taken before the patient arrives at the laboratory, the time of administration should be part of the record. Also, a request for pulmonary function test results for patients who regularly take bronchodilators should indicate whether the tests are to be done without interruption of the regular schedule of medications, whether bronchodilators are to be discontinued before the test is done, or whether regular bronchodilators are to be discontinued so that the effects of bronchodilation can be tested. Appropriate comments about bronchodilators are part of the report.

A major nonanalytical cause of misinterpreting results is the inappropriate application of predicted normal values to the patient population by the laboratory (see "Approach to Interpreting Commonly Performed Pulmonary Function Tests," below). For example, normal values based on data obtained using physically fit hospital personnel do not necessarily apply to those who have a sedentary existence. Noncomparable race, as well as lifestyle, may complicate comparisons.[18] Anthropologic differences among control and test populations are not easily reconciled. Extraordinary height, weight, or age cannot be easily extrapolated if corresponding subjects are not represented in the control group. Using patient-reported height, rather than making measurement of patient height, may introduce an error in the selection of appropriate normal values.[39] Comparison of control and test results at different altitudes can be invalid if due regard is not paid to the influence of hypoxia on certain measurements (e.g., diffusing capacity).

Analytical Factors in Quality Control

Performance of pulmonary function tests is replete with opportunities for error. The equipment, techniques, use of control values, and calculations are potential sources of error. In an attempt to minimize errors, standardization of techniques has been advocated. For example, with respect to performing the forced vital capacity maneuver, guidelines have been established for the number of attempts required, acceptable variability between efforts, and methods for selecting test data in order to arrive at acceptable results. To avoid misuse of spirometers, criteria have been set for minimal performance with respect to capacity, accuracy, and frequency response of various spirometers;[2] in addition, standards have been developed for determining the single-breath diffusing capacity.[1] Potential sources of discrepancies—such as breath-holding time, concentration of hemoglobin, dead space of the equipment and the patient, F_{IO_2}, volume of the alveolar sample, number of tests, and acceptable variability in results—are taken into account.

Unfortunately, setting standards is a long, tedious undertaking. For example, despite several publications that deal with quality control for the helium-dilution, nitrogen-washout, and body plethysmographic techniques, no official standards have yet been set, and no clear picture exists of the differences in the results that these tests provide.

Quality Control of Test Results

Guidelines for standardization play a major role in reducing discrepancies between laboratories. However, measures are also required to ensure accuracy and reproducibility within any given laboratory. Among the elements of control that merit consideration are calibration, validation of calibration, and performance of a control measurement. *Calibration* is the adjustment of an instrument's output so that it validly reflects a known input. *Verification of calibration* entails introduction of the same known input and demonstration that the correct output is reproduced. *Performance of a control measurement* refers to the testing of a substrate that has known properties, similar to those usually tested, to prove the accuracy of the instrumentation. One example of the application of these principles is blood gas analysis. Use of control measurements derived from tonometered blood or commercially prepared buffer solutions is now widespread.

Unfortunately, similar controls do not exist for pulmonary function tests. Therefore, laboratory technologists have the responsibility for continuing to be alert, not only with respect to faithful observance of guidelines for standardization but also to

detect in-house sources of error—e.g., a leak in the system, malfunction of gas analyzers, faulty analog-to-digital converters, and faulty electronics that reduce frequency response.

Responsibility and Cost in Quality Control

All who work in the laboratory must be concerned with quality control, despite the frequent temptation to cut corners. Indeed, one common rationalization for not doing so is the misguided impression that quality control, as described above, is too expensive. Time has to be set aside for the technologist to care for and calibrate equipment, to establish proper control values for the laboratory, to search for inconsistencies in the data and interpretation, and to keep up with changing standards. Also, equipment and supplies, including calibrating syringes and calibrating gases, are expensive. However, when put into the balance, the cost and waste of producing erroneous results exceed, by far, the expense of practicing quality control.

Infection Control

Given the relatively close contact between patients and technical staff during performance of pulmonary function tests, the issue of infection control is one that must be carefully considered. To date, the role of pulmonary function equipment in transmission of disease appears to be minimal. Although the presence of potential pathogens on laboratory mouthpieces, valves, and tubing has been well documented, implication of these organisms in the transmission of disease has not been established. Nevertheless, the potential hazards should be recognized and appropriate care exercised.

Infection control begins with practice of the basic principles of hygiene. Handwashing between patients and use of protective gloves by staff when they are handling potentially contaminated equipment are important considerations. Care must be taken in working with mouthpieces, nose clips, and any other implements that come in contact with mucosal surfaces. These devices, if reused, should be disinfected or sterilized after each use. Other equipment—manifolds, tubing, etc.—should be sterilized on a regular basis. In fact, guidelines from the American Thoracic Society call for the disinfection or sterilization before reuse of any equipment surface with visible condensation from expired air.[1,52]

Because of recent growing concern over cross-contamination among patients and laboratory personnel, manufacturers now produce a variety of in-line filters and disposable pneumotachographs. Care should be taken, however, to assure that response characteristics of the test equipment are not driven to unacceptable levels by use of these devices. Current literature on this topic should be consulted regularly.

APPROACH TO INTERPRETING COMMONLY PERFORMED PULMONARY FUNCTION TESTS

A standard battery of pulmonary function tests is commonly used to identify and quantify abnormalities in the performance of the respiratory system. Once a patient's baseline values are established, the tests are valuable in tracking the course of the disorder and its response to treatment.

As a rule, results of pulmonary function tests are interpreted with respect to predicted values for normal subjects. Originally, predicted values were based on standard linear regression equations that used age, height, and weight in calculating normal values, treating the two sexes separately. Subsequently, curvilinear or exponential equations came into use for predicting normal values. Despite dedicated attempts to improve prediction formulas, however, many still fail to take into account important sources of discrepancy, such as the racial and ethnic backgrounds of the patients and the control population, the effects of altitude and exposure to air pollution, and effects of inordinate body size or old age. As a result, not all sets of predicted normals are applicable in pulmonary function laboratories outside the immediate vicinity of the patient populations from whom the data were collected.

For most pulmonary function tests, normal values fall in a broad range that is assumed to follow a normal (gaussian) distribution. Traditionally, but without sound statistical basis, most laboratories have arbitrarily set upper and lower limits of normal, as well as gradations of abnormality, using percentage of predicted normal mean values.

Two alternative methods for expressing results have been proposed. One, the *95 percentile method,* defines the lower limit of normal as the value above which lie the values for 95 percent of the normal population.[28] Too few data are available for the practical utility of this method to be determined. The other method uses 95 percent confidence intervals.[34]

The 95 percent confidence interval method defines the limits of normal as the predicted value plus or minus the 95 percent confidence interval. The degree of abnormality for a particular test is expressed in terms of the *number* of 95 percent confidence intervals above or below the predicted normal; this number is calculated as the predicted normal value minus the measured value, divided by the confidence interval. In the discussion and tables that follow, the magnitude of abnormality is expressed both in traditional terms (ranges with respect to percent of predicted normal mean values) and in 95 percent confidence intervals.

Classification of Abnormal Patterns

A number of different schemes have been proposed for sorting out patterns of abnormalities in pulmonary function tests. The following categories of patterns have proved to have practical value.

1. *Obstructive.* This pattern stems from narrowing of any portion of the airways—from upper airway to bronchioles less than 2 mm in diameter—that reduces airflow.
2. *Restrictive.* This pattern is elicited by diseases of the lung, chest wall, pleural space, or neuromuscular respiratory apparatus that reduce the vital capacity and lung volumes, particularly total lung capacity.
3. *Combined obstructive-restrictive.* This pattern results from pathologic processes that reduce lung volumes, vital capacity, and airflow, and that also include an element of airway narrowing.
4. *Abnormal gas transfer.* The abnormality is in the alveolar-capillary membrane. The impairment used as a marker is oxygen uptake from alveolar gas to pulmonary capillary

blood. The outstanding feature is a reduction in the diffusing capacity for carbon monoxide ($D_{L_{CO}}$).

Overlap among categories is not uncommon. For example, widespread interstitial disease of the lungs, as in sarcoidosis, often shows a pattern that indicates important components of both restrictive disease and abnormal gas transfer.

A standard approach is advisable for interpreting pulmonary function tests. One simple, but useful, sequence for analyzing a conventional battery of tests is illustrated in Fig. 36-39. Analysis of the results begins with assessment of respiratory muscle strength, using peak inspiratory and expiratory pressures. These tests are useful in "routine spirometry" as an index of the extent to which the patient has exerted himself or herself during the testing. In addition, a poor response calls attention to the possibility of neuromuscular or respiratory disease.

After peak pressures have been assessed, the $FEV_1/FVC\%$, FVC, and FEV_1 are examined in turn. The appraisal up to this juncture generally suffices to indicate whether an obstructive or restrictive pattern is likely. Indeed, this panel of studies is useful as "screening spirometry" and may suffice to exclude appreciable disease of the lungs or airways. If the results of the flow studies are abnormal, additional insight into the nature of the disorder may be gained from examination of the lung volumes.

Finally, the $D_{L_{CO}}$ is determined and interpreted with regard to any abnormalities that may have been uncovered by the tests.

This battery is exceedingly useful at first encounter. Once the predominant abnormality is defined, the whole battery may not be necessary in following the course of the disease or in assessing its response to treatment. Instead, particular determinations, such as the $FEV_1/FVC\%$, may suffice.

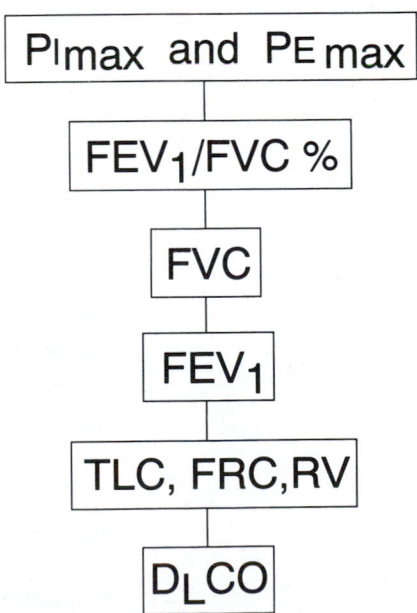

FIGURE 36-39 Proposed sequence of test review in the interpretation of pulmonary function tests. See text for discussion.

Assessing Respiratory Muscle Strength and Effort

The strength of the respiratory muscles is expressed in terms of peak inspiratory (PI_{max}) and peak expiratory (PE_{max}) pressures, determined under static conditions.[3] The technique was outlined in a previous section. Any of a number of factors may be responsible for low peak inspiratory or expiratory pressures (Table 36-16): suboptimal effort, fatigue, weakness of the respiratory muscles, deformity of the chest wall, or intrinsic diseases of the lungs or chest wall. Although the first three factors characteristically reduce both peak inspiratory and expiratory pressures, disease of the lungs or chest wall often reduces, selectively, one or the other peak pressure. Thus, diseases that reduce lung volumes (e.g., widespread interstitial fibrosis) and shorten the length of the expiratory muscles at the end-inspiratory position generally reduce maximal expiratory pressure. Conversely, diseases that increase lung volume, such as obstructive airway disease, by decreasing the inspiratory muscle length at end-expiration generally reduce maximal inspiratory pressure.

If airflow during spirometry is reduced, determination of the peak inspiratory and expiratory pressures may be helpful in suggesting the mechanism. Many pulmonary function tests depend on the cooperation of the patient. Poorly reproducible peak flows that are consistently subnormal raise the question of poor effort. Conversely, consistently low values that occur despite maximal effort may signal neuromuscular disease.

Obstructive Pattern

Included in this group of disorders (Table 36-17) are chronic obstructive diseases of the airways (chronic bronchitis and emphysema), cystic fibrosis, asthma, small-airway disease, and upper-airway obstruction.

Except for diseases confined to the small airways, the hallmark of the obstructive pattern is a reduction in the $FEV_1/FVC\%$ (Table 36-18). This measurement is also useful in quantifying

TABLE 36-16

Conditions Associated with Reduced Peak Inspiratory (PI_{max}) and Expiratory (PE_{max}) Pressures

Condition	PI_{max}	PE_{max}
Poor effort	↓	↓
Fatigue	↓	↓
Neuromuscular disease	↓	↓
Increased lung volume	↓	N
Decreased lung volume	N	↓

NOTE: ↓ = decreased; N = normal

the magnitude of the disorder (Table 36-19). In addition, the FEV_1 is consistently reduced and usually accompanied by a reduction in FVC. As a rule, the slow vital capacity is also abnormally low. A greater reduction in the forced vital capacity than in the slow vital capacity indicates air trapping.

Changes in lung volume commonly accompany the abnormal findings on spirometry. Frequently, but not invariably, lung volumes are abnormally high. Typically, all three lung volumes—residual volume, functional residual capacity, and total lung capacity—are increased. The increase in TLC or RV is useful in quantifying the degree of "hyperinflation" (Table 36-20).

In addition to uncovering the pattern of chronic obstructive airway disease described above, certain additional tests provide insight into the sites and mechanisms of obstructive airway disease.

REVERSIBLE VERSUS IRREVERSIBLE OBSTRUCTIVE AIRWAY DISEASE

The response to inhaled bronchodilators (Table 36-18) is helpful in distinguishing between chronic obstructive airway disease (chronic bronchitis and emphysema), in which airway resistance

TABLE 36-17

Causes of an Obstructive Pattern

Disease Process	Anatomic Location of Lesion	Cause of Reduced Airflow
Chronic obstructive pulmonary disease (COPD)		
Chronic bronchitis	Large and small (<2-mm diameter) airways	Narrowing of airways by fibrosis, secretions, edema
Emphysema	Lung parenchyma	Loss of lung elastic recoil
Cystic fibrosis	Large and small airways	Narrowing of airways by fibrosis, retained secretions, edema
		Loss of elastic recoil
Asthma	Large and small airways	Narrowing of airways by smooth-muscle contraction, edema, retained secretions
Small-airway disease	Small airways	Narrowing, stenosis of small airways
Upper-airway obstruction	Major, central airways (trachea, main bronchi)	Anatomic or functional narrowing of upper airway

TABLE 36-18

Distinguishing Features of Disorders Producing an Obstructive Pattern

Disorder	FEV_1	FVC	FEV_1/FVC%	Response of FEV_1 to Administration of Bronchodilator	Tests of Small-Airway Function	Lung Volumes	$D_{L_{CO}}$	Flow-Volume Loop
COPD								
Chronic bronchitis	↓	↓	↓	NC	ABN	↑	NL	ABN
Emphysema	↓	↓	↓	NC	ABN	↑	↓	ABN
Asthma	↓	↓	↓	↑	ABN	↑	NL	ABN
Small-airway disease	NL	NL	NL	NC	ABN	NL	NL	NL
Upper-airway obstruction	↓	↓	↓	NC	NL or ABN	NL or ↑	NL	ABN*

*Configuration frequently characteristic for upper airway obstruction.
NOTE: ↓ = decrease; ↑ = increase, NC = no significant change; NL = normal; ABN = abnormal.

TABLE 36-19

Categorization of Obstruction: Measurement of FEV₁/FVC%

	% Predicted Method	95% Confidence Interval (CI) Method		
			Predicted Minus Measured FEV_1/FVC%	
Category	Absolute FEV_1/FVC%	No. CIs Below Mean	Male	Female
Normal	>69	<1	<8.3	<9.1
Mild obstruction	61–69	(≥1–<2	8.3–16.5	9.1–18.1
Moderate obstruction	45–60	≥2–<4	16.6–33.1	18.2–36.3
Severe obstruction	<45	≥4	≥33.2	≥36.4

SOURCE: Guidelines from Kanner and Morris: *Clinical Pulmonary Function Testing: A Manual of Uniform Laboratory Procedures.* Salt Lake City, Intermountain Thoracic Society, 1975; Morris et al.[34]

TABLE 36-20

Categorization of Hyperinflation: Measurement of TLC and RV

	% Predicted Method	95% Confidence Interval (CI) Method		
			Measured Minus Predicted TLC, L*	
Category	TLC or RV, % Predicted	No. CIs Above Mean TLC	Male	Female
Normal	≤120	<1.0	<1.61	<1.08
Mild hyperinflation	121–<134	≥1.0–<1.5	1.61–2.41	1.08–1.61
Moderate hyperinflation	135–<149	≥1.5–<2.0	2.42–3.21	1.62–2.15
Severe hyperinflation	≥150	≥2	≥3.22	≥2.16

*The classification of normal is based additionally on a difference between predicted and measured RV of <0.76 L for males and <0.78 L for females. Differences in RV exceeding these values when differences in TLC are normal are suggestive of hyperinflation.

SOURCE: Guidelines from Kanner and Morris: *Clinical Pulmonary Function Testing: A Manual of Uniform Laboratory Procedures.* Salt Lake City, Intermountain Thoracic Society, 1975; Morris et al.[34]

TABLE 36-21

Categorization of Bronchodilator Response: Measurement of Vital Capacity and Expiratory Flow Rates Before and After Bronchodilator Administration

| | Measurement* | | |
Category	FVC	FEV$_1$	FEF$_{25-75\%}$
Not responsive	<1.05	<1.05	<1.10
Not clearly responsive	1.05–1.14	1.05–1.11	1.10–1.44
Responsive	1.15–1.24	1.12–1.24	1.45–1.99
Markedly responsive	≥1.25	≥1.25	≥2.00

*Each value represents the ratio of the measurement made after administration of a bronchodilator to that made before.

SOURCE: Guidelines from Morris et al.[34]

is virtually fixed, and asthma, in which bronchoconstriction is a prominent feature. Inhalation of a bronchodilator significantly improves expiratory airflow in asthma but not in chronic bronchitis or emphysema. One indication of responsiveness to a bronchodilator is a decrease in lung volumes toward normal. The magnitude of the response to a bronchodilator can be expressed semiquantitatively (Table 36-21).

CHRONIC BRONCHITIS VERSUS EMPHYSEMA

Although chronic bronchitis and emphysema usually coexist, occasionally one or the other exists in virtually pure form. Two pulmonary function tests have proved valuable in distinguishing between the two: diffusing capacity (D$_{CO}$) and static lung compliance (Cst,L). Emphysema, characterized by a loss of alveolar units and a decrease in alveolar surface area, is associated with a low D$_{CO}$, whereas the D$_{CO}$ in chronic bronchitis is usually normal or near normal.

The loss of alveolar units in emphysema also causes a decrease in the elastic recoil pressure of the lungs (see Chapters 10 and 55). As a result, Cst,L is increased in emphysema, whereas it is usually not appreciably altered in chronic bronchitis.

SMALL AIRWAY DISEASE

In obstructive disease of the small airways (less than 2 mm in diameter), expiratory flow is usually normal, except at low lung volumes; i.e., the FEV$_3$ and FEF$_{25-75\%}$ are abnormally low. Other tests of small airway disease, including the helium-oxygen flow-volume loop, nitrogen washout test, and frequency dependence of dynamic compliance, are also usually abnormal. Lung volumes and D$_{CO}$ are normal. Bronchodilators are virtually without effect (Table 36-18).

The practical value of tests of small airway function is problematic. At one time, high hopes were held that early detection of small-airway disease

might reinforce measures, such as cessation of smoking, that would prevent or arrest progression to irreversible obstructive disease of the airways. However, enthusiasm for testing for small-airway disease has waned, since it is still unclear if small airway disease is a reversible phase in the evolution of clinically significant obstructive airway disease that affects larger bronchi.

UPPER-AIRWAY OBSTRUCTION

The designation *upper airway obstruction* is an umbrella for anatomic or functional narrowing of the large upper airways—the larynx, extra- and intrathoracic trachea, and lobar bronchi. Although upper-airway obstruction of any cause (see Chapter 52), may reduce expiratory or inspiratory airflow, an alteration in the contour of the flow-volume loop has proved to be the most reliable abnormality in conventional pulmonary function testing.

Upper-airway obstruction can be divided into three major types: (1) fixed obstruction, (2) variable extrathoracic obstruction, and (3) variable intrathoracic obstruction.[29]

A *fixed obstruction*, such as tracheal narrowing by scar tissue at the site of a previous tracheotomy, is one in which the geometry and cross-sectional area of the lesion do not change during the respiratory cycle. Characteristically, both inspiratory and expiratory flows are affected about equally (Fig. 36-40A).

A *variable obstruction* is one in which the configuration of the obstructive lesion changes with the phases of respiration. Depending on its location in the tracheobronchial tree (extra- or intrathoracic), this type of lesion usually affects predominantly either inspiration or expiration.

The inspiratory arm of the flow-volume loop is primarily af-

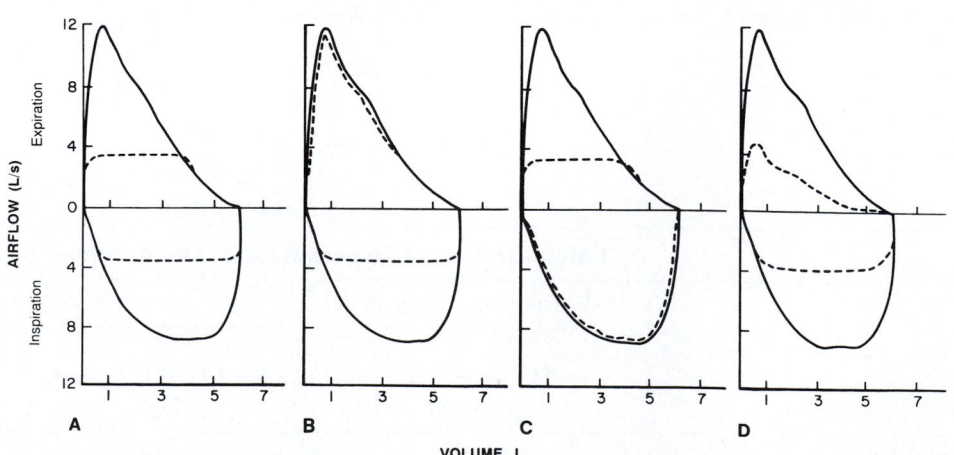

FIGURE 36-40   Schematic flow-volume loops in four pathologic conditions. *A.* In a fixed upper-airway obstruction, both inspiratory and expiratory limbs are truncated. *B.* In a variable extrathoracic obstruction, the inspiratory limb is flattened while the expiratory limb is not altered. *C.* In a variable intrathoracic obstruction, the expiratory limb is flattened while the inspiratory portion is unchanged. *D.* In chronic obstructive airway disease, although expiratory airflow is reduced, the tapering in airflow during expiration is generally maintained so that the configuration of the loop is different from that in variable intrathoracic obstruction.

fected by a *variable extrathoracic* obstruction, leaving the expiratory limb relatively unaffected (Fig. 36-40*B*). The abnormal configuration of the flow-volume loop is attributable to the following sequence: during forced expiration, tracheal pressure exceeds atmospheric, so that the degree of obstruction decreases; conversely, during forced inspiration, intratracheal pressure becomes less than atmospheric and the trachea tends to collapse.

The expiratory arm of the flow-volume loop is primarily affected by a *variable intrathoracic* obstruction (Fig. 36-40*C*). The following sequence is responsible for producing this abnormality in the flow-volume loop: during forced expiration, as pleural pressure reaches and then exceeds intratracheal pressure downstream from the lesion (i.e., toward the mouth), the obstruction tends to increase; conversely, during a forced inspiration, as intratracheal pressure exceeds pleural pressure, the intrathoracic obstruction decreases.

Not infrequently, variable intrathoracic lesions coexist with obstructive airway disease. In considering a variable intrathoracic lesion, we must distinguish between the respective roles played by obstructive disease of the airways (i.e., chronic bronchitis, emphysema, and asthma) and an obstructive upper-airway lesion (anatomic or functional) in deforming the flow-volume loop. Fortunately, this distinction is often possible. Although both upper-airway obstruction and obstructive airway disease (reversible and irreversible) do decrease maximal expiratory flow, the shapes of the flow-volume cures are frequently quite distinctive (Fig. 36-40*C* and *D*). Thus, in obstructive airway disease, despite a decrease in airflow, the expiratory limb of the loop generally retains its normal configuration (Fig. 36-40*D*)—i.e., an early peak in flow, followed by gradual tapering. In contrast, in upper-airway obstruction (fixed and variable intrathoracic), the expiratory limb is flat and flow is decreased throughout most of expiration (Fig. 36-40*C*).

In addition to changes in the shape of the flow-volume loop, clues from routine pulmonary function tests often alert the clinician to the possibility of upper-airway obstruction. The presence of any of the following indices should prompt the clinician to evaluate further the possibility of upper-airway obstruction: $FEF_{50\%}/FIF_{50\%}$ of at least 1, where $FEF_{50\%}$ and $FIF_{50\%}$ are the forced expiratory flow at 50 percent of FVC and the forced inspiratory flow at 50 percent of FIVC, respectively; $FEV_1/PEFR$ greater than 10 ml/L/min, where PEFR is the peak expiratory flow; $FIF_{50\%}$ less than 100 L/min; and $FEV_1/FEV_{0.5}$ at least 1.5.

Restrictive Pattern

The restrictive pattern (Table 36-22) characteristically occurs in several groups of disorders including: (1) a primary disorder of the lung parenchyma in which functional tissue is lost through disease (e.g., an alveolar filling process, such as pneumonia, tumor, atelectasis, or fibrosis); (2) surgical removal of lung tissue (e.g., lobectomy); (3) constrictive disease of the pleura and chest wall (e.g., extensive pleural fibrosis, large pleural effusion or pleural mass, kyphoscoliosis, obesity); and (4) neuromuscular diseases, notably those in which the generation of respiratory force is reduced (e.g., disorders of the spinal cord, peripheral nerves, neuromuscular junction, and muscle).

The hallmark of the restrictive pattern is a reduction in the vital capacity, accompanied by a proportional drop in the FEV_1. As a result, $FEV_1/FVC\%$ remains normal. Indeed, not uncommonly, because of an increase in elastic recoil pressure caused by many of the disease processes that evoke a restrictive pattern, $FEV_1/FVC\%$ is greater than normal.

Characteristically, lung volumes are reduced. However, different compartments are primarily affected in the four categories enumerated above. TLC generally is reduced in all. However, while FRC is usually preserved in disorders characterized by decreased respiratory force (e.g., the neuromuscular disorders), it is reduced in the others. In the neuromuscular disorders, expiratory reserve volume is decreased because of loss of expiratory force, so that RV is often increased. In the other types of restrictive disorders, RV is usually reduced. Both the VC and lung volumes have been used to categorize the degree of restriction (Table 36-23).

Whether or not the D_{LCO} is reduced in the restrictive disorders depends on the underlying disease process. Primary parenchymal disorders and removal of lung tissue decrease the diffusing surface area and reduce D_{LCO}. Diseases of the pleura and chest wall that limit thoracic excursion during the inspiratory vital capacity maneuver, which is part of the technique for determining D_{LCO}, also reduce this measurement.

TABLE 36-22

Causes of a Restrictive Pattern

Disease Process	Anatomic Location of Lesion	Cause of Pulmonary Function Test Abnormality
Primary parenchymal disease	Lung parenchyma	Loss of lung tissue → reduced volumes and flows
Surgical removal of lung tissue	Lung parenchyma	Loss of lung tissue → reduced volumes and flows
Diseases of pleura and chest wall	Pleura, chest wall	Limited expansion of thoracic cavity → reduced volumes and flows
Reduced generation of expiratory force	CNS, peripheral nerves, neuromuscular junction, muscles of respiration	Reduced muscle tension → reduced expiratory flow, atelectasis

TABLE 36-23

Quantitation of Restriction: Measurement of VC and TLC

| | *% Predicted Method* | | | | *95% Confidence Interval (CI) Method* | | | |
| | | | *No. CIs Below Mean* | | *Male* | | *Female* | |
Category	*VC, % Predicted*	*TLC, % Predicted*	*VC*	*TLC*	*VC*	*TLC*	*VC*	*TLC*
Normal	≥81	≥81	<1	<1	<1.12	<1.61	<0.68	<1.08
Mild restriction	66–80	66–80	≥1–1.75	≥1–1.5	1.12–1.95	1.61–2.41	0.68–1.18	1.08–1.61
Moderate restriction	51–65	51–65	≥1.75–2.5	≥1.5–2	1.96–2.79	2.42–3.21	1.19–1.69	1.62–2.15
Severe restriction	≤50	≤50	≥2.5	≥2	≥2.80	≥3.22	≥1.70	≥2.16

SOURCE: Guidelines from Kanner and Morris: *Clinical Pulmonary Function Testing: A Manual of Uniform Laboratory Procedures.* Salt Lake City, Intermountain Thoracic Society, 1975; Morris et al.[34]

Mixed Obstructive-Restrictive Pattern

Occasionally, the battery of pulmonary function tests will demonstrate features of both obstructive and restrictive patterns. Most often, the mixed pattern is characterized by a low $FEV_1/FVC\%$ (indicating obstructive airway disease) and small lung volumes (indicating coexisting restrictive disease).

A number of disorders can produce the mixed obstructive-restrictive pattern. Sarcoidosis and interstitial fibrosis, when severe, generally result in this pattern because the parenchymal disease causes restriction and narrowing of the airways by adjacent fibrosis, evoking signs of airway obstruction. The mixed pattern also occurs in complicated situations when there is more than one cause—e.g., a lobar pneumonia or large pleural effusion occurring in a patient with underlying chronic bronchitis or emphysema.

Isolated Decrease in the Efficiency of Gas Transfer

An isolated reduction in the $D_{L_{CO}}$ suggests one of two possible abnormalities: (1) interstitial lung disease that is so mild as not to affect measurements of airflow or lung volume, or (2) widespread occlusive disease of the pulmonary microcirculation (e.g., due to an inflammatory process or multiple small emboli). In occlusive vascular disorders, tests of airflow and lung volume are usually normal. Although other disorders can also decrease $D_{L_{CO}}$, almost invariably they also reduce airflow, lung volumes, or both. Quantification of the degree to which the $D_{L_{CO}}$ is reduced by any of these processes is indicated in Table 36–24.

Summary of Approach to Interpretation

Pulmonary function tests are designed to detect widespread disorders. Test interpretation relies heavily on recognition of major patterns of abnormality (Table 36–25). These patterns often suggest pathogenetic mechanisms and are helpful to the clinician in arriving at a diagnosis. The degree of abnormality provides a quantitative measure of the extent of involvement at a particular time. Moreover, repeated testing makes it possible to pace and quantify the course of the illness and to assess the effects of therapeutic interventions.

TABLE 36-24

Categorization of Reduction in Efficacy of Gas Transfer: Measurement of $D_{L_{CO}}$

| | | *95% Confidence Interval (CI) Method* | | |
| | | | *Predicted Minus Measured $D_{L_{CO}}$, ml/min/mmHg* | |
Category	*% Predicted Method*	*No. CIs Below Mean*	*Male*	*Female*
Normal	81–140	<1	<8.2	<6.1
Mild reduction	61–80	≥1–1.75	8.2–14.3	6.1–10.6
Moderate reduction	41–60	≥1.75–2.5	14.4–20.4	10.7–15.2
Severe reduction	≤41	≥2.5	≥20.5	≥15.3

SOURCE: Guidelines from Kanner and Morris: *Clinical Pulmonary Function Testing: A Manual of Uniform Laboratory Procedures.* Salt Lake City, Intermountain Thoracic Society, 1975; Morris et al.[34]

TABLE 36-25

Characteristic Alterations in Pulmonary Function Tests According to the Major Patterns of Abnormality

Pattern	Airflow (FEV$_1$/FVC%)	Airflow Response to Bronchodilators	Lung Volumes	D_{LCO}
Obstructive				
Irreversible	↓	↔	↑	↔ or ↓
Reversible	↓	↑	↑	↔
Small airway disease	↓	↔	↔	↔
Upper airway obstruction	↓	↔	↔ or ↑	↔
Restrictive				
Parenchymal disease	↔ or ↑	↔	↓	↓
Surgical resection	↔	↔	↓	↓
Pleural, chest wall disease	↔	↔	↓	↔
Reduced expiratory force generation	↔	↔	↓	↔
Mixed obstructive-restrictive	↓	↔ or ↑	↓	↓
Isolated reduction in efficiency of gas transfer	↔	↔	↔	↓

NOTE: ↓ = decreased; ↑ = increased; ↔ = no change or normal.

REFERENCES

1. ATS Statement: Single breath carbon monoxide diffusing capacity (transfer factor): Recommendations for a standard technique—1995 update. *Am J Respir Crit Care Med* 152:2185–2198, 1995.

2. ATS Statement: Standardization of spirometry—1994 update. *Am J Rev Respir Crit Care Med* 152:1107–1136, 1995.

3. Black LF, Hyatt RE: Maximal respiratory pressures: Normal values and relationship to age and sex. *Am Rev Respir Dis* 99:696–702, 1969.

4. Briscoe WA, DuBois AB: The relationship between airway resistance, airway conductance, and lung volume in subjects of different age and body size. *J Clin Invest* 37:1279–1285, 1958.

5. Britton J, Pavord I, Richards K, et al: Factors influencing the occurrence of airway hyperreactivity in the general population: The importance of atopy and airway calibre. *Eur Respir J* 7:881–887, 1994.

6. Clausen JL (ed): *Pulmonary Function Testing: Guidelines and Controversies.* New York, Academic Press, 1982.

7. Cosio M, Ghezzo H, Hogg JC, et al: The relations between structural changes in small airways and pulmonary-function tests. *New Engl J Med* 298:1277–1281, 1978.

8. Cotes JE, Dabbs JM, Elwood PC, et al: Iron deficiency anaemia: Its effect on transfer factor for the lung (diffusing capacity) and ventilation and cardiac frequency during sub–maximal exercise. *Clin Sci* 42:325–335, 1972.

9. Darling RC, Cournand A, Richards DW Jr: Studies on the intrapulmonary mixture of gases: III. An open circuit method for measuring residual air. *J Clin Invest* 19:609–618, 1940.

10. Despas PJ, Leroux M, Macklem PT: Site of airway obstruction in asthma as determined by measuring maximal expiratory flow breathing air and a helium–oxygen mixture. *J Clin Invest* 51:3235–3243, 1972.

11. Dollfuss RE, Milic-Emili J, Bates DV: Regional ventilation of the lung, studied with boluses of ^{133}xenon. *Respir Physiol* 2:234–246, 1967.

12. Dosman J, Bode F, Urbanetti J, et al: The use of a helium-oxygen mixture during maximum expiratory flow to demonstrate obstruction in small airways in smokers. *J Clin Invest* 55:1090–1099, 1975.

13. DuBois AB, Botelho SY, Bedell GN, et al: A rapid plethysmographic method for measuring thoracic gas volume: A comparison with a nitrogen washout method for measuring functional residual capacity in normal subjects. *J Clin Invest* 35:322–326, 1956.

14. DuBois AB, Botelho SY, Comroe JH Jr: A new method for measuring airway resistance in man using a body plethysmograph: Values in normal subjects and in patients with respiratory disease. *J Clin Invest* 35:327–335, 1956.

15. Edelman NH, Epstein PE, Lahiri S, Cherniack NS: Ventilatory response to transient hypoxia and hypercapnia in man. *Respir Physiol* 17:302–314, 1973.

16. Filley GF, MacIntosh DJ, Wright GW: Carbon monoxide uptake and pulmonary diffusing capacity in normal subjects at rest and during exercise. *J Clin Invest* 33:530–539, 1954.

17. Fowler WS: Lung function studies: III. Uneven pulmonary ventilation in normal subjects and in patients with pulmonary disease. *J Appl Physiol* 2:283–299, 1949.

18. Glindmeyer HW, Lefante JJ, McCollister C, et al: Blue-collar normative spirometric values for Caucasian and African-American men and women aged 18 to 65. *Am J Respir Crit Care Med* 151:412–422, 1995.

19. Hankinson JL, Das MK: Frequency response of portable PEF meters. *Am J Respir Crit Care Med* 152:702–706, 1995.

20. Hankinson JL, Viola JO: Dynamic BTPS correction factors for spirometric data. *J Appl Physiol* 55:1354–1360, 1983.

21. Hoppin FC, Green M, Morgan MS: Relationship of central and peripheral airway resistance to lung volume in dogs. *J Appl Physiol* 44:728–737, 1978.

22. Horsley JR, Sterling IJ, Waters WE, Howell JB: How common is increased airway reactivity amongst the elderly? *Gerontology* 39:38–48, 1993.

23. Huang YCT, MacIntyre NR: Real-time gas analysis improves the measurement of single-breath diffusing capacity. *Am Rev Respir Dis* 146:946–950, 1992.

24. Hutcheon M, Griffin P, Levison H, Zamel N: Volume of isoflow: A new test in the detection of mild abnormalities of lung mechanics. *Am Rev Respir Dis* 110:458–465, 1974.

25. Johnson LR, Enright PL, Voelker HT, Tashkin DP: Volume spirometers need automated internal temperature sensors. *Am J Respir Crit Care Med* 150:1575–1580, 1994.

26. Kelman GR, Nunn JF: Nomograms for correction of blood P$_{O_2}$,

PCO$_2$ pH, and base excess for time and temperature. *J Appl Physiol* 21:1484–1490, 1966.

27. Knudson RJ, Clark DF, Kennedy TC, Knudson DE: Effect of aging alone on mechanical properties of the normal adult human lung. *J Appl Physiol* 43:1054–1062, 1977.

28. Knudson RJ, Lebowitz MD, Holberg CJ, Burrows B: Changes in the normal maximal expiratory flow-volume curve with growth and aging. *Am Rev Respir Dis* 127:725–734, 1983.

29. Kryger M, Bode F, Antic R, Anthonisen N: Diagnosis of obstruction of the central and upper airways. *Am J Med* 61:85–93, 1976.

30. Lloyd BB, Cunningham DJC: A quantitative approach to the regulation of human respiration, in Cunningham DJC, Lloyd BB (eds), *The Regulation of Human Respiration.* Oxford, Blackwell, 1963, pp. 331–349.

31. Malmberg P, Larsson K, Sundblad BM, Zhiping W: Importance of the time interval beween FEV1 measurements in a methacholine provocation test. *Eur Respir J* 6:680–686, 1993.

32. Mead J, Lindgren I, Gaensler EA: The mechanical properties of the lungs in emphysema. *J Clin Invest* 34:1005–1016, 1955.

33. Milic-Emili J, Mead J, Turner JM, Glauser EM: Improved technique for estimating pleural pressure from esophageal balloons. *J Appl Physiol* 19:207–211, 1964.

34. Morris AH, Kanner RE, Crapo RO, Gardner RM (eds): *Clinical Pulmonary Function Testing: A Manual of Uniform Laboratory Procedures,* 2d ed. Salt Lake City, Intermountain Thoracic Society, 1984.

35. Neas LM, Schwartz J: The determinants of pulmonary diffusing capacity in a national sample of U.S. adults. *Am J Respir Crit Care Med* 153:656–664, 1996.

36. O'Connor GT, Sparrow D, Weiss ST: A prospective longitudinal study of methacholine airway responsiveness as a predictor of pulmonary-function decline: The Normative Aging Study. *Am J Respir Crit Care Med* 152:87–92, 1995.

37. Ogilvie CM, Forster RE, Blakemore WS, Morton JW: A standardized breath holding technique for the clinical measurement of the diffusing capacity of the lung for carbon monoxide. *J Clin Invest* 36:1–17, 1957.

38. Paoletti P, Carrozzi L, Viegi G, et al: Distribution of bronchial responsiveness in a general population: Effect of sex, age, smoking, and level of pulmonary function. *Am J Respir Crit Care Med* 151:1770–1777, 1995

39. Parker JM, Dillard TA, Phillips YY: Impact of using stated instead of measured height upon screening spirometry. *Am J Respir Crit Care Med* 150:1705–1708, 1994.

40. Phagoo SB, Watson RA, Silverman M, Pride NB: Comparison of four methods of assessing airflow resistance before and after induced airway narrowing in normal subjects. *J Appl Physiol* 79:518–525, 1995.

41. Pincock AC, Miller MR: The effect of temperature on recording spirograms. *Am Rev Respir Dis* 128:894–898, 1983.

42. Rahn H, Otis AB, Chadwick LE, Fenn WO: The pressure volume diagram of the thorax and lung. *Am J Physiol* 146:161–178, 1946.

43. Read DJC: A clinical method for assessing the ventilatory response to carbon dioxide. *Aust Ann Med* 16:20–32, 1966.

44. Rebuck AS, Campbell EJM: A clinical method for assessing the ventilatory response to hypoxia. *Am Rev Respir Dis* 109:345–350, 1974.

45. Ringqvist T: The ventilatory capacity in healthy subjects: An analysis of causal factors with special reference to the respiratory forces. *Scand J Clin Lab Invest* 18(Suppl 88):5–179, 1966.

46. Rodenstein DO, Stanescu DC: Reassessment of lung volume measurement by helium dilution and by body plethysmography in chronic airflow obstruction. *Am Rev Respir Dis* 126:1040–1044, 1982.

47. Sandqvist L, Kjellmer I: Normal values for the single breath nitrogen elimination test in different age groups. *Scand J Clin Lab Invest* 12:131–135, 1960.

48. Schilder DP, Roberts A, Fry DL: Effect of gas density and viscosity on the maximal expiratory flow-volume relationship. *J Clin Invest* 42:1705–1713, 1963.

49. Shore S, Milic-Emili J, Martin JG: Reassessment of body plethysmographic technique for the measurement of thoracic gas volume in asthmatics. *Am Rev Respir Dis* 126:515–520, 1982.

50. Smith L, McFadden ER Jr: Bronchial hyperreactivity revisited. *Ann Allergy Asthma Immunol* 74:454–470,1995.

51. Sorbini CA, Grassi V, Solinas E, Muiesan G: Arterial oxygen tension in relation to age in healthy subjects. *Respiration* 25:3–13, 1968.

52. Tablan OC, Williams WW, Martone WJ: Infection control in pulmonary function laboratories. *Infect Control* 6:442–444, 1985.

53. Townley RG, Bewtra AK, Nair NM, et al: Methacholine inhalation challenge studies. *J Allergy Clin Immunol* 64:569–574, 1979.

54. Ulrik CS: Bronchial responsiveness to inhaled histamine in both adults with intrinsic and extrinsic asthma: The importance of prechallenge forced expiratory volume in 1 second. *J Allergy Clin Immunol* 91:120–126, 1993.

55. Weil JV, Byrne–Quinn E, Sodal IE, et al: Hypoxic ventilatory drive in normal man. *J Clin Invest* 49:1061–1072, 1970.

56. Whitelaw WA, Derenne JP, Milic-Emili J: Occlusion pressure as a measure of respiratory center output in conscious man. *Respir Physiol* 23:181–199, 1975.

57. Wilson AF (ed): *Pulmonary Function Testing: Indications and Interpretations.* Orlando, Grune and Stratton, 1985.

58. Woolcock AJ, Vincent NJ, Macklem PT: Frequency dependence of compliance as a test for obstruction in the small airways. *J Clin Invest* 48:1097–1106, 1969.

CHAPTER 37

PRINCIPLES AND APPLICATIONS OF CARDIOPULMONARY EXERCISE TESTING

Karl T. Weber

Cardiopulmonary exercise testing draws on the recognition that the thorax represents a metabolic gas transport unit, the function of whose requisite components—diaphragm, heart, lungs, rib cage, and corresponding skeletal muscles—is to transport O_2 to and CO_2 from metabolizing tissues. Unit O_2 and CO_2 transport must adjust to physiological and pathophysiological stresses that augment the body's consumption of oxygen ($\dot{V}_{O_2}$) and carbon dioxide production ($\dot{V}_{CO_2}$). During strenuous levels of muscular work, for example, $\dot{V}_{O_2}$ may rise eightfold, accompanied by in-

creased $\dot{V}_{CO_2}$. Cardiovascular or ventilatory disease can disrupt the unit's functional integrity. With severe disease, an abnormality in respiratory gas transport may be apparent at rest, when the body's O_2 requirements are modest. Resting function is preserved with less severe expressions of disease, but abnormal respiratory gas transport becomes apparent when the unit is stressed by an elevation in $\dot{V}_{O_2}$.

Cardiopulmonary exercise testing includes the monitoring of respiratory gas exchange ($\dot{V}_{O_2}$ and $\dot{V}_{CO_2}$), minute ventilation ($\dot{V}_E$), and its components, tidal volume and respiratory rate, together with blood pressure, heart rate, and the electrocardiogram. Cardiopulmonary exercise testing represents a useful approach in the clinical evaluation of a whole host of disorders and circumstances. This chapter addresses physiological principles and the clinical application of cardiopulmonary exercise testing in the evaluation of major disorders that impair heart or lung function. The chapter is by no means an exhaustive review. For a more detailed discussion of specific entities, the interested reader is referred to several other textbooks.[30,33]

PRINCIPLES, DEFINITIONS, AND CLINICAL APPLICATION OF CARDIOPULMONARY EXERCISE TESTING

The metabolic gas transport unit, also referred to as the "cardiopulmonary unit," links metabolizing tissues to the atmosphere and its supply of O_2. O_2 transport to tissues must be precise and based upon prevailing need. CO_2 produced by tissues must be eliminated into the atmosphere in an equally efficient manner.

Resting Oxygen Uptake and Transport

Concepts and calculations pertaining to $\dot{V}_{O_2}$ and O_2 content, transport, and extraction are reviewed in Table 37-1. The heart and lungs accommodate to the metabolic requirements of tissues; they must do so on a moment-to-moment basis, according to physiological priorities. Tissue requirements for O_2 dictate a cer-

TABLE 37-1

Oxygen Utilization, Content, Transport, and Extraction

O$_2$ utilization 250 ml/min	$\begin{cases} = \text{Cardiac output} \cdot (\text{arterial } O_2 \text{ content} - \text{venous } O_2 \text{ content}) \\ = 5000 \text{ ml/min} \cdot (19 \text{ ml/dl} - 14 \text{ ml/dl}) \end{cases}$
Arterial O$_2$ content 19 ml/dl	$\begin{cases} = \text{Hemoglobin} \cdot \% \text{ saturation} \cdot O_2 \text{ combining capacity} \\ = 14 \text{ gm/dl} \cdot 0.96 \cdot 1.34 \text{ ml/gm} \end{cases}$
Venous O$_2$ content 14 ml/dl	$= 14 \text{ gm/dl} \cdot 0.96 \cdot 1.34 \text{ ml/gm}$
Arteriovenous O$_2$ difference 5 ml/dl	$\begin{cases} = \text{Arterial } O_2 \text{ content} - \text{venous } O_2 \text{ content} \\ = 19 \text{ ml/dl} - 14 \text{ ml/dl} \end{cases}$
O$_2$ transport 950 ml/min	$\begin{cases} = \text{Cardiac output} \cdot \text{arterial } O_2 \text{ content} \\ = 5000 \text{ ml/min} \cdot 19 \text{ ml/dl} \end{cases}$
O$_2$ extraction 25%	$\begin{cases} = \dfrac{\text{Arteriovenous } O_2 \text{ difference}}{\text{Arterial } O_2 \text{ content}} \cdot 100\% \\ = \dfrac{19 - 14}{19} \cdot 100\% \end{cases}$

SOURCE: Reproduced from Weber KT: Gas transport and the cardiopulmonary unit, in Weber KT, Janicki JS (eds), *Cardiopulmonary Exercise Testing: Physiologic Principles and Clinical Applications.* Philadelphia, Saunders, 1986, pp 15–33.

tain $\dot{V}_E$ and cardiac output. In an average-sized person, resting $\dot{V}_{O_2}$ averages 250 ml/min or 3.5 ml/min/kg body weight (one metabolic equivalent) and is associated with a $\dot{V}_E$ of 8 to 10 L/min and cardiac output of 4 to 6 L/min. O$_2$ transport, also termed O$_2$ delivery, ranges between 730 and 1040 ml/min and is more than adequate to satisfy resting $\dot{V}_{O_2}$. On average, 25 percent of arterial O$_2$ content is extracted by tissues. O$_2$ delivery and extraction each increase during physiological stress in proportion to the elevation in O$_2$. Factors that normally determine O$_2$ availability at rest and during exercise include cardiac output, hemoglobin concentration and its percent saturation, and O$_2$ extraction.

Exercise Oxygen Uptake and Transport

$\dot{V}_E$ and O$_2$ delivery must each rise during exercise. Strenuous work can raise $\dot{V}_E$ eight to 10 times its resting level. Ventilation normally poses no limitation on the ability of tissues to carry out aerobic work. By contrast, the extent to which cardiac output rises during progressive work is less dramatic. In untrained subjects, cardiac output increases four to five times its resting value. Cardiac output rises 600 ml/min for every 100-ml/min increment in $\dot{V}_{O_2}$. This is considered the normal "gain" setting between the heart and its cardiac output and $\dot{V}_{O_2}$. O$_2$ availability

during physical activity is further ensured by enhanced O$_2$ extraction and circulatory autoregulation. Reflexive and humoral influences produce vasoconstriction in less metabolically active tissues, permitting a greater apportionment of blood flow to exercising muscle.

Physiological limits to the elevation in cardiac output (i.e., cardiac reserve) and O$_2$ extraction (approximately 75 to 80 percent of arterial O$_2$ content) determine aerobic capacity of untrained subjects to incremental exercise. Beyond these physiological limits, any additional increment in work is not accompanied by an elevation in O$_2$; a plateau in $\dot{V}_{O_2}$ is attained and is termed the *maximal oxygen uptake* ($\dot{V}_{O_2max}$). Cardiopulmonary exercise test results, including $\dot{V}_{O_2max}$, are shown in Fig. 37-1 for a 40-year-old man without clinically apparent heart or lung disease. Shown are individual responses in $\dot{V}_{O_2}$, $\dot{V}_{CO_2}$, $\dot{V}_E$, and heart rate during progressive increments in treadmill work. A $\dot{V}_{O_2max}$ of 2198 ml/min (27.2 ml/min/kg) was attained. This is a true plateau in $\dot{V}_{O_2}$, with $\dot{V}_{O_2}$ remaining invariant for 2.5 stages (5 min) of exercise.

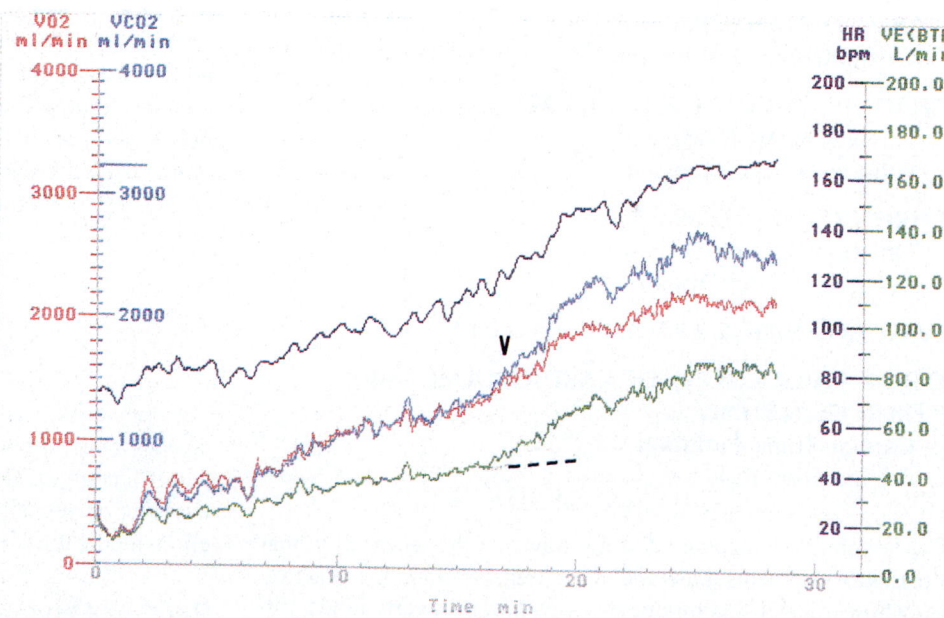

FIGURE 37-1 Cardiopulmonary exercise response in a 40-year-old man without heart or lung disease. Shown are 2 min of standing rest, followed by incremental treadmill exercise. Individual responses (color coded) include oxygen uptake ($\dot{V}_{O_2}$), carbon dioxide production ($\dot{V}_{CO_2}$), minute ventilation ($\dot{V}_E$), and heart rate (HR). Maximal O$_2$ uptake, a plateau in $\dot{V}_{O_2}$ was attained after the crossover of $\dot{V}_{CO_2}$ and $\dot{V}_{O_2}$ (arrowhead), representing the anaerobic threshold and accompanied by a disproportionate (broken line) rise in $\dot{V}_E$.

$\dot{V}_{O_2max}$ should not be equated or used synonymously with peak $\dot{V}_{O_2}$ achieved during symptom-limited exercise. $\dot{V}_{O_2max}$ reflects a person's aerobic capacity—a physiological capacity of the cardiovascular system. In an average-sized, untrained person whose maximum cardiac output and arteriovenous oxygen difference are 20 L/min and 12 ml/dl, respectively, a $\dot{V}_{O_2max}$ of 2400 ml/min is expected. In athletes, a greater cardiac reserve and enhanced capacity for oxidative metabolism by trained skeletal muscle are available, providing for greater aerobic capacity. In patients with heart disease, whose ability to raise cardiac output during exercise is impaired, $\dot{V}_{O_2max}$ is proportionally reduced (see above).

Carbon Dioxide Production

The right heart "accepts" metabolically produced CO_2, and the alveolar exchange surface expels CO_2 into the atmosphere. CO_2 is a major respiratory stimulant that maintains eucapnia. Seventy-five to 80 percent of O_2 is converted to CO_2. Accordingly, resting $\dot{V}_{CO_2}$ averages 190 ml/min and represents a *metabolic source* of CO_2. The resting $\dot{V}_{CO_2}/\dot{V}_{O_2}$ ratio, or respiratory gas exchange ratio (R), typically ranges between 0.75 and 0.85. The absolute value of R depends on the proportion of carbohydrates and fats available from the diet. $\dot{V}_{O_2}$ and $\dot{V}_{CO_2}$ rise in proportion to one another during physical activity as long as an adequate amount of O_2 is available to sustain oxidative metabolism.

With strenuous levels of muscular work, $\dot{V}_{O_2}$ rises to a level where the heart is unable to provide O_2 at a commensurate rate. Consequently, tissue O_2 availability becomes inadequate. Working skeletal muscle enhances its use of less efficient anaerobic metabolism to derive energy. This leads to lactate production from working muscle beyond that normally produced. This *nonmetabolic source* of CO_2 is derived from rapid buffering of the lactate by bicarbonate; the CO_2 generated serves as a respiratory stimulant. The accompanying increase in $\dot{V}_E$ maintains eucapnia and raises the respiratory gas exchange ratio above that associated with aerobic metabolism. Anaerobic metabolism during a progressive exercise test is heralded by this disproportionate rise in $\dot{V}_E$ and $\dot{V}_{CO_2}$ relative to $\dot{V}_{O_2}$. The corresponding level of $\dot{V}_{O_2}$ at which anaerobic metabolism occurs is termed the *anaerobic threshold* (AT).[30] The point during exercise at which $\dot{V}_{O_2}$ exceeds $\dot{V}_{O_2}$ and $\dot{V}_E$ rises disproportionately is shown in Fig. 37-1. Anaerobiosis normally occurs when 60 percent or more of a person's aerobic capacity has been attained. For the 40-year-old man whose exercise response is shown in Fig. 37-1, the AT occurred at a $\dot{V}_{O_2}$ of 18.8 ml/min/kg, or 69 percent of his $\dot{V}_{O_2max}$.

Clinical Application of Cardiopulmonary Exercise Testing

Patients with cardiovascular or respiratory disease of mild to moderate severity frequently note limiting symptoms of fatigue or breathlessness during physical activity. Because their quality of life is compromised, they seek or are referred for medical evaluation. Re-creating muscular work in a monitored setting permits an evaluation of the nature and severity of such symptoms and the relative importance of abnormal heart or lung function. This strategy provides information surpassing that available from static measures of heart and lung function, such as ejection fraction, lung volumes, or airflows, determined at rest. The continuous monitoring of $\dot{V}_{O_2}$, $\dot{V}_{CO_2}$, $\dot{V}_E$, respiratory rate, and tidal volume during incremental exercise can be performed simply and on a breath-by-breath basis. Data shown in Fig. 37-1 are displayed throughout the test. The choice of a particular cardiopulmonary exercise test (see above) depends on the nature and expression of the clinical disorder and the particular problem to be addressed. For most clinical evaluations, isotonic forms of exercise are used. Isotonic work is an acceptable, negotiable, and reproducible form of exercise for patients with heart or lung disease.

It should be noted, however, that while noninvasive cardiopulmonary exercise testing may help determine the impairment in aerobic capacity, abnormalities in ventilation with exercise, and their severity in patients with lung disease, these parameters are not necessarily diagnostic. For example, $\dot{V}_{O_2max}$, AT, or exercise $\dot{V}_E$ does not identify the underlying structural defect responsible for a patient's abnormal response. This may require invasive monitoring during cardiopulmonary exercise testing to identify specific hemodynamic abnormalities. Echocardiography and specialized pulmonary function studies may be required. The physician must draw upon sound clinical judgment and complementary laboratory tests to derive an understanding of the nature and severity of the heart or lung disease.

Noninvasive Treadmill Exercise

Walking represents a common daily exercise rather than a specialized skill. A patient who walks into the physician's office or down a hospital corridor can walk on a treadmill at 1.0 or 1.5 mph, zero grade. Treadmills are programmable. The Bruce protocol, which employs marked increments in treadmill speed and slope over short periods in the evaluation of myocardial ischemia, may not be useful for patients with limited exercise tolerance. A modified Naughton protocol of gradually progressive exercise (Table 37-2) serves to stress the cardiopulmonary unit for patients with heart or lung disease who have a wide range of exercise tolerance. In this protocol, the first two stages of exercise represent very low work loads and are a warmup for patients with heart or lung disease of minor severity; the stages represent near-maximal exercise for patients with more advanced disease.

$\dot{V}_{O_2max}$ is defined as $\dot{V}_{O_2}$ that remains invariant (less than 1 ml/min/kg for 30 s or more) despite an increment in work load. An invariant $\dot{V}_{O_2}$ for at least two stages of exercise is preferred (Fig. 37-1). $\dot{V}_{O_2max}$ follows the AT, and this definition of $\dot{V}_{O_2max}$ presumes that the AT has already been achieved. The AT generally occurs at 60 percent of a patient's aerobic capacity. $\dot{V}_{O_2max}$ associated with incremental treadmill exercise provides a greater aerobic capacity than does cycle ergometry because it works a larger group of muscles.[21] A patient's aerobic capacity to incremental treadmill exercise is used to grade the functional impairment (Table 37-3). $\dot{V}_{O_2max}$ is an objective measure of functional status—in contradistinction to the New York Heart Association classification, which is based on perceptions and biases of the patient and physician. Treadmill O_2max determination is reproducible in patients with a wide variety of cardiovascular disorders.[33] A $\dot{V}_{O_2max}$ of under 20 ml/min/kg has been selected as the cutoff for grading impaired aerobic capacity; adult men and

TABLE 37-2

Modified Naughton Treadmill Exercise Protocol

Stage	Speed	Grade	Physical Activities
1	1.0	0	Driving a car
			Sitting and writing or eating
2	1.5	0	Dressing; knitting
			Walking to bathroom
			Light auto repair
3	2.0	3.5	Shave self in bathroom
			Wash entire body
			Food shopping
4	2.0	7.0	Sexual activity
			Raking leaves
			Plastering
5	2.0	10.5	Stacking firewood
			Mowing lawn (powered)
			Walking down stairs
6	3.0	7.5	Scrubbing floors
			Gardening
			Walking up stairs
7	3.0	10.0	Lifting and carrying 65–80 lb
			Carpentry
			Climbing hills (no load)
8	3.0	12.5	Digging
			Snow shoveling
			Climbing stairs (20-lb load)
9	3.0	15.0	Beyond this level, work loads are equal to very vigorous exercise (e.g., skiing, basketball)
10	3.4	14.0	
11	3.4	16.0	
12	3.4	18.0	
13	3.4	20.0	
14	3.4	22.0	

SOURCE: Reproduced from Weber KT, Janicki JS, McElroy PA: Cardiopulmonary exercise (CPX) testing, in Weber KT, Janicki JS (eds), *Cardiopulmonary Exercise Testing: Physiologic Principles and Clinical Applications.* Philadelphia, Saunders, 1986, pp 151–167.

women, including the elderly (over 65 years of age), have an expected $\dot{V}_{O_2max}$ of more than 20 ml/min/kg.[22]

The duration of symptom-free treadmill exercise should not be equated with $\dot{V}_{O_2max}$. Treadmill time suffers from not having an objective, quantitative end-point. Differences in gait and body weight create different levels of work for equivalent stages of treadmill exercise. Symptom-limited exercise time is subject to patient motivation and physician bias.[2] Peak heart rate attained with exercise is also a less precise measure of $\dot{V}_{O_2max}$. This is particularly true in patients with atrial fibrillation.

Determination of the AT can be defined according to one or more criteria.[30] These include (1) a disproportionate rise in $\dot{V}_{CO_2}$, $\dot{V}_E$, or R relative to $\dot{V}_{O_2}$ and (2) a disproportionate rise in end-

tidal O_2 relative to end-tidal CO_2. These criteria can best be applied to breath-by-breath respiratory gas exchange data. In our laboratory, a simpler strategy is used. The AT is identified as the level of $\dot{V}_{O_2}$ attained during treadmill work after the plots of $\dot{V}_{O_2}$ and CO_2 cross, when R exceeds 1.0. Fig. 37-1 depicts the crossover in $\dot{V}_{CO_2}$ and $\dot{V}_{O_2}$ from breath-by-breath gas exchange data monitored throughout incremental treadmill exercise. It also demonstrates the point at which $\dot{V}_E$ rises disproportionately. Measured days or weeks apart, this noninvasive determination of the AT is reproducible in a wide range of patients with cardiac or circulatory failure and correlates with lactate threshold (see above).[5,16,33]

The normal ventilatory response to incremental treadmill exercise consists of an increase in $\dot{V}_E$ created by an increase in respiratory rate and tidal volume. Ventilatory reserves, represented by maximal voluntary ventilation (MVV) and vital capacity determined during routine pulmonary function testing, are only partly utilized during light, moderate, and maximal exercise by normal persons. The ratio of maximal exercise $\dot{V}_E$ to MVV reflects use of this ventilatory reserve. Exercise $\dot{V}_E$ in normal subjects and patients with predominant cardiovascular disease rarely exceeds 50 percent of MVV.[34] The same is true of the ratio between maximal exercise tidal volume and vital capacity. These limitations in ventilatory responses are consistent with a ventilatory effort that can be voluntarily sustained at rest without the appearance of fatigue or breathlessness.

An oximeter, worn on either an earlobe or a finger, provides noninvasive monitoring of arterial O_2 saturation during exercise. This is a useful screening procedure in patients in whom O_2 desaturation might be anticipated (e.g., those with congenital heart disease with right-to-left shunt, restrictive or obstructive lung disease, or pulmonary vascular disease). Normal subjects and patients with chronic cardiac or circulatory failure do not develop arterial hypoxemia (arterial O_2 saturation under 90 percent) during exercise. In patients in whom O_2 desaturation is evident from oximetry, confirmatory evidence from direct measurement of arterial blood gases during repeat exercise may be advisable.

Thus, incremental treadmill exercise can be used to determine the following: the AT with a submaximal test, the AT and $\dot{V}_{O_2max}$ with a maximal test, the ventilatory response to submaximal or maximal exercise, and arterial O_2 desaturation during submaximal or maximal exercise.

TABLE 37-3
Classification of Cardiac and Circulatory Failure

Class	Severity	$\dot{V}_{O_2}max$ (ml/kg/min)	Anerobic Threshold (ml/kg/min)	Predicted Cardiac Index (L/m²/min)
A	Mild to none	>20	>14	>8
B	Mild to moderate	16 to 20	11 to 14	6 to 8
C	Moderate to severe	10 to 16	8 to 11	4 to 6
D	Severe	6 to 10	5 to 8	<4

SOURCE: Adapted from Weber KT, Janicki JS, McElroy PA: Cardiopulmonary exercise (CPX) testing, in Weber KT, Janicki JS (eds), *Cardiopulmonary Exercise Testing: Physiologic Principles and Clinical Applications.* Philadelphia, Saunders, 1986, pp 151–167.

Invasive Treadmill Exercise

Invasive hemodynamic monitoring may be necessary to better define the nature and severity of an underlying cardiopulmonary disorder.[33] A triple-lumen flotation catheter can be safely used for hemodynamic monitoring during upright exercise. The hemodynamic response to incremental treadmill exercise in normal subjects is characterized by a progressive rise in cardiac output, accomplished with minimal elevations in left and right ventricular filling pressures. The rise in cardiac output occurs because of an increment in stroke volume, which is most apparent at low and moderate work loads, and because of an elevation in heart rate, which accompanies the entire exercise response. Systemic O_2 extraction rises progressively with incremental exercise to exceed 70 percent at maximal work loads. A rise in mixed venous lactate concentration, as observed with pulmonary arterial blood sampling, occurs when O_2 extraction exceeds 60 percent and when the subject is working at greater than 60 percent of $\dot{V}_{O_2}max$.

Systolic and mean arterial pressures rise during upright exercise. Because of skeletal muscle vasodilatation, arterial diastolic pressure remains essentially invariant during exercise. Systemic vascular resistance falls by 50 percent to approximately 600 dynes · s · cm⁻⁵ during incremental, isotonic treadmill exercise. In normal persons, pulmonary artery systolic, mean, and diastolic pressures rise only minimally with exercise and only with higher work loads. Pulmonary vascular resistance, like systemic vascular resistance, falls 50 percent to about 60 dynes · s · cm⁻⁵ during incremental isotonic exercise.

CHRONIC CARDIAC FAILURE

In physiological terms, *cardiac failure* is defined as an impairment in cardiac output secondary to a disease process affecting the myocardium. Ischemic heart disease and dilated cardiomyopathies are examples of disease entities that can result in chronic cardiac failure. $\dot{V}_{O_2}max$ and the AT each predict cardiac reserve and, thereby, the severity of cardiac failure. These parameters further serve to objectively demonstrate a patient's functional capacity, which is not predicted from the cardiac ejection fraction. Patients with an ejection fraction of under 20 percent may still be able to swim.

Systolic Dysfunction

In patients with chronic cardiac failure, $\dot{V}_{O_2}max$ attained during incremental treadmill exercise is primarily a function of maximal cardiac output.[34,35] This conclusion has been confirmed by numerous studies.[3,6,18,27,37] An impairment in aerobic capacity is gauged according to the exercise AT and $\dot{V}_{O_2}max$ and assigned a functional class as reviewed in Table 37-3. These parameters are, in turn, used to predict maximal exercise cardiac index (or cardiac reserve). Examples of $\dot{V}_{O_2}max$ and the AT attained by two patients with chronic cardiac failure (one class B, the other class C) are given in Fig. 37-2. To measure $\dot{V}_{O_2}max$ in such patients, they must be exercised to exhaustion. The AT is achieved at submaximal work loads short of exhaustion; it, too, stratifies the degree of cardiac dysfunction.

Validation of these concepts was obtained during treadmill exercise using invasive measures of cardiac output and mixed venous lactate concentration.[31,32] Patients had chronic cardiac failure of varying severity (classes A to D), due to either ischemic or myopathic heart disease. In each exercise class, the arteriovenous O_2 difference rose to 12 ml/dl or more at maximum exercise, corresponding to a systemic O_2 extraction in excess of 70 percent, suggesting that O_2 extraction reached maximal physiological levels. The reduction in aerobic capacity of a patient with chronic cardiac failure is, therefore, due primarily to impaired cardiac reserve. The cardiac output–O_2 relation to progressive treadmill exercise for these patients is given in Fig. 37-3. For each exercise class, cardiac output is presented as a percentage of $\dot{V}_{O_2}max$ (set equal to 100 percent) that existed at rest and throughout each stage of exercise. Cardiac output rose by 600 ml/min/m² for each dl/min/m² increase in $\dot{V}_{O_2}$ in each class. This indicates that the heart responds to tissue O_2 requirements irrespective of the severity of heart failure, but it is limited by the maximal cardiac output it can attain. Differences in cardiac output achieved at peak exercise are seen between classes. Progressive reductions in cardiac reserve are responsible for different aerobic capacities observed in these patients. $\dot{V}_{O_2}max$, therefore, serves as a noninvasive measure of peak exercise cardiac output and is given for each functional class in Table 37-3.

The cardiac output response to exercise is a function of the rises in stroke volume and heart rate. Responses in stroke volume for patients with chronic cardiac failure are shown in

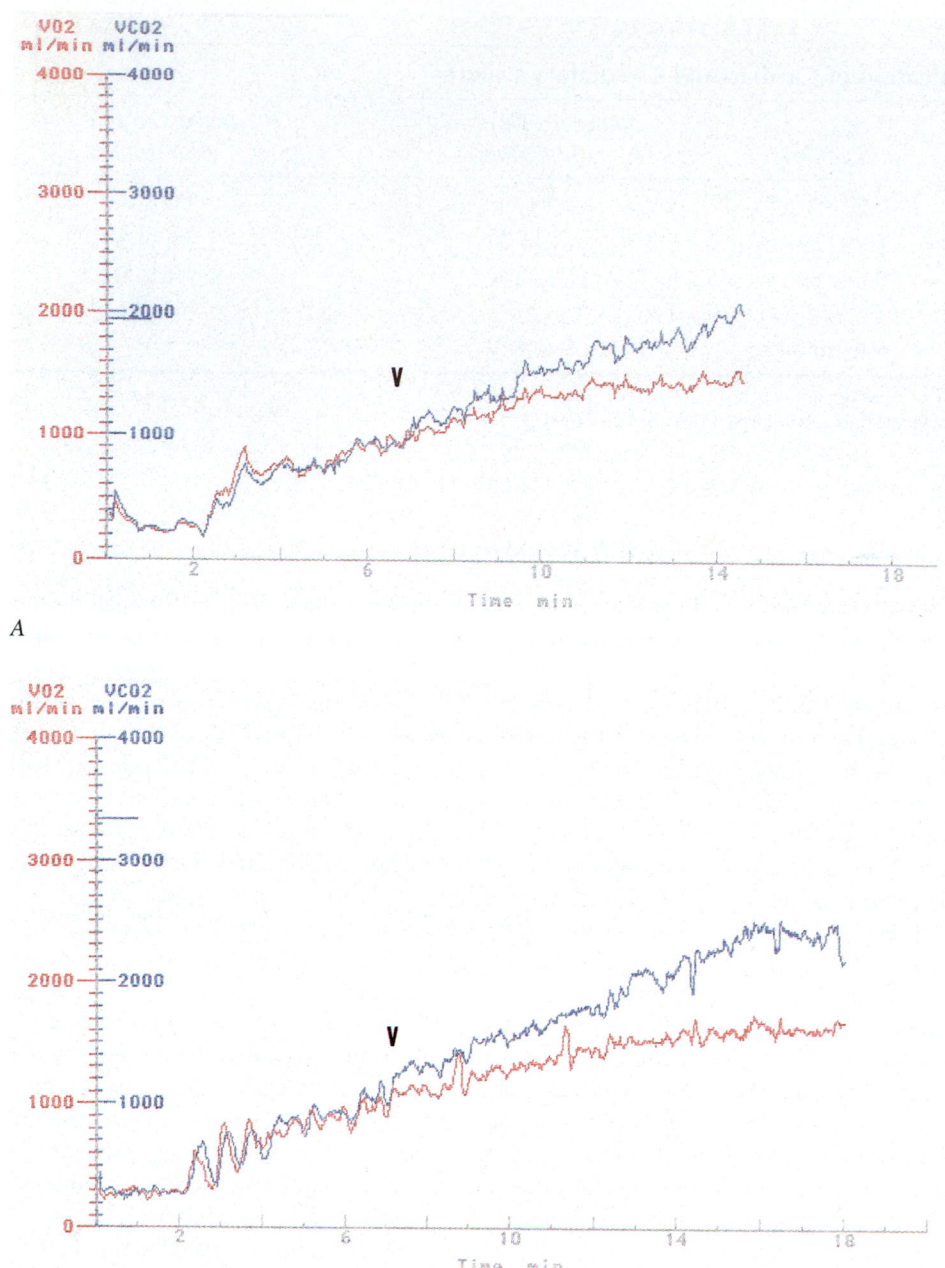

FIGURE 37-2 Cardiopulmonary exercise test results for a 45-year-old woman (*A*) and a 40-year-old man (right panel), each with ischemic heart disease and chronic cardiac failure. Only $\dot{V}_{O_2}$ and $\dot{V}_{CO_2}$ are shown, to better demonstrate the anaerobic threshold (AT) and $\dot{V}_{O_2max}$ attained by each patient. On the left, the AT was seen with a $\dot{V}_{O_2}$ of 11.6 ml/min/kg and a $\dot{V}_{O_2max}$ of 16.5 ml/min/kg. This represents a functional class B response. The AT and $\dot{V}_{O_2max}$ are 8.5 and 13.7 ml/min/kg, respectively. (*B*). This corresponds to functional class C.

For each functional class of chronic cardiac failure, the heart rate–$\dot{V}_2$ response to upright incremental exercise is represented by a common slope.[17] The average slope is 3.6 beats per minute for every 1-ml/min/kg increment in $\dot{V}_{O_2}$. Peak heart rate achieved is a function of maximal work load performed. Maximal exercise heart rate is, therefore, different for each class. In class D patients, the elevation in heart rate is the sole mechanism by which cardiac output rises during exercise.

Some patients with chronic cardiac failure deviate from this heart rate–$\dot{V}_{O_2}$ relation by having an inappropriate sinus tachycardia, either at rest and throughout exercise or simply during exercise. In the presence of a reduced ejection fraction and ventricular dilation, this inappropriately rapid heart rate further compromises exercise cardiac output and reduces aerobic capacity. β-Adrenergic receptor blockade is useful in attenuating resting or exercise heart rate under these circumstances.[36] Such chronotropic dysfunction (see below) to exercise may also apply to patients with chronic atrial fibrillation. An example of an inappropriate rapid heart rate relative to incremental treadmill exercise (Naughton protocol) is given in Fig. 37-5 for a patient with atrial fibrillation and dilated cardiomyopathy of uncertain origin.

As in normal persons, lactate production appears in patients with chronic cardiac failure when systemic O_2 extraction exceeds 60 percent. Mixed venous lactate concentration during exercise rises above resting values when 60 percent or more of $\dot{V}_{O_2max}$ is attained.[16,32] Given differences in aerobic capacity between exercise classes, different work loads are associated with this lactate threshold (Fig. 37-6). In class D patients whose cardiac output response is limited, the lactate threshold occurs at very light work loads ($\dot{V}_{O_2}$ of 5 to 8 ml/min/kg). Corresponding values for class C, B, and A patients are 8 to 11 ml/min/kg, 11 to 14 ml/min/kg, and more than 14 ml/min/kg, respectively. Thus, lactate threshold and $\dot{V}_{O_2max}$ reflect the severity of chronic cardiac failure as given in Table 37-3. A noninvasively determined AT based on measurements of respiratory gas exchange, as discussed previously, corresponds to the invasively measured lactate threshold.[16,18,26,32]

Exercise left ventricular filling pressure, as gauged from an occlusive wedge pressure recording, rises to a different degree in

Fig. 37-4 for each exercise class. In class A and B patients, stroke volume rises 50 percent during lighter work loads that represent less than 60 percent of $\dot{V}_{O_2max}$; at larger work loads, further increments in stroke volume are less apparent. A 25 percent rise in stroke volume occurs at submaximal exercise in class C patients, whereas in class D patients, exercise stroke volume is no different from its resting value. Exercise stroke volume is a result of several factors, including systolic wall stress, mitral or tricuspid regurgitation that may appear during exercise, and depressed myocardial contractility.

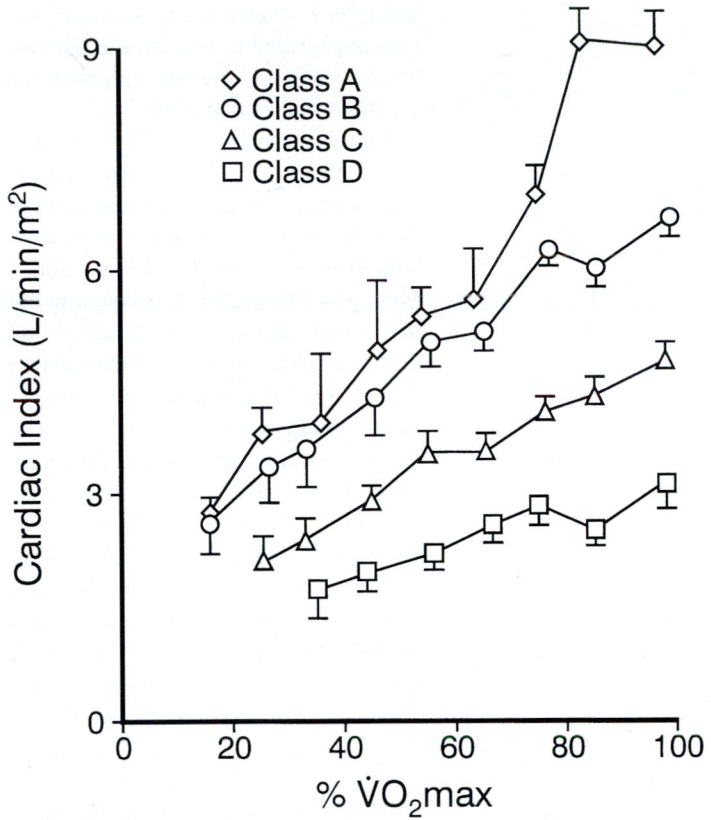

FIGURE 37-3 Relationship between treadmill exercise cardiac index and normalized aerobic capacity for patients with chronic cardiac failure of diverse origin and severity, subdivided according to each functional class. *(From Weber and Janicki.[31])*

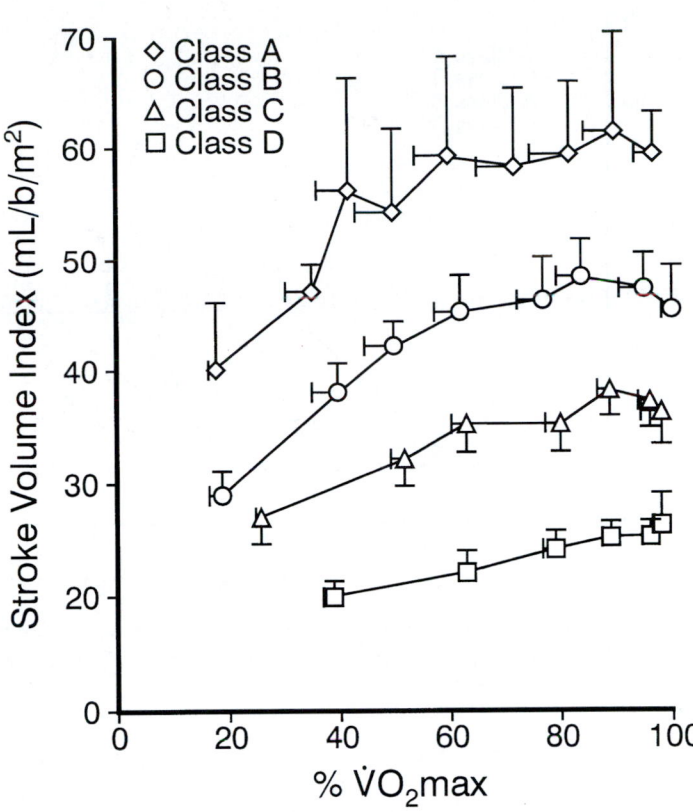

FIGURE 37-4 Relationship between treadmill exercise stroke volume index and normalized aerobic capacity for patients with chronic cardiac failure of varying severity, as expressed by each functional class. *(From Weber and Janicki.[31])*

each exercise class with chronic cardiac failure (Fig. 37-7). In class A patients, the rise in wedge pressure during isotonic exercise rarely exceeds 18 mmHg. This resembles a normal response. In class B patients, more dramatic elevations in exercise wedge pressure—to 25 mmHg or higher—are frequently noted. Resting filling pressure is increased in class C and D patients; a further rise may be seen during upright exercise, often to levels in excess of 30 mmHg. Despite these marked levels of pulmonary venous pressure, patients do not develop evidence of pulmonary congestion after exercise. Moreover, elevations in wedge pressure neither would predict exercise cardiac reserve and aerobic capacity nor are responsible for exertional dyspnea in these patients. Dyspnea corresponds with the lactate threshold and a disproportionate rise in $\dot{V}_E$ relative to $\dot{V}_{O_2}$.[13,25,32,34] Patients can be encouraged to exercise to exhaustion, attaining $\dot{V}_{O_2}$max in the presence of dyspnea. In patients with acute cardiac failure, pulmonary congestion and dyspnea correlate with the elevation in wedge pres-

sure; pulmonary edema occurs when hydrostatic pressure exceeds the colloidal osmotic pressure of 25 mmHg.

$\dot{V}_E$ rises appropriately during incremental exercise in patients with chronic cardiac failure. The response in $\dot{V}_E$ most closely

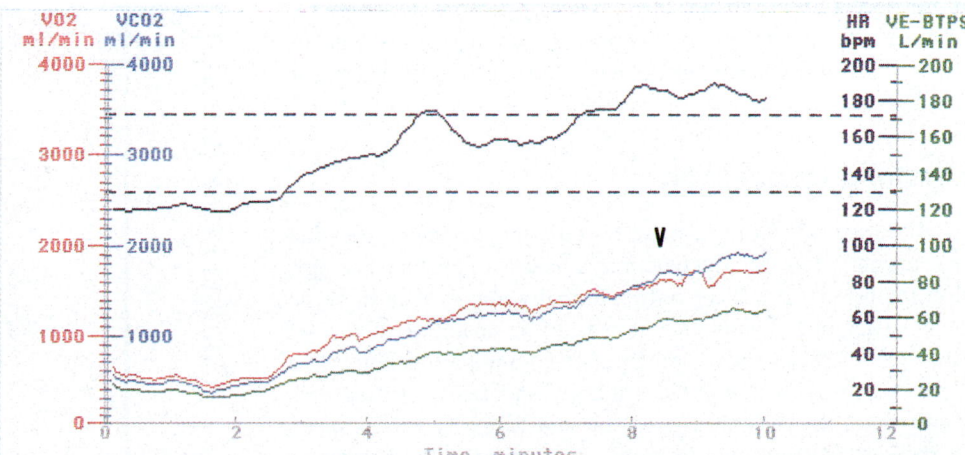

FIGURE 37-5 Cardiopulmonary exercise test results in a 48-year-old man with atrial fibrillation and dilated (idiopathic) cardiomyopathy. Note the rapid heart rate at rest and throughout incremental treadmill exercise. Predicted maximum heart rate range in this patient is shown by the broken lines. He achieved this rate during the first stage of exercise and exceeded it during the last stage of exercise. This is an inappropriate heart rate response. The AT is 13 ml/min/kg (arrow), in keeping with functional class B. He did not achieve $\dot{V}_{O_2}$max and, therefore, had a peak $\dot{V}_{O_2}$ of 15 ml/min/kg.

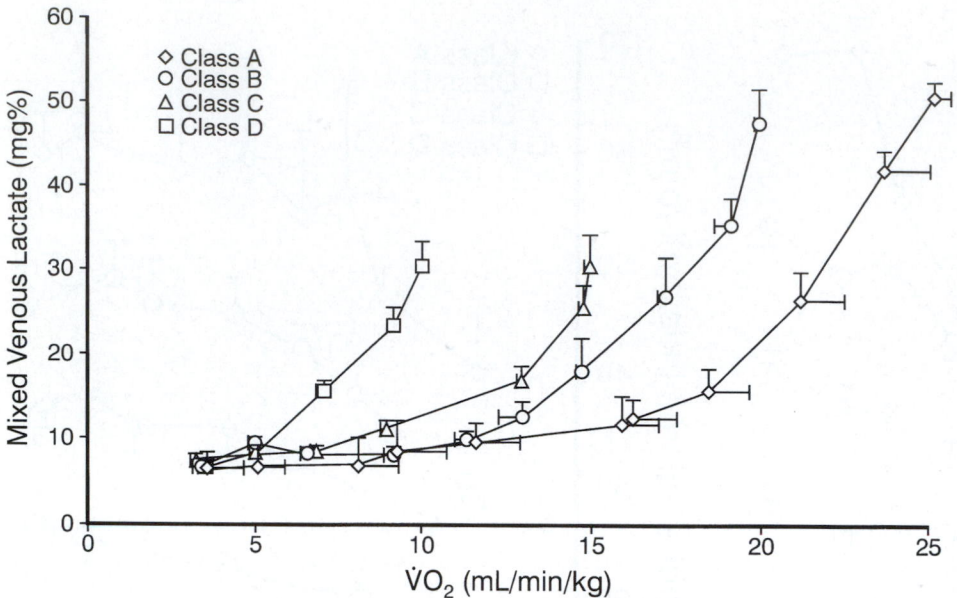

FIGURE 37-6 Relationship between mixed venous lactate concentration and $\dot{V}_{O_2}$ to incremental treadmill exercise for patients with chronic cardiac failure of varying severity, as expressed by each functional class. *(From Weber and Janicki.*[31]*)*

corresponds to $\dot{V}_{CO_2}$ throughout exercise (aerobic and anaerobic work) and is sufficient to sustain alveolar ventilation, thereby preventing hypoxemia and hypercapnia. Maximum $\dot{V}_E$ attained with exercise is less than 50 percent of MVV. Thus, these patients do not exhaust their ventilatory reserve in responding to exercise, even when their pulmonary compliance may be adversely elevated as a result of chronic pulmonary congestion and elevations in pulmonary venous pressure that appear with exercise. In order to minimize the work of breathing during exercise, class C and D patients use a pattern of rapid, shallow breathing to increase $\dot{V}_E$. Thus, the rise in tidal volume during exercise above its resting value is modest and compatible with a substantial portion of each breath being wasted in ventilation of anatomic dead space.[34] The response of class A and B patients more closely approximates that of healthy persons, in whom respiratory rate rises progressively during incremental exercise and the rise in tidal volume occurs early during the transition from rest to low level exercise.

Diastolic Dysfunction

In 30 percent or more of patients with symptomatic heart failure, primary diastolic dysfunction is held responsible. The ejection fraction is normal or only minimally impaired in these patients. Diastolic dysfunction relates to an inability of the left ventricle to accommodate left atrial and pulmonary venous blood flow during diastole without a marked increase in filling pressure. Abnormal diastolic relaxation and filling typically appear in patients with chronic ischemic heart disease (with previous myocardial infarction), in those with hypertensive heart disease, and in the elderly. Responsible mechanisms are thought to include abnormal tissue structure, as occurs with fibrous tissue accumulation or amyloid infiltration and abnormal calcium handling by sarcoplasmic reticulum. Factors extrinsic to the myocardium may also be contributory. Examples include the in-

teraction between the pressure or volume overloaded right ventricle with the left ventricle and the interplay between the heart and pericardium.

Invasive cardiopulmonary exercise testing, together with incremental bicycle exercise, has been used to address the hemodynamic response of patients with primary diastolic dysfunction.[11] Most patients studied had systemic hypertension, and many were elderly; all had a clinical history of pulmonary congestion. Peak exercise $\dot{V}_{O_2}$ was reduced, owing to a reduction in exercise cardiac output and stroke volume responses; arteriovenous O_2 difference rose above 10 ml/dl. The level of $\dot{V}_{O_2}$ achieved with exercise correlated with peak cardiac output response. In comparison to age-matched controls, expected exercise-associated increments in left ventricular end diastolic volume were not seen and were accompanied by increased left ventricular filling pressure. Thus, abnormalities in diastolic filling abrogated the Frank-Starling mechanism, thereby restricting the rise in exercise cardiac output; this finding may serve to explain symptoms of fatigue and breathlessness that these patients experience on exertion.

Primary diastolic dysfunction has been observed in patients following cardiac transplantation[10] in whom there is an abnormal blunting of stroke volume and heart rate responses to exer-

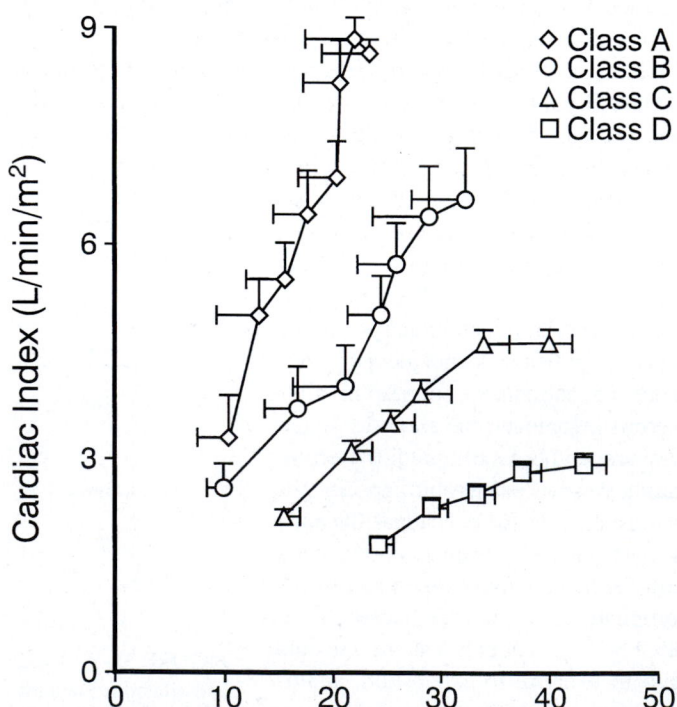

FIGURE 37-7 Relationship between treadmill exercise cardiac index and occlusion wedge pressure in patients with chronic cardiac failure, subdivided according to functional class. *(From Weber and Janicki.*[31]*)*

cise. Despite the slower exercise heart rate in the transplanted, denervated heart, in which diastolic filling periods would accordingly be longer, diastolic dysfunction is present, limiting the exercise cardiac output response. Abnormal diastolic function has also been observed in the elderly and contributes to impaired exercise cardiac output response.[9]

Chronotropic Dysfunction

Cardiac reserve in exercise depends not only on systolic and diastolic function but also on heart rate and rhythm, including a coordinated contraction of the atria and ventricles. Cardiopulmonary exercise testing has been used to address the contribution of abnormal heart rate and rhythm on the AT and $\dot{V}_{O_2}$max, broadly categorized here as chronotropic dysfunction. This includes abnormal sinus tachycardia, bradyarrhythmias, atrioventricular dissociation, and atrial fibrillation. Cardiopulmonary exercise testing has proved useful in the evaluation of pacemaker function and technique.[28] Improvements in the AT at submaximal levels of work have been demonstrated for single-chamber, activity-triggered pacing compared with fixed-rate atrial or ventricular pacing.

CHRONIC CIRCULATORY FAILURE

Circulatory failure, in physiological terms, refers to an inability of the heart to raise its cardiac output in a manner commensurate with prevailing $\dot{V}_{O_2}$. Responsible factors are extrinsic to the myocardium and include such entities as valvular heart disease, intrinsic pulmonary vascular disease, pericardial disease, and anemia.

Valvular Heart Disease

Mitral or aortic valve disease may alter the functional integrity of the cardiopulmonary unit by impairing the heart's ability to increase cardiac output in accordance with $\dot{V}_{O_2}$. Pathophysiological alterations within the unit that result from chronic valvular disease and that determine the clinical course and outcome following valve replacement include right heart overload and structural remodeling of the pulmonary vasculature and lung interstitium. The more marked the preoperative impairment in cardiac reserve, the poorer the long-term prognosis. Similarly, the greater the elevation in pulmonary vascular resistance, the more delayed is its return to normal levels and the slower the postoperative abatement of symptoms. The decision for surgical intervention requires an assessment of cardiopulmonary status—one that can be assessed noninvasively and monitored over time to detect a decline in cardiac reserve. Noninvasive cardiopulmonary exercise testing serves this purpose. Because of the heightened risk of syncope and the myocardial ischemia and arrhythmias that can occur during exercise in patients with aortic valvular stenosis, these patients should exercise with extreme caution, if at all.

Incompetence of the mitral and aortic valves is an example of a disorder that can result in chronic circulatory failure. Each creates a volume overload on the left ventricle. The onset of ventricular dysfunction is generally unpredictable and may initially

appear only during vigorous levels of physical activity. As dysfunction progresses, symptoms appear at lower levels of activity and, finally, at rest.

Resting cardiac output is often not distinguishable among class A, B, C, or D patients with mitral or aortic regurgitation. Cardiac reserve is reduced, however, and, accordingly, so is aerobic capacity.[33] No impairment in systemic O_2 extraction has been reported. Thus, as in chronic cardiac failure, any observed decrease in aerobic capacity must be due to a decline in maximal forward cardiac output. To the extent that cardiac output can rise, the exercise cardiac output–$\dot{V}_{O_2}$ relation is preserved among these classes, averaging 600 ml/min/m² for every dl/min/m² rise in $\dot{V}_{O_2}$. Responses in cardiac output and wedge pressure for each exercise class are given in Fig. 37-8. As in chronic cardiac failure, marked elevations in wedge pressure are seen in class C and D patients; this is also true for class B patients with mitral or aortic regurgitation. However, these patients do not develop clinical evidence of pulmonary congestion following exercise, and dyspnea correlates with the lactate threshold. Exercise wedge pressure does not presage aerobic capacity or functional class in these patients.

Anaerobic threshold can be used as an alternative measure in patients with valvular incompetence who are unable to attain $\dot{V}_{O_2}$max. The lactate threshold occurs at 60 to 70 percent of the patient's aerobic capacity and corresponds to a level of systemic O_2 extraction of 60 percent or more. Figure 37-9 depicts the response in mixed venous lactate concentration as a function of O_2 for each exercise class with mitral or aortic regurgitation. As in patients with chronic cardiac failure, the lactate threshold occurs at progressively lower levels of work as the severity of valvular disease increases.[33] The invasively measured lactate threshold correlates well with the valve obtained using noninvasive respiratory gas exchange measurements (see above).

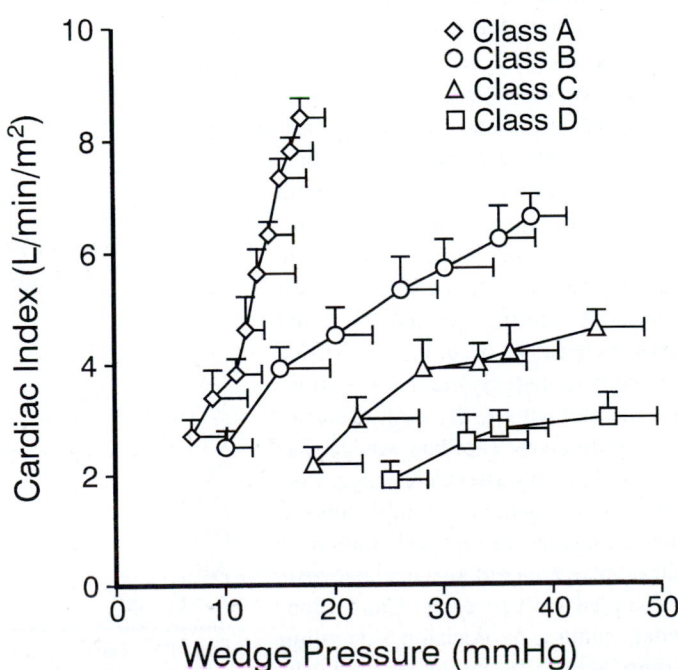

FIGURE 37-8   Relationship between treadmill exercise cardiac index and wedge pressure in patients with chronic mitral or aortic regurgitation, divided according to functional class. *(From Weber and Janicki.[33])*

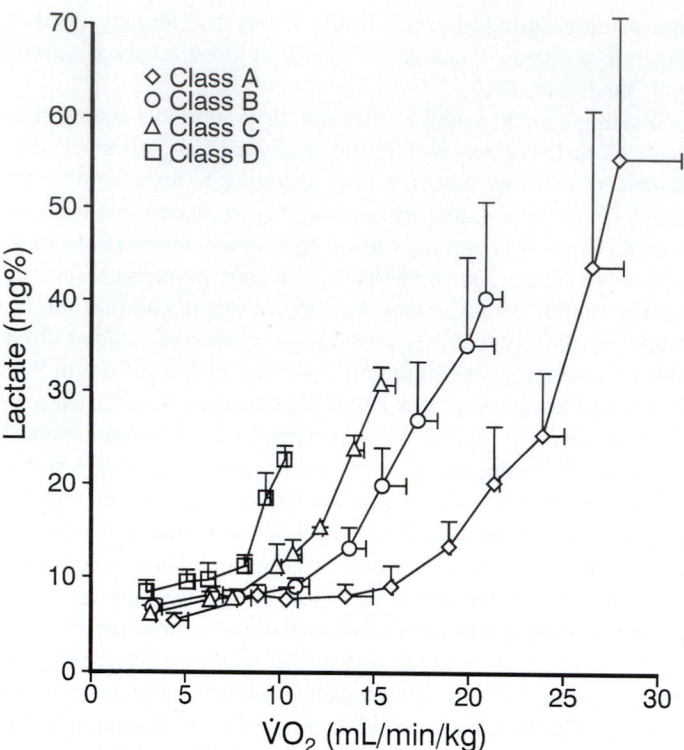

FIGURE 37-9 Relationship between mixed venous lactate concentration and $\dot{V}_{O_2}$ observed during incremental treadmill exercise in patients with chronic mitral or aortic regurgitation. As in chronic cardiac failure, the lactate threshold (lactate >12 mg/dl) occurs at different levels of $\dot{V}_{O_2}$, depending on functional class. *(From Weber and Janicki.[33])*

The reduced mitral valve orifice that accompanies rheumatic mitral valvular stenosis leads to left atrial chamber enlargement, pulmonary venous hypertension, and right heart pressure overload. Pulmonary vascular resistance in most patients ranges between 200 and 600 dynes · s · cm^{-5}. Mitral stenosis is responsible for reduced left ventricular filling at rest and during exercise. An exercise-associated rise in heart rate reduces the diastolic filling period to further curtail left ventricular filling.

Cardiac output fails to rise appropriately with exercise in patients with chronic circulatory failure due to mitral stenosis.[33] For most symptomatic patients, cardiac output fails to rise appropriately during symptom-limited exercise because of a limited stroke volume response. Systemic O_2 extraction increases markedly with exercise, as do pulmonary capillary wedge and mean pulmonary artery pressures. Preoperative assessment of mitral stenosis should include not only calculation of mitral valve area but also exercise test-determined cardiac reserve and functional status. A decision regarding surgery should be based on these objective measures and clinical judgment, not simply on a laboratory-based calculation of reduced valve area.

Pulmonary Hypertension

Pulmonary hypertension is expressed as an abnormal elevation in resting or exercise pulmonary artery pressure. Chronic left heart failure with attendant elevated left atrial pressure remains the most common cause of pulmonary *venous* hypertension. Pulmonary *arterial* hypertension (PAH) accompanies intrinsic pulmonary vascular disease or arteriolar vasoconstriction associated with hypoxemia due to intrinsic lung disease. PAH creates right ventricular pressure overload and an impediment to left ventricular filling. Accordingly, exercise cardiac output is compromised and aerobic capacity declines. PAH represents an example of chronic circulatory failure.

Patients with PAH have been studied with elective right heart catheterization using a triple-lumen flotation catheter and subsequent exercise testing.[33] Resting and peak treadmill exercise hemodynamic responses are given in Table 37-4. At rest, right heart and pulmonary arterial pressures exceeded the normal range. Right ventricular systolic pressure at rest was in excess of 50 mmHg, and in one-quarter of patients it approximated or exceeded left ventricular (and systemic arterial) systolic pressure. Resting wedge pressure was normal in these patients. Calculated pulmonary vascular resistance exceeded the upper range of normal (170 dynes · s · cm^{-5}) in all patients; in more than one-third, it was above 1000 dynes · s · cm^{-5}, approximating systemic vascular resistance.

Peak cardiac output attained with maximal exercise for each functional class (Table 37-3) is similar to that observed for chronic cardiac failure and valvular heart disease. The impairment in exercise cardiac output is related to the extent to which pulmonary vascular resistance is elevated. Patients with a markedly elevated resting pulmonary vascular resistance (above 1000 dynes · s · cm^{-5}) proved to be functional class D. In this group of patients with intrinsic pulmonary vascular disease, arterial O_2 desaturation during exercise was not observed, emphasizing the importance of compromised cardiac reserve—a function of the inability of the right ventricle to generate sufficient pulmonary blood flow to sustain left ventricular filling and,

TABLE 37-4

Resting and Peak Exercise Hemodynamics for Patients with Nonhypoxic Pulmonary Vascular Disease and Pulmonary Hypertension

		Resting	Exercise
PA	(mmHg)	29±9	47±20
RVSP	(mmHg)	52±30	86±37
RVDP	(mmHg)	7±4	16±10
PCW	(mmHg)	10±3	22±14
PVR	(dynes · s · cm^{-5})	412±319	302±331
CO	(L/m^2/min)	2.8±1.6	5.3±2.2
AP	(mmHg)	106±6	130±8
Art O_2 sat	(%)	97±2	96±2

NOTE: PA = mean pulmonary artery pressure; RVSP and RVDP = right ventricular systolic and diastolic pressures, respectively; PCW = wedge pressure; PVR = pulmonary vascular resistance; CO = cardiac output; AP = mean arterial pressure.
SOURCE: Reproduced from Weber KT, Janicki JS: Pulmonary hypertension, in Weber KT, Janicki JS (eds), *Cardiopulmonary Exercise Testing: Physiologic Principles and Clinical Applications.* Philadelphia, Saunders, 1986, pp 220–234.

thereby, systemic blood flow. Patients with PAH stopped exercising because of breathlessness or fatigue or both; none experienced retrosternal chest pain, light-headedness, or syncope; none developed arrhythmias. In most, it was possible to determine the $\dot{V}_{O_2max}$; in all, the AT could be attained (see above). Cardiopulmonary exercise test results for a 42-year-old woman with PAH are shown in Figure 37-10.

In patients with hypoxic pulmonary vasoconstriction, upright isotonic exercise also results in an increase in mean pulmonary artery and right ventricular systolic and diastolic pressures. In many of these patients, pulmonary vascular resistance rises during exercise because of marked hypoxemia, with arterial O_2 saturation ranging between 70 and 80 percent. This response can be attenuated with use of supplemental O_2. As a result, exercise mean pulmonary artery and right ventricular systolic and diastolic pressures rise less dramatically; resting pulmonary artery pressure is reduced.

CHRONIC LUNG DISEASES

In a normal subject performing maximal exercise, $\dot{V}_E$ rarely exceeds 50 percent of MVV; similarly, tidal volume uncommonly exceeds 50 percent of vital capacity. Given this large ventilatory reserve, exercise is not normally limited by ventilation. This changes in patients with lung disease, in whom ventilatory reserves are reduced. Other factors that may limit exercise in patients with lung disease are altered lung mechanics, impaired gas exchange with arterial hypoxemia and the appearance of pulmonary hypertension, and respiratory muscle fatigue.[7,15]

Obstructive Lung Disease

Exercise intolerance commonly accompanies chronic obstructive pulmonary disease (COPD), with dyspnea limiting physical activity to modest levels of work. Patients with COPD have a higher $\dot{V}_E$ for any given work load; this is largely due to increased dead space ventilation. Given their reduction in MVV and greater exercise $\dot{V}_E$, these patients often exercise with a $\dot{V}_E$/MVV ratio that exceeds 75 percent. Use of such a large portion of this ventilatory reserve cannot be sustained, accounting for breathlessness and termination of exercise. This generally occurs in patients with moderate to severe COPD before they have reached their AT, implying a ventilatory, rather than cardiac, limitation to exercise. The work load at which patients terminate exercise represents a peak $\dot{V}_{O_2}$; it is not their $\dot{V}_{O_2max}$, as can be attained in patients with chronic cardiac or circulatory failure in whom ventilatory responses pose no limitation to exercise.

In severe emphysema, DLCO is reduced in keeping with alveolar capillary destruction. In such patients, a significant fall in arterial O_2 saturation often appears during exercise. This is in contrast to patients with chronic bronchitis, in whom O_2 saturation may actually increase. The improvement in oxygenation in these patients is a result of improved ventilation in areas with low ventilation-perfusion ratios. DLCO portends exercise-induced arterial O_2 desaturation. Patients with a DLCO less than 55 percent of predicted are most likely to experience hypoxemia with exercise. Arterial hypoxemia limits effort tolerance, for several reasons: (1) reduced O_2 delivery to exercising muscle, including those associated with respiration; (2) increased chemical drive to respiration with a corresponding inappropriate $\dot{V}_E$ for a given level of work; and (3) secondary pulmonary vasoconstriction.

Restrictive Lung Disease

Patients with known interstitial lung disease, a diverse group of disease entities, experience limiting dyspnea on exertion. This may be secondary to reduced ventilatory reserve or development of arterial O_2 desaturation. The evaluation of exercise performance may also be useful in patients who complain of dyspnea out of proportion to their pulmonary function studies. Dyspnea may appear on exertion in a patient with an abnormal chest radiograph before pulmonary function studies are abnormal. Exercise testing may be indicated in these patients to detect abnormal ventilatory reserve and its response over time. Patients with interstitial lung disease tend to breathe at a higher respiratory rate and lower tidal volume than do normal subjects for any given $\dot{V}_{O_2}$. Because they have a reduced MVV, their ability to exercise is limited by nearly full utilization of their reduced ventilatory reserve.

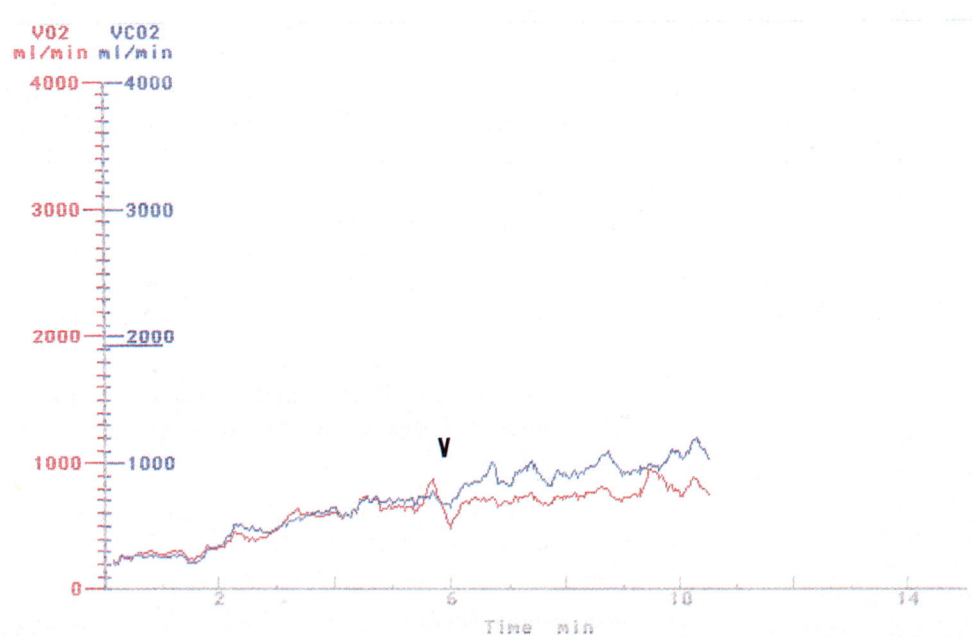

FIGURE 37-10 Cardiopulmonary exercise test results for a 42-year-old woman with pulmonary arterial hypertension of uncertain origin. The first 2 minutes represent standing rest. The patient attained the AT (7 ml/min/kg) during stage 2 of exercise (1.5 mph, 0 grade) and a $\dot{V}_{O_2max}$ of 10 ml/min/kg, corresponding to functional class D.

As in patients with airway disease, the DLCO is a good predictor of arterial O_2 desaturation during exercise in patients with interstitial lung disease. Most patients with a DLCO below 60 percent develop desaturation. If a patient has a normal DLCO, he or she is unlikely to develop exercise-induced arterial O_2 desaturation. Measurement of DLCO can be used to screen patients for exercise studies. Finally, the degree of arterial O_2 desaturation during exercise correlates with the reduction in DLCO.

EVALUATION OF EXERTIONAL DYSPNEA

Normally, a person is unaware of the act of breathing and the fact that 500 to 750 ml of air enters and leaves the lungs 10 to 15 times each minute. $\dot{V}$ increases secondary to normal or abnormal chemical stimuli (e.g., hypercapnia, hypoxemia, acidemia) or anxiety. When breathing is perceived to be inappropriate relative to the level of physical activity, it is considered an abnormal awareness of breathing that is termed breathlessness, shortness of breath, or dyspnea.[33] Dyspnea on exertion is common to patients with heart disease, pulmonary parenchymal or airway disease, and pulmonary vascular disease. Deformities of the chest wall and diseases associated with weakness of the respiratory muscles are also accompanied by exertional breathlessness. Dyspnea may seriously hinder a patient's ability to carry out muscular work, thereby compromising quality of life. The evaluation of dyspnea includes requisite historical information that characterizes its nature, onset, severity, relationship to exercise, and the patient's underlying physical condition and customary daily activity. Other associated symptoms—such as palpitations, anginal chest pain, and light-headedness—must be taken into consideration.

An objective and reliable estimate of dyspnea on exertion and its severity can be gauged from exercise testing. Dyspnea occurs when $\dot{V}_E$ is excessive relative to $\dot{V}_{O_2}$ and when $\dot{V}_E$ is driven by chemical stimuli or altered lung mechanics. Dyspnea with exercise can appear when $\dot{V}_E$ occupies an excessive proportion of MVV. An estimation of MVV can be derived by multiplying the patient's FEV_1 by 35. As a corollary, maximal encroachment on the vital capacity by exercise tidal volume cannot be sustained for long. Such ventilatory effort poses a substantial work load on respiratory muscles. An MVV maneuver during pulmonary function testing cannot be sustained for more than a few seconds, while more than 70 percent of the MVV cannot be sustained by normal subjects for more than several minutes. Hence, the ventilatory response to exercise that is associated with dyspnea in patients with heart or lung disease follows a similar pattern of short-lived, near-maximal ventilation.

The patient with pulmonary vascular disease or advanced interstitial lung disease may be unable to sustain exercise alveolar ventilation at a level commensurate with adequate arterial O_2 saturation. Consequently, hypoxemia may compound the patient's exercise response and be responsible for a heightened chemical drive to respiration. In the case of COPD, the need to move air through a partly obstructed tracheobronchial tree creates an added work load on respiratory muscles. Air flows in these patients are already compromised at rest and must increase with exercise; they may approach peak expiratory flows observed with maximal effort during pulmonary function testing.

Patients with mild, moderate, or severe cardiac or circulatory failure rarely use more than 50 percent of their ventilatory reserve at maximal exercise, and they do not experience arterial O_2 desaturation during exercise. If one estimates MVV from the FEV_1 (as noted above) for an FEV_1 of 1, 2, or 3 L, MVV is expected to equal 35, 70, or 105 L, respectively. In patients with chronic cardiac or circulatory failure, exercise maximum E has been found to range between 62 and 29 L per min for class A through D patients. Hence, unless there is a major reduction in MVV (or in FEV_1 to less than 3 L), these patients will not have a ventilatory limitation to exercise. Finally, patients are able to cross their AT and, if encouraged, may reach their point of exhaustion attaining $\dot{V}_{O_2max}$. By monitoring the breath-by-breath response in $\dot{V}_{O_2}$ and $\dot{V}_{CO_2}$ during exercise, the physician can immediately determine when the patient has achieved the AT and $\dot{V}_{O_2max}$. These end-points are not attained in the patients with lung disease or those with coexistent heart and lung disease in whom the respiratory system is the primary limitation to exercise. Table 37-5 summarizes the salient features used to differentiate primary ventilatory from cardiac or circulatory failure as the cause of exertional dyspnea, as detected by exercise testing.

OTHER APPLICATIONS OF CARDIOPULMONARY EXERCISE TESTING

Cardiopulmonary exercise testing, with its ability to foretell cardiac and ventilatory reserves, has proved useful in clinical decision making in a variety of circumstances, including assessment of a patient's candidacy for cardiac transplantation and preoperative assessment of preoperative risk.

Cardiac Transplantation

The severity of chronic cardiac and circulatory failure is gauged according to $\dot{V}_{O_2max}$ and the AT (Table 37-3) and is used to predict exercise cardiac reserve. This approach has been applied to patients with systolic dysfunction secondary to chronic ischemic heart disease or dilated (idiopathic) cardiomyopathy, who are considered potential candidates for cardiac transplantation. The ejection fraction or resting hemodynamic parameters (e.g., resting cardiac index or wedge pressure) do not help predict the severity of cardiac failure or functional capacity and are no longer a mainstay in decision making. The same is true

---

TABLE 37-5

Ventilatory Versus Cardiac/Circulatory Failure as the Predominant Cause of Exertional Dyspnea

Ventilatory Failure
1. Exercise maximum $\dot{V}_E$ utilizes >70% of MVV
2. Exercise-associated arterial hypoxemia
3. Failure to cross AT and to achieve $\dot{V}_{O_2max}$

Cardiac/Circulatory Failure
1. Cross AT and can achieve $\dot{V}_{O_2max}$
2. Maximum exercise $\dot{V}_E$ does not exceed 50% of MVV
3. Does not develop arterial hypoxemia with exercise

NOTE: AT = anaerobic threshold; MVV = maximal voluntary ventilation.

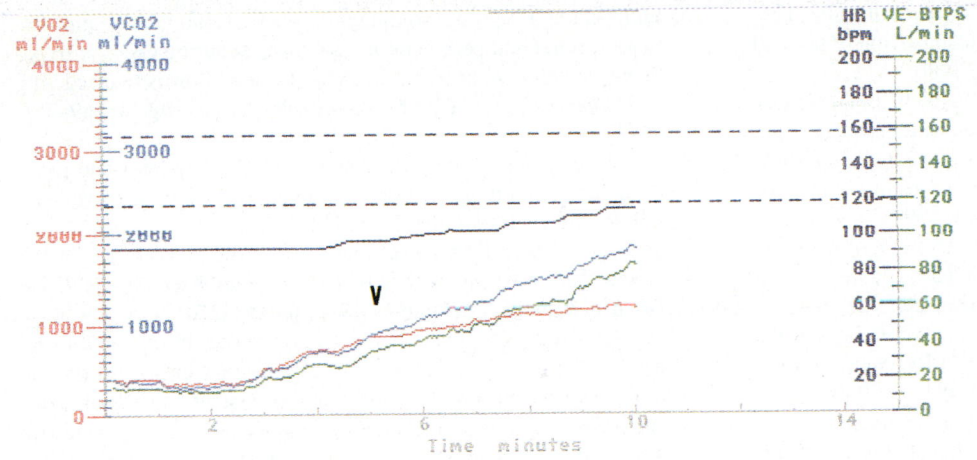

FIGURE 37-11 Cardiopulmonary exercise test results for a 62-year-old male cardiac transplant recipient. During this incremental treadmill test he attained an AT and $\dot{V}_{O_2}max$ of 8 and 11 ml/min/kg, respectively. Note the blunted heart rate response (predicted peak heart rate range shown as broken lines).

for subjective evaluation of functional status using the New York Heart Association criteria. Incremental exercise testing, with identification of AT and peak $\dot{V}_{O_2}$ achieved thereafter, has emerged as a valuable tool to objectively address cardiac reserve and functional capacity and which predicts survival.[4,12,14,24,29] In fact, consensus has been reached on recommending transplantation based on clinical criteria, in combination with functional stratification based on exercise test results.[19] Class D patients, having little or no cardiac reserve, have a marked reduction in 1- and 2-year survival and, therefore, are candidates for urgent transplantation. Class C patients with a modest increment in exercise cardiac output are probable candidates. On the other hand, class A and B patients in whom cardiac reserve remains intact, or class B patients in whom cardiac reserve is only minimally impaired, do not have an adequate indication for transplantation. Decision is deferred, and serial exercise studies are used to assess recovery or deterioration in the setting of optimal medical therapy.

Incremental exercise testing may also provide useful information after cardiac transplantation, including recovery of cardiac and ventilatory reserves. The importance of diastolic dysfunction in limiting exercise tolerance following cardiac transplantation was reviewed earlier. A blunted heart rate response to exercise is expected in these patients owing to cardiac denervation. Such chronotropic incompetence is demonstrated in Fig. 37-11, along with exercise test results.

Preoperative Risk

Preoperative incremental exercise testing has proved useful in assessing postoperative morbidity and mortality in the elderly and patients with underlying heart or lung disease who are scheduled for major intrathoracic or intraabdominal surgery. The premise underlying this approach is based on a recognition that during and after surgery, there may be a need to call on cardiac and ventilatory reserves—namely, the ability to increase cardiac output and maintain O_2 delivery, and to increase $\dot{V}E$ and prevent hypoxemia. Several studies have demonstrated the utility

of measuring the AT and peak $\dot{V}_{O_2}$, using exercise testing, in addressing these reserves and in identifying patients prone to postoperative complications.[1,20,23] Pulmonary function testing proved insensitive in forecasting postoperative course. Class C and D patients, with little or no cardiac reserve, had a greater number of morbid and mortal events following surgical interventions than did class A or B patients. Class A patients had few, if any, postoperative complications and no mortality. The risk of complications could, therefore, be gauged best by a patient's preoperative aerobic capacity.[1,8,20,23] The direct assessment of the AT or $\dot{V}_{O_2}max$ and prediction of cardiac reserve, and, by inference, ventilatory reserve supersede the value of an age-determined impairment in aerobic capacity.

REFERENCES

1. Bechard D, Wetstein L: Assessment of oxygen consumption as a preoperative criterion for lung resection. *Ann Thorac Surg* 44:344–349, 1987.
2. Clark AL, Poole-Wilson PA, Coats AJS: Effects of motivation of the patient on indices of exercise capacity in chronic heart failure. *Br Heart J* 71:162–165, 1994.
3. Cohen-Solal A: Cardiopulmonary exercise testing in chronic heart failure, in Wasserman K (ed), *Exercise Gas Exchange in Heart Disease.* Armonk, NY, Futura, 1996, pp 17–38.
4. Cohn JN, Rector TS: Prognosis of congestive heart failure and predictors of mortality. *Am J Cardiol* 62:25A–30A, 1988.
5. Dickstein K, Barvik S, Aarsland T, Snapinn S: Reproducibility of cardiopulmonary exercise testing in men following myocardial infarction. *Eur Heart J* 9:948–954, 1985.
6. Franciosa JA, Leddy CL, Wilen M, Schwartz DE: Relation between hemodynamic and ventilatory responses in determining exercise capacity in severe congestive heart failure. *Am J Cardiol* 53:127–134, 1984.
7. Gallagher CG: Exercise limitation and clinical exercise testing in chronic obstructive pulmonary disease. *Clin Chest Med* 15:305–326, 1994.
8. Gilbreth EM, Weisman IM: Role of exercise stress testing in preoperative evaluation of patients for lung resection. *Clin Chest Med* 15:389–403, 1994.
9. Higginbotham MB: Diastolic dysfunction and exercise gas exchange, in Wasserman K (ed), *Exercise Gas Exchange in Heart Disease.* Armonk, NY, Futura, 1996, pp 39–54.
10. Kao AC, Van Trigt P III, Shaeffer-McCall GS, et al: Central and peripheral limitations to upright exercise in untrained cardiac transplant recipients. *Circulation* 89:2605–2615, 1994.
11. Kitzman DW, Sheikh KH, Beere PA, et al: Age-related alterations of Doppler left ventricular filling indexes in normal subjects are independent of left ventricular mass, heart rate, contractility and loading conditions. *J Am Coll Cardiol* 18:1243–1250, 1991.
12. Likoff MJ, Chandler SL, Kay HR: Clinical determinants of mortality in chronic congestive heart failure secondary to idiopathic dilated or to ischemic cardiomyopathy. *Am J Cardiol* 59:634–638, 1987.

13. Lipkin DP, Canepa-Anson R, Stephens MR, Poole-Wilson PA: Factors determining symptoms in heart failure: Comparison of fast and slow exercise tests. *Br Heart J* 55:439–445, 1986.

14. Mancini DM, Eisen H, Kussmaul W, et al: Value of peak exercise oxygen consumption for optimal timing of cardiac transplantation in ambulatory patients with heart failure. *Circulation* 83:778–786, 1991.

15. Marciniuk DD, Gallagher CG: Clinical exercise testing in interstitial lung disease. *Clin Chest Med* 15:287–303, 1994.

16. Matsumura N, Nishijima H, Kojima S, et al: Determination of anaerobic threshold for assessment of functional state in patients with chronic heart failure. *Circulation* 68:360–367, 1983.

17. McElroy PA, Janicki JS, Weber KT: Physiological correlates of the heart rate response to upright isotonic exercise: Relevance to rate-responsive pacemakers. *J Am Coll Cardiol* 11:94–99, 1988.

18. Metra M, Raddino R, Dei Cas L, Visioli O: Assessment of peak oxygen consumption, lactate and ventilatory thresholds and correlation with resting and exercise hemodynamic data in chronic congestive heart failure. *Am J Cardiol* 65:1127–1133, 1990.

19. Mudge GH, Goldstein S, Addonizio LJ, et al: 24th Bethesda conference: Cardiac transplantation. Task Force 3: Recipient guidelines/prioritization. *J Am Coll Cardiol* 22:21–31, 1993.

20. Older P, Smith R, Courtney P, Hone R: Preoperative evaluation of cardiac failure and ischemia in elderly patients by cardiopulmonary exercise testing. *Chest* 104:701–704, 1993.

21. Page E, Cohen-Solal A, Jondeau G, et al: Comparison of treadmill and bicycle exercise in patients with chronic heart failure. *Chest* 106:1002–1006, 1994.

22. Pollock ML, Wilmore JH, Fox SM: *Health and Fitness Through Physical Activity.* New York, Wiley, 1978.

23. Smith TP, Kinasewitz GT, Tucker WY, et al: Exercise capacity as a predictor of post-thoracotomy morbidity. *Am Rev Respir Dis* 129:730–734, 1984.

24. Stevenson LW: Role of exercise testing in the evaluation of candidates for cardiac transplantation. In Wasserman K (ed), *Exercise Gas Exchange in Heart Disease.* Armonk, NY, Futura, 1996, pp 271–286.

25. Sullivan MJ, Higginbotham MB, Cobb FR: Increased exercise ventilation in patients with chronic heart failure: Intact ventilatory control despite hemodynamic and pulmonary abnormalities. *Circulation* 77:552–559, 1988.

26. Sullivan MJ, Knight JD, Higginbotham MB, Cobb FR: Relation between central and peripheral hemodynamics during exercise in patients with chronic heart failure. Muscle blood flow is reduced with maintenance of arterial perfusion pressure. *Circulation* 80:769–781, 1989.

27. Szlachcic J, Massie BM, Kramer BL, et al: Correlates and prognostic implication of exercise capacity in chronic congestive heart failure. *Am J Cardiol* 55:1037–1042, 1985.

28. Treese N: Exercise gas exchange to evaluate cardiac pacemaker function, in Wasserman K (ed), *Exercise Gas Exchange in Heart Disease.* Armonk, NY, Futura, 1996, pp 257–270.

29. van den Broek SAJ, van Veldhuisen DJ, de Graeff PA, et al: Comparison between New York Heart Association classification and peak oxygen consumption in the assessment of functional status and prognosis in patients with mild to moderate chronic congestive heart failure secondary to either ischemic or idiopathic dilated cardiomyopathy. *Am J Cardiol* 70:359–363, 1992.

30. Wasserman K (ed): *Exercise Gas Exchange in Heart Disease.* Armonk, NY, Futura, 1996.

31. Weber KT, Janicki JS: Cardiopulmonary exercise testing for evaluation of chronic cardiac failure. *Am J Cardiol* 55:22A–31A, 1985.

32. Weber KT, Janicki JS: Lactate production during maximal and submaximal exercise in patients with chronic heart failure. *J Am Coll Cardiol* 6:717–724, 1985.

33. Weber KT, Janicki JS (eds): *Cardiopulmonary Exercise Testing: Physiologic Principles and Clinical Applications.* Philadelphia, Saunders, 1986.

34. Weber KT, Kinasewitz GT, Janicki JS, Fishman AP: Oxygen utilization and ventilation during exercise in patients with chronic cardiac failure. *Circulation* 65:1213–1223, 1982.

35. Weber KT, Kinasewitz GT, West JS, et al: Long-term vasodilation therapy with trimazosin in chronic cardiac failure. *New Engl J Med* 303:242–250, 1980.

36. Weber KT, Likoff MJ, McCarthy D: Low-dose beta blockade in the treatment of chronic cardiac failure. *Am Heart J* 104:877–879, 1982.

37. Wilson JR, Ferraro N: Exercise intolerance in patients with chronic left heart failure: Relation to oxygen transport and ventilatory abnormalities. *Am J Cardiol* 51:1358–1363, 1983.

BRONCHOSCOPY, TRANSTHORACIC NEEDLE ASPIRATION, AND RELATED PROCEDURES

Michael Unger / Daniel Sterman

Gustav Killian reported his experience with the first bronchoscopy in 1898.[23] Technologic advances during the next century facilitated development of bronchoscopy as a pivotal diagnostic and therapeutic tool in pulmonary medicine. Although a number of bronchoesophagologists contributed to refinement of the technique based upon use of a rigid instrument, the advent of flexible fiberoptic bronchoscopy, pioneered by Ikeda in 1967, opened new horizons to clinicians.

More recently, transthoracic needle aspiration and biopsy have been added to the pulmonologist's diagnostic armamentarium. These techniques are particularly useful for evaluating localized or peripheral lung lesions. Transthoracic needle aspiration permits acquisition of material for cytologic and microbiologic analysis, while transthoracic needle biopsy provides tissue for histologic study.

This chapter comprises an overview of bronchoscopy, transthoracic needle aspiration and biopsy, and related techniques. Following a general discussion of bronchoscopy and associated general instrumentation, indications for the technique and patient preparation are considered. Specific applications of diagnostic and therapeutic bronchoscopy are discussed. Subsequently, safety factors related to bronchoscopy and complications of the technique are reviewed. Finally, transthoracic needle aspiration and biopsy are described.

TYPES OF BRONCHOSCOPY AND GENERAL INSTRUMENTATION

In the first three-quarters of the twentieth century, pulmonary endoscopy was performed with open-tube steel bronchoscopes. The advent of fiberoptic technology and, subsequently, miniaturized electronics permitted application of flexible endoscopy, as discussed below.

Rigid Bronchoscopy

The initial bronchoscope, developed by Killian in Europe and further perfected by Jackson in the United States, was a rigid metal tube that permitted either spontaneous or mechanical ventilation. Over the decades, rigid bronchoscopes of various lengths and sizes, which are adaptable for diverse applications in children and adults, have become available.[20] With development of fiberoptic and advanced electronic technology, the flexible bronchoscope has, to a large extent, replaced the rigid bronchoscope for both diagnostic and some therapeutic indications.

Both rigid and flexible modern systems are equipped with optic capabilities for airway observation alone. With the rigid bronchoscope, various types of telescopic rods, equipped with circumferential illumination, permit direct and magnified visualization. Specially designed telescopes allow viewing not only directly forward but also at oblique and lateral angles. Various diagnostic and therapeutic accessories can be inserted through the rigid bronchoscope while the patient remains ventilated.

In recent years, development of small cameras based on charged couple device (CCD) technology has facilitated transmission of bronchoscopic images to television monitors, enhancing the education of trainees and permitting improved documentation of bronchoscopic findings.

Flexible Fiberoptic and Videobronchoscopy

Although the optical resolution of early fiberoptic bronchoscopes was inferior to that of rigid devices, their flexibility, ease of manipulation, and simplicity of use, which permit rapid examination under topical anesthesia, have made flexible bronchoscopy the primary endoscopic procedure in pulmonary diseases.

Unlike the larger-bore rigid bronchoscope, the flexible bronchoscope varies from ultrathin, allowing for neonatal endoscopy, to larger, adult-size therapeutic devices. The diameter of the working channel permits aspiration of secretions or introduction of accessories required for diagnostic or therapeutic purposes (see below). With flexible bronchoscopy, the patient's ventilation is assured by airflow around the bronchoscope, between the external wall of the device and the tracheobronchial tree. Thus, the appropriate selection of bronchoscope size is crucial.

Recent technologic advances have permitted the replacement of fiberoptic systems by a miniaturized CCD camera at the tip of the scope that provides electronic transmission of images to a television monitor. Flexible bronchoscopes are more fragile and more prone to damage than are rigid metal instruments. Appropriate care and adherence to safety techniques during procedures, as well as during routine cleaning and maintenance of the instruments, help assure extended instrument life and reduce repair costs.

Diagnostic Bronchoscopy Accessories

The working channel of the fiberoptic or videobronchoscope, although of relatively small diameter, allows the insertion of various diagnostic and therapeutic accessories. Specially constructed accessories of larger caliber have been developed for use with the rigid bronchoscope.

BIOPSY FORCEPS

Simple visualization of lesions is usually not sufficient to determine a precise diagnosis and to guide management. Pathologic confirmation through biopsy is frequently required. A variety of instruments with improved distal control (i.e., control beyond the tip of the bronchoscope) have been developed that permit tissue cutting and retrieval of biopsy specimens.

The cutting cups of biopsy forceps may be round or elliptic and may have smooth or jagged edges. The use of nonserrated edges, however, seems to reduce tissue trauma and the concomitant risk of bleeding. The biopsy procedure is simple and generally associated with only minimal complications in the case of a visible lesion. Even peripheral lesions, which are not visible through the bronchoscope, may be biopsied.[33] With diffuse parenchymal or interstitial lung disease, specimens may be obtained without fluoroscopic guidance. With smaller or focal lesions, however, the diagnostic yield of biopsies increases when fluoroscopy is utilized.

BRONCHIAL BRUSHES

Lesions not accessible to direct biopsy with a forceps can be approached with a bronchial brush. This device consists of a rigid central wire surrounded by brushes of various sizes and shapes. To-and-fro movement of the brush against the adjacent tissue produces minor trauma but enables collection of ample specimens for cytologic or microbiologic analysis.

In some clinical circumstances, there is a need to obtain from the lower respiratory tract an uncontaminated specimen for microbiologic studies. A brush protected by an additional sheath and tip may be passed through the working channel of the bronchoscope (protected brush specimen, as discussed below). In these cases, special attention is needed not to use an excessive amount of local anesthetic or saline lavage, since these solutions contain bacteriostatic material that may inhibit microbial growth. The diagnostic yield depends on use of proper technique, appropriate choice of brush, and careful collection and preservation of the specimen.

NEEDLES FOR ASPIRATION AND BIOPSY

The first performance of a transbronchoscopic needle biopsy through a rigid bronchoscope was reported by Schieppati. Wang then developed a flexible needle technique, utilizing a fiberoptic bronchoscope. Initially, several models of needles were designed to obtain cytologic material; subsequently, histologic specimens from submucosal lesions and peribronchial mediastinal and hilar lymph nodes were obtained with larger-bore needles. These methods are useful in obtaining diagnostic material from areas that cannot be sampled with simple bronchoscopy forceps or brushes. The main indication for use of this type of cytology needle is staging of lung carcinoma.[51] The procedure is particularly useful for patients who are marginal or poor surgical candidates; in these patients, more invasive approaches, such as mediastinoscopy or mediastinotomy, may be obviated.

The tip of the needle is protected by a metal hub during the insertion and withdrawal to avoid damage to the flexible scope. Perforation of the working channel of the scope may occur if the needle is advanced in an exposed position. The diagnostic yield depends on two factors: optimization of the bend of the tip of the bronchoscope and proper performance of bronchial wall puncture by the needle through the intercartilaginous space. Familiarity with the type of needle used increases the success rate.

DEDICATED CATHETERS AND BALLOONS

Various investigational protocols for study of lung diseases utilize the technique of bronchoalveolar lavage (see below) and collection of uncontaminated specimens. In performing this procedure, selective aspiration catheters are necessary. These bronchoscopically guided, double-lumen catheters are wedged in the selected bronchus. After inflation of a balloon and isolation of the bronchus, instillation of fluid through the central lumen of the catheter is followed by aspiration of the fluid. In another application, the low-pressure balloon catheters contribute to estimation of airway diameter before the insertion of a stent (see below) (Fig. 38-1). Sometimes, inflation of the balloon at the tip of the bronchoscope permits enlargement of the lumen and eventual penetration of the bronchoscope beyond the area of stenosis, allowing exploration of peripheral airways.

ULTRASOUND PROBES

Recent technologic advances, including miniaturization of various instruments, have allowed for the integration of ultrasound equipment into the body of the bronchoscope and development of separate ultrasound probes that can be introduced through the working channel.[45] The integrated ultrasound bronchoscope may provide either linear array images, with sectional visualization of the bronchial wall and peribronchial structures, or circumferential pictures. Special attention is necessary to maintain close contact between the ultrasound probe and the bronchial wall. The presence of air understandably interferes with proper imaging. To avoid any interposition of air between the probe and the bronchus, specially designed fluid-filled balloons secure intimate contact with the airway wall, which allows better resolution and visualization of the peribronchial structures. Through improved image resolution, various histologic layers in bronchial structures can be delineated. With further refinements, these devices should provide better guidance for more precise biopsies, the potential

for in vivo diagnosis of infiltrative diseases of the bronchi, and more reliable delineation of clear surgical margins in lung cancer surgery.

PATIENT PREPARATION AND MONITORING DURING BRONCHOSCOPY

Most fiberoptic bronchoscopies are performed after patient premedication with sedative agents. The most frequently used are codeine, midazolam, hydroxyzine, and diazepam.[39] The sedatives are generally administered along with anticholinergic medication (e.g., atropine or glycopyrrolate) in order to reduce the risk of vasovagal reactions and to minimize airway secretions. Local anesthesia of the upper airway, larynx, and tracheobronchial tree is achieved with inhaled or bronchoscopically instilled lidocaine. This agent is generally preferred to cocaine because of the reduced risk of cardiac complications.

Although rigid bronchoscopy was performed initially with minimal anesthesia and later under general anesthesia, the recent trend has been to perform the procedure with patients either breathing spontaneously or ventilated with a jet ventilator. With appropriate monitoring, good oxygenation and adequate ventilation can be assured.[44]

Success of bronchoscopy, whether diagnostic or therapeutic, depends, in large part, on proper preparation of the patient, including relief of anxiety, muscle relaxation, cough suppression, and adequate anesthesia. Time spent in achieving these goals will be well worth it in reducing the risks of complications and in increasing the ease of performance of the procedure. As with any other procedure, analysis of the risk-benefit ratio helps reduce the complication rate. During and shortly after the procedure, appropriate monitoring of hemodynamic parameters (heart rate, rhythm, and blood pressure), oxygenation, and ventilation contributes to safety of bronchoscopy. Knowledge of the underlying disease process also has a significant influence on the choice of study procedures and risk of complications.

In the case of diffuse lung disease, use of fluoroscopy does not improve the yield of transbronchial biopsies. Fluoroscopy is useful, however, in providing information regarding the proximity of the forceps to the pleura and in more rapidly establishing the diagnosis of complications (e.g., pneumothorax). The role of fluoroscopy is essential in cases of localized peripheral lesions when attempts are made to obtain tissue by transbronchial (forceps or needle) biopsy.[33] Fluoroscopy provides the correct orientation of the instrument for tissue sampling from the affected area. In these cases, the risk of biopsy-induced pneumothorax is reduced with use of fluoroscopy.

Insertion of brachytherapy catheters and their precise localization must be accomplished with fluoroscopic guidance. Similarly, placement of various types of stents is facilitated by fluoroscopic control (see below).

APPLICATIONS OF DIAGNOSTIC BRONCHOSCOPY

Although the initial indications for bronchoscopy described by Killian and Chevalier Jackson centered primarily on therapeutic applications, both clinicians recognized the central role the tech-

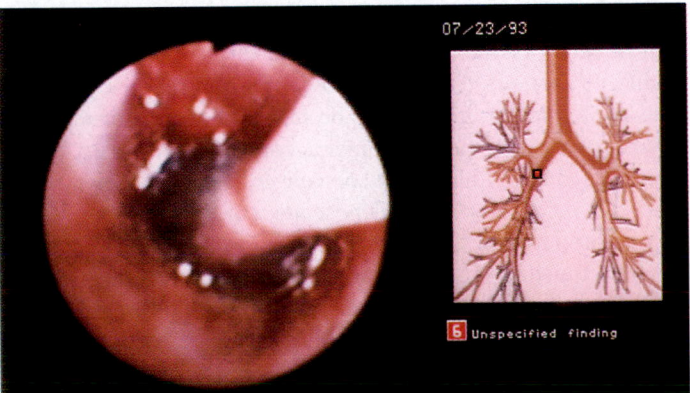

FIGURE 38-1   Use of a balloon catheter in measuring the diameter of an obstructed bronchus. The balloon also provides information regarding the firmness of the stenosis.

nique plays in visual examination of the tracheobronchial tree. Bronchoscopy is currently the primary means for diagnosing pulmonary malignancies.[7,42]

Development of the flexible bronchoscope and various accessory instruments that can be inserted via the working channel has extended bronchoscopic exploration to the lung periphery. The instrument permits acquisition of tissue biopsy specimens, selective mucosal brushings, and bronchoalveolar washings. In addition, a transbronchoscopic approach permits selective sampling of mediastinal structures,[48] as described below.

Assessment of Airway Anatomy and Function

Thorough bronchoscopic evaluation begins with examination of the upper airways. Special attention should be paid to the integrity of air passages and the function of the larynx. It is of paramount importance to distinguish among normal anatomy, anatomic variations without clinical significance, and frankly pathologic conditions. These considerations have important implications regarding potential diagnostic and therapeutic approaches. For example, finding an abnormal branching of a bronchus may be of no clinical significance. On the other hand, such an abnormality could explain symptoms of frequent infections due to impaired ventilation and drainage of the affected area. Special skills and observational experience are required for bronchoscopic examination after surgery, especially following creative bronchoplastic procedures or lung transplantation.

Assessment of airway integrity, with special attention to dynamic changes in airway caliber during either relaxed breathing or forced expiration and coughing, may be crucial in determining appropriate therapeutic maneuvers. Flexible bronchoscopy is superior to rigid bronchoscopy for this assessment. Relaxation and prolapse of the membranous portion of the trachea and main bronchi secondary to destruction of elastic connective tissue may account for exacerbations of expiratory airflow obstruction. On the other hand, finding localized, posttraumatic chondromalacia has very different therapeutic implications. On the basis of these bronchoscopic determinations, open surgical versus bronchoscopic therapeutic correction may be chosen.

Bronchoscopic examination generally permits evaluation and localization of congenital or postsurgical pathologic changes in bronchial integrity, such as tracheoesophageal or bronchopleural fistulas. Bronchoscopic observation and early diagnosis of bronchial rupture after chest trauma also greatly influence further therapy and prognosis. The same is true for evaluation of postsurgical anastomoses in reconstructive or posttransplantation surgery.

Advances in airway management in critically ill patients who require prolonged intubation or tracheotomy have resulted in reduction in the incidence of tracheal injuries. Delayed tracheal injuries documented by bronchoscopy are not rare, however. Such complications can have significant bearing on clinical outcome.

Evaluation of Tracheobronchial Mucosa

Careful examination of the mucosal surface is crucial in the formulation of differential diagnosis.[13] Rapid development of granulation tissue is frequently associated with reaction to a foreign body. Inflammatory mucosal reactions, although not very characteristic, should raise the possibility of mycobacterial infection, nonspecific viral and nonviral infections, and other granulomatous diseases, such as sarcoidosis.

The distinction between normal, pale-pink mucosa and hypervascular areas in the tracheobronchial tree may provide important diagnostic clues.[13] Most frequently, changes in mucosal coloration are associated with an inflammatory reaction due to bronchitis. These findings are, however, very distinctive from small hemangiomas or vascular distentions due to compression by enlarged, neoplastic lymph nodes. Similarly, a network of small mucosal lymphatics may be visible, with lymphatic interruption due to surgery, radiation therapy, fibrosis, or malignancy. This is most frequently associated with local edema, which contributes to airflow obstruction. In addition, distinct and characteristic mucosal discoloration can be observed in Kaposi's sarcoma.

Ulcerations of the mucosa are more characteristic of Wegener's granulomatosis or malignancy. Loss of the usual mucosal luster and presence of a roughened surface may alert the expert bronchoscopist to an early infiltrative or neoplastic process. Previously sustained injuries are characterized by the formation of mucosal and submucosal fibrosis, resulting in airway retraction or distortion.

Recently, various photosensitizers have been applied for the bronchoscopic evaluation of the tracheobronchial mucosa. Photosensitizers, such as hematoporphyrin derivative (HPD) and δ-aminoleveulinic acid (ALA), are retained more selectively by neoplastic tissues. When stimulated by blue light (wavelength, about 440 nm), tissues containing these photosensitizers (i.e., tumors but not normal tissues) emit weak fluorescence in the red spectrum (wavelength, about 630 nm). The low-intensity fluorescence can be captured by specially designed image intensifiers. The technique may be helpful in cancer detection or in the delineation of tumor limits.[10,25] Use of photosensitizers, however, is cumbersome and associated with skin photosensitivity and risk of sunburn. For these reasons, photosensitizer-mediated photodynamic techniques are not yet clinically practical.

Recent technologic developments permit observation and analysis of tracheobronchial mucosal surfaces using the discriminant characteristic of tissue autofluorescence.[26] It is well known that when stimulated with light of a specific wavelength, normal tissues emit specific fluorescence. Changes in the structural integrity of the same tissues due to pathologic processes modify or suppress the autofluorescence. The fluorescent emissions are too low in intensity to be seen by the human eye. With the use of a sophisticated camera, computer-controlled image analysis, and lung-imaging fluorescent endoscopy (LIFE system) attached to a fiberoptic bronchoscope, the airways can be examined for autofluorescence.

The acquisition of images is obtained in real time and helps in the detection of minute areas of change in normal tracheobronchial mucosal fluorescence. Biopsies from areas of abnormal fluorescence increase the rate of detection of small, premalignant (dysplasia) or early malignant (carcinoma in situ) lesions in the tracheobronchial tree. Confirmation is provided by biopsy of the suspect or abnormal areas under direct bronchoscopic control, followed by pathologic review. Attempts are under way to develop bronchoscopic spectrophotometric techniques for study of metabolic functions in vivo and performance of "optical biopsies," which provide information on specific tissue components—e.g., changes in intracellular concentrations of NADPH or other cellular constituents.

Evaluation of Hemoptysis

One of the most frequent indications for bronchoscopy is hemoptysis. Bronchoscopic evaluation can be of help in determining the precise location and the source of bleeding.[41] The choice of instrument (rigid versus flexible), as well as the timing of the procedure, should be dictated by clinical circumstances. Studies have shown that bronchoscopy is more effective in localizing the site of bleeding if performed early (91 percent yield) than if performed late (50 percent yield). In the case of a normal chest radiograph and hemoptysis, it is common to find traces of bleeding but not the site of origin. In these circumstances, examination with an ultrathin flexible instrument may be beneficial in identifying the source of bleeding in a peripheral airway. In some instances, bronchoscopy becomes useful not only as a diagnostic method but also as a therapeutic procedure (see below).

Evaluation of Peribronchial Structures

The trachea and bronchi are surrounded by mediastinal and parenchymal structures. Developmental or pathologic changes in these organs may be noted during bronchoscopic evaluation. An enlarged goiter or thymus can compress upper airways, resulting in airflow obstruction. Lymphadenopathy may produce structural changes, including widening of the carina due to subcarinal involvement and compression of other bronchi—as, for example, in the right-middle-lobe syndrome. Calcification of peribronchial lymph nodes may result in erosion of the bronchial wall and formation of a broncholith. These lesions are potential sources of obstruction, infection, or dangerous hemoptysis.

Development of the techniques of transbronchoscopic needle aspiration and biopsy has permitted sampling of the peribronchial lymph nodes. These transbronchial approaches provide us with diagnostic options that pose much less risk and a lower complication rate than mediastinoscopy; in addition, they are less costly. The transbronchial approach also facilitates, to a certain extent, more accurate staging of bronchogenic carcinoma.[48,52] Bronchoscopy with transbronchial needle aspiration and biopsy can be performed on an outpatient basis, through fiberoptic instruments, using real-time fluoroscopic or computed tomographic (CT) guidance.

New developments in bronchoscopic ultrasonography should further assist in the precise localization of lesions and guidance of diagnostic biopsies and needle aspirations.[45] With further technologic advances, integration of ultrasound is expected to provide higher resolution and better definition of fine bronchial structures and tissue layers, facilitating differential diagnosis.

Performance of Bronchial and Parenchymal Biopsies

Improvements in bronchoscopic instrumentation since the days of Chevalier Jackson have permitted performance of endo-

bronchial biopsies, as well as biopsy of peripheral lung lesions. Bronchoscopically visible lesions are generally biopsied with minimal risk; if bleeding occurs, it can usually be controlled easily. Transbronchial biopsies for diffuse parenchymal disease are usually of low risk and do not necessitate fluoroscopic guidance. In cases of small, peripheral, localized lesions, fluoroscopy is nevertheless mandatory to assure proper positioning of the brush, biopsy forceps, or needle.[33,42] Diffuse diseases, like sarcoidosis, can be diagnosed by transbronchial biopsy with a high rate of success and with minimal risk. The diagnosis of various infectious diseases can be established with a variety of transbronchoscopic sampling techniques. The role of bronchoscopic biopsy has been reaffirmed in immunocompromised hosts, in whom documentation of the precise pathogen is crucial for appropriate therapy. For example, while the presence of cytomegalovirus in bronchoalveolar lavage fluid may not be diagnostic, documentation of intracellular inclusion bodies on a biopsy specimen is practically pathognomonic. Simple, cost-effective transbronchoscopic tissue sampling can obviate much more complicated, expensive, and higher-risk transthoracic needle biopsy or thoracic surgical procedures.[42,48,52]

Sampling of Airway and Alveolar Constituents

Bronchoscopy provides easy and relatively safe access to material in the tracheobronchial tree and distal alveolar spaces. A variety of studies are routinely performed on specimens obtained from the airways and alveolar spaces with several techniques. For example, aspirated secretions can be sent for microscopy and for cultures to determine the offending organism in cases of infection or suspected infection.[12,31,46] Cytologic analysis of bronchoscopically obtained materials can provide proof of malignancy. With the advent of lung transplantation, the success of the procedure depends, in large measure, on the early diagnosis of rejection or infection in these immunocompromised subjects. The most commonly employed bronchoscopic techniques for sampling the airways and alveolar spaces include "bronchial washing," bronchial brushing (see above), and bronchoalveolar lavage.

BRONCHOALVEOLAR LAVAGE

A very useful bronchoscopic technique is bronchoalveolar lavage (BAL). BAL is safe, even in critically ill patients, when biopsy or brushings are not recommended because of the risk of bleeding.[36] Normal saline solution, devoid of any bacteriostatic material, is instilled into distal airspaces through the "wedged" bronchoscope and then aspirated through the instrument's suction channel. The fluid collected in this manner is analyzed for gross appearance to detect possible alveolar hemorrhage. The fluid may also be subjected to a variety of tests, depending on the clinical circumstances: microbiologic testing, specific cytologic analysis and cell count, immunologic parameters, presence of various biochemical mediators related to pathologic processes, tissue markers, polymerase chain reaction, electron microscopy, flow cytometry, and DNA probes.

The value of BAL is well documented in the diagnosis of diffuse parenchymal diseases such as eosinophilic pneumonia, eosinophilic granuloma, and pulmonary alveolar proteinosis. It remains investigational in the evaluation of many other diseases—e.g., sarcoidosis, hypersensitivity pneumonitis, and idiopathic pulmonary fibrosis. Overall, the diagnostic yield of BAL is very much dependent on specific patient characteristics, the underlying pathologic process, and many technical factors.

Application of Quantitative Microbiologic Techniques

Two bronchoscopic methods that are useful in the diagnosis of pulmonary infections are quantitative BAL and protected-specimen brushing (PSB). They are, perhaps, most useful in the setting of suspected ventilator-associated pneumonia (VAP), wherein a patient who is endotracheally intubated and receiving mechanical ventilation has signs of infection and an abnormal chest radiograph. Intubated patients experience colonization of their upper and lower airways with nosocomial organisms. Because of an abnormal mucociliary clearance mechanism, these patients are at greater risk for developing pulmonary infections. In addition, mechanically ventilated, intubated patients are often treated empirically with broad-spectrum antibiotics and, therefore, are at greater risk for infection with resistant organisms and unusual lower respiratory tract pathogens. Quantitative BAL and PSB aid tremendously in the distinction between benign distal airway bacterial colonization and clinically significant infection that warrants antibiotic therapy.

PROTECTED BRUSH CATHETER SPECIMEN

PSB utilizes a double-catheter system in which an outer cannula and distal, biodegradable plug protect the bronchoscopic brush within the inner cannula from contamination with secretions in the upper airway and suction channel of the bronchoscope. When the bronchoscope is positioned proximal to the segmental orifice of interest, the PSB inner cannula is advanced into a subsegment and the protective distal plug ejected. The brush is then advanced peripherally, rotated gently, and retracted into the inner cannula. The inner cannula is subsequently retracted into the outer cannula and the bronchoscope removed from the airway. The distal portion of the catheter is cleaned with 70 percent alcohol and the brush clipped into saline solution under sterile conditions. The PSB is then submitted for quantitative bacterial culture within 15 min of the performance of the procedure.[32] The threshold for diagnosis of VAP with PSB is 10^3 colony-forming units (CFU) per milliliter, which corresponds to an initial concentration of 10^5–10^6 organisms in the original respiratory sample.[28] In studies from various centers, PSB sampling has been shown to have a predictive value for the presence or absence of pneumonia of 72 to 100 percent.[30]

QUANTITATIVE BRONCHOALVEOLAR LAVAGE

Quantitative BAL entails the performance of a standardized BAL, with infusion of at least 120 ml of saline for adequate sampling of a pulmonary subsegment. Quantitative culture of the aspirated material is performed to determine the number of CFU recovered. For quantitative BAL, a threshold of 10^4 CFU per milliliter is used for the diagnosis of pneumonia, reflecting a concentration of 10^5–10^6 bacteria per milliliter in the original specimen.[15] Several groups have reported sensitivity and specificity rates for the detection of pneumonia by quantitative BAL culture in the range of 75 to 100 percent and 70 to 100 percent, respectively.[30]

Although PSB is more commonly used in bronchoscopic clinical investigations, quantitative BAL may be superior to PSB in the diagnosis of VAP, since BAL samples a much larger porportion of lung parenchyma and is estimated to recover 5 to 10 times as many organisms as PSB. Protected BAL, which requires the use of a balloon-tipped catheter with a distal ejectable plug inserted through the suction channel of the bronchoscope, has a greater specificity than standard BAL; its sensitivity is at least as good as that of PSB. Combining the techniques of PSB and quantitative BAL may significantly improve the sensitivity of diagnosing nosocomial pneumonia.[30]

APPLICATIONS OF THERAPEUTIC BRONCHOSCOPY

Since the introduction of bronchoscopy, the technique has been used not only for observation but also for treatment of local airway disorders. As with any clinical intervention, the guiding rule for treatment always remains, "If I can do no good, I will at least do no harm."

Removal of Foreign Bodies

One of the earliest uses of the bronchoscope was removal of aspirated foreign bodies. Ingenuity of the inventors arose from extensive experience in difficult clinical situations and resulted in the development of various types of grasping forceps, retrieval baskets, and magnetic devices.[21] Until the introduction of the flexible bronchoscope, all procedures were done through the rigid bronchoscope. Even at present, it is well accepted that the rigid bronchoscope is the tool of choice for the removal of foreign bodies, especially in children. The advantage of the rigid instrument resides in its larger access channel, permitting use of more adaptable retrieval tools, and the ability to provide and control the patient's ventilation. There are, however, situations in which rigid bronchoscopy cannot be performed because of limited neck mobility or danger of cervical hyperextension. Under these circumstances, use of the flexible bronchoscope has provided a safe approach.

Special attention should be paid to the period after removal of the foreign body—a time when complications can occur. Patients should be observed for any signs of hemoptysis or subglottic edema. Trauma inflicted during the extraction or forceful manipulation of instruments greatly accentuates the risk of postoperative complications, particularly if oversized instruments are used or if the bronchoscopy is prolonged.

Control of Hemoptysis

In cases of hemoptysis, bronchoscopy may be of value not only for diagnosis but frequently for emergency management of endobronchial bleeding as well. Because of difficulties with visualization, instruments with large and maximally effective suction channels should be used. Rigid bronchoscopy is generally preferred with massive bleeding, when the need to remove large clots is anticipated.

When continuous suctioning of blood fails to clear the airways, other means can be used. An iced saline solution can be instilled along with vasoactive drugs, such as epinephrine, to induce spasm of the bleeding vessels. The bronchoscope itself can also be used to stem the bleeding by tamponade of the bleeding site or to occlude the lumen of the bronchus from which the bleeding originates. The same effect, perhaps with better local control, can be achieved with bronchoscopic balloon catheters. Specially designed catheters have been developed for introduction through the working channel of the flexible bronchoscope, permitting subsequent removal of the scope while the tamponading balloon remains in place. Another effective method for control of visible sources of bleeding, particularly from endobronchial neoplasms, is neodymium-YAG laser photocoagulation (see below).

Aspiration of Secretions

According to a survey of bronchoscopists conducted in the United States, removal of retained secretions is cited as a leading indication for therapeutic bronchoscopy.[38] Bronchoscopic aspiration of secretions may be indicated in patients presenting with weakness of respiratory muscles (e.g., due to underlying neuromuscular disease or the postoperative state) or disorders leading to recurrent aspiration of food or excessive upper-airway secretions. In critically ill or mechanically ventilated patients, removal of secretions and mucous plugs usually can be rapidly achieved with the flexible bronchoscope.[54] A fiberoptic scope with a large-diameter suction channel should be chosen for this procedure. The nature of the retained material—its consistency and viscosity—may dictate frequent bronchoscopies to relieve segmental or lobar atelectasis due to inspissated mucous plugs.[47] Underlying pulmonary diseases, such as bronchiectasis, may aggravate the retention of airway secretions. Bronchoscopic aspiration of secretions should not be considered "routine" in the postoperative period or in other conditions where good chest physiotherapy and maintenance of adequate pulmonary toilet can be more effective.

Two specific disorders are worth highlighting in the context of therapeutic bronchoscopy: pulmonary alveolar proteinosis (PAP) and allergic bronchopulmonary aspergillosis (ABPA). In PAP, BAL for clearance of alveolar material is a time-honored therapeutic procedure that may be facilitated by use of a bronchoscopic approach.[38] In ABPA, lavage with saline solution may be insufficient to remove tenacious impactions (described as "plastic bronchitis"). In these circumstances, use of bronchoscopic forceps may prove helpful.

Treatment of Endobronchial Obstruction

Endobronchial tumors, granulation tissue, and other obstructive lesions may now be approached bronchoscopically. In general, with malignant tumors, therapy is palliative. Benign tracheo-

bronchial lesions may be treated endoscopically, with excellent long-term results.

THERMAL LASERS

Common endobronchial lesions include malignant and benign pulmonary tumors. Although attempts at removal with simple biopsy forceps, or debulking with the edge of the rigid bronchoscope, have been described, these procedures are fraught with significant risks, including fatal bleeding. The advent of laser technology has provided a new therapeutic tool.

The first laser used in treating lesions of the tracheobronchial tree was the CO_2 laser. Because of its far infrared (wavelength 10,600 nm) beam, this laser can be transmitted safely only by use of special mirror systems and a rigid bronchoscope. The usefulness of the CO_2 laser is based on the concept of tissue vaporization and cutting with a very high-energy source. Subsequent development of light sources of different wavelengths and, in particular, of neodymium doped crystal lasers, has permitted transmission of the beam through fiberoptic systems.

The neodymium-YAG laser has a wavelength of 1064 nm, which is in the near-infrared invisible spectrum. Because of its very high scattering coefficient in soft tissues, this laser can penetrate deeply. It also has a very strong thermal characteristic, leading to coagulation of blood vessels and other viable tissues. For these reasons, the neodymium-YAG laser can be used as a coagulating tool when placed at a distance from the target. With the use of a contact technique with specially designed sculpted or sapphire tips, the neodymium-YAG laser can be used bronchoscopically for coagulation of bleeding sources and preparation of a tumor before mechanical debulking.

Many reports have documented the significant beneficial effects of endobronchial neodymium-YAG laser photoradiation therapy, particularly in patients with obstruction of large airways by primary thoracic or metastatic malignant tumors (Fig. 38-2).[5,8,49] Treatment success rate is based on the appropriate selection of patients, as well as the experience and training of the endoscopist. Success rates and complications directly related to laser therapy are not different when the procedure is performed under general anesthesia through the rigid bronchoscope or under topical anesthesia through a flexible bronchoscope.[8,50]

PHOTODYNAMIC THERAPY

The concept of photodynamic therapy (PDT) is based on three independent factors: use of a photosensitizing substance, a light with a specific stimulating wavelength capable of activating the photosensitizer, and the presence of oxygen. Each of these factors is nontoxic when administered individually, at prescribed doses. In combination, however, these agents destroy tissue. As discussed previously, photosensitizers have a predilection to concentrate in neoplastic tissue. When, in the presence of oxygen, the tissue is exposed to stimulating energy from light at a specific wavelength, a photochemical reaction occurs, resulting in the release of oxygen free radicals. Oxygen free radicals are very toxic and destroy the tissue in which they are produced.

The concept of PDT, using a laser as a source of stimulating energy, is no longer based on thermal effects. Lasers of very low power in the red spectrum (wavelength of about 630 nm), when delivered with the flexible bronchoscope, are capable of stimulating photosensitivity and are effective in the treatment of early endobronchial lung cancer.

Patients selected for PDT are pretreated with an intravenous injection of a photosensitizing compound (e.g., hematoporphyrin derivative), which is preferentially localized and retained in neo-

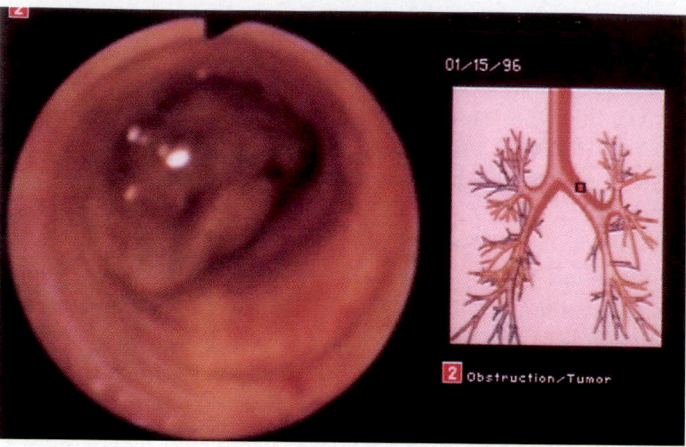

A

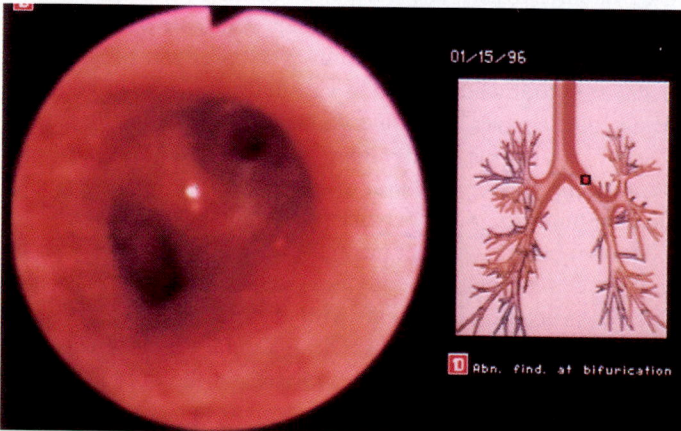

B

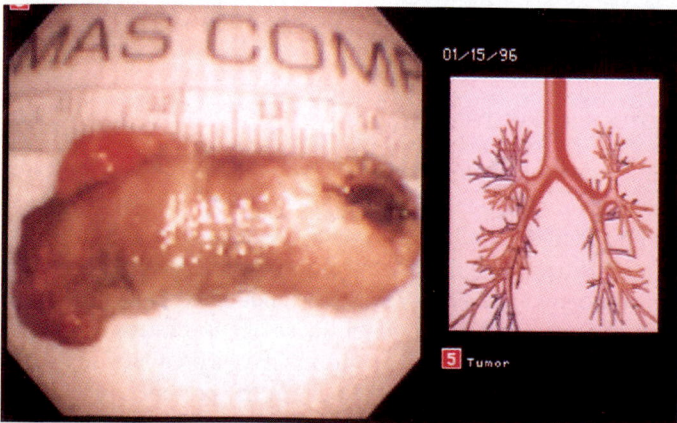

C

FIGURE 38-2 Left main-stem bronchial tumor. *A.* Total obstruction before YAG laser photoradiation therapy (PRT). *B.* Left upper and lower lobe bronchi are patent after PRT. *C.* Tumor removed en toto after coagulation of the base with PRT.

plastic tissue. About 48 h after injection, the patient undergoes bronchoscopy. The tumor, as well as surrounding normal tissues, is exposed to the red light generated by the argon dye, gold vapor, or copper vapor laser. In the protocols used, the currently accepted power is 200 to 400 mW/cm^2, with a total delivered dose of 100 to 400 j/cm^2. The treatment time is 500 s. Within 24 to 48 h after treatment, the malignant bronchial tumor becomes necrotic.[10,25] Generally, "cleanup" bronchoscopy is then required to remove the necrotic eschar, which would otherwise contribute to further obstruction of the airway.

Recent well-controlled studies from Japan have confirmed excellent results when this therapy is used in radiographically occult carcinoma; the complete response rate during a 5-year follow-up period is 95.2 percent. The diameter of successfully treated tumors was 1 cm or less.

The list of potential photosensitizers is growing rapidly, as are the energy delivery devices and their wavelengths. Additional trials of bronchoscopic PDT using other photosensitizers and different stimulating wavelengths are in progress. Among the more appealing photosensitizers for future clinical use is ALA, which can be given orally or topically. ALA has a shorter tissue half-life, decreasing the risk of prolonged photosensitivity.

BRACHYTHERAPY

Attempts to deliver a maximal therapeutic dose of radiation with minimal effects on unaffected surrounding tissues have fostered development of the technique of brachytherapy. In brachytherapy, the source of radiation is introduced as close as possible to the target.

Endobronchial irradiation for bronchial carcinoma, introduced in 1942, used implantable radioactive sources. Many isotopes have been tried in pulmonary medicine, including cobalt 60 and cesium 137. At present, most treatments are performed with iridium 192 (^{192}Ir).

The bronchial lesion is measured during a diagnostic bronchoscopy; then, under fluoroscopic guidance and direct bronchoscopic control, a special catheter is placed in proximity of the treated area. After appropriate calculation of the precise dose to be delivered, radioactive ^{192}Ir is introduced through the catheter. The radiation can be delivered either by high-dose-rate equipment or by a medium- or low-dose radioactive isotope, inserted manually.[1] The high dose rate (more than 12 Gy/h) delivered by a remote-control introducer requires an average of at least three bronchoscopic procedures, while the medium (2 to 12 Gy/h) and lower dose (0.4 to 2 Gy/h) rates can be completed in one session.

The cost of high-dose brachytherapy is much higher than the low- or medium-dose technique, owing to the high cost of the radiation source, the necessary special afterloading equipment, and the need for repeat bronchoscopies. Each treatment can be done in a few minutes, however, with less radioactive exposure risk to medical personnel. Recent studies suggest that lower dose rates are associated with a lower rate of complications. The effectiveness of brachytherapy in symptom palliation is most pronounced when the procedure is performed shortly after removal of most of the endobronchial tumor by photoradiation therapy with the neodymium-YAG laser.

ELECTROCAUTERY AND CRYOTHERAPY

Two other techniques of tissue destruction can be applied through the bronchoscope. Electrocautery has been used effectively in open "free-hand" surgery and gastrointestinal endoscopy. Tissue is destroyed by intense coagulation and vaporization.[19] The depth of penetration and resulting injury are, however, much more difficult to control. On the other hand, a specially designed bronchoscope had to be developed to prevent an electric current leak and potential injury to both the patient and the endoscopist. Also, creating an electric spark in an oxygen-enriched environment may result in combustion and severe burns. Although, theoretically, this technique appears less expensive than laser therapy, it remains investigational.

Even greater difficulties in precise control and prediction of depth of penetration are associated with cryotherapy.[18] Specially designed probes are inserted via the bronchoscope until they touch the target tissue. Through the channel in the probe, liquid nitrous oxide or nitrogen is introduced, resulting in the rapid creation of an "ice ball" (approximate temperature −20°C) at the end of the tip. This cooling effect is maintained for about 20 s; the area is then rewarmed, resulting in thawing. Inappropriate manipulations, excessively rapid thawing, or premature detachment of the probe may result in bleeding or tissue fracture. Cryotherapy is inappropriate for patients requiring rapid reopening of airways, since the beneficial effects of this method are delayed and are achieved only after subsequent removal of the sloughed necrotic tissue. Cryotherapy is also not very effective in poorly cellular lesions or those with a limited vascular supply—e.g., benign fibrotic structures and lipomas.

AIRWAY DILATION

The tracheobronchial tree is a dynamic structure composed of both rigid and flexible walls, in which cyclic changes occur during the respiratory cycle and with coughing. These changes include airway obstruction. Certain diseases can significantly aggravate airway obstruction, especially during expiration, by producing severe narrowing of the lumen and increased airflow resistance.

Rigid Scope Dilation

If obstruction is limited only to the proximal airways, correction of a short segment of narrowing can result in remarkable clinical and physiological improvement. Immediate, but generally temporary, results can be achieved by use of the rigid bronchoscope as a dilating instrument. In the case of posttraumatic stenosis, mechanical rupture of fibrous bands across the airway may provide immediate relief. The dilation may have to be done gradually, using bronchoscopes of progressively increasing diameters. This is particularly true when the stenosis occurs in the trachea. Once an acceptable bronchial lumen diameter is achieved, further consideration can be given to use of other methods, including insertion of endobronchial prostheses or additional dilation using special balloon catheters.

Stent Placement

Since early attempts at interventional bronchoscopy, various bronchoscopically placed prostheses have been tried, and most

have given rather disappointing long-term results. Initially the prostheses were rigid devices made of rubber, metal, plastic, or composite materials. More recently, however, technologic developments, including use of silicone or special alloys such as nitonol (a nickel-titanium alloy with shape and size memory capacity), have permitted placement of airway stents with very good results.[4]

Attempts at placing stents in the tracheobronchial tree should be guided by three basic principles: safe placement and fixation of the prosthesis, safe ventilation during the procedure, and safe handling of potential complications. The ideal indication for prosthetic placement is a short segment of stenosis (in two or three cartilaginous rings) in the left main-stem bronchus or the trachea, preferably due to tracheobronchomalacia or soft, compressible extrinsic compression (Fig. 38-3). The role of the prosthesis is prevention of airway collapse and maintenance of airway integrity and an acceptable airflow. This treatment technique should be considered, however, only as mechanical palliation, not as a cure for the underlying disease.[6]

The most popular tracheobronchial stents were developed in France by Dumon and colleagues, who also pioneered development of specially designed rigid bronchoscopes and stent intro-

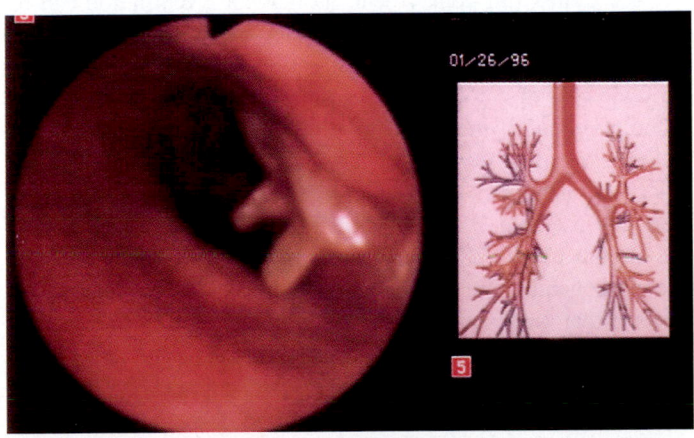

A

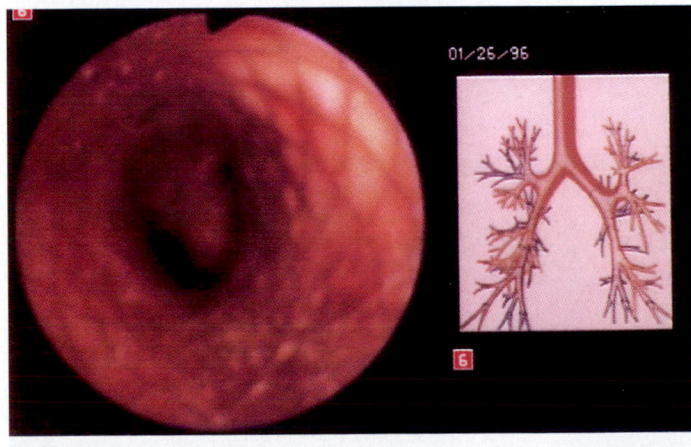

B

FIGURE 38-3 Expandable tracheobronchial stent. *A.* Severe tracheal stenosis with protruding broken cartilaginous rings. *B.* Same area after deployment of the covered "wall stent." The carina is now clearly visible from a distance.

ducers.[9] These endobronchial prostheses are of various lengths and diameters and are made of silicone. They have special external wall retention protrusions or studs, which maintain better endobronchial stability. Placement of the stents requires special training and dexterity, since placement must be accomplished without direct visualization and with some risk to ventilation. The advantage of these prostheses, however, is their ease of removal in case of complications. The most frequently reported complications are stent migration and overgrowth at the edge of the prosthesis of tumor or granulation tissue (Fig. 38-4). This abnormal growth may impede both ventilation and clearance of secretions. It may also result in increased bleeding.

Another recently developed endoprosthesis is the so-called dynamic stent. This stent is particularly suited for management of lower tracheal, carinal, and main-stem bronchial stenosis.[14] The stent is constructed from silicone and horseshoe-shaped metallic "scaffolding," which mimics the cartilaginous rings. The device has a soft posterior wall similar to the trachea's, and it should permit better mobility during coughing; expectoration of secretions is, theoretically, improved over that with standard Silastic stents. As with the dedicated Dumon stent, the dynamic stent has to be introduced with the help of a special introducer. During introduction of the dynamic stent through the stenotic area, and before the stent's full deployment, the patient's ventilation can be severely compromised; therefore, rapidity of placement is critical. There is much less risk of migration with this type of stent. As in the case of any synthetic prosthesis, however, there is a risk of the plugging of the lumen by secretions or necrotic debris.

Self-expanding stents were developed initially for vascular and biliary applications; only later were they modified for endobronchial use (Fig. 38-3). For this reason, their physical properties are not ideally adapted to the physiological demands of the tracheobronchial tree. The major advantage of self-expanding stents is that they can be introduced with the help of the fiberoptic bronchoscope and deployed under fluoroscopic and direct bronchoscopic guidance. There is much less impediment to ventilation during the deployment.[4] On the other hand, these prostheses also carry a higher risk of irritation of the tracheobronchial tree at their distal and proximal sharp edges. They can also contribute to airway obstruction by overgrowth through the metallic mesh of recurrent tumor or exuberant granulation tissue. Recently, improved models have been introduced that have the metallic mesh covered by either a polyethylene or polyurethane membrane in an attempt to prevent tissue overgrowth. The major risk with older, high-pressure, self-expanding metal stents is perforation of the tracheobronchial tree and fatal consequences. Because of their relatively rigid structure and overgrowth of tissue, removal of these stents is almost impossible.

Balloon Dilation

For fibrotic bronchial stenosis, another bronchoscopic approach of dilatation has been developed, borrowing from the technique and equipment used in angioplasty procedures.[2,3] After the nature, length, and initial diameter of bronchial stenosis have been determined, a high-pressure angioplasty balloon catheter is introduced through the working channel of the bronchoscope. The diameter of the inflated balloon should match the optimal dilatation of the stenotic segment (Fig. 38-5). The procedure must be performed under fluoroscopy and continuous bronchoscopic observation. During dilatation of the balloon, adequate ventilation and oxygenation of the remaining lung must be monitored constantly. The major risks of this technique are rupture of a bronchial wall, bleeding, and postprocedure airway edema. The advantage of the technique is that it obviates permanent introduction of foreign bodies into the tracheobronchial tree, which, by their presence, create a potential source of irritation, infection, or stasis of secretions.[22].

Closure of Bronchial Fistulae

Fiberoptic bronchoscopy can be a useful intervention in confirming the diagnosis of suspected bronchopleural fistula and specifying its precise location.[29] Depending on the location and the size of the fistula, it can be approached bronchoscopically and an attempt made to seal it. Simple tamponade using the body of the flexible bronchoscope or a balloon catheter provides only temporary relief. Many different techniques have been employed, including introduction of irritating substances—e.g., silver nitrate, which stimulates formation of reactive granulation tissue. Several potentially useful agents have been described, including Gelfoam, autologous blood patch, cryoprecipitate, and thrombin injection to create fibrin clot. Small bronchial openings in an otherwise normal bronchus following thoracic surgery respond much better, with a higher rate of success of bronchoscopic sealing. It is much more difficult to achieve good obliteration of the fistula when the fistula is infected or is due to an underlying malignancy.

Therapeutic Bronchoscopic Accessories

Growing clinical experience and many technologic advances have led to bronchoscopic accessories designed specifically for therapeutic applications. With the goal of minimizing aggressive, costlier, and riskier surgical procedures, new miniaturized therapeutic bronchoscopic accessories have been developed.

FOREIGN-BODY RETRIEVAL FORCEPS AND BASKETS

Aspiration of foreign bodies is much more common in children than adults. The reported diversity of objects retrieved from the

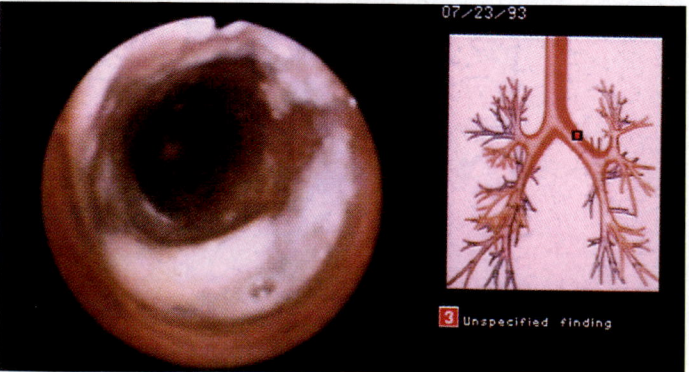

FIGURE 38-4   Silastic stent in the left main-stem bronchus. Accumulated secretions are visible at the proximal end.

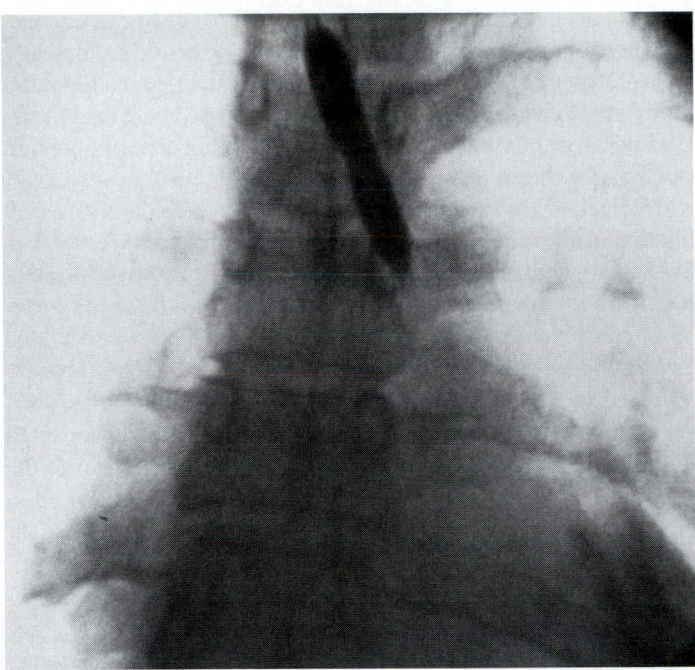

A

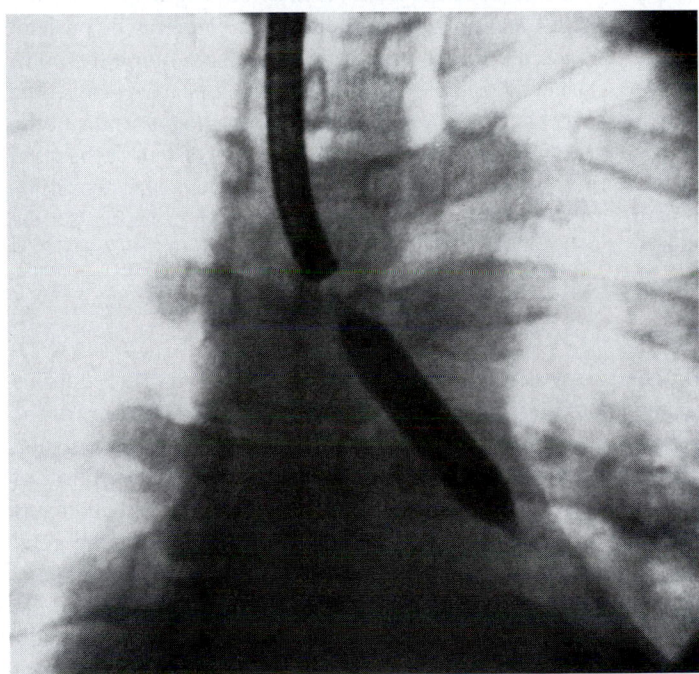

B

FIGURE 38-5 Balloon bronchoplasty of the left main-stem bronchus under fluoroscopic guidance. *A.* Visible indentation at the site of the firm stenosis. *B.* Smooth contour of the balloon after dilation.

tracheobronchial tree dictates particular vigilance on the part of the bronchoscopist and frequent need for improvisation during bronchoscopic removal. Ideally, a specialized bronchoscopic unit should be equipped with a large array of devices for foreign-body extraction. Unfortunately, however, removal of foreign bodies may need to be done on an emergency basis, in places where there is not ready access to specialized instrumentation.

Basic biopsy forceps may be of some value in foreign-body removal, particularly forceps with jagged edges or rough sur-

faces. These devices may be helpful in the retrieval of hard objects with an irregular surface. Smooth objects or organic materials (e.g., nuts, food particles) require more ingenious use of various expandable baskets or a combination of balloon catheters, suction devices, and grasping forceps. Under these circumstances, attempts are made to bypass the obstruction with a closed basket, which is then deployed distally, permitting anchoring and capturing of the foreign body within the closing arms of the device. Once this is achieved, the basket is pulled back gently until the entrapped, obstructing object is wedged between the top of the scope and the basket, permitting withdrawal of the scope and removal in toto. Special dexterity of the bronchoscopist is required to guide the retrieval forceps or basket at the proper angle, to avoid any additional perforation or injury to the tracheobronchial tree or upper airway during the withdrawal.

CONTACT AND NONCONTACT LASER FIBERS

Laser beams, which can be transmitted via nontoxic fiberoptic light guides, are useful for deep coagulation and, occasionally, for vaporization of tissue.[50] In the noncontact mode, the tip is maintained at a distance of 5 to 10 mm from the intended treatment area. Targeting is facilitated by another very-low-power helium-neon laser. The crucial aspects in this technique are the constant visualization of the aiming beam, maintenance of the tip of the laser guide free of debris, and observation of changes occurring in the targeted tissue during the procedure. Closure of the blood supply to a tumor results in reduction in tumor volume and progressive enlargement of the airway lumen. Specially designed sapphire or other sculpted contact tips require much lower (15 to 20 W) laser power. These devices provide improved tissue reaction control. Not only do they permit coagulation but they are also useful as cutting or debulking tools (Fig. 38-6). The disadvantage of the technique is that precise observation of tissue reaction is obscured. Judicious use of the contact tips in relation to the tumor type and location permits proper preparation of the region, with suppression of blood supply to the endobronchial portion of the tumor. Once this is achieved, rapid mechanical debulking can be accomplished without excessive risk of bleeding.

In response to specific needs of PDT, special light guides have been developed. For patients with small, superficial, well-circumscribed tumors, a microlens system can be utilized. Laser light is delivered by straightforward uniform illumination at the end of the quartz fiber. Fibers with radial light distribution patterns over a specified length at the tip, which are capable of affecting the lumen of the bronchus circumferentially, are preferred for treating more extensive tumors. The same fibers can also be used for interstitial insertion into large tumors. The output of the laser and the power density at the fiber tip are calibrated before insertion through the bronchoscope. The precise time of treatment and the total energy to be delivered to the tissues are calculated according to investigational protocols.

BALLOON CATHETERS

None of the widely used balloon catheters were developed specifically for bronchoscopic use. Fogarty catheters and angioplasty

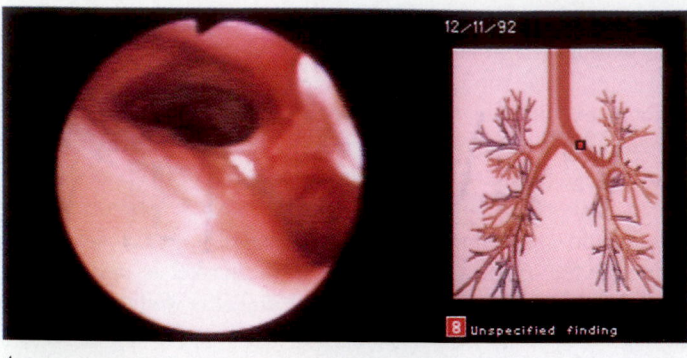

A

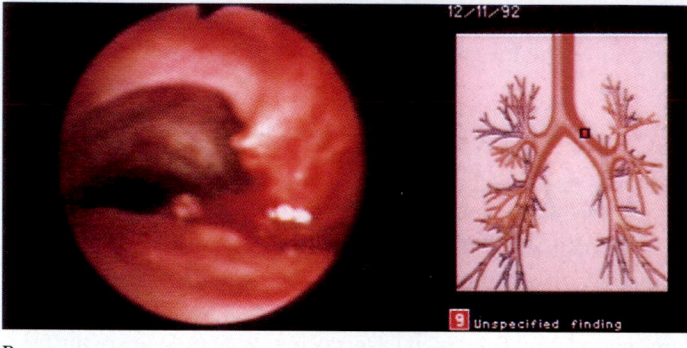

B

FIGURE 38-6 Web stenosis of the left main-stem bronchus. *A.* Approach with the laser contact probe. *B.* Findings after transection using the neodymium-YAG contact probe.

dilation catheters of various sizes, however, are utilized. These catheters have proved to be very helpful in removing accumulated secretions, blood clots, debris, and foreign bodies.

In the double-lumen catheter, the balloon is inflated for anchoring the catheter in place, and the central lumen is used for insertion of the radioactive source. Similarly, balloon-tipped catheters are very useful in selective obstruction of a bronchial lumen, for tamponading bronchial bleeding, or for temporary interruption of a bronchopleural communication. Selective delivery catheters have been used for endobronchial administration of antineoplastic drugs, antibiotics, radiolabeled monoclonal antibodies, and photosensitizers.

High-pressure angioplasty catheters with various balloon lengths and diameters have been used for airway dilation. These devices are inserted through the working channel of the flexible bronchoscope. Under fluoroscopic and direct visual guidance, the balloon, filled with radiopaque liquid, is inflated at the site of the stenosis until a smooth, uniform lumen of predictable diameter is attained (Fig. 38-5). Visualization of any indentation in the balloon signifies either an inappropriate diameter of the balloon or the presence of extrinsic pressure exceeding that of the balloon. Considering the potential risk of bronchial rupture, the general recommendation is to avoid exceeding a balloon pressure above 6 atm.

PROSTHESES INTRODUCERS

Ideally, endobronchial prostheses should be deployed under direct visual guidance and continuously preserved ventilation. This is possible with compressible, "self-expanding" stents, which can

be introduced through the working channel of the bronchoscope. Expansion can be observed simultaneously bronchoscopically and fluoroscopically. In some circumstances, when the diameter of the introducers exceeds the size of the working channel of the flexible bronchoscope, the catheter containing the compressed stent is introduced over a guidewire.

Dedicated tracheobronchial stents, however, are inserted blindly, using specially constructed introductory devices.[6,9] The Dumon stent first has to be folded, then compressed and introduced into a tube, which is then inserted through a rigid bronchoscope. Once the distal tip of this tube has reached beyond the estimated area of stenosis, the stent is pushed out from the proximal end with a special device. Only after removal of the introducer tube and the device can a telescope again be inserted through the bronchoscope to verify the correct placement of the stent. Proper positioning and deployment are corrected with a grasping forceps or balloon catheter. Modifications of this technique have been made in an attempt to provide better visual control and ventilation during deployment. The stents are placed over the external wall of a rigid bronchoscope, immobilized there during passage through the upper airways, and then advanced at the level of the stenosis by pressure from above.

Similarly, "the dynamic stent" is inserted over a specially designed double-function grasping forceps and integrated "pusher" device.[14] Once the forceps and pusher device holding the compressed, Y-shaped stent pass through the upper airways, the grasping forceps, which approximates the two small limbs of the Y, is opened. The integrated pusher anchors the stent at the level of the carina, while the introducer is withdrawn. The two Silastic arms remain in the left and right main-stem bronchi, and the main, "dynamic" part of the stent extends into the trachea.

SAFETY FACTORS IN BRONCHOSCOPY

Bronchoscopy is a specialized procedure that requires extensive training. Familiarity with both the physiology and anatomy of the airways is essential. Any diagnostic or therapeutic manipulation should be considered in relation to the underlying condition of the patient, localization of the area of investigation, and other surrounding structures in the thorax. It is essential to develop good communication between the bronchoscopist and other members of the team. While the bronchoscopist concentrates on the field of work—which, as seen through the bronchoscope, is two-dimensional—other team members are responsible for monitoring the patient (oxygen saturation, blood pressure, heart rhythm, etc.) and checking and maintaining the adequacy of ancillary equipment (suction, oxygenation, accessories such as forceps, balloons, catheters, laser light guides).[44] Risks are decreased if, for example, special attention is paid to the control of accessories during their manipulation beyond the tip of the bronchoscope. Premature deployment of the needle biopsy device or inappropriate bending of the bronchoscope while an instrument is inside the flexible portion can result in perforation of the bronchoscope. Activation of the laser with a broken light guide inside the bronchoscope or inadequate protrusion of the tip of the fiber beyond the bronchoscope may result in airway fires or severe burns to the patient. Attention to details and proper maintenance of the equipment, including accessories, enhance safety for the patient and staff. Diagnostic yield and therapeutic results are also improved. Last, but not least, proper knowledge and application of safety standards and maintenance procedures decrease the cost of bronchoscopy (see Table 38-1).

COMPLICATIONS OF BRONCHOSCOPY

Bronchoscopy is a potentially hazardous procedure. Complications are generally due to inappropriate preparation of patients before bronchoscopy, effects of local or general anesthesia, and manipulation of various instruments. Appropriate training and experience of the bronchoscopist and supporting team are crucial in reducing the rate of complications (see Table 38-2).

Anesthesia and Related Blood Gas Abnormalities

Approximately half of the life-threatening complications of diagnostic bronchoscopy are associated with premedication and use of topical anesthesia. Risk is significantly increased in the elderly. Predisposing factors include cardiovascular disease, chronic pulmonary disease, renal and hepatic dysfunction, seizures, and altered mental status. Mild sedation, anxiolysis, muscular relaxation, and anterograde amnesia increase patient cooperation and permit quicker and less traumatic procedures. Doses of benzodiazepines, opiates, anticholinergics, and topical anesthetics must be adjusted if there is underlying organ dysfunction. Conscious sedation techniques using short-acting benzodiazepines (e.g., midazolam), which offer significant antegrade amnesia but less muscle relaxation, seem to have reduced the incidence of potentially dangerous hypotension and respiratory depression.

Inadequate topical anesthesia potentiates coughing, gagging, and patient discomfort and increases the risk of injury during bronchoscopy. However, topical anesthetics such as lidocaine, the most frequently used agent, are absorbed systemically through the respiratory mucosa, increasing the risk of cardiac or CNS toxicity. These complications are more likely to occur in patients with underlying low cardiac output, hepatic dysfunction, and oropharyngeal candidiasis. Another, less frequent complication of lidocaine use is methemoglobinemia and tissue hypoxia.

Skillful manipulation of rigid and flexible bronchoscopes reduces the risk of injury to the upper airways, which can result in life-threatening laryngospasm during or after completion of the procedure. Particular caution must be exercised in patients with underlying bronchospastic disorders.

Introduction of the bronchoscope under general anesthesia or under conscious sedation with topical anesthesia frequently results in a decrease in oxygenation and in hypoventilation, with a significant increase in Pa_{CO_2}. In patients with underlying chronic lung disease, severe hypoxemia may occur, triggering life-threatening cardiac arrhythmias.

All patients undergoing bronchoscopic procedures should be monitored continuously (ECG, blood pressure, O_2 saturation, and, if indicated, expiratory CO_2 concentration). Use of supplemental oxygen during the procedure should be routine. Bronchoscopy probably should not be performed in patients who are unable to maintain a Pa_{O_2} of 65 mmHg while an F_{IO_2} of 1.0 and full ventilatory support are administered.

TABLE 38-1

Safety Measures to Avoid Bronchoscopic Complications

Attention to proper indications
Attention to contraindications
Experienced team and appropriate facilities
Appropriate instrumentation
Appropriate pre-, peri-, and postbronchoscopic monitoring
Proper preparation for emergencies

Significant oxygen desaturation may occur during BAL. The degree of desaturation is directly related to the duration of the procedure and the volume of lavage fluid used. Return to the prebronchoscopy level of O_2 saturation may be prolonged after removal of the bronchoscope, and supplemental O_2 should be continued throughout the procedure and during the postbronchoscopy observation period.

Fever and Infection

In patients with underlying valvular cardiac disease and those predisposed to endocarditis, the American Heart Association recommends use of prophylactic antibiotics before rigid bronchoscopy but not before flexible bronchoscopy. Antibiotic prophylaxis is mandatory, however, in patients with prosthetic valves, surgical vascular shunts, or a history of endocarditis.

Appearance of transient fever after bronchoscopy is not unusual and generally does not require any therapy. However, persistent fever in the setting of progressive radiographic infiltrates necessitates antibiotic therapy. The incidence of fever is in-

---

TABLE 38-2

Contraindications to Bronchoscopy

Cardiovascular
   Recent myocardial infarction
   Unstable angina
   Unstable cardiac arrhythmias
   Severe hypertension
   Severe carotid or cerebrovascular disease

Pulmonary
   Severe hypoxemia despite maximal oxygen supplementation
   Hypoventilation with hypercapnia
   Severe bronchospasm or unstable asthma

Neurologic
   Active seizures
   Increased intracranial pressure
   Severe agitation

Other medical conditions
   Bleeding diathesis
   Platelet dysfunction or thrombocytopenia
   Severe anemia
   Cirrhosis with portal hypertension
   Uremia

creased in the elderly, in those with underlying chronic pulmonary disease or documented endobronchial obstruction, and in those with bronchoscopic interventions for malignancy. The incidence of fever and extension of pulmonary infiltrates increase with the volume of BAL fluid and the total number of pulmonary segments lavaged. In most cases, these complications resolve spontaneously within 24 h. The incidence of postbronchoscopic infections is higher in immunocompromised hosts.

Airway Obstruction and Perforation

The advent of interventional bronchoscopy has resulted in complications not ordinarily seen with diagnostic bronchoscopy. Inappropriate use of lasers has resulted in endobronchial burns and bronchial perforations associated with catastrophic bleeding, pneumomediastinum, or pneumothorax. Endobronchial edema may also occur as a result of laser thermal effects.

Following photodynamic therapy, formation of a necrotic eschar, airway edema, or rapid, potentially complete airway obstruction should be anticipated and treated with "cleanup" bronchoscopy.

As noted previously, insertion of airway stents is associated with many potential complications. The Silastic stents may not be properly adapted to the diameter of the airway, resulting in either incomplete deployment of the stent or stent migration. Life-threatening airway obstruction may arise. The presence of this palliative foreign body in the airway may predispose to difficulties in clearing secretions and accumulation of inspissated mucus. Introduction of self-expanding metallic endobronchial prostheses may result in a severe local airway reaction, particularly at sharp edges of the device, producing granulation tissue, hemorrhage, or bronchial perforation.

Pneumothorax

Most of the serious complications directly due to bronchoscopic intervention have been reported in association with performance of transbronchial biopsies. Pneumothorax following transbronchial biopsy occurs in about 4 percent of cases, even when the procedure is done under fluoroscopic guidance. The incidence of pneumothorax increases when the procedure is done without fluoroscopy.

The risk of pneumothorax is not related to the size of the bronchoscopic biopsy forceps. The incidence of pneumothorax is increased greatly (three or four times), however, in immunocompromised hosts. The risk is also elevated in mechanically ventilated patients, with peripheral lung biopsies, and in the presence of bullous lung disease. For these reasons, a postbronchoscopic expiratory chest radiograph is performed routinely. In case of a significant pneumothorax, a chest tube should be inserted immediately to avoid tension pneumothorax.

Hemorrhage

One of the most frequently reported complications related to bronchoscopy is hemorrhage—a complication that can be largely avoided by proper evaluation of the patient before the procedure. An incidence of 45 percent has been reported in uremic patients.

For these reasons, a blood urea nitrogen (BUN) level above 30 mg/dl or a creatinine level above 3 mg/dl should be considered contraindications to bronchoscopy. Similarly, in patients with known underlying bleeding disorders, especially those caused by platelet dysfunction or thrombocytopenia, the risk of bleeding (epistaxis or hemoptysis) is increased during bronchoscopy. Bronchoscopy should not be performed if the platelet count is below $50,000/mm^3$, and transbronchial biopsy or aggressive interventional procedures (laser therapy, bronchoplasty, or stent placement) are probably safe only with platelet counts above $75,000/mm^3$.

Manipulation of the bronchoscope, mechanical trauma, vigorous suctioning, endobronchial brushing, and biopsy may result in bleeding in 1 to 4 percent of patients without underlying risks for hemorrhage. Hemorrhage can also occur with inadvertent perforation of pulmonary vessels during transbronchial needle aspiration or biopsy.

Overall, when bronchoscopy is performed by an experienced endoscopist, backed up by a well-trained team and appropriate facilities, mortality and morbidity are very low.

TRANSTHORACIC NEEDLE ASPIRATION AND BIOPSY

Transthoracic needle aspiration (TTNA) was first utilized for the diagnosis of pulmonary disease in 1883, when Leyden performed the procedure on three patients with pneumonia.[27] In 1886, Ménétrier reported the use of TTNA in the diagnosis of lung carcinoma.[34] Since that time, many published series have described the utility of TTNA for the diagnosis of a variety of benign and malignant thoracic lesions, using fluoroscopic, CT, or ultrasound guidance.[53,57,59] With the "reemergence" of thoracoscopy and recent development of video-assisted thoracic surgical techniques, patients can more easily undergo complete excision of pulmonary nodules. In the past, many pulmonologists performed TTNA as the initial diagnostic procedure for intrapulmonary lesions, especially those in the lung periphery. Physicians are now faced with the dilemma of whether to send patients directly to thoracoscopic biopsy for a definitive answer.

Transthoracic needle biopsy (TTNB) provides core biopsy material from pulmonary nodules for histologic examination. The ability to analyze histology is critical in establishing a definitive diagnosis for certain disease states (e.g., sarcoidosis) in which cytologic aspiration is inadequate in documenting the characteristic noncaseating granulomas. TTNB also provides improved diagnostic accuracy in lymphoma, both Hodgkin's and non-Hodgkin's varieties, in which anatomic structure is important in delineating the type of lymphoma and in distinguishing between clonal, neoplastic processes and inflammatory conglomerations of lymphocytes. TTNB plays a minor role in the diagnosis of suspected bronchogenic carcinomas, since most can be diagnosed accurately with cytologic analysis alone, and since subtyping of nonsmall carcinomas has little bearing on prognosis, therapeutic approach, or tumor response to therapy. Histologic specimens may improve the yield in the diagnosis of pulmonary hamartomas, characterized by the presence of cartilage or adipose tissue.

Indications and Contraindications

In 1989, the American Thoracic Society published guidelines for percutaneous needle aspiration biopsy.[16] The major indications include evaluation of solitary lung nodules and masses, mediastinal and hilar lesions, metastatic disease to the lung from a known extrathoracic malignancy, chest wall invasion by lung carcinoma, and pulmonary consolidation or infiltrates that are likely to be of infectious origin.[40] The most common indication for TTNA is evaluation of a solitary pulmonary nodule that arouses suspicions of bronchogenic carcinoma.

Establishment of a specific diagnosis with TTNA may play a major role in determining future interventions, particularly when findings indicate a definitive benign diagnosis, such as pulmonary hamartoma. TTNA may also profoundly affect therapeutic decisions by differentiating small-cell and non–small-cell carcinoma of the lung and distinguishing between primary and metastatic lung tumors. The latter distinction is often difficult, however, particularly in the case of adenocarcinomas. Diagnosis of benign disease, small-cell lung cancer, metastatic cancer, or synchronous primaries may obviate otherwise unnecessary thoracotomies.[55] One must also distinguish clinical circumstances in which transthoracic needle biopsy is more appropriate than transthoracic needle aspiration. A cytology sample may be inadequate for diagnosing certain pulmonary lesions, such as lymphoma and sarcoidosis. When these disorders are suspected, transthoracic needle biopsy is more appropriate.

Most of the original TTNA procedures were performed with thin, elongated (10- to 15-cm) needles, which permitted procurement of samples for cytologic analysis alone. Current indications for TTNA include diagnosis of thoracic malignancies and infections of unclear origin. A recent Spanish study of 45 HIV-positive patients with pulmonary infiltrates showed a 62 percent diagnosis rate for TTNA performed without fluoroscopy; a diagnostic rate of 88 percent for *Pneumocystis carinii* pneumonia was established.[11]

Few absolute contraindications to TTNA exist. These include an uncooperative patient or one with an intractable cough, as patients must be able to suspend respirations for 5 to 10 s while the needle crosses the pleura.[40] In addition, TTNA is absolutely contraindicated in patients with a suspected pulmonary hydatid cyst because of the risk of capsule rupture and systemic dissemination. Relative contraindications include bullous emphysema, pulmonary arterial hypertension, and coagulation or platelet disorders. Patients with bullous emphysema are at increased risk of developing symptomatic or tension pneumothoraces after TTNA, although most induced pneumothoraces are small and can be treated conservatively. Those with pulmonary hypertension who undergo TTNA have a higher chance of developing pulmonary hemorrhage and significant hemoptysis. Patients with prolonged prothrombin times secondary to warfarin administration should have their anticoagulation changed to heparin and stopped for 6 h before performance of TTNA.[40]

Technique

Proper technique in performing TTNA is critical in obtaining adequate material for reliable interpretation. In addition to the mechanics of needle insertion and aspiration, the choice of needle type and careful specimen processing are important aspects of the procedure.

CHOICE OF NEEDLE

Many needle types are available for TTNA. They vary in both length and width. In the early 1960s, TTNA was performed with large-bore cutting needles; significant hemmorhagic complications were reported. More recently, thin-needle aspiration has become standard; it uses devices ranging in size from 18 to 22 gauge. Coaxial needle systems have been introduced for the purpose of obtaining multiple samples from a single pleural penetration. These systems are also useful for procuring specimens for histologic evaluation.[40]

RADIOGRAPHIC GUIDANCE

Most transthoracic needle procedures are performed with fluoroscopic guidance, typically using a C-arm or biplane device capable of rotation of over 180° in a single plane. C-arm fluoroscopy allows for real-time imaging of pulmonary lesions during needle insertion and specimen retrieval. The instrumentation is readily available at most hospitals. CT has been used to guide TTNA of pulmonary lesions, most commonly lesions that are too small to be seen fluoroscopically or those that are centrally located and adjacent to major vascular structures. Because CT-guided TTNA is not performed with real-time visualization, the procedure takes longer to perform (60 to 90 min, compared with 15 to 20 min for fluoroscopy) and typically requires several passes to obtain diagnostic material. Not surprisingly, CT-guided TTNA is associated with an increased incidence of pneumothorax (up to 60 percent in some series).[40] Core biopsy for obtaining histologic specimens is commonly done with CT guidance. An automated biopsy system with a diagnostic sensitivity of 81 percent and a pneumothorax rate of 9 percent has been described.[58]

Ultrasound guidance of TTNA offers the advantage of real-time lesion imaging, easy portability, and absence of exposure to ionizing radiation for both the clinician and the patient. Ultrasound is used most commonly for peripheral lung lesions that extend to the pleural edge, or for the diagnosis of mediastinal masses. The sensitivity of ultrasound-guided TTNB of pulmonary and mediastinal lesions larger than 3 cm may be as high as 96.8 percent, with a pneumothorax rate less than 2 percent.[58]

NEEDLE INSERTION

The procedure is best performed with the patient lying on a table that is fluoroscopy compatible; positioning should be either supine or prone, depending on the location of the lesion. A lateral approach can be considered if the target lesion is large and apposed to the lateral pleural surface.

The lesion is localized by fluoroscopic guidance, and the overlying skin is marked and anesthetized with 1% lidocaine. Proper local anesthesia for TTNA requires injection of the subcutaneous tissues, including the parietal pleura, since the pleura is heavily innervated. Injection of anesthetic should follow a path bypassing the ribs, costal cartilages, and scapula, and traversing the inferior portion of the intercostal space, thereby avoiding the neurovascular bundle. Conscious sedation may be indicated for patients who are particularly anxious or agitated. Elevation of the arms over the head or alongside the body may help in moving the scapula out of the path of the aspiration needle.[56] Throughout the procedure, the patient's pulse, blood pressure, heart rate, cardiac rhythm, and oxyhemoglobin saturation should be monitored closely.

With the patient lying as still as possible, the aspiration needle is inserted perpendicularly through the anesthetized region into the lesion, as seen under fluoroscopy. Rotation of a C-arm fluoroscopy unit for visualization of the lesion in another plane aids in proper positioning of the needle. Appropriate placement of the needle can also be ascertained by a change in resistance to passage of the needle, indicating that the instrument has entered the lesion. However, inflammatory tissue surrounding malignant nodules can give the false impression of proper needle insertion. Under fluoroscopy, the needle may be seen to displace the lesion, or if properly positioned, the needle will move in concert with the lesion during quiet breathing. If the needle is seen to move independently of the lesion during respiration, it is positioned unsatisfactorily.

Ideal aspiration technique necessitates having the tip of the needle as close to the center of the lesion as possible. A 20-ml lockable syringe containing approximately 3 ml of sterile saline is attached to the needle hub, and the tip is maintained in proper position with fluoroscopic guidance. Suction is then applied by pulling the syringe plunger back and locking it into position with clockwise rotation. While suction is sustained with the locked syringe, the needle tip is advanced and withdrawn about 0.5 to 1 cm within the lesion under real-time fluoroscopic guidance. The needle is then removed from the chest, suction is released, and the aspirated material is flushed out into a specimen container. Several samples should be obtained, to increase the diagnostic yield. With a necrotic mass, aspiration should also be performed in peripheral locations of the lesion in order to obtain viable cells and to decrease the risk of false-negative results.

Noncoaxial transthoracic needles require an initial aspiration and immediate examination of a touch preparation to determine the adequacy of the specimen. If the aspirated material is insufficient, a second pleural puncture must be made, increasing the likelihood of pneumothorax or intraparenchymal hemorrhage. Fifty to 100 percent of TTNA procedures performed using noncoaxial thin needles require at least two passes through the pleural surface.[37] Coaxial TTNA systems allow for multiple aspirations with a single pleural puncture and, therefore, have a lower rate of pneumothorax without reduced diagnostic accuracy.[40]

The technique of TTNB is similar to that of TTNA and is performed primarily with a coaxial needle system. These systems typically consist of a 19-gauge, beveled-tip outer needle with a cutting edge and a 21-gauge inner needle that acts as a trocar, facilitating passage of the instrument toward the lesion. The inner needle may be used as a standard TTNA device to obtain multiple aspirates from the target lesion with a single puncture of the pleural surface. The distal lumen of the outer needle is used to core out and store the biopsy specimen. After retraction of the inner needle about 2 cm, the hollow outer needle is advanced and withdrawn 1 to 2 cm within the lesion while suction

is applied to the hub with a 20-ml lockable syringe containing 3 ml of sterile saline. The entire coaxial needle system is then removed from the thorax, suction is released, and the core biopsy is expelled from the hollow needle with the saline stored in the syringe. Occasionally, in patients who have a large amount of subcutaneous adipose tissue or muscle, insertion of a 14-gauge catheter proximal to the pleura as a guide for the TTNB needle is helpful in preventing alterations in the angle of the TTNB toward the lesion.[50]

Because of the need for complete withdrawal before a core biopsy is obtained, obtaining a second sample necessitates a second pleural puncture, increasing the risk of pneumothorax. In addition, by virtue of its larger diameter, the hollow outer needle carries a greater overall risk of complications than does the thinner cytology needle. TTNB has a higher pneumothorax rate per pleural puncture than does TTNA; TTNB is also associated with a greater chance of significant pulmonary hemorrhage.

TTNB is most useful for pulmonary lesions extending to the pleural surface, which are easily visualized fluoroscopically and are less likely to require multiple passes to obtain diagnostic material. In expert hands, the pneumothorax rate for TTNB may be as low as 21 percent, with negligible rates of pulmonary hemorrhage and air embolism.[53]

SPECIMEN PROCESSING

Specimens obtained with TTNA or TTNB can be placed into a glutaraldehyde solution for delayed analysis; however, evaluation is much more successful if a cytopathologist is present at the time of the procedure. Cytopathologists can immediately process the aspirated material with a modified Diff-Quik stain (Baxter Scientific Products) for on-site light microscopic examination. Cell blocks can also be created from multiple tissue fragments fixed in 95% ethanol.

With a high pretest probability for primary carcinoma of the lung, the primary goal of TTNA is to discriminate between small-cell and non–small-cell lung cancer, since this distinction has important therapeutic ramifications. Cytologic typing alone can often distinguish between metastatic and primary tumors of the lung, but occasionally, additional techniques may be required for proper diagnosis. Electron microscopy may be utilized to aid in identification of poorly differentiated tumors or to determine the primary malignancy of origin of a metastatic pulmonary lesion. Immunohistochemical analysis of aspirated cells can help differentiate epithelial from mesenchymal tumors, and can identify a specific tumor of origin through analysis of cell surface markers (e.g., estrogen or progesterone receptors in metastatic breast carcinoma).[56]

TTNA is commonly conducted as an outpatient procedure. It is standard to perform a chest radiograph 1 to 2 h after the procedure to rule out pneumothorax. Most clinically significant pneumothoraces necessitating medical intervention have been shown to occur within the first hour.[56] In one series of 673 TTNAs, only 9 percent of pneumothoraces were detected on chest radiographs 1 h after the procedure, and only 2 percent after 4 h. None of the 11 percent of pneumothoraces occurring after 1 h were clinically significant enough to warrant drainage or aspiration.[35] A patient with small, asymptomatic pneumothorax may be discharged home after an additional 1 to 2 h of observation if a repeat radiograph documents no interval enlargement of the pneumothorax.[40,56]

Results

TTNA and TTNB have excellent success rates in the diagnosis of primary or metastatic pulmonary malignancies; for TTNA, the sensitivity is 85 to 95 percent.[24,55] Major causes of false-negative results in malignant disease are inadequate sampling of the lesion and aspiration in an area of necrosis or postobstructive pneumonia. In addition, small, central malignant lesions may be difficult to diagnose accurately with TTNA. Aspiration of vascular tumors, such as angiosarcoma, carcinoid, or metastatic renal cell carcinoma, may yield a bloody aspirate with few, if any, malignant cells.[55] TTNA rarely leads to misclassification of primary pulmonary neoplasms, with a reported rate of misdiagnosis of small-cell carcinoma of 0 to 1.1 percent.[43] False-positive results are extremely rare (under 0.5 percent) and are typically reported in the setting of inflammatory processes, such as tuberculosis, radiation fibrosis, organizing pneumonia, and pulmonary infarction.[40]

Specific diagnosis of a benign lesion with TTNA is more problematic, with published sensitivities ranging widely, from 11.7 to 68 percent.[56] A TTNA that is negative for malignancy does not rule out the presence of neoplastic disease, especially if the aspirate was unsatisfactory. The degree of suspicion of malignancy in a particular clinical situation becomes extremely important in dictating the next step following a negative TTNA. For a smoker with a high risk of bronchogenic carcinoma, the proper course may lead to videothoracoscopic biopsy of the lesion, whereas in a young, otherwise healthy nonsmoker, close observation with serial chest radiographs may be the preferred option.

Complications

As mentioned previously, the most common complication of both TTNA and TTNB is pneumothorax; incidence rates reported in the literature vary from 8 to 61 percent. A small percentage of the pneumothoraces are clinically significant; only about 8 percent require thoracostomy tube drainage.[56] Most symptomatic pneumothoraces can be managed successfully with insertion of a pneumothorax catheter connected to a Heimlich valve. Tension pneumothoraces are true medical emergencies, typically occurring within minutes of the procedure; they should be treated with immediate decompression (e.g., with a 14-gauge catheter inserted in the second intercostal space in the midclavicular line). Preexisting lung disease—in particular, bullous emphysema—is the most significant predisposing factor to development of pneumothorax after TTNA or TTNB. Other risk factors are deep lesions, increased number of passes, more than one pleural surface crossed, and increased patient age. The vast majority of patients who develop clinically significant pneumothoraces after the procedure have an underlying diagnosis of COPD.[56]

Uncommon complications of TTNA and TTNB include hemorrhage and hemoptysis, although these are typically minor. Cases of fatal hemorrhage from tracheobronchial obstruction from clot and subsequent asphyxia after use of large-bore (18-gauge) cutting needles have been reported.[56]

Air embolism is a rare complication caused by creation of a communication between atmospheric air and a pulmonary vein. To minimize this risk, the needle should never be left open to air while in the chest, and the patient should be discouraged from deep breathing, straining, or coughing during the procedure. The procedure should be halted and the needle withdrawn if the patient is actively coughing. If an air embolism is suspected, 100 percent oxygen should be administered through a nonrebreather face mask and the patient placed in the left lateral decubitus position, with the head down; this position optimizes capture of air in the right atrium. The patient should be transferred immediately to a hyperbaric chamber.[56]

REFERENCES

1. Alberti WE: Endobronchial high dose rate brachytherapy. *Int J Radiat Oncol Biol Phys* 25:753–755, 1993.
2. Bagwell CE, Talbert JL, Tepas JJ: Balloon dilatation of long segment tracheal stenosis. *J Pediatr Surg* 26:153–159, 1991.
3. Ball JB, Delaney JC, Evans CC, et al: Endoscopic bougie and balloon dilatation of multiple bronchial stenoses: 10 year follow up. *Thorax* 46:933–935, 1991.
4. Becker H: Flexible versus rigid bronchoscopic placement of tracheobronchial prostheses (stent): Pro flexible bronchoscopy. *J Bronchol* 2:252–256, 1995.
5. Cavaliere S, Foccoli P, Farina PL: Nd:YAG laser bronchoscopy: A five-year experience with 1396 applications in 1000 patients. *Chest* 94:15–21, 1988.
6. Colt HG, Dumon JF: Tracheobronchial stents: Indications and applications. *Lung Cancer* 9:301–306, 1993.
7. Cordasco EM Jr, Mehta AC, Ahmad M: Bronchoscopically induced bleeding: A summary of nine years' Cleveland Clinic experience and review of the literature. *Chest* 100:1141–1147, 1991.
8. Cortese DA: Rigid versus flexible bronchoscopy in laser bronchoscopy. Pro rigid bronchoscopic laser application. *J Bronchol* 1:72–75, 1994.
9. Dumon JF, Cavaliere S, Diaz-Jimenez JP, et al: Seven-year experience with the Dumon prosthesis. *J Bronchol* 3:6–10, 1996.
10. Edell ES, Cortese DA: Photodynamic therapy in management of early superficial squamous cell carcinoma as an alternative to surgical resection. *Chest* 102:1319–1322, 1992.
11. Falguera M, Nogues A, Ruiz-Gonzalez A, et al: Transthoracic needle aspiration in the study of pulmonary infections in patients with HIV. *Chest* 106:697–702, 1994.
12. Feinsilver SH, Fein AM, Niederman MS, et al: Utility of fiberoptic bronchoscopy in non-resolving pneumonia. *Chest* 98:1322–1326, 1990.
13. Freitag L, Firusian N, Stamatis G, Greschuchna D: The role of bronchoscopy in pulmonary complications due to mustard gas inhalation. *Chest* 100:1436–1441, 1991.
14. Freitag l: Flexible versus rigid bronchoscopic placement of tracheobronchial prostheses (stent). Pro rigid bronchoscopy. *J Bronchol* 2:248–251, 1995.
15. Griffin JJ, Meduri GU: New approaches to the diagnosis of nosocomial pneumonia. *Med Clin North Am* 78:1091–1122, 1994.
16. Guidelines for percutaneous needle aspiration biopsy. *Am Rev Respir Dis* 140:255–256; 1989.
17. Haramati LB: CT-guided automated needle biopsy of the chest. *AJR Am J Roentgenol* 165:53–55, 1995.
18. Homasson JP: Bronchoscopic cryotherapy. *J Bronchol* 2:45–53, 1995.

19. Hooper RG, Jackson FN: Endobronchial electrocautery. *Chest* 94:595–598, 1988.

20. Jackson C, Jackson CL: Bronchoscopy, in *Bronchoesophagology*. Philadelphia, WB Saunders, pp 50–67, 1950.

21. Jackson C, Jackson CL: Bronchoscopy for foreign body, in *Bronchoesophagology*. Philadelphia, WB Saunders, pp 68–109, 1950.

22. Keller C, Frost A: Fiberoptic bronchoplasty: Description of simple adjunct technique for management of bronchial stenosis following lung transplantation. *Chest* 102:995–998, 1992.

23. Killian G: Ueber directe Bronchoscopie. *Munich Med Wochenschr* 27:844–847, 1898.

24. Lalli AF, McCormack LJ, Zelch M, et al: Aspiration biopsies of lung lesions. *Radiology* 127:35–40, 1978.

25. Lam S: Photodynamic therapy of lung cancer. *Semin Oncol* 21(Suppl 15):15–19, 1994.

26. Lam S, MacAulay C, LeRiche JC, et al: Detection of dysplasia and carcinoma in situ by lung imaging fluorescence endoscope (LIFE) device. *J Thorac Cardiovasc Surg* 105:1035–1040, 1993.

27. Leyden H: Ueber infectiöse Pneumonie. *Dtsch Med Wochenschr* 9:52, 1883.

28. Marquette CH, Ramon P, Courcol R, et al: Bronchoscopic protected catheter brush for the diagnosis of pulmonary infections. *Chest* 93:746–755, 1988.

29. McManigle JE, Fletcher GL, Tenholder MF: Bronchoscopy in the management of bronchopleural fistula. *Chest* 97:1235–1238, 1990.

30. Meduri GU: Diagnosis and differential diagnosis of ventilator-associated pneumonia. *Clin Chest Med* 16:61–93, 1995.

31. Meduri GU, Beals DH, Maijub AG, Baselski V: Protected bronchoalveolar lavage. *Am Rev Respir Dis* 143:855–864, 1991.

32. Meduri GU, Chastre J: The standardization of bronchoscopic techniques for ventilator-associated pneumonia. *Chest* 102(Suppl 1):557S–564S, 1992.

33. Mehta AL, Kathawalla SA, Chan CC, Arroliga A: Role of bronchoscopy in evaluation of solitary pulmonary nodule. *J Bronchol* 2:315–322, 1995.

34. Ménétrier P: Cancer primitif du poumon. *Bull Soc Anat Paris* 61:21–24, 1886.

35. Perlmutt LM, Braun SD, Newman GE, et al: Timing of chest film follow-up after transthoracic needle aspiration. *AJR Am J Roentgenol* 146:1049–1050, 1987.

36. Piscani RJ, Wright AJ: Clinical utility of bronchoalveolar lavage in immunocompromised hosts. *Mayo Clin Proc* 67:221–227, 1992.

37. Poe RH, Kallay MC: Transthoracic needle biopsy of lung in non-hospitalized patients. *Chest* 92:676–678, 1987.

38. Prakash UBS, Barham SS, Carpenter HA, et al: Pulmonary alveolar phospholipoproteinosis: Experience with 34 cases and review. *Mayo Clin Proc* 62:499–518, 1987.

39. Prakash UBS, Offord KP, Stubbs SE: Bronchoscopy in North America: The ACCP survey. *Chest* 100:1668–1675, 1991.

40. Sanders C: Transthoracic needle aspiration. *Clin Chest Med* 13:11–16, 1992.

41. Saumench J, Escarabill J, Padro L, et al: Value of fiberoptic bronchoscopy and angiography for diagnosis of the bleeding site in hemoptysis. *Ann Thorac Surg* 48:272–274, 1989.

42. Shure D: Transbronchial biopsy and needle aspiration. *Chest* 95:1130–1138, 1989.

43. Stanley JH, Fish GD, Andriole JG, et al: Lung lesions: Cytologic diagnosis by fine-needle biopsy. *Radiology* 162:389–391, 1987.

44. Stanopoulos IT, Pickering R, Beamis JF, Martinez FJ: Oximetric monitoring during routine oxygen-supplemental flexible bronchoscopy: What role does it have? *J Bronchol* 2:5–11, 1995.

45. Steiner RM, Liu JB, Goldberg BB, Cohn JR: The value of ultrasound-guided fiberoptic bronchoscopy. *Clin Chest Med* 16:519–534, 1995.

46. Torres A, De La Bellacana JP, Xaubet A, et al: Diagnostic value of quantitative cultures of bronchoalveolar lavage and telescoping plugged catheters in mechanically ventilated patients with bacterial pneumonia. *Am Rev Respir Dis* 140:306–310, 1989.

47. Tsao TC, Tsai YH, Lau RS, et al: Treatment for collapsed lung in critically ill patients: Selective intrabronchial air insufflation using the fiberoptic bronchoscope. *Chest* 97:435–438, 1990.

48. Turner JF, Wang KP: Staging of mediastinal involvement in lung cancer by bronchoscopic needle aspiration. *J Bronchol* 3:74–76, 1996.

49. Unger M: Nd:YAG laser therapy for malignant and benign endobronchial obstructions. *Clin Chest Med* 6:277–290, 1985.

50. Unger M: Rigid versus flexible bronchoscopy in laser bronchoscopy: Pro flexible bronchoscopic laser application. *J Bronchol* 1:69–71, 1994.

51. Wang KP: Staging of bronchogenic carcinoma by bronchoscopy. *Chest* 106:588–593, 1994.

52. Wang KP, Gonullu U, Baker R: Bronchoscopy needle aspiration versus transthoracic needle aspiration in the diagnosis of pulmonary lesions. *J Bronchol* 1:199–204, 1994.

53. Wang KP, Turner JF, Giargiana F: Transthoracic needle aspiration biopsy. *J Bronchol* 2:243–247, 1995.

54. Weinstein HJ, Bone RC, Ruth WE: Pulmonary lavage in patients treated with mechanical ventilation. *Chest* 72:583–587, 1977.

55. Weisbrod GL: Transthoracic percutaneous lung biopsy. *Radiol Clin North Am* 28:647–655, 1990.

56. Weisbrod GL: Transthoracic needle biopsy. *World J Surg* 17:705–711, 1993.

57. Westcott JL: Direct percutaneous needle aspiration of localized pulmonary lesions: Results in 422 patients. *Radiology* 137:31–35, 1980.

58. Yang PC, Chang DB, Yu CJ, et al: Ultrasound-guided core biopsy of thoracic tumors. *Am Rev Respir Dis* 146:763–767, 1992.

59. Zavala DC, Schoell JE: Ultrathin needle aspiration of the lung in infections and malignant disease. *Am Rev Respir Dis* 123:125–131, 1981.

THORACOSCOPY

Larry R. Kaiser

Thoracoscopy is a type of surgery in which a motivated medical specialist can develop a level of expertise that puts certain procedures well within his or her reach. These procedures are complementary to bronchoscopy in many instances and aid greatly in the diagnostic evaluation and potentially in therapy for a number of patients, especially those with pleural disease. Within the past several years, videothoracoscopy has, in many ways, changed the way pulmonary medicine and thoracic surgery are practiced, allowing us to alter the approach to a number of clinical problems.

HISTORICAL PERSPECTIVE

In the early 1920s, Jacobaeus, a Swedish physician, used a cystoscope in the pleural space to lyse pleural adhesions as an adjunct to collapse therapy in the treatment of pulmonary tuberculosis.[30] He subsequently used this technique of thoracoscopy to localize and diagnose benign and malignant lesions of the pleura and pulmonary parenchyma.[31] Despite the work of Jacobaeus, the procedure was performed only on a limited basis in the United States and was never truly endorsed. In one of the early textbooks of thoracic surgery, Lilienthal mentioned thoracoscopy but warned against its routine use in patients with tuberculosis because of the risk of significant bleeding and the perceived possibility of spreading infection within the pleural space.[43]

Thoracoscopy evolved mainly as "pleuroscopy," which was used as an adjunct to other procedures in the *diagnosis* of pleural pathology—specifically in cases of an effusion of unknown

cause, in which the thoracentesis was negative and a closed pleural biopsy was nondiagnostic. In many of these cases, the presence of malignancy was proved at the time of pleuroscopic examination. A number of instruments were used for thoracoscopic examination, including rigid bronchoscopes, mediastinoscopes, and flexible bronchoscopes, as well as rigid fiberoptic thoracoscopes. A mediastinoscope offered a large working channel and excellent visualization of the pleural space; an effusion could be drained, biopsies taken, and pleurodesis effected with talc.[32] The procedure was mainly of diagnostic utility and, other than pleurodesis, offered little in the way of therapeutic applications. It was possible to biopsy the lung, but only small pieces could be removed, and the area that was amenable to biopsy was limited.[40,42,50]

The availability of the charged coupling device, a silicon chip that is light sensitive, led to the sufficient miniaturization of a video camera so that, when coupled to a fiberoptic telescope, it was practical for use in the operating room by providing a magnified image projected on a video monitor that allowed the operating surgeon to work with an assistant (Fig. 39-1.) Previously, it was possible only for a single operator to work with the thoracoscope, but the videothoracoscope frees up the surgeon's hands and allows more complex procedures to be performed. The power of this technique has been amply demonstrated by the rapid rise of laparoscopic cholecystectomy, a procedure that changed the specialty of general surgery in a remarkably short time. It was not long before a number of thoracic surgeons began to adapt this new technique for work in the chest even though thoracoscopy had never been a mainstay in the practice of most such surgeons.

CURRENT TECHNIQUES

The term *video-assisted thoracic surgery* (VATS) encompasses all procedures performed with the thoracoscope, including those that are purely "thoracoscopic."

The bony thorax, as opposed to the abdomen, provides its own space once the lung is collapsed, so insufflation of gas, used in the abdomen to create a working space, is unnecessary and even slightly dangerous. The space in the chest is created simply by placing an endobronchial tube and collapsing the ipsilateral lung. This requires a general anesthetic, but certain procedures—namely, those involving the parietal pleura—may be performed with only regional anesthesia and intravenous sedation, since the lung collapses in the spontaneously breathing patient once the negative, intrathoracic pressure is lost.[56]

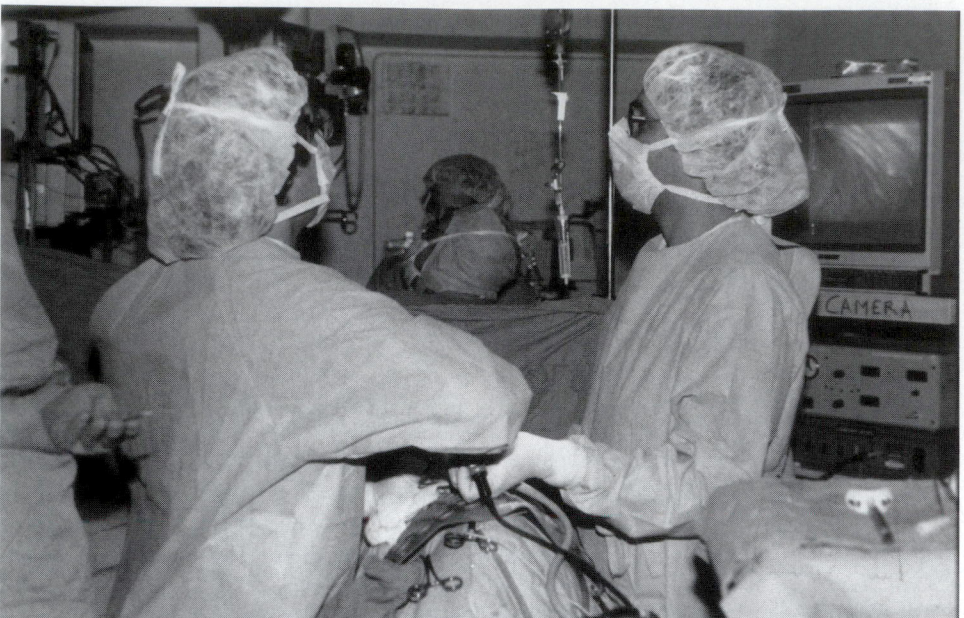

FIGURE 39-1 Surgeons carrying out a videothoracoscopic procedure. Note the video monitors, which allow the surgeon and assistants to view the surgical field. The work area is kept between the surgeon and the monitor.

The patient is placed on the operating table in the lateral decubitus position, and the chest is prepared and draped as for a thoracotomy. Incision placement depends somewhat on the procedure to be performed, but the location of the incision for insertion of the videothoracoscope remains constant in the seventh or eighth intercostal space aligned with the anterior superior iliac spine. A 1-cm incision is made, deepened to the intercostal muscles, as if one were inserting a chest tube; indeed, it is through this incision that the chest tube is placed at the conclusion of the surgical procedure. Entry into the chest is made with the index finger, to assure absolute safety. Occasionally, the lung is adherent to the chest wall, and these adhesions must be broken up with the index finger to allow for placement of the trocar sheath. Additional incisions are made as needed—usually arrayed in a triangular fashion, which facilitates instrument placement and allows one to work in coordination with an assistant (Fig. 39-2). It is best to work with two video monitors, which are placed at the head of the table on each side, so that both the operator and the assistant may have an unobstructed view of the surgical field. As long as one maintains the surgical field between oneself and the video monitor, the image is as it seems—that is, forward is forward, backward is backward, etc. It takes some adjustment to become accustomed to working in three dimensions while being able to see in only two.

The instrumentation available for thoracoscopy has been slowly improving. Instruments designed specifically for laparoscopy proved to be poor for this new application. Grasping the lung without teating the parenchyma proved to be especially difficult with these instruments. The most significant development in instrumentation, one that markedly expanded the utility of thoracoscopy, was the introduction of the endoscopic linear stapler. This instrument, more than any other, propelled thoracoscopy out of an alomost purely diagnostic realm into the mainstream of therapeutic applications.

SPECIFIC PROCEDURES

Pleural Disease

For many physicians, closed pleural biopsy has become a dying art—and perhaps it should be, with the emergence of videothoracoscopic techniques that allow one to biopsy specific areas of the parietal pleura under direct vision. The major, but certainly not the only, indication for thoracoscopy in the management of pleural disease remains the undiagnosed pleural effusion. In the past, the patient with an empyema often was forced to undergo thoracotomy for débridement and decortication to rid the space of infection and allow the lung to reexpand. With thoracoscopic techniques, many of these patients may now avoid thoracotomy, especially if they are seen early in the course of the empyema. Thoracoscopic débridement and decortication are indicated in the febrile patient with a pleural effusion in whom tube thoracostomy provides incomplete drainage. The fibrinous nature of the exudate precludes complete drainage with a tube alone, and mechanical débridement is required. Likewise, videothoracoscopic techniques have proved useful in the management of the organized posttraumatic hemothorax, in which a chest tube is unable to effectively drain the organized clot and debris.

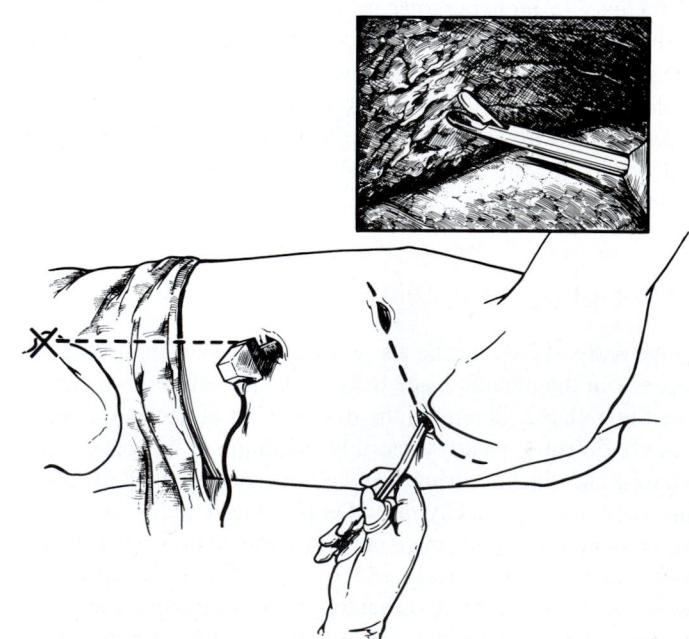

FIGURE 39-2 For most cases three incisions are used, as shown. The thoracoscope most commonly is placed through the inferior incision, allowing other instruments to be placed through the two opposed incisions. *Inset:* A view within the chest, as would be seen on the monitor, of a biopsy forceps in place to take a specimen of parietal pleura.

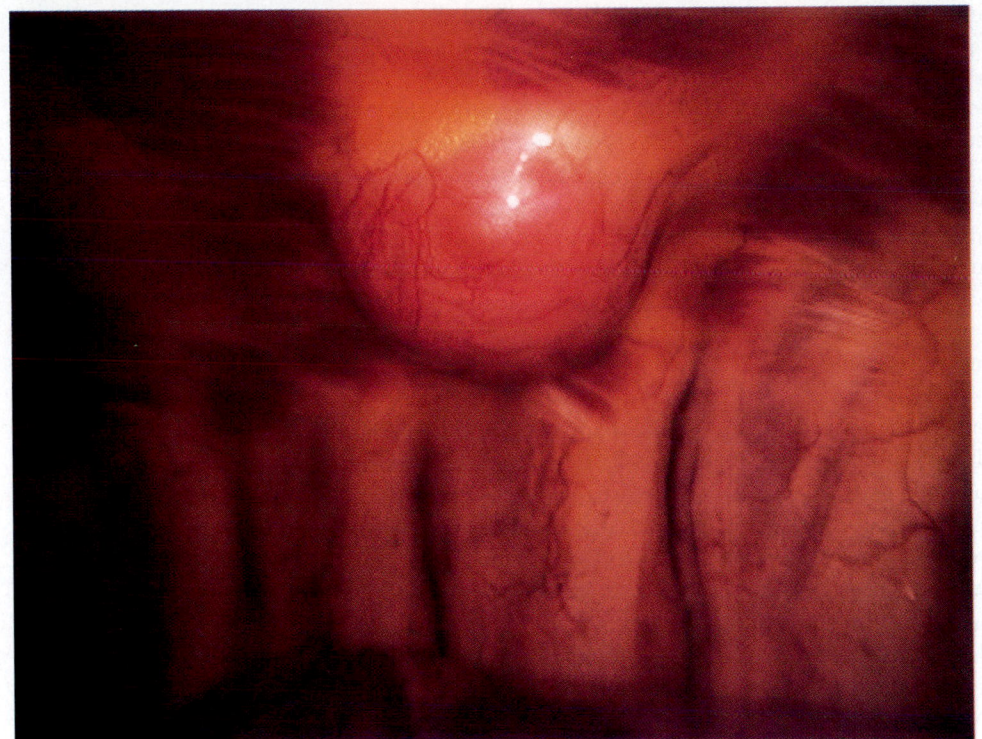

FIGURE 39-3   A benign schwannoma arising from the parietal pleural surface—a lesion that is easily amenable to thoracoscopic excision.

Benign pleural tumors, specifically solitary fibrous tumors, do occur; most commonly they arise from the visceral pleural surface and are ideal lesions for thoracoscopic resection (Fig. 39-3).

Videothoracoscopy also has increased our ability to deal successfully with malignant pleural effusions, especially those in which loculations are present. When tube thoracostomy results in incomplete drainage or one attempt at chest tube pleurodesis has failed, thoracoscopy—whereby the chest is evacuated under direct vision and talc is insufflated—is the procedure of choice. Hartman and colleagues compared the thoracoscopic insufflation of talc in patients who underwent tube thoracostomy and sclerosis with either tetracycline or bleomycin.[26] Talc pleurodesis was performed under local anesthesia supplemented with intravenous sedation. For patients in the talc group, there was a 97 percent rate of successful pleurodesis at 30 days and 95 percent at 90 days. This is significantly better than results seen in patients treated with the tube thoracotomy, only 33 percent of whom had achieved a successful pleurodesis at 30 days. The results were slightly better when bleomycin was used in the tube thoracostomy group. Patients sclerosed with talc seemed to have less pain following the procedure. The ability to perform thoracoscopic talc pleurodesis under local anesthesia may make the technique attractive for most patients with malignant effusions. Currently, a national prospective, randomized trial is in progress to determine if VATS pleurodesis offers advantages over tube thoracostomy.

Parenchymal Disease

Transbronchial lung biopsy often is successful in providing diagnostic material in patients with diffuse pulmonary infiltrates.

In situations in which a transbronchial biopsy fails to provide diagnostic material, a VATS procedure is indicated. Before the advent of videothoracoscopy, many of these patients were treated empirically, usually with steroids. Lung biopsy, which required a thoracotomy, albeit a "mini" one, was reserved for patients who either failed empiric therapy or were desperately ill and in intensive care. The empiric approach probably is warranted and may, in fact, be preferred in the non-neutropenic cancer patient with acute pneumonitis, for whom broad-spectrum antibiotic therapy usually is the treatment of choice.[52] In the non-immunocompromised patient, usually with a chronic interstitial process, serious consideration must be given to obtaining a piece of lung tissue. The pulmonologist must make a judgment as to whether a transbronchial lung biopsy is indicated—a decision that must take into account the most likely diagnostic possibility and whether a transbronchial specimen will be adequate to establish that diagnosis and the small but very real risks of bleeding and pneumothorax.[60] VATS lung biopsy will always provide diagnostic material. Burt and colleagues found a 94 percent diagnostic yield from open lung biopsy versus 59 percent for transbronchial biopsy in a series of 20 patients subjected to both procedures.[5]

Before the introduction of videothoracoscopy, a thoracotomy was required solely for the purpose of obtaining a piece of lung tissue.[22] The thoracotomy usually consisted of a small inframammary incision into the chest through the fourth or fifth intercostal space, a procedure that can be done expeditiously and allows one to obtain enough lung parenchyma to make a diagnosis. There should be minimal morbidity with this approach, and it still represents the best approach to lung biopsy in the critically ill, hemodynamically fragile patient who is ventilator dependent (requiring high peak airway pressures and high inspired oxygen concentration), for whom transport to the operating room represents a substantial risk. The "mini" anterior thoracotomy does not require single-lung ventilation and thus avoids the potential morbidity and mortality associated with exchange of the endotracheal tube for an endobronchial tube in these high-risk patients. However, the surgical exposure achieved by this approach can significantly limit the area of lung that may be accessible for biopsy. It is also difficult to obtain tissue from more than one site of the lung with this approach.

In most patients, however, VATS wedge lung biopsy, which we and others have referred to as "closed lung biopsy," represents the best alternative to the "mini" thoracotomy. It offers the advantage of excellent visualization of the entire lung so that suspect areas can be biopsied under direct vision and all areas of the lung can be reached with relative ease. The technique avoids spreading of the ribs, which seems to be one of the factors responsible for the pain that results following thoracotomy, including anterior thoracotomy. It may be that thoracoscopic biopsy causes less postoperative pain, which may be important in weaning patients from a ventilator in the immediate postoperative period, and results in a shorter hospital stay. In a non-randomized, retrospective study using historical controls, Ferson and colleagues from two other centers compared a group of 47 patients undergoing thoracoscopic lung biopsy with a group of 28 patients who had had open wedge resection via limited thoracotomy.[19] Adequate tissue for diagnosis was obtained for all patients in both groups. Mean surgical time was significantly longer in the thoracoscopic group (69 versus 93 min), but, as would be expected, the time decreased as additional experience was gained. The authors excluded from the study patients requiring mechanical ventilation and still found that hospital stay was significantly shorter in the group undergoing thoracoscopic biopsy (4.9 versus 12.2 days). There were significantly more complications in the open group (50 percent incidence) than in the VATS group (19 percent), a finding that no doubt explains the variation in duration of hospital stay. All surgeons engaged in the study believed that thoracoscopic biopsy provided better visualization of the entire lung than a "mini" thoracotomy.

Our own experience with 80 thoracoscopic lung biopsies in non–ventilator-dependent patients confirms the above-mentioned findings. Diagnostic tissue was obtained in all cases, and in several our ability to provide tissue from different areas of the lung greatly aided in establishing a diagnosis. The mean hospital stay in our series was 1.9 days, significantly shorter than that of Ferson and colleagues.[19] There was no mortality and no significant morbidity, including no prolonged air leaks. When lung biopsy is indicated, thoracoscopic biopsy is our procedure of choice for nonventilated patients. For patients requiring mechanical ventilation, in most cases we prefer a limited anterior thoracotomy with minimal rib spreading—a simple procedure that can be performed expeditiously and avoids the need for single-lung ventilation.

Of interest is that thoracoscopic lung biopsies were reported before the advent of VATS techniques and before the linear stapler was available.[2,17] With a cup biopsy forceps, pieces of lung parenchyma were obtained, and an insulated electrocautery provided the only means of hemostasis. Daniel and colleagues compared results obtained in the era before the advent of video technology with those obtained by current methods.[12] In 30 patients undergoing thoracoscopic cup biopsy, there were 10 deaths and one prolonged air leak that required a thoracotomy for repair. Mean hospital stay was 16.6 days. In contrast, 11 patients underwent videothoracoscopic biopsy with only one death and a mean hospital stay of 8.2 days. The significantly better hemostatic as well as aerostatic qualities of the linear stapler than those of a cup biopsy forceps and the larger amount of tissue obtained using a stapler clearly are advantageous. These authors also noted no advantage to either endoscopic approach over limited thoracotomy in patients requiring mechanical ventilation.

The availability of VATS lung biopsy should prompt earlier referral for lung biopsy of patients with interstitial disease who either would be treated empirically and not referred for biopsy or would be referred in desperation at the time of marked de-

compensation, usually after being intubated and ventilated. Utilizing these techniques to obtain an earlier tissue diagnosis in patients with interstitial lung disease should improve management and, it is hoped, improve the long-term outlook.

VATS techniques have also had a major impact on the management of spontaneous pneumothorax in the two major groups of patients who present with this problem: young patients with apical blebs and older patients with bullous emphysema. Primary spontaneous pneumothorax in a young person typically can be managed nonsurgically, with the likelihood of recurrence being approximately 30 percent.[4] Surgical treatment for a first-time pneumothorax classically has been reserved for patients with persistent air leaks (longer than 1 week), those whose occupations require them to experience extremes in atmospheric pressure, and those who live in isolated areas without access to medical care.[16] Otherwise, surgery is indicated after a first recurrence or for the patient who has experienced bilateral pneumothoraxes. Surgery for a spontaneous pneumothorax has required either a thoracotomy with stapling of apical blebs and, at times, a pleurectomy[4] or, more recently, a transaxillary thoracotomy with excision of blebs and pleural ablation or pleurectomy to create pleural symphysis.[15] These are both substantial procedures for what is really a trivial problem in terms of what needs to be done intraoperatively. An alternative approach to management, mentioned only to be dismissed, involves installation of talc or other sclerosant via tube thoracostomy.[1,41]

VATS management of spontaneous pneumothorax provides a simple surgical alternative that is associated with minimal morbidity. With recognition that in young patients the pneumothorax usually results from rupture of a bleb located at the lung apex or occasionally in the apical portion of the superior segment of the lower lobe, the surgical maneuvers include resection of the apical blebs and mechanical pleural abrasion to effect a pleural symphysis (Fig. 39-4). The blebs are easily visualized with the thoracoscope and excised with several applications of the linear stapler. The parietal pleural surface is mechanically abraded with

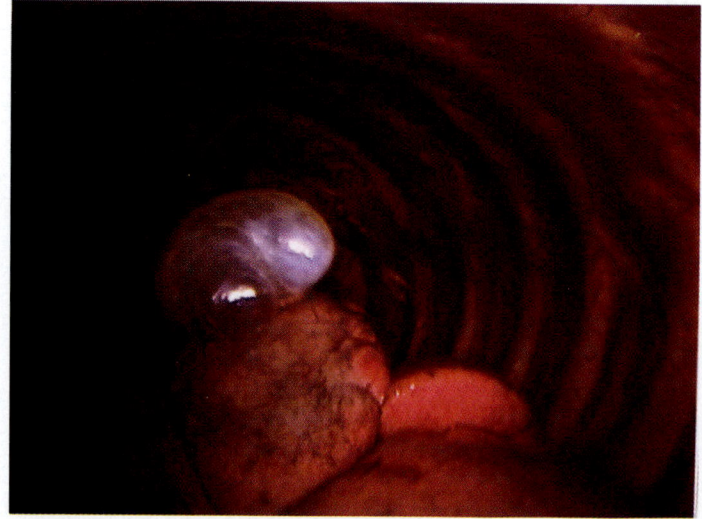

FIGURE 39-4 Thoracoscopic appearance of a typical apical bleb responsible for a spontaneous pneumothorax, usually in a young person. These are most commonly found at the lung apex, but they can also occur at the apex of the superior segment of the lower lobe.

a gauze sponge, which creates enough inflammation to cause pleurodesis. Talc or other sclerosing agents are not recommended for these young patients. Obliteration of the apical blebs alone probably would be sufficient, and the contribution of the pleurodesis is probably minimal. One would expect a very low recurrence rate (less than 5 percent) following this procedure, similar to that achieved after a transaxillary procedure or formal thoracotomy; the handling of the blebs is identical no matter which approach is used.

Cannon and associates performed thoracoscopic excision of apical blebs in nine patients with primary spontaneous pneumothorax and noted one recurrent small apical pneumothorax that resolved without treatment.[6] We performed 70 thoracoscopic procedures for primary spontaneous pneumothorax over a 4-year period. We noted three recurrences, two in patients with catamenial pneumothorax, at the time of their first menstrual period following the procedure, and one in a patient with routine apical blebs. The lesion responsible for catamenial pneumothorax is unknown, and we were unable to detect any pathology at the time of the procedure.[45] These patients experienced recurrence despite the performance of what was believed to be adequate pleurodesis, but the recurrences were early, probably before the development of pleural adhesions. Allen's team reported on 46 patients who underwent wedge excision and pleurodesis for spontaneous pneumothorax.[2] Only one patient required conversion to an open procedure. Seven patients had persistent air leaks (more than 10 days), and two of these required thoracotomy for correction. No recurrences have been seen with a median follow-up time of 25 months. Median hospital stay was 5 days. Our own experience, along with that of other groups, suggests that hospital stay after VATS operation for spontaneous pneumothorax is closer to 2 days; prolonged air leaks following the procedure, causing longer hospital stays, are rare.[14]

Indications for surgery for spontaneous pneumothorax have not changed significantly despite the availability of the VATS technique, which allows most patients to leave the hospital on the first or second postoperative day. Patients with primary pneumothorax are managed with either aspiration of the pneumothorax or chest tube placement. We used to wait 7 days for an air leak to seal before proceeding with surgery. We now wait only 48 to 72 h before recommending the thoracoscopic procedure, which allows the patient to leave the hospital sooner than if treated in the conventional fashion. The decision for earlier surgery is justified by the decreased morbidity associated with the VATS procedure when compared with an open procedure, even the transaxillary approach.[13] In a patient treated conservatively for a first-time pneumothorax, recurrence on the same side or a pneumothorax on the opposite side is an indication for surgery. If the pneumothorax occurs on the same side as the first one, we operate only on that side. With a contralateral pneumothorax, both sides should be operated on, since the consequences of spontaneous bilateral pneumothoraxes may be devastating. Bilateral VATS procedures conducted with a single anesthetic may be performed without significant additional morbidity, especially in young patients. If necessary, thoracic epidural analgesia may be used in the early postoperative period. VATS excision of apical blebs and mechanical pleural abrasion constitute the procedure of choice when surgery is indicated in a patient with spontaneous pneumothorax.

Pneumothorax occurring secondarily to a process other than the apical blebs seen in young people can also be managed with a VATS approach. In these situations, the pathology may be somewhat more complex, and one needs to search for the air leak and repair it, usually by stapling; but fibrin glue, the neodynium-YAG laser, and the argon beam coagulator have also been used with success. Over a recent 2-year period, we performed 13 procedures for so-called secondary pneumothorax—seven in patients with emphysema who presented in respiratory distress after developing a pneumothorax, two for persistent air leaks following thoracotomy and lobectomy, one in a patient with AIDS and bilateral pneumothoraxes secondary to *Pneumocystis carinii* infection causing necrotic parenchymal cavitary lesions, and three in patients with metastatic sarcomas. We were successful in managing the air leak in 12 patients; one patient was converted to open thoracotomy. Cannon and colleagues operated on six patients with secondary pneumothorax, two of whom subsequently required a thoracotomy to deal with persistent air leaks following the thoracoscopic procedure.[6] Although recognizing that some patients still may require thoracotomy, we prefer to attempt a VATS approach for an air leak because these patients often have significantly compromised pulmonary function and avoidance of a thoracotomy is advantageous. If a surgeon develops an interest and gains experience with VATS techniques, the frequency of conversion to an open procedure should remain low. It requires a commitment on the part of the surgeon, however, especially early in one's experience, to take the extra time that may be required to complete some of the more complex procedures rather than quickly converting to an open operation.

The management of bullous lung disease has also changed with the introduction of VATS techniques. The standard indication for surgery in patients with bullous emphysema is the presence of a giant bulla causing significant compression of adjacent, relatively normal lung parenchyma (Fig. 39-5). These giant bullae are readily recognizable on plain chest radiograph, and a CT scan helps to define the presence and extent of compressed

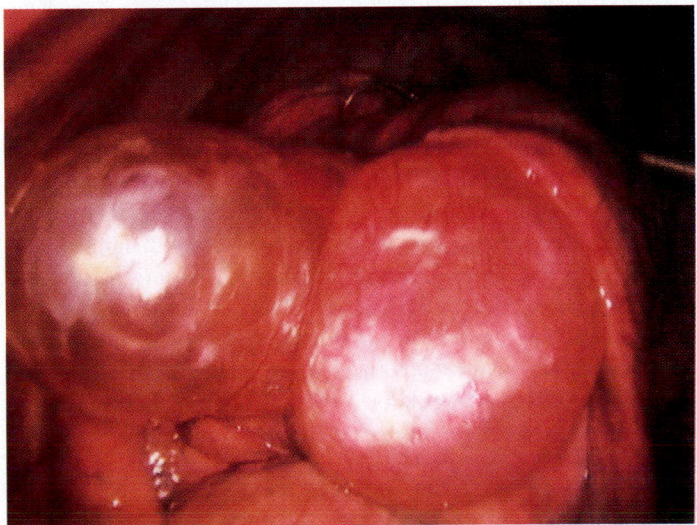

FIGURE 39-5 A giant bulla occurring as an isolated finding, resulting in compression of adjacent lung parenchyma. Excision usually offers significant relief of symptoms.

lung tissue. The major factor that enters into a decision on whether bullectomy is likely to result in improvement in a patient's condition relates to the compressed lung parenchyma and whether there is significant compressed parenchyma to expand and fill the pleural space after bullectomy. A residual space after bullectomy promotes the development of a persistent air leak and, in a small percentage of cases, an empyema, with resultant devastating consequences and usually a prolonged hospital stay. Reviewing a series of chest radiographs performed over the preceding several years to determine the progression in the size of the bullae allows for an assessment of the amount of compressed adjacent lung tissue. Pulmonary function studies should document a decrease in function, and the patient should note a decrease in exercise tolerance. Patients who fulfill these criteria are ideal candidates for VATS bullectomy.

The procedure itself requires obliteration of the bulla with the avoidance of air leaks, if possible. We prefer to use the argon beam coagulator, which, when applied at a low power setting, causes the wall of the bulla to shrivel although the bulla is not entered. Once the bulla has shrunk, the base may be delineated and then stapled in an attempt to minimize air leak. The walls of the bulla may be used as a buttress for the staple line. Alternatively, a piece of prosthetic material, specifically bovine pericardium (PeriGuard, Biovascular Medical, St. Paul, MN), may be used to reinforce the staple line to prevent air leaks. Performing a VATS procedure rather than open thoracotomy in these markedly compromised patients, most of whom are oxygen dependent and have FEV_1 well under 1 L, seems to be preferable. Still, in the early postoperative period these patients are most at risk of secretion retention and pneumonia—which, for many, would be a terminal event. Thus, postoperative pain management and aggressive chest physiotherapy are of major importance. We use thoracic epidural analgesia provided by a continuous infusion of narcotic for pain management in the early postoperative period so that patients may cough more effectively. Patients are extubated as soon as possible, ideally at the completion of the surgical procedure.

Unfortunately, giant bullae do occur in some patients with bullous emphysema. Wakabayashi identified 17 cases of giant bullous disease among more than 500 cases of bullous emphysema seen over a 3-year period.[58,59] Of more than 2000 thoracoscopic cases reported to the Video Assisted Thoracic Surgical Study Group (VATSSG) Registry, only 33 (1.8 percent) were for excision of giant bullae.[28]

Diffuse emphysema, with or without a bullous component, is a significantly greater clinical problem in terms of numbers of patients affected. Until recently, the therapeutic options of these patients were extremely limited, with oxygen therapy and bronchodilators being the mainstay for those with a reversible airway component. The reintroduction of a surgical procedure, volume reduction, which has been shown to be efficacious in some cases, may offer many of these desperate patients some relief from their symptoms.[10] Although the initial procedure of volume reduction for diffuse emphysema, as described by Cooper and colleagues, entailed a median sternotomy and bilateral excision of lung parenchyma, other authors have reported on either unilateral or bilateral VATS procedures to accomplish essentially the same outcome.[35,49] Kotloff and associates compared a series of patients from the University of Pennsylvania who underwent volume reduction via sternotomy with a group undergoing the procedure via a VATS approach.[39] Patients who underwent a bilateral VATS procedure fared as well as those undergoing sternotomy in terms of functional improvement. There were fewer postoperative deaths in the VATS group, but the difference was not statistically significant. A multi-institution, federally funded prospective trial to evaluate lung volume reduction surgery will further compare these two methods for performing the procedure, but it is reasonable to conclude that the same type of excision of emphysematous lung that can be accomplished with a median sternotomy can be achieved with a VATS technique. Questions that remain to be answered have to do with differences in procedure-related morbidity and mortality, as well as differences in overall functional improvement.

PULMONARY NODULES

The solitary indeterminate pulmonary nodule is a problem confronted routinely by pulmonologists. In light of the emergence of VATS as a minimally invasive procedure that can be performed with low morbidity even in compromised patients, we must examine closely the current management of a patient who presents with an indeterminate nodule. Whereas in the past definitive management required open thoracotomy, with its attendant morbidity, this no longer is the case. Thoracoscopy offers the opportunity both to definitively make the diagnosis and to treat many of these lesions and, therefore, causes a refocus in our thinking.

The salient question posed by the presence of a pulmonary nodule is a very simple one: Is it malignant? If a previous radiograph demonstrates a lesion that has not changed in size over several years, one can be reasonably certain of the benign nature of that lesion. Depending on the series, approximately 40 percent of resected nodules are malignant, and primary carcinoma of the lung accounts for the majority of malignant nodules.[44] A number of factors point to a benign diagnosis, although none are absolute. We may be far less suspicious of a nodule occurring in a nonsmoker, especially if the person is 35 years of age or younger. Lesions larger than 3 cm in diameter are likely to be malignant.[63] Specific patterns of calcification may also be associated with benign lesions, and CT comparison with a phantom of known density may further support a benign diagnosis. Even when all these factors have been taken into consideration, a histologic diagnosis is required in most cases. If benignity cannot be proved, malignancy must be assumed.

The diagnostic procedures available to the pulmonary physician are very good at establishing a diagnosis of malignancy but fall short in obtaining a "positive" diagnosis of benign disease. The diagnostic yield from fiberoptic bronchoscopy varies from 20 to 80 percent, but a specific benign diagnosis is made only 10 percent of the time.[11,20,61] With these figures, it is hard to justify the performance of a bronchoscopy if one is looking to make a diagnosis of benign disease. Unfortunately, percutaneous needle aspiration biopsy does not fare much better. Although its sensitivity in making the diagnosis of malignancy is high (64 to 97 percent),[57] a specific benign diagnosis can be made only about as often as the rate achieved bronchoscopically.[38] A "negative" needle biopsy is of no help and necessitates a further diagnostic procedure, while a diagnosis of malignancy essentially tells us what we already know: The lesion has to be excised.

Mack and colleagues, in a multicenter study, have looked closely at the role of thoracoscopy in the diagnosis of the indeterminate solitary pulmonary nodule.[46] Over an 18-month period, 242 patients with solitary nodules were treated. A wedge excision of the lesion that included some surrounding normal lung parenchyma was accomplished with an endoscopic stapler alone in most cases. A definite diagnosis was obtained in all cases; there was no mortality or major morbidity, and minor complications (atelectasis, pneumonia, prolonged air leak) occurred in only nine patients (3.6 percent). In two patients, the nodule could not be located and a thoracotomy was required; otherwise, a benign diagnosis was obtained in 127 patients (52 percent), while malignancy was found in 115 (48 percent). When a primary lung cancer was identified, formal open thoracotomy and anatomic resection were carried out in patients with adequate pulmonary reserve. The average hospital stay for the patients undergoing thoracoscopy alone was 2.4 days.

In a series of 771 VATS procedures at the Mayo Clinic, wedge excision of a pulmonary nodule was performed in 234 patients.[2] There were no deaths in this group of patients, and the most common complication was a prolonged air leak, which occurred in 3.0 percent of patients. The median hospital stay was 3 days. The lesion was found to be malignant in 107 patients, and all patients found to have bronchogenic carcinoma underwent an open thoracotomy for anatomic pulmonary resection and lymph node sampling.

It is hard to argue against a technique that has a sensitivity and specificity of 100 percent and can be done with no mortality and minimal morbidity. But is it necessary to excise so many benign lesions? If we could be certain of the benignity of a lesion, there would be no reason to excise it. It is the uncertainty of the benign diagnosis in most cases that presents the most compelling argument for thoracoscopic excision of most solitary pulmonary nodules. All questions are answered and the uncertainty disappears with one procedure.

Certain lesions are not considered for VATS excision. For lesions greater than 3 cm in diameter, the likelihood of malignancy is so high (greater than 90 percent) that in the absence of metastatic disease, thoracotomy and anatomic resection—i.e., lobectomy—should be the first procedure undertaken.[62] The CT scan aids greatly in localizing the nodule, and we have found it to be the only localizing study that is required. Even deep-seated lesions may be palpated and located, a technique that becomes easier with experience. In our experience with 400 thoracoscopic excisions of pulmonary nodules, we have failed to locate the nodule in only four cases, all early in our experience. Our technique relies heavily on instruments, specifically designed for thoracoscopy, that greatly facilitate the procedure, especially in grasping or moving the lung to the palpating finger (Fig. 39-6). Centrally located lesions, which lie in close proximity to hilar structures, are not suitable for VATS wedge excision and require open thoracotomy.

There is some controversy regarding the optimal management of the solitary nodule that proves to be a carcinoma. Is a VATS wedge excision sufficient treatment for a T1 (less than 3 cm) primary lung carcinoma? Based on current knowledge, we believe

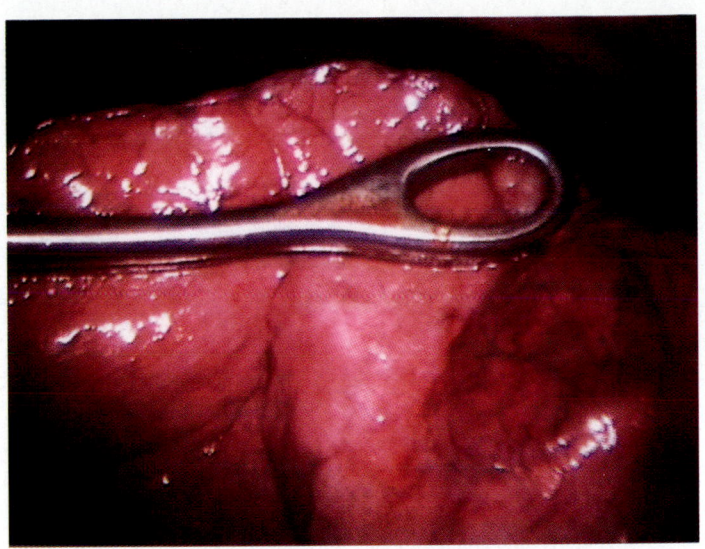

FIGURE 39-6   A modified ring forceps grasping the lung and moving the lung into position either for wedge excision of a nodule or for palpation of the area to identify the nodule. The forceps is able to grasp the lung without tearing the pulmonary parenchyma, a situation that commonly occurs if the lung is grasped with an instrument with a small surface area.

that wedge excision is not optimal treatment for primary lung cancer, even a small T1 lesion. A wedge excision is a compromise procedure that is acceptable only for the patient who otherwise cannot tolerate a thoracotomy and anatomic resection. Among other factors, a wedge excision removes no regional lymph nodes and thus staging is inadequate. Local recurrence is significantly higher after wedge excision than after lobectomy. Several authors have performed large series of nonanatomic resections for patients with marginal pulmonary function, and VATS excision, with its low morbidity, may offer another alternative.[18,48,53] The Lung Cancer Study group addressed the question of limited resection versus lobectomy for T1 N0 lesions in a prospective, randomized trial.[23] In this study of carefully staged patients proven conclusively to have N0 disease, there was a significantly higher incidence of local recurrence in those who underwent limited resection, but at 3 years there was no survival difference between the two groups. However, a reexamination of the data at 5 years showed a statistically significant survival advantage for the lobectomy group.[24] Wedge excision for bronchogenic carcinoma as a definitive procedure, whether carried out via a VATS approach or open thoracotomy, must be considered a compromise and should be reserved for patients whose pulmonary function is so marginal as to preclude lobectomy.

Anatomic resections (mainly lobectomy) have been performed using a VATS technique that requires a small (6 cm) "utility" incision, but usually without the need for rib spreading—which, theoretically, should minimize postoperative pain (Fig. 39-7).[36] A randomized trial comparing VATS lobectomy with standard muscle-sparing thoracotomy and lobectomy failed to show significant enough differences to justify the routine use of the VATS approach—which probably subjects the patient to a slightly greater risk of intraoperative catastrophe, although no intraoperative deaths have been reported.[37] Roviaro and colleagues

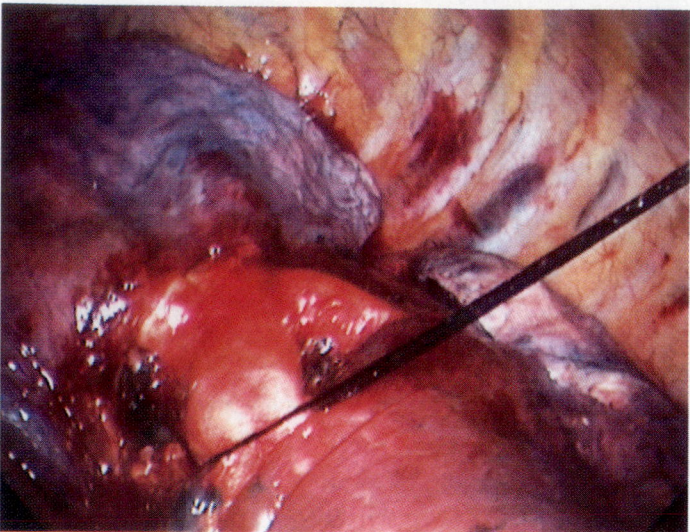

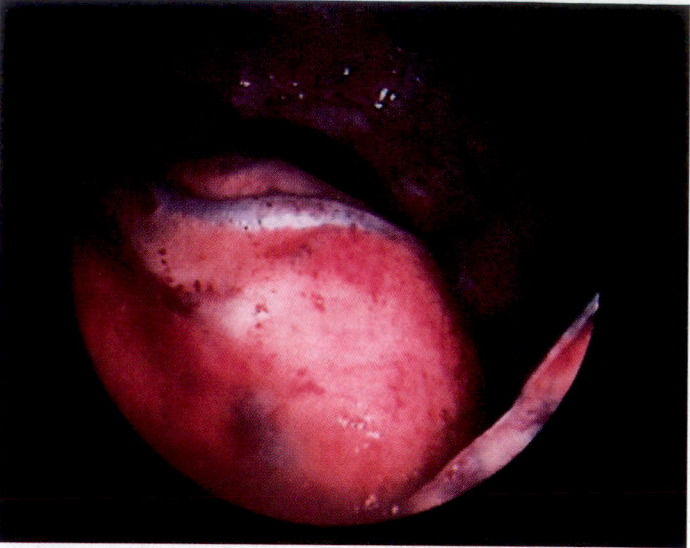

FIGURE 39-7 View of a video-assisted lobectomy showing the pulmonary artery in the fissure of the left lung. Note the basilar segmental trunk and the branch to the superior segment of the lower lobe. The procedure is performed with visualization provided by the video camera and access via a small utility incision through which regular instruments are inserted but without spreading the ribs.

FIGURE 39-8 The aortopulmonary window, a common site for lymph node involvement when the primary tumor is in the left upper lobe (level 5, subaortic, and level 6, para-aortic). These lymph node locations cannot be reached by standard cervical mediastinoscopy, and videothoracoscopy provides an ideal way both to visualize this area and, when appropriate, to take biopsies.

performed 52 VATS lobectomies and four pneumonectomies in patients with T1 N0 or T2 N0 lesions.[55] In seven patients it was necessary to convert to an open procedure, three for bleeding during the dissection. There were no deaths related to the procedure. Others have reported the feasibility of performing VATS lobectomy or segmentectomy.[14] A large randomized trial demonstrating the superiority of a VATS approach over an open procedure is lacking. VATS lobectomy has not found widespread acceptance, nor is the public demanding it. A few centers continue to perform the procedure regularly.

MEDIASTINAL PROCEDURES

VATS has proved useful as an adjunct to more conventional procedures used in the invasive staging of lung cancer. Mediastinoscopy remains the gold standard for invasive staging of the mediastinum, but lymph nodes in the posterior subcarinal space (level 7) and in the aortopulmonary window (level 5) are not accessible. VATS offers an unmatched ability to visualize the aortopulmonary window and sample lymph nodes in this region (Fig. 39-8); the same is true for the subcarinal space when it is approached from the right side. A VATS staging procedure is not a substitute for mediastinoscopy, but in certain situations directed by findings on the chest CT scan, it may add valuable staging information. This is particularly important because of the interest in preoperative therapy (neoadjuvant) for patients proven to have N2 (mediastinal) lymph node disease.

The utility of VATS is limited for assessing resectability, especially if one is trying to document direct invasion of mediastinal structures (either T3 or T4), but it is occasionally of use.[55] Dissection often proves difficult and potentially hazardous, and there is no substitute for putting one's hand on a lesion of questionable resectability. VATS proves extremely useful, however, in documenting the absence of diffuse pleural metastatic disease

if this possibility has been raised (usually by the presence of a pleural effusion).

Many primary lesions of the mediastinum prove to be ideal for VATS management. Lesions in all compartments of the mediastinum are easily accessible, and whether biopsy only or complete excision is the intent, VATS techniques save many patients from having to undergo thoracotomy.

To approach a lesion in the anterior mediastinum, the patient is positioned with the side to be operated on tilted up at approximately 30 degrees instead of in the full lateral position. Of-

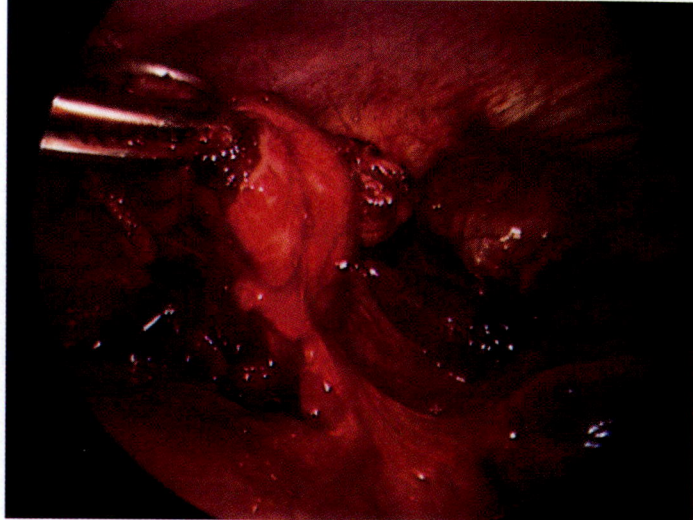

FIGURE 39-9 A well-encapsulated thymoma being dissected off the pericardium. The cervical portions of the thymus gland have been mobilized by a transcervical approach so that a total thymectomy—the goal of the operation in patients with myasthenia gravis—could be carried out.

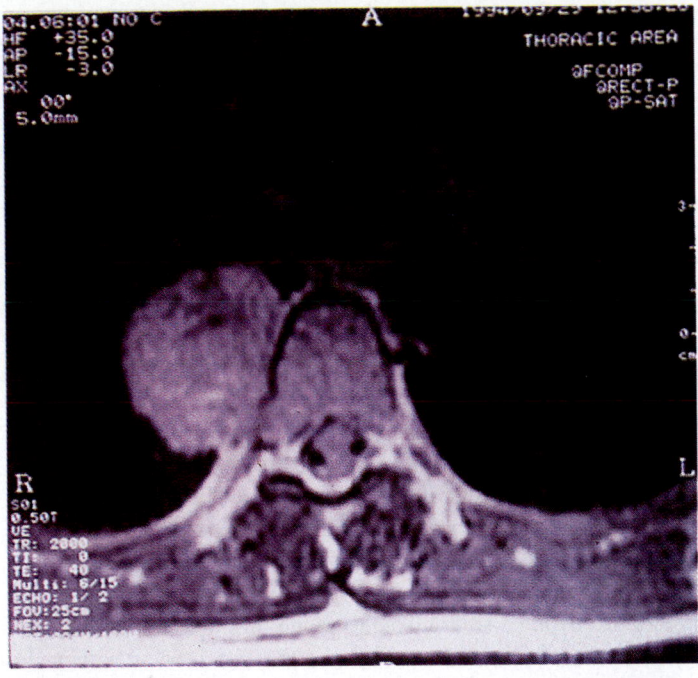

A

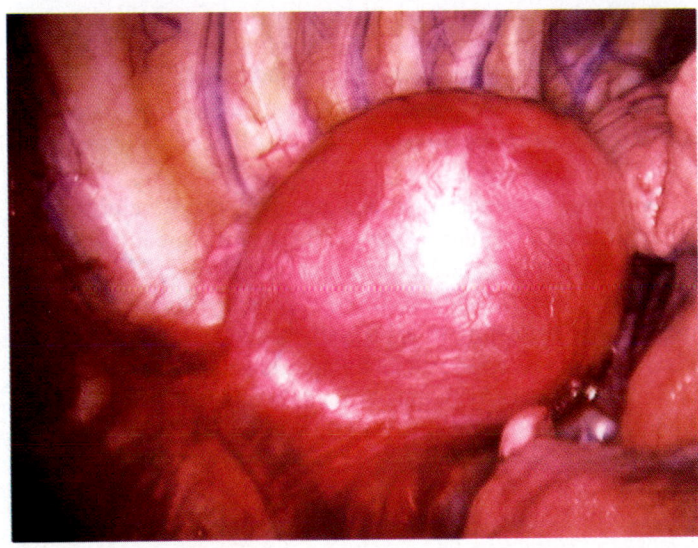

B

FIGURE 39-10 *A.* MRI scan showing a posterior mediastinal mass sitting in a paravertebral location. Lesions in this location usually are neurogenic, and this lesion proved to be a ganglioneuroma. *B.* View at the time of the videothoracoscopy showing the lesion seen in *A.* This lesion was able to be completely excised with a videothoracoscopic approach.

ten a small inframammary incision is employed. We have utilized a VATS approach to accomplish 15 thymectomies, nine of them for encapsulated thymomas (Fig. 39-9). A VATS procedure is contraindicated for presumed invasive thymomas. In patients with myasthenia gravis and a thymoma, a total thymectomy is mandatory and may be facilitated by combining a transcervical approach with the VATS exposure.[34] The thymus gland is initially mobilized in the neck, and branches to the innominate vein are divided. The mobilized gland is then tucked down into the

mediastinum, the neck closed, and the patient positioned for VATS. The thymoma is mobilized and the dissection completed with the removal of the gland and tumor through one of the chest incisions. Attempting to excise the tumor and perform a total thymectomy with a VATS approach alone is possible but more difficult, because of the need to extend the dissection well up into the neck.

The patient with a large, diffuse mediastinal mass from which tissue is required for diagnosis may also, at times, benefit from a VATS approach. Many of these lesions are more readily accessed for biopsy through an extrapleural, parasternal approach by excision of the costal cartilage (usually the second). Lesions that are not close to the anterior chest wall may be approached and readily sampled with a VATS approach.

The posterior mediastinum is also the site of either solid or cystic lesions that are amenable to VATS resection. We have resected eight posterior mediastinal lesions, including schwannomas (four) and bronchogenic cysts (four) (Fig. 39-10). Incisions used to approach these posterior or mediastinal lesions differ slightly from those used for access to the anterior mediastinum. Overall, we have performed a total of 85 VATS procedures for mediastinal pathology without mortality and with minimal morbidity.

OTHER PROCEDURES

Pericardial Drainage

A pericardial drainage procedure, so-called pericardial window, may be accomplished through either the right or left chest with a VATS procedure. It is, in fact, often easier to perform this procedure from the right side, where a larger area of pericardium is visible and there is more space in which to work. That being said, a subxiphoid approach to pericardial window usually is simpler, less invasive, and more expeditious, and accomplishes the same goals without the need to insert a double-lumen endobronchial tube and place the patient in the lateral decubitus position. If a large window is believed necessary, there may be an advantage to the VATS approach.

Sympathectomy

The sympathetic chain is easily visualized, as it lies along the vertebral bodies (Fig. 39-11). The magnification provided by VATS facilitates the performance of a sympathectomy. Either dorsal or lumbar sympathectomy may be performed, and bilateral procedures may be accomplished under the same anesthetic, with minimal morbidity. Dorsal sympathectomy may be indicated for palmar hyperhidrosis, reflex sympathetic dystrophy, or other upper-extremity pain syndromes. The superior cervical (stellate) ganglion is readily visualized and preserved, in order to avoid producing a case of Horner's syndrome. Lumbar sympathectomy may be useful for the management of pancreatic pain, particularly when caused by malignant disease. This requires a bilateral procedure to achieve maximal symptom relief.

In the treatment of chylothorax, VATS may be employed to ligate the thoracic duct. The thoracic duct is most readily identified in the right chest just as it courses through the aortic hiatus. In most patients, at this level it is still a single trunk running

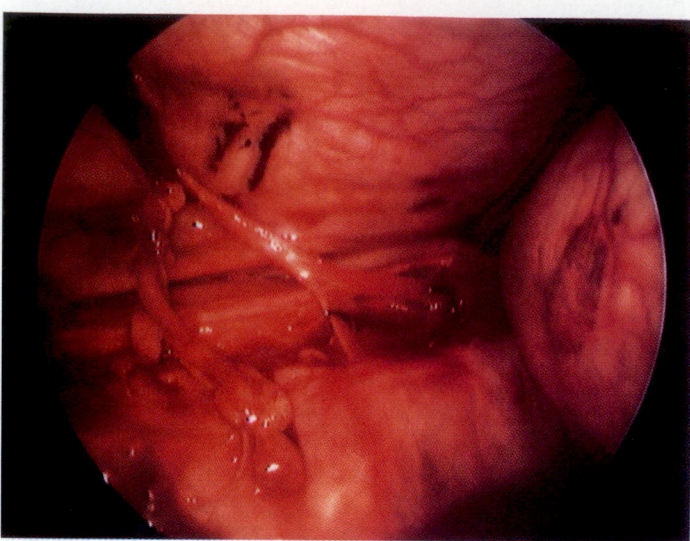

FIGURE 39-11 The sympathetic chain being mobilized off the vertebral bodies. Ganglia are easily seen as are the various branches of the nerve.

along the vertebral bodies between the aorta and the esophagus. We have performed 10 thoracic duct ligations for chyle leaks; in two patients, it was necessary to convert to an open procedure to successfully ligate the duct.

VATS provides excellent exposure to the thoracic spine, and procedures such as drainage of abscesses, biopsy of vertebral bodies, discectomy, and anterior releases for kyphoscoliosis have all been carried out successfully, thereby avoiding thoracotomy.[47] Because of the early success and significantly less morbidity in these patients, this technique is becoming the approach of choice in many centers.

COMPLICATIONS

We reviewed the complications that resulted from our initial 266 VATS procedures.[33] There were no deaths, and complications were not life-threatening. Ten patients had air leaks lasting longer than 7 days. Eleven patients were electively converted to an open procedure when the intended VATS procedure could not be completed successfully. Bleeding requiring blood transfusion occurred in five patients, and five patients developed superficial wound infections. Data collected on 1358 patients from the VATSG Registry show a similar spectrum of complications, along with a 2 percent mortality.[28] As in our series, prolonged air leakage was the most frequent complication; significant bleeding requiring transfusion occurred in only 15 cases (1 percent). To date, no consistent pattern of major complications resulting from VATS has been reported. DeCamp and coauthors list 127 complications occurring in 121 of 595 patients undergoing videothoracoscopy at Brigham and Women's Hospital.[14] Most of the complications were either prolonged air leakage or supraventricular dysrhythmias. We are aware of at least 10 instances of tumor seeding of VATS incisions, and there is at least one report of a death as a result.[21] There appears to be a slightly higher incidence, though still around 3 percent, of recurrent pneumothorax following VATS procedures for spontaneous pneumothorax. Whether this is sim-

ply a function of the "learning curve" remains to be determined. The fact that VATS procedures in general have been performed with minimal major morbidity is commendable, since the technology and skills are relatively new to most surgeons.

CONCLUSIONS

Video-assisted thoracic surgical procedures have proved to be extremely useful in the diagnosis and treatment of various thoracic problems. Improvements in video technology have made it feasible for a surgeon and an assistant to work together, and developments in instrumentation, especially staplers, have made many procedures commonplace that previously seemed impossible. Cost issues still need to be carefully examined. Are the more sophisticated techniques and more expensive equipment saving money or expending more resources? If we are expending greater resources, is there a significant enough benefit to the patient to justify the added expense in this time of cost consciousness? In at least one study, the cost of a thoracoscopic wedge excision (n = 45) was less than that of a wedge excision done via thoracotomy (n = 31), but the difference was not statistically significant.[27] Disposable instrument costs were significantly higher in the thoracoscopy group. There was no significant difference in the length of hospital stay for the two groups, but in the thoracoscopy group the length of stay was longer than expected. Cost savings potentially should come from a shorter length of stay, and, ultimately, if patients return to work sooner, the overall cost to society should be less, though admittedly this is difficult to measure.

With the tremendous strides made in the development of equipment for videothoracoscopy, there was a great rush on the part of thoracic surgeons to perform as many types of procedures as possible with this new technique. Now that the initial rush is over, we are beginning to appreciate just where these techniques have the greatest application. Some procedures for which there was tremendous early enthusiasm are being performed with less frequency; others have withstood the early shakedown period and have proved their worth over the conventional open procedure, resulting in a benefit to patients.

REFERENCES

1. Adler RH: A talc powder aerosol method for the prevention of recurrent spontaneous pneumothorax. *Ann Thorac Surg* 5:474–477, 1968.
2. Allen MS, Deschamps C, Jones DM, et al: Video-assisted thoracic surgical procedures: The Mayo experience. *Mayo Clin Proc* 71:351–359, 1996.
3. Boutin C, Viallat JR, Cargnino P, Rey F: Thoracoscopic lung biopsy: Experimental and clinical preliminary study. *Chest* 82:44–48, 1982.
4. Brooks JW: Open thoracotomy in the management of spontaneous pneumothorax. *Ann Surg* 177:798–805, 1973.
5. Burt ME, Flye MW, Webber BL, et al: Prospective evaluation of aspiration needle, cutting needle, transbronchial, and open lung biopsy in patients with pulmonary infiltrates. *Ann Thorac Surg* 32:146–151, 1981.
6. Cannon WB, Vierra MA, Cannon A: Thoracoscopy for spontaneous pneumothorax. *Ann Thorac Surg* 56:686–687, 1993.
7. Clark TA, Hutchinson DE, Deaner RM, Fitchett VH: Spontaneous

pneumothorax. *Am J Surg* 124:728–731, 1972.

8. Collard J-M, Lengele B, Otte J-B, Kestens P-J: En-bloc and standard esophagectomies by thoracoscopy. *Ann Thorac Surg* 56:675–679, 1993.

9. Cooper JD: Perspectives on thoracoscopy in general thoracic surgery. *Ann Thorac Surg* 56:697–700, 1993.

10. Cooper JD, Trulock EP, Triantafillou AN, et al: Bilateral pneumectomy (volume reduction) for chronic obstructive pulmonary disease. *J Thorac Cardiovasc Surg* 109:106–119, 1995.

11. Cortese DA, McDougall JC: Biopsy and brushing of peripheral lung cancer with fluoroscopic guidance. *Chest* 75:141–145, 1979.

12. Daniel TM, Kern JA, Cargnino P, Rey F: Thoracoscopic surgery for diseases of the lung and pleura. *Ann Surg* 217:566–575, 1993.

13. DeCamp MM, Jaklitsch MT, Harpole DH, et al: An improved video-thoracoscopic technique proves superior to axillary thoracotomy in the surgical management of spontaneous pneumothorax (abstract). *Am J Respir Crit Care Med* 4:A511, 1994.

14. DeCamp MM Jr, Jaklitsch MT, Mentzer SJ, et al: The safety and versatility of video-thoracoscopy: A prospective analysis of 895 consecutive cases. *J Am Coll Surg* 181:113–120, 1995.

15. Deslauriers J, Beaulieu M, Depres JP, et al: Transaxillary pleurectomy for treatment of spontaneous pneumothorax. *Ann Thorac Surg* 30:569–574, 1980.

16. Deslauriers J, LeBlanc P, McClish A: Bullous and bleb diseases of the lung, in Shield TW (ed), *General Thoracic Surgery*. Philadelphia, Lea and Febiger, 1989, pp 744–747.

17. Dijkman JH, van der Meer JWM, Bakker W, et al: Transpleural lung biopsy by the thoracoscopic route in patients with diffuse interstitial pulmonary disease. *Chest* 82:76–83, 1982.

18. Erret LE, Wilson J, Chiu RC, et al: Wedge resection as an alternative procedure for peripheral bronchogenic carcinoma in poor-risk patients. *J Thorac Cardiovasc Surg* 90:656–661, 1985.

19. Ferson PF, Landreneau RJ, Dowling RD, et al: Comparison of open versus thoracoscopic lung biopsy for diffuse infiltrative pulmonary disease. *J Thorac Cardiovasc Surg* 106:194–199, 1993.

20. Fletcher EC, Levin DC: Flexible fiberoptic bronchoscopy and fluoroscopically guided transbronchial biopsy in the management of solitary pulmonary nodules. *West J Med* 136:477–483, 1982.

21. Fry WA, Siddiqui A, Pensler JM, Mostafavi H: Thoracoscopic implantation of cancer with a fatal outcome. *Ann Thorac Surg* 59:42–45, 1995.

22. Gaensler EA, Carrington CB: Open biopsy for chronic diffuse infiltrative lung disease: Clinical, roentgenographic, and physiological correlations in 502 patients. *Ann Thorac Surg* 30:411–426, 1980.

23. Ginsberg RJ, Rubinstein L: A randomized comparative trial of lobectomy vs limited resection for patients with T1 N0 non-small cell lung cancer. *Lung Cancer* 7:304–309, 1991.

24. Ginsberg RJ, Rubinstein LV, and the Lung Cancer Study Group: Randomized trial of lobectomy versus limited resection for T1 N0 non-small cell lung cancer. *Ann Thorac Surg* 60:615–622, 1995.

25. Gossot D, Fourquier P, Celerier M: Thoracoscopic esophagectomy: Technique and initial results. *Ann Thorac Surg* 56:667–670, 1993.

26. Hartman DL, Gaither JM, Kesler KA, et al: Comparison of insufflated talc under thoracoscopic guidance with standard tetracycline and bleomycin pleurodesis for control of malignant pleural effusions. *J Thorac Cardiovasc Surg* 105:743–748, 1993.

27. Hazelrigg SR, Nunchuck SK, Landreneau RJ, et al: Cost analysis for thoracoscopy: Thoracoscopic wedge resection. *Ann Thorac Surg* 56:633–635, 1993.

28. Hazelrigg SR, Nunchuck SK, LoCicero J, and the Video Assisted Thoracic Surgery Study Group: Video-assisted thoracic surgery study group data. *Ann Thorac Surg* 56:1039–1044, 1993.

29. Jacobaeus HC: Possibility of the use of the cystoscope for investigation of serous cavities. *Munch Med Wochenschr* 57:2090–2092, 1910.

30. Jacobaeus HC: The cauterization of adhesions in pneumothorax treatment of tuberculosis. *Surg Gynecol Obstet* 32:493–500, 1921.

31. Jacobaeus HC: The practical importance of thoracoscopy in surgery of the chest. *Surg Gynecol Obstet* 34:289–296, 1922.

32. Kaiser LR: Diagnostic and therapeutic uses of pleuroscopy (thoracoscopy) in lung cancer. *Surg Clin North Am* 67:1081–1086, 1987.

33. Kaiser LR, Bavaria JE: Complications of thoracoscopy. *Ann Thorac Surg* 56:796–798, 1993.

34. Kaiser LR: Thoracoscopic resection of mediastinal tumors and the thymus. *Chest Surg Clin North Am* 6:41–52, 1996.

35. Keenan RJ, Landreneau RJ, Sciurba F, et al: Unilateral thoracoscopic surgical approach for diffuse emphysema. *J Thorac Cardiovasc Surg* 111:308–316, 1996.

36. Kirby TJ, Mack MJ, Landreneau RJ, Rice TW: Initial experience with video-assisted thoracoscopic lobectomy. *Ann Thorac Surg* 56:1248–1253, 1993.

37. Kirby TJ, Mack MJ, Landreneau RJ, Rice TW: Lobectomy: Video-assisted thoracic surgery versus muscle-sparing thoracotomy: A randomized trial. *J Thorac Cardiovasc Surg* 109:997–1001, 1995.

38. Khouri NF, Mezisne MA, Zerhouni EA, Siegelman SS: The solitary pulmonary nodule: Assessment, diagnosis and management. *Chest* 91:128–133, 1987.

39. Kotloff RM, Tino G, Bavaria JE, et al: Bilateral lung volume reduction surgery for advanced emphysema: A comparison of median sternotomy and thoracoscopic approaches. *Chest* 110:1399–1406, 1996.

40. Krasna MJ, McLaughlin JS: Thoracoscopic lymph node staging for esophageal cancer. *Ann Thorac Surg* 56:671–674, 1993.

41. Larrieu AJ, Tyers GFO, Williams EH, et al: Intrapleural instillation of quinacrine for treatment of recurrent spontaneous pneumothorax. *Ann Thorac Surg* 28:146–150, 1979.

42. Lewis RJ, Kunderman PJ, Sisler GE, Mackenzie JW: Direct diagnostic thoracoscopy. *Ann Thorac Surg* 21:536–539, 1975.

43. Lilienthal H: *Thoracic Surgery*. Philadelphia, WB Saunders, 1925.

44. Lillington GA: Management of solitary pulmonary nodules. *Dis Mon* 37:271–318, 1991.

45. Lillington GA, Mitchell SP, Wood GA. Catamenial pneumothorax. *JAMA* 219:1328–1331, 1972.

46. Mack MJ, Hazelrigg SR, Landreneau RJ, Acuff TE: Thoracoscopy for the diagnosis of the indeterminate solitary pulmonary nodule. *Ann Thorac Surg* 56:825–832, 1993.

47. Mack MJ, Regan JJ, Bobechko WP, Acuff TE: Application for thoracoscopy for diseases of the spine. *Ann Thorac Surg* 56:736–738, 1993.

48. Miller JI, Hatcher CR: Limited resection of bronchogenic carcinoma in the patient with marked impairment of pulmonary function. *Ann Thorac Surg* 44:340–343, 1987.

49. Naumheim KS, Keller CA, Krucylak PE, et al: Unilateral video-assisted thoracic surgical lung reduction. *Ann Thorac Surg* 61:1092–1098, 1996.

50. Oakes DD, Sherck JP, Brodsky JB, Mark JBD: Therapeutic thoracoscopy. *J Thorac Cardiovasc Surg* 87:269–273, 1984.

51. Pellegrini CA, Leichter R, Patti M, et al: Thoracoscopic esophageal myotomy in the treatment of achalasia. *Ann Thorac Surg* 56:680–682, 1993.

52. Potter D, Pass HI, Brower S, et al: Prospective randomized study of open lung biopsy versus empirical antibiotic therapy for acute pneumonitis in nonneutropenic cancer patients. *Ann Thorac Surg* 40:422–428, 1985.

53. Read RC, Yoder G, Schaeffer RC: Survival after conservative re-

section for T1 N0 M0 non-small cell lung cancer. *Ann Thorac Surg* 49:391–400, 1990.

54. Rice TW, Boyce GA, Siall MV: Esophageal ultrasound and the preoperative staging of carcinoma of the esophagus. *J Thorac Cardiovasc Surg* 101:536–543, 1991.

55. Roviaro G, Varoli F, Rebuffat C, et al: Videothoracoscopic staging and treatment of lung cancer. *Ann Thorac Surg* 59:971–974, 1995.

56. Rusch VW, Mountain C: Thoracoscopy under regional anesthesia for the diagnosis and management of pleural disease. *Am J Surg* 154:274–278, 1987.

57. Shulkin AN: Management of the indeterminate solitary pulmonary nodule: A pulmonologist's view. *Ann Thorac Surg* 56:743–744, 1993.

58. Wakabayashi A: Thoracoscopic technique for management of giant bullous lung disease. *Ann Thorac Surg* 56:708–712, 1993.

59. Wakabayashi A, Brenner M, Kayalek RA, et al: Thoracoscopic carbon dioxide laser treatment of bullous emphysema. *Lancet* 337:881–883, 1991.

60. Wall CP, Gaensler EA, Carrington CB, Hayes JA: Comparison of transbronchial and open biopsies in chronic infiltrative lung diseases. *Am Rev Respir Dis* 123:280–285, 1981.

61. Wallace JM, Deutsch AI: Flexible fiberoptic bronchoscopy and percutaneous needle lung aspiration for evaluating the solitary pulmonary nodule. *Chest* 81:665–671, 1982.

62. Westcott JL: Percutaneous transthoracic needle biopsy. *Radiology* 169:593–601, 1988.

63. Zerhouni EA, Stitik FP, Siegelman SS, et al: CT of the pulmonary nodule: A cooperative study. *Radiology* 160:319–327, 1986.

CHAPTER 40

PERIOPERATIVE RESPIRATORY CONSIDERATIONS IN THE SURGICAL PATIENT

Horace M. DeLisser / Michael A. Grippi

Postoperative pulmonary complications constitute a significant cause of morbidity and mortality following surgery. Managing patients at risk for postoperative pulmonary problems requires an understanding of the predictable changes in pulmonary physiology that occur with surgery and anesthesia, as well as knowledge of factors associated with development of postsurgical respiratory compromise. Despite the availability of several screening tests, a careful history and physical examination continue to be the cornerstone of preoperative pulmonary evaluation. Although a number of measures can be employed before and after surgery to minimize the risk of respiratory complications, close patient monitoring and early detection are essential.

This chapter focuses initially on changes in pulmonary function with surgery. Pulmonary risk factors before, during, and after surgery are reviewed prior to discussion of preoperative evaluation of the patient for surgery, including lung resectional surgery. Finally, recommendations are made regarding preoperative preparation and postoperative prophylactic measures.

CHANGES IN PULMONARY FUNCTION WITH SURGERY

Many postoperative respiratory complications relate to exaggerations of the expected postoperative changes in pulmonary function that occur as a result of the surgery itself, anesthesia, or various pharmacologic interventions. Hence, an appreciation of normal postoperative pulmonary physiology is useful in understanding a number of pulmonary problems seen following surgery. Five principal categories of change in pulmonary function with surgery may be considered: (1) lung volumes, (2) diaphragm function, (3) gas exchange, (4) control of breathing, and (5) lung defense mechanisms (Table 40-1).

Lung Volumes

The pattern of pulmonary function abnormalities following thoracic and abdominal surgery is restrictive, characterized by moderate to severe reductions in vital capacity (VC) and smaller, but more important, reductions in functional residual capacity (FRC).[8,10,12] The degree of impairment is similar after upper

---

TABLE 40-1

Changes in Pulmonary Function with Surgery

Reduction in lung volumes

Diaphragm dysfunction

Impaired gas exchange

Respiratory depression due to residual effects of anesthesia or postoperative narcotics

Impaired cough and mucociliary clearance

SOURCE: From Goldmann DR, Brown FH, Guarnieri DM (eds): *Perioperative Medicine.* New York, McGraw-Hill, 1994, with permission.

---

abdominal and thoracic surgery. Smaller changes in VC and FRC are noted with lower abdominal surgery; superficial or extremity surgery is usually unassociated with any significant or persistent changes in lung volumes.[1,2] During the first 24 h following upper abdominal surgery, VC and FRC may be reduced by more than 70 percent and 50 percent, respectively, and they may remain depressed for more than a week.[1,2,29] Consequently, it is not surprising that pulmonary complications are seen more often with thoracic and upper abdominal procedures than with surgery involving the lower abdomen or extremities (see discussion of intraoperative risk factors, below).

Reductions in other lung volumes, including total lung capacity (TLC), inspiratory capacity (IC), expiratory reserve volume (ERV), and residual volume (RV) have been noted. While the forced expiratory volume in 1 s (FEV_1) is decreased, the ratio of FEV_1 to the forced vital capacity (FEV_1/FVC%) remains unchanged, indicating that major airway obstruction does not occur.[10]

Since patients undergoing superficial or extremity surgery do not experience major changes in lung volumes, residual or carryover effects from general anesthesia do not appear to play a primary role in this regard. In fact, studies show that in many patients, FRC in the early postoperative period is unchanged from baseline. An alternative proposal for the reduction is that postsurgical pain and associated muscle splinting may impair lung mechanics. However, since effective pain control using epidural anesthesia or intercostal nerve block fails to fully restore VC or FRC to preoperative levels, other causes must be operative.[37,49] A growing consensus is that diaphragm dysfunction is an important contributing factor (see below).

The reduced FRC is of major physiologic significance postoperatively. Its importance can be understood when the phenomenon of airway closure and the concept of closing capacity (CC) are considered.[10] FRC is the lung volume at the end of a normal tidal expiration. CC is the lung volume at which small airways in the lung bases begin to close during expiration because of a reduction in airway radial traction. The rela-

tionship between the two is a key factor in the development of postoperative changes in lung function (Fig. 40-1).

In a normal lung, FRC is always greater than CC, and the airways remain open throughout a tidal breath. However, when CC is greater than FRC, lung volume fails to increase sufficiently during tidal breathing to open all the airways and, consequently, some alveolar units remain closed during a breath. Such regions constitute areas of atelectasis. An intermediate state exists when CC exceeds lung volume for part of the time during each tidal breath. Under these circumstances, the airways open for only a portion of the respiratory cycle, creating areas of low ventilation relative to perfusion. In summary, any circumstance that reduces FRC below CC or which increases CC above FRC produces regions of reduced ventilation and atelectasis (Table 40-2).

Diaphragm Function

Diaphragm dysfunction has been recognized as an important factor contributing to the postoperative reduction in lung volumes.[13]

TABLE 40-2

Conditions That Alter the Relationship between Functional Residual Capacity (FRC) and Closing Capacity (CC)

Decrease FRC	*Increase CC*
Supine position	Advanced age
Obesity	Smoking
Pregnancy	COPD
General anesthesia	Pulmonary edema
Abdominal pain	

SOURCE: From Goldmann DR, Brown FH, Guarnieri DM (eds): *Perioperative Medicine.* New York, McGraw-Hill, 1994, with permission.

FRC > CC   CC > FRC+V_T FRC < CC < FRC+V_T

NORMAL LUNG   ATELECTATIC LUNG   REGION OF LOW $\dot{V}/\dot{Q}$

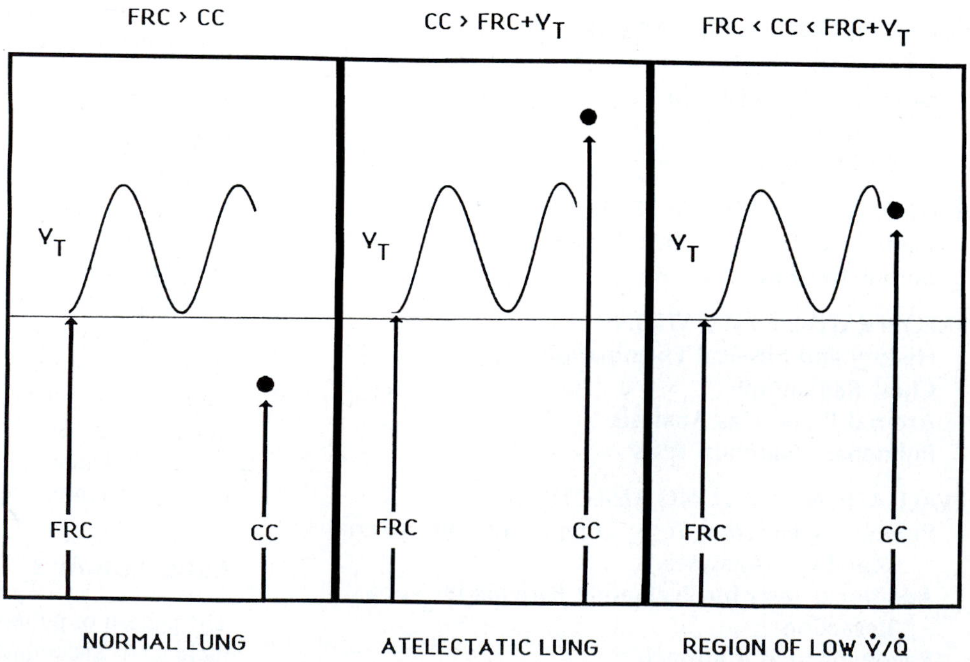

FIGURE 40-1 The relationship between functional residual capacity (FRC) and closing capacity (CC). See text. (*From Goldmann DR, Brown FH, Guarnieri DM (eds): Perioperative Medicine. New York, McGraw-Hill, 1994, with permission.*)

In patients undergoing cholecystectomy, the diaphragm's contribution to quiet tidal breathing after surgery is reduced.[12] This impairment is not due to postoperative pain.[37] Measurements of transdiaphragmatic pressure during maximal phrenic nerve stimulation following upper abdominal surgery indicate that decreased central nervous system output to the phrenic nerves, possibly as a result of inhibitory reflexes arising from sympathetic, vagal, or splanchnic receptors, may be the important etiologic factor.[9]

Gas Exchange

Postoperative arterial hypoxemia occurs commonly. There are two phases in its development.[11,28] The initial phase occurs in the first several hours following anesthesia and surgery. The underlying mechanisms are related largely to the residual effects of the anesthesia and include ventilation-perfusion mismatch, anesthetic-induced inhibition of hypoxic pulmonary vasoconstriction, right-to-left shunting, alveolar hypoventilation, depressed cardiac output, and increased oxygen consumption by peripheral muscle. This phase resolves within 24 h following superficial surgery.

A second phase of hypoxemia that may persist for several days or weeks is seen after thoracic and upper abdominal surgery. This phase correlates with reductions in FRC and changes in the FRC-CC relationship. Although alterations in the FRC-CC relationship predominate, other processes may contribute to late postoperative hypoxemia: (1) alveolar hypoventilation (see discussion of control of breathing below); (2) increased dead space ventilation due to rapid, shallow breathing; and (3) decreased mixed venous oxygen tension due to increased oxygen consumption, impaired cardiac output, and reduced oxygen carrying capacity.

Control of Breathing

Respiratory depression is a common feature of the postoperative period. Two factors are responsible. First, residual effects of preanesthetic or anesthetic agents inhibit respiratory drive and reduce the ventilatory response to hypercapnia, hypoxia, and acidemia.[23] Second, narcotics given for postoperative analgesia depress both hypercapnic and hypoxic ventilatory drives, resulting in decreased tidal volume, reduced minute ventilation, and increased $PaCO_2$.[46] Narcotics also alter the pattern of breathing, reducing the frequency of sighs or eliminating them entirely; in susceptible patients, narcotics may precipitate sleep apnea.

Lung Defense Mechanisms

Several mechanisms protect the lung from environmental and infectious insults. Two of the most important—cough and mucociliary transport—are compromised after surgery, contributing to an increased risk of pulmonary infection.[5,10] Postoperative pain or the excessive use of narcotics may inhibit coughing; in addition, altered lung mechanics decrease the expulsive force generated with each cough. Mucociliary clearance is impaired for up to a week following upper abdominal surgery. Although an ineffective cough reflex contributes significantly to reduced mucociliary clearance, several additional mechanisms are involved. These include: (1) cilia damage from endotracheal intubation and inhalation of dry, hyperoxic gas mixtures; (2) reduced tracheal mucus velocity due to the presence of an endotracheal tube; (3) anesthetic-induced inhibition of mucociliary transport; and (4) atelectasis.

PULMONARY COMPLICATIONS

The criteria used for defining postoperative pulmonary morbidity have varied considerably in published reports, although it is clear that, from a broad perspective, five major categories of complications may be considered: (1) atelectasis; (2) infection, including acute tracheobronchitis and pneumonia; (3) exacerbation of underlying chronic lung disease; (4) prolonged mechanical ventilation and respiratory failure; and (5) thromboembolic disease. With thoracic surgery, several additional unique problems have been noted (Table 40-3).

The variability in defining postoperative pulmonary complications has resulted in reported incidences in the literature ranging from 5 to 90 percent. In general, a healthy, young nonsmoker of normal weight has a very low risk of postoperative pulmonary complications (1 percent or less). However, a number of factors have been identified which are associated with the development of postoperative pulmonary complications (Table 40-4). They include preoperative factors (chronic lung disease, smoking, general state of health, age, obesity, nutritional status, and antecedent respiratory tract infection), intraoperative factors (type and duration of anesthesia, surgical site of operation, and type of surgical incision), and postoperative factors (immobilization and inadequate pain control).

TABLE 40-3

Pulmonary Complications Associated with Thoracic Surgery

Procedure	Complication	Incidence
Coronary artery bypass grafting	Phrenic nerve damage	10%
	Late pleural effusions (arising after discharge)	Not reported in literature
Thoracotomy with lung resection	Bronchopleural fistula or empyema*	5–20%
Median sternotomy	Sternal wound infection (mediastinitis or osteomyelitis)	1–2%
Esophagectomy, gastrectomy	Anastamotic leak	3–6%

*Higher for patients with sarcoidosis and aspergilloma
SOURCE: From Goldmann DR, Brown FH, Guarnieri DM (eds): *Perioperative Medicine*. New York, McGraw-Hill, 1994, with permission.

TABLE 40-4

Factors Associated with Development of Postoperative Pulmonary Complications

Preoperative	Intraoperative	Postoperative
Chronic lung disease	Type of anesthesia	Immobilization
Smoking	Duration of anesthesia	Inadequate pain control
General state of health	Surgical site	
Age	Type of surgical incision	
Obesity		
Nutritional status		
Antecedent respiratory tract infection		

PREOPERATIVE RISK FACTORS

A number of patient-related factors have been implicated in the development of postoperative respiratory complications. Chronic lung disease (particularly obstructive airway disease), cigarette smoking, and the patient's overall state of health are the most important preoperative risk factors. In addition, age and obesity are relatively minor factors. The precise risks associated with malnutrition and recent viral infections are unknown.

Chronic Lung Disease

The following discussion focuses on the operative risks in patients with three common categories of chronic lung disease: (1) chronic obstructive pulmonary disease, (2) restrictive lung diseases, and (3) pulmonary vascular diseases.

CHRONIC OBSTRUCTIVE PULMONARY DISEASE

Since chronic obstructive pulmonary disease (COPD) is the most common chronic pulmonary disorder, most studies addressing the impact of preexisting lung disease on surgical risk have focused on this entity. The reported incidence of postoperative pulmonary complications in patients with COPD varies from 25 to 100 percent and is influenced by type of surgery, magnitude of preexisting respiratory impairment, and criteria used to define complications.[25,47] Although not precisely quantified in the literature, the risk for postoperative respiratory complications appears to increase significantly (>50 percent) when the FEV_1 is below 65 percent of predicted.[25] The risk is also increased in patients who are hypercapnic.[31,38]

In patients with severe disease, an important issue is whether a critical level of lung function exists below which the risk of developing a major, potentially life-threatening pulmonary complication is so high as to make anesthesia and surgery too dangerous. In the 1950s, such a prohibitive threshold or level was proposed. More recent studies, however, have failed to support this hypothesis.[48] Patients with an FEV_1 as low as 450 ml have been found to tolerate surgery safely.[31] Hence, patients should not be denied necessary operative procedures solely on the basis of marginal lung function. As with all medical interventions, the potential benefits of the operative procedure must be weighed against the operative risk.

The increased incidence of postoperative pulmonary complications in patients with COPD is due, in part, to an increase in the closing capacity, favoring the development of areas of low ventilation-to-perfusion ratios and atelectasis. In addition, in patients who continue to smoke, impaired ciliary function and chronic tracheobronchitis may be contributing factors.

RESTRICTIVE LUNG DISEASES

The risk of pulmonary complications in patients with restrictive lung diseases who undergo surgery is unknown. Although some experience has been reported with patients undergoing thoracic and corrective orthopedic surgery (see below), very little data exist with regard to abdominal and extremity surgery. One might expect a higher incidence of postoperative respiratory complications in these patients for two reasons: (1) FRC is reduced, favoring the formation of areas of poor ventilation and atelectasis. (2) Coughing, and thus the ability to clear respiratory secretions, is impaired.

Experience with postoperative pulmonary complications has been reported in three relatively common situations for patients with restrictive disorders: (1) sarcoidosis complicated by aspergilloma and hemoptysis; (2) corrective surgery for kyphoscoliosis; and (3) myasthenia gravis with associated thymoma.

Sarcoidosis may progress to diffuse interstitial fibrosis and cavitary changes, primarily involving the upper lobes (see Chapter 69). These cavities are prone to infection with aspergillus species and aspergilloma formation, with subsequent development of recurrent and, at times, life-threatening hemoptysis. These patients generally have very poor lung function and, hence, are managed conservatively. However, if supportive medical therapy fails, patients may require thoracotomy and lung resection. Unfortunately, the postoperative course is rarely problem-free and is often complicated by the development of a bronchopleural fistula or empyema.

There are several indications for corrective surgery in patients with kyphoscoliosis, including deterioration of pulmonary function. Postoperative pulmonary complications have been reported to occur in approximately 20 percent of these patients.[3] Complications involving the pleural space (e.g., pneumothorax, pleural effusion, bronchopleural fistula, empyema) are particularly common. Important risk factors include: (1) nonidiopathic scoliosis, (2) anterior spinal fusion procedures, (3) age greater than 20 years, (4) mental retardation, (5) preoperative hypoxemia, and (6) obstructive pulmonary function tests.[3]

Most patients with myasthenia gravis will, during the course of their disease, undergo thymectomy. Up to 30 percent of patients will require mechanical ventilation for more than 3 days following the surgery.[18,50] A reduced preoperative maximal static expiratory pressure (<66 percent of predicted) appears to be the best predictor of the need for prolonged postoperative ventilatory support, and clinical severity of disease is only marginally predictive; the preoperative vital capacity is not helpful.[50] Virtually all patients with myasthenia are treated with anticholinesterases, which are usually discontinued prior to surgery to minimize tracheobronchial secretions. However, controversy exists regarding whether these agents should be restarted immediately after surgery or withheld for 24 to 48 h following thymectomy.

PULMONARY VASCULAR DISEASES

The risk of postoperative pulmonary complications in patients with underlying pulmonary vascular disease and intact respiratory mechanics is not known. However, one might anticipate an exaggeration of, or prolongation in, the hypoxemia seen postoperatively (see discussion of gas exchange above). In addition, pulmonary reserve in these patients is usually reduced; hence, additional pulmonary insults are less likely to be tolerated.

Smoking History

Smoking increases the risk of postoperative respiratory complications, independent of the association of smoking with chronic obstructive pulmonary disease.[14,17] Given the well-documented adverse changes in respiratory epithelium and pulmonary function which correlate with the degree of tobacco consumption, such an association is not surprising. In individuals undergoing coronary artery bypass graft surgery, the risk of smoking becomes significant when tobacco use exceeds 20 pack-years.[45] A statistically significant reduction in complications occurs only when patients discontinue smoking for at least 8 weeks prior to surgery. This finding is consistent with studies showing that abnormalities in pulmonary function may persist for up to several months after smoking cessation.

General State of Health

Overall clinical status, as categorized by the American Society of Anesthesiologists' (ASA) classification (Table 40-5), has correlated with the development of postoperative pulmonary complications.[21] For patients undergoing abdominal surgery, an ASA classification of II or higher is a powerful predictor of increased risk of respiratory problems after surgery.

Age

Based primarily on retrospective data from the 1950s and 1960s, advanced age has long been considered a major risk factor for postoperative pulmonary complications. However, recent work suggests that age may not be as significant as originally believed, once other confounding variables are controlled. For example, in a study of 520 patients undergoing elective thoracic or abdominal surgery, no association between age and postoperative pneumonia was found.[14] These findings appear to hold true even when lung tissue is resected. In addition, in a study of patients undergoing thoracotomy for lung cancer, despite a somewhat higher 30-day postoperative mortality in patients over age 70 years, the incidences of postoperative pulmonary complications and hospital stay were not increased and actual survival was not decreased in the older group.[36]

Obesity

A number of changes in respiratory mechanics and pulmonary function occur with obesity.[32] The accumulation of fat in the chest wall, diaphragm, and abdomen may reduce total respiratory compliance by more than 60 percent—a change which is amplified when the patient assumes the supine position. The reduced compliance, in turn, increases the work of breathing. Consequently, minute ventilation, oxygen consumption, and carbon dioxide production are further increased beyond baseline values, which are already elevated as a result of increased metabolic demands imposed by the obese state.

Normally, spirometry in obese patients does not indicate airway obstruction. However, a reduction in ERV is found consistently. The magnitude of the reduction correlates with the degree of obesity. Areas of low ventilation relative to perfusion and atelectasis are seen (see discussion of lung volumes above). In addition to these mechanical changes, obese patients appear to have a larger gastric volume and lower pH than do nonobese patients and may be predisposed to aspiration.

Despite what might be predicted based on the changes in lung function described above, retrospective reviews of obese patients undergoing abdominal surgery do not show an increased incidence of pneumonia or atelectasis compared to nonobese patients undergoing similar procedures. The few prospective studies on the risk in obesity of postoperative pulmonary complications have yielded conflicting results. However, in these studies, small numbers of patients have been studied, liberal definitions of obesity have been employed, patient height has not been routinely considered, and the degree of obesity has not been noted precisely. In studies that have shown a correlation between obe-

TABLE 40-5

American Society of Anesthesiologists' (ASA) Clinical Classification

ASA I:	Otherwise healthy patient undergoing elective surgery
ASA II:	Patient with single system or well-controlled disease which does not affect daily life
ASA III:	Patient with multisystem or well-controlled major system disease which limits daily activity
ASA IV:	Patient with severe, incapacitating disease which is poorly controlled or end-stage
ASA V:	Patient who is in imminent danger of death and is not expected to survive 24 hours

sity and postoperative respiratory morbidity, the principal complication has been atelectasis. Thus, although obesity may increase the risk of some postoperative pulmonary complications, the precise magnitude and significance of the risk are unknown.

Obesity is, however, clearly a risk factor for obstructive sleep apnea syndrome, which may be unmasked or exacerbated because of use of postoperative analgesics or narcotics. Since sleep apnea occurs in individuals of normal weight, all patients should be questioned about symptoms of the disorder (see Chapter 102).

Nutritional Status

The effects of malnutrition and severe starvation on the respiratory system include a reduced ventilatory response to hypoxia, decreased diaphragmatic muscle function, impaired cell-mediated and humoral immunity, and alterations in the elastic properties of the lung (see Chapter 178). Some evidence of malnutrition can be found in many hospitalized patients, but it is unclear whether the degree of malnutrition usually noted produces clinically significant changes in pulmonary function. In addition, although patients whose nutritional status is compromised may be at higher risk for developing postoperative pulmonary complications, aggressive preoperative nutritional support has not been shown to decrease postsurgical pulmonary morbidity.[44]

Antecedent Respiratory Tract Infection

Enhanced airway reactivity and increased airway resistance may persist for several weeks beyond resolution of the acute symptoms of a viral respiratory tract infection.[20] In addition, diaphragmatic dysfunction has been shown to be impaired during viral infections.[30] Although no published studies have addressed the effect of concurrent viral infections on postoperative pulmonary morbidity, a delay in elective surgery is generally advised, given the changes in airway reactivity and diaphragm function in this setting.

INTRAOPERATIVE RISK FACTORS

Several operative factors have have been associated with the development of pulmonary complications after surgery. These include the type of anesthesia, the length of the procedure (as determined by the duration of anesthesia), the surgical site, and the type of surgical incision.

Type of Anesthesia

The pulmonary effects of general anesthesia are addressed in detail elsewhere (see Chapters 170 and 179). They include impairment of oxygenation and carbon dioxide elimination. These effects result from anesthetic-induced changes in the shape and motion of the chest wall and diaphragm, which, in turn, lead to increases in alveolar dead space, shunt fraction, and ventilation-perfusion mismatching.[11,41] The alterations in lung function may contribute to pulmonary morbidity.

Because of the effects of general anesthesia on gas exchange, regional anesthesia has been used as an alternative in patients with underlying pulmonary disease.[35] Indeed, epidural anesthe-

sia to a T4 sensory level does not appear to alter FRC, VC, FEV_1, the alveolar-arterial oxygen gradient, shunt fraction, or cardiac output. Many clinicians have the impression that these strategies lower the incidence of postoperative respiratory complications. However, with the exception of several reports showing a reduced risk of postoperative thromboembolism, studies to date have not been well designed and have not consistently demonstrated that regional anesthesia results in a lower incidence of other postoperative pulmonary complications.

Duration of Anesthesia

The incidence of pulmonary complications increases significantly for procedures lasting longer than 3 to 4 h.[7,14,22,25,33] Patients whose procedure lasts 4 h or more are five times more likely to suffer postoperative pneumonia than those whose procedures last less than 2 h.[14]

Surgical Site

The development of postoperative pulmonary complications correlates strongly with the anatomic site of operation. The complication rate (excluding thromboembolic disease) is less than 1 percent for nonthoracoabdominal procedures, less than 5 percent for lower abdominal surgery, and greater than 5 percent for upper abdominal surgery (with reported complication rates ranging from 7 to 76 percent).[17,21,25,47] For thoracotomy with lung resection, the complication rate also depends on a number of other factors, including: (1) the presence of underlying lung disease, (2) the amount of functional lung removed, and (3) the extent to which the "bellows" function of the lung is impaired (see discussion of evaluation for lung resection below).

Type of Surgical Incision

For abdominal procedures, vertical laparotomy incisions carry a higher incidence of postoperative complications than do horizontal incisions.[19] Recently, the techniques of laparoscopic cholecystectomy and thoracoscopic lung resection have gained widespread acceptance because of reduced patient discomfort, shortened length of hospitalization, and faster patient return to full activity. Since the magnitude of incisional pain is usually less, and since patients typically ambulate sooner, the incidence of postoperative respiratory problems is expected to be much lower than that associated with conventional surgical approaches. However, studies confirming this expectation are lacking.[13]

POSTOPERATIVE RISK FACTORS

Inadequate pain control, prolonged bedrest, and inactivity contribute to the development of respiratory complications following surgery.

Inadequate Postoperative Analgesia

Effective pain control is vital in the early postoperative period, since pain inhibits coughing and deep breathing and discourages early mobilization—factors which contribute to an increased risk of pulmonary complications. Obstacles to good postoperative analgesia include hesitancy of the patient to report pain for fear of being labeled a "bad" patient and anxiety of caregivers in administering narcotics because of side effects.

Immobilization

Prolonged bed rest and inactivity following surgery impact the risk of postoperative respiratory complications in several ways. FRC decreases by 500 to 1000 ml in moving from the upright to the supine position, favoring the development of atelectasis.[11] Increased ambulation is associated with better patient mobilization and clearance of secretions. As discussed elsewhere (see Chapter 84), the lack of patient movement in the postsurgical period is a major risk factor for deep venous thrombosis and pulmonary embolism.

PREOPERATIVE EVALUATION

The principal elements in preoperative evaluation of the surgical patient are: (1) the history and physical examination, (2) the chest radiograph, (3) arterial blood-gas analysis, and (4) pulmonary function tests (Fig. 40-2).

History and Physical Examination

A careful history is an essential component of the preoperative evaluation. The following issues should be reviewed: (1) smoking history; (2) history of respiratory symptoms (e.g., cough, chest pain, dyspnea), including symptoms of sleep apnea; (3) extent of preexisting lung disease; and (4) history of recent respiratory tract infection. The physical examination is rarely helpful in identifying pulmonary risk factors. When the history is negative, the physical examination is typically unremarkable. However, the initial physical examination supplements the history and provides a baseline for future comparisons.

Chest Radiograph

The preoperative chest radiograph is usually unrevealing if risk factors and abnormal physical findings are absent.[42] Although the admission or screening chest radiograph is more likely to show an abnormality in individuals with known cardiopulmonary disease, the study usually simply confirms the presence of previously known abnormalities; only occasionally does it result in an alteration in management. Thus, a preoperative chest radiograph is indicated when there are new or unexplained symptoms or signs, when there is a history of underlying lung disease and no recent chest radiograph, or when thoracic surgery is planned.[42]

Arterial Blood-Gas Analysis

Since an elevated $PaCO_2$ is associated with an increased incidence of postoperative respiratory morbidity in patients with significant chronic lung disease, an arterial blood-gas analysis should be done preoperatively in these patients. It is also recommended that an arterial blood-gas specimen be obtained in patients who, by either history or physical examination, have a new significant pulmonary process or who are undergoing lung resection. Data do not support use of arterial blood-gas analysis as a routine preoperative screening test.[34]

Pulmonary Function Tests

An increased risk of respiratory complications has been demonstrated only in the obstructive category of pulmonary disorders. Although there are theoretical reasons to expect a higher incidence of postoperative respiratory problems in patients with restrictive lung diseases (see discussion of preoperative risk factors above), currently, no data correlate the degree of restriction (as assessed by lung volumes) with subsequent pulmonary morbidity. Hence, although a complete battery of pulmonary function tests is useful in evaluating suspected restrictive lung disease, spirometry to evaluate for airway obstruction is all that is required to screen patients at risk.

Indications for preoperative pulmonary function testing include the presence of cough or unexplained dyspnea, a history of chronic lung disease, a history of cigarette smoking (greater than 20 pack-years), and planned lung resection (discussed below).[15,51] Current data do not support the routine use of these studies to evaluate the pulmonary risks of advanced age, obesity, malnutrition, or abdominal surgery.[24] Finally, normal pulmonary function tests do not guarantee a complication-free postoperative course and do not lessen the need for diligent and attentive respiratory care following surgery.

EVALUATION FOR LUNG RESECTION

In evaluating patients for lung resection, the clinician must consider two issues: (1) What are the surgical morbidity and mortality for the patient with significant underlying chronic lung disease? (2) Will postoperative lung function be adequate? A number of approaches have been used over the years to address these questions. Sev-

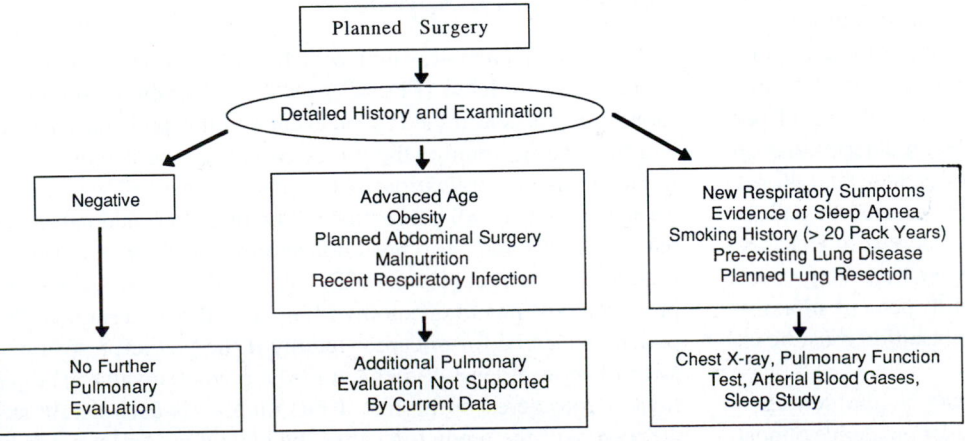

FIGURE 40-2 Algorithm for preoperative pulmonary evaluation. See text for discussion.

eral, including pulmonary function tests, lung scans, and arterial blood-gas analyses are used routinely; others are used less commonly.

Pulmonary Function Tests, Lung Scans, and Arterial Blood-Gas Analyses

Studies have shown that the risk of postoperative respiratory complications following lung resection (especially pneumonectomy) increases significantly when the FEV_1 is less than 2 L or when the FVC or maximal voluntary ventilation (MVV) is less than 50 percent predicted.[15] For these "high risk" patients, a number of additional tests have been used to estimate postoperative pulmonary function. The most helpful have been quantitative perfusion and ventilation scintigraphy.[27]

Ventilation and perfusion lung scans are equally accurate in calculating the postoperative FEV_1 although perfusion scanning is more commonly used because it is technically easier to perform.[26] These scans measure the relative blood flow or ventilation to one lung or lung region and can be used to predict postoperative FEV_1.

For pneumonectomy, the predicted postoperative FEV_1 is calculated as

$$\text{Predicted postoperative } FEV_1 = \text{preoperative } FEV_1 \times \text{percent perfusion to remaining lung} \quad (1)$$

For lobectomy, regional quantitative perfusion scans may be used. Alternatively, the postoperative FEV_1 may be predicted using the following equation:

$$\text{Predicted postoperative } FEV_1 = \text{preoperative } FEV_1 \times \text{(number of lung segments remaining after resection divided by total number of segments in both lungs)} \quad (2)$$

Equation (2) appears to provide information as accurate as that obtained from perfusion studies. When these calculations are inaccurate, they tend to *underestimate* the predicted postoperative FEV_1.

A predicted postoperative FEV_1 of 800 ml has been used as a cutoff for withholding resectional lung surgery, based on the clinical impression that below 800 ml many patients are disabled and develop CO_2 retention. Indeed, studies employing this threshold report "acceptable" surgical and postoperative morbidity and mortality.[27] However, no prospective studies have confirmed the significance of this value. Furthermore, the physiologic implications of an FEV_1 of 800 ml depend upon a number of factors, including the patient's body size. Therefore, calculation of percent predicted FEV_1 may be of greater value in determining operability. A predicted postoperative FEV_1 of greater than 40 percent predicted has been proposed as a safe criterion in patients undergoing pulmonary resection.[26] Finally, recognizing that most patients who undergo resectional lung surgery have lung cancer and that this malignancy has virtually a 100 percent mortality without surgery (for non-small cell tumors), caution must be exercised in applying exclusionary criteria.

Finally, as noted previously, hypercapnia in the setting of chronic lung disease is associated with a higher incidence of postoperative respiratory morbidity.[31,38] Hypoxemia is, however, not as good a predictor of subsequent pulmonary morbidity. In fact, resection of areas of the lung having significant ventilation-perfusion mismatch may *improve* the level of oxygenation postoperatively. A preoperative arterial blood-gas analysis should be obtained in all patients with preexisting lung disease undergoing pulmonary resection. Although supportive data are lacking, it is common practice to obtain an arterial blood-gas sample in all patients undergoing resectional surgery, even those without significant underlying lung disease. This determination serves as a basis for comparison with subsequent intra- and postoperative measurements.

Additional Tests for Evaluating Patients for Lung Resection

Several additional tests, including exercise testing, measurement of diffusing capacity, bronchospirometry, the lateral position test, and unilateral pulmonary artery occlusion have been advocated in the preoperative evaluation of the candidate for lung resection.[27]

A number of investigators have found measurement of maximal oxygen consumption ($\dot{V}O_{2max}$) to be useful in predicting postoperative morbidity and mortality. A $\dot{V}O_{2max}$ of less than 1 L/min (or 20 ml/kg/min) is associated with an increased incidence of postoperative complications.[27] In addition, exercise-induced arterial oxygen desaturation (greater than 2 percent decline) appears to predict postoperative complications, including death and respiratory failure.[26]

Measurement of the diffusing capacity ($D_{L_{CO}}$) has generally not proved helpful in assessing operative risk.[26,27] However, determination of predicted postoperative $D_{L_{CO}}$, using a formula similar in concept to Eq. (1), may have value. A predicted postoperative $D_{L_{CO}}$ of less than 40 percent appears to be associated with a high risk of operative morbidity and mortality.[26]

Bronchospirometry (the measurement of oxygen uptake in each lung, individually), the so-called lateral position test, and measurement of pulmonary artery pressure during temporary, unilateral pulmonary artery occlusion are techniques used in the past to assess the risk of thoracotomy in borderline patients. These tests are now of historical interest because of technical problems and concerns over reproducibility of results.[27]

Recommended Approach

In evaluating patients for lung resection, the following approach should be considered (Fig. 40-3).[15,26,27] Operability for pneumonectomy is determined in the event that this procedure is necessary, either to remove the tumor completely or because of an intraoperative complication. If the preoperative FEV_1 is 2 L or greater, or at least 80 percent of the predicted normal value, the patient is "cleared" for pneumonectomy; no further testing is required. If the preoperative FEV_1 is less than these values, the predicted post-pneumonectomy FEV_1 should be determined. The patient is cleared for pneumonectomy if the predicted postoperative FEV_1 is at least 40 percent of the predicted value. The patient is considered borderline if this number is between 30 and 40 percent of the predicted value; the patient is considered to be at high risk for pneumonectomy if the value is below 30 percent.

For the borderline patient, or for the patient with significant dyspnea or disability despite an "operable" FEV_1 or predicted postoperative FEV_1, the predicted post-pneumonectomy D_{LCO} should be determined. The patient is cleared for pneumonectomy if this value is at least 40 percent of the predicted value.

If confirmatory evidence of operability is required, an exercise test should be performed. The patient is cleared for pneumonectomy if the $\dot{V}O_{2max}$ is at least 20 ml/kg/min and arterial oxygen saturation declines less than 2 percent.

If the patient cannot tolerate a pneumonectomy but, from a technical standpoint, appears to be a good candidate for lobectomy, the appropriate steps in Fig. 40-3 should be followed for calculation of the predicted post-lobectomy FEV_1 and D_{LCO}.

When respiratory insufficiency occurs as a result of pulmonary resection, it is manifest early, i.e., within the first several weeks following operation. After 3 months, respiratory insufficiency directly attributable to the surgery is rare.

PREOPERATIVE PREPARATION

Surprisingly, few studies have specifically addressed the question of whether aggressive, preoperative pulmonary preparation decreases postoperative pulmonary morbidity and mortality. Although data on preoperative preparation are limited, for patients with significant obstructive airway disease, intensive preoperative respiratory therapy (bronchodilators, corticosteroids, antibiotics, and chest physiotherapy) does appear to reduce the incidence of postoperative respiratory complications by more than 50 percent.[17,21,39,43]

Several preoperative prophylactic measures should be considered in patients undergoing elective surgery (Table 40-6).

Pulmonary function in patients with obstructive airway disease should be optimized. Therapy may include any or all of the following: bronchodilators, corticosteroids, antibiotics (when there is evidence of infection), and chest physiotherapy (if excessive secretions are present). When possible, these interventions should be implemented 48 to 72 h prior to surgery.

Ideally, for at least 8 weeks prior to surgery, smoking should be discontinued.

In severely obese patients, if patient compliance can be achieved, weight reduction should be attempted.

Finally, patient education on the importance of coughing and pain control, proper use of an incentive spirometer, and deep breathing exercises should take place preoperatively.

POSTOPERATIVE PROPHYLACTIC MEASURES

Several postoperative measures may be employed in an attempt to prevent respiratory complications (Table 40-7).

Early patient mobilization and ambulation should be encouraged. As noted previously, these measures are important postoperatively in reducing the incidence of atelectasis, in promot-

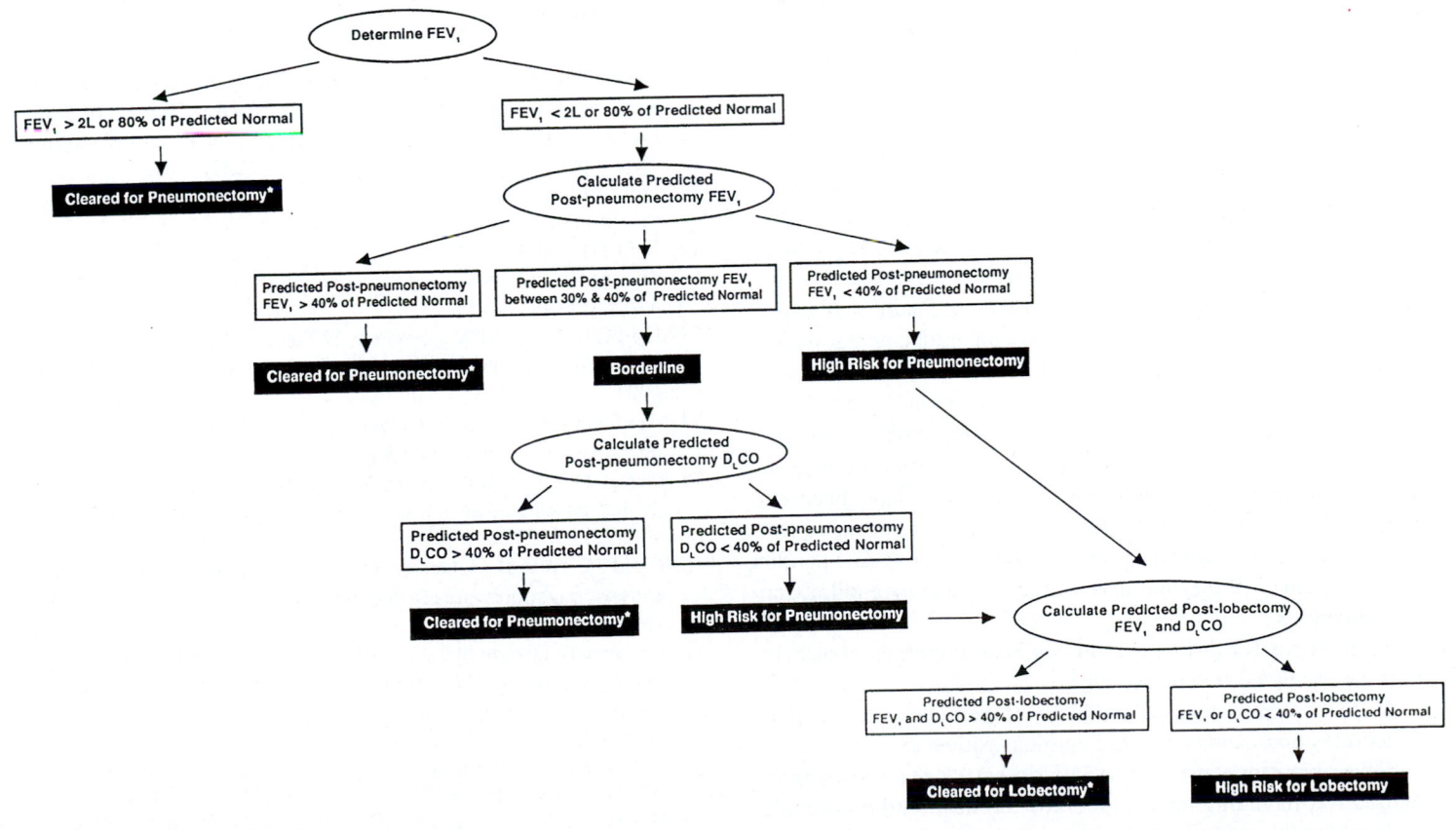

FIGURE 40-3   Algorithm for preoperative evaluation for lung resection. See text for discussion.

TABLE 40-6

Preoperative Pulmonary Preparation

Optimization of airway function in patients with obstructive lung disease (bronchodilators; corticosteroids, antibiotics, and chest physiotherapy, when indicated)

Smoking cessation (ideally, a minimum of 8 weeks prior to surgery)

Weight reduction for severely obese individuals

Patient education (deep breathing exercises, importance of coughing and pain control, use of incentive spirometry)

SOURCE: From Goldmann DR, Brown FH, Guarnieri DM (eds): *Perioperative Medicine.* New York, McGraw-Hill, 1994, with permission.

TABLE 40-7

Postoperative Measures for the Prevention of Respiratory Complications

Early patient mobilization and ambulation

Prophylatic lung expansion maneuvers (incentive spirometry, deep-breathing exercises, CPAP)

Provision of adequate analgesia (including patient-controlled analgesia, intercostal nerve blocks, and epidural anesthesia)

Prophylaxis against thromboembolism

ing the clearance of secretions, and in decreasing the risk of thromboembolic disease.

Prophylactic lung expansion maneuvers should be initiated.[4] Two equally effective measures are deep breathing exercises and incentive spirometry.[40] Intermittent positive pressure breathing (IPPB) is generally ineffective and costly and is associated with several adverse effects.[4] Recent reports of intermittent continuous positive airway pressure (CPAP) applied by face mask indicate that it is at least equivalent to deep breathing exercises and incentive spirometry in preventing and treating atelectasis.[40] However, while CPAP may be useful in the patient who cannot cooperate with inspiratory maneuvers, its role in the management of patients capable of taking deep breaths is unclear.

Adequate analgesia should be provided. Traditionally, parenteral narcotics have been used for postoperative analgesia, despite the risk of respiratory depression. Unfortunately, concerns over adverse respiratory effects may lead to inadequate dosing and inadequate pain relief. To overcome this problem, alternative approaches, including use of patient-controlled analgesia, epidural analgesia, and intercostal nerve blocks, have been employed. These alternative techniques provide analgesia equivalent or superior to parenteral narcotics, but published data conflict as to how effective they are in reducing postoperative pulmonary complications.

Prophylaxis for thromboembolism is an important consideration, as discussed in Chapter 84.

Finally, careful monitoring for postoperative complications constitutes a key element in all surgical patients.

Several postoperative interventions have been shown to be ineffective, including the use of "blow bottles," carbon-dioxide-induced hyperventilation,[4] chest physiotherapy in the absence of excessive secretions or sputum production, and routine application of positive end-expiratory pressure in mechanically ventilated patients.[16]

REFERENCES

1. Alexander JI, Spence AA, Parikh RK, Stuart, B: The role of airway closure in postoperative hypoxaemia. *Br J Anaesth* 45:34–40, 1973.
2. Ali J, Weisel RD, Layug AB, et al: Consequences of postoperative alterations in respiratory mechanisms. *Am J Surg* 128:376–382, 1974.
3. Anderson PR, Puno MR, Lovell SL, Swayze, CR: Postoperative respiratory complications in non-idiopthic scoliosis. *Acta Anasthesiol Scand* 29:186–192, 1985.
4. Bartlett RH, Gazzaniga AB, Geraghty TR: Respiratory maneuvers to prevent postoperative pulmonary complications. A critical review. *JAMA* 224:1017–1021, 1973.
5. Brain JD: Anesthesia and respiratory defense mechanisms. *Int Anesthesiol Clin* 15:169–198, 1977.
6. Catley DM: Postoperative analgesia and respiratory control. *Int Anesthesiol Clin* 22:95–111, 1984.
7. Celli BR, Rodriguez KS, Snider GL: A controlled trial of intermittent positive pressure breathing, incentive spirometry, and deep breathing exercises in preventing pulmonary complications after abdominal surgery. *Am Rev Respir Dis* 130:12–15, 1984.
8. Craig DB: Postoperative recovery of pulmonary function. *Anesth Analg* 60:46–52, 1981.
9. Dureuil B, Vires N, Cantineau J, et al: Diaphragmatic contractility after upper abdominal surgery. *J Appl Physiol* 61:1775–1780, 1986.
10. Fairshter RD, Williams JH: Pulmonary physiology in the postoperative period. *Crit Care Clin* 3:287–306, 1987.
11. Foltz BD, Benumof JL: Mechanisms of hypoxemia and hypercapnea in the perioperative period. *Crit Care Clin* 3:269–286, 1987.
12. Ford GT, Whitelaw WA, Rosenal TW, et al: Diaphragm function after upper abdominal surgery in humans. *Am Rev Respir Dis* 127:431–436, 1983.
13. Ford GT, Rosenal TW, Clergue F, Whitelaw WA: Respiratory physiology in upper abdominal surgery. *Clin Chest Med* 14:237–252, 1993.
14. Garibaldi RA, Britt MR, Coleman ML, et al: Risk factors for postoperative pneumonia. *Am J Med* 70:677–680, 1981.
15. Gass GD, Olsen GN: Preoperative pulmonary function testing to predict postoperative morbidity and mortality. *Chest* 89:127–135, 1986.
16. Good JT, Wolz JF, Anderson JT, et al: The routine use of positive end-expiratory pressure after open heart surgery. *Chest* 76:397–400, 1979.
17. Gracey DR, Diverte MB, Didier EP: Preoperative pulmonary preparation of patients with chronic obstructive pulmonary disease. A prospective study. *Chest* 76:123–129, 1979.
18. Gracey DR, Divertie MB, Howard FM, Payne WS: Postoperative respiratory care after transsternal thymectomy in myasthenia gravis. A 3-year experience in 53 patients. *Chest* 86:67–71, 1984.
19. Halasz NA: Vertical vs. horizontal laparotomies. *Arch Surg* 88:911–914, 1964.
20. Hall WJ, Hall CB, Speers DM: Respiratory syncytial virus infection in adults. Clinical, virologic, and serial pulmonary function studies. *Ann Intern Med* 88:203–205, 1978.

21. Hall JC, Tarala RA, Hall JL, Mander J: A multivariate analysis of the risk of pulmonary complications after laparotomy. *Chest* 99: 923–927, 1991.

22. Hansen G, Drablos PA, Steinert R: Pulmonary complications, ventilation and blood gases after upper abdominal surgery. *Acta Anaesth Scand* 21:211–215, 1977.

23. Kafer ER, Marsh HM. The effect of anesthetic drugs and disease on the chemical regulation of ventilation. *Int Anesthesiol Clin* 15: 1–38, 1977.

24. Lawrence VA, Page CP, Harris GD: Preoperative spirometry before abdominal operations. A critical appraisal of its predictive value. *Arch Intern Med* 149:280–285, 1989.

25. Latimer RG, Dickman M, Day WC, et al: Ventilatory patterns and pulmonary complications after upper abdominal surgery determined by preoperative and postoperative computerized spirometry and blood gas analysis. *Am J Surg* 122:622–632, 1971.

26. Markos J, Mullan BP, Hillman DR, et al: Preoperative assessment as a predictor of mortality and morbidity after lung resection. *Am Rev Respir Dis* 139:902–910, 1989.

27. Marshall MC, Olsen GN: The physiologic evaluation of the lung resection candidate. *Clin Chest Med* 14:305–320, 1993.

28. Marshall BE, Wyche MQ: Hypoxemia during and after anesthesia. *Anesthesiology* 37:178–209, 1972.

29. Meyers JR, Lembeck L, O'Kane H, Baue AE: Changes in functional residual capacity of the lung after operation. *Arch Surg* 110: 576–583, 1975.

30. Mier-Jedrzejowicz A, Brophy C, Green M: Respiratory muscle weakness during upper respiratory tract infection. *Am Rev Respir Dis* 138:5–7, 1988.

31. Milledge JS, Nunn JF: Criteria of fitness for anaesthesia in patients with chronic obstructive lung disease. *Br Med J* 3:670–673, 1975.

32. Pasulka PS, Bistrian BR, Benotti PN, Blackburn GL: The risk of surgery in obese patients. *Ann Intern Med* 104:540–546, 1986.

33. Pederson T, Eliasen K, Henriksen E: A prospective study of risk factors and cardiopulmonary complications associated with anesthesia and surgery: Risk indications of cardiopulmonary morbidity. *Acta Anaesthiol Scand* 34:144–155, 1990.

34. Raffin TA: Indications for arterial blood gas analysis. *Ann Intern Med* 105:390–395, 1986.

35. Scott NB, Kehlet H: Regional anaesthesia and surgical morbidity. *Br J Surg* 75:299–304, 1988.

36. Sherman S, Guidot CE: The feasibility of thoracotomy for lung cancer in the elderly. *JAMA* 258:927–930, 1987.

37. Simonneau G, Vivien A, Sartene R, et al: Diaphragm dysfunction induced by upper abdominal pain. Role of postoperative pain. *Am Rev Respir Dis* 128:899–903, 1983.

38. Stein M, Koota GM, Simon M, Frank HA: Pulmonary evaluation of surgical patients. *JAMA* 181:765–770, 1962.

39. Stein M, Cassara EL: Preoperative pulmonary evaluation and therapy for surgery patients. *JAMA* 211:787–790, 1970.

40. Stock MC, Downs JB, Gauer PK, et al: Prevention of postoperative pulmonary complications with CPAP, incentive spirometry and conservative therapy. *Chest* 87:151–157, 1985.

41. Sykes LA, Bowe EA: Cardiorespiratory effects of anesthesia. *Clin Chest Med* 14:211–226, 1993.

42. Tape TG, Mushlin AI: The utility of routine chest radiographs. *Ann Intern Med* 104:663–670, 1986.

43. Tarhan S, Moffitt EA, Sessler AD, et al: Risk of anesthesia and surgery in patients with chronic bronchitis and chronic obstructive pulmonary disease. *Surgery* 74:720–726, 1973.

44. The Veterans Affairs Total Parenteral Nutrition Cooperative Study Group. Perioperative total parenteral nutrition in surgical patients. *N Engl J Med* 325:525–532, 1991.

45. Warner MA, Divertie MB, Tinker JH: Preoperative cessation of smoking and pulmonary complications in coronary artery bypass patients. *Anesthesiology* 60:380–383, 1984.

46. Weil JV, McCullough RE, Kline JS, Sodal IE: Diminished ventilatory response to hypoxia and hypercapnia after morphine in normal man. *New Engl J Med* 292:1103–1106, 1975.

47. Wightman JAK: A prospective survey of the incidence of postoperative pulmonary complications. *Br J Surg* 55:85–91, 1968.

48. Williams CD, Brenowitz JB: "Prohibitive" lung function and major surgical procedures. *Am J Surg* 132:763–766, 1976.

49. Wahba WM, Don HF, Craig DB: Postoperative epidural analgesia: Effects on lung volumes. *Can Anaesth Soc J* 22:519–527, 1975.

50. Younger DS, Braun NMT, Jaretzki A, et al: Myasthenia gravis: Determinants for independent ventilation after transsternal thymectomy. *Neurology* 34:336–340, 1984.

51. Zibrack JD, O'Donnell CR, Marton K: Indications for pulmonary function testing. *Ann Intern Med* 112:703–771, 1990.

CHAPTER 41

IMPAIRMENT AND DISABILITY EVALUATION IN LUNG DISEASE

Paul E. Epstein

METHODS OF EVALUATION

MEDICAL HISTORY

PHYSICAL EXAMINATION

RADIOGRAPHIC STUDIES

PULMONARY FUNCTION TESTING

IMPAIRMENT AND DISABILITY ACCORDING TO AMERICAN MEDICAL ASSOCIATION GUIDELINES

AMERICAN THORACIC SOCIETY CRITERIA FOR EVALUATION OF IMPAIRMENT AND DISABILITY

DISABILITY EVALUATION UNDER SOCIAL SECURITY

WORKERS' COMPENSATION PROGRAM

AMERICANS WITH DISABILITIES ACT

NONMEDICAL FACTORS THAT INTERFERE WITH ACCURATE ASSESSMENT OF IMPAIRMENT OR DISABILITY

The process of evaluating physical status is a familiar and comfortable activity for most physicians. The usual purposes of such an evaluation are to differentiate between health and disease, to define the type of disease that might be present, and to evaluate the severity of the disease process in preparation for planning treatment. The evaluation of impairment or disability applies the same type of diagnostic reasoning to a regulatory and legal system that has been developed largely for social rather than medical purposes. The overarching reason for this type of analysis is to help individuals cope with injuries that have limited their full participation in occupational activities or activities of daily living. In this sense, the physician's responsibility is no different than in any other type of medical assessment. Other factors, however, peculiar to the quasi-legal aspects of disability evaluation set this activity apart from the physician's usual role.[22,31] Whereas the physician ordinarily acts solely as the patient's advocate, the role of the independent evaluator of impairment or disability requires fairness to all parties involved, whether governmental, commercial, or personal.

Injuries of any sort carry both physical and emotional components, and it is the responsibility of the evaluating physician to define clearly which portion of the inability to work is due to physical factors as opposed to other factors. Since this role of the physician differs from the usual therapeutic relationship, the injured worker often feels that the evaluating physician is "working for the other side" in any dispute. Suspicion on the part of the examinee often hampers the evaluation process.

Another difference between the usual activities of the physician and assessment of impairment or disability is that the medical evaluation is only one component of the many to be considered in reaching a final conclusion regarding ability to work.[1,33] For example, inability to perform heavy manual labor may be vocationally devastating to an uneducated, unskilled worker, but it may have little or no effect on job possibilities for a financial analyst. Assessment of education, job retraining possibilities, and local availability of alternative work are not within the expertise of the physician, yet these issues are critically important in evaluating the effect of an injury on an individual's life. For these reasons, the physician plays an important, but supporting, role in the process of deciding whether financial benefits will be awarded on the basis of an injury.

Finally, in an attempt to promote uniformity and fairness to the process of evaluation, professional societies and government agencies have set standards by which decrements of function can be judged. These considerations have led to the development of specific definitions to deal with the concepts described above. The American Thoracic Society[5] has defined *impairment* as a purely medical condition resulting from a functional abnormality. A worker may also be considered impaired if an environmental sensitivity exists that makes it impossible to perform in a specific job, if a lethal disease is present that is not amenable to therapy, or if the worker presents a public health hazard such as active, untreated tuberculosis. According to the American Thoracic Society, *disability* refers to the total effect of the impairment on the individual's life and requires consideration of many nonmedical factors. It is clear then, that impairment is evaluated by a physician, and disability is determined by a nonmedical adjudicator who depends heavily upon the physician's assessment of impairment. This chapter reviews the methods used for evaluation, the standards commonly applied for interpretation, and some of the important programs available for compensation.

METHODS OF EVALUATION

In order to make the evaluation process accessible to large numbers of people, the tools used for assessment must be widely available, standards for equipment reliability must be enforced, and schemes for interpretation must be standardized. The goal of physiological testing in the laboratory is to predict an individual's ability to carry out the duties required of a particular job and to assess the limits imposed by an injury or loss of function. Implicit in the evaluation of impairment or disability is the assumption that some test or combination of tests, whether simple or sophisticated, can adequately reproduce the effort and pattern of physical exertion required in performance of a real-world job. This attractive concept is only partially realistic for at least three reasons. First, measuring the actual physical requirements of any specific job is difficult, since the individual's method of performance has a large effect on the amount of effort required. For instance, a particular job may require 60 min of arduous effort during an 8-h work shift. An employee may be able to do the job if the work can be distributed over the whole day, but he or she may be unable to do so if all the hard work is required at one time. Although the examiner may be evaluating a worker for the ability to perform a particular job, the broader purpose of the evaluation is to test the individual's ability to function more generally in the workplace. Since the character of different jobs varies so widely, the type of judgment required is more abstract than it is precise. Second, unless studies have been performed at a particular work site, it is usually difficult to determine the specific energy output required by the job. Third, a surprisingly reliable predictor of an individual's ability to work is the motivation to do so. It is not uncommon to see workers holding fairly arduous jobs who are moderately or even severely impaired according to usual criteria. Conversely, unmotivated workers may have test results that are normal or very close to normal but, nonetheless, complain of intolerable dyspnea and fatigue during moderate exertion.

In order to produce useful information, methods of appraisal of functional ability must be standardized so that two or more physicians can agree on the extent of impairment. The findings must be presented in a manner that can be used for vocational, financial, and legal decisionmaking. These impairments can then be roughly translated into ability to perform in specific job categories according to previously published energy requirements for a wide variety of jobs.[28]

Most evaluations of impairment or disability are performed to assess permanent limitations of function, although certain exceptions occur in workers' compensation actions where temporary or partial disability may be evaluated. As a result, evaluations are best performed when the disease process is stable and after appropriate therapy has produced the maximal expected improvement.

MEDICAL HISTORY

Although determination of impairment or disability is approached in a quantitative fashion, the physician must begin the analysis by gaining a clear understanding of the disease process under evaluation and the subjective symptoms experienced. This is important for planning appropriate testing and assessing the clinical plausibility of an observed abnormality. A complete medical and occupational history should be obtained and recorded, paying particular attention to the potential workplace exposures that may have a bearing on loss of pulmonary function. In view of the long latency period between onset of exposure to certain deleterious substances and the manifestation of disease caused by those substances, the occupational history should start with the first job ever held by the individual and proceed chronologically up to the time of examination.[35] Job titles and specific duties should be described in conjunction with any known contact with hazardous materials. Onset of symptoms should be described along with any temporal relationship to workplace exposures. Prior medical evaluations should be reviewed in order to confirm the consistency of findings and to ensure that the severity of symptoms fits the recognized pattern of disease progression.

Various attempts have been made to quantitate subjective symptoms such as the sensation of dyspnea. One of the most widely used dyspnea scales has been proposed by the American Thoracic Society.[12] The scale grades dyspnea as mild, moderate, severe or very severe based on the level of common, everyday activity that causes breathlessness. The scale was adapted from the British Medical Research Council scale.[27]

Although a dyspnea scale is not sufficiently accurate to use for objective assessment of impairment, its utility lies in detecting inordinately severe symptoms when compared with objective findings on pulmonary function testing. This disparity sometimes leads to the discovery of disease in another organ system that contributes to the dyspnea. In addition, incongruence of symptoms with pulmonary function test results helps guide the need for further, more sophisticated testing. Finally, if no other cause can be found for disproportionate dyspnea, the evaluating physician must consider the possibility that the applicant is exaggerating discomfort for the purpose of financial gain.

Cough and sputum production have long been recognized as important symptoms of pulmonary disease. However, documentation of the frequency and severity of cough, as well as quantitation of sputum production, have proved so difficult that none of the commonly employed evaluation schemes uses these symptoms as cardinal indicators of impairment.

PHYSICAL EXAMINATION

A complete physical examination should be performed in order to confirm the presence of respiratory tract disease and to detect disease in other organs whose symptoms may affect respiratory function. Abnormalities of the vital signs such as tachycardia, bradycardia, irregular pulse beat, hypertension, pulsus paradoxus, wide pulse pressure, and tachypnea may direct further evaluation toward the heart, thyroid, or lungs. Conjunctival pallor suggests the possibility of anemia as a cause of dyspnea, and cyanosis suggests either respiratory or cardiac disease. Evidence of valvular heart disease, congestive heart failure, pulmonary hypertension, and cor pulmonale also help define the systems requiring further investigation in the evaluation of dyspnea.

The character of adventitious sounds in the lungs is helpful in defining the type of abnormality causing respiratory symptoms. Expiratory wheezing may be heard in chronic obstructive pulmonary disease as well as during exacerbations of asthma. Crackles, particularly at the posterior lung bases, may be indicative of interstitial fibrosis, but their presence may also indicate congestive heart failure, pulmonary infection, or other inflammatory conditions. Crackles are also often present during the first few deep breaths during the physical examination and, in this circumstance, do not indicate any disease when they disappear after continued deep breathing or coughing. Rhonchi indicate the presence of mucus in the bronchi which can be associated with infection, inflammation, or altered ability to clear the airways.

Whereas physical examination is necessary for diagnostic purposes, its use in evaluating impairment or disability is quite limited because of difficulty in quantifying the findings. For this reason, physical examination plays a supportive, rather than a definitive, role.

RADIOGRAPHIC STUDIES

The chest radiograph is often the initial indication of an abnormality that triggers impairment or disability evaluation, particularly when a pneumoconiosis is suspected. The International Labor Organization has devised a highly detailed classification system for grading the radiographic severity of pneumoconioses based on a set of standard films which are used for comparison purposes.[21] Qualified physicians can be certified by the National Institute of Occupational Safety and Health (NIOSH) as being expert in the classification system by passing an examination known as the *B-reader examination.* In view of the ability to classify and quantify the radiographic abnormalities with relative precision, it is disappointing to find that there is poor correlation between the severity of pulmonary function abnormalities and the radiographic readings among patients with pneumoconiosis.[18] The correlation between chest radiograph findings and pulmonary function abnormalities is even poorer in patients with obstructive lung disease. For this reason, radiographic findings are not generally considered reliable indicators of impairment or disability.

PULMONARY FUNCTION TESTING

Assessment of impairment on the basis of pulmonary function test abnormalities depends on several factors, including choice of laboratory equipment, standards of calibration, technician training and skill, patient cooperation, reproducibility of serial test results, and choice of standards of normal function. The American Thoracic Society has periodically published standards for equipment characteristics and test performance that are widely accepted in the medical community.[3,4,8]

The reference value used to compare an individual's test results against a normal standard is an important factor in deciding whether impairment is present. For this reason, care must be taken to chose an appropriate set of reference values.[10] Factors to be considered include methodologic, epidemiologic, and statistical criteria.[7] From a methodologic standpoint, the equipment and techniques recommended by the American Thoracic Society should be used in data collection. Epidemiologic considerations are somewhat more complex. Several large studies have been performed over the last few decades to evaluate pulmonary function test variability among normal individuals (i.e., those without respiratory tract symptoms, history of pulmonary or cardiac disease, abnormal physical examination findings, or history of cigarette smoking); these form the basis for the commonly used prediction formulae. Despite the excellent quality of data collection in many of these studies, a potential problem arises when they are used for comparative purposes because most of the studies were performed using a population restricted to a particular geographic location or connected to a well-defined affinity group such as employment in a particular industry or veterans' group.[16,25,26,30] These groups may differ in important ways from the population being tested for impairment in a particular laboratory, since geography, socioeconomic conditions, and ethnic makeup may differ widely and may affect pulmonary function test results. In choosing a reference population for comparative purposes, it is wise to attempt to match the characteristics of a reference group with those of the group being tested.

Another important issue in the interpretation of pulmonary function test results is deciding on the lower limit of normal. The older practice of judging FVC and FEV_1 as abnormal if the result is less than 80 percent of predicted does not appear to be justified, since there is no statistical support for such a classification (see Chapter 36). A statistically more defensible plan is to define the lowest 5 percent of a reference population as below the lower limit of normal.[7] Although 5 percent of normal individuals may be misclassified by this procedure, such a low rate of error is generally considered acceptable, particularly since there is likely to be overlap with abnormal test subjects in this range. It should be recognized, however, that certain entitlement programs for the evaluation of impairment mandate specific test results as cutoff points between normal and abnormal based on sex, height, and age.

Many authorities on evaluation of impairment or disability evaluation recommend performance of cardiopulmonary exercise testing in order to delineate the highest level of exertion that can be performed by the individual being studied.[15,34] Although earlier attempts to include cardiopulmonary exercise testing in the evaluation were hampered by the availability of testing only in larger medical centers, these studies have become more routine as result of technical developments that make computerized calculations of ventilatory, cardiac, and gas exchange data feasible for community-based laboratories.

In exercise testing, the highest level of exertion obtainable is indicated by the patient's maximal oxygen utilization ($\dot{V}_{O_2max}$). The underlying reason for the recommendation to use cardiopulmonary exercise testing is that the information obtained by this technique is much closer to the functional reality of work than is the surrogate information obtained by routine pulmonary function testing. When testing is performed, the individual can describe which symptom limited further exertion and can often differentiate between dyspnea, muscle fatigue, or chest pain as the cause of the cessation of exercise. In addition to a subjective description of symptoms, measurements made during cardiopulmonary exercise testing provide objective assessment of organ function. The results can be helpful in distinguishing among various causes of limitation, including cardiac dysfunction, pulmonary dysfunction, peripheral vascular disease, poor physical conditioning, and poor effort. Another attractive aspect of the study is the possibility of matching exercise capacity with the requirements of a particular job.

Most of the common protocols for exercise testing utilize a treadmill or bicycle ergometer to perform exertion, since these devices require use of large muscle groups in the legs. This allows for more rapid achievement of maximal exertion, increasing the efficiency of the testing process. Several different incrementally graded exercise protocols have been described, but all depend on increasing the work rate either minute-by-minute or continuously during the performance of the study. Most exercise protocols aim for achieving voluntary, symptom-limited cessation of exertion within 8 to 12 min of starting the test.

Measurements made during an exercise test include work rate, oxygen consumption ($\dot{V}_{O_2}$), carbon dioxide production ($\dot{V}_{CO_2}$), expired minute ventilation ($\dot{V}_E$), end-tidal P_{O_2}, end-tidal P_{CO_2}, heart rate, blood pressure, and oxygen saturation by pulse oximetry or, sometimes, by arterial blood-gas analysis (see Chapter 37).

Measured $\dot{V}_{O_2max}$ may be compared to normal predicted values for the individual's age, sex, and body surface area. This information indicates whether the individual can perform a normal amount of exertion. The level of exertion at which lactate begins to accumulate in the blood is also an important indicator of work capacity. This point is reached significantly before the $\dot{V}_{O_2max}$, but it indicates that less efficient anaerobic pathways are being used to produce energy. The level of exertion at which anaerobic pathways develop is known as the *anaerobic threshold* and is marked by an increase in blood lactate level above the normal resting value of less than 1 to 2 mmol/L. Noninvasive methods of measuring the anaerobic threshold are frequently used in the performance of cardiopulmonary exercise testing. Measurement of $\dot{V}_{O_2}$ at the anaerobic threshold helps in evaluating the level of exertion that can be sustained for long periods, since the anaerobic exertion clearly cannot be sustained indefinitely.[36]

Cardiopulmonary exercise testing may also provide other information about the cause of exercise limitation. *Ventilatory reserve* is the difference between the measured maximum voluntary ventilation (MVV) and ventilation achieved during exercise. If ventilation during exercise ($\dot{V}_E$) does not approximate the MVV, one can assume that ventilatory problems did not cause the individual to cease exertion. Similarly, assessment of cardiac reserve, the difference between predicted heart rate and observed heart rate during exercise, can help rule out a cardiac cause of exercise limitations if the achieved heart rate is much lower than the predicted heart rate. Lung ventilation-perfusion abnormalities as a cause of ventilatory dysfunction are suggested by an abnormally elevated ratio of dead space to tidal volume (V_{DS}/V_T), which can be calculated from the measurements made during cardiopulmonary exercise testing. In addition, abnormalities of arterial P_{O_2} during exercise are indicative of gas exchange abnormalities.

Although cardiopulmonary testing provides a great deal of information about an individual's ability to sustain exertion, certain limitations of the technique must be considered. Both the American Thoracic Society criteria for impairment and those of the American Medical Association suggest that cardiopulmonary exercise testing should not be performed if pulmonary function test results are normal, or if severe impairment is evident according to other criteria. Similarly, exercise studies should not be performed if other medical conditions exist that make maximal exertion dangerous, such as severe cardiac arrythmias or unstable angina. Even when none of these contraindications is present, exercise testing is rarely indicated if there is no disparity between symptoms and the observed pulmonary function test abnormalities.

From a practical standpoint, performing cardiopulmonary exercise testing in workers' compensation actions is often difficult because of the adversarial nature of the proceeding and a financial disincentive on the part of the claimant to perform maximal exertion. In addition, the cost of these studies is a significant factor in the decision to defer or proceed. Finally, one must consider how accurately the results of such testing reflects the reality of the work environment. Although knowledge of the energy requirements of various occupations provides a useful guide in decisionmaking, the only way to be certain about the requirements of a particular job is to test the individual at the work station. Although this is often impractical, standard cardiopulmonary exercise testing, even when performed to submaximal levels, may provide enough information to allow an individual to return to work if performance exceeds the usual requirements of the job. However, submaximal performance should not be used to decide that a worker is incapable of returning to the job.

IMPAIRMENT AND DISABILITY ACCORDING TO THE AMERICAN MEDICAL ASSOCIATION GUIDELINES

According to the American Medical Association (AMA) *Guides to the Evaluation of Permanent Impairment*,[1] the disease under evaluation should be stable, fully treated, and not amenable to additional treatment that might be expected to change the patient's condition. The first phase of evaluation is the *diagnostic phase* described earlier.

The *quantitative phase* of evaluation requires spirometry and diffusing capacity measurement. In this evaluation scheme, results are provided as "percent predicted," using the standards of normality proposed by Crapo and colleagues.[16] If there is reason to believe that spirometry and diffusing capacity results have underestimated the true severity of the disease process, the evaluating physician may choose to perform cardiopulmonary exercise testing.

The AMA standards provide a method of judging the relative severity of the impairment, rather than simply drawing an arbitrary line between normal and abnormal or between able and disabled. As noted in Table 41-1, the functional categories range from class I (normal) to class IV (severely impaired), depending on the degree of functional abnormality identified by the studies. As long as the tests have been performed properly, the most abnormal test result determines the class of impairment, even if all the other studies suggest a lesser degree of impairment. Inspection of Table 41-1 indicates that the physician is allowed a great deal of discretion within each class for the designation of specific percent of impairment on the basis of the study results. The reason for this discretionary latitude is that there is little scientific support for assigning an exact numerical decrement in function to a specific finding on pulmonary function or cardiopulmonary testing. In reality, the broad range of possibilities within each class reflects the physician's subjective judgment as well as the relative degree of test result abnormality.

In addition to the specific test results noted in Table 41-1, a number of disease processes are recognized by the AMA *Guides* to produce impairment, even though they are difficult to quantitate. These include diseases such as asthma, sleep apnea, pneumoconiosis, hypersensitivity pneumonitis, and lung cancer.

According to the AMA *Guides,* the severity of impairment in patients with asthma is judged on the basis of pulmonary function abnormalities documented on three separate occasions, at least 1 week apart, while the patient is receiving optimal medical treatment. The assessment of impairment may be modified by the examining physician, depending upon the frequency of asthma attacks.

Sleep apnea, whether classified as obstructive or central, is considered a severely impairing illness in the untreated patient because of the secondary effects of the illness on job performance. In those who have received treatment, the results of formal polysomography are used to determine the severity of persistent impairment.

Pneumoconiosis is a disease class that commonly presents a disparity between diagnosis and functional assessment. The diagnosis of pneumoconiosis is often made by recognizing characteristic patterns of abnormality on the chest radiograph. Although one of the guiding principles of impairment and disability

assessment is the requirement for strict evaluation of functional ability, another important facet of the problem involves the potential for further damage if the affected individual remains in his or her current position. It is well recognized that some, but not all, workers with pneumoconiosis may have progression of the disease even if no further dust exposure occurs. If the potential for further dust accumulation exists, the individual who has already shown susceptibility to the damaging effects of fibrogenic material should be removed from the workplace. The requirement for removal becomes less clear when ambient dust control has eliminated significant risk for additional dust exposure. In evaluating an individual for impairment or disability, it is prudent to restrict future employment to jobs that eliminate any further fibrogenic dust exposure and to evaluate residual pulmonary function for the individual's ability to perform other types of work. Conceivably, an individual with simple pneumoconiosis may be prohibited from pursuing usual employment but may be able to hold another job that requires the same level of physical exertion.

Hypersensitivity pneumonitis is usually a disease that relapses upon exposure to the offending agent. In between attacks, the affected individual may have normal pulmonary function. However, repeated attacks may lead to pulmonary fibrosis and restrictive lung disease. The rating of impairment in patients with hypersensitivity pneumonitis may be based on the test results noted in Table 41-1, but subjects may also be considered impaired for specific jobs involving exposure to the causative agent, even if pulmonary function is normal. In these cases, impairment depends on accurate diagnosis, rather than on pulmonary function test results.

All patients with lung cancer are considered to be severely impaired at the time of diagnosis. Following therapy, the patient may be reevaluated 1 year later. If there has been recurrence of the cancer, the designation of severe impairment is continued. If there is no recurrence, assessment is made on the basis of physiological findings, as noted in Table 41-1.

TABLE 41-1

Classes of Respiratory Impairment According to AMA *Guides to the Evaluation of Permanent Impairment*

	Class 1 (0%, no impairment of the whole person)	*Class 2* (10–25%, mild impairment of the whole person)	*Class 3* (16–50%, moderate impairment of the whole person)	*Class 4* (51–100%, severe impairment of the whole person)
FVC, FEV_1, $FEV_1FVC\%$, D_{LCO}	FVC ≥ 80% predicted, *and* FEV_1 ≥ 80% predicted, *and* $FEV_1/FEC\%$ ≥ 70, and D_{LCO} ≥ 70% predicted	FVC between 60 and 79% predicted, *or* FEV_1 between 60 and 79% predicted, *or* D_{LCO} between 60 and 69% predicted	FVC between 51 and 59% predicted, *or* FEV_1 between 41 and 59% predicted, *or* D_{LCO} between 41 and 59% predicted	FVC ≤ 50% predicted, *or* FEV_1 ≤ 40% predicted, *or* D_{LCO} ≤ 40% predicted
	or	or	or	or
$\dot{V}_{O_2max}$	>25 ml/(kg·min) *or* >7.1 METS	Between 20 and 25 ml/(kg·min); *or* 5.7–7.1 METS	Between 15 and 20 ml(kg·min); *or* 4.3–5.7 METS	<15 ml/(kg·min); *or* <1.05 L/min; *or* <4.3 METS

SOURCE: Reproduced with permission from *Guides to the Evaluation of Permanent Impairment,* American Medical Association, Copyright 1994.

AMERICAN THORACIC SOCIETY CRITERIA FOR EVALUATION OF IMPAIRMENT OR DISABILITY

The American Thoracic Society periodically issues official statements regarding impairment or disability evaluation.[5,6] The recommendations have generally paralleled those of the AMA, although there are some important differences, particularly with regard to evaluation of asthmatic conditions. According to the American Thoracic Society, a majority of individuals can be assessed adequately by using spirometry and diffusing capacity measurements, even though selected cases may benefit from additional studies such as exercise testing. The ATS recognizes that abnormalities of pulmonary function fall on a continuum that allows judgments to be made about the relative severity of respiratory dysfunction and does not assign a specific percentage of impairment as is found in the AMA *Guides*.

According to the ATS, individuals with an FVC $\geq$ 80 percent predicted, an $FEV_1 \geq$ 80 percent predicted, an $FEV_1/FVC\% \geq$ 75 percent, and a $D_{L_{CO}} \geq$ 80 percent predicted are considered normal. Those with decreased function are rated in terms of both severity of impairment and the expected effect of the impairment on ability to function in the workplace. Those with an FVC of 60 to 79 percent predicted, an FEV_1 of 60 to 79 percent predicted, an $FEV_1/FVC\%$ of 60 to 74 percent, or a $D_{L_{CO}}$ of 60 to 79 percent predicted are considered mildly impaired; however, these mild decrements in pulmonary function are not expected to diminish the ability to perform most jobs. Moderate impairment, defined as an FVC of 51 to 59 percent predicted, an FEV_1 of 41 to 59 percent predicted, an $FEV_1/FVC\%$ of 41 to 59 percent, or a $D_{L_{CO}}$ of 41 to 59 percent predicted is correlated with diminished ability to perform many jobs. Severe impairment is considered an FVC $\leq$ 50 percent predicted, an $FEV_1 \leq$ 40 percent predicted, an $FEV_1/FVC\% \leq$ 40, or a $D_{L_{CO}} \leq$ 40 percent predicted. Severe impairment suggests that the individual cannot perform most jobs and probably cannot even travel to the workplace.

The ATS specifically recommends that certain tests, such as maximal voluntary ventilation and measurements considered to be indicators of small airway dysfunction (e.g., $FEF_{25-75\%}$) not be used for evaluation of impairment, since abnormal findings on these tests do not provide additional useful information.

Arterial blood-gas analysis is not generally recommended by the ATS for evaluation of impairment and disability, since most patients with exercise-induced hypoxia already have impairment on the basis of less invasive tests, such as spirometry or $D_{L_{CO}}$ measurements. Even when a decision to perform arterial blood-gas measurements is made, abnormalities must be interpreted with caution. Arterial blood-gas analysis requires rigid control of laboratory techniques, consideration of the altitude at which the study is performed, and confirmation by repeated study with an interval of at least 4 weeks between measurements in clinically stable patients. Hypoxemia, either at rest or on exercise, is not considered evidence of severe impairment unless it is accompanied by cor pulmonale. According to the ATS statement, the presence of cor pulmonale is, in and of itself, proof of severe impairment, regardless of the spirometric results.

The ATS has recently updated its guidelines on the evaluation of impairment due to asthma.[2] By its very nature, asthma must be evaluated differently than either chronic obstructive lung disease or restrictive lung disease. Whether their asthma is caused by workplace exposures or arises spontaneously, some asthmatics are unable to work as a result of their impairment. Since airflow limitation occurs episodically in asthma and is either partially or completely reversible with appropriate therapy, it has been difficult to set acceptable and reproducible standards for specific levels of impairment. Furthermore, some individuals with asthma have no airflow limitation at the time of pulmonary function testing; rather, they have airway hyperresponsiveness when exposed by inhalation challenge to provocative agents such as methacholine or histamine.[14,24]

Current ATS recommendations for the evaluation of impairment due to asthma include a multistep process. The diagnosis must be confirmed using standard criteria. In the individual complaining of symptoms suggestive of asthma, spirometry is performed. If the $FEV_1/FVC\%$ is below normal, an inhaled beta-adrenergic agonist is administered before spirometry is repeated. A rise of 12 percent or more in the FEV_1 is indicative of asthma, while a rise of less than 12 percent is further evaluated by corticosteroid administration (beclomethasone by inhalation at a dose of >800 per day, or prednisone at 30 to 40 mg per day) and repeat spirometry after 1 to 2 weeks. If the spirometric results following corticosteroid administration show a rise in the FEV_1 of 20 percent or more, the diagnosis of asthma is confirmed.

If initial spirometry performed on a patient with asthmalike symptoms shows an $FEV_1/FVC\%$ above the lower limit of normal, methacholine or histamine challenge testing should be performed using standardized methods. Airway hyperresponsiveness is confirmed by a positive result, indicated by a fall in FEV_1 of 20 percent or greater when the concentration of the provocative agent administered by the tidal breathing method is $\leq$ 8 mg/ml (see Chapter 36).

The ATS recognizes that impairment or disability resulting from asthma may be either temporary or permanent, depending upon whether full treatment objectives have been achieved. These objectives have been published by the National Asthma Expert Panel in the United States[20] and by similar panels in the United Kingdom, Australia, New Zealand, and Canada.[11,37] If the treatment objectives have not been achieved, only a rating for temporary impairment can be assigned according to the ATS criteria, as shown in Tables 41-2 and 41-3. Reevaluation should be performed for assessment of permanent impairment when the treatment objectives are achieved or after 6 months, whichever is shorter.

Table 41-2 lists the parameters to be considered in rating impairment due to asthma. Table 41-3 classifies the impairment on the basis of a combined consideration of the parameters by adding the numerical scores achieved for each separate parameter. The stated goal of this classification system is to quantify the effects of the illness on the individual's life, rather than to focus primarily on the severity of the asthma itself.

DISABILITY EVALUATION UNDER SOCIAL SECURITY

The U.S. Social Security Administration is responsible for programs that provide benefits to the individuals who are unable to work based on physical or mental disability.[22] The legal defini-

TABLE 41-2

Factors to be Considered in Rating Impairment Due to Asthma

Score	Postbronchodilator FEV_1, % Predicted	Reversibility of FEV_1 or Degree of Airway Hyperresponsiveness		Minimum Medication Need
		% FEV_1 Change	PC_{20}, mg/ml or Equivalent	
0	>Lower limit of normal	<10	>8	No medication
1	Between 70 and lower limit of normal	10–19	Between 8 and 0.5	Occasional bronchodilator (not daily) and/or occasional cromolyn (not daily)
2	60–69	20–29	Between 0.5 and 0.125	Daily bronchodilator and/or daily cromolyn and/or daily low-dose inhaled corticosteroid (<800 mg beclomethasone or equivalent)
3	50–59	>30	<0.125	Bronchodilator on demand and daily, high-dose inhaled corticosteroid (>800 μg beclomethasone or equivalent), or occasional course (1–3 times annually) systemic corticosteroid
4	<50	—	—	Bronchodilator on demand and daily high-dose, inhaled corticosteroid (>1000 mg beclomethasone or equivalent) and daily systemic corticosteroid

SOURCE: American Thoracic Society. Modified with permission.

tion of disability under Social Security is the inability to engage in any substantial gainful activity over a period that has lasted (or can be expected to last) for at least 12 months or that is expected to result in death. In other words, individuals who are currently working are not eligible for Social Security benefits

TABLE 41-3

Impairment Rating Classes for Evaluation of Asthma

Impairment Class*	Total Score
0	0
I	1–3
II	4–6
III	7–9
IV	10–11
V	Asthma not controlled despite maximal treatment; i.e., FEV_1 remaining <50% despite use of >20 mg prednisone/day.

*The impairment rating is calculated as the sum of the patient's scores from each vertical column in Table 41-2.
SOURCE: American Thoracic Society.[2] Modified with permission.

under these programs. One of the Social Security–sponsored programs is Social Security Disability Insurance that is available to workers who have contributed to the Social Security Trust Fund through Social Security tax on their earnings. The other program, known as Supplemental Security Income (SSI), does not require prior contributions and is based on disability in individuals who have limited income and resources. Under both programs, medical evidence must be provided to field offices known as Disability Determination Services (DDSs).

The claimant's own treating physician is the preferred source of medical information for determination of eligibility for Social Security benefits. If insufficient medical evidence is available, the Social Security Administration may authorize additional data gathering through the purchase of a consultative examination. Part of this examination may consist of pulmonary function testing or other appropriate medical studies. In addition to the usual medical history, the consultant must also provide a statement about what the claimant can still do, despite his or her impairment. The Social Security Administration provides a listing of impairments that are considered severe enough to prevent an individual from engaging in any gainful activity. The criteria are identical for Social Security Disability Insurance and SSI. If an applicant meets the severity of impairment set forth in the listings, that information is usually sufficient to establish that the individual is disabled under Social Security regulations and eligible for benefits.

In order to evaluate respiratory impairment under Social Security guidelines, the applicant must undergo a chest radiograph examination and spirometry with postbronchodilator assessment, if there is evidence of airway obstruction. If these studies indicate obstructive lung disease, no further studies may be required. If interstitial lung disease or cor pulmonale is suspected, the spirometric evaluation may underestimate the degree of impairment, and additional testing, including diffusing capacity measurement or arterial blood-gas analysis, may be performed. Exercise testing with collection of arterial blood-gas measurements is also occasionally allowed by the Social Security Administration. Prior performance of right-sided heart catheterization may also be considered in decisionmaking, although the Social Security Administration does not compensate for such testing for the purpose of decisionmaking.

If the abnormalities identified by testing do not reach the level of listed impairments, the Social Security Administration considers whether the impairment or combination of impairments are medically equivalent to the listings. In addition, other factors such as active pulmonary infections lasting for more than 12 consecutive months, recurrent exacerbations of cystic fibrosis, bronchiectasis, substantial hemoptysis, chronic asthmatic bronchitis, or severe asthma may also be considered as disabling, depending on their severity. In addition, a sleep-related breathing disorder may qualify as a listed impairment if it has caused chronic cor pulmonale, pulmonary hypertension, or impaired cognitive function, or if there is morbid obesity.

Cardiopulmonary exercise testing is generally discouraged, but it may be performed if chronic pulmonary disease has been documented and other studies have failed to meet the required listings.

Asthma severity is judged under Social Security guidelines on the basis of the occurrence of severe episodes, despite adherence to a prescribed therapeutic regimen, occurring at least six times a year and requiring intensive treatment in a hospital emergency room or its equivalent, or hospitalization for longer than 24 h. Each hospitalization is counted as the equivalent of two attacks.

Abnormalities accepted as evidence of inability to work under Social Security guidelines are shown in Table 41-4 for chronic obstructive pulmonary disease, restrictive ventilatory disease, and hypoxemia at an altitude of less than 3000 feet above sea level.

WORKERS' COMPENSATION PROGRAM

The legal right to compensation for injury resulting from employment is a relatively recent phenomenon.[32] In the United States, the first legislation dealing with occupational injuries was developed in the early decades of the twentieth century and followed the example of the British Workers Compensation Statute of 1897. Most of the earliest legislation dealt with traumatic injuries. The concept of occupational illness, as opposed to occupational injury, was adapted slowly within the legal system. The U.S. federal government did not take any role in the development of these laws, and each state generated its own standards individually.

Although a few states enacted legislation of this type during the 1920s, it was not until hundreds of workers sickened and died as a result of acute silicosis from drilling operations at the Hawk's Nest Tunnel at Gauley Bridge, West Virginia,[13] in the early 1930s that the situation changed significantly. Public outrage at the circumstances of the disaster led to legislative action. Most states then began to enact their own standards, but the states often restricted the type of disease and the circumstances of exposure that were accepted as being compensable.

By 1978, all states had enacted workers' compensation laws covering occupational illnesses. State legislation was based on a compromise between labor and industry as a "no fault" liability

TABLE 41-4

Social Security Listings for Respiratory Disability

Evaluation of Chronic Obstructive Pulmonary Disease

Height without Shoes, in.	FEV_1 Equal to or Less than (L, BTPS)
60 or less	1.05
61–63	1.15
64–65	1.25
66–67	1.35
68–69	1.45
70–71	1.55
72 or more	1.64

Evaluation of Chronic Restrictive Ventilatory Disease

Height without Shoes, in.	FEV_1 Equal to or Less than (L, BTPS)
60 or less	1.25
61–63	1.35
64–65	1.45
66–67	1.55
68–69	1.65
70–71	1.75
72 or more	1.85

Evaluation of Arterial Hypoxemia at Various Levels of Arterial P_{CO_2} (Applicable at Test Sites Less than 3000 ft above Sea Level)

Arterial P_{CO_2} (mmHg)	Arterial P_{CO_2} Equal to or Less than (mmHg)
30 or below	65
31	64
32	63
33	62
34	61
35	60
36	59
37	58
38	57
39	56
40 or above	55

SOURCE: Modified from *Disability Evaluation under Social Security.* SSA Pub No 64-039.

insurance program. Injured workers received wage relief, full medical coverage, and full rehabilitation services without the necessity for lengthy and expensive litigation; industry received substantial protection from further litigation by the employee. Insurance payments were provided either through a state-administered workers' compensation fund or directly to the employee by self-insured companies.

Although workers compensation programs provide a great deal of protection for the injured employee, proof of occupational injury is still required. Disputes regarding causation of injury are adjudicated in an adversarial hearing before a referee who is appointed by the workers' compensation board. The lawyer representing the claimant usually presents testimony by a medical expert who has examined the injury worker. The employer has a right to have the worker reevaluated by an independent medical examiner and the results of that examination are also presented at the hearing. The hearing referee has the right to decide on acceptance or rejection of the claim, although he or she may or may not have any specialized knowledge of the scientific and medical issues under consideration. Decisions are made on the basis of arguments presented by the attorneys as well as the medical testimony.

In view of the fact that respiratory illness may be multifactorial in origin and may be caused in part, or in whole, by nonoccupational diseases, as well as by personal habits or aging, it has been estimated that up to 90 percent of respiratory claims are litigated in this fashion.

The first federal program for workers' compensation was enacted as the Federal Coal Mine Health and Safety Act of 1969.[19] This program provides for benefits as a result of coal worker's pneumoconiosis and is based on length of service in the coal industry and chest radiograph findings as assessed by the ILO International Classification of Pneumoconioses. Once having qualified for the diagnosis of pneumoconiosis, the miner is considered "totally disabled" if the disease prevents him from working in the immediate area of his residence using skills and abilities comparable to those he used in the coal mine. Medical criteria for total disability are arbitrarily stated in the Act and include such spirometric findings as an $FEV_1 \leq 1.6$ L for a man 66 in. tall, 1.8 L for a man 70 in. tall, and 1.9 L for a man 73 (or more) in. tall. No age requirement for the spirometric findings are listed. Since FEV_1 normally decreases with age, qualification for black lung benefits becomes easier as the miner grows older. Even if the miner fails to qualify through spirometric testing, he can still be judged totally disabled on the basis of a medical opinion furnished by one or more physicians designated by the Administration.

Workers' compensation claims in countries other than the United States are usually processed in a nonadversarial fashion by national agencies.[17] These agencies often obtain medical consultation from recognized experts or boards of experts who have previously been unassociated with the case under review. Lists or schedules of specific diseases accepted as being caused by employment are used to determine when compensation will be allowed. Such a system is used in the United Kingdom and France, as well as other Western European countries and some provinces of Canada. Disabled individuals who do not qualify for benefits under workers' compensation schedules are often covered by secondary sources of health and disability insurance that provide similar levels of support.

AMERICANS WITH DISABILITIES ACT

In the United States, the evaluation of whether an individual can perform a job has been substantially altered by enactment of the Americans with Disabilities Act (ADA) of 1990.[9,23] Prior to passage of this law, businesses were permitted to perform pre-employment physical examinations, ostensibly to evaluate physical fitness. However, it was quite apparent that many prospective employees were being excluded because of handicaps that had little or nothing to do with ability to perform the specific job being offered. To protect against this potential injustice, the ADA established rules for the evaluation of prospective workers.

According to ADA regulations, initial evaluation for a job must be performed on the basis of nonmedical criteria. The employer is specifically prohibited from asking any questions regarding health or physical impairment and may not perform medical examinations until an actual offer of employment has been made. Following an offer of employment, the prospective employer is allowed to perform a "fitness for duty" examination prior to the start of work. Any withdrawals of job offers following examinations must be supported by convincing evidence that valid medical data conclude that the individuals involved cannot perform the jobs or that the prospective employees would pose a substantial danger to themselves or coworkers in the performance of a particular job. It is not sufficient to conclude that workers with a particular disease in general cannot perform such a job, but rather, that the specific worker being considered cannot perform the specific job being offered. Furthermore, as long as the worker can perform most of the essential tasks of the job, the employer is obligated to make reasonable accommodations to the employee's handicap.

As an example, consider a worker who is being hired to perform a job that consists mostly of observing a conveyor belt in a factory to prevent jam-ups. Occasionally, however, the worker is required to lift 50-lb bags from floor level to shoulder level. Further, assume that the employee has chronic obstructive lung disease with an FEV_1 of 60 percent predicted and an $FEV_1/FVC\%$ of 59. The employer may comply with the law by providing a coworker to help with the lifting duties, but the employer may not refuse to employ the worker. However, if the job consists primarily of constant lifting of 100-lb bags, the employer could reasonably refuse to hire the job applicant. Similarly, a prospective employee with pulmonary fibrosis and normal oxyhemoglobin saturation at rest but desaturation on moderate exertion cannot be refused a job on that basis if the employment duties are clerical. The prospective employee could be refused employment if the job involved climbing to the top of water towers.

The physician's obligation under the provisions of ADA is to evaluate the physical condition of the job applicant in terms of his or her ability to perform specific tasks. The decision to hire does not belong to the physician but is solely the responsibility of the company requesting the evaluation. Embedded in the physician's professional obligation is the explicitly stated legal requirement according to the ADA to maintain confidentiality regarding all other aspects of the applicant's health. Medical files must be kept separate from other employment files, and only health professionals may have access to this information. The physician must supply enough information for the personnel office to judge fitness to perform a particular job, but he or she must not disclose other health-related information.

NONMEDICAL FACTORS THAT INTERFERE WITH ACCURATE ASSESSMENT OF IMPAIRMENT OR DISABILITY

No discussion of impairment or disability evaluation is complete without consideration of the issues of personal gain, fear of the unknown, and suboptimal effort.[29] For the physician honestly attempting to distinguish between health and impairment, the assessment of physiological normality appears clear-cut. Although techniques and opinions may vary among experts, the questions to be answered are quite simple: Do test results fall within normal range? If results are not normal, how severely has function been reduced? What effect has the reduction in function had upon the individual's ability to perform a particular job?

From the standpoint of an applicant applying for benefits or a litigant in a claim of injury, the issues are much more complicated. Financial considerations do not lend themselves easily to scientific analysis, but they are often imperatives that affect effort and performance on test procedures. Obviously some individuals are frankly dishonest and attempt to deceive the evaluating physician, but other, more subtle and less nefarious, motivations can often be discerned. Fear of a poorly understood but highly publicized potential danger (such as asbestos) frequently leads to an exaggeration of symptoms and assignment of those symptoms to a specific cause, regardless of the truth of such an assertion. Similarly, some workers are convinced that there has been a conspiracy to defraud them of their rightful compensation and feel justified in embellishing symptoms and decreasing their test performance in order to "even the score." Even when real symptoms are present, it is not unusual to find individuals who attempt to conceal other possible causations. A particularly common example of attempted concealment is the individual who firmly states that he or she has not smoked cigarettes for many years but who, nonetheless, has the odor of tobacco smoke on the breath and heavy nicotine stains on the index and middle fingers of the dominant hand.

The examiner should recognize that most respiratory testing requires the active cooperation of the examinee and that accurate interpretation of results requires an assessment of the possibility of poor effort. Numerical results cannot be accepted at face value in impairment or disability evaluations without assessing the quality of the underlying data. It is not at all unusual to detect evidence of poor effort on spirometric curves or early discontinuation of exertion on exercise testing. The examining physician should not assume that there has been an attempt at deception, but that possibility should routinely be ruled out by careful inspection of the raw data obtained during test sessions.

REFERENCES

1. American Medical Association: *Guides to the Evaluation of Permanent Impairment,* 4th ed. Chicago, American Medical Association, 1993.

2. American Thoracic Society: Guidelines for evaluation of impairment/disability in patients with asthma. *Am Rev Respir Dis* 147:1056–1061, 1993.

3. American Thoracic Society: Snowbird workshop on standardization of spirometry. *Am Rev Respir Dis* 119:831–838, 1979.

4. American Thoracic Society: Standardization of spirometry: 1987 update. *Am Rev Respir Dis* 136:1285–1298, 1987.

5. American Thoracic Society: Evaluation of impairment/disability secondary to respiratory disorders. *Am Rev Respir Dis* 133:1205–1209, 1986.

6. American Thoracic Society: Evaluation of impairment/disability secondary to respiratory disease. *Ann Rev Respir Dis* 126:945–951, 1982.

7. American Thoracic Society: Lung function testing: selection of reference values and interpretative strategies. *Am Rev Respir Dis* 144:1202–1218, 1991.

8. American Thoracic Society: Single breath carbon monoxide diffusing capacity (transfer factor). Recommendations for a standard technique. *Am Rev Respir Dis* 136:1299–1307, 1987.

9. Americans with Disabilities Act of 1990. 42 USC S 12101 et seq.

10. Becklake M: Concepts of normality applied to the measurement of lung function. *Am J Med* 80:1158–1164, 1986.

11. British Thoracic Society: Guidelines for management of asthma in adults: I. Chronic persistent asthma. *Br Med J* 301:651–653, 1990.

12. Brooks SM (Chairman): Task group on surveillance for respiratory hazards in the occupational setting. Surveillance for respiratory hazards. *ATS News* 8:12–16, 1982.

13. Cherniack M: *The Hawk's Nest Incident.* New Haven and London, Yale University, 1968.

14. Cockcroft DW, Killian DN, Mellon JJ, Hargreave FE: Bronchial reactivity to inhaled histamine. A method and clinical survey. *Clin Allergy* 7:235–243, 1977.

15. Cotes JE, Reed JW, Elliott C: Breathing and exercise requirements of the work place, in Whipp BJ, Wasserman K (eds), *Exercise, Pulmonary Physiology and Pathophysiology.* New York, Dekker, 1991.

16. Crapo RO, Morris AH, Gardner RM: Reference spirometric values using techniques and equipment that meets ATS recommendations. *Am Rev Respir Dis* 123:659–664, 1981.

17. Dewitte JD, Chan-Yeung M, Malo JL: Medicolegal and compensation aspects of occupational asthma. *Eur Respir J* 7:969–980, 1994.

18. Epler G, Saber F, Gaensler E: Determination of severe impairment (disability) in interstitial lung disease. *Am Rev Respir Dis* 121:647–659, 1980.

19. Federal Coal Mine Health and Safety Act of 1969 (Pub L91-173), enacted Dec 30, 1969, as amended by the Black Lung Benefits Act of 1972 (Pub L92-303), enacted May 19, 1972. 20 C.F.R. 410.101 et seq.

20. National Institute of Health Guidelines for the diagnosis and management of asthma. Expert panel report. National Asthma Education Program, Bethesda, MD: National Heart, Lung and Blood Institute. Pub no 91-3042A, 1991.

21. International Labour Office: *Guidelines for the Use of ILO International Classification of Radiographs of Pneumoconiosis,* rev ed. Geneva, 1980.

22. Hadler M: Medical ramifications of the federal regulation of the Social Security Disability Insurance Program. *Ann Intern Med* 96:665–669, 1982.

23. Harber P, Fedoruk, MJ: Work placement and worker fitness: implications of the Americans with Disabilities Act for pulmonary medicine. *Chest* 105:1565–1571, 1994.

24. Hargreave FE, Ryan G, Thomson NC, et al: Bronchial responsiveness to histamine or methacholine in asthma: measurement and clinical significance. *J Allergy Clin Immunol* 68:347–355, 1981.

25. Knudson RJ, Slatin RC, Lebowitz MD, Burrows B: The maximum expiratory flow-volume curve. *Am Rev Respir Dis* 113:587–600, 1976.

26. Kory RC, Callahan R, Boren HG, Syner JC: The Veterans Administration–Army Cooperative study of pulmonary function. Clinical spirometry in normal men. *Am J Med* 30:243–258, 1961.

27. Medical Research Council: *Questionnaire on Respiratory Symptoms.* London, Medical Research Council, 1966.

28. Miller WF, Scacci R: Pulmonary function assessment for determination of pulmonary impairment and disability evaluation. *Clin Chest Med* 2:327–341, 1981.

29. Morgan WKC: Clinical significance of pulmonary function tests. Disability or disinclination? Impairment or importuning. *Chest* 75:712–715, 1979.

30. Morris JF, Koski A, Johnson LC: Spirometric standards for healthy nonsmoking adults. *Am Rev Respir Dis* 103:57–67, 1971.

31. Rosenstock L, Hagopian A: Ethical dilemmas in providing health care to workers. *Ann Intern Med* 107:575–580, 1987.

32. Seligman PJ, Bernstein IL: Medicolegal and compensation aspects, in Bernstein IL, Chan-Yeung M, Malo JL, Bernstein DI (eds), *Asthma in the Workplace.* New York, Decker, 1993, pp 323–340.

33. Social Security Administration: *Disability Evaluation under Social Security.* SSA Pub No 64-039. Washington, DC, US Government Printing Office, 1995.

34. Sue DY: Exercise testing in the evaluation of impairment and disability. *Clin Chest Med* 15:369–387, 1994.

35. The Occupational and Environmental Health Committee of the American Lung Association of San Diego and Imperial Counties: Taking the occupational history. *Ann Intern Med* 99:641–651, 1983.

36. Wasserman K: The anaerobic threshold to evaluate exercise performance. *Am Rev Respir Dis* 129(suppl):S35, 1984.

37. Woolcock A, Rubinfeld AR, Seale JP, et al: Asthma management plan, 1989. *Med J Aust* 151:650–653, 1989.

PART FOUR

OBSTRUCTIVE LUNG DISEASES

SECTION 8

CHRONIC OBSTRUCTIVE PULMONARY DISEASE

CHAPTER 42

CHRONIC OBSTRUCTIVE LUNG DISEASE: OVERVIEW

Alfred P. Fishman

THE GROWTH OF IDEAS
   Chronic Obstructive Pulmonary Disease
   Cigarette Smoking

DEFINITIONS
   Emphysema
   Chronic Bronchitis
   Chronic Obstructive Pulmonary Disease
   Asthma
   Bronchiectasis
   Small-Airway Disease
   Bronchiolitis Obliterans (and BOOP)
   Lung Volume Reduction Surgery

THE GROWTH OF IDEAS

Chronic Obstructive Pulmonary Disease

The beginnings of modern chest medicine can be traced to the classic volume by Laennec, *A Treatise on the Diseases of the Chest*, which appeared in 1821.[36] This book, based on an enormous clinical experience and 18 years of clinicopathologic follow-up at the autopsy table, laid the cornerstone of modern chest medicine. Together with Auenbrugger's invention of auscultation, it established the role of physical diagnosis in medicine.

Laennec (Fig. 42-1) was not the first to relate morbid anatomy to clinical medicine. In 1760, Morgagni published his work *De sedibus et causis morborum* ("On the sites and causes of diseases"), which was based on his vast personal experience in performing postmortem examinations. In this tome, the findings at autopsy are related, case by case, to the patient's clinical history and course, and an attempt is made to relate symptoms to lesions. Morgagni was the first to describe the pathology of many diseases, including solidification of the lung in pneumonia.

After Morgagni, Corvisart (1755–1821) and Bichat (1771–1802), distinguished clinicians in Paris, used clinicopathologic correlations as the bases of their clinical practices and teachings. But it fell to Laennec not only to enlarge the horizons of chest medicine by inventing the stethoscope but also to explore the physical signs of many chest diseases. He showed that it was possible in the living to anticipate the physical changes in internal organs that would be found at autopsy. According to Forbes, translator of the English edition, a unique contribution by Laennec was that "he not only traces the progressive change of structure in the organ, but connects every successive step of the change with external signs indicative of its existence."[36]

In his treatise, Laennec devoted one chapter to "pulmonary catarrh or bronchitis" and another to emphysema. The chapter on bronchitis distinguishes between acute and chronic forms and subdivides chronic bronchitis into two types, the "humid" ("copious expectoration") and "dry" ("scarcely any expectoration"). Failure to observe this distinction, promulgated by Laennec in the nineteenth century, was destined to becloud twentieth-century attempts at determining the prevalence of chronic bronchitis in the United States.

chronic bronchitis was the same disease on both sides of the ocean but that the disease in Europe (e.g., Great Britain and the Netherlands) was generally more severe and characterized by greater production of sputum. Along with this reconciliation came insights into why some instances of chronic bronchitis were more of a nuisance than incapacitating: cough and sputum, the hallmarks of chronic bronchitis, were not responsible for high morbidity and mortality unless lung function, as manifested by limitation in airflow, was also impaired. Uncertainty about the clinical diagnosis of emphysema was not as readily dispelled: clinicians made the diagnosis of emphysema when cough and sputum were associated with breathlessness on exertion. Unfortunately, autopsy studies were subsequently to prove that these clinical hallmarks were unreliable predictors of findings at autopsy.

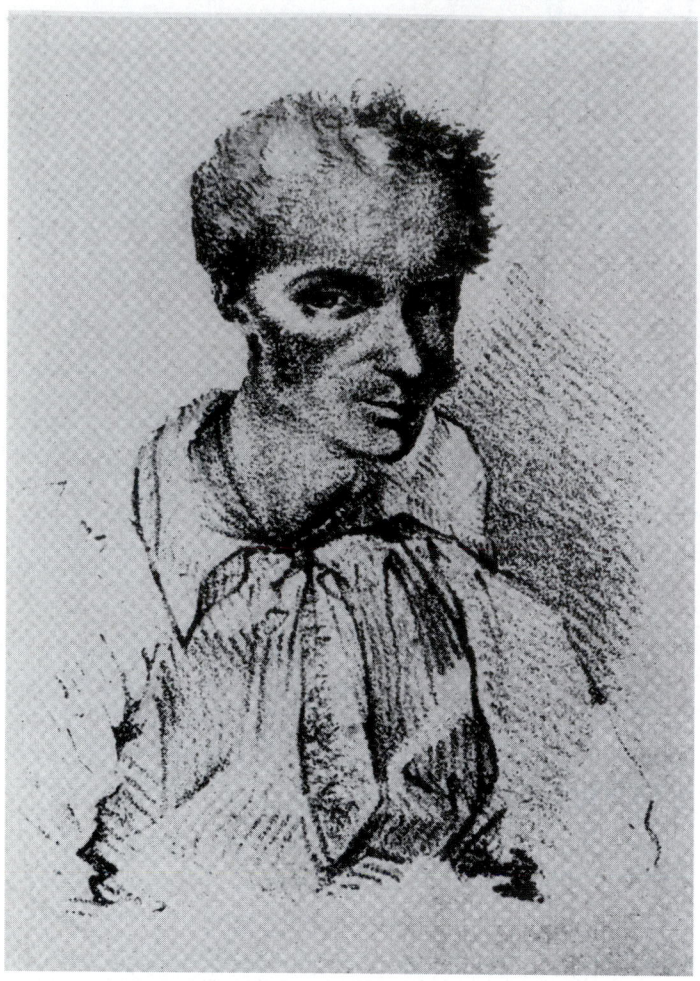

FIGURE 42-1 René-Théophile-Hyacinthe Laennec (1781–1826). Drawing and lithograph by Laennec are from about 1820, while he was undergoing rest treatment for tuberculosis. *(From Long ER: Selected Readings in Pathology. Springfield, IL, Charles C Thomas, 1929, p 144.)*

Laennec's chapter on emphysema draws together his personal observations and those of his predecessors into a remarkable depiction not only of structure but also of function. After giving due credit to those, such as Bonet (1620–1689) and Morgagni (1682–1771), who described isolated aspects of emphysema, he identified "dilatation of the air cells" as the essential feature of emphysema. The importance of disruption of alveolar walls in the functional consequences of emphysema was to come much later[11] (Fig. 42-2).

Recognition of chronic bronchitis as a potentially grave illness rather than as a trivial but nondisabling disease had to await the London fog of 1952. This fog, brought about by bad weather and air pollutants, carried with it a surge in morbidity and mortality due to chronic lung disease. Epidemiologists in the United States, the Netherlands, and elsewhere began to take serious stock of the prevalence of chronic bronchitis and emphysema and to wonder why the diagnosis of "emphysema" rarely appeared on death certificates in Great Britain and why the diagnosis of chronic bronchitis *never* appeared on death certificates in the United States.[7–9,18–20]

By applying standardized questionnaires in the United States and Europe, cooperative epidemiologic studies showed that

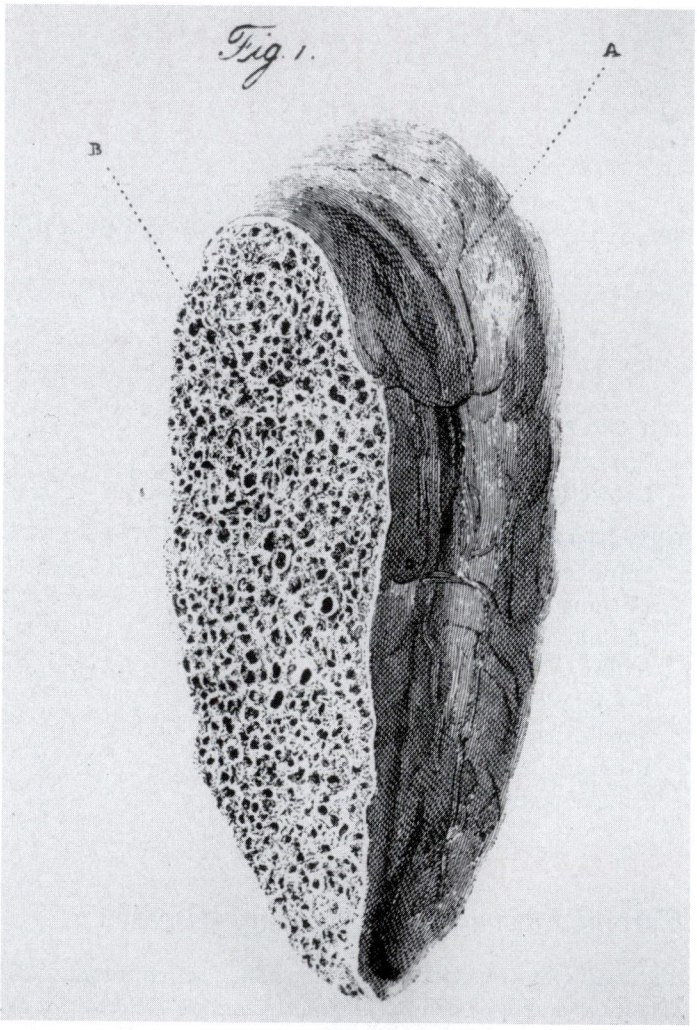

FIGURE 42-2 The emphysematous lung of Samuel Johnson, lexicographer. In 1793, in the original edition of his classic text, . . . *The Morbid Anatomy of Some of the Most Important Parts of the Human Body*, Baille provided the following description: "The lungs are sometimes, although I believe very rarely, formed into pretty large cells, so as to resemble somewhat the lungs of an amphibious animal. . . ." He also notes that the person from whom the lung had been obtained (presumably Samuel Johnson) "had been very long subject to difficulty of breathing."[4,41]

After World War II, clinical investigation of pulmonary diseases intensified, and clinicians were provided with a new diagnostic armamentarium: pulmonary function tests were extended beyond simple spirometry, and innovative techniques were developed for assessing the distribution of gases within the lungs; the regulation of breathing in chronic pulmonary disease began to be systematically explored; arterial blood-gas tensions became available, and right heart catheterization made it possible to record pulmonary arterial pressures and to apply the Fick principle for the determination of pulmonary blood flow (the cardiac output).

Because of lingering uncertainties about the differential diagnosis of chronic obstructive airway diseases, a CIBA symposium was convened in 1958 in an attempt to sort out its subsets.[11] Four major proposals at the CIBA meeting were destined to make a lasting impression on chest medicine: (1) instead of reliance on clinical findings for the diagnosis of emphysema, emphysema was to be defined in anatomic terms; (2) chronic bronchitis was to be defined as "chronic or recurrent excessive mucus secretion in the bronchial tree" that is manifested clinically by cough and expectoration and for which no other specific lung disease can be identified; (3) the concept of airflow limitation was introduced and used as a basis for distinguishing between nuisance bronchitis (Laennec's "catarrh") and the incapacitating bronchitis of chronic obstructive pulmonary disease; and (4) distinction was drawn between reversible obstructive airway disease (as in asthma) and persistent obstructive airway disease (as in "chronic obstructive pulmonary disease").[21] A major advance in the years following the CIBA symposium was the general awareness that the limitation to airflow caused by emphysema could be as severe as that caused by chronic bronchitis even though the mechanisms for increases in resistance to airflow were different: pulling on terminal airways by overdistended lungs in emphysema versus bronchoconstriction and mucous hypersecretion in large airways in chronic bronchitis.[1]

The advent of Gough sections (Fig. 42-3), which provided thin sagittal sections of the entire lung, helped to categorize two pathologic subtypes of emphysema based on the location of the lung destruction: (1) *centrilobular* (centriacinar), characterized by lung destruction in the center of the lung lobule and greater involvement of the upper lobes than of the lower lobes, and (2) *panlobular* (panacinar), characterized by uniform lung destruction within the lung lobule and greater involvement of the lower lobes than of the upper lobes (Figs. 42-4 and 42-5).[25,26,38] Cigarette smoking is commonly associated with both, but more often with centrilobular emphysema.[29] α_1-Antiprotease deficiency is usually associated with panlobular emphysema (Fig. 42-6). Frequently the centrilobular and panlobular types overlap, and the severity of involvement can vary greatly not only from lobe to lobe but also within a lobe. Moreover, both types of emphysema may be associated with bullae—i.e., emphysematous spaces greater than 1 cm in diameter when fully distended. Despite the overlap found at autopsy (Fig. 42-7), it seems likely that the pathogenetic mechanisms at work in the two types of emphysema are different. In support of this supposition is the observation on the lungs of cigarette smokers that for the same decrease in elastic recoil, the distensibility in the two types may differ.[45]

Up to this juncture, studies of chronic obstructive pulmonary disease had relied heavily on clinical-pathologic-physiological correlations.[44] A novel approach to the understanding of the

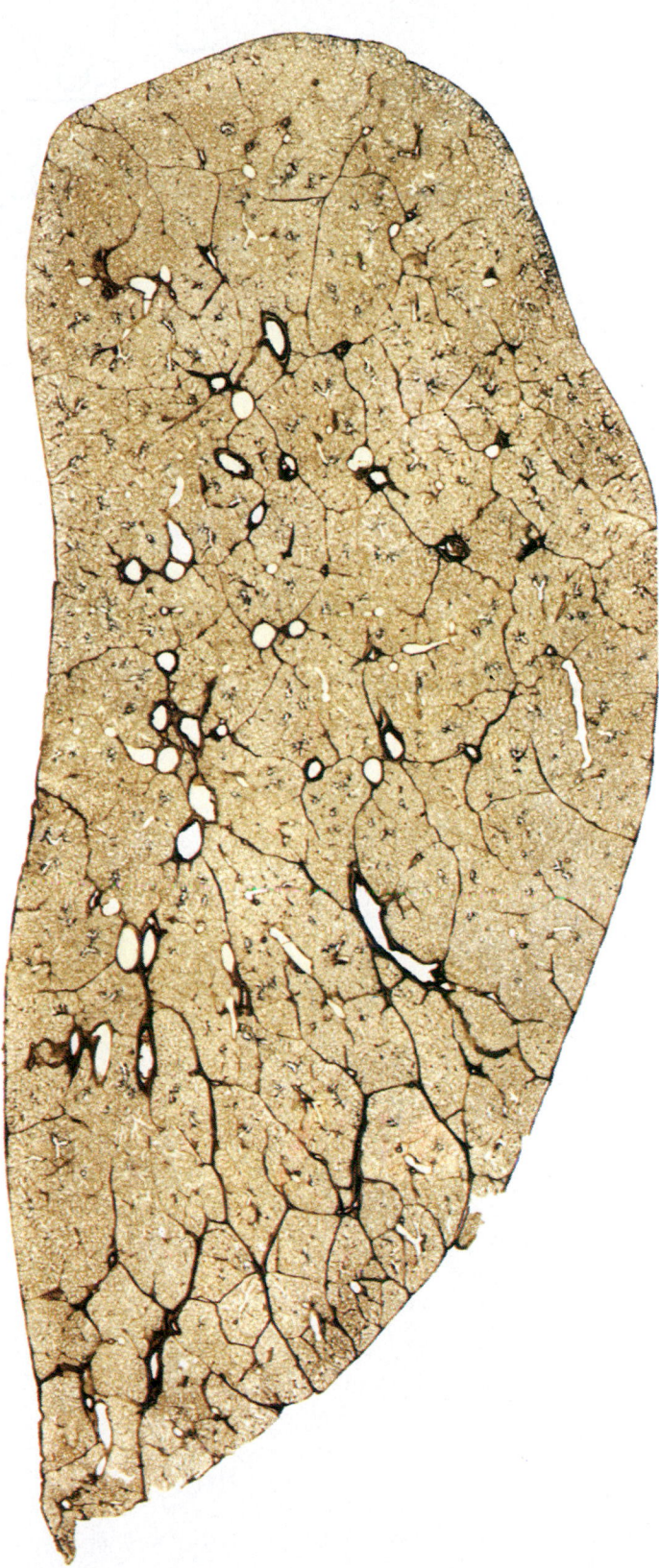

FIGURE 42-3 Gough sagittal section. Paper mount. Normal lung. *(This section and subsequent sagittal sections courtesy of Dr. S. Moolton.)*

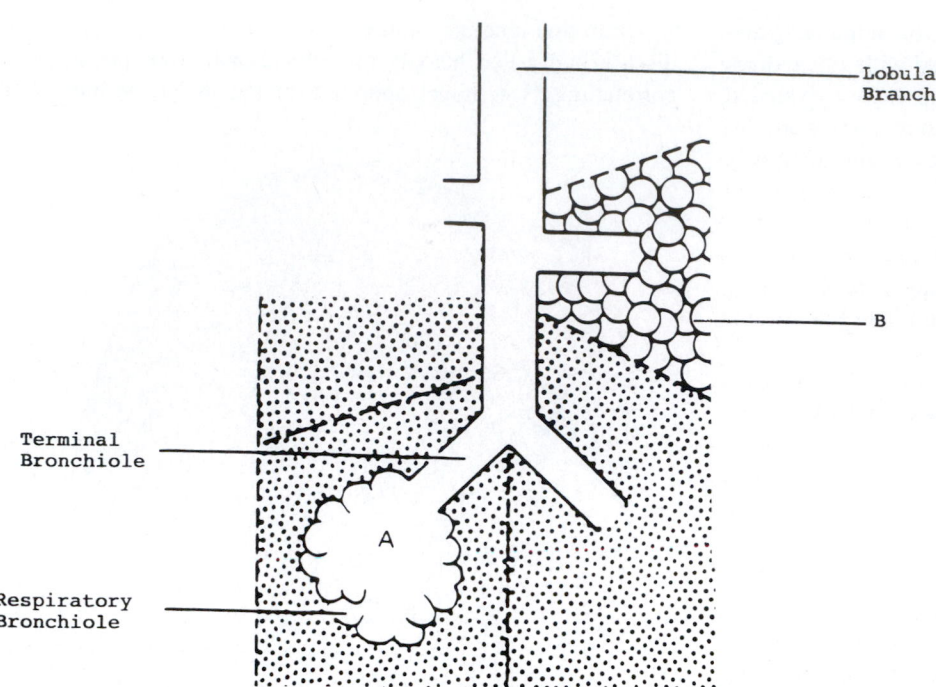

FIGURE 42-4 Anatomic varieties of emphysema. *A.* Centrilobular (centriacinar). *B.* Panlobular (panacinar). Dashed lines mark the edge of an acinus. *(Modified from Reid LM in Fishman.*[18]*)*

pathogenesis of emphysema began with the identification of the association of α_1-antitrypsin deficiency with panlobular emphysema. This association has since pointed the way to the study of the various elements operating to preserve the integrity of pulmonary architecture.[16]

Cigarette Smoking

The role of smoking in the pathogenesis of chronic obstructive lung disease received considerable attention in the 1960s. By the late 1970s, it was clear that the earliest lesions demonstrable in smokers affected the small airways—i.e., small bronchi and bronchioles.[30,31] Inflammation and fibrosis are cardinal elements contributing to limitation in airflow. Abnormalities in the larger airways contribute to a lesser degree. The harmful effects of smoking can be manifested primarily by catarrh as well as by limitation of airflow. Of these two

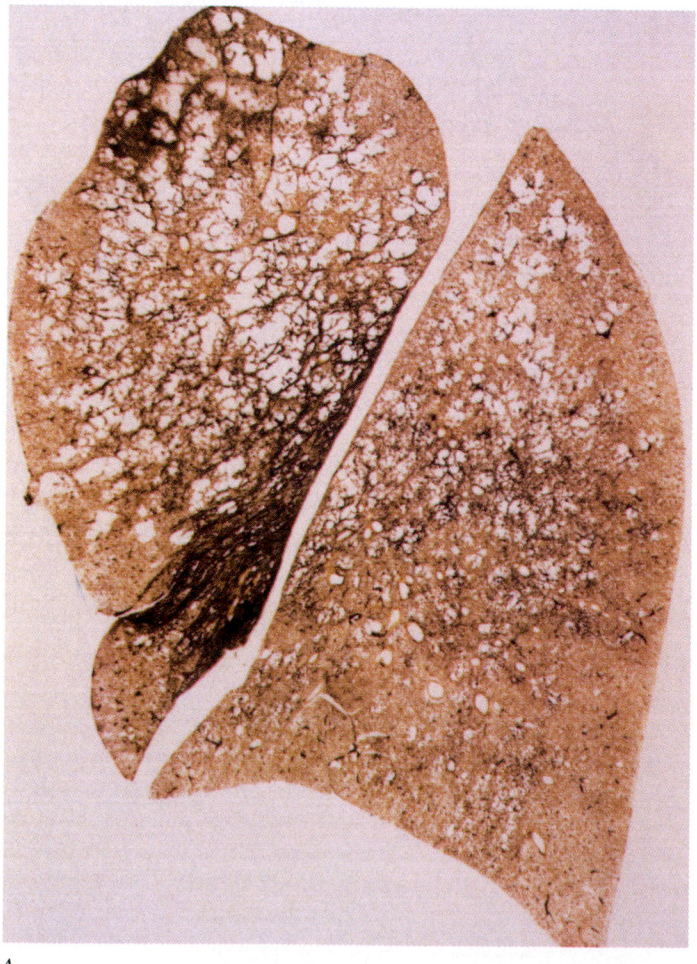

A

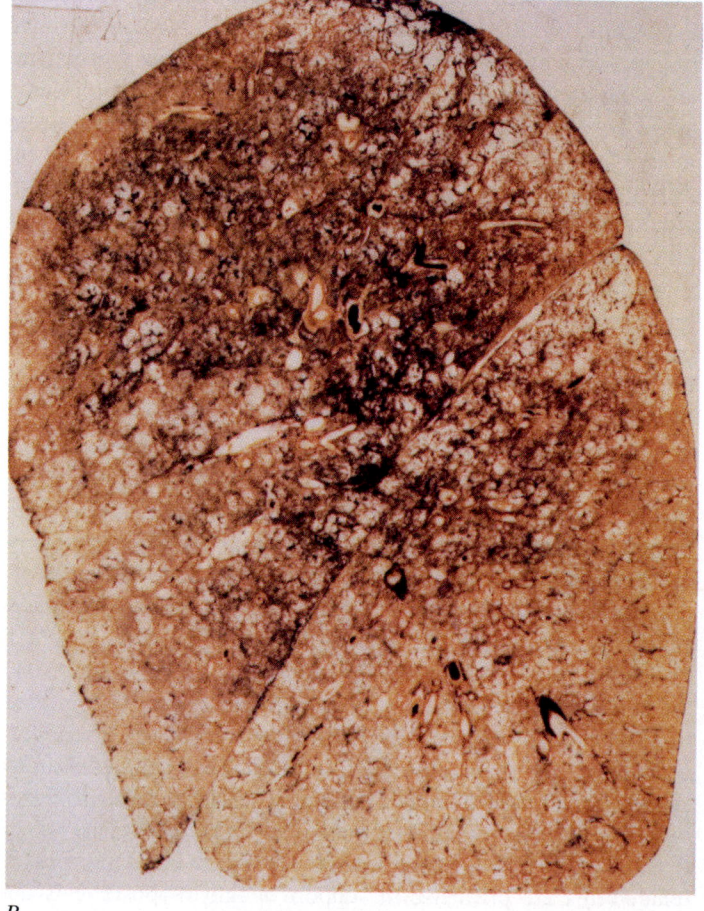

B

FIGURE 42-5 Pathologic subtypes of emphysema. *A.* Predominantly centrilobular emphysema. Chronic bronchitis at autopsy. Emphysema is more severe in upper lobes. *B.* Predominantly panlobular emphysema. Emphysema is more severe in lower lobes.

types, the catarrhal is more common; it occurs in about 80 percent of smokers. Also, the volume of sputum production is not directly related to limitation of airflow.[19,28]

Identification of the separate clinical pathways, one leading to disability due to airflow limitation and the other to nuisance due to excess sputum production, directed attention to the ability of cigarette smoke, a complex mixture of air pollutants, to injure different parts of the airways and pulmonary parenchyma. The sites and nature of the injury proved to depend not only on the composition of the smoke but also on the vulnerability, possibly genetic predisposition to injury, of different individuals. Thus, in some persons, the predominant effect of smoking may be hypertrophy of mucous glands and hypersecretion; in others, it may damage small airways, destroy alveolar walls, and modify elastic recoil of the lungs.

DEFINITIONS

Ever since Laennec, the lack of precise definitions has handicapped the study of chronic obstructive pulmonary diseases.[52,53] Scadding pointed out that Laennec appreciated that "nothing hurts the progress of science more than to divert terms from their customary meaning without sufficient reason, or to create new bad ones."[46] During the past half-century, definitions of chronic obstructive diseases have been refined repeatedly as the result of fresh clinical observations, new diagnostic tools, and sophisticated epidemiologic studies.[6,20,52]

Emphysema

This entity continues to be defined in anatomic terms—i.e., abnormal permanent enlargement of the gas-exchanging units of the lungs (acini) in association with destruction of alveolar walls and without obvious fibrosis.[1,2,44,48,49] The predominant physiological consequence of these anatomic abnormalities is a decrease in the elastic recoil of the lungs—which, in turn, causes outward displacement of the chest wall and flattening of the diaphragm, hyperinflation of the lungs, and increased resistance to airflow due to circumferential traction on the small airways by the overdistended lungs. The hyperinflation places the respiratory muscles at mechanical disadvantage, increasing the work and the oxygen cost of breathing. Although imbalances in ventilation–perfusion are seldom as marked as those in chronic (clinically significant) bronchitis, derangements sufficient to cause arterial hypoxemia are common.

Despite the emphasis on anatomic changes as the basis for the definition of emphysema, the clinical consequences of the decrease in elastic recoil (noted above) have enabled the diagnosis to be made, with considerable assurance, on clinical grounds. The conventional chest radiograph can be particularly helpful in this regard, especially when emphysema is marked. Computed tomography has sharpened this diagnostic capability.[24] Recent advances in imaging techniques hold promise of extending the capability of visualizing emphysematous areas and of localizing them three-dimensionally (Fig. 42-8).

The recently rekindled interest in lung reduction surgery has underscored the importance of distinguishing between the respective roles of emphysema and chronic bronchitis in the clinical syndrome of chronic obstructive lung disease, since the operation holds promise of successful outcome only if the airflow limitation is due to the decrease in elastic recoil and not to obstruction originating within the airways. Lung reduction surgery has also directed attention to the size and distribution of the emphysematous area because "lung trimming" may be most effective if discrete areas of emphysema can be identified for surgical removal (see below).

Chronic Bronchitis

As has been pointed out, chronic bronchitis is not a single clinical entity, and it is the airflow limitation that it produces that leads to serious morbidity and mortality.[5,43,49] This limitation has been identified traditionally from a decrease in the FEV_1. In recent years, more sophisticated tests (e.g., measurements made during a forced expiration at timed segments in the recording of flow-volume patterns) have made it possible to identify airflow limitation at stages earlier than that marked by a subnormal FEV_1. Such tests have raised the possibility of even recognizing the stages of mild airflow limitation that precede clinical manifestations.[41] However, the problem remains that chronic bronchitis is often associated with emphysema and that the relative contributions of each to limitation in airflow can be difficult to distinguish.

Chronic Obstructive Pulmonary Disease

The designation *chronic obstructive pulmonary disease* (COPD) is a clinical refuge. It recognizes that chronic bronchitis and emphysema generally coexist but that generally it is not possible, until the respiratory disease is extreme in one aspect or another, to quantify the relative contributions of each to the clinical syndrome (Fig. 42-9). The most recent definition, sponsored by the American Thoracic Society, defines "chronic obstructive pulmonary disease (COPD) as a disease state characterized by the presence of airflow obstruction due to chronic bronchitis or emphysema; the airflow obstruction is generally progressive, may be accompanied by airway hyperreactivity, and may be partially reversible."[3] Diagnostic features of this inclusive nonspecific entity are chronic productive cough, breathlessness on exertion, physiological evidence of airflow limitation (e.g., reduced $FEV_{1.0}$), and poor reversibility (e.g., response to bronchodilators).[47,53]

Attempts have been made to sort out on clinical and functional grounds the predominantly bronchitic from the predominantly emphysematous patient (Tables 42-1 and 42-2). One attempt along this line has been the distinction between the "pink puffer" and the "blue bloater" (Fig. 42-10). The pink puffer is thin, breathes through pursed lips, and maintains normal levels of P_{CO_2}; as a rule, the patient is breathless and lives longer than the blue bloater. In contrast, the blue bloater is generally better fed, evinces less pursed-lip breathing, presents with clinical evidence of inadequate ventilatory drive and chronic CO_2 retention, and is on the verge of right heart failure.[14]

This type of separation has been challenged largely on the ground that at autopsy, most patients have a combination of air-

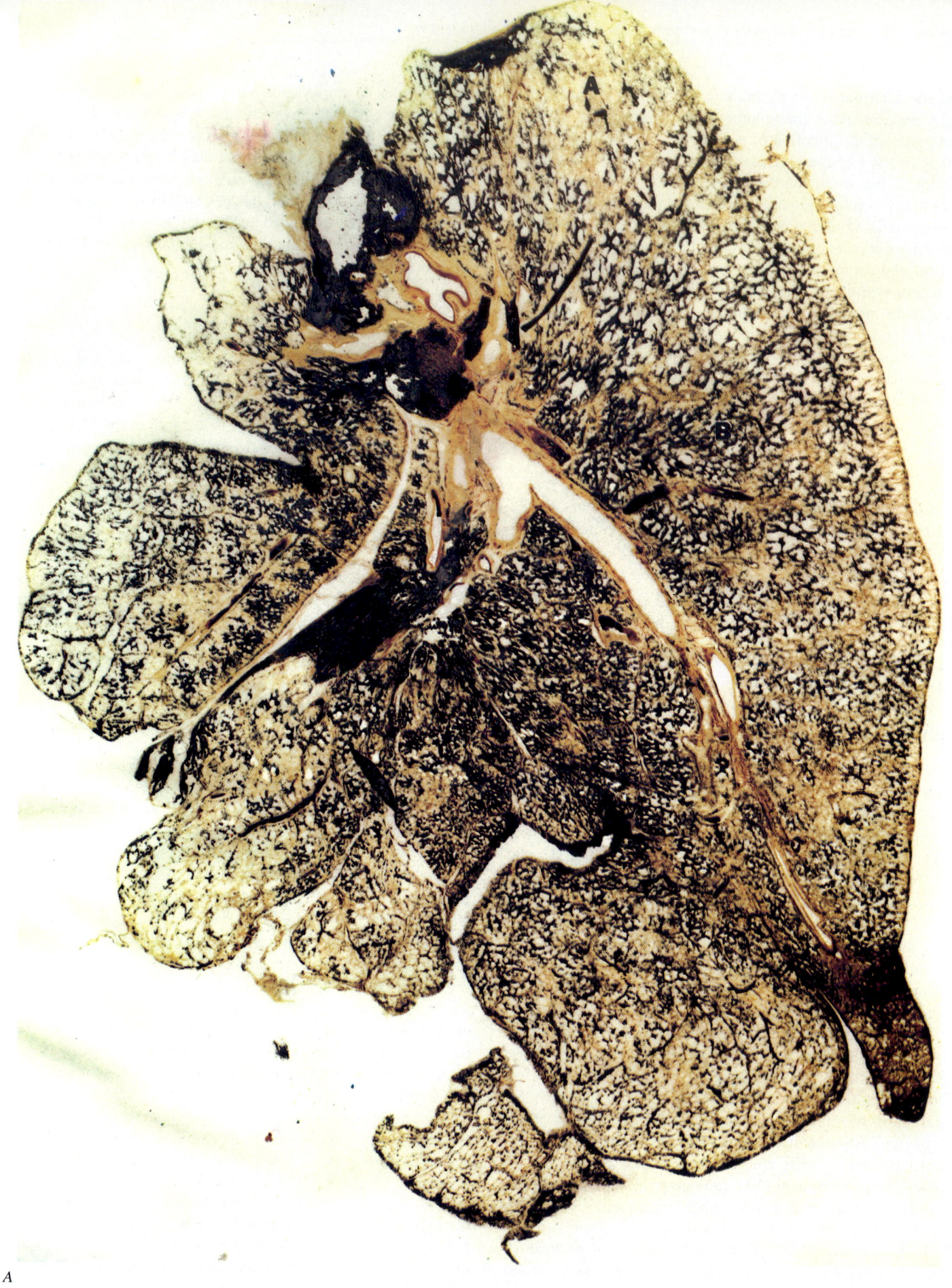

A

FIGURE 42-6 Proteinase = antiproteinase imbalance; severe widespread panlobular emphysema. *A.* α-1 antitrypsin deficiency. *B.* PiZ type α-1 antitrypsin deficiency.

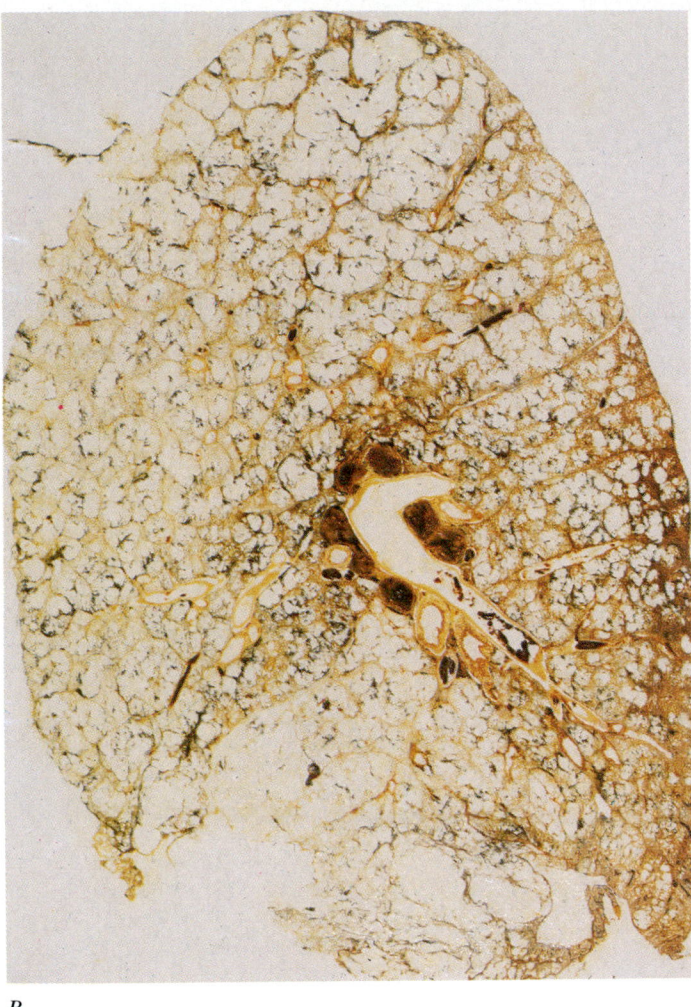

B

FIGURE 42-6   *(cont.)*

way and alveolar disease,[49] so it is not possible to pinpoint the morbid anatomy in the living patient (e.g., to equate the blue bloater with chronic bronchitis and the pink puffer with emphysema). Nonetheless, some clinics have found pink puffers and blue bloaters to be distinctive clinical entities—i.e., the stereotypical pink puffer is undeniably different in appearance, natural history, and longevity from the blue bloater—even though distinctions tend to blur in many instances, particularly when the pink puffer develops a severe upper respiratory infection and CO_2 retention supervenes; at that time, the two are clinically indistinguishable until the infection subsides.

Asthma

As a rule, clinicians believe that they can identify most patients with atopic or "extrinsic" asthma that begins in childhood and those with "intrinsic" asthma of middle age.[10] However, uncertainty creeps in when wheezing accompanies limitation to airflow in some patients with an acute exacerbation of bronchitis in the course of COPD. As indicated in Chapter 6, key elements in the differential diagnosis are the reversibility in asthma of the obstruction to airflow (either by treatment or

spontaneously) and hyperresponsiveness of the airways to diverse inciting influences. The diverse causes of asthma are reflected in a variety of qualifiers, such as "atopic," "occupational," "cardiac," and "cold induced." It is the hypersensitivity of asthma that is responsible for the episodes of widespread, but reversible, narrowing of the airways. Although the inflammatory component of asthma has attracted increasing attention in recent years, bronchoconstriction is recognized to play a critical role in evoking limitation to airflow.[50]

In asthma, the larger bronchi are predominantly affected: goblet cells undergo hyperplasia, bronchial glands hypertrophy, the basement membrane thickens, airway smooth muscle hypertrophies, and the lumina and walls are invaded by eosinophils. The inflammatory process extends to the distal airways: the inflammatory changes there vary in intensity; in severe inflammation, plugs may form of mucus and of shed necrotic bronchiolar epithelium. The inflammatory changes, coupled with submucosal edema, contribute to the airway obstruction.[32,42]

Bronchiectasis

Localized bronchiectasis is often present in patients with COPD. As a rule, however, bronchiectasis is characterized by dilation of airways rather than by narrowing (see Chapter 121). Bronchiectasis does not contribute to obstruction of airflow. In cystic fibrosis, bronchiectasis is a consistent concomitant. Characteristically, proximal airways are dilated and distal airways are obstructed by mucopurulent exudate and by narrowed, obliterated terminal airways (Fig. 42-11).

Small-Airway Disease

The designation *small-airway disease* began with observations made at autopsy. It refers to obstruction of small airways (less than 2 mm in diameter)—i.e., a combination of small bronchi and bronchioles—by inflammation and mucous plugs. This label has been carried over into in vivo measurements of small-airway function that are more localizing than the FEV_1 (e.g., closing volume).[30,39]

Bronchiolitis Obliterans (and BOOP)

The designation *bronchiolitis obliterans* was coined in 1901,[15] along with the description of an acute respiratory illness of unknown cause that resulted in the death of two patients. The lesions affected the terminal branches of the bronchial tree, where bronchi became devoid of cartilage in their walls. During the following decade, individual case reports appeared in rapid succession as different causes of bronchiolitis obliterans were uncovered (e.g., idiopathic, fume related, postinfectious).[27,35]

Between the 1940s and 1960s, there was an outpouring of papers that enlarged these categories by adding examples of novel toxic inhalants. A common feature at autopsy was partial or complete obliteration of the lumina by organizing connective tissue and peribronchiolar fibrous proliferation. In 1966, Liebow and Carrington described the entity of *bronchiolitis interstitial pneumonia*, in which pathologic changes in the bronchioles resembled

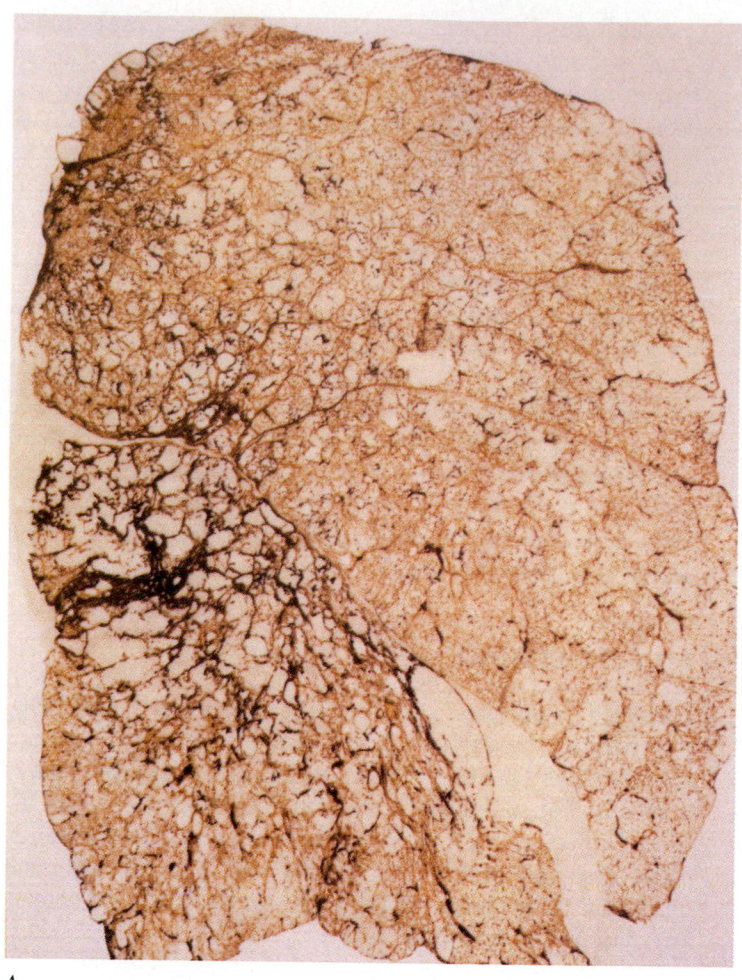

A

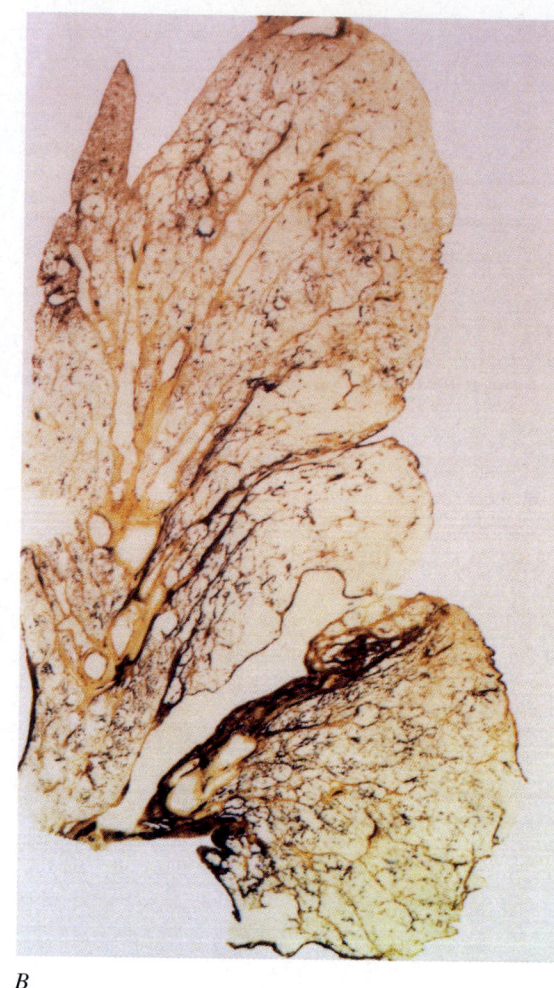

B

FIGURE 42-7   Widespread overlapping emphysema. *A.* "Pink puffer" who died in respiratory insufficiency precipitated by a viral infection.   *B.* "Blue bloater" with severe chronic bronchitis and emphysema.

those in the alveoli. Thus, by the 1970s, it was appreciated that bronchiolitis obliterans could be caused by one or more of three processes: plugging of the terminal bronchioles (1) from within by organizing exudate, (2) by constriction of the bronchioles due to inflammation and fibrosis within their walls, and (3) as part of a bronchiolar–alveolar process in which terminal bronchioles and adjacent alveoli are part of the same pathologic process.

During the 1970s, the rate at which new causes of bronchiolitis obliterans were uncovered accelerated: Connective-tissue disorders, toxic inhalants, and cigarette smoking attracted particular attention. In the 1980s, the focus of interest in bronchiolitis obliterans widened from preoccupation with the pathologic findings at autopsy to include clinical manifestations and pulmonary function testing. The span of causes increased greatly with the inclusion of immunologic disorders and infections in immunocompromised hosts. For example, in 1982, graft-versus-host disease was identified as the cause of bronchiolitis obliterans after allogeneic bone transplantation for aplastic anemia. In 1984, reports began to appear of bronchiolitis obliterans in patients who had undergone heart–lung or lung transplantation but had no evidence of graft-versus-host disease. Whether chronic lung allograft rejection or vi-

ral infection (i.e., cytomegalic inclusion virus or adenovirus) was the cause began to be debated. The debate concerning the respective roles of rejection and infection continues to the present.[15]

In 1985, the entity of bronchiolitis obliterans organizing pneumonia (BOOP) was described.[15] Its hallmarks were the presence of plugs of granulation tissue in the small airways, often with extension of the granulation tissue into alveolar ducts and alveoli. Distinctions were drawn between BOOP and other entities, such as usual interstitial pneumonia. A wide variety of causes were also identified for BOOP; among these were idiopathic infections and connective-tissue disorders. Currently, in part because of experiences with lung transplantation and in part because of those with BOOP, interest remains high in bronchiolitis obliterans, its etiology, its pathogenesis, and its management.

Lung Volume Reduction Surgery

As indicated above, emphysema, characterized anatomically by enlargement of airspaces distal to the terminal bronchioles in conjunction with destruction of alveolar walls, is characterized phys-

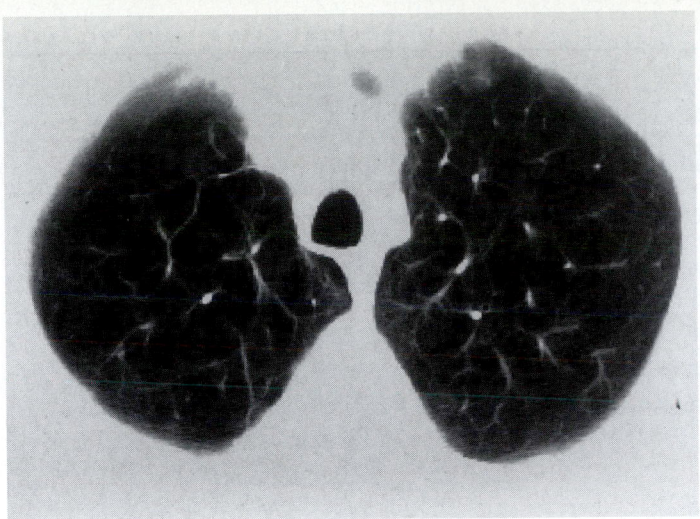

A

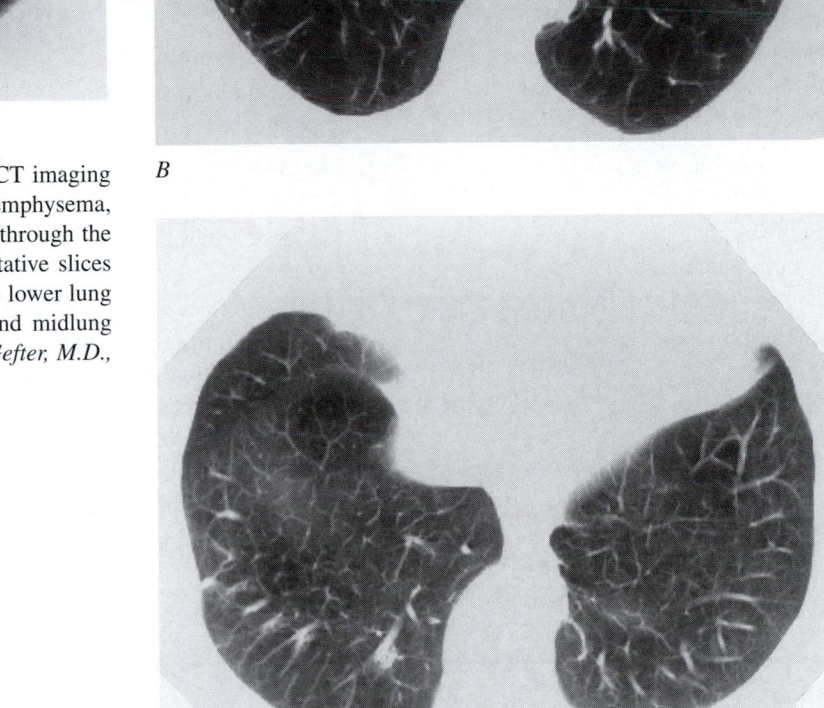

B

FIGURE 42-8 Distribution of emphysema displayed by CT imaging of the lungs. Helical CT scan of a 58-year-old man with emphysema, performed before lung volume reduction surgery. Imaging through the lungs was acquired during a single breath hold. Representative slices are shown: *(A)* upper lung zone, *(B)* midlung zone, and *(C)* lower lung zone. Centrilobular emphysema is present in the upper and midlung zones; the lung bases are spared. *(Courtesy of Warren B. Gefter, M.D., and Jean-Marc David.)*

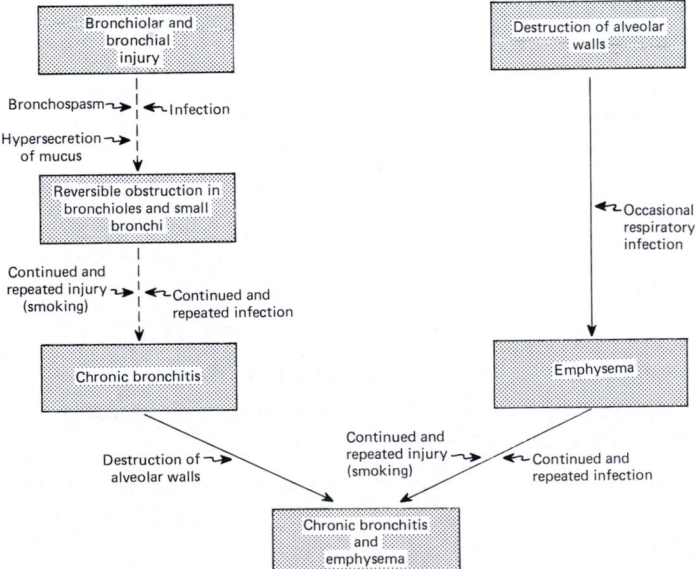

C

FIGURE 42-9 Schematic representation of the evolution of chronic bronchitis (left) and emphysema (right). Although both can culminate in chronic bronchitis and emphysema, the pathways are different, and either one or the other may predominate. The dashed arrows on the left reflect uncertainty about the origins of chronic bronchitis in small-airway disease (bronchiolar inflammation and obstruction).

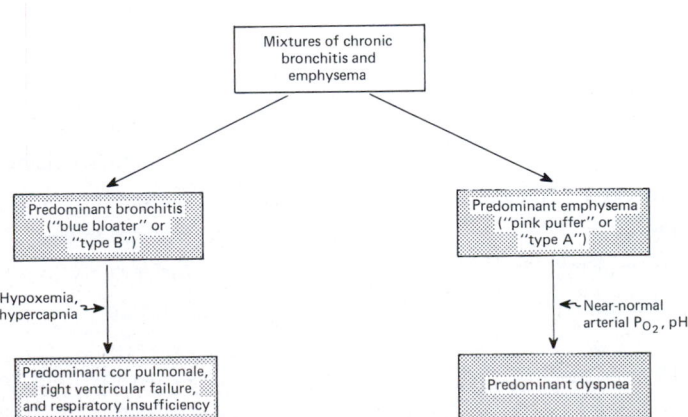

FIGURE 42-10 Blue bloater versus pink puffer. The blue bloater is pictured as predominantly bronchitic. A relatively hyporesponsive respiratory center blunts the ventilatory response to CO_2, resulting in chronic hypoxemia, hypercapnia, and respiratory acidosis.

TABLE 42-1

Clinical Hallmarks: Predominant Bronchitis Versus Predominant Emphysema

	Predominant Bronchitis	*Predominant Emphysema*
General appearance	Mesomorphic; overweight; dusky with suffused conjunctivae; warm extremities	Thin, often emaciated; pursed-lip breathing; anxious, prominent use of accessory muscles; normal or cool extremities
Age, years	40–55	50–75
Onset	Cough	Dyspnea
Cyanosis	Marked	Slight to none
Cough	More evident than dyspnea	Less evident than dyspnea
Sputum	Copious	Scanty
Upper respiratory infections	Common	Occasional
Breath sounds	Moderately diminished	Markedly diminished
Cor pulmonale and right-sided heart failure	Common	Only during bout of respiratory infection, and terminally
Radiograph	Normal diaphragm position; cardiomegaly; lungs normal or with increased bronchovascular markings	Small, pendulous heart; low, flat diaphragms; areas of increased radiolucency
Course	Ambulatory but constantly on verge of right-sided heart failure and coma	Incapacitating breathlessness punctuated by life-threatening bouts of upper respiratory infections; prolonged course, culminating in right-sided heart failure and coma

TABLE 42-2

Functional Hallmarks: Predominant Bronchitis Versus Predominant Emphysema

	Predominant Bronchitis	*Predominant Emphysema*
FEV_1/VC	Reduced	Reduced
FRC	Mildly increased	Markedly increased
TLC	Normal or slightly increased	Considerably increased
RV	Moderately increased	Markedly increased
Lung compliance	Normal or low	Normal or low
Recoil pressure	Normal or high	Low
MVV	Moderately decreased	Markedly decreased
Airway resistance	Increased	Normal or slightly increased
D_{CO}	Normal or low	Low
Arterial P_{O_2}	Moderately to severely reduced	Slightly to moderately reduced
Arterial hypercapnia	Chronic	Only during acute respiratory infection
Hematocrit	Generally high, may reach 70%	Normal or slightly high, rarely above 55%
Pulmonary artery pressure	Generally increased	Normal or slightly increased

NOTE: TLC = total lung capacity; RV = residual volume; D_{CO} = diffusing capacity of carbon monoxide.

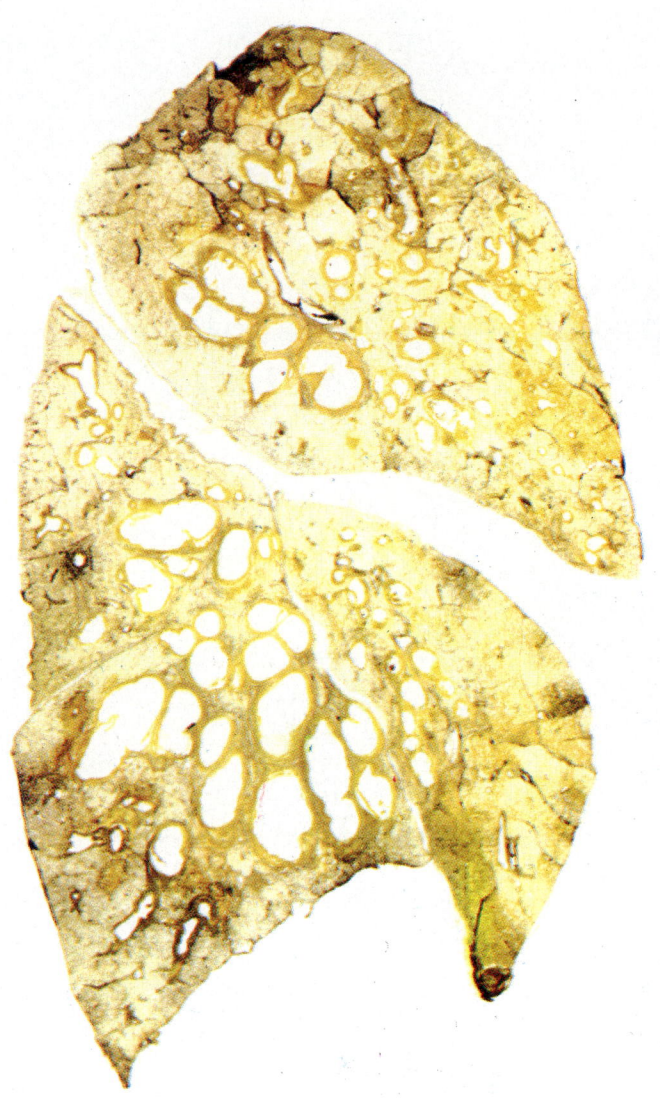

FIGURE 42-11 Bronchiectasis. Cystic fibrosis. The bronchi are greatly dilated and deformed by the inflammatory process. Mucopurulent exudate was removed during fixation of the lung.

iologically by loss of elastic recoil—which, in turn, leads to limitation of airflow during expiration and hyperinflation. Advanced stages of this disease lead to incapacitation—largely because of dyspnea on mild exertion, which imposes severe restrictions on daily activity and the quality of life. Intensive medical therapy—including administration of bronchodilators by inhalation, supplemental oxygen, and pulmonary rehabilitation—often proves ineffective in coping with severe forms of the disease. Because of the large number of affected persons and the prospect that surgical removal of local areas of overdistended and malfunctioning lung might be helpful when medical therapy fails, attempts have been made during the past 40 years to provide "surgical trimming" of the lungs, which might improve the lot of these patients by reducing total lung volume by 20 to 30 percent.

Lung reduction surgery is based on a different conceptual and practical framework than is surgical removal of large bullae,

which had become standard procedure by the mid-1950s.[37] In the late 1950s, Brantigan and Mueller reported a series of patients who had undergone resection of lung tissue that was emphysematous rather than the seat of bullae.[6] The rationale underlying the procedure was that with the excision of wedges of emphysematous lung tissue, lung volume would be reduced with several desirable consequences: (1) improvement in elastic recoil of the thorax and patency of the intrathoracic airways, (2) improvement in the mechanical function of the muscles of respiration by diminishing the expansion of the thoracic cage and repositioning the diaphragm, and (3) relief of compression of normal lung caused by localized areas of emphysema. It was anticipated that with removal of emphysematous lung that was nonfunctional, dyspnea would decrease, exercise tolerance would increase, and pulmonary function would improve. Although the surgical intervention did improve the clinical state of most of the patients, the high rate of postoperative morbidity and mortality precluded wide acceptance of this procedure.

Approximately 40 years later, Cooper and colleagues reintroduced bilateral lung resection for severe emphysema.[12] Cooper's criteria for surgery included marked airway obstruction due to emphysema, marked hyperinflation, and regional heterogeneity in the distribution of the emphysema.[13] Since the work of Brantigan and Mueller, anesthesia, perioperative care, and surgical techniques had improved dramatically and important lessons had been learned from experience with lung transplantation.[22] At present, a considerable number of "lung-trimming" operations are being done at different institutions, mostly via a midsternotomy thoracotomy but also by thoracoscopy coupled with laser technology or stapling.[3,17,23,33,34]

Experience to date indicates that the procedure helps certain patients with emphysema. The surgical outlook seems to be better for the person with heterogeneous distribution of emphysema than for the person with more homogeneous distribution (Fig. 42-12). New imaging techniques hold promise of improving the preoperative assessment of the extent and distribution of destroyed lung (Fig. 42-8).[51]

The reported mortality from the surgical procedure is on the order of 5 to 10 percent, the most common complication being persistent air leak. Less frequent, but still appreciable, have been a variety of complications, including pneumonia, sepsis, myocardial infarction, and stroke.

Because of the uncontrolled nature of the experience to date with lung volume reduction surgery and the widespread interest in its use, the National Institutes of Health has created 18 centers to evaluate the efficacy and safety of the surgical approaches, to establish criteria by which suitable candidates for the procedure will be chosen, and to compare the outcomes of medical and surgical management. The medical regimens provide for controlled pulmonary rehabilitation. Provision is also made for evaluating midsternotomy thoracotomy and thoracoscopy as surgical approaches. Cost-effectiveness of the surgical procedures will be included in the overall assessment. At present, the Health Care Financing Administration has indicated that Medicare will pay for lung volume reduction surgery only in patients enrolled in the clinical trial being conducted by the National Heart, Lung, and Blood Institute for the National Institutes of Health.

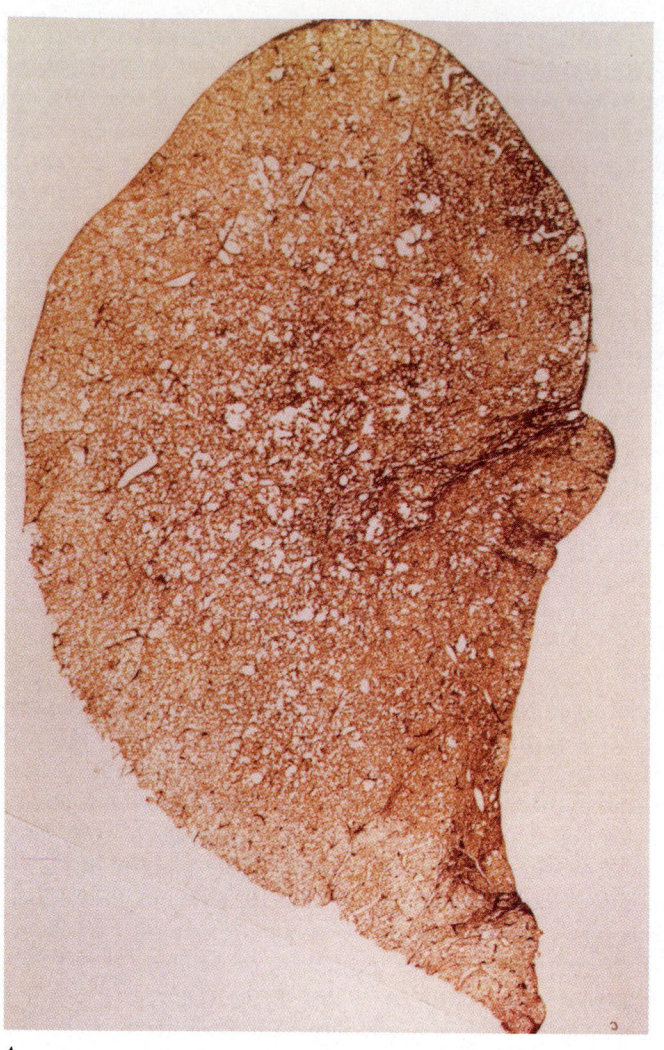

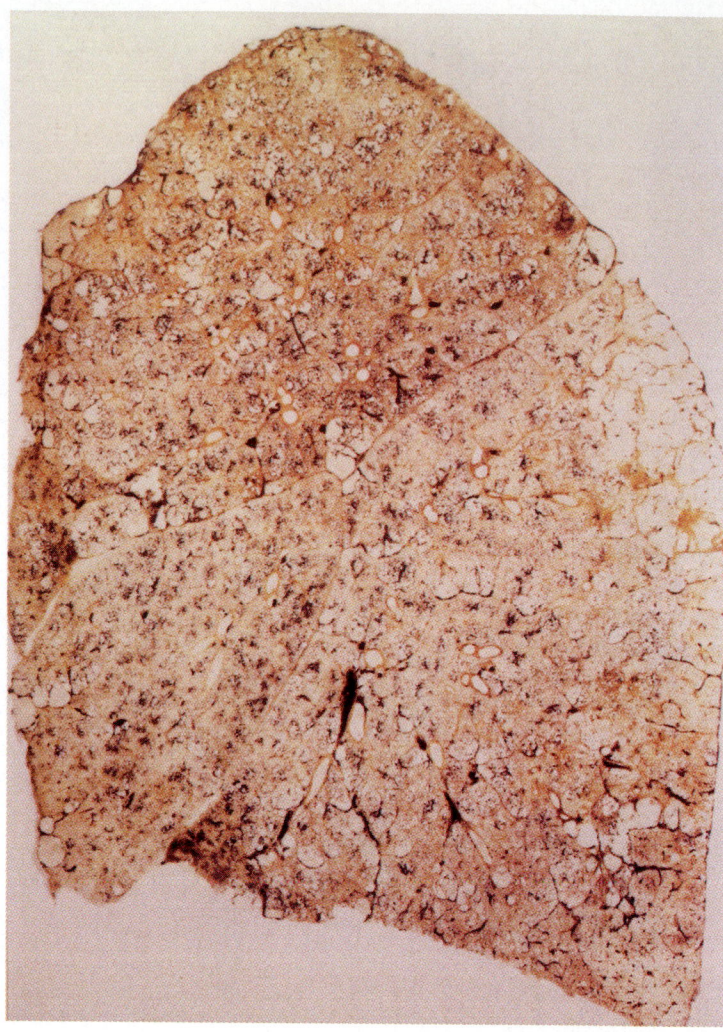

A   *B*

FIGURE 42-12 Homogeneous and heterogeneous distributions of emphysema. *A.* Homogeneous. The emphysematous process is evident throughout the lung, with relatively few localized areas of marked pulmonary destruction. *B.* Heterogeneous. Large areas of destroyed lung abut on the surface of the lung, while other areas are less severely affected.

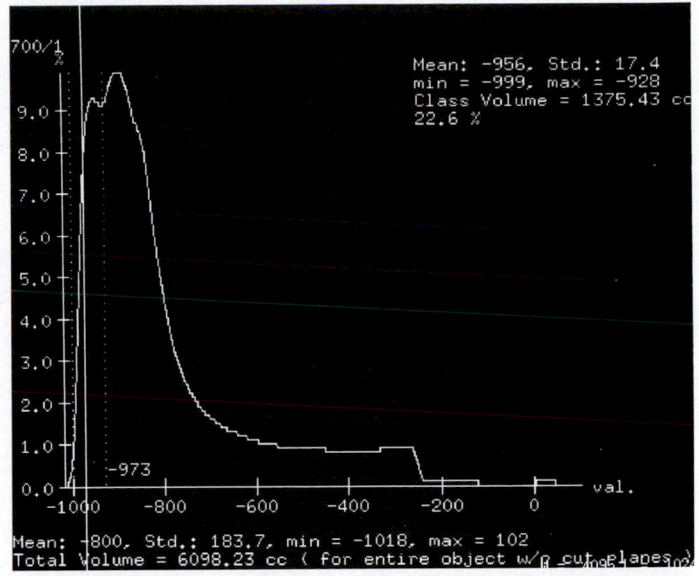

A

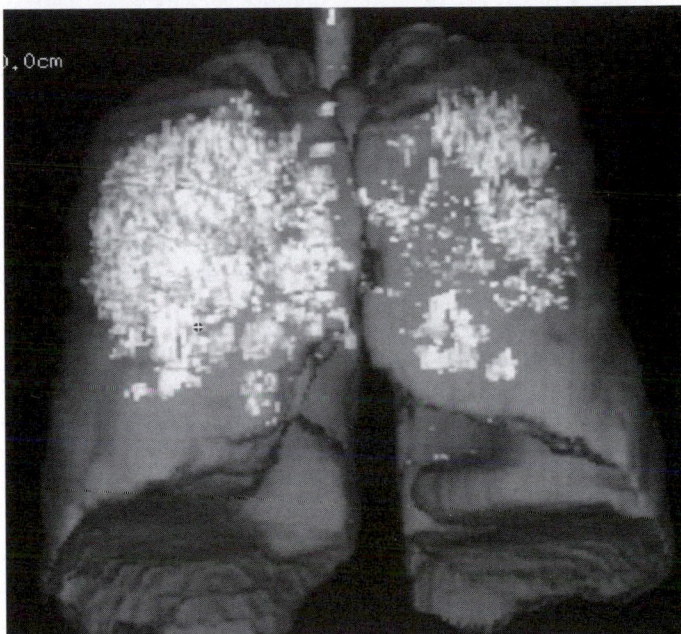

B

C

FIGURE 42-13   Determination of the volume of emphysematous lung. *A.* Segmented CT image of the right lung. Using a threshold-based image segmentation algorithm, image analysis software was used to automatically identify the borders of the lungs, in the process removing the chest wall and mediastinum. The segmentation program also allows the trachea and central airways to be subtracted from the images. Within the segmented volume of the lungs, the full range of pixel attenuation values is generated. *B.* Histogram showing the frequency distribution of pixel attenuation values (along x axis) within the lung as illustrated at *A* in Fig. 42-2. Pathologic studies have shown that pixel values at or below a threshold of −950 Hounsfield units (HU) are highly correlated with emphysematous lung. The area under the curve is proportional to lung volume. Based on the known pixel volume, the volume of emphysematous lung as well as the percent volume of emphysema/volume of normal lung can be calculated for any given lung region. *C.* Regional distribution of emphysema in the lungs. 3D display of the entire lungs showing the anatomic distribution of emphysema. Using the image-linked histograms described above, pixels with attenuation values ≤ −950 HU, corresponding to emphysematous lung, have been selected and are displayed as the white areas in the image. Note predominant involvement of the upper and midlung zones, with greater involvement of the right lung. This volumetric image analysis technique thus provides quantitative maps of the regional distribution of emphysema. *(Courtesy of Warren B. Gefter, M.D., and Jean-Marc David.)*

REFERENCES

1. American Thoracic Society: Chronic bronchitis, asthma and pulmonary emphysema: Definitions and classification. *Am Rev Respir Dis* 85:762–768, 1962.

2. American Thoracic Society: Standards for the diagnosis and care of patients with chronic obstructive pulmonary disease. *Am J Respir Crit Care Med* 152(Suppl):S78–S79, 1995.

3. American Thoracic Society: Official statement: Lung volume reduction surgery. *Am J Respir Crit Care Med* 154:1151–1152, 1996.

4. Baille M: *A Series of Engravings Intended to Illustrate the Morbid Anatomy of Some of the Most Important Parts of the Human Body.* London, W. Bulmer, 1803.

5. Bates DV: *Respiratory Function in Disease,* 3d ed. Philadelphia, Saunders, 1989, pp 172–235.

6. Brantigan OC, Mueller E: Surgical treatment of pulmonary emphysema. *Am Surg* 23:789–804, 1957.

7. Burrows B: An overview of obstructive lung diseases. *Med Clin North Am* 65:455–471, 1981.

8. Burrows B, Bloom JW, Traver GA, Cline MG: The course and prognosis of different forms of chronic airways obstruction in a sample from the general population. *New Engl J Med* 317:1309–1314, 1987.

9. Burrows B, Niden AH, Fletcher CM, Jones NL: Clinical types of chronic obstructive lung disease in London and in Chicago. *Am Rev Respir Dis* 90:14–27, 1964.

10. Cherniack RM: Physiologic diagnosis and function in asthma. *Clin Chest Med* 16:567–581, 1995.

11. CIBA. Terminology, definition and classification of chronic pulmonary emphysema and related conditions: A report of the conclusions of a CIBA guest symposium. *Thorax* 14:286, 1959.

12. Cooper JD, Patterson A, Sundaresan RS, et al: Results of 150 consecutive bilateral lung volume reduction procedures in patients with severe emphysema. *J Thoracic Cardiovasc Surg* 112:1319–1330, 1996.

13. Cooper JD, Trulock EP, Triantafillou AN, et al: Bilateral pneumectomy (volume reduction) for chronic obstructive pulmonary diseases. *J Thorac Cardiovasc Surg* 109:106–119, 1995.

14. Dornhorst AC: Respiratory insufficiency. *Lancet* 1:1185–1187, 1955.

15. Epler GR: *Diseases of the Bronchioles.* New York, Raven Press, 1994.

16. Eriksson S: A 30-year perspective on α_1-antitrypsin deficiency. *Chest* 110(Suppl):237S–242S, 1996.

17. Eugene J, Ott RA, Gogia HS, et al: Video-thoracic surgery for treatment of end-stage bullous emphysema and chronic obstructive pulmonary disease. *Am Surg* 61:934–936, 1995.

18. Fishman AP: *Pulmonary Diseases and Disorders,* 2d ed. New York, McGraw-Hill, 1988, p 1260.

19. Fletcher C, Peto R: The natural history of chronic airflow obstruction. *Br Med J* 1:1645–1648, 1977.

20. Fletcher C, Peto R, Tinker C, Speizer FE: *The Natural History of Chronic Bronchitis and Emphysema.* London and New York, Oxford University Press, 1976.

21. Fletcher CM, Pride NB: Definitions of emphysema, chronic bronchitis, asthma, and airflow obstruction: 25 years on from the CIBA symposium (editorial). *Thorax* 39:81–85, 1984.

22. Gaissert HA, Trulock EP, Cooper JD, et al: Comparison of early functional results after volume reduction or lung transplantation for chronic obstructive pulmonary disease. *J Thorac Cardiovasc Surg* 111:296–307, 1996.

23. Gelb AF, Brenner M, McKenna RJ Jr, et al: Lung function 12 months following emphysema resection. *Chest* 110:1407–1415, 1996.

24. Gevenois PA, de Maertelaer V, de Vuyst P, et al: Comparison of computed density and macroscopic morphometry in pulmonary emphysema. *Am J Respir Crit Care Med* 152:653–657, 1995.

25. Gough J: Pathological diagnosis of emphysema. *Proc R Soc Med* 45:576, 1952.

26. Gough J, Wentworth J: Thin sections of entire organs mounted on paper. *Harvey Lect* 53:182–185, 1957–1958.

27. Guerry-Force ML, Müller NL, Wright JL, et al: A comparison of bronchiolitis obliterans with organizing pneumonia, usual interstitial pneumonia, and small airways disease. *Am Rev Respir Dis* 135:705–712, 1987.

28. Hale KA, Ewing SL, Gosnell BA, Niewoehner DE: Lung disease in long-term cigarette smokers with and without chronic airflow obstruction. *Am Rev Respir Dis* 130:716–721, 1984.

29. Hall WJ, Hyde RW, Schwartz RH, et al: Pulmonary abnormalities in intermediate alpha$_1$-antitrypsin deficiency. *J Clin Invest* 58:1069–1077, 1976.

30. Hogg JC: Bronchiolitis in asthma and chronic obstructive pulmonary disease. *Clin Chest Med* 14:733–740, 1993.

31. Hogg JC, Macklem PT, Thurlbeck WM: Site and nature of airway obstruction in chronic obstructive lung disease. *New Engl J Med* 278:1355–1360, 1968.

32. Jeffery PK: Comparative morphology of the airways in asthma and chronic obstructive pulmonary disease. *Am J Respir Crit Care Med* 150(Suppl):S6–S13, 1994.

33. Kennan RJ, Landreneau FJ, Sciurba FC, et al: Unilateral thoracoscopic surgical approach for diffuse emphysema. *J Thorac Cardiovasc Surg* 111:308–316, 1996.

34. Kotloff RM, Tino G, Bavaria JE, et al: Bilateral lung volume reduction surgery for advanced emphysema. *Chest* 110:1399–1406, 1996.

35. Kraft M, Mortenson RL, Colby TV, et al: Cryptogenic constrictive bronchiolitis: A clinico-pathologic study. *Am Rev Respir Dis* 148:1093–1101, 1993.

36. Laennec RTH: *A Treatise on the Diseases of the Chest* (John Forbes, trans). New York, Hafner, 1962.

37. Laurenzi GA, Turino GM, Fishman AP: Bullous disease of the lung. *Am J Med* 32:361–378, 1962.

38. Leopold JG, Gough J: The centrilobular form of hypertrophic emphysema and its relation to chronic bronchitis. *Thorax* 12:219–235, 1957.

39. Macklem PT, Mead J: Resistance of central and peripheral airways measured by retrograde catheter. *J Appl Physiol* 22:395–401, 1967.

40. Macklem PT, Permutt S: *The Lung in the Transition Between Health and Disease.* New York, Marcel Dekker, 1979, pp 1–41.

41. McHenry LC: Dr. Samuel Johnson's emphysema. *Arch Intern Med* 119:98–105, 1967.

42. Ollerenshaw SL, Woolcock AJ: Characteristics of the inflammation in biopsies from large airways of subjects with asthma and subjects with chronic airflow limitation. *Am Rev Respir Dis* 145:922–927, 1992.

43. Reid L: Measurement of the bronchial mucus gland layer: A diagnostic yardstick in chronic bronchitis. *Thorax* 15:132–141, 1960.

44. Reid L, Millard FJC: Correlation between radiological diagnosis and structural lung changes in emphysema. *Clin Radiol* 15:307–311, 1964.

45. Saetta M, Kim WD, Izquierdo JL, et al: Extent of centriilobular and panacinar emphysema in smokers' lungs: Pathological and mechanical implications. *Eur Respir J* 7:664–671, 1994.

46. Scadding JG: Definition and clinical categories of asthma, in Clark TFH, Godfrey S (eds), *Asthma,* 2d ed. London, Chapman and Hall, 1983, pp 1–11.

47. Snider GL: Chronic obstructive pulmonary disease—a continuing challenge. *Am Rev Respir Dis* 133:942–944, 1986.

48. Snider GL, Kleinerman JL, Thurlbeck WM, Bengali ZH: The definition of emphysema. Report of a workshop of the National Heart, Lung, and Blood Institute. *Am Rev Respir Dis* 132:182–185, 1985.

49. Thurlbeck WM: Chronic airflow obstruction, in Thurlbeck WM, Churg AM (eds), *Pathology of the Lung,* 2d ed. New York, Thieme, 1995, pp 739–826.

50. Toelle BG, Peat JK, Salome CM, et al: Towards a definition of asthma for epidemiology. *Am Rev Respir Dis* 145:633–637, 1992.

51. Weinmann GG, Hyatt R: Evaluation and research in lung volume reduction surgery. *Am J Respir Crit Care Med* 154:1913–1918, 1996.

52. Weiss ST, Ware JH: Overview of issues in the longitudinal analysis of respiratory data. *Am J Respir Crit Care Med* 154(Suppl):S208–S216, 1996.

53. Woolcock AJ: The search for words to describe the bad blowers. *Chest* 85(Suppl):73S–74S, 1984.

CHAPTER 43

CHRONIC OBSTRUCTIVE PULMONARY DISEASE: EPIDEMIOLOGY, PATHOPHYSIOLOGY, AND PATHOGENESIS

Robert M. Senior / Steven D. Shapiro

The American Thoracic Society defines chronic obstructive pulmonary disease (COPD) as "a disease state characterized by the presence of airflow obstruction due to chronic bronchitis or emphysema; the airflow obstruction is generally progressive, may be accompanied by airflow hyperreactivity, and may be viewed as partially reversible."[3] This definition excludes other causes of chronic airflow obstruction, such as bronchiolitis obliterans and cystic fibrosis. It also excludes asthma. At times, the distinction between asthma and COPD can be difficult.

Since the definition of COPD includes the presence of chronic bronchitis or emphysema, the implication is that COPD can result from diseases of either the airways or the lung parenchyma. While this may be true, COPD is usually due to a mixture of pathology and dysfunction of both airways and lung parenchyma. Another complicating aspect of the definition of COPD relates to chronic bronchitis. The accepted diagnostic criteria for chronic bronchitis are cough and sputum on most days for at least 3 months for at least 2 consecutive years, without another explanation.[3] The criteria do not include airflow obstruction. Many people who meet the criteria for chronic bronchitis do not have COPD, although some evidence indicates that chronic bronchitis is a risk factor for COPD.[30]

EPIDEMIOLOGY

COPD occurs worldwide, but it is a major health problem principally in societies where cigarette smoking is common and the average lifespan extends into the sixth decade or beyond. Although smokers are, by far, the main group who develop COPD, the disorder does occur in nonsmokers. Nonsmokers in occupations associated with high levels of particulates in the inspired air and women in undeveloped countries who have long-term exposures to indoor open fires for cooking and heating are examples of groups who are prone to COPD without smoking cigarettes.[23] With the current large-scale marketing of tobacco products to developing countries, an increased prevalence of COPD can be expected throughout the world in the future.

The number of people in the United States afflicted with COPD has been rising sharply in recent decades. Estimates are that about 14 million people in the United States have COPD, a number that has increased 41 percent since 1982.[3] Approximately 12.5 million have chronic bronchitis, and 1.65 million have emphysema. Among those with chronic bronchitis, the number who actually have airflow obstruction is unknown. From other analyses, it is estimated that 4 to 6 percent of white male adults and 1 to 3 percent of white female adults have emphysema or chronic airflow obstruction. These figures may be underestimates. For example, in elderly persons, particularly those with low incomes, COPD may be unrecognized.[25]

The death rate from COPD in the United States has been rising in recent decades and contrasts with the falling death rates from heart and cerebrovascular diseases over the same interval. COPD is now the fourth most common cause of death in the United States, accounting for nearly 4.5 percent of all deaths; in 1993, associated mortality was 100,000.[16] This figure may well be low, since death certificates commonly do not include COPD, despite reviews of the medical records suggesting this diagnosis. Moreover, COPD may be a contributory factor in another 4.3 percent of deaths. The mortality from COPD in the United States varies between men and women and among Caucasians, Hispanics, and African Americans.[17] In each of these groups, men have a higher mortality than women. The highest mortality exists among white men, and the lowest rate is among Hispanic women. African Americans have death rates that are intermediate between Caucasians and Hispanics.

The percentage of smokers in the adult population in the United States has dropped from more than 50 percent to approximately 25 percent over the past 30 years; the drop has been particularly dramatic among males.[6] Accordingly, morbidity and mortality from COPD may decline in the years ahead, reflecting these favorable trends in smoking practices in recent decades. However, COPD will continue to be common into the foreseeable future, since in the United States there are 48 million smokers, and 3000 people, mostly teenagers, take up the habit daily.[33] In fact, smoking is increasing among teenagers.

RISK FACTORS

Table 43-1 lists proposed factors associated with risk of development of COPD. Three points about this list should be stressed. First, with the ex-

ceptions of smoking and α_1-antitrypsin (α_1-AT) deficiency, the mechanisms by which the risk factors lead to COPD are not at all clear. Second, even with smoking and α_1-AT deficiency, which carry the highest levels of risk, it is not possible to predict which persons with the proposed risk factors will actually develop COPD. Third, even though smoking and α_1-AT deficiency dominate the list, there are clearly other risk factors for developing COPD; low socioeconomic status is such a factor.[4] One might speculate that the basis for this proposed risk has to do with inadequate medical care for respiratory infections, increased occupational exposure to inhaled particulates, and exposure to household allergens. However, the exact reasons are obscure. The pathogenetic basis of COPD is still very poorly understood at a cellular and molecular level. Genetic factors, in concert with environmental influences, are almost certainly at work. In the fol-

TABLE 43-1

Proposed Risk Factors for COPD

Risk Factor	Comment
Increasing age	Ventilatory impairment primarily reflects cumulative lifetime smoking history
Gender	After standardization for smoking, males more at risk than females
Smoking habit	Some relation to number of cigarettes smoked per day and cumulative pack-years
Environmental pollution	Large differences in urban and rural death rates; particulates more important than photochemical pollutants
Occupation	Many dusts cause mucus hypersecretion; persistent obstruction develops in coal and gold miners, farmers, grain handlers, and cement and cotton workers; cadmium workers have increased risk of emphysema
Socioeconomic status	More common in persons of low socio-economic status
Diet	High fish intake may reduce risk in smokers
Genetic factors	Homozygous α_1-antitrypsin deficiency is the strongest single risk
Birth weight and childhood respiratory illness	Low birth weight presages low FEV_1 and high COPD mortality in later life; chronic childhood disease predisposes to chronic adult disease
Recurrent bronchopulmonary infections	Cause short-term decline in lung function, but not shown to accelerate long-term decline in otherwise healthy smokers
Allergy and airway hyperresponsiveness	Increased blood IgE and eosinophils and hyperresponsiveness found in smokers, but significance as risk factors may be confined to a subgroup of smokers

SOURCE: Reproduced with permission from Pride, Burrows: Development of impaired lung function: Natural history and risk factors, in Calverley, Pride (eds), *Chronic Obstructive Pulmonary Disease.* London, Chapman & Hall. 1995, Chap. 4.

lowing section, smoking, occupation, and airway hyperresponsiveness are discussed as risk factors. α_1-AT deficiency is considered in the section on the pathogenesis of emphysema.

Smoking

Accelerated deterioration of ventilatory function is common among smokers.[12,59] However, its magnitude is relatively small in most smokers. In males, the reduction in forced expiratory volume in 1 s (FEV$_1$) per year above the normal decline in adults for each pack-year of smoking is 9 ml; in females, the excess rate of decline is 6 ml. Based on these rates of decline, a man who has smoked one pack daily for 30 years will have an FEV$_1$ that is 270 ml less than it would have been had he not smoked. In a 40-year follow-up of British physicians, the annual mortality per 100,000 from COPD was 10 for those who never smoked and 225 for those who smoked more than 25 cigarettes daily; rates were intermediate for former smokers and those who smoked fewer than 25 cigarettes per day.[22] Similarly, there is a decreased average percentage of predicted normal FEV$_1$ associated with increasing pack-years of smoking (Fig. 43-1). However, the relationship between amount of smoking and risk of COPD is quite unpredictable on an individual basis. Many people with a significant number of pack-years still have a normal or near-normal FEV$_1$, while some people have a reduced FEV$_1$ with a relatively modest smoking history. Whether low-tar cigarette brands produce less COPD (analogous to their lower risk of causing bronchogenic cancer) is unclear. In addition, the relationship between the pattern of inhalation and the risk of developing COPD is not known. Smokers are not a reliable source of information about their own smoke inhalation, and there is no simple means of quantifying smoking patterns to determine the connection between patterns of smoke inhalation and development of COPD.

Among smokers who have already sustained reductions in FEV$_1$, the consequences of continued smoking on ventilatory function are much more impressive than when all smokers are lumped together. The Lung Health Study (Fig. 43-2) revealed that among middle-aged smokers with an FEV$_1$ between 55 and 90 percent of predicted, differences of several hundred milliliters in FEV$_1$ developed within 5 years between those who quit and those who did not quit.[3a] Thus, not surprisingly, in this group of smokers who have demonstrated an increased susceptibility to the effects of smoking on ventilatory function, the rate of decline of FEV$_1$ is much larger than that seen in the average middle-aged smoker who has normal or near-normal ventilatory function. The deleterious effects of smoking in these susceptible smokers is further evident in the trends in ventilatory function among those who stopped smoking. Their rate of decline of FEV$_1$ matches rates seen in nonsmokers, clearly showing the benefits of smoking cessation in this group.

Young adult smokers commonly show nonuniform distribution of ventilation and small-airway dysfunction while their FEV$_1$ is still normal.[11] However, it is not possible to predict which of these persons will be among the approximately 15 percent of smokers who go on to develop clinical COPD.

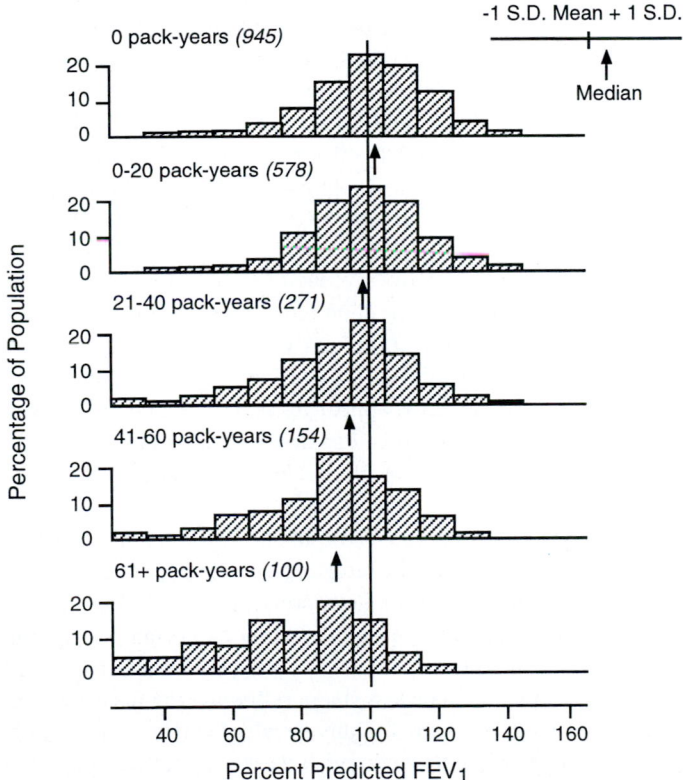

FIGURE 43-1 Distribution of percent predicted forced expiratory volume in 1 s (FEV$_1$) in adults with varying pack-years of smoking. Subjects with "respiratory trouble" before age 16 are excluded. The proportion of smokers with normal expiratory airflow decreases with increasing pack-years. Nevertheless, many smokers have a normal FEV$_1$ despite large cigarette-smoking histories. Means, medians, and +/− standard deviation of the data for each group are shown in the abscissas. The numbers in parentheses are the numbers of subjects. *(From Burrows, Knudson, Cline, Lebowitz: Am Rev Respir Dis 115:195–205, 1977, with permission.)*

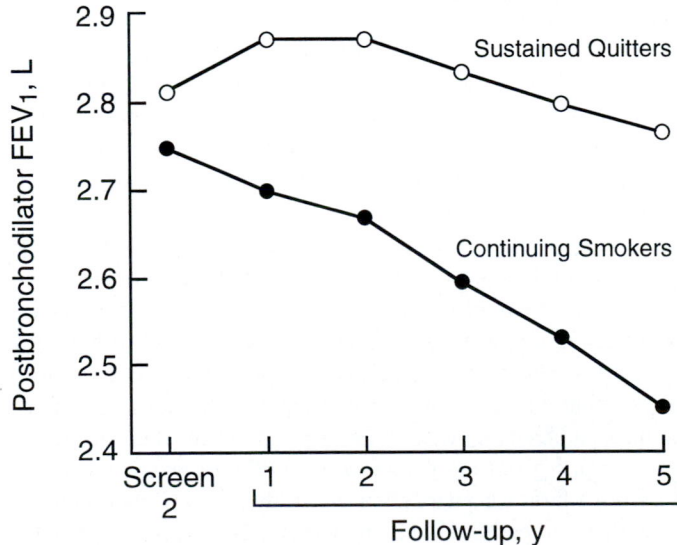

FIGURE 43-2 Mean postbronchodilator forced expiratory volume in 1 s (FEV$_1$) for participants in the Lung Health Study who were sustained quitters (open circles) and continuous smokers (closed circles) during 5 years of follow-up. The rate of decline of FEV$_1$ for quitters is significantly less than for continuous smokers. *(From Anthonisen et al,[3a] with permission.)*

Occupation

Although chronic inhalation of tobacco smoke as a risk factor for COPD has been completely accepted for several decades, the likelihood that chronic inhalation of other types of particulates and gases also carries a risk factor for COPD has been slow in finding acceptance. However, the delay in establishing the association is understandable, since ascertaining the risk of COPD in relation to occupation is difficult for several reasons. The high prevalence of smoking among workers has been a major confounding factor. Also, workers beginning jobs with a high risk of causing lung disease typically have better lung function than normal (the "healthy worker" phenomenon), obscuring work-related effects among relatively young workers.[7] In addition, among cohorts of workers, those with COPD may drop out, causing an underestimate of risk in follow-up studies confined to those still working.

Despite these difficulties, studies from different groups around the world, both urban and rural, workforce based and community based, clearly implicate occupations producing exposures to dusts, gases, and fumes as risk factors for COPD. Dusts appear to be most significant.[8,13,44] Similar to the experience with exposure to tobacco smoke, the presence or absence of chronic bronchitis does not necessarily imply the presence or absence of airflow obstruction. The risk generally relates to the intensity of exposure, but there is considerable individual variability, indicating the importance of host factors in determining susceptibility. The magnitude of the effect of occupational exposures on FEV_1 for groups of workers tends to match the effects produced by smoking. For example, among gold miners in South Africa, the annual loss of FEV_1 attributable to mining was 8 ml per year, compared to 6.9 ml per year for persons smoking 20 cigarettes per day.[18]

Airway Hyperresponsiveness

Airway hyperresponsiveness is difficult to analyze as a risk factor for COPD. It calls into play the so-called Dutch hypothesis, which ascribes a role to allergy and airway hyperresponsiveness in susceptibility to COPD.[3] What makes this area problematic is the question of whether the airway hyperresponsiveness that is common in COPD *precedes* or *follows* the development of COPD. An observation that argues against a causal relationship is that, unless they are also asthmatic, smokers do not show hyperresponsiveness until their baseline FEV_1 is already reduced. Furthermore, animal studies show the development of hyperresponsiveness after enzyme-induced emphysema.[9] Also confusing the relationship is the fact that smoking is not rare among asthmatic subjects, so that some asthmatics are likely to be included among groups of people with COPD. However, recent results from a large 25-year follow-up study in the Netherlands indicate that increased airway hyperresponsiveness, defined by measured responses to inhaled histamine, is an independent risk factor for an accelerated decline in FEV_1.[45] It seems likely that there are two different contexts for development of COPD in relation to airway hyperresponsiveness. In one, COPD develops out of an asthmatic predisposition that may include childhood respiratory problems and allergic features, such as an elevated

serum IgE and eosinophilia. In the other, airway hyperresponsiveness does not predispose to COPD, but rather is a consequence of COPD.

PATHOPHYSIOLOGY

Many pulmonary function abnormalities occur in COPD, but persistent reduction in forced expiratory flow rates is the most typical finding. Increases in residual volume and the residual volume/total lung capacity ratio (RV/TLC), nonuniform distribution of ventilation, and ventilation-perfusion mismatching are also typical.

Airflow Obstruction

Reductions in FEV_1 and FEV_1/FVC percent are the characteristic physiological abnormalities of COPD. In contrast to asthma, the reduced FEV_1 in COPD seldom shows large responses to inhaled bronchodilators, although improvements up to 15 percent are common. Maximal inspiratory flow may be relatively well preserved in the presence of a markedly reduced FEV_1. Such discrepancies between inspiratory and expiratory flow indicate that the reduction in forced expiratory flow is not simply due to fixed narrowing or obliteration of airways, but that there is also a dynamic component due to airway instability during forced exhalation.

Airflow during forced exhalation is the result of the balance between the elastic recoil of the lungs promoting flow and the resistance of the airways limiting flow (see Chapter 10). In normal lungs, as well as in lungs affected by COPD, maximal expiratory flow diminishes as the lungs empty, because the lung parenchyma provides progressively less elastic recoil and the cross-sectional area of the airways falls; resistance to airflow increases. The decrease in flow, coincident with the decrease in lung volume, is readily apparent on the expiratory limb of a flow-volume curve (Fig. 43-3). In the early stages of COPD, the abnormality in airflow is evident only at lung volumes at or below functional residual capacity, appearing as a "scooped out" lower part of the descending limb of the flow-volume curve (Fig. 43-3). In more advanced disease, the entire curve demonstrates decreased expiratory flow.

The relative contributions of diminished elastic recoil and increased airway resistance in reducing maximal expiratory airflow can be quantified from flow-pressure curves (Fig. 43-4). With decreased elastic recoil the curve has a normal slope, but it terminates prematurely. In contrast, with increased airway resistance the slope becomes less steep, reflecting the necessity for increased driving pressure for any level of airflow. In theory, therefore, it is possible to distinguish between emphysema ("decreased elastic recoil") and bronchitis ("increased airway resistance") as the cause for the reduced FEV_1. The situation is more complex, however, because most people with COPD have both emphysema and bronchitis. Moreover, elastic recoil and airway resistance are not necessarily separable. Elastic recoil affects the stiffness of small airways. When elastic recoil is reduced, the curve may be shifted to the right because of increased airway collapsibility. Because flow-pressure data are difficult to collect and interpret and are of little help in patient management, sorting among decreased elastic recoil, airway collapsibility, and in-

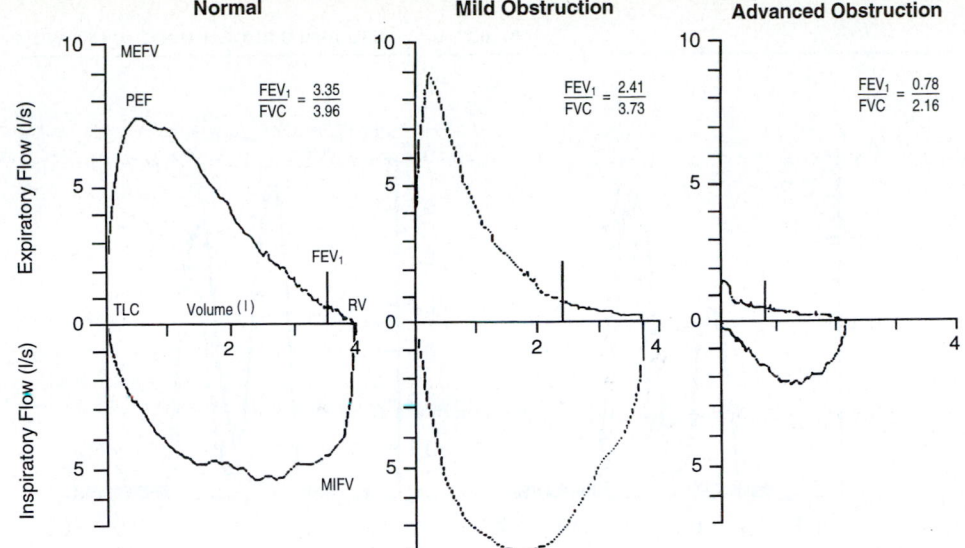

FIGURE 43-3 Maximum expiratory and inspiratory flow-volume (MEFV, MIFV) curves in a normal subject (left), a subject with mild airway obstruction (middle), due to COPD and a subject with advanced obstruction (right) due to COPD. The forced expiratory volume in 1 s (FEV_1) is indicated on the volume axis by a vertical bar. TLC = total lung capacity, RV = residual volume, FVC = forced vital capacity. Note the development of convexity of flow to the volume axis in mild obstruction, despite preservation of a large peak expiratory flow, a normal FVC, and only a small reduction in FEV_1/FVC ratio. Inspiratory flow is normal. In advanced COPD there is marked decrease of FEV_1, FVC, and maximal expiratory airflow generally. Inspiratory flow is also markedly reduced, but spared relative to expiratory flow. *(From Pride, Milic-Emili: Lung mechanics, in Calverley, Pride [eds], Chronic Obstructive Pulmonary Disease. London, Chapman & Hall, 1995, with permission.)*

The multiple inert gas elimination technique (MIGET), which enables quantification of the ventilation-perfusion ($\dot{V}_A/\dot{Q}$) profile, has demonstrated different $\dot{V}_A/\dot{Q}$ patterns among patients with advanced COPD (Fig. 43-5). In one pattern, so-called type A ("pink puffer") COPD, there is a substantial amount of ventilation distributed to high $\dot{V}_A/\dot{Q}$ regions. In a second pattern, called type B ("blue bloater") COPD, there is a substantial amount of pulmonary blood flow perfusing low $\dot{V}_A/\dot{Q}$ regions. There are important limitations to this simple classification. First, persons with the clinical features of type A or type B (that is, emphysema or chronic bronchitis) do not necessarily have the expected $\dot{V}_A/\dot{Q}$ pattern. Of perhaps greater importance, most people with COPD are not easily classified as either type A or type B. They have both high and low $\dot{V}_A/\dot{Q}$ regions. MIGET has also revealed that an increased dispersion of $\dot{V}_A/\dot{Q}$ values is already present in the early stage of COPD.[5]

creased airway resistance as the mechanism of airflow obstruction in COPD is rarely done in clinical practice. In addition, other data, such as the total lung capacity and computed chest tomography, may provide estimates of the severity of emphysema.

Although there is considerable variability in the relationships between the FEV_1 and other physiological abnormalities in COPD, certain generalizations may be made. The arterial P_{O_2} (Pa_{O_2}) usually remains near normal until the FEV_1 is decreased to about half of the predicted level; even a much lower FEV_1 may be associated with a normal Pa_{O_2}, at least at rest. An elevation of arterial P_{CO_2} (Pa_{CO_2}) is not expected in COPD until the FEV_1 is less than about one-fourth of predicted; even then an elevation in Pa_{CO_2} may not occur. Pulmonary hypertension due to COPD that is severe enough to cause cor pulmonale and right ventricular failure occurs only in persons who have a marked decrease in FEV_1 (one-fourth of predicted or less) and chronic hypoxemia (Pa_{O_2} under 55 mmHg), although some elevation of pulmonary artery pressure, particularly with exercise, is common with less advanced COPD.

Nonuniform Ventilation and Ventilation-Perfusion Mismatching

Nonuniform ventilation and ventilation-perfusion mismatching are characteristic of COPD[2] and reflect the heterogeneous nature of the disease process as it affects the airways and lung parenchyma. Nitrogen washout during breathing of 100 percent oxygen is delayed because of regions that are poorly ventilated, and the profile of the nitrogen washout curve is consistent with many parenchymal compartments having different washout rates because of regional differences in compliance and airway resistance. Radioisotopic ventilation scanning with ^{133}xenon reveals regional heterogeneity of ventilation in COPD.

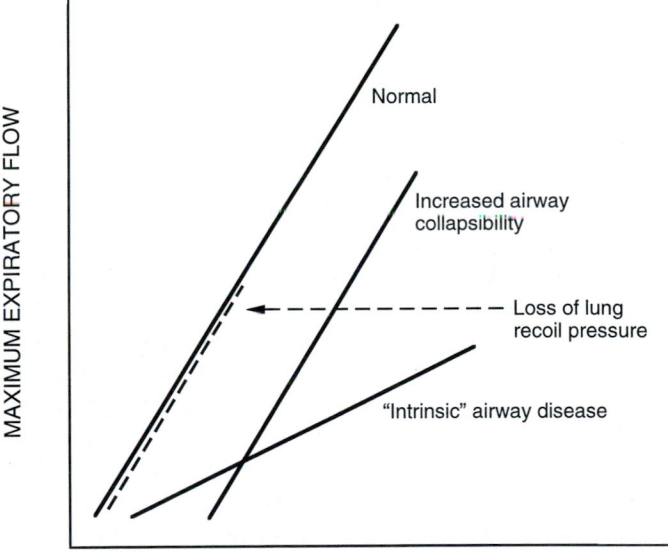

STATIC TRANSPULMONARY PRESSURE

FIGURE 43-4 Analysis of reduced maximum expiratory flow in COPD from maximum expiratory flow versus lung recoil pressure curves. With loss of lung recoil pressure—i.e., "emphysema" (heavy interrupted line)—the slope of the flow-pressure curve remains normal, but the curve terminates at lower pressure than normal. With intrinsic airway obstruction—i.e., "bronchitis"—the slope is reduced. Increased airway collapsibility, which may be a result of decreased elastic recoil, causes the curve to be displaced to the right. Commonly in COPD, the flow-pressure curve has premature termination and a decreased slope and is shifted rightward, indicating that decreased elastic recoil, increased airway resistance, and increased airway collapsibility are all involved in causing the reduced maximum expiratory flow. *(From Pride, Milic-Emili: Lung mechanics, in Calverley, Pride [eds], Chronic Obstructive Pulmonary Disease. London, Chapman & Hall, 1995, with permission.)*

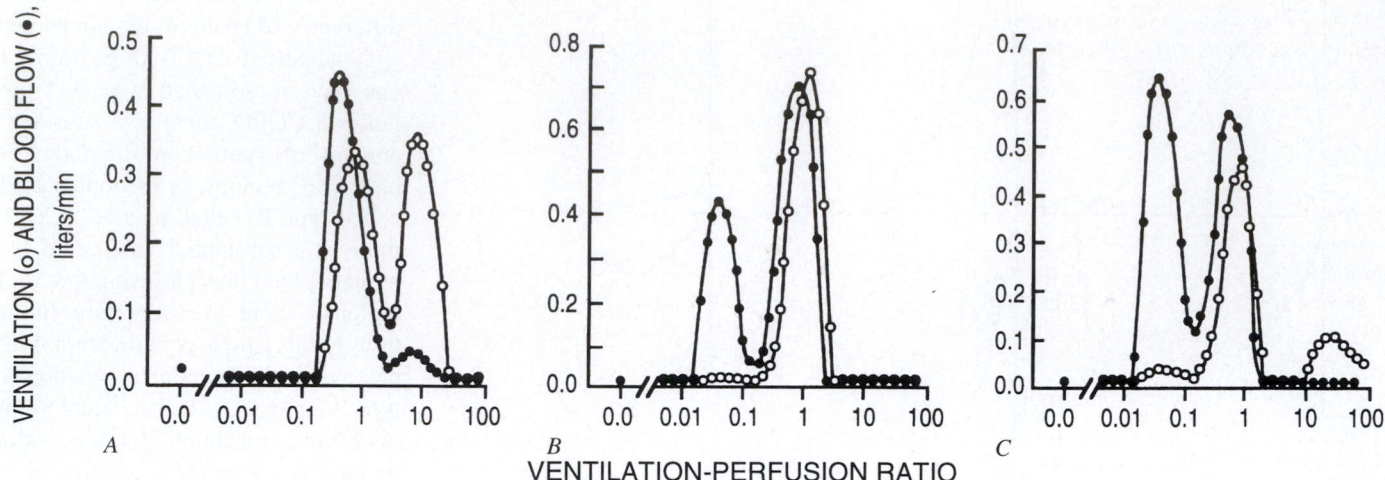

FIGURE 43-5   Ventilation-perfusion ($\dot{V}A/\dot{Q}$) distributions in three persons with COPD determined by the multiple inert gas elimination technique. *A.* Regions of high $\dot{V}A/\dot{Q}$, characteristic of "emphysematous," type A COPD. *B.* Regions of low $\dot{V}A/\dot{Q}$, characteristic of "chronic bronchitis," type B COPD. *C.* Regions of both high and low $\dot{V}A/\dot{Q}$, characteristic of many people with COPD. In the normal person, not shown, $\dot{V}A$ and $\dot{Q}$ virtually overlap and peak at about a $\dot{V}A/\dot{Q}$ of 1. *(From Wagner et al,[55] with permission.)*

One of the important contributions of MIGET has been the demonstration that $\dot{V}A/\dot{Q}$ mismatching accounts for essentially all of the reduction in Pa_{O_2} that occurs in COPD; shunting is minimal.[2,55] This finding explains the effectiveness of modest elevations of inspired oxygen in treating hypoxemia due to COPD and, therefore, the need to consider problems other than COPD when hypoxemia is difficult to correct with modest levels of supplemental oxygen.

Hyperinflation

Increases in residual volume and the ratio of residual volume to total lung capacity are characteristic of COPD. Total lung capacity is also often increased. Hyperinflation of the thorax during tidal breathing favors preservation of maximum expiratory airflow, because as lung volume increases, elastic recoil pressure increases and airways enlarge; airway resistance decreases. In effect, hyperinflation helps to compensate for airway obstruction. When the thoracic gas volume is expanded, however, the ventilatory bellows is less efficient and the work of breathing is increased, both of which contribute to dyspnea.

Hyperinflation may push the diaphragm into a flattened position and, thereby, create a number of adverse effects (Fig. 43-6). First, because the zone of apposition between the diaphragm and the abdominal wall is lost, positive abdominal pressure during inspiration is not applied as effectively to the chest wall, hindering rib cage movement and impairing inspiration. Second, because the muscle fibers of the flattened diaphragm are shorter than those of a more normally curved diaphragm, they are less capable than normal of generating inspiratory pressures. Third, the flattened diaphragm must generate greater tension to develop the transpulmonary pressure required to produce tidal breathing. This follows from Laplace's law, $P = 2T/r$. As the radius of diaphragm curvature (r) increases with diaphragm flattening, the tension (T) required to develop a transpulmonary pressure (P) to generate tidal breathing must increase. Also, with hyperinflation, the

thoracic cage, in general, may operate at a mechanical disadvantage. Because the thoracic cage is distended beyond its normal resting volume, during tidal breathing the inspiratory muscles must do work to overcome the resistance of the thoracic cage to further inflation, instead of gaining the normal assis-

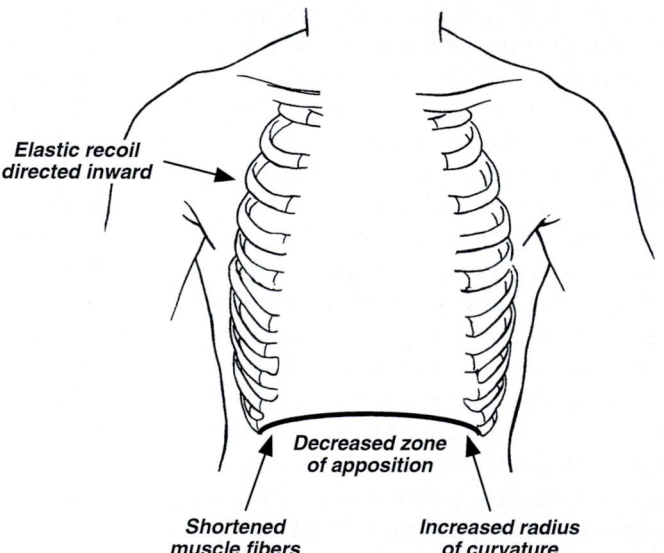

FIGURE 43-6   Detrimental effects of hyperinflation on diaphragmatic function. Hyperinflation causes flattening of the diaphragm, which (1) decreases the zone of apposition between the diaphragm and the abdominal wall, hindering rib cage movement; (2) shortens diaphragmatic muscle fiber length, decreasing the force that can be generated by the diaphragm; (3) increases the radius of curvature of the diaphragm, thereby decreasing transpulmonary pressure (at constant tension); and (4) directs diaphragmatic muscle fibers medially, impairing inflation with diaphragmatic contraction. In addition, hyperinflation prevents the thorax from assisting inspiration during tidal breathing because the resting volume of the thorax is above the volume at which the rib cage recoils outward during inspiration. *(From Yusen, Lefrak, and the Washington University Emphysema Surgery Group: Semin Thorac Cardiovasc Surg 8:1–12, 1996, with permission.)*

tance from the chest wall recoiling outward toward its resting volume. (See Chapter 46 for a detailed discussion of the respiratory muscles in COPD.)

Dyspnea

Most people with COPD seek medical care because of dyspnea. Dyspnea compromises their activities and quality of life. Dyspnea is seldom a complaint until the FEV_1 has fallen below about 60 percent of predicted, and some people with COPD are relatively free of dyspnea with impressively low levels of FEV_1.

The mechanisms of dyspnea in COPD are clearly complex and not fully understood.[37] Neural signals relating to abnormalities of chest wall and airway mechanics appear to be important. Specifically, an increased sense of effort relating to the pressures needed from the respiratory muscles relative to their maximum pressure-generating capacity is thought to be one factor in producing dyspnea. Signals of "length-tension inappropriateness" from the respiratory muscles due to hyperinflation constitute another. Also, impulses from airways undergoing abnormal dynamic compression during exhalation have been described. Hypercapnia and hypoxemia play only a small role, except in acute situations. Oxygen administration may decrease breathlessness by reducing ventilation during exertion and through poorly understood direct effects not associated with changes in ventilation.

PATHOLOGIC CORRELATIONS

Approximately 30 years ago, Hogg and associates made a finding of major importance when they observed that airways 2 mm or less in diameter contribute only a minor part of the total airway resistance normally, but that these airways become the principal sites of increased airway resistance in COPD.[28] These studies gave rise to the concept that COPD is a "small-airway disease."[57] The partitioning of airway resistance between small and large airways, originally found in autopsy specimens, has been confirmed in living subjects with bronchoscopic techniques.[54,60]

Although, from a physiological standpoint, the obstruction to airflow in COPD is in the small airways, the relative importance of emphysema versus intrinsic abnormalities of the small airways as the physical basis for the obstruction is not clear. The difficulties that researchers have had in resolving these issues over the past several decades make it evident that there is not a single pathologic feature that accounts for the obstruction in every person with COPD.[53] Emphysema and small-airway pathology are both present in most persons with COPD; their relative contributions to obstruction probably vary from one patient to another. In the following sections, the pathologic findings in COPD are considered. Large airways are discussed because they are commonly abnormal in COPD, but they rarely contribute to the abnormal pathophysiology.

Large Airways

Cigarette smoking often results in mucous gland enlargement and goblet cell hyperplasia in large airways. These changes are proportional to cough and mucus production that define chronic bronchitis, but the abnormalities are not related to airflow limitation. Goblet cells are increased in number as well as in peripheral extent through the bronchial tree. Moreover, they secrete a more acidic, highly sulfated mucus. Bronchi also undergo squamous metaplasia, which not only predisposes to carcinogenesis but also disrupts mucociliary clearance. Although not as prominent as in asthma, smooth-muscle hypertrophy and bronchial hyperreactivity may lead to airflow limitation. Atrophy of cartilage has also been described. This finding is not common in COPD, but if present, it may cause decreased airflow.

Histologic studies of bronchial mucosa have demonstrated increased numbers of macrophages and T lymphocytes in the airways of smokers. Smokers' mononuclear inflammatory cells also show markers of activation, including the cytokines TNF-α and IL-1β, which induce expression of the cell adhesion markers ICAM-1 and E-selectin.[21] These adhesion molecules are present on submucosal vessels and serve as ligands for leukocytes, initiating cell migration into the airway. A subgroup of ex-smokers appear to maintain expression of these cytokines and adhesion markers, perpetuating the inflammatory response for years after smoking cessation. Neutrophil influx has been associated with purulent sputum of upper respiratory tract infections that hamper patients with COPD. Detrimental effects of neutrophil influx include release of neutrophil elastase and cathepsin G. Independent of their proteolytic activity, these proteinases are among the most potent secretogogues identified.[50]

Small Airways

As stated previously, studies on lungs removed at surgery and postmortem, as well as data from bronchoscopic techniques applied in living subjects, indicate that the major site of increased resistance in most patients with COPD is in airways 2 mm in diameter or less. However, the nature of the lesions responsible for increased resistance in small airways is unresolved. Initial studies pointed to inflammatory and fibrotic changes; more recent studies highlight airway wall thickening, although the significance of this finding is uncertain.

Irrespective of their role in the pathophysiology of COPD, smokers' small airways typically do show abnormalities. Characteristic cellular changes include goblet cell metaplasia and replacement of surfactant-secreting Clara cells with mucus-secreting and infiltrating mononuclear inflammatory cells. Smooth-muscle hypertrophy may also be present. These abnormalities may cause luminal narrowing by excess mucus, edema, and cellular infiltration. Reduced surfactant may increase surface tension at the air-tissue interface, predisposing to airway narrowing or collapse. Fibrosis in the wall may cause airway narrowing in some patients; the fibrosis might also be beneficial, however, stabilizing the patency of the small airways, which lack cartilaginous support.

Because small-airway patency is maintained by the surrounding lung parenchyma that provides radial traction on bronchioles at points where alveolar septa attach, loss of bronchiolar attachments as a result of extracellular matrix destruction may cause airway distortion and narrowing in COPD (Fig. 43-7). In

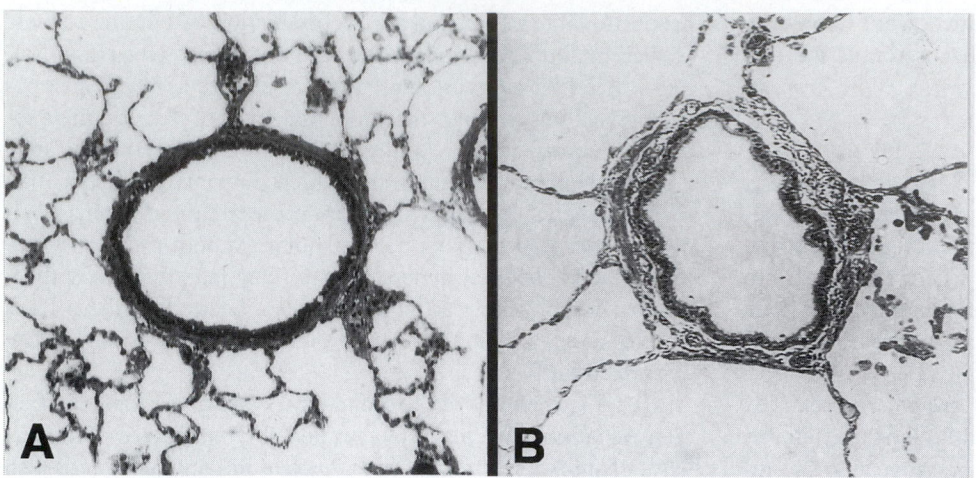

FIGURE 43-7 Reduced alveolar attachments to small airways in emphysema. Photomicrographs of two small airways cut in cross-section. *A.* Small bronchiole from a normal, nonsmoking person. Note the attachments of the bronchiole to adjacent alveolar walls, which provide support and maintain the patent circular shape. *B.* Small airway from a smoker with mild panacinar emphysema. Note the reduction in the alveolar wall attachments and consequent mildly elliptic, less patent profile of the bronchiole. *(From Lamb: Pathology, in Calverley, Pride [eds], Chronic Obstructive Pulmonary Disease. London, Chapman & Hall, 1995, with permission.)*

some correlative studies of preoperative pulmonary function with morphometric analyses of resected lungs, reduced FEV$_1$ was related to mean interalveolar attachment distance, airway ellipticality, and airspace wall surface area per unit volume, but not bronchiolar diameter.[35] However, similar types of analysis have not found a relationship between FEV$_1$ and alveolar attachments. Instead, decreased airflow was correlated with microscopic emphysema and decreased elastic recoil.[38] Although the significance of alveolar attachments is not resolved, the concept of decreased alvolar attachments leading to small-airway obstruction is appealing because it underscores the mechanistic relationship between loss of elastic recoil and increased resistance to airflow in small airways.

Accumulation of macrophages in respiratory bronchioles is a characteristic finding in young adult cigarette smokers.[49] Bronchoalveolar lavage (BAL) fluid from such persons contains roughly fivefold more macrophages than lavage from nonsmokers. In smokers' lavage fluid, macrophages constitute more than 95 percent of the total cell count, and neutrophils, nearly absent in nonsmokers' lavage, account for 1 to 2 percent of the cells.[40] Neutrophils appear to be sequestered within the microcirculation of smokers' lungs as a result of decreased neutrophil deformability in response to cigarette smoke and up-regulation of adhesion molecules on both endothelium and leukocytes.[24] Increased numbers of T lymphocytes have also been associated with emphysema.[26]

Respiratory bronchiolitis may be of importance in susceptible persons. Mononuclear inflammatory cells collecting in distal airway tissues may cause proteolytic destruction of elastic fibers in the respiratory bronchioles and alveolar ducts, where the fibers are concentrated as rings around alveolar entrances. The resulting distortion and narrowing of these structures may be responsible for the early airflow obstruction in cigarette smoking–related COPD.

Lung Parenchyma

From the standpoint of COPD, emphysema is the pathologic process affecting the lung parenchyma. Emphysema is defined "as a condition of the lung characterized by abnormal, permanent enlargement of airspaces distal to the terminal bronchiole, accompanied by destruction of their walls, and without obvious fibrosis."[3] Several aspects of this definition deserve further elaboration. First, it specifies that emphysema is a structural abnormality of the lung

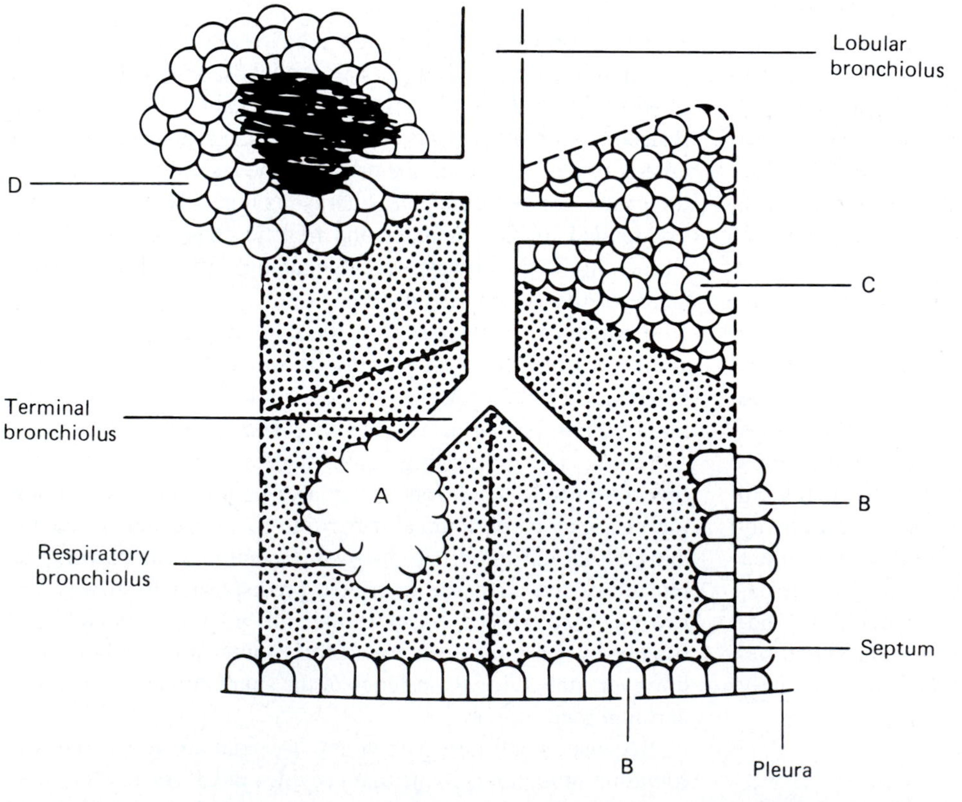

FIGURE 43-8 Anatomic varieties of emphysema. *A.* centriacinar (centrilobular). *B.* periacinar or paraseptal emphysema. *C.* panacinar emphysema. *D.* irregular (scar). The dashed lines mark the edge of the acinus. Only centriacinar and panacinar emphysema are commonly observed in COPD.

that affects the gas-exchanging airspaces—that is, the respiratory bronchioles, alveolar ducts, and alveoli. Second, it considers emphysema a destructive process in which airspace walls are obliterated or become perforated, with coalescence of small distinct airspaces into abnormal and much larger ones. Finally, the definition excludes enlarged airspaces due to fibrosis, to acknowledge that primary fibrotic processes can enlarge airspaces. Although fibrosis may not be a predominant histologic finding, recent studies indicate increased collagen per unit volume of airspace wall in emphysematous lungs from smokers.[36] These findings, which may require some adjustment in the definition of emphysema, suggest that the concept of emphysema formation as purely destructive may be in error.

Emphysema is classified into distinct pathologic types; the most important types are centriacinar and panacinar (Fig. 43-8). *Centriacinar emphysema,* the type most frequently associated with cigarette smoking, is characterized by enlarged airspaces

found (initially) in association with respiratory bronchioles (Fig. 43-9A and B). Centriacinar emphysema is most prominent in the upper lobes and superior segments of lower lobes and is often quite focal. *Panacinar emphysema* refers to abnormally large airspaces evenly distributed within and across acinar units (Fig. 43-9C and D). Panacinar emphysema is usually observed in patients with α_1-AT deficiency, which has a predilection for the lower lobes. An increase in airspace size, most prominent in the alveolar ducts, is also observed with aging, but this airspace enlargement does not appear to be associated with lung destruction (breaks in alveolar walls) and, therefore, is not emphysema. Distinctions between centriacinar and panacinar emphysema are interesting, and may ultimately be shown to have different mechanisms of pathogenesis. However, garden-variety, smoking-related emphysema is usually mixed, particularly in advanced cases. These pathologic classifications are not helpful in the care of patients with COPD.

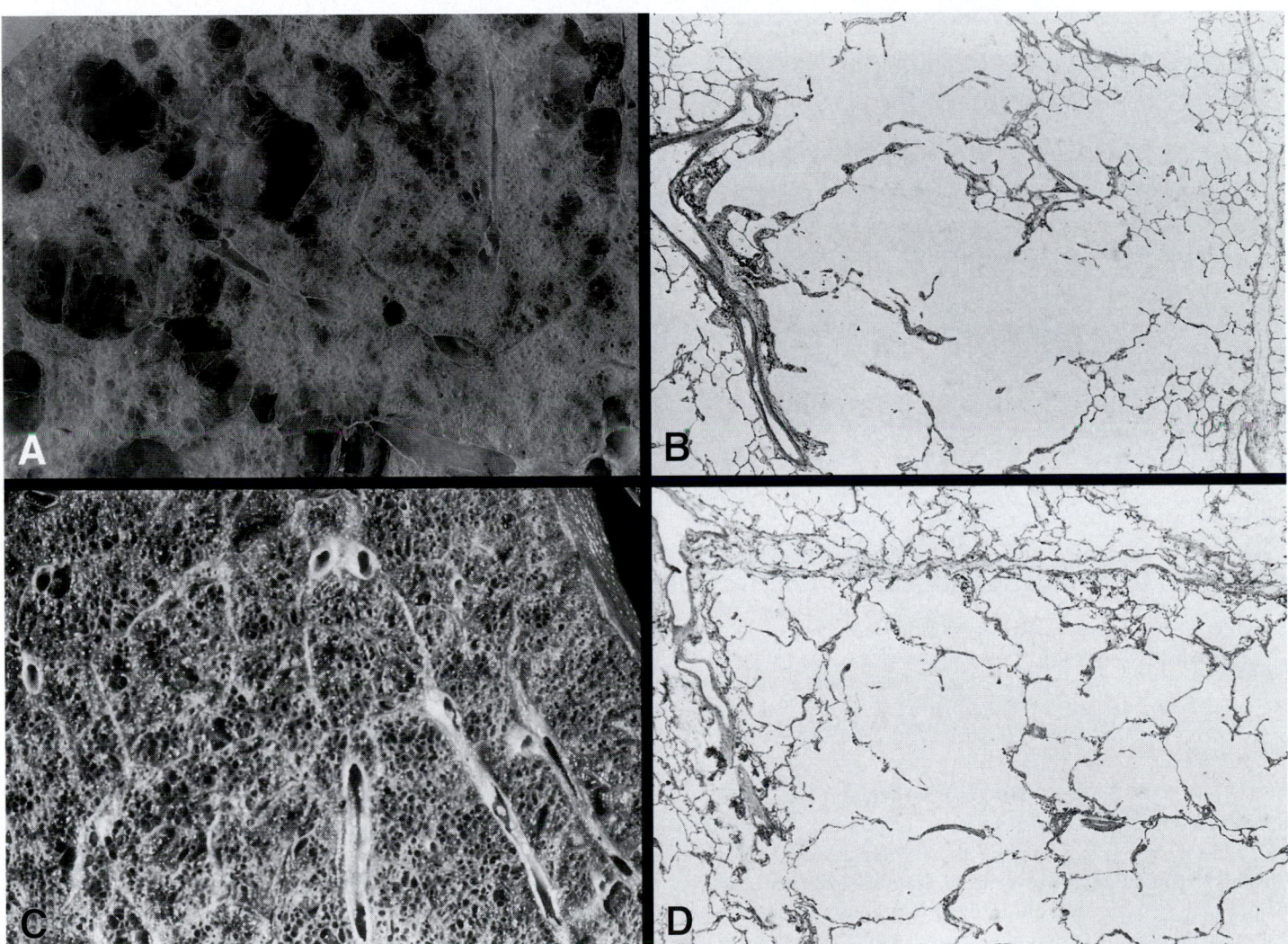

FIGURE 43-9   Histologic sections illustrating centriacinar emphysema (*A* and *B*) and panacinar emphysema (*C* and *D*). *A.* Cut surface from a lung with centriacinar emphysema, showing holes in the center of lobules surrounded by relatively normal parenchyma. The severity varies among lobules. *B.* Microscopic section showing that the airspace enlargement in centriacinar emphysema is most marked adjacent to the abnormal respiratory bronchiole that corresponds to the center of the lobule. Also, some of the alveolar walls of the abnormal airspaces are thickened and fibrotic. (H&E, ×16). *C.* Cut surface of a lung slice, showing how the entire lobule is uniformly affected in panacinar emphysema. *D.* Microscopic section demonstrating that in panacinar emphysema the airspaces adjacent to the lobular septa are enlarged to the same degree as those in the center of the lobule. (H&E, ×16) (*From Wright,[57] with permission.*)

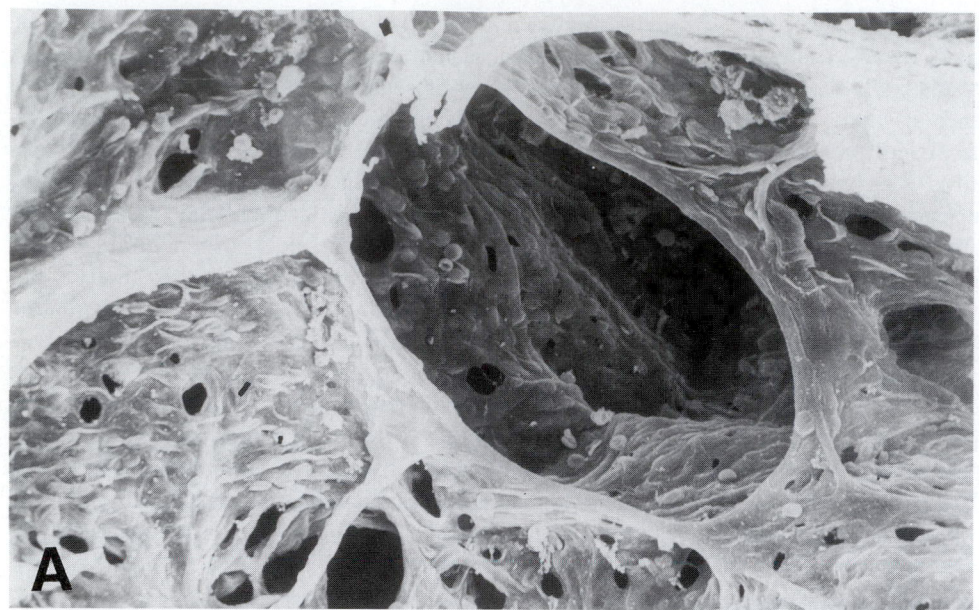

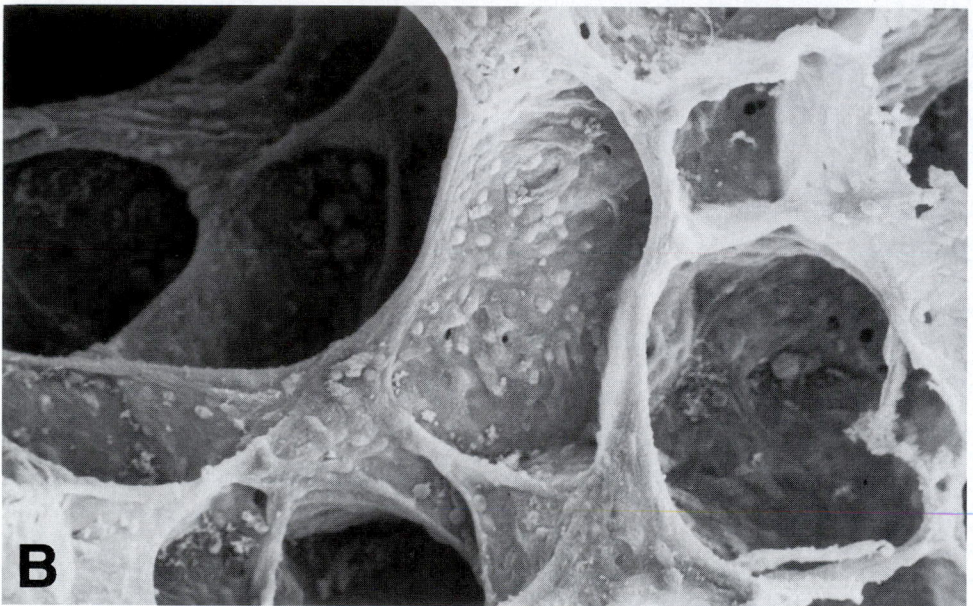

FIGURE 43-10   Holes in alveolar walls in early emphysema. Scanning electron micrographs of alveolar walls from surgically resected specimens: lung with mild emphysema *(A)* and nonemphysematous lung *(B)*. Holes are more numerous in alveolar walls in the emphysematous lung than in the normal lung. Original magnification ×250. *(From Nagai, Inano, Matsuba, Thurlbeck: Am J Respir Crit Care Med 150:1411–1415, 1994, with permission.)*

ume and alveolar surface area.[38] Also, the number and sizes of holes in alveolar walls in alveolar tissue adjacent to macroscopic emphysema show a correlation with lung function tests, including elastic recoil at total lung capacity (Fig. 43-10). These types of microscopic analyses indicate that physiological abnormalities characteristic of emphysema are sensitive to changes in alveolar structure that are not evident macroscopically. These studies also provide quantitative support for earlier concepts that discrete defects in alveolar walls are a feature of early emphysema.

PATHOGENESIS OF EMPHYSEMA

From the time of Laennec, in the first half of the nineteenth century, through the 1950s, mechanical explanations of airspace enlargement and destruction dominated thinking about the pathogenesis of emphysema.[49] In 1963, Laurell and Eriksson reported an association of chronic airflow obstruction and emphysema with deficiency of serum α_1-AT; in 1964, Gross and associates described the first reproducible model of emphysema created in experimental animals by injecting the lungs with the plant protease papain. Together, these two observations indicated that emphysema could be induced by proteolytic injury to the lung extracellular matrix; eventually, they led to the proteinase-antiproteinase hypothesis of emphysema, which has been the prevailing concept of the pathogenesis of emphysema.

Proteinase-Antiproteinase Hypothesis

As currently defined, emphysema may be diagnosed and quantified only by direct inspection of lung tissue, although computed chest tomography may be an alternative. One widely used means of estimating the severity of emphysema entails making whole-lung sections of fixed-inflated lung removed at surgery or autopsy and grading the sections by eye, comparing them to published pictures of paper-mounted whole-lung section lung slices demonstrating a range of emphysema. Thus, the grading is for macroscopic emphysema. This scoring system has appeal for its simplicity, but it may not be the most meaningful method from the standpoint of correlation with lung function. Recent studies suggest that elastic recoil and diffusing capacity correlate with microscopic measures of airspace wall per unit of alveolar vol-

According to the proteinase-antiproteinase hypothesis, there is a steady or episodic release of proteolytic enzymes into the lung parenchyma (Fig. 43-11). Normally, plasma proteinase inhibitors, especially α_1-AT, permeate lung tissue and prevent proteolytic enzymes from digesting structural proteins of the lungs. Proteinase inhibitors synthesized locally in the lungs also contribute to the antiproteinase "shield." Emphysema results from an augmentation of proteinase release in the lungs, a reduction in the antiproteinase defense within the lungs, or a combination of both increased proteinase burden and decreased proteinase inhibitory capacity. Accordingly, emphysema occurs when there is an imbalance between proteinases and antiproteinases in favor of proteinases. The proteinase burden is thought to derive from

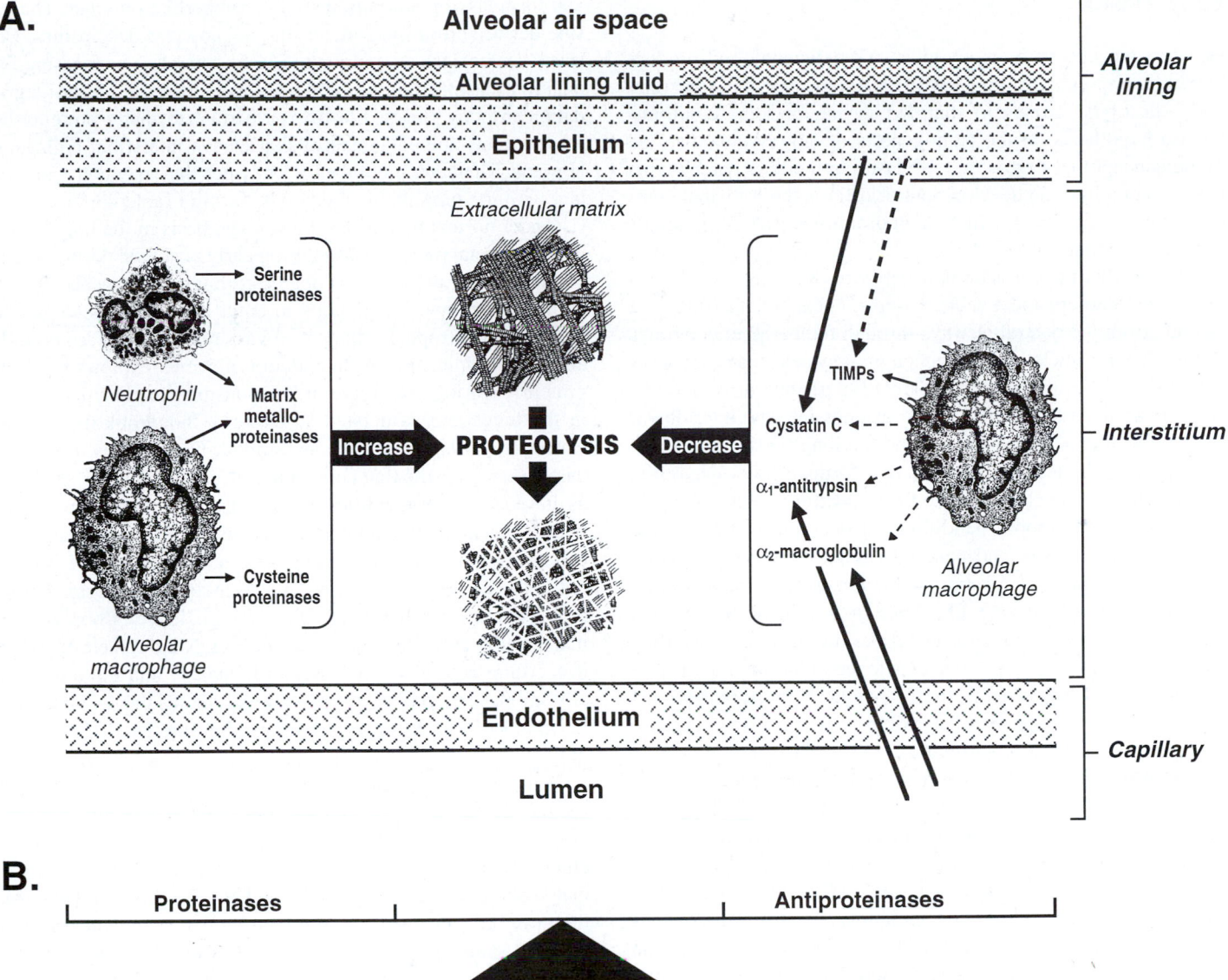

FIGURE 43-11 Proteinase-antiproteinase balance in the lung parenchyma determines the risk of proteolytic degradation of lung extracellular matrix. *A.* Proteinases released by neutrophils, macrophages, and, perhaps, resident cells have the capacity to degrade lung extracellular matrix components, including elastin, thus predisposing to emphysema. Matrix proteolysis is limited by the presence of inhibitors to each class of proteinases. Some inhibitors are locally derived (TIMP, cystatin C), while others arrive via the bloodstream (α_1-AT, α_2-macroglobulin). The predominant sources are depicted by solid arrows; lesser sources are indicated by dashed arrows. *B.* The balance of proteinases and antiproteinases determines the susceptibility of the lung to destruction. *(Adapted from Evans, Pryor: Am J Physiol 266 [Lung Cell Mol Physiol 10] L593–L611, 1994, with permission.)*

inflammatory cells, since these cells are known to release many proteinases that degrade extracellular matrix. In addition, the lungs of smokers have a greatly expanded population of inflammatory cells in the peripheral airways and gas-exchanging regions.

Although the proteinase-antiproteinase hypothesis has remained intact for 30 years, many fundamental questions related to the hypothesis are still unanswered. Inflammatory cells are the presumed source of injurious proteinases, but specifically which cells are the culprits? Is it possible that resident cells of the lungs, such as fibroblasts, also cause alveolar septal injury? What are the signals that initiate and perpetuate inflammation in the lungs during the development of emphysema? Which en-

zymes are active in lung destruction, and how do they make contact with the lung extracellular matrix and maintain their catalytic activity in the presence of an abundance of proteinase inhibitors?

During study of these questions, an appreciation has developed that events controlling proteolytic injury to the extracellular matrix of the lung do not necessarily operate throughout the lungs as a whole. In fact, important events are tightly controlled and occur at or near the cell membrane of inflammatory cells. Thus, the proteinase-antiproteinase hypothesis has been modified to account for an "imbalance" between proteinases and their inhibitors in compartments as small as the microenvironments immediately surrounding inflammatory cells.

Lung Elastin

The seminal observations about α_1-AT deficiency and production of emphysema in animals with elastolytic enzymes (and only with elastolytic enzymes) that led to the proteinase-antiproteinase hypothesis on the pathogenesis of emphysema also led to the concept that destruction of elastin in the lung parenchyma is key to emphysema development. Elastin is the principal component of elastic fibers, which are a prominent part of the lung's extracellular matrix.[39]

Structurally, the extracellular matrix of the lung is organized into three interdependent cable systems: (1) an axial system that extends from the central airways through the peripheral airways to the alveolar ducts; (2) a parenchymal system that comprises the matrix of the alveolar septae; and (3) a peripheral system that arises from the visceral pleura and extends into the interlobular septae, forming a fibrous sac around the lung. Distal to the respiratory bronchioles, the axial system forms a helix encircling the alveolar ducts, extending into the interstitium of alveolar septae. Elastic fibers loop around alveolar ducts, form rings at the mouths of the alveoli, and penetrate as wisps into the alveolar septae, where they are concentrated at bends and junctions (Fig. 43-12). Otherwise, elastic fibers are sparse in alveolar septa. Elastic fibers, which possess rubberlike reversible extensibility, come under tension and provide elastic recoil throughout the respiratory cycle. Unlike elastic fibers, the interstitial collagen fibers in alveolar septa are nondistensible and have high tensile strength. They can be thought of as relaxed ropes that straighten during inspiration and become taut at total lung capacity.

Elastin is secreted as a soluble protein of 60 to 70 kDa called tropoelastin (Fig. 43-13). Encoded by a gene on chromosome 7 in the human, tropoelastin molecules are deposited into the extracellular space and aligned on a "scaffold" of microfibrils consisting of a number of proteins, including fibrillins, microfibril-associated proteins, and latent TGF-β–binding proteins. In the extracellular space, lysyl oxidase modifies most of the lysine residues in tropoelastin monomers, causing them to cross-link

and form elastin, a highly insoluble rubberlike polymer. The lysine-derived cross-links in elastin are known as desmosines. Because desmosines are unique to elastin, they can be measured to quantify elastin in tissues and used as markers of elastin degradation in body fluids. Elastin is resistant to many proteinases, most notably the collagenases that cleave interstitial collagens. However, there are a number of enzymes that may come in contact with the lung that can degrade elastin (Table 43-2).

Under normal conditions, elastin synthesis in the lung begins in the late fetal period, peaks during early postnatal development, continues to a much lesser degree through adolescence (paralleling lung growth), and stops in adult life. There is some evidence that the tropoelastin gene always remains transcriptionally active, but rapid mRNA degradation prevents expression of the protein.[52] Various cell types are responsible for elastin synthesis in the lungs and associated structures. Chondroblasts produce elastin in cartilaginous airways. Smooth-muscle cells in the vasculature and mesothelial cells in the pleura are sources of elastin at those sites. The identities of the cells that make elastin in the lung parenchyma are not certain because of the large number of cell types present and the changes in the phenotypes of interstitial cells during development. As alveolar septae form, myofibroblasts near capillaries produce elastin. There is no evidence that alveolar epithelial cells make elastin. Although elastic fibers in the lung normally last a human lifespan[47] and there is virtually no elastin synthesis in the normal adult lung, animal studies indicate that elastin synthesis can be reinitiated in the adult lung.

Although destruction of lung elastin appears to be necessary for the development of emphysema due to smoking, how the breakdown of elastin translates into the deformity recognized as emphysema remains unknown. Even establishing that emphysematous lungs are deficient in elastin has been difficult. However, this was accomplished not long ago by careful characterization of small samples of lung tissue for severity of emphysema and the taking of adjacent slices for analysis of elastin content.[14] Elastin depletion was restricted to the sites of emphysema, rather than extending throughout the lung.

Just as it has been difficult to document elastin depletion in the emphysematous lung, obtaining direct evidence of active breakdown of lung elastin in association with emphysema is problematic. In some patients with COPD, elevations of elastin peptides and desmosine levels in blood and urine, presumably derived from elastin breakdown in the lungs, are suggestive,[51] as are data showing elevated levels of elastin peptides in BAL fluid of smokers.[10] However, documentation of elastin breakdown products coming from the lungs, along with quantification of progressive development of emphysema, has yet to be obtained.

Inflammatory Repair Hypothesis

Although elastases and elastin destruction occupy a preeminent position in our thinking about the pathogenesis of emphysema, reports over the past decade have suggested that alveolar septal collagen destruction and aberrant collagen repair also contribute to pathogenesis. These reports have led to the "inflammatory repair hypothesis."[56] In this context, mice expressing a human collagenase transgene in the lungs were found to have enlarged air-

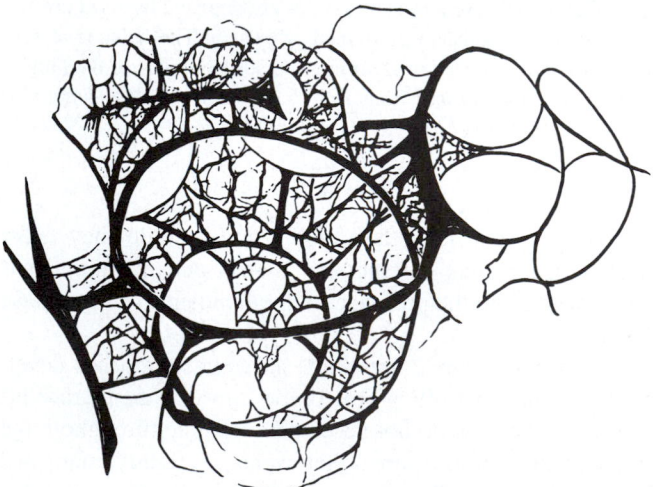

FIGURE 43-12 Alveolar elastic fiber network. Artist's sketch of the elastic fibers in the parenchyma of human lung, showing how elastic fibers form a helix encircling the alveolar ducts and penetrate into alveolar septae. (*From Pierce, Ebert: Thorax 20:469–476, 1965.*)

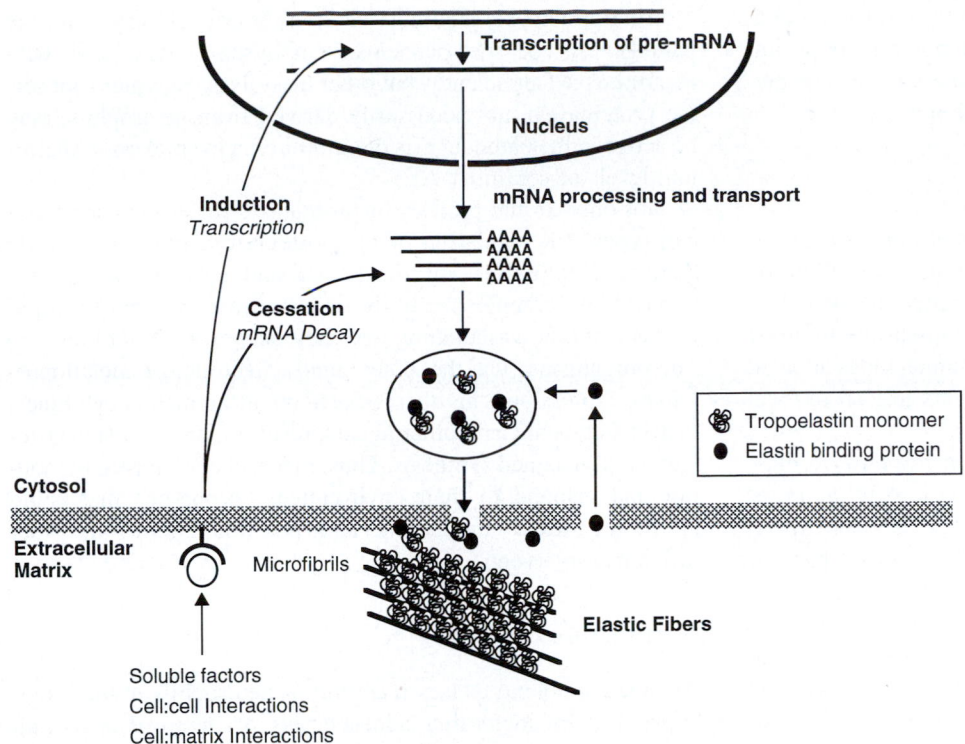

FIGURE 43-13 Synthesis of tropoelastin and assembly of the elastic fiber. Under the influence of extracellular and intracellular factors, tropoelastin pre-mRNA is transcribed within the nucleus of the elastogenic cell. Differential splicing of tropoelastin pre-mRNA leads to different tropoelastin mRNAs and tropoelastin isoforms. After tropoelastin is secreted from the cell, it associates with microfibrils adjacent to the cell surface. Uncertainty exists about whether there is a carrier protein that facilitates the secretion of tropoelasin. Microfibrils are thought to be a scaffold on which tropoelastin monomers align. On the microfibril, most of the lysines in tropoelastin monomers are modified by lysyl oxidase to form covalent cross-links (desmosines) between the monomers. The resultant polymer is elastin. *(Courtesy of William C. Parks, Ph.D.)*

spaces.[20] It is not certain, however, whether the alveolar disease in these animals is due to destruction of collagen in mature lung or whether expression of the transgene during development interferes with normal elastic fiber assembly, perhaps through destruction of the microfibrillar scaffold. In addition, in a guinea pig model of cigarette smoke–induced emphysema, a progressive increase in the volume proportion of collagen in alveolar septae after 6 and 12 months of smoke exposure, following an initial period of subnormal collagen content, was demonstrated.[58] Also, rats exposed to hyperoxia demonstrated airspace enlargement and increased compliance without showing evidence of degradation of lung elastin.[46] Recent observations in human emphysema of increased alveolar septal collagen and focally thickened alveolar walls, indicative of localized fibrosis, fit with these data from experimental animals.[56]

As noted previously, a feature of emphysema is an increased number of holes in alveolar walls and the holes are larger than those seen in normal alveolar septa. Over time, these alveolar septal holes enlarge, and alveoli coalesce into large, abnormal structures. The mechanisms of formation of these

TABLE 43-2

Elastases Present in the Lung Parenchyma

Elastase	Molecular Mass* (kDa)	Cell of Origin	Other Matrix Substrates	Elastolytic Capacity (pH 7.5)
Neutrophil elastase	27–31	Neutrophil (Monocyte)	bm components+	100%
Proteinase 3	28–34	Neutrophil (Monocyte)	bm components+	40%
Cathepsin G	27–32	Neutrophil (Monocyte) (Mast cell)	bm components+	20%
92-kDa gelatinase	92–95	Macrophage, neutrophil, eosinophil	Denatured collagens, Collagen types IV, V, and VII	30%
Metalloelastase	54	Macrophage	bm components+	35%
Cathepsin L	29	Macrophage	(Inactive at pH 7.5)	0‡
Cathepsin S	28	Macrophage	(Unknown)	80%‡

NOTE: Parentheses denote minor cellular sources.
*Denotes pre-proenzyme forms.
†Basement membrane (bm) components include fibronectin, laminin, entactin, vitronectin, and type IV collagen (nonhelical domains).
‡These enzymes are significantly more potent than neutrophil elastase at pH 5.5.

septal holes are not known. However, because interstitial collagens and basement membrane collagens are much more prominent in septal walls than are elastic fibers, these components presumably undergo degradation in the formation of the holes.

Parenchymal Repair

As stated previously, the elastin in the normal human lung has no detectable turnover. It is not known whether normal elastic fibers can be properly formed in the lung after the period of growth and development. Nothing is known about the turnover of other extracellular matrix components in human lungs affected by COPD. As noted, collagen turnover appears to lead to focal areas of fibrosis.

What little is known about lung repair in response to elastolytic proteinases derives from animal research. After an intratracheal injection of human neutrophil elastase into an experimental animal, acute depletion of elastin, followed by a burst of extracellular matrix synthesis, is noted. Over a few weeks, the elastin content of the lungs returns to normal, although the lungs develop emphysema. However, the newly synthesized elastic fibers, like the elastic fibers in human emphysema, appear disorganized.[27] To date, there is no information about elastogenesis in adult human lung parenchyma. Even if tropoelastin expression can be reinitiated in the adult human lung, the production of a functional elastic fiber entails temporally and physically coordinated expression of the microfibrillar scaffold and lysyl oxidase, along with synthesis of tropoelastin. Smoking may have direct deleterious effects on lung elastic fiber synthesis. Tobacco smoke inhibits lysyl oxidase, the enzyme that catalyzes the first step in the formation of lysine-derived crosslinks between elastin molecules during the formation of elastic fibers. To further complicate matters, repair must proceed within the dynamic environment of the lung. Apart from the biochemical issue, it is difficult to conceive of repair of holes in alveolar septa (Fig. 43-10).

Inflammatory Cells and Their Proteinases in the Lungs

Cigarette smoking leads to neutrophil retention in the pulmonary microcirculation and deposition in the lung parenchyma. Cigarette smoking also causes activation and marked accumulation of alveolar and, perhaps, interstitial macrophages. These cells are capable of producing a variety of metallo- and cysteine proteinases that can degrade all components of the extracellular matrix. Other immune and inflammatory cells—such as eosinophils, T lymphocytes, and mast cells—may also contribute to lung destruction, and resident cells within the lung, such as fibroblasts and alveolar type II cells, may be induced to synthesize proteolytic enzymes in response to cigarette smoking.

Defining the cells and proteinases responsible for destruction of lung extracellular matrix associated with cigarette smoking is critical for development of appropriate proteinase inhibitors for future application in treatment of COPD. For example, neutrophils produce predominantly serine proteinases, while macrophages synthesize a variety of metallo- and cysteine proteinases, as well as some serine proteinases. Neutrophil elastase,

a serine proteinase, is almost certainly a critical enzyme in the pathogenesis of the panacinar emphysema associated with marked α_1-AT deficiency, but other elastolytic enzymes (not serine proteinases), not necessarily derived from neutrophils, may be active in the pathogenesis of emphysema in smokers with normal levels of serum α_1-AT.

Not only do the profiles of proteinases differ between these cell types, but regulation of the proteinase expression is quite distinct. Neutrophils are short-lived and package active proteinases into granules ready for quick release, optimal for rapid egress from the vasculature, and they deliver a "lethal blow" to microorganisms. On the other hand, macrophage metalloproteinase expression is highly regulated by inflammatory cytokines, matrix fragments, and other agents, resulting in much slower release and sustained synthesis. Thus, macrophages appear to monitor and respond to their environment—properties that could allow for tissue remodeling and possible control of other inflammatory events.

NEUTROPHILS

As noted, smoking causes retention of neutrophils in the lungs, apparently by increasing adhesiveness of neutrophils to pulmonary microvascular endothelium. Smoking may also increase neutrophil stiffness so that the cells do not deform enough to get through pulmonary capillaries normally. BAL fluid from smokers shows more neutrophils than lavage fluid from nonsmokers, indicating that smoking leads to recruitment of neutrophils into lung tissue. Although these findings, together with evidence that the main function of α_1-AT is inhibition of neutrophil elastase, have suggested an important role for the neutrophil in emphysema, recent data point to alveolar macrophages and T lymphocytes as the predominant inflammatory cells in emphysematous lung tissue.[26]

The fact that neutrophil serine proteinases have a pH optimum of about 7.4 suggests that these enzymes could damage lung tissue if liberated from the neutrophil. In addition, because activated neutrophils can concentrate active neutrophil elastase and cathepsin G on their plasma surface,[43] these enzymes may function in the extracellular environment despite large excesses of α_1-AT and other inhibitors. Apart from digesting lung elastin and other extracellular matrix, neutrophil proteinases may participate in regulation of the inflammatory response via stimulation or activation of cytokines. For example, neutrophil elastase in bronchial fluid from patients with cystic fibrosis induces interleukin-8 (IL-8) transcription in airway epithelial cells in culture, and the cathepsin G–α_1-antichymotrypsin complex promotes transcription of interleukin-6 (IL-6).[34]

Neutrophil Serine Proteinases

Serine proteinases have diverged evolutionarily from a single gene product undergoing duplication and mutations. The result is a group of enzymes with diverse biologic functions, including digestive enzymes of exocrine glands, clotting factors, and leukocyte granule–associated proteinases, some of which degrade extracellular matrix proteins and are of relevance in emphysema. Serine proteinases are characterized by conserved histidine, asparagine, and serine residues that form a charge relay system that functions by transfer of electrons from the carboxyl group of asparagine to the oxygen of serine. Serine then becomes a powerful nucleophile that is able to attack the carbonyl carbon atom of the peptide bond of the substrate. All these enzymes are synthesized as pre-proenzymes in the endoplasmic reticulum and are processed by cleavage of the signal peptide (pre-) and removal of a dipeptide (pro-) by cathepsin C; they are stored in granules as active packaged proteins. Distinct subsets of serine proteinases are expressed in a lineage-restricted manner in immune and inflammatory cells. Serine proteinases are also expressed in a developmentally specific manner. For example, neutrophil elastase, proteinase 3, and cathepsin G are major components of primary or azurophil granules that are formed during a very specific stage in the development of myeloid cells.

Neutrophil Elastase

Human neutrophil elastase (HNE) has activity against a broad range of extracellular matrix proteins, including elastin (Table 43-2). Following the discovery of α_1-AT deficiency and the capacity of HNE to cause emphysema in experimental animals, HNE has been considered of primary importance in the pathogenesis of pulmonary emphysema. Further evidence supporting involvement of HNE in this disease includes (1) the presence of HNE and neutrophils in the lung tissue and BAL of patients with emphysema in some studies; (2) the acute increase in a specific peptide released by HNE action on fibrinogen with smoking; and (3) the oxidation of a methionine residue in the reactive center of α_1-AT by cigarette smoke, resulting in inactivation of α_1-AT and altering the HNE–α_1-AT balance (see below). Whether this inactivation occurs in vivo is uncertain. However, there are no studies directly linking HNE to the pathogenesis of the common form of emphysema related to cigarette smoking.

Proteinase 3

Proteinase 3 (PR3) is roughly 40 percent as potent as HNE against elastin. PR3 has been shown to cause emphysema in experimental animals. This molecule has been identified as the autoantigen target of cytoplasmic-staining antipolymorphonuclear neutrophil autoantibody in Wegener's granulomatosis.

Cathepsin G

Cathepsin G (CG) is stored in neutrophil primary granules and, to a lesser degree, in mast cells and a subset of peripheral blood monocytes. CG is chymotryptic. It also has matrix-degrading activity, with nearly 20 percent of the elastolytic capacity of HNE. Moreover, CG has been reported to increase elastolytic activity of HNE and may facilitate neutrophil penetration of epithelial and endothelial barriers by increasing their permeability.

Neutrophil Metalloproteinases

Neutrophils contain two matrix metalloproteinases (MMPs), the 92-kDa gelatinase (gelatinase B) and neutrophil collagenase. In the neutrophil, these MMPs are stored within specific granules. Neutrophil collagenase can degrade interstitial collagens, but is relatively inactive against other extracellular matrix components. Gelatinase B is active against a number of substrates, including denatured collagens (gelatins), basement membrane components, and elastin.

MONOCYTES

Blood monocytes resemble neutrophils in that they contain HNE and CG in peroxidase-positive granules that are similar to the azurophil granules of neutrophils. These proteinases are synthesized by monocyte precursors in the bone marrow, and can be rapidly released by the circulating cell, perhaps for transvascular migration. As monocytes differentiate into macrophages in tissues, they lose their HNE and CG but acquire the capacity to synthesize and secrete metalloproteinases. Expression of both the serine proteinases is limited to a subset of "proinflammatory" monocytes (about 15 percent of total) that appear to be those capable of tissue penetration.[42]

MACROPHAGES

Alveolar macrophages are the most abundant defense cells in the lung both under normal conditions and particularly during states of chronic inflammation. Alveolar macrophages are prominent in the respiratory bronchioles of cigarette smokers, where emphysematous changes are first manifested. Because it is capable of producing factors that both promote destruction of extracellular matrix and protect against matrix destruction, it is apparent that the macrophage may have a complex role in the pathogenesis of emphysema. Clearly, alveolar macrophages do have the capacity to degrade elastin by means of several proteolytic enzymes.

Macrophage Cysteine (Thiol) Proteinases

Cysteine proteinases[15] represent a large, diverse group of plant and animal enzymes with amino acid homology at the active site only. Human alveolar macrophages produce the lysosomal thiol proteinases and cathepsins B, H, L, and S. These enzymes have similar sizes (24 and 32 kDa) and high mannose side chains, typical of proteins that are targeted for lysosomal accumulation. Cathepsins B and H have little endopeptidase activity and may function to activate other proteins similar to interleukin-converting enzyme, another cysteine proteinase. Cathepsins L and S have large active pockets with relatively indiscriminate substrate specificities that include elastin and other matrix components. These enzymes have their maximum activity at acidic pH, but cathepsin S retains about 25 percent of its elastolytic capacity at neutral pH, making it approximately equal to neutrophil elastase. Thus, these enzymes clearly have the capacity to cause lung destruction if they are targeted to the cell surface or extracellular space, especially if macrophages can acidify their microenvironment. These properties are plausible, but remain to be proven.

Macrophage Matrix Metalloproteinases

Macrophage MMPs constitute a family of matrix-degrading enzymes believed to be essential for normal development and physiological tissue remodeling and repair. Abnormal expression of metalloproteinases has been implicated in many destructive processes, including tumor cell invasion and angiogenesis, arthritis, atherosclerosis, arterial aneurysms, and pulmonary emphysema.[41] MMP family members share about 40 percent identity at the amino acid level, and they possess common structural domains. MMPs are secreted as inactive proenzymes, which are activated at the cell membrane surface or within the extracellular space by proteolytic cleavage of the N-terminal domain. Catalytic activity is dependent on coordination of a zinc ion at the active site and is specifically inhibited by members of another gene family, tissue inhibitors of MMPs (see below). Optimal activity of MMPs is at a pH of about 7.4. All MMPs except matrilysin have a carboxyl terminal hemopexinlike domain that is important for conferring substrate specificity and for tissue inhibitor binding. The 92- and 72-kDa gelatinases have an additional fibronectinlike domain, which mediates their high binding affinity to gelatins and elastin.

Individual members of the MMP family can be loosely divided into groups based on their matrix-degrading capacity. As a whole, they are able to cleave all extracellular matrix components. The *collagenases* have the unique capacity to cleave native triple helical interstitial collagens but have a restricted substrate specificity and are unable to degrade elastin or basement membrane molecules. There are two *gelatinases,* of 72 kDa (gelatinase A) and 92 kDa (gelatinase B), which differ in their cellular origin and regulation; however, they share the capacity to degrade gelatins (denatured collagens), type IV collagen, elastin, and other matrix proteins. *Stromelysins* have a broad spectrum of susceptible substrates, including most basement membrane components. *Matrilysin,* the smallest MMP (28 kDa as a proenzyme) has the broad substrate specificity of stromelysin; in addition, it has some elastase activity. *Macrophage metalloelastase* also has a potent broad substrate specificity, which includes elastin. The MMP family continues to grow. The newest members are membrane-type matrix metalloproteinases (MT-MMPs). MT-MMP–1 activates the 72-kDa gelatinase; however, the MT-MMP spectrum of cellular expression and susceptible substrates is currently unknown. MMPs are active against a variety of proteins besides extracellular matrix. They cleave and activate latent tumor necrosis factor–α (TNF-α), thereby regulating inflammation. MMPs degrade and inactivate α_1-AT, indirectly enhancing the activity of HNE.

Alveolar macrophages produce several MMPs, including significant amounts of metalloelastase, interstitial collagenase, 92-kDa gelatinase, and smaller amounts of stromelysin-1 and matrilysin. Expression of these MMPs is highly regulated. Under basal conditions—in normal mature lung tissue, for instance—MMPs are essentially not expressed. They are induced, and their production and activity are carefully controlled during normal repair and remodeling processes. With chronic inflammation, regulation of MMPs may go awry, and MMPs may be overexpressed and produced at inappropriate sites. There is evidence that expression of metalloelastase and, to a lesser degree, matrilysin is up-regulated in alveolar macrophages of cigarette smokers. As mentioned previously, overexpression of interstitial collagenase in the lungs of transgenic mice leads to enlarged airspaces characteristic of emphysema.

EXPRESSION OF MATRIX METALLOPROTEINASES BY OTHER LUNG CELLS

Many cells in the lung have the capacity to produce MMPs. Eosinophils produce significant amounts of the 92-kDa gelatinase. T lymphocytes interacting with endothelial cell vascular adhesion molecule–1 (VCAM-1) are induced to express the 72-kDa gelatinase. Various resident lung cells can produce MMPs—including fibroblasts, which are a potential prominent source of interstitial collagenase, stromelysin, 72-kDa gelatinase, and the 66-kDa MT-MMP. Type II alveolar epithelial cells produce matrilysin and, perhaps, other MMPs in culture; they may also produce these enzymes in vivo. Considering the variety of lung cells capable of producing MMPs, it seems plausible that MMPs participate in the lung destruction resulting in emphysema.

Proteinase Inhibitors in Plasma

Human plasma contains at least six proteins that function as proteinase inhibitors (Table 43-3). Together, they make up about 10 percent of the total plasma protein. At a concentration of 150 to 350 mg/dl, α_1-AT is present in the highest concentration of all of the plasma inhibitors. α_1-AT belongs to a family of serine proteinase inhibitors called the *serpins.* Serpins have considerable sequence homology, particularly around their reactive sites. They are important for homeostasis, since they exert some control over such major proteolytic cascades as the complement system and coagulation. Another major inhibitor is α_2-*macroglobulin,* a large protein that is usually restricted to the circulation because of its mass (725,000 kDa). α_2-*Macroglobulin* inhibits proteinases of several classes by "entrapping" proteinases following cleavage of susceptible regions of the molecule.

α_1-ANTITRYPSIN

α_1-AT is a glycoprotein of 52 kDa synthesized primarily by the liver; it consists of a single polypeptide chain of 394 amino acids.[19] Fully processed α_1-AT has three carbohydrate side chains that account for 12 percent of the molecular mass. The gene for α_1-AT is 12.2 kb. It is located on chromosome 14, near the gene for α_1-antichymotrypsin, the inhibitor for cathepsin G—which, like neutrophil elastase, is a proteinase contained in the azurophil granules of neutrophils. The α_1-AT gene has seven exons and six introns. Exons four through seven code for the mature protein. Of interest is that the first two exons and a 5'-segment of exon three are encoded in the transcript expressed in macrophages, but not in hepatocytes. α_1-AT is an acute-phase reactant; plasma levels rise with trauma, estrogen therapy, and use of birth-control pills, and during pregnancy.

Proteolytic inhibition of neutrophil elastase and other serine proteinases by α_1-AT involves cleavage of the "strained" reactive, open center of α_1-AT between methionine[358] and serine[359]. The result is in an altered, "relaxed" α_1-AT conformation in complex with the proteinase. Formation of the complex renders the proteinase inactive, and because the complex is quite stable, inactivation is essentially permanent. α_1-AT inhibits many serine proteinases and does so on a 1:1 molar basis. However, α_1-AT associates with neutrophil elastase much faster than with trypsin or other serine proteinases. Indeed, the association with neutrophil elastase is so fast in comparison with other serine proteinases that inhibition of neutrophil elastase appears to be the primary function of α_1-AT. The capacity of α_1-AT to inhibit neutrophil elastase and other serine proteinases besides trypsin has led some authors to prefer the designations α_1-proteinase in-

TABLE 43-3

Proteinase Inhibitors Present in the Lung Parenchyma

Proteinase Inhibitor	Molecular Mass (kDa)	Cell of Origin	Proteinases Inhibited
α_1-AT	52	Hepatocyte (Macrophage)	Serine proteinases*
SLPI	12	Large-airway epithelial cells Type II pneumocytes	Serine proteinases†
Elafin	12	Large-airway epithelial cells	Serine proteinases
α_2-macroglobulin	725	Hepatocytes Lung fibroblasts (Macrophages)	Serine proteinases, MMPs, cysteine proteinases
TIMP-1	27.5	Macrophages Lung parenchymal resident cells	MMPs
Cystatin C	13	Bronchial epithelial cells (Macrophages)	Cysteine proteinases

NOTE: Parentheses denote minor cellular sources.
*α_1-AT has greater affinity for neutrophil elastase than PR3 and CG.
†SLPI does not inhibit neutrophil elastase.

hibitor or α_1-antiproteinase, but the name α_1-AT is still commonly used for historical reasons. When α_1-AT is complexed with a proteinase, the complex binds to serpin-enzyme complex receptors on hepatocytes and monocytes.[31]

The genetic aspects of α_1-AT have been elucidated in detail. α_1-AT is transmitted in a co-dominant fashion. Thus, the gene product from each parent is expressed in the offspring. More than 75 different α_1-AT alleles are known, most of which result in single amino acid changes that do not alter expression of the protein or its function and, therefore, have little clinical significance. In broad terms, the states produced by these different alleles are referred to as: *normal,* in which there is a normal serum concentration of functional α_1-AT; *deficient,* in which the serum α_1-AT level is lower than normal; *null,* in which there is no measurable serum α_1-AT; and *dysfunctional,* in which there is a normal serum concentration of α_1-AT, but the α_1-AT does not have the normal antiproteinase activity.

The nomenclature for α_1-AT polymorphism uses letters to specify the allelic variants. When a letter is not available, the letter of the nearest anodal variant, together with the city of birth of the oldest person with the variant, is used. The original letters were chosen to reflect electrophoretic mobility: F = fast, M = medium, S = slow, and Z = ultraslow. The normal phenotype, Pi M, exists in more than 90 percent of the population, with the MS and MZ phenotypes being the next most common. The MS, MZ, and SS phenotypes are associated with only modest deficiencies of α_1-AT (about half of the normal serum concentration). They do not present an increased risk of emphysema, although in family studies and surveys of some patients with COPD, there has been an increased incidence of Pi MZ phenotype. People with Pi MS phenotype may have an increased frequency of airway hyperreactivity. Because people with Pi SZ,

who have an average of 37 percent of the normal α_1-AT serum concentration, rarely develop emphysema, serum levels α_1-AT greater than 35 percent of normal are thought to provide protection.

As mentioned previously, cigarette smoke can oxidize a methionine residue in the reactive center of α_1-AT, inactivating its capacity as a proteinase inhibitor. The potential consequences of this reaction were demonstrated in a dog model. Animals treated with chloramine-T, an agent that profoundly depresses α_1-AT functional activity, developed pulmonary emphysema.[1] However, the initial studies in smokers, which demonstrated oxidatively inactivated α_1-AT in the BAL fluid, have not been corroborated.

Tissue-Derived Inhibitors

Although study of proteinase inhibition in lung disease has tended to focus on α_1-AT, a circulating proteinase inhibitor produced mainly by the liver, a number of proteinase inhibitors originate in the lung and may serve an important function within lung tissue.

SERINE PROTEINASE INHIBITORS

Low-molecular-weight serine proteinase inhibitors are abundant in airway fluid and, hence, are thought to represent the primary defense against proteinase-mediated airway damage (Table 43-3). *Secretory leukoprotease inhibitor* (SLPI) is a 12-kDa protein produced by mucus-secreting and epithelial cells in the airway, as well as type 2 pneumocytes. SLPI inhibits HNE and CG and many other serine proteinases, but not PR3. *Elafin,* also produced by airway secretory and epithelial cells, is released as a 12-kDa precursor that is processed to a 6-kDa form that specifically inhibits HNE and PR3. These inhibitors are able to inhibit HNE bound to substrate, giving them an added dimension that α_1-AT lacks.

Airway mucus contains several other substances that partly inhibit HNE, including polyanionic molecules, such as mucins, other glycosaminoglycans, and fatty acids. DNA, released from inflammatory leukocytes, binds to SLPI, greatly enhancing its rate of association with HNE. The relative contribution of each of these molecules to proteinase inhibition is unknown.

TISSUE INHIBITORS OF METALLOPROTEINASES

Tissue inhibitors of metalloproteinases (TIMPs), noted previously, make up a family of proteins (three to date) with molecular masses ranging between 21 (TIMP-2, nonglycosylated) and 27.5 (TIMP-1, glycosylated).[41] Each TIMP inhibits MMPs via tight, noncovalent binding with 1:1 stoichiometry. TIMP-1 binds

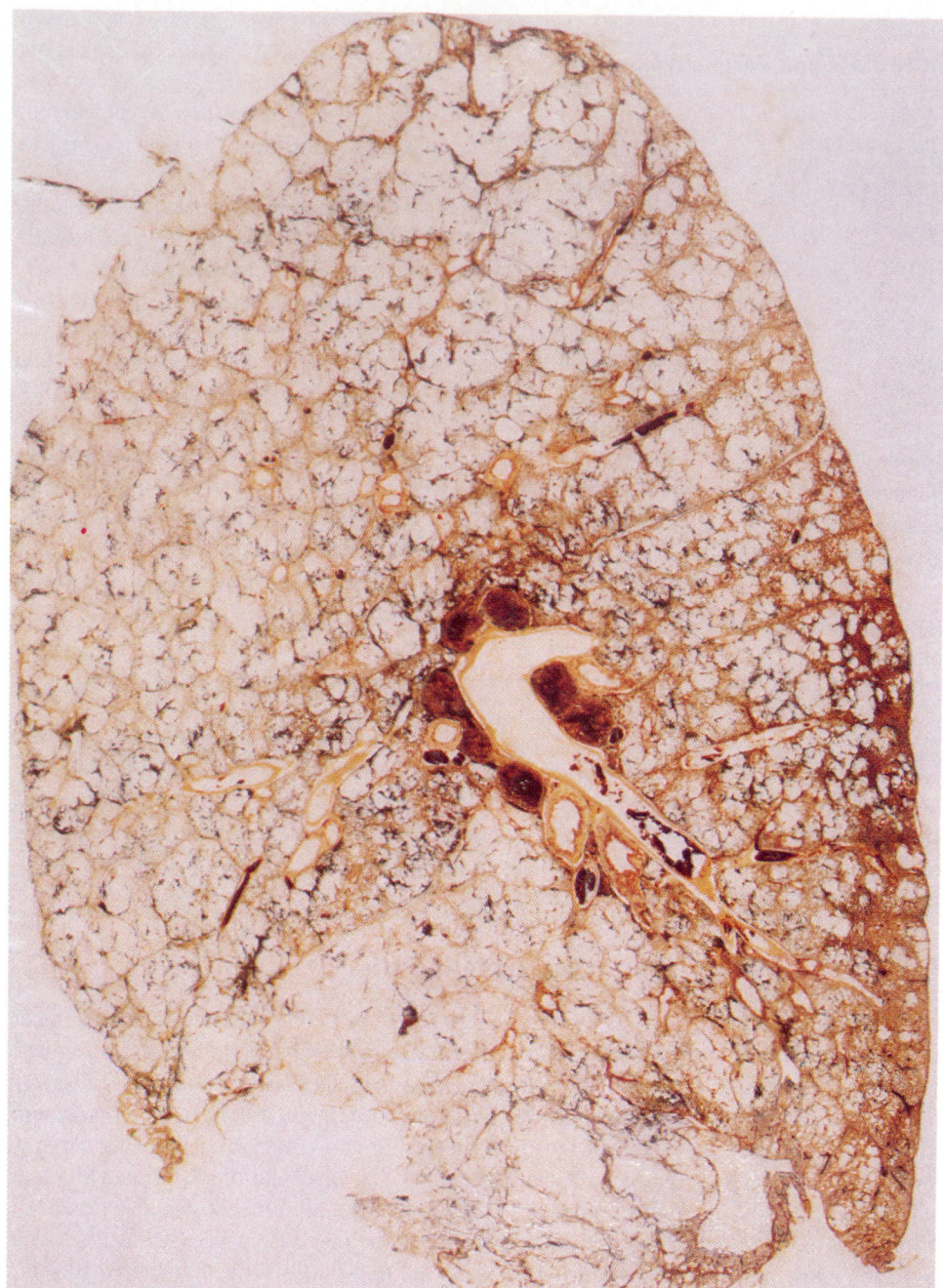

FIGURE 43-14   The pathology of Pi Z–type α_1-AT deficiency. Panacinar emphysema, worst in the lung base. Paper-mounted whole lung section.

as interferon-γ, inhibit collagenase and metalloelastase expression in macrophages, with little effect on TIMPs. Thus, depending on the inflammatory stimulus, MMPs and TIMPs may be coordinately regulated, perhaps limiting tissue injury during normal remodeling associated with inflammation. Alternatively, regulation may be discoordinate, potentially leading to tissue injury.

CYSTATINS

Cystatins represent families of cysteine proteinase inhibitors, some of which are strictly intracellular, while others, such as cystatin C, possess a signal peptide and are secreted by a variety of cells into the extracellular fluid. Cystatin C, composed of a single, nonglycosylated, 120-amino-acid peptide chain (13 kDa), forms reversible 1:1 complexes with enzymes in competition with substrates. Cystatin C is the most ubiquitous cystatin. It has been found in all human tissues and body fluids tested, providing general protection against tissue destruction by intracellular cathepsin enzymes leaking from dying cells. It is also a product of alveolar macrophages.

Emphysema Associated with α_1-Antitrypsin Deficiency

The clearest example of the association of proteinase-antiproteinase imbalance and emphysema occurs with inherited deficiency of α_1-AT. Several α_1-AT phenotypes are associated with very low serum concentrations of α_1-AT and emphysema. Of these, the Pi Z phenotype is, by far, the most common, accounting for more than 95 percent. The small remainder consist of Pi SZ, Pi null-null, or Pi null-Z phenotypes. Pi Z individuals have about 15 percent of the normal serum concentration of α_1-AT. The prevalence of the Pi Z phenotype in the United States is about one in 3000 people. The Z allele is rare in Asians and African Americans.

Most people with PiZ phenotype eventually become symptomatic with COPD, but there is considerable variation. Some people reach advanced age with minimal symptoms. In a group of subjects of Pi Z phenotype and their families, Silverman and colleagues confirmed the wide variability in pulmonary function among subjects. They found evidence for familial factors that segregated with deterioration in pulmonary function.[48] This striking variability in COPD between individuals of Pi Z phenotype

to the C-terminal domain of MMPs; how this binding leads to inhibition of catalysis is unknown. MMPs that lack the C-terminal domain, including matrilysin and the fully processed form of metalloelastase, are still susceptible to TIMP inhibition, although they require more TIMP to achieve inhibition than other MMPs. TIMP-2 is secreted complexed to the 72-kDa gelatinase in fibroblasts and is believed to interact specifically with the 72-kDa gelatinase.

TIMPs are secreted from many cell sources and are abundant in tissues. It is interesting to note that alveolar macrophages secrete a variety of metalloproteinases, as well as TIMP-1 and TIMP-2. Endotoxin induces synthesis of macrophage MMPs and TIMP-1, but it inhibits TIMP-2 production. Other cytokines, such

is a vivid illustration of how little is known about the mechanistic basis for COPD. Smoking has a marked effect on the age at which shortness of breath appears. The average smoker of Pi Z phenotype has symptoms by age 40, about 15 years earlier than a nonsmoker of Pi Z phenotype. The basis for COPD is panacinar emphysema (Fig. 43-14A), which is often worst in the basal parts of the lungs.

In addition to the association between α_1-AT deficiency and COPD, polymorphisms of the α_1-AT gene not associated with deficiency have been associated with COPD. These polymorphisms involve *Taq* I or *Hind* III susceptible sites in the 3' flanking region of the α_1-AT gene.[32] The basis for this possible association is not known, but one speculation is that these sites are specific to responsiveness of the gene to cytokines. According to this notion, the normal acute-phase response of increased synthesis of α_1-AT expression might not occur in some persons, making them relatively deficient in times of stress.

The diagnosis of marked deficiency of α_1-AT can be made in clinical laboratories by protein electrophoresis. Inspection of the electrophoretogram reveals a low, flat baseline in the α_1-globulin region, instead of the normal small peak (Fig. 43-15A). For precise quantification of α_1-AT concentration, radial immunodiffusion or other immunoassays are performed. For confirmation of the Pi Z phenotype, as well as determination of other phenotypes, isoelectric focusing of plasma in the pH range of 4.0 to 5.0, in which the protein focuses into several bands, is currently the procedure most widely used (Fig. 43-15B). Table 43-5 indicates the clinical situations in which screening for α_1-AT deficiency is advised.

The abnormality leading to the Pi Z phenotype is a point mutation in a single nucleotide at codon 342; the mutation results in coding for lysine instead of glutamic acid. This amino acid substitution changes the charge attraction between the amino acids normally present in positions 342 and 290 in α_1-AT and

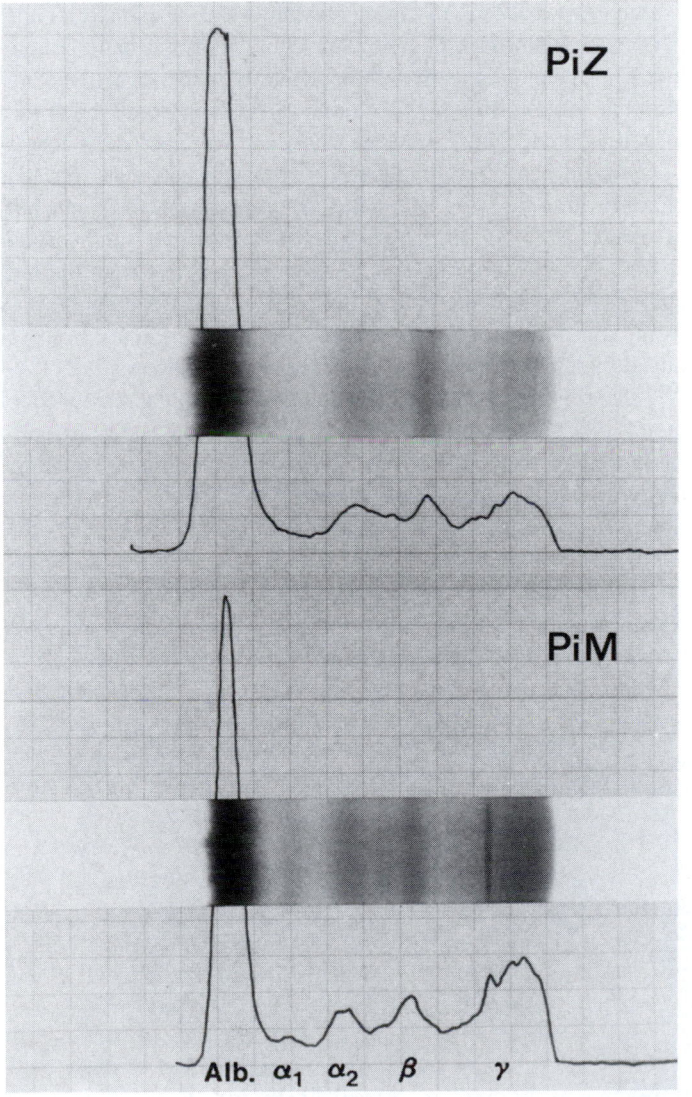

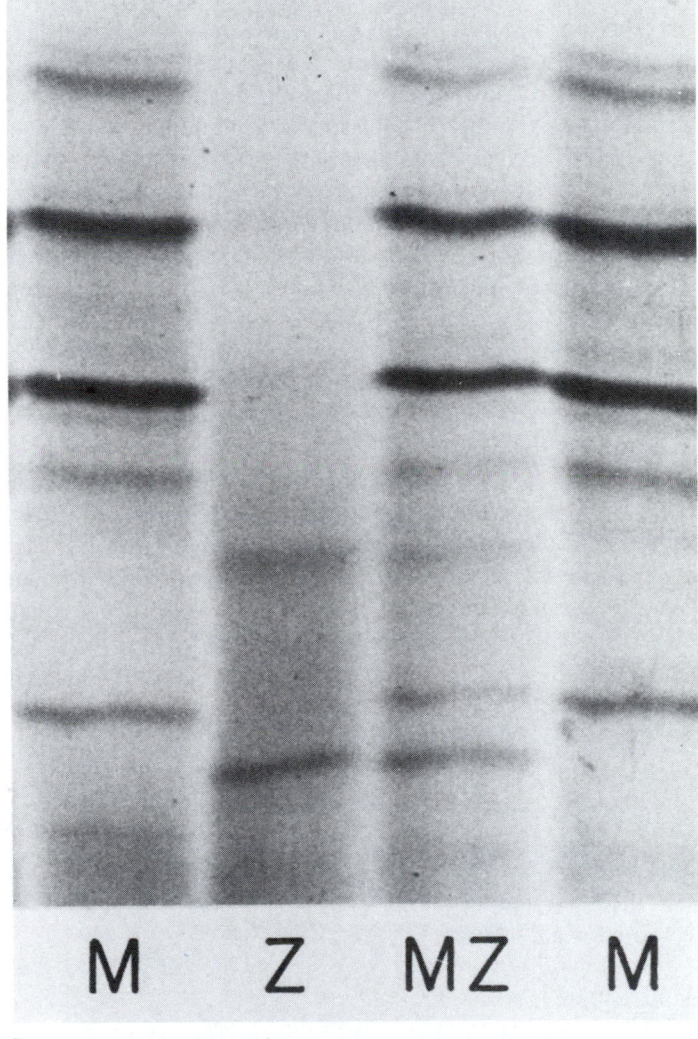

FIGURE 43-15 Detection of α_1-AT deficiency and determination of α_1-AT phenotype. A. Serum protein electrophoresis in Pi Z and Pi M, showing the absence of the normal peak in the α_1-globulin region in Pi Z. B. Patterns of Pi M, Pi Z, and Pi MZ on isoelectric focus. By this analysis, α_1-AT has microheterogeneity and thus appears as multiple bands. Pi M and Pi Z have distinctly different band patterns, while Pi MZ has a pattern that combines the patterns of both Pi M and Pi Z. *(Courtesy of John A. Pierce, M.D.)*

Screening for α_1-Antitrypsin Deficiency: Indications

Chronic bronchitis with airflow obstruction in a never-smoker

Bronchiectasis, especially in the absence of clear risk factors for the disease

Premature onset of COPD, with moderate or severe impairment by age 50

A predominance of basilar emphysema

Development of unremitting asthma, especially in a person under age 50 (screening is indicated even in the presence of atopy)

A family history of α_1-antitrypsin deficiency or COPD onset before age 50

Cirrhosis without apparent risk factors

source: From the American Thoracic Society,[3] with permission.

prevents the formation of a fold in the molecule. With this change in tertiary structure, the molecule is susceptible to dimerization with another α_1-AT molecule; the dimerization produces aggregation of α_1-AT in the endoplasmic reticulum that impedes secretion of the protein from the cell (Fig. 43-16A and B). Inability to secrete α_1-AT from the hepatocyte explains the low levels of the protein in plasma and other body fluids.

The Z form of α_1-AT has a second abnormal feature. Its rate of association with neutrophil elastase is significantly slower than the association rate of normal α_1-AT with neutrophil elastase. Thus, not only do persons with the Pi Z phenotype have a deficiency of α_1-AT protein, but the α_1-AT they do have is less effective than normal α_1-AT as an inhibitor of neutrophil elastase.

In contrast to the Z variant, the S variant of α_1-AT, which involves a single nucleotide alteration leading to substitution of glutamic acid[264] with valine, does not accumulate in the liver. This protein is less stable, presumably owing to loss of a salt bridge between the glutamic acid in position 264 and the lysine in position 387. The Pi null phenotype arises either because the α_1-AT gene is missing or because of a mutation in the α_1-AT gene that results in premature termination of the gene's transcription.

Other Mechanisms of Cigarette Smoking–Induced Lung Destruction

As noted above, cigarette smoke generates an inflammatory response, and products of inflammatory cells then unleash factors that perpetuate inflammation and cause a number of harmful effects. Apart from producing lung injury indirectly via inflammatory cells, cigarette smoke may affect the lungs directly (see Chapter 45).

OXIDANTS

Oxidants generated in cigarette smoke or produced by activated leukocytes recruited to the lungs by smoking represent potential direct and indirect sources of lung injury (see Chapter 45). For example, up to 20 mg of tar may be deposited in a smoker's lung per cigarette smoked. Cigarette tar contains more than 10^{17} stable, long-lived radicals per gram, primarily in the form of a semiquinone in equilibrium with quinones and hydroquinones in a viscous matrix. These radicals may lead to superoxide formation, which can then dismutate to hydrogen peroxide. The gas phase of tobacco smoke contains 10^{15} organic radicals per puff of smoke, although, in general, these small oxygen- and carbon-centered species are more short-lived and reactive than the radicals in the particulate phase. Collectively, the oxidants derived from both phases of tobacco smoke, as well as the species produced by leukocytes, may oxidize the methionine residue of α_1-AT, thereby inactivating this antiprotease. In the presence of metal ions such as iron, hydrogen peroxide may be reduced to form the hydroxyl radical (OH·), which is capable of "nicking" DNA strands. Hydroxyl radical may participate in the degradation of hyaluronic acid, as well as other glycosaminoglycans that coat elastic fibers. Desmosine and isodesmosine may be degraded through photo-oxidation, which is believed to be a hydroxyl radical–driven process. Hydroxyl radical may also participate in nonenzymatic degradation of type I collagen.

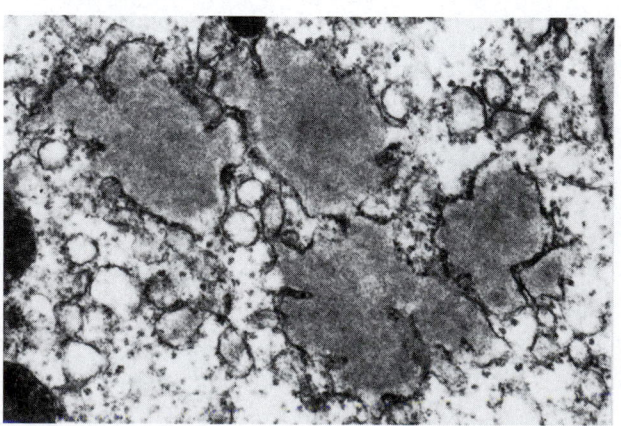

A

B

FIGURE 43-16 *A*. Globular cytoplasmic inclusions in hepatocytes in Pi Z α_1-AT. Periodic acid–Schiff stain after diastase digestion (×1250). *B*. Electron micrograph showing dilated cisterns of endoplasmic reticulum containing α_1-AT in a hepatocyte. These correspond to the globular inclusions in *A* (×25,000). *(Courtesy of Charles Kuhn III, M.D.)*

Oxidants may also facilitate proteinase-mediated extracellular matrix degradation by modification of matrix molecules, enhancing their susceptibility to proteolytic cleavage. Preexposure of elastin, collagen, or intact basement membrane to oxidants facilitates subsequent proteinase-driven degradation. The combination of cigarette smoke and elastase leads to greater emphysema in experimental animals than either insult alone.[29] Oxidants may also blunt the cells that synthesize matrix.

Inflammatory cells recruited to the lung may also be a source of oxidative injury. Although neutrophil chemotactic factors are recovered in the BAL fluid of oxidant-exposed rats, whether or not specific cigarette smoke constituents, such as nicotine, are chemotactic remains unclear. Components of tobacco smoke do, however, appear to "prime" neutrophils and alveolar macrophages to generate elevated amounts of reactive oxidants, such as hydrogen peroxide, hydroxyl radicals, and superoxide radicals. This increased activity is diminished with smoking cessation. Furthermore, in smokers, stimulation of alveolar macrophages in vivo is probably repetitive, with recurrent stimulation of the respiratory burst. The lung parenchyma of smokers also contains significantly more iron than that of nonsmokers, providing a catalyst for the production of hydroxyl radicals from H_2O_2. Additionally, smokers demonstrate increased production of neutrophil myeloperoxidase, which is capable of modifying H_2O_2, yielding oxidized halogens such as hypochlorous acid (HOCl). As a consequence, oxidants, regardless of their source, may act through a variety of mechanisms to produce lung tissue injury directly or indirectly.

ANTIOXIDANTS

Just as antiproteases provide an effective shield against local and circulating proteases, a system of antioxidant enzymes protects the intracellular—and, to a lesser extent, extracellular—environment from oxidative injury. Intracellular oxidant concentrations are maintained at acceptable levels by copper- and zinc-dependent superoxide dismutase in the cytoplasm and a manganese-dependent form in mitochondria. H_2O_2 is eliminated by catalase and glutathione peroxidase. Additional antioxidants include α-tocopherol and ascorbate. In the extracellular milieu, iron is prevented from participation in radical-generating reactions through its sequestration by transferrin, uric acid, and haptoglobin. Additionally, ceruloplasmin and albumin regulate relevant oxidants in the serum. Although it would appear that in the face of increased oxidative stress from exogenous and endogenous sources, the antioxidant defense system could be compromised, the available data are inconclusive. In fact, some evidence suggests that protective mechanisms are enhanced. The antioxidant capability of alveolar macrophages culled from smokers is increased. Moreover, the levels of glutathione in alveolar lining fluid are elevated. Measurements of ascorbate and α-tocopherol levels in smokers are difficult to interpret, however, with increased levels reported in macrophages and decreased quantities noted in serum and alveolar lining fluid. The bronchoalveolar and plasma concentrations of vitamin E are also reduced; systemic repletion does not increase these levels, suggesting local consumption. Given the available data to date, the physiological significance of selective increases or decreases in the antioxidant defense of cigarette smokers remains unclear.

TOBACCO CONSTITUENTS

In addition to oxidant-mediated injury discussed above, several specific cigarette constituents may play a role in the acute and chronic injury that follows exposure to tobacco smoke (see Chapter 45). The acute irritant response to cigarette smoke has been attributed to ammonia, acrolein, and nitrogen oxides. Chronic lung injury may be due, in part, to cadmium present in tobacco smoke. The question of cadmium's role was raised when survivors of vaporized cadmium salt inhalation were observed to develop airspace enlargement and fibrosis. Cadmium has also been found in emphysematous lungs in direct proportion to the degree of emphysema present, although it may simply represent a nonspecific marker of tobacco smoke exposure. Aerosolized $CdCl_2$ delivered to experimental animals results in lesions resembling human centriacinar emphysema. This is a neutrophil-independent process in which elastic fiber destruction does not seem to be a party. Unlike centriacinar emphysema in smokers, this emphysema carries a prominent fibrotic response.

Another cigarette smoke constituent capable of inducing airspace enlargement experimentally is nitrogen dioxide (NO_2). While the dominant nitrogen oxide in tobacco smoke is nitric oxide (NO), significant amounts of the more potent oxidant, NO_2, are present. Continuous generation of NO_2 is possible through the slow oxidization of NO. A hamster animal model utilizing inhalational NO_2 exposure led to decreased lung elastin and collagen content at 4 and 10 days, respectively. While total collagen content returned to normal after 14 days of exposure, elastin content did not return to a baseline level until NO_2 exposure ceased. Neutrophils were seen to accumulate in the lung after NO_2 exposure, however, suggesting that these inflammatory cells may have contributed to the reductions in collagen and elastin demonstrated. In summary, although data suggest that cigarette smoke may directly injure the lung or generate a chronic inflammatory response leading to emphysema or the airway changes of bronchitis, the specific components are not known.

CONCLUDING COMMENTS

Unchecked intrapulmonary elastase activity, released from inflammatory cells, that degrades lung elastin is generally accepted as the predominant mechanism for emphysema in smokers. Although elastin degradation may be the key element in the pathway to emphysema, the biology of emphysema is clearly complex (Fig. 43-17) and still poorly understood. It includes inflammatory cell recruitment, proteinase-antiproteinase balance, and oxidant-antioxidant balance, as well as responses of lung structural cells to proteinases and oxidants from inflammatory cells and to constituents of tobacco smoke. Degradation of extracellular matrix components besides elastin, particularly collagens, may also be an essential feature. The relative importance of chemotactic factors, proteinases, proteinase inhibitors, oxidants, antioxidants, repair processes, and other elements in the puzzle of emphysema is likely to vary on a genetic basis among different individuals with emphysema.

In an age when the entire human genome will soon be sequenced, unique opportunities arise to determine genetic factors that lead to emphysema in some smokers and protect other smok-

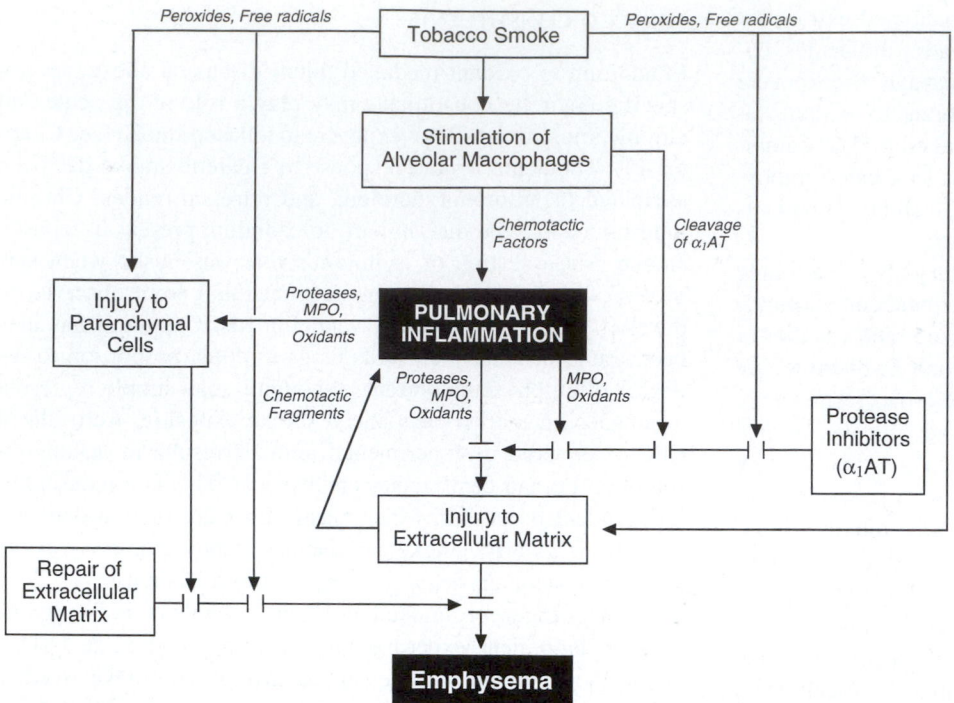

FIGURE 43-17   Schematic of concepts of the pathogenesis of emphysema due to smoking. Smoking causes an accumulation of inflammatory cells in peripheral tissues of the lungs. The inflammatory cells release proteinases and oxidants that damage or degrade extracellular matrix in the walls of alveoli, alveolar ducts, and respiratory bronchioles. Agents from inflammatory cells also inactivate intrapulmonary proteinase inhibitors, injure lung cells that make extracellular matrix, and interfere with the normal processing of lung extracellular matrix molecules. Components of tobacco smoke may have some of the same detrimental effects as products of inflammatory cells.

ers from this disorder. To probe the relative contribution of individual proteins in the development of emphysema, investigators are taking advantage of transgenic mice technology. Although mice are obviously quite different from humans, these animals are the closest species that can be rapidly genetically manipulated and used for controlled experiments. Researchers can generate strains of mice genetically deficient in individual proteinases by introducing targeted mutations of these genes into germline DNA. From these studies, it should be possible to pinpoint, more precisely than ever before, the proteins involved in the pathogenesis of smoking-induced emphysema.

REFERENCES

1. Abrams WR, Cohen AB, Damiano VV, et al: A model of decreased functional α-1-proteinase inhibitor: Pulmonary pathology of dogs exposed to chloramine T. *J Clin Invest* 68:1132–1139, 1981.

2. Agusti AGN, Barbera JA: Chronic pulmonary diseases: Chronic obstructive pulmonary disease and idiopathic pulmonary fibrosis. *Thorax* 49:924–932, 1994.

3. American Thoracic Society: Standards for the diagnosis and care of patients with chronic obstructive pulmonary disease. *Am J Respir Crit Care Med* 152:S77–S121, 1995.

3a. Anthonisen N, Connett J, Kiley J, et al: Effects of smoking intervention and the use of an inhaled anticholinergic bronchodilator on the rate of decline of FEV$_1$: The Lung Health Study. *JAMA* 272:1497–1505, 1994.

4. Bakke PS, Hanoa R, Gulsvik A: Educational level and obstructive lung disease given smoking habits and occupational airborne exposure: A Norwegian community study. *Am J Epidemiol* 141:1080–1088, 1995.

5. Barbera JA, Ramirez J, Roca J, et al: Lung structure and gas exchange in mild chronic obstructive pulmonary disease. *Am Rev Respir Dis* 141: 895–901, 1990.

6. Bartecchi C, MacKenzie T, Schrier R: The human costs of tobacco use. *New Engl J Med* 330:907–912, 975–980, 1994.

7. Becklake M, Lalloo U: The "healthy smoker": A phenomenon of health selection? *Respiration* 57:137–144, 1990.

8. Becklake MR: Occupational exposures: Evidence for a causal association with chronic obstructive pulmonary disease. *Am Rev Respir Dis* 140: S85–S91, 1989.

9. Bellofiore S, Eidelman DH, Macklem PT, Martin JG: Effects of elastase-induced emphysema on airway responsiveness to methacholine in rats. *J Appl Physiol* 66:606–612, 1989.

10. Betsuyaku T, Nishimura M, Yoshioka A, et al: Elastin-derived peptides and neutrophil elastase in bronchoalveolar lavage fluid. *Am J Resp Crit Care Med* 154:720–724, 1996.

11. Buist AS, Vollmer WM, Johnson LR, Mccamant LE: Does the single-breath N$_2$ test identify the smoker who will develop chronic airflow limitation? *Am Rev Respir Dis* 137:293–301, 1988.

12. Buist AS, Vollmer WM, Wu Y, et al: Effects of cigarette smoking on lung function in four population samples in the People's Republic of China. *Am J Respir Crit Care Med* 151:1393–1400, 1995.

13. Burge P: Occupation and chronic obstructive pulmonary disease (COPD). *Eur Respir J* 7:1032–1034, 1994.

14. Cardoso WV, Sekhon HS, Hyde DH, Thurlbeck WM: Collagen and elastin in human pulmonary emphysema. *Am Rev Respir Dis* 147:975–981, 1993.

15. Chapman HA Jr, Munger JS, Shi G-P: The role of thiol proteases in tissue injury and remodeling. *Am J Respir Crit Care Med* 150:S155–S160, 1994.

16. Centers for Disease Control and Prevention: Advance report of final mortality statistics, 1993. *Monthly Vital Statistics Report* 44:1–15, 1996.

17. Coultas DB, Gong H Jr, Grad R, et al: Respiratory diseases in minorities of the United States. *Am Rev Respir Dis* 149:S93–S131, 1993.

18. Cowie RL, Mabena SK: Silicosis, chronic airflow limitation, and chronic bronchitis in South African gold miners. *Br J Ind Med* 49:472–479, 1991.

19. Cox DW: α_1-Antitrypsin deficiency, in Scriver CR, Beaudet AL, Sly WS, Valle D (eds), *The Metabolic and Molecular Bases of Inherited Disease,* 7th ed. New York, McGraw-Hill, 1995, pp 4125–4158.

20. D'Armiento J, Dalal SS, Okada Y, et al: Collagenase expression in the lungs of transgenic mice causes pulmonary emphysema. *Cell* 71:955–961, 1992.

21. Di Stefano A, Maestrelli P, Roggeri A, et al: Upregulation of adhesion molecules in the bronchial mucosa of subjects with chronic obstructive bronchitis. *Am J Respir Crit Care Med* 149:803–810, 1994.

22. Doll R, Peto R, Wheatley K, et al: Mortality in relation to smoking: 40 years' observations on male British doctors. *Br Med J* 309:901–911, 1994.

23. Døssing M, Khan J, Al-Rabiah F: Risk factors for chronic obstructive lung disease in Saudi Arabia. *Respir Med* 88:519–52, 1994.

24. Drost EM, Shelby C, Lannan S, et al: Changes in neutrophil deformability following in vitro smoke exposure: Mechanism and protection. *Am J Respir Cell Mol Biol* 6:287–295, 1992.

25. Enright P, Kronmal R, Higgins M, et al: Prevalence and correlates of respiratory symptoms and disease in the elderly. *Chest* 106:827–834, 1994.

26. Finkelstein R, Fraser RS, Ghezzo H, Cosio MG: Alveolar inflammation and its relation to emphysema in smokers. *Am J Respir Crit Care Med* 152:1666–1672, 1995.

27. Fukuda Y, Masuda Y, Ishizaki M, et al: Morphogenesis of abnormal elastic fibers in panacinar and centriacinar emphysema. *Hum Pathol* 20:652–659, 1989.

28. Hogg JC, Macklem PT, Thurlbeck WM: Site and nature of airway obstruction in chronic obstructive lung disease. *New Engl J Med* 278:1355–1360, 1968.

29. Hoidal JR, Niewoehner DE: Cigarette smoke inhalation potentiates elastase-induced emphysema in hamsters. *Am Rev Respir Dis* 127:478–481, 1983.

30. Jørgen V, Prescott E, Lange P: Association of chronic mucus hypersecretion with FEV$_1$ decline and chronic obstructive pulmonary disease morbidity. *Am J Respir Crit Care Med* 153:1530–1535, 1996.

31. Joslin G, Fallon RJ, Bullock J, et al: The SEC receptor recognizes a pentapeptide neodomain of alpha$_1$-antitrypsin-protease complexes. *J Biol Chem* 266:11282–11288, 1991.

32. Kalsheker NA, Morgan K: Regulation of the α_1-antitrypsin gene and a disease-associated mutation in a related enhancer sequence. *Am J Respir Crit Care Med* 150(Suppl):S183–S189, 1994.

33. Kessler D: Nicotine addiction in young people. *New Engl J Med* 333:186–189, 1995.

34. Kurdowska A, Travis J: Acute phase protein stimulation by α_1-antichymotrypsin–cathepsin G complexes: Evidence for the involvement of interleukin-6. *J Biol Chem* 265:21023–21026, 1990.

35. Lamb D, McLean A, Gillooly M, et al: Relation between distal airspace size, bronchiolar attachments, and lung function. *Thorax* 48:1012–1017, 1993.

36. Lang M, Fiaux G, Gillooly M, et al: Collagen content of alveolar wall tissue in emphysematous and non-emphysematous lungs. *Thorax* 49:319–326, 1994.

37. Manning HL, Schwartzstein RM: Pathophysiology of dyspnea. *New Engl J Med* 333:1547–1553, 1995.

38. McLean A, Warren PM, Gillooly M, et al: Microscopic and macroscopic measurements of emphysema: relation to carbon monoxide gas transfer. *Thorax* 47:144–149, 1992.

39. Mecham RP, Davis EC: Elastic fiber structure and assembly, in Yurchenko P, Birk D, Mecham R (eds), *Extracellular Matrix Assembly and Structure.* Academic Press, San Diego, 1994, pp 281–314.

40. Merchant RK, Schwartz DA, Helmers RA, et al: Bronchoalveolar lavage cellularity. *Am Rev Respir Dis* 146:448–453, 1992.

41. Murphy G, Docherty AJP: The matrix metalloproteinases and their inhibitors. *Am J Respir Cell Mol Biol* 7:120–125, 1992.

42. Owen CA, Campbell MA, Boukedes SS, et al: A discrete subpopulation of human monocytes expresses a neutrophil-like proinflammatory (P) phenotype. *Am J Physiol* 267:775–785, 1994.

43. Owen CA, Campbell MA, Sannes PL, et al: Cell surface–bound cathepsin G on human neutrophils: A novel non-oxidative mechanism by which neutrophils focus and preserve catalytic activity of serine proteinases. *J Cell Biol* 131:776–789, 1995.

44. Oxman A, Muir D, Shannon H, et al: Occupational dust exposure and chronic obstructive pulmonary disease: A systematic overview of the evidence. *Am Rev Respir Dis* 148:38–48, 1993.

45. Rijcken B, Schouten J, Xu X, Rosner B, Weiss S: Airway hyperresponsiveness to histamine associated with accelerated decline in FEV$_1$. *Am J Respir Crit Care Med* 151:1377–1382, 1995.

46. Riley DJ, Kramer MJ, Kerr JS, et al: Damage and repair of lung connective tissue in rats exposed to toxic levels of oxygen. *Am Rev Respir Dis* 135:441–447, 1987.

47. Shapiro SD, Endicott SK, Province MA, et al: Marked longevity of human parenchymal elastic fibers deduced from prevalence of D-aspartate and nuclear weapons–related radiocarbon. *J Clin Invest* 87:1828–1834, 1991.

48. Silverman EK, Pierce JA, Province MA, et al: Variability of pulmonary function in alpha-1-antitrypsin deficiency: Clinical correlates. *Ann Intern Med* 111:982–991, 1989.

49. Snider GL: Emphysema: The first two centuries—and beyond: A historical overview, with suggestions for future research: Parts 1 and 2. *Am Rev Respir Dis* 146:1334–1344, 1615–1622, 1992.

50. Sommerhoff CP, Nadel JA, Basbaum CB, Caughey GH: Neutrophil elastase and cathepsin G stimulate secretion from cultured bovine airway gland serous cells. *J Clin Invest* 85:682–689, 1990.

51. Stone PJ, Gottlieb DJ, O'Conner GT, et al: Elastin and collagen degradation products in urine of smokers with and without chronic obstructive pulmonary disease. *Am J Respir Crit Care Med* 151:952–959, 1995.

52. Swee MH, Parks WC, Pierce RA: Developmental regulation of elastin production: Expression of tropoelastin pre-mRNA persists after down-regulation of steady-state mRNA levels. *J Biol Chem* 270:14899–14906, 1995.

53. Thurlbeck W: Letters to the editor: Lung structure and function in cigarette smokers. *Thorax* 49:1276, 1994.

54. Wagner EM, Bleeker ER, Permutt S, Liu MC: Peripheral airways resistance in smokers. *Am Rev Respir Dis* 146:92–95, 1992.

55. Wagner PD, Dantzker DR, Dueck R, et al: Ventilation-perfusion inequality in chronic obstructive pulmonary disease. *J Clin Invest* 59:203–216, 1977.

56. Wright JL: Emphysema: Concepts under change—A pathologist's perspective. *Mod Pathol* 8:873–880, 1995.

57. Wright JL, Cagle P, Churg A, et al: State of the art: Disease of the small airways. *Am Rev Respir Dis* 246:240–262, 1992.

58. Wright JL, Churg A: Smoke-induced emphysema in guinea pigs is associated with morphometric evidence of collagen breakdown and repair. *Am J Physiol* 268:L17–L20, 1995.

59. Xu X, Dockery DW, Ware JH, et al: Effects of cigarette smoking on rate of loss of pulmonary function in adults: A longitudinal assessment. *Am Rev Respr Dis* 146:1345–1348, 1992.

60. Yanai M, Sekizawa K, Ohrui T, et al: Site of airway obstruction in pulmonary disease: Direct measurement of intrabronchial pressure. *J Appl Physiol* 72:1016–1023, 1992.

CHAPTER 44

CHRONIC OBSTRUCTIVE PULMONARY DISEASE: CLINICAL COURSE AND MANAGEMENT

Ronald B. George / Gerardo S. San Pedro

Chronic obstructive pulmonary disease (COPD), a diagnosis devised and accepted by clinicians, refers to a constellation of clinical and pathologic findings that, individually or in combination, produce chronic airflow obstruction, disability, and, sometimes, death. The American Thoracic Society defines COPD as a disorder characterized by abnormal tests of expiratory flow (on a structural or functional basis) that do not change markedly over several months' observation. The diagnosis usually refers to the presence of chronic obstructive bronchitis associated with varying degrees of emphysema and bronchospasm (asthmatic bronchitis).

This chapter addresses the epidemiology, natural history, prevention, and treatment of COPD. Related diseases such as cystic fibrosis (see Chapter 53), asthma (see Chapter 50), bronchiectasis (see Chapter 132), and hypersensitivity pneumonitis (see Chapter 71) are not considered in detail here; only features that allow their differentiation are highlighted. The relevant anatomy and pathophysiology are covered in Chapters 42 and 43.

DEFINITIONS

Discussion of COPD begins with consideration of important differences among the most commonly recognized categories of disease, including chronic bronchitis, emphysema, and asthmatic bronchitis.

Chronic Bronchitis

Chronic bronchitis is a clinical diagnosis based on the symptoms of chronic cough and sputum production. The American Thoracic Society defines chronic bronchitis as the persistence of cough and excessive mucus secretion on most days over a 3-month period for at least 2 successive years. The closest pathologic correlate to this clinical syndrome is mucous gland hypertrophy, as assessed with the Reid index, which is the ratio of the width of the mucous glands to the thickness of the bronchial walls.

Most patients with chronic bronchitis do not have airflow obstruction and, hence, do not have COPD. However, about 10 to 15 percent of cigarette smokers are susceptible to a more rapid decline in airflow than normal.[19] Patients who have chronic productive cough and normal airflow are diagnosed as having *simple chronic bronchitis;* those who demonstrate a progressive abnormal decline in airflow have *chronic obstructive bronchitis.* The latter group constitutes the majority of patients with COPD.[19]

Emphysema

The diagnosis of *emphysema* is based on pathologic, rather than clinical, criteria. The American Thoracic Society defines emphysema as airspace enlargement distal to the terminal bronchiole and destruction of the alveolar wall; later refinements of the definition include the requirements that the airspace enlargement is permanent and that fibrosis is not a feature. Various subtypes of emphysema have been identified, based on the pattern of destruction within the acinus. These subtypes include *centrilobular* (proximal), *panacinar,* and *paraseptal* (distal) emphysema. The three patterns of emphysema have somewhat different etiologies and clinical presentations. Correlation of clinical patterns with pathologic changes is frequently inaccurate, and much overlap exists among the three types.

Centrilobular emphysema is the classic form associated with cigarette smoking. Frequently, it affects the lung apices and peripheral areas of the lungs. Marked hyperinflation and air flow obstruction are observed.

Panacinar emphysema more often affects the lower lung zones; it is the pattern associated with deficiency of α_1-antitrypsin.

Paraseptal emphysema (distal emphysema) affects the periphery of the acinus and is a cause of spontaneous pneumothorax in young adults. Since proximal portions of the acinus are spared in paraseptal emphysema, airflow obstruction may not be prominent.

Asthmatic Bronchitis

Marked reversibility of airway obstruction over relatively brief periods is the pathophysiological hallmark separating asthma from COPD. However, some patients with otherwise typical chronic obstructive bronchitis who are smokers or ex-smokers have significant changes in airflow following bronchodilator administration. Data from the Intermittent Positive Pressure Breathing Trial show that some patients with COPD have responses to inhaled bronchodilators that are comparable with those seen in patients with asthma.[5] Ten percent of patients in this trial demonstrated an improvement in 1-s forced expiratory volume (FEV_1) of 25 percent or more following inhalation of a β-adrenergic

agent. This patient subgroup appears to respond better to long-term therapy, including administration of corticosteroids.[36]

Little agreement exists on the precise definition of *asthmatic bronchitis,* although it is clear that emphysema and asthmatic bronchitis represent opposite ends of the clinical spectrum of COPD. Patients with emphysema have lower values for gas transfer in the lungs (DL_{CO}), exhibit more fixed obstruction, and respond less well to bronchodilator administration. Those with asthmatic bronchitis have more significant bronchospasm and little alteration in gas transfer. In addition, patients with asthmatic bronchitis may have wheezing on physical examination and increased numbers of eosinophils in the blood and sputum; the patient or family members may be atopic. Although the disease has not been defined by consensus, a reasonable working definition of asthmatic bronchitis is the presence of significant reversibility of airway obstruction (i.e., an increase in FEV_1 of 20 percent or more following bronchodilator administration) in a current or former cigarette smoker who has other symptoms of chronic obstructive bronchitis.

INCIDENCE AND SIGNIFICANCE

Currently, more than 14 million Americans are afflicted with COPD.[48] While chronic bronchitis is, by far, the most common component, most patients have a combination of chronic bronchitis and emphysema. Recent trends indicate that although the incidence of emphysema appears to be rising slightly, the incidence of chronic bronchitis has risen dramatically over the past 30 years.[48]

COPD and related disorders (including asthma, bronchiectasis, and hypersensitivity pneumonitis) currently rank as the fourth leading cause of death in the United States, having surpassed accidental deaths. In 1991, COPD accounted for 4.2 percent of all deaths (for a total of 90,650 deaths), with an age-adjusted mortality of 20.1 per 100,000.[38] Of greater significance from a public health standpoint is the chronic, progressive nature of the disorder, which may culminate in severe, prolonged disability. From a financial perspective, the estimated impact of COPD on the United States economy in 1986 was nearly $10 billion.[48] As the United States evolves a system of affordable, universal health care, prevention and treatment of COPD will become an increasingly important public health issue.

CLINICAL COURSE

Among the most important contributions to our knowledge of the natural history of chronic bronchitis and emphysema is a study of transport workers in the London area conducted by Fletcher and colleagues.[20] Nearly 800 working men, both smokers and nonsmokers, were studied over an 8-year period with serial recordings of FEV_1. The rate of decline in FEV_1, which normally begins at about age 25 years, was markedly increased among the 10 to 15 percent of susceptible cigarette smokers. Clinical disability did not occur until late in the course of the disease, when the FEV_1 had declined by about 70 percent. Typically, disability developed at approximately 65 years of age, when smoking cessation prolonged life only slightly; disability persisted lifelong (Fig. 44-1).

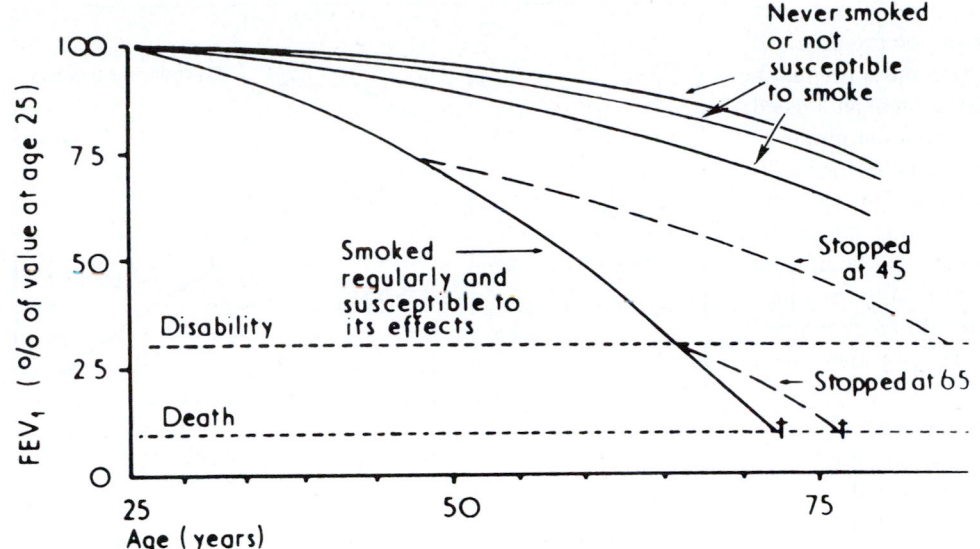

FIGURE 44-1   The effects of smoking and of smoking cessation on the forced expiratory volume in one second (FEV_1) in men aged 25 years and older. The top three solid lines indicate the average and range of values for decline in FEV_1 in men who were nonsmokers or who were not suceptible to the effects of smoking. The lower solid line represents a typical course in a smoker who was susceptible to developing COPD. Crosses indicate death from respiratory causes. Disability occurs at about age 65 years, when airflow is already markedly decreased. At that time, smoking cessation will prolong life by a few years, but disability will persist. In order to effect a major improvement in life expectancy, smoking cessation must occur at an earlier age. (*Based on data of Fletcher and Peto,*[19] *with permission.*)

In order to improve longevity and quality of life, smoking cessation must occur at an early age, before disability is evident. This underscores the importance of undertaking periodic evaluations of patients who smoke and vigorous attempts at breaking the smoking habit before disability occurs. As shown in Fig. 44-1, smoking cessation will decrease the accelerated rate of decline in lung function to a normal rate, but pulmonary function will not return to the age-adjusted range for nonsmokers.[20] Hence, ex-smokers revert to a normal rate of decline in FEV_1, but they manifest a lower level of lung function at the time of smoking cessation.

The findings in Fletcher's study have been confirmed.[2] The most recent confirmatory, longitudinal study is the COPD Early Intervention Trial, or Lung Health Study, a 5-year multicenter study sponsored by the National Heart, Lung, and Blood Institute;[2] details of the study are discussed below. The Lung Health Study evaluated the effects of smoking cessation and use of bronchodilators in early, mild COPD. As expected, in this population of adults with mild disease, smoking cessation resulted in a significant delay in the decline in FEV_1 with age.

Late Stages of Chronic Obstructive Pulmonary Disease

The late stages of COPD are characterized by a marked decline in pulmonary function and a decrease in reversibility of obstruction following administration of inhaled bronchodilators. Initially, patients are dyspneic during exertion. However, as disease progresses, lower levels of routine activity result in dyspnea; finally, dyspnea occurs at rest. Activities of daily living, such as bathing and dressing, become burdensome. During the very late stages of COPD, appetite is decreased and weight loss occurs. The weight loss is thought to be due to several factors, including decreased caloric intake and increased work of breathing; the latter is due to airway obstruction and a marked increase in physiological dead space (wasted ventilation), as discussed in Chapter 43. As lung function declines, the alveolar-arterial gradient for oxygen increases, primarily because of an increase in abnormal ventilation-perfusion relationships. Hypoxemia, pulmonary hypertension, and cor pulmonale develop. Psychological effects of advanced COPD may be observed, including anxiety and depression.

Respiratory infections are common in patients with COPD. Late in the course of the disease, the infections are associated with episodes of severe hypoxemia, with or without hypercapnia. Acute exacerbations require intensive therapy, often in a hospital; sometimes mechanical ventilation is necessary. During the final stages of the disease, weaning from mechanical ventilation becomes a major problem. The patient and family should be consulted in advance regarding their wishes on the use of mechanical ventilation to prolong life under these circumstances.

PREVENTION

The focus in prevention of COPD has been on smoking cessation and use of pharmacologic agents. Each is considered below, along with a brief review of additional prophylactic measures.

Smoking Cessation

The major cause of chronic bronchitis is cigarette smoking; in fact, the United States Surgeon General has stated that tobacco use is the single most important risk to human health in this country. Despite a significant decrease in cigarette smoking in the United States over the past 25 years, about 50 million Americans continue to smoke. While chronic bronchitis is rare among nonsmokers, the risk of COPD is increased up to 30-fold in smokers. Furthermore, a dose response relationship exists between the number of cigarettes smoked and the rate of decline in airflow in patients with chronic obstructive bronchitis.[20] In addition to the detrimental effects of active smoking, passive smoking among household members and workers exposed to cigarette smoke increases the normal rate of decline in pulmonary function with aging.[50]

In the COPD Early Intervention Trial, begun in 1986, 5887 adult smokers, 35 to 60 years of age, who had mild airway obstruction (with an average FEV_1 of 75 percent of predicted) were studied over a 5-year period. Subjects were entered randomly into three treatment groups: a smoking intervention program and regular use of an inhaled bronchodilator (ipratropium bromide), a smoking intervention program and administration of an inhaled placebo, and usual care with no smoking intervention program. The smoking intervention program consisted of behavior modification, group therapy, and nicotine replacement. Subjects who quit smoking entered a maintenance program aimed at preventing recidivism. Initial results of the study, which was completed in 1994, have been reported.[2] Consistent with results from previous investigations, smoking cessation resulted in a significant decrease in the age-related decline in FEV_1, even in patients with mild COPD (Fig. 44-2).

Based on the studies cited, an organized approach to smoking cessation counseling should be considered an essential component of the management of all smokers, especially those with COPD. However, fewer than 50 percent of cigarette smokers are advised by their physicians to smoke less or to stop smoking.[22] Intervention at an early age, when it is most effective, is rarely undertaken.

A simple office-based smoking cessation program can produce success rates as high as 50 percent in highly motivated patients. Direct, unequivocal advice to stop smoking has itself been shown to result in abstinence in up to 10 percent of patients. A simple, useful tactic is to establish a quitting date when the patient's stress level is low, and to have the patient sign a one-sentence contract (e.g., "I, John Doe, agree to quit smoking on the following date:_____") written in the progress notes and witnessed by the physician. Most patients who quit smoking do so on their own, with advice and support from their physician and members of the office staff. The patient's efforts should be supported by visits to the office 2 weeks after quitting, 1 month later, and, thereafter, as necessary. Several self-help programs are available at minimal cost from volunteer and government agencies, some of which are listed in Table 44-1. These programs assist the patient during the first few critical weeks of smoking withdrawal.

Commercial smoking cessation programs are available in most areas; however, they tend to be relatively expensive. Results from these programs are not superior to those of well planned office-based programs. A variety of methods should be made available to patients, and patients should be encouraged to choose the plan that best suits their needs.

Nicotine is a highly addictive drug that is thought to be a major factor in relapse following smoking cessation. In 1992, transdermal nicotine delivery systems ("patches") were introduced in the United States. In one multicenter trial, 61 percent of patients who used the nicotine patch had quit smoking at 6 weeks.[49] Long-term cessation of cigarette smoking achieved through use of nicotine patches alone is much less likely, and only about one-fourth remain abstinent at 6 months.

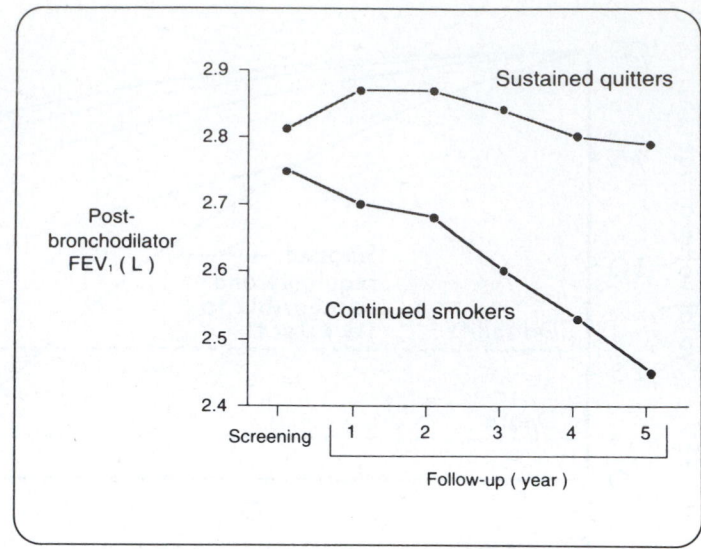

FIGURE 44-2   Mean postbronchial FEV_1 for participants in the Lung Health Study who were in the smoking intervention group; sustained quitters (open circles) and continued smokers (closed circles) are shown. The two curves diverse sharply from baseline. (*Based on data of Anthonisen et al,*[2] *with permission.*)

The importance of a "packaged approach" to smoking cessation has been emphasized, including counseling and follow-up visits.[17] The "four As" approach entails (1) **a**sking patients about their smoking status, (2) **a**dvising patients to quit, (3) **a**ssisting in setting a quit date, and (4) **a**rranging follow-up visits. Failure to adhere to a comprehensive program essentially guarantees failure, and patients should be encouraged not to depend on the nicotine patch alone to stop smoking.

Bronchodilators

Other "host" factors have been implicated in the abnormal decline of airflow in susceptible subjects, since most smokers do

TABLE 44-1

Sources for Self-Help Guides for Smoking Cessation

Title	Source
Smoker's Self-Testing Kit	PHS Publication No. 1904 Office of Smoking and Health Department of Health and Human Services Atlanta, GA 30341
Freedom from Smoking in 20 Days, and *A Lifetime of Freedom from Smoking*	American Lung Association 1740 Broadway New York, NY 10019
Quit for Good	National Cancer Institute National Institutes of Health Bethesda, MD 20892
I Quit Kit	American Cancer Society 90 Park Avenue New York, NY 10016

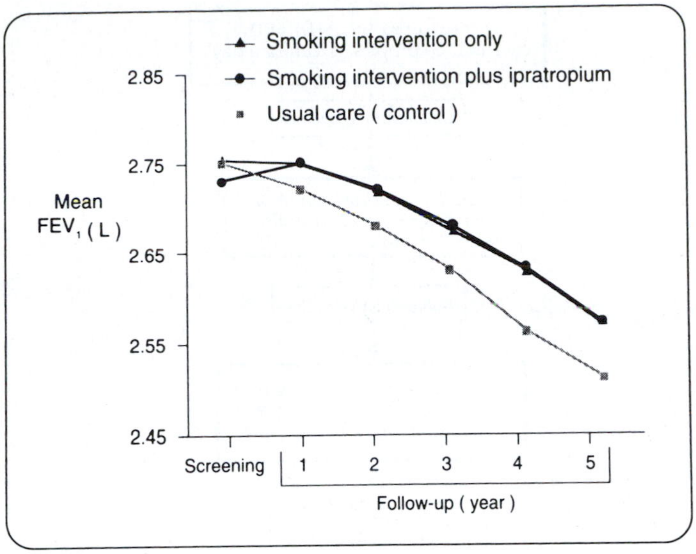

FIGURE 44-3   Mean postbronchodilator FEV_1 for all participants in the Lung Health Study in whom measurements were made over the 5-year period. The solid line represents the smoking intervention plus ipratropium bromide group. The dotted line with circles represents the smoking intervention plus placebo group. The dashed line with squares represents the usual care (control) group. The addition of ipratropium bromide in the smoking cessation group resulted in an early increase in FEV_1, which disappeared when the bronchodilator was stopped. The addition of a bronchodilator did not have a longterm effect on the decline in FEV_1. (*Based on data of Anthonisen et al,[2] with permission.*)

not develop COPD.[20] Prominent among these factors is airway hyperreactivity,[42] although the influence of bronchospasm on the decline in FEV_1 remains controversial.[34] According to the "Dutch hypothesis," smokers who have hyperreactive airways are more likely to develop symptomatic COPD than are smokers without airway hyperreactivity.[47] Indeed, some studies have shown a more rapid decline in lung function in smokers with hyperreactive airways.[51] Whether use of an inhaled bronchodilator in these patients will slow the rate of decline is unclear. Although early studies demonstrated that regular use of a bronchodilator might slow the decline in patients with hyperreactive airways,[5] results of the COPD Early Intervention Trial do not confirm this.[2] The addition of regular use of ipratropium bromide to a smoking cessation program produced a small increase in FEV_1 that disappeared after the bronchodilator was discontinued. Bronchodilator use did not affect the long-term decline in FEV_1 (Fig. 44-3).

Corticosteroids

Based on the common pathologic finding of airway inflammation in COPD, use of corticosteroids in preventing decline in lung function has been investigated. In one retrospective study, daily oral doses of at least 10 mg of prednisone produced a reduction in the rate of decline of FEV_1 over 14 to 20 years in patients with COPD.[43] More recently, results from an ongoing study indicate that addition of regular use of an inhaled corticosteroid to a bronchodilator regimen may delay the expected decline in FEV_1 in patients with COPD.[14] In this study, which includes patients with reversible airway obstruction, long-term inhaled cor-

ticosteroids appear to be most effective in subjects with the greatest variability of airflow. The addition of inhaled beclomethasone to regular bronchodilator therapy produced an initial improvement in FEV_1. Furthermore, although the decline in FEV_1 continued over time, airflow started from a "new," higher level and declined at a slightly slower rate than in controls. Hence, the anti-inflammatory effects of corticosteroids may affect the long-term decline in FEV_1 in COPD. Several studies of the effects of long-term inhaled corticosteroids on the course of COPD are currently under way.

Other Measures

Secondary preventive measures in COPD include administration of influenza and pneumococcal vaccinations. A general exercise plan and nutritional supplementation are also important adjunctive treatments for improving patients' functional status. These general measures are discussed further in the following sections on management of COPD.

THERAPY OF STABLE CHRONIC OBSTRUCTIVE PULMONARY DISEASE

A suggested approach to the continuing outpatient care of the patient with COPD is illustrated in Fig. 44-4.[11] Individual components are discussed in greater detail below.

Bronchodilators

Several classes of bronchodilator agents are used routinely in the management of COPD, including β-adrenergic agonists, anticholinergic agents, and methylxanthines.

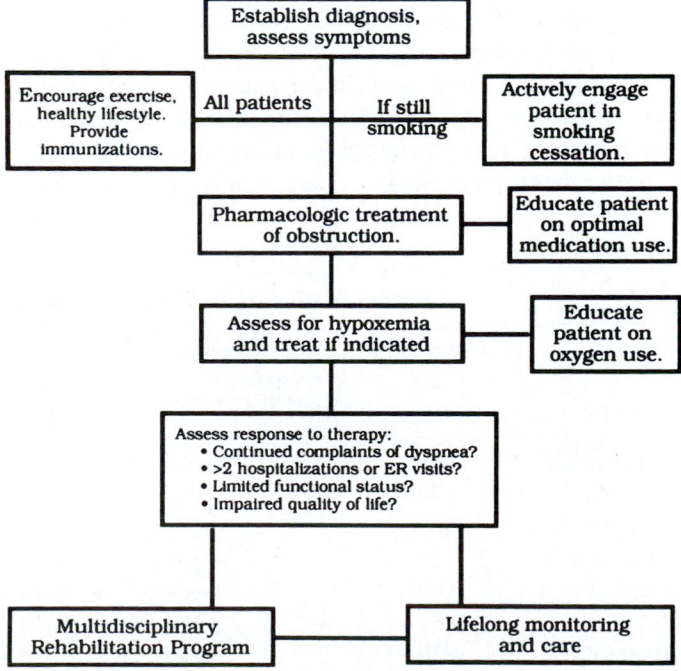

FIGURE 44-4   General outline for the outpatient management of stable COPD. (*Based on data of Celli et al,[11] with permission.*)

β-ADRENERGIC AGONISTS

β-Adrenergic agonists have been the mainstay of treatment of obstructive lung disease. These agents increase cyclic adenosine monophosphate (cAMP) formation, which, in turn, results in a change in intracellular calcium ion concentration and a reduction of bronchomotor tone. Onset of action is more rapid than for inhaled ipratropium bromide, but duration of action is shorter. Characteristics of the available agents are presented in Table 44-2.

Several agonists are available in various forms; because of their high incidence of side effects, oral formulations generally are not used unless patients are unable to use the inhaled forms. The various agents provide similar bronchodilation in equivalent doses, and the choice of agent depends on such factors as patient preference, physician experience, availability, and cost. The drugs are best taken on an "as needed" basis; hence, they may be used as primary therapy in patients who have dyspnea only intermittently. They may be added to regular doses of ipratropium when patients have daily symptoms. Excessive use of beta agonists may result in tachyphylaxis via a down-regulation of β_2 receptors, resulting in decreased bronchodilation. An algorithm for the proposed use of these and other therapeutic agents in patients with COPD is shown in Fig. 44-5.[16]

The side effects of beta agonists are numerous, and most stem from activation of β_1 receptors. Cardiovascular effects include tachycardia, dysrhythmias, exacerbation of myocardial ischemia, and hypo- or hypertension. Nervous system effects include tremor, agitation, and insomnia. Fortunately, tolerance to most subjective side effects develops within days, without loss of bronchodilation. Hypokalemia has been noted in patients receiving large doses.[16]

Reports on the incidence of serious adverse events during daily use of beta agonists by asthmatics have raised concerns about the safety of these drugs. Asthma exacerbations, both fatal and nearly fatal, have been linked to routine daily use of beta agonists; however, there is no clear cause-and-effect relationship. The increased use of the agents may simply identify patients with more severe disease who have an increased likelihood of more frequent and severe exacerbations. No data exist on the association between beta agonist use and adverse

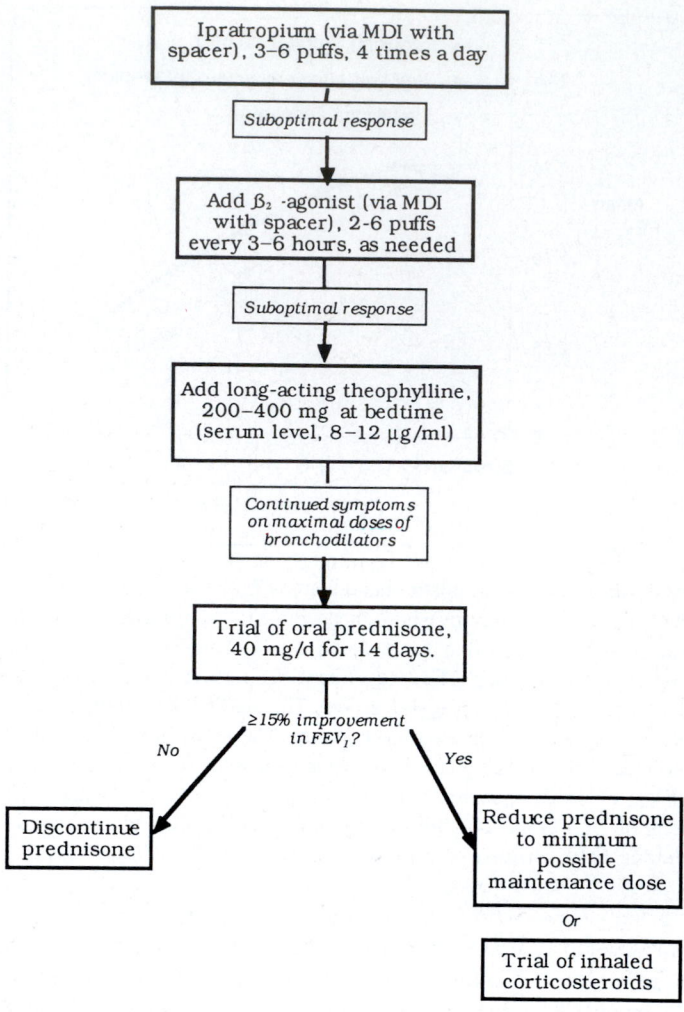

FIGURE 44-5 Proposed algorithm for the pharmacologic management of stable COPD. (*Based on data of Ferguson and Cherniak,[16] with permission.*)

events in COPD. At present, standard doses of the drugs are considered to be useful and safe in the management of patients with COPD.

TABLE 44-2

Characteristics of β-Adrenergic Agonists

Drug	Dose/puff (mg)	Beta-Receptor Activity β_1	Beta-Receptor Activity β_2	Time of Effect (min) Onset	Time of Effect (min) Peak	Time of Effect (min) Duration
Isoproterenol	0.08	+++	+++	3–5	5–10	60–90
Isoetharine	0.34	++	++	3–5	5–20	60–150
Metaproterenol	0.65	+	+++	5–15	10–60	60–180
Terbutaline	0.20	+	++++	5–30	60–120	180–360
Albuterol	0.09	+	++++	5–15	60–90	240–360
Bitolterol	0.37	+	++++	5–10	60–90	300–480
Pirbuterol	0.20	+	+++	5–10	30–60	240–480
Salmeterol	0.025	+	++++	10–20	~180	600–720

SOURCE: Adapted from Ferguson and Cherniak.[16]

ANTICHOLINERGIC AGENTS

Anticholinergic agents are among the oldest drugs known and were some of the first drugs to be used to treat respiratory disorders. These agents inhibit the action of acetylcholine at parasympathetic cholinergic nerve endings by competing for acetylcholine receptors. As a result, intracellular guanosine 3′,5′-cyclic monophosphate (cGMP) levels are reduced, resulting in a decrease in bronchial smooth-muscle tone.

Atropine sulfate has long been available in aerosolized and oral forms; however, its use has been limited by excessive side effects. Atropine is distributed rapidly in total-body water and readily crosses the blood-brain barrier, making unpleasant side effects—including dry mouth, tachycardia, blurred vision, urinary retention, and mental status changes—common and dose dependent. Atropine should not be given to patients with narrow-angle glaucoma or symptomatic prostatic hypertrophy.

New quaternary ammonium atropine derivatives have less mucosal absorption and fewer side effects. Currently, ipratropium bromide is the only such agent commercially available in the United States. Ipratropium bromide is available in a metered-dose inhaler and as a solution for nebulization. The drug has a relatively slow onset (60 to 90 min); however, it has a longer duration of bronchodilation (6 to 8 h) than do most β-adrenergic agonists. Hence, it is more suitable for use on a regular rather than an "as needed" basis. Submaximal bronchodilation has been demonstrated using the recommended dose of two puffs four times daily; consequently, the number of inhalations may be doubled or tripled, without notable side effects.[16] Ipratropium bromide also reduces sputum volume without altering sputum viscosity.

In some studies, ipratropium bromide has been reported to produce greater bronchodilation in chronic bronchitis than do conventional doses of beta agonists.[16] However, other investigations show that maximal doses of beta agonists produce the same degree of bronchodilation. A recent large, multicenter, double-blind clinical trial compared the efficacy of the beta agonist albuterol with that of ipratropium and a combination of the two agents in 534 patients with severe COPD.[12] The combination of drugs resulted in a greater change in FEV_1 from baseline than did either drug alone; the benefit persisted over the 85 days of the study. The additive effects may derive from the agents' disparate mechanisms and sites of action, as well as their differing time courses for bronchodilation.

Other studies have demonstrated a prolonged benefit (over 3 months) of ipratropium bromide. The incidence of side effects is low, and the side effects are generally minor. No tachyphylaxis has been reported, even when ipratropium bromide was used for as long as 5 years. Extended use of the agent does not appear to influence the long-term decline in FEV_1.[11] Given its effectiveness as a bronchodilator, prolonged duration of effect, wide therapeutic range, low incidence of side effects, and freedom from tachyphylaxis, ipratropium bromide has been recommended as a first-line agent for patients with COPD who have daily symptoms.[16]

METHYLXANTHINES

Methylxanthines are drugs with a long tradition of use in respiratory disease. Despite this history, the exact mechanism of action for theophylline, the prototype methylxanthine, remains unclear. The drug relaxes bronchial smooth muscle (although only to relatively mild degrees) and increases diaphragmatic contractility and endurance. Theophylline also improves cardiac output, reduces pulmonary vascular resistance, and improves perfusion to ischemic myocardium.[11] It has a narrow therapeutic window, with minimal improvement in lung function at serum levels less than 10 μg/ml; significant toxic effects are observed at levels

greater than 20 μg/ml. Theophylline's unique multisystem effects, additive actions with other bronchodilators, and availability in sustained-release oral formulations provide a role for the agent in maintenance regimens for patients with COPD.[44] Nevertheless, the potential for serious side effects (nausea, vomiting, insomnia, agitation, seizures, cardiac dysrhythmias) requires that serum levels be carefully monitored. This is especially true in the elderly and in patients with underlying medical disorders, including acute and chronic hepatic dysfunction, congestive heart failure, and febrile illnesses. In addition, a number of drugs commonly prescribed for patients with COPD (e.g., macrolide and quinolone antibiotics, H_2 blockers, propranolol) may prolong theophylline half-life, resulting in toxic side effects.

Corticosteroids

Several studies addressing use of systemic corticosteroids in patients with stable COPD have been conducted. Unfortunately, drug doses, routes of administration, duration of therapy, and end-points have varied from one study to another. A meta-analysis of all English-language, placebo-controlled trials of oral corticosteroids in COPD published between 1966 to 1989 has been performed.[8] Ten of the 15 studies evaluated met all nine prospectively defined, explicit quality standards. Response to oral corticosteroids was defined as a 20 percent improvement in baseline FEV_1. Response rate was defined as the proportion of patients who responded to corticosteroid therapy minus the proportion who responded to placebo. Only 10 percent of patients fulfilled the criteria for response. No association was found between steroid responsiveness and clinical factors, such as age and baseline FEV_1.

With only a limited number of patients demonstrating an objective response to corticosteroid therapy, is it possible to predict prospectively which patients will benefit from corticosteroids? Two measures that may be indicative are an increase in FEV_1 (at least 15 percent) following administration of an inhaled beta agonist[36] and the presence of sputum eosinophilia.[34]

The significant side effects associated with prolonged administration of systemic corticosteroids necessitate careful observation and documentation of the efficacy of therapy. If chronic oral therapy is required, alternate-day dosing, if possible, is recommended;[11] however, the efficacy of such a regimen has not been evaluated in patients with COPD. The recommended use of corticosteroids in patients with severe COPD is noted in Fig. 44-5. To date, use of nonsteroidal anti-inflammatory drugs, such as cromolyn and nedocromil, has not been evaluated in patients with severe COPD.[11]

Other Therapeutic Agents

Chronic cough is the defining symptom in chronic bronchitis. However, cough may be a sign of associated diseases, such as cancer and acute respiratory infection. In most patients, the cause is readily identified. Therapy should be directed at the specific cause once it has been identified. Antitussives and expectorants may be used to control the cough if it is a nuisance or results in other medical problems. Patients with ineffective, exhausting coughs can be trained to cough more effectively.

Mucolytics are of questionable benefit in the management of COPD. In one large multicenter, randomized, placebo-controlled clinical trial of iodinated glycerol, subjective measures—such as cough frequency, cough severity, chest discomfort, ease of expectoration, and overall health status—were improved in patients treated for 8 weeks. Objective evidence of benefit was considered insufficient, however, and the Food and Drug Administration mandated discontinuation of marketing of the drug. Other agents, including aerosolized water and acetylcysteine, have not been demonstrated to benefit patients with COPD.[11]

PULMONARY REHABILITATION

As the FEV_1 falls below 50 percent of predicted value in patients with COPD, essential activities of daily living become restricted. This limitation develops against a background of an already compromised quality of life due to shortness of breath and psychosocial disability. A vicious cycle ensues in which the patient performs less exercise and becomes more disabled and more depressed. Pulmonary rehabilitation is aimed at interrupting the cycle (see Chapter 46).

Pulmonary rehabilitation comprises a constellation of therapeutic methods that have been shown to improve survival and quality-of-life indices, reduce respiratory symptoms, increase length and intensity of exercise tolerance, decrease need for hospitalization, and improve psychological function. In addition, pulmonary rehabilitation is geared to reducing anxiety and depression and to increasing feelings of hope, control, and self-esteem.[11,45] Patients with COPD are candidates for a comprehensive rehabilitation program if, despite optimal medical therapy, they continue to complain of dyspnea, have had several emergency room visits or hospital admissions in the past year, exhibit limited functional status, or complain of impaired quality of life. Individual components of rehabilitation programs vary and may be tailored to the needs of the patient. Basic elements include patient education, nutritional assessment, exercise training, breathing retraining, and psychosocial support.

Patient Education

Education is a key factor in the routine care of the patient with advanced COPD. Educational goals include having patients understand the basic pathophysiology of their disease, modifying high-risk behaviors such as smoking, and making sure that medications are used properly. Patients who are educated about their disease generally demonstrate an increased ability to recognize and treat symptoms and develop practical ways of coping with disabling symptoms; they also manifest better adherence to the prescribed therapeutic regimen.[11]

The educational program should be offered along with other components of pulmonary rehabilitation, including physical reconditioning and smoking cessation. Improvements in disease status, daily functional status, mental health, and quality of life in patients with COPD completing a relatively short (6 to 12 h) health education program cannot be demonstrated when other components of comprehensive care are not provided.[29]

As part of patient education, the physician should explain the disease process and outline a management plan. The physician need not conduct the entire educational program, as studies have shown that nurses, respiratory therapists, physical therapists, and other allied health personnel may be better than physicians at educating patients. These medical professionals often spend more time with the patient than the physician does.

Since adults vary in their learning styles, a diversity of learning techniques should be made available, including printed materials (e.g., self-help programs for smoking cessation); videos, slides, or overheads for office and home use; didactic presentations; and group discussions. The patient should be encouraged to participate actively in the program; to maintain a healthy, active lifestyle; to obtain appropriate vaccines; and to avoid smoke and other irritants.[11] Emotional support and encouragement are important, especially during periods of frustration and depression. The management team must accept the fact that some functional changes are irreversible; the goal is prevention rather than cure. In patients with advanced disease, the physical therapist or respiratory therapist may approach the patient about a living will or limited power of attorney. The physician must be available for advice about advance directives. Whenever possible, these issues should be discussed before the patient is hospitalized for worsening respiratory failure.

Nutritional Assessment

About 25 percent of patients with COPD suffer from undernutrition (body weight less than 90 percent of ideal).[16] These patients have reduced respiratory muscle function and increased mortality. Even when receiving nutritional supplementation, many patients are unable to gain weight, perhaps because of an underestimation of caloric needs or an inability to maintain adequate caloric intake. Dyspnea may play a role in limiting intake. In patients with chronic hypercapnia, excess production of carbon dioxide due to increased carbohydrate intake was once thought to increase Pa_{CO_2}; however, recent studies have shown that this is not a problem unless the total caloric intake markedly exceeds caloric needs. Hypercapnic patients do not need to avoid carbohydrates, but should maintain a normal nutritious diet and optimum weight, eating foods they enjoy.

Exercise

Exercise is generally considered an important component of pulmonary rehabilitation programs. Reviews[10] of published studies of general exercise conditioning in chronic lung disease highlight consistent improvement in exercise endurance or maximum exercise tolerance. However, the optimal methods of training and the mechanisms underlying the improvements have not been clearly defined.[45] Principles of exercise physiology derived from normal subjects or cardiac patients cannot be applied to patients with COPD, owing to the different limitations to exercise performance and coexisting problems of training in older patients.

The intensity of exercise training may be important, and recent reports suggest that high-intensity training is beneficial for COPD patients. In a study comparing the training response in patients with moderate COPD who performed high-intensity bicycle ergometry with that in a control group who trained at a lower intensity, the high-intensity group showed a greater decrease in lactate levels and heart rate at a given level of work and similar levels of oxygen consumption. The lower lactate levels resulted in less CO_2 generation from bicarbonate buffering and a lower ventilatory demand at any given workload.[9]

Finally, it should be noted that exercise training is largely muscle group specific. Hence, it is unlikely that lower-extremity bicycle or treadmill training will affect performance with the arms. Indeed, a training program that utilizes both arm and leg exercise results in a greater improvement in activities of daily living than does a program limited to leg exercise.

Breathing Retraining

Breathing retraining includes instruction in techniques of chest physiotherapy, diaphragmatic breathing, and pursed-lip breathing.

Many patients with COPD have abnormalities in lung clearance mechanisms that make them more susceptible to problems related to retained secretions (e.g., infection and atelectasis). Rehabilitation programs teach coughing and chest physiotherapy techniques for secretion control. However, the benefit of the individual techniques is difficult to determine, and many clinicians remain skeptical of their efficacy. Available evidence suggests that postural drainage and controlled coughing may be the most effective techniques,[45] especially in patients who produce a large amount of sputum (more than 30 ml per day).

Diaphragmatic breathing is a maneuver in which the patient attempts to coordinate outward abdominal wall movement with inspiration and to slow expiration by pursed-lip breathing (see below). Respiratory rate slows and, supposedly, tidal volume increases. In studies evaluating this technique, patients report subjective improvement, but objective results are mixed.[45] In a recent study of patients with severe COPD studied before, during, and after training in diaphragmatic breathing, no change in tidal volume or respiratory frequency was observed.[25] Moreover, chest wall motion became discoordinated, mechanical efficiency of breathing declined, and the sensation of dyspnea increased.

In pursed-lip breathing, a technique often assumed naturally by some patients with COPD, the lips are tensed during expiration, resulting in airway narrowing and prolongation of the expiratory phase. Pursed-lip breathing results in increased tidal volume, reduced respiratory rate, improved ventilation-perfusion matching, and increased arterial oxygen saturation, as measured by pulse oximetry.[45]

Psychosocial Support

Patients with COPD develop a variety of psychosocial symptoms that reflect their progressive feeling of hopelessness and their inability to cope with their disease. Depression is common. Successful pulmonary rehabilitation programs attend to the patient's psychosocial problems as well as physical ones. Patients who respond to rehabilitation, both early and long-term, have less severe psychological symptoms (e.g., depression, anxiety, body preoccupation, fear of dyspnea) than do nonresponders.[45] Family members and friends should be included in program activities so that they can understand and cope better with the patient's disease. Patients with severe psychological disorders may benefit from individual counseling and psychotherapy. Psychotropic drugs should be reserved for patients who have severe psychological dysfunction.

OXYGEN THERAPY

In 1995, about 616,000 patients in the United States were treated with supplemental home oxygen, at an estimated annual cost of $1.4 billion.[40] The value of long-term supplemental oxygen therapy for hypoxemic patients with severe COPD has been demonstrated in major controlled trials. In the National Heart, Lung, and Blood Institute's Nocturnal Oxygen Therapy Trial,[39] patients with COPD and hypoxemia while breathing room air (Pa_{O_2} under 55 mmHg) were randomly assigned to receive oxygen for either 12 h a day (nocturnal group) or 24 h a day (continuous group); all patients received oxygen during sleep. At 26 months, overall mortality in the continuous group (who actually received oxygen for an average of 19 h a day) was approximately one-half that of the nocturnal group. In addition, morbidity in the continuous group was less than that of the nocturnal group. These findings, along with those reported in a study from the British Medical Research Council,[35] serve as the basis for current recommendations regarding supplemental oxygen use in patients with COPD (see below).

Indications for Oxygen Therapy

Indications for long-term supplemental oxygen include a resting Pa_{O_2} of 55 mmHg or less or evidence of tissue hypoxia and organ damage, such as cor pulmonale, secondary polycythemia, edema from right heart failure, or impaired mental status. Evaluation for nocturnal oxygen use should also be considered, since patients with COPD may have episodic arterial desaturation during sleep in the absence of daytime hypoxemia. These episodes are not always associated with sleep disturbances and may be related to abnormalities in gas exchange. In a study evaluating the long-term effects of nocturnal oxygen administration in patients with COPD who had nocturnal hypoxemia and a daytime Pa_{O_2} of 60 mmHg or more, a group treated with nasal oxygen was compared with another receiving compressed air via nasal cannula.[18] Over a 3-year period, mean pulmonary artery pressure decreased by 3.7 mmHg in patients receiving oxygen and increased by 3.9 mmHg in those receiving compressed air ($p < 0.02$). Mortality was similar in the two groups. Finally, patients with COPD who are normoxemic at rest may become hypoxemic during exercise; exercise capacity and endurance may be improved with oxygen supplementation.

Techniques of Administration of Supplemental Oxygen

Home oxygen can be supplied with an oxygen concentrator, a compressed oxygen cylinder, or a source of liquid oxygen. The most cost-effective and reliable method is the oxygen concentrator, since it requires only an electrical source and periodic maintenance; backup sources of oxygen, such as a cylinder or liquid oxygen, should be available for extenuating circumstances (e.g., electrical power failure). Liquid oxygen and compressed oxygen cylinders permit patient mobility.

Oxygen is usually delivered by nasal cannula at continuous flows of 0.5 to 4 L/min. Oxygen-conserving devices use reservoirs that allow delivery of a higher F_{IO_2} at lower flows. The goal of oxygen therapy is to achieve a Pa_{O_2} of 60 mmHg; using higher flows to achieve a significantly higher Pa_{O_2} will accomplish little clinically. The patient should be reevaluated with arterial blood gases after 1, 6, and 12 months; follow-up arterial blood gases are important, since about 20 percent of patients initially eligible for supplemental oxygen no longer need it after aggressive bronchodilator therapy.[39]

Other techniques of oxygen administration have been developed in an attempt to reduce supplemental oxygen requirements and improve cosmesis. Transtracheal oxygen delivery via a small-bore catheter offers several advantages over use of nasal cannula, including a 50 percent reduction in supplemental oxygen requirement, decreased dyspnea, improved exercise tolerance, and decreased rate of hospitalization.[26] In a comparison of clinical outcomes in 20 stable patients with COPD who received oxygen for 6 months by either nasal cannula or transtracheal catheter, those treated with the transtracheal technique had reduced flow requirements, increased 12-min walk distance, and fewer hospital days.[27] Minor complications of the transtracheal technique include catheter displacement and mucous ball formation at the catheter tip.

A number of factors may be operative to account for the beneficial clinical and arterial blood gas effects achieved with transtracheal oxygen. For example, the oxygen "jet" may flush CO_2 from the upper airway; in addition, dead-space volume is reduced. Furthermore, the trachea acts as a reservoir, reducing the amount of supplemental oxygen wasted during expiration. Other potential benefits of the technique are better patient compliance and avoidance of hypoxemia during obstructive sleep disturbances, since the nose and glottis are bypassed. Because the device can be easily covered by clothing, patient satisfaction is increased.

MANAGEMENT OF ACUTE EXACERBATIONS

Acute decompensation of COPD is characterized by increased dyspnea, cough, and purulent sputum production. The decision to hospitalize a patient with an acute exacerbation is usually based on the physician's subjective interpretation of clinical symptoms, including severity of dyspnea, short-term response to therapeutic efforts, and the presence of other conditions—e.g.,

---

TABLE 44-3

Indications for Hospitalization of Patients with COPD

Acute exacerbation (increased dyspnea, cough, or sputum production), plus one or more of the following:

　Inadequate response to outpatient management

　In a patient previously mobile, inability to ambulate due to dyspnea

　Inability to eat or sleep due to dyspnea

　Inadequate home care resources

　Serious co-morbid condition

　Prolonged progressive symptoms before emergency visit

　Altered mentation

　Worsening hypoxemia

　New or worsening hypercapnia

New or worsening cor pulmonale unresponsive to outpatient management

Planned invasive surgical or diagnostic procedure requiring analgesics or sedatives that may worsen pulmonary function

Co-morbid condition—e.g., severe steroid myopathy or acute vertebral compression fractures—that has worsened pulmonary function

SOURCE: Adapted from Celli et al.[11]

---

bronchitis, pneumonia, or other co-morbidities. Notably, up to 28 percent of patients with an acute exacerbation of COPD who are discharged from an emergency department (rather than admitted) have recurrent symptoms within 14 days;[37] 17 percent of patients discharged after emergency department management will relapse and require hospitalization.[11] The American Thoracic Society has devised guidelines for hospitalization (Table 44-3) and ICU admission (Table 44-4) of patients with an acute exacerbation of COPD.[11]

Mortality for patients who require hospitalization is substantial. In one study of 590 patients, the mortality was 14.4 percent. Using multivariate, logistic regression analysis, the investigators identified several independent variables that predicted mortality: increased age, an alveolar-arterial oxygen gradient greater than 41 mmHg, and presence of atrial fibrillation or ventricular dysrhythmias.[23]

Bronchodilators

Pharmacologic therapy for acute exacerbations of COPD centers on the use of beta agonists. Aerosol delivery is the most effective route of administration; delivery using a metered-dose inhaler (MDI) or nebulizer has been employed. Studies confirm the equal

---

TABLE 44-4

Indications for ICU Admission of Patients with Acute Exacerbation of COPD

Severe dyspnea that responds inadequately to initial emergency therapy

Confusion or lethargy

Respiratory muscle fatigue (especially, paradoxical diaphragmatic motion)

Persistent or worsening hypoxemia despite supplemental oxygen or severe/worsening respiratory acidosis (pH < 7.30)

Need for noninvasive or invasive assisted mechanical ventilation

SOURCE: Adapted from Celli et al.[11]

efficacy of the two techniques.[33] The safety and efficacy of continuous nebulization of beta agonists have not been established in COPD.[11] The slow onset of action of ipratropium bromide has relegated this drug to a minor role in the acute setting; however, its apparent additive effects with beta agonists[12] should be considered. High doses are generally well tolerated; an upper dosage limit has not been established. Ipratropium bromide may be combined with a beta agonist for nebulizer delivery.

In addition to beta agonists, theophylline has been used in the management of acute exacerbations of COPD. The efficacy of theophylline (or aminophylline) in this setting is uncertain.[44] If it is used, levels of the agent should be monitored closely so that overdosage can be averted. Serum levels of 8 to 12 μg/ml are appropriate for most patients, although some patients may tolerate higher levels (up to 18 to 20 μg/ml).

Corticosteroids

Controlled, double-blinded studies evaluating the effects of corticosteroids in the treatment of exacerbations of COPD have been relatively few; the results are conflicting.[30] In a double-blind, randomized, placebo-controlled parallel study of 44 consecutive patients hospitalized for an exacerbation of COPD and acute respiratory insufficiency, patients received intravenous methylprednisolone (0.5 mg/kg every 6 h for 72 h) or placebo.[1] All patients were given intravenous aminophylline, inhaled isoproterenol, supplemental oxygen, and antibiotics. The corticosteroid-treated group showed a statistically significant increase in postbronchodilator FEV_1 at every 6- to 8-h time point from 12 to 72 h; 12 of the 22 patients receiving methylprednisolone had a 40 percent or greater improvement in prebronchodilator FEV_1 by 72 h, compared with only 3 of 21 receiving placebo ($p < 0.05$). No differences were noted in arterial blood gases. In a more recent controlled study,[15] no differences in FEV_1 or hospitalization rates were noted among 96 patients with COPD who were randomized to receive either 100 mg intravenous methylprednisolone or placebo during acute exacerbations.

Treatment of Infection

Bronchial infection is the most common precipitating factor for an acute exacerbation of COPD. *Streptococcus pneumoniae* and *Hemophilus influenzae* are the most common pathogenic bacteria isolated in the sputum of patients experiencing an acute exacerbation. However, the same bacteria can be isolated from stable patients. Thus, there has been an ongoing debate over the efficacy of antibiotic therapy during acute flares. The most comprehensive study addressing this issue is a randomized, double-blinded, crossover trial in which 362 exacerbations in 173 outpatients were treated.[3] Ten-day courses of either trimethoprim-sulfamethoxazole (one double-strength tablet twice daily), amoxicillin (250 mg four times daily), or doxycycline (200 mg initially, followed by 100 mg twice daily) were administered. Patients treated with antibiotics had a higher clinical success rate—defined as resolution of all acute symptoms—within 21 days, than those receiving placebo. Patients receiving placebo were twice as likely to experience deterioration of symptoms. There was no difference in efficacy among the three antibiotic regimens. Peak expiratory flow rates (measured on day 6 of the trial)

were significantly more improved in antibiotic-treated patients. The incidence of side effects was similar in patients treated with antibiotics and those receiving placebo. On the basis of these findings, antibiotics appear to have a beneficial effect in patients experiencing an acute exacerbation of COPD. Indeed, a recent meta-analysis of the randomized trials of antibiotics in exacerbations of COPD published in English from 1955 to 1994 confirm a small but statistically and clinically significant improvement with antibiotic therapy in this patient population—especially for those hospitalized with severe disease (manifested by low peak expiratory flow).[46]

Other Measures

Supplemental oxygen should be administered to most patients with an exacerbation of COPD, since deterioration usually leads to increased ventilation-perfusion inequalities and worsening hypoxemia. Sputum may be tenacious and copious, so adequate hydration should be provided. Two to 3 L of fluid daily should be supplied by mouth or parenterally, unless cardiac or renal insufficiency is of concern.

SURGERY FOR EMPHYSEMA

Although removal of localized large bullae (bullectomy) has long been recognized as potentially beneficial in a carefully selected group of patients with emphysema and local bullous disease,[24] recent medical and surgical advances have prompted use of other surgical techniques in treating patients with generalized emphysema. These techniques include lung transplantation and volume reduction surgery.

Lung Transplantation

With the advent of improved methods of immunosuppression, lung transplantation has become a reasonable alternative for some patients with end-stage lung disease. For patients with emphysema, early recommendations were for double, rather than single, lung transplantation, owing to concerns about mediastinal shift and postoperative compression of the transplanted lung by the remaining, overinflated native lung. Recent experience has demonstrated, however, that single lung transplantation is feasible; mediastinal shift rarely has any clinically significant impact. As a consequence, lung transplantation for emphysema has increased in frequency, and, at present, emphysema (including that due to an α_1-antitrypsin deficiency) accounts for about 60 percent of all single lung transplants performed in the United States.[28] Patients with obstructive lung diseases complicated by chronic respiratory infections—e.g., cystic fibrosis and bronchiectasis—receive double lung transplantation, owing to the potential of cross infection from native to donor lung.

Selection criteria for lung transplantation in emphysema include age less than 60 years; life expectancy without transplantation of 2 years or less; progressive deterioration of clinical status; emotional stability; adequate nutrition; and a history of compliance with medical regimens, including abstinence from cigarette smoking. Coronary artery disease and renal or hepatic dysfunction should be absent. With increasing transplantation experience, some of these restrictions (e.g., age limit) are becoming less rigid.

Actuarial survival curves following single lung transplantation for emphysema demonstrate a 2-year survival of 77 percent and a 3-year survival of 75 percent.[28] The survival rate following transplantation for emphysema is significantly higher than for interstitial fibrosis or primary pulmonary hypertension (Fig. 44-6). Cost of the procedure and lack of an adequate supply of donor lungs remain problematic.

Volume Reduction Surgery

In the 1950s, Brantigan and colleagues attempted wedge resection of lung tissue in patients with diffuse emphysema in an attempt to improve radial traction on small airways.[6] Their patients were poor surgical risks, however, and complications, especially prolonged air leaks, were frequent. The consensus at that time was that widespread emphysema was not relieved by removal of lung tissue, some of which was functional.[24] Advances in anesthesiology and surgical techniques have led to renewed interest in volume reduction surgery. Cooper et al[13] have shown that the procedure, as currently performed in carefully selected patients, is associated with acceptable morbidity and mortality. Bilateral pneumectomy or lung volume reduction surgery consists of removal of 20 to 30 percent of each lung through a median sternotomy. The lung suture line is reinforced by stapling with a device fitted with strips of bovine pericardium; with this technique, the incidence of postoperative air leak is reduced. Early results from 20 patients followed for a mean of 6.4 months have shown a reduction in measured lung volumes, improvement in airflow, relief

TABLE 44-5

Results of Volume Reduction Surgery

	Preoperative	Postoperative	% Change	P Value
FEV_1, L (% predicted)	0.77 (25)	1.4 (44)	+82	<0.001
FVC, L (% predicted)	2.2 (56)	2.8 (73)	+27	<0.05
TLC, L (% predicted)	8.5 (140)	6.6 (110)	−22	<0.001
RV, L (% predicted)	5.9 (288)	3.6 (177)	−39	<0.001
Trapped gas, L	2.4	1.2	−50	<0.001
Pa_{O_2} (room air)	64*	70		<0.05
Pa_{CO_2} (room air)	40*	39		NS

*Two patients receiving oxygen excluded.
NOTE: FEV_1 = forced expiratory volume in one second; FVC = forced vital capacity; TLC = total lung capacity; RV = residual volume; NS = not significant.
SOURCE: From Cooper et al.[13]

of dyspnea, improved exercise tolerance, and improved quality of life (Table 44-5).[13]

Laser resection of emphysematous bullae via thoracoscopy has been described.[52] Unfortunately, prolonged postoperative air leaks complicate the procedure, and patient improvement following surgery has been limited. The current status of lung volume reduction surgery for emphysema remains to be elucidated; long-term effects are unknown. Prospective studies performed in carefully selected centers are necessary.

PROGNOSIS IN SEVERE CHRONIC OBSTRUCTIVE PULMONARY DISEASE

Given the increasing incidence of COPD in our aging population, the chronic, debilitating nature of the disease, and its economic impact, it is not surprising that substantial research on the natural history of COPD has been performed. On the basis of studies conducted over the past 40 years, especially in the United States, the United Kingdom, and the Netherlands, the natural history of COPD has been fairly well elucidated. A few areas of controversy persist, and these are discussed briefly below.

As shown in Fig. 44-1, patients who smoke experience a more rapid decline in FEV_1 over time—approximately 40 to 80 ml per year for smokers versus 20 to 30 ml per year for nonsmokers.[19] While smoking is, by far, the most important risk factor for an accelerated decline in FEV_1, other factors must be operative, since not all smokers are affected equally. As noted previously, only 10 to 15 percent of smokers experience an accelerated decline in FEV_1.[19] The factors potentially operative in this subgroup have been sought and are listed in Table 44-6.

Data on the effects of passive cigarette smoking on airway disease have been summarized in a report of the U.S.

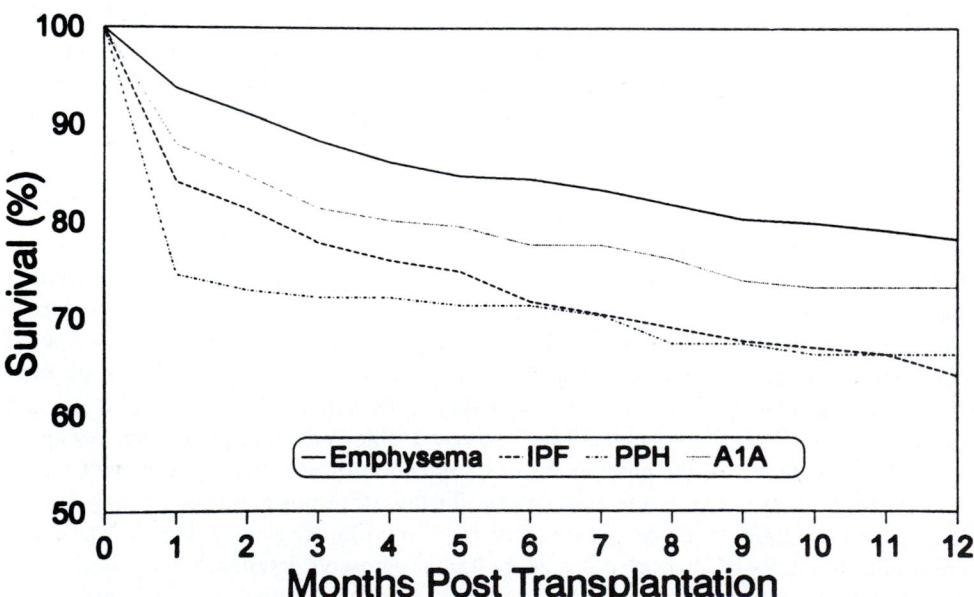

FIGURE 44-6 Actuarial survival following single lung transplantation in patients with emphysema, idiopathic pulmonary fibrosis (IPF), primary pulmonary hypertension (PPH), and α_1-antitrypsin deficiency (A1A). Average survival is significantly longer for patients undergoing transplantation for emphysema (including A1A) than for those undergoing transplantation for IPF or PPH. (*Based on data of Hosenpud et al,*[28] *with permission.*)

Surgeon General.[50] Most studies on passive smoking address exposure in the home or workplace. Children appear to be particularly susceptible to passive smoking if the mother smokes. The incidence of respiratory infections in children exposed to passive smoke is increased, and there may be an associated temporary decline in FEV_1. In addition, workplace exposure to passive cigarette smoke has been associated with increases in the frequency of respiratory infections and loss of work time.[53] The long-term effects of passive exposure to cigarette smoke remain to be determined.

Age has an independent effect in all long-term studies of survival. In addition, the effect of age on survival is greater in older people.[4,31] In studies of younger people, age per se appears not to be an important predictor of survival. Based on the previously noted study conducted by Fletcher and Peto, the onset of respiratory disability occurs late in the course of COPD, after the FEV_1 has decreased by about 70 percent.[19] Since the magnitude of response to bronchodilators may be related to survival (see below), longitudinal studies have examined the correlation between postbronchodilator FEV_1 and disease course.[5] The studies demonstrate that the degree of fixed obstruction is the strongest determinant of survival in these patients.

Hypercapnia, hypoxemia, cor pulmonale, and weight loss are late findings in patients with COPD; their presence correlates with significant disability and limited survival.[21,31,32,35,41,54] Associated findings—e.g., resting tachycardia—are due to hypoxemia, pulmonary hypertension, and right heart failure. Recent reports on administration of supplemental oxygen to hypoxemic patients with COPD suggest that the reduction in pulmonary artery pressure with oxygen administration is a better predictor of survival than the FEV_1 or degree of hypoxemia or hypercapnia.[41] Treatment of chronic hypoxemia with supplemental oxygen results in improved survival in COPD;[35,39] survival rates may be similar to those of patients with similar levels of FEV_1 without hypoxemia.[41]

Finally, the type of obstructive disease—chronic bronchitis, asthmatic bronchitis, or emphysema—may relate to prognosis.[6,34,42,51] As mentioned previously, these three forms of COPD are distinguished by reversibility of airflow obstruction, or lack thereof, following administration of a bronchodilator. While some studies[5,7] show that bronchodilator responsiveness correlates with a slower decline in FEV_1 and increased survival, others[51] demonstrate that bronchodilator responsiveness is associated with a more rapid decline in FEV_1. The relationship between reversibility of airflow obstruction and survival has been a subject of controversy for many years. The Dutch hypothesis, described earlier, contends that bronchial hyperresponsiveness results in mucus hypersecretion and mucosal edema, which are followed by irreversible bronchial obstruction. In contradistinction, the British propose that mucus hypersecretion is the primary inciting factor, rather than bronchial hyperresponsiveness. Mucus retention leads to recurrent bronchial infections (bronchitis) and destruction of lung parenchyma (emphysema).

Finally, analysis of the relationship between bronchial hyperresponsiveness and prognosis in chronic bronchitis should incorporate the results from some recent studies suggesting that the presence of sputum eosinophilia correlates with a poorer prognosis.[34] Sputum eosinophilia, bronchial hyperresponsiveness, and recurrent wheezing may reflect an active inflammatory process within bronchi that leads to a more rapid decline in

TABLE 44-6

Factors Associated with Clinical Course and Survival in Patients with COPD

Factor	Reference(s)
Cigarette smoking	18, 31
Passive smoking exposure	50
Age	4, 31
Rate of decline of FEV_1	31
Hypercapnia	31, 32
Pulmonary artery pressure	21, 32, 41
Resting heart rate	4
Weight loss	54
Type of lung disease (reversibility)	7, 34, 42, 51

airflow. Under these circumstances, hyperresponsiveness and sputum eosinophilia may denote a poor prognosis. Since the inflammatory process is treatable, however, use of anti-inflammatory therapy may slow the decline in FEV_1 over time. Early diagnosis and treatment of bronchial responsiveness would be expected to result in a better prognosis. Studies using inhaled corticosteroids in patients with COPD[14] may provide an answer to this important question.

REFERENCES

1. Albert RK, Martin TR, Lewis SW: Controlled clinical trial of methylprednisolone in patients with chronic bronchitis and acute respiratory failure. *Ann Intern Med* 92:753–758, 1980.
2. Anthonisen NR, Connett JE, Kiley JP, et al: Effects of smoking intervention and the use of an inhaled anticholinergic bronchodilator on the rate of decline of FEV_1: The Lung Health Study. *JAMA* 272:1497–1505, 1994.
3. Anthonisen NR, Manfreda J, Warren CPW, et al: Antibiotic therapy in exacerbations of chronic obstructive pulmonary disease. *Ann Intern Med* 106:196–204, 1987.
4. Anthonisen NR, Wright EC, Hodgkin JE: Prognosis in chronic obstructive pulmonary disease. *Am Rev Respir Dis* 133:14–20, 1986.
5. Anthonisen NR, Wright EC, IPPB Trial Group: Bronchodilator response in chronic obstructive pulmonary disease. *Am Rev Respir Dis* 133:814–819, 1986.
6. Brantigan OC, Mueller E, Kress MB: A surgical approach to pulmonary emphysema. *Am Rev Respir Dis* 80:194–202, 1959.
7. Burrows B, Bloom JW, Traver GA, Cline MG: The course and prognosis of different forms of chronic airways obstruction in a sample from the general population. *New Engl J Med* 317:1309–1314, 1987.
8. Callahan CM, Dittus RS, Katz BP: Oral corticosteroids therapy for patients with stable chronic obstructive pulmonary disease: A meta-analysis. *Ann Intern Med* 114:216–223, 1991.
9. Casaburi R, Patessio A, Ioli F, et al: Reductions in exercise lactic acidosis and ventilation as a result of exercise training in patients with obstructive lung disease. *Am Rev Respir Dis* 143:9–18, 1991.
10. Casaburi R: Exercise training in chronic obstructive lung disease, in Casaburi R, Petty TL (eds), *Principles and Practice of Pulmonary Rehabilitation*. Philadelphia, WB Saunders, 1993, pp 204–224.
11. Celli BR, Snider GL, Heffner J, et al: Standards for the diagnosis and care of patients with chronic obstructive pulmonary disease. *Am J Respir Crit Care Med* 152(Suppl).S77–S120, 1995.

12. COMBIVENT Inhalational Aerosol Study Group: In chronic obstructive pulmonary disease, a combination of ipratropium and albuterol is more effective than either agent alone: An 85-day multicenter trial. *Chest* 105:1411–1419, 1994.

13. Cooper JD, Trulock EP, Triantafillou AN, et al: Bilateral pneumectomy (volume reduction) for chronic obstructive pulmonary disease. *J Thorac Cardiovasc Surg* 109:106–119, 1995.

14. Dompeling E, van Schayck CP, van Grunsven PM, et al: Slowing the deterioration of asthma and chronic obstructive pulmonary disease observed during bronchodilator therapy by adding inhaled corticosteroids: A 4-year prospective study. *Ann Intern Med* 118:770–778, 1993.

15. Emerman CL, Connors AF, Lukens TW, et al: A randomized controlled trial of methylprednisolone in the emergency treatment of acute exacerbations of COPD. *Chest* 95:563–567, 1989.

16. Ferguson GT, Cherniak RM: Management of chronic obstructive pulmonary disease. *New Engl J Med* 328:1017–1022, 1993.

17. Fiore MC, Jorenby DE, Baker TB, Kenford SL: Tobacco dependence and the nicotine patch: Clinical guidelines for effective use. *JAMA* 268:2687–2694, 1992.

18. Fletcher EC, Luckett RA, Goodnight-White S, et al: A double-blind trial of nocturnal supplemental oxygen for sleep desaturation in patients with chronic obstructive pulmonary disease and daytime PaO_2 above 60 mmHg. *Am Rev Respir Dis* 145:1070–1076, 1992.

19. Fletcher C, Peto R: The natural history of chronic airflow obstruction. *Br Med J* 1:1645–1648, 1977.

20. Fletcher C, Peto R, Tinker C, Speizer FE: *The Natural History of Chronic Bronchitis and Emphysema: An Eight-Year Study of Early Chronic Obstructive Lung Disease in Working Men in London.* New York, Oxford University Press, 1976.

21. France AJ, Prescott RJ, Biernacki W, et al: Does right ventricular function predict survival in patients with chronic obstructive lung disease? *Thorax* 43:621–626, 1988.

22. Frank E, Winkleby MA, Altman DG, et al: Predictors of physicians' smoking cessation advice. *JAMA* 266:3139–3144, 1991.

23. Fuso L, Incalzi RA, Pistelli R, et al: Predicting mortality of patients hospitalized for acutely exacerbated chronic obstructive pulmonary disease. *Am J Med* 98:272–277, 1995.

24. Gaensler EA, Cugell DW, Knudson RJ, Fitzgerald MX: Surgical management of emphysema. *Clin Chest Med* 4:443–463, 1983.

25. Gosselink RAAM, Wagenaar RC, Rijswijk H, et al: Diaphragmatic breathing reduces efficiency of breathing in patients with chronic obstructive pulmonary disease. *Am J Respir Crit Care Med* 151:1136–1142, 1995.

26. Heimlich HJ, Carr GC: The Micro-Trach: A seven-year experience with transtracheal oxygen therapy. *Chest* 95:1008–1012, 1989.

27. Hoffman LA, Wesmiller SW, Sciurba FC, et al: Nasal cannula and transtracheal oxygen delivery: A comparison of patient response after 6 months of each technique. *Am Rev Respir Dis* 145:827–831, 1992.

28. Hosenpud JD, Novick RJ, Breen TJ, Daily OP: The registry of the International Society for Heart and Lung Transplantation: Eleventh Official Report—1994. *J Heart Lung Transplant* 13:561–570, 1994.

29. Howland J, Nelson EC, Barlow PB, et al: Chronic obstructive pulmonary disease: Impact of health education. *Chest* 90:233–238, 1986.

30. Hudson LS, Monti CM: Rationale and use of corticosteroids in chronic obstructive pulmonary disease. *Med Clin North Am* 74:661–690, 1990.

31. Kanner RE, Renzetti AD Jr, Stanish WM, et al: Predictors of survival in subjects with chronic airflow limitation. *Am J Med* 74:249–255, 1983.

32. Kawakami Y: Prognostic factors in COPD: The importance of pulmonary hemodynamic variables. *Pract Cardiol* 11:124–137, 1985.

33. Kuhl DA, Agiri OA, Mauro LS: Beta-agonists in the treatment of acute exacerbation of chronic obstructive pulmonary disease. *Ann Pharmacother* 28:1379–1388, 1994.

34. Lebowitz MD, Postma DS, Burrows B: Adverse effects of eosinophilia and smoking on the natural history of newly diagnosed chronic bronchitis. *Chest* 108:55–61, 1995.

35. Medical Research Council Working Party: Long-term domiciliary oxygen therapy in chronic hypoxic cor pulmonale complicating chronic bronchitis and emphysema. *Lancet* 1:681–686, 1981.

36. Mendella LA, Manfreda J, Warren CPW, Anthonisen NR: Steroid response in stable chronic obstructive pulmonary disease. *Ann Intern Med* 96:17–21, 1982.

37. Murata GH, Gorby MS, Chick TW, Halperin AK: Use of emergency medical services by patients with decompensated obstructive lung disease. *Ann Emerg Med* 18:501–506, 1989.

38. National Center for Health Statistics: Advance report of final mortality statistics, 1991. *Monthly Vital Statistics Report* 42(Suppl), 1993.

39. Nocturnal Oxygen Therapy Trial Group: Continuous or nocturnal oxygen therapy in hypoxemic chronic obstructive lung disease: A clinical trial. *Ann Intern Med* 93:391–398, 1980.

40. O'Donohue WJ Jr, Plummer AL: Magnitude of usage and cost of home oxygen therapy in the United States. *Chest* 107:301–302, 1995.

41. Oswald-Mammosser M, Weitzenblum E, Quoix E, et al: Prognostic factors in COPD patients receiving long-term oxygen therapy: Importance of pulmonary artery pressure. *Chest* 107:1193–1198, 1995.

42. Postma DS, de Vries K, Koëter GH, Sluiter HJ: Independent influence of reversibility of air-flow obstruction and nonspecific hyperreactivity on the long-term course of lung function in chronic airflow obstruction. *Am Rev Respir Dis* 134:276–280, 1986.

43. Postma DS, Peters I, Steenhuis EJ, Sluiter HJ: Moderately severe chronic airflow obstruction: Can corticosteroids slow down obstruction? *Eur Respir J* 1:22–26, 1988.

44. Ramsdell J: Use of theophylline in the treatment of COPD. *Chest* 107(Suppl):206S–209S, 1995.

45. Ries AL: Position paper of the American Association of Cardiovascular and Pulmonary Rehabilitation: Scientific basis of pulmonary rehabilitation. *J Cardiopulm Rehab* 10:418–441, 1990.

46. Saint S, Bent S, Vittinghoff E, Grady D: Antibiotics in chronic obstructive pulmonary disease exacerbations: A meta-analysis. *JAMA* 273:957–960, 1995.

47. Sluiter HJ, Koeter GH, deMonchy JGR, et al: The Dutch hypothesis (chronic nonspecific lung disease) revisited. *Eur Respir J* 4:474–489, 1991.

48. Statistical Compendium on Adult Lung Diseases: New York, American Lung Association, 1987.

49. Transdermal Nicotine Study Group: Transdermal nicotine for smoking cessation: Six-month results from two multicenter controlled clinical trials. *JAMA* 266:3133–3139, 1991.

50. U.S. Department of Health and Human Services: *The Health Consequences of Involuntary Smoking: A Report of the Surgeon General.* Rockville, MD, Office on Smoking and Health, 1986.

51. Vollmer WM, Johnson LR, Buist AS: Relationship of response to a bronchodilator and decline in forced expiratory volume in one second in population studies. *Am Rev Respir Dis* 132:1186–1193, 1985.

52. Wakabayashi A, Brenner M, Kayaleh RA, et al: Thoracoscopic carbon dioxide laser treatment of bullous emphysema. *Lancet* 337:881–883, 1991.

53. White JR, Froeb HF, Kulik JA: Respiratory illness in nonsmokers chronically exposed to tobacco smoke in the workplace. *Chest* 100:39–43, 1991.

54. Wilson DO, Rogers RM, Wright EC, Anthonisen NR: Body weight in chronic obstructive pulmonary disease: National Institutes of Health IPPB Trial. *Am Rev Respir Dis* 139:1435–1438, 1989.

CIGARETTE SMOKING AND DISEASE

Stephen I. Rennard / David M. Daughton

Native Americans discovered the use of the tobacco plant, *Nicotiana tabacum,* during antiquity. By the time Columbus arrived in America, tobacco use was widespread in the Western Hemisphere and was well integrated into Native American cultures. Production of tobacco and its trade represented a major economic activity in the pre-Columbian Americas. Early European explorers learned of the tobacco plant from Native Americans, and by the middle of the seventeenth century, tobacco was widely used in Europe.

Nicotine is the active psychopharmaceutical drug contained in the leaves of the tobacco plant. This alkaloid represents a major metabolic product of the tobacco plant and probably evolved as protection against insect predators, since nicotine is a potent insect neurotoxin. In fact, nicotine has been exploited in this regard as a commercial insecticide. Nicotine is also active on the mammalian nervous system.

Nicotine is a potent euphoriant. On a molar basis, nicotine is more active than such euphoria-inducing drugs as cocaine, amphetamine, and morphine. Nicotine also has a number of other effects on the central nervous system. For example, nicotine may improve task performance and attention time measurably in non-habituated subjects. Nicotine may also alleviate anxiety and depression and induce a sense of well-being, while causing a state of arousal. Unfortunately, nicotine is also an addicting substance.

NICOTINE ADDICTION

Evidence supporting the addictive potential of nicotine includes the well-described withdrawal syndrome (Table 45-1), the clear association of nicotine withdrawal with drug-seeking behavior, and the increase in dosage that occurs early in the habitual use of nicotine. Current concepts suggest that both the psychoactive effects of nicotine and its potential for addiction depend on its pharmacokinetics.[4] As with many other addicting drugs, the CNS effects of nicotine depend on both the absolute level of the drug and the rate of rise in drug concentration at brain receptors. Smoking is a particularly effective means of delivering nicotine

TABLE 45-1

Nicotine Withdrawal Symptoms

Dysphoric or depressed mood
Insomnia
Irritability, frustration, or anger
Anxiety
Difficulty concentrating
Restlessness
Decreased heart rate
Increased appetite or weight gain

to induce psychoactive effects. After inhalation, the drug, because of its lipid solubility, is quickly absorbed across the alveolar surface into pulmonary capillary blood, causing a rapid increase in nicotine levels in the arterial circulation. Consequently, the nicotine concentration at the receptors in the brain increases rapidly. The pharmacodynamics maximize the psychoactive potential of nicotine and are important in determining its addictive potential. Alternative forms for delivering nicotine that do not achieve such rapid increments in blood levels are associated with a smaller psychoactive effect and a lower addictive potential. These pharmacodynamic principles are important in use of nicotine replacement as an aid to smoking cessation (see "Nicotine Replacement Therapies").

Nicotine addiction appears to be a pediatric problem. Most people who become addicted do so before adulthood. In the United States, the peak incidence for developing a regular nicotine habit is in adolescence. Persons who do not acquire a nicotine habit before age 20 years are very unlikely to do so as adults.[21] The demographics of smoking initiation are, undoubtedly, well known in the tobacco industry. Marketing campaigns to promote the image of specific brands of cigarettes have been carefully designed and are exceedingly effective. For example, a high degree of logo recognition for "Joe Camel" has been achieved among American kindergartners. This campaign has possibly also contributed to brand selection among American adolescents.

Most children who begin to smoke do so on an occasional basis. Within a few years, however, a regular habit may develop. Most often the habit is characterized by smoking only a few cigarettes daily. The number of cigarettes smoked, however, generally increases for the first 8 to 10 years. Once a smoker achieves a "mature" addiction, cigarette consumption typically remains constant. It is interesting that the smoker appears to adjust to nicotine intake. If supplemental nicotine is administered, smokers often reduce their nicotine consumption.[5] Alternatively, if smoking is restricted (e.g., by decreasing the number of cigarettes available), smokers alter their smoking strategy (e.g., by smoking each cigarette more deeply) in order to maintain a relatively constant nicotine intake.

While the pathogenetic mechanisms underlying withdrawal symptoms are incompletely understood, it is generally believed that some withdrawal symptoms are related to decreases in nicotine blood levels below certain thresholds. For example, smokers may experience nicotine withdrawal at night, when sleep interferes with nicotine intake. The concept that nicotine replacement may help alleviate withdrawal symptoms by maintaining nicotine blood levels is also an important concept underlying nicotine replacement as an aid to smoking cessation (see "Nicotine Replacement Therapies").

Why some children experiment with cigarettes but eventually remain abstinent is an important and largely unanswered question. The experience that a child has with initial attempts at smoking appear to be important. Other factors that may play a role are attitude toward smoking—i.e., the "image" of the smoker, peer pressure, parental cigarette use, and cigarette availability.[24] Several studies have suggested that a genetic component may also exist. In particular, studies of identical twins raised apart suggest that there is a higher than expected concordance for smoking.[14] Risk for smoking also appears to be associated with other behaviors, suggesting that some personality characteristics may predispose some persons to smoking. Thus, although it is clear that nicotine is a highly addicting psychoactive substance, nicotine addiction is also a complex biologic process that depends not only on the drug but also on the host and social situation. This complexity suggests that various smokers may smoke for different reasons; some may be relatively "casual" smokers, while others are "hard core." Understanding the nature of the addiction is likely to become more important as cessation techniques become increasingly sophisticated.

SOCIAL AND CULTURAL ASPECTS OF SMOKING

As in ancient America, use of tobacco products has become well integrated into modern cultures worldwide. Tobacco is a multibillion-dollar industry. In some regions, tobacco is a crucial cash crop in an agricultural economy. In addition, the manufacture, distribution, marketing, and sale of tobacco products employ many people worldwide. Taxation on tobacco products has become an important means for the support of many governments. Thus, any change in tobacco usage will have an economic as well as health impact.

The use of tobacco also serves a cultural role. In some societies (e.g., certain Native American tribes), tobacco usage has religious significance. In other groups, tobacco usage is associated with a strong cultural "image." Often this image may have been created through direct efforts of the tobacco industry to market their product. In this regard, at the turn of the century, a cigarette brand was successfully marketed in association with an advertising program promoting the image of the cigarette smoker as rugged, independent, and masculine. This was followed by a campaign for another brand suggesting that cigarette usage in women was a mark of independence and sophistication. Perhaps unfortunately, this image led the feminist movement to adopt the cigarette as a symbol—"the torch of freedom." More recently, marketing campaigns for popular brands of cigarettes have promoted rugged independence in males and sophisticated maturity among young women. The latter campaign may be one cause for the rise in smoking prevalence among younger women. Finally, the recent advertising campaign based on the cartoon character "Joe Camel" has promoted to American children the image of cigarette smoking as associated with urbane sophistication. Although these images of cigarette smoking have their origins in advertising, the effectiveness of marketing programs cannot be underestimated. Whatever the reasons, cigarettes clearly have a cultural significance. The social and economic impact of tobacco usage, therefore, must be considered when one is attempting to deal with smoking as a public health problem.

SMOKING AS A PUBLIC HEALTH PROBLEM

Cigarette smoking is a major public health problem. In fact, cigarette smoking can be considered *the* major public health problem. The number of deaths attributed to cigarette smoking in the United States is estimated to be more than 400,000 annually, a number vastly exceeding that attributable to other specific causes. The health costs of smoking are significant not only in the United States but throughout the developed and the developing world as well. Not surprisingly, health hazards attributable to smoking parallel smoking prevalence. As a result, smoking-induced disease is becoming more common in the developing world, where smoking prevalence is increasing. Smoking is also increasing in subpopulations—e.g., young women[45]—in the developed world, and it can be expected that smoking-related disease will also increase in these groups.

Smoking may cause disease through a myriad of mechanisms. Cigarette smoke contains more than 6000 compounds. Detailed toxicity studies have been done on relatively few of the potential toxins. Some toxins are present in the tobacco plant; others are generated during tobacco leaf processing or pyrolysis of processed tobacco. Tobacco smoke contains compounds that can disrupt DNA, causing mutations and altering gene expression. In addition, compounds may bind to, and disrupt, proteins and alter cellular lipids. Because of the diversity of the toxins, the many biochemical and cellular elements with which they may interact, and the variability in individual susceptibilities, the heterogeneous ill effects of cigarette smoke are not surprising. Among the most prevalent diseases with which cigarette smoking has been implicated are atherosclerotic cardiovascular disease, cancer, and chronic obstructive pulmonary disease. The epidemiologic and mechanistic evidence linking cigarette smoking and these diseases is substantial. A variety of other adverse health effects have also been associated with smoking. Table 45-2 provides a list of diseases that have been reported to be associated with smoking.

SMOKING AND CHRONIC OBSTRUCTIVE PULMONARY DISEASE

Cigarette smoking is the major risk factor associated with the development of chronic obstructive pulmonary disease (COPD) (see Chapters 43 and 44). Nearly all patients with clinically significant emphysema are smokers. Smoking is also a major risk factor for development of chronic bronchitis. Heavy smokers are at greater risk of developing COPD than are moderate smokers,[20] but low exposures to cigarette smoke, as may be encountered during "passive smoking," also seem to be harmful.

On average, the rate of expiratory airflow in cigarette smokers decreases twice as fast in smokers (40 ml a year) as in nonsmokers (20 ml a year).[20] Nonetheless, most smokers do not develop symptomatic COPD, probably because of the large physiological reserve of the lung and the relatively sedentary lifestyle in most developed countries. However, some smokers (perhaps 15 percent) do experience accelerated loss of lung function and develop clinically significant disease. Although the basis for heightened susceptibility in this group is unknown, it is important to pinpoint the rapid decline in these smokers, since their condition is apt to continue to deteriorate rapidly.

A number of interacting mechanisms appear to be operative in the pathogenesis of COPD caused by cigarette smoke. Emphysema appears to develop from lung damage, which can be caused either by direct injury inflicted by cigarette smoke–induced oxidants or by inflammatory mediators recruited into the lung as a consequence of exposure to smoke. Chronic bronchitis appears to result from similar mechanisms in the airways. Inflammation induced by cigarette smoke is capable of both stimulating acute production of airway secretions and inducing persistent anatomic changes in the airway. For example, goblet cell metaplasia may predispose to a hypersecretory state and peribronchial fibrosis may result in airflow obstruction. The clinical heterogeneity of COPD probably results from varied host responses to cigarette smoke.

SMOKING AND MALIGNANCY

The risk of developing lung cancer is about 20-fold greater in smokers than in nonsmokers.[46,47] Indeed, smoking is the major risk factor associated with lung cancer. The attributable risk for the development of lung cancer is estimated to be 79 percent in women and 90 percent in men. As in the case of COPD, epidemiologic evidence supports a dose dependency between cigarette smoking and lung cancer. Thus, the risk of lung cancer increases with the amount smoked and the duration of smoking. The risk of lung cancer among passive smokers also seems to be increased, suggesting that even low-dose exposure to cigarette smoke carries significant risk.

Considerable experimental evidence has implicated cigarette smoke in the development of lung cancer. A multistage process seems to be at work in the carcinogenesis. Tumor initiators and tumor promoters are present in cigarette smoke, and epithelial cell abnormalities in smokers have been observed to progress from mild metaplastic changes to severe dysplasia; these changes are believed to progress to cancer. Lesions are also often widespread, raising the possibility that development of lung cancer in the smoker may be a multifocal process.

Many substances present in cigarette smoke—in particular, the polycyclic aromatic hydrocarbons—may contribute to carcinogenesis. In turn, the development of cancer may depend on host factors. For example, some potential carcinogens must be activated in the lung by the action of mixed-function oxidases. Since these enzymes are under genetic control, differences in the capability of inducing such enzymes may contribute to differences in the risk of cancer. As noted above, although it would be highly desirable to identify smokers at high risk of developing cancer, such identification is not yet possible. Therefore, all smokers should be considered to be at significantly increased risk for the development of lung cancer.

Both respiratory and nonrespiratory malignancies are associated with cigarette smoking. Thus, cigarette smoking not only is

TABLE 45-2

Diseases Associated with Cigarette Smoking

Cardiovascular diseases
Atherosclerotic cardiovascular
disease
  Coronary artery disease
  Carotid vascular disease
  Mesenteric, renal, iliac disease
  Abdominal aortic aneurysm
Other cardiac diseases
  Coronary artery spasm
  Arrhythmias
Peripheral vascular diseases
  Thromboangiitis obliterans
    (Berger's disease)
  Deep venous thrombosis
  Pulmonary embolus

Malignant diseases
Respiratory tract malignancies
Lung cancer
  Squamous cell
  Adenocarcinoma
  Large cell
  Small cell
Laryngeal cancer
Oral cancer
Other Malignancies
  Esophagus
  Pancreas
  Bladder
  Uterine cervix
  Breast
  Kidney
  Anus
  Penis
  Stomach
  Liver
  Leukemia

Nonmalignant lung diseases
Chronic obstructive pulmonary
  disease (COPD)
Asthma
Eosinophilic granuloma of lung
Respiratory bronchiolitis
Goodpasture's syndrome
Sleep apnea
Pneumothorax

**Gastrointestinal
diseases**
Peptic ulcer disease
  Gastric
  Duodenal
Gastroesophageal reflux
Chronic pancreatitis
Crohn's disease
Colonic adenomas

Dermatologic diseases
Skin wrinkling
Psoriasis

Reproductive diseases
Ovarian failure
Pregnancy-related
  Prematurity
  Premature rupture of membranes
  Spontaneous abortion
Decreased sperm quality
Fetal effects
  Low birthweight
  Impaired lung growth
  Sudden infant death syndrome
    (SIDS)
  Febrile seizures
  Reduced intelligence
  Behavioral disorders
  Atopic disease/asthma

Effects on children of parental smoking
Asthma
Rhinitis
Otitis
Pneumonia
Increased risk to begin smoking

Rheumatologic diseases
Osteoporosis
Rheumatoid arthritis

Psychiatric diseases
Depression
Schizophrenia

Oral diseases
Periodontal disease
Loss of taste

Loss of olfaction

Infectious diseases
Tuberculosis
Pneumococcal infection
Meningococcal infection

Endocrine diseases
Altered hormonal secretion
Grave's disease
Antidiuresis
Goiter

Renal diseases
Glomerulonephritis

**Benign prostatic
hypertrophy**

Cataracts

deemed to be a major cause of both oral and laryngeal cancer but also has been associated with a number of other malignancies (Table 45-2). As a rule, the mechanisms underlying these associations are not understood. In the case of carcinoma of the bladder, however, it seems reasonable to implicate concentration of carcinogens in the urine as a contributing factor.

SMOKING AND CARDIOVASCULAR DISEASE

Cigarette smoking is also a major risk factor for the development of cardiovascular disease.[47,48] Indeed, the impact of cigarette smoking is similar in magnitude to that of the other two major risk factors: hypertension and hypercholesterolemia. From a public health perspective, however, because cigarette smoking is more prevalent than either hypertension or hypercholesterolemia, it is more important as a risk factor than either of these two disorders. As with other smoking-related diseases, heavier smokers are at greater risk.

Cigarette smoking may contribute to the development of chronic cardiac diseases by a variety of mechanisms: direct endothelial injury, tachycardia, hyperlipidemia with increased levels of LDL, increase in circulating neutrophils, and increased blood coagulability. Cigarette smoking not only is the major risk factor for thromboangiitis obliterans but also accelerates the development of microvascular disease in persons with diabetes mellitus.

Cigarette smoke has also been postulated to contribute to acute cardiac events in a variety of ways. For example, myocardial ischemia can result from an increase in myocardial oxygen requirements, increased concentrations of carbon monoxide in blood (which impair oxygen delivery), increase in blood viscosity that predisposes to a hypercoagulable state, and increase in circulating catecholamines (which can evoke coronary vasospasm). A second category of mechanisms is induction of cardiac arrhythmias.

OTHER ADVERSE HEALTH EFFECTS OF SMOKING

Cigarette smoking has been implicated in a variety of nonmalignant lung diseases, including eosinophilic granuloma and spontaneous pneumothorax. Also, as indicated in Table 45-2, cigarette smoking has been associated with a large number of nonrespiratory diseases (e.g., peptic ulcer disease).[47] These associations have often been made in epidemiologic studies, and although some associations are well established, some remain to be confirmed. Cause-and-effect relationships are generally not fully elucidated for most of these associations. In some cases (e.g., depression), the association may be a result of a beneficial (i.e., antidepressant) effect of nicotine. Of interest is that many of the diseases listed in Table 45-2 may share mechanistic features (e.g., activation of inflammation, connective-tissue matrix destruction, activation of cell proliferation).

SMOKING CESSATION BACKGROUND

Since 1964, when Dr. Luther Terry released the first Surgeon General's report on smoking and health, the prevalence of adult smokers in the United States has dropped from 40 to 25 percent and smoking bans have become commonplace in hospitals, restaurants, and office buildings and on public transportation. In 1984, Surgeon General C. Everett Koop proclaimed that the number one health goal in the United States was to achieve a "smoke-free society by the year 2000."[30] Unfortunately, this goal is not likely to be achieved, since the overall incidence of smokers in the adult population has stagnated at roughly 25 percent during the past several years. Although smoking rates have decreased steadily among black, Asian, and Hispanic adolescents,[33] the prevalence of smoking among white adolescents has increased in recent years.

SMOKING CESSATION: BEHAVIORAL TECHNIQUES

A wide spectrum of behavioral techniques have been used to treat cigarette addiction. These include education, individual and group counseling, adversive conditioning, psychotherapy, transcendental meditation, sensory deprivation, hypnosis, and desensitization.[42] Although it is beyond the scope of this chapter to discuss these methods in detail—particularly since most behavioral approaches have been marked by poor overall success rates—several deserve special mention.

Patient Education

For years, cigarette smoking was viewed as largely a social or psychological habit. As such, the ability to quit was considered a measure of personal motivation and willpower. Motivation to stop smoking, combined with sufficient psychological resources, was seen as a driving force behind successful cigarette abstinence. Thus, if smokers could be educated about the health risks of cigarette smoking, they could theoretically become sufficiently motivated and psychologically empowered to quit. Unfortunately, the anticipated benefits of achieving smoking cessation through education were overoptimistic and simplistic. More than 80 percent of current smokers indicate they would like to quit but can't.[13] Educational programs to aid smoking cessation have produced disappointing results and high long-term failure rates.[42]

Hypnosis

The goal of hypnosis in smoking cessation is to enable the smoker to achieve an altered state of consciousness that enhances the ability to quit. However, the hypnotic trance is generally not measurably different from deep muscle relaxation. The effects of hypnosis are often short-lived. Controlled trials of hypnosis have generally not documented long-term efficacy for smoking cessation.[42] Hypnosis is of low reliability, with published quit rates ranging between 0 and 88 percent.[42] Although of uncertain value, hypnosis remains a commercially popular stop-smoking method. The primary advantage of hypnosis is that it may be an attractive alternative for people who have failed to quit with other methods.

Adversive Conditioning

Adversive conditioning is based on the premise that smoking is a learned response that can be extinguished by creation of an association between smoking and a negative sensation. Among the adversive techniques utilized for smoking cessation are electric shock; nausea-inducing drugs; hot, smoky air treatments; and rapid smoking.[42] High quit rates were reported in some of the early smoking cessation trials using adversive conditioning. However, these high rates may be attributed, in part, to factors relating to patient selection, since only the most highly motivated persons are, arguably, willing to undergo therapies such as electric shock or the breathing of hot, smoky air. Additionally, adversive conditioning techniques may represent a health hazard.

For example, the rapid inhalation of hot, smoky air may induce bronchospasm in asthmatics. Finally, adversive conditioning techniques have proved to be of limited value, since impressive quit rates are generally not seen unless these techniques are combined with other methods, such as individual or group counseling programs.[42]

Group Counseling

Group counseling programs for smoking cessation are offered by several commercial and voluntary health organizations. These programs are similar in content and typically include lectures, group interactions, exercises on recognition of one's habit, some form of tapering method leading to a quit day, development of coping skills, and suggestions for relapse prevention. Group counseling programs sponsored by voluntary health organizations, such as the American Lung Association, are the best value for smokers. These programs are generally limited to large metropolitan areas, however, and may be offered on a sporadic basis. One-year success rates associated with group counseling programs are typically in the range of 15 to 35 percent.[42]

Gradual Reduction Versus Abrupt Abstinence

Gradual reduction or tapering appears to offer smokers the least abrasive way to stop smoking. However, gradually cutting down can be stressful when smokers attempt to reduce the cigarette use below their critical blood nicotine threshold. At this stage, smokers often begin to experience tobacco withdrawal symptoms. Rather than suffer prolonged discomfort, most taperers gradually return to their customary cigarette levels and do not succeed in quitting. One of the negative consequences of tapering is that the method can strongly reinforce smokers' belief of their underlying need for cigarettes. Abrupt abstinence is often stressful and can lead to tobacco withdrawal symptoms. Within a few weeks of total abstinence, however, complete abstainers experience less frequent cigarette cravings than do taperers and are less prone to relapse.[50] Cigarette tapering is often a component of many group programs in which gradual cigarette reduction is used as a preparatory stage leading toward a target quit day. Under these circumstances, the tapering approach may prove beneficial to some smokers.

SMOKING CESSATION: PHARMACOLOGIC APPROACHES

The concept of utilizing a pharmacologic deterrent for cigarette smoking is not new: chemical antismoking agents were used before 1900. Perhaps the best investigated of the early smoking cessation drugs was lobeline sulfate, which was developed in tablet form in 1936. In the past few decades, a broad spectrum of pharmaceutical agents have been investigated as antismoking aids. These include tranquilizers, antidepressants, topical anesthetics, antianxiety agents, silver nitrate, anticholinergics, clonidine, and nicotine replacement therapy.[42] Several of these agents are discussed below.

Lobeline Sulfate

Lobeline was selected as a stop-smoking agent because of its pharmacologic similarities to nicotine.[8] It was hoped that the drug might serve as a nicotine substitute for smokers who wished to quit. Clinical trials have produced mixed results.[8] Interest in lobeline declined in the 1970s and 1980s as the smoking cessation value of the drug was questioned. More recently, a sublingual formulation of the drug has been tested as a stop-smoking aid for highly dependent smokers.

Amphetamines

Amphetamines, similar to nicotine, may induce euphoria, serve as a "pick-me-up," and improve concentration in fatigued subjects.[43] For these reasons, amphetamines were once believed to have some cigarette replacement value. Unfortunately, amphetamines do not work as stop-smoking agents, and their use may result in increased, rather than decreased, cigarette use.[8] Amphetamines may also exacerbate tobacco withdrawal symptoms, particularly anxiety and depression. High doses of amphetamines can produce anxiety, and the initial mood-enhancing qualities of amphetamines may be followed by dysphoria and depression.[43]

Mecamylamine

Mecamylamine is a nicotine antagonist capable of blocking the reinforcing effects of nicotine.[8] Because of its mechanism of action, mecamylamine may be of limited or no value in alleviating tobacco withdrawal symptoms associated with smoking cessation. As with amphetamines, the initial response to mecamylamine is increased smoking.[8] Mecamylamine, however, may have potential as a relapse prevention drug. Thus, mecamylamine may prove useful in combination therapy with nicotine replacement products that can be used to treat tobacco withdrawal and enhance early abstinence.

Antidepressants

Early studies on the use of antidepressants for smoking cessation produced disappointing results.[42] The mechanisms of action for antidepressant medications, however, vary considerably. Ongoing trials to evaluate the smoking cessation value of selected antidepressant drugs are still promising.

Clonidine

Clonidine is an antihypertensive agent that has proved beneficial in diminishing opiate withdrawal symptoms, particularly craving, irritability, and restlessness.[23] Early studies with clonidine suggested that the drug might reduce some tobacco withdrawal symptoms and enhance quit rates.[22] The value of transdermal clonidine with respect to smoking cessation, however, was not supported in a five-center trial revealing that although transdermal clonidine administration is associated with decreased anxiety and irritability during the initial week of quitting, it does not improve 12-week abstinence rates.[37]

Nicotine Replacement Therapies

The earliest form of nicotine replacement therapy was a nicotine lozenge used in stop-smoking clinics in Stockholm in the 1950s. Why the nicotine lozenge did not achieve widespread use is not well documented. Nicotine tablets are, once again, available as a nicotine replacement product, along with nicotine polacrilex, transdermal nicotine, nicotine nasal spray, nicotine aerosols and vapors, and nicotine toothpicks.[27] Although several forms of nicotine replacement therapies are available, only two forms currently can be purchased over the counter in the United States: nicotine polacrilex and transdermal nicotine.

NICOTINE POLACRILEX

Nicotine polacrilex was the first nicotine replacement therapy to gain FDA approval. It is now commercially available in 2-mg and 4-mg doses. Nicotine is bound to a resin that contains a buffering agent to improve delivery of the nicotine through the buccal mucosa. Mouth pH and rate of chewing influence the rate of nicotine absorption. Ad lib use of 2 mg of nicotine polacrilex is associated with blood nicotine levels less than 40 percent of those associated with customary smoking.[3] At this level of nicotine replacement, many patients using nicotine gum still experience discomforting symptoms of tobacco withdrawal. A fixed dosage regimen of nicotine gum may produce higher blood nicotine levels.

Nicotine gum has proved effective in reducing tobacco withdrawal symptoms and in improving quit rates. However, proper use of the gum is imperative to maximize benefits with respect to smoking cessation. In general-practice settings, the results observed from the use of nicotine gum have been disappointing—perhaps, in part, because of the difficulty of using this pharmaceutical agent.

TRANSDERMAL NICOTINE

Transdermal systems have been utilized to administer several drugs, including nitroglycerin, estrogen, clonidine, scopolamine, and nicotine. The primary advantages of patch delivery systems are ease of use and controlled drug delivery.

Transdermal nicotine systems have repeatedly been found to reduce tobacco withdrawal symptoms and to significantly enhance smoking cessation rates.[17] Although variations in study design make cross-study comparisons difficult, abstinence rates associated with use of the nicotine patch are generally double those of placebo controls.[17] Unlike nicotine polacrilex, transdermal nicotine systems have consistently improved quit rates in the primary care setting. This difference is probably due to the ease of patch use in this setting.

Plasma nicotine concentrations obtained by use of nicotine patches that deliver 21 mg per day provide about 40 to 50 percent of the nicotine levels achieved by customary smoking.[34] The recommended use period for patches varies according to manufacturers' recommendations, but a minimum of 4 weeks of therapy is probably required to help achieve long-term abstinence. The 6-month rates of abstinence are generally around 20 to 40 percent.[17]

Perhaps because the replacement of nicotine is only partial, most smokers who use patches still experience some tobacco withdrawal symptoms during the first few days of quitting. Although symptoms are less severe than those occurring with quitting abruptly, some patients are tempted to smoke *and* to wear patches. The first 2 weeks of wearing the patches is critical: patients who continue to smoke and use patches after the 2-week period are unlikely to achieve abstinence. For this reason, the simultaneous wearing of nicotine patches while smoking is continued should be strongly discouraged.

SMOKING INTERVENTION MODELS

According to one popular model, the smoking cessation process consists of five stages: *precontemplation, contemplation, preparation, action,* and *maintenance.*[36] These stages are viewed as a continuum; smokers progress sequentially through each stage. In the *precontemplation stage,* smokers are not interested in quitting smoking and are unresponsive to direct intervention. In the *contemplation stage,* smokers are considering quitting and may be receptive to physician advice about the risks and benefits. In the *preparation stage,* smokers are actively preparing to quit. The *action stage* encompasses both initial abstinence and the 6-month postcessation period. The *maintenance period* commences after the 6-month abstinence period. It is rare for a smoker to progress successfully through these stages in the initial attempt at quitting. The cycle will probably be repeated several times before smoking cessation is ultimately achieved.

National Cancer Institute Model for Smoking Intervention

The model recommended by the National Cancer Institute (NCI) for smoking intervention is based, in part, on five NCI-supported trials that included more than 30,000 subjects.[31] The NCI approach, popularly referred to as the "four As," emphasizes the role of medical professionals to *ask* patients about their smoking status, to *advise* smokers to stop, to *assist* them in their stop-smoking efforts, and to *arrange* for follow-up visits to support the patients' efforts. The approach utilizes brief intervention techniques and emphasizes the role of physicians as facilitators in the quitting process.

Pragmatic Approaches to Smoking Cessation

There is no single "best" approach for smoking cessation. While nicotine replacement therapy may help one smoker quit, the identical regimen may be of absolutely no benefit to another. In the past, 95 percent of all successful quitters stopped smoking on their own, without outside intervention. Many (approximately 25 percent) stop smoking without developing tobacco withdrawal symptoms.[8,10] However, many other people who quit by themselves develop withdrawal symptoms, although the discomfort is not sufficiently powerful to overwhelm the desire to quit. These people obviously have a strong reason for stopping that can help sustain their quitting efforts during challenging times. Thus, one of the two critical ingredients required for successful abstinence is that smokers have a *reason for quitting*. The second component is equally important: the *ability to quit*.

REASON FOR QUITTING

Presumably, almost any smoker in today's society should be able to mention a number of reasons for quitting smoking, such as serious health risks, expense, social unacceptability, and prevalence of smoke-free environments. However, the question is not whether a smoker can provide reasons for quitting but, rather, whether these reasons are *sufficient* to drive the smoker to quit. General information about the health risks of smoking, for example, is not likely to compel any smoker to stop. However, personal information about the immediate health risks of smoking and long-term benefits of quitting for that person may make a difference. Patients who have recently experienced a myocardial infarction or recurrent pneumonia are likely to be very receptive to the physician's antismoking message. Many patients at risk will make a genuine effort to quit when they have an immediate reason for quitting. Unfortunately, having a reason to quit does not ensure successful abstinence.

ABILITY TO QUIT

Strongly motivated persons should, arguably, be able to quit smoking. However, many people fail to quit smoking even though they have extraordinarily powerful reasons to do so. All too common is the severely disabled patient with emphysema and serious heart disease who continues to smoke.

Two categories of smokers experience considerable difficulty in quitting. One group are those with significant psychiatric disorders. The incidence of smoking among such patients is notoriously high.[26] For these people, not only is their ability to quit compromised but smoking may provide a treatment for their underlying condition. In this regard, nicotine may function as an antidepressant, aid in anger control, or enhance relaxation.[8]

Heavily nicotine-dependent smokers constitute the second group of those whose ability to quit on their own may be compromised. For some, abrupt abstinence results in severe tobacco withdrawal symptoms that are unmanageable on a prolonged basis. While this group may experience considerable difficulty with a "cold turkey" approach, they may be excellent candidates for pharmaceutical intervention.

Evaluation Process

In the evaluation process, patients are questioned about their motivation or reason to quit and their ability to stop smoking. For patients who indicate that they are not currently interested in quitting, the goal is simple: provide a reason for quitting. For example, if an unmotivated patient has recently been found to have hypercholesteremia, the results can be framed to encourage the patient not to smoke: "With your high cholesterol level, you are at increased risk for heart attack or stroke. If you quit smoking, your health risk will decrease by 50 percent within 2 years." Providing smokers with a personal reason to quit may move some of them to stop smoking.

The second component of the evaluation process assesses the smoker's ability to quit on his or her own. The effectiveness of smoking intervention is contingent, in part, on accurate and thorough assessments of the smoker's habit. With a modicum of time, this evaluation can be conducted by the primary care physician, nurse, or member of the support staff. The decision whether to recommend pharmacologic therapy is contingent on whether the patient actually needs this therapy.

A simple, easy-to-use measure, the Fagerström test for nicotine dependence (Table 45-3),[25] provides a brief assessment of the patient's nicotine dependency. Patients with Fagerström scores of 7 or greater make up a group of persons likely to benefit from nicotine replacement therapy. Patients with low Fagerström scores should be encouraged initially to quit on their own. Moreover, patients who are able to cope with smoke-free environments for an extended period (more than 4 h) without developing uncomfortable withdrawal symptoms may not require nicotine replacement therapy.

TABLE 45-3

The Fagerström Tolerance Questionaire

1. How soon after you wake do you smoke your first cigarette? ____ 1 = Within 30 minutes / 0 = After 30 minutes
2. Do you find it difficult to refrain from smoking in places where it is forbidden; e.g., in church, at the library, in cinemas, etc? ____ 1 = Yes / 0 = No
3. Which cigarette would you most hate to give up ____ 1 = The first one in the morning / 0 = Any other
4. How many cigarettes a day do you smoke? ____ 2 = 26 or more / 1 = 16–25 / 0 = 15 or fewer
5. Do you smoke more frequently during the early morning than the rest of the day? ____ 1 = Yes / 0 = No
6. Do you smoke if you are so ill that you are in bed most of the day? ____ 1 = Yes / 0 = No
7. What is the nicotine level of your usual brand of cigarettes? ____ 2 = More than 1.0 mg / 1 = 0.61 mg–1.0 mg / 0 = 0.6 mg or fewer
8. Do you inhale? ____ 2 = Always / 1 = Sometimes / 0 = Never

TOTAL SCORE ____

SOURCE: Used with permission of Karl-Olov Fagerström.[25]

Preparing Smokers for Quitting

Several obstacles challenge smokers during their first 3 months of quitting. By anticipating the problems smokers will likely encounter, clinicians can help guide patients through the pitfalls that await them. Problems vary somewhat from smoker to smoker, but underlying similarities exist in the quitting process. The process begins with the setting of a target quit day, when the smoker will make an all-out effort to stop smoking.

TOBACCO WITHDRAWAL PERIOD

The first 3 days of abstinence are usually the most difficult. Symptoms of tobacco withdrawal (Table 45-1) generally peak during the first 72 h and then gradually subside over a 3- to 4-week period.[8,10] The symptoms include restlessness, anxiety, difficulty concentrating, irritability, frustration, depression, and an almost relentless craving for cigarettes.[13] Common suggestions to help smokers cope with these early withdrawal symptoms, in addition to nicotine replacement therapy, include the following: 1. Be active. Increased activity may curtail some of the drive to smoke. 2. Avoid caffeine. Caffeine is a stimulant that, theoretically, may exacerbate withdrawal symptoms. 3. Use deep-breathing exercises. The simplest breathing exercise requires nothing more than extended breath-holding, followed by slow exhalation through pursed lips. 4. Avoid high-risk situations for smoking during the first 3 weeks of quitting. 5. Use plenty of gum or chewable candies. 6. Combat strong urges to smoke by repeatedly reminding yourself that the urge to smoke will go away, whether you smoke or not.

During the second and third weeks of abstinence, the craving waves usually occur less frequently, but they sometimes catch smokers off guard because of their unexpected intensity.

DEPRESSION

At some time during the first 3 months of abstinence, some smokers experience depression. For many, the depression is mild and transient. For very few, quitting smoking may produce clinical depression that requires antidepressant therapy, counseling, or a return to smoking.

WEIGHT GAIN

One of the most disheartening components of quitting smoking is weight gain. Rapid weight gain is common during the first 6 to 8 weeks of cigarette abstinence. This is followed by a more gradual increase in weight to roughly 4 kg at 6 months. Average weight gain at 10 years after cessation is 4.4 kg for men and 5.0 kg for women.[19] However, the health risks associated with the weight gain that follows smoking cessation are clearly surpassed by the health benefits of stopping smoking.

DESIRE FOR AN OCCASIONAL CIGARETTE

The desire for an occasional cigarette may extend beyond the first year of abstinence. Strong urges to smoke periodically recur during times of extreme stress or while drinking alcohol with friends who smoke. Smoking one cigarette is a reliable predictor of relapse. Therefore, ex-smokers should remind themselves that they are "smoke-aholics" and will not be able to limit themselves to just one cigarette.

HEALTH BENEFITS OF SMOKING CESSATION

Data on the health benefits of smoking cessation are derived largely from studies of former smokers.[12] In many cases, these are people who have quit smoking because of the development of disease; therefore, they represent a highly selected group. Also, many studies involve more than one intervention for smoking cessation, so the effects of individual interventions are difficult to assess.[2] Nevertheless, smoking cessation is clearly associated with health benefits: mortality from all causes is decreased significantly among former smokers; moreover, the decrease in mortality is observed in all age groups and in both men and women. Thus, little doubt exists that all smokers, regardless of age or sex, are likely to benefit from smoking cessation.[12]

Cardiovascular Risk Reduction

Most of the reduction in mortality with smoking cessation is due to decreased mortality from cardiovascular causes. Smoking cessation is associated with a very rapid reduction in acute myocardial events and a more gradual reduction in complications of atherosclerotic cardiovascular disease.[12] The effects are consistent with the concept that smoking contributes to cardiovascular disease by several mechanisms. The rapid reduction in acute events may be due to removal of the acute stresses that smoking places on the heart. The longer-term, gradual effects may be associated with alteration of the atherosclerotic disease process.

Reduced Risk of Malignancy

Smoking cessation is also associated with significantly reduced risks of both respiratory and nonrespiratory malignancies.[12] Lung cancer risk appears to decrease gradually after smoking cessation, approaching that of the nonsmoker after 10 to 15 years. However, the risk of lung cancer risk shows a clear dependency on age. Thus, for both smokers and nonsmokers, risk of development of lung cancer increases with age. Whereas ex-smokers have an initial decrease in cancer risk approaching that of nonsmokers, it has been suggested that with advancing age, their risk can again exceed that of the never-smoker.

Impaired Lung Function

In subjects with relatively mild impairment, improvements in FEV_1 may be observed in the first 6 months to 1 year after smoking cessation.[2] In the Lung Health Study, which included nearly 6000 subjects, participants were assigned to three groups: no special intervention, smoking cessation with the addition of the bronchodilator ipratropium, and smoking cessation without ipratropium. The subjects who quit successfully in the intervention program manifested significant improvement in FEV_1 in the first year after cessation; this change was dramatically different from the continued decline observed in continuing smokers in the same treatment group. Smaller trials than the Lung Health Study have demonstrated that smoking cessation is associated with improvement in measures of small-airway function, including closing volume, closing capacity, and the slope of phase III of the nitrogen washout curve.[12]

Several studies have suggest that smoking cessation may be associated with partial improvement in the diffusion capacity (DLCO).[12] This physiological effect may relate to the cellular changes associated with smoking cessation: the number of alveolar macrophages recoverable by bronchoalveolar lavage is markedly decreased after smoking cessation.

Although, as noted above, cigarette smoking is associated with an accelerated loss of lung function, only some smokers develop symptomatic disease.[20] Cross-sectional studies clearly demonstrate that former smokers lose lung function at a rate comparable to that of nonsmokers, suggesting that smoking cessation can slow the accelerated rate of decline. Whether smoking cessation per se is responsible for this effect was addressed in the Lung Health Study.[2] In the study, the rate of decline of lung function was clearly reduced among smokers who successfully quit—i.e., 20 percent of participants in the intervention program. However, the improvement in the rate of decline in lung function for the entire treatment group was relatively small, suggesting that better cessation regimens are needed.

Effects on Other Respiratory Disorders

Smoking is the major risk factor for respiratory bronchiolitis, and smoking cessation is usually associated with dramatic abatement of this disease. Smoking cessation is also associated with relief of respiratory symptoms, including cough, sputum production, dyspnea, and wheezing.[44] Improvement may be manifest in the first few months.

Eosinophilic granuloma of the lung occurs almost exclusively in smokers. Smoking cessation is generally regarded as an important therapeutic goal for such people. Instances of complete radiographic resolution of eosinophilic granuloma of the lung have been reported after smoking cessation.[49]

Other Beneficial Health Effects

Data on the effect of smoking cessation on other diseases associated with smoking are limited. Former smokers have a reduced incidence of peptic ulcer disease and a more rapid rate of ulcer healing than do current smokers.[44] Similarly, the ovarian function of women who are former smokers appears to resemble more closely that of never-smokers than that of smokers.

RISKS OF SMOKING CESSATION

In some persons, smoking cessation may be hazardous. Depression is a well-recognized manifestation of the nicotine withdrawal syndrome. At times, this depression can be of major clinical importance. Nicotine may have a significant antidepressant effect, and many people who are inherently depressed may have found empirically that smoking helps alleviate symptoms.

Smoking, and nicotine in particular, may also have a salutary effect on ulcerative colitis. In this context, exacerbations of ul-

cerative colitis have been associated with acute smoking cessation.[32]

Thus, although cigarette smoking is a major health hazard, the numerous physiological effects associated with nicotine may have potential benefits. However, such benefits should not deflect from the desirability of smoking cessation. Instead, such observations have introduced the concept that nicotine may, in selected circumstances, have a pharmaceutical role.

OTHER APPROACHES TO PREVENTING SMOKING RISKS

Smoking cessation remains an important therapeutic goal. Unfortunately, only a small percentage of persons who wish to stop are successful in quitting. In addition, many people do not wish to give up smoking completely. The limited applicability and success of current smoking cessation techniques have led to a number of other approaches to prevent the health hazards of smoking. These approaches fall into three general categories: administration of agents to counteract the effects of cigarette smoking, smoking reduction, and development of a less toxic cigarette.

Since cigarette smoking is thought to produce its effects through pathogenetic mechanisms that are at least partly defined, it is appealing to devise mechanisms for therapeutic intervention. In this regard, use of antioxidants to alleviate the oxidant-induced injury caused by cigarette smoke and protease inhibitors to bolster antiprotease defenses constitutes potential therapeutic strategies. Although this is conceptually appealing, however, no data exist to suggest that either approach is of benefit in continuing smokers.

The observation that most smokers maintain a relatively constant nicotine intake suggests the possibility that nicotine replacement may help sustain smoking reduction. In a group of heavy smokers, short-term smoking reduction has been associated with abatement of lower respiratory tract inflammation, as assessed with bronchoscopy and bronchoalveolar lavage.[39] However, in a group of lighter smokers with less airway inflammation, a benefit of smoking reduction is more difficult to demonstrate. Nevertheless, these studies, coupled with observations that smoking-induced disease shows a clear dose dependency on numbers of cigarettes smoked, suggest that smoking reduction might be a reasonable strategy for persons who cannot or do not wish to quit. Finally, nicotine replacement and concurrent smoking may have health risks. Initial reports of an increased frequency of myocardial infarction among nicotine patch users who continue to smoke have not been substantiated.[28,51] However, the many forms of nicotine currently available have a potential risk that cannot be ignored.

Cigarette smoke contains numerous potential toxins. Reducing toxin delivery, while still providing the smoker with a satisfactory cigarette, has been an important commercial goal.[38] A number of problems in developing such a cigarette have arisen, since cigarette filters that have been designed to remove tar have also removed nicotine. Because smokers strive to maintain a constant intake of nicotine, many smokers compensate for reduced nicotine inhalation by simply smoking more. By altering smoking strategies, filtered cigarettes may actually deliver more toxins. Many of the cigarette-derived toxins are generated as a result of pyrolysis. As a result, cigarettes that burn tobacco differently have offered promise for delivering less toxins. A number of these cigarettes have been found unacceptable as commercial products because of problems with taste. Other products, however, are currently under investigation.[38] These products appear to deliver smaller amounts of toxins, but whether they are associated with any realistic health benefits remains to be determined. Finally, reduced-risk cigarettes may have unforeseen problems. For example, they might be particularly appealing for persons beginning to smoke, since they may be easier to smoke and are not perceived as having significant risks. The availability of these products may increase the number of smokers.

Cigarette smoking can, at least to some extent, be prevented. As noted previously, smoking initiation is generally a pediatric problem.[21] Precisely why some children begin to smoke is not fully understood. A number of factors are thought to contribute, including the child's social environment and attitude toward smoking, which appears to be based, in large part, on the smoking behavior of parents, friends, and peer-group role models.[18,41] Reasons for initiating smoking, however, are not entirely environmental; studies on twins suggest a genetic basis for smoking.[14] A limited number of interventions have suggested that altering the social milieu may be of benefit. For example, active participation in sporting activities may decrease smoking initiation.[15] Control of affective disorders may also be beneficial.[7] Finally, restrictions on tobacco advertising may have an important impact.[16] Attitudes toward smoking appear to be key factors leading to smoking initiation,[24] and these attitudes can depend, in part, on advertising and marketing programs.[6]

A second approach to limiting smoking initiation is to restrict the sale of tobacco products to minors. Many states have legal restrictions on tobacco sales.[40] In many cases, however, the laws are not enforced. Current evidence clearly demonstrates that active enforcement of tobacco restrictions may lead to a decrease both in experimental smoking and in regular cigarette use among younger smokers.[29] For such measures to be effective, they must be uniformly enforced in the community, and vending machines must be made inaccessible to minors.

Taxation constitutes another approach to restrict tobacco usage by minors. Increased tobacco taxes have been suggested as a means of decreasing tobacco use—an effect that will be particularly prominent among less addicted smokers. Since adolescents may have less disposable income, the effect may be even greater. Although such an approach is appealing, the magnitude of price changes required is unclear. Data in the United States suggest that adolescent smoking initiation has increased over the past decade, when the real price of cigarettes has also increased.[45]

Measures aimed at restricting tobacco sales to minors may lead simply to a deferral of smoking initiation. Current data suggest that if a smoker does not develop a regular habit by young adulthood, he or she is unlikely to become a smoker. On the other hand, such observations are based on our current social milieu. Efforts aimed at deferring smoking initiation among children and adolescents may leave the same people at risk at later ages. Thus, if measures are effective at delaying smoking initiation among children, parallel measures may also be required to affect smoking initiation among older adolescents and young adults.[11]

CONCLUSION

Cigarette smoking is a complex social and medical issue. The physician has a particularly important role in the debate and needs to participate not only as a citizen but also as a protector of the public health. The physician must take an active role in health promotion, including discouraging smoking initiation among younger patients, encouraging and assisting smoking patients to quit, and participating in social efforts designed to curb smoking at various levels. A number of policy statements have been prepared regarding the role of the physician.[1,9] Perhaps, through such efforts, cigarette smoking, the number one preventable cause of death in the developed world, may be effectively controlled.

REFERENCES

1. American College of Chest Physicians, American Thoracic Society, Asia Pacific Society of Respirology, Canadian Thoracic Society, European Respiratory Society, International Union Against Tuberculosis and Lung Disease: Smoking and health: A physician responsibility. A statement of the joint committee on smoking and health. *Eur Respir J* 8:1808–1811, 1995.
2. Anthonisen NR, Connett JE, Kiley JP, et al: Effects of smoking intervention and the use of an inhaled anticholinergic bronchodilator on the rate of decline of FEV$_1$. *JAMA* 272:1497–1505, 1994.
3. Benowitz NL: Pharmacologic aspects of cigarette smoking and nicotine addiction. *New Engl J Med* 319:1318–1330, 1988.
4. Benowitz NL: Pharmacokinetic considerations in understanding nicotine dependence. *Ciba Found Symp* 152:186–200, 1990.
5. Benowitz NL, Jacob P: Intravenous nicotine replacement suppresses nicotine intake from cigarette smoking. *J Pharmacol Exp Ther* 254:1000–1005, 1990.
6. Botvin GJ, Goldberg CJ, Botvin EM, Dusenbury L: Smoking behavior of adolescents exposed to cigarette advertising. *Public Health Rep* 108:217–224, 1993.
7. Carmody TP: Affect regulation, nicotine addiction, and smoking cessation. *J Psychoactive Drugs* 24:111–122, 1992.
8. Centers for Disease Control: *The Health Consequences of Smoking, Nicotine Addiction: A Report of the Surgeon General.* U.S. Department of Health and Human Services, Public Health Service, Center for Health Promotion and Education, Office on Smoking and Health. Rockville, Maryland, U.S. Government Printing Office, 1988.
9. Cigarette smoking and health (editorial). *Am J Respir Crit Care Med* 153:861–865, 1996.
10. Daughton DM, Rennard SI: The tobacco withdrawal syndrome: Recognition of the physiological rebound phenomenon and treatment implications. *Monaldi Arch Chest Dis* 48:574–575, 1993.
11. Dawley HH: A comprehensive worksite smoking control, discouragement and cessation program. *Int J Addict* 26:685–696, 1991.
12. Department of Health and Human Services: *Health Benefits of Smoking Cessation: A Report of the Surgeon General.* Washington, DC, DHHS Publication (CDC) 90-8416, 1990.
13. *Diagnostic and Statistical Manual of Mental Disorders, 4th ed.* Washington, DC, American Psychiatric Association, 1994.
14. Edwards KL, Austin MA, Jarvik GP: Evidence for genetic influences on smoking in adult women twins. *Clin Genet* 47:236–244, 1995.
15. Escobedo LG, Marcus SE, Holtzman D, Giovino GA: Sports participation, age at smoking initiation, and the risk of smoking among US high school students. *JAMA* 269:1391–1395, 1993.

16. Evans N, Farkas A, Gilpin E, et al: Influence of tobacco marketing and exposure to smokers on adolescent susceptibility to smoking. *J Natl Cancer Inst* 87:1538–1545, 1995.

17. Fiore MC, Jorenby DE, Baker TB: Tobacco dependence and the nicotine patch: Clinical guidelines for effective use. *JAMA* 268:2687–2694, 1992.

18. Flay BR, Hu FB, Siddiqui O, et al: Differential influence of parental smoking and friends' smoking on adolescent initiation and escalation of smoking. *J Health Soc Behav* 35:248–265, 1994.

19. Flegal KM, Troiano RP, Pamuk ER, et al: The influence of smoking cessation on the prevalence of overweight in the United States. *New Engl J Med* 333:1165–1170, 1995.

20. Fletcher C, Peto R, Tinker C, Speizer F: *The Natural History of Chronic Bronchitis and Emphysema.* New York, Oxford University Press, 1976, p 272.

21. Gilpin EA, Lee L, Evans N, Pierce JP: Smoking initiation rates in adults and minors: United States, 1944–1988. *Am J Epidemiol* 140:535–543, 1994.

22. Glassman AH, Jackson WK, Walsh BT, et al: Cigarette craving, smoking withdrawal and clonidine. *Science* 226:864–867, 1984.

23. Gold MS, Redmond DE, Kleber HD: Clonidine blocks acute opiate withdrawal symptoms. *Lancet* 2:599–602, 1978.

24. Headen SW, Bauman KE, Deane GD, Koch GG: Are the correlates of cigarette smoking initiation different for black and white adolescents? *Am J Public Health* 81:854–858, 1991.

25. Heatherton TF, Kozlowski LT, Frecker RC, Fagerström K-O: The Fagerström Test for Nicotine Dependence: A revision of the Fagerström Tolerance Questionnaire. *Br J Addict* 86:1119–1127, 1991.

26. Hughes JR: Possible effects of smoke-free inpatient units psychiatric diagnosis and treatment. *J Clin Psychiatry* 54:109–114, 1993.

27. Hughes JR: Risk-benefit assessment of nicotine preparations in smoking cessation. *Drug Saf* 8:49–56, 1993.

28. Hwang SL, Waldholz M: Heart attacks reported in patch users still smoking. *Wall Street Journal,* June 19, 1992, p B1.

29. Jason LA: Active enforcement of cigarette control laws in the prevention of cigarette sales to minors. *JAMA* 266:3159–3161, 1991.

30. Koop CE: 80th Annual Meeting of American Lung Association. Miami Beach, Florida, 1984.

31. Manley M, Epps RP, Husten C, et al: Clinical interventions in tobacco control. *JAMA* 266:3172–3173, 1991.

32. Motley RJ, Rhodes J, Ford GA, et al: The relationship between cessation of smoking and onset of ulcerative colitis. *Digestion* 37:125–127, 1987.

33. Nelson DE, Giovino GA, Shopland DR, et al: Trends in cigarette smoking among U.S. adolescents, 1974 through 1991. *Am J Public Health* 85:34–40, 1995.

34. Palmer KJ, Buckley MM, Faulds D: Transdermal nicotine: A review of its pharmacodynamic and pharmacokinetic properties, and therapeutic efficacy as an aid to smoking cessation. *Drugs* 44:498–529, 1992.

35. Peto R, Speizer FE, Cochrane AL, et al: The relevance in adults of air-flow obstruction, but not of mucus hypersecretion, to mortality from chronic lung disease: Results from 20 years of prospective observation. *Am Rev Respir Dis* 128:491–500, 1983.

36. Prochaska JO, DiClemente CC: Stages of change in the modification of problem behaviors. *Prog Behav Modif* 28:183–218, 1992.

37. Prochazka AV, Petty TL, Nett L, et al: Transdermal clonidine reduced smoke withdrawal symptoms but did not increase smoking cessation. *Arch Intern Med* 152:2065–2069, 1992.

38. RJ Reynolds Tobacco Company: *New Cigarette Prototypes that Heat Instead of Burn Tobacco.* Winston-Salem, NC, RJ Reynolds Tobacco Company, 1988.

39. Rennard SI, Daughton D, Fujita J, et al: Short-term smoking reduction is associated with reduction in measures of lower respiratory tract inflammation in heavy smokers. *Eur Respir J* 3:752–759, 1990.

40. Rigotti NA: No-smoking laws in the United States. *JAMA* 266:3162–3167, 1991.

41. Santi S, Best JA, Brown KS, Cargo M: Social environment and smoking initiation. *Int J Addict* 25:881–903, 1991.

42. Schwartz JL: *Review and Evaluation of Smoking Cessation Methods: The United States and Canada, 1978–1985.* NIH Publication 87-2940, 1987, pp 125–156.

43. Segal DS, Kuczenski R: Behavioral pharmacology of amphetamine, in Cho AK, Segal DS (eds), *Amphetamine and Its Analogs.* San Diego, Academic, 1994, pp 115–150.

44. Sifers RN, Brashears-Macatee S, Kidd VJ, et al: A frameshift mutation results in a truncated alpha 1–antitrypsin that is retained within the rough endoplasmic reticulum. *J Biol Chem* 263:7330–7335, 1988.

45. Trends in smoking initiation among adolescents and young adults—United States, 1980–1989. *MMWR* 44:521–525, 1995.

46. US Department of Health and Human Services: *The Health Consequences of Smoking: Cancer. A Report of the Surgeon General.* DHHS Publication (PHS)82-50179, 1982.

47. US Department of Health and Human Services: *The Health Consequences of Smoking. A Report of the Surgeon General.* DHHS Publication (PHS) 84-50205, 1984.

48. US Department of Health and Human Services: *The Health Consequences of Smoking: Cardiovascular Disease. A Report of the Surgeon General.* DHHS Publication (PHS)84-50204, 1983.

49. Von Essen S, West W, Sitorius M, Rennard SI: Complete resolution of roentgenographic changes in a patient with histiocytosis X. *Chest* 98:765–767, 1990.

50. West DW, Graham S, Swanson M, Wilkinson G: Five-year follow-up of a smoking withdrawal clinic population. *Am J Public Health* 67:536–544, 1977.

51. Working Group for the Study of Transdermal Nicotine in Patients with Coronary Artery Disease: Nicotine replacement therapy for patients with coronary artery disease. *Arch Intern Med* 154:989–995, 1994.

REHABILITATION IN CHRONIC OBSTRUCTIVE PULMONARY DISEASE AND OTHER RESPIRATORY DISORDERS

Andrew L. Ries

Rehabilitation for patients with chronic lung diseases is well established as a means of enhancing standard pharmacologic and other therapies in controlling and alleviating symptoms and optimizing functional capacity.[1–3,11,21,27,40] The primary goal of any rehabilitation program is to restore the patient to the highest possible level of independent function. This goal is accomplished by helping patients and significant others learn more about the underlying disease, treatment options, and coping strategies. Patients are encouraged to participate actively in providing their own health care, to become more independent in daily activities, and to be less dependent on health professionals and expensive medical resources. Rather than addressing solely reversal of the disease process, rehabilitation focuses on improving disability from disease.

Historically, pulmonary rehabilitation strategies were developed and have been used primarily for patients with chronic obstructive pulmonary disease (COPD). However, pulmonary rehabilitation has also been applied successfully to patients with other chronic lung conditions, including interstitial diseases, cystic fibrosis, bronchiectasis, and thoracic cage abnormalities.[17] It has been used successfully in the evaluation and preparation of patients for surgery, such as lung transplantation and volume reduction lung surgery, and in maximizing recovery after surgery.[7,13,16] Pulmonary rehabilitation has been used to facilitate patient recovery from acute processes such as acute lung injury or from exacerbations of chronic lung disease requiring mechanical ventilation or acute hospital care. Pulmonary rehabilitation is appropriate for any patient with stable lung disease who is disabled by respiratory symptoms. Even patients with advanced disease may benefit if they are selected appropriately and realistic goals are set.

This chapter defines pulmonary rehabilitation and outlines issues related to patient selection and evaluation. Key components of a pulmonary rehabilitation program are described and results of rehabilitation programs reviewed. Finally, the role of rehabilitation prior to and following lung surgery is reviewed.

DEFINITION

In 1974, the American College of Chest Physicians' Committee on Pulmonary Rehabilitation adopted the following definition of pulmonary rehabilitation:

> Pulmonary rehabilitation may be defined as an art of medical practice wherein an individually tailored, multidisciplinary program is formulated which through accurate diagnosis, therapy, emotional support, and education, stabilizes or reverses both the physio- and psychopathology of pulmonary diseases and attempts to return the patient to the highest possible functional capacity allowed by his pulmonary handicap and overall life situation.[2]

This definition focuses on three important features of successful rehabilitation. First, the program is tailored to the *individual*. Patients with disabling lung disease require individual assessment of needs, individual attention, and a program designed to meet realistic individual goals. Second, the program is *multidisciplinary*. Pulmonary rehabilitation programs utilize expertise from various health care disciplines that is integrated into a comprehensive, cohesive program tailored to the needs of each patient. Third, the program addresses *physio-* and *psychopathology*. To be successful, pulmonary rehabilitation must address the psychological and emotional problems as well as seek to optimize medical therapy to improve lung function.

A newer definition of pulmonary rehabilitation proposed by a National Institutes of Health (NIH) Workshop on Pulmonary Rehabilitation Research emphasizes, as key aspects of any program, multidimensional services, an interdisciplinary team, involvement of patients and families, and individual goals for patient independence and function in the community:

> Pulmonary rehabilitation is a multidimensional continuum of services directed to persons with pulmonary disease and their families, usually by an interdisciplinary team of specialists, with the goal of achieving and maintaining the individual's maximum level of independence and functioning in the community.[16]

The interdisciplinary team of health care professionals in pulmonary rehabilitation includes physicians, nurses, respiratory and physical therapists, psychologists, exercise specialists, and others with appropriate expertise. The specific team makeup depends upon the resources and expertise available, but it usually includes at least one full-time staff member. Responsibilities of team members generally cross disciplines.

Within this general framework, successful pulmonary rehabilitation programs have been established in both outpatient and inpatient settings and with different formats. A key to success is a dedicated, enthusiastic staff that is familiar with respiratory problems and can relate well to pulmonary patients and motivate them.

PATIENT SELECTION

Any patient with symptomatic chronic lung disease is a candidate for pulmonary rehabilitation (Table 46-1). Appropriate patients are aware of disability from their disease and are motivated to participate actively in their own care in order to improve their health status. Patients with mild chronic disease may not

TABLE 46-1

Patient Selection Criteria for Pulmonary Rehabilitation

Symptomatic chronic lung disease

Stable on standard therapy

Functional limitation from disease

Relationship with primary care provider

Motivated to be actively involved in and take responsibility for own health care

No other interfering or unstable medical conditions

No arbitrary lung function or age criteria

perceive their symptoms to be severe enough to warrant a comprehensive care program. On the other hand, patients with severe disease who are bed bound may be too limited to benefit greatly.

Criteria based on arbitrary lung function parameters or age alone should not be used in selecting patients.[1,40] Pulmonary function is not a good predictor of symptoms, function, or improvement after rehabilitation.[33] Older patients with chronic lung diseases may live many years with pulmonary disability. In general, selection should be based upon a person's disability and functional limitation from respiratory symptoms, potential for improvement, and motivation to participate actively in a comprehensive self-care program.

Other factors are also important in evaluating candidates. Pulmonary rehabilitation is not a primary mode of therapy. Patients should be evaluated and stabilized on standard medical therapy before beginning a program. They should not have other disabling or unstable conditions that might limit their ability to participate fully in the program and to concentrate on the necessary tasks.

The ideal patient for pulmonary rehabilitation, then, is one with functional limitation from moderate to severe lung disease who is stable on standard therapy, not distracted or limited by other serious or unstable medical conditions, willing and able to learn about his or her disease, and motivated to devote the time and effort necessary to benefit from a comprehensive care program.

PATIENT EVALUATION

The initial step in pulmonary rehabilitation is screening patients to ensure appropriate selection and to set realistic individual and program goals. The evaluation process includes the following components: an interview, the medical evaluation, psychosocial assessment, diagnostic testing, and goal setting (Table 46-2).

Interview

The screening interview is an important first step. It serves to introduce the patient to the program, review the medical history, and identify psychosocial problems and needs. Family members and significant others should be included in the interview. Communication with the primary care physician is also important to

TABLE 46-2

Components of a Comprehensive Pulmonary Rehabilitation Program

Patient evaluation
    Interview
    Medical evaluation
    Diagnostic testing
        Pulmonary function
        Exercise
        Arterial blood gases/oximetry
    Psychosocial assessment
    Goal setting
Program content
    Education
    Respiratory and chest physiotherapy instruction
    Exercise
    Psychosocial support

establish the vital link for the rehabilitation staff in clarifying medical questions prior to initiation of the program and in facilitating recommendations during and after treatment. Care and attention in this initial evaluation helps in setting goals compatible with everyone's expectations as well as appropriate programmatic objectives.

Medical Evaluation

A review of the medical history helps to identify the patient's lung disease and to assess its severity. Other medical problems that might preclude or delay participation may be identified. Available laboratory data should be reviewed, including pulmonary function and exercise tests, rest and exercise arterial blood gas measurements, chest radiographs, the electrocardiogram, and pertinent blood tests. Program staff can then determine the need for additional information or take action before the program begins.

Diagnostic Testing

Planning an appropriate rehabilitation program requires accurate, current information. The complexity of the testing procedures performed depends upon individual patient and program goals as well as the facilities and expertise available.

Pulmonary function testing is used to characterize lung disease and quantify impairment. Spirometry and lung volume measurements are most useful; other tests (e.g., diffusing capacity, airway resistance, and maximal respiratory pressures to assess muscle strength) can be added as needed.

Exercise testing helps to assess the patient's exercise tolerance and to evaluate changes in arterial blood gases (e.g., development of hypoxemia or hypercapnia) with exercise. This may also uncover coexisting diseases (e.g., heart disease). The exercise test is also used to establish a safe and appropriate prescription for subsequent training.

Maximal exercise of patients with chronic lung disease is limited largely by their breathing reserve. Simple pulmonary function tests such as spirometry can be used to estimate a patient's capacity for sustained breathing (maximal ventilation) during exercise. The forced expiratory volume in 1 s (FEV_1) is most useful in this regard.[43] However, an individual patient's maximum work capacity can only be estimated from lung function. Exercise tolerance depends also on the patient's perception and tolerance of the subjective symptom of breathlessness. Therefore, it is important to exercise patients to assess their physical function and symptom tolerance.

Exercise evaluation for rehabilitation is most easily performed with the type of activity planned for training (e.g., treadmill for a walking training program). Variables measured or monitored during testing should include workload, heart rate, electrocardiogram, arterial oxygenation, and symptoms (e.g., breathlessness). Other measures, such as ventilation or expired gas analysis to calculate oxygen uptake ($\dot{V}O_2$) and related variables may be obtained depending on the interest and expertise of the program staff and laboratory.[43]

Measurement of arterial blood gases at rest and during exercise is important because of the frequent but unpredictable occurrence of exercise-induced hypoxemia.[44] Arterial blood gas sampling during exercise makes testing more complex. The noninvasive estimate of arterial oxygen saturation by cutaneous (e.g., pulse) oximetry is useful for continuous monitoring, but it has limited accuracy (95 percent confidence limits, ±4 to 5 percent).[31,43]

Psychosocial Assessment

Successful rehabilitation requires attention not only to the patient's physical problems but also to his or her psychological, emotional, and social issues. Patients with chronic illnesses experience psychosocial difficulties as they struggle to deal with symptoms they may not fully understand.[14]

Neuropsychological impairment is common in patients with chronic lung diseases and cannot be accounted for solely on the basis of age, depression, or organic disease.[29] Commonly, such patients become depressed, frightened, anxious, and more dependent on others to care for their needs. Progressive dyspnea is a frightening symptom and may lead to a vicious "fear-dyspnea" cycle: with progressive disease, less exertion results in more dyspnea, which produces more fear and anxiety, which, in turn, lead to more dyspnea. Ultimately, the patient avoids any physical activity associated with both of these unpleasant symptoms.

In addressing these problems, the initial evaluation should include an assessment of the patient's psychological state and attention should be directed to "psychosocial clues" that may be apparent during the screening interview (e.g., the level of family and social support and the patient's living arrangement, activities of daily living, hobbies, and employment potential). Important clues in initial interviews may be evident in nonverbal communication, such as facial expression, physical appearance, handshake, and "body space." Cognitive impairment that may limit the patient's ability to participate fully in the rehabilitation program may be identified. Family members and significant others may provide valuable insight and should be included in the screening process and program whenever possible.

Goals

After a patient's medical, physiologic, and psychosocial state has been evaluated, specific goals should be set that are compatible with his or her disease, needs, and expectations. Goals should be realistic in light of the objectives of the program. Family members and significant others should be included in this process so that everyone understands what can and cannot be achieved.

PROGRAM CONTENT

Comprehensive pulmonary rehabilitation programs typically include several key components: education, instruction in respiratory and chest physiotherapy, psychosocial support, and exercise training (Table 46-2). Often, the various components are provided simultaneously; for example, during an exercise session, a patient may learn and practice breathing techniques for symptom control while being encouraged and supported by staff or other patients.

Education

Successful pulmonary rehabilitation depends upon an understanding of lung disease and active involvement by patients and those important in providing their social support. Education is an integral component; even patients with severe disease can gain a better understanding of their disease and learn specific means to deal with problems.[32] Instruction can be provided individually or in small groups, but it should be adapted to different patient learning abilities. Topics discussed commonly include normal lung function, chronic lung disease, medications, nutrition, travel, stress reduction and relaxation, reasons to call the physician, and planning a daily schedule. Individual instruction and coaching may be provided on the use of respiratory therapy equipment and supplemental oxygen, breathing techniques, bronchial drainage, chest percussion, energy-saving techniques, and self-care tips. The general philosophy is to encourage patients to assume responsibility for their own care and to become partners with their physician in providing the care.[42]

Despite the importance of education, it is unlikely that increased patient knowledge alone will lead to improved health status. It is more difficult to change patient attitudes and behaviors. Patients require specific, individualized treatment strategies, instruction, and reinforcement. Thus, education is a necessary but not sufficient component of pulmonary rehabilitation.

Respiratory and Chest Physiotherapy Techniques

Patients with chronic lung disease use, abuse, and are confused about respiratory and chest physiotherapy techniques. In pulmonary rehabilitation, each patient's needs for respiratory care techniques should be assessed and instruction provided in proper use. These techniques may include chest physiotherapy to control secretions; breathing retraining techniques to relieve and control dyspnea and improve ventilatory function; and proper use and care of respiratory equipment, including nebulizers, metered dose inhalers, and supplemental oxygen.[27]

Bronchial Hygiene

Patients with chronic lung diseases frequently have abnormal lung clearance mechanisms that increase susceptibility to problems with retained secretions and infection. Therefore, rehabilitation programs entail the teaching of a variety of chest physiotherapy techniques for secretion control (e.g., coughing, postural drainage, and chest vibration and percussion).[42,46] These methods are important for patients who experience excess mucus production during exacerbations of their lung disease as well as for those who chronically produce sputum. The use of mucolytic agents to reduce viscosity of secretions is of questionable benefit.[36]

Breathing Retraining Techniques

Pulmonary rehabilitation typically includes instruction in breathing techniques, such as diaphragmatic and pursed lips breathing—techniques aimed at helping patients relieve and control breathlessness, improve their ventilatory pattern (i.e., achieve a slower respiratory rate and increased tidal volume), prevent dynamic airway compression, improve respiratory synchrony of the abdominal and thoracic musculature, and improve gas exchange.[3,5,9,31,42,46] Review of studies evaluating these techniques indicates that improvement in symptoms (e.g., dyspnea) is a more consistent finding than are measurable changes in physiological parameters. The diaphragmatic breathing technique, described by Barach[5] and Miller[31] is a maneuver in which the patient coordinates abdominal wall expansion with inspiration and slows expiration through pursed lips. The primary effect is to slow the respiratory rate and increase the tidal volume.

Pursed-lips breathing is a technique commonly taught to pulmonary patients, particularly those with COPD.[5,31] This technique was observed by Laennec as early as 1830 and was advocated as a physical exercise for pulmonary patients in the early part of the twentieth century. As a maneuver assumed naturally by many patients with respiratory disease, pursed-lips breathing is characterized by tensing of the lips and narrowing of the opening of the mouth during expiration. The aim is to slow the expiratory phase and maintain positive airway pressure in order to "stent the airways open," thereby improving ventilatory efficiency.

Oxygen

When chronic oxygen therapy is required, the available delivery methods should be reviewed with the patient to help select the best system for his or her needs. Supplemental oxygen is beneficial for patients who have severe resting hypoxemia (see Chapter 172). Long-term continuous oxygen therapy has been clearly shown to improve survival and reduce mortality and morbidity in hypoxemic patients with COPD.[3,30,34,49] In fact, this is the only treatment modality that has been proved to prolong survival in these patients. The benefits of supplemental oxygen for nonhypoxemic patients or those with intermittent hypoxemia (e.g., during exercise or sleep) are less clearly defined.

Although continuous oxygen therapy is feasible and safe, maintaining patients on supplemental oxygen presents several challenges. Handling equipment is particularly difficult for physically disabled and frail patients. Therefore, it is important to assess each person's oxygen needs and to provide instruction on appropriate techniques.

Several new developments have improved the efficiency of gas delivery systems and patient compliance in using continuous oxygen therapy.[48,49] Liquid oxygen provides more gas with less weight than do tanks of compressed gas, particularly in portable systems. Also, transtracheal delivery of oxygen (see Chapter 172) may increase the efficiency of delivery, reducing flow requirements and prolonging the life span of portable gas sources. In addition, compliance may be improved and problems with nasal catheters avoided. However, patients must be instructed carefully in caring for and maintaining the catheter.

Exercise

Exercise is important in pulmonary rehabilitation.[1,2,11,21,27] Considerable evidence exists demonstrating favorable responses to exercise training in patients with chronic lung diseases.[6,11,40] Benefits are both physiological and psychological. Patients may increase their maximum capacity and endurance for physical activity, even though objective measures of lung function do not usually change. Patients may also benefit from learning to perform physical tasks more efficiently. Exercise training provides an ideal opportunity for patients to learn their capacity for physical work and to use and practice methods for controlling dyspnea (e.g., breathing and relaxation techniques). Of all the components in a comprehensive pulmonary rehabilitation program, exercise is probably the most costly and labor-intensive, considering the personnel, equipment, and expertise required. Principles of exercise testing and training for patients with lung disease differ from those based on normals or other patient populations because of differences in the limitations to exercise and the problems encountered in training.[6]

Many approaches have been used in rehabilitation to train the person with chronic lung disease. To be successful, the program should be tailored to the individual's physical abilities, interests, resources, and environment. For general application, techniques should be simple and inexpensive. As in normals and other patients, benefits are largely specific to the muscles and tasks involved in training. Patients tend to do best with activities and exercises for which they are trained. Walking programs are particularly useful. They have the added benefit of encouraging patients to expand social horizons. In inclement weather, many can walk indoors (e.g., at shopping malls). Other types of exercise (e.g., cycling, swimming) are also effective. Patients should be encouraged to incorporate regular exercise into daily activities they enjoy (e.g., golf, gardening). Since many persons with chronic lung disease have limited exercise tolerance, emphasis during training should be placed on increasing endurance. Changes in endurance with rehabilitation are often greater than changes in maximal exercise tolerance.[33,41] This allows patients to become more functional within their physical limits. Increase in maximum exercise is also possible as patients gain experience and confidence in their exercise program.

Exercise Prescription

Selecting a training target based upon a predetermined percentage of predicted maximal heart rate or $\dot{V}O_2$ is a well-established practice for normals or patients without underlying pulmonary disease. However, in patients with chronic lung diseases, the best method of choosing an appropriate training prescription is less clearly defined. Exercise tolerance in pulmonary patients is typically limited by maximal achievable ventilation and breathlessness. Such patients frequently do not reach their limits of cardiac or peripheral muscle performance.

Much controversy exists regarding the appropriate training intensity target for patients with chronic lung disease. Use of a target heart rate has been advocated by some, although it is recognized that such a target may not be reliable for patients with more severe disease.[6,45] Many patients with lung disease can be trained at a high percentage of their maximal activity level, with work levels approaching or even exceeding the maximal level reached on the initial exercise test. In a study of 52 patients with moderate to severe COPD, patients were able to perform endurance exercise testing at an average workload of 95 percent of their baseline maximal exercise tolerance.[37] After 8 weeks in a training program, these patients were training at 86 percent of the baseline maximal workload. In fact, many patients with severe COPD were exercising at levels exceeding their baseline maximum. In a study that examined 59 patients with moderate to severe COPD who trained at levels near their ventilatory limits, a mean peak exercise ventilation of 100 percent of measured maximal voluntary ventilation was achieved after 12 days of training and at 3 months of follow-up.[10] These findings suggest that even patients with advanced disease can be trained successfully at or near maximal exercise levels.

Based on the findings noted previously, some pulmonary rehabilitation programs define exercise targets and progression during training more by symptom tolerance than by heart rate, work level, or other physiological measurements.[6,45] Ratings of perceived symptoms (e.g., breathlessness) help teach patients to exercise to "target" levels of breathing discomfort.[8,28] A typical approach is to begin training at a level that the patient can sustain with reasonable comfort for several minutes and then to increase the time or exercise level according to symptom tolerance. Patients are encouraged to exercise daily and to increase exercise duration up to 15 to 30 min of continuous activity. This graduated program helps patients to achieve a goal of improved tolerance for tasks of daily living, which often require a period of sustained activity.

Blood-Gas Changes

A major problem in planning a safe exercise program for patients with lung disease is the potential for worsening of hypoxemia with exercise. Patients who are not hypoxemic at rest may develop changes in arterial oxygenation that cannot be predicted reliably from resting measurements of pulmonary function or gas exchange. Normal individuals do not become hypoxemic with exercise. In patients with obstructive lung disease, Pa_{O_2} changes unpredictably during exercise.[4] In patients with mild COPD, Pa_{O_2} typically does not change with exercise; in fact, it may even improve. However, in patients with moderate to severe COPD, Pa_{O_2} may increase, decrease, or remain the same. Patients with interstitial lung disease commonly develop worsening oxygenation with exercise.

Based on these observations, it is important to evaluate a patient's oxygenation status both at rest and during exercise. Such testing is also used to prescribe oxygen therapy at rest and with physical activity. With the availability of convenient, portable systems for ambulatory oxygen delivery, hypoxemia is not a contraindication to safe exercise training.

Other Types of Exercise

Exercise programs for pulmonary patients typically emphasize lower extremity training (e.g., walking or cycling). Exercise conditioning is largely specific to the muscles and tasks involved in training. Therefore, other forms of exercise may be particularly valuable for persons with chronic lung diseases.

UPPER EXTREMITY TRAINING

Many patients with chronic lung disease report disabling dyspnea with daily activities involving the upper extremities (e.g., lifting, grooming) at work levels that are much lower than activities involving the lower extremities.[12] Upper extremity exercise is accompanied by a higher ventilatory demand for a given level of work than is lower extremity exercise. Given the aforementioned muscle specificity of training, upper extremity exercises may be important in helping pulmonary patients cope better with common daily activities.[15]

VENTILATORY MUSCLE TRAINING

The potential role of ventilatory muscle fatigue as a cause of respiratory failure and ventilatory limitation in patients with chronic lung disease has stimulated attempts to train the ventilatory muscles.[47] Techniques of isocapnic hyperventilation, inspiratory resistive loading, and inspiratory threshold loading have been shown to improve function of the respiratory muscles in both normals and patients. In normals, respiratory muscle function does not limit exercise tolerance; therefore, specific respiratory muscle training is unlikely to be of clinical benefit. In patients with COPD, the patient group most extensively studied, improvement in general exercise performance from ventilatory muscle training alone has not been demonstrated consistently.[19,47] Thus, the role of respiratory muscle training as a routine component of pulmonary rehabilitation has not been clearly established.

Psychosocial Support

An essential component of pulmonary rehabilitation is psychosocial support, the goal of which is to help patients combat symptoms reflective of progressive feelings of hopelessness and an inability to cope with chronic, progressive disease.[3,14,27] Depression is common in patients with chronic pulmonary disorders, as are anxiety (especially anxiety over dyspnea), denial, anger, and isolation. Patients become sedentary and dependent upon family members, friends, and medical services to provide

for their needs. Excessive concern over other physical problems and psychosomatic complaints arises. Sexual dysfunction and fear are common and represent often unspoken consequences of chronic lung disease. Patients may also demonstrate cognitive and neuropsychological dysfunction, possibly related to or exacerbated by the effects of hypoxemia on the brain.

Psychosocial support is provided best by a warm and enthusiastic staff who can communicate effectively with patients and devote the time and effort necessary to understand and motivate them. Family members and significant others should be included in activities so that they can understand the disease and help the patient cope. Support groups are also effective. Patients with severe psychological disorders may benefit from individual counseling and therapy. Psychotropic drugs should generally be reserved for patients with more severe psychological dysfunction.

Because breathlessness is associated closely with fear and anxiety, techniques of relaxation training have been used successfully in pulmonary rehabilitation. In a controlled study of 10 patients with COPD, progressive muscle relaxation, a technique in which patients are taught to sequentially tense and then relax 16 different muscle groups, resulted in a greater reduction in dyspnea and anxiety in the experimental group than in the controls. Furthermore, the magnitude of the change in dyspnea was significantly correlated with the magnitude of the change in anxiety.[39]

RESULTS OF PULMONARY REHABILITATION

Several comprehensive reviews provide support and extensive references in substantiating the practices and expected results of pulmonary rehabilitation (Table 46-3).[3,11,21,27,40]

Randomized Clinical Trials

Three recently published, randomized clinical trials demonstrate important and significant benefits of pulmonary rehabilitation for

TABLE 46-3
Results of Pulmonary Rehabilitation

Decreases in:
  Medical resource utilization (e.g., hospitalizations, emergency room visits)
  Respiratory symptoms (e.g., breathlessness)
  Psychological symptoms (e.g., depression, fear)
Increases in:
  Quality of life
  Physical activity
    Exercise tolerance (endurance or maximal level of activities of daily living)
  Knowledge
  Independence
Return to work possible
No change in lung function
Possible prolonged survival

patients with COPD, including improvements in exercise performance, symptoms, and key elements of quality of life.

In a randomized clinical trial of rehabilitation versus education alone in 119 patients with COPD, a highly significant improvement in exercise endurance in the rehabilitation group was noted; the beneficial effect was maintained up to 18 months later (Fig. 46-1A).[41] The rehabilitation group also experienced a significant decrease in perceived symptoms of breathlessness (Fig. 46-1B) and muscle fatigue (Fig. 46-1C) during exercise as well as improvements in maximal exercise tolerance, reported breathlessness with daily activities, and self-efficacy with walking.

In two other randomized trials, short-term benefits of pulmonary rehabilitation over conventional treatment have also been reported. Significant improvement in exercise tolerance, dyspnea, and quality of life after 6 months was noted in a study in which 45 patients, who received 8 weeks of inpatient pulmonary rehabilitation followed by 16 weeks of supervised outpatient care, were compared with 44 patients who received conventional care from their own physicians.[18] Similarly, in another investigation in which 28 patients who were randomly allocated to a home pulmonary rehabilitation program for 12 weeks were compared to 15 patients who received no rehabilitation, significant improvements in exercise tolerance and quality of life were reported.[51]

Hospitalizations and Medical Resources

Pulmonary rehabilitation has been shown to produce cost-effective benefits for patients with chronic lung disease. Several studies have analyzed hospital and medical resource utilization before and after rehabilitation. Given the high cost of hospitalization for acute care for these often sick patients, the potential savings from a reduction in inpatient days alone is significant. In one study, an average decrease of 20 hospital days per year from pulmonary rehabilitation was described;[27] in another, a 38 percent reduction in hospital days from the previous year was noted among 85 patients with COPD 1 year after rehabilitation.[35]

Several reports have examined longer-term results of pulmonary rehabilitation. In one study of hospitalization rates following rehabilitation for COPD, for 44 of 64 patients alive 4 years following initiation of the program, hospital days were reduced from 529 days in the year prior to the program to 145, 270, 278, and 207 days in years 1, 2, 3, and 4, respectively.[22] The benefit was most striking in the 14 patients hospitalized during the year prior to the program; hospital days in this group decreased from an average of 38 to 10 days per patient.

In another study of 96 patients with severe COPD (mean FEV_1, 0.87 L), a 55 percent decrease in hospital days was noted in the year following institution of the program;[23] in a follow-up study of 193 patients with COPD who underwent pulmonary rehabilitation, the estimated reduction in hospital days was 21 days per surviving patient per year.[24] Finally, for 80 patients with COPD, an average reduction from 19 to 6 hospital days was noted following the first year of a rehabilitation program. The improvement was maintained for 8 years of follow-up.[21]

Quality of Life

After rehabilitation, improvements have been noted in several aspects of quality of life, including respiratory and psychological symptoms, exercise tolerance, and social activity. Several quality-of-life instruments that incorporate aspects of physical, emotional, and psychological function into one or a small number of measures have been used increasingly in the evaluation of patients with chronic lung diseases.

A disease-specific measure that has been used frequently for patients with chronic lung diseases is the Chronic Respiratory

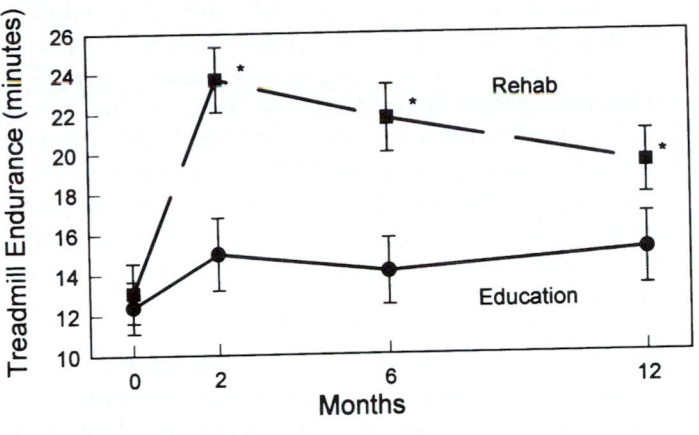

A

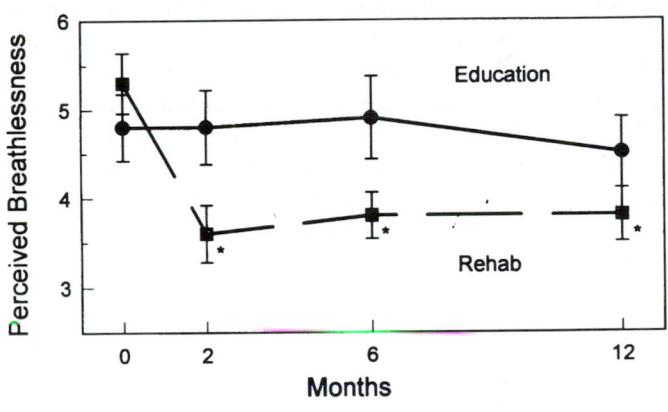

B

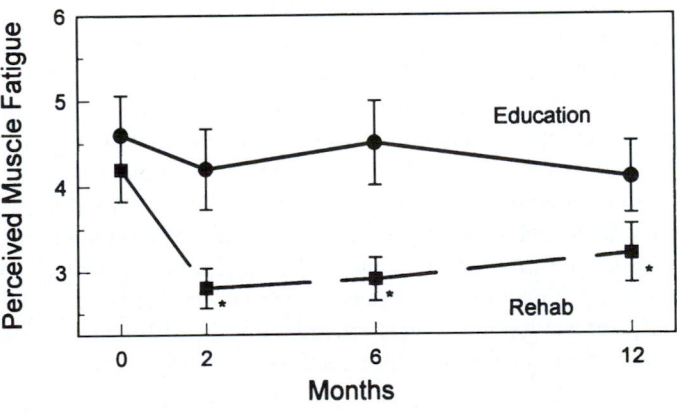

C

FIGURE 46-1 Benefits of comprehensive pulmonary rehabilitation (Rehab) versus education program (Education) in 119 subjects with COPD. Significant increases in treadmill exercise endurance (*A*) and corresponding decreases in ratings of perceived breathlessness (*B*) and muscle fatigue (*C*) were observed for up to 12 months of follow-up. (*From Ries et al,[41] with permission.*)

Questionnaire (CRQ).[20] In studies utilizing this questionnaire, long-term improvements in all four measured dimensions of quality of life—dyspnea, fatigue, emotional function, and mastery—have been reported following a program of multidisciplinary pulmonary rehabilitation.[20,38]

Another reliable, valid, disease-specific measure of health-related quality of life is the St. George's Respiratory Questionnaire (SGRQ).[25] This self-administered questionnaire contains 76 items. A completed questionnaire permits calculation of a composite score which, in turn, includes three component scores: symptoms, activity, and impacts on daily life. Good correlation appears to exist between changes in the SGRQ and changes in measures of severity of COPD, including spirometry, 6-min walk distance, anxiety, depression, dyspnea, and the Sickness Impact Profile.[25]

The Quality of Well-Being Scale (QWB) is a comprehensive measure of health-related quality of life shown to have validity as an outcome measure for evaluating interventions that affect general health status.[26] Using the QWB, investigators have demonstrated that in a randomized, controlled trial of behavioral intervention on exercise in patients with COPD, greater changes are observed in the interventions groups than in controls; furthermore, the treatment appears to be cost-effective.[4] However, in another randomized trial of pulmonary rehabilitation in patients with COPD, no significant changes were observed in the QWB, despite marked improvements in exercise tolerance and breathlessness following rehabilitation.[41]

Another general health measure, the Rand Health Survey instrument (equivalent to the SF-36), which was developed as part of the Medical Outcomes Study, includes 36 items which can be combined into eight dimensions of health status.[50] This instrument has only recently begun to be used in studies of pulmonary rehabilitation.

Exercise

Exercise plays an important and well-established role in pulmonary rehabilitation, producing both physiological and psychological benefits.[6,11,40] Review of 37 published studies of exercise training in more than 900 patients with COPD[11] indicates that, almost uniformly, pulmonary rehabilitation results in improvement in exercise endurance or maximal exercise tolerance.

Several controlled trials of exercise training, including three recently published randomized clinical trials of rehabilitation that included exercise as a central component,[18,41,51] support the beneficial effects of exercise in patients with chronic lung disease. In the largest clinical trial to date comparing rehabilitation with an education program as control, Ries and coworkers reported highly significant improvements in exercise endurance and maximal exercise tolerance after rehabilitation in 119 patients with COPD; the effects were maintained for up to 18 months.[41]

Pulmonary Function and Symptoms

Pulmonary rehabilitation does not result in any consistent changes in lung function in chronic lung disease if the patient is on a good medical regimen prior to beginning the program. Nevertheless, many patients report improvement in respiratory symptoms, particularly the troubling sensation of breathlessness. Decreased dyspnea has been reported consistently in experimental studies.[40,41] Improvement in psychological symptoms has also been demonstrated consistently after rehabilitation.[40]

Education

Pulmonary rehabilitation emphasizes educating patients, family members, and significant others to be actively involved in the patient's care, improving their understanding of disease, and learning practical ways of coping with disabling symptoms. Studies that have examined the effects of education in rehabilitation programs have shown that even patients with severe disease can learn to understand their disease better.[32,40] However, education alone typically does not lead to improved health status. Patients also require specific, individual strategies for changing behavior, along with encouragement, practice, and positive feedback.

Survival

Studies of the survival of patients with chronic lung disease after pulmonary rehabilitation have shown variable results. In a randomized trial with 6 years of follow-up, there was no statistically significant difference in survival between rehabilitation and education groups, although there was a nonsignificant trend of improved survival in the rehabilitation subjects (67 versus 56 percent survival).[41]

PULMONARY REHABILITATION AND LUNG SURGERY

Pulmonary rehabilitation has been applied primarily as part of the medical management of patients with stable, chronic pulmonary disease. In recent years, surgical options for patients with severe, disabling lung disease have been used more frequently. Lung surgery in these patients represents new challenges and may further compromise already reduced lung function. The use of pulmonary rehabilitation in preparing the patient for surgery or in the postsurgery recovery phase has been found to be a valuable adjunct.

Lung Transplantation

Pulmonary rehabilitation is recommended and used commonly in both the preoperative and postoperative phases of lung transplantation programs.[7,13] Although the general strategies of rehabilitation may be similar, the individual and program goals and specific program components differ.

Pretransplant Rehabilitation

Patients with advanced lung disease who are candidates for lung transplantation are usually initially evaluated by the transplant team and then referred for pulmonary rehabilitation after their transplant candidacy is approved. Rehabilitation staff evaluate the patient to assess needs and plan an appropriate program that can be maintained throughout a waiting period which may last months to years. Since these patients have advanced disease with limited life expectancy, the goals in the preoperative period differ from those that typically apply to rehabilitation in chronic lung disease (Table 46-4).

TABLE 46-4

Goals of Pulmonary Rehabilitation in Lung Transplantation

Pretransplant

Maintain/increase mobility and exercise tolerance

Monitor disease progression

Prevent complications

Provide education about:

Underlying disease

Transplantation procedures

Self-care and self-assessment

Provide psychosocial support during waiting period for patients and families

Posttransplant

Improve physical work tolerance

Monitor clinical status/assess symptoms and oxygenation

Prevent complications

Reinforce self-care and self-assessment

Encourage compliance with medical regimen

Provide psychosocial support for adaptation to new demands and expectations

---

The overall goals of pulmonary rehabilitation in the pretransplant setting are to maintain function, monitor disease progression, prevent complications, provide education about the underlying lung disease and lung transplantation, and offer psychosocial support for patients and families in coping with the stresses of waiting for a potentially lifesaving procedure.

The exercise training program may be similar to that provided to other chronic lung disease patients with the exception that patients with primary pulmonary vascular diseases do not typically participate in exercise or other physical activities because of the increased risk of sudden death. Although patients may have some initial improvement in exercise tolerance or endurance as they begin rehabilitation, the primary goal for these patients with advanced, progressive lung disease is to maintain mobility and exercise capacity. Exercise sessions also provide an excellent means to monitor disease progression and to detect, at an earlier stage, problems that commonly occur (e.g., increased breathlessness or reduced arterial oxygenation with exercise).

The goals of education in the pretransplant period are to teach patients about their underlying lung disease, the transplant procedure itself, and expectations following transplantation. Patients can also be taught techniques for self-care and self-assessment that will be useful before and after surgery.

The psychosocial stresses of waiting for transplantation are considerable. Many patients feel as though their lives were "on hold." Some may have moved away from family and their usual social support network to live close to the transplant center. Providing support for patients and family members during this time, whether through formal group support sessions or informal contact with supportive staff and other patients, helps patients cope better with these problems.

Posttransplant Rehabilitation

After undergoing lung transplantation, patients must learn to cope with a new level of function, new expectations, and a new set of problems. Rehabilitation for patients in this phase can facilitate physical reconditioning, help implement self-care and assessment techniques, and facilitate coping with the psychosocial adaptations to a new life-style.

Goals of exercise training after rehabilitation are improved physical work tolerance and continued assessment of symptoms and oxygenation as early warning signs of complications, including rejection and infection. Educational goals are focused on self-care and assessment and the importance of compliance with a new medical regimen. Psychosocial support can assist with adaptation to a new set of stresses related to additional demands and expectations that patients have of themselves and their significant others. Patients who are used to being sick, disabled, and cared for by others may now be expected to be well, to be independent, to return to work, and to provide support for others.

Volume Reduction Lung Surgery

Recently, there has been a resurgence of interest in volume reduction lung surgery for treatment of patients with severe emphysematous obstructive lung disease (see Chapter 44). Pulmonary rehabilitation has been recommended as an important modality in evaluating patients and preparing them for this procedure. In addition, rehabilitation has been employed in the postoperative recovery phase. Since these patients have severe, disabling chronic lung disease, they are typically good candidates for pulmonary rehabilitation. Enrolling patients in rehabilitation prior to surgery has several advantages: (1) optimizing functional status, (2) improving physical and psychological symptoms, (3) helping patients to learn more about their disease and alternative treatment options, and (4) improving patient skills for coping and actively co-managing their disease. Patients can then make informed decisions about surgical treatment, based upon their optimal level of baseline function.

Just as in the posttransplant period, rehabilitation following volume reduction surgery helps patients to adapt to new levels of function and to reassess symptoms and needs for supplemental oxygen.

Although it is promising, to date there has been little published experience with volume reduction lung surgery. As practitioners gain more experience, the expertise of pulmonary rehabilitation professionals in assessing patients and evaluating health outcomes will be useful in developing guidelines for appropriate patient selection and determining the ultimate usefulness of this procedure.

Rehabilitation after Lung Resection

Patients who undergo pulmonary resection frequently experience a significant increase in symptoms and reduction in functional status. This is particularly true for patients with underlying chronic lung disease. Most commonly, surgery is used in treatment of patients with thoracic neoplasms who are deemed to have resectable disease and are operative candidates. Following resection, these patients with already limited lung function have to learn to adapt to a new, lower level of function.

Similar changes may be observed in patients who undergo radiation therapy. Patients who are in a stable phase of their treatment or who are in remission may be appropriate candidates for pulmonary rehabilitation. Improvement in health status, physical and psychological symptoms, exercise tolerance, and quality of life—as well as reduction in health care burdens—are potential benefits. These patients' survival may be as limited by their underlying lung disease as by their treated malignancy.

SUMMARY AND FUTURE OF PULMONARY REHABILITATION

Pulmonary rehabilitation has been well established as a means of improving functional status and reducing the disability and economic burden of the growing number of patients with chronic lung diseases. In adopting a broad rehabilitation medicine perspective, such programs provide interdisciplinary expertise directed toward the needs of the individual disabled patient.

Much of the experience in pulmonary rehabilitation has been with patients who have COPD. However, it is clear that similar benefits can result for patients with other disabling pulmonary conditions. Pulmonary rehabilitation may also play an important role in the preoperative evaluation, preparation, and postoperative recovery of patients undergoing surgical procedures, including lung transplantation, volume reduction lung surgery, and lung resection.

REFERENCES

1. American Association of Cardiovascular and Pulmonary Rehabilitation: *Guidelines for Pulmonary Rehabilitation Programs.* Champaign, IL, Human Kinetics, 1993.
2. American Thoracic Society: Pulmonary rehabilitation. *Am Rev Respir Dis* 124:663–666, 1981.
3. American Thoracic Society: Standards for the diagnosis and care of patients with chronic obstructive pulmonary disease (COPD) and asthma. *Am Rev Respir Dis* 152:S78–S121, 1995.
4. Atkins CJ, Kaplan RM, Timms RM, et al: Behavioral exercise programs in the management of chronic obstructive pulmonary disease. *J Consult Clin Psychol* 52:591–603, 1984.
5. Barach AL: Breathing exercises in pulmonary emphysema and allied chronic respiratory disease. *Arch Phys Med Rehabil* 36:379–390, 1955.
6. Belman MJ: Exercise in patients with chronic obstructive pulmonary disease. *Thorax* 48:936–946, 1993.
7. Biggar D, Malen J, Trulock E, Cooper J: Pulmonary rehabilitation before and after lung transplantation, in Casaburi R, Petty T (eds): *Principles and Practice of Pulmonary Rehabilitation.* Philadelphia, Saunders, 1993, pp 459–467.
8. Borg GAV: Psychophysical bases of perceived exertion. *Med Sci Sports Exerc* 14:377–381, 1982.
9. Campbell EJM, Friend J: Action of breathing exercises in pulmonary emphysema. *Lancet* 268:325–329, 1955.
10. Carter R, Nicotra B, Clark L, et al: Exercise conditioning in the rehabilitation of patients with chronic obstructive pulmonary disease. *Arch Phys Med Rehabil* 69:118–122, 1988.
11. Casaburi R, Petty T: *Principles and Practice of Pulmonary Rehabilitation.* Philadelphia, Saunders, 1993.
12. Celli BR, Rassulo J, Make BJ: Dyssynchronous breathing during

arm but not leg exercise in patients with chronic airflow obstruction. *New Engl J Med* 314:1485–1490, 1986.
13. Craven JL, Bright J, Dear CL: Psychiatric, psychosocial, and rehabilitative aspects of lung transplantation. *Clin Chest Med* 11:247–257, 1990.
14. Dudley D, Glaser E, Jorgenson B: Psychosocial concomitants to rehabilitation in chronic obstructive pulmonary disease: Part 1. Psychosocial and psychological considerations; Part 2. Psychosocial treatment; Part 3. Dealing with psychiatric disease (as distinguished from psychosocial or psychophysiologic problems). *Chest* 77:413–420, 544–551, 677–684, 1980.
15. Ellis B, Ries A: Upper extremity exercise training in pulmonary rehabilitation. *J Cardiopulm Rehabil* 11:227–231, 1991.
16. Fishman A: Pulmonary rehabilitation research. *Am J Respir Crit Care Med* 149:825–833, 1994.
17. Foster S, Thomas HM: Pulmonary rehabilitation in lung disease other than chronic obstructive pulmonary disease. *Am Rev Respir Dis* 141:601–604, 1990.
18. Goldstein R, Gort E, Avendano M, Guyatt G: Randomized controlled trial of respiratory rehabilitation. *Lancet* 344:1394–1397, 1994.
19. Guyatt G, Keller J, Singer J, et al: Controlled trial of respiratory muscle training in chronic airflow limitation. *Thorax* 47:598–602, 1992.
20. Guyatt G, Berman L, Townsend M, et al: A measure of quality of life for clinical trials in chronic lung disease. *Thorax* 42:773–778, 1987.
21. Hodgkin JE, Connors GL, Bell CW: *Pulmonary Rehabilitation Guidelines to Success,* 2d ed. Philadelphia, Lippincott, 1993.
22. Hudson LD, Tyler ML, Petty TL: Hospitalization needs during an outpatient rehabilitation program for severe chronic airway obstruction. *Chest* 70:606–610, 1976.
23. Johnson HR, Tanzi F, Balchum OJ, et al: Inpatient comprehensive pulmonary rehabilitation in severe COPD. *Respir Ther* May/June: 15–19, 1980.
24. Johnson N, DeFlorio G, Einstein H: Cost/benefit outcomes of pulmonary rehabilitation in severe COPD. *Am Rev Respir Dis* 127: A111, 1983.
25. Jones P, Quirk F, Baveystock C, Littlejohns P: A self-complete measure of health status for chronic airflow limitation. *Am Rev Respir Dis* 145:1321–1327, 1992.
26. Kaplan RM, Anderson JP: Quality of life: Assessment and application, in Walker SR and Rosser RM: *The Quality of Well-Being Scale: Rationale for a Single Quality of Life Index.* London, MTP Press, 1988, pp 51–77.
27. Lertzman MM, Cherniack RM: Rehabilitation of patients with chronic obstructive pulmonary disease. *Am Rev Respir Dis* 114: 1145–1165, 1976.
28. Mahler D: The measurements of dyspnea during exercise in patients with lung disease. *Chest* 101:242S–247S, 1992.
29. McSweeney AJ, Grant I (eds): *Chronic Obstructive Pulmonary Disease: A Behavioral Perspective.* New York, Marcel Dekker, 1988, pp 39–57.
30. Medical Research Council Working Party: Long-term domiciliary oxygen therapy in chronic hypoxic cor pulmonale complicating chronic bronchitis and emphysema. *Lancet* 1:681–686, 1981.
31. Miller WF: Physical therapeutic measures in the treatment of chronic bronchopulmonary disorders: Methods for breathing training. *Am J Med* 24:929–940, 1958.
32. Neish CM, Hopp JW: The role of education in pulmonary rehabilitation. *J Cardiopulm Rehabil* 11:439–441, 1988.
33. Niederman MS, Clemente PH, Fein AM, et al: Benefits of a multidisciplinary pulmonary rehabilitation program: Improvements are independent of lung function. *Chest* 99:798–804, 1991.

34. Nocturnal Oxygen Therapy Trial Group: Continuous or nocturnal oxygen therapy in hypoxemic chronic obstructive lung disease: A clinical trial. *Ann Intern Med* 93:391–398, 1980.

35. Petty TL, Nett LM, Finigan MM, et al: A comprehensive care program for chronic airway obstruction: Methods and preliminary evaluation of symptomatic and functional improvement. *Ann Intern Med* 70:1109–1120, 1969.

36. Pierson DJ: Drugs used in respiratory care, in Pierson DJ, Kacmarek RM (eds): *Foundations of Respiratory Care.* New York, Churchill Livingstone, 1992, pp 175–193.

37. Punzal P, Ries A, Kaplan R: Maximum intensity exercise training in patients with chronic obstructive pulmonary disease. *Chest* 100: 618–623, 1991.

38. Reardon J, Patel K, ZuWallack R: Improvement in quality of life is unrelated to improvement in exercise endurance after outpatient pulmonary rehabilitation. *J Cardiopulm Rehabil* 13:51–54, 1993.

39. Renfroe KL: Effect of progressive relaxation on dyspnea and state anxiety in patients with chronic obstructive pulmonary disease. *Heart Lung* 17:408–413, 1988.

40. Ries AL: Position paper of the American Association of Cardiovascular and Pulmonary Rehabilitation: Scientific basis of pulmonary rehabilitation. *J Cardiopulm Rehabil* 10:418–441, 1990.

41. Ries AL, Kaplan RM, Limberg TM, Prewitt LM: Effects of pulmonary rehabilitation on physiologic and psychosocial outcomes in patients with chronic obstructive pulmonary disease. *Ann Intern Med* 122:823–832, 1995.

42. Ries AL, Moser KM, Sassi-Dambron DE, et al: *Shortness of Breath: A Guide to Better Living and Breathing,* 5th ed. St. Louis, Mosby–Year Book, 1995.

43. Ries A: The role of exercise testing in pulmonary diagnosis. *Clin Chest Med* 8:81–89, 1987.

44. Ries A, Farrow J, Clausen J: Pulmonary function tests cannot predict exercise-induced hypoxemia in chronic obstructive pulmonary disease. *Chest* 93:454–459, 1988.

45. Ries A: The importance of exercise in pulmonary rehabilitation. *Clin Chest Med* 15:327–337, 1994.

46. Rochester DF, Goldberg SK: Techniques of respiratory physical therapy. *Am Rev Respir Dis* 122(suppl):133–146, 1980.

47. Smith K, Cook D, Guyatt G, et al: Respiratory muscle training in chronic airflow limitation: A meta-analysis. *Am Rev Respir Dis* 145: 533–539, 1992.

48. Tiep BL, Lewis MI: Oxygen conservation and oxygen-conserving devices in chronic lung disease: A review. *Chest* 92:263–272, 1987.

49. Tiep B: Long-term home oxygen therapy. *Chest* 11:505–521, 1990.

50. Ware J, Sherbourne C: The MOS 36-item short form health survey (SF-36): I. Conceptual framework and item selection. *Med Care* 30: 473–483, 1992.

51. Wijkstra PJ, van Altena R, Kraan J, et al: Quality of life in patients with chronic obstructive pulmonary disease improves after rehabilitation at home. *Eur Respir J* 7:269–273, 1994.

CHAPTER 47

THE BIOLOGY OF ASTHMA

William W. Busse / David E. Parry

Asthma is characterized by intermittent airflow obstruction, airway inflammation, and bronchial hyperresponsiveness. This disorder affects an estimated 5 to 10 percent of the population, and as such is a major health-care issue in most countries. A precise definition of asthma remains elusive, partly because the cause of this disease has yet to be found. Moreover, it is entirely possible that asthma is not a distinct disease, with a discrete etiology, but rather a "syndrome" in which various precipitating factors result in similar clinical and pathologic manifestations. This approach to understanding asthma may explain its varied patterns and presentations, while explaining the common development of intermittent airflow obstruction, bronchial hyperresponsiveness, and inflammation.

Until recently, the focus on asthma definition, study, and treatment had emphasized the mechanisms of acute bronchospasm and the control of airway smooth muscle tone. With the exception of "severe asthma," the consideration of bronchial inflammation as an essential component of the disease had been largely neglected. However, the preponderance of investigations and information on the mechanisms of inflammation in asthma, as well as renewed therapeutic emphasis on "anti-inflammatory" medications, led to the current belief that airway bronchoconstriction, hyperresponsiveness, and inflammation are not mutually exclusive. Rather, acute and chronic inflammation, including airway edema and mucus secretion, are important, if not central, to the airflow obstruction and overall "reactivity" of the airways in asthma. Further, it has been recognized that although asthma covers a wide spectrum of clinical severity, inflammatory changes may be seen in the airways of even asymptomatic asthmatics. This chapter will detail our understanding of the mechanisms of acute and chronic inflammation in the asthmatic airway. We shall focus on the cellular components of the asthmatic inflammatory response and elucidate how the properties of these cells, and the mediators they produce, contribute to the pathophysiology of asthma.

MEDIATORS AND AIRWAY CELLS IN THE BIOLOGY OF ASTHMA

The inflammatory response in the asthmatic airway is extremely complex. It is characterized by varying degrees of mononuclear cell and eosinophil infiltration, epithelial desquamation, mucus hypersecretion (and airway plugging), smooth muscle hyperplasia, and airway remodeling with subepithelial fibrosis.[16,32] Studies of this response have implicated a multitude of cells in its generation. Similarly, a wide variety of mediators and cytokines are dysregulated at sites of asthmatic inflammation, suggesting that these moieties may play a role in the pathogenesis of the asthmatic diathesis. These cells and mediators are reviewed below.

Cytokines

Cytokines participate in the cell-to-cell communications essential to growth, development, and function. They are low-molecular-weight protein molecules that are produced and secreted by virtually all nucleated cells. Cytokines regulate inflammation and the immune response. They are generally categorized as *interleukins* (more than 20 reported thus far), *interferons, tumor necrosis factors, transforming growth factors, colony-stimulating factors,* or *chemokines,* with the recognition that the respective descriptive names do not preclude particular cytokines from having many and varied potential actions and functions. Cytokine secretion is usually a brief, self-limited event. It may, however, require new mRNA and protein synthesis, which takes place over a matter of hours rather than seconds or minutes. Furthermore, the effects of cytokines, which generally act locally, in an autocrine or paracrine fashion, are often redundant or different, depending on the particular cellular microenvironment. Cytokines may induce the expression of receptors on the producing cell or neighboring cells, which may result in a change in the responsiveness of both the secreting cell and target cells. A variety and range of cytokines have been implicated in the regulation of airway inflammation and thus in the pathogenesis of asthma. Support for each is obtained by the detection of cytokines in the airways of patients with chronic asthma, particularly in lavage fluid after airway allergen challenge, and/or by in situ hybridization of retrieved cells or biopsy materials. Of the cytokines identified, several are linked closely with allergic inflammation in asthma.

PRINCIPAL CYTOKINES IMPLICATED IN ASTHMA PATHOGENESIS

Interleukin-1β (IL-1β) is produced by macrophages and monocytes and activates airway epithelial cells to produce *granulocyte-macrophage colony–stimulating factor* (GM-CSF) and *regulated on activation normal T cell expressed and secreted* (RANTES), chemokines that recruit eosinophils to the airways. IL-1β also increases endothelial cell adhesion protein expression, which enhances inflammatory cell migration into the airways. IL-3 and IL-5 from mast cells and T lymphocytes, along with GM-CSF, promote eosinophil recruitment, activation, and survival, perpetuating eosinophilic inflammation in asthma.

Like IL-3 and IL-5, IL-4 is produced by a lymphocyte subset (T helper [TH]$_2$–like cells) and mast cells. IL-4 is a critical early signal for B lymphocyte switching to IgE synthesis, which is important in allergic inflammation. IL-4 also promotes mast cell survival and increases adhesion molecule (vascular cell adhesion molecule–1, or VCAM-1) expression on endothelium. This endothelial event contributes to the recruitment of inflammatory cells, particularly eosinophils, to the airways. Last, IL-4 plays a crucial role in the development of TH$_2$ lymphocytes, which are increasingly appreciated to play a regulatory role in asthmatic inflammation (see below).

Tumor necrosis factor–α (TNF-α) is synthesized by macrophages, mast cells, and epithelial cells and increases the expression of the adhesion molecules intercellular adhesion molecule–1 (ICAM-1) and VCAM-1, in addition to promoting GM-CSF production by epithelial cells.

Interferon-γ (IFN-γ) is produced by TH$_1$ cells and inhibits the formation and function of TH$_2$ cells. Since TH$_2$ cells produce IL-3, IL-4, IL-5, and GM-CSF, which have been implicated in the asthmatic diathesis, this inhibition can potentially decrease the asthmogenic activities of these cytokines. However, IFN-γ can also activate epithelial cells to release cytokines, promote eosinophil survival, and increase ICAM-1 expression, all of which are proinflammatory, potentially asthmogenic effects.

The overall effect of the complex cytokine network in the airway depends on a number of factors, including the relative abundance of the various cytokines, their ability to recruit and perpetuate the actions of inflammatory cells such as eosinophils and lymphocytes, and their ability to amplify inflammation by interacting with structural cells such as fibroblasts, endothelial cells, and epithelial cells. There is no question, however, that cytokines are key mediators in the pathogenesis of the chronic inflammation characteristic of asthma.

Mast Cells

Mast cells, like basophils and other cells that circulate through the blood, are derived from a pluripotent bone marrow progenitor cell. Basophils are derived from the myeloid lineage, whereas nonmyeloid precursors are the source of mast cells. Mast cells, unlike basophils, leave the bone marrow as immature, undifferentiated cells and are eventually seen as two distinguishable types in tissue. A bone marrow–associated cytokine, stem cell factor, as well as IL-3, influences both the initial development and the phenotypic modulation of mast cells.[27] Furthermore, local factors in mucosal and connective tissues contribute to the maturation and differentiation of mast cells. Originally, two types of mast cells were found in rodents. The cell subtypes were based primarily on their tissue location and biochemical characteristics: mucosal mast cells (atypical) and connective-tissue mast cells (typical). In humans, a similar differentiation can be made, with the currently preferred nomenclature referring to the distinct neutral protease compositions of the two types of mast cells. MC$_T$ refers to mast cells containing the neutral protease tryptase alone, while MC$_{TC}$ denotes mast cells containing chymase in addition to tryptase and the other neutral proteases, carboxypeptidase and cathepsin G–like proteins (Table 47-1).

Mast cells can be identified in essentially all vascularized tissues of the body, with major concentrations found in the skin and mucosal surfaces of the respiratory and gastrointestinal tracts. Although one type of mast cell may be predominant in any given tissue, the relative abundance may change with tissue damage or inflammation. MC$_{TC}$ predominate in the skin and in the submucosa of the small intestine, while MC$_T$ are found in histologically normal small intestinal mucosa. In the normal human lung, alveoli-associated mast cells are almost exclusively of the MC$_T$ type, which also predominate in the subepithelium

TABLE 47-1

Human Mast Cell Characteristics

	MCT_T	MC_{TC}
Neutral proteases	Tryptase	Tryptase
		Chymase
		Carboxypeptidase
		Cathepsin G–like protein
Predominant location	Bronchi/bronchioles	Skin
	Intestinal mucosa	Small-intestinal submucosa
	Nasal epithelium	

of the bronchi and bronchioles. Although mast cells are found throughout the lung, they tend to associate most closely with endothelial and epithelial cell layers.

Mast cells and basophils are important effector cells in allergic diseases. For many years, mast cells have been thought to play a central role in the pathogenesis of asthma in both allergic and nonallergic patients. The evidence for this, as for the other cells and mediators we discuss in this chapter, is largely circumstantial, as the precise connections between these cells and molecules have yet to be elucidated.

MAST CELL PRODUCTS

A variety of mediators are associated with mast cells and may have a role in the pathogenesis of asthma (Fig. 47-1). These mediators are either preformed molecules, found within mast cell granules (histamine, neutral proteases, and proteoglycans) or newly generated molecules (prostaglandins, leukotrienes, and cytokines). Histamine is primarily a product of synthesis from histidine in the Golgi apparatus of mast cells and basophils, and it is secreted spontaneously at low levels by these cells. As a preformed mediator, released on activation of mast cells primarily through IgE-receptor interaction, histamine has direct vasoactive and smooth muscle spasmogenic effects. The half-life of histamine is short, and its effects are localized primarily to the sites of release, such as the skin or airways of susceptible subjects,

although elevated plasma or urine histamine levels can be found in anaphylaxis and within minutes after allergen inhalation in atopic asthmatics. Even though inhaled histamine is a potent inducer of bronchoconstriction in asthmatics, histamine antagonists have been remarkably unsuccessful in alleviating either acute or chronic symptoms of asthma, implying that other mediators are also important in asthma pathogenesis.

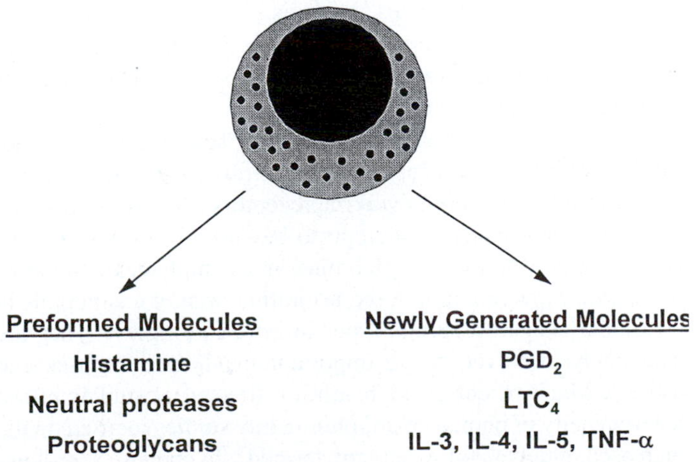

As the term implies, neutral proteases are enzymes that catalyze peptide bond cleavage best at neutral pH. Nearly half of the entire mast cell protein content may be tryptase, which is a helpful marker for human mast cells and is released along with histamine during mast cell degranulation. The enzymatically active tryptase is stored in secretory granules and stabilized by heparin. Although proof of a specific role for tryptase in the pathogenesis of asthma remains elusive, in vitro studies indicate that tryptase increases airway smooth muscle responsiveness to histamine.[47] Recently, tryptase has been identified as a potent growth factor for epithelial cells and inducer of IL-8 production.[7]

Unlike tryptase, which is found in both subtypes of human mast cells, chymase is a neutral protease confined to the MC_{TC} subset found prominently in skin and intestinal submucosa. Chymase has been implicated as a potent enhancer of glandular mucus secretion in airways.[48] Both tryptase and chymase degrade neuropeptides, such as vasoactive intestinal peptide (VIP), a molecule that may be active in bronchial smooth muscle relaxation.[50]

The metachromatic staining by basic dyes of the secretory granules of human mast cells is due to the presence of sulfated proteoglycans, which, in humans, are heparin and chondroitin sulfate E. Heparin is found selectively concentrated in all human mast cells. Another proteoglycan, chondroitin sulfate A, is found in human basophils. Heparin helps stabilize intracellular tryptase. Chondroitin sulfate E is less effective in this manner. Endogenous proteoglycans may be important in regulating enzyme function[45] and modulating matrix protein–cell adhesion properties.

Arachidonic acid metabolites, prostaglandins and leukotrienes, are produced by various inflammatory cell types, including mast cells. Arachidonic acid is found in intracellular lipid stores incorporated with neutral lipids and phospholipids. Hydrolysis of these membrane-bound molecules by lipases results in free arachidonate, which can then proceed down one of two main enzymatic pathways. The cyclooxygenase pathway yields prostaglandins and thromboxanes, while the lipoxygenase route leads to production of leukotrienes (Fig. 47-2).

Prostaglandin D_2 (PGD_2) is formed by mast cells following IgE receptor stimulation. Elevated levels of PGD_2 have been found in bronchoalveolar lavage (BAL) fluid after airway antigen challenge.[35] PGD_2 and its metabolites have very potent bronchospastic activity[23] and potentiate airway hyperresponsiveness to inhaled histamine and methacholine.[19]

Leukotriene B_4 (LTB_4) is a precursor to the sulfidopeptide or cysteinyl leukotrienes LTC_4, LTD_4, and LTE_4. Leukotrienes cause vascular permeability, smooth muscle constriction, and

Preformed Molecules

Histamine

Neutral proteases

Proteoglycans

Newly Generated Molecules

PGD_2

LTC_4

IL-3, IL-4, IL-5, TNF-α

FIGURE 47-1   Mast cell mediators.

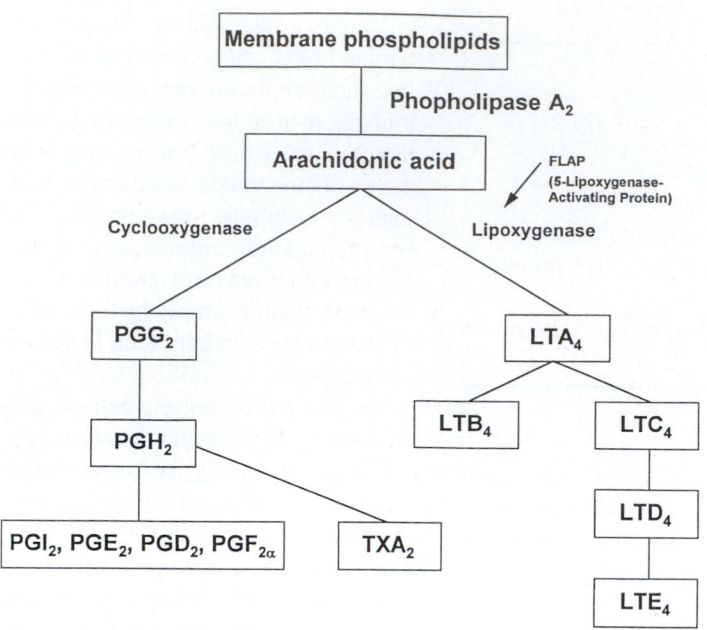

FIGURE 47-2 Pathways in the formation of prostaglandins, thromboxanes, and leukotrienes.

bronchial mucus secretion. LTB_4, along with the sulfidopeptide leukotrienes, is thought to increase airway mucus production. LTC_4, which is produced by eosinophils, basophils, and monocytes in addition to mast cells, increases the adhesiveness of leukocytes to endothelial cells. Both leukotriene production and receptor antagonists have shown some therapeutic promise in early studies in asthma patients. These observations suggest that these mediators have a role in the pathogenesis of asthma.

MAST CELLS IN ASTHMA

To establish the involvement of mast cells in asthma, studies of isolated cells, bronchial biopsies, and BAL fluid have been performed and, when possible, correlated with pulmonary physiology. The cellular studies have demonstrated that mast cell activation can occur either through the cross-linking of high-affinity IgE receptors on the cell surface or the interaction of other stimuli (such as the neuropeptide substance P) with the mast cell membrane. Each results in mast cell degranulation, with the generation and release of vasoactive, inflammatory, and smooth muscle active mediators including histamine, leukotrienes, prostaglandins, and the cytokines TNF-α, IL-3, IL-4, and IL-5. BAL fluid samples have generally, although not consistently, shown increases in mast cell numbers in asthma. In contrast to the airways of normal individuals, however, partly degranulated mast cells have been found in BAL fluid samples and the bronchial lamina propria from the airways of even asymptomatic asthma patients, indicating ongoing mast cell activation.

Additional insights into the kinetics and importance of mast cell mediators have been obtained from measurements of the levels of BAL histamine and tryptase (a fairly specific marker of mast cell activation). These studies have demonstrated that mast cell activation is an early event, with elevated BAL histamine and tryptase levels being seen 12 min after endobronchial

antigen challenge and the levels of tryptase returning to normal by 48 h. The levels of histamine remain elevated after 48 h, raising the possibility that non–mast cells (for example, basophils) are activated and produce histamine at these later points.[46]

Measurements of BAL histamine and tryptase before and after endobronchial allergen challenge in allergic and nonallergic patients with and without asthma have also provided interesting information.[54] These studies demonstrated similar baseline histamine levels in all groups, with elevated levels after allergen challenge in both asthmatic and nonasthmatic allergic patients. Of the four study groups, allergic asthmatic subjects had only moderately elevated levels of tryptase at baseline but the highest concentration of tryptase after antigen challenge. Others have demonstrated a higher level of spontaneous histamine release from BAL mast cells of asthmatics, which also suggests that mast cells are active in chronic asthma. The potential importance of mast cell mediators in the generation of the physiological abnormalities characteristic of asthma can also be appreciated from the correlations that have been noted between the levels of bronchial hyperresponsiveness and elevated levels of BAL mast cell mediators and cytokines (IL-3, IL-4, GM-CSF).[46] These cytokines may also contribute to the generation of chronic airway inflammation, with IL-3 and GM-CSF stimulating eosinophil recruitment and activation and IL-4 stimulating IgE synthesis and TH2 lymphocyte proliferation and development.

Eosinophils

Eosinophils and basophils derive from a common progenitor cell in the bone marrow. Cytokines such as IL-3, GM-CSF, and IL-5 are intimately involved in the stimulation of eosinophil production, growth, and maturation. IL-5 is particularly important in the development and terminal differentiation of eosinophils. Eosinophils enter the circulation from the bone marrow as mature, differentiated cells. From the circulation, eosinophils migrate into body tissues. Normally, there are an estimated hundredfold more eosinophils in tissues than in the circulation. Under normal conditions, however, eosinophils are rarely found in the lungs and skin. The transmigration of eosinophils from the blood into tissues is a complex process that entails the adherence of eosinophils to blood vessel endothelial cells by the interaction of adhesion molecules, such as VCAM-1, found on endothelial cell surfaces, and eosinophil cell surface ligands such as very late antigen–4 (VLA-4).[44] This process will be discussed in more detail later.

Eosinophils have a variety of cell surface receptors, including low-affinity IgE receptors (in contrast to the high-affinity mast cell IgE receptors), cytokine receptors such as the IL-5 receptor (IL-5R), which is thought to be specific for eosinophils, and receptors for immunoglobulins and complement. Some of these molecules function in the primordial role of eosinophils in host defense against certain types of infectious agents. They are also likely, however, to be important in allergic diseases and asthma. Much recent effort has been directed at studies of the heterogeneity of human eosinophils. Early studies focused on the increased numbers of what are termed "hypodense," or low-density, eosinophils, which were identified variably in the blood of patients with eosinophilia-associated diseases, including allergy. Our current understanding of eosinophil heterogeneity focuses on functional differences between circulating and airway eosinophils. Compared to circulating eosinophils, airway eosinophils have increased functional activity, including increased surface receptor expression, degranulation with the release of the mediators discussed below, and increased cytotoxicity. Furthermore, the activated-eosinophil products IL-3, IL-5, and GM-CSF enhance the recruitment of eosinophils to the airways, perpetuating eosinophilia in asthma.

EOSINOPHIL PRODUCTS

Eosinophils contain primary and secondary granules. The primary granules, seen principally in less mature eosinophils, house membrane-derived Charcot-Leyden crystal protein, whose major component is lysophospholipase. The secondary, or specific, granules contain four principal cationic proteins: major basic protein (MBP) in the dense core, along with the matrix proteins eosinophil cationic protein (ECP), eosinophil-derived neurotoxin (EDN), and eosinophil peroxidase (EPO) (Table 47-2). Most evidence suggests that the eosinophil is the primary if not sole source of MBP *synthesis,* even though MBP has also been found in basophils. MBP is the principal protein constituent of eosinophil granules. It is toxic for epithelial tissues, induces airway hyperresponsiveness, and—in contrast to ECP, EDN, and EPO—causes histamine release from basophils. ECP is more cytotoxic to respiratory epithelium than MBP and damages target cells by membrane pore formation. Its expression is a useful marker for eosinophil activation. EDN is not restricted to eosinophils and, as the name implies, damages myelinated neurons. EPO differs from neutrophil and monocyte myeloperoxidases. It decreases LTC_4 and LTD_4 degradation and causes histamine release from mast cells. Eosinophils also produce a variety of cytokines, including IL-4, IL-5, TNF, and GM-CSF. IL-5 and GM-CSF can further perpetuate airway eosinophilia, TNF-α can regulate eosinophil effector function, and IL-4 plays a key role in initiating IgE synthesis and TH_2 lymphocyte development.

EOSINOPHILS AND ASTHMA

Peripheral blood eosinophilia is a prominent feature of asthma. Autopsy airway samples from asthma patients, even those who died of nonasthma causes, and biopsies from asthmatics, even some with mild disease, also contain eosinophilic inflammatory cell infiltrates.[15,32] Similarly, eosinophils are prominent features of the BAL and tissue response after segmental antigen challenge.[3,14] Immunohistochemical studies have also demonstrated eosinophils and their granule products in the asthmatic airway, and elevated levels of ECP have been found in the BAL and sputum of asthmatics.[5,38,51] A number of lines of evidence speak to the importance of the eosinophil in the asthmatic process. Among the most striking is the positive correlation between the levels of blood and airway eosinophilia and the severity of asthma.[4,5]

The finding of eosinophils in the asthmatic airway is important because it is likely that eosinophils contribute, in a major way, to the pathogenesis of asthma. As noted above, eosinophil activation releases granule-derived proteins and cytokines. The precise stimuli for and mechanisms of eosinophil degranulation are not certain but are thought to involve immunoglobulin complexes, with enhancement of this process by IL-3, IL-5, and GM-CSF. The cationic proteins are cytotoxic for epithelial cells, and concentrations of ECP and MBP that can cause injury are actually present in asthmatic airways. The observation that asthmatic airways contain injured and sloughed airway epithelium, eosinophilia, and cytotoxic proteins led Reed to refer to asthma as "chronic desquamating eosinophilic bronchitis."[40] Cationic proteins also regulate the function of the airways. MBP enhances tracheal and bronchial smooth muscle contraction, reduces airway cell ciliary activity, induces bronchial hyperresponsiveness,[11] and may interrupt the anionic barrier normally present on the luminal side of the epithelium. Damage to airway epithelium may also expose sensory nerve endings, resulting in activation of neurogenic inflammatory peptides.[2,31]

In addition to cytokines and granule proteins, eosinophils produce important lipid mediators, including LTC_4, platelet-activating factor (PAF), and thromboxane A_2 (TXA_2). PAF can increase bronchial hyperresponsiveness and perpetuate airway eosinophilia, while the lipoxygenase pathway product TXA_2 is a short-lived yet potent airway smooth muscle constrictor. The importance to asthma of these and various other mediators derived from eosinophils has yet to be fully elucidated.

Neutrophils

Neutrophils are granulocytic cells of the bone marrow myeloid lineage that share only a very early precursor cell with eosinophils and basophils. The multilobed nucleus neutrophils, normally found in the bloodstream and tissues, are terminally differentiated cells that are notable morphologically

---

TABLE 47-2

Eosinophil Granules

Type of Granule	Protein Constituents	Properties
Primary	Charcot-Leyden crystal protein	Lysophospholipase
Secondary	Major basic protein (MBP)	Cytotoxic (epithelium)
		Promotes histamine release from mast cells and basophils
	Eosinophil cationic protein (ECP)	Cytotoxic (epithelium)
	Eosinophil-derived neurotoxin (EDN)	Damages myelinated neurons
	Eosinophil peroxidase (EPO)	Histamine release from mast cells

for their granules, whose synthesis and assembly occur only during early stages of neutrophil development. Primary (azurophilic) and secondary (specific) granules contain various microbial enzymes, neutral proteases, and acid hydrolases. Many of these molecules participate in the host defense function of neutrophils and are also potentially injurious to normal tissues, including airway epithelium. The primary granules contain neutrophil myeloperoxidase and lysozyme as well as hydrolases and proteinases, which are important in tissue penetration by neutrophils. Secondary granules also contain lysozyme and collagenases, which can potentially damage airway tissue.

NEUTROPHILS AND ASTHMA

The possible role of neutrophils in the pathogenesis of asthma remains to be established. IL-1, TNF-α, and GM-CSF are chemoattractants for neutrophils in vivo. However, airway specimens obtained from BAL, bronchoscopy, and lung biopsies usually fail to show a consistent pattern of neutrophilia in asthma. One exception is the finding of increased neutrophils in lung autopsy specimens from patients who died in sudden-onset status asthmaticus compared with fatal cases of slow-onset status asthmaticus, in which eosinophils predominate.[49] This represents a very small number of asthmatics. In addition, airway neutrophilia can be observed during nocturnal exacerbations of asthma, and increased numbers of neutrophils can be found in the BAL fluid of atopic asthmatics 4 h, but not 24 h, after inhaled allergen challenge.[33] However, neutrophils, in contrast to eosinophils, are natural residents of the lung, particularly lung parenchyma. Thus, their mere presence in asthma is far from conclusive evidence for their involvement in the disorder. Nonetheless, neutrophils contain or synthesize a number of molecules with the potential to damage airway tissue and, perhaps more importantly, to act as chemotactic factors or mediators for other inflammatory cells.

Upon activation, neutrophils release the contents of their granules, including a number of cationic proteins, which may damage airway epithelium in a manner similar to that discussed for eosinophils. Furthermore, neutrophils synthesize and release the arachidonic acid product LTB_4, a potent neutrophil chemoattractant that could perpetuate airway neutrophilia. Neutrophils also generate superoxide radicals, alone and in combination with nitrogen oxide anions, which can disrupt airway epithelial tissue. Perhaps the greatest potential role for neutrophils in asthma is in their contribution to the development of the late-phase reaction (LPR), so called because it represents an exacerbation of airway symptoms that begins after the immediate bronchoconstriction associated with inhaled allergen has subsided. The LPR, which has not been shown in all patients with asthma, generally begins 4 to 6 h after allergen challenge and resolves by 24 to 48 h.[29] Increased levels of serum neutrophil chemotactic activity correlate with the development of the LPR in asthma, and airway neutrophilia is found 24 to 48 h after bronchial allergen challenge. Thus, neutrophils have the ability to contribute to asthma. However, our current understanding does not give them a key role in asthma pathogenesis.

Monocytes and Macrophages

Monocytes and macrophages are derived from a granulocyte-monocyte progenitor cell in the bone marrow. The precursor promonocytes leave the bone marrow and further differentiate into mature monocytes in the bloodstream. Some monocytes are deposited at various sites in the body as the larger, more mature macrophages that are known by various names in different tissues such as the liver, kidney, brain, and connective tissue. In the lung, the terms *alveolar* and *interstitial* macrophages refer to the location of these cells of the mononuclear phagocyte system. Macrophages residing in the luminal airways are called *airway macrophages* and are the predominant cells in BAL fluid.

MACROPHAGE PRODUCTS AND ASTHMA

As normal residents of the lung and airways, macrophages are found in great numbers in either tissue samples or BAL fluid from normal subjects. In these locations they play a major role in host defense mechanisms. They accomplish this by their ability to release a variety of cytokines (IL-1, IL-6, IL-8, GM-CSF, TNF-α), lipid mediators (TXA_2, LTB_4, LTC_4, LTD_4 and PGD_2), reactive oxygen species, lysosomal enzymes, PAF, and histamine-releasing factors.[39] They are also professional antigen-presenting cells that interact with and stimulate T-lymphocyte proliferation and cytokine production.[18] After antigen challenge, the percentage increase in airway macrophages exceeds that of eosinophils, neutrophils, and lymphocytes. Furthermore, in contrast to the high-affinity IgE receptors on mast cells and basophils, subpopulations of macrophages express low-affinity IgE receptors. These receptors are increased in patients with atopic asthma, and antigen IgE-dependent mechanisms may lead to the release of inflammatory mediators by these cells.

Basophils

Basophils are bone marrow–derived cells that originate from myeloid precursors and contain metachromatic granules. They are activated by the interaction of membrane high-affinity IgE receptors with antigen. Airway-associated cytokines, including IL-1, IL-3, IL-5, and GM-CSF, can all potentiate the IgE-dependent activation process. Complement fragments (C5a and C3a) and histamine-releasing factors can also activate basophils through IgE-independent perturbation of the cell membrane. Upon activation, basophils release a number of mediators, including both preformed and newly formed molecules. Preformed mediators include histamine (not tryptase) and chondroitin sulfate A. Like eosinophils, basophils contain some MBP, although it is not certain that this molecule is actually synthesized by the cell. Basophils also generate lipid mediators (LTC_4, LTD_4, LTE_4, and PAF) and a number of cytokines, including IL-4, IL-5, and possibly IL-13. Although some similarities exist, basophils are physiologically distinct from mast cells, particularly in regard to the basophil's heightened ability to be activated and to release mediators, such as histamine.

Normally, there are comparatively few basophils in circulation or tissues, and only recently has it been possible to quantify their existence in diseases such as asthma. Increased numbers of basophils have been found in the blood and sputum of asthma patients during clinical exacerbations of the disease. Enhanced spontaneous release of mediators (histamine, LTC_4) from basophils is seen in asthmatics when compared with normal subjects. The most striking increase in basophil number has been noted in BAL fluid obtained 24 h after inhaled allergen challenge. This rise in basophils corresponds to the LPR seen in some asthmatics. Furthermore, histamine-releasing factors[26] and basophil chemotactic activators (IL-3, GM-CSF) have been found in BAL fluid in conjunction with the LPR, providing a potential mechanism for basophil recruitment and activation in this setting. The prevailing concept, at present, is that basophils are not associated with the acute asthmatic reaction but function primarily in the development of chronic allergic inflammation such as that in the LPR. Their contribution in this setting is believed to result from their release of mediators and the cytokines IL-4, IL-5, and IL-13, which can enhance allergic inflammation with effects on IgE synthesis, TH_2 lymphocyte development, and eosinophil recruitment.

Lymphocytes

Lymphocytes are long-lived cells that have immune memory. They can be divided into B lymphocytes and T lymphocytes, with the remaining cells being mostly *natural killer* cells. Lymphocytes arise from a common precursor in the bone marrow and circulate in the bloodstream with more specifically defined functions. Immunoglobulin molecules on B-cell surfaces interact with antigens, resulting in B-cell activation and ultimately B-cell maturation into effector cells that secrete antibody molecules. Such cells actively produce antibody when stimulated by antigen exposure. T-cell maturation occurs in the thymus, resulting in two broad populations distinguished by membrane markers, the $CD4^+$ "helper" and $CD8^+$ "cytotoxic" T lymphocytes. T lymphocytes are also active in antigen recognition and response, albeit through different cellular mechanisms than B cells.

LYMPHOCYTE SUBSETS AND ASTHMA

The realization that lymphocytes may play a key role in the complex inflammatory reaction in asthma is a recent and important development. It is based on the work of a number of investigators looking for correlations between proinflammatory lymphocytes and clinical and pathologic features of asthma. Although both T and B cells are found in the airways, most of the lymphocytes are T cells, with the $CD4^+$ population predominating, particularly in the airways of atopic asthmatics. $CD8^+$ T cells may also be increased in patients with asthma, especially in nonatopic subjects.[1] $CD4^+$ cells have the capacity to secrete a select profile of proinflammatory cytokines in response to various stimuli. Both allergic and nonallergic asthmatics have an increase in activated airway T cells, marked by the expression of CD25 (the IL-2 receptor).[4] Others[10] have also observed increased $CD4^+$ cells in the peripheral blood of patients experiencing severe asthma episodes; they noted that these T cells were activated as manifest by the enhanced expression of CD25 and two other "activation markers," VLA-1 and human leukocyte antigen–DR. Furthermore, increased numbers of activated BAL T cells

have been correlated with increased bronchial responsiveness and numbers of eosinophils.[52] Activated T lymphocytes in the airways are most evident approximately 24 h after inhaled allergen challenge. Since not all asthma is obviously associated with allergen exposure, it is intriguing to consider the possible activation of T lymphocytes by other stimuli, such as respiratory viruses.

Of increasing interest, and perhaps importance, in the study of T lymphocytes and their relationship to inflammation is the discovery of "helper" $CD4^+$ T-cell subsets called T helper $(TH)_1$ and TH_2 cells. These subsets, which are distinguishable on the basis of their patterns of cytokine production, were first confirmed in mice (Table 47-3). Murine TH_1 cells secrete IFN-γ, IL-2, and lymphotoxin, whereas TH_2 lymphocytes notably produce IL-4, IL-5, IL-6, IL-10, and IL-13. Both subsets release IL-3, TNF-α, and GM-CSF. The probable existence of these subsets in humans has been noted.[42] Human TH_1 and TH_2 cells produce similar patterns of cytokines, although their synthesis of IL-2, IL-6, IL-10, and IL-13 is not as tightly restricted to a single cell subset. TH_1 and TH_2 cells are thought to be derived from a common uncommitted precursor lymphocyte called a TH_0 cell. The TH_2 cells proliferate and develop in response to IL-4, while TH_1 cells develop in response to IL-12, IFN-γ, or transforming growth factor-β (TGF-β). It follows that TH_2 cells, by virtue of their associated cytokines, enhance IgE synthesis and eosinophil activation and accumulation. Conversely, TH_1 cells are believed to play a key role in cell-mediated immune responses. Which response predominates depends on the local cytokine profile, with TH_1 cells inhibiting TH_2 activity by the release of IFN-γ, and TH_2 cells inhibiting TH_1 activity by the production of IL-4 and possibly IL-10 and IL-13. It has been proposed that allergic inflammation represents the activation of TH_2 lymphocytes and release of their proinflammatory cytokines. In accord with this proposal, cells in the BAL fluid from patients with asthma have shown increased mRNA expression for both IL-4 and IL-5. This and other observations suggest, but do not prove, that TH_2-like cells and their associated cytokines play a major role in orchestrating the inflammatory response in the asthmatic airway, in particular its IgE production (IL-4, IL-13) and eosinophilia (IL-5).

TABLE 47-3

Cytokine Profiles of Classic T Cell Subsets

	TH_0	
TH_1		**TH_2**
−	IL-4	+
+	IFN-γ	−
+	GM-CSF	+
+	TNF-α	+
+	IL-2	+/−
+	IL-3	+
−	IL-5	+
+/−	IL-10	−
+	Lymphotoxin (TNF-β)	−

NOTE: TH_0 = common uncommitted precursor lymphocyte; TH_1, TH_2 = "helper" $CD4^+$ T-cell subsets.

Epithelial Cells

The airway lumen is lined by epithelial cells, which form a barrier between inhaled substances and the inner components of the airways. Almost all epithelial cell types form a single layer, with a basal surface adherent to the underlying basement membrane and an apical surface contacting the luminal space. Histologically, normal proximal airway epithelial cells are arranged in a pseudostratified columnar configuration, with most luminal airway cells possessing apical cilia. Additionally, secretory epithelial cells (mucous goblet, Clara, and serous) may contribute to the excessive mucus production in asthma when stimulated by IL-4 or neuropeptides such as substance P. There are various forms of cell-to-cell adhesion and epithelium-to-extracellular matrix adhesion, including tight junctions, intermediate junctions, and desmosomes. These structures not only serve to maintain cell adherence but also contribute to intercellular communication. Airway epithelium functions as much more than a simple anatomic barrier. These cells actively regulate fluid and ion transport in the airway as well as mucus production. One of the most important activities of the airway epithelium is mucociliary clearance of secretions in conjunction with foreign particles.

The initial interest in airway epithelial involvement in asthma stemmed from epithelial cell clusters (Creola bodies) noted in the sputum of asthma patients,[36] and from the observation of denuded epithelium in autopsy lung specimens of patients who died in status asthmaticus.[16] Although possible artifactual damage to structural airway cells during bronchoscopy has been a concern, it is now clear that airway epithelial damage is a hallmark feature of asthma[24] that can be seen even in mild clinical disease.[28]

Increased mucus production is an important component of asthma, primarily in status asthmaticus. The presence of mucus in the small airways, along with airway wall thickening, contributes to decreased airway cross-sectional area and the increased bronchial hyperresponsiveness seen in asthma.[6] In asthma, hypertrophy and hyperplasia of goblet cells and submucosal glands, as well as microvascular leakage of fluid secondary to increased vascular permeability, add to excessive mucus production. The airway secretions in asthma patients are often thick and contain proteins, shed airway epithelial cells, and eosinophils.[15] Mucociliary clearance is decreased in asthma, compounding the retention of airway mucus. Both structural and functional damage of the mucociliary cells may be responsible for the decreased mucus removal seen in patients with asthma.

Although irreversible airflow obstruction is not a typical feature of asthma, fibrosis has been noted in the airways of patients with asthma, even those with mild disease. Decreased airway elastic tissue and increased collagen deposition beneath the true basement membrane are also noted in asthma.[15] The "basement membrane thickening" described in asthma patients is thought to represent this increase in connective tissue intimately associated with the basement membrane. Many of the structural abnormalities noted in asthmatic airways are considered the result of ongoing airway "remodeling" that occurs in conjunction with airway epithelial damage and the presence of inflammatory cells. This continual process of epithelial injury and repair may lead to irreversible abnormalities in the airway tissue in asthma.

It has become increasingly clear that the airway cells not only serve as a structural support and anatomic barrier but also are sources of inflammatory mediators. Epithelial cell–derived factors include lipid mediators (e.g., 15-hydroxyeicosatetraenoic acid and PGE_2), the potent bronchoconstrictor *endothelin*, fibronectin, and a variety of cytokines, including IL-1, IL-6, TGF-β, RANTES, IL-11, macrophage inflammatory protein–1α (MIP-1α), and GM-CSF.[12] Tissue fibroblasts also secrete a variety of cytokines, including GM-CSF. The release of IL-8, RANTES, and MIP-1α by epithelial cells may contribute to the influx of cells—including eosinophils, neutrophils, lymphocytes, and monocytes—to the asthmatic airway.

The role of nitric oxide (NO) in epithelial function is intriguing. NO is continually synthesized at low levels in the airways of normal subjects and has similarities to the previously described *epithelial-derived relaxing factor.* Cell sources of NO in the respiratory tract include airway epithelial cells, smooth muscle cells, sensory nerves, endothelial cells, and macrophages. At low levels, NO is a bronchodilator and vasodilator that antagonizes endothelin and has protective effects in the airway. Higher levels of NO are found in asthma, secondary to increased inducible NO synthase expression[21] by the action of proinflammatory cytokines IL-1, TNF-α and IFN-γ. Higher levels of NO production may be detrimental to airway epithelium. This may be mediated by the ability of NO to react with superoxide anion in inflamed tissue to produce biologic oxidants that could contribute to ongoing tissue damage and chronic asthmatic inflammation.[37]

Airway Smooth Muscle

Bronchospasm remains an important component of asthma, particularly acute asthma. Despite this long-standing recognition, the details of airway smooth muscle function, both in normal and in asthmatic persons, are still under investigation.[41] Smooth muscle is innervated by branches of both the parasympathetic (cholinergic) and sympathetic (adrenergic) nervous systems. The parasympathetic system is "excitatory" and maintains bronchial smooth muscle tone with vagal nerve fibers. Vagal stimulation narrows the airways. The sympathetic system is "inhibitory," and stimulation of this system's β-receptors results in smooth muscle relaxation.

Nonadrenergic, noncholinergic (NANC) neural pathways have increasing importance in airway smooth muscle function. The NANC system has both inhibitory and excitatory components, mediated by neurotransmitters. There is actually little direct sympathetic innervation of the airways, and the inhibitory NANC system exerts the most prominent neural bronchodilatory effect, by the neurotransmitter vasoactive intestinal peptide and NO. Excitatory neurotransmitters of the NANC system include substance P, neurokinins A and B, and calcitonin gene-related peptide (CGRP). Nerve injury secondary to ongoing inflammation in asthma may result in increased neuropeptide release. Substance P, neurokinins A and B, and CGRP all increase bronchoconstriction and vascular permeability. Substance P also contributes to asthma pathogenesis by enhancing mucus secretion.

Asthma is characterized by bronchial hyperresponsiveness. This is manifest as an *exaggerated* constrictive response to a given amount of a nonspecific (methacholine, histamine) or specific (antigen) stimulus. The mechanistic explanation for this hyperresponsiveness is poorly understood. It is thought, however, to be largely the result of the ongoing asthmatic inflammatory response, with its release of hyperresponsiveness-engendering mediators (histamine, PGD_2, $PGF_{2\alpha}$, etc.), and possibly the structural alterations (epithelial sloughing, airway remodeling, etc.) that this response causes.

ROLE OF ADHESION MOLECULES IN INFLAMMATION

The activation of cells in the airways and recruitment of cells from the circulation entail cell-cell and cell-extracellular matrix communication, a process that is facilitated and regulated by adhesion molecules and cytokines. It is currently held that the epithelial and endothelial cells, along with leukocytes, are active participants in the inflammatory process. Adhesion molecules are cell surface proteins that have been grouped according to structural and functional similarities. Several categories have thus far been identified, including the selectins, integrins, and members of the immunoglobulin (Ig) gene superfamily. The various molecules interact with complementary binding sites (ligands) on respective cells, allowing them to adhere to epithelial or endothelial surfaces and, in some cases, enter the pulmonary interstitium.

Selectins

The selectins are also called LECAMs (*Lectin, Epidermal growth factor, Complement-related* Cell Adhesion Molecules) in deference to their structural homologies. Three members of the group have been identified: endothelial (E)-selectin, platelet (P)-selectin, and leukocyte (L)-selectin. E-selectin is also called endothelial-leukocyte adhesion molecule–1 (ELAM-1). Both E- and P-selectin are found on endothelial cells, while L-selectin is located only on leukocytes, including lymphocytes, eosinophils, monocytes, basophils, and neutrophils. L-selectin can also be shed from leukocytes and, like P-selectin, may be found in a circulating soluble form, in which it is potentially available to participate in inflammatory reactions.

Integrins

Integrins are found on the surfaces of leukocytes but not endothelial cells. They are classified according to the composition of their various subunits, including several different alpha and beta chains. One line of evidence for the importance of integrins in human disease is the finding that partial or total absence of a β_2-integrin subunit leads to a crucial defect of neutrophil recruitment to sites of inflammation and recurrent, potentially life-threatening bacterial infections in patients with leukocyte adhesion defect syndromes. The integrins most likely to be important in leukocyte–endothelial cell signaling include VLA-4 and lymphocyte function–associated antigen–1 (LFA-1), also known as CD11a/CD18, a ligand for intercellular adhesion molecule–1 (ICAM-1) and ICAM-2. Not surprisingly, integrins have been implicated in tissue repair, platelet aggregation, and tumor invasion, in addition to their other, more general roles in leukocyte binding and recruitment. Integrins are the primary mediators of cell-extracellular matrix adhesion.[43] In asthma, integrins are also important to transendothelial migration of inflammatory cells into the airways.

Ig Gene Superfamily Members

Endothelial proteins of the immunoglobulin gene superfamily share functional as well as structural similarities with immunoglobulin domains. ICAM-1, ICAM-2, vascular cell adhesion molecule–1 (VCAM-1), platelet–endothelial cell adhesion molecule–1 (PECAM-1), and mucosal addressin cell adhesion molecule–1 (MadCAM-1) are all active in later steps of leukocyte–endothelial cell adhesion. These interactions are not final random events, but represent a coordinated effort of cells, cell surface molecules, and cytokines.

Mechanisms of Cellular Migration

There are three major interrelated steps in leukocyte recruitment from the circulation into tissues. They are categorized as adhesion, diapedesis, and chemotaxis (Fig. 47-3).[9] Although the specific molecules and cytokines associated with these processes may be somewhat different, depending on the particular cells involved, the following general steps for leukocyte–endothelial cell and extracellular matrix interaction are proposed. As leukocytes move through capillary vessels, they initially contact the endothelial cell walls in a random fashion. In vascular beds in the region of inflammation, endothelial cells are "activated," with in-

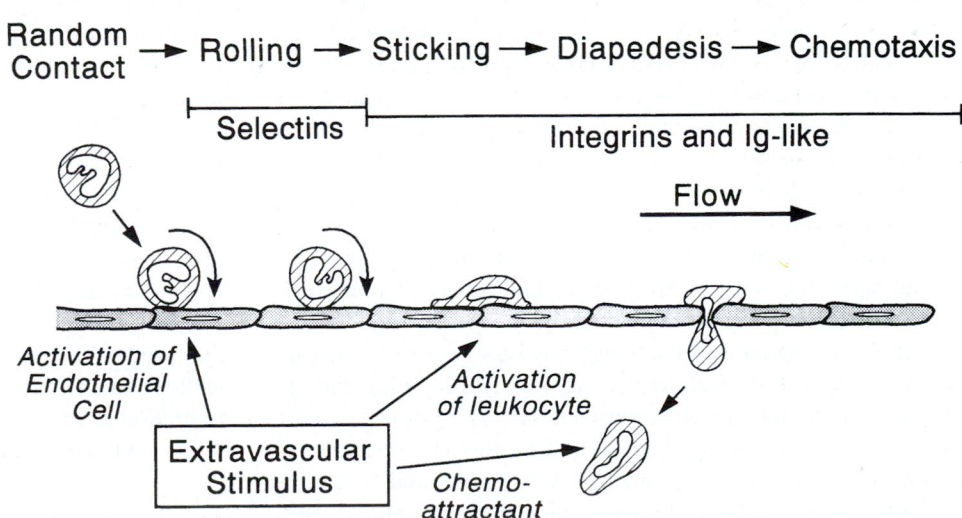

FIGURE 47-3   Mechanism of leukocyte vascular adhesion and migration into tissues and airways. Leukocytes "roll" along endothelial cell layer and then selectively adhere firmly to endothelium near inflammatory sites. The adhering leukocytes then migrate into subendothelial tissue. Cell surface molecules (selectins, integrins, Ig superfamily members) facilitate the process. *(Based on data of Carlos and Harlan,[9] with permission.)*

creased expression of adhesion molecules, such as E-selectin, on their cell surfaces. During flow through vessels with activated endothelial cells, leukocytes begin to "roll" along the endothelial cell luminal surfaces as a consequence of the interactions of these selectins and ligands on leukocyte and endothelial cell surfaces. As leukocytes travel near sites of inflammation, locally produced cytokines act on them to up-regulate expression of cell surface proteins, including those active in cell adhesion and migration. These activated leukocytes then participate in firm adhesion, much of which is mediated through interactions of leukocyte integrins (VLA-4, CD11a/CD18) and endothelial cell surface Ig gene superfamily members (ICAM-1, VCAM-1).

The next step is transmigration of leukocytes across endothelial cells and between endothelial cells (diapedesis) into the surrounding tissues. For actual migration of leukocytes to occur through the endothelial cell barrier, the firm adhesion must loosen somewhat. This process of transmigration and diapedesis involves cell adhesion molecules that are important in firm adhesion. In some cases, the particular adhesion molecules expressed on a given cell type, and their binding to specific cell ligands, help confer selectivity in leukocyte recruitment. For example, endothelial cell VCAM-1 binds mononuclear leukocytes and eosinophils, but not neutrophils. In contrast, both neutrophil and eosinophil migration across endothelial cells is enhanced by binding to ICAM-1.[44] Various inflammatory mediators induce either an increased or de novo expression of cell surface adhesion molecules and ligands. Furthermore, various chemoattractants, or *chemokines,* may be present that aid in the preferential recruitment of particular cell types into the tissues. The consequence of these interactions is the recruitment of inflammatory cells into target tissues (i.e., the airway) and, frequently, the activation of these cells during their transit.

Adhesion Molecules and Asthma

The appearance of specific cytokines or chemoattractants during the inflammatory process appears key to the delivery of an activated cell population to sites of asthmatic inflammation. The expression of specific cell adhesion molecules and ligands also permits or directs certain cell types to areas of tissue inflammation, even though the various and redundant cytokines released by cells at inflammatory sites may not seem to favor the infiltration of a specific cell type.

Communication between cells and their environment is critical to the development of airway inflammation. The importance of cell surface molecules in these interactions is becoming obvious from studies performed largely in animal models. For example, chronic antigen challenge has been shown to increase ICAM-1 expression and induce airway eosinophilia and increased bronchial hyperresponsiveness in monkeys. These processes were ICAM-1 dependent, since the administration of monoclonal antibodies against ICAM-1 inhibited both the eosinophilia and airway hyperresponsiveness to inhaled antigen.[53] Further, in a primate model of extrinsic asthma, antigen-challenged animals manifested rapid up-regulation of endothelial E-selectin (ELAM-1) that temporally correlated with neutrophil infiltration and the onset of late-phase airway obstruction. Treatment with monoclonal antibodies against ELAM-1 ab-

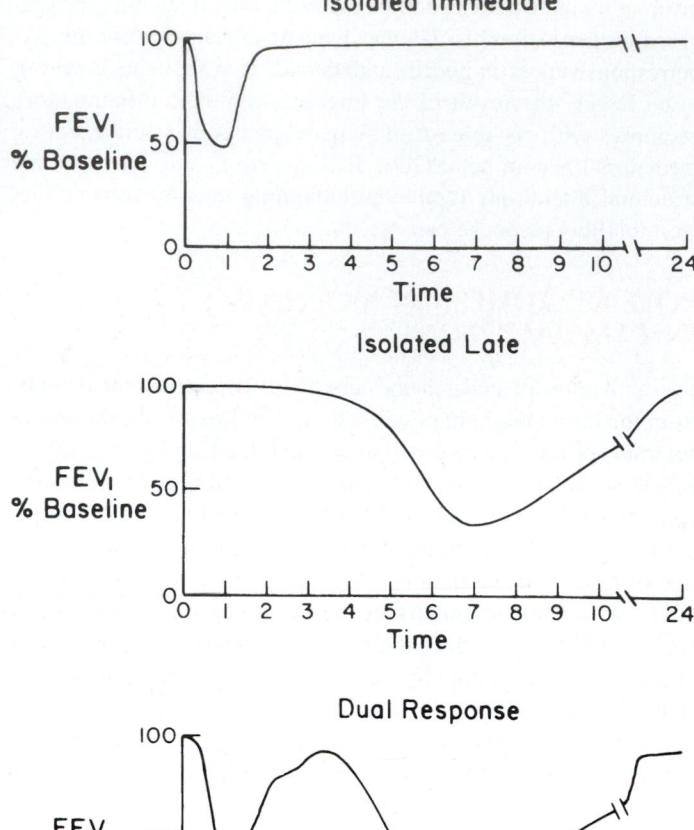

FIGURE 47-4   Acute and late phases of asthmatic responses (time in hours). *(Based on data of Lemanske and Kaliner,[29] with permission.)*

rogated this neutrophil influx and physiological dysregulation, demonstrating the ELAM-1 dependence of the pathophysiology of this model.[20] The induction of these adhesion molecules may be cytokine mediated, since IL-1 and TNF (cytokines present in asthmatic airways) augment endothelial cell expression of E- and P-selectin, ICAM-1, ICAM-2, and VCAM-1, while IL-2 augments VCAM-1 expression on endothelial cells. In human asthma, Hakansson and associates found increased functional eosinophil adhesion to VCAM-1 and ICAM-1.[22] This priming of eosinophil adhesion might contribute to the selective eosinophil recruitment in this disorder. Collectively, these observations suggest that cytokines released during the inflammatory process increase the expression of adhesion proteins on both leukocytes and endothelial surfaces that attract and facilitate the migration of the leukocytes into the airway, where they produce injury and perpetuate the process of allergic inflammation.

MODELS OF MECHANISMS OF ASTHMA PATHOGENESIS

The bronchoconstriction and airway inflammation of asthma can be elicited by allergens, respiratory infections, and occupational exposures. Two models have been particularly instructive in our efforts to further understand the pathogenesis of asthma in these settings. They are the late-phase asthmatic response to antigen and the airway changes seen with viral respiratory infections.

Late Phase Asthmatic Response

If an allergic asthmatic patient inhales antigen, several patterns of airway limitation can occur (Fig. 47-4). In the acute phase response (APR), inhalation of allergen causes an immediate fall in lung function. This airway response is characterized by wheezing, coughing, and/or shortness of breath. The APR usually resolves within 1 h and may be followed by a late phase response (LPR), beginning about 4 to 6 h after allergen challenge. The LPR often persists for 24 to 48 h. An isolated LPR is rare and is found primarily in occupational asthma.

Late asthmatic reactions share a number of features with chronic asthma: increased airway responsiveness, decreased responsiveness to bronchodilator therapy, and bronchial inflammation.[29] In asthma patients who exhibit the dual-phase features of an APR followed by the LPR, the later reaction is not only more prolonged but more intense as well. This is true even though the original apparent stimulus (allergen exposure) for bronchoconstriction has been removed.

The LPR is associated with the recruitment of inflammatory cells into the airway. Many have used bronchoscopy and lavage to examine the cellular and mediator composition of the airways both before and after allergen challenge. BAL fluid from the APR shows increased levels of histamine and tryptase, reflecting mast cell activation. Airway eosinophilia begins 4 to 6 h after allergen challenge in LPR subjects. The eosinophils and lymphocytes in the airway are activated, as indicated by the expression of cell surface activation markers and release of eosinophil granule proteins. Airway macrophage numbers also increase. The increase in eosinophils is greater in asthma patients who exhibit the LPR than in controls and isolated acute-phase responders. Increased numbers of eosinophils, neutrophils, and T lymphocytes (especially "helper" T cells) are seen in BAL fluid 48 h after segmental antigen challenge.[34] On repeat bronchoscopy 96 h after the initial allergen challenge, neutrophil numbers have returned to baseline, while the elevation in eosinophils and lymphocytes

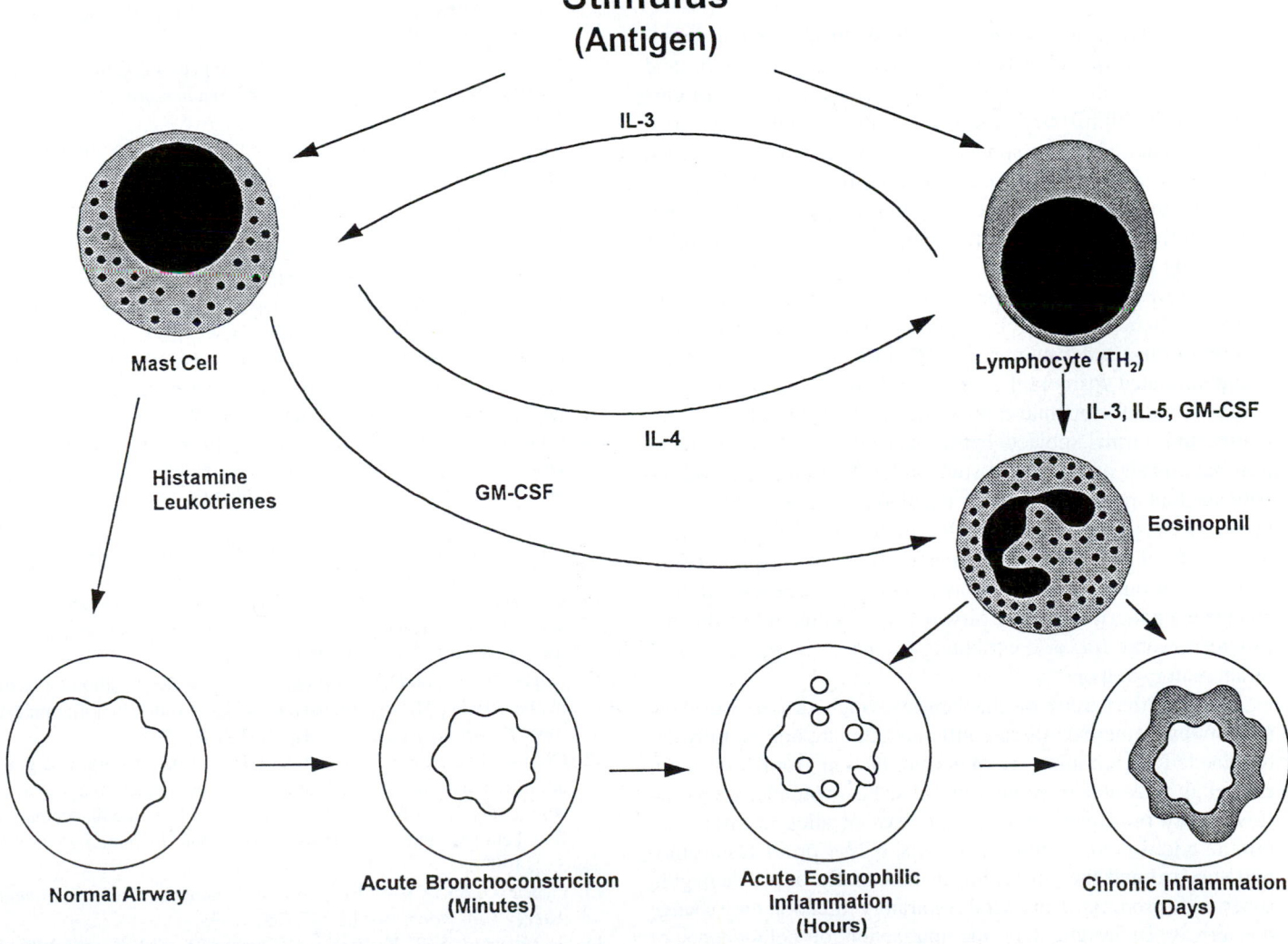

FIGURE 47-5 Stimulus (antigen) initiates mast cell and lymphocyte activation with release of mediators and cytokines, which promote both bronchoconstriction and airway inflammation.

persists. There is a striking correlation between the airway eosinophilia and IL-5 found in BAL samples during the LPR. These observations suggest that allergen challenge activates a series of airway events, including early mast cell degranulation, eosinophil recruitment, and lymphocyte activation, with release of TH$_2$-like cytokines such as IL-5. They also suggest that the IL-5 that is produced is the major stimulus for eosinophil recruitment to the asthmatic airway (Fig. 47-5).

Respiratory Viruses and Asthma

Viral respiratory infections increase asthma symptoms in many patients, particularly children. The viruses most typically associated with asthma in epidemiologic studies are respiratory syncytial virus (RSV) and rhinoviruses (RV).[13] Infection with "cold viruses" normally occurs in the upper airway and entails viral entry into a minority of bronchial epithelial cells. It has been difficult to determine the extent to which actual viral infection and replication occur in the lower airway or whether viruses adversely affect asthma by indirect means.[25] Experimental infection of subjects with respiratory viruses provides a useful model to establish the mechanisms in the pathogenesis of asthma.

Airway hyperresponsiveness to inhaled histamine may be increased in normal subjects as well as in allergic rhinitis and asthma patients during acute infection with RV. When patients with allergic rhinitis were voluntarily infected with rhinovirus, the heightened airway response to inhaled histamine remained elevated for as long as 4 weeks after virus inoculation.[30] Furthermore, the immediate response to inhaled allergen during RV infection was enhanced and, more importantly, the likelihood of developing a LPR to inhaled antigen was increased. In a subsequent investigation of allergic patients who underwent segmental bronchoscopy and antigen bronchoprovocation 1 month before, during, and 1 month after RV infection, the viral infection potentiated eosinophilic airway inflammation.[8] In addition, comparisons of bronchial biopsy specimens from allergic asthmatics and normal subjects before, during, and after RV infection have been made. These studies demonstrated that asthma patients had persistent airway eosinophilia, compared to the transient airway eosinophilia noted in control subjects.[17] Thus, the results of several studies suggest that viral respiratory infections not only increase airway hyperresponsiveness but also change the pattern of allergic airway response, including the factors responsible for, or contributing to, the eosinophilic allergic inflammatory response.

Although the precise mechanisms by which viruses contribute to the enhancement of allergic inflammation are not yet determined, RVs stimulate cytokine production from respiratory epithelial cells and mononuclear cells. For example, increased IFN-γ may propagate some components of allergic inflammation, in addition to its antiviral effects. IFN-γ promotes eosinophil survival and the generation of potentially tissue-damaging superoxide products. Thus, viral respiratory infection may change the airway environment or the interaction of components of airway inflammation, including cells and mediators, to promote factors responsible for allergic inflammation.

SUMMARY

Asthma is a complex and varied disorder with variable airflow obstruction, bronchial hyperresponsiveness, and the presence of acute and chronic bronchial inflammation. The orchestration of this inflammatory response comprises the participation of airway cells, mast cells, and lymphocytes; the generation of proinflammatory cytokines; the recruitment and activation of eosinophils; and the development of factors in the lung that sustain these events to cause persistent airway obstruction and injury. Many questions remain to be answered, including the genetic factors at work in the initiation and regulation of this process and the individual subject's susceptibility to this process. What has been learned is the importance of airway inflammation to altered airway physiology in asthma and the relevance of this component of asthma as a principal therapeutic target.

REFERENCES

1. Azzawi M, Bradley B, Jeffery PK, et al: Identification of activated T lymphocytes and eosinophils in bronchial biopsies in stable atopic asthma. *Am Rev Respir Dis* 142:1407–1413, 1990.
2. Barnes PJ: Neuropeptides and asthma. *Am Rev Respir Dis* 143: S28–S32, 1991.
3. Beasley R, Roche WR, Roberts JA, Holgate ST: Cellular events in the bronchi in mild asthma and after bronchial provocation. *Am Rev Respir Dis* 139:806–817, 1989.
4. Bentley AM, Menz G, Storz C, et al: Identification of T lymphocytes, macrophages, and activated eosinophils in the bronchial mucosa in intrinsic asthma: Relationship to symptoms and bronchial responsiveness. *Am Rev Respir Dis* 146:500–506, 1992.
5. Bousquet J, Chanez P, Lacoste JY, et al: Eosinophilic inflammation in asthma. *New Engl J Med* 323:1033–1099, 1990.
6. Brown RH, Zerhouni EA, Mitzner WJ: Airway edema potentiates airway reactivity. *J Appl Physiol* 79:1242–1248, 1995.
7. Cairns JA, Walls AF: Mast cell tryptase is a mitogen for epithelial cells: Stimulation of IL-8 production and intercellular adhesion molecule–1 expression. *J Immunol* 156:275–283, 1996.
8. Calhoun WJ, Dick EC, Schwartz LB, Busse WW: A common cold virus, rhinovirus 16, potentiates airway inflammation after segmental antigen bronchoprovocation in allergic subjects. *J Clin Invest* 94:2200–2208, 1994.
9. Carlos TM, Harlan JM: Leukocyte-endothelial adhesion molecules. *Blood* 84:2068–2101, 1994.
10. Corrigan CJ, Kay AB: CD4 T-lymphocyte activation in acute severe asthma: Relationship to disease severity and atopic status. *Am Rev Respir Dis* 141:970–977, 1990.
11. Coyle AJ, Uchida D, Ackerman SJ, et al: Role of cationic proteins in the airway: Hyperresponsiveness due to airway inflammation. *Am J Respir Crit Care Med* 150:S63–S71, 1994.
12. Cromwell O, Hamid Q, Corrigan CJ, et al: Expression and generation of interleukin-8, IL-6 and granulocyte-macrophage colony–stimulating factor by bronchial epithelial cells and enhancement by IL-1 beta and tumour necrosis factor–alpha. *Immunology* 77:330–337, 1992.
13. Cypcar D, Busse WW: Role of viral infections in asthma. *Immunol Allergy Clin North Am* 13:745–766, 1993.
14. de Monchey JGR, Kauffman HF, Venge P, et al: Bronchoalveolar eosinophilia during allergen-induced late asthmatic reactions. *Am Rev Respir Dis* 131:373–376, 1985.

15. Djukanovic R, Roche WR, Wilson JW, et al: Mucosal inflammation in asthma. *Am Rev Respir Dis* 142:434–457, 1990.

16. Dunnill MS, Massarella GR, Anderson JA: A comparison of the quantitative anatomy of the bronchi in normal subjects, in status asthmaticus, in chronic bronchitis, and in emphysema. *Thorax* 24:176–179, 1969.

17. Fraenkel DJ, Bardin PG, Sanderson G, et al: Lower airways inflammation during rhinovirus colds in normal and in asthmatic subjects. *Am J Respir Crit Care Med* 151:879–886, 1995.

18. Fuller RW: Macrophages. *Br Med Bull* 48:65–71, 1992.

19. Fuller RW, Dixon CMS, Dollery CT, Barnes PJ: Prostaglandin D_2 potentiates airway responsiveness to histamine and methacholine. *Am Rev Respir Dis* 133:252–254, 1986.

20. Gundel RH, Wegner CD, Torcellini CA, et al: Endothelial leukocyte adhesion molecule–1 mediates antigen-induced acute airway inflammation and late-phase airway obstruction in monkeys. *J Clin Invest* 88:1407–1411, 1991.

21. Guo FH, De Raeve HR, Rice TW, et al: Continuous nitric oxide synthesis by inducible nitric oxide synthase in normal human airway epithelium in vivo. *Proc Natl Acad Sci USA* 92:7809–7813, 1995.

22. Hakansson L, Bjornsson E, Janson C, Schmekel B: Increased adhesion to vascular cell adhesion molecule–1 and intercellular adhesion molecule–1 of eosinophils in patients with asthma. *J Allergy Clin Immunol* 96:941–950, 1995.

23. Hardy CC, Robinson C, Tattersfield AE, Holgate ST: The bronchoconstrictor effect of inhaled prostaglandin D_2 in normal and asthmatic men. *New Engl J Med* 311:209–213, 1984.

24. Jeffery PK, Wardlaw AJ, Nelson FC, et al: Bronchial biopsies in asthma: An ultrastructural, quantitative study and correlation with hyperreactivity. *Am Rev Respir Dis.* 140:1745–1753, 1989.

25. Johnston SL: Natural and experimental rhinovirus infections of the lower respiratory tract. *Am J Respir Crit Care Med* 152:S46–S52, 1995.

26. Kaplan AP, Baeza M, Reddigari S, Kuna P: Histamine-releasing factors. *Int Arch Allergy Appl Immunol* 94:148–153, 1991.

27. Kirshenbaum AS, Goff JP, Kessler SW, et al: Effect of IL-3 and stem cell factor on the appearance of human basophils and mast cells from CD34+ pluripotent progenitor cells. *J Immunol* 148:772–777, 1992.

28. Laitinen LA, Laitinen A, Haahtela T: Airway mucosal inflammation even in patients with newly diagnosed asthma. *Am Rev Respir Dis* 147:697–704, 1993.

29. Lemanske RF Jr, Kaliner MA: Late phase allergic reactions, in Middleton E Jr, Reed CE, Ellis EF, et al (eds), *Allergy: Principles and Practice,* Vol 1. St. Louis, Mosby–Year Book, 1993, pp 320–361.

30. Lemanske RF Jr, Dick EC, Swenson C, et al: Rhinovirus upper respiratory infection increases airway hyperreactivity and late phase asthma. *J Clin Invest* 83:1–10, 1989.

31. McFadden ER Jr, Gilbert IA: Asthma. *New Engl J Med* 327:1928–1937, 1992.

32. Messer JW, Peters GA, Bennett WA: Causes of death and pathologic findings in 304 cases of bronchial asthma. *Dis Chest* 38:616–624, 1960.

33. Metzger WJ, Richerson HB, Worden K, et al: Bronchoalveolar lavage of allergic asthmatic patients following allergen bronchoprovocation. *Chest* 89:477–483, 1986.

34. Metzger WJ, Zavala D, Richerson HB, et al: Local allergen challenge and bronchoalveolar lavage of allergic asthmatic lungs: De-

35. Murray JJ, Tonnel AB, Brash AR, et al: Release of prostaglandin D_2 into human airways during acute antigen challenge. *New Engl J Med* 315:800–804, 1986.

36. Naylor B: The shedding of the mucosa of the bronchial tree in asthma. *Thorax* 17:69–72, 1962.

37. Nijkamp FP, Folkerts G: Nitric oxide and bronchial hyperresponsiveness. *Arch Int Pharmacodyn* 329:81–96, 1995.

38. Pin I, Gibson PG, Kolendowicz R, et al: Use of induced sputum cell counts to investigate airway inflammation in asthma. *Thorax* 47:25–29, 1992.

39. Rankin JA: The contribution of alveolar macrophages to hyperreactive airway disease. *J Allergy Clin Immunol* 83:722–729, 1989.

40. Reed CE: New therapeutic approaches in asthma. *J Allergy Clin Immunol* 77:537–543, 1986.

41. Rodger IW: Airway smooth muscle. *Br Med Bull* 48:97–107, 1992.

42. Romagnani S: Biology of human TH_1 and TH_2 cells. J Clin Immunol 15:121–129, 1995.

43. Ruoslahti E: Integrins. *J Clin Invest* 87:1–5, 1991.

44. Sano H, Nakagawa N, Nakajima H, et al: Role of vascular cell adhesion molecule–1 and platelet-activating factor in selective eosinophil migration across vascular endothelial cells. Int Arch Allergy Immunol 107:533–540, 1995.

45. Schwartz LB, Bradford TR: Regulation of tryptase from human lung mast cells by heparin: Stabilization of the active tetramer. *J Biol Chem* 261:7372–7379, 1986.

46. Sedgwick JB, Calhoun WJ, Gleich GJ, et al: Immediate and late airway response of allergic rhinitis patients to segmental antigen challenge: Characterization of eosinophil and mast cell mediators. *Am Rev Respir Dis* 144:1274–1281, 1991.

47. Sekizawa K, Caughey GH, Lazarus SC, et al: Mast cell tryptase causes airway smooth muscle hyperresponsiveness in dogs. *J Clin Invest* 83:175–179, 1989.

48. Sommerhoff CP, Caughey GH, Finkbeiner WE, et al: Mast cell chymase: A potent secretagogue for airway gland serous cells. *J Immunol* 142:2450–2456, 1989.

49. Sur S, Crotty TB, Kephart GM, et al: Sudden-onset fatal asthma: A distinct entity with few eosinophils and relatively more neutrophils in the airway submucosa? *Am Rev Respir Dis* 148:713–719, 1993.

50. Tam EK, Caughey GH: Degradation of neuropeptides by human lung tryptase. *Am J Respir Cell Mol Biol* 3:27–32, 1992.

51. Virchow J-C Jr, Hölscher U, Virchow C Sr: Sputum ECP levels correlate with parameters of airflow obstruction. *Am Rev Respir Dis* 146:604–606, 1992.

52. Walker C, Kaegi MK, Braun P, Blaser K: Activated T cells and eosinophilia in bronchoalveolar lavages from subjects with asthma correlated with disease severity. *J Allergy Clin Immunol* 88:935–942, 1991.

53. Wegner CD, Gundel RH, Reilly P, et al: Intercellular adhesion molecule–1 (ICAM-1) in the pathogenesis of asthma. *Science* 247:456–459, 1990.

54. Wenzel SE, Fowler AA III, Schwartz LB: Activation of pulmonary mast cells by bronchoalveolar allergen challenge. *Am Rev Respir Dis* 137:1002–1008, 1988.

CHAPTER 48

ASTHMA: EPIDEMIOLOGY

Scott T. Weiss

Asthma is a clinical syndrome that affects approximately 10 million Americans. Two-thirds of those afflicted with asthma are children under the age of 18 years. It is estimated that roughly half of these children received their diagnosis prior to the age of 6 years. As a result, the origins of asthma are believed to have a clear genetic component that is often manifest in early childhood. The clinical course of this illness is influenced greatly by environmental exposures, particularly indoor allergens and maternal cigarette smoke. It is becoming increasingly recognized that childhood asthma also has important consequences for maximal growth in lung function and the potential development of chronic obstructive lung disease in later adult life. Thus, this clinical disease has important consequences in childhood and may have important consequences for adult obstructive lung disease.

Asthma is an extremely common clinical problem and the most common cause of hospitalization for children in the United States.

The estimated cost of asthma care exceeds $6 billion per year in the United States.[27] The paradox of this common clinical illness is that, in recent years, important strides have been made in discovering etiologic environmental factors that cause the airway inflammation characteristic of the syndrome. Despite this new knowledge and improved treatments, the prevalence and morbidity of asthma, particularly in children under the age of 6 years, is increasing in industrialized countries. Thus, these worrisome epidemiologic trends are occurring in the face of greater knowledge of disease pathophysiology and more effective therapies.

The purpose of this chapter is to describe trends in asthma epidemiology, specifically prevalence, hospitalization, and mortality. In so doing, we examine potential reasons for these trends, including changes in diagnostic classification by physicians, changes in health care and medication use, and changes in asthma risk factors. We also examine the relationship of the intermediate phenotypes of airway hyperresponsiveness and allergy to the asthma syndrome and consider a variety of risk factors for asthma occurrence. We conclude with a review of asthma natural history.

DEFINITIONS AND PREVALENCE

In 1991, the National Asthma Education Program Expert Panel Report from the National Institutes of Health defined asthma as "a lung disease with the following characteristics: (1) airway obstruction that is reversible, either spontaneously or with treatment; (2) airway inflammation; and (3) increased airway responsiveness to a variety of stimuli" (National Asthma Education Program).

Because asthma is a clinical syndrome, there is no gold standard for its diagnosis. As such, physicians employ nonstandardized algorithms for making the diagnosis. It is not uncommon for physicians to utilize a history of wheezing or parental history of asthma in conjunction with a response to a bronchodilator as the sole criteria for making an asthma diagnosis. Frequently age, gender, and other patient characteristics such as smoking status or response to allergen may influence a physician's diagnosis. Rarely are tests of airway responsiveness systematically used to investigate symptomatic patients in the clinical setting.

In general, epidemiologic surveys have tended to rely on historical or questionnaire sources to identify patients with asthma. Asthma cases have been identified, either by physicians or by surveys of population groups in whom the definition of who is asthmatic has been left to the patients themselves, parents of pa-

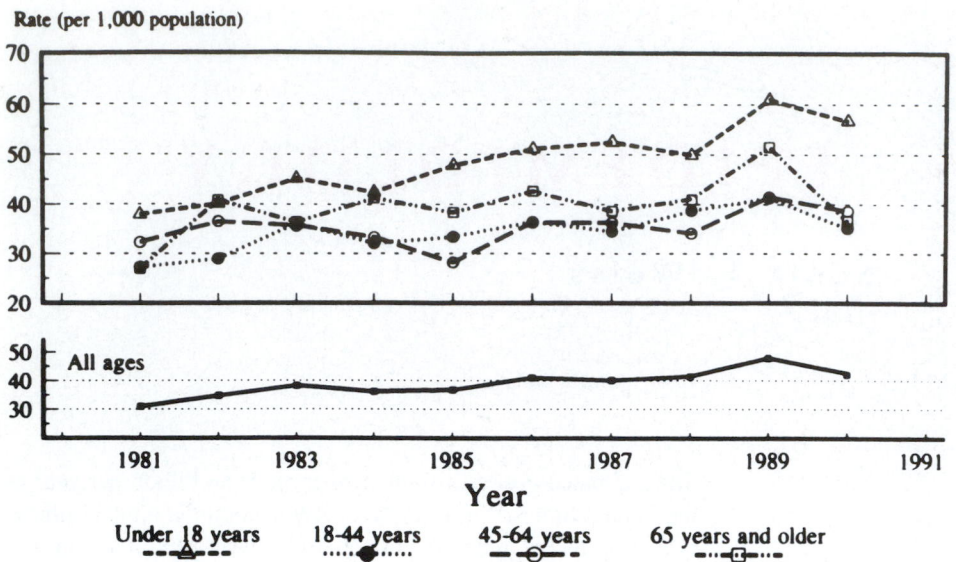

Rate (per 1,000 population)

Under 18 years   18-44 years   45-64 years   65 years and older

Notes: ICD-9 = 493, all age crude rates.
SOURCE: National Health Interview Survey

FIGURE 48-1   The trend in prevalence over a 10-year period is depicted for various age groups. The greatest increase is in the under-18 group. *(From Weiss et al,[29] with permission.)*

tients, or the report of the diagnosis having been made by the patient's physician. Clearly, each of these methods of identifying asthma patients has inherent weaknesses. One must, therefore, assume that some bias in the reporting of cases is present and that the biases in each method of gathering data are different.

The National Health Interview Survey (NHIS) is a random population household interview survey that provides information on asthma prevalence in the United States. Previous reports using NHIS data suggested that there was a 23 percent increase in the prevalence of asthma in children under 17 years between 1970 and 1980. Figure 48-1 illustrates trends in U.S. asthma prevalence from 1981 to 1990, based on the NHIS. It is clear from this figure that asthma prevalence continued to increase among children under the age of 18 years during this time period. The increase from 1981 to 1988 has been from 3.2 to 4.3 per 100 population, or 39 percent. This increase, noted in the NHIS data, has been confirmed in other population surveys in the United States, such as the National Health and Nutrition Examination Survey (NHANES). Current data suggest that asthma prevalence over all ages is 4.1 per 100 population, with the rates for children under 18 years being 5.7 per 100 population. These prevalence rates are based on responses to a question as to whether the individual had seen a physician for asthma within the past year. There does not appear to be substantial regional variation with regard to prevalence rates.

Although no incidence studies have been performed in the United States in the last 10 years, older investigations suggest that roughly half of all asthma cases are diagnosed before the age of 10 years.[2] There does appear to be significant modification of prevalence by gender, in that males tend to predominate in this younger age group, whereas gender ratios equalize in puberal age range, and females predominate throughout the rest of the adult life. Thus, gender and age play an important role in modifying disease incidence.

HOSPITALIZATIONS

Data from the National Hospitalization Discharge Survey suggest that hospitalization rates for asthma have been reasonably stable throughout the 1980s (Fig. 48-2). The apparent increase from 1978 to 1979 is most likely due to a change in the International Classification of Disease (ICD) coding for hospitalizations. There has been a very mild increase in hospitalizations, most notable in children under the age of 5 years, where rates have increased from 3.2 per 1000 in 1979 to 5.5 per 1000 in 1990.

TRENDS IN ASTHMA MORTALITY

Perhaps the most notable feature about asthma mortality rates in the United States is that they are quite low. Figure 48-3 reports the trends in asthma mortality in the United States between 1929

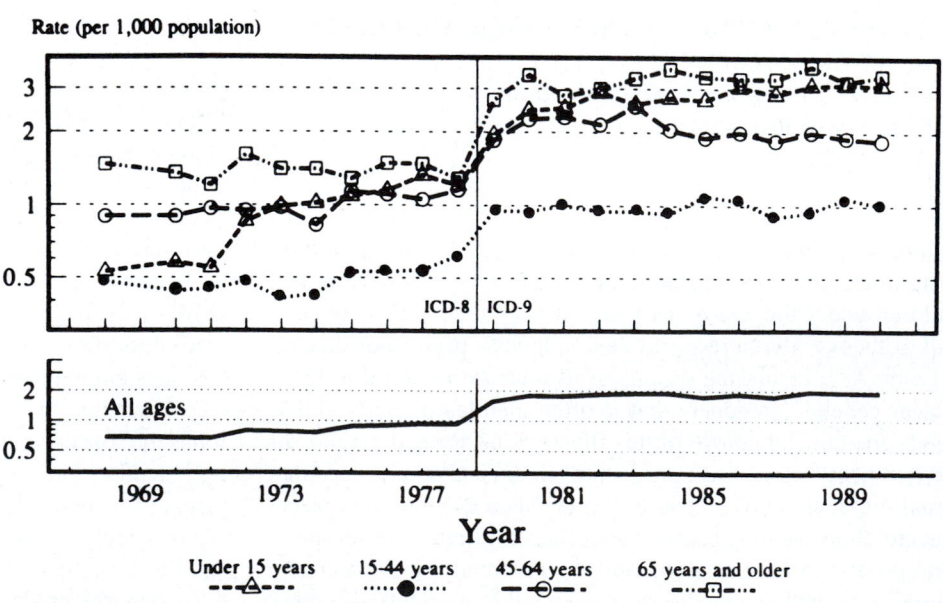

Rate (per 1,000 population)

Under 15 years   15-44 years   45-64 years   65 years and older

Notes: ICD-8 and ICD-9 = 493, all ages crude rate.
SOURCE: National Hospital Discharge Survey

FIGURE 48-2   The trend in hospitalizations for asthma is depicted over a 20-year period for various age groups. The increase is in the under-18 group. *(From Weiss et al,[29] with permission.)*

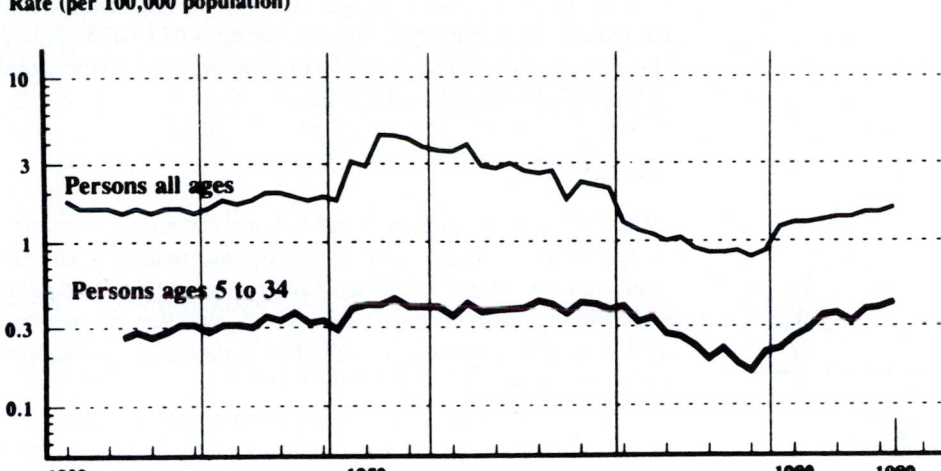

Rate (per 100,000 population)

Persons all ages

Persons ages 5 to 34

Note: crude rates.
Source: NCHS VSS

FIGURE 48-3 Asthma mortality rates are depicted over a 60-year period. The vertical lines represent ICD coding changes. *(From Weiss et al,[29] with permission.)*

and 1989. Vertical lines represent ICD coding changes. Although the rates appear to have increased since 1975, the absolute rates still remain extremely low. Again, these overall trends in countrywide asthma mortality tend to belie pockets of very high prevalence, morbidity, and mortality in inner-city minority populations.

The low mortality rates do not represent a public health concern in an absolute sense as the number of deaths is still very low. However, the rates represent a concern in a clinical sense in that most experts agree that almost all asthma deaths are preventable, and certain urban and minority areas have extremely high mortality rates suggesting inadequate care practices.

INTERMEDIATE PHENOTYPES

There are two intermediate phenotypes that contribute to the asthmatic syndrome: airway responsiveness and allergy. Both of these intermediate phenotypes have a genetic component, and both are influenced by environmental factors. We will discuss each of these phenotypes below and then consider their interrelationship to each other and to asthma.

Airway Responsiveness

Airway responsiveness is measured using increasing doses of a bronchoconstrictive stimulus, and then quantitating the decline in lung function caused by the stimulus. The most common pharmacologic stimuli are histamine and methacholine. Increasing bronchoconstrictive doses of histamine or methacholine are administered, and when the patient's FEV_1 decreases by 20 percent from its initial value, the test is terminated. The dose at which this drop occurs is called the *provocative dose,* or PD_{20}. Individuals that manifest a PD_{20} at a low dose of stimulus are said to have increased airway responsiveness and are hyperresponsive to the inhaled agent.

Cross-sectional population-based surveys of children and adults conducted in many different countries and using a variety of techniques for measuring airway responsiveness have shown that the prevalence of airway hyperresponsiveness is roughly 20 percent in the general population.[28] The prevalence of increased airway responsiveness exceeds the prevalence of asthma by anywhere from two- to fivefold.

These studies have also demonstrated that airway responsiveness is log normally distributed in the general population. An example of this is given in Fig. 48-4.[18] In this population-based study of the distribution of histamine airway responsiveness, symptomatic or asthmatic subjects appear at the more responsive end of the distribution, but there is considerable overlap with asymptomatic subjects. This phenomenon has been repeatedly demonstrated in population-based studies in which a large number of asymptomatic subjects have been found to manifest airway hyperresponsiveness to this agent.

It has now been well demonstrated in studies of both children and adults that airway hyperresponsiveness antedates and predicts the development of asthma. Recent data from the Childhood Respiratory Disease Study suggest that increased airway responsiveness has a two- to threefold risk for predicting the development of asthma in children and young adults.[7] This risk is somewhat lower than that found by other investigators who noted that subjects with increased airway responsiveness had a four- to fivefold greater risk of developing asthma than subjects without increased airway responsiveness.[30]

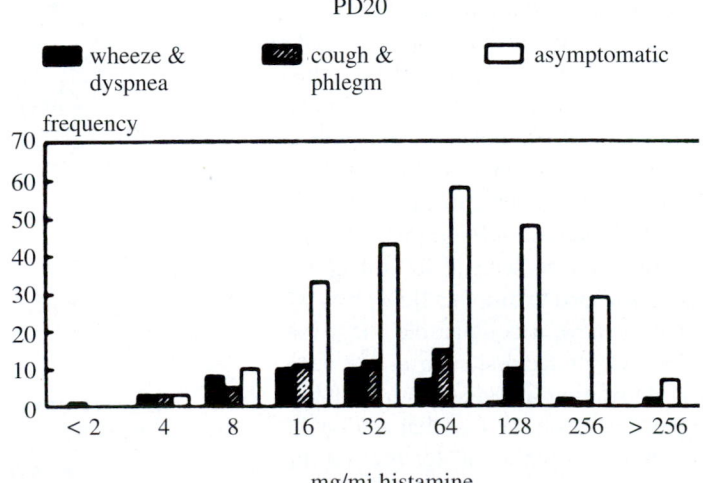

FIGURE 48-4 The log-transformed distribution of histamine airway responsiveness from a random population of subjects in the Netherlands. Note that symptomatic subjects are more common in the responsive end of the distribution. *(From Rijcken et al,[18] with permission.)*

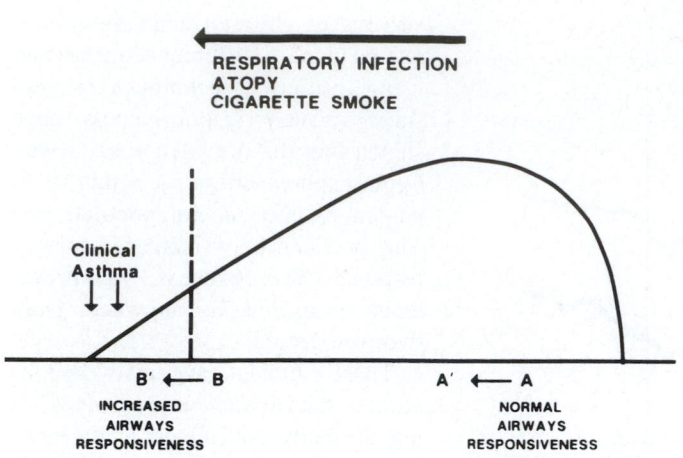

FIGURE 48-5 The effect of environmental exposures on the population distribution of airway responsiveness acting to move people in a more responsive direction. *(From Brown and Weiss,[3] with permission.)*

Taken together, these data suggest that increased airway responsiveness is a necessary but not a sufficient condition for the development of asthma. In all likelihood, subjects who are genetically predisposed have increased airway responsiveness. They then encounter environmental stimuli that generate airway inflammation. The inflammation then moves them in the direction of greater responsiveness and the development of respiratory symptoms. This theoretical paradigm is graphically depicted in Fig. 48-5.

A variety of mechanical factors influence airway responsiveness. First, and most important, is the level of lung function. Individuals with lower levels of lung function are more likely to have increased airway responsiveness. In part, this is simply a mathematical phenomenon. Since airway responsiveness is expressed as a percent change from baseline, baseline value will obviously be important in determining the level at which an individual would be considered responsive (i.e., have a PD_{20}). This can be best understood with a simple mathematical example. A man with a 5-L FEV_1 would be required to drop his prechallenge level of lung function by 1 L to achieve a PD_{20} for FEV_1. In contrast, a man with a 500-ml FEV_1 will only need to drop his FEV_1 by 100 ml to achieve a comparable PD_{20} for FEV_1. Other factors, such as the central deposition and distribution of the inhaled aerosol, the fact that airflow is inversely proportional to the fourth power of the airway radius, and baseline bronchomotor tone all contribute to the relationship of lung function to airway responsiveness.[9] For this reason, airway responsiveness is likely to be increased at the extremes of age (i.e., in children and older adults) and reduced in young adults between the ages of 15 and 45 years. This may account, in part, for the reduction in symptomatic asthma with aging seen in some individuals.

Allergy

Allergy refers to immediate (type 1) hypersensitivity to environmental antigens encountered by inhalation, ingestion, or cutaneous contact. Atopy is characterized by an immediate type hypersensitivity skin reaction with wheal and flare to common environmental antigens and familial aggregation. Atopic subjects represent a subset of allergic subjects.

To briefly summarize the pathophysiology of the allergic response, serum IgE antibody is secreted by B cells in response to signaling from two distinct T-cell populations. CD-4 positive (helper/inducer) T cells induce and enhance IgE synthesis, whereas CD-8 positive (suppressor) T cells inhibit IgE synthesis. These T-cell regulators are controlled by a variety of self-signaling cytokines and by the level and mode of presentation of environmental antigen. A key cytokine in the regulation of IgE production is IL-4, which instructs B lymphocytes to "switch" to IgG-1 and IgE production. IL-4 is produced by T-helper (TH) 2 cells which are, most commonly, a subset of CD-4 positive T lymphocytes. Figure 48-6 depicts the complex interactions between inhaled antigen, dendritic cells in the airway (marked *DC*), and TH2 lymphocytes. The dendritic cells present antigen to TH2 lymphocytes which secrete IL-4. The IL-4 then stimulates B cells to produce IgE.[9] This immune response can be influenced by cytokines such as interferon-γ that are produced by a different subset of CD-4 positive T cells (called *TH1 cells*) and inhibit IgE production.

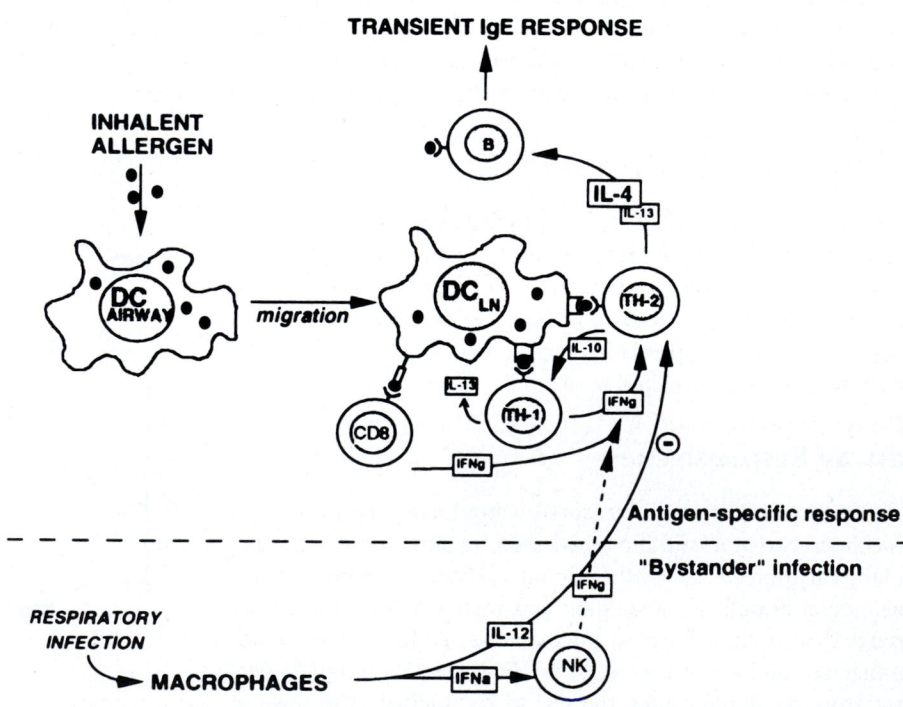

FIGURE 48-6 Dendritic cells (DC) present antigen to T lymphocytes which in turn secrete and are influenced by a variety of cytokines that determine the child's immune phenotype. The sources of the antigens are diverse and include both bacterial and viral infections as well as environmental antigens. *(From Holt,[9] with permission.)*

A variety of allergy markers have been utilized in epidemiologic studies of asthma. Serum-total and -specific IgE measurements have been utilized, along with skin testing, particularly prick testing, to provide some measure of the prevalence of allergic responsiveness. Both total serum IgE levels and skin test reactivity measure sensitization as well as recent exposure to environmental antigens. Skin test reactivity depends on at least three separate factors: an intact immune system, the presence of a mast cell-basophil complex that can combine with IgE and release mediators when exposed to antigen, and skin that can respond to histamine with the development of an inflammatory response, including erythema and induration. Although these manifestations of an allergic response depend on prior exposure to environmental antigen, they do not measure or take into account the level of exposure in the environment.

Skin test reactivity and total serum IgE levels are closely correlated and appear to be equal in males and females. There is an increase in these allergy markers with age that appears to be maximal at approximately age 15 years. After this time, there is a progressive decline, both in skin test reactivity and total serum IgE, although the decline in skin test reactivity is greater than the decline in IgE, related to local factors in the skin.

The processes that lead to the development of a TH2 as opposed to a TH1 phenotype in early life are complex and poorly understood. It is currently believed that IgE responses to inhalant allergens are commonly set in early childhood. It is now believed that sensitization to environmental antigens is not just a function of genetic susceptibility, dose, timing, and duration of exposure but also may reflect exposure to other environmental antigens, particularly microbial or viral organisms. Respiratory or gastrointestinal infections may stimulate macrophages to produce interferon alpha and IL-12 and then stimulate NK cells to produce interferon gamma, which would inhibit the development of a TH2-type response. Recently, the Tucson Epidemiologic Study[15] noted that children who had a nonwheezing lower respiratory tract illness before 9 months of age had lower total IgE levels at 9 months and 6 years of age when compared to children who had no lower respiratory illnesses before 9 months of age. These children were also less likely to be atopic than those who had no lower respiratory tract illnesses. This study suggests that it is not simply the exposure to environmental aeroallergens but the total antigen exposure in the first year of life that sets the immune system to develop a TH1 or a TH2 phenotype.

Relationship of Airway Responsiveness and Allergy to Asthma

Atopy and increased airway responsiveness are separate but related factors, both of which contribute to the development of the asthma phenotype. Over 80 percent of childhood asthmatics are atopic. Epidemiologic studies have shown that asthma is more closely related to serum IgE levels than to skin test reactivity[5] and that increased airway responsiveness, even in nonasthmatic children, is strongly related to total serum IgE levels.[20] Individuals appear to inherit these two intermediate phenotypes separately. It is determined relatively early in childhood whether exposure to environmental antigens results in the development of a TH2-predominant response. A child who develops a TH2-type phenotype may then manifest susceptibility to appropriate environmental aeroallergens. Thus, sensitization and exposure are linked.

Relatively few studies have examined the relationship between exposure to allergen and the development of asthma. One study described an 11-year follow-up of 67 children of atopic parents, approximately half of whom were atopic (skin test positive) to common aeroallergens.[22] Seventeen of the children went on to develop asthma. Sixteen of these 17 were in the atopic group. All 16 were sensitized to house dust mite. The level of house dust mite in the home at age 1 year correlated directly with the degree of sensitization at age 11 years. However, the level of house dust mite did not correlate with the degree of sensitization at age 5 years. All but one of the children with asthma at age 11 years were exposed to more than 10 μg of house dust mite per gram of dust in the first year of life. These children had a relative risk of 4.8 of developing asthma by age 11 years. This study also demonstrated that the age at which the first episode of wheezing occurred was inversely related to level of exposure at age 1 year for all children, with an especially strong relationship being noted for atopic children. Prevalence of allergy in Western populations, as measured by skin test reactivity, varies from 15 to 40 percent, depending on the age, gender, and definition of a positive skin test. There is an imperfect correlation between skin test reactivity, total serum IgE level, and peripheral blood eosinophil count, such that no single phenotypic marker completely defines the atopic state. It would appear that changes in atopy, both as a result of increased sensitization and higher levels of indoor allergens, may be an important risk factor that has changed in the past 20 years, potentially accounting for the increased prevalence of asthma. There is some evidence from Scandinavia that thermally tighter homes have been associated with higher indoor allergen levels. In addition, increased home carpeting may also contribute to higher house dust mite levels. At the present time, incomplete characterization of the number and level of allergens in homes and a lack of clear data demonstrating that this has changed have hampered studies that have focused on increased allergen exposure as a causal factor for the increased development of asthma. Other risk factors, notably maternal cigarette smoking and childhood respiratory infection, may also contribute to the development of a TH2 phenotype and, hence, an increased predisposition to allergy and asthma.

RISK FACTORS

Age

Asthma and airway responsiveness are increased in very young and very old individuals. Individuals at the extremes of age have lower levels of lung function, such that milder degrees of airway inflammation and smaller changes in lung function may precipitate symptoms and, hence, the diagnosis of asthma. No studies have examined the relationship of age to asthma, independent of level of lung function.

Gender

Asthma in childhood is predominantly a male disease. The gender ratio for a doctor's diagnosis of asthma is approximately 2 to 1, male to female, until puberty, at which time the gender ratio equalizes. Following puberty, asthma incidence is greater in females. Virtually all diagnosed cases of asthma in subjects after age 40 years are female, and there is now evidence that estrogen use is a risk factor for asthma in adult individuals.

Race

Asthma prevalence is higher in blacks than in whites. In addition to higher prevalence, hospitalization and mortality rates are also consistently higher in blacks than in whites. Whether these racial differences in asthma prevalence, hospitalization, and mortality are solely due to inadequate treatment and access to medical care remains unclear. Alternatively, genetic differences or environmental factors, such as urban crowding or indoor air pollution, could contribute to these findings.

Socioeconomic Status

In the United States, lower socioeconomic status is associated with an increase in asthma prevalence. The factors underlying this association are unknown, although indoor air pollution, maternal cigarette smoking, allergen exposure, and decreased access to medical care may all contribute to this relationship.

Young Maternal Age

Some reports in the literature suggest that infants born to mothers who are very young (i.e., less than 20 years) have an increased incidence of asthma.[14] It is known that prematurity and low birth weight are more common in these younger mothers, but the association of young maternal age is independent of any relationship to prematurity. It is also unrelated to lower socioeconomic status. The reasons for this association are unclear but may relate to IgE hypersensitivity in the mother and a subsequent transfer or development in the fetus.

Breastfeeding

There is no conclusive evidence that breastfeeding is beneficial in the prevention of atopic sensitization.[11] Although the benefits of breast milk relate to the passive transfer of maternal antibody to the fetus, maternal transfer of foreign proteins such as cows milk protein ingested by the mother may induce allergy. Furthermore, there is no evidence for secular trends in breastfeeding practices that parallel the increases in asthma prevalence.

Prematurity

Infants born prematurely carry a fourfold increased risk of development of asthma.[25] Prematurity also is associated with bronchopulmonary dysplasia, a disease characterized by increased airway responsiveness and asthma symptoms. Some investigators have found that low birth weight, independent of prematurity, also contributes to asthma risk. Note that African Americans have lower birth weights and higher rates of prematurity than whites, and thus prematurity may contribute to racial differences in asthma prevalence and morbidity.

Cigarette Smoking

Maternal cigarette smoking is clearly a risk factor for the development of asthma in the first year of life.[26] The risk is roughly twofold in infants born to smoking mothers without an allergic history but increases to almost fourfold in infants of allergic parents with mothers who smoke. The predominant effect of maternal cigarette smoking is due to in utero exposure with decreased lung function at birth. Thus, early life effects of maternal cigarette smoking are predominantly mechanical in nature. Several studies have suggested that maternal cigarette smoke exposure may also alter the development of the allergic response. Specifically, maternal cigarette smoking has been associated with an increase in peripheral blood eosinophilia, serum IgE levels, and skin test reactivity. It is also clear that maternal cigarette smoke exposure is associated with a greater occurrence of lower respiratory tract infections. To date, the extent to which maternal cigarette smoke exposure influences the development of atopy in children remains unclear. In adults, active cigarette smoking is associated with increased airway responsiveness, elevations in total serum IgE level, and peripheral blood eosinophilia. Although there are no data to suggest that active cigarette smoking is associated with the development of skin test reactivity or sensitization to aeroallergens, there is clear evidence suggesting that active cigarette smoking does lead to the development of asthma in adults.

Respiratory Illness

The relationship between asthma and respiratory illness has been investigated at a number of levels. Among the most important is the relationship between respiratory infection, childhood wheezing, and the development of asthma in later life. These studies have demonstrated a prominent association between lower respiratory tract viral infections in early life and wheezing illnesses.[6] Respiratory syncytial virus (RSV) has drawn particular attention, since it is the major cause of bronchiolitis in children and RSV infection is associated with IgE production, airway inflammation, and increased airway responsiveness. These studies also noted that RSV bronchiolitis in childhood is associated with the development of chronic wheezing in later life.[21] In a recent study, asthma, defined as three episodes of bronchial obstruction verified by a physician, was found in 23 percent of patients who had experienced infantile RSV bronchiolitis as versus 1 percent of controls when evaluated at age 3 years.

Most children who wheeze before 2 years of age rarely wheeze after that age, and only a minority still have symptoms 3 to 5 years after their original illness. As a result, investigators have attempted to identify the features that differentiate children with wheezing-associated lower respiratory tract illnesses that resolve over time from those that likely presage chronic airway symptomatology. These groups cannot be differentiated based on their symptomatology or socioeconomic background.[6] Lung function and atopic status, however, appear to be important. Children who wheeze only in the first 2 years of life had lower levels of lung function when evaluated at age 2 and 6 years. In contrast, children who wheezed early in life and who were still wheezing at age 6 years had normal levels of lung function but statistically elevated IgE levels during the first year of life. They also had elevated levels of IgE at 6 years of age, but their levels of lung function had deteriorated and were now below those of individuals who had never wheezed.[15] This has led to the hypothesis that there are two wheezing syndromes associated with lower respiratory tract infection in young children. One is mainly the result of small airway caliber, lacks bronchial hyperresponsiveness, and has an excellent prognosis. The other, which can be equated with early-onset asthma, is associated with increased prevalence of allergic markers, bronchial hyperreactivity, and a significant decrease in lung function over the first 6 years of life.[6] Support for the importance of an interaction between viral infection and atopy in this pathogenic schema comes from studies that noted that RSV bronchiolitis is most prominently associated with the development of asthma in patients with a concomitant family history of atopy and/or asthma.[19,21]

Although the association between viral respiratory tract infections and asthma is well documented, it is still not clear that this relationship is based on cause and effect. The alternative possibility is that patients with abnormal lung function or an underlying asthmatic or atopic diathesis may be predisposed to viral respiratory tract infections in childhood. The importance of early sensitization to aeroallergens and a predisposition to high-serum IgE levels[12] is noted above. However, the effect that viral infection has on the development of atopic sensitization is poorly understood. It has been proposed that viral and bacterial infections in early life are protective in terms of the long-term development of allergic sensitization.[9] However, a recent study reported that children who have had infantile RSV bronchiolitis manifest enhanced allergy to food and inhalant allergens diagnosed by skin prick test and analysis of specific serum IgE at 3 years of age.[21] Additional investigation will be required to clarify the relationship among viral infection, atopy, and the subsequent development of asthma.

Another important relationship between respiratory illness and asthma relates to the ability of respiratory illnesses to trigger asthmatic exacerbations. A number of studies have demonstrated a close temporal relationship, at the individual and population level, between virus infection and asthma exacerbations.[1,17,23] These studies have also demonstrated that: (1) in contrast to viruses, bacterial infections are not associated with asthmatic exacerbations; (2) different viruses exacerbate asthma in patients of different ages with RSV and parainfluenza virus being most common in young children and rhinovirus predominating in older children and adults; (3) viruses are the precipitants of an even higher percentage of severe (versus mild) asthmatic exacerbations; and (4) viral infections can induce nonspecific increases in airway responsiveness and airway obstruction in children. The importance of viruses in asthmatic exacerbations was recently highlighted by studies employing sensitive polymerase chain reaction (PCR) viral detection techniques in addition to traditional techniques of viral isolation.[10] These studies demonstrated the presence of respiratory virus in approximately 80 percent of acute asthmatic exacerbations in 9- to 11-year-old children in the United Kingdom. Interestingly, the studies also noted a seasonality to the occurrence of these episodes that might otherwise have been attributed to aeroallergens. Thus, although the impact of atopy on asthma increases throughout childhood with increasing age, it is now also clear that viral respiratory infections are important triggers of acute asthmatic symptomatology.

REASONS FOR TRENDS IN PREVALENCE, MORBIDITY, HOSPITALIZATIONS

Changes in Diagnostic Classification

There is little question that public awareness of asthma as a public health problem has increased and that this has been coupled with an increased willingness on the part of physicians to diagnose asthma in children under the age of 5 years. Physicians appear to be more willing to diagnose asthma in young children and perhaps to substitute a diagnosis of asthma for a diagnosis of bronchitis or bronchiolitis in this age group. However, when one examines bronchitis rates relative to asthma rates, there has been no concomitant decrease in bronchitis to offset the increase in asthma. This suggests that diagnostic transfer (i.e., physicians calling bronchitis patients asthmatic) cannot be the explanation for the increase in asthma prevalence and morbidity seen in young children. Although increased asthma awareness among physicians and the public may account for some of the increase, it seems unlikely that all the increase can be due to this factor alone. Similarly, although ICD coding changes have been responsible for increases in asthma prevalence and mortality in subjects over the age of 45 years, coding changes have had little influence on asthma in the very young. This suggests that the increase in the prevalence and morbidity of asthma observed in industrialized countries is not the result of diagnostic alterations and is due instead to alterations in the risk factors for the disease (discussed below).

Changes in Risk Factors

It remains unknown whether the very real increases in asthma prevalence are due in some measure to changes in the above-noted risk factors. Viewed from the perspective of the ontogeny of IgE immunity, the sum total of exposure to respiratory infections (both bacterial and viral), allergens, maternal cigarette smoke, and possibly other air pollutants may interact to determine T-cell phenotype. In addition, other, relatively unstudied factors such as diet may contribute to T-cell phenotype and immune function. Conclusive data linking trends in any of these risk factors to trends in asthma prevalence are lacking.

PROGNOSIS

Recently, the prognosis of asthma in early childhood has been clarified substantially by data from the Tucson Epidemiologic Study.[15] These investigators followed a cohort of children through the first 6 years of life. They characterized these children into four groups: persistent wheezers (children who wheezed both before and after the age of 3 years); transient early wheezers (infants who wheezed before the age of 3 years and then stopped); transient late wheezers (infants who wheezed after age 3 years but not before); and "never wheezers." Fully 40 percent of all children in the Tucson Epidemiologic cohort wheezed in the first year of life.

Significant predictors of persistent wheezing, and hence children at risk for the development of chronic asthma, were young maternal age, IgE level at 9 months, parents with asthma, maternal cigarette smoke exposure in utero, abnormal lung function at birth, and male gender. It is likely that early-life wheezing is predominantly a mechanical factor and less due to severe and chronic airway inflammation. It also seems unlikely that allergen exposure predominates as a factor in early childhood.

The characteristics of older children who wheeze are atopy, female gender, and active and passive cigarette smoking. By preadolescence, atopy and environmental allergen exposure are important risk factors for wheezing in children.

Roughly half of all childhood asthmatics will have their symptoms decrease or disappear by late adolescence and early adulthood. Characteristics that suggest a good prognosis include male gender, precipitation of attacks by viral respiratory illness, and children with airway parenchymal dysynapsis (i.e., large lungs but small airways).[30] These children are predominantly male, and, although often atopic, still are likely to outgrow their asthma. In a longitudinal study of children initially 5 to 9 years of age followed over a 13-year period, the effect of asthma on lung growth was different for boys than for girls. Boys with asthma had larger growth in vital capacity than boys without asthma and tended to have mild disease. This was associated with fewer hospitalizations for asthma, despite somewhat greater prevalence than in girls. Asthmatic girls, however, had persistent reductions in FEV_1 and were more likely to be hospitalized for asthma, despite an initially reduced prevalence relative to the boys. These data are consistent with asthma being milder in boys in that the boys are more likely to "outgrow" their asthma. Existing data suggest that atopy per se is not a risk factor for asthma persistence. In older adults, airway responsiveness predicts the development of asthma and antedates and predicts accelerated decline in lung function. Active cigarette smoking also predicts the development of asthma in older adults.[8] Several studies suggest that asthma in adults with or without active cigarette smoking is associated with the development of fixed airflow obstruction.[4] The severity of adult asthma is clearly predicted by the severity of childhood asthma and the persistence of symptoms in childhood and early adulthood is associated with reduced lung function and more severe disease in later adult life.

REFERENCES

1. Bjornsdottir US, Busse WW: Respiratory infections and asthma. *Clin Allergy* 76:895–915, 1992.
2. Broder I, Higgins NW, Matthews KP, et al: Epidemiology of asthma and allergic rhinitis in a total community: Tecumseh, Michigan. III: Second survey of the community. *J Allergy Clin Immunol* 53:127, 1974.
3. Brown RW, Weiss ST: The influences of lower respiratory illness on childhood asthma: Defining risk and susceptibility. *Semin Respir Infect* 6:225–234, 1991.
4. Burrows B, Lebowitz MD, Barbee RA, Cline MG: Findings before diagnoses of asthma among the elderly in a longitudinal study of a general population sample. *J Allergy Clin Immunol* 88:870, 1991.
5. Burrows B, Martinez FD, Halonen M, et al: Association of asthma with serum IgE levels and skin-test reactivity to allergens. *New Eng J Med* 320:271–275, 1989.
6. Busse WM, Banks-Schlegel SP, Larsen GL: NHLBI workshop summary. Childhood- versus adult-onset asthma. *Am J Respir Crit Car Med* 151:1635–1639, 1995.
7. Carey VJ, Weiss ST, Tager IB, et al: Airway responsiveness, wheeze onset and recurrent asthma episodes in young adolescents: The East Boston childhood respiratory disease cohort. *Am J Respir Crit Care Med* 153:356–361, 1996.
8. Dodge RR, Burrows B: The prevalence and incidence of asthma and asthma-like symptoms in a general population sample. *Am Rev Respir Dis* 122:567–571, 1980.
9. Holt PG: Environmental factors and primary T-cell sensitization to inhalant allergens in infancy: reappraisal of the role of infections and air pollution. *Pediatr Allergy Immunol* 6:1–10, 1995.
10. Johnston SL, Pattemore PK, Sanderson G, et al: Community study of role of viral infections in exacerbation of asthma in 9–11 year old children. *Br J Med* 310:1225–1228, 1995.
11. Kramer MS: Does breast feeding help protect against atopic disease? Biology, methodology, and a golden jubilee of controversy. *J Pediatr* 112:181–190, 1988.
12. Martinez FD: Viral infections and the development of asthma. *Am J Respir Crit Care Med* 151:1644–1648, 1995.
13. Martinez FD, Morgan WJ, Wright AL, et al: Diminished lung function as a predisposing factor for wheezing respiratory illness in infants. *New Eng J Med* 319:1112–1117, 1988.
14. Martinez FD, Wright AL, Holberg CJ, et al: Maternal age as a risk factor for wheezing lower respiratory illnesses in the first year of life. *Am J Epidemiol* 136:1258, 1992.
15. Martinez FD, Wright AL, Taussig LM, et al: Asthma and wheezing in the first six years of life. *N Eng J Med* 322:133–137, 1995.
16. National Asthma Education Program, Expert Panel Report. *Guidelines for the Diagnosis and Management of Asthma.* Bethesda, MD, US Dept of Health and Human Services, Pub no 91-3042.
17. Pattemore PK, Johnston SL, Bardin PG: Viruses as precipitants of asthma symptoms: I. Epidemiology. *Clin Exp Allergy* 22:325–336, 1992.
18. Rijcken B, Schouten JP, Weiss ST, et al: The distribution of nonspecific bronchial responsiveness in symptomatic and asymptomatic subjects: a population based analysis of various indices of responsiveness. *Am Rev Respir Dis* 140: 615–623, 1989.
19. Rooney JC, Williams HE: The relationship between proved viral bronchiolitis and subsequent wheezing. *J Pediatr* 79:744–747, 1971.
20. Sears MR, Burrows B, Flannery GP, et al: Relation between airway responsiveness and serum IgE in children with asthma and in apparently normal children. *New Eng J Med* 325:1067–1071, 1991.
21. Sigurs N, Bjarnason R, Sigurbergsson F, et al: Asthma and immunoglobulin E antibodies after respiratory syncytial virus bronchiolitis: a prospective cohort study with matched controls. *Pediatrics* 95:500–505, 1995.
22. Sporik R, Holgate ST, Platts-Mills TAE, Cogswell JJ: Exposure to house-dust mite allergen (Der p1) and the development of asthma in childhood: a prospective study. *N Eng J Med* 323:502–507, 1990.
23. Stark JM, Graziano FM: Lower airway response to viruses, in Busse WW, Holgate ST (eds), *Asthma and Rhinitis.* Boston, Blackwell, 1995, pp 1229–1243.
24. Troisi RJ, Speizer FE, Willett WC, et al: Menopause, postmenopause estrogen preparations, and the risk of adult-onset asthma. A prospective cohort study. *Am J. Respir Crit Care Med* 152:1183–1188, 1995.
25. Von Mutius E, Nicolai T, Martinez FD: Prematurity as a risk factor for asthma in preadolescent children. *J Pediatr* 123:223, 1993.
26. Weiss ST: Smoking and asthma. *Compr Ther* 20:606–610, 1994.
27. Weiss KB, Geigen PJ, Hodgson TA: An economic evaluation of asthma in the United States. *New Eng J Med* 326:862–866, 1992.

28. Weiss ST, O'Connor GT, Sparrow D: The role of allergy and airways responsiveness in the natural history of chronic airflow obstruction, in Weiss ST, Sparrow D (eds), *The Relationship of Airways Responsiveness and Atopy to the Development of the Obstructive Airways Diseases.* New York, Raven, 1989, pp 181–240.

29. Weiss KB, Geigen PJ, Wagener DK: Breathing better or wheezing worse? The changing epidemiology of asthma morbidity and mortality. *Am Rev Pub Health* 14:491–513, 1993.

30. Weiss ST, Segal MR, Tager IB, et al: Effects of asthma on pulmonary function in children: a longitudinal population-based study. *Am Rev Respir Dis* 145:58–64, 1992.

31. Zhong NS, Chang CR, Yang MO, et al: Is asymptomatic bronchial hyperresponsiveness an indication of potential asthma? *Chest* 102:1104–1109, 1992.

CHAPTER 49

ASPIRIN- AND EXERCISE-INDUCED ASTHMA

Gregory P. Geba

Asthma is well known to be triggered by specific immune factors such as aeroallergen exposures. There are, however, several important nonallergic triggers for the development of asthmatic bronchial obstruction. Two of the most important of these are aspirin-induced asthma and exercise-induced asthma. Both of these airway responses can occur in the setting of established aeroallergen-induced asthma or, in some cases, seem to occur in isolation. These two nonspecific triggers may also share some pathophysiological mechanisms, including possible mast cell and leukotriene mediation and the contribution of vascular responses to the airway narrowing.

ASPIRIN-INDUCED ASTHMA

Introduction

It is believed that aspirin-induced asthma (AIA) was first reported by Hirschberg in 1902. More than 60 years later, the association between aspirin sensitivity, asthma, and nasal polyps was recognized in a classic paper by Samter and Beer.[35] As early as 1928, the clinical importance of sensitivity to aspirin was highlighted by van Leewen, who challenged 100 asthmatics with aspirin, provoking bronchoconstriction in 16. Several others[37,50] have made similar observations, noting that the prevalence of aspirin sensitivity in asthmatics ranges from 5 percent to as high as 30 percent, depending on the characteristics of the asthmatics studied (severity increases risk) and the criteria applied to make the diagnosis.

Aspirin was originally recognized as the most important drug capable of precipitating asthma. With the development of other analgesic and nonsteroidal anti-inflammatory drugs (NSAIDs) after 1950, these related agents were also found to be implicated in asthma exacerbations. In a study of 781 asthmatics observed over a period of 2 years, drugs were noted to precipitate asthma in 10.5 percent of patients.[21] Reactions to NSAIDs were thought to be responsible for 77 percent of all cases, with aspirin accounting for two-thirds of the reactions to NSAIDs, or nearly 50 percent of all cases of drug-induced asthma. Thus, although aspirin is the most common drug to induce asthma and the most common NSAID to cause asthma, other NSAIDs are responsible for an important number of these reactions.

Clinical Presentation

Reactions to aspirin can take two distinct forms: *cutaneous,* leading to urticaria and angioedema, and *respiratory,* resulting in rhinoconjunctivitis and bronchospasm.[43] In the former, a subpopulation of patients with established urticaria experience cutaneous flares of hives with or without angioedema after ingesting NSAIDs. Almost all of these patients were able to ingest the same NSAIDs before the development of urticaria, suggesting that the NSAIDs interact with an underlying urticarial process but do not directly and independently cause the hives. Therefore, avoiding NSAID ingestion does not eliminate the urticarial syndromes experienced by these patients. In contrast, only a small subgroup of patients has hives exclusively *after* exposure to these drugs, without a history of underlying chronic urticaria. It is postulated, although not proven, that such patients manifest IgE-mediated immune responses to some NSAID-related antigen. NSAID avoidance is an effective treatment for urticaria in these patients.

The upper (nasal) and lower (asthma) respiratory manifestations of aspirin sensitivity are generally linked, although sometimes upper respiratory symptoms precede the development of lower respiratory asthmatic reactions to these agents. Patients usually develop a viruslike upper respiratory tract illness. This is followed by inflammation of the nasal mucosa and paranasal sinuses, which becomes chronic. This chronic inflammation is characterized by impressive eosinophilic infiltration and, with time, may lead to the development of nasal polyps. Although nasal polyps are noted as part of the classic triad, it is becoming increasingly evident that polyps are at times *absent,* and almost all cases present with sinusitis. Opacification of one or more sinuses on plain radiographs can be seen in more than 90 percent of these patients.[41,43]

Contrasting with classic atopic asthma, which patients usually develop before the age of 20, AIA generally occurs in people in the fourth decade of life. In general, these patients do not have a history of sensitivity to NSAIDs. Familial predisposition is also rare, with one study noting a positive family history in only 2 of 500 patients.[44] Men and women are affected equally. No confirmed association has been made to HLA type, although one study showed an increase in the expression of HLA-DQw2 in one group of such patients.[30] Aeroallergen skin testing of these patients is usually negative, and IgE levels are normal. The search for NSAID-specific IgEs has been unsuccessful. After acute challenge with aspirin, such patients do not develop blood eosinophilia and fail to produce detectable elevations of blood histamine or complement activity, as seen with acute allergen challenge of atopic asthmatics. All of this suggests that nonatopic mechanisms are responsible for the development of this syndrome.

The typical reaction after aspirin ingestion by these patients is the slow development (within one-half to 4 h, mean 50 min) of nasal congestion with profuse rhinorrhea, cutaneous flushing of the head and neck, mild conjunctivitis, and bronchial obstruction, usually manifested as wheezing. A typical reaction provoked by an oral challenge under laboratory conditions is illustrated in Fig. 49-1. In severe reactions, headache, nausea, and vomiting and acute hypercarbic respiratory failure culminating in death can occur. Life-threatening responses with faster kinetics have also been reported with systemically administered NSAIDs such as ketorolac.[20] Combined cutaneous and respiratory reactions (i.e., true urticarial eruptions in association with asthma) occur in less than 3 percent of cases.[41]

Cross-Reactivity

Cross-reactivity of aspirin with other NSAIDs was first recognized in 1967 by Vanselow and Smith.[49] This was followed by reports of reactions to other structurally unrelated NSAIDs, which suggested that these reactions were not atopic. It was subsequently shown that the ability of these drugs to provoke asthma in susceptible patients was related to their ability to inhibit cyclooxygenase and that the degree of cross-reactivity with aspirin was related to the degree to which these agents inhibited cyclooxygenase in vitro.[45,46] Conversely, drugs that do not inhibit cyclooxygenase but are structurally related to aspirin (e.g., sodium salicylate) do not provoke AIA. A partial list of NSAIDs reported to provoke asthma is given in Table 49-1.

A number of analgesics have long been thought to be well tolerated in patients with AIA. They are listed in Table 49-1. However, some analgesics formerly considered safe for use by these patients have recently been shown to be capable of provoking bronchospasm if given in large doses. For example, in doses of 600 to 1000 mg, acetaminophen can provoke significant declines in FEV_1 in some aspirin-sensitive asthmatics. Of interest is that desensitization with increasing doses of aspirin *prevented* bronchospasm after ingestion of these agents.[41,43] This suggests that the reactions are also mediated by the weak ability of these agents to inhibit cyclooxygenase.

Although it was initially believed that tartrazine dyes were capable of provoking asthma exacerbations in patients with AIA, this has not been confirmed on further study.[38] Tartrazine doses of 25 to 50 mg, on double-blind challenge of patients with proven AIA, did not provoke detectable changes in lung function. This supports the view that tartrazine intolerance is extremely rare and that true cross-reactivity with aspirin probably does not exist. Similar conclusions can be drawn regarding the cross-reactivity of other FD&C dyes, sodium benzoate, other benzoic acid derivatives, monosodium glutamate, and sodium and potassium sulfites.

An interesting association of AIA with sensitivity to hydrocortisone has been made. Several case reports[8,11,24] were followed by two larger studies[12,13] demonstrating that a small percentage of patients with aspirin-induced asthma may experience acute bronchospasm (15 to 30 min) after the intravenous or intramuscular injection of hydrocortisone. The vehicles and diluents used in the hydrocortisone preparations could

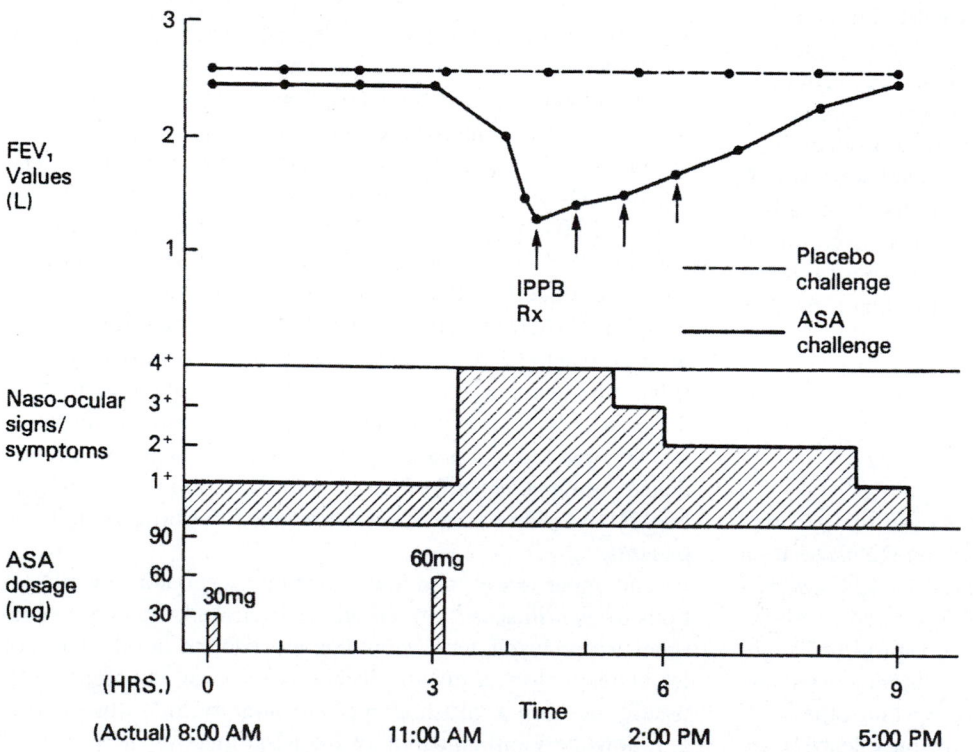

FIGURE 49-1   Typical reaction to aspirin in AIA. The time line illustrates the kinetics of respiratory compromise and naso-ocular symptoms after graded aspirin or placebo challenge. IPPB = intermittent positive-pressure ventilation with beta-adrenergic agonist bronchodilator. *(Based on data of Stevenson DD, Simon RA,[43] with permission.)*

TABLE 49-1

NSAIDs in Aspirin-Induced Asthma

NSAIDs That Can Provoke Airway Narrowing in AIA
  Carboxylic Acids
    Salicylates
      Acetylsalicylic acid (aspirin, Easpirin, Zorpin)
    Acetic Acids
      Indomethacin (Indocin)
      Sulindac (Clinoril)
      Tolmentin (Tolectin)
      Dicolfenac (Voltaren)
      Ketorolac (Toradol)
      Zomepirac (Zomax)
    Proprionic acids
      Ibuprofen (Motrin, Advil, Nuprin)
      Naproxen (Naprosyn)
    Fenamates
      Meclofenamate (Meclomen)
      Mefenamic acid (Ponstel)
    Enolic acids
      Piroxicam (Feldene)
NSAIDs and Analgesics That Appear to Be Well Tolerated in AIA
  Sodium salicylate
  Choline salicylate
  Salicylamide
  Dextropropoxyphene
  Acetaminophen in low doses

clooxygenase-dependent pathways of arachidonic acid metabolism (Fig. 49-2). Others are based on the release of other mediators, most likely from mast cells, basophils, or platelets. These theories include up-regulation of mast cell–basophil mediator releasability by substances not yet identified that affect mast cell membranes, increased histamine production by basophils of patients with aspirin-induced asthma in comparison to normal subjects, decreased production of prostaglandin E2 (PGE2) and enhanced production of leukotriene B4 (LTB4) by AIA basophils, and enhanced aspirin-induced release of serotonin and other mediators by AIA platelets.[1,43] It has been proposed that complement activation[48] may be important in these processes. However, the role of complement activation in AIA has been questioned by data showing no significant changes in CH50 and C4 levels in patients experiencing asthma exacerbation after acute oral aspirin challenge.[33]

Alterations in arachidonic acid metabolism appear to play a central role in AIA. The major pathways of cyclooxygenase and lipoxygenase metabolism of arachidonic acid are illustrated in Fig. 49-2. Arachidonic acid is derived from membrane phospholipids by phospholipase A2. It is then metabolized via the cyclooxygenase pathway to prostaglandins and thromboxanes or via the lipoxygenase pathway to sulfidopeptide (cysteinyl) leukotrienes. The leukotrienes have a variety of effects, including the induction of contraction of bronchial smooth muscle. In contrast, the prostaglandins, in particular PGE2, act as bronchodilators and may inhibit T cell–mediated inflammatory responses in the lung. Aspirin and the other NSAIDs that cause AIA inhibit cyclooxygenase activity. A shift occurs after the administration of aspirin or appropriate doses of these other agents, shunting approxi-

not be linked to the reactivity. One of these studies showed no bronchoconstrictor response to methylprenisolone, dexamethasone, or betamethasone given intravenously,[47] demonstrating that these potent anti-inflammatory steroid preparations, related to hydrocortisone and differing in side chain chemical structure, could be used safely. The mechanism of this reaction is not known.

Pathogenesis

The pathophysiological basis of aspirin-induced asthma has been a subject of considerable study. As a result, our knowledge of the pathogenesis of the disorder has improved immensely, and new therapeutic approaches that may be useful in the treatment of AIA have been identified. Several theories have been proposed to account for the phenomenon. The major theory is based on alterations in the balance between leukotrienes and prostaglandins generated by the lipoxygenase- and cy-

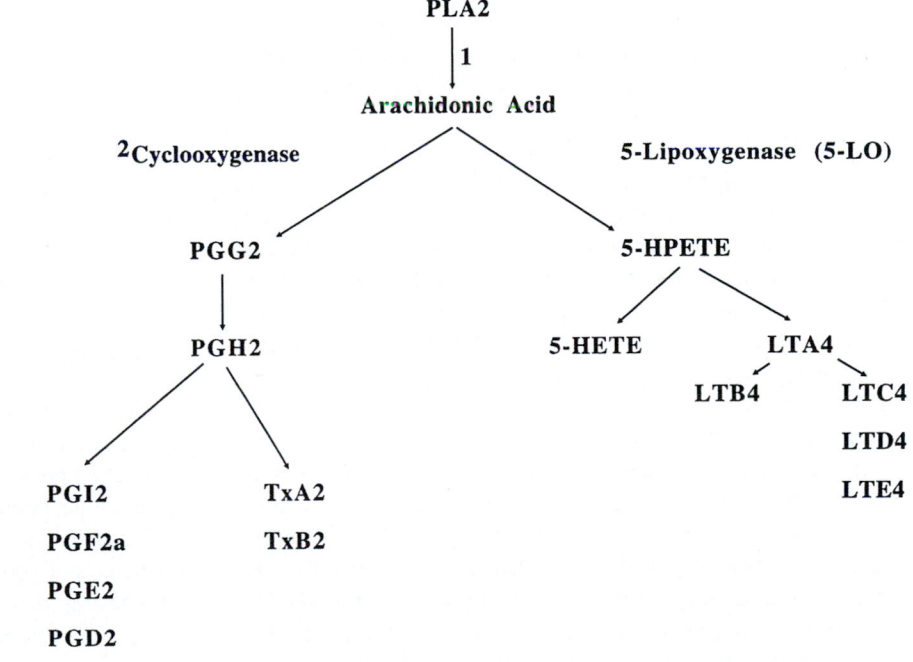

1 Locus of action of corticosteroids

2 Locus of action of NSAIDS that inhibit cyclooxygenase

FIGURE 49-2   Major pathways of arachidonic acid metabolism. The loci of action of corticosteroids (1) and NSAIDs that induce AIA (2) are noted.

mately 90 percent of the arachidonic acid metabolism to the 5-lipoxygenase pathway, decreasing prostaglandin and thromboxane production, and increasing leukotriene generation. In comparison to normal persons, patients with AIA generate leukotrienes in exaggerated quantities after aspirin challenge. They may also be more sensitive than normal subjects to the bronchoconstrictor properties of leukotrienes (particularly LTE_4) and more susceptible to the loss of the bronchodilating and potentially anti-inflammatory effects of PGE_2. The data supporting these conclusions are briefly summarized below.

Several groups have analyzed the nasal lavage fluid from aspirin-sensitive and control patients and found inducible levels of cysteinyl leukotrienes and plasma proteins when patients with AIA received oral or nasal aspirin challenges.[17,26] One study[26] found that LTC_4 and LTD_4 levels were not significantly induced in normal subjects, but could be mildly induced in patients with allergic rhinitis and in those with isolated nasal polyps (rising 93 and 69 percent above baseline levels, respectively). In contrast, the levels rose most dramatically in patients with AIA (211 percent above baseline levels). Similarly, although histamine levels rose significantly in the AIA, nasal polyp, and allergic rhinitis groups, the rise was highest in the AIA group. The protein levels also rose in the AIA group (greater than threefold increase in total protein) but did not rise significantly in the control groups. Analysis of the nasal lavage fluids showed impressive increases in lactoferrin and lysozyme, suggesting that submucosal glands are stimulated in this process.

In a follow-up study,[17] the cellular source of these nasal abnormalities was investigated by analysis of nasal lavage fluids induced by aspirin challenge for the presence of mast cell tryptase and eosinophil cationic protein (ECP). Significant increases in nasal tryptase, histamine, and cysteinyl leukotrienes were observed after AIA was provoked in these patients. ECP levels at baseline were variable and did not increase significantly after challenge. These results support the notion that after aspirin challenge, the leukotrienes in the nasal secretions of patients with AIA are probably of mast cell origin. They also suggest that eosinophils are not as important as mast cells in the pathogenesis of the nasal manifestations of AIA. These findings are consistent with earlier work[20] that showed similar increases in *blood* tryptase (4 h) and *urinary* LTE_4 levels (6 h) and decreases in blood eosinophil counts ($p < 0.01$) (6 h) after aspirin challenge.

The metabolism of arachidonic acid in the lung has not been studied as extensively. The available data show both similarities and differences with findings in the nose and circulation. For example, bronchoalveolar lavage fluid (BALF) obtained 30 min after inhalation of threshold doses of lysine-aspirin contained depressed levels of cyclooxygenase-dependent mediators [PGE_2, PGD_2, thromboxane B_2 (TXB_2), and $PGF_{2\alpha}$]. However, only small increases in LTE_4 and 5-hydroxyeicosatetraenoic acid (HETE) levels were noted. Lysine-aspirin inhalation also did not produce a significant rise in tryptase levels in BALF and led to a significant fall in ECP levels despite baseline eosinophil and ECP levels, which were higher in the AIA group than in the placebo-treated nonasthmatics.[38] The authors postulated that the altered pulmonary eicosanoid production might be related to the unequivocal eosinophilic inflammation in the airways of patients with AIA.

To further dissect the mechanism of bronchospasm in AIA, a number of investigators have used newly developed inhibitors of leukotriene effector function. The first administered a specific sulfidopeptide leukotriene receptor antagonist via inhalation and noted that it attenuated aspirin-induced asthma in five of six subjects by 43 to 74 percent.[8] This was followed by a double-blind, placebo-controlled, crossover study that showed that a specific leukotriene receptor antagonist given as a single oral dose 1 h before peri-threshold lysine-aspirin inhalant provocative challenge could almost completely block the development of aspirin-induced bronchospasm.[11] This was achieved without evidence of any direct bronchodilatory effect of the drug before lysine-aspirin challenge, confirming that leukotriene antagonism could prevent AIA. Similarly, another leukotriene receptor antagonist has been shown to be effective in preventing analgesic-induced (dipyrone) bronchospasm.

Leukotriene effects in the lung can also be modulated by blocking 5-lipoxygenase activity. The efficacy of this approach was demonstrated in a randomized, double-blind, crossover study in which the 5-lipoxygenase inhibitor Zileuton (600 mg orally, four times a day, for 6 to 8 days before aspirin challenge) led to a greater than 70 percent reduction in baseline urinary LTE_4 excretion, a greater than 60 percent reduction in mean maximal urinary concentration of LTE_4 after aspirin challenge, and almost complete suppression of subthreshold and threshold oral aspirin–induced bronchospasm.[24] In addition, naso-ocular, gastrointestinal, and dermal symptoms were reduced to the levels of symptoms produced by placebo challenge.

In summary, although the mechanism of AIA remains incompletely understood, there appears to be a clear role for lipoxygenase products in the pathogenesis of the disorder. The available data also suggest that mast cells, stimulated by aspirin directly or indirectly, discharge their leukotriene mediators in large amounts into nasal secretions but may not play a similarly significant role in the lung. The presence of increased numbers of eosinophils is also a feature of the airways of these patients. This probably reflects their recruitment secondary to the release of mast cell–derived mediators, including leukotrienes and cytokines. These cells may also contribute to the pathogenesis of the airway symptoms experienced by these patients.

Diagnosis

Although some promise exists for the development of in vitro tests to identify patients with this disorder based on differential platelet responses to aspirin and NSAIDs in vitro, these methods have not yet been validated for routine use.[1] For this reason, AIA is still diagnosed by in vivo testing with placebo-controlled oral challenges of persons suspected to have this disorder (Table 49-2). This testing can be performed according to published protocols using single-blind or double-blind approaches. These protocols generally begin with 3-mg doses of aspirin; the dosage is then increased to a maximum of 650 mg over a 3-day period. Spirometric pulmonary function is serially monitored during the challenge to assess the degree of bronchial obstruction. Airway reactivity to methacholine is not a viable surrogate for spirometry, since aspirin does not consistently alter methacholine sensitivity. The protocol can be individualized by the physician with

TABLE 49-2

Diagnosis of Aspirin-Induced Asthma: Aspirin Challenge Protocols

Single-Blind Oral 3-Day Aspirin Challenge

Time	1	2	3
		Test days	
0	Placebo	ASA 3 or 30 mg	ASA 150 mg
+3 h	Placebo	ASA 60 mg	ASA 325 mg
+6 h	Placebo	ASA 100 mg	ASA 600 mg

Double-Blind Oral Aspirin Challenge

Both tester and patient are blinded to eliminate potential bias.

Bronchial Challenge with Lysine-Aspirin

Time (Minutes)	Challenge (Lysine-aspirin in mg/ml)
0	Placebo
45	Placebo
90	11.25
135	22.5
180	45
225	90
270	180
315	360
350	360 (10 breaths)

Patients receive four breaths of all doses of lysine-aspirin unless otherwise indicated.

SOURCE: Data from Stevenson DD, Simon RA: Sensitivity to aspirin and nonsteroidal antiinflammatory drugs, in Middleton E Jr, Reed CE, Ellis EF (ed), *Allergy: Principles and Practice.* St. Louis, CV Mosby, 1993; Phillips GD, Foord R, Holgate ST: Inhaled lysine-apirin as a bronchoprovocation procedure in aspirin-sensitive asthma: Its repeatibility, absence of a late-phase reaction, and the role of histamine. *J Allergy Clin Immunol* 84:232–241, 1989.

respect to the doses of aspirin given and their timing. This challenge procedure should probably be reserved for use in research centers experienced in its application and adverse effects. An alternative to oral challenge, used in some centers in Europe for the diagnosis of AIA, is the inhalation of stabilized lysine-aspirin (discussed above). Inhalation is administered in increasing doses, and sequential spirometric and clinical evaluation is made akin to that used for methacholine challenge. However, this drug is not currently available for clinical use in the United States.

Treatment

Optimal treatment of patients with AIA requires knowledge of the proper approaches to treat acute aspirin-induced bronchial symptoms and associated nasal and sinus pathology. No specific therapy can yet be recommended for the routine treatment of acute bronchospasm provoked by NSAIDs. It has been stated that corticosteroids are not effective after acute aspirin ingestion, and that theophylline and cromolyn sodium play no definite role.[43] Treatment of symptoms after acute ingestion relies mainly on beta-adrenergic agonists to reverse bronchospasm, and topical vasoconstrictors for both nasal congestion and eye symptoms. Frequent applications of these agents usually are

necessary to maintain nasal and airway potency over the 2- to 6-h reaction duration.

On a chronic basis, the treatment of AIA depends on the correct diagnosis and avoidance of aspirin and other cyclooxygenase inhibitors that could cross-react to induce acute bronchospasm. Patients should be instructed that many over-the-counter medications contain aspirin or other NSAIDs, and they should carefully read package inserts before using any medication. Currently there also appears to be no clear role for systemic corticosteroids or theophylline in the prevention of AIA.

Drug treatment of AIA should focus on treating the underlying asthma and the strict avoidance of aspirin and cross-reacting NSAIDs. Some investigators have found that antihistamines such as clemastine and mast cell stabilizers such as ketotifen and cromolyn can have prophylactic efficacy. However, not all subjects on these drugs are protected against bronchoconstriction after aspirin challenge. The new leukotriene receptor antagonists and 5-lipoxygenase inhibitors, still in phase three trials, will soon be available for use in the prevention of aspirin-induced symptoms. Whether these drugs will prove to be useful in the routine management of these patients remains to be seen.

In cases in which aspirin (or cross-reacting NSAIDs) cannot be avoided or the efficacy of prophylactic measures cannot be assured, aspirin "desensitization" can be considered. Protocols are available for selected patients (Fig. 49-3).[34] These methods can effectively protect many patients from experiencing symptoms on exposure to aspirin or NSAIDs and will maintain this level of desensitization as long as aspirin is ingested indefinitely at doses of 325 to 650 mg a day. In a study of 25 aspirin-sensitive asthmatics, such therapy has been shown to reduce nasal symptoms by 67 percent and asthma severity by 48 percent.[34,42] Larger studies are planned to confirm this finding. It is interesting to note that although there are some reports of increased methacholine reactivity developing in patients soon after aspirin challenge,[8] baseline methacholine responsiveness does not seem to be successfully down-regulated by aspirin desensitization. Also, there is no evidence that aspirin desensitization leads to abatement in skin disease in those with aspirin-urticaria syndrome.

The ability of chronic sinusitis to contribute to asthmatic exacerbations is well established. Aspirin sensitivity, chronic sinusitis, and nasal polyposis are well documented to coexist in AIA. Thus, the presence of these upper-airway disorders must be considered in patients with AIA and effective treatment instituted if they are identified. High-dose topical intranasal corticosteroids can shrink polyp tissue and prevent obstruction of nasal passageways. In the setting of chronic sinusitis, standard approaches—including topical vasoconstrictors, antihistamines, and antibiotics–should also be utilized. Surgery to drain sinuses and remove polyps has been shown to be effective in the short term; however, polyps can regrow and the sinusitis often recurs.[40]

EXERCISE AND ASTHMA

Introduction

The first report of exercise-induced asthma (EIA) is attributed to John Floyer in 1698.[18] After a lull of nearly 300 years, interest in this subject grew when it was recognized that exercise or hy-

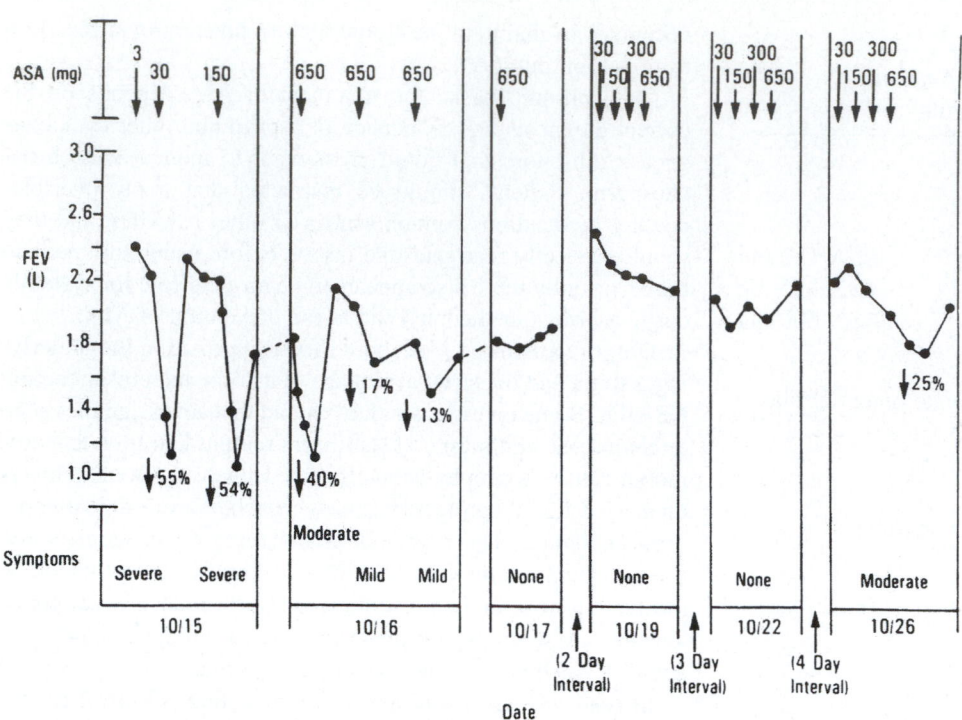

FIGURE 49-3 Airway desensitization to aspirin challenge in AIA. Timeline of respiratory function and overall symptoms after serial aspirin dosing. The reappearance of respiratory compromise and symptoms after 4 days without aspirin shows the need for continuous aspirin administration to maintain desensitized state. *(Based on data of Pleskow WW et al,*[34] *with permission.)*

perventilation could provoke asthma attacks. EIA can be defined as a condition in which vigorous physical activity triggers acute airway narrowing in persons with heightened airway reactivity.[29] It appears that EIA is always associated with an asthmatic diathesis, although EIA can be seen before other characteristic features of asthma emerge. Various reports indicate that EIA is common, affecting between 50 and 90 percent of all asthmatics[25] and 40 percent of patients with allergic rhinitis without known asthma.[10] Some have suggested that all asthmatics can be shown to manifest airway narrowing to thermal provocations of sufficient intensity, whether induced by exercise or hyperventilation. Other susceptible persons are first-degree relatives of asthmatics, atopic "nonasthmatics," and patients with cystic fibrosis. In contrast, airway narrowing to similar stimuli does not occur in normal subjects.

Clinical Presentation

Patients with EIA generally manifest a series of fairly predictable symptoms and alterations in pulmonary function that can be assessed by laboratory testing (Fig. 49-4). Normal persons and asthmatics generally first respond to exercise by bronchodilation, probably mediated by the release of catecholamines.[5] This response is short-lived, peaking at midexercise, and is followed by return of normal baseline airway tone at the end of exercise. In patients with EIA, the transient bronchodilation and reversal are followed by bronchoconstriction coincident with symptoms of cough, wheezing, dyspnea, and chest tightness typical of asthmatic attacks. Typically, when they are provoked with a brief,

intense exercise period in the laboratory, maximal bronchoconstriction occurs 5 to 10 min after the cessation of exercise and lasts for 30 to 60 min (Fig. 49-4). Rarely does this form of bronchconstriction result in ventilatory failure, although it can limit the performance of trained athletes.

In addition to asthma after exercise, many athletes describe dyspnea during exercise. If these athletes are able to continue to exercise despite the initial airway obstruction, especially if they are able to increase their level of activity, relief of bronchoconstriction often occurs. This is associated with symptomatic improvement with time that is described as "running through the attack." The development of dyspnea during exercise is ostensibly related to the development of bronchoconstriction at lower work intensities (simulating a postexercise state), which is reversed by interval training at higher intensities (simulating an exercise state). This has been taken as evidence that airway function during exercise reflects a balance between bronchoconstrictor and protective bronchodilator influences, and that this balance can be influenced by rapid changes in exercise intensity.[5]

The reproducibility of EIA is highly dependent on the specific characteristics of the stimulus and patient-related factors. The net influence of exercise intensity, the temperature and humidity of the inspired air, and the patient's baseline airway reactivity are fundamental in determining whether exercise will lead to bron-

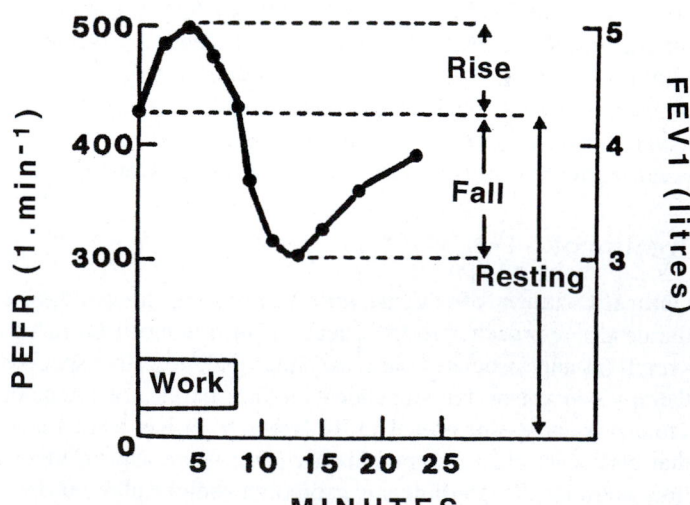

FIGURE 49-4 Typical pulmonary function changes induced by exercise in EIA. Transient bronchodilitation during exercise and bronchospasm after exercise are noted. *(Based on data of Anderson SD,*[2] *with permission.)*

choconstriction. If asthma is better controlled at baseline, EIA may be more difficult to provoke. If climatic conditions vary, even though asthma is not well controlled, EIA may fail to develop. Classic work has shown that for a fixed minute ventilation, cold, dry air inspired during exercise is more likely to provoke EIA than warm, humid air.[4] Thus, EIA is more likely to occur with jogging during the winter than with swimming indoors.

It is interesting that about 50 percent of patients with EIA will not manifest a bronchoconstrictor response after exercise if rechallenged with the same stimulus within 60 min. Neither baseline airway obstruction nor the degree of obstruction provoked by exercise can be used to determine who will be refractory to repeated exercise challenges. After 3 h, even patients who are refractory to repeated challenge will again respond to exercise with bronchoconstriction.

Pathophysiology

The mechanisms associated with exercise-induced bronchoconstriction have been studied intensively over the past 2 decades. Despite this intense scrutiny, the pathophysiology of this response is still a subject of considerable debate. Three principal, non–mutually exclusive, potential pathogenetic schema have emerged from these studies. They focus on the roles of heat exchange and water loss, inflammation, and leukotriene mediators.

Heat Exchange and Water Loss   During tidal breathing, heat (via conduction and evaporation) and water (via evaporation) are transferred from the mucosa of the upper airways to the entering air. Since exercise requires marked increases in minute ventilation, surpassing the volume of air that can be inspired through nasal structures, air enters directly through the mouth, bypassing the normal warming and conditioning function of the nose. The lower respiratory mucosa then attempts to compensate for the function of the bypassed nose. Heat and water fluxes first occur. The lower airways are then subject to rewarming by warm blood carried by the bronchial circulation.

In the late 1970s, a number of investigators postulated that EIA was the result of increased heat loss in the airway. This was based on the observation that cold, dry air caused a greater fall in FEV_1 than did hot, dry air[13] and on correlations between heat exchange and the degree of bronchoconstriction. Others, however, showed that the temperature of the inspired air was not crucial to inducing bronchoconstriction and that temperatures of dry inspired air varying as much as 60° could still provoke airway narrowing.[3,19] This suggested that airway evaporative water loss might be more important than airway cooling. The water loss was predicted to change the osmolarity of the cellular and extracellular components of the airway wall, stimulating increased bronchial blood flow in order to increase the delivery of water.[2] Additionally, bronchial wall hyperosmolarity was hypothesized to increase the release of proinflammatory mediators from resident airway inflammatory cells such as mast cells.[13] This concept was supported by work that demonstrated that changes in the humidity of inspired air, and not temperature, determine the magnitude of EIA. Further support came from studies using cold gas mixtures with different water-carrying capacities, which showed a significant correlation between evaporative heat loss

but not total heat loss or temperature gradient on the airway response.[22] In apparent contrast to these data is the considerable body of work that does not support the concept that osmolar changes precipitate EIA. The most important of these showed that increasing minute ventilation at constant humidity increases the severity of EIA.[10]

An important theory that also remains to be unequivocally proven is that offered by McFadden.[28] He proposed that the process of airway rewarming is active in the pathogenesis of the airway narrowing that occurs in EIA. This theory postulates that loss of heat associated with exercise transiently leads to decreased bronchial blood flow. At the end of exercise, the bronchi undergo reactive hyperemia characterized by vascular engorgement, which leads to airway caliber compromise and airway wall edema. The strongest support for this theory arises from studies showing that the severity of EIA could be controlled by regulation of the thermal gradient during exercise and the rate of rewarming after exercise.

In summary, there is evidence that associates exercise-induced bronchoconstriction with a sequence of events that includes heat loss, water loss, and airway rewarming. The degree to which these temperature and water alterations contribute to the pathogenesis of EIA is still, however, a topic of significant controversy.

Inflammation and EIA   Theories postulating a role for inflammatory mediators in the pathogenesis of EIA follow in the wake of evidence supporting a role for inflammation in the pathogenesis of other forms of asthma. The data as they relate to EIA still should be regarded as controversial, however, since there is considerable discrepancy in the protocols employed and the findings reported by various groups. One study analyzing the characteristics of BALF from patients with EIA 12 min after exercise failed to find evidence for mast cell mediator release since BAL histamine, tryptase, LTC_4, and PGD_2 levels were not altered. Similarly, studies performed 1 h and 25 h after exercise did not reveal significant differences in BAL cellularity or in histamine or tryptase levels. In contrast, BAL studies performed 3 h after exercise showed mildly increased airway eosinophilia and mast cell degranulation. Interpretation of these findings is confounded by the limited amount of information that is available and the incomplete kinetic evaluations that have been performed to date. Additional investigation will be required to directly assess the presence and potential role of inflammatory cells in EIA.

Leukotrienes in EIA   To determine whether leukotrienes play a role in the pathogenesis of EIA, LTD_4 receptor antagonists and 5-lipoxygenase inhibitors have been employed. Studies using an intravenous LTD_4 receptor antagonist 20 min before exercise demonstrated significant attenuation of the maximal provoked bronchconstriction and mean time to recover from bronchoconstriction (8 min for the treatment group versus 33 min for placebo).[27] Similar results were noted by others using oral or inhaled leukotriene antagonists. In general, although the protection was relatively small, it was significant and equivalent in potency to inhaled cromolyn.

The results obtained with peptidoleukotriene antagonists are consistent with those obtained when the effects of a 5-lipoxygenase inhibitor on bronchoconstriction induced by cold, dry air were evaluated. In the most important study of this kind,[23] a 5-lipoxygenase antagonist was as effective as cromlyn or tert-butaline in augmenting respiratory heat exchange. Thus, leukotrienes may well be active in the pathogenesis of EIA.

Differential Diagnosis

The diagnosis of EIA is accomplished most accurately by employing well-established exercise protocols coupled with pulmonary function testing. However, patients are commonly given a presumptive diagnosis based on their history and physical examination. Important points in the history include the level and type of exercise that provokes asthma, the timing of symptom onset, situations that modify symptom onset, and the precise symptoms experienced. Many of the symptoms of EIA can mimic other conditions that would require an entirely different therapeutic approach (Table 49-3). For example, chest tightness with exercise should be unequivocally distinguished from coronary ischemia. Other cardiac disorders that can mimic EIA are arrhythmias, cardiomyopathies, atrial myxoma, and mitral valve prolapse, all of which can manifest with dyspnea and wheezing. The presence of a murmur, click, or other findings on physical examination should help to identify patients with these conditions. Exercise-induced anaphylaxis can also mimic EIA but will generally exhibit skin manifestations (urticaria), and respiratory symptoms will be less prominent. Two other conditions that have been reported to mimic EIA are fixed glottal and tracheal obstruction, which become noticeable with the increased ventilation of exercise and exercise-induced vocal cord/arytenoid dysfunction that is not present at rest. Some have also suggested that panic disorders and the excessive tachypnea associated with deconditioning can be confused with EIA, especially in atopic or asthmatic subjects.[10] In contrast to EIA, symptoms due to these other conditions generally are greatest *during* exercise provocation rather than afterward, when airflow limitation due to EIA usually reaches its peak.

Exercise-induced cough is another phenomenon that can mimic EIA. Both may be induced by changes in the osmolarity of the airways reflecting water loss from the respiratory tract during exercise.[6] The inhalation of humid air also prevents both phenomena. However, EIA and exercise-induced cough respond differently to beta-adrenergic agonists, suggesting that they are mediated by different underlying mechanisms. It is postulated that exercise-induced cough is the direct result of the osmolarity changes provoked by airway drying, whereas EIA is due to the mediator release that results from the process of airway drying. Therefore, although nearly all patients with EIA cough with exercise provocation, there are patients who have exercise-induced cough without bronchospasm, and thus do not have EIA.

Physiological Documentation

To formally diagnose EIA, the clinician needs to document airflow obstruction that reaches a peak just after provocation, during the recovery period. Two basic methods of provocation have been used, exercise and the inhalation of dry air (isocapnic hyperventilation, ISH). The latter is an acceptable surrogate for exercise, since the bronchoconstriction it induces is similar to that induced by exercise in terms of magnitude, time course, and refractory period. However, significant differences exist between the two provocation techniques. Exercise provocation, whether performed on an ergometer or a treadmill, leads to significantly greater increases in heart rate, metabolic rate, and oxygen consumption. Exercise, but not ISH, is accompanied by increased numbers of circulating basophils and increased circulating catecholamines and cAMP.[3] The differences in the last two parameters probably explain why the bronchodilatory response that characterizes exercise is not provoked by ISH. ISH does, however, have a number of advantages over exercise. The first relates to the ease with which the ISH protocol can be standardized; the other relates to the finding that oxygen consumption and heart rate are not increased with ISH. As a result, ISH is useful in differentiating EIA from occult cardiac disease and is especially valuable when elderly or cardiac patients are being evaluated.

The most commonly used protocol for the diagnosis of EIA in the United States is that published by O'Byrne and colleagues[31] and modified by Philips and coworkers (Fig. 49-5).[32] This is accomplished by registering changes in pulmonary function in response to varying rates of ventilation using dry air with a fixed CO_2 content of 4.9 percent to maintain isocapnia. Each ventilatory challenge is performed for 3 min, with spirometry performed at intervals thereafter (usually 2, 5, and 10 min after the end of hyperventilation). Serial increases in hyperventilation are performed until maximal voluntary ventilation is reached. If the FEV_1 falls 10 to 20 percent after provocation, the test is considered positive, confirming the diagnosis of EIA. Although some have pointed out that it is not necessary to condition air to subfreezing temperatures in order to perform the test, Scandinavian investigators showed that assessing bronchoconstrictor responses to whole-body exposure to very cold air resulted in a significant increase in the number of asthmatic patients who experienced bronchconstriction.

In order to optimize the validity, repeatability, and practicality of exercise testing for the diagnosis of EIA, a variety of testing protocols have been pursued. Unfortunately, the criteria used to define a positive test in these different studies were, at times,

---

TABLE 49-3

Differential Diagnosis of Exercise-Induced Asthma

Cardiac disease	Functional abnormalities
Coronary ischemia	Vocal cord dysfunction
Mitral valve prolapse	Panic disorders
Atrial myxoma	
Cardiomyopathy	General
Arrythmias	Deconditioning
	Anemia
Lung disease	
Fixed airway obstruction	
Interstitial lung disease	
Exercise-induced cough	

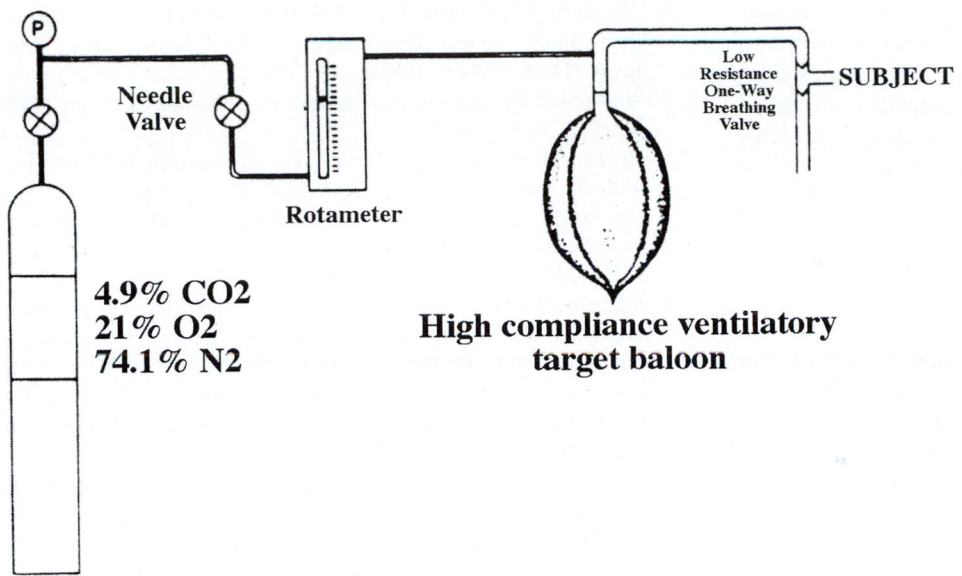

FIGURE 49-5   Apparatus for isocapnic hyperventilation challenge to diagnose EIA. (*Based on data of Philips YY et al,[32] with permission.*)

arbitrary. This has confounded interpretation of these evaluations and comparisons between patient populations. This suggests that the optimal diagnostic algorithm for the assessment of EIA is still lacking.[9]

In addition to the difficulties inherent in the standardization of the challenge protocol, the clinician must be aware of situations that can lead to false-negative evaluations. Specifically, it is important that all drugs that can potentially attenuate bronchoconstrictor responses—such as calcium channel blockers, methylxanthines, cromolyn, and beta-adrenergic agonists—are discontinued for a sufficient period before the evaluation.

Treatment

The treatment of EIA depends, in part, on the treatment of the underlying asthma, since, in general, patients with more severe baseline asthma are most inconvenienced by EIA (Table 49-4). It has been shown that inhaled steroids attenuate the development of EIA on laboratory provocation and increase the threshold for the development of EIA clinically. Prophylactic measures to prevent EIA include avoiding exercises that expose the patient to cold, dry air and favoring those that expose the patient to humid air during exercise. Patients can reduce the severity of their EIA by breathing through the nose rather than through the mouth during exercise. Face masks (e.g., 3M Cold Weather Mask) can be used by the many people who find it impossible to breathe through the nose during intense exer-

cise. It is still unclear whether physical training and improvement in work capacity can relieve symptoms of EIA. They ought to be useful, at least theoretically, since a better-trained athlete may require a lower mandatory minute volume—which may lead to less water loss from the airways and less severe EIA. Preexposure of patients with EIA to air high in ozone in two studies performed in Los Angeles and Toronto showed that EIA was not enhanced. This suggests that choosing a day to exercise on the basis of ozone will not help prevent EIA. A series of repeated short sprints has been shown to be effective in inducing the refractory state, which might then allow the athlete to maximally exercise without developing EIA.[36] A warmup period to induce the refractory period has been advocated by some to improve performance in the competitive athlete.[14] However, this effect may not last longer than 40 min.[29]

Several classes of drugs have been shown to prevent EIA if administered just before (10 to 15 min) exercise. The list includes beta-adrenergic agonists, cromolyn sodium, anticholinergics, and possibly rapid-release theophylline (Table 49-4).[3,42] Beta-adrenergic agonists are the most effective drugs for use against EIA. They are 90 percent effective in preventing EIA when used just before exercise. They are especially useful if the patient has some reversible airway obstruction, since they also improve lung function before exercise. Longer-acting beta-adrenergic agonists, such as salmeterol, have also been found to be effective in preventing EIA. The duration of protection they confer may approach 10 h. It is interesting that the cough so often associated with EIA appears to occur independent of the bronchospasm provoked by exercise. Although exercise-induced airway narrowing is prevented by the inhalation of beta-adrenergic agonists before exercise, the cough is not.

Cromolyn sodium also has been shown to attenuate bronchoconstriction in most patients with EIA. This medication

TABLE 49-4

Treatment of EIA

Treatment Immediately Before Exercise (10–20 min before)	Treatment of Underlying Disease (days before)
Beta-adrenergic agonists	Goal: Improved asthma control
Cromolyn sodium	Inhaled corticosteroids
Nedocromil	Systemic corticosteroids
? Anticholinergics	? Theophylline
? Inhaled furosemide	
? Leukotriene receptor antagonists	

will not be effective in those who seek reversal of pre-exercise bronchoconstriction, since it is not a direct bronchodilator. Cromolyn does, however, have two advantages over other agents. First, it does not contribute to tachycardia and is therefore useful in elderly patients or patients with cardiac compromise. In addition, cromolyn has been shown to prevent the late bronchoconstrictor response to exercise. Related drugs (including nedocromil, minocromil, and oxatomide, but not ketotifen) have been shown to be similarly effective against EIA.

Anticholinergics, such as ipratropium bromide, prevent airway narrowing after exercise in a high percentage of patients with EIA. They are especially useful in those who experience a rapid bronchodilating effect of the drug. The slow onset of action for most patients, however, limits their utility.

Theophylline with its weak bronchodilatory effects, high side-effect profile, and slow onset of action, is not recommended for routine use as pretreatment for EIA. However, it has been shown to confer protection against EIA if 100 to 200 mg is taken 2 h before exercise. Other orally administered drugs that are not commonly used, but have the potential to be helpful in preventing EIA, are terbutaline, albuterol (2 h before exercise), some alpha-adrenergic agonists, verapamil, and sublingual nifedipine (the last two if taken one-half hour before exercise), as well as the inhaled antihistamine clemastine.[3] In addition, terfenadine was shown by one group to prevent EIA.[16] For the elite athlete, of the above drugs, only a few are approved for use in competition by the International Olympic Committee. They include inhaled albuterol, terbutaline, cromolyn, and nedocromil and oral theophylline. Salmeterol and all oral sympathomimetics are not approved.

New directions in drug therapy for EIA hold promise for the future. Diuretics are known to be of some use in the prevention of EIA in adults.[7] The most recent use of these agents indicates that inhaled furosemide (20 to 30 mg by inhalation 20 min before exercise) also attenuates EIA in children and can be combined with nedocromil to increase the protective effects of the drug. Leukotriene antagonists, which have been developed over the past few years, also appear to have potential for the treatment of EIA. Because of their low side-effect profile, leukotriene antagonists would appear to be well suited for use against EIA. However, additional studies showing efficacy during exercise will be required before these agents can be recommended over inhaled beta-adrenergic agonists in routine prophylaxis against EIA.

REFERENCES

1. Ameisen JC, Capron A, Joseph M, et al: Aspirin-sensitive asthma: Abnormal platelet response to drugs inducing asthma attacks: Diagnostic and pathophysiological implications. *Int Arch Allergy Appl Immunol* 78:438–448, 1985.

2. Anderson SD: Is there a unifying hypothesis for exercise-induced asthma? *J Allergy Clin Immunol* 73:660–665, 1984.

3. Anderson SD. Exercise-induced asthma, in Middleton E, Reed CE, Ellis EF (eds), *Allergy: Principles and Practice,* 5th ed. St. Louis, CV Mosby, 1993, p 1342.

4. Anderson SD, Schoffel RE, Black JI, Daviskas E: Airway cooling as a stimulus to exercise-induced asthma: A re-evaluation. *Eur J Respir Dis* 67:20–30, 1985.

5. Anderson SD: Exercise-induced asthma: The state of the art. *Chest* 87:191S–195S, 1985.

6. Banner AS, Chausow A, Green J: The tussive effect of hyperpnea with cold air. *Am Rev Respir Dis* 131:362–367, 1985.

7. Bianco S, Vaghi A, Robuschi M, Pasargilian M: Prevention of exercise-induced bronchoconstriction by inhaled furosemide. *Lancet* 2:252–255, 1988.

8. Christie PE, Smith CM, Lee TH: The potent and selective sulfidopeptide leukotriene antagonist SK&F 104353 inhibits aspirin-induced asthma. *Am Rev Respir Dis* 144:957–958, 1991.

9. Custovic A, Arifhodzic N, Robinson A, Woodcock A: Exercise testing revisited: The response to exercise in normal and atopic children. *Chest* 105:1127–1132, 1994.

10. Cycar D, Lemanske RF Jr: Asthma and exercise. *Clin Chest Med* 15:351–368, 1994.

11. Dahlen B, Kumlin M, Margolskee DJ, et al: The leukotriene receptor antagonist MK-0679 blocks airway obstruction induced by bronchial provocation with lysine aspirin in aspirin-sensitive asthmatics. *Eur Respir J* 6:1018–1026, 1993.

12. Dajani BM, Sliman NA, Shubair KS, Hamzeh YS: Bronchospasm induced by intravenous hydrocortisone sodium succinate (Solu-Cortef) in aspirin-sensitive asthmatics. *J Allergy Clin Immunol* 68: 201–206, 1981.

13. Deal EC Jr, McFadden ER Jr, Ingram RH Jr, et al: Role of respiratory heat exchange in production of exercise-induced asthma. *J Appl Physiol* 46:467–475, 1979.

14. Eggleston PA: Exercise-induced asthma, in *Clinical Immunology: Principles and Practice.* St. Louis, CV Mosby, 1996, pp 526–527.

15. Eggleston PA, Kagey-Sobotka A, Schleimer RP, Lichtenstein LM: Interaction between hyperosmolar and IgE-mediated histamine release from basophils and mast cells. *Am Rev Respir Dis* 130:86–91, 1984.

16. Finnerty JP, Harvey A, Holgate ST: The relative contribution of histamine and prostanoids to bronchoconstriction provoked by isocapnic hyperventilation in asthma. *Eur Respir J* 5:323–330, 1992.

17. Fischer AR, Rosenberg MA, Lilly CM, et al: Direct evidence for a role of the mast cell in the nasal response to aspirin in aspirin-sensitive asthma. *J Allergy Clin Immunol* 94:1046–1056, 1994.

18. Floyer JA: *Treatise of Asthma.* London, R. Wilkens and W. Innis, 1698.

19. Hahn A, Anderson SD, Morton AR, et al: A reinterpretation of the effect of temperature and water content of the inspired air in exercise-induced asthma. *Am Rev Respir Dis* 130:575–579, 1984.

20. Hebert WG, Scopelitis E: Ketorolac precipitated asthma. *South Med J* 87:282–283, 1994.

21. Iamandescu IB: NSAIDS-induced asthma: Peculiarities related to background and association with other drug or non-drug etiological agents. *Allergol Immunopathol (Madr)* 17:285–290, 1989.

22. Ingenito E, Solway J, Lafleur J, et al: Dissociation of temperature gradient and evaporative heat loss during cold gas hyperventilation in cold-induced asthma. *Am Rev Respir Dis* 138:540–546, 1988.

23. Israel E, Dermarkarian R, Rosenberg M, et al: The effects of a 5-lipoxygenase inhibitor on asthma induced by cold, dry air. *New Engl J Med* 323:1740–1744, 1990.

24. Israel E, Fischer AR, Rosenberg MA, et al: The pivotal role of 5-lipoxygenase products in the reaction of aspirin-sensitive asthmatics to aspirin. *Am Rev Respir Dis* 148:1447–1451, 1993.

25. Kawabori I, Pierson WE, Conquest LL, Bierman CW: Incidence of exercise induced asthma in children. *J Allergy Clin Immunol* 58: 447–455, 1976.

26. Kowalski ML, Sliwinska-Kowalska M, Igarishi Y, et al: Nasal secretions in response to acetylsalicylic acid. *J Allergy Clin Immunol* 91:580–598, 1993.

27. Manning PJ, Watson RM, Margolskee DJ, et al: Inhibition of exercise-induced bronchconstriction by MK-571, a potent leukotriene D4-receptor antagonist. *New Engl J Med* 323:1736–1739, 1990.

28. McFadden ER Jr: Exercise-induced asthma: Assessment of current etiologic concepts. *Chest* 91:1515–1575, 1987.

29. McFadden ER Jr: Exercise-induced airway obstruction. *Clin Chest Med* 16:671–682, 1995.

30. Mullarkey MF, Thomas PS, Hansen JA, et al: Association of aspirin-sensitive asthma with HLA-DQW2. *Am Rev Respir Dis* 133:261–263, 1986.

31. O'Byrne PM, Ramsdale EH, Hargreave FE: Isocapnic hyperventilation for measuring airway hyperresponsiveness in asthma and chronic obstructive pulmonary disease. *Am Rev Respir Dis* 143:1444–1445, 1991.

32. Phillips YY, Jaeger JJ, Laube BL, Rosenthal RR: Eucapnic voluntary hyperventilation of compressed gas mixture: A simple method for bronchial challenge by respiratory heat loss. *Am Rev Respir Dis* 131:31–35, 1985.

33. Pleskow WW, Chenoweth DE, Smith RA, et al: The absence of detectable complement activation in aspirin sensitive patients during aspirin challenge. *J Allergy Clin Immunol* 72:462–468, 1983.

34. Pleskow WW, Stevenson DD, Mathison DA, et al: Aspirin desensitization in aspirin-sensitive asthmatic patients: Clinical manifestations and characterization of the refractory period. *J Allergy Clin Immunol* 69:11–19, 1982.

35. Samter M, Beer RF: Intolerance to aspirin: Clinical studies and consideration of its pathogenesis. *Ann Intern Med* 68:975–983, 1968.

36. Schnall RP, Landau LI: Protective effects of repeated short sprints in exercise-induced asthma. *Thorax* 3:828–832, 1980.

37. Settipane GA: Asthma, aspirin intolerance and nasal polyps. *New Engl Reg Allergy Proc* 7:32–37, 1986.

38. Sladek K, Dworski R, Soja J, et al: Eicosanoids in bronchoalveolar lavage fluid of aspirin-intolerant patients with asthma after aspirin challenge. *Am J Respir Crit Care Med* 149:940–946, 1994.

39. Sladek K, Szczelik A: Cysteinyl leukotrienes overproduction and mast cell activation in aspirin-provoked bronchospasm in asthma. *Eur Respir J* 6:391–399, 1993.

40. Slavin RG: Nasal polyps and sinusitis, in Middleton E Jr, Reed CE, Ellis EF, et al (eds), *Allergy: Principles and Practice.* St. Louis, CV Mosby, 1993, p 1459.

41. Spector SL, Wangaard CH, Farr QS: Aspirin and concomitant idiosyncrasies in adult asthmatic patients. *J Allergy Clin Immunol* 64:500–506, 1979.

42. Stevenson DD, Pleskow WW, Simon RA: Aspirin-sensitive rhinosinusitis asthma: A double-blind crossover study of treatment with aspirin. *J Allergy Clin Immunol* 73:500–507, 1984.

43. Stevenson DD, Simon RA: Aspirin sensitivity: Respiratory and cutaneous manifestations, in Middleton E Jr, Reed CE, Ellis EF, et al (eds), *Allergy: Principles and Practice.* St. Louis, CV Mosby, 1993, pp 1747–1767.

44. Szczelik A: Analgesics, allergy and asthma. *Br J Clin Pharamacol* 10:4015–4055, 1980.

45. Szczelik A, Gryglewski RJ, Czerniawska-Mysik G: Relationship of inhibition of prostaglandin biosynthesis by analgesics to asthma attacks in aspirin-sensitive patients. *Br Med J* 1:67–69, 1975.

46. Szczelik A, Gryglewski RJ, Czerniawska-Mysik G: Clinical patterns of hypersensitivity to nonsteroidal anti-inflammatory drugs and their pathogenesis. *J Allergy Clin Immunol* 60:276–284, 1977.

47. Szczelik A, Nizankowska E, Czerniawska-Mysik G, Sek S: Hydrocortisone and airflow impairment in asprin-induced asthma. *J Allergy Clin Immunol* 76:530–536, 1985.

48. Van Oss CJ, Friedman JC, Fontaine M: Anticomplementary action of aspirin. *Nature* 189:147, 1961.

49. Vanselow NA, Smith Jr: Bronchial asthma induced by indomethacin. *Ann Intern Med* 66:568–572, 1967.

50. Weber RW, Hoffman M, Raine DA, Nelson RS: Incidence of bronchoconstriction due to aspirin, azo dyes, non-azo dyes and preservatives in a population of perennial asthmatics. *J Allergy Clin Immunol* 64:32–37, 1979.

CHAPTER 50

ASTHMA: CLINICAL PRESENTATION AND MANAGEMENT

James E. Fish / Stephen P. Peters

Asthma can be defined operationally as a disorder characterized by variable airflow obstruction, airway hyperresponsiveness to specific and nonspecific stimuli, and symptoms of wheezing, chest tightness, cough, and, occasionally, dyspnea. Although asthma is frequently referred to as a disease, as if it were a single nosologic entity with a unique pathogenesis, experienced clinicians recognize that this is not the case. Asthma is more likely a syndrome, one that comprises multiple disorders manifesting common symptoms but having distinct and probably different pathogenetic and etiologic mechanisms. Phenotypic heterogeneity is evident not only in terms of the etiologic factors involved but also in terms of the severity and natural history of the disorder among different patients. This chapter, like most discussions on diagnosis and management, addresses asthma as a single disease, not out of naïveté but because there is insufficient knowledge to relate different clinical phenotypes to more fundamental pathogenetic processes that define the clinical presentation and response to therapy.

CLASSIFICATION OF ASTHMA

For many years, asthma has been classified as *extrinsic* or *intrinsic*, depending on the suspected role of allergens as etiologic factors. By convention, atopic subjects are considered to have extrinsic asthma, while nonatopic subjects have intrinsic asthma. However, this nomenclature has been used with diminishing frequency, because it lacks sufficient discriminative power to aid in establishing an etiologic diagnosis or to help in defining treatment strategies. The presence of atopy, often defined by the presence of skin test sensitivity to aeroallergens, does not, by itself, indicate that allergens are important triggers of asthma, since a large percentage of skin-sensitive persons report no allergic symptoms. Moreover, exercise and viral respiratory infections may play a more prominent role than allergens as triggers of symptoms in some atopic subjects. Classifying patients as having intrinsic asthma is problematic also, since it implies that all possible allergens in the environment have been excluded as etiologic factors—a task that is nearly impossible to achieve.

Although allergens are often triggers of acute asthma, there is a growing appreciation of their role as inducers of subclinical inflammation that may lead to enhanced airway responsiveness and greater susceptibility to the provocative effects of exercise and viral infections. In this regard, it is important to understand the distinction between triggers and etiologic factors. Whereas triggers may lead to symptoms, they do so only in susceptible persons who already possess the underlying asthmatic diathesis. In cases of occupational asthma, the disease can often be classified according to its etiology. In these circumstances, not only is the specific agent that triggers symptoms known but the same agent is usually the underlying cause of asthma.

Another category of asthma is that which is exercise induced. The term *exercise-induced asthma* is somewhat misleading, however, in that it suggests that exercise is the cause of the asthma. In fact, exercise is not a cause of asthma. Rather, it is one of many nonimmunologic triggers that produce symptoms in patients who already have the disease. Having useful etiologic or mechanism-based diagnostic classifications that help in disease management will require a greater understanding of the heterogeneity of asthma phenotypes, their corresponding mechanisms and causes, and, in some cases, their genotypes.

Perhaps the most useful classification of asthma is that based on levels of severity. This approach has facilitated the development of rational treatment guidelines that have been endorsed by expert physicians throughout the world. This classification, as well as management strategies that are based on it, is discussed later in this chapter.

CLINICAL PRESENTATION AND DIAGNOSIS

The diagnosis of asthma is made clinically, usually on the basis of a history of typical symptoms and confirmatory, objective evidence of variable airflow obstruction. In the authors' view, asthma is a relatively underdiagnosed disorder, although those who have gone undiagnosed are likely to have relatively mild disease. The diagnosis of asthma is usually made accurately, although the degree of diagnostic accuracy is probably patient age dependent. For example, asthma diagnosis in young adults is usually not difficult, since there are few other conditions that mimic asthma or confound its clinical presentation. With increasing age, however, cardiovascular disease and other forms of chronic lung disease are more common, and the differential diagnosis of episodic chest symptoms is more extensive. The frequent finding of an irreversible component of airway obstruction in older asthmatics[8] also adds to the challenge of distinguishing between asthma and tobacco-related chronic obstructive pulmonary disease (COPD), particularly in current and ex-smokers. Because the predictive value of clinical and laboratory findings in establishing the diagnosis of asthma appears to decline with advancing age, the probability of misdiagnosis is highest in the elderly, who have the same high asthma prevalence (4 to 7 percent) as younger adults.[35] The following clinical and laboratory manifestations are important in consideration of the diagnosis of asthma.

History

The history of symptoms, their pattern of occurrence, precipitating or aggravating factors, and the profile of a typical exacerbation are important elements of the clinical evaluation. During an acute episode, usual complaints include wheeze and a sensation of chest tightness. Breathlessness may also occur, although this symptom is often interpreted as a sensation of having difficulty inspiring, or "getting air in." This sensation is probably due to tonic inspiratory muscle activity that accompanies acute asthma episodes. Tonic inspiratory muscle contraction holds the lungs in a state of relative hyperinflation, in which further inspiratory efforts are made against a higher respiratory system recoil pressure. Cough may also be present; on occasion, it may be the sole presenting manifestation of an episode of asthma. These symptoms may occur abruptly or may evolve slowly over days or weeks. The frequency and severity with which symptoms occur vary considerably within the asthmatic population, although most patients are thought to have mild, intermittent disease.

Although no single symptom is specific for asthma, wheezing is a useful sign, since most asthmatics complain of more than just rare episodes of wheezing, and nonasthmatics rarely report frequent wheezing. The symptom of chest tightness is also helpful, since it occurs more often in association with asthma than with other pulmonary or cardiac disorders.

Perhaps more important than the asthmatic symptoms themselves is their pattern and triggering factors. For example, chest symptoms that vary by season and are accompanied by symptoms of irritation of other mucous membranes, such as conjunctivitis and rhinitis, are typical of allergic asthma. Whereas pollens and mold spores are likely to provoke seasonal symptoms, indoor allergens, such as house dust mites, cockroaches, and animal dander proteins, are more apt to result in perennial symptoms.

Early-morning symptoms or nocturnal episodes are very common in adult asthmatics. It is important to distinguish whether nocturnal symptoms are due to asthma, gastroesophageal reflux, or cardiovascular events, such as angina or left ventricular dysfunction. Typically, nocturnal asthma symptoms occur between 4:00 and 6:00 A.M.; usually they are relieved with administration of inhaled bronchodilators. This contrasts with gastroesophageal reflux, which causes similar symptoms soon after the patient reclines at night, or cardiovascular symptoms, which can occur at any time of night. Although the cause of symptoms of nocturnal asthma is unknown, putative mechanisms include circadian variations in blood levels of catecholamines, cortisol, and chemical mediators capable of causing airway obstruction.

ROLE OF RESPIRATORY INFECTIONS

Viral respiratory infections are a common cause of exacerbations of asthma in adults. Approximately 36 percent of severe asthma exacerbations are associated with viral infection, and almost 60 percent of viral infections in asthmatics are associated with exacerbations. The viruses most commonly implicated are respiratory syncytial virus, rhinovirus, influenza virus, and parainfluenza virus. *Mycoplasma* and *Chlamydia* are also associated with exacerbations of asthma, although bacterial infections are not. It should be noted that viral respiratory infections can evoke an increase in airway responsiveness in otherwise healthy persons, causing self-limited episodes of chest tightness, cough, and wheezing that may last for up to 8 weeks. Although these episodes are frequently diagnosed as asthma, the disappearance of symptoms after 8 weeks suggests that the illness was due to a temporary, postviral increase in airway responsiveness.

EXERCISE-INDUCED ASTHMA

A history of symptoms after heavy exertion, especially in cold air, is highly suggestive of exercise-induced asthma.[33] Typically, the patient experiences symptoms at the end of exercise, rather than during its performance. Excessive coughing, in the absence of wheezing, after exercise may also be a sign of asthma. Patients with COPD or heart failure may experience exertional dyspnea, but, as a rule, these patients do not develop symptoms of chest tightness, cough, and wheeze.

ASTHMA AND ASPIRIN SENSITIVITY

The association of asthma and sensitivity to aspirin and other nonsteroidal anti-inflammatory drugs (NSAIDs) is well established. Of particular note is the triad of asthma, nasal polyps, and aspirin intolerance. This condition is thought to affect 2 to 3 percent of all asthmatic patients and up to 20 percent of patients with severe asthma.[60] In this syndrome, the first symptom is usually rhinitis. This is followed several years later by the development of aspirin intolerance and asthma symptoms and finally, much later, by the development of nasal polyps. Nasal polyps are usually bilateral and originate from the turbinates, as well as the paranasal sinuses. Aspirin-induced asthma has been associated with enhanced leukotriene production and mast cell activation, but mechanisms responsible for these events are unclear.

Although aspirin-induced asthmatic episodes often resemble allergic reactions in that they have an abrupt onset and affect both the upper and lower respiratory tract, there is no evidence that IgE-related immunologic mechanisms are at work. In fact, most patients with this disorder are nonatopic. Patients with aspirin intolerance may also be sensitive to other NSAIDs and tartrazine dye–containing substances. As a rule, aspirin intolerance is associated with severe asthma that is often resistant to therapy, including glucocorticoid therapy. The diagnosis of aspirin intolerance and asthma is made on the basis of the history and clinical findings of sinusitis and nasal polyps; it can be confirmed by aspirin challenge procedures. β-Adrenergic receptor–blocking drugs, including those contained in topical ophthalmic preparations, can also precipitate severe, acute, and, sometimes, fatal asthmatic episodes. Accordingly, beta blockers are contraindicated in asthmatic patients.

OCCUPATIONAL ASTHMA

Asthma related to occupational exposure can often be identified on the basis of a typical history of symptoms during the work week and improvement over the weekend. Symptoms may occur during exposure to the etiologic substance, or they may be delayed until the evening or night after the workday. It is important to distinguish between occupational asthma that is triggered by nonspecific irritants in patients with preexisting or concurrent asthma and asthma that arises de novo as a consequence of exposure to a specific etiologic agent. A number of natural and synthetic chemicals are known to cause asthma by IgE-mediated mechanisms, as well as by nonallergic mechanisms of unknown origin. The diagnosis of occupational asthma is based on a history of typical symptoms, the presence of variable airflow obstruction, and a demonstrable link between asthma and workplace exposure.

OTHER FACTORS

Heightened airway responsiveness is a characteristic, if not pathognomic, feature of asthma. Clinically, increased airway responsiveness is manifest as intolerance to air pollution, smoke, strong odors or fumes, and particulate matter such as dust. Exposure to these agents typically results in transient symptoms of cough and chest tightness. Although emotional factors are not a cause of asthma, they may exacerbate symptoms in a large number of patients.

Physical Examination

The physical examination is useful for confirming the presence of airway obstruction and for distinguishing among conditions that cause asthmalike symptoms. Wheezing, the most characteristic physical finding in asthma, is caused by high-velocity, turbulent airflow through narrowed airways. In asthma, wheezing is usually present during expiration, although it may be present during inspiration as well. Wheezing is typically polyphonic;

variations in quality are noted throughout the chest, reflecting nonuniformity of airflow. Although the loudness and pitch of wheezing have been shown to correlate with peak expiratory flow, these associations are primarily of statistical interest; the quality of wheezing should not be considered predictive of the degree of obstruction in an individual patient. Patients who are asymptomatic, or who complain only of cough, may demonstrate end-expiratory wheezing, although this is a nonspecific and insensitive sign of asthma. It is important to note that wheezing of any character is not specific for asthma; in cases of very mild or very severe airway obstruction, wheezing may be absent.

Clinical signs of rhinitis, sinusitis, and nasal polyps are seen more commonly in patients with asthma than in those with other chronic lower respiratory tract disorders or congestive heart failure. Chronic sinus disease may be difficult to diagnose on clinical grounds, however, and specialized imaging studies may be required. Marked weight loss or severe wasting, pursed-lip breathing, chest hyperinflation, and diminished breath and heart sounds reflect a phenotype most characteristic of severe emphysema. Although patients with asthma may show signs of hyperinflation and diminished breath and heart sounds, these fundings are usually seen during an acute exacerbation. Use of accessory muscles of respiration and the presence of pulsus paradoxus are signs of severe airway obstruction and are usually observed during acute episodes. Pulsus paradoxus, which is an exaggerated fall in systolic blood pressure during inspiration, is a consequence of generation of a markedly negative inspiratory pleural pressure reflecting the degree of airway obstruction, air trapping, and ventilatory effort. Because ventilatory effort can be diminished with respiratory muscle fatigue, the absence of pulsus paradoxus does not preclude severe airway obstruction. Grossly audible inspiratory and expiratory wheezes, heard best with auscultation over the upper airways, should prompt a further search for causes of upper-airway obstruction, including vocal cord dysfunction, vocal cord paralysis, upper-airway tumors, and airway narrowing due to thyroid enlargement.

Laboratory Studies

The use of laboratory studies in the diagnosis of asthma is largely restricted to pulmonary function studies—particularly spirometry and peak flow measurements, which are employed to confirm the clinical diagnosis. Skin testing and serologic studies may also be useful in defining allergic triggers of asthma in some patients, although the clinical history often provides more clinically relevant information regarding the relation between symptoms and exposure. Radiographic studies, blood tests, and more extensive lung function studies are used to exclude other conditions that may mimic asthma or complicate its clinical presentation.

PULMONARY FUNCTION TESTS

Pulmonary function tests are important for confirming the diagnosis of asthma, for establishing the severity of the disease, and for monitoring the response to therapy. The diagnosis of asthma is usually confirmed by objective demonstration of airway obstruction by spirometry. In addition, there should be evidence of significant improvement in the 1-s forced expired volume (FEV_1)

acutely after bronchodilator administration, or with repeated measurement over time. Unfortunately, there are no standard criteria for judging the degree of reversibility after bronchodilator administration for diagnostic purposes. Although a postbronchodilator increase in FEV_1 of 15 percent is often considered evidence of reversible airway obstruction, this level is quite arbitrary and lacks sensitivity for detecting asthma. Based on studies of variability in interindividual measurements, a change in FEV_1 of 12 percent would exceed the 95 percent confidence limits.[42] Hence, while a 12 percent increase in FEV_1 may be statistically significant, this level of improvement does not discriminate between asthma and other forms of chronic airway obstruction.

In a study of 287 asthmatics and 108 patients with COPD,[27] average postbronchodilator responses of 16.4 percent and 10.7 percent, respectively, were found. Because of the overlap between the two groups, no single degree of reversibility provided a high level of both specificity and sensitivity for the diagnosis of asthma. On the other hand, an increase in FEV_1 of 20 percent, with a minimum volume change of 200 ml, was found to be highly specific, although not sensitive, for asthma (Table 50-1). Thus, while a marked spirometric response to inhaled bronchodilator confirms reversibility of airway obstruction and is strongly indicative of asthma, the lack of an acute bronchodilator response does not rule out asthma.

Some asthmatics, especially elderly patients, demonstrate persistent airway obstruction even when optimally treated and in remission.[8] An empiric trial of oral glucocorticoids, with spirometric monitoring before and after treatment, is often necessary to identify patients with reversible airway obstruction. As a rule, we administer the equivalent of 0.4 to 0.5 mg per kg of prednisone daily for 2 weeks. Although the dose and duration of treatment are largely empiric, limited studies suggest that the response to systemic glucocorticoids is usually achieved within 8 days.[58] Documentation of significant deterioration in lung function during an exacerbation, followed by improvement after treatment, is also evidence for a diagnosis of asthma.

Peak Expiratory Flow

Although peak expiratory flow (PEF) measurements before and after a bronchodilator may be useful for detecting reversible airway obstruction, little is known about the magnitude of change required for a reasonable degree of diagnostic precision. Since office spirometry is inexpensive and easy to perform, there seems to be little justification for sacrificing diagnostic sensitivity and specificity by using peak flow measurements made in the office. Conversely, home monitoring of variability in PEF may be of diagnostic use, especially in patients with mild, intermittent symptoms who often demonstrate normal spirometry during physician visits.

Asthma is characterized by increased variability in PEF. Owing to circadian variation in lung function, PEF is usually lowest in the early morning and highest in the late afternoon. When variability in PEF is defined as the ratio of the difference between evening and morning values to the mean of the evening and morning values (i.e., amplitude divided by mean), the 95 percent confidence limit in a normal population is 19 percent. When it is measured in a population with an asthma prevalence rate of 9 percent, a variability in PEF of at least 20 percent provides approximately 70 percent specificity and 61 percent sensitivity in the detection of asthma.[44]

Lung Volumes

Complete pulmonary function studies, including lung volumes, are often useful for excluding restrictive lung disease. In asthma, an increase in residual volume is typically seen, reflecting airway closure at a lung volume that is higher than normal. During acute asthmatic episodes, functional residual capacity and total lung capacity may also be increased. The mechanism of hyperinflation is not entirely understood, but a decrease in lung elastic recoil and increases in airway obstruction and inspiratory muscle tone are thought to play a role. Inspiratory and expiratory flow-volume curves may be helpful in detecting upper-airway problems that mimic asthma.

Diffusing Capacity

Measurement of diffusing capacity of the lung (D_{LCO}) deserves mention because of its value in identifying patients with emphysema. Airspace enlargement, alveolar septal destruction, and loss of effective alveolar surface area in emphysema correlate with a reduction in D_{LCO} (Chapter 36). By contrast, the D_{LCO} is usually normal in asthma.[29]

ARTERIAL BLOOD GASES

Arterial blood gases are typically normal in patients with chronic, stable asthma. During an acute episode, hypoxia is often present; in rare instances, the arterial P_{O_2} is less than 50 mmHg. Arterial P_{CO_2} is typically reduced owing to hyperventilation. With severe obstruction, arterial P_{CO_2} may rise because of respiratory muscle fatigue and an inability to maintain the required alveolar ventilation. On occasion, the pH may be lower than predicted from the elevation in arterial P_{CO_2}; in these cases, lactic acidosis may be observed.

RADIOGRAPHY

Because the chest radiograph is generally unremarkable in patients with uncomplicated asthma, it is used primarily to exclude other causes of respiratory symptoms.[22] Nonspecific radio-

---

TABLE 50-1

Sensitivity and Specificity of Postbronchodilator Changes in FEV_1 and FVC for the Diagnosis of Asthma

% increase	Sensitivity (%)	Specificity (%)
Minimum of 200 ml change in FEV_1		
≥10	58	77
≥15	43	81
≥20	29	87
No minimum change in FEV_1		
≥10	63	58
≥15	44	72
≥20	29	84

SOURCE: Adapted from Kesten and Rebuck.[27]

graphic findings, such as overinflation and prominent hilar vessels, have been reported in up to 31 percent of patients between the ages of 15 and 65 years who first developed asthmatic symptoms before age 15 years.[22] Overinflation has also been reported in asthmatics with severe disease, in those with chronic, persistent, rather than intermittent, symptoms, and during acute exacerbations. Because asthma may coexist with chronic bronchitis in elderly patients who have significant smoking histories, findings thought to be typical of chronic bronchitis may be present—e.g., increased bronchovascular markings ("dirty lung" appearance).

ELECTROCARDIOGRAM

Asthma in remission is usually not associated with electrocardiographic abnormalities. During an acute exacerbation, however, several abnormalities can occur, including sinus tachycardia, P pulmonale, right-axis deviation, right bundle branch block, right ventricular strain, repolarization abnormalities, and a variety of arrhythmias. Signs of right ventricular overload occur, however, only during a severe episode or with additional underlying cardiovascular or pulmonary disorders. The electrocardiogram can sometimes be helpful in ruling out cardiac disease as the cause of chest symptoms and in assessing the risks of theophylline and beta-agonist therapy in patients with asthma as well as cardiac disease.

BLOOD TESTS

The blood tests most useful in evaluating asthma are the white blood cell count and serum immunoglobulin E level.

Eosinophilia

Peripheral blood eosinophilia (greater than 4 percent or 300 to 400 per mm^3) may be seen in both allergic and nonallergic asthmatics. When present, eosinophilia may be used to support a diagnosis of asthma; however, its absence is of no value in excluding asthma. Unusually high eosinophil counts (greater than 800 per mm^3) suggest the presence of other disorders, such as allergic bronchopulmonary aspergillosis, Churg-Strauss syndrome, tropical eosinophilia, and Loeffler's syndrome. It should be noted that eosinophilia may not be present if the patient is taking corticosteroids. Moreover, corticosteroids may induce a leukocytosis, with a relative increase in polymorphonuclear leukocytes.

Immunoglobulin E Level

Epidemiologic studies have demonstrated an association between asthma and total serum immunoglobulin E (IgE) levels, standardized for age and sex. Whether this association signifies that aeroallergens are prominent etiologic factors, or that immunologic processes in the pathogenesis of asthma are capable of stimulating IgE production as an unrelated phenomenon, needs further definition. Studies have shown a relationship between total serum IgE and asthma in patients with negative skin tests.[9] In addition, other studies have reported that elevations in total IgE are strongly associated with asthma, whereas skin test reactivity is more closely related to allergic rhinitis.[54] These findings suggest that IgE levels may be more a marker of disease than a critical etiologic factor.

The association between asthma and IgE levels is more of statistical interest than of diagnostic value. Elevated total IgE levels (greater than 100 IU) are frequently seen in allergic patients, but the finding is not specific for asthma; furthermore, an elevated level does not confirm an allergic origin for respiratory symptoms. Finally, a normal IgE level cannot be used to exclude the diagnosis of asthma.

Other Tests

Other blood tests, such as autoantibody levels and specific antifungal IgG levels, may be useful for ruling out vasculitic processes and allergic bronchopulmonary fungal disease. However, these tests should be employed only when clinical suspicion warrants pursuit of uncommon causes of asthma symptoms. Severe, acute episodes of asthma are often associated with increases in blood lactate and creatine phosphokinase, but these measurements are not of much diagnostic importance; they simply reflect the severity of the acute episode.

SPUTUM EXAMINATION

Although sputum eosinophilia is more characteristically found in asthmatics than in patients with COPD, and neutrophils are found more often in patients with an acute exacerbation of chronic bronchitis, sputum eosinophils can be seen in both disorders. Studies using bronchoalveolar lavage have shown that there are more eosinophils in the airways of asthmatic subjects than in those of normal subjects, even during times of remission. During exacerbations, sputum examination may reveal an increase in eosinophil numbers, as well as Charcot-Leyden crystals, which are composed of eosinophil granule membranes. Creola bodies, consisting of fragments of degenerated epithelial cells and Curschmann spirals or twisted strands of mucus, are also seen in sputum during an acute exacerbation (see Chapter 22).

ALLERGY TESTS

Tests to determine whether the patient is allergic and to investigate the role of specific allergens as a cause of asthma are of value in some patients, although specific allergens are thought to play a diminishing role with increasing age. An allergic evaluation may be appropriate when the clinical history suggests that specific aeroallergens are important triggers in a particular patient and when asthma symptoms are accompanied by other symptoms typical of allergic disease, such as rhinitis and conjunctivitis. In selected populations, evaluations for perennial or indoor allergens, such as dust mite, cockroach, and animal dander, have become increasingly important.

The components of an allergic evaluation include a detailed history of the patient's environment and possible triggers, followed by tests of allergic sensitivity. Sensitivity to a particular allergen (or the presence of specific IgE antibody) can be verified by skin tests or by in vitro serum antibody studies. In general, it is necessary to demonstrate specific IgE antibodies in order to confirm the presence of allergy. On the other hand, the presence of IgE antibodies does not, by itself, signify that the patient has clinically significant allergic disease. Because of the high prevalence of positive skin tests in persons with no allergic symptoms, the clinical history is essential for making sound judgments concerning the importance of allergic triggers. Allergy evaluation is useful for developing avoidance treatment strategies or, in selected cases, for developing immunotherapy regimens.

BRONCHIAL CHALLENGE TESTING

For several centuries, clinicians have appreciated that asthma symptoms are largely an expression of abnormal airway responsiveness. Indeed, the concept of airway responsiveness evolved primarily in the context of asthma and the recognition that virtually all symptomatic asthmatic patients demonstrate increased airway responsiveness, as measured by objective airway challenge tests. Abnormal airway responsiveness is detected in the laboratory by an exaggerated response to inhaled pharmacologic agents, such as histamine and methacholine, or to physical stimuli, such as exercise and hyperventilation (Chapter 49). To the extent that these different stimuli appear to act through distinct mechanisms, it is reasonable to question whether hyperresponsiveness elicited by a pharmacologic agent, such as methacholine, has the same underlying pathophysiology as hyperresponsiveness evoked by isocapnic hyperventilation. Nevertheless, the correlation between different airway challenge tests is remarkably good, especially between histamine and methacholine and, to a lesser extent, between pharmacologic agents and exercise and cold air hyperventilation.

Physical Measures

Physical measures to assess airway responsiveness include exercise and isocapnic hyperventilation. Both stimuli induce airway obstruction as a consequence of cooling or drying of the airway mucosa.[33] Because heat and water loss from the airways is determined primarily by the level of minute ventilation, as well as the temperature and humidity of inspired air, the level of the challenge stimulus can be regulated by adjusting the physical workload (to change minute ventilation) or by altering conditions of the inspired air. The prevalence of exercise-induced bronchospasm in an asthmatic population and, hence, the sensitivity of exercise testing have been reported to vary from 60 to 90 percent. This wide range is related to variations in the magnitude of the stimulus applied, as determined by workload and the conditions of inspired air. While it is possible that by adjusting the intensity of the stimulus, exercise or isocapnic hyperventilation challenges could achieve the same degree of sensitivity as pharmacologic challenges, the requirement for strenuous physical work limits the use of such challenges to persons who are physically capable of performing them.

Pharmacologic Measures

The most widely employed methods for airway challenge are based on administration of aerosolized solutions of methacholine or histamine. Methacholine aerosol challenge was first used as a diagnostic test for asthma by Parker and colleagues in 1965.[40] Since then, protocols using standard methods of dosing and aerosol delivery have been developed, and normal limits of airway responsiveness have been defined.[51]

The largest experience with pharmacologic challenge testing is with intermittent and continuous aerosol generation techniques. The two techniques give remarkably similar results when airway responsiveness is expressed as the concentration of methacholine or histamine causing a 20 percent fall in FEV_1 (PC_{20}), as determined from dose-response curves.

Some studies have shown that 100 percent of patients with current asthma symptoms demonstrate a PC_{20} at histamine concentrations $\leq$ 8 mg/ml,[11] while others, using methacholine, have reported a sensitivity of approximately 85 percent at the same PC_{20} threshold.[23] Differences in reported sensitivity rates are likely to reflect differences in the definition of "current" symptoms of asthma. For example, in reporting a 100 percent sensitivity rate, investigators defined current asthmatic patients as those with active disease at the time of testing.[11] On the other hand, a lower sensitivity was noted if current asthma was defined as the patient's having had at least three wheezing episodes in the preceding year.[23] Thus, false-negative results can be obtained in patients who experience only intermittent symptoms and who are tested when they are asymptomatic. Indeed, atopic patients with seasonal asthma symptoms may demonstrate PC_{20} greater than 8 mg/ml when tested "out of season." False-negative challenge responses may also occur in patients with occupational asthma if tests are performed remote in time from exposure to the etiologic agent. Whereas diagnostic tests are more likely to be performed in patients who have had recent symptoms, pharmacologic challenges are generally conceded to have a low false-negative rate. Thus, when a diagnostic threshold PC_{20} of $\leq$ 8 mg/ml is used, pharmacologic challenges are sensitive tests with a high negative predictive value (i.e., a PC_{20} greater than 8 mg/ml excludes a diagnosis of asthma with a high degree of accuracy).

Most surveys indicate that the specificity of pharmacologic challenge testing is approximately 90 percent when a PC_{20} of $\leq$ 8 mg/ml is used as the diagnostic threshold. In a survey of 154 subjects, age 19 to 42 years, we found a specificity rate of 91 percent; i.e., 9 percent of "normal" subjects demonstrated a PC_{20} $\leq$ 8 mg/ml. A specificity rate of approximately 95 percent has been reported in children,[23] while 91 percent specificity has been noted for current asthma in a random sample of 500 university students (Table 50-2).[11]

It is estimated that approximately 10 percent of asymptomatic persons with a history of asthma retain elevated airway responsiveness.[11] Likewise, approximately 10 to 15 percent of atopic subjects without asthma demonstrate abnormal airway responsiveness.[11] The prevalence of abnormal responsiveness in nonatopic, nonasthmatic subjects who have no history of prior respiratory problems ranges from 5 to 10 percent.[11] While these studies reveal an approximately 10 percent false-positive rate of abnormal responsiveness among nonasthmatics, the term "false-positive" should be used with caution. The significance of abnormal responsiveness in this population is uncertain. For example, it is not known whether the retention of abnormal responsiveness in former asthmatics predisposes to relapse later in life. Likewise, it is not known whether abnormal airway responsiveness predisposes to the subsequent development of asthma or COPD.

TABLE 50-2

Prevalence of Airway Hyperresponsiveness

Disease	Number	PC_{20} <8 mg/ml	%
Asthma			
Current	17	17	100
Seasonal	16	6	38
Past	19	2	11
Total	52	25	48
Rhinitis			
Atopic	77	11	14
Nonatopic	81	9	11
Total	158	20	13
Normal subjects			
No asthma or rhinitis	290	13	4.5
Total	500	58	11.6

SOURCE: Adapted from Cockcroft et al.[11]

Clinical Application of Bronchial Challenge Tests

The specificity of bronchial challenge tests in the diagnosis of asthma is compromised further by the finding that abnormal airway responsiveness is associated with a number of other disorders, including cystic fibrosis, COPD, and heart failure. Moreover, conditions associated with airway injury or inflammation—such as viral respiratory infections, exposure to pollutants, and exposure to aeroallergens—can induce a temporary state of abnormal responsiveness.

As a rule, abnormal airway responsiveness found in association with acute airway inflammation tends to be transient and, in the case of viral respiratory infections, may return to baseline within several weeks. A number of studies indicate that abnormal responsiveness in COPD correlates with the level of pulmonary function decline, and that the degree of abnormal responsiveness typical of asthma (i.e., $PC_{20} \leq 8$ mg/ml) is usually not observed in COPD until the FEV_1 has declined below 70 percent of the predicted value.[53] Accordingly, pharmacologic challenges are not useful for discriminating between asthma and COPD in patients with abnormal spirometry. In these cases, the spirometric response to bronchodilator therapy or an empiric course of glucocorticoid therapy is often the best approach to ascertain the degree of reversibility and, hence, variability of the underlying pathology. In contrast to patients with COPD, asthmatics demonstrate abnormal airway responsiveness even when spirometry results are normal. For this reason, airway challenge testing is used, perhaps most gainfully, in evaluating patients who have unexplained chest symptoms and normal spirometry results.

The clinical history, by itself, has little value in establishing a diagnosis of asthma in patients with atypical symptoms. For example, wheezing may be absent, and cough or dyspnea alone may be the sole manifestation of disease in some asthmatic patients. In these cases, bronchial provocation testing may be especially useful for excluding a diagnosis of asthma because of the low false-negative rate and high negative predictive value. Conversely, the finding of abnormal responsiveness in such patients may not be diagnostic of asthma because of the test's poor positive predictive value and the possibility that hyperrespon-

siveness may also reflect self-limited pathology that occurs with transient airway inflammation secondary to viral infections. In any event, the demonstration of abnormal airway responsiveness may be taken as presumptive evidence of an association between symptoms and abnormal responsiveness, thus providing an objective basis for asthma therapy.

Finally, while many studies on bronchial reactivity have been conducted in adult populations, there is limited information on testing in the elderly. Because the distribution of airway responsiveness in the elderly population is not known, the standards established for interpreting challenge tests in younger patients may or may not be applicable to the elderly. Furthermore, the higher prevalence of COPD and cardiovascular disease in the elderly can compromise the discriminative power of methacholine challenge testing, since both COPD and congestive heart failure are associated with abnormal airway responsiveness.

Differential Diagnosis

A variety of respiratory and cardiac disorders constitute the differential diagnosis of asthma.

OTHER OBSTRUCTIVE AIRWAY DISEASE

The most common conditions to consider in the differential diagnosis of asthma include other forms of chronic airway disease, such as chronic bronchitis, emphysema, and bronchiectasis. Difficulties in diagnosis arise from the fact that these other conditions not only can mimic asthma in clinical presentation but also may coexist with asthma as co-morbid conditions. In addition, a component of irreversible airway obstruction may prevail in asthma patients, and a significant proportion of smokers who meet diagnostic criteria for chronic obstructive bronchitis (i.e., productive cough for 3 months of the year for 2 consecutive years and demonstrable airflow limitation) experience episodic bronchospasm with cough, wheezing, and dyspnea. Such episodes may even improve clinically, as well as physiologically, following administration of bronchodilators or glucocorticoids. The term *asthmatic bronchitis* has been used to describe such patients, although it is recognized that this label more nearly reflects diagnostic confusion than an understanding of pathogenesis. Thus, when asthma symptoms develop in a person who has smoked, traditional nosologic categories become indistinct, and the ability to discriminate asthma from chronic bronchitis becomes more challenging. On the other hand, symptoms of episodic airway obstruction in a nonsmoker are almost always due to asthma. Other factors that favor a diagnosis of asthma are a history of childhood asthma or allergies, a family history of allergies, and blood eosinophilia.

CONGESTIVE HEART FAILURE

Acute increases in left atrial pressure and pulmonary vascular pressures can lead to narrowing of the airways, dyspnea, and wheezing. The underlying cause of airway obstruction is uncertain, but it probably relates to reflex bronchoconstriction mediated by afferent and efferent nerve fibers, as well as changes in airway geometry associated with increased interstitial pressures in the lung. Mitral stenosis, a disorder that is still found with some frequency in the elderly, is commonly mistaken for asthma, especially when typical heart sounds and murmurs are not audible. Abrupt increases in airway resistance associated with acute heart failure are reversed by bronchodilator administration and by resolution of the hemodynamic abnormality.

Diagnostic confusion in patients with left ventricular dysfunction can arise because such patients do not always present with overt manifestations of congestive heart failure. Peripheral edema and basal inspiratory rales may be absent, and typical radiographic signs of vascular congestion may be subtle or absent, especially in patients with coexistent COPD with altered lung architecture. Spirometric measurements obtained in patients with left ventricular failure may demonstrate reductions in FVC, FEV_1, $FEV_1/FVC\%$, and flow at low lung volumes. The major physiological abnormality, however, is a restrictive, rather than an obstructive, defect. Moreover, experience suggests that the degree of symptoms appears to be out of proportion to the degree of airway obstruction in left ventricular failure, whereas in asthma there is a greater correspondence between symptoms and physiological impairment. In both COPD and congestive heart failure, daytime dyspnea is almost always associated with exertion. If dyspnea and wheezing occur at rest, asthma should be suspected.

CHRONIC SINUSITIS AND GASTROESOPHAGEAL REFLUX

Persistent cough can sometimes be the first and only manifestation of asthma. Chronic cough in nonsmoking patients with normal chest radiographs is commonly due not only to asthma but also to postnasal drainage (chronic rhinosinusitis) or gastroesophageal reflux. Although 24-h esophageal pH monitoring, sinus imaging procedures, and airway challenge procedures may help establish the presence of these disorders, they do not establish the cause of cough. However, the cause of cough can often be identified on the basis of the response to a therapeutic trial with bronchodilators or inhaled glucocorticoids, decongestants or topical nasal glucocorticoids, or histamine (H_2) blockers or protein pump inhibitors. If symptom relief is obtained, the therapy itself suggests the diagnosis.

The association between asthma and gastroesophageal reflux disease (GERD) is well established. Up to 60 percent of asthmatic adults demonstrate acid reflux on either pH monitoring or gastroesophageal scintiscanning. The nature of the association is complex, as asthma is thought to lead to exacerbations of GERD, and vice versa. Asthma may worsen GERD by mechanisms of low, flat diaphragms, a thoracoabdominal pressure gradient favoring reflux during acute exacerbations, and use of bronchodilators, which lower esophageal sphincter tone.[48] The mechanisms whereby GERD exacerbates asthma are unclear. While intraesophageal acid infusion can reduce lung function, the presence of gastric acid in the distal esophagus may also increase airway responsiveness. Although it is important to distinguish between asthma and GERD in patients with wheezing, it is also important to recognize that the two disorders often coexist.

LARYNGEAL DYSFUNCTION

Laryngeal dysfunction masquerading as asthma is an increasingly recognized problem.[16] The condition appears to reflect a spectrum of disorders that have been reported under various names, including Munchausen's asthma, emotional laryngeal wheezing, factitious asthma, and vocal cord dysfunction. While Munchausen's asthma is, by definition, induced voluntarily, most cases of laryngeal dysfunction masquerading as asthma are thought to represent involuntary adduction of the true and false vocal cords during the respiratory cycle. Normally, the glottic chink widens with inspiration and narrows with expiration. With vocal cord dysfunction mimicking asthma, the anterior two-thirds of the vocal cords adduct, leaving a narrow, posterior diamond-shaped chink. Typically, this occurs during inspiration, but it also may occur throughout the respiratory cycle; it has been observed, in some cases, to be more pronounced during the expiratory phase.

Patients with vocal cord dysfunction typically present with acute episodes of dyspnea and wheezing that appear out of proportion to what is expected on the basis of pulmonary function testing between episodes. Wheezing is heard best over the larynx—although this is not a consistent finding, since breath sounds are often transmitted throughout the thorax. Patients may also present with clear evidence of stridor and use of accessory muscles of respiration. In our experience, hoarseness or a "barking" cough is often a prelude to acute episodes. The typical patient is a woman between the age of 20 and 45 years; frequently, the patient is employed in the health professions.[10] A high incidence of psychiatric disorders is observed in afflicted patients, although the spectrum of psychiatric disorders and their etiologic link to vocal cord dysfunction are unclear.

Vocal cord dysfunction frequently goes unrecognized until after the patient has been treated for a number of acute episodes. In some cases, the patient has undergone several intubations or even tracheotomy. As a rule, acute episodes of upper-airway obstruction do not respond to antiasthmatic therapy. On the other hand, the syndrome can often be distinguished from asthma because its resolution is inordinately abrupt and not associated with the residual airway obstruction typically seen with a resolving exacerbation of asthma. A useful diagnostic sign in this condition is the disappearance of wheezing after the upper airway is bypassed by endotracheal intubation.

The definitive diagnosis of vocal cord dysfunction is usually made from fiberoptic laryngoscopic observation of adduction of the cords during an acute episode. Between episodes, vocal cord function is usually normal, and attempts to voluntarily reproduce the abnormality are unsuccessful.[10] Full inspiratory and expiratory flow volume loops may suggest a diagnosis if a plateau of inspiratory flow, indicating variable extrathoracic airway obstruction, is evident during an acute episode. As a rule, arterial blood gases are remarkably normal in relation to the apparent degree of airflow obstruction. In some cases, a pattern of hypoxemia and hypercapnia with a normal alveolar-arterial oxygen gradient is observed. Hypoxemia and a widened alveolar-arterial oxygen gradient suggest ventilation-perfusion mismatching and the presence of intrathoracic airway obstruction. This has been reported in patients who are thought to have both laryngeal dysfunction and coexisting asthma.[16] In our experience, the coexistence of asthma and vocal cord dysfunction is not uncommon.

Patients with vocal cord dysfunction are treated most successfully with a combination of speech therapy and psychiatric counseling. Unfortunately, most patients go unrecognized and are treated with high doses of inhaled, or even systemic, corticosteroids, bearing the consequences of corticosteroid toxicity. Because of the difficulty in establishing a diagnosis of vocal cord dysfunction, the prevalence of this disorder is unknown and is probably underestimated.

OTHER CONSIDERATIONS

Other conditions to consider in the differential diagnosis of asthma are mechanical obstruction of the airways, anatomic obstruction of major airways, pulmonary embolism, eosinophilic pneumonias, and herpes simplex tracheobronchitis.

MANAGEMENT OF ASTHMA

Successful management of the asthmatic patient requires an appreciation of two basic principles. First is an understanding that asthma is characterized by considerable heterogeneity with respect to etiology, clinical presentation, severity, natural history, and response to therapy. Because of this heterogeneity, it is unlikely that a single management approach will work for all patients. Thus, therapy must be tailored to the individual patient.

The second principle recognizes that in each patient, symptom severity may vary considerably over time. For example, some patients may experience a remission of symptoms during adolescence, only to have them recur with even greater severity later in life. Even when the disease remains relatively stable over long intervals, intercurrent flares that arise as a result of seasonal allergies or infection are the rule in asthma. Thus, the patient should be monitored regularly, and treatment should be modified on an ongoing basis to meet the patient's current needs.

A number of comprehensive treatment guidelines drafted by multidisciplinary expert committees have been published over the past decade, the most recent of which represents a global initiative.[15] In the following discussion, no attempt is made to recapitulate published guidelines; rather, there is an effort to summarize the recommended general approaches, to point out gaps in information, and to highlight areas where controversy exists.

Nonpharmacologic Therapy

Although pharmacologic therapy has been an unexpendable component of good asthma management, nonpharmacologic management strategies, including patient education and avoidance of asthma triggers, are also important. These strategies are increasingly emphasized in asthma disease management programs designed to improve adherence to medication regimens and reduce hospitalizations for exacerbations. Recent studies suggest that patient education and environmental control programs are effective in reducing asthma morbidity, although additional research is needed to better determine which methods are the most effective and which patients benefit the most.

EDUCATION

The goal of asthma education is to improve patient understanding of the disease and its management and, consequently, to improve adherence to treatment recommendations. Another aim is to engage the patient in self-management practices, especially in terms of identifying and avoiding asthma triggers and recognizing and treating exacerbations of asthma in their earliest stages.

Controlled trials evaluating structured education and self-management programs for adult asthmatics generally show that such programs result in better asthma control and decreased emergency room visits and hospitalizations.[3,59] The success of patient education programs is, to a large extent, dependent on their format. For example, individual one-on-one educational sessions and sessions with small groups of patients have been shown to be of comparable efficacy; both are more effective than provision of written materials alone in terms of symptom control, use of proper inhaler technique, application of environmental control practices, and encouragement of physical activity.[59] However, the provision of written materials alone may be sufficient to decrease hospital and emergency room use.[3] Audiotapes may be substituted for written materials, but personal contact with a knowledgeable professional is considered superior to provision of either audiovisual or written materials. Because of the wide variation in personal learning skills and interest in participating in self-management, it is unlikely that any single educational format could suit the entire asthmatic population. Like drug therapy, the educational program, as well as the method and frequency of reinforcement, should be tailored to the individual.

With respect to the content of the educational program, the patient must first have an understanding of the disease. Included in this understanding is the knowledge that symptoms are a product of airflow obstruction and that therapy is designed to both prevent and relieve the obstruction. An understanding that asthma is a chronic disorder that is unlikely ever to go into complete remission is of primary importance. The patient should appreciate that symptoms will fluctuate and that occasional exacerbations are to be expected. In addition, reassurance should be provided that, with proper treatment, these events can be minimized; in most cases, a relatively normal lifestyle and normal life expectancy can be anticipated.

Educational programs should also encompass a discussion of the patient's individual treatment plan, including the purpose of different drugs, as well as their side effects. Distinguishing between drugs that control or prevent symptoms and those that relieve symptoms is necessary to reinforcing the importance of "controller" medications that offer no immediate relief of symptoms. Instruction in the proper use of inhaled medications is of obvious importance; so, too, is a description of likely triggers of episodes of asthma and ways to avoid such triggers. Finally, teaching the patient to recognize and intervene in exacerbations during their earliest stages can be helpful in avoiding more serious morbidity and, in some cases, mortality. Educating the patient in self-administration of oral glucocorticoids and providing a telephone number where professional assistance is available around the clock are, in our experience, the most crucial elements of a management program designed to reduce morbidity and hospitalizations.

ENVIRONMENTAL CONTROL

An important, often overlooked part of the management plan for all asthmatics, especially those with severe asthma who remain symptomatic despite intensive drug therapy, consists of measures to control environmental triggers. Avoidance of aeroallergens, viral respiratory pathogens, air pollution, and certain drugs (beta blockers, aspirin, etc.) can prevent exacerbations, reduce the need for drug treatment, and decrease utilization of emergency facilities. Of perhaps greater importance is avoidance of factors that may contribute to longer-term, subclinical airway inflammation responsible for abnormal airway responsiveness. Allergens from house dust mites, cockroaches, molds, and pets, particularly cats and dogs, have been associated with asthma. While the house dust mite is recognized as a significant cause of asthma throughout the developed world, the relative importance of different indoor allergens may vary among populations. For example, cockroach allergen may play a more prominent role in asthma in inner-city populations. Cat dander may be more important among suburban and rural dwellers or in areas where house pets are common and levels of mite and cockroach allergens are low.

Complete removal from exposure to house dust mites has been shown to reduce asthma severity and to reduce airway hyperresponsiveness.[43] However, incomplete or partial reductions of dust mite counts are of questionable benefit in improving asthma control.[12] Occupational asthma due to low-molecular-weight chemicals is also more likely to abate if patients are completely removed from exposure to the offending agent early in the course of their disease. Most patients with chronic asthma have numerous triggers. Therefore, the impact of avoidance of any single trigger is likely to vary considerably from patient to patient.

Other preventive measures also appear to be worthwhile. Influenza vaccination has been shown to reduce the incidence of upper respiratory illnesses in people of all ages. It seems likely that influenza vaccination would decrease the incidence of exacerbations of asthma, although we are not aware of studies that address this issue specifically. Allergen immunotherapy also appears to be of benefit in highly selected patients with defined allergic triggers.[1] As a rule, patients who have many allergic triggers tend to benefit less from immunotherapy than those with a single trigger. Furthermore, because of a high incidence of adverse systemic reactions, persons whose FEV_1 is less than 70 percent of predicted should be considered at high risk for immunotherapy.

Pharmacologic Management

Although most drugs now used to treat asthma have been in use for many years, only recently have there been large-scale, controlled trials to evaluate the efficacy of various regimens. This trend toward large, well-designed controlled trials is, in part, related to the development of treatment guidelines that have created both a structure and a demand for better information about asthma management. The structure for investigating asthma therapy evolved from a careful attempt to classify asthma according to clinical severity using symptoms, lung function, and drug use as variables. The demand for more information emerged from the realization that treatment guidelines could not be based on the results of well-designed studies. Rather, they could only reflect the opinion of experts. Controlled multicenter clinical trials have also been promoted by advances in drug development, including improved formulations of existing drugs, as well as novel classes of experimental compounds.

Drugs currently available to treat asthma are often classified as bronchodilator or nonbronchodilator agents, although there have been recent attempts to reclassify these agents as "reliever" or "controller" agents on the basis of their principal pharmacodynamic effect. Thus, short-acting bronchodilators such as inhaled beta agonists or anticholinergics are considered reliever medications. Corticosteroids, cromolyn sodium, nedocromil sodium, sustained-release theophylline, and long-acting beta agonists are considered controller medications, since they are used to achieve and maintain control of symptoms and are used daily on a long-term basis. Nomenclature that classifies drugs according to whether or not they have anti-inflammatory properties is discouraged, since some medications (e.g., theophylline) may have anti-inflammatory as well as bronchodilator properties.

β-ADRENERGIC AGENTS

Inhaled β_2-adrenergic agonists are the drugs of choice for relief of symptoms due to acute airway obstruction. Activation of the β_2-adrenergic receptor leads to activation of adenylate cyclase, an increase in cyclic AMP concentrations, and activation of protein kinase A. Protein kinase A lowers intracellular calcium concentrations by inhibiting myosin phosphorylation, resulting in relaxation of smooth muscle. Although there is evidence that beta agonists inhibit mast cell and eosinophil secretory function in vitro, the clinical importance of these effects is unknown. Short-acting beta agonists have a rapid onset of action and a 3- to 6-h duration of activity. At recommended doses, inhaled beta agonists have few adverse effects. Tachycardia, palpitations, and tremor are the most common side effects, and they often disappear during chronic administration; i.e., tolerance develops. Hypokalemia may occur at higher doses of inhaled beta agonists. Long-acting inhaled beta agonists, which have at least a 12-h duration of action, are available in some countries. These agents are not recommended for the short-term relief of acute symptoms. Rather, they are viewed as controller or maintenance medications and should be given twice daily on a long-term basis.

THEOPHYLLINE

For many years, long-acting preparations of theophylline were considered the first-line treatment of choice for asthma in the United States. Recently, their role in management has been redefined, and their use now is primarily as adjunctive therapy in patients whose symptoms fail to abate with inhaled corticosteroids. Although theophylline is generally considered a bronchodilator, it has relatively weak bronchodilator activity in therapeutic doses. Recent evidence suggests that theophylline may also have anti-inflammatory properties.[28]

The mechanisms underlying the effects of theophylline are unknown, although inhibition of the phosphodiesterase (PDE) isoenzyme PDE IV, with consequent increases in cyclic AMP, may be at work. The dose-related adverse effects of theophylline are well known, as are the drug interactions that lead to altered theophylline metabolism (Table 50-3). Although nausea is usually cited as the first sign of theophylline toxicity, in our experience, nervousness, anxiety, and tachycardia are more often the earliest manifestations of toxicity.

ANTICHOLINERGIC AGENTS

Anticholinergic agents induce airway smooth-muscle relaxation by blocking muscarinic receptors on airway smooth muscle, thus inhibiting vagally mediated cholinergic tone. In general, anticholinergic agents are not as effective as beta agonists in asthma. Although they have a slower onset of action than beta agonists, the duration of their activity is more prolonged, usually lasting 6 to 8 h. Because anticholinergic agents have a different side-effect profile than beta agonists, they are often given in combination with beta agonists in the management of severe acute asthma. Side effects are uncommon when quartenary ammonium compounds, such as ipratropium bromide, are used.

GLUCOCORTICOIDS

Glucocorticoids are the most effective agents available for treating moderate to severe asthma.[4] Although steroid efficacy is generally attributed to anti-inflammatory effects, the mechanisms whereby these agents suppress inflammation in asthma are unknown. Glucocorticoids are available for systemic or inhalational use. The major systemic side effects include adrenal suppression, osteoporosis, growth suppression, weight gain, hypertension, diabetes, dermal thinning, cataracts, myopathy, and psychotic reactions. These effects are dose related and are usually seen with systemic administration. Local side effects, including oral candidiasis and dysphonia, may occur at lower doses of inhaled glucocorticoids.

TABLE 50-3

Factors That Alter Theophylline Clearance

Increase Clearance
  Cigarette smoking
  Rifampin
  Phenytoin
  Barbiturates
Decrease Clearance
  Cirrhosis
  Heart failure
  Febrile viral illness
  Cimetidine
  Ciprofloxacin
  Erythromycin
  Troleandomycin
  Oral contraceptives
  Propranolol
  Allopurinol

CROMOLYN SODIUM AND NEDOCROMIL SODIUM

Cromolyn sodium and nedocromil sodium are classified as controller agents. Although these agents are chemically unrelated, they have similar clinical profiles and are believed to inhibit the release of chemical mediators from mast cells. Whereas cromolyn sodium and nedocromil sodium may inhibit bronchoconstriction induced by neurally mediated events, they may have other beneficial properties as well. Because they are remarkably safe, these drugs are considered first-line agents in the treatment of children with asthma. In adults, however, the drugs are most often prescribed for patients with mild disease, since responses are unpredictable.

TREATMENT REGIMENS BASED ON CLASSIFICATION

The classification of asthma as mild, moderate, or severe, as presented in published treatment guidelines, allows for a stepwise approach to drug therapy.[15] This approach recognizes that severity may vary with time and facilitates treatment as a dynamic process, with increments and decrements in drug dosages dictated by changes in severity of illness. Although errors in management are most often related to undertreatment with drugs, overtreatment can also be a problem, especially in patients with moderate to severe asthma. In such patients there is a tendency to maintain a static treatment regimen, even after symptoms are controlled and clinical stability is achieved.

Mild Asthma

A large percentage of asthmatic patients experience only mild, intermittent symptoms that are easily reversed by inhaled bronchodilators or are of brief duration and, hence, well tolerated. In fact, in a review of drug utilization records from a large health maintenance organization with a pharmacy benefit plan, we found that approximately 70 percent of patients with asthma use fewer than four canisters of a short- or intermediate-acting beta agonist per year (unpublished observations). The use of inhaled beta agonists on an as-needed basis as sole therapy is likely to provide satisfactory results and no major side effects for most asthmatics. Similarly, for patients whose symptoms occur under predictable circumstances—e.g., with exercise or exposure to airborne allergens such as danders and occupational agents—preventive treatment with an inhaled beta agonist or cromolyn sodium may be adequate. The use of inhaled beta agonists on an as-needed basis as sole therapy is usually recommended for patients who have normal or near-normal lung function (FEV_1 more than 80 percent predicted), little variability in peak flow (less than 20 percent), and symptoms that occur infrequently. For those who develop symptoms after exposure to allergens or occupational agents, the treatment of choice is, of course, avoidance of the offending agent, although that is not always possible.

Current treatment guidelines recommend the addition of a "controller" medication when mild symptoms are no longer intermittent.[15] Controller medications are those that are assumed to alleviate the underlying inflammatory basis of asthma. Included in this group are the inhaled glucocorticoids. There is general agreement that inhaled glucocorticoids are indicated in the patient with persistent asthma symptoms. However, there is no consensus on the frequency with which symptoms must occur before asthma is no longer considered mild and intermittent and additional therapy beyond as-needed beta agonists is indicated. This uncertainty is evident in the varied recommendations offered in different treatment guidelines. Some guidelines recommend additional treatment if symptoms occur more than once per week or if nocturnal symptoms occur more than twice per month. In our experience, few physicians prescribe inhaled glucocorticoids until "rescue" beta agonists are needed more than once daily to control symptoms. Thus, it is important to ask whether current treatment guidelines are too conservative in urging the use of medications that have unknown long-term side effects, or whether many physicians are withholding appropriate treatment. Guideline recommendations are intended not only to alleviate symptoms but also to prevent longer-term complications of asthma. With regard to the latter, recommendations appear to be predicated on the following assumptions: inhaled beta agonists will have adverse effects on airways if they are used on a frequent basis, and symptoms of only modest frequency suggest the presence of underlying airway inflammation, which will have long-term adverse consequences if left untreated.

Use of Inhaled Beta Agonists   Whether frequent use of inhaled beta agonists adversely affects the airways is a subject of considerable controversy. The controversy has several facets, the first of which pertains to the effects of regular beta-agonist use on asthma control. Although some studies have shown that regular use of beta agonists four times daily can lead to poor control of asthma symptoms, reduced lung function, and increased airway responsiveness,[47] others have failed to confirm these findings.[41] Much of the concern over possible adverse effects of beta agonists is based, unfortunately, on retrospective analysis of studies that were not designed to assess the adverse effects of regular beta-agonist use.

The second issue regarding safety of beta agonists pertains to the observation that regular use of inhaled beta agonists four times daily—or twice daily in the case of longer acting beta agonists—can lead to a decrease in the degree of protection that these agents afford against the bronchoconstrictor effects of exercise, allergens, and inhaled autocoids such as histamine or methacholine.[39] Loss of the protective effect can be seen as early as 7 days after regular administration of beta agonists. How long this phenomenon persists, once the drug is discontinued, is unknown.

The mechanism responsible for this loss of protection is not known, nor is the clinical importance of the phenomenon. If frequent beta-agonist use causes β-adrenergic receptor desensitization, it could lead to loss of functional antagonism—the putative mechanism of "bronchoprotection." Alternatively, regular beta-agonist use could lead to β-adrenergic receptor desensitization on mast cells, eosinophils, and other effector cells. By augmenting cell secretory function, such desensitization could cause an increase in airway inflammation. For example, regular treatment with terbutaline has been demonstrated to augment the airway response to adenosine, a compound that causes airway obstruction by mast cell stimulation.[39]

Issues related to regular use of beta agonists remain in the forefront of asthma management, despite practice guideline recommendations that beta agonists be used on an as-needed basis only. Pharmacy records suggest that physicians frequently prescribe short-acting beta agonists to be taken regularly, four times daily. Moreover, there are probably significant numbers of patients who are de facto, regular users because the frequency of their symptoms demands it. Equally important is the growing use of long-acting beta agonists that are intended to be used on a regular basis. Prospective clinical trials using measures of asthma control and airway responsiveness as primary endpoints are needed to resolve these issues.

Use of Anti-inflammatory Agents   Whether untreated airway inflammation leads to long-term adverse consequences is an unsettled issue. Of concern is the possibility that untreated airway inflammation may lead to airway remodeling and chronic, persistent airway obstruction. Examination of tissue from autopsies performed in elderly patients with long-standing asthma who died from unrelated causes has demonstrated narrowing of small airways in association with peribronchial fibrosis.[49] The fact that elderly patients with long-standing asthma have significant airway obstruction, even when asymptomatic, coupled with a lower level of reversibility of obstruction,[8] supports the hypothesis that long-standing inflammation might have adverse effects. Conversely, some elderly asthmatics who have had lifelong disease still demonstrate normal or near-normal lung function. This suggests that the natural history of asthma may be one of chronic persistent obstruction in some, but not all, patients. How these diverse natural histories reflect differences in pathogenesis is unknown.

If persistent airway obstruction is a consequence of untreated chronic airway inflammation, it is important to understand how inflammation becomes a chronic process. For example, it is not known whether chronicity is related to continued exposure to aggravating factors (e.g., allergens) or whether inflammation is sustained through self-perpetuating processes that are unrelated to exposures. If the former mechanism is operative, avoidance measures should be given higher priority than they are now given by most physicians. It is also important to know whether glucocorticoid therapy can prevent or alter such events. Inhaled glucocorticoids can alleviate symptoms and decrease airway responsiveness over a period of 1 year in patients with mild, intermittent asthma.[26] Moreover, the improvement in airway responsiveness has also been shown to occur in association with evidence of decreasing airway inflammation.[30]

On the basis of these observations, it might seem prudent to treat all patients, including those with the mildest disease, as early as possible with inhaled glucocorticoids. However, it should be noted that while glucocorticoid therapy reduces markers of inflammation, the improvement is not complete. Evidence of inflammation may persist even after 3 to 4 months of therapy.[7] Furthermore, if glucocorticoids are discontinued after long-term therapy, asthma will recur,[20] suggesting that underlying inflammation is not eradicated but rather only partly suppressed; airway remodeling may still occur.

A compelling argument for early treatment of patients with mild asthma can be made on the basis of studies comparing inhaled glucocorticoids with regularly scheduled beta agonists in patients with newly detected mild asthma.[19,20] In a trial spanning 2 years, inhaled glucocorticoids were found to be superior to beta agonists in improving peak expiratory flow, reducing symptoms and rescue beta-agonist medication use, and improving histamine responsiveness (Fig. 50-1). When inhaled glucocorticoids were discontinued or reduced in dosage, increases in symptoms and rescue beta-agonist use, as well as decreases in peak flow and spirometry, were noted (Fig. 50-1).[20] Moreover, when patients taking beta agonists were switched to inhaled glucocorticoids after 2 years, asthma abated, as measured by decreased symptoms, less rescue medication use, and slight increases in lung function. Of particular interest was the fact that patients who were switched to inhaled glucocorticoids after 2 years of beta-agonist use had much less improvement in airway responsiveness and morning peak flow than those initially given

inhaled glucocorticoids as first-line therapy. These results suggest that earlier intervention with inhaled glucocorticoids may result in better lung function and better symptom control over a 3-year period.

Although these studies tend to support the early use of glucocorticoids in all patients with mild asthma, ultimately the decision to treat is based on risk-benefit considerations, some of which are unknown. The short-term benefits of inhaled glucocorticoids—reduction in symptoms and inhaled beta-agonist use and improved lung function—are clear. In adults, the risks relate primarily to pituitary-adrenal suppression and osteoporosis. Studies of the effects of inhaled glucocorticoids on pituitary-

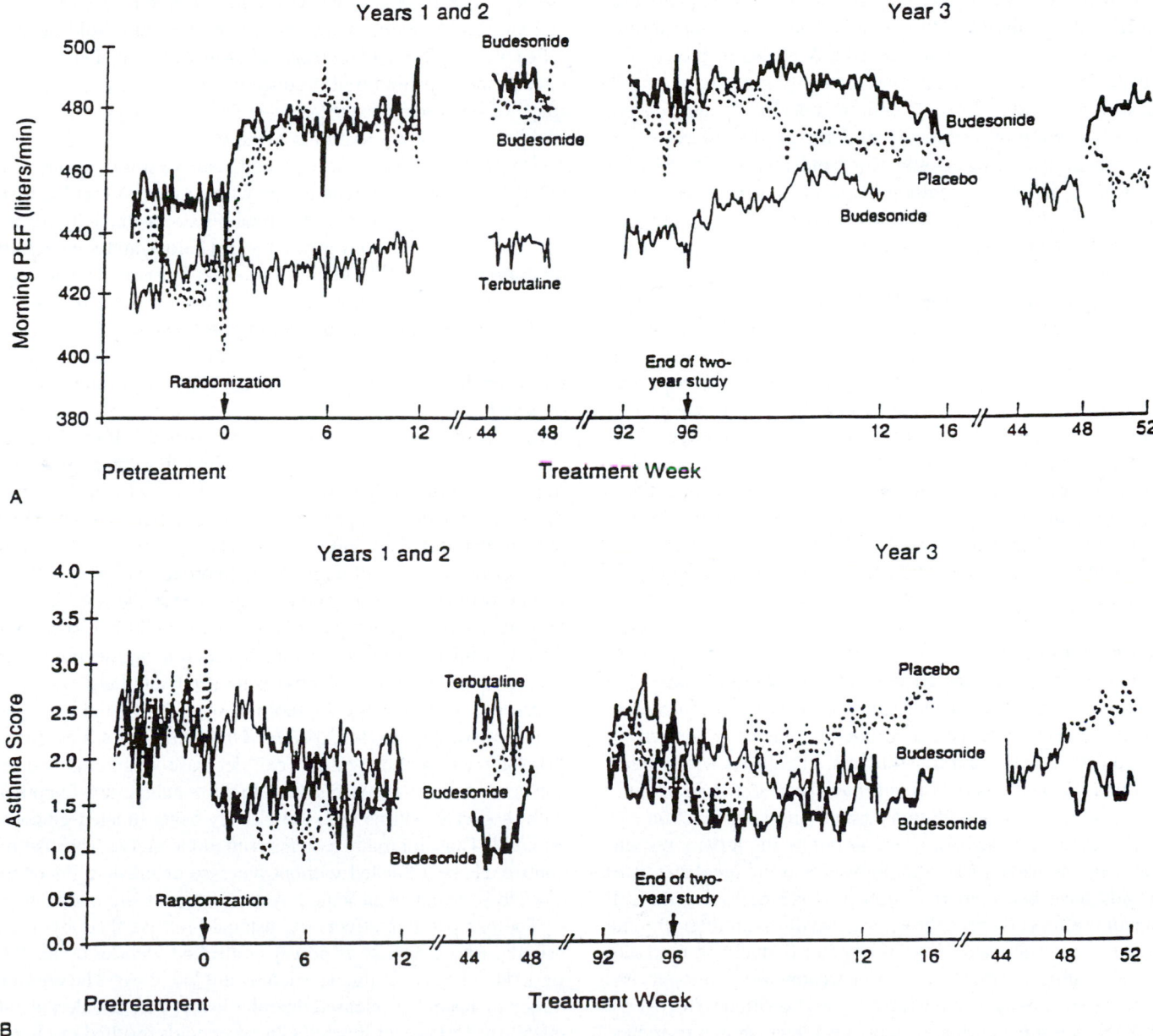

FIGURE 50-1 Day-to-day mean peak expiratory flow (PEF) (A) and asthma symptom scores (B) during a 3-year study comparing regular inhaled terbutaline with the inhaled glucocorticoid budesonide. During the first 2 years, patients were assigned to either terbutaline, 375 μg twice daily (n=53), or budesonide, 600 μg twice daily (n=50). After 2 years, 37 patients who received terbutaline were crossed over (open label) to budesonide, 600 μg twice daily. Of those treated with budesonide for the first 2 years, 19 patients were crossed over to treatment with budesonide, 200 μg twice daily, and 18 patients were assigned to placebo. The figure includes only patients completing all 3 years of the study. *(Based on data of Haahtela et al,[20] with permission.)*

adrenal function have yielded conflicting results due to differences in methods of measuring adrenal function, in techniques of aerosol delivery, and in treatment regimens. For similar reasons, the effects of inhaled glucocorticoids on bone mineral density are unclear. The risk of these adverse events is clearly related to dose; in the case of osteoporosis, risk is related to duration of therapy.

As a rule, doses below 1000 μg daily are considered safe for most patients taking currently available formulations of beclomethasone dipropionate, triamcinolone acetonide, or flunisolide. The safety profile of newer, more potent agents and the effects of newer delivery systems on dosing are now under investigation. Whether inhaled glucocorticoids, at doses now considered safe, will lead to skeletal complications in high-risk patients (e.g., post-menopausal women) remains to be seen. Furthermore, whether starting treatment during childhood, when bone formation is occurring, poses any additional risk is also unknown. The fact that inhaled glucocorticoids are currently not used in all patients with mild asthma reflects both the uncertainty and concern over the possibility of insidious, long-term adverse effects.

We recommend inhaled glucocorticoid therapy for any patients who experience symptoms requiring rescue beta-agonist use on a daily basis, or for patients who have moderately impaired lung function (FEV_1 less than 75 percent predicted). Glucocorticoids are used more selectively if symptoms are less frequent but still troublesome. Nonsteroidal anti-inflammatory alternatives, such as cromolyn or nedocromil, or even long-acting beta agonists are alternative approaches to achieving symptom control in mild asthmatics. Cromolyn and nedocromil may alleviate symptoms, reduce beta-agonist use, and, in the case of nedocromil, reduce airway responsiveness;[6,57] they might be of benefit in patients with mild asthma whose symptoms are increasing in frequency but occur less than once daily. In patients with more frequent or severe symptoms, inhaled glucocorticoids provide more favorable results. Cromolyn and nedocromil have a remarkable safety profile, and concerns over long-term effects are nonexistent.

Moderate Asthma

Moderate asthma is characterized by a symptom frequency that necessitates inhaled beta agonists several times daily; moderate asthma may also be defined as asthma in which frequent use of beta agonists fails to control symptoms. In patients with moderate asthma, inhaled glucocorticoids have been shown to be quite effective in controlling symptoms, improving lung function, decreasing rescue beta-agonist use, and improving airway responsiveness to methacholine.[19] Salutary effects of inhaled glucocorticoids have been reported after a single dose, but the full therapeutic effects of these drugs are usually seen after chronic administration. The major benefits of inhaled glucocorticoids are achieved within the first 2 weeks of treatment,[19] although improvement in airway responsiveness may continue for over a year.[26] Inhaled glucocorticoids have also been shown to reduce bronchial inflammation, as reflected by reductions in airway mast cells and eosinophils.[30] Because some markers of inflammation are not altered by either high- or low-dose inhaled glucocorticoids,[8] these effects of glucocorticoids are of uncertain clinical significance.

Although glucocorticoids are quite effective for controlling symptoms and improving lung function, they do not provide a cure for asthma. Patients whose condition is stabilized after a course of inhaled glucocorticoids can often undergo a reduction in dosage without loss of stability.[20] However, abrupt discontinuation of glucocorticoids after long-term treatment may result in clinical deterioration. The interval between complete discontinuation of therapy and deterioration is quite variable and may range from several days to more than a year.[20,56]

Although a few investigations have demonstrated efficacy of inhaled glucocorticoids at low doses,[19,26] most efficacy studies reported in the literature have examined high doses. The threshold dose at which efficacy can be demonstrated is likely to vary considerably within the asthmatic population. Thus, choosing a starting dose is largely empiric and not aided by current prescribing information. While there may be a threshold dose for efficacy in a given patient, it is not clear that an increase in dose beyond the threshold will produce greater salutary effects. As a rule, we recommend starting at higher doses and reducing the dose after symptom control is achieved.

Unfortunately, there is little comparative information on inhaled glucocorticoid preparations with respect to relative therapeutic or toxic potencies in the treatment of asthma. Table 50-4 lists the commonly used inhaled formulations and their relative binding affinities and potencies in other systems. Whereas different products are not equivalent on a puff-per-puff basis, by convention they are considered more or less equivalent on a microgram-per-microgram basis. The comparisons are crude and unproven, however, and the drugs may not be equivalent in terms of toxicity.

Inhaled glucocorticoids in usual doses (under 1000 μg a day) may not be sufficient to control symptoms in some patients. Options for additional therapy are usually limited to an increase in the dose of inhaled glucocorticoid or the addition of another medication, particularly a long-acting beta agonist or sustained-release theophylline. Although either approach is likely to result in improvement, recent studies suggest that the addition of a long-acting beta agonist provides greater benefit than does an increase in inhaled glucocorticoid. Symptoms are decreased; the need for rescue beta-agonist use is reduced; and lung function is improved, including higher morning peak flow and decreased peak flow variability (Fig. 50-2).[17] Other studies have confirmed that long-acting beta agonists can decrease symptoms and rescue beta-agonist use when given as additional therapy to patients with moderate asthma who are already using inhaled glucocorticoids.[41] Thus, for many patients with moderately severe asthma, control can be achieved without increase of inhaled glucocorticoid doses to levels at which systemic effects are encountered.

The comparative effects of sustained-release theophylline in patients whose disease is poorly controlled with less than 1000 μg a day of inhaled glucocorticoids are less clear. The administration of sustained-released theophylline to patients already taking 500 to 1500 μg of inhaled glucocorticoids resulted in a higher morning peak flow rate than did the addition of salbutamol (albuterol) four times daily.[45] The salutary effects of theophylline include bronchodilatation, enhanced mucociliary clearance, and improved diaphragmatic muscle contractility. Recent evidence also suggests that theophylline has anti-inflammatory activity.[28]

TABLE 50-4

Characteristics of Inhaled Glucocorticoids

Glucocorticoid	Relative Binding Affinity*	Relative Blanching Potency†	Inhaled Dose (µg/puff)
Beclomethasone dipropionate‡	0.4	600	50,100‖
Beclomethasone monopropionate‡	13.5	450	—
Triamcinolone	3.6	330	100¶
Flunisolide	1.8	330	250
Budesonide§	9.4	980	50, 100, 200
Fluticasone	18.0	1200	44, 110, 220

*Values are for binding affinity to human glucocorticoid receptors in vitro, relative to that of dexamethasone.
†Blanching potency on human skin indicates topical potency, relative to that of dexamethasone.
‡Beclomethasone dipropionate is converted in the liver to the more active beclomethasone monopropionate.
§Not available in the United States.
‖Larger doses (200, 250 µg per puff) are available in Europe, Asia, and Australia but are not available in the United States.
¶The dose delivered by the metered-dose inhaler is 200 µg, but 100 µg is delivered by spacer.
SOURCE: Adapted from Reed: *Am Rev Respir Dis* 140(suppl):S82–S88, 1990, and Barnes: *New Engl J Med* 332:868–875, 1995.

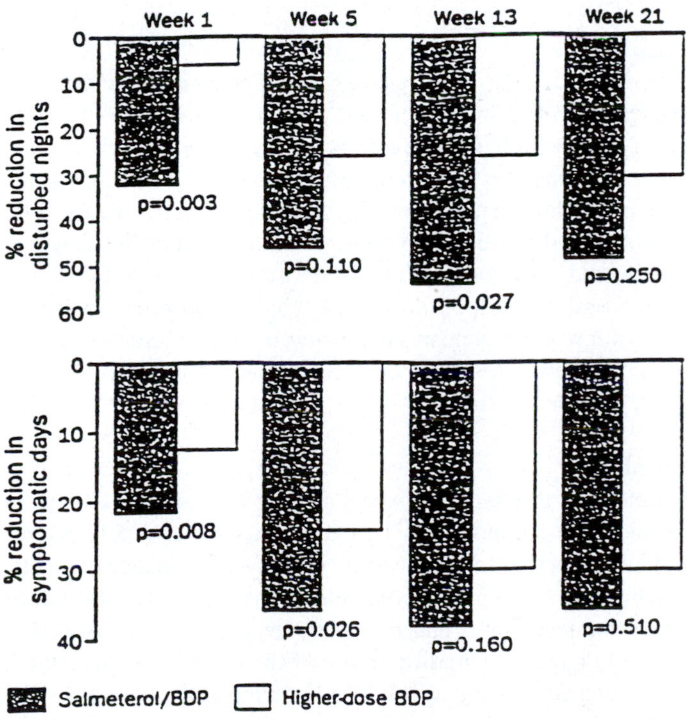

sustained-released theophylline in controlling symptoms, increasing peak flow, and reducing the need for rescue beta-agonist use; in addition, the incidence of side effects was lower.[14] Longer-term comparisons of long-acting beta-agonists and sustained-release theophyllines in patients whose disease is not controlled by inhaled glucocorticoids are of potential value, since theophylline is less costly and offers an alternative route of administration for patients who prefer, or are better able to use, oral medications than metered-dose inhalers. Although encouraging anecdotes exist, the role of nedocromil or cromolyn as additional therapy in patients with asthma not controlled by inhaled glucocorticoids has not been established.

FIGURE 50-2   The effects of added salmeterol versus higher-dose inhaled glucocorticoid in patients with asthma symptoms while taking beclomethasone dipropionate (BDP), 200 µg twice daily. Patients randomly received either salmeterol (50 µg twice daily) or increased BDP (500 µg twice daily) for 6 months. *(Based on data of Greening et al,[17] with permission.)*

There is little question that theophylline is efficacious in patients with asthma. However, because of a low therapeutic index and high potential for severe toxicity, the role of sustained-released theophylline in asthma management is unclear. In a 2-week comparative trial that was confounded by failure to maintain theophylline blood levels of at least 10 µg/ml in many patients, long-acting beta agonists were shown to be superior to

Severe Asthma

For purposes of discussion, severe asthma can be defined as asthma in which symptoms persist despite treatment with inhaled glucocorticoids (at or under 1000 µg daily) and additional therapy, in the form of either long-acting beta agonists or theophylline. Severe asthma is frequently caused by poor adherence to drug regimens or exposure to environmental factors or drugs, such as aspirin or beta blockers. A thorough investigation of these factors is indicated before the start of additional drug therapy.

For the patient with severe asthma, chemotherapeutic options are quite limited. Although doses of inhaled glucocorticoids can be increased, dosages of theophylline and long-acting beta agonists are limited because of the risk of toxicity. Options include increasing the dose of inhaled glucocorticoids, adding sustained-release theophylline in patients already taking inhaled glucocorticoids and long-acting beta agonists, and adding a long-acting beta agonist to the regimen for patients already taking inhaled glucocorticoids and theophylline. Patients who fail to achieve symptom control, despite treatment with inhaled glucocorticoids in doses up to 2000 µg daily and one or more long-acting bronchodilators, are often considered candidates for systemic glucocorticoid therapy.

Oral glucocorticoids are favored over parenteral formulations and, in principle, should be given in the lowest dose possible every other morning. However, it is recognized that daily or even twice-daily doses are required in some patients. Oral glucocorticoids may be given in moderate to high doses (0.5 mg/kg per day) for 8 to 21 days, followed by a tapering course to the lowest dose that maintains control. This approach is often sufficient to modify the underlying disease process and to permit better control at lower doses. Although a "threshold dose" of glucocorticoids is required to maintain stability in some patients, this approach may achieve results that are good enough to permit complete discontinuation of oral glucocorticoids.

Whereas potent and higher-dose formulations of inhaled glucocorticoids are now available, it is reasonable to ask whether the administration of increasing doses of inhaled glucocorticoids is more appropriate than prescribing oral steroids. For equivalent therapeutic effects, inhaled glucocorticoids have been shown to produce fewer steroid-related side effects than oral glucocorticoids.[55] Moreover, comparisons of oral prednisolone (40 mg a day) with budesonide (3.2 mg a day) have demonstrated greater systemic toxicity with prednisolone, despite greater efficacy with budesonide.[21] Others have shown that high doses of fluticasone (1000 μg twice daily) can improve asthma control and measures of quality of life. At the same time, the high doses permit a reduction in oral prednisone in severe cases with abnormal lung function and symptoms despite intensive therapy.[38] Thus, improved formulations of inhaled glucocorticoids may obviate chronic oral prednisone.

Patients who require high doses of oral glucocorticoids to maintain control of symptoms are referred to as *steroid-dependent* asthmatics. This is in contrast to *steroid-resistant* patients, who fail to demonstrate an improvement in lung function on reasonably high doses of systemic steroids, despite demonstrable improvement with inhaled beta agonists. Steroid resistance may be a primary defect due to an unknown intrinsic abnormality, or it may be secondary defect related to increased steroid metabolism or the effects of drugs that alter steroid activity. Steroid dependence, on the other hand, is thought to be a reflection of severe disease with intense airway inflammation. In fact, these may simply be semantic differences, since intense airway inflammation itself may alter steroid responsiveness, and steroid dependence may be nothing more than an intermediate form of true resistance. Glucocorticoid resistance in asthma and its potential mechanisms have been reviewed.[5] In patients with severe asthma manifesting steroid dependence or resistance, consideration should be given to the use of alternative anti-inflammatory agents.

ALTERNATIVE ANTI-INFLAMMATORY THERAPY

Because of the complex array of inflammatory mechanisms putatively at work in asthma, there has been hope that agents such as gold salts, methotrexate, cyclosporine, and others might prove effective in management.

Gold Salts

In a short-term, blinded, placebo-controlled trial, oral gold salts have been found to decrease symptoms and increase FEV_1.[37] A reduction in average daily prednisone dosage from 9.3 to 5.3 mg was achieved in gold-treated patients, whereas no prednisone reduction was achieved in placebo-treated patients. The side effects of gold treatment included serious eczema (in 16 percent of patients) and nausea and diarrhea (in 25 percent). Parenteral gold has also been found to be superior to placebo in terms of relieving symptoms and reducing oral corticosteroid requirements, although side effects are frequent and patient tolerance is rather poor. Unfortunately, no studies have examined the longer-term effects of gold in steroid-dependent asthmatics. Based on current information, gold therapy appears to be associated with considerable risk, especially when administered parenterally, and its usefulness in the management of asthma should be considered unproven on the basis of risk-benefit considerations.

Methotrexate

Several controlled studies of the efficacy of methotrexate in the management of severe asthma have been carried out; results are mixed. In general, the discordant results obtained from these trials suggest that the benefits of methotrexate are not universal and are, perhaps, of questionable significance, particularly in light of the potential for significant adverse reactions to the drug. On the other hand, given the probability that asthma pathogenesis is heterogeneous, it would not be surprising to find a select group of steroid-dependent asthmatics who might derive benefit from methotrexate or another anti-inflammatory agent.

Macrolide Antibiotics

Studies of the steroid-sparing effects of macrolide antibiotics in asthma management have yielded discordant results. While macrolide therapy has been reported to achieve steroid dose reductions in some patients, or to allow alternate-day dosing in others, at least some of these effects appear to be caused by alterations in steroid metabolism.[52] Thus, while steroid dose reductions may be achieved, systemic effects may be enhanced, leading to increased steroid-related side effects.

Cyclosporine

Few clinical studies have examined the effects of cyclosporine in asthma. In the only controlled trial of cyclosporine (5 mg/kg a day) in steroid-dependent asthmatics,[2] peak flow improved and fewer exacerbations occurred in the treated group during the 12-week trial. However, the treated group experienced frequent side effects, including headache, hypertension, hypertrichosis, paresthesias, and infections with herpes zoster. No significant reduction in oral prednisone dose was achieved. Further controlled trials of low-dose cyclosporine, using frequency asthma exacerbations rather than steroid dose reductions as the primary endpoint, may be warranted.

Colchicine

Another anti-inflammatory agent of interest in asthma therapy is colchicine, a compound that inhibits microtubular polymerization and that has a wide array of anti-inflammatory effects. Colchicine has been shown to relieve symptoms and to reduce rescue bronchodilator usage in patients with allergic asthma.[46] We are not aware of studies on use of this drug in severe asthma or as a steroid-sparing agent. The beneficial effects of fish oils, chloroquine, and hydroxychloroquine also remain unproved.

FUTURE THERAPIES

Several new types of antiasthmatic compounds are currently undergoing clinical trials and are expected to be approved for general use in the near future.

Lipoxygenase Inhibitors and Leukotriene Receptor Antagonists

Compounds that alter the pathophysiological effects of leukotrienes derived from the 5-lipoxygenation of arachidonic acid are likely to be the first novel drugs available. Two classes of agents are under investigation: inhibitors of the 5-lipoxygenase (5-LO) enzyme and leukotriene D_4 (LTD_4) receptor antagonists. Clinical studies have shown that the 5-LO inhibitors and the LTD_4 receptor antagonists can inhibit the bronchospastic effects of allergens, exercise, cold dry air, and aspirin challenge. Both strategies have been found efficacious in alleviating symptoms and improving pulmonary function during 4 to 6 weeks of therapy in patients with moderately severe asthma.[25,50]

Since most efficacy studies of the antileukotriene products have, thus far, entailed comparisons with placebo only, the position of 5-LO inhibitors and LTD_4 receptor antagonists in asthma management is still speculative. There are no published studies comparing the effects of either class of compound with inhaled corticosteroids in the management of patients whose disease is poorly controlled with only a beta agonist used on an as-needed basis. Furthermore, there are no studies of these agents as added therapy in patients with more severe disease. Because of the perceived importance of cysteinyl peptide leukotrienes in asthma pathogenesis, further clinical trials examining these questions, as well as the role of antileukotrienes in the management of severe acute asthma, are warranted.

Other Agents

Agents designed to inhibit the effects of cytokine products, such as IL-4 and IL-5, are nearing the stage of clinical trials. Other approaches under investigation entail regulation of IgE synthesis, anti-IgE antibodies, and cytokines that down-regulate allergic inflammation. Most of these novel compounds have a highly specific biologic target or mode of action. Availability of the agents will furnish a unique opportunity to test hypotheses concerning the role of specific proinflammatory pathways in asthma pathogenesis and, perhaps, provide new and effective modes of therapy. Because of the specificity of newer agents, it is likely that some agents will prove more effective in certain patients than others, and that the variability in response will reflect differences in the relative importance of different pathogenetic pathways.

Treatment of Associated Conditions

Successful management of asthma often requires treatment of conditions that are thought to aggravate asthmatic symptoms. Although asthma may coexist with a number of disorders that affect lung function, especially in the elderly, gastroesophageal reflux disease and chronic sinusitis are the most common disorders associated with poorly controlled asthma.

GASTROESOPHAGEAL REFLUX DISEASE

The widely accepted notion that gastroesophageal reflux disease (GERD) can aggravate asthma is, to a large extent, based on empiric observations that antireflux therapy often improves asthma control. A review of the medical literature tends to support this notion, but the evidence is not strong and is somewhat discordant.[48] In general, most studies have employed small numbers of subjects and have suffered from poor study design. Ambulatory intraesophageal pH monitoring is a sensitive and specific diagnostic test to verify the diagnosis of GERD. While a negative study is valuable in excluding GERD as a cause of asthma symptoms, a positive study does not indicate that GERD

is the cause of asthma symptoms. As a rule, an empiric course of antireflux therapy is necessary to establish a causal relationship. Antireflux therapy should be offered to patients with GERD who complain of reflux symptoms (heartburn, water brash, regurgitation, dysphagia, hoarseness, and choking) in association with wheezing; patients with worsening asthma symptoms after meals or with reclining; and patients with intractable nocturnal asthma. Patients whose disease is poorly controlled on antiasthma medications, those who require either systemic or high-dose inhaled glucocorticoid therapy, and elderly patients with new-onset asthma should also be considered candidates for antireflux therapy.

Medical management of GERD consists of conservative antireflux measures, such as antacids, blockers of the histamine$_2$ receptor (H$_2$RA), protein pump inhibitors, such as omeprazole, and prokinetic agents, such as cisapride. While studies suggest that the use of any of these agents may relieve asthma symptoms in some patients, recent work indicates that the proper management of GERD requires higher doses of medications than are usually recommended, especially H$_2$RA agents.

Recent studies have demonstrated the efficacy of surgical approaches to GERD.[31] Although the relative benefits of medical versus surgical approaches are yet to be defined, we consider surgery only as a long-term alternative in patients who have demonstrated abatement of asthma symptoms on adequate medical therapy. Recently developed less invasive laparoscopic fundoplication procedures may prove useful as a therapeutic alternative in these patients.

CHRONIC SINUSITIS

The relationship between asthma and chronic sinusitis is well established,[36] although the underlying mechanisms are not clear. In general, the association between asthma and chronic sinusitis is limited to patients with extensive disease, as determined by patency of the nasal passages and osteomeatal complex and thickening of the sinus mucosa.[36] Although aggressive treatment of chronic sinusitis is generally believed to result in improved asthma control, there is little published supportive evidence. The treatment of choice for sinusitis includes antibiotics, decongestants, and intranasal topical glucocorticoids. Patients who fail to respond to medical therapy may benefit from endoscopic sphenoethmoidectomy. It should be noted, however, that the results of endoscopic sinus surgery are poorest in patients with asthma, especially those with aspirin sensitivity and polyposis.

Patient Monitoring

In an individual patient, severity may fluctuate with time, owing to changes in environmental exposure or improved disease management, or because of the natural history of the disease. Ongoing treatment should remain consistent with disease severity. Hence, just as therapy is "stepped up" to gain control in symptomatic patients, a gradual reduction in medications, starting with the medication with the greatest toxicity, should be attempted once stability is achieved and sustained for several months.

SYMPTOMS, PEAK FLOW, AND SPIROMETRY

Long-term monitoring of the asthmatic patient is essential for proper adjustment of the management plan. Published guidelines have emphasized the importance of objective measurements over symptoms because of poor patient perception of airway obstruction, especially in patients with long-standing asthma.[15] On the other hand, for some patients, symptoms may be a more sensitive indicator of deterioration than are peak expiratory flow measurements. Clearly, the best strategy for monitoring asthma on a long-term basis is to use both objective and subjective measures. The amount of rescue beta agonist used on a daily basis is also a useful barometer of asthma control.

Whereas spirometry is recommended to diagnose airway obstruction in the initial assessment of the asthmatic patient, we believe that spirometry and peak flow measurements provide comparable information for monitoring patients on a long-term basis. The historical advantage of peak flow measurements has been their relative ease of performance and lack of expense with self-monitoring on a daily basis. The recent development of hand-held, automated spirometers providing digital output of FEV_1 and data storage capability may offer an alternative for home monitoring. It remains to be determined, however, whether self-administered spirometry is as reliable as peak flow measurements. The goal of monitoring symptoms, along with objective measures of lung function, is to achieve a balance in the control of symptoms and physiology with an acceptable level of drug therapy. For example, using high-dose glucocorticoids to achieve a normal FEV_1 in a patient who has tolerable symptoms with a lower FEV_1 may be counter to the best interests of the patient.

Asthma treatment guidelines have included an enthusiastic recommendation that patients use peak expiratory flow measurements not only to monitor their course but also to dictate self-administered treatment regimens. This recommendation is based on studies showing improvement in subjective, as well as objective, measures of asthma control when patients used peak flow measurements to adjust medication usage. The combination of home peak flow monitoring and a comprehensive education and self-management program has been shown to increase pulmonary function, to reduce physician visits and emergency room admissions, and to reduce use of inhaled beta agonists and prednisone when compared with a program of minimal education and no self-management.[24] It is difficult to ascertain from these studies, however, how much benefit is derived from peak flow monitoring compared with the other interventions. In addition, the relative benefits of comprehensive education and symptom-guided self-management are unclear. Notably, in a study of integrated asthma care, the benefits of routine peak flow monitoring as part of a self-management plan over a program of conventional peak flow monitoring without self-management could not be demonstrated.[13]

Given the variable nature of asthma and the people it afflicts, it seems unlikely that peak flow-guided self-management would benefit all patients at all times. Clearly, no single treatment algorithm is apt to be the best therapeutic plan for all patients with the same change in peak flow. Likewise, not all patients are capable of executing, or even comprehending, complicated treat-ment plans. Future studies should focus on whether the benefits of peak flow–guided self-management, if any, outweigh the risks of overtreatment that might result from its use. Severely asthmatic patients using home peak flow monitoring tend to use more oral glucocorticoids.[13] Although this may be viewed as a potential benefit of peak flow monitoring, it is unclear whether the increased use is appropriate or medically warranted. Although the correspondence between peak expiratory flow and its variability and symptoms or other measures of asthma severity is quite good, it is not absolute. Future studies comparing home peak flow monitoring with other means of grading disease activity, such as rescue bronchodilator use, or more quantitative assessments of asthma symptoms may be useful.

Although the role of peak flow monitoring in asthma management needs to be more clearly defined, the practice of self-monitoring is beneficial to some, if not most, patients. When there are striking discrepancies between reported symptoms and physiological findings, peak flow monitoring can be useful in establishing a diagnosis and in defining the severity of disease. Peak flow measurements, whether used for monitoring purposes only or for patient-induced adjustments in the medical regimen, can improve medication adherence and prompt earlier physician contact during an exacerbation. In our practice, peak flow meters are offered to all patients for home monitoring. However, the use of peak flow measurements to dictate patient-initiated dosage adjustments is offered on a more selective basis.

MARKERS OF AIRWAY INFLAMMATION

The importance of using markers of airway inflammation to monitor disease activity is uncertain. While asthma symptoms, airway responsiveness, and numbers of airway inflammatory cells correlate, the correlations are primarily of statistical interest and are not predictive of one another in an individual patient. For example, there is considerable overlap in airway responsiveness between patients who require only occasional therapy and those who are steroid dependent. That asymptomatic asthmatics with normal lung function have evidence of ongoing airway inflammation is also well established. The important unanswered question is whether untreated airway inflammation leads to chronic and persistent airway obstruction. If so, treatment of asymptomatic patients with normal lung function may be indicated; under these circumstances, markers of airway inflammation will be important in long-term monitoring. Defining the marker that best reflects the inflammatory diathesis of asthma is an important scientific challenge.

EOSINOPHIL COUNTS

Eosinophil counts have been shown to correlate with peak flow measurements in asthmatics whose disease is poorly controlled.[18] In our experience, however, eosinophil counts may be low in patients with severe, uncontrolled disease. In addition, they may be elevated in some patients with severe allergic rhinitis and rather mild asthma. Because of their poor sensitivity and specificity, blood eosinophil counts are not recommended in routine monitoring of asthma severity or as a barometer of airway inflammation.

Eosinophil cationic protein (ECP), an eosinophil granule protein, has also been shown to correlate with peak flow and is thought to reflect not only eosinophil numbers but eosinophil activity as well.[18] Although ECP serum levels have been of value in studies of large groups of patients, it is not clear that they are of value in monitoring individual patients.

NITRIC OXIDE LEVELS

Levels of nitric oxide (NO) in mixed expired gas have been found to be elevated in asthmatics as compared with normal subjects. The level may reflect the degree of underlying airway inflammation. Mixed expired concentrations of NO have been shown to fall during glucocorticoid therapy in patients with severe exacerbations of asthma, suggesting a possible role for NO as an index of disease severity or treatment efficacy.[32] Further studies are needed to assess the value of measurements of NO in patients with less severe disease.

REFERENCES

1. Abramson MJ, Puy RM, Weiner JM: Is allergen immunotherapy effective in asthma? *Am J Respir Crit Care Med* 151:969–974, 1995.
2. Alexander AG, Barnes NC, Kay AB: Trial of cyclosporin in corticosteroid-dependent chronic severe asthma. *Lancet* 339:324–328, 1992.
3. Bailey WC, Richards JM Jr, Brooks CM, et al: A randomized trial to improve self-management practices of adults with asthma. *Arch Intern Med* 150:1664–1666, 1990.
4. Barnes PJ, Pedersen S: Efficacy and safety of inhaled corticosteroids in asthma. *Am Rev Respir Dis* 148(Suppl):S1–S26, 1993.
5. Barnes PJ, Greening AP, Crompton GK: Glucocorticoid resistance in asthma. *Am J Respir Crit Care Med* 152(Suppl):S125–S142, 1995.
6. Bel EH, Timmers MC, Hermans J, et al: The long-term effects of nedocromil sodium and beclomethasone dipropionate on bronchial responsiveness to methacholine in nonatopic asthmatic subjects. *Am Rev Respir Dis* 141:21–28, 1990.
7. Booth H, Richmond I, Ward C, et al: Effect of high dose inhaled fluticasone propionate on airway inflammation in asthma. *Am J Respir Crit Care Med* 152:45–52, 1995.
8. Braman SS, Kaemmerlen JT, Davis SM: Asthma in the elderly: A comparison between patients with recently acquired and long-standing disease. *Am Rev Respir Dis* 143:336–340, 1991.
9. Burrows B, Barbee RA, Cline MG, et al: Characteristics of asthma among elderly adults in a sample of the general population. *Chest* 100:935–942, 1991.
10. Christopher KL, Wood RP, Eckert RC, et al: Vocal cord dysfunction presenting as asthma. *New Engl J Med* 308:1566–1570, 1983.
11. Cockcroft DW, Murdock KY, Berscheid BA, Gore BP: Sensitivity and specificity of histamine PC_{20} determination in a random selection of young college students. *J Allergy Clin Immunol* 89:23–30, 1992.
12. Dietemann A, Bessot J-C, Hoyet C, et al: A double-blind, placebo controlled trial of solidified benzyl benzoate applied in dwellings of asthmatic patients sensitive to mites: Clinical efficacy and effect on mite allergens. *J Allergy Clin Immunol* 91:738–746, 1993.
13. Drummond N, Abdalla M, Beattie JAG, et al: Effectiveness of routine self-monitoring of peak flow in patients with asthma. *Br Med J* 308:564–567, 1994.
14. Fjellbirkeland L, Gulsvik A, Palmer JB: The efficacy and tolera-
15. Global initiative for asthma. Global strategy for asthma management and prevention. NHLBI/WHO Workshop Report. Bethesda, MD, Department of Health and Human Services. Publication No. 95-3659, 1995.
16. Goldman J, Muers M: Vocal cord dysfunction and wheezing. *Thorax* 46:401–404, 1991.
17. Greening AP, Ind PW, Northfield M, Shaw G: Added salmeterol versus higher-dose corticosteroid in asthma patients with symptoms on existing inhaled corticosteroids. *Lancet* 344:219–224, 1994.
18. Griffin E, Hkansson L, Formgren H, et al: Blood eosinophil number and activity in relation to lung function in patients with asthma and eosinophilia. *J Allergy Clin Immunol* 87:548–557, 1991.
19. Haahtela T, Järvinen M, Kava T, et al: Comparison of a β_2-agonist, terbutaline, with an inhaled corticosteroid, budesonide, in newly detected asthma. *New Engl J Med* 325:388–392, 1991.
20. Haahtela T, Järvinen M, Kava T, et al: Effects of reducing or discontinuing inhaled budesonide in patients with mild asthma. *New Engl J Med* 331:700–705, 1994.
21. Hodsman AB, Toogood JH, Jennings B, et al: Differential effects of inhaled budesonide and oral prednisolone on serum osteocalcin. *J Clin Endocrinol Metab* 72:530–540, 1991.
22. Hodson ME, Simon G, Batten JC: Radiology of uncomplicated asthma. *Thorax* 29:296–303, 1974.
23. Hopp RJ, Bewtra AK, Nair NM, Townley RG: Specificity and sensitivity of methacholine inhalation challenge in normal and asthmatic children. *J Allergy Clin Immunol* 74:154–158, 1984.
24. Ignacio-Garcia JM, Gonzalez-Santos P: Asthma self-management education program by home monitoring of peak expiratory flow. *Am J Respir Crit Care Med* 151:353–359, 1995.
25. Israel E, Rubin P, Kemp JP, et al: The effect of inhibition of 5-lipoxygenase by zileuton in mild-to-moderate asthma. *Ann Intern Med* 119:1059–1066, 1993.
26. Juniper EF, Kline PA, Vanzieleghem MA, et al: Effect of long-term treatment with an inhaled corticosteroid (budesonide) on airway hyperresponsiveness and clinical asthma in nonsteroid-dependent asthmatics. *Am Rev Respir Dis* 142:832–836, 1990.
27. Kesten S, Rebuck AS: Is the short-term response to inhaled β-adrenergic agonist sensitive or specific for distinguishing between asthma and COPD? *Chest* 105:1042–1045, 1994.
28. Kidney J, Dominguez M, Taylor PM, et al: Immunomodulation by theophylline in asthma. *Am J Respir Crit Care Med* 151:1907–1914, 1995.
29. Knudson RJ, Kaltenborn WT, Burrows B: Single breath carbon monoxide transfer factor in different forms of chronic airflow obstruction in a general population sample. *Thorax* 45:514–519, 1990.
30. Laitinen LA, Laitinen A, Haahtela T: A comparative study of the effects of an inhaled corticosteroid, budesonide, and a β_2-agonist, terbutaline, on airway inflammation in newly diagnosed asthma: A randomized, double-blind, parallel-group controlled trial. *J Allergy Clin Immunol* 90:32–42, 1992.
31. Larrain A, Carrasco E, Galleguillos F, et al: Medical and surgical treatment of nonallergic asthma associated with gastroesophageal reflux. *Chest* 99:1330–1335, 1991.
32. Massaro AF, Gaston B, Kita D, et al: Expired nitric oxide levels during treatment of acute asthma. *Am J Respir Crit Care Med* 152:800–803, 1995.
33. McFadden ER Jr, Gilbert IA: Exercise-induced asthma. *New Engl J Med* 330:1362–1367, 1994.
34. McFadden ER Jr, Lyons HA: Arterial-blood gas tension in asthma. *New Engl J Med* 278:1027–1032, 1968.

35. National Health Interview Survey Series 10, No. 166. DHHS Publication No. (PHS) 88–1594, 1987, p 85.

36. Newman LJ, Platts-Mills TAE, Phillips CD, et al: Chronic sinusitis: Relationship of computed tomographic findings to allergy, asthma, and eosinophilia. *JAMA* 271:363–367, 1994.

37. Nierop G, Gijzel WP, Bel EH, et al: Auranofin in the treatment of steroid dependent asthma: A double blind study. *Thorax* 47:349–354, 1992.

38. Noonan M, Chervinsky P, Busse WW, et al: Fluticasone propionate reduces oral prednisone use while it improves asthma control and quality of life. *Am J Respir Crit Care Med* 152:1467–1473, 1995.

39. O'Connor BJ, Aikman SL, Barnes PJ: Tolerance to the nonbronchodilator effects of inhaled β_2-agonists in asthma. *New Engl J Med* 327:1204–1208, 1992.

40. Parker CD, Bilbo RE, Reed CE: Methacholine aerosol as test for bronchial asthma. *Arch Intern Med* 115:452–458, 1965.

41. Pearlman DS, Chervinsky P, LaForce C, et al: A comparison of salmeterol with albuterol in the treatment of mild-to-moderate asthma. *New Engl J Med* 327:1420–1425, 1992.

42. Pennock BE, Rogers RM, McCaffree: Changes in measured spirometric indices—what is significant? *Chest* 80:97–99, 1981.

43. Platts-Mills TAE, Mitchell EB, Nock P, et al: Reduction of bronchial hyperreactivity during prolonged allergen avoidance. *Lancet* 2:675–678, 1982.

44. Quackenboss JJ, Lebowitz MD, Krazyzanowski M: The normal range of diurnal changes in peak expiratory flow rates. *Am Rev Respir Dis* 142:323–330, 1991.

45. Rivington RN, Boulet L-P, Côté J, et al: Efficacy of Uniphyl, salbutamol, and their combination in asthmatic patients on high-dose inhaled steroids. *Am J Respir Crit Care Med* 151:325–332, 1995.

46. Schwarz YA, Kivity S, Ilfeld DN, et al: A clinical and immunologic study of colchicine in asthma. *J Allergy Clin Immunol* 85:578–582, 1990.

47. Sears MR, Taylor DR, Print CG, et al: Regular inhaled beta-agonist treatment in bronchial asthma. *Lancet* 336:1391–1396, 1990.

48. Simpson WG: Gastroesophageal reflux disease and asthma. *Arch Intern Med* 155:798–803, 1995.

49. Sobonya RE: Quantitative structural alterations in long-standing allergic asthma. *Am Rev Respir Dis* 130:289–292, 1984.

50. Spector SL, Smith LJ, Glass M, Accolate Asthma Trialists Group: Effects of 6 weeks of therapy with oral doses of ICI 204,219, a leukotriene D_4 receptor antagonist, in subjects with bronchial asthma. *Am J Respir Crit Care Med* 150:618–623, 1994.

51. Sterk PJ, Fabbri LM, Quanjer PH, et al: Airway responsiveness: Standardized challenge testing with pharmacological, physical and sensitizing stimuli in adults. *Eur Respir J* 16(Suppl):53–83, 1993.

52. Szefler SJ, Rose JQ, Elliot EF, et al: The effect of troleandomycin on methylprednisolone elimination. *J Allergy Clin Immunol* 66:447–451, 1980.

53. Tashkin DP, Altose MD, Bleecker ER, et al: The lung health study: Airway responsiveness to inhaled methacholine in smokers with mild to moderate airflow limitation. *Am Rev Respir Dis* 145(2 Pt 1):301–310, 1992.

54. Tollerud DJ, O'Connor GT, Sparrow D, Weiss ST: Asthma, hay fever, and phlegm production associated with distinct patterns of allergy skin test reactivity, eosinophilia, and serum IgE levels. *Am Rev Respir Dis* 144:776–781, 1991.

55. Toogood JH, Baskerville J, Jennings B, et al: Bioequivalent doses of budesonide and prednisone in moderate and severe asthma. *J Allergy Clin Immunol* 84:688–700, 1989.

56. van Schayck CP, van den Broek PJJA, den Otter JJ, et al: Periodic treatment regimens with inhaled steroids in asthma or chronic obstructive pulmonary disease. *JAMA* 274:161–164, 1995.

57. Wasserman SI, Furukawa CT, Henochowicz SI, et al: Asthma symptoms and airway hyperresponsiveness are lower during treatment with nedocromil sodium than during treatment with regular inhaled albuterol. *J Allergy Clin Immunol* 95:541–547, 1995.

58. Webb J, Clark TJH, Chilvers C: Time course of response to prednisolone in chronic airflow obstruction. *Thorax* 36:18–21, 1981.

59. Wilson SR, Scamagas P, German DF, et al: A controlled trial of self-management education for adults with asthma. *Am J Med* 94:564–576, 1993.

60. Zeitz HJ: Bronchial asthma, nasal polyps, and aspirin sensitivity: Samter's syndrome. *Clin Chest Med* 9:567–576, 1988.

CHAPTER 51

ALLERGIC BRONCHOPULMONARY ASPERGILLOSIS AND HYPERSENSITIVITY REACTIONS TO FUNGI

Roy Patterson

The first case of allergic bronchopulmonary aspergillosis (ABPA) was reported in England in 1952.[6] This was followed by a number of significant descriptions of the disorder.[12] The first case report of ABPA in the United States appeared in 1968.[9] The patient described in that report is alive and well despite having had corticosteroid-dependent asthma (stage IV) for 27 years (Table 51-1).[9] This patient illustrates some characteristics of ABPA. The disease is often indolent and may be present for years before diagnosis. When the diagnosis is made sufficiently early—i.e., before irreversible lung damage—the prognosis for control of ABPA is very good.

Although typical ABPA initially presents with asthma, fleeting pulmonary infiltrates, and marked eosinophilia, there are many other ways in which the disease may be first manifested. The asthma may be extremely mild, there may be no symptoms, and pulmonary infiltrates with eosinophilia may not be noted. The first presentation may be in the form of collapse of a lung or end-stage fibrotic lung disease. End-stage lung disease is rarely seen now, since most cases of ABPA are recognized and progression of the disease is prevented. A patient with cystic fibrosis may also have ABPA, which may be difficult to distinguish from other manifestations of the disease.

The full-blown picture of ABPA consists of asthma, peripheral blood eosinophilia, sputum eosinophilia, fleeting pulmonary infiltrates, golden-brown sputum plugs with hyphae in the sputum, and positive sputum cultures for *Aspergillus fumigatus.* This full-blown picture is not often seen because the diagnosis is generally made in an early stage, recurrences are treated, and progression to end-stage lung disease is prevented. In a recent study of 14 patients seen during 214 patient-years of ABPA, no progression of disease has occurred. This observation underscores that the appropriate approach to the diagnosis of ABPA entails the exclusion of the disease in every patient with asthma or cystic fibrosis by skin tests performed for immediate-type hypersensitivity. When these tests are positive, ABPA must be ruled in or out by appropriate serologic studies.

DEFINITION OF ALLERGIC BRONCHOPULMONARY ASPERGILLOSIS

ABPA is a disease in which the fungus *Aspergillus fumigatus* colonizes sputum plugs in the bronchi of asthmatics, with little or no tissue invasion by the organism. Antigens released from the fungus stimulate an immune response of the host, resulting in production of IgE, IgG, and IgA antibodies against the organism and an intense production of nonspecific IgE. The presence in the bronchi of both *A. fumigatus* antigens and the various antibodies is accompanied by inflammatory reactions in the bronchial mucosa and the surrounding pulmonary tissue. If it goes undetected and untreated, damage to bronchial mucosa and pulmonary tissue will occur. If the diagnosis of ABPA is made, however, treatment with prednisone controls the asthma and causes the sputum to disappear—i.e., the culture medium for *A. fumigatus* is gone and the organism no longer colonizes the

TABLE 51-1

Classification and Staging of ABPA

Classification	Stage	Description
Acute	I	Findings at time of diagnosis, usually including pulmonary infiltrates, eosinophilia, asthma in varying degrees, with positive serology
Remission	II	Follows treatment with prednisone with clearing of radiograph (if infiltrates are present), decline in eosinophilia and total serum IgE, and disappearance of asthma; remission may persist for months or years.
Recurrent exacerbation	III	Manifestations of acute phase reappear, and total serum IgE rises; reversal of all manifestations occurs with prednisone therapy
Corticosteroid-dependent asthma	IV	Patient requires corticosteroids for control of asthma: systemic or topical, irrespective of whether ABPA is stage I, II, or III
Fibrotic end-stage	V	Severe fibrotic lung disease; rarely seen in last decade, as early diagnosis and therapy may have prevented progression to stage V disese
Other Useful Classifications		
Serologic ABPA		Patient with positive serology and no other manifestations of ABPA; patient at risk for progression of ABPA; observation is required
Central bronchiectasis		Present or absent in stages I–IV; always present in stage V; demonstrates structural damage to bronchi

bronchi. The prednisone also eliminates the inflammatory reactions of the bronchi and pulmonary tissue so that the patient's condition improves clinically. Inflammatory pulmonary infiltrates on the chest radiographs also disappear.

CLASSIFICATION AND STAGING

Observations made on patients over 20 years have led to the classification of the stages of ABPA indicated in Table 51-1.[10] These stages are useful in managing ABPA, since they allow one to determine whether the disease has progressed or lung damage has occurred.

In the acute phase (stage I), all of the typical findings of ABPA described above may be present. Treatment of the patient with prednisone, as described below, will improve all of the findings suggestive of ABPA, including the resolution of inflammatory pulmonary infiltrates, decline in total serum IgE (by at least 35 percent), and alleviation or disappearance of eosinophilia. However, the precipitating antibody and IgE and IgG antibody indices may remain positive for months or even years.

After control of the acute phase, the patient enters the remission phase (stage II), which may persist for months or years. Alternatively, there may be recurrent exacerbations (stage III), characterized by respiratory symptoms, a doubling (at least) of total serum IgE, and usually pulmonary infiltrates. An exacerbation of ABPA will again respond to prednisone. Recurrent exacerbations may occur in no apparent pattern, although these may relate to poorly controlled asthma and regional mold seasons—October

and November in the upper Midwest, for example.

Stage IV is the phase in which corticosteroids are required for control of the patient's asthma. In this stage, high-dose corticosteroids may be administered by inhalation, with or without alternate-day prednisone. In any patient, the acute stage (stage I) may be followed by stage II, stage III, or stage IV. When the diagnosis of the acute stage is made, it is impossible to predict which stage will follow. The particular stage is established by close observation and treatment of the patient.

Patients with stage V disease have end-stage fibrotic lung disease. In our clinic, most of these patients were identified as having stage V disease 15 to 25 years ago, and have since died from progressive fibrotic lung disease or cardiac complications. We have not seen patients in earlier stages (stage I, II, III, or IV) progress to stage V, suggesting that diagnosis and control of ABPA can prevent progression to fibrotic lung disease.

DIAGNOSIS

The diagnosis of ABPA is easily made in a patient presenting with the typical constellation of findings: asthma, fleeting pulmonary infiltrates, eosinophilia, *A. fumigatus* in sputum cultures, increase in total serum IgE and rapid clearing of clinical symptoms and radiographic lesions, and decrease in total serum IgE in response to prednisone therapy. In contrast, low-grade, indolent ABPA with mild asthma and a normal chest radiograph may be overlooked unless every patient with asthma or cystic fibrosis is evaluated to exclude ABPA. This is accomplished by skin testing for immediate-type hypersensitivity to *A. fumigatus*. This is a simple and safe procedure that initially entails a prick test to *A. fumigatus*. If this is negative, an intradermal test with *A. fumigatus* is done. If the skin tests are negative, ABPA has been ruled out. If either skin test is positive, ABPA must be excluded with appropriate serologic tests performed by a qualified laboratory. Four serologic tests are necessary (Table 51-2). The diagnosis of

TABLE 51-2

Serologic Studies of Value in Diagnosis of ABPA

Serologic Test	Positive
Total serum IgE	>1000 ng/ml
Precipitation test	Precipitin band present
IgE antibody index	>2 compared with asthma pool
IgG antibody index	>2 compared with asthma pool

Four results positive, diagnostic of ABPA
Three results positive, consistent with ABPA
Two results positive, possible ABPA; repeat serology in 3 to 6 months
All negative or one positive, ABPA excluded

ABPA is supported by the following criteria: total serum IgE greater than 1000 ng/ml, IgE and IgG indices more than twice the prick test–positive asthma control pool (see below), and precipitins against *A. fumigatus.* If three of four tests are positive, ABPA is likely. If two of four tests are positive, the serologic tests should be repeated three to six months later. A positive serologic result should prompt evaluation for central bronchiectasis to determine whether damage to bronchi has occurred. There are few causes of central bronchiectasis other than ABPA. These serologic analyses have recently been reviewed.[13] Of importance is that the serologic analysis be done by a diagnostic laboratory that is experienced and competent in the diagnosis or exclusion of ABPA.

The IgE and IgG antibody indices play an important role in the diagnosis of ABPA. They are calculated with the enzyme-linked immunosorbent assay (ELISA). Initially, a reading is obtained for IgE antibody activity in the test serum against *A. fumigatus* antigen. A similar reading is obtained for a sample from a pool of serum samples from patients who are skin test positive to *A. fumigatus* but in whom ABPA has been excluded (asthma pool). The ELISA reading for the IgE antibody activity in the test sample is then divided by the reading for the asthma pool. A value greater than 2 is consistent with ABPA. A similar process is carried out for IgG antibody activity; again, a reading greater than 2 is consistent with ABPA. Of the serologic tests for ABPA, the most variable is the total serum IgE, which decreases in response to prednisone therapy.

The diagnosis of ABPA-serologic (S) is made in the patient with asthma in whom skin tests for *A. fumigatus* and serology are positive but who has no other features of ABPA. Treatment with prednisone until the total IgE level decreases to a plateau is an option for these patients.

Once the diagnosis of ABPA has been established, subsequent evaluation should focus on the extent of lung damage. If it has not already been done, the presence or absence of central bronchiectasis should be established. Pulmonary function tests and chest radiograph evaluations may also provide evidence of pulmonary damage. Comparisons of pulmonary status before and after treatment of the acute phase of ABPA with prednisone will give the clinician an idea of the reversibility versus irreversibility of the pulmonary abnormalities.

A flow diagram for the diagnosis and management of ABPA is shown in Fig. 51-1.

MANAGEMENT

The management of ABPA depends on the stage of the disease. In the acute stage (stage I), prednisone at a dose of 0.50 mg/kg daily for two to four weeks clears the radiographic lesions, controls the asthma, and decreases the total serum IgE. Control of asthma causes clearing of the mucus, which is the culture medium for *A. fumigatus,* and the disease undergoes remission. The program of prednisone therapy is then switched to an alternate-day regimen, gradually reduced thereafter, and then terminated. In the course of treatment with prednisone, the IgE level will drop at least 35 percent and probably more before reaching a plateau. Instead of using prednisone therapy in an attempt to get the total serum IgE to a normal level, therapy is directed only at reaching the plateau, whose level varies with each patient. Attempts to normalize IgE can cause overtreatment with prednisone, inducing significant side effects from the steroid.

The frequency with which total serum IgE is determined in patients with ABPA is tailored to the individual patient. After the

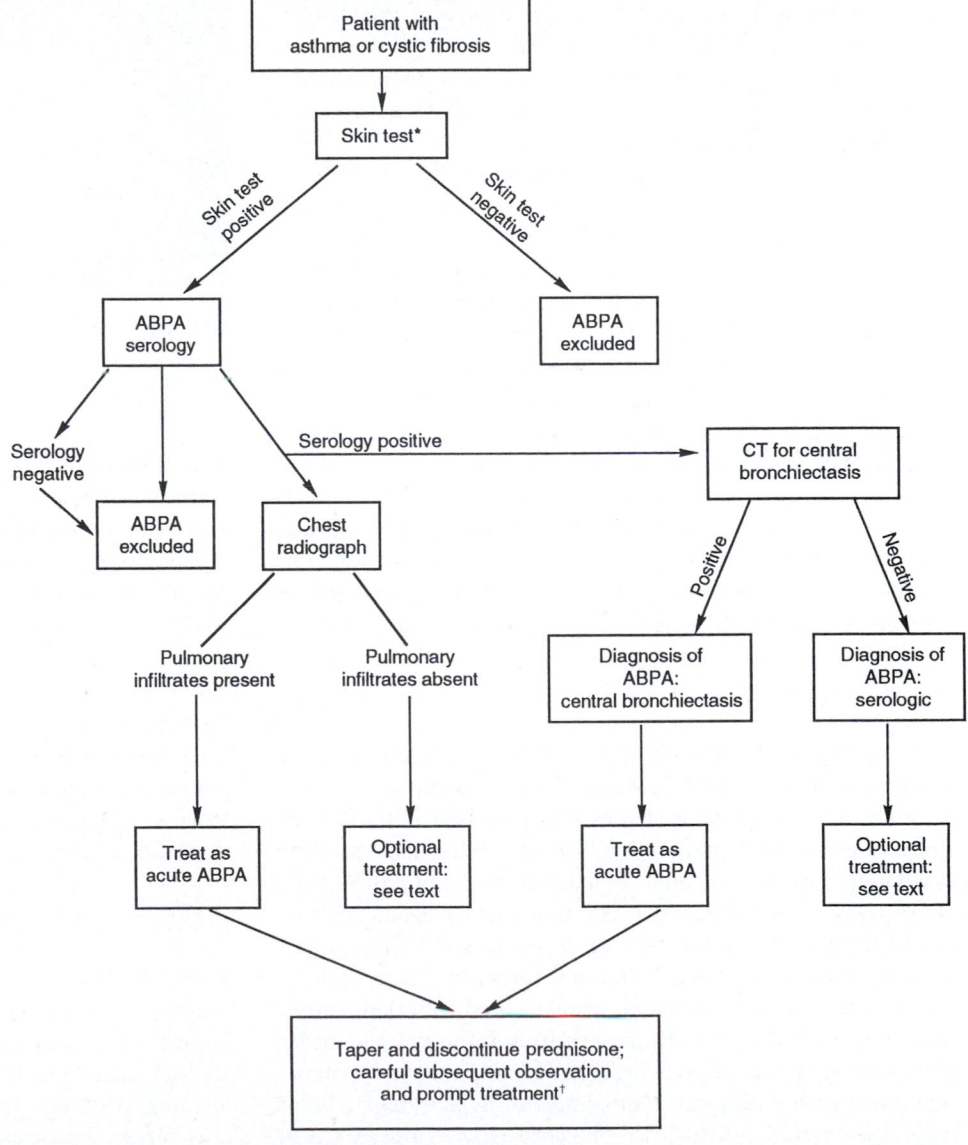

FIGURE 51-1 Flow diagram for the diagnosis and management of ABPA.

*With *Aspergillus fumigatus.* Prick test followed by intradermal test.
†Early diagnosis and management is designed to prevent stage V disease (end-stage fibrotic lung disease).

diagnosis of ABPA and initiation of prednisone therapy, IgE levels are determined monthly until they reach a plateau. After the IgE level has plateaued and the patient's condition is stable, testing every 3 months for the first year is advisable. These intervals may be extended if the patient's condition remains stable and the disease is in remission.

Further management depends on the stage of ABPA. Patients who have achieved remission are in stage II. These remissions may persist for months to years, but frequently they end with exacerbations manifest by an increase in total serum IgE and a return of clinical symptoms, radiographic infiltrates, and eosinophilia. Prednisone therapy is again required on a temporary basis. In stage IV (the corticosteroid-dependent asthma stage), chronic administration of corticosteroids is required to control the asthma. Treatment may consist of inhaled steroids alone or inhaled steroids and prednisone. As a rule, the dosage of prednisone is moderate and administered according to an alternate-day regimen. In stage IV, exacerbations may take the form of bouts of asthma or recurrences of ABPA, as manifested by a doubling of the IgE level. Both are treated with prednisone. The exacerbation of ABPA requires a longer course of prednisone, using the decrease in IgE level as a guide.

The number of cases of stage V ABPA has decreased in the last quarter of this century—probably because ABPA is diagnosed earlier and treated, preventing progression to end-stage fibrotic lung disease. Treatment of stage V ABPA usually does not require high-dose prednisone, since the inflammatory process is probably no longer active. Instead, the primary goal of therapy is the management of recurrent respiratory infections, usually bacterial, and supportive management of irreversible fibrotic lung disease. Severe central bronchiectasis generally accounts for the recurrent respiratory infections. These patients are often colonized with the same organisms seen in patients with cystic fibrosis.

The natural history of patients with ABPA-serologic (S) is poorly defined. It is believed, however, that these patients are at increased risk for the development of active ABPA. As a result, the optimal management of these patients is somewhat uncertain. Close observation is obviously required. A treatment regimen comparable with that used for stage I ABPA—i.e., the administration of prednisone until IgE levels plateau—should be considered.

RADIOGRAPHIC STUDIES

The radiographic manifestations of ABPA are very important in diagnosis and management. Although chest radiographs are sometimes normal, radiographic abnormalities provide important information about the activity of the disease and the damage it has caused in respiratory structures. In the acute phase of ABPA, variable degrees of parenchymal infiltration usually occur, with or without respiratory symptoms. The infiltrates can be fleeting or persistent. Progression to cavitation can also occur. Because these abnormalities are not distinctive, parenchymal infiltration from ABPA may be difficult to distinguish from infiltrates caused by other parenchymal diseases. Plugging of first-, second-, or third-order bronchi with plugs containing mucus, hyphae, and cellular debris can provide a distinctive "finger-in-glove" appearance in ABPA (Fig. 51-2). These obstructions can be fleeting or persistent and may be associated with local atelectasis. Less common

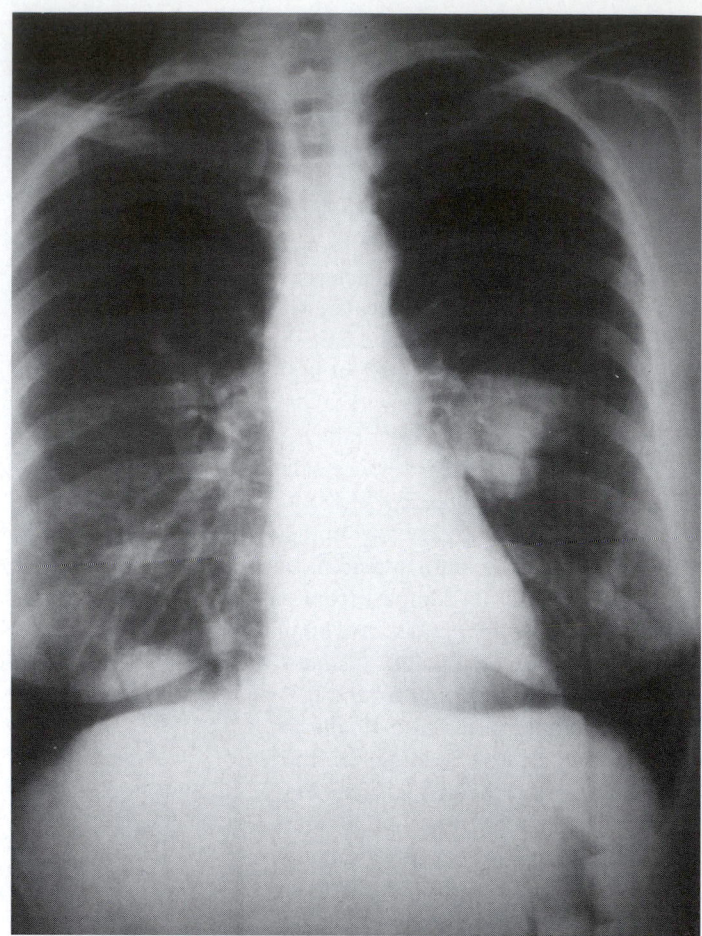

FIGURE 51-2   Chest radiograph of a patient with ABPA with peripheral infiltrates and "finger-in-glove" mucoid impaction. *(Courtesy of Dr. Jack A. Elias, Yale University School of Medicine.)*

than in previous years are manifestations of pulmonary fibrosis: scarring, volume loss, and local retraction. Hyperinflation has also been noted and ascribed to collateral air flow.[2]

The documentation of central bronchiectasis with normal peripheral airways is important in the diagnosis and staging of ABPA. In previous years, bronchography was the gold standard for the diagnosis of central bronchiectasis. However, this procedure is invasive, unpleasant, difficult, and potentially risky to perform in patients with asthma. The recent demonstration that high-resolution computed tomography (HRCT) can establish the presence of central bronchiectasis in ABPA with a high degree of sensitivity and specificity has made HRCT the test of choice when evaluations for central bronchiectasis are required (Fig. 51-3).[1,8]

IMMUNOPATHOGENESIS

When *A. fumigatus* colonizes the sputum of a patient with asthma, the organism releases *A. fumigatus* antigens into the bronchi. The host reacts with a variety of immunologic responses, including IgE, IgG, and IgA antibodies against *A. fumigatus*. Although less clearly defined, lymphocyte reactivity also occurs. The result is the presence of *A. fumigatus* antigens and immunologic reactions, which can result in three types of hypersensitivity reactions: IgE-mediated, IgA-mediated, and

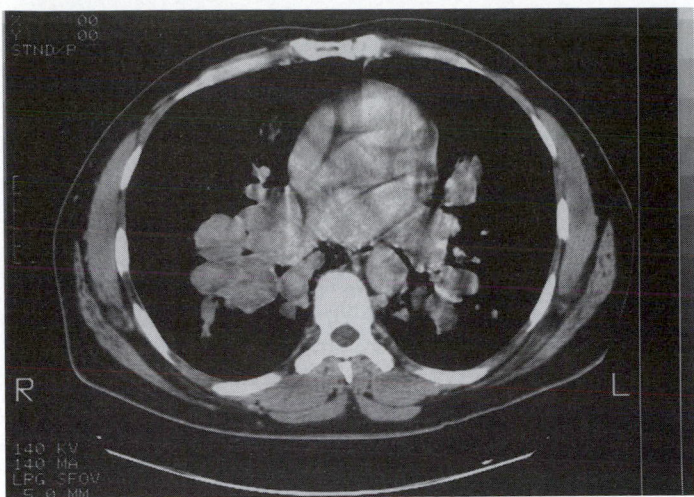

FIGURE 51-3   HRCT demonstrating mucus-filled central bronchiectasis in a patient with ABPA. (*Courtesy of Dr. Coralie Shaw, Yale University School of Medicine.*)

IgG-mediated antigen-antibody complex reactions. The result is an immunologic inflammatory reaction in the bronchial mucosa and surrounding pulmonary parenchyma. This inflammation, if uncontrolled, leads to central bronchiectasis and fibrotic lung disease. With appropriate anti-inflammatory prednisone therapy, the inflammation is suppressed, the asthma is controlled, and mucus production of the bronchi is arrested so that the culture medium for *A. fumigatus* is eliminated. Thus, the entire process is reversed. Permanent damage occurs only if ABPA has progressed to the point of central bronchiectasis and fibrosis of parenchyma. Even in such instances, however, further progression can be prevented by prednisone therapy.

OTHER ALLERGIC BRONCHOPULMONARY MYCOSES

In some patients with typical ABPA (fleeting pulmonary infiltrates, eosinophilia, asthma, elevated IgE, and bronchial plugs or casts), all serologic tests to demonstrate antibody against *A. fumigatus* are negative. Often such patients have other allergic bronchopulmonary mycoses. In these instances, the disease may be due to a variety of fungi.[7] The most common of these are *Candida, Curvularia,* and *Helminthosporium* species. Identification of the species of fungus can be difficult unless recurrent sputum cultures demonstrate the organism. Nevertheless, these patients respond to the prednisone regimen useful for ABPA: radiographic lesions clear along with clinical improvement and decreases in total serum IgE. Thus, the patient can be managed effectively without extensive studies, which may not be productive in defining the organism because of the complexity of this type of analysis.

CYSTIC FIBROSIS AND ABPA

The major organisms that cause bronchopulmonary infections in patients with cystic fibrosis include *Pseudomonas* species, *Hemophilus influenzae, Staphylococcus aureus,* and *Klebsiella.* Aspergillus species are often found in the respiratory secretions of patients with cystic fibrosis. In some patients with cystic fibrosis, the complete spectrum of the ABPA syndrome is seen.[4] Treatment with prednisone, as in the asthma patient with ABPA, results in reversal of the ABPA process, leaving the residual problem of cystic fibrosis.[5] Recurrent ABPA in this population, as in asthma patients, is always a potential problem.

HYPERSENSITIVITY REACTIONS TO FUNGI

To put ABPA and the other bronchopulmonary mycoses into proper perspective, it is important to appreciate that inhaled fungi also cause other hypersensitivity responses in the lungs. Two of the most important are hypersensitivity pneumonitis and immediate-type hypersensitivity reactions.

Hypersensitivity Pneumonitis due to Inhaled Fungi

The usual causes of hypersensitivity pneumonitis are inhaled foreign organic antigens such as pigeon proteins. However, fungal antigens also cause hypersensitivity pneumonitis.[12] One such example is hypersensitivity pneumonitis due to *A. flavus* inhalation.[11]

The diagnosis of hypersensitivity pneumonitis due to mold spores is often complex. Suspicion is based on pulmonary infiltrates that are not due to infection, decreased diffusing capacity, and, at times, a lung biopsy consistent with hypersensitivity pneumonitis. The histologic appearance is usually that of granulomatous infiltrates with or without bronchiolitis obliterans. Further evaluation includes a careful history of occupational and other environmental exposures. Possible sources, such as home or work humidifiers, must be considered. The expertise of mycologists and immunologists is often required to identify the potential organisms.

Immediate-Type Hypersensitivity Reactions to Fungi

IgE antibody–mediated reactions to fungi are common. Fungal antigens are important causes of allergic rhinitis and allergic conjunctivitis and triggers of allergic asthma. Fungi are more likely to trigger asthma than are pollens because the larger size of many pollens inhibits their deposition in the lower airway, whereas fungal spores can reach the smaller bronchi. Moreover, counts of fungal spores may greatly exceed those of pollen grains, and people in the natural environment can be exposed to as many as 100 species of fungi. These reactions are also exceedingly complex in terms of diagnosis, correlation with exposure, avoidance, and treatment.

Natural exposure to fungal antigens varies markedly with climate, humidity, and geography. Significant snow cover in the northern United States sharply reduces exposure to fungi. Even exacerbations of ABPA are reduced in such circumstances.

The diagnosis of IgE-mediated rhinitis and asthma due to mold spores is based on history and physical examination and the presence of symptoms during mold season, when pollens are not prevalent (e.g., in October in the upper Midwest). IgE antibody against mold antigens can be demonstrated by immediate-type skin tests using appropriate antigens.

Fungi that are important in evoking bronchopulmonary hypersensitivity reactions, based on skin test reactivity and atmospheric surveys, include *Aspergillus, Alternaria, Cladosporium,* and *Penicillium.* Positive skin tests and perennial symptoms that are exacerbated during mold seasons suggest mold allergy. Negative skin tests are of value, since appropriate negative prick and intradermal tests to fungi can exclude fungal antigens as triggers of IgE-mediated reactions. In the patient with asthma, negative tests for *A. fumigatus* exclude ABPA.

The treatment of mold allergy is based on pharmacologic control of rhinitis and asthma. When other aeroallergens are part of the stimulus to the allergic response, immunotherapy, including mold allergens, is a reasonable approach.[3]

REFERENCES

1. Angus RM, Davies M-L, Cowan MD, et al: Computed tomographic scanning of the lung in patients with allergic bronchopulmonary aspergillosis and in asthmatic patients with a positive skin test to *Aspergillus fumigatus. Thorax* 49:586–589, 1994.
2. Aquino SL, Kee ST, Warnock ML, Gamsu G: Pulmonary aspergillosis: Imaging findings with pathologic correlation. *AJR Am J Roentgenol* 163:811–815, 1994.
3. Bush RK: Allergens and other factors important in atopic disease, in Patterson R et al (eds), *Allergic Diseases Diagnosis and Management,* 5th ed. Philadelphia, JB Lippincott. In press.
4. Ditto AM, Patterson R, Sider L: Allergic bronchopulmonary aspergillosis, idiopathic anaphylaxis and cystic fibrosis in a 9-year-old: A case report. *Pediatr Asthma Allergy Immunol* 9:107–115, 1995.
5. Fink JN: Allergic bronchopulmonary aspergillosis and cystic fibrosis, in Patterson R, Greenberger PA, Roberts ML (eds), *Allergic Bronchopulmonary Aspergillosis.* Providence, RI, Oceanside Publications, 1995, pp 69–70.
6. Hinson KFW, Moon AJ, Plummer NS: Bronchopulmonary aspergillosis. *Thorax* 7:317–333, 1952.
7. Hogan MB: Other allergic bronchopulmonary mycoses, in Patterson R, Greenberger PA, Roberts ML (eds), *Allergic Bronchopulmonary Aspergillosis,* Providence, RI, Oceanside Publications, 1995, pp 57–59.
8. Panchal N, Pant C, Bhagat R, Shah A: Central bronchiectasis in allergic bronchopulmonary aspergillosis: Comparative evaluation of computed tomography of the thorax with bronchography. *Eur Respir J* 7:1290–1293, 1994.
9. Patterson R, Golbert TM: Hypersensitivity disease of the lung. *Univ Mich Med Center J* 34:8–11, 1968.
10. Patterson R, Greenberger PA, Radin RC, Roberts M: Allergic bronchopulmonary aspergillosis: Staging as an aid to management. *Ann Intern Med* 96:286–291, 1982.
11. Patterson R, Sommers H, Fink JN: Farmer's lung following inhalation of *Aspergillus flavus* growing in moldy corn. *Clin Allergy* 4:79–86, 1974.
12. Pepys J: Hypersensitivity diseases of the lungs due to fungi and organic dusts, in Kallos P (ed), *Monographs in Allergy.* New York, Karger, 1969.
13. Roberts M, Greenberger PA: Serologic analysis of allergic bronchopulmonary aspergillosis, in Patterson R, Greenberger PA, Roberts ML (eds), *Allergic Bronchopulmonary Aspergillosis.* Providence, RI, Oceanside Publications, 1995, pp 11–15.

SECTION 10

OTHER OBSTRUCTIVE DISORDERS

CHAPTER 52

UPPER AIRWAY OBSTRUCTION

Sidney S. Braman / Henning A. Gaissert

The upper airway is defined as the segment of the conducting airways between the nose (during nasopharyngeal breathing) or the mouth (during oropharyngeal breathing) and the main carina, located at the end of the distal trachea. Air passes through five compartments on its way to the lung: oral cavity and nose, pharynx, larynx, and trachea. Physiological points of narrowing are the nostrils, the velopharyngeal valve at the passage between the naso- and oropharynx, and the glottis. Clinically significant obstruction may occur within any compartment, and its recognition and treatment can be lifesaving. This chapter provides a brief overview of upper airway anatomy and focuses on clinical features, assessment, etiology, and management of upper airway obstruction.

HISTORICAL PERSPECTIVE

Obstruction of the upper airway and its treatment have concerned physicians for centuries. Asclepiades, a surgeon living in Rome during the first century B.C., is credited with performing the first tracheostomy to relieve upper airway obstruction. A translation of Galen's *Introductio seu Medicus* mentions his name, although a description of the procedure is not preserved. In a historical review of tracheostomy, Goodall[14] found a total of 28 successful operations—with recovery—before the year 1825. No single reason accounts for this paucity of reports, but failure to understand the essential function of breathing, the commonly fatal outcome when the procedure was attempted, and a lack of proper training may all have played a role at different times.

The French physician Bretonneau established the modern use of tracheostomy when diphtheria became increasingly prevalent in France in the first quarter of the nineteenth century. An English report in 1859 on 88 tracheostomies performed over a 5-year period detailed indications and success rates.[34] With 37 tracheostomies performed for laryngeal obstruction due to syphilis, acute laryngitis, and pharyngeal obstruction, 20 patients died. Eleven of 14 children undergoing tracheostomy for scalding injuries died. Eleven of 15 patients with croup died, as did 5 of 13 patients with foreign bodies in the airway. Eight of 9 patients undergoing tracheostomy for a variety of other indications died. Thus, the mortality for tracheostomy was remarkably high at 62 percent, with death often occurring during the operation. Improving socioeconomic conditions in Europe and North America, and the introduction of effective antitoxin and antibiotic therapy for diphtheria and other infectious diseases, changed the role of tracheostomy.

In recent decades, new causes of upper airway obstruction and different strategies of treatment have evolved. Smoking habits and exposure to modern environmental toxins have led to an ever-increasing incidence of airway malignancies in the oropharynx, larynx, and tracheobronchial tree. Care of civilian and military victims of fires has facilitated an understanding of the pathophysiology of inhalation injury. The increasing use of endotracheal tubes and tracheostomy for long-term ventilation has led to characteristic injuries of the trachea (see Chapter 174). Patients with rare congenital diseases or severe injuries survive their acute illness only to present with the chronic sequelae of airway disease. Interventions for airway obstruction today occur earlier, often obviating emergency conditions. Sophisticated surgical techniques for reconstruction of the larynx, trachea, and bronchi offer a cure or successful palliation for many patients.

UPPER AIRWAY ANATOMY

Functional or anatomic obstruction can occur at any level of the upper airway. Because of their parallel arrangement, the mouth and nose are rarely the site of obstruction except in massive facial trauma. Obstruction to airflow through the nose leads to discomfort and a sensation of congestion or stuffiness, which necessitates mouth breathing. Common causes of nasal obstruction are local infection, allergy, nasal polyposis, and hypertrophied adenoids. In rare instances, foreign bodies and tumors restrict airflow.

From an anatomic perspective, the upper airway may be considered to comprise two areas. Structures located above the thoracic inlet constitute the extrathoracic airway; the portion of the trachea below the thoracic inlet makes up the intrathoracic upper airway. Occasionally, the pharynx may be the site of clinically significant airflow obstruction. The oropharynx and hypopharynx are a muscular tube formed by superior, middle, and inferior pharyngeal constrictors located in the lateral and posterior walls. The anterior border of the pharynx is composed of muscular, bony, and cartilaginous elements. In descending order, these are the uvula, base of the tongue, salpingoepiglottic folds, epiglottis, and larynx. The normal pharynx provides an unrestricted airway; however, the loose attachment of the pharyngeal wall to the prevertebral fascia and lateral parapharyngeal structures provides a potential space that, when occupied, may compromise the lumen as a result of bleeding, edema, or infection. Infection of the anatomic spaces surrounding the pharynx can rapidly lead to life-threatening obstruction. Examples include abscesses of the retropharyngeal space and the submandibular space (the site of Ludwig's angina; see below) and deep neck infections. Similarly, trauma to the neck can lead to fulminant obstruction of the upper airway, and patients with multiple trauma must be carefully assessed for life-threatening hemorrhage into these tissues. A ring of lymphatic conglomerates located at the entry to the oropharynx—the pharyngeal, lingular, and palatine tonsils, with additional lymphatic tissue in the posterior pharyngeal wall—may enlarge and obstruct the airway. Strictures caused by ingestion of corrosive materials, foreign bodies, and tumors can also cause significant pharyngeal obstruction.

The larynx extends from the root of the tongue to the inferior border of the cricoid cartilage. The larynx is located anterior to the third to sixth cervical vertebrae in men and is more cranial in women and children. The epiglottis covers the laryngeal inlet as a thin elastic fibrocartilage suspended by two ligaments from the thyroid cartilage anteriorly, and in its midportion from the hyoid bone. The lateral margins of the epiglottis are formed by the aryepiglottic folds. The interior of the larynx extends from the inlet to the cricoid cartilage and is divided into three parts by the vestibular folds (false vocal cords) and vocal folds (true vocal cords). The space between inlet and vestibular folds is called the *vestibule,* the space between vestibular and vocal folds is the *ventricle,* and that between the vocal folds and cricoid is the *subglottic space.* An unrestricted airway through the glottis is maintained by contraction of the posterior cricoarytenoid muscles, which abduct the vocal cords. This position is preserved except during phonation and deglutition.

The airway is protected from aspiration during swallowing by three laryngeal sphincters. Following laryngeal elevation, the aryepiglottic muscles pull the epiglottis posteriorly and the aryepiglottic folds medially. The epiglottis does not close the larynx completely during swallowing. Adduction of the false and true vocal cords completes the act of laryngeal closure. The laryngeal mucosa of the vocal folds, the medial surface of the arytenoid cartilage, and the dorsal surface of the epiglottis consist of squamous epithelium. A ciliated, cuboidal respiratory epithelium lines the subglottic larynx. Greater vulnerability of the respiratory mucosa is thought to explain the profound epithelial damage after inhalation injury that often begins just below the glottis.

Obstruction of the larynx can occur rapidly with foreign-body aspiration, angioneurotic edema, postintubation trauma, inhalation injuries, external trauma, and infections such as croup or acute epiglottitis. More gradual obstruction of the larynx occurs with malignant and benign tumors, following vocal cord paralysis, and secondary to laryngeal involvement in a variety of systemic diseases, such as tuberculosis, sarcoidosis, eosinophilic granuloma, and histoplasmosis.

The trachea joins the larynx at the cricoid cartilage and measures 10 to 11 cm in length. Less than half of the tracheal length extends above the suprasternal notch. There are 16 to 20 horseshoe-shaped hyaline cartilages, which make the trachea circular or slightly ovoid. The posterior wall, the *membranous portion,* is composed of an outer fibrous sheath and transversely organized smooth-muscle fibers. The range of the normal coronal tracheal diameter is 13 to 25 mm in men and 10 to 21 mm in women. During inspiration, both tracheal length and diameter change in size, thereby decreasing resistance to airflow. The trachea terminates at the bifurcation into the main-stem bronchi. The carina is located to the right of the midline, at the level of the fourth or fifth thoracic vertebra.

Enlargement of the thyroid gland, which surrounds the anterior and lateral walls of the extrathoracic trachea, may result in upper airway obstruction.[21] Generalized tracheal abnormalities associated with an increase in tracheal caliber can cause significant airflow obstruction due to excessive dynamic compression during forced expiration. Examples include tracheobronchiomegaly (Mounier-Kuhn syndrome) and tracheobronchomalacia. Diseases causing airflow obstruction because of a decrease in tracheal caliber may be associated with diffuse or localized narrowing of the tracheal lumen. Rare causes of diffuse narrowing include the saber-sheath trachea, amyloidosis, relapsing polychondritis, tracheobronchopathia osteochondroplastica, scleroderma, and Wegener's granulomatosis. Localized tracheal abnormalities, such as postintubation strictures and benign and malignant tracheal tumors, occur more commonly.

CLINICAL FEATURES

While disorders affecting the upper airway are considerably less common than lower airway diseases such as chronic obstructive pulmonary disease (COPD) and asthma, they are no less important, for several reasons. First, the symptoms, and often the clinical signs, are identical for upper and lower airway diseases. Since COPD and asthma are much more common than diseases of the upper airways, they are often assumed to be the cause of the patient's symptoms. Significant upper airway obstruction may be obscured for a considerable period, resulting in a delay of diagnosis. Since diseases of the upper airway are usually associated with obstruction to airflow, they assume great importance for an additional reason. When the obstruction happens acutely, as it does with acute epiglottitis, angioneurotic edema, sudden aspiration and trauma, acute asphyxia, and death may result within minutes to hours. When upper airway obstruction occurs more slowly, as is seen with tracheal tumors or postintubation tracheal stenosis, a delay in diagnosis may predispose a patient to unnecessary complications, such as bleeding or respiratory failure or, in the case of an upper airway malignancy, to advanced and incurable disease.

The main symptoms of upper airway obstruction are dyspnea and noisy breathing. These symptoms are especially associated with exercise and may also be aggravated by a change in body position. The patient may complain that breathing is labored in the recumbent position and may have a severely disrupted sleep pattern. The upper airway obstruction in such patients causes the sleep apnea syndrome (see Chapter 52), which may resolve completely when the obstruction is relieved.[42] Daytime somnolence, therefore, may be a prominent feature of upper airway obstruction. In severely affected patients, cor pulmonale may occur.

Typically, significant anatomic obstruction precedes overt symptoms. For example, if exertional dyspnea occurs, the airway diameter is probably reduced to about 8 mm. Dyspnea at rest develops when the airway diameter reaches 5 mm, coinciding with the onset of stridor. Stridor is a loud, musical sound of constant pitch that usually connotes obstruction of the larynx or upper trachea. Although it should be easy to distinguish stridor from lower airway sounds, recordings from the neck and chest have shown that the sound signals from the asthmatic wheeze and stridor are of similar frequency.[1] This explains why errors in diagnosis can be made and an upper airway obstruction due to a tumor or foreign body mistakenly treated for asthma. However, unlike wheezing, which is characteristic of diffuse lower airway narrowing and occurs predominantly during expiration, the musical sounds of stridor usually occur during inspiration and are heard loudest in the neck. Maneuvers that increase flow, such as voluntary hyperventilation, accentuate stridor. Stridor that varies in intensity with neck flexion suggests a thoracic outlet obstruction. When the obstructing lesion is below the thoracic inlet, both inspiratory and expiratory stridor may be heard. At times, the character of a patient's voice may be a clue to an upper airway obstruction. Hoarseness may be a sign of a laryngeal abnormality. Muffling of the voice without hoarseness may represent a supraglottic process.

PHYSIOLOGICAL ASSESSMENT

Just as upper airway obstruction must be quite advanced before symptoms occur, physiological abnormalities also do not become apparent on lung function testing until severe obstruction occurs. Studies of subjects breathing through orifices having a range of diameters[35] suggest that an upper airway obstruction must narrow the lumen of the airway to less than 8 mm in diameter to produce abnormalities on the flow-volume loop. This would correspond to an obstruction of more than 80 percent of the tracheal lumen. In these studies, the 1-s forced expiratory volume (FEV_1), determined from the spirogram, remained above 90 percent of control until a 6-mm orifice was created. Therefore, spirometry, which is often the first screening test for pulmonary symptoms, may not be an effective way to detect upper airway abnormalities. The peak expiratory flow rate (PEFR) and maximal voluntary ventilation (MVV) are more sensitive tests for detecting obstruction than the FEV_1.

The flow-volume loop is a recording of maximal inspiratory and expiratory flow at various lung volumes and is the most important tool for the diagnosis of upper airway obstruction.[24,34] The configuration of the normal flow-volume loop is seen in Fig. 52-1. During a forced expiratory maneuver from total lung capacity (TLC), which is the total amount of air in the lungs after maximal inspiration, the maximal flow achieved during the first 25 percent of the forced vital capacity is dependent on patient effort. An increase in driving pressure (effort) may result in increased flow. During the remaining 75 percent of the forced vital capacity maneuver, flow is determined by the mechanical properties of the lungs and is not effort dependent. During this portion of forced exhalation, a linear deceleration of flow is caused by dynamic compression of the intrathoracic airways

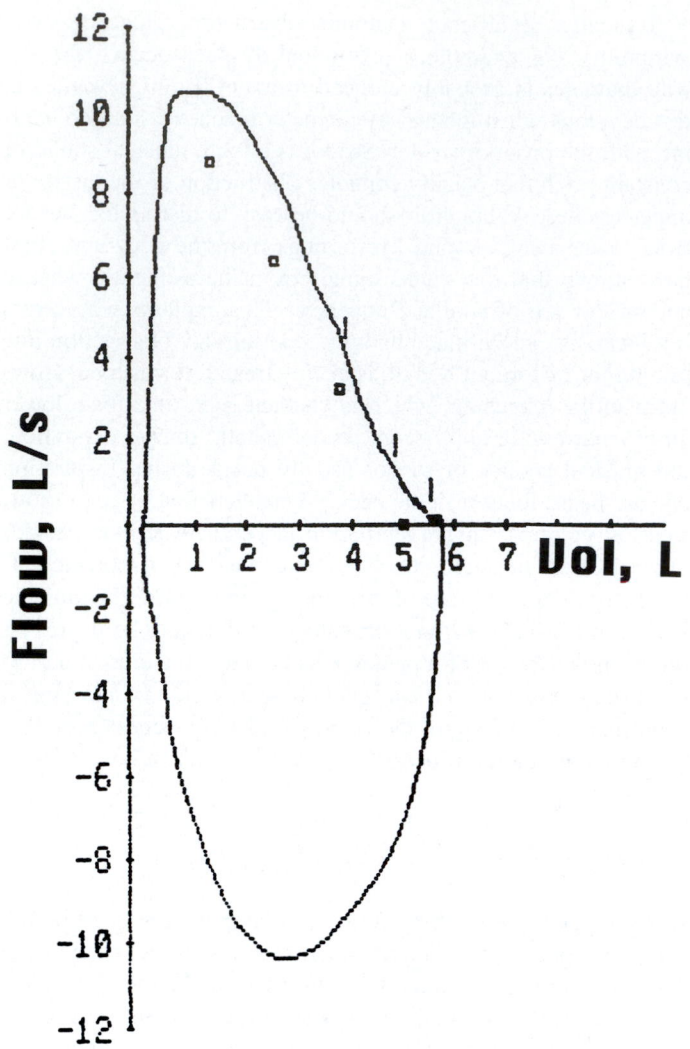

FIGURE 52-1 Normal flow-volume loop following maximal expiratory (above) and inspiratory (below) effort. Small vertical lines denote seconds.

(Fig. 52-2*A*). An increase in effort and, therefore, pleural pressure causes further compression of the intrathoracic airways and a further limitation of airflow. At higher lung volumes, flow may be limited by an upper airway obstruction. At low lung volumes, flow may not be affected by an upper airway obstruction, since measurement of flow in this effort-independent portion of the curve reflects the function of the peripheral airways. Since the FEV_1 reflects a large portion of flow at these lower lung volumes, it is not a sensitive test for upper airway obstruction. PEFR does reflect flow at higher lung volumes and, therefore, may be abnormal when the FEV_1 is not.

Forced inspiratory flow is also measured with simultaneous volume measurements to constitute the inspiratory curve of the flow-volume loop. Forced inspiratory flow is limited by effort during the entire inspiratory maneuver. Flow increases from residual volume (the amount of air left in the lungs during a maximal forced exhalation) to near the midportion of the curve, where it becomes maximal at the peak inspiratory flow rate. Flow then declines until TLC is reached. The pressure surrounding the extrathoracic portion of the upper airway is atmospheric. The turbulent nonlaminar airflow, which occurs during forced inspiration

Inspiration

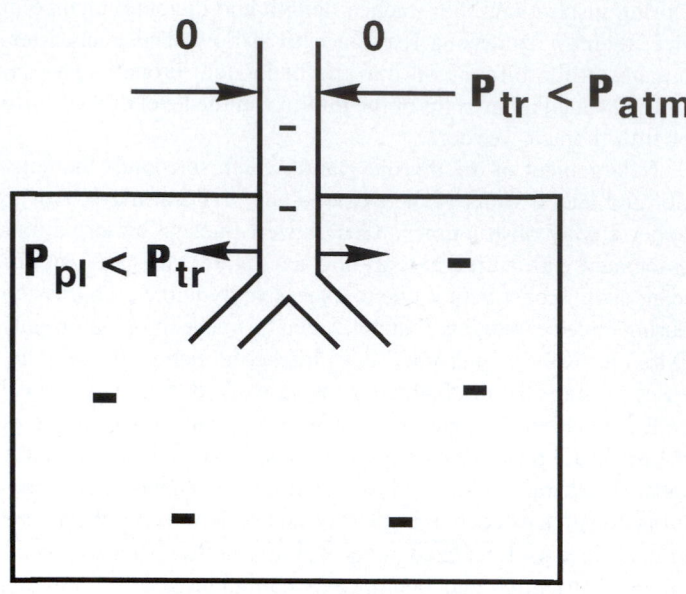

A

Expiration

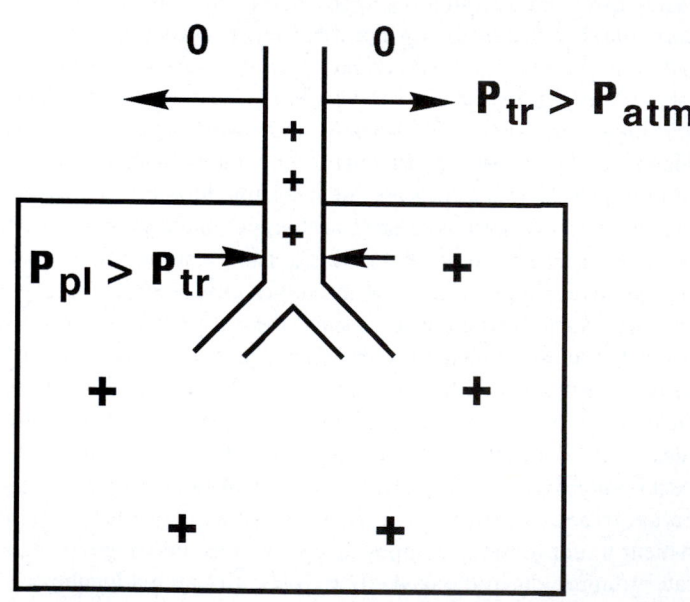

B

FIGURE 52-2 Forces acting on intra- and extrathoracic airway walls during inspiration and expiration. 0 denotes atmospheric pressure; + and − denote positive and negative pressures, respectively. *A.* During inspiration, extrathoracic tracheal pressure (P_{tr}) falls below atmospheric pressure (P_{atm}), favoring narrowing of the lumen (arrows). Intrapleural pressure (P_{pl}) becomes negative, favoring airway enlargement (arrows). *B.* During expiration, the extrathoracic tracheal pressure (P_{tr}) becomes positive and, therefore, greater than P_{atm}, favoring enlargement of the lumen (arrows). Intrapleural pressure (P_{pl}) is positive, causing dynamic compression of the intrathoracic trachea (arrows).

TABLE 52-1

Physiological Classification of Upper Airway Obstruction

Type	Clinical Examples	Flow Characteristics	$FEF_{50\%}/FIF_{50\%}$
Variable extrathoracic	Vocal cord paralysis, glottic stricture, tumors	Forced inspiration increases obstruction and causes decrease in inspiratory flow. Forced expiration decreases the obstruction.	>2
Variable intrathoracic	Malignant tumors, tracheomalacia	During forced expiration, positive pleural pressure causes decrease in airway diameter and increases obstruction. During inspiration, the negative pleural pressure decreases obstruction.	Very low (~0.3)
Fixed extra- or intrathoracic	Goiter, postintubation stricture	No change in airway diameter; fixed flow with inspiration and expiration.	~1

and causes airway pressure in this portion of the airway to fall, slightly favors narrowing of the extrathoracic airway (Fig. 52-2B). Peak inspiratory flow is, therefore, less than peak expiratory flow in normal subjects. Because of dynamic compression of the intrathoracic airways that occurs during exhalation, flow during the middle of inspiration, the forced inspiratory flow at 50 percent of the forced vital capacity ($FIF_{50\%}$), is usually greater than flow during the middle of forced expiration, the forced expiratory flow at 50 percent of the forced vital capacity ($FEF_{50\%}$).

Typical patterns of the flow-volume loop may be seen, depending on whether the obstruction to flow is "fixed" or "variable" and whether the site of the obstruction is above or below the thoracic outlet or suprasternal notch (Table 52-1).

Fixed obstructions of the upper airway are those whose cross-sectional area does not change in response to transmural pressure differences during inspiration or expiration. A fixed obstruction may occur in either the intrathoracic or extrathoracic airways; irrespective of the site of the obstruction, a fixed lesion results in the flattening of the flow-volume loop. A variable obstruction is one that responds to transmural pressure changes, eliciting varying degrees of obstruction during the respiratory cycle. Since the stresses on the intrathoracic and extrathoracic airways are different, changes seen in the flow-volume loop vary according to the site of the obstruction.

A number of conditions have been associated with nondistensible narrowing of the upper airway and fixed airway obstruction. The most common cause is a benign stricture resulting from prolonged endotracheal intubation. Other causes are tracheal compression from a large goiter, posttracheostomy tracheal stenosis, benign and malignant tumors, foreign-body aspiration, hypertrophied tonsils and adenoids, and postinjury fixation of the vocal cords. Maximal inspiratory and expiratory flow-volume loops with fixed obstruction show constant flow represented by a plateau during both inspiration and expiration (Fig. 52-3). On the expiratory curve, the plateau effect is seen

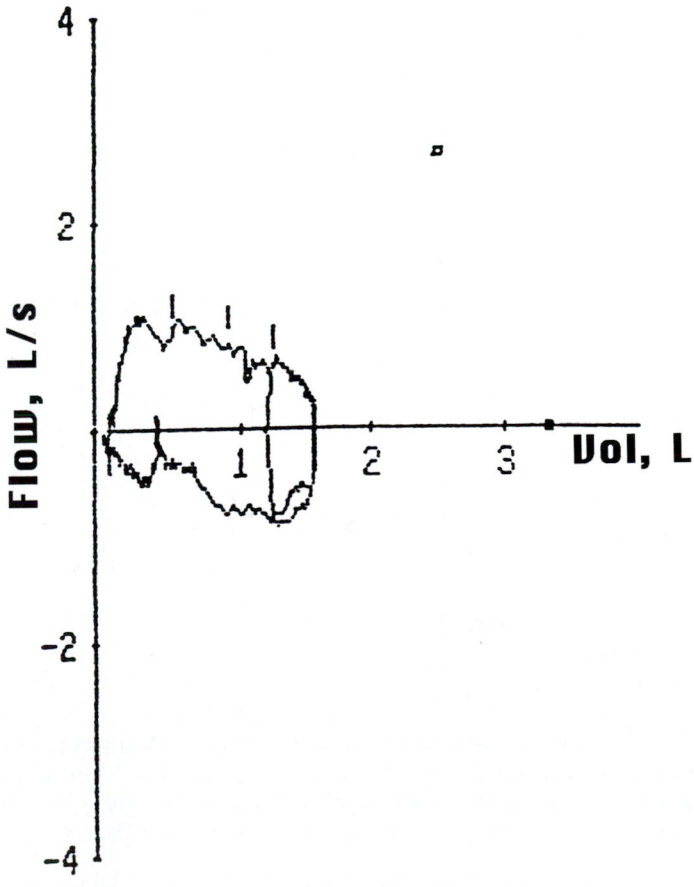

FIGURE 52-3 Flow-volume loop in fixed upper-airway obstruction due to tracheal stenosis. Prolonged translaryngeal intubation and tracheostomy were required in this patient, who had been injured in a motor vehicle accident. The flow-volume loop demonstrates a plateau of flow during inspiration and expiration; the $FEF_{50\%}/FIF_{50\%}$ ratio is near 1.

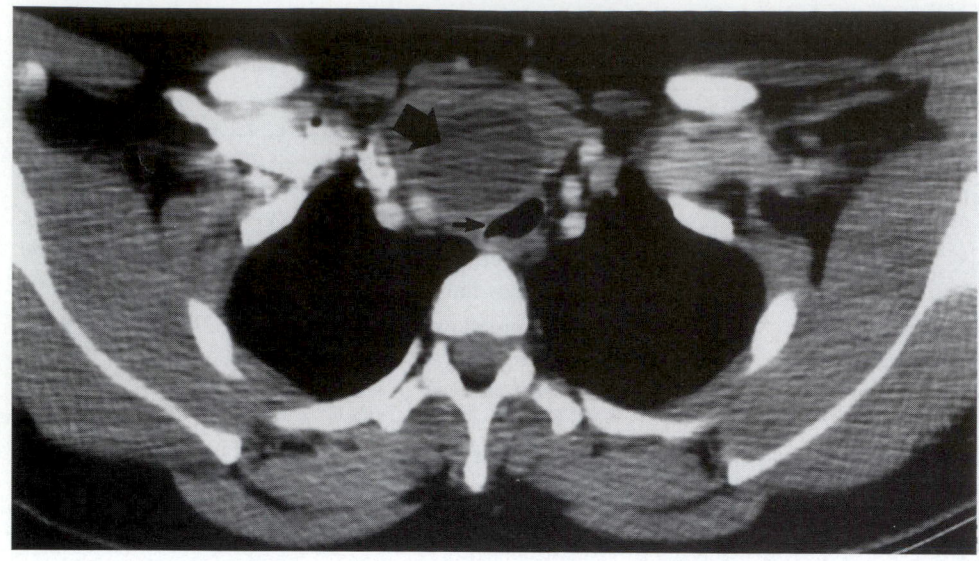

A

B

FIGURE 52-4   Variable extrathoracic obstruction due to thyroid cyst in a 32-year-old woman with dyspnea on exertion. *A.* CT of the neck shows a 10×4-cm cystic mass (large arrow) in the thyroid gland compressing the trachea (small arrow). *B.* Flow-volume loop shows inspiratory obstruction. $FEF_{50\%}/FIF_{50\%}$ is very high, and the inspiratory curve is flattened.

the same in fixed upper airway obstruction.

A variable extrathoracic obstruction is caused most commonly by vocal cord paralysis. Other causes are epiglottitis, chemical burns, adhesions, malignancies, enlarged lymph nodes, and large fat deposits. A variable extrathoracic airway obstruction increases the turbulence of inspiratory flow, and intraluminal pressure falls markedly below atmospheric pressure. This leads to partial collapse of an already narrowed airway and a plateau of the inspiratory flow loop (Fig. 52-4). Expiratory flow is not significantly affected, since the markedly positive pressure in the airway tends to decrease the obstruction. The ratio of $FEF_{50\%}$ to $FIF_{50\%}$ is high (usually greater than 2). Similarly, the FEV_1 is greater than the FIV_1.

When a variable obstruction occurs in the intrathoracic airways, the situation is reversed. A predominant reduction in maximal expiratory flow is noted, with relative preservation of maximal inspiratory flow. This occurs because during forced expiration, intrapleural pressure becomes markedly positive and causes dynamic compression of the intrathoracic airways. The obstruction caused by an intrathoracic lesion is accentuated, and a plateau in expiratory flow on the flow-volume loop is noted (Fig. 52-5). A plateau of flow suggests that the lesion has caused the airway lumen to reach its minimal size. A flow peak may precede the plateau, suggesting that the obstruction may not affect flow until a certain lung volume is reached. During inspiration, intrapleural pressure is markedly negative and the obstruction is, therefore, lessened. The ratio of $FEF_{50\%}$ to $FIF_{50\%}$ is very low and may approach 0.3. Similarly, the FEV_1 is considerably lower than the FIV_1. While the flow ratios are similar to those seen in patients with COPD and chronic asthma, these disorders can often be distinguished by the appearance of the flow-volume loop. The expiratory curve seen in patients with COPD and asthma is mainly altered in the effort-independent portion of the curve, leading to a characteristic shape—unlike the plateau configuration of an upper airway obstruction (Fig. 52-6).

in the effort-dependent portion of the curve near TLC; very little change is noted in the effort-dependent portion near residual volume. Since the inspiratory curve shows a similar appearance, the ratio of $FEF_{50\%}$ to $FIF_{50\%}$ is normal (close to 1). The forced inspiratory volume in 1 s (FIV_1) and FEV_1 is nearly

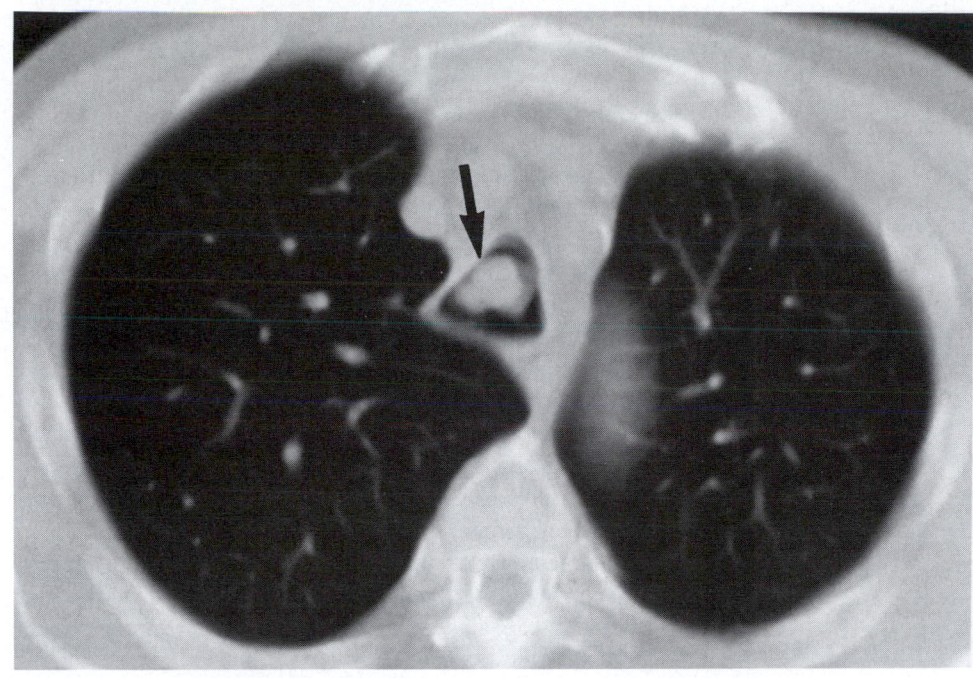

A

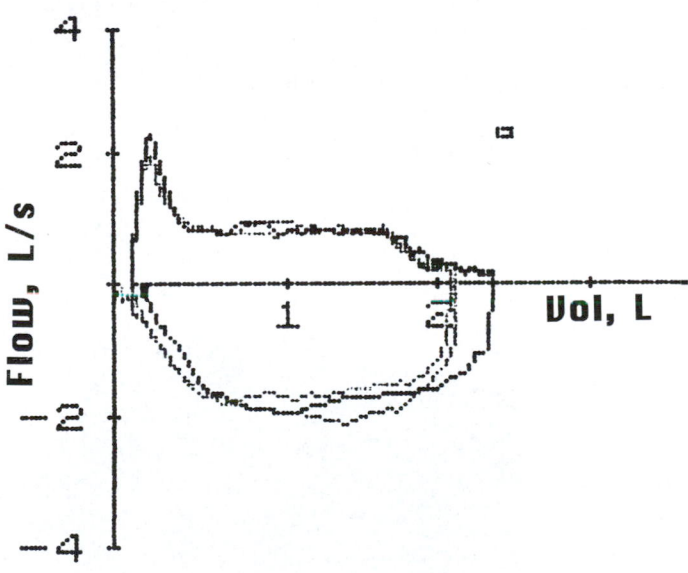

B

FIGURE 52-5   Variable intrathoracic obstruction due to squamous cell carcinoma of the trachea. *A.* CT of the chest shows a tracheal lesion (arrow), which was not readily apparent on plain chest radiograph. *B.* Superimposed flow-volume loops show a plateau of expiratory flow preceded by a peak of flow at higher lung volumes. The forced inspiratory flow is preserved in comparison to expiratory flow, but it is also reduced. $FEF_{50\%}/FIF_{50\%}$ is 0.4.

than 1 and an FEV_1 that is decreased to the same degree as the $FEF_{25-75\%}$. The MVV may also be a useful test, since it measures both inspiratory and expiratory flows. A ratio of MVV to FEV_1 of less than 25 percent is often found with upper airway obstruction. Whenever the MVV is reduced in the presence of a normal FEV_1, a diagnosis of upper airway obstruction should be considered. In contrast to the situation in patients with diffuse obstructive disease of the lower airways (COPD, asthma), the distribution of ventilation in the lungs is normal, and ventilation-perfusion mismatch does not occur.

Hypercarbia is not seen unless the degree of obstruction is very severe, although nocturnal hypercarbia may be seen with normal daytime levels of P_{CO_2}. Hypoxemia is also not present except during exercise, when it may occur in response to increases in the level of P_{CO_2}. In contrast to asthma and many cases of COPD, the airflow obstruction caused by an upper airway lesion does not resolve following the inhalation of a bronchodilator. On the other hand, flow does improve after the patient breathes a mixture of helium and oxygen.[25] The resistance caused by turbulent flow in the upper airway is reduced by the low-density helium, whereas the laminar flow in more peripheral airways is not improved (see Chapter 36).

ETIOLOGY

The causes of upper airway obstruction include infection, angioedema, tumors, trauma, vascular abnormalities, foreign-body aspiration, neuromuscular disorders, and iatrogenic causes. In addition, functional wheezing and stridor may simulate upper airway obstruction.

Infection

Three major infections of the upper airway may lead to acute upper airway obstruction: acute epiglottitis, laryngotracheobronchitis (croup), and Ludwig's angina.

ACUTE EPIGLOTTITIS

Acute epiglottitis was originally thought to be a disease of children. A case review from all hospitals in Rhode Island has shown that epiglottitis continues to occur through adulthood at an inci-

When a hospital laboratory or physician's office is not equipped to perform flow-volume loops, results of other tests, such as routine spirometry,[40] may be useful. If the forced spirogram shows that the PEFR is reduced disproportionately more than the FEV_1, an upper airway obstruction should be suspected. Findings that suggest the diagnosis also include a ratio of the inspiratory flow between 25 and 75 percent of the inspired vital capacity ($FIF_{25-75\%}$) and the expiratory flow between 25 and 75 percent of the expired vital capacity ($FEF_{25-75\%}$) of less

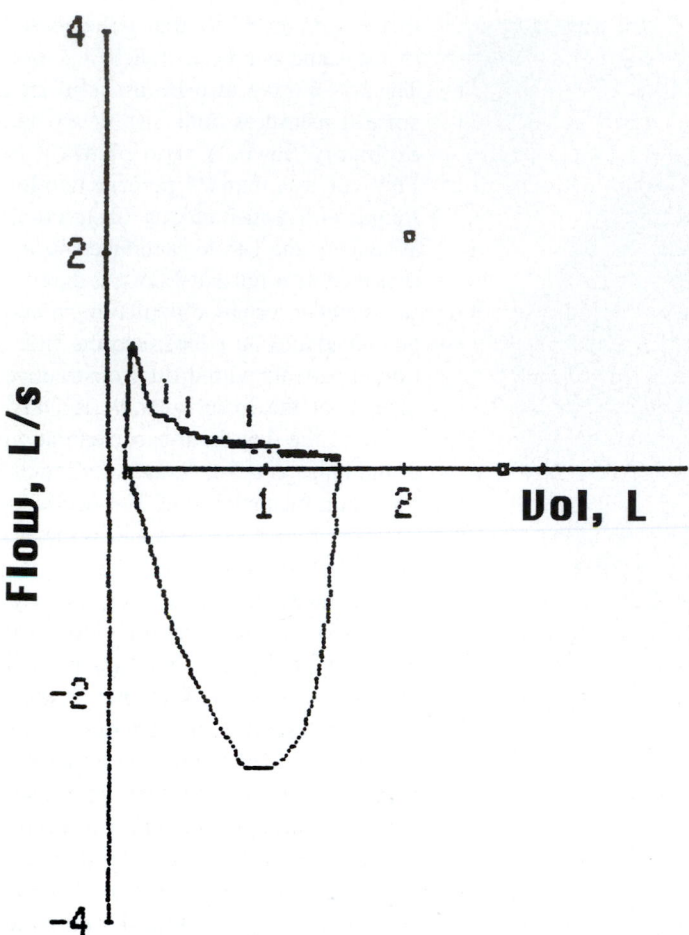

FIGURE 52-6 Flow-volume loop typical of chronic obstructive lung disease. Very low $FEF_{50\%}/FIF_{50\%}$ and typical curvilinear shape are noted.

goscopy has been shown to be safe. Fiberoptic laryngoscopy through the nose is not likely to provoke laryngospasm. On inspection, numerous anatomic sites in the larynx and oropharynx are involved, and the infection may more appropriately be labeled *supraglottitis*. In fact, the epiglottis may be the least affected site or may not even be affected at all. Lateral soft-tissue radiographs of the neck may be helpful if abnormal, but this finding occurs in only 64 percent of cases (Fig. 52-7).

The most frequent causative agent in acute epiglottitis is *Hemophilus influenzae*. Disease prevention should now be possible with the availability of anti–*H. influenzae* type b vaccine. Bacteremia is present in about half of the cases in children, but the incidence is somewhat lower in adults. A wider range of pathogens is seen in adults, including *Streptococcus pneumoniae*, group A or group F streptococcus, *Staphylococcus aureus*, *Staphylococcus pyogenes,* and *Streptococcus viridans*. With careful airway management and antibiotics, mortality is quite low. Because ampicillin-resistant strains of *H. influenzae* are becoming more common, third-generation cephalosporins and the second-generation cephalosporin cefuroxime are the antimicrobials

dence of about 10 cases per million;[31] this is low compared to the rate of more than 100 cases per million each year reported in children. In adults, epiglottitis may occur at any age, although it is more common in younger adults.[12] In children, 75 percent of cases occur after age 2 years. The disease is more common in the colder winter months and is usually seen in drier, temperate regions.

The clinical features of acute epiglottitis are similar in children and adults, except that the larger size of the adult larynx accounts for a less fulminant presentation. In most adults, symptoms are present for more than 24 h. In children, dysphagia, dysphonia, respiratory distress, and drooling are the "four Ds" that accompany stridor, fever, and generalized toxicity. In adults, fever, sore throat, and pain on swallowing are the usual presenting symptoms, and as many as half of patients develop respiratory difficulties. The latter complication may be predicted from the presence of stridor, but not from the duration of symptoms.

The diagnosis of acute epiglottitis is suspected on clinical grounds; the definitive diagnosis is made at laryngoscopy. Before any diagnostic testing is done, an adequate airway must be assured. Most pediatricians avoid direct inspection of the upper airway, in order to prevent trauma and to reduce the risk of precipitating acute airway obstruction. Rather, direct laryngoscopy under general anesthesia is advised, and the physician should be prepared to perform an emergency tracheostomy. In adults, laryn-

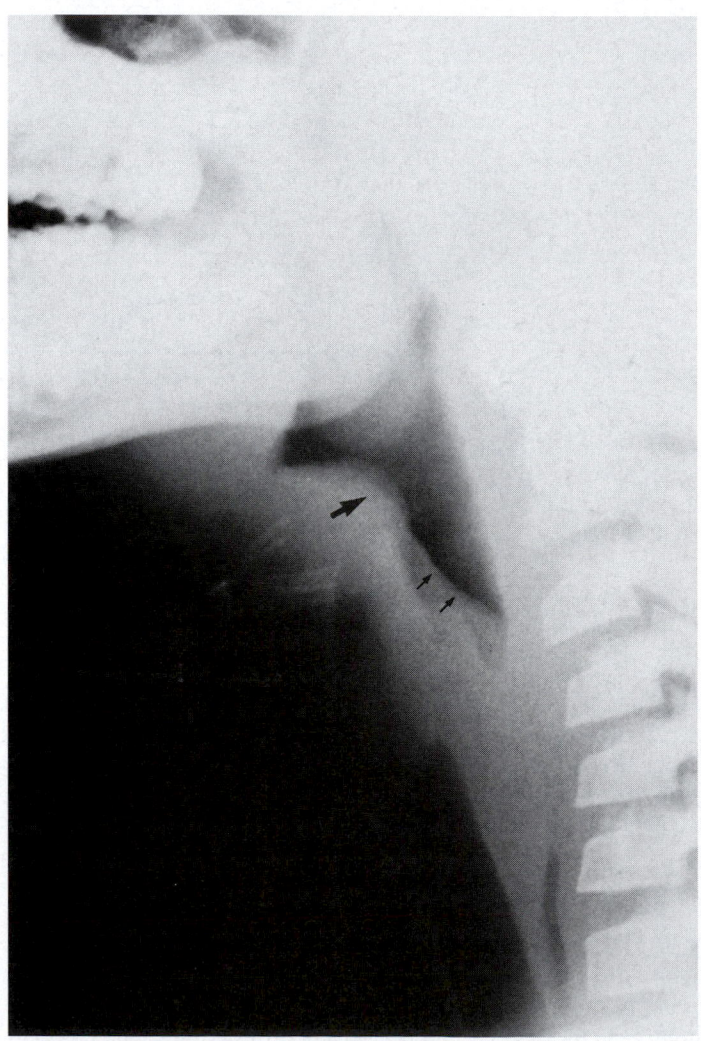

FIGURE 52-7 Acute epiglottitis. Lateral soft-tissue radiograph of the neck of a patient with stridor shows swelling of the epiglottis (large arrow) and loss of normal convexity of the edematous aryepiglottic folds (small arrow).

of choice. Corticosteroids are often used, but they are of no proven benefit. Nebulized racemic epinephrine is purported to help obviate intubation, based on anecdotal case reports.

LARYNGOTRACHEOBRONCHITIS

Laryngotracheobronchitis (croup) is an acute viral respiratory illness commonly seen in children. The most common agents responsible for croup, in order of frequency, are parainfluenza virus, respiratory synsytial virus, adenovirus, and influenza A and B viruses.

Croup is characterized by narrowing of the subglottic trachea, causing symptoms of inspiratory stridor, barking cough, and hoarseness. Typically, symptoms occur several days after the onset of a cold in a child under the age of 4 years.

LUDWIG'S ANGINA

Ludwig's angina is an uncommon, potentially lethal infection of the floor of the mouth and submandibular space.[36] Most patients were previously healthy, but have a history of dental disease, external facial trauma, or oropharyngeal instrumentation. Neck swelling, pain, sore throat, drooling, and dysphagia are the most common symptoms. Acute upper airway obstruction may occur. Soft-tissue radiographs of the neck are usually helpful in showing the extent of the bilateral cellulitis typical of Ludwig's angina. Antibiotics, maintenance of the airway, and, frequently, surgical drainage are the mainstays of therapy.

Other infections of the upper airway have been reported to cause upper airway obstruction. Acute tonsillitis and pharyngitis, usually caused by β-hemolytic streptococci, with or without an associated retropharyngeal abscess, represent one example; acute uvulitis and acute lingular cellulitis are others. Acute suppurative parotitis, most commonly caused by *S. aureus,* may lead to severe edema of the face and neck, with glottic obstruction. Bacterial tracheitis is an uncommon disorder that can also be potentially fatal. Usually, fever, dry cough, and inspiratory stridor are the presenting symptoms. *S. aureus* is the typical pathogenic organism, and an antecedent viral respiratory infection is common. Subglottic edema and mucopurulent secretions are thought to contribute to the airway obstruction. Tuberculosis is a rare cause of upper airway obstruction.

Angioedema

The syndrome of angiodema was described by Quinke in 1882 and is characterized by well-demarcated swelling of the face, lips, tongue, and mucous membranes of the nose, mouth, and throat. Involvement of the larynx may result in upper airway obstruction and death in as many as 25 percent of cases. In most instances, the cause is unclear, and antecedent exposure to common allergens such as drugs, chemical additives, and insect bites should be suspected. While IgE-mediated reactions are thought to be the most common causes of angioedema, the most commonly identified causes are not IgE initiated. These include reactions to histamine-releasing drugs, such as narcotics and radiocontrast materials, to aspirin and other nonsteroidal anti-

inflammatory drugs, and to angiotensin-converting enzyme inhibitors. In rare instances, C1 esterase inhibitor deficiency (see below) is the cause. Physical stimuli (cold, heat, stress) and circulating immune complex diseases (serum sickness, systemic lupus erythematosus) are also known to cause angioedema.

Angioneurotic edema following ingestion of angiotensin-converting enzyme inhibitors such as captopril, enalapril, and lisinopril occurs in 0.1 to 0.2 percent of patients and usually begins within hours or, at most, within 1 week after the drug is taken.[19] The onset does not appear to be dose related, and the findings resolve spontaneously within hours after discontinuation of the drug. When the upper airway is compromised by angioedema, emergency measures may be necessary. Subcutaneous injection of epinephrine and intravenous or intramuscular injection of the antihistamine diphenhydramine are effective immediately, while corticosteroids are useful for associated late-phase reactions. The mechanisms by which the angiotensin-converting enzyme inhibitors cause angioedema are unknown, but non–IgE-mediated immunologic mechanisms are suspected. Patients with a history of idiopathic angioedema are at increased risk for this complication and should probably avoid this class of drugs.

Hereditary angioedema is a rare cause of upper airway obstruction that is transmitted by autosomal dominance in both sexes; it occurs in all races.[38] Hereditary angiodema is characterized by painless nonpitting edema of the face and upper airway, which usually begins in childhood and becomes more prominent in adolescence. Typically, the swelling progresses over many hours and then spontaneously resolves over 1 to 3 days. Despite this slow progression, deaths have occurred because of laryngeal obstruction.

Hereditary angioedema is caused by a deficiency in the production or function of C1 esterase inhibitor, a serum protease inhibitor that regulates the complement, fibrinolytic, and kinin pathways. A deficiency of this inhibitor allows for nonphysiological and inappropriate activation of these pathways. As a result, products of the complement cascade or, possibly, bradykinin accumulate and, because of their vasoactive qualities, cause tissue edema and other inflammatory reactions. When a patient with angioedema reports a family history or repetitive attacks with minor trauma or surgery, the diagnosis should be suspected and a C4 blood level should be determined. The C4 level is almost always low during and between attacks, since this complement component is depleted by cascade activation. If the C4 level is low, the C1 esterase inhibitor level should be measured. Eighty-five percent of patients with hereditary angioedema have abnormally low levels, usually below 30 percent of the levels seen in normals; such patients are considered to have type I disease. The remaining patients have abnormal functional assays (type II disease). Another group of patients with acquired C1 esterase inhibitor deficiency have been described. These patients typically present after the fourth decade and demonstrate an increased rate of metabolism, rather than a decreased rate of synthesis of the inhibitor. Most cases described have had an associated B-cell proliferative disorder, such as chronic lymphocytic leukemia, Waldenström's macroglobulinemia, or lymphocytic lymphoma.

Although little efficacy has been demonstrated for epinephrine, antihistamines, or corticosteroids in treating hereditary angiodema, these agents are often used for the limited benefit they may offer. Airway protection should be foremost in mind, as intubation is sometimes required. Infusion of C1 inhibitor concentrate, when available, may resolve the attack within hours. The attenuated androgens stanozolol and danazol, which may increase C1 production by the liver, are used for prophylaxis.

Tumors

Benign or malignant tumors of the pharynx, larynx, trachea, or bronchi may produce upper airway obstruction.

PHARYNX

Because gradually enlarging pharyngeal tumors ordinarily interfere with swallowing first, they are usually discovered before airflow restriction occurs and do not present with obstruction unless untreated or advanced at initial presentation.

LARYNX

Benign and malignant tumors of the larynx may obviously lead to upper airway obstruction. These include submucosal lesions—e.g., hemangiomas of the subglottis and carcinomas of the supraglottic, glottic, and subglottic regions.

TRACHEA AND BRONCHI

Tumors of the trachea, carina, and bronchi produce a gradual decrease in airway diameter. Therefore, patients often present with signs and symptoms of chronic airflow obstruction and wheezing for weeks to months and, in some cases, for years, misleading the physician into establishing a diagnosis of asthma. A diagnosis of asthma of recent onset should provoke closer scrutiny of the upper airways. Bronchogenic carcinomas are the most common primary and secondary tumors of the trachea. In a large surgical series comprising 198 patients, squamous cell carcinoma (36 percent) was slightly less common than adenoid cystic carcinoma (40 percent), followed by a variety of benign and malignant tumors.[15] Secondary tracheal involvement occurs with local advancement of bronchogenic, laryngeal, esophageal, and thyroid carcinomas, or Hodgkin's lymphoma. A distant solid tumor metastasis to the trachea may cause upper airway obstruction (Fig. 52-8).

Primary resection and reconstruction constitute the preferred treatment for localized lesions.[15,41] The extent of tracheal and main bronchial involvement is determined with computed tomography (CT), conventional tomography of the trachea, and careful bronchoscopy. Resection is often precluded by tumor extent or metastatic spread and is rarely indicated for secondary tracheal invasion; thyroid carcinomas are an exception.[17] Adjuvant therapy is less well defined; however, either preoperative[41] or postoperative[15] irradiation, or a combination of the two,[41] is used after resection of malignant airway tumors, because of the narrow margins obtained in the mediastinum.

Acute palliation may be accomplished with several techniques. If conservative measures fail, rigid bronchoscopy with mechanical debridement[31] or bronchoscopic laser vaporization[46] restores airway patency. Radiotherapy, instituted immediately in patients with well-compensated obstruction, may lead to rapid improvement of airway diameter within days. Consolidation of such improvement is then achieved with a completed course of

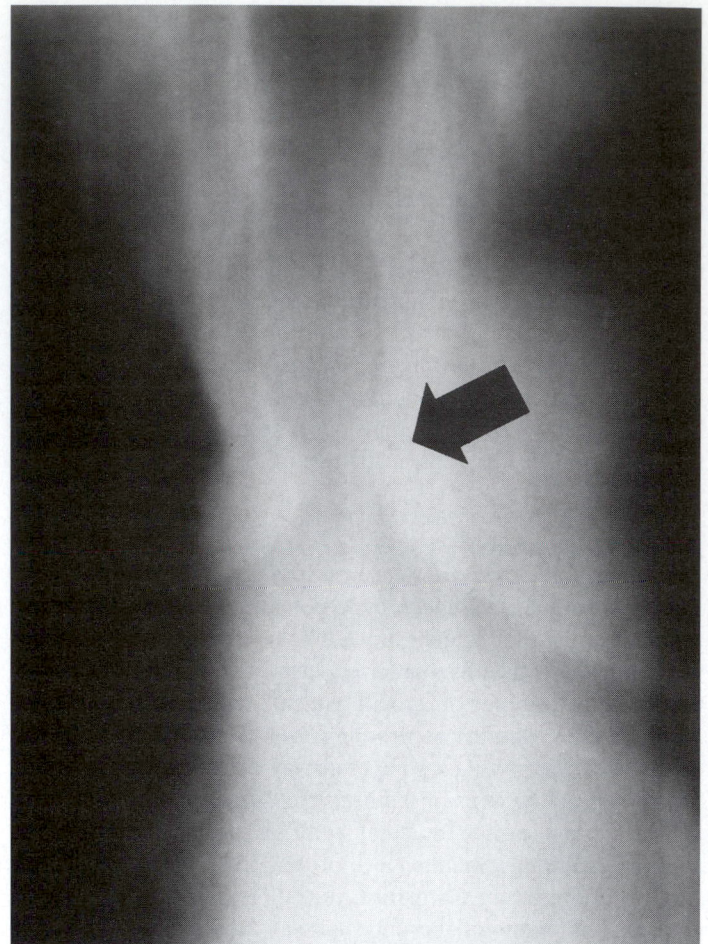

FIGURE 52-8 Tomogram showing tracheal obstruction (arrow) caused by endobronchial metastases from a breast carcinoma.

radiation. Airway stents, such as the silicone T tube, have been used successfully to palliate airway obstruction.[7] The stent must bridge the entire length of affected airway in order to avoid recurrence of the obstruction.

Trauma

Acute obstruction of the airway may be caused by blunt or penetrating trauma to the face, neck, or chest, or by inhalation of noxious gases. Often, airway compromise is only one of several injuries sustained in an accident and may not be recognized immediately. Natural protection of the airway is provided by the facial skeleton, the thoracic cavity, and a voluntary defensive posture in which the chin and anterior chest are approximated to shield the neck. This protection is overcome by high speed, severe force, or offensive aim. Motor vehicle accidents are the most common cause of blunt injury. Penetrating injuries are typically caused by knife or gunshot wounds. Airway obstruction caused by inhalation of noxious fumes and burns is discussed below.

FACIAL TRAUMA

Crush injuries of the face, particularly when associated with fractures of the midface or mandible and CNS trauma, may present with acute airway obstruction. Loss of airway patency results from edema in the oro- or hypopharynx, posterior displacement of the base of the tongue, or intrapharyngeal collection of blood or secretions. Further compromise of the pharyngeal airway is caused by subcutaneous emphysema, mucosal edema following pharyngeal perforation, or large neck hematomas. Endotracheal intubation may be difficult or impossible, and the urgency of the situation may be compounded by the absence of spontaneous breathing due to neurologic injury or pharmacologic paralysis. A safe procedure in patients with significant facial trauma is the construction of a cervical tracheostomy utilizing local anesthesia. A cricothyroidotomy is substituted in an emergency.

LARYNGEAL TRAUMA

The larynx is exposed to injury during extension of the neck from rapid deceleration or direct assault. Compression of the larynx and trachea against the rigid spine results in fractures of the laryngeal cartilage and laceration of the mucosa. The neurovascular structures and the esophagus are usually protected by their flexibility; however, concomitant spinal fractures may exist. Presenting symptoms include dyspnea and stridor, dysphonia or aphonia, neck pain, cough, aspiration, hemoptysis, and dysphagia. Glottic closure may be incomplete during the Valsalva maneuver. The laryngeal prominence is lost, and the contour of the neck is flat. Subcutaneous emphysema originating from mucosal tears may be subtle or prominent. Development of edema or a hematoma in the submucosal planes of the larynx leads to further reduction of airway patency. Contamination with oropharyngeal organisms in the deeper fascial compartments of the neck introduces infection and associated edema.

Physical examination should include an assessment of quiet respiration and the patient's speech. The hyoid bone and laryngeal cartilages should be palpated and any fractures noted. Radiographs of the cervical spine are useful in ruling out a fracture. Neck radiographs may demonstrate subtle subcutaneous air. CT has probably supplanted other radiologic tests. Indirect and direct laryngoscopy should be performed to evaluate the laryngeal lumen and glottic function.

Laryngeal trauma is rare, and no unified approach to its treatment exists. Because translaryngeal intubation carries the risk of enlarging mucosal tears and creating false passages, it should be performed only under direct vision by an experienced physician. A tracheostomy under local anesthesia creates a more secure airway. Early repair appears to afford the best chance for recovery; however, associated injuries may warrant a delay.[4,5] Surgical exploration is indicated for a palpable or displaced fracture of the cartilage and extensive mucosal tears with exposed cartilage. The ultimate clinical outcome depends on the extent and severity of the initial injury. With surgical reconstruction, more than 80 percent of patients achieve decannulation and a good voice.[43]

Tracheobronchial Injuries

Blunt trauma of trachea and bronchi is uncommon. A review of 1178 autopsy reports of blunt trauma victims revealed only 33 ruptures of major airways.[3] The tracheobronchial segment within 2 cm of the carina is the region most susceptible to laceration from blunt trauma.[2,45] The cervical trachea and main-stem bronchi are the segments next most commonly affected. Patients present with subcutaneous emphysema and hemoptysis. However, associated injuries may receive more immediate attention and may require early endotracheal intubation. A review of the recent literature found 183 reported cases over a 20-year period.[45] Of these, 10 percent were located in the cervical trachea, 22 percent in the thoracic trachea, 27 percent in the right main bronchus, 17 percent in the left main bronchus, and 16 percent in a lobar bronchus. Transverse ruptures were found in 74 percent, while 18 percent had longitudinal tears and 8 percent had complex injuries. A small tear may induce a massive pneumothorax after institution of positive-pressure ventilation; however, subtle injuries may be overlooked unless specifically sought. Airway obstruction is uncommon, but it may occur with complete transection of the trachea above the carina. The chest radiograph demonstrates one-sided or bilateral pneumothorax and pneumomediastinum. The diagnosis is made with bronchoscopy; a rigid bronchoscope should be used if the airway is not secure. Immediate reconstruction with direct repair or segmental resection of the airway (with cardiopulmonary bypass, if necessary) generally produces excellent results.

Inhalation Injuries

Fires in closed spaces, such as buildings or cars, release concentrations of noxious fumes sufficient to induce injury even after brief exposure. The initial insult to the airway is caused by irritant gases, such as aldehydes, ammonia, and hydrochloride acid, and by local effects of heat.[8] A severe tracheobronchitis ensues, which may result in sloughing of the mucosa. In the presence of an intact basal cell layer in the airways, early repair is accomplished rapidly.[29,44] If the basal membrane is destroyed by the original injury or by additional trauma, delayed healing may result in granulation tissue formation, scarring, and stenosis. The effects of inhalation and intubation are often impossible to separate, since intubation is performed early in the presence of respiratory symptoms in order to prevent acute airway obstruction.

Acute inhalation injury is diagnosed on the basis of exposure history or the presence of oropharyngeal soot associated with hoarseness and stridor, or with bronchoscopy. Liberal use of endotracheal intubation decreases the risk of delayed obstruction due to glottic edema. Late strictures of larynx and trachea are common following inhalation injury, particularly after long-term intubation. Among 99 patients with inhalation injury and tracheostomy, major airway complications developed in 28, and 6 of 25 survivors had tracheal stenosis.[20] If not severely symptomatic, laryngotracheal stenosis may not come to medical attention unless specifically investigated. In a study in which 17 survivors of inhalation burns were screened for late airway sequelae, four patients with tracheal stenoses and five with tracheal granulomas were noted.[28] Inhalation burns cause a transmural inflammation that does not subside for several years. Confluent laryngotracheal strictures are common (Fig. 52-9). Tracheal resection soon after injury often results in stenosis and should be avoided. Subglottic reconstruction may be performed earlier,[11] however, and stenting with the silastic tracheal T tube has proved particularly helpful.[13] Most patients regain a functional airway and voice following prolonged treatment.

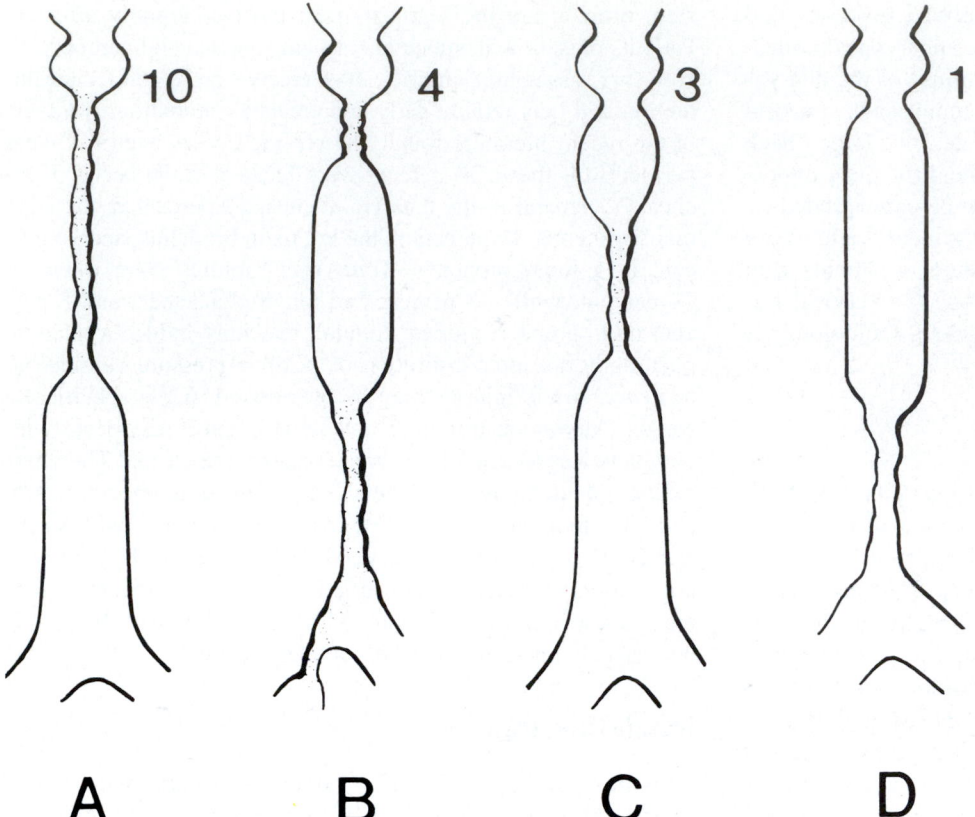

FIGURE 52-9   Distribution of upper airway lesions in 18 patients with inhalation injuries. *A.* Subglottic and upper tracheal stenosis. *B.* Subglottic stenosis and lower tracheal stenosis, with or without extension into main bronchi. *C.* Upper tracheal stenosis. *D.* Lower tracheal stenosis. The number of patients in each category is noted. *(Based on data of Gaissert et al,[13] with permission.)*

Vascular Causes

Vascular compression of the airway arises typically in infancy or childhood as a developmental disorder. Narrowing of the adult airway from vascular causes is uncommon and may occur as a result of enlarging aneurysms of the thoracic aorta. The following three entities all occur in children.

INNOMINATE ARTERY SYNDROME

Pressure of the innominate artery on the anterior wall of the trachea may cause stridor and airway collapse, possibly owing to an intrinsic weakness of the tracheal wall and tracheomalacia, as no structural abnormalities of the aortic arch or the innominate artery have been identified. Only mild obstruction occurs during quiet breathing; however, coughing and swallowing lead to partial or total tracheal collapse. Most children get better without therapy. Cyanotic spells, with apnea, bradycardia, or even cardiac arrest, may occur during bottle feeding and are an indication for surgical intervention. The operative treatment consists of suspending the innominate artery and aortic arch behind the sternum in order to alter the tracheal diameter to a more circular shape and to abolish the pressure of a full esophagus.

DOUBLE AORTIC ARCH

This anomaly is the most common cause of a true vascular ring and is due to persistence of the right and left fourth aortic arches. The smaller left aortic arch passes anterior to the trachea (Fig. 52-10). The descending aorta is usually located on the left side. The tightness of the ring determines the severity of symptoms and time of presentation. Symptoms include stridor, aspiration with recurrent pneumonia, and dysphagia. Surgical correction consists of division of the anterior left arch through a left thoracotomy and division of the ligamentum arteriosum. Acute respiratory compromise may require intubation and urgent correction.

ABERRANT LEFT PULMONARY ARTERY SLING

In the anomaly known as aberrant left pulmonary artery sling, the left pulmonary artery arises from the right pulmonary artery and passes behind the trachea to the left hilum. In 50 percent of patients there is a coexisting congenital tracheal stenosis, which does not resolve after division of the sling. Therefore, in these patients, both lesions require separate correction.

Foreign-Body Aspiration

This cause of upper airway obstruction occurs in both children and adults. Children are likely to aspirate toys, coins, and hard candy, while adults more commonly aspirate food and dental appliances (Fig. 52-11). The *café coronary syndrome* is the name given to the sudden aspiration of a bolus of food, usually meat, into the hypopharynx and upper portion of the larynx. Unlike a patient with a true coronary, the victim suffers sudden respiratory embarrassment while eating and is suddenly unable to talk or breathe. Emergency measures using a food extractor or the Heimlich maneuver may be lifesaving. In performing the Heimlich maneuver, the rescuer stands behind the victim with both arms locked into a fist in the victim's upper abdomen. A sudden backward thrust of the fist causes sudden exhalation and, it is hoped, dislodgment of the bolus of food. Risk factors for foreign-body aspiration include advanced age, altered state of consciousness due to alcohol or drugs, poor dentition, and neurologic disorders such as Parkinson's disease and stroke. Institutionalized patients are particularly at risk. A large foreign body lodged in the esophagus may also cause upper airway obstruction by compressing the trachea. Endoscopic removal may be necessary.

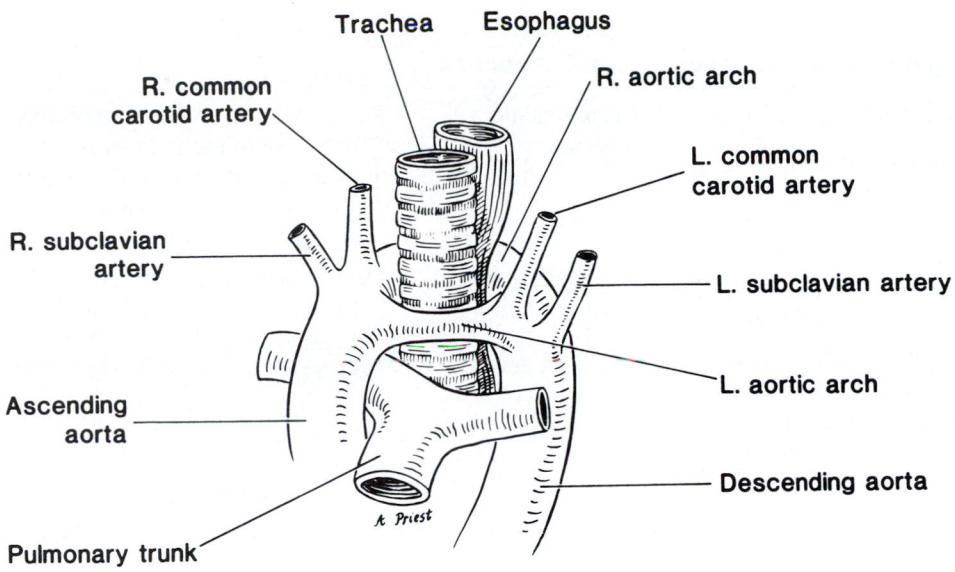

FIGURE 52-10   Double aortic arch. The larger right arch gives rise to the carotid and subclavian arteries and is located posterior to the esophagus, whereas the smaller left arch courses to the trachea. The lumen of the esophagus and trachea is compressed between the two arches. Note the left-sided descending aorta. Not depicted is the ligamentum arteriosum, which may contribute to tracheal compression. *(Based on data of Humphrey et al,[18] with permission.)*

Neuromuscular Disorders

Neuromuscular disorders may affect the bulbar muscles, many of which surround the upper airway. When this occurs, resistance to airflow is increased and the flow-volume loop often shows an inspiratory flow plateau typical of a variable extrathoracic upper airway obstruction.[47] This may also be associated with flow oscillations during inspiration ("sawtooth pattern"). The abnormal flow pattern was first noted in patients with sleep apnea, but it is commonly seen with extrapyramidal disorders, myasthenia gravis, and motoneuron disease. It is also observed in patients who have functional stridor and wheezing (see below). In extrapyramidal disorders, the flow oscillations correspond to vocal cord tremor.[48] In motoneuron diseases, muscle denervation causes irregular muscle fasciculations, which result in tremor of the upper airway muscles.

Upper airway symptoms have been seen in Shy-Drager syndrome with extrapyramidal involvement and in Parkinson's disease. Patients may present with symptoms of chronic dyspnea or with stridor and respiratory failure that are relieved by endotracheal intubation. Bilateral vocal cord paralysis also results in abnormalities of inspiratory flow and a characteristic flow-volume loop. Bilateral vocal cord paralysis may be a cause of nocturnal stridor, oxygen desaturation, and sleep disruption or, in extreme cases, acute respiratory failure. In children, vocal cord paralysis may be a complication of Dandy-Walker syndrome and Arnold-Chiari malformation. In adults, causes include familial bulbar spinal muscle atrophy, postpoliomyelitis syndrome, Parkinson's disease, multiple sclerosis, acute poliomyelitis, amyotrophic lateral sclerosis, Guillain-Barré syndrome, brain-stem stroke, and a large cerebral hemisphere stroke. Nonneurologic causes include laryngeal nerve injury following neck surgery, endotracheal intubation injury, laryngeal trauma, infection, trauma, and thoracic aortic aneurysm. Dystonic extrapyramidal reactions due to neuroleptic medications, such as haloperidol, may cause significant upper airway obstruction. The usual reactions to these medications are akathisia, dyskinesia, dysarthria, and dystonic reactions such as torticollis. Laryngeal-pharyngeal dystonia may cause severe upper airway dysfunction. If not reversed, symptoms can last for days or lead to respiratory arrest.

Iatrogenic Causes

The iatrogenic causes of upper airway obstruction are listed in Table 52-2. The most common complications affect the larynx or trachea as a result of prolonged endotracheal intubation (see Chapter 174). Complications from tracheostomy may lead to acute airway obstruction soon after the procedure, as well as delayed obstruction months or years afterward.[26] Injury to the glot-

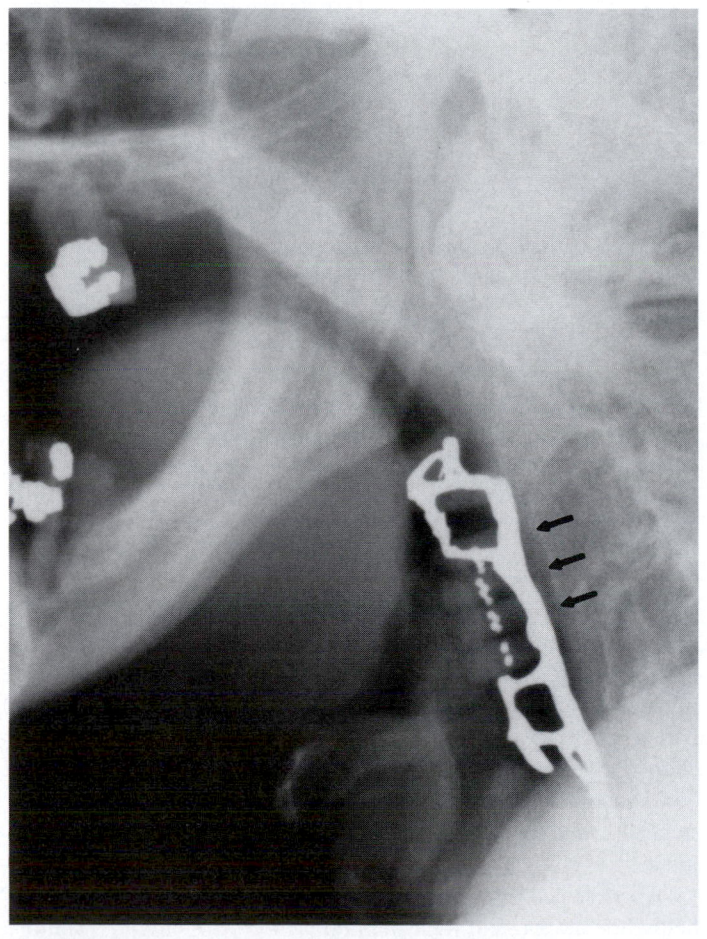

FIGURE 52-11   Foreign-body aspiration. Lateral soft-tissue radiograph of the neck showing aspirated portion of denture (arrows) that caused upper airway obstruction in an elderly patient.

TABLE 52-2

Iatrogenic Causes of Upper Airway Obstruction

Airway Complications of Tracheal Intubation	
Vocal cord granuloma	Vocal cord ulcerations, edema, and granuloma are the most common complications of prolonged intubation; usually resolve spontaneously within 12 weeks; a cause of postextubation hoarseness and stridor
Glottic stenosis	Reported to occur in 4–12 percent of patients; incidence increases with duration of intubation; other risk factors are large tube caliber, oral vs. nasal intubation, and severe respiratory failure
Vocal cord paralysis	May result from vocal cord trauma, surgery, or recurrent laryngeal nerve injury; a cause of postextubation airway obstruction
Laryngospasm	Can be caused by mechanical trauma to the vocal cords; rare cause of post-extubation stridor
Tracheal stenosis	Can occur at subglottic area, stoma or cuff level; incidence reduced by low-pressure, high-volume cuffs; commonly occurs 2–3 months after tracheostomy removal; may occur years later
Bleeding	A complication of tracheostomy; early bleeding (within hours) occurs from thyroid isthmus or anterior jugular system; late bleeding occurs from tracheal–innominate artery fistula when stoma is placed too low
Tracheal tube displacement	An early complication (<4 days); tracheostomy tube becomes displaced anteriorly into the mediastinum and compresses the trachea; inhalation of a tracheostomy tube has also been reported
Tracheal mucoid impaction	Desiccated mucus plug can obstruct distal portion of the tube; can result in ball-valve obstruction to airflow; can also occur with transtracheal oxygen catheters
Faulty placement of endotracheal tube	Occurs most frequently in association with emergency intubations
	Endotracheal tube may be misplaced in the esophagus or main bronchi
Complications of Medical Therapy	
Drug induced	Allergic laryngospasm has been reported following oral propranolol therapy
	Excessive anticoagulation can result in upper airway obstruction due to hematoma formation in the laryngeal, retropharyngeal, submaxillary, or sublingual spaces
	Angioedema is a rare but potentially fatal complication of several commonly used drugs by IgE and non-IgE mechanisms (aspirin, NSAIDs, ACE inhibitors, and radiocontrast materials)
Venous catheterization	Percutaneous central venous catheterization may be complicated by laceration of neck vessels and resulting hemorrhage or extravasation of IV fluids that cause tracheal compression

tis is caused by posterior displacement of the endotracheal tube by the tongue and the forward convexity of the cervical spine. While damage to the vocal cords is common, these milder pressure-induced lesions usually regress spontaneously within 8 to 12 weeks.[6] The more serious complication of stenosis at the posterior glottic commissure occurs in 6 to 12 percent of cases. In a prospective study of 200 intubations, stenosis at this site was shown to correlate with the duration of translaryngeal intubation.[49] For patients intubated for more than 10 days, the incidence was 12 percent. Such statistics have prompted clinicians at many medical centers to proceed with tracheostomy when ex-

tubation does not appear to be imminent after 10 days of intubation.[30] However, the decision regarding the timing of tracheostomy remains controversial because of the early and late complications, particularly tracheal stenosis. Many centers delay tracheostomy for up to 3 weeks of prolonged airway management.[30]

Tracheal stenosis typically occurs at the cuff site, 1.0 to 3.5 cm below the stoma, and measures up to 4 cm in length.[50] The incidence has decreased in recent years with the advent of high-volume, low-pressure tracheostomy tube cuffs. Overinflation of the cuffs is still a cause of tracheal strictures. Stenosis at the level of the stoma is caused by an overlarge stoma or excessive traction on the tracheostomy tube. Stenosis of the subglottic trachea may also occur, usually from a stoma placed too high. Last, tracheomalacia due to thinning of the tracheal cartilage may occur, by itself or in combination with tracheal stricture, and may lead to upper airway obstruction (Fig. 52-12).

Airway injury caused by translaryngeal intubation can result in immediate symptoms, seen with postextubation glottic edema or laryngospasm, or delayed symptoms, as in the case of glottic stenosis or tracheal stenosis. The routine chest radiograph is usually unrevealing. Lateral neck films may show glottic or subglottic stenosis. Tomograms of the trachea in both posteroanterior and lateral views are usually diagnostic. Fluoroscopy can be used to evaluate laryngeal function and to demonstrate tracheomalacia during a forced expiratory maneuver. CT may offer little additional information with benign strictures. If time permits, postextubation stridor can be evaluated with transnasal fiberoptic laryngoscopy. Endoscopic examination of the airway with a flexible fiberoptic bronchoscope may be diagnostic, but the procedure may be hazardous in uncontrolled environments.[50] Acute airflow obstruction may be precipitated by the presence of blood, airway secretions, airway wall trauma, or the bronchoscope itself. The rigid bronchoscope may be useful in dilating the stricture in preparation for definitive surgery. Long-term results with laryngotracheal resection and reconstruction are good to excellent in more than 80 percent of patients.[16] If resection is not feasible or has to be delayed, placement of a silicone tracheal T tube can offer tracheal patency. Laser therapy may also provide temporary relief, but long-term success with this form of therapy is limited. More than 70 percent of the procedures fail within 6 to 8 weeks.

Vocal Cord Dysfunction

The glottis plays an active role in adjusting airflow, both voluntarily and through reflex control from laryngeal and pulmonary receptors. Normally, the glottic opening widens during inspiration and narrows with expiration. Occasionally, the glottis can become dysfunctional in the absence of any organic disease. The disorder, called *vocal cord dysfunction,* is characterized by paradoxical closure of the vocal cords intermittently during inspiration. The mechanism is unknown, but psychogenic factors seem more likely than a disordered processing of neural input to the larynx.

The signs and symptoms resemble those of laryngeal edema, laryngospasm, vocal cord paralysis, or asthma. Wheezing or stridor and shortness of breath are typical and are often so dramatic that they suggest acute asphyxia and respiratory failure. Intubation and other emergency measures are frequently used. A review of 95 cases of vocal cord dysfunction showed that 53 patients also had asthma.[37] Patients without asthma were predominantly women who had been misdiagnosed with asthma an average of 5 years earlier and were taking large doses of oral corticosteroids. Medical treatment for the entire group was very common, with frequent emergency room visits, hospitalizations, and endotracheal intubations.

Psychiatric disorders are common in these patients. Major psychiatric disorders, personality disorders, and sexual and

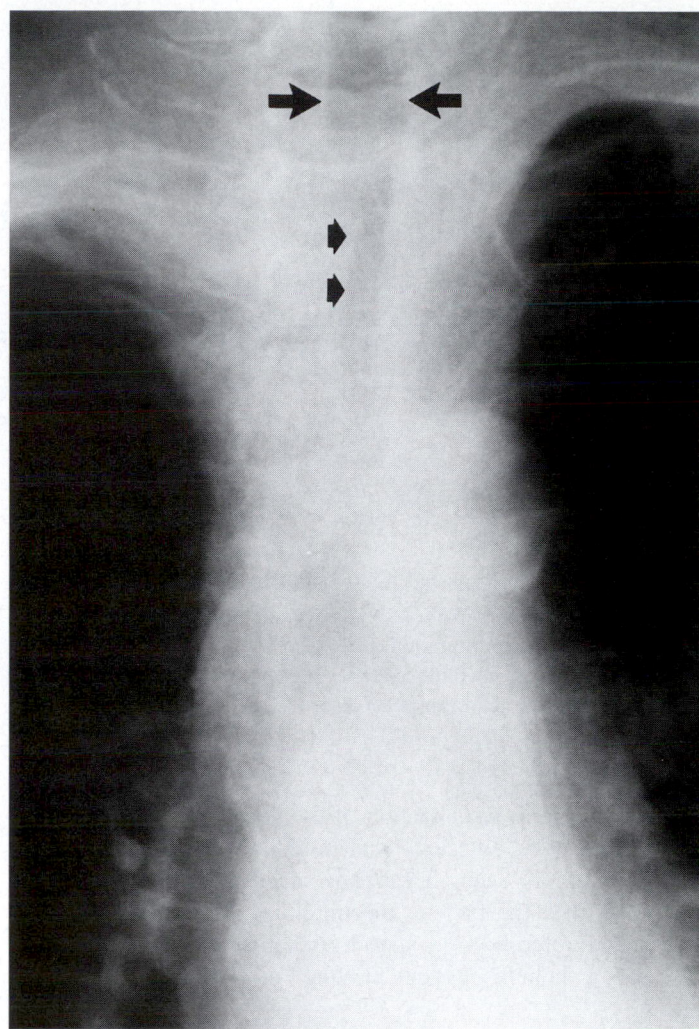

FIGURE 52-12   Tracheomalacia. Radiograph demonstrates a tracheal air column that shows diffuse narrowing of the intrathoracic trachea (small arrows) compared with the extrathoracic trachea (large arrows).

physical abuse are commonly discovered. Whereas many patients are unaware of their self-induced wheeze or stridor, others appear to derive secondary gain from their symptoms and manifest factitious illness.[9] A high index of suspicion of this disorder should be present when a patient presents with wheezing, stridor, or both, and the adventitious sounds heard are loudest over the neck. The response to bronchodilator therapy is usually poor. Despite their respiratory distress, patients often have little difficulty completing full sentences, can hold their breath, and will abolish the laryngeal-induced sounds during a panting maneuver. On pulmonary function testing, a pattern of variable extrathoracic airway obstruction is found, resulting in an increase in the ratio of $FEF_{50\%}$ to $FIF_{50\%}$.

Another pattern seen in some patients is "sawtoothing," or fluttering of the inspiratory limb, representing fluctuations in the abnormal cord motion (Fig. 52-13). Often, attempts to perform the flow-volume loop maneuver give variable results from test to test. A normal alveolar-arterial oxygen gradient and absence of bronchial hyperresponsiveness are other clues to the diagnosis. The diagnosis of vocal cord dysfunction is

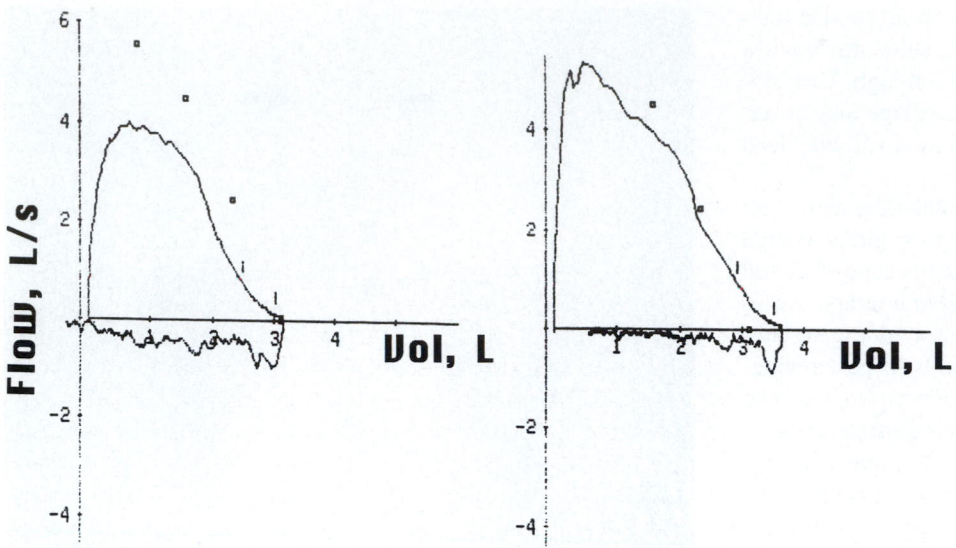

FIGURE 52-13 Variable extrathoracic obstruction due to vocal cord dysfunction. Two consecutive flow-volume loops from a young woman with inspiratory stridor. Variable effort accounts for the differences in configuration. FEF$_{50\%}$/FIF$_{50\%}$ in each is very high. The inspiratory loop is flat and demonstrates a sawtooth pattern. This pattern has also been associated with sleep apnea syndrome and various neuromuscular disorders.

made from direct visualization of the vocal cords during an attack. Inspiratory, anterior vocal cord closure with a posterior glottic chink is seen. Treatment includes discussion of the diagnosis with the patient, discontinuing unnecessary medications, and referral to a speech therapist or psychotherapist. Use of a helium-oxygen mixture may alleviate an acute attack.

Miscellaneous Causes

A variety of other causes may result in upper airway obstruction.

COLLAGEN VASCULAR DISEASES

Relapsing polychondritis is a rare, autoimmune connective-tissue disease that affects cartilage throughout the body.[10] When the larynx and trachea are affected, the prognosis is poor. Airflow obstruction is caused by flaccidity and increased compliance of the airway so that it collapses during a forced expiratory maneuver. No laboratory tests are specific for the diagnosis. Evidence of recurrent inflammation of two or more cartilaginous sites, usually the ear and nose, is sufficient for the diagnosis. Corticosteroids, anti-inflammatory agents, and immunosuppresive drugs have been used with some success to control the disease. Life-threatening upper airway obstruction has also been noted in patients with Sjögren's syndrome as a result of compressing mediastinal lymph nodes, and with Wegener's granulomatosis due to tracheal stenosis. Hoarseness, inspiratory stridor, and dyspnea may result from rheumatoid arthritis, resulting in midline fixation of the arytenoid cartilages at their articulations with the cricoid cartilage. Hyperostosis of the cervical spine in ankylosing spondylitis may produce upper airway obstruction.

TRACHEAL ABNORMALITIES

Tracheobronchiomegaly is a rare familial disorder that is associated with marked dilatation of the respiratory tract; it may affect the airways from the larynx down to the smaller airways. Tracheal compliance is increased; tracheal diameter may measure 30 to 50 mm or more, owing to thin, atrophied muscular and elastic tissue. This can result in flaccidity and airflow obstruction. An irregular, corrugated appearance of the trachea may be seen on routine chest radiography. Bronchiectasis may result from poor airway clearance. Occasionally, the coronal diameter of the trachea is markedly reduced, and the sagittal diameter is correspondingly increased. This disorder is called the *saber sheath trachea*. Its only significance may be that it is a sign of underlying chronic obstructive pulmonary disease. *Tracheobronchopathia osteochondroplastica* is a degenerative disease of the trachea and bronchi of older men that is characterized by nodules of cartilage and bone within the submucosa of these structures. These nodules present as polypoid masses that may narrow the airway lumen and cause dyspnea and wheezing.

NONCARDIOGENIC PULMONARY EDEMA AS A COMPLICATION OF ACUTE UPPER AIRWAY OBSTRUCTION

Noncardiogenic pulmonary edema as a complication of upper airway obstruction was first recognized in children following acute epiglottis and foreign-body aspiration. It has since been reported as a result of hanging, strangulation, thyroid goiter, hypothyroidism, upper airway tumors, acromegaly, mediastinal tumors, and insertion of a peroral dental prosthesis. The most common cause in adults is postanesthetic laryngospasm. Risk factors include an anatomically difficult intubation, nasal or laryngeal surgery, obesity, short neck, and obstructive sleep apnea.[23]

The mechanism of this unusual complication appears to be multifaceted and includes the accumulation of alveolar fluid due to hydrostatic forces, as well as an acquired defect in alveolar-capillary permeability. The main mechanism proposed is the generation of negative intrathoracic and transpulmonary pressures from attempted inspiration against an obstructed airway. This maneuver (Müller's maneuver) results in an increase in pulmonary blood volume and a decrease in pulmonary capillary perivascular pressure. The increase in blood volume and changes in hydrostatic pressure gradients are factors favoring the accumulation of pulmonary edema fluid. In some patients, pulmonary edema fluid protein has been measured and found to be high relative to serum concentrations. This finding suggests the presence of an acquired defect in membrane permeability—a possibility that is also supported by the fact that pulmonary edema formation may be delayed for several hours in some patients following acute upper airway obstruction. Most patients with pulmonary edema following upper airway obstruction have a relatively benign course and experience rapid improvement with supportive care and supplemental oxygen. Vigorous diuresis can be deleterious and lead to hypotension. Noninvasive ventilatory support with nasal ventilation can be helpful when the pulmonary edema is more severe and profound hypoxemia occurs.

ACUTE MANAGEMENT

Several medical and surgical measures constitute the basic management strategy for upper airway obstruction.

General Measures

The patient with acute obstruction presents a formidable challenge to the judgment and skills of the responsible physician.[22] The situation requires that the physician immediately assess the condition of the patient, take a history (however brief), perform a physical examination, and make the right management decision. Endotracheal intubation is not the standard procedure for relief of all causes of airway obstruction, and an improperly planned and hastily performed intubation may result in the loss of an airway that might otherwise have been reasonably compensated.

If the level and cause of obstruction are not obvious, diagnostic efforts should be pursued before intubation is attempted, unless there is complete obstruction or impending respiratory arrest. Conservative measures are instituted in the interval to improve breathing. The patient is placed in upright sitting position or mildly reclined. Inspired air is humidified and supplemental oxygen is provided to maintain an oxygen saturation greater than 90 percent. If stridor is present or laryngeal edema is suspected, racemic epinephrine and a helium-oxygen mixture may decrease airflow resistance.[40] Racemic epinephrine reduces inflammation and edema. An aerosolized solution (0.5 ml in 2.5 ml saline) is administered and may be repeated every 4 h. Helium decreases turbulence of the inspired air and improves laminar flow across a stenosis.[39] Oxygen concentrations above 40 percent render helium ineffective; typically, concentrations of 70 percent helium and 30 percent oxygen are used. The usefulness of corticosteroids has been shown in treating croup. These agents may obviate intubation and decrease length of hospital stay. No such advantage has been shown with acute epiglottitis, hereditary angioedema, or postextubation laryngeal edema. Corticosteroids are indicated for allergic, IgE-mediated angioedema.

The level of obstruction is of importance and determines which intervention will provide relief. When there is oropharyngeal obstruction, secretions are removed with suction; an attempt is made to lift the base of the tongue from a posterior position with jaw thrust and chin lift maneuvers, and an oropha-

ryngeal airway is inserted. If any of these steps fail to improve the airway, and if, on laryngoscopy, the vocal cords are not visualized, a tracheostomy is performed. Laryngeal obstruction is approached in a similar manner. Except in the case of an emergency, endotracheal intubation should be planned in advance. Pharmacologic muscle relaxation should be avoided, in order to maintain spontaneous breathing. The cessation of spontaneous respirations in the presence of airway obstruction creates an unnecessary emergency. Alternatively, local mucosal anesthesia is provided or inhalational anesthesia instituted if the procedure is done in an operating room. Endotracheal tubes of different sizes, from 5 to 8 mm in internal diameter, and, particularly for tracheal or carinal obstruction, fiberoptic and rigid bronchoscopy should be available. For lesions located above the cricoid cartilage, the inability to intubate indicates the need for tracheostomy. A tracheostomy is rarely helpful in tracheal lesions, however, and either intubation with a small (5-mm) endotracheal tube in a dire emergency or, under more controlled circumstances, rigid bronchoscopy is preferred.

Cricothyroidotomy

When seconds count, access through the cricothyroid membrane affords the shortest distance between skin and airway with few, if any, interposed structures. When this procedure is used, local anesthesia should not matter. A 2-cm transverse incision is made over the cricothyroid membrane, which is incised close to the prominent cricoid cartilage (Fig. 52-14). Either the handle of the scalpel or, more appropriately, a 7-mm endotracheal (or tracheostomy) tube is inserted carefully. Once the immediate emergency is resolved (usually after 24 to 48 h), the airway stoma is relocated to the trachea to prevent damage to the subglottic space and the cricoid cartilage.

Tracheostomy

Tracheostomy is best performed in an operating room by a surgeon or otolaryngologist. A tracheostomy is performed under general anesthesia or after application of a local anesthetic agent. The patient is placed in a supine position with elevation of the shoulders and extension of the neck. A 4-cm transverse incision is made midway between cricoid cartilage and the upper manubrial edge. The platysma is incised transversely, while the further dissection is conducted in the midline. The strap muscles are separated, and the anterior trachea is exposed. If the thyroid isthmus precludes exposure, it is divided between clamps and suture ligatures. If a rapid airway is desired, the thyroid is pushed upward. A vertical incision is made in the second and third tracheal rings. Under retraction of the tracheal wall, a 7- or 8-mm tracheostomy tube is inserted. The tube is secured to the skin with a heavy monofilament suture; however, no attempt is made to close the skin incision. Usually a tract forms around the tracheostomy by the seventh day, and the tube can then be changed. Accidental removal before that time requires reinsertion in the operating room or endotracheal intubation.

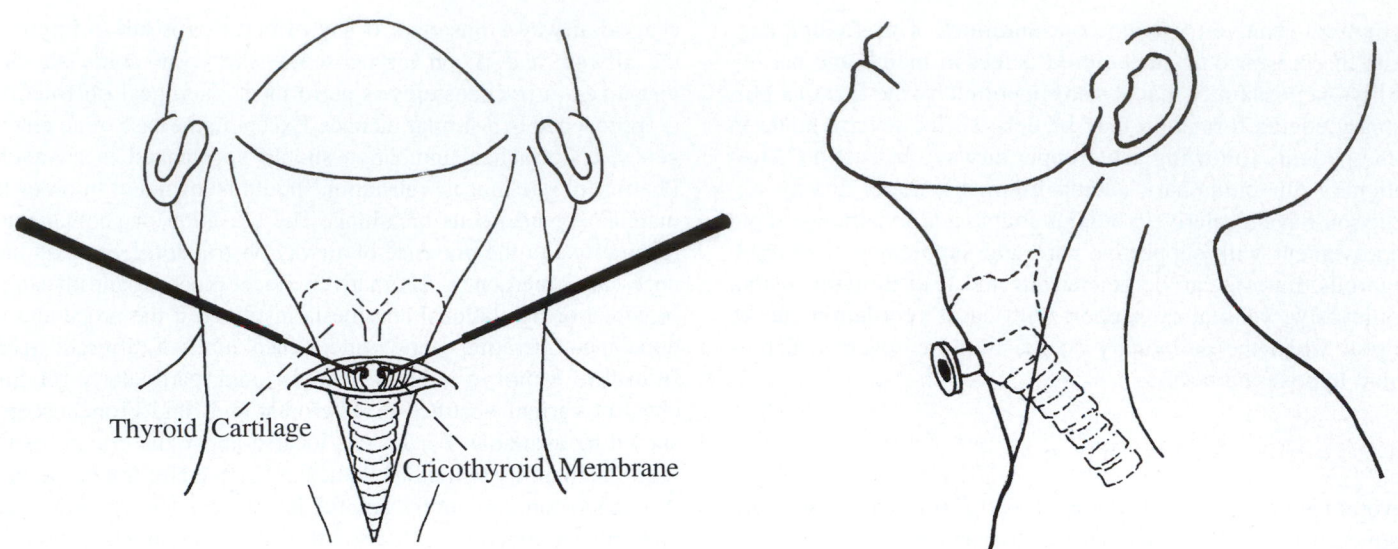

FIGURE 52-14   Cricothyroidotomy. Hyperextension of the neck facilitates exposure, but is avoided in trauma patients with suspected cervical spine injury.

REFERENCES

1. Baughman RP, Loudon RG: Stridor: Differentiation from asthma or upper airway noise. *Am Rev Respir Dis* 139:1407–1409, 1989.
2. Baumgartner F, Sheppard B, de Virgilio C, et al: Tracheal and main bronchial disruptions after blunt chest trauma: Presentation and management. *Ann Thorac Surg* 50:569–574, 1990.
3. Bertelsen S, Howitz P: Injuries of the trachea and bronchi. *Thorax* 27:188–194, 1972.
4. Biller HF, Lawson W: Management of acute laryngeal trauma, in Bailey BJ, Biller HF (eds), *Surgery of the Larynx.* Toronto, WB Saunders, 1985, p 149.
5. Casiano RR, Goodwin WJ: Restoring function to the injured larynx. *Otolaryngol Clin North Am* 24:1215–1226, 1991.
6. Colice GL, Stukel TA, Dain B: Laryngeal complications of prolonged intubation. *Chest* 96:877–884, 1989.
7. Cooper JD, Pearson FG, Patterson GA, et al: Use of silicone stents in the management of airway problems. *Ann Thorac Surg* 47:371–378, 1989.
8. Crapo RO: Causes of respiratory injury, in Haponik EF, Munster AM (eds), *Respiratory Injury: Smoke Inhalation and Burns.* New York, McGraw-Hill, 1990, pp 47–60.
9. Downing ET, Braman SS, Fox MJ, Corrao WM: Factitious asthma. *JAMA* 248:2878–2881, 1982.
10. Eng J, Sabanathan SS: Airway complications in relapsing polychondritis. *Ann Thorac Surg* 51:686–692, 1991.
11. Flexon PB, Cheney ML, Montgomery WW, et al: Management of patients with glottic and subglottic stenosis resulting from thermal burns. *Ann Otol Rhinol Laryngol* 98:27–30, 1989.
12. Frantz TD, Rasgon BM, Quesenberry CP: Acute epiglottitis in adults. *JAMA* 272:1358–1360, 1994.
13. Gaissert HA, Lofgren RH, Grillo HC: Upper airway compromise after inhalation injury: Complex strictures of the larynx and trachea and their management. *Ann Surg* 218:672–678, 1993.
14. Goodall EW: The story of tracheotomy. *Br J Child Dis* 31:167–176, 253–272, 1934.
15. Grillo HC, Mathisen DJ: Primary tracheal tumors: Treatment and results. *Ann Thorac Surg* 49:69–77, 1990.
16. Grillo HC, Mathisen DJ, Wain JC: Laryngotracheal resection and reconstruction for subglottic stenosis. *Ann Thorac Surg* 53:54–63, 1992.
17. Grillo HC, Suen HC, Mathisen DJ, Wain JC: Resectional management of thyroid carcinoma invading the airway. *Ann Thorac Surg* 55:476–481, 1993.
18. Humphrey PW, Spadone DP, Silver D: Vascular disorders of the upper torso. *Curr Probl Surg* 30:817–920, 1993.
19. Israili ZH, Hall WD: Cough and angioneurotic edema associated with angiotensin-converting enzyme inhibitor therapy. *Ann Intern Med* 117:234–242, 1992.
20. Jones WG, Madden M, Finkelstein J, et al: Tracheostomies in burn patients. *Ann Surg* 209:471–474, 1988.
21. Karbowitz SR, Edelman LB, Nath S, et al: Spectrum of advanced upper airway obstruction due to goiters. *Chest* 87:18–21, 1985.
22. Kharasch M, Graff J: Emergency management of the airway. *Crit Care Clin* 11:53–66, 1995.
23. Kollef MH, Pluss J: Noncardiogenic pulmonary edema following upper airway obstruction: 7 cases and a review. *Medicine (Baltimore)* 70:91–98, 1991.
24. Kryger M, Bode F, Antic R, Anthonisen N: Diagnosis of obstruction of the upper and central airways. *Am J Med* 61:85–93, 1976.
25. Lavelle TF Jr, Rotman HH, Weg JG: Isoflow-volume curves in the diagnosis of upper airway obstruction. *Am Rev Respir Dis* 117:845–852, 1978.
26. Lewis RJ: Tracheostomies: Indications, timing and complications. *Clin Chest Med* 13:137–149,1992.
27. Lund T, Goodwin CW, McManus WF, et al: Upper airway sequelae in burn patients requiring endotracheal intubation or tracheostomy. *Ann Surg* 201:374–382, 1985.
28. Mallory TB, Brickley WJ: Pathology, with special reference to the pulmonary lesions. *Ann Surg* 117:865–884, 1943.
29. Marsh HM, Gillespie DJ, Baumgartner AE: Timing of tracheostomy in the critically ill patient. *Chest* 96:190–193, 1989.
30. Mathisen DJ, Grillo HC: Endoscopic relief of malignant airway obstruction. *Ann Thorac Surg* 48:469–473, 1989.
31. MayoSmith MF, Hirsch PJ, Wodzinski SF, Schiffman FJ: Acute epiglottitis in adults. *New Engl J Med* 314:1133–1139, 1986.

32. *Medical Times and Gaz* 2:357, 379, 404, 430, 457. 1859; *cit.* Gurlt E. Jahresbericht für 1859. *Arch Klin Chir* 1:191, 1861.

33. Miller RD, Hyatt RE: Obstructing lesions of the larynx and trachea: Clinical and physiologic characteristics. *Mayo Clin Proc* 44:145–161, 1969.

34. Miller RD, Hyatt RE: Evaluation of obstructing lesions of the trachea and larynx by flow-volume loops. *Am Rev Respir Dis* 108:475–481, 1973.

35. Mittleman RE, Wetli, CV: The fatal cafe coronary. *JAMA* 247:1285–1288, 1982.

36. Moreland LW, Corey J, McKenzie R: Ludwig's angina. *Arch Intern Med* 148:461–466, 1988.

37. Newman KB, Mason UG III, Schmaling KB: Clinical features of vocal cord dysfunction. *Am J Respir Crit Care Med* 152:1382–1386, 1995.

38. Orfan NA, Kolski GB: Angioedema and C1 inhibitor deficiency. *Ann Allergy* 60:167–172, 1992.

39. Orr JB: Helium-oxygen gas mixtures in the management of patients with airway obstruction. *Ear Nose Throat J* 67:866–869, 1988.

40. Owens GR, Murphy DMF: Spirometric diagnosis of upper airway obstruction. *Arch Intern Med* 143:1331–1334, 1983.

41. Pearson FG, Todd TRJ, Cooper JD: Experience with primary neoplasms of the trachea. *J Thorac Cardiovasc Surg* 88:511–516, 1984.

42. Randall CS, Braman SS, Millman RP: Rapid development of cor pulmonale following acute tonsillitis in adults. *Chest* 95:462–463, 1989.

43. Schaefer SD: The acute management of external laryngeal trauma: A 27-year experience. *Arch Otolaryngol Head Neck Surg* 118:598–604, 1992.

44. Shimazu T, Yukioka T, Hubbard GB, et al: A dose-responsive model of smoke inhalation injury. *Ann Surg* 206:89–97, 1987.

45. Symbas PN, Justicz AG, Ricketts RR: Rupture of the airways from blunt trauma: Treatment of complex injuries. *Ann Thorac Surg* 54:177–183, 1992.

46. Unger M: Neodymium:YAG laser therapy for malignant and benign endobronchial lesions. *Clin Chest Med* 6:277–290, 1985.

47. Vincken W, Elleker G, Cosio MG: Detection of upper airway muscle involvement in neuromuscular disorders using the flow-volume loop. *Chest* 90:52–57, 1986.

48. Vincken WG, Gauthier SSG, Dollfuss RE, et al: Involvement of upper airway muscles in extrapyramidal disorders. *New Engl J Med* 311:438–442, 1984.

49. Whited RE: A prospective study of laryngotracheal sequelae in long-term intubation. *Laryngoscope* 94:367–377, 1984.

50. Wood DE, Mathisen DJ: Late complications of tracheotomy. *Clin Chest Med* 12:597–609, 1991.

CHAPTER 53

CYSTIC FIBROSIS

Cynthia Robinson / Thomas F. Scanlin

Cystic fibrosis (CF) is a common inherited disease that has a high frequency in Caucasians. The disorder affects all exocrine glands, with symptoms involving the lungs and pancreas usually dominating the clinical picture. Two aspects of the disease make CF particularly difficult to both diagnose and manage: tremendous variability in the degree and pattern of involvement of organs in different persons and lack of information about the precise details of the molecular and cellular pathogenesis of the disease even though the gene responsible for CF and its gene product, an integral membrane glycoprotein, have been identified.[52] This chapter focuses on the pathophysiology and management of CF. Our current understanding of the genetics and underlying molecular biology are highlighted. Complications of the disorder are addressed, and a brief discussion of relevant psychosocial and reproductive issues is provided. Finally, potential future directions in treatment are described, including gene therapy.

GENETICS

CF demonstrates an autosomal recessive pattern of inheritance. In the United States, the incidence of the disease in Caucasians is approximately 1 in 3300 live births and in African Americans, 1 in 15,300. The frequency of unaffected heterozygote carriers of a CF mutation is 1 in 25 in persons of Northern European ancestry.

CF is caused by mutations in a single gene named the *cystic fibrosis transmembrane conductance regulator* (CFTR).[39] This gene was identified with an approach known as positional cloning, which permitted mapping of the gene without prior knowledge of the biochemical defect through the use of polymorphic DNA markers. The first genetic marker that was found to be linked to CF was paraoxonase. In 1985, the demonstration of the linkage of CF to two DNA markers, D7S15 and D7S8, and to the *met* oncogene established the localization of the CF gene to the long arm of chromosome 7. Following a series of molecular cloning experiments, which included "chromosome walking" and "jumping," a candidate gene was identified. This was proved to be the CF gene in 1989, largely through the discovery of a frequent mutation.[40] Formal proof that this was the CF gene came in 1990 with correction of the chloride secretory defect in CF cells in vitro following transfection of the CFTR gene.[15]

The CF gene spans approximately 230 kb of DNA and contains 27 exons. The mRNA is 6.5 kb and is detected in a variety of tissues, including lungs, pancreas, and sweat glands, which are predominantly affected in pathogenesis of the disease. The deduced polypeptide was predicted to be an integral membrane glycoprotein containing 1480 amino acids (Fig. 53-1; see "Pathogenesis"). Several major and minor splicing variants in the transcripts have been described in both persons with and those without CF. In most cases, however, the significance of the alternative splicings is not clear.[54]

The most common CF mutation, and the first to be described, is a three-base pair deletion in exon 10 that causes a deletion of phenylalanine from position 508 (ΔF508) of the CFTR glycoprotein. This mutation accounts for 66 percent of CF mutations. More than 600 CF mutations have now been reported, however, and the list continues to grow. In addition, a number of benign sequence variations have been described. A listing of the most common mutations and their relative frequency is included in Table 53-1. The large number of mutations makes accurate detection of a satisfactory percentage of carriers extremely difficult, and carrier screening for the general population has not been recommended or implemented. Testing for 32 of the most common mutations is commercially available; such testing will detect approximately 90 percent of the carriers in Caucasians of northern European descent. In families with an affected individual and known mutations, prenatal diagnosis and carrier testing using direct detection of mutations is accurate and available. In families with a member diagnosed as having CF but with undetected mutations, use of restriction fragment length polymorphism analysis using linked DNA markers can be informative in a high percentage of cases.

PATHOGENESIS

Discovery of the gene responsible for CF and description of its product, CFTR, have provided the necessary foundation for understanding the pathogenesis of the disorder at the molecular and cellular levels. CFTR is an integral membrane glycoprotein of approximately 170 kD that is expressed in epithelial cells of affected organs. CFTR contains 1480 amino acids, which are arranged in 12 transmembrane domains, two nucleotide binding domains, and a putative regulatory domain (Fig. 53-1). The most common mutation, ΔF508, is a three-base deletion that causes deletion of phenylala-

nine from position 508, located in the proposed first nucleotide-binding domain. The original structural model, which was based on hydrophobicity plots, has proved to be essentially correct in its main features. CFTR shares many structural features with the "ATP-binding cassette" transporter family, which includes P glycoproteins, as well as a number of bacterial transporters. CFTR has been clearly shown to function as an apical chloride channel in airway epithelial cells.

The role of CFTR as an apical chloride channel fits nicely with the simplest hypothesis to account for the pathogenesis of pulmonary disease in CF: Decreased secretion of chloride and water by airway epithelial cells results in dehydrated mucus. However, electrophysiological studies have also shown an increased reabsorption of sodium ions by airway epithelial cells in

TABLE 53-1

Most Common CFTR Mutations in the World

Name of Mutation	Frequency (%)	Population with High Prevalence
ΔF508	28,948 (66)	
G542X	1062 (2.4)	Spanish
G551D	717 (1.6)	English
N1303K	589 (1.3)	Italian
W1282X	536 (1.2)	Jewish-Ashkenazi
R553X	322 (0.7)	German
621+1G→T	315 (0.7)	French-Canadian
1717−1G→A	254 (0.6)	Italian
R117H	133 (0.3)	
R1162X	125 (0.3)	Italian
R347P	106 (0.2)	
3849+10kbC→T	104 (0.2)	Jewish-Ashkenazi, Hispanic
Δ1507	93 (0.2)	
394delTT	74 (10–30)*	Nordic, Finnish
G85E	67	
R560T	67	
A455E	62	Dutch
1078delT	57	Celtic
2789+5G→A	54	Spanish
3659delC	54	
R334W	53	
1898+1G→T	53	
711+1G→T	49	French-Canadian
2183AA→G	49	Italian
3905insT	38 (6–17)*	Swiss, Amish, Acadian
S549N	30	
2184delA	29	
Q359K/T360K	(87.5)*	Jewish-Georgian
M1101K	(69)*	Hutterite
Y122X	(48)*	French, Reunion Island
1898+5G→T	(30)*	Chinese, Taiwan
3120+1G→A	(11)*	African-American
I148T	(9.1)	French-Canadian

Numbers based on screening of 43,849 CF chromosomes (not all tested for the indicated mutations). Mutations found in Caucasians, except where indicated. Geographic location (or ethnic group) with highest prevalence indicated for some of the mutations. A rough relative frequency (%)* is given for mutations studied in samples of relatively small size or in indicated populations only.

SOURCE: Data from CF Genetic Analysis Consortium and Zielinski and Tsui.[54]

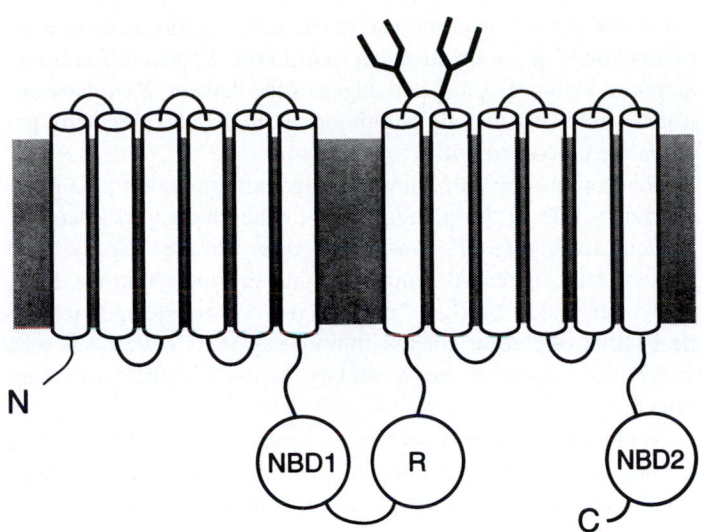

FIGURE 53-1 Domain model of the cystic fibrosis transmembrane conductance regulator (CFTR). Based on hydrophobicity plots, CFTR has 12 transmembrane spanning domains, two nucleotide (N) binding domains (NBD 1 and NBD 2), and a regulatory (R) domain. The 12 transmembrane domains form the ion channel "pore." In the closed state, the "R" domain is believed to obstruct the channel. Channel opening requires binding of two ATPs to the nucleotide binding domains. This model is similar to other ATP-binding cassette transporter proteins that bind ATP and transport ions or micronutrients. *(Modified from Riordan.[39])*

CF (Fig. 53-2). Among other abnormalities of airway epithelium in CF is increased sulfation of respiratory mucins, with decreased sialylation and increased fucosylation of both secreted and membrane glycoproteins.[30] These findings, as well as the propensity for *Pseudomonas* colonization of the airway in CF, are not easily explained by the presence of dehydrated secretions alone.

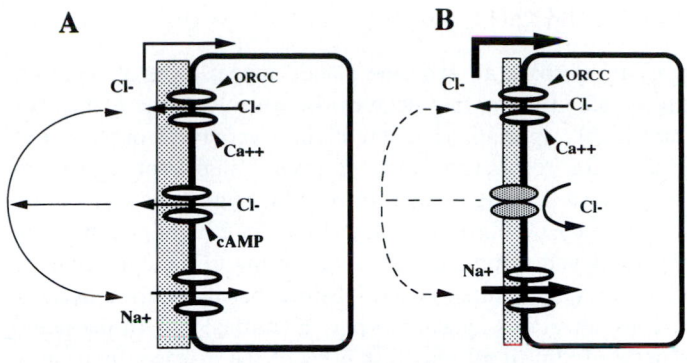

FIGURE 53-2 Simplified model of ion transport in airway epithelium. *A.* Normal airway cell with multiple apical ion channels. At the top, two different chloride channels are represented, the outwardly rectifying chloride channel (ORCC) and the Ca^{++}-gated chloride channel. In the center, cAMP-gated CFTR is shown. The apical sodium channel is depicted at the bottom. Experimental data suggest that CFTR interacts with the other channels, although the type of interaction is not clear (solid arcs). *B.* CF cell with nonfunctioning cAMP-gated apical chloride transport. The function of the other channels is affected in an unknown manner (dashed arcs). The net result of ion channel activity on the pericellular fluid composition (hatched area) is under investigation. Many questions remain concerning the function of CFTR and ion transport in the airway.

CFTR mutations have been grouped into four or five classes, depending on the effect of the mutation on the expression, processing, and function of the protein (Fig. 53-3).[10] The most common mutation, ΔF508, is a processing mutation in which very little of the mutant protein reaches the apical surface. If the mutant protein escapes normal intracellular processing, however, ΔF508 protein functions normally in the apical membrane. Furthermore, only 25 percent of normal CFTR transcripts are properly processed and transported to the cell surface. The remaining 75 percent are degraded before being processed. These data suggest that one therapeutic strategy to overcome the defect in CF is to disrupt normal intracellular processing mechanisms.

Several other functions have been proposed for CFTR, providing potential mechanisms to explain some of the diverse manifestations of CF. CFTR is thought to play a role in regulation of endosomal pH. The defect may be responsible for altered function of glycosyltransferases—which, in turn, causes the altered glycosylation characteristic of the CF phenotype. CFTR has also been shown to transport ATP, perhaps accounting for CFTR's proposed interactions with outwardly rectifying chloride channels and sodium channels. CFTR may also have a major functional role in *intracellular* membranes (e.g., endoplasmic reticulum, endosomes, and clathrin-coated vesicles).[51]

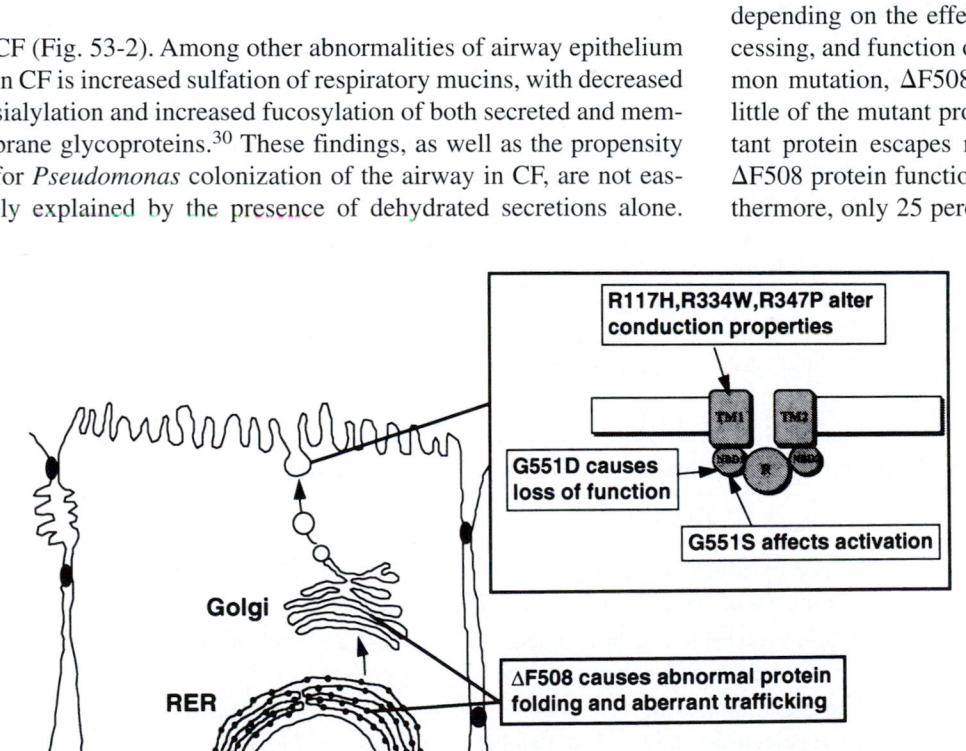

FIGURE 53-3 Types of CFTR mutations. CFTR mutations can affect synthesis of the resultant protein and, thereby, profoundly affect CFTR function. As shown, some mutations (e.g., G542X) produce a truncated transcript and no protein, while other mutations (e.g., R117H) produce proteins that have impaired conduction properties. *(Based on data of Collins, 1992,[8] with permission.)*

PATHOPHYSIOLOGY

In cystic fibrosis, all exocrine glands appear to be affected primarily, albeit to varying degrees. Because exocrine glands perform highly specialized functions in a variety of organs—e.g., in the skin, respiratory tract, gastrointestinal tract, and reproductive system—the number of possible symptoms and complications in cystic fibrosis is large. Table 53-2 highlights the complications and symptoms of CF according to the age groups in which they most often occur. Obstruction of exocrine ducts by viscous secretions appears to play a cardinal role in the pathogenesis of almost all manifestations of the disease. In 10 to 20 percent of patients, the initial manifestation is often *meconium ileus*[13]—i.e., obstruction of the intestine by thick, viscous meconium stool. Chronic pulmonary disease, pancreatic insufficiency, and focal biliary cirrhosis progress gradually throughout the course of the disease, albeit at different rates in different patients. Progressive obstruction of exocrine ducts is a regular feature of the disease except in sweat glands, where obstruction of ducts has not been implicated in pathogenesis.

Respiratory Tract

In the lungs, hypersecretion of viscid mucus and chronic bacterial infection combine to produce a progressive and distinctive type of chronic obstructive airway disease that eventually leads to diffuse, severe bronchiectasis. The earliest pathologic lesions are found in the distal bronchioles, although the highest levels of CFTR expression are in submucosal glands in the large airways. Whether the viscid secretions are primary or are secondary to chronic bacterial infections remains unsettled. In favor of a primary disturbance is the demonstration of hyperplasia of the mucus-secreting cells in the airways of neonates with CF, who have not yet developed any evidence of bacterial infection or chronic colonization of the airways. With the use of sophisticated culture methods, bacterial pathogens can almost invariably be isolated from the respiratory tract of patients with CF. The most common pathogens isolated from sputum cultures are *Staphylococcus aureus* and *Pseudomonas aeruginosa*. Less commonly found are mucoid *Escherichia coli*, *Klebsiella*, and *Hemophilus influenzae*. In later stages of the disease, *Pseudomonas* usually predominates. By adulthood, more than 80 percent of patients are colonized with *P. aeruginosa*.

Neutrophil-dominated lower-airway inflammation also plays a primary role in the pathogenesis of the characteristic central bronchiectasis of CF. Bronchoalveolar lavage (BAL) fluid demonstrates increased neutrophils and various cytokines, especially interleukin 8 (IL-8), even in infants whose BAL is sterile.[2] Other alterations in the immune systems have been seen in CF and appear to be secondary to the chronic pulmonary infections.

Typically, respiratory secretions increase when a patient with CF, already chronically colonized with *Pseudomonas*, develops a viral respiratory tract infection. In turn, the increase in secretions leads to a gradual increase in cough and sputum production and then to an exacerbation of the pulmonary disease, usually manifested by increase in respiratory rate; retraction of the chest during inspiration; and diffuse, coarse inspiratory crackles. Fever and leukocytosis are common. The chest radiograph demonstrates worsening hyperinflation. Both peribronchial thickening and nodular or cystic densities are more marked than usual. Pulmonary function tests show a worsening over baseline. Usually, residual volume (RV) increases; forced vital capacity (FVC) and forced expiratory volume in 1 s (FEV_1) decrease; the forced expiratory flow between 25 and 75 percent of the exhaled vital capacity ($FEF_{25-75\%}$) also decreases. Treatment using antipseudomonal antibiotics and chest physiotherapy generally succeeds in restoring most indices of pulmonary function to, or almost to, baseline. However, *Pseudomonas* persists in sputum cultures.

The most attractive hypothesis to account for the pattern of response to treatment is that therapy reduces the number and, probably, virulence of organisms. Despite the virtual return to baseline after an exacerbation, however, the cumulative effect of repeated episodes is progressive bronchiectasis or atelectasis, or a combination of the two, accompanied by a gradual and irre-

TABLE 53-2

Complications and Presenting Symptoms of Cystic Fibrosis by Age Group

Infancy	Childhood	Adolescence/Adulthood
Meconium ileus	Pulmonary infections with *Staphylococcus* and *Pseudomonas*	Chronic bronchitis
Obstructive jaundice	Malnutrition with steatorrhea and pancreatic insufficiency	Pansinusitis
Edema with hypoproteinemia, anemia, and hypoprothrombinemia	Heat prostration with hypoelectrolytemia and metabolic alkalosis	Hemoptysis
Failure to thrive	"Atypical asthma" with clubbing and/or bronchiectasis	Chronic abdominal pain
Intussusception	Esophageal varices	Delayed sexual development
Volvulus	Hypersplenism	Obstructive aspermia
Rectal prolapse	Nasal polyps	
Recurrent pneumonia/bronchiolitis		

versible decrease in pulmonary function. The striking degree of airway destruction and relative sparing of the pulmonary parenchyma at autopsy are shown in Fig. 53-4. A simplified scheme illustrating the evolution of the process is shown in Fig. 53-5.

Gastrointestinal Tract

Although pancreatic function may be either normal or abnormal at birth, it gradually becomes increasingly abnormal in most CF patients as the pancreatic ducts become progressively obstructed by thick, viscous secretions from the exocrine portion of the organ; pancreatic enzymes that are trapped within the ducts lead to autodestruction of the pancreas. A cycle of destruction and obliteration of the ducts is set into motion, leading to cystic dilatation of ducts proximal to sites of obstruction and fibrosis of the body of the pancreas. In advanced stages of the disease, pancreatic fibrosis sometimes causes obliteration of the islets of Langerhans and, consequently, diabetes mellitus.

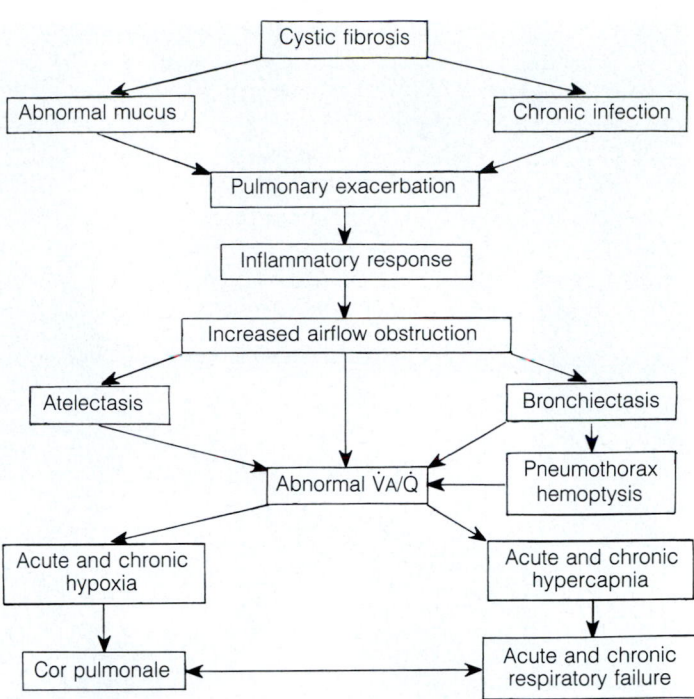

FIGURE 53-5   Simplified scheme for pathogenesis and progression of pulmonary disease in CF.

The liver and biliary tract are also affected in CF. Here too, the primary mechanism appears to be obstruction of ducts by abnormally viscid secretions. The earliest pathologic change is focal biliary cirrhosis that may be present in early infancy. In some patients, focal cirrhosis progresses to diffuse cirrhosis and portal hypertension. Some newborn infants with CF develop the *inspissated bile syndrome,* characterized by prolonged obstructive jaundice starting at 2 to 8 weeks of age. The jaundice often clears without therapy. In approximately 20 to 30 percent of patients, the gallbladder is small, presumably because of underdevelopment due to obstruction by viscid secretions. Compared with age-matched controls, the risk of cholelithiasis and cholecystitis is increased in adults with CF.

The most striking pathologic change in the intestines is hyperplasia of the mucous glands and globlet cells. Biochemical abnormalities in intestinal mucins may contribute to malabsorption of specific nutrients and bile acids. Much of the malabsorption in CF can be corrected by administration of pancreatic enzymes. However, the abnormal mucins may lead to slowing of intestinal transit time; the slowing, combined with maldigestion of food substances, sometimes causes fecal impaction in the terminal ileum and ileocecal area, a condition referred to as *meconium ileus equivalent* or distal intestinal obstruction syndrome. The fecal impaction, in turn, occasionally causes volvulus or intussusception of the bowel (Fig. 53-6).

Reproductive Organs

Except for an increase in viscosity and an abnormal midcycle ferning pattern in cervical mucus, no consistent pathologic changes occur in the female reproductive tract in patients with CF. In the male reproductive tract, however, the vas deferens is

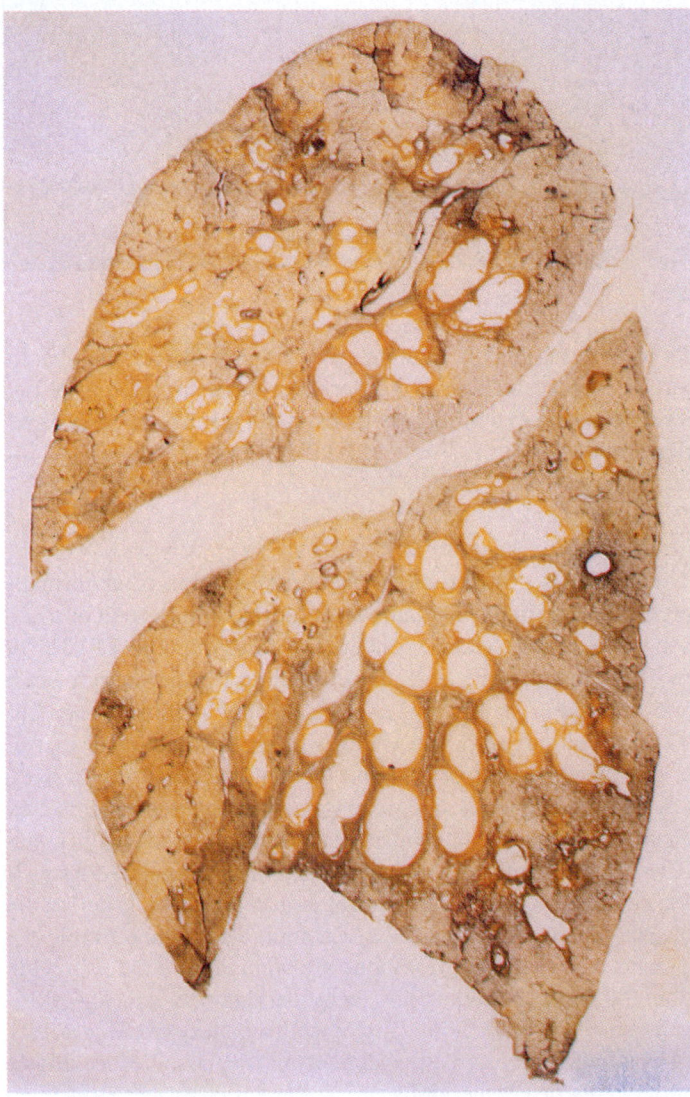

FIGURE 53-4   Section of lung from autopsy of a patient with CF, demonstrating remarkable dilation of large airways and preservation of intervening pulmonary parenchyma. *(Courtesy of Dr. S. Moolten.)*

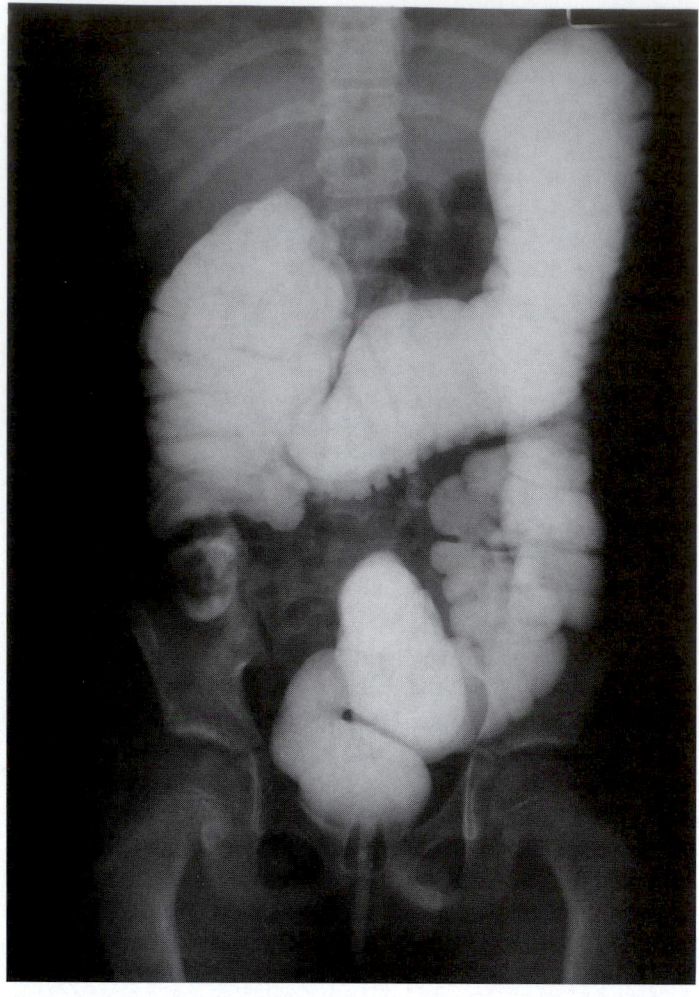

A

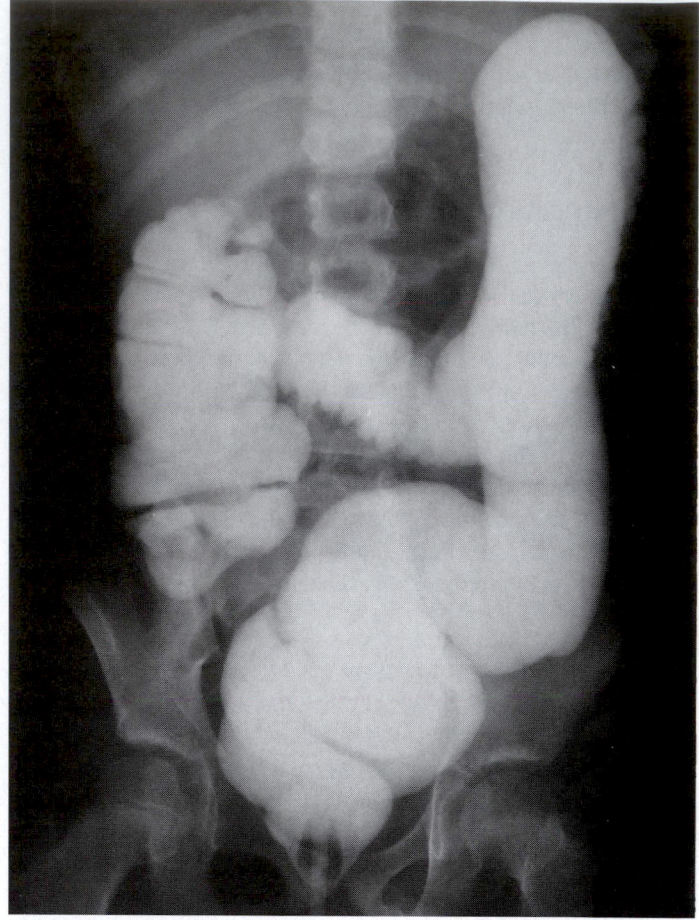

B

FIGURE 53-6   Distal intestinal obstruction syndrome (DIOS). *A*. Presenting Gastrografin enema of a child who had crampy abdominal pain and a right lower-quadrant mass. Fecal impaction with intussception is demonstrated. *B*. Partial resolution of the obstruction following Gastrografin administration. *C*. Complete resolution of the intussception and fecal impaction.

either atretic or absent at birth. Although the pathogenesis of this lesion is not certain, viscous secretions may contribute to obstruction in utero, followed by failure of development of the vas deferens. Spermatogenesis and testicular development are otherwise normal. Because of either partial or complete obstruction of the vas deferens, approximately 98 percent of males with CF are aspermic.

Sweat Glands

The sweat glands of patients with CF manifest no distinctive histologic changes. Nonetheless, their function is abnormal. Micropuncture experiments have shown that the precursor solution secreted by the sweat glands is isotonic to plasma, both in CF patients and in normal subjects. In normal persons, as the sweat flows along the duct of the gland, sodium and chloride are reabsorbed, so that by the time that the opening at the skin surface is reached, sweat is hypotonic to plasma with respect to both sodium and chloride concentrations. The relative impermeabil-

ity to chloride ions is thought to be responsible for the characteristic increase in potential differences across isolated, perfused sweat glands and epithelial cells from the respiratory tract of patients with CF.

DIAGNOSIS

The diagnosis of CF requires the demonstration of abnormally high concentrations of sodium and chloride in the sweat of a person who has the characteristic history and symptoms of CF. The most prominent clinical features are chronic pulmonary disease and pancreatic insufficiency. The most compelling family history for the diagnosis is CF in a sibling. If the clinical picture and/or the family history support the diagnosis, and if two sweat tests using the quantitative pilocarpine iontophoresis method are clearly positive, the diagnosis of CF can be made with assurance. Identification of two pathologic mutations, in addition to the characteristic clinical picture, is accepted as a criterion for the diagnosis. However, CF is a complex syndrome (Table 53-2) whose clinical manifestations are sometimes subtle. In addition, the family history is not always straightforward. Therefore, a high index of suspicion, coupled with a battery of clinical tests, is sometimes required to establish the diagnosis, especially in adolescents or young adults.

Since CF occurs with a high frequency in the general population, the diagnosis should be considered routinely in a broad array of differential diagnoses. Although Table 53-2 categorizes symptoms according to the age at which they occur most often,

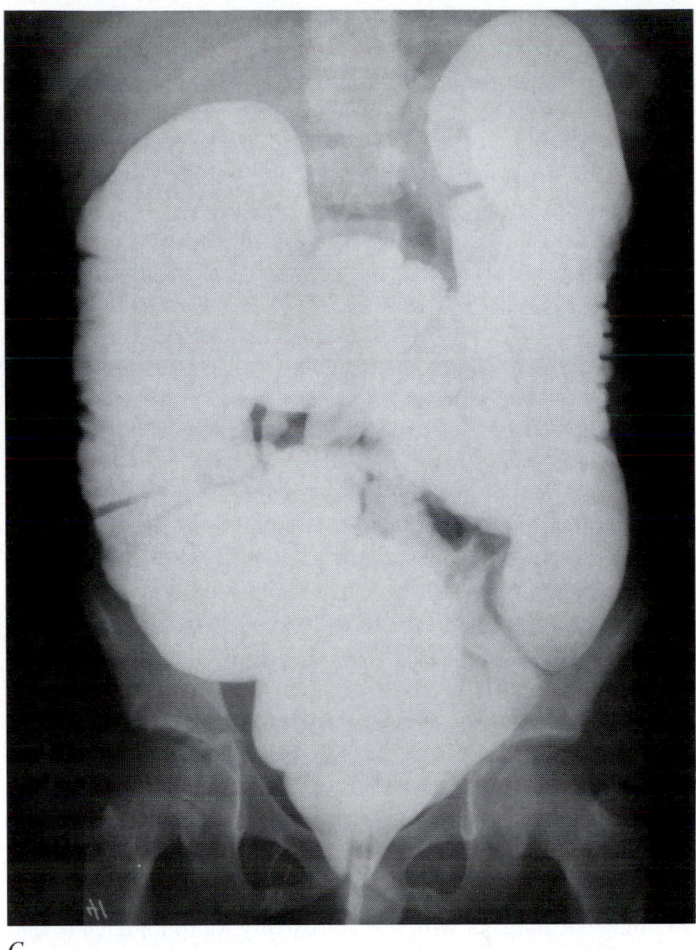

C

FIGURE 53-6   (*Cont.*)

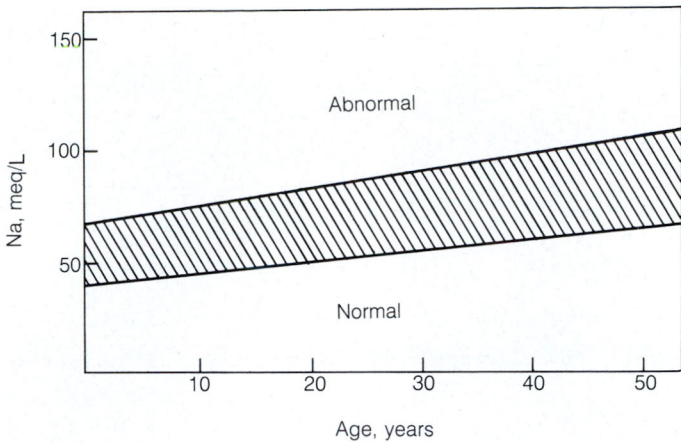

FIGURE 53-7   Graph of sweat test results versus age; normal, elevated, and borderline (stippled).

symptoms at any age should prompt consideration of the diagnosis of CF.

The most consistent feature of CF is an abnormally high concentration of sodium and chloride in sweat. The only reliable sweat test is based on iontophoresis of pilocarpine, followed by quantitative determination of the concentration of either chloride or sodium in an adequate, measured volume of sweat. Seventy-five milligrams of sweat is the minimum acceptable amount. When a preweighed, measured pad is used, this amount ensures that an adequate sweat flow rate (1 g/m^2 per min) has been achieved and that the sample is large enough for the determination of sodium by flame photometry and of chloride by titration. In children, concentrations of sodium and chloride of less than 40 meq/L are usually regarded as normal. However, the average of values for sodium and chloride concentrations are about 20 meq/L for normal subjects and 95 meq/L for those with CF. In children, values between 40 and 60 meq/L are borderline elevated; such values call for repetition of the sweat test until a clear pattern emerges.

The concentration of sodium and chloride in sweat increases gradually with age. An age-corrected scale of normal, abnormal, and borderline values of sodium concentration in sweat is available (Fig. 53-7). Conditions other than CF in which the concentrations of sodium and chloride in sweat are abnormally high include malnutrition, adrenal insufficiency, hereditary nephrogenic diabetes insipidus, ectodermal dysplasia, and fucosidosis. Except in some instances of malnutrition, these conditions are readily distinguished from CF. The finding of abnormal concentrations of sodium and chloride in sweat should automatically prompt evaluation of the patient to determine if, and to what extent, other organs are affected.

Genetic analysis can be used to confirm the diagnosis of CF. In patients with minimal symptoms, the diagnosis of CF can be made with certainty if two CF-associated alleles are present. As mentioned previously, screening for 32 of the most common alleles yields an overall sensitivity of 90 percent due to undetected alleles. Therefore, a negative mutation analysis does not rule out a diagnosis of CF, and atypical patients should be followed carefully.

CLINICAL EVALUATION

The evaluation of patients with CF includes chest radiography, tests of pulmonary performance, sputum culture, and assessment of pancreatic, hepatic, and reproductive functions. Each is described below.

Chest Radiography

Rarely is the chest radiograph completely normal in CF. In the person with minor pulmonary symptoms, the manifestations may be questionable (e.g., mild hyperinflation and minimal peribronchial thickening). However, the radiographic findings become more distinctly abnormal as the disease increases in severity. Peribronchial thickening, which is often most prominent in the upper lobes of the lungs early in the course of the disease, usually progresses to affect all lobes. In the advanced stage of pulmonary involvement, ring shadows, cystic lesions, and nodular densities are increasingly apparent, as are areas of bronchiectasis and atelectasis. The central pulmonary artery often enlarges in the middle stages of the disease, but the cardiac silhouette remains within normal limits until the disease is far advanced. The variability in the chest radiograph is illustrated in Fig. 53-8 for three siblings with cystic fibrosis when each was 17 years old.

High-resolution CT scans are more sensitive than plain radiographs. The most common abnormalities described are "ground glass opacities." Early bronchiectasis is easily detected on the

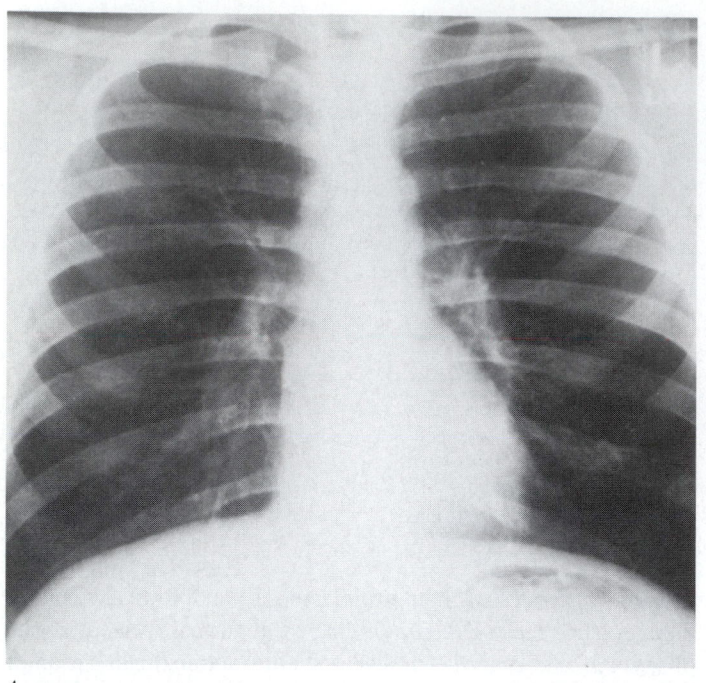

A

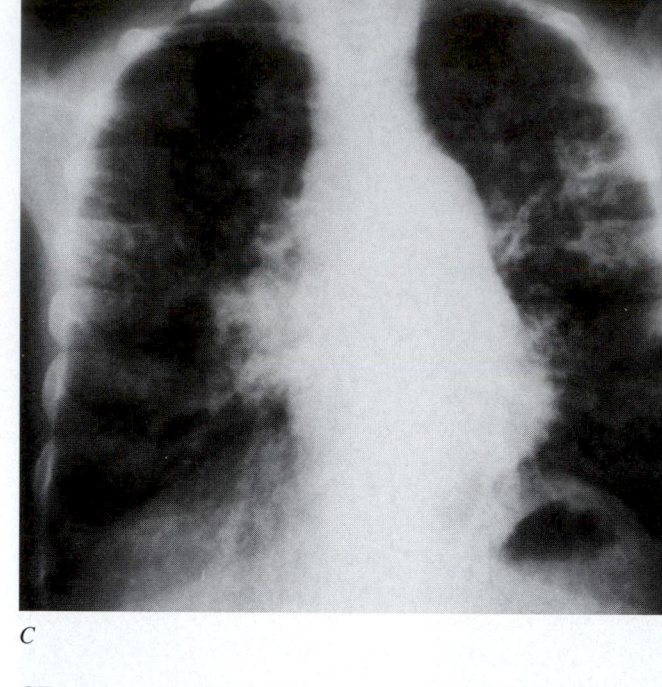

C

CT scan, even when routine chest radiographs are normal, as seen in Fig. 53-9.

Pulmonary Performance

The lungs of patients with CF are usually morphologically and functionally normal at birth. Over time, accumulation of tracheobronchial secretions and recurrent infections progressively impair pulmonary function in almost all patients.[19] In the fully developed clinical syndrome, all the pulmonary function abnormalities seen in chronic bronchitis, emphysema, and asthma may occur. However, one complicating regular feature of cystic fibrosis—bronchiectasis—modifies pulmonary performance. Chronic, local infection and airway damage increase the com-

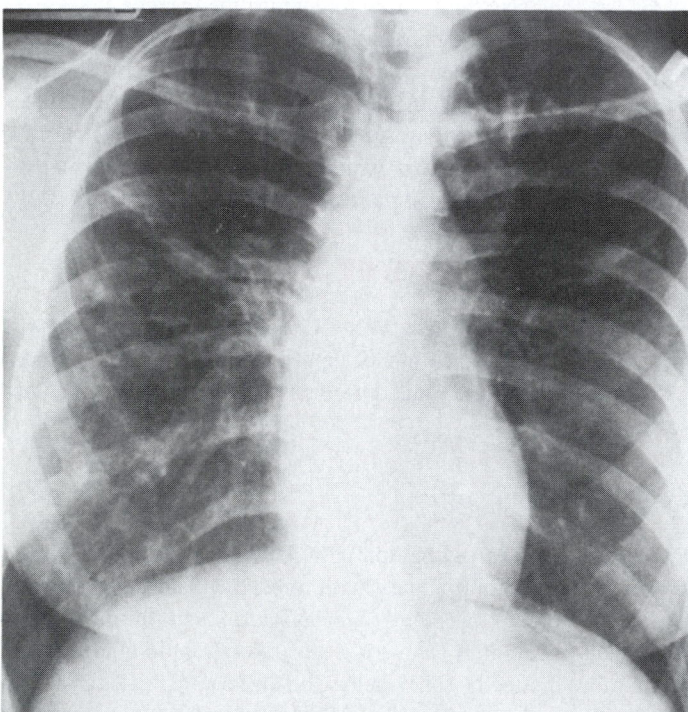

B

FIGURE 53-8　Chest radiographs of three siblings with CF taken when the patients were 17 years of age. *A.* Mild hyperinflation; otherwise normal. Patient is now 32 years old and has been hospitalized once for treatment of electrolyte depletion. *B.* Diffuse peribronchial thickening, mild hyperinflation, and cystic changes in both upper lobes. The patient was hospitalized seven times for pulmonary exacerbations, once for diabetes, and once for hemoptysis. She died at age 34 following complications from lung transplantation. *C.* Severe hyperinflation, diffuse peribronchial thickening, multiple infiltrates, and increased pulmonary vascular markings and heart size. The patient died 1 month later from respiratory failure complicated by congestive heart failure.

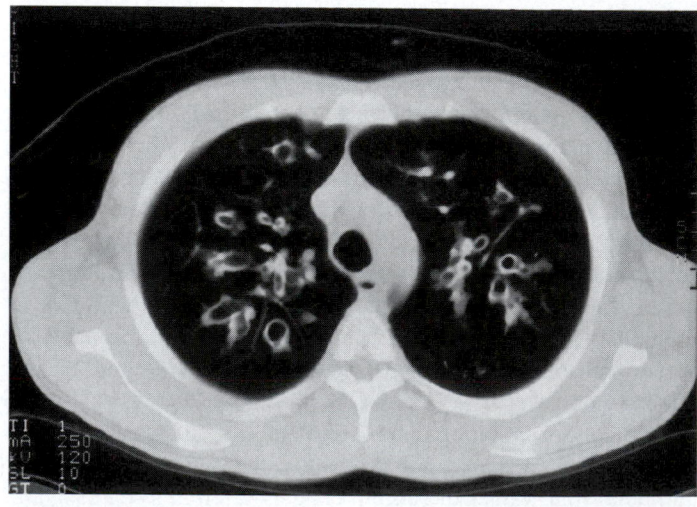

FIGURE 53-9　High-resolution chest CT scan from a patient with CF. Marked bronchiectasis with peribronchial thickening is shown in the upper lobes.

pliance of bronchiectatic airways, resulting in airway collapse during rapid expirations or cough.

The usefulness of pulmonary function testing in CF is twofold: tracing the natural history of the disease and assessing the value of therapeutic interventions.

The earliest stages of the pulmonary disorder are the most difficult to quantify. In infants, tests are limited almost entirely to those that do not depend on the patient's understanding and cooperation. A variety of methods to measure infant pulmonary function have been devised, although none are readily adaptable to routine clinical use.[45]

In some infants, despite clinically and radiographically normal lungs, both residual volume and airway resistance are abnormally high and dynamic compliance is low. An intercurrent pulmonary infection accentuates test abnormalities; subsidence of the infection correlates with restoration of test results toward normal. Because of the uncertainties associated with pulmonary function testing in infancy, variations in time and severity of onset of the disease, and variable effect of recurrent pulmonary infections, the early stages of evolution of pulmonary abnormalities in CF are poorly documented.

Until age 6 years, determination of arterial blood gases can be used as a measure of overall pulmonary function, both in the stable state and during an intercurrent infection. This test is neither easy to perform nor simple to interpret in the early years of life, however, because of the ventilatory and metabolic changes that often accompany anxiety and crying. Noninvasive measurement of oxygen saturation is a valuable and widely used test to assess the severity of pulmonary abnormalities during acute exacerbations.

After age 6 years, pulmonary function tests originally designed for adults may be performed quite readily on children. Changes in pulmonary performance throughout the natural history of CF can be described with confidence.

OBSTRUCTION IN SMALL AIRWAYS

The small airways—i.e., the bronchioles—are vulnerable to obstruction early in the course of CF. At this stage, as in cigarette smokers, results of tests for small-airway disease are apt to be abnormal, while those of tests for obstruction of large airways are still normal. Three factors interact in causing the obstruction: (1) intrinsic disease of the smaller airways, often in association with bronchiectasis in the proximal, larger airways; (2) viscid secretions, impaired ciliary action, and impaired cough; and (3) progressive decrease in lung elastic recoil.

The progressive reduction in lung elastic recoil in CF is predominantly a function of overinflation due to intrinsic airway disease, rather than loss of pulmonary parenchyma. This mechanism differs from that in chronic bronchitis and emphysema, in which the combined effects of parenchymal destruction and overinflation are responsible for the decrease in elastic recoil. Emphysema is not a regular feature of cystic fibrosis. In some patients, emphysema occurs only late in the course of the disease (Fig. 53-4).

Airway smooth-muscle tone increases only slightly in CF. Exercise elicits bronchodilation, followed shortly thereafter by bronchoconstriction. Both the bronchodilation and bronchoconstriction are far less impressive in CF than in asthma. Indeed,

exaggerated bronchomotor responses in CF raise the possibility of superimosed asthma. In distinguishing between contributions to airway obstruction by intrinsic airway disease caused by CF and asthma, maximal expiratory flow-volume curves are sometimes helpful. In severe CF, the tracing is curvilinear because of high flow at the start of expiration, followed by an abrupt decrease in flow—a pattern consistent with early emptying of "fast" lung compartments followed by emptying of slower compartments (see Chapter 36). In asthma, peak expiratory flows are reduced, and the fall-off with time is relatively linear.

A useful test for detecting small-airway disease is the relative decrease in V_{max} when an inspired mixture of helium (80%) and oxygen (20%) is substituted for air (see Chapter 36).[17] An abnormal density dependence of V_{max} signifies small-airway obstruction. Another manifestation of obstruction of small airways is the superimposition of the two curves at larger lung volumes than in normal persons. Because of the bronchiolar locus of the early lesions in cystic fibrosis, abnormalities in breathing frequency–dependent tests (e.g., dynamic lung compliance), in volume-dependent tests (e.g., closing volume), and in maximal expiratory flow ($V_{E_{max}}$) at low lung volumes are demonstrable, even though results of tests of large airway function (e.g., FEV_1 and airway resistance) are still normal.

CHANGE IN LUNG VOLUMES

As with chronic bronchitis, emphysema, and asthma, residual volume in CF increases. Thereafter, an increase in functional residual capacity and, sometimes, in total lung capacity is seen.

ABNORMALITIES IN GAS EXCHANGE

Early in the evolution of the pulmonary abnormalities in CF—i.e., when tests of small-airway function alone are abnormal—ventilation-perfusion abnormalities usually result in widening of the alveolar-arterial oxygen gradient and an increase in the ratio of dead space to tidal volume (V_D/V_T). These abnormalities portend increasing inhomgeneities in alveolar ventilation and blood flow as the affected child grows to adulthood. The diffusing capacity for carbon monoxide ($D_{L_{CO}}$) is low at rest and does not increase normally during exercise. This observation is difficult to reconcile with the preservation of the gas-exchanging surface of the lungs (in the absence of emphysema) until late in the course of the disease (Fig. 54-3).

As obstructive disease of the airways progresses and exaggerates the imbalances between alveolar ventilation and blood flow, arterial hypoxemia develops; pulmonary hypertension, cor pulmonale, and right ventricular failure follow, in turn. Late in the course of the disease, hypercapnia and respiratory acidosis contribute to the final picture of respiratory failure. At this juncture, the ventilatory response to inhaled CO_2 is depressed. Evidence of acute CO_2 retention supervenes, and respiratory depression caused by administration of supplemental oxygen or sedatives may bring the patient closer to the brink of respiratory depression and coma. Bouts of infection punctuate the course of the illness; during each episode, pulmonary function deteriorates, but it usually returns toward baseline, except in the preterminal stages of the disorder.

Sputum Culture

The unique respiratory flora isolated from sputum cultures from patients with CF are helpful in establishing the diagnosis and in guiding the antimicrobial therapy for acute exacerbations. In many patients with CF, *P. aeruginosa* and *S. aureus* are found alone, or in combination, in the sputum. Once present, the organisms, especially *Pseudomonas,* are rarely eradicated, despite use of intermittent or continuous antibiotics administered intravenously, orally, or by nebulization. Although these organisms are sometimes found in sputum cultures from patients with pulmonary diseases other than CF, their association with the disorder is so consistent that a dedicated attempt to obtain a sputum culture is an integral part of the evaluation of all patients, including infants and young children, suspected of having CF. Conversely, isolation of *S. aureus* or *P. aeruginosa* in sputum in a child or young adult should raise the suspicion of CF.

Pancreatic Function

The evaluation of pancreatic function is an important part of establishing the diagnosis of CF, since almost 90 percent of patients have pancreatic insufficiency. In infants with pancreatic insufficiency due to CF, the most striking feature of the history and physical examination is often failure to thrive; the record of bowel movements may disclose only loose or frequent stools. In the older child, whose diet includes more fat and protein, a history of bulky, foul, malodorous stools is often easier to elicit. Documentation of malabsorption is best accomplished by collection of stools for 72 h while the patient is ingesting a known quantity of fat (approximately 100 g per day) and measurement of the stool fat content. A malabsorption coefficient of greater than 7 percent is usually considered abnormal; in patients with CF, the malabsorption coefficient often is around 20 to 30 percent.

In infants and young children, the determination of trypsin or chymotrypsin activity in a properly collected stool specimen is an accurate way to determine the content of pancreatic enzymes. In older patients, however, trypsin or chymotrypsin activity in a stool sample may be artificially low because of a delayed transit time that causes partial inactivation of the enzyme. In some instances, a secretin stimulation test may be helpful in demonstrating pancreatic insufficiency. For this purpose, a triple-lumen tube is introduced into the duodenum. The response to secretin is usually abnormal: the volume of secretion is small, the fluid is viscid, and the bicarbonate ion concentration is low. This test is not often used in children because it is cumbersome to perform.

For infants, the serum immunoreactive assay for trypsin is used in some centers as a screening test for pancreatic insufficiency. As a rule, serum levels of trypsin are abnormally high in CF, usually reflecting ongoing destruction of the pancreas. However, the assay does not provide an accurate measure of pancreatic function. Another approach is based on measurements of metabolic products of compounds that are ingested orally and hydrolyzed by pancreatic enzymes. For example, the hydrolysis of *N*-benzyl-L-tyrosil-*p*-aminobenzoic acid is quantified by determining the amount of aminobenzoic acid present in serum or excreted in the urine. This test is a useful test for assessment of pancreatic function in CF.

Endocrine function of the pancreas is usually preserved in children, but approximately 50 percent of all adult patients are overtly diabetic by age 30 years.

Liver Function

Evaluation of liver function is an important part of the evaluation of CF. In infants and children, the concentrations of bilirubin and transaminases in serum sometimes increase transiently. However, concentrations of these substances are usually normal, even in patients with mild or moderate focal biliary cirrhosis. The prothrombin time is sometimes prolonged, owing to a combination of malabsorption and decreased synthesis of clotting factors by the liver. Occasionally, patients present with bleeding esophageal varices from advanced cirrhosis; endoscopy and upper gastrointestinal contrast studies are often helpful in demonstrating the varices.

Semen Analysis

Occasionally, a man who is found to have aspermia during the course of an evaluation for infertility is found to have CF. In men with CF, a complete semen analysis is part of the evaluation. Azoospermia is found in more than 97 percent of men with the disorder.

Mutation Analysis

Numerous attempts have been made, with limited success, to characterize phenotype on the basis of genotype. In general, homozygotes for ΔF508 have pancreatic insufficiency; patients with CF who have pancreatic insufficiency tend to have a worse prognosis. Several mutations, including R117H, are associated with pancreatic sufficiency and a mild phenotype.[21] However, a direct association of a particular genotype with progression of the pulmonary disease has not been found.

An interesting genotype-phenotype correlation is the increased frequency of genotype R117H in males with congenital bilateral absence of the vas deferens (CBAVD).[1] Males affected with this recessive disorder lack a vas deferens, but they are otherwise completely healthy and have normal sweat test results. Approximately 35 percent of chromosomes of patients with CBAVD carry a CF-associated mutation. To complicate this phenotype-genotype correlation further, 8 percent of patients with CBAVD without clinical CF have two CF-associated mutations. Genetic testing is not required to establish or confirm the diagnosis of CF when a compatible history and physical examination and abnormal sweat test results are found. Genetic testing is useful in identifying patients who have a compatible history and physical examination but whose sweat test results are negative. Certain alleles associated with CF (e.g., 3849 + 10kbC → T) are associated with nasal polyposis and bronchiectasis but normal sweat test results. The diagnosis of CF can be made with confidence in these patients. More problematic are persons with atypical presentations, normal sweat test results, and at least one CF-associated mutation. Since complete screening for the second allele is impractical, these patients' diseases remain undiagnosed; however, they should be followed carefully. Mutation analysis may become clinically relevant in all patients with CF if specific therapies depend on the types of mutations present (see "Genetics" and "Future Directions").

ATYPICAL CLINICAL PRESENTATIONS

Atypical clinical presentations confound the diagnosis of CF in adults; a high index of suspicion is required to establish the diagnosis. Approximately 6 percent of all CF is diagnosed after age 18 years. Late presentations of CF tend to occur in persons with pancreatic sufficiency; indeed, overweight or well-nourished persons may have CF.

Recovery of unusual gram-negative organisms, mucoid *Pseudomonas* species, or *S. aureus* from sputum of asthmatics with persistent sputum production, chest radiographic abnormalities, or clubbing should prompt referral for sweat testing.

Recurrent sinusitis and nasal polyposis may be the only manifestations of CF in a mildly affected person. Isolation of *P. aeruginosa* from deep nasal cultures should raise the suspicion of CF. Frequently, the sinus findings on computed tomography mimic fungal sinusitis, demonstrating concentric, inhomogeneous material.[11] Occasionally, persistent inflammation produces bony destruction that is mistaken for previous surgical intervention.

Sweat testing and referral to a CF center should be considered for men with azoospermia or CBAVD.

TREATMENT

Intensive, comprehensive CF treatment programs designed to deal with particular symptoms, correct deficiencies, and prevent progression and complications of the disease have led to a dramatic increase in the median age of survival (Fig. 53-10). Although the value of comprehensive treatment is beyond question, far less certain are the utility of each component of the treatment plan and the level of each component necessary in a given patient. At present, the best approach still appears to be determination of the type and degree of abnormality in individual patients and design of a treatment program that will improve or maintain function of the organ systems affected.

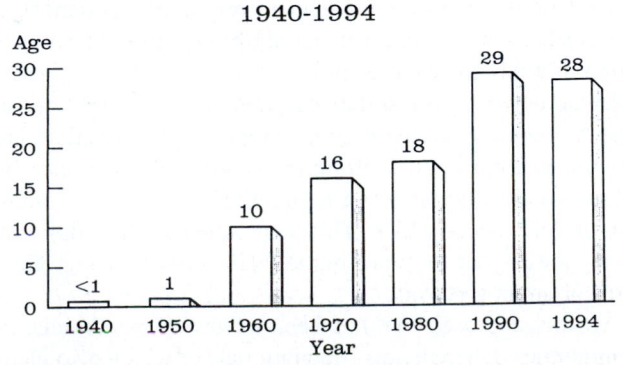

MEDIAN SURVIVAL AGE
IN PATIENTS WITH CYSTIC FIBROSIS

FIGURE 53-10   Median survival in patients with CF. (*Data from the Cystic Fibrosis Foundation Data Registry, 1994, with permission.*)

To ensure that the treatment regimen meets the needs of the individual patient, that necessary treatment is not omitted, or that side effects of prescribed treatments do not go unnoticed, it is often desirable to hospitalize the patient for diagnosis and evaluation. Hospitalization also provides an excellent opportunity for counseling the patient, parents, and family about the diverse aspects of the diagnosis, treatment, prognosis, and inheritance pattern of CF. Hospitalization provides the opportunity to monitor the response of individual patients to each component of the therapeutic program.

An important aspect of the care of patients with CF is the network of more than 100 CF centers that exist throughout the United States and the larger network throughout the world. Most larger centers use a team approach to the care of patients. A CF care team usually includes physicians, nurses, respiratory therapists, physical therapists, nutritionists, social workers, and genetic counselors.

Management of the Pulmonary Disease

More than 90 percent of the patients with CF die from respiratory failure or pulmonary complications. The goals of treating the pulmonary disorder in CF are to prevent and treat the complications of airway obstruction and infection. Although management of the pulmonary disorder consists of many components applied in combination, the individual components of therapy are discussed separately below.[37]

CHEST PHYSIOTHERAPY

Almost all treatment programs for CF include a strategy intended to clear pulmonary secretions in order to prevent complications arising from airway plugging by viscous secretions. Chest physiotherapy—i.e., "percussion and postural drainage"—performed regularly, is the most widely prescribed method. In infants and young children, chest physiotherapy is generally performed routinely, twice daily. In older patients, manual chest physiotherapy is often replaced by use of vibrators and mechanical percussors, or a combination of exercise and forced expirations or forced coughing maneuvers. Although the latter approaches are widely held to constitute a reasonable program for improving clearance of secretions and maintaining pulmonary function, objective proof is not available. However, in patients with moderate pulmonary disease who do not receive chest physiotherapy for a period of 3 weeks, pulmonary function deteriorates; in these patients, reinstitution of percussion and postural drainage for a 3-week period restores pulmonary function to baseline levels.[14] At present, most CF centers recommend that all patients with CF attempt to maintain clearance of pulmonary secretions with a method that is applied regularly (e.g., twice daily). An additional recommendation is that chest physiotherapy be applied more often during an exacerbation of the chronic pulmonary infection. Unfortunately, the recommendation of chest physiotherapy on a regular basis—a time-consuming and often arduous form of treatment—is difficult to implement without considerable support and encouragement from family and health professionals.

Several new methods for clearance of pulmonary secretions in CF have been developed. The first of these is autogenic drainage, which has been widely used in Europe and is currently being introduced in the United States. Proper performance usually requires at least 4 h of personal instruction by a physical therapist specifically trained to teach this technique. Another method uses the Flutter, a small pipelike device that produces an oscillating resistance during a forced expiratory maneuver. It has been reported to be effective in allowing patients to expectorate large quantities of sputum. One important limitation of these alternative airway clearance techniques is that patients must have an FEV_1 greater than 30 percent of predicted in order to have sufficient expiratory time to operate the devices.

Several inflatable vests that provide high-frequency chest compression have also been developed. However, the one most rigorously tested is a large and expensive machine and has had limited usage. One advantage to vest therapy is that it can be used on patients with limited airflow, but none of these techniques have been demonstrated to maintain and improve pulmonary function in a rigorous crossover trial—as has been done for chest physiotherapy, which remains the standard technique.[50]

ANTIBIOTICS

During the past few decades of treatment of CF, antibiotics have proved to be the key element responsible for increased survival. However, antibiotic regimens are not standardized. At one end of the spectrum are centers that treat all patients with antistaphylococcal antibiotics, uninterruptedly, from the time of diagnosis; during an exacerbation, additional antibiotics are administered orally or intravenously. At the other end of the spectrum are centers that reserve the use of antibiotics solely for severe exacerbations of pulmonary infection because of concern over promoting emergence of new and more resistant strains of *Pseudomonas*.

A reasonable compromise between the aforementioned approaches balances the dangers of overzealous administration of antibiotics against progressive airway damage and bronchiectasis resulting from untreated infection. The approach is based on sputum culture at the time of diagnosis and at regular intervals thereafter. When signs and symptoms herald worsening of the pulmonary infection (i.e., increased cough or sputum production) or new abnormalities on the physical examination, the chest radiograph, or pulmonary function tests, use of percussion and postural drainage is increased and appropriate antibiotics are given orally.

Currently useful agents for treating staphylococcal infections include dicloxacillin, cephalexin, the newer cephalosporins, clavulinic acid combinations, and chloramphenicol. Early in the course of the pulmonary disease, a small fraction of *Pseudomonas* strains may be sensitive to tetracycline, trimethoprim-sulfamethoxazole, or chloramphenicol. Occasionally, even *Pseudomonas* strains considered resistant according to laboratory sensitivity tests apparently respond to these antibiotics. A mechanism that has been proposed to account for this phenomenon is that even though the antibiotic is not bactericidal, it may inhibit either growth of the organism or its production of exotoxin and proteases. Ciprofloxacin, a quinolone derivative that can be given orally, is initially effective against many strains of

Pseudomonas and has gained widespread use in the outpatient management of CF. A major disadvantage in its use is that resistance often develops after a few courses of treatment.

For treatment of a pulmonary exacerbation of CF caused by *Pseudomonas,* a combination of an aminoglycoside given intravenously and a semisynthetic penicillin is generally used. This combination is presumed to act synergistically on *Pseudomonas,* and the *Pseudomonas* is less likely to become resistant to either antibiotic.

The most popular antibiotic combination currently in use is tobramycin and ticarcillin. In order to achieve high levels of antibiotics in the airways and in secretions, the aminoglycoside is generally administered in higher doses and more often than usual. For example, tobramycin, 10 mg/kg per day in four divided doses, is given instead of 7.5 mg/kg per day in three divided doses. The resulting concentrations in serum are monitored. Instead of the usual therapeutic serum levels for gentamicin and tobramycin of 4 to 8 μg/ml, the goal in treating patients with CF is a serum level of 8 to 10 μg/ml; some centers advocate even higher levels. Serum antibiotic concentrations, renal function, and hearing acuity are monitored to avoid toxic reactions. The higher serum levels of 8 to 10 μg/ml do not seem to elicit greater toxicity than the usual levels. No advantage has been demonstrated for further increments in dosage.

Some of the newer antibiotics—e.g., piperacillin, azlocillin, and ceftazidime—are also quite effective against *Pseudomonas*. Although they may be effective at first when given alone, resistance often develops quickly. Usually, these agents are used in combination with an aminoglycoside. Because the sensitivity and resistance patterns of the *Pseudomonas* often change, various combinations are tried at different times, with clinicians relying on sensitivities from recent isolates to determine which is most effective for the particular strain of *Pseudomonas*.

Pseudomonas, once found in the sputum, is rarely eradicated. However, most other manifestations of an exacerbation of pulmonary disease abate during a 2-week course of antibiotics administered intravenously; i.e., the densities seen on the chest radiograph decrease, the white blood cell count decreases, fever and respiratory rate decrease, and pulmonary function test results, which often deteriorate at the start of an exacerbation, return to their previous baseline. Although many patients begin to show improvement after 5 to 7 days, most CF centers continue antibiotics intravenously for at least 2 weeks in order to decrease the relapse rate and to avoid a decrease in the interval between exacerbations. Indeed, some centers routinely recommend a 3- to 4-week course of intravenous antibiotics to treat an exacerbation of a pulmonary infection.

In the occasional hospitalized patient who experiences a relapse or manifests an increase in symptoms shortly after administration of intravenous antibiotics is stopped, long-term intravenous administration of an aminoglycoside can be continued with use of a heparin lock. This technique may be helpful in allowing the patient to return home while still receiving effective doses of aminoglycosides.

Another approach that has been advocated is administration of antibiotics by inhalation—the rationale of which is to increase antibiotic concentrations in airways infected by *Pseudomonas*.

Although it has been argued that inhalation will not deliver effective concentrations to diseased portions of the lungs because of interference with ventilation by local airway obstruction, inhaled antibiotics appear to be helpful in some instances. Gentamicin or tobramycin, 20 to 40 mg/ml given in 1 to 2 ml of inhaled solution two or three times per day, is often used. As a rule, inhalation of antibiotics is reserved for patients who have been hospitalized repeatedly for exacerbations of pulmonary symptoms that recur at increasing frequency and after shorter intervals between exacerbations. Often, if inhalation therapy is started after completion of a course of intravenous antibiotics, the interval before the next exacerbation is prolonged.

It should be emphasized that all the aforementioned practices are based more on the individual experiences of different cystic fibrosis centers than on controlled clinical trials. In one study, a 600-mg dose of inhaled, preservative-free tobramycin was given three times daily for 28 days to a group of 71 stable patients with CF who had mild to moderate pulmonary function abnormalities at baseline. A modest but statistically significant improvement in FEV_1 of 9.7 percent was noted in the treatment group; virtually no side effects were noted, and serum levels were undetectable.[37] However, questions regarding selection of patients, timing and duration of treatment, and advisability of using this mode of therapy during an acute exacerbation when ventilatory abnormalities are increased remain unanswered.

MIST AND MUCOLYTICS

Mist therapy, delivered by having the patient sleep in a mist tent or through intermittent inhalation of an aerosol, was a common form of treatment of CF several decades ago. The goal was to "liquefy" respiratory secretions. However, the treatment could not be demonstrated to be helpful, and the use of mist tents has largely been discontinued. Intermittent aerosols are still used to deliver bronchodilators and mucolytics.

A number of mucolytic agents have been tried over the years. One that has endured is *N*-acetylcysteine. In the test tube, this agent is quite effective in dissolving mucin components and in decreasing the viscosity of sputum from patients with cystic fibrosis. Although some centers have found this agent to be a useful adjunct to therapy in CF, others have encountered an inordinate frequency of complicating bronchospasm or tracheitis. Some difficulties noted in the past can now be attributed to the use of a 20 percent (undiluted) solution of *N*-acetylcysteine, which can be irritating because of its extremely high osmolarity. The incidence of side effects may be decreased greatly by use of a 5 percent solution; during an exacerbation, when cough and sputum production increase, the 5 percent solution is inhaled two or three times per day, before chest physiotherapy. Should the patient develop bronchospasm, demonstrated by physical examination or by pulmonary function testing, a bronchodilator is used. If successful, the bronchodilator and the *N*-acetylcysteine are administered jointly by inhalation. However, should the bronchospasm persist despite use of the bronchodilator, *N*-acetylcysteine is not administered.

In 1994, Pulmozyme, a DNA-cleaving enzyme, was approved for use in patients with CF following a large phase III multicenter trial.[18] More than 900 patients were enrolled for a 6-month period. Three dosing regimens were employed: placebo, 2.5 mg inhaled once daily, and 2.5 mg inhaled twice daily. The treatment groups showed a 5 percent improvement in FEV_1 over placebo, as well as a slightly lower relative risk of exacerbation of lower respiratory tract infection after 6 months. There was no difference between the once- and twice-daily treatment groups. Currently, this drug is in fairly widespread use for CF. However, questions regarding patient selection and timing and duration of use of this expensive drug remain unanswered. Studies to determine the safety and efficacy in patients under 6 years of age are in progress.

The use of inhaled amiloride to change electrolyte concentrations in the sputum of patients with CF has been studied; very modest benefits have been documented. Use of this agent in combination with uridine 5'-triphosphate has been proposed as potentially more efficacious. Other inhalational agents that are under development as potentially useful are a compound that, in vitro, reduces viscosity of CF sputum by interfering with actin binding of mucins and protease inhibitors, such as serum leukocyte protease inhibitor.

BRONCHODILATORS AND ANTI-INFLAMMATORY AGENTS

Bronchodilators are often used in treating the pulmonary manifestations of CF. Their use should be individualized. For example, in many patients, bronchospasm that is reversible with bronchodilators at one point in the course of the illness may prove refractory a short time later. Some patients undergo deterioration in pulmonary function following use of bronchodilators. In infants who are audibly wheezing, a bronchodilator can be tried. In older patients, pulmonary function testing provides a more objective and quantitative measure of bronchodilator effectiveness.

Corticosteroids have been used with good results in infants with severe obstructive airway disease that does not respond to antibiotics and bronchodilators and in patients with CF in whom the pulmonary disease is complicated by severe asthma or allergic bronchopulmonary aspergillosis. Preliminary observations initially suggested that patients with CF would benefit from long-term administration of alternate-day corticosteroids,[3] based on the presumption that corticosteroids would decrease the airway inflammatory response. However, in a large, placebo-controlled, multicenter trial of alternate-day corticosteroids administered in two dosage regimens (1 mg/kg and 2 mg/kg), the development of many side effects precluded a general recommendation for long-term corticosteroid treatment in CF. Subgroup analysis led to the suggestion that patients with moderately severe obstructive airway disease and those with chronic *Pseudomonas* infection might benefit from treatment for periods of less than 1 year.[42] Beneficial effects were sufficient to prompt further studies of anti-inflammatory agents in CF. A controlled 4-year trial of high doses of ibuprofen in 40 patients with CF showed improvement in the rate of decline of pulmonary function in children.[24] Questions remain whether side effects that might accrue with continued therapy will justify the gains. In concert, these two studies suggest that future development of a lung-specific anti-inflammatory agent with fewer systemic side effects may offer a promising approach.

Nutritional Support

Patients with CF require careful evaluation to determine if partial or complete pancreatic insufficiency is present and to design a nutritional program to correct any deficiencies. The mainstay in managing the pancreatic insufficiency of CF is use of pancreatic enzyme preparations currently available in the form of enteric-coated capsules containing coated microspheres. These pancreatic enzymes are ingested along with any food that contains protein, fat, or complex carbohydrates. The dosage is adjusted to ensure a relatively normal pattern of bowel movements, adequate weight gain or maintenance of ideal weight for height, and a decrease in bowel symptoms, such as cramping and flatulence.

The development of colonic strictures was first noted following the introduction of pancreatic enzymes with lipase contents of 25,000 units per capsule. Capsules with more than 20,000 units are no longer available. Subsequent recommendations urge caution in prescribing high total doses of lipase with any preparation. Recommendations are for use of not more than 2500 units/kg per meal. Since strictures have apparently developed in several patients using doses as low as 6000 units/kg per meal, it has been recommended that for patients who require higher doses to maintain nutritional status or to control bowel symptoms, the enzyme requirement be documented by measuring the coefficient of fat absorption and other causes pursued to account for symptoms.

As a rule, patients with CF are advised to consume a double dose of a multivitamin preparation and a vitamin E supplement each day. Infants, those in whom the prothrombin time is prolonged, and those who take antibiotics uninterruptedly require supplemental vitamin K. Vitamin A supplementation is required in children with significant fat malabsorption and failure to thrive; however, care must be taken to avoid hypervitaminosis A. Supplemental salt is needed by patients in order to prevent electrolyte depletion, metabolic alkalosis, and heat prostration. For infants, 1 to 2 g of salt per day is added to the feeding formula; children and adults are encouraged to salt their foods liberally and to take salt-containing liquids and snacks during hot weather.

Although it is true that pulmonary function is the predominant factor in determining morbidity and mortality in CF, it is becoming increasingly clear that overall patient status is closely tied to nutritional status. Data from the national CF Registry indicate that 40 percent of patients with CF are below the fifth percentile of weight for age and that mortality is increased in this group.

Despite use of pancreatic enzyme replacement, the correction of pancreatic insufficiency is incomplete; accordingly, patients require more than 100 percent of recommended caloric intake. In some, an even greater caloric intake is necessary because of increased energy expenditure due to increased work of breathing secondary to chronic pulmonary infection. Aggressive nutritional supplementation, using either oral supplements or nocturnal nasogastric feeding of hydrolyzed formulas, has been helpful in the short term in promoting weight gain at this stage of disease. Hyperalimentation is occasionally required in infants with meconium ileus and in other special circumstances.

NATURAL HISTORY AND PROGNOSIS

A comprehensive treatment program for CF has unequivocally improved overall survival of patients. Thirty years ago, the median survival was only a few years of age; currently, it is about 30 years (Fig. 53-10). However, because CF is a complex disorder that affects different organs to different degrees, it is difficult to describe a "typical course" for a patient with CF. Some patients die in childhood or adolescence, while others survive beyond age 40 years.

An important determinant of the natural history of CF is the severity of the pulmonary disease and the rate at which it progresses. Although most patients' condition improves in response to therapy, skillful management does less to influence the course of the severely affected than that of the mildly affected patient.

A variety of scoring systems have been devised for CF. The clinical scoring system devised by Shwachman and Kulczycki[46] and the chest radiograph scoring system devised by Brasfield and associates are widely used.[5] However, although these and more elaborate scoring systems are useful in categorizing patients according to the severity of illness, none has proved useful in prognosticating the course of an individual patient.

Because CF is a genetic disease, the question of a familial pattern of severity is often raised. Figure 53-8 shows chest radiographs of three siblings with CF; the radiographs demonstrate mild, moderate, and severe disease in individuals in the same family. The capsule histories, which are included in the figure legend, also illustrate the variability in courses experienced.

Patients with CF can be categorized not only with respect to severity of illness but also with regard to survival. For example, more than one-half of patients with CF who underwent surgery for meconium ileus before 1965 died in the first 2 months of life. Although this situation had improved markedly by 1976, the survival rate for patients with meconium ileus was still not as good as for all other patients with CF. In addition, the survival rate was much lower for females than for males, especially in adolescents. In recent years, differences between the patients in these groups have declined or disappeared. Because of improvements in the collection of mortality statistics, comparison of current data with those from previous years may be somewhat misleading. However, 50 percent survival age has not been increasing as rapidly in recent years as in the 1970s and 1980s (Fig. 53-10). Indeed, it appears that the average duration of life for patients with CF may be approaching a plateau.

COMPLICATIONS

The course of CF is often characterized by a gradual decrease in pulmonary function, punctuated by further abrupt declines during exacerbations. Malnutrition, when present despite therapy, usually correlates best with the severity of the pulmonary disease. However, the course of CF may be suddenly altered by certain complications of the disease.

Hypoelectrolytemia and Metabolic Alkalosis

Hypoelectrolytemia and metabolic alkalosis are serious complications that are especially apt to occur during periods of hot

TABLE 53-3

Hypoelectrolytemia and Metabolic Alkalosis in Two Cystic Fibrosis Patients

Patient	*Serum Electrolytes, meq/L*				
	Na	*K*	*Cl*	*CO$_2$*	*Serum pH*
No. 1	123	2.2	49	48	7.60
No. 2	125	2.4	55	41	7.63

SOURCE: Modified from Scanlin TF, Cystic fibrosis, in Fleisher G, Ludwig S (eds), *Textbook of Emergency Pediatrics.* Baltimore, Williams & Wilkins, 1983, pp 532–556, with permission.

weather, when losses of sodium and chloride increase. Electrolyte depletion may be life-threatening, especially in infants and young children (Table 53-3). Prompt fluid replacement with isotonic saline is critical.

Intestinal Obstruction

Acute or chronic crampy abdominal pain attributable to some degree of intestinal obstruction is common in patients with CF. If the obstruction is incomplete and manifested soley by a tender right lower-quadrant mass, medical therapy using oral *N*-acetylcysteine and mineral oil is recommended. Alternatively, adequate oral intake or nasogastric tube administration of Go-Lytely may be used. If these measures are unsuccessful, hyperosmolar enemas using an agent such as meglumine diatrizoate (Gastrografin) may dislodge the fecal mass. Patients with a history of crampy abdominal pain are occasionally noted to have radiographic evidence of intestinal obstruction, manifested by dilated bowel loops and air-fluid levels. After the neonatal period, intestinal obstruction is referred to as *meconium ileus equivalent.* An impacted fecal mass may serve as the leading edge for a volvulus or intussusception (Fig. 53-6). If either of these is present and not resolved with hyperosmolar enema, surgery is required. Careful pre- and postoperative management is essential to avoid the deterioration in pulmonary function that may follow the use of anesthesia.[34]

Esophageal Varices

Although cirrhosis occurs in fewer than 5 percent of people with CF, esophageal varices and portal hypertension may cause upper gastrointestinal bleeding in these patients. Once bleeding has been identified as due to varices and hemoptysis has been excluded, therapeutic endoscopy with a sclerosing agent is undertaken. For patients with severe involvement, transjugular intrahepatic portosystemic shunting can effectively decompress esophageal varices by decreasing portal pressure. This procedure is likely to supplant surgical portosystemic shunts.

Liver transplantation is another option for many patients with CF who have end-stage liver disease. Bleeding esophageal varices or vitamin K–resistant prolongation of the prothrombin time should prompt evaluation for liver transplantation. Criteria for priority transplantation include bleeding varices not responsive to sclerosis, severe ascites, and encephalopathy. Ideal candidates are those with an FEV$_1$ of at least 50 percent of predicted. Colonization with a multidrug-resistant or panresistant strain of *Pseudomonas* is a relative contraindication to transplantation. In patients in whom poor pulmonary function or drug-resistant pulmonary infection is an issue, double organ (liver and lung) transplantation may be considered. However, this surgery has been successfully accomplished only several times to date. Despite concerns about worsening airway infection during transplant-associated immunosuppression, liver transplantation in patients with CF does not worsen their pulmonary status.

Atelectasis

Atelectasis of a lung segment or lobe sometimes occurs in CF. Acute atelectasis is generally associated with few symptoms (Fig. 53-11*A*). If it is untreated, however, the end result of atelectasis is a severely bronchiectatic segment or lobe (Fig. 53-11*B*). Vigorous chest physiotherapy, in conjunction with antibiotics, is often successful in reexpanding the affected lung region. Bronchoscopy is occasionally helpful. As a rule, however, bronchoscopy is no more effective than chest physiotherapy and pulmonary pharmacotherapy. Resection of a persistently atelectic or bronchiectatic lobe is undertaken only when the remaining areas of the lung are in relatively good condition, overall pulmonary function is good, and the evidence convincing that the affected segment is responsible for intolerable symptoms (fever, cough, or sputum production).[48]

Pneumothorax

Recurrent pneumothorax is common in CF, particularly in older patients (Fig. 53-11*C*). Tension pneumothorax occurs in up to 30 percent of patients with CF who develop pneumothorax. Tube thoracostomy is indicated when the pneumothorax occupies more than 10 percent of the area of the hemithorax seen on the posteroanterior chest radiograph. Because the frequency of recurrence of pneumothorax is high, attempts are often made at the time of the initial event to achieve chemical or surgical pleurodesis.[33] Surgical pleurodesis is more effective at preventing recurrence of a pneumothorax and is no longer considered a contraindication to lung transplantation.

Hemoptysis

Expectoration of a small amount of blood-streaked sputum is a fairly common ocurrence in CF and is generally managed by intensifying home therapy for pulmonary infection. In contrast, hemoptysis (the expectoration of at least 30 to 60 ml of fresh blood) requires hospitalization, even with a chest radiograph that is virtually unchanged (Fig. 53-11*D*). The probable mechanism underlying most instances of hemoptysis in CF is the erosion of an area of localized infection into a bronchial vessel. Massive hemoptysis (blood loss of 300 to 2500 ml) is uncommon in CF. However, it represents a potentially life-threatening situation. Bronchoscopy, and sometimes thoracic surgery, may be required to control the hemorrhage. Bronchial artery embolization has been used successfully in patients with CF and is now the treatment of choice when a physician experienced in the procedure is available.[4]

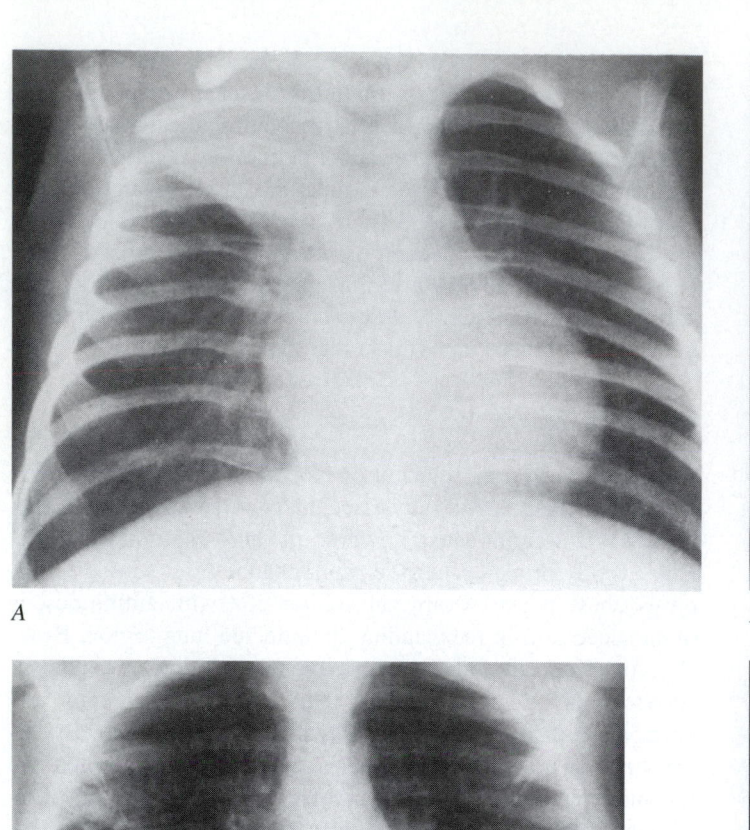

A

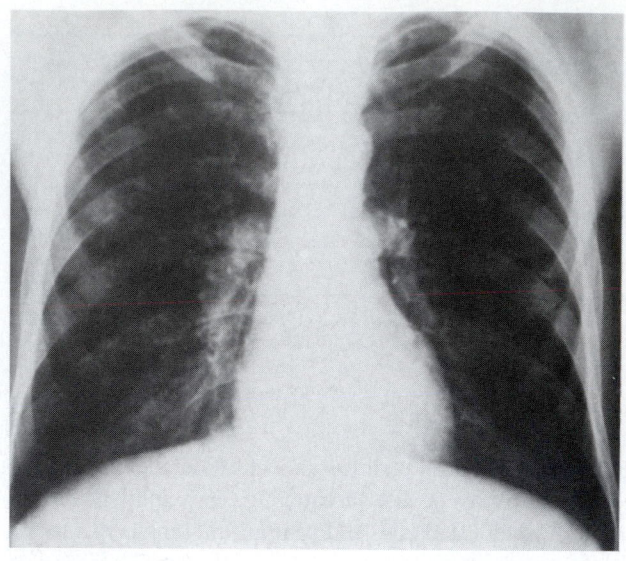

D

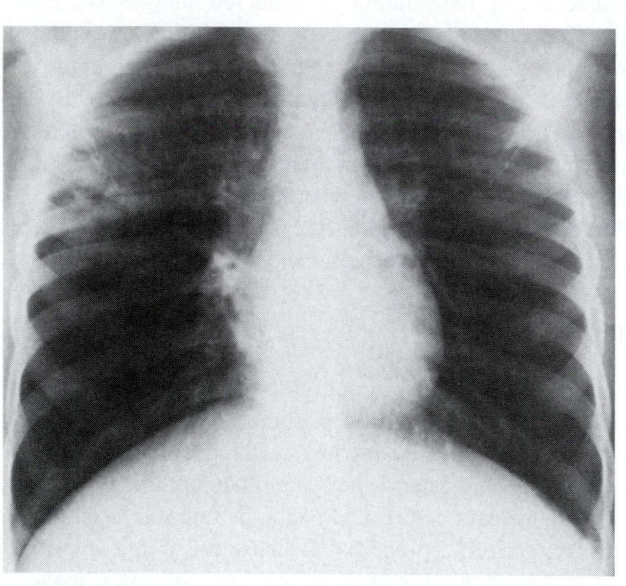

B

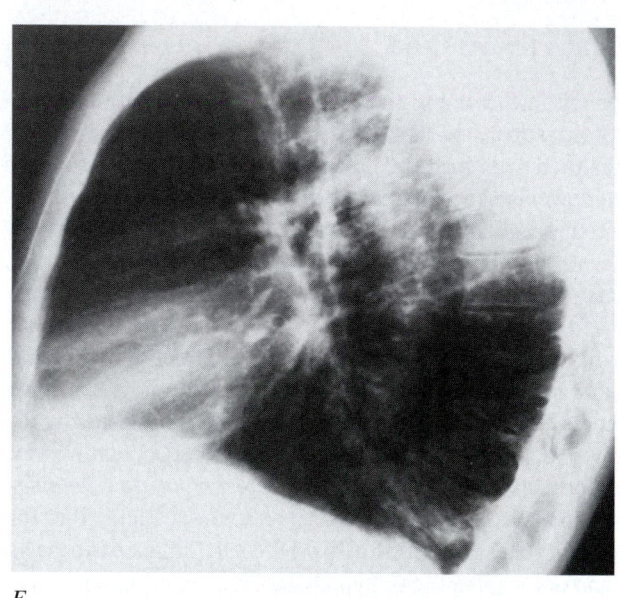

E

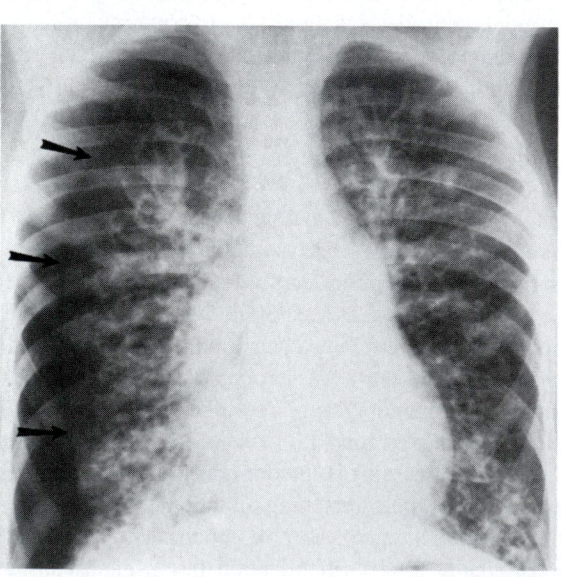

C

FIGURE 53-11 Chest radiographs of patients with pulmonary complications of CF. *A.* Atelectasis of the right upper lobe in a 4-month-old male. The atelectasis resolved with antibiotics and chest physiotherapy. *B.* The same patient at 9 years of age with mild hyperinflation, central bronchiectasis, resolving right upper lobe infiltrate. The diagnosis of allergic bronchopulmonary aspergillosis was made, and the patient improved after treatment with prednisone. *C.* Pneumothorax of the right lung (arrows) in a 13-year-old male. The pneumothorax resolved after tube thoracostomy and tetracycline sclerosis. The patient died 3 years later from respiratory failure with congestive heart failure. There were no recurrences of the pneumothorax. *D* and *E.* A 43-year-old male showing hyperinflation and diffuse peribronchial thickening. The radiograph was taken during an episode of significant hemoptysis, and no acute changes were seen on the radiograph. He works full-time and has not had another episode of hemoptysis in the last 12 years.

Infection with Unusual Organisms

CF produces central bronchiectasis, even though the disease initially is in the small bronchioles. Bronchiectatic airways are frequently colonized with unusual organisms, including *Aspergillus* and atypical mycobacteria. As is the case with pathogenic bacteria, eradication of these organisms from the airways is virtually impossible. The focus of therapy is directed toward verifying that the organisms are resulting in worsening of the disease and controlling the infection, rather than effecting a microbiologic cure.

MYCOBACTERIA

The prevalence of infection with mycobacteria in CF is approximately 12 to 15 percent. Frequently, the sputum culture is overgrown with pathogenic bacteria; accordingly, the culture should be handled specially to enhance isolation. Patients with CF should be screened for *M. tuberculosis* infection with yearly PPD skin tests. Prophylaxis and treatment of *M. tuberculosis* in CF are the same as for patients without CF. A decision about therapy for isolation of atypical mycobacteria is based on the likelihood that the organism is contributing to airway infection and a decline in pulmonary function. Isolation of the same organism on several occasions, positive smears, presence of progressive chest radiographic changes, further decline in pulmonary status decline despite vigorous antipseudomonal (or antistaphylococcal) therapy, persistent night sweats, and fever are clinical clues that the atypical mycobacteria are contributing to disease. Demonstration of tissue infection with transbronchial lung biopsy is rarely recommended. A clinical database has been established by the CF Foundation to track results of treatment for atypical mycobacterial infections in patients with CF.

ASPERGILLUS

In an analogous fashion, molds, especially *Aspergillus,* are occasionally isolated from patients with CF. Approximately 5 to 15 percent of patients have allergic bronchopulmonary aspergillosis (ABPA).[29] The diagnosis of ABPA in CF is difficult because of overlapping symptoms between the two disorders. Diagnostic criteria for ABPA are (1) reversible airway obstruction, (2) proximal bronchiectasis, (3) history of pulmonary infiltrates, (4) skin test positivity to aspergillus antigens, (5) precipitating serum antibodies to *A. fumigatus,* (6) elevated total serum IgE, (7) elevated specific serum IgE and serum IgG to *Aspergillus,* and (8) peripheral eosinophilia. A negative skin test for *Aspergillus* effectively rules out the diagnosis of ABPA. During the active phase of ABPA, elevations in total IgE and eosinophil count are seen. Rises in *Aspergillus*-specific titers (IgE and IgG) are more specific for ABPA than are serum precipitins. ABPA in patients with CF is also treated with corticosteroids, despite colonization of the lower airways with pathogenic bacteria.

GRAM-NEGATIVE BACTERIA

In the late 1970s and early 1980s, the importance of *Burkholderia cepacia* (formerly *Pseudomonas cepacia*) was recognized. *B.* *cepacia* is a gram-negative, oxidase-positive rod that is uniformly resistant to polymixin and, frequently, panresistant. Isolation of *B. cepacia* requires plating on special OFPBL (oxidative fermentive polymixin B bacitracin lactose) or PC (*P. cepacia*) agar plates to retard growth of other gram-negative rods and enhance growth of *B. cepacia*. The plates must be maintained for a minimum of 4 days. *B. cepacia* colonization has been associated with septicemia, which is very rarely seen with *P. aeruginosa*. The clinical course after acquisition of *B. cepacia* may be fulminant, with death occurring in a matter of months. However, most patients' disease follows a more benign course. Carefully controlled epidemiologic studies are needed to better define risk factors and to establish the true virulence of *B. cepacia*. Experimental evidence exists that at least one strain of *B. cepacia* may be transmitted in an epidemic fashion.[49] The combination of a poor clinical course after acquisition of *B. cepacia* and the evidence supporting epidemic transmission has led to cohorting or isolation of patients with CF infected with *B. cepacia,* as recommended by the CF Foundation and the CDC.

In addition to being colonized with *Pseudomonas* and *Burkholderia* species, patients with CF may be colonized with other gram-negative, oxidase-positive organisms, such as *S. maltophilia, F. oryzihabitans,* and *A. xylosidans.* These are pathogenic organisms, similar in importance to *P. aeruginosa.* Antibiotic therapy should be directed toward these bacteria when they are isolated from the patient with CF who is experiencing an acute exacerbation. The prolonged, prophylactic, aggressive use of antibiotics in CF has led to emergence of resistant organisms. A multiply resistant *Pseudomonas* is an organism that is resistant to all agents in at least two different classes of antibiotics. Resistance to oral fluoroquinolones occurs after about 3 weeks of therapy; if the agent is withheld, the organism occasionally becomes sensitive again.

Cor Pulmonale

As the pulmonary disease of CF progresses and the degree of hypoxia increases, patients eventually develop pulmonary hypertension and cor pulmonale. An increase in hypoxia during exacerbations of the pulmonary disease often precipitates overt right ventricular failure. During the acute episode, antibiotic treatment for the underlying pulmonary disorder is intensified and supplemental oxygen and diuretics are added. Digitalis and pulmonary vasodilators have not proved to be of benefit in CF. Although clear indications for and benefits of the use of oxygen in CF have not been established, in our experience, expectant monitoring and aggressive treatment of nocturnal hypoxemia (maintaining Sa_{O_2} at 95% or more) delay the onset of cor pulmonale.

Respiratory Failure

When development of respiratory failure in CF—i.e., hypercarbia (Pa_{CO_2} at least 55 mmHg) in addition to hypoxemia—management becomes extremely difficult. As a rule, patients do not respond as well to mechanical ventilation as those without CF; in addition, patients with CF have more complications from mechanical ventilation than do those with other forms of chronic obstructive airway disease.

Mechanical ventilation is generally instituted when an acute episode, such as viral pneumonia or status asthmaticus, thrusts the patient into respiratory failure. This approach is particularly indicated in the patient who has had good pulmonary function before the acute episode. Mechanical ventilation is less apt to be successful if the patient has previously experienced a bout of respiratory failure. When respiratory failure marks the end of a chronic course of progressive pulmonary insufficiency despite adequate medical therapy, mechanical ventilation is usually unhelpful. None of the indications or contraindications for mechanical ventilation are absolute, however, and the clinical outcome depends, to a large extent, on the availability of a dedicated and skilled intensive care team experienced in caring for patients with CF.

Noninvasive mechanical ventilation using bilevel positive airway pressure has been used successfully in relatively stable end-stage patients with CF, most of whom have been evaluated and listed for lung transplantation. Studies are necessary to determine precise criteria for the use of this technique in CF.

Complications Related to Lung Transplantation

Lung transplantation has emerged as an option for patients with end-stage CF.[27] Despite initial concerns about immunosuppression in patients with suppurative lung disease, the outcome for those with CF who undergo lung transplantation is among the best reported for this procedure. Two major problems prevent lung transplantation from becoming widely recommended for CF. One is the lack of suitable organs for transplantation. Forty percent of patients with CF who are awaiting transplantation die before an organ is made available. The attrition is due, in part, to the allocation of lungs on the basis of wait list time *alone*, rather than on the basis of severity of disease. The median waiting time is currently more than 12 months, but wide variability exists. The organ shortage, especially from pediatric donors, has driven the development of living related donor transplants.

The second major problem with lung transplantation for CF is the occurrence of obliterative bronchiolitis following transplantation. Obliterative bronchiolitis is a progressive occlusion of the bronchiolar lumina by inflammatory cells and submucosal fibrosis. The cause is probably chronic allograft rejection; transient improvement in airflow is seen following augmentation of immunosuppression. About 50 percent of transplant patients develop obliterative bronchiolitis after the second year following the procedure. The disease pursues a relentless downhill course, with a median survival of about 2 years following the initial diagnosis.

The poor prognosis associated with obliterative bronchiolitis has several important implications for patient selection and timing of referral for transplantation. First, the main reason for seeking lung transplant is to improve the quality of life, rather than to improve survival. Second, the timing of referral for lung transplantation necessitates weighing the risks of dying while on the waiting list against the possibility of developing obliterative bronchiolitis.

Appropriately timed referral for transplantation includes consideration of (1) the priority given solely to time on the list, (2) the average length of waiting time, (3) the natural history of the disease, (4) the natural history of lung transplantation, and (5) the requirement that the patient be fully ambulatory. Therefore, ideal candidates for lung transplantation are those who have less than 2 years to live and have significant functional impairment but are capable of participating in a pulmonary rehabilitation program.

Results from clinical studies may aid with proper timing of referral for lung transplantation in CF. A study of 673 patients with CF revealed that patients with an FEV_1 less than 30 percent of predicted have a 50 percent 2-year mortality.[22] Other important clinical parameters useful in determining the timing of transplantation are the presence of hypoxemia (Pa_{O_2} under 55) and hypercarbia (Pa_{CO_2} above 50). Of interest, in both single and multivariate analyses, female sex is associated with an increased relative risk, suggesting that for female patients, referral for lung transplantation should be considered at an even earlier stage.

Because CF is a multisystem disorder, both management and proper selection of patients are more complicated than for other diseases managed with lung transplantation. Among the most difficult challenges presented by patients with CF before transplantation is the microbiology of their lower airways. As discussed previously, colonization with multidrug-resistant *B. cepacia* has been associated with a poor clinical outcome. In a study of patients with CF who were colonized with *B. cepacia*, including 10 patients who were colonized before transplant and 5 de novo after transplant, 7 died; the median survival was 28 days.[47] This miserable outcome has led to great reluctance to list patients with *B. cepacia* for transplantation.

For poorly understood reasons, patients with CF metabolize drugs differently from those without CF, complicating the dosing of medications, including cyclosporine. The difficulties in achieving an optimal drug dose may be related to malabsorption or enhanced excretion of the drug.

Nutritional issues also complicate the posttransplantation management of patients with CF. About 50 percent of all patients with CF over 30 years of age are overtly diabetic, and administration of corticosteroids induces diabetes in another 10 percent. Maintenance of proper nutrition is important in CF, especially for rapid postoperative recovery. The importance of nutrition is underscored by the fact that if patients are less than 75 percent of their ideal body weight, they are not listed for transplantation.

Despite all the special challenges to successful lung transplantation posed by patients with CF, their actuarial survival is quite good (Fig. 53-12). The 4-year survival is about 50 percent, reinforcing the tenet that lung transplantation is done principally to improve quality of life.

PSYCHOSOCIAL ISSUES

A number of psychosocial issues are important in the management of patients with CF. Special circumstances should be recognized for adults with the disorder.

General

Careful attention to the emotional, social, and financial well-being of the patient with CF and his or her family has considerable value in favorably influencing the course of the disease. At the time of diagnosis, it is important to strike an optimistic note while educating the patient about the illness and its management. As part of the early encounter with the patient, the importance

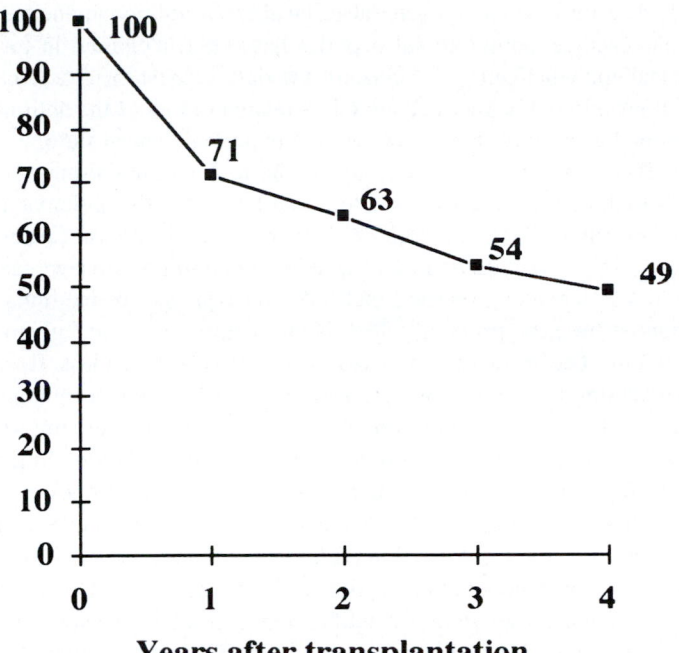

FIGURE 53-12 Actuarial survival following lung transplantation for CF. The numbers along the ordinate indicate the percentage surviving at each time point. *(Data from the St. Louis Organ Transplant Data Registry, 1995.)*

of identifying and reinforcing the emotional and financial strengths of the family, as well as weaknesses that will need buttressing, should be recognized. Medical care for CF patients is costly, especially if hospital admissions are required. Many states have crippled-children's programs that provide support for patients and families. Several states have also established special programs for adults with CF.

As the disease runs its course, counseling and feedback about disease progression are essential. As the patient and family go about setting educational, career, and family goals, they need guidance in realistic planning. It is vital that the physician develop and maintain a positive attitude. The patient who gives up hope is liable to undergo rapid deterioration. Conversely, even patients with severe pulmonary disease can continue to function well and be productive. At the stage when medical therapy is of no further avail, however, the patient and family require considerable emotional support to accept the inevitable. In recent years, many CF centers have allowed patients to die at home, rather than in the hospital. The family requires specific instructions about how to provide physical and emotional comfort for the patient in the home. Usually, home visits by some members of the CF team are required. Not all families have the strength or resources to care for the patient dying at home.

Special Considerations in Adult Patients

In 1995, the median life expectancy for patients with CF was about 30 years. Managing a chronic illness becomes more complicated when patients must also begin to manage their independence and make life decisions regarding education, marriage, children, careers, insurance, and self-care. Intense support for both patients and their families is required. Patients who enjoy a relatively mild clinical course form healthy and satisfying relationships in a manner similar to that of their healthy, age-matched peers. With advanced disease, patients with CF have more difficulty in forming intimate relationships. Disturbances in body image, decreased mobility, and lack of opportunity to meet suitable partners are cited as reasons for the decreased ability to form intimate relationships in the severely affected young adult with CF.

The adult patient with CF faces unique problems with self-care. Families of patients with CF provide a tremendous amount of care that is expensive and time-consuming to replace for the independently living adult. When the disease flares, patients must "step up" their level of care at precisely the time when they are least able to do so. Judicious use of hospitalization and home care must be provided if the patient is to recover. The trend toward home management of a pulmonary exacerbation using intravenous antibiotics alone ignores the obvious contributions of nutrition, airway clearance, and rest toward resolution of the problem.

REPRODUCTIVE ISSUES

More than 97 percent of male patients with CF are sterile, secondary to bilateral absence of the vas deferens. Microsurgical epididymal sperm aspiration (MESA), coupled with in vitro fertilization, has been successful in producing pregnancies in a few carefully selected patients.[31] Not all males with CF are sterile, however. In addition to counseling, these men should be offered sperm analysis.

Pregnancy for women with CF is increasingly common, and several important issues remain unsolved. In 1994 alone, 58 women with CF gave birth. This stands in marked contrast to the total of 13 pregnancies in 10 patients recorded from 1960 to 1966 (data from the 1994 CF Foundation Data Registry).

Maternal clinical status before pregnancy is the most important sign of maternal outcome.[26] In a study of 25 women with 38 pregnancies, no significant difference was seen between pre- and postgravid gas exchange or nutritional status. A small but statistically significant decline in spirometry was noted. However, the decline was not outside the range of expected decline for the natural progression of the disease. More severely affected women suffer an irreversible decline in clinical status during pregnancy. Without an appropriately matched control group of nongravid women with CF, it is impossible to determine whether pregnancy per se is responsible for the decline or whether the decline is a reflection of the natural history of the disease.

Recommendations about pregnancy for women who are either mildly affected or severely affected is straightforward. For the woman with moderately compromised pulmonary status (i.e., FVC under 50 to 60 percent of predicted), an overall assessment of the clinical situation is recommended, although no firm guidelines can be given. Increased incidence of fetal prematurity is noted in women with a pregravid FVC below 50 percent of predicted, lending additional weight against recommending pregnancy to women with moderate to severe airflow obstruction. In any woman with CF who is contemplating pregnancy, thorough evaluation and treatment of nutritional deficiencies and pulmonary exacerbations are required. Frequent use of antibiotics is unavoidable, and the teratogenic risk of many antibiotics is unknown. Despite this theoretical risk, good maternal and fetal health depend on aggressive management of pulmonary exacerbations, including use of antibiotics. Management of the gravid patient with CF is best accomplished in a CF center that has a program in high-risk obstetrics.

For men with CF who opt for MESA and for women with CF who are contemplating pregnancy, all offspring are obligate heterozygotes for CF. These offspring need to be counseled that their risk of having a child with CF is about 1 in 50 if the genotype of the spouse is not known. Although genetic testing of children from affected parents is not recommended, they should receive genetic counseling on reaching adolescence. Parents with CF also need to consider the ethical issues of a premature parental death and its effect on the family.

Discovery of the CF gene in 1989 led to the hope that prenatal diagnosis would eventually decrease the incidence of the disease. However, affected families either are choosing not to test at-risk pregnancies or, if tested and found to be affected, are choosing to continue the pregnancy. Similarly, there has not been a large increase in the number of therapeutic abortions of fetuses with CF among women with the disorder who have a good clinical status. Obviously, the expected survival and quality of life for the child with CF must be sufficiently promising to explain these parents' decisions.

FUTURE DIRECTIONS

Concern exists that the marked improvement in survival of patients with CF noted over the past 2 decades is approaching a plateau. To further enhance survival in CF, physicians must look to insights gained from basic research. Although much work needs to be done, much has already been accomplished, warranting a realistic expectation that major breakthroughs will soon occur in the treatment of the disorder. Important areas for future development include new pharmacologic approaches and gene therapy.

Pharmacologic Approaches

Infection with *Pseudomonas* organisms is a critical aspect of CF that has attracted a great deal of attention. To date, *Pseudomonas* species have demonstrated a remarkable capacity to change expression of phenotype and to develop resistance to new antibiotics. One management strategy that is being employed more frequently is performance of synergy testing on isolates of *Pseudomonas* that are resistant to multiple antibiotics. Frequently, such testing directs the use of nontraditional combinations and doses of antibiotics with good therapeutic results. However, this strategy may be successful for only a limited period before panresistance develops. New classes of antibiotics, originally called magainins and defensins, offer hope as alternative drug choices in the near future. One synthetic magainin, MS843, has been shown to be effective in vitro against a tobramycin-resistant strain of *P. aeruginosa*. Further progress can be anticipated if clinical trials of safety and efficacy are successful.

Increased electrolyte concentrations have been measured in the apical fluid from airway epithelial cells in CF. This hypertonic

fluid permits increased bacterial survival.[46a] In addition, inducible, salt-sensitive, antimicrobial peptides have been identified in tracheal epithelial cells.[43] In concert, the data suggest that bacterial colonization of airway cells in CF is related to loss of the antimicrobial activity of these peptides in a hypertonic apical fluid.

Pharmacologic approaches to the basic defect in CF may offer treatment alternatives or additional benefit to the anticipated use of directed gene therapy (see below). As described earlier, many of the mutations in CF have been classified into five categories, depending on the functional consequences of the mutation on the gene product, which is an integral membrane glycoprotein. The most common mutation, ΔF508, is a class II or processing mutation in which most of the gene product remains in the endoplasmic reticulum, with only a very small amount localized to the surface membrane prior to degradation. Since CFTR has been shown to interact with several chaperones during processing, these molecules provide an attractive theoretical target for pharmacologic intervention, although, to date, there has been no functional correction with this approach. However, two agents, 4-phenylbutyric acid and glycerol, have been shown to increase cell surface localization of CFTR in vitro by an unknown mechanism. Since analogs of 4-phenylbutyric acid have been employed clinically in treatment of sickle cell disease, a phase I clinical trial is under way, based on sweat test values as a measure of efficacy.

Other classes of compounds have been shown to increase the chloride conductance of cells with the ΔF508 mutation by increasing intracellular levels of cAMP. These compounds include the methylxanthine derivative IBMX (3-isobutyl-1-methylxanthine), amrinone, and milrinone, each of which increases intracellular levels of cAMP by either direct or indirect action on intracellular phosphodiesterases. Further understanding of the processing and function of CFTR should lead to additional, potentially useful pharmacologic therapies.

Finally, since inflammation plays a critical role in the pathophysiology of the lung disease of CF, efforts have been directed at decreasing airway inflammation. The approaches are both pharmacologic (e.g., use of ibuprofen and prednisone) and physiological (e.g., prevention of *Pseudomonas* binding to airway cells and immunization against *Pseudomonas*).

Gene Therapy

Improvements in gene transfer technology represent an important future direction in CF. Because the disease is inherited as an autosomal recessive trait, only one normal copy of the gene needs to be provided to cells. Suitable vectors to date for carrying the normal CFTR gene include replication-deficient adenovirus, adeno-associated virus, cationic liposomes, and DNA-protein complexes.[41]

Several human clinical trials of gene therapy in CF have been initiated, based on use of adenoviral vectors and cationic liposome-mediated gene transfer.[53] Results have been remarkably similar among the trials. In a few patients, patchy expression of the transgene has been demonstrated in both the nose and lung using immunohistochemistry or in situ hybridization. Dose-dependent inflammation has been encountered at very high infection rates in the nose; in one study, a patient became acutely ill for several days following instillation in the lung of a high titer of replication-deficient adenovirus. Physiological correction of cAMP-mediated chloride secretion in the nose has not been convincingly demonstrated after gene transfer, although a trend toward correction of the basal potential difference has been observed.

Finally, because the immune response to viral vectors constitutes a significant impediment to successful gene transfer, several approaches are currently being developed. These include production of less immunogenic viral vectors, immune suppression, and development of nonimmunogenic, nonviral vectors.[25]

Progress toward cure of CF will require a multidisciplinary approach. Management of the lung disease in CF will probably be based on combined methods. However, the momentum gained from recent improvements in our understanding of basic pathogenetic mechanisms provides a basis for realistic optimism that specific therapy will result in better outcomes for patients with CF.

REFERENCES

1. Amos JA, Oates RD, Dean M, et al: Congenital absence of the vas deference: A primarily genital form of cystic fibrosis. *Pediatr Pulmonol* 14:142–143, 1992.

2. Armstrong DS, Grimwood K, Carlin JHB, et al: Bronchoalveolar lavage or oropharyngeal cultures to identify lower respiratory pathogens in infants with cystic fibrosis. *Pediatr Pulmonol* 21:267–275, 1996.

3. Auerbach HS, Williams M, Kirkpatrick JA, Colten HR: Alternate-day prednisone reduces morbidity and improves pulmonary function in cystic fibrosis. *Lancet* 2:686–688, 1985.

4. Baker MD, Scanlin TF: Pulmonary emergencies, in Fleisher GR, Ludwig S (eds), *Synopsis of Pediatric Emergency Medicine.* Baltimore, Williams & Wilkins, 1995, pp 489–501.

5. Brasfield D, Hicks G, Soong S, Tiller RE: The chest roentgenogram in cystic fibrosis: A new scoring system. *Pediatrics* 63:24–29, 1979.

6. Canny GJ, Corey M, Livingstone RA, et al: Pregnancy and cystic fibrosis. *Obstet Gynecol* 77:850–853, 1991.

7. CF Genotype-Phenotype Consortium: Correlation between genotype and phenotype in patients with cystic fibrosis. *New Engl J Med* 329:1308–1313, 1993.

8. Collins FS: Cystic fibrosis: Molecular biology and therapeutic implications. *Science* 256:774–779, 1992.

9. Cropp GJ, Pullano TP, Cerny FJ, Nathanson IT: Exercise tolerance and cardiorespiratory adjustments at peak work capacity in cystic fibrosis. *Am Rev Respir Dis* 126:211–216, 1982.

10. Cutting GR: Genotype defect: Its effect on cellular function and phenotypic expression. *Semin Respir Crit Care Med* 15:356–361, 1994.

11. Davidson TM, Murphy C, Mitchell M, et al: Management of chronic sinusitis in cystic fibrosis. *Laryngoscope* 105:354–358, 1995.

12. Davis PB: *Cystic Fibrosis.* New York, Dekker, 1993.

13. Del Pin CE, Czyrko C, Ziegler MM, et al: Management and survival of meconium ileus: A 30-year review. *Ann Surg* 215:179–185, 1992.

14. Desmond KJ, Schwenk WF, Thomas E, et al: Immediate and long-term effects of chest physiotherapy in patients with cystic fibrosis. *J Pediatr* 103:538–542, 1983.

15. Drumm ML, Pope HA, Cliff WH, et al: Correction of the cystic fibrosis defect *in vitro* by retrovirus-mediated gene transfer. *Cell* 62:1227–1233, 1990.

16. Fellows K, Khaw KT, Schuster S, Shwachman H: Bronchial artery embolization in cystic fibrosis: Technique and long-term results. *J Pediatr* 95:959–963, 1979.

17. Fox WW, Bureau MA, Taussig LA, et al: Helium flow-volume curves in the detection of early small airway disease. *Pediatrics* 54:293–299, 1974.

18. Fuchs HJ, Borowitz DS, Christiansen DH, et al: Effect of aerosolized recombinant human DNase on exacerbations of respiratory symptoms and on pulmonary function in patients with cystic fibrosis. *New Engl J Med* 331:637–673, 1994.

19. Ingram RH Jr, McFadden ER Jr: Pulmonary performance in cystic fibrosis, in Fishman AP (ed), *Pulmonary Diseases and Disorders.* New York, McGraw-Hill, 1980, pp 614–617.

20. Kerem BS et al: Identification of the cystic fibrosis gene: Genetic analysis. *Science* 245:1073–1080, 1989.

21. Kerem E, Corey M, Kerem B, et al: The relation between genotype and phenotype in cystic fibrosis—Analysis of the most common mutation (ΔF508). *New Engl J Med* 323:1517–1522, 1990.

22. Kerem E, Reisman J, Corey M, et al: Prediction of mortality in patients with cystic fibrosis. *New Engl J Med* 326:1187–1191, 1992.

23. Khan TZ, Wagener JS, Bost T, et al: Early pulmonary inflammation in infants with cystic fibrosis. *Am J Respir Crit Care Med* 151:1075–1082, 1995.

24. Konstan MW, Byard PJ, Hoppel CL, et al: Effect of high-dose ibuprofen in patients with cystic fibrosis. *New Engl J Med* 332:848–887, 1995.

25. Kollen WJW, Midoux P, Erbacher P, et al: Gluconoylated and glycoylated polylysine as vectors for gene transfer into cystic fibrosis airway epithelial cells. *Hum Gene Ther* 7:1577–1586, 1996.

26. Kotloff RM, FitzSimmons SC, Fiel SB: Fertility and pregnancy in patients with cystic fibrosis. *Clin Chest Med* 13:623–635, 1992.

27. Kotloff RM, Zuckerman JB: Lung transplantation for cystic fibrosis: Special considerations. *Chest* 109:787–789, 1996.

28. Knowles MR, Hohnecker KW, Zhou Z, et al: A controlled study of adenoviral-mediated gene transfer in the nasal epithelium of patients with cystic fibrosis. *New Engl J Med* 133:823–831, 1995.

29. Laufer P, Fink J, Bruns T, et al: Allergic bronchopulmonary aspergillosis sin cystic fibrosis. *J Allergy Clin Immunol* 73:44–48, 1984.

30. Lazatin JO, Glick MC, Scanlin TF: Fucosylation in cystic fibrosis airway epithelial cells. *Glycosylation Dis* 1:263–270, 1994.

31. Liu J, Lissens W, Silber SJ, et al: Birth after preimplantation diagnosis of the cystic fibrosis ΔF508 mutation by polymerase chain reaction in human embryos resulting from intracytoplasmic sperm injection with epididymal sperm. *JAMA* 272:1858–1860, 1994.

32. Matthews LW, Dearborn DG, Tucker AS: Cystic fibrosis, in Fishman AP (ed), *Pulmonary Diseases and Disorders.* New York, McGraw-Hill, 1980, pp 600–613.

33. McLaughlin FJ, Matthews WJ, Strieder DK, et al: Pneumothorax in cystic fibrosis: Management and outcome. *J Pediatr* 100:863–869, 1982.

34. Olsen MM, Gauderer MW, Girz MK, Izant RJ Jr: Surgery in patients with cystic fibrosis. *J Pediatr Surg* 22:613–618, 1987.

35. Orenstein DM, Franklin BA, Doershuk CF, et al: Exercise conditioning and cardiopulmonary fitness in cystic fibrosis. *Chest* 80:392–397, 1981.

36. Ramsey BW: Management of pulmonary disease in patients with cystic fibrosis. *New Engl J Med* 335:179–188, 1996.

37. Ramsey BW, Dorkin JL, Eisenberg JD, et al: Efficacy of aerosolized tobramycin in patients with cystic fibrosis. *New Engl J Med* 328:1740–1746, 1993.

38. Redding GJ, Restuccia R, Cotton EK, Brooks JG: Serial changes in pulmonary functions in children hospitalized with cystic fibrosis. *Am Rev Respir Dis* 126:31–36, 1982.

39. Riordan JR, Rommens JM, Kerem B, et al: Identification of the cystic fibrosis gene: Cloning and characterization of the complementary DNA. *Science* 245:1066–1073, 1989.

40. Rommens JM, Iannuzzi MC, Kerem B, et al: Identification of the cystic fibrosis gene. Chromosome walking and jumping. *Science* 245:1059–1065, 1989.

41. Rosenfeld MA, Collins FS: Gene therapy for cystic fibrosis. *Chest* 109:241–252, 1996.

42. Rosenstein BJ, Eigen JH: Risks of alternate-day prednisone inpatients with cystic fibrosis. *Pediatrics* 87:245–246, 1991.

43. Russell JP, Diamond G, Tarver AP, et al: Coordinate induction of two antibiotic genes in tracheal epithelial cells exposed to the inflammatory mediators lipopolysaccharide and tumor necrosis factor alpha. *Infect Immun* 64:1565–1568, 1996.

44. Saiman L: Treatment of infections in patients with cystic fibrosis. *Infect Med* 10:37–43, 1993.

45. Schramm CM, Grunstein MM: Infant pulmonary function testing, in Chernick V (ed), *Kendig's Disorders of the Respiratory Tract in Children,* 5th ed. Philadelphia, WB Saunders, 1990, pp 127–147.

46. Shwachman H, Kulczycki LL: Long-term study of one hundred five patients with cystic fibrosis. Study made over a five to fourteen year period. *J Dis Child* 96:6–15, 1958.

46a. Smith JJ, Travis SM, Greenberg EP, Welsh MJ: Cystic fibrosis airway epithelia fail to kill bacteria because of abnormal airway surface fluid. *Cell* 85:229–236, 1996.

47. Snell GI, Hoyos A, Krajden M, et al: *Pseudomonas cepacia* in lung transplant recipients with cystic fibrosis. *Chest* 103:466–471, 1993.

48. Stern RC, Boat TF, Orenstein DM, et al: Treatment and prognosis of lobar and segmental atelectasis in cystic fibrosis. *Am Rev Respir Dis* 118:821–826, 1978.

49. Sun L, Jiang R-Z, Steinbach S, et al: Emergence of a highly transmissible lineage of cbl+ *Burkholderia cepacia* causing CF centre epidemics in North America and Britain. *Nature Med* 1:661–666, 1995.

50. Thomas J, Cook DJ, Brooks D: Chest physical therapy management of patients with CF: A meta-analysis. *Am J Respir Crit Care Med* 151:846–850, 1995.

51. Wei X, Eisman R, Xu J, et al: Turnover of the cystic fibrosis transmembrane conductance regulator (CFTR): Slow degradation of wild-type and ΔF508 CFTR in surface membrane preparations of immortalized airway epithelial cells. *J Cellular Physiol* 168: 373–384, 1996.

52. Welsh MJ, Tsui L-C, Boat TF, Beaudet AL: Cystic fibrosis, in Scriber CL, Beaudet AL, Sly WS, Fiel SB (eds), *The Metabolic and Molecular Bases of Inherited Disease,* 7th ed. New York, McGraw-Hill, 1995, pp 3799–3876.

53. Wilson JM: Gene therapy for cystic fibrosis: Challenges and future directions. *J Clin Invest* 96:2547–2554, 1995.

54. Zielinski J, Tsui L-C: CF genotype and phenotypic variations. *Annu Rev Genet* 29:777–807, 1995.

BRONCHIOLITIS

Talmadge E. King, Jr.

Commonly occurring diseases with prominent involvement of the small airways (asthma, bronchitis, bronchiectasis) are described elsewhere in this book. However, several additional, uncommon small-airway diseases are important to recognize and treat. Interest in these "bronchiolar syndromes" has increased markedly in the past 2 decades, largely because of recognition that bronchiolar injury (bronchiolitis, with or without obliterans) frequently accompanies infections, drug reactions, connective-tissue diseases, toxic gas or fume exposure, and organ transplantation. In addition, several new (or better-clarified) syndromes that involve the small airways have been identified, including idiopathic bronchiolitis obliterans organizing pneumonia and respiratory bronchiolitis–associated interstitial lung disease. This chapter reviews the clinical, radiographic, and histopathologic findings of the bronchiolar syndromes.

DEFINITION AND CLASSIFICATION

Although bronchiolitis has been recognized since the 1800s, it was not until 1901 that the first detailed description of the clinicopathologic syndrome appeared and the phrase *bronchiolitis obliterans* was applied. Bronchiolitis is an inflammatory reaction that follows damage to the bronchiolar epithelium of the small conducting airways. Subsequent healing leads to excessive proliferation of granulation tissue within the airway walls, lumen, or both. Depending on disease stage, the repair process may cause narrowing and distortion of the small airways (constrictive bronchiolitis) or complete obliteration (bronchiolitis obliterans). Alveoli adjacent to the injured small airways are almost always affected, but a considerable portion of the pulmonary interstitium is often spared. Repair occurs in numerous clinical settings, with a variable clinical course and histologic appearance. Consequently, a clear understanding of pathogenesis is lacking.

The nomenclature applied to the bronchiolar syndromes has been confusing. The following terms have been used: *bronchiolitis obliterans, bronchiolitis fibrosa obliterans, bronchiolitis obliterans and interstitial pneumonia, bronchiolitis obliterans with organizing pneumonia* (BOOP), *cryptogenic organizing pneumonia,* and *follicular bronchiolitis.* Unfortunately, the terms are often used interchangeably to describe what are now believed to be separate and distinct clinical entities. Before the description of BOOP in 1985, most cases described as idiopathic bronchiolitis obliterans were actually cases of BOOP. Since some degree of inflammation, narrowing, and obliteration of the small airways is present in most patients, we have chosen the term *bronchiolitis* to refer to the broad spectrum of histopathologic processes. *Bronchiolitis obliterans* refers to histologic lesion characterized by polypoid obliteration of the lumen of bronchioles, without involvement of the distal lung parenchyma by inflammation or organizing pneumonia—i.e., constrictive bronchiolitis. "BOOP" refers to disorders characterized histologically by intraluminal polyps in the respiratory bronchioles, alveolar ducts, and alveolar spaces, accompanied by organizing pneumonia in the more distal parenchyma. In BOOP, the alveolar walls show a mild to moderate chronic inflammatory infiltrate, type II cell hyperplasia, and foamy macrophages in the alveolar spaces; a "proliferative" bronchiolitis is present. Since only a minority of cases showing the "BOOP pattern" represent the idiopathic syndrome described in 1985, and since patients with idiopathic BOOP manifest a distinctive clinical syndrome, this group is referred to as "cryptogenic organizing pneumonia," in order to distinguish this syndrome from other causes of the BOOP pattern.

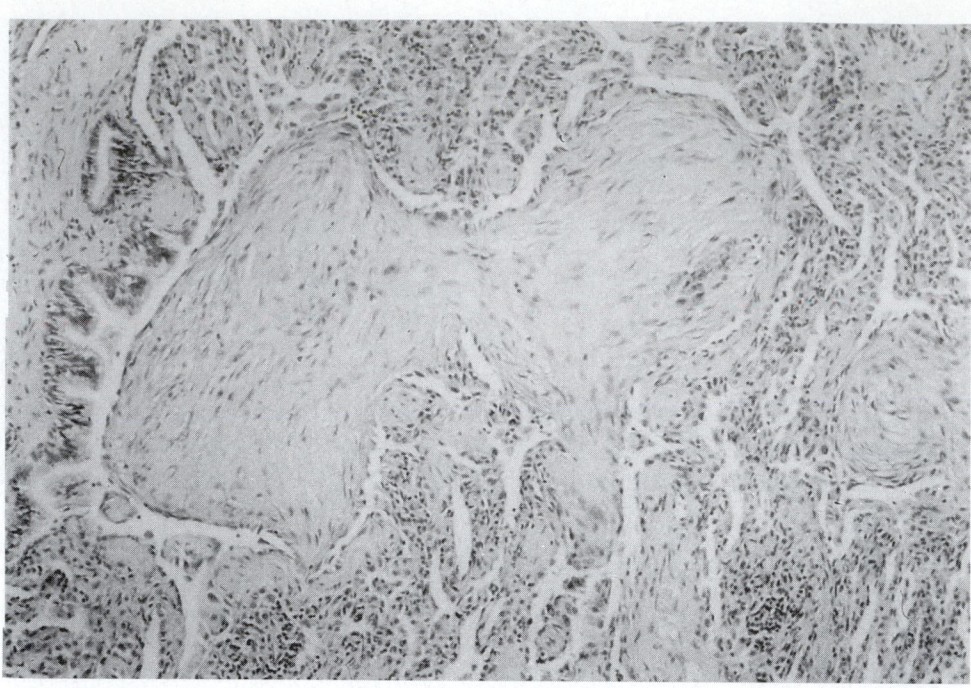

FIGURE 54-1   Bronchiolitis obliterans–organizing pneumonia. Photomicrograph of open lung biopsy from a patient with cryptogenic organizing pneumonia. Polypoid masses of granulation tissue fill the lumens of a respiratory bronchiole and alveolar ducts. Adjacent alveolar interstices are broadened by a lymphoplasmacytic inflammatory infiltrate. (Pentachrome stain, ×156.)

Two classification schemes appear useful in defining cases of bronchiolitis: (1) a clinical classification based on the etiology and (2) a histopathologic classification that includes two major morphologic types: proliferative bronchiolitis and constrictive bronchiolitis.[8,9] The histopathologic classification appears more useful, since pathologic changes correlate best with clinical manifestations.

Clinical Classification

The clinical classification of bronchiolitis is based on etiology (Table 54-1): inhalation injury, infections, drug reactions, and idiopathic causes. The first three categories are frequently recognized from their association with an acute illness or known exposure before the onset of disease. Idiopathic cases often have a more insidious onset, characterized by cough or dyspnea; initially, they may be confused with more common problems, such as chronic obstructive pulmonary disease or interstitial lung disease, depending on the predominant histopathologic pattern.

Histopathologic Classification

The histopathologic classification (Table 54-2) of bronchiolitis includes proliferative and constrictive varieties. Each type, including the presumed pathogenesis, is described below.

PROLIFERATIVE BRONCHIOLITIS

Proliferative bronchiolitis—the "BOOP pattern"—is characterized by an organizing intraluminal exudate[9] and is found, to some degree, in a variety of pulmonary disorders. It is particularly extensive and prominent in cryptogenic organizing pneumonia (also called idiopathic BOOP). The intraluminal fibrotic buds (Masson bodies) are seen in respiratory bronchioles, alveolar ducts, and alveoli (Fig. 54-1). Proliferative bronchiolitis most frequently is associated with diffuse infiltrates on chest radiograph and a restrictive defect on pulmonary function testing, especially when cryptogenic organizing pneumonia is present.

CONSTRICTIVE BRONCHIOLITIS

Constrictive bronchiolitis is characterized by alterations in the walls of membranous and respiratory bronchioles which cause concentric narrowing or complete obliteration of the airway lumen (Fig. 54-2). Often these lesions occur without extensive changes in alveolar ducts or alveolar walls. The changes of constrictive bronchiolitis may be extremely subtle, and frequently they are identified only after step-sectioning and special staining (e.g., use of stains to identify remnants of airway walls) of the lung biopsy. The range of histopathologic changes includes (1) subtle cellular infiltrates around the small airways; (2) extensive cellular infiltrates and smooth-muscle hyperplasia; (3) bronchiolectasia with mucous stasis, distortion, and fibrosis; and (4) total obliterative bronchiolar scarring.[9] These lesions are seen most often in patients with progressive obstructive lung disease.

TABLE 54-1

Clinical Syndromes Associated with Bronchiolitis

Inhalational injury	*Drug-induced reactions*
Toxic gases (e.g., oxides of nitrogen)	Penicillamine
Grain dusts	Hexamethonium
Irritant gases (e.g., chlorine)	L-Tryptophan
Mineral dusts	Busulfan
Organic dusts (hypersensitivity pneumonitis)	Gold
Cigarette smoke	Cephalosporin
Free-base cocaine	Sulfasalazine
Fire smoke	Amiodarone
	Acebutolol
Postinfectious (mostly in children)	Sulindac
Acute bronchiolitis	Paraquat poisoning
Common	
Respiratory syncytial virus	*Idiopathic*
Parainfluenza (types 1, 2, and 3)	No associated disease
Adenovirus (types 1, 2, 3, 5, 6, 7, and 21)	Cryptogenic constrictive bronchiolitis
Mycoplasma pneumoniae	Respiratory bronchiolitis-associated interstitial lung disease
Uncommon	Cryptogenic organizing pneumonia (also called idiopathic
Coronavirus	bronchiolitis obliterans–organizing pneumonia, BOOP)
Rubeola	Diffuse panbronchiolitis
Mumps	Primary diffuse hyperplasia of pulmonary neuroendocrine
Varicella zoster	cells
Influenza	Associated with other disease
Rhinovirus	Associated with organ transplantation
Parvovirus B_{19}	Bone marrow
Enteroviruses	Heart-lung
Bronchiolitis obliterans	Lung
Herpes simplex virus	Associated with connective-tissue diseases
Human immunodeficiency virus (HIV)	Rheumatoid arthritis
Cytomegalovirus	Sjögren's syndrome
Rubeola	Systemic lupus erythematosus
Parainfluenza (type 3)	Polymyositis dermatomyositis
Adenovirus	Distal to bronchial obstruction ("obstructive pneumonitis")
Mycoplasma pneumoniae	Ulcerative colitis
Klebsiella	Chronic eosinophilic pneumonia
Hemophilus influenzae	Other rare associations
Legionella pneumophila	Radiation pneumonitis
Serratia marcescens	Aspiration pneumonitis
Bordetella pertussis	Idiopathic pulmonary fibrosis
Streptococcus group B, beta-hemolytic	Malignant histiocytosis
Cryptococcus neoformans	Acute respiratory distress syndrome
Nocardia asteroides	Vasculitis, especially Wegener's granulomatosis
Pneumocystis carinii	Chronic thyroiditis

SOURCE: Data from King[35] and Penn and Liu.[47]

A normal chest radiograph may be present. Cases of constrictive bronchiolitis are very rare.

Pathogenesis

A similar sequence of events may lead to both histopathologic patterns of bronchiolitis. However, differences appear to relate to the type of insult, extent and severity of the initial insult, and predominant site of the injury (bronchioles, alveolar ducts, or both). In some diseases associated with bronchiolitis, varying degrees of both proliferative and constrictive bronchiolitis can be found on histologic examination.

The initial lesion in constrictive bronchiolitis usually involves airway epithelial injury and destruction (Fig. 54-3). An inflammatory response follows, with accumulation of neutrophils at the site of injury. Neutrophils cause further injury to the airway epithelium and matrix by release of inflammatory mediators. Persistence of the injury may determine whether there is resolution and recovery

TABLE 54-2

Comparison of Key Pathologic, Radiologic and Physiologic Features in Proliferative and Constrictive Bronchiolitis

Feature	Proliferative Bronchiolitis	Constrictive Bronchiolitis
Histopathologic manifestations	Common finding Nonspecific reparative reaction to bronchiolar injury Organizing intraluminal exudate Most prominent in alveolar ducts Inflammatory changes in surrounding alveolar walls Foamy macrophages in alveoli	Very uncommon finding Obliterans not a constant feature Variety of histologic changes: bronchiolar inflammation to progressive concentric fibrosis; smooth-muscle hyperplasia, bronchioloectasia with mucous stasis; distortion and fibrosis of small-airway walls with bronchial metaplasia extending onto peribronchiolar alveolar septa Follicular bronchitis (lymphoid hyperplasia) Cellular bronchiolitis Diffuse panbronchiolitis
Radiographic abnormalities	Bilateral patchy airspace opacities Interstitial opacities Small rounded opacities Opacities may be recurrent and migratory	May be normal Progressive increase in lung volume on serial radiographs HRCT scan may show marked heterogeneity of lung density
Pulmonary function	Restrictive defect (a mixed pattern may be seen)	Obstructive defect with hyperinflation
Clinical syndromes	Cryptogenic organizing pneumonia (idiopathic BOOP) Collagen vascular disease (e.g., rheumatoid arthritis, dermatomyositis, SLE) Organizing acute infection (especially influenza or *Nocardia asteroides,* Mycoplasma, *Pneumocystis carinii, Legionella pneumophila,* cytomegalovirus, or HIV infection) Chronic eosinophilic pneumonia Hypersensitivity pneumonitis Organizing diffuse alveolar damage/adult respiratory distress syndrome (ARDS) Vasculitides, especially Wegener's granulomatosis Organ transplantation (rare) Drug-induced reactions (hexamethonium, L-tryptophan, busulfan, free-base cocaine, gold, cephalosporin, sulfasalazine, amiodarone, acebutolol, sulindac) Other uncommon associations: chronic thyroiditis, ulcerative colitis, irradiation pneumonitis, aspiration pneumonitis, distal to bronchial obstruction, "obstructive pneumonitis," chronic heart or renal failure, common variable immunodeficiency syndrome	Allograft recipients (bone marrow, heart-lung, lung) Collagen vascular disease (especially rheumatoid arthritis) Postinfectious (especially respiratory syncytial virus, adenovirus, influenza, parainfluenza, Mycoplasma) Inhaled toxins (e.g., nitrogen dioxide, sulfur dioxide, ammonia, chlorine, phosgene) Drugs (e.g., penicillamine, lomustine) Cigarette smoke Mineral dust airway disease (asbestosis, silica, iron oxide, aluminum oxide, talc, mica, and coal) Idiopathic Hypersensitivity reactions
Natural history	Corticosteroid responsive and usually reversible	Relatively corticosteroid unresponsive and usually progressive with the development of irreversible airflow obstruction and air trapping

SOURCE: Adapted from King.[34]

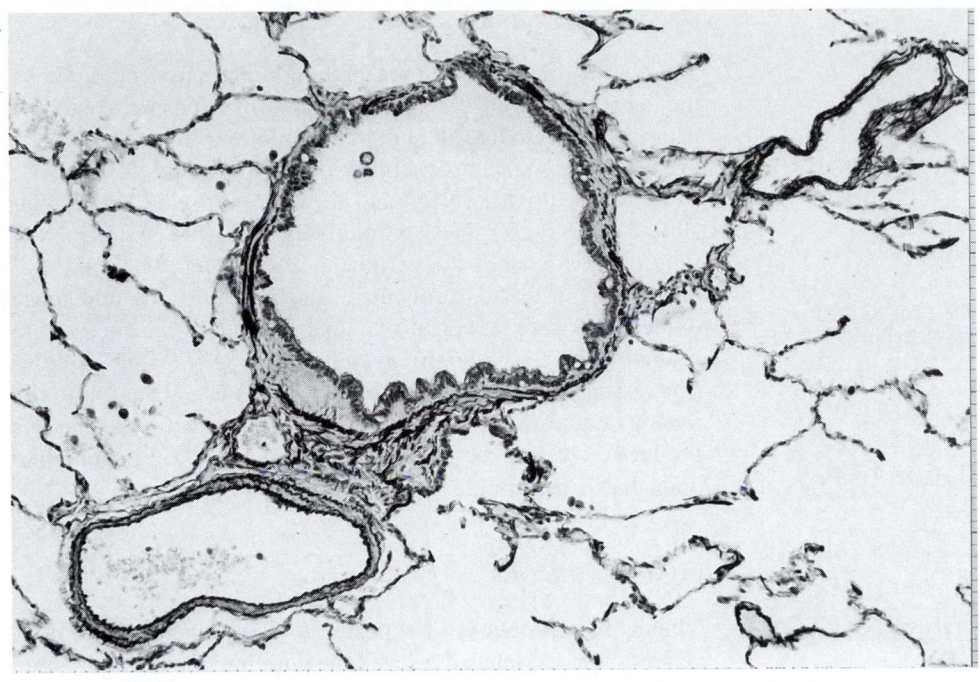

A

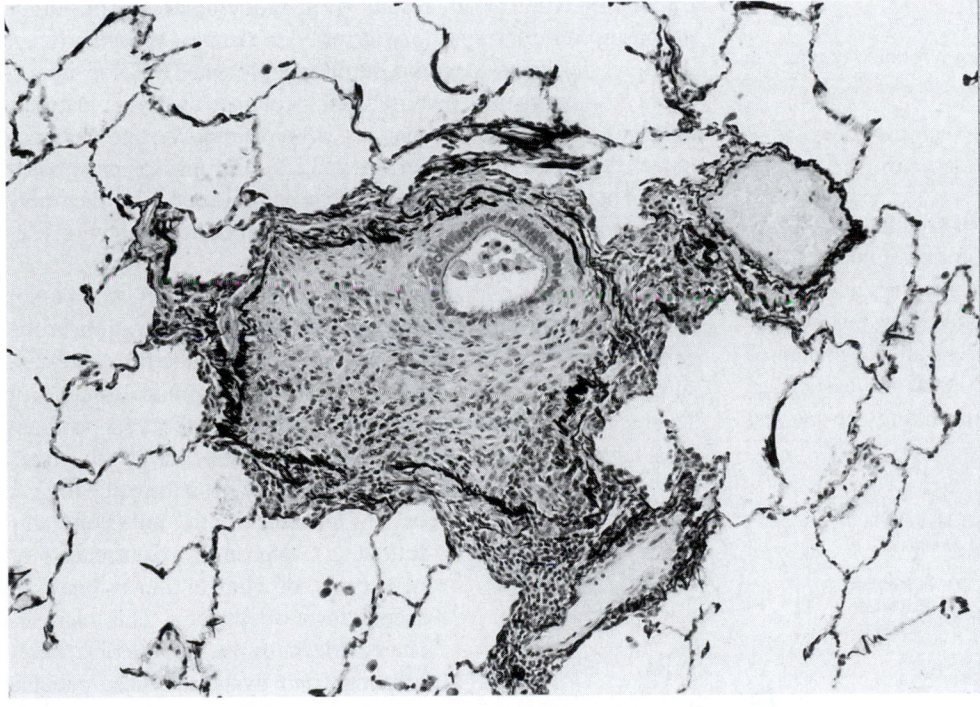

B

FIGURE 54-2   Constrictive bronchiolitis. Photomicrograph of open lung biopsy from a patient with constrictive bronchiolitis following toxic gas exposure. *A.* Slightly dilated but otherwise normal bronchiole with normal intervening lung. (Pentachrome stain, ×156.) *B.* Step-section of specimen. Marked concentric narrowing of the bronchiolar lumen due to fibrosis is apparent. (Pentachrome stain, ×156.)

termediary steps in the development of intraluminal, extracellular matrix synthesis have been clarified (Fig. 54-4).[39,40,48] First, a florid alveolitis with edema occurs as a result of damage to the alveolar lining. The degree of alveolar lining destruction and disruption of the basal lamina, with resulting gaps on the basement membrane, appears to determine the extent of intra-alveolar fibrosis.[39] Although the alveolar basement membrane is most frequently damaged, minor changes are also noted in the endothelial basement membrane.[48] The alveolitis coincides with the presence of inflammatory proteins in the airspace, including immunoglobulins (IgG, IgA, and IgM), fibronectin, and procoagulant factors (fibrinogen and factors VII and X). The cellular response includes neutrophils, eosinophils, macrophages, and lymphocytes. Many mast cells are also present in the septal and intra-alveolar compartments.[48]

After development of the alveolitis, fibroblasts migrate into the lesion, proliferate, and secrete matrix proteins. This results in the formation of Masson bodies, polypoid buds of fibroblasts, and extracellular matrix projecting into the lumina of respiratory bronchioles, alveolar ducts, and alveoli. The matrix of the Masson bodies stain positive for type III collagen and fibronectin (cell and plasma in origin). The fibroblasts in the Masson bodies also stain strongly for procollagen type I. Delicate fibrils within the matrix of some Masson bodies contain type IV collagen.[39] Inflammatory changes in the surrounding alveolar walls, including prominent foamy macrophages in the alveoli spaces (i.e., organizing pneumonia), are commonly present.[39,40,48]

INHALATIONAL LUNG INJURY CAUSING BRONCHIOLITIS

The inhalation of fumes, gases, mists, mineral dusts, or organic material constitutes a significant industrial and environmental hazard in many settings (Table 54-3). Exposure can result in subtle or severe clinical illness, usually associated with immediate development of pulmonary edema and late development of constrictive bronchiolitis with airflow limitation.

or progression to a less reversible state, manifested by intramural and intraluminal fibrosis. The repair process results in the characteristic obliterative bronchiolar lesions.

In general, "proliferative" bronchiolitis appears to be a common "early" lesion that may resolve completely or partly. In-

Insult

Injury or destruction of small airway epithelium

Acute and chronic inflammatory response

Repair by proliferation of granulation tissue

Intramural and intraluminal fibrosis

Airway obliteration

FIGURE 54-3 Proposed pathogenetic mechanism for airway injury in constrictive bronchiolitis. (See text for details).

Toxic Gases

The inhalation of gases or fumes (i.e., fine particulates) is a rare cause of bronchiolitis, with or without obliterans. Oxides of nitrogen are the most common and best-described agents leading to acute and chronic lung injury. Silo filler's disease is a well-studied example (Fig. 54-5).[17,65] The estimated annual incidence of silo filler's disease is 5.0 cases per 100,000 silo-associated farm workers per year.[65] Most cases occur during the harvest period (September and October).

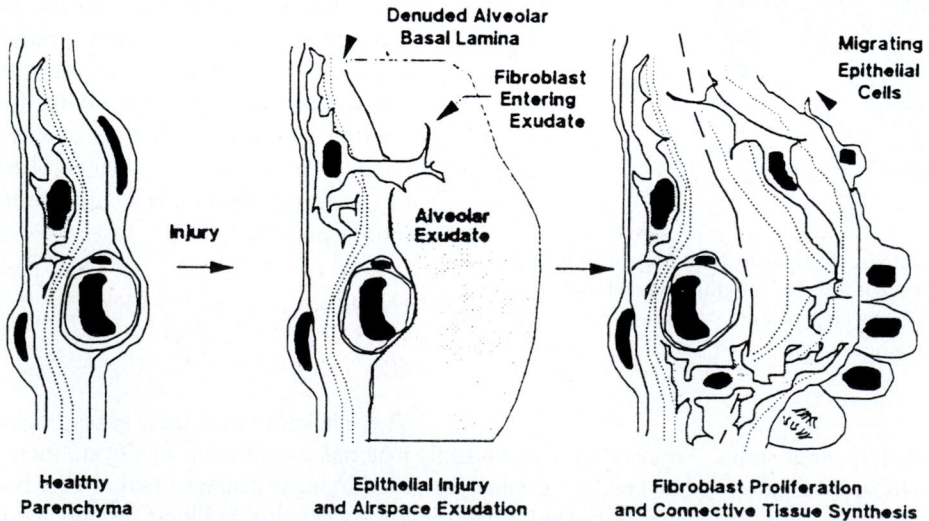

FIGURE 54-4 Schematic illustration of focal intraluminal extracellular matrix synthesis in chronic pulmonary fibrosis. (*Based on data from Kuhn et al,[39] with permission.*)

MECHANISM OF INJURY

The distribution and extent of the lung injury are determined by the concentration of the agent, duration of exposure, route and pattern of breathing, solubility and biologic reactivity of the agent, and biologic susceptibility of the individual.[16]

Nitrogen dioxide (NO_2) and nitrogen tetroxide are responsible for the injury. NO_2 is relatively insoluble. After inhalation, the gas reaches the periphery of the lung, where it combines with water to form nitric and nitrous acids and nitric oxide, which are powerful oxidants capable of causing severe tissue injury. Unlike highly water-soluble gases, such as chlorine, ammonia, and sulfur dioxide, NO_2 is less irritating to the mucous membranes of the nasal and upper airways. The gas produces a yellow to brown haze and an acrid, ammonialike odor that is irritating.

CLINICAL FINDINGS

Clinical manifestations of exposure to NO_2 depend on the concentration of the inhaled gas and the duration of exposure. Three clinical patterns or phases may follow exposure.[35]

Sudden death may occur in persons exposed to high concentrations of NO_2. Death results from bronchiolar spasm, laryngospasm, reflex respiratory arrest, or simple asphyxiation.[28] Acutely, during milder exposures, people may develop upper-airway and visual disturbances, cough, dyspnea, fatigue, cyanosis, vomiting, hemoptysis, hypoxemia, vertigo, somnolence, headache, emotional difficulties, and loss of consciousness. These findings usually resolve within hours, but they may persist for several weeks; complete recovery without obvious sequelae is usually observed.

At higher concentrations of exposure, pulmonary edema (so-called chemical pneumonitis) is a frequent complication in the early stages. Patients may be asymptomatic at the time of exposure, only to later develop (in 3 to 30 h) the clinical picture of severe acute respiratory distress syndrome. Recovery without long-term sequelae is usual, but death may occur at this stage.

After recovery from the acute illness, or in patients with no symptoms following exposure, recurrence or new onset of clinical illness may be seen 2 to 6 weeks later. This phase is characterized by the progressive onset of cough and dyspnea. These patients may be identified in an early, asymptomatic stage from the appearance of mild hypoxemia. Tachypnea is present, and rales are usually heard. Widespread proliferative bronchiolitis with marked intraluminal fibrous tissue proliferation arising in the bronchiolar wall (without organizing pneumonia) is found, especially in those with preceding pulmonary edema; however, these findings may occur as the initial manifestation of previous exposure.

TABLE 54-3

Toxic Exposures Associated with Bronchiolitis, with or without Obliterans

Nitrogen dioxide ("nitrous fume")*

Spillage of nitric acid (component of jet and missile fuels)

Metal pickling

Silo gas

Chemical manufacturing (explosives, dyes, lacquers, celluloid)

Detonation of explosives

Electric arc or acetylene gas welding

Contamination of anesthetic gases (nitrous oxide gas cylinder)

Nitrocellulose combustion

Tobacco smoke

Fire smoke (firemen, astronauts, others exposed to burning materials)*†

Sulfur dioxide†

Burning of sulfur-containing fossil fuels

Bleaching of wool, straw, wood pulp

Sugar refining, fruit preserving

Fungicides

Refrigerants

Ore smelting

Acid production

Ammonia†

Fertilizer and explosives, production, refrigeration

Chlorine‡

Bleaching, disinfectant and plastic making

Phosgene*

Chemical industry, dye and insecticide manufacturing

Chloropicrin

Trichlorethylene

Ozone

Arc welding and air, sewage, and water treatment

Cadmium oxide

Ore smelting, alloying, and welding

Methyl sulfate

Hydrogen sulfide

Natural gas retrieval, paper pulp, sewage treatment, tannery work

Hydrogen fluoride

Etching, petroleum industry, silk working

Talcum powder (hydrous magnesium silicate)

Stearate of zinc powder

Oxygen toxicity

Asbestos (chrysotile and amphibole)

Iron oxide§

Aluminum oxide§

Silica§

Sheet silicates (talc, mica, etc.)§

Coal§

Activated charcoal

Talc

Free-base cocaine*

*These agents have been associated with the development of bronchiolitis obliterans (intraluminal polyps).[28]
†These agents have been associated with the development of constrictive bronchiolitis.[28]
‡These agents have been associated with the development of histologic focal bronchiolitis without significant clinical disease.[28]
§These agents have been associated with the development of respiratory bronchiolitis.
SOURCE: Data from King.[35]

In the acute phase, patients who develop pulmonary edema and acute respiratory distress syndrome have significant pulmonary dysfunction. Hypoxemia is secondary to ventilation-perfusion mismatching as a result of altered airway dynamics and interstitial and alveolar edema, impaired diffusing capacity, and methemoglobinemia that occurs when nitrate ions react with hemoglobin. Severe metabolic acidosis occurs because of the dissolution of NO_2 in body fluids, resulting in formation of nitrous and nitric acid, as well as the lactic acidosis resulting from tissue hypoxia. Systemic hypertension may be present. The radiographic manifestations during this stage include pulmonary edema (i.e., alveolar filling). In survivors, these changes clear rapidly. Physiological studies reveal the simultaneous occurrence of restrictive and obstructive ventilatory defects; the former is manifest as a shift in the static pressure-volume curve downward and to the right. These abnormalities gradually resolve in survivors. Histopathologic findings, as determined from autopsy studies, include marked intra-alveolar edema and exudation, as well as thickening of the alveolar walls with lymphocytic cellular infiltrates.

In patients who progress to the second phase, physiological disturbances include hypoxemia at rest or with exercise and associated restrictive or obstructive pulmonary function abnormalities. The radiographic pattern in this late stage may be variable. A normal chest film may be seen; however, a miliary, or discretely nodular, pattern is thought to be characteristic of bronchiolitis obliterans. Occasionally, only pulmonary hyperinflation is seen, usually accompanied by a progressive and irreversible obstructive ventilatory defect noted on lung function testing.

MANAGEMENT

The treatment of patients exposed to NO_2 or other toxic gases or fumes should include observation in the hospital for 48 h, followed by weekly or biweekly evaluations for 6 to 8 weeks. When

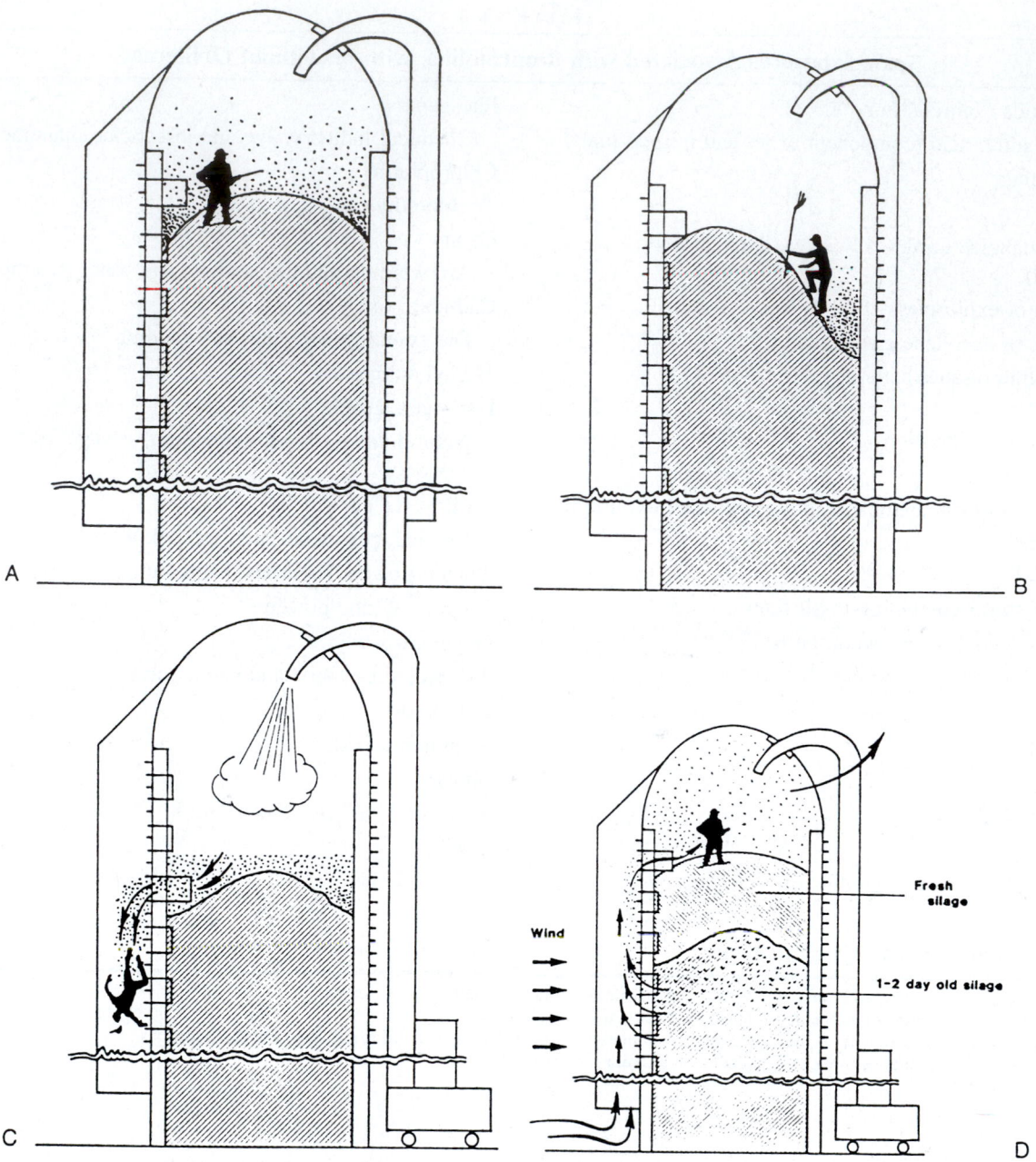

FIGURE 54-5 Exposure to nitrogen oxides and silo filler's disease. The upright concrete stave silo is the most common type of silo. Chopped silage is blown through the filling pipe (on right of silo) to the top of the silo and dispersed evenly. *A.* Exposure usually occurs 1 to 4 days after silo filling, when the farmer enters to level the silage, to prepare for unloading, or to spread a plastic sheet over the top. *B.* Silo gas is heavier than air and accumulates in low places within the silo. Descent into these areas may be fatal. *C.* Opening a door just above the silage may result in concentrated exposure, causing rapid loss of consciousness and a fall down the silo chute. *D.* Entry immediately after completion of silo filling may not be safe, since gas from 1- to 2-day-old silage may leak out through the silo doors and be drawn into the working spaces by a chimneylike updraft. *(Based on data from Douglas and Colby,[16] with permission.)*

dysfunction occurs, treatment with corticosteroids should be started immediately. Corticosteroid therapy has been demonstrated to be useful in the management of both the acute phase (pulmonary edema) and the late phase (bronchiolitis obliterans). Corticosteroids should be continued for a minimum of 8 weeks, since relapses have been reported with the earlier cessation of therapy. Bronchodilators are occasionally helpful, but antibiotics should be used only when clinically indicated; they should be

directed at a specific pathogen. If methemoglobinemia is present, methylene blue should be administered at a dose of 2 mg/kg intravenously, followed by doses titrated according to the concentration of methemoglobin in the blood. For patients in whom this diagnosis is suspected, and for whom open lung biopsy or general anesthesia is planned, some have suggested that nitrous oxide not be used as an anesthetic because of concern that it might lead to disease progression.

PROGNOSIS

In general, the prognosis for survivors of toxic gas or fume inhalation (fewer than one-third die acutely) is good. Some authors have suggested that lasting pulmonary disability is uncommon in silo filler's disease; others have identified a wide variety of functional derangements. What functional abnormalities result from chronic, low-level exposure to NO_2 are not clear. Education is key in preventing this disease, since simple measures to reduce the NO_2 levels and use of approved respiratory protection equipment will eliminate the risk of injury.

Other Irritant Gases

A number of irritant gases have occasionally been associated with bronchiolitis, with or without obliterans (Table 54-3). Since lung biopsies have not been performed in all cases, it is not always clear that the pulmonary injury associated with these inhalation exposures is only bronchiolitis obliterans. However, sulfur dioxide, chlorine gas, "smoke inhalation" or inhalation burns, hydrogen chloride, ammonia, phosgene, and chloropicrin produce a disease with clinical, physiological, and radiographic manifestations similar to those described for NO_2 exposure. Respiratory bronchiolitis after exposure to photochemical air pollutants, ozone, and NO_2, has been reviewed.[58]

Mineral Dusts

Pathologic changes in the small airways (respiratory bronchiolitis) may be found secondary to exposure to inorganic mineral dusts, including asbestos, silica, iron oxide, aluminum oxide, several different sheet silicates, and coal.[59] Clinical relevance of the changes remains to be better defined. Nonetheless, development of an obstructive, rather than restrictive, pattern is increasingly recognized in subjects with inorganic mineral dust exposure.

Pathologically, these lesions are characterized by marked abnormalities in the small airways, particularly in the membranous and respiratory bronchioles. The principal finding is fibrosis in small-airway walls and, occasionally, in alveolar ducts. The lesions appear to extend down into the airway and often are accompanied by pigment deposition. Abnormalities are seen in nonsmokers, but occur most commonly in heavily exposed workers who are cigarette smokers. The pathogenesis is unclear, but a synergistic role for cigarette smoking appears likely. The injury appears to result from the inflammatory response that follows deposition of mineral particles or fibers in the walls of the small airways.[6]

Organic Dusts

Numerous agents are associated with the development of hypersensitivity pneumonitis, a topic discussed elsewhere (see Chapter 71). Interstitial pneumonitis is seen in virtually 100 percent, and granulomas in approximately 70 percent, of patients with hypersensitivity pneumonitis; unappreciated is that bronchiolar lesions are also seen in essentially all cases. The bronchioles contain granulomas within the walls or lumina—or show tufts of granulation tissue, as seen in bronchiolitis obliterans. A reversible restrictive process is the most common physiological abnormality in hypersensitivity pneumonitis. However, small-airway dysfunction may be present in patients with early hypersensitivity pneumonitis. As the disease progresses, either obstructive or restrictive physiology may arise, depending on the predominant histopathologic process present.

INFECTIOUS CAUSES OF BRONCHIOLITIS

Infection is the most common cause of acute bronchiolitis, although infectious causes are more frequent in children than adults. The usual agents include viruses and *Mycoplasma pneumoniae*—organisms that have a propensity to infect and injure epithelial cells of the respiratory tract. Constrictive bronchiolitis is the most common histopathologic pattern observed after bronchiolar infection.

Infectious Bronchiolitis in Children

Acute bronchiolitis is a common illness in infants and young children, occurring primarily as a result of a viral infection. Pathogens include respiratory syncytial virus (approximately 34 percent of cases), parainfluenza virus types 1, 2, and 3 (approximately 30 percent of cases), adenoviruses (approximately 7 percent of cases), influenza A and B, and *M. pneumoniae* (approximately 11 percent of cases) (Table 54-1). Males are more commonly affected with respiratory syncytial virus than are females (1.5–1.8:1 male-to-female ratio). Reviews of bronchiolitis in children have been published recently.[25,47,57] Infectious bronchiolitis obliterans is rarely seen in persons older than 2 years. Adenovirus types 3, 7, and 21 are the most common etiologic agents. Other causes are measles, whooping cough due to *Bordetella pertussis, M. pneumoniae,* and influenza A. Severe infectious bronchiolitis obliterans leading to hospitalization and death is rare.

CLINICAL FINDINGS

The usual presentation is an acute virallike illness with mild coryza and sneezing occurring during the winter months. Several days later, cough, dyspnea, tachypnea, tachycardia, fever, chest wall retractions, sibilant and sonorous rales, expiratory wheezing, and, in severe cases, cyanosis develop. Prostration and respiratory failure are unusual.

RADIOGRAPHIC FINDINGS

The radiographic pattern of childhood bronchiolitis is variable. The chest radiograph may be normal or show hyperinflation with increased bronchial markings. Subsegmental consolidation and collapse may be seen. A pattern similar to that of diffuse interstitial pneumonia, often in association with hyperinflation, is seen. Some patients demonstrate a diffuse nodular or reticulonodular pattern, whereas others may show patchy alveolar or ground-glass opacities. Those with a nodular pattern frequently have "pure" bronchiolitis obliterans on lung biopsy; those with a reticulonodular pattern are likely to have more interstitial inflammation and scarring. The role of high-resolution computed tomography (HRCT) has not been adequately defined, but it is thought to be important in ruling out other diagnoses, especially bronchiectasis. Ventilation-perfusion lung scans may be very helpful, since a markedly abnormal pattern of patchy, matched ventilation and perfusion defects is often seen, even when the plain chest film is unremarkable. Bronchography may reveal saccular bronchiectasis and ballooning of the airways at the blind end when the airways are distended by positive pressure; passage of contrast medium into the alveoli does not occur. Bronchography has largely been abandoned with the advent of HRCT.

PHYSIOLOGIC FINDINGS

Tests of lung function may be normal. However, obstructive changes with air trapping can often be documented. Pulmonary function testing has not been well studied in infants with this disease. Resting hypoxemia is frequently present.

HISTOPATHOLOGIC FINDINGS

In this setting, open lung biopsy is the gold standard for the diagnosis of bronchiolitis obliterans. The earliest change is necrosis of the respiratory epithelium, followed by epithelial proliferation. Dense plugs of alveolar debris and strands of fibrin are seen within small bronchi and bronchioles, causing partial or complete obstruction. These findings may develop as soon as 8 days after the onset of the illness. A lymphocytic infiltrate, including collections with germinal centers, may be seen in the airway wall. Severe and widespread destruction of the respiratory epithelium may cause denudation and a pronounced inflammatory response that involves the adjacent peribronchial space and alveolar walls. Depending on the stage at which the biopsy is obtained, findings consistent with proliferative bronchiolitis ("early"), constrictive bronchiolitis ("late"), or both may be seen. The pathogenetic mechanisms in development of obliterative bronchiolitis secondary to infections and the reason for the predilection in infants are unknown.

MANAGEMENT

Treatment is symptomatic, including administration of supplemental oxygen and adequate hydration. Bronchodilators, antibiotics, antiviral agents, and corticosteroids are frequently used in management, but few controlled clinical trials on their efficacy have been performed. Mechanical ventilation is rarely required; it may be necessary if progressive respiratory failure ensues. Lung transplantation has been performed in severe cases.

PROGNOSIS

Recovery is usual and occurs in days or weeks. Whether or not bronchiolitis in infancy predisposes to asthma or chronic obstructive pulmonary disease (COPD) in later life remains unproved.

Swyer-James (MacLeod) syndrome—unilateral hyperlucent lung—is a long-term complication of bronchiolitis in children, especially after adenoviral infection occurring in infancy. The affected child may be asymptomatic, but more often he or she has recurrent pulmonary infections and eventually develops bronchiectasis. Dyspnea on exertion, hemoptysis, and chronic productive cough are seen. Patients may have localized, unilateral, or bilateral involvement. The chest radiograph demonstrates lobar or unilateral hyperlucent lung; normal or reduced volume of the affected lung is noted on full inspiration. Severe airway obstruction occurs during expiration. The affected lung has a diminished pulmonary vascular bed, decreased pulmonary blood flow, and reduced peripheral vascular markings. Bronchography demonstrates diffuse bronchiectasis with absence of filling of the terminal bronchioles ("pruned tree" appearance) (see Chapter 132). HRCT is the procedure of choice for identifying the characteristic changes in Swyer-James syndrome.[42]

The final size of the affected lung in Swyer-James syndrome relates to the age of the patient at the time bronchiolitis occurs. If it occurs early in life, the lung fails to grow normally and appears smaller than the opposite lung. If the bronchiolitis occurs later in childhood, the lung may be of normal size. Pulmonary function tests reveal airflow obstruction and a reduced total lung capacity in cases where concomitant pulmonary fibrosis exists. The syndrome has been reported with a number of etiologic agents and must be distinguished from congenital absence of the pulmonary artery, pulmonary artery occlusion, partial obstruction of a lobar or main bronchus, and congenital lobar emphysema. Computed tomography and pulmonary angiography are helpful in distinguishing among these conditions.

Infectious Bronchiolitis in Adults

Acute bronchiolitis in older children and young adults has been associated primarily with M. pneumoniae; however, a number of other viruses (e.g., respiratory syncytial virus, especially in the elderly) and bacterial agents have been identified (Table 54-1). Only sporadic cases of bronchiolitis obliterans secondary to infections have been reported in adults (Fig. 54-6).[12,47]

The clinical presentation of infectious bronchiolitis in adults is ill defined; no systematic study has been reported. Most patients have a history of an upper respiratory tract illness that precedes the onset of dyspnea with exertion, cough, tachypnea, fever, and wheezing. Measles, varicella-zoster, and pertussis have been reported to cause bronchiolitis obliterans in adults. A number of adults have developed an acute or subacute diffuse ventilatory obstruction that has occasionally been fatal.

IDIOPATHIC FORMS OF BRONCHIOLITIS

Several clinicopathologic syndromes associated with prominent bronchiolar impairment have been reported recently. Although no specific origins have been identified, the constellation of find-

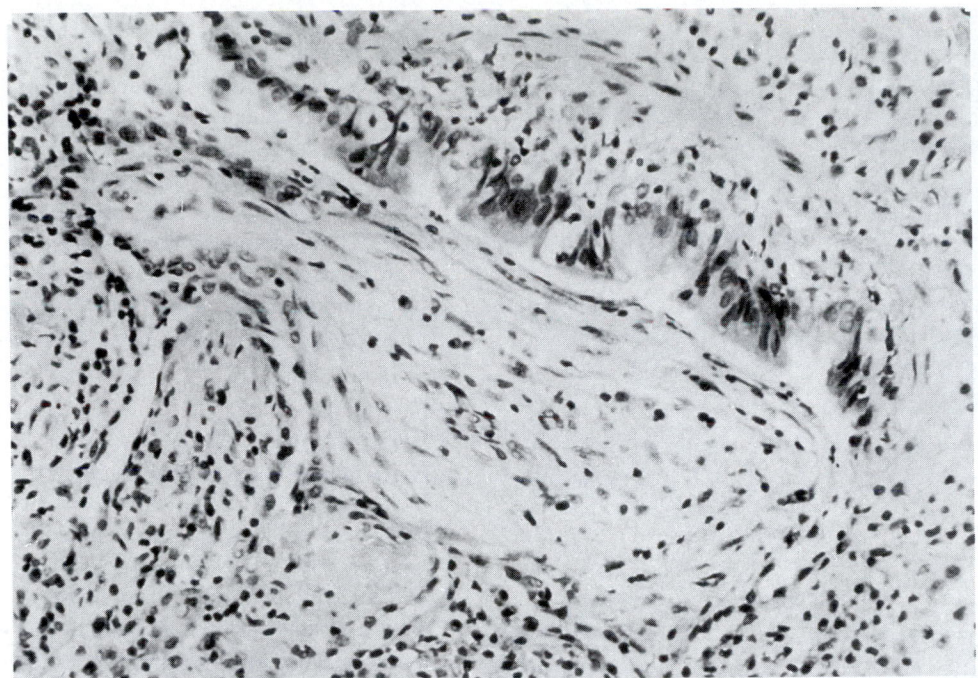

FIGURE 54-6   Acute infectious bronchiolitis. Photomicrograph showing acute bronchiolitis in a patient with adenovirus infection. An intraluminal infiltrate associated with epithelial necrosis (lower left) is present. In addition, a peribronchiolar infiltrate of acute and chronic inflammatory cells is demonstrated. (H&E stain, ×156.)

CLINICAL FINDINGS

Most patients are middle-aged women who have a nonproductive cough, shortness of breath, or other nonspecific chest complaints, usually of relatively short duration (6 to 24 months). Most are identified because of an accelerated, severe obstructive respiratory disorder that is clinically distinct from the more commonly encountered obstructive disorders. A history of cigarette smoking, chronic sputum production, frequent chest infections, wheezing, known connective-tissue disorder, and immunoglobulin deficiency are absent. No association with inhalation injury or viral infection has been identified. Physical findings are unremarkable, although wheezing or crackles may be heard.

DIAGNOSTIC STUDIES

The chest radiographic findings are normal or nonspecific. Increased bronchial wall thickening may be seen. Hyperinflation (without marked flattening or hyperlucent areas) may be the only abnormality noted. HRCT scanning is normal or shows airway dilatation.

Pulmonary function testing yields a variety of results. Most patients have increased lung volumes and airflow limitation. A few patients who have had pressure-volume curves performed show an upward shift and a normal slope, consistent with airflow limitation. The diffusing capacity is reduced, and resting hypoxemia may be present. Exercise testing shows gas exchange abnormalities associated with an abnormal V_D/V_T.

Bronchoalveolar lavage (BAL) studies demonstrate marked neutrophilia associated with an increase in the specific neutrophil products, collagenase and myeloperoxidase. Most patients have a neutrophil level over 25 percent (normal for nonsmokers, under 4 percent); some have levels exceeding 90 percent.

ings in reported cases suggests that these syndromes are unique and must be distinguished from more common problems, including COPD, pneumonia, and pulmonary fibrosis. In the discussion below, three syndromes are highlighted: cryptogenic adult bronchiolitis, respiratory bronchiolitis–associated interstitial lung disease (RB-ILD), and cryptogenic organizing pneumonia (COP) or idiopathic BOOP.

Cryptogenic "Adult" Bronchiolitis

Cryptogenic adult bronchiolitis is a rare clinicopathologic syndrome that must be distinguished from asthma, chronic bronchitis, emphysema, cystic fibrosis, bronchiectasis, and α_1-antitrypsin deficiency. Few cases have been reported, and it is not entirely clear that all of those reported are the same entity. For example, many patients have had a significant cigarette smoking history and may have smoker's bronchiolitis. Despite these concerns, the constellation of findings in reported cases is unique and suggests that adult bronchiolitis represents a distinct, definable clinicopathologic entity that is a diagnostic challenge to clinicians and pathologists.[15,18,33,38]

The pathogenesis of cryptogenic adult bronchiolitis is unknown. The true incidence of the disease is also unknown, but has been estimated to be approximately 4 percent of all causes of obstructive lung diseases. The disorder is diagnosed largely by exclusion and requires a high index of suspicion, along with an awareness of its unique clinical features.

PATHOLOGIC FINDINGS

Lung biopsies reveal a cellular constrictive bronchiolitis, often quite subtle, with both acute and chronic inflammatory changes, primarily in the membranous bronchioles (Fig. 54-7). Few cases examined have shown airway obliteration and mucous stasis. The pulmonary parenchyma is normal or shows only mild hyperinflation. Mild focal interstitial fibrosis has been identified in a few subjects. No vascular lesions have been described.

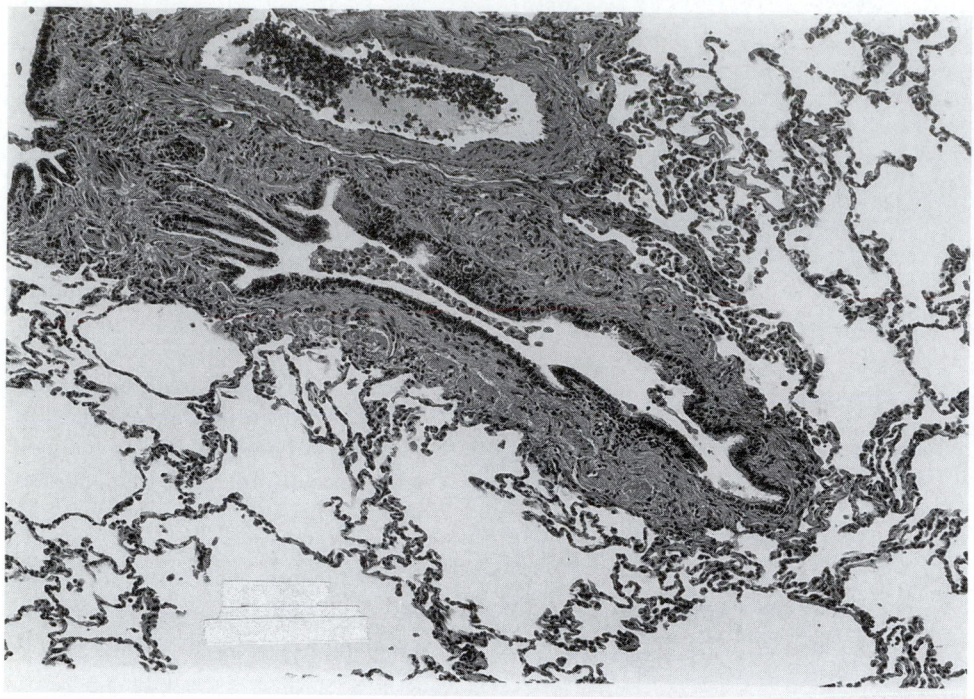

A

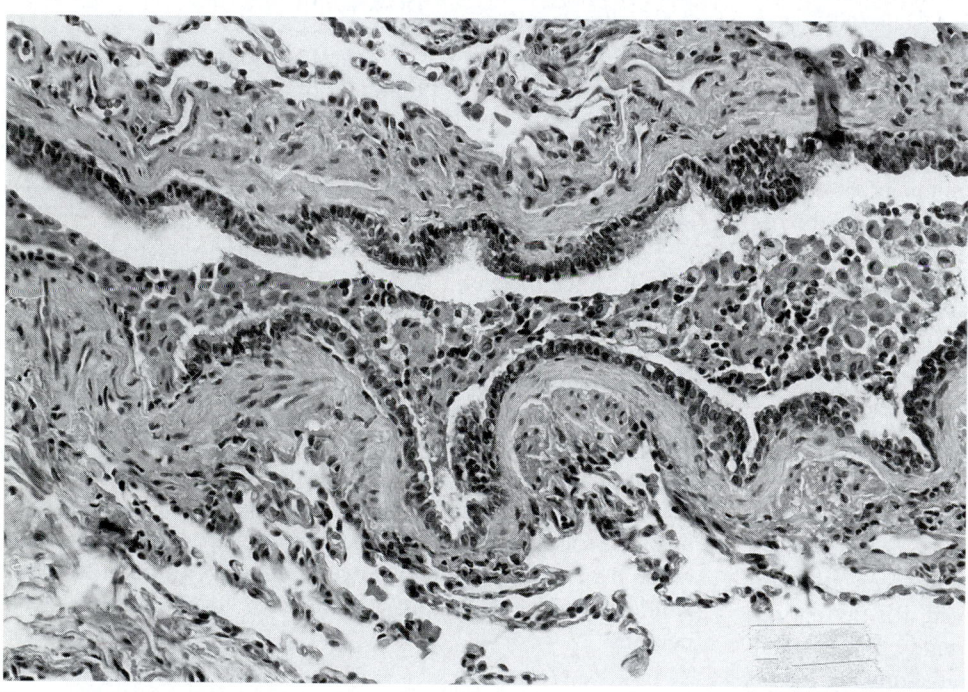

B

FIGURE 54-7   Cryptogenic constrictive bronchiolitis. *A.* Constrictive bronchiolitis with bronchiolar smooth-muscle hyperplasia and mild submucosal and adventitial bronchiolar scarring. Alveolar parenchyma architecture is preserved; no significant interstitial inflammation or fibrosis is present. (H&E stain.) *B.* Histiocytes in the lumen of some bronchioles. While intraluminal histiocytes are common in smokers, their presence in nonsmokers suggests airway pathology analogous to mucus stasis. (H&E stain.) *(Based on data from Kraft et al,[38] with permission.)*

TREATMENT

Steroids may be of benefit in many patients with adult bronchiolitis. Early treatment may be important, since irreversible structural changes and persistent, progressive breathlessness may de-velop, often with recurrent bouts of respiratory infection. BAL neutrophilia returns toward normal in patients who respond to treatment. Thus, recognition of these cases and distinction from other small-airway disorders (e.g., RB-ILD, asthma, chronic bronchitis, emphysema, bronchiolitis associated with connective-tissue disease, and diffuse panbronchiolitis) are possible and important.

Respiratory Bronchiolitis–Associated Interstitial Lung Disease

Bronchiolitis has been demonstrated in patients exposed to cigarette smoke. The inflammation and fibrosis lead to distortion and narrowing of small airways. Because respiratory bronchiolitis was initially found at autopsy in young cigarette smokers without known disease, the lesions were considered to be clinically insignificant. Later, it was hypothesized that the lesions in the respiratory bronchioles could explain the mild abnormalities in lung function seen in cigarette smokers—so-called small-airway disease (i.e., elevated airflow resistance, airway hyperresponsiveness, and subsequent airflow limitation). More recently, RB-ILD has been recognized as a distinct clinical syndrome found in current or previous cigarette smokers.[24,37,44,60,64] This disease may be confused with chronic diffuse interstitial fibrosis, desquamative interstitial pneumonia, and eosinophilic granuloma of the lung (pulmonary histiocytosis X). The last two disorders also develop almost exclusively in cigarette smokers.

CLINICAL FINDINGS

The male-to-female ratio is 1.6:1. Most are current or former smokers in the fourth or fifth decade of life. The average exposure is more than 30 pack-years of cigarette smoking. The incidence of RB-ILD is unknown. Patients commonly present with dyspnea (70 percent) and cough (58 percent). Coarse rales are often heard (33 percent) and occur throughout inspiration; sometimes they continue into expiration. Finger clubbing has not been reported. Routine laboratory studies are usually normal.

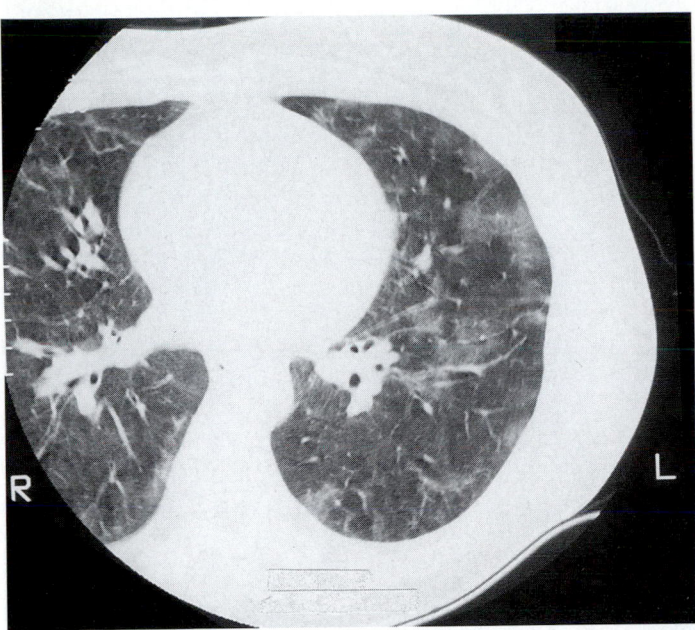

FIGURE 54-8   Respiratory bronchiolitis-associated interstitial lung disease. HRCT in a 35-year-old woman with a heavy smoking history and progressive dyspnea with exertion. Extensive ground-glass opacities are demonstrated. The plain chest film was normal. The diagnosis was confirmed by open lung biopsy. Symptoms improved after smoking cessation.

Diffuse, fine reticulonodular interstitial infiltrates are found on the chest radiograph in most patients (80 percent), usually with normal lung volumes. Bronchial wall thickening, prominence of peri-bronchovascular interstitium, small regular and irregular opacities, and small peripheral ring shadows are distinctive features of respiratory bronchiolitis. Diffuse or patchy ground-glass opacities or fine nodules are found on HRCT (Fig. 54-8). Mild emphysema, atelectasis, or linear and reticular interstitial abnormalities are also detected. In a study correlating pathologic findings with CT abnormalities, areas of ground-glass attenuation were related to three main histologic features: (1) accumulation of pigmented macrophages and mucus in alveolar spaces, associated with mild interstitial inflammation or fibrosis; (2) thickening of alveolar walls by inflammatory cells; and (3) presence of organizing alveolitis. The parenchymal micronodules corresponded to bronchiolectases with peribronchiolar fibrosis.

Pulmonary function may be normal; however, a mixed obstructive-restrictive pattern is most commonly found. Normal TLC and FRC are commonly present, but the RV is usually increased. A normal or slightly reduced D_{LCO} is frequently present. Hypoxemia may be present at rest or with exercise.

HISTOPATHOLOGIC FINDINGS

An inflammatory process in the membranous and respiratory bronchioles is the characteristic histopathologic feature of RB-ILD. Tan-brown pigmented macrophages within respiratory bronchioles, neighboring alveolar ducts, and alveoli dominate the pathologic findings (a "DIP-like" reaction) (Fig. 54-9). These macrophages stain strongly with diastase-predigested periodic acid–Schiff.[64] The bronchiole may be ectatic with mucous stasis; the walls are mildly thickened. There is frequently evidence of extension of the bronchiolar metaplastic epithelium into the immediately surrounding alveoli. Most of the interstitium is usually normal; alternatively, it may demonstrate mild hyperinflation. The findings are sometimes so subtle as to be missed during routine evaluation. On occasion, examination of multiple-step sections may be required. Many cases of respiratory bronchiolitis have actually been misclassified as "desquamative interstitial pneumonia." Similar pathologic findings have been demonstrated in other conditions.

TREATMENT

The clinical course and prognosis of RB-ILD are unknown. Most studies suggest a favorable response to corticosteroids, with documented improvement in the chest radiograph and in lung function. Since smoking appears to play a role in pathogenesis, smoking cessation is considered to be important in management.

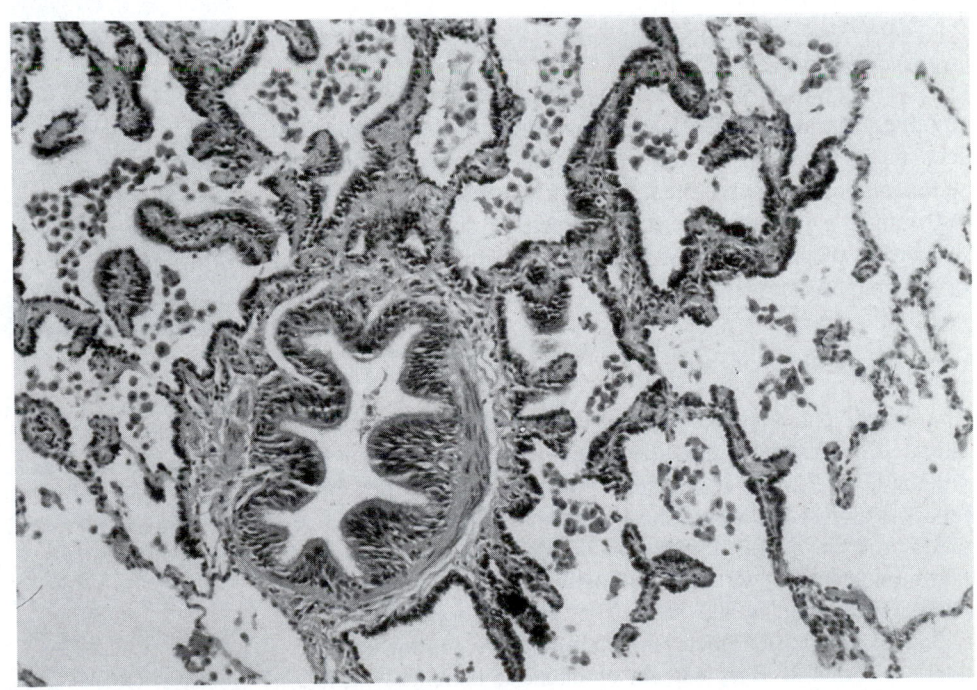

FIGURE 54-9   Respiratory bronchiolitis-associated interstitial lung disease. Photomicrograph shows inflammatory process in the membranous and respiratory bronchioles. Bronchiole wall is thickened, and bronchiolar metaplastic epithelium extends into immediately surrounding alveoli. Macrophages are present within the peribronchiolar alveolar spaces (DIP-like reaction). (H&E stain.) *(Based on data from King and Mortenson,*[37] *with permission.)*

Cryptogenic Organizing Pneumonia

Cryptogenic organizing pneumonia (COP), or idiopathic BOOP, is a distinct clinical entity that was described in 1901 by Lange.[41] However, recognition of COP increased in the early 1980s, as several investigators highlighted the characteristic clinical course and suggested that COP is a distinct entity with features of a pneumonia, rather than a primary airway disorder.[14,19,23] The true incidence and prevalence of COP are unknown; a prevalence of 6 to 7 per 100,000 admissions has been reported.[2]

CLINICAL FINDINGS

Disease onset is usually in the fifth or sixth decade, with a mean age of 58 years; men and women are affected equally. Almost three-quarters of patients have symptoms for less than 2 months; few have symptoms for more than 6 months before diagnosis. Cigarette smoking is not a precipitating factor, since approximately 50 percent of subjects are never smokers, 25 percent are ex-smokers, and only 25 percent are current smokers.[35]

A persistent and usually nonproductive cough is the most common presenting symptom (72 percent of subjects). Frequently, patients experience dyspnea with exertion (66 percent). Disease onset is usually described as a flulike illness, with fever (51 percent), malaise (48 percent), fatigue, and cough. Weight loss of greater than 10 lb is a common complaint (57 percent). The clinical presentation may mimic that of community-acquired pneumonia. Physical examination reveals inspiratory crackles (74 percent); wheezing is rare and is usually present in conjunction with crackles. Clubbing is rare (fewer than 5 percent of patients). Twenty-eight percent of patients in one series had normal pulmonary function.[19]

LABORATORY FINDINGS

Routine laboratory studies are nonspecific. A leukocytosis is seen in approximately half of patients. The initial erythrocyte sedimentation rate is elevated, frequently reaching or exceeding 100 mm/h; a positive C-reactive protein is observed in 70 to 80 percent of patients.[10,30] Autoantibodies are usually negative or only slightly positive.

CHEST IMAGING STUDIES

The radiographic manifestations of COP are quite distinctive: bilateral, diffuse alveolar opacities in the presence of normal lung volume (Fig. 54-10). This pattern was present in 79 percent of reported subjects for whom the radiographic appearance was detailed.[35] A peripheral distribution of opacities, very similar to that thought to be "virtually pathognomic" for chronic eosinophilic pneumonia, is also seen. The alveolar opacities may be unilateral. In addition, recurrent and migratory pulmonary opacities are common. Fifty percent of Japanese patients with idiopathic BOOP demonstrated migration of radiographic shadows.[31] Irregular linear or nodular interstitial infiltrates were rarely present as the sole radiographic manifestation. Honeycombing is rarely seen at presentation and is discussed only as a late manifestation in the few patients who have progressive

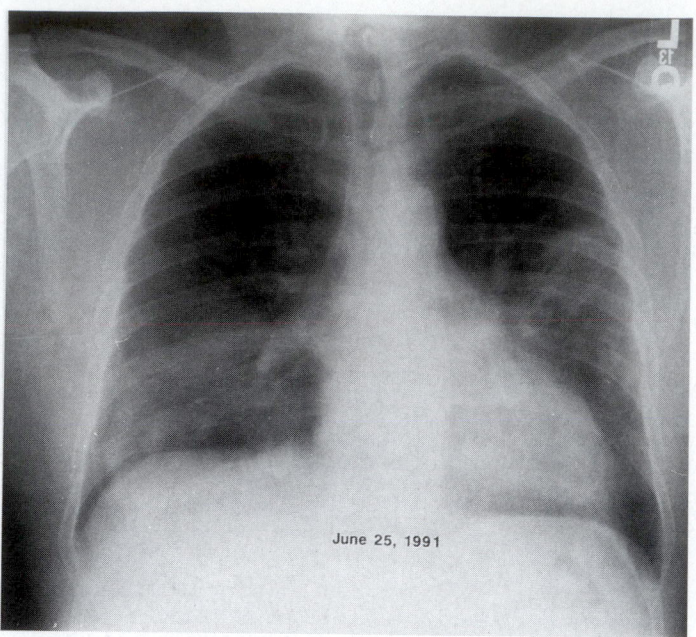

A

June 25, 1991

B

FIGURE 54-10 Cryptogenic organizing pneumonitis in a 62-year-old man with a 1-month history of dyspnea with exertion, fatigue, and weight loss. *A.* Posteroanterior radiograph reveals bilateral patchy alveolar opacities. *B.* CT shows bilateral patchy airspace consolidation in the right and left lower lobes. Air bronchograms are present on the right. Corticosteroid therapy resulted in complete resolution.

disease. Other radiographic abnormalities—such as pleural effusion, pleural thickening, hyperinflation, and lung cavities—seldom occur. Severity of the radiographic abnormalities correlates with the extent of histologic involvement of the respiratory bronchioles and alveolar ducts, but not of the larger terminal bronchioles.

Computed tomography of the lung reveals patchy airspace consolidation, ground-glass opacities, small nodular opacities, and bronchial wall thickening and dilation. These patchy opacities occur more frequently in the periphery of the lung and are often in the lower lung zones (Fig. 54-10). CT may reveal much more extensive disease than is expected from review of the plain chest radiograph.

PHYSIOLOGICAL FINDINGS

Pulmonary function is usually impaired; a restrictive defect is the most common finding.[36] An obstructive defect ($FEV_1/FVC\%$ less than 70 percent) is found uncommonly (in fewer than 21 percent of cases) and is seen mostly in patients who are current or former smokers. Lung function is occasionally normal. The pressure-volume curve is shifted downward and to the right, consistent with noncompliant lungs. The maximal transpulmonary pressure and the coefficient of elastic recoil (maximal transpulmonary pressure divided by total lung capacity) are increased. Gas exchange abnormalities are extremely common. The diffusing capacity ($D_{L_{CO}}$) is reduced in most patients (72 percent). Widening of the resting alveolar arterial oxygen gradient (greater than 20 mmHg) and exercise-related hypoxemia are common abnormalities (83 percent).

BRONCHOALVEOLAR LAVAGE CELLULAR FINDINGS

BAL studies have been reported in only a few subjects with COP. The percentage of instilled fluid recovered from patients with COP is lower than that from healthy volunteers. However, the total number of cells recovered is greater in patients with COP. The proportion of macrophages is lower, while the proportion of lymphocytes, neutrophils, and eosinophils is higher in COP. Patients with COP tend to have higher lymphocyte counts than those with idiopathic pulmonary fibrosis.[45] Other BAL abnormalities in COP include presence of foamy macrophages and, occasionally, mast cells and plasma cells; decreased ratio of CD4 to CD8 cells; normal percentage of CD57$^+$ cells; increased activated T-cells, as reflected in human HLA-DR expression; and, occasionally, interleukin-2 receptor (CD25) expression.[11] The findings are similar to those in hypersensitivity pneumonitis; in hypersensitivity pneumonitis, however, CD25 expression is normal, and CD57$^+$ cells are increased. This "mixed pattern" of increased cellularity is thought to be characteristic of COP, especially when associated with multiple alveolar opacities on the chest radiograph.[10]

HISTOPATHOLOGIC FINDINGS

The histopathologic lesion characteristic of COP is an excessive proliferation of granulation tissue within small airways (i.e., proliferative bronchiolitis) and alveolar ducts, along with chronic inflammation in surrounding alveoli. This organizing pneumonia is the most important basis for the clinical and radiographic manifestations of COP. Several additional key features are notable: (1) the distribution of lesions is usually patchy and peribronchiolar; (2) the lesions are usually located predominantly within the airspace; (3) there is a uniform, recent temporal appearance to the changes in that all the lesions look similar, with an inflamed, edematous-appearing stroma with little collagen deposition; (4) the intraluminal buds of granulation tissue consist of loose, collagen-embedding fibroblasts and myofibroblasts that extend through the pores of Kohn from one alveolus to another, giving rise to the characteristic "butterfly" pattern; (5) the bronchiolar lesions are usually secondary to intraluminal plugs of granulation tissue occurring in association with plugs in the alveolar ducts and alveolar spaces; (6) severe fibrotic changes (honeycombing) are unusual at the time of diagnosis; (7) foamy macrophages are very common in alveolar spaces, presumably secondary to the bronchiolar occlusion; (8) giant cells are rare or absent, and no granuloma or vasculitis is present; and (9) the lung architecture is not severely disrupted.[9,10,32]

DIAGNOSIS

The clinical and histopathologic features of COP may be present in other disorders, such as bacterial pneumonia, hypersensitivity pneumonitis, chronic eosinophilic pneumonia, viral infection, drug reactions, and connective-tissue disorders. Thus, the diagnosis of COP depends on both the clinical setting and characteristic pathologic features, including the prominent finding of the BOOP pattern in the absence of features suggestive of an underlying process.

An open or thoracoscopic lung biopsy is recommended to confirm the diagnosis. Ample lung tissue must be obtained and carefully reviewed to rule out other diseases, especially idiopathic pulmonary fibrosis, hypersensitivity pneumonitis, chronic eosinophilic pneumonia, and diffuse alveolar damage seen in the acute respiratory distress syndrome.

Transbronchial lung biopsies are generally inadequate in confirming COP *and* ruling out other disorders. The histopathologic features of bronchiolitis obliterans associated with areas of organizing pneumonia can be seen in a number of settings; therefore, small biopsies increase the chance of missing the central diagnosis. Step-sectioning of transbronchial biopsies is useful in identifying the lesions of COP.

The biopsies must be reviewed by an experienced lung pathologist who has been given adequate clinical information to guide the search for specific lesions supporting the diagnosis. Once the characteristic findings of proliferative bronchiolitis are confirmed, the clinician must ensure that a thorough search has been performed to rule out the many other diagnostic considerations. Indeed, the clinicopathologic syndrome of COP is a diagnosis of exclusion.

TREATMENT AND CLINICAL COURSE

Corticosteroid therapy is the most common treatment. Complete clinical recovery, physiological improvement, and normalization of the chest film are seen in two-thirds of patients. Approximately one-third demonstrate persistent disease.

In general, clinical improvement is rapid, within several days or a few weeks. Occasionally, recovery is quite dramatic. Relapses occur commonly when corticosteroids are withdrawn after 1 to 3 months. Most patients who relapse show improvement when re-treated with corticosteroids. Spontaneous improvement in a few patients appears to occur over 3 to 6 months.[19,61]

Patients with airspace opacities on the chest radiograph have a much better outcome than those with interstitial opacities. The overall prognosis for COP is much better than for other interstitial lung diseases (e.g., idiopathic pulmonary fibrosis). Rapidly fatal COP is uncommon.

Based on our clinical experience and that of others, high-dose oral corticosteroid therapy should be used to treat COP. Therapy is usually initiated with prednisone in a dose of 1 to 1.5 mg/kg per day (using ideal body weight), not to exceed 100 mg daily. The drug is given as a single oral dose in the morning, and the dose is maintained for 4 to 8 weeks. If, after 5 to 8 weeks, the patient's condition is stable or improved, the dose is gradually tapered to 0.5 to 1 mg/kg per day for the ensuing 4 to 6 weeks. High-dose parenteral corticosteroid therapy (e.g., methylprednisolone, 125 to 250 mg intravenously every 6 h for 3 to 5 days) has been recommended as initial treatment for patients with rapidly progressive COP.

For the patient in stable or improved condition, the prednisone is gradually tapered off after 3 to 6 months of therapy. A chest radiograph and pulmonary function tests should probably be performed every 6 to 8 weeks during the first year, and therapy should be reinstituted aggressively with any sign of recurrence. Although therapy with corticosteroids is usually well tolerated, side effects are common; some patients develop side effects more readily than others.

If the patient's condition deteriorates despite corticosteroid therapy, a cytotoxic agent should be considered while low-dose (0.25 mg/kg per day) therapy with prednisone is continued. Cyclophosphamide in a single daily dose of 1 to 2 mg/kg has been used, although the optimal dose in COP is unknown. A daily dose of 50 mg may be used at the start of treatment; the dose is slowly increased over 2 to 4 weeks. Maximal dose should not exceed 150 mg per day. A trial of at least 3 to 6 months is needed to ensure an adequate opportunity for clinical response. The hematologic effects of cyclophosphamide are common and frequently require a dose adjustment; the total white blood count should be maintained above 4000/mm^3. Leukopenia is the most commonly reported hematologic toxicity; anemia and thrombocytopenia are noted less often. In some cases, the hematologic effects may persist for several months after discontinuation of the drug. Urologic complications of hemorrhagic cystitis and bladder carcinoma are recognized, although they are thought to be less common in the dose range utilized in treating COP than with the higher dosages used in cancer treatment regimens.

Localized Bronchiolitis Obliterans–Organizing Pneumonia

Occasionally, localized areas BOOP are found at open lung biopsy, usually performed to rule out carcinoma. These lesions present radiographically as irregular nodules or irregular sublobar areas of airspace consolidation. Surgical resection usually resolves this problem. The origin of the lesions is unknown and may be secondary to resolving pneumonia.

CONNECTIVE-TISSUE DISEASES

Pulmonary impairment is common in many of the connective tissue disorders. In most cases, the pulmonary dysfunction is related to alveolar, rather than airway, pathology. Bronchiolitis appears to occur infrequently and varies in its manifestations among the connective-tissue diseases. Further, most of the current understanding of bronchiolar disease in this setting is based largely on anecdotal case reports or small case series. This section reviews the characteristics of bronchiolitis in rheumatoid arthritis, Sjögren's syndrome, systemic lupus erythematosus, progressive systemic sclerosis, and polymyositis, dermatomyositis.

Rheumatoid Arthritis and Constrictive Bronchiolitis

Obstructive pulmonary disease is remarkably prevalent in rheumatoid arthritis. In particular, bronchiolitis obliterans with airway obstruction is an increasingly recognized complication of this connective-tissue disorder. The basic lesion is fibrous narrowing and obliteration of the bronchioles and smallest bronchi. The role of prior penicillamine therapy as a potential etiologic factor remains to be confirmed.

CLINICAL FINDINGS

Most patients are middle-aged women with long-standing seropositive rheumatoid arthritis. This finding is consistent with the increased incidence of rheumatoid arthritis in women, but it is inconsistent with the increased frequency of pulmonary disease in rheumatoid arthritis reported among men. The clinical manifestations of bronchiolitis obliterans associated with rheumatoid arthritis help to distinguish it from other pulmonary processes associated with this disorder. Clinical findings include the rather abrupt onset of dyspnea and dry cough, often associated with inspiratory crackles and a midinspiratory "squeak."

The chest radiograph is typically normal. HRCT usually excludes the presence of bronchiectasis. Pulmonary function studies reveal airflow obstruction and normal pulmonary compliance. Arterial blood gases show moderate hypoxemia and a respiratory alkalosis. The rapid rate of progression in airflow obstruction is atypical for COPD.

HISTOPATHOLOGIC FINDINGS

A "constrictive" bronchiolitis is most common. Lymphoplasmocytic infiltration of small-airway walls is noted. The lumina are gradually obliterated, and the bronchiolar wall is destroyed by granulation tissue. Lesions are usually confined to the small bronchi and bronchioles. Parenchymal involvement is generally localized to areas surrounding the bronchiolitis. Lesions may be at different stages of development or may appear uniform. Immunofluorescence studies show granular depositions of IgM and a striking linear deposition of IgG in the alveolar wall, suggesting possible direct immune-mediated lung injury.

TREATMENT AND PROGNOSIS

Treatment with antibiotics and bronchodilators is ineffective. Corticosteroid therapy appears effective in some patients. The use of intravenous cyclophosphamide and oral prednisone has been suggested. The prognosis is poor, with early deaths reported. Most patients' disease has a chronic course.

Rheumatoid Arthritis and Bronchiolitis Obliterans–Organizing Pneumonia

Occasionally, patchy organizing pneumonia with granulation tissue plugs extending into the alveolar ducts (BOOP) is the predominant lesion. Rheumatoid arthritis with BOOP appears to have a worse prognosis than rheumatoid arthritis with constrictive bronchiolitis. In fact, rheumatoid patients with BOOP are prone to develop a rapidly progressive and fatal form of pneumonia.

Penicillamine-Associated Bronchiolitis Obliterans

Pulmonary complications of penicillamine therapy are uncommon. Use of this agent has been implicated in the pathogenesis of four diffuse lung processes: (1) bronchiolitis obliterans, (2) interstitial infiltrates, (3) Goodpasture's syndrome, and (4) bronchospasm.[4,56] Whether there is a cause-and-effect relationship between penicillamine therapy and development of bronchiolitis obliterans in patients with rheumatoid arthritis is unclear. This form of bronchiolitis obliterans may be characterized by a rapidly deteriorating course and pulmonary insufficiency.

Most patients with penicillamine-associated bronchiolitis are women who never smoked. Breathlessness and cough begin within 3 to 14 months after initiation of the drug. Radiographic abnormalities are unusual, except for mild hyperinflation. Pulmonary function abnormalities are characteristically obstructive. The histopathology is thought to be distinct from other causes of bronchiolitis obliterans, since penicillamine-associated cases usually show a concentric, constrictive form of bronchiolar obstruction. Death from progressive respiratory failure occurs in one-third of patients.

The implication of penicillamine as the etiologic agent is less tenable because bronchiolitis obliterans has not been reported in other diseases treated with penicillamine for prolonged periods—for example, Wilson's disease.[20,52] Although conclusive proof of an association between bronchiolitis obliterans and penicillamine therapy is lacking, when confronted with a dyspneic patient with rheumatoid arthritis on penicillamine therapy, one should stop the drug, consider open lung biopsy, and then administer corticosteroids to prevent disease progression. Cyclophosphamide and prednisone may constitute a useful treatment approach.

Rheumatoid Arthritis and Follicular Bronchiolitis

Follicular bronchitis and bronchiolitis may occur in patients with rheumatoid arthritis, Sjögren's syndrome, juvenile rheumatoid arthritis, immunodeficiency syndromes, familial lung disorders, chronic infection, and a heterogeneous group of patients with a hypersensitivity-type reaction.[22,63]

Patients with rheumatoid arthritis always present with dyspnea; fever and cough occur occasionally. A positive rheumatoid factor is present, often at high levels (1:640 to 1:2560). The

chest film is abnormal, showing bilateral reticulonodular opacities. Arterial blood gases demonstrate hypoxemia, hypocapnia, and a widened alveolar-arterial oxygen gradient. Both obstructive and restrictive patterns have been identified by spirometry, but the restrictive pattern appears to be more common. Immunofluorescence studies are negative.

The lesions of follicular bronchiolitis produce obstruction by external compression of the bronchioles rather than by direct luminal occlusion, as is characteristic for proliferative bronchiolitis obliterans. In almost all cases, a concentric inflammatory infiltrate of lymphocytes and plasma cells surrounds the bronchiole. Abundant germinal centers in the peribronchiolar regions are present and are characterized by hyperplastic follicles located between bronchioles and pulmonary arteries. The bronchiolar lumen is often compressed into a slitlike or fish-mouth shape. Some have suggested that follicular bronchiolitis may be the precursor of interstitial lymphoid pneumonia or pseudolymphoma. Treatment with corticosteroids has yielded variable results.

Sjögren's Syndrome

Obstructive airway disease has been reported in patients with Sjögren's syndrome, often in association with other connective-tissue diseases, particularly rheumatoid arthritis. Desiccation of the tracheobronchial tree is very common in Sjögren's syndrome and no doubt accounts for the obstructive findings. Atrophic rhinitis, xerostomia, xerotrachea (manifested by chronic, dry cough), chronic bronchitis (with cough and production of tenacious sputum), atelectasis (with frequent middle-lobe collapse), and recurrent bronchopneumonia are manifestations of the severe mucosal dryness that can occur within the tracheobronchial tree. Secondary BOOP has been reported as a rare complication of Sjögren's syndrome.

The clinical impact of the obstructive airway dysfunction in Sjögren's syndrome is rarely severe. Most symptomatic patients complain only of a dry cough and mild dyspnea. Adequate studies addressing pulmonary function and pathology are limited. However, lung biopsy has revealed a mononuclear cell infiltration around narrowed small airways (constrictive bronchiolitis).

Systemic Lupus Erythematosus

Fewer than 5 percent of patients with systemic lupus erythematosis (SLE) have airflow obstruction. A patient with SLE who developed rapidly progressive airway obstruction and early obliterative bronchiolitis on open lung biopsy has been reported. Hence, this lesion may account for the obstructive dysfunction occasionally seen in SLE. BOOP has also been reported in two patients with SLE. Although one patient responded to corticosteroid therapy, the other died, despite treatment with corticosteroids and cyclophosphamide.

Progressive Systemic Sclerosis

Clinically significant small-airway disease is not frequently found in nonsmokers with progressive systemic sclerosis, even in the presence of interstitial pulmonary involvement. Focal lymphoid hyperplasia (follicular bronchiolitis) was identified in 23 percent of the open lung biopsies from patients with progressive systemic sclerosis. Interstitial lung disease is the most important pulmonary complication of this disorder.

Polymyositis and Dermatomyositis

BOOP, usual interstitial pneumonia, and diffuse alveolar damage are the most common histologic patterns identified in patients with polymyositis and dermatomyositis. BOOP may occur de novo. Patients with polymyositis or dermatomyositis and BOOP present with cough, fever, and dyspnea, in addition to the proximal muscle weakness, malaise, and rash commonly found in this disease. The pulmonary lesion is responsive to corticosteroid therapy.

ORGAN TRANSPLANTATION

Pulmonary disease is a common complication of organ transplantation and consequently is a significant source of morbidity and mortality in transplant recipients. Bronchiolitis, manifested by progressive airflow obstruction, is increasingly becoming one of the most frequent noninfectious posttransplant respiratory complications.

Bone Marrow Transplantation

Pulmonary disease is a common complication of bone marrow transplantation, occurring in 40 to 60 percent of patients. Furthermore, pulmonary complications are a significant source of morbidity and mortality in transplant recipients. The disease usually results from an infectious pneumonia (bacterial, fungal, or viral, especially cytomegalovirus) or idiopathic interstitial pneumonitis. Lymphocytic bronchitis and lymphoplasmacytic infiltrates of the trachea and large bronchi are among the earliest pulmonary problems encountered after bone marrow transplantation. Progressive airflow obstruction secondary to bronchiolitis obliterans is one of the most frequent noninfectious posttransplant respiratory complications. Cases appear after the first 100 days following transplantation, usually in the setting of chronic graft-versus-host disease (GVHD). GVHD has been postulated to play a role in the development of this lung disease. Bronchiolitis obliterans is most prevalent in patients after allogeneic transplantation, but it has been recently reported with autologous bone marrow transplantation as well.

CLINICAL FINDINGS

Approximately 10 to 17 percent of long-term survivors with chronic GVHD develop severe obstructive pulmonary disease. Risk factors include older age, recurrent sinusitis, chronic GVHD, methotrexate prophylaxis for GVHD, and acquired hypogammaglobulinemia.[5,13] Patients usually present with nonproductive cough (60 percent), dyspnea with exertion (51 percent), and nasal congestion. Scattered wheezes are heard in 40 percent of patients; expiratory "squeaks" are also frequently noted. Bibasilar crackles are uncommon.

RADIOGRAPHIC FINDINGS

The chest radiograph may show diffuse interstitial infiltrates; in approximately 80 percent of cases, the lung fields are normal. Hyperventilation may also be seen. Pneumothoraces may complicate the course of advanced disease. HRCT can be helpful in supporting the diagnosis. In established bronchiolitis obliterans, the most striking CT feature is lobular or segmental areas of lung attenuation, associated with narrowing of pulmonary vessels. The attenuation is presumed to represent areas of air trapping and oligemia.

PHYSIOLOGIC FINDINGS

The development of a new obstructive pattern on pulmonary function testing is a significant signal that bronchiolitis obliterans is developing, especially when noted in the presence of GVHD. Reduced flow, often with hyperinflation and air trapping, is the most common manifestation. Bronchial hyperreactivity also has been identified in some patients after transplantation, but most have fixed obstruction unresponsive to bronchodilators. The presence of bronchial hyperreactivity before transplantation has not been associated with the subsequent development of either clinical or pathologically proven posttransplantation bronchiolitis obliterans. The diffusing capacity is reduced, and hypoxemia is common.

HISTOPATHOLOGIC FINDINGS

Lung biopsy findings are quite variable. The major changes are in and around the bronchioles. In most patients with rapidly progressive obstruction, marked lymphocytic, plasmacytic, or neutrophilic infiltration of the walls of the terminal respiratory bronchioles and obliteration of the bronchiolar lumina with fibrous tissue and surrounding interstitial fibrosis (i.e., "pure" bronchiolitis obliterans) are found. A moderate lymphocytic infiltrate may invade the adjacent pulmonary parenchyma. Other changes characteristic of constrictive bronchiolitis are frequently noted (see above).

DIAGNOSIS

Transbronchial lung biopsies are usually inadequate for a definitive diagnosis to be made. An open or thoracoscopic lung biopsy is often necessary. Since infections are frequent, they should be diagnosed and treated promptly. In this setting, BAL analysis is useful only in ruling out infections. A lymphocytic (i.e., 30 to 50 percent lymphocytes in BAL fluid) or mixed lymphocyte-neutrophil predominance is usual.

MANAGEMENT

The appropriate treatment of bronchiolitis obliterans associated with bone marrow transplantation is questionable. In most cases, bronchodilators and corticosteroids have not improved airflow limitation. Furthermore, use of immunosuppressive agents for the treatment of chronic GVHD has had no consistent beneficial effect on pulmonary function. Consequently, it appears that early recognition and management are required if treatment is to be successful.

The prognosis is variable. A significant number of reported patients have had progressive or persistent disease; many have died secondary to respiratory failure (40 to 65 percent of subjects) (Fig. 54-11). Increasing recognition, early treatment, and the introduction of cyclosporine have resulted in a reduction of the incidence of posttransplantation obstructive airway disease.

Heart-Lung Transplantation

The main pulmonary complication in long-term survivors of heart-lung transplantation is a life-threatening obstructive ventilatory defect—bronchiolitis obliterans. The incidence of obliterative bronchiolitis in this setting has declined in recent years from 50 percent to 10 to 23 percent.[3]

CLINICAL FINDINGS

Bronchiolitis obliterans is noted clinically several months to several years after heart-lung transplantation. Cough productive of mucopurulent sputum is most often seen. Progressive dyspnea follows. Most patients experience repeated upper respiratory tract infections, both viral and bacterial. Occasionally, disease onset is identified only from abnormalities in routine pulmonary function testing (Fig. 54-12). With advanced disease, wheezing on exertion is common.

The development of bronchiolitis obliterans frequently is preceded by acute organ rejection. Often, patients have a history of prior lung infection with cytomegalovirus, *Pneumocystis*, or Epstein-Barr virus. Chest examination reveals diffuse, coarse crackles and expiratory rhonchi.

On physical examination, scattered, late inspiratory high-pitched rhonchi (inspiratory squeaks) are frequently heard.

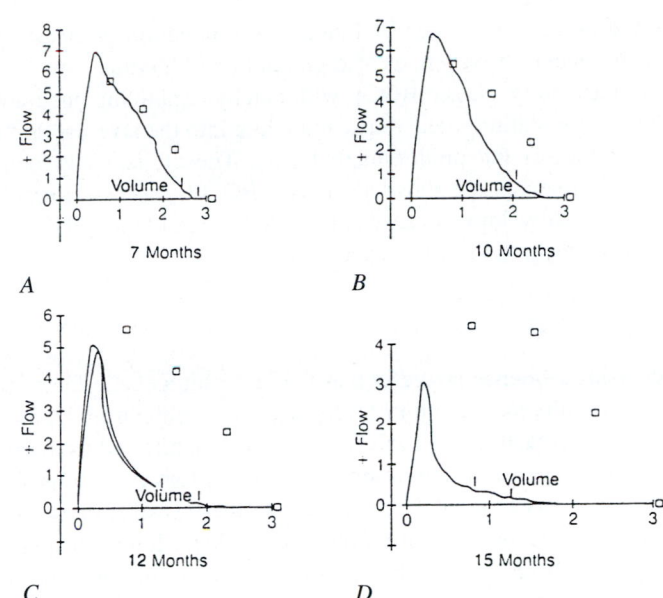

FIGURE 54-12 Segmented changes in flow-volume loops in bronchiolitis obliterans associated with heart-lung transplantation. Curves are from a 33-year-old woman 7, 10, 12, and 15 months after transplantation. *A.* Upper left figure is essentially normal curve. *B.* Upper right curve shows early "coving" of the expiratory flow limb over the middle 50 percent of the forced vital capacity. *C* and *D.* Progressive obstruction is present at 12 (lower left) and 15 months (lower right). Small boxes in each panel represent normal flow. Flow is expressed in L/s; volume is expressed in L. *(Based on data from Theodore et al,[55] with permission.)*

Bibasilar crackles are uncommon, but they may be heard late in the course of the disease. The classic signs of severe airflow obstruction and hyperinflation are seen in advanced, end-stage disease.

RADIOGRAPHIC FINDINGS

The chest radiograph may be normal in early stages of the disease, but frequently it reveals diffuse, nonspecific peribronchial and interstitial infiltrates and variable pleural thickening. Bronchography and CT reveal central bronchiectasis.

PHYSIOLOGIC FINDINGS

Pulmonary function tests show largely irreversible airflow obstruction; however, total lung capacity is reduced. The $D_{L_{CO}}$ is moderately depressed. Hypoxemia and hypocapnia are universally present.

HISTOPATHOLOGIC FINDINGS

Histopathologic changes affect all areas of the lung, but they are frequently patchy. Inspissated mucus and distal obstructive airway changes are often noted. Diffuse increases in peribronchial and interstitial fibrosis are present in most biopsies. Pleural, venous, and arteriosclerotic vascular changes are common. These changes are different from those in acute pulmonary rejection, which is characterized by perivascular lymphocytic cuffing and

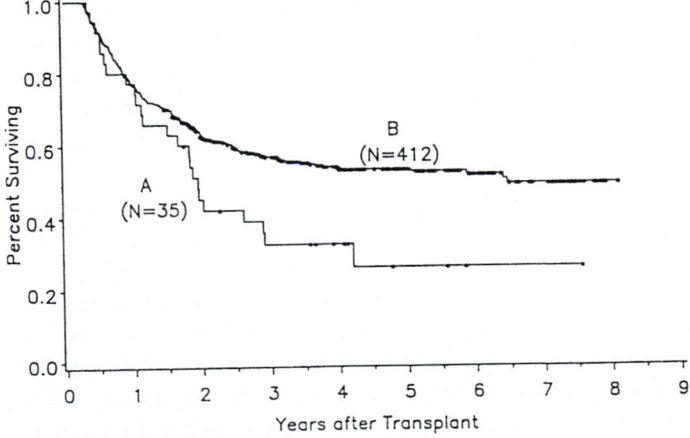

FIGURE 54-11 Bronchiolitis obliterans associated with bone marrow transplantation. Curve A shows posttransplant survival of 35 patients who developed obstructive lung disease. Curve B shows posttransplant survival of 412 concurrent patients (age 16 years or over) with chronic graft-versus-host disease who survived at least 80 days after transplantation and who had no evidence of obstructive lung disease. *(Based on data from Clark et al,[7] with permission.)*

diffuse alveolar damage.[62] Clinical acute rejection predisposes to subsequent development of bronchiolitis obliterans.

Occasionally, classic BOOP with patchy organizing pneumonia and granulation tissue plugs extending into the alveolar ducts is observed as the predominant lesion. The clinical and radiographic features are those seen with BOOP (discussed previously). Usually, known causes of this lesion are identified—e.g., infection, aspiration, drug reaction, etc.

PATHOGENESIS

Increasing evidence suggests that the key pathogenetic factor is a form of alloreactive injury to the bronchial epithelium. Donor-specific alloreactivity of BAL lymphocytes, manifested by a proliferative response to donor spleen cells, appears to be a useful marker for this process.[50] A number of other possible causes or associations of bronchiolitis obliterans in heart-lung transplantation have been described: (1) recurrent, persistent bacterial or viral infections; (2) immunoreaction to the transplanted lung (e.g., "host-versus-graft" disease or transplant rejection); (3) altered mucociliary clearance and impaired ciliary function from injury to the pulmonary nerve supply or from abnormal mucus chemistry and viscosity; (4) bronchial artery ligation and resulting alteration in repair of injured bronchi and bronchioles; (5) reaction to immunosuppressive drugs (especially cyclosporine, which has been shown to have fibroproliferative properties that could cause progressive narrowing and obliteration of affected bronchioles); and (6) loss of cough reflex and aspiration, creating a milieu favorable to continued growth of infectious agents.[62]

DIAGNOSIS

Open or thoracoscopic lung biopsy is required to confirm the diagnosis of bronchiolitis obliterans and to rule out other causes of pulmonary dysfunction in patients who have undergone heart-lung transplantation. With increased recognition of this potential complication, early detection of the disorder through use of serial pulmonary function tests, BAL, and repeated transbronchial lung biopsies can be achieved and may decrease the need for surgical lung biopsy to confirm the diagnosis.

MANAGEMENT

No clearly useful treatment protocol has been established. Efforts at preventing repeated episodes of rejection seem most important. Prompt diagnosis and treatment of acute rejection and any infectious complications are paramount. Routine serial lung function testing and fiberoptic bronchoscopy with transbronchial biopsy and BAL are helpful. The best medical regimen for prevention of bronchiolitis obliterans remains to be defined. Nonetheless, experience suggests that optimal maintenance of immunosuppression requires a regimen that includes azathioprine and cyclosporine. Prednisone is also commonly included. Use of corticosteroids, bronchodilators, antibiotics, antithymocyte globulin, or OKT3 monoclonal antibody has resulted in documented stabilization or reversal of disease in some patients. Retransplantation has been successful. Spontaneous improvement does not occur.

Lung Transplantation

Initially, lung transplant recipients were thought not to develop bronchiolitis obliterans. However, this complication is now recognized as the major factor limiting long-term success with this procedure. The incidence of bronchiolitis obliterans among single-lung recipients is approximately 20 percent; in double or bilateral sequential single-lung recipients, the incidence is 12 percent.[43] Risk factors include recurrent episodes of acute rejection, severe acute rejection, inadequate or fluctuating levels of maintenance immunosuppression, recurrent infections, and ischemic airway injury occurring early after lung transplantation.[43,46]

CLINICAL FINDINGS

The clinical presentation is similar to that described in heart-lung transplantation. Nonproductive cough, mild malaise, and fatigue are common symptoms. Eventually, all subjects develop dyspnea. Results of physical examination are usually normal, but inspiratory squeaks may be heard. Crackles are uncommon.

RADIOGRAPHIC FINDINGS

Decreased peripheral vascular markings, slight volume loss, and subsegmental atelectasis may be early changes. A common radiographic finding in long-standing disease is the gradual progression of pleural-based densities in the middle and upper lung zones. Biopsy reveals subpleural parenchymal fibrosis without active inflammation. The scarring may result from relative ischemia in areas of affected lung.

HRCT shows lobular or segmental areas of lung attenuation and narrowing of pulmonary vessels, representing regions of air trapping and oligemia.

HISTOPATHOLOGIC FINDINGS

Three major kinds of airway injury may be seen in lung allografts: acute rejection, bronchiolitis obliterans, and lymphocytic bronchitis or bronchiolitis.[46] The lesions of bronchiolitis obliterans affect the membranous and respiratory bronchioles. They are characterized by the features of constrictive bronchiolitis (see above). If a submucosal mononuclear cell infiltrate is present, the lesions are considered "active." Their absence may indicate "inactive" disease. Vascular changes are often found and usually consist of fibrointimal thickening of arteries and veins, with or without an active inflammatory component.

A BOOP pattern, with patchy organizing pneumonia and granulation tissue plugs extending into the alveolar ducts, has been reported in some lung transplant recipients.[43] The clinical and radiographic features are progressive respiratory failure, acute or subacute alveolar opacities noted on chest radiograph, and a restrictive pattern of pulmonary function tests. Usually, known causes of this lesion are identifiable, especially infection. Patients respond well to corticosteroid therapy.

MANAGEMENT

No effective treatment has been found. Prevention of repeated episodes of rejection appears important. Prompt diagnosis and treatment of acute rejection and infectious complications are key. A regimen of immunosuppression that includes azathioprine, cyclosporine, and prednisone is most commonly employed. This regimen appears to slow the rate of decline in lung function; however, the overall prognosis remains poor. Approximately 50 percent of all deaths after the first year following transplant are due to bronchiolitis obliterans. Retransplantation has been successfully employed in several patients.

DIFFUSE PANBRONCHIOLITIS

Diffuse panbronchiolitis is a distinctive form of small airway disease that is relatively common in Japan, China, and Korea; it is rare in other parts of the world.[27,29,53] A few case reports of the disease in non-Asians have appeared in the literature.[21,26,49,51] A familial occurrence has been described, with a significant increase in HLA Bw54 (63 percent frequency).[54] Because HLA Bw54 or its related haplotype are confined primarily to some Mongoloid races—e.g., Japanese, Chinese, and Koreans—the genetic and ethnic background observed with this unique syndrome may be explained. HLA Bw54 may also be a useful marker in the differential diagnosis of diffuse panbronchiolitis, since the frequency of this antigen in the general population is very low (11.8 percent).[54] A similar pulmonary lesion has been demonstrated in ulcerative colitis and adult T-cell leukemia. Environmental factors also appear important, since the disorder is very uncommon in persons of Asian ancestry living abroad.

Clinical Findings

Diffuse panbronchiolitis is more prevalent in men, with a 2:1 male-to-female ratio. The peak incidence occurs between the fourth and seventh decades of life; mean age at presentation is 50 years. Chronic sinusitis is present in 75 to 100 percent of cases. Sinus symptoms often precede chest symptoms by years or decades. Chronic cough with expectoration of copious purulent sputum, exertional dyspnea, and wheezing are the most common clinical manifestations. Cigarette smoking or occupational exposures have not been shown to be predisposing factors. Physical examination reveals coarse crackles; clubbing is not a feature.

The most characteristic laboratory abnormality is persistent, marked elevation of serum cold agglutinins; mycoplasma antibody titers are negative. Rheumatoid factor may be elevated. Immunoglobulin levels are usually normal. BAL studies reveal marked neutrophilia.

Radiographic Findings

The chest radiograph often reveals small nodular opacities up to 2 mm in diameter; the opacities are seen diffusely throughout the lung fields. A reticular "airway" pattern may be evident with more advanced disease. Hyperinflation may also be present. HRCT yields more information about the location and distribution of the pulmonary disease than do conventional radiographic techniques. HRCT also better reflects the clinical stages and pathology. On HRCT, the nodular shadows are distributed in a centrilobular fashion, often extending to small, branching linear areas of attenuation. The nodular and linear densities correspond to thickened and dilated bronchiolar walls with intraluminal mucus plugs. Inhomogeneity in lung density may be apparent as a result of peripheral air trapping. Bronchiectasis may be prominent in advanced disease.

Physiological Findings

Pulmonary function tests reveal marked obstruction. Arterial blood gases show hypoxemia, with or without hypercapnia. In rare instances, a restrictive ventilatory defect is present. The diffusing capacity is variably reduced. In general, patients with diffuse panbronchiolitis exhibit less bronchodilator responsiveness than do patients with COPD.

Histopathologic Findings

Thickening of the walls of the respiratory bronchiole, infiltration with lymphocytes, plasma cells, and histiocytes, and extension of the inflammatory changes into peribronchiolar tissue are noted on biopsy. Advanced disease is manifested by secondary ectasia of proximal bronchioles.

Management and Outcome

The optimal therapy for diffuse panbronchiolitis is unclear. Low-dose erythromycin (200 to 600 mg a day) is adequate for most patients. Erythromycin impairs neutrophil chemotaxis, neutrophil superoxide production, and neutrophil-derived elastolytic activity, and it decreases the number of neutrophils in BAL fluid following challenge with gram-negative bacteria. In addition, erythromycin may cause a reduction in mucus production by decreasing glycoconjugate secretion. Finally, erythromycin has been shown to reduce the circulating pool of T lymphocytes bearing HLA-DR, a marker of cellular activation.

Corticosteroids are utilized commonly in treatment regimens, but there is no evidence supporting their efficacy. Nonsteroidal anti-inflammatory drugs (NSAIDs) may have a role in controlling the bronchorrhea associated with this disease by altering airway epithelial ion and water transport. No controlled trials with NSAIDs have been performed. Routine use of β_2-agonists or ipratropium bromide should be encouraged to promote mucociliary clearance and bronchodilation in patients with a component of reversible airway disease and as a part of routine pulmonary toilet. In addition, treatment of coexisting sinus disease may help in control of airway disease.

Prompt treatment of bronchial infections is also important. The choice of antibiotics should be guided by results of sputum gram stain and culture. The disease progresses insidiously, and the prognosis is often poor, with fatalities due to repeated respiratory infections (particularly with *Pseudomonas aeruginosa*) that result in respiratory failure.

PRIMARY DIFFUSE HYPERPLASIA OF PULMONARY NEUROENDOCRINE CELLS

Primary diffuse hyperplasia of pulmonary neuroendocrine cells is a clinicopathologic entity characterized by diffuse hyperplasia and dysplasia of neuroendocrine cells primarily affecting the distal bronchi and bronchioles. The disorder is seen primarily in women in their fifth or sixth decade. Clinical findings include nonproductive cough and long-standing dyspnea (usually of more than 10 years' duration). All reported cases are in never-smokers. The chest examination is unrevealing. Chest radiographs show diffuse reticulonodular opacities in most; multiple nodules are seen in a few cases. HRCT demonstrates diffuse small-airway thickening, with patchy areas of hyperlucency, suggesting air trapping. The most common physiological abnormality is irreversible airflow obstruction. Open or thoracoscopic lung biopsy is required for diagnosis. The spectrum of histopathologic changes includes diffuse hyperplasia and dysplasia of neuroendocrine cells, numerous neuroepithelial bodies, prominent carcinoid tumorlets, and even typical carcinoid tumors in the distal bronchi and bronchioles. Pathogenesis, treatment, and prognosis of the syndrome are unknown. Most patients have a relatively benign course characterized by many years of symptoms.

REFERENCES

1. Aguayo SA, Miller YE, Waldron JA Jr: Idiopathic diffuse hyperplasia of pulmonary neuroendocrine cells and airway disease. *New Engl J Med* 327:1285–1288, 1992.
2. Alasaly K, Muller N, Ostrow D, et al: Cryptogenic organizing pneumonia: A report of 25 cases and a review of the literature. *Medicine* 74:201–211, 1995.
3. Burke CM, Yousem SA, Corris PA: Heart-lung transplantation, in Epler GR (ed), *Diseases of the Bronchioles.* New York, Raven, 1994, pp 259–274.
4. Camus P: The respiratory complications of D-penicillamine therapy (author's translation). *Rev Fr Mal Respir* 10:7–20, 1982.
5. Chan CK: Bone marrow transplantation bronchiolitis obliterans, in Epler GR (ed), *Diseases of the Bronchioles.* New York, Raven, 1994, pp 247–257.
6. Churg A: Small airways disease associated with mineral dust exposure. *Semin Respir Med* 13:140–148, 1992.
7. Clark JG, Crawford SW, Madtes DK, Sullivan KM: Obstructive lung disease after allogeneic marrow transplantation: Clinical presentation and course. *Ann Intern Med* 111:368–376, 1989.
8. Colby TV, Churg AC: Patterns of pulmonary fibrosis, in Sommers SC, Rosen PP, Fechner RE (eds), *1986 Pathology Annual,* vol 21. Norwalk, CT, Appleton-Century-Crofts, 1986, pp 277–309.
9. Colby TV, Myers JL: The clinical and histologic spectrum of bronchiolitis obliterans including bronchiolitis obliterans organizing pneumonia (BOOP). *Semin Respir Med* 13:119–133, 1992.
10. Cordier JF: Cryptogenic organizing pneumonitis. *Clin Chest Med* 14:677–692, 1993.
11. Costabel U, Teschler H, Guzman J: Bronchiolitis obliterans organizing pneumonia (BOOP): The cytological and immunocytological profile of bronchoalveolar lavage. *Eur Respir J* 5:791–797, 1992.
12. Coultas DB, Funk LM. Postinfectious bronchiolitis obliterans, in Epler GR (ed), *Diseases of the Bronchioles.* New York, Raven, 1994, pp 215–229.
13. Crawford SW, Clark JG: Bronchiolitis associated with bone marrow transplantation. *Clin Chest Med* 14:741–749, 1993.
14. Davison AG, Heard BE, McAllister WAC, Turner-Warwick MEH: Cryptogenic organizing pneumonitis. *Q J Med* 52:382–394, 1983.
15. Dorinsky PM, Davis WB, Lucas JG, et al: Adult bronchiolitis: Evaluation by bronchoalveolar lavage and response to prednisone therapy. *Chest* 88:58–63, 1985.
16. Douglas WW, Colby TV: Fume-related bronchiolitis obliterans, in Epler GR (ed), *Diseases of the Bronchioles.* New York, Raven, 1994, pp 187–213.
17. Douglas WW, Norman G, Hepper G, Colby TV: Silo-filler's disease. *Mayo Clin Proc* 64:291–304, 1989.
18. Edwards C, Cayton R, Bryan R: Chronic transmural bronchiolitis: Non-specific lesion of small airways. *J Clin Pathol* 45:993–998, 1992.
19. Epler GR, Colby TV, McLoud TC, et al: Bronchiolitis obliterans organizing pneumonia. *New Engl J Med* 312:152–158, 1985.
20. Epler GR, Snider GL, Gaensler EA, et al: Bronchiolitis and bronchitis in connective tissue disease: A possible relationship to the use of penicillamine. *JAMA* 242:528–532, 1979.
21. Fitzgerald JE, King TE Jr, Lynch DA, et al: Diffuse panbronchiolitis in the United States. *Am J Respir Crit Care Med* 154:497–503, 1996.
22. Fortoul TI, Cano-Valle F, Oliva E, Barrios R: Follicular bronchiolitis in association with connective tissue diseases. *Lung* 163:305–314, 1985.
23. Grinblat J, Mechlis S, Lewitus Z: Organizing pneumonia–like process: An unusual observation in steroid responsive cases with features of chronic interstitial pneumonia. *Chest* 80:259–263, 1981.
24. Guerry-Force ML, Mueller NL, Wright JL, et al: A comparison of bronchiolitis obliterans with organizing pneumonia, usual interstitial pneumonia, and small airways disease. *Am Rev Respir Dis* 135:705–712, 1987.
25. Hardy KA. Childhood bronchiolitis obliterans, in Epler GR (ed), *Diseases of the Bronchioles.* New York, Raven, 1994, pp 415–426.
26. Homer R, Khoo L, Walker Smith G: Diffuse panbronchiolitis in a Hispanic man with travel to Japan. *Chest* 107:1176, 1995.
27. Homma H, Yamanaka A, Tanimoto S, et al: Diffuse panbronchiolitis: A disease of the transitional zone of the lung. *Chest* 83:63–69, 1983.
28. Horvath EP, Colico DGA, Barbee RA, Dickie HA: Nitrogen dioxide–induced pulmonary disease. *J Occup Med* 20:103–110, 1978.
29. Izumi T: A nation-wide survey of diffuse panbronchiolitis in Japan, in Grassi C, Rizzato G, Pozzi E (eds), *Sarcoidosis and Other Granulomatous Disorders.* New York, Elsevier, 1988, pp 753–757.
30. Izumi T: The global view of idiopathic bronchiolitis obliterans organizing pneumonia, in Epler GR (ed), *Diseases of the Bronchioles.* New York, Raven, 1994, pp 307–312.
31. Izumi T, Kitaichi M, Nishimura K, Nagai S: Bronchiolitis obliterans organizing pneumonia: Clinical features and differential diagnosis. *Chest* 102:715–719, 1992.
32. Katzenstein ALA, Myers JL, Prophet DW, et al: Bronchiolitis obliterans and usual interstitial pneumonia. *Am J Surg Pathol* 10:373–381, 1986.
33. Kindt GC, Weiland JE, Davis WB, et al: Bronchiolitis in adults: A reversible cause of airway obstruction associated with airway neutrophils and neutrophil products. *Am Rev Respir Dis* 140:483–492, 1989.
34. King TE Jr: Bronchiolitis. *Clin Chest Med* 14:607–772, 1993.
35. King TE Jr: Bronchiolitis obliterans, in Schwarz MI, King TE Jr (eds), *Interstitial Lung Disease,* 2d ed. St. Louis, Mosby–Year Book, 1993, pp 463–495.
36. King TE Jr, Mortenson RL: Cryptogenic organizing pneumonia: The North American experience. *Chest* 102:8S–13S, 1992.
37. King TE Jr, Mortenson RL: Syndromes that mimic idiopathic pulmonary fibrosis. *Immunol Allergy Clin North Am* 12:461–489, 1992.
38. Kraft M, Mortenson RL, Colby TV, et al: Cryptogenic constrictive bronchiolitis. *Am Rev Respir Dis* 148:1093–1101, 1993.

847

39. Kuhn C III, Boldt J, King TE Jr, et al: An immunohistochemical study of architectural remodeling and connective tissue synthesis in pulmonary fibrosis. *Am Rev Respir Dis* 140:1693–1703, 1989.

40. Kuhn C III, McDonald JA: The roles of the myofibroblast in idiopathic pulmonary fibrosis: Ultrastructural and immunohistochemical features of sites of active extracellular matrix synthesis. *Am J Pathol* 138:1257–1265, 1991.

41. Lange W: Ueber eine eigenthumliche Erkrankung der kleinen Bronchien und Bronchiolen (Bronchitis et bronchiolitis obliterans). *Dtsch Arch Klin Med* 70:342–364, 1901.

42. Marti-Bonmati L, Perales FR, Catala F, et al: CT findings in Swyer-James syndrome. *Radiology* 172:477–480, 1989.

43. Maurer JR: Lung transplantation bronchiolitis obliterans, in Epler GR (ed), Diseases of the bronchioles. New York, Raven, 1994, pp 275–289.

44. Myers JL, Veal CF, Shin MS, Katzenstein ALA: Respiratory bronchiolitis causing interstitial lung disease: A clinicopathologic study of six cases. *Am Rev Respir Dis* 135:880–884, 1987.

45. Nagai N: The value of BALF cell findings for differentiation of idiopathic UIP, BOOP, and interstitial pneumonia associated with collagen vascular disease, in Harasawa M, Fukuchi Y, Morinari H (eds), *Interstitial Pneumonia of Unknown Etiology*. Tokyo, University of Tokyo Press, 1989, pp 131–136.

46. Paradis I, Yousem S, Griffith B: Airway obstruction and bronchiolitis after lung transplantation. *Clin Chest Med* 14:751–763, 1993.

47. Penn CC, Liu C: Bronchiolitis following infection in adults and children. *Clin Chest Med* 14:645–654, 1993.

48. Peyrol S, Cordier JF, Grimaud JA: Intra-alveolar fibrosis of idiopathic bronchiolitis obliterans–organizing pnemonia: Cell-matrix patterns. *Am J Pathol* 137:155–170, 1990.

49. Poletti V, Patelli M, Poletti G, et al: Diffuse panbronchiolitis observed in an Italian (letter). *Chest* 98:515–516, 1990.

50. Rabinowich H, Zeevi A, Paradis IL, et al: Proliferative responses of bronchoalveolar lavage lymphocytes from heart-lung transplant patients. *Transplantation* 49:115–121, 1990.

51. Randhawa P, Hoagland MH, Yousem SA: Diffuse panbronchiolitis in North America: Report of three cases and review of the literature. *Am J Surg Pathol* 15:43–47, 1991.

52. Sternlieb I, Bennet B, Scheinberg IH: D-Penicillamine–induced Goodpasture's syndrome in Wilson's disease. *Ann Intern Med* 82:673–676, 1975.

53. Sugiyama Y: Diffuse panbronchiolitis. *Clin Chest Med* 14:765–772, 1993.

54. Sugiyama Y, Kudoh S, Maeda H, et al: Analysis of HLA antigens in patients with diffuse panbronchiolitis. *Am Rev Respir Dis* 141:1459–1462, 1990.

55. Theodore J, Starnes VA, Lewiston NJ: Obliterative bronchiolitis. *Clin Chest Med* 11:309–321, 1990.

56. Turner-Warwick M: Adverse reactions affecting the lung: Possible association with D-penicillamine. *J Rheumatol* 7:166–168, 1981.

57. Wohl MEB. Bronchiolitis in children, in Epler GR (ed), *Diseases of the Bronchioles*. New York, Raven, 1994, pp 397–407.

58. Wright JL: Inhalational lung Injury causing bronchiolitis. *Clin Chest Med* 14:635–644, 1993.

59. Wright JL, Cagle P, Churg A, et al: Diseases of the small airways. *Am Rev Respir Dis* 146:240–262, 1992.

60. Wright JL, Lawson LM, Pare PD, et al: Morphology of peripheral airways in current smokers and ex-smokers. *Am Rev Respir Dis* 127:474–477, 1983.

61. Yamamoto M, Ina Y, Kitaichi M: Bronchiolitis obliterans organizing pneumonia (BOOP): Profile in Japan, in Harasawa M, Fukuchi Y, Morinari H (eds), *Interstitial Pneumonia of Unknown Etiology*. Tokyo, University of Tokyo Press, 1989, pp 61–70.

62. Yousem SA, Burke CM, Billingham ME: Pathologic pulmonary alterations in long-term human heart-lung transplantation. *Hum Pathol* 16:911–923, 1985.

63. Yousem SA, Colby TV, Carrington CB: Follicular bronchitis/bronchiolitis. *Hum Pathol* 16:700–706, 1985.

64. Yousem SA, Colby TV, Gaensler EA: Respiratory bronchiolitis-associated interstitial lung disease and its relationship to desquamative interstitial pneumonia. *Mayo Clin Proc* 64:1373–1380, 1989.

65. Zwemer FL, Pratt DS, May JJ: Silo filler's disease in New York State. *Am Rev Respir Dis* 146:650–653, 1992.

CHAPTER 55

BULLOUS DISEASES OF THE LUNG

David M. Murphy / Alfred P. Fishman

A bulla is a large, air-containing space within the substance of the lungs that results from destruction, dilatation, and confluence of airspaces distal to terminal bronchioles (Fig. 55-1B). By definition, a bulla is larger than 1 cm in diameter.[5,37] Its walls are made up of attenuated and compressed parenchyma (Fig. 55-2).

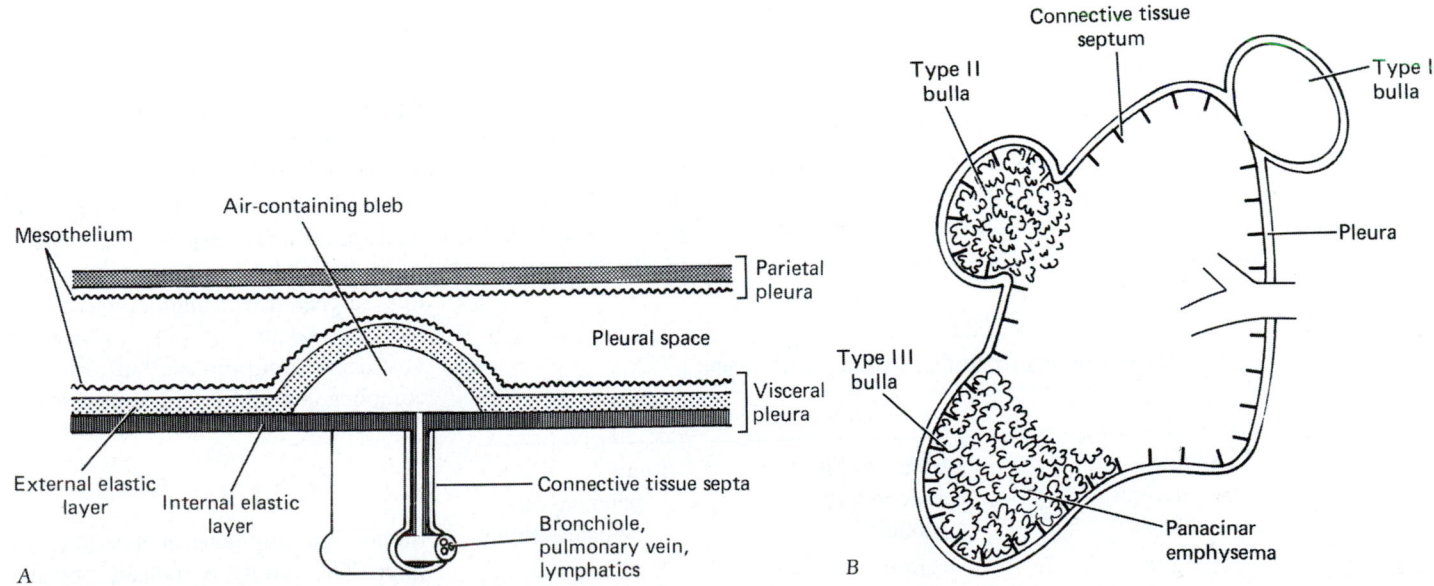

FIGURE 55-1 Blebs and bullae. A. Development of a bleb. A bleb is an accumulation of air within the pleura that is not confined by connective-tissue septa within the lung. Air that escapes within the substance of the lungs makes its way to the surface, separating the internal from the external elastic layers on the visceral pleura. B. Different types of bullae. In contrast to a bleb, a bulla is confined by connective-tissue septa of the lung and is deep to the internal elastic layer of the visceral pleura. Three different types of bullae are shown arising from a lung that has been removed from within the chest wall. A type I bulla is shown at the apex, a type II in the middle zone, and type III arising at the base. The short dark lines denote connective-tissue septa. Panacinar emphysematous parenchyma is present within the types II and III bullae. (Based on data of Reid,[32] with permission.)

Bullae occur in a variety of disorders: (1) emphysema ("bullous emphysema"), most often in association with acinar (paraseptal) emphysema;[40,9] (2) fibrosis, as in the late stages of sarcoidosis or complicated pneumoconiosis; and (3) "vanishing lung," in which the parenchyma is rapidly replaced by multiple bullae.[3,34] Bullae also occur in lungs that are otherwise normal (bullous disease), suggesting a mechanism different from that of bullae that occur in conjunction with the three types of emphysema (Table 55-1).

Distinctions are drawn between bullae, blebs, and cysts (Table 55-2). A bleb is an accumulation of air between the layers of the visceral pleura. The thin covering of a bleb predisposes to rupture and the entry of air into the pleura (Fig. 55-1A).

Cysts are epithelial-lined cavities that may resemble bullae on the chest radiograph. Many fall into the category of hamartomas (i.e., developmental anomalies containing mixtures of mesenchymal and epithelial components that are normally present in the lung). The pathologic nature of cystic lesions is generally reflected in their names: "cystic adenomatoid malformations," "peripheral bronchogenic cysts," "congenital polycystic disease," "atypical bronchopulmonary sequestrations."

The designation *bullous disease* is reserved for multiple bullae in lungs that are otherwise normal. This entity is different in origin and pathogenesis from that in which bullae occur in conjunction with underlying chronic obstructive pulmonary disease (COPD) with bullae.

Confusion occasionally arises between the two entities because some pathologists are inclined to regard bullous disease as

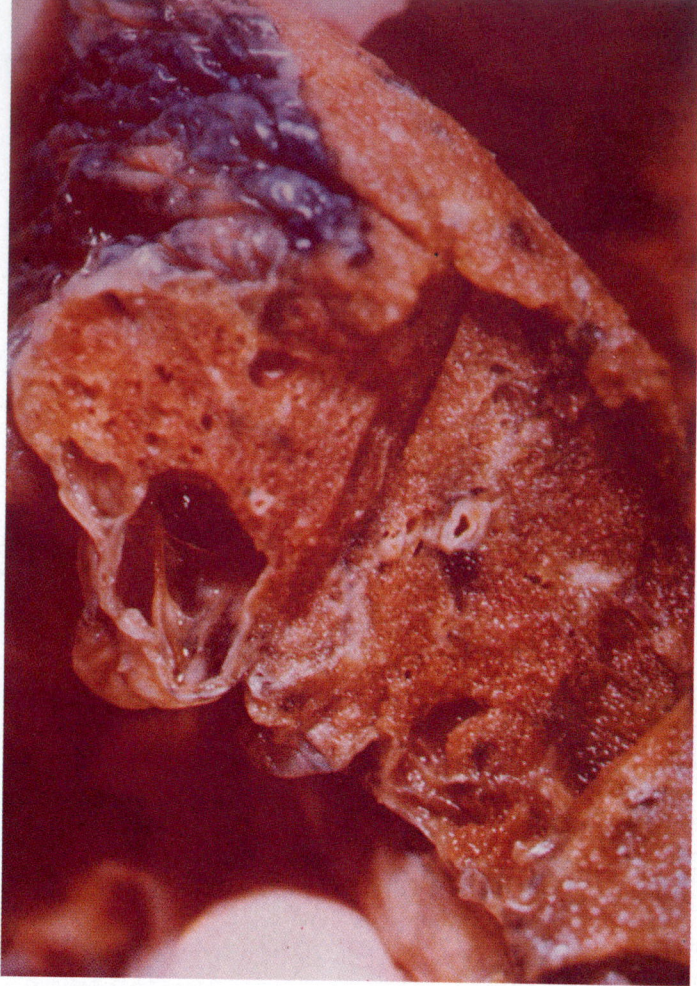

FIGURE 55-2 Bullae projecting from the cut surface of the lung. *(Courtesy of Dr. I. Gordon.)*

a subset of panacinar emphysema. However, this view is not useful clinically on at least three counts: (1) panacinar emphysema tends to occur in the lower lobes, whereas bullous disease favors the upper lobes; (2) the natural history of the two disorders is quite different; and (3) panacinar emphysema has certain distinctive features not shared by bullous disease (e.g., a "winter-tree" appearance on angiography). Bullae may occur not only as part of obstructive lung disease but also as a complication of fibrotic lung disease.

ETIOLOGY OF BULLAE

Bullae can originate in a variety of ways. The variety is indicated by the many clinical entities with which it is associated: (1) emphysema of distal acini[9,32,36] (Fig. 55-3); (2) cigarette smoking; (3) scar formation, which traps some parenchymal areas of normal lung or enlarges airspaces by traction on surrounding intact alveoli or by

TABLE 55-2

Characteristics of Blebs, Bullae, and Cysts

	Bleb	Bulla	Cyst
Site	Within visceral pleura	Arises within secondary lobule	Lung parenchyma or mediastinum
Size	1–2 cm	1 cm to >75% of a lung	2–10 cm
Lining	Elastic laminae of the pleura	Connective tissue septa	Epithelium
Associated condition	Spontaneous pneumothorax		Respiratory infection

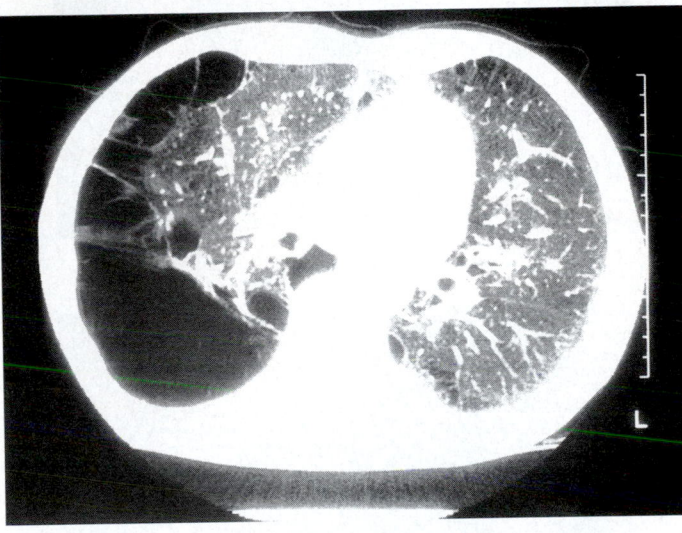

A

B

FIGURE 55-3 *A.* Computer tomographic image of the lungs of a patient with bullous emphysema showing a bulla in the right lung. *B.* Similar images from the same patient showing associated paraseptal emphysema.

retraction or shrinkage of the intact walls of adherent alveoli; (4) intravenous drug abuse;[12] (5) experimental production of emphysema in rabbits using Caledon blue dye injected intravenously;[38] (6) chronic inflammation and destructive changes in the terminal and first-order respiratory bronchioles, which causes overdistention of airspaces by delaying their emptying;[38] and (7) α_1-antitrypsin deficiency in the elderly.[16]

CLASSIFICATION

Bullae are classified into three main types (Fig. 55-1B).[32]

Type I bullae are characterized by a narrow neck that connects the bulla with the pulmonary parenchyma. This type of bulla may be caused by overinflation of a volume of flawed lung tissue. The bullae behave like a paper bag—which is extremely compliant until full, when it becomes tense.[41] The walls of type I bullae are thin, and their interiors are empty. Type I bullae are

usually found at the apices of the lung and along the edges of the lingua and middle lobes. They occur often in association with paraseptal emphysema. Scanning electron microscopy has disclosed not only that the thin neck is a consistent feature of these bullae but also that the pleural mesothelial cells on the external surface are either reduced in number or completely absent, revealing bundles of collagen fibers lying naked and separated from each other by small pores or crevices.[30]

In contrast, type II bullae arise from the subpleural parenchyma and are characterized by a neck of panacinar emphysematous lung tissue. Also, the interior of these airspaces consists of emphysematous lung in which blood vessels are still present. In contrast to the type I bulla, the type II bulla has an outer wall that is formed by pleura covered with intact mesothelial cells. Although connective-tissue septa are present within the bullae, they are not found in the wall. Type II bullae may occur anywhere in the lung but are most frequently found in the upper lobe, on the anterior surface of the middle lobe, and over the diaphragm.

Type III bullae consist of slightly hyperinflated lung connected to the rest of the lung by a broad base that extends deep into the parenchyma. This type is believed to represent an atrophic form of emphysema.

PATHOGENESIS

How bullous disease develops is still unclear. Several hypotheses have been tendered over the years, but none have been proved. Among these are the following: 1. Weakness of the alveolar walls predisposes to the formation of bullae—particularly at the apices of the lungs, where pleural pressures are most negative. This theory underscores the proclivity of bullae for the upper lobes and stresses the influence of mechanical forces acting upon flawed tissue. 2. Inflammatory disease of a bronchiole leads to progressive air trapping and "tension airspaces." 3. Disordered collateral ventilation is responsible. 4. The same mechanisms as those responsible for generalized emphysema underlie the formation of bullae. 5. Underlying paraseptal emphysema is the cause.

Of all the hypotheses, that of underlying paraseptal emphysema is the most popular.[9] It envisages destruction of alveoli adjacent to connective-tissue septa or the pleura (Fig. 55-3), with small "bubbles" developing along the edges of the lung. This pattern may be related to the fact that the capillaries in the alveolar walls that abut connective-tissue septa are less numerous than in other alveolar walls because of a sparse network of arterioles and arteries to these peripheral alveoli. As a result, these regions of the acinus have less vascularity and greater compliance.[9] Small bullae rarely become visible on the chest radiograph but are usually easily visualized with computed tomography (Fig. 55-3). As a rule, small bullae produce no symptoms, signs, or discernible alteration in pulmonary function. But rupture of one or more bullae leads to spontaneous pneumothorax. Recurrent pneumothorax secondary to paraseptal emphysema or small bullae may be an indication for surgical resection of the affected area.

Recently, dynamic computed tomography and intrabullous pressure measurements have questioned the belief that bullae are formed by positive pressure within the airspace. The basis for this challenge is that the lung surrounding a bulla is less compliant than the bulla itself; accordingly, the pressure necessary to inflate the surrounding lung is greater than that necessary to inflate the bulla. Therefore, when a bulla and its surrounding lung are exposed to the same negative pleural pressure, the bulla fills preferentially and completely before the surrounding lung does.[26] Further inspiration increases the elastic recoil pressure—exerting a greater retractive force on the lung parenchyma, which enlarges the airspace.[19,26]

Bullae within the intact chest are molded and compressed to fit adjacent anatomic configurations. However, should the lung be released from these constraints, as when removed from the chest cavity, bullae will project as shiny bubbles from the lung surface (Fig. 55-2). Large bullae cause crowding of adjacent lung parenchyma, and structures such as bronchi are displaced, stretched, and narrowed over its surface. Very large airspaces can expand across the midline or even extend into the neck. Bullae represent more than just overexpanded alveoli because the remnants of bronchioles and their accompanying vessels sometimes persist as trabeculae within the bulla (Fig. 55-2). Interlobular septae also can become incorporated into the wall as the airspace expands from within the secondary lobule.

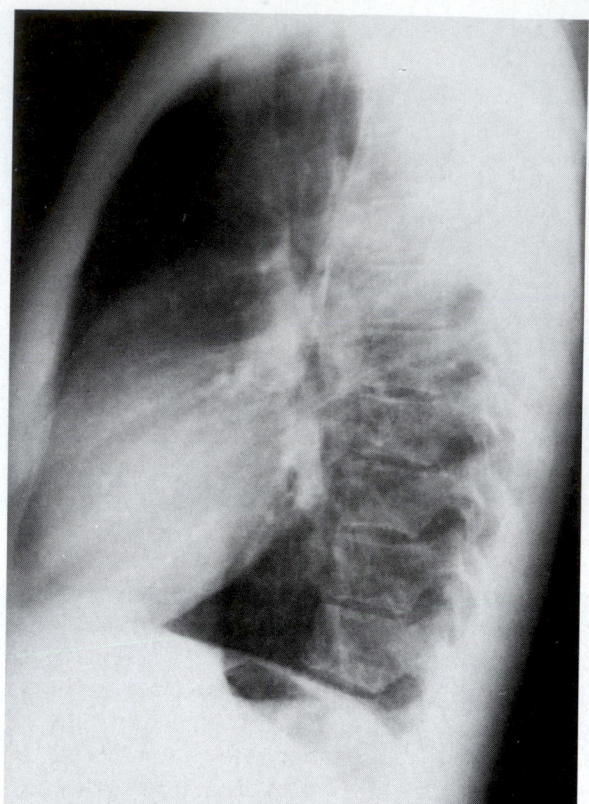

B

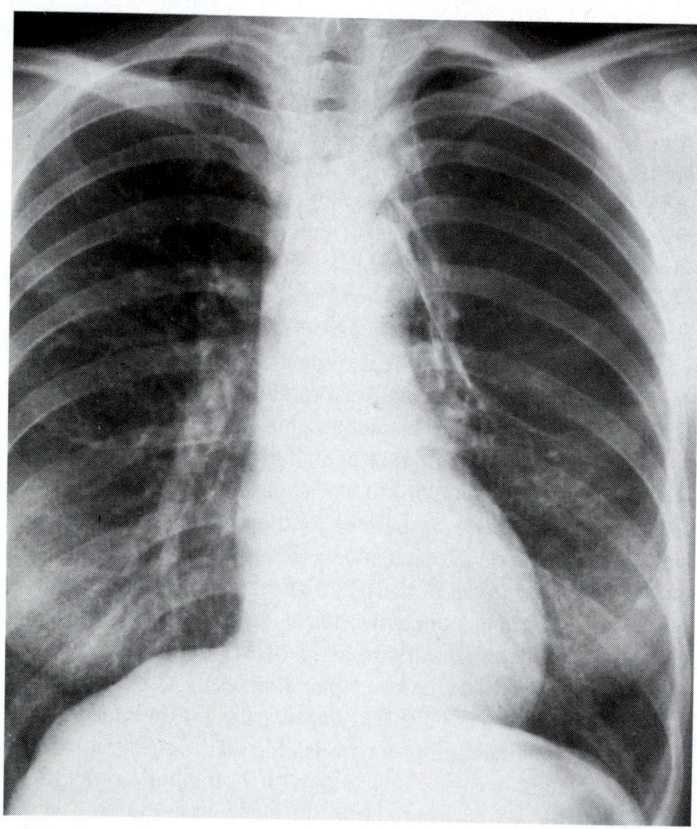

A

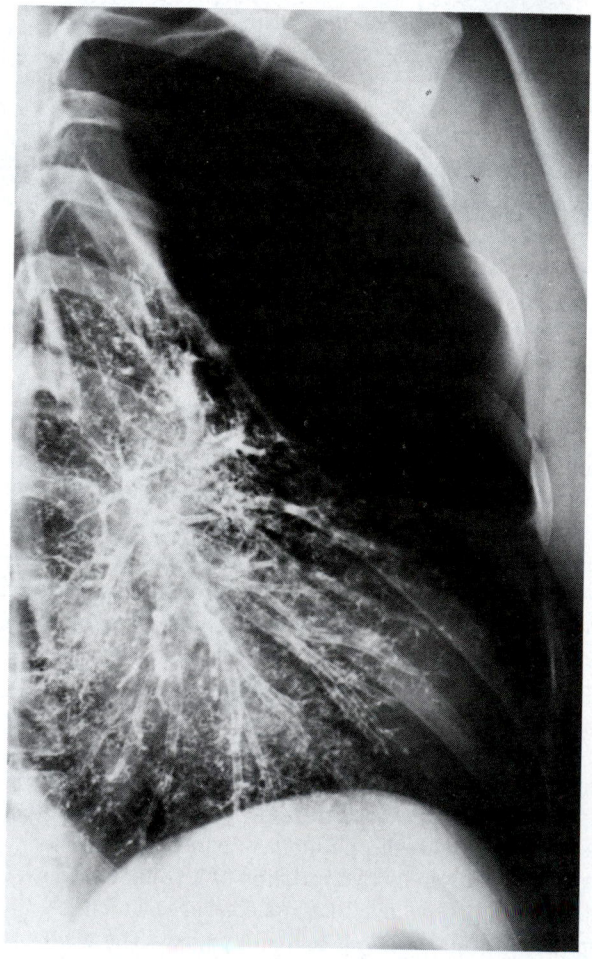

C

FIGURE 55-4 Large bulla in a 35-year-old woman admitted because of chest pain and increasing dyspnea. *A.* Chest radiograph (PA view). A large translucent area in the left upper lung represents a bulla that is causing compression of adjacent lung. *B.* Chest radiograph (lateral view). A hairline shadow outlines a large bulla in the left upper lobe. *C.* Bronchogram of left lung. Compression of the bronchial tree by the large bulla is evident.

DISTRIBUTION OF BULLAE

As noted above, the tendency for bullae to occur in the upper lobes is usually attributed to the greater mechanical stresses imposed on the apices than on the bases of the lungs. Because intrapleural pressure is more negative near the apices of the lungs than at the bases, apical alveoli are subjected to greater expanding stresses than are basal alveoli. Radioactive gas studies and in situ freezing techniques have demonstrated that the alveoli in the upper zones of the lungs are considerably larger than those in the lower zones. As indicated elsewhere in this book, gravity also plays a role in this feature of the upright lung, behaving like a coiled spring that, when allowed to dangle in the upright position, shows larger gaps between coils at its top than at its bottom.

Engineering techniques used to study the distribution of stresses in aircraft have been applied to the analysis of stresses on the lung. These have shown that the larger expanding stresses at the apices are directed primarily in a vertical direction and also, to lesser extent, laterally.[50] These stresses tend to increase with expansion of the lung, but they are also present when the lung volume decreases below functional residual capacity. The increase in apical stress at low lung volumes has been attributed to an increase in the rigidity of the lungs as the residual volume is approached.

CLINICAL FEATURES OF BULLOUS DISEASES

In asymptomatic subjects, bullae may be detected in the course of routine chest radiography. In some patients, however, bullae give rise to progressive dyspnea or chest pain (Fig. 55-4). On occasion, a patient with bullous disease of the lungs develops sudden severe breathlessness due to the development of a spontaneous pneumothorax (Fig. 55-5) or sudden increase in the size of a bulla due to air trapping. The development of bullae in patients with obstructive airway disease tends to aggravate breathlessness, presumably by further reducing expiratory flow rates (Fig. 55-6).

In the person known to have bullous disease, the onset of fatigue, generally accompanied by an increase in coughing and sputum production, usually heralds the presence of infection in a bulla[31] (Fig. 55-7). Pleuritic chest pain is occasionally part of the syndrome. Fever and leukocytosis are often not prominent, and Gram's stain of the sputum often shows only mixed flora without a predominant organism. Radiographically, infection is usu-

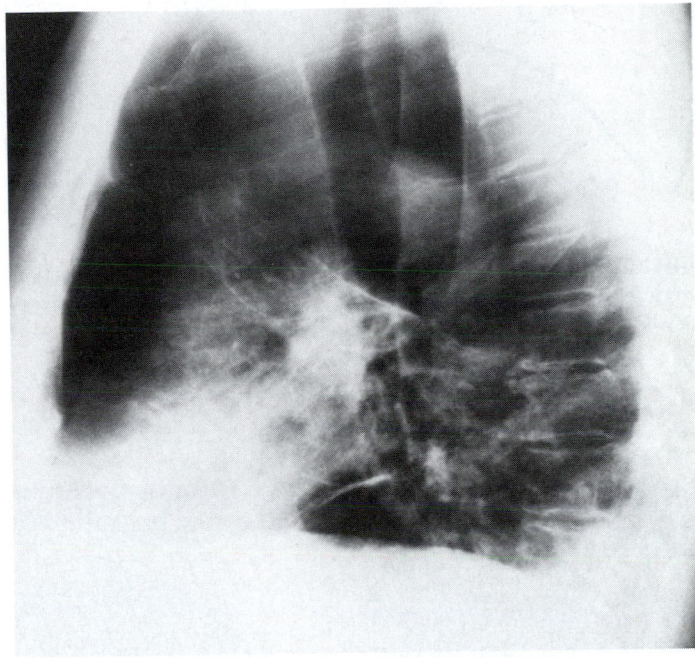

B

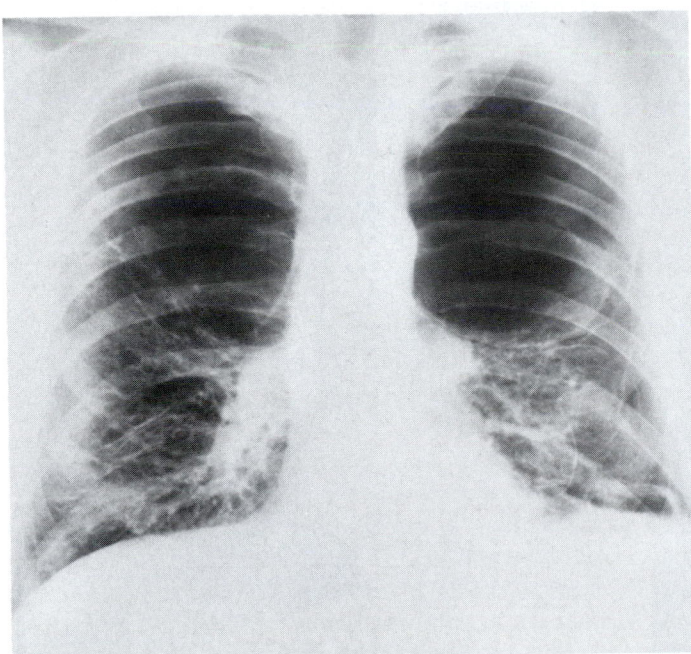

A

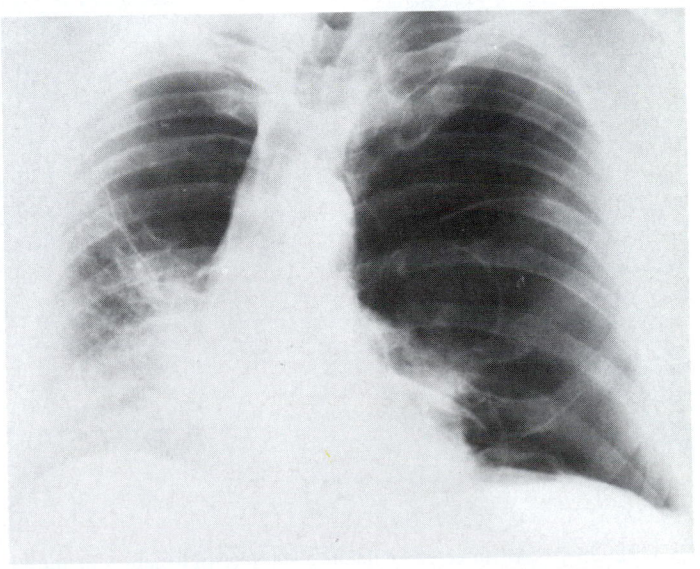

C

FIGURE 55-5   Bullous disease in a 53-year-old man. *A.* Chest radiograph (PA view) showing upper zonal areas of increased radiolucency. *B.* Chest radiograph (lateral view) showing hairline borders of multiple bullae. *C.* Chest radiograph showing a left-sided pneumothorax with residual inflated bullae. (*Courtesy of Dr. S. Flicker.*)

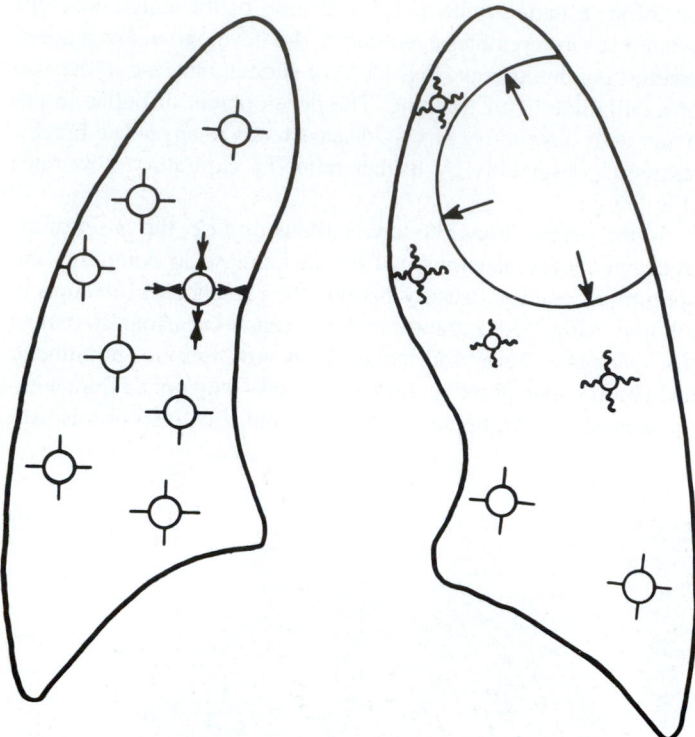

FIGURE 55-6   The effects of an enlarging airspace on radial traction exerted by elastic tissue on the airways. The reduction in lumen diameter is associated with an increase in airway resistance.

ally identified on the appearance of an air-fluid level (Fig. 55-7). Alternatively, the occurrence of fluid has been attributed to impeded drainage of the contents of the bulla due to obstruction of microscopic communications between the airspace and the pulmonary parenchyma. On occasion, infection of a bulla causes it to disappear completely;[18] more often, the air-fluid level persists for weeks or months after the infection has cleared.

The physical findings in a patient with one or more bullae usually reflect the state of the lungs overall, or in the immediate vicinity of the bulla. Only infrequently do giant bullae reach a size sufficient to cause a localized decrease or absence of breath sounds and the associated increase in resonance to percussion over the bulla.

RADIOLOGIC FEATURES

Although routine chest radiography is the most practical method for identifying the presence of bullae, this technique discloses only about 15 percent of bullae identified at autopsy. In a given patient, serial radiographs taken over years are invaluable in tracing the evolution of the disease. The presence of the disease is suggested by areas of increased radiolucency sharply delineated by fine radiopaque lines that delineate the walls of the bullae. These lines, or "hairline shadows," are composed of compressed and fused interlobular septae or pleura.[36] Because these hairline shadows appear incomplete on the chest radiograph, they display only segments of the wall of the bulla (Fig. 55-5). It is usually not difficult to distinguish the hairline shadows produced by a bulla from the thicker, sometimes irregular walls of a cavity.

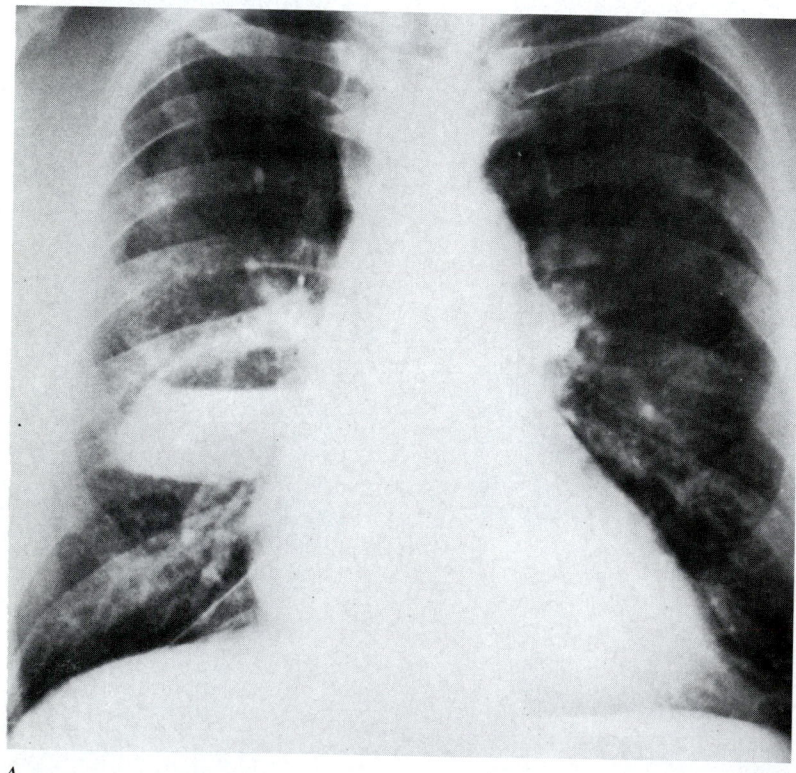

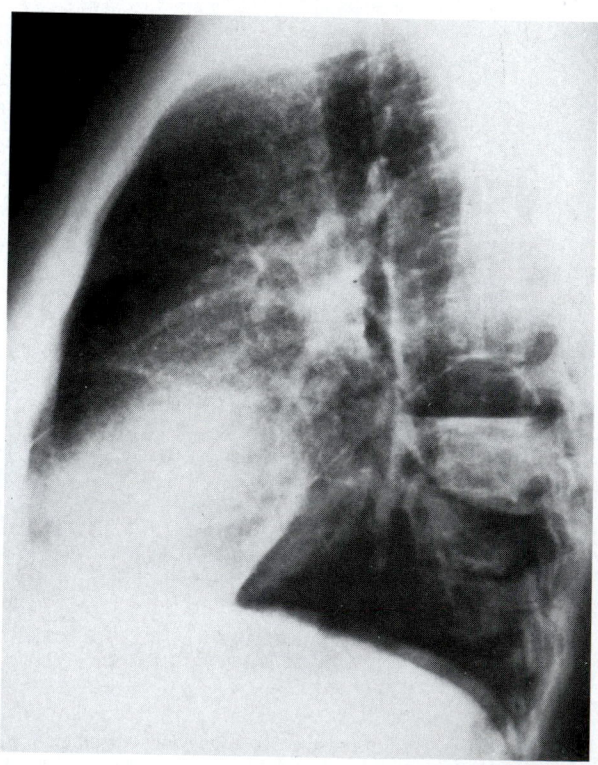

A

B

FIGURE 55-7   An infected bulla in a 44-year-old man with mitral stenosis. *A.* Chest radiograph (PA view). A translucent area is visible in the right midzone with a clearly defined air-fluid level. *B.* Lateral radiograph.

More troublesome is the distinction between bullae and cysts. In favor of bullae is the presence of other radiologic signs of emphysema or fibrotic lung disorders. The differential diagnosis of multiple enlarged thin-walled airspaces on the chest radiograph in adults is shown in Table 55-3.

Fluid in a Bulla

Although a localized air-fluid level on the chest radiograph raises the prospect of infection,[23] the differential diagnosis includes lung abscess, pulmonary tuberculosis, pulmonary fungal disease, cavitary lung carcinoma, pulmonary hemorrhage within a bulla, congestive heart failure, and carcinoma arising from a bulla (Fig. 55-8). The superimposition of a chronic infiltrate in association with an existing bulla raises the possibility of a concomitant fungal or tuberculous infection.

The presence of a fluid level within a bulla, especially if the bulla is located subpleurally, occasionally prompts the mistaken diagnosis of a loculated hydropneumothorax. Computed tomography is helpful in separating these two conditions: when locules within the bulla fill with fluid, the bulla shows characteristic

strands or septa sometimes in a "stepladder" configuration; in contrast, a loculated hydrothorax shows no septae. Sometimes it is difficult to distinguish between a large bulla and a pneumothorax.

Special Techniques

A forced expiration is sometimes helpful in demonstrating the presence of bullae on the chest radiograph: air trapping during the expiratory maneuver accentuates their outline by preventing a decrease in size as the surrounding lung empties. Large bullae sometimes displace the mediastinum contralaterally and may even compress the opposite lung.

Occasionally, angiography is necessary to provide previous information about the state of the pulmonary vasculature[17] (see Fig. 55-11B, on p. 857). A regional bronchogram at the time of bronchoscopy is also sometimes helpful in assessing the state of the airways in the region of lung compression (Fig. 55-4).

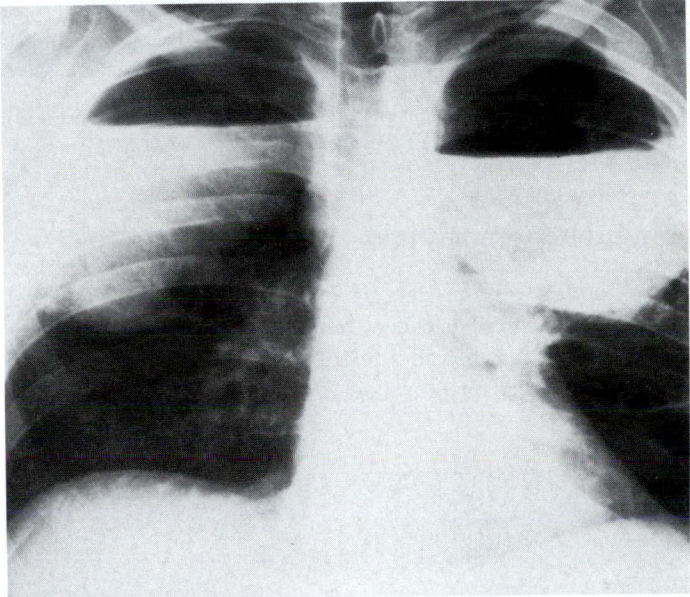

B

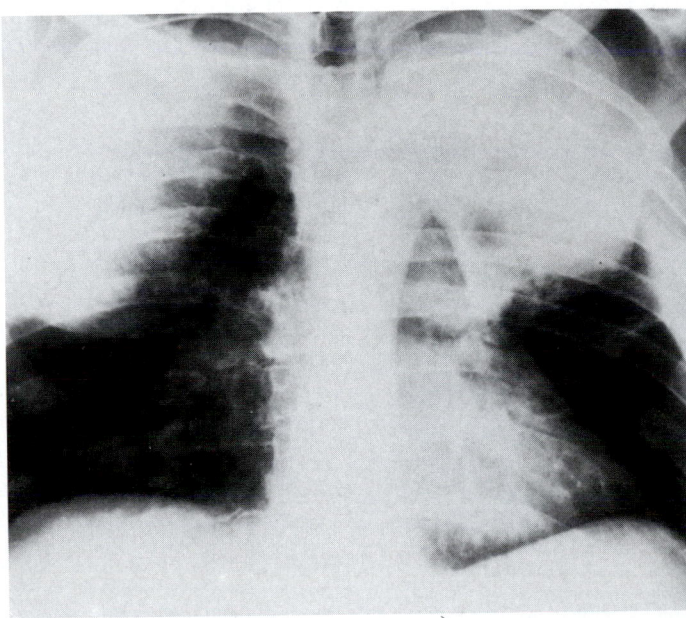

A

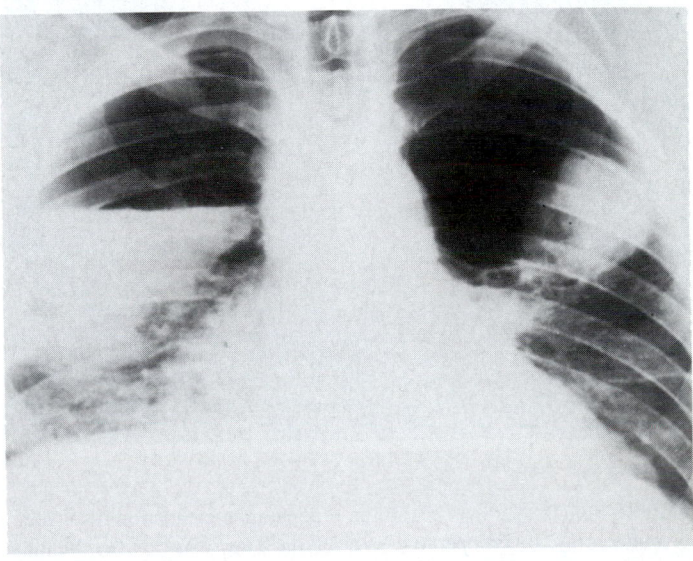

C

FIGURE 55-8 Infected bullae. *A.* Bilateral infected bullae in a 62-year-old man. *B.* Fluid levels in both bullae. *C.* Clearing of the infection revealed a bronchogenic carcinoma on the left. *(Courtesy of Dr. M. Feierstein.)*

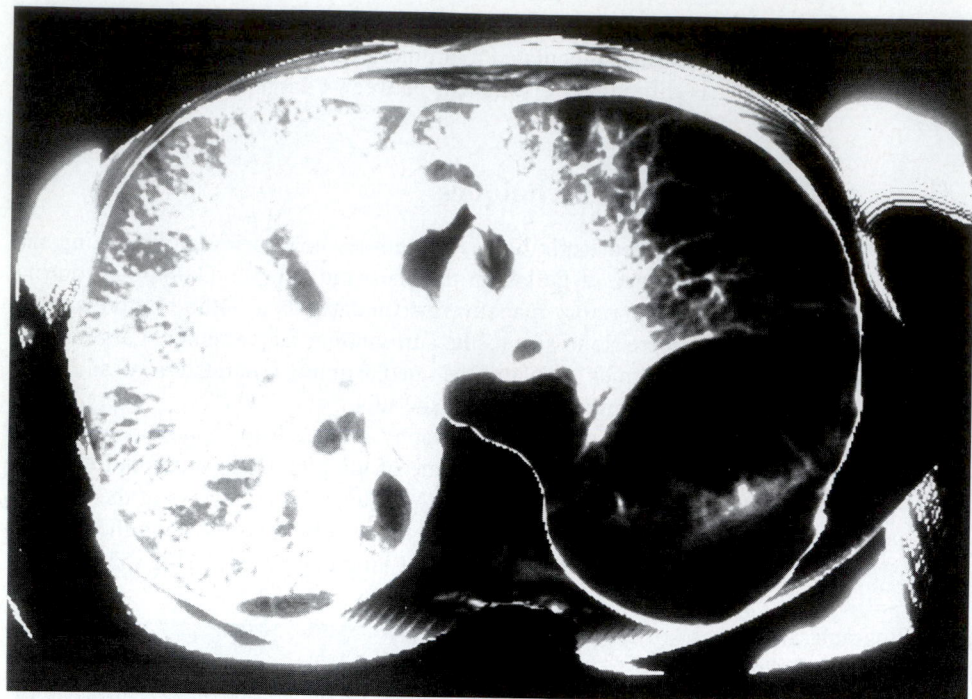

FIGURE 55-9   Three-dimensional reconstruction of the lung using computed tomography images. A large bulla can be seen in the right lung. *(Courtesy of K. Carr.)*

Computed Tomography

Linear tomography has largely been succeeded by computed tomography, which provides valuable anatomic information about the size, number, and relationships of bullae, as well as crowding of adjacent lung and disposition of the pulmonary

vasculature (Fig. 55-3). Bullae are identified as areas of transradiancy that usually do not contain blood vessels and are confined by visible walls. High-resolution computed tomography shows that large bullae (bullous emphysema) are frequently associated not only with distal acinar (paraseptal) emphysema but also with centriacinar emphysema, the type of emphysema usually associated with cigarette smoking.[27] These observations are consistent with the hypothesis, noted above, that peripheral airspaces of paraseptal emphysema may coalesce to form larger bullae that can crowd normal adjacent lung. Also, computed tomography has shown that when bullae occur in the context of general emphysema, the extent of bullous emphysema correlates poorly with measurements of pulmonary function and that the main determinant of respiratory function is the severity of emphysema in the bullous-free parts of the lung. In contrast, the severity of emphysema in nonbullous lung, assessed by computed tomographic density histograms of the lung, does correlate well with measurements of airflow limitation and diffusing capacity.[14]

Computed tomography has also been used to create three-dimensional reconstructions of bullae (Fig. 55-9), which can be

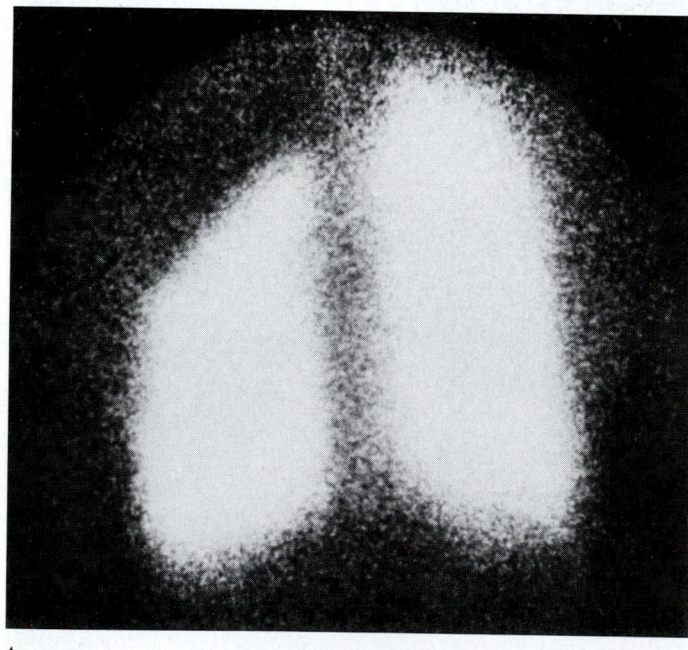

A

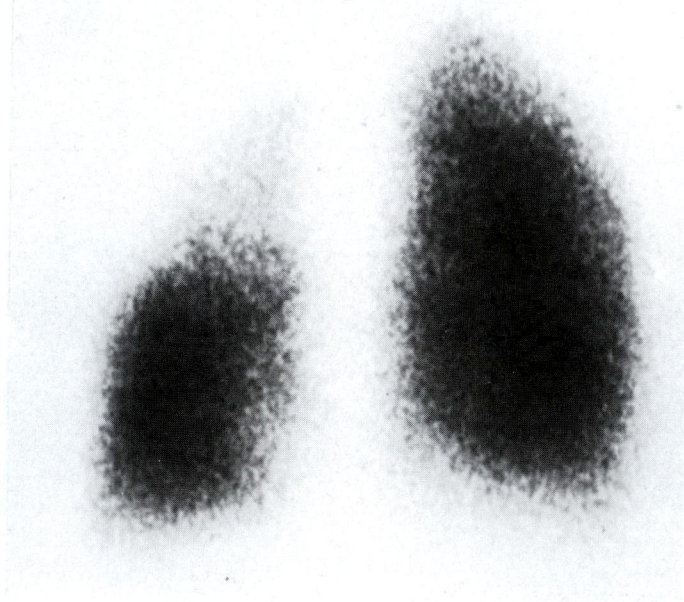

B

FIGURE 55-10   Lung scans in the preoperative evaluation of patients for bullectomy. *A.* Preoperative ventilation lung scan (^{133}Xe). Ventilation is absent in the left upper zone. *B.* Preoperative perfusion lung scan using ^{131}I-macroaggregated albumin. Blood flow is absent in the left upper zone while it is maintained at the left base. *(Courtesy of Dr. A. Alavi.)*

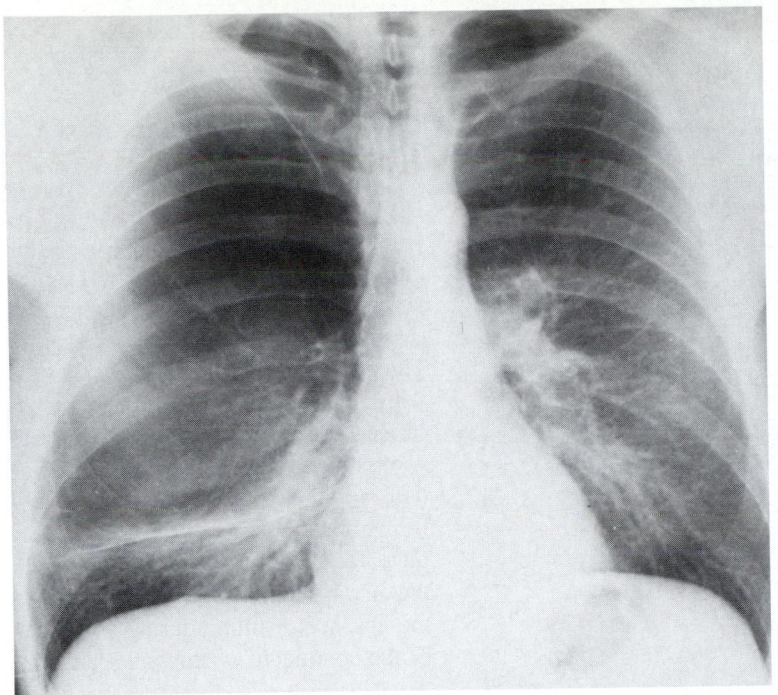

A

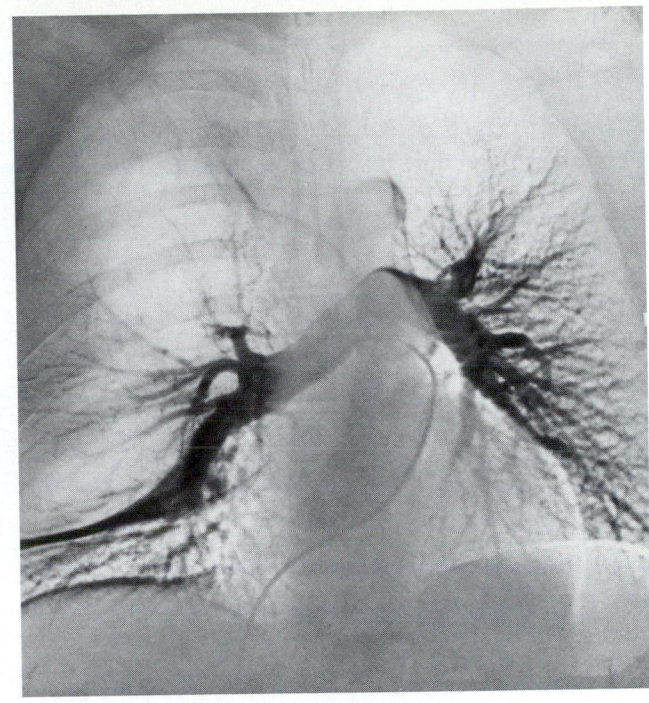

B

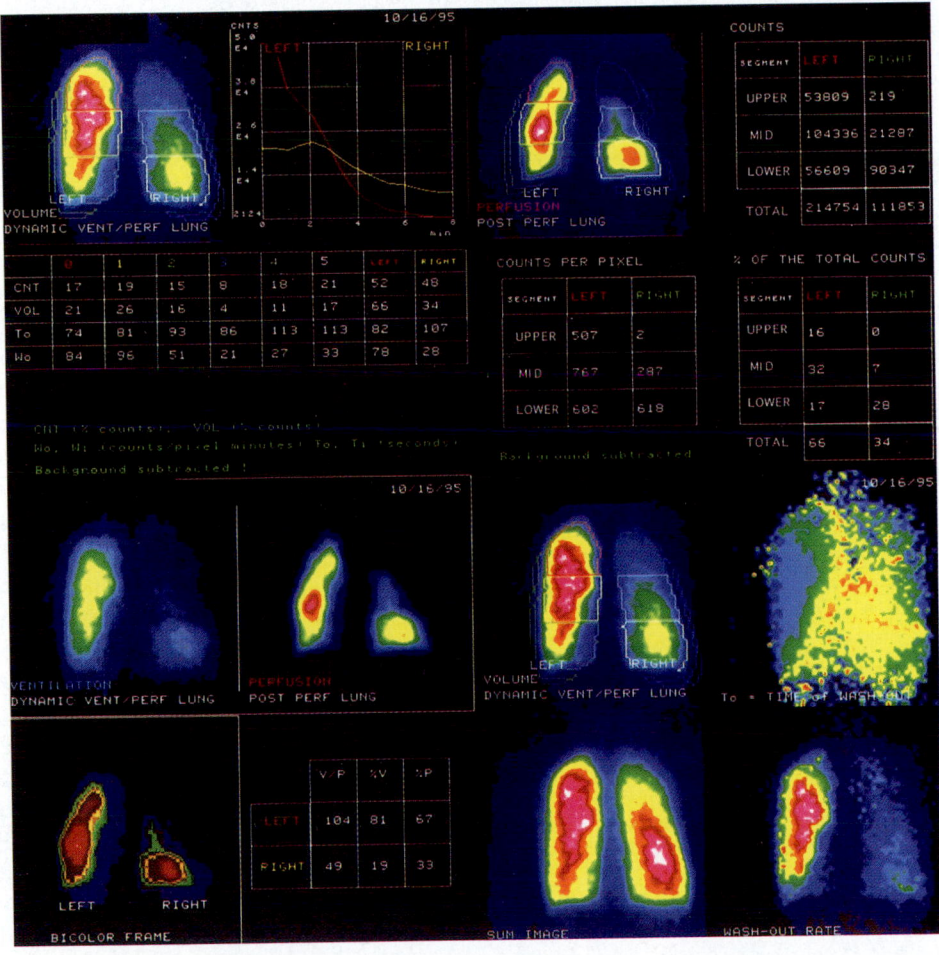

C

FIGURE 55-11 Large bulla in a 38-year-old man admitted because of increasing dyspnea. *A.* A chest radiograph (PA view). A large translucent area in the right upper lung represents an enlarging bulla that is causing compression of adjacent lung. *B.* Pulmonary arteriogram, subtraction technique. The pulmonary vasculature is compressed by the large bulla. *C.* Lung scans in the preoperative evaluation of patients for bullectomy. The ventilation lung scan (^{133}Xe) shows decreased ventila-

tion to the left upper lung zone. The perfusion lung scan using ^{131}I macroagglutinated albumin shows blood flow is decreased on the left upper zone while it is maintained at the left base. Quantitative regional ventilation and perfusion obtained from the lung scans of this patient. Ventilation is markedly reduced in the right upper zone. Perfusion is absent in the right upper zone while it is present at the base. *(A and B courtesy of Dr. M. Ora; C courtesy of Dr. B. Paczolt.)*

TABLE 55-4

Pulmonary Function Tests in a 65-Year-Old Black Man with Bullous Lung Disease

Spirometry	Prebronchodilator		
	Actual	% Pred.	Pred.
FVC, L	1.21	38	3.16
FEV_1, L	0.74	30	2.46
FEV_3, L	1.03	35	2.94
$FEV_1/FVC\%$	61		80
$FEV_3/FVC\%$	85		97
FEF_{25-75}, L/s	0.34	11	3.21
PEFR, L/s	3.05	46	6.57
FIF_{25-75}, L/s	1.30	23	5.67
SVC, L	1.42	38	3.72
IC, L	1.13	48	2.38
ERV, L	0.28	21	1.33
FRC, L	1.60	44	3.59
RV, L	1.31	58	2.26
TLC, L	2.73	47	5.85
RV/TLC%	48.11	123	39.00
D_{LCO}, single breath, ml/min/mmHg	10.06	40	25.18
Pulmonary vascular pressures			
Pulmonary artery, mmHg	60/22		30/16
Mean, mmHg	27		20

used to calculate their volume and vital capacity.[25] For example, at full expansion there is little change in the volume of bullae. Also, although the RV/TLC ratios of most bullae are usually high, the VC of bullae, expressed as a proportion of overall VC, is often less than 8 percent.

TABLE 55-5

Pulmonary Function Tests

Test	Bullous Disease	Obstructive Airways Disease and Bullae
TLC, L	N	N ↑
RV, L	N	↑
FRC, L	N	↑
FRC,* L	↑	↑
RV/TLC%	N	↑
FEV_1, L	N ↓	↓
FVC, L	N ↓	↓
$FEV_1/FVC\%$	N	↓
MVV, L/min	N	↓
D_{CO}/V_A, (ml/min/mmHg)/L	N	↓
Raw, cmH_2O/L/s	N ↑	↑
Cst, exp, L/cmH_2O	N ↑	↑
Pst, TLC, cmH_2O	N ↓	↓

*FRC determined by body plethysmography.
NOTE: N = normal, ↑ = increased, ↓ = decreased.

Nuclear Medicine Techniques

Useful preoperative information can be obtained from lung scanning using radioisotopes (Figs. 55-10 and 55-11C). A perfusion scan provides a qualitative assessment of the pulmonary vasculature. The results of ventilation scans vary with the technique: a single-breath ^{133}Xe scan often fails to demonstrate ventilation of a bulla, whereas a continuous ventilation scan often shows slow filling and emptying of the bulla. Complete lack of communication between the airways and the bulla is reflected in the absence of filling during all phases of the continuous ventilation scan.

PATHOPHYSIOLOGY OF BULLOUS DISEASES

Pulmonary Function Tests

Pulmonary function tests have considerable practical value in distinguishing between localized bullae with normal intervening lung (bullous disease) and localized bullae as part of obstructive airway disease (Tables 55-4 and 55-5). This distinction is important because patients with obstructive airway disease are generally poor surgical candidates owing to impaired pulmonary function.[21]

In patients with bullous disease, the volume of air in the lungs can be estimated by radiography, computed tomography, body plethysmography, or closed-circuit methods (helium dilution) and open-circuit methods (nitrogen washout). The volume of air trapped in bullae can be determined as the difference between the functional residual capacities determined plethysmographically and by open- or by closed-circuit methods (Table 55-6); the difference is due to the inability of the inert gas used in the method to enter the bullae. Pulmonary function is generally normal as long as the bullae occupy one-third or less of the volume of the lung. Expansion of a large bulla that crowds intervening normal lung may produce a restrictive pattern.

Although the nitrogen washout curve is usually normal, the concentration of N_2 in alveolar gas at the close of 7 min of breathing 100 percent O_2 is often abnormal.

TABLE 55-6

Pulmonary Function Tests in a 44-Year-Old Man with a Large Noninfected Bulla and Mitral Stenosis

Spirometry	Prebronchodilator		
	Actual	% Pred.	Pred.
FVC, L	2.67	57	4.70
FEV$_1$, L	1.57	42	3.76
FEV$_3$, L	2.31	52	4.47
FEV$_1$/FVC%	59		
FEV$_3$/FVC%	87		
FEV$_{25-75}$, L/s	0.76	16	4.69
PEFR, L/s	3.86	43	9.50
FIF$_{25-75}$, L/s	2.41	34	7.03
MVV, L/min	59	43	137
SVC, L	2.89	62	4.70
IC, L	2.27	65	3.47
ERV, L	0.62	51	1.23
FRC, L	2.86	87	3.29
TGV*	4.71		3.29
RV, L	2.24	109	2.06
TLC, L	5.13	76	6.71
RV/TLC%	43.63	137	31.79
D$_{LCO}$, single breath, ml/min/mmHg	17.65	60	29.45
Gaw/V$_L$, cmH$_2$O/s	0.07		0.13–0.34

*Measured by body plethysmography.

Pulmonary Mechanics

As large bullae distend, acting as expanding space-occupying lesions, they first relax adjacent lung tissue and then compress it. Relaxation of the surrounding pulmonary parenchyma decreases radial traction on the airway, increasing resistance to airflow[11] (Fig. 55-6). The effects of bullectomy on mechanics are inconsistent: in some patients, removal of a large bulla increases the static recoil pressure of the lungs and decreases both airways and upstream resistances;[35] in others, bullectomy decreases the elastic recoil pressure.

Distinction between widespread obstructive airway disease with bullae, on the one hand, and bullous disease, on the other, has practical significance because resection in the presence of generalized emphysema offers a less certain therapeutic response than does resection of large bullae in the absence of widespread obstructive lung disease. However, since both reduce the static elastic recoil pressure of the lungs, the diffusing capacity is usually determined to aid in distinguishing between widespread emphysema and localized bullae.[21] The reason for resorting to measurement of the diffusing capacity is that it correlates better with morphologic estimates of emphysema than do most other tests. Although the combination of a significant decrease in diffusing capacity and in static elastic recoil does favor the diagnosis of widespread emphysema and would tend to discourage attempts at surgical bullectomy, it must be kept in mind that both the elastic recoil and the diffusing capacity can be decreased by bullae that compress the lungs.

Respiratory muscle strength assessed by measurements of maximal inspiratory and transdiaphragmatic pressures improves after bullectomy in some patients with bullous emphysema.[42]

Exercise

Both progressive and steady-state exercise testing have been used to determine if the tracheobronchial tree and the lung tissue between bullae are normal or abnormal.[39] Exercise is invariably used as part of a constellation of tests to determine the state of the airways and parenchyma, keeping in mind the distortions introduced by the space-occupying bullae.

In patients with a few circumscribed bullae but otherwise normal lungs, exercise reveals that the alveolar-arterial difference in P$_{O_2}$, the VD/VT ratio, the D$_{LCO}$, and the arterial oxygenation remain normal or near normal.

Patients in whom bullae are associated with panacinar emphysema differ in that the alveolar-arterial difference in P$_{O_2}$ is widened, both at rest and during exercise, and they develop arterial hypoxemia during exercise. The arterial Pa$_{CO_2}$ tends to hover around the upper limits of normal at rest and during exercise; the VD/VT ratio is higher in this group than in the group with normal intervening lung; also, steady-state diffusing capacities are reduced in this group and fail to increase normally during exercise. In many of these patients, the D$_{LCO}$ is reduced at rest and arterial hypoxemia develops during exercise.

Patients in whom bullae are associated with chronic bronchitis show a widened alveolar-arterial difference in P$_{O_2}$ and an increased VD/VT ratio at rest. However, the decrease in arterial P$_{O_2}$ during exercise is only modest even though arterial Pa$_{CO_2}$ at rest is abnormally high and increases further during exercise, indicating progressive alveolar hypoventilation.

Pulmonary Circulation

As a rule, pulmonary arterial pressures and blood flow are within normal limits in patients with bullous disease at rest (i.e., the bullae act like amputated segments of lung), limiting the volume of the vascular bed available for recruitment as cardiac output increases. However, in patients in whom the extent of the pulmonary vascular bed has been severely curtailed by widespread bullous disease, the pulmonary arterial pressures tend to rise, at rest and during exercise, and in a few instances reach levels of

TABLE 55-7

Preoperative and Postoperative Pulmonary Function Tests in Bullous Disease*

Spirometry	Preoperative			Postoperative
	Actual	% Pred.	Pred.	Actual
FVC, L	3.97	77	5.15	4.64
FEV_1, L	2.72	66	4.14	3.36
FEV_3, L	3.60	73	4.93	4.25
PEFR, L/s	6.05	63	9.60	7.07
FEV_{25-75}, L/s	1.68	33	5.08	2.41
$FEV_1/FVC\%$	69		83	72
$FEV_3/FVC\%$	91		97	91
FIF_{25-75}, L/s	5.67	74	7.61	5.92
MVV, L/min	98	76	128	129
SVC, L	4.28	83	5.15	9.73
IC, L	2.88	91	3.16	3.36
ERV, L	1.29	65	1.99	1.37
RV, L	0.81	39	2.04	1.90
TLC, L	5.08	71	7.17	6.63
RV/TLC%	16		29	28.63
FRC, L	2.10	52	4.03	3.27
D_{LCO}, single breath, ml/min/mmHg	21.04	64	32.93	26.43

*Thirty-eight-year-old man who underwent successful bullectomy. Second study done 20 months after surgery.

pulmonary hypertension that lead to cor pulmonale. Exercise in patients with bullous disease is generally associated with abnormally high increments in pulmonary arterial pressure as the normal increases in pulmonary blood flow are accommodated in the restricted vascular bed. Underlying pulmonary disease exaggerates the increments in pulmonary arterial pressure during exercise.

COMPLICATIONS

The major complications of bullous disease of the lungs are infection of the bulla, chest pain, hemorrhage, spontaneous pneumothorax, and lung cancer.[8] Recurrent spontaneous pneumothorax also may be a complication of paraseptal emphysema.

Infections within bullae are rare. In most bullae, air-fluid levels are the result of peribullous pneumonitis. The fluid within the airspace, which is usually sterile,[31] is often reabsorbed and may be associated with shrinkage and complete resolution of the bulla. Chest pain is attributed to overdistention, has an anginalike quality, and is located retrosternally. This symptom is sometimes of sufficient severity to be an indication for surgical intervention. Hemoptysis, which is occasionally massive, can result from rupture of blood vessels within the walls of bullae. Pneumothorax secondary to rupture of a bulla into the pleural space can severely compromise a patient's ventilatory reserve in the setting of generalized emphysema. The rate of recurrence of pneumothoraces (50 percent) is generally higher for patients who have experienced rupture of a bulla than for those who have experienced a spontaneous pneumothorax due to rupture of blebs. Patients with ruptured bullae also tend to have prolonged air leaks, with increased pleural and parenchymal infections.[8]

Primary lung cancer has been reported to be associated with bullous lung disease[1,13,29,43] (Fig. 55-8). In many instances, the bullae are detected only by computed scanning. The high incidence of lung cancer may be due to the fact that lung cancer occurs more frequently in lung scars that predispose to the development of bullae. Explanations also include dystrophic changes in the lung parenchyma caused by bullous disease and the behavior of bullae as poorly ventilated spaces where carcinogens may linger.

TREATMENT

Many patients with bullous disease of the lungs can be managed medically. Because the natural history of a bulla is unpredictable, the patient with bullous disease should be monitored by chest radiography at regular intervals to ensure that the situation is stable. Bullae occasionally enlarge suddenly and rapidly for no apparent reason.

Medical Treatment

The finding of a bulla in an asymptomatic patient calls for reassurance, a recommendation for annual chest radiography, advice to stop smoking, and an alert to the need for a prompt visit to a physician should symptoms develop. Activities that promote rupture of bullae (e.g., contact sports and scuba diving) should be proscribed. Chronic bronchitis, asthma, and emphysema associated with bullae require treatment in their own right.

Infection of a bulla requires sputum specimens for culture and Gram's stain. Fiberoptic bronchoscopy is usually done if sputum studies fail to disclose the nature of the infection; sterile sheathed catheters are sometimes helpful in obtaining uncontaminated respiratory tract secretions for culture. Direct sampling of fluid from within the bulla is rarely useful in making the diagnosis.[31] Once the diagnosis of an infected bulla has been established, treatment is begun with antibiotics and chest physiotherapy. The choice of antibiotic depends on the Gram's stain and sputum cultures. Treatment is prolonged, since poor drainage of the bulla inevitably slows resolution of the disease process. The course of the infection can be followed with intermittent chest radiographs (Fig. 55-8). Most infections of bullae eventually respond to medical therapy. Infected bullae with large amounts of fluid may require surgical intervention because of the risk that fluid from the infected bulla may empty into the contralateral lung, flooding the airways.

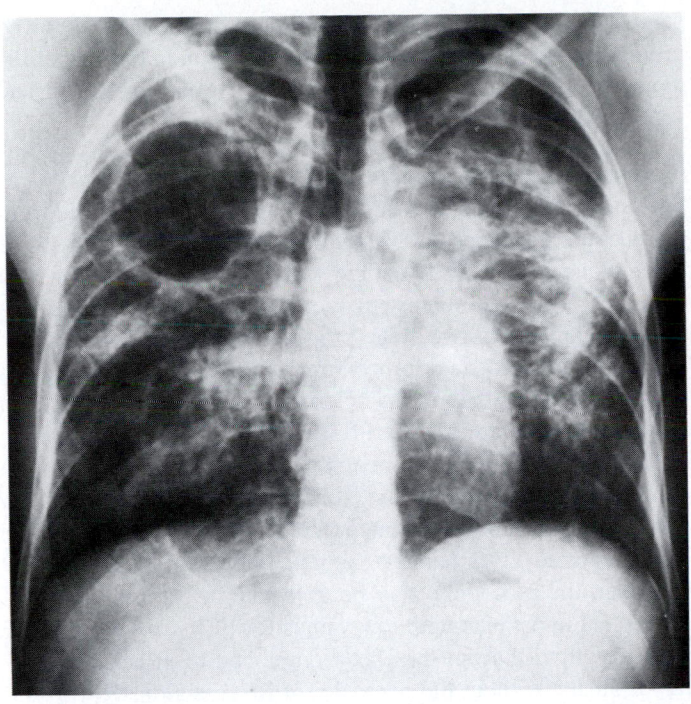

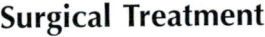

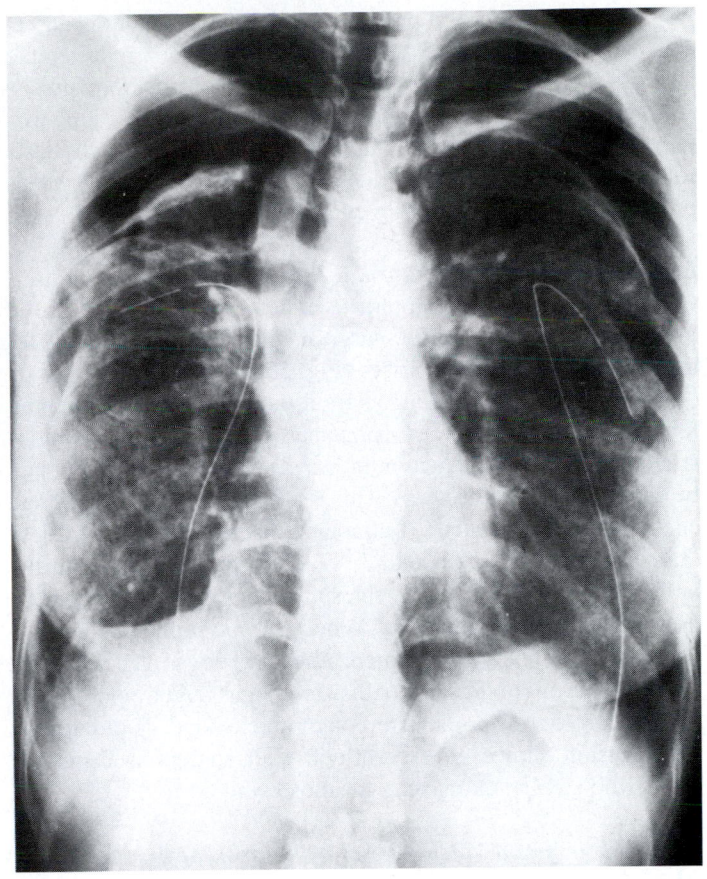

FIGURE 55-12   Bullae in sarcoidosis. *A.* A bulla in a 27-year-old man with sarcoidosis. *B.* Bilateral pneumothorax in a 26-year-old woman with sarcoidosis. A large bulla was found at the right apex.

Surgical Treatment

GENERAL

In some patients carefully selected for localized disease and well-preserved pulmonary function, surgical intervention may provide symptomatic relief, improved exercise tolerance, and improvement on pulmonary function testing, such as spirometry, diffusingcapacity, and ventilation perfusion matching (Table 55-7).[20,33]

In general, surgical outcome depends on the size and number of the resected bullae, the condition of the compressed lung,[6] the condition of the contralateral lung, and the incidence of postoperative complications.[8] Radionucleotide scanning and computed tomography can be helpful in preoperative assessment of the compressed lung,[4,25] but on occasion, pulmonary angiography may be required for this purpose (Fig. 55-11*B*).

Localized Bullae with Normal Intervening Lung (Bullous Lung Disease)

In this subgroup there are definite indications for surgical intervention. For example, certain acute complications (e.g., spontaneous pneumothorax or massive hemorrhage) demand urgent surgical intervention even though the bullae may be small. In less urgent circumstances, the indications for operation in bullae that coexist with relatively normal surrounding parenchyma are as follows: (1) bullae that have become large enough to cause dyspnea, (2) bullae that are increasing in size or have become large enough to compress surrounding lung tissue, (3) bullae that are responsible for recurrent pneumothoraces, (4) infected bullae that fail to respond to medical treatment, (5) acute respiratory insufficiency attributable to the bullae, (6) acute distention of a bulla, (7) severe chest pain attributed to a change in bulla size, and (8) primary lung cancer occurring in association with bullae.

The surgical approach depends on the location of the bullae. Median sternotomy, which results in less postoperative morbidity than does the standard thoracotomy incision, may be appropriate for bilateral upper-lobe bullae.[46] As a rule, small-wedge excisions or plications of large bullae have brought about larger increments in expiratory flow rates than has lobectomy.[10]

The size of the bulla is an important selection criterion in determining the outcome of surgery, as the best functional improvement occurs when the bulla constitutes 50 to 100 percent of the hemithorax (Fig. 55-9); in such patients, postoperative increments in FEV$_1$ range from 50 to 200 percent.[10] Good results may be anticipated when the invaded lung contributes little to overall ventilation, when large volumes of trapped air exist, and when there is crowding of normal lung parenchyma. Attention to postoperative management is critical to a good surgical outcome and includes underwater thoracostomy suction and vigorous bronchial toilet. Regular postoperative chest radiographs identify residual airspaces that may require supplemental tube thoracostomy.

The overall mortality in this type of surgery is about 1.5 percent, with the most common causes being infection and respiratory failure.[51] Sudden development of a contralateral pneumothorax or herniation of a bulla across the mediastinum is an occasional cause of death. Postoperative complication rates tend to be high (between 14 and 44 percent). Not surprisingly, persistent air leaks and pleuropulmonary infections have been the major causes. Prolonged follow-up shows that benefit usually lasts for about 5 years, with no evidence that the bullectomy hastens progression of the underlying emphysematous process.[15,28]

Localized Bullae with Abnormal Intervening Lung

Generally, bullae that complicate either obstructive or fibrotic lung disease do not require surgical intervention unless a life-threatening complication arises (Fig. 55–12).

When bullae occur in association with abnormal intervening lung—as with widespread panacinar emphysema, as demonstrated by a marked reduction in $D_{L_{CO}}$—little improvement can be expected from bullectomy. This is particularly true in the presence of chronic obstructive pulmonary disease if the FEV_1 is less than 35 percent of predicted.[10,51] Elderly patients in whom the bullae are associated with widespread emphysema frequently have a high surgical mortality. When chronic bronchitis is associated with bullae, improvement after surgery is generally not sustained for more than 6 months. Two signs augur a poor prognosis: a prolonged productive cough and secondary pulmonary hypertension. However, the outlook after surgery is better for those who stop smoking than for those who do not.[15]

Laser Surgery and Video-Assisted Thoracoscopy

Recently, laser surgery in conjunction with thoracoscopy using video assistance has been used to ablate bullae.[7] Thoracoscopy requires general anesthesia, with introduction of a double-lumen endotracheal tube to permit collapse of one lung. Three thoracoports are made in the chest wall to introduce the surgical instruments. Once a bulla has been identified, the lung is deflated and the bulla excised with a stapling device.

Current laser surgical techniques have evolved since 1989, when a low-energy CO_2 laser was used to ablate pleural blebs in the treatment of spontaneous pneumothorax.[47] As it was observed that subpleural bullae also collapse when exposed to the laser, multiple bullae in lungs with widespread emphysema also have been treated by ablation with the CO_2 laser. In the initial report, 20 of 22 patients survived the procedure. Of 11 patients followed for 3 months, significant postoperative increases in FVC and FEV_1 were recorded. Maximal treadmill exercise time also increased. Complications included postoperative air leaks, bleeding, and acute lung injury.[48] In a prospective study,[2] patients with large bullae associated with crowding of adjacent lung structures, upper-lobe predominance, and minimal underlying emphysema showed the greatest improvement, with increases in FVC, FEV_1, MVV, and specific conductance and decreases in residual volume. Both the argon beam coagulator[22] and the YAG laser[49] have also been used in conjunction with video-assisted thoracoscopy to ablate bullae in the treatment of bullous emphysema. The mortality from these procedures has been 0 to 4.7 percent, respectively.

In contrast to surgical bullectomy, some patients with bullae and abnormal intervening lung who underwent CO_2 laser ablation demonstrated improvements in pulmonary function even though there was no evidence of crowding of adjacent lung

parenchyma by the bullae. The authors suggested that improved mechanical advantage resulting from reduction in the size of the thoracic cavity leads to improved respiratory muscle function and ventilatory capacity.[2]

External Drainage—Monaldi Procedure

The open intubation and external drainage of bullae evolved from a procedure described by Monaldi in 1938 for the treatment of tuberculous cavities.[24] Later the technique was adapted to the treatment of intrapulmonary pyogenic abscesses and bullae. Initially proposed as a two-stage procedure, it is now usually performed as a single-stage procedure, with resection of a portion of a rib and instillation of a sclerosing agent into the bulla to produce rapid contraction and fibrosis. Continuous drainage using a Foley catheter maintained in place by a purse-string suture completes the procedure. The technique is sometimes useful in patients whose pulmonary function precludes thoracostomy. One study reported a 22 percent median improvement in FEV_1.[45] However, the procedure may be associated with a mortality of 15 percent in patients with low values for FEV_1 or hypercapnia. Recently, thoracoscopy has been employed to effect intracavitary drainage without the necessity of rib resection.[44]

REFERENCES

1. Aaronberg DJ, Sagel SS, LeFrak S, et al: Lung carcinoma associated with bullous lung disease in young men. *AJR* 134:249, 1980.
2. Brenner M, Kayaleh RA, Milne EN, et al: Thorascopic laser ablation of pulmonary bullae: Radiographic selection and treatment response. *J Thorac Cardiovasc Surg* 107:883, 1994.
3. Burke RM: Vanishing lung: A case report of bullous emphysema. *Radiology* 28:367, 1937.
4. Carr DH, Pride NB: Computed tomography in preoperative assessment of bullous emphysema. *Clin Radiol* 35:43, 1984.
5. CIBA Guest Symposium: Terminology, definitions and classifications of chronic pulmonary emphysema and related conditions. *Thorax* 14:286, 1959.
6. Connolly JE, Wilson A: The current status of surgery for bullous emphysema. *J Thorac Cardiovasc Surg* 97:351, 1989.
7. Daniel TM, Wyatt, DA: Pneumothorax and bullous disease, in Kaiser LR, Daniel TM (eds), *Thoracoscopic Surgery*. Little, Brown, 1993, pp 85–96.
8. DesLauriers J, Leblanc P: Management of bullous disease. *Chest Surg Clin North Am* 4:539, 1994.
9. Edge J, Simon G, Reid L: Periacinar (paraseptal) emphysema: Its clinical, radiological and physiological features. *Br J Dis Chest* 60:10, 1966.
10. Fitzgerald MX, Keelan PJ, Cugell DW, Gaensler EA: Long-term results of surgery for bullous emphysema. *J Thorac Cardiovasc Surg* 68:566, 1974.
11. Gelb AF, Gold WM, Nadel JA: Mechanisms limiting airflow in bullous lung disease. *Am Rev Respir Dis* 107:571, 1973.
12. Goldstein DS, Karpel JP, Appel D, Williams MH Jr.: Bullous pulmonary damage in users of intravenous drugs. *Chest* 89:266, 1986.
13. Goldstein MJ, Snider GL, Liberson M, Roske RM: Bronchogenic carcinoma and giant bullous disease. *Am Rev Respir Dis* 97:1062, 1967.
14. Gould GA, Redpath AT, Ryan M, et al: Parenchymal emphysema measured by CT lung density correlates with lung functions in patients with bullous disease. *Eur Respir J* 6:698, 1993.

15. Hughes JA, MacArthur AM, Hutchinson DCS, Hugh-Jones P: Long-term changes in lung function after surgical treatment of bullous emphysema in smokers and ex-smokers. *Thorax* 39:140, 1984.

16. Jack CIA, Evans CC: Three cases of alpha-1-antitrypsin deficiency in the elderly. *Postgrad Med J* 67:840, 1991.

17. Jensen KM, Miscall L, Steinberg I: Angiography in bullous emphysema—Its role in selections of the case suitable for surgery. *Am J Roentgenol* 85:229, 1961.

18. Khan MA, Dulfano MJ: Disappearance of a giant bulla following acute pneumonitis. *Chest* 68:746, 1975.

19. Kinner WJM, Tattersfield AE: Emphysematous blebs (editorial). *Br Med J* 300:208, 1990.

20. Klingman RR, Angelillo VA, DeMasters TR: Cystic and bullous lung disease. *Ann Thorac Surg* 52:576, 1991.

21. Laurenzi GA, Turino GM, Fishman AP: Bullous disease of the lung. *Am J Med* 32:361, 1962.

22. Lewis RJ, Caccavale RJ, Sisler GE: Vats argon beam coagulator treatment of diffuse end-stage bilateral bullous disease of the lung. *Ann Thorac Surg* 55:1394, 1994.

23. Mahler DA, D'Esopo ND: Periemphysematous lung infection. *Clin Chest Med* 4:51, 1981.

24. Monaldi V: Tentativi di aspirazione endocavitaria nelle caverne tubercolari del pulmone. *Lotta Contro la Tuberculosi* 9:910, 1938.

25. Morgan MDL, Denison DM, Strickland B: Value of computed tomography for selecting patients with bullous lung disease for surgery. *Thorax* 41:855, 1986.

26. Morgan MDL, Edwards CW, Morris J, Matthews HR: Origin and behavior of emphysematous bullae. *Thorax* 44:533, 1989.

27. Morgan MDL, Strickland B: Computed tomography in the assessment of bullous lung disease. *Br J Dis Chest* 78:10, 1984.

28. Nickoladze GD: Functional results of surgery for bullous emphysema. *Chest* 101:119, 1992.

29. Nickoladze GD: Bullae and lung cancer (letter). *J Thorac Cardiovasc Surg* 106:186, 1993.

30. Ohata M, Suzuki H: Pathogenesis of spontaneous pneumothorax with special reference to the ultrastructure of emphysematous bullae. *Chest* 77:771, 1980.

31. Peters JI, Kubitschek KR, Gotleib MS, Awe RJ: Lung bullae with air-fluid levels. *Am J Med* 82:759, 1987.

32. Reid L: *The Pathology of Emphysema*. Chicago, Year Book, 1967, pp 211–240.

33. Ribet ME: Cystic and bullous disease. *Ann Thorac Surg* 53:1147, 1992.

34. Richards DW: The aging lung. *Bull NY Acad Med* 32:407, 1956.

35. Rogers RM, DuBois AB, Blakemore WS: The effect of removal of bullae on airway conductance and conductance volume ratios. *J Clin Invest* 47:2569, 1968.

36. Sanders C: The radiographic diagnosis of emphysema. *Radiol Clin North Am* 29:1019, 1991.

37. Snider GL: The definition of emphysema. Report of the National Heart, Lung, and Blood Institute, National Institutes of Health, Division of Lung Diseases Workshop. *Am Rev Respir Dis* 132:182, 1985.

38. Spencer H: *Pathology of the Lung,* 4th ed. New York, Pergamon Press, 1984, p 557.

39. Tenholder MF, Jones PA, Matthews JI, Hooper RG: Bullous emphysema: Progressive incremental exercise testing to evaluate candidates for bullectomy. *Chest* 77:801, 1980.

40. Thurlbeck MM: Chronic airflow obstruction in lung disease, in Bennington JL (ed), *Major Problems in Pathology,* vol 5. Philadelphia, Saunders, 1976, p 181.

41. Ting EY, Klopstock R, Lyons HA: Mechanical properties of pulmonary cysts and bullae. *Am Rev Respir Dis* 87:538, 1963.

42. Travaline JM, Addonizio VP, Criner GJ: Effect of bullectomy on diaphragm strength. *Am J Respir Crit Care Med* 152:1697, 1995.

43. Tsutsue M, Araki Y, Shikakusa T, et al: Characteristic radiographic features of pulmonary carcinoma associated with large bullae. *Ann Thorac Surg* 46:679, 1988.

44. Urschel JD, Dickout WJ: Thorascopic intracavitary drainage for pneumothorax secondary to bullous emphysema. *Can J Surg* 36:548, 1993.

45. Venn GE, Williams PR, Goldshaw TR: Intracavitary drainage for bullous emphysematous lung disease: Experience with the Bromptom technique. *Thorax* 43:998, 1988.

46. Vishnevsky AA, Nickoladze GD: One stage operation for bilateral bullous lung disease. *J Thorac Cardiovasc Surg* 99:30, 1990.

47. Wakabayashi A: Thoracoscopic ablation of blebs in the treatment of recurrent or persistent spontaneous pneumothorax. *Ann Thorac Surg* 68:651, 1989.

48. Wakabayashi A, Brenner M, Kayaleh RA, et al: Thoracoscopic carbon dioxide laser treatment of bullous emphysema. *Lancet* 337:881, 1991.

49. Wakabayashi A: Video assisted laser resection is the best treatment for bullous emphysema, in Proceedings of the 79th Annual Clinical Congress of the American College of Surgery Thoracic Surgery Postgraduate Course. San Francisco, October 1993, pp 46–48.

50. West JB: Distribution of mechanical stress in the lung, a possible factor in localization of pulmonary disease. *Lancet* 1:839, 1971.

51. Witz JP, Roeslin N: La chirurgie de l'emphyseme bulleux chez l'adulte ses resultats éloignés: *Rev Fr Mal Respir* 8:121, 1980.

PART FIVE

OCCUPATIONAL AND ENVIRONMENTAL DISORDERS

CHAPTER 56

OCCUPATIONAL LUNG DISORDERS: GENERAL PRINCIPLES AND APPROACHES

Carrie A. Redlich

The past decade has seen a marked increase in concern about the adverse health effects of hazardous exposures in the workplace and elsewhere in the environment.[1] The lung—with its extensive surface area, high blood flow, and thin alveolar epithelium—is an important site of contact with substances in the environment. Because of the seemingly endless array of substances that can affect the lung, physicians must be prepared to recognize, diagnose, and treat occupational lung diseases. Physicians must also be prepared to provide preventive advice and to address patients' concerns regarding occupational and environmental, exposures. Since many respiratory diseases may be caused or exacerbated by factors in the workplace or environment, knowledge of the basic approaches used in the diagnosis and management of occupational and environmental disorders is essential for all medical practitioners. This chapter provides an overview to these approaches. Additional information can be obtained from several excellent recent texts on this topic.[4,16,21,26,27]

CLASSIFICATION OF OCCUPATIONAL AND ENVIRONMENTAL LUNG DISEASE

Environmentally induced lung diseases can be classified according to several schemes. One useful approach is to classify them by clinical presentation or disease, as shown in Table 56-1. One should remember that a given exposure (asbestos, cobalt, etc.) can cause more than a single disorder. When one is examining a patient, it can also be helpful to classify occupational lung diseases by types of exposures that can cause lung disease, such as mineral dusts (asbestos, silica, coal), biologic factors (animal exposures, microbial agents), metals (beryllium, nickel, cobalt, aluminum), or inorganic gases (carbon monoxide, chlorine, nitrogen oxides), or by the type of industry potentially associated with respiratory diseases, such as mining, agriculture, forestry, or welding.

Occupational and environmental exposures play an important role in many lung disorders. Accurate estimates of the contribution of such factors to specific lung diseases are, however, difficult to find. It is generally believed that underrecognition and underreporting of occupational lung diseases are widespread.[28] Although historically the pneumoconioses have been the most commonly diagnosed occupational lung diseases, occupational asthma has become the most prevalent occupational lung disease in developed countries.[6,7] Worldwide, silicosis remains the most common occupational lung disease.[10] In a few instances, such as the rare tumor mesothelioma, most cases can be attributed to occupational exposure to asbestos. However, the contribution of occupational and environmental factors to most other lung diseases is much harder to determine. For example, estimates of the proportion of lung cancers attributable to occupational exposures have ranged from 1 percent to over 40 percent,[13,33] and estimates of the prevalence of occupational asthma in adult asthmatics have ranged from 2 percent to over 20 percent.[4,16,30]

BASIC PRINCIPLES OF OCCUPATIONAL AND ENVIRONMENTAL LUNG DISEASE

Certain principles apply broadly to the full range of respiratory disorders caused by inhalational exposure to agents in the workplace or environment:

1. While a few environmental and occupational lung diseases may present with pathognomonic features, most are difficult to distinguish from disorders of nonenvironmental origin. In addition, most lung disorders can be caused or exacerbated by environmental or occupational exposures. Thus, environmental and occupational triggers must be constantly sought in the evaluation and management of pulmonary disorders.

2. A given substance in the workplace or environment can cause more than one clinical or pathologic entity. For example, cobalt can cause interstitial lung disease and airway disease (see Chapter 68).

3. The etiology of many lung diseases may be multifactorial, and occupational factors may interact with other factors. For example, the risk of developing lung cancer in asbestos-exposed workers who smoke is much greater than in those exposed to either asbestos or cigarettes alone.

4. The dose of exposure is an important determinant of the proportion of people affected or the severity of disease. Higher doses of exposure usually result in more affected individuals or greater disease severity. Dose generally correlates with severity in patients experiencing nonimmunologic direct toxicity, such as chemical toxic pneumonitis, asbestosis, or silicosis. In those with malignant or immune-mediated disorders, dose more commonly affects incidence than severity.

5. Individual differences in susceptibility to exposures do exist. Adverse effects may occur in some persons, while others with similar exposure are spared. Host factors that determine susceptibility to environmental agents are poorly understood but probably include both inherited, genetic factors and acquired factors such as diet, and the presence of other lung diseases and other exposures.[12,32] Occupational diseases, especially immune-mediated processes such as chronic beryllium disease or low-molecular-weight occupational asthma, can occur or progress at low levels of exposure, even those below government-set exposure standards.[7,11]

6. The effects of a given occupational or environmental lung exposure occur after the exposure with a predictable latency interval. For acute diseases such as toxic pneumonitis, there is a short and usually predictable period between exposure and resultant clinical manifestations. This brief interval facilitates the recognition of a causal relationship between the exposure and the disease. When symptoms or signs are recurrent with repeated exposures, as with occupational asthma, this temporal relationship can help establish the diagnosis. For chronic diseases such as cancer or most pneumoconioses, long

TABLE 56-1

Classification of Occupational Lung Disorders

Major Disease Category	Representative Causative Agents
Upper respiratory tract irritation	Irritant gases, solvents
Airway disorders	
Occupational asthma	
Sensitization	
Low molecular weight	Diisocyanates, anhydrides, wood dusts
High molecular weight	Animal-derived allergens, latex
Irritant-induced, RADS	Irritant gases
Byssinosis	Cotton dust
Grain dust effects	Grain
Chronic bronchitis / COPD	Mineral dusts, coal
Acute inhalation injury	
Toxic pneumonitis	Irritant gases, metals
Metal fume fever	Metal oxides: zinc, copper
Polymer fume fever	Plastics
Smoke inhalation	Combustion products
Hypersensitivity pneumonitis	Bacteria, fungi, animal proteins
Infectious disorders	Tuberculosis, viruses, bacteria
Pneumoconioses	Asbestos, silica, coal, beryllium, cobalt
Malignancies	
Sinonasal cancer	Wood dust
Lung cancer	Asbestos, radon
Mesothelioma	Asbestos

NOTE: RADS = reactive airway dysfunction syndrome; COPD = chronic obstructive pulmonary disease.

latency periods between the first exposure and subsequent clinical manifestations are common. Consequently, the patient's exposure to the offending agent(s) may have ceased long before the onset of disease, making the diagnosis of such diseases more challenging.

IMPORTANCE OF OCCUPATIONAL AND ENVIRONMENTAL LUNG DISEASES

There are several compelling reasons to pursue the search for an occupational or environmental cause in all cases of pulmonary disease. First, knowledge of cause may affect patient management and prognosis, and may prevent further disease progression in the affected person. Second, establishment of cause may have significant legal, financial, and social implications for the patient. Third, the recognition of occupational and environmental risk factors can also have important public health and policy consequences. For example, a larger population at risk may benefit from preventive measures that can be initiated. In addition, new associations between exposure and disease may be identified, such as new agents that can cause occupational asthma. Last, occupational and environmental lung diseases can also serve as important disease models. For example, exposure to sensitizing agents such as isocyanates in the workplace may serve as a model for antigen-induced asthma.

ESTABLISHING A CAUSE

Diagnostic Criteria

To establish whether a lung disease has an occupational or environmental origin, it must first be defined and characterized, and then the degree to which occupational or environmental exposures are causative or contributory must be determined. The degree of uncertainty in diagnosing occupational illnesses is generally significantly greater than in other medical settings—a source of uneasiness for many clinicians. For example, in the United States, for most workers' compensation systems, a disease is considered occupational if "more probably than not" (greater than 50 percent chance) it is work-related.

The following criteria are used to determine whether a disease is caused or exacerbated by agents in the workplace or environment:

1.   The clinical presentation and workup are consistent with the diagnosis.
2.   A causal relationship between the exposure and the diagnosed condition has been previously established or strongly suggested in the medical, epidemiologic, or toxicologic literature (see below).
3.   There is sufficient exposure to cause the disease (see below).
4.   The details of the particular case, such as the temporal relationship between exposure and disease, are consistent with known information about the exposure-disease association.
5.   There is no other, more likely diagnosis.

In addition, for acute diseases such as occupational asthma, improvement away from the exposure and reproduction of the disease manifestations by reexposure to the suspected agent may provide compelling evidence to support the diagnosis.

Determination of Causal Relationship

Three main types of information can be used to establish a causal relationship between an exposure and a respiratory condition: case series or reports, epidemiologic studies, and toxicologic studies. Clinical studies or case reports of similarly exposed patients can be used to determine the adverse effects of an exposure. Case series and disease cluster reports have played an important role in identifying potential occupational causes of lung disease, which have then undergone further epidemiologic investigation.[15] The clinical practice of occupational and environmental lung disease relies heavily on the fields of epidemiology and toxicology to provide databases for diagnostic decision making.

EPIDEMIOLOGY

Epidemiology focuses on the causes of disease in populations. Occupational and environmental epidemiologic studies (such as cohort or case control studies) can demonstrate associations between certain exposures or jobs and adverse effects.[8] Such studies may also provide useful information about the magnitude of the risk, the amount of exposure necessary for disease, and the latency between exposure and disease. Such research has been pivotal in determining whether certain occupational and environmental exposures increase the risk of disease, the magnitude of the risk at different exposure levels, and whether control measures are effective in reducing the risk of disease. There are three basic study designs of epidemiologic studies: (1) cross-sectional observation of a population at one point in time, (2) longitudinal observation of a group (or cohort) over time, and (3) case control studies comparing cases with the disease to controls. All give some measure of the relative risk of disease in the exposed group compared to the nonexposed group. Most common, especially in the study of nonmalignant respiratory disease, have been cross-sectional studies, which measure disease prevalence at one point or period in time, or the prevalence odds ratio. Longitudinal cohort studies provide information on the incidence rate of disease over time in the exposed group compared to the nonexposed group. Case control studies compare a group of cases with the disease to controls without the disease and provide an odds ratio—the ratio of the odds of exposure in the cases compared to the controls. A relative risk or odds ratio greater than 2 implies that, more probably than not, the abnormality observed can be attributed to the exposure in question.

TOXICOLOGY

Data from animal toxicologic studies can also be helpful in determining whether the patient's respiratory problem may be due to an occupational exposure, especially when human data are limited.[19] Such studies can provide information on the adverse effects due to exposures, dose-response relationships, and the primary organ of toxicity for a given exposure. Serious limitations include potential differences between species and the use in animals of single or high-dose exposures that do not simulate the long-term, chronic, lower-level exposures seen with humans. Animal studies also may use a convenient route of exposure, such as intraperitoneal injection, rather than the most common human route.

CLINICAL APPROACH TO THE PATIENT

General Approach

As noted above, there are two important phases in the workup of any patient with a potential occupational or environmental lung disease. First, as with any patient presenting with a potential disorder of the respiratory tract, its nature and extent must be defined and characterized, regardless of the suspected origin. Although knowledge of exposures may guide the order of the diagnostic workup, it is crucial to establish the basic disorder before proceeding to investigate the etiology of the process. Second, the extent to which the disease or symptom complex is caused or exacerbated by an exposure at work or in the environment must be determined.

The initial approach to all such patients includes a detailed history, physical exam, appropriate laboratory testing, chest radiograph, and pulmonary function testing (PFT). Initial exposure information can be used to direct the sequence of the workup and to obviate unnecessary procedures when the diagnosis is fairly straightforward. If the initial evaluation does not fully explain the patient's symptoms, other tests are available to better characterize the nature and extent of the respiratory disorder, including computed chest tomography, cardiopulmonary exercise studies, nonspecific inhalation challenge, bronchoscopy, open lung biopsy, and various immunologic studies. However, few are specific for any given occupational or environmental diagnosis.

Prior medical records can be extremely helpful in the evaluation of a patient with a potential occupational or environmental lung disease. Such records can establish the patient's complaints at earlier points in time, may provide objective data such as prior PFT or chest radiographs for comparison, and may clarify temporal relationships between exposure and effect—an important factor in establishing cause.

The Occupational and Environmental History

The occupational and environmental history is the single most helpful tool to determine whether a respiratory problem may be related to an occupational or environmental exposure.[16,23,29] A detailed occupational history includes a chronologic list of all jobs, including job title, a description of job activities, potential toxins at each job, and an assessment of the extent and duration of exposure. An approach focusing on the jobs and exposures of greatest concern is very useful, especially given most clinicians' time constraints. Such an approach can provide key information on whether exposure to one or more environmental agents has occurred, the magnitude and extent of the exposure, and the timing of the exposure in relationship to symptoms or the disease (Table 56-2). A thorough description of the job process or work done is key. The length of time (hours to years) of exposure to the agent, the nature and use of personal protective equipment

---

TABLE 56-2

Taking an Occupational and Environmental History

General health history

Does the patient think symptoms/problem is related to anything at work?

When was the onset of symptoms, and how are they related to work?

Has patient missed days of work, and why?

Prior pulmonary problems

Medications

Cigarette use

Current or most relevant employment

Job/process: title and description

Type of industry and specific work

Name of employer

Years employed

Exposure information

General description of job process and overall hygiene

Materials wed by worker and others

Ventilation/exhaust system

Use of respiratory protection

Are other workers affected?

Industrial hygiene samples/OSHA data

Environmental nonoccupational factors

Cigarettes

Diet

Hobbies

Pets

Specific workplace exposures

Fumes/dusts/fibers

Gases

Metals

Solvents

Other chemicals: plastics, pesticides, corrosive agents

Infectious agents

Organic dusts: cotton, wood

Physical factors

Noise

Repetitive trauma

Radiation

Emotional factors, stress

Past employment

List jobs in chronologic order

Job title

Exposures

Military service

---

such as respirators, and a description of the ventilation and overall hygiene are all helpful in attempting to quantify exposure from the patient's history. Patients should be asked whether they think their problem is related to anything in the environment, and the presence of similar symptoms among coworkers should be determined. Information about potential exposures outside the workplace, such as in the home or with hobbies, should also be obtained.

PHYSICAL EXAMINATION

With occupational lung diseases, the physical exam is generally unrevealing about specific cause. It is most helpful in ruling out nonoccupational causes of respiratory symptoms or diseases such as cardiac problems or connective-tissue diseases.

Diagnostic Tests

A number of tests can be helpful in the diagnosis of occupational lung disorders, such as chest radiography and PFT. The use of these diagnostic tests in the occupational setting is discussed below.

CHEST RADIOGRAPHY

The chest radiography is the most important diagnostic test for occupational pneumoconioses. It is critical that radiographs of high technical quality be obtained. Under certain circumstances, the chest radiograph can be unique or highly suggestive of an occupational disorder and may be sufficient, along with an appropriate exposure history, to establish a diagnosis. For example, silicosis, coal workers' pneumoconiosis, and asbestosis with pleural disease all have characteristic radiographic findings strongly suggestive of the specific occupational diagnosis. The finding of small rounded opacities, progressive massive fibrotic lesions in the upper zones, and

"eggshell" calcification is highly suggestive of silicosis (Fig. 56-1). Similarly, the finding of bilateral pleural plaques and diffuse small irregular linear opacities in the lower lung zones is highly suggestive of asbestosis (Fig. 56-2). However, the chest radiography findings can also be nonspecific, as with asbestosis without pleural plaques, hard-metal disease, or beryllium disease. Chest radiographs can also be normal in patients with symptomatic pneumoconiosis.[14]

Under the auspices of the International Labour Office (ILO) in Geneva, Switzerland, a uniform classification system has evolved to evaluate chest radiographs for epidemiologic studies, clinical evaluation, and screening.[18] The system requires a posteroanterior radiograph and comparison to a standard set of radiographs. Parenchymal opacities are classified according to size, shape, extent, and profusion (concentration). There are two major types of opacities, large (greater than 10 mm in diameter) and small. Small opacities are further classified on the basis of shape (rounded or irregular) and size. The profusion of small opacities is rated on a 12-category scale in comparison to standard radiographs, which range from 0/0 to 3/3 (greatest intensity). The 12-point scale is as follows:

0/–	0/0	0/1
1/0	1/1	1/2
2/1	2/2	2/3
3/2	3/3	3/+

The first number is the major category: 0 is normal, and 1 to 3 are grades of abnormality. The second number is a "hedge" to suggest whether the film resembles a higher (e.g., 1/2), a lower (e.g., 3/2), or no other category (e.g., 2/2). Examples of ILO readings are shown in Figs. 56-1 and 56-2. Pleural changes are also graded according to site, pleural thickening, and pleural calcification.

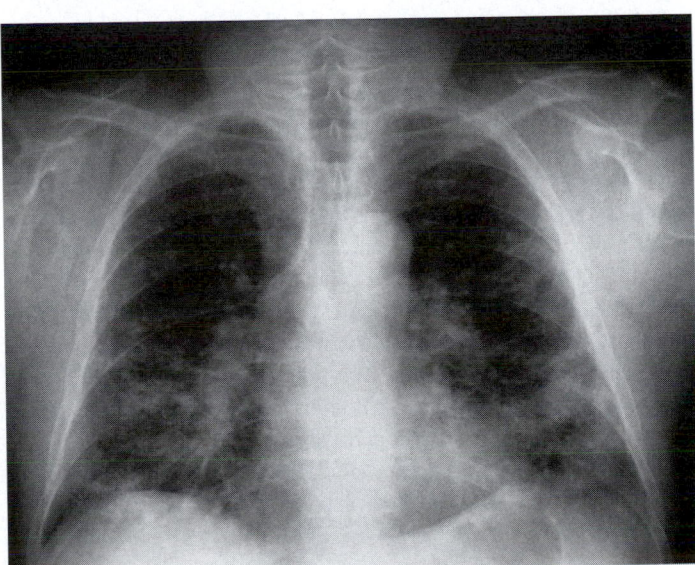

FIGURE 56-1   Posteroanterior chest radiograph of a patient with silicosis. Multiple small nodular densities are seen throughout both lungs. Bilateral conglomerate masses of progressive massive fibrosis are also seen. ILO classification of the film is category 3/3 showing category C large opacities.

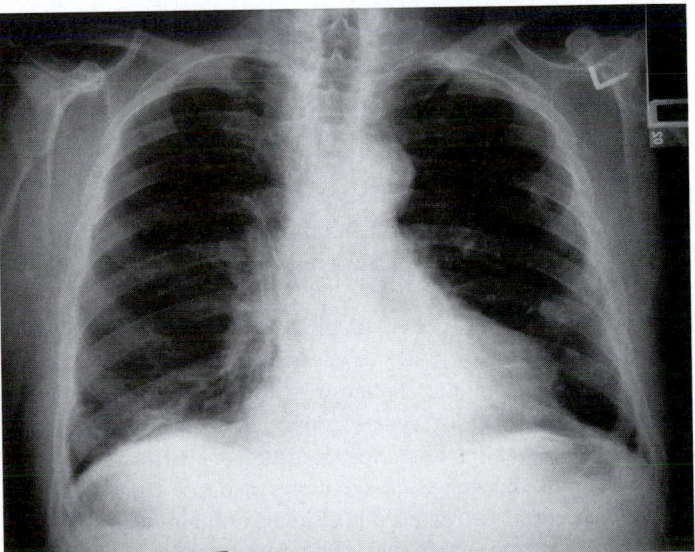

FIGURE 56-2   Posteroanterior chest radiograph of a patient with asbestosis and pleural plaques. Calcified pleural plaques are seen on the diaphragms bilaterally, *en face* in the left thorax, and on the right medial pleural surface. Increased reticular markings greatest at the lung bases are also seen. ILO classification of the film is category 1/1 small irregular opacities predominantly in the lower lung fields.

COMPUTED TOMOGRAPHY

There is a growing scientific literature about the role of computed tomography (CT) scanning in the evaluation of patients with occupational interstitial lung disease, primarily asbestosis.[3,25] This has arisen because conventional chest radiography is insensitive, missing as many as 10 to 15 percent of cases with pathologically documented disease.[25a] Conventional CT scanning (8- to 10-mm-thick slices) and high-resolution computed tomographic (HRCT) scanning (1- to 3-mm-thick slices) can be used to better evaluate pleural and parenchymal abnormalities. Conventional CT scanning is more sensitive than chest radiography for the diagnosis of pleural disease and is helpful in distinguishing subpleural fat from pleural fibrosis. It is most useful for evaluating focal pulmonary masses, but should not be ordered routinely.

HRCT scanning allows improved visualization of the lung parenchyma. HRCT can identify parenchymal abnormalities not evident on standard radiographs and is being increasingly used in the evaluation of patients with asbestosis and other interstitial diseases. However, the clinical significance and utility of HRCT scanning in most patients remain unclear. In most cases in which the diagnosis of an occupational interstitial lung disease is clear on the basis of the chest radiograph and history, HRCT scanning is not indicated. Unexplained dyspnea or abnormal physiology (restrictive lung function, abnormal gas exchange, or abnormal response to exercise) should raise the suspicion for interstitial lung disease. In patients with suspected interstitial lung disease but a normal chest radiograph, HRCT may be helpful in identifying parenchymal abnormalities. The specific features and distribution of the HRCT changes may occasionally be suggestive of a specific cause and help narrow the differential diagnosis.

PHYSIOLOGICAL METHODS

Resting PFTs—including spirometry, lung volumes, and diffusing capacity—are the most important tool to assess functional respiratory status in patients with occupational lung disease, especially interstitial processes.[16,34] PFT findings are generally not specific for a particular cause but are important for evaluating dyspnea, for differentiating obstructive from restrictive airway defects, and for assessing the degree of pulmonary impairment.

In addition, several other methods are particularly useful in the diagnosis of obstructive airway disorders. When spirometry is normal, methacholine challenge testing is helpful in demonstrating the presence of hyperreactive airways. For the diagnosis of occupational asthma, demonstration of airflow limitation on exposure to the suspected agent and of improvement with removal is key. This can be accomplished by obtaining preshift and postshift FEV_1 measurements, serial measurements of peak expiratory flow rates, or specific inhalation challenge.[4,5,22] Specific challenge testing with the suspected agent(s) is considered the "gold standard" for diagnosing occupational asthma.[4,7] A 20 percent fall in FEV_1 after exposure to the offending agent is diagnostic of occupational asthma. However, such testing requires a specialized chamber, carries certain risks, is time-consuming, and is not widely available, and false negatives can occur. Specific challenge is not necessary for the diagnosis of most cases of occupational asthma.

CARDIOPULMONARY EXERCISE TESTING

Cardiopulmonary exercise testing is being used increasingly to assess functional impairment and disease progression in patients with certain occupational respiratory disorders.[34] Exercise testing can help distinguish among cardiac, pulmonary, and deconditioning causes of dyspnea. In patients with significant interstitial lung disease, exercise results in an increase in the alveolar-arterial oxygen gradient and arterial hypoxemia. Cardiopulmonary exercise testing is helpful in evaluating a select group of patients with dyspnea and normal pulmonary function tests or dyspnea that appears out of proportion to the changes in lung function. However, cardiopulmonary exercise testing is not helpful in determining the specific origin of the pulmonary disease.

BRONCHOSCOPY

Although the diagnosis of occupational lung disease can usually be made on the basis of the occupational history, chest radiograph, and PFT, under certain circumstances, such as the evaluation of beryllium disease, bronchoscopy with transbronchial biopsy and bronchoalveolar lavage (BAL) may be helpful diagnostically.[20] Transbronchial biopsies yield small tissue samples that may be adequate to diagnose disorders such as interstitial fibrosis, but are often unable to shed light on the reason for the pathology that is noted. Transbronchial biopsies are most helpful in diagnosing granulomatous interstitial processes such as sarcoidosis, beryllium disease, and hypersensitivity pneumonitis, or diffuse malignant processes. Sufficient tissue is usually not obtained for performance of extensive analyses for dust content.

Under certain circumstances, BAL can be diagnostically helpful. A predominance of lymphocytes suggests certain diagnoses such as sarcoidosis, hypersensitivity pneumonitis, or beryllium disease, but is not by itself diagnostic. The diagnosis of beryllium disease can be established with the finding of a positive lymphocyte transformation test in the BAL cells of exposed patients (see Chapter 58). Characteristic multinucleated giant cells may be seen in the BAL cells of patients with hard-metal lung disease. Cells obtained from BAL may contain dust particles, which may reflect current and possibly also past exposures. Such particles can be identified and counted. For example, uncoated asbestos fibers and asbestos bodies (asbestos particles coated with iron) have been quantitated from BAL fluid. However, it is unclear how well such assays correlate with other measures of exposure or with disease, and at present such assays are rarely used clinically.

PATHOLOGIC EXAMINATION OF TISSUES

Thoracoscopic and open lung biopsy techniques are usually not needed to make a diagnosis of occupational interstitial lung disease. However, when there is no clear cause or exposure history, lung biopsies can be helpful. They can assist in establishing the diagnosis, and can rule in or out certain nonoccupational causes of lung disease, such as pulmonary vascular disease, infection, or bronchiolitis obliterans.[9] Both biopsy techniques obtain a more adequate size of tissue for histologic and mineralogic (qualitative and quantitative) analysis than does transbronchial biopsy. The thoracoscopic approach is, however, less invasive and more easily tolerated by the patient. Thus it is the procedure of choice for specimen sampling of appropriately situated pulmonary abnormalities.

A number of methods have been used to analyze the dust content of lung tissue.[9] Light microscopic evaluation with polarization is widely available and can provide a qualitative assessment of the presence of dust particles and ferruginous bodies. It does not, however, identify the specific dust particles or enable quantification. Bulk and microanalytic techniques that allow more definitive identification and quantification of minerals and dusts are also available. They include radiographic fluorescence scanning electron microscopy and energy dispersion radiographic spectroscopy.[9] These methods can be used to identify and quantify specific minerals in sections or tissue digests. When a patient with interstitial lung disease of unclear origin in whom an occupational or environmental pathogen is being considered or a patient with an unclear occupational history undergoes open lung biopsy, more extensive particle analysis should be considered if light microscopic histologic examination is not diagnostic. There are some serious limitations that should be remembered. First, only particulates that are insoluble and retained in tissue at sufficient concentration will be detected. More soluble agents, such as cobalt, can be underestimated with these techniques. Second, these analytic methods can be tedious, and there can be significant differences in results from different laboratories. Most important, a positive finding documents biologically detectable exposure but does not demonstrate disease or establish a causal relationship.

OTHER LABORATORY TESTS

Few specific laboratory tests exist to diagnose occupational lung diseases. IgG and IgE antibody assays to specific antigens such as isocyanates or large-molecular-weight antigens such as animal or plant proteins may confirm that exposure has occurred and that the patient has responded to the agent. It should be remembered, however, that a positive finding indicates an immunologic reaction, not clinical disease, and a negative finding does not rule out either exposure or disease. BAL and peripheral blood lymphocyte blast transformation in response to beryllium represent one of the few highly sensitive and specific laboratory assays available to diagnose an occupational lung disease.

Exposure Assessment

As noted above, the occupational and environmental exposure history is frequently the best and only source of information regarding exposures. However, for many reasons, including inadequate information about specific exposures or the extent of exposure and various biases in reporting the exposure history, it is frequently helpful to obtain additional exposure information. A number of sources are available and are summarized below.[16,27]

OTHER SOURCES OF EXPOSURE INFORMATION

In the United States, employers are required by federal law to provide employees with information about the potential toxicity of all materials used in the workplace, called Material Safety Data Sheets (MSDS).[17,23] Your patient should obtain an MSDS on any substances of concern for your review. For recent or current exposures, a site visit is usually most helpful in providing information about the nature and extent of potential exposures and other exposed workers. A number of methods and sampling strategies exist to measure particular exposures in either the work or home environment. They include personal or work site sampling devices that absorb the contaminants, direct air sampling devices, and direct monitoring devices. When such data are reviewed, it should be remembered that sampling variability and analytic errors can occur, and that the exposure information obtained usually reflects only the narrow window of time during which monitoring was performed. Employers are required to make available to patients any available information about exposure dose, such as the results of air sampling.

Another potential source of information is the results of inspections by health and regulatory agencies such as the Occupational Safety and Health Administration (OSHA). Unions, insurance groups, and community groups may also provide exposure information. In addition, epidemiologic data on coworkers or workers with similar types of jobs can be used to assess the nature and extent of exposure for a given patient.

Recently there has been great interest in developing biologic markers that attempt to more accurately identify and quantify exposure(s), or an early effect of the exposure, such as sensitization to a specific antigen. Such markers can be measured in the target organ, such as the lung or BAL fluid, or in blood or urine. Examples of possible markers of exposure include the radioallergosorbent test (RAST) or skin tests to a specific antigen or tissue mineralogic analysis. In general, although of great research interest, most markers have relatively limited use in the clinical practice of occupational and environmental medicine.

Once the available information is obtained, the clinician has to make a final determination about whether occupational or environmental exposures are causing or contributing to the patient's disease process. Although some diagnoses such as asbestosis are fairly straightforward, others may be diagnostically more challenging and easily overlooked. As noted above, making the diagnosis of an occupational lung disease frequently entails a greater degree of diagnostic uncertainty than physicians are generally used to in other settings. In most workers' compensation cases in the United States, the standard of certainty is a greater than 50 percent likelihood that the disorder is related to an occupational or environmental exposure. Thus, occupational or environmental diseases are diagnosed even in the presence of a significant degree of uncertainty.

PREVENTION

Social, Economic, and Public Health Considerations

It is important for the clinician to remember that making the diagnosis of an occupational or environmental respiratory disease almost invariably has important social, economic, legal, and public health considerations. Many countries require some form of reporting of occupational illnesses and injuries. For the individual patient, such a diagnosis can have a profound impact on the patient's work, income, and social situation. When one is evaluating a patient with a suspected occupational or environmental lung disease, it is extremely helpful to determine the patient's agenda and the agenda of others (such as referring physician, employer, attorney, insurance companies) engaged in the patient's care. In addition, related broader public health issues may be concerned, such as prevention of disease among other exposed workers.

Prevention is central to the practice of occupational and environmental medicine. There are two main strategies for prevention: primary prevention, which entails removal or modification of the hazardous risk or exposure before disease has occurred, and secondary prevention, early detection, and prompt treatment after some adverse effect of the exposure has occurred. Primary prevention entails improving work practices such as engineering controls to reduce exposures. Sampling and monitoring of exposures are necessary to determine levels and compliance. The physician can play an important role in prevention, especially secondary prevention, through monitoring of patients to detect early abnormalities, through early diagnosis and removal from further exposures, and through modification of potential disease complications. Reporting of occupational illnesses is critical in identifying problem areas that need further investigation and improved preventive strategies.

Regulatory Issues

In the United States, a number of federal and state laws and agencies regulate hazardous substances in the environment and workplace, including the Environmental Protection Agency and OSHA, which was established in 1970 by the Occupational Safety and Health Act to reduce the risk of injury and illness to workers. The National Institute for Occupational Safety and Health, also established in 1970, is charged with performing research and teaching, and evaluating occupational safety and health hazards. Some states require reporting of occupational diseases and have ongoing surveillance programs. The recent Americans with Disabilities Act prohibits discrimination in employment if the worker has a physical or mental disability, and it can affect physician decision making regarding employability.

The United States workers' compensation system consists of a series of state and federal laws that establish "no-fault" insurance to provide medical, lost work time, and other benefits for workers with work-related injuries and illnesses. Physicians are obligated to diagnose and treat work-related illness, to inform the patient of such an illness, and to assist with documentation.

Respirators

The best strategy for reducing inhalational exposures is to prevent or contain the exposure, or substitute a less harmful material for a toxic one. Respiratory protective devices (respirators) are used to provide protection from exposure by inhalation when adequate engineering control of airborne contaminants is not feasible, or in an emergency or temporary situation. There are two main types of respirators: air-purifying respirators, which remove contaminants from the air using filters or chemical absorbents, and atmosphere supply respirators, which supply breathable air from another source, such as an air cylinder (Fig. 56-3).[24] Types of air-purifying respirators include dust masks, cartridge respirators, and high-efficiency particulate air (HEPA) filters. Atmosphere supply respirators can deliver air from an air-supplied respirator or from a self-contained source (self-contained breathing apparatus). The choice of respirator depends on characteristics of both the exposure (i.e., type of chemical or dust) and the workplace (i.e., the ventilation system and oxygen supply.) For example, HEPA respirators can significantly reduce exposure to droplet nuclei carrying *Mycobacterium tuberculosis* (TB) bacilli. However, an effective TB control program for health-care and other TB-exposed workers involves not only HEPA or other particulate respirators but also administrative controls such as the isolation of patients with active disease, employee TB skin testing, and engineering controls such as negative-pressure TB isolation rooms.

Respirators are effective only if the proper device is chosen, it fits properly and is maintained properly, and the worker has been trained in its use. Respirators do not provide absolute protection; rather, they serve to reduce exposure. In the United States, federal regulations set by OSHA include specific rules for respirator use, and they require the employer to provide an acceptable respirator protection program, including fit testing, correct choice of respirator, and worker education and training.

Physicians may be asked to determine a worker's fitness for respirator use. OSHA regulations require that a worker not be assigned to a job requiring use of a respirator unless the worker is able to perform the work with a respirator. It should first be determined whether appropriate engineering controls and an appropriate respiratory protection program are in place. No spirometric or other specific criteria exist to determine respirator fitness. The physician must use clinical judgment in determining whether a given worker will be able to use a respirator. Respirators can increase the work of breathing, and they can interfere with the worker's ability to perform the job (by reducing vision, range of motion, and hearing). In addition, respirators are generally not pleasant to wear for prolonged periods. Factors that can limit respirator use include facial hair, inability to tolerate the respirator, claustrophobic reactions, and particular medical conditions, such as pulmonary or cardiovascular disease. Reassessment after a brief trial of respirator use is indicated if the patient is having problems or concerns. Excellent reviews are available for physicians who will be doing respirator evaluations.[2,24]

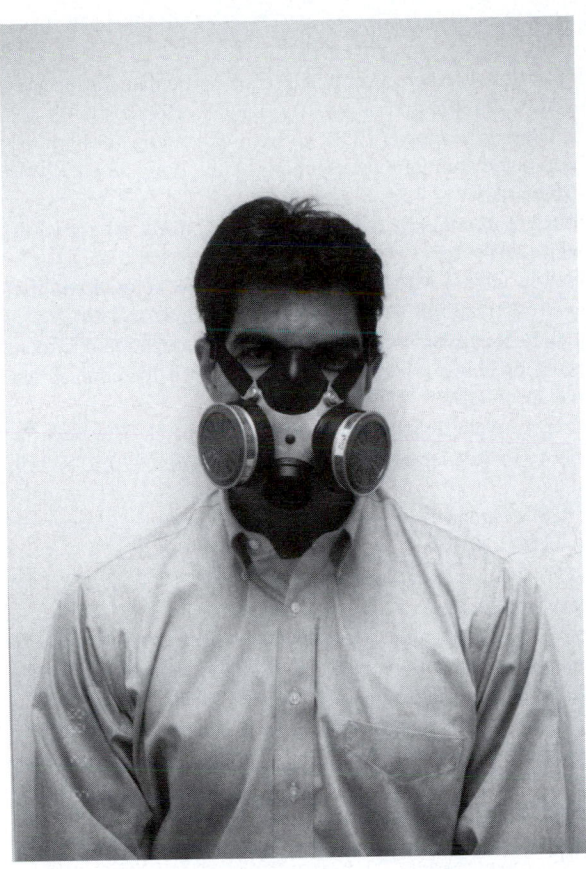

A

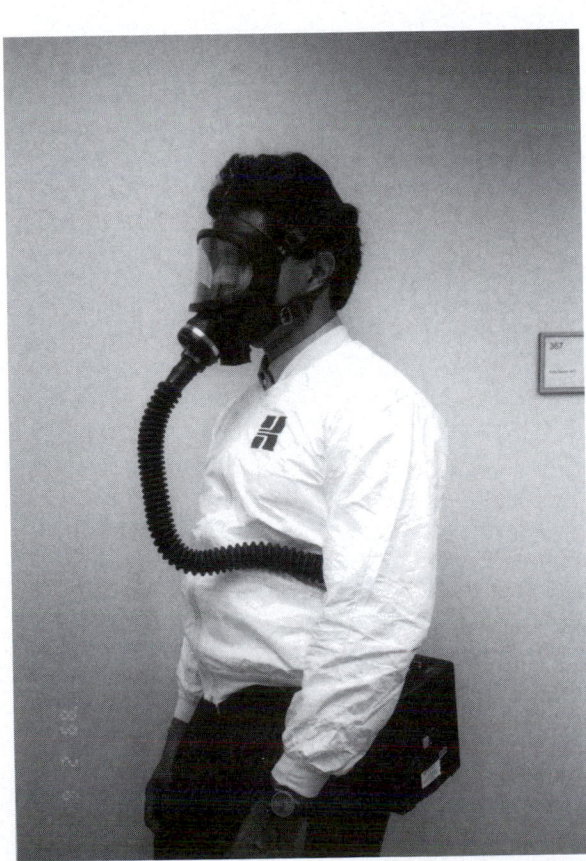

C

FIGURE 56-3   Examples of three common respirators. *A.* An air-purifying cartridge respirator. *B.* A high-efficiency particulate air filter (HEPA). *C.* A self-contained breathing apparatus providing clean air under positive pressure.

B

REFERENCES

1. American College of Physicians: Occupational and environmental medicine: The internist's role. *Ann Intern Med* 113:974–982, 1990.
2. Beckett WS: Certifying the worker for respirator use. *Semin Occup Med* 1:119–124, 1986.
3. Begin R: Computed tomography in the early detection asbestosis. *Br J Ind Med* 50:689–698, 1993.
4. Bernstein IL, Chan-Yeung M, Malo J-L, et al (eds): *Asthma in the Workplace.* New York, Dekker, 1993.
5. Burge PS: Use of serial measurements of peak flow in the diagnosis of occupational asthma. *Occup Med* 8:279–294, 1993.
6. Chan-Yeung M, Malo JL: Aetiological agents in occupational asthma. *Eur Respir J* 7:346–371, 1994.
7. Chan-Yeung M, Malo JL: Occupational asthma. *New Engl J Med* 333:107–112, 1995.
8. Checkoway HA, Pearce NE, Crawford-Brown DJ: *Research Methods in Occupational Epidemiology.* New York, Oxford University Press, 1989.
9. Churg A, Green FHY (eds): *Pathology of Occupational Lung Disease.* New York, Igaku-Shoin, 1988.
10. Cullen MR, Cherniack MG, Rosenstock L: Medical progress: Occupational medicine. *New Engl J Med* 322:594–601, 675–683, 1990.
11. Cullen MR, Kominsky JR, Rossman MD, et al: Chronic beryllium disease in a precious metal refinery: Clinical epidemiologic and

immunologic evidence for continuing risk from exposure to low level beryllium fume. *Am Rev Respir Dis* 135:201–208, 1987.

12. Cullen MR, Redlich CA: Significance of individual sensitivity to chemicals: Elucidation of host susceptibility by use of biomarkers in environmental health research. *Clin Chem* 41:1809–1813, 1995.

13. Doll R, Peto R: The causes of cancer: Quantitative estimates of avoidable risks of cancer in the United States today. *J Natl Cancer Inst* 66:1192–1308, 1981.

14. Epler GR: Normal chest roentgenograms in chronic diffuse infiltrative lung disease. *New Engl J Med* 27:934–939, 1978.

15. Fleming LE, Ducatman AM, Shalat SL: Disease clusters: A central and ongoing role in occupational health. *J Occup Med* 33:818–825, 1991.

16. Harber P, Schenker M, Balmes J (eds): *Occupational and Environmental Respiratory Disease.* St. Louis, Mosby–Year Book, 1995.

17. Himmelstein JS, Frumkin H. The right to know about toxic exposures: Implications for physicians. *New Engl J Med* 312:687–690, 1985.

18. International Labour Office. Guidelines for the use of ILO International Classification of Radiographs of Pneumoconioses. *Occupational Safety and Health Series,* no 22 (revised). Geneva, ILO, 1980.

19. Klaassen CD (ed): *Casarett and Doull's Toxicology: The Basic Science of Poisons,* 5th ed. New York, McGraw-Hill, 1996.

20. Kreiss K, Miller F, Newman LS, et al: Chronic beryllium disease—From the workplace to cellular immunology, molecular immunogenetics, and back. *Clin Immunol Immunopathol* 71:123–129, 1994.

21. Morgan W, Keith C: *Occupational Lung Diseases.* Philadelphia, WB Saunders, 1995.

22. Moscato G, Godnic-Cvar J, Maestrelli P, et al: Statement on self-monitoring of peak expiratory flows in the investigation of occupational asthma. *Eur Respir J* 8:1605–1610, 1995.

23. Newman LS: Occupational illness. *New Engl J Med* 333:1128–1134, 1995.

24. NIOSH guide to the selection and use of particulate respirators. DHHS (NIOS) Publication no 96-101, January 1996.

25. Padley S, Gleeson F, Flower CDR: Current indications for high resolution computed tomography scanning of the lungs. *Br J Radiol* 68:105–109, 1995.

25a. Parkes WR: *Occupational Lung Disorders.* Oxford, Butterworth-Heinemann, 1994.

26. Rosenstock L, Cullen MR: *Textbook of Clinical Occupational and Environmental Medicine.* Philadelphia, WB Saunders, 1994.

27. Rosenstock L, Rest KM, Benson JA Jr, et al.: Occupational and environmental medicine: Meeting the growing need for clinical services. *New Engl J Med* 325:924–927, 1991.

28. Schwartz DA, Wakefield DS, Fieselmann JF, et al: The occupational history in the primary care setting. *Am J Med* 990:315–319, 1991.

29. Timmer S, Rosenman K. Occurrence of occupational asthma. *Chest* 104:816–820, 1993.

30. U.S. Code of Federal Regulations, Title 29, Part 1910, 134(A) (1), Respiratory Protection.

31. Van Damme K, Casteleyn L, Heseltine E, et al: Individual susceptibility and prevention of occupational diseases: Scientific and ethical issues. *J Occup Environ Med* 37:91–99, 1995.

32. Vineis P, Lorenzo S: Proportion of lung and bladder cancers in males resulting from occupation: A systemic approach. *Arch Environ Health* 46:6–15, 1991.

33. Weiderman HP: Evaluating pulmonary impairment: Appropriate use of pulmonary function and exercise tests. *Cleve Clinic J Med* 58:148–152, 1991.

CHAPTER 57

ASBESTOS-RELATED LUNG DISEASE

William N. Rom

TYPES OF EXPOSURE

NONMALIGNANT PLEURAL MANIFESTATIONS
Pleural Plaques
Diffuse Pleural Thickening
Rounded Atelectasis
Acute Benign Pleural Effusions

ASBESTOSIS
Pathology
Pathogenesis
Epidemiology
Natural History
Clinical and Physiological Features
Radiographic Features
Diagnosis
Treatment and Prognosis

MALIGNANT MESOTHELIOMA
Pathology
Natural History
Epidemiology
Pathogenesis
Clinical and Radiographic Features
Diagnosis
Treatment and Prognosis

LUNG CANCER
Epidemiology
Pathology
Pathogenesis
Clinical Features
Radiographic Features
Diagnosis
Treatment and Prognosis

EFFORTS AT ASBESTOS CONTROL

Asbestos is a fibrous hydrated magnesium silicate with more than 3000 commercial uses due to its indestructible nature, fire resistance, and spinnability. It has been used for centuries: the ancient Greeks called asbestos *amiantos,* and the Greek biographer Plutarch (A.D. 46–120) commented on its use in wicks for oil lamps and napkins that could be cleansed in a fire.[41] Mining and milling that began in the late nineteenth century used asbestos in textiles and insulation materials. Cooke described the first case of asbestosis in 1924 in a 33-year-old textile worker with 25 years of exposure to asbestos and extensive pulmonary fibrosis.[41]

Approximately 98 percent of the asbestos used in the United States has been chrysotile, a serpentine form of asbestos. Other asbestos types are the amphiboles—notably amosite, mined in South Africa, and crocidolite, mined in the Cape Province of South Africa and in Western Australia. Anthophyllite in minimal amounts has been used commercially in Finland. These asbestos fiber types have strikingly different physical characteristics: chrysotile tends to be wavy and long, and occurs in bundles; crocidolite is needle shaped with many long fibers; and amosite is similar to crocidolite but generally thicker.

Initially, asbestos was widely used in fireproof textiles and later as insulation for boilers and pipes. Thereafter, asbestos was used in yarn, felt, paper, millboard, shingles, paints, cloth, tape, filters, and wire insulation. More recently, asbestos has been used in cement pipes for potable water, in gaskets, and in friction materials, including brake linings, and roofing and floor products. Asbestos was extensively used for ship construction during World War II. World consumption of asbestos declined in the 1990s to approximately 50 percent of the peak in 1973. In 1994, approximately 2.7 million tons were produced, with the United States consuming less than 27,000 metric tons. Worldwide production by mining in 1994 was led, in order, by Russia, Canada, Kazakhstan, China, and Brazil.

TYPES OF EXPOSURE

Asbestos exposure has occurred in a variety of settings. Primary exposures occurred in miners and millers. Secondary exposures occurred in manufacturing plants using asbestos in the production of textiles, friction materials, tiles, and insulation materials. Epidemiologic studies focused on cohorts in these plants, since asbestos fiber type was often specified and dust measurements were obtained. These studies demonstrated that intensity and duration of exposure play an important role in the prevalence of asbestos-related disease. In a study of 1584 insulation workers and 1330 sheet-metal workers, 83.5 percent of the insulators had abnormal chest radiographs (55 percent with parenchymal opacities), whereas 42 percent of the sheet-metal workers had abnormal chest radiographs (17 percent with parenchymal opacities).[21]

Although measurements of airborne asbestos fibers were seldom made, the most significant exposures appear to have occurred in the construction trades. These trades included asbestos insulators (called "laggers" in the United Kingdom), who mixed asbestos cement on site to insulate joints and elbows on pipes; boilermakers and sheet-metal workers, who worked adjacent to the asbestos workers; and electricians, carpenters, plumbers, and others who worked in the vicinity of work requiring asbestos exposure. These exposures were mainly to chrysotile asbestos, since practically no crocidolite was imported into the United States, and only small amounts of amosite were admixed.

Asbestos workers and other construction workers wore their asbestos-covered clothes home, so their wives and children were exposed either upon greeting them or while washing their garments. These household contact exposures are often referred to as *indirect exposures,* and those exposed while working near asbestos workers are called *bystander exposures.* In the United States, approximately 14 million persons who were exposed to asbestos in the workplace between 1940 and 1979 were alive in 1980. From this cohort, estimates have been projected for the late 1990s of a peak incidence of approximately 3000 mesothelioma deaths and 5000 asbestos-related lung cancer deaths. Pleural fibrosis remains a relatively common finding among asbestos-exposed blue-collar workers, whereas asbestosis is becoming increasingly uncommon.

NONMALIGNANT PLEURAL MANIFESTATIONS

Pleural disease is the most common manifestation of asbestos exposure. The nonmalignant manifestations of asbestos exposure in the pleural space include circumscribed pleural plaques, diffuse pleural thickening, rounded atelectasis, and asbestos-related pleural effusions.

Pleural Plaques

PATHOLOGY

Pleural plaques are the most common manifestation of asbestos exposure. They are focal, irregular, raised white lesions found on the parietal and, rarely, the visceral pleura. The plaques may be small or extensive; commonly they occur in the lateral and posterior midlung zones, where they may follow rib contours and the diaphragm. They commonly enter lobar fissures and can invade the mediastinum or pericardium; rarely do they invade the apices or costophrenic sulci. Histologically, asbestos-related pleural plaques are characterized by a paucity of cells, extensive collagen fibrils arranged in a basket-weave pattern, and a thin covering of mesothelial cells. The parietal pleura is uniformly involved, with minimal thickening of the visceral pleura. The two pleural surfaces are free of adhesions. Pleural calcifications frequently develop in these fibrohyaline lesions as the length of time from exposure increases. Exposure to asbestos is the most frequent cause of pleural plaques. These plaques, although typical of asbestos, are not specific for asbestos exposure.

PATHOGENESIS

Two theories have been proposed for the pathogenesis of pleural plaques. The most plausible is based on the direct effects of fibers that reach the pleural space. Asbestos fibers—the short, thin ones in particular—have been shown to be transported by subpleural lymphatics to the pleural space. In the pleural space, it is believed that they scratch, injure, and irritate the pleural surface, leading to hemorrhage, inflammation, and eventually fibrosis. The plaques are submesothelial. Cell-cell interactions appear to play an important role in this response. In the absence of macrophages, pleural reactions tend to be disorganized and widespread. Mesothelial cells also appear to play an important role in the pathogenesis of these lesions: they internalize asbestos fibers via an integrin receptor that recognizes vitronectin; in vitro pleural mesothelial cells also can synthesize collagens (types I, III, and IV), elastin, laminin, and fibronectin. In keeping with the submesothelial location of the plaques, cultured mesothelial cells can organize these macromolecular connective-tissue components into an assemblage of extracellular matrix that is limited to the base of the cell.

EPIDEMIOLOGY AND NATURAL HISTORY

In the 1960s, hyaline and calcified pleural plaques were noted to be an index of exposure to asbestos. In shipyard workers, the frequency of pleural abnormalities was approximately 10 times that of parenchymal disease. The greater the exposure, the more likely the worker was to have extensive calcified pleural plaques as well as parenchymal fibrosis. The intensity of the exposure has been noted to be an important determinant of the prevalence of these abnormalities. For example, among British shipyard workers, 36 percent of those with continuous exposure as "laggers" developed pleural plaques, while extensive pleural thickening and pulmonary fibrosis were seen in 5 and 7 percent, respectively.[43] In contrast, those with intermittent exposure had a 6 percent prevalence of plaques and no pulmonary fibrosis. On average, the latency time for the appearance of plaques is 30 years, but the time can vary greatly. This variation can also be appreciated from studies of British shipyard workers in whom the prevalence of pleural plaques increased from 17 percent at 10 years after the first exposure to 70 percent at 30 years among those with continuous exposure; for those with intermittent exposures, the prevalence increased from 1 percent at 10 years to 16 percent at 30 years.

All asbestos fibers are equally capable of inducing pleural plaques: pleural plaques are found in American insulators or shipyard workers exposed to chrysotile or amosite, as well as miners in Western Australia who were exposed to crocidolite. Circumscribed pleural plaques are not associated with pleural effusions. They increase in size slowly, usually over decades, and rarely if ever give rise to diffuse malignant mesothelioma.

In addition to occupational exposures, domestic and residential exposures have, on rare occasions, been implicated in the production of pleural plaques. Evidence for the latter is the remarkably high rates of pleural calcification (up to 30 percent) in some rural areas of Greece, Bulgaria, and Turkey.

CLINICAL AND PHYSIOLOGICAL FEATURES

In the absence of concomitant asbestosis or obliteration of the costophrenic angle, pleural plaques are usually asymptomatic. Most often they are incidental findings on chest radiographs. In addition, they do not cause significant abnormalities such as pleural rubs, rales, or rhonchi on auscultation of the chest.

Pleural disease has been recognized as a cause of reduced pulmonary function since the 1970s. Among 998 shipyard workers in Groton, Connecticut, who had 15 or more years of asbestos exposure, 17 percent of those with pleural changes had a forced vital capacity (FVC) under 80 percent of predicted; for those with normal chest radiographs, 9 percent had decreased vital capacities ($p < 0.05$). In those with normal chest radiographs, the values were significantly reduced only among smokers and ex-smokers. Recent studies that have applied stepwise regression analysis to data from insulation workers have disclosed a significant inverse relationship between FVC and an integrative pleural index for patients with circumscribed pleural plaques.[23] Even among those with pleuroparenchymal abnormalities, the pleural index was found to make a significant contribution to decrements in FVC, independent of that due to parenchymal abnormalities.

In nonsmoking asbestos workers with circumscribed or diaphragmatic pleural plaques, flow rates (FEV_1, $FEF_{25-75\%}$, and $FEF_{75-85\%}$) have been reported to be reduced. In an epidemiologic study of 1211 sheet-metal workers, pleural fibrosis was detected in 334 and was related to age, duration of exposure, more pack-years of smoking, and the presence and degree of interstitial fibrosis.[37] After controlling for these confounders, multivariate regression analysis found that both plaques and diffuse thickening were independently associated with decrements in FVC, but not with decrements in the FEV_1/FVC ratio. Furthermore, diffuse pleural thickening was associated with a decrement in FVC twice as great as that seen with circumscribed pleural plaques. After confounding variables such as age, height, smoking status, and the presence of parenchymal abnormality as assessed by chest radiography and gallium scintography were taken into account, there was a significant decrease in FEV_1 and FVC (222 and 402 ml, respectively) among workers who had pleural plaques or diffuse pleural fibrosis.[37]

RADIOGRAPHIC FEATURES

The visualization of plaques on routine chest radiography depends on their thickness, location, and the orientation of the radiographic beam. As a result, they can be viewed in profile along the lateral chest wall or on *en face* with a rolled or holly leaf pattern, especially if calcified (Fig. 57-1). Only a modest proportion of plaques detected at autopsy can be seen on standard posteroanterior (PA) chest radiograph. Oblique views and computed tomographic (CT) scanning increase plaque detection.

The CT scan can recognize plaques at a much earlier and less well-defined state than the conventional chest radiograph. The CT scan is particularly useful for perivertebral and pericardiac plaques, and high-resolution CT scanning (HRCT)

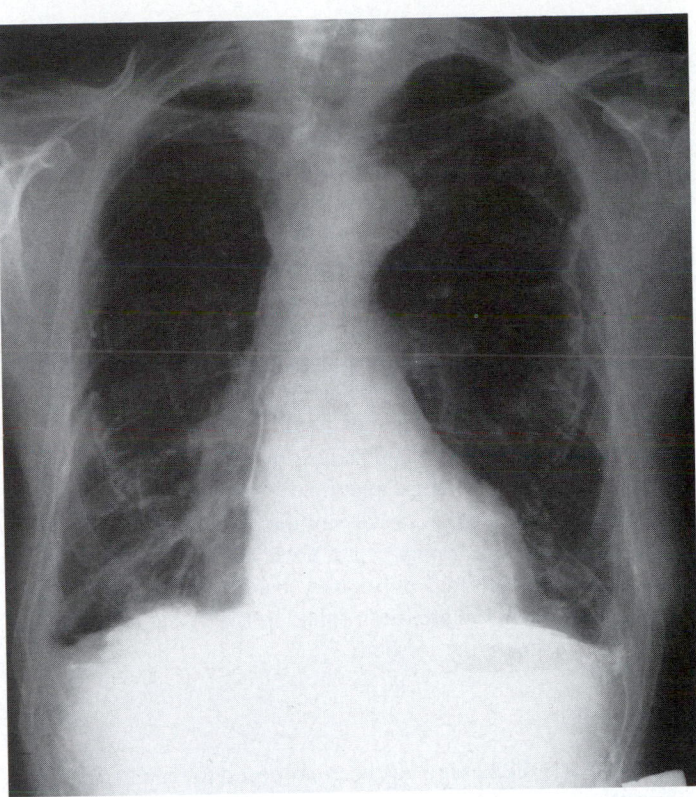

FIGURE 57-1   Posteroanterior (PA) chest radiograph of a 75-year-old man who worked in a shipyard during World War II insulating ships. The radiograph shows bilateral calcified pleural plaques *en face* and on top of the diaphragm. The pleura is diffusely thickened bilaterally and the costophrenic angles are blunted. Mediastinal pleural calcification is present on the right. (*Courtesy of Dr. Timothy Harkin.*)

helps to establish the presence of diaphragmatic lesions. In all cases, the CT scan can help to differentiate plaques from extrapleural fat pads and can detect concomitant parenchymal abnormalities that may be difficult or impossible to see on the PA chest radiograph.

DIAGNOSIS

Pleural plaques due to asbestos exposure are usually bilateral (80 percent of the time), whereas unilateral pleural plaques may be due to trauma, previous tuberculosis, or, rarely, other causes, such as collagen vascular disease. The lesions are usually stable and will remain the same size for months. This helps to differentiate plaques from pleural tumors. Histologic tissue examination is not necessary for diagnosis the vast majority of the time.

TREATMENT

No specific treatment is required for asbestos pleural plaques. Since they are markers of asbestos exposure and identify patients at risk for other asbestos-related disorders,[17] medical surveillance, including periodic chest radiographs, is recommended.

Diffuse Pleural Thickening

PATHOLOGY

Pleural fibrosis in persons who have been exposed to asbestos has been well described. The fibrotic responses can be localized or diffuse and either unilateral or bilateral. Macroscopically, the lesions vary in thickness from a whitish discoloration of the lung surface to a thick white peel that can encase significant pulmonary structures. Diffuse pulmonary thickening is most often seen as a continuous sheet that is 5 to 10 cm in craniocaudal extent, and in 90 percent of the patients it affects the costophrenic angle. Interlobar and interlobular fissures are commonly involved. Whereas pleural plaques predominantly affect the parietal pleura, diffuse pleural thickening or fibrosis is a disease of the visceral pleura. Diffuse pleural fibrosis occurs most commonly as part of a fibrotic process of the visceral pleura and subadjacent interstitium. It may occur, however, and be quite severe, in patients with minimal pulmonary parenchymal fibrosis. Asbestos bodies or fibers are often found in the visceral pleura, the underlying parenchyma, or both.

PATHOGENESIS

Diffuse pleural thickening has been proposed to result from three different mechanisms. The first is the confluence of large pleural plaques. This is believed to account for 10 to 20 percent of the cases. The second is the extension of subpleural fibrosis to the visceral pleura. This probably accounts for 10 to 30 percent of cases. The most common pathogenic mechanism is thought to be the fibrotic resolution of a benign pleural effusion, producing diffuse pleural thickening. The importance of this mechanism is highlighted by the finding that about one-third of patients with diffuse pleural thickening have had a prior benign asbestos-related pleural effusion diagnosed by thoracentesis or on serial chest radiographs. The pathogenic mechanisms differentiating diffuse pleural thickening from circumscribed pleural plaques are not well defined. However, the fundamental irritative mechanism of asbestos fibers is likely to be important in both. In the case of diffuse pleural responses, these fibers are deposited mainly in the parenchymal subpleural areas of the lung.

CLINICAL AND PHYSIOLOGICAL MANIFESTATIONS

Diffuse pleural fibrosis most often occurs long after short-term heavy exposure to asbestos. When mild, diffuse pulmonary fibrosis can be asymptomatic and discovered as an incidental finding on a chest radiograph obtained for another reason. The diffuse nature of the lesion, however, often leads to pulmonary symptoms, including dyspnea on exertion, chronic dry cough, and chest pain. As noted above, diffuse pleural thickening can, per se, cause a restrictive physiological abnormality. The degree of physiological abnormality varies with the degree of fibrotic response. On rare occasions, in patients with severe bilateral disease, respiratory insufficiency and death have occurred. Diffuse pleural fibrosis can increase in severity over time. In miners heavily exposed to crocidolite asbestos, however, progression of diffuse pleural thickening has been noted to level off as much as 15 years after the initial exposure.

RADIOGRAPHIC FEATURES

On the routine chest radiograph, diffuse pleural fibrosis presents as a continuous pleural opacity extending over more than 25 percent of the pleural surface of a lung, often blunting the costophrenic angle. It can be unilateral or bilateral and seen in the presence or absence of concomitant asbestosis and pleural calcifications. Rarely, the pleural fibrosis will produce a fibrotic pseudotumor with a pleural basis (rounded atelectasis) (see below). CT scanning is particularly useful in delineating the relationship between diffuse fibrosis and other pleural abnormalities and differentiating pleural fibrosis from fat deposits.

DIAGNOSIS

The diagnosis of diffuse pleural fibrosis is usually based on the clinical presentation and chest radiograph. In more than 30 percent of cases, a history of asbestos-related pleuritis can be obtained. The lesions of diffuse pleural fibrosis are not unique to asbestos-exposed persons and can represent old inflammatory reactions from tuberculosis, thoracic surgery, hemorrhagic chest trauma, or drug reactions. Differentiation among these causes is frequently based on a careful clinical history. Radiographic patterns are also helpful, since bilateral interstitial changes in the lower lung zones in association with pleural plaques or calcifications strongly support a diagnosis of asbestos exposure. A biopsy may be required when the thoracic lesion is progressing or when malignancy is in the differential.

TREATMENT

As seen with circumscribed pleural plaques, there are no specific therapies for asbestos-related diffuse pleural fibrosis. Medical surveillance is required to detect disease progression and observe for other asbestos-related disorders. In the rare extremely severe case, pleurectomy may be required.

Rounded Atelectasis

Rounded atelectasis is a rare complication of asbestos-induced pleural disease. It is caused by scarring of the visceral and parietal pleura and the adjacent lung, with the pleural reaction folding over on itself. The pleural surfaces then fuse to one another, trapping the underlying lung and leading to atelectasis. As a result of this alteration, a mass lesion that mimics lung cancer can be seen on the PA chest radiograph (Fig. 57-2). This lesion is most easily appreciated to be a pseudotumor with use of CT scanning. HRCT can noninvasively demonstrate continuity to areas of diffuse pleural thickening, evidence of volume loss in the adjacent lung, or a characteristic comet tail of vessels and bronchi sweeping into a wedge-shaped mass (Fig. 57-2).

CT scanning can also demonstrate stability over time (from months to years), which supports the diagnosis of a benign lesion, and pleural plaques or parenchymal changes, which support a diagnosis of asbestos exposure. In one clinical series of 74 patients with rounded atelectasis, 64 had significant asbestos exposure, and the lingula or right middle lobe was affected in 49 (62 percent) of the patients.[16] HRCT scans localized most cases of rounded atelectasis to the lower, posterior portion of the lung

(Fig. 57-2); moreover, in one-third of the patients, the lesions were multiple. In most patients, rounded atelectasis occurs suddenly on a background of only plaques or a normal chest radiograph. In others, a slowly increasing pleural effusion may precede its appearance. If the benign nature of the lesion cannot be assured by chest radiography, the patient may require fiberoptic bronchoscopy with a transbronchial biopsy or transthoracic needle aspiration to rule out a malignant process.

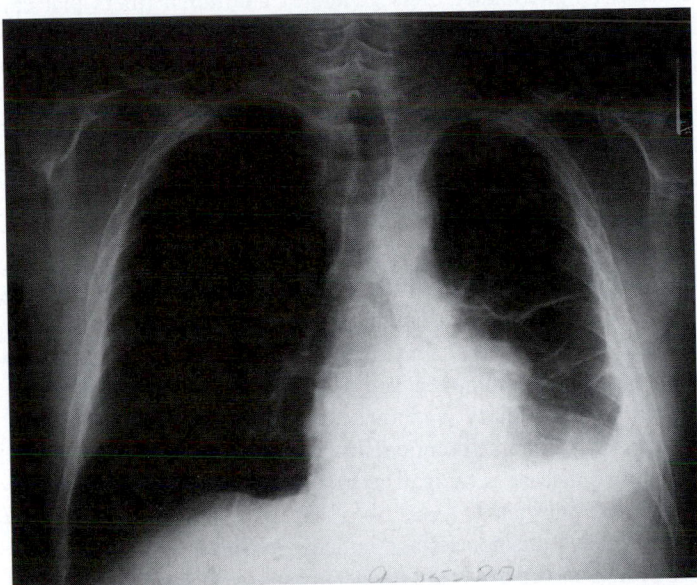

A

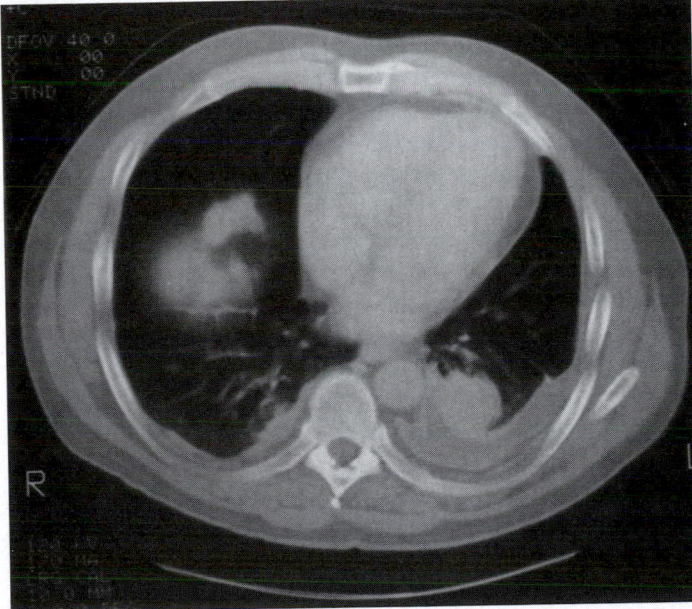

B

FIGURE 57-2   Rounded atelectasis and other pleural abnormalities in an asbestos worker. The chest radiograph *(A)* shows a left-sided pleural effusion, bilateral pleural thickening, greater on the left than on the right, and a mass in the left midlung field. HRCT *(B)* demonstrates the mass to be rounded atelectasis, with bronchovascular structures entering the trapped lung. It also reveals the pleural effusion, bilateral pleural thickening, and pleural plaques, one of which is on the right hemidiaphragm. *(Chest radiograph and HRCT courtesy of Dr. Coralie Shaw.)*

Acute Benign Pleural Effusions

Acute benign pleural effusions are common pleural manifestations in asbestos-exposed persons between 20 and 40 years of age. The latency period for these effusions is shorter than for pleural plaques, malignant mesotheliomas, or pulmonary malignancies. Benign pleural effusions generally occur earlier after exposure than do other asbestos-related processes—12 to 15 years after the first asbestos exposure. However, benign effusions can also occur as long as 30 years after first exposure.[18] The effusions may be small to moderate in size or may be manifested as an increase in the extent or severity of an existing pleural reaction.

About 50 percent of the patients with acute benign pleural effusions are asymptomatic. When patients are symptomatic, the manifestations may be those of a pleurisy (chest pain, chest tightness, dyspnea, cough, and fever). Physical examination reveals the signs of a pleural effusion; a pleural friction rub may be heard. The effusions are exudative and often bloody; glucose concentrations are normal. Mesothelial cells are found in about 50 percent of patients. In about 25 percent of patients, the fluid is eosinophilic. Rarely are asbestos bodies found even though they may be present in underlying lung tissue.

The designation "benign" refers to the lack of evidence of malignancy. The collections may persist for 6 months or more. They frequently clear spontaneously, only to recur on the contralateral side. Benign asbestos pleural effusions do not presage the development of malignant mesotheliomas. Moreover, patients with effusions have the same risk of developing asbestosis as do patients with chronic pleural fibrosis. However, a benign asbestos pleural effusion is a risk factor for the development of pleural thickening, especially diffuse pleural fibrosis. The diagnosis of acute benign pleural effusions is one of exclusion. Thoracentesis is essential. Pleural biopsy is frequently required to rule out other causes of pleural effusions, including mesothelioma. The usual pathologic findings are a chronic fibrous pleurisy with minimal cellularity. Long-term follow-up is also a diagnostic requirement, since the diagnosis of a benign pleural effusion cannot be fully established until a tumor-free interval of 3 years has elapsed.[6]

ASBESTOSIS

Pathology

Asbestosis is the interstitial pneumonitis and fibrosis caused by exposure to asbestos fibers. Early lesions are characterized by discrete areas of fibrosis in the walls of respiratory bronchioles. The septi adjacent to the respiratory bronchioles are often thickened, and the fibrosis sometimes appears to spread outward from the bronchioles. In addition to the peribronchiolar fibrosis, there is an intense peribronchiolar cellular reaction that may narrow and obstruct the airway lumen. Macrophage accumulation is a prominent feature of this cellularity. Proliferation of type II alveolar epithelial cells is enhanced. The interstitium may contain collections of lymphocytes; smooth-muscle proliferation may be prominent in areas of remodeling; and buds of loose connective tissue may be seen within the alveoli (Fig. 57-3). Initially, the

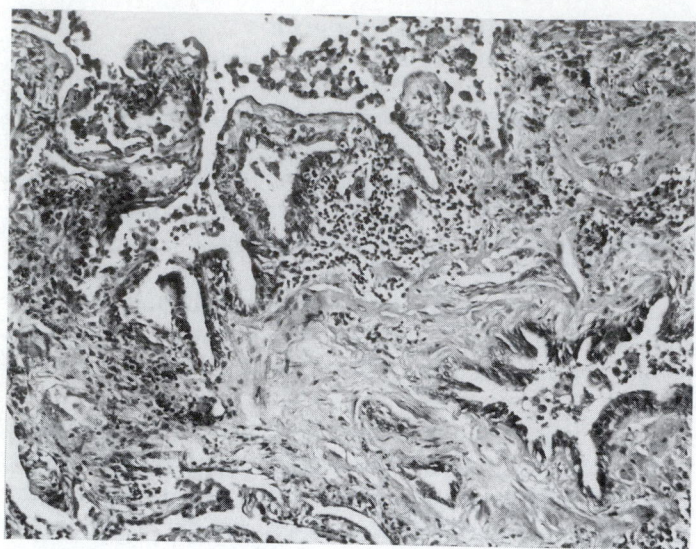

FIGURE 57-3 Lung tissue from a 64-year-old asbestos insulator with 46 years of exposure to asbestos while insulating pipes. His chest radiograph revealed extensive irregular opacities and bilateral pleural thickening. The figure illustrates peribronchiolar fibrosis, interstitial chronic inflammation, accumulation of macrophages in the airspaces, and proliferation of type II pneumocyte. *(Based on data of Rom et al, 1991,[35] with permission.)*

disease usually involves first-order bronchioles; subsequently, second- and third-order bronchioles are affected. As the disease progresses, the fibrosis becomes diffuse, the architecture of the lung undergoes extensive remodeling, and honeycombing supervenes. In contrast to other pneumoconioses, lymph node enlargement and progressive massive fibrosis do not occur. Pathologically, the alterations seen in asbestosis cannot be differentiated from many other interstitial fibrotic disorders except for the presence of asbestos bodies and uncoated asbestos fibers.

Pathogenesis

Asbestos fibers are deposited at airway bifurcations and in respiratory bronchioles and alveoli by impaction, sedimentation, and interception. Fibers then migrate into the interstitium, in part via an uptake process involving type I alveolar epithelial cells. This causes alveolar macrophages to accumulate in the alveolar ducts, peribronchiolar interstitium, and alveolar spaces, constituting an alveolar macrophage alveolitis.[34] Following this initial macrophage alveolitis, most fibers are cleared, leaving the lungs unscarred. If clearance is incomplete, fibrosis can ensue. The degree of fibrosis in asbestosis relates, in general, to the lung dust burden. If the dust load is small, the tissue reaction may be limited and the disease may be mild and not progress. If the retained dust load is great, tissue reaction and macrophage alveolitis are proportionately more intense, greater injury occurs, and chronic and progressive lung disease can develop.

The macrophage alveolitis that is seen in early stages of asbestosis results from monocyte recruitment from the blood and in situ macrophage replication. These cells appear to play an important role in the pathogenesis of the inflammation and fibrosis seen in this disorder.[45] Morphologically, they express an activated phenotype characterized by cellular multinucleation and a striking increase in membrane ruffling, surface blebbing, and lysosomes and phagolysosomes. These macrophages are presumably attempting to engulf and clear the asbestos fibers. This process is not uniformly successful, however. First, the fibers induce apoptosis in the cells. Although the coating of asbestos fibers to form asbestos bodies makes them less toxic, the vast majority of fibers in the lung remain uncoated. Second, the long fibers cannot be completely phagocytosed. Finally, chrysolite asbestos fibers tend to split longitudinally. This generates additional fibers that can multiply the asbestos effect even after exposure has ceased. As a result, asbestos has a prolonged residence and surprising mobility and penetrates the interstitium of the distal lung.

These characteristics probably contribute to the pathogenesis of the disease, since—in contrast to inert particles, which can be ingested by macrophages and cleared without generating a significant response—asbestos fibers stimulate macrophages to produce a variety of important moieties. These include cytokines, such as platelet-derived growth factor (PDGF), insulin-like growth factor–1 (IGF-1),[33] interleukin 1β (IL-1β), tumor necrosis factor (TNF), and IL-8, the matrix molecule fibronectin,[34] oxygen free radicals, and plasminogen activators. The oxygen radicals contribute to tissue injury via direct cell cytotoxicity and lipid peroxidation of membrane components. The IL-8 recruits granulocytes to sites of disease activity. The PDGF, IGF-1, IL-1, TNF, and fibronectin contribute to tissue fibrosis by stimulating fibroblast proliferation and chemotaxis and collagen biosynthesis.

Bronchoalveolar lavage (BAL) in asbestosis has demonstrated an alveolar macrophage alveolitis with a modest increase in neutrophils.[34,35,50] This neutrophilia correlates with the finding of rales on physical examination and oxygenation parameters[50] and is apt to be more pronounced in patients with advanced disease.[35] In patients with asbestosis, gallium 67 lung scans may also be positive. Clinically apparent asbestosis occurs only after a significant latent period. However, studies using BAL, CT scanning, and gallium 67 scanning have demonstrated that inflammatory events occur well before the onset of clinical disease. Thus, it is likely that the initial exposure induces inflammation and injury that persist through the latent or subclinical phase and develops into the clinical disease diagnosed by classic radiography and other techniques. Current concepts of the pathogenesis of the disease link inflammation and fibrosis in a causal fashion.

Epidemiology

The prevalence of parenchymal asbestosis among asbestos workers increases as the length of employment increases. This is nicely illustrated in an early report in which investigators analyzed the chest radiographs of 1117 New York and New Jersey asbestos insulation workers.[41] They found asbestosis in 10 percent of the workers who had been employed for 10 to 19 years, in 73 percent of those who had worked for 20 to 29 years, and in 92 percent of those who had worked 40 or more years. A similar dose-response relationship was found in the asbestos cement industry. Among "bystanders"—i.e., among sheet-metal workers who worked in close proximity to insulation workers[47]—the overall prevalence of asbestos-related changes was 31 percent, including 9 percent who had only pleural abnormalities and 12 percent who had parenchymal abnormalities. Among those who had been in the trade for 40 years or more, 41.5 percent had radiographic signs of asbestos-related disease.

Cigarette smoking can affect the expression of asbestosis. Smokers without dust exposure may have a few irregular radiographic opacities, probably representing acute or chronic bronchitis or bronchiectatic changes in the lung parenchyma. Both smokers and ex-smokers have a higher frequency of asbestos-related irregular opacities on their chest radiographs than do their nonsmoking colleagues.[24] Among asbestos insulation workers, lower grades of radiographic small opacities predominated.[24] Smoking does not alter the expression of asbestos-induced pleural fibrosis. The effects of smoking on asbestosis may be clinically important, since the mortality from asbestosis is higher in asbestos workers who have smoked than in their nonsmoking coworkers. This risk declines if the worker quits smoking. The mechanism of interaction of asbestos and cigarette smoking is poorly understood. However, cigarette smoking may interfere with the clearance of inhaled asbestos, thereby potentiating the effects of the dust in the lung.

Natural History

Following asbestos exposure, asbestosis becomes evident only after an appreciable latent period. The duration of exposure and its intensity influence the prevalence of radiographically evident parenchymal pulmonary fibrosis. Because work sites around the world increasingly meet recommended control levels, high-level exposure to asbestos is now uncommon and clinical asbestosis is becoming a less severe disease that manifests after a longer latent interval. In Western Australian crocidolite workers, a median of 14 years elapsed before asbestosis was detectable radiographically (range, 2 to 34 years). In retired Quebec chrysotile miners and millers, the frequency of pleuroparenchymal lesions was 31 percent, and progression of parenchymal opacities occurred in 9.3 percent; progression was confined to the more heavily exposed group.[3]

One approach to the study of low-level exposure is to evaluate the outcome from short-term exposure. In such a study in an amosite asbestos factory, employment for even as little as 1 month resulted in a 20 percent prevalence of parenchymal opacities[37]: one-third of the participants had pleural abnormalities after 20 years of follow-up;[13] it is significant that both "first attacks" and progression of established radiographic abnormalities occurred 20 and more years after exposure had ceased.

Radiographic asbestosis, once established, may remain static or progress. Rarely has regression been recorded. The factors that determine the outcome are poorly understood. The level and duration of exposure (i.e., cumulative exposure) appear to be prognostic factors. Progression is also considerably more common in persons who already have radiographic abnormalities. This fact provides the basis for the advice that further exposure is to be avoided once the diagnosis of parenchymal asbestosis has been made.

Clinical and Physiological Features

Dyspnea on exertion is the earliest, most consistently reported, and frequently the most distressing symptom of asbestosis. Often dyspnea is accompanied by a persistent cough, which can be spasmodic, and sputum production. Chest tightness is not uncommon, and wheezing also can occur. In a cross-sectional survey of 816 asbestos-exposed workers using the respiratory symptom questionnaire of the American Thoracic Society, cough, phlegm, wheeze, and dyspnea were inversely related to pulmonary function.[7] Cough, phlegm, and chronic bronchitis were associated with a 2 to 8 percent reduction in FVC and FEV_1; the reduction in these measurements was more significant with wheeze and dyspnea, which caused an 11 to 17 percent reduction. Similarly, based on the British Medical Research Council questionnaire for dyspnea, the prevalence of grade 3 dyspnea among asbestos insulators increased in stepwise fashion from 19.4 percent in patients with category 1 chest radiographic abnormalities (1/0–1/2 abnormalities by ILO classification) to 34.5 percent in patients with category 2 chest radiographs and to 49.4 percent in patients with category 3 radiographic abnormalities.

Rales are a distinctive feature of asbestosis. They are usually bilateral, late to paninspiratory in timing, heard best at the posterior lung bases, and not cleared by coughing. They differ in quality and timing from the crackles of bronchitis, which tend to be fewer and earlier. The crackles of asbestosis appear first at the bases in the midaxillary line and tend to spread toward the posterior bases. In prevalence surveys, approximately 83 percent of patients with higher radiographic categories of asbestosis have bilateral rales.[27] In a study of 42 patients with a clinical diagnosis of asbestosis, in 40 the chest radiograph showed at least 1/0 profusion of irregular opacities, 36 had rales, 36 had dyspnea, and 22 had digital clubbing.[30] Rales and clubbing were almost as common among those with less as those with more advanced categories of asbestosis.

In years past, asbestosis-induced respiratory failure was a frequent cause of death in patients with this disorder. In recent years, as the severity of asbestosis appears to have attenuated, cancer has become an increasingly common terminal event. It is important to appreciate that the clinical features of asbestosis and the findings on physical examination are not unique to this disorder and resemble those of a variety of other diffuse interstitial inflammatory and fibrotic processes.

The characteristic pulmonary function changes of asbestosis are a restrictive impairment with a reduction in lung volumes (especially FVC and total lung capacity), decreased diffusing capacity D_{LCO}), and arterial hypoxemia.[25,36] Large-airway function, as reflected in the FEV_1/FVC ratio, is generally well preserved. In one of the earliest studies,[40] approximately 50 percent of asbestos workers had a reduced FVC and the vital capacity was decreased, on the average, by 18 percent as predicted over the next 10 years. Among the 1117 asbestos insulators in New York and New Jersey, the frequency of an abnormal FVC increased to more than 50 percent as follow-up was prolonged. In a larger cohort of 2611 asbestos insulators, the FVC percent predicted decreased as the profusion of irregular opacities on the chest radiograph increased; pleural thickening exaggerated the decrease for each category of profusion.[25] For each category of profusion, diffuse pleural thickening caused a further decrease (at least 10 percent) in FVC percent predicted compared to circumscribed plaques.

Mild airway obstruction can also be seen in nonsmokers with asbestosis. These patients usually have a restrictive pattern of lung function, increased isoflow volume, and increased upstream resistance at low lung volumes.[4] Open lung biopsies from a limited number of these patients suggest that these obstructive findings may be due to peribronchiolar fibrosis, since they revealed peribronchiolar infiltrates with macrophages and fibrosis that extended into the adjacent interstitium. Therefore, it is not surprising that lesser grades of asbestosis can show a mixed restrictive and obstructive abnormality.

Long-term medical surveillance is recommended for all asbestos-exposed persons, especially those with radiographic abnormalities. Periodic physiological assessments play an important role in these evaluations. Although complex physiological abnormalities can be seen in these patients, for prospective assessments of asbestosis carried out in the clinical context, simple measurements of lung volume, such as the forced vital capacity, seem to be the most useful.

Radiographic Features

In asbestosis, the standard PA chest radiograph reveals bilateral diffuse reticulonodular opacities, predominantly in the lower lung zones. In 1980, the International Labor Organization (ILO) revised the International Classification of the Radiographs of the Pneumoconioses to make provisions for reading the radiographic features of asbestosis. It used the term *small irregular opacities* to describe the irregular linear shadows that develop in the lung parenchyma and obscure the normal bronchovascular branching pattern seen in disease-free lungs. This schema categorized the irregular rounded opacities found on PA chest radiographs according to size and expressed them on a 12-point scale. Category 0 was defined as a normal radiograph and category 1 as mild asbestosis. Typically, a profusion of irregular opacities at the level of 1/0 is taken as the break point between normal and abnormal. Moderate asbestosis and advanced asbestosis were defined as category 2 and 3 chest radiographs, respectively. As duration from onset and intensity of exposure increase, there is an increase in prevalence and severity of asbestosis as reflected in the chest radiograph.

CT scanning has improved the sensitivity for detecting asbestos-related lesions (Fig. 57-4). It eliminates a common problem with PA chest radiographs—i.e. the superimposition of pleural abnormalities over parenchymal lesions. It also enhances the attenuation discrimination for parenchymal opacities. As a result of more than 300 HRCT evaluations of persons with asbestos exposure, five HRCT features of asbestosis have been identified: curvilinear subpleural lines, increased intralobular septa, dependent opacities, parenchymal bands and interlobular core structures, and honeycombing.[15] These changes have recently been corroborated by histologic examination. This spectrum of radiographic findings[15] stands in contrast to the fine irregular opacities that are so prominent on the PA chest radiographs of these persons. In asbestos-exposed workers, abnormal HRCT has been shown to correlate with restrictive physiological abnormalities and abnormal diffusing capacities.[44] HRCT is also extremely sensitive in documenting the asbestos-related pleural abnormalities discussed above. The presence of

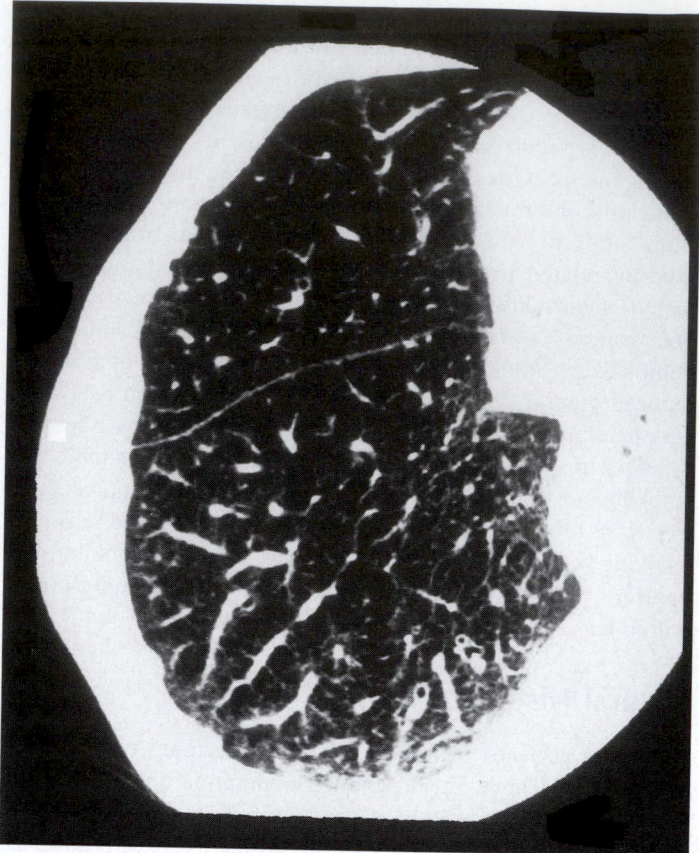

FIGURE 57-4   HRCT scan with irregular opacities of the lung parenchyma and interlobar structure. The PA chest radiograph was graded 2/1 on the ILO International Classification of the Radiographs of the Pneumoconioses. *(Courtesy of Dr. David Naidich.)*

pleural plaques (particularly if they are bilateral) provides useful evidence that the parenchymal process is asbestos related. Hilar node enlargement is not a feature of asbestosis, and progressive massive fibrosis is also uncommon.

Diagnosis

Asbestosis is defined as parenchymal fibrosis, with or without pleural thickening, usually associated with dyspnea, bibasilar rales, and pulmonary function changes.[1] To diagnose this disorder, one must establish the presence of pulmonary fibrosis and determine whether exposure has occurred of a duration and intensity sufficient to put the person at risk for developing this syndrome. The PA chest radiograph and its interpretation are the most important factors in the former. As noted above, a profusion of irregular opacities at the level of 1/0 is used as the break point between normal and abnormal in the evaluation of lung fields on the chest radiographs of asbestos-exposed persons. When radiographic or lung function changes are marginal, CT scanning often reveals characteristic parenchymal abnormalities as well as pleural plaques and/or pleural fibrosis. These lesions, particularly when bilateral, are strongly suggestive of asbestos exposure.

The diagnosis of asbestosis must always be based on an appropriate exposure history. The features of the history that need to be defined include the duration, onset, type, and intensity of exposure experienced by the patient. Convincing occupational exposures include manufacture of asbestos products, asbestos mining and milling, construction trade worker (insulator, sheet-metal worker, electrician, plumber, pipe fitter, carpenter), power plant worker, boilermaker, and shipyard worker. In performing this evaluation, it is important to keep in mind that intensity of exposure can be heavy even if duration of exposure is short. For example, heavy exposures were experienced by shipyard workers engaged in insulation application or removal in contained areas for brief periods aboard ship and by asbestos insulators during their apprenticeship when they unloaded asbestos sacks into troughs and mixed asbestos cement. Short, intense exposures of this sort, which lasted from several months to 1 or 2 years, can be sufficient to cause asbestosis. Exposures over 10 to 20 years are, however, usually necessary. The timing of the exposure is also relevant. Industrial hygiene controls in the 1950s and 1960s, especially in the construction trades, were not widely applied or enforced. Thus, workers exposed during these periods may have received a heavy asbestos load. Time since onset of exposure is also crucial. Cohort studies have identified latency to be an important factor, with the prevalence of asbestosis increasing with time since the onset of exposure.

The specificity of the diagnosis of asbestosis increases as the number of clinical criteria (symptoms, signs, chest radiograph, pulmonary function) increase. In addition, as the accuracy of the diagnosis increases, the more significant the asbestos exposure. The more trivial the asbestos exposure, the less likely it is to be causal. Misclassification and diagnostic difficulty occur in patients with a heavy cigarette-smoking history and concurrent emphysema (which also reduces the diffusing capacity). Patients with idiopathic pulmonary fibrosis (IPF) may have a history of asbestos exposure. These patients tend to be younger, however, and their asbestos exposure is usually casual, brief, and recent and can often be discounted. Since patients with IPF require a lung biopsy for confirmatory diagnosis, an asbestos fiber count per milligram of dry lung can be helpful (see below). An open lung biopsy is not required in most cases when a significant exposure history can be identified.

In the absence of an adequate exposure history or in the presence of a confusing clinical presentation, biopsy material may be helpful in identifying the nature of the disease. It allows the pulmonary interstitial process to be compared to the known features of asbestosis and other interstitial disorders. It also allows the pathologist to look for the presence of asbestos materials. Asbestos fibers exist in the lung in two forms: uncoated or bare fibers, which, for practical purposes, are visible only on electron microscopy, and coated fibers, which are also called asbestos bodies. The latter are visible by light microscopy (Fig. 57-5). Uncoated fibers are much more common, exceeding the frequency of coated fibers by anything from 5- to 10,000-fold. Although other inhaled particles may also become coated, most coated fibers found in human lungs have an asbestos core. Thus, the presence of asbestos bodies or asbestos fibers is considered the hallmark of exposure, past or current. The presence of more than one coated fiber has been cited as a necessary criterion for the pathologic diagnosis of asbestosis, even in a subject with an obvious exposure history. This may be inappropriate, however, since asbestos bodies may not be able to be detected even after

heavy exposure. Cases have been described in which the load of uncoated fibers was high in the absence of asbestos bodies, and asbestos bodies have been noted in the tissues of people without significant asbestos exposure. Thus, although asbestos bodies probably reflect exposure, their absence by no means excludes it.

Asbestos bodies can also be detected in BAL samples. In some studies, these asbestos bodies correlate with heavy exposure and asbestosis. This is nicely illustrated in a large series of 563 patients: those with asbestosis had a mean of 120 asbestos bodies per milliliter; those with pleural disease, 5 asbestos bodies per milliliter; and those with malignant mesothelioma or lung cancer, 8 asbestos bodies per milliliter of lavage fluid.[11] Of 49 patients with more than 100 asbestos bodies per milliliter of lavage fluid, 30 had asbestosis, 8 had pleural disease, 13 had mesothelioma or lung cancer, and 3 had an exposure history only. Others have estimated that one asbestos body per milliliter of BAL fluid correlates with 1000 to 3000 asbestos bodies per gram of dry lung tissue.[38] The problems inherent in counting asbestos bodies in an attempt to establish a diagnosis of asbestosis were noted above. Thus, the utility of BAL asbestos body counts in diagnosing asbestos awaits further definition.

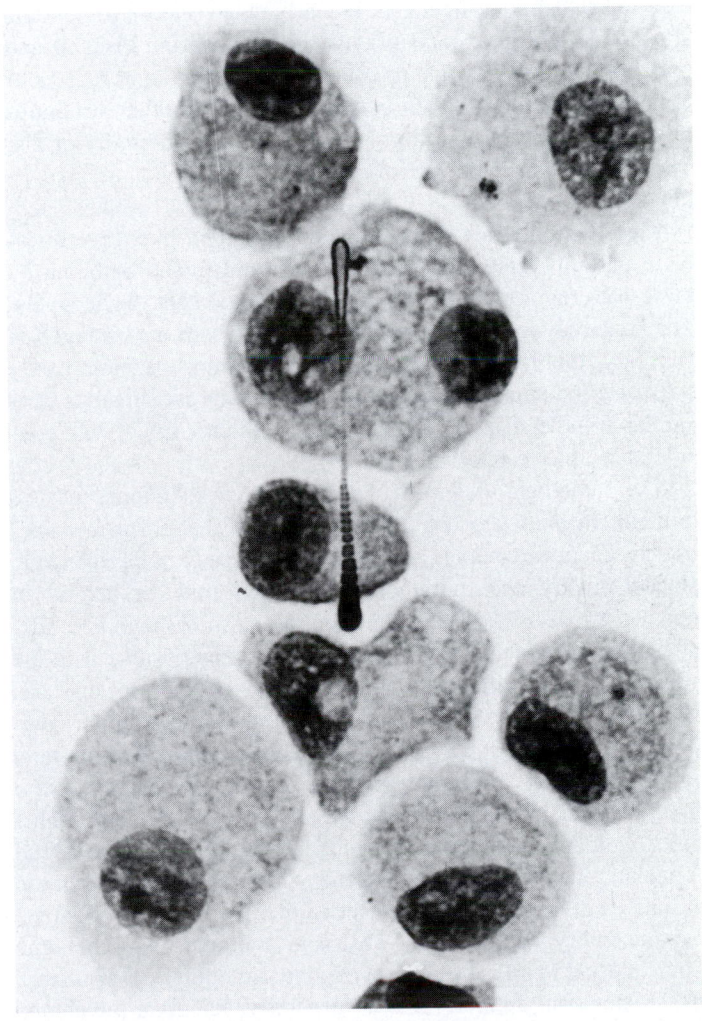

FIGURE 57-5 Light microscopic appearance of an asbestos body in a cytocentrifuged preparation of alveolar macrophages lavaged from a nonsmoking asbestos insulator. Wright-Giemsa stain, ×400. *(Courtesy of Dr. T. Takemura and Dr. V. Ferrans.)*

Treatment and Prognosis

Major causes of morbidity and mortality in patients with asbestosis include the progression of the underlying lung disease and the development of lung cancers and malignant mesotheliomas. Longitudinal observations of asbestos-exposed trade workers have demonstrated accelerated declines in pulmonary function. In a study of 77 workers with a mean of 31 ± 1 years of occupational exposure, linear regression demonstrated a mean annual decline of 92 ± 28 ml per year in FVC, 66 ± 22 ml per year in FEV_1, and 14 ± 53 ml per year in total lung capacity.[32] Although corticosteroids and colchicine have been used for the treatment of IPF, they have not been demonstrated to be beneficial in asbestosis. At present, there is no established treatment for this disorder. Because of the risk of lung cancer and mesothelioma, however, medical surveillance is recommended.

MALIGNANT MESOTHELIOMA

Pathology

Most instances of mesothelioma occur in persons who have been exposed to asbestos fibers. In its early stage, the mesothelioma appears as multiple small grayish nodules on the visceral and parietal pleura that evolve to coalesce and form larger masses of tumors. These tumors then invade thoracic and other structures by direct extension, causing the morbidity and mortality of disease. Fewer than 25 percent of malignant mesotheliomas are peritoneal in origin.

Mesotheliomas are conventionally classified into three histologic patterns: epithelial, sarcomatous, and mixed or biphasic; these patterns account for 50, 20, and 30 percent, respectively. The epithelial variant—in which neoplastic cells are arranged in papillary, tubular, or solid nest configurations—is most easily confused with metastatic adenocarcinoma. The sarcomatous variant has spindle-shaped cells that may be pleomorphic, with considerable mitotic activity.

The pathologic diagnosis of malignant mesothelioma may be difficult. In particular, the differentiation of malignant mesotheliomas, adenocarcinomas, and other tumors may be problematic. Histochemistry and immunohistochemistry may be helpful in making the distinction. Thus, in contrast to mesotheliomas, adenocarcinomas contain neutral mucin that stains positive with the periodic acid–Schiff stain and is often resistant to diastase. Hyaluronic acid, the major acid mucopolysaccharide in mesotheliomas, can be identified with the alcian blue or colloidal iron stain. Removal by prior digestion with hyaluronidase increases the specificity of the reaction. In contrast, adenocarcinomas are alcian blue and colloidal iron negative. Mesothelial cells contain cytoskeletal filaments, including cytokeratin and vimentin; staining for these structures is not specific, since other tumor types are also positive. Carcinoembryonic antigen is absent in malignant mesothelioma but is present in up to 90 percent of adenocarcinomas.[35] Similarly, the monoclonal antibody B72.3, generated against a membrane fraction of human metastatic breast cancer, was positive in 19 of 22 pulmonary adenocarcinomas but none of 20 mesotheliomas.[35] Monoclonal antibody Leu MI is frequently positive in lung carcinomas and nonreactive with mesotheliomas.

The ultrastructural features of malignant mesotheliomas are also noteworthy. Malignant mesotheliomas contain abundant tonofilaments, often organized into perinuclear bundles, and long, sinuous, slender surface microvilli. The microvilli sometimes show secondary and tertiary branching and may interdigitate with stromal collagen. Malignant mesothelial cells produce collagen, a prominent feature of the sarcomatous variant.

Natural History

Malignant mesotheliomas are locally invasive, spreading along the pleural wall and invading the lung, mediastinal lymph nodes, and other thoracic and nearby structures. At autopsy, tumor may be found in the diaphragm, heart, liver, spleen, adrenals, gastrointestinal tract serosa, bone, pancreas, and kidneys. Fifty to 80 percent of patients also have metastases.

About 10 percent of patients with a malignant mesothelioma are alive at 24 months. Survival is significantly longer for patients with an epithelial subtype or with a pleural rather than a peritoneal mesothelioma, and for those under 65 years of age.

The incidence of mesothelioma is increasing because of the cohort exposed to asbestos between 1940 and 1970. Incidence rates vary from a low of 11 to 13 per million per year in the United States to 33 per million per year in South Africa and to 66 per million per year in Western Australia. These rates reflect mining and manufacturing industries and the location of crocidolite mines. Although the peak incidence in the United States may have passed since imports decreased after 1945, imports of asbestos in the United Kingdom reached their peak in the 1960s to 1970s. Thus, the peak of mesothelioma deaths in the United Kingdom is expected to occur in 2020, when up to 1 percent of men may die of the disease. Chrysotile was the major asbestos import to the United Kingdom, and half of this material went into the construction industry. Amosite was the leading amphibole import, and most of it went into insulation board. Thus, workers in the construction industry in the United Kingdom seem to be at greatest risk.[29]

Epidemiology

In 1960, Wagner and colleagues published a landmark paper demonstrating an association between malignant mesothelioma and asbestos exposure.[46] They reported on 33 patients from South Africa, 28 of whom were exposed in the crocidolite mining region and 4 of whom were exposed in asbestos factories. They observed that mesotheliomas occurred 20 to 40 years after exposure to asbestos dust and found asbestos bodies in lung tissue from 8 of 10 patients from whom lung tissue was available for study. Subsequently, the importance of direct asbestos exposure was confirmed and the potential importance of indirect exposure to asbestos was recognized.[28,40]

Evaluations of asbestos fiber content have shown a clear association between asbestos exposure and the occurrence of mesothelioma.[48] Epidemiologic studies have shown that crocidolite may be the more potent fiber type among asbestos miners. Most mesotheliomas have occurred from chrysotile-amphibole mixtures, since chrysotile is the most common fiber in commercial use.[29] Few controversies in medicine are as intense as the disagreements concerning the relation between asbestos fiber type and carcinogenic risk.[26] Nonetheless, associations between malignant mesothelioma and other (noncrocidolite) fiber types have been reported. For example, the incidence of malignant mesotheliomas among chrysotile workers who came before the Workers' Compensation Board of Quebec was similar to that in Western Australian crocidolite miners.[5] Studies of Canadian cohorts have also indicated that high concentrations of chrysotile, or an amphibole contaminant, are required to cause mesothelioma,[9] suggesting that chrysotile has weaker biopersistence than does tremolite, which is merely a contaminant in most ores.[3] In the United States, amosite is the predominant amphibole found in lung tissue: in one study it was identified in 81 percent of 90 patients with mesothelioma; in this population, it accounted for 58 percent of all fibers at least 5 μm in length.[31]

Cigarette smoking is a confounding variable in studies that relate asbestos-exposed persons to cancer risk. The contribution that cigarettes make to the risk of lung cancer is impressive (see below). It is universally accepted, however, that mesothelioma is not associated with cigarette smoke per se.

Pathogenesis

Insight into the pathogenesis of malignant mesothelioma has come from experiments in which asbestos fibers were introduced into the pleural space of animals. These studies have demonstrated that amosite, anthophyllite, crocidolite, and Canadian chrysotile can all cause these pleural malignancies. Studies of fiber size have shown that the most carcinogenic fibers in the pleural space are 1.5 μm or less in diameter and more than 8 μm in length. Inspection of electron micrographs of asbestos fibers has shown that crocidolite and amosite possess needlelike characteristics, whereas anthophyllite has a more boxlike appearance and chrysotile has a long, curly appearance. These variations in size are also consistent with epidemiologic studies indicating that crocidolite and amosite may have greater risk for mesothelioma than do other types of asbestos, although these studies are often confounded by intense exposures to these amphibole types.

One theory concerning the mechanism of asbestos-induced carcinogenesis focuses on the observation that asbestos fibers become entangled in the mitotic spindle during interphase, thereby causing chromosomal abnormalities. Electron microscopic evaluations have shown fibers penetrating between multiple lobes of the nucleus and associating, along their length, with the outer surface of the nuclear envelope. Structural chromosomal abnormalities in mesothelioma are clonal and complex, and include both chromosomal gains (chromosome 22) and losses (chromosome 7). Deletions of the short arm of chromosome 3, the break point 1p11–p22, chromosome 17, and structural and numeric changes in chromosome 7 have been described. The last is quite interesting, since the tumor suppresser gene *p53* is located in the region of 17p13. In asbestos insulators, sister chromatid exchanges in circulating lymphocytes are increased: larger chromosomes are more susceptible, and in the largest chromosome group, there is a significant interactive effect between asbestos exposure and cigarette smoking.[35]

Cell lines established from malignant mesotheliomas have been shown to constitutively upregulate the PDGF B-chain gene and, to a lesser extent, the PDGF A-chain gene. High levels of transforming growth factor–β1 (TGF-β_1), TGF-β_2, and TGF-β_3 mRNA and bioactivity have been reported for cell lines derived from malignant mesotheliomas. These TGF-β moieties may be involved in the considerable matrix formation that accompanies mesothelial tumors. Mesothelioma cell lines also release IGF-1 and express mRNA for the IGF-1 receptor. This is consistent with an IGF-1–based autocrine loop for mesothelioma cell proliferation.

Clinical and Radiographic Features

Pleural mesotheliomas are found mainly in males (ratio, between 3 and 4 to 1) and are most commonly diagnosed in patients between 50 and 70 years of age. Chest pain is the most common symptom experienced by patients with mesotheliomas. Dyspnea is next in frequency. Less common symptoms are cough, weight loss, and fever. A pleural effusion is usually present and can be massive. The effusion is an exudate, can be hemorrhagic, and may have high levels of hyaluronic acid (Fig. 57-6). Malignant mesothelioma is locally invasive, spreading along the pleural wall and invading the lung and nearby structures. Metastases are less common but can give rise to symptoms due to tumor in the diaphragm, heart, liver, spleen, adrenals, gastrointestinal tract, bone, pancreas, and kidneys. The syndrome of inappropriate ADH secretion, clubbing, or hypoglycemia is rare. Thrombocytosis is common—in 90 percent of cases in one series—and thromboembolic complications can occur. Ascites and weight loss are characteristic features of peritoneal mesothelioma.

A variety of radiographic abnormalities are found in malignant mesothelioma. They include a thick pleural peel along the lateral chest wall that can extend to the apex with an irregular nodular surface, multiple pleural nodules or masses, plaquelike opacities, and pleural effusion(s). As the disease progresses, the lung parenchyma may be involved, the affected hemithorax may decrease in size, and the mediastinum or hilar may be invaded.

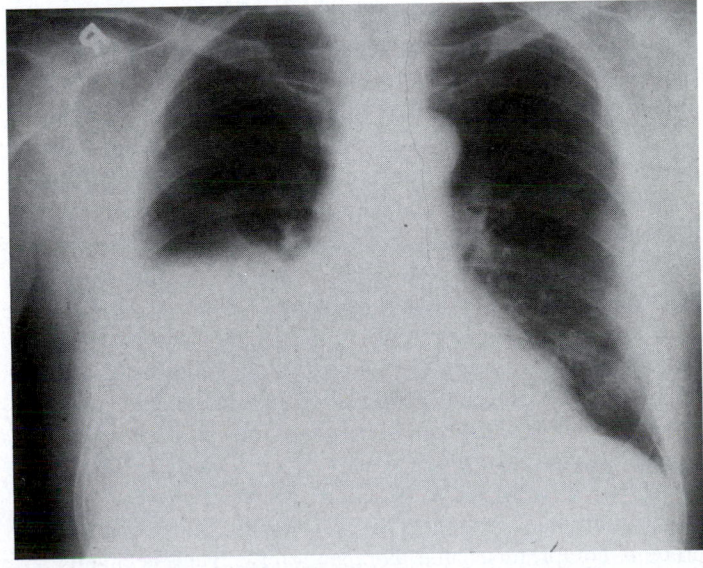

FIGURE 57-6 Large pleural effusion in an asbestos-exposed worker with an underlying malignant mesothelioma. *(Courtesy of Dr. J. Elias.)*

Pericardial thickening or effusion, abdominal extension, and chest wall invasion are common. The HRCT can help in differentiating pleural effusion from tumor and in determining the extent of tumor progression. The presence of asbestosis or of pleural plaques on the opposite side can assist in establishing the diagnosis of malignant mesothelioma.

Diagnosis

The diagnosis of malignant mesothelioma requires cytologic or histologic validation. Obtaining a cytologic diagnosis from the pleural exudate is difficult because reactive mesothelial cells and malignant cells are not easy to distinguish. Biopsy is required. Because mesothelioma has been shown to invade the track of the needle on about 20 percent of patients in whom biopsy was performed by transthoracic needle, open biopsy is preferable. Thoracoscopy is probably the procedure of choice in establishing the diagnosis of mesothelioma. Its diagnostic rates are greater than 80 percent—a value similar to that of open pleural biopsy. Local radiation after biopsy significantly reduces spread in needle tracks or incisions.

Treatment and Prognosis

Median survival time is approximately 8 to 12 months for all patients with malignant mesothelioma. Overall, fewer than 20 percent of patients are alive at 2 years. Pleurectomy or pneumonectomy, combined with radiation therapy, has failed to significantly influence survival rates. Chemotherapy with doxorubicin (Adriamycin) has shown variable responses without prolonging survival.

Interventions, such as gene therapy or the use of cytokines, for the treatment of malignant mesothelioma are currently being investigated. Thus, in 89 patients, the intrapleural instillation of γ-interferon twice weekly for 8 weeks resulted in eight histologically confirmed complete responses and nine partial responses, with at least a 50 percent reduction in tumor size. The overall response rate was 20 percent, increasing to 45 percent in stage I disease. In 15 patients, a phase I clinical trial of continuous infusion into the pleural space of recombinant IL-2 for 5 days, when evaluated at 36 days after infusion, revealed one complete remission and six partial remissions. The main side effect was fluid retention, no greater than 10 percent, in one-third of the patients. In mice with severe combined immune-deficiency, gene therapy, using a replication defective adenovirus carrying the herpes simplex–thymidine kinase gene followed by the antiviral drug ganciclovir, was used successfully to treat malignant mesothelioma. A significant antitumor effect occurred with clinically achievable dose ranges, even in bulky tumors. The virus did not spread from the serosal cavity following instillation. In mice with subcutaneously implanted mesothelioma, tumor regression occurred when only 10 percent of cells were infected—a result consistent with a *bystander effect.* A phase I clinical trial has shown this therapy to be safe. However, humoral and cell-mediated immune responses that developed against viral surface proteins compromised the therapeutic effectiveness of this approach. Also, the thymidine kinase gene in vivo had no effect on promoting regression of the tumor. These promising areas of research need further development before they can be applied as standard therapy.

LUNG CANCER

Epidemiology

The association between asbestos exposure and the development of lung cancer is based on a number of successive epidemiologic investigations. Case reports of lung cancer and asbestos deaths occurred as early as 1935. Series of patients with asbestosis who went to autopsy were reported by 1947. In 1955, an epidemiologic cohort study of 113 men exposed to asbestos for 20 years disclosed 11 deaths due to cancer (compared with 0.8 expected), all of which had evidence of asbestosis.[12] In 1965, a retrospective cohort study in two asbestos insulator unions in the United States reported that deaths from lung cancer were 6.8 times the expected rate and that the incidence of lung cancer increased with time after exposure.[40] In 1968, a follow-up of men in this cohort demonstrated an important synergy between asbestos exposure and cigarette smoking, since the risk of lung cancer was almost entirely borne by those who had a history of cigarette smoking.[41]

The largest survey of asbestos-related deaths looked at a North American asbestos insulator cohort.[42] This study demonstrated a threefold excess of cancer deaths that were due primarily to pulmonary malignancies. Comparatively few of these excess deaths were observed among those less than 25 years after the start of exposure. Lung cancer peaked at 40 years from exposure and mesothelioma at 45 years. In contrast, death rates from asbestosis increased progressively with time. This study confirmed the multiplicative effect of smoking plus asbestos exposure on the risk of lung cancer. Moreover, it showed that deaths from lung cancer dropped by almost two-thirds for asbestos insulators who subsequently stopped smoking.

Additional insights were provided by a study of amosite workers who were exposed to concentrations of 50 fibers per milliliter.[39] These patients experienced a fivefold increase in lung cancer. Long-term follow-up showed: (1) a latency period of about 20 years before the increase in cancer occurred; (2) the greater the dose or the longer the exposure, the greater risk of developing lung cancer; and (3) the greater the dose or exposure time, the shorter the latency period before the tumor developed. Malignancies were also noted in the wives and children of these workers who were exposed to asbestos in the household, primarily on workclothes. In addition, men employed for less than 1 month between 1941 and 1945 developed lung cancer at an increased rate. Studies of a variety of other cohorts have confirmed the increased incidence of lung cancer in asbestos-exposed populations.[10,14,19,28] They have also demonstrated an increased frequency of digestive cancers and cancer of the larynx; in the latter, asbestos has been found in laryngeal tissue. As in the case of cancer of the lung, cigarette smoking has a strong association with the occurrence of these laryngeal malignancies.

Epidemiologic studies have also provided information about dose-response relationships and about the importance of asbestos-processing techniques and fiber type in the pathogenesis of pulmonary malignancies. A number of investigators have observed linear dose-response relationships for lung cancer.[10,19] Different dose-response relationships have, however, been found in other studies.[14] These differences may be the result of differences in processing techniques. For example, studies in a South Carolina plant demonstrated that the steeper dose-response relationship of miners versus millers was probably due to the manufacturing process, which resulted in high levels of brief exposure during the opening of asbestos bags and the sudden separation of the asbestos fibers.[10] Similarly, differences in lung cancer mortality in asbestos cement product plants in Louisiana were found to be associated with the addition, in one of these plants, of crocidolite to the asbestos cement pipe mixture.[19] Other risk factors in the work place—such as concomitant metals, ionizing radiation, and other chemicals—may also contribute to the differences that have been noted. It has been argued that there is a difference in lung cancer risk for different asbestos fiber types; however, the risk of lung cancer increases most clearly with cumulative asbestos exposure. Despite these uncertainties, however, it is clear that each of the asbestos fiber types causes lung cancer.

Pathology

Asbestos-related lung cancers are not distinct from lung cancers that occur in cigarette smokers and otherwise normal persons in type, nature, or location. All histologic types of lung cancer occur with increased frequency, but adenocarcinoma has the highest incidence. In the vast majority of patients, there is histologic evidence of asbestosis and asbestos bodies are frequently found. Whether asbestos-related lung cancers occur in the absence of asbestosis is debatable (see below).

Pathogenesis

Animal experiments using several types of asbestos have succeeded in reproducing pulmonary malignancies. In one study, approximately one-third of rats exposed by inhalation to asbestos (amosite, anthophyllite, crocidolite, Canadian chrysotile, or Rhodesian chrysotile) for periods ranging from 1 day to 24 months developed adenocarcinomas or squamous cell carcinomas of the lung. In these experiments, a clear dose-response relationship existed between asbestos dose and the occurrence of tumors. The mechanisms responsible for the induction of these malignancies are poorly understood. However, DNA injury and activation of nuclear transcription factors may play an important role. The former appears to relate to the physical properties of the asbestos fibers, which enable DNA, RNA, and chromatin to bind to asbestos.[2] Reactive oxygen species may also play an important role in this process, since chrysotile asbestos, along with cigarette smoke, synergistically increases the number of breaks in DNA strands, and oxidant scavengers—such as mannitol, catalase, iron chelators, and dimethylsulfoxide—prevent this DNA damage. Asbestos also induces nuclear factor–κB (NF-κB) DNA binding in tracheal epithelial cells in vitro. NF-κB is an important transcription factor for cytokines, growth factors, and proto-oncogenes that could contribute in a variety of ways to malignant transformation.

Clinical Features

The patterns of presentation of lung cancer among asbestos workers are similar to those of high-risk patient populations: cough, chest pain, dyspnea, hemoptysis, recurrent bouts of pneumonia, and localized wheezing are major symptoms that frequently bring patients to medical attention. However, patients can also be asymptomatic at the time of initial discovery, the abnormality being noted on a routine or screening chest radiograph. Other manifestations of carcinoma—such as rib invasion, shoulder-arm pain, and paraneoplastic syndromes—can also occur in asbestos-related malignancies.

One of the most vexing questions in asbestos-related lung cancers is the relationship between the lung cancer and asbestosis. Asbestosis can be detected radiographically or histologically in the vast majority of patients with asbestos-related lung cancer. Most, but not all, lung cancer patients in the Quebec asbestos mining district had small parenchymal opacities on the chest radiograph before death. In addition, in amphibole miners from South Africa with carcinoma of the lung who were evaluated by stepwise regression analysis for exposure variables, asbestosis was by far the most striking variable. Moreover, a dose-response relationship was found between the severity of asbestosis and the frequency of lung cancer. However, in keeping with the high frequency of asbestosis that cannot be seen on the chest radiograph—i.e., asbestosis that can be detected only in vivo by HRCT or biopsy—it is clear that radiographic evidence of asbestosis cannot be detected in all patients with asbestos-related lung cancer. Thus, in the North American insulator cohort, 18 percent of the patients who died of lung cancer did not have radiographic evidence of parenchymal fibrosis.[20] Similarly, in a case control study of 271 lung cancer patients, a small but definite increase in cancer risk was noted in patients whose chest radiographs were not definitely abnormal (0/1 or less by ILO classification). This study indicated that asbestos exposures that do not cause small opacities on the chest radiograph may nevertheless increase the risk of lung cancer.[49]

Radiographic Features

The radiographic manifestations of asbestos-induced lung cancers do not differ, per se, from those of lung cancers associated with other carcinogens. Mass lesions, atelectasis, postobstructive pneumonia, and pleural effusions are all seen. As noted above, these lesions are frequently superimposed on a background of asbestosis or asbestos-induced pleural abnormalities. Confusion with lung cancer may arise from *en face* pleural plaques or rounded atelectasis. In contrast to lung cancer, however, these abnormalities are stable over time. Newer techniques, such as the helical CT scan, which can evaluate the chest in a single breath, may increase the early detection rate of lung cancer in this high-risk patient population.

Diagnosis

The principles employed in the diagnosis of lung cancer in asbestos workers are identical to those in the diagnosis of pulmonary malignancies in patients exposed to other carcinogenic agents. Appropriate cytologic or histologic specimens are required. This can be accomplished by sputum analysis or by bronchoscopy with brushings, biopsy, or lavage. Transthoracic needle aspirates, thoracoscopic parenchymal biopsies, or open lung biopsies may be required for definitive diagnosis.

Treatment and Prognosis

The therapeutic approaches utilized for asbestos-related lung cancers are similar to those employed for lung cancers induced under other circumstances. When one is dealing with non–small cell malignancies, patient operability and resectability need to be evaluated and, if appropriate, surgical extirpation undertaken. The impact of other asbestos-related pulmonary processes must always be taken into account. For example, severe asbestosis may limit operability, and diffuse pleural thickening may make surgical intervention problematic. Overall, however, lung cancer has a dismal prognosis—8 to 10 percent survival at 5 years.

EFFORTS AT ASBESTOS CONTROL

In order to control the risk of exposure to asbestos, the U.S. Occupational Safety and Health Administration regulates the usage of all types of asbestos fibers.

Industrial hygiene efforts to control exposure have focused on engineering controls, including enclosure of the process lines, especially all sites where asbestos is introduced into a system, increasing ventilation, and the use of wet manufacturing methods. Personal respirators are used as a last resort in achieving control of exposure in the workplace. Most of the insulation-manufacturing industry has switched to alternative materials, especially fibrous glass, rock and slag wool, and refractory ceramic fibers. Animal experiments have generally shown these asbestos substitutes to be safe, except that refractory ceramic fibers were able to produce mesotheliomas in hamsters. Asbestosis and asbestos-related cancers may occur at increased rates in the future, owing to the increased use of asbestos in developing countries.

REFERENCES

1. American Thoracic Society: The diagnosis of nonmalignant diseases related to asbestos. *Am Rev Respir Dis* 134:363–368, 1986.
2. Appel JD, Fasy TM, Kohtz DS, et al: Asbestos fibers mediate transformation of monkey cells by exogenous plasmid DNA. *Proc Natl Acad Sci USA* 85:7670–7674, 1988.
3. Becklake M: Fiber burden and asbestos-related lung disease: Determinants of dose-response relationships. *Am J Respir Crit Care Med* 150:1488–1492, 1994.
4. Bégin R, Cantin A, Berthiaume Y, et al: Airway function in lifetime-nonsmoking older asbestos workers. *Am J Med* 75:631–638, 1983.
5. Bégin R, Guntier JJ, Desmeules M, Ostiguy G: Work-related mesothelioma in Quebec, 1967–1990. *Am J Ind Med* 22:531–542, 1992.
6. Bégin R, Samet JM, Shaikh RA: Asbestos, in Harber P, Schenker MB, Balmes JR (eds), *Occupational and Environmental Respiratory Disease.* St. Louis, Mosby–Year Book, 1996, pp 293–321.
7. Brodkin CA, Barnhart S, Anderson G, et al: Correlation between respiratory symptoms and pulmonary function in asbestos-exposed workers. *Am Rev Respir Dis* 148:32–37, 1993.
8. Brody AR, Hill LH, Adler KB: Actin-containing microfilaments of pulmonary epithelial cells provide a mechanism for translocation asbestos to the interstitium. *Chest* 83(Suppl):11–12, 1983.
9. Churg A, Vedal S: Fiber burden and patterns of asbestos-related disease in workers with heavy mixed amosite and chrysotile exposure. *Am J Respir Crit Care Med* 150:663–669, 1994.
10. Dement JM, Harris RL, Symons MJ, Shy CM: Exposures and mortality among chrysotile asbestos workers: Part II. Mortality. *Am J Ind Med* 4:421–433, 1983.
11. de Vuyst P, Dumortier P, Moulin E, et al: Diagnostic value of asbestos bodies in bronchoalveolar lavage fluid. *Am Rev Respir Dis* 136:1219–1224, 1987.
12. Doll R: Mortality from lung cancer in asbestos workers. *Br J Ind Med* 12:81–86, 1955.
13. Ehrlich R, Lilis R, Chan E, et al: Long-term radiological effects of short-term exposure to amosite asbestos among factory workers. *Br J Ind Med* 49:268–275, 1992.
14. Finkelstein MM: Mortality among employees of an Ontario asbestos cement factory. *Am Rev Respir Dis* 129:754–761, 1984.
15. Gamsu G, Salmon CJ, Warnock ML, Blanc PD: CT quantification of interstitial fibrosis in patients with asbestosis: A comparison of two methods. *AJR Am J Roentgenol* 164:63–68, 1995.
16. Hillerdal G: Rounded atelectasis. *Chest* 95:836–841, 1989.
17. Hillerdal G: Pleural plaques and risk for bronchial carcinoma and mesothelioma. *Chest* 105:144–150, 1994.
18. Hillerdal G, Ozesmi M: Benign asbestos pleural effusion: 73 exudates in 60 patients. *Eur J Respir Dis* 71:113–121, 1987.
19. Hughes JM, Weill H, Hammad YY: Mortality of workers employed in the asbestos cement manufacturing plants. *Br J Ind Med* 44:161–174, 1987.
20. Kipen HM, Lilis R, Suzuki Y, et al: Pulmonary fibrosis in asbestos insulation workers with lung cancer: A radiological and histopathological evaluation. *Br J Ind Med* 44:96–100, 1987.
21. Lilis R, Miller A, Godbold J, et al: Comparative quantitative evaluation of pleural fibrosis and its effects on pulmonary function in two large asbestos-exposed occupational groups—insulators and sheet metal workers. *Environ Res* 59:49–66, 1992.
22. Lilis R, Miller A, Godbold J, et al: Radiographic abnormalities in asbestos insulators: Effects of duration from onset of exposure and smoking: Relationships of dyspnea with parenchymal and pleural fibrosis. *Am J Ind Med* 20:1–15, 1991.
23. Lilis R, Miller A, Godbold J, et al: Pulmonary function and pleural fibrosis: Quantitative relationships with an integrative index of pleural abnormalities. *Am J Ind Med* 20:145–161, 1991.
24. Lilis R, Selikoff IJ, Lerman Y, et al: Asbestosis: Interstitial pulmonary fibrosis and pleural fibrosis in a cohort of asbestos insulation workers: Influence of cigarette smoking. *Am J Ind Med* 10: 459–470, 1986.
25. Miller A, Lilis R, Godbold J, et al: Relationship of pulmonary function to radiographic interstitial fibrosis in 2611 long-term asbestos insulators. *Am Rev Respir Dis* 145:263–270, 1992.
26. Mossman BT, Gee JBL: Asbestos-related diseases. *New Engl J Med* 320:1721–1730, 1989.
27. Murphy RLH, Gaensler EA, Holford SK, et al: Crackles in the early detection of asbestosis. *Am Rev Respir Dis* 129:375–379, 1984.
28. Newhouse ML, Berry G, Wagner JC: Mortality of factory workers in east London, 1933–80. *Br J Ind Med* 42:4–11, 1980.
29. Peto J, Hodgson JT, Matthews FE, Jones JR: Continuing increase in mesothelioma mortality in Britain. *Lancet* 345:535–539, 1995.
30. Picado C, Rodríguez-Roisín R, Sala H, Agusti-Vidal A: Diagnosis of asbestosis: Clinical, radiological and lung function data in 42 patients. *Lung* 162:325–335, 1984.

31. Roggli V, Pratt PC, Brody AR: Asbestos fiber type in malignant mesothelioma: An analytical scanning electron microscopic study of 94 cases. *Am J Ind Med* 23:605–614, 1993.

32. Rom WN: Accelerated loss of lung function and alveolitis in a longitudinal study of non-smoking individuals with occupational exposure to asbestos. *Am J Ind Med* 21:835–844, 1992.

33. Rom WN, Basset P, Fells G, et al: Alveolar macrophages release an insulin-like growth factor I–type molecule. *J Clin Invest* 82:1685–1693, 1988.

34. Rom WN, Bitterman PB, Rennard SI, et al: Characterization of the lower respiratory tract inflammation of nonsmoking individuals with interstitial lung disease associated with chronic inhalation of inorganic dusts. *Am Rev Respir Dis* 136:1429–1434, 1987.

35. Rom WN, Travis WD, Brody AR: Cellular and molecular basis of the asbestos-related diseases: State of the art. *Am Rev Respir Dis* 143:408–422, 1991.

36. Rosenstock L, Barnhart S, Heyer NJ, et al: The relation among pulmonary function, chest roentgenographic abnormalities, and smoking status in an asbestos-exposed cohort. *Am Rev Respir Dis* 138:272–277, 1988.

37. Schwartz DA, Galvin JR, Yagla SJ, et al: Restrictive lung function and asbestos-induced pleural fibrosis. *J Clin Invest* 91:2685–2692, 1993.

38. Sebastién P, Armstrong B, Monchaux G, Bignon J: Asbestos bodies in bronchoalveolar lavage fluid and in lung parenchyma. *Am Rev Respir Dis* 137:75–78, 1988.

39. Seidman H, Selikoff IJ, Gelb SK: Mortality experience of amosite asbestos factory workers: Dose-response relationships 5 to 40 years after onset of short-term work exposure. *Am J Ind Med* 10:479–514, 1986.

40. Selikoff IJ, Churg J, Hammond EC: Asbestos exposure and neoplasia. *JAMA* 188:22–26, 1964.

41. Selikoff IJ, Lee DH: Asbestos and its distribution: Historical background, in Selikoff IJ, Lee DH (eds), *Asbestos and Disease* (Environmental Science Series). New York, Academic Press, 1978, pp 3–32.

42. Selikoff IJ, Seidman H: Asbestos-associated deaths among workers in the United States and Canada, 1967–1987. *Ann NY Acad Sci* 643:1–14, 1991.

43. Sheers G, Templeton AR: Effect of asbestos on dockyard workers. *Br Med J* 3:574–579, 1968.

44. Staples CA, Gamsu G, Ray CS, Webb NR: High resolution computed tomography and lung function in asbestos-exposed workers with normal chest radiographs. *Am Rev Respir Dis* 139:1502–1508, 1989.

45. Takemura T, Rom WN, Ferrans VJ, Crystal RG: Morphological characterization of alveolar macrophages from individuals with occupational exposure to inorganic particles. *Am Rev Respir Dis* 140:1674–1685, 1989.

46. Wagner JC, Sleggs CA, Marchand P: Diffuse pleural mesothelioma and asbestos exposure in the northwestern Cape province. *Br J Ind Med* 17:260–271, 1960.

47. Welch LS, Michaels D, Zoloth SR: The national sheet metal worker asbestos disease screening program: Radiologic findings. *Am J Ind Med* 25:635–648, 1994.

48. Whitwell F, Scott J, Grimshaw M: Relationship between occupations and asbestos fibre content of the lungs in patients with pleural mesothelioma, lung cancer, and other disease. *Thorax* 32:377–386, 1977.

49. Wilkinson P, Hansell DM, Janssens J, et al: Is lung cancer associated with asbestos exposure when there are no small opacities on the chest radiograph? *Lancet* 345:1074–1078, 1995.

50. Xaubet A, Rodríguez-Roisín R, Bombi JA, et al: Correlation of bronchoalveolar lavage and clinical and functional findings in asbestosis. *Am Rev Respir Dis* 133:848–854, 1986.

CHAPTER 58

CHRONIC BERYLLIUM AND HARD-METAL LUNG DISEASE

Milton D. Rossman / Jeffrey D. Edelman

CHRONIC BERYLLIUM DISEASE

History

Beryllium is the lightest metal, with an atomic number of 4. It was discovered as an element in 1798 by the French chemist Vauquelin, and reduced to its metallic form and named beryllium in 1828 by the German metallurgist Wohler. The commercial uses of beryllium stem from its light weight, thermal and electrical conductivity, high melting point, and tensile strength. This usage began after World War I, when it was used as an alloy, first with aluminum and later with copper, nickel, and cobalt. The industry grew in the 1930s because of the increased use of beryllium-copper products during World War II and the use of beryllium oxide in the refractory and fluorescent lamp industries. During and after World War II, beryllium was used in the nuclear industry because of its ability to function as a neutron multiplier. As a result, beryllium is used both for civilian nuclear reactors and for military weapons.

Coincident with the increased industrial usage of beryllium, acute beryllium disease was noted, first by Weber and Engelhardt in Germany in 1933 and then in the United States by Van Ordstrand and colleagues in 1943.[35] This disorder is a toxic, dose-related injury syndrome that commonly affects the upper respiratory tract. With high-level exposure, it is also associated with a chemical pneumonitis, with involvement of bronchi, bron-

chioli, and alveoli. The disorder peaked in the 1940s. As the result of the implementation of industrial hygiene standards, it is now seen only if there are plant explosions or other serious lapses in industrial hygiene procedures. The last reported possible case of acute beryllium disease in the United States occurred in the early 1980s.

A second pulmonary complication of beryllium exposure was first described by Hardy and Tabershaw in 1946.[14] This disease differed from acute beryllium disease because of the delayed onset, granulomatous response, and chronic course. Now known as chronic beryllium disease, the disorder is a hypersensitivity reaction to beryllium and is the major hazard facing beryllium workers.

Clinical Presentation

Chronic beryllium disease (CBD) is primarily a pulmonary granulomatous disorder. Although involvement of other organ systems has been reported (e.g., lymph node, skin, and liver), the lungs are the principal organ affected and account for the morbidity and mortality of the disorder. In its early stages, CBD may be asymptomatic. A positive blood proliferative response to beryllium (evidence for beryllium hypersensitivity) may be the earliest sign of CBD.[16] Radiologic abnormalities on routine chest radiographs may also be detected, and pulmonary function tests early in the disease may be normal or have an isolated diffusing capacity (DLCO) abnormality.[34] Symptomatic disease usually begins with nonspecific respiratory complaints, such as exertional dyspnea and cough. As the disease progresses, symptoms become more characteristic of chronic interstitial lung disease, with a nonproductive cough, substernal burning pain, and progressive exertional dyspnea. At this stage, dry bibasilar crackles are observed on physical examination. A few patients may have asthmatic-type complaints and physical findings. With advanced disease, progressive weakness, easy fatigability, dyspnea at rest, anorexia, and weight loss may occur, and acrocyanosis and clubbing may be observed. As cor pulmonale develops, peripheral edema, hepatomegaly, and distended neck veins are seen. Fever is unusual but may be seen. Hypercalcemia and nephrocalcinosis, joint pains, and severe cachexia have been described. Severe liver impairment has not been seen, but liver granulomas with mild abnormalities of liver function tests

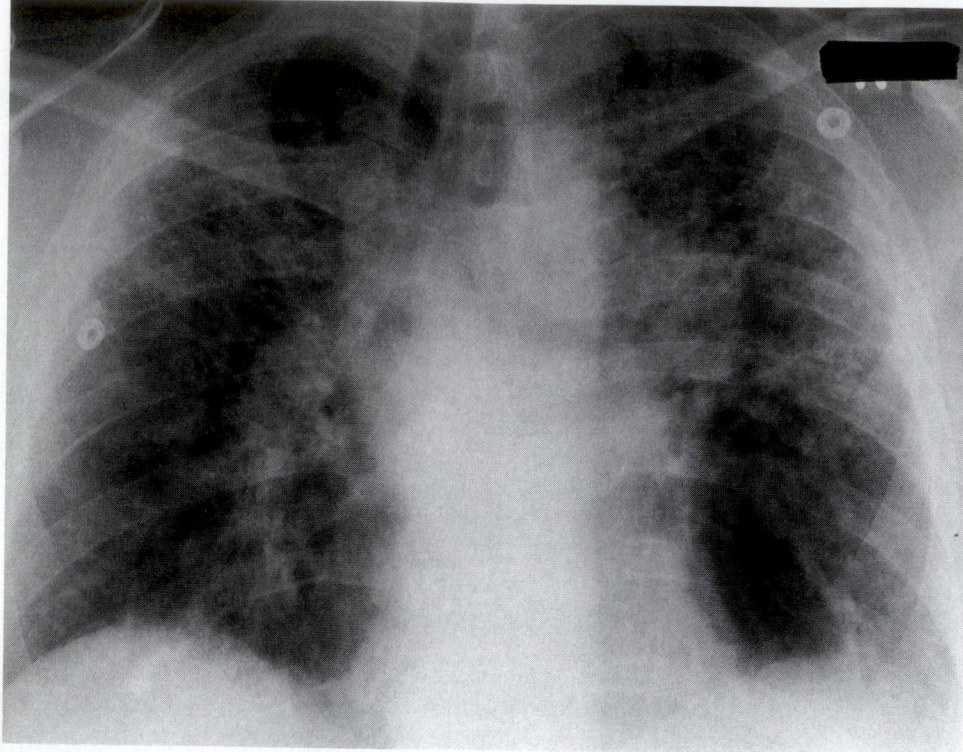

A

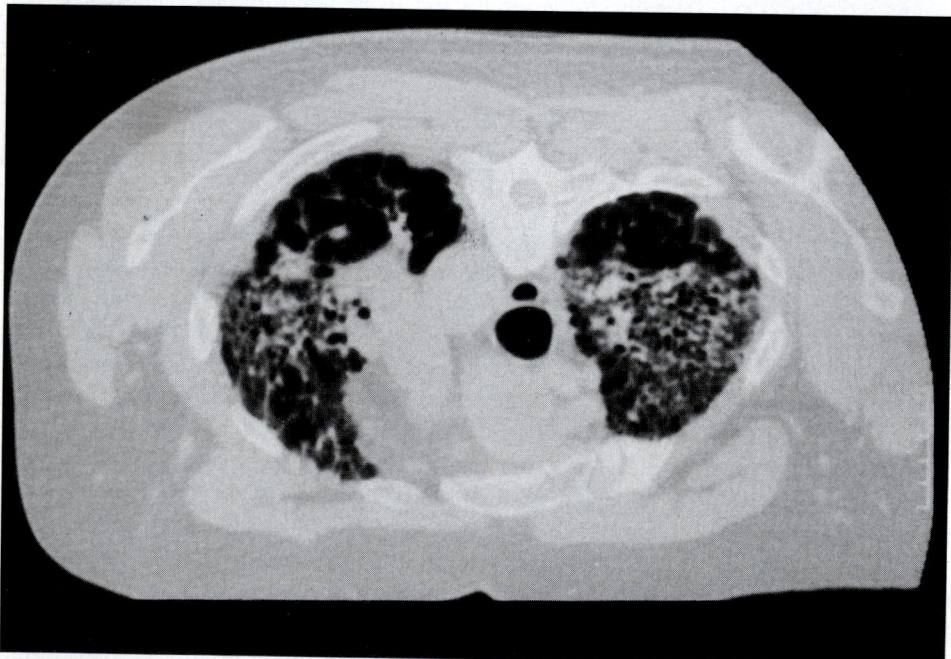

B

FIGURE 58-1 A 49-year-old man with extensive chronic beryllium disease demonstrating upper-lobe predominance, hilar adenopathy, and pleural involvement. The patient had been exposed between 1968 and 1974 at a Department of Defense facility and first became sick in 1985 with a cough. The initial diagnosis was idiopathic pulmonary fibrosis, and he was treated with steroids. Transbronchial biopsy in 1991 demonstrated granuloma, and bronchial lavage showed 28.6 percent lymphocytes and an abnormal lymphocyte proliferative response to beryllium (blood = 4.4, lung = 32.2, nl = <5.0). *A.* Chest radiograph at diagnosis demonstrating upper-lobe fibrosis, hilar adenopathy, and pleural thickening. *B.* High-resolution CT scan of the chest of the same patient demonstrates vesicular pattern of interstitial lung disease and pleural disease.

have been noted to occur. Skin involvement occurs in 10 to 30 percent of cases and frequently manifests as small granulomatous nodules on the hands, arms, and chest.

Radiography

Radiographic changes in CBD are non-specific and cannot be differentiated from those of sarcoidosis (Fig. 58-1). The most common radiographic abnormalities are diffuse round and reticular abnormalities.[3] Although most patients have both round and reticular nodules, opacities may be only round or only reticular. These opacities are usually present diffusely throughout the lung but may be confined to the upper lobes. Hilar adenopathy similar to what is commonly observed in sarcoidosis may also be seen in up to 50 percent of cases. However, the large "potato-type" node involvement that can be seen in sarcoidosis is not seen in CBD. As the disease advances, radiologic evidence of scarring and retraction can be seen. The hila are retracted upward, and conglomerate masses and emphysematous bullae may be present. Gross architectural distortion can occur from severe fibrosis. Pleural thickening can be seen in the presence of long-standing disease. In early disease, complete resolution of radiographic abnormalities can occur secondarily to corticosteroid therapy. Recurrences are common as the corticosteroids are tapered. Complete spontaneous disappearance of the radiographic lesions of CBD has not been observed.

Immunopathogenesis

There are three important characteristics of chronic beryllium disease. First, the disease occurs only after an industrial exposure to beryllium. The only cases that have been seen in nonindustrial workers have been in persons who lived near beryllium plants and were exposed to airborne emissions from the plant or from family members who were exposed to contaminated work clothes. All other cases have been seen in persons who have been engaged in the heating, grinding, abrading, or handling of beryllium metals, alloys, salts, or oxides. In addition, workers not directly handling beryllium may be exposed from processes occurring near them. In some cases, the exposure can be slight. For example, secretaries with apparently little exposure who worked in industry for less than 1 year have been noted to develop CBD years later. As a result, current industrial hygienic practices include efforts to remove potential airborne beryllium at the source to prevent beryllium from becoming airborne, thereby limiting the number of workers with potential exposure.

The second important characteristic of chronic beryllium disease is the long interval or latency that occurs between initial exposure and the onset of disease. The average time to the onset of clinical symptoms is 10 years.[9] This fact, combined with the lack of a clear-cut dose-response relationship to CBD, has hampered efforts to determine a safe level of beryllium. Thus, it is uncertain whether the peak exposure level or a total accumulated dose is more important for the development of CBD. At present, standards set by the Occupational Safety and Health Administration (OSHA) preclude exposure to levels greater than 2 $\mu g/m^3$ per 8-h shift as a threshold weighted average.

The third important characteristic of CBD is that only 1 to 5 percent of exposed workers will develop the disease. Of interest is that this percentage appears to have remained stable despite dramatic efforts by industry to reduce the potential exposure in workers. The tendency for CBD to occur in only a subgroup of exposed people may be due to a genetic predisposition (see below).

An evolving body of data suggests that CBD is the result of an immunologic reaction to beryllium. This perception is based on the following observations: 1. Beryllium can be used as a patch test reagent, which elicits delayed-type hypersensitivity reactions in patients with CBD.[7] (However, because of the concern that patch testing could sensitize persons to beryllium, skin testing has not been widely used.) 2. CBD is associated with an "immunologic" granulomatous response. 3. Animals can be sensitized to beryllium, and this hypersensitivity can be passed to naïve animals by cell transfers.[1]

The observations noted above suggest that cell-mediated immune responses play a prominent role in CBD. The development, in the 1970s, of in vitro studies that simulated patch testing provided further support for this concept. They demonstrated that the blood cells from a large percentage of patients with CBD had positive proliferative responses to beryllium.[8,22] In addition, after stimulation with beryllium, blood cells from many patients with CBD released the lymphokine macrophage inhibition factor.[10] However, not all patients with CBD manifested these positive responses.

The confirmation that CBD was due to a cell-mediated immune response to beryllium came in the 1980s, when cells harvested from the bronchoalveolar lavage (BAL) fluid of patients with CBD were examined.[6,10,29] Not only was a marked increase in the number and percent of CD4$^+$ T lymphocytes in the BAL fluid noted, but also a positive proliferative response of bronchoalveolar lymphocytes to beryllium was observed. Positive proliferative responses to beryllium were observed in all cases of CBD, and negative responses were noted in beryllium workers with biopsy-proven nonberyllium lung disease, in patients with sarcoidosis and no history of beryllium expo-

sure, and in normal volunteers. Not only did all patients with CBD have a positive proliferative response of their bronchoalveolar cells to beryllium, but this response was more pronounced in their lung cells than in their blood cells. Thus, there was an accumulation of beryllium-specific lymphocytes in the lungs of all patients with CBD. Further studies demonstrated that only CD4$^+$ T cells of beryllium-sensitive subjects proliferate in response to beryllium in vitro and that this beryllium response could be blocked by antibodies against the interleukin-2 receptor on T cells or against major histocompatibility complex (MHC) class II molecules.[30] These observations suggest that the beryllium-induced lymphocyte proliferative response in these patients is a normal immunologic response, since the T-cell receptor on CD4$^+$ T cells recognizes antigen in the context of MHC class II molecules. It also appears to be antigen driven, since the beryllium-sensitive T cells from these patients could be cloned and shown to retain their specific reactivity for beryllium but not for other antigens. In contrast, when other antigen sensitive cells from the same patients were cloned, these cells did not react to beryllium.

The above-described studies suggest the following model for the pathogenesis of chronic beryllium disease. Beryllium is inhaled and deposited in the periphery of the lung. In genetically predisposed persons (see below), beryllium, acting as a hapten, combines with a normal lung protein(s), causing it to be recognized as a foreign antigen (sensitization). The beryllium protein is poorly digestible and cannot be removed by the immune response. The host response to this antigen leads to persistent inflammation and to granuloma formation, which results in tissue destruction and fibrosis.

Genetic Predisposition

As noted above, only a fraction of exposed subjects develop CBD. To determine whether a genetic predisposition to CBD exists, investigators have characterized the MHC class II molecules in patients with CBD.[27] By heteroduplex analysis, certain human leukocyte antigen (HLA)–DP alleles were shown to be associated with CBD. HLA-DPB1*0201 was positively associated with beryllium disease, while HLA-DPB1*0401 was negatively associated with CBD. When a specific amino acid, glutamic acid, at position 69 was studied, it was found to be present on HLA-DPB1*0201 but not on HLA-DPB1*0401. Overall, 97 percent of patients with CBD expressed this motif, while only 30 percent of the control population expressed the same motif.[27] This study has recently been confirmed and extended to also demonstrate an association between HLA-DRB1*0901 and CBD. These studies demonstrate impressive associations between HLA motifs and CBD, implying that a genetic predisposition is required in the acquisition of the disorder.

Diagnosis

A diagnosis of CBD requires the demonstration of a granulomatous reaction and beryllium hypersensitivity. Because of the frequent need to treat patients with CBD, the former requires biopsy material. The latter can be most convincingly demonstrated by testing the proliferative response of bronchoalveolar cells to beryllium. If BAL cells cannot be easily or safely obtained, assessing the proliferative response of blood cells to beryllium is a reasonable alternative. Laboratories performing these tests are listed in Table 58-1.

Because immunologic tests of beryllium hypersensitivity have been available only since the late 1980s, their proper use for screening workers is not clear. However, studies indicate that assessments of blood lymphocyte proliferative responses to beryllium constitute the most sensitive screening test for CBD.[16,17] The major difficulty with the use of this assessment as a screening tool is the number of positive responses seen in asymptomatic, otherwise normal subjects. It is not known whether these are false-positive responses or represent early CBD. It is also not known whether all persons with a positive blood response to beryllium will develop CBD. Until the natural course of blood lymphocyte proliferative responses to beryllium is characterized, it will be difficult to establish definitive recommendations for screening workers. Nevertheless, because the risk of developing CBD is not temporally limited, lifelong surveillance may be necessary for all workers with exposure to beryllium or beryllium sensitivity.

Differential Diagnosis

The major challenge to making the diagnosis of CBD is to think of the possibility of beryllium exposure. Most cases of CBD that are misdiagnosed are diagnosed as sarcoidosis because either the exposure to beryllium was not known by the patient or the physician failed to elicit an occupational history. The confusion of CBD and sarcoidosis is not surprising, since many of the radiographic and clinical manifestations of the diseases are similar (Table 58-2). As in sarcoidosis, the dif-

ferential diagnosis of CBD includes other granulomatous and inflammatory disorders (Table 58-3). In the final analysis, the differential among CBD, sarcoidosis, and the other disorders often depends on the result of in vitro beryllium proliferation testing. Patients with sarcoidosis and other lung disorders do not manifest a blood proliferative response to beryllium, while CBD patients do. Sarcoidosis and other granulomatous disorders can be diagnosed in beryllium workers in this manner. Caution should always be exercised, however, and repeated assessments of blood and lung cell proliferative responses to beryllium should always be obtained before a granulomatous lung disease is diagnosed in a beryllium worker as a disorder other than CBD.

Natural History

The long-term prognosis for CBD is uncertain. Follow-up of cases that were diagnosed in the 1940s and 1950s suggests that the mortality of the disease might be as high as 30 percent.[34] Whether a similar mortality will be present in patients with disease diagnosed in the 1980s or 1990s is not certain. Newer techniques to diagnose CBD (immunologic testing) enable the disease to be detected earlier. The natural history of the disease detected at the presymptomatic stage is, however, unknown.

TABLE 58-2

Comparison of Chronic Beryllium Disease and Sarcoidosis

Manifestations	Sarcoidosis	Chronic Beryllium Disease
Erythema nodosum	10–20%	Absent
Hilar adenopathy	50–75%	<50%
Peripheral adenopathy	Occasional	Rare
Hypercalcemia	Occasional	Rare
Nephrocalcinosis	Rare	Rare
Bone changes	In chronic disease	Absent
Parotid involvement	Occasional	Absent
Posterior uveitis	Occasional	Absent
Liver involvement	Common	Frequent
Splenomegaly	Rare	Rare
Skin	Uncommon	Unusual
CNS	Occasional	Absent
Response to steroids	Only active disease	Only active disease

TABLE 58-1

Laboratories Performing Beryllium Proliferation Testing

1. Immunopathology Laboratory
   Cleveland Clinic Foundation
   Cleveland, Ohio

2. National Jewish Center for Immunology
   and Respiratory Medicine
   Denver, Colorado

3. Pulmonary Immunology Laboratories
   Hospital of the University of Pennsylvania
   Philadelphia, Pennsylvania

4. Oak Ridge Institute for Science and Education
   Oak Ridge, Tennessee

5. Specialty Laboratories, Inc.
   Santa Monica, California

TABLE 58-3

Differential Diagnosis of Chronic Beryllium Disease

Sarcoidosis
Hypersensitivity pneumonitis
Tuberculosis
Histoplasmosis
Silicosis
Talc granulomatosis
Eosinophilic granuloma
Idiopathic pulmonary fibrosis

Specifically, we do not know whether this early disease is inevitably progressive or particularly amenable to corticosteroid therapy.

Treatment

Corticosteroids are the first line of therapy for patients with CBD. However, no standard approach to the use of corticosteroids has been adopted in the treatment of this disorder. Because of their side effects, corticosteroids should be reserved for patients with documented pulmonary impairment or those with progressive deterioration. Corticosteroids should also be tapered to the lowest dose that controls signs of active disease. Monitoring of patients with chest radiographs, pulmonary function tests, and exercise tests may be useful. Some patients with CBD have elevated serum angiotensin-converting enzyme (ACE) levels. In these patients, ACE levels may also be a useful gauge of disease activity. Most cases of CBD will be arrested with corticosteroid treatment. In cases of corticosteroid resistance or end-stage disease, lung transplantation may be a reasonable approach.

Beryllium and Lung Cancer

Animal studies have clearly indicated that beryllium is carcinogenic.[13] Whether beryllium is carcinogenic in humans is not clear. The most recent study undertaken by the National Institute for Occupational Safety and Health (NIOSH) suggests that a small increase in lung cancer (standardized mortality ratio [SMR] = 1.26) may occur in beryllium workers.[36] This finding has been challenged, however, because of potential confounding issues related to cigarette smoking.[21] This issue will remain controversial until additional studies are performed. Whatever the risk of cancer is in beryllium workers, the more significant medical concern is CBD.

HARD-METAL LUNG DISEASE

Introduction and Overview

Hard metal is a sintered alloy containing mainly tungsten carbide and cobalt, with smaller amounts of chromium, molybdenum, nickel, niobium, tantalum, titanium, and vanadium. These components are milled to a fine powder, mixed together, pressed into the desired shape, and heated under pressure to between 800 and 1000°C, yielding a product with a chalklike consistency. The material may then undergo additional machining before being baked at 1500°C, which is above the melting point of cobalt and leads to the formation of an alloy that is 90 to 95 percent as hard as a diamond. Because of this property, hard metal is an important component in cutting tools, drill bits, armor plate, and jet engine parts.

Hard metal was developed in the 1920s, and interstitial lung disease was first reported in hard-metal workers in 1940. Lung disease has been noted to occur in those working in both the initial production of hard metal and the machining and maintenance of hard-metal tool components. In addition, although hard metal is not used in the diamond-polishing industry, a similar spectrum of disease has been reported in diamond polishers using steel polishing disks whose cutting surfaces consist of microdiamonds

cemented into a fine cobalt mesh. In contrast, workers in the cobalt-producing industry, who are more likely to be exposed to cobalt alone, may develop occupational asthma but appear to be much less likely to develop interstitial lung disease.

The industrial processes associated with hard-metal lung disease produce respirable fine metallic dust particles. They also produce metallic ions that accumulate in the coolants used in the metalworking procedure and are absorbed through the skin or inhaled in vaporized coolant fluids. To counteract these exposures, the American Conference of Government Industrial Hygienists (ACGIH), NIOSH, and OSHA have established current permissible exposure limits for cobalt metal, dust, and fumes at an 8-h threshold-weighted average of 0.05 mg/m^3.

Mechanisms of Injury

The pathogenesis of the hard-metal–associated lung diseases is poorly understood. Tungsten carbide and cobalt are, however, felt to be the main components of hard metal active in the pathogenesis of these disorders. Of interest is that a number of lines of evidence suggest that these agents contribute to the pathogenesis of these disorders by their individual effects and their ability to interact with one another. First, while cobalt is known to cause contact dermatitis and occupational asthma in humans, the incidence of interstitial lung disease after pure cobalt exposure is extremely low. Second, in vitro studies using peritoneal and alveolar macrophages from rats and mice have demonstrated that the combination of tungsten carbide and cobalt is highly cytotoxic, while cobalt and tungsten carbide alone produce minimal or no cytotoxicity.[20] Lastly, the acute lung toxicity of tungsten carbide plus cobalt is much higher than that of each component after intratracheal instillation in rats.[18]

The events that mediate the responses of the lung to tungsten or cobalt have not received significant attention. The limited information that is available suggests that both humoral and cellular mechanisms play a role, since elevated levels of IgE directed against cobalt-conjugated serum albumin[31] and in vitro lymphocyte transformation after cobalt stimulation have been observed in cobalt exposed patients. Similarly, localized contact dermatitis has been noted in response to patch testing with cobalt salts. Because of experiences with berylliosis, whereby patch testing has been shown to cause sensitization, the use of cobalt skin testing as a screening tool is not recommended.[5]

Clinical Manifestations in Hard-Metal– and Cobalt-Exposed Persons

Work-related illnesses in hard-metal– and cobalt-exposed persons include the interstitial lung disease described as *hard-metal disease* and airway syndromes compatible with asthma and bronchitis. In both, the development of asthma and interstitial lung disease appears to require inhalation rather than ingestion or absorption.

INTERSTITIAL LUNG DISEASE

Interstitial lung disease has been seen in hard-metal workers and diamond polishers. In recent studies, the prevalence of fibrosis in hard-metal workers has ranged up to 2.6 percent. Although interstitial lung disease may occur after a short duration and low levels of exposure, longer duration or higher levels of exposure are associated with increased risk.[33] Nonsmokers and former smokers also appear to be at higher risk.[2] Interstitial disease is more common in workers engaged in the grinding of hard metal where there is exposure to ionized cobalt in the grinding coolants in addition to hard-metal dust.[33] It is possible that ionized cobalt, which is highly protein bound, acts as a hapten in this setting.

In some patients, hard-metal disease presents as a hypersensitivity pneumonitis, or allergic alveolitis. These patients manifest fever, anorexia, cough, dyspnea, inspiratory crackles, and fine reticulonodular infiltrates on chest radiograph. Pulmonary function testing typically shows a restrictive pattern, with a reduced DLCO. Symptoms may resolve when exposure is discontinued but may recur with reexposure. Over time, progressive dyspnea, lung function impairment, and interstitial fibrosis may develop. Fibrosis may also occur in the absence of antecedent symptoms. Patients with advanced disease exhibit weight loss, hypoxemia, digital clubbing, pulmonary hypertension, and cor pulmonale. Patients with alveolitis or fibrosis related to cobalt often have positive skin patch tests to cobalt.

The histopathologic manifestations of the interstitial disease in these patients can be varied, with findings consistent with bronchiolitis, desquamative interstitial pneumonitis, usual interstitial fibrosis, and giant-cell interstitial pneumonitis (GIP). Granuloma formation does not occur. Lung biopsies may show heterogeneous patchy involvement, with foci of active alveolitis, fibrosis, and normal parenchyma. Bronchiolitis may be seen in areas with and without active alveolitis. GIP is characterized by lymphoplasmocytic infiltration, epithelial desquamation, and the presence of numerous multinucleated giant cells in the alveolar spaces.[26] These giant cells are formed by both actively phagocytic alveolar macrophages and type II pneumocytes.[2] Infiltration with eosinophils has also been described. Analysis of BAL fluid may demonstrate hypercellularity, with increased numbers of macrophages and giant cells. A relative or absolute increase in the number of lymphocytes, with a reduced CD4/CD8 ratio as well as increased numbers of neutrophils, eosinophils, and mast cells, may also be seen.[11]

Electron microscopy with energy dispersive x-ray analysis (EDAX) of the particulate material present in biopsy specimens may demonstrate the presence of the elements used to form hard metal. Because of its high solubility, significant amounts of cobalt may not always be present.[2] Neutron activation analysis of BAL fluid yields similar results.[28] Such findings in clinical specimens are suggestive of hard-metal exposure but do not necessarily indicate disease.

Treatment for this disease consists of discontinuation of exposure and administration of systemic corticosteroids. Although no clinical trials have been performed, dosage and duration of treatment similar to those used in other forms of active alveolitis or fibrosis should be considered. Patients with active alveolitis may show a dramatic response to steroids, whereas patients with more prominent fibrosis may show minimal response despite prolonged steroid treatment.[5] GIP has been observed to recur after lung transplantation despite cessation of occupational exposure.[12]

OCCUPATIONAL ASTHMA

The reported prevalence of asthma or wheezing related to cobalt or hard-metal exposure ranges from less than 1 percent to 10.9 percent. This variation may be attributed to different levels of exposure and the criteria used by various authors to define occupational asthma. As with other forms of occupational asthma, patients may note cough, wheezing, dyspnea, chest tightness, conjunctivitis, and rhinitis. Throughout the workday, symptoms may increase in severity, and a progressive decline in peak flow may be demonstrated. Symptoms usually abate during weekends or vacations and often resolve when exposure is discontinued. Upper-airway symptoms may result from either direct airway irritation or atopic responses.

In addition to demonstrating an association between workplace exposure and symptoms, the diagnosis may be confirmed by bronchoprovocation testing (BPT) with cobalt or cobalt salts. Testing with cobalt salts is preferable, as it is much easier to control dosage and delivery of soluble ion solutions than those of particulate substances. Immediate or delayed airway reactivity to cobalt chloride may be observed after BPT.[31] Tungsten carbide has not been shown to produce bronchoconstriction. A positive radioimmunosorbent test (RAST) to cobalt-conjugated human serum albumin has also been reported in some patients, suggesting a type I allergic response.[31] Patients with hard-metal asthma may have positive RAST and BPT responses to both nickel and cobalt.[32] Skin patch testing with cobalt salts does not appear to be of use in diagnosing hard-metal asthma.

The dose-response relationship between heavy-metal or cobalt exposure and asthma has been looked at in a number of studies. A twofold increase in the relative odds ratio for work-related wheezing was noted when cobalt exposure exceeded 0.05 mg/m^3.[33] Two recent studies in hard-metal workers and diamond grinders demonstrated statistically significant reductions in FEV$_1$ and FVC values, whereas measured cobalt levels were well below the allowable limit of 0.05 mg/m^3. This suggests that the current permissible exposure limit may not protect all workers against the development of cobalt-induced asthma.[15,24] Because of findings of this sort, baseline evaluations and employee screenings should be performed in workers exposed to hard-metal dust. A reasonable strategy would include assessments for symptoms of rhinitis, conjunctivitis, wheezing, dyspnea, or chest tightness; the relationship of symptoms to work hours; smoking history; physical examination; pulmonary function testing; and chest radiography. In patients with symptoms or findings suggestive of occupational asthma, peak flow monitoring during working and nonworking hours should be performed and other causes of pulmonary function deterioration ruled out. Specific BPT and RAST results may provide additional positive criteria for diagnosis. Personal employee air sampling and measurement of urinary cobalt levels can provide information about ongoing exposure. The workplace should also be examined for levels of cobalt exposure and employee protective practices.

Treatment for occupational asthma related to cobalt includes control of exposure as well as medical therapy with bronchodilators and inhaled corticosteroids. Systemic corticosteroid treatment is usually not required.[5]

LUNG CANCER

Cobalt and cobalt-containing compounds have been shown to cause cancer in rats after local injection and intratracheal instillation. The International Agency for Research on Cancer reviewed the evidence for the carcinogenicity of cobalt in 1991 and concluded that although there was sufficient evidence for the carcinogenicity of cobalt metal powder and cobalt oxide in experimental animals, there was inadequate evidence for the carcinogenicity of cobalt and cobalt compounds in humans.[4] To date, a link between cobalt or hard metal and the development of lung cancer in humans has not been clearly demonstrated. This controversy can be appreciated in three studies from the literature. One study, of 1148 workers in an electrochemical plant producing cobalt and nickel in France from 1950 to 1988, failed to demonstrate a statistically significant increase in the standardized mortality ratio (SMR) for lung cancer among workers exposed to cobalt.[23] In contrast, a second study, of 709 workers exposed to hard-metal dust, showed an increase in the SMR for lung cancer,[19] while a third study, evaluating 3163 Swedish workers exposed to hard metal, found a statistically significant increase in the SMR for lung cancer only in workers with more than 10 years' exposure time and more than 20 years since first exposure.[25]

REFERENCES

1. Alekseeva OG: Ability of beryllium compounds to produce delayed allergy. Gig Tr Prof Zabol 11:20–25, 1965.
2. Antila S, Sutinen S, Paananen M, et al: Hard metal lung disease: A clinical, histological, ultrastructural and x-ray microanalytical study. Eur J Respir Dis 69:83–94, 1986.
3. Aronchick JM, Rossman MD, Miller WT: Chronic beryllium disease: Diagnosis, radiographic findings and correlation with pulmonary function tests. Radiology 163:677–682, 1987.
4. Chlorinated drinking water, chlorination by-products, some other halogenated compounds. IARC Monographs on the Evaluation of Carcinogenic Risks to Humans 52, 1991.
5. Cugell DW: The hard metal diseases. Clin Chest Med 13:269–279, 1992.
6. Cullen MR, Kominsky JR, Rossman MD, et al: Chronic beryllium disease in a precious metal refinery: Clinical epidemiologic and immunologic evidence for continuing risk from exposure to low level beryllium fume. Am Rev Respir Dis 135:201–209, 1987.
7. Curtis GH: Cutaneous hypersensitivity due to beryllium: A study of 13 cases. Arch Dermatol Syph 64:470–482, 1951.
8. Deodhar SD, Barna B, Van Ordstrand HS: A study of the immunologic aspects of chronic berylliosis. Chest 63:309–313, 1973.
9. Eisenbud M, Lisson J: Epidemiological aspects of beryllium-induced nonmalignant lung disease: A 30 year update. J Occup Med 25:196–202, 1983.
10. Epstein PE, Dauber JH, Rossman MD, Daniele RP: Bronchoalveolar lavage in a patient with chronic berylliosis: Evidence for hypersensitivity pneumonitis. Ann Intern Med 97:213–216, 1982.
11. Forni A: Bronchoalveolar lavage in the diagnosis of hard metal disease. Sci Total Environ 150:69–76, 1994.
12. Frost AE, Keller CA, Brown RW, et al: Giant cell interstitial pneumonitis disease recurrence in the transplanted lung. Am Rev Respir Dis 148:1401–1404, 1993.
13. Groth DH: Carcinogenicity of beryllium: Review of the literature. Environ Res 21:56–62, 1980.
14. Hardy HL, Tabershaw IR: Delayed chemical pneumonitis occurring in workers exposed to beryllium compounds. J Ind Hyg Toxicol 28:197–211, 1946.
15. Kennedy SM, Chan-Yeung M, Marion S, et al: Maintenance of stellite and tungsten carbide saw tips: Respiratory health and exposure-response evaluations. Occup Environ Med 52:185–191, 1995.
16. Kreiss K, Mroz MM, Zhen B, et al: Epidemiology of beryllium sensitization and disease in nuclear workers. Am Rev Respir Dis 148:985–991, 1993.
17. Kreiss K, Wasserman S, Mroz MM, Newman LS: Beryllium disease screening in the ceramics industry. J Occup Med 35:267–274, 1993.
18. Lasfargues G, Lison D, Maldague P, Lauwerys R: Comparative study of the acute lung toxicity of pure cobalt powder and cobalt-tungsten carbide mixture in rat. Toxicol Appl Pharmacol 112:41–50, 1992.
19. Lasfargues G, Wild P, Moulin JJ, et al: Lung cancer mortality in a French cohort of hard metal workers. Am J Ind Med 26:585–595, 1994.
20. Lison D, Lauwerys R: In vitro cytotoxic effects of cobalt-containing dusts on mouse peritoneal and rat alveolar macrophages. Environ Res 52:187–198, 1990.
21. MacMahon B: The epidemiological evidence on the carcinogenicity of beryllium in humans. J Occup Med 36:15–24. 1994.
22. Marx JJ Jr, Burrell R: Delayed hypersensitivity to beryllium compounds. J Immunol 111:590–598, 1973.
23. Moulin JJ, Wild P, Mur JM, et al: A mortality study of cobalt production workers: An extension of the follow-up. Am J Ind Med 23:281–288, 1993.
24. Nemery B, Casier P, Roosels D, et al: Survey of cobalt exposure and respiratory health in diamond polishers. Am Rev Respir Dis 145:610–616, 1992.
25. Nordberg G: Assessment of risks in occupational cobalt exposures. Sci Total Environ 150:201–207, 1994.
26. Ohori NP, Sciurba FC, Owens GR, et al: Giant-cell interstitial pneumonia and hard metal pneumoconiosis. Am J Surg Pathol 13:581–587, 1989.
27. Richeldi L, Sorrentino R, Saltini C: HLA-DPB1 glutamate 69: A genetic marker of beryllium disease. Science 262:242–244, 1993.
28. Rizzato G, Fraioli P, Sabbioni E, et al: The differential diagnosis of hard metal lung disease. Sci Total Environ 150:77–83, 1994.
29. Rossman MD, Kern JA, Elias JA, et al: Proliferative response of bronchoalveolar lymphocytes to beryllium. Ann Intern Med 108:687–693, 1988.
30. Saltini C, Winestock D, Kirby M, et al: Maintenance of alveolitis in patients with chronic beryllium disease by beryllium-specific T cells. New Engl J Med 320:1103–1109, 1989.
31. Shirakawa T, Kusaka Y, Fujimura N, et al: Occupational asthma from cobalt sensitivity in workers exposed to hard metal dust. Chest 95:29–37, 1989.
32. Shirakawa T, Kusaka Y, Fujimura N, et al: Hard metal asthma: Cross immunological and respiratory reactivity between cobalt and nickel? Thorax 45:266–271, 1990.
33. Sprince NL, Oliver LC, Eisen EA, et al: Cobalt exposure and lung disease in tungsten carbide production. Am Rev Respir Dis 138:1220–1226, 1988.
34. Stoeckle SD, Hardy HL, Weber AL: Chronic beryllium disease. Am J Med 46:545–561, 1969.
35. Van Ordstrand HS, Hughes R, Carmody MG: Chemical pneumonia in workers extracting beryllium oxide: Report of three cases. Cleve Clin Q 10:10–18, 1943.
36. Ward E, Okun A, Ruder A, et al: A mortality study of workers at seven beryllium processing plants. Am J Ind Med 22:885–904, 1992.

CHAPTER 59

COAL WORKERS' LUNG DISEASES AND SILICOSIS

John E. Parker / Edward L. Petsonk

COAL WORKERS' LUNG DISEASES

Introduction and History

Coal miners are at risk for developing several distinct clinical illnesses in relation to their occupational exposures. Historically, some names applied to these disorders were miners' asthma, phthisis, anthracosis, and, in Scotland, miners' black lung. It was recognized early that these afflictions were related to the occupation of mining. However, it wasn't until the development of specialized techniques such as chest radiography and pulmonary function testing, the discovery of the tubercle bacillus, and the sophisticated histologic examination of tissue that respiratory diseases affecting miners could be differentiated and defined.

Coal workers' pneumoconiosis (CWP) is the parenchymal lung disease that results from the inhalation and deposition of coal mine dust and the tissue's reaction to its presence. This occupational lung disease was first defined in the early 1800s. In addition to CWP, coal mine dust exposure increases a miner's risk of developing chronic bronchitis and pathologic emphysema and accelerates loss of ventilatory lung function.

For a long time, the pneumoconiosis that affected coal miners was thought to be silicosis. In the 1930s, however, it was argued for the first time that silicosis, CWP, and bronchitis were distinct clinically and pathologically. Unfortunately, it was also suggested that coal dust was not harmful, despite reports of the adverse effects from coal dust among coal trimmers. It was not until washed coal that was free of silica was shown to produce a dust disease in the lungs of stevedores leveling coal in the holds of ships that CWP was widely accepted as a distinct pathologic entity.

In the United States, little attention was given to coal miners' respiratory diseases until the Public Health Service (USPHS) conducted a pilot prevalence study of CWP in the early 1900s. Since then, a large number of studies, performed by the National Institute for Occupational Safety and Health, have greatly increased our knowledge of the lung diseases associated with coal mining in the United States.[11]

Coal and Coal Mining

Coal is not a pure mineral. It is a conglomeration of carbonaceous rocks derived from the accumulation of vegetation sedimented under swampy conditions and subjected to extreme pressure over long periods. Coals are characterized by rank (which relates to geologic age), hardness, carbon content, and the amount of heat released (BTUs) when burned. Peat is the lowest-rank (softest) and geologically newest type of coal, while anthracite is the highest-rank (hardest) and oldest coal.

Since coal may be found in outcroppings and in seams that are only a few feet below the surface, it can often be readily obtained by simply scraping off the surface, or overburden, and mined with large earth-moving equipment. This type of mining, called strip mining, currently accounts for most U.S. coal production. Occasionally, surface mining is also performed by boring into coal outcrops with an auger. Dust levels in the air at surface mines are generally considerably lower than in underground mines, with a few notable exceptions (see below).

When coal seams are buried deep within the earth's crust, it is not economically feasible to strip away the overburden. The only practical way of mining the coal is to sink shafts from the surface to the coal seam and then follow the seam with a series of more or less horizontal tunnels. In the past, shaft mines of this sort were the most common type of coal mine in the world. They still represent an important source of coal and produce slightly less than half of the coal mined in the United States.

Not all coal-mining jobs are equally exposed to respiratory hazards. In underground mines, airborne dust concentrations are highest at the coal cutting face, where coal is removed from the intact seams. Face jobs include the loading of coal into transportation vehicles or train cars and, depending on the techniques used in the mine, operation of continuous or long wall mining machines. Exposure to crystalline silica and thus the risk of silicosis also occur in underground mines, particularly in miners engaged in roof support, called roof bolting (Fig. 59-1), or drilling operations, and in motormen who operate underground coal trains and use sand for traction on the rails. Workers in some exclusively aboveground coal-mining operations also may have important exposure to dusts. These include workers at tipples and preparation plants, where crushing, sizing, washing, and blending of coal are done and coal is stored and loaded into ships, railroad cars, or river barges. Workers at surface coal mines who operate the drilling rigs (drillers), to make holes in which explosives are placed, are exposed to silica and are at risk for the development of silicosis rather than CWP.[1,6]

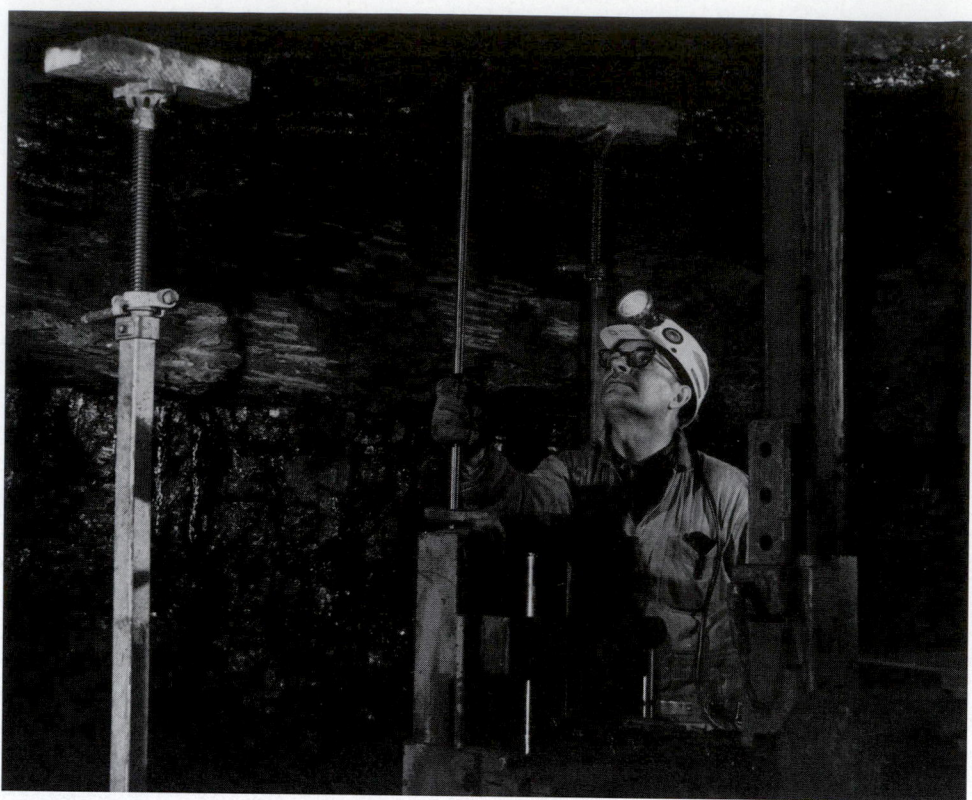

FIGURE 59-1   Roof bolting in underground coal mine. A potentially high-risk operation for respiratory exposures to airborne silica. *(Photo courtesy of U.S. Bureau of Mines.)*

Epidemiology of Lung Diseases in U.S. Coal Miners

The first major survey of the health of American coal workers was conducted by the USPHS from 1969 to 1971, evaluating symptoms, lung function, and chest radiographic findings.[34] This study included more than 9000 miners at two anthracite and 29 bituminous mines. Participation in the survey was over 90 percent. The mines were chosen to represent different geographic areas, coal seams, and mining methods. Since this initial study, subsequent surveys have studied miners at these and other U.S. mines.

RADIOGRAPHIC FINDINGS

Radiographic data from the initial survey showed an overall prevalence of simple and complicated CWP of nearly 30 percent. There was variation by region of the country and the type (rank) of coal mined. Among eastern Pennsylvania anthracite (high-rank) coal miners, 46 percent had simple and 14 percent had complicated CWP. In contrast, among miners in the western plateau of Colorado and Utah mining a lower-rank coal, only 5 percent had simple CWP and none had the complicated form.[34] Among underground miners, those working at the coal face and exposed to higher concentrations of coal mine dust had higher prevalences of CWP than surface workers or those whose jobs caused them to enter the face area intermittently.

After this initial survey, many miners with CWP became eligible to retire, and follow-up studies have demonstrated a decline in the prevalence of CWP in active US miners.[11] Enforcement of and compliance with dust control measures, adopted in 1969 and introduced about the time of the initial survey, also resulted in a reduced attack rate of CWP. This was confirmed in the periodic chest radiograph surveillance program in U.S. miners. In 1970–73, CWP was found in 28 percent of participants with 25 years or more underground. By 1992–95, fewer than 10 percent showed radiographic evidence of CWP (Fig. 59-2).[11] Compliance with lower exposure standards probably also reduced the risk of disease progression among miners with CWP who continued to work in mines that were in compliance with mandated dust standards.

Data from the U.S. studies noted above clearly demonstrated that the prevalence of radiographic changes of simple CWP is related to the duration and intensity of dust exposure, even at current dust levels.[5] Data from studies of British miners also demonstrated that the attack rate (incidence of new cases) and

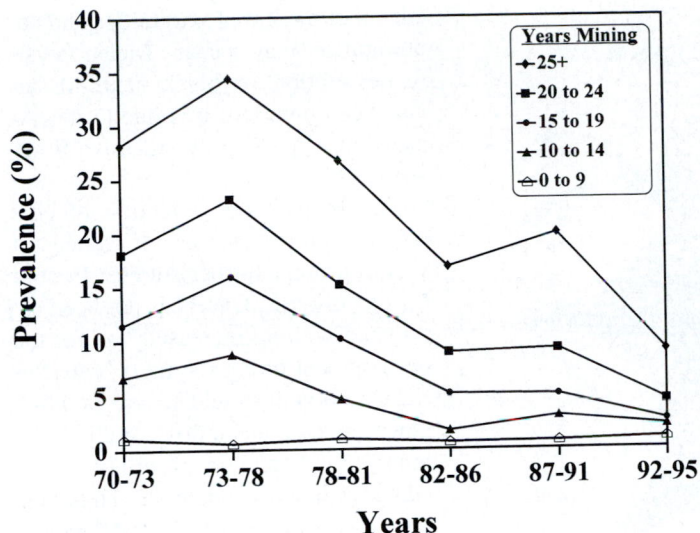

the probability of disease progression in simple CWP were related to the mass of respirable dust to which the miner was exposed during his or her lifetime.[24] The same cannot be said for the complicated form of CWP—progressive massive fibrosis (PMF). Once a person has inhaled sufficient coal mine dust into the lungs for the chest radiograph to be classified with at least ILO category 2 pneumoconiosis (see below), the probability of its progressing to the complicated form appears to be independent of any further dust exposure. The rate of progression to PMF appears to be influenced chiefly by the age at which the miner begins to show radiographic changes of CWP. Progression may also be influenced by the presence of a rheumatoid diathesis (see below).[30]

VENTILATORY LUNG FUNCTION

Ventilatory function was also evaluated in the large studies of U.S. miners mentioned above. Initial reports examined miners' lung function in comparison to their *radiographic findings*. Miners with complicated CWP were found to consistently show an important defect in lung function. This defect could be restrictive or obstructive, depending on the contributions of fibrosis and bronchitis, respectively. In contrast to the ventilatory findings associated with progressive massive fibrosis, mild obstructive abnormalities were often noted in miners with simple pneumoconiosis. However, the findings were not consistent, and with increasing category of simple CWP, the average functional decrement was small and quite variable.[33] Subsequent studies in the United States and Great Britain helped to clarify the adverse effects of dust on coal miners' lung function by evaluating lung function with respect to the miners' *cumulative dust exposure.*[29] They noted that miners manifest a progressively greater risk of lung function loss with increasing cumulative dust exposure and

that this deterioration was independent of the chest radiographic findings of CWP.[3] The FEV_1 loss was most severe in those who worked for many years at the dustiest jobs. Among smoking miners, the effects of tobacco smoke appeared to be additive to the dust effect.[4] The studies also noted that miners experience a more rapid loss of lung function over their first few years of mining, with slower dust-related declines after that time.[41]

In summary, epidemiologic data have shown that coal miners experience ventilatory lung function loss with increasing exposure to dust, either in the presence or in the absence of CWP. Among smoking miners, the effects of tobacco and dust appear to be additive. Although, on average, functional losses associated with dust are small, it is estimated that 35 years of work at the current dust limit will cause a clinically important FEV_1 loss in eight of 100 nonsmoking coal miners.[36] When complicated CWP is present, an additional restrictive or obstructive ventilatory deficit is often noted.

MORTALITY

Studies of mortality in coal miners have been reported from the United States and Britain. The findings from both nations have been generally consistent, revealing that miners experience increased mortality attributable to pneumoconiosis, emphysema, and chronic bronchitis. Radiographic findings of advanced CWP (i.e., PMF) are consistently associated with mortality, especially in categories B and C (see below). Among miners with simple CWP, decreases in survival were significantly smaller.[26,31] Of interest is that miners' risks of dying from emphysema and chronic bronchitis exhibited a geographic pattern different from that associated with their mortality from CWP, suggesting that these dust effects may be mediated by different mechanisms.[13]

Pathology of Coal Miners' Lung Diseases

The coal macule is the primary lesion of simple CWP and is essential for the pathologic diagnosis of the disorder.[25] The lesion consists of a focal collection of coal dust in pigment-laden macrophages around respiratory bronchioles, tapering off toward the alveolar duct (Fig. 59-3). A fine network of reticulin is present in the early lesion. Macules may also contain a small amount of collagen, depending on the character of the initiating dust. Centriacinar emphysema, the dilation and injury of lung gas exchange units, is also observed with increased prevalence in the lungs of coal miners. The severity of this lesion is proportional to the miner's cumulative dust exposure and retention. Focal emphysema is the form of centriacinar emphysema that is seen as an integral part of the lesion of simple CWP. It is characterized by enlargement of the airspaces immediately adjacent to the dust macule (Fig. 59-3). Muscular thickening of pulmonary arteries can be observed in both simple and complicated CWP. In severe cases, especially when CWP is complicated or associated with other disorders, cor pulmonale with hypertrophy of the right ventricle is noted. Pathologic changes in the airways consistent with chronic bronchitis, including enlargement of mucous glands, have also been noted in miners' lungs.

With increasing dust exposure, owing to the overwhelming of the normal clearance mechanisms of the lung, coal-induced le-

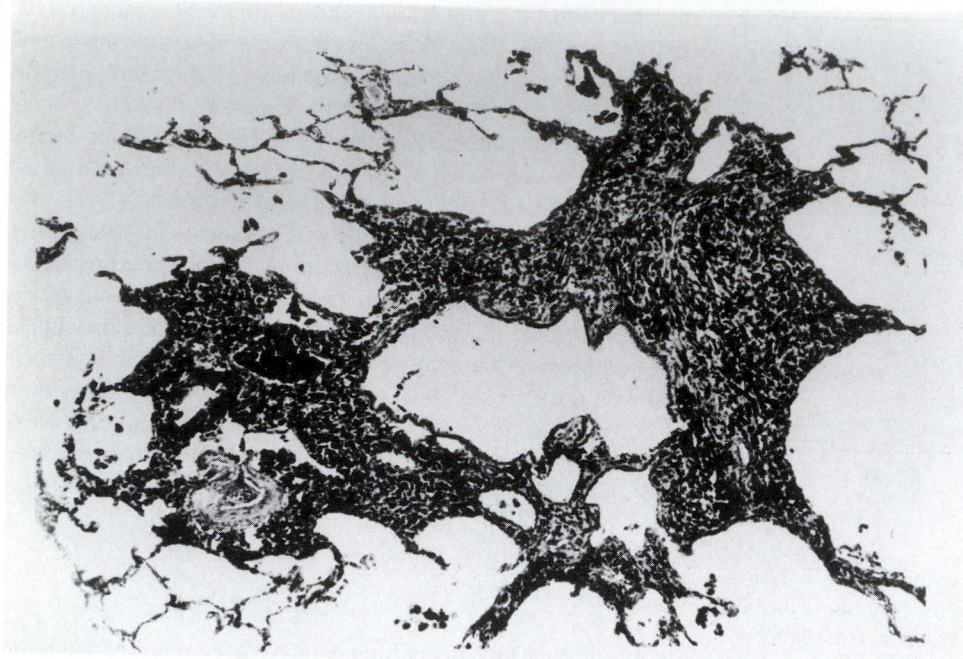

FIGURE 59-3   A coal macule, microscopic section. *(Courtesy of Dr. Val Vallyathan, National Institute for Occupational Safety and Health, Morgantown, WV.)*

sions increase in size and number. These larger fibrotic lesions are called *coal nodules* and are palpable in lung specimens. Palpable coal nodules are classified as micronodular up to 7 mm in diameter and macronodular if they are 7 mm or larger (Fig. 59-4).[25]

Complicated CWP or PMF is diagnosed when one or more nodules in a lung specimen are noted to attain a size of 2 cm or greater in diameter. The 2 cm cutoff is an arbitrary choice of a minimal diameter that permits better correlation with clinical and radiographic measurements.[25] Radiographically, PMF is said to be present when coal-induced radiographic shadows are at least 1 cm in diameter. These lesions are solid, heavily pigmented, and rubbery to hard, and they occur most commonly in the apical posterior portions of upper lobes or the superior segments of lower lobes (Fig. 59-5). They tend to occur symmetrically, but they may be asymmetric and cavitate. Airways and vessels adjacent to the lesions may be distorted, and within the lesions, they are destroyed. PMF generally occurs in association with background pathologic changes of simple CWP.

Clinical Features of Coal Workers' Lung Diseases

Some coal-exposed workers, even those with simple pneumoconiosis, do not manifest respiratory signs or symptoms. Others experience a variety of respiratory problems, with chronic cough and sputum production being the most common. These symptoms are more common with increasing dust exposure and can be seen in the presence or absence of simple pneumoconiosis. The symptoms are probably related to bronchitic changes in the large airways, including thickening of the airway wall and mucous gland enlargement and hypersecretion. These findings result from continued inhalation of dust particles, presenting a chronic burden to the mucociliary escalator. With more severe airflow obstruction or advanced pneumoconiosis, dyspnea can be noted, cough and sputum production are more frequent, and

edema of the lower extremities and cor pulmonale may occur. Melanoptysis (expectoration of black sputum) has also been reported; it is due to the excavation of progressive massive fibrosis lesions.

Clubbing is not a feature of coal miners' lung diseases; if noted, it should prompt further studies. In contrast to silicosis, CWP has not been associated with an increased risk for the development of coexisting mycobacterial infection. It should be kept in mind, however, that in autopsy studies, the lungs of 12 percent of miners show classic silicotic nodules.[18] Thus, the appearance of a cavity in PMF should prompt examination of the sputum for typical and atypical mycobacteria.

RADIOLOGY AND DIAGNOSIS OF CWP

The diagnosis of CWP can be made with confidence, without histologic confirmation, in the presence of an adequate history (at least five to ten years) of coal mine dust exposure and a characteristic chest radiograph. The radiograph in simple pneumoconiosis shows small opacities, ranging in size from a pinhead up to 1 cm in diameter. Rounded nodules predominate and tend to appear first in the upper zones and invaded middle and lower zones as the number of opacities increase. Progressive massive fibrosis is characterized by one or more large opacities greater than 1 cm in diameter. An upper-lobe predominance is typical of this complicated pneumoconiosis. Lower-lobe emphysema is also commonly noted, and atelectisis and consolidation can be appreciated. High-resolution computed tomographic scanning appears to be the most sensitive radiologic technique in coal workers, since it can reveal parenchymal nodules and emphysema when standard radiographs are normal.[14]

Several schemes have been used to classify the radiographic shadows of pneumoconiosis in epidemiologic studies. Currently, the 1980 classification of the International Labour Office (ILO) is the most widely accepted.[23] When the ILO system is used, simple pneumoconiosis is divided into major categories 1, 2, and 3, according to the profusion of small opacities in the lung fields. Category 0 represents a normal radiograph. Each major category, including 0, is subdivided into 3 minor categories, providing a range of 12 categories for simple CWP. A reading of category 1/0 indicates the definite presence of opacities consistent with pneumoconiosis (see Chapter 56). Complicated CWP (PMF) is divided into categories A, B, and C, based on the size of the large opacities.

The clinician may be presented with the diagnostic dilemma of distinguishing a primary or metastatic neoplasm from an unusual presentation of progressive massive fibrosis or Caplan's syndrome. When typical large opacities of PMF occur symmetrically and bilaterally on a background of simple CWP, one can be confident that the lesions are unlikely to represent neoplastic disease. Prior radiographs from medical screening pro-

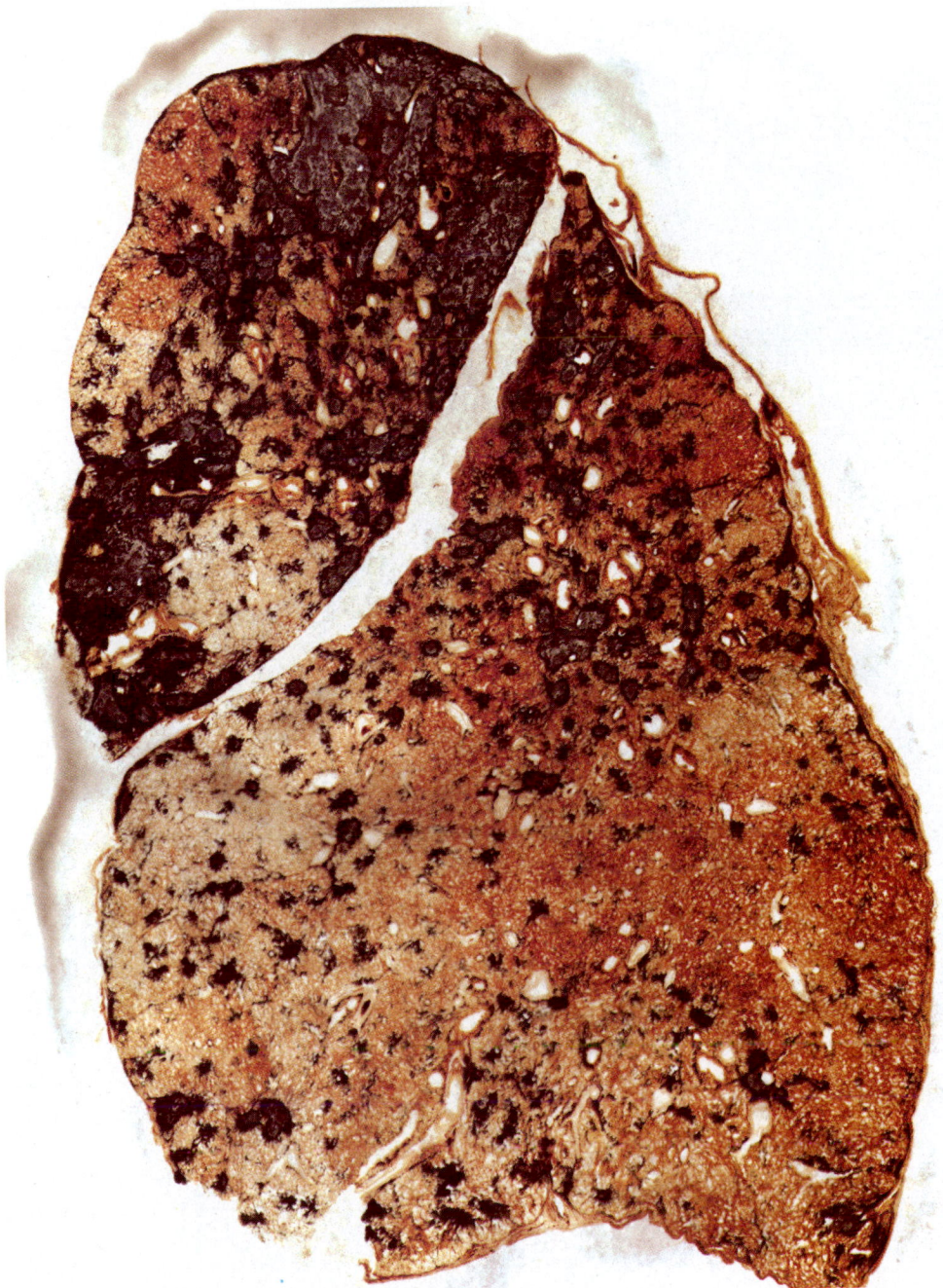

FIGURE 59-4   Simple coal workers' pneumoconiosis, sagittal section. *(Courtesy of Prof. J. Gough.)*

have adverse physiological consequences. In an individual miner, the pattern and severity of impairment will be related to such recognized factors as the intensity and duration of respirable dust exposure, geologic factors (e.g., coal rank, silica content), residence time of dust in the lung, and exposure to other respiratory hazards (e.g., tobacco smoke). In miners with airway hyperresponsiveness, greater functional deficits and an increased risk of symptoms may be expected.[37] Other factors that are also hypothesized to affect the lung function of coal workers, but have not been adequately investigated, are childhood respiratory diseases, home heating fuels, and variations in the subject's immunologic, biochemical (e.g., antiprotease), and inflammatory responses to dust inhalation.

VENTILATORY FUNCTION

A variety of studies have focused on the lung function abnormalities in patients with CWP. They have characterized the abnormalities in simple and complicated CWP and investigated the natural history of these disorders. In keeping with the bronchitic and fibrotic features of PMF, prominent obstructive and restrictive abnormalities have been noted in this disorder. Similarly, the mild obstructive abnormalities seen in nonsmokers with simple CWP[20] are frequently the result of small-airway dysfunction—a finding that correlates nicely with the pathologic features of dust deposition in this disorder.[50]

The epidemiologic studies, as discussed above, have extensively documented the occurrence of exposure-related decreases in FEV_1 and FVC in coal miners. The magnitude of the average dust effect has varied between studies. Over a working lifetime, average predicted losses in FEV_1 under current U.S. dust standards ranged from 124 ml[3] to 610 ml,[40] with 6 to 8 percent of miners being expected to develop clinically significant airflow limitation.[36] Subgroups of miners may, however, experience a more severe effect. For example, a much more severe effect of dust on loss of lung function was observed in a group 199 men who had chosen to leave coal mine work.[21] The magnitude of the effects coal dust has on pulmonary function can be appreciated when they are compared to those caused by cigarette smoking. In one study evaluating the lung function of 1072 miners over an 11-year period, work at coal face jobs resulted in lung function losses essentially similar to those due to smoking. When tenure in less dusty work

grams are often obtainable, and they can help confirm stability or progression over a long time. If the background of simple CWP is sparse or absent, the lesion is unilateral, or there are multiple peripherally situated nodules (Caplan's syndrome), the differentiation from a neoplasm may indeed be impossible without a biopsy.

Lung Function and Respiratory Impairment in Coal Miners

Coal mine exposures may result in several pathologic processes, including simple and complicated CWP, chronic bronchitis, emphysema, and dust-related airflow limitation. Each of these may

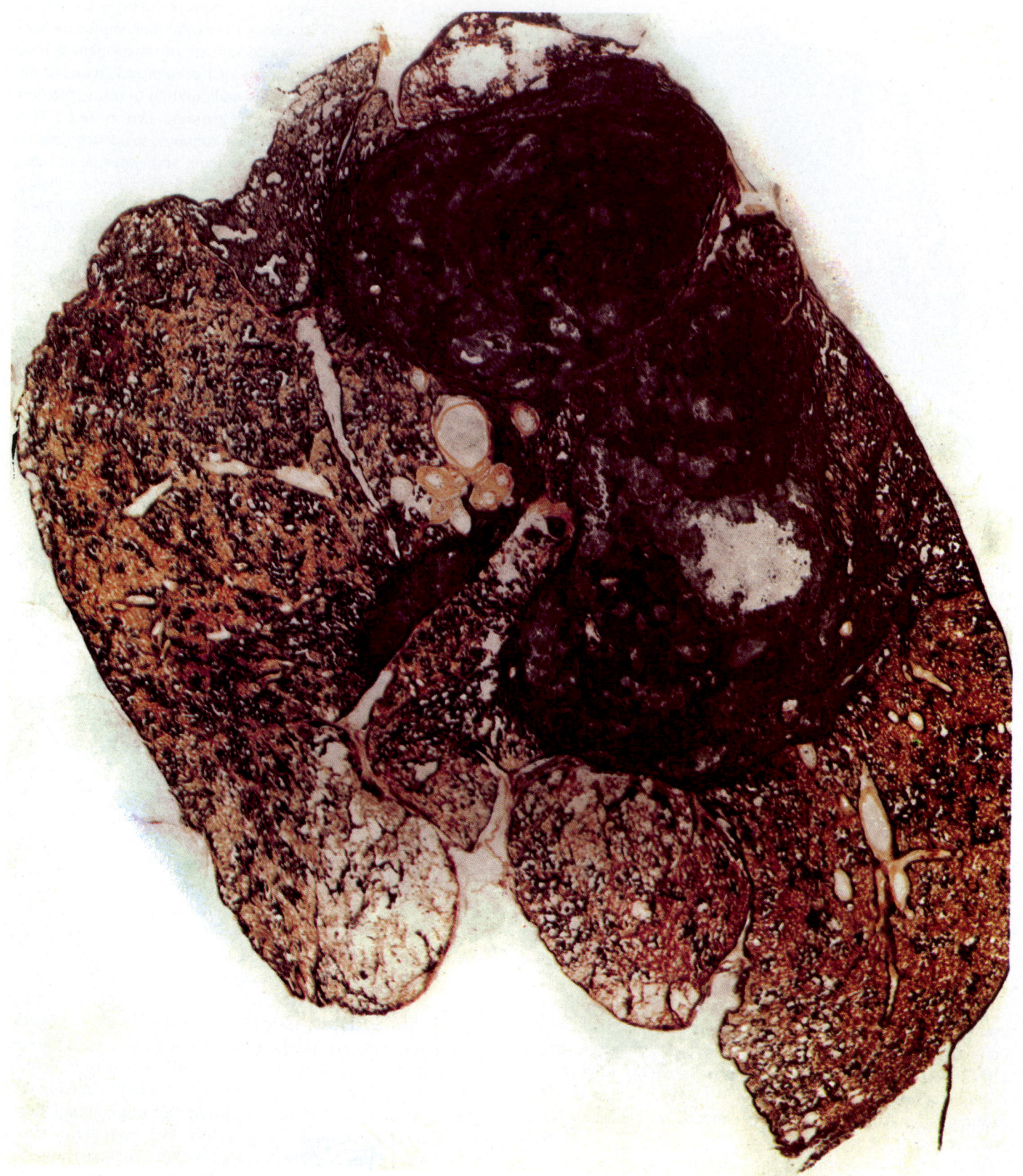

FIGURE 59-5 Complicated coal workers' pneumoconiosis or progressive massive fibrosis, Sagittal section. *(Courtesy of Prof. J. Gough.)*

was included in the analysis, mine dust exposure resulted in lung function losses about 38 percent of that attributable to smoking (average 13 cigarettes per day).[2]

GAS EXCHANGE

Diffusing capacity has been studied in relation to the radiographic changes of CWP. In general, the small rounded opacities seen in miners with simple CWP have not been associated with measurable reductions in DLCO. However, subgroups of miners do have abnormal diffusing capacities that correlate with radiographic alterations. Gas transfer is often low when the large opacities of complicated CWP are present, and it may also be reduced in miners who show either predominantly pinpoint opacities ("p" type by the ILO classification) or small irregular opacities on their chest radiographs.[12,39]

Gas exchange on exercise has also been used in studying coal miners. Many of the reports have been based on patients referred for disability evaluations, and thus suffer from ill-defined selection biases. Exposure-response relationships are also unclear with respect to findings in these series. Exertional hypoxia, pulmonary arterial hypertension, and excess ventilation have frequently been observed in miners, particularly those with complicated CWP or airflow obstruction.[27,35] However, the proportion of miners who show exertional gas exchange abnormalities in the absence of either PMF or clinically important airflow obstruction is still a topic of investigation.[17]

Caplan's Syndrome

In 1953, Anthony Caplan described an association between distinctive nodular opacities in the lungs of Welsh coal miners and rheumatoid arthritis.[9] The pulmonary nodules were 0.5 to 5 cm in diameter, bilateral, and located peripherally. They often developed rapidly (over weeks) in the presence of a mild pneumoconiosis and could cavitate or calcify. In many cases, the pulmonary opacities preceded the onset of the arthritis by months to years. In others, the pulmonary nodules and arthritis appeared coincidentally or the pulmonary lesions appeared only after the arthritis was full-blown. In its early stages, the opacities of Caplan's syndrome and progressive massive fibrosis are readily distinguishable. They are not mutually exclusive, however: Caplan's lesions and PMF lesions have been found in the same subjects. Although Caplan's syndrome was originally seen in coal miners, its definition has since been broadened to include patients with rheumatoid arthritis, similar radiographic abnormalities, and a variety of other pneumoconioses, including silicosis and asbestosis.

Immunology of CWP

The potential role of immunologic factors in the pathogenesis of mineral dust pneumoconioses was first noted with the description of Caplan's syndrome. A number of lines of evidence have provided additional support for this concept. First, a Caplan's-like syndrome has been noted in miners without arthritis but with circulating rheumatoid factor (RF), and coal workers with rheumatoid arthritis have been noted to have an increased prevalence of progressive massive fibrosis. In addition, patients with CWP have a high prevalence of autoantibodies, with RF and antinuclear antibody (ANA) evaluations being positive in 9 to 10 percent and 17 to 34 percent of patients, respectively.[28,43] It is interesting to note that the prevalence of these autoantibodies varies with the stage of CWP, with a positive ANA or RF being detected in 13 percent of patients with simple CWP and 45 percent of patients with stage C CWP.[28,43,47]

To further understand the mechanisms of injury and repair in CWP, a variety of serum parameters have been examined in patients with simple and complicated CWP and Caplan's syndrome.[19] These studies noted significantly higher serum concentrations of C3, α_1-antitrypsin, IgA, and IgG in anthracite miners than in bituminous miners with PMF. Compared to normal controls, the miners' C3, α_1-antitrypsin, IgG, and IgA values were also elevated. The significance of these findings is not clear, since the authors did not find any association between the elevated immunoglobulins and FEV$_1$. The IgA antibodies may play a role, however, since IgA autoantibodies against collagen and reticulin have been detected in the sera of patients with CWP.[8]

A reproducible feature of CWP is the variability in the responses manifested by different persons with similar levels of dust exposure. As a result, it has been suggested that constitutional differences contribute, in a major way, to important facets of this response, such as attack rates and rates of disease progression. To date, however, no definite associations between personal or genetic factors and CWP have been noted.

Bronchoalveolar Lavage Evaluations

The development of bronchoalveolar lavage (BAL) has provided a means for sampling lung cells and fluids in a variety of pulmonary disorders. When it is applied to the pulmonary reactions in CWP, somewhat divergent results have been noted. Early studies of symptomatic, nonsmoking coal miners with simple CWP found no significant difference between miners with CWP and controls in the number or differential of cells recovered by BAL or their release of superoxide anion or hydrogen peroxide. They did, however, note elevated levels of production of fibronectin and alveolar macrophage–derived growth factor, providing insight into potential mechanisms that could contribute to fibrogenesis in this disorder.[38] In contrast, others have noted that BAL in miners with simple and complicated CWP yields increased numbers of lung cells, alveolar macrophages, lymphocytes, and neutrophils, and alveolar cells that produce significantly more superoxide than controls.[48]

Management of Coal Workers' Lung Diseases

There is no specific therapy for CWP. Thus, management is best directed at prevention, early recognition, and treatment of complications. The primary prevention of lung disease in miners must include continuing efforts at reducing exposure to coal mine dust. The major clinical challenges are the recognition and management of airflow obstruction, respiratory infection, hypoxemia, respiratory failure, cor pulmonale, arrhythmias, and pneumothorax.

Improved mining methods and lower dust levels appear to be reducing exposure and the number of new cases of both simple and complicated pneumoconiosis. Medical surveillance programs, using chest radiographs, allow early recognition of workers with simple pneumoconiosis. Workers with simple pneumoconiosis should be encouraged to exercise transfer rights to low-dust jobs. Any worker with the unexpected finding of PMF should be carefully advised about the hazards of further dust exposures.

Workers presenting with respiratory symptoms should have a careful evaluation. The history and physical examination should be supplemented by chest radiography, spirometry with lung volume and diffusing capacity assessments, an evaluation of bronchodilator responsiveness (if the patient has airway obstruction), and resting arterial blood gas measurement as indicated. A thorough initial database allows accurate assessment of the worker's respiratory health and serves as a starting point for observing the response to therapy or progression of disease.

Symptomatic reversible airflow obstruction may benefit from treatment with inhaled and oral bronchodilators. Patients with severe obstruction and inadequate improvement from the usual measures should be considered for a monitored trial of corticosteroids. If improvement is objectively documented, continuation of inhaled and, rarely, oral steroids may be of benefit. When it is an issue, smoking cessation needs to be strongly encouraged.

Hypoxemia can be a serious complication in advanced, complicated pneumoconiosis, categories B and C. It may be present at rest, with exercise, or during sleep. Chronic hypoxemia can lead to additional complications, including polycythemia, pulmonary hypertension, cor pulmonale, and cerebral dysfunction. Therapy with low-flow oxygen is indicated when arterial oxygen tension is less than 55 mmHg. Oxygen therapy in this setting may improve exercise tolerance, reduce dyspnea, and prevent arrhythmias, polycythemia, and heart failure.

Patients with significant airflow obstruction or PMF should receive appropriate immunization with influenza and pneumococcal vaccines. Bacterial and viral episodes of bronchitis or pneumonia should be promptly recognized and appropriately treated.

Patients with complicated CWP, especially those who have been exposed to silica as well as coal mine dust, deserve special attention with regard to mycobacterial infection. Patients with a history of weight loss, fever, sweats, or malaise should be promptly investigated with chest radiographs and their sputum examined for AFB with stains and cultures. Occasionally, fiberoptic bronchoscopy with brushings and washings is required to establish the diagnosis. Active tuberculosis in patients with CWP can usually be successfully treated with the usual drug regimens, provided rifampin is one of the drugs employed.[16] In coal miners with a significant history of concurrent silica exposure (such as motormen, roof bolters, and shaft development workers), some authorities suggest that the treatment for tuberculosis should be more aggressive (see silicosis section below). Long-term follow-up is also indicated in view of several reports of recurrent pulmonary tuberculosis in patients with PMF after completion of apparently adequate therapy.[32]

Respiratory failure may complicate advanced disease in coal miners, as it does in other chronic obstructive respiratory disorders. Ventilatory support measures are indicated when the fail-

ure is precipitated by a treatable complication. The application of ventilatory support measures should be discussed with the patient before the need arises.

Clinicians may need to assess the contribution of coal dust exposure to the ventilatory impairments of their patients. Factors that can assist in this evaluation include a careful work history, with documentation of the mining region, duration and categories of coal mine employment, as well as the duration and intensity of any tobacco smoking. Factors associated with an increased risk of a clinically significant dust effect are a history of prolonged exposures in dusty jobs, exposures to higher-rank coals, a younger age at first employment, and the finding of radiographic changes of CWP.

SILICOSIS

Introduction and High-Risk Occupations

Silicosis is a fibrotic disease of the lungs caused by the inhalation, retention, and pulmonary reaction to crystalline silica. Despite knowledge of the cause of this disorder—respiratory exposures to silica-containing dusts—this serious and potentially fatal occupational lung disease remains prevalent throughout the world. Silica, or silicon dioxide, is the predominant component of the earth's crust. It is particularly important in sandstone, granite, and slate, as it makes up 20 to 100 percent of these rock formations. When the earth's crust is disturbed or silica-containing rock is used or processed, there are potential respiratory risks for workers. Occupational exposure to silica particles of respirable size (aerodynamic diameter of 0.5 to 5 μ) is associated with mining, quarrying, drilling, tunneling, and abrasive blasting with quartz-containing materials (sandblasting). Silica exposure also poses a hazard to stonecutters (Fig. 59-6) and pottery, foundry, ground silica, and refractory workers. The silicon dioxide that is inhaled is usually crystalline and most often quartz. Cristobalite and tridymite are other crystalline forms of silica. These three crystalline forms are also called "free silica" to distinguish them from silicates, such as asbestos and talc.

The development and progression of silicosis frequently occur after exposure has ceased. Because of this latency, the true prevalence of the disease is unknown. However, crystalline silica exposure is so widespread, and silica sand is such an inexpensive and versatile component of so many manufacturing processes, that millions of workers throughout the world are at risk of the disease. This is reflected in the fatal cases of silicosis, multiple cases of silicosis from the same work site, and epidemics of silicosis that continue to be recognized, even in developed countries.[6,10,46]

Forms of Silicosis

EXPOSURE HISTORY AND CLINICOPATHOLOGIC DESCRIPTIONS

Chronic, accelerated, and acute forms of silicosis have been well characterized. These clinical and pathologic expressions of the disease reflect differing exposure intensities, latency periods, and natural histories. The chronic or classic form usually follows one or more decades of exposure to respirable dust containing quartz. The accelerated form results from heavier exposures, often with a du-

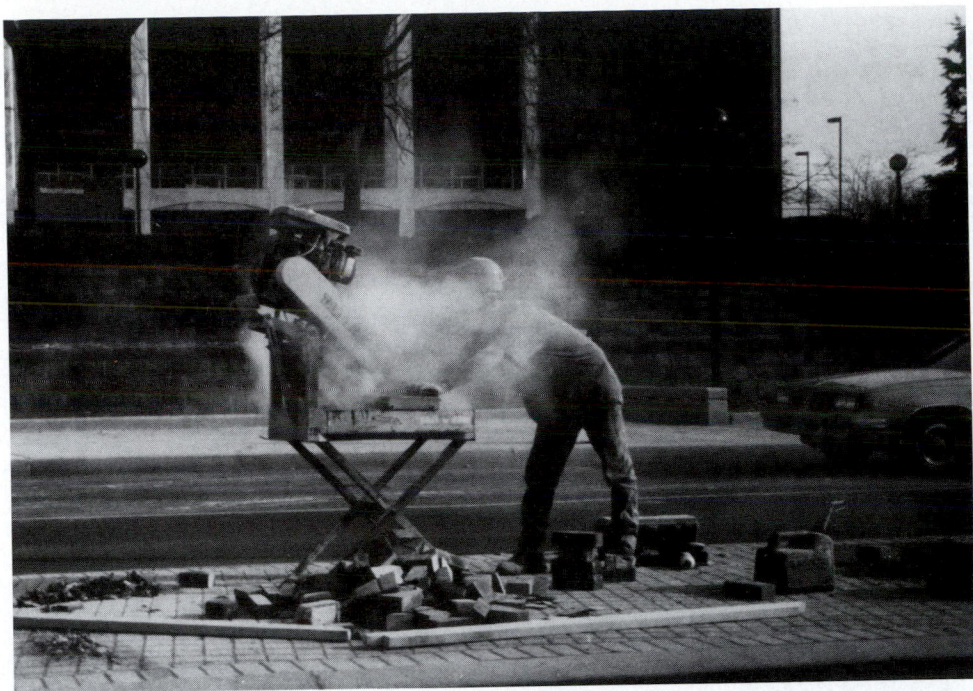

FIGURE 59-6 Masonary cutting. Note the potential for respiratory exposure to excessive silica-containing dusts. *(Courtesy of Kenneth Linch, National Institute for Occupational Safety and Health, Morgantown, WV.)*

associated with basilar emphysema. This progressive illness may occur even after exposure to silica-containing dust has ceased. The result is a clinically significant compromise of lung structure and function and, as a consequence, symptoms of exertional dyspnea and reduced functional status. Common laboratory findings include a diminished carbon monoxide–diffusing capacity, reduced arterial oxygen tension at rest or with exercise, and a demonstrable restrictive pattern on pulmonary function evaluation. Concomitant dust-induced bronchitis or distortion of the bronchial tree may also result in productive cough or airflow obstruction. Recurrent bacterial infections, not unlike those seen in bronchiectasis, may occur. Weight loss and cavitation of the large opacities should prompt concern for tuberculosis or other mycobacterial infections. Pneumothorax may be a life-threatening complication, since the fibrotic lung may be difficult to reexpand. Hypoxemic respiratory failure with cor pulmonale and congestive heart failure can be terminal findings.

Accelerated Silicosis Accelerated silicosis results from exposures that are more intense and of shorter (5 to 10 years) dura-

ration of 5 to 10 years. Accelerated silicosis develops more rapidly than the chronic form and in general progresses inexorably even after silica exposure is interrupted. The acute form of silicosis is a consequence of intense exposures to high levels of respirable dust that contain a significant proportion of silica. The reported exposure period is usually from several months up to about 5 years, and the clinical course is usually one of rapid progression.

Chronic (or Classic) Silicosis Chronic silicosis may be asymptomatic or result in insidiously progressive exertional dyspnea or cough. A latency of 15 years or more since onset of exposure is common. Radiographically, it presents with small (less than 10 mm) rounded opacities, predominantly in the upper lung zones (Fig. 59-7). The pathologic hallmark in the lungs of patients with the chronic form is the silicotic nodule (Fig. 59-8). The lesion is characterized by a cell-free central area of concentrically arranged whorled, hyalinized collagen fibers, surrounded by cellular connective tissue with reticulin fibers. When it is examined under polarized light, birefringent particles are typically seen most prominently in the periphery of the silicotic nodule. Electron microscopy utilizing specialized techniques can help to identify the specific mineral content of the nodules, but it is rarely needed for routine diagnostic purposes. Silicotic nodules in the visceral pleura, in regional lymph nodes, and occasionally in other organs may also result from silica exposure.

Progressive Massive Fibrosis Progressive massive fibrosis (PMF) or conglomerate silicosis occurs when one or more groups of the small nodules in the lungs of a patient with chronic silicosis coalesce to form larger (over 10 mm) shadows on the chest radiograph (Fig. 59-9). The chest radiograph often contains multiple nodules that are bilateral, located in upper lung zones, and

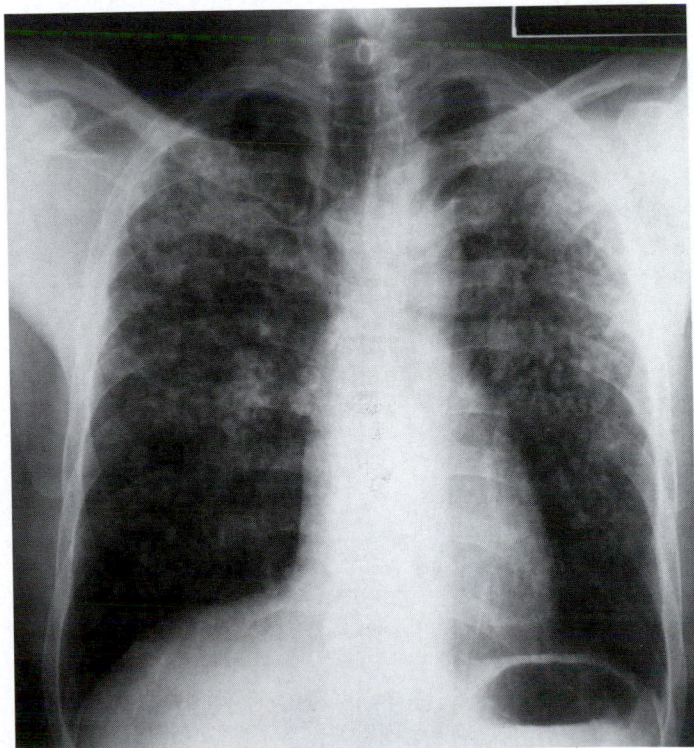

FIGURE 59-7 Chronic silicosis, ILO profusion category 2/3 with typical "r" size rounded opacities.

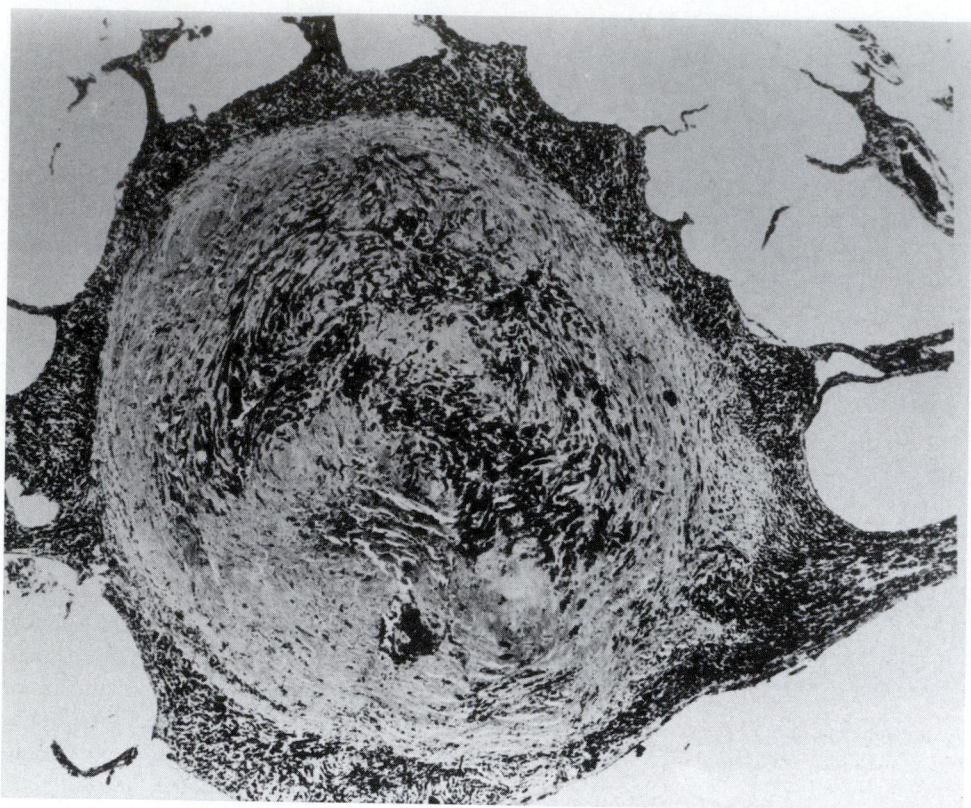

FIGURE 59-8　A silicotic nodule, microscopic section. *(Courtesy of Dr. Val Vallyathan, National Institute for Occupational Safety and Health, Morgantown, WV.)*

of disease progression is more rapid for accelerated silicosis, and workers with accelerated disease may develop superimposed mycobacterial infection. Findings consistent with autoimmune diseases such as scleroderma are also more frequent in the accelerated form of silicosis. When these autoimmune findings are present, the progression of radiographic abnormalities and functional impairment can be quite striking.

Acute Silicosis. Acute silicosis develops within a few months up to about 5 years after a massive inhalation of silica.[6] Dramatic dyspnea, weakness, and weight loss are often presenting symptoms. The radiographic findings differ from those in the more chronic forms of silicosis, and are dominated by a diffuse alveolar filling pattern with a lower lung zone predominance (Fig. 59-10). Air bronchograms may be present. Histologic findings similar to those of pulmonary alveolar proteinosis have been described, and extrapulmonary (renal and hepatic) abnormalities are occasionally reported. The usual clinical course of this rare form of silicosis is rapid progression to severe hypoxemic ventilatory failure and death.

tion than in the chronic form. The symptoms, radiographic findings, physiological measurements, and lung pathology of chronic and accelerated silicosis are quite similar. However, rate

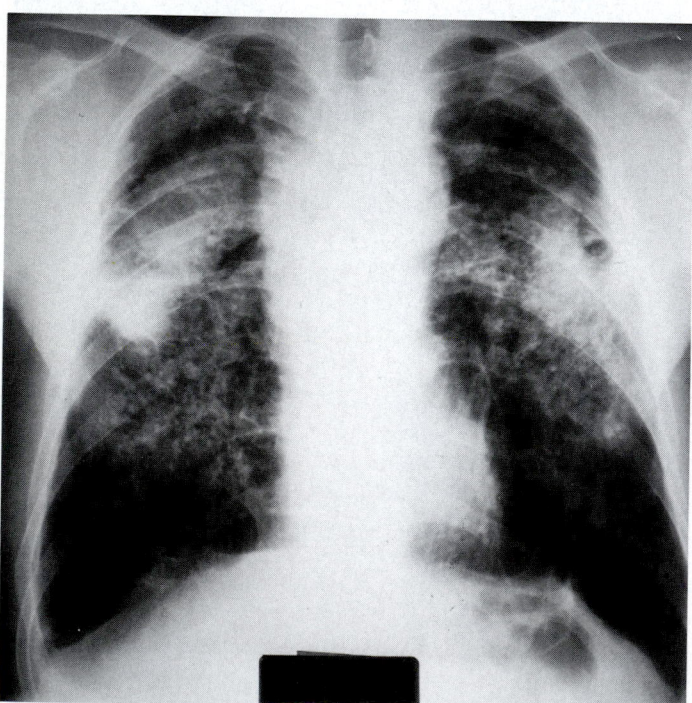

FIGURE 59-9　Complicated silicosis demonstrating progressive massive fibrosis.

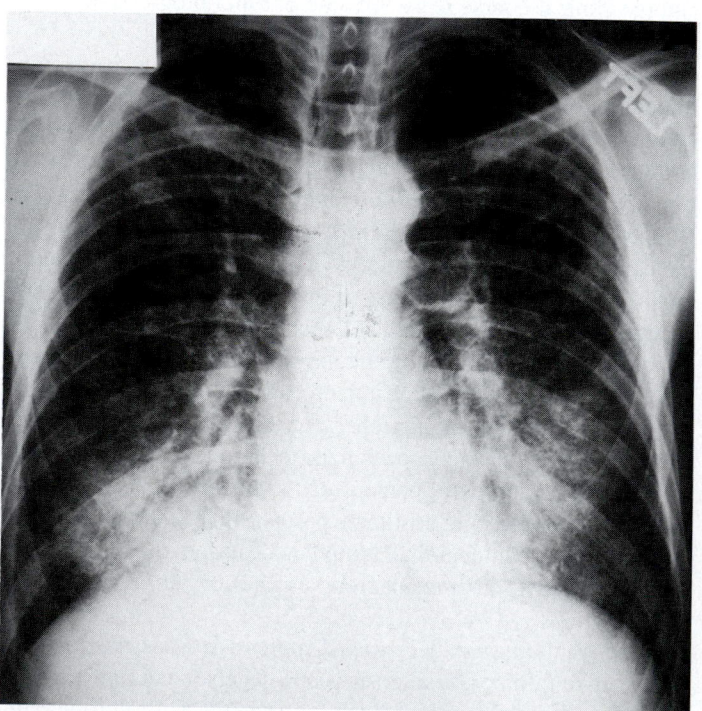

FIGURE 59-10　Acute silicosis, silicoproteinosis pattern, in a surface coal miner. *(Courtesy of Drs. Daniel E. Banks and N. LeRoy Lapp, University of West Virginia, Morgantown, WV.)*

Other Disorders   Even in the absence of radiographic silicosis, silica-exposed workers may develop chronic bronchitis and emphysema from their occupational dust exposure. Progressive declines in lung function have also been documented in workers exposed to silica and other occupational mineral dusts.

Pathogenesis

The precise pathogenesis of silicosis is uncertain. An abundance of evidence, however, suggests that interactions between pulmonary alveolar macrophages and silica particles play a major role in the pathogenesis of this disorder. Surface properties of the silica particle appear to promote macrophage activation. These cells then release chemotactic factors and inflammatory mediators that elicit cellular responses by polymorphonuclear leukocytes, lymphocytes, and additional macrophages. Fibroblast-stimulating factors are also released; they promote hyalinization and collagen deposition. The resulting pathologic lesion is the hyaline nodule, which contains a central acellular zone, with free silica surrounded by whorls of collagen and fibroblasts, and an active peripheral zone composed of macrophages, fibroblasts, plasma cells, and additional free silica.[15]

The precise properties of the silica particles that evoke the pulmonary response described above are not known. The nature and the extent of the biologic response are, in general, related to the intensity of the exposure. The surface characteristics of the dust also appear to be important. For example, there is growing evidence that freshly fractured silica may be more toxic than aged silica-containing dusts, perhaps because of reactive radical groups on the cleavage planes of the freshly fractured moiety.[45] This may offer a pathogenic explanation for the more frequent observation of cases of advanced disease in both sandblasters and rock drillers, in whom exposures to recently fractured silica are particularly intense.

The initiating toxic insult in silicosis may occur with minimal immunologic reaction. However, a sustained immunologic response to the insult may be important in the generation of some of the chronic manifestations of the disease. For example, the antinuclear antibodies that are noted in the accelerated form of silicosis associated with scleroderma and other collagen vascular disorders may contribute to the pathogenesis of this syndrome. Indeed progressive systemic sclerosis and other autoimmune phenomena have been noted in patients with silicosis.[44]

Association with Tuberculosis

The propensity for people with silicosis to get tuberculosis has been recognized for nearly a century.[42] Tuberculosis can complicate all forms of silicosis. Patients with the acute and accelerated forms of the disease appear to be at the highest risk of infection. Silica exposure alone, even without silicosis, may predispose to this infection. *Mycobacterium tuberculosis* is the usual organism, but atypical mycobacteria (and, less often, *Nocardia asteroides*) can also be seen. The mechanism of this susceptibility is poorly understood. It may, however, be related to the toxic effects of silica on alveolar macrophages.

Clinical Manifestations of Silicosis

Patients with silicosis can be asymptomatic and present with abnormal chest radiographs. They can also be minimally symptomatic in spite of advanced radiographic abnormalities. When silicosis is symptomatic, the primary symptom is usually dyspnea. It is first noted with activity or exercise and later, as the pulmonary reserve of the lung is lost, also reported at rest. The appearance or progression of dyspnea may herald the development of complications, including tuberculosis, airway obstruction, or PMF. Productive cough is often present, secondary to chronic bronchitis from occupational dust exposure, tobacco use, or both. Cough may, at times, also be attributed to pressure from large masses of silicotic lymph nodes on the trachea or main-stem bronchi.

Other chest symptoms are less common than dyspnea and cough. Hemoptysis is rare and should raise concern for complicating disorders, such as pulmonary neoplasms or mycobacterial infection. Wheeze and chest tightness may occur in the presence of silicosis, but they occur more commonly as part of associated obstructive airway disease or bronchitis. Chest pain and finger clubbing are not features of silicosis. Systemic symptoms, such as fever and weight loss, suggest complicating infection or neoplastic disease. Advanced forms of silicosis are associated with progressive respiratory failure with or without cor pulmonale. Few physical signs may be noted unless complications are present.

Radiographic Patterns in Silicosis

The earliest radiographic signs of uncomplicated silicosis are generally small rounded opacities. These can be categorized using the ILO International Classification of Radiographs of Pneumoconioses by size, shape, and profusion category.[23] In silicosis, rounded opacities of the "q" and "r" type dominate (Fig. 59-7). Other patterns have also been described, including linear or irregular shadows. The opacities seen on the radiograph represent the summation of pathologic silicotic nodules. They are usually found to predominate initially in the upper lung zones and may progress to invade other zones. Hilar lymphadenopathy is also noted, sometimes in advance of nodular parenchymal shadows. Eggshell calcification of the lymph nodes is strongly suggestive of silicosis, although this feature is seldom seen (Fig. 59-11).

PMF is characterized by the formation of large opacities. These are generally categorized by size, using the ILO classification, as category A, B, or C. The large fibrotic lesions of PMF tend to contract to the upper lung zones, leaving areas of compensatory emphysema at their margins and in the lung bases (Fig. 59-9). As a result of this process, small rounded opacities that previously were evident on the radiograph may become less visible or at times disappear. Pleural abnormalities are not a frequent radiographic feature with silicosis but do occur, particularly in association with conglomerate lesions. Large opacities also frequently pose a concern regarding neoplasm. The radiographic distinction between PMF lesions and lung malignancies may be difficult, particularly if previous chest films are unavailable for comparison. Although ischemic necrosis may occur

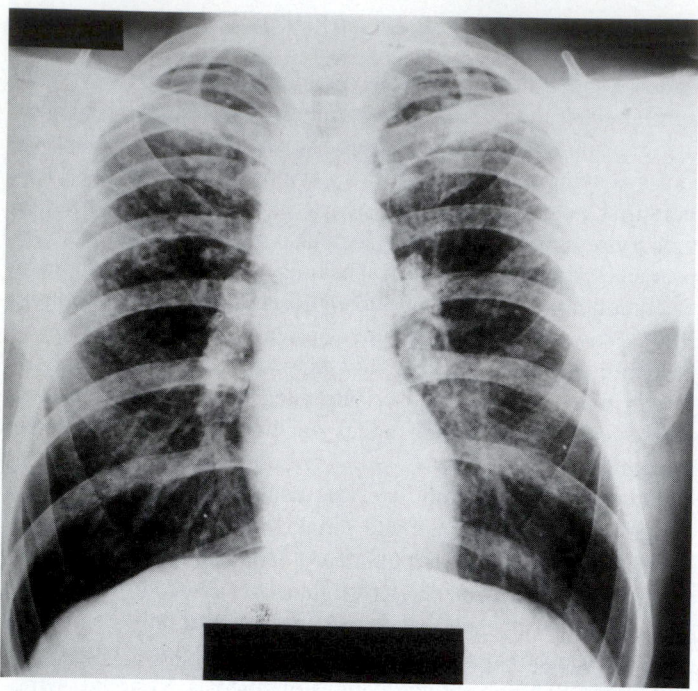

FIGURE 59-11　Eggshell calcification of hilar lymph nodes in silicosis.

in large silicotic lesions, the onset of cavitation or a rapid change in the radiographic appearance should prompt a search for active mycobacterial disease. Acute silicosis may present with a radiologic alveolar filling pattern (Fig. 59-10) and progress rapidly to PMF or complicated mass lesions.

Lung Function Abnormalities in Silicosis

Pulmonary function tests, such as spirometry and diffusing capacity, are helpful for the clinical evaluation of people with suspected silicosis. Spirometry may also be of value in the early recognition of the health effects from occupational dust exposures, as it can detect physiological abnormalities that may precede radiographic changes. No specific or characteristic pattern of ventilatory impairment is present in silicosis. Spirometry may be normal; when it is abnormal, the tracings may show obstruction, restriction, or a mixed pattern. Obstruction may indeed be the more common finding. Silica and mixed dust exposures[7] may lead to clinically significant airflow limitation independent of radiographic abnormality.[36]

In general, workers experience lung function loss proportionate to the duration and intensity of silica dust exposure. In addition, functional changes tend to be more marked with advanced radiologic categories. However, no good correlation exists between radiographic abnormalities and ventilatory impairment. Diffusing impairment may also occur in the absence of ventilatory impairment. In acute and accelerated silicosis, functional changes generally occur earlier, are more marked, and progress more rapidly than in the chronic form of the disease. In acute silicosis, radiographic progression is accompanied by increasing ventilatory impairment and gas exchange abnormalities, which lead to respiratory failure and eventually to death from intractable hypoxemia.

Complications and Special Diagnostic Issues in Silicosis

With a history of exposure and a characteristic radiograph, the diagnosis of silicosis is generally not difficult to establish. Challenges arise only when the radiologic features are unusual or the history of exposure is not recognized. Lung biopsy is rarely required to establish the diagnosis. However, tissue samples are helpful in some clinical settings when complications are present or the differential diagnosis includes tuberculosis, neoplasm, or PMF. Biopsy material should be sent for culture, and in research settings, dust analysis may be a useful additional measure. When tissue is required, open or thoracoscopic lung biopsies are generally necessary for adequate material for examination.

Vigilance for infectious complications, especially tuberculosis and other mycobacteria, cannot be overemphasized. New onset or a change in cough, hemoptysis, fever, or weight loss should trigger a workup to exclude this treatable problem. Nocardial and fungal infections are also reported in association with acute silicosis.

Lung Cancer and Silicosis

Substantial concern and interest about the relationship between silica exposure, silicosis, and cancer of the lung continue to stimulate debate. The International Agency for Research on Cancer[22] has classified crystalline silica as a 2A carcinogen on the basis of "sufficient" evidence of carcinogenicity in experimental animals and "limited" evidence of carcinogenicity in humans. Uncertainty over the pathogenic mechanisms for the development of lung cancer in silica-exposed populations exists, and the possible relationship between silicosis (or lung fibrosis) and cancer in exposed workers continues to be studied.

Prevention of Silicosis

Prevention remains the principal goal in dealing with this occupational lung disease. Exposures can be reduced through the use of improved ventilation and local exhaust, process enclosure, wet abrasive techniques, personal protection (including the proper selection of respirators), and, when possible, substitution of industrial agents less hazardous than silica. The education of workers and employers regarding the hazards of silica dust exposure and measures to control exposure are also important.

If silicosis is recognized in a worker, termination of exposure is advisable. Unfortunately, the disease can progress even without further silica exposure. Additionally, the finding of a case of silicosis, especially in the acute or accelerated form, should prompt a thorough evaluation of workplace exposures and industrial hygiene measures, with the goal of recognizing the hazardous operation and protecting other workers who may be at risk.

Medical Screening and Surveillance in Silicosis

Workers exposed to silica and other mineral dusts should undergo periodic screening for adverse health effects as a supplement to, but not a substitute for, dust exposure control. Such screening commonly includes evaluations for respiratory symptoms, spirometric abnormalities, radiographic changes, and neoplastic disease. Evaluation for tuberculosis infection with intradermal skin testing should also be performed. In addition to the reporting of results to the individual workers, screening health data from all workers in a plant or operation should be periodically assembled and evaluated for surveillance and prevention activities.

Therapy, Management of Complications, and Control of Silicosis

Over the years, a variety of treatments for silicosis have been attempted. However, aerosolized aluminum did not prove successful in the treatment of the disorder, and polyvinyl pyridine-N-oxide, a polymer that has protective effects in experimental animals, is not available for use in humans. In addition, tetranidine, an agent that diminishes fibrosis in silica-exposed animals, has not been shown to be effective in humans and is highly teratogenic. As a result of this unsuccessful search, therapy for silicosis is directed largely at complications of the disease. Therapeutic measures are similar to those commonly used in the management of airflow obstruction, infection, pneumothorax, hypoxemia, and respiratory failure complicating other pulmonary disorders. For workers with a diagnosis of silicosis, further exposure to silica-containing dusts is undesirable. If the disease is advanced, or has occurred after a relatively short exposure (less than 15 years), further dust exposure should be assiduously avoided. Advice on job reassignment should be considered in the context of the worker's age, symptoms, and functional status and the current working conditions and measured silica exposures.

In the medical management of silicosis, vigilance for complicating infection, especially tuberculosis, is critical. This entails yearly chest radiographs and PPD evaluations. The use of prophylactic isoniazid for tuberculin-positive silicotic subjects is recommended. The use of bacillus Calmette-Guérin in the tuberculin-negative silicotic patient is not recommended.

The diagnosis of active tuberculosis infection in patients with silicosis can be difficult. Clinical symptoms of weight loss, fever, sweats, and malaise should prompt radiographic evaluation and sputum acid-fast bacilli stains and cultures. Radiographic changes with infection may be subtle and atypical. Enlargement and cavitation in conglomerate lesions or nodular opacities are of particular concern. Bacteriologic studies on expectorated sputum may not always be reliable in silicotuberculosis. Fiberoptic bronchoscopy for additional specimens for culture and study may be helpful in establishing a diagnosis of active disease. The use of multidrug therapy for suspected active disease in patients with silicosis is justified at a lower level of suspicion than in the nonsilicotic subject, owing to the difficulty in firmly establishing evidence for active infection. To obtain satisfactory results in the presence of silicosis, antituberculous treatment must be more prolonged, with regimens lasting at least 8 months.

Ventilatory support for respiratory failure is indicated when precipitated by a treatable complication. Pneumothorax, spontaneous and ventilator related, is usually treated by chest tube insertion. Bronchopleural fistula may develop, and surgical intervention may be required.

Acute silicosis may rapidly progress to respiratory failure. When this disease resembles pulmonary alveolar proteinosis and severe hypoxemia is present, aggressive therapy has included massive whole-lung lavage with the patient under general anesthesia in an attempt to improve gas exchange and remove alveolar debris. Although it is appealing in concept, the efficacy of whole-lung lavage has not been established.[49] Glucocorticoid therapy has also been used for acute silicosis. However, it is still of unproven benefit.

The rare young patient with end-stage silicosis may be considered candidates for lung or heart-lung transplantation in centers experienced with this expensive and high-risk procedure. Early referral and evaluation for this intervention may be offered to selected subjects.

The discussion above underscores the serious and potentially fatal nature of silicosis. The lack of a specific therapy for silicosis further emphasizes the crucial role of primary prevention in our therapeutic approach to this disorder. The control of silicosis ultimately depends on the control of workplace dust exposures. This is accomplished by rigorous and conscientious application of fundamental occupational hygiene and engineering principles, with a commitment to the preservation of worker health.

REFERENCES

1. Amandus HE, Petersen MR, Richards TB: Health status of anthracite surface coal miners. *Arch Environ Health* 44:75–81, 1989.
2. Attfield MD: Longitudinal decline in FEV$_1$ in United States coalminers. *Thorax* 40:132–137, 1985.
3. Attfield MD, Hodous TK: Pulmonary function of U.S. coal miners related to dust exposure estimates. *Am Rev Respir Dis* 145:605–609, 1992.
4. Attfield MD, Hodous TK: Does regression analysis of lung function data obtained from occupational epidemiologic studies lead to misleading inferences regarding the true effect of smoking? *Am J Ind Med* 27:281–291, 1995.
5. Attfield MD, Seixas NS: Prevalence of pneumoconiosis and its relationship to dust exposure in a cohort of U.S. bituminous coal miners and ex-miners. *Am J Ind Med* 27:137–151, 1995.
6. Banks DE, Bauer MA, Castellan RM, Lapp NL: Silicosis in surface coalmine drillers. *Thorax* 38:275–278, 1983.
7. Becklake MR: Chronic airflow limitation: Its relationship to work in dusty occupations. *Chest* 88:608–617, 1985.
8. Burrell R: Immunological aspects of coal workers' pneumoconiosis. *Ann NY Acad Sci* 200:94–105, 1972.
9. Caplan A: Certain unusual radiological appearances in the chest of coal miners suffering from rheumatoid arthritis. *Thorax* 8:29–37, 1953.
10. CDC: Silicosis: Cluster in sandblasters—Texas, and Occupational Surveillance for Silicosis. *MMWR* 39:433–437, 1990.
11. CDC/NIOSH: *Criteria for a Recommended Standard, Occupational Exposure to Respirable Coal Mine Dust.* DHHS (NIOSH) Publication No. 95-106, September 1995.
12. Cockcroft A, Berry G, Cotes JE, Lyons JP: Shape of small opacities and lung function in coalworkers. *Thorax* 37:765–769, 1982.
13. Coggon D, Inskip H, Winter P, Pannett B: Contrasting geographical distribution of mortality from pneumoconiosis and chronic bronchitis and emphysema in British coal miners. *Occup Envir Med* 52:554–555, 1995.

14. Collins LC, Willing S, Bretz R, et al: High-resolution CT in simple coal workers' pneumoconiosis: Lack of correlation with pulmonary function tests and arterial blood gas values. *Chest* 104:1156–1162, 1993.

15. Craighead JE, Kleinerman J, Abraham JL, et al: Diseases associated with exposure to silica and nonfibrous silicate minerals: Silicosis and Silicate Disease Committee. *Arch Pathol Lab Med* 112:673–720, 1988.

16. Dubois P, Gyselen A, Prignot J: Rifampicin-combined chemotherapy in coal worker's pneumoconio-tuberculosis. *Am Rev Respir Dis* 115:221–228, 1977.

17. Fields CL, Roy TM, Dow FT, Anderson WH: Impact of arterial blood gas analysis in disability evaluation of the bituminous coal miner with simple pneumoconiosis. *J Occup Med* 34:410–413, 1992.

18. Green FHY, Althouse R, Weber KC: Prevalence of silicosis at death in underground coal miners. *Am J Ind Med* 16:605–615, 1989.

19. Hahon N, Morgan WKC, Petersen M: Serum immunoglobulin levels in coal workers' pneumoconiosis. *Ann Occup Hyg* 23:165–174, 1980.

20. Hall DR, Lapp NL, Reger R, Seaton A: Small airways disease in coal miners: A longitudinal study. *Bull Physiopathol Respir (Nancy)* 11:863–877, 1975.

21. Hurley JF, Soutar CA: Can exposure to coal mine dust cause a severe impairment of lung function? *Br J Ind Med* 43:150–157, 1986.

22. International Agency for Research on Cancer: IARC monographs on the evaluation of the carcinogenic risk of chemicals to humans: *Silica and Some Silicates,* vol 42. Lyon, France, World Health Organization, International Agency for Research on Cancer, pp 49, 51, 73–111, 1987.

23. International Labour Office: *Guidelines for the Use of ILO International Classification of Radiographs of Pneumoconiosis,* revised ed. Geneva, International Labour Office, 1980.

24. Jacobsen M, Rae S, Walton WH, Rogan JM: The relation between pneumoconiosis and dust-exposure in British coal mines, in Walton WH (ed), *Inhaled Particles,* vol III. Woking, Surrey, Unwin Brothers, 1971, pp 903–917.

25. Kleinerman J, Green F, Lacquer W, et al: Pathology standards for coal workers' pneumoconiosis. *Arch Path Lab Med* 103:374–432, 1979.

26. Kuempel ED, Stayner LT, Attfield MD, Buncher CR: Exposure-response analysis of mortality among coal miners in the United States. *Am J Ind Med* 28:167–184, 1995.

27. Lapp NL, Seaton A, Kaplan KC, et al: Pulmonary hemodynamics in symptomatic coal miners. *Am Rev Respir Dis* 104:418–426, 1971.

28. Lippmann M, Eckert HL, Hahon N, Morgan WKC: Circulating antinuclear and rheumatoid factors in United States coal miners. *Ann Intern Med* 79:807–811, 1973.

29. Marine WM, Gurr D, Jacobsen M: Clinically important respiratory effects of dust exposure and smoking in British coal miners. *Am Rev Respir Dis* 137:106–112, 1988.

30. McLintock JS, Rae S, Jacobsen M: The attack rate of progressive massive fibrosis in British coal miners, in Walton WH (ed), *Inhaled Particles,* vol III. Woking, Surrey, Unwin Brothers, 1971, pp 933–950.

31. Miller BG, Jacobsen M: Dust exposure, pneumoconiosis, and mortality of coalminers. *Br J Ind Med* 42:723–733, 1985.

32. Morgan EJ: Silicosis and tuberculosis. *Chest* 75:202–203, 1979.

33. Morgan W, Handelsman L, Kibelstis J, et al: Ventilatory capacity and lung volumes of U.S. coal miners. *Arch Environ Health* 28:182–189, 1974.

34. Morgan WKC, Burgess DB, Jacobsen G, et al: The prevalence of coal workers' pneumoconiosis in U.S. coal miners. *Arch Environ Health* 27:221–226, 1973.

35. Nemery B, Veriter C, Brasseur L, Frans A: Impairment of ventilatory function and pulmonary gas exchange in non-smoking coalminers. *Lancet* 2:1427–1430, 1987.

36. Oxman AD, Muir DC, Shannon HS, et al: Occupational dust exposure and chronic obstructive pulmonary disease. A systematic overview of the evidence (see comments). *Am Rev Respir Dis* 148:38–48, 1993.

37. Petsonk EL, Daniloff EM, Mannino DM, et al: Airway responsiveness and job selection: A study in coal miners and non-mining controls. *Occup Environ Med* 52:745–749, 1995.

38. Rom WN, Bitterman PB, Rennard SI, et al: Characterization of the lower respiratory tract inflammation of nonsmoking individuals with interstitial lung disease associated with chronic inhalation of inorganic dust. *Am Rev Respir Dis* 136:1429–1434, 1987.

39. Seaton A, Lapp NL, Morgan WK: Relationship of pulmonary impairment in simple coal workers' pneumoconiosis to type of radiographic opacity. *Br J Ind Med* 29:50–55, 1972.

40. Seixas NS, Robins TG, Attfield MD, Moulton LH: Exposure-response relationships for coal mine dust and obstructive lung disease following enactment of the Federal Coal Mine Health and Safety Act of 1969. *Am J Ind Med* 21:715–734, 1992.

41. Seixas NS, Robins TG, Attfield MD, Moulton LH: Longitudinal and cross sectional analyses of exposure to coal mine dust and pulmonary function in new miners. *Br J Ind Med* 50:929–937, 1993.

42. Snider DE: The relationship between tuberculosis and silicosis. *Am Rev Respir Dis* 118:455–460, 1978.

43. Soutar CA, Turner-Warwick M, Parkes WR: Circulating antinuclear antibody and rheumatoid factor in coal pneumoconiosis. *Br Med J* 3:145–147, 1974.

44. Steenland K, Goldsmith DF: Silica exposure and auto-immune diseases. *Am J Ind Med* 28:603–608, 1995.

45. Vallyathan V, Shi X, Dalal NS, et al: Generation of free radicals from freshly fractured silica dust. *Am Rev Respir Dis* 138:1213–1219, 1988.

46. Wagner GR: The inexcusable persistence of silicosis (editorial). *Am J Public Health* 85:1346–1347, 1995.

47. Wagner JC, McCormick JN: Immunological investigations of coalworkers' disease. *J R Coll Physicians Lond* 2:49–56, 1967.

48. Wallaert B, Lassalle P, Fortin F, et al: Superoxide anion generation by alveolar inflammatory cells in simple pneumoconiosis and in progressive massive fibrosis of non-smoking coal workers. *Am Rev Respir Dis* 141:129–133, 1990.

49. Wilt JL, Banks DE, Weissman DN, et al: Reduction of lung dust burden in pneumoconiosis by whole lung lavage. *J Occup Environ Med* 38:619–624, 1996.

50. Wright JL, Cagle P, Churg A, et al: State of the art: Diseases of the small airways. *Am Rev Respir Dis* 146:240–262, 1992.

CHAPTER 60

OCCUPATIONAL ASTHMA, BYSSINOSIS, AND INDUSTRIAL BRONCHITIS

J. Allen D. Cooper, Jr.

Inhalation of foreign material at the workplace can cause a number of pulmonary syndromes. The lung, next to the skin, is the second most common organ affected by occupation-related toxic reactions. Lung parenchyma and airways as well as the pleura can be affected by inhalation of toxic material. This chapter discusses reactions of the airway to toxic inhalation of substances occurring at the workplace.[17,18,45] Lung parenchymal and pleural reactions as well as obliterative bronchiolitis in response to inhaled materials are discussed in other locations in this text. Occupational airway disease can manifest as chronic bronchitis without airway hyperreactivity (industrial bronchitis) or asthma with hyperreactive airways (occupational asthma). Two major differences between these syndromes are that (1) industrial bronchitis generally occurs without a latent period while occupational asthma develops after a latency time period of exposure and (2) occupational asthma occurs after the airway has become sensitized to a substance, so that a very small amount of that substance will induce bronchospasm.[18] Cotton dust is the most common substance causing industrial bronchitis without causing any well-documented cases of occupational asthma. Although grain dust can cause industrial bronchitis, exposure to grain can also result in development of asthma. In this chapter general and specific issues regarding industrial bronchitis and occupational asthma are discussed.

INDUSTRIAL BRONCHITIS

Byssinosis

HISTORY

Adverse reactions in cotton workers have been recognized for more than 100 years. In 1831, Kay described chest tightness and fever that commonly occurred on Monday after workers had been off work over the weekend.[30] It was because of this observation that the term *Monday morning fever* was coined. The term *Byssinosis* was proposed by the French physician Proust and is derived from the Greek word meaning linen or fine flax.[31] Over the years, as cotton mills appeared in more and more countries, the association of chronic bronchitis with cotton dust exposure was confirmed.

EPIDEMIOLOGY

There is no doubt that recurrent exposure to cotton dust results in chronic bronchitis. In a prospective study, 16 percent of cotton mill workers in South Carolina developed symptoms of chronic bronchitis, as compared to only 1 percent of appropriate controls in the region.[5] In another study,[44] 4.5 percent of 2000 cotton workers screened by questionnaires and pulmonary function testing complained of Monday morning chest tightness and showed physiologic impairment. The percentage of subjects with symptoms varied according to their work area and was as high as 26 percent in certain areas.

There are over 800,000 textile workers in the United States.[49] These are the individuals who are primarily at risk for developing symptoms due to inhalation of cotton dust.[49] Flax and hemp workers are also at risk for developing the problem. Clinical studies suggest that approximately 65 percent of the general population will react significantly to de novo inhalation of components of cotton dust. Therefore the majority of those who begin employment involved with cotton, flax, or hemp processing are at risk for developing respiratory symptoms. The reason why some individuals are more susceptible than others to the effects of cotton dust are unclear.

Certain jobs in the textile mill are associated with a higher risk for development of bronchitis. Ginning, opening, or carding work carry a higher degree of risk.[46] In addition, workers who clean out or maintain the various machines that divide up and clean the cotton are especially prone to develop symptoms. These are particularly high-risk jobs because of the high levels of cotton dust generated during the cleaning procedure. Strippers and grinders, who maintain the carding machinery that cleans and aligns the cotton, are particularly at risk for development of symptoms. In fact, byssinosis has been termed "strippers' asthma" in the past.

CLINICAL PRESENTATION, RISK FACTORS, AND STAGES OF BYSSINOSIS

Shortness of breath often occurs on the day back to work after several days of absence, as on a Monday after being off work over the weekend. Subsequently, workers can develop more persistent symptoms. These have been graded by Schilling[47] (Table 60-1) to allow comparison of symptomatology with physiological parameters. Using this grading system, it has been established that workers with a higher grade of symptoms tend to have a more rapid decline in pulmonary function.[29] Risk factors for developing higher grades of byssinosis include (1) length of employment in a cotton mill and (2) dust exposure level. Tobacco smoking has also been shown to be synergistic with cotton dust exposure for producing chronic bronchitis.[45] Although it is controversial whether cotton dust exposure results in chronic pulmonary disability in the absence of cigarette smoking, it appears that 7 percent of exposed individuals will develop irreversible airway obstruction that cannot be explained by smoking.[7]

PULMONARY FUNCTION TEST ABNORMALITIES

Byssinosis is associated with a reduction in the forced vital capacity (FVC) and forced expiratory volume in 1 s (FEV_1) characteristically seen on the day of return to work after an absence. The degree of reduction in these parameters increases over the workday. This change will generally be more severe on the first day of work after an absence than on subsequent days.[49] The

mechanism by which this developed tolerance occurs is unknown. Whether subjects with byssinosis have airways that are hyperreactive to methacholine challenge is controversial. One study has also shown a significant decrease in arterial oxygen tension after exposure to hemp dust.[34]

PATHOLOGY AND PATHOGENESIS OF BYSSINOSIS

The histopathology of byssinosis appears to be similar to that associated with tobacco smoke–induced bronchitis, with mucous gland hyperplasia and polymorphonuclear neutrophil infiltration into bronchi.[49] Several animal studies have demonstrated that different components of cotton dust can recruit neutrophils into bronchi. In addition, components of cotton dust can also stimulate resident pulmonary cells, such as mast cells and macrophages, to release molecules that attract neutrophils.[20]

There is now a large amount of information pointing to a lipopolysaccharide (endotoxin) produced by bacterial contaminants of cotton as the causative agent of byssinosis.[15,44] The evidence for this is listed in Table 60-2. The most compelling study examining this issue was presented by Castellan and colleagues,[15] who demonstrated that ambient concentrations of endotoxin in a simulated carding room correlated with reduction in airway flow rates in a time frame similar to that occurring after exposure to cotton dust at the workplace. An interesting related finding is that byssinosis is less prevalent in Australia, probably because of the lower level of endotoxin on cotton grown in this drier climate.[44] The acquired tolerance over the work week displayed in patients with byssinosis can be simulated with multiple aerosols of endotoxin in animals. Because airborne levels of endotoxin have appeared to be directly related to the pathogenesis of byssinosis, mechanisms to control this and other airborne components of cotton dust have been implemented in the textile industry. This has met with success in controlling industrial bronchitis due to cotton dust.

There have also been reports implicating other components of cotton dust in the pathogenesis of byssinosis. An extract of cotton bract has been shown to induce bronchoconstriction in approximately 60 percent of normal volunteers.[20] The level of this low-molecular-weight (MW) compound tends to parallel the

---

TABLE 60-1

Clinical Grading of Byssinosis as Proposed by Schilling

Grade 0:	No symptoms on first day of work
Grade 1/2:	Occasional chest tightness or irritation of respiratory tract on the first work day of week
Grade 1:	Chest tightness on every first day of work week
Grade 2:	Chest tightness on first and other days of work week
Grade 3:	Chest tightness on first and other days of work week and physiologic evidence of permanent disability

---

TABLE 60-2

Evidence that Bacterial Endotoxin Is the Causative Agent in Byssinosis

1. Measurable levels of endotoxin can be detected in cotton dust.
2. Inhaled endotoxin can induce airway inflammation in animals and humans.
3. In a controlled setting, ambient levels of endotoxin correlate with degree of airflow reduction occurring in a simulated carding room.
4. Repeated inhalation of endotoxin results in an attenuation of the airway response similar to that noted in patients with byssinosis.
5. Measures that reduce levels of ambient endotoxin reduce the incidence of byssinosis.

endotoxin level in certain cotton dust preparations, but it is not a component of endotoxin. Other reports have documented significant histamine levels in cotton dust extracts. In addition, clinical studies have suggested that workers with byssinosis have elevated serum histamine levels. The role(s) that these other components of cotton dust (including cotton bract and histamine) play in the pathogenesis of byssinosis is not clear, since none have held up under scrutiny as well as endotoxin as a cause of this disorder.

TREATMENT AND PREVENTION

The most important treatment for byssinosis is removal of the individual from the offending work environment. Screening pulmonary function testing at the workplace is important to identify individuals who exhibit airflow abnormalities. In addition, since the 1970s, measures have been taken in developed countries to control cotton dust levels in textile mills. One measure has been to steam-clean cotton while it is still in the bale. In 1970, Burlington Industries began a program for dust control and annual medical surveillance. With this program, the incidence of symptoms consistent with byssinosis dropped from 4.5 percent in 1970 to 0.6 percent in 1979.[44]

In addition, the number of employees who had a significant decrease in FEV_1 over the work shift decreased from 18 percent in 1971 to 3.5 percent in 1979. Similar measures have been taken in other textile plants, with good success in controlling byssinosis.

Grain Dust–Induced Industrial Bronchitis

Exposure to grain dust can also result in the development of chronic bronchitis. Between 4 and 11 percent of grain workers show a reduction in FEV_1 of 10 percent or greater over the work shift. This reduction in flow rates is directly related to the amount of dust in the air. Studies have suggested that the component of grain dust responsible for causing airway symptoms is endotoxin,[20] the apparent active component of cotton dust (see above). Grain dust extract, possibly its endotoxin contaminant, can activate complement, and this may be a mechanism by which grain dust induces inflammation in bronchi. However, in contrast to cotton dust, grain dust can, in sensitive individuals, also precipitate an acute drop in airway flow rates rather than only the slow reduction in flow rates similar to that precipitated by cotton dust. This finding suggests that airway reactions to grain dust may be heterogeneous. Grain dust also tends to produce skin abnormalities in affected individuals, in contrast to cotton dust, which generally does not cause skin reactions.

OCCUPATIONAL ASTHMA

Definition and List of Offending Agents

Occupational asthma is characterized by variable airway obstruction resulting from exposure to ambient dusts, vapors, gases, or fumes incidentally present at a workplace.[4,17,18] Bronchial hyperresponsiveness to agents such as methacholine or histamine is usually present. In this setting, asthma may be caused de novo by the offending agent, as in the case of isocyanate-induced

asthma, or underlying asthma may be exacerbated by the offending agent. The subcommittee on occupational allergy of the European Academy of Allergology and Clinical Immunology has proposed five steps in the diagnosis of this disorder: (1) a history supporting the reaction, (2) evidence of variable obstructive airway disease, (3) confirmation of bronchoconstriction at the workplace, (4) documentation of bronchial sensitization to the suspected agent, and (5) establishment of a causal connection by bronchial challenge with the agent.[50] Bronchial challenge should be performed only by experienced clinicians in a controlled setting. This usually entails the use of an environmental chamber or comparable facility for the challenge.

Agents that have been associated with induction of occupational asthma can be conveniently grouped into categories of high- and low-MW compounds (Table 60-3). All of these agents tend to sensitize the individual, so that low ambient concentrations of the substance can ultimately cause significant bronchoconstriction. In addition, certain agents can cause direct irritant-related bronchoconstriction and airway hyperreactivity.

Risk Factors

Atopy appears to be the major risk factor for developing occupational asthma, particularly when the inciting agent is a high-MW compound.[18] Family or personal history of atopy appears to put the subject at risk. Because low-MW agents can induce asthma through nonallergic as well as allergic mechanisms, atopy may not be as important. Smoking is also a risk factor for the development of occupational asthma. There have been several studies documenting that workers who smoke have a higher incidence of asthmatic reactions to specific airborne agents, possibly due to overall higher IgE levels in smokers as compared with nonsmokers.[56]

Clinical Presentations

Occupational asthma presents in a similar manner as other forms of asthma. If the physician does not maintain a high index of suspicion, symptoms will be treated but the inciting agent will not be identified. Recently two general forms of occupational asthma have been identified.[18] Patients most commonly develop symptoms after a period of exposure to the inciting agent (occupational asthma with latency) or, less commonly, will develop immediate symptoms with exposure to the agent (occupational asthma without latency).

OCCUPATIONAL ASTHMA WITH LATENCY

Most commonly patients who develop occupational asthma do so after a period of exposure to the inciting agent. Agents that induce this sort of pattern include high- and low-MW molecules. Subjects usually are exposed to the agent for weeks to months prior to development of symptoms. With the appearance of symptoms, nonspecific airway hyperreactivity, determined by methacholine or histamine challenge, is present. Also with appearance of symptoms, the subject is hypersensitive to low ambient concentrations of the implicated agent. Therefore exposure to very low concentrations of the material at the workplace can precipitate severe bronchoconstriction. Controlled exposure with the

TABLE 60-3

Categories of Agents That Commonly Cause Occupational Asthma

Categories	Occupations at Risk	Major Putative Component
High-MW compounds		
Animal products	Animal handlers Veterinarians	Pelt or urinary proteins
Seafoods	Crab or prawn processors Oyster farmers	Water-extractable proteins
Insects	Entomologists Grain workers Laboratory workers River workers Flight crews	Insect proteins
Plants	Grain handlers Bakers Tea workers Brewery chemists Tobacco manufacturers	Extractable plant proteins
Biologic enzymes	Detergent industry workers Pharmaceutical workers Bakers	*Bacillus subtilis,* trypsin, pancreatin, papain, pepsin
Latex	Health care workers Doll manufacturers Glove makers	Latex rubber extract
Gums	Printers Gum manufacturers	Gum acacia Gum tragacanth
Low-MW compounds		
Diisocyanates	Polyurethane workers Plastic workers Foundry workers Spray painters	Isocyanate-protein complex
Anhydrides	Epoxy resin workers Plastics workers	Phthalic anhydride-protein complexes
Wood dust	Carpenters Sawmill workers	Plicatic acid (western red cedar) Wood dust extracts
Fluxes	Aluminum solderers Electronics workers	Aminoethylethanolamine
Pharmaceuticals	Pharmaceutical manufacturers	Antibiotics, psyllium, piperazine
Fixatives	Hospital workers	Formaldehyde, glutaraldehyde

offending agent will elicit bronchoconstriction in patients with this syndrome, especially when asthma is due to a high-MW molecule.

OCCUPATIONAL ASTHMA WITHOUT LATENCY

This syndrome is less common. Symptoms develop within hours of the exposure. Pathological changes are generally similar to those that occur in the syndrome of occupational asthma with latency, although epithelial changes such as desquamation and subepithelial fibrosis may be more prominent. Agents that commonly cause this syndrome are irritant gases or fumes such as chlorine or ammonia. In addition, certain agents such as acid anhydrides and isocyanates can cause occupational asthma with and without latency.

Mechanisms and Pathology

HIGH-MOLECULAR-WEIGHT COMPOUNDS

Most commonly, high-MW compounds, usually proteins, produced at the workplace induce asthma through IgE-dependent classic immediate hypersensitivity reactions. Specific serum IgE antibodies to the protein can usually be demonstrated and skin tests using extracts of the substance show positive results. Atopic individuals are more at risk for developing the syndrome. Because specific IgE antibodies must be produced in this setting, the latent period for developing the reaction can be long, sometimes several months or years. Pathologically, asthma due to high-MW compounds is associated with bronchial infiltration of lymphocytes and eosinophils, indistinguishable from other forms of allergic asthma. Specific IgE antibodies to occupation-related allergens trigger mast cell degranulation in a similar manner as in the nonoccupational setting. In severe cases, bronchial epithelial desquamation and subepithelial fibrosis are exhibited.

LOW-MOLECULAR-WEIGHT COMPOUND

These agents also tend to cause IgE-dependent bronchoconstriction. However, in contrast to higher-MW agents, specific IgE or IgG antibodies produced in these individuals are directed at the low-MW compound coupled to a protein within the serum. There is also some evidence that low-MW compounds induce asthma through IgE-independent mechanisms, possibly by affecting T lymphocytes directly. Evidence for this mechanism exists for cobalt and nickel salts as well as isocyanates.[18] Interestingly, the bronchial pathology is similar whether or not the response is an IgE-dependent reaction. In addition, certain low-MW compounds can directly affect chemical pathways that are involved in airway tone. For example, organophosphates have been shown to induce bronchoconstriction through anticholinergic effects.[54] Other agents may cause asthma simply through irritation of the airways.

Diagnosis

HISTORY

A high index of suspicion must always be present when patients with new-onset asthma are being evaluated. Because asthma can be induced by remote exposure to a substance, the current and previous occupational history is very important.[4] Computerized lists of exposures that occur at various workplaces are available, and these facilitate this process. Included in the history should be documentation of specific jobs for the individual at the specific workplace as well as potential exposures during performance of those jobs. The history can be verified through the use of material safety data sheets as well as industrial hygiene data and employee health records from the workplace. Historical factors that suggest occupation-related asthma include symptoms that occur at work and improve when the patient is away from work for a period of time, as during vacations. The duration of symptoms prior to removal from the offending environment is important for predicting prognosis. Those subjects who have had symptoms for a longer period of time are more likely to develop chronic symptoms that do not remit after exposure has been discontinued.[18] It should be noted that many compounds induce a late reaction, several hours after exposure. Therefore the relationship between the exposure and symptoms may not be entirely apparent to the patient.

Questions should also be asked regarding other causes of obstructive pulmonary disease. Questions regarding a history of tobacco abuse are important. A past history or family history of asthma may suggest that the patient's symptoms are not occupation-related. Therefore, questions to establish the degree of respiratory symptomatology prior to beginning a particular job are important. Questions aimed at assessing cardiac or upper airway abnormalities are also very important.

PHYSICAL EXAMINATION

Signs of atopy should be assessed. As in cases of asthma due to other causes, the pulmonary examination may be entirely normal when the patient presents outside the workplace. However, wheezing, either during quiet respiration or on a forced maneuver, suggests airflow obstruction. Signs of dermatitis may support the diagnosis of work-related disease.

SKIN AND IMMUNOLOGIC TESTS

General atopy appears to be a risk factor for developing certain forms of occupational asthma when it is due to high-MW compounds. Therefore routine skin testing, using a panel of allergens, for wheal-and-flare reactions can be useful. In addition, extracts of a compound that is suspected to cause occupational asthma in a particular patient can be used for skin testing. Extracts from flour, animal by-products, coffee, and other sources have been used for skin testing in various studies.[17] Specific IgE antibodies to extracts containing high-MW compounds or to low-MW compounds coupled to a serum protein, such as albumin, can also be detected by the radioallergosorbent test (RAST) or enzyme-linked immunoadsorbent assay (ELISA). In addition, specific IgE antibodies to low-MW compounds have been detected in patients with asthma due to these compounds. However, positive results in all of these tests do not necessarily indicate that disease is due to the specific agent; they simply suggest sensitization. All of these tests must be evaluated in the context of the individual patient.

PULMONARY FUNCTION TESTS

Patients with workplace-induced asthma may present with normal pulmonary function tests when they are away from the inciting agent. For this reason pulmonary function tests should be assessed in the light of the time elapsed since the patient was exposed to a suspected agent. Pulmonary function tests pre- and postwork can be very helpful in objectively evaluating respiratory function in relation to work.

Peak-flow monitors are also useful in the assessment of workplace-related symptoms because they can be used on the job. Initially, peak-flow measurements should be determined at least four times per day: on awakening, at the beginning and end of work, and before bed.[19] Similarly timed measurements should also be performed on days that the subject is off work. Three measurements at each time period should be made and recorded; two of these should be within 20 L/min of each other to demonstrate reproducibility. Measurements should be performed each day over a 3- to 4-week period. In addition to this regimen, a more intense regimen of peak flow measurements every 2 h has been proposed by Burge,[11] but this schedule may be too cumbersome to be practical, and studies have suggested that a protocol using measurements performed four times a day is as predictive.

Because peak flow measurements are very effort-dependent, they should be supplemented by other methods for assessing the degree of impairment. In this regard it is always important to document that patients who are being evaluated for occupational asthma are not malingering to obtain compensation for their disorder. When pulmonary function is assessed in these patients, technicians should be alerted that a work-related disorder is suspected, so that they can evaluate the patient's effort. In addition, reproducibility of the repeated maneuvers can be useful in determining degree of effort. If peak flow measurements suggest that there is an airway reaction to a substance at the workplace, a technician with a portable spirometer can be sent to the workplace to measure FVC and FEV_1 at hourly intervals during work.

BRONCHIAL PROVOCATION TESTS

Patients who develop occupational asthma invariably develop bronchial hyperreactivity to nonspecific agents such as methacholine and histamine. In fact, in those patients with normal spirograms at presentation, a bronchial challenge with either of these agents may be necessary for diagnosis. Such a challenge can also be used to choose the concentration(s) of specific allergen that should be employed in a specific bronchial provocation test, since studies have shown a good correlation between the degree of nonspecific bronchial reactivity and responses to specific allergens.

Specific bronchoprovocation can be a valuable tool to determine whether a subject's symptoms are due to a particular agent. This maneuver should be performed only by an experienced physician because it carries some risks. Bronchodilator and anti-inflammatory medication should be withheld prior to the exposure, which should be performed in a whole-body chamber if possible. This allows more reproducibility of the work situation. Exposure levels should start low and gradually increase to levels that are consistent with ambient levels at the subject's workplace.

Patterns of bronchoconstriction after exposure to specific agents can differ. The two most common patterns are an immediate reaction, occurring within a few minutes of challenge and peaking at 10 to 15 min after challenge, and a late reaction, occurring several hours after challenge and peaking at 5 to 8 h (Fig. 60-1). These responses can be seen individually or together in a given patient. Less frequent patterns have also been noted. One involves a reduction in flow rates 1 h after challenge, with resolution 3 to 4 h after exposure. In another, a reduction in flow rates occurs much later, the day after the exposure, and occasionally recurrent abnormalities can be manifest for several days. Recurrent symptoms of nocturnal asthma for several days have also been reported after exposure to a number of agents.[18]

Management

Once it has been determined that an individual has developed asthma due to workplace exposure, he or she should be removed from the offending environment. Although some studies have suggested use of certain therapeutic agents, such as cromolyn for bakers' asthma,[52] can inhibit physiological changes triggered by the offending agent, protection is not complete. Because it is sometimes difficult to convince the patient to change jobs, an alternative to this is the use of a protective mask to prevent airway exposure to the offending agent. The inciting agent dictates the

type of protective headgear employed. For example, subjects working with low-MW compounds require helmet respirators with an isolated air source to prevent exposure. If the subject continues to work in the implicated environment, pulmonary function tests should be done frequently to rule out progressive physiological impairment.

DISABILITY DETERMINATION

Documentation of impairment associated with objective physiological changes occurring primarily at the workplace suggests an occupation-related disorder. Patients with asthma due to an occupational exposure should be referred to the appropriate compensation or review board. The American Thoracic Society[1] has developed guidelines for the evaluation of impairment and disability due to this disorder. Determination of initial impairment should be made after optimal treatment of the asthma has been given. Impairment should be assessed using lung function tests, or measurements of airway hyperresponsiveness using (1) methacholine or histamine; (2) documentation of the type and amount of medication required to treat the patient; and (3) observation of the effect of the disease on the patient's life-style.

Specific Examples

ANIMAL HANDLERS' ASTHMA

For several years it has been known that there is a high incidence of asthma and rhinitis among workers in animal care facilities.[24] Development of symptoms tends to occur following a period of months or years of exposure. Symptoms of asthma are often preceded by rhinitis, conjunctivitis, or urticaria occurring primarily at work. In one study,[9] 56 percent of individuals who had been exposed to laboratory animals for 3 months or more complained of respiratory symptoms. Skin testing to animal-associated allergens may be helpful in determining individuals at risk for developing this syndrome. In addition, a prior history of atopy, elevated serum IgE levels, and positive skin tests against nonanimal environmental allergens also predict the development of asthma in animal handlers.[43] Approximately one-third of individuals with a history of atopy will develop asthma when exposed to laboratory animals for more than 3 months.[48] Although multiple allergens—including molecules found in the pelt, serum, and urine of the animal—may be involved, a major allergen is the rat urinary allergen.[43] In one study, specific IgE antibody to this protein correlated very well with reported asthmatic symptoms in animal handlers.[43] Serum IgG antibody to this protein was also present in animal handlers with symptoms, but it was present in a significant number of asymp-

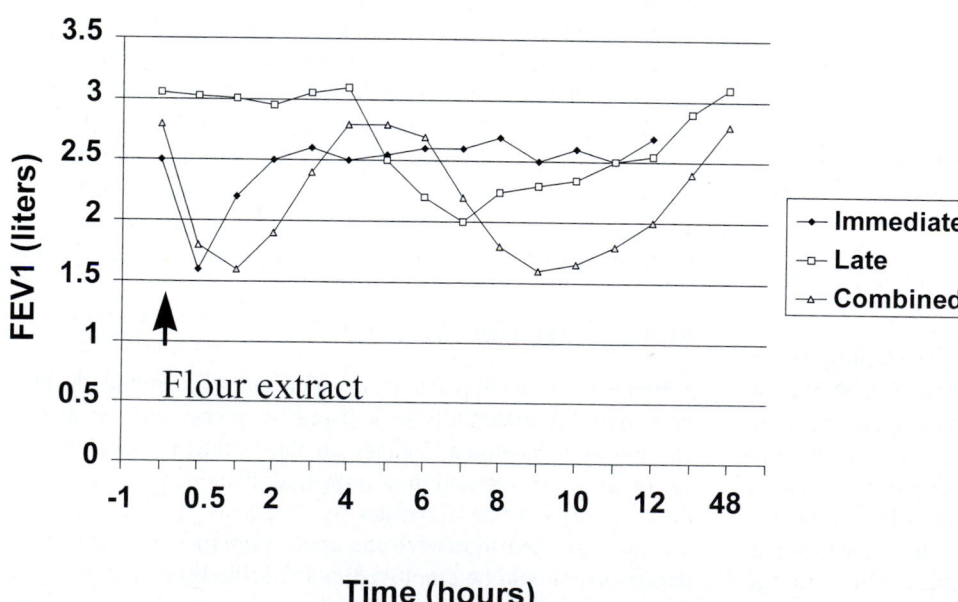

FIGURE 60-1 Examples of early, late, and combined reactions to inhalation of a specific agent (in this case, flour extract) implicated in causing occupational asthma. Flow rates are plotted versus time after inhalational exposure.

tomatic subjects as well. Antirat urinary protein IgG antibody appeared to be simply a marker of exposure, while IgE antibody was integrally associated with onset of asthma.

Avoidance of exposure to laboratory animals is the best treatment for this condition. Although one study[36] has documented that airway reactivity does not tend to worsen in these individuals even if they remain on the job, chronic exposure most likely perpetuates airway inflammation. If the individual cannot avoid the exposure, use of a helmet respirator, enabling him or her to completely avoid inhalation of the protein allergen, can prevent symptoms. Worker education regarding avoidance of airborne allergens can also be useful in controlling symptoms.[6]

SOY DUST ASTHMA

In 1981, an epidemic of emergency room visits for asthmatics was noted in Barcelona, Spain.[53] The increase in the number of visits was sporadic; it occurred in a well-defined period of time, after which visits decreased to baseline numbers, followed by another increase in numbers. Several theories regarding the cause of the apparent regional epidemic were proposed. It was not until 1987[2] that the increase in emergency room visits was connected to unloading of soybeans into a defective silo. This silo had a defective filtration system, resulting in inadequate protection of the ambient air from the soybean dust. Subsequently studies showed that asthmatics involved in the outbreaks had a much higher incidence (74 percent) of IgE antibodies to soybean extracts when compared to controls (5 percent).[51] After adequate filters were placed in the defective silo, epidemics of asthma exacerbations disappeared in Barcelona. Although this is not a pure example of occupational asthma because nonworkers as well as workers were involved, it demonstrates how airborne substances related to industrial activity can cause significant disease.

ASTHMA IN CRAB PROCESSORS

Approximately 16 percent of workers who process snow crabmeat will develop asthma due to work exposure.[12] The majority of individuals who develop this problem exhibit nonspecific airway hyperreactivity at the time of diagnosis. Studies have suggested that asthma in this setting is due to an immediate hypersensitivity reaction to a component of the crab. One study showed that immediate hypersensitivity skin reactivity or the appearance of specific IgE antibody to crabmeat extracts or the cooking water used in crab processing correlated with the development of asthma.[13] Water extracts were more potent than the meat extract.

Much as in other forms of occupational asthma, the syndrome in crabmeat processors can become chronic even after removal of the individual from the implicated work environment. In one study,[27] 19 of 31 subjects with the syndrome continued to have symptoms of asthma after being removed from exposure for an average of 1 year. The propensity to develop chronic symptoms appeared to correlate with the time of employment in the crab processing plant. As with other causes of occupational asthma, it is important to identify susceptible individuals early, so that they can be removed from the offending environment.

BAKERS' ASTHMA

Cereal flours can induce a specific IgE reaction in a high percentage of exposed subjects. Epidemiologic studies of bakers' asthma have been most complete in Germany, where it has been shown that IgE-mediated immediate skin test reactivity in bakers is directly related to their time in service. One study[26] has shown that 20 percent of bakers' apprentices develop positive skin tests after 5 years of service. Exposed individuals can develop specific IgE antibodies and skin test reactivity to flour antigens without developing asthma symptoms. Thus, these tests are mainly a parameter of exposure. However, in one study, the percentage of bakers with documented occupation-related airway disease had a much higher concentration of IgE antibody than did unselected bakers who had been employed for a similar period of time.[3] Overall, 7 to 20 percent of bakers developed allergic symptoms, including asthma, that manifest primarily at the workplace.[52] Symptoms can be minimized by using properly occlusive masks, although most subjects find these devices difficult to wear during the entire work shift. Airway reactions to inhaled flour dust allergens can also be reduced by pretreatment with cromolyn sodium.[52] However, no studies have documented that cromolyn can reduce symptoms at the workplace or prevent chronic respiratory abnormalities from developing.

BIOLOGIC ENZYME—INDUCED ASTHMA

Detergents containing proteolytic enzymes from bacteria were first noted to cause asthma in 1966.[25] Biologic enzymes associated with asthma include trypsin, pancreatin, papain, pepsin, flaviastase, and bromelain. These proteins appear to induce an immediate hypersensitivity reaction, as specific IgE antibodies have been demonstrated in some instances. Attempts to reduce this problem have included changes in the detergent preparations so that the molecules will be less readily inhaled.

ASTHMA DUE TO LATEX GLOVES

Urticaria and asthma occur in a small number of subjects who are exposed to rubber latex by wearing gloves[28] or working in doll factories.[38] Risk factors for developing sensitization to latex are (1) frequent use of disposable gloves, (2) the presence of prior atopic disease, and (3) prior or current hand dermatitis.[28] Approximately 80 percent of patients with asthma due to latex develop contact urticaria upon wearing gloves. A large percentage of patients also report rhinitis and conjunctivitis upon exposure to latex gloves. Skin tests using extracts of latex are usually positive in affected individuals. Treatment is limited to avoidance of latex-based products.

ASTHMA DUE TO ACID ANHYDRIDES

These low-MW compounds are used in numerous industries, including the curing of epoxy and alkyl resins, production of plasticizers and adhesives, and the manufacture of drugs.[17] Specific acid anhydride compounds used include trimellitic acid (TMA), phthalic acid (PA), tetrachlorophthalic acid (TCPA), and malic acid (MA). All of these compounds have been associated with induction of asthma. TMA exposure has been associated with several different syndromes: (1) an irritant syndrome, (2) early asthma and rhinitis, (3) late-onset dyspnea with systemic symptoms ("TMA flu"), and (4) pulmonary infiltrates with hemoptysis.[55] The irritant syndrome does not require a latency period, while the other three syndromes require a period of exposure to the acid anhydride prior to development. Asthma caused by these compounds appears to be due to the development of specific antibodies to the acid anhydride coupled to a body protein. Specific IgE and IgG antibodies to TMA coupled to human serum albumin have been noted.[40,41,55] In one study,[41] total IgE levels were a good parameter of exposure, while specific IgE levels correlated with symptoms of asthma and skin test positivity. The absence of a specific IgE antibody to TMA strongly argues against that agent as the cause of asthma in a specific patient. Another study has shown that IgG in serum from sensitized patients can trigger histamine release by basophils. In contrast to asthma caused by high-MW compounds, atopy does not appear to be a definite risk factor for development of asthma due to acid anhydrides. However, a history of smoking may be a risk for the development of asthma due to these agents.[24] Removal of the employee from the environment is the most efficacious form of therapy for the disorder. Employee education regarding exposure can also be useful. Even with removal from the offending environment, affected subjects may continue to have symptoms for as many as 5 years after changing work.[37] Specific IgE antibody may also be detected several years after discontinuation of exposure.[37]

ISOCYANATE-INDUCED ASTHMA

Isocyanates are highly reactive chemicals used in a number of industries. Prominent in this regard is their use in the production of polyurethane, which is found in paints, varnishes, flexible foams, and adhesives.[17] Major forms of isocyanates include toluene diisocyanate (TDI), diphenyl methane diisocyanate (MDI), and hexamethylene diisocyanate (HDI). Exposure to TDI has been most associated with the development of asthma, and TDI is also the most chemically reactive isocyanate. Overall 5 to 30 percent of exposed workers develop airway symptoms.[8] There is some evidence that HLA class II alleles are associated with increased risk for the development of isocyanate-induced asthma. Isocyanates can cause an irritation syndrome similar to that due to acid anhydrides, which occurs without significant latency. In one reported case, a subject was exposed to large concentrations of TDI and developed airway symptoms within hours of the exposure.[35] Twelve years after exposure, the patient continued to manifest TDI as well as nonspecific airway hyperreactivity. More commonly, isocyanates induce an asthma syndrome that develops after exposure to the substance for weeks to years.[33] When subjects develop asthma due to these agents, they will also manifest bronchoconstriction after exposure to the substances in a controlled setting, such as an exposure chamber, and will usually manifest nonspecific airway reactivity to methacholine or histamine. Isocyanates may also induce chronic airway abnormalities in the absence of symptoms. One study, which examined the decremental fall in flow rates in workers exposed

to TDI, predicted a 2-L greater loss in FEV_1 over 40 years in these workers as compared with appropriate controls.[21]

Isocyanates cause asthma by inducing intense airway inflammation.[22] Bronchoalveolar lavage studies have demonstrated increased numbers of neutrophils and eosinophils in the airways of subjects with asthma due to isocyanates, particularly those that manifest a late airway reaction upon controlled exposure. Bronchial biopsies of affected patients also show intense inflammation, much of which is lymphocytic. Why inflammation is induced by these agents is controversial. There are studies suggesting that isocyanates may interact directly with elements that modulate inflammation. Because these compounds are very reactive, they may affect membrane receptors or enzymes involved in inflammatory pathways.[24] However, because of the latency period that is commonly required prior to the development of isocyanate-induced asthma, an immunologic mechanism is likely. Lymphocyte-mediated and humoral responses have been proposed. One study has demonstrated specific IgE and IgG antibodies to isocyanates coupled to human serum albumin in sera of individuals with symptoms and positive inhalation challenge tests with isocyanates.[14] Although the levels of both of these subclasses of immunoglobulins tends to correlate with airway responsiveness to the isocyanate, the IgG level tends to be more predictive.

As with other forms of occupational asthma the most efficacious treatment for individuals affected with isocyanate-induced asthma is removal from the offending environment. Once the individual has become sensitized, very low concentrations of the particular agent can induce bronchospasm,[24] so transfer of the individual to an area that is in close proximity to isocyanate use is not effective management. Bronchoconstriction following controlled isocyanate exposure can be attenuated by inhaled or oral corticosteroids.[23] However, use of these agents should not replace removal of the patient from the work exposure. Use of respirators prophylactically in areas with high concentrations of isocyanates is important to prevent the development of asthma. There have been reports of persistent isocyanate-induced asthma even after removal of the subject from the offending environment. One study[32] reported persistent respiratory symptoms in 83 percent of workers who had been away from isocyanate exposure for 4 years. Another study[24] demonstrated that 7 of 12 subjects with TDI-induced asthma continued to have nonspecific airway hyperreactivity 2 years after removal from the work environment.

ASTHMA DUE TO WESTERN RED CEDAR WOOD DUST

Workers are at risk for developing asthma due to wood dust exposure.[17,24] Although a number of woods are associated with this problem, the syndrome due to western red cedar is best characterized and the causative agent within the dust has been identified. Overall 5 percent of workers who are exposed to western red cedar dust develop symptoms of wheezing and cough after a latency period of months to years.[16] The mean latency period prior to development of symptoms is 50 months.[16] Workers who develop the syndrome usually have nonspecific airway hyperreactivity to methacholine or histamine. In addition, a specific airway reaction to plicatic acid, a component of the wood dust, manifest by an early or late reduction in flow rates after exposure, is usually present.

Mechanisms of western red cedar–induced asthma are not totally defined. Plicatic acid, which makes up approximately 50 percent of the total extractable fraction of the wood dust, induces bronchoconstriction in affected subjects.[39] Those subjects who manifest an early and late airway response to inhalation of plicatic acid generally have had a longer exposure to the western red cedar dust. Specific IgE antibodies to plicatic acid coupled to human serum albumin have also been detected in 28 to 40 percent of subjects with the syndrome.[39]

Like other forms of occupational asthma due to low-MW compounds, subjects with the syndrome due to western red cedar can continue to have symptoms even when they are removed from the offending environment. In one study, 60 percent of affected individuals continued to have symptoms after leaving the industry.[17] For this reason, the identification of individuals and specific jobs that place individuals at risk is important. Use of protective devices may reduce exposure and subsequent development of asthma due to this dust, but this has not been systematically addressed.

ASTHMA DUE TO METAL SALTS

Platinum used in electroplating, platinum refinery, and jewelry making has been noted to cause asthma.[17] Smoking is a definite risk factor for development of asthma due to this metal. Airway responses to preparations of complex salts of platinum have been documented in affected workers.[42] In addition, positive skin-prick tests and specific IgE antibodies to platinum conjugated to albumin have also been found.[24] There has been one report of hyposensitization being useful for prevention of symptoms, but this has not been verified.[18] Exposure to nickel, chromium, cobalt, vanadium, and tungsten carbide has also been associated with development of asthma. Welders are commonly exposed to nickel fumes when welding stainless steel.[17]

SOLDERING FLUX ASTHMA

Various fluxes—including aluminum solder flux, which contains aminoethylethanolamine, and colophony—have been associated with and felt to cause asthma.[17] One study documented occupational asthma in 21 percent of workers in the plant of a consumer electronics manufacturer.[10] Colophony fumes can also induce bronchoconstriction in affected individuals when given as a controlled exposure. However, skin tests and RAST evaluations using extracts of colophony have failed to show positive results in affected workers.[17] Thus, the mechanism(s) of these reactions is unknown. They may very well be secondary to the irritant properties of the fumes.

REFERENCES

1. American Thoracic Society Ad Hoc Committee on Impairment/ Disability Evaluation in Subjects with Asthma: Guidelines for the evaluation of impairment/disability in patients with asthma. *Am Rev Respir Dis* 147:1056–1061, 1993.
2. Anto JM, Sunyer J, Rodriguez-Roisin R, et al: Community outbreaks of asthma associated with inhalation of soybean dust. *New Engl J Med* 320:1097–1102, 1989.
3. Baldo BA, Krilis S, Wrigley CW: Hypersensitivity to inhaled flour allergens. *Allergy* 35:45–56, 1980.
4. Bardana EJ Jr: Occupational asthma and related respiratory disorders. *Dis Mon* 41:143–199, 1995.
5. Beck GJ, Schachter EN, Maunder LR, Schilling RSF: A prospective study of chronic lung disease in cotton textile workers. *Ann Intern Med* 97:645–651, 1982.
6. Bothan PA, Davis GE, Teasdale EL: Allergy to laboratory animals: A prospective study of its incidence and the influence of atopy in its development. *Br J Ind Med* 44:627–632, 1987.
7. Bouhuys A, Schoenberg JB, Beck GJ, Schilling RSF: Epidemiology of chronic lung disease in a cotton mill community. *Lung* 154:167–187, 1977.
8. Brooks SM: Bronchial asthma of occupational origin. *Scand J Work Environ Health* 3:53–72, 1977.
9. Bryant DH, Boscato LM, Mboloi PN, Stuart MC: Allergy to laboratory animals among animal handlers. *Med J Aust* 163:415–418, 1995.
10. Burge PS, Edge G, Hawkins R, et al: Occupational asthma in a factory making flux-cored solder containing colophony. *Thorax* 36:828–834, 1981.
11. Burge PS: Single and serial measurements of lung function in the diagnosis of occupational asthma. *Eur J Respir Dis Suppl* 123:47–59, 1982.
12. Cartier A, Malo JL, Forest F, Lafrance M: Occupational asthma in snow crab processing workers. *J Allergy Clin Immunol* 74:261–269, 1984.
13. Cartier A, Malo JL, Ghezzo H, et al: IgE sensitization in snow crab–processing workers. *J Allergy Clin Immunol* 78:344–348, 1986.
14. Cartier A, Grammer L, Malo JL, et al: Specific serum antibodies against isocyanates: Association with occupational asthma. *J Allergy Clin Immunol* 84:507–514, 1989.
15. Castellan RM, Olenchock SA, Kinsley KB, Hankinson JL: Inhaled endotoxin and decreased spirometric values. *New Engl J Med* 317:605–610, 1987.
16. Chan-Yeung M, Lam S, Koener S: Clinical features and natural history of occupational asthma due to western red cedar (*Thuja plicata*). *Am J Med* 72:411–415, 1982.
17. Chan-Yeung M, Lam S: Occupational asthma. *Am Rev Respir Dis* 133:686–703, 1986.
18. Chan-Yeung M, Malo J-L: Occupational asthma. *New Engl J Med* 333:107–112, 1995.
19. Chan-Yeung M, Brooks SM, Alberts WM, et al: Assessment of asthma in the workplace. *Chest* 108:1084–1117, 1995.
20. Cooper JAD Jr, Buck MG, Gee JBL: Vegetable dust and airway disease: Inflammatory mechanisms. *Environ Health Perspect* 66:7–15, 1986.
21. Diem JE, Jones RN, Hendrich DJ: Five-year longitudinal study of workers employed in a new toluene diisocyanate manufacturing plant. *Am Rev Respir Dis* 126:420–428, 1982.
22. Fabbri CM, Boschetto P, Zocca E: Bronchoalveolar neutrophilia during late asthmatic reactions induced by toluene diisocyanate. *Am Rev Respir Dis* 136:36–42, 1987.
23. Fabbri LM, DiGiacomo R, Dal Vecchio C: Prednisone, indomethacin and airway responsiveness in toluene diisocyanate sensitized subjects. *Bull Eur Physiopathol Respir* 21:421–426, 1985.
24. Fine JM, Balmes JR: Airway inflammation and occupational asthma. *Clin Chest Med* 9:577–590, 1988.

25. Flindt MLH: Pulmonary disease due to inhalation of derivatives of *Bacillus subtilis* containing proteolytic enzyme. *Lancet* 1:1177–1181, 1969.

26. Herxheimer H: The skin sensitivity to flour of bakers' apprentices. *Acta Allergol* 28:42–49, 1973.

27. Hudson P, Cartier A, Pineau L, et al: Follow-up of occupational asthma caused by crab and various agents. *J Allergy Clin Immunol* 76:682–688, 1985.

28. Hunt LW, Fransway AF, Reed CE, et al: An epidemic of occupational allergy to latex involving health care workers. *J Occup Environ Med* 37:1204–1209, 1995.

29. Kamat SR, Kamat GR, Salpekar VY, Lobo E: Distinguishing byssinosis from chronic obstructive pulmonary disease: Results of a prospective 5 year study of cotton mill workers in India. *Am Rev Respir Dis* 124:31–40, 1981.

30. Kay JP: Trades producing phthisis. *0 Med Surg* 1:357, 1831.

31. Proust A: *Traite d'hygiene publique et privee.* Paris, Masson, 1877, p 171.

32. Lozewicz S, Assoufi BK, Hawkins R: Outcome of asthma induced by isocyanates. *Br J Dis Chest* 81:14–22, 1987.

33. Mapp CE, Polato R, Maestrelli P: Time course of the increase in airway responsiveness associated with late asthmatic reactions to toluene diisocyanate in sensitized subjects. *J Allergy Clin Immunol* 75:568–572, 1985.

34. Merino VL, Lombart RL, Marcon RF, et al: Arterial blood gas tensions and lung function during acute responses to hemp dust. *Am Rev Respir Dis* 107:809–812, 1973.

35. Moller DR, McKay RT, Bernstein IL: Persistent airways disease caused by toluene diisocyanate. *Am Rev Respir Dis* 134:175–176, 1986.

36. Newill CA, Eggleston PA, Prenger VL, et al: Prospective study of occupational asthma to laboratory animal allergens: Stability of airway responsiveness to methacholine challenge for one year. *J Allergy Clin Immunol* 95:707–715, 1995.

37. Newman Taylor AJ, Venables KM, Durham SR: Acid anhydrides and asthma. *Int Arch Allergy Appl Immunol* 82:435–439, 1987.

38. Orfan NA, Reed R, Dykewicz MS, et al: Occupational asthma in a latex doll manufacturing plant. *J Allergy Clin Immunol* 94:826–830, 1994.

39. Paggiaro PL, Chan-Yeung M: Patterns of specific airway response in asthma due to western red cedar (*Thuja plicata*): Relationship with length of exposure and lung function measurements. *Clin Allergy* 17:333–339, 1987.

40. Patterson R, Addington W, Banner A: Anti-hapten antibodies in workers exposed to trimellitic anhydride fumes: A potential immunopathogenetic mechanism for the trimellitic anhydride pulmonary disease-anemia syndrome. *Am Rev Respir Dis* 120:1259–1267, 1979.

41. Patterson R, Zeiss CR, Roberts M, et al: Human antihapten antibodies in trimellitic anhydride inhalation reactions: Immunoglobulin classes of anti-trimellitic anhydride antibodies and hapten inhibition studies. *J Clin Invest* 62:971–978, 1978.

42. Pepys J, Pickering CAC, Hughes EG: Asthma due to inhaled chemical agents: Complex salts of platinum. *Clin Allergy* 2:391–396, 1972.

43. Platts-Mills TAE, Longbottom J, Edwards JL: Airborne allergens associated with asthma: Particle sizes, carrying dust mite and rat allergens measured with a cascade impactor. *J Allergy Clin Immunol* 77:850–857, 1986.

44. Rylander R: Diseases associated with exposure to plant dusts: Focus on cotton dust. *Tubercle Lung Dis* 73:21–26, 1992.

45. Schachter EN: Occupational airway disease. *Mt Sinai J Med* 58:483–493, 1991.

46. Schilling RSF, Goodman N: Cardiovascular disease and cotton workers: Part I. *Br J Ind Med* 8:77–82, 1951.

47. Schilling RSF: Worldwide problems of byssinosis. *Chest* 79:3S–5S, 1981.

48. Slovak AJM, Hill RN: Laboratory animal allergy: A clinical survey of an exposed population. *Br J Ind Med* 38:38–41, 1981.

49. Spencer H: *Pathology of the Lung,* 2d ed. New York, Pergamon Press, 1968.

50. Subcommittee on "Occupational Allergy" of the European Academy of Allergology and Clinical Immunology: Guidelines for the diagnosis of occupational asthma. *Clin Exp Allergy* 22:103–108, 1992.

51. Sunyer J, Anto JM, Rodrigo MJ, Morell F: Case-control study of serum immunoglobulin-E antibodies reactive with soybean in epidemic asthma. *Lancet* 1:179–182, 1989.

52. Thiel H, Ulmer WT: Bakers' asthma: Development and possibility for treatment. *Chest* 78(suppl):400–405, 1980.

53. Ussetti P, Roca J, Augusti AGN, et al: Asthma outbreaks in Barcelona. *Lancet* 2:280–281, 1983.

54. Weiner A: Bronchial asthma due to organic phosphate insecticide. *Ann Allergy* 19:397–401, 1961.

55. Zeiss CR, Patterson R, Pruzansky JJ, et al: Trimellitic anhydride-induced airway syndromes: Clinical and immunologic studies. *J Allergy Clin Immunol* 60:96–103, 1977.

56. Zetterstrom O, Ostermann K, Machado L: Another smoking hazard: Raised serum IgE concentrations and increased risk of occupational allergy. *Br Med J* 283:1215–1217, 1981.

TOXIC INHALATIONS

David A. Schwartz / Christine A. Blaski

Many fumes, gases, vapors, dusts, and other inhaled substances have potentially toxic effects that are manifested by pulmonary as well as extrapulmonary injury. Exposure by inhalation occurs in industrial settings as well as in the home, in public places, and in other environments. This chapter describes the pathology and pathophysiology relating to various inhaled toxins and specifically addresses a number of common and medically significant inhalation exposures. It focuses primarily on accidental inhalation exposures without addressing intentional inhalation of toxic agents. The scope of the chapter is limited to the acute and long-term effects of inhaled agents that manifest pulmonary and extrapulmonary injury through predominantly irritant mechanisms.

Finally, several inhalation exposures that result in systemic illness through other mechanisms are discussed.

DETERMINANTS AND MECHANISMS OF IRRITANT-INDUCED PULMONARY INJURY

Inhaled toxins exist in many forms and may be categorized according to their physical properties. General categories include gases, vapors, fumes, aerosols, and smoke. Tables 61-1 and 61-2 summarize the physical properties of these inhalants. The initial pathologic responses to a harmful inhaled agent depend on a number of factors, including the concentration of the substance in the ambient air, the pH of the inhaled substance, the presence and size of particles, the relative water solubility of the inhaled agent, the duration of exposure, and whether the exposure occurs in an enclosed space or in an area with adequate ventilation and free circulation of fresh air. In addition, an undetermined number of host factors—including age, smoking status, the presence of preexisting pulmonary or extrapulmonary disease, and the use of respirators or other protective breathing apparatus—all affect a person's response to the inhalation of a toxic substance.[27,44]

Inhaled gases with potential irritant effects manifest their actions at different anatomic locations in the respiratory system.[27,44] In general, substances that are highly water soluble—such as ammonia, sulfur dioxide, and hydrogen chloride—can cause immediate irritant injury to the upper airway. The acute effects of highly water-soluble irritants on the upper airway, exposed skin, and other mucous membranes often produce such unpleasant symptoms that exposed persons quickly leave the area of exposure, and avoid continued inhalation of the harmful toxins. In contrast, inhaled toxins that have low water solubility, such as phosgene, ozone, and oxides of nitrogen, often have little or no acute effect on the upper airway, and instead produce irritant effects at the level of the terminal bronchiole and alveolus. Because agents of low water solubility do not produce immediately noticeable upper-airway irritation (except in episodes of massive acute exposure), exposed persons may inadvertently remain in the area of exposure, and thus increase their duration of exposure to harmful inhalants. Agents that exhibit intermedi-

TABLE 61-1

Definitions of Types of Inhaled Substances

Gas:	A formless state of matter in which molecules move freely about and completely occupy the space of enclosure
Aerosol:	A relatively stable suspension of liquid droplets or solid particles in a gaseous medium
Vapor:	The gaseous form of a substance that normally exists as a liquid or solid and generally can be changed back to a liquid or solid by either an increase in ambient pressure or a decrease in the temperature
Fume:	An aerosol of solid particles generally less than 0.1 μm in size that arises from a chemical reaction or condensation of vapors, usually after volatilization from molten materials
Smoke:	The volatilized gaseous and particulate products of combustion whose particles are generally less than 0.5 μm in size and do not settle readily

SOURCE: Adapted from Kizer.[27]

TABLE 61-2

Physical Properties and Mechanisms of Lung Injury of Gaseous Respiratory Irritants

Irritant Gas	Water Solubility	Mechanism of Injury
Ammonia	High	Alkali burns
Chlorine	Intermediate	Acid burns, reactive oxygen species
Hydrogen chloride	High	Acid burns
Oxides of nitrogen	Low	Acid burns, reactive oxygen species
Ozone	Low	Reactive oxygen species
Phosgene	Low	Acid burns
Sulfur dioxide	High	Acid burns

SOURCE: Adapted from Schwartz.[44]

ate water solubility, such as chlorine, can have pathologic effects throughout the respiratory system. However, extreme exposure to any one of these irritants may result in upper and lower respiratory tract involvement. Absorption of any one of these irritants on particulate matter may also alter the area of involvement.

In addition to solubility, the size of inhaled particles is important in the pathogenesis of the toxic inhalation injury.[27] Aerosols, dusts, fumes, and smoke can produce upper-airway injury as well as parenchymal damage. The location and extent of injury depend on the size of the inhaled particles as well as the intensity of the exposure. Particles that are 5.0 μm or less in diameter have the ability to penetrate into the lower respiratory tract, and often produce significant injury at the level of the terminal bronchioles and alveoli. Zinc chloride (hexite) particles, for example, have an average diameter of 0.1 μm, and it is estimated that up to 20 percent of the inhaled zinc reaches the bronchiolar level, with the remainder deposited in more proximal airways.[21] The particles themselves may have direct toxic effects, or they may serve as vehicles for adsorbed gaseous agents that are carried more distally into the lungs and do harm when they interact with terminal bronchioles and alveolar cells.

Irritants directly injure cells through nonimmunologically me-

diated mechanisms of injury and inflammation. Cell injury involves the deposition or formation of an acid (chlorine, hydrogen, chloride, oxides of nitrogen, phosgene, and sulfur dioxide), alkali (ammonia), or reactive oxygen species (ozone, oxides of nitrogen, and possibly chlorine).[2,44] The primary injury is localized in airway epithelial tissues, but extensive damage may also occur in subepithelial and alveolar regions. Acid injury results in coagulation of the underlying tissue, while acute injury due to alkali results in liquefaction of the mucosa and deep penetrating lesions in the airways. Reactive oxygen species include oxygen-derived metabolites (such as hydrogen peroxide and hydrochlorous acid) and oxygen-derived free radicals (such as superoxide anions and hydroxyl radicals). These reactive oxygen species may injure tissues and cells through lipid peroxidation that can directly injure cells and lead to elaboration of inflammatory mediators that can perpetuate the initial damage.[2] Regardless of the initial mechanism of irritant injury, inflammatory mechanisms that involve networks of proinflammatory cytokines may be subsequently initiated. The resultant inflammation may be important with regard to perpetuation of the acute injury as well as long-term sequelae. In addition, disruption and eventual repair of the airway epithelia may decrease the host's ability to defend against future inhaled infectious or irritant substances.

PATHOGENESIS AND CLINICAL PRESENTATION OF TOXIC INHALATION INJURY

Upper Airway

ACUTE INJURY

The potential for an inhaled substance to acutely injure the upper airway depends largely on that substance's irritant qualities. Water solubility and particle size, as well as duration and intensity of exposure, influence the host response to a specific exposure. Upper-airway injury due to the inhalation of toxic agents entails a number of pathophysiological mechanisms. Irritants produce injury through direct contact with the skin and mucous membranes. Tissue and cellular damage can result from the injurious effects of acid, alkali, or reactive oxygen species. Acidic substances or those that react to form acids coagulate the underlying tissue. In contrast, alkalotic substances cause liquefaction of the surface mucosa and lead to further penetrating injury of deeper structures.[44] Reactive oxygen species are engaged in a variety of cellular and tissue disruptions through lipid peroxidation.[2] The cellular injuries that result from the actions of acids, alkali, and reactive oxygen species may include loss of epithelial cell layer integrity, influx of inflammatory cells and mediators, and leakage of interstitial fluid. The initial insult to the airway epithelia decreases their ability to function as a protective barrier between the environment and the subepithelial layers. Disruption of the epithelium by inhaled toxins exposes underlying inflammatory cells, nerves, muscles, and blood vessels. The resulting inflammation, edema, and stimulation of neuronal afferent receptors may all contribute to the clinical manifestations.

Persons exposed to irritants that injure the upper airway often have associated injury to exposed mucous membranes and skin. Clinical presentations include burns of exposed skin and corneas, rhinitis, conjunctivitis, tracheobronchitis, and oral mucositis. Persons exposed to upper airway irritants may experience burning sensations of the eyes, nasal passages, and throat; profuse lacrimation and copious sputum production may also occur. Coughing and sneezing may be prominent symptoms. Upper-airway injury from irritant inhalants is generally acute and self-limited. Life-threatening upper-airway obstruction due to mucosal edema, large amounts of secretions and sloughed epithelial cells, or laryngospasm can occur in cases of massive acute exposure. Hoarseness or stridor may warn of impending airway compromise, and patients presenting with either of these physical findings must be carefully observed and may require emergency management of acute upper-airway obstruction.

Treatment for most inhaled substances is not specific; instead, it addresses removal of the patient from the exposure. Basic principles of airway management are paramount because the most likely acute life-threatening manifestation of this injury is upper-airway obstruction due to a combination of tissue edema, thick secretions, and laryngospasm. Frequent suctioning of secretions is often required. Provision of adequate supplemental oxygen is necessary if there is evidence of hypoxemia. Inhaled racemic epinephrine may be useful for patients susceptible to upper-airway obstruction, but it should not be employed as a substitute for emergency airway management by endotracheal intubation or tracheotomy if that is necessary. Corticosteroids have not been conclusively shown to influence outcome, but they are suggested in cases with extensive upper-airway edema. Toxic substances that remain on the skin or mucosal surfaces should be removed by irrigation with large amounts of water. Basic principles of burn management should be applied to skin and mucosal surface burns. Ophthalmologic consultation is recommended for management of injuries to the corneas or other eye structures.

Conducting Airways

ACUTE INJURY

Inhaled irritants that penetrate to the conducting airways are capable of inducing immediate as well as long-lasting injury through a variety of mechanisms. The airway epithelium provides a barrier that protects inflammatory cells and submucosal structures (nerves, vessels, and muscle) from direct exposure to environmental agents. Disruption of the integrity of this protective barrier can be caused by a variety of environmental agents and may result in edema, inflammation, direct smooth-muscle contraction, and stimulation of neuronal afferent receptors. Moreover, this primary lesion in the airway epithelium can facilitate stimulation by subsequent agents that come in contact with the denuded epithelial surface.

The tight junction between epithelial cells appears to be the primary site of injury after exposure to a variety of gases and aerosols. For instance, cigarette smoke has been shown to damage the airway epithelium by disrupting the tight junctions between epithelial cells, resulting in increased permeability to other unrelated irritants, such as horseradish peroxidase.[6] Similarly, hamsters exposed to nitrogen dioxide gradually develop severe disruption of tight junctions between bronchial epithelial cells.[9] Ozone[30] has also been shown to increase airway epithelial permeability. Thus, damage to the airway epithelium, particularly at tight junctions, renders the respiratory mucosa permeable to other inhaled substances, which are then able to penetrate the subepithelial mucosal region. These agents may directly interact with effector cells in subepithelial mucosa. Thus, they may have direct smooth-muscle bronchoconstrictive effects; they may also stimulate parasympathetic sensory afferent nerve endings, resulting in extensive bronchoconstriction.[22]

Inhalation of irritant gases and aerosols may cause airway hyperresponsiveness by initiating a localized inflammatory response. Inhalation studies with allergens and specific environmental irritants have demonstrated that neutrophils and eosinophils are recruited within a few hours to the airway and alveolar surface, and this response has been shown to persist for at least 48 h after this type of challenge.[31] Moreover, the number of mast cells, eosinophils, and airway epithelial cells obtained by bronchoalveolar lavage (BAL) following an aerosol challenge has been found to correlate strongly with the degree of airway hyperreactivity in mildly atopic asthmatics.[49] Inflammatory cells such as neutrophils appear to be critical elements in the development of airway hyperreactivity after exposure to ozone.[16]

Damage to the airway epithelium and inflammation of the subepithelial mucosa may contribute to the development of airway disease in persons exposed to irritant gases and aerosols. Inhaled agents, either allergens or irritants, may cause mucosal inflammation that subsequently results in increased epithelial permeability. The altered epithelial permeability exposes subepithelial irritant receptors, which are subsequently at risk of being stimulated by a variety of agents, including cold air, changes in humidity and temperature (exercise), and cigarette smoke. Damage to the airway epithelium from cigarette smoke is associated with increased epithelial permeability and an inflammatory reaction characterized by mucosal edema and infiltration of neutrophils.[20] In addition, direct damage to the airway epithelium may result in decreased production of epithelial-derived bronchodilating substances and neutral endopeptidases that would normally serve to reduce the effects of bronchoconstricting agents.[20]

The inflammatory response in the epithelial and subepithelial regions can result in chronic remodeling of the underlying airway architecture. Striking inflammatory changes—such as extensive collagen deposition beneath the epithelial basement membrane, eosinophil infiltration, and mast cell degranulation—are seen in transbronchial biopsy specimens obtained from asthmatic persons following aerosol challenges.[4] Chronic bronchitis, an inflammatory state characterized by neutrophil infiltration, is strongly associated with airway hyperresponsiveness and has been demonstrated in animals after exposure to irritant gases.[44] Release of mediators—such as histamine, leukotrienes, prostaglandins, neutrophil chemotactic factors, platelet-activating factor, tachykinins, cytokines, and growth factors—from a variety of structural and inflammatory cells in the airway and subepithelial region may significantly contribute to the chronic inflammatory response that has been well documented in asthma and in other forms of chronic airway disease.

Changes in the structure of the airways may significantly enhance the development of airway reactivity and contribute to the development of respiratory symptoms. Baseline airway caliber appears to be an important determinant of airway hyperresponsiveness.[37] The airway caliber can be influenced by a variety of factors, including the tone of the airway smooth muscle and the overall thickness of the subepithelial region. The thickness of the subepithelial region is influenced by edema and inflammation. Of interest is that inflammation and edema of the submucosal region not only may decrease airway caliber but also may alter airway smooth-muscle mechanics, resulting in maximal contraction following stimulation of the airway smooth muscle. Similarly, chronic changes in the architecture of the basement membrane may also alter smooth-muscle length-tension relations.

Lower-airway injury resulting from irritant toxic inhalation can be manifested as transient or long-lasting intrathoracic airflow obstruction. The precise mechanism of the obstruction is not clear, but it probably entails one or more inflammatory mechanisms. Exposed persons who are cigarette smokers or who have preexisting airway obstruction may be at increased risk for the persistence of toxin-induced airflow obstruction. Significant clinical manifestations of lower airway injury may not be initially recognizable, but may develop and worsen over the first 24 to 48 h after exposure. Hospitalization for observation is indicated for initially asymptomatic exposed subjects with any objective evidence of respiratory compromise, such as decreased airflow, abnormalities of gas exchange, or an abnormal chest radiograph, or whose exposure history is suggestive of a relatively intense exposure. In addition, persons who report respiratory symptoms including dyspnea or chest tightness should be hospitalized, followed closely with objective measures of pulmonary function, and treated symptomatically, even in the absence of objective abnormalities.

Spirometry findings may initially be normal, but in some cases progressive airflow obstruction develops; thus, a case can be argued for obtaining baseline airflow indices and following the exposed subject with spirometry over the first 24 to 48 h after exposure. For persons without significant decrements in airflow but with symptomatic chest tightness or wheezing, inhaled steroids are essential and bronchodilators may be useful. In cases that demonstrate airflow obstruction (FEV$_1$ of 80 percent or less than predicted, or 10 percent or less than the patient's initial baseline), a short course of systemic corticosteroids may be beneficial in addition to the use of inhaled steroids and bronchodilators. However, there is no definitive evidence that treatment with parenteral corticosteroids substantially relieves the airflow obstruction or prevents the onset of bronchiolitis obliterans.

CHRONIC INJURY

Obstructive Airway Disease

Previously healthy people who experience acute toxic inhalation may go on to develop clinical and pathologic features of chronic obstructive pulmonary disease (COPD). Inhaled irritants most often implicated in the development of chronic bronchitis, emphysema, or reversible airflow obstruction are chlorine[33] and sulfur dioxide.[10] However, definitive evidence that demonstrates a causal relationship between a toxic exposure and resultant chronic respiratory disease is at times difficult to elicit. This is often because of the frequent concomitant presence of potentially confounding factors, most prominently cigarette smoking, that independently increase any person's risk for the development of COPD. Nevertheless, there is some evidence that acute exposure to a number of inhaled irritants may produce conditions in the conducting airways that lead to a complex interaction of inflammation, smooth-muscle activity, and neuronal inputs that are active in the creation and perpetuation of varying degrees of fixed and reversible airflow obstruction. The initial irritant insult to epithelial cells appears to be central to subsequent abnormal function and continuing injury processes that invade the epithelium as well as subepithelial structures. Repair of the acute injury may also contribute to resultant chronic airflow obstruction by scarring and other mechanical factors. Disruption of normal protective structures and mechanisms may also predispose exposed persons to chronic pulmonary infections. In addition, damage to and destruction of functional alveoli may affect ongoing inflammatory and repair processes that have been initiated by the acute irritant exposure.

The development of irritant-induced COPD appears to depend on the intensity of the exposure. In addition, underlying host factors, including cigarette smoking and preexisting pulmonary disease, may increase a person's likelihood of developing COPD. It is extremely difficult to accurately assess the potential contribution of acute irritant inhalation to chronic lung disease in cigarette smokers. Baseline measures of pulmonary function can help determine the presence of preexisting disease, but unfortunately this information is often unavailable, especially in cases of accidental acute exposure. Evaluation of possible irritant-induced COPD includes a thorough history, physical examination, radiographic evaluation, and objective measures of pulmonary function, including spirometry, measurement of lung volumes, determination of diffusing capacity, and assessment of gas exchange. Frequent measurement of spirometry may help determine progression or regression of airflow abnormalities. Treatment is as for COPD due to causes other than acute irritant exposure and includes bronchodilators, corticosteroids, smoking cessation, and, if necessary, supplemental oxygen.

Reactive Airway Dysfunction Syndrome

The persistence of airway reactivity after acute exposure to respiratory irritants has been termed reactive airway dysfunction syndrome (RADS).[8] A variety of inhaled irritants have been associated with this syndrome, including sulfuric acid, chlorine, ammonia, household cleaners, and smoke. Most often, the initial inhalation injury is due to a single acute, high-intensity exposure. Symptoms of airflow obstruction, including cough, dyspnea, and wheezing, are reported immediately or several hours after the end of the exposure, and may persist for months to years. Previous exposure or sensitization to the toxic agent does not appear to be necessary. By definition, persons who develop RADS have no history of respiratory illness. Pulmonary function test results may be normal, or they may demonstrate airflow obstruction. Persons with RADS have persistent positive responses to methacholine challenge testing, even in the presence of normal pulmonary function test results. Nonspecific bronchial reactivity may persist for months to years after the initial inhalation injury.

Bronchial biopsies of patients with RADS demonstrate an inflammatory response characterized by epithelial desquamation and mucous cell hyperplasia. The exact mechanisms of the pathophysiology of RADS are unclear, but implicated mechanisms include altered neural tone and vagal reflexes, modified β-adrenergic sympathetic tone, and influences of a number of proinflammatory mediators. The direct irritant injury may expose and damage subepithelial irritant receptors. Subsequently, repair mechanisms that are not fully understood may result in alteration of the irritant receptor threshold and lead to airway hyperreactivity. Changes in epithelial permeability may also contribute to the resultant hyperreactivity. None of these proposed mechanisms is completely understood at this time.

Treatment of RADS includes the use of corticosteroids to help minimize inflammatory mechanisms, and bronchodilators to reverse bronchospasm. There is limited, mostly anecdotal, evidence for the efficacy of corticosteroids. Bronchodilators may only partly alleviate airflow obstruction—especially in later, chronic stages of the syndrome.[18] Despite treatment with corticosteroids and bronchodilators, many exposed persons may be left with persistent asthmalike symptoms, airflow obstruction, and nonspecific bronchial hyperreactivity.

Pulmonary Parenchyma

ACUTE INJURY

Toxic inhaled agents that have relatively low water solubilities, such as phosgene, ozone, and nitrogen oxides, produce most of their irritant damage distal to the upper airway. Because of the relatively low solubilities of these substances, inhalation does not typically result in upper-airway irritation and its associated symptoms. As a result, subjects may endure continued exposure to the toxic gases and thus increase the total time and amount of exposure. In addition, massive acute inhalation of gases and aerosols that have intermediate (chlorine) or high water solubilities (ammonia, sulfur dioxide) can overwhelm the absorptive capacity of the upper airway and injure more distal structures (Fig. 61-1). Damage may be particularly severe when particulates form part of the inhaled substance. The reasons for this are not fully understood, although it is possible that particle deposition in the alveoli provides a nidus for ongoing inflammation and subsequent severe injury. Respirable particles with diameters in the range of 0.3 to 0.5 μm can bypass the upper airways and can be deposited in the more distal airways and alveoli.[27] The clinical consequences of these injuries include diffuse bronchiolar inflammation and obstruction as well as alveolar filling (pulmonary edema). Atelectasis may result from destruction or disruption of the surfactant layer. Persons who have sustained an initial toxic

insult to the lower airways and lung parenchyma may be more susceptible to subsequent pulmonary infections because of damage to inflammatory cells, including alveolar macrophages, that provide host defense against infectious agents.

The lower respiratory tract and alveoli are susceptible to injury from many inhaled toxins. In general, the extent and severity of acute lung injury due to a toxic inhalant appear to be dose related. The clinical and histopathologic features of toxin-associated pulmonary edema and adult respiratory distress syndrome (ARDS) are not unique to any particular inhalant. Instead, many different inhaled toxins can damage the pulmonary parenchyma via what appear to be common pathways that are identical or at least qualitatively similar to those that cause acute lung injury secondary to causes other than toxin inhalation. Unlike some focal processes that progress to ARDS, however, the initial inhalation of toxins is more likely to produce a diffuse, relatively homogeneous acute lung injury.

Regions of the lower respiratory system that are susceptible to toxin injury include the airway epithelium, subepithelial mucosa, alveolar lining cells, and vascular endothelium. Alveolar type I epithelial cells seem particularly susceptible to acute injury from inhaled substances. Some of the mechanisms engaged in the general epithelial injury described in the previous section also apply to injury to the epithelia of the lower airway and alveoli. Damage can result in focal and confluent areas of edema with protein-rich fluid in the alveolar spaces, hyaline membrane formation, and denudation of the alveolar epithelium. Mucous membranes of the bronchial and bronchiolar walls may be destroyed or denuded.

Pulmonary parenchymal injury that results from inhalation of irritant substances runs the spectrum of acute lung injury and includes pneumonitis, pulmonary edema, and ARDS. Pneumonitis is the most frequent parenchymal manifestation of inhalation injury. Clinical features include dyspnea, productive or dry cough, hypoxemia, mild restriction of ventilation, decreased alveolar gas diffusion, and diffuse bilateral infiltrates on the chest radiograph. Generally, pneumonitis caused by toxic inhalation is a self-limited process, with clinical improvement mirrored by rapid clearing of infiltrates seen on the chest radiograph. Treatment is supportive, usually includes supplemental oxygen, and may require mechanical ventilation. The use of corticosteroids has not been shown to be of significant benefit in the treatment of pneumonitis secondary to the inhalation of irritant gases such as chlorine, ozone, and phosgene, but may be indicated in cases of known inhalation of fumes from some metals, such as mercury, cadmium and zinc, which have been reported to progress to severe and sometimes fatal acute lung injury. As it is for toxic pneumonitis, the treatment of toxin-induced pulmonary edema and ARDS remains largely supportive, and may include hemodynamic monitoring and mechanical ventilation.

CHRONIC INJURY

Bronchiolitis Obliterans
Bronchiolitis obliterans can occur as a late consequence of the inhalation of several toxins (Fig. 61-2). Exposures to ammonia, mercury, oxides of nitrogen, and sulfur dioxide have been associated with bronchiolitis obliterans.[17,26,29,40] High-intensity inhalation exposures can be followed by acute pulmonary edema

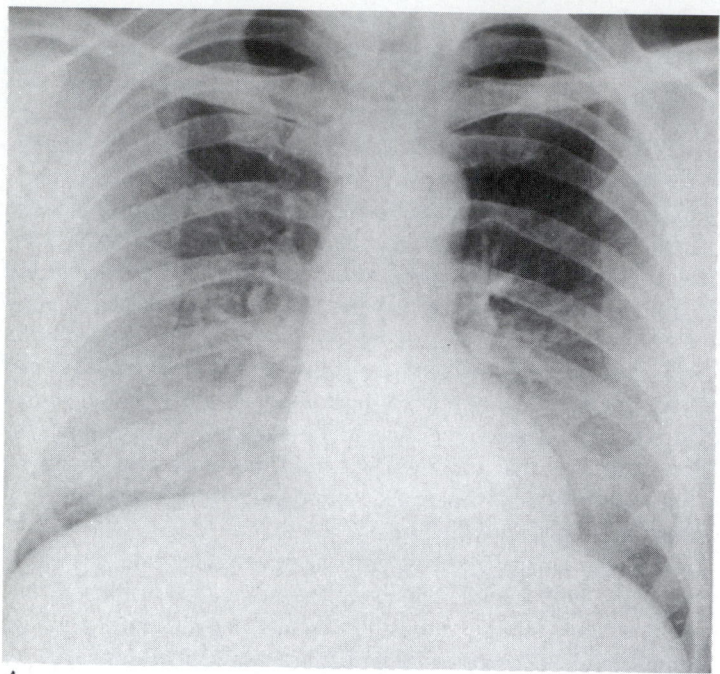

A

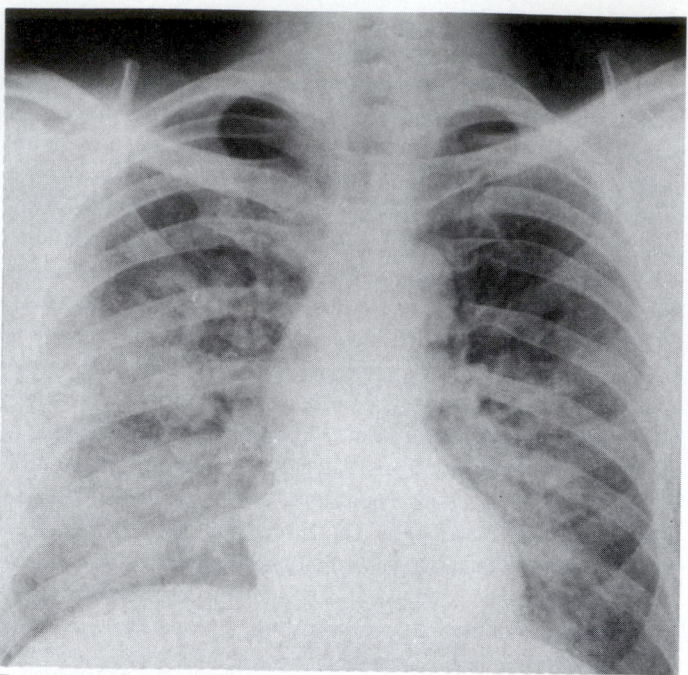

B

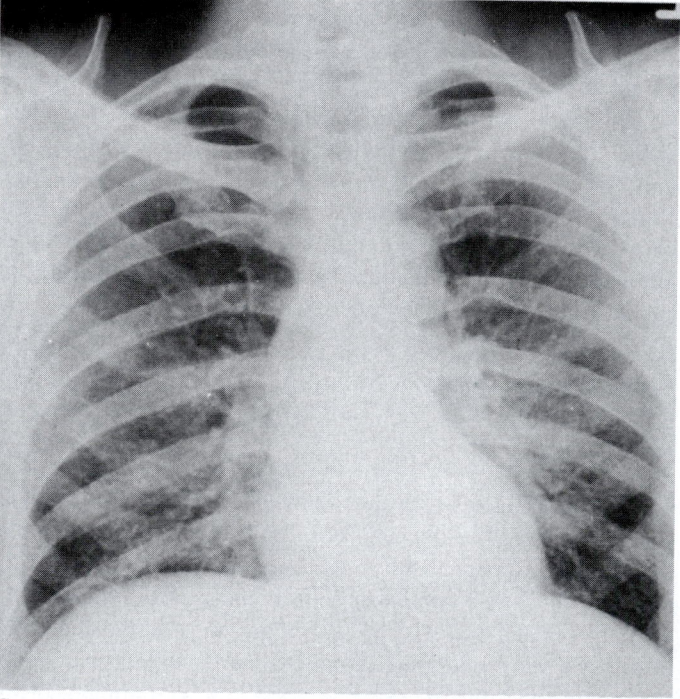

C

FIGURE 61-1 Accidental exposure of 55-year-old mechanic to spill of liquid Cl_2, followed immediately by coughing and dyspnea. *A.* Day of exposure. Bilateral alveolar infiltrates, most marked on right. *B.* Two days later. Progression of alveolar infiltrates. *C.* Seven days later. Incomplete resolution of infiltrates associated with persistent shortness of breath.

and ARDS. Survivors of the acute lung injury may experience a relatively asymptomatic period that is followed by the development of irreversible airflow obstruction, which often presents 1 to 3 weeks after the initial injury. Early inspiratory crackles are a characteristic physical exam finding. The appearance of the chest radiograph is variable, and may demonstrate the degree of clinical severity. Patients with mild cases can have normal chest radiographs, while more severely affected persons may demonstrate hyperinflation. Infiltrates are generally absent. Pulmonary function tests typically demonstrate airflow obstruction that may in some cases also be associated with restrictive defects. The histologic picture is characterized by the presence of granulation tissue plugs within the lumen of small airways and occasionally alveolar ducts, as well as by the destruction of small airways with obliterative fibrous scarring.

The pathophysiology of bronchiolitis obliterans due to toxin inhalation is not well understood. The predominance of neutrophils in the BAL fluid of some patients with bronchiolitis obliterans clearly identifies an active inflammatory process, but the exact mechanisms at work are not well defined. The process may not respond to treatment with corticosteroids; however, a 6-month trial of corticosteroids should be given. Bronchodilators may be efficacious in some symptomatic patients, although clearcut evidence of this potential benefit is not available.

Bronchiolitis Obliterans–Organizing Pneumonia

Bronchiolitis obliterans–organizing pneumonia (BOOP) may also be a late or delayed consequence of the inhalation of toxic substances.[14,15] The clinical presentation is characterized by a persistent, nonproductive cough, fever, sore throat, and malaise.

The lung exam typically reveals late inspiratory crackles but no wheezes; many patients have no abnormalities on physical exam. The characteristic chest radiograph findings include bilateral, patchy, "ground glass" densities, which start as focal lesions but may coalesce with time. In contrast to patients with bronchiolitis obliterans, those with BOOP present with restrictive ventilatory physiology and decreased diffusing capacity.

The histology of BOOP includes the presence of granulation tissue in the small airways and alveolar ducts, as in bronchiolitis obliterans. In addition, however, the granulation tissue extends into the alveoli and may result in interstitial scarring. This distinction between the histologic features of BOOP and those of "pure" bronchiolitis obliterans (without organizing pneumonia)

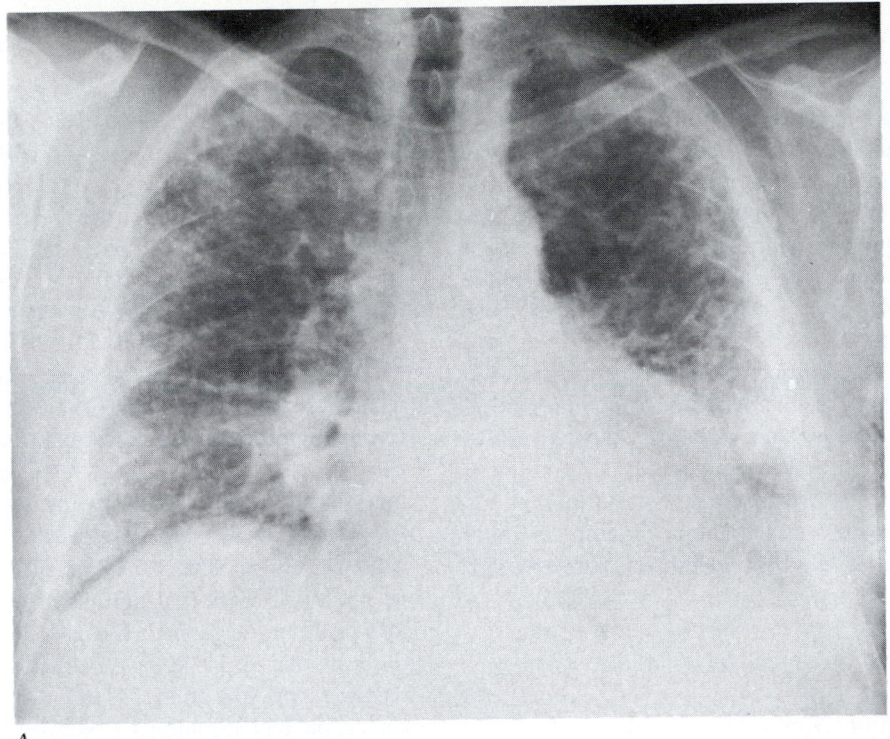

A

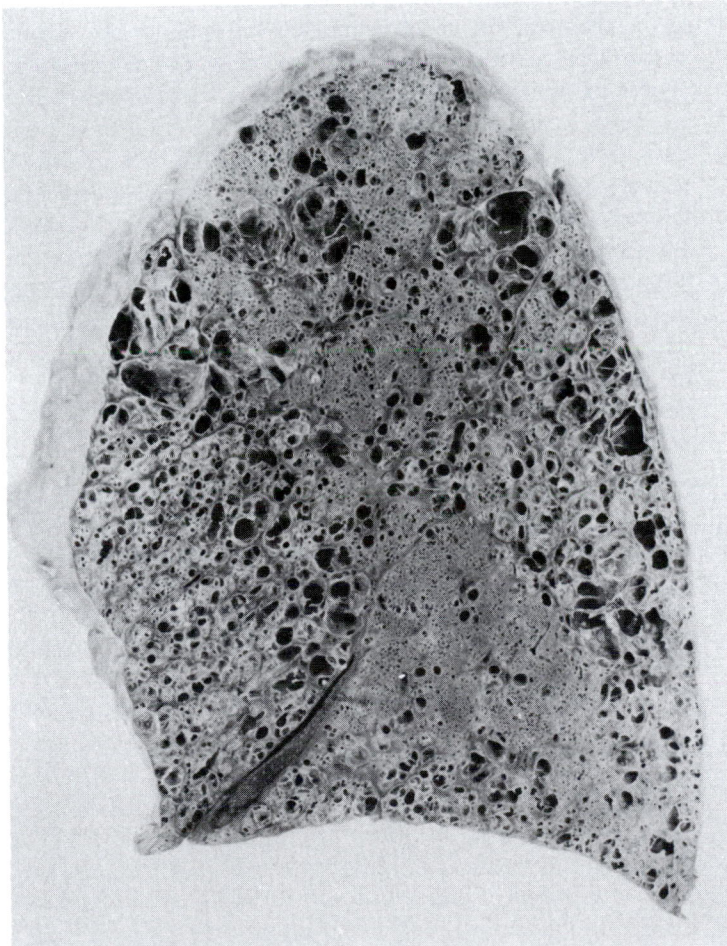

B

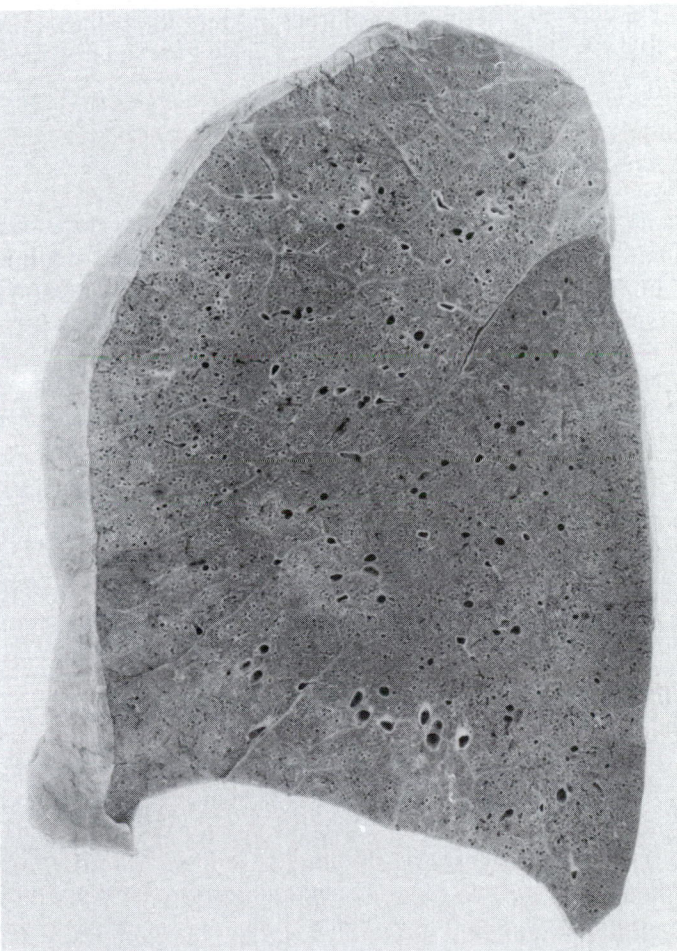

C

FIGURE 61-2 Bronchiolitis obliterans in a 63-year-old man who had been exposed to a wide variety of unidentified fumes in his jobs, which included welding. *A.* Chest radiograph. Diffuse pulmonary fibrosis and honeycombing, most marked in the peripheral portions of the lungs. *B.* Sagittal section of lung from same patient showing markedly dilated airspaces. Microscopic sections revealed bronchiolitis obliterans and chronic interstitial pulmonary fibrosis. *C.* Normal lung from a 43-year-old man who died suddenly. The difference between *B* and *C* in the alveolar portions of the lungs is striking. *(Courtesy of Dr. R. Ochs.)*

may reflect different host responses to similar inhaled toxins.[14] Examination of the granulation tissue plugs from patients with BOOP demonstrates temporal uniformity in a patchy distribution with the preservation of background architecture. BAL fluid demonstrates a neutrophilic alveolitis; lymphocytes may also be prominent. These findings suggest that the pathologic process results from an initial insult (e.g., an inhaled toxin), with subsequent inflammatory and reparative processes.

Treatment of BOOP with corticosteroids often results in dramatic clinical improvement. Pulmonary function abnormalities can lessen considerably, and in some cases may rapidly resolve. The radiographic abnormalities also rapidly clear. A small number of patients may not respond to corticosteroid therapy and may develop progressive fibrosis. Duration of therapy is generally at least 6 months but should be guided by the rate and completion of the clinical response.

EFFECTS OF SPECIFIC INHALED TOXINS ON THE RESPIRATORY SYSTEM

The following sections specifically address the pulmonary effects of a number of inhaled toxins. Table 61-3 summarizes the acute and long-term manifestations.

Ammonia

Ammonia is a highly water-soluble substance that is extensively used in the manufacturing, chemical, and agricultural industries. Its uses are many, and include the manufacture of explosives, cyanides, synthetic fibers, and plastics. It also has applications in petroleum refining, as a cleaning agent, and as a refrigeration system coolant. Its high nitrogen content makes ammonia a commonly used soil fertilizer; it can be applied in its liquid form or dissolved in water. Most inhalation exposures are the result of accidental releases, including tank leaks and transportation mishaps.[1,32,40]

Exposure to ammonia gas or vapors causes immediate irritation of the mucosal surfaces of the eyes, skin, nasopharynx, oropharanx, larynx, and trachea. Ammonia reacts with water that is present on mucosal surfaces to form ammonium hydroxide, which in turn forms hydroxyl ions. This exothermic reaction contributes to thermal burns that form part of the initial injury. In addition, chemical injury results from alkali burns that are deeply penetrating and result in tissue liquefaction. Cutaneous burns, which may be disfiguring, are deepest in areas with the highest moisture content. Burn injuries to the eyes may result in permanent visual impairment and include damage to the corneal endothelium, corneal stroma, iris, and lens; these burns are often more severe than those caused by other alkalis because of ammonia's ability to deeply penetrate tissues. Initial injury to the mucosa of the oropharynx may result in edema, hemorrhage, and sloughing of tissue and can result in fatal upper-airway obstruction.

The severity of ammonia-induced injury depends on the concentration and duration of exposure. Lower airway and pulmonary parenchymal injury can occur acutely with high-intensity exposures. It is characterized by pulmonary edema, hemorrhage, and atelectasis. A biphasic pattern of pulmonary response to ammonia inhalation has been reported, characterized by initial, acute pneumonitis that may clear over the next 2 to 3 days, followed in some patients by the gradual development of airway obstruction and respiratory failure.[1] Bronchopneumonia due to superinfection with bacterial organisms is common. Bronchiectasis and focal bronchiolitis obliterans have been associated with this late phase; although the mechanism of this delayed injury is unclear, there is speculation that the acute injury may result in impaired host defenses that subsequently lead to the delayed, sometimes life-threatening, or chronic and debilitating abnormalities.

TABLE 61-3

Pulmonary Manifestations of Toxin Inhalation

| Substance | Onset | Acute Clinical Manifestations | | Chronic Clinical Manifestations | | |
		Upper Airway Irritation	Pneumonitis, ARDS	Bronchiolitis Obliterans, BOOP	Obstructive Lung Disease	RADS
Irritant						
Gases						
Ammonia	Minutes	Severe	+	+	+	+
Chlorine	Minutes to hours	Moderate	+	−	+	+
Hydrogen chloride	Minutes	Severe	+	−	−	+
Oxides of nitrogen	Hours	Mild	+	+	+	+
Ozone	Minutes to hours	Mild	+	−	−	−
Phosgene	Hours	Mild	+	−	+	−
Sulfur dioxide	Minutes	Severe	+	+	+	+
Metals						
Cadmium	Hours	Mild	+	−	+	−
Mercury	Hours	Mild	+	+	−	−
Zinc chloride	Minutes	Mild	+	−	−	−
Zinc oxide	Hours	Mild	+	−	−	−

NOTE: + = exposure reported to be associated with clinical entity;
− = exposure as yet not reported to be associated with clinical entity.

Initial treatment of persons exposed to ammonia gas or vapors includes immediate irrigation of all exposed surfaces, especially eyes, with copious amounts of water. The airway must be secured, and in some persons emergency tracheotomy is necessary. Evidence of lower airway and pulmonary parenchymal injury is best assessed initially by physical exam. The presence of rales determines the subsequent hospital course, even in the absence of hypoxemia and chest radiograph abnormalities.[1] Treatment of pulmonary impairment is supportive, and includes supplemental oxygen and mechanical ventilation with positive pressure if indicated. The use of corticosteroids is controversial, and prophylactic antibiotics have not been shown to clearly improve outcome.

Chlorine, Chloramine, and Hydrochloric Acid

Chlorine (Cl_2) is a highly reactive gas that is widely found in industrial, environmental, and home settings. One of its earliest recognized uses was as a chemical warfare agent. Its nonmilitary uses are as a bleaching agent in the textile and paper industries and as part of water purification processes at swimming pools and sewage systems. Episodes of toxic inhalation exposure are most often the result of accidental releases and spills. Common settings for chlorine exposure are secondary to transportation accidents, industrial mishaps, and accidental spills or releases at swimming pools and sewage treatment facilities.[13,43]

Chlorine reacts with water to form hydrochloric acid (HCl) and hypochlorous acid (HOCl). These products, as well as elemental chlorine itself, exert various irritative effects on the respiratory system. Chlorine has intermediate water solubility, and its inhalation can therefore result in irritation of the upper and lower respiratory tracts. Its mechanism of cellular injury appears to entail the generation of oxygen free radicals. HCl and HOCl, on the other hand, are highly water soluble, and thus exert significant irritative effects on the mucous membranes of the upper respiratory tract and ocular conjunctivae. Lower respiratory irritation is less common with these acids, although it has been reported following acute, high-intensity exposures. The mechanisms of injury proposed for HOCl may have to do with the inhibition of enzymes, reactions in vitro with sulfhydryl groups in cysteine, and formation of N-chloroderivatives. HCl is an irritant and acts to coagulate underlying tissues.

The clinical manifestations of the inhalation of chlorine and its derivatives are similar to those of other inhaled gases that have similar solubility profiles. Because chlorine has intermediate water solubility, its irritant effects are manifested throughout the respiratory system, and include immediate rhinitis, conjunctivitis, and skin irritation, as well as cough, dyspnea, and chest tightness.

In addition to the toxic effects of chlorine and its derivatives discussed above, a significant number of toxic inhalation exposures are of products that result from the mixing of chlorine compounds and other substances. Many of these exposures are to household cleaning agents.[41] Chloramine gas is formed when chlorine or hypochlorous acid is mixed with ammonia. Chloramine gas, in turn, decomposes to ammonia and HOCl or HCl when it comes into contact with water. Ammonia, HOCl, and HCl are all highly water soluble, and therefore have primarily upper respiratory tract irritative effects. Household bleach (which contains HOCl, or hypochlorite) reacts to form chlorine gas when it is mixed with phosphoric acid or HCl. The resultant chlorine gas subsequently produces irritative symptoms throughout the respiratory tract.

Chlorine gas was one of several chemical warfare agents used in World War I. Several follow-up studies of exposed military personnel report long-lasting pulmonary impairments, including chronic bronchitis and airflow obstruction, in some victims. Others, however, apparently fully recovered from similar degrees of chlorine gas exposure. Total amount of exposure is probably the most significant determinant of long-term adverse respiratory effects following acute chlorine inhalation, although host factors that are currently not well defined may also contribute to chronic debility.[33]

Sulfur Dioxide

Sulfur dioxide is a heavy, colorless gas that is widely used in many industrial processes. Occupational settings in which sulfur dioxide is encountered include mining, ore smelting, sugar refining, and the bleaching of wool and wood pulp. Persons who experience acute, high-intensity exposure report the immediate onset of symptoms that include burning of the eyes, nose, and throat, rhinorrhea, tearing of the eyes, dyspnea, chest tightness, and cough. Extremely high-intensity, acute exposures can lead to death within minutes from respiratory failure due to a combination of alveolar hemorrhage and edema, possible reflex vagal stimulation, and the asphyxiating effect of high concentrations of sulfur dioxide.[10] Significant extrapulmonary injuries include corneal injuries, which can range in severity from superficial burns that resolve completely in days to weeks to permanent opacification; these injuries appear to be dose dependent. Less intense acute exposures can produce a broad range of upper and lower respiratory tract injuries that also appear to occur in a dose-dependent manner. Acute pneumonitis can progress to ARDS. Survivors of the acute lung injury may experience a relatively asymptomatic period that is followed several weeks later by the onset of irreversible airflow obstruction due to bronchiolitis obliterans.[50] Other victims may demonstrate immediate, persistent airflow obstruction and nonspecific bronchial hyperreactivity consistent with RADS.[8]

Sulfur dioxide is highly water soluble and hydrolyzes to sulfuric acid upon contact with water on mucous membranes. While the acid injury to cellular components is not fully understood, it appears to cause direct damage via irritant mechanisms. In addition, subacute inflammation may contribute to long-term respiratory sequelae. Injury to the respiratory tract occurs in a dose-dependent manner. Acute, high-intensity exposures irritate the upper and lower airways. Injury to the proximal airways is characterized by acute denudation of the mucosa without inflammatory cell infiltrates. Alveoli may become filled with fluid, but the alveolar architecture is preserved, and the clinical picture is consistent with ARDS. Subjects who survive the initial acute injury may die weeks later with bronchiolitis obliterans. Characteristic fibrosis of the terminal bronchioles is seen on autopsy, and the alveoli are distended with alveolar septal disruption. Irritant injury to the bronchial epithelium may result in tracheobronchitis and obstructive lung disease.

Treatment of inhalation injury due to sulfur dioxide and sulfuric acid is supportive and includes supplemental oxygen, maintenance of a patent airway, and, if necessary, mechanical ventilation. Corticosteroids have not been shown to positively influence the course of ARDS due to this toxic inhalation, and they rarely provide significant benefit for patients who have developed bronchiolitis obliterans. However, a trial course of corticosteroids is not unreasonable. Bronchodilators may be helpful for patients with symptomatic airflow obstruction, but this has not been systematically studied. Prevention of acute exposure can be problematic because many serious exposures occur as industrial accidents. Persons working with or near sulfur dioxide or sulfuric acid should be aware of the potential for serious inhalation injury, should recognize initial symptoms of the irritant injury, and should have appropriate respiratory protective equipment. Workers should take particular care when entering confined, poorly ventilated areas, such as tanks, where sulfur dioxide or sulfuric acid may be present. Industrial processes that may liberate either of these substances should be administered by well-trained persons who are aware of the potential dangers.

Nitrogen Oxides

Nitrogen oxides are major components of air pollution. In addition, accidental releases of nitrogen oxide gases can occur in occupational settings and result in high-intensity exposures. Oxides of nitrogen are present in a number of industrial settings, including mining, acetylene welding, and explosives manufacturing. These gases can also be present in closed or poorly ventilated areas in which engines are operated. Perhaps the best-recognized occupational exposure to nitrogen oxides occurs in agricultural workers ("silo-filler's disease") who are exposed to silo gas that is formed by the decomposition of organic matter.[36] Clinical manifestations of toxicity include signs and symptoms of a chemical pneumonitis, the severity of which is dose dependent and is influenced by both the time and concentration of the exposure. Severe cases progress to ARDS and sometimes lethal acute lung injury, whereas less severe cases can completely resolve or result in varying degrees of chronic airway obstruction and RADS. Bronchiolitis obliterans can be a late cause of death, and may develop following a relatively asymptomatic period after the resolution of ARDS.

The mechanism of injury due to the inhalation of nitrogen dioxide is the production of nitric acid from the hydrolysis of nitrogen dioxide and water; this acid production occurs at the levels of the terminal bronchioles and alveolar membranes. Nitric acid can subsequently dissociate to nitrates and nitrites that can cause tissue injury through direct local cytotoxicity and inflammation, as well as by the formation of free oxygen radicals that can be engaged in the peroxidation of lung lipids, with resultant disruption of cellular membranes. This constellation of toxin damage may explain the clinically recognized pulmonary edema and lower airway obstruction that often result from nitrogen oxide inhalation. Animal models suggest that vascular endothelial cells may be among the first to be damaged. This initial injury may lead to increased capillary permeability, the release of vasoactive substances, and, possibly, damage to other cellular components of the pulmonary interstitium, such as fibroblasts. Hypoxemia may result from ventilation-perfusion mismatch that is due to a combination of redistribution of pulmonary perfusion and increased airway resistance.

Medical personnel who treat victims of acute inhalation exposure to oxides of nitrogen must be aware of the potential for the development of clinical manifestations of ARDS several hours after the inhalation. The treatment of the acute lung injury is supportive and includes supplemental oxygen and mechanical ventilation. In addition, awareness of the potential for the development of obstructive lung disease, including bronchiolitis obliterans, several weeks after initial apparent recovery is important. Persons who survive the acute lung injury are at risk for these later complications and should be followed closely with serial assessment of pulmonary mechanics and gas exchange. Asymptomatic hypoxemia or decrements in airflow should be closely monitored, since these patients may develop bronchiolitis obliterans. Corticosteroids may be helpful in preventing or decreasing the severity of progressive airflow obstruction, and should be considered in asymptomatic subjects who demonstrate spirometric or gas exchange abnormalities.

Prevention of exposure includes the provision of adequate ventilation and appropriate respiratory protective equipment in all environments in which nitrogen oxides may be encountered. Agricultural workers should be aware that the hazard from oxides of nitrogen in silos is greatest during the first week to 10 days after green silage has begun fermenting. Poorly ventilated silos should not be entered unless adequate respiratory protection is available, including air-supplied respirators when the oxygen level is low. Engineering controls, such as horizontal open silo designs and active ventilation of silos by air blowers, may minimize the accumulation of harmful nitrogen oxides. In addition, extra workers who may be utilized as rescue personnel should be available whenever coworkers enter silos.[36]

Phosgene

Phosgene, another gaseous toxin that has relatively low water solubility, is perhaps most notorious for its role as a war gas. Its use in World War I reportedly led to as many as 80 percent of all the gas deaths during that conflict. In modern times, phosgene is used to catalyze a number of industrial reactions. Its contemporary industrial uses include roles in the production of polyurethane resin, toluene diisocyanate, pesticides, pharmaceutical products, and dyes. In addition, it is produced from heat decomposition of various solvents, paint removers, dry-cleaning fluids, and methylene chloride.[7]

As for other inhaled toxins that have low water solubilities, phosgene produces its most recognized clinical effects through injury to the lower airway and lung parenchyma. A clinical picture of pneumonitis that can progress to ARDS results. Phosgene is hydrolyzed to HCl, and injury may occur from direct cytotoxicity or enzymatic poisoning. Damage to small airways and alveoli is manifested as epithelial necrosis. Eventually, alveolar membranes become increasingly permeable, alveolar flooding occurs, and the clinical manifestations of ARDS can be seen. Phosgene is a colorless gas that at a concentration of 1 ppm has the odor of newly mown grass or hay. At higher concentrations it has a more pungent odor and can be mildly irritating to the upper airway. Concentrations of 5 to 10 ppm inhaled for as little as 5 to 10 s can cause immediate cough, lacrimation, and mucosal irritation. A latent period of 30 min to 8 h can precede the onset of symptoms of lower airway and parenchymal irritation. The duration of the latent period is inversely proportional to the severity of exposure and is also thought to be inversely proportional to the subsequent severity of disease. Clinical manifestations of the lower airway and parenchymal effects include dyspnea, chest tightness, cough, and increasing respiratory distress. Physical exam may reveal cyanosis and rales. Chest radiographs can show diffuse bilateral infiltrates consistent with pulmonary edema. Hypoxia and decreased vital capacity are observed. Treatment is supportive, and may include mechanical ventilation with positive pressure, supplemental oxygenation, and hemodynamic monitoring. Persons who survive the acute injury can be left with chronic bronchitis or emphysema, although others may experience no long-lasting adverse clinical sequelae.[7]

Ozone

Ozone is recognized as a major constituent of environmental smog and is also present as a naturally occurring gas in the upper atmosphere, where it has a protective effect against ultraviolet radiation from the sun. It is a colorless, odorless gas that has relatively low water solubility. Chronic and acute adverse health effects from the concentrations of ozone (0.05 to 0.8 ppm) that are commonly found in ambient air have been well described and include a myriad of respiratory symptoms, as well as evidence of upper and lower airway irritation, inflammation, and airflow obstruction.[30] In the occupational setting, ozone has been implicated as a toxic inhalant in airplane cabins during high-altitude flight, in industries where it is used as an oxidizing agent, and in arc welding, where it can occur in association with oxides of nitrogen.[47]

The mechanism of respiratory injury from ozone is not fully understood, although the clinical responses suggest initial irritant effects that may ultimately implicate cytokine-mediated inflammatory pathways in the airways as well as at the alveolar level. Animal exposure response studies have suggested that the acute inhalation of ozone at a concentration of 2 ppm may directly affect alveolar type II epithelial cells and result in the production of reactive nitrogen and oxygen intermediates and other cytotoxic and inflammatory mediators. Alveolar macrophages may also contribute to the ozone-initiated inflammatory cascade.[30]

Cadmium

Cadmium is a highly corrosion-resistant metal that has many industrial applications. It is used in solder and brazing rods as well as in the manufacture of batteries, alkaline accumulators, steel alloys for electric cables, bearings, and marine hardware. It is commonly used to electroplate or galvanize metal surfaces. Cadmium is also present in many metal ores. In addition, cadmium-containing pigments are used in paints, artists' colors, rubber, plastics, printing inks, wallpaper, leather, glass, and enamels. Toxic inhalation exposures may be encountered by workers who do soldering, brazing, smelting, and refining. Plumbers, copper-

smiths, and electronic equipment assemblers may be exposed, as may be persons who engage in hobbies that include working with sheet metal.[3]

Most toxic exposures have been reported following exposure to cadmium vapors in enclosed spaces or poorly ventilated areas. Heating of cadmium-containing materials can release vapors and cadmium oxide fumes. The typical clinical presentation is similar to that for metal fume fever, and includes an initial asymptomatic period that lasts several hours and is followed by fevers, chills, and myalgias. These constitutional symptoms are often accompanied or soon followed by respiratory distress, including cough, chest tightness, and dyspnea. The chest radiograph reveals bilateral infiltrates consistent with pneumonitis. Initial pulmonary function tests can show a restrictive ventilatory defect and decreased diffusion. Fatal cases have been remarkable for initial pneumonitis that relentlessly progresses to ARDS and eventual death from respiratory failure.[39] Victims who survive the acute lung injury may be left with persistent ventilatory restriction.

The mechanisms of acute lung injury due to cadmium inhalation are not well defined. Postmortem examinations of persons who died after accidental acute inhalation exposure have revealed tracheobronchitis, consolidated lungs, denuded bronchial epithelium, intra-alveolar hemorrhage, and the presence of macrophages in the alveolar spaces.[39] Rats exposed to cadmium fumes and cadmium chloride aerosols develop pulmonary edema and on necroscopy show increased numbers of alveolar type II cells.[3]

Treatment of acute lung injury due to the inhalation of cadmium fumes is supportive and similar to treatment for other forms of acute lung injury and ARDS. Corticosteroids may help improve outcome, but their efficacy is not well established. Elevated blood and urine cadmium levels may help establish cadmium as the likely etiologic agent in cases in which the nature of the exposure is not clear. Blood levels may reflect acute exposure, while urine levels better reflect the total body burden. Monitoring of blood or urine levels during treatment has not been shown to influence the clinical outcome.[3]

Mercury

Acute mercury vapor inhalation occurs in occupational settings, including metal reclamation processing, fur and felt hat making, and dentistry. A number of other exposures—including several that resulted in fatal outcomes—have occurred in the home during amateur attempts to extract precious metals from amalgams that also contain mercury.[35,42] Common to episodes of toxic mercury inhalation is vapor generation in closed spaces or poorly ventilated areas.

Mercury vapor has little or no immediate upper airway or mucosal surface irritant effects; as a result, exposed persons may unknowingly remain in an area where the harmful vapors are present. Typical clinical presentations include symptoms of cough, dyspnea, and respiratory distress that develop 12 to 24 h after exposure. These initial symptoms are sometimes accompanied by fever, nausea, vomiting, diarrhea, and a metallic taste in the mouth, similar to what is often experienced by patients with metal fume fever and associated transient pneumonitis. In fact, mercury vapor inhalation can be mistaken for metal fume fever or influenza. Symptoms of mercury vapor inhalation do not, however, spontaneously resolve in a pattern similar to that for metal fume fever. Instead, the pneumonitis may progress to ARDS. Death due to progressive respiratory failure may ensue; pneumothorax has been reported to be a preterminal event in several cases. The severity of the injury appears to depend on the intensity of exposure and, possibly, the size and age of the exposed person. Children and small household pets seem especially vulnerable to life-threatening acute lung injury after the inhalation of mercury, but death due to respiratory failure has also been reported in exposed adults.[42] Adults who survive the acute lung injury usually experience resolution of their symptoms 2 to 7 days after onset, although longer courses of resolution have been reported for those who have sustained more severe injury.

The acute effects of inhaled mercury are usually confined to the respiratory system, although renal impairment with acute tubular necrosis has been reported.[26] The acute gastrointestinal and renal injuries that are seen after mercury ingestion are not typical of acute inhalation exposure. Chronic, low-intensity inhalation exposure may be associated with central nervous system and systemic symptoms and injury similar to that observed after ingestion.

The metabolism of inhaled mercury entails initial uptake by red blood cells and subsequent release to plasma and other tissues. Mercury produces direct irritant injury at the alveolar and bronchiolar levels. It coagulates protein, blocks cellular metabolism of carbohydrates at the pyruvic oxidase level, and, as a result, produces a metabolic acidosis.[35] The acute lung injury can be characterized by stages that include capillary damage, pulmonary edema, the desquamation and proliferation of alveolar cells, obliteration of airspaces, formation of hyaline membranes, intra-alveolar hemorrhage, and micro- and macroatelectasis. Mercury is stored in the kidneys, CNS, and other organs. Excretion occurs in exhaled breath, urine, and feces. Blood levels of mercury may reflect acute uptake, and urine levels can monitor chronic stores.

Treatment of mercury inhalation is supportive and addresses the acute lung injury. Mechanical ventilation, including positive-pressure and high-frequency oscillating ventilation, may be beneficial in the treatment of mercury-induced ARDS.[34] Corticosteroids have no proven benefit. Chelating agents, such as dimercaprol and penicillamine, frequently used to increase the rate of mercury excretion after ingestion, have not been shown to affect the outcome of the acute lung injury.[42]

Smoke Bombs (Zinc Chloride)

Zinc chloride ($ZnCl_2$, or hexite) is a major ingredient of smoke bombs.[21,23] Oxides and chlorides of zinc and chloride are formed by the ignition of hexachloroethane, zinc oxide, and calcium chloride and are produced by some of the smoke-generating devices used by the military, in firefighter training, and for the generation of special effects in the entertainment industry. Toxic inhalations have occurred when people have breathed in smoke in confined spaces, in most instances without functional protective breathing apparatus (Fig. 61-3). The smoke effect tends to contribute to the duration of exposure by obscuring vision, sometimes resulting in directional disorientation and the inability to escape quickly from the area of exposure.

$ZnCl_2$ is a hygroscopic, caustic salt that forms HCl and zinc oxychloride upon contact with water on mucous membranes and other surfaces. The severity of injury appears to be related to the intensity of the exposure, and depends both on the duration of exposure and on the concentration of zinc chloride in the smoke. Irritation and burning of the eyes, skin, and mucous membranes result. $ZnCl_2$ is present in particulate form, and the average size has been reported as 0.1 μm. This size makes it possible for relatively large amounts of the inhaled hexite to penetrate into the lower respiratory tract, and as much as 20 percent of the total may reach beyond the level of the respiratory bronchioles, while the remainder settles throughout the tracheobronchial tree. Deposition of particles in the lungs and subsequent formation of HCl may be primarily responsible for the diffuse lung injury.[23]

Signs and symptoms of tracheobronchitis and pneumonitis are common after inhalation of smoke that contains $ZnCl_2$. Initial chest radiographs can be normal, but can also show diffuse bilateral infiltrates that are consistent with pneumonitis. Hypoxemia may not be present initially, but can develop over the course of several days after the exposure as signs and symptoms of pneumonitis become more predominant. Progression to ARDS following an initial period of clinical stabilization or partial resolution has been reported. Pneumothorax is a frequent complication of the acute lung injury due to subpleural emphysema.

The treatment of $ZnCl_2$ inhalation includes oxygen supplementation and mechanical ventilatory support with positive pressure if indicated. Corticosteroids have been used, but it is unclear whether they significantly alter the clinical course. N-Acetylcysteine may minimize oxidant-induced lung injury, but it is not clear whether this influences the clinical outcome.[21] Exposed persons who survive may have persistent ventilatory and diffusion defects.

Mace and Tear Gas

Chloroacetophenone (Mace) and orthochlorobenzamalonitrile are crowd control agents commonly used by the military and law enforcement agencies. These inhaled agents, often referred to as "tear gas," have immediate, profound irritant effects on exposed mucous membranes and lacrimal glands and are used to incapacitate people. Exposure to either of these agents produces acute rhinorrhea, oral mucositis, conjunctivitis, and lacrimation. The severity of the effect is apparently related to the intensity of the exposure, and thus depends on the concentration of the agent in the ambient air, duration of exposure, and presence or absence of ventilation and protective breathing apparatus. Initial physical examination performed within hours of the inhalation exposure demonstrates irritant injury to mucous membranes and lacrimal glands, but no evidence of lower airway or parenchymal damage. Auscultation of the chest is typically clear, and the chest radiograph usually shows no abnormality. However, several case reports describe varying degrees of pneumonitis and pulmonary edema, typically developing hours to several days after the inhalation exposure. The cases reported were in persons who were exposed to tear gas for prolonged periods in poorly ventilated structures.[38,46] Controlled animal studies have also demonstrated delayed-onset pulmonary parenchymal injury and

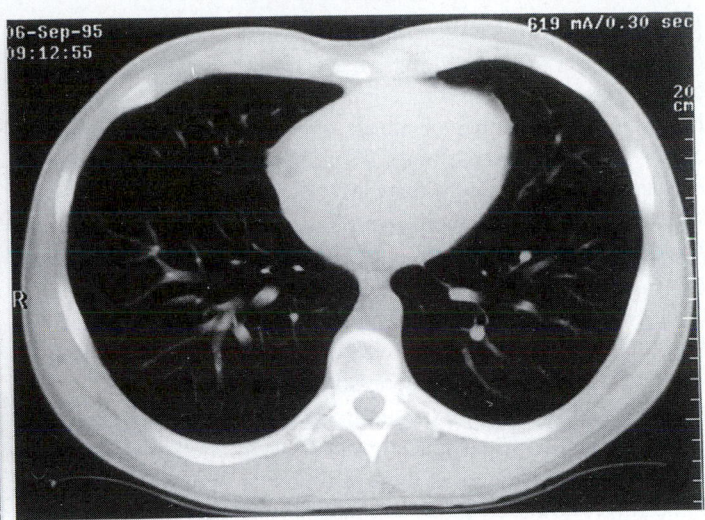

1 Week

12 Weeks

	1 week	3 weeks	12 weeks
FVC	2.5 (54%)	3.2 (68%)	5.7 (119%)
FEV$_1$	2.2 (52%)	3.0 (69%)	4.7 (107%)
FEV$_1$/FVC	88%	75%	83%
TLC	3.6 (61%)	4.9 (82%)	6.9 (114%)
RV	1.1 (90%)	1.3 (106%)	1.2 (94%)
DLCO	14 (44%)	19.1 (58%)	48.7 (141%)

FIGURE 61-3   Chest CT scan and pulmonary function tests obtained on a person with inhalation injury after a smoke bomb was ignited in an underground cave. The CT scans were obtained 1 week and 12 weeks after the accident and demonstrated extensive interstitial lung disease, which resolved on radiographs. The pulmonary function tests obtained 1, 3, and 12 weeks after the exposure demonstrated marked restrictive lung function and abnormal gas exchange, which also resolved within 3 months of exposure.

respiratory failure, with postmortem findings of pulmonary edema as well as hemorrhagic and atelectatic lungs, following exposure to high concentrations of tear gas.[12]

Treatment of inhalation injury due to tear gas is supportive and includes management of the immediate mucous membrane irritant effects, with particular attention to maintenance of a patent upper airway and frequent suctioning if necessary. Infants and small children may be at particular risk for acute airway obstruction due to copious oral and nasal secretions. Humidified supplemental oxygen may be helpful in the treatment of inadequate oxygenation due to the acute lung injury. The use of corticosteroids has not been studied in a controlled manner, and no clear evidence exists regarding its efficacy in this situation. Awareness of the potential for delayed evidence of acute lung injury is essential. Persons who have experienced relatively high-intensity inhalation exposures may benefit from hospital admission and close medical observation of their pulmonary status for several days, regardless of whether or not they demonstrate any objective evidence of lower airway and parenchymal damage at the time of initial presentation.

SYSTEMIC ILLNESS FROM INHALED TOXINS

A number of inhaled substances can cause extrapulmonary illness and injury. Metal fumes, fumes composed of heat-degraded fluorocarbons, and organic dusts have been implicated as causative agents in self-limited systemic syndromes (metal fume fever, polymer fume fever, and the organic dust toxic syndrome) that are notable for influenza-like illness with complete resolution within hours to days of exposure.[19,45,48] While some exposed persons experience only constitutional symptoms, there appears to be a continuum of illness that extends to include significant pulmonary parenchymal injury in others. The mechanisms of these syndromes are currently unknown, although recent human exposure response studies have implicated cytokine-mediated inflammation as central to the pathogenesis of metal fume fever[5] and the organic dust toxic syndrome. There is some suggestion that immune-mediated mechanisms may be responsible for the tolerance that occurs in some people who are chronically exposed to metal fumes, but the evidence for this is anecdotal and is not based on controlled studies.

Metal Fume Fever

Metal fume fever is a self-limited syndrome characterized by the delayed onset of fever, chills, myalgias, and generalized malaise after exposure to fumes that contain metal oxides. The syndrome has acquired a number of names over time, including brazier's disease, spelter shakes, brass chills, zinc chills, welder's ague, copper fever, and foundry fever. Metalworkers with the syndrome sometimes describe their symptoms as being "galvanized." Welders are the workers most often reported to experience metal fume fever, although a variety of other metalworking occupations—including soldering, brazing, cutting, metallizing, forging, melting, and casting—have been associated with exposures to metal fumes that are responsible for the syndrome. A common scenario is that of exposure to metal oxide fumes generated by welding in a closed space or poorly ventilated area. Zinc oxide is often implicated as the toxic agent responsible for metal fume fever; however, fumes composed of oxides of copper, cadmium, mercury, aluminum, antimony, selenium, iron, magnesium, nickel, silver, and tin have also been implicated.[19]

Constitutional symptoms are often preceded or accompanied by complaints of dry throat and a sweet or metallic taste in the mouth. The characteristic fever, chills, and myalgias, which are sometimes accompanied by headache and nausea, usually develop 4 to 8 h after exposure to metal fumes, and spontaneously resolve over the next 24 to 48 h. Laboratory findings are remarkable for transient leukocytosis. Tachyphylaxis appears to occur in some people who are repeatedly exposed to metal oxide fumes, usually in occupational settings. These workers often report recurrent "Monday fever" after returning to the workplace following weekend or vacation absences. Metal fume fever has been mistaken for influenza, atypical or community-acquired pneumonia, and a malaria-like illness because of overlapping presenting symptoms.

Some, but not all, affected subjects also complain of chest tightness, cough (usually nonproductive), and varying degrees of dyspnea. The chest radiograph is typically normal, but in persons with respiratory symptoms a radiographic picture consistent with pneumonitis has been reported. Pulmonary function is usually normal, although in those with symptomatic and radiographic evidence of pneumonitis, obstructive and restrictive defects, as well as abnormalities of diffusion, have been reported. Human studies that have examined the systemic and pulmonary responses to exposure to zinc oxide fumes generated by welding in an environmental chamber suggest that cytokine-mediated inflammatory mechanisms are at work.[5] There appears to be a continuum of clinical severity that ranges from the classic, self-resolving, constitutional symptoms of metal fume fever, to transient pulmonary impairment, and to more severe, sometimes even life-threatening, pulmonary injury. The predisposition to developing these more serious manifestations of metal fume exposure appears to be related to the duration and concentration of the inhalation exposure, and is most frequently reported after inhalation of fumes from zinc, mercury, and cadmium. The treatment of metal fume fever is supportive, and includes antipyretics and analgesics. Prevention includes provision of adequate ventilation, fume removal devices, and respiratory protection for workers in environments where metal oxide fumes are generated.

Polymer Fume Fever

Polymer fume fever is a syndrome with many clinical similarities to metal fume fever. It results from the inhalation of pyrolosis products of fluoropolymers, the most often reported of which is polytetrafluoroethylene (PTFE, or Teflon).[45] In addition to their popularly recognized use as nonstick coatings on cooking equipment, fluorocarbon polymers are widely used in industrial settings as mold release sprays, lubricants, and fabric or leather treatments. Heating of fluoropolymers to high temperatures results in the production of fumes composed of a vapor phase that can contain or ultimately produce carbonyl fluoride, perfluorinated alkanes, hydrofluoric acid, and carbon dioxide. Respirable particles may also contribute to the toxic elements in the heat-generated fumes.[45] The fumes produced may lead to the systemic and pulmonary toxicities through mechanisms that are not well understood.

The clinical presentation of polymer fume fever includes initial, sometimes immediate, symptoms of upper-airway irritation: dry throat, rhinitis, chest tightness, and conjunctivitis. Typically, constitutional symptoms consisting of fever, chills, and myalgias occur 4 to 8 h after exposure and spontaneously resolve over the next 24 h. Laboratory features include a transient leukocytosis. There is no consistent pattern of pulmonary function studies. However, persons with preexisting obstructive lung disease may experience worsening obstruction after recurrent exposures to polymer fumes.[25] Cough and dyspnea that are associated with wheezing and sometimes radiographic evidence of parenchymal consolidation are common. Pneumonitis accompanies constitutional symptoms more often than is reported in cases of metal fume fever. The reasons for this difference are unknown, but may relate to the release of hydrofluoric acid. Unlike the decline in the severity of metal fume fever symptoms that is observed with frequent, repeated exposures to metal fumes, tolerance does not appear to develop in people repeatedly exposed to pyrolized fluoropolymers, implying possible qualitative differences in the mechanisms of injury and host response in these two syndromes.[25]

Exposure to pyrolized fluoropolymers occurs in home and industrial settings, often in poorly ventilated areas. Humans as well as animals may suffer the effects of this form of toxic inhalation; several case reports of polymer fume fever in humans also mention the sudden deaths of pet birds that were similarly exposed. It is interesting to note that many workers who experience symptoms consistent with polymer fume fever are cigarette smokers, some of whom have reported the abrupt onset of symptoms immediately after smoking tobacco products that they have carried into the work environment. Several reports have suggested that these workers may have directly contaminated their smoking products with inert fluoropolymers that are subsequently pyrolized and inhaled in concentrated form along with the tobacco smoke. Alternatively, cigarette smoking may independently predispose persons to the development of polymer fume fever and associated acute lung injury.

Treatment of polymer fume fever is supportive and similar to that for metal fume fever. Prevention includes provision of adequate ventilation. In addition, workers should adhere to strict handwashing habits after handling products containing fluoropolymers, should not eat, drink, or smoke in the work environment, and should not carry smoking materials into work.

Organic Dust Toxic Syndrome

Organic dust toxic syndrome (ODTS), also referred to as silo unloader's syndrome, atypical farmer's lung, or pulmonary mycotoxicosis, is a self-limited illness characterized by fever, chills, myalgias, dry cough, headache, and dyspnea that occurs 4 to 8 h after exposure to large amounts of organic dusts.[48] These symptoms, although uncomfortable and sometimes transiently debilitating, usually spontaneously resolve with no long-term adverse sequelae over the next 36 to 48 h. The etiologic agents have not been fully characterized, but probably are substances that are present in moldy organic material, including fungal spores, actinomyces, endotoxin, and other components of grain dusts. These airborne substances are often encountered after the uncapping of silos that contain hay or corn silage, during the removal of layers of spoiled animal feed, or in work in swine confinement facilities. Agricultural workers are understandably at the highest risk for the development of ODTS, but others who are exposed to environments where large amounts of grains, hay, straw, or wood chips are present can also develop this syndrome. Although prior sensitization does not appear to be a characteristic feature in people who develop ODTS, those who have a history of atopy may manifest more severe symptoms than nonatopics.[24]

The physical exam in patients with ODTS is usually normal but can show the presence of bibasilar crackles and scattered wheezes. Laboratory studies reveal a neutrophil-predominant leukocytosis. Mild hypoxemia and infiltrates on chest radiograph have been reported. BAL performed early in the course of the illness may reveal a predominance of neutrophils; with time, lymphocytes may dominate the BAL cellular population.[48] Open lung biopsy in ODTS patients reveals multifocal areas of acute inflammation, with neutrophils and macrophages in terminal bronchioles, alveoli, and interstitial areas, but no evidence of granulomas. Human exposure response studies have reproduced the characteristic symptoms and laboratory abnormalities and have also demonstrated transient airflow obstruction.[11,28]

The initial symptoms of ODTS are sometimes confused with those of hypersensitivity pneumonitis. However, unlike hypersensitivity pneumonitis, ODTS is transient, can occur in previously unexposed persons, and requires a relatively intense exposure. BAL consistent with an acute neutrophilic alveolitis is different from the BAL lymphocytic predominance that has been reported throughout the entire course of hypersensitivity pneumonitis. In contrast to what is often found in cases of hypersensitivity pneumonitis, serum allergic precipitins are usually negative in persons with ODTS.[48]

The course of ODTS is benign, with spontaneous resolution of symptoms as well as laboratory and radiographic abnormalities within days of the exposure. Treatment is symptomatic. Long-term sequelae of repeated high-intensity exposures that lead to recurrent episodes of ODTS may be associated with chronic bronchitis and decrements in airflow, but these have not been clearly established. Prevention requires education of agricultural workers and other potentially exposed subjects regarding practices related to the handling of moldy hay, grains, and

other organic materials. In addition, people who engage in activities known to produce large quantities of potentially harmful airborne organic substances—such as weighing of swine and the intense handling of moldy grain, hay, straw, or wood chips—should be advised to wear respiratory protection.

SUMMARY

Inhalation exposure to a number of irritant substances produces a spectrum of pulmonary and systemic injuries. Physicians and other health-care professionals often encounter people who have experienced acute inhalation exposure to unknown types or doses of toxic substances. Treatment is generally supportive and is not specific to any particular exposure. This chapter has described typical presentations of injury resulting from a number of inhaled toxins. Awareness of the patterns of presentation and potential consequences of irritant-induced inhalation injury can help guide initial and subsequent management. Since the clinical course of these accidental inhalations is often unpredictable, it is prudent to carefully monitor, follow, and be ready to hospitalize these patients. This chapter has provided an overview of frequently encountered inhaled toxins as well as specific references to more detailed case reports, studies, and discussions. Materials safety data sheets can furnish concise information about specific substances or products. Additional information is available through computerized library search tools and on-line information services.

REFERENCES

1. Arwood R, Hammond J, Ward GG: Ammonia inhalation. *J Trauma* 25:444–447, 1985.
2. Barnes PJ: Reactive oxygen species and airway inflammation. *Free Radic Biol Med* 9:235–243, 1990.
3. Barnhart S, Rosenstock L: Cadmium chemical pneumonitis. *Chest* 86:789–791, 1984.
4. Beasley R, Roche WR, Roberts JA, Holgate, ST: Cellular events in the bronchi in mild asthma and after bronchial provocation. *Am Rev Respir Dis* 139:806–817, 1989.
5. Blanc PD, Boushey HA, Wong H, et al: Cytokines in metal fume fever. *Am Rev Respir Dis* 147:134–138, 1993.
6. Boucher RC, Johnson J, Inoue S, et al: The effect of cigarette smoke on the permeability of guinea pig airways. *Lab Invest* 43:94–100, 1980.
7. Bradley BL, Unger KM: Phosgene inhalation: A case report. *Tex Med* 78:51–53, 1982.
8. Brooks SM, Weiss MA, Bernstein IL: Reactive airways dysfunction syndrome (RADS). *Chest* 88:376–384, 1985.
9. Case BW, Gordon RE, Kleinerman J: Acute bronchiolar injury following nitrogen dioxide: A freeze fracture study. *Environ Res* 29:399–413, 1982.
10. Charan NB, Myers CG, Lakshminarayan S, Spencer TM: Pulmonary injuries associated with acute sulfur dioxide inhalation. *Am Rev Respir Dis* 119:555–560, 1979.
11. Clapp WD, Becker S, Quay J, et al: Grain dust-induced airflow obstruction and inflammation of the lower respiratory tract. *Am J Respir Crit Care Med* 150:611–617, 1994.
12. Cucinell SA, Swentzel KC, Biskup R, et al: Biochemical interactions and metabolic fate of riot control agents. *Fed Proc* 30:86–91, 1971.

13. Das R, Blanc PD: Chlorine gas exposure and the lung: A review. *Toxicol Ind Health* 9:439–455, 1993.

14. Epler GR, Colby TV, McLoud TC, et al: Bronchiolitis obliterans organizing pneumonia. *New Engl J Med* 312:152–158, 1985.

15. Epler GR: Bronchiolitis obliterans organizing pneumonia: Definition and clinical features. *Chest* 102:2S–6S, 1992.

16. Fabbri LM, Aizawa H, Alpert SE, et al: Airway hyperresponsiveness and changes in cell counts in bronchoalveolar lavage after ozone exposure in dogs. *Am Rev Respir Dis* 129:288–291, 1984.

17. Galea M: Fatal sulfur dioxide inhalation. *Can Med Assoc J* 91:345–347, 1964.

18. Gautrin D, Boulet L-P, Boutet M, et al: Is reactive airways dysfunction syndrome a variant of occupational asthma? *J Allergy Clin Immunol* 93:12–22, 1994.

19. Gordon T, Fine JM: Metal fume fever. *Occup Med* 8:505–517, 1993.

20. Hay DWP, Muccitelli RM, Wilson KA, et al: Agonist specificity in the effects of epithelium removal on contractions of the guinea pig trachea produced by leukotrienes, 5-hydroxytryptamine, and U-44069. *Pharmacologist* 28:141–148, 1986.

21. Hjortso E, Qvist J, Bud MI, et al: ARDS after accidental inhalation of zinc chloride smoke. *Intensive Care Med* 14:17–24, 1988.

22. Holgate ST, Beasley R, Twentyman OP: The pathogenesis and significance of bronchial hyperresponsiveness in airways disease. *Clin Sci* 73:561–572, 1987.

23. Homma S, Jones R, Qvist J, et al: Pulmonary vascular lesions in the adult respiratory distress syndrome caused by inhalation of zinc chloride smoke: A morphometric study. *Hum Pathol* 23:45–50, 1992.

24. Jacobs RR, Boehlecke B, van Hage-Hamsten M, Rylander R: Bronchial reactivity, atopy, and airway response to cotton dust. *Am Rev Respir Dis* 148:19–24, 1993.

25. Kales SN, Christiani DC: Progression of chronic obstructive pulmonary disease after multiple episodes of an occupational inhalation fever. *J Occup Med* 36:75–78, 1994.

26. Kanluen S, Gottlieb CA: A clinical pathologic study of four adult cases of acute mercury inhalation toxicity. *Arch Pathol Lab Med* 115:56–60, 1991.

27. Kizer KW: Toxic inhalations. *Emerg Clin North Am* 2:649–666, 1984.

28. Larsson K, Eklund A, Hansson L-O, et al: Swine dust causes intense airways inflammation in healthy subjects. *Am J Respir Crit Care Med* 150:973–977, 1994.

29. McAdams AJ, Krop S: Injury and death from red fuming nitric acid. *JAMA* 158:1022–1024, 1955.

30. Menzel DB: Ozone: An overview of its toxicity in man and animals. *J Toxicol Environ Health* 13:183–204, 1984.

31. Metzger WJ, Richerson HB, Worden K, et al: Bronchoalveolar lavage of allergic asthmatic patients following allergen provocation. *Chest* 89:477–483, 1986.

32. Montague TJ, Macneil AR: Mass ammonia inhalation. *Chest* 77:496–498, 1980.

33. Moore BB, Sherman M: Chronic reactive airway disease following acute chlorine gas exposure in an asymptomatic atopic patient. *Chest* 100:855–856, 1991.

34. Moromisato DY, Anas NG, Goodman G: Mercury inhalation poisoning and acute lung injury in a child: Use of high-frequency oscillatory ventilation. *Chest* 105:613–615, 1994.

35. Moutinho ME, Tompkins AL, Rowland TW, et al: Acute mercury vapor poisoning. *Am J Dis Child* 135:42–44, 1981.

36. NIOSH: *Criteria for a Recommended Standard: Occupational Exposure to Oxides of Nitrogen (Nitrogen Dioxide and Nitric Oxide).* Cincinnati, U.S. Dept. of Health Education and Welfare, 1976.

37. O'Connor G, Sparrow D, Tayler D, et al: Analysis of dose-response curves to methacholine. *Am Rev Respir Dis* 136:1412–1417, 1987.

38. Park S, Giammona ST: Toxic effects of tear gas on an infant following prolonged exposure. *Am J Dis Child* 123:245–246, 1972.

39. Patwardhan JR, Finckh ES: Fatal cadmium-fume pneumonitis. *Med J Aust* 1:962–966, 1976.

40. Price SK, Hughes JE, Morrison SC, Potgieter PD: Fatal ammonia inhalation: A case report with autopsy findings. *S Afr Med J* 64:952–955, 1993.

41. Reisz GR, Gammon RS: Toxic pneumonitis from mixing household cleaners. *Chest* 89:49–52, 1986.

42. Rowens B, Guerrero-Betancourt D, Gottlieb CA, et al: Respiratory failure and death following acute inhalation of mercury vapor: A clinical and histologic perspective. *Chest* 99:185–190, 1991.

43. Sabonya R: Fatal anhydrous ammonia inhalation. *Hum Pathol* 8:293–299, 1977.

44. Schwartz DA: Acute inhalational injury, in Rosenstock L (ed), *Occupational Medicine: Occupational Pulmonary Disease,* vol 2, no. 2. Philadelphia, Hanley and Belfus, 1987, pp 297–318.

45. Shusterman DJ: Polymer fume fever and other fluorocarbon pyrolysis–related syndromes. *Occup Med* 8:519–531, 1993.

46. Stein AA, Kirwan WE: Chloracetophenone (tear gas) poisoning: A clinico-pathologic report. *J Forensic Sci* 9:374–382, 1964.

47. Tashkin DP, Coulson AH, Simmons MS, Spivey GH: Respiratory symptoms of flight attendants during high-altitude flight: Possible relation to cabin ozone exposure. *Int Arch Occup Environ Health* 52:117–137, 1983.

48. Von Essen S, Robbins RA, Thompson AB, Rennard SI: Organic dust toxic syndrome: An acute febrile reaction to organic dust exposure distinct from hypersensitivity pneumonitis. *J Toxicol Clin Toxicol* 28:389–420, 1990.

49. Wardlaw AJ, Dunnette S, Gleich GJ, et al: Eosinophils and mast cells in bronchoalveolar lavage in subjects with mild asthma. *Am Rev Respir Dis* 137:62–69, 1988.

50. Woodford DM, Coutu RE, Gaensler EA: Obstructive lung disease from acute sulfur dioxide exposure. *Respiration* 38:238–245, 1979.

SECTION 12

ENVIRONMENTAL DISORDERS

CHAPTER 62

INDOOR AND OUTDOOR AIR POLLUTION

Jonathan M. Samet / Mark J. Utell

Both indoor and outdoor air pollution are of concern to pulmonary physicians. Exposures to indoor and outdoor air pollutants may both exacerbate and cause respiratory diseases and also increase the population's risk for morbidity and mortality from malignant and nonmalignant diseases. This chapter provides a broad introduction to indoor and outdoor air pollution. It begins with a brief review of the emergence of indoor and outdoor air pollution as clinical and public health issues. The chapter then considers general principles and concepts related to inhalation injury, exposure, and health outcomes. The health consequences of indoor and outdoor air pollution are covered separately, although this distinction is artificial, given the penetration of outdoor pollutants into indoor environments and the overlap between the pollutants found in indoor and outdoor locations. The chapter concludes by considering two issues of direct concern to clinicians: susceptible populations and control strategies.

OVERVIEW

Air pollution has probably had adverse effects on health throughout history. The use of fire for heating and cooking brought exposure to smoke, and the rise of cities concentrated the emissions of pollutants from dwellings and from manufacturing facilities within restricted locales. Industrialization and electric power generation brought new point sources of pollution, that is, localized sources such as power plants, and sometimes immense emissions of combustion by-products, particles, nitrogen oxides, and sulfur oxides into adjacent areas where people lived and worked. During the twentieth century, mobile sources, including cars, trucks, and other fossil fuel–powered vehicles, created a new type of pollution—photochemical pollution, or "smog," first recognized in the Los Angeles air basin. The unprecedented growth of some urban areas to form "megacities," such as Mexico City, São Paulo, and Shanghai, has led to unrelenting air pollution from massive vehicle fleets and snarled traffic and from polluting industries and power plants. During the twentieth century, there has also been increasing recognition that the problem of air pollution extends into indoor environments. In the less developed countries, exposure to smoke from biomass fuel combustion is widespread, as it was in past centuries. In the more developed countries, indoor pollutants are generated by human activities and released from the materials used for construction and in furnishings, and often maintained at unhealthy concentrations by building designs that seal pollutants within.

Health effects of air pollution have long been of concern. During the reign of Edward I (1272–1307), the pollution of London by coal smoke prompted a royal proclamation banning burning of "sea-coal" in open furnaces.[15] In 1661, John Evelyn published *Fumifugium or the Aer and Smoake of London Dissipated*, describing an approach to the control of air pollution in London. However, air pollution was not regulated in England until approximately two centuries later with the passage of the Smoke Nuisance Abatement Act and the Alkali Act, directed at industrial pollution. In the United States, recognition of the public health dimensions of air pollution began in the middle of the twentieth century, driven by the rising problem of smog in southern California and the 1948 air pollution episode in Donora, Pennsylvania, which caused 20 excess deaths and thousands of illnesses. The first national legislation, the Air Pollution Control Act, was passed in the mid-1950s; the original Clean Air Act was passed in 1963 and most recently revised in 1990.

The modern era of air pollution research and control dates to the episodes in Donora and other cities, during which extremely high levels of pollution caused clearly evident excess deaths. The most dramatic episode was the London Fog of 1952, which caused approximately 4000 excess deaths.[7] These episodes led to regulations for the control of outdoor air pollution and to the conduct of research designed to develop evidence on the health effects of outdoor air pollution as a foundation for control measures. The research included characterization of the pollutants in outdoor air as to their sources, concentrations, and chemical and physical properties; toxicologic investigation on the injury caused by air pollutants and the underlying mechanisms; and epidemiologic studies of the health effects of air pollution in the community. These approaches remain fundamental to research on air pollution. We now have a large body of evidence on the health effects of air pollution gained over nearly 50 years of investigation and complex regulations that limit emissions and control concentrations of key pollutants in outdoor air.

The health effects of indoor air pollution are a more recent concern.[52] Only limited measurements were made of indoor air contaminant levels before the 1970s, and the findings of the first large-scale studies of the health effects of indoor air pollution were not reported until the late 1960s and early 1970s. Pollutants of initial interest included environmental tobacco smoke (ETS), the mixture of side-stream smoke and exhaled mainstream smoke inhaled involuntarily by nonsmokers, and nitrogen dioxide (NO$_2$) generated by gas cooking stoves and ranges and by

space heaters. Research soon broadened to biologic agents, volatile organic compounds, and two respiratory carcinogens—radon and asbestos. Concern about the potential health effects of indoor air pollution was heightened by the design and construction of buildings with reduced exchange of indoor with outdoor air for the purpose of energy conservation; the reduction of air exchange was anticipated to diminish dilution and thereby increase indoor air pollutant concentrations. Beginning in the 1970s, outbreaks of nonspecific complaints started to occur among workers, who attributed their symptoms to the indoor environments where they worked. Now referred to as *sick-building syndrome*, these outbreaks continue—and in seemingly increasing incidence. Another new syndrome, *multiple chemical sensitivity*, has also been linked to indoor air pollution; persons with this syndrome, who may obtain consultation from pulmonary specialists, often report debilitating symptoms after exposure to indoor air contaminants, even at levels that may be considered generally safe.

Control of indoor air pollution has been enacted primarily through nonregulatory approaches,[52] as the Environmental Protection Agency (EPA) does not directly regulate the levels of pollutants in indoor air. The cornerstone of the control of indoor air pollution has been education of the public, manufacturers, and employers on approaches for reducing exposures and for reducing emissions from indoor sources. The EPA has given a guideline value for an acceptable indoor radon concentration; it has also proposed that all homes be tested for radon and the homes modified if the concentration is above the guideline. The handling of asbestos in schools was regulated under the Asbestos Hazard Emergency Reduction Act, and the Agency has classified ETS as a class A carcinogen. The Occupational Safety and Health Administration published Proposed New Rules on indoor air quality in 1994; these rules have general provisions for indoor air quality and specific provisions related to ETS. As of this writing, the rule making was still in progress.

The literature on air pollution is now voluminous and has been published in a broad array of journals and technical reports. Of necessity, this chapter is selective in its review and citation of the evidence; emphasis has been placed on the most relevant findings for clinicians and on the newer literature. The documents prepared by the EPA on the six "criteria" pollutants (sulfur dioxide [SO$_2$], particulate matter, NO$_2$, carbon monoxide [CO], ozone [O$_3$], and lead) offer encyclopedic reviews that are updated periodically (Table 62-1). The American Thoracic Society (ATS) has occasionally published summary statements for health professionals on the health effects of outdoor air pollution, with several published in 1996.[2,3,48] Several books address the topic of indoor air pollution generally or address specific aspects of indoor air pollution.[17,18,24,42] The EPA has published an introductory primer on indoor air pollution.[58] Key documents on specific pollutants are cited within the appropriate sections of this chapter.

GENERAL PRINCIPLES AND CONCEPTS

Adverse responses to air pollutants reflect exposure and the delivery of the dose of the injurious agent to the target site within the respiratory tract. Air pollutants cause disease through various mechanisms. This section of the chapter covers principles of

TABLE 62-1

Criteria Pollutants, Sources, and National Ambient Air Quality Standards (NAAQS)

Pollutant	Sources	Primary Standards	Averaging Time
Sulfur dioxide	Coal and petroleum combustion, smelting and other manufacturing	0.14 ppm (365 μg/m^3) 0.03 ppm (80 μg/m^3)	24 h Annual (arithmetic mean)
PM$_{10}$	Coal and petroleum combustion, vehicles, industry, surface dust	150 μg/m^3 50 μg/m^3	24 h Annual (arithmetic mean)
Nitrogen dioxide	Coal and petroleum combustion, vehicles, industry	0.053 ppm (100 μg/m^3)	Annual (arithmetic mean)
Carbon monoxide	Coal and petroleum combustion, vehicles	35 ppm (40 μg/m^3) 9 ppm (10 μg/m^3)	1 h 8 h
Ozone	Secondary formation from NO$_2$ and hydrocarbons	0.12 ppm (235 μg/m^3)	Maximum daily 1-h average
Lead	Gasoline, lead-containing dust	1.5 mg/m^3	Maximum quarterly average

inhalation injury and the related spectrum of adverse health effects; it also covers principles of exposure assessment. The research methods used to characterize the effects of air pollutants are also detailed.

Principles of Inhalation Injury

Atmospheric pollutants, whether indoors or outdoors, exist in both gaseous and particulate forms. In evaluating clinical consequences of specific exposures, the clinician should recognize that penetration into and retention within the respiratory tract of toxic gases can vary widely, depending on the physical properties of the gas (e.g., solubility), the concentration of the gas in the inspired air, the rate and depth of ventilation, and the extent to which the material is reactive. Gases that are highly water soluble, such as SO$_2$, are almost completely extracted by the upper airways of healthy subjects during brief exposures at rest. In contrast, removal of less water-soluble gases, such as NO$_2$ or O$_3$, is much less complete, and these gases may penetrate to the airways and alveoli of the respiratory tract. CO is poorly soluble in water and is not removed in the upper airways. On reaching the lung, CO diffuses across the alveolar-capillary membrane and then binds avidly to hemoglobin.

Exercise greatly augments penetration of gases into the deep lung and, thus, the total dose of pollutants delivered to targets in the airways. Exercise increases the dose directly by increasing minute ventilation; also, because many people switch from the nasal to the oral breathing route during moderate to heavy exercise, the more efficient pollutant removal in the nasal passages is replaced by the less efficient removal in the oral airway.

Particulate pollutants usually occur in nature as aerosols. Small liquid droplets or solid particles are dispersed in the atmosphere with sufficient stability to remain in an aerosol suspension. Examples of common aerosols are sulfuric acid mists and sulfate and nitrate salts formed from SO$_2$ and NO$_2$, respectively. Deposition of inhaled particles depends on many factors, including the aerodynamic properties of the particle (primarily size), airway anatomy, and breathing pattern. Particles larger than 10 μm are effectively filtered out in the nose and nasopharynx, where these relatively large particles are deposited efficiently be-

cause of impaction against surfaces and gravitational forces. Particles trapped in the nose and nasopharynx are cleared in secretions and coughed out or swallowed. Particles less than 10 μm in aerodynamic diameter (PM$_{10}$) may be deposited in the tracheobronchial tree; deposition in the lung's alveoli is maximal for particles 1 to 2 μm in diameter. Particles smaller than 0.5 μm move by diffusion to the alveolar level, where they collide with gas molecules by Brownian movement and are impacted on alveolar surfaces. Removal of particles from the larger airways by the mucociliary apparatus is efficient and occurs within hours of deposition; clearance from the deep lung by alveolar macrophages is much slower, requiring days to months.

The mechanisms by which inhaled gases and particles injure the lung are diverse and not yet fully understood.[2,3] Oxidant gases, O$_3$ and NO$_2$, cause inflammation of the respiratory epithelium, presumably through the production of toxic oxidant species and release of potent mediators. SO$_2$ is also an irritant gas. The response to particles depends on the chemical nature of the particles. Acidic compounds on particles may dissolve into tissue fluids and induce an inflammatory response. Organic materials on particles may also produce inflammation or act as initiators or promoters of cancer.

Adverse Health Effects of Air Pollution: Clinical and Public Health Concerns

The spectrum of adverse effects of air pollution is broad, ranging from the consequences of acute and dramatic exposures, which may cause death, to far more subtle and chronic effects on disease risk and well-being. This spectrum has been conceptualized as a pyramid with mortality at its tip and an increasingly common set of morbidities as the base. Perhaps the most common "adverse" effect is a loss of well-being from the diminished aesthetic value of a polluted environment. Clinicians are more likely to be concerned with the less common, more acute effects with clinical consequences—acute responses, often in asthmatics, for which a link to air pollution exposure may be made by history or challenge testing; the more subtle and long-term consequences are typically a focus for public health researchers and regulators. Nevertheless, clinicians may be asked to assess risks of long-term exposures or to estimate the contribution of exposures to disease causation in a particular patient. They may also be asked to guide their communities in evaluating air pollution as a local public health problem.

To interpret the scientific evidence on the effects of air pollution, clinicians need a framework for determining whether an effect is "adverse." Judgment on the adversity of responses is societal and reflective of prevalent valuations and perceptions of risk. The Clean Air Act uses the term "adverse" without definition. If a broad construct of health is used that includes a state of well-being as a component, adverse effects of air pollution include not only clinically evident disease but also more subtle symptom responses and physiological effects that may compromise well-being or increase the risk of disease. In a 1985 report, a committee of the ATS offered guidelines for defining adverse respiratory health effects in epidemiologic studies of outdoor air pollution.[5] The committee turned to a medical basis for this determination, defining adverse respiratory health effects as "medically significant physiologic or pathologic changes. . . ."

Indoor air pollution has a broad range of effects as well (Table 62-2).[44] Cases of clinically evident disease caused by indoor air pollution occur, and an unquestionable causal link can often be established for specific persons from a careful history or appropriate diagnostic testing, as with hypersensitivity pneumonitis. Indoor air pollution can also exacerbate chronic respiratory diseases—e.g., house dust mite antigen and asthma in house-dust mite–allergic persons. More subtle effects have become of increasing concern as we have learned that indoor air pollution can adversely affect comfort and increase risk for future disease; con-

---

TABLE 62-2

A Classification of the Adverse Effects of Indoor Air Pollution

Clinically evident diseases: Diseases for which the usual methods of clinical evaluation can establish a causal link to an indoor air pollutant

Exacerbation of disease: The clinical status of already established disease is exacerbated by indoor air pollution

Increased risk for diseases: Diseases for which epidemiologic or other evidence establishes increased risk in exposed persons; however, the usual clinical methods indicative of injury typically cannot establish the causal link in an individual patient

Physiological impairment: Transient or persistent effects on a measure of physiological functioning that are of insufficient magnitude to cause clinical disease

Symptom responses: Subjectively reported responses that can be linked to indoor pollutants or are attributed to indoor pollutants

Perception of unacceptable indoor air quality: Sensing of indoor air quality as uncomfortable to an unacceptable degree

Perception of exposure to indoor air pollutants: Awareness of exposure to one or more pollutants with an unacceptable level of concern about exposure

SOURCE: Data from Samet.[44]

---

sequently, even the perception of exposure to indoor pollutants may adversely affect well-being. Radon and asbestos, for example, are respiratory carcinogens, which are presumed to increase risk of lung cancer.

Concepts of Time-Activity and Total Personal Exposure

Definitions of concentration, exposure, and dose are fundamental to considering the health effects of air pollution.[34] *Concentration* refers to the amount of material present in air. *Exposure* constitutes contact with a material at a portal of entry into the body—the respiratory tract, the gastrointestinal tract, and the skin. For the lung, exposure would constitute time spent in contaminated air. Exposure is the unit of concentration multiplied by time. *Dose* refers to the amount of material that enters the body; *biologically effective dose* is the amount of material reaching target sites for injury—e.g., the mass of respirable particles delivered to the small airways. For example, the concentration of particles less than 10 mm in aerodynamic diameter (PM_{10}) might be 100 mg/m^3; a person spending 10 h at this concentration would have an exposure of 10 h times 100 mg/m^3, or 1000 mg/m^3-h. Assuming lung deposition to be 50 percent of the total mass and a minute volume of 10 L/min, the dose of PM_{10} would be 600 mg. For most inhaled pollutants, dose will vary with activity level as ventilation rises and falls with the demands imposed by activities.

With regard to impact on health, *total personal exposure* to a pollutant is the relevant index of exposure, not the exposures received separately within indoor and outdoor environments. The total personal exposure of a person to a pollutant can be conceptualized as the time-weighted average pollutant concentration in the "microenvironments" where the person spends time (Fig. 62-1).[33] The microenvironments are locations having relatively constant concentration of the pollutant during the time spent there. The principal microenvironments contributing to total personal exposure are those with relatively high concentrations or where relatively large amounts of time are spent. For example, for exposure to particles, key microenvironments might include an office where smoking is allowed and an urban environment where a home is located and time is spent outdoors and indoors.

Studies of time-activity patterns indicate that residents of more developed countries spend most of their time indoors and, consequently, personal exposures to many pollutants take place largely in indoor microenvironments. However, pollutants generated by outdoor sources do penetrate indoors, so indoor microenvironments can contribute to exposures to pollutants typically considered outdoor pollutants, such as particles and CO. Data on time use in a number of countries showed that people spend an average of 65 to 75 percent of their time inside their residences and more than 90 percent of time indoors, counting time at home, work, and elsewhere. Recent data from a 1987–88 survey of Californians show a similar pattern, with employed adults averaging 15 h per day indoors at home and 6 h per day in other indoor settings.[27] In the California study, school-age children spent an average of 18 h indoors at home. While these data emphasize the predominance of indoor microenvironments in determining exposures to many pollutants, exposure outdoors may

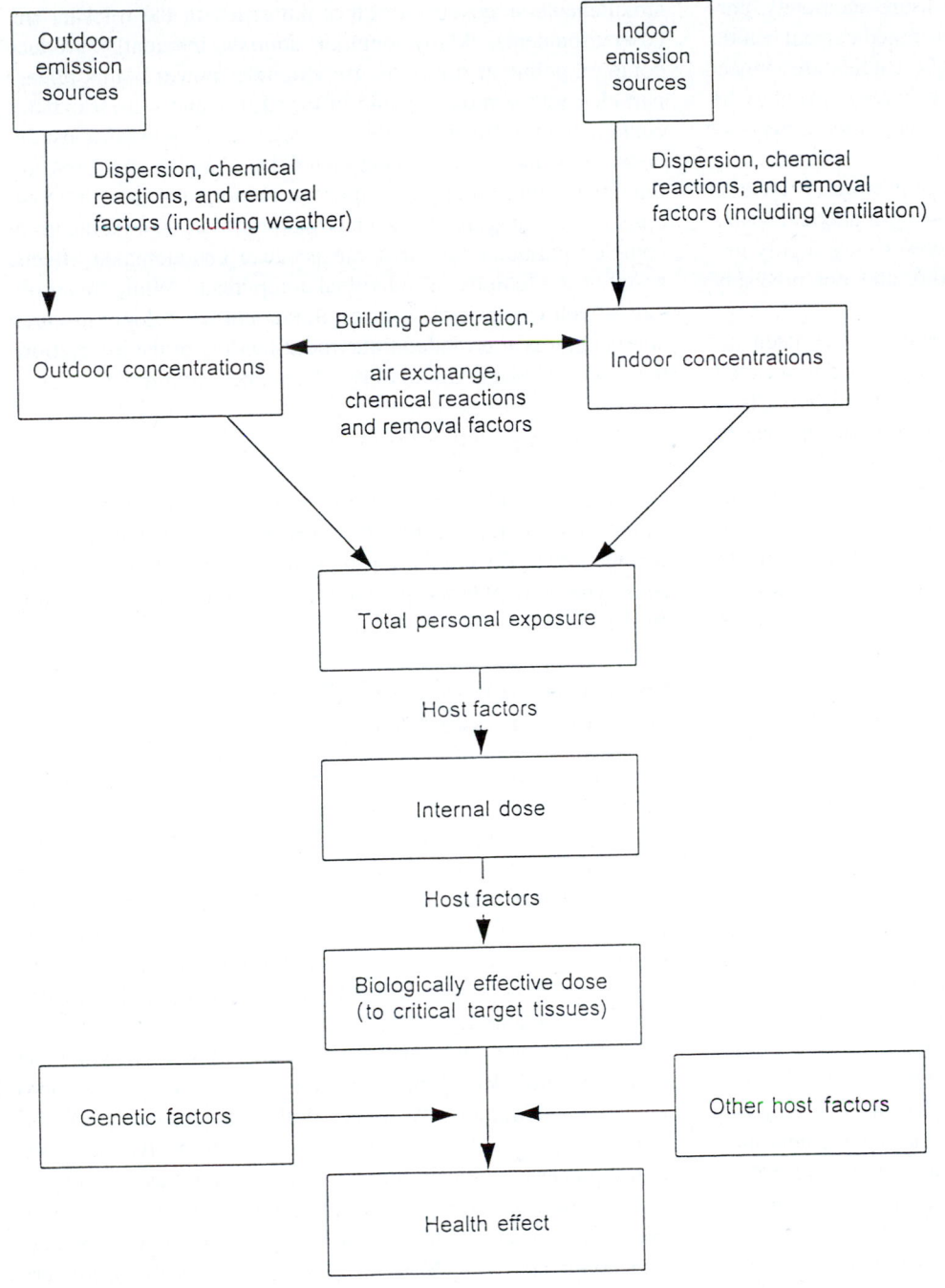

FIGURE 62-1   Framework for conceptualizing exposure, dose, and health effects from outdoor and indoor air pollution. *(Based on NRC data,[33] with permission.)*

properties of air pollutants. Recently, exposure assessment has emerged as a separate research discipline. The tools of the exposure assessor include questionnaires that capture activities and time use, personal and area monitors, statistical models for estimating exposures, and biomarkers of exposure and dose.[34]

Toxicologic studies are often conducted to characterize the hazards of air pollutants; research may entail exposures of animals to one or more pollutants to assess patterns of injury and disease risk. Increasingly, toxicologic approaches are used to characterize the relationship between exposure and dose and the mechanisms underlying injury. This mechanistic information addresses the appropriateness of extrapolating from animal studies to humans, particularly if parallel data from humans are available on dosimetry and mechanisms. Toxicologic studies in which volunteers are exposed to pollutants, often referred to as *clinical studies,* have proved to be an informative approach for investigating the acute consequences of pollution exposure. In addition to healthy volunteers, groups in the population considered susceptible to the effects of the pollutant(s) of concern may be selected for investigation—e.g., persons with asthma, chronic obstructive pulmonary disease (COPD), or coronary artery disease. Of necessity, exposures in clinical studies are of brief duration and ethically limited to levels that will have limited, transient effects. In addition to monitoring symptoms and physiological measures, clinical studies may be strengthened by more invasive collection of biologic specimens, using phlebotomy, nasal lavage, or fiberoptic bronchoscopy with biopsy of the mucosa or bronchoalveolar lavage, to elucidate mechanisms of injury.

Epidemiologic studies provide an assessment of the adverse effects of pollution exposures under the circumstances of "real world" exposure.[33] The findings of epidemiologic studies of air pollution have direct public health and regulatory relevance. The exposures are inherently representative of those received in the community, and the pollutants are inhaled in the form of the complex mixtures that actually exist in indoor and outdoor air. Additionally, the community members in a study can be selected from the full spectrum of potentially susceptible subjects. There are, however, weaknesses to the epidemiologic approach. Expo-

be the predominant determinant of dose for some pollutants. For example, the dose of O_3 (which generally has low indoor levels) received by the lung's airways may be dominated by exposure received outdoors, particularly for people exercising outdoors.

Research Approaches to Air Pollution

Our understanding of the health effects of air pollution derives from a tripartite research approach: characterization of atmospheric pollutants and exposures, toxicologic studies, and epidemiologic studies. These approaches are complementary. There has long been research on the physical and chemical

sures to pollutants may be difficult to measure accurately, particularly past exposures that may have determined current health; hence, exposure estimates in epidemiologic studies are subject to substantial error. The effects of other exposures relevant to the health outcome of interest, termed *confounding factors*, may not be sufficiently controlled, and these extraneous exposures may artifactually increase or decrease the apparent effect of air pollution exposure. Epidemiologic studies having inadequate sample size and, therefore, limited statistical power may supply imprecise and uninformative estimates of risk and not precisely answer public health questions.

The technique of quantitative risk assessment has been increasingly applied to estimate the burden of disease associated with air pollution, particularly carcinogens.[36] The 1990 Clean Air Act amendments include specific provisions on the use of risk assessment, particularly in regard to the hazardous air pollutants regulated under Section 112 of the Act. This process integrates the information on exposure and dose response to provide a characterization of the impact of an environmental agent on the population's health; as the evidence is systematically reviewed in the conduct of a risk assessment, gaps in the evidence and attendant uncertainties are identified, and assumptions are made to fill the gaps.[36]

Risk assessment can be conceptualized as comprising the four steps outlined in the seminal 1983 report of the National Research Council (Table 62-3).[38] A full risk assessment can be a large undertaking, requiring review of all relevant data and mathematical modeling to characterize the risk. In a risk assessment, gaps in the scientific evidence, which are sources of uncertainty, are catalogued and used to estimate the level of confidence attached to the risk characterization. The findings of risk assessment guide *risk management*, the process by which decisions are made about the need for risk reduction and the approaches to be implemented to reduce risks. Risk management means choosing among the options to control risk and balancing risk reduction, costs, and technologic capability for reducing exposure. Uncertainties in the scientific information that have been catalogued in the risk assessment process may cloud risk management and introduce ambiguity regarding the optimum strategy. Nevertheless, risk managers need to make decisions in the face of uncertainty.

Understanding the effects of complex mixtures of pollutants in indoor and outdoor air has proved particularly daunting for researchers. Exposures to pollutants rarely occur singly, without

TABLE 62-3

Steps in Risk Assessment

Hazard identification: The determination of whether an agent is causally linked to the health effect of concern

Dose-response assessment: The determination of the relation between level of exposure and risk of the health effect

Exposure assessment: Description of the extent of human exposure

Risk characterization: Description of the human risk, including uncertainties

SOURCE: Data from National Research Council.[38]

simultaneous exposures to other pollutants in the relevant microenvironments. Many outdoor sources inherently produce complex pollutant mixtures; for example, power plants release particles, nitrogen oxides, and sulfur oxides, and vehicle exhaust contains CO, nitrogen oxides, particles, and hydrocarbons. Indoor air is inevitably contaminated by complex mixtures, reflecting the multiplicity of sources in indoor environments. Synergistic or antagonistic interactions between components of complex pollutant mixtures can produce unanticipated effects, based on the toxicity of individual components. While this problem is well recognized, epidemiologic and toxicologic research approaches have provided little understanding of the interactions that may determine the toxicity of complex mixtures.[41]

OUTDOOR AIR POLLUTION

Outdoor air pollutants have diverse sources, both man-made and natural. This section begins with a review of the sources and then considers the effects of the principal man-made outdoor pollutants. The pollutants are grouped according to their designation by the EPA.

Overview: Sources and Classification of Outdoor Air Pollution

Many pollutants, from both man-made and natural sources, can be found in outdoor air. Some naturally occurring pollutants in outdoor air are well documented as causing or exacerbating pulmonary diseases—e.g., pollens and fungi. This chapter does not address these biologic agents but considers the man-made pollutants. Researchers have focused more attention on the effects of man-made pollutants, which may reach potentially hazardous levels in urban areas or near point sources, such as power plants, smelters, or manufacturing facilities. In the United States, the principal outdoor pollutants are generally classified within the framework provided by the Clean Air Act, which identifies two sets of air pollutants, "criteria" pollutants (Table 62-1) and "toxic" air pollutants. The term *criteria* refers to the standard-setting process for these pollutants, which requires preparation of a criteria document reviewing all relevant evidence every 5 years. The criteria pollutants include primarily combustion-related pollutants (SO_2, NO_2, CO, and particles), the secondary pollutant O_3, and lead. The toxic pollutants are predominantly carcinogens; the sources are diverse but principally comprise industrial emissions and waste products. Examples of these pollutants are benzene, chlordane, ethylene oxide, hydrochloric acid, methane, parathion, propylene oxide, toluene, and vinyl chloride.

These two groups of pollutants are regulated through different mechanisms. For the criteria pollutants, National Ambient Air Quality Standards (NAAQS) are set after extensive review of all relevant evidence; the standards must afford protection to the entire population, including those with heightened susceptibility, and offer an "adequate margin of safety." The hazardous pollutants are predominantly carcinogens, such as asbestos and radionuclides, and standards for maximum concentrations are also intended to provide a margin of safety. The Act includes mechanisms for achieving levels within the standards and for enforcement. In spite of existing federal standards for ambient air quality, excesses are common in many areas of the country, particularly for O_3. Although the pollutants are considered in the following section on an individual basis, it should be reemphasized that exposures of the population occur most often to mixtures.

Outdoor Air Pollutants: Exposures and Health Effects

The pollutants covered in this section are of public health significance throughout the world. Sulfur oxides, particles, nitrogen oxides, and CO are generated by combustion and are typically found together in the complex air pollutant mixtures in outdoor environments. O_3 is a secondary pollutant. While the pollutants are considered individually, exposures to them typically occur in the form of inhaled mixtures.

SULFUR DIOXIDE

Sulfur oxides are produced by combustion of fuels containing sulfur, such as coal from the eastern United States and crude petroleum. Smelting of ores containing sulfur is also a prominent source in some regions, such as the southwestern United States. In the past, scientific research and regulatory concern in relation to the sulfur oxides were directed primarily at the health effects of SO_2, the criteria pollutant regulated by the EPA. SO_2 is a water-soluble gas that is effectively scrubbed from inspired air by the upper airway; exercise, however, may increase the inhaled dose by its effect on minute ventilation and the switch to the oral breathing route. This pollutant has been shown to have adverse effects without concomitant exposures to other pollutants.[2,3] In fact, exposures of volunteers to SO_2 alone show that the gas may have adverse respiratory effects; asthmatics are particularly sensitive, with some showing exquisite sensitivity. Significant exposures to SO_2 alone might result from plumes released by smelters processing sulfur-containing ores or from other industrial processes.

Exposures to SO_2 in outdoor air occur primarily with simultaneous exposures to other combustion-related pollutants, including nitrogen oxides and particles. Heavy industry and coal-burning power plants are predominant sources for this type of pollutant mixture. Tall smokestacks for power plants, increasingly used to control local pollutant concentrations, release sulfur oxides and nitrogen oxides high into the atmosphere, where residence time is prolonged. Through a series of chemical reactions, the sulfur oxides and nitrogen oxides form acidic sulfate and nitrate particles, which may undergo long-range transport.[51] These acidic particles represent a regional air pollution problem—blanketing, for example, the central and northeastern United States and portions of Canada. The effects of particulate air pollution and acidic aerosols are considered separately below; this section considers the effects of gaseous SO_2.

Asthmatics are particularly susceptible to SO_2, responding to exposure in chambers with increased airway resistance and reduced levels of lung function. With exercise and hyperventilation, which increase the dose delivered to the respiratory tract, some asthmatics are adversely affected at levels common in ambient air and well below those that might occur transiently with direct exposure to the plume from a power plant or factory.[2,3,47] Inhalation of SO_2 produces an immediate response and does not provoke delayed reactions or repetitive nocturnal attacks. The decrements in lung function on breathing of SO_2 may be sufficient to produce symptoms of dyspnea, wheezing, and chest tightness. The bronchoconstriction resolves within an hour of exposure, and peak bronchoconstrictor responses may lessen on repeated challenge after a short recovery period. Responses to SO_2 can be partly blocked by pretreatment with cromolyn sodium and anticholinergics and can be reversed by β-adrenergic agonists. Sequential exposures to SO_2 and oxidant gases (O_3 and NO_2) have been performed in asthmatics; these clinical studies have provided little evidence of synergistic interactions in reducing airway function. Although some asthmatics have been shown to be affected by SO_2 with exposure at low concentrations in the laboratory,[47] complementary epidemiologic data have not been reported that document parallel community morbidity.

NITROGEN DIOXIDE

Nitrogen oxides, like sulfur oxides, are produced by combustion processes and contribute to the formation of acid aerosols.[2,3,51] Even though NO_2 is regulated by the EPA as a criteria pollutant, most personal exposure in the United States occurs in indoor microenvironments contaminated by unvented gas stoves and space heaters. The principal source of NO_2 in outdoor air is motor vehicle emissions, but power plants and industrial sources may also contribute. There have been few locations where point sources were strong enough to make NO_2 alone a source of concern. The health effects of NO_2 released into outdoor air probably arise principally from the formation of secondary pollutants. NO_2 is an essential precursor of O_3, and one of the principal pathways by which NO_2 in outdoor air adversely affects respiratory health may be through the formation of O_3. The nitrogen oxides also secondarily form acidic nitrate particles.

NO_2 is an oxidant gas of low solubility that penetrates to the small airways and alveoli of the lung.[2,3] The toxicologic evidence at exposures far greater than typically sustained in indoor and outdoor environments suggests that NO_2 exposure can impair lung defenses against respiratory pathogens and cause airway inflammation, with associated effects on lung function and respiratory symptoms.[43] In animal models, exposure to NO_2 increases mortality after challenge with bacterial respiratory pathogens. Therefore, a wide range of health effects are of concern, including increased risk for respiratory infections, respiratory symptoms, reduced lung function, and exacerbation of chronic respiratory diseases. However, there have been only limited epidemiologic data, largely derived from studies of children exposed to indoor sources of NO_2; these studies and other evidence on indoor exposures are considered separately in the section on indoor air pollution.

A number of clinical studies have been performed to investigate the acute effects of NO_2 by itself on the status of persons with asthma.[43] These studies were performed to assess the need for a short-term standard for outdoor NO_2 concentration, as the present NAAQS provide only an annual standard for NO_2. NO_2 could plausibly affect airway responsiveness by causing airway inflammation. The findings of the clinical studies have been inconsistent, and the discrepancies between the "positive" and "negative" studies have not been readily explained. One study showed consistent responses to NO_2 of some asthmatics, suggesting that there might be a susceptible group among persons having asthma in general, but this susceptibility has not been found in other studies.[43] The epidemiologic evidence remains inconclusive, largely because of methodologic problems arising in attempting to separate the effects of NO_2 from those of other pollutants. Persons with COPD may represent a group with increased susceptibility to short-term exposure to NO_2 outdoors.

PARTICLES

Particles in outdoor air have numerous natural and man-made sources, including the same combustion processes that produce SO_2 and NO_2.[2,3] Particles are suspended in air by the action of wind on crustal material. The man-made sources are diverse and include power plants, industry, and motor vehicles. Diesel-powered vehicles emit particles in the inhalable size range. Particles, of course, are present in indoor and outdoor air; consequently, personal exposures to particles reflect both indoor and outdoor microenvironments. Additionally, outdoor particles, particularly those of smaller size, penetrate indoors, so indoor microenvironments may contribute to exposure to outdoor particles.

Large numbers of people in the United States and other industrialized countries are exposed to acid aerosols arising from primary combustion pollutants. As previously discussed, tall stacks release SO_2, NO_2, and particles high into the atmosphere, where transformations yield acid particles containing sulfate and nitrate species.[51] This problem of acid aerosols predominantly affects the central and eastern United States and adjacent portions of Canada, but point sources can produce local problems. Of course, acid particles are a threat in many industrialized locations worldwide.

Historically, particle concentrations in outdoor air have been measured with several different techniques. Until 1987, the EPA specified the measurement of total suspended particulates (TSP), which included particles well above the inhalable size range. In 1987, the reference method for NAAQS was changed to particulate matter less than 10 mm in aerodynamic diameter (PM_{10}). This size range includes some particle masses in the coarse particle size range above the 2.5-mm boundary between respirable and nonrespirable particles. The standard makes no provision with regard to the chemical composition of the particles. Consequently, equivalent mass concentrations of particles may have differing toxicity, depending on acidity, content of metals, or carcinogenic potency. The size distribution below the 10-mm cutoff may also affect toxicity through its effect on sites of deposition.

There has been extensive epidemiologic investigation of the effects of particles on health since the air pollution disasters at midcentury.[2,3,48] These studies have addressed the relationship between exposures to particles and short- and long-term variation of mortality, both from all causes and from cardiovascular causes. The studies have also addressed the relationship between exposures to particles and diverse indicators of respiratory morbidity, including the frequency of respiratory symptoms and illnesses, level of lung function and rate of lung function growth

and decline, and outpatient visits and inpatient admissions. In the early studies of particulate air pollution, the measures of exposure were general; some studies covered only surrogate measures of exposure, such as residence location. In spite of such crude exposure measures, these studies found adverse effects of exposure to particulate air pollution and became the basis for establishing air quality standards for particles. The standards were generally considered to be sufficiently protective of public health. Studies linked particulate air pollution to a number of adverse health effects (Table 62-4).[14]

As levels of air pollution were reduced in the United States and other Western countries, readily evident excess mortality was no longer observed at times of higher concentrations, and the focus of research and of public health concern generally shifted to morbidity. However, recent studies of daily variation in mortality, facilitated by new techniques for longitudinal data analysis, have shown statistically significant positive associations between measures of particle concentration, primarily TSP and PM_{10}, and daily mortality counts for some regions in the United States.[14] Similar positive reports have been based on data from cities throughout the world. Some complementary studies of morbidity have also been reported. These findings suggest that the present NAAQS for particulate matter may not be protecting against adverse health effects with the "adequate margin of safety" mandated by the Clean Air Act; they also call other national and international standards into question. However, the toxicologic mechanisms by which inhaled particulate matter could lead to cardiopulmonary morbidity and mortality are yet to be established, and this gap tempers the interpretation of these data. It would be premature to offer specific clinical recommendations with regard to particulate air pollution until mechanisms of toxicity are better understood and the rate of outdoor exposures is clarified.

Epidemiologic data indicate associations of acid aerosol levels with mortality and respiratory symptoms in children.[2,3] Asthmatics also appear sensitive to acid aerosols. The evidence on acid aerosols and health was recently reviewed by a committee of the ATS.[6] Persons considered to be at greatest risk were those working outdoors and, consequently, highly exposed and those with increased airway responsiveness or asthma. Health effects of concern included increased respiratory symptoms and decreased lung function.

CARBON MONOXIDE

Carbon monoxide (CO) is an invisible gas formed by incomplete combustion of fossil fuels and other organic materials. The most prominent outdoor source is vehicle exhaust; consequently, outdoor concentrations are highly variable in place and time, changing with vehicle density and traffic patterns. Urban locations with high traffic density tend to have the highest concentrations. CO, of course, also has indoor sources, such as cooking stoves and tobacco smoke.[11] Exposures to CO can be conveniently assessed by using the level of carboxyhemoglobin as a biomarker of exposure or by measuring the concentration of CO in an end-tidal breath sample, following a breath hold.

In regard to outdoor air, acute effects of CO on susceptible persons have been of particular concern, and the current U.S.

TABLE 62-4

Health Effects of Particulate Air Pollution

	% Change in Health Indicator per Each $10\text{-}\mu g/m^3$ Increase in PM_{10}
Increase in daily mortality	
Total deaths	1.0
Respiratory deaths	3.4
Cardiovascular deaths	1.4
Increase in hospital usage (all respiratory)	
Admissions	0.8
Emergency department visits	1.0
Exacerbation of asthma	
Asthmatic attacks	3.0
Bronchodilator use	2.9
Emergency department visits*	3.4
Hospital admissions	1.9
Increase in respiratory symptom reports	
Lower respiratory	3.0
Upper respiratory	0.7
Cough	1.2
Decrease in lung function	
Forced expired volume	0.15
Peak expiratory flow	0.08

*One study only.
SOURCE: Data from Dockery and Pope.[14]

standard is intended to protect susceptible persons with coronary artery disease. Inhaled CO binds to hemoglobin with high affinity (more than 200 times greater than for oxygen) to form carboxyhemoglobin (COHb) (see Chapter 13). The COHb complex is very stable; depending on ambient levels of CO, level of activity, and lung function, the half-life of CO in the body ranges from about 2.5 to 4 h. The rate of accumulation of ambient CO in the body above endogenous levels is affected by ambient CO concentrations, alveolar ventilation, lung diffusivity, total hemoglobin mass, and COHb level.[11] People with impaired gas exchange (e.g., persons with COPD) have compromised ability to excrete CO.

The binding of CO to hemoglobin reduces oxygen transport by red blood cells to tissues. The binding also displaces oxygen and causes an allosteric change in the hemoglobin molecule, increasing the affinity for oxygen carried by heme groups. Persons with cardiovascular disease are considered to be at greatest risk from CO exposure. Standard exercise tests on subjects with ischemic heart disease have demonstrated a decreased time interval to the onset of angina at COHb levels ranging from 2 to 6 percent.[1] The 1-h 35-ppm and 8-h 9-ppm federal standards for outdoor air (Table 62-1) were selected to prevent COHb levels from rising above 1.5 percent, thereby protecting persons with ischemic heart disease from aggravation of myocardial ischemia with onset of angina and attendant loss of exercise capacity. Recent evidence indicates that controlled CO exposure during exercise of patients with stable coronary artery disease can induce subjective and objective evidence of myocardial ischemia earlier in the exposure than without CO.[1] This effect can be induced at COHb levels as low as 2 to 4 percent. These studies are relevant

to the urban environment, where people may be exposed to sufficient CO to reach blood COHb levels in this range. Furthermore, moderate exercise results in even greater CO loading. In addition, at a COHb level of 6 percent, patients with coronary artery disease have an increased frequency of arrhythmias.[2,3] Fetuses, as well as persons with COPD, may also be susceptible to CO, and normal persons may have reduced oxygen uptake during exercise at low levels of CO exposure.

OZONE

Photochemical pollution, or "smog," is a complex oxidant mixture produced by the action of sunlight on hydrocarbons and nitrogen oxides in vehicle exhaust.[2,3,48] Ozone (O_3) is invariably present in photochemical pollution, and its concentration serves as an index of the level of this mixture. The problem of tropospheric O_3 pollution is distinct from the problem of depletion of the stratospheric ozone layer. Photochemical pollution was first recognized nearly 50 years ago in southern California, where the combination of sunlight and heavy vehicle travel promotes its formation. O_3 has now become a problem in many other locations, including western cities with similar sprawling growth and heavy vehicle traffic and the eastern United States during the summertime. O_3 is also produced naturally, but the exposure of concern for health almost exclusively reflects the O_3 created by human activities.

The toxicology of O_3 has been extensively investigated.[2,3] Low-level exposures cause damage to the small airways of experimental animals; the demonstration of subtle fibrosis in one animal model raises concern for permanent structural alteration in exposed populations. Volunteers exposed to O_3 at concentrations in the range of the present standard, often present during pollution episodes, have transient reductions of lung function; normal subjects have a range of responsiveness that is broad but repeatable for individuals. Recently, evidence of an inflammatory response and biochemical changes in BAL fluid has been detected 18 h after an experimental exposure to O_3 at a level below the current standard. Taken together, the progressive decrements in pulmonary mechanics during exposure, coupled with the persistent biochemical changes many hours after cessation of exposure, indicate the potential for chronic effects from repeated inhalation. Surprisingly, in clinical studies, asthmatics have not been shown to have increased susceptibility to O_3 compared with nonasthmatics. The evidence for short-term effects of O_3 exposure on the lung function of normal volunteers has raised concern about possible long-term effects of living in southern California and other locations with sustained photochemical pollution. Relevant epidemiologic data are suggestive of chronic effects of O_3, but these data are not definitive. Studies are in progress to address the long-term effects of O_3 exposure on children.

LEAD

The population may be exposed to lead through many environmental media, including ambient air. Ingestion is, of course, the principal pathway of concern at present in the United States. Fortunately, in the United States the importance of ambient air as a source of population exposure to lead has diminished with the removal of lead from gasoline. Children are particularly vulnerable to lead exposure. Even levels previously considered safe have been associated with adverse neurologic effects, and there has been a progressive tightening of recommendations of blood lead levels by the Centers for Disease Control and Prevention.

TOXIC AIR POLLUTANTS

The toxic air pollutants are predominantly carcinogens, but they demonstrate a variety of other toxicities. Approximately 200 "hazardous pollutants" are listed as air toxics in the 1990 Clean Air Act amendments. Examples of the hazardous pollutants are asbestos, benzene, cadmium compounds, chlorine, formaldehyde, and nickel. Although the sources are diverse, emission releases tend to be localized, often at industrial sites, or from municipal incinerators or waste sites.

Only a small proportion of lung cancers can be attributed to air pollution,[50] even though carcinogens are found widely in outdoor air. For example, polycyclic aromatic hydrocarbons (PAHs), found in diesel exhaust, are widely dispersed and present in urban air throughout the world. The PAHs possess mutagenic and carcinogenic activity, but to date, only limited epidemiologic data on risks in humans are available. Analyses of occupational cohorts exposed to diesel exhaust for years are suggestive of a small excess risk of lung cancer.[10] Given the difficulties of measuring exposure, confounding by cigarette smoke and by other occupations, and the small excess numbers of lung cancers, it is difficult to reach any definitive conclusion on the role of diesel exhaust in causing lung cancer in the general population. Nevertheless, as the percentage of light-duty vehicles powered by diesel fuel in the United States increases, there will be an increasing imperative to determine the carcinogenicity of the PAHs and diesel exhaust. There is

TABLE 62-5

Sources of Common Air Contaminants

Contaminant	Source
Asbestos	
Chrysotile	Some wall and ceiling insulation installed between 1930 and 1950
Crocidolite	Old insulation on heating pipes and equipment
Amosite	Old wood stove door gaskets
Tremolite	Some vinyl floor tiles
	Drywall joint-finishing material and textured paint purchased before 1977
	Cement-asbestos millboard and exterior wall shingles
	Some sprayed and troweled ceiling finishing plaster installed between 1945 and 1973
	Sprayed onto some structural steel beams as fire retardant
Combustion by-products	
Carbon monoxide	Gas range
Nitrogen dioxide	Wood and coal stoves
Sulfur dioxide	Gas and propane engines
Particulate soot	Fireplaces
Nitrogenated compounds	Backdrafting of exhaust flues
	Candles and incense
Tobacco smoke	
Carbon monoxide	Cigarettes
Nitrogen dioxide	Pipes
Carbon dioxide	Cigars
Hydrogen cyanide	
Nitrosamines	
Aromatic hydrocarbons	
Benzo[a]pyrene	
Particles	
Benzene	
Formaldehyde	
Nicotine	
Formaldehyde	Some particle board, plywood, pressed board, paneling
	Some carpeting and carpet backing
	Some furniture and dyed materials
	Urea-formaldehyde insulating foam
	Some household cleaners and deodorizers
	Combustion (gas, tobacco, wood)

also current concern that new types of fuels may introduce additional carcinogens into outdoor air.

INDOOR AIR POLLUTANTS AND HEALTH EFFECTS

Indoor environments are contaminated by numerous air pollutants, including outdoor air pollutants that have penetrated indoors and indoor air pollutants generated by the numerous indoor sources. This section reviews exposures and health effects of the principal indoor pollutants. The organic compounds and biologic agents include myriad individual agents that may adversely affect health. As for outdoor air pollution, clinicians should consider that exposures to indoor air pollutants typi-

TABLE 62-5

Sources of Common Air Contaminants (Cont.)

Contaminant	Source
Formaldehyde *(cont.)*	Some glues and resins
	Tobacco smoke
	Cosmetics
	Permanent-press textiles
Biologic organisms	
Fungal spores	Mold, mildew, and other fungi
Bacteria	Humidifiers with stagnant water
Virus	Water-damaged surfaces and materials
Pollens	Condensing coils and drip pans in HVAC systems
Arthropods	Drainage pans in refrigerators
Protozoa	Some thermophilics on dirty heating coils
	Animals
	Rodents
	Insects
	Humans
Radon	
Radon gas and	Radon gas emanating from soil, rocks, and water
radon progeny	that diffuses through cracks and holes in the
	foundation and floor
	Radon in well water
	Radon in natural gas used near the source wells
	Some building materials such as granite
Volatile organic compounds	
Alkanes	Solvents and cleaning compounds
Aromatic hydrocarbons	Paints
Esters	Glues and resins
Alcohols	Spray propellants
Aldehydes	Fabric softeners and deodorizers
Ketones	Combustion
	Dry-cleaning fluids
	Some fabrics and furnishings
	Stored gasoline
	Outgasing from water
	Some building materials
	Waxes and polishing compounds
	Pens and markers
	Binders and plasticizers

SOURCE: Data from Turner et al.[55]

cally occur as exposures to mixtures, rather than as single agents.

Overview: Sources and Classification of Indoor Air Pollution

Indoor air pollution has myriad sources, including the materials from which the space is constructed, its furnishings, processes operating within the environment, biologic agents, and even the occupants. Outdoor air pollutants can also penetrate indoors, as can soil gas. The broad source headings are combustion, evaporation, abrasion, biologic, and radon (Table 62-5).[55] The principal combustion sources are gas cooking stoves, burning cigarettes, fireplaces and wood stoves, and unvented space heaters.

Evaporation of volatile organic compounds from materials and products leads to ubiquitous contamination by these agents. Abrasion of friable asbestos is a principal source of this indoor contaminant. The biologic agents are heterogeneous, extending from infectious organisms to pets and the occupants themselves. Radon comes primarily from soil gas.

The concentration of an indoor contaminant depends on the strength of its source, the rate of removal, the volume of the space, and the rate of exchange of air between the space and outdoors. This *mass-balance* formulation indicates that the concentration of a contaminant might be reduced by limiting source strength, increasing removal rate, or increasing exchange between indoor and outdoor air.

In the typical modern building, the exchange of indoor with outdoor air is accomplished by a central heating, ventilating, and air-conditioning (HVAC) system. These systems are diverse, although all have the same purpose: the delivery of air of acceptable quality to building occupants.[55] The volume of air to be delivered follows the recommendation of standards set by the American Society of Heating, Refrigerating, and Air-Conditioning Engineers. In most new buildings, occupants can no longer control the temperature of the work environment and cannot open windows to increase air exchange. Most residences, however, still rely on natural ventilation.

Carbon Monoxide

Carbon monoxide, a by-product of combustion of fuels, is released indoors by cooking and heating devices and also by smoking. Surveys of urban population exposures in Denver, Colorado, and Washington, D.C., indicate that residential concentrations of CO are typically low, ranging from 2 to 4 ppm during the winter, when windows of homes are generally closed and the homes heated.[11] People living in homes with gas cooking ranges and those living with smokers have slightly higher levels of personal exposure. Measurements of CO in commercial and institutional buildings in the surveys showed concentrations in the same range as in residences. The CO in residences and public buildings without combustion sources primarily reflects entry of motor vehicle exhaust from outdoor air into buildings through natural and mechanical ventilation. Intake vents at street level bring co-contaminated air into buildings. Elevated levels have been measured in commercial buildings with drive-in window operations (e.g., banks), buildings with underground parking garages, and enclosed ice rinks with ice-resurfacing machines without emission controls.

Acute and chronic health effects may be caused by CO exposure. About 900 accidental deaths in the United States are attributed annually to asphyxiation by CO inhalation.[9] Although most of them occur from the operation of motor vehicles, some deaths occur in residences, with a small proportion occurring in public buildings having faulty, unvented, or improperly ventilated combustion sources such as charcoal stoves.[19]

The level of CO in the blood is a useful biomarker of dose, and the health effects of exposure to CO can be related to COHb levels. In nonsmokers who are not exposed to CO in the environment, COHb levels are approximately 0.5 percent. This endogenous COHb comes from catabolism of hemoglobin and heme-containing enzymes of the liver. In comparison, COHb levels of cigarette smokers average about 4 percent and may be much higher. Frank CO poisoning, as manifest in headache, loss of motor control, and coma, generally occurs with COHb levels above 20 percent. Clinicians have proposed the concept of "occult" CO poisoning, arising from persistent exposure to low levels of CO in indoor environments. Headache and dizziness, early symptoms of CO poisoning, have been associated with COHb levels greater than 10 percent. Elevated COHb levels resulting from indoor exposures may, at times, extend to values at which clinical testing has demonstrated cardiovascular and neurobehavioral effects.

Nitrogen Dioxide

In the United States, with the exception of a few urban areas where outdoor NO_2 levels are high, indoor environments are the predominant determinant of total personal exposure.[45] Residential exposures from unvented gas cooking stoves and kerosene space heaters are the major sources contributing to total personal exposure. Although vented to the outside by building codes, gas furnaces and water heaters may pollute residences because of flue-gas spillage and backdrafting caused by improper installation, maintenance, and weather conditions.

Levels in residences and the determinants of these levels have been characterized in many regions of the United States. Indoor NO_2 levels are generally increased during the winter, when homes are closed; they may also be high in the summer, when homes are closed for air conditioning. During cooking, concentrations may reach 1000 ppb while the stove is in use, resulting in substantial, but brief, exposures for persons near the stove. High indoor NO_2 concentrations have been documented in small inner-city apartments and when the oven is used for heating. Data on NO_2 levels in commercial and institutional buildings are very limited, but they generally show low levels consistent with the lack of indoor sources. High concentrations of NO_2 have been measured in ice-skating rinks, contaminated by emissions from resurfacing machines without emissions controls.

Oxidant injury has been postulated to be the principal mechanism by which NO_2 damages the lung. Inhaled NO_2 is thought to combine with water in the lung to form nitric acid (HNO_3) and nitrous acid (HNO_2). At high concentrations, NO_2 causes extensive lung injury in animals and humans. Fatal pulmonary edema and bronchopneumonia have been reported at extremely high concentrations; lower concentrations are associated with bronchitis, bronchiolitis, and pneumonia.

Experimental evidence indicates that NO_2 exposure adversely affects lung defense mechanisms.[43,45] In experimental models, NO_2 effects mucociliary clearance, the alveolar macrophage, and the immune system. In animal experiments employing challenge with respiratory pathogens, exposure to NO_2 reduces clearance of infecting organisms and increases the mortality of the experimental animals. Adverse effects in these animal experiments have been demonstrated at concentrations that are an order of magnitude greater than those typically found in indoor environments.

The health effects of indoor NO_2 have been investigated primarily in studies directed at the consequences of exposures indoors for children.[43,45] The toxicology of NO_2 implies that a wide variety of health effects are of potential concern, including reduced efficacy of host defenses against infectious organisms and consequent increased risk of infection, exacerbation of asthma and chronic obstructive pulmonary disease, and respiratory tract inflammation with manifestations of respiratory symptoms and reduction of lung function. In spite of extensive investigation using laboratory and epidemiologic approaches, the evidence still remains inconclusive in regard to each of these health outcomes.

The hypothesis that NO_2 increases the risk for respiratory infection has received the most intensive investigation. A number of epidemiologic studies have compared the occurrence of respiratory infections in children in homes having gas stoves and higher concentrations of NO_2 with that in children in homes with electric stoves and lower concentrations of NO_2.[43,45] The findings of these studies have been inconsistent, largely because of the methodologic complexities of investigating this association.[43] Experimental exposures have also failed to provide consistent evidence that NO_2 increases infectivity in humans.

Inflammation of the airways by NO_2 could plausibly be associated with increased respiratory symptoms and reduced lung function. These potential adverse effects of NO_2 have been examined using data from epidemiologic studies of children and adults.[43,45] Many of these studies have included large numbers of participants studied cross-sectionally. The health outcome measures (e.g., reports of symptoms and levels of spirometric lung function) have been compared for participants living in homes with NO_2 sources, such as gas stoves and space heaters, and participants living in homes without such sources. Despite the number of such studies, there is no clear pattern. A meta-analysis using data from 11 studies found that a long-term increase in NO_2 exposure of approximately 15 ppb, consistent with the presence of a gas stove in the home, is associated with a 20 percent increase in the risk of respiratory illness in children.[21] On the other hand, a large study of children under the age of 2 years in Albuquerque found no association between indoor NO_2 exposure and respiratory illness.

Inflammation of airways would be expected to worsen the status of persons with asthma. Short-term effects of NO_2 exposures on asthmatics have been studied by exposing volunteers and following pulmonary function level and nonspecific airway responsiveness. The evidence has been conflicting,[43] and the findings are of limited generality because of the inclusion of relatively mild asthmatics in most studies. The NO_2 exposures typically found in indoor and outdoor environments are not likely to cause clinically relevant effects for most persons with asthma. However, recent studies indicate that exposure to NO_2 in combination with allergens may adversely affect persons with asthma. Two studies showed that exposure to NO_2 increases the response to challenge with specific allergen at levels as low as 0.40 ppm.[13,54] Thus, for persons with asthma, indoor NO_2 from unvented combustion sources could increase the adverse effects of exposure to common indoor allergens, such as those associated with house-dust mites, cats, and cockroaches. There is little information on the effects of NO_2 exposure on persons with COPD.

Environmental Tobacco Smoke

Although the prevalence of smoking has decreased among adults to approximately 25 percent in the United States,[57] smoking remains common in public places and homes. *Environmental tobacco smoke* (ETS) is a term now widely used to refer to the combination of side-stream smoke that is released from the cigarette's burning end and the mainstream smoke exhaled by the smoker. The available data on ETS exposure for nonsmokers and children, while limited, suggest widespread exposures. If smokers are present, exposure received indoors at home may dominate total personal exposures of involuntary smokers for particles and some gaseous pollutants, such as benzene.[60]

Hundreds of chemical compounds have been identified in cigarette smoke; the indicators most often used to quantify its presence in the environment are respirable suspended particles (RSP), which are particles of mean aerodynamic diameter of less than 2.5 μm, CO, and nicotine, which is in the vapor phase of ETS.[18,57] Nicotine is a highly specific marker for the presence of tobacco smoke; it can be monitored with both active and passive techniques. Largely because RSP can be readily monitored with area and personal sampling methods, levels of RSP have been widely used as a marker for ETS. The data show that smoking in the home approximately doubles the 24-h average indoor RSP concentration.[56] Far higher short-term exposures, not reflected in these longer-term integrated measurements, must occur in homes when smoking is actually taking place. Data on ETS levels in public buildings have shown high short-term measurements in bowling alleys, at cocktail parties, in bars, and in other locations with a high density of smokers.[18,57]

The adverse effects of ETS have been assessed in the context of the voluminous evidence on active smoking and health and of the detailed characterizations that have been made of the composition and toxicology of mainstream and side-stream cigarette smoke. Associations of ETS with disease and other adverse outcomes have been demonstrated (Table 62-6). The evidence has been reviewed by a number of expert panels, with the repeated conclusion that ETS causes both malignant and nonmalignant diseases in nonsmokers.[25,35,56,57]

Studies of children of smoking parents provided the first warning of the adverse effects of ETS on nonsmokers. Maternal smoking was found to increase risk of infants for lower respiratory tract illnesses, and smoking by household members, particularly the mother, was shown to increase the incidence of chronic res-

TABLE 62-6

Established and Potential Health Effects of Involuntary Exposure to Tobacco Smoke

Established
    Increased lower respiratory infections in children
    Increased respiratory symptoms in children
    Reduced lung growth in children
    Increased lung cancer risk in nonsmokers
    Irritation of the eyes, nose, throat, and lower respiratory tract
    Increased risk for cardiovascular disease
Potential
    Increased respiratory symptoms in adults
    Reduced lung function in adults
    Exacerbation of asthma
    Increased risk for nonrespiratory cancers
    Earlier age at menopause
    Increased risk for sudden infant death
    Reduced birth weight

piratory symptoms and reduce the rate of lung growth in children.[56,57] Children with asthma whose parents smoke have heightened airway responsiveness and increased morbidity, as documented by indexes of medical care utilization.[57] Exposure to ETS is also a suspect cause of asthma,[57] and infants of smoking parents have increased airway responsiveness shortly after birth. Epidemiologic studies show that parental smoking is associated with persistent middle-ear effusions.[57]

Exposure to ETS was first linked to lung cancer in never-smokers in two reports published in 1981. Numerous epidemiologic studies have addressed this association,[40,57] and the weight of the evidence shows a positive association between living with a smoker and risk of lung cancer. In a 1992 risk assessment published by the EPA,[57] epidemiologic studies were systematically reviewed and a meta-analysis was performed. The number of studies showing a positive association could not be completely explained by potential sources of bias, including confounding by other causes of lung cancer and misclassification of smoking status (never or ever smoking). The risk of lung cancer was increased by approximately 20 percent for never-smoking women married to smokers.

Based on review of the epidemiologic evidence, as well as the supporting toxicologic data, the EPA classified ETS as a class A carcinogen, a designation applied to agents causally linked to cancer.[57] This designation mirrored the earlier conclusions of the International Agency for Research on Cancer,[25] the U.S. Surgeon General, and the U.S. National Research Council.[35] The EPA estimated that ETS exposure causes approximately 2000 lung cancer deaths annually in never-smokers.[57]

Additional health effects of ETS remain under investigation. A number of epidemiologic studies have shown that marriage to a smoker increases risk for ischemic heart disease. Although the evidence is not so extensive as for the respiratory consequences of ETS exposure, the American Heart Association has concluded that ETS exposure is a major preventable cause of cardiovascular disease and death.[53] The Council on Cardiopulmonary and Critical Care of the American Heart Association offered the estimate that 35,000 to 40,000 cardiovascular disease–related deaths occur annually because of ETS exposure. Cited mechanisms include promotion of atherosclerosis, increased platelet aggregation, endothelial cell damage, and the consequences of CO exposure. ETS exposure at home and in the workplace has been linked to reduced lung function in some studies. Other proposed associations of ETS with disease are increased risk for cancers at sites other than the lung, younger age at menopause, increased risk for sudden infant death syndrome, reduced birth weight, and worsening of cystic fibrosis.

Wood Smoke

The presence of wood smoke indoors can be assessed by measurements of particles, organic compounds, and CO. Available data suggest that the routine operation of a properly installed and maintained wood stove does not directly affect indoor air quality, and outdoor air contaminated with wood smoke of neighbors can enter and pollute the interior air of homes without wood stoves.

Wood smoke is a complex mixture, both in its physical and chemical characteristics and in its toxicologic properties. The toxicology of some components of wood smoke, such as benzo[a]pyrene, other polycyclic organic compounds, and nitrogen oxides, has been extensively studied. Little research, however, has addressed the toxicology of wood smoke as a complex mixture.

Most of the available epidemiologic evidence on the health effects of wood smoke is derived from investigations in developing countries, where intense smoke exposure results from the use of cooking fires in poorly ventilated dwellings.[49] The studies from less developed countries suggest that smoke exposure adversely affects children and adults, increasing the occurrence of acute respiratory illness in children and chronic respiratory morbidity in children and adults. The occurrence of COPD in never-smoking women exposed to wood smoke has been described as well. Data from more developed countries are sparse and do not clearly indicate adverse effects at the lower concentrations of wood smoke generally present.

Organic Compounds

Organic compounds are ubiquitous indoors, where they are released from furnishings and equipment, construction materials, and consumer and office products (Table 62-7).[60] The organic

TABLE 62-7

Common Organic Chemicals and Their Sources

Chemicals	Measured Peak Nonoccupational Exposure (μg/m³)	Major Sources of Exposure
Volatile chemicals		
Benzene	1000	Smoking, auto exhaust, passive smoking, driving, pumping gas
Tetrachloroethylene	1000	Wearing or storing dry-cleaned clothes, visiting dry cleaners
p-Dichlorobenzene	1000	Room deodorizers, moth cakes
Chloroform	250	Showering (10-min average)
	50	Washing clothes, dishes
Methylene chloride	500,000	Paint stripping, solvent usage
1,1,1-Trichloroethane	1000	Wearing or storing dry-cleaned clothes, aerosol sprays, fabric protectors
Trichloroethylene	100	Unknown (cosmetics, electronic parts)
Carbon tetrachloride	100	Industrial strength cleansers
Aromatic hydrocarbons	1000	Paints, adhesives, gasoline, combustion sources
Toluene, xylenes, ethylbenzene, trimethylbenzenes		
Alphatic hydrocarbons	1000	Paints, adhesives, gasoline, combustion sources
Octane, decane, undecane		
Terpenes	1000	Scented deodorizers, polishes, fabrics, fabric softeners, cigarettes, food, and beverages
Limonene, a-pinene		
Semivolatile chemicals		
Chlorpyrifos (Dursban)	10	Insecticide
Chlordane, heptachlor	100	Termiticide
Diazinon	100	Insecticide
Polychlorinated biphenyls (PCBs)		Transformers, fluorescent ballasts, ceiling tiles
Polycyclic aromatic hydrocarbons (PAHs)	1	Combustion products (smoking, wood burning, kerosene heaters)

SOURCE: Data from Wallace.[60]

compounds found in indoor air can be grouped by boiling point range as volatile (0 to 240°C), semivolatile (240°C to 380°C), and particulate (over 380°C).[31,62] The volatile and semivolatile organic compounds are most relevant to human health. Volatile organic compounds exist as vapors over the normal range of air temperatures and pressures, whereas semivolatile organic compounds are liquids or solids but also evaporate.

Hundreds of organic compounds have been identified in indoor air.[31,60] Although many of these agents are also released by outdoor sources such as chemical plants, indoor concentrations and sources have been shown to determine personal exposures to most of the organic compounds.[60] The Total Exposure Assessment Methodology (TEAM) study conducted by the EPA showed the dominant contributions of indoor sources to personal exposures, even in locations with outdoor air polluted by industry.[61] For example, benzene, a human carcinogen, may be emitted into outdoor air by industry and from gasoline. Among cigarette smokers in the TEAM study, however, the main source of personal exposure was benzene in mainstream cigarette smoke; passive smokers are also exposed to benzene.

Formaldehyde, used in hundreds of products, is one of the most ubiquitous indoor organic compounds.[60] The largest use of formaldehyde is in urea and phenol-formaldehyde resins, which are used to bond laminated wood products and to bind the wood chips in particle board. Formaldehyde-containing wood products are used as shelving, counters, bookcases, cabinets, floors, and wall coverings in homes, offices, and public buildings. Formaldehyde resins are also used to treat paper products and fabrics and are constituents of numerous other consumer products.

The health risks of the organic compounds are diverse; the organics found in indoor air include several dozen carcinogens and mutagens (e.g., benzene), irritants (e.g., formaldehyde and terpenes), and neurotoxins (e.g., aromatic compounds).[60] Despite the potential risks of the organic compounds in indoor air, few studies have shown specific exposure-disease associations, largely because of the difficulty of characterizing exposures and identifying effects of components of complex mixtures in indoor air. Indoor exposures to organics may contribute to the risks for several cancers, although few epidemiologic studies have been directed specifically at assessing cancer risk in relation to indoor exposures to organics.

Irritation of mucosal surfaces and neurotoxic effects may contribute to the symptom complex widely referred to as *sick-building syndrome*.[31] In an investigation of the effects of a mixture of volatile organic compounds on lung function of 11 subjects with bronchial hyperactivity,[20] at the highest concentration studied (25 mg/m³) there was evidence of a significant decline of forced expiratory volume 1 s (FEV$_1$) after exposure, although histamine responsiveness was unchanged.

Radon

Radon-222, a noble gas, is in the decay chain of naturally occurring uranium-238. It decays with a half-life of 3.8 days into a series of short-lived progeny: polonium-218, lead-214, bismuth-214, and polonium-214. Irradiation of respiratory epithelial cells by alpha particles released by polonium-218 and polonium-214 is considered to damage cellular DNA and lead to lung cancer. The principal source of radon in buildings is entrance of

naturally occurring gas in soil.[39] The driving pressure for entry of soil gas into a building is the pressure gradient established by a structure across the soil. The soil gas enters through openings such as sump pump wells, drains, cracks, and utility access holes. In most locales, building materials and water used in the home do not contribute significantly to concentrations of radon indoors. Because radium, the parent radioisotope for radon, is ubiquitous, radon is present in outdoor air and in higher concentrations in indoor environments.

Extensive data on radon concentrations in homes in the United States show that the average value is about 1.5 picocuries per liter (pCi/L). Homes with high concentrations have been identified in all states, although the proportion exceeding the EPA's action guideline of 4 pCi/L is variable among the states. In a national survey conducted from 1988 through 1991, the EPA measured radon concentration in 6000 randomly selected homes in the United States. About 4 percent of homes were estimated to exceed the guideline of 4 pCi/L annual average.

Exposure to radon progeny, the short-lived decay products of radon, has been causally linked to increased risk of lung cancer in uranium miners and other underground workers.[57] Measurements made since the 1970s have shown that radon is present in most homes and can reach high concentrations—as high as those in underground mines—with a documented excess of lung cancer. Current risk models imply that even values under current guidelines cause a significant number of lung cancer cases, as the risk is assumed in these models to follow a linear nonthreshold relationship. Thus, any exposure is assumed to convey some risk.[30,37]

The hazard posed by radon progeny exposure in indoor air has been addressed primarily through risk estimation procedures. In the most widely applied risk assessment approach, the risks for the general population are projected by extrapolating risks observed in the studies of miners to the general population. Use of such models leads to the conclusion that radon contributes significantly to the burden of lung cancer in the population, causing an estimated 10,000 to 20,000 cases annually in the United States.[12] The burden of radon-related lung cancer in the general population reflects, in part, the synergism between radon and cigarette smoking assumed in the models.

The most recent risk model is based on a pooled analysis of data from 11 epidemiologic studies of male miners, including 68,000 among whom there were more than 2700 cancer deaths.[30] The analysis showed a positive linear relationship between the risk of lung cancer and occupational radon exposure, down to exposures only a fewfold greater than average lifetime exposure from indoor radon. Lung cancer risk was found to decline with increasing age and time since exposure; the risk was also found to increase as the rate of exposure decreased—the so-called inverse-dose rate effect. When the model was applied to the U.S. population, indoor exposure to radon at home was estimated to be responsible for about 12 percent of lung cancer deaths in the United States. Of the 18,200 lung cancer deaths attributed to radon in 1993, 12,400 were assigned to smokers and 5800 to never-smokers.

The substantial lung cancer burden attributed to indoor radon has led to programs for exposure reduction. The program in the United States, conducted by the EPA, calls for voluntary measurement of radon levels in single-family homes and modification if the annual concentration exceeds the Agency's guideline level of 4 pCi/L.[59] Two types of passive measurement devices are available: short-term devices, which make measurements for a few days, and long-term devices, which make measurements for periods of months up to a year. The short-term devices, primarily charcoal canisters, are often used when a measurement is quickly needed during a real estate transaction; the longer-term devices incorporate a piece of plastic that is etched by alpha particles released by progeny.

Fortunately, elevated radon concentrations can be lowered, often by such simple measures as sealing basement cracks and sump holes. Approaches also include ventilating the basement to the outside and, for homes built on concrete slabs, providing a system to exhaust the soil gas from beneath the slab. In areas having a high potential for indoor radon problems, there are radon-resistant construction techniques that can be applied in anticipation of high levels.

The success of the EPA's program for managing the indoor radon problem rests on voluntary action by the public. To engage the public, the Agency has developed a risk communication strategy that uses the media, voluntary health agencies (e.g., the American Lung Association), and health-care providers. Its pamphlet, "A Citizen's Guide to Radon," informs readers about the risks and the recommended approaches for managing them.[59]

Asbestos and Man-Made Fibers

Asbestos, comprising several fibrous inorganic materials characterized by chemical formulation and crystalline structure, has been extensively used in building materials since the beginning of the century because of high tensile strength and thermal properties. The broad categories of use are thermal and acoustic insulation, fire protection, and the reinforcement of building products. In addition to its use in acoustic ceiling tiles and vinyl floor tiles, asbestos has been used in paints and wall and ceiling plaster; until banned in the late 1970s, asbestos materials were used to coat pipes, boilers, and steel structural beams.

Asbestos-containing materials are present in homes, offices, and schools. The EPA has estimated that 20 percent of the nation's buildings, or about 733,000 buildings (not including schools and residential dwellings with fewer than 10 units), contain some asbestos materials.[22]

Asbestos was widely used in ceiling tiles, pipe wrap, plaster, floor tiles, shingles, and sprayed-on insulation, among other applications. Release of fibers from these materials may result from impact, abrasion, fallout, vibration, air erosion, and fire damage.[22] Water damage and the normal aging of binders, leading to the friability of the material, increase the likelihood of release. Asbestos-contaminated surface dust may contribute to airborne concentrations in buildings.

Man-made mineral fibers are now used increasingly as substitutes for asbestos in building materials. These are fibrous inorganic substances made primarily from rock, clay, slag, or glass; the three principal types are glass fibers (comprising glass wool and glass filaments), rock wool, and slag wool and ceramic fibers.[22] Fiberglass and glass wool refer to silica-based vitreous fibers manufactured by a number of different processes. The different types of fibers vary in their chemistry and dimensions, as well as in their durability in vivo.[22] Because they are physically fibrous, there is concern about the same health effects as for asbestos.

An enlarging database on airborne asbestos concentrations in buildings demonstrates extremely low average values under the conditions of normal building use.[22,32] Occupant risk is determined by exposures to airborne fibers, rather than the presence of asbestos-containing materials in the building. Surveys of asbestos concentrations in commercial buildings demonstrate very low fiber concentrations under normal conditions.[22] The Literature Review Panel Report published by the Health Effects Institute, Asbestos Research Committee,[22] compiled all published data, as well as previously unpublished information on buildings sampled for litigation and for other purposes. The total data set included 1377 measurements made by transmission electron microscopy in 198 buildings. For fibers greater than 5 mm in length, which are considered most relevant to disease risk,[29] the mean and median concentrations were low, at approximately 0.001 fiber per milliliter, or three or more orders of magnitude lower than concentrations in the occupational settings of the past. Individual buildings with levels much higher than the typical values in the data assembled by the Health Effects Institute, Asbestos Research Committee, have been reported.

For office workers, visitors to buildings, and schoolchildren and teachers, mesothelioma and lung cancer are the principal health effects of concern; asbestosis would not be expected at usual exposures for these building occupants.[22] The risks of indoor asbestos for the general population have been estimated by extrapolation of risks for occupationally exposed persons. Uncertainty is inherent in this approach, but the risks cannot be directly investigated by epidemiologic methods. The Literature Review Panel Report of the Health Effects Institute, Asbestos Research Committee, has estimated risks for various scenarios of exposure (Table 62-8).[22]

Custodial and maintenance workers in buildings with asbestos-containing materials may be exposed to higher levels of asbestos than other building occupants, as their activities disturb the materials and release fibers. These workers may be at particular risk if they are unaware that asbestos-containing materials are present or are untrained in dealing with these materials. Several studies have shown that custodial and maintenance workers may have pleural plaques and possibly asbestosis, causing concern that a "third wave" of asbestos-caused disease could occur in such workers.[28]

Because of the morphologic and toxicologic comparability of asbestos and man-made mineral fibers, there has been concern that exposure to man-made mineral fibers could produce the same diseases caused by asbestos.[29] The relevant epidemiologic data from exposed workers are less extensive than for asbestos. There is an indication of increased lung cancer risk in workers who produced rock and slag wool in the early years of the industry; data on levels of exposure are unavailable, however, and other carcinogens may have contributed to the increased risk.[26,29] Animal studies have shown the fibers that are long and thin to be carcinogenic.[22] Lippmann concluded from the epidemiologic evidence and toxicologic properties of the materials that the health risk of man-made mineral fibers is likely to be negligible for exposures of building occupants.[29]

TABLE 62-8

Estimated Lifetime Cancer Risks for Different Scenarios of Exposure to Airborne Asbestos Fibers*

Conditions	Premature Cancer Deaths (Lifetime Risks) per Million Exposed Persons
Lifetime, continuous outdoor exposure	
0.00001 fiber/ml from birth (rural)	4
0.00001 fiber/ml (high urban)	40
Exposure in a school containing ACM, from age 5 to 18 years (180 days/year, 5 h/day)	
0.0005 fiber/ml (average)†	6
0.005 fiber/ml (high)†	60
Exposure in a public building containing ACM, from age 25 to 45 years (240 days/year, 8 h/day)	
0.0002 fiber/ml (average)†	4
0.002 fiber/ml (high)†	40
Occupational exposure from age 25 to 45	
0.1 fiber/ml (current occupational levels)‡	2000
10 fiber/ml (historical industrial exposures)	200,000

*This table represents the combined risk (average for males and females) estimated for lung cancer and mesothelioma for building occupants exposed to airborne asbestos fibers under the circumstances specified. These estimates should be interpreted with caution because of the reservations concerning the reliability of the estimates of average levels and of the risk assessment models.
†The "average" levels for the sampled schools and buildings represent the means of building averages for the buildings reviewed herein. The "high" levels for schools and public buildings, shown as 10 times the average, are approximately equal to the average airborne levels of asbestos recorded in approximately 5% of schools and buildings with asbestos-containing materials. If the single highest sample value is excluded from calculation of the average indoor asbestos concentration in public and commercial buildings, the average value is reduced from 0.00021 to 0.00008 fiber/ml, and the lifetime risk is approximately halved.
‡The concentration shown (0.1 fiber/ml) represents the permissible exposure limit proposed by the U.S. Occupational Safety and Health Administration. Actual worker exposure, expected to be lower, will depend on a variety of factors, including work practices and use and efficiency of respiratory protective equipment.
SOURCE: Data from Health Effects Institute.[22]

Biologic Agents

Indoor allergens and microbes—the principal biologic agents in indoor air relevant to human health—have diverse sources, both indoors and outdoors (Table 62-9). Indoor levels of allergens and microbes may be elevated by accumulation of materials indoors, such as human and animal dander, and growth of fungi and bacteria on interior surfaces or in air-conditioning systems. Indoor pollen is derived almost entirely from outdoor plants, and fungus spores from outdoors may also enter the indoor environment on air infiltration or inadvertently on people, animals, or objects.

The most severe and prevalent indoor biologic pollution problems result from the growth of microorganisms on interior surfaces that are wet and moist. Substrates providing a source of both carbon and water can support the growth of microorganisms. High relative humidity, in excess of 70 percent, promotes condensation on interior surfaces (e.g., cool exterior walls or windowsills).[16] Leaks from water pipes and roofs can also provide consistent sources of moisture. Other moisture sources are humidifiers, vaporizers, and air conditioners; once contaminated, these devices can distribute fungal fragments, spores, and dissolved allergens into room air.

There is limited information on levels of microbial particles in air. Indoor levels and, hence, personal exposure are highly variable and are probably affected by activities such as vacuuming, sweeping, dusting, making beds, scrubbing contaminated surfaces, and using electric fans. Further, airborne and dust concentrations of allergens probably have limited value for assessing the contribution of a particular allergen in causing disease. Factors such as aerodynamic behavior, respirability, solubility, and cross-reactivity with other allergens are also important in the process of immunologic sensitization and the development of allergic disease.[24]

Dust mites (*Dermatophagoides pteronyssinus*, *D. farinae*, and *Euroglyphus maynei*) are commonly found in houses and are important sources of allergens, particularly for persons with asthma.[24] These mites are approximately 0.3 mm in length and live in carpets, upholstered furniture, mattresses, and bedding, where they eat skin scales. Two major dust mite allergens have been identified, *Der p* I and *Der p* II. These proteins are derived from digestive enzymes in the gut of the mite and are found in high concentrations in the fecal pellets. Vacuum sampling and immunologic assays indicate that in the home, the highest levels of allergen occur in the bedroom in carpeting, mattresses, and bedding.

Domestic cockroaches, including the German cockroach, *Blattella germanica,* are commonly found indoors and represent another source of allergen in residences, particularly in infested inner-city housing. Fecal material and saliva contain large amounts of the allergens *Bla g* I and *Bla g* II.

Cats and dogs are prevalent sources of allergen exposures. *Fel d* I is the most significant allergen associated with cats, and high levels of this protein are found in cat dander and fur and also in saliva and urine. The median level of *Fel d* I in samples of settled household dust in homes with a cat are reported to range from 2 to 130,000 mg per gram of dust, with a median level of 90 ng of *Fel d* I per gram of dust.[63] In homes without a cat, much lower levels are observed, ranging from 2 to 7500 mg of *Fel d* I per gram of dust; the antigen is persistent in indoor environments for long periods after a cat is no longer indoors. The presence of the allergen in the dust of homes and buildings in which cats are not kept suggests that the allergen can be transported on clothing. The major dog allergen, *Can f* I, is present in dog fur and saliva and is a relatively stable protein that may persist in dust for a long time. The content of *Can f* I in household dust from homes with a dog range from 10 to 10,000 mg per gram of dust, compared with 0.3 to 23 mg per gram of dust in homes without a dog.[46]

Fungi are present in the air of virtually all homes and public buildings. Commonly isolated genera include *Cladosporium,*

TABLE 62-9

Sources of Biologic Air Pollutants

Acarids
  Dust mites and spiders
Insects
  Cockroaches, crickets, beetles, fleas, moths, flies, and midges
Domestic animals
  Cats, dogs, other mammals, and birds
Rodents
  Wild
    Mice and rats
  Pets
    Mice, gerbils, and guinea pigs
Fungi
  Indoors (growing on interior surfaces or in air-conditioning systems)
    Penicillium, Aspergillus, Rhizopus, and *Cladosporium*
  Outdoors
    Numerous species entering with incoming air
Pollens
  Derived from outdoor plants or plant materials brought inside
Bacteria
  Legionella (introduced into ventilation systems by cooling towers and standing water reservoirs)

Penicillium, Alternaria, Epicoccum, Aspergillus, and *Drechslera.*

Biologic agents in indoor air may cause disease through various mechanisms, including direct toxicity, infections, and immune hyperresponsiveness. A complete review of these diverse effects is beyond the scope of this chapter. Selected examples of diseases caused by biologic agents are given; more extensive information is available in recently published reviews.[8,24]

Home dampness and mold, determined by questionnaire, have been associated with upper respiratory symptoms and eye irritation in large studies of children in the United States[8,24] and Canada. These associations were adjusted for known determinants of respiratory symptoms, including maternal smoking, city, child's age and sex, and parent education. Because the exposure and outcome variables were based on parental report, the findings are limited by the subjective nature of the study designs.

Allergic rhinitis, or "hay fever," is common, affecting approximately 20 percent or more adults in the United States. Identification of the specific indoor allergen associated with the symptoms may be accomplished by skin testing and in vitro measurement of antibody [radioallergosorbent test (RAST)]. Many persons with asthma are sensitive to specific antigens from pollens, animal fur, fungi spores, and house dust. The risk of acute or severe attacks of asthma is increased in residences with levels of *Der p* I in excess of 10 mg per gram of house dust, and asthmatic patients have been reported to show a 25 percent prevalence of skin test positively to cat or dog allergen extracts. Building-related allergic respiratory disease and epidemic asthma have been reported in office buildings in association with air-handling systems and humidifiers contaminated with bacteria and fungi.[17]

Avian proteins are present in bird excreta (e.g., the droppings of pet birds such as parakeets), and fungal spores of thermophilic actinomycetes, *Aspergillus* species, *Penicillium* species, and *Aureobasidium* species may contaminate the indoor environment and cause hypersensitivity pneumonitis. A careful review of symptom pattern in relation to home and work environments and site evaluation may be needed to identify the source of exposure.

The bacterium *Legionella pneumophila,* the agent of legionnaires' disease, causes an often fatal pneumonia associated with exposure to the bacterium in aerosols of cooling towers and air-handling systems and in humidifiers and spas. It exemplifies a respiratory pathogen associated primarily with indoor environments, in both source and transmission. Of course, indoor environments are the locus of transmission of many infectious respiratory diseases, including influenza and tuberculosis. The risk of diseases depends on the strength of sources and the level of ventilation. A recent report has shown, for example, that a low air exchange rate increased the risk for pneumococcal infection among inmates in a large county jail.[23]

SUSCEPTIBLE POPULATIONS

The legislative history of the Clean Air Act mandated that the primary NAAQS were to be set low enough to protect the health of all susceptible groups within the population except those requiring life-support systems. Only two diseases, asthma and emphysema, were specifically identified in the Clean Air Act as associated with increased susceptibility. Other groups in the population, accounting for large numbers of people, are also considered to be at increased risk from air pollutants: persons with coronary artery disease and, possibly, peripheral vascular disease; infants and the elderly in general; and children with chronic pulmonary ailments such as cystic fibrosis and bronchopulmonary dysplasia.

In this section we consider the evidence on these susceptible groups (Table 62-10). Pulmonologists are likely to be asked about the consequences of pollution exposures by persons with chronic lung diseases. Patients may report being adversely affected by exposures and may request guidance concerning control measures—e.g., purchase of an air-cleaning device or additional medication use when exposed.

Clinical Studies in Asthma and COPD

Clinical studies have provided much of the evidence on the effects of pollutants on persons with chronic respiratory diseases. Controlled laboratory studies of volunteers have attempted to identify specific effects of individual pollutants, as assessed primarily by pulmonary mechanics; however, other end points, including symptoms, have been assessed.

The most striking effect of acute exposure to SO_2 at concentrations under 1.0 ppm is the induction of bronchoconstriction in asthmatics after exposures lasting only 5 min. In contrast, inhalation of concentrations of SO_2 in excess of 5 ppm causes only small decrements in airway function in normal subjects. Lung function responses to SO_2 in asthmatics are greater when SO_2 exposure is accompanied by increased ventilation, usually stimulated by exercise. SO_2-induced bronchoconstriction can be exacerbated by breathing cold or dry air and oral (versus nasal) breathing. The SO_2 bronchoconstrictor response can be reduced or inhibited in asthmatics by anticholinergic agents such as atropine, mast cell stabilizers such as cromolyn, and β-agonist bronchodilators such as metaproterenol.

Inhalation of acidic aerosols generally produces little alteration of pulmonary function in normal subjects, even at the workplace Permissible Exposure Limit of 1 mg/m^3. As with SO_2, asthmatic subjects have been found susceptible to the effects of acidic aerosol exposure, although different laboratories have found differing threshold exposure concentrations. Adult asthmatics exposed to 450 and 1000 μg/m^3 of H_2SO_4 aerosols demonstrated decrements in specific airway conductance. Adolescent asthmatics appear to be more sensitive to the effects of acidic aerosols than adult asthmatics. Functional decrements have been observed in adolescents at levels as low as 70 μg/m^3, occasionally noted in outdoor air, and an order of magnitude lower than the level at which effects are observed in normal subjects. The apparent difference in sensitivity of adult and adolescent asthmatics may also be due to differences in the research protocols. In these studies, young asthmatics showed functional decrements at exposure levels near peak outdoor levels in the northeastern United States. Field studies in summer camps of both normal and asthmatic children reported decrements in pulmonary function during pollution episodes that included increased levels of acidic aerosols, supporting the concern that children and adolescents may be particularly susceptible to effects of acidic atmospheres.

Although several controlled human studies have found asthmatics to be responsive to low levels of NO_2, the findings have not been consistent. The conflicting results among these studies are probably related to the differences in subject selection and exposure protocols. Persons with COPD may represent a group with increased susceptibility to short-term NO_2, but further study of the issue is needed.

Consonant with the provisions of the Clean Air Act and with its legislative history, a group that appears to be at potential risk from exposure to ozone would also be the group characterized as having preexisting respiratory disease. In the case of asthmatics, however, emerging data from controlled studies indicate no greater responsiveness to ozone in mild asthmatics than in normal, healthy populations. Pretreatment of healthy volunteers with β-adrenergic agents before O_3 exposure and exercise did not prevent bronchoconstriction, whereas pretreatment with atropine or indomethacin reduced the decrement in lung function. Since exercise greatly potentiates the response to ozone, the best strategy would be to avoid outdoor exercise during periods of high O_3 pollution.

Clinical Studies in Heart Disease

Persons with coronary heart disease have also been identified as a group at risk from elevated air pollution levels. In the presence of coronary artery disease, there is limited ability to increase coronary blood flow in response to increased myocardial oxygen consumption during exercise. When myocardial blood flow is not sufficient to meet oxygen demand, the myocardium becomes ischemic, resulting in angina pectoris, ECG changes, or both. Several recent studies conducted at relatively low COHb levels have investigated the effects of CO exposure on exercise capacity and on the occurrence of myocardial ischemia. These studies found a decrease in the time to the occurrence of myocardial ischemia in persons with coronary artery disease during exercise after CO exposure. The lowest CO dose to produce a decrease in time to the onset of angina was associated with a 2 percent COHb level. In this study, there was a mean decrease of 4.2 percent in the time to angina and a mean decrease of 5.1 percent in the time to ECG changes indicative of myocardial ischemia at 2 percent COHb compared to control (air exposure) days; greater effects were noted at 3.9 percent COHb.[1] The clinical studies have shown a significant dose-response relationship for the individual differences in time to the onset of ECG changes at increasing COHb levels. In addition, at a COHb level of 6 per-

TABLE 62-10

Populations Considered Susceptible to Air Pollution

Population	Potential Mechanism	Consequences
Asthmatics	Increased airway responsiveness	Increased risk for exacerbation and respiratory symptoms
Cigarette smokers	Impaired defense and clearance, lung injury	Increased damage through synergism
Elderly	Impaired respiratory defenses, reduced functional reserve	Increased risk for respiratory infection, increased risk for clinically significant effects on function
Infants	Immature defense mechanisms of the lung	Increased risk for respiratory infection
Persons with coronary heart disease	Impaired myocardial oxygenation	Increased risk for myocardial ischemia
Persons with COPD	Reduced level of lung function	Increased risk for clinically significant effects on function

cent, patients with coronary artery disease have an increased frequency of arrhythmias. It is interesting that, at the same low levels of COHb, adverse effects have been observed in humans but have not been found in animal studies.

CONTROL STRATEGIES

Controlling the health effects of indoor and outdoor air pollution requires strategies oriented toward populations and toward patients. Clinicians can make practical recommendations to their patients in order to reduce risk for disease and for exacerbation of established disease. Clinicians may serve as consultants or as advocates in seeking to reduce the effects of indoor and outdoor air pollutants through population-oriented control approaches.

Patient-Oriented Strategies

Approaches for limiting the health risks of breathing polluted ambient air have received little investigation. Present understanding of the determinants of exposure suggests that modifying time-activity patterns to limit time outside during episodes of pollution represents the most effective strategy. The levels of some reactive pollutants tend to be lower indoors than outdoors. O_3 levels in buildings are lower than outdoor levels, but they can be driven upward by increasing the rate of exchange of indoor with outdoor air. Fine acid aerosols can penetrate indoors, but neutralization by ammonia produced by occupants, pets, and household products may reduce concentrations. Other types of particles in outdoor air may also enter indoor air. Nevertheless, health-care providers can reasonably advise patients to stay indoors during pollution episodes. Vigorous exercise outdoors, which increases the dose of pollution delivered to the respiratory tract, should also be avoided at such times.

Susceptible patients should be counseled concerning the nature and degree of their susceptibility. The use of medication should follow the usual clinical indications, and therapeutic regimens should not be adjusted because of the occurrence of a pollution episode without evidence of an adverse effect on symptoms or function. In the laboratory, inhalation of cromolyn sodium and bronchodilating agents blocks the response to some pollutants, but use of these drugs solely because of exposure to air pollution cannot be advised.

Respiratory protective equipment has been developed for use in the workplace to minimize exposure to toxic gases and particles. Many of these devices, particularly those likely to be most effective, add to the work of breathing and cannot be tolerated by persons with respiratory disease. Under most circumstances, health-care providers should not suggest respiratory protection as a method for reducing the risks of ambient air pollution. Similarly, air cleaners have not been shown to have health benefits, whether directed at indoor pollutants generated by indoor sources or at those brought in with outside air.[4]

Pulmonologists may be concerned with diverse issues related to the control of indoor air pollution, ranging from answering the questions of individual patients concerning pollutant health effects and control to the management of complex problems in large buildings. Some commonly asked questions and answers that reasonably reflect the state of the evidence are provided in Table 62-11. The clinically relevant microenvironments are numerous, including the home, the workplace, public buildings, and places where leisure time is spent.

Workplace problems, such as the sick-building syndrome, may be particularly challenging. The health-care provider needs to establish the connection between the workplace and the occurrence of symptoms and then seek a solution that includes identifying and remediating the responsible factors in the workplace. The diagnostic task requires a sufficient awareness of the possible causal role of the indoor environment (Fig. 62-2). Resolution may require an evaluation and intervention by indoor air quality professionals.[4] The physician may be unable to resolve the patient's symptoms without motivating a building evaluation and resolution of underlying problems. Guidance for the clinician has been offered by the ATS.[4]

Community-Oriented Strategies

Frequently, communities become concerned about the effect of particular local sources—e.g., a power plant or manufacturing facility. Concern about the health risks may quickly lead to controversy and litigation. Thus, understanding the health risks posed by local sources may be difficult and may require skills in community health, as well as in epidemiology and toxicology. Local physicians may become active through concerns about the health of their patients or as advocates for the community's environment or for the polluting facility. Most often the dimensions of such complex problems exceed the skills of local physicians. Involvement may be appropriate, but guidance should be obtained from appropriate public health and environmental agencies.

TABLE 62-11

Questions and Answers About Indoor Air Pollution

Question	Answer
Do air cleaners work?	Air cleaners have not yet been shown to have direct health benefits.
Should the radon concentration in my home be measured?	Yes, radon can be readily measured at relatively low cost, and mitigation is feasible.
Should the air ducts in my home be cleaned?	There is no evidence on health benefits of air cleaning.
Will controlling mites be beneficial?	Controlling mite levels is beneficial for persons with mite-sensitive asthma.
Should my home be humidified?	Humidification may increase allergen levels.

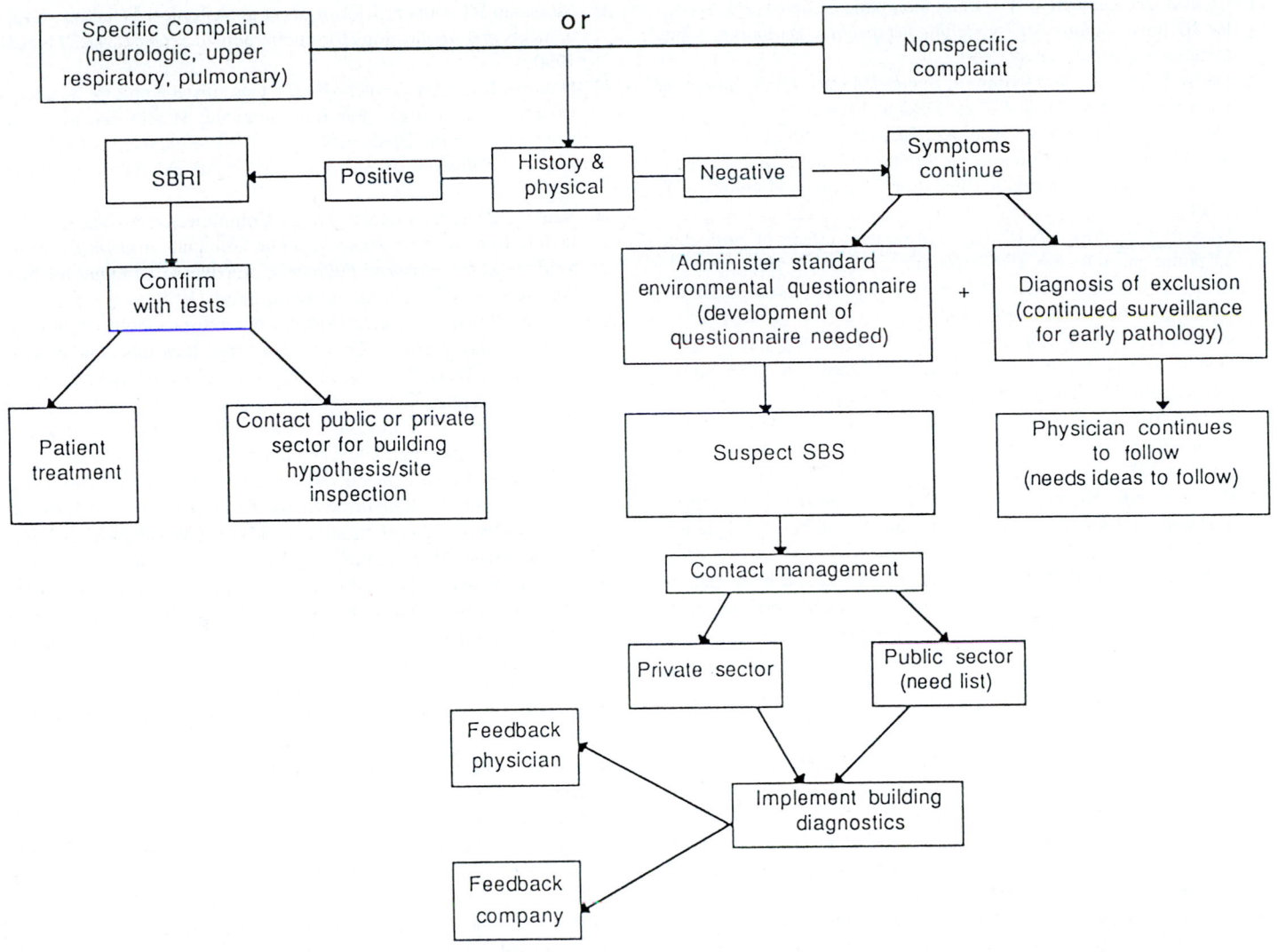

FIGURE 62-2 Medical approach to patient with complaints possibly related to indoor air pollution without an antecedent diagnosis. SBRI = Specific building-related illnesses; SBS = sick building syndrome. *(Based on ATS data,[4] with permission.)*

In 1976, the EPA proposed cautionary statements for public reporting of outdoor air quality—the Pollutant Standards Index—for criteria pollutants. The actions taken when "alert levels" are reached or expected to be reached include the issuance of health advisories (or cautionary statements) to the public. The EPA's advice is intended to be applied by local air pollution agencies in preparing daily air quality summaries to be disseminated to the media. Although the cautionary statements require some revisions, especially as related to ozone exposures, useful guidelines are offered for the physician and public health officials.

REFERENCES

1. Allred EN, Bleecker ER, Chaitman BR, et al: Short-term effects of carbon monoxide exposure on the exercise performance of subjects with coronary artery disease. *New Engl J Med* 321:1426–1432, 1989.
2. American Thoracic Society, Committee of the Environmental and Occupational Health Assembly: Health effects of outdoor air pollution. Part 1. *Am J Respir Crit Care Med* 153:3–50, 1996.
3. American Thoracic Society, Committee of the Environmental and Occupational Health Assembly: Health effects of outdoor air pollution. Part 2. *Am J Respir Crit Care Med* 153:477–498, 1996.
4. American Thoracic Society: Environmental controls and lung disease. *Am Rev Respir Dis* 142:915–939, 1990.
5. American Thoracic Society: Guidelines as to what consitutes an adverse respiratory health effect, with special reference to epidemiologic studies of air pollution. *Am Rev Respir Dis* 131:666–669, 1985.
6. American Thoracic Society: Health effects of atmospheric acids and their precursors. *Am Rev Respir Dis* 144:464–467, 1991.
7. Brimblecombe P: *The Big Smoke.* London, Routledge, Chapman & Hall, 1987.
8. Burge H: Center for Indoor Air Research (Ed): *Bioaerosols.* Boca Raton, FL, Lewis, 1995.
9. Cobb N, Etzel RA: Unintentional carbon monoxide-related deaths in the United States, 1979 through 1988. *JAMA* 266:659–663, 1991.
10. Cohen AJ, Higgins MWP: Health Effects of Diesel Exhaust: Epidemiology. Anonymous Diesel Exhaust: A Critical Analysis of Emissions, Exposure, and Health Effects. A Special Report of the Institute's Working Group. Cambridge, MA, Health Effects Institute, 1995.

11. Coultas DB, Lambert WE: Carbon monoxide, in Samet JM, Spengler JD (eds), *Indoor Air: A Health Perspective.* Baltimore, Johns Hopkins University Press, 1991.

12. Darby SC, Samet JM: Radon, in Samet JM (ed), *Epidemiology of Lung Cancer.* New York, Marcel Dekker, 1994.

13. Devalia JL, Rusznak C, Herdman MJ, et al: Effect of nitrogen dioxide and sulphur dioxide on airway responses of mild asthmatic patients to allergen inhalation. *Lancet* 344:1668–1671, 1994.

14. Dockery DW, Pope CA III: Acute respiratory effects of particulate air pollution. *Annu Rev Public Health* 15:107–132, 1994.

15. Elsom DM: *Atmospheric Pollution, a Global Problem,* 2d ed. Cambridge, MA, Blackwell, 1992.

16. Godish T: *Indoor Air Pollution Control.* Chelsea, MI, Lewis, 1989.

17. Godish T: *Sick Buildings: Definition, Diagnosis and Mitigation.* Boca Raton, FL, Lewis (CRC Press), 1995.

18. Guerin MR, Jenkins RA, Tomkins BA (eds): *The Chemistry of Environmental Tobacco Smoke: Composition and Measurement.* Chelsea, MI, Lewis, 1992.

19. Hampson NB, Kramer CC, Donford RG, Norkool DM: Carbon monoxide poisoning from indoor burning charcoal briquettes. *JAMA* 271:52–53, 1994.

20. Harving H, Dahl R, Molhave L: Lung function and bronchial reactivity in asthmatics during exposure to volatile organic compounds. *Am Rev Respir Dis* 143:751–754, 1991.

21. Hasselblad V, Kotchmar DJ, Eddy DM: Synthesis of environmental evidence: Nitrogen dioxide epidemiology studies. *J Air Waste Manage Assoc* 42:662–671, 1992.

22. Health Effects Institute, Asbestos Research Committee, and Literature Review Panel: *Asbestos in Public and Commercial Buildings: A Literature Review and a Synthesis of Current Knowledge.* Cambridge, MA, Health Effects Institute, 1991.

23. Hoge CW, Reichler MR, Dominguez EA, et al: An epidemic of pneumococcal disease in an overcrowded, inadequately ventilated jail. *New Engl J Med* 331:643–648, 1994.

24. Institute of Medicine, Committee on the Health Effects of Indoor Allergens, Division of Health Promotion and Disease Prevention: *Indoor Allergens: Assessing the Controlling Adverse Health Effects.* Washington, DC, National Academy Press, 1993.

25. International Agency for Research on Cancer: IARC monographs on the evaluation of the carcinogenic risk of chemicals to humans: Tobacco Smoking. Lyons, France, World Health Organization, 1986.

26. International Agency for Research on Cancer: IARC monographs on the evaluation of carcinogenic risks of chemicals to humans: Man-Made Mineral Fibers and Radon. Lyons, France, World Health Organization, 1986.

27. Jenkins PL, Phillips TJ, Mulberg EJ, Hui SP: Activity patterns of California: Use and proximity to indoor pollutant sources. *Atmos Environ* 26:2141–2148, 1992.

28. Landrigan PJ, Kazemi H: *The Third Wave of Asbestos Disease: Exposure to Asbestos in Place. Public Health Control.* New York: New York Academy of Sciences, 1991, p 1.

29. Lippmann M: Asbestos and other mineral fibers, in Lippmann M (ed), *Environmental Toxicants: Human Exposures and Their Health Effects.* New York, Van Nostrand Reinhold, 1992.

30. Lubin JH, Boice JD Jr, Edling C, et al: *Radon and Lung Cancer Risk: A Joint Analysis of 11 Underground Miners Studies.* Bethesda, MD, U.S. Department of Health and Human Services, Public Health Service, National Institutes of Health, 1994.

31. Molhave L: Volatile organic compounds and the sick building syndrome, in Lippmann M (ed), *Environmental Toxicants: Human Exposures and Their Health Effects.* New York, Van Nostrand Reinhold, 1992.

32. Mossman BT, Bignon J, Corn M, et al: Asbestos: Scientific developments and implications for public policy. *Science* 247:294–301, 1990.

33. National Research Council (NRC), Commission on Life Sciences, Board on Toxicology and Environmental Health Hazards, and Committee on the Epidemiology of Air Pollutants: *Epidemiology and Air Pollution.* Washington, DC, National Academy Press, 1985, p 1.

34. National Research Council (NRC), Committee on Advances in Assessing Human Exposure to Airborne Pollutants: *Human Exposure Assessment for Airborne Pollutants: Advances and Opportunities.* Washington, DC, National Academy Press, 1991.

35. National Research Council (NRC), Committee on Passive Smoking: *Environmental Tobacco Smoke: Measuring Exposures and Assessing Health Effects.* Washington, DC, National Academy Press, 1986.

36. National Research Council (NRC), Committee on Risk Assessment of Hazardous Air Pollutants: *Science and Judgment in Risk Assessment.* Washington, DC, National Academy Press, 1994.

37. National Research Council (NRC), Committee on the Biological Effects of Ionizing Radiation: *Health Risks of Radon and Other Internally Deposited Alpha-Emitters: BEIR IV.* Washington, DC, National Academy Press, 1988.

38. National Research Council (NRC), Committee on the Institutional Means for Assessment of Risks to Public Health: *Risk Assessment in the Federal Government: Managing the Process.* Washington, DC, National Academy Press, 1983.

39. Nero AV Jr: Radon and its decay products in indoor air: An overview. In Nazaroff WW, Nero AV Jr (eds), *Radon and Its Decay Products in Indoor Air.* New York, Wiley, 1988.

40. Pershagen G. Passive smoking and lung cancer, in Samet JM (ed), *Epidemiology of Lung Cancer.* New York, Marcel Dekker, 1994.

41. Samet JM, Speizer FE: Introduction and recommendations: Working Group on Indoor Air and Other Complex Mixtures. *Environ Health Perspect* 101:143–147, 1994.

42. Samet JM, Spengler JD: *Indoor Air Pollution: A Health Perspective.* Baltimore, Johns Hopkins University Press, 1991.

43. Samet JM, Utell MJ: The risk of nitrogen dioxide: What have we learned from epidemiological and clinical studies? *Toxicol Indust Health* 6:247–262, 1990.

44. Samet JM: Indoor air pollution: A public health perspective. *Indoor Air* 3:219–226, 1993.

45. Samet JM: Nitrogen dioxide, in Samet JM, Spengler JD (eds), *Indoor Air Pollution: A Health Perspective.* Baltimore, Johns Hopkins University Press, 1991.

46. Schou C, Hansen GN, Lintner T, Løwenstein H: Assay for major dog allergen, *Can f* I: Investigation of house dust samples and commercial dog extracts. *J Allergy Clin Immunol* 88:847–853, 1991.

47. Sheppard D, Saisho A, Nadel JA, Boushey HA: Exercise increases sulfur dioxide-induced bronchoconstriction in asthmatic subjects. *Am Rev Respir Dis* 123:486–491, 1981.

48. Shy CM, Goldsmith JR, Hackney JD, et al: Health effects of air pollution. *ATS News* 6:1–63, 1978.

49. Smith KR: *Biofuels, Air Pollution, and Health: A Global Review.* New York, Plenum, 1987.

50. Speizer FE, Samet JM: Air pollution and lung cancer, in Samet JM (ed), *Epidemiology of Lung Cancer.* New York, Marcel Dekker, 1994.

51. Spengler JD, Brauer M, Koutrakis P: Acid air and health. *Environ Sci Technol* 24:946–956, 1990.

52. Spengler JD, Samet JM: A perspective on indoor and outdoor air pollution, in Samet JM, Spengler JD (eds), *Indoor Air Pollution: A Health Perspective.* Baltimore, Johns Hopkins University Press, 1991.

53. Taylor AE, Johnson DC, Kazemi H: Environmental tobacco smoke and cardiovascular disease: A position paper from the council on cardiopulmonary and critical care, American Heart Association. *Circulation* 86:1–4, 1992.

54. Tunnicliffe WS, Burge PS, Ayres JG: Effect of domestic concentrations of nitrogen dioxide on airway responses to inhaled allergen in asthmatic patients. *Lancet* 344:1733–1736, 1994.

55. Turner WA, Bearg DW, Brennan T: Ventilation, in Seltzer JM (ed), *Effects of the Indoor Environment on Health.* Philadelphia, Hanley & Belfus, 1995.

56. U.S. Department of Health and Human Services (USDHHS): *The Health Consequences of Involuntary Smoking: A Report of the Surgeon General.* Washington, DC, U.S. Government Printing Office, 1986.

57. U.S. Environmental Protection Agency, Office of Research and Development, and Office of Air and Radiation: *Respiratory Health Effects of Passive Smoking: Lung Cancer and Other Disorders.* Washington, DC, U.S. Government Printing Office, Monograph 4, 1993.

58. U.S. Environmental Protection Agency: *Indoor Air Pollution.* Washington, DC, U.S. Government Printing Office, 1991.

59. U.S. Environmental Protection Agency: *Technical Support Document for the 1992 Citizen's Guide to Radon.* Washington, DC, U.S. Government Printing Office, 1992.

60. Wallace LA: Volatile organic compounds, in Samet JM, Spengler JD (eds), *Indoor Air Pollution: A Health Perspective.* Baltimore, Johns Hopkins University Press, 1991.

61. Wallace LA: *The Total Exposure Assessment Methodology (TEAM) Study: Summary and Analysis.* Washington, DC, Office of Research and Development, U.S. Environmental Protection Agency, 1987.

62. Wolkoff P: Volatile organic compounds—Sources, measurements, emissions, and the impact on indoor air quality. *Indoor Air* 3:9–73, 1995.

63. Wood RA, Eggleston PA, Lind P, et al: Antigenic analysis of household dust samples. *Am Rev Respir Dis* 137:358–363, 1988.

PULMONARY ADAPTATION AND CLINICAL DISORDERS RELATED TO HIGH ALTITUDE

S u k h a m a y   L a h i r i / J a m e s   S.   M i l l e d g e

Ascent to high altitude presents an interesting physiological challenge to humans. The response of oxygen-sensing organs, the pulmonary circulation, and the ventilatory control system lie at the core of the adaptations that take place with ascent to high altitude. This chapter focuses on these physiological adaptations. In addition, important clinical disorders associated with high altitude are discussed, including acute mountain sickness, high-altitude pulmonary edema, high-altitude cerebral edema, and chronic mountain sickness. Finally, the effect of high altitude on preexisting pulmonary conditions is reviewed.

ARTERIAL CHEMORECEPTORS AND CONTROL OF RESPIRATION

Only since the late 1920s and early 1930s have we recognized that the ventilatory response to hypoxia originates from peripheral chemoreceptors located in the carotid and aortic bodies. Previously, the central chemoreceptors, as CO_2-sensing organs, were the focus of investigation of the respiratory control system. Even Haldane believed that hypoxia acted centrally by producing acid. Eventually, the basis of the hypoxic stimulus to breathing was uncovered, employing simple cross-circulation experiments in dogs. Cyanide injected into the donor dog stimulated ventilation in the recipient dog. However, when the carotid sinus regions of the recipient dog were denervated, the response in the recipient dog was eliminated and in the donor dog maintained. Additional studies have elucidated the structural basis of carotid body function[12] (Fig. 63-1).

Nonrespiratory and Respiratory Hypotheses

The carotid body has innervated cells (type I cells) which respond to hypoxia and to hypercapnia.[19] The mechanism underlying the response is not completely understood. At present, two hypotheses prevail: the *nonrespiratory* or *membrane hypothesis* and the *respiratory or metabolic hypothesis* (Fig. 63-2).

In both the nonrespiratory and respiratory hypotheses, ionized calcium (Ca^{2+}) entry into cells is a key step, although chemoreception occurs preceding the entry. In the nonrespiratory scheme, K^+ currents in the type I cell membrane are suppressed during hypoxia.[12,41] Depolarization and opening of Ca^{2+} channels follow.[53] In the respiratory scheme, hypoxia increases intracellular $[Ca^{2+}]$ by acting on intracellular stores, such as the endoplasmic reticulum and mitochondria; however, the exact mechanism is unclear. With depletion of stored calcium, Ca^{2+} entry occurs. In both the nonrespiratory and respiratory schemes, Ca^{2+} entry is followed by secretion of neurotransmitters and neural discharge. Other hypotheses subsidiary to the nonrespiratory and respiratory ones have also been described.

Other Hypotheses

Nicotinamide adenine dinucleotide phosphate (NADPH) oxidase catalyzes reactions which produce H_2O_2. During hypoxia, decreased production of H_2O_2 by NADPH-oxidase-catalyzed reactions may suppress K^+ currents and neural discharge.[1] H_2O_2 generation by NADPH oxidases associated with cell membranes is ubiquitous; generation of H_2O_2 is prominent in macrophages and

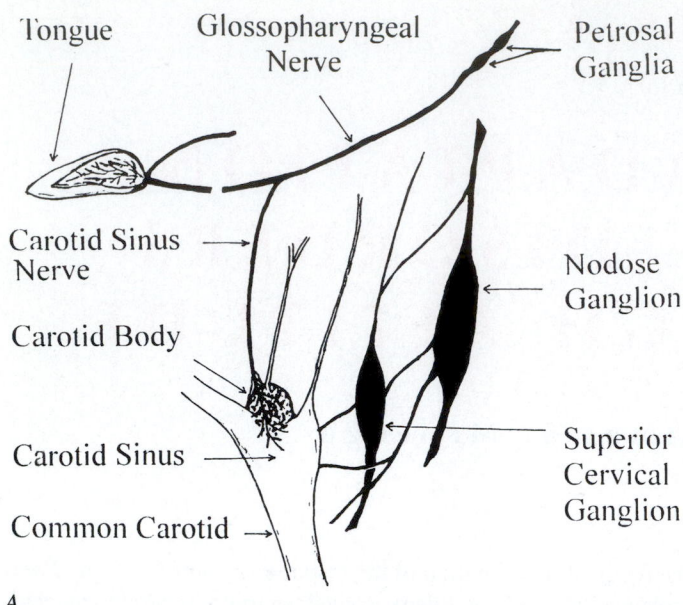

A

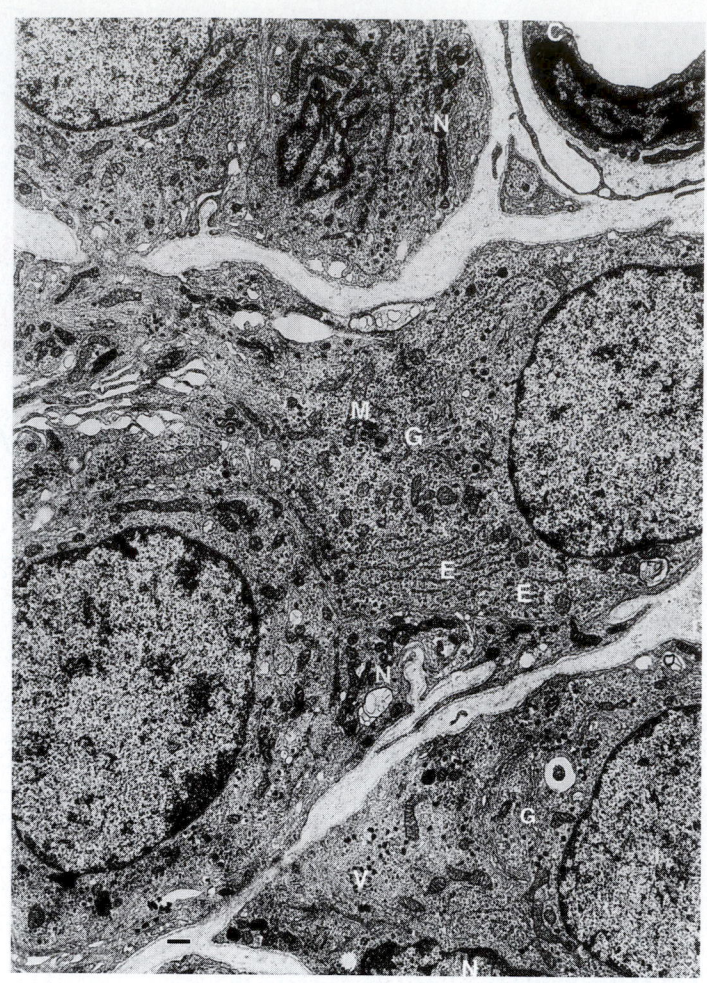

B

FIGURE 63-1 *A.* Region of carotid sinus area and carotid body. *B.* Electron micrograph ($\times 10000$) of chinchilla carotid body. I, glomus cell; II, sustentacular cell; C, capillary; E, endoplasmic reticulum; G, Golgi apparatus; M, mitochondria; N, nerve ending in apposition to glomus cell membrane; V, dense-cored vesicles.

neutrophils.[48] The oxidase is insensitive to the inhibitors of the respiratory chain,[11] unlike the carotid chemoreceptors[12] and pulmonary arterial smooth muscle cells,[11] indicating that different mechanisms operate.

Nitric oxide (NO) decreases chemoreceptor excitation through an increase in (cGMP).[7] By decreasing NO production, hypoxia increases chemosensory excitation. However, whether cGMP is crucial in chemoreceptor activity is unknown (see below).

The arterial chemoreceptors also respond to acid; chemoreceptor fibers are activated by increased [H^+] which suppresses K^+ currents.[42] Whether hypoxia and H^+ interact at the cellular level is unknown, although such interaction does exist at the fiber level.[29] Furthermore, the sensitivity of the aortic body to H^+ is feeble compared to that in the carotid chemoreceptors[32] (Fig. 63-3). Whether the type I cells of the aortic body also show a blunted response to acid is unknown.

Finally, neuroepithelial bodies (NEB), which are clusters of innervated cells scattered throughout the airway mucosa, are sensitive to hypoxia. Recently, these cells were studied in isolation and were shown to have the properties of glomus cells, including serotonin secretion.[59] However, their function and the final destination of their afferent innervation are unknown.

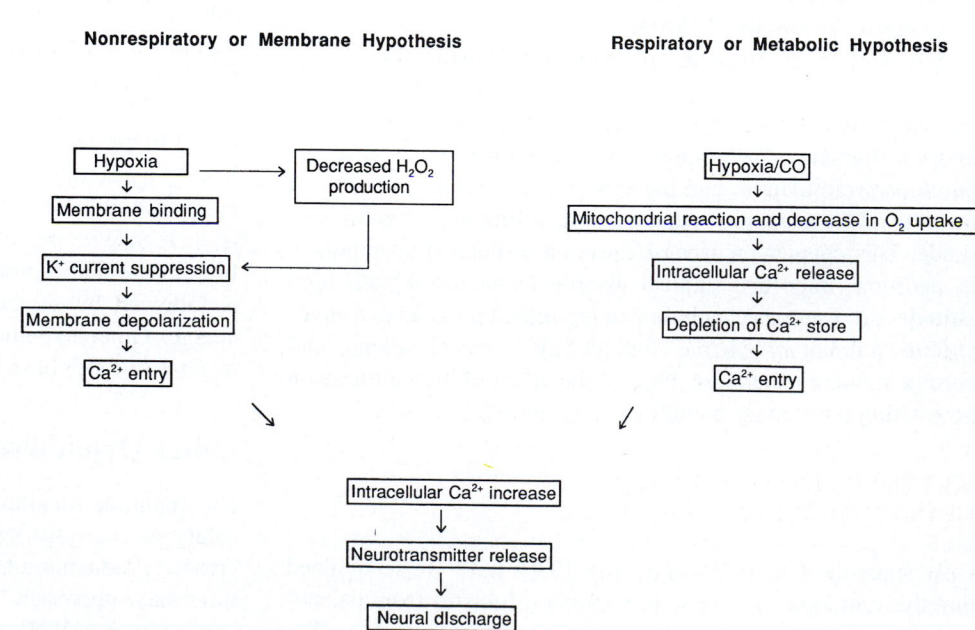

FIGURE 63-2 Chemoreception in the carotid body. See text.

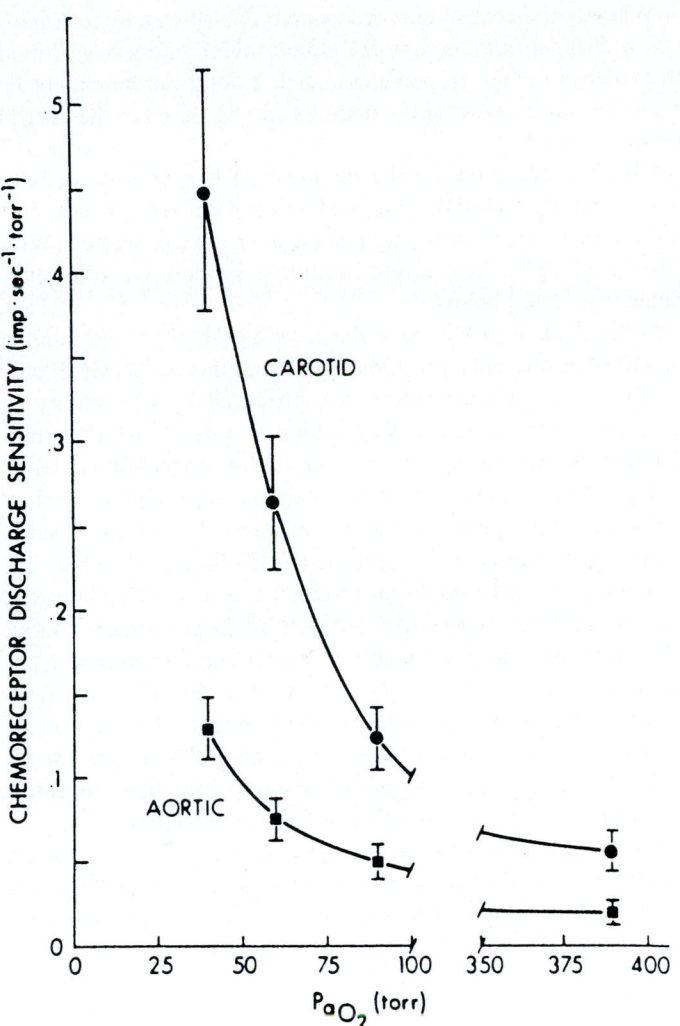

FIGURE 63-3   Effect of Pa_{O_2} on aortic and carotid chemoreceptor discharge rates. Data are mean ±SE. *(From Peñaloza et al.[44])*

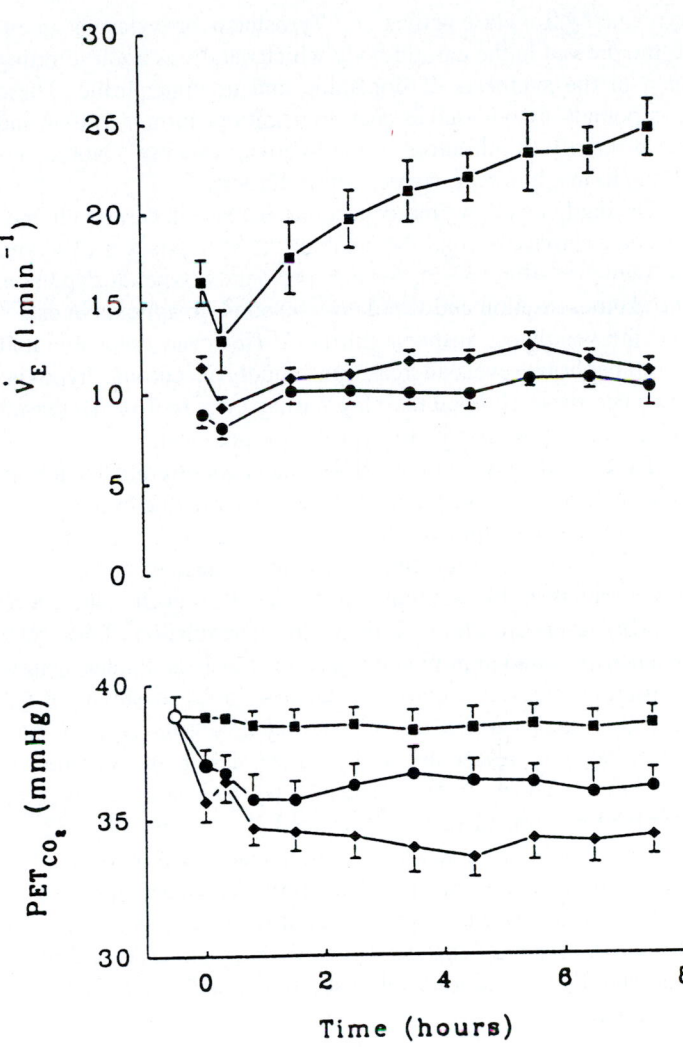

FIGURE 63-4   Changes in $\dot{V}E$ and end-tidal P_{CO_2} (PET_{CO_2}). See text for details. ■, isocapnic hypoxia; ◆, poikilocapnic hypoxia; ●, mean resting value of PET_{CO_2}. *(From Howard and Robbins.[20])*

The Carotid Body and Ventilatory Acclimatization

The ventilatory increase to acute hypoxia often shows a "roll-off" response (Fig. 63-4) in which the initial ventilatory increase due to hypoxia is not sustained; rather, the increase "rolls back" somewhat after about a minute. With sustained hypoxia, ventilation continues to increase further over several hours or days, a process known as *ventilatory acclimatization*.[20,30,46,57] During acclimatization, alveolar P_{CO_2} decreases as alveolar P_{O_2} diminishes with ascent (Fig. 63-5).

A large body of evidence demonstrates that the carotid bodies are essential for ventilatory acclimatization to hypoxia.[3,4] Bilateral denervation of the carotid bodies limits the altitude to which safe ascent can be made and makes survival at high altitudes precarious.[4,28] In addition, studies using the isolated perfused carotid body have shown that acclimatization does not occur during systemic hypoxia when the carotid bodies remain normoxic. Hypercapnic stimulation of the isolated carotid body does not induce acclimatization. These findings are consistent with the observation that hypoxia, but not hypercapnia, induces

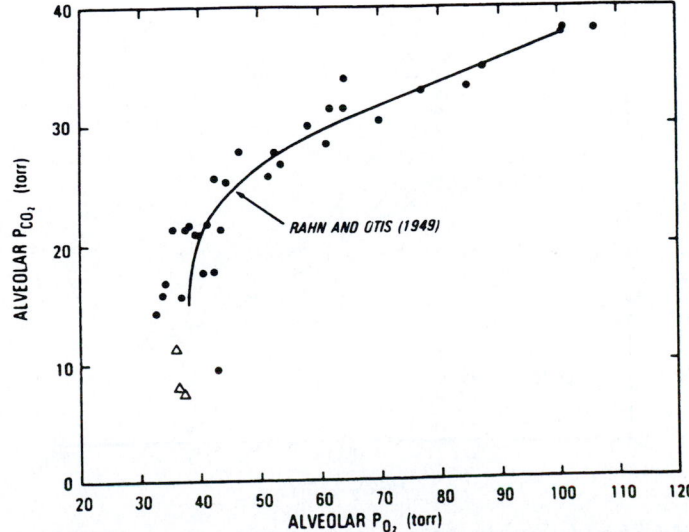

FIGURE 63-5   Oxygen-carbon dioxide diagram showing alveolar gas values at low altitude (●) and at extreme altitude (△). *(From West.[56])*

tyrosine hydroxylase activation.[9] Tyrosine hydroxylase is an enzyme present in the carotid body which catalyzes a rate-limiting step in the synthesis of dopamine and norepinephrine. These compounds are released as neurotransmitters during hypoxia and act primarily as inhibitors of the hypoxic response.[4] Not all investigations, however, support these findings.[12]

During hypoxia, a time-dependent increase in carotid chemoreceptor activity beyond the acute effect of hypoxia is observed in animals[2,4] (Fig. 63-6). Severe, prolonged hypoxia depresses the chemosensation and ventilatory response to hypoxia in cats[52] and the ventilatory response in rats.[59] However, dopamine and norepinephrine levels increase profoundly in chronic hypoxia; the roles these compounds play during increased or decreased chemosensory responses to hypoxia are not clear.

The carotid body glomus cell size increases several-fold in both intact animals[36] and cell cultures exposed to chronic hypoxia.[51,59] A consequence of this increase is a decrease in K^+ current density, since whole-cell K^+ current remains unchanged and cells are more excitable. In addition, adenosine $3',5'$-cyclic phosphate (cAMP) levels are elevated, mediating upregulation of the Na^+ channel, a calmodulin-binding protein which facilitates neurotransmitter release.[51] However, a decrease in the sensitivity of the carotid chemoreceptors during prolonged, severe hypoxia may mean that cells are not able to depolarize, despite the presence of potassium channels.[59] The decrease may be due to the lack of charibdotoxin-sensitive, Ca^{2+}-activated K^+ current (Fig. 63-7).

Upon returning to sea level, a major decrease in ventilation occurs immediately, but a similar time-dependent decrease in ventilation also occurs.[4] This residual hyperventilation may be attributed, in part, to changes in carotid body structure and function which take time to develop at altitude and which decline at sea level.

Whether the central nervous system contributes to acclimatization channel is controversial. Some investigators have found no evidence for it.[4] Nonetheless, such a contribution cannot be ruled out, since O_2-sensitive neurons can be found in the central nervous system.[24]

Efferent inhibition can be demonstrated in afferent activity before and after partial section of the carotid sinus nerve, i.e., afferent nerve activity is augmented after such a section. With chronic hypoxia, the efferent inhibition is reported to be augmented, as noted below.

Nitric oxide is produced in the carotid body[7,13,54] and inhibits carotid sinus afferents, presumably through increased cGMP production.[7] Carbon monoxide (CO), produced by the activity of heme oxygenase II, also has an inhibitory effect[45] which is mediated by cGMP. During hypoxia, the rate of production of cGMP is low[45,54]; consequently, cGMP's chemosensory inhibitory effect is low (i.e., the chemoreceptors are excited). The vascular bed is innervated by nitric oxide synthase (NOS) fibers,[13,54] which are vasodilatory. In addition, H_2O_2 production is less during hypoxia, resulting in decreased cGMP production[6] in pulmonary arterial smooth muscle and, presumably, in increased chemosensory excitation. Thus, cGMP is a key substance in this scheme. However, how the inhibitory effects of these endogenous compounds relate to the efferent nerve output of the carotid bodies is not yet clarified. Furthermore, how chronic hypoxia modifies concentrations of the compounds and their effects is unknown.

The enhancement of dopamine production in chronic hypoxia is well known.[16] The balance of evidence suggests that dopamine is inhibitory to chemosensory discharge.[2,52] Although the mech-

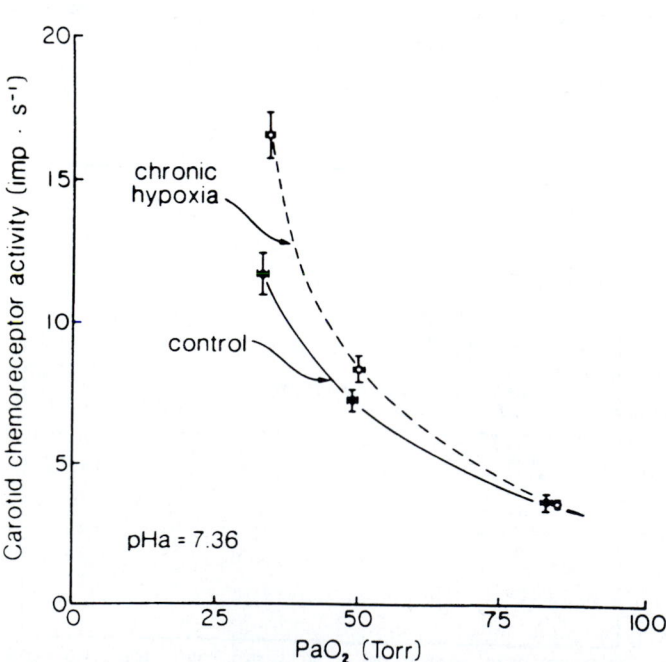

FIGURE 63-6   Steady-state activity of carotid chemoreceptor afferents in cats at sea level exposed to air (solid symbols) and to 10% O_2 (open symbols). Data are mean ±SD. (*From Barnard et al.[2]*)

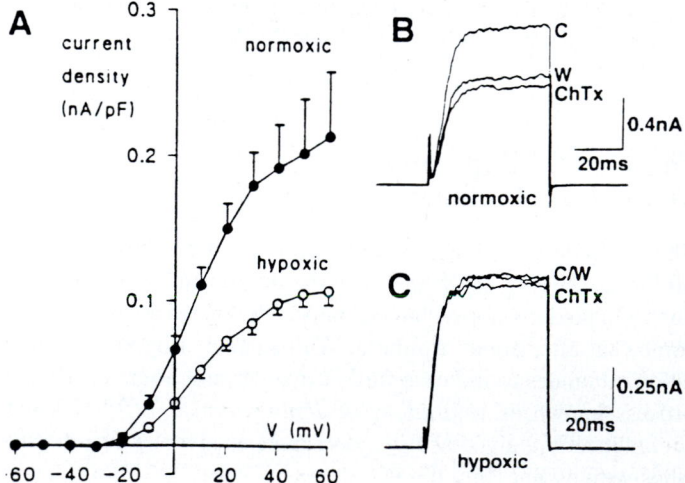

FIGURE 63-7   Whole-cell K^+ current density (nA/pF) and sensitivity to charibdotoxin (ChTx) in type I cells. *A.* Plot of mean K^+ current density (± SEM) versus membrane potential (mV) for type I cells isolated from normoxic (filled circles) and chronically hypoxic (open circles) neonatal rats. *B.* K^+ currents evoked by step depolarizations from −70 mV to +30 mV in normoxic type I cell before, during, and after bath application of 20 nM ChTx. *C.* K^+ currents evoked as in panel *B,* but from type I cell from a chronically hypoxic neonatal rat. Note the smaller effect of ChTx, as compared with the effect on cells from the normoxic rats. C, control; W, wash. (*From Wyatt et al.[59]*)

anism of inhibition is not known, it may be related to increased cGMP production. We do know that during chronic hypoxia, efferent inhibition is augmented; dopamine receptor blockade eliminates the efferent inhibition. Hence, the efferent inhibition is dopaminergic.[33] If afferent inhibition is related to NO, efferent nerves must influence the vascular bed via a dopaminergic mechanism. However, proof of this is lacking.

The ventilatory response to acute hypoxia remains blunted in natives at high altitude compared to humans at sea level (Fig. 63-8). The blunted response is presumably due to an attenuated response in carotid chemosensory discharge; a central integration effect has not been excluded.

CONTROL OF VASCULAR TONE IN THE PULMONARY CIRCULATION

In contrast to the systemic circulation, the pulmonary circulation is a high-flow, low-pressure system. Because of the low pressure, gravity has a marked effect on pulmonary blood flow (see Chapter 12). In the upright position, pulmonary arterial pressure is just sufficient to maintain perfusion to the lung apex. Perfusion increases progressively from lung apex to base. Ventilation also increases from apex to base, but relatively less steeply. As a result, the ratio of ventilation to perfusion decreases from the apex to the base of the lungs. Because of these ventilation-perfusion relationships, the apex of the lung has a lower alveolar P_{CO_2} and a higher alveolar P_{O_2}. At high altitude, although lung mechanics do not change appreciably, development of pulmonary hypertension may affect gas exchange significantly.

Pulmonary blood vessels are supplied extensively with fibers from the autonomic nervous system, including sympathetic vasoconstrictor nerves and, to a lesser extent, parasympathetic vasodilator fibers. Despite this innervation, the regulation of pulmonary vasomotor tone is largely mediated by the local effects of P_{O_2} and P_{CO_2}. When a bronchiole is obstructed, hypoxia develops in underventilated alveoli, and the resulting regional hypoxia acts directly on the vascular smooth muscle, constricting blood vessels and shunting blood away from the hypoxic area. Local CO_2 accumulation leads to a decline in pH, which, in turn, leads to vasoconstriction. (In other tissues, local increases in P_{CO_2} result in vasodilation.)

The sensing of local P_{O_2} in vascular smooth muscle has been investigated with regard to the role of cytochrome a_3 oxidase-dependent and noncytochrome oxidase-dependent mechanisms.[25] With heme-based mechanisms, following O_2 sensing, K^+ current is suppressed in pulmonary arterial smooth muscle cells, resulting in depolarization and opening of Ca^{2+} channels, followed by muscle contraction. In contrast, in systemic arteries, hypoxia decreases opening of ATP-dependent K^+ channels and increases K^+ outflow, resulting in membrane hyperpolarization and smooth-muscle relaxation.[55]

Recent studies[6] have demonstrated that H_2O_2 generated via NADPH oxidases elicits pulmonary arterial relaxation and activation of guanylate cyclase. Hypoxia decreases H_2O_2 production, guanylate cyclase activity, and cGMP production. H_2O_2 production is linked to K^+ current,[23] decreasing with hypoxia; pulmonary arterial smooth muscle K^+ current is inhibited by reduced glu-

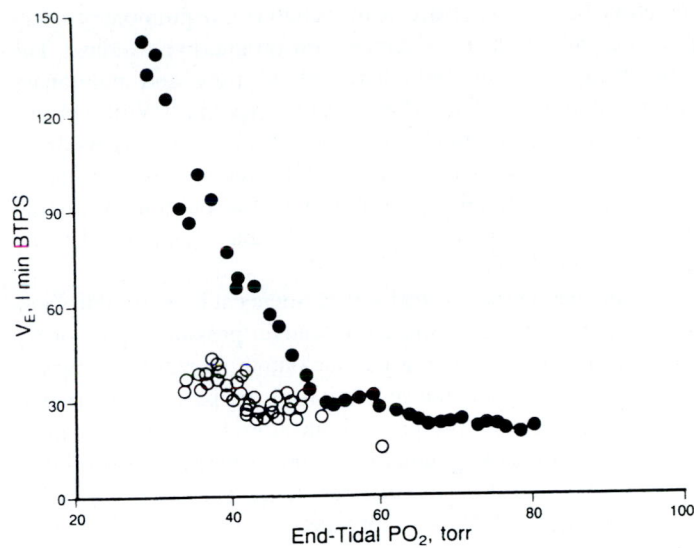

FIGURE 63-8 The hypoxic ventilatory response (HVR). Response of acclimatized lowlander (filled circles) compared with that of a lifelong native of Cerro de Pasco (open circles). Note that there is no significant increase in $\dot{V}E$ with progressive hypoxia in the high-altitude dweller. (*From Winslow and Monge.*[52])

tathione (GSH) and enhanced by oxidized glutathione (GSSG). These findings suggest that a redox-based O_2 sensor is operative in the pulmonary circulation.[1] All these reactions are heme- and O_2-based, and the chronic hypoxia of high altitude should be expected to influence these reactions.

Pulmonary hypertension (systolic and diastolic) at high altitude has been well documented.[48] More prevalent in younger than older individuals, altitude-related pulmonary hypertension is due to pulmonary vasoconstriction; its magnitude is accentuated by exercise. With relief of hypoxia, regression of both pulmonary hypertension and the resultant muscularization of the pulmonary arterial tree occurs. Right ventricular hypertrophy associated with pulmonary hypertension also regresses with return to sea level. Pulmonary hypertension due to acute hypoxia reverses promptly if the hypoxia is only of a few hours' duration; however, pulmonary hypertension with hypoxia of several days' duration does not reverse immediately with relief of the hypoxia.

EXERCISE AT ALTITUDE

Ventilation increases with exercises. In the steady state, ventilation increases in proportion to oxygen uptake, so that alveolar P_{CO_2} remains essentially unchanged. During heavy exercise, the generation of lactic acid results in a further increase in ventilation, so that alveolar P_{CO_2} may fall. With increasing altitude and the resulting decrease in inspired P_{O_2}, resting ventilation increases, determining the set point for the increase in ventilation during exercise. The mechanism by which alveolar P_{CO_2} is maintained constant during exercise is not clear. It is known, however, that carotid chemoreceptor output is not altered during exercise, with or without hypoxia. Natives at high altitude show a blunted ventilatory response to acute hypoxia.[8,26]

The entire cardiac output passes through the lungs. At sea level, the low-pressure pulmonary circulation accomodates the increased blood flow easily, with a small rise in pulmonary artery pressure and vascular resistance with progressive exercise. The relationship between pulmonary blood flow and pulmonary artery pressure is altered during acute hypoxia.[48] With chronic hypoxia, structural remodeling of pulmonary arterioles results in increases in resting pulmonary arterial pressure and resistance, resulting in a parallel, upward shift of the pulmonary arterial pressure-flow relationship, presumably due to increased resistance in the microcirculation.

Compared to those at sea level, residents at high altitude show a widened pulmonary-arterial-to-wedge pressure (pulmonary artery occlusion) gradient as cardiac output increases during exercise, suggesting that the regulation of the pulmonary circulation is significantly different at high altitude. At high altitude, control of pulmonary vascular resistance is in the lung arterioles; at sea level, control of vascular resistance is at the level of the left side of the heart.[48] Thus, altitude resets the regulation of the pulmonary circulation according to the structural remodeling of the lungs; exercise makes the difference obvious.

NONRESPIRATORY LUNG FUNCTION

Pulmonary type II cells manufacture and secrete surfactant, which lowers surface tension and maintains alveolar inflation (Chapter 7). The lung also produces many other substances[55] that are synthesized, stored, and released into the blood (e.g., prostaglandins, histamine, and kallikrein) or partially removed from the blood (e.g., prostaglandins, bradykinin, adenine nucleotides, serotonin, norepinephrine, and acetylcholine). The lungs also convert angiotensin I to angiotensin II, releasing it to the pulmonary circulation. The responsible enzyme, angiotensin converting enzyme (ACE), is located primarily in small pits in the endothelial cells of the pulmonary capillary. Many of the hormones pass through the lungs without being metabolized. In addition, biologically active peptides, including vasoactive intestinal peptide (VIP), substance P, and opioid peptides are found in the lungs. The effects of altitude on production of these compounds is not known.

SLEEP AND PERIODIC BREATHING

During sleep, alveolar P_{O_2} decreases and alveolar P_{CO_2} increases. At altitude, these changes become critically important, stimulating breathing. The resulting stimulation increases P_{O_2} and decreases P_{CO_2}, which, in turn, decrease ventilation, triggering periodic breathing.

At an altitude above 3000 m, normal people manifest periodic breathing, particularly during sleep.[15,30,56,57] The sleep state determines the characteristics of the breathing pattern, and altitude changes the characteristics of sleep. At altitude, the quality of both REM and non-REM sleep becomes impaired. With acclimatization, the sleep pattern tends to become more normal. However, periodic breathing during non-REM sleep continues at high altitudes.

The periodic breathing and apnea with ascent to high altitude disappears in subjects who take acetazolamide but not in those who take almitrine[15] (Fig. 63-9). Almitrine stimulates peripheral chemoreceptors, whereas acetazolamide stimulates central chemo-

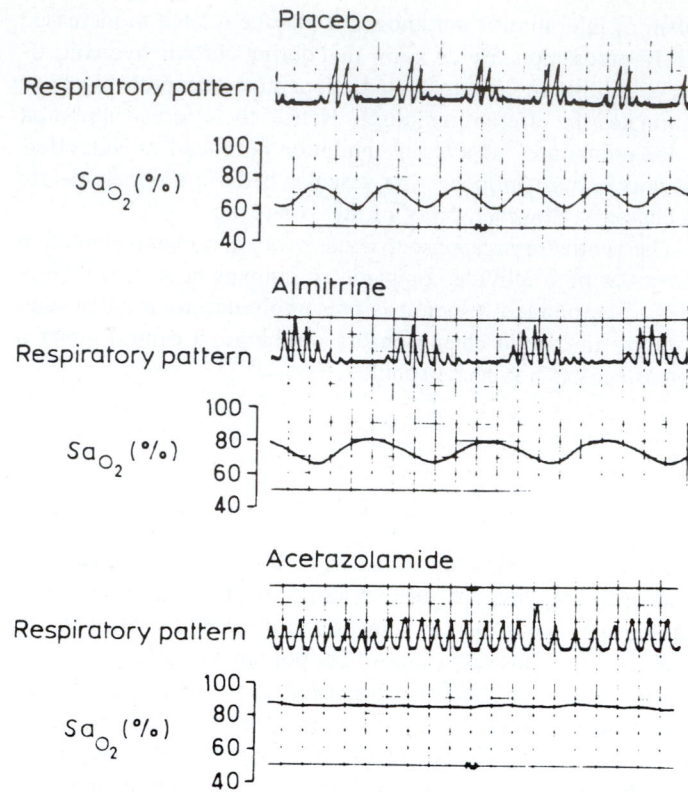

FIGURE 63-9 Effects of placebo, almitrine, and acetazolamide on respiratory pattern (periodic breathing) and arterial oxygen saturation (SaO_2) at an altitude of 4400 m. Acetazolamide abolished the apneic periods, and almitrine exaggerated them. *(From Hackett et al.[15])*

receptors through a rise in central CO_2. Thus, the hypothesis that the augmented peripheral chemoreceptor gain gives rise to oscillations in breathing pattern and apnea because of lack of central chemoreceptor stimulation is substantiated. The high-altitude native with a blunted hypoxic drive seldom manifests periodic breathing and apnea at altitude[30] (Fig. 63-10).

ERYTHROPOIESIS AT HIGH ALTITUDE

Erythropoietin is found in blood of anemic animals[10] in the setting of hypoxia of erythropoietic tissue, including the kidney and liver.[23] Levels are increased at high altitude[57] because of chronic hypoxia, leading to increased numbers of erythrocytes. Hypoxia also increases ventilation, decreases alveolar and arterial P_{CO_2} and arterial [H^+], and increases 2, 3-diphosphoglycerate (2,3-DPG). The decreased P_{CO_2} and [H^+] increase hemoglobin affinity for O_2, and the increased 2,3-DPG diminishes the affinity for O_2. Hence, loading and unloading of O_2 depend on these factors. Normally, loading also depends on the exercise level and degree of O_2 extraction. For unknown reasons, there is a decreased hypoxic ventilatory drive from the carotid body at high altitude, which is followed by a decreased arterial P_{O_2}. In addition, polycythemia, pulmonary hypertension, and impaired lung function follow, resulting in right ventricular hypertrophy, decreased cardiac output, and right-side heart failure. This constellation constitutes classic chronic mountain sickness, which is relieved by descent to sea level (see below).

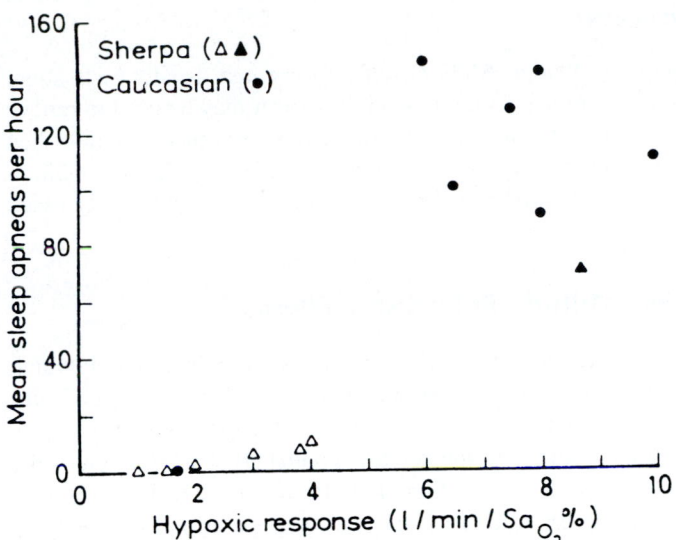

FIGURE 63-10 Relationship between frequency of sleep apnea and ventilatory response to hypoxia in awake acclimatized, lowlander caucasians (solid circles); high-altitude Sherpas (open triangles); and lower-altitude Sherpas (solid triangles). One lowlander did not have period of apnea; the low-altitude Sherpa showed periodic breathing. *(From Lahiri et al.[30])*

Although much work has been done on erythroprotein production, including identification of the regions of DNA to which transcription factors bind in response to hypoxia, identification of the O_2 sensor itself remains elusive.[11]

FLUID HOMEOSTASIS

In healthy individuals, the normal response to ascent to high altitude is a diuresis that persists during the stay at high altitude.[18] The diuresis is accompanied by suppression of voluntary sodium and water intake. Peripheral arterial chemoreflexes may play a role.[18] Lung edema, cerebral edema, and peripheral edema may be seen (see below), with elevated levels of aldoserone and antidiuretic hormone.

CLINICAL DISORDERS RELATED TO HIGH ALTITUDE

A spectrum of maladaptation, with associated clinical manifestations, may develop with ascent to high altitude. In the short term, these include acute mountain sickness, high-altitude pulmonary edema, and high-altitude cerebral edema. The likelihood of developing symptoms depends on the speed of ascent, elevation, length of stay at altitude, and on individual susceptibility. In the long term, chronic mountain sickness may be observed. Each of these disorders is considered below.

Acute Mountain Sickness

Acute mountain sickness (AMS) affects previously healthy individuals who ascend rapidly to high altitude. Symptoms develop a few hours to 2 days after ascent and include headache (usually frontal), nausea, vomiting, irritability, malaise, insomnia, and poor climbing performance. The simple or benign form of the condition is self-limiting, lasting 3 to 5 days. The disorder does not recur at the altitude at which it appears, although it may develop if the subject goes to a higher altitude. In a small proportion of individuals, progression to a malignant form of AMS may be seen, including high-altitude pulmonary edema (HAPE), high-altitude cerebral edema (HACE), or a mixed form of these two disorders. If not treated, these conditions are frequently fatal in a matter of hours.[14]

INCIDENCE

The incidence of AMS depends upon the altitude and the rate of ascent. With the increased accessibility of high-altitude resorts and the possibility of ascending high mountains in a very few days, the incidence of AMS is probably greater than in the more leisurely days of old. A recent survey of alpine huts showed an incidence of 9 percent at 2850 m, 13 percent at 3050 m, 34 percent at 3650 m, and 53 percent at 4559 m.[35] Among trekkers on their way to Everest base camp, an incidence of 43 percent was found at 4300 m[14]; the incidence was higher in those who had flown into an airstrip at 2800 m than in those who had walked all the way (49 percent versus 31 percent).

RISK FACTORS

Clearly, hypoxia of more than a few hours' duration is required for the development of AMS, and speed of ascent is an important determinant of AMS; however, there is great variation in susceptibility. Among a group of people ascending to high altitude, some will be unaffected, some mildly affected, and some severely affected. At present, susceptibility cannot be predicted, although past performance at altitude may be an index. As Ravenhill observed in his classic paper of 1913,[47] "There is in my experience no type of man of whom one can say he will or will not suffer from puna [the South American term for AMS]. Most cases I have instanced were young men to all appearances perfectly sound. Young, strong and healthy men may be completely overcome. Stout, plethoric individuals . . . may not even have a headache."

People of all ages and either sex seem to be equally affected. Fitness is no protection; indeed, the fit are likely to ascend faster and therefore may be at greater risk. Any respiratory infection is probably a risk factor and may account for illness in the subject who has previously acclimatized well. A brisk hypoxic ventilatory response would be expected to be protective; although some studies seem to support this, others do not.[37] Certainly, high-altitude residents who have a blunted hypoxic ventilatory response are less prone to AMS than are lowlanders. A brisk pulmonary artery pressor response to hypoxia may well be a risk factor for HAPE.

MECHANISMS

Although hypoxia is obviously the standing point in the genesis of AMS, it is not the immediate cause of symptoms, which are delayed by several hours after ascent and onset of hypoxia. The symptoms of AMS are similar to those associated with raised intracranial pressure seen on neurosurgical wards; at least in cases of high-altitude cerebral edema, good evidence exists for increased intracranial pressure. The most popular view is that even in simple AMS, a degree of cerebral edema (and often subclinical pulmonary edema) exists which causes symptoms of AMS. Frequently, dependent or periorbital edema exists as well. These findings point to a disturbance of fluid balance or capillary permeability throughout the body.

Other factors which may operate in development of AMS include changes in ventilation on arrival at altitude. Earlier studies suggested that individuals with the highest P_{CO_2} on arrival at altitude (who have failed to lower their P_{CO_2} by hyperventilation) were likely to develop AMS, although more recent studies have failed to confirm this. Exercise is thought to be a risk factor, although this has not yet been rigorously tested. Prolonged exercise performed by mountaineers causes retention of sodium and water through activation of the renin-aldosterone system,[38] which may place subjects at risk for AMS.

PREVENTION

A slow rate of ascent is the best way to prevent AMS. In general, above 300 m (10,000 ft), ascent should be no more than 300 m (1000 ft) per day, with a "rest" day every three days, during which no further ascent is made. This rate of ascent will be too fast for some and unnecessarily slow for others. If symptoms of AMS develop, the individual should go no higher. If symptoms become severe, the individual should descend to lower altitude.

It is often not possible or practicable to plan for this rate of ascent. No camp site may exist between the valley floor and a pass 500 m higher. Those ascending who know themselves to be slow acclimatizers may not wish to delay their companions. Under these circumstances, the use of acetazolamide is justified. The drug is a carbonic acid anhydrase inhibitor which probably acts as a respiratory stimulant. Its administration results in an increase in Pa_{O_2} and a decrease in Pa_{CO_2}, providing a sort of "artificial respiratory acclimatization." Double-blind controlled trials have shown that AMS is reduced in those taking acetazolamide.[54] Of course, AMS, and even HAPE or HACE, are still possible while taking the drug, and common sense is required. The dose used in trials has usually been 250 mg every 8 h, but 250 mg or 125 mg twice daily is currently recommended. The drug should be started at least 24 h prior to a major ascent. Side effects include a mild diuresis which tends to decrease if the drug is continued; paresthesias of the fingers and toes is almost universal. Flushing, thirst, headache, rash, and blood dyscrasias have been described but are rare. Finally, beer and all carbonated beverages taste flat. The drug has been very widely used for prolonged periods in the treatment of glaucoma, often at higher doses than are recommended for AMS prophylaxis, supporting the impression of its relative safety.

Dexamethasone has been shown to be an effective prophylactic drug, but most would consider it unjustified to use for this purpose.

TREATMENT

Simple or benign AMS is self-limiting and usually lasts about 3 days; treatment is not essential. Aspirin may be used to relieve headache, but it is not very efficacious. In a placebo-controlled trial,[5] ibuprofen has been shown to be effective. If the condition progresses to HAPE or HACE, treatment is urgent, as discussed below.

High-Altitude Pulmonary Edema

In the great majority of cases, AMS is a minor affliction which resolves in a few days. However, in a small proportion of subjects, the potentially lethal conditions of acute pulmonary edema (HAPE) or high-altitude cerebral edema (HACE) develop; some may develop a combination of HAPE and HACE. The incidence depends on the rate of ascent and the population examined. An incidence of 0.5 to 2.0 percent has been reported. Individuals with a previous history of HAPE are at greater risk of developing the syndrome.

Both lowlanders and high-altitude residents who reascend to altitude are susceptible. Men and women of all ages may be victims, although young males appear to be more at risk than others. Athletic fitness affords no protection.

CLINICAL MANIFESTATIONS

The typical patient who develops HAPE is a previously fit young man who has climbed rapidly to altitude and has been very energetic on arrival. At least a moderate degree of AMS is observed. The subject becomes more breathless than his companions. A cough develops, which is dry at first but which becomes productive of frothy white sputum which is later blood-tinged. Chest discomfort may develop. Crackles are heard at the lung bases, and increases in pulse and respiratory rates are noted. Peripheral edema and increased jugular venous pressure may be noted. A right ventricular heave and accentuated pulmonary second heart sound may be detected. Over a few hours, the condition deteriorates. Pulse and respiratory rates rise; breathing becomes "bubbly," and cyanosis develops. Without intervention, coma and death develop.

LABORATORY INVESTIGATION

The chest radiograph typically shows asymmetric, patchy opacities which clear in a few days if the patient recovers. A neutrophil-predominant leucocytosis is present. Arterial blood gases show a reduced P_{O_2} and arterial oxygen saturation compared with fit individuals at the same altitude. The P_{CO_2} is variable, but it is not significantly different from controls. The electrocardiogram reveals tachycardia, peaked P waves, right axis deviation, and, in some cases, ST segment elevation changes which are suggestive of pulmonary hypertension. Cardiac catheterization confirms the presence of a high pulmonary artery and normal pulmonary artery occlusion pressures. The cardiac output is normal. Pulmonary edema fluid has a high protein content, with a concentration approaching that of plasma.[48]

In fatal cases, postmortem findings show the lungs to be edematous; the edema is very patchy, with areas of normal lung adjacent to areas of edema. Other areas show hemorrhagic edema in a pattern corresponding with the radiograph appearance. Many thrombi and fibrin clots are seen in small arteries and veins. The alveoli contain fluid, red blood cells, polymorphonuclear white cells, and macrophages; hyaline membrane formation may be noted.

MECHANISMS

The mechanism of HAPE is not clear. Despite its clinical similarity to acute left ventricular failure, HAPE is not due to ventricular dysfunction; cardiac catheterization reveals a normal wedge pressure. The most popular hypothesis on pathogenesis was proposed originally by Hultgren and coworkers.[21] According to this hypothesis, susceptible subjects, who have been shown to have a brisk hypoxic pulmonary artery pressor response, demonstrate nonhomogeneous areas of vasoconstriction throughout the lung. Areas with a greater degree of vasoconstriction have reduced blood flow and are "protected" from edema formation. Areas with less vasoconstriction have greatly increased blood flow. The increased flow may cause capillary damage, perhaps through sheer stress on vessel walls or through increased capillary pressure. The result is patchy pulmonary edema in the setting of pulmonary hypertension. A variety of kinins are found in the edema fluid[48] and may account for a further increase in permeability, as well as leukocyte recruitment.

TREATMENT

The most important intervention in HAPE is evacuation of the patient to a lower altitude. A reduction in altitude of as little as 300 m (1000 ft) may result in significant clinical improvement. If descent is not possible, administration of supplemental oxygen will help. Supplemental oxygen should also be administered while the patient is awaiting evacuation.

A portable, lightweight, rubberized canvas hyperbaric chamber (Gamow bag) is commercially available for the treatment of HAPE. The patient can be placed in the chamber and its pressure increased by 2 psi using a foot pump. Use of this device effectively reduces the patient's altitude by almost 2000 m (6000 ft). Cases have been reported in which dramatic clinical improvement in HAPE (and HACE) has been observed with use of the chamber. Considerable effort is required to maintain pumping if limited help is available. The device may result in sufficient patient improvement to allow unaided descent.

In a randomized controlled trial of 64 cases of AMS treated with 1 h of pressurization in the Gamow bag at either 193 mbar of 20 mbar (control), pressure treatment resulted in greater immediate clinical improvement. However, in the 12-h follow-up period at 4600 m, no differences in use of analgesics or in symptom scores were noted.[3]

Since pulmonary vasoconstriction is thought to be important in the genesis of HAPE, vasodilators have been tried as therapy. The calcium channel blocker, nifedipine, has been shown to be beneficial.[41] A sublingual dose of 10 mg, in conjunction with a slow-release oral dose of 20 mg, has been used. However, since the sublingual drug may cause systemic hypotension, the oral formulation alone is advised unless the situation is critical.

Diuretics have been advocated in treatment of HAPE, but their use appears to be losing favor among those who see many cases of HAPE. Similarly, morphine and digoxin have been suggested, but evidence from controlled trials to support their use is lacking.

OUTCOME

In fully established cases of HAPE where patient evacuation is impossible, the result is usually death within a few hours. When victims are evacuated promptly, signs and symptoms usually resolve within minutes or hours, although the chest radiograph may take several days to clear. Patients should be warned to be cautious in reascent since they are at greater risk for recurrence. However, many have been able to go back to high altitude without problems.

HAPE is a life-threatening condition. It may be avoided by following the rules for avoiding AMS: slow ascent, no further ascent if symptoms occur, and descent if symptoms persist or worsen. If HAPE is diagnosed, descent as soon as possible is the first priority. Use of supplemental oxygen or nifedipine is likely to be beneficial, and a pressure bag may be useful as a temporary measure.

High-Altitude Cerebral Edema

The other malignant form of AMS is high-altitude cerebral edema (HACE). In its early stages, HACE is indistinguishable from simple AMS, with headache, nausea, and vomiting as prominent symptoms. When ataxia occurs, "malignant AMS," or HACE, is present. Truncal ataxia, hallucinations, clouding of consciousness, and a variety of neurological signs, including extensor plantar reflexes and papilledema, may follow. Signs of pulmonary edema are often present as well. Finally, the patient may become unconscious and die, if not treated.

The incidence of HACE is lower than that of HAPE. An incidence of 1.8 percent (compared with 2.5 percent for HAPE) has been reported in 278 trekkers passing through Pheriche (4243 m) on their way to Everest base camp.[14,54]

The mechanism of HACE is presumably the same as that underlying simple AMS (see above). However, why few individuals progress to this lethal complication, while the majority suffer only a self-limiting, reversible condition, is unclear. As with HAPE, both lowlanders and highlanders, as well as men and women of any age, may be victims.

In the few cases of HACE in which postmortem examination has been conducted, evidence of cerebral edema, increased intracranial pressure, and petechial hemorrhages have been noted. Venous thrombi have also been reported.[54]

TREATMENT

Treatment for HACE is similar to that for HAPE. The most important measure is descent to a lower altitude. While awaiting evacuation, administration of supplemental oxygen and use of a pressure bag (see above) may help, but the beneficial effect may be slower to develop than in HAPE, especially in more severe cases. Dexamethasone, 4 mg intramuscularly in severe cases or orally in milder cases, helps reduce cerebral edema and should be used while awaiting patient evacuation.

OUTCOME

As in HAPE, descent often leads to rapid improvement in HACE. However, in some cases, recovery is delayed for several days. Permanent or long-lasting neurologic defects may be observed.[19]

Chronic Mountain Sickness

In the 1920s, Carlos Monge reported cases of polycythemia in high-altitude residents of the Andes. Monge's disease, or chronic mountain sickness (CMS), is quite different from AMS. This disorder is more common in males and develops in middle and later life. The defining feature of CMS is extreme polycythemia. In 1942, detailed observations of eight cases, including symptomatology and hematologic changes, were published in the English literature.[22] Since then, CMS has been reported in North America and Asia.

SYMPTOMS

Patients with CMS typically have rather vague neuropsychological complaints, including headache, dizziness, somnolence, fatigue, difficulty in concentration, and loss of mental acuity. Irritability, depression, and hallucinations may be present. Dyspnea on exertion is not a common complaint, but poor exercise tolerance is frequent. Patients may also gain weight. A characteristic feature of CMS is that symptoms disappear with descent to sea level, only to reappear upon return to altitude.

Although normal individuals are mildly cyanotic at an altitude of 4000 m, patients with CMS are particularly affected, since with a high hemoglobin concentration and low oxygen saturation, the concentration of reduced hemoglobin is high. In Andean natives—the population with the greatest incidence of CMS—signs may be florid. As has been noted, "The combination of virtually black lips and wine-red mucosal surfaces against the greenish tinge of the Indian skin gives the patient with Monge's disease a striking appearance."[17] The conjunctivae are congested, and the fingers may be clubbed. In Caucasians and at lower altitudes, e.g., Leadville, Colorado (3100 m), the appearance is less striking. Individuals look similar to patients with polycythemia secondary to hypoxic lung disease at sea level. Some individuals with CMS have few clinical signs of disease.

LABORATORY INVESTIGATION

The red blood cell count, hemoglobin concentration, and packed red cell volume are increased; hemoglobin values as high as 28 g/dl and hematocrits as high as 83 percent have been recorded.[22] Like secondary polycythemia at sea level, and unlike polycythemia rubra vera, white blood cell counts are not increased. Arterial blood-gas values, compared with those of healthy individuals as controls at the same altitude, show a higher Pa_{CO_2},

lower Pa_{O_2}, and lower O_2 saturation. The lower Pa_{O_2} is partly due to hypoventilation, as indicated by the increased Pa_{CO_2}. In many cases, the alveolar-arterial oxygen gradient is increased. In some cases, standard pulmonary function tests show abnormalities consistent with obstructive or restrictive defects, suggesting that patients have coexisting chronic lung disease.

HEMODYNAMICS AND PATHOPHYSIOLOGY

The very high hematocrit increases the blood viscosity enormously. Systemic blood pressure may be moderately elevated, and the pulmonary artery pressure is significantly higher than in healthy high-altitude residents. Cardiac output is not significantly changed, so calculated pulmonary vascular resistance is high. As might be expected, the hemodynamic alterations lead to right ventricular hypertrophy and associated electrocardiographic changes. Thickening of the peripheral pulmonary arteries to a greater degree than that observed in normal residents at high altitude is also present.

TREATMENT

As noted previously, symptoms and signs of CMS clear with descent to sea level. However, many patients wish to remain at altitude for family or economic reasons. In these cases, phlebotomy is beneficial. Phlebotomy not only lowers the hematocrit, but it also improves many of the neuropsychological symptoms. Phlebotomy also improves pulmonary gas exchange and exercise performance in some subjects.

An alternative to phlebotomy for residents at high altitude is long-term use of respiratory stimulants. Medroxyprogesterone has been used with some success, but side effects, including loss of libido, are a limitation. Reported trials of other stimulants, such as acetazolamide, an agent which has been shown to be effective in preventing acute mountain sickness (see above), are lacking.

EPIDEMIOLOGY

CMS is found most commonly in the Andes,[57] where it was first described. Populations affected primarily include the local Native Americans, especially the Quechuan population living on the Altiplano at altitudes from about 3300 to 4500 m. Men are affected far more commonly than women. The incidence increases with increasing age; most patients present in late middle age. Occasionally, cases are seen in expatriots working for mining companies. Previously, CMS was thought to be virtually confined to the Andes; however, this is not the case.

Until recently, few cases of CMS in the Himalayas have been reported. However, studies now describe the occurrence of CMS in Lhasa (3600 m).[58] CMS is not uncommon among male, cigarette-smoking Han Chinese. These subjects immigrated years before becoming polycythemic and have subsequently displayed the usual signs and symptoms of CMS. In one report, in a 12-mo period, 24 patients were admitted to a hospital with CMS. All were male; 23 were Han and only one was Tibetan. Six were nonsmokers, and the remainder, including the one Tibetan, were smokers. The mean duration of altitude exposure in the lowlanders was 26 years. Although the incidence of CMS in Tibetans may be less than in Han immigrants, CMS has now been reported in this population. Typical symptoms of CMS have been reported in 26 native-born Tibetans living at an altitude between 3680 and 4179 m.[58] A mean hemoglobin concentration of 22.2 g/dl was noted, compared with 16.5 g/dl in healthy individuals as controls at the same altitude.

Although more evidence is needed, people of Tibetan stock appear less at risk for CMS than Andean highlanders and lowland Han subjects who are long-time residents at high altitude. Genetic adaptation to high altitude over very many generations may be operative.

TERMINOLOGY

Opinions differ with regard to the hemoglobin value required for a diagnosis of CMS. A value of 23 g/dl has been used, but it is probably advisable to consider the normal value and range for the particular altitude. Some argue that CMS does not represent a distinct entity. Rather, hemoglobin values may represent merely the "tail" of a normal distribution curve. For practical purposes, however, a value of two standard deviations above the mean for the altitude can be considered the cutoff for "normal." The "tail" population may be considered abnormal and polycythemic for that altitude. Since symptoms occur at this value, treatment is indicated. Therefore, this definition has practical implications.

There has also been debate about whether to exclude individuals with lung disease as having CMS. The problem is how rigorous one must be in excluding any lung disease. The final assessment is a postmortem examination. Most clinicians are content to apply the diagnosis of CMS (Monge's disease or polycythemia of high altitude) to any patient with a hemoglobin higher than 23 g/dl, with or without overt lung disease.

MECHANISMS

Clearly, hypoxemia is the crucial factor in development of CMS. Contributing factors include: (1) altitude (the higher the altitude, the greater the incidence of CMS); (2) lung function (which, in turn, is affected by smoking, atmospheric pollution—many patients are miners working in dusty environments, chest infections, and so on); (3) hypoxic ventilatory response (patients in Peru with CMS were found to have a very low hypoxic ventilatory response,[49] although this finding could not be confirmed in patients in Leadville, Colorado; (4) age (the incidence increases with age, possibly because lung function and hypoxic ventilatory response decline with age); (5) gender (females appear to be protected, perhaps by the respiratory-stimulating effects of female sex hormones, as well as menstrual blood loss); (6) hyperventilation or apneas during sleep.

EFFECT OF HIGH ALTITUDE ON PREEXISTING DISORDERS

With increasing numbers of people going to high altitudes for adventure holidays, expeditions, and skiing, doctors are more frequently asked for advice about avoiding and treating potential medical consequences. Furthermore, these trips are frequently pursued in later life; hence, individuals are more likely to be suffering from chronic diseases that may prompt questions as to their fitness for ascent to altitude.

The effect of any condition that interferes with oxygen transport is exaggerated by altitude. As a general rule, individuals should be as fit as possible before leaving for a trip to high altitude, although fitness is no protection from acute mountain sickness.

Those who have health problems should find out as much as possible about their condition before setting out on the trip. The action of specific medicines must be understood and an adequate supply taken, particularly when regular doses are necessary, as in diabetes mellitus or asthma.

All bodily functions, including maximal oxygen uptake, decline with age, both at sea level and at altitude. One's ability to safely ascend to altitude depends more on one's degree of fitness than age. Fit, lowland men of 75 years of age have spent months at 5000 m without difficulty; an 80 year-old mountaineer has climbed a peak of 6000 m. No one should be discouraged from ascending to altitude on the grounds of age alone; however, rapid ascent and undue exertion place more strain on older individuals. In general, the greater experience of the elderly enables them to appropriately pace themselves.

Increasing numbers of middle-aged and elderly people are visiting high altitudes to ski, trek, climb, and attend conferences. The effects of altitude on cardiovascular and pulmonary disorders have been studied. A recent survey of over 1900 visitors to Keystone, Colorado (2783 m), revealed that 48 percent were between 40 and 60 years of age and 15 percent were over 60 years of age. Approximately 10 percent of trekkers in Nepal were 50 years of age or older[21]; a few mountaineers of this age have climbed Everest using supplemental oxygen.

ASTHMA

Asthma is a very common disorder, and the question of the advisability of an asthmatic individual undertaking a trip to high altitude is frequent. Although an asthma attack may be provoked by cold air or exercise, many asthmatic patients have less trouble at altitude than at home, possibly because of freedom from inhaled allergens. In addition, the associated increased sympathetic and adrenocortical activity may counter the bronchoconstrictor effects of cold air and exercise in the first few days at altitude. The importance of taking a sufficient supply of asthma medication and using it regularly must be stressed. No evidence exists that asthmatics are at greater risk of acute mountain sickness than nonasthmatics, although it must be presumed that poorly controlled patients may be at some risk. Acetazolamide helps to prevent acute mountain sickness in asthmatic patients.[39]

OBSTRUCTIVE PULMONARY DISEASES

In patients with significant chronic obstructive pulmonary disease (COPD), ventilatory capacity may be reduced and oxygen uptake impaired. If patients are short of breath with exercise at sea level, they will certainly be worse at altitude. Patients with even mild COPD will find their exercise performance markedly diminished at altitude. The reserve capacity of the lung may be further diminished by infection; therefore, antibiotics should be started at the first sign of infection. Patients with COPD should probably be advised to avoid trips to high altitude.

Patients with cystic fibrosis and bronchiectasis have airway obstruction and abnormal gas exchange. Two patients with cystic fibrosis have been described in whom ascent to altitude appeared to precipitate cor pulmonale.[50] In all but the mildest cases, patients with cystic fibrosis should be advised against ascending to high altitude.

Patients with stable cystic fibrosis who wish to ascend to altitude or to fly in commercial aircraft can be tested in the laboratory by breathing a hypoxic gas mixture (15 percent oxygen in nitrogen) for 10 min. Arterial oxygen saturation measured by pulse oximetry provides a good indication of oxygen saturation at altitude.[40] Other patients with stable lung disease might also benefit from the test prior to ascent.

INTERSTITIAL LUNG DISEASE

In patients with interstitial lung disease, lung volumes are reduced, and gas exchange is abnormal. Altitude has a marked effect on gas exchange, and patients with interstitial lung disease will find themselves much more short of breath following ascent.

HIGH-ALTITUDE PULMONARY EDEMA

A previous attack of high-altitude pulmonary edema indicates susceptibility to recurrence and the need for caution on future ascents. However, many individuals are able to make subsequent ascents without trouble. The prophylactic use of acetazolamide should be discussed, and nifedipine should be included in the first aid kit.

OTORHINOLARYNGOLOGIC CONDITIONS

Nasal polyps or a deviated nasal septum which interferes with breathing should be treated prior to ascent. Patients with perennial rhinitis and sinusitis should have adequate supplies of their usual medications. Like those with asthma, patients with these disorders may have less trouble at high altitude than in their home environment.

OTHER MEDICAL CONDITIONS

Consideration of the effect of altitude on other medical conditions, including heart disease, diabetes mellitus, and gastrointestinal disorders has been recently reviewed.[51]

REFERENCES

1. Archer SL, Huang J, Henry T, et al: A redox-based O_2 sensory in rat pulmonary vasculature. *Circ Res* 73:1100–1172, 1993.
2. Barnard P, Andronikou S, Pokorski M, et al: Time-dependent effect of hypoxia on carotid body chemosensory function. *J Appl Physiol* 63:685–691, 1987.
3. Bartsch P, Merki B, Hofstetter D, et al: Treatment of acute mountain sickness by simulated descent: A randomized controlled trial. *Br Med J* 306:1098–1101, 1993.
4. Bisgard GE, Forster HV: Ventilatory responses to acute and chronic hypoxia, in Fregly MJ, Blatteis CM (eds), *Handbook of Physiology: environmental physiology.* New York, Oxford University Press, 1996, pp 1207–1249.
5. Broom JR, Stoneham MD, Beeley JM, et al: High altitude headaches: Treatment with ibuprofen. *Aviat Space Environ Med* 65:19–20, 1994.
6. Burke TM, Wolin MS: Hydrogen peroxide elicits pulmonary arterial relaxation and guanylate cyclase activation. *Am J Physiol* 252:H721–H732, 1987.
7. Chugh DK, Katayama M, Mokashi A, et al: Nitric oxide-related inhibition of carotid chemosensory nerve activity in the cat. *Respir Physiol* 97:147–156, 1994.
8. Curran LS, Zhuan J, Croma T, Moore LG: Hypoxic ventilatory responses in Tibetan residents of 4400 m compared with 3658 m. *Respir Physiol* 100:223–230, 1995.
9. Czyzyk MF, Bayliss DA, Lawson EE, Milhorn DE: Regulation of tyrosine hydroxylase gene expression in the rat carotid body by hypoxia. *J Neurochem* 58:1538–1546, 1992.
10. Erslev AJ, Caro J, Besarab A: Why the kidney? *Nephron,* 41:413–416, 1985.
11. Fandrey J, Frede S, Jelkman W: Role of hydrogen peroxide in hypoxia-induced erythropoiekin production. *Biochem J* 303:507–510, 1994.
12. Gonzalez C, Almaraz L, Obeso A, Rigul R: Carotid body chemoreceptors: from natural stimuli to sensory discharges. *Physiol Rev* 74:829–900, 1994.
13. Grimes PA, Mokashi A, Stone RA, Lahiri S: Nitric oxide synthase in autonomic innervation of the cat carotid body. *J Autonom Nerv Syst* 54:80–86, 1995.
14. Hackett PH, Rennie D, Levine HD: Rales, peripheral edema, retinal hemorrhage and acute mountain sickness. *Am J Med* 67:214–218, 1979.
15. Hackett PH, Roach RC, Harrison GL, et al: Respiratory stimulants and sleep periodic breathing at high altitude. *Am Rev Respir Dis* 135:896–898, 1987.
16. Hanbauer I, Karoum E, Hellstrom S, Lahiri S: Effects of hypoxia lasting up to one month on the catecholamine content in rat carotid body. *Neuroscience* 6:81–86, 1981.
17. Heath D, Williams D: *High Altitude Medicine and Pathology,* 4th ed. Oxford, Oxford Medical Pub, 1995.
18. Honig A: Peripheral arterial chemoreceptors and reflex control of sodium and water homeostasis. *Am J Physiol* 257:R1282–R1302, 1989.
19. Houston CS, Dickenson J: Cerebral form of high-altitude illness. *Lancet* 2:758–761, 1985.
20. Howard LSGE, Robbins PA: Alterations in respiratory control during eight hours of isocapnic and porkilocapnic hypoxia in humans. *J Appl Physiol* 78:1092–1097, 1995.
21. Hultgren HN, Robison MC, Wuerflein RD: Over perfusion pulmonary edema. *Circulation* 34:132–133, 1966.
22. Hurtado A: Chronic mountain sickness. *JAMA* 120:1278–1282, 1941.
23. Jelkman W: Erythropoietin: structure, control of production, and function. *Physiol Rev* 72:449–489, 1992.
24. Jiang C, Haddad GG: A direct mechanism for sensing low oxygen levels by central neurons. *Proc Natl Acad Sci* 91:7198–7201, 1994.
25. Katayama Y, Coburn RF, Fillers WS, Baron CB: Oxygen sensors in vascular smooth muscle. *J Appl Physiol* 77:2086–2092, 1994.
26. Lahiri S: Blood oxygen affinity and alvolear ventilation in relation to body weights in mammals. *Am J Physiol* 22:529–536, 1975.
27. Lahiri S, Brody JS, Velaquez T, et al: Pulmonary adaptation to high altitude: genetic vs. environment. *Nature* 261:133–135, 1978.
28. Lahiri S, Cherniack NS, Edelman NH, Fishman AP: Regulation of respiration in goat and its adaptation to chronic and life-long hypoxia. *Respir Physiol* 12:388–403, 1971.

29. Lahiri S, Delaney RG: Stimulus interaction in the responses of carotid body chemoreceptor single afferent fibers. *Respir Physiol* 24:249–266, 1975.

30. Lahiri S, Maret K, Sherpa MG: Dependence of high altitude sleep apnea on ventilatory sensitivity to hypoxia. *Respir Physiol* 52:281–301, 1983.

31. Lahiri S, Milledge JD: Sherpa physiology. *Nature* 207:610–612, 1965.

32. Lahiri S, Mokashi A, Nishino T, Mulligan E: Comparison of aortic and carotid chemoreceptor responses to hyperapcapnea and hypoxia. *J Appl Physiol* 51:55–61, 1981.

33. Lahiri S, Smatresk N, Pokorski M, et al: Dopaminergic efferent inhibition of carotid body chemoreceptors in chronically hypoxic cats. *Am J Physiol* 247:R24–R28, 1984.

34. Maggiorini M, Buhler B, Walter M, Oelz O: Prevalence of acute mountain sickness in the Swiss Alps. *Br Med J* 301:853–855, 1990.

35. Maly FE, Schürer-Maly CC: How and why cells make superoxide: the "phogocytic" NADPH oxidase. *NIPS* 10:233–238, 1995.

36. McGregor KH, Gil J, Lahiri S: A morphometric study of the carotid body in chronically hypoxic rats. *J Appl Physiol* 57:1430–1438, 1984.

37. Milledge JS, Thomas PS, Belley JM, English JSC: Hypoxic ventilatory response and acute mountain sickness. *Eur Resp J* 1:948–951, 1988.

38. Milledge JS: Sodium balance, fluid homeostasis and the renin-aldosterone system during the prolonged exercise of hill walking. *Clin Sci* 62:595–604, 1982.

39. Mirrakhimov M, Brimjulov N, Cieslick J: Effect of acetazolamide on overnight oxygenation and acute mountain sickness in patients with asthma. *Eur Resp J* 6:536–640, 1993.

40. Oades PJ, Buchdahl RM, Bush A: Prediction of hypoxemia at high altitude in children with cystic fibrosis. *Br Med J* 308:15–18, 1994.

41. Oelz O, Maggiorini M, Ritter M, et al: Nifedipine for high altitude pulmonary oedema. *Lancet* 2:1241–1244, 1989.

42. Peers C: Ionic channels in type I carotid body cells, in O'Reagan R, Nolan P, McQuen DS, Patterson D: *Arterial Chemoreceptors: Cell to System.* New York, Plenum Press, 1994, pp 29–40.

43. Pei SX, Chen XJ, Si Ren BZ, et al: Chronic mountain sickness in Tibet. *Q J Med* 71:555–574, 1989.

44. Peñaloza D, Sime F, Banchero N, et al: Pulmonary hypertension in healthy man born and living at high altitudes. *Am J Cardiol* 11:50–57, 1963.

45. Prabhakar NR, Dinerman JL, Againi FH, Solomon S: Carbon monoxide: A role in carotid body chemoreception. *Proc Natl Acad Sci* 92:1994–1997, 1995.

46. Rahn H, Otis AB: Man's respiratory response during and after acclimatization to high altitude. *Am J Physiol* 157:445–462, 1949.

47. Ravenhill TH: Some experiences of mountain sickness in the Andes. *Trop Med Hyg* 20:313–322, 1913.

48. Schoene RB, Hackett PH, Hornbein TF: High altitude, in Murray JF, Nadel JD (eds), *Textbook on Respiratory Medicine.*

49. Severighaus JW, Bainton CK, Carcelen A: Respiratory insensitivity to hypoxia in chronically hypoxic man. *Respir Physiol* 1:308–334, 1966.

50. Speechley-Dick ME, Rimmer SJ, Hodson ME: Exacerbations of cystic fibrosis after holidays at high altitude—a cautionary tale. *Respir Med* 86:55–56, 1992.

51. Stea A, Jackson A, Nurse CA: Hypoxia and $N^6O^{2'}$ dibutyladenosine $3',5'$-cyclic monophosphate, but not nerve growth factor, induces Na^+ channels and hypertrophy in chromaffin-like arterial chemoreceptors. *Proc Natl Acad Sci* 89:9469–9473, 1992.

52. Tatsumi K, Pickett CK, Weil JV: Decreased carotid body hypoxic sensitivity in chronic hypoxia: Role of dopamine. *Respir Physiol* 101:4–57, 1995.

53. Ureña J, Fernández-Chacón R, Benot AR, et al: Hypoxia induces voltage-dependent Ca^{2+} entry and quantal dopamine secretion in carotid body glomus cells. *Proc Natl Acad Sci* 91:10208–10211, 1994.

54. Ward MP, Milledge JS, West JB: *High Altitude Medicine and Physiology,* 2d ed. London, Chapman and Hall Medical, 1995.

55. Weir EK: The mechanisms of acute hypoxix pulmonary vasoconstriction: The tale of no channels. *FASEB J* 9:183–189, 1995.

56. West JB: Man on the summit of Mount Everest, in West JB, Lahiri S (eds), *High Altitude and Man.* Washington, DC, American Physiological Society, 1984, pp 5–17.

57. Winslow RM, Monge CC: *Hypoxia, Polycythermia, and Chronic Mountain Sickness.* Baltimore, Johns Hopkins University Press, 1987.

58. Wu TY, Zhang Q, Jin B, et al: Chronic mountain sickness (Monge's disease): an observation in Quinghai-Tibet plateau, in Ueda G, Reeves JT, Sekiguchi M (eds), *High Altitude Medicine.* Matsumoto, Sunshu University Press, 1992, pp 314–324.

59. Wyatt CN, Wright C, Bee D, Peers C: O_2-sensitive K^+ currents in carotid body chemoreceptor cells from normoxic and chronically hypoxic rats and their roles in hypoxic chemotransduction. *Proc Natl Acad Sci* 92:295–299, 1995.

60. Youngson C, Nurse C, Yeger H, Cutz E: Oxygen sensing in airway chemoreceptors. *Nature* 365:153–155, 1993.

DIVING INJURIES AND AIR EMBOLISM

James M. Clark

The adverse effects of diving upon the lung and other organs originate from two major sources: (1) compression of gas within the lungs and other body spaces as ambient pressure is increased, with later expansion of that gas upon return to normal atmospheric pressure; and (2) solution of excess quantities of inert gas in blood and body tissues during exposure to increased ambient pressures, followed by evolution of venous and tissue bubbles when decompression occurs too rapidly. The former condition can cause pulmonary barotrauma, with arterial gas embolism as its most serious sequela, while the latter can result in decompression sickness with manifestations ranging from localized pain in a joint to massive neurologic deficits from spinal cord infarction.[14]

With the increasing popularity of sport diving in the United States, the yearly incidence of diving accidents has increased progressively since 1986, which is the first year that statistics reported by the Divers Alert Network became available. Among the currently estimated 2.5 to 3.2 million divers in the United States, the number of reported accidents involving gas lesions increased progressively from 562 in 1986 to 1164 in 1994, with an average annual fatality rate of about 90 for the same period.[10] Although the incidence of arterial air embolism caused iatrogenically is not reported annually, it is likely that such statistics, if available, would add significantly to the morbidity and mortality of gas lesion diseases related to diving accidents.

PULMONARY BAROTRAUMA

If a diver were to descend while holding his or her breath, the gas within the lungs would be compressed progressively while maintaining a volume that is inversely proportional to the increasing pressure (Fig. 64-1). In order to prevent collapse of the lung to less than residual volume, with tearing of pulmonary parenchyma and blood vessels, the diver is obliged to breathe an oxygen-containing gas mixture at a pressure equal to that of the surrounding water. During return to normal atmospheric pressure, compressed gas within the lungs expands exponentially and must be exhaled if alveolar rupture is to be avoided.

The greatest danger of alveolar bursting occurs within the last 33 ft of ascent to the surface, because the relative gas volume doubles during that transition (Fig. 64-1). Theoretically, a critical threshold for alveolar rupture could be reached by ascent from as shallow a depth as 4 ft (1.2 m) after full inspiration at that depth. Fatal arterial gas embolism has occurred following ascent from a depth of 7 ft (2 m).[19]

Possible Sequelae of Alveolar Rupture during Decompression

The sequelae of pulmonary overpressure accidents are determined by the nature and severity of associated tissue trauma as well as by the volume of expanding extraalveolar gas.[17,19] Following rupture of alveolar septa, expanding gas enters the interstitial spaces and dissects along perivascular sheaths to enter the mediastinum. Gas may also enter the pleural space to cause pneumothorax. Mediastinal gas may further dissect into the pericardial sac, the retroperitoneal space, or the subcutaneous tissues of the neck.

Mediastinal emphysema is often associated with mild substernal discomfort that may be described as a dull ache or a feeling of tightness. Deep inspiration, coughing, or swallowing may exacerbate symptoms, and mild pain may radiate to the shoulders, neck, or back. Unless extensive, mediastinal emphysema is usually not associated with dyspnea, tachypnea, or other signs of respiratory distress. Clinically significant volumes of mediastinal gas have a distinctive appearance on the chest radiograph.

Subcutaneous emphysema from pulmonary barotrauma causes swelling and crepitance in the neck and supraclavicular fossae. These signs may be associated with sore throat, dyspha-

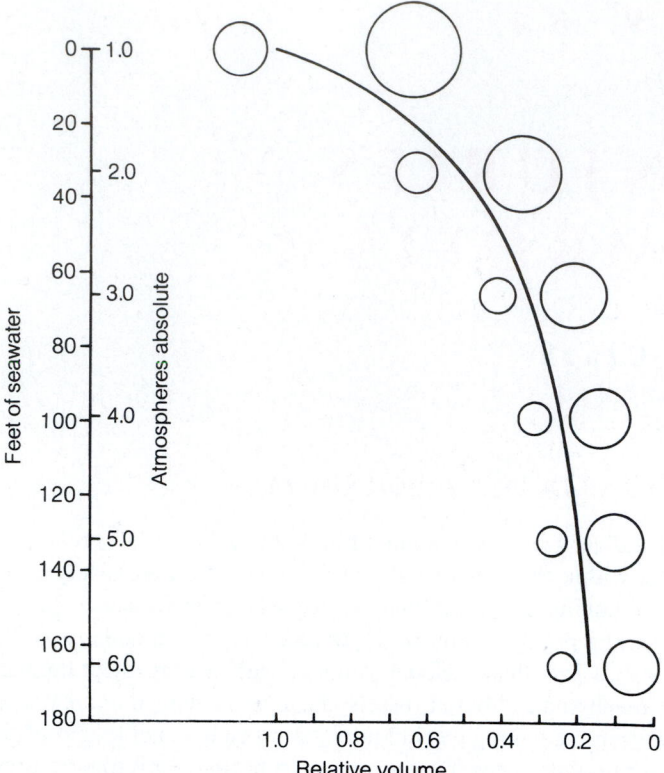

FIGURE 64-1 Relationship of relative gas volume to ambient pressure during compression from 1.0 to 6.0 atm (surface to 165 ft of sea water). Boyle's law states that, at constant temperature, the volume of a gas is inversely proportional to its pressure. Bubbles on the left show the decrease in diameter that would occur during compression without access to a gas source at ambient pressure. Bubbles on the right show expansion that would occur during decompression after restoration of unit volume at a depth of 165 ft. Similar lung volume changes during diving are prevented by inhalation of compressed gas during descent and exhalation of expanding gas during ascent.

gia, or a change in voice tone. Subcutaneous gas can also be demonstrated radiographically. Recompression therapy is not needed for uncomplicated cases of mediastinal or subcutaneous emphysema. If symptoms are bothersome, resolution of gas can be hastened by breathing 100% oxygen at normal atmospheric pressure. Gas volumes within the pericardial sac or retroperitoneal space are seldom large enough to be clinically significant.

Pneumothorax is not a frequent complication of pulmonary barotrauma. In one series of submarine escape ascents, pneumothorax occurred in about 10 percent of the divers who had lung overinflation syndromes.[36] Recompression of an individual who is known to have a pneumothorax should be avoided if at all possible. Nevertheless, it must be carried out if neurologic symptoms or any other manifestations of arterial gas embolism are present.

Conversion from a simple to a tension pneumothorax will occur if a tear in the visceral pleura remains open during descent, thereby allowing compressed gas to enter the pleural space, and then becomes effectively sealed prior to ascent. Upon decompression, the gas in the pleural space will expand to compress the lung and interfere with venous return. Severe dyspnea, cyanosis, and hypotension may occur, especially when the infe-

rior vena cava is kinked at the diaphragmatic hiatus. This is an emergency that will require immediate recompression to relieve symptoms and insertion of a chest tube before decompression is resumed. Smaller pneumothoraxes can be managed by inserting a large, 10- to 14-gauge catheter (Angiocath) through the appropriate intercostal space and attaching it to a flutter valve made from a Penrose drain or some other suitable material.

Arterial Gas Embolism

When expanding extraalveolar gas is forced down a pressure gradient into torn septal vessels, it traverses the pulmonary veins to the left atrium and left ventricle, from which it is ejected into the systemic circulation as foamy particles.[19] Distribution of the gas emboli is determined by their buoyancy relative to blood and orientation of the body with respect to gravity. It may also be influenced by local factors such as turbulence and eddy currents. With the body in the head-up, erect position, most of the embolic air travels to the brain, while the coronary vessels are embolized more frequently with the body in a feet-up, inverted posture.

Cerebral air embolism is a relatively frequent component of lung overinflation syndromes. In a series of 88 divers with pulmonary barotrauma, the incidence of neurologic signs and symptoms was about 75 percent.[13] Electroencephalographic evidence of abnormal neuronal activity after submarine escape training ascents in the absence of associated clinical manifestations indicates that the true incidence of cerebral gas embolism may be even higher than that established on the basis of positive historical and physical findings.[22]

The pathogenesis of cerebral gas embolism involves as a primary event—the lodging of embolic gas in arteries and arterioles—causing circulatory arrest with ischemia of the distal tissues.[47] Demonstration of abnormal permeability to protein tracers such as Evans Blue dye within 1 to 2 min of air embolism indicates that the bubbles also cause direct endothelial damage at the site of obstruction.[23] Endothelial interaction with active bubble surfaces has been proposed as the basis for this damage.[19]

Clinical manifestations of dysbaric arterial gas embolism have been grouped into two categories, based on the initial presentation.[14,19] The smaller group encompasses critically injured divers who develop apnea, unconsciousness, and cardiac arrest during ascent or immediately after surfacing from a dive. Most of these individuals die even when recompression is initiated within minutes. It is presumed that at least some of these catastrophes are caused by direct embolization of the coronary arteries. Experimental evidence also indicates that autonomic influences on the heart and lung can be initiated by brainstem embolization.[16]

The majority of patients with dysbaric arterial gas embolism present with neurologic signs and symptoms, but spontaneous respiration and heart rate are maintained. Just as in the more seriously injured divers, onset of symptoms occurs during ascent or within minutes after surfacing. The clinical spectrum of neurologic disturbances ranges from focal signs, such as monoparesis or discrete sensory deficits, to diffuse brain dysfunction, as manifest by confusion, stupor, or coma. In response to prompt recompression, most patients undergo complete resolution of all neurologic deficits. For reasons that are not well understood, some fail to respond completely or experience initial improvement followed by recurrence of the presenting signs and symptoms. The probability of incomplete response or recurrence is increased as the time between onset of symptoms and initiation of definitive therapy is prolonged.

Iatrogenic Arterial Gas Embolism

Accidental arterial gas embolism is a serious and sometimes lethal complication of many procedures that are widely used in modern medicine.[37] It is often misdiagnosed or recognized only after a delay of several hours. Even when the diagnosis of arterial gas embolism is correctly made, many physicians who are not specifically trained in diving medicine are apparently unaware that hyperbaric oxygenation is the definitive and highly efficacious therapy for this condition. No other useful therapy exists. As an example of such unawareness, there are no references to hyperbaric oxygen therapy in at least two surgical texts that contain discussions of cerebral gas embolization as a complication of open-heart surgery.

Arterial gas embolism has been reported in association with a variety of procedures including cardiac surgery; intravenous therapy, especially with the use of central venous catheters; neurosurgery; pulmonary diagnostic or surgical procedures; surgery of the aorta or cervical arteries; surgical procedures involving the head and neck; hemodialysis; arterial catheterization, especially for arteriography; mechanical ventilation; abdominal or retroperitoneal gas insufflation; liver transplantation; and uterine catheterization or insufflation, usually during criminal abortion (i.e., if performed under nonmedical, unsterile conditions). Most cases of accidental arterial gas embolism present with focal or diffuse manifestations of brain ischemia. Management is often made more difficult by the existence of concurrent medical or surgical complications. In many patients, hyperbaric oxygen therapy, if administered promptly, completely reverses all neurologic deficits. It is generally remarkably efficacious even when initiated after a delay of several hours.

DECOMPRESSION SICKNESS

Decompression sickness, which is characterized by a broad clinical spectrum with multiple manifestations, occurs when ambient pressure is reduced too rapidly to allow the inert gas dissolved in blood and body tissues to remain in physical solution.[17,19] It usually occurs in the diver after inadequate decompression from prolonged exposure to increased ambient pressures, but it can also occur in the aviator or astronaut who is exposed to high altitude or space with blood and body tissues that are saturated with inert gas at normal atmospheric pressure.

Although the precipitating cause of decompression sickness is the evolution of dissolved inert gas from body fluids, neither the physical mechanisms nor the locations of bubble formation are completely understood.[17,19] Both intravascular and extravascular bubbles have been found in animals exposed to severe decompression stress. Intravascular bubbles are more likely formed in veins than in arteries, due to the greater hydrostatic pressure in the latter vessels. Primary effects caused by the physical presence of undissolved gas in vivo include the obstruction of blood vessels and the mechanical disruption of tissue. In addition, there are secondary effects, caused by tissue reactions to intravascular or extravascular bubbles, that include the concurrent activations of cellular components, such as leukocytes and platelets, and biochemical pathways, such as the complement, coagulation, and kinin systems. It is also possible during or after decompression from a dive to have circulating venous bubbles, as detected by Doppler ultrasonography, without precipitating the onset of decompression sickness.

Clinical Manifestations of Decompression Sickness

Musculoskeletal pain in one or more extremities is the most common symptom of decompression sickness in military divers, commercial divers, and caisson workers.[14] Sport divers, in contrast, more commonly present with neurologic symptoms or signs. These apparent patterns may reflect both the reluctance of professional divers to report neurologic symptoms due to the related occupational penalties and the tendency of many recreational divers to delay seeking medical assistance until neurologic symptoms occur. However, neurologic and pain-only manifestations of decompression sickness also appear to have different latencies. Among divers who present with neurologic involvement, about 50 percent become symptomatic within 10 min of surfacing, and over 90 percent are symptomatic within 3 h.[14] In about 90 percent of divers who present with musculoskeletal pain only, symptoms occur within 6 h after the dive. Onsets of decompression sickness 36 h or more after the dive have been reported, but delays exceeding 24 h are extremely rare. Relatively long delays prior to symptom onset sometimes occur during flights in commercial aircraft that are not pressurized to 1.0 atm and may have cabin altitudes as high as 8000 ft. It is generally recommended that flying should be delayed for at least 24 h after diving.

Clinical manifestations of neurologic decompression sickness usually reflect involvement of the spinal cord at the lower thoracic or upper lumbar levels. Paresthesias and sensory deficits may occur with or without associated weakness or paralysis. Transient or persistent abdominal pain may be present. Bladder or bowel dysfunction may occur alone or with associated signs. A form of decompression sickness that is characterized by vestibular involvement may present with the sudden onset of vertigo and severe impairment of balance. Associated symptoms often include nausea, vomiting, nystagmus, tinnitus, and sometimes hearing loss. Vestibular decompression sickness can be unusually difficult to treat, as manifest by a slow or incomplete response to aggressive hyperbaric oxygen therapy.

Pulmonary Decompression Sickness

The pulmonary form of decompression sickness occurs most frequently after short, deep dives or altitude decompressions.[19] This condition, known to divers as the "chokes," is manifest by substernal pain, cough, and dyspnea, often associated with extreme malaise. The onset of symptoms is often within minutes after decompression, but it may be delayed for several hours. In some instances, there is only a mild sensation of chest "tightness" that resolves spontaneously. Patients who are more severely affected characteristically manifest a progressive exacerbation of symptoms, entailing rapid, shallow breathing to avoid substernal pain and paroxysmal coughing whenever deep inspiration is attempted. If untreated by hyperbaric oxygenation, pulmonary decompression sickness can terminate in asphyxia, shock, and death.

Although the pathogenesis of pulmonary decompression sickness is not well understood, it apparently involves accumulation in the lung of embolic bubbles along with entrapped aggregates of platelets, fibrin, leukocytes, and erythrocytes.[19] In dogs, either pulmonary gas embolism or severe decompression stress increased pulmonary arterial and right ventricular pressures, reduced cardiac output, and decreased arterial oxygenation.[2] Pulmonary microvascular permeability was increased in rabbits exposed to extreme decompression profiles.[4] Divers exposed to a single air decompression dive had significant reductions in arterial P_{O_2} and pulmonary diffusing capacity for carbon monoxide concurrently with the detection of venous bubbles by precordial Doppler monitoring.[12] The occurrence of the adult respiratory distress syndrome following accidental venous air embolism in a patient has been reported.[15]

CONTINUOUS PULMONARY EMBOLISM AS A MODEL OF PULMONARY DISEASE

Development of a unique experimental model of lung disease was stimulated by a series of unexpected observations during deep diving research in human subjects exposed in a hyperbaric chamber to ambient pressures equivalent to depths up to 1200 ft of seawater.[29] When the respired inert gas was nitrogen or neon, with helium as the ambient inert gas at constant ambient pressure, the subjects experienced intense itching in association with maculopapular skin lesions and, on some occasions, developed severe vestibular derangements, with vertigo and nystagmus. The skin lesions were found to be caused by gas bubbles in the skin and subcutaneous tissues. The vestibular derangements were attributed to counterdiffusion of inert gases through the eardrum and middle ear to the inner ear.

Subsequent experiments in pigs and in vitro systems[18,21] revealed that the development of skin and subcutaneous tissue gas bubble lesions at constant pressure was caused by the more rapid inward diffusion of helium from the ambient atmosphere into skin capillaries than outward diffusion of nitrogen or neon from capillaries to atmosphere. The process has been designated "isobaric counterdiffusion gas lesion disease," and Fig. 64-2 illustrates schematically its probable pathogenetic mechanism. In vivo systems are obviously much more complex than the simple two-layer system shown in Fig. 64-2.

Continuous, steady-state venous gas embolism can be produced in an anesthetized pig by administration of a normoxic nitrous oxide–oxygen inspired gas mixture with all or part of the pig's body enclosed in a helium-filled bag.[38] This inert gas counterdiffusion model can be used to study adverse effects of gas embolization, interactions of bubble surfaces with blood and vascular constituents, and various methods of therapeutic intervention.

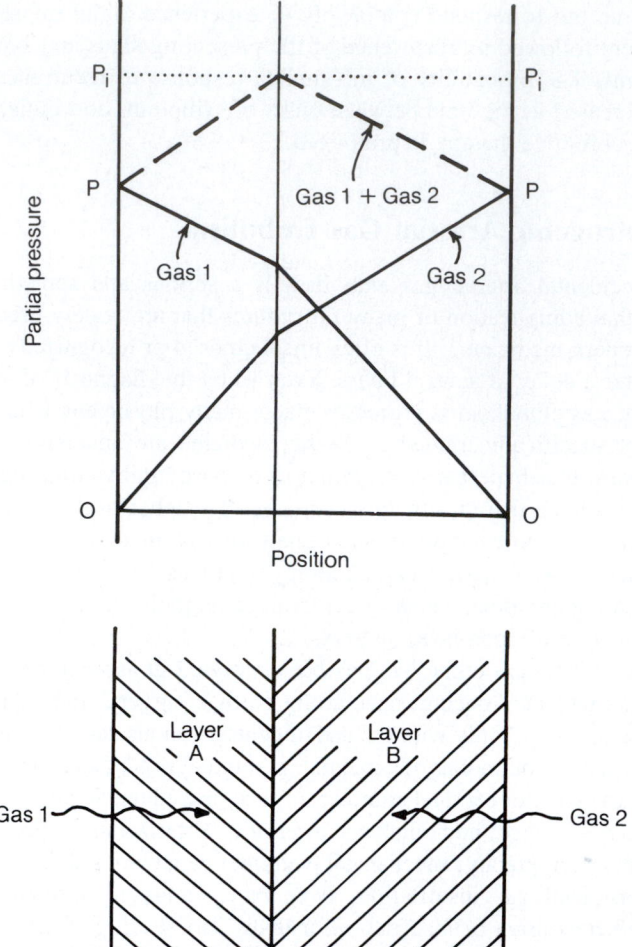

FIGURE 64-2   Supersaturation and bubble formation by countercurrent diffusion at the interface of a two-layer system. The two gas reservoirs are large, and their contents are well mixed. In this model, gas 1 (helium) diffuses more rapidly than gas 2 (nitrogen) through layer A (water), and the relative diffusivities of gases 1 and 2 are reversed in layer B (oil). Total gas pressure at any point in the system is the sum of partial pressures of both gases. Bubbles will form at the interface if suitable nuclei are present and if at least one of the two layers is a liquid. *(From Graves et al.,[18] with permission.)*

HYPERBARIC OXYGEN THERAPY

In apparently the first medical application of hyperbaric oxygenation in diving, the British navy began using oxygen inhalation during the early 1930s to hasten inert gas elimination during the final stages of decompression from dives to 300 ft.[1] However, even though it was known by then, from animal experiments, that oxygen exerts toxic effects on the lungs and central nervous system, the introduction of oxygen decompression as a routine form of treatment was handicapped by the paucity of data concerning oxygen tolerance in humans. This stricture was significantly diminished within the same decade by a series of studies on oxygen toxicity in humans and animals and of oxygen recompression therapy of decompression sickness in anesthetized dogs conducted by A. R. Behnke and colleagues at the Harvard laboratories of Cecil Drinker and Louis Shaw.

Use of oxygen diving for underwater surveillance and demolition during the closing years of World War II greatly stimulated investigation of effects and mechanisms of oxygen toxicity. During the mid-1940s, the times of onset of the signs and symptoms of neurologic oxygen poisoning were observed by K. W. Donald in hundreds of British divers exposed to oxygen pressures ranging up to nearly 4 atm.[11] Working concurrently on different continents, Dickens[9] in London and Stadie and coworkers[39] in Philadelphia studied biochemical effects of oxygen toxicity in brain slices and other tissue preparations. Many enzymes, especially those with active sulfhydryl groups, were found to be inactivated by increased oxygen pressures.

In a series of investigations during the 1950s,[27,28,30–32] Lambertsen and many collaborators at the University of Pennsylvania obtained extensive data describing, in humans, the effects of hyperbaric oxygenation on blood-gas transport, pulmonary ventilation, cerebral circulation, and cerebral metabolism. Arterial blood-gas measurements, showing the large increments in oxygen pressure and content that could be achieved in a hyperbaric environment (Fig. 64-3), provided a physiological basis for later clinical applications of hyperbaric oxygenation. Medical uses of hyperbaric oxygen therapy now extend considerably beyond its initial applications in diving. Several conditions in which there is a physiological and/or experimental basis for its use and in which its clinical efficacy has been demonstrated are listed in Table 64-1.

Therapeutic Effects of Hyperbaric Oxygenation

The oxygen environment of any organ or tissue depends on several interacting factors that influence the balance between oxygen supply and its metabolic utilization. Arterial oxygen content is

TABLE 64-1

Current Indications for Hyperbaric Oxygen Therapy Approved by the Hyperbaric Oxygen Committee of the Undersea and Hyperbaric Medical Society

Gas lesion diseases
  Decompression sickness
  Gas embolism

Infections
  Clostridial myonecrosis
  Necrotizing soft tissue infections
  Chronic refractory osteomyelitis

Vascular insufficiency states
  Radiation necrosis of bone or soft tissue
  Healing enhancement in problem wounds
  Compromised skin grafts or flaps
  Acute traumatic ischemias
  Thermal burns

Postischemic reperfusion injury
  Carbon monoxide poisoning

SOURCE: Modified after Clark,[6] with permission.

determined by oxygen partial pressure, hemoglobin concentration, and oxyhemoglobin percent saturation. Oxygen supply to any organ is also highly dependent on the blood flow. Diffusion distance between any individual cell and the nearest capillary is determined by the density of the capillary network. Finally, at the mitochondrial end of the oxygen pathway, tissue requirements for oxygen are determined by the level of metabolic activity.

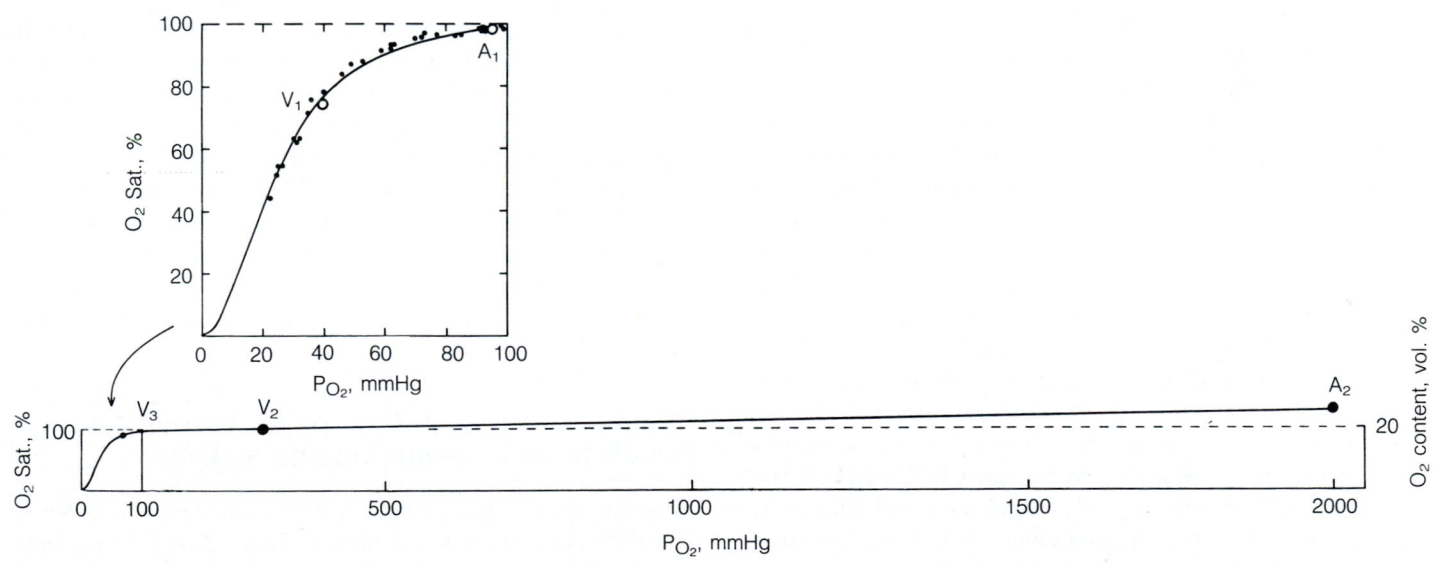

FIGURE 64-3 Hemoglobin-bound and physically dissolved oxygen in the arterial blood of normal men. *Top:* A typical range of arterial to mixed venous P_{O_2} (A_1 to V_1) during air breathing and its relationship to oxyhemoglobin percent saturation. The points through which the curve is drawn represent measurements in arterial blood of normal men breathing air or low oxygen/gas mixtures. Hemoglobin is an important source of oxygen transport at this level of P_{O_2}. *(From Lambertsen et al.,[27] with permission.) Bottom:* The increase in arterial P_{O_2} and the additional oxygen uptake over that bound to hemoglobin when inspired P_{O_2} is increased to 3.5 atm. The additional oxygen is transported as gas physically dissolved in blood water. Fall in P_{O_2} from A_2 to V_2 indicates the decrement across brain capillaries predicted on the basis of same oxygen extraction that occurs during air breathing. Direct measurement shows that brain venous P_{O_2} actually falls to V_3, because brain blood flow is reduced prominently during oxygen breathing at 3.5 atm. *(From Lambertsen,[26] with permission.)*

Many of the therapeutic benefits of hyperbaric oxygenation are associated with its capacity for increasing oxygen delivery to hypoxic tissues (Fig. 64-3).[26] Although little additional oxygen can be combined with hemoglobin, which is 97 to 98 percent saturated at normal arterial P_{O_2}, the quantity of physically dissolved oxygen increases linearly with arterial P_{O_2} elevation (about 2.4 ml O_2 per 100 ml blood per atmosphere-inspired P_{O_2}). This important increment in arterial oxygen content is associated with a much larger elevation of the oxygen partial pressure gradient from capillary blood to metabolizing cell. The combined increments in oxygen content and diffusion gradient facilitate oxygen delivery to tissues that, due to ischemia or some other cause, remain hypoxic during air breathing. In many of these states, oxygen breathing at 1.0 atm would also be beneficial, but the associated increments in oxygen content and P_{O_2} are often insufficient to ensure resumption of normal metabolic function in ischemic tissues.

In addition to enhancing oxygen delivery, hyperbaric oxygenation has other therapeutic effects in specific disease states.[6,25,42] Resolution of bubbles in decompression sickness and air embolism is greatly hastened by breathing oxygen at increased pressure, because the associated elimination of nitrogen from all body tissues and concurrent bubble compression combine to maximize the outward diffusion gradient for bubble nitrogen.[6] Hyperoxygenation is also a valuable adjunct in the therapy of clostridial myonecrosis (gas gangrene) because it inhibits multiplication of the anaerobic organisms and, even more importantly, prevents formation of the toxic lecithinase that causes necrotizing myositis.[20]

The antibacterial actions of polymorphonuclear leukocytes are decreased under hypoxic conditions,[3] presumably by an impaired generation of oxygen radicals. When the oxygen tension of a hypoxic area is elevated to normal or slightly increased levels, leukocyte function is improved.[3] Improved antibiotic efficacy by restoration of normal P_{O_2} levels has also been demonstrated in a rabbit osteomyelitis model.[3]

Patients who receive high-dose radiation therapy for cancer experience a delayed-injury response in nonmalignant irradiated tissues that is apparently caused by the progressive destruction of microcirculation secondary to obliterative radiation endarteritis.[33] Many of these patients develop varying degrees of radiation necrosis in bone and soft tissues that is associated with delayed or arrested healing in response to accidental or surgical trauma. Related sequelae—such as nonhealing wounds, fistula formation, and pathological fractures—can be avoided or ameliorated by the adjunctive use of hyperbaric oxygenation to increase fibroblast activity and induce capillary angiogenesis in the irradiated tissues.[33] Nonhealing foot wounds in diabetic patients who have significant microvascular impairment with little or no large vessel disease often respond favorably to hyperbaric oxygen therapy.[34] As a component in the comprehensive care of thermal burns, adjunctive hyperbaric oxygen therapy can significantly reduce morbidity and mortality, decrease the required number of surgical procedures, and reduce the length of hospitalization.[5] Potential mechanisms for these beneficial effects include increased capillary angiogenesis and rate of epithelialization, edema reduction, decreased extravasation of fluid, and reduced incidence of infection.

In carbon monoxide poisoning, hyperbaric oxygenation rapidly decreases blood carboxy-hemoglobin concentration and may also oppose CO effects on the cytochrome chain. However, any therapeutic advantage related to reducing the half-time for carboxy-hemoglobin dissociation from about 90 min on 100% O_2 at 1.0 atm to about 23 min on O_2 at 3.0 atm[42] is frequently lost due to the time required to transport a patient from the CO exposure site to a hyperbaric chamber. Nevertheless, in a recent prospectively randomized trial of hyperbaric versus normobaric oxygen therapy for patients who had CO poisoning without loss of consciousness, none of 30 patients who received hyperbaric oxygen developed delayed neuropsychological sequelae, whereas a statistically significant 23 percent incidence (7 of 30) occurred in the patients who received oxygen at 1.0 atm.[45]

Additional support for the use of hyperbaric versus normobaric oxygen therapy for CO poisoning is provided by the recent demonstration that 45 min of oxygen breathing at 3.0 atm, but not at 1.0 atm, prevented a CO-induced oxidative brain injury in rats.[40] In this model of CO poisoning, many of the biochemical changes in the brain induced by CO exposure were characterized as a postischemic reperfusion injury that involved the postexposure sequential occurrence of the following: (1) leukocyte sequestration in the brain microcirculation; (2) leukocyte adherence to endothelium by the action of B_2 integrins; (3) release of proteases that convert xanthine dehydrogenase to xanthine oxidase; and (4) brain lipid peroxidation by reactive oxygen species.[43] Related studies of hyperoxic antagonism of the CO-induced oxidative brain injury showed that the above sequence of events was blocked by functional inhibition of leukocyte B_2 integrins.[41] Clinical relevance of this observation was confirmed by the subsequent demonstration that leukocyte B_2 integrin function in humans was inhibited for at least 8 but less than 12 h by 45 min of oxygen breathing at 2.8 or 3.0 atm.[44]

Beneficial actions of hyperbaric oxygen therapy against the pathological effects of postischemic reperfusion injuries have also been demonstrated in skeletal muscle as well as cerebral and cardiac tissues.[6] In one of the skeletal muscle models of this injury,[48] functional inhibition of leukocyte B_2 integrins has been identified as the basis for the beneficial effects of hyperbaric oxygenation.[49] Given the known involvement of postischemic reperfusion injuries over a wide range of disease states,[24] it can be expected that this reversible action of hyperbaric oxygenation will have broader therapeutic applications than are now employed.

Hyperbaric Oxygen Therapy of Arterial Gas Embolism and Decompression Sickness

Although arterial gas embolism and decompression sickness have different etiologies and clinical presentations, similar therapeutic principles are applied in both conditions.[35] Primary aims of therapy in both cases are reduction in bubble size, acceleration of bubble resolution, and maintenance of tissue oxygenation. The pressure-oxygenation profile used to accomplish these aims in arterial gas embolism is shown in Fig 64-4.

The rationale for initial compression to 165 ft is that reduction in bubble size to one-sixth of their original volume will allow at least some bubbles to traverse capillaries and enter the

Minutes
0 20 40 60 80 100 120 140 160 180 200 220 240 260 280 300 320
Feet of seawater
0 20 40 60 80 100 120 140 160 180
Atmospheres absolute
1.0 2.0 3.0 4.0 5.0 6.0
Start 100% O2
Air
Air
Air
Air
Air
50% O2/50% N2

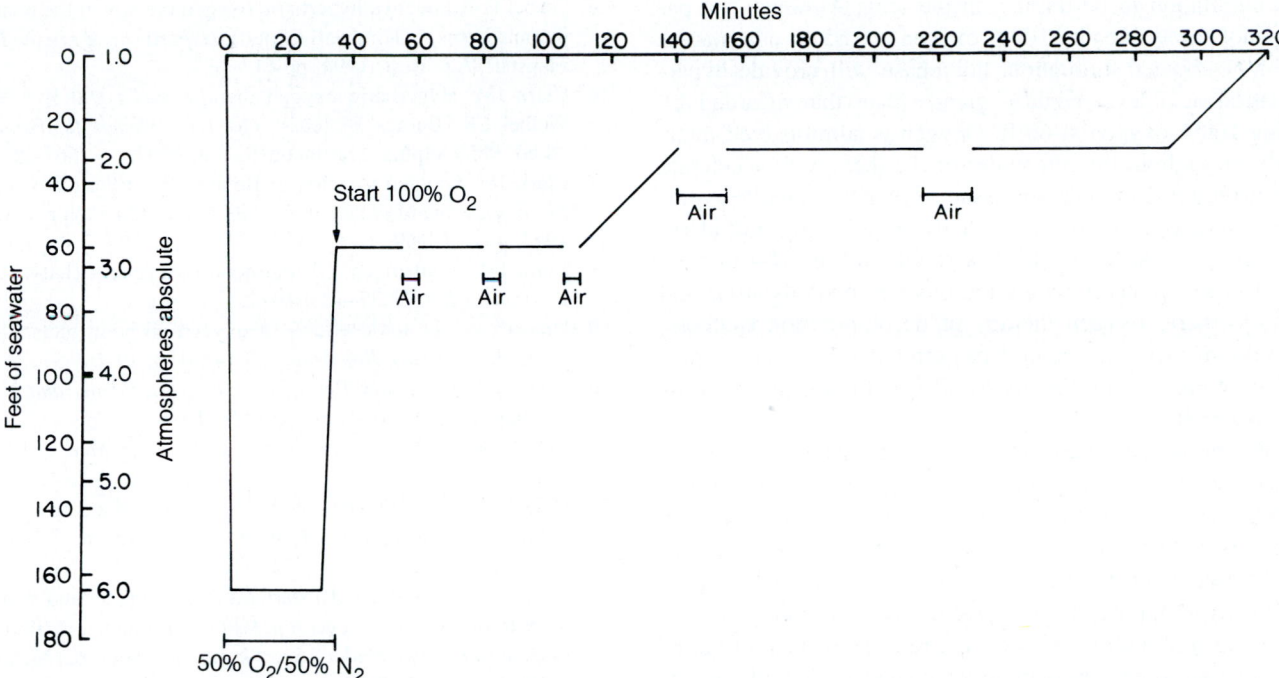

FIGURE 64-4 Pressure-time profile for hyperbaric oxygen therapy of arterial gas embolism and severe decompression sickness. During the initial period of compression to a pressure equivalent to a depth of 165 ft, 50% O_2 in N_2 is administered to the patient for up to 30 min. Upon decompression to 60 ft over a 4-min interval, the patient breathes 100% O_2 and chamber air intermittently for at least 75 min. After a 30-min period of decompression on oxygen to 30 ft, the patient breathes oxygen and air intermittently for at least 150 min, followed by another 30-min decompression on oxygen to normal ambient pressure. *(Modified after* U.S. Navy Diving Manual,[46] *with permission.)*

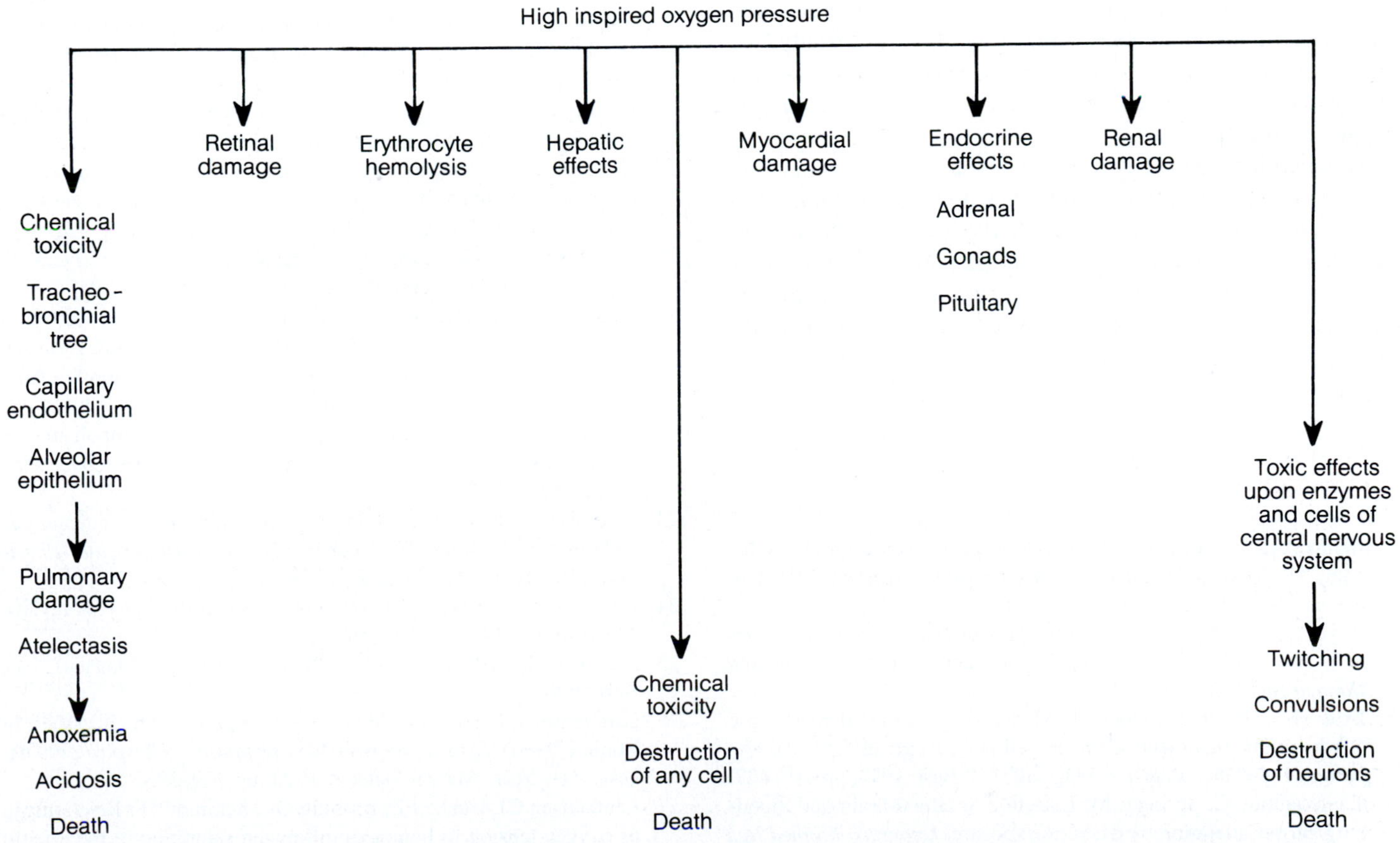

High inspired oxygen pressure
Chemical toxicity
Tracheo-bronchial tree
Capillary endothelium
Alveolar epithelium
Pulmonary damage
Atelectasis
Anoxemia
Acidosis
Death
Retinal damage
Erythrocyte hemolysis
Hepatic effects
Chemical toxicity
Destruction of any cell
Death
Myocardial damage
Endocrine effects
Adrenal
Gonads
Pituitary
Renal damage
Toxic effects upon enzymes and cells of central nervous system
Twitching
Convulsions
Destruction of neurons
Death

FIGURE 64-5 Manifestations of oxygen poisoning in specific organs and functions. *(Modified after Clark,[7] with permission.)*

venous circulation to be trapped in the lung. Although the patient cannot safely breathe 100% oxygen at 165 ft, administration of 50% oxygen throughout this phase will provide hyperoxygenation at a level slightly greater than that afforded by breathing 100% oxygen at 60 ft. Oxygen is administered intermittently throughout the remainder of the therapy to accelerate bubble resolution and maintain tissue oxygenation, while avoiding harmful effects of oxygen toxicity by allowing partial recovery during the air intervals. The profile in Fig. 64-4 may be extended in severe cases by adding oxygen intervals at 60 and 30 ft. Hyperbaric oxygen therapy of decompression sickness, which seldom involves cerebral gas embolism, is usually performed by compressing directly to 60 ft without prior pressurization to 165 ft.

In both arterial gas embolism and decompression sickness, increased blood viscosity, hypovolemia, and other systemic effects of bubble interactions with blood components and vessels occur concurrently with the localized tissue ischemia caused by mechanical vascular obstruction. Isotonic fluids are administered intravenously to oppose at least some of these secondary effects. If the patient has other conditions that require medical or surgical intervention, such care is provided concurrently with the administration of hyperbaric oxygenation.

LIMITATIONS IMPOSED BY OXYGEN TOXICITY

During oxygen breathing at increased ambient pressures, rate of intoxication increases progressively in proportion to inspired P_{O_2} elevation. Duration of oxygen exposure at 1.0 to 2.0 atm is limited primarily by pulmonary effects of oxygen toxicity.[8] At oxygen pressures of 3.0 atm or higher, visual impairment and convulsions usually occur before development of prominent pulmonary intoxication.[7]

Although the toxic effects of oxygen are numerous and varied (Fig. 64-5), they can be avoided by appropriate administration of hyperbaric oxygen therapy. Early stages of intoxication, even when associated with symptoms and detectable functional alterations, are fully reversible upon termination of exposure. The onset of toxic effects is delayed effectively by periodic interruption of oxygen exposure with scheduled "air breaks" (Fig. 64-4).

REFERENCES

1. Behnke AR: A brief history of hyperbaric medicine, in Davis JC, Hunt TK (eds): *Hyperbaric Oxygen Therapy.* Bethesda, MD, Undersea Medical Society, 1977, pp 3–10.
2. Bove AA, Hallenbeck JM, Elliott DH: Circulatory responses to venous air embolism and decompression sickness in dogs. *Undersea Biomed Res* 1:207–220, 1974.
3. Britt M, Calhoun J, Mader JT, Mader JP: The use of hyperbaric oxygen in the treatment of osteomyelitis, in Kindwall EP (ed): *Hyperbaric Medicine Practice.* Flagstaff, AZ, Best, 1994, pp 419–427.
4. Chryssanthou C, Springer M, Lipschitz S: Blood-brain and blood-lung barrier alteration by dysbaric exposure. *Undersea Biomed Res* 4:117–129, 1977.
5. Cianci P: Adjunctive hyperbaric oxygen therapy in the treatment of thermal burns, in Kindwall EP (ed): *Hyperbaric Medicine Practice.* Flagstaff, AZ, Best, 1994, pp 613–631.
6. Clark JM: Hyperbaric oxygen therapy, in Crystal RG, West JB, Weibel ER, Barnes PJ (eds): *The Lung: Scientific Foundations,* 2d ed. Philadelphia, Lippincott-Raven, 1997, pp 2667–2676.
7. Clark JM: Oxygen toxicity, in Bennett PB, Elliott DH (eds): *The Physiology and Medicine of Diving,* 4th ed. Philadelphia, Saunders, 1993, pp 121–169.
8. Clark JM, Lambertsen, CJ: Pulmonary oxygen toxicity: A review. *Pharmacol Rev* 23:37–133, 1971.
9. Dickens F: The toxic effects of oxygen on brain metabolism and on tissue enzymes. *Biochem J* 40:145–186, 1946.
10. *Divers Alert Network Report on Diving Accidents and Fatalities.* Durham, NC, Divers Alert Network, 1996.
11. Donald KW: Oxygen poisoning in man. *Br Med J* 1:667–672, 712–717, 1947.
12. Dujic Z, Eterovic D, Denoble P, et al: Effect of a single air dive on pulmonary diffusing capacity in professional divers. *J Appl Physiol* 74:55–61, 1993.
13. Elliott DH, Harrison JAB, Barnard EEP: Clinical and radiological features of 88 cases of decompression barotrauma, in Shilling CW, Beckett MW (eds): *Underwater Physiology.* Bethesda, MD, FASEB, 1978, vol 6, pp 527–535.
14. Elliott DH, Moon RE: Manifestations of the decompression disorders, in Bennett PB, Elliott DH (eds): *The Physiology and Medicine of Diving,* 4th ed. Philadelphia, Saunders, 1993, pp 481–505.
15. Ence TJ, Gong H: Adult respiratory distress syndrome after venous air embolism. *Am Rev Respir Dis* 119:1033–1037, 1979.
16. Evans DE, Kobrine AI, Weathersby PK, Bradley ME: Cardiovascular effects of cerebral air embolism. *Stroke* 12:338–344, 1981.
17. Francis TJR, Gorman DF: Pathogenesis of the decompression disorders, in Bennett PB, Elliott DH (eds): *The Physiology and Medicine of Diving,* 4th ed. Philadelphia, Saunders, 1993, pp 454–480.
18. Graves DJ, Idicula J, Lambertsen CJ, Quinn JA: Bubble formation in physical and biological systems: A manifestation of counterdiffusion in composite media. *Science* 179:582–584, 1973.
19. Hallenbeck JM, Andersen JC: Pathogenesis of the decompression disorders, in Bennett PB, Elliott DH (eds): *The Physiology and Medicine of Diving,* 3d ed. San Pedro, CA, Best, 1982, pp 435–460.
20. Heimbach RD: Gas gangrene, in Kindwall EP (ed): *Hyperbaric Medicine Practice.* Flagstaff, AZ, Best, 1994, pp 373–394.
21. Idicula J, Graves DJ, Quinn JA, Lambertsen CJ: Bubble formation resulting from the steady counterdiffusion of two inert gases, in Lambertsen CJ (ed): *Underwater Physiology.* Bethesda, MD, FASEB, 1976, vol 5, pp 335–340.
22. Ingvar DH, Adolphson J, Lindemark C: Cerebral air embolism during training of submarine personnel in free escape. *Aerospace Med* 44:628–635, 1973.
23. Johansson B: Blood-brain barrier dysfunction in experimental gas embolism, in Shilling CW, Beckett MW (eds): *Underwater Physiology.* Bethesda, MD, FASEB, 1978, vol 6, pp 79–81.
24. Kerrigan CL, Stotland MA: Ischemia reperfusion injury: A review. *Microsurgery* 14:165–175, 1993.
25. Kindwall EP (ed): *Hyperbaric Medicine Practice.* Flagstaff, AZ, Best, 1994.
26. Lambertsen CJ: Effects of hyperoxia on organs and their tissues, in Robin ED (ed): *Extrapulmonary Manifestations of Respiratory Disease.* New York, Marcel Dekker, 1978, pp 239–303.
27. Lambertsen CJ, Bunce PL, Drabkin DL, Schmidt CF: Relationship of oxygen tension to hemoglobin oxygen saturation in the arterial blood of normal men. *J Appl Physiol* 4:873–885, 1952.

28. Lambertsen CJ, Ewing JH, Kough RH, et al: Oxygen toxicity: Arterial and internal jugular blood gas composition in man during inhalation of air, 100% O_2 and 2% CO_2 in O_2 at 3.5 atmospheres ambient pressure. *J Appl Physiol* 8:255–263, 1955.

29. Lambertsen CJ, Idicula J: A new gas lesion syndrome in man, induced by "isobaric gas counterdiffusion." *J Appl Physiol* 39:434–443, 1975.

30. Lambertsen CJ, Kough RH, Cooper DY, et al: Comparison of relationship of respiratory minute volume to pCO_2 and pH of arterial and internal jugular blood in normal man during hyperventilation produced by low concentrations of CO_2 at 1 atmosphere and by O_2 at 3.0 atmospheres. *J Appl Physiol* 5:803–813, 1953.

31. Lambertsen CJ, Kough RH, Cooper DY, et al: Oxygen toxicity. Effects in man of oxygen inhalation at 1 and 3.5 atmospheres upon blood gas transport, cerebral circulation and cerebral metabolism. *J Appl Physiol* 5:471–486, 1953.

32. Lambertsen CJ, Stroud MW, Gould RA, et al: Oxygen toxicity: Respiratory responses of normal men to inhalation of 6 and 100 percent oxygen under 3.5 atmospheres pressure. *J Appl Physiol* 5:487–494, 1953.

33. Marx RE: Radiation injury to tissue, in Kindwall EP (ed): *Hyperbaric Medicine Practice.* Flagstaff, AZ, Best, 1994, pp 447–503.

34. Matos LA, Nunez AA: Enhancement of healing in selected problem wounds, in Kindwall EP (ed): *Hyperbaric Medicine Practice.* Flagstaff, AZ, Best, 1994, pp 589–612.

35. Moon RE, Gorman DF: Treatment of the decompression disorders, in Bennett PB, Elliott DH (eds): *The Physiology and Medicine of Diving,* 4th ed. Philadelphia, Saunders, 1993, pp 506–541.

36. Moses J: *Casualties in Individual Submarine Escape.* New London, CT, Navy Submarine Medical Research Laboratory Report No 438, 1964.

37. Pierce EC: Cerebral gas embolism (arterial) with special reference to iatrogenic accidents. *HBO Rev* 1:161–184, 1980.

38. Pisarello J, Fried M, Fisher DG, Lambertsen CJ: Superficial isobaric counterdiffusion gas lesion disease: Effects leading to mortality, in Bachrach AJ, Matzen MM (eds): *Underwater Physiology.* Bethesda, MD, Undersea Medical Society, 1984, vol 8, pp 101–106.

39. Stadie WC, Riggs BC, Haugaard N: Oxygen poisoning. *Am J Med Sci* 207:84–114, 1944.

40. Thom SR: Antagonism of carbon monoxide-mediated brain lipid peroxidation by hyperbaric oxygen. *Toxicol Appl Pharmacol* 105:340–344, 1990.

41. Thom SR: Functional inhibition of leukocyte B_2 integrins by hyperbaric oxygen in carbon monoxide-mediated brain injury in rats. *Toxicol Appl Pharmacol* 123:248–256, 1993.

42. Thom SR: Hyperbaric oxygen therapy. *J Intens Care Med* 4:58–74, 1989.

43. Thom SR: Leukocytes in carbon monoxide-mediated brain oxidative injury. *Toxicol Appl Pharmacol* 123:234–247, 1993.

44. Thom SR, Mendiguren II, Nebolon M, et al: Temporary inhibition of human neutrophil B_2 integrin function by hyperbaric oxygen (HBO). *Clin Res* 42:130A, 1994.

45. Thom SR, Taber RL, Mendiguren II, et al: Delayed neuropsychologic sequelae after carbon monoxide poisoning: Prevention by treatment with hyperbaric oxygen. *Ann Emerg Med* 25:474–480, 1995.

46. *U.S. Navy Diving Manual,* vol 1. Flagstaff, AZ, Best, 1993, chap 8, p 46.

47. Waite CL, Mazzone WF, Greenwood ME, Larsen RT: Dysbaric cerebral air embolism, in Lambertsen CJ (ed): *Proceedings of the Third Symposium on Underwater Physiology.* Baltimore, Williams & Wilkins, 1967, pp 205–215.

48. Zamboni WA, Roth AC, Russell RC, et al: Morphologic analysis of the microcirculation during reperfusion of ischemic skeletal muscle and the effect of hyperbaric oxygen. *Plast Reconstr Surg* 91:1110–1123, 1993.

49. Zamboni WA, Stephenson LL, Roth AC, et al: Ischemia-reperfusion injury in skeletal muscle: CD18 dependent neutrophil-endothelial adhesion. *Undersea Hyperbaric Med* 21(suppl):53, 1994.

THERMAL LUNG INJURY AND ACUTE SMOKE INHALATION

Jacob S. Loke

THE FIRE ENVIRONMENT

PARTICULATES, TOXIC GASES, AND CHEMICALS
Carbon Monoxide
Hydrogen Cyanide
Hydrogen Chloride
Aldehydes

THERMAL INHALATION LUNG INJURY

PATHOPHYSIOLOGY OF ACUTE SMOKE INHALATION
AND THERMAL INHALATION INJURY

RESPIRATORY TRACT PATHOLOGY

SPECTRUM OF CLINICAL MANIFESTATIONS
Acute Manifestations
Subacute/Chronic Manifestations

CLINICAL EVALUATION
Assessment of Oxygenation/Ventilation
Quantification of Toxic Gases
Anatomic Evaluation of the Airways
Physiological Evaluation

TREATMENT
Airway Patency and Ventilation
Oxygenation
Bronchodilators
Antibiotics
Corticosteroids

The adverse respiratory effects of smoke inhalation and thermal injury have been recognized for centuries. Their appreciation in the United States has been accentuated by a number of unfortunate disasters. The 1942 Coconut Grove nightclub fire in Boston highlighted the importance of respiratory injuries, since many of the 491 people who died did so in the absence of cutaneous burns. The Las Vegas MGM Grand Hotel fire in 1980 focused attention on the particular problems of smoke inhalation posed by modern construction practices. Studies of these fires and others have demonstrated that morbidity and mortality are increased in fire victims with respiratory smoke inhalation and thermal injury. These studies have also demonstrated that the heat, flame, smoke, and gases generated by the fire can all contribute to these adverse consequences.

Smoke inhalation can trigger a wide variety of clinical manifestations. They range from minor exacerbations of preexisting asthma or bronchitis following transient smoke exposure to tragic and lethal respiratory failure. The degree of pulmonary injury from acute smoke inhalation depends on the magnitude of the smoke and thermal exposure. The fire environment is also a major variable, since, in addition to heat and smoke, fires produce a variety of different toxic gases and particulates when different materials burn. Some of the features of the fire scene may give fire investigators and physicians clues about the cause of the fire and the combustible materials and toxic gases involved. However, physicians in emergency rooms, intensive care units, and burn centers must often treat a patient with acute smoke inhalation without knowledge of the particular materials and gases to which the patient was exposed. Thus, an appreciation of the different types of toxic gases and adverse exposures that are common in fire environments is required to allow smoke inhalation and thermal injury to be understood and treated appropriately.

THE FIRE ENVIRONMENT

Many materials in the home are potentially combustible. The floor, walls, and ceiling may be constructed with wood and covered with plastic paneling, foam material padding, wallpaper, or carpeting. Paints and varnish are used for the finishing materials. In addition, the normal contents of residential dwellings include wood furniture, kitchen cabinets, mattresses, clothing, paper and books, plastic, upholstery, carpets, rugs, and polyurethane materials (e.g., telephones, television cabinets, cups, foam-rubber pillows). Some workplace environments also contain chemicals and other hazardous physical agents that have the potential to become toxic if safety features are not followed. When fire occurs, smoke, flames, and heat are generated, a variety of toxic gases and chemical products of combustion are produced, and oxygen is utilized (Table 65-1). The smoke is a suspension of visible particles in air and toxic gases. The combustion or smoldering of carbonaceous substances produces carbon or soot to which organic acids and aldehydes adhere, producing initially a gray-white and later a dark-gray vapor. If significant quantities of hydrocarbon materials are available, the smoke is black in the initial stages of fire. White smoke may indicate the combustion of plastic polymers. The type of flame that is present at a fire location may also provide information on the types of combustion that are taking place. Yellow flame may be due to the combustion of cloth, wood, and paper; red flame may result from flammable liquids and hydrocarbon by-products; and blue flame is produced by alcohol and natural gas.

A large number of toxic gases and chemicals can be generated in the fire environment.[1,8,23,33] The combustion of a variety of products, including polyvinyl chloride–containing materials (floor coverings, etc.) and wood and petroleum products, can generate carbon monoxide and other toxic gases. The polyvinyl chloride materials can produce hydrogen chloride. The combustion of polyurethane (in the upholstery of chairs and sofas) produces isocyanates and hydrogen cyanide, while the combustion of nylon (in carpets) releases cyanide and ammonia. Nitrocellulose film and other fabrics produce oxides of nitrogen. The combustion of acrylic and nylon materials also releases acrolein. Sulfur-containing products produce sulfur dioxide, and fluorinated resins produce hydrogen fluoride and hydrogen bromide. In a study of controlled low-energy fires using a combination of wood, paper, clothing, polyvinyl chloride, and other synthetic materials, free radicals with the equivalent oxidative power of chlorine gas were also produced.[34]

Since the materials that are burning differ from fire scene to fire scene, the toxic gases, fumes, and hazardous chemicals that are produced differ in each fire setting. The types and amounts of toxic gases produced by a fire also depend on whether the materials are decomposed in the pyrolysis (nonflaming or smoldering) stage of the fire, in the combustion (flaming) stage of the

TABLE 65-1

Features of the Fire Environment

Smoke
    Particulates
    Organic acids
    Aldehydes
    Hydrocarbon material

Flame
    Yellow color
        Often due to combustion of cloth, wood, paper
    Red color
        Often due to combustion of flammable liquids and
            hydrocarbon by-products
    Blue color
        Often due to combustion of alcohol or natural gas

Heat

Gases/chemicals
    Carbon monoxide
    Cyanide
    Hydrogen chloride
    Chlorine
    Phosgene
    Ammonia
    Isocyanates
    Oxides of nitrogen
    Hydrogen fluoride
    Hydrogen bromide
    Sulfur dioxide
    Benzene

Decreased inspired oxygen concentration

fire, or in both.[28] In addition, the spread rate of the fire and the amount of smoke produced by the fire depend on the ignition source, the quantity and type of combustible material present, as well as the structure, interior configuration, and ventilation and sprinkler systems of the burning structure. For example, in a one-story building, fire spreads horizontally unless there is ventilation through windows or openings in the ceiling. In a multistory building, fire spreads upward to the top floors and will spread rapidly through vertical elevator shafts, air-conditioning ducts, pipe shafts, and open stairways.

Acute smoke inhalation is a major cause of morbidity and mortality in fire-exposed persons. The severity of this injury, however, can be modulated by a number of factors. One of the important factors is the water solubility of the gases that are inhaled. Highly water-soluble agents (e.g., ammonia, sulfur dioxide, hydrogen fluoride, and acrolein) have a propensity to injure proximal airways. Since they are quite noxious, the irritation they cause is usually noted by the fire victims. In contrast, agents with low levels of water solubility—such as chlorine, phosgene, and nitrogen oxide—are more likely to cause insidious injury and thus more delayed and severe respiratory damage.[22]

During pyrolysis and combustion, oxygen is consumed and carbon monoxide and carbon dioxide are produced. The concentration of oxygen and carbon dioxide at a fire depends on the supply of air, the ventilation in the vicinity of the fire, and the burning rate of the combustible material. An ambient oxygen concentration of as low as 17.5% has been recorded in a confined-space wood fire.[47] During the flashover phase of a fire (when a room bursts into flame), it is estimated that inspired oxygen concentrations can decrease to 10 to 15%.[10] Motor coordination is impaired when the ambient air oxygen concentration is about 17%; faulty judgment and fatigue occur when the oxygen concentration is 10 to 14%, and unconsciousness and death result when the oxygen concentration is 6 to 10%.[25] Thus, the fire environment can contribute, in a major way, to the oxygenation abnormalities experienced by fire victims.

PARTICULATES, TOXIC GASES, AND CHEMICALS

The particulates, toxic gases, and chemicals present in smoke play important roles in the pathogenesis of smoke inhalation. The particulates are generally cleared by the respiratory tract. They may cause traumatic injury, nonspecific mechanical irritation, and, with massive exposure, anatomic obstruction of the airways. The toxic gases account for most of the clinically recognized effects of smoke inhalation. Important gases and chemicals are highlighted below.

Carbon Monoxide

Carbon monoxide is the most dangerous gas produced in fires. It is the leading cause of death at the fire scene or during the first 24 h after the fire. Many accidental[7,17] and intentional deaths have been linked to carbon monoxide poisoning. The incomplete combustion of carbon-containing materials and a decrease in available oxygen or a lack of ventilation can contribute to the buildup of carbon monoxide. High and even lethal levels of carbon monoxide may occur in basements and other small, confined spaces, making these areas especially hazardous to fire victims and firefighters without self-contained compressed air breathing devices.[31]

Carbon monoxide is an odorless, colorless gas that competes with oxygen for binding sites on the hemoglobin molecule. The affinity of carbon monoxide for hemoglobin is about 210 times greater than that of oxygen. Carbon monoxide poisoning causes a shift of the oxygen-hemoglobin dissociation curve to the left, thereby decreasing oxygen release at the tissue level causing tissue hypoxia. Tissue hypoxia due to carbon monoxide poisoning is most frequently manifest in the central nervous system and the cardiovascular system, in which oxygen utilization is high. The central nervous system (CNS) manifestations include headache, dizziness, psychomotor impairment, behavioral incapacitation, decreased visual discrimination, confusion, ataxia, convulsion, central hypoventilation, and unconsciousness. Headache, confusion, and collapse may occur when the blood carboxyhemoglobin (COHb) level is 40 to 50%. A COHb level of 60 to 70% causes unconsciousness, intermittent convulsions, respiratory failure and death if exposure continues.[53]

The myocardial manifestations of acute carbon monoxide poisoning result from its ability to increase heart rate and cardiac output and decrease myocardial oxygen delivery. The clinical manifestations of these alterations depend on the severity of the poisoning and of underlying coronary artery disease. Even low levels of carbon monoxide exposure can be important, since decreased exercise tolerance and increased myocardial ischemia have been noted in patients with coronary artery disease with COHb levels of 4.5%.[2] In addition, the number and complexity of ventricular arrhythmias have been noted to increase in patients with coronary artery disease who were exposed to carbon monoxide during exercise, with COHb levels approximating 6%.[43] Chest pain, dyspnea, myocardial infarction, and myocardial ischemia have been noted in patients with severe carbon monoxide poisoning with underlying coronary artery disease.[26]

Carbon monoxide also has toxic effects outside the central nervous and cardiovascular systems. Although it is not generally considered to be directly toxic to the lungs or other tissues, studies in animals suggest that carbon monoxide may cause tissue damage.[18,19,44] For example, an ultrastructural study of the lungs of rabbits exposed to carbon monoxide showed epithelial and endothelial cell swelling, interstitial edema, and depletion of lamellar bodies in alveolar type II cells.[18] In addition, carbon monoxide poisoning can be associated with cutaneous skin blisters, retinal hemorrhages, disseminated intravascular coagulation, myonecrosis, hyperglycemia, and diabetes insipidus.

Hydrogen Cyanide

Hydrogen cyanide is produced by the smoldering and combustion of polyurethane foam in upholstered seats and furniture as well as nylon, wool, silk, and Acrilan. Although it is not a major component of toxic gases in some fires, fire victims who died have been shown to have increased cyanide levels,[50] and lethal blood cyanide levels have been found in victims of fatal airplane crashes.[36] Significant levels of cyanide have also been detected

in survivors of fires who sustained smoke inhalation, with a concomitant increase in COHb levels.[6]

Hydrogen cyanide is a colorless gas with the odor of bitter almonds—an odor that is difficult to detect at a fire scene. Hydrogen cyanide is a histotoxic asphyxiant that interferes with cellular utilization of oxygen and inhibits cytochrome-c oxidase in mitochondria. Cyanide poisoning results in anaerobic metabolism and lactic acidosis.[20] Poisoning initially stimulates respiration by causing hypoxia of the central nervous system; later it causes CNS depression. The clinical manifestations of cyanide poisoning depend on the blood cyanide levels.[21] Flushing and tachycardia occur when the blood cyanide level is 0.5 to 1.0 mg/L. Severe poisoning occurs at or above 2.5 mg/L. Patients affected at this level may be obtunded and hypotensive, with slow, labored breathing and dilated pupils. They often have a pink face and nail beds, bright-red venous blood despite poor oxygen utilization, and a severe metabolic lactic acidosis with an anion gap. Dyspnea and tachycardia are frequently noted. At times, pulmonary edema is seen, followed by bradycardia, apnea, coma, and death. Hydrogen cyanide and carbon monoxide interact in an additive or synergistic manner to depress the central nervous system, preventing fire victims from escaping. The half-life of cyanide is 1 h.[6] Since most hospital clinical laboratories cannot measure whole-blood cyanide levels, the cyanide antidote should be given if cyanide poisoning is suspected clinically.

Hydrogen Chloride

Plastic and its polymers cause significant morbidity and mortality among fire victims.[16] The combustion of the polyvinyl chloride in many plastic polymers produces hydrogen chloride, a hydroscopic agent that, in combination with water vapor, forms an aerosol of hydrochloric acid. Hydrochloric acid is a mucosal irritant that can produce severe alterations of the mucous membranes of the eyes, nose, and respiratory tract. Fire victims without surface burns and with nonlethal levels of carbon monoxide have died of severe pulmonary injury from the acute inhalation of smoke containing hydrogen chloride. The degree of emission of toxic gases from plastic polymers may be greater when the material is smoldering than when it is undergoing combustion.

Aldehydes

The aldehydes—formaldehyde, acetaldehyde, and acrolein—are dermal and mucosal irritants that affect the skin, eyes, nose, and mucous membranes of the lung. When these agents are present in significant concentrations in the fire environment, pulmonary edema and death have resulted. Airway manifestations may also occur, since experimental animals exposed for 62 days to an acrolein concentration of 4.0 ppm developed obstruction of the small and large airways.[9] Aldehydes are present in greater amounts in wood smoke than in kerosene smoke.[55] Acrolein is also present in small amounts in cigarette smoke and photochemical smog and in significant amounts in fires that burn polyethylene, polypropylene, acrylic, and nylon materials. Thus, the Occupational Safety and Health Administration (OSHA) sets the threshold limit of acrolein for an 8-h exposure period at 0.1 ppm.

THERMAL INHALATION LUNG INJURY

Although smoke and toxic gases are the leading causes of respiratory morbidity and mortality in fire victims, heat and flames can also be important causes of pulmonary injury. High temperatures may cause surface burns and thermal injury to the airways.[22,45] These lesions are usually limited to the upper airways because the trachea and upper airways are an efficient heat sink that protects the lower respiratory tract from thermal injury. There are, however, a number of settings in which burns of the subglottic airways or lung parenchyma should be suspected. They include overwhelming heat exposures (see below), the inhalation of steam, with its increased heat-carrying capacity; and the respiratory aspiration of hot liquids, which causes direct pulmonary injury. In addition, pulmonary burns have been caused by the inhalation of the ignited ether vehicle used with crack cocaine.

Although thermal inhalation injury occurs in a minority of burn patients, respiratory complications and lung infection are the leading cause of death in patients with burns and inhalation injury. For example, inhalation injury was noted in only 66 of 2297 burn patients (2.9 percent) at the Brooke Army Medical Center in Texas.[14] Of these patients, 32 (48.5 percent) also had burns over more than 50 percent of their total body surface area, 95 percent had facial burns, and 55 percent had edema of the oropharynx. The overall mortality in this study was 58 percent. At the Shriners' Burn Institute in Galveston, Texas, between 1981 and 1984, 88 of 1018 patients had inhalation injury diagnosed bronchoscopically. The mortality of these patients was 56 percent, in contrast to 4.1 percent in patients without inhalation injury.[52] In a study of 1058 consecutive burn patients treated at the U.S. Army Institute of Surgical Research in Fort Sam Houston, Texas, 373 patients (35.3 percent) had inhalation injury diagnosed by bronchoscopy or ventilation perfusion lung scan. One hundred forty-one of these patients (38 percent) had pneumonia, whereas only 60 of 685 patients (8.8 percent) without inhalation injury had pneumonia.[46] In these studies, thermal inhalation injury was noted to occur most commonly in victims who were exposed in an enclosed environment or were close to the flames or heat. These patients commonly had shortness of breath, hoarseness, wheezing, carbonaceous sputum, and burns of the face and oropharyngeal area.

PATHOPHYSIOLOGY OF ACUTE SMOKE INHALATION AND THERMAL INHALATION INJURY

In burn patients, systemic and local manifestations of cutaneous and respiratory injuries are often evident. They manifest as metabolic alterations, changes in the surface barrier of the skin, complex pathophysiological alterations in respiratory structure and function, and, in some, a systemic dysfunction of a variety of visceral organs—including the lung, liver, and kidney—referred to as the systemic inflammatory response syndrome (SIRS). The metabolic alterations consist of a hypermetabolic state with an increase in plasma levels of catecholamines, glucagon, cortisol, and growth hormone. This state is also manifested by an increase in oxygen consumption, body temperature, protein catabolism,

and hyperglycemia. The increase in catecholamines leads to systemic vasoconstriction and an increase in systemic vascular resistance. The cutaneous alterations are seen in severe second- and third-degree burns and result from the loss of the protective barrier of the skin. Patients with these lesions experience heightened evaporative heat loss, the third spacing of bodily fluids, and, when the lesions are severe, hypothermia or hypotension.

Studies in animal models and humans have provided evidence for a variety of mechanisms in the mediation of smoke- and heat-induced pulmonary injury. They include direct coagulative necrosis at sites of frank burns, the generation of toxic oxygen– and nitric oxide–derived free radicals[24] that damage cells by causing lipid peroxidation,[42] the elicitation of a local inflammatory response with mediator release, and complement activation. Some of these responses may be activated in the absence of obvious respiratory injury, because it has been shown that granulocytes are recruited to and sequestered in the lung after cutaneous burns alone.[12] This presumably primes respiratory structures for a potentially catastrophic response when other stimuli (such as infection) are superimposed.

Acute smoke inhalation and thermal injury have a number of important effects in the lung, including (1) impairment of mucociliary function; (2) mucus hypersecretion; (3) tissue inflammation with tracheobronchitis, bronchitis, laryngitis, and/or pneumonitis; (4) epithelial sloughing; (5) biochemical alterations with surfactant inactivation; (6) increased vascular permeability with bronchorrhea and pulmonary edema; and (7) bronchoconstriction.[31] The mucociliary dysfunction may occur in the presence or absence of airway burns, since studies in experimental animals have shown that the acute inhalation of wood smoke alone disrupts the mucociliary blanket of the tracheobronchial tree.[32] The propensity of these injuries to damage ciliated epithelium further compromises particulate clearance (Fig. 65-1). This dysfunction may contribute to the high frequency of respiratory infection experienced by victims of smoke inhalation. The mucus hypersecretion, airway sloughing, bronchorrhea, and bronchoconstriction can significantly compromise airway function. In addition, the lower respiratory tract permeability alterations and surfactant inactivation lead to atelectasis, restrictive physiological alterations, and, when severe, respiratory failure due to the adult respiratory distress syndrome (ARDS).

Studies of tissues and investigations using bronchoalveolar lavage (BAL) have provided insights into the inflammatory response seen after smoke inhalation and thermal injury. These studies have demonstrated the augmented release of inflammatory mediators, the activation of complement, and changes in pulmonary immunoglobulin levels. Most important, they have demonstrated that an acute inflammatory response occurs within hours of exposure to smoke. Although the yield of inflammatory cells varies with the timing of the BAL and the injury, the BAL is most often characterized by an increase in BAL granulocytes and macrophages. Experimental investigations have provided evidence that the neutrophils may contribute to the pathogenesis of these respiratory lesions. Specifically, their release of nitric oxide–derived oxidants augments the lung permeability alterations and indices of oxidative injury seen in animals exposed to smoke from nonflaming pyrolysis products of combined Douglas fir wood and polyvinyl chloride.[24] The macrophages in these le-

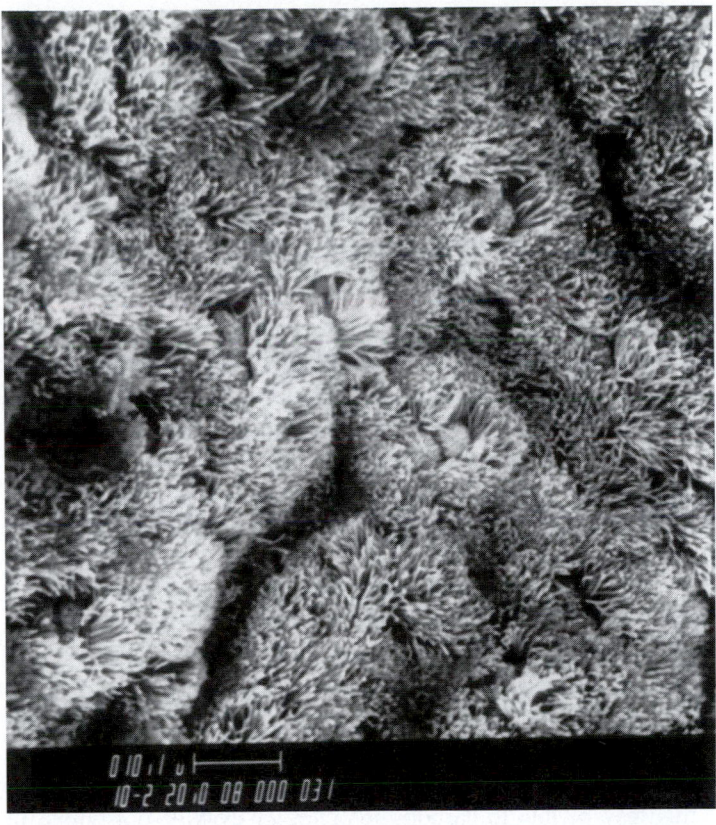

A

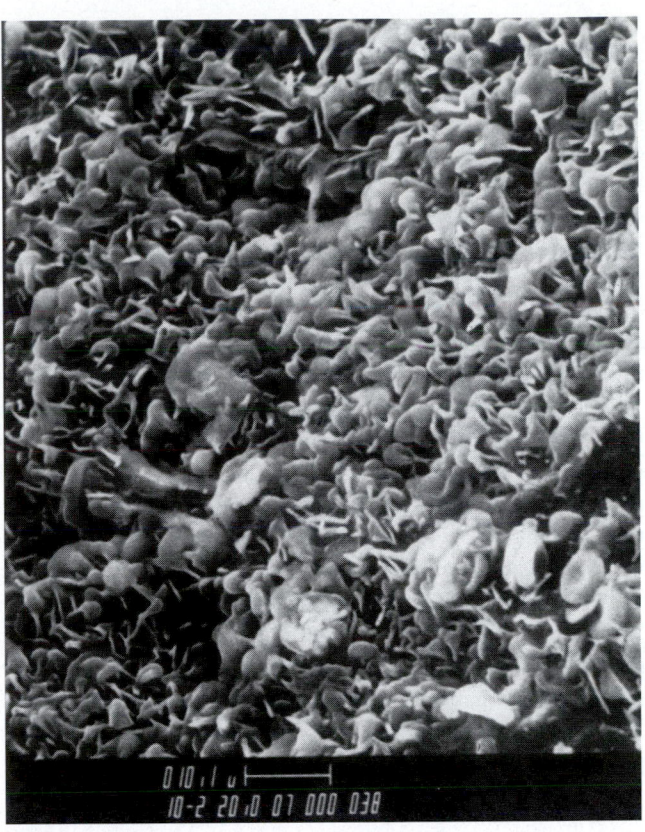

B

FIGURE 65-1 Experimental demonstration of damage to type I ciliated epithelial cells after smoke inhalation. Scanning electron micrographs were obtained from tracheas of control and smoke-exposed animals. The surface of the trachea from the control animal (*A*) demonstrates abundant normal ciliated epithelial structures and normal nonciliated areas (×1000). The trachea from the smoke-exposed rabbit (*B*) shows denuded areas focally with red blood cells apparent on the epithelial surface and abnormal cilial structure (×1000). *(Based on data of Loke et al,[32] with permission.)*

sions show evidence of both activation and deactivation. Their activation is manifest as enhanced chemoluminescence (indicating activation of oxidative metabolism) and enhanced cytokine elaboration.

In contrast, alveolar macrophage chemotactic dysfunction has been observed in experimental animals exposed to a variety of pyrolysis products, and the alveolar macrophages from smoke-exposed animals manifest cytoplasmic and structural alterations, decreased surface adherence, and decreased phagocytic and bactericidal function. The enhanced ability of alveolar macrophages (and probably other cells) to produce cytokines likely contributes to the elevated levels of tumor necrosis factor (TNF),[48] interleukin 1 (IL-1),[4] IL-8, and IL-6 that have been noted after smoke inhalation and thermal injury. These mediators may play a major role in disease pathogenesis, since TNF and other cytokines have been implicated in the generation of SIRS and related disorders, including infection, bacteremia, sepsis, septic shock, and the multiple-organ dysfunction syndrome (MODS).[40] The changes in the structure and function of the alveolar macrophages may simultaneously decrease lung defense barriers and contribute to the increased susceptibility of smoke inhalation victims to pulmonary infection.[31]

Bronchoconstriction and increased airway resistance are prominent features of smoke inhalation and thermal injury. Enhanced bronchomotor tone, edema, mucus hypersecretion, bron-

chorrhea, and mucosal sloughing can contribute to these alterations. The bronchospasm and bronchorrhea may be due to the direct effects of the smoke or irritation-induced reflex responses. Bronchoconstrictive mediators,[11] including histamine and thromboxane A_2, are also produced at these sites of injury. In the initial phases of acute smoke inhalation, the major site of obstruction is the large airways. Subsequently large- or small-airway dysfunction can be present, depending on the severity and location of the injury. These changes, along with confounding issues such as alveolar injury, carbon monoxide poisoning, and cyanide toxicity, can all contribute to the generation of severe arterial hypoxemia in smoke and thermal inhalation injury victims.

RESPIRATORY TRACT PATHOLOGY

Smoke inhalation and thermal injury can cause alterations that extend from the upper respiratory tract to the distal lung parenchyma. The upper-tract lesions have been characterized in experimental models and human victims. In experimental animals, the inhalation of hot air (350° and 500°C) caused inflammation of the upper trachea without injury to the lower trachea. However, when the animals inhaled flame from a blast burner, severe inflammation, mucosal edema, ulcers, and necrosis occurred in the upper and lower trachea.[37] Autopsies of the fire victims from the Coconut Grove nightclub fire in Boston characterized the lesions in lethal smoke inhalation and thermal injury. They showed that the larynx could be completely blocked by black charred material extending into the trachea.[35] In addition, one victim had diffuse bronchostenosis and in three victims there was a diffuse hemorrhagic and necrotizing membranous inflammatory infiltrate in the lower trachea and airways, as well as laryngotracheobronchitis. Gross examination of the trachea revealed severe edema of the mucous membranes, a fibropurulent exudate, carbonaceous material, and petechial hemorrhages. Light microscopy revealed that the epithelium of the trachea was desquamated with edema and hemorrhage and the lumen of the bronchus was obstructed by desquamated cells, fibrin, and leukocytes.

The histopathologic evolution of experimental smoke inhalation–induced parenchymal injury is similar to that observed in postmortem human tissues. The sequence of events that has been noted is also similar to that seen in acute lung injury from a variety of pulmonary insults. There is an early exudative phase, in which interstitial and alveolar edema, hemorrhage, granulocyte influx, and type I pneumocyte alterations are prominent. This is followed by a degenerative phase, characterized by type I pneumocyte injury, denuding of basement membranes, tissue necrosis, and the generation of hyaline membranes. Proliferative and repair responses are then seen. Initially they are characterized by type II pneumocyte hyperplasia, which reepithelializes the alveolar basement membrane. The type II pneumocytes subsequently evolve into type I cells, and fibroblast proliferation and matrix production attempt to restore architectural integrity.[22] In survivors of acute smoke inhalation, bronchiolitis obliterans, atelectasis, coagulation necrosis of alveoli, and alveolar soot may be present on lung biopsy (Figure 65-2).

SPECTRUM OF CLINICAL MANIFESTATIONS

Burn victims come to medical attention with a variety of presentations. This is due, in part, to the combination of respiratory and nonrespiratory injuries these patients can experience. Prominent nonrespiratory lesions include cutaneous burns and crush and traumatic injuries. Alcohol intoxication must also be kept in mind, since up to 40 percent of residential fires in some cities are alcohol related.

The respiratory tract injuries and alterations noted in fire victims can be most easily thought of as those affecting the nervous system, upper airway, lower airways, and lung parenchyma. Syndromes associated with specific toxins must also be kept in mind. The neurologic manifestations include altered sensorium, obtundation, and coma, with associated alveolar hypoventilation and compromised protection of the upper airway. As noted above, this may be due to carbon monoxide or cyanide poisoning. In the lung, the airways are the major site of respiratory injury, with upper-airway invasion being more common and more severe than lower-airway invasion. The types of airway and parenchymal injuries experienced by these patients can be classified as those that are acute (occurring within the first 24 to 48 h of presentation) and those that occur in a subacute or chronic fashion (Tables 65-2 and 65-3).

Acute Manifestations

Upper airway obstruction due to pharyngeal edema, laryngeal edema, and, rarely, mucosal sloughing, airway obstruction due to bronchitis and bronchospasm, and an alveolar level permeability alteration leading to pulmonary edema are the major acute manifestations of smoke inhalation and thermal injury. Risk factors for these manifestations include exposure in a closed space, victim entrapment, unconsciousness or other neurologic alterations, and the presence of respiratory signs and symptoms on presentation (Table 65-4) (see below). The presence of facial or cervical burns, especially lesions in the nasal vibrissae, eyebrows, nose, lips, the circumoral area or the upper cervical area, are of major concern. The expectoration of carbonaceous sputum, sore throat, and stridor may be present. When one is evaluating patients who may have thermal injury of the upper airways, it is important to remember that upper airway edema may not be clinically evident on presentation and may be noted only after fluid resuscitation. Upper airway edema usually resolves in 2 to 4 days.

Acute pulmonary edema is not commonly seen after smoke inhalation and thermal injury. When noted, it is a marker of disease severity. In the acute setting, pulmonary edema may be the result of alveolar capillary injury or a cardiac complication resulting from asphyxia or hypoxia.

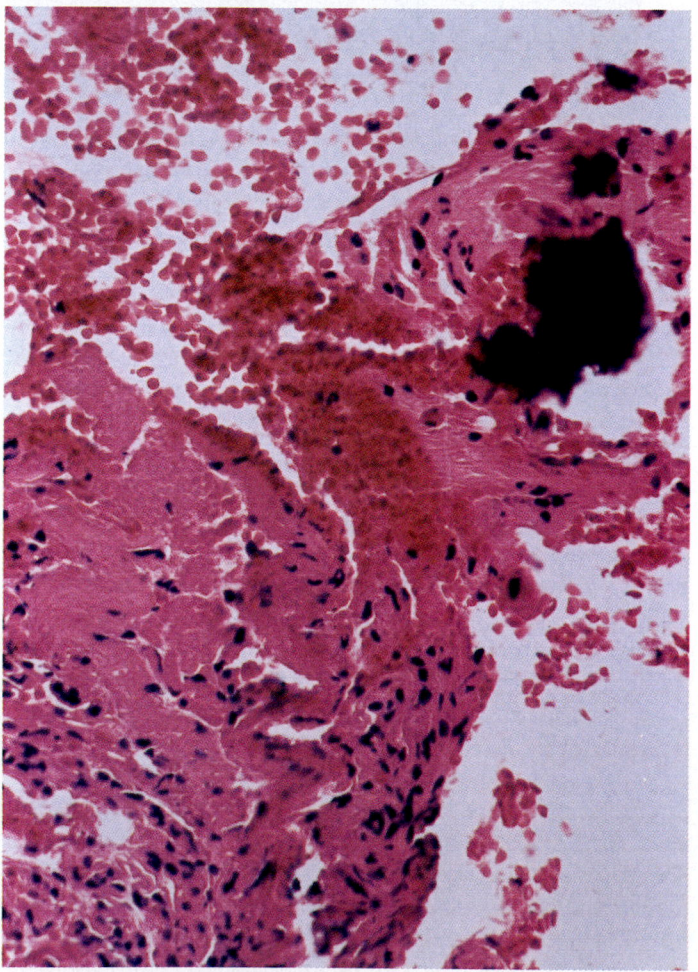

FIGURE 65-2 Transbronchial biopsy obtained 7 months after fire exposure demonstrating coagulation necrosis, collapse of alveoli, and soot in the alveoli (dark area in lower right). *(Based on data of Loke and Matthay,[30] with permission.)*

TABLE 65-2

Acute Respiratory Complications of Smoke Inhalation and Thermal Injury

Site/Type	Description
Neurologic	Altered sensorium, obtundation, coma Alveolar hypoventilation Compromised ability to protect upper airway
Toxic	Carbon monoxide intoxication Cyanide intoxication
Upper-airway obstruction	Oropharyngeal and laryngeal edema
Airway obstruction	Bronchitis Bronchospasm Airway inflammation/edema Atelectasis
Alveolar	Capillary membrane permeability alteration Pulmonary edema, ARDS

Subacute/Chronic Manifestations

The subacute and chronic complications experienced by fire-exposed subjects may represent delayed manifestations of the initial injury, dysregulated healing, or complications of patient management (Table 65-3). Important manifestations of the initial injury include delayed-onset upper airway obstruction and airway obstruction, inflammation, and bronchospasm. The delayed onset of upper-airway obstruction is caused most commonly by airway edema and occurs most commonly after fluid resuscitation has been performed. It can also be caused by mucosal sloughing, which occurs most commonly 3 to 4 days after the original injury. The air-

TABLE 65-3

Subacute/Chronic Manifestations of Smoke Inhalation and Thermal Injury

Pathogenesis/Etiology

Manifestations of injury and inflammation
   Delayed upper airway edema/mucosal
      sloughing
   Delayed pulmonary edema, ARDS
   Airway obstruction/bronchospasm
   Bronchitis
   Atelectasis
   MODS sequelae

Manifestations of abnormal repair
   Pulmonary fibrosis
   Bronchiolitis obliterans
   Bronchiectasis
   Endobronchial polyposis
   Hyperactivity of the airways, asthma

Complications of patient management
   Pneumonia
   Pulmonary embolus
   Tracheal stenosis

way obstruction can be the result of airway inflammation and edema, epithelial injury, and associated hyperreactivity of the airways.[31] Over time, an asthmalike syndrome may follow smoke inhalation and thermal injury.

Delayed-onset pulmonary edema or respiratory failure can also be seen in fire victims. It may be the result of ARDS due to irritant gases or secondary to hypotension, superimposed sepsis, or diffuse pneumonia. In these patients, ARDS can sometimes be associated with MODS.[40] MODS is characterized by the concurrent onset of abnormalities in renal, hepatic, hematologic, and CNS function in the presence of the pulmonary injury of ARDS.

In the vast majority of cases, even severe acute fire-induced injuries to the upper airway, tracheobronchial tree, and parenchyma heal with minimal sequelae. Some patients experience mild nonspecific and self-limited symptoms—including cough, nasopharyngitis, and sinusitis—after smoke exposure. In a minority of cases, there may be pulmonary fibrosis, bronchiolitis obliterans, bronchiectasis (Fig. 65-3), or endobronchial polyposis.

Patients with smoke inhalation and thermal injury may have prolonged hospitalizations requiring supportive measures, including mechanical ventilation. Pneumonia is a frequent complication in these patients. Similarly, pulmonary emboli commonly occur in these immobilized and often instrumented patients. Trauma due to intubation is the most common cause of tracheal stenosis seen following smoke inhalation.

CLINICAL EVALUATION

Patients with smoke inhalation and thermal injury can present with trivial exposures and minimal injury or with complicated multiorgan dysfunction. Their clinical picture can be further complicated by traumatic injuries caused by building collapses or jumps from burning structures, alcohol intoxication, and illicit or recreational drug use. From the respiratory perspective, the evaluation of fire victims needs to shed light on the extent and severity of the patient's injury. Historical facts that, when possible, should be elicited include details of the types of combustion in the fire environment and details of the patient's exposure. The latter includes the patient's location, duration of exposure, presence or absence of entrapment, state of consciousness, and the use, or lack of use, of protective clothing and breathing devices. In addition, paramedics and fire personnel should be questioned about specific toxic gases and chemicals that may have been involved in the fire. This evaluation should allow medical personnel to determine whether the patient is at significant risk for smoke inhalation or thermal injury (Table 65-4). Respiratory symptoms—including dyspnea, cough, and chest pain—are seen in 25 to 75 percent of patients in different studies. The expectoration of carbonaceous sputum, an increase in nasal and oral secretions, headache, and dizziness are also fre-

Exposure in closed spacez
Victim entrapment
Unconsciousness or other neurologic alterations
Facial or cervical burns
Respiratory signs or symptoms

quently noted. Hemoptysis is seen less frequently. A history of hoarseness, change in voice quality, or painful swallowing should always be sought. When present, they raise the possibility of severe upper-airway injury.

Objective signs of respiratory dysfunction—including tachypnea, labored breathing, stridor, wheezing, and rales—should be documented in all fire victims. If stridor is present on quiet breathing or forced expiration, critical pharyngeal edema may exist. When rales are present, they generally reflect severe lung injury. Similarly, when bronchospasm is noted in a nonasthmatic, significant respiratory exposure is likely. The importance of facial and cutaneous burns as a precursor of lung injury has been discussed (Table 65-4). Severe third-degree burns of the chest

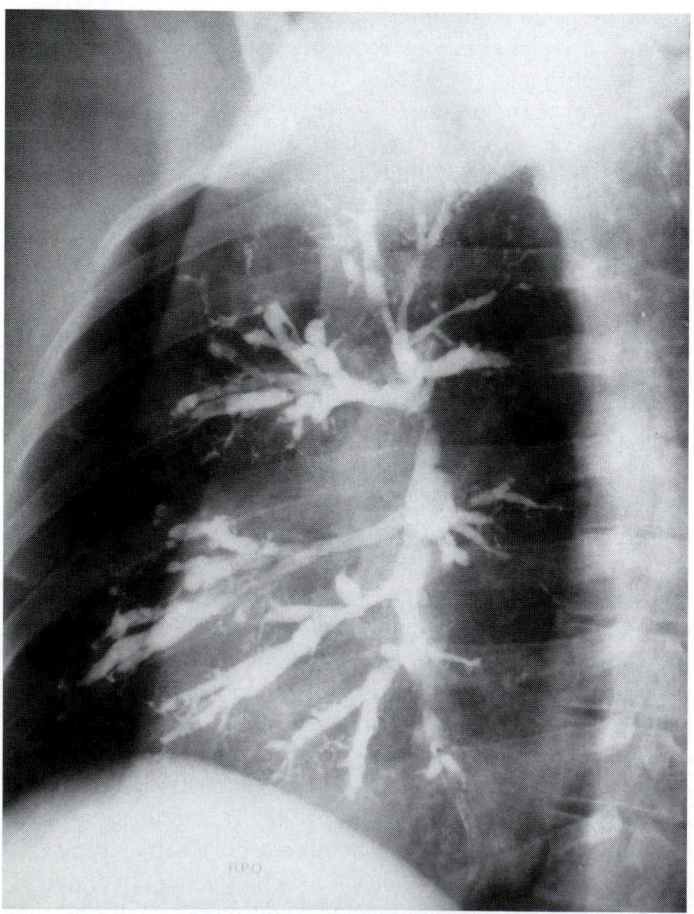

FIGURE 65-3 Diffuse saccular bronchiectasis demonstrated on a bronchogram of the right lung of a firefighter 9 months after smoke inhalation injury. *(Based on data of Putman et al,[39] with permission.)*

wall can also limit respiratory excursions, causing a restrictive ventilatory defect.

Depending on the patient's presentation and available resources, arterial blood gas evaluations, carbon monoxide and cyanide determinations, chest radiographs, and pulmonary function testing (including serial flow-volume loop studies) may be required to provide information about the anatomy and severity of the injury. When clinically appropriate, alcohol levels and drug toxicology screens should be performed. Anatomic evaluations of the upper and lower airways can also provide useful information.

Assessment of Oxygenation/Ventilation

Hypoxemia is a common finding in smoke inhalation and thermal injury victims. It is usually mild when patients have isolated upper airway damage or mild parenchymal abnormalities. Ventilation-profusion mismatching is the major cause of this decrease in oxygenation. Shunt physiology with severe hypoxia can be seen. This pathophysiological profile is noted in patients with severe pulmonary edema (ARDS versus cardiogenic) or significant atelectasis. One of the quickest ways to assess oxygenation is by bedside pulse oximetry. In fire victims, however, these readings may be problematic. Dermal soot and peripheral vasoconstriction may alter the accuracy of these readings. In addition, carbon monoxide poisoning may yield normal calculated levels of oxygen saturation but diminished arterial oxygen content and low levels of actual oxygen saturation as measured by an arterial blood gas CO oximeter.[3] Carbon monoxide poisoning can also be seen in patients with normal arterial P_{O_2} values. Thus, in hospitals where arterial oxygen saturation can be measured, this parameter should be monitored in patients with elevated levels of COHb.

Smoke inhalation and thermal injury are dynamic processes, with patients experiencing acute, delayed onset and late-phase manifestations. A normal early P_{O_2} does not ensure that lung injury has not occurred or that significant hypoxia will not be present at a later phase of the disease. Thus, serial arterial blood gas evaluations or pulse oximetry monitoring of oxygen saturation is often needed.

Most chest radiographs of fire victims are normal on initial presentation. When abnormalities are noted, a spectrum of alterations can be seen, including focal atelectasis, diffuse interstitial changes, and alveolar filling processes such as pulmonary edema.[39] Patients with smoke inhalation and thermal injury may manifest focal and patchy lung infiltrates as late as 24 to 48 h after smoke inhalation,[5] and diffuse alveolar infiltrates may be seen as late as 96 h after presentation. Thus, a normal early chest radiograph does not accurately predict a lack of inhalation injury. In evaluating the chest radiographs of fire victims, the physician must also look for signs of the thoracic trauma that can be experienced by these patients. This includes careful observation for pneumothoraces, hemothoraces, pulmonary contusions, and rib and spinal fractures.

Quantification of Toxic Gases

In all but patients with the most trivial of smoke exposures, COHb levels should be measured, since these levels cannot be inferred reliably from clinical signs or symptoms. In interpreting the data that are obtained, one must note that the COHb levels measured in the hospital are lower than those at the fire scene, since most fire victims are treated with high concentrations of oxygen during their resuscitation and transport to the hospital. In patients with arterial hypoxemia and a severe metabolic acidosis, significant carbon monoxide poisoning should be suspected. Similar findings can occur in cyanide poisoning. Cyanide and thiocyanide levels should be measured when cyanide poisoning is suspected. Interpretation of arterial blood gases can be difficult in patients with an increase in COHb. In these patients, a normal PaO_2 and a normal calculated oxygen saturation may be seen in the presence of a reduced measured arterial oxygen saturation and arterial oxygen content. Thus, serial measurements of actual arterial oxygen saturation are especially useful in monitoring patients with significant carbon monoxide poisoning. The therapeutic approach to elevated COHb levels is discussed below.

Anatomic Evaluation of the Airways

Unrecognized, untreated upper-airway injury can lead to severe and sudden airway obstruction with catastrophic results. Unfortunately, clinical evaluations do not rule out significant upper-airway injury with sufficient accuracy. Thus, the anatomic definition of upper- (and at times lower-) airway injury is frequently required. In patients with very mild smoke exposure and no other significant injury, simple oropharyngeal and nasal inspection may suffice. In all patients in whom serious injury is an issue, more extensive evaluation is required. This is most readily accomplished with laryngoscopy[22] or fiberoptic bronchoscopy.[45] The spectrum of findings ranges from mild erythema to the documentation of soot, carbonaceous materials, secretions, blisters, hemorrhage, ulcers, dynamic airway abnormalities (laryngospasm), and ischemia and edema of the hypopharyngeal, supraglottic, and glottic areas. In rare cases, large bronchial casts composed of sloughed necrotic mucosa, inflammatory exudate, and carbon particles are noted.[45] These casts may need to be removed with a rigid bronchoscope, since dislodgment may result in potentially life-threatening acute airway obstruction.

Physiological Evaluation

The airways are the major site of injury in patients with smoke inhalation and thermal injury. Thus, obstructive ventilatory defects characterized by reduced expiratory volumes and flow rates and a reduced FEV_1/FVC ratio are the major findings in these patients. When pulmonary edema, atelectasis, pneumonia, or other major parenchymal abnormalities occur, or large surface burns are present, restrictive ventilatory defects with decreased lung volumes can be superimposed.

Maximal inspiratory and expiratory flow-volume curves are used to evaluate upper-airway lesions. Studies of these curves have demonstrated a number of characteristic flow-volume loop abnormalities. They include patterns compatible with variable extrathoracic obstruction (a predominant reduction in inspiratory flow rates or a plateau pattern in the inspiratory loop), fixed upper-airway obstruction (reductions in expiratory and inspiratory flow rates), variable intrathoracic obstruction (reduction in ex-

piratory flow rates), and sawtoothing of normally smooth curves, reflecting upper airway instability. Serial flow-volume curves are useful in the detection of delayed-onset upper airway obstruction and late-onset subglottic stenosis in fire victims.

TREATMENT

The treatment of fire injury victims must include management of respiratory dysfunction and associated medical and traumatic problems.[30] This treatment focuses on general supportive measures designed to maximize respiratory function. Prominent in this regard are the maintenance of airway patency, ventilation, and oxygenation. Fluid replacement, nutritional supplementation, and burn wound management are also essential. Specific therapies directed against asphyxiant gas exposures (carbon monoxide/cyanide), bronchospasm, and infection may also be required.

Airway Patency and Ventilation

The maintenance of airway patency and alveolar ventilation is a crucial aspect of the management of smoke and thermal respiratory injury. Fire victims may hypoventilate and may be unable to protect their airway owing to altered neurologic function. Patients may also experience upper airway obstruction, which can present as a medical emergency or arise insidiously over time. Patients with hypoventilation, severe hypoxemia, and carbon dioxide retention should be intubated and ventilated with 100% oxygen. Similarly, patients who cannot protect their airway should be intubated. A low threshold for intubation is also warranted for patients with established or evolving upper-airway obstruction and patients with respiratory failure and coexisting chronic obstructive pulmonary disease (COPD). This is particularly true for patients with respiratory distress, stridor, or significant burns of the face and neck. In evaluating patients at risk for smoke inhalation and thermal injury, it is important to note that patients can present without an obvious upper-airway problem and may develop upper airway obstruction as a delayed, rapid, and at times dramatic response to fluid resuscitation. In patients with upper airway dysfunction that is not immediately life-threatening, the status of the upper airway can be assessed with serial flow volume studies, laryngoscopy, or fiberoptic bronchoscopy. In addition, inhaled racemic epinephrine (1% solution) may be useful in decreasing upper airway edema.

Oxygenation

Oxygenation is always a major concern in treating fire victims. Hypoxia can result from intrinsic pulmonary abnormalities or agents such as carbon monoxide. Patients with hypoxia need to be treated with increasing doses of supplemental O_2 until an adequate level of oxygenation is achieved. When adequate oxygenation cannot be achieved with 100% O_2 delivered by face mask, the patient needs to be intubated and positive end-expiratory pressure (PEEP) may need to be instituted.

CARBON MONOXIDE TOXICITY

Carbon monoxide poisoning must be considered in all patients with smoke inhalation. The prognosis in carbon monoxide poisoning depends on the level of COHb, the rapidity of therapeutic intervention, the nature of the therapeutic intervention (100% O_2 alone versus hyperbaric hyperoxia), and the spectrum of end-organ consequences experienced by the patient. Blood pH has been reported to be prognostic in some series[27] but not in others.[49]

Carbon monoxide poisoning causes a hypoxic insult with varied acute and chronic neurologic and psychological sequelae. The psychological events may occur up to a reported 240 days after carbon monoxide exposure.[54] and emergency hyperbaric oxygen therapy may prevent the development of these delayed neuropsychological manifestations.[51] The half-life of COHb is reduced to approximately 80 min by breathing 100% oxygen; it can be reduced even further with hyperbaric oxygen. At 3 atm, hyperoxia causes a 50% clearance of carbon monoxide from the blood within 25 min,[13] and at 2.5 atm the COHb level is reduced to an acceptable 20% of its greater than 50% pretreatment level in about 50 min.[53]

In severe carbon monoxide poisoning (COHb level at least 40 percent), hyperbaric oxygen therapy is the most efficacious method to reduce the COHb level and thereby prevent neuropsychological sequelae. In a prospective randomized study of 65 patients with mild to moderate carbon monoxide poisoning, 32 were treated with ambient-pressure 100% oxygen and 33 patients were treated with hyperbaric oxygen (2.8 atm for 30 min, followed by 2.0 atm for 90 min). Seven of the 30 patients (23 percent) treated with ambient pressure 100% oxygen developed delayed neuropsychiatric sequelae, whereas no such complications developed in the 30 patients treated with hyperbaric oxygen.[51] Thus, when possible, all fire victims with significant exposure should be resuscitated with and transported on 100% oxygen. In hospitals, which hyperbaric oxygen therapy is available, it is the treatment of choice for severe carbon monoxide poisoning. The alternative treatment is the continued administration of 100% oxygen. This may require elective intubation, mechanical ventilation, and the addition of 5 cm of PEEP. These interventions should be undertaken in patients with elevated COHb levels and evidence of end-organ toxicity or in patients with COHb levels greater than 40% even without obvious symptoms. In comatose patients with severe arterial hypoxemia and metabolic acidosis, emergency endotracheal intubation and mechanical ventilation with 100% oxygen (and 5 cm H_2O PEEP) should be initiated before the results of the COHb measurement are available.

CYANIDE TOXICITY

Cyanide toxicity must also be considered in all patients with smoke inhalation. It is particularly problematic in patients with carbon monoxide poisoning. In patients with cyanide poisoning, specific antidotes (Lilly Cyanide Antidote Kit) with inhaled amyl nitrite pearls, 10% sodium nitrite, and 25% sodium thiosulfate solutions are given.[21]

Bronchodilators

Bronchospasm is a well-characterized feature of smoke inhalation and thermal airway injury. A variety of bronchodilators—including oral and intravenous theophyline, inhaled β_2-sympathometics, and anticholinergic agents—have been administered to patients with smoke- or thermal injury–induced acute or chronic airway obstruction. In wheezing and burned patients with a history of COPD or asthma, these agents have well-documented efficacy. These therapies may also be useful in patients without preexisting obstructive lung disease.

Antibiotics

Empiric antibiotic therapy is not recommended for patients with thermal inhalation injury and acute smoke inhalation. Clinical evaluations, chest radiographic findings, white blood cell counts, and examinations and cultures of sputum should guide the use of intravenous antibiotics. Fire victims who are smokers with a history of chronic bronchitis may require antibiotic therapy earlier than nonsmokers. Aerosolized gentamicin therapy was formerly used to control infections in burn patients. However, this treatment has been shown not to significantly affect morbidity or mortality.[29] The choice of antibiotics (and/or antifungal agents) should be guided by the results of sputum culture sensitivity evaluations. When there is a significant increase in bronchorrhea with negative bacterial sputum cultures, or there is worsening hypoxemia in patients with diffuse lung infiltrates, quantitative bronchoscopic cultures may be useful in documenting nosocomial infection in the lung.

Corticosteroids

Corticosteroid therapy is not indicated for fire victims with dermal burns and thermal inhalation injury.[11,45] This statement is based on a variety of lines of evidence, including a prospective study comparing dexamethasone to placebo in which corticosteroid therapy did not reduce pulmonary complications or mortality[29] and a double-blind study comparing methylprednisolone (30 mg/kg a day by bolus for 2 days) and placebo in which corticosteroid-treated patients had mortality and infection rates four and three times higher, respectively, than the placebo control group.[38] However, in patients with acute smoke inhalation only, the role of corticosteroids is somewhat less clear. In experimental animals exposed acutely to white pine smoke, both methylprednisolone and dexamethasone (but not hydrocortisone) decreased mortality.[15] In contrast, corticosteroid therapy (equivalent dose of 10 mg of dexamethasone every 6 h for 48 h) did not affect the morbidity or mortality of patients with isolated smoke inhalation injury.[41] Thus, in acute isolated smoke inhalation injuries, corticosteroid therapy is not a standard recommendation. There are, however, centers that advocate short courses (48 to 72 h) of empiric corticosteroid intervention. Physicians using this approach have cited the small possibility that steroid-treated patients may develop asthma, bronchiolitis obliterans, or some other long-term adverse effect less frequently than untreated patients with similar injuries. They also point to experiences with irritant gases, such as nitrogen oxides, in which steroid therapy is associated with improved physiological and radiologic parameters.[22] Additional investigation will be required, however, to determine the role, if any, of empiric corticosteroids in treatment of isolated smoke inhalation injury.

Although there are no clinical trials demonstrating the effectiveness of corticosteroids in the routine treatment of smoke inhalation and thermal injury, there are situations where corticosteroids are important and need to be administered. The most common is the use of corticosteroids as anti-inflammatory agents for patients with underlying asthma or severe bronchospastic responses. Corticosteroids are also used to treat bronchiolitis obliterans, which has been diagnosed as a long-term consequence of smoke inhalation. Lastly, systemic or inhaled steroids may be useful for patients with upper-airway edema who fail extubation.

REFERENCES

1. Alarie YC, Anderson RC: Toxicologic and acute lethal hazard evaluation of thermal decomposition products of synthetic and natural polymers. *Toxicol Appl Pharmacol* 51:341–362, 1979.

2. Anderson EW, Andelman RJ, Strauch JM, et al: Effect of low-level carbon monoxide exposure on onset and duration of angina pectoris: A study in ten patients with ischemic heart disease. *Ann Intern Med* 79:46–50, 1973.

3. Buckley RG, Aks SE, Eshom JL, et al: The pulse oximetry gap in carbon monoxide intoxication. *Ann Emerg Med* 24:252–255, 1994.

4. Cannon JG, Friedberg JS, Gelfand JA: Circulating interleukin-1 beta and tumor necrosis factor–alpha concentrations after burn injury in humans. *Crit Care Med* 20:1414–1419, 1992.

5. Chiles C, Hedlund LW, Putman CE: Diagnostic imaging in inhalation lung injury, in Jacob L (ed), *Lung Biology in Health and Disease: Pathophysiology and Treatment of Inhalation Injuries,* vol 34. New York, Dekker, 1988, pp 187–206.

6. Clark CJ, Campbell D, Reid WH: Blood carboxyhaemoglobin and cyanide levels in fire survivors. *Lancet* 1:1332–1335, 1981.

7. Cobb N, Etzel RA: Unintentional carbon monoxide-related deaths in the United States, 1979 through 1988. *JAMA* 266:659–663, 1991.

8. Committee on Fire Toxicology Fire and Smoke: Understanding the hazards. National Research Council, Board on Environmental Studies and Toxicology. Washington, DC, National Academy Press, 1986.

9. Costa DL, Kutzman RS, Lehmann JR, Drew RT: Altered lung function and structure in the rat after subchronic exposure to acrolein. *Am Rev Respir Dis* 133:286–291, 1986.

10. Crapo RO: Some inhalation injuries. *JAMA* 246:1694–1696, 1981.

11. Demling RH: Burns, in Greenfield LJ (ed), *Surgery-Scientific Principles and Practice,* Philadelphia, JB Lippincott, 1993, pp 368–389.

12. Demling RH, LaLonde C, Liu Y, Zhu D: The lung inflammatory response from thermal injury (relationship between physiological and histological changes). *Surgery* 106:52–59, 1989.

13. Dinman BD: The management of acute carbon monoxide intoxication. *J Occup Med* 16:662–664, 1974.

14. DiVincenti FC, Pruitt BA Jr, Reckler JM: Inhalation injuries. *J Trauma* 11:109–117, 1971.

15. Dressler DP, Skornik WA, Kupersmith S: Corticosteroid treatment of experimental smoke inhalation. *Ann Surg* 183:46–52, 1976.

16. Dyer RF, Esch VH: Polyvinyl chloride toxicity in fires: Hydrogen chloride toxicity in fire fighters. *JAMA* 235:393–397, 1976.

17. Ely EW, Moorhead B, Haponik EF: Warehouse workers' headache: Emergency evaluation and management of 30 patients with carbon monoxide poisoning. *Am J Med* 98:145–154, 1995.

18. Fein A, Grossman RF, Jones JG, et al: Carbon monoxide effect on alveolar epithelial permeability. *Chest* 78:726–731, 1980.

19. Fisher AB, Hyde RW, Baue AE, et al: Effect of carbon monoxide on function and structure of the lung. *J Appl Physiol* 26:4–12, 1969.

20. Graham DL, Lawson D, Theodore J, Robin ED: Acute cyanide poisoning complicated by lactic acidosis and pulmonary edema. *Arch Intern Med* 137:1051–1055, 1977.

21. Hall AH, Rumack BH: Clinical toxicology of cyanide. *Ann Emerg Med* 15:1067–1074, 1986.

22. Haponik EF: Clinical smoke inhalation injury: Pulmonary effects. *Occup Med* 8:431–468, 1993.

23. Hartzell GE, Packham SC, Switzer WG: Toxic products from fires. *Am Indust Assoc J* 44:248–255, 1983.

24. Ischiropoulos H, Mendiguren I, Fisher D, et al: Role of neutrophils and nitric oxide in lung alveolar injury from smoke inhalation. *Am J Respir Crit Care Med* 150:337–341, 1994.

25. Kimmerle MG: Aspects and methodology for the evaluation of toxicological parameters during fire exposure. *JFF/Combust Toxicol* 1:4–51, 1974.

26. Landa J, Avery WG, Sackner MA: Some physiologic observations in smoke inhalation. *Chest* 61:62–64, 1972.

27. Larkin JM, Brahos GJ, Moylan JA: Treatment of carbon monoxide poisoning: Prognostic factors. *J Trauma* 16:111–114, 1976.

28. Levin BC, Paabo M, Fultz ML, Barley CS: Generation of hydrogen cyanide from flexible polyurethane foam decomposed under different combustion conditions. *Fire Mater* 9:125–134, 1985.

29. Levine BA, Petroff PA, Slade CL, Pruitt BA Jr: Prospective trials of dexamethasone and aerosolized gentamicin in the treatment of inhalation injury in the burned patient. *J Trauma* 18:188–193, 1978.

30. Loke JA, Matthay RA: Managing victims of smoke inhalation. *J Respir Dis* 2:87–98, 1981.

31. Loke J, Matthay RA, Walker Smith GJ: The toxic environment and its medical implications with special emphasis on smoke inhalation, in Loke J (ed), *Lung Biology in Health and Disease: Pathophysiology and Treatment of Inhalation Injuries,* vol 34. New York, Dekker, 1988, pp 453–504.

32. Loke J, Paul E, Virgulto JA, Walker Smith GJ: Rabbit lung after acute smoke inhalation. Cellular responses and scanning electron microscopy. *Arch Surg* 119:956–959, 1984.

33. Lowry WT, Juarez L, Petty CS, Roberts B: Studies of toxic gas production during actual structural fires in the Dallas area. *J Forensic Sci* 30:59–72, 1985.

34. Lowry WT, Peterson J, Petty CS, Badgett J: Free radical production from controlled low-energy fires: Toxicity considerations. *J Forensic Sci* 30:73–85, 1985.

35. Mallory TB, Brickley WJ: Pathology: With special reference to the pulmonary lesions. *Ann Surg* 117:865–884, 1943.

36. Mohler SR: Air crash survival: Injuries and evacuation toxic hazards. *Aviat Space Environ Med* 46:86–88, 1975.

37. Moritz AR, Henriques FC Jr, McLean R: The effects of inhaled heat on the air passages and lung. *Am J Pathol* 21:311–331, 1945.

38. Moylan JA: Supportive therapy in burn care: Smoke inhalation—Diagnostic techniques and steroids. *J Trauma* 19(Suppl):917, 1979.

39. Putman CE, Loke J, Matthay RA, Ravin CE: Radiographic manifestations of acute smoke inhalation. *Am J Roentgenol* 129:865–870, 1977.

40. Rinaldo JE: Multiple organ dysfunction syndrome (MODS) in the context of ARDS, in Stein JH (ed), *Internal Medicine,* 4th ed. St. Louis, Mosby–Year Book, 1994, pp 1646–1649.

41. Robinson NB, Hudson LD, Riem M, et al: Steroid therapy following isolated smoke inhalation injury. J Trauma 22:876–879, 1982.

42. Sasaki J, Cottam G, Baxter C: Lipid peroxidation following thermal injury. *J Burn Care Rehabil* 4:251–255, 1983.

43. Sheps DS, Herbst MC, Hinderliter AL, et al: Production of arrhythmias by elevated carboxyhemoglobin in patients with coronary artery disease. *Ann Intern Med* 113:343–351, 1990.

44. Shimazu T, Ikeuchi H, Hubbard GB, et al: Smoke inhalation injury and the effects of carbon monoxide in the sheep model. *J Trauma* 30:170–175, 1990.

45. Shirani KZ, Moylan JA, Pruitt BA Jr: Diagnosis and treatment of inhalation injury in burn patients, in Loke J (ed), *Pathophysiology and Treatment of Inhalation Injuries.* vol 34. New York, Dekker, 1988, pp 239–280.

46. Shirani KZ, Pruitt BA Jr, Mason AD Jr: The influence of inhalation injury and pneumonia on burn mortality. *Ann Surg* 205:82–87, 1987.

47. Sidor R, Peterson NH, Burgess WA: A carbon monoxide–oxygen sampler for evaluation of fire fighter exposures. *Am Ind Hyg Assoc J* 34:264–274, 1973.

48. Strieter RM, Kunkel SL, Bone RC: Role of tumor necrosis factor–α in disease states and inflammation. *Crit Care Med* 21(suppl):S447–S463, 1993.

49. Strohl KP, Feldman NT, Saunders NA, O'Connor N: Carbon monoxide poisoning in fire victims: A reappraisal of prognosis. *J Trauma* 20:78–80, 1980.

50. Symington IS, Anderson RA, Thomson I, et al: Cyanide exposure in fires. *Lancet* 11:91–92, 1978.

51. Thom SR, Taber RL, Mendiguren II, et al: Delayed neuropsychologic sequelae after carbon monoxide poisoning: Prevention by treatment with hyperbaric oxygen. *Ann Emerg Med* 25:474–480, 1995.

52. Thompson PB, Herndon DN, Traber DL, Abston S: Effect on mortality of inhalation injury. *J Trauma* 26:163–165, 1986.

53. Winter PM, Miller JN: Carbon monoxide poisoning. *JAMA* 236:1502–1504, 1976.

54. Yang ZD: Observation of hyperbaric oxygen in 160 patients with later manifestations after acute carbon monoxide poisoning. *J Hyperbar Med* 1:188, 1986.

55. Zikria BA, Ferrer JM, Floch HF: The chemical factors contributing to pulmonary damage in "smoke poisoning." *Surgery* 71:704–709, 1972.

PART SIX

DRUG-INDUCED
LUNG DISEASES

CHAPTER 66

PULMONARY TOXICITY ASSOCIATED WITH CHEMOTHERAPEUTIC AGENTS

Lynn T. Tanoue

Toxicities related to medications make up a major category of iatrogenic illness. More than a hundred medications, including many chemotherapeutic agents, are known to have the potential for pulmonary toxicity. As the horizons for treating malignancies broaden, the problem of treatment-induced illness also increases. Drug-induced lung disease is therefore an area of growing concern. Chemotherapeutic agents, therapeutic radiation, and biologic response modifiers are used in a wide range of regimens, further complicated by the use of hematopoietic support and bone marrow or stem cell transplantation. All can be directly or indirectly associated with pulmonary toxicity. An estimated 5 to 10 percent of patients undergoing chemotherapy ultimately develop therapy-related pulmonary disease.[34]

APPROACH TO THE PATIENT WITH SUSPECTED CHEMOTHERAPY-INDUCED PULMONARY TOXICITY

The diagnosis of drug-induced pulmonary toxicity is one of exclusion. Patients most often present with nonspecific constitutional or respiratory complaints. In many cases, symptoms and physical signs may be minimal or absent. In these situations, the only evidence of an ongoing pulmonary process may be an abnormal chest radiograph. In this setting, however, abnormalities on the chest radiograph can be caused by a variety of other processes (Table 66-1).

The diagnosis of lung disease caused by chemotherapeutic agents poses a particular challenge to the clinician, as several additional complicating features are inherent in the oncologic patient population. First, treatment may be given in multidrug regimens or in combination with other modalities, such as radiation therapy or bone marrow transplantation. Therefore, assigning pulmonary toxicity to a single drug within such a regimen is often impossible. Moreover, the combined toxicity of two or more drugs or a single drug with radiation therapy may exceed the individual toxicities of those drugs. Second, patients undergoing chemotherapy are often immunosuppressed, either from the malignancy itself or from myelosuppressive or immunosuppressive effects of therapy. These patients are therefore susceptible to opportunistic infections, which may be mimicked by drug toxicity. It should be remembered that the lung is the most common site of serious infection in patients with cancer. A relative minority (5 to 30 percent) of pulmonary complications in the immunocompromised host are actually due to drug toxicity.[34] Third, cancers themselves may mimic lung disease. This is particularly true when there is lymphangitic tumor spread or metastasis to the parenchyma or pleura. Fourth, pulmonary toxicity due to a single chemotherapeutic agent may present with several different syndromes that vary clinically, radio-

TABLE 66-1

Differential Diagnosis of Radiographic Abnormalities in Cancer Patients

Infection
Primary malignancy
Lymphangitic tumor, metastatic disease, leukemic infiltration
Drug toxicity
Radiation injury
Pulmonary edema
ARDS
Pulmonary hemorrhage
Pulmonary emboli
Leukoagglutinin reaction
Pulmonary fibrosis

graphically, and temporally. While a severe pulmonary reaction acutely following drug administration will usually raise suspicion of drug toxicity, it is becoming increasingly clear that toxicity due to some chemotherapeutic agents may appear months to years after the treatment. In such situations, clinical suspicion of drug toxicity may be low. Last, toxicity from some drugs appears to be related to cumulative dosage levels. However, adverse reactions may occur even with a low cumulative dose, when clinical suspicion for toxicity is low.

Monitoring for pulmonary toxicity in the patient undergoing chemotherapy requires ongoing clinical vigilance. Symptoms such as cough, dyspnea, or chest discomfort may be mild or absent. Radiographic findings may be equally subtle. Even if clinical symptoms and radiographic abnormalities are present and severe, they are usually nonspecific. The possibility of adverse drug effects must be considered within the complex medical context inherent to the patient with cancer undergoing therapy that may be physically taxing and immunosuppressive.

Pulmonary Physiological Testing

Pulmonary physiological testing has received significant attention as a potential screening tool for drug-induced pulmonary disease. A multitude of investigations have studied the utility of pulmonary function tests (PFT) in monitoring chemotherapy. The most common physiological abnormalities are decreases in lung volumes and diffusing capacity for carbon monoxide (DL_{CO}). The extent to which these findings apply to clinical management has been the subject of much debate. Most of the clinical investigations using PFT as a screening and monitoring tool have been done in patients undergoing therapy with bleomycin or busulfan, with the results extrapolated to many other chemotherapeutic agents. Whether this practice is valid has yet to be determined. Even with a drug such as bleomycin, which has been extensively studied, pulmonary physiological testing may yield confusing results. In one series of patients, successive doses of bleomycin led to progressive decreases in DL_{CO}.[48] The decrements did not, however, correlate with the cumulative dose of bleomycin. In addition, clinical and radiographic abnormalities were not seen, suggesting that subclinical lung damage had occurred. Conversely, in some well-documented cases of bleomycin toxicity,

there have been no abnormalities in pulmonary function. Moreover, in bleomycin toxicity associated with abnormalities in PFT, clinical recovery has not necessarily been paralleled by improvement in the physiological parameters.

A number of other factors complicate the practice and interpretation of PFT in oncologic patients. Many physiological parameters are effort dependent. The ability of a patient to perform test maneuvers in a consistent way may be compromised by weakness, pain, or the use of analgesic or sedating medication. Therefore, it may be difficult to obtain reproducible results in patients whose functional status and strength may be impaired by their malignancy or its treatment. In many patients, anemia is induced by the malignancy, medication, or chronic illness. Since DL_{CO} is affected by hemoglobin concentration, it is critical that appropriate corrections be made. Patients with cancers may also be subject to processes other than drug toxicity that will affect pulmonary function tests. A wide variety of other clinical conditions—such as primary pulmonary malignancy, metastatic lung disease, infection, and thoracic or abdominal surgical procedures—can cause variation in physiological measurements. Therefore, identification of pulmonary physiological abnormalities specific to drug effects may be extremely difficult.

Despite the uncertainties in interpretation of PFT, it seems likely that most clinicians will continue to rely on such testing as a screening and monitoring tool in the hope of identifying toxicity early enough to prevent serious pulmonary disease. Unfortunately, the predictive value of baseline or serial PFT remains unclear. Moreover, there are no definitive data to indicate that toxicity can be avoided on the basis of serial monitoring. Although the detection of subclinical abnormalities does not mean that patients will develop irreversible lung disease, such abnormalities often lead to the withdrawal of a drug. Conversely, normal PFT results do not ensure that pulmonary toxicity will not occur. As always, the clinical application of pulmonary physiological findings must be made in the context of the patient's entire clinical situation.

Diagnostic Evaluation

Given the potential impact of pulmonary drug toxicity on treatment, it is important to establish this diagnosis as firmly as possible. The thoughtful and judicious use of invasive procedures plays an important role in that evaluation.

In the cancer patient in whom drug toxicity is suspected, the diagnostic approach is the same as that used for any immunocompromised patient with diffuse or localized lung disease. Because clinical features are usually not specific, sampling of respiratory tract secretions and/or lung tissue may be critical in this evaluation. Direct examination or culture of sputum may yield malignant cells or specific pathogens or may be diagnostic of infections—with *Pneumocystis carinii* or tuberculosis, for example.

In the absence of diagnostic findings in sputum, invasive procedures may be necessary. For a focal lesion, fine-needle aspiration of the lung may be useful. In contrast, the value of this procedure in diffuse lung disease is relatively low. Fiberoptic bronchoscopy, with bronchoalveolar lavage and transbronchial biopsy, has become central in the evaluation of both diffuse and localized lung disease in the immunocompromised host. The frequency of major complications associated with this procedure is low (under 1 percent), whereas the diagnostic yield ranges from 37 to 72 percent.[42,45] This broad variation in yield probably reflects the wide range of disease processes that can affect the lung in the immunocompromised patient. The highest diagnostic yields are obtained in patients with infections; lower yields are seen in interstitial inflammatory processes, which may include toxicity from drugs. Even in situations where a specific cause is not identified, however, exclusion of infection by bronchoscopy often provides clinically useful information. Open or thoracoscopic lung biopsy is associated with the highest diagnostic yield and can be performed with low complication rates, even in critically ill patients. If drug-induced pulmonary injury is suspected, surgical biopsy may be necessary to definitively exclude other causes of lung disease.

As part of thorough evaluation and management of patients receiving chemotherapeutic regimens, awareness of potential iatrogenic complications related to drug therapy is essential. The major pulmonary toxicities associated with chemotherapeutic agents are reviewed below.

CYTOTOXIC ANTIBIOTICS

Bleomycin

Bleomycin is a cytotoxic antibiotic (Table 66-2) used in the treatment of various malignancies, including lymphomas, germ cell tumors, and cancers of the head and neck. The drug is concen-

TABLE 66-2

Cytotoxic Antibiotics

Drug	Pulmonary Syndrome	Treatment	Comments
Bleomycin	1. Chronic pneumonitis/ pulmonary fibrosis	Corticosteroids Discontinue drug	Most common syndrome of bleomycin toxicity "Radiation recall" effect Risk factors: Cumulative dose > 400u Oxygen therapy Therapeutic radiation Renal insufficiency Older age ? Concurrent use of other cytotoxic drugs
	2. Hypersensitivity-type lung disease	Corticosteroids Discontinue drug	Dyspnea, cough, skin rash, eosinophilia May not recur with rechallenge
	3. Chest pain syndrome	Discontinue drug	Associated with IV infusion of drug
Mitomycin-C	1. Chronic pneumonitis/ pulmonary fibrosis	Corticosteroids Discontinue drug	Most common syndrome of mitomycin-induced lung toxicity Risk Factors: Oxygen therapy Therapeutic radiation Concurrent use of other cytotoxic drugs
	2. Acute dyspnea/bronchospasm Noncardiogenic pulmonary edema	Supportive care Discontinue drug Corticosteroids	Occurs in patients also receiving vinca alkaloids Risk Factors: Concurrent use of vinca alkaloids
	3. Hemolytic-uremic syndrome	Supportive care Discontinue drug	Microangiopathic hemolytic anemia, thrombocytopenia, renal insufficiency, noncardiogenic pulmonary edema
Actinomycin-D	Exacerbation of radiation-induced injury	Discontinue drug	Radiosensitizing effect may be long-standing Risk factors: Therapeutic radiation

trated in skin and lung, with its major toxicities manifested in these organs. Limitation in its use usually hinges on its potential for pulmonary toxicity. The overall incidence of bleomycin-induced lung injury varies from 3 to 40 percent.[51] One to 2 percent of patients who receive this drug will succumb to pulmonary toxicity.[22,34]

PATHOGENESIS

Unlike those for most chemotherapeutic agents, the pulmonary toxicities and mechanisms of injury, inflammation, and scarring associated with bleomycin have been studied extensively in animal models. Although not necessarily applicable to all drug-induced disorders, bleomycin serves as a model for the mechanisms by which chemotherapeutic agents can injure the lung. The initiation of lung injury by bleomycin appears to be oxidant mediated. Bleomycin is known to generate reactive oxygen metabolites, including superoxide and hydroxyl radicals. These

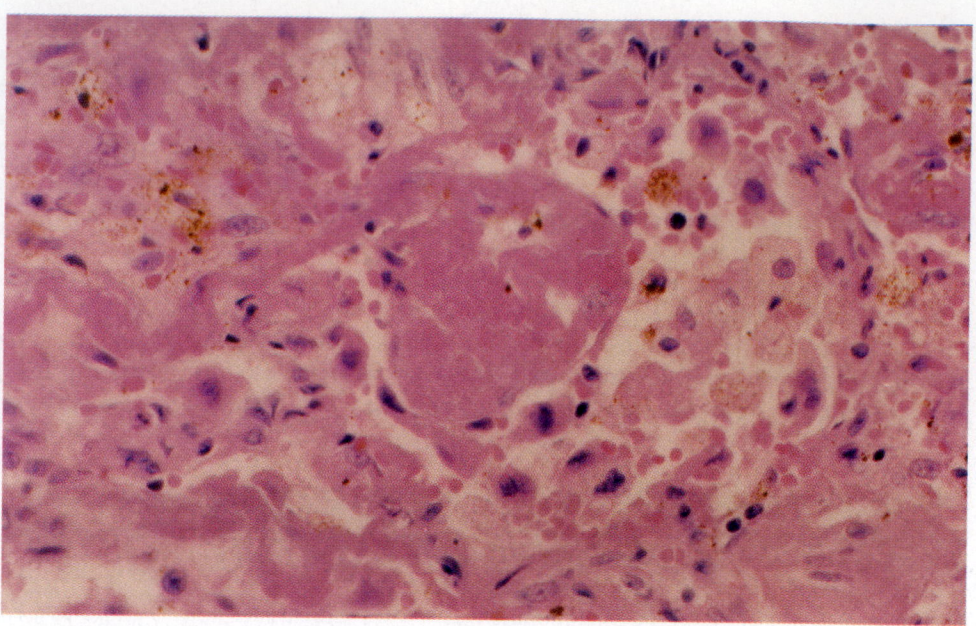

FIGURE 66-1   Lung biopsy specimen from a patient with clinical and radiographic evidence of bleomycin-induced pulmonary toxicity shows drug effect with acute and chronic changes. The alveolus contains an exudate of fibrin, which is undergoing organization and is surrounded by alveolar macrophages. The large and atypical cells are markedly reactive alveolar type II pneumocytes. The alveolar wall itself is scarred with collagen deposition by the spindle-shaped fibroblasts. *(Courtesy of Dr. Darryl Carter, Professor of Pathology, Yale University School of Medicine.)*

reactive species have a number of effects, including DNA injury, lipid peroxidation, alterations in lung prostaglandin synthesis and degradation, and increase in lung collagen synthesis. The major sites of injury appear to be the type I alveolar epithelial cell and the pulmonary capillary endothelial cell. Type I pneumocyte destruction in the alveolar epithelium is generally followed by type II pneumocyte hyperplasia and dysplasia. This repair process appears to be more delayed in cytotoxic drug–induced lung injury than in injury produced by inhalational toxins, such as air pollutants.[9] Subsequent infiltration, initially by granulocytes and later by lymphocytes, eosinophils, and plasma cells, results in inflammation and cytokine release.

A variety of cytokines have been implicated in the pathogenesis of bleomycin-induced injury and scarring, including transforming growth factor–β (TGF-β), tumor necrosis factor (TNF), interleukin-1 (IL-1), IL-5, IL-6, platelet-derived growth factor, and a variety of chemokine cytokines.[40] TGF-β, IL-1, and TNF are prominent examples of cytokines that play roles in this type of injury. In bleomycin-treated mice, TGF-β mRNA accumulates in alveolar macrophages, and the administration of anti-TGF-β antibodies minimizes the drug-induced pulmonary response.[16,20,23] Similarly, increased amounts of IL-1 and TNF are produced in bleomycin-sensitive animals, and treatment with the IL-1 receptor antagonist, anti-TNF antibodies, or soluble TNF receptors diminishes bleomycin-induced pulmonary fibrosis.[30–32,40]

As a result of the injury, inflammation, and cytokine dysregulation that occur after bleomycin administration, fibroblasts are activated, fibroblast and myofibroblast proliferation is augmented, and collagen production is stimulated while collagen degradation is inhibited and fibrosis occurs.[24] The resulting picture, interstitial inflammation and fibrosis (Fig. 66-1), is a hallmark of cytotoxic drug–induced pulmonary injury.

CLINICAL MANIFESTATIONS

The clinical presentation of bleomycin toxicity is usually subacute and insidious, occurring within a few weeks to 6 months after treatment. A more fulminant presentation with acute respiratory failure does occur but is less common. Patients generally present with dyspnea, nonproductive cough, and low-grade fever. Substernal or pleuritic chest pain occurs but is infrequent. Up to 20 percent of patients are asymptomatic. Chest radiographs usually show bilateral reticular or fine nodular infiltrates with a basilar predominance, often beginning at the costophrenic angles (Fig. 66-2). Decrease in lung volume accompanied by elevation of the diaphragm is also commonly seen. However, various radiographic patterns—including alveolar infiltrates, lobar consolidation, asymmetric lung involvement, and even lung nodules—have been described. Computed tomographic scanning appears to be more sensitive in the evaluation of radiographic abnormalities and may be useful in patients who have spirometric or clinical evidence of toxicity but negative chest radiographs (Fig. 66-3).

Several risk factors have been identified for the development of bleomycin-induced pulmonary toxicity. These include the following: 1. *Total dose.* Toxicity appears to correlate with higher cumulative dosages, the risk escalating significantly when total doses exceed 400 units. However, pulmonary injury has been observed after administration of as little as 20 units.[3] 2. *Oxygen.* Oxygen is clearly a synergistic toxin in patients with prior bleomycin therapy. Hypoxia appears to be protective in animal models.[5] 3. *Radiation.* Thoracic irradiation before, during, or after bleomycin administration has been associated with an increase in toxicity.[10] This injury may extend beyond the original port of irradiation. This "radiation recall" effect may last for years

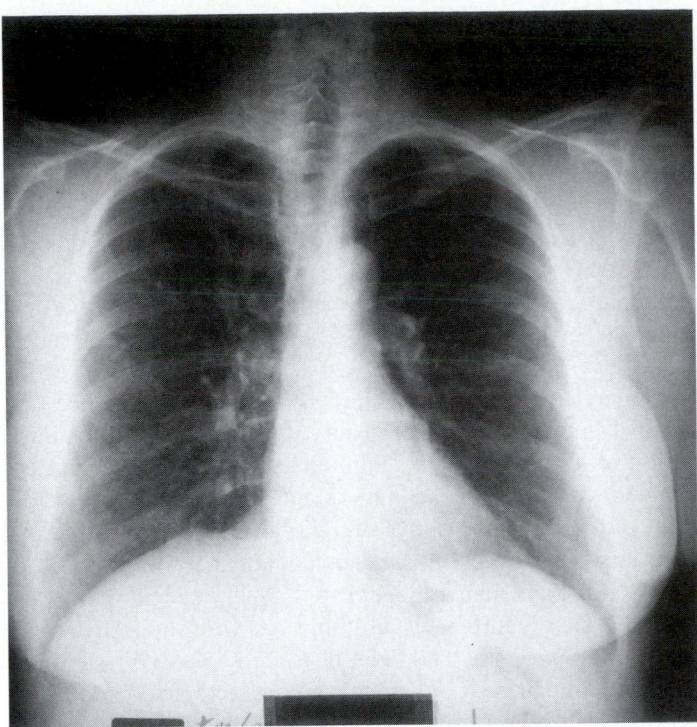

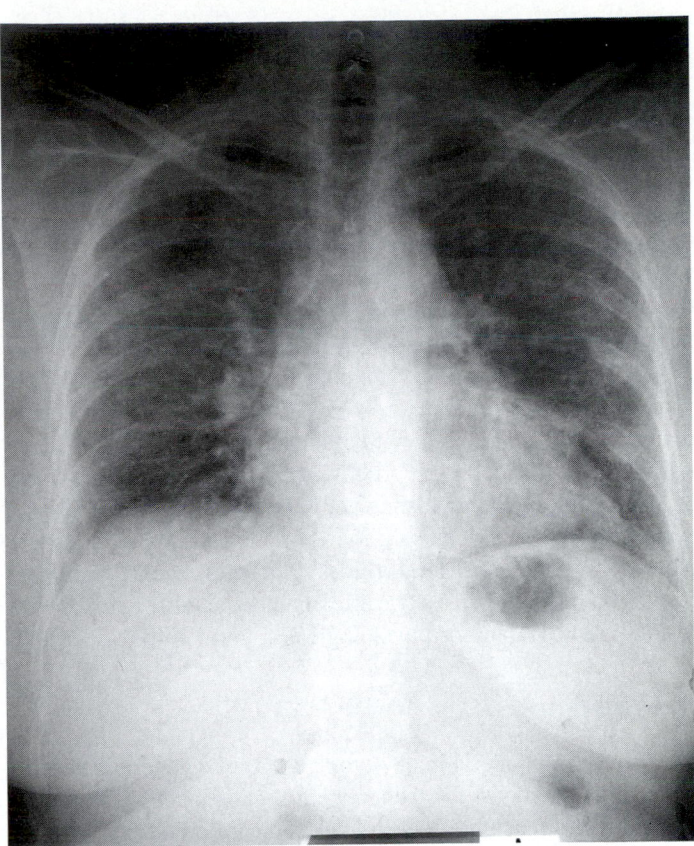

A

B

FIGURE 66-2   PA chest radiographs of a 56-year-old woman with cervical carcinoma before *(A)* and after *(B)* chemotherapy with a bleomycin-containing regimen. Note the decrease in lung volume and diffusely increased interstitial lung markings in the postchemotherapy radiograph.

after bleomycin therapy. 4. *Renal function*. Abnormal renal function is a risk factor for pulmonary toxicity. Bleomycin is excreted by the kidneys. Drug half-life increases when creatinine clearance decreases below 35 ml per minute. 5. *Age*. Older persons, especially those over 70, appear to be more susceptible to toxicity. 6. *Concurrent use of other cytotoxic agents*. The possibility has been raised that concurrent use of other chemotherapeutic agents can confer synergistic toxicity. Drugs implicated have included doxorubicin, cyclophosphamide, vincristine, and methotrexate. However, this synergistic effect has not been consistently reproducible. It is therefore unclear whether concurrent use of other drugs represents a true increase in risk.[22,24]

Bleomycin has also caused an acute syndrome of dyspnea, cough, and rash immediately after administration of the drug.[50] Lung biopsy in these cases has shown eosinophilic infiltration and changes consistent with a hypersensitivity response. Rechallenge with drug

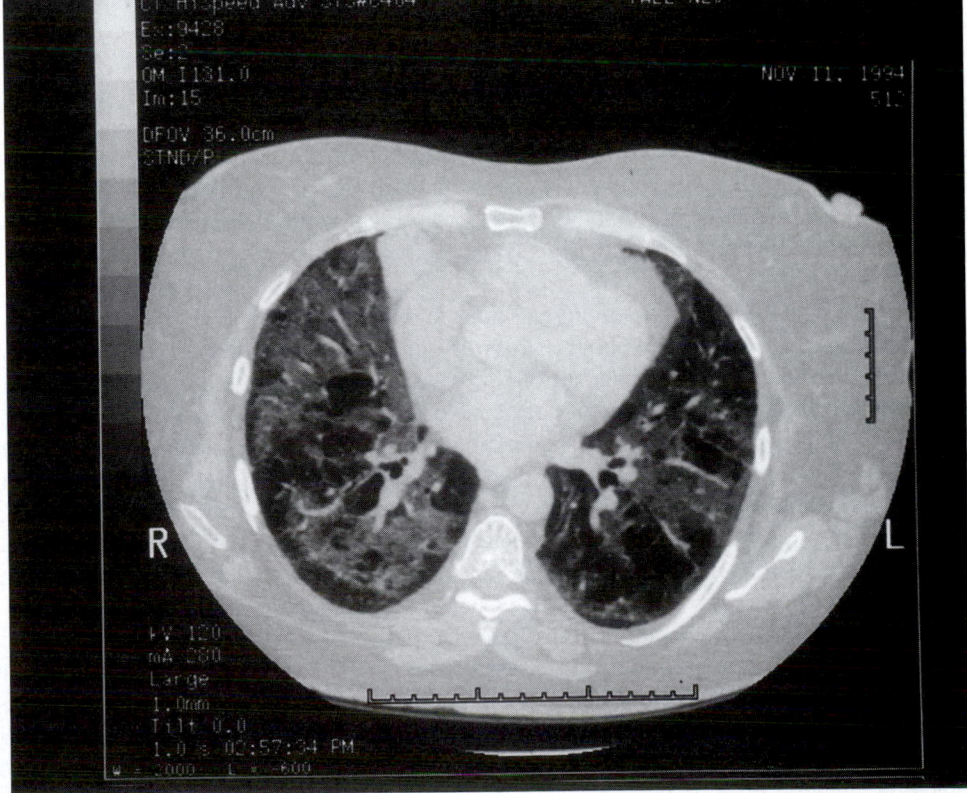

FIGURE 66-3   Chest CT scan of same patient as in Fig. 66-2, taken at the time of radiograph in Fig. 66-2*B*. Note the patchy distribution of bilateral infiltrates, whose extent is clearly delineated by CT.

has not consistently caused recurrence of the syndrome, suggesting that this syndrome is not a true immune reaction.

Bleomycin toxicity may also present with acute chest pain. In one series of 286 patients, the incidence of severe chest pain was 2.8 percent.[47] Chest pain in these patients was concurrent with bleomycin infusion and resolved after the drug was stopped. Clinical and radiographic evidence of pleuropericarditis are common.

The overall mortality due to drug toxicity in patients receiving bleomycin is 1 to 2 percent.[22,51] In patients who develop pulmonary toxicity, mortality varies from 10 to 83 percent.[22,51] In patients with mild toxicity, stopping the drug may suffice to reverse the abnormalities. However, corticosteroids are generally recommended for patients with clinically significant bleomycin-induced toxicity. Doses of corticosteroids are usually in the range of 60 to 100 mg of prednisone per day; tapering is done slowly, according to the clinical stability of the patient. When improvement does occur, it generally does so within weeks. Complete resolution may take up to 2 years. Some patients will be left with residual radiographic or physiological abnormalities.

Mitomycin

Mitomycin is an alkylating cytotoxic antibiotic generally used in multidrug regimens for solid organ malignancies, including breast, gastrointestinal, gynecologic, and lung cancers. The incidence of pulmonary toxicity due to mitomycin is variably reported as between 3 and 39 percent.[12,34] This variation may be due in part to two factors. First, the drug is rarely given alone, and toxicity seems dependent to some extent on concurrent administration of other agents or therapies. Although agreement about synergistic toxicity is not universal, pulmonary toxicity may be potentiated when mitomycin is used in conjunction with bleomycin, vinca alkaloids, cisplatin, 5-fluorouracil, cyclophosphamide, and doxorubicin.[10,13,51] Therapeutic thoracic irradiation and oxygen may also be cotoxins.[10,13] Second, mitomycin-induced lung injury presents with at least three clinically distinct syndromes: an interstitial pneumonitis with fibrosis, an acute lung syndrome with bronchospasm, and a hemolytic-uremic syndrome.

The most common form of mitomycin-induced lung toxicity is a chronic pneumonitis with pulmonary fibrosis similar to that seen with bleomycin. The mechanism of this syndrome is unknown, although several have been proposed, including lipid peroxidation, a hypersensitivity reaction, and immune complex generation.[24,29] Toxicity is believed to be potentiated by oxygen supplementation and therapeutic radiation. Toxicity does not appear to be dose related. Although it has been suggested that patients receiving doses greater than 30 mg/m² are at increased risk of pulmonary injury, this dose dependency has not been substantiated.[27] Pulmonary toxicity usually occurs after 2 to 12 months of therapy but may occur after a single dose.[24,51] Clinically, patients present with a subacute syndrome of cough and progressive dyspnea, often with fatigue and sometimes with pleuritic chest pain. Fever is less common. Chest radiographs usually show bilateral interstitial infiltrates, occasionally with alveolar or fine nodular patterns. Histologically, biopsy specimens show mononuclear cell infiltration, alveolar lining cell hyper-

trophy, collagen deposition, and alveolar septal thickening. Type II pneumocyte enlargement and lymphocytic or eosinophilic infiltration have also been seen. Patients develop a clinical picture of interstitial pneumonitis and fibrosis. This syndrome generally responds to discontinuation of drug and institution of corticosteroids.[8]

The second syndrome of mitomycin-induced pulmonary toxicity is seen in patients who have also received vinca alkaloids. While drugs of the latter category confer little risk of pulmonary toxicity when used as single agents, vinblastine and vindesine given along with or after administration of mitomycin have been reported to precipitate a syndrome of acute pulmonary toxicity.[19,25,33] Clinically, patients experience onset of dyspnea or bronchospasm within hours after administration of a vinca alkaloid. Pulmonary symptoms may be associated with hypoxia and bilateral interstitial infiltrates on the chest radiograph. In a series of 126 patients, 6 percent developed this syndrome.[25] A smaller number may develop respiratory failure and noncardiogenic pulmonary edema. While the acute dyspnea syndrome usually subsides with supportive care, withdrawal of drug, and administration of corticosteroids, long-term impairment of clinical and physiological parameters may persist. Rechallenge with a vinca alkaloid causes recurrence of symptoms in most patients.

The third syndrome associated with mitomycin toxicity is a hemolytic uremic syndrome, which consists of microangiopathic-hemolytic anemia, thrombocytopenia, and renal failure. Approximately half of these patients develop noncardiogenic pulmonary edema. Pulmonary alveolar hemorrhage is another manifestation of mitomycin toxicity. The mechanism of toxicity appears related to pulmonary vascular endothelial injury. The prognosis for patients with this syndrome is poor. In a series of 39 patients, overall mortality was 72 percent.[39] In patients who also developed pulmonary edema, mortality increased to 95 percent. A variety of therapies have been tried in attempts to reverse this toxicity, including the administration of corticosteroids, plasmapheresis, heparin, and cytotoxic agents. None have had clear benefit.

Dactinomycin

Dactinomycin is an antitumor antibiotic used in the treatment of sarcomas, Wilson's tumor, and gestational choriocarcinoma. It can occasionally be associated with pulmonary toxicity, usually presenting as an interstitial pneumonitis with pulmonary fibrosis. Like bleomycin and mitomycin, dactinomycin may exacerbate radiation-induced injury. This radiosensitizing effect may be long-standing.

ALKYLATING AGENTS

Administered as single agents, the alkylating agents cyclophosphamide, busulfan, chlorambucil, melphalan, and ifosfamide (Table 66-3) are associated with less pulmonary toxicity than any other class of chemotherapeutic agents. As with bleomycin, synergistic pulmonary toxicity may occur in the setting of radiation therapy, oxygen supplementation, or combination treatment with other cytotoxic agents.

TABLE 66-3

Alkylating Agents

Drug	Pulmonary Syndrome	Treatment	Comments
Busulfan	Chronic pneumonitis/ pulmonary fibrosis	Discontinue drug Corticosteroids	Toxicity may occur several years after treatment Fibrosis may occur without symptoms
Cyclophosphamide	Chronic pneumonitis/ pulmonary fibrosis	Discontinue drug Corticosteroids	Toxicity may occur several years after treatment Toxicity may increase with very high doses of drug Risk factors: Concurrent use of other cytotoxic drugs Therapeutic radiation
Chlorambucil Melphalan Ifosfamide	Chronic pneumonitis/ pulmonary fibrosis	Discontinue drug	Clinical pulmonary toxicity uncommon

Busulfan

Busulfan is used in the treatment of chronic myeloproliferative disorders. Because of the nature of these hematologic malignancies, patients may require therapy for months to years. Cumulative dosage is therefore of concern, although a threshold dose for toxicity has not been evident. Busulfan is usually well tolerated. Histologically, up to 46 percent of patients treated with busulfan may have evidence of pulmonary fibrosis; most of them have no clinical symptoms.[10,18]

Symptoms of busulfan lung injury usually present insidiously, often weeks to even years after initiation of therapy. Symptoms include cough, fever, fatigue, weight loss, and progressive dyspnea. Chest radiographs usually show bilateral interstitial infiltrates with basilar predominance. Pathologic findings are consistent with other cytotoxic drug–induced pulmonary injury syndromes, with an interstitial pneumonitis, type II pneumocyte hyperplasia, dysplasia, and desquamation into alveolar spaces. Fibroblast proliferation, collagen deposition, and fibrosis are usually evident. Scattered cases of pulmonary ossification and pulmonary alveolar proteinosis have also been reported.

When clinically evident busulfan-induced pulmonary toxicity does occur, prognosis for recovery is poor. The overall mortality is estimated at 50 to 80 percent.[10,34] Corticosteroids have anecdotally been reported to be of benefit, but, as with most chemotherapeutic agents, no prospective studies are available.

Cyclophosphamide

Cyclophosphamide is widely used in the treatment of a variety of malignancies, including lymphomas and breast and ovarian cancers. It is also used in the treatment of nonneoplastic inflammatory disorders such as Wegener's granulomatosis. Although the incidence of pulmonary toxicity is reported to be less than 1 percent, the broad indications for its use make it likely that cyclophosphamide-induced lung injury will be encountered by the practicing pulmonologist.

Cyclophosphamide is metabolized to two active compounds, phosphoramide mustard and acrolein. Both of these metabolites have been shown in animal studies to deplete hepatic glutathione stores. This depletion may render cells more susceptible to oxidant injury. Intratracheal or intraperitoneal administration of cyclophosphamide in animals causes lung injury manifested by type II cell abnormalities, inflammatory pneumonitis, and progressive interstitial fibrosis. However, the exact mechanism of cyclophosphamide-induced pulmonary toxicity is unknown.

Clinically, the onset of cyclophosphamide-induced pulmonary toxicity is usually insidious, with symptoms of cough and progressive dyspnea, often accompanied by fever. The timing of the onset of pulmonary toxicity is exceedingly variable, occurring 2 weeks to 13 years after initiation of treatment.[24] However, most patients develop symptoms soon after exposure to the drug. No definite dose-response relationship has been established for cyclophosphamide. Chest radiographs usually show an interstitial pattern with basilar predominance. In patients who present with very late onset of lung fibrosis, the upper zones may be predominantly affected.[51] Histologic findings are similar to those seen with toxicity from other cytotoxic drugs.

Cyclophosphamide-induced lung injury carries significant morbidity. When cyclophosphamide is used to treat nonneoplastic lung disease, the underlying pulmonary process may be compounded by superimposed drug toxicity. The distinction between the two processes may be difficult to delineate. When cyclophosphamide is used as a chemotherapeutic agent, its identification as the specific cause of lung injury may be difficult, since it is seldom used alone. As with all multidrug or multimodality regimens, pinpointing specific toxicity to a single agent may be impossible. Moreover, it is recognized that cyclophosphamide appears to have synergistic toxicity with therapeutic thoracic radiation as well as with other chemotherapeutic agents.[27,43] Prognosis of the patient with symptomatic drug toxicity ascribed to cyclophosphamide is poor; mortality is approximately 50 percent.[51] Most authors recommend treatment with corticosteroids even though there is no definitive evidence that cyclophosphamide toxicity is reversed by this intervention.

Although cyclophosphamide administered at conventional dosage poses relatively low risk for pulmonary injury, treatment with high doses may cause significant toxicity. In one study of patients with small-cell lung cancer, treatment with radiation therapy and very high doses of cyclophosphamide was complicated by a 74 percent incidence of pulmonary fibrosis.[43] A similar situation has been described with the use of high-dose carmustine in conditioning regimens for bone marrow transplantation. By extrapolation, patients undergoing new dose-intensive regimens using drugs generally thought to be "safe" at conventional doses from a pulmonary standpoint merit careful follow-up for signs of pulmonary toxicity.

Other Alkylating Agents

Chlorambucil and melphalan are slow-acting nitrogen mustards. Chlorambucil has an important role in the treatment of lymphoreticular malignancies, including chronic lymphocytic leukemia. Like cyclophosphamide, this drug has also been used in the treatment of nonneoplastic diseases, including sarcoidosis. Pulmonary toxicity is fairly uncommon, occurring in less than 5 percent of patients.[34] As with busulfan, treatment may encompass long time spans. Pulmonary toxicity may appear months to years after initiation of therapy and may be related to cumulative dosage. Clinical and histologic manifestations of drug toxicity are similar to those seen with other alkylating agents.

Melphalan has been used in the treatment of multiple myeloma as well as solid tumors, including breast cancer. Mel-

phalan-induced pulmonary toxicity is rare and resembles that caused by other cytotoxic drugs with respect to clinical radiographic and pathologic findings. Of note is that radiographic findings of predominantly upper-lobe infiltrates in mephalan toxicity contrast with the more typical bibasilar pattern seen with most of the other cytotoxic drug–induced pulmonary disorders.

Ifosfamide is structurally related to cyclophosphamide. Limitation of dosage is usually related to bladder toxicity. Clinically evident pulmonary toxicity induced by iphosfamide appears to be rare, but interstitial pneumonitis has been reported.

ANTIMETABOLITES

Methotrexate

Methotrexate (Table 66-4) is a folate antagonist used as a chemotherapeutic agent as well as for the treatment of nonneoplastic inflammatory diseases. When the agent is used in high doses for the treatment of cancers, the incidence of pulmonary toxicity is estimated at 7 percent.[10] Toxicity does not appear to have dose dependency but may be related to frequency of administration. In one study, daily or weekly treatment carried more risk of pulmonary injury than did treatment every 2 to 4 weeks.[15] Synergistic toxicity has been reported with combination therapy using cyclophosphamide. Tapering of corticosteroid therapy or adrenalectomy may also increase the risk of methotrexate-induced toxicity.[10,46]

The mechanism of methotrexate-induced lung injury is unknown. Clinically, toxicity presents with several syndromes. The most common of these is characterized by fever, dyspnea, cough,

TABLE 66-4

Antimetabolites

Drug	Pulmonary Syndrome	Treatment	Comments
Methotrexate	1. Chronic pneumonitis/ pulmonary fibrosis	Corticosteroids Discontinue drug	Most common syndrome of methotrexate-induced lung toxicity
	2. Hypersensitivity-type lung disease	Corticosteroids Discontinue drug	May resolve even if drug is continued, but can progress to fibrosis
	3. Acute chest pain syndrome	Discontinue drug	Often accompanied by pleural effusions
	4. Noncardiogenic pulmonary edema	Supportive care Discontinue drug	Associated with intrathecal administration
Cytosine arabinoside	Noncardiogenic pulmonary edema	Supportive care Discontinue drug	Onset of symptoms usually occurs within days of initiation of treatment Risk factors: Toxicity increases with cumulative dose
Fludarabine	1. Hypersensitivity reaction	Discontinue drug	Associated with increased incidence of opportunistic infections
	2. Interstitial pneumonitis	Discontinue drug	Toxicity is uncommon
6-Mercaptopurine	Chronic pneumonitis/ pulmonary fibrosis	Discontinue drug	Toxicity is uncommon

malaise, and myalgias, usually within weeks of the initiation of therapy. Chest radiographs usually show diffuse interstitial infiltrates. Occasionally, chest radiographs may show unilateral or bilateral effusions or a nodular appearance; they may even look normal.[41] Additionally, hilar and mediastinal adenopathy have been observed. Skin rash is present in up to 17 percent of patients, and peripheral blood eosinophilia is noted in up to 40 percent.[41]

Although bronchoalveolar lavage may indicate a lymphocytic alveolitis, suggestive of a hypersensitivity reaction, the illness may resolve even though the drug is continued. Moreover, rechallenge does not necessarily result in relapse. These findings suggest that the disorder is not due to an immune mechanism of injury. This presentation of methotrexate-induced pulmonary toxicity parallels the hypersensitivity-type syndrome that is sometimes observed with bleomycin.[46] Since some patients will go on to develop chronic pneumonitis and pulmonary fibrosis, the drug is generally withdrawn when toxicity occurs.

Pulmonary toxicity from methotrexate may also present as a more insidious subacute syndrome of interstitial lung disease. Symptoms—including cough, fever, dyspnea, headache, and malaise—typically occur within 4 months after the initiation of treatment. Radiographically and clinically, this syndrome more closely resembles the type of chronic pneumonitis seen with other cytotoxic drugs and has been described as complicating all routes of methotrexate administration (oral, intravenous, intrathecal). In contrast to that from many other chemotherapeutic agents, the pneumonitis caused by methotrexate appears in general to be responsive to corticosteroids.

As seen with other cytotoxic drugs, interstitial and alveolar inflammation and fibrosis are the predominant lesions in the lungs of patients with methotrexate pulmonary toxicity. Additionally, eosinophilic infiltration of the interstitium and granuloma formation may occur.[41]

Methotrexate-induced lung injury may also appear as an acute syndrome with pleuritis and pleural effusion. Respiratory distress progressing to noncardiogenic pulmonary edema has been seen after intrathecal administration of drug and may be neurogenic.[17]

The prognosis with methotrexate-associated lung toxicity is generally favorable. As noted above, symptoms and radiographic abnormalities may resolve despite continuation of treatment. The use of corticosteroids is generally recommended, although prospective trials of this treatment are not available. The overall mortality with methotrexate-induced pneumonitis is approximately 10 percent.[41]

Cytosine Arabinoside

Cytosine arabinoside, or cytarabine (ara-C), is a pyrimidine nucleoside analog that rapidly inhibits DNA synthesis. It is important in the treatment of acute leukemias and non-Hodgkin's lymphoma. Pulmonary toxicity parallels intensity of treatment. High-dose regimens have been associated with a 5 to 44 percent incidence of acute or subacute respiratory insufficiency.[1,34,51] Symptoms include fever, cough, dyspnea, and tachypnea and may either coincide with the chemotherapeutic treatment or be delayed for up to several weeks after treatment is initiated. Hy-

poxemia may be present. Chest radiographs generally show a diffuse interstitial or alveolar pattern.

The pathogenesis of pulmonary toxicity due to ara-C is unknown. The syndrome induced by the drug does appear, however, to be a form of noncardiogenic pulmonary edema. Its importance can be appreciated in an autopsy series of 181 patients who died of acute leukemia. In this series were 42 patients who had received ara-C within 30 days of death and who had moderate to severe pulmonary edema with highly proteinaceous infiltrates in both alveoli and interstitium.[21] Twenty-eight of these 42 patients had no other identifiable cause for the pulmonary edema, leading to the belief that ara-C had precipitated their pulmonary disorder.

Treatment for ara-C lung toxicity is standard supportive care for noncardiogenic pulmonary edema. Administration of corticosteroids has been recommended by some authors, but this form of therapy is of uncertain benefit. Clinical and radiographic resolution may take 7 to 21 days. Overall mortality associated with ara-C–induced pulmonary toxicity ranges from 6 to 13 percent.[51]

Fludarabine

Fludarabine phosphate is a purine nucleoside analog used in the treatment of chronic lymphoproliferative disorders. As the drug is generally used after failure of standard alkylating agent therapy, experience with toxicities has been limited and sometimes difficult to evaluate because of prior treatment with other drugs. Both a hypersensitivity-type pulmonary reaction and interstitial pneumonitis have been reported after fludarabine administration.[7,11] It should be noted that therapy with fludarabine has been associated with a high incidence of opportunistic infections, including pneumocystis carinii pneumonia. The drug is immunosuppressive, and its effects may persist for months after initiation of treatment. The risk of opportunistic infection appears to be increased by the use of corticosteroids before, during, or after fludarabine administration.[6]

Azathioprine/Mercaptopurine

Azathioprine is used as an immunosuppressive agent in the treatment of nonneoplastic diseases and in the medical management of organ transplantation. Its metabolic product, mercaptopurine, is used as an antineoplastic agent. These drugs are rarely associated with pulmonary toxicity. Interstitial pneumonitis, eosinophilic pneumonitis, and fibrosis have been reported.[27] In one series of seven renal transplant patients, a more fulminant course of respiratory toxicity associated with diffuse alveolar damage was described.[4]

NITROSOUREAS

The nitrosourea group of agents (Table 66-5) includes carmustine, or BCNU (1,3-bis-[2-chloroethyl]-1-nitrosourea), lomostine, or CCNU (1-[2-chloroethyl]-3-cyclohexyl-1-nitrosourea), semustine, or methyl-CCNU, and chlorozotocin. These cytotoxic drugs are active against a variety of neoplasms. The ability of these drugs to cross the blood-brain barrier makes them particularly useful in the treatment of central nervous system malignancies.

TABLE 66-5

Nitrosoureas

Drug	Pulmonary Syndrome	Treatment	Comments
BCNU	Chronic pneumonitis/ pulmonary fibrosis	Supportive care Discontinue drug	Toxicity may be delayed years after therapy Risk factors: Preexisting pulmonary disease Abnormal baseline pulmonary physiology Cumulative dose > 1500 mg/m^2
CCNU Semustine Chlorozotocin	Chronic pneumonitis/ pulmonary fibrosis	Supportive care Discontinue drug	By extrapolation, toxicities and risk factors probably parallel BCNU

Carmustine

Of the nitrosoureas, carmustine (BCNU) has been most extensively studied. Like bleomycin, this drug has been used in animal models of lung injury. Intraperitoneal injection of BCNU in rats results in granulomatous inflammation and interstitial fibrosis that progress even after the drug is withdrawn. Oxidant lung injury may play a role in the pathogenesis of toxicity, since BCNU is known to inhibit glutathione reductase in pulmonary macrophages and reduces lung glutathione stores. As with bleomycin, the toxicity of BCNU appears to be dose related. At cumulative doses of greater than 1500 mg/m^2, the incidence of BCNU-induced lung toxicity ranges from 39 to 50 percent.[24] Doses of 900 to 1200 mg/m^2 are associated with pulmonary toxicity in approximately 20 percent of patients, but pulmonary toxicity has been seen with doses as low as 240 mg/m^2.[38] It has been suggested that simultaneous treatment with cyclophosphamide or radiation therapy potentiates BCNU toxicity. In general, however, these reports are limited to small series of patients. Synergistic toxicity of BCNU with other chemotherapeutic agents or methods has therefore not been firmly established.

The onset of symptoms related to BCNU pulmonary toxicity is highly variable, occurring from a few days to up to 17 years after the initiation of chemotherapy.[28] A number of factors that increase the risk of BCNU pulmonary toxicity have been delineated, including the total cumulative dose of BCNU, the duration of treatment, and a history of preexisting lung disease.[2] As a result, it is recommended that the cumulative dose of BCNU be limited to 1400 mg/m^2 and that frequent pulmonary physiological testing be done during treatment. It has also been recommended that BCNU be excluded from use in patients with preexisting symptomatic pulmonary disease or with baseline pulmonary physiological abnormalities, particularly an abnormal vital capacity or $D_{L_{CO}}$.

The clinical presentation of BCNU-induced lung toxicity is variable. It may present fulminantly as acute respiratory failure, but more commonly it presents insidiously with asymptomatic physiological abnormalities or radiographic evidence of pulmonary fibrosis. Symptoms of the latter, subacute course include cough, fatigue, and progressive dyspnea. The chest radiograph is rarely normal in symptomatic patients, usually showing bilateral interstitial infiltrates with a basilar predominance. Patients with an acute presentation may present with confluent alveolar infiltrates. Pneumothorax may occur and may be bilateral. PFT generally shows a restrictive ventilatory defect with diffusion abnormalities and eventually hypoxia. As with bleomycin, $D_{L_{CO}}$ may decrease without radiographic or clinical evidence of disease. While it has been suggested that a decrease in $D_{L_{CO}}$ may be the earliest sign of pulmonary toxicity, prospective evaluations of screening pulmonary function studies in the diagnosis of BCNU-induced lung toxicity are not yet available.

Pathologic changes in the lung resemble those seen with other cytotoxic agents. Type II pneumocyte hyperplasia and dysplasia, fibroblast proliferation, and deposition of proteinaceous material in alveoli have been described. However, the cardinal feature of BCNU-induced lung toxicity appears to be interstitial fibrosis, which may be patchy and often occurs without clinical evidence of inflammation. Angiocentric necrotizing granulomatous inflammation has been noted in some patients.[38] In two patients, pulmonary veno-occlusive disease has accompanied BCNU-induced pulmonary toxicity.[26]

The prognosis for patients with BCNU-induced lung injury is poor. Estimates of mortality range as high as 90 percent.[10] Administration of corticosteroids simultaneously with BCNU does not appear to prevent pulmonary toxicity. Likewise, institution of corticosteroid therapy after the onset of symptoms does not consistently result in improvement. The primary approach to BCNU toxicity is to withdraw the drug immediately as soon as signs of toxicity appear. Long-term treatment remains supportive. In light of the long latent period that can exist between treatment and the onset of signs of toxicity, long-term follow-up is also warranted.

OTHER NITROSOUREAS

The other nitrosoureas used as chemotherapeutic agents, lomustine (CCNU), semustine (methyl CCNU), and chlorozotocin, have also been associated with pulmonary toxicity. In general, these drugs have been less widely used than BCNU, and in smaller cumulative doses. As with BCNU, toxicity tends to become manifest insidiously with interstitial pneumonitis and pulmonary fibrosis. These drugs have been thought to confer a lower risk of pulmonary toxicity than BCNU. Because of their close chemical relation to BCNU, however, the potential for severe lung toxicity must be considered when these or other drugs of this class are used.

BIOLOGIC RESPONSE MODIFIERS

Retinoic Acid

All-*trans* retinoic acid is a biologically active agent (Table 66-6) that has proven benefit in the treatment of acute promyelocytic leukemia. In contrast to conventional cytotoxic chemotherapy, activity of this drug occurs through the promotion of the differentiation of malignant into mature neutrophils. In up to 25 percent of treated patients, this therapy has been associated with a constellation of symptoms termed the "retinoic acid syndrome."[14]

The retionic acid syndrome is characterized by fever, dyspnea, and pleural or pericardial effusions, often in association with hypertension or renal insufficiency. Chest radiographs show interstitial infiltrates and pleural effusions. Leukocytosis, which is common during treatment, is often, though not invariably, associated with the syndrome. In a series of 35 patients treated with all-*trans* retinoic acid for promyelocytic leukemia, nine developed the retinoic acid syndrome.[14] More than 50 percent of these patients required mechanical ventilation, and 33 percent died of complications related to the syndrome. The cause of the syndrome is unclear but must be linked to the differentiation process induced by the drug. Several different mechanisms have been proposed: maturing leukemic cells may release vasoactive cytokines, resulting in a "capillary leak" syndrome, fever, and hypotension; persistent dysfunction of the differentiated leukemic cells may trigger acute injury to the lungs or kidneys; or up-regulation by all-*trans* retinoic acid of genes encoding leukocyte adhesion receptors may cause impaired leukocyte adhesion to the capillaries or loss of integrity of the pulmonary vascular endothelium.

Recent reports indicate that the severity of the retinoic acid syndrome may be decreased by treatment with corticosteroids. However, in patients who develop leukocytosis and therefore appear to be at increased risk of retinoic acid syndrome, management is unclear. Full-dose cytotoxic chemotherapy has been suggested as a therapeutic strategy in this circumstance, although this approach remains uncertain on two accounts: fewer than half of the patients who develop leukocytosis will develop retinoic acid syndrome, and cytotoxic chemotherapy has inherent risks. At present, regimens using all-*trans* retinoic acid should also include corticosteroids.

Interleukin-2

Interleukin 2 (IL-2) is a glycoprotein secreted by activated lymphocytes. IL-2 therapy, alone or in conjunction with lymphokine-activated killer (LAK) cells, has proved beneficial in patients with metastatic renal cell carcinoma or melanoma. However, significant treatment-related pulmonary toxicities have been observed. In a series of 54 patients who received high-dose IL-2 and LAK therapy, 80 percent were noted to have focal or diffuse parenchymal lung opacities.[37] Pleural effusions were also common. The spectrum of pulmonary toxicities ranges from subclinical restrictive and obstructive physiological abnormalities, often associated with a decline in the $D_{L_{CO}}$, to more severe clinically evident respiratory insufficiency. The latter generally presents as a syndrome of noncardiogenic pulmonary edema and may be associated with hypotension and renal insufficiency.[49]

Several mechanisms have been proposed to explain the increase in capillary permeability caused by IL-2. IL-2–activated lymphocytes produce a variety of cytokines, including TNF and IL-1. These moieties may alter pulmonary endothelial permeability in a fashion analogous to the role they are believed to play in the septic shock syndrome.[37] IL-2 may also promote the ad-

	TABLE 66-6		
	Biologic Response Modifiers		
Drug	*Pulmonary Syndrome*	*Treatment*	*Comments*
All-*trans* retinoic acid	"Retinoic acid syndrome"	Corticosteroids Discontinue drug Supportive care	Treatment regimens using all-*trans* retinoic acid should include corticosteroids
Interleukin 2	1. Pleural effusions Focal or diffuse radiographic abnormalities	Supportive care Discontinue drug	Radiographic abnormalities uncommon Usually reversible Risk factors: Increasing cumulative dose Administration of LAK cells IL-2-induced cardiac toxicity may contribute to pulmonary edema
	2. Noncardiogenic pulmonary edema	Supportive care Discontinue drug	

TABLE 66-7

Miscellaneous

Drug	Pulmonary Syndrome	Treatment	Comments
Doxorubicin	Noncardiogenic pulmonary edema	Supportive care Discontinue drug	Increases risk of radiation pneumonitis Risk factors: Therapeutic radiation
Procarbazine	1. Hypersensitivity-type pneumonitis	Discontinue drug	Pulmonary toxicity uncommon
	2. Chronic pneumonitis/ pulmonary fibrosis	Discontinue drug	Pulmonary toxicity uncommon
Vinca Alkaloids Vindesine Vinblastine	Noncardiogenic pulmonary edema, interstitial pneumonitis bronchospasm	Supportive care Discontinue drug Corticosteroids	Risk factors: Concurrent treatment with mitomycin-C
Taxines Paclitaxel	Dyspnea, bronchospasm	Discontinue drug Supportive care	Pretreatment with histamine antagonists and corticosteroids reduces incidence of toxicity
Docetaxel	Noncardiogenic pulmonary edema	Discontinue drug Supportive care	Toxicity is related to cumulative dose

hesion of natural killer cells to the capillary endothelium, thus altering vascular integrity. Last, IL-2 also has toxic effects in other organs, including the heart. IL-2–induced cardiac dysfunction may contribute to the development of pulmonary interstitial edema.

IL-2 appears to have a cumulative dose-dependent lung toxicity, which seems to be compounded by LAK cell administration.[44] Lung toxicity does appear to be reversible. In most cases, clinical and radiographic abnormalities will resolve within several days after cessation of therapy.[44,51]

MISCELLANEOUS AGENTS

Doxorubicin

The use of the anthracycline doxorubicin (Table 66-7) is usually limited by cardiac toxicity. While direct pulmonary toxicity has not been described for this drug, the combination of the drug and therapeutic thoracic radiation, either during or preceding doxorubicin therapy, increases the incidence of radiation pneumonitis in 10 percent of patients. In severe cases, a capillary leak syndrome and noncardiogenic pulmonary edema may develop. Of note is that in contrast to conventional radiation-induced lung injury, radiographic abnormalities in cases of combined doxorubicin and radiation therapy may be observed outside the ports of radiation—a situation similar to that seen with bleomycin.

Procarbazine

Procarbazine is a cytotoxic drug used primarily in the treatment of lymphoma. Procarbazine has been associated with a hypersensitivity type of pneumonitis, as well as with the more usual cytotoxic drug–induced interstitial pneumonitis. The incidence of pulmonary toxicity with procarbazine appears to be low.

Vinca Alkaloids

The vinca alkaloids given as sole agents are generally not associated with pulmonary toxicity. However, the combination of vinblastine or vindesine with mitomycin has been reported to be associated with noncardiogenic pulmonary edema, interstitial pneumonitis, and bronchospasm.[19,25,33] This synergistic toxicity is discussed in more detail in the preceding section on cytotoxic antibiotics.

Taxines

PACLITAXEL

Paclitaxel (Taxol) is the first of a new class of anticancer agents known as taxines. It is approved for use in the therapy of ovarian and breast cancers and is currently undergoing clinical trials for the treatment of other malignancies, including cancer of the lung. Paclitaxel inhibits the disassembly of microtubules. This disruption of normal microtubular function ultimately results in cell death.[35] The incidence of major hypersensitivity reactions—including dyspnea, bronchospasm, urticaria, and hypotension—is high (25 to 30 percent). The administration of histamine (H_1 and H_2) antagonists and corticosteroids before treatment with paclitaxel has reduced the incidence of such reactions to a more acceptable 1 to 2 percent.[36]

Paclitaxel has not been associated with any specific syndromes of lung injury. This may not be the case with other drugs of this group. Docetaxel, like paclitaxel, is associated with hypersensitivity reactions. Unlike paclitaxel, docetaxel is also associated with cumulative pulmonary toxicity, including a syndrome of noncardiogenic pulmonary edema.[35]

REFERENCES

1. Andersson BS, Cogan BM, Keating MJ, et al: Subacute pulmonary failure complicating therapy with high-dose Ara-C in acute leukemia. *Cancer* 56:2181–2184, 1985.
2. Aronin PA, Mahaley MS, Rudnick SA, et al: Prediction of BCNU pulmonary toxicity in patients with malignant gliomas: An assessment of risk factors. *New Engl J Med* 303:183–188, 1980.
3. Bechard DE, Fairman RP, DeBlois GG, Via CT: Fatal pulmonary fibrosis from low-dose bleomycin therapy. *South Med J* 80:646–649, 1987.
4. Bedrossian CWM, Sussman J, Conklin RH, Kahan B: Azathioprine-associated interstitial pneumonitis. *Am J Clin Pathol* 82:148–154, 1984.
5. Berend N: Protective effect of hypoxia on bleomycin lung toxicity in the rat. *Am Rev Respir Dis* 130:307–308, 1984.
6. Byrd JC, Hargis JB, Kester KE, et al: Opportunistic pulmonary infections with fludarabine in previously treated patients with low-grade lymphoid malignancies: A role for *Pneumocystis carinii* pneumonia prophylaxis. *Am J Hematol* 49:135–142, 1995.
7. Cervantes F, Salgado C, Montserrat E, Rozman C: Fludarabine for prolymphocytic leukaemia and risk of interstitial pneumonitis (letter). *Lancet* 336:1130, 1990.
8. Chang AY, Kuebler JP, Pandya KJ, et al: Pulmonary toxicity induced by mitomycin C is highly responsive to glucocorticoids. *Cancer* 57:2285–2290, 1986.
9. Cherniack RM, Abrams J, Kalica AR: Pulmonary disease associated with breast cancer therapy. *Am J Respir Crit Care Med* 150:1169–1173, 1994.
10. Cooper JAD Jr, White DA, Matthay RA: Drug-induced pulmonary disease. Part 1: Cytotoxic drugs. *Am Rev Respir Dis* 133:321–340, 1986.
11. Devlin JW, Wass H, Waters CI: Fludarabine associated pulmonary hypersensitivity. *Can J Hosp Pharm* 47:125–127, 1994.
12. Doll, DC, Weiss RB, Issel BF: Mitomycin: Ten years after approval for marketing. *J Clin Oncol* 3:276–286, 1985.
13. Doyle LA, Ihde DC, Carney DN, et al: Combination chemotherapy with doxorubicin and mitomycin in non–small cell bronchogenic carcinoma: Severe pulmonary toxicity from q 3 weekly mitomycin C. *Am J Clin Oncol* 7:719–724, 1984.
14. Frankel SR, Eardley A, Lauwers G, et al: The "retinoic acid syndrome" in acute promyelocytic leukemia. *Ann Intern Med* 117:292–296, 1992.
15. Ginsberg SJ, Comis RL: The pulmonary toxicity of antineoplastic agents. *Semin Oncol* 9:34–51, 1982.
16. Giri SN, Hyde DM, Hollinger MA: Effect of antibody to transforming growth factor beta on bleomycin induced accumulation of lung collagen in mice. *Thorax* 48:959–966, 1993.
17. Hamous JE, Guffy MM, Aschenbrener CA: Fatal acute respiratory failure following intrathecal methotrexate administration. *Cancer Treat Rep* 67:1025–1026, 1983.
18. Heard BE, Cooke RA: Busulfan lung. *Thorax* 23:187–193, 1968.
19. Hoelzer KL, Harrison BR, Luedke SW, Luedke DW: Vinblastine-associated pulmonary toxicity in patients receiving combination therapy with mitomycin and cisplatin. *Drug Intell Clin Pharm* 20:287–289, 1986.
20. Hoyt DG, Lazo JS: Alterations in pulmonary mRNA encoding procollagens, fibronectin and transforming growth factor–β precede bleomycin-induced pulmonary fibrosis in mice. *J Pharmacol Exp Ther* 246:765–771, 1988
21. Hupt HM, Hutchins GM, Moore GW: Ara-C lung: Non-cardiogenic pulmonary edema complicating cytosine arabinoside therapy of leukemia. *Am J Med* 70:256–261, 1981.
22. Jules-Elysee K, White DA: Bleomycin-induced pulmonary toxicity. *Clin Chest Med* 11:1–20, 1990.
23. Khalil N, Bereznay O, Sporn M, Greenberg A: Macrophage production of transforming growth factor β and fibroblast collagen synthesis in chronic pulmonary inflammation. *J Exp Med* 170:727–737, 1989.
24. Kreisman H, Wolkove N: Pulmonary toxicity of antineoplastic therapy. *Semin Oncol* 19:508–520, 1992.
25. Kris MG, Pablo D, Graller J, et al: Dyspnea following vinblastine or vindesine administration in patients receiving mitomycin plus vinca alkaloid combination therapy. *Cancer Treat Rep* 68:1029–1031, 1984.
26. Lombard CM, Churg A, Winokur S: Pulmonary veno-occlusive disease following therapy for malignant neoplasms. *Chest* 92:871–876, 1987.
27. Matthay RA, Twohig K: Pulmonary effects of cytotoxic agents other than bleomycin. *Clin Chest Med* 11:31–54, 1990.
28. O'Driscoll BR, Hasleton PS, Taylor PN, et al: Active lung fibrosis up to 17 years after chemotherapy with carmustine (BCNU) in childhood. *New Engl J Med* 323:378–382, 1990.
29. Orwoll ES, Kiessling PJ, Patterson JR: Interstitial pneumonia from mitomycin. *Ann Intern Med* 89:352–355, 1978.
30. Phan SH, Kunkel SL: Inhibition of bleomycin-induced pulmonary fibrosis by nordihydroguiaretic acid: The role of alveolar macrophage activation and mediator production. *Am J Pathol* 124:343–352, 1986.
31. Piguet PF, Collart MA, Grau GE, et al: Tumor necrosis factor/cachectin plays a key role in bleomycin-induced pneumopathy and fibrosis. *J Exp Med* 170:655–663, 1989.
32. Piguet PF, Vesin C, Grau GE, Thompson RC: Interleukin 1 receptor antagonist (IL-1ra) prevents or cures pulmonary fibrosis elicited in mice by bleomycin or silica. *Cytokine* 5:57–61, 1993.
33. Rivera AP, Kris MG, Gralla RJ: Syndrome of acute dyspnea related to combined mitomycin plus vinca alkaloid chemotherapy. *Am J Clin Oncol* 18:245–250, 1995.
34. Rosenow EC III: Drug-induced pulmonary disease. *Dis Mon* 40:253–310, 1994.
35. Rowinsky EK, Donehower RC: Paclitaxel (Taxol). *New Engl J Med* 332:1004–1014, 1995.
36. Rowinsky EK, Eisenhauer EA, Chaudhry V, et al: Clinical toxicities encountered with paclitaxel (Taxol). *Semin Oncol* 20(Suppl 3):1–15, 1993.
37. Saxon RR, Klein JSB, Bar MH, et al: Pathogenesis of pulmonary edema during interleukin-2 therapy: Correlation of chest radiographic and clinical findings in 54 patients. *Am J Radiol* 156:281–285, 1991.

38. Selker RG, Jacobs SA, Moore PB, et al: 1,3-Bis-(2-chloroethyl)-1-nitrosourea (BCNU)–induced pulmonary fibrosis. *Neurosurgery* 7:560–565, 1980.

39. Sheldon R, Slaughter D: A syndrome of microangiopathic hemolytic anemia, renal impairment, and pulmonary edema in chemotherapy-treated patients with adenocarcinoma. *Cancer* 58:1428–1436, 1986.

40. Smith RE, Strieter RM, Zhang K, et al: A role for C-C chemokines in fibrotic lung disease. *J Leukoc Biol* 57:782–787, 1995.

41. Sostman HD, Matthay, RA, Putnam CE: Methotrexate-induced pneumonitis. *Medicine* 55:371–388, 1976.

42. Stover DA, Zaman MB, Hajdu SI, et al: Bronchoalveolar lavage in the diagnosis of diffuse pulmonary infiltrates in the immunosuppressed host. *Ann Intern Med* 10:1–7, 1984.

43. Trask CWL, Joannides T, Harper PG, et al: Radiation-induced lung fibrosis after treatment of small cell carcinoma of the lung with very high-dose cyclophosphamide. *Cancer* 55:57–60, 1985.

44. Villani S, Galinberti M, Rizzi M, et al: Pulmonary toxicity of recombinant interleukin-2 plus lymphokine-activated killer cell therapy. *Eur Respir J* 6:828–833, 1993.

45. Wallace RH, Kolbe J: Fiberoptic bronchoscopy and bronchoalveolar lavage in the investigation of the immunocompromised host. *New Zealand Med J* 105:215–217, 1992.

46. White DA, Orenstein M, Godwin TA, Stover DE: Chemotherapy-associated pulmonary toxic reactions during treatment for breast cancer. *Arch Intern Med* 144:953–956, 1984.

47. White DA, Schwartzberg LS, Kris MG, et al: Acute chest pain syndrome during bleomicin infusions. *Cancer* 59:1582–1585, 1987.

48. White DA, Stover DE, Smith G, Beck G: Serial pulmonary function studies during bleomycin therapy (abstract). *Am Rev Respir Dis* 135(Suppl):A39, 1987.

49. White RL Jr, Schwartzentruber DJ, Guleria A, et al: Cardiopulmonary toxicity of treatment with high dose interleukin-2 in 199 consecutive patients with metastatic melanoma or renal cell carcinoma. *Cancer* 74:3212–3222, 1994.

50. Yousem SA, Lifson JD, Colby TV: Chemotherapy-induced eosinophilic pneumonia: Relation to bleomycin. *Chest* 88:103–106, 1985.

51. Zitnik RJ. Drug-induced lung disease: Cancer chemotherapy agents. *J Respir Dis* 16:855–865, 1995.

CHAPTER 67

DRUG-INDUCED LUNG DISEASE DUE TO NONCHEMOTHERAPEUTIC AGENTS

Ralph J. Zitnik

Drug-induced pulmonary disease has been recognized since the beginning of the modern era of medicine. In 1880, William Osler described a case of pulmonary edema in a drug addict and postulated that opiates were implicated in the pathogenesis of the patient's lung infiltrates. A comprehensive review of this topic that appeared 25 years ago listed approximately 20 agents that were clearly associated with lung injury.[45] Since then, the number of implicated drugs has more than doubled. In the future, it is certain that as the diversity of available pharmacologic therapies increases, the list of drugs causing pulmonary toxicity will also continue to grow.

Although the clinical presentations of most forms of drug-induced pulmonary toxicity are well characterized, the epidemiology of these disorders is often poorly defined. There are no generally accepted criteria to determine whether an untoward pulmonary reaction has been caused by a given drug. For most drugs, risk factors that predispose patients to develop toxicity are not clearly identified, and pulmonary reactions often occur idiosyncratically, rather than in a dose- or time-dependent manner. Much of the literature in this area consists of case reports and small series, and in many instances, case descriptions are incomplete. Because of these problems, accurate epidemiologic data are available for only the more commonly observed forms of drug-induced pulmonary disease. In many cases, such data are found only in the description of adverse effects published in reports of clinical trials using a particular drug or as unpublished reports available only from the drug's manufacturer.

Establishing the diagnosis of a drug-induced pulmonary disease may be difficult. Frequently there are no pathognomonic signs, symptoms, laboratory tests, or pathologic findings. In addition, the clinical manifestations of such disorders often mimic those of other lung diseases. Thus, the diagnosis of drug-induced pulmonary toxicity always rests on the exclusion of a variety of other pathologic conditions, including neoplasm, infection, pulmonary thromboembolism, and congestive heart failure. Drug toxicity can also be difficult to distinguish from progression of the underlying disease for which the patient was originally treated. Finally, agents that cause pulmonary toxicity are commonly used in multidrug regimens, often in combination with toxic concentrations of oxygen or lung-damaging radiation. These factors, individually and in combination, contribute to the difficulty the clinician frequently encounters in attempting to attribute causation to a single agent.

From a therapeutic standpoint, there are few specific forms of treatment for pulmonary drug toxicities. In most cases, the mainstay of therapy consists of drug withdrawal. In many, a trial of corticosteroids is warranted if gas exchange abnormalities are severe. Unfortunately, there are few controlled studies available to guide these pharmacologic interventions.

CLINICAL SYNDROMES IN DRUG-INDUCED PULMONARY DISORDERS

The clinical presentations of patients with drug-induced lung diseases typically fall into a fairly small group of syndromes. None are drug specific, however, since all are frequently caused by processes other than drug toxicity (Table 67-1). Despite this lack of specificity, it is important to summarize these syndromes because drug toxicity must be carefully considered whenever these constellations of signs and symptoms are encountered. Unfortunately, the diagnosis of drug-induced pulmonary toxicity is often missed because the possibility of a drug reaction was not given appropriate consideration.

Interstitial Lung Disease   A wide variety of drugs can cause interstitial lung disease. As a result, interstitial disorders are the most common and well-recognized form of pulmonary drug toxicity. These disorders fall into two general patterns. The first is a subacute to chronic form of interstitial disease that resembles idiopathic pulmonary fibrosis, designated *chronic alveolitis/fibrosis syndrome.* The second pattern, termed *hypersensitivity lung disease,* has a more acute presentation and is often associated with peripheral or tissue eosinophilia.[9,10] In both syndromes, chest radiographs reveal interstitial or mixed interstitial-alveolar infiltrates. Pulmonary function studies, in both, also show a restrictive ventilatory defect, with decreased diffusing capacity. The chronic alveolitis/fibrosis and hypersensitivity lung disease designations represent the ends of a spectrum of drug-induced interstitial lung disease. Not surprisingly, patients with features encompassing both categories have been encountered.

Acute Noncardiogenic Pulmonary Edema   A variety of drugs—including opiates, aspirin, amiodarone, and tocolytic agents—can cause pulmonary vascular permeability alterations resulting in pulmonary edema. In all cases, widespread bilateral alveolar or alveolar-interstitial infiltrates are noted. The severity and outcome of these cases are quite variable. Most often the pulmonary edema is rapidly reversible. In some patients, however, severe

lung injury occurs, and the clinical course progresses to the point where the case fulfills criteria for adult respiratory distress syndrome (ARDS).

Alveolar Hypoventilation   Respiratory depression is a well-known side effect of many centrally acting therapeutic agents, particularly sedatives and opiates. Alveolar hypoventilation can also be caused by drugs that impede neuromuscular transmission or diaphragmatic muscle function. Usually, the effects of these agents are clinically insignificant. However, these drugs can cause hypercarbic respiratory failure in normal persons and can be particularly problematic in patients with underlying pulmonary or neuromuscular disease.

Bronchospasm   Drug-induced wheezing and bronchospasm can occur as a direct pharmacologic effect of the drug, as in the case of β-adrenergic receptor–blocking agents. Other mechanisms can also be operative—as exemplified by aspirin-induced bronchospasm in asthmatics and the bronchospasm that can be caused by adenosine and protamine.

Drug-Induced Systemic Lupus Erythematosus   A disorder that exhibits many of the features of idiopathic systemic lupus erythematosus can be caused by a wide variety of drugs. Patients with this toxicity frequently experience arthralgias, arthritis, fever, and/or pericarditis. The most common pulmonary manifestations are pleurisy and pleural effusions which are sometimes associated with parenchymal infiltrates.

Bronchiolitis Obliterans   A number of drugs have been reported to produce bronchiolitis obliterans without pathologic features of organizing pneumonia. Patients with this reaction manifest severe, progressive fixed obstructive ventilatory defects. Drug-induced bronchiolitis obliterans often occurs during treatment for rheumatoid arthritis, a disease that itself can be complicated by bronchiolitis obliterans as a systemic manifestation. Thus, the distinction between collagen vascular and drug-associated bronchiolitis is sometimes difficult.

Alveolar Hemorrhage   Acute alveolar hemorrhage and recurrent alveolar hemorrhage have been reported to occur in response to some drugs. Patients present with hemoptysis and, on chest radiographs, with alveolar infiltrates. In some cases, the alveolar hemorrhage occurs as part of a pulmonary-renal syndrome that is very similar to Goodpasture's disease.

Pulmonary Infiltrates with Eosinophilia   Eosinophilic infiltration is a well-documented manifestation of a variety of pulmonary drug toxicities. These eosinophilic syndromes can resemble acute or chronic eosinophilic pneumonia. Most commonly, a Loeffler's syndrome is noted, with dyspnea, cough, blood eosinophilia, and transient pulmonary infiltrates.

It is important to note that each of these clinical syndromes can be caused by a variety of drugs. For example, intravenous terbutaline, opiates, and aspirin can all cause acute noncardiogenic pulmonary edema. Conversely, a single drug can also cause several forms of pulmonary toxicity, as exemplified by the ability of nonsteroidal anti-inflammatory drugs (NSAIDs) to cause

TABLE 67-1

Major Clinical Syndromes Associated with Pulmonary Drug Toxicity

Interstitial Lung Disease
  Chronic alveolitis/fibrosis
    Amiodarone
    Gold
    Nitrofurantoin
    Methotrexate
    Mexiletine
    Penicillamine
    Tocainide
  Hypersensitivity lung disease
    Beta-lactam and sulfa antibiotics
    Carbamazepine
    Diphenylhydantoin
    Gold
    Methotrexate
    Nitrofurantoin
    NSAIDs
    Penicillamine

Noncardiogenic Pulmonary Edema
  Amiodarone
  Aspirin and NSAID overdose
  Opiate and sedative/hypnotic agent overdose
  Tocolytic therapy
    Terbutaline
    Isoxuprine
    Ritodrine

Alveolar hypoventilation
  Aminoglycosides
  Polymyxins
  Opiates and sedative-hypnotic agents

Bronchospasm
  Adenosine and dipyridamole
  Aspirin and NSAIDs
  β-Adrenoreceptor antagonists
  Sotalol

Drug-Induced SLE
  Hydralazine
  Isoniazid
  Procainamide
  Quinidine

Bronchiolitis Obliterans
  Gold
  Penicillamine

Alveolar Hemorrhage
  Cocaine
  Penicillamine

Pulmonary Infiltrates with Eosinophilia
  Beta-lactam antibiotics
  Sulfa antibiotics
  Fluoroquinolones
  Tetracycline and derivatives
  Erythromycin and derivatives
  Nitrofurantoin
  Anti-TB medications (isoniazid, PAS, ethambutol)
  NSAIDs

Isolated Cough
  ACE Inhibitors

pulmonary edema, bronchospastic exacerbations, and hypersensitivity lung disease.

The large number of drugs that can have adverse effects in the lung and the large number of clinical situations in which drug toxicity must be considered make a thorough understanding of drug-induced pulmonary disorders essential for all medical practitioners and students of pulmonary biology. To accomplish this, we will discuss the drug-induced lung diseases caused by agents used to treat cardiovascular and ophthalmic disorders, tocolytics, antibiotics, anticonvulsants, and anti-inflammatory drugs. In addition, a summary of the pulmonary complications of illicit drug use will be presented.

DRUGS USED TO TREAT CARDIOVASCULAR DISORDERS

The evaluation and treatment of drug-induced pulmonary dysfunction in patients with cardiovascular disease present a number of specific challenges. First, fever and hypoxemia associated with drug toxicity are very poorly tolerated in patients with coronary artery disease and left ventricular dysfunction. Many of the deaths ascribed to drug toxicity in this population are caused by secondary cardiac ischemia or arrhythmias rather than primary respiratory failure. Second, the worsening cough and pulmonary infiltrates seen in these patients can be misattributed to congestive heart failure rather than drug toxicity. Similarly, since obstructive airway disease and cardiovascular disease often coexist, drug-induced bronchospastic exacerbations may not be appropriately recognized. Third, patients with congestive heart failure, angina, or claudication often become sedentary. This can mask pulmonary symptoms; it also increases the risk of developing venous thrombosis and pulmonary embolism, which can further confound diagnosis. Finally, even after drug toxicity is determined to be the cause of the patient's respiratory problem, immediate withdrawal of the causative agent is not always possible. This is especially true with medications used in the treatment of life-threatening disorders such as ventricular arrhythmias. Often a second antiarrhythmic medication must be started before the offending drug is withdrawn. The choice of this agent sometimes necessitates further invasive cardiac electrophysiological evaluation.

Amiodarone

Amiodarone is used to treat severe ventricular arrhythmias and selected refractory supraventricular arrhythmias. In addition to pulmonary disease, the drug causes ophthalmic, cutaneous, hepatic, and thyroid toxicities. Pulmonary toxicity occurs with an incidence of approximately 5 percent, and case fatality rates are in the range of 10 to 20 percent.[15,32,33]

Pharmacology and Potential Mechanisms of Toxicity Amiodarone is an iodine-containing amphipathic compound with high lipid solubility. As a result, it becomes concentrated in cell membranes, especially those in the lung, skin, and liver. The drug has a high volume of distribution and an elimination half-life of approximately 30 to 60 days. Thus, even after amiodarone is discontinued, measurable serum levels and a continued antiarrhythmic effect can persist for weeks to months before the drug is completely excreted. In addition to its antiarrhythmic effects, amiodarone is a potent phospholipase inhibitor. This inhibition causes undigested surfactant phospholipids to accumulate within the lung, forming inclusions within alveolar macrophages and other cells.[32,33]

The mechanism of amiodarone toxicity is not known; however, several possibilities have been put forth. In some patients, the cellular phospholipidosis induced by amiodarone may cause direct cellular injury, resulting in secondary pulmonary inflammation. In addition, many patients develop a cell-mediated immunologic response to amiodarone. Finally, there is some evidence that the injury may be due, in part, to damage caused by toxic oxygen metabolites. Whether different mechanisms or combinations of mechanisms are operative in different patient subgroups has yet to be determined.

Clinical Features Amiodarone pulmonary toxicity has several clinical manifestations. The most common is an alveolitis/fibrosis syndrome that may be either subacute or chronic. The chronic form occurs in about two-thirds of patients, and is characterized by the insidious onset of cough, dyspnea, and weight loss. These symptoms are associated with interstitial infiltrates and a restrictive ventilatory defect. The more acute form presents with fever, chest pain, and alveolar or mixed alveolar-interstitial infiltrates on chest radiograph. This presentation occurs in the remaining one-third of patients and may mimic an infectious process. A peripheral leukocytosis and elevated erythrocyte sedimentation rate are features of both presentations. Peripheral eosinophilia is uncommon.[32,33]

Amiodarone use has been associated with episodes of acute noncardiogenic pulmonary edema, often culminating in ARDS. This complication occurs after pulmonary angiography and several types of cardiac and noncardiac surgery.[29,37,49] There is frequently a 24- to 48-h lag between the onset of ARDS and the uneventful surgical procedure that preceded it. At present, it is unclear whether the reports represent a true clinical syndrome or the coincidental occurrence of ARDS after surgery in severely ill patients. However, a recent retrospective series noted a much higher incidence of ARDS in patients on amiodarone than in very similar control groups undergoing identical cardiac surgical procedures.[37] In addition, a prospective, randomized study of amio-

darone in the treatment of postpneumonectomy atrial arrhythmias was prematurely terminated because of a substantial increase in the incidence of ARDS among patients treated with the drug postoperatively.[49] These data suggest that this syndrome is a real clinical entity.

Risk Factors for Toxicity The risk factors for amiodarone pulmonary toxicity are not well defined. Some studies report that a daily amiodarone dose of less than 400 mg is associated with a lower risk of toxicity. However, pulmonary toxicity can occur at lower doses, and higher doses are often well tolerated. Total cumulative dose and serum levels of amiodarone and its metabolite, desethylamiodarone, do not reliably presage toxicity. Whether baseline pulmonary function or radiographic abnormalities portend subsequent toxicity is also very controversial.[34] Finally, several prospective studies of patients treated with amiodarone have shown that a decrement in diffusing capacity is a poor indicator of toxicity.[34] Thus, a decreased diffusing capacity is not by itself reason to discontinue the drug in the absence of clinical signs and symptoms or a worsening chest radiograph.

Radiographic and Pathologic Features Patients with the subacute and chronic forms of amidarone pneumonitis typically have diffuse bilateral interstitial or mixed interstitial-alveolar infiltrates (Fig. 67-1). Patients with noncardiogenic pulmonary edema have diffuse alveolar infiltrates. Several less common radiographic manifestations have also been described, including isolated pleural effusions, pleura-based or parenchymal mass lesions, solitary nodules, and lobar or segmental infiltrates. Computed tomography (CT) during episodes of toxicity shows nonspecific interstitial and alveolar infiltrates in accord with the chest radiographic findings. However, both localized and diffuse areas of very high CT attenuation can also be seen.[44] Pathologic-radiographic correlation studies have shown that these regions correspond to areas of focal accumulation of foamy macrophages. These cells contain large amounts of amiodarone, which is 37 percent iodine by weight, accounting for the high CT attenuation. Since these findings are also seen in patients taking amiodarone without clinical toxicity, the presence of these high attenuation areas is not diagnostic of toxicity.[44] Gallium[67] scanning is positive in most cases of toxicity, and typically reverts to negative after clinical resolution. Gallium scanning cannot differentiate amiodarone toxicity from other causes of lung inflammation. A positive scan along with other supportive clinical evidence may be helpful in excluding other diagnostic entities.

The pathologic features of amiodarone toxicity are variable. In the acute form, intra-alveolar hemorrhage, type II alveolar epithelial cell proliferation, and hyaline membrane formation can be seen. The chronic form is characterized by alveolar septal thickening due to infiltration with lymphocytes, monocytes, and plasma cells. In later stages, alveolar and septal fibrosis occurs. Abundant intra-alveolar macrophages are seen; they are described as being "foamy." When examined by electron microscopy, the cytoplasm of these macrophages contains "lamellar" inclusions, filled with undigested phospholipids. Foamy macrophages are seen in the lungs of virtually all patients taking amiodarone, and therefore their presence is not diagnostic of toxicity.

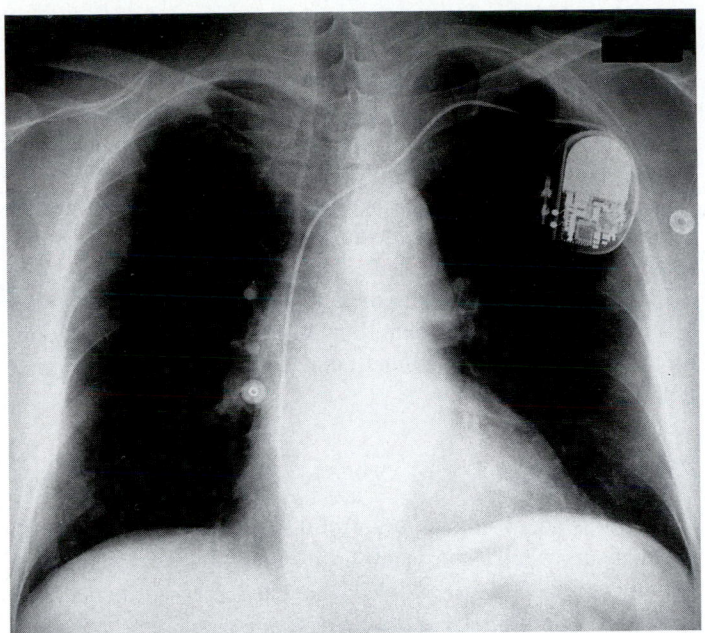

A

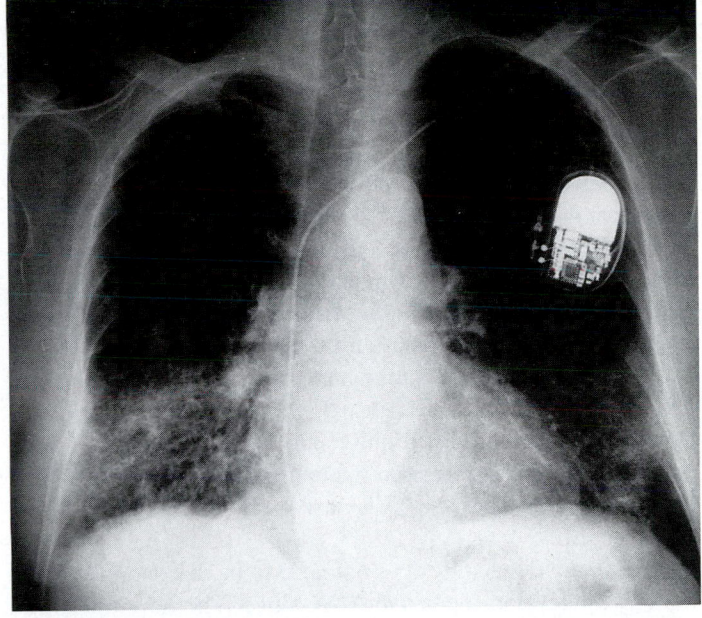

B

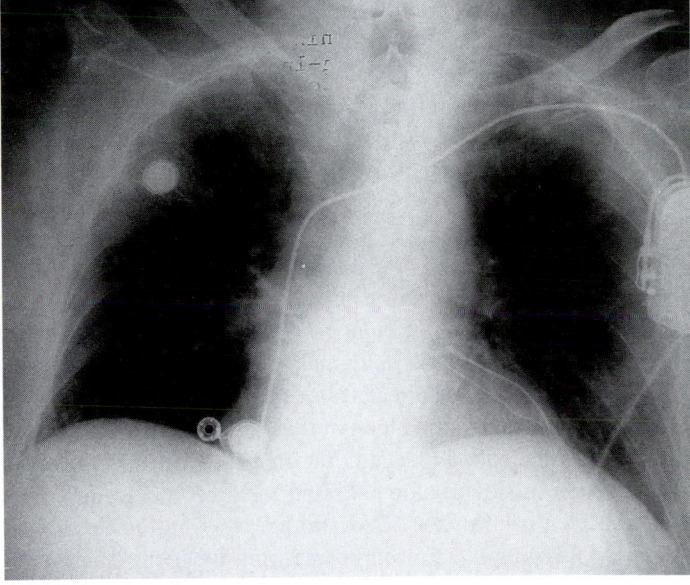

C

Bronchoalveolar lavage (BAL) findings are quite variable in amiodarone toxicity. Red blood cells and elevated neutrophil counts are seen early in the course of the response. In some patients, a BAL lymphocytosis occurs, with an increase in the proportion of lymphocytes bearing the CD8 surface marker. In most patients, the only abnormality is an increased number of alveolar macrophages. As is the case with lung biopsies, "foamy macrophages" can be seen in the BAL of patients taking amiodarone who have no clinical evidence of toxicity; thus, their presence is not diagnostic of a toxic response to the drug.[11]

Diagnostic and Therapeutic Management   The diagnosis of amiodarone toxicity can often be made clinically, although bronchoscopy may sometimes be necessary to exclude infection. Once the diagnosis of amiodarone toxicity is established, the drug should be discontinued and a new antiarrhythmic agent begun. Although there are no controlled studies to support the use of corticosteroids, they are frequently initiated. Responses are well documented, and a recrudescence of symptoms can occur during corticosteroid tapering. Courses of treatment longer than 6 months in duration are sometimes necessary.

Procainamide

Procainamide is commonly used to treat supraventricular and ventricular arrhythmias. It is also commonly implicated as a cause of drug-induced systemic lupus erythematosus (SLE). Remarkably, between 50 and 90 percent of patients taking procainamide for more than 2 months develop serum antinuclear antibodies (ANAs). Ten to 20 percent of these ANA-positive patients will develop symptomatic drug-induced SLE, and 40 to 80 percent of them will have pulmonary manifestations. As in other types of drug-induced SLE, the ANA is positive in a homogeneous or diffuse pattern, and antihistone antibodies are present. Unlike the case with idiopathic SLE, anti–double-stranded DNA antibodies are absent. The mechanism responsible for the

FIGURE 67-1   The radiographic appearance of amiodarone pulmonary toxicity. *A.* The chest radiograph before the onset of toxicity shows no abnormalities other than the presence of a permanent transvenous pacemaker. *B.* A chest film taken during the episode of toxicity reveals bilateral basilar interstitial markings. *C.* After discontinuation of amiodarone and corticosteroid therapy, the infiltrates have resolved. Note the automatic implantable cardiac defibrillator (AICD), whose leads are now visible over the left ventricular shadow. The AICD was placed to treat intractable arrhythmias that occurred after amiodarone was discontinued. *(From Zitnik RJ: Drug-induced lung disease: Antiarrythmic agents. J Respir Dis 17:254–270, 1996. Case courtesy of Dr. William Batsford, Division of Cardiovascular Medicine, Yale University School of Medicine.)*

development of autoimmunity is unknown. In addition, it is not clear that the autoantibodies actually play a direct pathogenetic role in the generation of the disorder. Procainamide, hydralazine, and isoniazid all have the capacity to cause drug-induced SLE, and all are metabolized by acetylation. The rate at which acetylation occurs is genetically determined, and there is evidence that "slow acetylators" develop ANAs and clinical SLE more rapidly than "fast acetylators."[52]

Clinically, arthralgias and fever are common presenting symptoms, while renal and CNS impairment is rare. Pleural effusions and pleuritic chest pain are the most common pulmonary findings. Parenchymal pulmonary infiltrates are seen in up to 40 percent of patients with pulmonary impairment. In contrast, parenchymal infiltrates are unusual in SLE caused by drugs other than procainamide. Other pulmonary manifestations of idiopathic SLE—such as chronic interstitial fibrosis, alveolar hemorrhage, and progressive atalectasis—are quite rare in drug-induced SLE.

Procainamide therapy does not need to be discontinued in patients who develop a positive ANA alone. The development of rheumatologic symptoms should, however, prompt drug withdrawal. The response after the discontinuation of the drug is rapid, and symptoms frequently resolve within 2 to 3 weeks. When corticosteroids are added, the improvement is even more rapid, sometimes occurring within days. Despite rapid clinical resolution, the ANA can remain positive for months to several years after drug withdrawal. In contrast to the situation with idiopathic SLE, once the drug is withdrawn, persistent or relapsing rheumatologic symptoms do not occur.

Quinidine

Quinidine has been in use for many decades in the treatment of ventricular and supraventricular arrhythmias. During this time, it has been found to cause pulmonary toxicity only rarely. It has most commonly been implicated as a cause of drug-induced SLE, although this link is much less well established than with other drugs. Most patients with quinidine-induced SLE have positive ANAs. Their most common pulmonary manifestations are pleuritis and pleural effusions. Drug withdrawal and corticosteroid treatment commonly result in prompt improvement.[35]

Tocainide

Tocainide, an oral agent used to treat ventricular arrhythmias, causes adverse nonpulmonary effects in up to 50 percent of patients. Pulmonary toxicity occurs far less frequently. The most common respiratory side effect is an interstitial pneumonitis/fibrosis syndrome, which occurs in approximately 0.3 percent of patients. No apparent risk factors for the development of tocainide-induced lung disease have been described. Radiographically, interstitial infiltrates are seen, while high-resolution CT scanning shows interstitial septal thickening and patchy airspace disease. Biopsy typically reveals interstitial mononuclear cell infiltration, which can progress to interstitial fibrosis.[48] In most reported cases, the prognosis after drug withdrawal and treatment with steroids is good, although deaths have been reported.

Mexiletine

Mexiletine is used to treat ventricular arrhythmias. In the process, it can also cause pulmonary toxicity. Four cases have been reported in the literature, and the incidence in a manufacturer's compassionate-use trial was one in 11,000. Mexiletine causes an alveolitis/fibrosis syndrome with reticulonodular infiltrates on chest radiograph. The prognosis is usually good; however, respiratory failure and death have been reported.[6] Mexiletine also interferes with theophylline metabolism. Thus it can also raise serum theophylline concentrations to toxic levels. Theophylline levels should be followed and adjusted during the initiation of mexiletine therapy.

Adenosine

Intravenous adenosine is very useful in the diagnosis and treatment of supraventricular tachycardias that do not respond to vagal maneuvers. The use of adenosine has increased markedly in recent years, especially in the emergency room and "prehospital" settings. Adverse effects occur in 30 to 60 percent of patients. These side effects tend to be well tolerated because the drug is extremely short-acting. The most common pulmonary side effect is acute dyspnea during the infusion. This occurs in 5 to 10 percent of patients. Much less commonly, adenosine infusions can precipitate acute bronchospasm in patients with a history of asthma or chronic obstructive pulmonary disease (COPD). The mechanism of adenosine-induced bronchospasm is uncertain. It may induce mast cells to release bronchoconstrictive mediators such as leukotrienes and histamine.[7] Inhaled adenosine causes a dose-dependent drop in FEV_1 in asthmatics. However, it is not possible to determine which patients will have adverse reactions when given the intravenous preparation of the drug.[13] Although some reactions can be severe enough to precipitate respiratory failure, adenosine-induced bronchospasm typically responds quickly to intravenous aminophylline. In this setting, the aminophylline probably acts as a direct adenosine receptor antagonist. A history of COPD or asthma is not an absolute contraindication to the use of intravenous adenosine; however, it should be administered with extreme caution.

Sotalol

Sotalol is an agent with both class III antiarrhythmic and nonselective β-adrenoreceptor blocking effects that is used to treat ventricular and selected supraventricular arrhythmias. Sotalol causes respiratory symptoms in up to 2 percent of patients. Most commonly, it exacerbates bronchospasm in patients with preexisting obstructive airway disease.[22] Because of this problem, the use of sotalol should be avoided in patients with asthma and COPD.

Angiotensin-Converting Enzyme Inhibitors

Angiotensin-converting enzyme (ACE) inhibitors are in widespread use for the treatment of hypertension and congestive heart failure. The major adverse pulmonary effect of ACE inhibitors is a chronic nonproductive cough. ACE inhibitors also cause angioneurotic edema, a rare side effect characterized by transient edema of the skin, lips, tongue, and upper airway. The episodes are usually self-limited and respond to epinephrine and steroid treatment. When severe, they can cause airway obstruction resulting in respiratory failure and death. Finally, some studies suggest that ACE inhibitors may exacerbate bronchospasm in a subgroup of asthmatics; however, this finding is quite controversial.

Nonproductive cough occurs to an approximately equal extent with all ACE inhibitors. The incidence of cough varies widely, but in most studies it has been noted to occur in 5 to 15 percent of patients. The cough typically begins after 1 to 2 months, but it can occur up to 1 year after the initiation of treatment. After drug withdrawal, improvement typically occurs within 1 to 2 weeks. Patients without a history of asthma who develop a cough are slightly more sensitive to methacholine challenge than those who do not. However, ACE inhibitors do not reproducibly diminish airflow, and known asthmatics are not at increased risk for developing ACE inhibitor–induced cough.[27] The cough recurs with rechallenge, and patients who develop a cough in response to one ACE inhibitor also cough when "cross-challenged" with other ACE inhibitors.[43]

Several mechanisms have been proposed to explain ACE inhibitor–induced cough. However, none has clearly been proved to be responsible. The most attractive theory focuses on the ability of ACE inhibitors to block the metabolism of neuropeptides such as substance P and bradykinin. This results in neuropeptide accumulation, and the bronchoconstrictor and irritating effects of these moieties may generate the clinical syndrome.[25]

In most cases, the occurrence of ACE inhibitor–induced cough is an indication to withdraw the drug. In patients for whom no alternative therapy is practical, one can "treat through" the cough. In these cases, the cough will occasionally resolve spontaneously despite continued exposure.[43] ACE inhibitor–induced cough can also be treated with inhaled cromolyn sodium.[19]

β-Adrenergic Receptor Blockers

β-Adrenergic receptor blockers continue to be used in the treatment of a variety of cardiovascular diseases, including essential hypertension, unstable angina, and myocardial infarctions. Unfortunately, β-adrenergic blockers have a number of adverse effects in the lung. They have been implicated as a very rare cause of pulmonary fibrosis and drug-induced SLE. Most important is that they commonly precipitate bronchospastic exacerbations in patients with asthma or worsen chronic airway obstruction in patients with COPD.

In asthma and COPD patients with chronic stable hypertension, nonselective β-adrenergic blockers such as propranolol cause substantial, dose-dependent decreases in FEV_1. They often precipitate episodes of clinically significant bronchospasm and therefore should not be used.[51] While $β_1$ receptor-selective blockers, drugs with intrinsic sympathomimetic effect, and the mixed α/β-antagonist labetolol are better tolerated, these agents are still capable of causing severe bronchospasm, and should be used carefully if at all. In contrast, esmolol, an intravenous β-adrenergic blocker often used in ICUs, is well tolerated in most asthma and COPD patients because its "ultrashort" half-life allows treatment to be immediately withdrawn in case of a significant reaction. It is currently the agent of choice when beta blockade is required in patients with a history of asthma or COPD who develop unstable angina.

Dipyridamole

In the evaluation of patients with suspected coronary artery disease who are not capable of performing standard treadmill exercise tests, cardiac nuclear imaging with thallium[201] is often carried out after infusion of intravenous dipyridamole. Dipyridamole induces tachycardia and acts as a coronary vasodilator, thereby simulating the effect of exercise on the heart. Its mechanism of action is to prevent cellular reuptake of adenosine. This increases adenosine concentrations within the lung and other organs in a manner similar to a direct adenosine infusion. Dipyridamole-thallium stress testing precipitates acute bronchospasm in about 0.15 percent of patients.[42] Most of these patients have a history of asthma. As is the case in bronchospastic exacerbations caused directly by adenosine, dipyridamole-induced bronchospasm responds to intravenous aminophylline. While a history of obstructive airway disease is not an absolute contraindication to dipyridamole stress testing, the study should be performed with extreme caution.

Hydralazine

Hydralazine is an antihypertensive agent and vasodilator. It causes SLE in approximately 5 percent of patients when used in antihypertensive doses and in up to 15 percent of patients when used at higher vasodilator doses. As with procainamide, "slow" acetylation status may be a risk factor for the occurrence of drug toxicity. The clinical presentation is similar to that seen in SLE caused by other drugs, although renal disease occurs more commonly. Pleural disease is the most common pulmonary manifestation. Parenchymal infiltrates occur in only 3 percent of patients.[12]

Protamine

Protamine is a cationic polypeptide that binds to and neutralizes heparin. It is frequently given intravenously to reverse anticoagulation during cardiac catheterization and cardiopulmonary bypass. Transient, mild pulmonary hypertension and systemic hypotension occur during approximately 5 percent of infusions. Systemic anaphylaxis, urticaria, angioedema, and bronchospasm occur in 0.2 percent of patients, usually within 1 h of infusion. In rare cases, protamine causes a severe delayed reaction, with progressive and refractory pulmonary hypertension, cor pulmonale, and systemic hypotension. This syndrome carries a 30 percent mortality rate.[31,50]

The mechanisms underlying protamine toxicity are not fully understood. Protamine is capable of inducing anaphylaxis by cross-linking antibodies on mast cell surfaces. In addition, protamine-heparin complexes can activate the classic complement pathway, which directly damages the pulmonary vascular system and recruits activated neutrophils to the lung. Finally, protamine can increase pulmonary levels of thromboxane A_2, a potent vasoconstrictor.

Several purported risk factors for protamine toxicity have been described. Insulin-dependent diabetics often develop antiprotamine antibodies as a result of exposure to the protamine present in NPH insulin preparations. Similarly, since protamine is prepared from the testicular tissue of fish, patients with fish allergies and those who have undergone vasectomy may develop immunologic cross reactivity to the agent. While no large retrospective study has confirmed that these patients are at increased risk, protamine should be used with caution in such cases.[31] Treatment of protamine toxicity is supportive, including H_1 and H_2 histamine receptor blockers, fluid resuscitation and inotropic agents.

TOPICAL OPHTHALMIC AGENTS

In addition to their use in cardiovascular diseases, β-adrenergic receptor blockers are used in the treatment of ophthalmic disorders. By lowering intraocular pressures, these topical agents have become very useful in the treatment of open-angle glaucoma. When applied to the corneal surface, they can, however, be absorbed across mucosal membranes. This results in substantial serum levels and systemic beta blockade. Significant decreases in FEV_1 occur even in asymptomatic patients. Severe bronchospastic exacerbations with sporadic fatalities have been reported in asthmatics using these agents. Most of these exacerbations have been attributed to the nonselective agent timolol. The cardioselective agent betaxolol is purported to be better tolerated. The presence of asthma is a strong relative contraindication to the use of either drug. Patients with glaucoma who experience unexplained pulmonary symptoms should be specifically questioned regarding the use of ophthalmic drugs, as they often do not consider them to be "medicines."

TOCOLYTIC AGENTS

β-Adrenergic agonists suppress uterine contractions, and are used therapeutically to delay premature delivery. Terbutaline is the most commonly employed agent, while ritodrine, isoxuprine, and salbutamol are used less often. Acute pulmonary edema occurs during tocolytic therapy, with an incidence of up to 4.4 percent.[40] Most commonly, the pulmonary edema occurs approximately 2 days into the course of therapy. The onset of pulmonary edema can, however, be delayed for up to 12 h after the tocolytic agent is discontinued.

The pathogenesis of this disorder is not known. Since β-adrenergic agonists do not cause pulmonary edema in asthmatics, the physiological changes that occur during pregnancy probably contribute in some fashion. Most patients are volume overloaded as a result of the intravenous infusion superimposed on the chronic volume and salt retention caused by pregnancy. However, in most cases of tocolytic-induced pulmonary edema, left ventricular filling pressures and echocardiographic assessments of left ventricular systolic function are normal. Thus, a cardiac mechanism alone is unlikely. Other proposed pathophysiological mechanisms may be increased pulmonary capillary permeability, postcapillary venoconstriction, and—much less likely—a direct toxic effect of the β-adrenergic agonists.

Clinically, patients with tocolytic-induced pulmonary edema present with acute-onset chest pain, dyspnea, cough, and the expectoration of frothy pink sputum. These symptoms are associated with tachypnea, tachycardia, hypoxemia, and bilateral alveolar infiltrates on the chest radiograph. In addition to tocolytic-induced pulmonary edema, the differential diagnosis of acute respiratory compromise in the peripartum period includes pulmonary thromboembolism, gastric aspiration, amniotic fluid embolism, peripartum cardiomyopathy, and Valsalva-induced pneumomediastinum—all of which must be excluded. In most cases the syndrome is mild, with only 3 to 10 percent of patients requiring intubation and mechanical ventilation. The pulmonary edema usually resolves quickly with diuresis and discontinuation of the tocolytic. The mortality from this syndrome is 3 percent or less. Most of the fatalities occur in patients whose course is complicated by sepsis or acute respiratory distress syndrome.[40]

ANTIBIOTICS

Antibiotic-Induced Hypersensitivity Lung Disease

Hypersensitivity reactions caused by antibiotics typically present as *pulmonary infiltrates with eosinophilia,* or "PIE" syndromes. These reactions are idiosyncratic, and there are no known risk factors for their occurrence. Although the precise incidence of antibiotic-associated pulmonary eosinophilia is not known, these reactions are rare. In some cases, these toxic responses are severe or prolonged and resemble either acute or chronic eosinophilic pneumonia.[1] The most common antibiotic-associated PIE syndrome is simple pulmonary eosinophilia, or *Loeffler's syndrome.* β-Lactam and sulfa antibiotics (including antimalarials) are most often associated with this type of reaction. Fluoroquinolones, tetracycline and erythromycin derivatives, and nitrofurantoin can also cause this syndrome. The antituberculosis drugs isoniazid, para-aminosalicylic acid, and ethambutol have also been implicated. Loeffler's syndrome is characterized by dyspnea, cough, fever, and peripheral blood eosinophilia with transient, patchy pulmonary infiltrates. It is usually acute in onset and from 1 to 4 weeks in duration. In general, patients are not very ill, and respiratory symptoms are mild. Spontaneous resolution often occurs when the drug is withdrawn, and the response to a brief course of corticosteroids is usually excellent.

Nitrofurantoin Pulmonary Toxicity

Nitrofurantoin has been used for several decades in the treatment of acute urinary tract infections and in chronic suppression therapy for asymptomatic bacteriuria. Nitrofurantoin was one of the first drugs to be implicated as a cause of pulmonary disease. Although ARDS and alveolar hemorrhage have been reported, most cases of nitrofurantoin toxicity fall into one of two distinct categories: an acute form, which typically fits the pattern of hypersensitivity lung disease, and a chronic alveolitis/fibrosis syndrome. The exact incidence of nitrofurantoin pulmonary toxicity is not known. Studies during the 1960s concluded that toxicity seldom occurred. In a more recent HMO-based study, however, acute toxicity severe enough to warrant hospitalization occurred in approximately one in 5000 new administrations, while one in

750 patients on long-term suppression therapy developed chronic pulmonary toxicity.[10,26]

Acute Nitrofurantoin Toxicity. The onset of acute nitrofurantoin toxicity occurs less than 1 month after the first dose in 86 percent of cases, and reoccurs with rechallenge. The acute syndrome is characterized by fever, dyspnea, cough, chest pain, and a maculopapular rash. An elevated erythrocyte sedimentation rate is common, and peripheral blood eosinophilia occurs in 83 percent. Radiographically, mixed interstitial and alveolar infiltrates are seen. Pleural effusions are observed in approximately 16 percent of patients. Of interest is that the chest radiograph is normal in up to 18 percent of patients. Pulmonary function testing reveals a restrictive ventilatory defect, with decreased diffusing capacity. Since most of these cases do not require biopsy, pathologic studies are somewhat scarce and reflect the severest end of the clinical spectrum. Typical findings include interstitial infiltration with lymphocytes and plasma cells and, in the most severe cases, alveolar edema, hyaline membranes, and alveolar hemorrhage. Although infectious causes must be ruled out, in most cases the diagnosis can be made clinically. Drug withdrawal alone usually results in rapid improvement. Corticosteroid treatment is sometimes necessary. In general, the prognosis is good, although some patients develop respiratory failure and ARDS. Most patients will experience either full normalization or at least improvement in chest radiograph and pulmonary function parameters and alleviation of symptoms. The mortality in acute nitrofurantoin pulmonary toxicity is 0.5 percent.[23]

Chronic Nitrofurantoin Toxicity Chronic nitrofurantoin toxicity often occurs in elderly patients undergoing chronic oral suppression therapy for bacteriuria. As in the acute form, cyanosis, dyspnea, and cough are seen. However, fever and rash are less common as presenting symptoms. Unlike the situation with acute toxicity, fatigue, weight loss, and other constitutional symptoms are often observed.[23] Peripheral blood eosinophilia occurs but is less common than in the acute form. Low-level positive titers of ANAs and rheumatoid factor and elevated serum gamma globulins have also been noted. The chest radiograph usually shows bilateral, predominantly interstitial infiltrates. Pleural effusions are uncommon. The mechanism of this response is unknown. There is some evidence, however, that toxic oxygen metabolites play a role in inducing lung injury. Lung biopsies show chronic interstitial inflammation, interstitial and alveolar fibrosis, and "honeycomb" changes in end-stage disease. In most cases a clinical diagnosis can be made, although BAL and occasionally lung biopsy may be necessary. The prognosis is substantially worse than that for patients with acute toxicity. Most patients (73 percent) either fail to improve at all or show significant residual chest radiograph or pulmonary function testing abnormalities. The overall mortality in patients with chronic nitrofurantoin toxicity is approximately 8 percent.[23]

Isoniazid-Induced Systemic Lupus Erythematosus

While a large number of patients taking isoniazid will develop ANAs, most patients will not progress to clinically significant SLE. The exact incidence of the disease is not known. However, SLE is caused less frequently by isoniazid than by hydralazine or procainamide.[46] "Slow acetylators" have been purported to be at higher risk to develop both ANA positivity and clinical lupus, although this is controversial and not as well established as with other SLE-inducing drugs.

The typical clinical presentation of isoniazid-induced SLE includes fever, anemia, rash, arthralgias, and arthritis. Pleuritis and pericarditis with associated pleural and pericardial effusions are the most common chest findings. Renal, CNS, and parenchymal pulmonary impairment are unusual. In patients on isoniazid, a tuberculous effusion may be difficult to differentiate from isoniazid-induced SLE with pleuritis. The presence of a positive ANA and antihistone antibodies is helpful diagnostically. Thoracentesis and even pleural biopsy may be necessary for TB to be adequately excluded TB. Withdrawal of isoniazid results in the rapid resolution of symptoms. Improvement can be hastened by corticosteroids.

Antibiotic-Induced Alveolar Hypoventilation

Antibiotics can induce alveolar hypoventilation and precipitate acute hypercarbic respiratory failure by either causing or potentiating neuromuscular blockade.[3] This form of toxicity occurs in four major clinical scenarios: First, patients can have postoperative and postanesthetic respiratory dysfunction. This is often manifest as an unexplained inability to be extubated postoperatively, an enhancement of the normal effects of neuromuscular blocking agents given during anesthesia, or delayed-onset postoperative respiratory depression in patients who have already recovered from the effects of anesthesia (the so-called recurarization phenomenon).[3] Second, patients with underlying, previously unrecognized myasthenia gravis can have their myasthenia "unmasked" by neuromuscular blockade due to antibiotics. Third, patients with known myasthenia gravis can have an acute "myasthenic crisis" precipitated by antibiotics. Finally, acute weakness and respiratory failure can, in rare instances, occur as part of a "myasthenialike syndrome" in normal patients.

Aminoglycosides are the class of antibiotics that most commonly cause neuromuscular blockade. Neomycin, gentamicin, streptomycin, tobramycin, and kanamycin have all been implicated. Polymyxins, tetracyclines, ampicillin, and fluoroquinolones have been reported to cause this type of toxicity only rarely. This complication is the result of "presynaptic" events, which decrease acetylcholine release and "postsynaptic" events that block the effects of acetylcholine at the receptor itself. Respiratory failure has often been reported after intraperitoneal lavage with aminoglycosides during laparotomy. However, it can also occur after intravenous or intramuscular administration. Toxicity is potentiated by conditions, such as renal insufficiency, that decrease aminoglycoside clearance, and by concomitant treatment with other neuromuscular blocking agents. Treatment is mainly supportive, including intubation and mechanical ventilation when necessary. Cholinesterase inhibitors such as neostigmine and pyridostigmine are also indicated, especially in cases of drug-induced myasthenic crisis. Intravenous calcium infusion has been anecdotally reported to be useful as well.[3,41]

ANTICONVULSANTS

Diphenylhydantoin

Diphenylhydantoin (DPH) causes several forms of pulmonary toxicity that vary in their presentation and severity. They include asymptomatic physiological abnormalities, a DPH hypersensitivity syndrome, lymphocytic interstitial pneumonitis, and a "pseudolymphoma" syndrome. The physiological abnormalities stem from reports of restrictive ventilatory defects, mildly decreased diffusing capacities, and mildly increased alveolar-arterial oxygen gradients with exercise in patients on DPH. These findings are controversial, however, and these physiological abnormalities rarely cause clinically significant impairment.

In contrast to this mild toxicity, a generalized *dilantin hypersensitivity syndrome* has been described that is often accompanied by substantial, life-threatening pulmonary disease.[36] The exact incidence of this rare syndrome is unknown. In addition, there are no established risk factors for its occurrence. A genetically determined inability to adequately detoxify metabolic intermediates of DPH may, however, predispose some patients to develop this toxic response.

DPH hypersensitivity reactions typically occur within 1 month after beginning the drug. They are heralded by the onset of fever, lymphadenopathy, skin rash, and peripheral eosinophilia. The rash can progress from a simple maculopapular eruption to severe exfoliation. A multiorgan system reaction often ensues, including hepatitis, acute renal failure, myositis, aseptic meningitis, and granulocytopenia. Pulmonary manifestations include the acute onset of wheezing, dyspnea, and interstitial or mixed alveolar-interstitial radiographic infiltrates. They can be of sufficient severity to cause either hypoxemic or hypercarbic respiratory failure. Pathologically, a mixed inflammatory infiltrate is seen in both the pulmonary interstitium and alveolar space, and increased numbers of lymphocytes and eosinophils are recovered in BAL fluid. A subgroup of patients with DPH hypersensitivity reactions develop a systemic vasculitis affecting the skin and visceral organs, including the lung. A spectrum of pathologic features have been noted in these patients, including lesions consistent with polyarteritis nodosum and hypersensitivity vasculitis.[53] Although a rapid response to drug withdrawal and steroids is typical in cases of DPH hypersensitivity, the clinical course may continue to worsen for many days before improvement is seen. Fatalities are common, especially in cases that manifest this systemic vasculitis.

Based on isolated case reports, DPH has also been associated with an interstitial lung disease resembling lymphocytic interstitial pneumonitis.[8] Patients with this presentation have interstitial chest radiographic abnormalities without fever or peripheral eosinophilia. In one case, BAL cell counts revealed a marked lymphocytosis, and transbronchial biopsy showed a lymphocytic infiltrate with mild epithelial hyperplasia and fibrosis. Although the infiltrates resolve after DPH withdrawal, pulmonary function test abnormalities can persist.

DPH may also cause a "pseudolymphoma" syndrome, which mimics malignant lymphoma clinically and pathologically.[21] DPH-induced pseudolymphoma can occur as an isolated entity but more often presents at the same time as a systemic DPH hypersensitivity reaction. Patients manifest fever, skin rash, diffuse peripheral lymphadenopathy, hepatosplenomegaly, and, in many cases, radiographic evidence of hilar and mediastinal lymphadenopathy. In addition to pseudolymphoma syndrome, some retrospective studies have linked DPH use with true Hodgkin's and non-Hodgkin's lymphomas, although this association has not been clearly proved. DPH-induced pseudolymphoma recurs with rechallenge; anecdotally, it responds well to drug withdrawal and steroid treatment.

Carbamazepine

Carbamazepine causes an acute hypersensitivity syndrome similar to that induced by DPH.[39] Fever, peripheral eosinophilia, exfoliative dermatitis, hepatitis, and generalized lymphadenopathy occur in association with interstitial pulmonary infiltrates. Histologically, the interstitium is infiltrated with eosinophils and plasma cells. The syndrome recurs with rechallenge and cross challenge with other agents, including both diphenylhydantoin and phenobarbital. The propensity to develop this hypersensitivity may, in part, be caused by a genetically determined inability to adequately detoxify arene hydroxide intermediates, which are produced as the drug is metabolized.

ANTI-INFLAMMATORY AGENTS

Salicylates

Aspirin-Induced Asthma   Aspirin sensitivity occurs in approximately 5 percent of a general population of asthmatics. In asthmatics who have nasal polyposis and chronic sinusitis, or "Sampter's triad," the incidence of aspirin sensitivity approaches 30 percent. Episodes of asthma exacerbation induced by aspirin usually occur 30 min to 2 h after ingestion. In addition to bronchospasm, profuse rhinorrhea, facial flushing, angioedema, and gastrointestinal symptoms can be observed. The diagnosis is made from a careful exposure history. Unfortunately, a history of aspirin use may be be difficult to elicit because many over-the-counter aspirin-containing medications are not clearly labeled. Occasionally, a controlled diagnostic aspirin challenge is required to establish the diagnosis.[17]

Insight into the mechanism of aspirin-induced asthma has recently been obtained. Aspirin and most other nonsteroidal anti-inflammatory drugs (NSAIDs) inhibit the activity of cyclooxygenase, an enzyme active in the metabolism of arachidonic acid into prostaglandins. As a result, arachidonic acid is shunted toward metabolism by the 5-lipoxygenase pathway—increasing the production of leukotrienes, which have a potent bronchoconstricting effect. The importance of this mechanism is evidenced by two recent findings. Measurement of urinary leukotriene E_4 excretion is a standard means of assessing changes in serum leukotriene levels. Following a diagnostic aspirin challenge, patients with aspirin-sensitive asthma have a much greater increase in urinary leukotriene E_4 levels than do nonsensitive asthmatics. Moreover, the clinical symptoms and airflow reduction induced by aspirin are attenuated by the 5-lipoxygenase inhibitor zileuton.[24]

In aspirin-sensitive asthmatics, symptoms of nasal polyposis are managed with inhaled corticosteroids, and episodes of acute sinusitis are treated with antibiotics. Surgical excision of the polyps may also be necessary to obtain symptomatic control. The most important aspect of management is aspirin avoidance. For patients with rheumatologic disorders or other conditions that necessitate the use of aspirin or NSAIDs, symptoms can sometimes be managed with zileuton. In addition, choline magnesium trisalicylate and salicylsalicylic acid are much weaker inhibitors of cyclo-oxygenase, and are safe in all but the most sensitive patients.[17]

Salicylate-Induced Pulmonary Edema   Salicylate-induced pulmonary edema was first recognized during the 1950s in patients with rheumatic fever treated with high-dose aspirin. In these early cases, the difficulty in differentiating drug-induced pulmonary edema from congestive heart failure due to rheumatic valvular disease was noted by many authors. With the advent of modern ICU techniques, it became clear that aspirin-induced pulmonary edema is not cardiogenic.[54] Several reports of adult patients with salicylate toxicity have established that pulmonary edema complicates approximately 10 to 15 percent of severe salicylate overdoses. Patients with salicylate-induced pulmonary edema fall into two general categories: younger patients who purposefully ingest large quantities of salicylates during suicide attempts and older patients on chronic salicylate therapy who overdose inadvertently.[2,20]

Salicylate-induced pulmonary edema is usually apparent on presentation, but it can be delayed by up to 24 h. In addition to dyspnea and tachypnea, mental status alterations are very common. A simple respiratory alkalosis, or a mixed anion gap metabolic acidosis and respiratory alkalosis are seen in almost all patients. Significant proteinuria with an otherwise unremarkable urinary sediment is another common feature. Although there is no clear relationship between the serum salicylate level and the development of pulmonary edema, this complication is unusual in patients with levels below 40 mg/dl. The chest radiographs of these patients show bilateral perihilar alveolar infiltrates, usually without pleural effusion or cardiomegaly. Left ventricular filling pressures and systolic function are normal. Because of the generally good prognosis, the pathologic features of this toxicity are poorly described. Early autopsy reports relate only the finding of "fluid-filled lungs."

Although animal models have shown that aspirin-induced pulmonary edema is due to increased capillary permeability, the mechanism underlying this abnormality is not known. Salicylate-induced alterations in platelet-vascular interaction and deranged metabolism of arachidonic acid metabolites have been proposed. However, these assertions are mainly speculative.

Treatment includes supportive measures such as intubation, mechanical ventilation, and positive end-expiratory pressure when needed. Alkaline diuresis decreases the free salicylate level by increasing its albumin binding, and also increases renal salicylate excretion. In young and otherwise healthy patients, with prompt recognition of the overdose, mortality is 1 to 2 percent or less. Conversely, older patients with numerous medical problems in whom the diagnosis is delayed suffer death rates as high as 25 percent.

Nonsteroidal Anti-inflammatory Drugs

NSAIDs are a structurally heterogeneous group of medications used as first-line agents for a wide spectrum of rheumatologic disorders, as well as for minor musculoskeletal pain in otherwise healthy persons. Since they are among the most commonly prescribed drugs and are also available in several over-the-counter preparations, it is important to recognize the different forms of pulmonary toxicity caused by these agents. Like salicylates, NSAIDs can induce noncardiogenic pulmonary edema after overdose. Because NSAIDs inhibit cyclooxygenase activity, they can also exacerbate bronchospasm in aspirin-sensitive asthmatics. Last, NSAIDs can also cause a PIE syndrome.

NSAID-Induced PIE Syndrome   Virtually all currently available NSAIDs can cause acute pulmonary hypersensitivity reactions.[54] This rare form of toxicity is idiosyncratic, and there are no clear risk factors or predisposing conditions for its occurrence. The pathogenetic mechanism that mediates this response is unknown. However, it is known that NSAID-induced PIE syndromes reoccur with controlled or inadvertent rechallenge, as well as cross challenge with a second NSAID.

The onset of NSAID toxicity is variable, occurring in some cases after less than 1 week, and in others up to 3 years after first exposure to the drug. Patients with this syndrome experience cough, dyspnea, fever, chest pain, and rash. These symptoms are accompanied by peripheral blood eosinophilia and an elevated erythrocyte sedimentation rate. Bilateral interstitial infiltrates are the most common radiographic manifestation. Patchy alveolar infiltrates, dense peripheral infiltrates with central sparing ("radiographic-negative pulmonary edema"), pleural effusions, and hilar adenopathy are noted less frequently. Gallium[67] lung scans are typically positive during the acute illness, and become negative after clinical resolution. It is interesting that the scan becomes positive once again with PIE syndrome recurrence after NSAID rechallenge. Unfortunately, a positive gallium[67] scan does not differentiate NSAID pulmonary hypersensitivity from other causes of pulmonary inflammation.

BAL in patients with NSAID-induced PIE syndromes reveals marked eosinophilia. Pathologic findings include thickening and fibrosis of the alveolar septum, type II alveolar epithelial cell hyperplasia, and infiltration of the interstitium and alveolus by polymorphonuclear leukocytes, lymphocytes, monocytes, and eosinophils.

The symptoms and radiographic abnormalities of these patients resolve rapidly after discontinuation of the NSAID. Although improvement may be hastened by corticosteroid therapy, such treatment is usually not needed. In rare cases, a severe reaction including acute respiratory distress syndrome and multiorgan system failure ensues. Patients with this presentation have a high mortality. However, in the vast majority of NSAID-associated pulmonary hypersensitivity reactions, resolution is complete and the prognosis is excellent.

Methotrexate

Methotrexate is an inhibitor of dihydrofolate reductase and is used as an antitumor and immunosuppressive agent. Pulmonary toxicity due to methotrexate was initially found only after high-

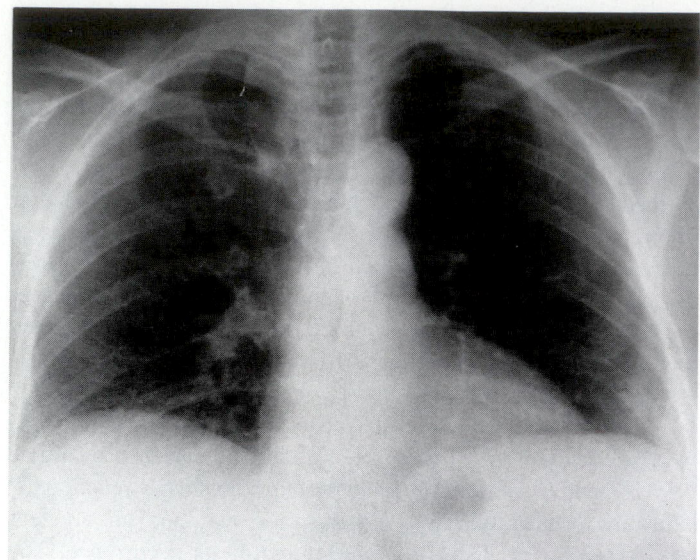

A

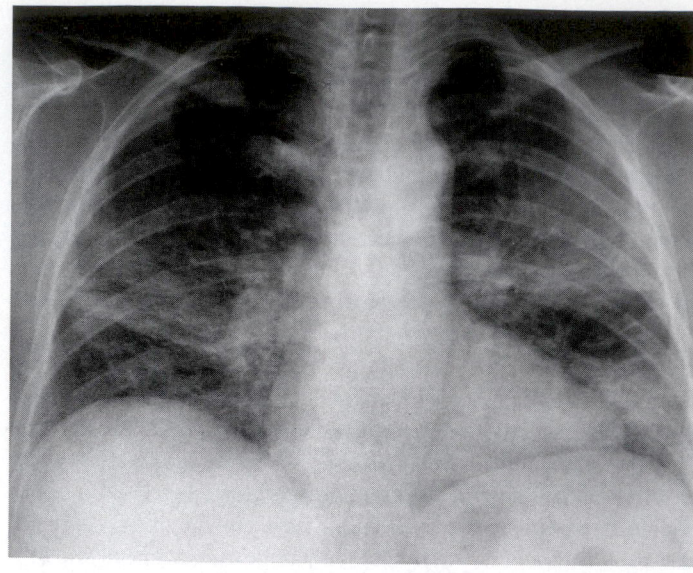

B

dose regimens given during cancer chemotherapy. In the early 1980s, as the drug came into wider use for the treatment of rheumatoid arthritis, it became clear that toxicity also occurred during low-dose oral therapy in an outpatient setting.[54] Pulmonary toxicity has been reported to complicate the treatment of asthma, psoriasis, primary billiary cirrhosis, and most other disorders for which methotrexate has been used. Methotrexate pulmonary toxicity occurs in 1 to 5 percent of patients with rheumatoid arthritis and as many as 14 percent of patients treated for primary billiary cirrhosis.[5,47] A number of factors have been proposed to increase risk for the development of pulmonary toxicity, including higher daily and cumulative doses, renal insufficiency, concomitant high-dose aspirin or NSAID therapy, and preexisting lung disease. None of these risk factors have been definitively established.

The pathogenesis of methotrexate pneumonitis is not known. A hypersensitivity mechanism is suggested by the frequent finding of a BAL lymphocytosis and peripheral eosinophilia. In many cases, however, rechallenge with methotrexate does not cause recurrence of pulmonary disease. Moreover, BAL lymphocyte CD4:CD8 ratios may be decreased, increased, or normal. Both of these findings suggest that different mechanisms may be operative in different subjects.

The typical clinical presentation of methotrexate pulmonary toxicity is subacute, occurring 1 to 5 months into therapy. Fever, cough, dyspnea, and inspiratory rales are noted. They are accompanied by hypoxemia and a peripheral leukocytosis. Periph-

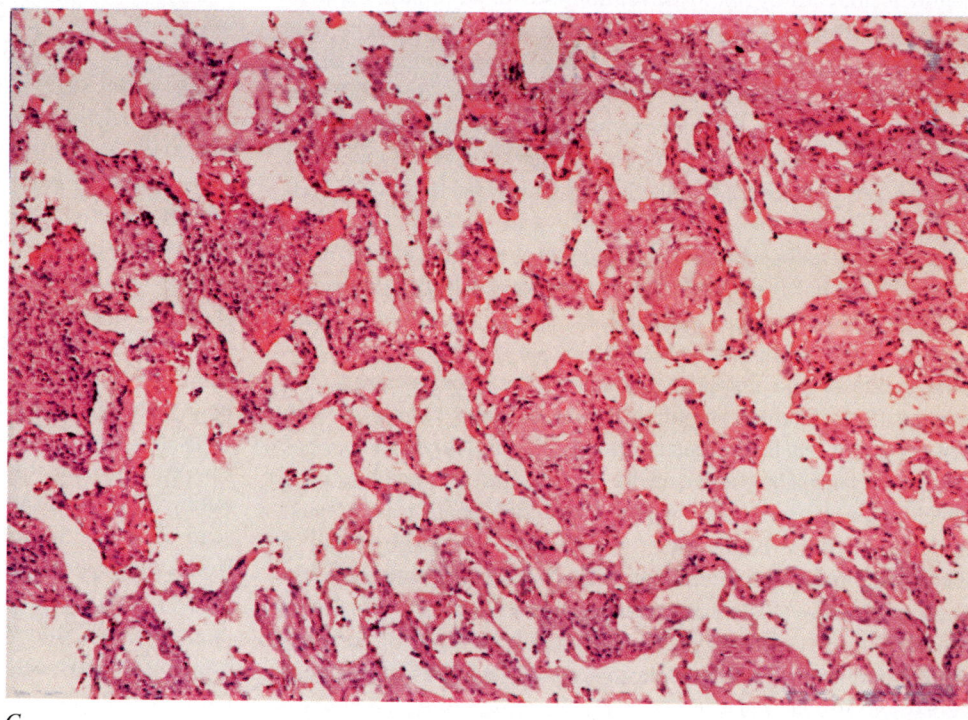

C

FIGURE 67-2 Methotrexate pulmonary toxicity in a patient with rheumatoid arthritis. *A.* Normal radiographic appearance before the onset of toxicity. *B.* Bilateral diffuse interstitial infiltrates seen during the acute episode of toxicity. *C.* Open lung biopsy taken at the time of the chest film shown in panel *B,* showing thickened intra-alveolar septae and infiltration with mononuclear inflammatory cells. *(Courtesy of Dr. Peter Rogol, Division of Pulmonary and Critical Care Medicine, Yale University School of Medicine.)*

eral eosinophilia is seen in one-third to one-half of the patients experiencing this complication. Radiographically, a bilateral interstitial or mixed interstitial-alveolar pattern occurs, in some cases accompanied by a pleural effusion or hilar adenopathy (Fig. 67-2). Pulmonary function studies reveal a restrictive ventilatory defect with decreased diffusing capacity. Histologically, mononuclear cell interstitial infiltration is accompanied in acute cases by type II pneumocyte hyperplasia and in more chronic cases by interstitial fibrosis (Fig. 67-2). Isolated areas of bronchiolitis obliterans may also be noted. In contrast to most other forms of drug-induced lung disease, noncaseating granulomas are sometimes present.

Patients taking low-dose methotrexate are at increased risk for opportunistic infections.[30] It is interesting to note that there is an especially high frequency of infectious complications in rheumatoid arthritis patients taking methotrexate compared to rheumatoid patients on other immunosuppressive regimens. *Pneumocystis carinii* pneumonia is the most common complication. Disseminated histoplasmosis, herpes zoster, and a variety of other infections can occur. In contrast to the clinical features of *P. carinii* pneumonia in AIDS patients, peripheral CD4-positive lymphocyte counts do not clearly identify patients at increased risk for this complication. Therefore, exclusion of opportunistic pathogens is especially important in the differential diagnosis of methotrexate pneumonitis.

The treatment of methotrexate pneumonitis includes withdrawal of the drug and supportive care. Corticosteroids may also be useful and are generally initiated after infection has been excluded. However, there are no clear guidelines for the optimal dose or duration of therapy. Although fatalities can occur, the outcome is generally favorable.

Gold

Gold compounds have been used in the treatment of rheumatoid arthritis since 1929. The first case of pulmonary toxicity in this setting was recognized in 1948.[54] Gold can be given parenterally (gold sodium thiomalate) and in an orally absorbable form (auranofin). Both preparations can cause pulmonary toxicity. In addition to rheumatoid arthritis, gold-induced pulmonary toxicity has been reported during the treatment of asthma, osteoarthritis, and pemphigus. Although more than 60 cases have been reported, the overall incidence of this side effect is less than 1 percent. There are no proven risk factors for the development of gold pneumonitis. There is, however, a strong association between this disorder and the HLA-B40 and -B35 haplotypes. Gold typically causes an interstitial pneumonitis. A small number of patients with bronchiolitis obliterans have also been noted. However, the association between bronchiolitis obliterans and gold use is much more tenuous than that with penicillamine therapy.

Clinically, gold toxicity usually occurs after 2 to 4 months of therapy. Patients with this toxicity present with dyspnea, cough, fever, skin rash, and peripheral eosinophilia. Radiographically, the most common pattern is a diffuse interstitial infiltrate. Less commonly, mixed infiltrates or purely alveolar patterns are seen. Lung biopsy findings include alveolar septal thickening, interstitial fibrosis, and interstitial mononuclear cell infiltration. Gold particles are often observed within macrophage lysosomes.

The precise pathogenesis of gold-induced lung disease is not known. Evidence in favor of an immune mechanism includes the presence of elevated serum IgE levels and peripheral eosinophilia, the ability of gold to induce in vitro lymphocyte proliferation, and the appreciation of a BAL lymphocytosis with decreased CD4:CD8 ratios in many patients.

The mainstays of treatment of gold toxicity include drug withdrawal and corticosteroids. Improvement without steroid treatment is rare. Since relapse is sometimes observed after rapid steroid withdrawal, a treatment duration of at least 1 to 3 months is recommended.

Penicillamine

The anti-inflammatory, antifibrotic, and copper-chelating effects of penicillamine make it an attractive agent for the treatment of a variety of disorders, including rheumatoid arthritis, primary biliary cirrhosis, scleroderma, and Wilson's disease. In the course of its utilization, it has been documented to cause a wide variety of systemic toxicities, including membranous glomerulonephritis, a myasthenia gravis–like syndrome, and drug-induced systemic lupus erythematosus. The pulmonary manifestations of penicillamine toxicity include interstitial lung disease, bronchiolitis obliterans, and alveolar hemorrhage occurring as part of a pulmonary-renal syndrome.[54]

Penicillamine-Associated Interstitial Lung Disease Penicillamine use is associated with both the chronic alveolitis/fibrosis and hypersensitivity varieties of interstitial lung disease. Unlike the other forms of penicillamine-associated lung toxicity, interstitial lung disease has been reported only in patients being treated for rheumatoid arthritis. Thus it is somewhat difficult to differentiate the contributions that penicillamine and the underlying collagen vascular disease make to the genesis of this toxic reaction.

Patients with penicillamine-induced interstitial disease usually have nonspecific respiratory complaints. They also manifest a restrictive ventilatory defect with decreased diffusing capacity and chest radiographs with diffuse interstitial infiltrates. In the subgroup of patients with hypersensitivity reactions, elevated serum IgE levels and peripheral eosinophilia are observed. In the few cases with well-documented pathologic findings, type II alveolar epithelial hyperplasia, desquamative changes, and interstitial fibrosis have been reported. This form of toxicity is characterized by a favorable response to corticosteroids, a lack of residual pulmonary function derangements, and a low mortality.

Penicillamine-Associated Bronchiolitis Obliterans Bronchiolitis obliterans in the absence of organizing pneumonia occurs as a pulmonary complication of rheumatoid arthritis and as a sequela of viral pneumonia and inhalational injury. In addition to these causes, there is a strong association between penicillamine therapy and bronchiolitis obliterans. While it is possible that this association is artifactual, reflecting only the severity of the rheumatoid arthritis in patients taking penicillamine, a single case that occurred in a patient taking penicillamine for eosinophilic fasciitis supports the concept that this is a separate process.

The incidence of penicillamine-induced bronchiolitis obliterans is not known. It is known to be rare, however, occurring in slightly less than 1 percent of the rheumatoid arthritis patients on this therapy. There are no clearly defined risk factors that contribute to the frequency of this toxic response. Patients who develop bronchiolitis obliterans in this setting note the subacute onset of cough, wheeze, and dyspnea. On auscultation, severe expiratory wheezes and a high-pitched "midinspiratory squeak" are often appreciated. Chest radiographs reveal increased lung volumes in the absence of pulmonary infiltrates. Pulmonary function findings include an obstructive ventilatory defect without bronchodilator reversibility, markedly increased lung volumes due to air trapping, and a normal diffusing capacity when corrected for alveolar volume. Biopsies from these patients are remarkable for bronchiolar narrowing caused by mononuclear inflammation and fibrosis. This narrowing is usually concentric, rather than eccentric or polypoid.

Drug withdrawal and supportive therapy are the mainstays of treatment for penicillamine-induced bronchiolitis obliterans. Corticosteroids, azathioprine, and cyclophosphamide have also been used in the treatment of this disorder. However, it is unclear whether any of these agents have a substantial impact on outcome. Unfortunately, the prognosis of this form of penicillamine toxicity is poor. Approximately 50 percent of reported cases have had a fatal outcome, and in patients who survive, severe residual obstructive impairment is common.

Penicillamine-Associated Pulmonary Renal Syndrome   Goodpasture's syndrome is characterized by diffuse alveolar hemorrhage and rapidly progressive glomerulonephritis, caused by the production of autoantibodies to glomerular and alveolar basement membrane constituents. Although most cases of Goodpasture's syndrome are idiopathic, a pulmonary-renal syndrome with similar features can occur as a complication of penicillamine therapy. This complication is rare, and fewer than a dozen cases have been reported. It has been reported to occur during penicillamine chelation therapy for Wilson's disease as well as in the treatment of rheumatoid arthritis, indicating that this syndrome is not merely a manifestation of the underlying collagen vascular disease.

There are no defined risk factors for the development of this pulmonary-renal syndrome. In addition, the mechanism in the pathogenesis of the disorder is unknown. The syndrome may occur after a wide variety of dosing regimens and treatment durations. Patients with this syndrome experience the rapid onset of cough, dyspnea, hemoptysis, and hematuria. These symptoms are associated with acute renal failure and severe hypoxemia. Progressive respiratory failure requiring mechanical ventilatory support is common. Chest radiographs show diffuse alveolar infiltrates without cardiomegaly or pleural effusions.

Unlike the situation with idiopathic Goodpasture's syndrome, circulating anti–glomerular basement membrane (GBM) antibodies have been reported only rarely in the penicillamine-induced disorder. Serum antinuclear antibodies are often present at high titer, but in contrast to idiopathic systemic lupus erythematosus, anti–double-stranded DNA antibodies are negative and complement levels are normal. Pathologically, the acute renal failure is the result of a crescentic glomerulonephritis. Linear anti-GBM immunofluorescence, a typical finding in idiopathic Goodpasture's syndrome, is seen only in rare cases. Instead, complement and immunoglobulin deposits with a "lumpy" appearance are noted in glomerular regions. BAL in these patients reveals red blood cells and hemosiderin-laden macrophages. Open

lung biopsies show alveolar hemorrhage in the absence of linear anti-GBM staining or pulmonary vasculitis.

The prognosis of this complication of penicillamine therapy is poor, with a mortality of about 50 percent and a high incidence of progression to chronic renal insufficiency and dialysis. In patients who recover, a residual restrictive ventilatory defect with decreased diffusing capacity is common. Drug withdrawal and high-dose steroids are always employed in treatment. Although anti-GBM antibodies are almost never detected, plasmapheresis has been attempted in many cases. In addition, cyclophosphamide or azathioprine is often used as an adjunctive immunosuppressive agent. Although there are no controlled trials that demonstrate the safety or efficacy of this aggressive management strategy, the apparent anecdotal success and the generally poor prognosis of the pulmonary-renal syndrome support the use of these measures.

COMPLICATIONS OF ILLICIT DRUG USE

The use of illicit drugs has reached epidemic proportions in many countries. Since there are a variety of pulmonary complications associated with illicit drug use, these drugs have become major causes of respiratory morbidity (Table 67-2). Many of these complications have been appreciated for decades. They include the ability of sedative and hypnotic agents to diminish respiratory drive, resulting in alveolar hypoventilation and, when severe, hypercarbic respiratory failure, and to decrease patients' level of consciousness and alter their gag reflex, putting them at high risk for gastric aspiration and aspiration pneumonia. In addition, intravenous injections commonly cause right heart endocarditis and other endovascular infections, which can result in septic pulmonary emboli and pulmonary infarction. It has recently been appreciated that the incidence of HIV infection is high even among users of illicit drugs who do not inject intravenously. Therefore HIV-associated opportunistic pulmonary infections are a concern in these patients. Finally, intravenous drug abusers are at high risk for community-acquired pneumonia, as well as drug-sensitive and multidrug-resistant tuberculosis. Each of these processes must be considered in the differential diagnosis of lung abnormalities in patients who use illicit drugs. In addition to these complications, there are several other pulmonary disorders associated with illicit drug abuse that need to be considered. They are summarized below.

Complications of Central Venous Cannulation

Intravenous drug users who have destroyed the peripheral vessels of their extremities will often attempt to obtain vascular access by using their internal jugular and subclavian veins. They will attempt to cannulate these vessels themselves or with the help of others, who are paid to perform the injections. These attempts can be complicated by symptomatic pneumothoraces, sometimes requiring chest tube drainage. The incidence of pleural space infection is surprisingly low in these patients. In contrast, soft-tissue and endovascular infections occur quite commonly. In addition, aneurysms and dissections following inadvertent arterial cannulation are well documented.

TABLE 67-2

Complications of Illicit Drug Use

Alveolar hypoventilation, hypercarbic respiratory failure
Gastric aspiration, aspiration pneumonia
Endocarditis, intravascular infections, septic emboli
HIV-associated infections
Tuberculosis
Complications of central cannulation
   Pneumothorax
   Intravascular infections
   Soft-tissue infections
   Arterial aneurysm and or dissection
Foreign-body granulomatosis
Opiate-induced pulmonary edema
Cocaine "crack" lung
   Bronchospasm
   Pneumothorax, pneumomediastinum, pneumopericardium
   Airway burns
   Noncardiac pulmonary edema
   Pulmonary infiltrates with eosinophilia
   Acute alveolar hemorrhage syndrome

Foreign-Body Granulomatosis

Foreign-body granulomatosis results from the injection of insoluble material during intravenous drug abuse. It can be caused by particulate contaminants used to "cut" street heroin. It also occurs as a result of the injection of crushed tablets, meant for oral ingestion, that contain substantial amounts of filler substances such as talc (magnesium silicate) and methyl cellulose. The injected material lodges in pulmonary arterioles and initiates a thrombogenic response. The foreign material is indigestible by phagocytic cells and thus elicits a granulomatous inflammatory response, causing chronic pulmonary vascular and parenchymal destruction. Amphetamine tablets, as well as opiates such as methadone, pentazocine, and hydromorphone, are often abused in this fashion.

Patients with foreign-body granulomatosis can be asymptomatic. However, they more commonly experience relentlessly progressive dyspnea. During the early phase, chest radiographs show nodular interstitial infiltrates. Over several years, these nodules can coalesce to form large infiltrates resembling the *progressive massive fibrosis syndrome* that sometimes complicates inhalational silicosis. These large fibrotic masses are surrounded by cystic and bullous spaces—which can rupture, producing pneumothoraces. Surprisingly, the early phase is characterized by a mild obstructive ventilatory defect rather than restrictive physiology. As the disorder progresses, the bullous and cystic changes are accompanied by worsening airflow obstruction, air trapping, and a markedly decreased diffusing capacity.[38]

In addition to the radiographic similarity to silicosis, foreign-body granulomatosis has some clinical features that are reminiscent of sarcoidosis.[16] As with sarcoidosis, pulmonary gallium[67] scanning is positive, and serum ACE levels can be elevated. In contrast, other features of sarcoidosis—such as cutaneous anergy, BAL lymphocytosis, and alterations in the BAL

lymphocyte CD4:CD8 ratio—are often absent. Lung biopsies from patients with foreign-body granulomatosis reveal vascular, perivascular, and interstitial noncaseating giant-cell granulomas containing birefringent material. These birefringent talc particles are often greater than 10 μm in length—a size much larger, on average, than particles that can be deposited into the distal lung parenchyma after inhalation. The granulomatous inflammation induced by these particles progresses, causing pulmonary hypertension, parenchymal destruction, and scarring—ultimately resulting in respiratory failure and cor pulmonale. Corticosteroids have little effect on the poor outcome seen in most cases of foreign-body granulomatosis.[38]

Opiate-Induced Pulmonary Edema

Acute pulmonary edema is a common complication of serious heroin overdoses.[14] Pulmonary edema has been seen following inadvertent and intentional overdoses with a wide variety of oral and intravenous narcotics in addition to heroin. Opiate antagonists such as naloxone are also capable of causing pulmonary edema, often paradoxically when they are used during the treatment of an overdose or intoxication. In addition, pulmonary edema occurs after overdoses with nonopiate sedative and hypnotic agents such as ethchlorvynol and chlordiazepoxide.

There are no known risk factors for the development of opiate-induced pulmonary edema. The pulmonary edema is noncardiogenic; however, the pathogenetic mechanisms responsible for its generation are unknown. Altered alveolar-capillary permeability caused by an increase in catechol production (similar to the mechanism proposed for neurogenic pulmonary edema) has been postulated. Direct opiate cytotoxicity, drug hypersensitivity, hypoxemic alveolar injury, and negative-pressure injury caused by transient upper-airway obstruction have also been proposed. However, none of these mechanisms have been adequately investigated in either animal models or human studies. Autopsies of patients with opiate-induced pulmonary edema reveal alveolar edema and hemorrhage, often with interstitial polymorphonuclear inflammatory infiltrates. Diffuse alveolar damage with hyaline membranes and pneumocyte hyperplasia can be seen in severe cases. Pulmonary edema is usually apparent on presentation, but it can occur up to 24 h after the initial episode of intoxication. Patients with this complication experience dyspnea and appear cyanotic. These symptoms are accompanied by a typical perihilar alveolar infiltrate on the chest radiograph. In some cases, a depressed sensorium caused by the CNS effects of the opiate may mask the dyspnea. In addition, the clinical picture can be clouded by the presence of fever, especially when gastric aspiration has occurred. In some cases, opiate-induced pulmonary edema progresses to ARDS. Such patients have a more protracted course, with a longer duration of mechanical ventilation. However, if ARDS, pneumonia, or other complications of intravenous drug abuse do not supervene, the pulmonary edema usually resolves with supportive care over 48 to 72 h.

Pulmonary Complications of Cocaine Use

Cocaine is a sympathomimetic that acts as a topical anesthetic and CNS stimulant. The salt, cocaine hydrochloride, can be injected intravenously and is also rapidly absorbed across the nasopharyngeal mucosa. The mucosal vasoconstriction caused by cocaine can result in ischemic necrosis and perforation of the nasal septum. Cocaine hydrochloride is not heat stable and thus cannot be smoked. Free-base cocaine is prepared by alkaline precipitation of the hydrochloride salt. Free-base cocaine is thermally stable and vaporizes when heated, allowing rapid absorption of large quantities of the drug across the pulmonary epithelial surface. The term "crack" refers to the popping sound made by the cocaine crystals as they are heated.[18]

While the pulmonary toxicities of intravenous cocaine are similar to those of intravenous opiates, free-base cocaine smoking causes a distinct spectrum of pulmonary disorders often referred to as "crack lung."[28] Complaints of cough, chest pain, dyspnea, hemoptysis, wheezing and expectoration of soot are typical among cocaine smokers. Other common sequelae are thermal burns of the upper airway and trachea, and pneumothorax, pneumomediastinum, or pneumopericardium caused by strong Valsalva maneuvers during the act of smoking. Whether or not chronic cocaine use has an effect on baseline pulmonary function values is controversial. A reduction in diffusing capacity has been observed in some studies, whereas others have shown no abnormalities. Crack smoking is, however, associated with acute pulmonary edema, pulmonary infiltrates with eosinophilia, and acute alveolar hemorrhage.

Cocaine-induced pulmonary edema is usually noncardiogenic and often culminates in hypoxemic respiratory failure. The acute lung injury that underlies this syndrome is probably caused by direct toxic effects of cocaine on the alveolar epithelium and pulmonary vasculature. However, in many cases a cardiogenic component to the edema may also be present owing to cocaine-induced myocardial infarction or severe systemic hypertension. In most uncomplicated cases, the infiltrates and hypoxemia resolve within 24 to 48 h.

An acute pulmonary hemorrhage syndrome with chest pain, hemoptysis, and fleeting interstitial or alveolar infiltrates is also commonly noted in cocaine abusers. The clinical presentation ranges in severity from recurrent low-grade hemoptysis, resulting in iron deficiency anemia, to massive hemoptysis and fatal asphyxiation. Pathologically, alveolar hemorrhage and hemosiderin-laden macrophages are seen in the absence of pulmonary vasculitis. Of interest is that pathologic evidence of pulmonary hemorrhage is found coincidentally at autopsy in up to 70 percent of free-base cocaine smokers regardless of the direct cause of death.[4] Some patients with cocaine-induced pulmonary hemorrhage develop severe disease with fatal respiratory failure. In most cases, however, the outcome is favorable, with radiographic and clinical resolution in 2 to 5 days.

REFERENCES

1. Allen JN, Davis WB: Eosinophilic lung diseases. *Am J Respir Crit Care Med* 150:1423–1438, 1994.
2. Anderson RJ, Potts DE, Gabow PA, et al: Unrecognized adult salicylate intoxication. *Ann Intern Med* 85:745–748, 1976.
3. Argov Z, Mastaglia FL: Disorders of neuromuscular transmission caused by drugs. *New Engl J Med* 301:409–413, 1979.
4. Bailey ME, Fraire AE, Greenberg SD, et al: Pulmonary histopathology in cocaine abusers. *Hum Pathol* 25:203–205, 1994.
5. Barrera P, Laan RFJM, van Riel PLCM, et al: Methotrexate-related pulmonary complications in rheumatoid arthritis. *Ann Rheum Dis* 53:434–439, 1994.
6. Bero CJ, Rihn TL: Possible association of pulmonary fibrosis with mexiletine. *DICP* 25:1329–1331, 1991.
7. Bjorck T, Gustafsson LE, Dahlen S-E: Isolated bronchi from asthmatics are hyperresponsive to adenosine, which apparently acts indirectly by liberation of leukotrienes and histamine. *Am Rev Respir Dis* 145:1087–1091, 1992.
8. Chamberlain DW, Hyland RH, Ross DJ: Diphenylhydantoin-induced lymphocytic interstitial pneumonia. *Chest* 90:458–460, 1986.
9. Cooper JAD Jr, White DA, Matthay R: Drug-induced pulmonary disease. Part 1: Cytotoxic drugs. *Am Rev Respir Dis* 133:321–340, 1986.
10. Cooper JAD Jr, White DA, Matthay R: Drug-induced pulmonary disease. Part 2: Non-cytotoxic drugs. *Am Rev Respir Dis* 133:488–505, 1986.
11. Coudert B, Bailly F, Lombard JN, et al: Amiodarone pneumonitis: Bronchoalveolar lavage findings in 15 patients and review of the literature. *Chest* 102:1005–1012, 1992.
12. Cush JJ, Goldings EA: Drug-induced lupus: Clinical spectrum and pathogenesis. *Am J Med Sci* 290:36–45, 1985.
13. Cushley MJ, Tattersfield AE, Holgate ST: Adenosine-induced bronchoconstriction in asthma: Antagonism by inhaled theophylline. *Am Rev Respir Dis* 129:380–384, 1984.
14. Duberstein JL, Kaufman DM: A clinical study of an epidemic of heroin intoxication and heroin-induced pulmonary edema. *Am J Med* 51:704–714, 1971.
15. Dusman RE, Stanton MS, Miles WM, et al: Clinical features of amiodarone-induced pulmonary toxicity. *Circulation* 82:51–59, 1990.
16. Farber HW, Fairman RP, Glauser F: Talc granulomatosis: Laboratory findings similar to sarcoidosis. *Am Rev Respir Dis* 125:258–261, 1982.
17. Fischer AR, Israel E: Identifying and treating aspirin-induced asthma. *J Respir Dis* 16:304–317, 1995.
18. Haim DY, Lippmann ML, Goldberg SK, Walkenstein MD: The pulmonary complications of crack cocaine: A comprehensive review. *Chest* 107:233–240, 1995.
19. Hargreaves MR, Benson MK: Inhaled sodium cromoglycate in angiotensin-converting enzyme inhibitor cough. *Lancet* 345:13–16, 1995.
20. Heffner JE, Sahn SA: Salicylate-induced pulmonary edema: Clinical features and prognosis. *Ann Intern Med* 95:405–409, 1981.
21. Heitzman ER: Lymphadenopathy related to anticonvulsant therapy: Roentgen findings simulating lymphoma. *Radiology* 89:311–312, 1967.
22. Hohnloser SH, Meinertz T, Stubbs P, et al: Efficacy and safety of *d*-sotalol, a pure class III antiarrythmic compound, in patients with symptomatic complex ventricular ectopy. *Circulation* 92:1517–1525, 1995.
23. Holmberg L, Boman G: Pulmonary reactions to nitrofurantoin. *Eur J Respir Dis* 62:180–189, 1981.
24. Israel E, Fischer AR, Rosenberg MA, et al: The pivotal role of 5-lipoxygenase products in the reaction of aspirin-sensitive asthmatics to aspirin. *Am Rev Respir Dis* 148:1447–1451, 1993.
25. Israili ZH, Hall WD: Cough and angioneurotic edema associated with angiotensin-converting enzyme inhibitor therapy. *Ann Intern Med* 117:234–242, 1992.
26. Jick S, Jick H, Walker A, Hunter J: Hospitalizations for pulmonary reactions following nitrofurantoin use. *Chest* 96:512–515, 1989.

27. Kaufman J, Casanova JE, Riendl P, Sclueter DP: Bronchial hyperreactivity and cough due to angiotensin-converting enzyme inhibitors. *Chest* 95:544–548, 1989.

28. Kissner DG, Dwayne LW, Selias JE, Flint A: Crack Lung: Pulmonary disease caused by cocaine abuse. *Am Rev Respir Dis* 136:1250–1252, 1987.

29. Kupferschmid JP, Rosengart TK, McIntosh CL, et al: Amiodarone-induced complications after cardiac operation for obstructive hypertrophic cardiomyopathy. *Ann Thorac Surg* 48:359–364, 1989.

30. Lemense GP, Sahn SA: Opportunistic infection during treatment with low dose methotrexate. *Am J Respir Crit Care Med* 150:258–260, 1994.

31. Levy JH, Schwieger IM, Zaidan JR, et al: Evaluation of patients at risk for protamine reactions. *J Thorac Cardiovasc Surg* 98:200–204, 1989.

32. Martin WJ, Rosenow EC: Amiodarone pulmonary toxicity: Recognition and pathogenesis (Part I). *Chest* 93:1067–1074, 1988.

33. Martin WJ, Rosenow EC: Amiodarone pulmonary toxicity: Recognition and pathogenesis (Part II). *Chest* 93:1242–1248, 1988.

34. Mason JW: Prediction of amiodarone-induced pulmonary toxicity. *Am J Med* 86:2–3, 1989.

35. McCormack GD, Barth WF: Quinidine induced lupus syndrome. *Semin Arthritis Rheum* 15:73–79, 1985.

36. Michael JR, Rudin M: Acute pulmonary disease caused by phenytoin. *Ann Intern Med* 95:452–454, 1981.

37. Mickleborough LL, Maruyama H, Mohamed S, et al: Are patients receiving amiodarone at increased risk for cardiac operations? *Ann Thorac Surg* 58:622–629, 1994.

38. Pare JP, Cote G, Fraser RS: Long-term follow-up of drug abusers with intravenous talcosis. *Am Rev Respir Dis* 139:233–241, 1989.

39. Pirmohamed M, Graham A, Roberts P, et al: Carbamazepine-hypersensitivity: Assessment of clinical and in vitro chemical cross-reactivity with phenytoin and oxcarbazepine. *Br J Clin Pharmacol* 32:741–749, 1991.

40. Pisani RJ, Rosenow EJ: Pulmonary edema associated with tocolytic therapy. *Ann Intern Med* 110:714–718, 1989.

41. Pittinger CB, Eryasa Y, Adamson R: Antibiotic-induced paralysis. *Anesth Analg (Cleve)* 49:487–501, 1970.

42. Ranhosky A, Kempthorne-Rawson J: The safety of intravenous dipyridamole thallium myocardial perfusion imaging. *Circulation* 81:1205–1209, 1990.

43. Ravid D, Lishner M, Lang R, Ravid M: Angiotensin-converting enzyme inhibitors and cough: A prospective evaluation in hypertension and in congestive heart failure. *J Clin Pharmacol* 34:1116–1120, 1994.

44. Ren H, Kuhlman JE, Hruban RH, et al: CT-pathology correlation of amiodarone lung. *J Comp Assist Tom* 14:760–765, 1990.

45. Rosenow EC: The spectrum of drug-induced pulmonary disease. *Ann Intern Med* 77:977–991, 1972.

46. Rothfield NF, Bierer WF, Garfield JW: Isoniazid induction of antinuclear antibodies: A prospective study. *Ann Intern Med* 88:650–652, 1978.

47. Sharma A, Provenzale D, McKusick A, Kaplan MM: Interstitial pneumonitis after low-dose methotrexate therapy in primary biliary cirrhosis. *Gastroenterology* 107:266–270, 1994.

48. Stein MJ, Demarco T, Gamsu G, et al: Computed tomography: Pathologic correlation in lung disease due to tocainide. *Am Rev Respir Dis* 137:458–460, 1988.

49. Van Mieghem W, Coolen L, Malysse I, et al: Amiodarone and the development of ARDS after lung surgery. *Chest* 105:1642–1645, 1994.

50. Wakefield TW, Lindblad B, Stanley TJ, et al: Heparin and protamine use in peripheral vascular surgery: A comparison between surgeons of the Society for Vascular Surgery and the European Society for Vascular Surgery. *Eur J Vasc Surg* 8:193–198, 1994.

51. Wallin JD: Beta-adrenergic blockers in the hypertensive asthmatic patient. *Chest* 88:801–802, 1985.

52. Woosley RL, Drayer DE, Reidenberg MM, et al: Effect of acetylator phenotype on the rate at which procainamide induces antinuclear antibodies and the lupus syndrome. *New Engl J Med* 298:1157–1159, 1978.

53. Yermakov VM, Hitti IF, Sutton AL: Necrotizing vasculitis associated with diphenylhydantoin: Two fatal cases. *Hum Pathol* 13:182–184, 1983.

54. Zitnik RJ, Cooper JAD: Pulmonary disease due to antirheumatic agents. *Clin Chest Med* 11:139–150, 1990.

PART SEVEN

INTERSTITIAL AND INFLAMMATORY LUNG DISEASES

CHAPTER 68

INTERSTITIAL LUNG DISEASE: A CLINICAL OVERVIEW AND GENERAL APPROACH

Ganesh Raghu

EPIDEMIOLOGY

CLINICAL APPROACH AND DIFFERENTIAL DIAGNOSIS
   Chest Radiographic Patterns
   Pulmonary Physiology Testing
   Computed Tomography and High-Resolution CT
      Images
   Bronchoalveolar Lavage
   Bronchoscopy with Transbronchial Biopsy
   Surgical Lung Biopsy: Thoracoscopy-Guided and Open
      Lung Biopsy
   Treatment

It has been nearly 65 years since Hamman and Rich described the first case of progressive pulmonary fibrosis that resulted in death.[9] Since then, several acute and chronic lung disorders with variable degrees of pulmonary fibrosis have been described and are commonly referred to as the *interstitial lung diseases* (ILDs). *Diffuse parenchymal lung disease* is, perhaps, a more appropriate descriptive term for this heterogeneous group of lung diseases, since the term *interstitium* actually refers to the microscopic anatomic space bounded by the basement membranes of epithelial and endothelial cells. Within this interstitial space, fibroblastlike cells (mesenchymal and connective tissue cells) and

extracellular matrix components (interstitial collagens, elastin, proteoglycans) are present. It is clear that the disease is not restricted to the interstitium, as it involves epithelial, endothelial, and mesenchymal cells, macrophages and recruited inflammatory cells, secreted proteins, and aberration of matrix components within the alveolar walls. In addition, the disease process extends into the alveolar space, acini, bronchiolar lumen, and bronchioles. The initial host response is inflammation of the alveolar walls, airspace, and terminal bronchioles, leading to irreversible pulmonary fibrosis in some patients. Thus, the entire pulmonary parenchyma is affected in ILD. Despite this misnomer, it seems appropriate to continue to use the term as long as the scope of these diseases is appreciated.

In the apparently normal, immunocompetent host, clinicians recognize the heterogeneous group of ILD as a syndrome with the following common clinical features: (1) exertional dyspnea; (2) bilateral diffuse infiltrates on chest radiographs; (3) physiological abnormalities with a restrictive lung defect, decreased diffusing capacity (D_{LCO}), and abnormal alveolar–arterial oxygen gradient (P_{AO_2}–P_{aO_2}) at rest or with exertion; (4) absence of pulmonary infection and neoplasm; and (5) histopathology with varying degrees of fibrosis and inflammation, with or without evidence of granulomatous or secondary vascular changes in the pulmonary parenchyma. Idiopathic pulmonary fibrosis (IPF), a distinct clinical entity, is considered the prototypic ILD. Since there are no pathognomonic features for IPF, it is often diagnosed by careful elimination of other interstitial disorders.

The term *fibrosing alveolitis* has also been used to describe ILDs in general. The term *cryptogenic fibrosis alveolitis* (CFA— "cryptogenic" meaning hidden) has been used for diseases, such as IPF, in which the pathogenesis of the alveolitis and pulmonary fibrosis is still unclear. Since the clinical course and prognosis of CFA and ILD associated with collagen vascular disease differ, the term *lone CFA* has been introduced to refer specifically to IPF.

In some ILDs, the small airways—the respiratory and terminal bronchioles—are primarily affected. Respiratory bronchiolitis–associated interstitial lung disease (RBILD) is an idiopathic inflammatory condition of respiratory bronchioles and adjacent alveolar structures, occurring almost exclusively in cigarette smokers. While RBILD is physiologically characterized by a restrictive lung defect (with or without coexisting airflow obstruction), bronchiolitis obliterans (BO—also referred to as obliterative bronchiolitis), a disorder localized to the walls of the small airways, is physiologically characterized by obstructive airflow defect. BO may occur as an idiopathic entity or as a result of exposure to toxic gases, viral infection, complication of bone marrow or lung transplantation, or may be associated with collagen vascular diseases (especially rheumatoid arthritis). Since there is no alveolar inflammation in BO, it should not be confused with bronchiolitis obliterans organizing pneumonia (BOOP) that is characterized by a restrictive lung defect and histologically by an organizing noninfectious pneumonia associated with an inflammatory exudative and fibrotic process within the small airways. (Bronchiolitis obliterans syndrome [BOS], a distinct clinical entity occurring in the transplanted lung, also involves the small airways primarily and should not be confused with BO or BOOP that occurs in nontransplant situations.) BOOP can manifest in several clinical situations, including pulmonary disorders associated with collagen vascular diseases and drug and environmental causes. The term *cryptogenic organizing pneumonia* (COP) has also been used to describe BOOP. When a cause or associated clinical disorder (such as a collagen vascular disease) cannot be identified, the term *idiopathic BOOP* or *lone COP* has been used.

In thinking of the ILDs, it is important to differentiate terms used to define clinical entities and terms describing the pathologic lesions of these disorders. IPF, CFA, lone CFA, idiopathic BOOP/lone COP, RBILD, BO, BOS, and acute interstitial pneumonia of unknown origin (probably the previously described Hamman-Rich syndrome) are descriptions of clinical syndromes. Pathologic descriptions include usual interstitial pneumonia, desquamative interstitial pneumonia, lymphocytic interstitial pneumonia, giant cell interstitial pneumonitis, diffuse alveolar damage, nonclassifiable interstitial pneumonia, and BOOP. Identical pathologic lesions can be seen in a variety of clinical syndromes, and a variety of pathologic entities can be seen in a single lung biopsy. In addition, the boundaries between these clinical and pathologic entities are not always clear. For example, desquamative interstitial pneumonia, originally thought to represent the early cellular stage of IPF, is known to aptly describe RBILD. In contrast, usual interstitial pneumonia, initially

described as the late fibrotic phase of IPF, remains a characteristic histologic feature of this disorder. Nevertheless, these clinical and pathologic terms have informational features in their own right. Each is useful as long as its relationship to other entities is appropriately acknowledged.

EPIDEMIOLOGY

Relatively little is known about the epidemiology of ILD in general populations. Recent epidemiologic studies suggest that the incidence of ILD is more frequent than previously recognized. Specifically, the incidence ranges from 3 to 26 per 100,000 per year.[3,29] Among these, IPF is the most common, representing at least 30 percent of the incident cases. Furthermore, the prevalence of preclinical and undiagnosed ILD in the community is estimated to be 10 times that of the clinically recognized disease.[3]

CLINICAL APPROACH AND DIFFERENTIAL DIAGNOSIS

The clinician confronted with a patient with possible ILD faces a significant challenge. He or she must first determine if the patient has ILD. This requires the consideration and appropriate elimination of a variety of other pathologic processes that can mimic the interstitial disorders. This is particularly important in the setting of acquired immunosuppression (drug or virus induced) and transplantation, where opportunistic lung infection, neoplasm, and transplant-related immunologic problems need to be primarily addressed. Similarly, diffuse neoplasia, congestive heart failure, pulmonary infection, occupational exposure, and pulmonary vascular disorders (such as Wegener's granulomatosis) must be suspected in appropriate clinical settings. Even when appropriate screening has taken place, the clinician must be aware that the clinical diagnosis of ILD in the apparently normal immunocompetent host is not always accurate. This can be appreciated by a look at the specific diagnoses made by open lung biopsy in patients with this syndrome (Table 68-1). In one large series of 1234 patients with ILD accumulated over several years, 502 (40 percent) underwent open lung biopsy.[6] IPF was the diagnosis in more than one-third of patients subjected to open lung biopsy.[6,7] Appreciable frequencies of neoplasia, infection, congestive heart failure, pneumoconioses, and pulmonary vascular disease were also noted.

ILD presents a clinical conundrum to the physician confronted with a given patient. First, the physician has to amass specific knowledge relating to the common causes of ILD (some of which are reviewed in Table 68-2). The physician also has to be aware of at least 150 other clinical entities and situations associated with ILD. Second, owing to the broad differential diagnoses and the availability of various ever-evolving invasive and noninvasive diagnostic techniques, the best approach to use to establish a specific diagnosis is frequently difficult to determine. Third, in a significant portion of patients, a conclusive cause cannot be ascertained even when the most invasive diagnostic pathways are taken. Often, the lung biopsy reveals nonspecific inflammation or end-stage fibrosis potentially attributable to the chronic progression of a variety of pulmonary inflammatory responses. Fi-

TABLE 68-1

Diagnostic Groups in 502 Patients with ILD Subjected to Open Lung Biopsy

Diagnosis	Number of patients	(%)
Idiopathic pulmonary fibrosis*	175	(34.9)
Granulomatous (sarcoid, Wegener's, etc.)	83	(16.6)
Pneumoconioses	74	(14.7)
Unusual, specific (eosinophilic granuloma, alveolar proteinosis, etc.)	43	(8.6)
"Allergic" (eosinophilic pneumonia, allergic alveolitis, etc.)	34	(6.8)
Malignant neoplasm	26	(5.2)
Pulmonary vascular disease	19	(3.8)
Infections	16	(3.2)
Bronchiolitis obliterans	11	(2.2)
Pleural disease only	11	(2.2)
Cardiac (passive congestion)	6	(1.2)
Normal lung	4	(0.8)
Total	502	

*Includes usual interstitial pneumonia, desquamatative interstitial pneumonia, acute interstitial pneumonia, honeycombing, nonspecific pulmonary fibrosis.
SOURCE: Modified from Gaensler and Carrington.[6]

nally, even when a specific diagnosis is made, an effective therapeutic regimen is not available for many patients with ILD, as the specific cause and curative treatment of these disorders remain to be determined.

The heterogeneous group of acute and chronic ILD can be broadly categorized under six main groupings (Fig. 68-1). Establishing a diagnosis from within these groups requires a knowledge of the spectrum of ILD and the judicious use of invasive and noninvasive diagnostic approaches. It is important not to underestimate the value of the noninvasive approaches, as they have the ability to obviate the need to subject some patients to surgery to obtain relatively large lung specimen for diagnostic purposes. In addition, without the clinical information gathered by the clinician, the nonspecific histologic features in the lung biopsy may be meaningless.

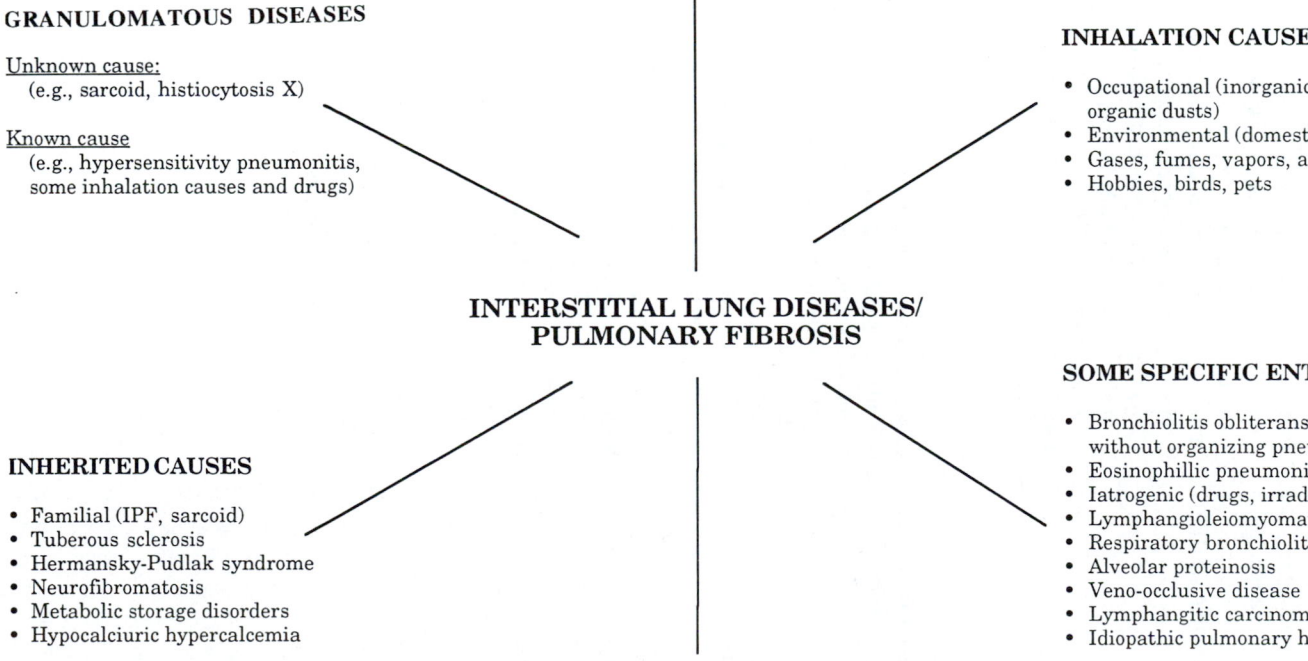

*COLLAGEN VASCULAR/CONNECTIVE TISSUE DISEASES
AND PULMONARY–RENAL SYNDROMES

GRANULOMATOUS DISEASES

Unknown cause:
(e.g., sarcoid, histiocytosis X)

Known cause
(e.g., hypersensitivity pneumonitis, some inhalation causes and drugs)

INHALATION CAUSES

- Occupational (inorganic and organic dusts)
- Environmental (domestic included)
- Gases, fumes, vapors, aerosols
- Hobbies, birds, pets

**INTERSTITIAL LUNG DISEASES/
PULMONARY FIBROSIS**

SOME SPECIFIC ENTITIES

- Bronchiolitis obliterans (with or without organizing pneumonia)
- Eosinophillic pneumonia
- Iatrogenic (drugs, irradiation)
- Lymphangioleiomyomatosis
- Respiratory bronchiolitis
- Alveolar proteinosis
- Veno-occlusive disease
- Lymphangitic carcinomatosis
- Idiopathic pulmonary hemosiderosis

INHERITED CAUSES

- Familial (IPF, sarcoid)
- Tuberous sclerosis
- Hermansky-Pudlak syndrome
- Neurofibromatosis
- Metabolic storage disorders
- Hypocalciuric hypercalcemia

*IDIOPATHIC PULMONARY FIBROSIS
(IPF)

* Both grouped as Cryptogenic Fibrosing Alveolitis in Europe

FIGURE 68-1 Six main groups of interstitial lung diseases. (*Based on Raghu,[26] with permission.*)

TABLE 68-2

Salient Clinical Features in Selected Interstitial Lung Diseases

Disease	Associated Selected Clinical Findings	Histology (Type of Biopsy)	Requirements for Diagnosis
Drug induced (e.g., chemotherapeutic agents, amiodarone, nitrofurantoin, methotrexate)	Exposure history—temporal cause-and-effect relationship; acute, subacute, and chronic disease; eosinophilia	Nonspecific pulmonary inflammation and fibrosis (loose noncaseating granuloma in methotrexate pneumonitis)	History, clinical response to cessation of offending drug and treatment with corticosteroids
Idiopathic pulmonary fibrosis (IPF)	Adult disease (5th, 6th decades); insidious onset of exertional dyspnea; finger clubbing; relentlessly progressive disorder; predominantly lower lobes (chest radiograph and HRCT)	Usual interstitial pneumonia (surgical lung biopsy)	Process of elimination; histology (surgical lung biopsy)
Sarcoidosis	Bilateral hilar adenopathy with or without iridocyclitis or arthritis; anergy	Multiple, tightly formed, uniform noncaseating granuloma in the affected tissue	Lofgren's syndrome: clinical diagnosis. Others: compatible clinical picture, characteristic histology, no other explanation, absence of infection (fungi, mycobacteria)
Hypersensitivity pneumonitis (extrinsic allergic alveolitis)	Exposure history to known antigen (inhaled, ingested); acute, subacute, chronic; peripheral eosinophilia unusual; precipitating antibodies merely indicate exposure	Interstitial inflammation with lymphocytes and mononuclear cells; loosely formed noncaseating granuloma	Histology (transbronchial or surgical lung biopsy)
Collagen vascular diseases	ILD similar to IPF;		
Progressive systemic sclerosis	Associated skin and digital changes and other, systemic symptoms	Nonspecific (surgical lung biopsy) indistinguishable from usual interstitial pneumonia/IPF	Clinical features of PSS; serology: +SSA, SSB, SM and RNP
Rheumatoid arthritis	Polyarticular arthritis	Nonspecific (surgical lung biopsy)	Rheumatoid factor >1:80
Systemic lupus erythematosus	Multisystem disorder	Nonspecific (surgical lung biopsy)	Positive ANA; >15% DNA binding
Polymyositis-dermatomyositis	Skin rash; muscle tenderness and weakness (symmetrical); elevated muscle enzymes	Nonspecific (surgical lung biopsy); specific (muscle)	Positive Sm Ab, elevated muscle enzymes; electromyogram, abnormal muscle biopsy
Sjögren's syndrome	Associated clinical features of collagen vascular disease: polyarticular arthritis; dryness in eyes, mouth; recurrent bronchopneumonia	Lymphocytic interstitial pneumonia; pseudolymphoma (surgical lung biopsy)	Clinical features of Sjögren's syndrome
Chronic eosinophilic pneumonia	Middle-aged women; fever; night sweats, dyspnea; asthma (50%); peripheral eosinophilia ($\frac{2}{3}$); elevated sedimentation rate; "photographic negative" of pulmonary edema in chest radiograph; BAL eosinophilia	Eosinophilic pneumonia; absence of infection, vasculitis, granuloma (surgical lung biopsy)	Typical clinical features; peripheral eosinophilia (may be absent in $\frac{1}{3}$ of patients); dramatic therapeutic response to corticosteroids within a few days

Disease	Clinical Features	Pathology	Diagnosis
Acute interstitial pneumonia of unknown origin	Similar to ARDS, but not associated with known risk factors for ARDS; rapid-onset; progressive respiratory failure	Diffuse alveolar damage (nonspecific) (surgical lung biopsy)	Process of elimination of infection, other known causes of acute lung injury; surgical lung biopsy
Langerhans' cell granulomatosis (pulmonary histiocytosis X; eosinophilic granuloma)	Young male; cough, dyspnea; cigarette smokers (~95%); recurrent pneumothorax; diffuse ILD, "ILD with large lung volumes"; HRCT scan: cystic lesions	Granulomatous inflammation with Langerhans' cells detected by electron microscopy or S100 protein by light microscopy (surgical or transbronchial lung biopsy)	Langerhans' cells by BAL/lung biopsy (light microscopy; +S100 protein)
Lymphangioleiomyomatosis (LAM)	Woman of reproductive age; exertional dyspnea, pneumothorax, hemoptysis chylothorax; ILD with preserved or large lung volumes; obstructive airflow defect with decreased $D_{L}CO$ (±coexisting restrictive lung defect); HRCT: numerous thin-wall cysts (<20 mm) *throughout* the pulmonary parenchyma	Bundles of smooth muscle in walls of cysts, peribronchial, perilymphatic areas; positive HMB 45 by immunocyto-chemistry (surgical or transbronchial lung biopsy)	Typical clinical and histologic features
Idiopathic bronchiolitis obliterans organizing pneumonia (BOOP)	Subacute illness; cough, dyspnea ± fever; localized or patchy alveolar infiltrates (unilateral or bilateral); HRCT: patchy, alveolar ground-glass attenuation; restrictive lung defect	Inflammatory and fibrotic infiltration of the terminal bronchioles, obliteration of small airways, and associated finding of organizing pneumonia in the absence of infection (surgical lung biopsy)	Clinical features; requires elimination of infection by BAL/lung biopsy (surgical or transbronchial)
Obliterative bronchiolitis (OB) (constrictive bronchiolitis)	Dyspnea; obstructive airflow defect; "clear lungs," air trapping by HRCT; clinical situations: viral infections, toxic gas inhalations, bone marrow or lung transplant, rheumatoid arthritis; idiopathic	Disease limited to small airways with patent lumen: bronchioles constricted (surgical lung biopsy)	Clinical setting and features
Respiratory bronchiolitis associated ILD (RBILD)	Smokers (almost exclusively); cough; dyspnea; "dirty lungs" on chest radiograph; may have normal HRCT	Inflammation: resp. bronchioles, alveolar ducts; mild interstitial fibrosis; pigmented alveolar macrophages within airways (distal), air sacs, and alveoli; desquamative interstitial pneumonia (surgical lung biopsy)	Clinical and histologic features

A suggested diagnostic algorithm for evaluating a patient with ILD is schematically shown in Fig. 68-2. The diagnostic process should start with a very thorough medical history that must include a review of environmental factors, occupational exposures, medication and drug usage, and family medical history. A review of the medical records of family members with apparent breathing problems may provide evidence for familial pulmonary fibrosis or another inherited ILD. Risk factors for HIV infection or immunosuppression should also be identified, since a diagnosis of HIV infection and associated pulmonary diseases and opportunistic lung infection will require appropriate evaluation.

The patient's age, cigarette-smoking status, and sex may provide useful clues. IPF is almost always an adult disorder, typically occurring in patients beyond 50 years of age. Although pulmonary sarcoidosis can manifest in the elderly patient, it is more common in young adults and middle-aged people. Langerhans' cell granulomatosis (also known as pulmonary histiocytosis X and eosinophilic granuloma) typically occurs in young cigarette-smoking males. RBILD is seen almost exclusively in cigarette smokers, but it can occur in both men and women of all ages. Lymphangioleiomyomatosis is a very rare disorder occurring exclusively in women of childbearing age.

Although ILD associated with tuberous sclerosis appears to occur predominantly in women, this very rare disorder can occur in men as well.

The clinician's index of suspicion for the diagnosis of hypersensitivity pneumonitis is generally raised by a history of at-risk employment (such as farming) or exposure to known causes of hypersensitivity pneumonitis, including birds, drugs, humidifiers, etc. In such instances, it is important to establish the relationship between the exposure and the timing of symptom onset. The history should also include a careful review of medication and therapeutic interventions to identify iatrogenic causes of ILD.

Several drugs are well known to cause ILD (Table 68-3). These include chemotherapeutic and cytotoxic agents, anti-inflammatory agents (nonsteroidal), antibiotics, narcotic analgesics, antiarrhythmics (amiodarone), hydralazine, tricyclic antidepressants, methotrexate, and penicillamine. The list continues to increase; thus, any new medication that the patient may have taken before the onset of ILD must be considered as a potentially attributable cause. Use of over-the-counter medications and "alternative medicines" ("herbal" medicines, naturopathics, and vitamins and mineral supplements) must not be overlooked.

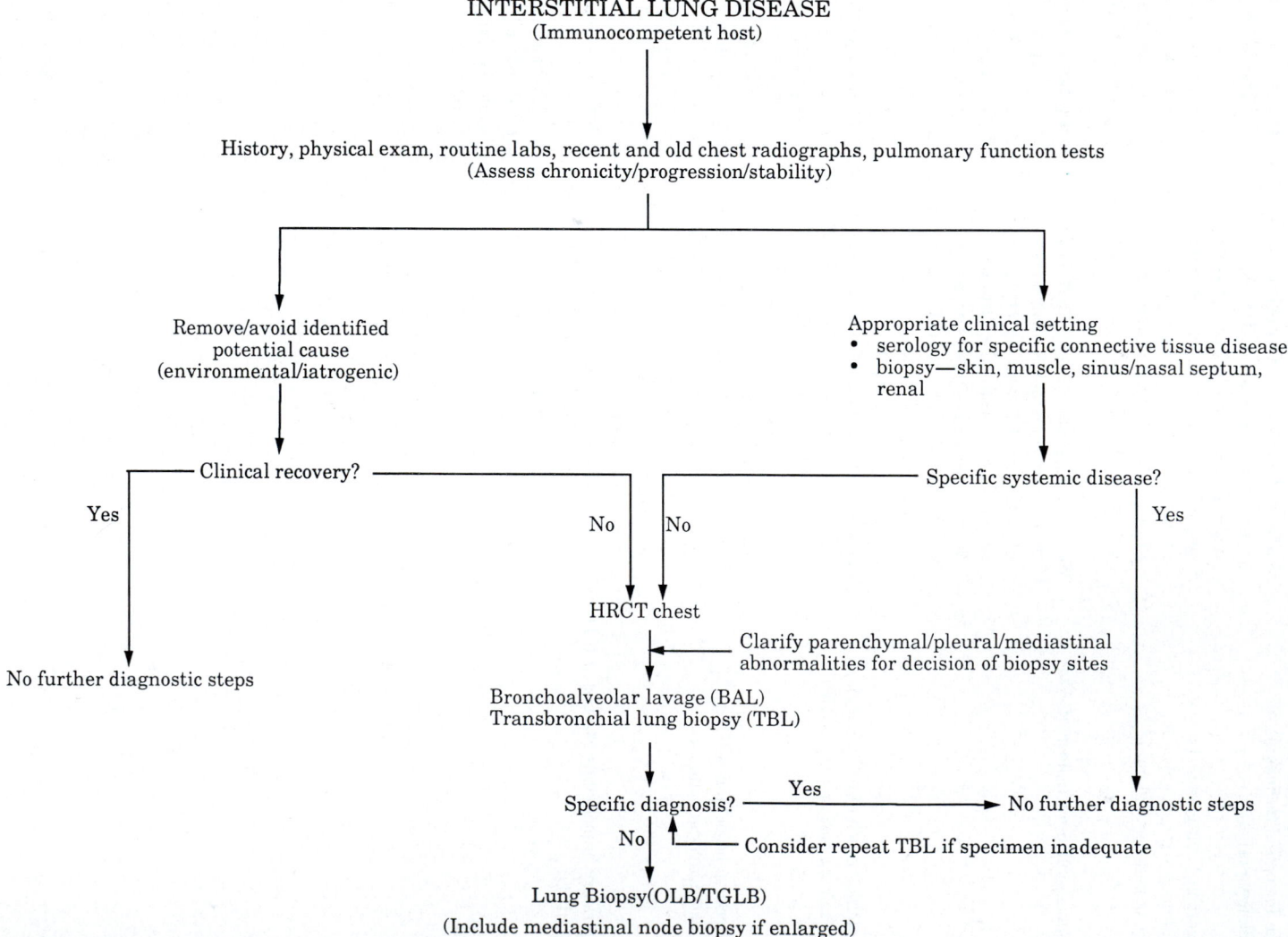

FIGURE 68-2 Suggested diagnostic evaluation of a patient with ILD: A rational approach. (*Based on Raghu,*[26] *with permission.*)

TABLE 68-3

Iatrogenic Interstitial Lung Diseases (Partial List)

Cytotoxic drugs
   Bleomycin, mitomycin
   Busulfan, cyclophosphamide, chlorambucil
   BCNU
   Methotrexate
Noncytotoxic drugs
   Antibiotics
      Nitrofurantoin, sulfasalazine
   Anti-inflammatory agents
      Nonsteroidal (NSAIDs)
   Analgesics
      Aspirin
   Opiates
      Heroin, methadone
   Anticonvulsants
      Carbamazepine, dilantin
   Diuretics
      Hydrochlorthiazide
   Tranquilizers
      Haloperidol
   Antiarrythmics
      Amiodarone, beta blockers
   Vasodilators
      Hydralazine
   Miscellaneous
      Gold salts, penicillamine, colchicine, tricyclic
         antidepressants
Radiation-induced lung disease

An occupational history is also essential, as it may lead to a specific inhalation cause for ILD. People in at-risk occupations and associated diseases include miners (pneumoconioses); sandblasters and granite workers (silicosis); dental workers (dental workers' pneumoconioses); welders, shipyard workers, pipe fitters, electricians, mechanics, and workers with brakes (asbestosis); farmworkers (hypersensitivity pneumonitis); poultry workers; bird fanciers, bird breeders (hypersensitivity pneumonitis); and workers in aerospace, nuclear, computer, and electronic industries (berylliosis).

The presenting illness of a patient with ILD should be characterized with particular attention to the onset and duration of symptoms, rate of disease progression, and association with hemoptysis, fever, and extrathoracic symptoms. Symptoms lasting 4 weeks or less and the presence of fever suggest BOOP, drug-induced pulmonary injury, and hypersensitivity pneumonitis. This acute presentation is atypical in IPF, pulmonary histiocytosis X, and ILD associated with connective tissue disease. Patients with sarcoidosis may also present with a brief illness and fever. They often have accompanying erythema nodosum and arthritis (Lofgren's syndrome).

A number of extrapulmonary symptoms provide useful clues in the differential diagnosis of ILD. A history of aspiration or dysphagia suggests aspiration pneumonia, scleroderma, or mixed connective tissue disease; arthritis suggests a collagen vascular disease or sarcoidosis; recurrent sinusitis suggests Wegener's granulomatosis; pneumothorax can be seen with a variety of interstitial lung diseases, particularly eosinophilic granuloma and lymphangioleiomyomatosis; muscle and skin symptoms suggest polymyositis or dermatomyositis; dry and gritty eyes and dry mouth (sicca syndrome) suggest sarcoidosis, Sjögren's syndrome, or other collagen vascular disorders; and hemoptysis suggests alveolar hemorrhage syndromes such as Goodpasture's syndrome, Wegener's granulomatosis, pulmonary capillaritis, and systemic lupus erythematosus. When present, these symptoms will direct the clinician to appropriate laboratory tests that may lead to a specific diagnosis other than IPF. For example, elevated levels of creatinine kinase, aldolase, and cytoplasmic antineutrophil antibody, glomerular basement membrane antibody, or specific antinuclear antibodies may offer specific diagnostic clues in the appropriate clinical setting.

Physical examination of the respiratory system is rarely helpful in the diagnostic evaluation of ILD. In contrast, extrathoracic findings can be insightful. For example, skin abnormalities, peripheral lymphadenopathy, and hepatosplenomegaly are commonly associated with sarcoidosis. Characteristic skin rashes and lesions also occur in collagen vascular diseases, disseminated histiocytosis X, tuberous sclerosis, and neurofibromatosis. Muscle tenderness and proximal muscle weakness raise the possibility of coexisting polymyositis. Signs of arthritis may be associated with sarcoidosis or collagen vascular disease. Patients with IPF also often have arthralgias. However, they rarely show active synovitis or arthritis on physical examination. Sclerodactyly, Raynaud's phenomenon, and telangiectatic lesions are characteristic features of scleroderma and CREST syndrome. Iridocyclitis, uveitis, or conjunctivitis may be associated with sarcoidosis and collagen vascular syndromes. Abnormalities of the central nervous system suggest the diagnosis of sarcoidosis (cranial nerves abnormalities, diabetes insipidus, anterior pituitary dysfunction), Langerhans cell granulomatosis (diabetes insipidus), and tuberous sclerosis (epilepsy, mental retardation).

Routine laboratory tests should include complete blood count, leukocyte differential, erythrocyte sedimentation rate, chemistry profile (calcium, liver function tests, electrolytes, renal function tests), screening for collagen vascular diseases, and urinalysis. When appropriate, creatinine kinase, aldolase, and angiotensin-converting enzyme levels should be measured. Abnormalities in some laboratory tests, although nonspecific, may be present in some ILDs (Table 68-4).

Chest Radiographic Patterns

The pulmonary clinician should make every effort to obtain all previous chest radiographs for review. This allows the clinician to ascertain the onset, progression, chronicity, and stability of the patient's disease. A rare patient with ILD will present with a normal chest radiograph. When radiographic abnormalities are noted, their distribution and appearance are useful in narrowing the differential diagnosis of the ILD (Table 68-5). A pattern of upper-lobe/zone predominance (Fig. 68-3A) suggests sarcoidosis, berylliosis, Langerhans' cell granulomatosis (eosinophilic granuloma), cystic fibrosis, silicosis, and ankylosing spondylitis.

TABLE 68-4

Interstitial Lung Diseases: Laboratory Associations (Blood and Urine)

Erythrocyte sedimentation rate (>50 mm/h)
  Collagen vascular diseases (pulmonary–renal syndromes)
  Systemic vasculitis
  Wegener's granulomatosis
  Chronic eosinophilic pneumonia
  Malignancy
Complete blood count
  Anemia
    Iron deficiency
      Diffuse alveolar hemorrhage syndromes
    Normocytic
      Lymphangitic carcinomatosis, collagen vascular
        diseases
    Hemolytic
      Drugs, collagen vascular diseases
      (Rare: sarcoidosis, idiopathic pulmonary fibrosis)
  Leukopenia
    Sarcoidosis, collagen vascular diseases, lymphoma, drug
      induced (cytotoxic)
  Thrombocytopenia
    Drug induced; collagen vascular disease
    (Rare: idiopathic pulmonary fibrosis, sarcoidosis)
  Leukocytosis
    Systemic vasculitis
    Hypersensitivity pneumonitis
    Eosinophilic pneumonia
    Acute interstitial pneumonia
    Bronchiolitis obliterans organizing pneumonia (BOOP)
  Eosinophilia
    Eosinophilic pneumonias
    Drugs
    Sarcoidosis
    Systemic vasculitis
Antibodies, gammaglobulins, circulating immune complexes
  Hypergammaglobulinemia and serum autoantibodies (RF,
    ANA):
    Sarcoidosis
    Idiopathic pulmonary fibrosis
    Lymphocytic interstitial pneumonias
    (Hypogammaglobulinemia has been described
    as well)
    Collagen vascular disease (RF, ANA, SS-A, SS-B,
      anti-ds DNA)
    Systemic vasculitis
    Asbestosis
    Silicosis

  Circulating immune complexes
    Idiopathic pulmonary fibrosis
    Langerhans cell granulomatosis
    Systemic vasculitis
    Collagen vascular diseases
    Lymphocytic interstitial pneumonias
  Anti–basement membrane antibody (anti–glomerular
    basement membrane anti-GBM)
    Goodpasture's syndrome
  Antineutrophil cytoplasmic antibody (C-ANCA)
    Wegener's granulomatosis
    Systemic necrotizing vasculitis
    Pulmonary capillaritis
    Allergic granulomatosis of Churg and Strauss
  AntiJo₁
    Polymyositis/dermatomyositis
Chemistry
  Abnormal liver function tests
    sarcoid
    systemic lupus erythematosis
    interstitial lung disease associated with hepatitis/cirrhosis
    drug induced
    malignancy
  Elevated blood urea nitrogen
    creatinine
    pulmonary–renal syndromes and collagen vascular
      diseases
    drug induced
    Goodpasture's syndrome
    systemic vasculitis
  Elevated calcium
    sarcoidosis
    malignancy
  Elevated ceatinine phosphokinase, aldolase
    polymyositis/dermato-myositis
  Increased angiotensin-converting enzyme
    sarcoidosis
    hypersensitivity pneumonitis
    silicosis
    berylliosis
    adult respiratory distress syndrome
    Gaucher's disease
Abnormal Urinary Sediment
  systemic vasculitis
  collagen vascular diseases and pulmonary-renal syndromes
  Goodpasture's syndrome
  drug induced

SOURCE: Modified from MKSAP (American College of Physicians: with permission) and adapted from Schwarz MI, King JE (eds): *Interstitial Lung Disease,* 2d ed. Philadelphia, Mosby Year Book, 1993.

In contrast, the abnormalities of lymphangitic carcinomatosis, subacute eosinophilic pneumonias, IPF, asbestosis, and pulmonary fibrosis associated with rheumatoid arthritis or scleroderma are predominantly concentrated in the middle and lower lung zones (Fig. 68-3*B*).

The presence and the pattern of adenopathy may provide additional clues. The coexistence of paratracheal and symmetric bilateral hilar adenopathy strongly suggests sarcoidosis. This pattern may, however, be seen in metastatic tumor and lymphoma as well. The presence of eggshell calcification suggests sarcoidosis or silicosis. Kerley B lines and ILD in association with a normal heart size suggest lymphangitic carcinomatosis. However, if concomitant radiographic evidence of pulmonary hypertension is present in the same setting, pulmonary veno-occlusive disease must be considered.

The pattern of peripherally located pulmonary infiltrates in the upper and middle zones with relatively clear perihilar or central zones (often described as "photographic negative of pulmonary edema") is highly suggestive of chronic eosinophilic pneumonia. Bilateral infiltrates that recur in the same anatomic

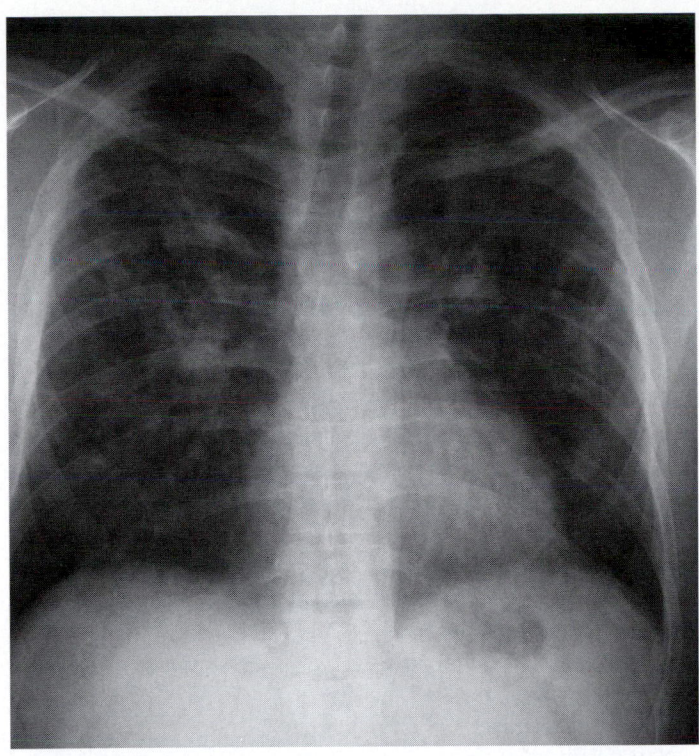

A

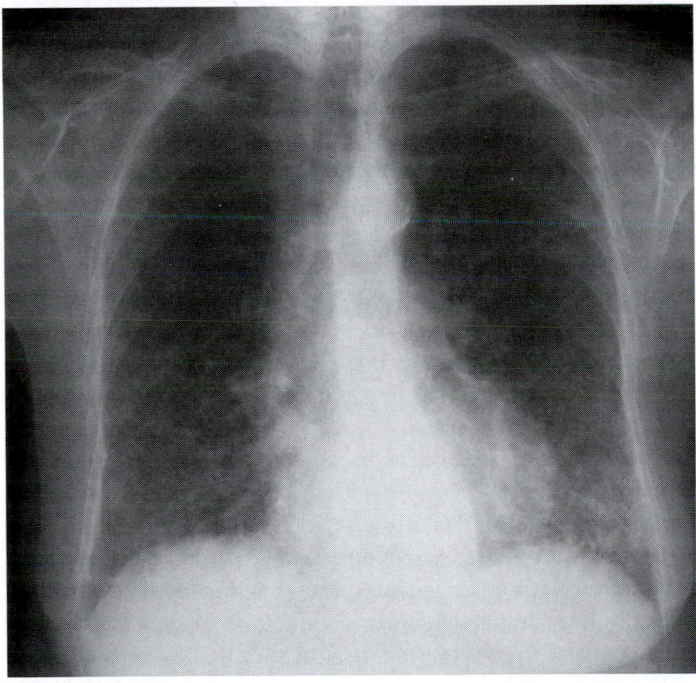

B

FIGURE 68-3 Posteroanterior view of chest radiographs revealing bilateral diffuse pulmonary infiltrates predominantly in (*A*) upper lobes and (*B*) lower lobes. (See Table 68-5 for differential diagnoses.)

The presence of pleural plaques or localized thickening in the setting of ILD predominantly affecting the lower lobes suggest asbestosis. Diffuse pleural thickening can result from asbestos pleurisy, rheumatoid arthritis, scleroderma, or malignancy. The coexistence of pleural effusion raises the possibility of rheumatoid arthritis, systemic lupus erythematosis, a drug reaction, asbestos-related lung diseases, amyloidosis, lymphangioleiomyomatosis, or lymphangitic carcinomatosis. Apparently normal (preserved lung volume) and increased lung volumes on the chest radiograph in the context of ILD suggest the coexistence of an obstructive airflow defect and a few specific disease entities (Table 68-5). Prominent in this regard are lymphangioleiomyomatosis, eosinophilic granuloma, hypersensitivity pneumonitis, tuberous sclerosis, and sarcoidosis. In interpreting these findings, it is important to realize that the chest radiograph provides only a semiquantitative assessment of lung volume and often correlates poorly with estimates of histologic and functional impairment.[7,20] Despite these limitations, when the clues provided by the chest radiograph are combined with those from the history, physical examination, laboratory tests, and pulmonary function evaluation, the clinician is often able to narrow the differential diagnoses to a few possibilities.

Pulmonary Physiology Testing

Regardless of the cause, a restrictive lung defect and decreased diffusing capacity ($D_{L_{CO}}$) are the predominant physiological abnormalities seen in ILD. The forced expiratory volume in 1 s (FEV_1) and forced vital capacity (FVC) are decreased proportionally, so the ratio of the two remains normal. The total lung capacity and lung volumes are reduced. The P_{A_O}–P_{a_O} difference, at rest or with exercise, may be normal or increased, depending on disease severity. Similarly, the $D_{L_{CO}}$, corrected for hemoglobin concentration, may be normal or low. However, the $D_{L_{CO}}$, although highly nonspecific, is believed to be a relatively sensitive parameter in detecting the presence of pulmonary dysfunction and may be the only abnormality seen in early stages of interstitial lung disease. Additionally, it can be useful in the monitoring of disease progression or response to therapy. Significant changes in FVC, $D_{L_{CO}}$, and resting $P_{A_{O_2}}$–$P_{a_{O_2}}$ at the end of 1 year correlate with survival.[10,25]

Typically, static pulmonary function tests identify the presence of clinically significant restrictive physiology and quantify the severity of impairment, but do not aid in the differential diagnosis.[1,5,7] However, a number of patterns can be seen that are of diagnostic utility. Diseases such as polymyositis, scleroderma, and systemic lupus erythematosus should come to mind when tests performed on a cooperative patient demonstrate reproducibly a decrease in the maximal voluntary ventilation out of proportion to the decrease in FEV_1 and a decrease in maximal inspiratory pressures in association with respiratory muscle weakness. When an obstructive airflow abnormality is present, the diagnostic possibilities are also narrowed. A mixed pattern of obstructive and restrictive abnormalities may be present when ILD coexists with chronic obstructive pulmonary disease or asthma. ILDs associated with asthma or recurrent bronchospasm include Churg-Strauss syndrome, ABPA, sarcoidosis (endobronchial), and tropical pulmonary interstitial eosinophilia.

location raise the possibility of BOOP, chronic eosinophilic pneumonia, drug-induced ILD, or a relapse/recall radiation pneumonitis. In contrast, fleeting or migratory infiltrates suggest Churg-Strauss syndrome (allergic angiitis and granulomatosis), allergic bronchopulmonary aspergillosis (ABPA), BOOP, tropical eosinophilic pneumonia, or Loeffler's syndrome.

TABLE 68-5

Interstitial Lung Disease: Helpful Radiographic Patterns

Upper-lobe/zone predominance
  Sarcoidosis
  Berylliosis
  Langerhans cell granulomatosis (pulmonary histiocytosis X;
    eosinophilic granuloma)
  Pneumoconiosis (silicosis, coal worker's)
  Rheumatoid arthritis
  Ankylosing spondylitis
  Radiation fibrosis
  Chronic hypersensitivity pneumonitis
    (Cystic fibrosis, tuberculosis are also upper-lobe–
      predominant diseases that are not generally
      included in the category of ILD)

Lower-lobe/zone predominance
  Idiopathic pulmonary fibrosis (including familial idiopathic
    pulmonary fibrosis)
  Collagen vascular diseases (progressive systemic sclerosis,
    polymyositis, rheumatoid arthritis)
  Asbestosis
  Acute hypersensitivity pneumonitis

**Midzone/perihilar ground-glass/diffuse alveolar filling
(usually with preserved lung volumes)**
  Pulmonary alveolar proteinosis
  Diffuse alveolar hemorrhage syndromes
  Lupus pneumonitis

Photographic negative of pulmonary edema
  Chronic eosinophilic pneumonia

Diffuse micronodular pattern
  Sarcoidosis
  Silicosis
  Hypersensitivity pneumonitis
  Respiratory bronchiolitis–associated interstitial lung disease
  Langerhans cell granulomatosis (pulmonary histocytosis X)
  Pulmonary microlithiasis (fine calcified lesions)
  Amyloidosis (may calcify)
  Infectious granulomatous disease (miliary tuberculosis;
    varicella pneumonia, histoplasmosis, coccidiomylosis)
  Miscellaneous (metastic malignant disease: thyroid
    carcinoma, hypernephroma, adenocarcinoma of breast,
    malignant melanoma)

Preserved or increased lung volumes
  Lymphangioleiomyomatosis
  Tuberous sclerosis
    Langerhans cell granulomatosis (pulmonary histiocytosis X;
      eosinophilic granuloma)
  Neurofibromatosis
  Idiopathic pulmonary fibrosis and cigarette smoker (with or
    without associated COPD)
  Hypersensitivity pneumonitis
  Sarcoidosis
  Respiratory bronchiolitis
  Bronchiolitis obliterans
  (Cystic fibrosis)

Decreased or low lung volumes
  Idiopathic pulmonary fibrosis
  Chronic hypersensitivity pneumonitis
  Collagen vascular diseases (especially systemic lupus
    erythematosis, progressive systemic sclerosis,
    polymyositis)
  Asbestosis

Associated pneumothorax
  Langerhans cell granulomatosis (pulmonary histiocytosis X;
    eosinophilic granuloma)
  Lymphangioleiomyomatosis
  Tuberous sclerosis
  Neurofibromatosis
  (Cystic fibrosis)

**Associated pleural involvement (pleural thickening; pleural
effusion)**
  Asbestosis
  Collagen vascular diseases (especially rheumatoid arthritis,
    systemic lupus erythematosis)
  Lymphangitic carcinomatosis
  Lymphangioleiomyomatosis (chylous effusion)
  Drug induced (especially nitrofurantion)
  Radiation fibrosis (late stages)
  Malignancy
  Amyloidosis
  Sarcoidosis (very rare)

Associated with Kerley B lines
  Chronic left ventricular failure
  Mitral valve disease
  Lymphangitic carcinomatosis
  Lymphoma
  Lymphangioleiomyomatosis
  Pulmonary veno-occlusive disease

**Associated with enlarged pulmonary arteries (secondary
pulmonary hypertension)**
  Pulmonary veno-occlusive disease

Even though a number of precipitants of acute hypersensitivity pneumonitis can cause bronchospasm, acute hypersensitivity pneumonitis is not typically associated with an asthmalike syndrome. In the absence of asthma, the differential diagnosis of ILD in association with pulmonary function tests of combined obstructive and restrictive lung defects narrows further. It includes the disorders whose airflow obstruction and the associated air trapping cause the patient to have normal or expanded lung volumes by chest radiograph (Table 68-5). It also includes patients with severe ILD with secondary bronchiectasis. Thus, resting pulmonary function tests document the existence, gauge the severity, and provide clues that are useful in the differential

diagnosis of ILD. In addition, they provide simple tools that are useful in the monitoring of clinical progression of the disease.

A major strength of pulmonary function testing in ILD is in the functional assessment of physiological impairment by single or serial evaluations during exercise. Such evaluations can play an important role in the management of patients with ILD. The degree of arterial hypoxemia induced by exercise and the alveolar–arterial difference in P_{O_2} (the "A–a O_2 gradient") correlate well with the degree of pulmonary fibrosis.[1,5] Exercise also affords the most sensitive diagnostic and physiological test for ILD, since in some patients with biopsy-proven ILD, the physiological responses to exercise (see below) are distinctly abnormal even

Mixed connective tissue disease; CREST syndrome; progressive systemic sclerosis

Mitral valve disease

Idiopathic pulmonary fibrosis (advanced stages)

Chronic secondary pulmonary fibrotic disorders (advanced stages)

Associated with hilar or medastinal lymphadenopathy

Sarcoidosis (may be calcified)

Lymphoma

Lymphangitic carcinomatosis

Berylliosis (may be calcified)

Silicosis (may be calcified)

Collagen vascular disease (occasional)

Drug induced (dilantin)

Amyloidosis (may calcify)

Metastatic tumor

(Associated chronic infection: tuberculosis, histoplasmosis: may be calcified)

Associated with hilar nodal eggshell calcification

Silicosis

Sarcoidosis

Associated with subcutaneous calcinosis

Scleroderma (CREST)

Dermatomyositis/polymyositis

Associated subsegmental migratory infiltrates

Churg-Strauss syndrome

Allergic bronchopulmonary aspergillosis

Tropical/pulmonary interstitial eosinophilia

Bronchiolitis obliterans organizing pneumonia

Recurrent infiltrates in same anatomic location(s)

Chronic eosinophilic pneumonia (upper lobes/peripheral)

Idiopathic BOOP

Drug induced

Relapse/recall radiation pneumonitis

Normal chest radiograph

Idiopathic pulmonary fibrosis (early, cellular stages)

Sarcoidosis

Hypersensitivity pneumonitis

Other ILDs (including collagen vascular diseases)

Respiratory bronchiolitis

Bronchiolitis obliterans

SOURCE: Modified from MKSAP (American College of Physicians), with permission.

though pulmonary function tests (including D_{LCO} and arterial blood gases), chest radiographs, and HRCT scans are all normal.[21]

The exercise-induced physiological abnormalities in ILD[11,27] include a decrease in work rate and maximal oxygen consumption, abnormally high minute ventilations at submaximal work rates (high ventilatory equivalents), decreased peak minute ventilations, failure of tidal volumes to increase at submaximal levels of work while respiratory rates increase disproportionately, increased heart rates, low O_2 pulses, progressive arterial hypoxemia and widening of the P_{AO_2}–Pa_{O_2} difference, and persistent respiratory alkalosis. In advanced pulmonary fibrosis, progressive exercise may be associated with an initial failure of Pa_{CO_2} to decrease, followed by progressive increase in Pa_{CO_2} in the terminal stages of exercise. As the level of exercise increases pro-

gressively, in patients with advanced pulmonary fibrosis, the physiological dead space remains elevated and a low O_2 pulse (oxygen uptake/heart rate) may be present.

The exercise response patterns described above are not specific for pulmonary parenchymal involvement and cannot be distinguished from those seen with pulmonary vascular disease, primary or secondary pulmonary hypertension, or thromboembolic disease. They do, however, provide useful information. A correlation between reduction in the maximal oxygen consumption and the degree of fibrosis has been shown.[5] In addition, they can point to cardiac dysfunction in some patients. In the earlier stages of ILD, patients rarely have ventilatory limitation despite the restrictive abnormalities demonstrated by the static pulmonary function tests. Indeed, a ventilatory reserve can still be shown to exist at peak exercise.[11,27] In advanced ILD, patients quit the exercise test because of leg fatigue, suggesting cardiac dysfunction associated with a low output state.[27] This apparent cardiac limitation with progressive exercise is similar to that noted in patients with primary pulmonary hypertension and cardiac myopathy. The exact mechanism for this apparent cardiac dysfunction is unclear.

Computed Tomography and High-Resolution CT Images

CT and HRCT scans are more sensitive and have a greater ability to detect anatomic abnormalities than do chest radiographs.[16,20,22] This power may have ramifications for the staging and diagnosis of ILD. The ability of these scans to be useful in staging comes from their perceived ability to differentiate between predominantly active and reversible versus fibrotic and irreversible disease (see below).[33] Preliminary studies suggest that some HRCT patterns, particularly when combined with clinical and radiographic findings,[8] can have diagnostic utility. If confirmed, these diagnostic techniques may allow invasive diagnostic procedures to be obviated in a small subset of ILD patients. Most important, these techniques can serve to identify areas of nonfibrotic, active disease and relatively unaffected areas to guide appropriate site selection for biopsy.[26]

Because of the impressive sensitivity of CT-based methods, investigators have evaluated their utility both in ruling out a diagnosis of ILD and in defining the parenchymal, pleural, and mediastinal abnormalities in these disorders. These studies have demonstrated that a normal HRCT does not exclude the presence of microscopic ILD in patients with a high pretest probability of the disorder.[12,21,22] They have also demonstrated that pathology can be demonstrated by CT that cannot be appreciated on the chest radiograph. For example, before the CT era, IPF and ILD were thought to affect the pulmonary parenchyma only. At present, CT-based evaluations have shown that hilar and mediastinal adenopathy may be present in IPF and the ILD that accompany collagen vascular diseases.

Enthusiasm has been increasing about the utility of HRCT in identifying "active inflammation" in ILD.[32,33] Thus, it has been proposed that ground-glass attenuation on HRCT represents histologically "active" and reversible pulmonary inflammation (Fig. 68 4A). Unfortunately, increasing experience has shown that ground-glass attenuation is not as specific as was hoped (Table

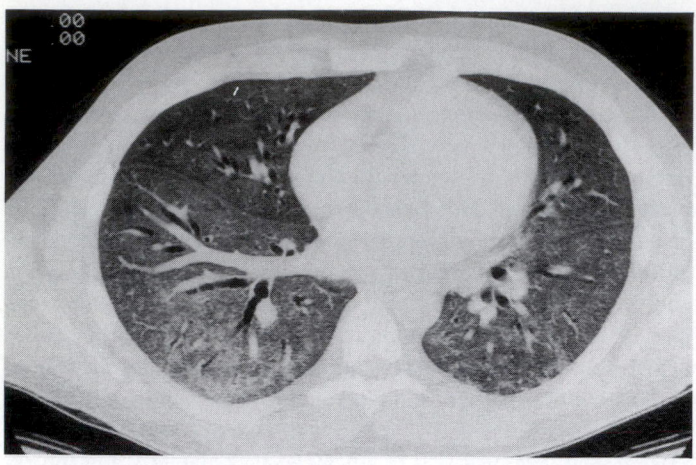

A

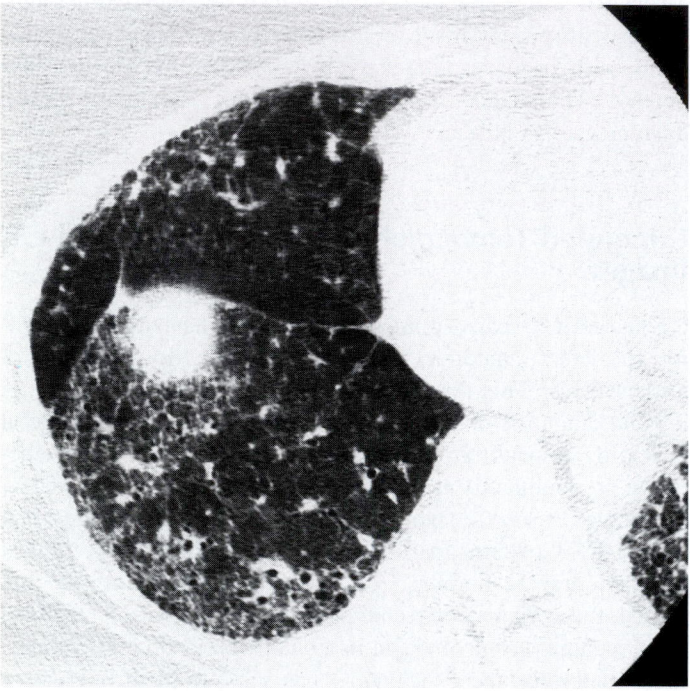

B

FIGURE 68-4   HRCT features of (*A*) ground-glass attenuation, suggestive of active inflammatory process; (*B*) subpleural reticular fibrotic pattern with honeycombing, suggestive of advanced pulmonary fibrosis.

"fibrotic" changes suggest end- or advanced-stage disease with limited potential for therapeutic response. Findings of this sort might preclude an invasive diagnostic approach or a prolonged therapeutic trial that could be toxic, particularly in elderly patients with co-morbid disease.

A number of HRCT patterns are suggestive of specific interstitial disorders. HRCT images provide valuable information on the fine architecture of pulmonary secondary lobules. As a result, HRCT has the potential for differentiating sarcoidosis, lymphangitic carcinomatosis, and bronchiolitis (Table 68-6). The presence of *cystic images* within the parenchyma raises the possibilities of three major "cystic" ILDs: lymphangioleiomyomatosis, tuberous sclerosis, and Langerhans cell granulomatosis (Fig. 68-5). In lymphangioleiomyomatosis and tuberous sclerosis, the cysts are numerous, thin walled, typically less than 2 cm in diameter, and distributed throughout the pulmonary parenchyma. In Langerhans' cell granulomatosis, by contrast, cysts are distributed predominantly in the upper lobes and tend to be bizarrely shaped. In acute hypersensitivity pneumonitis, a frequent diagnostic clue is a markedly abnormal HRCT with multifocal ground-glass attenuation despite a normal chest radiograph and significant clinical symptoms.[31] Similarly, smokers with symptomatic RBILD typically have patchy ground-glass attenuation on HRCT in the setting of bilateral interstitial radiographic infiltrates and normal lung volumes.[12] Finally, IPF is characterized by patchy subpleural and basilar fibrosis (Fig. 68-4*B*).

Based on promising preliminary data,[32] a prospective multicenter study has been initiated to evaluate the utility of HRCT in the diagnosis of IPF. However, enthusiasm for this study has been somewhat dampened by a recent report indicating that CT was not reliable in distinguishing between chronic hypersensitivity pneumonitis and IPF.[17] Thus, the degree to which HRCT will provide diagnostic information that will reduce the need for invasive tissue diagnosis in IPF or in other ILD remains to be seen. Currently, there are no data available regarding the impact of HRCT on cost and outcome in managing patients with ILD.

68-6).[2] In a recent study, ground-glass attenuation corresponded to inflammation in only 65 percent of patients with ILD and to fibrosis in as many as 54 percent.[28] Another study, in patients with sarcoidosis, showed no correlation between ground-glass attenuation and active alveolitis.[19] On the other hand, the presence of traction bronchiectasis and bronchiolectasis on HRCT does correlate with tissue fibrosis.[28] Honeycombing is also believed to represent an irreversible fibrotic manifestation.

Diagnostic or treatment decisions should not be made solely on the basis of the presence or absence of ground-glass attenuation on HRCT. Instead, the strength of HRCT lies in its ability to give an overall assessment on the severity of honeycombing and fibrotic changes that are, in general, irreversible. Extensive

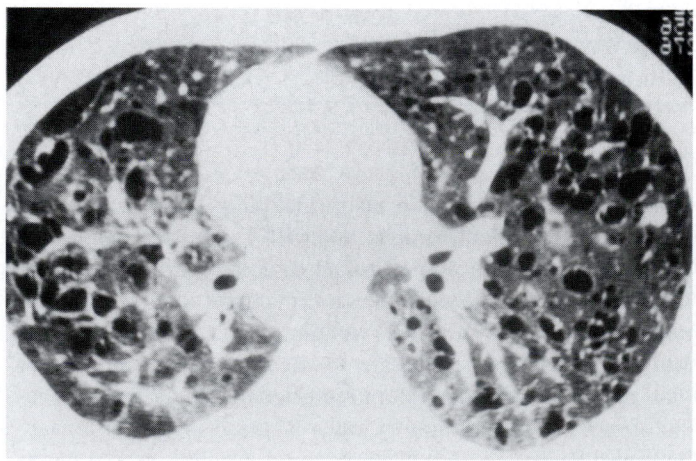

FIGURE 68-5   HRCT features of a patient with Langerhans cell granulomatosis. Note the multiple bizarre-shaped thin- and thick-wall cysts within the pulmonary parenchyma. Differential diagnosis includes lymphangioleiomyomatosis and tuberous sclerosis.

....TABLE 68-6

Anatomic/Pathologic Patterns and HRCT Features of Some Interstitial Lung Diseases

Lung Disease	Anatomic/Pathologic Pattern	HRCT
IPF (UIP)	Peripheral acinar fibrosis Subpleural, honeycombing	Patchy basilar subpleural reticular infiltrates; interlobular + intralobular thickening; ground glass (reversible ?); honeycombing (end stage)
RBILD	Bronchiolocentric ± parenchymal DIP	Multifocal ground glass; indistinguishable from DIP; mild linear/reticular abn.
Idiopathic BOOP	Patchy; mixed interstitial + parenchymal infiltrates/consolidation	Bilateral, multifocal regions of consolidations + ground glass; nodular opacities
CEP	Parenchymal consolidation, sharp demarcation of septa	Indistinguishable from BOOP; ground glass
Acute HP (EAA)	Bronchiolocentric/diffuse interstitial granulomatous interstitial pattern; BOOP pattern	Diffuse or patchy ground glass; may consolidate; diffuse small nodules
Histiocytosis X (also called eosinophilic granuloma and Langerhans' cell granulomatosis)	Bronchiolocentric/fibrotic nodules Cellular ± fibrotic Cystic changes within nodules	Upper-lobe predominance; thin- and thick-wall cysts, some bizarre shaped; small nodules
LAM	Diffuse holes/cystic spaces with fascicular smooth muscle cells in the wall	Diffuse cysts, uniform thin walled (< 20 mm)
Sarcoidosis	Lymphatic/peribronchiolar noncaseating granuloma	Adenopathy; central, perihilar, peribronchovascular changes; ground glass (early); occasional honeycombing
Silicosis	Dust-filled histocytes, perilymphatics (early); fibrotic nodules (late); weakly birefringent silica particles	Diffuse small nodules; upper-zone/dorsal predominance; conglomerate masses (advanced disease)
Lymphangitic carcinoma	Lymphatics	Thickening along bronchovascular bundles; thickened interlobular septa

IPF = idiopathic pulmonary fibrosis; UIP = usual interstitial pneumonia; RBILD = respiratory bronchiolitis–associated interstitial lung disease; BOOP = bronchiolitis obliterans organizing pneumonia; CEP = chronic eosinophilic pneumonia; HP (EAA) = hypersensitivity pneumonitis (extrinsic allergic alveolitis); LAM = lymphangioleiomyomatosis.
SOURCE: Modified from Colby and Swenson.[2]

Perhaps the most important aspect of HRCT is its potential utility in determining the most appropriate sites for obtaining lung biopsies. It is believed that HRCT will increase the probability of making a definitive diagnosis by helping the surgeon sample relatively unaffected, actively inflamed, and densely fibrotic areas of the lung. Additionally, enhanced definition of coexisting pleural or mediastinal and hilar nodal abnormalities will guide appropriate surgical diagnostic approaches and optimize the overall management plan.[26] Although the cost-effectiveness of the routine use of HRCT in diagnostic evaluation has not been established, it seems appropriate and justifiable, for the sake of selecting the optimal sites for biopsy, to obtain an HRCT scan of the chest before a patient is subjected to lung biopsy (Fig. 68-2).

Bronchoalveolar Lavage

The role of bronchoalveolar lavage (BAL) in the diagnosis and staging of ILD has been the subject of intense study. The results indicate that BAL can be diagnostic if an infectious agent or neoplastic cell is present in the specimen. Occasionally, special stains for Langerhans cells and surfactant material may also reveal sufficient abnormalities in the BAL specimen to enable the diagnosis of Langerhans cell granulomatosis or pulmonary alveolar proteinosis, respectively. In the absence of infection, an increase in T lymphocytes with an increased CD4:CD8 ratio (in the absence of an increase in neutrophils and eosinophils) is suggestive of sarcoidosis.[23,34] However, the CD4:CD8 ratio can be highly variable in sarcoidosis,[15] and other diseases are associated with similar BAL findings (Table 68-7).

Bronchoscopy with Transbronchial Biopsy

Bronchoscopy with transbronchial lung biopsy may provide additional information in some patients with ILD, especially when tissue abnormalities tend to be distributed in peribronchovascular areas. For instance, sarcoidosis, lymphangioleiomyomatosis, and lymphangitic carcinomatosis are typically bronchocentric disorders in that their infiltrative lesions tend to be located along the peribronchovascular bundles. Transbronchial lung biopsies may disclose certain distinctive abnormalities (e.g., the tight, uniform, well-formed noncaseating granulomas of sarcoidosis, the smooth muscle proliferation of lymphangioleiomyomatosis, or the lymphatic metastasis of malignant cells). The presence of giant cell granulomas is suggestive of hard-metal pneumoconiosis.

A transbronchial lung biopsy specimen is diagnostic if an infectious agent or malignancy is detected. In an appropriate clinical setting, a transbronchial lung biopsy that reveals granulomas without mycobacteria or fungi can support a diagnosis of sarcoidosis or hypersensitivity pneumonitis. At times, the diagnosis of Langerhans cell granulomatosis or lymphangioleiomyomatosis may be made if characteristic microscopic features are present in the transbronchial lung biopsy. However, a lack of these findings in such specimens does not necessarily exclude these diseases, since the possibility of sampling error poses a problem. Thus, when transbronchial lung biopsies or bronchoalveolar lung specimens fail to confirm the clinically suspected disease, the ultimate diagnostic step—thoracoscopic or open lung biopsy—may be necessary to obtain a larger and more representative lung biopsy to clarify or confirm the diagnosis.

Surgical Lung Biopsy: Thoracoscopy-Guided and Open Lung Biopsy

As noted above, despite a thorough clinical evaluation and detailed analysis of the specimens obtained by transbronchial lung biopsy, the specific diagnosis for a patient with ILD may remain unclear (Fig. 68-2). Thoracoscopy-guided lung biopsy (TGLB) or open lung biopsies merit consideration as the final diagnostic step. The question then emerges: Which patients are suitable candidates for these procedures? Unexplained dyspnea on exertion or abnormal results on pulmonary function testing favor such interventions. Normal chest radiographs or HRCT scans do not, in themselves, negate the need for tissue diagnosis.

On the other hand, not all patients with typical clinical features compatible with IPF require surgical lung biopsy for definitive diagnosis.[26] In selected patients, such as those who are elderly with co-morbidity, it may be appropriate to make a clinical diagnosis of IPF after a thorough clinical, radiographic, and HRCT assessment even though bronchoscopy with BAL and transbronchial biopsies have proved nondiagnostic. The same approach merits consideration in patients more than 65 years of age with typical and long-standing chest radiographic findings (i.e., stable or slow progression of bibasilar interstitial abnormalities over several years, fibrotic changes in the lower zones, small lung volumes despite adequate inspiratory effort, absence

of hilar or mediastinal adenopathy, and pleural abnormalities) who also have one of the following: (1) no other explanation for exertional dyspnea; (2) lack of extrapulmonary manifestations (except finger clubbing); (3) documented collagen vascular disease; (4) typical HRCT evidence of IPF; and (5) typical physiological abnormalities (restrictive lung defect, decreased $D_{L_{CO}}$, with or without hypoxemia at rest).

Among younger patients (under 65 years of age), however, surgical lung biopsy is indicated in the functionally impaired patient when the diagnosis is unclear despite thorough clinical evaluation (inclusive of bronchoscopic assessment). This is especially so when clinical features are suggestive of a diagnosis other than, or in addition to, IPF. In the following associated clinical situations, histologic clarification by surgical lung biopsy is desirable to ascertain a specific diagnosis: (1) history of fever, weight loss, sweats, and hemoptysis; (2) family history of apparent familial ILD and IPF; (3) history of pneumothorax; (4) symptoms and signs of peripheral vasculitis; (5) atypical radiographic features of IPF (inclusive of normal chest radiographs); (6) unexplained extrapulmonary manifestations; (7) unexplained pulmonary hypertension; (8) unexplained cardiomegaly at the time of presentation; (9) rapidly progressive disease; and (10) rapid deterioration or new symptoms with new radiographic abnormalities in focal areas superimposed on long-standing "stable" diffuse radiographic changes.

The current clinical practice for subjecting patients with ILD to surgical lung biopsy is highly variable. This is understandable because the ILDs are a diverse group of diseases, each with a variable natural course. In addition, the therapies for these disorders vary in effectiveness and potential toxicity. Some diseases (e.g., sarcoidosis) may respond promptly to intervention, whereas others respond minimally, if at all. Studies are needed to determine whether surgical lung biopsy is indeed essential to make the diagnosis of diseases such as IPF before treatment is started in all symptomatic or functionally impaired patients who manifest typical clinical features but whose clinical assessment yields otherwise negative results.

Once the decision for surgical lung biopsy is made, the options are open lung biopsy and TGLB. There is increasing evidence supporting the routine use of TGLB, since it entails a less morbid surgical procedure. Adequate TGLB specimens are readily obtained by experienced surgeons. A concerted interaction of the pulmonary clinician, thoracic surgeon, and pathologist is needed, since many, often appropriately chosen biopsies need to be obtained, and the handling and processing of the lung specimens need to be coordinated to maximize and optimize the diagnostic yield.[26]

Treatment

The therapeutic regimens used for patients with ILD need to be tailored to the patient and the disease process. In a small number of situations, the natural history of the disease is so favorable that disease-specific interactions may not be necessary and only symptomatic therapies need to be utilized. Stage I sarcoidosis usually falls into this category. In most patients with ILD, however, disease-specific intervention is warranted. When an offending agent is known to cause or exacerbate the disease, treatment should begin with avoidance of the offending agent or

TABLE 68-7

Bronchoalveolar Lavage Cellular Profile

Normal adults (nonsmokers)
  Marked uniformity in differential cellular analysis
  Alveolar macrophages   ≥85%
  Lymphocytes   10–15%   (T4:T8 ratio 0.9–2.5)*
  Neutrophils   ≤1%
  Eosinophils   ≤1%
  Ciliated columnar epithelial cells   ≤2%

Interstitial lung disease
  Increased total number of nucleated cells, but of no clinical value
  Increased percentage of inflammatory cells

T Lymphocytes	Eosinophils	Neutrophils
Sarcoidosis†	Sarcoidosis (±)	Sarcoidosis (±)
Berylliosis		
Hypersensitivity pneumonitis†		Hypersensitivity pneumonitis (±)
Collagen vascular diseases	Systemic lupus erythematosis	Collagen vascular diseases
Idiopathic pulmonary fibrosis‡	Idiopathic pulmonary fibrosis§	Idiopathic pulmonary fibrosis
Drug induced	Drug induced	
Radiation pneumonitis	Eosinophilic pneumonias	Aspiration pneumonia
Lymphoma/pseudolymphoma	Hodgkin's disease	
Silicosis		
Lung rejection	Bone marrow transplant	
AIDS	AIDS	
Infection: tuberculosis, viral	Infection: bacterial, fungal helminthic, pneumocystis	Infection: bacterial, fungal
	Bronchitis	Bronchitis
	Asthma	
	Churg-Strauss syndrome	
	Allergic bronchopulmonary aspergillosis	
		Asbestosis
		Adult Respiratory Distress Syndrome

Diagnostic
  Infectious agent
  Malignant cell
Diagnosis aided by additional, special stains or studies
  Langerhans cell granulomatosis
  Lymphangioleiomyomatosis
  Pneumoconioses
  In vitro lymphocyte proliferative response to specific antigen (e.g., berylliosis)
  Alveolar proteinosis

*Individual labs should have their own reference values.
†Both increased and decreased CD4:CD8 T-cell ratios have been described. The increased ratio is most common in sarcoidosis.
‡Associated with favorable prognosis.
§Associated with poor prognosis.

its environment. The particular regimens for specific disease categories are discussed elsewhere (see Chapter 71). Since the exact etiology and pathogenesis of most ILD are unclear, currently available therapeutic regimens are nonspecific and essentially aimed at diminishing inflammation, with the belief that this will halt or decrease the rate of progression of pulmonary fibrosis. The clinical response to these currently available therapeutic regimens[18] is variable and unpredictable. Some ILDs generally have a better prognosis and respond more favorably to available treatment regimens than do others (Table 68-8). In this category are several acute and granulomatous ILDs. For example, the prognosis is excellent in acute hypersensitivity pneumonitis, since most patients respond to removal of the offending agent and treatment with corticosteroids (usually for 3 to 6 months). A dramatic clinical response and radiographic clearance of pulmonary infiltrates are also seen when corticosteroids are given to patients with chronic eosinophilic pneumonia.

In chronic fibrotic lung disorders, however, the prognosis is generally poor (Table 68-8). The use of corticosteroids, alone or in combination with immunosuppressives (azathioprine, cy-

TABLE 68-8

Clinical Response to Currently Available Therapeutic Regimens in ILD

Generally Favorable	Generally Unfavorable*
Sarcoidosis	IPF
Acute hypersensitivity pneumonitis (extrinsic allergic alveolitis)	Chronic secondary and advanced pulmonary fibrosis
	Chronic sarcoidosis (minor subset of sarcoidosis)
Drug induced (acute)	Chronic hypersensitivity pneumonitis
Environmental/occupational/inhalation causes (less exposure/mild disease)	Chronic drug/environmental/occupational/inhalation exposure
Idiopathic pulmonary capillaritis	Associated with collagen vascular diseases (rheumatoid arthritis, progressive systemic sclerosis, systemic lupus erythematosis, polymyositis/dermatomyositis)
Idiopathic BOOP	
Respiratory bronchiolitis–associated ILD (RBILD)	
Chronic eosinophilic pneumonia	Chronic aspiration
Primary alveolar proteinosis	Chronic radiation fibrosis
Acute radiation pneumonitis	Pulmonary fibrosis coexisting/associated with pulmonary hypertension
Lymphocytic interstitial pneumonia	
Nonspecific/nonclassifiable interstitial pneumonia	Chronic idiopathic BOOP (subset of idiopathic BOOP)
Other disorders with components of ILD with a favorable prognosis are Wegener's granulomatosis, Goodpasture's syndrome, and acute pulmonary capillaritis associated with collagen vascular/autoimmune disorders; see pulmonary vasculitis chapters	BOOP associated with collagen vascular diseases
	Chronic pulmonary hemorrhage syndromes
	Pulmonary veno-occlusive disease
	Obliterative bronchiolitis with or without associated ILD (idiopathic, rheumatoid arthritis, progressive systemic sclerosis, transplanted lung, toxic gas/fume inhalation)
	Acute interstitial pneumonia of unknown origin
	Langerhans cell granulomatosis (eosinophilic granuloma, histocytosis X)
	Lymphangioleiomyomatosis
	Tuberous sclerosis
	Pulmonary fibrosis associated with other inherited disorders
	Familial idiopathic pulmonary fibrosis

*Currently available therapy ineffective; clinical course progressive; "response": minimal improvement in only 20–30% of cases; no further deterioration (stability) is considered "response" as well.

clophosphamide), is currently recommended for most of these patients. A good clinical outcome may be possible only if these treatment regimens are initiated early in the course of the disease. Even in this circumstance, however, a favorable response may be seen in only 20 to 30 percent of patients with chronic pulmonary fibrosis, especially in those with IPF.[18,24]

Since the use of corticosteroids and immunosuppressives is associated with significant adverse effects, there appears to be an evolving consensus to discontinue the prolonged use of these drugs if stability or improvement has not been objectively shown after 6 to 12 months of available therapy. The dose and duration of corticosteroid use are less clear. Plasmapheresis is indicated in intractable and severe cases of alveolar hemorrhage syndromes resistant to corticosteroids and immunosuppressives. Supplemental oxygen is indicated for patients with hypoxia or demonstrating oxygen desaturation to maintain adequate oxygen saturation. In addition, unless contraindicated, all patients should receive pneumococcal and periodic influenza vaccinations.

Lung transplantation is a viable surgical option for selected patients who do not respond to currently available therapeutic regimens. Other supportive measures, such as rehabilitation, are indicated in appropriate patients.[18] It is to be hoped that better therapeutic regimens will become available in the near future.[13]

REFERENCES

1. Cherniack RM, Colby TV, Flint A, et al: Correlation of structure and function in idiopathic pulmonary fibrosis. *Am J Respir Crit Care Med* 151:1180–1188, 1995.
2. Colby TV, Swenson SJ: Anatomic distribution and histopathologic patterns in diffuse lung disease: Correlation with HRCT. *J Thorac Imaging* 11:1–26, 1996.
3. Coultas DB, Zumwalt RE, Black WC, Sobonya RE: The epidemiology of interstitial lung diseases. *Am J Respir Crit Care Med* 150:967–972, 1994.
4. Davis GS: Bronchoalveolar lavage in interstitial lung disease. *Semin Respir Crit Care Med* 15:37–60, 1994.
5. Fulmer JD, Roberts WC, von Gal ER, Crystal RG: Morphologic-physiologic correlates of the severity of fibrosis and degree of cellularity in idiopathic pulmonary fibrosis. *J Clin Invest* 63:665–676, 1979.
6. Gaensler EA, Carrington CB: Open biopsy for chronic diffuse infiltrative lung disease: Clinical, roentgenographic and physiological correlations in 502 patients. *Ann Thorac Surg* 30:411–426, 1980.

7. Gaensler EA, Carrington CB, Coutu RE, Fitzgerald MX: Radiographic-physiologic-pathologic correlations in interstitial pneumonias. *Prog Respir Res* 8:223–241, 1975.

8. Grenier P, Chevret S, Beigelman C: Chronic diffuse infiltrative lung disease: Determination of the diagnostic value of clinical data, chest radiography, and CT with Bayesian analysis. *Radiology* 191:383–390, 1994.

9. Hamman L, Rich AR: Clinical pathologic conference. *Int Clin* 1:196–231, 1933.

10. Hanson D, Winterbauer RH, Kirtland SH, Wu R: Changes in pulmonary function test results after 1 year of therapy as predictors of survival in patients with idiopathic pulmonary fibrosis. *Chest* 108:305–310, 1995.

11. Hansen JE, Wasserman K: Pathophysiology of activity limitation in patients with interstitial lung disease. *Chest* 109:1566–1576, 1996.

12. Holt RM, Schmidt RA, Godwin JD, Raghu G: High resolution CT in respiratory bronchiolitis–associated interstitial lung disease. *J Comput Tomogr* 17:46–50, 1993.

13. Hunninghake GW, Kalica AR: Approaches to the treatment of pulmonary fibrosis. *Am J Respir Crit Care Med* 151:915–918, 1995.

14. Johnson MA, Kwan S, Snell NJ, et al: Randomised controlled trial comparing prednisolone alone with cyclophosphamide and low dose prednisolone in combination in cryptogenic fibrosing alveolitis. *Thorax* 44:280–288, 1989.

15. Kantrow S, Meyer KC, Calhoun WJ, et al: The T helper:suppressor ratio in bronchoalveolar lavage is highly variable in sarcoidosis (abstract). *Am J Respir Crit Care Med* 149:A606, 1994.

16. Leung AN, Miller RR, Müller NL: Parenchymal opacification in chronic infiltrative lung diseases: CT-pathologic correlation. *Radiology* 188:209–214, 1993.

17. Lynch DA, Newell JD, Logan PM, et al: Can CT distinguish hypersensitivity pneumonitis from idiopathic pulmonary fibrosis? *AJR Am J Roentgenol* 165:807–811, 1995.

18. Meier-Sydow J, Weiss SM, Buhl R, et al: Idiopathic pulmonary fibrosis: Current clinical concepts and challenges in management. *Semin Respir Crit Care Med* 15:77–96, 1994.

19. Nishimura K, Itoh H, Kitaichi M: Pulmonary sarcoidosis: Correlation of CT and histopathologic findings. *Radiology* 189:105–109, 1993.

20. Nugent KM, Peterson MW, Jolles H: Correlation of chest roentgenograms with pulmonary function and bronchoalveolar lavage in interstitial lung disease. *Chest* 96:1224–1227, 1989.

21. Orens JB, Kazerooni EA, Martinez FJ, et al: The sensitivity of high-resolution CT in detecting idiopathic pulmonary fibrosis proved by open lung biopsy: A prospective study. *Chest* 108:109–115, 1995.

22. Padley SPG, Hansell DM, Flower CDR, Jennings P: Comparative accuracy of high resolution computed tomography and chest radiography in the diagnosis of chronic diffuse infiltrative lung disease. *Clin Radiol* 44:222–226, 1991.

23. Peterson MW, Nugent KM, Jolles H: Uniformity of bronchoalveolar lavage in patients with pulmonary sarcoidosis. *Am Rev Respir Dis* 137:79–84, 1988.

24. Raghu G, DePaso WJ, Cain K, et al: Azathioprine combined with prednisone in the treatment of idiopathic pulmonary fibrosis: A prospective double-blind, randomized, placebo-controlled clinical trial. *Am Rev Respir Dis* 144:291–296, 1991.

25. Raghu G, Cain K, Hammer S, Winterbauer R: Improved forced vital capacity (FVC), DLCO$_{SB}$ and resting P[A-a]O$_2$ measurements at one year predict long term survival in idiopathic pulmonary fibrosis (IPF) (abstract). *Am Rev Respir Dis* 143:A57, 1991.

26. Raghu G: Interstitial lung disease: A diagnostic approach. Are CT scan and lung biopsy indicated in every patient? *Am J Respir Crit Care Med* 151:909–914, 1995.

27. Ralph D, Robertson HT, Raghu G: Exercise limitation in patients presenting with interstitial lung disease (abstract). *Am J Respir Crit Care Med* 149:A876, 1994.

28. Remy-Jardin M, Giraud F, Remy J, et al: Importance of ground-glass attenuation in chronic diffuse infiltrative lung disease: Pathologic-CT correlation. *Radiology* 189:693–698, 1993.

29. Roelandt M, Demedts M, Callebaut W, et al: Epidemiology of interstitial lung disease (ILD) in Flanders: Registration by pneumologists in 1992–1994. Working group on ILD, VRGT. Vereniging voor Respiratoire Gezondheidszorg en Tuberculosebestrijding. *Acta Clin Belg* 50:260–268, 1995.

30. Schwarz MI, King TE: *Interstitial Lung Disease,* 2d ed. St. Louis, Mosby–Year Book, 1993.

31. Trentin L, Marcer G, Chilosi M: Longitudinal study of alveolitis in hypersensitivity pneumonitis patients. *J Allergy Clin Immunol* 82:577–585, 1988.

32. Tung KT, Wells AU, Rubens MB, et al: Accuracy of the typical computed tomographic appearances of fibrosing alveolitis. *Thorax* 48:334–338, 1993.

33. Wells AU, Hansell DM, Rubens MB, et al: The predictive value of appearances on thin-section computed tomography in fibrosing alveolitis. *Am Rev Respir Dis* 148:1076–1082, 1993.

34. Winterbauer RH, Lammert J, Selland M, et al: Bronchoalveolar lavage cell populations in the diagnosis of sarcoidosis. *Chest* 104:352–361, 1993.

SYSTEMIC SARCOIDOSIS

David R. Moller

Sarcoidosis is a multisystem granulomatous disorder of unknown origin characterized by activation of T lymphocytes and mononuclear phagocytes at sites of disease. Although any organ can be involved, the disease most commonly affects the lungs and intrathoracic lymph nodes. Eye and skin involvement is seen in approximately 20 percent of patients; symptomatic involvement of other organs occurs less frequently. Since the cause of sarcoidosis is unknown, a diagnosis is most securely established from a compatible clinical history together with histologic evidence of widespread, noncaseating granulomas in more than one organ and the absence of a competing diagnosis, such as tuberculosis, fungal disease, or malignancy. Clinical, epidemiologic, and fam-

ily studies support the hypothesis that sarcoidosis is caused by exposure to an environmental, possibly infectious, agent and that there may be genetic susceptibility to the disease. Corticosteroids remain the mainstay of treatment when patients need to be treated because of threatened organ failure or chronic progressive disease.

HISTORICAL PERSPECTIVE

Hutchinson was the first to describe a case of sarcoidosis; he called it Mortimer's malady, after one of his patients who presented with face and limb skin lesions.[19] In 1889, Besnier of Paris described a 34-year-old man with violaceous skin lesions of the nose, ear lobules, and central face; he proposed that the lesions were a variant of lupus erythematosis, leading to its designation as "lupus pernio."[3] In 1899, Boeck became the first investigator to describe the characteristic noncaseating granulomas in a patient with swollen peripheral lymphadenopathy and skin nodules. He proposed the term *multiple benign sarkoids of the skin* because he thought the granulomatous changes resembled sarcomatous tissue.[5] Subsequently, descriptions of sarcoid-type lesions in the eyes, bones, lungs, and salivary glands were made, but the systemic and unifying nature of sarcoidosis was not recognized for almost 20 years.

The view that sarcoidosis is a systemic disorder is based on the work of Schaumann, a Swedish dermatologist, who in 1914 presented a prizewinning essay on lupus pernio.[38] In his treatise, he expressed the view that Besnier's lupus pernio and Boeck's multiple sarcoids were manifestations of the same disease. He suggested that the disease might affect the lymph nodes, nasal mucosa, tonsils, bones, and lungs with a "tuberculoid granulomatous process." Following these observations, hundreds of cases of sarcoidosis affecting almost every organ system were reported.

The next major breakthrough in understanding sarcoidosis was based on the pioneering observations of Löfgren of Sweden in the 1940s and '50s. Löfgren noted that sarcoidosis frequently begins with asymptomatic bilateral hilar adenopathy or acute erythema nodosum and that these presentations have favorable prognoses.[26] Widespread chest radiography screenings demonstrated that clinically symptomatic sarcoidosis represents only a small proportion of all cases of sarcoidosis. During this period, studies of the Kveim-Siltzbach reaction provided support for a unifying pathogenesis of both spontaneously resolving and progressive sarcoidosis.

More recently, the tools of modern cell and molecular biology have led to remarkable advances in our understanding of the immunopathogenesis of sarcoidosis. Bronchoalveolar lavage (BAL) has been an important research tool in this effort, having allowed investigators to study the local cellular mechanisms underlying granulomatous inflammation in pulmonary sarcoidosis. Although advances in our understanding of the pathogenesis of sarcoidosis continue, the next major breakthrough awaits elucidation of the etiology of the disease.

EPIDEMIOLOGY

Although the frequency and clinical presentation of sarcoidosis vary among geographic regions, there are more similarities than differences throughout the world.[15,40,43] Since many people with sarcoidosis are asymptomatic, estimates of annual incidence rates and prevalence figures depend heavily on the extent with which mass screening chest radiography is performed. In addition, the prevalence of sarcoidosis is particularly difficult to estimate in regions where tuberculosis is common. Prevalence rates of between 10 and 40 cases per 100,000 population have been reported in North America, southern Europe, and Japan. Higher prevalence rates have been noted in Sweden (64/100,000). In the United States the prevalence is estimated to be 10 to 17 times higher among African-Americans than in Caucasian-Americans. Worldwide, the disease is reported to be slightly more frequent in women. More than 80 percent of cases occur in persons between 20 and 45 years. In a small number of people, the disease begins in the preadolescent period or in the sixth or seventh decade. Erythema nodosum is more common among young, childbearing women, often after pregnancy and lactation, as originally noted by Löfgren. Irish women in London and Puerto Rican women in New York City have a particularly high frequency of erythema nodosum, while this clinical presentation is less common among African-Americans. In contrast, lupus pernio, a condition associated with chronic disease, appears more frequently in African-Americans.

ETIOLOGY

Despite the tools of modern medicine, the cause of sarcoidosis remains unknown. The clinical similarities to tuberculosis led Boeck as early as 1905 to conclude that sarcoidosis is an infectious disease similar or identical to tuberculosis. Investigators in the 1960s reported the presence of a transmissible agent in sarcoid tissue.[31] These studies could not be reproduced, however, and despite many attempts, no mycobacterial or other infectious organisms have been reproducibly cultured from sarcoid tissue. More recently, reports of mycobacterial nucleic acids in biopsy specimens and BAL detected by highly sensitive molecular biologic techniques have also not been confirmed by other investigators.[4,37] High titers of antibodies against lymphotropic DNA viruses (Epstein-Barr virus, cytomegalovirus, human herpesvirus type 6), rubella, parainfluenza, and HTLV1 have been described in patients with sarcoidosis, but a viral origin has not been substantiated by viral cultures or tissue analysis. The presence of virus-specific antibodies probably reflects generalized B-cell activation and not a causal relationship. Although direct demonstration of an infectious origin remains unproven, support for an infectious or environmental cause derives from several epidemi-

ologic studies that demonstrate seasonal, time-space, or occupational clusters of sarcoidosis cases.

The absence of convincing evidence for a primary infectious agent in sarcoidosis has led to the hypothesis that sarcoidosis is the result of an aberrant or autoimmune response to a persistent infectious or environmental agent or an autoantigen. The presence of antinuclear antibodies, rheumatoid factor, hypergammaglobulinemia, and immune complexes in sarcoidosis may reflect a generalized immune dysregulation that is consistent with this possibility.

Kveim-Siltzbach Test

The hypothesis that sarcoidosis might be caused by an infectious agent led to attempts to develop skin tests similar to that of Mendel and Mantoux for tuberculosis. In 1935, Williams and Nickerson reported that intradermal inoculation of a suspension of sarcoid tissue resulted in firm red papules in patients with suspected sarcoidosis but not in normal control subjects. Kveim, a dermatologist in Oslo, demonstrated that these papules contained sarcoidlike granulomas when biopsied 1 to 4 weeks after injection. In the 1950s, Siltzbach and others demonstrated, in worldwide studies, that a single, validated reagent was positive (showed a granuloma on biopsy 4 weeks after application) in up to 80 percent of patients with early sarcoidosis and manifested under 1 percent false-positive responses.[16,22,31] To date, however, attempts to identify the component in the Kveim-Siltzbach reagent responsible for inducing sarcoid granulomas have been unsuccessful.

GENETICS

Family studies support the concept that genetic factors may predispose to sarcoidosis or determine clinical expression of the disease.[31,43] One retrospective study reported that familial clustering of sarcoidosis occurred in 16 percent of African-American patients with sarcoidosis referred to a tertiary-care hospital in the United States.[13] Within the same family, sibling pairs are most common and mother-daughter pairs are more frequent than father-son pairs. Monozygotic twins appear more likely to both have sarcoidosis than dizygotic twins, strongly suggesting a genetic component to the disease. The lack of a clear genetic pattern suggests that susceptibility to sarcoidosis is likely to be polygenic and associated with important environmental factors.

HLA studies have been performed in many population groups, with inconsistent results. HLA-B8 is associated with spontaneous remission and erythema nodosum in some studies, whereas other haplotypes have been associated with either favorable or unfavorable prognoses in different populations.[14] Newer techniques for molecular genotyping may better identify major histocompatibility complex (MHC) genes important in determining disease susceptibility, as illustrated by the association of susceptibility to chronic beryllium disease with HLA-DP haplotypes containing glutamate in position 69 of the β chain.[34]

PATHOLOGY

The pathologic hallmark of sarcoidosis is the presence of discrete, noncaseating, epithelioid cell granulomas typically at different stages of development (Fig. 69-1). The dominant cell in

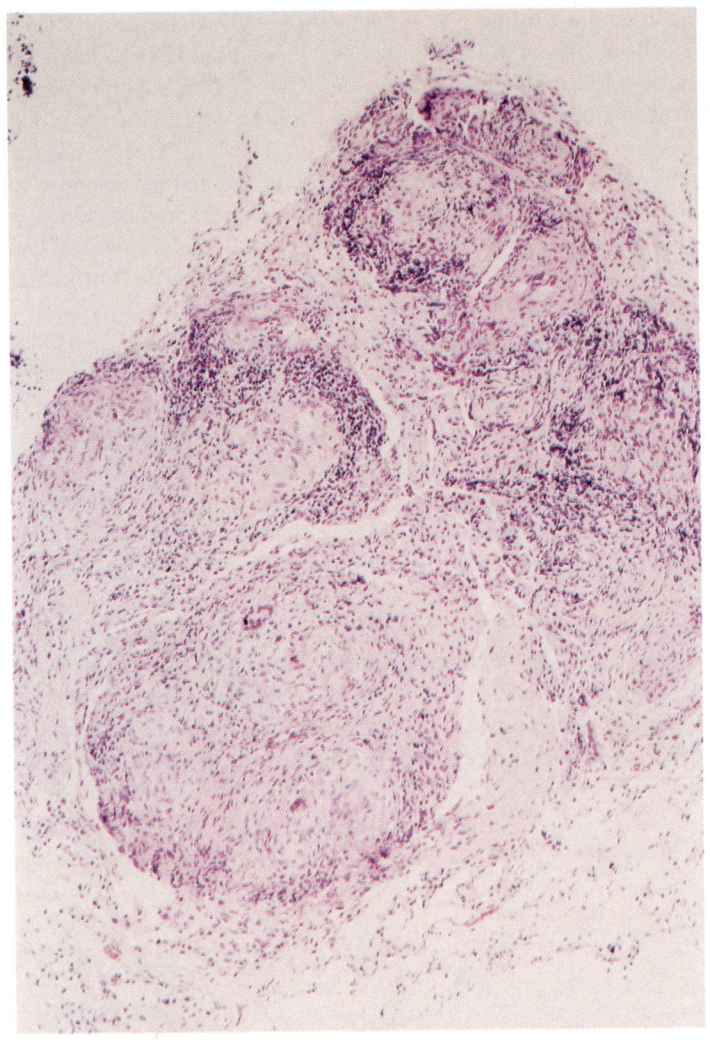

A

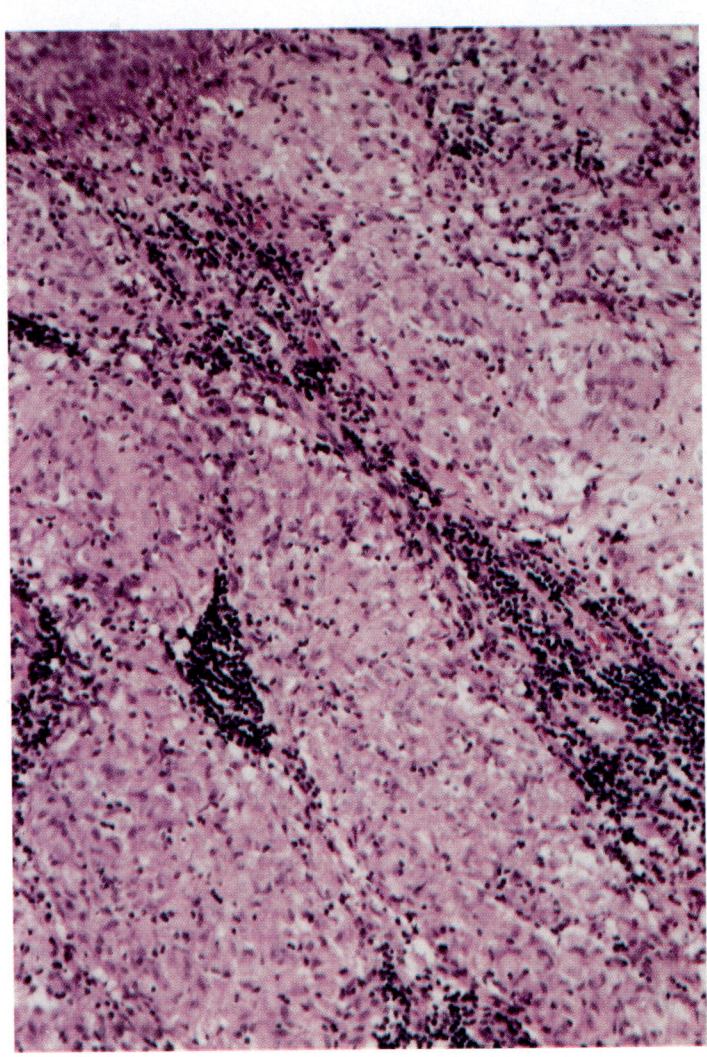

B

FIGURE 69-1   Photomicrographs of tissue demonstrating noncaseating granulomatous inflammation in patients with sarcoidosis. *A.* Thoracoscopic lung biopsy showing extensive parenchymal involvement with granulomas, multinucleated giant cells, and mononuclear cell in-flammation (×80). *B.* Mediastinal lymph node biopsy showing typical discrete epithelioid granulomas (×200). *C.* Extensive granulomatous in-flammation of the myocardium in a fatal case of cardiac sarcoidosis (×100).

the central core is the epithelioid cell (thought to be a differentiated form of a mononuclear phagocyte), which contains abundant eosinophilic cytoplasm and a pale staining nucleus. CD4+ lymphocytes and mature macrophages are typically interspersed throughout the epithelioid core, whereas both CD4+ and CD8+ lymphocytes may be seen in the periphery of the granuloma. Giant cells, often containing cytoplasmic inclusions such as calcium and iron-laden Schaumann bodies, are scattered throughout the inflammatory locus. These features are not specific for sarcoidosis, as similar histopathologic findings can be seen in beryllium disease, tuberculosis, leprosy, Crohn's disease, primary biliary cirrhosis, fungal disease, foreign-body material, and local "sarcoid reactions" that occur in lymph nodes near neoplastic or chronic inflammatory areas.

In the lung, granulomas tend to form along perivascular and peribronchial regions, areas rich in lymphatic vessels. Frequently, a mononuclear cell infiltration composed predominantly of lymphocytes is present in the adjacent interstitium. Ultrastructural studies of active pulmonary inflammation demonstrate disrupted type I epithelial cells with damage to the alveolar basement membrane that correlate with parameters of interstitial cellular inflammation. Granulomas in sarcoidosis may resolve, leaving few residual changes, or may undergo fibrosis, leaving a stellate scar or hyalinized ghost of a former granuloma.

IMMUNOPATHOGENESIS

Granulomatous inflammation in sarcoidosis is regulated by a complex interplay of T cells, mononuclear phagocytes, fibroblasts, B cells, dendritic cells, and other accessory cells (Fig. 69-2).[6,7,39,44] Interaction among these cells is regulated in large part by cytokines released by immunocompetent cells, as well as by direct cell-cell communication. The result is a tightly orchestrated process culminating in the formation of compact granulomatous structures. This inflammatory process results in pathologic changes in organ function by damaging local tissues, disrupting normal architecture, and producing cytokines and chemical mediators with local and systemic effects.

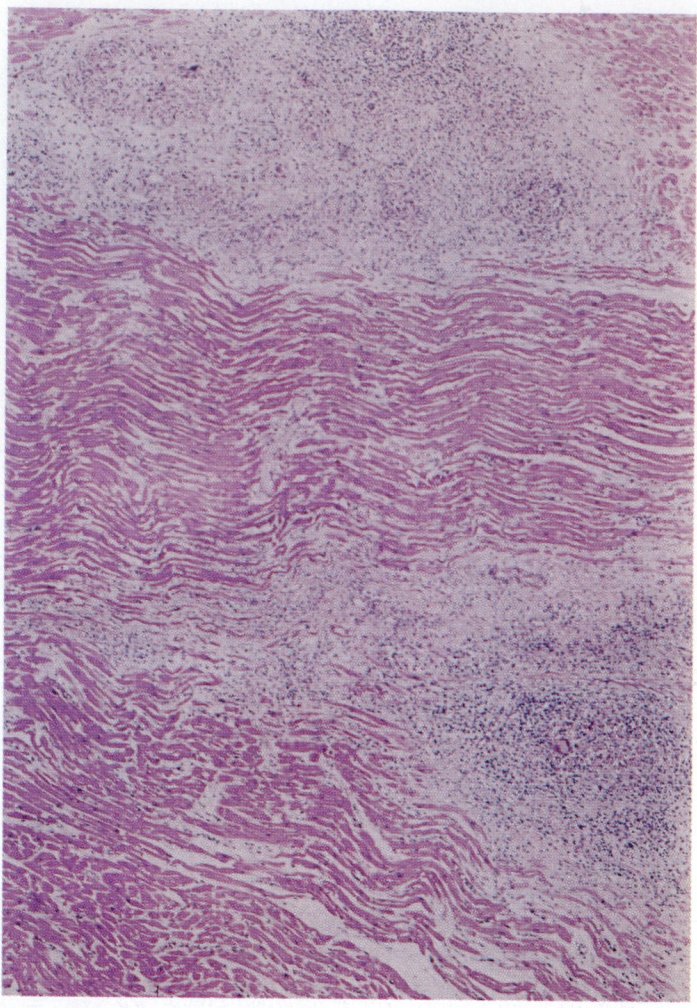

C

FIGURE 69-1   *(Cont.)*

T Lymphocytes

T-cell activation is a central feature of granulomatous inflammation in sarcoidosis.[39] There is a marked preponderance of T cells at sites of disease, including lymph nodes, skin, spleen, and lung. Morphologically, the T lymphocytes are large, have features of activated cells, and are predominantly of the CD4+ phenotype. Lung T cells recovered from the lower respiratory tract by BAL have similar features, including an increased proportion of CD4+ T lymphocytes that frequently express interleukin-2 receptor (IL-2R) p55 protein, very late activation antigen–1 (VLA-1), and class II major histocompatibility complex (MHC) molecules.[6,7,17] Lung T cells demonstrate reduced surface density of the CD3 component of the T-cell receptor complex, a hallmark of T cells activated through the T-cell antigen receptor pathway. Consistent with these findings, T cells recovered by BAL are proliferating at an increased rate and frequently express the cell cycle–related nuclear antigen Ki-67. Lung T cells in sarcoidosis spontaneously produce lymphokines, including interleukin (IL-2), γ-interferon (IFNγ), and molecules that function in monocyte chemotaxis and migration inhibition (Fig. 69-2).[36,44] IFNγ is critical to the development of T-cell–mediated responses that are characteristic of many granulomatous processes.

In contrast to the general activation and expansion of CD4+ T cells at sites of inflammation, peripheral blood of patients with sarcoidosis typically demonstrates CD4+ T-cell lymphopenia, which is occasionally profound. Cytokine expression by blood T cells is generally reduced compared with lung T cells, consistent with compartmentalization of the inflammatory response to affected tissues. Blood lymphocytes do express higher than normal levels of IL-2 receptor genes, suggesting that a subset of circulating T cells are not truly quiescent but may be trafficking from sites of inflammation.

In order to determine whether the accumulation of T cells at sites of disease in sarcoidosis is a direct result of antigen stimulation, the molecular structure of T-cell receptor genes expressed in patients with sarcoidosis has been investigated.[10,32] Most T cells express a T-cell antigen receptor composed of an α and a β chain. A minor subset of T cells have a T-cell receptor with γ and δ subunits. Each of these chains has variable and constant regions analogous to immunoglobulin genes. Antigen specificity of T cells is created by the imprecise rearrangement of specific variable (V), joining (J), and diversity (D) (in β and δ chains only) gene segments. Appropriate stimulation of the T-cell receptor by antigenic peptide-MHC molecular complexes results in clonal T-cell activation and proliferation that can bias the distribution of T-cell receptor gene expression. In sarcoidosis, sub-

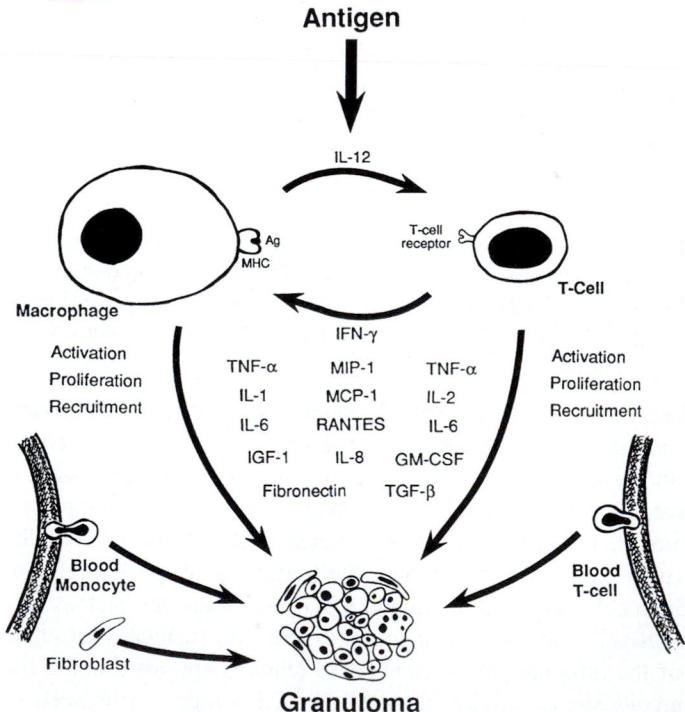

FIGURE 69-2   Mechanisms underlying granuloma formation in sarcoidosis. Antigenic stimulation in sarcoidosis results in activation of T cells with production of Th1 cytokines such as IFNγ and IL-2. Macrophages, activated directly by the inciting agent and by IFNγ, produce IL-12, TNFα, IL-6, and other cytokines important in cell activation, proliferation, and recruitment. Activated macrophages and T cells along with other effector cells, such as fibroblasts, orchestrate the complex process of granuloma formation under the regulatory influence of local cytokine production.

groups are characterized by biased expression of specific $V\beta$, $V\alpha$, or $\gamma\delta^+$ T-cell receptor genes in the lung or blood. For example, T cells bearing $V\beta8$ or $V\alpha2.3$ are dramatically increased in the lungs of subgroups with pulmonary sarcoidosis.[10,32] An increase in the proportions of $V\alpha2.3^+$ lung T cells in Swedish patients correlates with the DR3 haplotype, supporting the concept that these T cells are being preferentially expanded by a conventional antigen. The observation that the expansion of specific $\alpha\beta^+$ T-cell subsets in the lung and at sites of Kveim-Siltzbach skin reactions is oligoclonal provides additional evidence that sarcoidosis is an antigen-driven disorder.

Mononuclear Phagocytes

Macrophages are clearly at work in the development of granulomatous inflammation in sarcoidosis.[39,44] Sarcoid alveolar macrophages appear activated, containing increased amounts of lysozyme and angiotensin-converting enzyme. These cells produce higher levels of reactive oxygen species and more frequently express transferrin receptors and IL-2 receptors than normal alveolar macrophages. A high level of surface class II MHC molecules and other accessory molecules on sarcoid alveolar macrophages probably contribute to their enhanced ability to present antigen to T cells compared with normal alveolar macrophages[24] Alveolar macrophages from patients with sarcoidosis demonstrate enhanced production of TNFα, IL-6, IL-12, and possibly IL-1, cytokines known to be important in granuloma formation (Fig. 69-2). In contrast, sarcoid alveolar macrophages produce less than normal amounts of prostaglandin E_2, a potent inhibitor of many proinflammatory cytokines. A relative lack of PGE_2 and other anti-inflammatory molecules may contribute to the maintenance of chronic inflammation.

Multiple proinflammatory chemotactic cytokines (chemokines), including monocyte chemotactic protein (MCP)-1, RANTES, macrophage inflammatory protein (MIP)-1, IL-2, and IL-8, are found in BAL or tissue specimens in sarcoidosis.[39] These chemokines probably play important roles in the recruitment and activation of T cells, monocytes, and granulocytes to inflammatory loci in sarcoidosis. A higher than normal proportion of sarcoid alveolar macrophages have an immature phenotype typical of circulating monocytes, consistent with trafficking of blood monocytes into the lung. Alveolar macrophages from patients with sarcoidosis also release increased amounts of fibronectin and fibroblast growth factors, such as insulinlike growth factor–1 (IGF-1), which are important in fibroblast recruitment and replication. Along with these cytokines, tumor necrosis factor–α (TNF-α) and transforming growth factor-β (TGF-β) are expressed at sites of sarcoid granulomas. These factors no doubt contribute to pulmonary fibrosis in this disorder.

Th1 Cytokines

A current paradigm in immunology is that the nature of an immune response to an antigenic stimulus is determined largely by the pattern of cytokines produced by activated CD4$^+$ (and CD8$^+$) T cells. T helper 1 (Th1) cells express IFNγ and IL-2, cytokines important in macrophage activation and delayed-type hypersensitivity responses. T helper 2 (Th2) cells express IL-4 and IL-5,

cytokines important in macrophage deactivation, antibody-mediated responses, and eosinophilia. The subsets show cross-regulation, with IFNγ down-regulating cytokine production and proliferation of Th2 cells, and IL-4 providing a similar function for Th1 cells. Cytokines such as IL-12 and IL-10 play an important role in the regulation of these responses. IL-12, produced by macrophages and dendritic cells, is critical to Th1 development and directly stimulates production of IFNγ by T cells and NK cells. IL-10, produced by macrophages and both Th1 and Th2 cells, is a potent macrophage deactivator that down-regulates Th1 responses by inhibiting IL-12 and IFNγ production.

There is increasing evidence that granulomatous inflammation in sarcoidosis is characterized by a type 1 (or Th1) cytokine profile.[36,46] BAL studies demonstrate increased levels of IFNγ, IL-2, and IL-12 and low or undetectable levels of IL-4, IL-5, and IL-10 in patients with active, recently diagnosed pulmonary sarcoidosis compared with normal persons. The known dependence of granulomatous inflammation on type 1 cytokines such as IFNγ and IL-12 in many experimental models makes it likely that these cytokines function in a similar fashion in the initiation and maintenance of granulomatous inflammation in sarcoidosis.

A hypothetical model of the pathogenesis of sarcoidosis can be based on these clinical and experimental data (Fig. 69-3). In many patients with sarcoidosis, granulomatous inflammation resolves with few residua—an outcome probably based on a Th1-dependent immune response that is effective in removing the inciting agent. Apoptotic bodies have been documented in sarcoid granulomas, suggesting that programmed cell death (apoptosis) is a major mechanism of granuloma resorption. If the immune response is ineffective in removing the inciting stimulus, dysregulated cytokine production may result in the persistence of granulomatous inflammation driven initially by dominant Th1 cytokine production. In some cases, chronic granulomatous inflammation may be associated with progressive fibrosis. The mechanisms underlying these processes are unknown but may involve tissue injury from the local release of reactive oxygen species and potent proteases, lipases, and lysosomal products from macrophages and other effector cells at sites of inflammation. Conceivably, cytokines such as TGFβ, IL-10, and IL-4, which have been implicated in fibrotic responses in experimental models of granulomatous diseases, play a role in pulmonary fibrosis in sarcoidosis, though this has not yet been established. A fibrotic outcome may theoretically be prevented by suppressing the inflammatory response early in the course of the disease.

CLINICAL FEATURES

The clinical presentation and natural course of sarcoidosis vary greatly.[1,27,30,31,33,40] Although almost any organ of the body can be affected, the lungs or intrathoracic lymph nodes are involved in more than 90 percent of patients with the disease (Table 69-1). Up to two-thirds of patients are asymptomatic but have sarcoidosis diagnosed after an incidental radiographic finding of bilateral hilar adenopathy (Fig. 69-4). Occasionally, interstitial infiltrates are seen in association with intrathoracic adenopathy in asymptomatic patients, most commonly in Caucasians. Symptomatic presentations of sarcoidosis most frequently involve the respiratory system, usually associated with pulmonary infiltrates.

TABLE 69-1

Major Clinical Manifestations of Sarcoidosis

Organ System	Clinical Feature
Pulmonary	Restrictive and, less often, obstructive disease, fibrocystic disease, bronchiectasis, endobronchial granulomas, mycetomas, hemoptysis, lobar atelectasis
Upper airway	Hoarseness, laryngeal or tracheal obstruction, nasal congestion, sinusitis, saddle nose deformity
Ocular	Anterior and posterior uveitis, chorioretinitis, conjunctivitis, optic neuritis, glaucoma, catarracts
Skin	Erythema nodosum, chronic nodules and plaques, lupus pernio, alopecia
Hepatic	Hepatomegaly, jaundice, cirrhosis
Cardiac	Arrhythmias, heart block, cardiomyopathy, sudden death
Central nervous	Facial and other cranial neuropathies (e.g., Bell's palsy), aseptic meningitis, brain mass, seizures, obstructing hydrocephalus, myelopathy, polyneuropathy, mononeuritis multiplex
Salivary and lacrimal gland	Salivary, lacrimal, and parotid gland enlargement, sicca syndrome
Hematologic	Mediastinal, peripheral, and retroperitoneal lymphadenopathy, splenomegaly, hypersplenism, anemia, lymphopenia, thrombocytopenia
Joints and musculoskeletal	Polyarthritis, Achilles tendinitis, heel pain, polydactylitis, bone cysts, myopathy
Endocrine	Hypercalciuria, hypercalcemia, hypopituitarism, diabetes insipidus, epididymitis
Renal	Renal calculi, nephrocalcinosis, renal failure

Eye and skin impairment is seen in approximately 20 percent of patients; symptomatic involvement of other organs occurs less frequently.

Patients may demonstrate an acute, a subacute, or a chronic presentation. One classification scheme with prognostic information categorizes patients based on their initial presentation as follows: asymptomatic, acute sarcoidosis with erythema nodosum (Löfgren's syndrome), subacute sarcoidosis with symptoms or signs of pulmonary disease for less than 2 years, chronic sarcoidosis with evidence of pulmonary disease for more than 2 years, fibrocystic sarcoidosis, and dominant extrapulmonary sarcoidosis. Two years represents an arbitrary but useful reference point for distinguishing patients with chronic disease, since remissions, if they occur, usually do so within this period.

Acute Sarcoidosis with Erythema Nodosum

Sarcoidosis may present in patients with an acute onset of erythema nodosum and bilateral hilar adenopathy, usually associated with fevers, polyarthritis, and uveitis, known as Löfgren's syndrome. Erythema nodosum is characterized by tender reddish nodules several centimeters in diameter, usually located on the lower extremities. The polyarthritis is often severe and incapacitating. Typically the ankles, feet, knees, and, occasionally, wrists

and elbows are affected. Approximately 10 percent of patients with this syndrome will have a normal chest radiograph. Löfgren's syndrome is more common in European and Caucasian populations than in African-American.[40,43] The onset is usually abrupt, but the prognosis is excellent, with resolution of symptoms typically occurring within weeks to several months.

Pulmonary Sarcoidosis

Respiratory symptoms occur in 40 to 60 percent of patients. The most common symptoms are cough and shortness of breath, usually of a progressive, insidious nature. The cough is usually nonproductive and may be severe. Dyspnea is typically worse with exertion. Sputum production and hemoptysis are frequent in patients with fibrocystic sarcoidosis, a condition that is often associated with bronchiectasis and recurrent respiratory infections. Ill-defined chest pain is a frequent complaint, possibly caused by nerve irritation from inflammation, scarring, and lymph node enlargement in the chest. Chest tightness and wheezing are not uncommon, particularly with endobronchial disease or fibrocystic changes, but are rarely the only manifestation. These symptoms are usually poorly responsive to bronchodilators, except in a subgroup of patients with bronchial hyperresponsiveness and reversible airway obstruction. Segmental atelectasis and bronchial or tracheal stenosis are rare but have been reported. Pulmonary hypertension and cor pulmonale may be the result of chronic, severe fibrocystic sarcoidosis. Rarely, dyspnea from severe pulmonary hypertension occurs without extensive interstitial lung disease, presumably from granulomatous vasculitis of pulmonary vessels.

Extrapulmonary Sarcoidosis

Many patients have clinically important affliction of one or more organ systems with or without significant pulmonary disease (Table 69-1).[27,30] Systemic constitutional symptoms such as fever, malaise, fatigue, and weight loss are seen in about 20 percent of patients and may be disabling.

Sarcoidosis of the upper respiratory tract occurs in 5 to 10 percent of patients, usually in those with long-standing disease. Severe nasal congestion and chronic sinusitis may result in considerable morbidity. Typically, these symptoms are unresponsive to decongestants and inhaled steroids. Chronic disease or surgical intervention may result in destruction of the nasal septum and a "saddle nose" deformity. Laryngeal sarcoidosis may present with severe hoarseness, stridor, and acute respiratory failure sec-

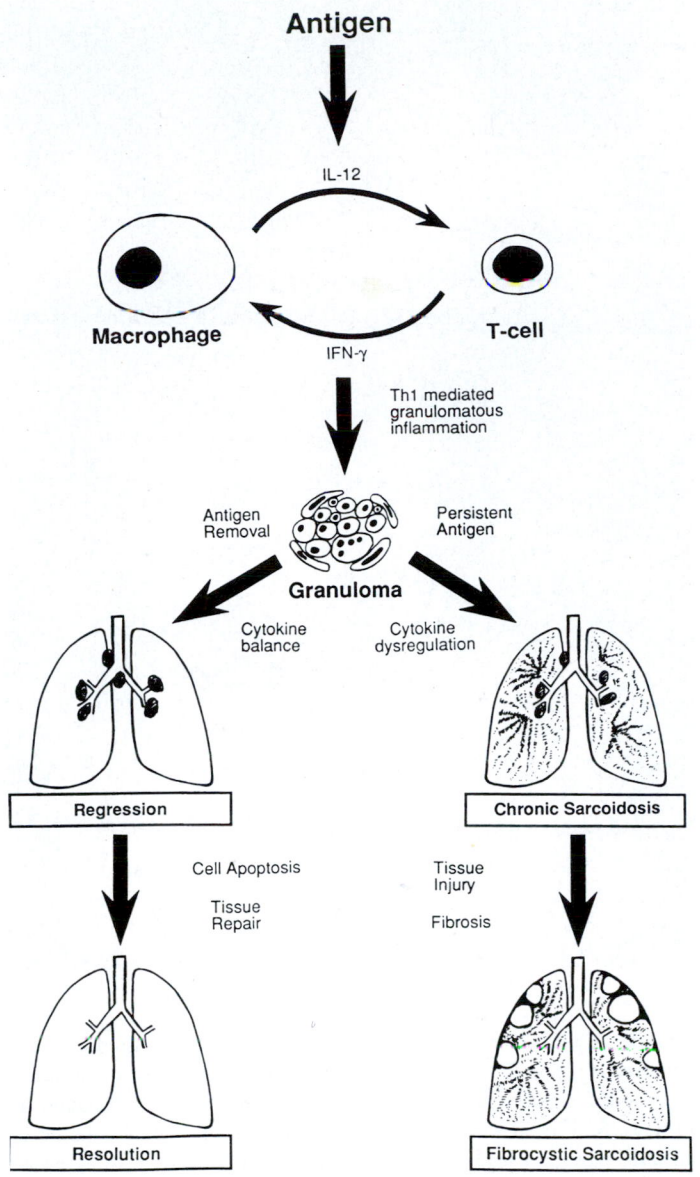

Antigen

IL-12

Macrophage   **T-cell**

IFN-γ

Th1 mediated
granulomatous
inflammation

Antigen   Persistent
Removal   Antigen

Granuloma

Cytokine   Cytokine
balance   dysregulation

Regression   **Chronic Sarcoidosis**

Cell Apoptosis   Tissue
                                  Injury
Tissue
Repair   Fibrosis

Resolution   **Fibrocystic Sarcoidosis**

FIGURE 69-3 Hypothetical model of the pathogenesis of sarcoidosis. An inciting agent induces antigen-specific Th1 mediated granulomatous inflammation and stimulates mononuclear phagocytes to produce IL-12. Removal of the inciting agent with return to cytokine homeostasis results in granuloma regression, probably by cell apoptosis. Persistent antigenic stimulation results in cytokine dysregulation and chronic disease. If untreated, persistent inflammation may result in prominent tissue damage and fibrosis.

ondary to upper-airway obstruction. Frequently, laryngeal sarcoidosis is associated with chronic skin lesions, particularly lupus pernio.

Uveitis is the most common eye lesion in sarcoidosis and may be the initial presenting manifestation. The uveitis is more commonly anterior, may be unilateral or bilateral, and is frequently associated with bilateral hilar adenopathy. Severe chorioretinitis occurs uncommonly. Optic neuritis may present dramatically with blindness. Granulomatous conjunctivitis appears as a granular or cobblestonelike appearance of the conjunctivae. Chronic uveitis occurs in as many as 20 percent of patients with chronic sarcoidosis and may be more frequent in African-Americans. Ad-

hesions between the iris and lens, glaucoma, and cataracts are potential complications of sarcoid eye inflammation.

Chronic sarcoidosis of the skin usually manifests as plaques and subcutaneous nodules. Typically, the plaques are located around the hairline, eyelids, ears, nose, mouth, and extensor surfaces of the arms and legs. Lesions in the scalp are sometimes associated with alopecia. Occasionally, the skin lesions are pruritic or tender and may be either hyper- or hypopigmented. The main complaint is usually cosmetic. Lupus pernio is a particularly disfiguring form of cutaneous sarcoidosis of the face, with violaceous plaques and nodules covering the nose, nasal alae, malar areas, and areas around the eyes. Chronic skin lesions are more common and severe in African-Americans. Hilar adenopathy, pulmonary, upper respiratory tract, and bone involvement is commonly associated with severe cutaneous sarcoidosis.

The liver is frequently affected in sarcoidosis, but hepatic involvement is rarely the sole manifestation of the disease.[29] Active hepatic inflammation may be associated with fever and tender hepatomegaly. Pruritus can be severe and disabling in a small number of patients. In these cases, hepatic sarcoidosis may mimic primary biliary cirrhosis, except that antimitochondrial antibodies are absent. On biopsy, liver granulomas in all stages of development are typical for sarcoidosis but are nonspecific. Characteristically, the serum alkaline phosphatase and γ-glutamyltransferase are elevated proportionately higher than the transaminases or bilirubin, though all patterns can be seen. Elevated serum liver function frequently reverts to normal spontaneously or after treatment with corticosteroids. Progressive cirrhosis may occur if chronic, granulomatous inflammation of the liver is not treated. Symptomatic gastrointestinal impairment in sarcoidosis is rare.

Although myocardial sarcoidosis is clinically apparent in 5 percent or less of cases, it remains a major cause of mortality in young adults with sarcoidosis.[35] Arrhythmia, heart block, or sudden death can be the presenting clinical manifestation due to granulomatous inflammation of the conduction system. Extensive involvement of the myocardium can lead to cardiomyopathy and congestive heart failure or angina. Endomyocardial biopsy can establish the diagnosis when there is clinical uncertainty, but it is positive in only 60 percent of cases, owing to sampling inefficiencies. Holter monitoring is used to exclude serious arrhythmias in persons with suspected cardiac sarcoidosis. Electrophysiological testing may be indicated to exclude arrhythmias undetected by routine studies. Echocardiography is useful in assessing physiological abnormalities such as abnormal myocardial wall motion.

Neurologic symptoms occur in less than 5 percent of patients with sarcoidosis. The most common manifestation is cranial neuropathy. All cranial nerves have been implicated, though most commonly the seventh and fifth nerves are affected. Eighth nerve involvement may cause hearing loss and vestibular dysfunction. Often the palsies resolve spontaneously or with corticosteroids, but they sometimes recur years later. Manifestations of central nervous system involvement include mass lesions that may mimic meningioma, aseptic meningitis, obstructive hydrocephalus, and hypothalamic or pituitary dysfunction. Seizures, headache, change in mental status, confusion, and diabetes in-

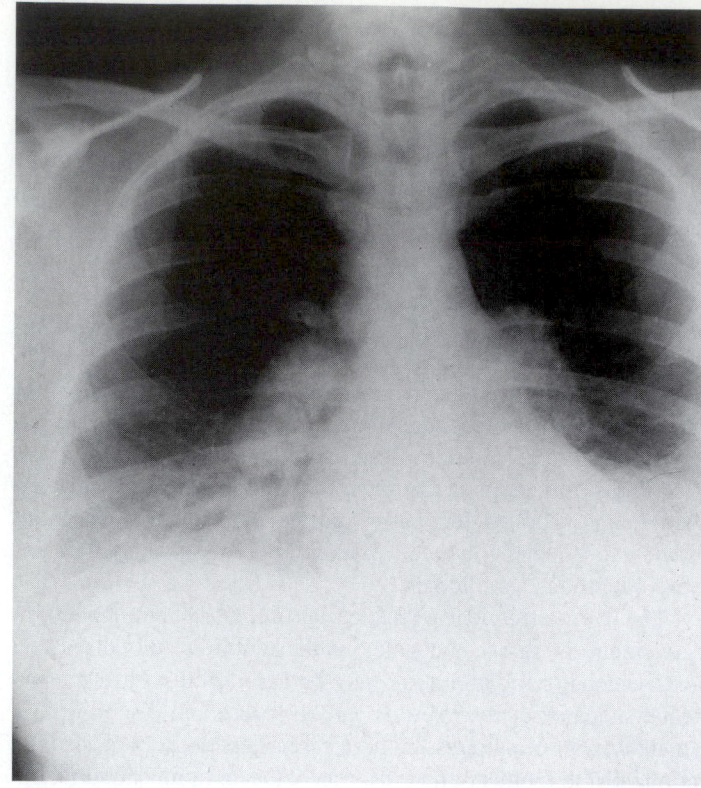

A

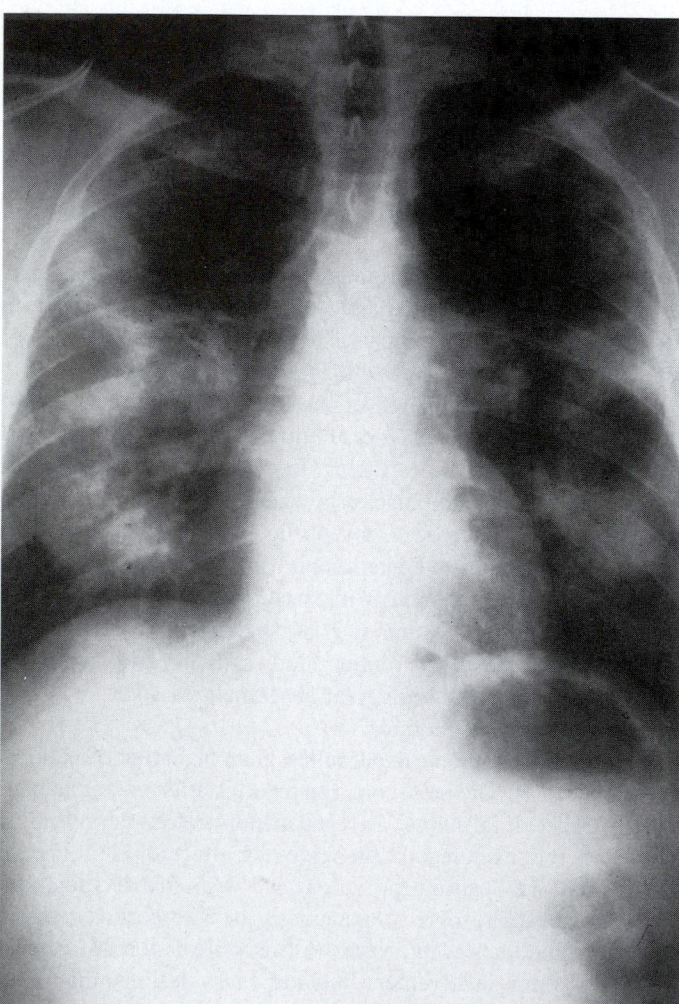

B

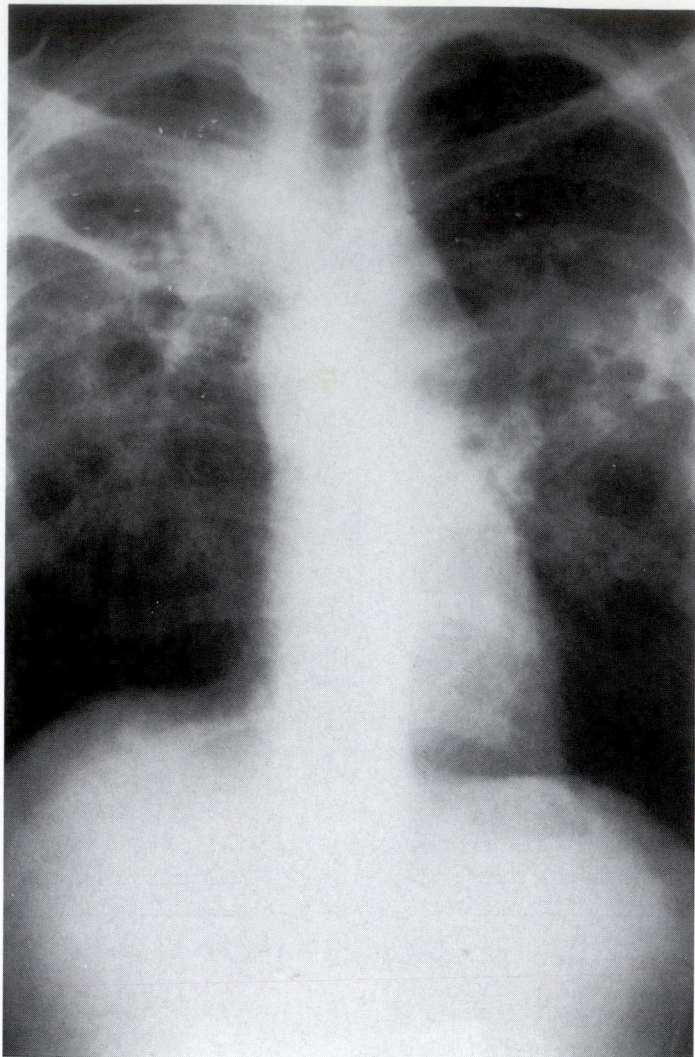

C

FIGURE 69-4 Chest radiographs of patients with pulmonary sarcoidosis. *A.* Type II sarcoidosis with prominent, discrete "stand-away" hilar nodes, right paratracheal adenopathy, and fine reticulonodular infiltrates. *B.* Type II sarcoidosis with an unusual pattern of large nodular and coalescent infiltrates. *C.* Fibrocystic sarcoidosis with extensive scarring, bullous and cystic changes, hilar retraction, and parenchymal infiltrates.

sipidus may be presenting symptoms. Cerebrospinal fluid characteristically demonstrates elevated protein levels with a lymphocytic pleocytosis. Magnetic resonance imaging with gadolinium enhancement or contrast-enhanced computed tomography (CT) may demonstrate inflammatory lesions with a propensity for the leptomeningeal and periventricular areas. Spinal cord compression syndromes may result in hemiparesis. Peripheral neuropathies account for about 15 percent of cases of neurosarcoidosis, typically presenting as mononeuritis multiplex or a predominant sensory deficit.

Granulomatous inflammation of salivary, parotid, and lacrimal glands results in enlarged, tender glands and/or sicca syndrome with dry mouth and dry eyes in less than 5 percent of patients with sarcoidosis. The association of fever, parotid enlargement, facial palsy, and uveitis is known as uveoparotid fever, or Heerfordt's syndrome, and is usually accompanied by bilateral hilar adenopathy.

Peripheral lymph node enlargement is usually minimal in sarcoidosis and often regresses spontaneously. A pattern of bilateral, symmetric lymphadenopathy in the cervical, supraclavicular, axillary, and epitrochlear nodes is most frequently seen. Bulky, disfiguring adenopathy is seen in less than 5 percent of patients.

Splenomegaly occurs in 10 to 20 percent of patients, often associated with hepatomegaly and, less frequently, hypercalcemia. Occasionally, splenic enlargement may be massive. Hypersplenism with anemia and thrombocytopenia occurs but is uncommon. Peripheral blood leukopenia is common in sarcoidosis, probably more often as a result of altered trafficking of lymphocytes than splenic trapping. Splenic rupture rarely occurs.

Granulomas in the bone marrow are found in about 20 percent of patients who come to autopsy but rarely cause symptoms during the course of the disease. Granulomas in the bone marrow are nondiagnostic and require the strict exclusion of other conditions, such as malignancy and infectious granulomatous diseases.

Arthralgias are a frequent complaint in sarcoidosis. A short-lived polyarthritis is typical of early-onset joint disease, which is usually associated with erythema nodosum. Joint disease is found in less than 5 percent of patients with chronic sarcoidosis.[11] Signs of arthritis or synovitis of the knees, phalanges of the hands, shoulders, or ankles are most commonly seen. Joint erosion is rare, but "punched out" bony lesions with cystic changes and loss of bony trabeculae may be seen on radiograph. Cystic lesions of the long bones, pelvis, sternum, skull, and vertebrae occur rarely.

Although random muscle biopsies demonstrate muscle granulomas in most patients with sarcoidosis, symptomatic myopathy in sarcoidosis with weakness and tenderness is uncommon. In rare cases, a polymyositis presenting as profound weakness is observed and is associated with marked elevation of serum creatine phosphokinase.

Abnormal calcium metabolism is found in sarcoidosis, with hypercalciuria more frequent than hypercalcemia. Evidence supports the concept that these abnormalities are due primarily to increased conversion of vitamin D metabolites to active $1,25(OH)_2$ vitamin D by tissue macrophages and epithelioid cells at sites of granulomatous inflammation.[2] Higher serum levels of active vitamin D result in increased calcium absorption from the gut and reduced serum parathyroid hormone.

Kidney stones are the most frequent manifestation of renal sarcoidosis, usually related to abnormal calcium metabolism. Renal failure due to nephrocalcinosis may result from chronic, often asymptomatic hypercalcemia or hypercalciuria. Nephrotic syndrome and chronic glomerulonephritis are also associated with sarcoidosis. Granulomatous involvement of the kidneys occurs but is rarely the cause of significant renal dysfunction.

Sarcoidosis has been found in association with a variety of disorders of the immune system, such as common variable immunodeficiency, primary biliary cirrhosis, rheumatoid arthritis, systemic lupus erythematosus, Sjögren's syndrome, autoimmune thrombocytopenic purpura, hemolytic anemia, and autoimmune endocrinopathies. Given the rarity of some of these disorders, it is reasonable to postulate that these associations are the result of immune disturbances that may predispose to both disorders.

CLINICAL ASSESSMENT

An initial evaluation routinely includes a chest radiograph, pulmonary function tests with lung volumes, spirometry and diffusing capacity, liver function tests, calcium level, complete blood count, urinalysis, ECG, and a purified protein derivative (PPD) skin test. An initial slit-lamp examination is recommended in all cases of sarcoidosis in order to exclude uveitis that may not be clinically apparent. Other tests may be indicated if the clinical history or physical examination suggests specific organ involvement. For example, a Holter monitor or echocardiogram may be indicated if cardiac sarcoidosis is suspected.

Chest Radiography

The chest radiograph is important in the initial evaluation of patients with sarcoidosis, since it is abnormal in more than 90 percent of known cases and carries prognostic information.[9,15,40] By international convention, the chest radiograph is divided into stages or types (Fig. 69-4). A normal chest radiograph, or type 0, is found in 5 to 10 percent of patients with sarcoidosis, who frequently present with extrapulmonary manifestations of sarcoidosis. Intrathoracic adenopathy may be demonstrated by CT in some patients without obvious adenopathy by plain chest radiograph.

A type I chest radiograph is characterized by hilar adenopathy without evidence of interstitial infiltrates and is seen in approximately 40 percent of patients, many of whom are asymptomatic. Hilar adenopathy has typically a discrete, symmetric "potato node" appearance. Paratracheal adenopathy, particularly on the right side, is frequently present. CT may also demonstrate anterior or posterior mediastinal and subcarinal adenopathy. Asymmetric adenopathy suggests the possibility of malignancy, tuberculosis, or fungal disease. Patients presenting with a type I chest radiograph have the best overall prognosis, with a high likelihood of spontaneous remission.

A type II chest radiograph, characterized by bilateral hilar adenopathy and pulmonary infiltrates, is seen in 30 to 50 percent of patients on initial presentation (Fig. 69-4A). Commonly, the infiltrates demonstrate fine linear markings and small reticulonodules, particularly of the upper lobes. The infiltrates tend to be central, following bronchovascular structures. Occasionally, the infiltrates consist of discrete nodules or areas of fluffy "alveolar" consolidation that can mimic eosinophilic pneumonia, tumor, Wegener's granulomatosis, or infection (Fig. 69-4B). A miliary pattern can also be seen resembling miliary tuberculosis, hypersensitivity pneumonitis, chronic beryllium disease, or lymphangitic carcinomatosis. Calcification of hilar lymph nodes is very uncommon, but can occur with long-standing disease. Patients with a type II chest radiograph have an intermediate prognosis, with fewer spontaneous remissions.

When interstitial infiltrates are seen without evidence of hilar adenopathy, the chest radiograph is designated as type III. This is the pattern that is seen in 15 percent of patients on initial presentation. Differential diagnosis includes infections, idiopathic pulmonary fibrosis, and collagen vascular lung disease.

Patients with extensive fibrocystic changes and scarring on chest radiograph are often grouped separately (e.g., type IV) because of their poor prognosis. These patients demonstrate cephalad hilar retraction, volume loss, coarse fibrous strands, small and large bullae, cystic changes, and honeycombing from destructive inflammation and retraction of scar tissue (Fig. 69-4C). Tuberculosis and fungal disease can mimic this radiographic picture.

Unusual radiographic signs of sarcoidosis include pneumothorax, which is rare except when fibrocystic changes are present. Pleural effusions are rare and warrant investigation to exclude such causes as congestive heart failure, tuberculosis, and malignancy.

CT of the chest is usually not needed in the evaluation of patients with suspected sarcoidosis unless it is needed to help plan bronchoscopic biopsy of subcarinal, paratracheal, or other mediastinal lymph nodes. Sometimes this study is helpful in defining unusual radiographic features or to assess the extent of fibrocystic disease or bronchiectasis in advanced pulmonary sarcoidosis. The further utility of CT of the chest in clinical staging is under investigation.

Pulmonary Function Tests

Pulmonary function may be normal even when the chest radiograph demonstrates pulmonary infiltrates.[9,48] However, restrictive impairment with reduction in lung volumes, FVC and FEV_1, is common, particularly when pulmonary infiltrates are present on chest radiograph. Reduction in diffusing capacity can be seen in association with restrictive impairment or as an isolated deficit. Obstructive impairment is common in advanced fibrocystic disease, but can also be caused by endobronchial disease, laryngeal involvement, or tracheal and bronchial stenosis. A subgroup of patients have bronchial hyperresponsiveness to methacholine and airway obstruction that may respond to bronchodilators. Resting hypoxemia and exercise O_2 desaturation are typical when there is severe obstructive or restrictive impairment. CO_2 retention is unusual except in advanced pulmonary disease.

Cutaneous Anergy

A well-recognized feature of sarcoidosis is the impaired cutaneous response to common antigens that elicit delayed-type hypersensitivity reactions, seen in 30 to 70 percent of patients.[31] Since anergy to PPD is common in sarcoidosis, active tuberculosis must be strongly considered in any patient who develops a positive tuberculin skin test. Postulated mechanisms underlying the cutaneous anergy include a redistribution of T cells to sites of inflammation and the presence of local inhibitors of delayed-type hypersensitivity reactions, though additional mechanisms are also likely to be important.

DIAGNOSTIC APPROACH

A diagnosis of sarcoidosis is established on the basis of a compatible clinical and radiographic picture, evidence of widespread noncaseating granulomas, and exclusion of other granulomatous disorders. Although histologic evidence is needed from only a single site, clinical involvement of more than one system is necessary to exclude local granulomatous reactions to foreign bodies, infections, or tumor.

In some instances, the clinical presentation alone may be highly suggestive of sarcoidosis. For example, the acute onset of erythema nodosum, fever, uveitis, and polyarthritis with bilateral hilar adenopathy is highly suggestive of Löfgren's syndrome. When the possibility of infections such as histoplasmosis is low, it may be reasonable to observe without biopsy confirmation. There is controversy over the need for tissue confirmation in persons presenting with isolated bilateral hilar adenopathy. In the absence of symptoms and with a negative physical examination, this presentation is almost always a manifestation of sarcoidosis, and a period of observation is often justified.[47] When the adenopathy is asymmetric, massive, or located in the posterior or anterior mediastinum, or symptoms such as fever, chest pain, or constitutional symptoms are present, the increased risk of malignancy or infectious granulomatous disease favors biopsy. Some authorities recommend biopsy for all cases of bilateral hilar adenopathy to exclude malignancy.

In general, the easiest accessible biopsy site is used to confirm a diagnosis of sarcoidosis. Biopsy of a skin nodule, superficial lymph node, lacrimal gland, conjunctivae, or salivary gland can often help to establish a diagnosis but has a reasonable yield only if the tissue is grossly abnormal (Fig. 69-1). A liver biopsy can support a diagnosis in the proper clinical context despite the nonspecificity of hepatic granulomas. A positive Kveim-Siltzbach test may be used to support a diagnosis of sarcoidosis in centers possessing validated reagent. The scarcity of appropriately standardized extracts and concerns over the injection of human materials has, however, greatly diminished the utility of this approach. When superficial abnormalities are not apparent or if there is a need to exclude infectious or malignant chest disease, bronchoscopic biopsy is usually performed.

Biopsy by fiberoptic bronchoscopy is frequently used to confirm a diagnosis of pulmonary sarcoidosis because of the high yield and relative safety of the procedure.[23] The yield approaches 90 percent when pulmonary infiltrates are seen radiographically and at least four transbronchial biopsies are taken. When hilar adenopathy alone is present, the yield of transbronchial biopsy may still exceed 50 percent, indicating that granulomatous inflammation is present despite an absence of radiographic infiltrates. By sampling intrathoracic lymph nodes, transbronchoscopic needle aspiration biopsy can increase the probability of making a diagnosis when the location of the adenopathy makes the procedure technically feasible. Widespread endobronchial nodules with a cobblestone appearance are highly suggestive of sarcoidosis and, when biopsied, often demonstrate granulomas. Wegener's granulomatosis, fungal disease, or tuberculosis is less likely to cause this appearence. Bronchoscopic biopsy in advanced fibrocystic sarcoidosis has a low yield, owing to extensive fibrotic changes in the lung parenchyma.

Mediastinoscopy is rarely required to establish a diagnosis of sarcoidosis but should be considered in cases in which lymphoma, metastatic disease, or infection cannot be reasonably excluded.

Landmark studies in the early 1980s established that active pulmonary sarcoidosis is characterized by a marked increase in the proportion of lymphocytes recovered by BAL.[6,7] Lymphocytes recovered by bronchoalveolar lavage are typified by a dominance of $CD4^+$ T cells, in contrast to the $CD8^+$ lymphocytosis seen in hypersensitivity pneumonitis, viral infections, and many drug reactions.[17] However, there is wide variability in the proportions of lymphocytes and the ratio of $CD4^+$ to $CD8^+$ T cells found in pulmonary sarcoidosis, with considerable overlap in findings from some infectious, inflammatory, and malignant diseases.[44,45] In the proper clinical context, these nonspecific findings support but do not establish a diagnosis of sarcoidosis.

Serum angiotensin-converting enzyme (ACE) levels are elevated in 30 to 80 percent of patients with clinically active disease.[25] This protein has been detected in sarcoid granulomas, BAL fluid, tears, and cerebrospinal fluid, probably originating from activated epithelioid cells and macrophages at sites of inflammation. Although it was originally proffered as a potential diagnostic marker, elevated levels are seen in a variety of disorders, including infectious granulomatous diseases, lymphoma, hepatitis, and diabetes. The low specificity and wide variability of ACE levels militate against their use as a diagnostic marker.

Gallium 67 scans almost always demonstrate enhanced uptake in the lungs or hilar or mediastinal regions in patients with active pulmonary sarcoidosis.[6,22] These findings correlate with active inflammation but are not specific. Extrapulmonary sites such as the parotid, salivary, and lacrimal glands ("panda" sign) may also demonstrate positive uptake. Recent data from many centers suggest that routine use of gallium scanning is not warranted as a diagnostic aid or for clinical staging, owing to the lack of specificity, wide variability, expense, and radiation exposure of the test.

MONITORING CLINICAL ACTIVITY

The term *active* or *inactive* is used to describe a perception of the presence or absence of ongoing granulomatous inflammation in a patient with sarcoidosis. Although conceptually useful, measurements of disease activity do not equate with a need for treatment, since asymptomatic or low levels of granulomatous inflammation may not need to be treated if organ function is not compromised. Currently, treatment decisions are best based on repeated clinical examinations and direct measurement of organ function.

Several serologic tests have been promoted as potential clinical and prognostic aids, most notably serum ACE levels. Studies demonstrate that elevated serum ACE levels usually decrease as the disease regresses or in response to corticosteroids.[25] Although levels tend to correlate with extent of granulomatous inflammation throughout the body, the marked variability of this test in different studies has made the clinical utility of ACE levels uncertain.[45] Since the test does not assess dysfunction of any single organ and does not presage future course, it is generally agreed that ACE levels should not be used to make therapeutic decisions. Serum concentrations of lysozyme, β_2-microglobulin, neopterin, and soluble IL-2 receptor have also been suggested as biochemical markers of disease "activity," since they are elevated in many patients with clinically apparent disease. Although these measurements provide insight into immunologic activation in sarcoidosis, the clinical utility of these tests is unproven.

Recognition that BAL samples lung inflammation in pulmonary sarcoidosis led to studies that compared BAL measurements with disease activity.[6,44,45] Some studies found that the degree of $CD4^+$ lymphocytosis or the $CD4^+$:$CD8^+$ ratio of lung lymphocytes correlates with disease activity or clinical course. However, other studies found wide variation and considerable overlap of these parameters in different patient groups. A recent consensus view suggests that no single parameter or battery of bronchoalveolar measurements has sufficient predictive value to serve as a basis for making clinical decisions. Although a role for BAL in clinical management has not been established, this technique remains an extremely valuable research tool.

CLINICAL COURSE AND PROGNOSIS

Prognosis in sarcoidosis is strongly influenced by the initial disease presentation.[1,9,15,33,40,42] Patients with Löfgren's syndrome generally have an excellent prognosis, with symptoms regressing within weeks to months. Patients with asymptomatic hilar adenopathy also generally experience complete spontaneous recovery within several years. Overall, 60 to 80 percent of patients presenting with a type I chest radiograph undergo spontaneous remission. When taken together with the large group of patients with unrecognized sarcoidosis who also have a high incidence of complete spontaneous remission, the prognosis for most patients with sarcoidosis is excellent.

Patients presenting with type II chest radiographs have a somewhat poorer outcome, with spontaneous resolution occurring approximately 50 to 60 percent of the time. When treated with corticosteroids, they usually respond promptly, though treatment may need to be continued for an extended interval to prevent progressive fibrosis. Patients with type III chest radiographs undergo spontaneous remission less frequently and do not uniformly respond to corticosteroid therapy. Dramatic improvement can be noted, however, in some cases. Progression to pulmonary insufficiency and cor pulmonale is particularly common in patients with advanced fibrocystic disease. This group of patients has a particularly poor prognosis, since all have irreversible lung damage that may progress despite treatment. Although some patients clearly demonstrate sequential evolution in radiographic type during the course of their disease, others have resolution or no change in their chest radiograph over prolonged periods.

Anecdotal experience suggests that initial severity of symptoms provides important prognostic information.[1] Extrathoracic disease that is asymptomatic and detected as part of an initial evaluation may not indicate a poor prognosis, since it probably reflects incidental granulomatous inflammation. When extrathoracic impairment is symptomatic and severe on presentation, the disease tends to be persistent and usually requires treatment. The pattern of organ involvement typically declares itself during the first year of clinical disease and does not change with time. Peripheral adenopathy, salivary gland enlargement, and Bell's palsy generally subside spontaneously or with treatment and usually do not recur.

In general, pregnancy has little effect on the long-term course of sarcoidosis. Sometimes, spontaneous abatement of chronic sarcoidosis occurs in pregnant patients, allowing a temporary reduction in steroid dosage. After pregnancy, however, an exacerbation often occurs, requiring a return to the original maintenance dose.

Estimates from available hospital statistics suggest that sarcoidosis may be directly responsible for the death of 4 to 5 percent of persons with the disease.[40] Major causes of death include respiratory insufficiency and cor pulmonale, massive hemoptysis, cardiac arrest, and uremia from chronic renal failure. Several centers in the United States and Britain suggest that race is an important prognostic indicator, with African-American and West Indian patients being most likely to have chronic persistent disease and to suffer from the morbidity and mortality of the disorder.

TREATMENT

Indications

The need for treatment must be balanced against the overall excellent prognosis for most patients with sarcoidosis.[1] This is particularly true for patients with stage I disease, for whom systemic therapy is rarely required. As a result, it is generally believed that symptomatic or local therapy should be utilized whenever possible. Examples include analgesics and antipyretics for systemic symptoms, topical steroids for anterior occular lesions, and the avoidance of calcium and sunlight for patients with disordered calcium metabolism. Persistently, symptomatic or progressive pulmonary disease is generally accepted to be an indication for a course of systemic therapy. Threatened organ failure such as severe ocular, CNS, or cardiac disease should also be treated with systemic corticosteroids. Similarly, persistent hypercalcemia, renal or hepatic dysfunction, posterior uveitis or anterior uveitis not responding to local steroids, pituitary disease, myopathy, palpable splenomegaly, or evidence of hypersplenism such as thrombocytopenia should be treated. Severe fatigue and weight loss, disfiguring skin disease, and lymphadenopathy are among the other indications for treatment.

Corticosteroid Therapy

Corticosteroids are the mainstay of therapy for sarcoidosis. Although controversy exists regarding their overall effectiveness in altering the long-term course of the disease, there is no disagreement that corticosteroids can provide prompt symptomatic relief and often reverse organ dysfunction.[1,8,18,21] Furthermore, anecdotal experience from many centers around the world attests to the clinical impression that corticosteroids favorably affect the course of the disease, preventing or delaying progressive pulmonary fibrosis and organ dysfunction in chronic cases.[21,40]

Initial treatment of pulmonary and systemic sarcoidosis with corticosteroids usually does not require more than 40 mg per day of prednisone. Some have even proposed initiating therapy with a q.o.d. regimen or lower daily doses of prednisone in patients without life- or organ-threatening diseases. A reasonable regimen for treating pulmonary sarcoidosis with corticosteroids is outlined in Table 69-2.[1] Treatment should ordinarily be continued for a minimum of 6 to 12 months, since premature attempts to taper off steroids are likely to result in relapse of disease. A main-

tenance dose of 5 to 15 mg per day of prednisone is usually sufficient to suppress persistent pulmonary disease. A small dose of daily prednisone may be helpful in patients with advanced fibrocystic disease in an attempt to prevent further progression. Inhaled steroids do not appear to be effective in preventing progressive pulmonary disease and are not recommended.

Special Circumstances

High doses of oral corticosteroids or high-dose pulse intravenous therapy may be indicated for serious ocular or CNS disease. Anterior uveitis can usually be treated with topical ophthalmologic steroid drops; posterior uveitis and chronic eye disease usually need oral therapy. CNS sarcoidosis tends to be chronic, requiring long-term therapy.

Erythema nodosum (Löfgren's syndrome) is usually managed with bed rest and aspirin or nonsteroidal anti-inflammatory drugs. Corticosteroids are almost immediately effective but are recommended only in cases in which symptoms are disabling and persistent. In this situation, corticosteroids are usually needed for only several weeks.

Chloroquine is efficacious in many patients with mucocutaneous sarcoidosis.[41] This drug is particularly useful in lupus pernio and severe nasal sarcoidosis, diseases that are often poorly responsive to corticosteroids. Hypercalcemia has also been reported to respond to this drug. Chloroquine may be useful in chronic laryngeal sarcoidosis, though steroids are usually used initially to reduce airway obstruction. Ocular toxicity has limited its use but is rare when low doses are employed (Table 69-2). Hydroxycholorquine appears to be less effective, but its lower toxicity may make this agent a useful alternative to chloroquine. These drugs are generally not effective in pulmonary or systemic sarcoidosis.

Treatment of cardiac sarcoidosis consists of antiarrhythmic therapy, diuretics, and afterload-reducing agents for specific cardiac abnormalities. Automatic implantable defibrillators may

---

TABLE 69-2

Oral Drug Regimens for the Treatment of Sarcoidosis

Pulmonary and Systemic Sarcoidosis

	Initial Dose	Duration
Prednisone:	40 mg/day	2 weeks
	30 mg/day	2 weeks
	25 mg/day	2 weeks
	20 mg/day	2 weeks
	15 mg/day	6–8 months

Taper 2.5 mg/day every 2–4 weeks; assess for relapse.

Mucocutaneous Sarcoidosis

Chloroquine:	500 mg/day	2 weeks
	250 mg/day	5½ months
	0 mg/day	6 months

Repeat as needed at 6-month intervals.

prevent sudden death in patients with serious arrhythmias. In addition, corticosteroids in moderate doses are generally recommended, even when extensive myocardial fibrosis is present, in an attempt to reduce ongoing inflammation and prevent further fibrosis.

Fibrocystic sarcoidosis may be complicated by mycetomas, bronchiectasis, and recurrent, occasionally massive hemoptysis.[20] *Aspergillus fumigatus* is the usual organism to colonize preexisting cystic spaces. Spontaneous resolution of mycetomas may be seen. Antifungal agents are not recommended, since they are not effective and the fungi rarely cause invasive disease. Bronchiectasis is usually present in these patients and is often associated with chronic and acute bacterial infections and episodes of hemoptysis. Rotating chronic antibiotics and low-dose steroid therapy are often effective in treating symptoms. Massive hemoptysis may be life-threatening, requiring therapeutic embolization of the appropriate bronchial or collateral artery for control. Surgery is usually not feasible because of severe underlying restrictive lung disease.

Management of cor pulmonale includes supplemental oxygen, diuretics, and bronchodilators for obstructive impairment. Aggressive antibiotic treatment of bronchitis and bronchiectasis is indicated to reduce the frequency of infectious episodes. Corticosteroids in low to moderate doses are also indicated in an attempt to prevent progressive pulmonary insufficiency.

Alternative Agents

Methotrexate has been used to treat severe sarcoid skin disease with anecdotal success. Recently, methotrexate in low weekly doses has been proposed as an alternative therapy for refractory pulmonary and systemic sarcoidosis. Experience with this drug in sarcoidosis is limited, however, and the long-term toxicity of the drug in these patients is not known. Clear advantages of methotrexate over low-dose corticosteroids in the routine management of pulmonary or systemic sarcoidosis have not been established. Other immunosuppressive agents, such as azathioprine, chlorambucil, and cyclophosphamide, have had anecdotal successes in treating progressive sarcoidosis refractory to corticosteroids, though the potential toxicity of these drugs has limited their usefulness. Clinical experience with cyclosporine, a drug known to inhibit T-cell activation, has proved disappointing.

Heart-Lung Transplantation

Successful lung and heart-lung transplantations have been performed in a small number of patients with advanced pulmonary sarcoidosis and respiratory insufficiency. Although noncaseating granulomas have been found in some transplanted lungs, it is not apparent that these findings portend a poor outcome. Indications for single- or double-lung transplantation in patients with advanced pulmonary sarcoidosis are still being debated, and as experience grows, it is likely that specific guidelines will emerge. Heart transplantation for end-stage sarcoid cardiomyopathy has also been successful in a small number of patients, though experience remains limited.

REFERENCES

1. Bascom R, Johns CJ: The natural history and management of sarcoidosis. *Adv Intern Med* 31:213–241, 1986.
2. Bell NH, Stern PH, Pantzer E, et al: Evidence that increased circulating 1 α, 25-dihydroxyvitamin D is the probable cause for abnormal calcium metabolism in sarcoidosis. *J Clin Invest* 64:218–225, 1979.
3. Besnier E: Lupus pernio de la face. *Ann Dermatol Syph (Paris)* 10:333–336, 1889.
4. Bocart D, Lecossier D, de Lassence A, et al: A search for mycobacterial DNA in granulomatous tissues from patients with sarcoidosis using the polymerase chain reaction. *Am Rev Respir Dis* 145:1142–1148, 1992.
5. Boeck C: Multiple benign sarkoids of the skin. *J Cutan Dis* 17:543–550, 1899.
6. Crystal RG, Roberts WC, Hunninghake GW, et al: Pulmonary sarcoidosis: A disease characterized and perpetuated by activated lung T-lymphoctyes. *Ann Intern Med* 94:73–94, 1981.
7. Daniele RP, Dauber JH, Rossman MD: Immunologic abnormalities in sarcoidosis. *Ann Intern Med* 92:406–416, 1980.
8. DeRemee RA: The present status of treatment of pulmonary sarcoidosis: A house divided. *Chest* 71:388–393, 1977.
9. DeRemee RA: The roentgenographic staging of sarcoidosis: Historic and contemporary perspectives. *Chest* 83:128–133, 1983.
10. Grunewald J, Olerup O, Persson U, et al: T-cell receptor variable region gene usage by CD4$^+$ and CD8$^+$ T cells in bronchoalveolar lavage fluid and peripheral blood of sarcoidosis patients. *Proc Natl Acad Sci USA* 91:4965–4969, 1994.
11. Gumpel JM, Johns CJ, Shulman LK: The joint disease of sarcoidosis. *Ann Rheum Dis* 26:194–205, 1967.
12. Hance AJ, Couches S, Winchester RJ, et al: Characterization of mononuclear phagocyte subpopulations in the human lung by using monoclonal antibodies: Changes in alveolar macrophage phenotype associated with pulmonary sarcoidosis. *J Immunol* 134:284–292, 1985.
13. Harrington DW, Major M, Rybicki B, et al: Familial sarcoidosis: Analysis of 91 families. *Sarcoidosis* 11:240–243, 1994.
14. Hedfors E, Lindström F: HLA-B8/DR3 in sarcoidosis: Correlation to acute onset disease with arthritis. *Tissue Antigens* 22:200–203, 1983.
15. Hillerdal G, Nou E, Osterman K, Schmekel B: Sarcoidosis: Epidemiology and prognosis, a 15-year European study. *Am Rev Respir Dis* 130:29–32, 1984.
16. Hirsch JG, Cohen ZA, Morse SI, et al: Evaluation of the Kveim reaction as a diagnostic test for sarcoidosis. *New Engl J Med* 265:827–830, 1961.
17. Hunninghake GW, Crystal RG: Pulmonary sarcoidosis: A disorder mediated by excess helper T-lymphocyte activity at sites of disease activity. *New Engl J Med* 305:429–434, 1981.
18. Hunninghake GW, Gilbert S, Pueringer R: Outcome of the treatment of sarcoidosis. *Am J Respir Crit Care Med* 149:893–898, 1994.
19. Hutchinson J: Cases of Mortimer's malady. *Arch Surg (London)* 9:307–314, 1898.
20. Johns CJ: Management of hemoptysis with pulmonary fungus balls in sarcoidosis. *Chest* 82:400–401, 1982.
21. Johns CJ, Zachary JB, Ball WC Jr: A 10-year study of corticosteroid treatment of pulmonary sarcoidosis. *Johns Hopkins Med J* 134:271–283, 1974.
22. Johns CJ (ed): Tenth International Conference on Sarcoidosis and Other Granulomatous Disorders, Sept 17–22, 1984, Baltimore, MD. *Ann NY Acad Sci* 465:1–749, 1986.
23. Koerner SK: Transbronchial lung biopsy for the diagnosis of sarcoidosis. *New Engl J Med* 293:268–270, 1975.

24. Lem VM, Lipscomb MF, Weissler JC, et al: Bronchoalveolar cells from sarcoid patients demonstrate enhanced antigen presentation. *J Immunol* 135:1766–1771, 1985.

25. Lieberman, J: Elevation of serum angiotensin-converting-enzyme (ACE) level in sarcoidosis. *Am J Med* 59:365–372, 1975.

26. Löfgren S: Primary pulmonary sarcoidosis. *Acta Med Scand* 145:424–474, 1953.

27. Longcope WT, Freiman DG: A study of sarcoidosis: Based on a combined investigation of 160 cases including 30 autopsies from the Johns Hopkins Hospital and Massachusetts General Hospital. *Medicine* 31:1–132, 1952.

28. Lower EE, Baughman RP: The use of low dose methotrexate in refractory sarcoidosis. *Am J Med Sci* 299:153–157, 1990.

29. Maddrey WC, Johns CJ, Boitnott JK, Iber FL: Sarcoidosis and chronic hepatic disease: A clinical and pathological study of 20 cases. *Medicine* 49:375–395, 1970.

30. Mayock RL, Bertrand P, Morrison CE, Scott JH: Manifestations of sarcoidosis: Analysis of 145 patients with a review of nine series selected from the literature. *Am J Med* 35:67–89, 1963.

31. Mitchell DN, Scadding JG: Sarcoidosis. *Am Rev Respir Dis* 110:774–802, 1974.

32. Moller DR, Konishi K, Kirby M, et al: Bias toward use of a specific T cell receptor beta-chain variable region in a subgroup of individuals with sarcoidosis. *J Clin Invest* 82:1183–1191, 1988.

33. Neville E, Walker AN, James DG: Prognostic factors predicting the outcome of sarcoidosis: An analysis of 818 patients. *Q J Med* 208:525–533, 1983.

34. Richeldi L, Sorrentino R, Saltini C: HLA-DPB1 Glutamate 69: A genetic marker of beryllium disease. *Science* 262:242–244, 1993.

35. Roberts WC, McAllister HA Jr, Ferrans VJ: Sarcoidosis of the heart: A clinicopathologic study of 35 necropsy patients (group I) and review of 78 previously described necropsy patients (group II). *Am J Med* 63:86–108, 1977.

36. Robinson BWS, McLemore TL, Crystal RG: Gamma interferon is spontaneously released by alveolar macrophages and lung T lymphocytes in patients with pulmonary sarcoidosis. *J Clin Invest* 75:1488–1495, 1985.

37. Saboor S, Johnson N, McFadden J: Detection of mycobacterial DNA in sarcoidosis and tuberculosis with polymerase chain reaction. *Lancet* 339:1012–1015, 1992.

38. Schaumann J: Étude sur le lupus pernio et ses rapports avec les sarcoides et la tuberculose. *Ann Dermatol Venereol* 6:357–373, 1917.

39. Semenzato G, Agostini C: Immunology in sarcoidosis, in Schwartz MI, King TE (eds), *Interstitial Lung Disease,* St. Louis, Mosby–Year Book, 1993.

40. Siltzbach LE, James DG, Neville E, et al: Course and prognosis of sarcoidosis around the world. *Am J Med* 57:847–852, 1974.

41. Siltzbach LE, Teirstein AS: Chloroquine therapy in 43 patients with intrathoracic and cutaneous sarcoidosis. *Acta Med Scand* 425:S302–308, 1964.

42. Sones M, Israel HL: Course and prognosis of sarcoidosis. *Am J Med* 29:84–93, 1960.

43. Teirstein AS, Lesser M: Worldwide distribution and epidemiology of sarcoidosis, in Fanburg BL (ed), *Sarcoidosis and Other Granulomatous Diseases of the Lung.* New York, Dekker, 1983.

44. Thomas PD, Hunninghake GW: Current concepts of the pathogenesis of sarcoidosis. *Am Rev Respir Dis* 135:747–760, 1987.

45. Turner-Warwick M, McAllister W, Lawrence R, et al: Corticosteroid treatment in pulmonary sarcoidosis: Do serial lavage lymphocyte counts, serum angiotensin converting enzyme measurements and gallium-67 scans help management? *Thorax* 41:903–913, 1986.

46. Walker C, Bauer W, Braun RK, et al: Activated T cells and cytokines in bronchoalveolar lavages from patients with various lung diseases associated with eosinophilia. *Am J Respir Crit Care Med* 150:1038–1048, 1994.

47. Winterbauer RH, Belic N, Moores KD: A clinical interpretation of bilateral hilar adenopathy. *Ann Intern Med* 78:65–71, 1973.

48. Winterbauer RH, Hutchinson JF: Use of pulmonary function tests in sarcoidosis. *Chest* 78:640–647, 1980.

IDIOPATHIC PULMONARY FIBROSIS

Joseph P. Lynch III / Galen B. Toews

Idiopathic pulmonary fibrosis (IPF), is an inflammatory interstitial lung disease of unknown origin. Cryptogenic fibrosing alveolitis and diffuse interstitial fibrosis are synonymous terms. IPF typically affects people late in life, presenting with nonspecific symptoms of cough or dyspnea. Symptoms inexorably worsen over a period of several months to years. Gradual deterioration, progressing to end-stage respiratory insufficiency or death within 3 to 8 years from the onset of symptoms, is characteristic.[1,5,24,39,40,47] Corticosteroids or immunosuppressive/cytotoxic agents are the mainstay of therapy, but fewer than 30 percent of patients respond to existing therapies and toxicities are substantial.[17,24,27,31,39,40,47] Cardinal histologic features on lung biopsy include a mixture of fibrosis and inflammatory cell infiltration of the pulmonary interstitium and alveolar spaces.[6,8]

In the early phases of the disease, collections of inflammatory cells within the alveolar septa and in the alveoli (termed an "alveolitis") are believed to injure the alveolar epithelium and interstitium. Persistence of this alveolitis causes progressive disruption and destruction of the alveolar architecture, which can result in end-stage fibrosis or honeycomb lung. Although the inciting factors responsible for the disorder have not been elucidated, the clinical features and course are sufficiently distinctive to represent a distinct entity. However, pulmonary fibrosis indistinguishable from IPF may complicate collagen vascular disease and may result from certain genetic disorders.[30] Optimal therapy of IPF is controversial, as objective determinants of prognosis or therapeutic responsiveness are lacking. Clinical symptoms, chest radiographs, and pulmonary function studies do not portend therapeutic responsiveness. Ancillary techniques—including radionuclide scans, bronchoalveolar lavage, and high-resolution thin-section computed tomographic scans—have been used to assess prognosis and "activity" of the disease. Their role remains controversial.

CLINICAL PRESENTATION

Clinical Features

IPF usually presents insidiously, with the gradual onset of nonproductive cough and dyspnea.[27] The dyspnea is the most prominent and disabling symptom for most patients. The paroxysmal dry cough is often refractory to antitussive agents and may be the most distressing symptom for others. Bilateral infiltrates on chest radiographs and a restrictive ventilatory defect on pulmonary function tests are characteristic. During physical examination, crackles can be detected on chest auscultation in more than 80 percent of patients. These are typically dry and end-inspiratory, and are most prevalent in the lung bases. With progression of the disease, rales may extend to the apices. Bronchial breath sounds may reflect alveolar consolidation. Digital clubbing is noted in 25 to 50 percent of patients. Cyanosis, cor pulmonale, an accentuated pulmonic second heart sound, right ventricular heave, and peripheral edema may be observed in the late phases of the disease.[27,28] Extrapulmonary involvement does not occur, but weight loss, malaise, and fatigue may be noted. Fever is rare, and suggests an alternative diagnosis.

Epidemiology

In 1988, 30,000 hospitalizations and 4851 deaths in the United States were attributed to interstitial pulmonary diseases.[9] By contrast, more than 665,000 patients are hospitalized annually for chronic obstructive lung disease. The prevalence of IPF is difficult to determine. Open lung biopsy, the gold standard for the diagnosis of IPF, is not performed in large population-based epidemiologic studies. Studies from tertiary care centers cite prevalence rates of three to six cases per 100,000 in the general population.[16] A comprehensive epidemiologic study from a single county in New Mexico noted a prevalence of 27 to 29 cases per 100,000.[9] The incidence increased substantially with age. Most patients present after age 50, with a peak incidence in the seventh decade. Prevalence for adults 35 to 44 years of age was 2.7 per 100,000. By contrast, prevalence exceeded 175 per 100,000 for patients older than 75 years.[9] IPF is rare in children; it is slightly more common in males. Exposure to dusts, metals, or organic solvents, residence in agricultural or polluted urban areas, and a history of cigarette smoking are associated with an increased risk.[16] Up to 70 percent of patients with IPF are current or former smokers.[16,38,40] Workers at increased risk include painters, miners, metalworkers, woodworkers, laundry workers, beauticians, or those in occupations resulting in inhalation of hazardous dusts, or chemicals.[16]

Familial and Genetic Factors

No clear genetic basis or predisposition has been found for IPF. Inherited or familial IPF is rare.[30] The clinical presentation and course of familial IPF are similar to those of the nonfamilial variant. The mode of transmission has not been elucidated, but is believed to be autosomal dominant with variable penetrance. The presence of specific genes on chromosome 14 may be associated with an increased risk of IPF. HLA antigens, located on chromosome 6, do not correlate with IPF risk.[32]

Natural History and Prognosis

The natural history of IPF is characterized by gradual but inexorable loss of lung function over months to years.[28,31,32,37] In rare cases the course is fulminant, progressing to fatal respiratory failure within 6 to 12 months. This variant has been termed acute interstitial pneumonitis or Hamman-Rich syndrome. Occasionally, the process stabilizes after an initial period of decline. Spontaneous resolution rarely occurs (fewer than 1 percent of cases). Mean survival from the onset of symptoms to death is for 3 to 5 years. The 5-year mortality of IPF exceeds 40 percent. The major cause of death is respiratory insufficiency. Severe derangements in pulmonary function or chest radiographic scores and male sex have been associated with a worse survival. A lymphocytosis on bronchoalveolar lavage (BAL) is associated with a higher rate of responsiveness to corticosteroids. Low BAL lym-

phocyte counts are associated with increased mortality. Early institution of therapy may maximize the chances of averting progressive fibrosis and fatal respiratory insufficiency. Other causes of death of IPF patients are ischemic cardiac disease, cerebrovascular events, pulmonary embolism, neoplasia, and infections. Lung cancer complicates IPF in 9 to 11 percent of patients.

Differential Diagnosis

The differential diagnosis of IPF is extensive. Important considerations include congestive heart failure, lymphangitic carcinomatosis, sarcoidosis, hypersensitivity pneumonitis, pneumoconiosis, asbestosis, pulmonary alveolar proteinosis, bronchiolitis obliterans–organizing pneumonia, pulmonary infection, malignancy, eosinophilic granuloma, and drug-induced interstitial lung disorders. Serologic studies are useful to exclude alternative diagnoses. Serum angiotensin-converting enzyme levels are not elevated—in contrast to sarcoidosis. High titers of antinuclear antibody may suggest an associated collagen vascular disease and serum precipitating antibodies to *Aspergillus* species, *Thermoactinomyces* species, *Micropolyspora faeni,* or pigeon products may identify cases of hypersensitivity pneumonitis.[21]

DIAGNOSTIC STUDIES

Chest Radiographs

Chest radiographs are abnormal in 95 percent of patients with IPF. The most common radiographic abnormalities are bibasilar reticular or reticulonodular infiltrates with small lung volumes (Fig. 70-1).[27,37] The process is usually diffuse and relatively symmetric. Strictly unilateral disease is rare. The infiltrates are distributed preferentially in the peripheral or subpleural regions of the lung.[25,30,43] With progression of the disease, extension of the infiltrates to the apices and progressive shrinking of lung vol-

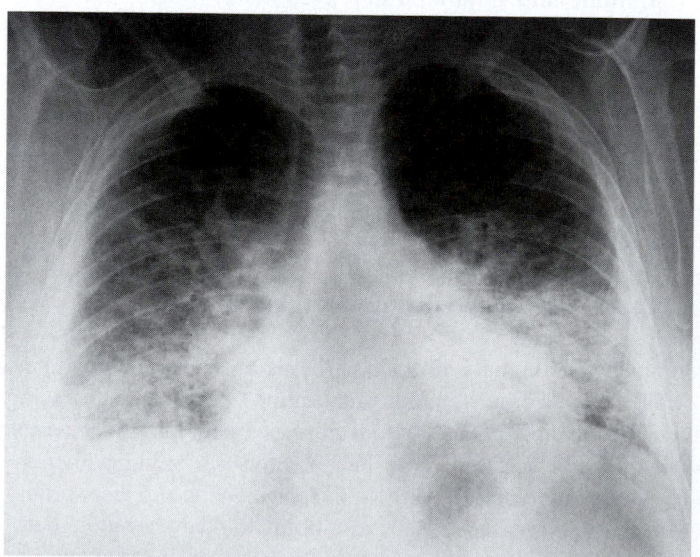

FIGURE 70-1 Idiopathic pulmonary fibrosis (IPF). PA chest radiograph of a 37-year-old woman with extensive alveolar and mixed alveolar-interstitial infiltrates bilaterally, predominantly in lower and middle lung fields.

umes occur. The presence of cystic radiolucencies ranging in size from 3 to 15 mm in diameter (honeycomb cysts) correlates with fibrosis, destruction of the alveolar architecture, and poor responsiveness to therapy (Fig. 70-2).[30,43] Overlapping features, with areas of interstitial infiltrates, alveolar (ground glass) opacities, and honeycomb cysts, may be present in individual patients. Pleural effusions or intrathoracic lymphadenopathy is not a part of the radiographic presentation. The International Labor Organization (ILO) classification system for occupational lung disease has been applied to IPF, but has no advantage over conventional chest radiographs.[43] ILO scores are complex, require an expert "B reader," and do not correlate with extent of alveolar inflammation, prognosis, or responsiveness to therapy. Conventional chest radiographs cannot discriminate alveolitis from fibrosis, and cannot reliably determine prognosis or responsiveness to corticosteroid therapy.[43] Asymptomatic patients with abnormal chest radiographs or mildly symptomatic patients with normal chest radiographs should be examined thoroughly. These presentations may represent early and potentially therapeutically reversible phases of IPF.

High-Resolution Computed Tomographic Scanning

High-resolution computed tomographic (HRCT) scanning, employing 1 to 2 mm sections of the lung parenchyma, is more sensitive and specific for the detection of idiopathic pulmonary fibrosis than is chest radiography.[11,25,30,33,43,48] HRCT is noninvasive, does not require contrast, and provides useful information about the extent and nature of the disease. It has demonstrated that the pulmonary impairment in IPF is patchy and heterogeneous. It has also demonstrated the propensity for IPF to involve the peripheral (subpleural) and basilar regions of the lung in a disproportionate fashion. The characteristic features of IPF on HRCT include focal alveolar (ground glass) opacifications, cystic airspaces, air bronchograms, ragged pleural surfaces, irregular or thickened bronchial walls or pulmonary vessels, and increased lung attenuation. Of these, the ground-glass, reticular, and honeycombing patterns appear to be the major abnormalities that are noted.[25,48] In most patients with IPF, mixtures of these patterns are noted. Pleural effusions are not a feature of IPF.

The HRCT abnormalities seen in IPF correlate with histopathologic manifestations of the disease. The ground-glass opacities are hazy zones of increased alveolar attenuation that do not obscure vascular markings. These areas of alveolar (ground glass) opacification correlate with a cellular biopsy (active alveolitis) (Fig. 70-3). A reticular pattern, characterized by in-

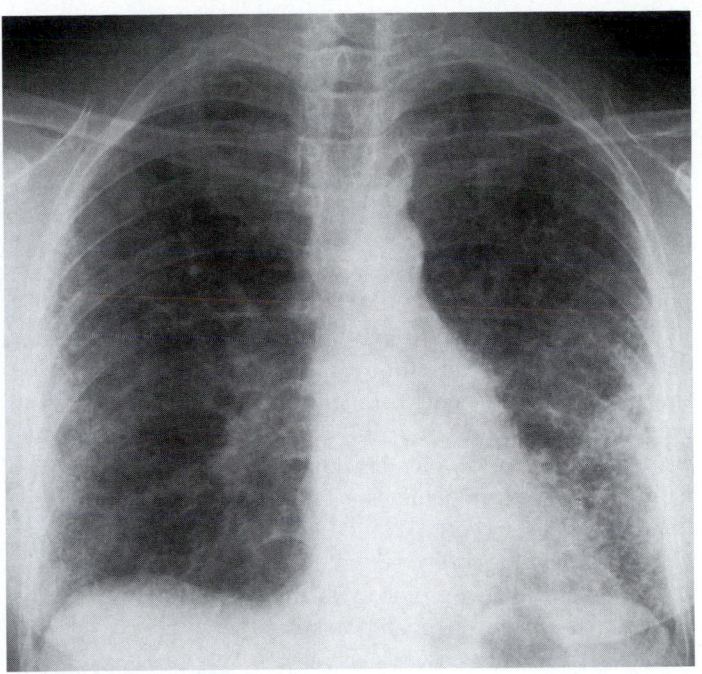

FIGURE 70-2   IPF. PA chest radiograph from a 47-year-old woman with extensive reticulonodular infiltrates, with a bibasilar predominance. Multiple cystic radiolucencies, consistent with honeycombing, are evident.

tersecting fine or coarse lines, reflects fibrosis, small (less than 5 mm) honeycomb cysts, or inflammation within alveolar septa, ducts, and airspaces. Air bronchograms (1 to 2 mm in diameter) on HRCT represent dilated peripheral airways surrounded by fibrotic lung tissue. Cystic lesions on HRCT greater than 5 mm

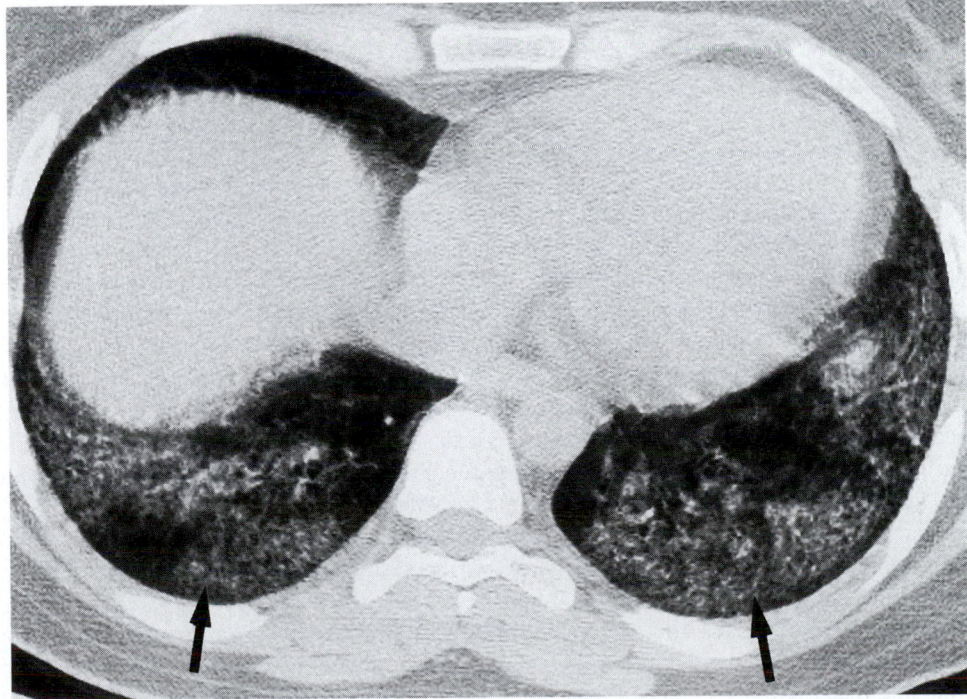

FIGURE 70-3   IPF. Thin-section high-resolution computed tomographic scan (HRCT) taken at the level of the lower lobes from a 29-year-old woman. Focal alveolar (ground glass) opacities (see arrows) are seen at the posterior aspects of both lung bases. The patchy and subpleural nature is characteristic of IPF.

in diameter correspond to macroscopic honeycombing on open lung biopsy (Fig. 70-4). Pathologic and HRCT evaluations also reveal traction bronchiectasis, severe volume loss, anatomic distortion, and dilated pulmonary arteries in end-stage IPF. Zones of emphysema (particularly in the upper lobes) may be present concomitantly in smokers with IPF.

The predictive value of HRCT in determining the response to treatment and prognosis is uncertain. Extensive ground-glass opacities and little honeycombing on HRCT are associated with improvement in pulmonary functional parameters (FVC, DLCO, FEV1%) following corticosteroid therapy. By contrast, honeycomb cysts are seen in end-stage disease, and suggest minimal or no response to therapy. Only a minority of patients with a predominant reticular pattern show a response to therapy. Serial HRCTs in patients being treated for IPF showed that a ground-glass pattern can either resolve or progress to a reticular pattern (unresponsive patients). Reticular patterns usually failed to regress and were often associated with disease progression. A honeycomb pattern was almost always associated with disease progression and unresponsiveness to therapy. Thus, HRCT provides useful clinical and prognostic information in IPF. Additional studies are required, however, to further define the prognostic value of HRCT and the role of sequential HRCT in the management of IPF patients.

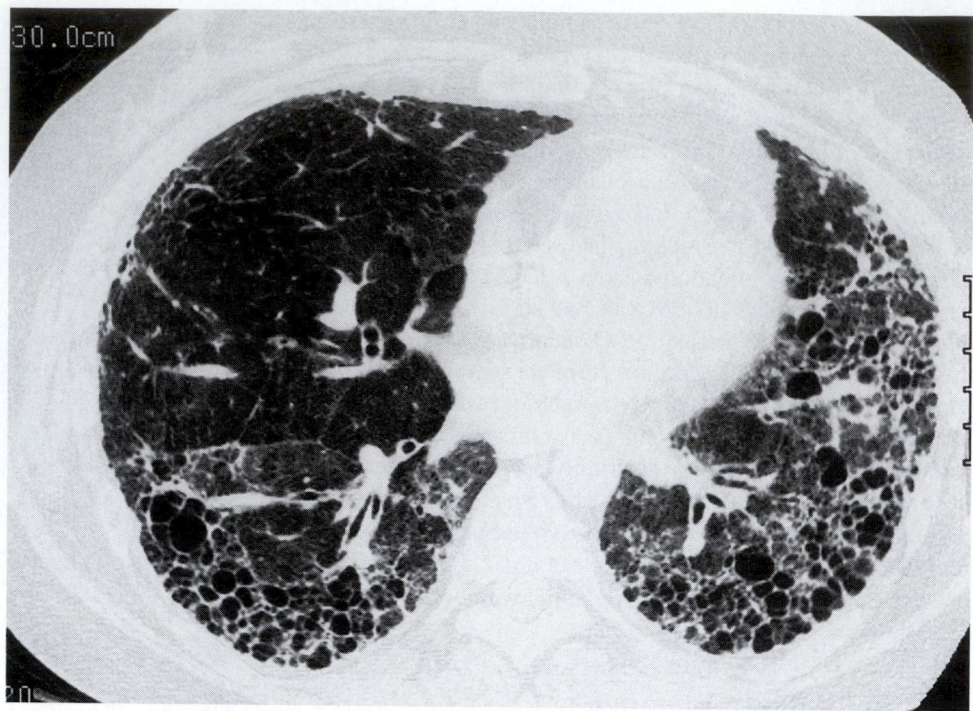

FIGURE 70-4   IPF. HRCT scan showing extensive cystic radiolucencies (honeycombing). No significant areas of ground-glass opacification are identified. Note the patchy nature of the disease, and predominant involvement of the peripheral (subpleural) regions.

Pulmonary Function Tests/Exercise Tests

Pulmonary Function Testing   Characteristic physiological aberrations in IPF include reductions in lung volumes (e.g., vital capacity and total lung capacity), impaired single-breath diffusing capacity for carbon monoxide (D_{LCO}), and impaired oxygenation (either at rest or with exercise).[7,27,35] Expiratory flow rates are preserved, and the FEV_1/FVC (1-s forced expiratory volume/forced vital capacity) ratio is usually increased. An increased number of pack-years of cigarette smoking is associated with worsening gas exchange and increased lung volumes. These functional changes probably reflect a component of emphysema in addition to pulmonary fibrosis. The diagnosis of IPF may be suspected from spirometry or flow-volume loop, on the basis of reduced vital capacity and normal or supranormal expiratory flow rates (Fig. 70-5). More sophisticated tests, including lung volumes, diffusing capacity (D_{LCO}), and cardiopulmonary exercise tests, are more sensitive than spirometry and may be helpful in monitoring the course of the disease. The D_{LCO} is the most sensitive of the static pulmonary functional parameters, and may be reduced even when lung volumes are preserved. The D_{LCO} is an indirect mea-

sure of the pulmonary vasculature, with reductions reflecting destruction or loss of integrity of alveolar walls or capillary units. The diffusing capacity can be normalized to lung volume (V_A), yielding the D_{LCO}/V_A ratio. However, the histologic severity of disease correlates better with D_{LCO} than with D_{LCO}/V_A ratio.

Pulmonary function tests are useful to assess extent of disease and to serve as a baseline to gauge efficacy of therapy. Correlations have been made between specific measures of pulmonary function and histologic findings or responsiveness to therapy. Reductions in vital capacity (below 60 percent predicted) have been associated with a worse prognosis and lower rate of response to therapy.[27,35,37] By contrast, others have noted higher response rates among patients with lower vital capacity.[45] Severe impairment or a declining D_{LCO} has been associated with a higher mortality.[7,31,35] The 3-year mortality exceeds 50 percent when the D_{LCO} falls below 45 percent of predicted values.[7,37] Changes in total lung capacity do not correlate with histology, prognosis, or survival.[35] None of these physiological parameters can distinguish alveolitis from fibrosis or portend responsiveness to therapy in individual patients.[28,32,35] The sequential evaluation of physiological parameters following institution of therapy is also valuable. Failure to respond at 3 months indicates a low likelihood of improvement with continued corticosteroid use.

Exercise Testing   Abnormal gas exchange (i.e., hypoxemia or a widened alveolar-arterial oxygen gradient) is a hallmark of IPF.[32,35] The resting alveolar-arterial O_2 gradient ($P_{AO_2}–P_{aO_2}$) is increased in more than 85 percent of patients with IPF and invariably worsens with exercise. The exercise-induced alveolar-arterial O_2 gradient correlates better with histologic abnormalities than do lung vol-

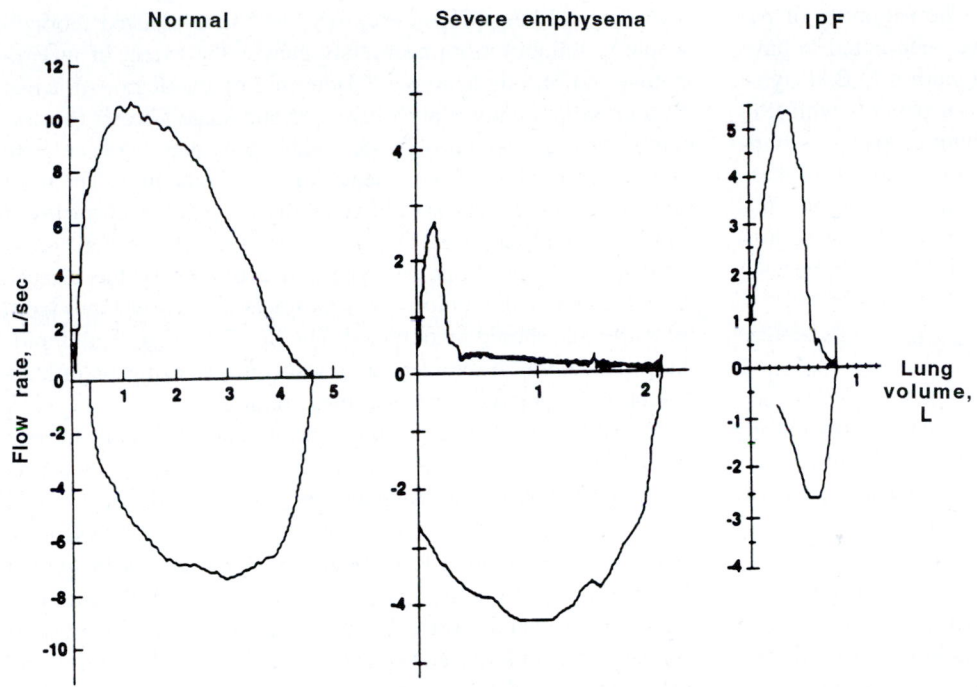

FIGURE 70-5 Flow-volume loops obtained from three different patients. Vertical (y) axis depicts expiratory flow rates in liters per second. Horizontal (x) axis depicts lung volume in liters. Scales are not the same for the three patients. The left panel depicts a normal curve. The middle panel (taken from a patient with severe emphysema) demonstrates marked reduction in peak flow rates, with severe reduction of expiratory flow rates. Note the abnormal shape of the flow-volume loop. The right panel demonstrates marked narrowing of the curve, indicating a small vital capacity (approximately 1 L). Peak expiratory flow rates are well preserved, and the shape of the loop does not reveal airways obstruction. This is a classical curve from a patient with IPF. *(From Lynch JP III, Standiford TJ: What are your best tools for diagnosing and managing idiopathic pulmonary fibrosis? J Intern Med 14:19–38, 1993, with permission.)*

Clinical-Radiographic Physiological Scores

Because clinical, radiographic, and physiological scores do not reliably correlate with histology or responsiveness to therapy, a clinical-radiographic-physiological (CRP) scoring system has been developed to more accurately gauge the extent of disease.[46] The CRP score incorporates seven clinical, radiographic, and physiological variables into a single composite score. Variables include grade of dyspnea, chest radiography, lung volume, spirometry, $D_{L_{CO}}$, resting $P_{A_{O_2}}$–Pa_{O_2}, and arterial O_2 saturation during exercise. Differential weighting of each of these variables allows determination of a single score to grade severity of the disease. The CRP score correlated better with histopathologic findings on open lung biopsy than any of the individual components. The CRP score does not indicate disease activity, but provides an objective quantifiable index of the extent and severity of disease. It may prove useful in assessing disease evolution when serially evaluated. Since HRCT scores correlate more closely with pathology than do chest radiographic scores, we have adopted a modified CRP score that replaces plain chest radiographic with HRCT criteria. Unfortunately, prospective studies are lacking to validate the use of any of these scoring systems.

umes or $D_{L_{CO}}$. These correlations are, however, imprecise. Normalizing $P_{A_{O_2}}$–Pa_{O_2} to oxygen consumption improves the correlations, but significant overlap and variability exist.

Exercise testing provides a reproducible and objective marker of extent of impairment.[35,46] Characteristic aberrations observed during exercise in patients with IPF include markedly limited exercise tolerance, widening $P_{A_{O_2}}$–Pa_{O_2}, respiratory alkalosis, reduced oxygen consumption, increased dead space (V_D/V_T), increased minute ventilation for the level of oxygen consumption, and low oxygen pulse.[13,35] Serial measurement of exercise gas exchange is the most sensitive physiological indicator of disease course. Exercise testing (particularly with arterial cannulation) is expensive, requires considerable technical support, is modestly uncomfortable, and may be difficult in elderly or debilitated patients. Less formalized tests (6-min walk test) may be acceptable for monitoring in some patients. Oximetry of the ear or finger is less accurate than direct measurement of arterial blood gases but is well tolerated. Despite its limitations, a 6-min walk test with oximetry may be acceptable as a quantifiable index of disease progression (or regression). More sophisticated measures, such as lung compliance or pressure-volume assessments, aid in assessing extent of impairment, but they are invasive and require expertise not available in many pulmonary function laboratories.

Laboratory Tests

Conventional laboratory and serologic tests are not specific for IPF. The erythrocyte sedimentation rate is elevated in 60 to 94 percent, circulating antinuclear antibodies or rheumatoid factor is positive in 10 to 20 percent, and circulating immune complexes are detected in 50 to 67 percent of patients with IPF.[21,27] These various tests do not correlate with the extent or activity of the disease and do not predict therapeutic responsiveness.

Bronchoalveolar Lavage

BAL has been enormously helpful in elucidating the key immune effector cells driving the inflammatory response in IPF.[22,47] Increases in polymorphonuclear neutrophils (PMNs), neutrophil products, activated alveolar macrophages, alveolar macrophage products, cytokines, growth factors, and immune complexes have been noted in patients with IPF. Despite its value as a research tool, BAL has limited clinical usefulness.[3] Increases in the percentage of PMNs or eosinophils (or both) in BAL fluid are noted in 67 to 90 percent of patients with IPF. The subgroup of patients with increased BAL eosinophils have been noted to have a worse prognosis in some[37,46] but not all studies.[45] BAL lymphocytosis, found in fewer than 15 percent of patients with IPF, has been associated with a more cellular lung biopsy, less honeycombing, and a greater responsiveness to corticosteroid therapy.[39,40,47] The clinical value of BAL for staging or monitoring of IPF is limited. Serial bronchoscopy with BAL cannot be justified as a diagnostic or evaluative approach. BAL should be considered primarily an investigational tool.

Radionuclide Imaging

Gallium-67 citrate has been used as an adjunctive measure of alveolitis, since activated alveolar macrophages and other inflammatory cells avidly take up Ga[67]. Increased intrapulmonary uptake of Ga[67] has been noted in idiopathic pulmonary fibrosis, sarcoidosis, and diverse inflammatory disorders, and may correlate with a more cellular lung biopsy. However, even with careful quantitation (which is logistically difficult), Ga[67] scans do not help predict therapeutic responsiveness or clinical course. Gallium scans are expensive and inconvenient (scanning is done 48 h after injection), and they expose patients and health-care personnel to radiation. Despite initial enthusiasm for their use, Ga[67] scans have no role in staging or monitoring disease activity in IPF.

Other radionuclide scans have been used to assess disease activity in IPF.[19] Positron-emission tomograph (PET) scans in patients with active interstitial lung disorders have demonstrated enhanced clearance of diethylenetriamine pentacetate (DTPA, a measure of alveolar epithelial permeability), increased levels of 18F-deoxyglucose metabolism, and increased pulmonary transcapillary escape rates for transferrin (a measure of pulmonary vascular permeability). In one study, increased clearance of Tc-DTPA and sustained increases or rising levels of 18F-deoxyglucose metabolism suggested subsequent clinical deterioration, whereas gallium scanning had no predictive value. PET is complex and expensive and should still be considered investigational.

Lung Biopsy

The optimal approach to biopsy in IPF is controversial. Surgical (open or thoracoscopic) lung biopsies are considered the diagnostic "gold standard." In some instances, transbronchial lung biopsies may be acceptable provided that clinical, radiographic, and physiological features are all consistent with IPF.[18,30,48] Transbronchial biopsies (TBBs), via a flexible fiberoptic bronchoscope, can be performed on outpatients, with low morbidity. Transbronchial biopsies should be performed on patients with interstitial lung disease before open or thoracoscopic lung biopsies, as TBBs alone may substantiate a variety of specific diagnoses (eosinophilic granuloma, sarcoidosis, malignancy, hypersensitivity pneumonitis, infections, bronchiolitis obliterans, eosinophilic pneumonia, pulmonary alveolar proteinosis, etc.) other than IPF. Because of the small sample size (2 to 5 mm), TBBs cannot be used to assess the degree of fibrosis or inflammation or to assess the prognosis in IPF.[8] When TBB is nondiagnostic, video-assisted thoracoscopic lung biopsy should be performed unless specific contraindications exist.[2]

A surgical lung biopsy (i.e., open or video-assisted thoracoscopic technique) more accurately gauges the extent of inflammatory and fibrotic lesions.[2,33] Determining the degree of active alveolar inflammation (alveolitis) and end-stage fibrosis (honeycombing) has some prognostic value, provided representative samples are obtained from at least two sites in the lung. The most severely affected areas should generally be avoided. Biopsies of both moderately affected and unaffected (grossly normal) areas yield information about the type and evolution of the disease process. Two or three biopsies from upper and lower lobes from the same side should be obtained. The tip of the lingula and middle lobe should be avoided, as nonspecific scarring or inflammation is frequently present in these regions.

Variability in the degree of cellularity and fibrosis from lobe to lobe (or even within the same lobe) within individual patients causes problems in assessing the prognosis of IPF even when surgical lung biopsies are available.[8,30] Semiquantitative scoring systems and morphometric analytic techniques have been applied to more accurately assess degrees of fibrosis or inflammation. These sophisticated scoring systems grade the overall degrees of fibrosis and cellularity and quantify the nature and extent of the inflammatory and fibrotic processes within specific sites (alveolar walls, alveolar spaces, airways). Certain histologic features (alveolar wall metaplasia and smooth-muscle and vascular changes) correlate with honeycombing and fibrotic lesions. Distinguishing young connective tissue from end-stage fibrosis (honeycombing) has been advocated. Significant interobserver variability is a problem, even among experienced pathologists. No studies have determined whether the use of such complex scoring systems improves the prognostic value of a lung biopsy.

Utility of Surgical Lung Biopsy   The open lung biopsy "gold standard" is performed in a minority of patients with chronic interstitial lung disease, in all likelihood reflecting the low likelihood that open lung biopsy will alter the course of treatment.[25,30,48] In the United Kingdom, transbronchial and open lung biopsies were performed in only 33 and 7.5 percent, respectively, of 200 patients with cryptogenic fibrosing alveolitis (CFA). The diagnosis of CFA was made on clinical grounds in most cases.[18] Clinical activities in the United States mirror this practice.[33] A survey of pulmonologists in California indicated that open lung biopsy was subsequently performed in only 42 percent of patients with a nonspecific transbronchial lung biopsy. Only 2 of 33 patients with IPF referred to a tertiary University Hospital had a prior open lung biopsy. This reluctance to subject patients to open lung biopsy is most evident in older patients with "classic" features of IPF on ancillary studies (rales on physical examination, a restrictive defect on pulmonary function tests, characteristic findings on HRCT, etc.).

A flexible approach to biopsy is appropriate. The potential risks and cost associated with surgical lung biopsy need to be balanced against the likelihood of altering treatment plan or efficacy. Algorithms to decide when open lung biopsy is appropriate have been developed,[30] but controlled studies delineating the role of open lung biopsy for chronic interstitial lung disease have not been performed. We believe that a surgical biopsy should be performed in most patients and that video-assisted thoracoscopic lung biopsy is the preferred technique. This technique has been associated with less morbidity, less prolonged chest tube drainage, and reduced length of hospital stay than open lung biopsy.[2] Fiberoptic bronchoscopy with transbronchial lung biopsies may be acceptable for patients at increased risk for surgical complications (e.g., age greater than 70 years, extreme obesity, concomitant cardiac disease, extreme impairment in pulmonary function) when other features are classic for IPF.

PATHOLOGY

Histologic analysis of lung biopsies is critical to exclude alternative diagnoses and objectively quantify the extent of fibrosis and inflammation. The cardinal histologic features of IPF include varying degrees of alveolar septal (interstitial) and intra-alveolar inflammation and fibrosis.[8] Because similar features may be observed with a host of other chronic inflammatory lung disorders, the presence of granulomas, vasculitis, minerals, or inorganic material must be excluded. The pathologic abnormalities in IPF are heterogeneous and patchy but exhibit a predilection for the peripheral (subpleural) regions of the lung. Some alveolar walls are spared, even within a heavily involved secondary lobule. Early in the course of the disease, the alveolar architecture is preserved but the alveolar walls are expanded by edema and interstitial collections of inflammatory cells. Mononuclear cells predominate (e.g., lymphocytes, plasma cells, monocytes, or macrophages), but scattered PMNs and eosinophils are observed (Fig. 70-6).

In the early phases of the disorder, focal aggregates of alveolar macrophages (termed desquamative interstitial pneumonitis) may be seen (Fig. 70-7). These intra-alveolar macrophages are absent in moderate or advanced disease. As the disease progresses, the chronic inflammatory infiltrates are less evident, and the alveolar structures are replaced by dense collagen. The alveolar walls are disrupted and destroyed, leading to dilated cystic airspaces (honeycombing) (Fig. 70-8). At this late phase, excessive lung collagen, extracellular matrix, and fibroblasts are apparent within the pulmonary interstitium, even though inflammatory cells may be sparse or absent. The alveolar epithelium also becomes hyperplastic, and squamous dysplasia may be observed in long-standing disease (Fig. 70-9). Marked reactive smooth-muscle hyperplasia occurs in some patients,

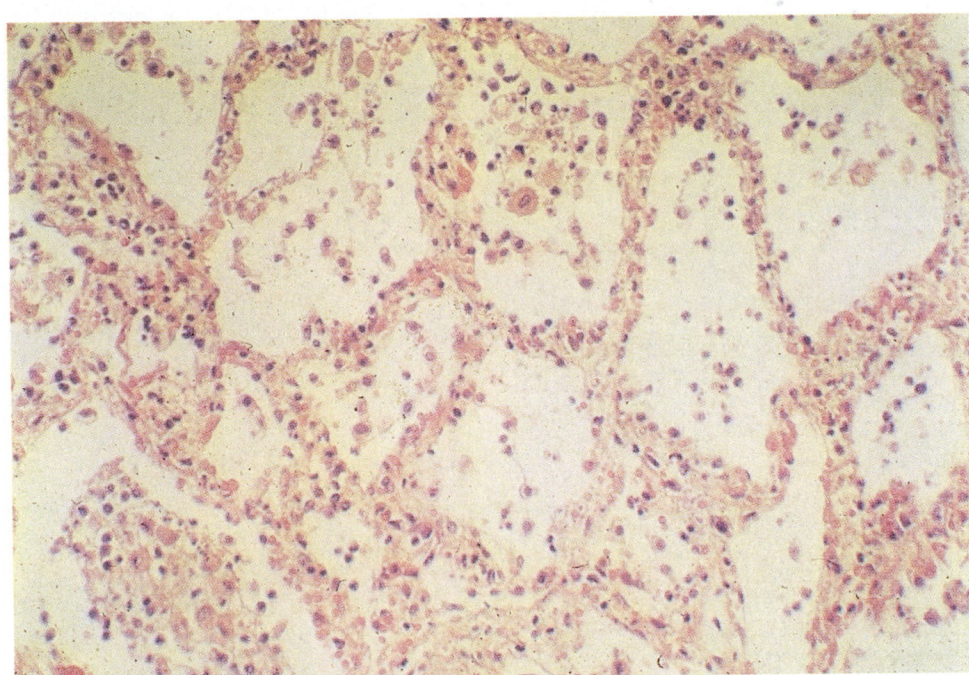

FIGURE 70-6   IPF. Alveolar architecture is preserved, but the alveolar walls are expanded by edema and interstitial collections of inflammatory cells. An increased number of macrophages and lymphocytes are noted in the alveolar spaces.

and enlarged pulmonary vessels and secondary pulmonary hypertensive changes may be present. Airspaces may also become distorted, and give rise to "traction bronchiectasis." Emphysematous changes may be observed concomitantly in smokers with IPF. Emphysema is distinguished from honeycombing by the presence of fibrosis around the honeycomb cysts.

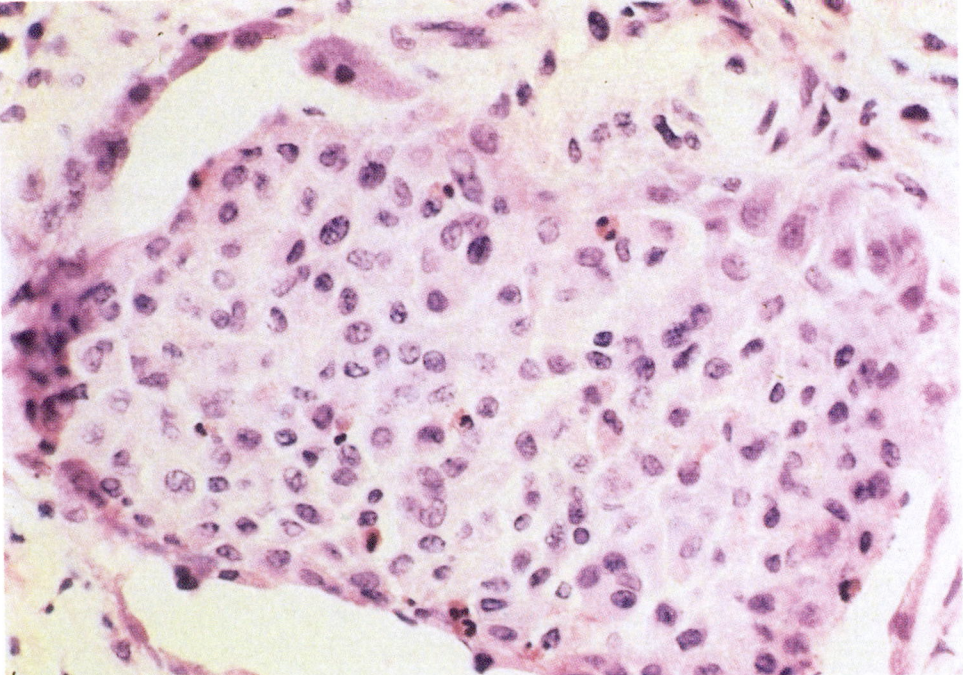

FIGURE 70-7   Desquamative interstitial pneumonia (DIP). Focal aggregates of alveolar macrophages are present within the alveolar space. These aggregates of macrophages almost completely fill the airspace.

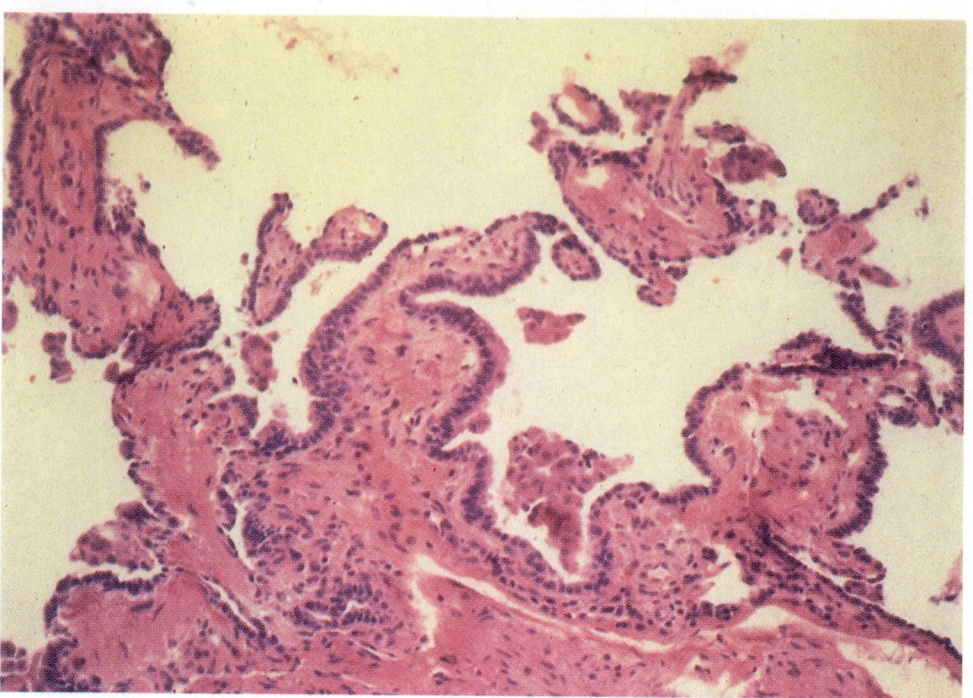

FIGURE 70-8   IPF. The alveolar walls are disrupted, leading to dilated cystic airspaces. Extensive lung collagen, extracellular matrix, and fibroblasts are apparent within the pulmonary interstitium. Inflammatory cells are sparse to absent.

Diffuse alveolar damage is not a feature of early IPF but may be seen in patients with rapidly progressive disease or at necropsy in patients with fatal respiratory insufficiency. Hyaline membranes, fibrinous exudates, epithelial cell necrosis, and interstitial and intra-alveolar edema may be prominent in this setting. As the process organizes and undergoes repair, type II cells proliferate along alveolar walls, hyaline membranes and airspace ex-

udates resorb, and fibroblasts proliferate within the alveolar interstitium and alveolar space. This variant has been termed "acute interstitial pneumonitis" and is similar to pathologic descriptions originally cited by Hamman and Rich more than 50 years ago. These histologic features are not specific for IPF but may be seen with a large number of other disorders, including adult respiratory distress syndrome (ARDS); inhalation-, radiation-, or drug-induced injury; collagen vascular disorders; and infections.

Subgroups of patients have been characterized on the basis of their pathologic findings. Usual interstitial pneumonitis (UIP), the classic histopathologic variant observed in patients with IPF, is observed in the vast majority of cases. Defining features include a prominent fibrotic component, dense interstitial inflammatory infiltration, a minimal intra-alveolar component, destruction of the alveolar architecture, and heterogeneous involvement.[8] UIP is characteristic of moderate to advanced disease and has been associated with a poor prognosis and low rate of responsiveness to corticosteroid therapy. By contrast, another histologic variant, desquamative interstitial pneumonitis (DIP), is associated with well-preserved alveolar architecture, minimal or absent fibrosis, a pronounced intra-alveolar inflammatory component, and a striking uniformity throughout the lung architecture. The striking heterogeneity and peripheral distribution characteristic of UIP are lacking in DIP. DIP correlates with ground-glass opacities on chest radiographs or CT scans and a high rate of therapeutic responsiveness. The relationship of DIP to UIP is controversial. The fact that foci of both UIP and DIP may be observed within the same biopsy in individual patients suggests that DIP could be an early phase of IPF, rather than a distinct disease. However, the remarkable dissimilarities in treatment responsiveness and rate of disease progression argue that these disorders are distinct entities. The uniformity of the lung lesion in DIP suggests a reaction to an inhaled stimulus or agent.

Nonspecific interstitial pneumonia/fibrosis is a third histo-pathologic variant of IPF.[20] Defining criteria include varying proportions of inflammation and fibrosis—which tend to be histologically uniform, suggesting that the lesions are of similar age and result

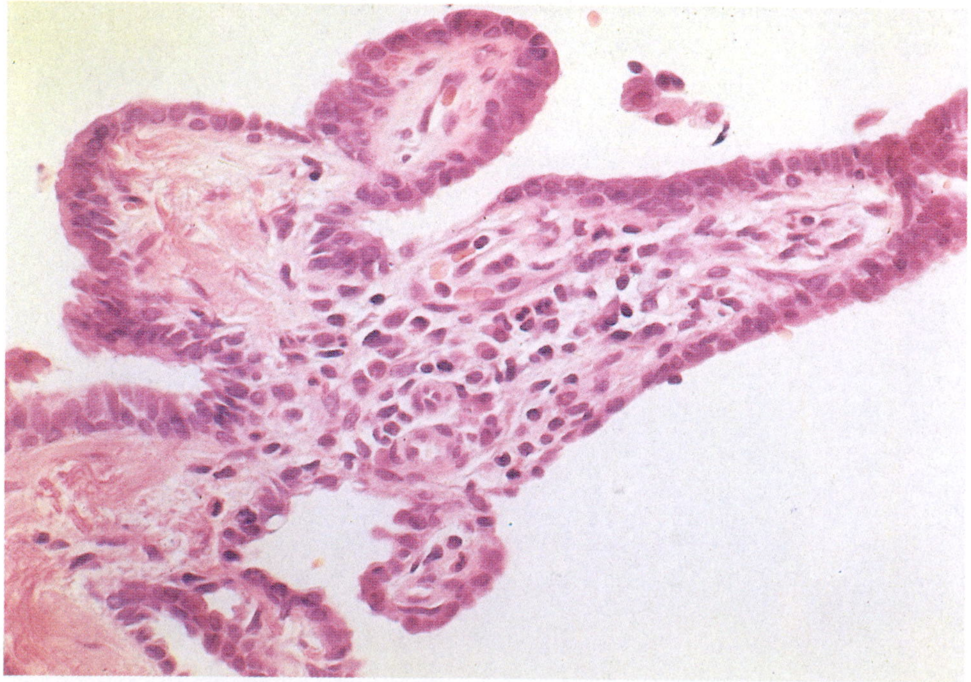

FIGURE 70-9   IPF. Hyperplastic alveolar epithelial cells cover the dilated cystic airspaces as well as the organizing intra-alveolar fibrin deposits.

from a single insult. The pathologic spectrum ranges from pure inflammation to dense fibrosis. The interstitial infiltrates contain primarily lymphocytes and plasma cells. Eosinophils and neutrophils are present in smaller numbers. The extent of fibrosis ranges from minimal to extensive, with honey-comb cysts. In its original description, scattered foci of bronchiolitis obliterans–organizing pneumonia were noted in 31 of the 64 patients with nonspecific interstitial pneumonia (NIP) and fibrosis. In addition, prominent accumulations of intra-alveolar macrophages were noted in 19 and loosely formed granulomas were noted in five of these patients. It is apparent that these histologic features overlap extensively with UIP and somewhat with DIP. The intra-alveolar cellular component is patchy in nonspecific interstitial pneumonitis but uniform in DIP. The interstitial component is lacking in DIP, and is overshadowed by the prominent intra-alveolar collections of macrophages.

The key feature distinguishing nonspecific interstitial pneumonitis from UIP is its histologic and presumed temporal uniformity. The clinical and radiographic features of NIP are similar to those of IPF, with bibasilar interstitial infiltrates, cough, dyspnea, and a subacute to chronic course. As with IPF, this histologic picture can also be seen in patients with collagen vascular disorders (10 of the 64 patients in the report providing its original description). The prognosis of NIP is considerably more favorable than UIP. In one series in which 48 patients were available for follow-up, five (11 percent) died of respiratory failure while nearly half recovered completely. Treatment regimens varied, but most patients received corticosteroids. Cyclophosphamide and azathioprine were used in six and two patients, respectively. All five deaths occurred in patients receiving cyclophosphamide (four) or azathioprine (one) in addition to corticosteroids.

The separation of pulmonary fibrotic disorders according to these histopathologic criteria is arbitrary. It is likely that UIP, DIP, and NIP represent stereotypical responses to diverse lung toxins or injuries. Additional studies assessing CT patterns, clinical features, and outcomes are required to determine the relationship between NIP and the other histologic variants.

PATHOGENESIS

The cause of IPF is unknown. Viruses, fungi, environmental agents, and toxic agents have all been implicated. These etiologic agents are presumed to interact with resident pulmonary immune cells to generate inflammatory or immune responses. They might also directly injure epithelial or endothelial cells. IPF probably results from the persistent superimposed processes of inflammation, tissue injury, and repair (Fig. 70-10).[4,10,22,41,42,44]

Immune and Inflammatory Responses

A lower respiratory tract inflammatory response is the earliest detectable lesion in IPF. Lymphocytes, macrophages, and neutrophils are present in increased numbers in the interstitium and within the alveolus. Antigen-specific immune responses are likely to be generated early in the course of IPF. T-lymphocyte activation requires the recognition of antigen in association with major histocompatibility complex on the surface of antigen-pre-

senting cells such as dendritic cells and recruited monocytes. The unknown agents that cause IPF may also lead to epithelial injury and the production of granulocyte-macrophage colony–stimulating factor, which is important in dendritic cell differentiation. The generation of an antigen-specific immune response depends on the migration of antigen-presenting dendritic cells to local lymph nodes, where clonal expansion of specific lymphocytes occurs. The activated lymphocytes then recirculate and eventually enter the lung.

T lymphocytes may play a dual role in IPF by contributing to both lung injury and the modulation of disease progression. The T lymphocytes obtained from the alveoli of patients with IPF are activated, expressing IL-2 receptors and constitutively secreting IFN-γ. T lymphocytes in the lungs of patients with IPF also provide excessive helper function to B cells. This excessive help might be important in the enhanced production of immune complexes observed in patients with this disorder. T-lymphocyte–secreted products may both inhibit and enhance fibrosis. The T lymphocytes from patients with IPF secrete soluble factors that inhibit fibroblast proliferation and soluble factors that increase fibroblast collagen synthesis.

The generation of a specific immune response within the pulmonary parenchyma is important in inducing the recruitment of inflammatory cells to affected pulmonary tissues. Inflammatory cell recruitment can be divided into four steps: (1) weak binding of inflammatory cells to the endothelium, (2) firm adherence of inflammatory cells to endothelial cells, (3) transmigration through the vascular wall, and (4) migration of leukocytes through extracellular matrix under the influence of a chemotactic gradient. Selectin adhesion molecules, integrin adhesion molecules, and members of the immunoglobulin supergene family all play crucial roles in inflammatory cell/endothelial cell interactions. Early response cytokines such as tumor necrosis factor–α (TNF-α) rapidly induce the expression of endothelial selectin molecules. The interaction of selectins with their ligands on leukocytes does not firmly anchor these cells against the shear forces generated by the flow of blood but instead causes them to roll along the endothelium as a result of continually making and losing contact with the endothelium.

Firm adhesion for many cells is dependent on the interaction between intercellular adhesion molecule–1 (ICAM-1) and leukocyte function antigen–1 (LFA-1). TNF-α induces ICAM-1 expression on endothelial cells. The extravasation of leukocytes involves LFA-1 and platelet endothelial cell adhesion molecule, which is expressed both on the leukocyte and at the junction of endothelial cells. The presence of urokinase-type plasminogen activator is also required for the development of pulmonary inflammatory responses. Urokinase-type plasminogen activator (u-PA) is probably in the proteolytic degradation of the varied tissue planes during the movement of inflammatory cells from the vasculature to the alveolar space. Directed migration of inflammatory cells in IPF depends on a variety of chemotactic agents. The chemotaxins include the cytokines interleukin-1 (IL-1), RANTES (regulated on activation normal T expressed and secreted), monocyte chemoattractant protein–1 (MCP-1), and macrophage inflammatory protein–1α (MIP-1α) for lymphocytes; the complement component C5a, cytokines (MCP-1, MIP-1α), and fibronectin fragments containing the RGD domain for

Immune Response

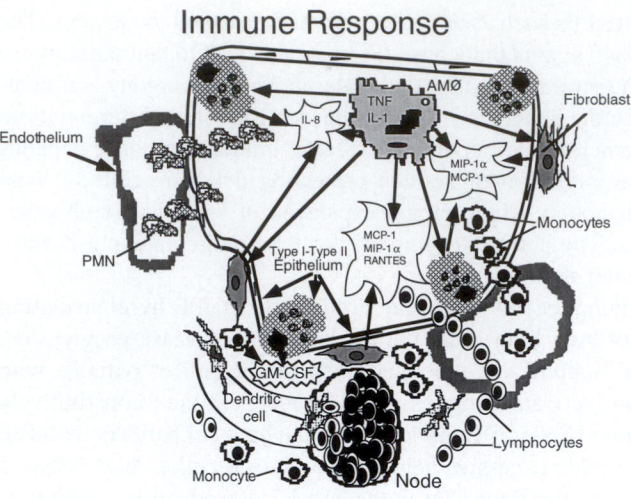

A

Injury

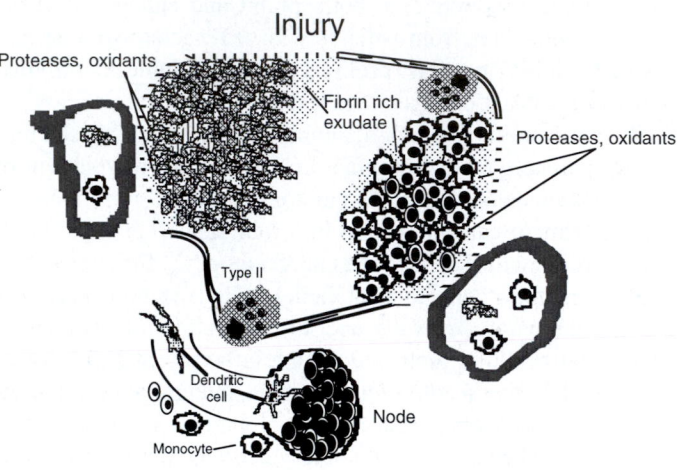

B

Repair/Reepithelialization

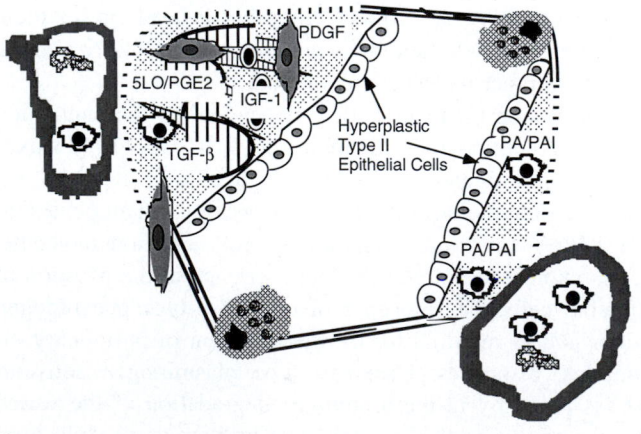

C

monocytes; and leukotriene B$_4$ (LTB$_4$), IL-8, and C5a for neutrophils.[4,22,41,42] T lymphocytes, alveolar macrophages, endothelial cells, epithelial cells, and fibroblasts are all important sources of these cytokines. The urokinase receptor (u-PAR; CD87) is necessary for chemotaxis of both monocytes and PMN. u-PAR probably affects leukocyte trafficking and activation by modulating the adhesive function of complement receptor 3.

FIGURE 70-10 Pathogenesis of IPF. IPF results from the superimposed processes of immune inflammation, tissue injury, and attempted repair. *A.* Immune response. Specific immune responses are initiated following migration of antigen-presenting cells such as the dendritic cells to local nodes, clonal expansion of specific lymphocytes, and recirculation of activated lymphocytes to the lung. Activated lymphocytes, alveolar macrophages, and parenchymal cells secrete chemokines (IL-8, MCP-1, MIP-1α, RANTES), which direct leukocyte immigration into the parenchyma and alveolar spaces. These cells also produce GM-CSF, which has an important role in dendritic cell differentiation and macrophage activation. Macrophage activation further amplifies this process via the production of the early-response cytokines IL-1 and TNF. *B.* Injury. Recruited inflammatory cells cause epithelial cell injury, epithelial cell loss, and basal lamina destruction. Proteases and oxidants play a major role mediating this injury. The result is a fibrin-rich exudate that forms within the alveolar spaces. *C.* Repair and reepithelialization. Successful repair of injured alveoli following the inflammatory response requires the clearance of plasma proteins that have leaked into the alveolar space and replacement of injured alveolar cells. Plasminogen activator (u-PA) is secreted by epithelial cells and alveolar macrophages. Its activity is regulated by the local concentration of plasminogen activator inhibitors (PAI). Active u-PA generates plasmin, which limits scar formation by dismantling the provisional matrix on which fibroblasts migrate and secrete interstitial collagens. If the fibrin-rich exudate cannot be cleared from the alveolar space, fibroblasts migrate into the matrix and multiply, producing matrix molecules that cause scar formation. The rate and magnitude of scar formation are regulated by a variety of factors, including the profibrotic cytokines PDGF, IGF-1, and TGF-β. In addition, increased 5-lypoxygenase products and decreased prostaglandin E$_2$ are noted; they enhance fibroblast proliferation. Alveolar type II epithelial cell migration and proliferation eventually cover the repaired basement membrane and scarified intra-alveolar thrombus, completing the process of intra-alveolar fibrosis. (*From Toews GB: Interstitial lung disease, in Bennett JC (ed), Cecil Textbook of Medicine, 20th ed. Philadelphia, Saunders, 1996, pp. 390–399, with permission.*)

Injury

Epithelial cell injury is a hallmark of IPF. Viral infections and effector molecules produced by immune and inflammatory cells (oxidants, proteases) have been proposed as mediators of this injury. Injury or loss of epithelial cells allows serum proteins to exude into the alveolar space. The alveolar basal lamina may also be destroyed during the injury. The persistence of activated inflammatory cells (lymphocytes, macrophages, PMNs) may contribute to ongoing alveolar wall injury.

Repair/Fibrosis

The successful repair of damaged alveoli requires clearance of plasma proteins that have entered the alveolar space, replacement of injured alveolar cells, and the restoration of damaged extracellular matrix. The alveolar exudate that forms during the inflammatory response contains cytokines and mediators not usually present within the alveolar space, including growth factors (platelet-derived growth factor, transforming growth factor–β, insulin-like growth factor–I) fibronectin, thrombin, and fibrinopeptides.

Alveolar epithelial cells and macrophages regulate both the formation and clearance of intra-alveolar fibrin.[10] The normal alveolar space has net fibrinolytic activity due to the presence of u-PA. However, the fibrinolytic activity in BAL fluid from patients with IPF is suppressed because of increased levels of inhibitors of plasminogen activators and plasmin such as plasminogen activator inhibitor–1 (PAI-1). Accordingly, fibrin collects within the alveolar space. The importance of this decreased fibrinolytic state can be appreciated from experimental studies that demonstrated a strong relationship between PAI-1 gene dose and the degree of pulmonary fibrosis in PAI-1 transgenic mice following bleomycin administration. PAI-1–overexpressing mice experienced greater fibrosis than wild-type mice, while mice homozygous deficient for PAI-1 were protected from fibrosis.[10] If the intra-alveolar exudate is not cleared, the exudate is invaded by fibroblasts and other cells. These cells proliferate and produce new matrix proteins, converting the fibrin-rich exudate into scar.

Arachidonic acid metabolites probably play important regulatory roles in the fibrotic response in patients with idiopathic pulmonary fibrosis.[49,50] Compared to homogenates of nonfibrotic control lungs, homogenates from IPF patients contain 15 times more LTB_4 and five times more LTC_4. Leukotrienes exert direct effects on fibroblasts and other mesenchymal cells. They stimulate fibroblast chemotaxis, proliferation, and collagen synthesis. Leukotrienes also augment the mitogenic effect of insulin-like growth factor. It is interesting to note that fibroblasts isolated from the lungs of patients with IPF have a diminished capacity to synthesize prostaglandin E_2 (PGE_2). The growth-promoting actions of leukotrienes on lung fibroblasts are enhanced when endogenous fibroblast production of PGE_2 is pharmacologically inhibited. Thus, defective PGE_2 production would tend to magnify the effects of increased leukotriene levels on fibroblast proliferation in the milieu of the IPF lung.

An important feature in alveolar repair is the reepithelialization of the alveolar basement membrane. To accomplish this, type II epithelial cells proliferate and eventually resurface the repaired basement membrane and local organized exudate. This process no doubt occurs under the influence of keratinocyte growth factor and hepatocyte growth factor, which regulate epithelial cell proliferation and migration.

During the course of IPF, alveolar surface area is also lost as a result of alveolar collapse. Alveolar collapse results from the loss of epithelial cells, allowing denuded basal lamina to directly contact and fibrose to one another. When this process incorporates numerous alveoli, the collapse leads to conglomerate scar formation.

THERAPY

Optimal therapy for IPF is a subject of contention. Treatment strategies are based on eliminating or suppressing the inflammatory component. Treatment options include corticosteroids, immunosuppressive/cytotoxic agents, and antifibrotic agents (colchicine or penicillamine), alone or in combination.[17,24,27,31,37,51] Only 10 to 30 percent of patients respond to existing therapies, and toxicity is substantial. Responses are usually partial and transient. Cures (sustained, complete remissions) are achieved in fewer than 5 percent of patients. Even among responders, relapses or progression of the disease following an *initial* response is common and suggest that these patients require prolonged treatment.[15]

Limited data exist regarding the determinants of responsiveness to treatment of IPF. Response rates may be higher when treatment is initiated early in the course of the disease, before irreversible fibrosis has developed. Factors associated with an improved prognosis and responsiveness to therapy include female sex, young age, less severe degrees of physiological or radiographic impairment, a shorter duration of symptoms, histologic pattern of desquamative interstitial pneumonitis on open lung biopsy, increased percentage of lymphocytes on BAL, and ground-glass opacities on chest radiographs or CT studies.[37,45,46,48] Objective, validated parameters to assess disease activity and response to therapy have varied among studies. Changes in pulmonary function parameters have typically been used to identify "responders" (or "nonresponders"), but criteria for assessing response have not been uniform. Increases of only 10 to 15 percent from pretreatment levels in even a single parameter of pulmonary function (V_C, DL_{CO}) have been deemed favorable responses. Lack of change, or "stabilization," has been considered to represent a response among patients previously exhibiting a rapid downhill course.

Patients being treated for IPF should be closely monitored for drug side effects and complications as well as for evidence of response to therapy. Patients should have a thorough evaluation 3, 6, and 12 months after diagnosis and initiation of therapy and at least annually thereafter. The assessment should include a careful history and physical exam, lung imaging (chest radiography or HRCT), pulmonary function testing (including diffusing capacity), and lung volume and gas exchange studies at rest and during exercise. "No further decline" in lung function or symptoms is a positive outcome, since IPF is usually progressive. Clinical deterioration is usually due to disease progression, but it may be caused by complications associated with IPF or adverse effects of therapy. Complications include heart failure, pneumothorax, pulmonary infections, bronchogenic carcinoma, and thromboembolic disease. Identification of the cause of deterioration is important so that therapeutic interventions can be appropriately directed.

Corticosteroids

Corticosteroids have been the cornerstone of therapy for IPF for more than 3 decades. Unfortunately, no more than 10 to 30 percent of patients respond to therapy, and complete remissions are rare.[24,27,37,39,40] In the vast majority of patients, the disease worsens in spite of therapy. Prospective studies assessing optimal dosage, rate of taper, and duration of therapy have not been done. Most investigators initiate therapy with high-dose corticosteroids (40 to 80 mg daily of prednisone or prednisolone) for 2 to 4 months, with a subsequent gradual taper.[24,17,37] Others advocate initial dosages of up to 1.5 mg/kg a day of prednisone (or equivalent).[27,47] If responses occur with corticosteroids, improvement is usually noted within 2 to 3 months. No studies have compared differing dosages or duration of corticosteroid therapy in matched patients. We initiate treatment with prednisone (60 mg daily for 1 month); the dosage is then reduced to 40 mg daily for an additional 2 months.

Maintenance corticosteroid therapy is reserved for patients exhibiting *objective* improvement on pulmonary function testing or HRCT. Corticosteroid-responsive patients are maintained on prednisone chronically (sometimes indefinitely), but with a tapering dose. The daily dose of prednisone is tapered to 30 mg by the fourth month, and to 15 to 20 mg (or an equivalent alternate day dose) by 6 months. The dose of corticosteroid and rate of tapering should be guided by clinical and physiological parameters. Since it is unlikely that corticosteroids completely eradicate the disease, treatment for a minimum of 1 to 2 years (and sometimes indefinitely) is reasonable for patients exhibiting unequivocal responses to therapy. In this context, chronic low-dose prednisone (15 to 20 mg every other day) may be adequate as maintenance therapy. Relapses or deterioration warrants an increase of the dose or the addition of an immunosuppressive agent. High-dose intravenous "pulse" methylprednisolone (1 to 2 G once weekly or biweekly) has been used, but it has no proven advantage over oral corticosteroids. Patients failing to respond to corticosteroids may be candidates for immunosuppressive or cytotoxic agents (see below). In these patients, azathioprine or cyclophosphamide is added, and the prednisone is tapered and discontinued over 4 to 6 weeks. In some patients, the disease may accelerate and their condition deteriorate as the steroids are tapered. In these patients, therapy with alternate-day prednisone (20 to 40 mg every other day), in addition to the immunosuppressive or cytotoxic agent, can be used.

Side effects of corticosteroid therapy are common and potentially disabling. Peptic ulcer disease, posterior capsular cataracts, and endocrine and metabolic alterations (hyperglycemia, hypocalemia, metabolic alkalosis, secondary renal insufficiency, impotence, menstrual irregularities, truncal obesity, and moon facies) all occur. Musculoskeletal complications include osteoporosis, vertebral compression fractures, aseptic necrosis of femoral and humeral heads, and myopathy. Corticosteroid-induced myopathies may impair diaphragmatic strength and complicate the assessment of therapeutic efficacy. Psychiatric side effects include depression, psychoses, and inappropriate euphorias. These side effects occur especially in elderly patients. Finally, corticosteroid therapy suppresses immune and inflammatory responses to microbes. Opportunistic infection with both T-cell– and neutrophil-dependent infectious agents may occur.

Immunosuppressive Agents

Immunosuppressive or cytotoxic agents (azathioprine or cyclophosphamide) should be considered as therapy for steroid nonresponders, patients experiencing serious adverse effects from corticosteroids, and patients at high risk for corticosteroid complications (e.g., age over 70 years, poorly controlled diabetes mellitus or hypertension, severe osteoporosis, or peptic ulcer disease). Favorable responses have been noted with azathioprine or cyclophosphamide in 15 to 50 percent of cases.[17,29,31,32,37] Few prospective or long-term studies have critically evaluated these agents. No studies have directly compared cyclophosphamide with azathioprine.

Cyclophosphamide Oral cyclophosphamide (Cytoxan, CTX) (1 to 2 mg/kg a day) has been associated with favorable re-

sponses in both idiopathic and collagen vascular–associated pulmonary fibrosis, even in patients previously not responding to corticosteroids.[37] However, data comparing cyclophosphamide with corticosteroids are limited. Only two randomized studies have evaluated cyclophosphamide therapy for IPF.[17,26] A 6-month trial at the National Institutes of Health randomized 28 patients with "midcourse" IPF to prednisone alone, prednisone plus oral CTX (1.5 mg/kg a day), or CTX alone.[26] Mean BAL neutrophil counts declined significantly at 3 and 6 months only in the patient groups receiving cyclophosphamide. These suppressive effects of CTX on neutrophils obtained with BAL were noted even in nine patients who had previously failed corticosteroid therapy. Despite these beneficial effects on measures of alveolitis, pulmonary function did not change in any group during the 6-month period.

A second randomized, prospective trial enrolled patients with *untreated* IPF. Patients were randomized to receive oral CTX (1 to 2 mg/kg a day) plus low-dose prednisolone (20 mg every other day) or high-dose prednisolone alone (60 mg a day with gradual tapering).[17] According to clinical, radiographic, and physiological criteria, results were generally similar in the two groups. Five of 21 patients (23 percent) receiving CTX plus prednisolone improved within the first 12 months as compared to 7 of 22 patients (31 percent) receiving prednisolone alone. At 3-year follow-up, only one CTX-treated patient had maintained improvement above pretreatment baseline, while 7 were in stable condition, and the condition of the remaining patients had deteriorated. By comparison, at 3-year follow-up, 2 of 22 treated with prednisolone were still in improved condition and 3 were in stable condition.

In this study, the kinetics of response differed between CTX and corticosteroid therapies. Responses to CTX were delayed for at least 3 months. While occasional patients responded to corticosteroids within 1 month, no patient receiving CTX therapy responded at this early time. A minimum of 4 to 6 months of therapy with CTX is required to judge efficacy. Mortality at 3 years was higher in the prednisolone group (10 of 22 deaths) than in the CTX group (3 of 21 deaths). However, this difference did not achieve statistical significance. In addition, it may have reflected a bias at the time of entry into the study, since a disproportionate number of patients with severe derangements in pulmonary function at study entry were randomized to the prednisolone arm.

In accord with this finding, initial pulmonary function was an independent indicator of outcome. All 12 patients with initial TLC less than 60 percent predicted failed therapy. Only three had been randomized to CTX. The survival advantage attributable to CTX (if any) may be limited to patients with moderate disease at entry (i.e., TLC greater than 60 percent but less than 80 percent predicted). Prognosis was poor in crossover patients who failed initial therapy with either agent. Only 3 of 16 patients failing initial treatment with prednisolone responded to treatment with CTX. Similarly, only one of eight responded to prednisolone after initially failing on CTX.

High-dose intravenous ("pulse") CTX administered every 2 to 4 weeks (dose range 500 to 1800 mg) has been tried in open trials of refractory IPF. Results have been generally unimpressive. In one study, pulmonary function improved modestly in some patients and prednisone was discontinued in 14 of 17 patients within 12 months. However, 13 patients died. In a second study, 12 patients with corticosteroid-refractory IPF received pulse CTX. Pulmonary function tests did not change, and seven patients (63 percent) died. No studies have compared oral with pulse CTX for IPF.

Toxicity associated with CTX remains a major impediment to the routine use of this agent for IPF.[23] Hematologic alterations are common and frequently require adjustment of dose. Leukopenia, anemia, and thrombocytopenia are the most common hematologic abnormalities. Bacterial and opportunistic infections can occur. Infections occur both in association with leukopenia and in the absence of leukopenia. Herpes zoster is frequently reported during cyclophosphamide therapy. In our clinic, trimethoprim-sulfamethoxazole (one single-strength tablet three times weekly) is added routinely as prophylaxis against *Pneumocystis carinii* infection in patients receiving CTX therapy. Urologic complications include hemorrhagic cystitis and carcinoma of the bladder. Infertility may occur in males, and ovarian fibrosis, follicular destruction, ovarian failure, and amenorrhea are well documented complications in females. GI symptoms of stomatitis, nausea, and diarrhea may occur. Therapy with CTX also increases the risk of subsequent leukemias and other hematologic neoplasms.

Determination of which patients should receive CTX is difficult. Because of its toxicity, CTX is usually reserved for patients failing corticosteroids or experiencing adverse effects from corticosteroids.

Azathioprine   Azathioprine (Imuran) is a purine analog that inhibits DNA synthesis in a variety of cell lines and exhibits global immunosuppressive effects on both humoral and cellular immunity. It has been used as therapy for IPF, primarily in patients resisting treatment with or experiencing adverse effects from corticosteroids.[24,37] Anecdotal responses have been noted in uncontrolled studies.[37] The combination of azathioprine and corticosteroids was associated with modest improvement in some patients in European studies. Only two prospective studies have evaluated azathioprine for IPF.[33,51] In both studies, azathioprine was combined with prednisone. In the first (uncontrolled) study, 20 patients with progressive IPF were initially treated with prednisone for 3 months.[51] At that point, azathioprine (3 mg/kg a day) was added and the *combination* of azathioprine and low-dose prednisone was maintained for 9 months or longer. Twelve of 20 patients (60 percent) responded favorably to this regimen. Since corticosteroids were administered concomitantly, the independent effect of azathioprine was difficult to assess.

A subsequent double-blind study enrolled 27 patients with newly diagnosed, previously untreated idiopathic pulmonary fibrosis who were randomized to receive azathioprine plus prednisone or prednisone plus placebo.[31] Both groups received prednisone 1.5 mg/kg a day (maximum dose 100 mg a day) for the first 2 weeks, which was then gradually tapered over several weeks to 20 mg a day or lower as a maintenance dose. Azathioprine (3 mg/kg a day, maximal dose 200 mg a day) was administered concomitantly. Mortality and pulmonary functional parameters (FVC, $D_{L_{CO}}$, A-a O_2 gradient) did not differ between groups when analyzed at 1 year. Four patients died in each group by the 12-month end point. Mortality was lower (43 percent versus 77 percent) at late (9-year) follow-up and mean survival was

longer (43 versus 34 months) among patients receiving prednisone plus azathioprine than in patients receiving prednisone plus placebo. These differences did not reach statistical significance.

Significant adverse drug reactions cause azathioprine to be discontinued in 20 to 30 percent of patients.[23] Nausea, vomiting, peptic ulcer disease, and diarrhea are the most frequent side effects. Leukopenia, anemia, thrombocytopenia, pure red cell aplasia, and pancytopenia also occur. Elevation of hepatic enzymes occurs in approximately 5 percent of patients treated with this immunosuppressive agent.

Current studies are inadequate to judge the efficacy of azathioprine either alone or in combination with corticosteroids as therapy for IPF. Azathioprine may be considered as an alternative to cyclophosphamide therapy in patients with progressive IPF that is refractory to corticosteroids or in patients experiencing the side effects of corticosteroids. The initial dose of 100 mg a day can be increased to a maximal dose of 200 mg a day if toxicity does not ensue. Blood counts should be monitored biweekly for the first 6 weeks and monthly thereafter. Care should be taken to maintain total leukocyte counts above 3000 per mm^3 and platelet counts above 100,000 per mm^3. Response to azathioprine may be delayed; accordingly, a 4- to 6-month trial is recommended.

Cyclosporin A   Cyclosporin A, a fungal decapeptide with potent inhibitory effects on T-cell activation and proliferation, has only rarely been used for IPF. Anecdotal responses have been noted, even in corticosteroid failures. However, sustained remissions have been rare and toxicity is high. Cyclosporin A is very expensive (typically more than $500 a month) and has been associated with numerous adverse effects (neurologic, renal, gastrointestinal, hypertrichosis).

Agents That Influence Collagen Synthesis or Fibrosis

Since therapeutic results achieved with immunosuppressive or antiinflammatory agents have been disappointing, strategies employing antifibrotic agents (colchicine)[29] and penicillamine[24] have been advocated. However, the value of these interventions is unproven.

Colchicine   Colchicine inhibits collagen formation and modulates the extracellular milieu in vitro and in animal models. It suppresses the release of alveolar-macrophage–derived growth factor and fibronectin by alveolar macrophages from patients with sarcoidosis or IPF cultured in vitro and reduces the concentration of neutrophil elastase in BAL fluid from ex-smokers.[34] Data regarding colchicine as therapy for idiopathic or collagen vascular disease–associated pulmonary fibrosis are limited to anecdotal case reports and one uncontrolled study.

A retrospective case series of 35 patients with IPF treated with colchicine (0.6 mg a day) reported beneficial results. Follow-up data were available in only 23 patients.[29] Vital capacity or $D_{L_{CO}}$ improved by at least 15 percent in 5 of 23 patients (22 percent) after 3 to 12 months of treatment with colchicine. The condition of nine patients (39 percent) remained stable, while that of nine others deteriorated during the period of follow-up. The independent effect of colchicine was impossible to ascertain, since 18 of 23 patients received concomitant prednisone, and azathioprine and cyclophosphamide were each used in one patient. Colchicine was given as sole therapy in only five patients, three of whom experienced improvement. The lack of a control group, the failure to evaluate pulmonary function tests (the major indicator of therapeutic efficacy) at consistent time points, and the exclusion of one-third of the patients from analysis are serious flaws in this study.

Thus, substantive data affirming the efficacy of colchicine as therapy for IPF are lacking. However, side effects attributed to colchicine are rarely severe. As a result, oral colchicine (0.6 mg once or twice daily) may be considered as adjunctive therapy for patients refractory to corticosteroids, either alone or in combination with immunosuppressive and cytotoxic agents.

Penicillamine   Penicillamine reduces collagen deposition in animal models (bleomycin- and radiation-induced pneumonitis) and may have beneficial effects in rheumatoid arthritis and collagen vascular disorders.[24] Anecdotal responses to penicillamine have been noted in idiopathic or collagen vascular disease–associated pulmonary fibrosis,[24,37] but controlled studies have not been performed. Penicillamine usage has been associated with a reduced rate of pulmonary function deterioration in patients with scleroderma-associated pulmonary fibrosis. However, penicillamine was associated with clinical improvement in only 3 of 21 patients with IPF previously resistant to corticosteroid treatment in three retrospective studies.[24,37] Penicillamine is toxic, and significant adverse effects (loss of taste, nausea, vomiting, stomatitis, nephrotoxicity, etc.) complicate its use in up to 50 percent of patients. In view of its toxicity and the lack of data affirming its efficacy, penicillamine has little value as therapy for idiopathic pulmonary fibrosis.

Ancillary Therapies

No randomized trials have demonstrated the benefits of supplemental oxygen therapy on survival in patients with IPF. It seems reasonable, however, to extrapolate from the proven benefits in hypoxic patients with obstructive disease. Standard established criteria from patients with chronic obstructive pulmonary disease can be used to determine when to begin supplemental oxygen. Supplemental oxygen alleviates exercise-induced hypoxemia and improves exercise performance.[13]

Severe paroxysms of cough may be among the most distressing features of IPF. A variety of antitussive agents have been used in IPF, but controlled studies assessing efficacy have not been performed. Rib fractures secondary to protracted episodes of coughing may occur in elderly persons with severe osteoporosis. Oral codeine or other antitussives may be helpful in some patients and can be used in patients with cough refractory to proprietary cough suppressants.

Pulmonary hypertension may complicate IPF in the late phases of the disease. However, administration of vasodilators to reduce pulmonary arterial pressure has not been shown to be beneficial and may cause serious adverse effects (including systemic hypotension).

Opioids have been used to reduce dyspnea in patients with severe chronic lung disease, but data affirming the efficacy of this practice are lacking. In a recent study, low-dose (2.5 to 5 mg) nebulized morphine failed to relieve dyspnea or improve exercise tolerance in patients with interstitial lung disease. As with all patients with chronic lung disease, pneumococcal vaccination and periodic influenza vaccinations are warranted.

Lung Transplantation

Single lung transplantation is an important treatment option for certain patients with end-stage pulmonary fibrosis refractory to medical therapy (Fig. 70-11).[14] The prognosis for patients with IPF who fail medical therapy is poor; most patients die within 2 to 3 years. Severe derangements in pulmonary function (vital capacity or total lung capacity less than 60 percent predicted or diffusing capacity less than 40 percent predicted) and oxygen dependency have been associated with a 2-year mortality exceeding 50 percent. Unless specific contraindications exist, patients with severe functional impairment, oxygen dependency, and a deteriorating course should be listed for lung transplantation. Owing to the limited donor availability, early listing is important, as waiting time for procuring a suitable donor organ may exceed 2 years. Unfortunately, patients with rapidly progressive or severe IPF may die while awaiting transplantation. Contraindications to lung transplantation include age over 60 years, unstable or inadequate psychosocial profile/stability, and significant extrapulmonary disorders (liver, renal, or cardiac dysfunction), which may negatively influence survival.

Consensus Conference on Novel Therapies

A recent Consensus Conference on therapy for pulmonary fibrosis underscored the marginal benefit of existing therapies and

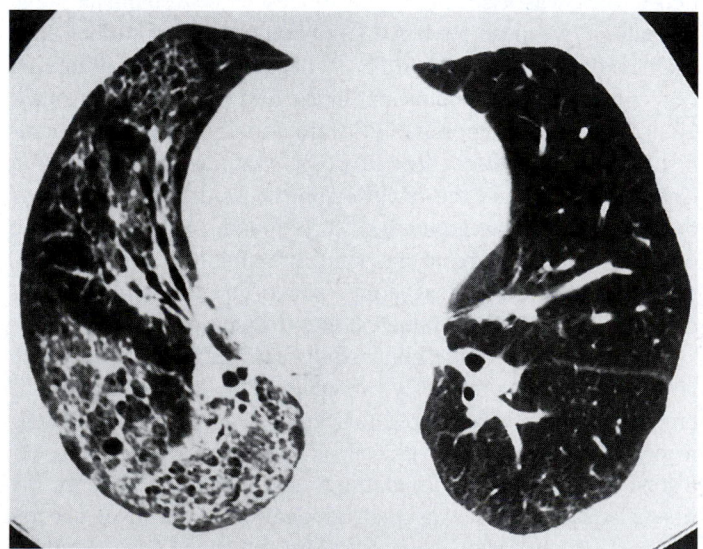

FIGURE 70-11   HRCT scan from a 47-year-old man with IPF 18 months following single (left) lung transplant. The native right lung is contracted with diffuse reticulonodular infiltrates and honeycombing consistent with IPF. The transplanted (left) lung allograft is well expanded with normal lung parenchyma.

suggested that major advances in survival awaited the development of novel therapies.[15] Possible future (and completely untested) therapeutic strategies include agents that inhibit cytokines, proteases, and/or oxidants; antifibrotic agents (platelet-activating factor receptor antagonists, pifenidone, proline inhibitors); dietary modifications; more efficient intrapulmonary drug delivery via liposomes; diphosphonates; inhibitors of leukocyte integrins; and gene therapy.[15] The generation of novel therapeutic strategies will require a better understanding of the pathogenesis of this difficult disorder.

REFERENCES

1. Agusti C, Xaubet A, Agusti AGN, et al: Clinical and functional assessment of patients with idiopathic pulmonary fibrosis: Results of a 3-year follow-up. *Eur Respir J* 7:643–650, 1994.

2. Bernsard DD, McIntyre RC, Simon JS, et al: Comparison of video thorascopic lung biopsy to open lung biopsy in the diagnosis of interstitial lung disease. *Chest* 103:765–770, 1993.

3. Boomars KA, Wagenaar SS, Mulder PG, et al: Relationship between cells obtained by bronchoalveolar lavage and survival in idiopathic pulmonary fibrosis. *Thorax* 50:1087–1092, 1995.

4. Carre PC, Mortensen RL, King TE Jr, et al: Increased expression of the interleukin 8 gene by alveolar macrophages in idiopathic pulmonary fibrosis: A potential mechanism for the recruitment and activation of neutrophils in lung fibrosis. *J Clin Invest* 88:1802–1810, 1991.

5. Carrington CB, Gaensler EA, Coutu RE, et al: Natural history and treated course of usual and desquamative interstitial pneumonia. *New Engl J Med* 298:801–809, 1978.

6. Cherniak RM, Colby TV, Flint A, et al: Correlation of structure and function in idiopathic pulmonary fibrosis. *Am J Respir Crit Care Med* 151:1180–1188, 1995.

7. Chinet T, Jaubert F, Dusser D, et al: Effects of inflammation and fibrosis on pulmonary function in diffuse lung fibrosis. *Thorax* 45:675–678, 1990.

8. Corrin B. Pathology of interstitial lung disease. *Semin Respir Crit Care Med* 15:61–76, 1994.

9. Coultas DB, Zumwalt RE, Black WC, Sobonya RE: The epidemiology of interstitial lung diseases. *Am J Respir Crit Care Med* 150:967–972, 1994.

10. Eitzman DT, McCoy RD, Zheng Z, et al: Bleomycin-induced pulmonary fibrosis in transgenic mice that either lack or overexpress the murine plasminogen activator inhibitor–1 gene. *J Clin Invest* 97:232–237, 1996.

11. Grenier P, Chevret S, Beigelman C, et al: Chronic diffuse infiltrative lung disease: Determination of the diagnostic value of clinical data, chest radiography and CT with Bayesian analysis. *Radiology* 191:383–390, 1994.

12. Hanley ME, King TE Jr, Schwarz MI, et al: The impact of smoking on mechanical properties of the lung in idiopathic pulmonary fibrosis and sarcoidosis. *Am Rev Respir Dis* 144:1102–1106, 1991.

13. Harris-Eze AO, Sridhar G, Clemens RE, et al: Oxygen improves maximal exercise performance in interstitial lung disease. *Am J Respir Crit Care Med* 150:1616–1622, 1994.

14. Hosenpud JD, Novick RJ, Breen TJ, Daily OP: The registry of the International Society for Heart and Lung Transplantation: Twelfth Official Report—1995. *J Heart Lung Transplant* 14:805–815, 1995.

15. Hunninghake GW, Kalica AR: Approaches to the treatment of pulmonary fibrosis. *Am J Respir Crit Care Med* 151:915–918, 1995.

16. Iawai K, Mori T, Yamada N, et al: Idiopathic pulmonary fibrosis: Epidemiologic approaches to occupational exposure. *Am J Respir Crit Care Med* 150:670–675, 1994.

17. Johnson MA, Kwan S, Snell NJ, et al: Randomised controlled trial comparing prednisolone alone with cyclophosphamide and low dose prednisolone in combination with cryptogenic fibrosing alveolitis. *Thorax* 44:280–288, 1989.

18. Johnston ID, Gomm SA, Kalra A, et al: The management of cryptogenic fibrosing alveolitis in three regions of the United Kingdom. *Eur Respir J* 6:891–893, 1993.

19. Kaplan JD, Trulock EP, Anderson DJ, Schuster DP: Pulmonary vascular permeability in interstitial lung disease: A positron emission tomographic study. *Am Rev Respir Dis* 145:1495–1498, 1992.

20. Katzenstein AA, Fiorelli RF: Nonspecific interstitial pneumonia/fibrosis: Histologic features and clinical significance. *Am J Surg Pathol* 18:136–147, 1994.

21. Lynch JP III, Chavis AD: Chronic interstitial pulmonary disorders, in Victor L. (ed), *Clinical Pulmonary Medicine.* Boston, Little, Brown, 1992, pp 193–264.

22. Lynch JP III, Standiford TJ, Rolfe MW, et al: Neutrophilic alveolitis in idiopathic pulmonary fibrosis: The role of interleukin-8. *Am Rev Respir Dis* 145:1433–1439, 1992.

23. McCune WJ, Vallance DK, Lynch JP III: Immunosuppressive drug therapy. *Curr Opin Rheumatol* 6:262–272, 1994.

24. Meier-Sydow J, Weiss SM, Buhl R, et al: Idiopathic pulmonary fibrosis: Current concepts and challenges in management. *Semin Respir Crit Care Med* 15:77–96, 1994.

25. Nishimura K, Kitaichi M, Izumi T, et al: Usual interstitial pneumonia: Histologic correlation with high-resolution CT. *Radiology* 182:337–342, 1992.

26. O'Donnell K, Keogh B, Cantin A, Crystal RG: Pharmacologic suppression of the neutrophil component of the alveolitis in idiopathic pulmonary fibrosis. *Am Rev Respir Dis* 136:288–292, 1987.

27. Panos RJ, King TE Jr: Idiopathic pulmonary fibrosis, in Lynch JP III, DeRemee RA (eds), *Immunologically Mediated Pulmonary Diseases.* Philadelphia, JB Lippincott, 1991, pp 1–39.

28. Panos RJ, Mortenson RL, Niccoli SA, King GE Jr: Clinical deterioration in patients with idiopathic pulmonary fibrosis: causes and assessment. *Am J Med* 88:396–404, 1990.

29. Peters SG, McDougall JC, Douglas WW, et al: Colchicine in the treatment of pulmonary fibrosis. *Chest* 103:101–104, 1993.

30. Raghu G: Interstitial lung disease: a diagnostic approach: Are CT scan and lung biopsy indicated in every patient? *Am J Respir Crit Care Med* 151:909–914, 1995.

31. Raghu G, DePaso WJ, Cain K, et al: Azathioprine combined with prednisone in the treatment of idiopathic pulmonary fibrosis: A prospective, double-blind, randomized, placebo-controlled trial. *Am Rev Respir Dis* 144:291–296, 1991.

32. Raghu G, Hert R: Interstitial lung diseases: Genetic predisposition and inherited interstitial lung diseases. *Semin Respir Med* 14: 323–332, 1993.

33. Remy-Jardin M, Giraud F, Remy J, et al: Importance of ground-glass attenuation in chronic diffuse infiltrative lung disease: Pathologic-CT correlation. *Radiology* 189:693–698, 1993.

34. Rennard SI, Bitterman PB, Ozaki T, et al: Colchicine suppresses the release of fibroblast growth factors from alveolar macrophages *in vitro:* The basis of a possible therapeutic approach to the fibrotic disorders. *Am Rev Respir Dis* 137:181–185, 1988.

35. Robertson HT: Clinical application of pulmonary function and exercise tests in the management of patients with interstitial lung disease. *Semin Respir Crit Care Med* 15:1–9, 1994.

36. Rochester CL, Elias JA: Cytokines and cytokine networking in the pathogenesis of interstitial and fibrotic lung disorders. *Semin Respir Med* 14:389–416, 1993.

37. Rudd RM, Haslam PL, Turner-Warwick M: Cryptogenic fibrosing alveolitis: Relationships of pulmonary physiology and bronchoalveolar lavage to response to treatment and prognosis. *Am Rev Respir Dis* 124:1–8, 1981.

38. Schwartz DA, Merchant RK, Helmers RA, et al: The influence of smoking on lung function in patients with idiopathic pulmonary fibrosis. *Am Rev Respir Dis* 144:504–506, 1991.

39. Schwartz DA, Helmers RA, Galvin JR, et al: Determinants of progression in idiopathic pulmonary fibrosis. *Am J Respir Crit Care Med* 149:450–454, 1994.

40. Schwartz DA, Van Fossen DS, Davis CS, et al: Determinants of progression in idiopathic pulmonary fibrosis. *Am J Respir Crit Care Med* 149:444–449, 1994.

41. Smith RE, Strieter RM, Zhang K, et al: A role for C-C chemokines in fibrotic lung disease. *J Leukoc Biol* 57:782–787, 1995.

42. Standiford TJ, Rolfe MW, Kunkel SL, et al: Macrophage inflammatory protein-1α expression in interstitial lung disease. *J Immunol* 151:2852–2863, 1993.

43. Terriff BA, Kwan SY, Chan-Yeung MM, Muller NL: Fibrosing alveolitis: Chest radiography and CT as predictors of clinical and functional impairment at follow-up in 26 patients. *Radiology* 184:445–449, 1992.

44. Toews GB: Pulmonary dendritic cells: Sentinels of lung-associated lymphoid tissues. *Am J Respir Cell Mol Biol* 4:204–205, 1991.

45. van Oortegem K, Wallaert B, Marquette CH, et al: Determinants of response to immunosuppressive therapy in idiopathic pulmonary fibrosis. *Eur Respir J* 7:1950–1957, 1994.

46. Watters LC, King TE, Schwarz MI, et al: A clinical, radiographic and physiologic scoring system for the longitudinal assessment of patients with idiopathic pulmonary fibrosis. *Am Rev Respir Dis* 133:97–103, 1986.

47. Watters LC, Schwarz MI, Cherniak RM, et al: Idiopathic pulmonary fibrosis: Pretreatment bronchoalveolar lavage cellular constituents and their relationships to lung histopathology and clinical response to therapy. *Am Rev Respir Dis* 135:696–704, 1987.

48. Wells AU, Rubens MB, du Bois RM, Hansell DM: Serial CT in fibrosing alveolitis: Prognostic significance of the initial patters. *Am J Roentgenol* 161:1159-1165, 1993.

49. Wilborn J, Crofford LJ, Burdick MD, et al: Cultured lung fibroblasts isolated from patients with idiopathic pulmonary fibrosis have a diminished capacity to synthesize prostaglandin E_2 and to express cyclooxygenase-2. *J Clin Invest* 95:1861–1868, 1995.

50. Wilborn J, Bailie M, Coffey M, et al: Constitutive activation of 5-lipoxygenase in the lungs of patients with idiopathic pulmonary fibrosis. *J Clin Invest* 97:1827–1836, 1996

51. Winterbauer RH, Hammar SP, Hallman KO, et al: Diffuse interstitial pneumonitis: Clinicopathological correlations in 20 patients treated with prednisone/azathioprine. *Am J Med* 65:661–672, 1978.

CHAPTER 71

HYPERSENSITIVITY PNEUMONITIS

Mark Schuyler

CLINICAL PRESENTATIONS: ACUTE AND CHRONIC

RADIOLOGY

EPIDEMIOLOGY

PATHOLOGY

DIFFERENTIAL DIAGNOSIS

LABORATORY FINDINGS

PATHOGENESIS

PROGNOSIS AND TREATMENT

Hypersensitivity pneumonitis (or *extrinsic allergic alveolitis,* the British term) is a group of lung diseases caused by inhalation of a wide variety of different materials that are usually organic and always antigenic. The stereotypical clinical events are transient fever, hypoxemia, myalgias, arthralgias, dyspnea, and cough that occur 2 to 9 h after exposure and resolve in 12 to 72 h without specific treatment.

Hypersensitivity pneumonitis was first clearly described in 1874 in Dr. Jon Finsen's doctoral thesis wherein he described *heykatarr* in Iceland in the following fashion:

> This is a chronic chest disease. I do not know its incidence, as my observations thereupon are incomplete. The disease occurs only in winter, or rather during the time when the animals are kept inside, and is found only in the man whose job it is to loosen the hay in the barn and handle it before it is fed to cattle. The hay is always more or less dusty and has to be shaken to eliminate the dust before it is used as fodder. When this dust is inhaled, especially when the harvesting has been difficult and the hay has molded in the barn, the man who works with the hay becomes ill with this disease, which lasts as long as he continues the same occupation, but usually disappears in summer. The disease expresses itself by cough, rather scant expectoration, and chest heaviness, especially in the evening (the hay is usually loosened in the afternoon, i.e., when it is intended to be given in the evening and the next morning). When examining the chest of those men, I have on a few occasions found signs of bronchitis, but in most cases I have never found anything abnormal. I have never had the occasion to examine a patient during an acute episode.[42]

This syndrome was seen again in British farmers in the 1930s by Campbell[6] and designated farmer's lung disease (FLD). Dr. Finsen's description is notable for the association of the illness with a particular environmental exposure, its relationship to the season of the year, its occurrence several hours after exposure, the nature of the symptoms, and even the association with bronchitis. Many other diseases have since been described that exhibit the same clinical features and are denoted as hypersensitivity pneumonitis (HP). Despite the terms *hypersensitivity* and *allergic,* HP is not an atopic disease and is not associated with increased IgE or eosinophils. Drug reactions are sometimes described as representing HP, usually because certain bronchoalveolar lavage (BAL) fluid findings resemble those in HP. However, these are not HP, as the inciting agent is administered systemically and the pathogenetic mechanisms are probably different from those of HP.

A large number of agents cause HP. This can be seen in Table 71-1, which is a list of currently described examples of HP. In interpreting this table, it is important to remember that there is a dynamic quality to the causes of HP. Some types of HP have apparently disappeared from their originally described clinical settings (e.g., bagassosis in Louisiana) but presumably exist in areas with similar agricultural or industrial settings. In addition, other forms of HP are being newly recognized (e.g., potato riddler's lung and machine operator's lung). Both the disappearance of previously described examples of HP and the appearance of new examples are due to changing agricultural or industrial practices that result in changes of exposure of subjects to antigenic material that can cause HP. At the present time FLD bird fancier's disease (BFD), ventilator lung, and Japanese summer-type HP are the most commonly recognized forms of HP.

Recognition of new examples of HP usually requires a cluster of new cases with a unifying exposure history. Since complete occupational and avocational histories are at times not obtained from patients with "pneumonia," it is likely that there are substantially more examples of HP that have not yet been recognized and described. For example, introduction of a new metalworking fluid led to recognition of machine operator's lung in an auto parts–manufacturing facility due to clustering of cases and a common unusual exposure (*Pseudomonas* in cooling fluid).[3]

CLINICAL PRESENTATIONS: ACUTE AND CHRONIC

There are two different clinical presentations of HP.

In *acute HP,* dyspnea, nonproductive cough, myalgias, chills, diaphoresis, lassitude, headache, and malaise occur 2 to 9 h

TABLE 71-1

Types of Hypersensitivity Pneumonitis

Disease	Antigen Source	Probable Antigen	References
Plant products			
Farmer's lung disease	Moldy hay	Thermophilic actinomycetes *M. faeni (S. rectivirgula)* *T. vulgaris* *Aspergillus* spp.	Pepys J et al. *Lancet* 2:607–611, 1963
Bagassosis	Moldy pressed sugarcane (bagasse)	Thermophilic actinomycetes *T. sacchari* *T. vulgaris*	Salvaggio J et al. *Am J Med* 46:538–544, 1969
Mushroom worker's disease	Moldy compost and mushrooms	Thermophilic actinomycetes *M. faeni* *T. vulgaris* *Aspergillus* spp. Mushroom spores	Cox A et al. *Eur Respir J* 1:466–468, 1988
Suberosis	Moldy cork	*Penicillium* spp.	Avila R et al. *Lancet* 1:620–621, 1968
Malt worker's lung	Contaminated barley	*Aspergillus clavatus*	Riddle HF et al. *Thorax* 23:271–280, 1968
Maple bark disease	Contaminated maple logs	*Cryptostroma corticale*	Emanuel D et al. *New Engl J Med* 274:1413–1418, 1966
Sequoisis	Contaminated redwood dust	*Graphium* spp. *Pullularia* spp.	Cohen HI et al. *Am J Med* 43:785–794, 1967
Soybean lung	Soybeans in animal feed	Soybean hull antigens	Zubeldia JM et al. *J Allergy Clin Immunol* 95:622–626, 1995
Wood pulp worker's disease	Contaminated wood pulp	*Alternaria* spp.	Schleuter D et al. *Ann Intern Med* 77:907–914, 1972
Wood dust HP	Contaminated wood dust	*Bacillus subtilis* *Alternaria*	Sosman AJ et al. *New Engl J Med* 281:977–980, 1969
Compost lung	Compost	*Aspergillus* spp. *T. vulgaris*	Vincken W et al. *Thorax* 39:74–75, 1984
Cheeseworker's disease	Cheese or cheese casings	*Penicillium* spp.	Campbell J et al. *Am Rev Respir Dis* 127:495–496, 1983
Wood trimmer's disease	Contaminated wood trimmings, at times in sawmills	*Rhizopus* spp. *Mucor* spp.	Belin L. *Int Arch Allergy Appl Immunol* 82: 440–443, 1987
Thatched roof disease	Dried grasses and leaves	*Saccharomonospora viridis*	Blackburn CR et al. *Lancet* 2:1396–1397, 1966
Greenhouse lung	Greenhouse soil	*Aspergillus* spp. *Penicillium* spp. *Cryptostroma corticale*	Yoshida K et al. *Arch Environ Health* 48: 260–262, 1993
Coffee worker's lung	Green coffee dust	Unknown	Van Toorn D. *Thorax* 25:399–405, 1970
Potato riddler's lung	Moldy hay around potatoes	Thermophilic actinomycetes *M. faeni* *T. vulgaris* *Aspergillus* spp.	Greene JJ et al. *Irish Med J* 78:282–284, 1985

TABLE 71-1   **(Continued)**

Disease	Antigen Source	Probable Antigen	References
Tobacco worker's disease	Mold on tobacco	*Aspergillus* spp.	Huuskonen MS et al. *Br J Ind Med* 41:77–83, 1984
Wine grower's lung	Mold on grapes	*Botrytis cinerea*	Popp W et al. *Prax Klin Pneumol* 41:165–169, 1987
Woodman's disease	Mold on bark and fuel chips	*Penicillium* spp.	Dykewicz MS et al. *J Allergy Clin Immunol* 81:455–460, 1988
Soy sauce brewer's lung	Fermentation starter for soy sauce	*Aspergillus oryzae*	Tsuchiya Y et al. *J Allergy Clin Immunol* 91:688–689, 1993
Domestic allergic alveolitis	Decayed wood	Fungi *Serpula lacrymans* *Leucogyrophana pinastri* *Paecilomyces variottii* *Aspergillus fumigatus*	Bryant DH et al. *Allergy Proc* 12:89–94, 1991
Riding school lung	Hay in horse stall	Thermophilic actinomycetes *M. faeni* (*S. rectivirgula*) *T. vulgaris*	Kristiansen JD et al. *Acta Paediatr Scand* 80:386–388, 1991
Stipatosis	Esparto grass (*Stipa tenacissima*), used to make plaster	Esparto grass antigens	Gamboa PM et al. *Allergol Immunopathol* 18:331–334, 1990
Animal products Pigeon breeder's disease	Pigeon droppings	Altered pigeon serum (probably IgA), pigeon bloom (derived from feathers)	Reed C et al. *JAMA* 193:261–265, 1965
Turkey handler's disease	Turkey products	Turkey proteins	Boyer RS et al. *Am Rev Respir Dis* 109:630–635, 1974
Chicken breeder's lung	Chicken feathers	Chicken feather proteins	Warren CP et al. *Am Rev Respir Dis* 109:672–677, 1974
Bird fancier's lung	Domestic and wild bird products	Bird proteins	Burdon JG et al. *Am Rev Respir Dis* 134:1319–1320, 1986
Duvet lung	Duvet and pillow	Goose proteins	Haitjema T et al. *Thorax* 47:990–991, 1992
Laboratory worker's HP	Rat fur	Rat urine protein	Carroll K et al. *Clin Allergy* 5:443–456, 1975
Pituitary snuff taker's disease	Pituitary powder	Vasopressin	Harper L et al. *Ann Intern Med* 73:581–584, 1970
Shell lung	Oyster or mollusk shell	Shell proteins	Orriols R et al. *Ann Intern Med* 113:80–81, 1990
Miller's lung	Grain weevils in wheat flour	*Sitophilus granarius* proteins	Lunn J et al. *Br J Ind Med* 24:158–162, 1967
Sericulturist's lung	Silkworm larvae	Silkworm larvae proteins	Nakazawa T et al. *Thorax* 45:233–234, 1990

TABLE 71-1   **(Continued)**

Disease	Antigen Source	Probable Antigen	References
Reactive chemicals			
TDI HP	Toluene di-isocyanate	Altered proteins (albumin + others)	Yoshizawa Y et al. *Ann Intern Med* 110: 31–34, 1989
MDI HP	Diphenylmethane di-isocyanate		Vandenplas O et al. *Am Rev Respir Dis* 147:338–346, 1993
HDI HP	Hexamethylene di-isocyanate		Selden AI et al. *Scand J Work Environ Health* 15:234–237, 1989
TMA HP	Trimetallic anhydride	Altered proteins	Baur X. *J Allergy Clin Immunol* 95:1004–1010, 1995
Other			
Ventilator lung	Contaminated humidifiers, dehumidifiers, air conditioners, heating systems	Thermophilic actinomycetes *T. candidus* *T. vulgaris* *Penicillium* spp. *Cephalosporium* spp. Amoebae *Klebsiella* spp. *Candida* spp.	Banaszak E et al. *New Engl J Med* 283:271–276, 1970
Basement lung	Contaminated basement (sewage or mold)	*Cephalosporium* spp. *Penicillium* spp.	Patterson R et al. *J Allergy Clin Immunol* 68: 128–132, 1981
Sauna taker's disease	Sauna water	*Aureobasidium* spp.	Metzger WJ et al. *JAMA* 236:2209–2211, 1976
Detergent worker's disease	Detergent enzymes	Bacillus subtilis	Berson SA et al. *New Engl J Med* 284:688–690, 1971
Japanese summer house HP	House dust, bird droppings(?)	*Trichosporon cutaneum*	Shimazu K et al. *Am Rev Respir Dis* 130:407–411, 1984
Hot-tub lung	Mold on ceiling	*Cladosporium* spp.	Jacobs RL et al. *Ann Intern Med* 105:204–206, 1986
Tractor lung	Contaminated tractor, cab air conditioner	*Rhizopus* spp.	O'Connell M et al. *J Allergy Clin Immunol* 95:779–780, 1995
Machine operator's lung	Contaminated metal working fluid	*Pseudomonas* spp.	Bernstein DI et al. *Chest* 108:636–641, 1995
Fertilizer lung	Contaminated fertilizer	*Streptomyces albus*	Kagen S et al. *J Allergy Clin Immunol* 68: 295–299, 1981
Sax lung	Saxophone mouthpiece	*Candida albicans*	Lodha S et al. *Chest* 93:1322, 1988

after a particular exposure. These symptoms typically peak between 6 and 24 h after exposure and resolve without specific treatment in 1 to 3 days (sometimes longer after a particularly intense exposure). Patients exhibit fever, tachypnea, bibasilar rales, and occasionally cyanosis. Figure 71-1 diagrams the course of acute HP. There is peripheral blood leukocytosis with neutrophilia and lymphopenia, but not eosinophilia, and BAL neutrophilia.

Chronic HP presents as progressively more severe dyspnea, nonproductive cough, weight loss, and often anorexia in a patient exposed to a recognized cause of HP. Symptoms are usually present for months to years. There is typically no fever, but tachypnea and bibasilar dry rales are usually present. Symptoms and signs of cor pulmonale are not uncommon at presentation. In general, clubbing seldom occurs,[24] although it has been reported in up to 50 percent of subjects with pigeon breeder's disease (PBD) in Mexico City.[41]

A proportion (20 to 40 percent) of patients with chronic HP present with symptoms of chronic bronchitis (e.g., chronic productive cough),[5,14] some even without radiologic parenchymal densities on standard chest radiographs. There is substantial morphologic evidence of bronchitis in the large airways of patients with FLD. Since most patients with HP are nonsmokers and have no other reason for the development of chronic bronchitis, these symptoms are probably a result of HP and may correlate with evidence of airway hyperreactivity in patients with chronic HP.

The reasons for the different clinical presentations (i.e., acute and chronic) of HP are not clear, but could include differences of intensity and duration of exposure (low-intensity long-duration exposure tending to cause chronic HP; high-intensity short-duration exposure tending to cause acute HP). This is most clearly demonstrated in HP due to bird exposure. BFD (chronic exposure to low amounts of bird antigens) is associated with chronic HP. PBD has different presentations in different geographic areas, manifesting as an acute HP in some and chronic HP in others. Intermittent exposure of pigeon breeders to large amounts of pigeon antigens in the United States and Europe is associated with acute disease and a good prognosis, whereas chronic exposure to a few household pigeons in Mexico is associated with chronic disease and a much poorer prognosis.[40] In the United States and Europe, pigeon breeders keep their animals in an enclosure separate from their living areas, which they visit periodically so that exposure is intermittent. In Mexico, birds are kept in living quarters so that exposure is constant. It is of interest that bird antigens can persist in a room for substantial lengths of time (more than 18 months) after removal of the birds,[11] so that Mexicans with PBD would be expected to be exposed to pigeon antigens for prolonged periods even after removal of the pigeons. Therefore, PBD in Mexico resembles BFD in the United States and Europe in type of exposure, clinical presentation, and prognosis. It differs greatly from the acute HP that characterizes the PBD in the United States and Europe. Since the relevant antigens are similar in these two examples of bird-associated HP, it is likely that the type of exposure, and not the antigen characteristics, determines clinical presentation and prognosis.

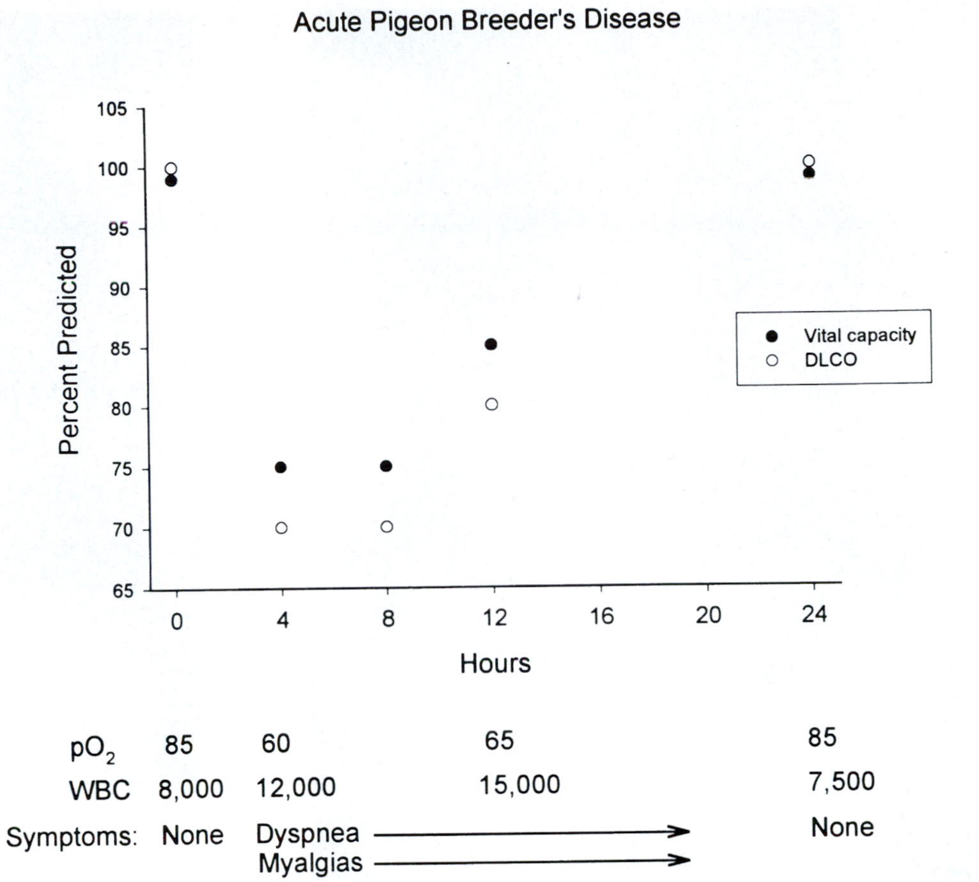

FIGURE 71-1   Diagram of a typical episode of acute pigeon breeder's disease induced by exposure to pigeon serum at 0 h.

Although the recognition of a new example of HP is usually associated with the acute form, most patients with well-recognized types of HP present with chronic disease.[31] This might be related to the difficulties in establishing a link between chronic disease and chronic exposure, as opposed to the relative ease in making the association of acute disease and acute exposure.

The above discussion indicates that HP, and particularly chronic HP, may be more prevalent than is readily apparent and may be confused with bronchitis or misdiagnosed as idiopathic pulmonary fibrosis (IPF). The latter may be particularly important because detailed histories are not always obtained from patients with IPF, the serum antibody levels to the agents responsible for HP tend to wane after cessation of exposure, and chest high-resolution computed tomography (CT) scans of chronic HP can resemble those of IPF.

RADIOLOGY

In accord with their differing clinical presentations, the chest radiographs of patients with acute and chronic HP differ significantly. In acute HP, chest radiographs demonstrate diffuse poorly defined nodular radiodensities, at times with areas of ground-glass radiodensities or even consolidation. These radiodensities tend to occur in the lower lobes and spare the apices. Linear radiodensities (presumably representing areas of fibrosis from previous episodes of acute HP) may also be present. The nodular and ground-glass densities tend to disappear after cessation

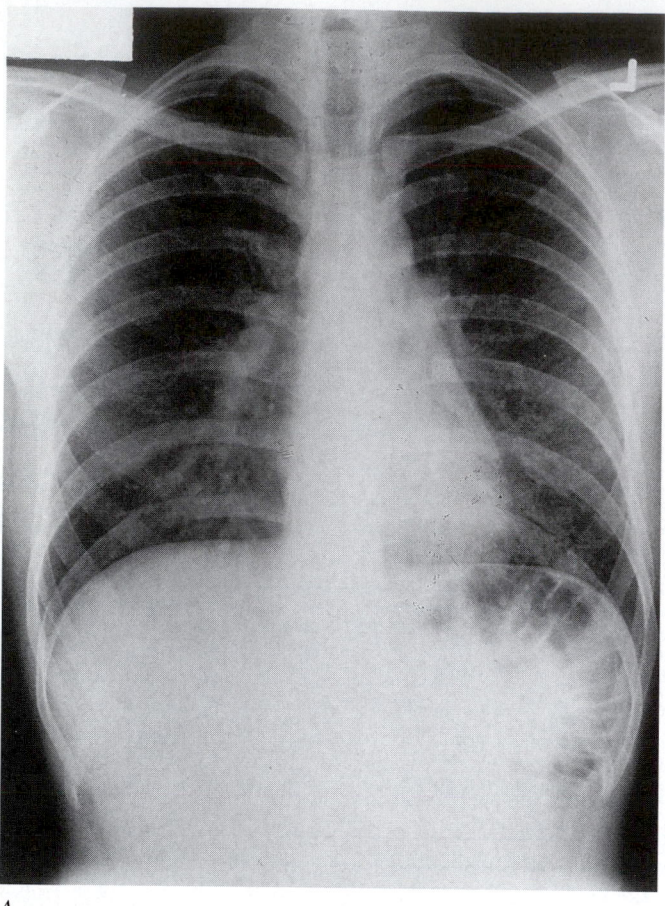

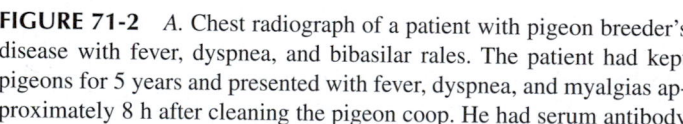

A

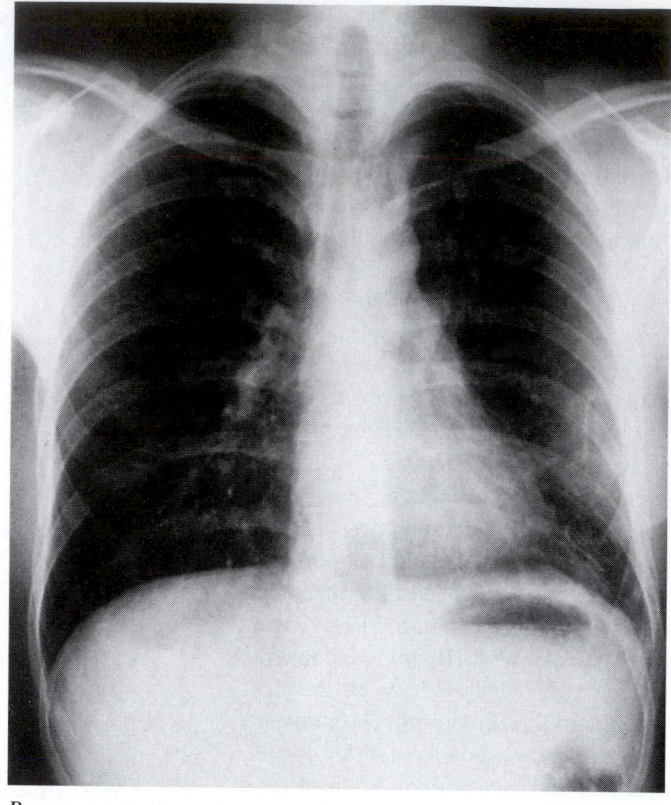

B

FIGURE 71-2   *A*. Chest radiograph of a patient with pigeon breeder's disease with fever, dyspnea, and bibasilar rales. The patient had kept pigeons for 5 years and presented with fever, dyspnea, and myalgias approximately 8 h after cleaning the pigeon coop. He had serum antibody to pigeon dropping extract. Note bilateral lower lobe 2- to 3-mm nodules. *B*. Chest radiograph of the same patient 2 weeks later without specific treatment. Note clearing of the lower-lobe nodules and the staples in the left chest from the open lung biopsy.

of exposure, so the chest radiograph may be normal after resolution of an acute episode of HP (Fig. 71-2). High-resolution CT scans often demonstrate ground-glass densities better than chest radiographs and at times reveal diffusely increased pulmonary radiodensities. They may also become normal after resolution of an acute episode. Pleural effusions or thickening, calcification, cavitation, atelectasis, localized radiodensities (coin lesions or masses), and intrathoracic lymphadenopathy are rare.

In chronic HP, chest radiographs are notable for diffuse linear and nodular radiodensities, with sparing of the bases and upper-lobe predominance, and volume loss (Fig. 71-3). Pleural effusions and thickening are very unusual, although subcutaneous emphysema (presumably as a consequence of pleural rupture due to bronchiolitis and lobular overinflation) has been reported.

High-resolution CT scans of patients with chronic HP demonstrate several patterns. Most commonly there are multiple centrilobular nodules 2 to 4 mm in diameter throughout the lung fields, with some areas of ground-glass radiodensities, especially in the lower lobes (Fig. 71-4).[29] Unlike sarcoidosis, the nodules are seldom attached to the pleura or bronchovascular bundles, and the border between the nodules and the surrounding lung is well demarcated. There are also well-delineated areas of increased radiolucency, which are presumably overinflated pul-

monary lobules subserved by partly occluded bronchioles. The ground-glass densities and micronodules tend to resolve after cessation of exposure. Although these findings are suggestive of HP, they are found in only a subset (50 to 75 percent) of patients with HP, and high-resolution CT scans of the lungs of patients with HP can resemble those of patients with IPF.[29] A substantial prevalence of mild to moderate emphysema is also detectable by high-resolution CT scans in nonsmoking patients with FLD.[27] It is not clear if this represents lobular overinflation or emphysema. Magnetic resonance imaging (MRI) is inferior to high-resolution CT scanning in demonstrating anatomic detail, but is the equal of CT in demonstrating ground-glass areas and may be useful in determining the course of ground-glass densities without radiation exposure.

EPIDEMIOLOGY

The prevalence of HP is quite variable in different populations, presumably because of differing intensity, frequency, and duration of inhalation exposure. Among pigeon breeders, 8 to 30 percent of members of pigeon-breeding clubs who participated in surveys exhibited PBD.[5,11] Among farmers, 0.5 to 5 percent have symptoms compatible with FLD.[14,22,50] The prevalence of symp-

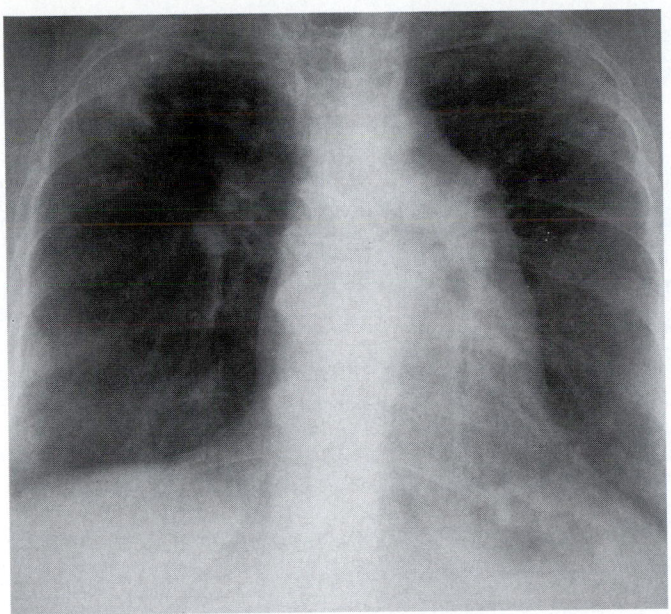

FIGURE 71-3 Chest radiograph of a patient with bird fancier's disease who presented with progressive dyspnea and weight loss. She had kept 2 to 3 parakeets in her home for 15 years and did not notice episodic fever or acute dyspnea. She had positive serum precipitins to parakeet serum, severe restrictive disease, and resting hypoxemia. Note the diffuse radiodensities, loss of volume of the upper lobes, and pulmonary hypertension.

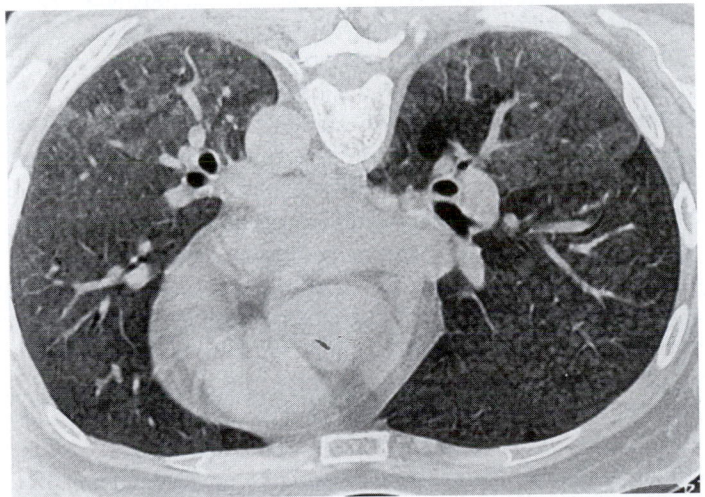

FIGURE 71-4 High-resolution CT scan of a nonsmoking patient with exposure to both birds and shells who presented with progressive dyspnea and weight loss and had hypoxemia and a restrictive ventilatory defect. Note the diffuse nodular radiodensities in the lower lobes, with areas of ground-glass densities posteriorly.

toms is lower in farms that use hay-drying methods that decrease exposure to the responsible antigens and increased after a wet summer season.[19]

The population at risk and the season of exposure vary with the type of HP. For example, most cases of FLD occur in cold, damp climates in late winter and early spring,[24] when farmers (usually male) use stored hay to feed their livestock. PBD occurs chiefly in men in Europe and the United States but pre-

dominantly in women in Mexico, owing to differing patterns of exposure,[40] but without a seasonal preference in either population. BFD in Europe and the United States occurs in subjects who keep domestic birds and does not exhibit a predilection to either sex. Japanese summer-type HP occurs mostly in women without an occupation outside the home in June to September in warm, moist parts of the country.[1]

In contrast to other pulmonary diseases, there is a remarkable predominance (80 to 95 percent) of nonsmokers in all examples of HP, which is substantially higher than the proportion of nonsmokers in similarly exposed but nonill subjects.[2,31,50] The mechanisms of this striking phenomenon are unknown, but could include smoking-induced alterations of lung defense mechanisms or immunologic reactivity. This clinical finding indicates that the presence of active smoking is substantial evidence against the diagnosis of HP.

An important feature of HP is the great variability of susceptibility among exposed populations and the apparent resistance to illness of most exposed persons. Possible reasons include differences of exposure or in the host, either inborn or acquired. There are no differences in the prevalence of atopy or HLA-A, B, C, or DR haplotypes in exposed subjects with and without HP.[50] There is an increased prevalence of HLA-DPβ_1 glutamate 69 in berylliosis, a disease with many similarities to HP, but HLA-DP haplotypes have not been reported in HP. The prevalence of HP, unlike most other lung diseases, is not increased but is substantially decreased by cigarette smoking.[2,31,50] This protection against development of HP in smokers extends to serum antibody, so that smokers have a lower prevalence of serum antibody than apparently equally exposed nonsmokers.[22] The reasons for these phenomena are unknown, but could include depression of immune responses to antigen delivered to the lung, which are well documented to occur in smokers.[20]

PATHOLOGY

Lung biopsies (almost always from patients with chronic HP) show chronic interstitial inflammation with infiltration of plasma cells, mast cells, macrophages, and lymphocytes, usually with poorly formed nonnecrotizing granulomas. There is often bronchiolitis and sometimes (in 25 to 50 percent of cases) bronchiolitis obliterans (Fig. 71-5).[19,45] Organizing pneumonia is often also present, so that 15 to 25 percent of patients with HP have bronchiolitis obliterans with organizing pneumonia (BOOP). Conversely, patients with recognized BOOP may have HP as the cause of their BOOP. Varying degrees of interstitial fibrosis are also often present. The granulomatous interstitial inflammatory responses of HP and sarcoidosis can be difficult to differentiate. In contrast to sarcoidosis, however, the interstitial inflammatory cell infiltrate in HP occurs distal as well as proximal to the granulomas. The granulomas of HP also do not occur in groups and do not tend to occur near bronchi or in subpleural locations. Instead, they are usually adjacent to bronchioles and often single. Giant cells, at times with Schaumann's or asteroid bodies or cholesterol clefts, are present both within and outside the granulomas in patients with HP.[7] Foamy alveolar macrophages are often observed in patients with HP due to bird exposure (Fig. 71-6). Vasculitis and eosinophils are not evident.

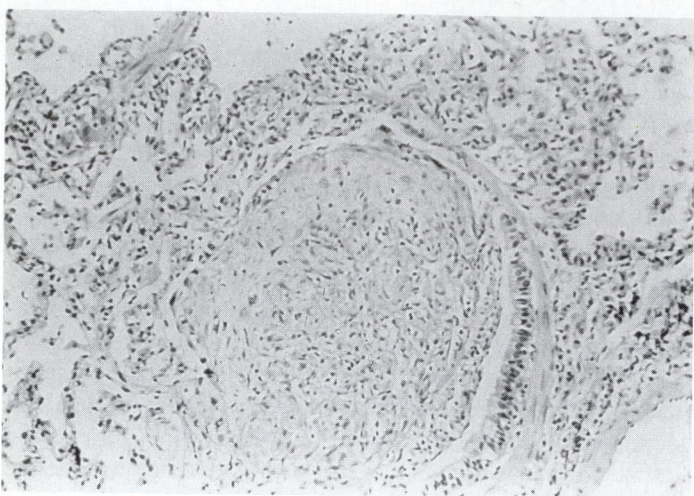

FIGURE 71-5 Bronchiolitis obliterans in the same patient with pigeon breeder's disease as in Fig. 71-2.

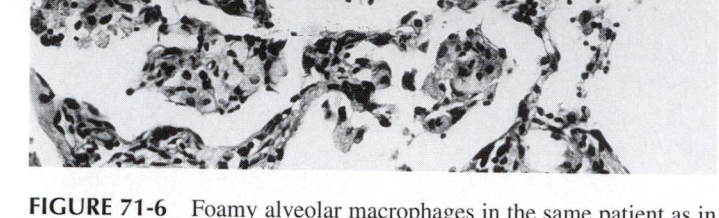

FIGURE 71-6 Foamy alveolar macrophages in the same patient as in Fig. 71-5.

The specific histologic changes of HP, when present, are quite helpful in making the diagnosis. However, the granulomas and respiratory bronchiolitis may not be present years after cessation of exposure, so only interstitial inflammation and fibrosis remain.

DIFFERENTIAL DIAGNOSIS

The symptoms, signs, and laboratory findings of acute HP can resemble those of many other lung diseases, including pulmonary edema, bronchoalveolar cell carcinoma, organic dust toxic syndrome, and some pneumoconioses. Acute HP is most often confused with infectious pneumonia (usually thought to be of viral or mycoplasmal origin and at times psittacosis in subjects exposed to birds).

Organic dust toxic syndrome (ODTS) has been seen in some of the same populations exposed to materials that cause HP. ODTS can occur in a larger proportion of the exposed population than HP and is characterized by transient fever, dyspnea, nonproductive cough, peripheral blood leukocytosis, and BAL fluid neutrophilia; unlike HP, however, it is not associated with chest radiographic changes, permanent lung damage or prior sensitization (as indicated by the absence of serum antibodies).[15] Endotoxin, complement activation, and cytokine release from alveolar macrophages have been implicated as mediators of ODTS. Patients presenting with ODTS tend to have more intense exposure of shorter duration than those who present with FLD.[30]

Another disease caused by exposure to the same agents that cause ventilator lung is humidifier fever. This is characterized by fever, chills, myalgias, arthralgias, headache, malaise, cough, dyspnea, peripheral blood leukocytosis, and arterial hypoxemia, which begin 4 to 12 h after exposure. Some investigators report decreased lung volumes with normal flow rates ("restrictive pattern") and decreased diffusing capacity,[35] whereas others report normal lung volumes and diffusing capacity. The clinical syndrome remits after 12 to 24 h without specific therapy. Symptoms and signs are exaggerated following an exposure that occurs after a period of nonexposure (such as vacations or weekends), but then become blunted despite continued exposure

("Monday illness"). Monday illness with tolerance to apparently the same exposure later in the workweek also occurs in byssinosis and metal fume fever. All signs and symptoms of humidifier fever remit after cessation of exposure, and there are no permanent physiological or radiographic changes. Serum antibodies to thermophilic organisms are rarely present, but antibodies are often present in extracts of humidifier water or slime, gram-negative and -positive bacteria (*Bacillus* species, *Flavobacterium* species, *Pseudomonas* species, *Streptomyces* species), fungi (*Cephalosporium, Penicillium, Sporotrichum, Aspergillus, Fusarium, Mucor, Phoma, Rhizopus*), or ameba.[35] In contrast to HP, there is evidence that some cases of humidifier fever may be caused by endotoxin. Many of the symptoms of humidifier fever can be reproduced by exposure to endotoxin, and investigators have noted high levels of endotoxin in humidifier water and in the atmosphere when a humidifier was operating in a plant with a large number of cases of the disease.[39] However, other investigators, using a pyrogen assay, have not detected endotoxin in humidifier water,[17] so the role of endotoxin in humidifier fever is uncertain.

Chronic HP resembles, and in some instances is impossible to distinguish from, IPF. The differential diagnoses also includes other causes of pulmonary fibrosis (chemotherapeutic agents, radiation, inhaled toxins, pneumoconiosis, etc.), granulomatous pneumonitis (sarcoidosis), and heart failure.

A thorough and complete occupational and avocational history is essential to the diagnosis of both forms of HP. The history should seek to establish a link between a particular exposure (at work, at home, or elsewhere) and previous episodes of "pneumonia." Knowledge of other exposed persons with similar symptoms should be sought.

If the history suggests a relationship between exposure and pulmonary symptoms, evidence of sensitization and the nature of the pulmonary inflammatory response should be determined. Sensitization is indicated by the presence of serum antibody to an agent known to cause HP. A large proportion of lymphocytes in BAL fluid (usually over 40 percent) is suggestive of HP, although many other pulmonary processes can cause a BAL fluid lymphocytosis.

Evidence of repetitive appropriate symptoms and laboratory and radiologic abnormalities associated with exposure to a particular environment is sufficient for diagnosis of HP. In questionable instances, a "natural exposure" (i.e., documentation of appropriate symptoms and laboratory abnormalities after exposure to an environment suspected of causing HP) can be used to diagnose HP. A "natural exposure" challenge should not be considered positive unless there is objective evidence of a change in temperature, total peripheral white blood cell count, chest radiograph or high-resolution CT scan, or increased A-a gradient as reflected by the development or worsening of decreased arterial P_{O_2}. In some patients, lung biopsy may be required to differentiate HP from other causes of diffuse pulmonary inflammation or fibrosis. Transbronchial lung biopsies often do not provide sufficient material to fully establish the presence and interrelationships of granulomas, bronchiolitis, and interstitial inflammation, so either open or thoroscopically obtained lung biopsies are often required.

Deliberate aerosol inhalation exposure to the suspected antigens should not be performed outside research settings, owing to the lack of standardized antigens, the possibility of severe adverse effects of the inhaled material in a sensitized subject, the necessity to demonstrate the nonreactivity of normal unexposed subjects to the same material, and the possible induction of sensitization in a previously nonsensitized subject.

Clearly, a variety of lines of evidence are used to substantiate a diagnosis of HP. In patients in whom FLD is a question, major and minor diagnostic criteria have been proposed.[49] An adaptation of these criteria to HP in general is given in Table 71-2. The diagnosis is confirmed if the patient fulfills all of the major criteria and at least four of the minor criteria and if all other diseases with similar symptoms (e.g., sarcoidosis) are ruled out. A normal chest radiograph is acceptable if pulmonary histology is compatible with HP. A normal high-resolution CT scan eliminates the possibility of active or chronic HP, but is possible between acute episodes, so a normal high-resolution CT scan is acceptable if there are compatible pulmonary histologic changes.

TABLE 71–2

Major and Minor Criteria Used to Substantiate a Diagnosis of HP

Major criteria for HP
- Evidence of exposure to appropriate antigen from history or detection of serum antibody
- Symptoms compatible with HP
- Findings compatible with HP on chest radiographs or high–resolution CT scan

Minor criteria for HP
- Bibasilar rales
- Decreased diffusing capacity
- Arterial hypoxemia, either at rest or during exercise
- Pulmonary histologic changes compatible with HP
- Positive "natural challenge"
- BAL fluid lymphocytosis

LABORATORY FINDINGS

Patients with acute HP have a peripheral blood leukocytosis with neutrophilia. Prominent cellular abnormalities are also seen in their BAL fluid. At time points less than 48 h after exposure, the lavage is characterized by BAL fluid neutrophilia.[16] At time points more than 5 days after the last exposure, a two- to fourfold increase in BAL fluid cell number and a BAL fluid lymphocytosis (typically 40 to 80 percent of total cells) are noted. This BAL fluid lymphocytosis, at least in dairy farmers, is related to continued antigenic exposure and not to the presence of disease, and it does not presage outcome.[10] In most instances of HP, the BAL fluid lymphocytes are virtually all CD3$^+$, with a relative increase of CD8$^+$ cells, so that the CD4:CD8 ratio is less than 1.[23] Many of the CD8$^+$ cells express CD57, a marker of cytotoxic cells, and also express CD25 (the IL-2 receptor) and other activation markers. However, the BAL fluid CD4:CD8 ratio is more than 1 in ventilator lung, some cases of BFD, and some cases of FLD in Japan,[33] although the BAL fluid CD4:CD8 ratio is less than 1 in Japanese summer-type HP.[23] These differences between Japanese and non-Japanese patients with some types of HP might be related to different types of exposure, differing times between the last important exposure, and BAL or genetic differences. In support of the importance of timing between last exposure and lavage, Soler's team demonstrated that cessation of exposure is associated with an increase of BAL fluid CD8$^+$ cells.[47] There is some suggestion that an increase of BAL fluid CD8$^+$ cells is associated with protection against pulmonary fibrosis.[33] There is increased BAL fluid natural killer (NK) cell activity in patients with HP who continue to be exposed to the responsible antigen.[13] The killer cell activity is found in cell populations with characteristics of both NK cells and non-NK cells, including lymphokine-activated killer cells.[46] Most of the CD3$^+$ cells are TCRα/β^+, but there is an increase of TCRγ/δ^+ cells and some tendency toward T-cell oligoclonality as demonstrated by increased Vβ8, Vβ6, and Vβ5 TCR usage in some patients with HP.[34] BAL fluid macrophages display many aspects of activation, including spontaneous secretion of TNFα and IL-1[13] and expression of CD25. Monokines, which can activate macrophages and cause chemotaxis of CD8$^+$ cells (e.g., MIP-1α, MCP-1, and IL-8), are present in BAL fluid and alveolar macrophages from patients with acute HP.[12] Mast cells, often with ultrastructural markers of degranulation, are increased in both the lung parenchyma and BAL fluid of patients with HP.[47] The concentration of IgG, IgM, IgG, and albumin is increased in BAL fluid, presumably as a result of pulmonary inflammation.[16] BAL fluid histamine and tryptase are increased in some patients with acute HP.[47]

Virtually all patients with HP have easily demonstrable antibodies (typically IgG, IgM, and IgA) to the offending material in serum and often also in BAL fluid. A multitude of methods have been used to demonstrate these antibodies (ELISA and variants, indirect immunofluorescence, complement fixation, latex agglutination, counterimmunoelectrophoresis, radioimmunoassay, Western blot). Since most clinical studies have used simple agar diffusion ("Ouchterlony") methods to detect antibody, this is the standard method, but other methods are also acceptable

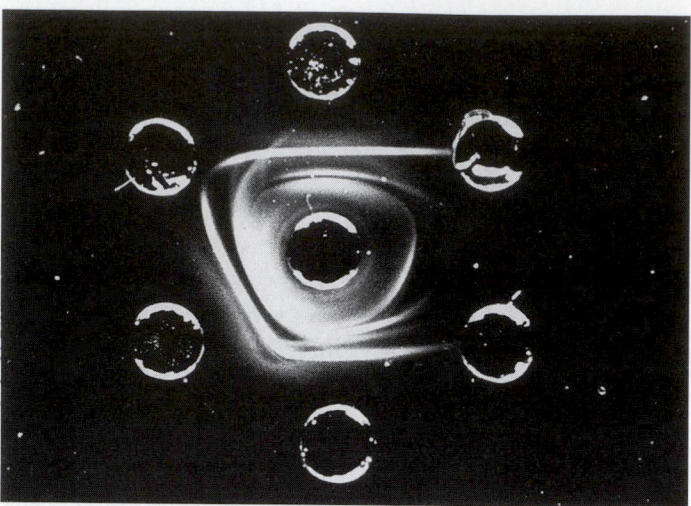

FIGURE 71-7 Precipitin lines to *Micropolyspora faeni* ("Ouchterlony," or double diffusion in agar technique). Central well contains serum from a patient with farmer's lung disease. Outer wells contain different preparations of *M. faeni* antigen. Note the multiple lines and lines of identity between the antigen preparations.

(Fig. 71-7). The key issue is the ability of the antigen to detect antibody in the serum of patients with HP. This varies with the method of antigen preparation and depends on a number of variables, such as the protocols of bacterial growth (for bacterial antigens) and extraction of soluble antigens from either cultured material or material that causes HP (hay in FLD, bird droppings in BFD, etc.). Since antigen preparations are not standardized, it is difficult to be confident of the meaning of a negative result unless the antigens have been tested against panels of sera from patients with and without HP. Even with this precaution, it is not always clear that the antigen used in the assay is the one the patient is reacting to. As a result, it is useful for some patients, particularly those with suspected ventilator lung, to use antigens prepared from the environment suspected to cause the HP. All in all, it is clear that reports of a negative "hypersensitivity pneumonitis panel" do not exclude the diagnosis of HP.

Serum antibody is also present in many exposed, but not ill, subjects in virtually the same amounts as in patients with HP. Therefore, the presence of antibody indicates exposure and sensitization and not necessarily disease. There is some suggestion that the presence of IgG and IgA antibody to *Trichosporon cutaneum* correlates with symptoms in subjects with Japanese type HP, whereas IgG antibody alone correlates with exposure but not symptoms. This correlation of exposure and symptoms with IgA antibody is not found in pigeon breeders or farmers. In asymptomatic pigeon breeders, the prevalence of antibody to pigeon antigens is 30 to 60 percent.[2] In farmers, the prevalence of anti–*Micropolyspora faeni* serum antibody is 2 to 27 percent.[8,22] The occurrence of serum antibody is not consistently related to apparent exposure (i.e., hours of exposure or intensity of exposure) in most instances of HP. This may be related to a threshold effect, so that most exposures are above the minimum required to induce antibody and increases above that threshold are not associated with increases of the prevalence of antibody. In addition, serum antibody tends to wane after cessation of exposure, so patients with chronic HP who have not been exposed for some time may not have demonstrable antibody. In FLD, approximately 50 percent of patients with initially positive serum antibody to *M. faeni* (*Saccharopolyspora rectivirgula*) lose demonstrable antibody 6 years after cessation of exposure.[21,24] Farmers who continue to farm also lose detectable antibody (35 to 50 percent in 5 years),[32] and some asymptomatic farmers who were initially negative later develop antibody[8] without FLD. In PBD and BFD, approximately 50 percent of patients with initially positive serum antibody to avian antigens lose demonstrable antibody 2 to 3 years after cessation of exposure.[28] Therefore, it is possible that patients with HP will have no detectable serum antibody owing to either use of an inappropriate antigen in the assay or the waning of antibody in time since the last exposure.

Nonspecific markers of inflammation, such as increased sedimentation rate and C-reactive protein, are often elevated during an acute episode of HP. There are a few reports of increased prevalence of rheumatoid factor in patients with HP. Antinuclear antibody or other autoantibodies are not present. There is increased uptake of gallium-67 in the lungs of patients with active HP, which declines with resolution of the disease. In contrast to sarcoidosis, the serum angiotensin-converting enzyme levels are usually not elevated.

Skin tests (either immediate or delayed type) to detect sensitization to the suspected antigens are not useful, since extracts of agents that cause HP produce nonspecific reactions that do not indicate sensitization and do not discriminate between sensitized and nonsensitized subjects. In addition, preparations of antigens that cause HP are not readily commercially available. Early reports indicated that some patients with HP demonstrate 4- to 8-h skin test reactivity ("arthus type"), which correlates with the presence of serum antibody. However, the presence of this reaction does not add to information important in the diagnosis of HP, as antibody can be readily detected in serum.

Tests designed to detect cell sensitization (most commonly antigen-induced lymphocyte proliferation or lymphokine secretion) are not useful in the clinical diagnosis of HP, although they have been performed in specialized research settings. Patients with HP have depressed delayed-type skin reactivity to recall antigens,[19] which is similar to that observed in patients with sarcoidosis.[36]

Pulmonary function tests typically demonstrate a restrictive ventilatory defect with small lung volumes, normal or increased flow rates, increased lung elastic recoil, and usually decreased diffusing capacity.[40] There is also the frequent occurrence of a mild obstructive defect and increased upstream airway resistance,[27] probably related to either bronchiolitis or emphysema. Arterial hypoxemia with hypocapnia reflecting an increased A-a oxygen gradient either at rest or after exercise is common.

Many patients with HP (20 to 40 percent) exhibit increased nonspecific airway reactivity,[31,32] which may be related to increased mast cells in the lung and BAL fluid or to bronchial epithelial damage. Some (5 to 10 percent) also develop clinical asthma.[26] The increased airway reactivity and asthma tend to diminish after cessation of exposure.

PATHOGENESIS

Multiple immunologic markers are present in subjects with HP, suggesting that immune mediation is important in the pathogenesis of this syndrome.[2,50] In addition, the necessity for previous sensitization (indicated by the presence of serum antibody in virtually all patients with HP) suggests immunologic mediation.

The presence of serum antibody in patients with HP and the timing of symptoms after exposure (2 to 9 h) led to the hypothesis that HP represents an example of immune complex–mediated lung disease.[37] However, the presence of antibody in exposed but not ill subjects, the lack of correlation of the presence of serum antibody and abnormal pulmonary function tests,[28] the lack of evidence of complement consumption during acute exposure, the pathology (which includes granulomatous changes), and findings from animal models strongly suggest that cell-mediated immune processes are very important in HP.

Many of the agents responsible for HP can act as adjuvants and are particulate (promoting retention of antigen within the lung for prolonged periods), persistent, and nondegradable. They can interact with humoral mediators (complement and antibody) and cells in the lung to produce inflammation. The agents can induce injury by causing polymorphonuclear leukocytes and macrophages to release phlogistic substances such as reactive oxygen compounds, proteolytic enzymes, and products of arachidonic acid metabolism such as prostaglandins and leukotrienes. The agents can also cause the production and release of IL-1, TNFα, and IL-6 from macrophages and lymphokines (IL-2, interferon-γ, and B-cell growth and differentiation factors) from lymphocytes. Injury to the lung caused by these factors could allow enhanced pulmonary exposure to inhaled antigen, which might promote immunologic sensitization and subsequent pulmonary damage. The result of all these processes is pulmonary inflammation.

In animal models of HP, T cells, macrophages, and adhesion molecules are central in the induction and expression of HP. Macrophage-derived cytokines such as IL-1α, IL-6, TGFβ, and TNFα play a central role in models that entail intrapulmonary administration of materials causing HP. In addition, cyclosporin A alleviates pulmonary lesions in animals subjected to airway challenges with *Thermoactinomyces vulgaris*, nude mice do not exhibit pulmonary lesions of HP after exposure to agents that produce lesions in thymus-intact littermates, and pulmonary lesions could be transferred with T cells from sensitized mice.[48] Lastly, the pulmonary fibrosis induced by repeated challenges with *M. faeni*, but not an increase of BAL fluid inflammatory cells, can be reduced by the administration of anti-CD11a, implicating integrins in the processes that lead to fibrosis in this model.

Adoptive transfer models of HP allow differentiation between direct lung damage (i.e., toxicity), sensitization (the development of antibody and cellular reactivity), and the results of immunologic reactions (the interaction of antigen with antibody or cells). We have developed such a model in inbred guinea pigs and mice, which allows transfer of susceptibility to intratracheal *M. faeni* by cultured cells from sensitized animals. The cells that transfer this susceptibility can be generated by the culture of peritoneal exudate, spleen, peripheral or lung-associated lymph node cells with a soluble extract of *M. faeni*, the agent that causes FLD. Once administered, they confer susceptibility to *M. faeni*–induced injury within 4 days. This pulmonary injury is characterized by increased numbers of mononuclear cells in the lungs in both perivascular and peribronchiolar locations. This phenomenon is dependent on the sensitization of the donor with *M. faeni*, culture with soluble *M. faeni*, and the number of transferred cells, and it persists for at least 8 weeks after cell transfer.

Serum from sensitized animals cannot transfer EHP. Three different mouse strains (C3H/HeJ, SJL/J, and C57Bl/6) do not differ in their response.[44] The postculture cells responsible for transfer are $CD3^+$, $CD4^+$, $CD8^-$, and surface IgM^- T cells. $CD3^+$, $CD4^+$, but not $CD8^+$ cells are required at the onset of culture to allow the development of this transferring population. The transferring cells are a mixture of naïve and memory (as defined by CD44, CD45RB, and LECAM-1 markers) $CD4^+$ cells. The presence of recipient $CD3^+$, $CD4^+$, but not $CD8^+$ cells is required for expression of adoptive EHP.[43] Interferon-γ and IL-2 are present in substantial quantities in culture supernatants, suggesting a predominance of Th1 $CD4^+$ cells. The presence of serum IgG_4 antibody to pigeon antigens correlates with lack of symptoms in pigeon breeders. Since IgG_4 is an immunoglobulin isotype that is induced by IL-4 and suppressed by IFNγ, this suggests that HP may be characterized by predominance of Th1-type immunologic reactivity.

PROGNOSIS AND TREATMENT

Prognosis varies considerably with the type of HP and even the geographic location. For example, FLD has a good prognosis in Quebec,[9] even in farmers who continue to farm. However, FLD in Finland often results in significant physiological impairment and even death.[25] PBD has a good prognosis in the United States and Europe, whereas the same disease in Mexico has a 30 percent 5-year mortality.[38] The reasons for these differences are not clear but probably include differences of the antigen and in the nature of the exposure.

Removal from exposure to the offending antigen(s) is usually sufficient to resolve symptoms and physiological abnormalities within a few days for acute HP and within a month for chronic HP.[26] In some patients, signs and symptoms of pulmonary fibrosis persist more than 6 months, suggesting a poor outcome.[24] Complete removal from exposure is most effective, but cleaning of the environment in situations when removal is impractical (Japanese summer-type HP) can prevent further episodes of HP. There is one report of resolution of symptoms of HP by installation of filters in an air-conditioning system, which greatly lowered mold colony counts. Pigeon lofts that do not use litter materials designed to absorb pigeon excreta have significantly fewer airborne pigeon antigens than lofts that use litter material.[18] It is not known whether avoidance of litter materials is associated with a decrease in PBD.

Systemic glucocorticosteroids are sometimes required to treat severe disease, although there is no formal evidence that such treatment is associated with long-term abatement of symptoms or radiologic or pulmonary function test abnormalities.[32] The usual treatment is prednisone or prednisolone, 40 to 60 mg a day for 2 weeks, followed by a gradual decrease over 1 to 2 months. Patients with FLD treated with prednisolone, compared to those not treated with prednisone, demonstrated slightly more rapid resolution of some radiologic (ground-glass opacities) and some physiological abnormalities than untreated patients (slight improvement of diffusing capacity, no difference in lung volumes or arterial P_{O_2}). However, there were no differences between the groups 6 months after the diagnosis of HP.[32] The above evidence suggests that systemic steroids may slightly increase the rate of resolution of acute pulmonary inflammation but have little or no effect on chronic residue of HP. Inhaled glucocorticosteroids, nonsteroidal anti-inflammatory drugs (e.g., cromolyn and nedocromil) or systemic immune modulators are not indicated in the treatment of HP.

If patients are removed from exposure before there are permanent radiologic or physiological abnormalities, the prognosis is excellent, with little evidence of long-term ill effects. If removal from exposure is impossible, the use of efficient masks during exposure can result in prevention of acute HP and an excellent prognosis. If exposure persists, some patients (proportion unclear, but probably 10 to 30 percent) will progress to diffuse pulmonary fibrosis, with resultant cor pulmonale and premature death.[9] Mortality from FLD is reported to be up to 20 percent and usually occurs after more than 5 years of recurrent symptoms,[19] although there are a few case reports of death after acute massive exposure to the antigen.[25] The prognosis varies considerably with different types of HP. In general, long-term, relatively low-level exposure seems to be associated with poorer prognosis, whereas short-term, intermittent exposure is associated with a better prognosis. This is well illustrated by PBD, which in the United States and Europe has an excellent prognosis, with most patients asymptomatic and no deaths reported 10 years after diagnosis in a group of 24 patients with PBD,[4] whereas in patients with PBD in Mexico City, the mortality was 30 percent after 5 years.[38] Unfortunately, many patients with chronic HP present with pulmonary fibrosis and physiological abnormalities that are only partly reversible after cessation of exposure.

Markers of pulmonary inflammation at the time of presentation, such as the proportion of BAL fluid lymphocytes, neutrophils, or mast cells[21] or the presence of procollagen III, hyaluronic acid, fibronectin, and fibroblast growth factors in BAL fluid, do not portend outcome.[27]

In conclusion, HP is an immunologically mediated lung disease with important roles for T cells and macrophages. It is diagnosed from a careful history and appropriate laboratory tests. Avoidance of exposure is usually associated with a good prognosis. Because of changing environmental exposure, new examples of HP are constantly being described, and they represent a continuing challenge to astute clinicians.

REFERENCES

1. Ando M, Arima K, Yoneda R, Tamura M: Japanese summer-type hypersensitivity pneumonitis: Geographic distribution, home environment, and clinical characteristics of 621 cases. *Am Rev Respir Dis* 144:765–769, 1991.

2. Banham SW, McSharry C, Lynch PP, Boyd G: Relationships between avian exposure, humoral immune response, and pigeon breeders' disease among Scottish pigeon fanciers. *Thorax* 41:274–278, 1986.

3. Bernstein DI, Lummus ZL, Santilli G, et al: Machine operator's lung: A hypersensitivity pneumonitis disorder associated with exposure to metalworking fluid aerosols. *Chest* 108:636–641, 1995.

4. Bourke SJ, Banham SW, Carter R, et al: Longitudinal course of extrinsic allergic alveolitis in pigeon breeders. *Thorax* 44:415–418, 1989.

5. Bourke SJ, Carter R, Anderson K, et al: Obstructive airways disease in non-smoking subjects with pigeon fanciers' lung. *Clin Exp Allergy* 19:629–632, 1989.

6. Campbell J: Acute symptoms following work with hay. *Br Med J* 2:1143–1144, 1932.

7. Coleman A, Colby TV: Histologic diagnosis of extrinsic allergic alveolitis. *Am J Surg Pathol* 12:514–518, 1988.

8. Cormier Y, Belanger J: The fluctuant nature of precipitating antibodies in dairy farmers. *Thorax* 44:469–473, 1989.

9. Cormier Y, Belanger J: Long-term physiologic outcome after acute farmer's lung. *Chest* 87:796–800, 1985.

10. Cormier Y, Belanger J, Laviolette M: Persistent bronchoalveolar lymphocytosis in asymptomatic farmers. *Am Rev Respir Dis* 133:843–847, 1986.

11. Craig TJ, Hershey J, Engler RJ, et al: Bird antigen persistence in the home environment after removal of the bird. *Ann Allergy* 69:510–512, 1992.

12. Denis M: Proinflammatory cytokines in hypersensitivity pneumonitis. *Am J Respir Crit Care Med* 151:164–169, 1995.

13. Denis M, Bedard M, Laviolette M, Cormier Y: A study of monokine release and natural killer activity in the bronchoalveolar lavage of subjects with farmer's lung. *Am Rev Respir Dis* 147:934–939, 1993.

14. Depierre A, Dalphin JC, Pernet D, et al: Epidemiological study of farmer's lung in five districts of the French Doubs province. *Thorax* 43:429–435, 1988.

15. doPico GA: Health effects of organic dusts in the farm environment: Report on diseases. *Am J Ind Med* 10:261–265, 1986.

16. Drent M, van Velzen-Blad H, Diamant M, et al: Bronchoalveolar lavage in extrinsic allergic alveolitis: effect of time elapsed since antigen exposure. *Eur Respir J* 6:1276–1281, 1993.

17. Edwards J, Cockcroft A: Inhalation challenge in humidifier fever. *Clin Allergy* 11:227–235, 1981.

18. Edwards JH, Trotman DM, Mason OF, et al: Pigeon breeders' lung—the effect of loft litter materials on airborne particles and antigens. *Clin Exper Allergy* 21:49–54, 1991.

19. Emanuel D, Wenzel F, Bowerman C, Lawton B: Farmer's lung: Clinical, pathologic and immunologic study of twenty-four patients. *Am J Med* 37:392–401, 1964.

20. Finklea J, Hasselblad V, Riggan W, et al: Cigarette smoking and hemagglutination inhibition response to influenza after natural disease and immunization. *Am Rev Respir Dis* 104:368–376, 1971.

21. Gariepy L, Cormier Y, Laviolette M, Tardi FA: Predictive value of BAL cells and serum preciptins in asymptomatic dairy farmers. *Am Rev Respir Dis* 140:1386–1389, 1989.

22. Gruchow HW, Hoffmann RG, Marx JJ Jr, et al: Precipitating antibodies to farmer's lung antigens in a Wisconsin farming population. *Am Rev Respir Dis* 124:411–415, 1981.

23. Hamagami S, Miyagawa T, Ochi T, et al: A raised level of soluble CD8 in bronchoalveolar lavage fluid in summer-type hypersensitivity pneumonitis in Japan. *Chest* 101:1044–1049, 1992.

24. Hapke EJ, Seal RM, Thomas GO, et al: Farmer's lung: A clinical, radiographic, functional, and serological correlation of acute and chronic stages. *Thorax* 23:451–468, 1968.

25. Kokkarinen J, Tukiainen H, Terho EO: Mortality due to farmer's lung in Finland. *Chest* 106:509–512, 1994.

26. Kokkarinen JI, Tukiainen HO, Terho EO: Recovery of pulmonary function in farmer's lung: A five-year follow-up study. *Am Rev Respir Dis* 147:793–796, 1993.

27. Lalancette M, Carrier G, Laviolette M, et al: Farmer's lung: Long-term outcome and lack of predictive value of bronchoalveolar lavage fibrosing factors. *Am Rev Respir Dis* 148:216–221, 1993.

28. Lee TH, Wraith DG, Bennett CO, Bentley AP: Budgerigar fancier's lung: The persistence of budgerigar precipitins and the recovery of lung function after cessation of avian exposure. *Clin Allergy* 13:197–202, 1983.

29. Lynch DA, Newell JD, Logan PM, et al: Can CT distinguish hypersensitivity pneumonitis from idiopathic pulmonary fibrosis? *AJR Am J Roentgenol* 165:807–811, 1995.

30. Malmberg P, Rask-Andersen A, Rosenhall L: Exposure to microorganisms associated with allergic alveolitis and febrile reactions to mold dust in farmers. *Chest* 103:1202–1209, 1993.

31. Mönkäre S: Clinical aspects of farmer's lung: Airway reactivity, treatment and prognosis. *Eur J Respir Dis* 137(Suppl):1–68, 1984.

32. Mönkäre S, Haahtela T: Farmer's lung—A 5-year follow-up of eighty-six patients. *Clin Allergy* 17:143–151, 1987.

33. Murayama J, Yoshizawa Y, Ohtsuka M, Hasegawa S: Lung fibrosis in hypersensitivity pneumonitis: Association with CD4+ but not CD8+ cell dominant alveolitis and insidious onset. *Chest* 104:38–43, 1993.

34. Murayama J, Yoshizawa Y, Sato T: A compartmentalized bias for T-cell receptor V beta usage in summer-type hypersensitivity pneumonitis. *Int Arch Allergy Immunol* 107:581–586, 1995.

35. Newman Taylor A, Pickering C, Turner-Warwick M, Pepys J: Respiratory allergy to a factory humidifier contaminant presenting as pyrexia of undetermined origin. *Br Med J* 2:94–95, 1978.

36. Orriols R, Morell F, Curull V, et al: Impaired non-specific delayed cutaneous hypersensitivity in bird fancier's lung. *Thorax* 44:132–135, 1989.

37. Pepys J: Hypersensitivity diseases of the lungs due to fungi and organic dusts. *Monogr Allergy* 4:1–147, 1969.

38. Pérez-Padilla R, Salas J, Chapela R, et al: Mortality in Mexican patients with chronic pigeon breeder's lung compared with those with usual interstitial pneumonia. *Am Rev Respir Dis* 148:49–53, 1993.

39. Rylander R, Haglind P: Airborne endotoxins and humidifier disease. *Clin Allergy* 14:109–112, 1984.

40. Sansores R, Pérez-Padilla R, Paré PD, Selman M: Exponential analysis of the lung pressure-volume curve in patients with chronic pigeon-breeder's lung. *Chest* 101:1352–1356, 1992.

41. Sansores R, Salas J, Chapela R, et al: Clubbing in hypersensitivity pneumonitis: Its prevalence and possible prognostic role. *Arch Intern Med* 150:1849–1851, 1990.

42. Schullian D: Notes and events. *J Hist Med Allied Sci* 37:440–443, 1982.

43. Schuyler M, Gott K, Edwards B, Nikula KJ: Experimental hypersensitivity pneumonitis: Effect of Thy1.2+ and CD8+ cell depletion. *Am J Respir Crit Care Med* 151:1834–1842, 1995.

44. Schuyler M, Gott K, Haley P: Experimental murine hypersensitivity pneumonitis. *Cell Immunol* 136:303–317, 1991.

45. Seal RM, Hapke EJ, Thomas GO, et al: The pathology of the acute and chronic stages of farmer's lung. *Thorax* 23:469–489, 1968.

46. Semenzato G, Trentin L, Zambello R, et al: Different types of cytotoxic lymphocytes recovered from the lungs of patients with hypersensitivity pneumonitis. *Am Rev Respir Dis* 137:70–74, 1988.

47. Soler P, Nioche S, Valeyre D, et al: Role of mast cells in the pathogenesis of hypersensitivity pneumonitis. *Thorax* 42:565–572, 1987.

48. Takizawa H, Ohta K, Horiuchi T, et al: Hypersensitivity pneumonitis in athymic nude mice: Additional evidence of T cell dependency. *Am Rev Respir Dis* 146:479–484, 1992.

49. Terho E: Diagnostic criteria for farmer's lung disease. *Am J Ind Med* 10:329–334, 1986.

50. Terho EO, Husman K, Vohlonen I: Prevalence and incidence of chronic bronchitis and farmer's lung with respect to age, sex, atopy, and smoking. *Eur J Respir Dis* 152(Suppl):19–28, 1987.

CHAPTER 72

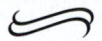

RADIATION PNEUMONITIS

Sara Rockwell / Kenneth B. Roberts

As of this writing, the discovery of x-rays is barely 100 years old. On January 27, 1896, within months after Roentgen's discovery, the use of x-rays was introduced into clinical practice in the treatment of malignant diseases in a totally empiric manner. Beneficial effects of radiation on tumors were quickly recognized, but detrimental effects on normal tissues also became apparent quite rapidly. Because of the low energy of the early x-ray and gamma-ray sources, radiotherapy in its early days was limited to using poorly penetrating radiations, which delivered much higher doses of radiation to skin than to even relatively superficial tumors. As a result, severe early radiation reactions in the skin limited the doses of radiation that could be delivered to tumors. Studies of these skin reactions led to the development of the concept of normal tissue tolerance and to an appreciation of the beneficial effects of "fractionated" radiotherapy, which used multiple treatments with small doses of radiation. The relative sensitivity of the lung to injury from radiation also became apparent early in the development of radiation oncology. The clinical syndromes of dyspnea, cough, fever, and radiographic infiltrates occurring weeks to months after irradiation of the thorax were dramatic enough to be described as early as 1922.[15]

The field of radiation oncology has matured immeasurably over the last century and has incorporated significant advances from fields as diverse as theoretical and applied physics, radiation biology, pathology, cell biology, and immunology.[3,4,19,21] The importance of advances in physics and engineering to the maturation of radiation oncology is especially notable.[21] These advances have led to the development of modern linear accelerators capable of delivering very high energy, deeply penetrating radiations, which can be used to deliver high radiation doses with great precision to tumors deep within the body. Precise systems for radiation dose measurement, or *dosimetry,* and precise algorithms for planning radiotherapy treatments have been developed. These advances have changed the dose-limiting radiation toxicities from painful early reactions in the skin to life-threatening late reactions in the normal tissues surrounding the tumors.[3] Radiation reactions in the lung therefore have acquired increasing importance with improvements in radiotherapy.

To the readers of this book, understanding radiation pneumonitis is important for two reasons. First, an understanding of radiation injury to the lung can be useful in understanding other lung diseases. Because the chemical mediators of radiation effects, both beneficial and harmful, are free radicals, the pathway leading to radiation injury overlaps with those leading to many other lung injuries. Second, understanding radiation pneumonitis has practical value to physicians in many areas of medicine. Approximately 1 in 4 people in the United States will be diagnosed with cancer at some point in their lifetimes. Over half of these patients will be permanently cured of their malignancies. Approximately 65 percent of all cancer patients now receive radiotherapy at some point in the treatment of their malignancies, and radiotherapy seems destined to remain an important component of cancer treatment for the foreseeable future. Because of this, every physician can expect to care for many patients who are receiving radiotherapy or have received radiotherapy at some point in the past. A working knowledge of the basics of radiobiology and radiation oncology is therefore important to every physician. An understanding of the potential toxicities of radiotherapy, including radiation pneumonitis, can be critical to patient care.

Many neoplasms involving the thorax are treated with regimens that include the use of radiotherapy to produce either cure or palliation. Radiotherapy is principally a localized and anatomically based modality. The success of radiotherapy hinges on delivering radiation selectively to the sites of malignant disease, while sparing to the maximal extent possible the uninvolved normal tissues of the patient.[3] To plan radiotherapy treatments effectively, the radiation oncologist must have a sophisticated appreciation of the malignancy being treated and must understand its biologic behavior, its patterns of local and metastatic spread, its radiosensitivity, and the factors that influence the responses of individual patients to therapy. The radiation oncologist must also consider the effects of radiation on the normal tissues within the treatment volumes. Many factors including the radiation dose, the fractionation pattern of the radiotherapy, the volume of the tumor and involved margins, the prior or planned use of other therapies such as surgery or systemic chemotherapy, and the presence of other diseases influence both the probability of controlling the neoplasm and the probability of producing toxic reactions. For cancers of the lung, esophagus, pleura, breast, and chest wall, as well as for lymphomas involving the thorax, optimal treatment frequently involves the use of multiple overlapping x-ray beams and possibly electron beams, planned to encompass

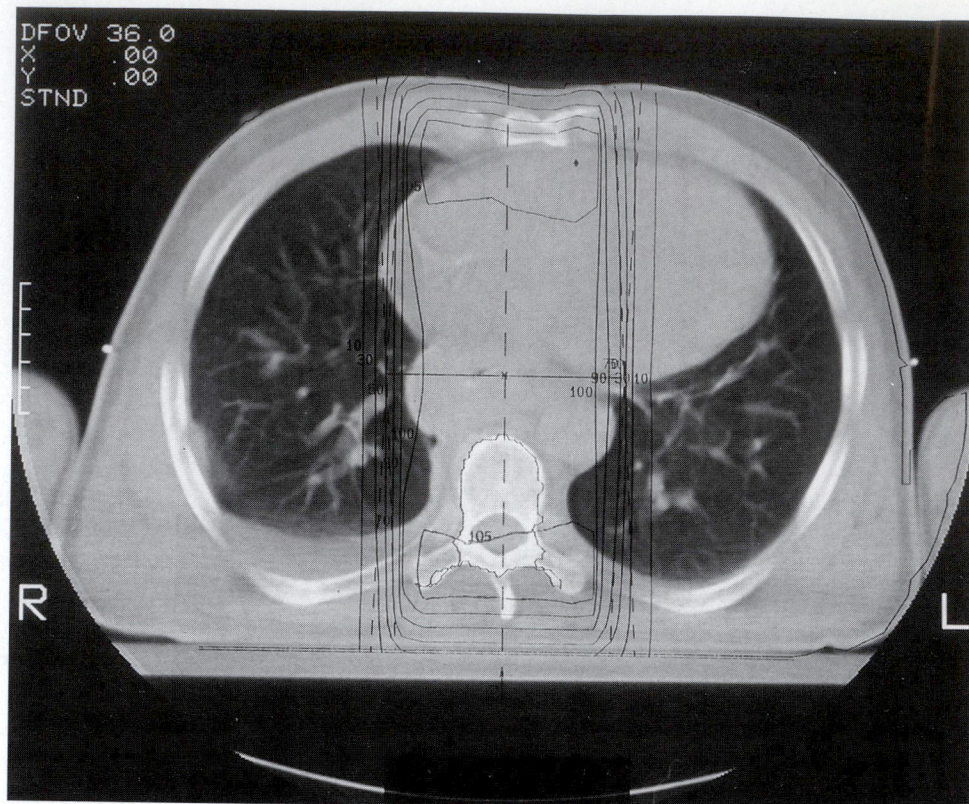

FIGURE 72-1 A 50-year-old male presented with dysphagia and was found to have an unusual low-grade non-Hodgkin's lymphoma of the esophagus, stage IVA, refractory to chemotherapy. He was treated with anterior and posterior external beam portals. A CT scan section is shown with the radiation isodose distribution superimposed.

all of the cancer-containing tissues. Although treatments are carefully planned to include the smallest possible amount of healthy normal tissue, some normal tissue will necessarily be included in the radiation fields. The radiation sensitivity of the specific tissues in the irradiated fields and the acceptable level of risk for complications combine to limit the dose of radiation that can be administered. The planning of radiotherapy always involves a balance of benefit and risk, because the probabilities of controlling the malignant disease increase with increasing radiation dose, but the probabilities and severities of the potential complications increase with dose as well.

To illustrate the mechanisms involved in planning radiotherapy treatments, a relatively straightforward treatment plan is depicted in Fig. 72-1, which shows the isodose distribution for treatment of an esophageal tumor. Such intrathoracic tumors are often treated initially using daily irradiations through both anterior and posterior portals. The volume of normal tissue, in particular the lung, within the region receiving a full dose of radiation is readily appreciated. A second example, shown in Fig. 72-2, shows the treatment fields for a patient receiving postoperative irradiation after resection of a non–small cell lung cancer invading the chest wall, with positive surgical margins. A follow-up chest radiograph (Fig. 72-2C) reveals a pattern of radiation-induced fibrotic changes corresponding to the high-dose region of the radiotherapy. In a case such as this, if the malignancy is cured or the patient experiences the desired improvement in the symptoms from the malignant disease with little or no toxicity from the radiotherapy, then the treatment has produced a desirable re-

sult despite radiographic changes or subclinical damage to the lung or other organs. Overt pulmonary toxicity is, however, a potential consequence of thoracic radiotherapy.

BRIEF OVERVIEW OF RADIOLOGIC PHYSICS

External-beam radiotherapy is generally delivered using x-rays or gamma rays. Both of these radiations are high-energy electromagnetic radiations.[21] The only difference between them lies in the manner in which they are produced: Gamma-ray photons are emitted from the nuclei during the decay of radioactive atoms, and x-rays are produced when high-energy electrons strike a target material and interact with the electron shells of atoms in that target, causing them to emit x-ray photons. After its emission, an individual x-ray photon would be indistinguishable from a gamma-ray photon. Thus, although our discussion will use x-rays for its examples, the discussions would be equally applicable to radiotherapy given using high-energy gamma rays, for example from cobalt teletherapy units.

The x-rays used for diagnostic imaging are in a relatively low energy range where the dominant interaction of the photons with matter is through the *photoelectric effect*. In this process, absorption of an x-ray photon causes an electron to be ejected from the inner shell of an atom. The probability of photoelectric interactions increases as a function of the cube of the atomic number, that is as Z^3. Because of this, large, heavy atoms absorb diagnostic x-rays much more efficiently than smaller, lighter atoms. Diagnostic radiologists capitalize on the large differences be-

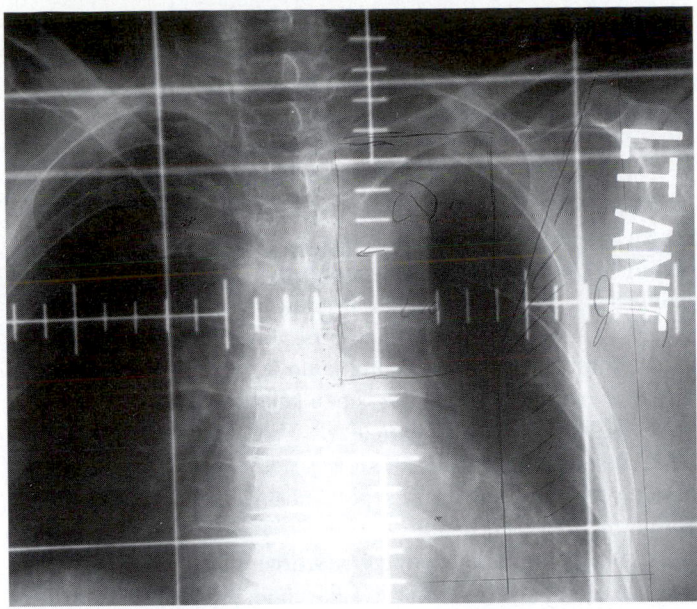

A

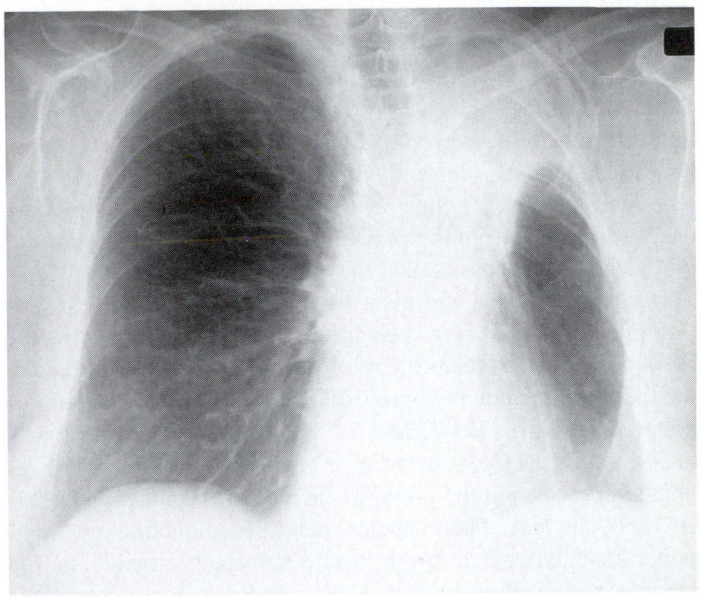

C

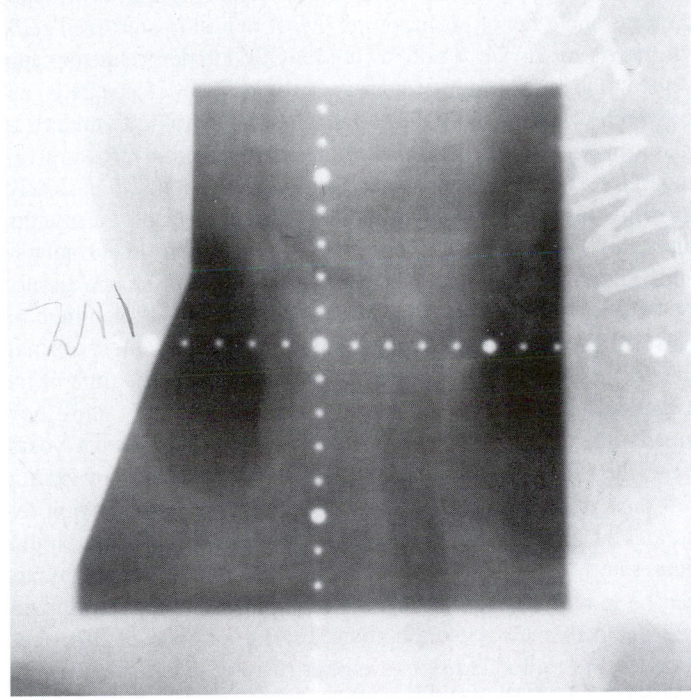

B

FIGURE 72-2   A 66-year-old female presented with left scapular pain and was found to have a localized adenocarcinoma of the left upper lobe invading the posterior chest wall. Positive surgical margins and negative mediastinal lymph nodes were found after an *en bloc* resection and lobectomy. The patient received postoperative radiotherapy using a shrinking field technique with 55 Gy in 26 fractions over 37 days. *A* shows the initial "simulation" field taken using low-energy diagnostic x-rays. *B* shows the "port" film of the initial anterior treatment field taken using high-energy x-rays from the linear accelerator used for radiotherapy. The differences in contrast in *A* and *B* reflect the differences in the absorption of low- and high-energy x-rays. Four years later, the patient remains asymptomatic despite a chest x-ray showing dense fibrotic changes in the irradiated area (*C*).

tween the absorption of these low-energy x-rays in materials with different compositions, e.g., air, soft tissue (which is 70 percent water and therefore comprised primarily of small atoms), bone (with its high calcium content), and administered contrast agents containing barium, iodine, or other heavy atoms, and use the difference in absorption to image anatomical structures. In contrast, the high-energy x-rays used in radiotherapy interact with matter primarily by a phenomenon called the "Compton effect" in which x-rays cause ionization of atoms via their interactions with the outer electron shells. The Compton effect is not dependent on the atomic number but is instead a function of the electron density. Because the electron densities of different biologic tissues are relatively uniform, it is a reasonable approximation for the purposes of most radiotherapy dosimetry to assume that a patient is of a uniform density, equivalent to water.

An important caveat to radiation dosimetry relevant to this chapter involves the standard specification of doses in tissues that have a large proportion of air, such as the lung. As a single x-ray beam penetrates through water or tissue, the dose received by the tissue attenuates progressively, generally as an exponential function of the depth. Because of its markedly lower density, air will attenuate radiation less than would tissue or water. With the quantitative knowledge of lung density which can now be derived from CT scanning, algorithms have been devised to estimate the inhomogeneity in the absorbed dose resulting from the differences in the density of lung and soft tissue.[21,49] These heterogeneity corrections show that routine dosimetric calculations, which assume uniform density, can underestimate the radiation doses to lung and to tissues beyond the lung by factors that range from 5 to 25 percent. Although this is a very important consideration when quantifying the radiation dose delivered to the lungs, remember that doses delivered to the thorax and the lungs historically have been reported in the medical literature *without* heterogeneity corrections. Moreover, because the preponderance of clinical data concerning lung tolerance has been reported using the older algorithms, which assume for dosimetric purposes that the lung has water-equivalent density, the impetus to change dose reporting is limited by a desire to avoid confusion between the new and older literature. The reader should therefore assume, unless explicitly stated otherwise, that the radiation doses given in this chapter, or for that matter any publication, are not corrected for lung density.

Radiation dose is currently reported using the unit of the System International (SI), the gray (Gy). The Gy is a measure of the energy absorbed from the radiation; 1 Gy = 1 J/kg. The former unit of absorbed dose, called the "rad" (an acronym for "radiation absorbed dose") was measured with the cgs system; by definition, 1 rad = 100 ergs per gram. To compare old and recent literature, one must therefore recall that 1 Gy = 100 rad. Despite the fact that it is not an approved SI unit, some radiotherapy literature avoids this conversion by giving the dose in centigray (cGy), where 1 cGy = 0.01 Gy = 1 rad. Other measures of radiation dose seen in the literature include the roentgen, the sievert, and the rem. The roentgen measures radiation exposure, rather than energy absorption, and refers specifically to the amount of ionization produced in air under standard conditions (1 R = 1 electrostatic unit/cc = 2.58×10^4 coulombs/kg of standard air). This unit is frequently encountered in the radiation dosimetry literature, not only because it was historically a measure of dose but also because many widely used radiation monitors (e.g., ionization chambers) directly measure radiation exposure at the surface of the body. The dose absorbed by tissue can then be calculated from this exposure. The radiation protection literature uses the unit of "equivalent dose," the sievert (Sv), which is calculated as the absorbed dose (in Gy) multiplied by a "weighting factor" that considers the differing biologic effects of different radiations. Although the weighting factors for some radiations, such as neutrons and alpha particles, can be as high as 20, the weighting factors for x-rays, gamma rays, and electrons are defined as 1. For most purposes in diagnostic and therapeutic radiology, therefore, 1 Sv = 1 Gy. The Sv replaces the older unit of equivalent dose, the rem (1 Sv = 100 rem). Unfortunately, the literature on radiation-induced lung injury includes papers using all these different units, creating great confusion for the casual reader. All doses given in this chapter have been converted to Gy.

RADIOBIOLOGY OF RADIOTHERAPY

When x-rays pass through tissue, a complex series of physical and chemical reactions occurs.[19,36] As the x-rays interact with atoms along their path, as described above, energy is absorbed, and energetic fast electrons are ejected. These fast electrons travel through tissue, producing secondary ionizations, which lead rapidly to the generation of a variety of highly reactive free-radical species. Because biologic materials are about 70 percent water, ions and free radicals derived from water (e.g., $H\cdot$, $OH\cdot$, H_2O^+, H_3O^+) are the main reactive species. These ions and radicals react with each other and with other nearby molecules, producing a wide variety of chemically reactive species and many kinds of damage in biologic macromolecules. Because the DNA contains information that is critical to the cell while most other molecules can be replaced, damage to DNA is the most important effect of radiation. Radiation produces a wide variety of lesions in DNA, including single and

double strand breaks, damaged bases, and loss of bases, as well as chromosomal breaks and rearrangements. If these lesions are not repaired, the result can be permanent mutations or changes in chromosomal structure that lead to injurious biologic effects or to the death of the cell.

The cytotoxic effects of radiation are the basis for both the antineoplastic effects and the toxicities of radiotherapy. A theoretical concern is that radiotherapy may produce a mutation in a previously normal cell that leads to the development of a new malignancy. Although radiation-induced malignancies do occur,[19,36] malignant transformation is, fortunately, a rare enough event at the doses used in radiotherapy that the risk of inducing a second cancer is acceptably small relative to the great benefit of curing the existing malignancy.[3] The greater risk to the patient lies in the fact that radiation is not selectively toxic to the tumor cells but instead kills both normal and malignant cells within the treatment field.

Although the radiochemical reactions that lead to cytotoxic damage are complete within milliseconds after the end of irradiation, cells dying from radiation injury do not die immediately. In fact, soon after irradiation, radiation-sterilized cells are indistinguishable from cells that will ultimately survive irradiation in their appearance, in their metabolic activities, and even in their patterns and rates of proliferation. Most radiation-sterilized cells ultimately die during a mitosis but may first undergo one or even several divisions, producing an abortive clone of sterile cells, all of which will ultimately die. This delayed cytotoxicity underlies many of the effects seen in radiotherapy. Rapidly growing tumors, for example, generally begin shrinking sooner than slowly growing tumors, and many tumors continue to shrink for months after radiotherapy. Analogously, radiation reactions in normal tissues reflect t' ..ormal patterns of cell turnover in the tissue. Nonprolifer .ng, terminally differentiated cells will continue to perform their differentiated functions throughout their normal life spans. Other cells that are not proliferating at the time of irradiation will likewise continue to function normally until they are recruited into proliferation, perhaps months or even years later; then they will die. Rapidly proliferating cells die within a few days of irradiation, leading to the familiar early radiation reactions of epilation, desquamation, mucositis, and hematologic depression.[3] There is increasing evidence that some cell types can be induced by radiation to enter a pathway of programmed cell death that leads to apoptosis; the importance of this phenomenon to radiotherapy is a matter of intensive current investigation.

A typical survival curve for mammalian cells, obtained using mouse lung cells, is shown in Fig. 72-3. To a first approximation, cell survival falls exponentially as the radiation dose increases. Statistically, this implies that each incremental dose of radiation has the same cytotoxic effect; that is, each incremental dose kills the same proportion of the viable cells present in the population at the beginning of that irradiation. Very low doses of radiation have somewhat lesser effects, which reflect the ability of the cells to accumulate and repair some radiation damage.

The effect of the repair of radiation damage can be seen when the radiation dose is divided into two or more treatments separated by hours or days, rather than being delivered in a large single dose. Dividing, or "fractionating," the radiation dose allows

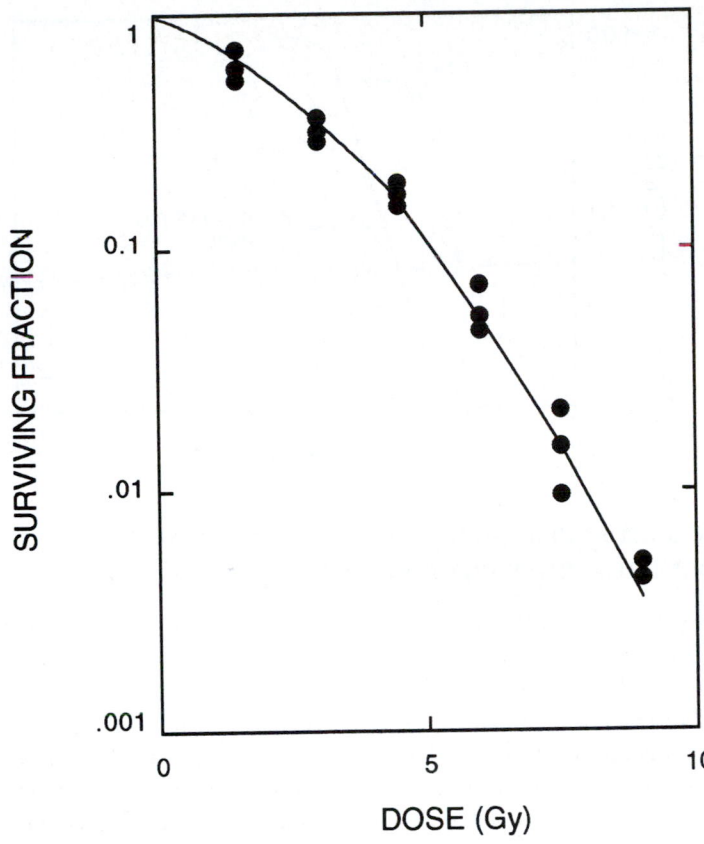

FIGURE 72-3   Survival of lung cells treated with different doses of radiation. Cells were explanted from mouse lungs, irradiated in vitro, and assayed for viability using a colony formation assay. *(Redrawn from Guichard et al,*[17] *with permission.)*

sensitivity of the critical cells and differences in the patterns of cell proliferation and cell loss, as well as differences in the ability of the cells to repair radiation damage. Empiric observations of patients treated with radiotherapy, laboratory experiments with tumors and normal tissues in rodents, and studies with cells in culture have all been used to guide the development of the clinical fractionation schedules now in use. This optimization process is ongoing and will undoubtedly continue, incorporating new information about the repair of radiation damage in normal and malignant cells and about the factors that modulate the development of radiation injuries in specific normal tissues. In this process, as in any change in cancer therapy, the parameter of critical importance is always the therapeutic ratio (Figure 72-5). A new treatment regimen will be superior only if it produces an increased effect on the tumor, without producing an equivalent increase in toxicities to critical normal tissues, thereby increasing the therapeutic ratio and producing therapeutic gain. The art of radiotherapy lies in the design of treatment fields that minimize radiation doses to normal tissues and in the development of treatment regimens that use all available information on the biology of the tumor and the critical normal tissues to design treatment protocols that will maximize the therapeutic ratio.

PATHOPHYSIOLOGY OF RADIATION PNEUMONITIS

Much of our current understanding of the pathophysiology of radiation injury to the lungs is derived from animal experimentation. Translation of animal data to human conditions is always tenuous, because differences in the biology and physiology of

cells to repair damage to their DNA between treatments.[19] As a result, there is less cytotoxicity from a fractionated treatment regimen than from the same total radiation dose delivered as a large single fraction (Fig. 72-4). Smaller fractions produce less cytotoxicity than larger fractions. Similarly, the cytotoxic effects of radiation are diminished when the radiation is delivered continuously at a low dose rate, over hours or days, to allow repair and proliferation to occur during irradiation (Fig. 72-4). Fractionating radiotherapy or delivering the radiation at low dose rates generally appears to increase the therapeutic ratio, by protecting normal tissues against radiation injury while producing a smaller increase in the radioresistance of the tumor, thereby improving the outcome of treatment. This increase in the therapeutic ratio is thought to reflect qualitative and quantitative differences between the normal and malignant cell populations, including differences in the intrinsic radio-

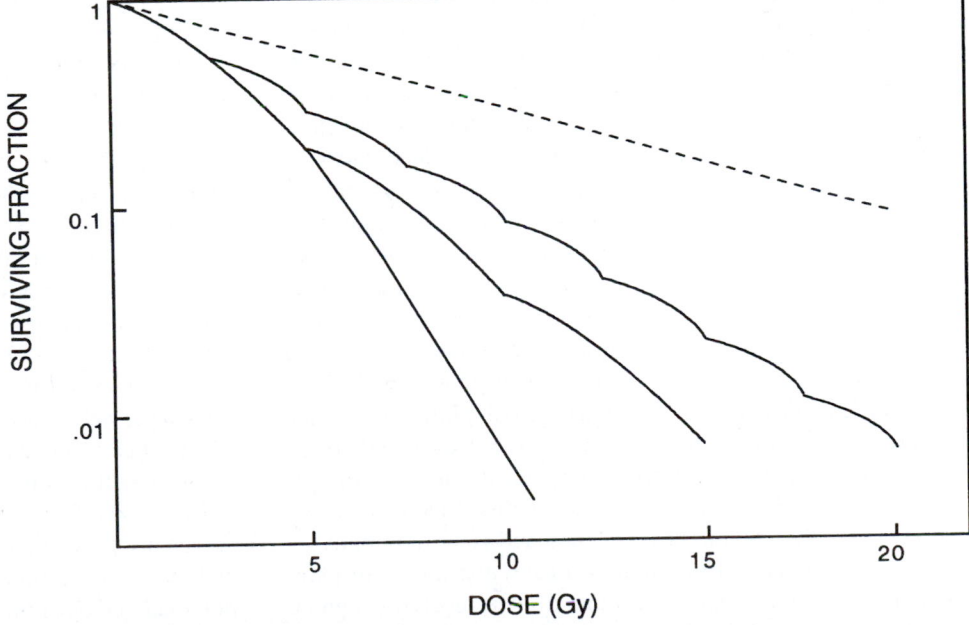

FIGURE 72-4   Effect of fractionated irradiation and low dose rate irradiation on cell survival. The survival curve for lung cells treated with a single dose of radiation is redrawn from Fig. 72-3. The calculated effect of dividing the radiation dose into several daily treatments with 5 Gy/fraction or 2.5 Gy/fraction is illustrated. The dashed line illustrates the survival curve that would be expected for irradiation delivered continuously at a low dose rate over several hours, allowing repair and proliferation to occur during treatment. Changes in the cytotoxicity of radiation with fractionation and at low dose rates lead to decreased injury in lungs irradiated with analogous regimens.

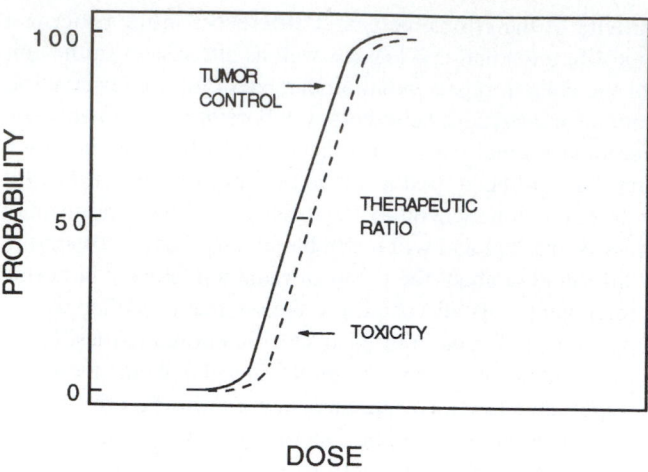
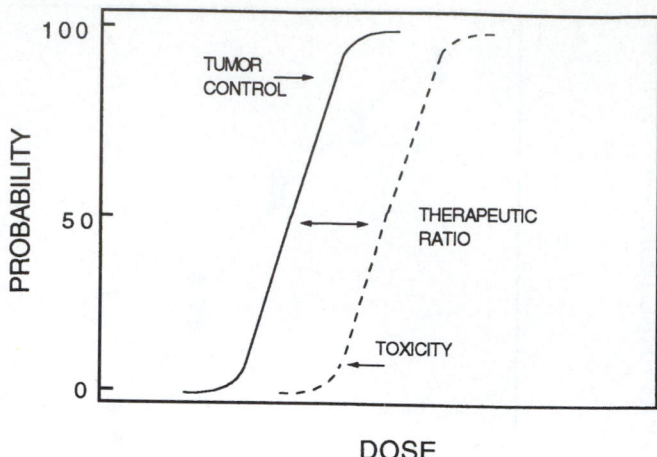

Increasing the therapeutic ratio, either by selectively increasing the effect on tumor or by selectively protecting normal tissues from injury, produces therapeutic gain.

FIGURE 72-5 The therapeutic ratio is the critical factor determining the success of cancer therapy.

different species may preclude direct extrapolation from animals to humans. Instead, studies with experimental animals must be designed to elucidate physiological factors and mechanisms that can be used to interpret clinical data and to suggest avenues for clinical investigations. Data on radiation pneumopathy in humans is fragmentary and is complicated by the variability in the patients treated with thoracic irradiation. Most studies of radiation pneumonitis include patients with a variety of malignancies, treated with different regimens that often include chemotherapy and surgery as well as radiation. Moreover, the patients vary widely in age and in the presence of other diseases and risk factors. Our current understanding of radiation injury to the lung therefore remains incomplete. What is known suggests a complex, multifactorial disease mechanism reflecting cytotoxic effects on both epithelial and endothelial tissues, inflammatory responses that include disordered cytokine and cellular signaling, and the induction of interstitial fibrosis.[30,39] Similarities to lung injuries resulting from cancer chemotherapy, other drugs, inhaled chemicals, oxygen toxicity, and idiopathic pulmonary fibrosis are intriguing, especially when one considers that many of these diseases include pathologic responses to free-radical chemical species and are likely to reflect similar underlying initial lesions.

Partial lung resection and localized irradiation have certain similarities, because their effects are largely localized to the treated areas and consequently depend on the number of pulmonary lobules or alveolar–capillary units functionally destroyed. Thus the volume of lung irradiated is an important determinant of toxicity. The radiation oncologist therefore plans the treatment to minimize the volume of lung receiving high radiation doses, just as the thoracic surgeon plans a lobectomy or pneumonectomy to consider the residual capacity of the lungs. Of course this simple analogy has its limitations. For example, radiation inactivation of enough lobules will increase the ventilatory dead space and could potentially lead to shunting and ventilation–perfusion mismatching. In clinical practice, extensive shunting generally is not observed. In fact, postradiation

radionuclide ventilation–perfusion scans tend to show underperfusion rather than underventilation in irradiated partial lung volumes.[35] In most cases, radiation injury in lung conforms to the radiation treatment fields, but in some instances effects outside the treated areas can be recognized, with localized radiation inducing a more generalized or diffuse hypersensitivity pneumonitis.[34]

The effects of radiotherapy on the lung reflect the proliferation patterns of the different cellular components of the terminal capillary–alveolar units.[48] Type I pneumocytes are the dominant epithelial cells of the lung, covering about 93 percent of the alveolar surface. Type I pneumocytes are normally nonproliferating and do not proliferate in response to injury. Because of this, they are thought to be relatively resistant to the cytotoxic effects of radiation. Type II pneumocytes, which comprise about 16 percent of the cells in the human lung, are the principal source for the surfactant that modifies alveolar surface tension to prevent atelectasis. Type II pneumocytes have turnover times of about 1 month. In response to certain injuries, these granular pneumocytes can be induced both to undergo rapid mitosis and to differentiate into type I pneumocytes. Endothelial cells comprise about 30 percent of the cells in human lungs and form a continuous layer between the blood and the lung tissue. Although endothelial cells are classified in most tissues as stromal cells, endothelial cells in lung are actually parenchyma, because they are critical to the function of this organ. Capillary endothelial cells are a constantly renewing population. The turnover time of these cells has been estimated to be on the order of 2 months. Endothelial cells can be induced into rapid compensatory proliferation after injury. Radiation therefore can result in the depletion of both type II pneumocytes and endothelial cells.

Several lines of evidence suggest that radiation injury is related primarily to cytotoxic damage, especially to the surfactant-producing type II pneumocytes and the vascular endothelial cells. Although clinical signs of pneumonitis require weeks to develop, laboratory studies reveal evidence of lung injury within hours after large single doses of radiation.[4,16,18,32,41] Shortly after irradiation, electron microscopy can detect abnormalities in surfactant-containing lamellar bodies. There is an increase in surfactant in bronchoalveolar lavage specimens within hours of irradiation that persists for several weeks. Ultrastructural evidence of endothelial cell damage is also seen soon after lung irradiation, and a rapid increase in capillary permeability occurs, reflecting loss of integrity of cell junctions, intracellular vacuolization, cellular pleiomorphism, and sloughing of the basement membrane. Capillary occlusion by cellular debris and microthrombi may occur at high doses.

The clinical course of lung injury occurs later and includes a pneumonitic phase, developing weeks to months after radiation, followed by a fibrotic phase, developing months to years later. To explain the two clinical phases, Rubin and Casarett's original model of radiation lung toxicity suggested that the pneumocytes and endothelium represented two separate and distinct cellular targets and that damage to pneumocytes led to pneumonitis, while vascular damage led to fibrosis. This older model is now thought to be incorrect. The current weight of evidence from Rubin and others[11,12,25,30,39–41,46–48] suggests that the pneumonitic and fibrotic processes both are manifestations of a common pathway of injury and response.

Histologically, one can recognize a typical sequence of events developing in the lung after large doses of radiation.[4,16] Within days to weeks, vascular congestion and intra-alveolar edema and exudation occur, followed by infiltration of inflammatory cells and epithelial desquamation. Weeks later, collagen fibrils are deposited within areas of injury and interstitial edema, leading to a thickening of alveolar septa similar to that in hyaline membrane disease. The probability and severity of these changes are quite variable and depend on such factors as the radiation dose and treatment volume. The severity of the damage and volume of tissue affected determine whether a pneumonitic picture will be evident clinically. Resolution of inflammatory infiltrates and alveolar exudates, which can be improved by anti-inflammatory agents such as glucocorticoids, will correlate with symptomatic improvement and with resolution of radiographic opacities in the affected lung.

Inflammatory cells, particularly alveolar macrophages, migrate into areas of radiation injury. This induces an ensuing cytokine cascade and mediates the host response,[39,41] as occurs in other inflammatory conditions that can lead to pulmonary fibrosis. Rubin and his collaborators have detected a biphasic increase in mRNA expression for the proinflammatory cytokines IL-1α, IL-1β, and TNF-α at 2 and 8 weeks after radiation. Beginning at 2 weeks, TGF-β, a cytokine that mediates fibrotic responses, increases. Collagen gene expression is also appreciably increased, corresponding to the fibrotic changes seen histologically. These studies suggest that early and persistent elevations of cytokine production and alterations of intercellular signaling are critical to the development of radiation reactions in the lung. Interestingly, there is increasing evidence from studies with inbred mice that genetic differences modulate the development and severity of fibrosis and hyaline membrane formation and thus determine the nature of the late toxic lesion and the time of development of radiation pneumotoxicity.[11,12]

The processes described above lead to pathologic changes that conform spatially to the areas where localized radiation was administered. Interestingly, it has recently been discovered that radiation can also induce an allergic alveolitis. This is observed infrequently as a diffuse pneumonitis or even more rarely as patchy, transient pneumonitis occurring outside the treated fields. In its most severe form, this leads to adult respiratory distress syndrome. Morgan and Breit[34] have suggested that this form of radiation pneumonitis be termed "sporadic"; however, the subclinical occurrence of this syndrome may actually be fairly common. Bronchoalveolar lavage in humans and in experimental animals frequently shows a significant increase in activated T-helper (CD4+) lymphocytes, temporally related to irradiation, occurring equally in the irradiated lung and in the contralateral, unirradiated lung. Gallium scanning in these subjects may also show bilateral uptake, not corresponding to the treated regions.[34] Frequent reports of autoantibodies, including antibodies to collagen, in the sera of human cancer patients even before treatment suggest the possibility that malignancy-associated autoimmune reactions may be involved in this syndrome.

CONFOUNDING EFFECTS OF CHEMOTHERAPY

Many cytotoxic drugs employed as antineoplastic agents can produce pulmonary toxicity.[6] Bleomycin, which kills cells by generating reactive free-radical species, can give rise to both pneumonitis and fibrosis. Mitomycin C and doxorubicin have both been associated with lung toxicity. As high-dose alkylating agent chemotherapy is used more frequently in the setting of bone marrow or peripheral stem cell transplantation, agents such as cyclophosphamide, BCNU, and busulfan have been increasingly associated with clinically significant pneumonitis. The direct toxicity of anticancer drugs to the lungs sounds a note of caution for those considering the development of treatment protocols combining systemic chemotherapy with lung irradiation.

Animal studies looking at changes in respiratory rates and/or death resulting from lung injury show that the severity of the lung injury can be increased when doxorubicin, bleomycin, cyclophosphamide, mitomycin C, dactinomycin, and vincristine are administered along with radiation.[22,50] No enhancement has been documented in studies with 5-fluorouracil, cis-platinum, carboplatinum, hydroxyurea, vinblastine, or methotrexate, despite reports of lung toxicity from methotrexate alone. As a variety of cytokines are now available for pharmacologic administration due to recombinant DNA technologies, interactions between radiation and these biologic agents have come under increasing study. Interferons have been shown both to increase and to decrease radiation lung toxicity, whereas interleukins 1 and 2 may have protective effects. Some radiation-drug interactions in the lung have been shown to be schedule dependent, with the effect of the combination varying with the sequence and with the time between treatments with the two agents.[22,50] Additive, subadditive, and even supra-additive toxicities may be observed in rodents when single treatments with the same dose of radiation and drug are given over a 24-h period, but with different sequences and different times between treatments. Such findings highlight the complexities of combined modality therapy and the difficulty of using animal data to plan clinical regimens.

Data from several specific clinical situations, described below, show that regimens combining radiation with multidrug chemotherapy can produce significant risks of pneumonitis. However, it is often difficult to identify which of the drugs is responsible. Clinical data strongly suggest that administration of concurrent adriamycin or actinomycin D with thoracic radiotherapy should generally be avoided or, alternatively, that the radiation doses should be significantly reduced. Sequential treatment with these drugs and radiation is less likely to produce lung injury. However, a phenomenon termed "radiation recall" has been well described, in which either of these two drugs given even several months after radiotherapy will produce an inflammatory reaction in the region corresponding to the radiation treatment fields.[26] Although this reaction is best known in skin, it has also been well documented in the lungs in several case reports, as well as in experimental animals. Radiation recall probably reflects the fact that the irradiated areas of the lung still retain residual, subclinical injury, which is exacerbated into clinical pneumonitis as a result of the additional injury from the drug. The biologic basis of the recall phenomenon is therefore analogous to that of the residual radiation injury, which decreases the ability of heavily irradiated lung tissue to tolerate a second course of radiotherapy delivered months or years later.[3,4,46]

CLINICAL SYNDROMES

Radiation oncologists conventionally divide clinical toxicities into acute and late effects,[3,4] with both radiation pneumonitis and fibrosis considered late toxicities.

Acute Manifestations

It is relatively uncommon to observe acute pulmonary toxicity during the administration of fractionated radiotherapy. At relatively high therapeutic doses (50 to 60 Gy), however, acute radiation injuries to the tracheobronchial tree can be expected. Bronchoscopic examination of these patients is likely to reveal erythematous mucosa, with thickened secretions that can accumulate in and obstruct the airways. Although a majority of patients remain asymptomatic, occasional patients experience an irritative, dry cough. Antitussive agents such as codeine, adequate hydration, and reassurance are usually all that are required to manage this problem. Once the radiotherapy has been completed, the bronchial epithelium regenerates and heals over several weeks with a corresponding resolution of any symptoms.

Late Manifestations

The clinical course of late radiation injury to the lungs is biphasic with both inflammatory and fibrotic components.[16,30,32]

RADIATION PNEUMONITIS

A pneumonitic process frequently becomes evident 2 to 6 months following radiotherapy. At this time radiographs show alveolar opacities that generally conform to the treatment portals. The severity of radiation pneumonitis varies dramatically from patient to patient, even in those receiving identical therapeutic reg-

imens. In most cases, the pneumonitis is asymptomatic, even though radiologic abnormalities are quite common, having been found in some prospective studies in as many as 50 percent of patients who have completed a course of thoracic radiotherapy. When symptomatic this syndrome is often characterized by the abrupt onset of fever, cough, and dyspnea. The severity of symptoms depends on the extent of radiotherapy, increasing with the treated volume and the radiation dose. Symptoms in patients irradiated to limited lung volumes or to relatively low doses may consist of low-grade fever, cough, congestion, and chest fullness or discomfort. Any hemoptysis tends to be minimal. In more severe situations, dyspnea, high fever, and cough occur. When more than three-quarters of the total lung volume is irradiated to doses of 45 Gy—a situation, in fact, to be avoided—acute radiation pneumonitis is highly likely and can be extremely severe, producing respiratory distress. The radiation oncologist is probably most likely to see clinically significant radiation pneumonitis that can be life-threatening when it occurs as a rare consequence of standard treatment despite appropriate treatment planning designed to minimize the volume of lung treated with high doses of radiation.

It is important to distinguish radiation pneumonitis from infection, recurrent tumor (particularly with lymphangitic spread), drug reactions, congestive heart failure, and other respiratory ailments. Bacterial, fungal, viral, and pneumocystis pneumonias can be quite difficult to differentiate from pneumopathy induced by chemotherapy or radiation. Aids in the differential diagnosis include the clinical course and the temporal relationship between therapy and the respiratory illness. The radiographic pattern of the infiltrate is also very useful, with radiation pneumonitis often conforming to the outline of the sharply demarcated radiation portal (Fig. 72-6). Bronchoscopy and lung biopsy can also be important diagnostic tools to direct therapeutic decisions. Ruling out infection is particularly important, because treatment of symptomatic radiation pneumonitis relies on supportive care in conjunction with steroids, which would be contraindicated with infection. Doses of glucocorticoids generally can be tailored to the severity of the symptoms. Asymptomatic pneumonitis can be managed with close observation. Severe cases generally warrant treatment with 0.5 to 1.0 mg/kg per day of prednisone (or its equivalent) in divided doses. Response rates to steroid therapy between 20 and 100 percent have been reported, and dramatic clinical and radiographic responses are not infrequently seen. Steroids should be tapered slowly after the patient is stabilized, because it is common to see a recrudescence of symptomatology when steroids are discontinued too rapidly. Failure to respond to steroid therapy carries the prospect of rapid disease progression.

RADIATION FIBROSIS

A more indolent fibrotic process can follow after either subclinical or symptomatic radiation pneumonitis.[16,30,32] This begins several months after radiotherapy and peaks in radiographic severity several years later. This fibrosis tends to occur in or adjacent to areas of prior pneumonitis,[12] but can also occur in the absence of clinically overt radiation pneumonitis. Fibrotic changes and the retraction of the lung parenchyma from scarring

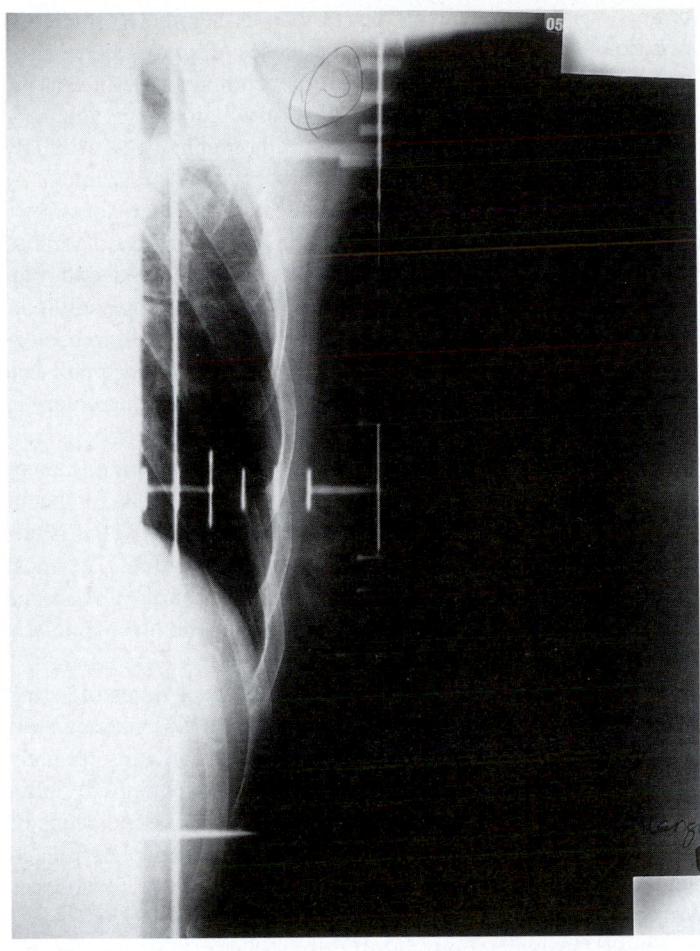

A

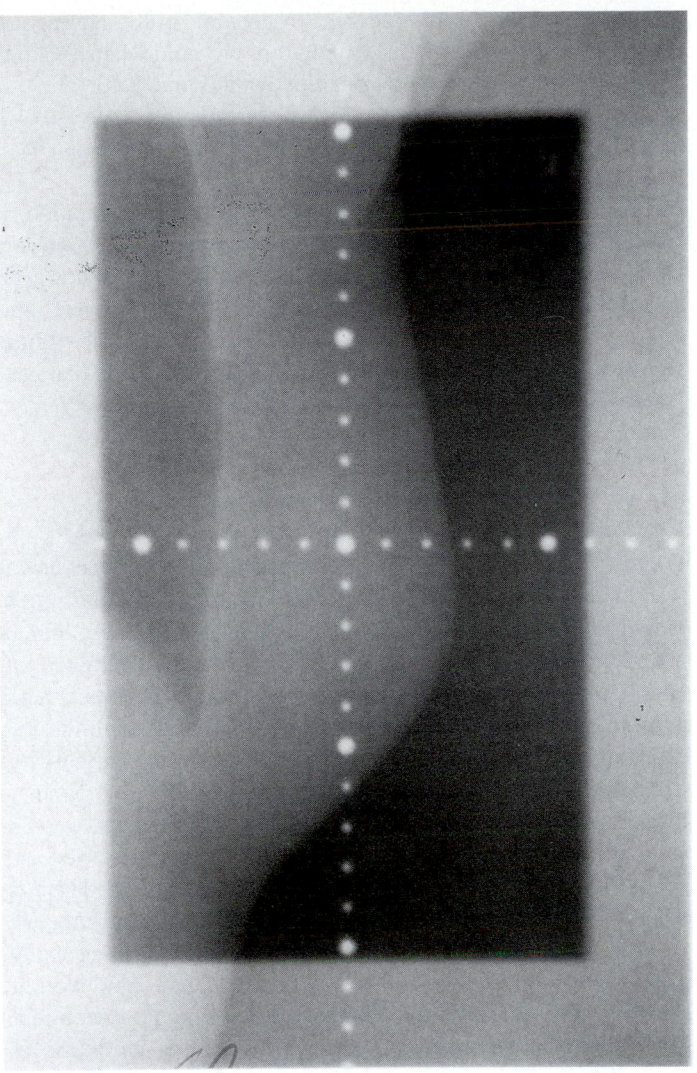

B

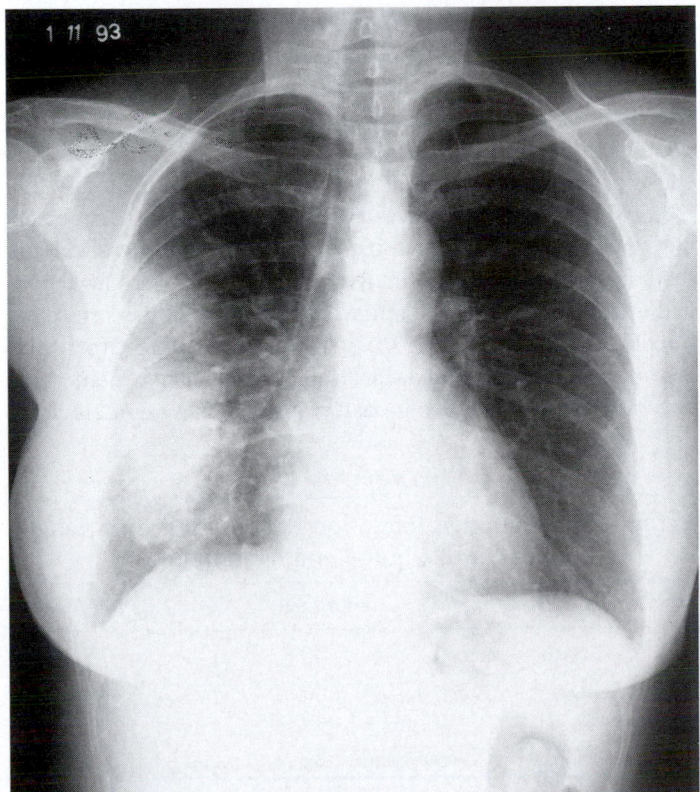

C

FIGURE 72-6   A 52-year-old female found a nontender lump in her right breast and subsequently underwent a lumpectomy for a localized 1.4-cm diameter infiltrating ductal carcinoma. The axillary lymph nodes were negative. The patient was placed on Tamoxifen and underwent radiotherapy to the right breast, using tangential fields, to 50 Gy in 25 fractions over 36 days. This was followed by boost radiation treatments to the surgical bed for an additional 14 Gy in 7 fractions. *A* and *B* show the simulation and port films, respectively, of the whole-breast treatments, again highlighting the different interactions of low-energy and high-energy x-rays with tissues. Four months after radiotherapy, the patient developed radiation pneumonitis characterized by fever, cough, and dyspnea requiring hospitalization. *C* shows a right-lung opacity that does not correspond to normal anatomic structures but does correspond to her treatment fields. The patient responded dramatically to steroids, with resolution of radiographic findings on follow-up chest radiographs.

occur in the irradiated regions (Fig 72-2*C*). When the volume of lung irradiated is relatively small and the remaining lung parenchyma contains sufficient respiratory surface area, these changes tend to be asymptomatic. With increasing relative volumes of pulmonary fibrosis, a spectrum of symptomatology is possible, ranging from mild dyspnea on exertion to severe fibrosis with respiratory compromise, chronic cor pulmonale, cyanosis, and finger clubbing. At this end of the spectrum the syndrome can be life-threatening. In general, in the absence of other underlying lung disease, symptoms are mild when less than 25 to 30 percent of total lung parenchyma is involved.

RADIATION-INDUCED PLEURAL REACTIONS

Pleuritis can also be seen 2 to 6 months following radiation. It can be associated with plueritic chest pain, a pleural friction rub, and an exudative pleural effusion. Large effusions are, however, distinctly unusual in the absence of other pathology. Like radiation pneumonitis, radiation-induced pleuritis can heal without significant residuae or proceed through a fibrotic phase that generates pleural thickening.

DEFINING THE RADIATION TOLERANCE OF THE LUNGS

Whereas we customarily speak of radiation doses that can be delivered safely either to the whole body or to a particular organ, radiation tolerance is often defined as the dose that will yield a 5 percent risk of late radiation injury.[10] When discussing the tolerance of the lungs, one must consider several different therapeutic situations. The tolerance of the lung varies with the volume of lung tissue irradiated.[25] In addition, single-dose irradiations, fractionated irradiations, and irradiations given at low dose rates have different risks of injury and must be considered separately.[44,47] Additional injury from surgery or chemotherapy or a prior course of radiotherapy must also be considered. Confounding effects of injury to lung tissue from coexisting cardiopulmonary disease and from the underlying malignancy must also be considered. Infections and immunologic reactions are also important. The clinical endpoints to define an index case of radiation pneumonitis also vary, because the severity of the lung injury spans a wide spectrum of diagnostic signs and clinical symptoms. Given the heterogeneity of clinical circumstances and biologic data in general, it is not surprising that the medical literature that defines the risks for radiation pneumonitis and fibrosis is extremely complex and often difficult to interpret.

WHOLE-LUNG IRRADIATION

A good starting point to discussing lung tolerance is to consider the effects of irradiating the entire lung. This has direct clinical relevance because there are several circumstances in which the entire lung would be irradiated. These include total body irradiation for hematopoietic transplantation, hemibody irradiation for palliation of widespread metastatic disease, and whole-lung irradiation electively or therapeutically for relatively radiosensitive tumors such as Wilms' tumor, Ewing's sarcoma, or Hodgkin's lymphoma. These are often circumstances in which chemotherapy is also being administered.

Published experience from the Princess Margaret Hospital in Toronto[13,23,27,28,49] provides some of the best data regarding lung tolerance. Investigators from that institution have an extensive experience with delivering upper hemibody irradiation to different doses and with varying fractionation patterns. They reported in 1978 on a cohort of 245 patients, most with metastatic solid tumors, who received single-fraction upper hemibody irradiation at dose rates of 0.3 to 0.8 Gy/min to doses of up to 10 Gy.[13] The actuarial incidence of acute radiation pneumonitis, defined as the sudden onset roughly 16 weeks after irradiation of cough, dyspnea, and opacities visible on chest radiographs, was strikingly dose dependent (Table 72-1). The doses shown in Table 72-1 were not corrected for density heterogeneity.[49] When doses were corrected for heterogeneity, producing an upward estimation of the doses actually received by the lungs, analysis yielded the sigmoid-shaped curve shown in Fig. 72-7. Using heterogeneity-corrected data, the incidence of pneumonitis is estimated to be negligible for single doses less than about 7.5 Gy. Other published data regarding upper hemibody single-fraction irradiation are in general agreement with these findings.

The careful reader would be struck by the fact that the single-fraction data might predict an unacceptable risk for pneumonitis when single-fraction, total-body irradiation (TBI) is utilized in the setting of bone marrow transplantation. The most important treatment factor making single-fraction TBI in the range of 8 to 10 Gy (uncorrected for heterogeneity) tolerable is that these treatments generally are given at a low dose rate (≤0.1 Gy/min), so that the treatment is delivered over times of 1 to 2 h.[9,47] In Seattle, where hundreds of patients with leukemia have undergone bone marrow transplantation (BMT) with total-body irradiation, using single fractions of 10 Gy (uncorrected) delivered at dose rates on the order of 0.08 Gy/min, the incidence of pneumonitis is roughly 25 percent. Review of transplant-related single-fraction TBI with variable dose rates shows incidences varying from 70 to 25 percent.[2,23,33,42]

Studies in mice show that the toxicities of TBI can be improved further by fractionating the irradiation as well as delivering radiation at low dose rate. This concept is supported by a randomized clinical trial comparing low-dose-rate single-fraction TBI (10 Gy) with low-dose-rate fractionated TBI (12 Gy in 6 fractions over 3 days) for patients with acute myelogenous leukemia in first remission, which showed a significant improvement in event-free survival with fractionation, mainly because of an improvement in early mortality.[9] Interstitial pneumonitis in these patients was decreased from 26 to 15 percent with fractionation. Ongoing trials are seeking to optimize irradiation regimens for TBI. Many fractionation patterns have been and are being tested, including daily fractions and 2 or 3 daily fractions with doses of 1.5 to 2.25 Gy per fraction. Other trials are testing different dose rates. At many transplant centers it has become common practice to utilize lung transmission blocks to

TABLE 72-1

Actuarial Incidence of Radiation Pneumonitis after Single-Fraction Whole-Lung Irradiation

Uncorrected Dose	Patients	Pneumonitis
< 6 Gy	49	2.7%
6 Gy	24	17.5%
8 Gy	149	35.6%
10 Gy	23	83.9%

SOURCE: Data from Fryer et al.[13] Doses are not corrected for heterogeneity in tissue density.

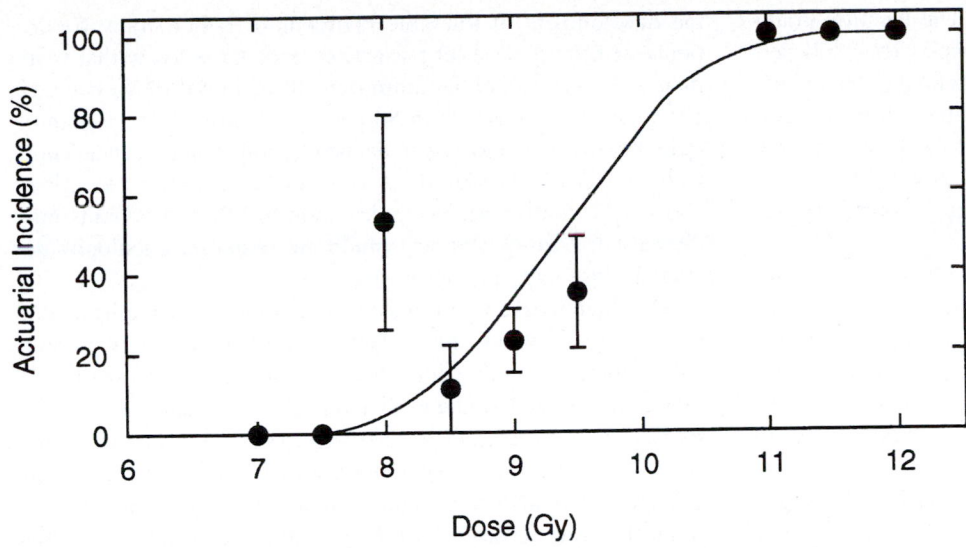

FIGURE 72-7   Incidence of radiation pneumonitis in patients receiving single-dose, whole-lung irradiation at dose rates of 0.3 to 0.8 Gy/min. Unlike most doses given in the text, doses on this figure *are* corrected for heterogeneity. The effect of this correction can be seen by comparing these data with those in Table 72-1, which were derived from an earlier analysis by the same group and are presented using uncorrected doses. (*Data are redrawn from Van Dyk et al.*[49])

attenuate the lung dose and thereby reduce the risk of pneumonitis, in effect by compensating for the heterogeneity in density within the lungs.[42]

Pneumonitis in the BMT setting has a multifactorial etiology, reflecting not only the effects of radiation but also the effects of chemotherapy, graft-versus-host disease (GVH), lung injury from tumor, opportunistic infections, and other risk factors.[2,42] Cyclophosphamide is almost universally given with TBI. The addition of other drugs is based on institutional treatment policies. Many anticancer drugs are known to injure the lung. BMT conditioning regimens that do not use TBI (which tend to use high-dose busulfan in place of radiation) in fact have rates of interstitial pneumonitis comparable to regimens including TBI. The presence of GVH is also important, not only because GVH causes direct lung injury but also because the drugs used to control this disease are toxic to the lung.

Whole-lung irradiation has also been used in the treatment of widespread lung metastases. In two published series a combined total of 70 patients with osteosarcoma who received elective whole-lung irradiation to prevent pulmonary metastases (which is not currently a standard practice pattern) received 15 to 17.5 Gy in 10 fractions. None of these patients developed pneumonitis.[30] Similarly, in a series of 40 patients who received 20 to 25 Gy of thoracic irradiation in 1.5-Gy fractions to treat pulmonary metastasis, there were no cases of pneumonitis reported.[30] This and other clinical experience with fractionated whole-lung irradiation in the nontransplant setting and in the absence of chemotherapy would indicate that the following dose schemes should have a relatively low risk (< 5 percent) for radiation pneumonitis: 25 Gy given in 20 fractions over 4 weeks or 20 Gy given in 10 fractions over 2 weeks. (As a reminder, all doses are given without heterogeneity corrections.)

Historically, radiotherapy for Hodgkin's disease has utilized whole-lung treatment in situations where there is massive medi-astinal adenopathy, hilar adenopathy, or overt pulmonary disease treated with chemotherapy. Risks of symptomatic pneumonitis ranging from 7 to 35 percent have been reported, with the risk highly dependent on the total radiation dose and the fractionation pattern.[30,45] When the whole lung is to be included, the available data suggest that the lungs should be treated through transmission blocks rather than with open fields. This reduces the total dose and the dose per fraction to the lungs, thereby reducing the risk of symptomatic pneumonitis to 4 to 7 percent, over a broad range of total lung doses of 10 to 20 Gy. There is a suggestion that the addition of mediastinal irradiation to fractionated whole-lung radiotherapy increases the risk of pneumonitis. To many chemotherapists, the risk of radiation pneumonitis from such treatment seems too great. As a result such patients are often treated primarily with chemotherapy (often with adjuvant low-dose radiotherapy), even though this, too, has significant risks for lung toxicity. In the setting of pulmonary metastases, the addition of low-dose radiotherapy to the whole lung after chemotherapy is controversial but is rational and has its advocates. There are few clinical data to quantify risks and benefits, but doses of 10 to 16 Gy, given in 0.7- to 1.5-Gy fractions, are associated with only modest risk.[20,45]

Lung radiotherapy using 12 to 14 Gy for pulmonary metastases in pediatric patients with Wilms' tumor (who also receive sequential doxorubicin and actinomycin D) is associated with a 10 percent incidence of pneumonitis.[14] Long-term follow-up in such children also shows restrictive lung disease, with total lung and vital capacities approximately 70 percent of the predicted values. In children receiving thoracic irradiation, inhibition of the normal growth and development of the lung parenchyma and bones from radiotherapy also produces significant morbidity. The effects of radiation on growth and development and the radiosensitivity of growing tissues raise special concerns in the treatment of pediatric patients.[3]

PARTIAL-LUNG IRRADIATION

Assessment of Risk

Estimating the risks of radiation pneumopathy for individual patients receiving fractionated external-beam radiotherapy is a daunting task, because so many confounding factors must be considered. With lung cancer, the tumor size and location influence the volume of adjacent normal lung that must be irradiated. The volume irradiated should determine the number of capillary–alveolar units destroyed and therefore influence the risk of symptomatic radiation pneumonitis and fibrosis.[48] This qualitative prediction is borne out by clinical experience, but quantifying the risks is not straightforward. The location irradiated is also important because the upper lobe is less well perfused and therefore less important to gas exchange. Irradiation of this region produces less change in lung function than irradiation of areas lower in the lung. Treatment-related factors such as total dose, dose per fraction, and overall treatment time are also important, as are the other confounding factors described above.[32]

Patients begin radiotherapy with a wide range of pulmonary functions, reflecting their age, smoking history, and the absence or presence of underlying cardiopulmonary disease. Because regional pulmonary fibrosis can be partially compensated by functional lung parenchyma, pretreatment lung status influences the severity of the symptoms. The clinical endpoints used to measure lung injury are quite varied and include symptom or quality-of-life scores, radiographic changes such as changes in CT-assessed lung density, pneumonitis, fibrosis, or other objective measures.[32]

Pulmonary function tests are global organ measures that correlate quite crudely with symptomatology after partial-lung irradiation. A large tumor mass can cause localized obstructive or restrictive changes in lung function or phrenic nerve dysfunction, any of which may either improve or worsen as the tumor shrinks with treatment. These factors add to the variability produced by patient-to-patient differences in the treatment volume, dose, fractionation, and so on. Thus the changes from radiotherapy in global lung function with regard to gas exchange, physiological dead space, shunting, $\dot{V}/\dot{Q}$ mismatch, and respiratory surface area as measured by arterial blood gases, spirometry, and CO diffusing capacity ($D_{L_{CO}}$) are complex and highly individualized. Several clinical studies have attempted to correlate predicted changes in FEV_1 from radiotherapy by superimposing radiation treatment portals on quantitative ventilation and perfusion scans.[1,5,8,38] The simple notion that the proportion of lung irradiated should match the drop in FEV_1, akin to the highly useful preoperative assessment of predicted postresection lung function, unfortunately has not been verified. In fact, a report from the Massachusetts General Hospital[5] examining global and regional pulmonary function in patients with lung cancer showed improvement in pulmonary function in 52 percent of patients, a mild decline in 37 percent, and the decline predicted from changes in radionuclide scans in only 11 percent. Similar observations have been made[8] in nonoperative lung cancer patients. Whereas the mean pretreatment FEV_1 of 1.71 ± 0.67 L declined in these patients to an average of 1.15 ± 0.43 L after treatment, the posttreatment FEV_1 was improved in 19 percent of the patients, unchanged in 53 percent, mildly decreased in 22 percent, and decreased below predicted levels in 5 percent. Thus, the technique of superimposing radiation treatment portals over quantitative lung perfusion scans is of limited utility in predicting pneumonitis in individual patients. In fact it has been suggested[1] that the diffusing capacity is a more sensitive indicator of tolerance to radiotherapy. Unfortunately, there are no firm tests or data to guide

the development of tolerable regimens of radiotherapy for patients with borderline lung function, except we know that treatment volumes should be minimized. If the initial FEV_1 is below 1.0 L or $D_{L_{CO}}$ is less than 50 percent of normal, large-volume radiotherapy (e.g., elective nodal irradiation for lung cancer) may well be excessively hazardous. Despite the limitations described above, quantitative perfusion scanning in selected patients may give a worst-case scenario to help the radiation oncologist decide on dose and volume of treatment.

The quantitative importance of the volume of lung irradiated vis à vis toxicity has only recently been studied in any systematic fashion. An interesting set of mouse data published by investigators at MD Anderson[25] showed a clear shift in dose response curves for changes in respiratory rate and pulmonary death as a function of volume irradiated. As expected, the site irradiated was also important: Effects were more pronounced when the well-perfused base of the lung was irradiated, rather than the less well perfused apex. The response to lung irradiation was quite heterogeneous, even within a single mouse strain, and histologic damage did not always predict morbidity in individual mice. In patients, preliminary dose–volume histogram analyses derived from detailed three-dimensional treatment evaluations and applied to an empirical normal-tissue complication model showed a fair to poor correlation between volume and complication risk.[31] Investigators at Duke[29] have attempted to refine the correlation of dose-volume histograms with toxicity by factoring out nonfunctioning lung using lung perfusion scans. In lung cancer patients, particularly with chronic obstructive pulmonary disease (COPD), areas of hypoperfusion separate from tumor are seen frequently; irradiation of such irreversibly hypoperfused lung may not contribute additional toxicity. Such a "functional" dose–volume histogram analysis has not yet been shown to be of clinical value but does provide an interesting and promising analytical framework.

Perhaps the most accurate and clinically relevant means to estimate risks for radiation pneumopathy is to study a large group of patients who receive a relatively standard dose and fractionation scheme for a given disease. As described above, the variability of the treatment volume for diseases such as lung cancer, as well as the frequent coexistence of other lung disease, especially COPD from tobacco use, makes this a difficult task. Nevertheless, one widely quoted expert consensus panel that reviewed the risks for late radiation toxicity using "conventionally" fractionated radiotherapy given in 1.8- to 2.0-Gy fractions developed the risk estimates depicted in Table 72-2 for radiation pneumonitis, stratifying by volume of lung irradiated.[10] These

TABLE 72-2

Dose Producing Clinically Apparent Radiation Pneumonitis after Conventionally Fractionated Radiotherapy

Lung Volume Irradiated	Dose (in Gy) Producing Pneumonitis	
	5% of Patients	50% of Patients
1/3	45	65
2/3	30	40
All	17.5	24.5

SOURCE: Data from Emami et al.[10] Doses are not corrected for heterogeneity in tissue density.

data reflect the incidence of clinically apparent radiation pneumonitis as defined by symptoms of cough and dyspnea, as well as radiographic opacities corresponding to the treatment areas. Similar data regarding the incidence of radiation fibrosis are quite difficult to obtain, largely because of the wide spectrum of severity in symptomatology. Clinical experience would suggest that radiographic fibrosis is rare below 20 Gy and common above 40 to 50 Gy, with symptoms of respiratory insufficiency dependent on the volume of injured lung and on the presence of coexisting lung disease.

Local Tumor Boosting

In the treatment of lung and esophageal cancer, it is quite standard to boost the primary tumor and a small volume of the lung to total cumulative doses beyond 50 Gy and commonly to 60 to 65 Gy. Clinical data, notably the dose-escalation lung cancer trials of the Radiation Therapy Oncology Group, suggest that increasing doses to small volumes from ~50 to ~65 Gy is not associated with a significant increase in lung toxicity,[7] probably because the number of nonfunctional alveoli is not increased by this increase in dose. In most series of patients receiving radical thoracic radiotherapy, the risk of symptomatic radiation pneumonitis is usually around 5 to 10 percent, and some degree of radiographic fibrosis is almost universal.

Breast Cancer

Breast cancer radiotherapy, whether after lumpectomy or mastectomy, typically uses opposed tangential beams as depicted in Fig. 72-7, which irradiate a volume of lung anterolateral to a plane demarcating the midchest to the lateral axillary line to doses of 45 to 50 Gy in 23 to 25 fractions. The volume of the ipsilateral lung irradiated can be estimated for individual patients from the simulator films and is typically about 20 percent of the lung volume. If supraclavicular and axillary nodes are irradiated as well, anterior treatment portals are matched to the tangential chest wall fields. As a result the apex of the lung (roughly another 10 to 15 percent of ipsilateral lung volume) is also irradiated. The incidence of symptomatic pneumonitis from tangential fields alone is roughly 0.5 percent, with some series documenting an increased risk with increasing lung volume.[24,37] It is desirable to keep the irradiated volume below ~25 percent, if possible. Nodal irradiation increases the risk for pneumonitis to 0.5 to 1.5 percent. Risk further increases to as high as 9 percent when chemotherapy is given concurrently. The risk of pneumonitis is much lower when chemotherapy and radiation are given sequentially.

Early-Stage Hodgkin's Disease

Radiotherapy for early-stage Hodgkin's lymphoma, using moderate doses (40 to 45 Gy in 1.5- to 2.0-Gy fractions) and large volumes to treat lymph node–bearing regions, has represented a remarkable success story in oncology.[3,20] Because it now has produced very high cure rates in a young patient population, allowing for extended follow-up over several decades, this experience has also produced considerable data regarding late radia-

tion toxicities. In these protocols, the chest is irradiated with treatment portals, generically called "mantle fields," as depicted in Fig. 72-8. With modern radiation techniques that use sequential shrinking fields, the incidence of symptomatic radiation pneumonitis is 3 to 4 percent. The risk of pneumonitis increases to roughly 10 percent when full doses of both chemotherapy (MOPP or ABVD-type combinations) and radiation to a mantle field are given sequentially. Studies on pulmonary function in Hodgkin's disease patients suggest that a transient reduction in FEV_1 and vital capacity, on the order of 5 to 20 percent, occurs 3 to 9 months after radiotherapy, corresponding to the period of pneumonitis. There tends to be some recovery by roughly one year. Late follow-up of pulmonary function in Hodgkin's disease patients at Stanford[20] further suggests that mantle field radiotherapy is associated with small, and for the most part clinically insignificant, reductions in vital capacity and D_{LCO}. These decreases in pulmonary function tests were associated with minor, if any, symptomatology, even for treatment regimens that included sequential chemotherapy with doxorubicin or bleomycin. In the setting where lower-dose (20 to 25 Gy) involved-field radiotherapy is delivered after chemotherapy, the incidence of clinical pneumonitis is quite low, although small changes in spirometric and diffusion capacity parameters can still be detected in up to 50 percent of the patients.

PROGNOSTIC ASSAYS AND FUTURE TRENDS

Our understandings of the molecular and cellular mechanisms of radiation injury in general and of radiation pneumonitis in particular are still evolving and improving. We hope increased understanding of these processes will lead to approaches for avoiding radiation injury to the lung, for modulating the development of injury or ameliorating its symptomatology, and for identifying patients at unusually high risk of injury. Several different lines of investigation leading to these ends are being pursued.

Innovations in radiation therapy techniques are under active investigation. These include modifications in the dose rates, in the fractionation patterns, and in the radiation dose distributions used in radiation therapy regimens for specific diseases. Improvements in diagnostic imaging that allow better identification of tumor-involved regions, computerized treatment planning and dosimetry systems, improved patient immobilization systems, and the use of multiple "noncoplanar, noncoaxial" radiation portals that lead to what has been termed "three-dimensional conformal radiotherapy" all are being explored in the hope that they will enable the radiotherapist to increase the dose to the tumor while decreasing the volume of surrounding normal tissue irradiated to high doses. Conformal radiotherapy will be more complex, and probably more costly, than current radiotherapy approaches. It may also be difficult to prove whether this technology results in improved clinical outcomes. Refinements in combined-modality therapy may lead to the development of regimens that decrease pulmonary toxicity and therefore increase the therapeutic ratio for the treatment of thoracic tumors. Improvements in the delivery of antineoplastic therapy therefore may decrease the risk and severity of radiation pneumonitis.

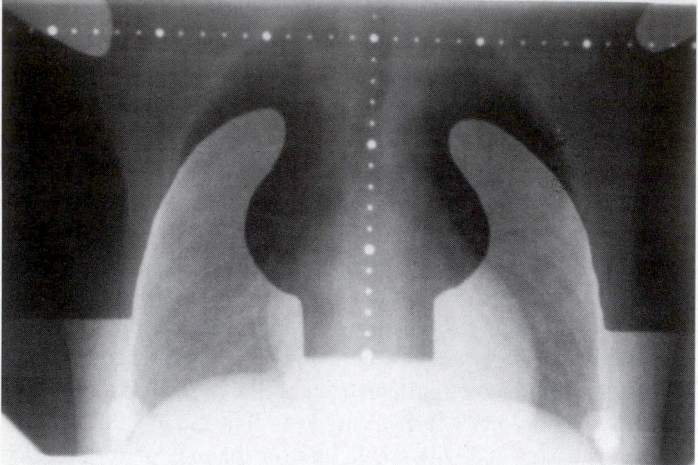

A

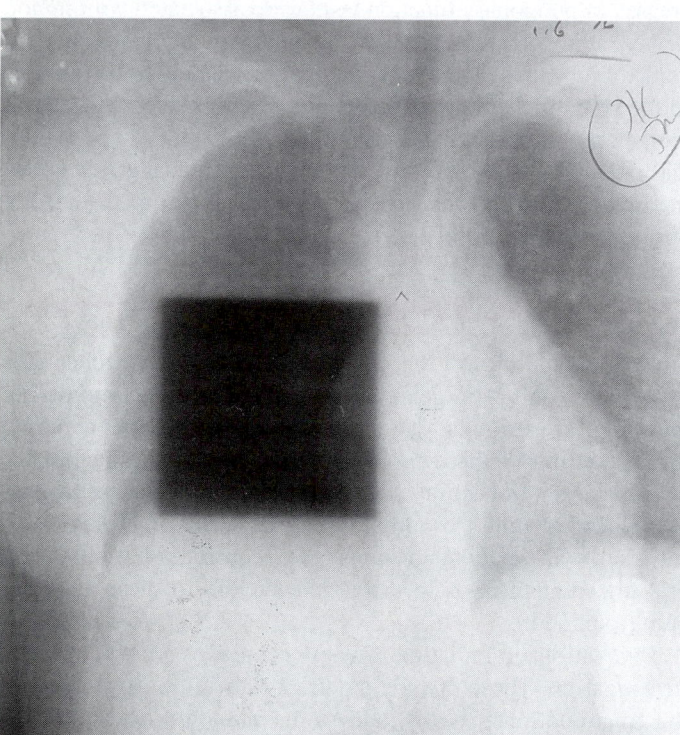

B

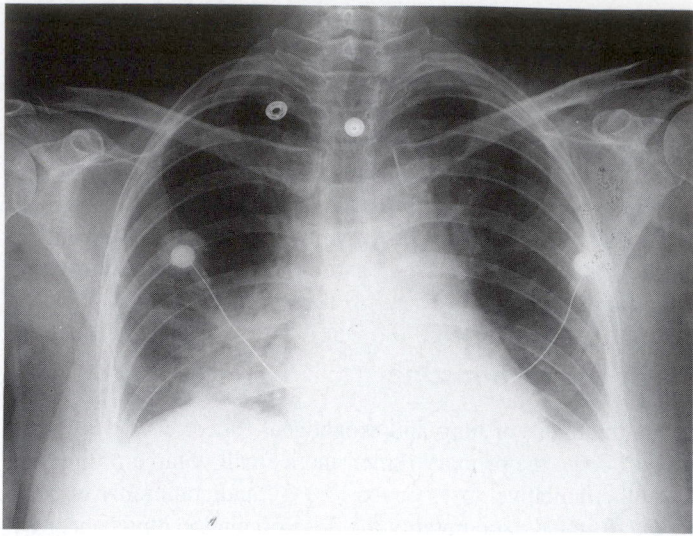

C

FIGURE 72-8 *A* shows the port film for a typical mantle used for treatment of a patient with Hodgkin's lymphoma. Note the effect of the lung blocks in reducing the dose to large volumes of the lung. (In this example, the whole heart/pericardium is not being treated.)

A 30-year-old female underwent mantle field and subdiaphragmatic radiotherapy (not shown) for early-stage Hodgkin's lymphoma. Ten years later, a recurrence in the right lower lobe and mediastinum was treated with MOPP-type chemotherapy and low-dose involved-field radiotherapy. The treatment field to the right lung, shown in *B*, was irradiated to 15 Gy in 10 fractions, in addition to the 40 Gy given to the mantle field ten years previous. Radiation pneumonitis occurred 6 months later, as seen in *C*. This responded to prednisone. Sixteen years later, the patient remains well and free of recurrence.

The risk of developing radiation pneumonitis varies dramatically in different patients. To a certain extent, increased risk can be predicted from identifiable risk factors, such as prior treatment with thoracic radiotherapy, treatment with pneumotoxic drugs, or the existence of lung disease from other causes. However, even when the known risk factors are considered, the risk of symptomatic injury after radiotherapy varies dramatically from patient to patient. Studies with mice indicate that genetic factors contribute to individual variability in the development of late radiation injury in the lung.[11] This raises the possibility that pretreatment measurements of enzyme or cytokine levels in the lung, analyses during treatment of changes in cytokine levels or of tissue response to cytokines, or some other relevant measure may be useful in predicting patients at high risk for the devel-

opment for pneumotoxicity.[40] Assays of surfactant levels shortly after irradiation predict radiation pneumonitis in some rodent studies but have not predicted radiation pneumonitis in individual patients in the clinical trials performed to date. TGF-β, a cytokine that mediates fibrosis, is currently the subject of intense investigation. Serum levels of TGF-β have been reported to predict toxicity after high-dose chemotherapy for breast cancer and might be expected to predict radiation toxicity as well.[32] Similarly, analyses of the intrinsic radiosensitivity in vitro of fibroblasts from patient biopsies have been suggested as a possible approach to measuring the general risks of individual patients for radiation injury. Such assays have proven useful in the treatment of patients with the genetic disease ataxia telangectasia, which leads to unusual radiosensitivity. Prognostic assays predicting high or low risk for radiation pneumopathy could be used to guide clinical decision making and to plan therapy to minimize risks for individual patients.

Insights into the physiology underlying the development of radiation pneumopathy may also lead to the development of regimens that prevent the development of disease or ameliorate its symptomology. The use of "radioprotectors" such as WR2721 during irradiation has thus far proven disappointing in clinical studies. The development of radiation pneumopathy has not been appreciably altered by the use of prophylactic steroids or anticoagulants. The use of gamma interferon in conjunction with radiation actually worsened pneumonitis in recent clinical trials.[43] Beta interferon is currently under clinical investigation. Nutritional factors merit further consideration, as vitamin A deficiency increases radiation injury in the mouse lung. Numerous other approaches are being investigated in laboratory studies, including the use of captopril, pentoxifylline, interleukin-11, and the modulation of TGF-β production. All attempts to modulate the development of radiation pneumonitis must be pursued cautiously, because these therapeutic strategies are based on biologic epiphenomena and on an incomplete understanding of the mechanisms by which radiation pneumopathies are produced. In testing such interventions, as with any alteration of cancer therapy, it will be critical to consider the effects of the intervention on the response of the malignancy, as well as its effects on normal tissue injury, because the intervention will be of value only if it increases the therapeutic ratio.

REFERENCES

1. Abratt RP, Willcox PA, Smith JA: Lung cancer in patients with borderline lung functions—zonal lung perfusion scans at presentation and lung function after high dose irradiation. *Radiother Oncol* 19:317–322, 1990.

2. Cardozo BL, Zoetelief H, van Bekkum DW, et al: Lung damage following bone marrow transplantation: I. The contribution of irradiation. *Int Radiat Oncol Biol Phys* 11:907–914, 1985.

3. Carter SK, Glatstein E, Livingston RB: *Principles of Cancer Treatment,* New York, McGraw-Hill, 1981.

4. Casarett GW: *Radiation Histopathology,* Boca Raton, FL, CRC Press, 1980.

5. Choi NC, Kanarek DJ, Kazemi H: Physiologic changes in pulmonary function after thoracic radiotherapy for patients with lung cancer and role of regional pulmonary function studies in predicting postradiotherapy pulmonary function before radiotherapy. *Cancer Treat Symp* 2:119–130, 1985.

6. Collis CH: Lung damage from cytotoxic drugs. *Cancer Chemother Pharmacol* 4:17–27, 1980.

7. Cox JD, Azarnia N, Byhardt RW, et al: A randomized phase I/II trial of hyperfractionated radiation therapy with total doses of 60.0 Gy to 79.2 Gy: Possible survival benefit with ≥ 69.6 Gy in favorable patients with Radiation Therapy Oncology Group Stage III non-small cell lung carcinoma: Report of radiation therapy oncology group 83-11. *J Clin Oncol* 8:1543–1555, 1990.

8. Curran WJ, Moldofsky PJ, Solin LJ: Observations of the predictive value of perfusion lung scans on post-irradiation pulmonary function among 210 patients with bronchogenic carcinoma. *Int Radiat Oncol Biol Phys* 24:31–36, 1992.

9. Deeg HJ, Sullivan KM, Buckner CD, et al: Marrow transplantation for acute nonlymphoblastic leukemia in first remission: Toxicity and long-term follow-up of patients conditioned with single dose or fractionated total body irradiation. *Bone Marrow Transplant* 1:151–157, 1986.

10. Emami B, Lyman J, Brown A, et al: Tolerance of normal tissue to therapeutic irradiation. *Int J Radiat Oncol Biol Phys* 21:109–122, 1991.

11. Franko AJ, Sharplin J, Ward WF, Hinz JM: The genetic basis of strain-dependent differences in the early phase of radiation injury in mouse lung. *Radiat Res* 126:349–356, 1991.

12. Franko AJ, Sharplin J: Development of fibrosis after lung irradiation in relation to inflammation and lung function in a mouse strain prone to fibrosis. *Radiat Res* 140:347–355, 1994.

13. Fryer CJH, Fitzpatrick PJ, Rider WD, Poon P: Radiation pneumonitis: Experience following a large single dose of radiation. *Radiat Oncol Biol Phys* 4:931–936, 1978.

14. Green DM, Finklestein JZ, Tefft ME, Norkool P: Diffuse interstitial pneumonitis after pulmonary irradiation for metastatic Wilms' tumor. *Cancer* 63:450–453, 1989.

15. Groover TA, Christie AC, Merrit EA: Observations on the use of the copper filter in roentgen treatment of deep-seated malignancies. *South Med J* 15:440, 1922.

16. Gross NJ: Pulmonary effects of radiation therapy. *Ann Intern Med* 86:81–92, 1977.

17. Guichard M, Deschavanne PJ, Malaise E-P: Radiosensitivity of mouse lung cells measured using an *in vitro* colony method. *Int J Radiat Oncol Biol Phys* 6:441–447, 1980.

18. Gurley LR, London JE, Tietjen GL, et al: Lung hyperpermeability and changes in biochemical constituents in bronchoalveolar lavage fluids following X irradiation of the thorax. *Radiat Res* 134:151–159, 1993.

19. Hall EJ: *Radiobiology for the Radiologist,* 4th ed. Philadelphia, Lippincott, 1994.

20. Horning SJ, Adhikari A, Rizk N, et al: Effect of treatment for Hodgkin's disease on pulmonary function: Results of a prospective study. *J Clin Oncol* 12:297–305, 1994.

21. Johns HE, Cunningham JRL: *The Physics of Radiology,* 4th ed. Springfield, Ill, Thomas, 1983.

22. Kallman RF: The importance of schedule and drug dose intensity in combinations of modalities. *Int J Radiat Oncol Biol Phys* 28:761–771, 1994.

23. Keane TJ, Van Dyk J, Rider WD: Idiopathic interstitial pneumonia following bone marrow transplantation: The relationship with total body irradiation. *Int J Radiat Oncol Biol Phys* 7:1365–1370, 1981.

24. Lingos TI, Recht A, Vicini F, et al: Radiation pneumonitis in breast cancer patients treated with conservative surgery and radiation therapy. *Int J Radiat Oncol Biol Phys* 21:355–360, 1991.

25. Liao Z-X, Travis EL, Tucker SL: Damage and morbidity from pneumonitis after irradiation of partial volumes of mouse lung. *Int J Radiat Oncol Biol Phys* 32:1359–1370, 1995.

26. Ma LD, Taylor GA, Wharam MD, Wiley JM: "Recall" pneumonitis: Adriamycin potentiation of radiation pneumonitis in two children. *Radiology* 187:465–467, 1993.

27. Mah K, Keane TJ, Van Dyk J, et al: Quantitative effect of combined chemotherapy and fractionated radiotherapy on the incidence of radiation-induced lung damage: A prospective clinical study. *Int J Radiat Oncol Biol Phys* 28:563–574, 1994.

28. Mah K, Van Dyk J, Keane T, Poon PY: Acute radiation-induced pulmonary damage: A clinical study on the response to fractionated radiation therapy. *Int J Radiat Oncol Biol Phys* 13:179–188, 1987.

29. Marks LB, Spencer DP, Sherouse GW, et al: The role of three dimensional functional lung imaging in radiation treatment planning: The functional dose-volume histogram. *Int J Radiat Oncol Biol Phys* 33:65–75, 1995.

30. Marks LB: The pulmonary effects of thoracic irradiation. *Oncology* 8:89–104, 1994.

31. Martel MK, Ten Haken RK, Hazuka MB, et al: Dose-volume histogram and 3-D treatment planning evaluation of patients with pneumonitis. *Int J Radiat Oncol Biol Phys* 28:575–581, 1994.

32. McDonald S, Rubin P, Phillips TL, Marks LB: Injury to the lung from cancer therapy: Clinical syndromes, measurable endpoints, and potential scoring systems. *Int J Radiat Oncol Biol Phys* 31:1187–1203, 1995.

33. Molls M, Budach V, Bamberg M: Total body irradiation: The lung as critical organ. *Strahlentherapie und Onkologie* 162:226–232, 1986.

34. Morgan GW, Breit SN: Radiation and the lung: A reevaluation of the mechanisms mediating pulmonary injury. *Int J Radiat Oncol Biol Phys* 31:361–369, 1995.

35. Prato FS, Kurdyak R, Saibil EA, et al: Physiological and radiographic assessment during the development of pulmonary radiation fibrosis. *Radiology* 122:389–397, 1977.

36. Rockwell S: Radiobiology. *Encycl Human Biol* 6:441–453, 1991.

37. Rothwell RI, Kelly SA, Joslin CA: Radiation pneumonitis in patients treated for breast cancer. *Radiother Oncol* 4:9–14, 1985.

38. Rubenstein JH, Richter MP, Moldofsky PJ, Solin LJ: Prospective prediction of postradiation therapy lung function using quantitative lung scans and pulmonary function testing. *Int J Radiat Oncol Biol Phys* 15:83–87, 1988.

39. Rubin P, Finkelstein J, Shapiro D: Molecular biology mechanisms in the radiation induction of pulmonary injury syndromes: Interrelationship between the alveolar macrophage and the septal fibroblast. *Int J Radiat Oncol Biol Phys* 24:93–101, 1992.

40. Rubin P, Finkelstein JN, Siemann DW, et al: Predictive biochemical assays for late radiation effects. *Int J Radiat Oncol Biol Phys* 12:469–476, 1986.

41. Rubin P, Johnston CJ, Williams JP, et al: A perpetual cascade of cytokines postirradiation leads to pulmonary fibrosis. *Int J Radiat Oncol Biol Phys* 33:99–109, 1995.

42. Shank B: Radiotherapeutic principles of bone marrow transplantation, in Forman S, Thomas ED, Blume K (eds): *Bone Marrow Transplantation.* Boston, Blackwell, 1994, pp 96–113.

43. Shaw EG, Deming RL, Creagan ET, et al: Pilot study of human recombinant interferon gamma and accelerated hyperfractionated thoracic radiation therapy in patients with unrespectable Stage IIIA/B nonsmall cell lung cancer. *Int J Radiat Oncol Biol Phys* 31:827–831, 1995.

44. Siemann DW, Rubin P, Penny DP: Pulmonary toxicity following multi-fraction radiotherapy. *Br J Cancer* 53:365–367, 1986.

45. Tarbell NJ, Thompson L, Mauch P: Thoracic irradiation in Hodgkin's disease: Disease control and long-term complications. *Int J Radiat Oncol Biol Phys* 18:275–281, 1990.

46. Terry NHA, Tucker SL, Travis EL: Residual radiation damage in murine lung assessed by pneumonitis. *Int J Radiat Oncol Biol Phys* 14:929–938, 1988.

47. Travis EL, Peters LJ, McNeill J, et al: Effect of dose-rate on total body irradiation: Lethality and pathologic findings. *Radiother Oncol* 4:341–351, 1985.

48. Travis EL, Tucker SL: The relationship between functional assays of radiation response in the lung and target cell depletion. *Br J Cancer* 53:304–319, 1986.

49. Van Dyk J, Keane TJ, Kan S, et al: Radiation pneumonitis following large single dose irradiation: A re-evaluation based on absolute dose to lung. *Int J Radiat Oncol Biol Phys* 7:461–467, 1981.

50. Von der Maase H, Overgaard J, Vaeth M: Effect of cancer chemotherapeutic drugs on radiation-induced lung damage in mice. *Radiother Oncol* 5:245–257, 1986.

CHAPTER 73

PULMONARY MANIFESTATIONS OF THE COLLAGEN VASCULAR DISEASES

Marvin I. Schwarz

HISTOLOGIC SPECTRUM OF PARENCHYMAL REACTIONS IN COLLAGEN VASCULAR DISEASE
  Interstitial Lung Disease
  Pulmonary Vascular Disease
  Diffuse Alveolar Hemorrhage
  Bronchiolitis
  Parenchymal Nodules

CLINICAL FEATURES OF THE COLLAGEN VASCULAR DISEASES
  Systemic Lupus Erythematosus
  Rheumatoid Arthritis
  Scleroderma
  Polymyositis-Dermatomyositis
  Mixed Connective Tissue Disease
  Sjögren's Syndrome
  Ankylosing Spondylitis

The pleuropulmonary complications associated with the collagen vascular diseases are frequent occurrences, and it would be the exception rather than the rule for an individual to avoid one of these during the course of such an illness. All the elements of the respiratory system are affected, either separately or in combination. This includes the respiratory muscles, the pleura, and the lung parenchyma—the small airways, the interstitium, or the pulmonary vessels. Moreover, these patients experience an increased incidence of community-acquired pneumonia as well as pneumonia associated with the immunosuppressive drugs employed for treatment. These cytotoxic drugs, particularly methotrexate and gold, can also induce various noninfectious interstitial reactions which are often difficult to distinguish from a primary interstitial complication of a collagen vascular disease.

Although most pulmonary complications appear in an established case of a collagen vascular disease, in some situations the lung disease precedes the more typical manifestations. For example, in both rheumatoid arthritis and polymyositis-dermatomyositis, the interstitial lung disease may precede the joint and muscle disease for several months to several years. This is also the case, but to a lesser extent, for scleroderma. In a recent study of 68 patients initially diagnosed as idiopathic pulmonary fibrosis, 19 percent over a period of 1 to 11 years developed a collagen vascular disease, primarily rheumatoid arthritis or polymyositis-dermatomyositis.[20] These individuals were younger and more likely to be women. Pleuritis with or without effusion sometimes heralds the onset of rheumatoid arthritis or systemic lupus erythematosus. An acute immunologic pneumonitis or diffuse alveolar hemorrhage has been reported to be the signal event in systemic lupus erythematosus, polymyositis-dermatomyositis, and mixed connective tissue disease.

The actual incidence of the pleuropulmonary complications (Table 73-1) is variable. For example, in some series, interstitial lung disease in scleroderma is reported to be as high as 60 percent in premortem and 100 percent in postmortem studies. In contrast, interstitial lung disease in ankylosing spondylitis is an uncommon event. The incidence of interstitial lung disease is increasing for most of the collagen vascular diseases. This is primarily due to increased recognition, aided by the use of high-resolution computed tomography and bronchoalveolar lavage, which will detect abnormalities in both asymptomatic as well as symptomatic patients with normal chest radiographs. Moreover, many of the earlier incidence studies relied on physiologic testing which included spirometry, lung volumes, and diffusing capacity but did not measure rest and exercise gas exchange which is the most sensitive physiologic marker of interstitial lung disease as well as pulmonary vascular disease.

HISTOLOGIC SPECTRUM OF PARENCHYMAL REACTIONS IN COLLAGEN VASCULAR DISEASE

Interstitial Lung Disease

Interstitial involvement is a common respiratory manifestation of the collagen vascular disorders. It can present with diffuse alveolar damage and/or with one of a number of inflammatory responses. Diffuse alveolar damage is the underlying histologic lesion which is also seen in the acute respiratory distress syndrome, idiopathic acute interstitial pneumonitis (Hamman-Rich Syndrome), and cytotoxicity from some drugs. This damage consists of a mixed interstitial inflammatory infiltrate, interstitial edema and fibrin deposition, and the characteristic intraalveolar hyaline membrane formation. Intraalveolar red blood cells (dif-

TABLE 73-1

Pulmonary Complications of the Collagen Vascular Diseases

Manifestation	Relative Frequency (0–4)						
	SLE	RA	SS	PM-DM	MCTD	AS	Sjögren's
Respiratory muscle dysfunction	2	0	0	2	1	0	0
Aspiration pneumonia	0	0	3	3	2	0	2
Primary pulmonary hypertension	2	1	4	1	2	0	0
Vasculitis	2	2	0	1	1	0	0
Interstitial lung disease	2	3	4	3	2	1	3
Capillaritis + DAH	2	1	1	1	1	0	0
Bland DAH	2	0	0	0	1	0	0
Diffuse alveolar damage	2	0	0	2	1	0	0
Cellular interstitial pneumonitis	2	3	2	3	3	0	1
Lymphocytic interstitial pneumonitis	1	2	1	0	0	0	3
Usual interstitial pneumonitis	2	3	4	3	2	1	1
Honeycomb lung	1	2	4	3	2	1	1
Bronchiolitis obliterans organizing pneumonia	1	3	1	3	2	0	1
Bronchiolitis	1	2	1	0	1	0	1
Obliterative bronchiolitis	0	2	0	0	0	0	1
Pleural effusion	2	3	1	0	2	0	1
Parenchymal nodules	0	2	0	0	0	0	1

Abbreviations: SLE = systemic lupus erythematosus; RA = rheumatoid arthritis; SS = systemic sclerosis (scleroderma); PM-DM = polymyositis-dermato-myositis; MCTD = mixed connective tissue disease; AS = ankylosing spondylitis; Sjögren's = Sjögren's syndrome; DAH = diffuse alveolar hemorrhage

fuse alveolar hemorrhage) may be present in severe cases. With progression, there is intraalveolar organization, intraalveolar and interstitial fibrosis, alveolar collapse, and the development of an end-stage fibrotic lung. An acute immunologic pneumonia in systemic lupus erythematosus (acute lupus pneumonia) and in polymyositis-dermatomyositis may demonstrate this underlying histologic appearance.

Cellular interstitial pneumonitis refers to a lymphoplasmocytic infiltration of the interstitium with minimal or no collagen deposition (Fig. 73-1). This pneumonitis probably represents an early phase of usual interstitial pneumonitis (see below) and is most frequently seen with rheumatoid arthritis, polymyositis-dermatomyositis, and mixed connective tissue disease.

Lymphocytic interstitial pneumonitis refers to a monotonous infiltration of the interstitium by mature lymphocytes (Fig. 73-2). These lymphocytes tend to form germinal centers within the interstitium as well as displaying an angiocentric distribution. Other features of lymphocytic interstitial pneumonia include macrophagic giant cells, granuloma formation, and amyloid deposition. If unresponsive to treatment, lymphocytic interstitial

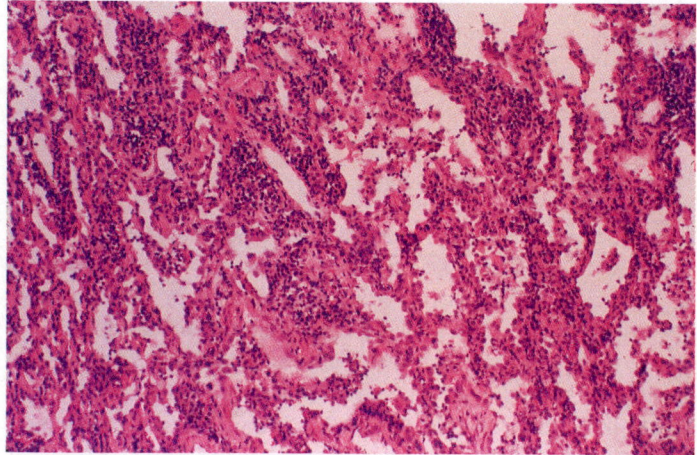

FIGURE 73-1 Cellular interstitial pneumonitis in rheumatoid arthritis. There is a lymphoplasmyocytic infiltration of the interstitial compartment with minimal collagen deposition.

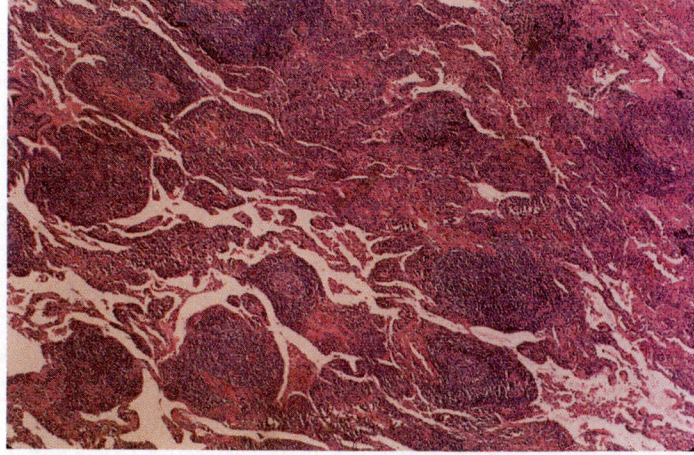

FIGURE 73-2 Lymphocytic interstitial pneumonitis in a patient with primary Sjogren's syndrome. There is a dense lymphocytic infiltrate, broadening the interstitium and lymphoid follicles.

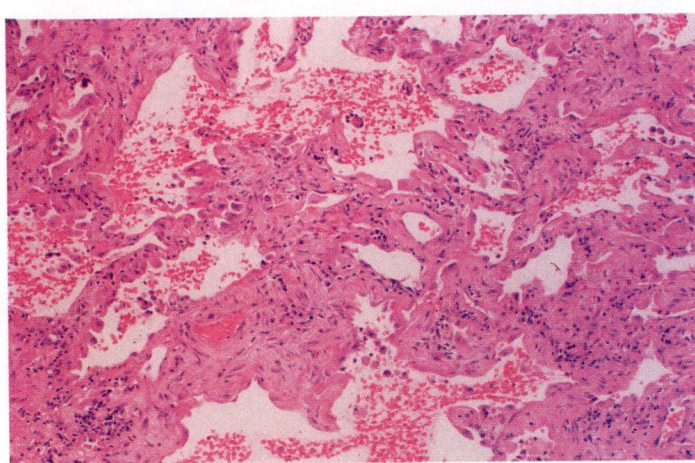

FIGURE 73-3   Usual interstitial pneumonia in a patient with rheumatoid arthritis. There is broadening of the interstitium by varying degrees of mononuclear cell infiltration and collagen deposition.

pneumonitis can progress to usual interstitial pneumonitis and end-stage honeycomb lung. Among the collagen vascular diseases, this pneumonitis most commonly accompanies the primary form of Sjogren's syndrome as well as a secondary form of Sjogren's syndrome appearing with other collagen vascular diseases, particularly rheumatoid arthritis.

Usual interstitial pneumonitis is the underlying lesion of idiopathic pulmonary fibrosis and can also appear in all the collagen vascular diseases, thereby representing the most common interstitial reaction in this group of diseases. It consists of varying degrees of mononuclear cell infiltration and fibroblastic proliferation leading to collagen deposition within the alveolar interstitium (Fig. 73-3). With progression, this fibrotic reaction results in marked distortion of the lung architecture and what remains are 2- to 3-mm cystic spaces lined by metaplastic epithelium, the so-called honeycomb lung (Fig. 73-4). Other features of usual interstitial pneumonitis include type II epithelial cell hyperplasia producing a hob-nailed appearance on the alveolar surface, collections of intraalveolar macrophages, and smooth-muscle proliferation within the interstitium.

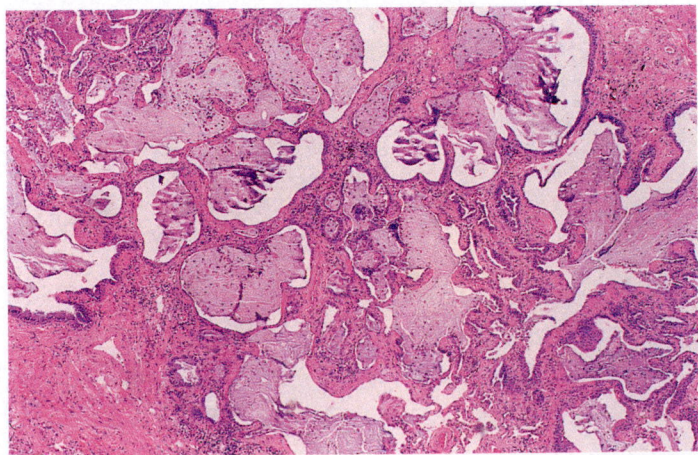

FIGURE 73-4   Advanced usual interstitial pneumonia in a patient with scleroderma (honeycomb lung). Normal alveolar tissue is replaced with broad bands of fibrous tissue lined by metaplastic epithelium and filled with inspissated mucus producing a cystlike network.

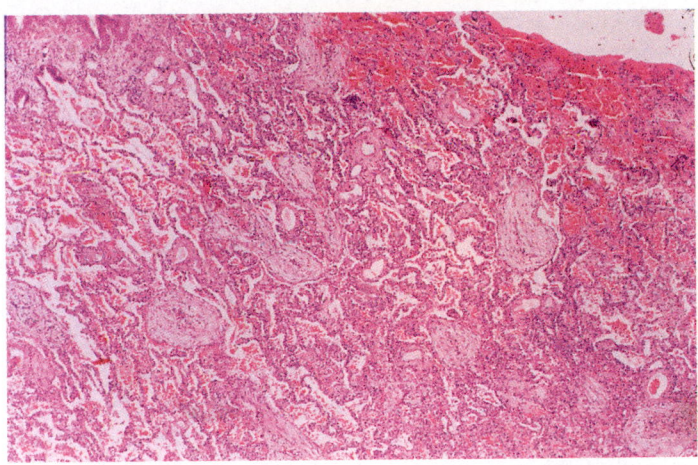

FIGURE 73-5   Bronchiolitis obliterans organizing pneumonia in a patient with rheumatoid arthritis. There is a mononuclear cellular infiltration of the interstitium without collagen deposition as well as alveolar duct and intraalveolar fibroblastic proliferation and early collagen production.

Bronchiolitis obliterans organizing pneumonia is a distinctive histologic lesion that follows a variety of insults to the alveolar structures including drugs, infection, radiation, and an idiopathic variety. Bronchiolitis obliterans organizing pneumonia can also complicate the collagen vascular diseases, particularly rheumatoid arthritis and polymyositis-dermatomyositis. Three features comprise the histologic picture: a cellular interstitial pneumonitis, intraalveolar space and intraalveolar ductal fibroblastic proliferation with early collagen deposition (Masson's bodies), and inflammatory polyps consisting of fibroblasts and mononuclear cells protruding into the lumens of respiratory and terminal bronchioles (Fig. 73-5). Bronchiolitis obliterans organizing pneumonia has the potential for being a completely reversible lesion; however, with continuing injury it may progress to usual interstitial pneumonia and honeycomb lung.

Pulmonary Vascular Disease

A form of idiopathic pulmonary hypertension which most commonly appears in patients with scleroderma and is now being increasingly recognized in systemic lupus erythematosus, rheumatoid arthritis, and mixed connective tissue disease is histologically identical to the syndrome of primary pulmonary hypertension seen in young women without collagen vascular disease. This is a proliferative disorder (plexogenic arteriopathy) affecting the arterioles and small muscular pulmonary arteries. This form of pulmonary hypertension must be differentiated from secondary forms as a result of hypoxic vasoconstriction induced by interstitial lung disease. In the idiopathic variety there is endothelial cell intimal proliferation and smooth-muscle cell proliferation causing medial thickening and producing an onion ring configuration. This results in luminal obliteration. With further endothelial cell proliferation, new vascular channels are eventually formed. In the secondary forms of pulmonary hypertension due to hypoxia, medial hypertrophy is the primary finding. Patients with systemic lupus erythematosus and the antiphospholipid syndrome may develop recurrent pulmonary emboli mimicking the clinical picture of idiopathic pulmonary hypertension.[10]

Vasculitis refers to an acute inflammatory angio-destructive process resulting in fibrinoid necrosis of the vascular wall. In the collagen vascular diseases this is most often a small-vessel vasculitis involving arterioles and small muscular pulmonary arteries. Although uncommon, this is seen with greatest regularity in systemic lupus erythematosus and less frequently in rheumatoid arthritis, polymyositis-dermatomyositis, and mixed connective tissue disease. Often accompanying the arteriolitis is the lesion of pulmonary capillaritis (see below).

Diffuse Alveolar Hemorrhage

Diffuse alveolar hemorrhage is recognized by the filling of the alveolar spaces with red blood cells, and with recurrent episodes, as is often the case, intraalveolar and interstitial hemosiderin is deposited. With recurrent episodes, the potential for interstitial fibrosis also exists. There are two histologic appearances of diffuse alveolar hemorrhage. One is devoid of inflammation and is referred to as *bland hemorrhage* (Fig. 73-6). It is therefore similar in histologic appearance to idiopathic pulmonary hemosiderosis. The other, pulmonary capillaritis, is a unique neutrophilic infiltration of the alveolar interstitium which results in necrosis and loss of integrity of the alveolar-capillary basement membrane, capillary destruction and thrombosis, and an outpouring of red blood cells into the alveolar space (Fig. 73-7). The unique feature of this reaction is that many of the infiltrating neutrophils are undergoing fragmentation (leucocytoclasis), and others appear as densely staining apoptotic cells. There is also deposition of nuclear dust within the interstitial and intraalveolar compartments. The interstitium is edematous and necrotic, and red blood cells are lying free within the interstitial matrix due to capillary destruction. This lesion is most commonly seen in the systemic vasculitides, particularly Wegener's granulomatosis and microscopic polyangiitis, the small-vessel variant of polyarteritis nodosa. Of the collagen vascular diseases, both bland pulmonary hemorrhage and diffuse alveolar hemorrhage secondary to pulmonary capillaritis appear most frequently in systemic lupus erythematosus.[26] Cases of pulmonary capillaritis

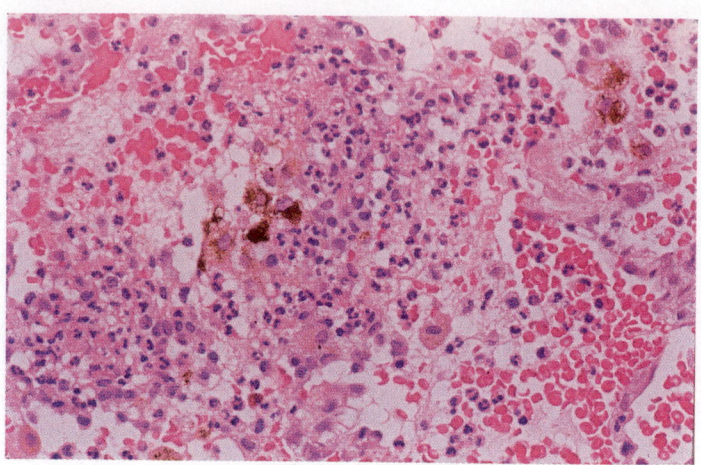

FIGURE 73-7   Low-power view of pulmonary capillaritis in a patient with systemic lupus erythematosus. There is marked thickening of the interstitial compartment and infiltration by acute and chronic inflammatory cells. The alveolar spaces are filled with red blood cells and neutrophils.

have also been reported to occur in rheumatoid arthritis, Sjogren's syndrome, polymyositis-dermatomyositis, and mixed connective tissue disease.

Bronchiolitis

Bronchiolitis refers to an inflammatory-fibrotic process involving the terminal and respiratory bronchioles and possibly the surrounding alveolar structures. Respiratory bronchiolitis is primarily seen in smokers with or without an associated collagen vascular disease. There is also a primary form of respiratory bronchiolitis which complicates the collagen vascular diseases, most often appearing in rheumatoid arthritis and Sjogren's syndrome. Histologically, there is a mononuclear cell infiltration of the wall of the bronchiole without impingement of the bronchiolar lumen. Bronchiolitis obliterans, or obliterative bronchiolitis, however, is a concentric fibrous obliteration of the bronchiolar lumen leading to a severe obstructive lung disease (Fig. 73-8).

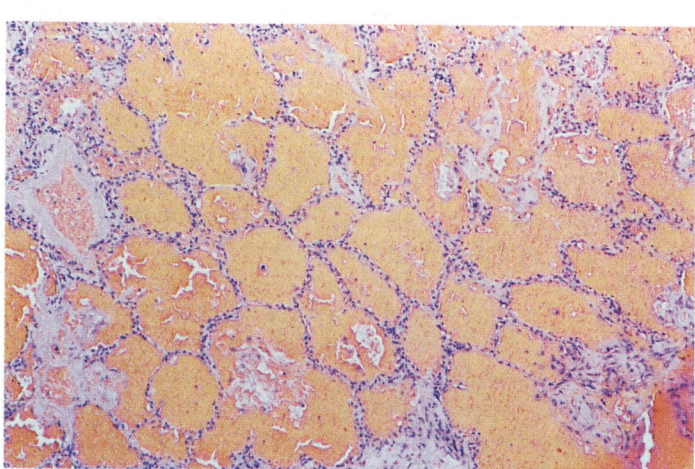

FIGURE 73-6   Bland diffuse alveolar hemorrhage in systemic lupus erythematosus. There is little if any interstitial reaction except for type II pneumocyte epithelial cell hyperplasia. The alveolar spaces are filled with red blood cells.

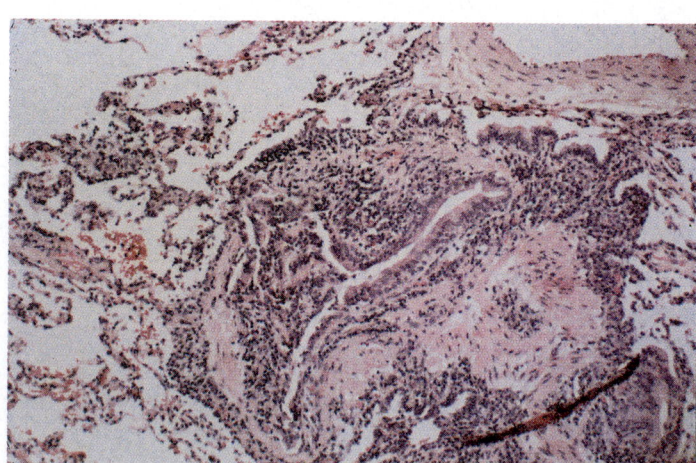

FIGURE 73-8   Obliterative bronchiolitis in rheumatoid arthritis. There is a marked reduction of the luminal diameter due to concentric fibrous obliteration and dense chronic inflammation. *(Reprinted with permission. Schwarz MI, Lynch DA, Tuder R: Bronchiolitis obliterans: The lone manifestation of rheumatoid arthritis. Eur Respir J 7:817–820, 1994.)*

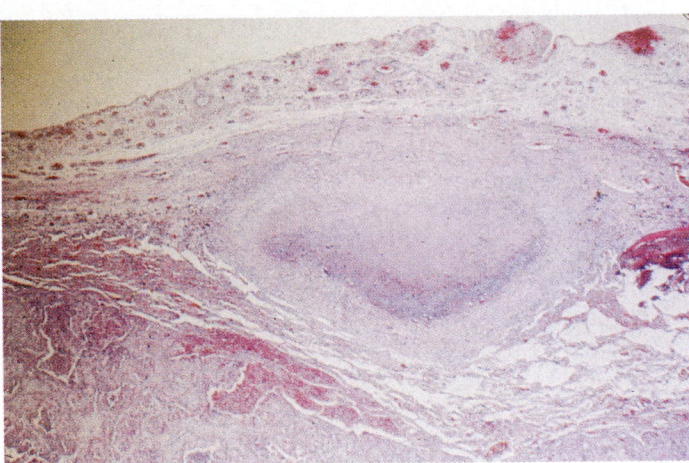

FIGURE 73-9 Typical subpleural location of a necrobiotic rheumatoid nodule. There is a central area of fibrinoid debris surrounded by palisading histiocytes.

Bronchiolitis obliterans is most often reported as a complication of rheumatoid arthritis.

Parenchymal Nodules

Noninfectious inflammatory parenchymal nodules occur in both rheumatoid arthritis and Sjogren's syndrome. In rheumatoid arthritis the nodules are referred to as the *necrobiotic* or *rheumatoid nodule*. This lesion is found both in the pleura and lung parenchyma and is identical in appearance to the subcutaneous rheumatoid nodule. In the lung parenchyma these nodules are located in the interlobular septa and in the subpleural parenchyma. The necrobiotic nodule is comprised of palisading histiocytes, giant cells, and other mononuclear cells surrounding an area of fibrinoid debris (Fig. 73-9). In Sjogren's syndrome a rounded lesion known as pseudolymphoma can occasionally be detected on the chest radiograph. Pseudolymphoma is considered to be a localized form of lymphocytic interstitial pneumonia and is made up of a dense infiltrate of lymphocytes and histiocytes with occasional granuloma formation. It has potential for lymphomatous transformation.

CLINICAL FEATURES OF THE COLLAGEN VASCULAR DISEASES

Systemic Lupus Erythematosus

Systemic lupus erythematosus is characterized by the production of antibodies against various cellular antigens derived from the nucleus, cytoplasm, and cell membrane. Tissue injury appears to be associated with the development of immune complexes, the presence of low serum complement levels, and the production of antibodies to native DNA. The pulmonary complications are thought to be the result of an immune-complex-induced injury. A number of situations (Table 73-2) can cause an acute respiratory type illness in systemic lupus erythematosus. A patient with systemic lupus erythematosus who presents with a febrile illness, cough with or without productive sputum, and new pulmonary infiltrates must be considered to have an infectious pneumonia, although acute lupus pneumonitis and diffuse alveolar hemor-

TABLE 73-2

Acute Lung Syndromes in Systemic Lupus Erythematosus

Community-acquired or immunocompromised pneumonias
Pulmonary embolization
Uremic pneumonitis
Cardiogenic pulmonary edema
Acute reversible hypoxemia syndrome
Acute lupus pneumonitis
Diffuse alveolar hemorrhage
Pleurisy

rhage may have a similar presentation. Infection can be community acquired or result from immunosuppressive treatment. Infectious pneumonia represents the most common cause of pulmonary disease in systemic lupus erythematosus, and infections in general represent the most common reason for death (33 to 77 percent) in these patients.[31] Bronchoalveolar lavage is often helpful in excluding an infectious pneumonia in the immunocompromised systemic lupus erythematosus patient.

Another important consideration in an acutely dyspneic systemic lupus erythematosus patient is pulmonary embolization, a complication reportedly occurring in up to 25 percent of patients and a significant cause of mortality.[22] The occurrence of thromboembolic disease correlates with the presence in the serum of acquired antiphospholipid antibodies (lupus anticoagulant and anticardiolipin). In large series, up to 34 percent of systemic lupus erythematosus patients have the antiphospholipid syndrome. Other clinical features associated with this syndrome are thrombocytopenia, recurrent venous thrombosis, hemolytic anemia, leg ulcers, and fetal loss.[2] Other causes for acute respiratory failure include a volume overload state due either to renal failure or to congestive heart failure secondary to myocarditis. Uremic pneumonitis with underlying diffuse alveolar damage is also a possible cause of an acutely dyspneic systemic lupus erythematosus patient.

A syndrome (acute reversible hypoxemia) occurring in acutely ill systemic lupus erythematosus patients who are experiencing systemic exacerbations has recently been described.[1] These patients have hypoxemia and a widened alveolar-arterial oxygen gradient, but both the chest radiograph and ventilation-perfusion lung scans are normal. It is postulated that there is complement-activated neutrophil aggregation in the pulmonary vasculature. With corticosteroid treatment of the acute exacerbation, the hypoxemia resolves.

ACUTE LUPUS PNEUMONITIS

Acute lupus pneumonitis is a clinical syndrome whose underlying histology is diffuse alveolar damage, bronchiolitis obliterans organizing pneumonia, cellular interstitial pneumonitis, or a combination of these. Acute lupus pneumonitis mimics an acute infectious pneumonia and may be the presenting manifestation of systemic lupus erythematosus in up to 50 percent of cases who have this complication.[24] It also appears during a flare of the other systemic components of systemic lupus erythematosus particularly pleuritis, pericarditis, arthritis and nephritis, but still is a relatively uncommon complication (less than 5 percent). It reportedly is more common in the postpartum period.[48] This pneumonitis tends to recur, and cases have been documented which have progressed to a more chronic interstitial lung disease (usual interstitial pneumonia). The resultant acute respiratory failure often requires assisted mechanical ventilation. The chest radiograph demonstrates bilateral alveolar infiltrates which can be patchy or densely consolidated and often accompanied by pleural effusions and cardiomegaly due to underlying pericardial effusion or myocarditis (Fig. 73-10A). White blood cell counts and sedimentation rates are elevated, and serum complement is often low. Immunopathologic studies reveal the presence of complement as well as antibodies to IgG and DNA in some patients, supporting the concept of an immune complex pathogenesis (Fig. 73-10B). Because of the difficulty in distinguishing acute lupus pneumonitis from an infectious pneumonia, a bronchoalveolar lavage and sometimes an open (thorascopic) lung biopsy are indicated prior to instituting anti-inflammatory and immunosuppressive therapy. Although recent data are not available, the mortality rate has been reported to be as high as 50 percent.[24] The causes of death in patients with acute lupus pneumonitis are either respiratory failure, another complication of systemic lupus erythematosus (nephritis, cerebritis), or a superimposed infectious problem.

DIFFUSE ALVEOLAR HEMORRHAGE

Although unusual, diffuse alveolar hemorrhage can sometimes be the presenting manifestation of systemic lupus erythematosus. In several recorded cases recurrent diffuse alveolar hemorrhage was present for years prior to the diagnosis of systemic lupus erythematosus.[11] In spite of this, the majority of cases, in contrast to acute lupus pneumonitis, first appear in a well-documented case of systemic lupus erythematosus. The underlying histopathology is either bland pulmonary hemorrhage or pulmonary capillaritis, and the incidence of diffuse alveolar hemorrhage (approximately 5 percent) in a systemic lupus erythematosus population appears to be increasing. In one series it was always accompanied by active glomerulonephritis.

Diffuse alveolar hemorrhage can also present with symptoms reminiscent of an infectious pneumonia or acute lupus pneumonitis, and the additional symptom of hemoptysis raises the possibility of this diagnosis. Not all patients with diffuse alveolar hemorrhage will have hemoptysis when first seen, but rather a falling hematocrit, an elevated diffusing capacity due to the availability of hemoglobin to combine with carbon monoxide, or a serosanguinous bronchoalveolar lavage may be the first clue to this diagnosis. The chest radiograph indicates diffuse alveolar infiltrates (Fig. 73-11), but pleuritis and pericarditis are not prominent features as they are in acute lupus pneumonitis. The mortality rate is approximately 50 percent and apparently does not depend upon the underlying histopathology (bland hemorrhage versus pulmonary capillaritis). Pathologic changes that are reminiscent of both acute lupus pneumonitis (diffuse alveolar damage and cellular interstitial pneumonitis) and diffuse alveolar hemorrhage with or without pulmonary capillaritis are not unusual in a single biopsy specimen. Recurrence is the rule.

There are no controlled clinical trials for the treatment of either acute lupus pneumonitis or diffuse alveolar hemorrhage.

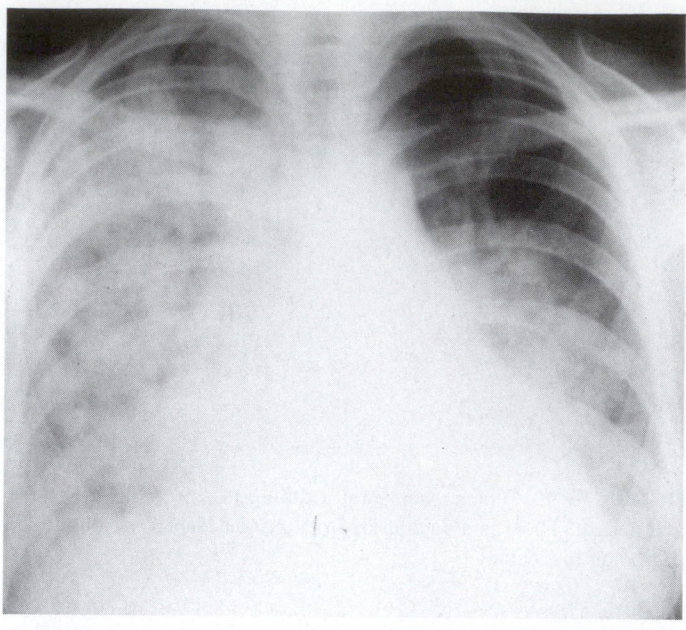

A

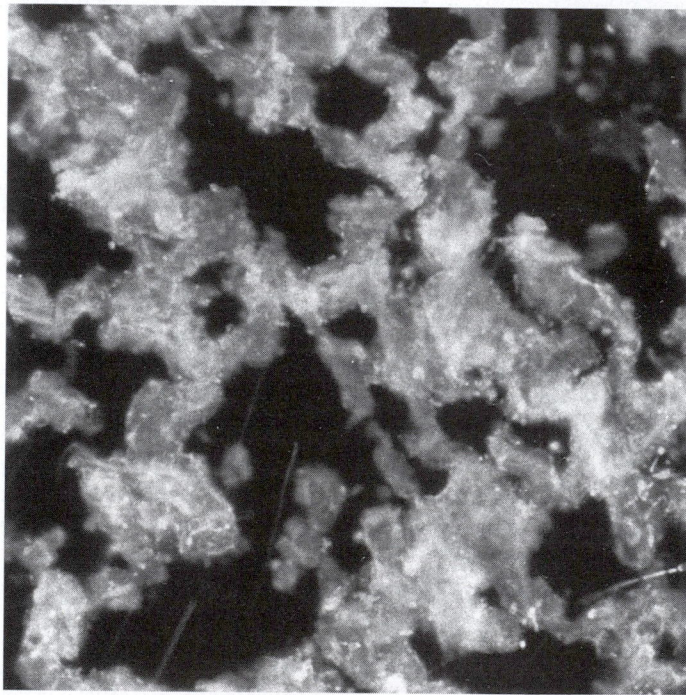

B

FIGURE 73-10 Acute lupus pneumonitis. The chest radiograph demonstrates diffuse alveolar filling with cardiomegaly (pericardial effusion versus myocarditis). *A.* There is also a left pleural effusion. *B.* The immunofluorescent study demonstrates granular immune complex deposition in the alveolar interstitium.

Corticosteroids, azathioprine, cyclophosphamide, and plasmapheresis in various combinations have been employed. Once infection has been excluded, we institute intravenous methyl prednisolone (1 to 2 grams daily in divided doses) for 3 to 4 days prior to tapering. Concomitantly, either oral or parenteral cyclophosphamide or azathioprine are administered and, in the case of cytoxan, continued as oral therapy (2 to 3 mg/kg daily) or monthly intravenous therapy. Azathioprine is continued as oral

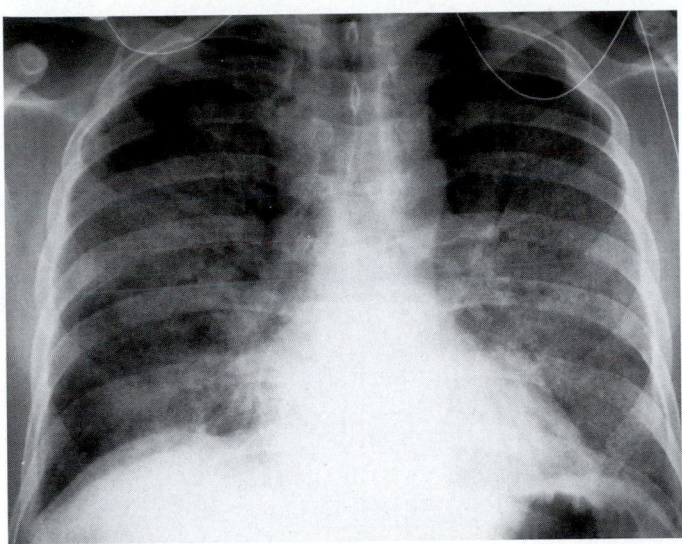

FIGURE 73-11 Diffuse alveolar hemorrhage in systemic lupus erythematosus. There are diffuse alveolar infiltrates without cardiomegaly or pleural effusions.

therapy (2 to 3 mg/kg daily). Plasmapheresis, although logical in lieu of the proposed immune complex pathogenesis, has no proven efficacy to date. The same is true for immune globulin therapy.

LUPUS PLEURITIS

Pleurisy and pleural effusion are the most common primary pulmonary complications of systemic lupus erythematosus, occurring in 50 to 80 percent.[18] Pleurisy and pleural effusion may also be the presenting and sole manifestation. It is usually recurrent and may accompany acute lupus pneumonitis. Examination of the pleural tissue reveals infiltration with plasma cells and lymphocytes, and, with repeated episodes, pleural fibrosis supervenes. Occasionally, a vasculitis of the pleural vessels is detected, and immune complex deposition has been reported. Patients complain of pleuritic pain, fever, and dyspnea. The chest radiograph may be normal (dry pleurisy) or demonstrate small to moderate pleural effusions (massive effusions are rare) which are bilateral in 50 percent of patients. When unilateral, there is no predilection for either side.

The effusion is clear or serosanguinous, is an exudate, and contains increased concentrations of protein and lactic dehydrogenase. The white cell counts range from 5 to 10,000 cells per cubic millimeter. Early on, neutrophils predominate, and with time mononuclear cells appear. These characteristics are nonspecific and are often seen with infectious parapneumonic effusions.

In distinction to rheumatoid arthritis, the pleural fluid glucose concentration is not reduced. As in rheumatoid pleural effusions, the rheumatoid factor may be positive, and the pleural fluid complement, both the total levels and the individual components, is reduced. A positive double-stranded pleural fluid DNA titer is nonspecific as opposed to the serum test, since it has been found in pleural effusions due to malignancy and tuberculosis. The most helpful measurement is the pleural fluid antinuclear antibody

titer. Levels greater than 1 : 160 are very suggestive of lupus pleuritis. Corticosteroid treatment is effective for relief of pleural pain, but time to resolution of the pleural effusion is quite variable and probably unaffected by this treatment. In the unusual case, recurrent lupus pleuritis may result in massive pleural fibrosis and lung entrapment, necessitating a pleural stripping procedure.

INTERSTITIAL LUNG DISEASE

It was previously held that, in contrast to scleroderma and rheumatoid arthritis, clinically apparent interstitial lung disease with underlying usual interstitial pneumonitis, lymphocytic interstitial pneumonitis, or bronchiolitis obliterans organizing pneumonia occurred in a small percentage of patients with systemic lupus erythematosus. Usual interstitial pneumonitis is known to appear following acute lupus pneumonitis and in some cases has been documented to appear as an independent insidious disease. The prior presumed low incidence of this complication is in part due to inadequate screening techniques such as chest radiographs and physiological testing which did not include gas exchange function. However, utilizing high-resolution computed tomography, 38 percent of 45 systemic lupus erythematosus patients with normal chest radiographs demonstrated pulmonary abnormalities consistent with some form of interstitial lung disease.[5] In a recent series, 25 percent (16 of 63) of systemic lupus erythematosus patients had interstitial lung disease by chest radiographic and physiological criteria, but only four had histologic confirmation.[9] Of these, seven had at least one previous episode of acute lupus pneumonitis and nine had an insidious onset of dyspnea. Anti-SSA(Ro) antibodies were found in 13/16 or 81 percent compared to 38 percent for the entire group of patients. The prevalence of interstitial lung disease is increased in a subset of systemic lupus erythematosus patients who also had sclerodermatous changes of the hands.

In patients who develop the insidious form of interstitial lung disease, the diagnosis of systemic lupus erythematosus is present for several years, and no other pattern of organ involvement predicts its appearance. These patients have progressive dyspnea and cough with interstitial infiltration on the chest radiograph. High-resolution computed tomography indicates combinations of ground glass attenuation, inter- and intralobular septal thickening, and honeycomb change. Pulmonary function tests reveal a restrictive pattern with reduction in the diffusing capacity and hypoxemia accentuated by exercise. Response to therapy, either corticosteroids alone or in combination with cyclophosphamide or azathioprine, depends upon the underlying histology. Those cases with underlying cellular interstitial pneumonitis or organizing pneumonia are more likely to respond to treatment than those who demonstrate excess collagen deposition and cystic honeycomb formation.

PULMONARY VASCULAR DISEASE

Idiopathic pulmonary hypertension due to plexogenic arteriopathy and therefore independent of interstitial lung disease was previously thought to be an unusual complication of systemic lupus erythematosus but is now being reported with increasing regularity. One study reported a 5 percent incidence.[4] This form of pulmonary hypertension is associated with Raynaud's phenomenon, digital vasculitis, serositis, antibodies to ribonucleoprotein, rheumatoid factor, antiphospholipid antibodies, and most recently antiendothelial cell antibodies. Patients complain of dyspnea and fatigue but have normal chest radiographs. In advanced cases, pulmonary arterial enlargement appears. Spirometry and lung volumes are normal, but there is often an isolated reduction of the diffusing capacity for carbon monoxide as well as gas exchange abnormalities. Ventilation-perfusion lung scanning and, occasionally, pulmonary arteriography are indicated, particularly in those patients with the antiphospholipid syndrome who have a potential for recurrent small pulmonary emboli. There is no effective treatment for idiopathic pulmonary hypertension, although oxygen and calcium channel blockers possibly delay the onset of cor-pulmonale. Continuous intravenous prostacyclin has recently been approved for patients with primary pulmonary hypertension as it appears to improve survival as well as functional status. It is likely that trials in collagen-vascular-disease-associated pulmonary hypertension are forthcoming.

Vasculitis in systemic lupus erythematosus is more likely to be discovered in lung biopsy specimens which demonstrate either diffuse alveolar hemorrhage or acute lupus pneumonitis as opposed to being an isolated finding. Autopsy series indicate small-vessel vasculitis in 20 percent of cases.

BRONCHIOLITIS

The primary lung physiological disturbance in systemic lupus erythematosus is restrictive. However, 5 percent of systemic lupus erythematosus patients are reported also to have obstructive physiology, but true concentric obliterative bronchiolitis has not been documented as it has for rheumatoid arthritis. Bronchiolitis obliterans organizing pneumonia with inflammatory polyps protruding into bronchiolar lumens is one of the interstitial patterns that occurs in acute lupus pneumonitis and in chronic interstitial lung disease in systemic lupus erythematosus, but this entity causes restrictive lung disease. Therefore a reduction in airflow rates in a minority of nonsmoking patients with systemic lupus erythematosus has no demonstrated anatomic correlation.

RESPIRATORY MUSCLE DYSFUNCTION

It is estimated that weakness of the diaphragm and other respiratory muscles is found in 25 percent of patients with systemic lupus erythematosus. This accounts for the previously unexplained findings of dyspnea without evidence of interstitial or pulmonary vascular disease. These patients have subsegmental atelectasis, an elevated diaphragm on chest radiograph (Fig. 73-12), and restrictive physiology. This has been referred to as *unexplained dyspnea and shrinking lungs syndrome*. Although there is a reduction in static lung volumes, the diffusing capacity when corrected for alveolar volume remains normal, thereby distinguishing respiratory muscle dysfunction from interstitial lung disease. The likely explanation for this is a reduction in the transdiaphragmatic pressure generated during maximal inspiration, which in turn reduces static lung compliance producing the linear atelectasis seen on the chest radiograph. Moreover, in the pa-

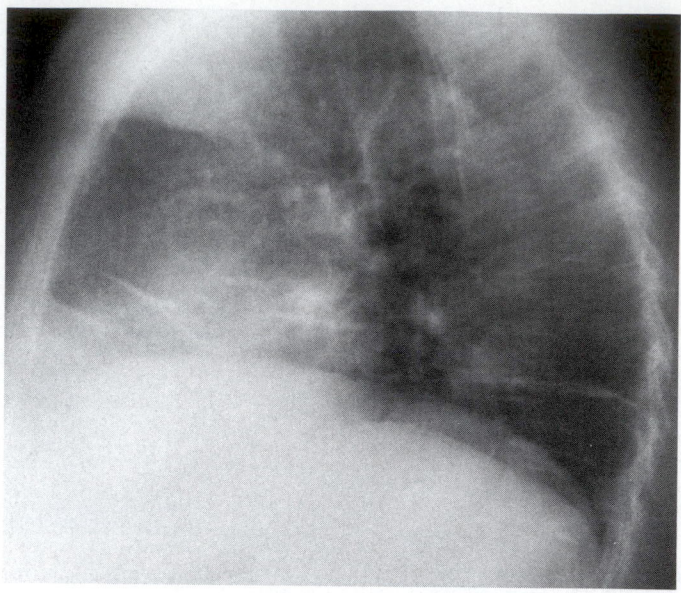

FIGURE 73-12 Diaphragmatic dysfunction in systemic lupus erythematosus. There is diaphragmatic elevation resulting in platelike atelectasis.

tients with respiratory muscle weakness, no evidence for a generalized neuromuscular disease can be found. The pathogenesis of respiratory muscle dysfunction remains unexplained, although phrenic nerve conduction abnormalities have been excluded.[49] Corticosteroids are not a frequently effective treatment modality for this disorder. Progression of this restrictive process is unusual. Although no information is available, it would seem that positive pressure ventilation (c-PAP or biPAP) particularly at night would improve these patients' daytime symptoms.

Rheumatoid Arthritis

Rheumatoid arthritis primarily affects the articular surfaces, but pleuropulmonary complications are responsible for an increased morbidity and mortality. Most often cited is a 50 percent incidence for these complications, but it is likely that this underestimates their frequency. Pleuropulmonary complications are more apt to occur in patients with more severe chronic articular disease, with high titers of rheumatoid factor, and in patients who have subcutaneous nodules as well as other systemic complications such as cutaneous vasculitis, myocarditis, pericarditis, ocular inflammation, and Felty's syndrome. Remember that pleuropulmonary disease may appear in seronegative patients and that both methotrexate and gold compounds, commonly employed for treatment, can induce an interstitial lung disease, which is often difficult to distinguish from the primary forms complicating rheumatoid arthritis. Moreover, interstitial lung disease, pleuritis, and occasionally obliterative bronchiolitis may be the first and only manifestation of the rheumatoid state, preceding the articular manifestations by months to years.

PLEURISY AND PLEURAL EFFUSION

Pleural disease in a postmortem series was found in 40 percent of patients with rheumatoid arthritis. The incidence of clinically apparent pleural disease is closer to 20 percent, and the majority of patients experience mild symptoms. Furthermore, in approximately 20 percent of the patients who develop pleural complications, they do so prior to the onset of articular disease. In patients with rheumatoid arthritis, pleural complications are more common in men and occur most frequently during episodes of active articular disease and in patients with subcutaneous rheumatoid nodules.

Pleural disease is often first discovered on routine chest radiograph, and both pleural fibrosis and effusions have been reported to occur in asymptomatic patients. The pleural effusion can be unilateral or bilateral and coexist with interstitial lung disease or necrobiotic nodules. Symptomatic patients present with pleuritic pain, dyspnea, and occasionally fever. The effusion is an exudate by protein and lactic dehydrogenase criteria, and, if chronic, cholesterol concentrations are increased. Other characteristics include a low pleural fluid pH (less than 7.2) thought to be due to impaired carbon dioxide exit from the pleural space. The leukocyte counts can be as high as 15,000 cells per cubic millimeter and consist of a mixture of neutrophils and mononuclear leukocytes. As in systemic lupus erythematosus, the total and individual complement components are low, and the rheumatoid factor activity is increased. The presence of rheumatoid factor in pleural fluid has also been reported with tuberculosis, malignancy, and other infectious diseases. A low pleural fluid glucose concentration, thought to be due to a defect in glucose transport, is characteristic of rheumatoid effusions. Up to 40 percent of patients have pleural fluid glucose levels less than 10 mg/dl, and 75 percent have levels under 50 mg/dl.[38] It has been stated that cytologic examination of the pleural fluid which demonstrates a background of necrotic debris, spindle-shaped macrophages, and multinucleated histiocytes is characteristic of a rheumatoid effusion. Necrobiotic nodules are thought to be involved in the pathogenesis of the pleural effusions, but transthoracic pleural biopsy only occasionally will demonstrate this finding rather than nonspecific acute and chronic inflammation.

Treatment is not indicated for asymptomatic cases; however, corticosteroids when utilized for active articular disease are also effective in hastening the resolution of the pleural effusion. Rarely, is any other form of intervention such as intrapleural corticosteroids necessary for these patients. In the unusual case, pleural fibrosis with resultant lung entrapment occurs requiring surgical intervention. Spontaneous pneumothorax due to rupture of a necrobiotic nodule, another uncommon complication, necessitates tube thoracostomy and with persistence of the bronchopleural fistula, surgical intervention is indicated.

PULMONARY VASCULAR DISEASE

In general, pulmonary vascular disease is the least common pleuropulmonary complication in rheumatoid arthritis. The fibroproliferative plexogenic arteriopathy typical of scleroderma and systemic lupus erythematosus is an infrequent complication. When it does occur, Raynaud's phenomenon is also present. The chest radiograph indicates normal lung fields and enlarged pulmonary arteries, and there is an isolated reduction of the diffusing capacity for carbon monoxide as well as hypoxemia. Response to a calcium channel blocker has been reported.

Small-vessel vasculitis in rheumatoid arthritis occurs in the setting of diffuse alveolar hemorrhage due to pulmonary capillaritis, and this is a very rare event in rheumatoid arthritis. Several cases have been well documented and, in one, antineutrophilic cytoplasmic antibody to myeloperoxidase (p-ANCA) was present in the serum. Treatment with intravenous followed by oral corticosteroid preparations in addition to cyclophosphamide is indicated for this complication.

NECROBIOTIC (RHEUMATOID) NODULE

Radiographically visible lung parenchymal rheumatoid nodules are infrequently seen in a rheumatoid population (less than 1 percent). When they do occur, they are more common in men with active articular disease and high rheumatoid factors and in those who have subcutaneous nodules.[44] The nodules are primarily a chest radiograph finding, since most are asymptomatic. The major problem is differentiating the necrobiotic nodule from either malignant or infectious granulomatous diseases. Occasionally, cough and hemoptysis are the presenting symptoms. Radiographically, the nodules can be single or multiple with upper and midzone predilection, and approximately 50 percent will undergo cavitation due to the large amounts of proteolytic enzymes in these lesions. The size is variable, and nodules up to 7 cm have been reported. Spontaneous resolution and recurrence are to be expected. Continuous growth, although possible, should prompt a more aggressive diagnostic approach. In most cases, no treatment is required.

Caplan's syndrome refers to a radiographic picture that developed in Welsh coal miners with rheumatoid arthritis.[12] It consists of the sudden appearance of discrete nodules primarily in the upper lobes that are histologically identical to the necrobiotic nodule (Fig. 73-13). The incidence of necrobiotic nodules

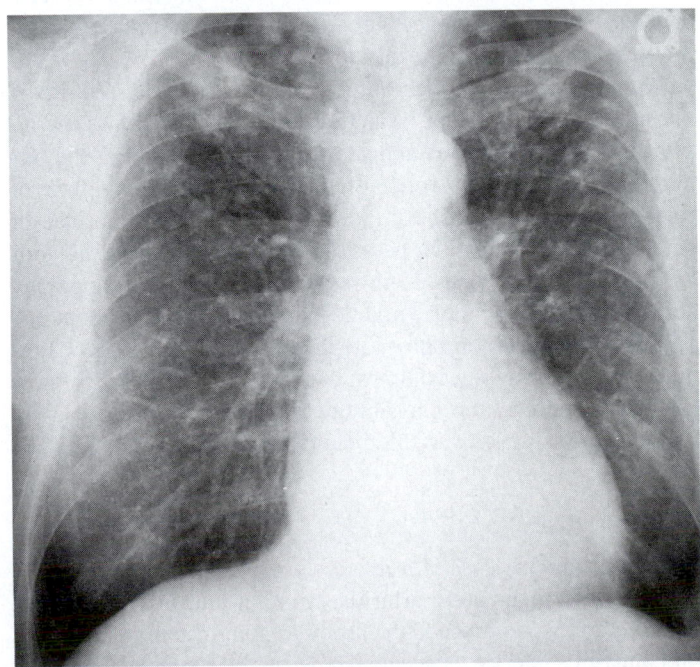

FIGURE 73-13 Caplan's syndrome in a patient with rheumatoid arthritis and silicosis (hard-rock miner). There are multiple small nodules in the middle and upper lung representing the silicosis. In addition, multiple upper-zone rheumatoid nodules are present.

is higher in rheumatoid patients with underlying pneumoconiosis, including coal workers' pneumoconiosis, silicosis, and asbestosis, than it is in a general rheumatoid population.

AIRWAY DISEASE

Upper airway involvement by the rheumatoid process is most likely to involve the cricoarytenoid joint, causing difficulty with inspiration and occasionally resulting in stridor. A sore throat, hoarseness, and fullness in the throat are other common complaints. The prevalence of this complication, although asymptomatic in the majority of cases, approaches 50 percent when screening by computed tomography scanning is employed. Clinically significant disease can be detected by performing flow volume loops which indicate a variable extrathoracic obstruction of the inspiratory loop.

Bronchiolitis obliterans or obliterative bronchiolitis is a well recognized cause of progressive and often severe obstructive lung disease in patients with rheumatoid arthritis.[17] This complication was first thought to be a consequence of either penicillamine or gold therapy, but many cases have appeared in the absence of either treatment. The onset of obliterative bronchiolitis is insidious, with patients complaining of progressive dyspnea and cough in the face of a normal or hyperinflated chest radiograph (Fig. 73-14A). Initially, it was thought that this complication was limited to women, but this is not the case. Physical examination reveals a generalized reduction of breath sounds and occasionally an inspiratory squeak. Physiological testing reveals varying degrees of airflow limitation and hyperinflation, and the diffusing capacity may be normal or reduced. High-resolution computed tomography demonstrates adjacent areas of decreased and increased attenuation (geographic pattern) (Fig. 73-14B). Some patients have responded to treatment with a combination of corticosteroids and cyclophosphamide, but the majority of cases progress to hypercapnic respiratory failure.

Another form of bronchiolitis seen in rheumatoid arthritis is a respiratory or follicular bronchiolitis consisting of a dense infiltration of lymphocytes and plasma cells surrounding the terminal and respiratory bronchioles. These patients complain of cough and dyspnea. Chest radiographs are either normal or demonstrate a fine nodular pattern more predominant in the middle and lower lung zones. High-resolution computed tomography demonstrates centrilobular nodules and bronchiectasis (Fig. 73-15). There is usually no physiological evidence for airflow limitation or reduced lung volumes, but rather gas exchange abnormalities dominate the physiological picture. Treatment with corticosteroids yields variable results.

INTERSTITIAL LUNG DISEASE

Interstitial lung disease is a relatively common complication in patients with rheumatoid arthritis. It is not unusual for interstitial lung disease to precede the articular manifestations for a significant time interval. The incidence of this complication in a rheumatoid population is difficult to determine, being reported in 5 to 40 percent of patients depending upon the methods of detection. The utility of bronchoalveolar lavage indicating alveolar inflammation and high-resolution computed tomographic

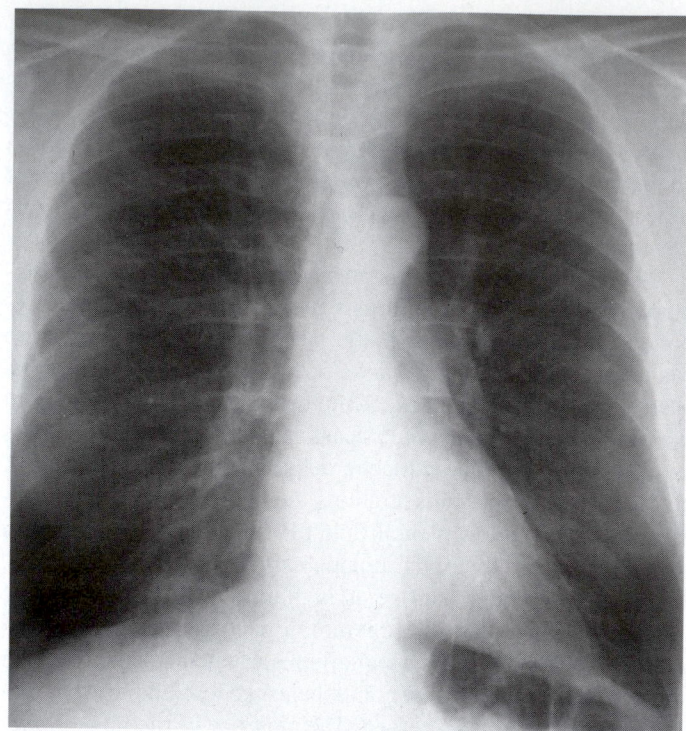

A

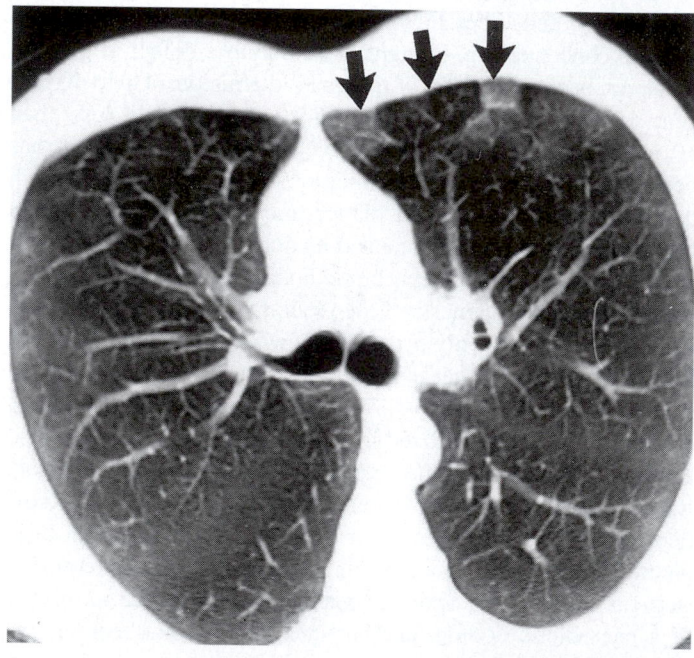

B

FIGURE 73-14 Obliterative bronchiolitis in a patient with rheumatoid arthritis. *A.* The chest radiograph is normal except for hyperinflation. *B.* A high-resolution tomographic scan demonstrating areas of increased and decreased attenuation (arrows).

scans indicating various interstitial changes, often in the face of a negative chest radiograph, are difficult to interpret. This is because follow-up studies determining whether these patients developed clinically apparent interstitial lung disease are lacking. Furthermore, some parenchymal changes described on computed tomography such as bronchiectasis have very little if any clinical significance. It is likely that clinically important interstitial

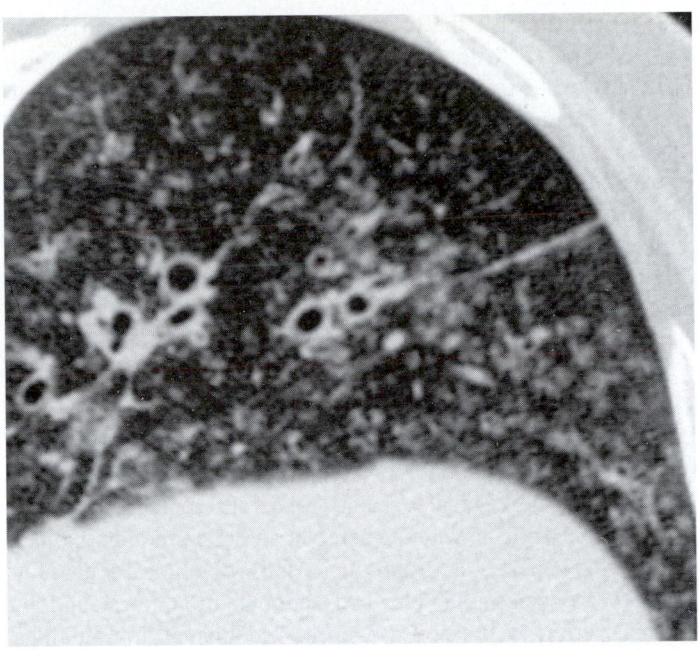

FIGURE 73-15 Respiratory bronchiolitis in rheumatoid arthritis. High-resolution computed tomography demonstrating multiple centrilobular nodules.

lung disease occurs in 5 to 10 percent of patients with rheumatoid arthritis, the most common form being usual interstitial pneumonitis with varying degrees of cellular interstitial pneumonitis. These patients are dyspneic and complain of cough. Physical examination reveals bibasilar crackles, clubbing of the digits in up to 75 percent, and evidence of cor-pulmonale when pulmonary hypertension appears secondary to hypoxic vasoconstriction. The chest radiograph and computed tomographic scan demonstrate varying degrees of interstitial infiltrates with predilection for the lung bases and lung periphery (Fig. 73-16A). Other features include ground glass attenuation on computed tomography with mixed alveolar-interstitial infiltrates on chest radiograph indicating a component of cellular interstitial pneumonitis. Both imaging studies in advanced disease reveal the presence of honeycomb lung (Fig. 73-16B).

Two other interstitial reactions which produce subacute or chronic symptoms complicate rheumatoid arthritis. The first is bronchiolitis obliterans organizing pneumonia, which can present with identical symptoms to usual interstitial pneumonia and preempt the onset of the articular disease as well. The chest radiograph (Fig. 73-17) and computed tomographic scan differ from that seen in usual interstitial pneumonia because the infiltrates are primarily alveolar and localized, patchy, or diffuse. The second interstitial reaction is lymphocytic interstitial pneumonia, which occurs when rheumatoid arthritis is complicated by Sjogren's syndrome. In addition to dyspnea and cough, these patients complain of dry mouth and eyes (keratoconjunctivitis sicca and xerostomia). The chest radiograph indicates patchy alveolar infiltrates primarily seen at the lung bases.

It is important to establish the underlying histology, since response to therapy and prognosis differs. Unless the imaging studies indicate end-stage honeycomb lung, which can also result from unresponsive or recurrent bronchiolitis obliterans organizing pneumonia and lymphocytic interstitial pneumonia as well as usual interstitial pneumonitis, further evaluation is indicated.

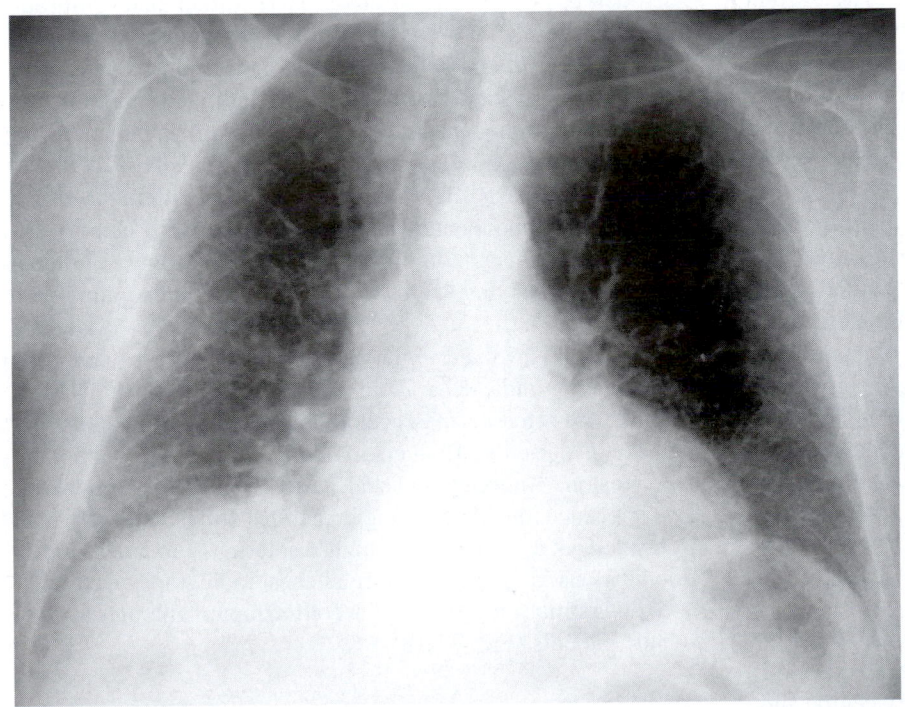

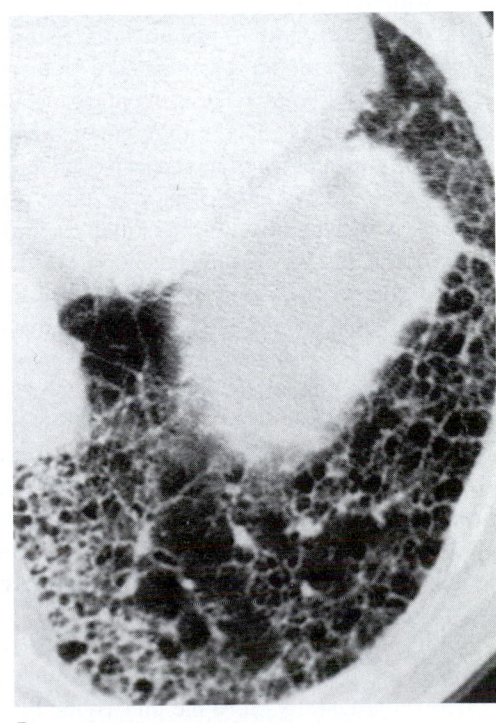

A

B

FIGURE 73-16 Usual interstitial pneumonitis in rheumatoid arthritis. *A.* Chest radiograph demonstrating lower zone and peripheral reticulonodular infiltrates. *B.* High-resolution computed tomography demonstrating a cystic network (honeycomb lung) at the lung base in a patient with advanced disease.

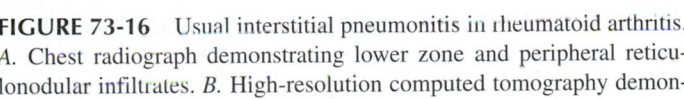

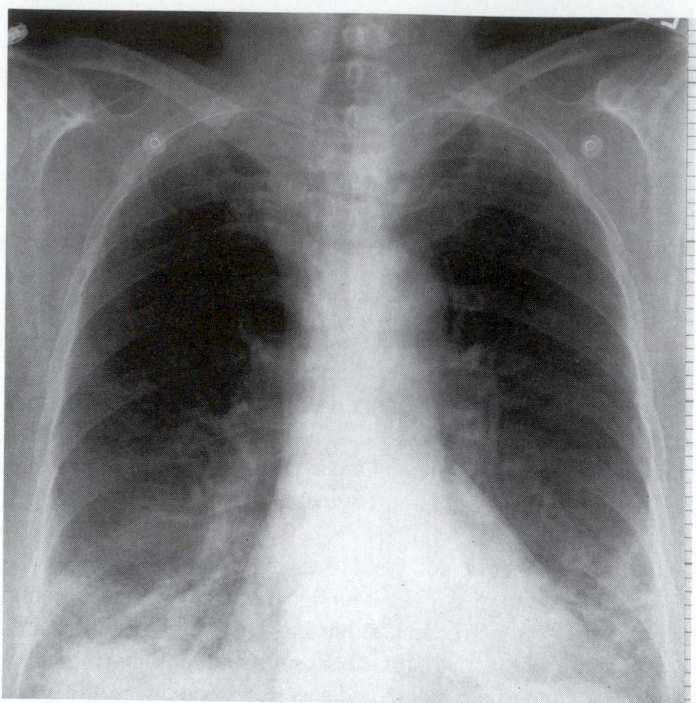

FIGURE 73-17 Bronchiolitis obliterans organizing pneumonia in rheumatoid arthritis. Chest radiograph demonstrating lower-zone mixed alveolar-interstitial infiltrates.

Bronchoalveolar lavage will not necessarily help differentiate between these three histologic pictures, but the finding of increased lymphocytic percentages as opposed to neutrophils and eosinophils indicates the potential for therapeutic responsiveness. Alveolar infiltrates and increased lymphocyte percentages are seen in lymphocytic interstitial pneumonitis. Bronchiolitis obliterans organizing pneumonia is associated with increases in neutrophil, eosinophil, and lymphocyte percentages as well as radiographic alveolar infiltrates. The finding of increased neutrophil and eosinophils percentages in suspected underlying usual interstitial pneumonitis is an indicator of poor prognosis. Therefore patients with lymphocytic interstitial pneumonitis and bronchiolitis obliterans organizing pneumonia are more treatment responsive when compared to those with usual interstitial pneumonitis. If imaging studies and bronchoalveolar lavage cellular analysis are not definitive, thorascopic open lung biopsy should be considered. Treatment consists of a corticosteroid preparation and often the addition of cytotoxic drugs in the nonresponsive cases. As opposed to the idiopathic variety of bronchiolitis obliterans organizing pneumonia, in which 66 percent of cases have favorable responses to corticosteroid medications, those associated with collagen vascular diseases are less responsive to treatment, often recur with tapering of the treatment regimen, and can progress to usual interstitial pneumonitis.

Gold-induced pneumonitis must be differentiated from the primary forms of interstitial lung disease in rheumatoid arthritis patients, particularly since the underlying histology can be similar indicating varying degrees of cellular interstitial pneumonitis and bronchiolitis obliterans organizing pneumonia.[22] Dyspnea and cough usually begin 4 to 6 weeks following initiation of therapy, and peripheral eosinophilia occurs in a minority of cases. Occasionally, the chest radiograph will demonstrate upper- as opposed to lower-zone mixed alveolar interstitial infiltration. Bronchoalveolar lavage indicates a predominance of lymphocytes, and differentiation from rheumatoid interstitial lung disease can only be made after withdrawal of the drug results in remission. In severe cases with marked gas exchange abnormalities, corticosteroid therapy will occasion prompt reversal.

Methotrexate given in relatively low weekly doses (10 to 20 mg) is associated with the development of an interstitial disease in rheumatoid patients.[6] No correlation with age, sex, duration of disease, or weekly or cumulative dose could be found. Conflicting data suggest that rheumatoid patients with underlying primary rheumatoid lung disease are predisposed to develop methotrexate pneumonitis. In rheumatoid patients treated with methotrexate the incidence of methotrexate pneumonitis is 1 to 11 percent. The clinical onset is relatively acute with cough, fever, dyspnea and new mixed alveolar and interstitial pulmonary infiltrates on chest radiograph. Increased white blood cell counts with mild eosinophilia, elevated sedimentation rates, and increased serum lactic dehydrogenase are nonspecific findings. Bronchoalveolar lavage indicates lymphocytosis and should be performed to rule out an infectious etiology. Lung tissue reveals a cellular interstitial pneumonitis, organizing pneumonia, and granuloma formation reminiscent of a hypersensitivity pneumonitis. In patients who develop this clinical syndrome while on methotrexate, the drug should be discontinued, since progression to end-stage fibrosis occurs. With life-threatening respiratory failure, corticosteroids given intravenously is an effective therapy.

Scleroderma

Scleroderma or systemic sclerosis is an inflammatory-fibrotic disease that results in the laying down of excessive extracellular matrix in the skin and some internal organs. Pulmonary disease contributes significantly to both the morbidity and mortality of patients. The pathogenesis, although not well understood, involves a complex interaction among immune cells, endothelial cells, and fibroblasts. Besides the excessive extracellular matrix which in the lung results in interstitial fibrosis, there is endothelial cell damage with intimal thickening leading to luminal obliteration. This results in a form of idiopathic pulmonary hypertension.

The lung is involved in the great majority of cases and postmortem series indicate a 70 to 100 percent incidence.[14] Most patients with scleroderma develop dyspnea during the course of their illness due either to interstitial lung disease or to pulmonary hypertension. Although unusual, both of these complications have preceded the dermatologic manifestations. Further, both bronchoalveolar lavage and high-resolution computed tomographic scans in the face of normal chest radiographs have indicated interstitial lung disease in both symptomatic and asymptomatic patients (Fig. 73-18).

PLEURAL DISEASE

Although pleural fibrosis and adhesions are reported to be present in 40 percent of patients with scleroderma in postmortem studies, clinically apparent pleural thickening or pleural effusions

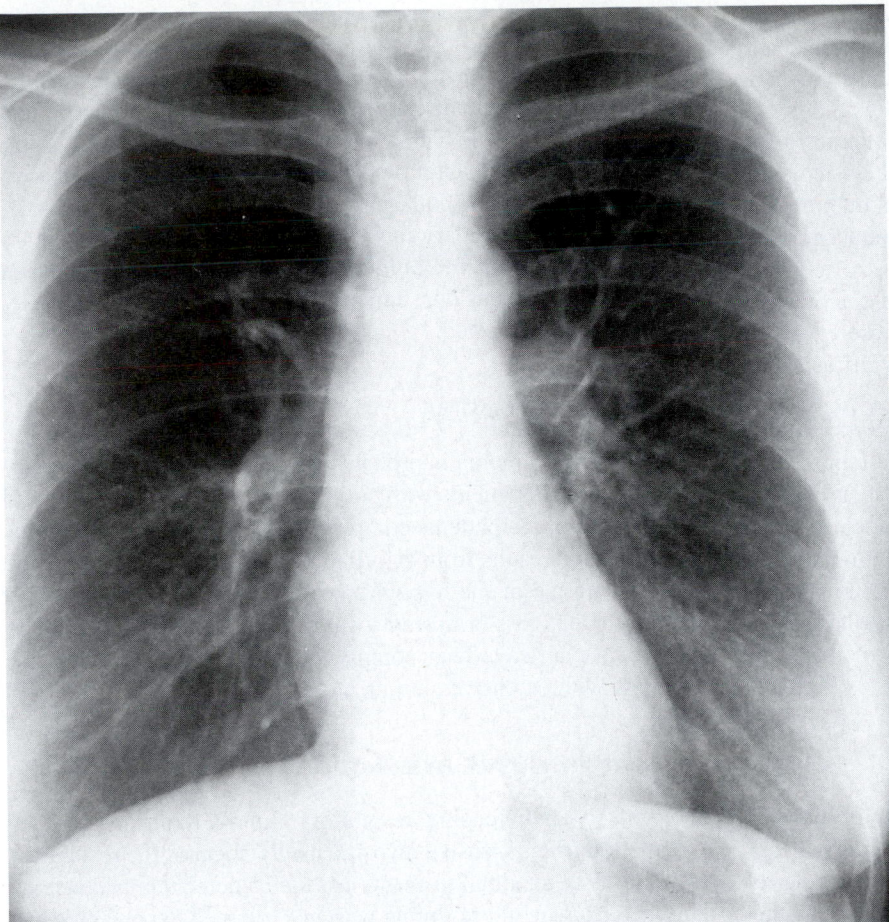

A

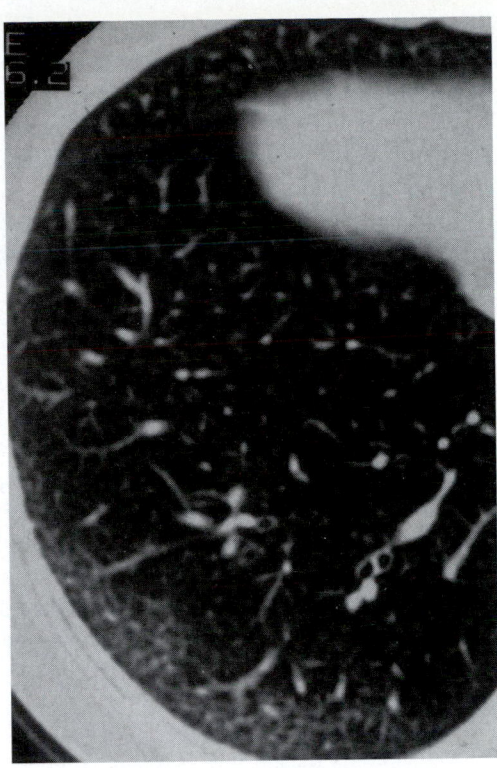

B

FIGURE 73-18 *A.* Normal chest radiograph in a dyspneic patient with scleroderma. *B.* High-resolution computed tomography of the same patient demonstrating reticular interstitial infiltrates.

on chest radiographs are considerably less frequent. The exception to this are pleural effusions secondary to congestive heart failure due to a scleroderma-associated constrictive cardiomyopathy.

INTERSTITIAL LUNG DISEASES

Usual interstitial pneumonitis progressing to honeycomb lung is the most common pulmonary complication of scleroderma, occurring in 30 to 100 percent of cases. A high-resolution computed tomographic study indicated a greater than 90 percent incidence of this abnormality. In this study, 66 percent of the cases had normal chest radiographs.[37] As many as 60 percent of patients who undergo bronchoalveolar lavage will demonstrate an abnormal inflammatory cell distribution. Clearly, chest radiographic and physiological screening indicate somewhat lower figures. The significance of the bronchoalveolar lavage and computed tomographic findings remain unclear, since no longitudinal follow-up is available. The predominant underlying histology is usual interstitial pneumonia and honeycomb lung, similar to that found in idiopathic pulmonary fibrosis. Interestingly, the survival of scleroderma patients with usual interstitial pneumonia from time of onset of dyspnea far exceeds that for idiopathic

pulmonary fibrosis.[47] It was previously thought that interstitial lung disease in scleroderma was primarily a fibrotic disorder. However, recent information derived from high-resolution tomography demonstrating ground glass attenuation which indicates more cellular disease, bronchoalveolar lavage revealing increased inflammatory cell populations, and biopsy material demonstrating cellular infiltration of the interstitium indicates the presence of a cellular inflammatory response which predates the development of fibrosis. It is likely that the inflammatory phase in most cases is clinically silent.

Usual interstitial pneumonitis is more likely to occur in the diffuse cutaneous forms of scleroderma although it may also complicate limited cutaneous system sclerosis formerly referred to as the CREST syndrome. As with other conditions associated with usual interstitial pneumonia, dyspnea with exertion and then at rest and cough are the predominant symptoms. Bibasilar crackles are heard, but clubbing is unusual due to the capillary destruction in the nail beds. Physical findings of cor-pulmonale eventually appear. Bibasilar interstitial infiltrates followed by more diffuse changes, loss of lung volume, honeycomb cysts, and pulmonary hypertension are the typical radiographic features. Scleroderma was the first interstitial lung disease in which scar carcinoma (adenocarcinoma or alveolar cell carcinoma) was reported. Physiological testing eventually reveals restrictive lung disease, preserved flow rates, and a reduced diffusing capacity. Early on, the aforementioned measurements may be normal, and hypoxemia and a widened alveolar-arterial oxygen gradient at rest and heightened by exercise may be the only physiologic abnormality. A disproportionally greater reduction of the diffusing capacity when compared to lung volumes most likely indicates the presence of idiopathic pulmonary hypertension due to plexogenic arteriopathy, particularly in the limited cutaneous form of systemic sclerosis.

Other forms of interstitial lung disease seen in scleroderma include lymphocytic interstitial pneumonitis in those cases associated with Sjogren's syndrome, and rare cases of diffuse alveolar hemorrhage have been reported.

Treatment is empiric, with beneficial effects in corticosteroid failures accorded to cyclophosphamide and penicillamine in a limited number of cases. Those cases in which therapeutic effect is expected are those demonstrating ground glass attenuation as compared to honeycomb change on high-resolution computed tomography, lymphocytic or even an eosinophilic predominance as opposed to neutrophil predominance on bronchoalveolar lavage, and cellular versus a fibrotic lung biopsy.

PULMONARY VASCULAR DISEASE

Idiopathic pulmonary hypertension due to a primary fibroproliferative process involving the pulmonary vessels occurs in approximately 10 percent of cases of scleroderma and is primarily seen in the limited cutaneous forms (CREST syndrome). In this form of scleroderma, idiopathic pulmonary hypertension may coexist with usual interstitial pneumonitis. Patients present with a gradual onset of dyspnea and increasing fatigue. Physical examination and chest radiograph may initially be normal, and, with disease progression, physical and radiographic signs of pulmonary hypertension appear. Lung volumes and airflow parameters are maintained unless there is concomitant interstitial lung disease. Typically there is an isolated reduction in the diffusing capacity as well as progressive hypoxemia. At present, treatment consists of supplemental oxygen, since the use of vasodilator compounds are generally unsuccessful. Survival past 5 years from the time of diagnosis is unusual. Trials with continuous intravenous prostacycline, which appears to be beneficial for other forms of primary pulmonary hypertension, are soon to commence for the collagen vascular diseases.

ASPIRATION PNEUMONIA

There is a high incidence of esophageal dilitation and decreased peristalsis in patients with scleroderma, particularly in the limited cutaneous variety. This leads to dysphagia, heartburn, gastroesophageal reflux, and recurrent aspiration pneumonia. It has long been held that aspiration contributes to the development of interstitial lung disease. A definitive study has indicated that direct measurements of gastroesophageal reflux did not correlate with physiological impairment (low lung volumes and diffusing capacity) in these patients.[42]

Polymyositis-Dermatomyositis

In polymyositis-dermatomyositis, pulmonary complications are common, are important causes of morbidity and mortality, and often predate or overshadow the muscle or skin manifestations. Pulmonary involvement has been reported in 40 percent of cases. In contrast to the other collagen vascular diseases, in polymyositis-dermatomyositis primary involvement of the airways and pleura do not occur. Idiopathic pulmonary hypertension has been seen on only several occasions, and in these cases crossover with scleroderma was suspected.

ASPIRATION PNEUMONIA

Aspiration pneumonia is probably the most common pulmonary complication in patients with polymyositis-dermatomyositis, and almost half of the patients complain of dysphagia as well.[15] This complication results from an inflammatory myositis affecting the striated muscle of the hypopharynx and upper esophagus. As a result, there is loss of normal swallowing function and failure to protect the airway. This complication is more likely in those patients with extensive skin or muscle involvement.

RESPIRATORY MUSCLE DYSFUNCTION

Fortunately, hypercapnic respiratory failure requiring assisted ventilation from extensive myositic involvement of the respiratory muscles is an uncommon event (less than 5 percent prevalence).[34] In fact, in a patient presenting with unexplained hypercapnic respiratory failure, this entity as well as other neuromuscular problems should be entertained. With less extensive involvement of these muscles, however, there is a reduction in cough generation and the potential for the development of hypostatic pneumonia and atelectasis due to mucous plugging. This weakness can also cause a restricted physiological defect with resulting tachypnea and dyspnea in the face of a normal diffusing capacity, normoxemia, and hyperventilation. Respiratory muscle dysfunction as the cause of restrictive lung disease can best be demonstrated by measurement of the maximal pressure generated during both phases of the respiratory cycle. Pressures are reduced, and sequential measurements are useful for monitoring the disease course and response to treatment.

INTERSTITIAL LUNG DISEASE

The prevalence of interstitial lung disease in polymyositis-dermatomyositis ranges from 5 to 30 percent. More recently, Japanese series indicate a much higher incidence (40 to 80 percent). As in the other collagen vascular diseases, the use of bronchoalveolar lavage and high-resolution computed tomography for screening will increase the incidence figures.

Usual interstitial pneumonitis is the histologic type of interstitial lung disease in polymyositis-dermatomyositis. However, diffuse alveolar damage, bronchiolitis obliterans organizing pneumonia, and diffuse alveolar hemorrhage secondary to pulmonary capillaritis may also occur.[35,36,41] All forms of interstitial lung disease may proceed, appear simultaneously with, or follow the muscle or skin manifestations. There is no relationship between interstitial lung disease and the extent of muscle or skin disease, the level of creatine phosphokinase elevation, or the presence of serum rheumatoid factor or antinuclear antibodies. There is, however, a relationship between interstitial lung disease and a serum antibody directed against the cellular enzyme histidyl-tRNA-synthetase, known as anti-Jo-1.[7] This antibody appears in 25 percent of patients with polymyositis-dermatomyositis and is present in 50 percent of patients with interstitial lung disease and in 13 percent of patients who do not have this complication. In a patient thought to have idiopathic pulmonary fibrosis who is also positive for anti-Jo-1 antibody, there is a good chance that polymyositis-dermatomyositis will develop at a later date.

All forms of interstitial lung disease in this disorder are more common in women. Several clinical syndromes occur depending on the underlying interstitial lung disease. The most common presentation is chronic cough and progressive dyspnea due to usual interstitial pneumonitis with varying degrees of cellular interstitial pneumonitis. Digital clubbing is rarely if ever seen. Chest radiographs demonstrate reticulonodular infiltrates, and with disease progression there is a reduction of the lung volume and the development of radiographic honeycomb lung and pulmonary hypertension. Physiological testing indicates a restrictive pattern with a low diffusing capacity. Response to treatment depends upon the underlying histology, the more cellular disease being more responsive.

There is also an acute pulmonary presentation whose clinical and radiographic picture is reminiscent of a diffuse infectious pneumonia. Here the underlying lesion is diffuse alveolar damage.[13,41] Severe respiratory failure occurs, and recovery is unusual in spite of aggressive anti-inflammatory and immunosuppressive therapy. Bronchiolitis obliterans organizing pneumonia may have either an acute or subacute presentation (Fig. 73-19). The differentiation from diffuse alveolar damage becomes important because of the marked disparity in treatment outcome and survival. In bronchiolitis obliterans organizing pneumonia, corticosteroid responsiveness with or without an additional agent is the rule rather than the exception. The most recently described interstitial reaction reported in polymyositis-dermatomyositis is diffuse alveolar hemorrhage due to pulmonary capillaritis.[36] This complication appears simultaneously with the onset of the muscle disease. Although alveolar hemorrhage was present on histologic sections, hemoptysis did not occur. As with other forms of pulmonary capillaritis, these patients responded to corticosteroid and cyclophosphamide.

Mixed Connective Tissue Disease

Patients with mixed connective disease have features of systemic lupus erythematosus, polymyositis-dermatomyositis, and scleroderma. Mixed connective disease is characterized by elevated titers of a specific antinuclear antibody directed against nuclear ribonucleoprotein. Because of the similarity of mixed connective tissue disease to the aforementioned collagen vascular diseases, pleuropulmonary complications are frequent, occurring in 20 to 80 percent of cases.[28]

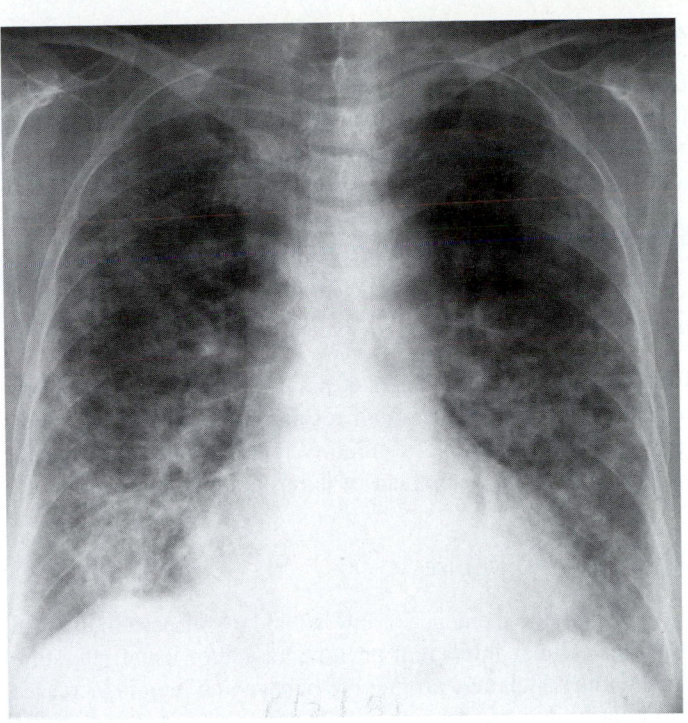

FIGURE 73-19   Bronchiolitis obliterans organizing pneumonia in a patient with polymyositis-dermatomyositis and acute symptoms. Chest radiograph demonstrating diffuse patchy alveolar infiltrates.

PLEURAL DISEASE

Although pleurisy has been reported to occur in 40 percent of cases, pleural effusion appears in approximately 5 percent.[39] It is an exudative effusion, but very little information concerning its characteristics is available in the literature.

PULMONARY VASCULAR DISEASE

Pulmonary hypertension may be caused by recurrent pulmonary emboli, hypoxic vasoconstriction secondary to interstitial lung disease, or idiopathic pulmonary hypertension due to a plexogenic arteriopathy as occurs in systemic lupus erythematosus and scleroderma. This is a significant problem for these patients; however, the incidence is unknown.[43] The pathologic features of the idiopathic variety are similar to those seen for systemic lupus erythematosus and scleroderma. These patients, primarily women, present with dyspnea and fatigue, normal chest radiographs except for pulmonary arterial enlargement, and an isolated reduction in the diffusing capacity for carbon monoxide. Survival, as with this form of pulmonary hypertension in the other collagen vascular disease, is rather dismal. There are a few reports of a medium-size pulmonary artery vasculitis in mixed connective tissue disease, and one patient had evidence for immune complex deposition (IgG, C_3) in the vascular walls.[46]

These patients may also have a circulating lupus anticoagulant (antiphospholipid syndrome), thereby making these women more susceptible to pulmonary embolism. Recurrent small pulmonary emboli may mimic the clinical picture of idiopathic pulmonary hypertension.[19]

ASPIRATION PNEUMONIA

In those patients with mixed connective tissue disease whose features resemble scleroderma or polymyositis-dermatomyositis, esophageal dysmotility and dilitation can be a significant problem leading to reflux esophagitis and recurrent aspiration pneumonia. The incidence of abnormal esophageal manometry in one series was greater than 50 percent.[29]

RESPIRATORY MUSCLE DYSFUNCTION

In those patients with features of polymyositis-dermatomyositis, an inflammatory myositis with respiratory muscle involvement may lead to hypercapnic respiratory failure or a restrictive lung disease with the development of hypostatic pneumonia.[39]

INTERSTITIAL LUNG DISEASE

As expected, the incidence of interstitial lung disease in the form of either cellular interstitial pneumonia and/or usual interstitial pneumonia which may progress to honeycomb lung is increased, particularly in those patients with the features of scleroderma. If one applies physiological as opposed to radiographic criteria, the incidence approaches 80 percent. As with the other connective tissue diseases, this interstitial lung disease manifests as progressive dyspnea, bibasilar reticulonodular infiltrates on chest radiograph, and physiological parameters which indicate low lung volumes and a reduction in the diffusing capacity for carbon monoxide.

Diffuse alveolar hemorrhage has been reported in a few cases of mixed connective tissue disease and is similar in presentation to this complication in systemic lupus erythematosus. Histologic evaluation of the lung was not available (bland hemorrhage versus pulmonary capillaritis).[32]

Sjögren's Syndrome

Sjögren's syndrome refers to a triad of keratoconjunctivitis sicca, xerostomia, and polyarthritis. This is an autoimmune exocrinopathy characterized by lymphocytic infiltration of the luminal and salivary glands. There is a primary form of this syndrome as well as a secondary form associated with one of the other collagen vascular diseases, most frequently rheumatoid arthritis. There is a strong female predominance (greater than 90 percent).[8] Positive rheumatoid factor (95 percent) and antinuclear antibodies in a speckled pattern (80 percent) are to be expected as well as positive tests for antibodies to extractable nuclear antigens (anti-SSA, anti-SSB) which are specific for the primary form of the syndrome.[3]

AIRWAY DISEASE

Because of lymphoid infiltration of the mucous glands resulting in dessication of the tracheobronchial tree, these patients develop hoarseness, cough, inspissation of secretions resulting in atelec-

tasis, recurrent pneumonias, and commonly bronchiectasis.[27] There is a high incidence of obstructive ventilatory dysfunction in these patients, and occasionally obliterative bronchiolitis occurs.

INTERSTITIAL LUNG DISEASE

This occurs more often in the secondary forms of Sjogren's syndrome and most likely represents a complication of the associated collagen vascular disease. Therefore, in secondary Sjogren's syndrome usual interstitial pneumonia, cellular interstitial pneumonitis, and bronchiolitis obliterans organizing pneumonia are not unusual. Usual interstitial pneumonia, however, is unusual in the primary form of Sjogren's syndrome.[21]

As lymphocytic infiltration of the upper airway typifies either type of Sjogren's syndrome, so does lymphoproliferation in the lung parenchyma. This occurs in two forms, lymphocytic interstitial pneumonitis and, less commonly, pseudolymphoma. Both of these lesions have the potential for lymphomatous conversion.[33] Lymphocytic interstitial pneumonitis is an interstitial lung disease, and therefore cough, dyspnea, and a restrictive lung disease are to be expected. Because lymphocytes also infiltrate the alveolar spaces as well as the interstitium, the radiologic studies indicate mixed alveolar and interstitial infiltrates. The development of pleural effusion or the appearance of hilar or mediastinal adenopathy often but not always indicates the development of a lymphoma. Lymphocytic interstitial pneumonia is quite responsive to anti-inflammatory agents, occasionally requiring immunosuppressive therapy. Cyclosporin has also been recommended in corticosteroid resistant cases.[25]

Pseudolymphoma is often difficult to distinguish from a malignant lymphoma. This tumorlike proliferation appears as single or multiple masses on the chest radiograph. It has been suggested that pseudolymphoma, which is considered to be a localized form of lymphocytic interstitial pneumonitis, is a premalignant lesion. If associated with a monoclonal gammopathy, malignant conversion probably has occurred.[45]

Ankylosing Spondylitis

Ankylosing spondylitis is one of the seronegative spondyloarthropathies which may eventually result in fixation of the chest wall and a mild to moderate restrictive lung disease. Since there is no muscular involvement, diaphragmatic function is preserved, so respiratory failure on the basis of the chest wall fixation does not occur.[16]

The incidence of interstitial lung disease complication is repordedly less than 2 percent.[31] In contrast to the other collagen vascular diseases, it has a predilection for the upper lung zones, only appears late in the course of the chronic spondylitis, and never precedes it. This complication often appears fibrocystic on the chest radiograph (Fig. 73-20) and is difficult to distinguish from tuberculosis. Histologically it is a fibrosing process with cystic formation. Progressive dyspnea and cough are the predominant symptoms, and treatment with corticosteroids is ineffective and therefore not indicated. The most serious complication of this apical fibrocystic disease is infection with invasive

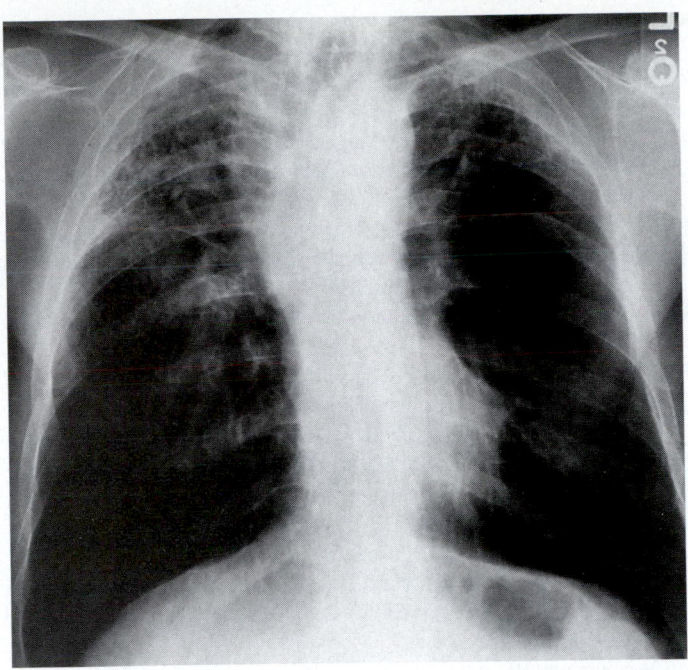

FIGURE 73-20 Ankylosing spondylitis. Chest radiograph demonstrating bilateral upper-zone fibronodular infiltrates.

aspergilla species as well as atypical mycobacteria. Further, saprophytic colonization of the cysts by aspergilla species (fungus balls) may induce life-threatening hemoptysis.[40]

REFERENCES

1. Abramson SB, Dobro J, Eberle MA, et al: Acute reversible hypoxemia in systemic lupus erythematosus. *Ann Intern Med* 114:941–947, 1991.
2. Alarcon-Segovia D, Deleze M, Oria CV, et al: Antiphospholipid antibodies and the antiphospholipid syndrome in systemic lupus erythematosus: a prospective analysis of 500 consecutive patients. *Medicine* 89:353–365, 1989.
3. Alspaugh MA, Tan EM: Antibodies to cellular antigen in Sjogren's syndrome. *J Clin Invest* 55:1067–1073, 1973.
4. Asherson RA, Higenbottam TW, Xuan D, et al: Pulmonary hypertension in a lupus clinic: experience with 24 patients. *J Rheumatol* 17:1292–1298, 1990.
5. Bankier AA, Kiener HP, Wiesmayr MN, et al: Discrete lung involvement in systemic lupus erythematosus: CT assessment. *Radiology* 196:835–840, 1995.
6. Barrear P, Laan R, vanRiel P, et al: Methotrexate related pulmonary complications in rheumatoid arthritis. *Ann Rheum Dis* 53:434–439, 1994.
7. Bernstein RM, Morgan SH, Chapman J, et al: Anti-Jo-1 antibody: a marker for myositis with interstitial lung disease. *Br Med J* 289:151–152, 1984.
8. Block KG, Buchanan WW, Wohl MJ, et al: Sjogren's syndrome. *Medicine* 44:187–231, 1965.
9. Boulware DW, Hedgpeth MT: Lupus pneumonitis and anti-SSA(Ro) antibodies. *J Rheumatol* 16:479–481, 1989.
10. Brucato A, Baudo F, Barberis M, et al: Pulmonary hypertension secondary to thrombosis of the pulmonary vessels in a patient with the primary antiphospholipid syndrome. *J Rheumatol* 21:942–944, 1994.
11. Byrd RB, Trunk G: Systemic lupus erythematosus presenting as pulmonary hemosiderosis. *Chest* 64:128–129, 1973.
12. Caplan A: Certain unusual radiographic appearances in the chest of coal miners suffering from rheumatoid arthritis. *Thorax* 8:19–37, 1953.
13. Clawson K, Oddis CV: Adult respiratory distress syndrome in polymyositis patients with the anti-Jo-1 antibody. *Arthritis Rheum* 35:1519–1523, 1995.
14. D'angelow W, Fries W, Masi A, et al: Pathologic observations in systemic sclerosis (Scleroderma). *Am J Med* 46:428–440, 1969.
15. Dickey BF, Myers AR: Pulmonary disease in polymyositis-dermatomyositis. *Semin Arthritis Rheum* 14:60–76, 1984.
16. Fisher LR, Lawley MI, Holgate ST: Relation between chest expansion, pulmonary function and exercise tolerance in patients with ankylosing spondylitis. *J Rheum Dis* 49:921–925, 1990.
17. Geddes DM, Corrin B, Brewerton DA, et al: Progressive airway obliteration in adults and its association with rheumatoid disease. *Q J Med* 46:427–444, 1977.
18. Gross M, Esterley R, Earle RH: Pulmonary alterations in systemic lupus erythematosus. *Am Rev Respir Dis* 105:572–577, 1972.
19. Hainaut P, Lavenne E, Magy JM, Lebacq EG: Circulating lupus type anticoagulant and pulmonary hypertension associated with mixed connective tissue disease. *Clin Rheumatol* 5:96–101, 1986.
20. Homma Y, Ohtsuka Y, Tanimura K, et al: Can interstitial pneumonia as the sole presentation of collagen vascular disease be differentiated from idiopathic interstitial pneumonia? *Respiration* 62:248–251, 1995.
21. Kadota J, Kusano S, Kawakami K, et al: Usual interstitial pneumonia associated with primary Sjogren's syndrome. *Chest* 108:1756–1758, 1995.
22. Levinson ML, Lynch JP, Bower JS: Reversal of progressive gold hypersensitivity pneumonitis by corticosteroids. *Am J Med* 71:908–912, 1981.
23. Love PE, Santoro SA: Antiphospholipid antibodies: anticardiolipin and the lupus anticoagulant systemic lupus erythematosus (SLE) and in non-SLE disorders. *Ann Intern Med* 112:682–698, 1990.
24. Matthay RA, Schwarz MI, Petty TL, et al: Pulmonary manifestations of systemic lupus erythematosis: review of 12 cases of acute lupus pneumonitis. *Medicine* 54:397–409, 1975.
25. Moolman JA, Bardin PG, Rossouw DJ, Joubert JR: Cyclosporin as a treatment for interstitial lung disease of unknown etiology. *Thorax* 46:592–595, 1991.
26. Myers JL, Katzenstein AL: Microangiitis in lupus-induced pulmonary hemorrhage. *Am J Clin Pathol* 85:552–556, 1986.
27. Newball HH, Brahim SA: Chronic obstructive airway disease in patients with Sjogren's syndrome. *Am Rev Respir Dis* 115:295–304, 1977.
28. Prakash UBS: Lungs in mixed connective tissue disease. *J Thorac Imaging* 7:55–61, 1992.
29. Prakash UBS, Luthra HS, Divertie MB: Intrathoracic manifestations of mixed connective tissue disease. *Mayo Clin Proc* 60:813–821, 1985.
30. Rosenow EC, Sirimlan CV, Muhm JR, et al: Pleuropulmonary manifestations of ankylosing spondylitis. *Mayo Clin Proc* 52:641–649, 1977.
31. Rosner S, Ginzler EM, Diamond HS, et al: A multicenter study of outcome in systemic lupus erythematosus: II. Causes of death. *Arthritis Rheum* 25:612–617, 1982.

32. Sanchez-Guerrero J, Cesarman G, Alarcon-Segovia D: Massive pulmonary hemorrhage in mixed connective tissue disease. *J Rheumatol* 16:1132–1134, 1989.

33. Schuurman HJ, Gooszen HC, Tan IW: Low grade lymphoma of immature T-cell phenotype in a case of lymphocytic interstitial pneumonia and Sjogren's syndrome. *Histopathology* 11:1193–1204, 1987.

34. Schwarz MI: Pulmonary and cardiac manifestations of polymyositis-dermatomyositis. *J Thorac Imaging* 7:46–54, 1992.

35. Schwarz MI, Matthay RA, Sahn SA, et al: Interstitial lung disease in polymyositis-dermatomyositis: analysis of 6 cases and review of the literature. *Medicine* 55:89–104, 1976.

36. Schwarz MI, Sutarik JM, Nick J, et al: Pulmonary capillaritis and diffuse alveolar hemorrhage: a primary manifestation of polymyositis. *Am J Respir Crit Care Med* 151:2037–2040, 1995.

37. Schurawitzki H, Stiglbauer R, Graninger W, et al: Interstitial lung disease in progressive systemic sclerosis: high resolution CT versus radiography. *Radiology* 176:755–759, 1990.

38. Shannon TM, Gale ME: Non-cardiac manifestations of rheumatoid arthritis in the thorax. *J Thorac Imaging* 7:19–29, 1992.

39. Sullivan WD, Hurst DJ, Harmen CE, et al: A prospective evaluation emphasizing pulmonary involvement in patients with mixed connective tissue disease. *Medicine* 63:92–107, 1984.

40. Tanoue L: Pulmonary involvement in collagen vascular disease: a review of the pulmonary manifestations of the Marrfan-Syndrome, ankylosing spondylitis, Sjogren's syndrome, and relapsing polychondritis. *J Thorac Imaging* 7:62–77, 1992.

41. Tazelaar HD, Viggiano RW, Pickersgill J, Colby TV: Interstitial lung disease in polymyositis and dermatomyositis: clinical features, and prognosis is correlated with histological findings. *Am Rev Respir Dis* 141:727–733, 1990.

42. Troshinsky MB, Kane GC, Varga J, et al: Pulmonary function and gastroesophogeal reflux in systemic sclerosis. *Ann Intern Med* 121:6–10, 1994.

43. Veda N, Mimura K, Maeda H, et al: Mixed connective tissue disease with fatal pulmonary hypertension and a review of the literature. *Virchows Arch [A]*. 404:335–340, 1984.

44. Walker WC, Wright V: Pulmonary lesions and rheumatoid arthritis. *Medicine* 47:501–520, 1968.

45. Walters MT, Stevenson FK, Herbert A, et al: Urinary monoclonal free light chaining in primary Sjogren's syndrome: an aid to the diagnosis of malignant lymphoma. *Ann Rheum Dis* 45:210–219, 1986.

46. Weiner-Kronish JP, Solinger AM, Warnock ML, et al: Severe pulmonary involvement in mixed connective tissue disease. *Am Rev Respir Med* 124:499–503, 1981.

47. Wells AU, Cullinan P, Hansell DM, et al: Fibrosing alveolitis associated with systemic sclerosis has a better prognosis than lone cryptogenic fibrosing alveolitis. *Am J Respir Crit Care Med* 149:1583–1590, 1994.

48. Wiedemann HP, Matthay RA: Pulmonary manifestations of systemic lupus erythematosus. *J Thorac Imaging* 7:1–18, 1992.

49. Wilcox PG, Stein HB, Clarke SD, et al: Phrenic nerve function in patients with diaphragmatic weakness and systemic lupus erythematosus. *Chest* 93:352–358, 1988.

CHAPTER 74

THE EOSINOPHILIC PNEUMONIAS

Carolyn L. Rochester

EOSINOPHILIC PNEUMONIAS WITH ACUTE PRESENTATIONS
  Loeffler's Syndrome (Simple Pulmonary Eosinophilia)
  Parasitic Infections
  Drug-Induced Pulmonary Eosinophilic Syndromes
  Idiopathic Acute Eosinophilic Pneumonia

TROPICAL PULMONARY EOSINOPHILIA

CHRONIC EOSINOPHILIC PNEUMONIA

ALLERGIC BRONCHOPULMONARY ASPERGILLOSIS (MYCOSIS)

CHURG-STRAUSS SYNDROME (ALLERGIC GRANULOMATOSIS AND ANGIITIS)

IDIOPATHIC HYPEREOSINOPHILIC SYNDROME

APPROACH TO THE EVALUATION OF EOSINOPHILIC PNEUMONIAS

In 1932, Loeffler first identified the association between pulmonary infiltrates and eosinophilia. Subsequently, Crofton separated the eosinophilic pneumonias into five groups on the basis of clinical criteria: Loeffler's syndrome, prolonged pulmonary eosinophilia, pulmonary eosinophilia associated with asthma, tropical eosinophilia, and periarteritis nodosa. In 1952, Reeder and Goodrich coined the term *pulmonary infiltrates with eosinophilia* (PIE syndrome) to refer to these disorders. However, it was subsequently appreciated that pulmonary infiltration with eosinophils can occur in the absence of peripheral blood eosinophilia. As a result, in 1969, Liebow and Carrington broadened the description of the term *eosinophilic pneumonia* to include all disorders characterized by infiltration of the lungs with eosinophils, with or without an excess of eosinophils in the peripheral blood. Subsequent studies also demonstrated that in numerous disorders, peripheral blood eosinophilia can occur without tissue eosinophilic infiltration. As a result, the eosinophilic pneumonias are now recognized as a heterogeneous group of disorders characterized by varying degrees of pulmonary parenchymal or blood eosinophilia.[1]

The precise role that eosinophils play in the pathogenesis of the different eosinophilic pneumonias is not clear. Our knowledge of the biology of eosinophils (see Chapter 22) does, however, suggest that they play a variety of roles, including initiation, perpetuation, and amplification of tissue inflammation and injury. These effector functions are no doubt the result of the ability of the eosinophils to release numerous soluble mediators, including granule-derived proteins, arachidonic acid metabolites, cytokines, superoxide anions, and hydroxyl radicals. The different roles of eosinophils in these disorders can be appreciated when comparisons are made of parasitic infections and disorders such as asthma or allergic bronchopulmonary aspergillosis. In the former, eosinophils play a crucial role in eradicating the infectious pathogen; in the latter, the eosinophils accumulate in the lung as a result of immune hypersensitivity and are prominent mediators of tissue injury.

The spectrum of diseases that can be primarily or secondarily associated with blood or pulmonary eosinophilia is shown in Table 74-1. It is beyond the scope of this chapter to discuss each of these disease entities in detail. Instead, discussion will focus on diseases in which eosinophilic infiltration of lung tissue is a characteristic feature, including acute eosinophilic pneumonias, tropical pulmonary eosinophilia, chronic eosinophilic pneumonia, allergic bronchopulmonary aspergillosis, Churg-Strauss syndrome, and idiopathic hypereosinophilic syndrome. Since eosinophilic granuloma of the lung is frequently seen in the absence of blood or tissue eosinophilia, it is considered separately in Chapter 76.

EOSINOPHILIC PNEUMONIAS WITH ACUTE PRESENTATIONS

Loeffler's Syndrome (Simple Pulmonary Eosinophilia)

In 1932, Loeffler first described a clinical syndrome characterized by mild respiratory symptoms, peripheral blood eosinophilia, and transient, migratory pulmonary infiltrates.[1] The term *Loeffler's syndrome,* or *simple pulmonary eosinophilia,* has been used to define the numerous similar cases reported subsequently. Immune hypersensitivity to *Ascaris lumbricoides* has been recognized as the likely cause of most of the earliest reported cases.[1] *A. suum,* a large roundworm endemic to pigs, can cause a nearly identical syndrome. Although several other parasitic infections and exposures to numerous drugs and other agents have also been recognized to induce a Loeffler's-like syndrome (see below and Table 74-2), an identifiable etiologic agent may be lacking in up to one-third of patients.[1]

TABLE 74-1

Diseases Associated with Pulmonary Infiltrates and Eosinophilia

Asthma/allergy
Bronchocentric granulomatosis
Bronchiolitis obliterans–organizing pneumonia
Infections
   Parasitic
   Fungal (esp. coccidioidomycosis, *Aspergillus*)
   Tuberculosis
   Pneumocystis carinii
Interstitial lung disease
   Idiopathic pulmonary fibrosis
   Collagen-vascular disease associated
   Sarcoidosis
   Eosinophilic granuloma (pulmonary histiocytosis X)
Malignancy
   Non–smallcell cancer of lung
   Non-Hodgkin's lymphoma
   Myeloblastic leukemia
Miscellaneous (e.g., ulcerative colitis)
Pulmonary eosinophilic syndromes
   Acute eosinophilic pneumonias (drugs, parasites, idiopathic, other)
   Tropical pulmonary eosinophilia
   Chronic eosinophilic pneumonia
   Allergic bronchopulmonary mycosis
   Churg-Strauss syndrome (allergic granulomatosis and angiitis)
   Idiopathic hypereosinophilic syndrome

tive until 8 weeks after the onset of the respiratory syndrome. Histologic evaluation of lung tissue is usually not required for confirmation of the diagnosis. When tissue has been obtained, a characteristic and striking eosinophilic infiltration of interstitium and alveolar-capillary units has been noted. Increased numbers of macrophages have also been appreciated. Tissue necrosis and vasculitis are not features of the disorder.[5]

Since Loeffler's syndrome may be induced by a variety of exposures, a search for an etiologic agent (e.g., parasitic infection or drug reaction) should be undertaken. In cases due to *Ascaris* species, treatment with oral mebendizole (100 mg twice a day for 3 days) is indicated to prevent late (e.g., 8 weeks after onset of respiratory symptoms) GI manifestations of *Ascaris* infestation, which may include malnutrition, diarrhea, abdominal pain, and/or intestinal obstruction. Since stool specimens are negative for ova and parasites early in the illness, clinical follow-up over a 2- to 3-month period is indicated.

When Loeffler's syndrome is due to *A. lumbricoides,* the pulmonary manifestations are believed to result from a hypersensitivity reaction to the *Ascaris* larvae.[1] Following ingestion of ova, larvae hatch within the small intestine, then cross the intestinal wall to enter the splanchnic and ultimately the pulmonary circulation. Subsequently, the larvae migrate across pulmonary capillaries into alveoli, mature into adult worms, ascend the large airways, and are swallowed into the gastrointestinal tract, where they complete their life cycle. The pulmonary manifestations of Loeffler's syndrome occur during the migration of larvae through the lung.

Loeffler's syndrome affects people of all ages. It is characterized clinically by the presence of low-grade fever, nonproductive cough, dyspnea (mild to severe), and occasionally hemoptysis.[1] The respiratory manifestations of Loeffler's syndrome are usually self-limited, typically resolving in 1 to 2 weeks. Laboratory examination of peripheral blood from patients reveals moderate to extreme eosinophilia, the peak levels of which may be present as respiratory symptoms resolve. Expectorated sputum, if present, frequently contains eosinophils. Transient, migratory nonsegmental interstitial and alveolar infiltrates (often peripheral or pleural based) are evident on the chest radiograph.[1] Pulmonary function evaluation typically reveals a mild to moderate restrictive ventilatory defect with a reduced diffusing capacity for carbon monoxide (D_{LCO}). During the pneumonic stage of the illness, *Ascaris* larvae may be identified in sputum or gastric aspirates. In keeping with the life cycle of *Ascaris,* stool examination for ova and parasites is typically nega-

TABLE 74-2

Drugs and Other Exposures Causing Eosinophilic Pneumonia

Ampicillin	Mephenesin carbamate
Acetaminophen	Methotrexate
Aluminum	Methylphenidate
Beclomethasone dipropionate	Minocycline
Bleomycin	Naproxen
Captopril	Nickel
Carbamazepine	Nitrofurantoin
Chlorpromazine	Para-aminosalicylic acid
Chlorpropamide	Penicillin
Clofibrate	Pentamidine (inhaled)
Cocaine (inhalation)	Phenytoin
Cromolyn (inhalation)	Piroxicam
Dapsone	Pyramethamine
Desipramine	Rapeseed oil
Diclofenac	Red spider antigens
Ethambutol	Sulfonamides
Fenbarbamate	Sulindac
Fenbufen	Tamoxifen
GM-CSF	Tetracycline
Heroin (inhalation)	Tolazamide
Ibuprofen	Tolfenamic acid
Iodinated contrast agents	L-Tryptophan
Maloprim	

Parasitic Infections

Infections with parasites other than *Ascaris* species are also commonly associated with pulmonary infiltrates and blood or pulmonary eosinophilia. The parasites associated with the development of pulmonary eosinophilic syndromes are listed in Table 74-3. The prevalence of infection with each of these organisms varies with geographic location, socioeconomic status, and host immunity. In addition to *Ascaris* species, *Strongyloides stercoralis* (an intestinal nematode), *Toxocara canis* (dog roundworm, "visceral larva migrans"), and *Ancylostoma brasiliensis* (cutaneous helminthosis, "creeping eruption") are the parasitic agents most commonly associated with pulmonary eosinophilia in the United States.

Pulmonary eosinophilia occurs in association with *Strongyloides* infection when it is complicated by the "hyperinfection syndrome."[1,22,52] This usually occurs in persons with defects in cell-mediated immunity (e.g., lymphomas, HIV infection), after chronic corticosteroid use, and in persons with underlying gastrointestinal disease, but it may also occur in healthy persons.[22] Respiratory manifestations include cough, dyspnea, chronic bronchitis, wheezing, hemoptysis, and pulmonary infiltrates, in association with blood eosinophilia. GI manifestations are also common, including abdominal pain, paralytic ileus, nausea and vomiting, bowel perforation, and secondary gram-negative sepsis. Cardiac and central nervous system (CNS) manifestations have also been noted.[22] The diagnosis of *Strongyloides* infection may be established by identification of larvae in sputum, bronchoalveolar lavage (BAL) fluid, bronchial brushings, or transbronchial biopsy specimens.[52] The hyperinfection syndrome associated with *Strongyloides* is difficult to cure, since thiabendizole treatment alone may not be adequate.[1,22] Ivermectin may be effective as an alternative or additional therapy for some patients.[22]

Ancylostomiasis is a nematodal infection endemic to the southeastern coastal regions of the United States, Mexico, and Central and South America. The organism is present in soil contaminated by stool from infected domestic animals. It penetrates human skin most commonly through the feet. This results in the development of the "creeping eruption" lesion—a raised, erythematous, serpiginous, tunnel-like, and often itchy lesion on areas of exposed skin.[1] A Loeffler's-like syndrome occurs in up to 50 percent of cases of "creeping eruption." Treatment includes thiabendizole, 25 mg/kg twice a day for 2 days, to be repeated after 1 week.[1]

TABLE 74-3

Parasitic Infections Associated with Eosinophilic Pneumonia

Ancylostoma spp.	*Opisthorchiasis* spp.
Ascaris spp.	*Paragonimus westermani*
Brugia malayi	*Schistosoma* spp.
Clonorchis sinesis	*Strongyloides stercoralis*
Dirofilaria immitis	*Toxocara gondii*
Echinococcus spp.	*Trichinella spiralis*
Entamoeba coli	*Trichosporon terrestre*
Necator americanus	*Wuchereria bancrofti*

Infection with *T. canis* leads to the clinical syndrome of "visceral larva migrans." This is characterized by hepatomegaly, leukocytosis, fever, hypergammaglobulinemia, and persistent blood eosinophilia.[44] Because the disease most commonly affects young children, a high degree of clinical suspicion is necessary to establish the diagnosis in adults. Respiratory symptoms, including cough and wheezing, may occur after ingestion of substantial numbers of larvae.[44] Laboratory evaluation reveals peripheral blood and BAL eosinophilia, elevated serum levels of IgE, and poorly defined, diffuse nodular alveolar infiltrates on chest radiograph.[1,44] Although the disease may be self-limited, treatment with mebendizole or corticosteroids may hasten recovery in severely ill patients.

Drug-Induced Pulmonary Eosinophilic Syndromes

A vast number of drugs have been associated with the development of pulmonary infiltrates and blood or pulmonary eosinophilia. A partial list of these medications is given in Table 74-2. The precise incidence of drug-induced pulmonary eosinophilia is difficult to assess, considering that most of the literature pertaining to these drug-induced syndromes is published in the form of case reports, rather than large series or controlled trials. For the same reason, the precise pathogenesis and the definition of the clinical syndromes associated with the use of individual agents are difficult to characterize. In general, drug-induced pulmonary eosinophilic syndromes have an acute onset and are not always related to either the cumulative dose of drug used or the duration of treatment.[12] Respiratory symptoms vary widely in severity, from a mild Loeffler's-like illness with dyspnea, cough, and fever to severe fulminant respiratory failure.[1,12] Wheezing may be present, but obstructive physiology is not common on pulmonary function testing. Interstitial or alveolar infiltrates are typically evident on chest radiograph (Fig. 74-1). The prognosis is favorable in most cases.[1,12] Elimination of exposure to the drug usually leads to resolution of symptoms, eosinophilia, and pulmonary infiltrates within a month.[1] Residual radiographic abnormalities exist in fewer than 10 percent of cases several months after clinical recovery.[12] Supplemental therapy with corticosteroids is not universally required, but it may hasten recovery in severely ill patients.[1,12]

Idiopathic Acute Eosinophilic Pneumonia

In contrast to the generally benign Loeffler's syndrome, a more severe idiopathic form of eosinophilic pneumonia termed *acute eosinophilic pneumonia* (AEP) has been recognized as a distinct clinical entity.[3,4] AEP may affect persons of either sex and any age, and occurs commonly in previously healthy persons.[1,3,4] Similar cases have been reported in persons with a history of chronic myelogenous leukemia or HIV infection. Although none of the patients in the original reported series had a history of atopy or asthma,[3,4] cases have since been described in persons with a history of allergic disease.[21]

Idiopathic AEP presents as an acute illness with fever, myalgias, cough, dyspnea, pleuritic chest pain, and hypoxemia (P_{O_2} under 60 mmHg).[1,3,4,21] Patients often have diffuse crackles on

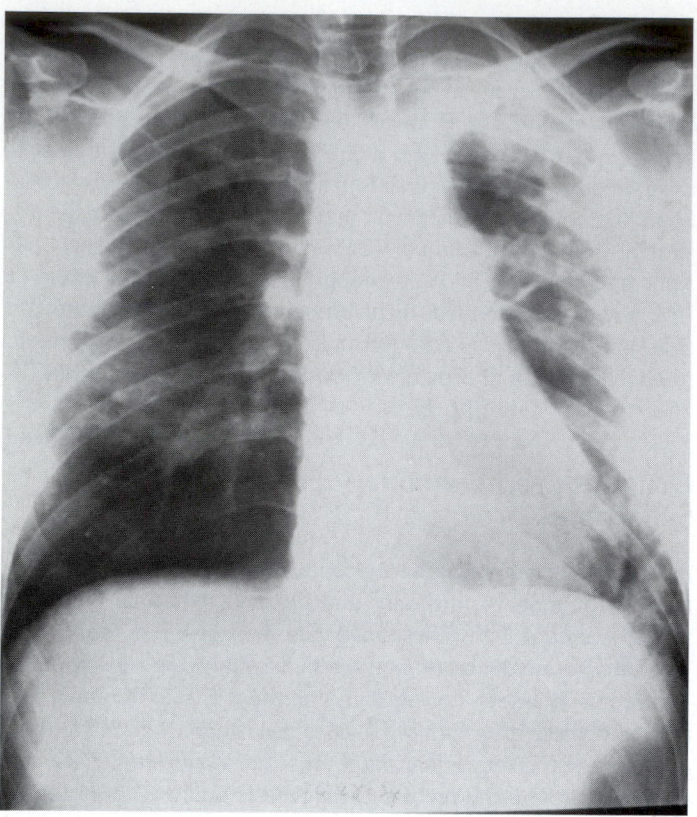

FIGURE 74-1   Chest radiograph of a 23-year-old woman with acute sulfasalazine-induced eosinophilic pneumonia. Bilateral interstitial and alveolar infiltrates are present.

chest auscultation or overt respiratory failure requiring mechanical ventilation.[1,3,4] A moderate leukocytosis is typical, but in contrast to other forms of acute eosinophilic pneumonia, blood eosinophilia is usually absent. Serum IgE levels may be moderately elevated in some cases. Early in the course of illness, the chest radiograph reveals subtle, patchy infiltrates with Kerley B lines.[1] Bilateral, diffuse, symmetric alveolar and interstitial infiltrates resembling adult respiratory distress syndrome (ARDS) with a ground-glass or micronodular appearance[21] develop within 48 h. Small to moderate bilateral pleural effusions with a high pH and marked eosinophilia may also be present. Computed tomographic (CT) scanning confirms the presence of diffuse parenchymal infiltrates, with prominence along bronchovascular bundles and septae.[1] Pulmonary function tests reveal a restrictive ventilatory defect, with a reduced $D_{L_{CO}}$. Striking eosinophilia (25 to 50 percent) is present in BAL fluid.[3] Light microscopic examination of lung tissue reveals prominent eosinophil infiltration in alveolar spaces, bronchial walls, and, to a lesser degree, the interstitium. There is no evidence of vasculitis or extrapulmonary involvement.[1,3]

Idiopathic AEP is a diagnosis of exclusion. A careful search must be undertaken for other causes of pulmonary infiltrates. Specimens of blood, sputum, stool, BAL, and often transbronchial biopsy specimens should be obtained for culture, Gram's and fungal staining, and serologic testing to rule out bacterial, mycobacterial, fungal, and parasitic infection.

The pathogenesis of idiopathic AEP is poorly understood. One case occurred in a person who had had a recent exposure to a dusty environment.[4] This and other features of the disease have led to the speculation that acute eosinophilic pneumonia is a hypersensitivity reaction to an unidentified antigen.[1,3] In addition, the role of the eosinophil in this disorder has not been elucidated. Specifically, it is not known whether the eosinophils initiate the disease process or are a secondary manifestation of the disorder.

Idiopathic AEP carries an excellent prognosis. Although fatalities have been reported, most patients demonstrate rapid dramatic responses to corticosteroid therapy, with abatement of fever and respiratory symptoms within hours and complete resolution of infiltrates within 1 to 2 weeks.[1,3,4] The optimal steroid regimen for the treatment of AEP has not been determined. However, success has been noted with initial doses of methylprednisolone 60 to 125 mg administered every 6 h, followed by 40 to 60 mg of prednisone per day for 2 to 4 weeks and a subsequent slow (over several weeks) taper.[3] Despite the apparent clinical success of steroid treatment, there exists no definitive proof that steroids alter the natural history of the disease. Spontaneous disease regression has been reported, and absence of clinical relapse is characteristic.[1,3,21]

TROPICAL PULMONARY EOSINOPHILIA

Tropical pulmonary eosinophilia (TPE) was first described in the early 1940s as a syndrome characterized by fevers, malaise, anorexia, weight loss, paroxysmal dry cough with dyspnea or wheezing, marked peripheral blood eosinophilia, and spontaneous resolution over several weeks' time.[35] In the 1950s and 1960s, filarial infections were recognized as the cause of this disorder. Tropical pulmonary eosinophilia is most prominent in India, Africa, and Southeast Asia, but it may be seen worldwide in filarial-endemic regions.[36] There is no known genetic or seasonal propensity to this disease. Most patients with TPE manifest the disease between the age of 25 and 40 years, although children and younger adults may also be affected.[35,50] Typical symptoms include a 1- to 2-week period of low-grade fevers, weight loss, fatigue, malaise, and a paroxysmal nocturnal hacking cough.[35] Dyspnea and wheezing, which can be severe, are common, and the clinical presentation may resemble status asthmaticus. Chest pain, muscle tenderness, and cardiac, pericardial, and CNS involvement have also been reported.[50] Rarely, patients remain asymptomatic. Physical examination of patients with TPE is notable for coarse rales or rhonchi and wheezing.[35] Generalized lymphadenopathy and hepatosplenomegaly may be present, but they are less common in adults than in children.[35,50]

Laboratory findings in TPE include extreme peripheral blood eosinophilia (up to 90 percent of the leukocyte differential; more than 3000 eosinophils per cubic millimeter)[35,36,50] that persists for several weeks and marked elevation of total serum IgE (usually more than 1000 U/ml).[35,36] The degree of eosinophilia generally does not correlate well with clinical disease severity or radiographic findings.[50] The erythrocyte sedimentation rate (ESR) may be moderately elevated, and eosinophils may be identified in the sputum.[50] Up to 50 percent of patients have an abnormal ECG.[50] High titers of filarial-specific IgE and IgG, measured by complement fixation and hemagglutination techniques, are the crucial diagnostic findings.[35,36] Microfilariae are not found in blood or sputum, and examination of stool or urine for ova and parasites is typically unrewarding. In contrast, microfilariae have been identified in lymph node tissue (especially when lymphadenopathy is present) and lung.[35] Pulmonary function tests reveal an obstructive ventilatory defect in up to 30 percent of patients, particularly when symptoms have been present less than 1 month. A restrictive ventilatory defect and reduced D_{LCO}, with or without a concomitant obstructive defect, are typical of long-standing disease.[35] Ill-defined, diffuse reticulonodular infiltrates with a mottled appearance are characteristic radiographic findings in TPE. The mid- to lower lung fields are most commonly affected, but disease may appear anywhere in the lung. Bronchovascular markings may be prominent, and hilar adenopathy and pleural effusions have been reported occasionally. The chest radiograph may be normal at the time of presentation.[1,35,36,50]

The histopathologic findings in TPE depend on the tissue examined, as well as the stage and duration of the disease.[1,35,45,50] Studies of lung pathology have shown that the early stage of the disease (within the first 2 weeks) is characterized by histiocytic inflammation in the alveolar, interstitial, peribronchial, and perivascular spaces, with preservation of lung architecture. Tiny nodules may be palpable within the lung tissue. One to 3 months after symptom onset, eosinophilic infiltration with eosinophilic bronchopneumonia and microabscesses is present in lungs of untreated patients. Degenerating microfilariae may be present within the center of the microabscesses, and some destruction of alveolar walls may be evident. Local bronchial walls are also edematous and inflamed, with evidence of epithelial disruption. Long-standing untreated disease is associated with the presence of chronic mixed cell inflammation in a nodular pattern and the development of pulmonary fibrosis.[1,35] Foreign body–type granulomatous lesions are often present.[45] Lymph node biopsies may reveal degenerating microfilariae or adult worms, surrounded by aggregates of eosinophils, their granule products, and giant cells.[35,50]

The clinical features of TPE are believed to result from an intense hypersensitivity reaction to microfilarial antigens. Although a broad spectrum of clinical disease may be caused by filaria, patients with TPE rarely have other systemic features of filariasis. Both human filariasis (*Wuchereria bancrofti*) and canine filarial forms (e.g., *Dirofilaria immitis*)[50] have been recovered from lung and lymph node specimens. Uncertainty exists, however, as to which species causes most of the disease. In both cases, larvae introduced into the body via insect bites develop into mature filariae. The adult worms, dwelling within the lymphatics, produce microfilariae, which are then trapped in the pulmonary vasculature. The release of antigens from degenerating microfilariae leads to an intense local and systemic inflammatory response.[36] A striking antibody and eosinophilic response, similar to that seen in peripheral blood, is present within the lung.[1,36,41] Increased numbers of total cells and eosinophils (up to 50 percent of differential), elevated levels of total IgE, and filaria-specific IgG, IgM, and IgE are present in fluid obtained by BAL.[36,41] Although little is known about the precise mechanisms by which filariae are cleared in patients with TPE, both antibody-dependent mechanisms and eosinophils probably play a role. In vitro, both granulocytes and macrophages can bind microfilariae in the presence of IgG, IgE, or complement, leading to the death of the organism.[50] The finding of an intense lymphocytic and plasma cell infiltrate around microfilariae in tissues suggests that lymphocytes may be important for clearance of the organism. In vitro lymphocyte transformation in response to stimulation with microfilarial antigens can be demonstrated in some cases.[50] The precise mechanisms by which eosinophils accumulate in the lung and contribute to tissue inflammation in patients with TPE are incompletely understood. IgE and eosinophil-, mast cell–, or basophil-derived products may contribute to the wheezing that occurs in this disorder.

The diagnosis of TPE is usually established on the basis of the clinical and laboratory findings described above. Lung biopsies are not typically required. The differential diagnosis includes Loeffler's syndrome, chronic eosinophilic pneumonia, allergic bronchopulmonary mycosis, drug reactions, other parasitic infections, hypereosinophilic syndrome, and lymphangitic spread of carcinoma.[35,50] In nonendemic areas, the disease may also masquerade as asthma, atypical pneumonia, sarcoidosis, Churg-Strauss syndrome, Wegener's granulomatosis, or tuberculosis. Biopsy of enlarged lymph nodes (e.g., scalene) may assist in establishing the diagnosis in some cases. A rapid treatment response may provide confirmatory evidence that the correct diagnosis has been made.

Diethylcarbamazine, a piperazine derivative used widely in the treatment of filarial infections, is the therapy of choice for TPE. When given for 1 to 3 weeks at a dose of 6 to 12 mg/kg a day, it leads to abatement of symptoms and improvement in pulmonary function, reduction in blood and BAL eosinophilia, a decrease in total and filaria-specific IgE and IgG, and radiographic clearing within 1 to 3 weeks of treatment.[1,35,36,41] Three full weeks of treatment is recommended for adult patients.[45] Clinical improvement following diethylcarbamazine treatment has been correlated temporally with the resolution of eosinophilic alveolitis.[41] Diethylcarbamazine acts by both direct and indirect mechanisms. It is directly filaricidal to both adult worms and microfilariae. It can also enhance the binding of granulocytes, macrophages, antibodies, and complement to the surface of microfilariae.[50]

The course and prognosis of the acute disease in patients treated with diethylcarbamazine are generally benign, and 3 weeks of diethylcarbamazine therapy is curative in most patients. However, acute relapses do occur. Patients who experience acute relapses often respond to additional treatment with diethylcarbamazine. Alternatively, mild, chronic inflammation may persist, causing chronic interstitial lung disease, with persistent respiratory symptoms, radiographic findings, and hematologic and serologic abnormalities.[35,45] Persistent clinical symptoms have been reported over 2- to 5-year follow-up periods in up to 13 percent of patients with TPE treated with a standard course of therapy.[45] BAL in these patients reveals a mild, persistent eosinophilia. Persons with symptoms of longer duration are less likely to have a favorable treatment response. Alternative antifilarial drugs (e.g., ivermectin) or a trial of corticosteroids may be useful therapies for the chronic variant of the disease.

Untreated disease usually persists for weeks to months. Untreated TPE may remit spontaneously, but it commonly recurs within months to years.[35] Although seldom fatal, TPE recognized several weeks to months after symptom onset often leads to the development of chronic interstitial lung disease.[45]

CHRONIC EOSINOPHILIC PNEUMONIA

Chronic eosinophilic pneumonia (CEP) was first described as a clinical entity by Carrington and coworkers in 1969.[7] Although CEP may develop in people of any age, the peak incidence occurs in persons 30 to 40 years of age. Women are affected approximately twice as often as men, and CEP has been reported during pregnancy. The female predominance is less obvious in patients whose disease begins after the age of 60.[23] Most cases occur in Caucasians. There is no consistent association with a history of cigarette smoking, but approximately one-third to one-half of patients have antecedent atopy, allergic rhinitis, or nasal polyps. In addition, up to two-thirds have adult-onset asthma preceding (by several months) or arising concurrently with other pulmonary symptoms. In contrast to idiopathic AEP, CEP has a subacute presentation, with symptoms typically present for several months before diagnosis.[2,16,23] Common presenting complaints include low-grade fevers, drenching night sweats, and moderate (10- to 50-pound) weight loss. Cough, often dry initially and later productive of small amounts of mucoid sputum, is a virtually universal finding. Two of the 9 patients described in Carrington's original series had minor hemoptysis. Patients ultimately develop progressive dyspnea, which may be associated with wheezing in those with adult-onset asthma. Although a subacute presentation is typical, some patients with CEP may also have severe acute respiratory failure or ARDS, with severe hypoxemia requiring mechanical ventilation. There are no major extrapulmonary manifestations of CEP.

Patients with CEP frequently manifest a moderate leukocytosis.[23] The majority (66 to 90 percent) have peripheral blood eosinophilia, with eosinophils constituting more than 6 percent of their leukocyte differential.[7,23] Leukocyte differentials with up to 90 percent eosinophils have been noted in this disorder.[7] However, a lack of peripheral blood eosinophilia does not rule out the diagnosis, since eosinophilia was absent in one-third of the cases originally described.[7] A moderate normochromic, normocytic anemia and thrombocytosis may be present, the ESR is typically elevated (greater than 20 mm an hour), and IgE levels are elevated in up to one-third of cases. The severity of pulmonary function abnormalities depends on the stage and severity of the disease. They typically reveal a moderately severe restrictive ventilatory defect, with reduced D_{LCO} and mildly elevated alveolar-arterial oxygen gradient. Persons with an asthmatic component may also have an obstructive defect. Blood and sputum cultures routinely fail to identify an infectious etiology in these patients.

In the original series, Carrington and colleagues described three radiographic features that are characteristic for chronic eosinophilic pneumonia: (1) peripherally based, progressive dense infiltrates; (2) rapid resolution of infiltrates following corticosteroid treatment, with recurrences in identical locations; and (3) the appearance of infiltrates as the "photographic negative of pulmonary edema."[7] In contrast to Loeffler's syndrome, the pulmonary infiltrates associated with CEP are nonmigratory and

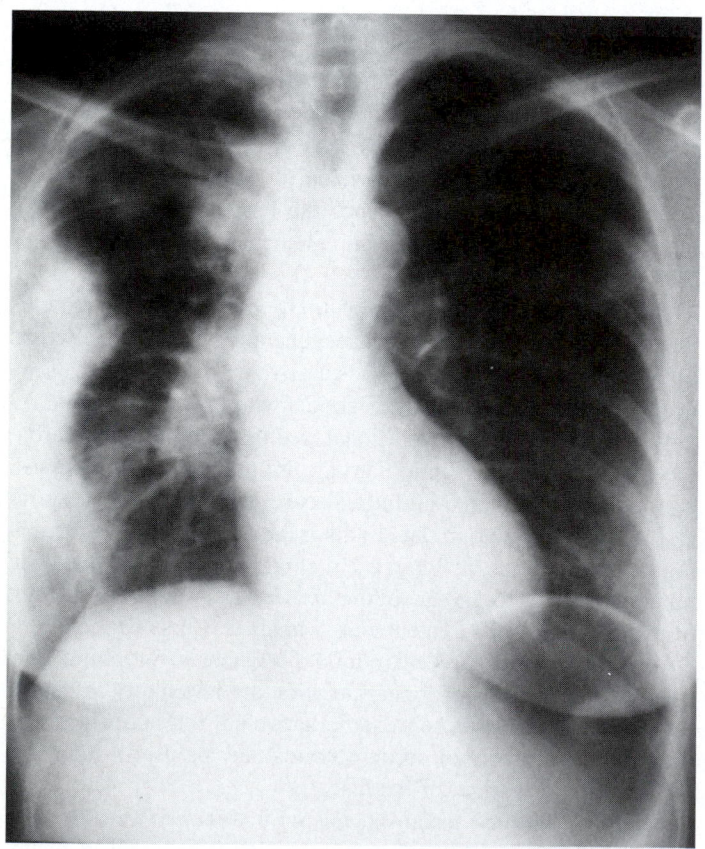

A

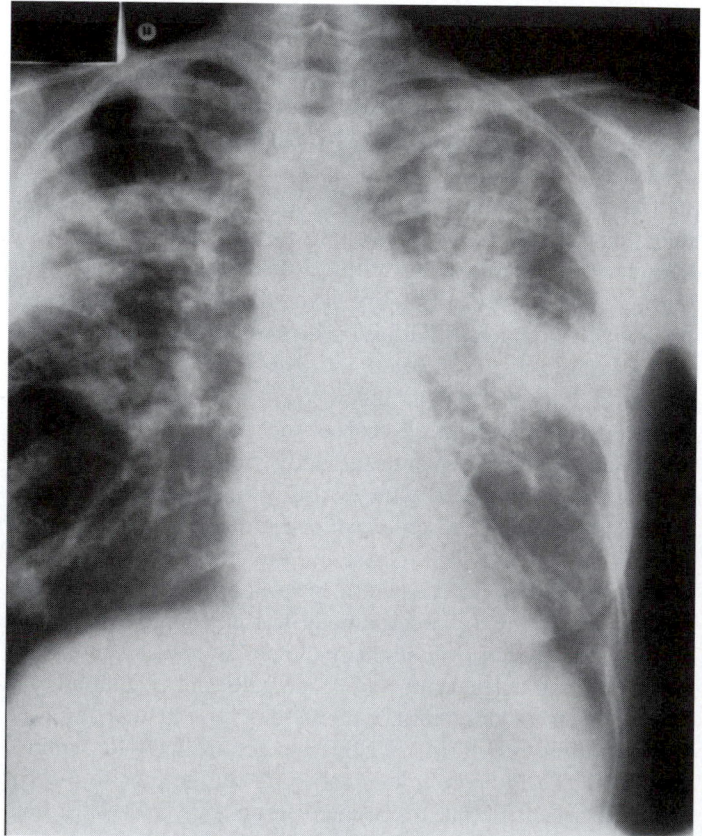

B

FIGURE 74-2 Chest radiographs in CEP. *A.* Extensive dense peripherally based infiltrates in right lung and peripheral infiltrate in left lung.

B. Dense, patchy, bilateral, predominantly peripheral infiltrates with ill-defined margins.

typically affect the outer two-thirds of the lung fields (Fig. 74-2).[16,23] The areas of consolidation are patchy and dense and can have ill-defined margins. They are frequently nonsegmental, subsegmental, or lobar in distribution and apposed to the pleura (Fig. 74-2).[16,31] Infiltrates are most commonly bilateral, are located in the mid- to upper lung zones, and may mimic loculated pleural fluid. The characteristic "photographic negative of pulmonary edema" appearance (which occurs in under 50 percent of cases) results if extensive infiltrates surround major portions of or the entire lung.[23] Less typical radiographic findings include nodular infiltrates, a diffuse ground-glass alveolar filling pattern, linear oblique or vertical densities, and areas of fibrosis unassociated with anatomic divisions. CT scanning may be a useful diagnostic adjunct in cases in which CEP is suspected clinically but typical radiographic features are lacking. Various abnormalities have been identified on CT in patients with CEP, depending on the timing of the CT relative to the onset of symptoms. Typical areas of dense, peripherally located airspace consolidation are found in most cases within the first several weeks of disease onset.[31] Streaky bandlike opacities may appear when symptoms have been present for more than 2 months. Mediastinal adenopathy, which may be evident on conventional chest radiograph, may also be identified on CT scan.[31]

The pulmonary lesions of CEP are characterized histopathologically by varying degrees of leukocytic infiltration of the alveolar airspaces and interstitium. These infiltrates are predominantly eosinophilic, with some associated macrophages, a small to moderate number of lymphocytes, and occasional plasma cells.[7] They disrupt alveolar wall architecture, usually without causing wall necrosis. Focal edema of the capillary endothelium, focal type II epithelial cell hyperplasia, proteinaceous alveolar exudates,[7] and multinucleated histiocytes within alveolar spaces can also be appreciated. Histologic evidence of proliferative bronchiolitis obliterans may occur in up to one-third of cases,[16] and a mild, nonnecrotizing microangiitis affecting predominantly the small venules may be seen.[7,16] A small percentage of lesions (less than 20 percent) may have frank intra-alveolar necrosis, eosinophilic microabscesses, or noncaseating granulomas.[7,23] Biopsy specimens of lymph nodes from patients with intrathoracic lymphadenopathy reveal lymphoid hyperplasia and eosinophil infiltration.

The cause of CEP is unknown. In addition, no specific genetic predisposition for the disease has been identified, although CEP has been reported in identical twins, raising the question of a familial tendency toward the disease. Although the precise immunopathogenesis of CEP is unknown, a variety of lines of evidence suggest that eosinophils play a primary pathogenetic role in the pulmonary tissue damage seen in this disorder. Increased numbers of eosinophils appear in the peripheral blood and bone marrow before the onset of clinical disease, and an eosinophilia is the predominant abnormality in BAL fluid.[13] These eosinophils appear to be activated, since eosinophil-derived granule proteins (EDGP) have been identified microscopically within the pulmonary parenchyma and microvasculature, increased concentrations of EDGP are identified in BAL fluid from patients with CEP compared to controls, and BAL-derived eosinophils express activation markers including class II major histocompatibility (MHC) antigens. The processes that regulate eosinophil activation and degranulation in CEP are not clear. Evidence showing that class II MHC and other activation markers are expressed by BAL- but not blood-derived eosinophils suggests the presence of an immune inflammatory response compartmentalized within the lung. Of interest are the findings that immunoglobulins can augment eosinophil chemotaxis and degranulation in vitro, and that circulating immune complexes and elevated titers of IgE are noted in the context of clinical flares of the disease. To date, however, no clear causal relationship has been established between immunoglobulins and eosinophil activation in CEP.

The differential diagnosis of CEP includes infection (especially TB and fungal diseases like cryptococcosis), sarcoidosis, Loeffler's syndrome, desquamative interstitial pneumonitis, bronchiolitis obliterans organizing pneumonia, chronic hypersensitivity pneumonitis, and eosinophilic granuloma.[7] The diagnosis of CEP is based on clinical, radiographic, and BAL findings, and on the inability to document pulmonary or systemic infection. The clinical signs and symptoms of CEP are nonspecific, however, and blood eosinophilia and typical radiographic features may be absent in some cases. BAL eosinophilia of 30 to 50 percent is typical of CEP.[1,13] A range of BAL eosinophilia from 14 to 75 percent has been reported.[13] In most reported series, open lung biopsy has been required only rarely to establish the diagnosis. Transbronchial biopsy, usually performed to rule out other diagnostic entities, may reveal eosinophil and mononuclear cell infiltrates. Because of the rapid and dramatic responsiveness of CEP to steroid treatment, a therapeutic trial of steroids is often useful in establishing the diagnosis. Failure to document rapid clinical improvement should alert the physician to consider other diagnoses.

Corticosteroids are the mainstay of therapy for CEP. Dramatic clinical, radiographic, and physiological improvements have been documented following steroid treatment in all series reported.[7,16,23] Even patients presenting with severe respiratory failure may respond well to steroid treatment. In most cases, treatment with prednisone (40 mg per day as the initial dose) leads to defervescence within 6 h,[16] reduced dyspnea, cough, and blood eosinophilia within 24 to 48 h,[23] resolution of hypoxia in 2 to 3 days,[7,16] radiographic improvement within 1 to 2 weeks, complete resolution of symptoms within 2 to 3 weeks,[23] and normalization of the chest radiograph within 2 months.

The prognosis of CEP is generally favorable. Spontaneous remissions seldom occur in untreated patients.[7,16] In steroid-treated patients (40 mg a day for 10 to 14 days, followed by tapering over 4 to 6 weeks), morbidity and mortality directly related to CEP are low. However, clinical, hematologic, or radiographic evidence of relapse occurs in most patients (58 to 80 percent) when steroids are tapered or discontinued.[23,33] These relapses commonly occur in the exact anatomic distribution of the original disease. Patients may require 1 to 3 years of initial steroid treatment to control the disease, and up to 25 percent may require long-term maintenance treatment (2.5 to 10 mg prednisone a day) to remain disease-free. The lowest possible dose of steroid that suppresses disease activity should be used. Although no obvious factors exist to identify persons who are likely to relapse or require long-term steroids, relapses are more common in persons treated initially with a short course (1 to 3 months) of steroids.[23,33]

Multiple recurrences may occur in anyone. The reinstitution of steroids generally leads to improvement during these relapses. In rare instances, patients develop pulmonary fibrosis and honeycombing.

ALLERGIC BRONCHOPULMONARY ASPERGILLOSIS (MYCOSIS)

Allergic bronchopulmonary aspergillosis (ABPA) was first described in 1952 by Hinson and coworkers.[1] In 1967, Scadding recognized an association of this disease with proximal bronchiectasis in areas previously affected by infiltrates, often in the upper lobes.[1] The first adult case of ABPA in the United States was described in 1968.[20] Although most cases entail hypersensitivity to *Aspergillus* species—especially *A. fumigatus*—the finding of a virtually identical clinical syndrome associated with immune sensitivity to *Candida albicans, Helminthosporium* species, *Curvularia lunata, Dreschlera hawaiiensis, Stemphylium languinosum,* and *Pseudoallescheria boydii* has led to the use of the term *allergic bronchopulmonary mycosis* to describe this syndrome. The precise prevalence of this syndrome is unknown, owing in part to variability in diagnostic criteria used in various studies and to delays in the diagnosis of patients with long-standing disease.[20] It is estimated that ABPA complicates approximately 1 to 2 percent of cases of chronic (often steroid-dependent) asthma[17] and 10 to 15 percent of cases of cystic fibrosis.[25] The disease has no predilection for either sex, and persons of any age may be affected. ABPA may have its onset in childhood or adolescence yet go unrecognized until adulthood. The peak age at disease recognition is in the third and fourth decades.[42] Most patients have a history of atopy with rhinitis, history of drug allergy, asthma onset before age 20, and/or allergic conjunctivitis.[42]

Typical presenting complaints include dyspnea, wheezing, poor asthma control, cough (commonly productive of thick, brown mucus plugs), malaise, low-grade fever, and hemoptysis.[42] There may be an antecedent history of asthma exacerbation in conjunction with pneumonia without a culture-identified bacterial source.[20] A number of schema have been proposed for the diagnosis of ABPA. One is based on an appropriate clinical history, a positive immediate hypersensitivity skin test to *Aspergillus,* total IgE levels, and IgG and IgE antibody indices (see Chapter 51). Another is based on major and minor diagnostic criteria as first proposed by Rosenberg's team (Table 74-4).[46] The major diagnostic criteria include (1) asthma (mild to severe), (2) peripheral blood eosinophilia, (3) serum IgG–precipitating antibody against *Aspergillus* (or other relevant fungus), (4) positive immediate hypersensitivity skin test to *Aspergillus,* (5) elevated serum total IgE, (6) history of pulmonary infiltrates, and (7) elevated serum *Aspergillus*–specific IgE and IgG.[20,46] Radiographic evidence of proximal bronchiectasis is also considered to be a diagnostic criterion by some authors. Its absence does not rule out the diagnosis, especially early in the course of the disease. Minor diagnostic criteria include the finding of brown mucus plugs, identification of *Aspergillus* in sputum, and dual (immediate and delayed) cutaneous reactions to challenge with *Aspergillus.* Rare cases lacking a history of asthma but meeting the other major diagnostic criteria have been reported.

TABLE 74-4

Diagnostic Criteria for Allergic Bronchopulmonary Aspergillosis

Major

    Asthma

    Peripheral blood eosinophilia

    Precipitating antibodies against *Aspergillus*

    Positive immediate hypersensitivity skin-prick test to *Aspergillus*

    Elevated total IgE

    Elevated serum *Aspergillus*–specific IgE, IgG

    History of pulmonary infiltrates

    (Proximal bronchiectasis)

Minor

    Mucous plugs containing *Aspergillus*

    Dual cutaneous reaction to *Aspergillus*

Five clinical stages of ABPA have been recognized, based on clinical, serologic, and radiographic characteristics.[1,20,40] Stage I, the *acute* stage, is characterized by symptoms of asthma, elevated total IgE (typically more than 1000 ng/ml),[20] positive immediate hypersensitivity skin reaction to *Aspergillus* challenge, infiltrate on chest radiograph (with or without proximal bronchiectasis), peripheral blood eosinophilia (frequently greater than 2000/mm[3]), and positive precipitating antibodies to *A. fumigatus* (up to fivefold concentration of serum may be required for detection of the precipitating antibodies). Treatment of stage I disease with corticosteroids typically results in decreased sputum production, improved control of bronchospasm, greater than 35 percent reduction in total IgE within 8 weeks,[43] clearing of precipitating antibodies,[20] and resolution of radiographic infiltrates.[1,40] IgE levels typically do not completely normalize.[1,20] Patients with stage II ABPA have disease that is in *remission.* This is characterized by the resolution of symptoms, radiographic clearing, and stabilization of total IgE levels. Remissions may last several months to years, and corticosteroid treatment can be tapered or discontinued. Patients with stage III ABPA have disease *exacerbations.* Their disease is characterized by the development of new pulmonary infiltrates or by a greater than 100 percent increase in total IgE.[1,20] An isolated increase in severity of bronchospasm does not constitute an exacerbation.[19] Disease exacerbation may occur in the presence or absence of a concomitant increase in symptoms. Since up to one-third of patients with radiographic infiltrates may be asymptomatic, evolving progressive lung damage may remain unrecognized.[47] As such, total serum IgE levels should be monitored every 1 to 2 months for at least a year after diagnosis. IgE levels fluctuate with disease activity, and a normal IgE level in a symptomatic untreated person virtually excludes the diagnosis.[1] *Aspergillus*-specific IgA levels may also be elevated in the acute or exacerbation stages of disease. Stage IV ABPA is defined as *steroid-dependent asthma.* In stage IV disease, total IgE, *Aspergillus* precipitins, and *Aspergillus*-specific IgE and IgG typically remain elevated despite chronic steroid therapy. Stage V is defined as *pulmonary fibrosis.* Stage V patients have prominent symptoms of dyspnea;

are often steroid dependent because of persistent bronchospasm; frequently have chronic sputum production, recurrent respiratory infections, and gas exchange abnormalities; and may have cyanosis or clubbing. The serologic profile of patients with stage IV disease persists during stage V.

Analysis of BAL fluid from patients with ABPA reveals a moderate eosinophilia and increased levels of *Aspergillus*-specific IgE and IgA but not IgG. Mucoid impaction may be evident, and bronchial brushings may reveal mucus containing aggregates of eosinophils, fungal hyphae, and eosinophil-derived Charcot-Leyden crystals. Pulmonary function tests typically reveal an obstructive ventilatory defect (due to bronchospasm or mucous impaction of the bronchi) during stages I, III, IV, and often V. These pulmonary function findings often do not correlate with the duration of ABPA or asthma. Persons with stage V disease typically also have a restrictive ventilatory defect with a reduced D$_{LCO}$.

The differential diagnosis of ABPA includes corticosteroid-dependent asthma without ABPA, TB, parasitic infections, hypersensitivity pneumonitis, Churg-Strauss syndrome, acute eosinophilic pneumonia, CEP, and cystic fibrosis (CF). The identification of ABPA in patients with mold-sensitive asthma and CF poses particular diagnostic difficulty. Serum precipitins to *Aspergillus* species may be present in up to 10 percent and positive immediate skin tests to *Aspergillus* in up to 25 percent of asthmatics.[42] Persons with mold-sensitive asthma or ABPA can have peripheral blood eosinophilia and/or elevated serum total IgE levels. However, persons with ABPA have 2- to 20-fold higher serum levels of *Aspergillus*-specific IgE and total IgE than do mold-sensitive asthmatics without ABPA.[20] In addition, proximal bronchiectasis is not seen in mold-sensitive asthma but is common in ABPA.[34] Likewise, it is difficult to establish the diagnosis of ABPA in patients with CF, because patients with CF alone can manifest chronic airflow obstruction, recurrent infections, underlying bronchiectasis, pulmonary infiltrates, chronic sputum production, *Aspergillus* colonization of the airways, and positive serum precipitins.[25] ABPA should be suspected in patients with CF who develop a greater than fourfold increase in total serum IgE (especially more than 500 U/ml) or who have positive *Aspergillus*-specific IgE or IgG.[25] Patients with CF and ABPA may derive some symptomatic or functional improvement from steroid treatment. CF patients on steroids should, however, be followed closely for development of invasive aspergillosis. It is unclear whether the development of ABPA alters the course of CF disease progression.

The typical radiographic manifestations of ABPA include parenchymal infiltrates and bronchiectasis. The infiltrates are often irregular and transient (1 to 6 weeks). They have a predilection for upper lobes, although all lobes may be affected.[1,20] The bronchiectasis is classically cylindric and proximal (central), occurring within the proximal two-thirds of the lung.[1,34,42] The characteristic (but nonspecific) radiographic appearances of ABPA may include the "gloved finger" infiltrate (bandlike densities with a rounded end, reflecting secretion-filled dilated bronchi), "tramline shadows" (extending from hilum in bronchial distribution and reflecting inflamed, edematous bronchi), "toothpaste shadows" (mucoid impaction of the bronchi), "parallel line shadows" (dilated bronchi), "ring shadows" (dilated bronchi seen on end), local consolidation, or lobar collapse (Fig. 74-3).[1,42] Less common radiographic findings include bullous changes, pneumothorax, and cavitating nodular lesions. High-resolution CT scanning is the most reliable noninvasive means of detecting proximal bronchiectasis.[34]

Open lung biopsy is usually not required to establish the diagnosis of ABPA. Histopathologic findings in this disease, however, include intense bronchocentric inflammation, with prominent eosinophilia, as well as lymphocytes, plasma cells, and monocytes. Regions of bronchocentric granulomatosis, eosinophilic pneumonia, eosinophilic microabscess, lymphocytic interstitial pneumonitis, desquamative interstitial pneumonitis, proliferative bronchiolitis, lipoid pneumonia, or interstitial fibrosis may also be seen.[1,6,20]

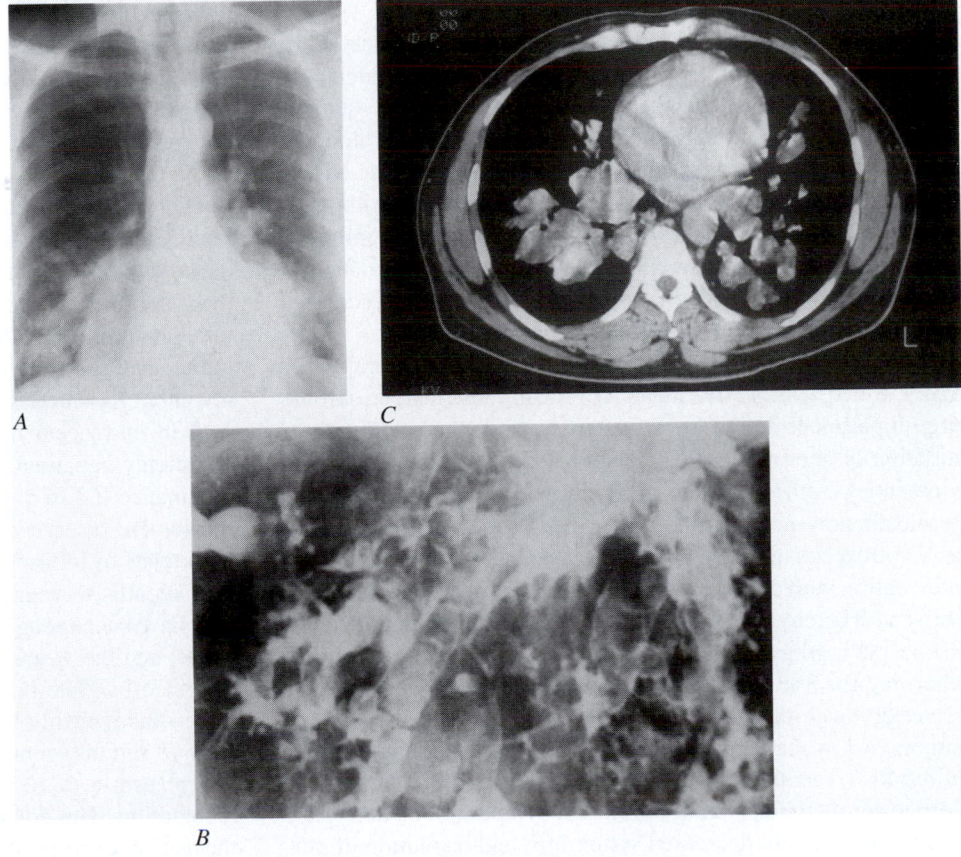

A

B

C

FIGURE 74-3 Radiographic appearance of ABPA. Extensive infiltrates with tubular configuration and "gloved finger" appearance are present, in this case predominantly in the lower lobes (*A*). The bronchogram (*B*) and CT of the chest (*C*) reveal extensive proximal bronchiectasis. Extensive mucoid impaction of the bronchi is evident on CT scan.

The features of ABPA are believed to result from a complex immunologic reaction to chronic airway colonization by *Aspergillus* (or other relevant fungal) species. *Aspergillus* species are ubiquitous, thermotolerant organisms[19] that reside in decaying organic matter. Inhaled spores colonize the airway, proliferate, and result in chronic antigenic stimulation of the airway.[42] This results in intense eosinophil and mononuclear cell inflammation that leads to airway injury and bronchiectasis.[24] The precise pathogenetic mechanisms are unclear. A role for type I hypersensitivity reactions is strongly suggested by the elevated levels of total and *Aspergillus*-specific IgE.[19,42] Type III hypersensitivity is suggested by the presence of *Aspergillus* precipitins and circulating immune complexes during disease exacerbations.[19,42] A type IV cell-mediated immune reaction may also be at work, based on the finding of dual (immediate and delayed) cutaneous reactions and in vitro lymphocyte transformation to *Aspergillus* antigen stimulation in some patients.[42] Eosinophils and basophils may contribute to local airway injury.[20] A pathogenetic role for T lymphocytes is suggested by a number of findings, including (1) the presence of increased numbers of airway T cells and increased levels of soluble interleukin 2 (IL-2) receptors (suggesting T-cell activation) in the circulation of persons with active ABPA; (2) the derivation of *Aspergillus*-specific T-cell clones with T helper–2 (Th2) patterns of cytokine production from the blood of patients with ABPA; (3) the correlations between activated T-cell number, the levels of the T cell–derived cytokines IL-4 and IL-5, and the number of airway eosinophils in the disease; and (4) the important role IL-5 plays in murine models of ABPA.

The fungus itself may also be of substantial pathogenetic importance. A variety of *Aspergillus*-derived antigens (including proteases, cytotoxins, and heat shock proteins) with demonstrated ability to bind IgE and IgG derived from the blood of patients with ABPA could potentially incite the immune hypersensitivity process. *Aspergillus*-derived proteinases with antibody-binding capacity can also cause direct epithelial injury in vitro. Fungus-induced epithelial injury may trigger immune hypersensitivity by inducing inflammation or by allowing increased penetration of fungal antigens into the airway.

Systemic corticosteroids are the mainstay of therapy for ABPA. Since, without treatment, ABPA can cause marked chronic lung impairment due to bronchiectasis or pulmonary fibrosis,[47] initiation of appropriate treatment early in the course of disease is essential. Although there is no definitive proof that corticosteroid therapy prevents the development of central bronchiectasis, retrospective studies have suggested that early therapeutic intervention with corticosteroids may prevent progression to lung fibrosis.[1] Therapy for stage I or III disease should include prednisone, 0.5 mg/kg a day for 2 weeks, followed by treatment every other day for 3 months.[1,38] A subsequent taper (by 5 mg every 2 weeks) over the ensuing 3 months is advocated by some authors. A low maintenance dose (e.g., 7.5 mg a day) may be required for 1 year to control the disease and prevent recurrence.[47] Corticosteroid therapy leads to relief of symptoms and decreased airflow obstruction, decreased serum IgE, and resolution of pulmonary inflammation and infiltrates.[19,43,47] Although not generally advocated, inhaled corticosteroids have occasionally been used as primary therapy and as steroid-sparing agents for the treatment of symptomatic exacerbations and pulmonary infiltrates. Inhaled steroids are, however, useful for control of bronchospasm and for minimizing the dose of systemic steroid necessary to control wheezing. Bronchodilators and antibiotics also help control bronchospasm and secondary respiratory infections. Although antifungal agents—including nystatin, amphotericin B, and natamycin—are generally ineffective in controlling ABPA, itraconazole had steroid-sparing effects in isolated case reports and an uncontrolled trial in six patients.[14]

With appropriate treatment, long-term control of ABPA is feasible. Progression of stage IV disease to pulmonary fibrosis can be prevented if patients are maintained on low-dose steroids,[39] and most patients with stage V disease have a stable course over several years' time.[28] Persons with an FEV$_1$ persistently less than 0.8 L have a worse prognosis.[28] In addition to severe airflow obstruction and pulmonary fibrosis, long-term complications of ABPA occasionally include the development of an aspergilloma, chronic or recurrent lobar atelectasis, allergic *Aspergillus* sinusitis,[1] or limited *Aspergillus* tissue invasion.

CHURG-STRAUSS SYNDROME (ALLERGIC GRANULOMATOSIS AND ANGIITIS)

In 1939, Rackemann and Greene reported a subgroup of patients with polyarteritis nodosa and concomitant allergic disease.[26] Similar findings were reported in the early 1940s by Harkavy. The histopathology and clinical features associated with this disease entity were first described in 1951 by Churg and Strauss. They reported a form of necrotizing vasculitis in several organs, associated with eosinophilic tissue inflammation and extravascular granulomas, occurring in asthmatics, with associated fever and peripheral hypereosinophilia. This disease entity, now recognized as Churg-Strauss syndrome (CSS), is an uncommon systemic disease. The precise incidence of CSS is uncertain. Only a few small series (ranging between 30 and 50 cases each) and many isolated case reports have been published. The true incidence of CSS may be higher than is generally recognized, since the syndrome has many clinical, radiographic, and histologic features in common with other vasculitic, eosinophilic, and granulomatous disease states. The diagnosis of CSS may be missed if not carefully entertained.[26]

CSS may occur in patients of any age, but it develops most commonly in patients age 38 to 50.[1,8] There is a slight male predominance (52 to 75 percent of patients in different series).[8,26] In women, disease onset has been reported during pregnancy. CSS tends to follow a subacute course, with symptoms ranging over months to years. Three distinct clinical phases of the disease have been recognized: the prodromal phase, the eosinophilic phase, and the vasculitic phase.[26] The prodromal phase is characterized by "late-onset" (usually after age 21) allergic disease in persons typically lacking a family history of atopy.[1,26] Severe allergic rhinitis, sinusitis, drug sensitivity, and asthma are usually present 8 to 10 years (up to 30 years) before CSS disease recognition. The eosinophilic phase is typified by the development of marked peripheral blood eosinophilia and eosinophilic tissue infiltration, most commonly of the lung, GI tract, and skin.[26] The onset of the vasculitic phase is often heralded by development of constitutional symptoms, including fever, malaise, weight loss, and increased allergic or asthmatic symptoms.[1,9] Although the vasculitis tends to occur years after the onset of allergic manifestations of the disease,[1,27] in some cases it develops within months of, or concomitant with, the onset of asthma. A short duration between the onset of asthma and vasculitis is associated with increased severity of vasculitis.[8] During the vasculitic stage, the asthma symptoms may persist and worsen,[27] or they may diminish. When asthma dissipates, it often flares later in the course of illness and may require prolonged steroid treatment. Although CSS typically affects multiple organ systems, more limited forms of disease have been described.[29] Although virtually every organ system may be affected with CSS, manifestations in the lungs, heart, skin, and nervous system are most common.[30]

Most of the respiratory manifestations of CSS occur in the prodromal and eosinophilic phases of the disease. All patients have asthma at some point in the illness. Upper-airway allergic disease, including sinusitis, rhinitis, and polyposis, is seen in 75 to 85 percent of patients.[26] The asthma and upper-airway disease usually are long-standing and often require steroid therapy (systemic or inhaled) to maintain control of symptoms. Spirometry may reveal an obstructive ventilatory defect. In rare instances, recurrent respiratory infection leads to bronchiectasis. A Loeffler's-like syndrome with eosinophilic infiltration of the lung parenchyma is seen in 38 to 40 percent of patients. These patients may develop dyspnea, cough, and wheezing. Their chest radiographs have transient, migratory nonlobar, nonsegmental, often peripheral pulmonary infiltrates, with no regional predilection.[1,8,26,30] Pulmonary function tests done in this setting may reveal a restrictive or obstructive ventilatory defect with a reduced $D_{L_{CO}}$. Up to 30 percent of patients develop pleural effusions, which may be associated with pleuritic chest pain. Less commonly, a radiographic pattern of diffuse nodularity or interstitial lung disease is seen.[1] In contrast to Wegener's granulomatosis, the CSS nodules rarely cavitate. Hilar lymphadenopathy may be present, and occasionally the chest radiograph may be normal. High-resolution CT screening has demonstrated patchy peribronchial thickening, pulmonary artery enlargement (in comparison to the corresponding bronchi), irregular stellate configuration of some vessels, areas of septal thickening, and scattered patchy parenchymal opacities. These findings have been reported to correlate with pathologic findings evident on open lung biopsy. Further studies are necessary to determine whether HRCT is useful to stage the disease or establish the diagnosis without tissue biopsy.

Cardiac manifestations generally are not present on initial presentation of CSS. However, they typically occur during the vasculitic phase of the disease[26] and are a major source of morbidity and the principal cause of death (in 33 to 48 percent of cases) from the disorder.[1,8,26] Progressive congestive heart failure (CHF) occurs in 47 percent of cases because of myocardial infiltration by eosinophils or ischemic cardiomyopathy resulting from necrotizing vasculitis of the coronary arteries. This coronary vasculitis is fatal up to 60 percent of the time.[26] Pericarditis is present in approximately one-third of cases, and cardiac tamponade has been reported.

A wide array of neurologic manifestations may develop in CSS.[1,8,30,32] Mono- or polyneuropathy (most notably mononeu-

ritis multiplex) is present in 69 to 75 percent of cases.[1,30] CNS manifestations occur in approximately two-thirds of patients and include cranial nerve impairment (especially optic neuritis), subarachnoid hemorrhage, and cerebral infarction.

Skin, GI, renal, and other systemic alterations in CSS have been well described in CSS. Skin findings are present in 70 percent of cases[1,26,30] and may develop in localized crops. They can manifest as nonthrombocytopenic purpura, tender cutaneous or subcutaneous nodules (which may ulcerate), urticaria, a maculopapular rash, or livedo reticularis. GI manifestations of CSS are present in up to 60 percent of cases. They can include diarrhea, abdominal pain, intestinal obstruction, cholecystitis, bleeding, liver function test abnormalities, and bowel perforation.[1] They may relate to visceral eosinophilic tissue infiltration or to overt vasculitis.[26] GI disease is the fourth leading cause of death in patients with CSS (after cardiac, CNS, and renal impairment). Renal insufficiency occurs in up to 50 percent of patients with CSS.[1,8,26] Interstitial nephritis, focal glomerulonephritis,[26,27] hematuria, and albuminuria are common. Severe, difficult-to-control hypertension is also a major sequela of CSS (in 25 to 75 percent of cases) and may be due to recurrent renal infarction.[26] In contrast to Wegener's granulomatosis, overt renal failure is not commonly seen in CSS. Mild lymphadenopathy (in 30 to 40 percent), rheumatologic manifestations (migratory polyarthralgias, myalgias, temporal arteritis), urologic disease (ureteral, urethral, prostatic),[8] and ocular manifestations have also been described.

Laboratory studies of CSS are notable for a striking but fluctuating degree of peripheral blood eosinophilia (20 to 90 percent of the differential) in virtually all patients.[1,8,26] The degree of eosinophilia may be suppressed by corticosteroid treatment of asthma. Serum total IgE levels are typically elevated (range, 500 to 1000 U/ml) and may parallel disease activity.[8,27] Most patients have a normochromic, normocytic anemia and moderate elevation of their ESR.[8,27] As many as 50 percent of patients have low titers of rheumatoid factor,[8,34] and 50 to 70 percent of patients have positive pANCA (perinuclear antineutrophil cytoplasmic antibody, antimyeloperoxidase antibody),[1] although the presence of the latter is not used to monitor disease activity or direct therapeutic intervention. Circulating immune complexes, hypergammaglobulinemia,[27] and elevated urinary levels of eosinophil-derived neurotoxin have been reported. Laboratory examination of pleural fluid reveals an acidotic eosinophilic exudate (pH under 3) with low glucose levels. Pleural biopsy reveals chronic pleuritis with eosinophilic infiltration. BAL reveals an increased percentage of eosinophils, the magnitude of which is generally less than that seen with CEP or idiopathic hypereosinophilic syndrome. However, patients have been described whose BAL fluid leukocyte differential contained 81 percent eosinophils.

In 1984, three diagnostic criteria for CSS were proposed: asthma, a peak blood eosinophil count greater than 1.5×10^9, and a systemic vasculitis affecting more than two extrapulmonary organs.[26] In 1990, following an analysis of 20 cases of CSS compared with 787 controls with other forms of vasculitis, the American College of Rheumatology published updated diagnostic criteria for CSS, based on assessments of the sensitivity and specificity of the diagnostic criteria used previously in establishing the diagnosis of the disorder.[30] The presence of at least four out of six of the following criteria yielded 85 percent sensitivity and 99.7 percent specificity in establishing the diagnosis: (1) asthma, (2) peripheral eosinophilia greater than 10 percent, (3) mono- or polyarthropathy, (4) migratory or transient pulmonary infiltrates, (5) paranasal sinus abnormality, and (6) extravascular eosinophils in a blood vessel on a biopsy specimen. In this study, the presence of asthma or allergy as well as more than 10 percent eosinophilia was 95 percent sensitive and 99 percent specific in distinguishing CSS among a subgroup of patients with well-documented systemic vasculitis. Open lung biopsy is the gold-standard site for tissue biopsy.[1] Biopsy of other sites (e.g., skin, pericardium, muscle, nerve, gut), with or without immunostaining, may assist in establishing the diagnosis in selected cases.

The histopathologic hallmarks of CSS include tissue (interstitial, blood vessel, and alveolar) infiltration by eosinophils; necrotizing vasculitis of small arteries, arterioles, and, to a lesser extent, small veins, venules, and capillaries;[1,29] and extravascular and interstitial eosinophilic granulomas (typically microscopic).[1,26,30] Both pulmonary and systemic vessels may be affected.[29] The precise histopathology of vascular impairment depends on the stage of the lesion. Early lesions demonstrate eosinophilic infiltration of the vessels and perivascular region (Fig. 74-4). Later lesions are characterized by necrotizing arteritis or vessel obliteration and scarring.[8] The extent of vascular impairment varies from mild, eosinophilic perivascular cuffing to severe transmural inflammation with necrotization.[26] Lesions may be sparse or widespread.

The differential diagnosis of CSS includes polyarteritis nodosa, Wegener's granulomatosis, CEP, idiopathic hypereosinophilic syndrome, Loeffler's syndrome, asthma, and disseminated fungal infection. The pathogenesis of CSS is poorly understood. Our lack of understanding is due, in large part, to the limited number of CSS cases reported and available for study. The strong association with allergy, atopy, and elevated levels of IgE (especially during the vasculitic phase of the disease) has raised the question of immune hypersensitivity. As a result, it has been proposed that repeated antigenic stimulation in patients with a heightened eosinophil response may be important in the development of the disorder.[26] Definitive proof of this theory is, however, lacking. In addition, no genetic predisposition or HLA association with the disease has been identified.

Patients in whom CSS goes untreated have a poor prognosis, with up to 50 percent dying within 3 months after the onset of vasculitis.[8] As such, efforts at early recognition and treatment are important. No large randomized, controlled trials exist comparing various treatment methods, largely because of the rarity of the disorder. Thus, it is difficult to define the optimal treatment for the disease. Nevertheless, it is clear that corticosteroid treatment generally leads to dramatic clinical improvement, with disease stabilization or cure. Prednisone, 40 to 60 mg per day, is given for several weeks, aiming to eliminate constitutional symptoms and cardiac, renal, neurologic, or other vasculitic manifestations.[1,8] Higher doses are occasionally required. Severe hypertension and mononeuritis multiplex often require prolonged steroid treatment. Once the vasculitic phase is controlled, steroids may be tapered, with doses titrated to maintain disease control. Low-dose prednisone is often given every day or every other day for up to 1 year. Although relapses are uncommon,[1] patients should be followed closely for evidence of clinical deterioration, and should have periodic screening of total WBC and differential, ESR, and IgE levels.

Patients with steroid-dependent asthma, in whom the diagnosis of CSS has not been demonstrated or entertained, should be monitored closely for evidence of CSS when steroid doses are tapered.[9] Treatment with azathioprine, cyclophosphamide, high-dose methylprednisolone, or chlorambucil may prove effective in patients whose condition fails to improve with steroid treatment.[1,8] Beta blockers should be avoided in the management of CSS-related hypertension, owing to the risk of bronchospasm and congestive heart failure (CHF).[26] In a series of 30 patients collected over the period 1950 to 1974, a median survival more than 9 years was reported in patients treated with steroids; 1-year survival was 90 percent, 3-year survival was 76 percent, and 62 percent survival was noted at 5 years.

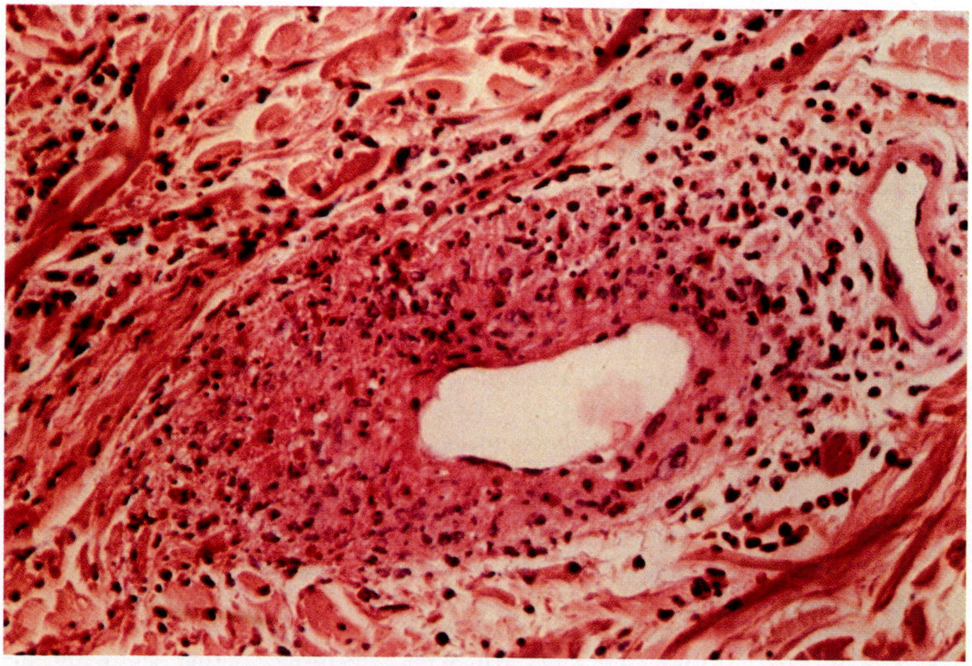

IDIOPATHIC HYPEREOSINOPHILIC SYNDROME

Idiopathic hypereosinophilic syndrome (IHS) is a rare disorder first described in 1968 by Hardy and Anderson.[53] Over the ensuing years, many case reports of severe peripheral eosinophilia and diffuse organ infiltration with eosinophils were described.

FIGURE 74-4 Pathologic appearance of small arteriole in Churg-Strauss vasculitis. Intense perivascular inflammation with eosinophilia is present.

Several names—including *eosinophilic leukemia, Loeffler's fibroplastic endocarditis,* and *disseminated eosinophilic cardiovascular disease*—were used to describe this disease entity. In 1975, Chusid and colleagues revised the definition of IHS to include only cases in which no other underlying cause of hypereosinophilia could be found.[10] IHS is now recognized as a clinically heterogeneous syndrome with a wide range of disease severity. Whereas some patients experience a mild, limited form of the disease with minimal involvement of noncritical organs (e.g., skin), others have life-threatening multiorgan dysfunction.[49]

IHS predominantly affects males, although the sex association is less prominent in older patients.[53] Persons of any age may be affected. Disease onset is, however, most common between 20 and 50 years of age. There is no known racial or ethnic predisposition.[53]

Symptoms vary according to the organ system(s) affected. Presenting complaints are often nonspecific and include weakness, fatigue, low-grade fevers, and myalgias.[15] Involvement of virtually every organ system has been described. Cardiac disease, which occurs in most cases, is the major cause of morbidity and mortality. The most common cardiac manifestations are relentlessly progressive CHF, intracardiac thrombi, and endocardial fibrosis. Mitral regurgitation, restrictive cardiomyopathy, and bacterial endocarditis have also been noted.[15,54] Involvement of the central or peripheral nervous system, which occurs in more than 60 percent of patients,[15] is also a major cause of morbidity. Neurologic manifestations of IHS include neuropsychiatric dysfunction, gait disturbances, peripheral neuropathies, visual changes, and sequelae of thromboembolic events, including hemiparesis.[10,15] The bone marrow is universally affected with a striking eosinophilia (up to 25 to 75 percent of the differential). Other hematologic manifestations are anemia, thrombocytopenia, elevated vitamin B_{12} levels, venous and arterial thromboembolism, hepatosplenomegaly, and lymphadenopathy (in 12 to 20 percent). GI (25 to 46 percent of patients), cutaneous (25 to 56 percent), renal (10 to 20 percent), musculoskeletal, ocular, and endocrine manifestations are all well described.

The respiratory system is affected in 40 to 60 percent of patients with IHS.[15,49] Up to 60 percent of patients develop a predominantly nocturnal cough, which is either nonproductive or productive of small quantities of nonpurulent sputum. Wheezing and dyspnea are also common, without an obstructive ventilatory defect on spirometric examination. Pulmonary hypertension, ARDS, and pleural effusions (which may be due to CHF) have been reported. In patients with pulmonary manifestations, the chest radiograph may reveal transient focal or diffuse pulmonary infiltrates[49,53] and/or pleural effusion(s). Histopathologic examination of affected lung specimens most commonly reveals intense interstitial infiltration with eosinophils.[10] Less commonly, necrotic areas of parenchyma are found. These are believed to be due to pulmonary microemboli. In contrast to CSS, significant vasculitis is not present.

The diagnosis of IHS is established by demonstrating multiorgan dysfunction, severe peripheral blood eosinophilia (greater than $1.5 \times 10^9/mm^3$) for at least 6 months (or with death before then), and an absence of any other known causes of peripheral blood eosinophilia.[15,53] Occasionally, the disease presents with the incidental finding of blood eosinophilia before development of other complications. The total peripheral leukocyte count is typically elevated to above 10,000 (typical range, 10,000 to 30,000), with a preponderance of eosinophils (up to 70 percent). The leukocytosis may be progressive. Eosinophilic blast transformation was reported to occur at some time during the course of the disease in 28 percent of 51 patients in one series.[10] Other laboratory findings are elevated total serum IgE (25 to 38 percent),[10,15] hypergammaglobulinemia, circulating immune complexes (32 to 50 percent),[15] and an ESR above 15 mm/h (68 percent).[10] Elevated serum B_{12} and leukocyte alkaline phosphatase levels are also noted. Fungal and parasitic serologies, as well as aspirates of body fluids for ova and parasites, are negative. Of interest is that whereas blood and BAL eosinophilia are both prominent in persons with pulmonary involvement,[49] blood eosinophilia is present and BAL eosinophilia is absent in persons lacking pulmonary manifestations of the disease. This finding has raised the question whether BAL eosinophilia may serve as a marker for the development of pulmonary disease associated with IHS. The differential diagnosis of IHS includes acute eosinophilic pneumonias, CEP, TPE, parasitic infection, tuberculous or fungal infection, allergic or autoimmune disease, and other lymphoproliferative disorders.[53]

The organ damage in IHS is believed to be due both to eosinophilic infiltration of tissues and to tissue injury caused by thromboembolic events. Eosinophils probably contribute to tissue damage via antibody-mediated cytotoxicity and the release of toxic granule products such as major basic protein and eosinophil cationic protein.[15] Elevated serum levels of eosinophil cationic protein and major basic protein have been reported, but they do not correlate universally with clinical disease severity.[15] The precise events inciting the extreme eosinophilia in IHS are unknown. A variety of chromosomal abnormalities (including the Philadelphia chromosome) have been described, and abnormal growth regulation may exist at the level of the eosinophil stem cell in the bone marrow.[53] A variety of other abnormalities of the immune system in IHS patients have been appreciated. Most notable are case reports describing the clonal expansion of Th2-like T cells with elevated serum levels of IL-4 and IL-5 (cytokines important for eosinophil growth, differentiation, and chemotaxis), which declined following steroid therapy for the disease.[11] Elevated levels of IL-5 messenger RNA are present in bone marrow or blood mononuclear cells from some but not all patients with IHS.[48] In several cases, the levels of bone marrow IL-5 correlated with the degree of blood eosinophilia. These findings suggest that dysregulated T-cell function may play a role in the pathogenesis of some cases of IHS.

Before the discovery of an effective therapy, the prognosis of IHS was poor. In one early series,[37] 81 percent of 48 patients died within 1 year of diagnosis. Overall, without therapy, average survival is 9 months, and 3- to 4-year survival is estimated at 10 to 12 percent.[10] Only rarely do patients exhibit long-term survival without therapy. The greatest mortality occurs within the first year after diagnosis.[10] Death may occur from refractory CHF, azotemia, hepatic failure, venous thromboembolism, a perforated abdominal viscus, or infection.[37] The advent of effective therapy for IHS has led to a marked improvement in median survival to more than 10 years.[10,37] The mainstay of therapy for IHS includes corticosteroids and the alkylating agent hydroxyurea. It has been suggested that patients without evidence of end-organ dysfunction but with the incidental finding of peripheral eosinophilia be followed closely at 3- to 6-month intervals.[15] Persons with progressive organ dysfunction should receive prednisone (1 mg/kg per day) for several weeks, followed by a change to alternate-day dosing.

If the disease stabilizes or resolves, alternate-day corticosteroids should be continued for approximately 1 year at the minimal dose that effectively controls disease activity. Hydroxyurea (0.5 to 1.5 g per day) should be added to the regimen if there is evidence of further disease progression, with the aim of reducing the peripheral leukocyte count to the range of 5000 to 10,000.[15] Vincristine may be used as a chemotherapeutic inducing agent in patients with extremely high peripheral WBC counts.[37] Etoposide and troleandomycin are effective alternative agents for cases that prove refractory to standard treatment. Interferon-α, a mediator that suppresses eosinophil function in vitro, has been beneficial in the management of some cases of chronic myelogenous leukemia. When administered at 4 to 8×10^6 units a day, it has been shown to induce long-term remissions (up to 2 years) in severe, refractory IHS.[54]

Allogeneic bone marrow transplantation has also been anecdotally reported to be successful in selected cases of IHS in which end-organ damage is potentially reversible. Leukapheresis affords no clear benefit unless there is elevated blood viscosity with associated coagulation. Antiparasitic agents and radiation therapy are ineffective. Factors associated with a poor prognosis include presence of total blood WBC greater than 100,000/mm³, myeloblasts in the peripheral blood, refractory CHF, basophilia above 3 percent, identifiable chromosomal abnormalities in bone marrow cells, and elevated serum B_{12} levels.[10,37] Favorable prognostic features include a rapid clinical response to treatment with reduction in blood eosinophilia and the presence of angioedema or an elevated IgE.[37] The mechanisms by which these features are associated with a given prognosis are largely unknown.

APPROACH TO THE EVALUATION OF EOSINOPHILIC PNEUMONIAS

In approaching the patient with pulmonary infiltrates and eosinophilia, one must first establish whether the patient has one of the eosinophilic disorders described in this chapter or a dis-

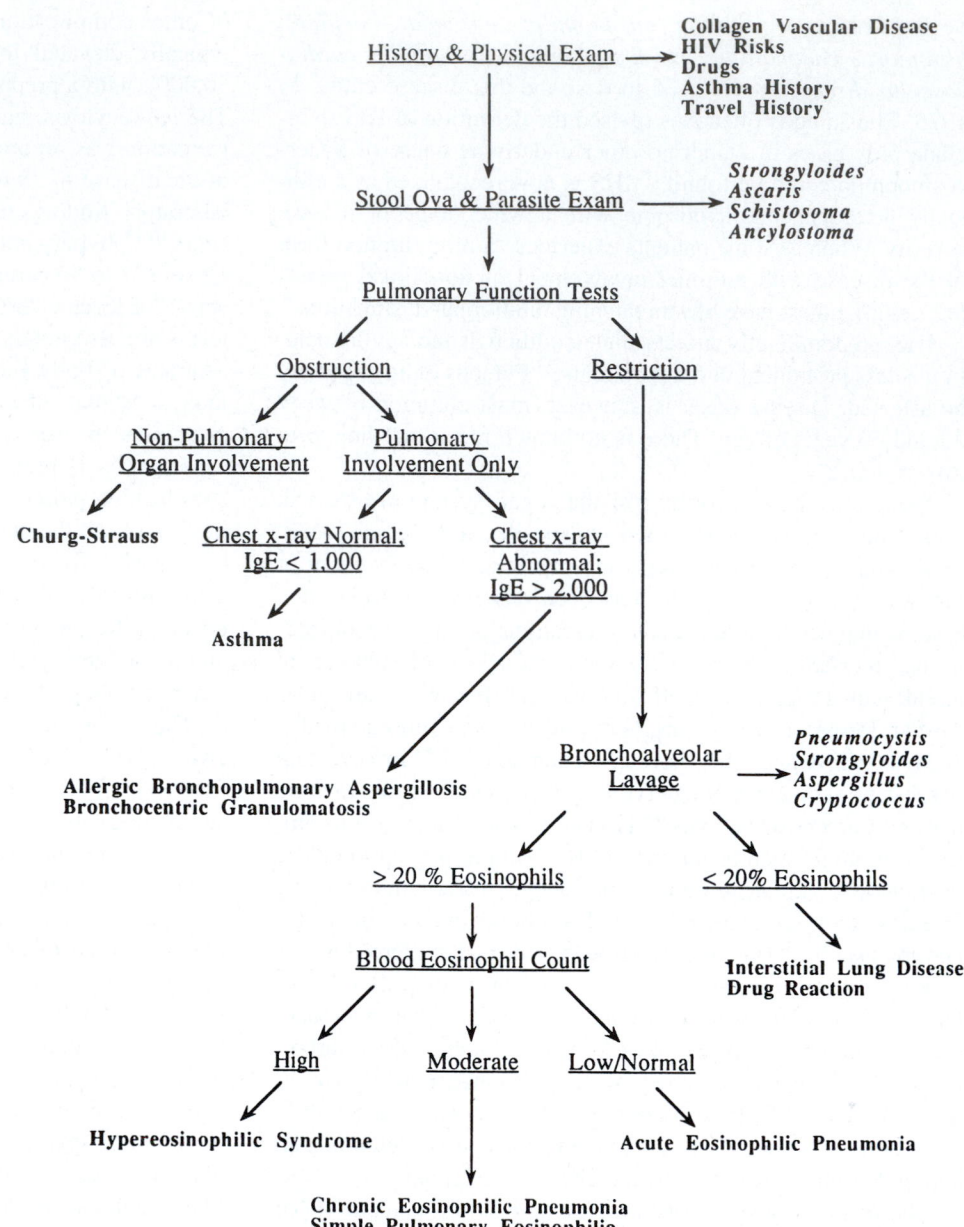

FIGURE 74-5 Algorithmic approach to evaluation of patients with pulmonary infiltrate and eosinophilia. *(Based on data of Allen and Davis,[1] with permission.)*

ease process that is secondarily associated with eosinophilia (Table 74-1). A useful algorithmic approach to the evaluation of patients with pulmonary infiltrates and eosinophilia (blood or lung) is shown in Fig. 74-5.[1] A careful search for the cause of the disease should be undertaken. A comprehensive medical history should be elicited, with particular attention paid to any antecedent illness (e.g., atopy, rhinitis, asthma, steroid use, immunosuppression), disease exposures, travel, and the duration and nature of the patient's symptoms. One should take special notice of the sequence and timing of events during the course of the illness. In addition to a careful chest examination, a search should be undertaken for physical findings suggestive of extrapulmonary disease (e.g., skin lesions, CHF, hypertension, neurologic abnormalities, musculoskeletal disorders, or GI illness). The nature, distribution, and duration of infiltrates on chest radiograph should be noted.

TABLE 74-5

Comparative Features of the Pulmonary Eosinophilic Syndromes

	Loeffler's	*AEP*	*TPE*
Clinical course	Acute	Acute	Acute, subacute, chronic
H/o allergic disease/asthma	—	+/–	—
Blood eosinophilia	Extreme, transient	Absent	Extreme >90 percent
Sputum/BAL eosinophilia	Prominent	Striking	Prominent
Elevated serum IgE	+/–	Moderate elev. in some	Highly elevated
Etiologic agent	*Ascaris* spp. (other parasites, drugs)	Unknown	Filarial infection
Radiographic infiltrates	Transient, migratory	Diffuse, alv. and interstitial	Diffuse, reticulonodular
PFTs	RVD	RVD	OVD early, RVD late
Characteristic diagnostic findings	*Ascaris* larvae in sputum, gastric asp.	None	Filaria-specific IgE, IgG, microfilaria in LN/lung
Vasculitis	None	None	None
Extrapulmonary manifestations	GI late, if untreated	None	Cardiac, central nervous system rare
Therapy	Mebendizole	Corticosteroids	DEC
Chronic/recurrent disease	None	None	Infrequent

NOTE: + = yes or present; – = no or not present; h/o = history of; RVD = restrictive ventilatory defect; OVD = obstructive ventilatory defect; LN = lymph node; DEC = diethylcarbamazine.

The workup should include the following additional laboratory data: CBC with differential, ESR, IgE level, ECG, BUN, creatinine, liver function tests, urinalysis, sputum cultures, and, when appropriate, sputum cytology. Serologies (e.g., *Aspergillus* precipitins, ANCA, antiparasite antibodies) are indicated in selected cases. Bronchoscopy with BAL or transbronchial biopsy is important in the evaluation of pulmonary eosinophilic syndromes. The advent of BAL has allowed diagnosis of most cases of eosinophilic pneumonia without open lung biopsy. Normally, BAL fluid contains less than 2 percent eosinophils. In contrast to diseases associated secondarily with eosinophilia, all the primary pulmonary eosinophilic syndromes are characterized by striking BAL eosinophilia (more than 20 percent of the BAL leukocyte differential). The finding of more than 20 percent BAL eosinophils, viewed in combination with appropriate clinical and radiographic features, is strongly suggestive of the diagnosis of one of these syndromes. BAL and transbronchial biopsy are also useful in ruling out infections (bacterial, fungal, tuberculous,

parasitic, and *Pneumocystis carinii*), malignancies, and other causes of eosinophil-associated disease. It must be kept in mind that in the context of the overall list of pulmonary diseases associated with more than 5 percent BAL eosinophilia, the true pulmonary eosinophilic syndromes are rare.[2]

The pulmonary eosinophilic syndromes are at times difficult to distinguish from one another, owing to the substantial amount of overlap among their clinical, radiographic, histologic, and therapeutic features. The comparative features of the eosinophilic pneumonias described in this chapter, with regard to several key features, are shown in Table 74-5. The clinical presentation may be acute, subacute, or chronic. Disease may range from mild, self-limited to severe and life-threatening illness. To varying degrees in all the pulmonary eosinophilic syndromes, dyspnea, malaise, low-grade fever, cough, and wheezing are common presenting complaints. Of the diseases considered in detail in this chapter, only CSS and IHS are consistently associated with significant extrapulmonary manifestations. Radiographic infiltrates

TABLE 74-5 *(Cont.)*

CEP	ABPA	CSS	IHS
Subacute	Acute, subacute, chronic	Acute, subacute, chronic	Subacute, chronic
+ (30–60 percent)	Nearly 100%	100%	—
Mild–mod. in most	Typical	Extreme, fluctuating	Extreme, persistent
Striking	In some	Prominent	Striking
Mod.–elev. in 30 percent	Marked elev., fluctuates w/ disease	Mod.–elev.	Mod.–elev. in some
Unknown	*Aspergillus* (or other fungus)	Unknown	Unknown
Periph., dense	Upper lobe predom.	Transient, migratory	Transient focal or diffuse
Nonmigratory, recur.	Prox. bronchiectasis	Peripheral, rarely diffuse	
RVD +/− OVD	OVD +/− RVD	OVD +/− RVD	Mild RVD in some
None	See Table 74-4	Histopathology plus approp. clinical setting	Extreme persistent eos. and multiorgan dysfunction (no other evident cause)
Occas. mild, non-necrotic	None	Characteristic (see text)	None
None	None	Typical of vasculitic phase	Cardiac, neurologic, gastrointestinal, hematol., other
Corticosteroids	Corticosteroids, bronchodilators, antibiotics	Corticosteroids, other immunosuppr.	Corticosteroids, hydroxyurea
Common	Typical	Infrequent after Rx	Chronicity typical

may be transient in Loeffler's syndrome, TPE, CSS, ABPA, and IHS. Blood eosinophilia is present in all the diseases discussed except idiopathic AEP. Variable degrees of elevation of serum IgE are also present. Pulmonary function abnormalities are not specific for these disorders. Except for the diseases caused by parasites, corticosteroids are the mainstay of therapy.

Although the eosinophilic pneumonias can, at times, pose diagnostic difficulties, it is crucial, whenever possible, to establish an accurate diagnosis. The importance of an accurate diagnosis results, in part, from the appreciation that the prognosis, dose, and duration of treatment and follow-up measures that these diseases require vary widely. Furthermore, chronic fibrotic lung disease may result from failure to accurately diagnose and treat some of these disorders in a timely fashion, and misdiagnosis with resultant inappropriate therapy (e.g., high-dose steroid treatment of invasive fungal infection masquerading as CEP) may be catastrophic.

REFERENCES

1. Allen JN, Davis WB: Eosinophilic lung diseases. *Am J Respir Crit Care Med* 150:1423–1438, 1994.
2. Allen JN, Davis WB, Pacht ER: Diagnostic significance of increased bronchoalveolar lavage fluid eosinophils. *Am Rev Respir Dis* 142:642–647, 1990.
3. Allen JN, Pacht ER, Gadek JE, Davis WB: Acute eosinophilic pneumonia as a reversible cause of noninfectious respiratory failure. *New Engl J Med* 321:569–574, 1989.
4. Badesch DB, King TE, Schwarz MI: Acute eosinophilic pneumonia: A hypersensitivity phenomenon? *Am Rev Respir Dis* 139:249–252, 1989.
5. Bedrossian CWM, Greenberg SD, Williams LJ Jr: Ultrastructure of the lung in Loeffler's pneumonia. *Am J Med* 58:438–443, 1975.
6. Bosken CH, Myers JL, Greenberger PA, Katzenstein ALA: Pathologic features of allergic bronchopulmonary aspergillosis. *Am J Surg Pathol* 12:216–222, 1988.

7. Carrington CB, Addington WW, Goff AM, et al: Chronic eosinophilic pneumonia. *New Engl J Med* 280:787–798, 1969.

8. Chumbley LC, Harrison EG Jr, DeRemee RA: Allergic granulomatosis and angiitis (Churg-Strauss syndrome): Report and analysis of 30 cases. *Mayo Clin Proc* 52:477–484, 1977.

9. Churg A, Brallas M, Cronin SR, Churg J: Formes frustes of Churg-Strauss syndrome. *Chest* 108:320–323, 1995.

10. Chusid MJ, Dale DC, West BC, Wolff SM: The hypereosinophilic syndrome: Analysis of fourteen cases with review of the literature. *Medicine* 54:1–27, 1975.

11. Cogan E, Schandene L, Crusiaux A, et al: Brief report: Clonal proliferation of type 2 helper T cells in a man with the hypereosinophilic syndrome. *New Engl J Med* 330:535–538, 1994.

12. Cooper JAD, White DA, Matthay RA: Drug-induced pulmonary disease, Part 2: Noncytotoxic drugs. *Am Rev Respir Dis* 133:488–505, 1986.

13. Dejaegher P, Demedts M: Bronchoalveolar lavage in eosinophilic pneumonia before and during corticosteroid therapy. *Am Rev Respir Dis* 129:631–632, 1984.

14. Denning DW, Van Wye JE, Lewiston NJ, Stevens DA: Adjunctive therapy of allergic bronchopulmonary aspergillosis with itraconazole. *Chest* 100:813–819, 1991.

15. Fauci AS, Harley JB, Roberts WC, et al: The idiopathic hypereosinophilic syndrome: Clinical, pathophysiologic, and therapeutic considerations. *Ann Intern Med* 97:78–92, 1982.

16. Gaensler EA, Carrington CB: Peripheral opacities in chronic eosinophilic pneumonia: The photographic negative of pulmonary edema. *Am J Roentgenol* 128:1–13, 1977.

17. Greenberger PA, Miller TP, Roberts M, Smith LL: Allergic bronchopulmonary aspergillosis in patients with and without evidence of bronchiectasis. *Ann Allergy* 70:333–338, 1993.

18. Greenberger PA, Smith LJ, Hsu CCS, et al: Analysis of bronchoalveolar lavage in allergic bronchopulmonary aspergillosis: Divergent responses of antigen-specific antibodies and total IgE. *J Allergy Clin Immunol* 82:164–170, 1988.

19. Greenberger PA, Patterson R: Diagnosis and management of allergic bronchopulmonary aspergillosis. *Ann Allergy* 56:444–448, 1986.

20. Greenberger PA, Patterson R: Allergic bronchopulmonary aspergillosis: Model of bronchopulmonary disease with defined serologic, radiologic, pathologic and clinical findings from asthma to fatal destructive lung disease. *Chest* 91(Suppl):165S–171S, 1987.

21. Hayakawa H, Sato A, Toyoshima M, et al: A clinical study of idiopathic eosinophilic pneumonia. *Chest* 105:1462–1466, 1994.

22. Jamil SA, Hilton E: The strongyloides hyperinfection syndrome. *NY State J Med* 92:67–68, 1992.

23. Jederlinic PJ, Sicilian L, Gaensler EA: Chronic eosinophilic pneumonia: A report of 19 cases and a review of the literature. *Medicine* 67:154–162, 1988.

24. Kauffman HF, Tomee JFC, van der Werf TS, et al: Review of fungus-induced asthmatic reactions. *Am J Respir Crit Care Med* 151:2109–2116, 1995.

25. Knutsen AP, Mueller KR, Hutcheson PS, Slavin RG: Serum anti–*Aspergillus fumigatus* antibodies by immunoblot and ELISA in cystic fibrosis with allergic bronchopulmonary aspergillosis. *J Allergy Clin Immunol* 93:926–931, 1994.

26. Lanham JG, Elkon KB, Pusey CD, Hughes GR: Systemic vasculitis with asthma and eosinophilia: A clinical approach to the Churg-Strauss syndrome. *Medicine* 63:65–81, 1984.

27. Leavitt RY, Fauci AS: Pulmonary vasculitis. *Am Rev Respir Dis* 134:149–166, 1986.

28. Lee TM, Greenberger PA, Patterson R, et al: Stage V (fibrotic) allergic bronchopulmonary aspergillosis: A review of 17 cases followed from diagnosis. *Arch Intern Med* 147:319–323, 1987.

29. Lie JT: Illustrated histopathologic classification criteria for selected vasculitis syndromes. *Arthritis Rheum* 33:1074–1087, 1990.

30. Masi AT, Hunder GG, Lie JT, et al: The American College of Rheumatology 1990 criteria for the classification of Churg-Strauss syndrome (allergic granulomatosis and angiitis). *Arthritis Rheum* 33:1094–1100, 1990.

31. Mayo JR, Muller NL, Road J, et al: Chronic eosinophilic pneumonia: CT findings in six cases. *Am J Roentgenol* 153:727–730, 1989.

32. Moore PM, Calabrese LH: Neurologic manifestations of systemic vasculitides. *Semin Neurol* 14:300–306, 1994.

33. Naughton M, Fahy J, Fitzgerald MX: Chronic eosinophilic pneumonia: A long-term follow-up of 12 patients. *Chest* 103:162–165, 1993.

34. Neeld DA, Goodman LR, Gurney JW, et al: Computerized tomography in the evaluation of allergic bronchopulmonary aspergillosis. *Am Rev Respir Dis* 142:1200–1205, 1990.

35. Neva FA, Ottesen EA: Current concepts in parasitology: Tropical (filarial) eosinophilia. *New Engl J Med* 298:1129–1131, 1978.

36. Nutman TB, Vijayan VK, Pinkston P, et al: Tropical pulmonary eosinophilia: Analysis of antifilarial antibody localized to the lung. *J Infect Dis* 160:1042–1050, 1989.

37. Parrillo JE, Fauci AS, Wolff SM: Therapy of the hypereosinophilic syndrome. *Ann Intern Med* 89:167–172, 1978.

38. Patterson R, Greenberger PA, Halwig JM, et al: Allergic bronchopulmonary aspergillosis: Natural history and classification of early disease by serologic and roentgenographic studies. *Arch Intern Med* 146:916–918, 1986.

39. Patterson R, Greenberger PA, Lee TM, et al: Prolonged evaluation of patients with corticosteroid-dependent asthma stage of allergic bronchopulmonary aspergillosis. *J Allergy Clin Immunol* 80:663–668, 1987.

40. Patterson R, Greenberger PA, Radin RC, Roberts M: Allergic bronchopulmonary aspergillosis: Staging as an aid to management. *Ann Intern Med* 96:286–291, 1982.

41. Pinkston P, Vijayan VK, Nutman TB, et al: Acute tropical pulmonary eosinophilia: Characterization of the lower respiratory tract inflammation and its response to therapy. *J Clin Invest* 80:216–225, 1987.

42. Richeson RB, Stander PE: Allergic bronchopulmonary aspergillosis: An increasingly common disorder among asthmatic patients. *Postgrad Med* 88:217–224, 1990.

43. Ricketti AJ, Greenberger PA, Patterson R: Serum IgE as an important aid in management of allergic bronchopulmonary aspergillosis. *J Allergy Clin Immunol* 74:68–71, 1984.

44. Roig J, Romeu J, Riera C, et al: Acute eosinophilic pneumonia due to toxocariasis with bronchoalveolar lavage findings. *Chest* 102:294–296, 1992.

45. Rom WN, Vijayan VK, Cornelius MJ, et al: Persistent lower respiratory tract inflammation associated with interstitial lung disease in patients with tropical pulmonary eosinophilia following conventional treatment with diethylcarbamazine. *Am Rev Respir Dis* 142:1088–1092, 1990.

46. Rosenberg M, Patterson R, Mintzer R, et al: Clinical and immunologic criteria for the diagnosis of allergic bronchopulmonary aspergillosis. *Ann Intern Med* 86:405–414, 1977.

47. Safirstein BH, D'Souza MF, Simon G, et al: Five-year follow-up of allergic bronchopulmonary aspergillosis. *Am Rev Respir Dis* 108:450–459, 1973.

48. Satoh T, Sun L, Li MS, Spry CJ: Interleukin-5 mRNA levels in blood and bone marrow mononuclear cells from patients with the idiopathic hypereosinophilic syndrome. *Immunology* 83:308–312, 1994.

49. Slabbynck H, Impens N, Naegels S, et al: Idiopathic hypereosinophilic syndrome–related pulmonary involvement diagnosed by bronchoalveolar lavage. *Chest* 101:1178–1180, 1992.

50. Spry CJF, Kumaraswami V: Tropical eosinophilia. *Semin Hematol* 19:107–115, 1982.

51. Weller PF: The immunobiology of eosinophils. *New Engl J Med* 324:1110–1118, 1991.

52. Williams J, Nunley D, Dralle W, et al: Diagnosis of pulmonary strongyloidiasis by bronchoalveolar lavage. *Chest* 94:643–644, 1988.

53. Winn RE, Kollef MH, Meyer JI: Pulmonary involvement in the hypereosinophilic syndrome. *Chest* 105:656–660, 1994.

54. Zielinski RM, Lawrence WD: Interferon-α for the hypereosinophilic syndrome. *Ann Intern Med* 113:716–718, 1990.

CHAPTER 75

DEPOSITIONAL DISEASES OF THE LUNGS

Richard H. Ochs / Alfred P. Fishman

AMYLOIDOSIS
    Nature of Amyloid
    Tracheobronchial Amyloidosis
    Pulmonary Parenchymal Amyloidosis
    Diagnosis of Amyloidosis

DIFFUSE PULMONARY CALCIFICATION

ALVEOLAR MICROLITHIASIS

ALVEOLAR HEMORRHAGE SYNDROMES
    Goodpasture's Syndrome
    Pulmonary Vasculitis and Capillaritis
    Antiphospholipid Antibody-Associated Alveolar
        Hemorrhage
    Hemorrhage Associated with Connective Tissue
        Disease
    Toxic Alveolar Hemorrhage
    Idiopathic Pulmonary Hemosiderosis

Deposits of endogenous body constituents or exogenous materials in amounts sufficient to deform structure and impair function can occur virtually anywhere in the body. Deposits of endogenous materials in the lungs or airways cause a variety of diseases (Table 75-1). These may have different clinical manifestations, depending on localization (i.e., pulmonary parenchyma or conducting airways).[11,24,29,37] This chapter deals with a few of these manifestations: amyloidosis; diffuse pulmonary calcification; alveolar microlithiasis and alveolar hemorrhage syndromes, in-

cluding Goodpasture's syndrome; pulmonary microvasculitis; and idiopathic pulmonary hemosiderosis. Others are dealt with elsewhere in this text.

AMYLOIDOSIS

Amyloidosis refers to the extracellular deposition of amyloid, a fibrillar proteinaceous insoluble crystalline material. The main fibrillar component can be derived from any one of 15 proteins, all of which share common morphologic features. When amyloid is deposited in tissues it may produce atrophy of parenchymal cells (e.g., glomeruli), interference with mechanical function (e.g., heart and lungs), or impaired vasoconstriction of blood vessels, leading to hemorrhage (e.g., lungs and gastrointestinal tract).

Amyloidosis may be a systemic disease with deposition of amyloid in multiple sites. In such cases, the amyloid is derived from a soluble circulating plasma precursor. Localized amyloid deposition, involving a single body site, is thought to be derived from protein produced at the site of deposition.

Amyloidosis may involve any portion of the respiratory tract. For example, deposits in the tongue may be extensive enough to cause obstructive sleep apnea. Deposits in the tracheobronchial tree may cause signs of bronchial obstruction or hemorrhage. Diffuse interstitial pulmonary amyloidosis may lead to dyspnea or pulmonary hemorrhage. Pleural deposition may be associated with pleural effusion. Diaphragmatic deposition may lead to respiratory failure. Tracheobronchial amyloid deposition and nodu-

TABLE 75-1

Depositional Diseases of the Lungs

Biological Material	Disease
Interstitium	
Amyloid	Amyloidosis
Water	Interstitial edema
Calcium	Metastatic calcification
Alveoli	
Surfactant	Alveolar proteinosis
Water	Alveolar edema
Calcium	Alveolar microlithiasis
Blood and hemosiderin	Alveolar hemorrhage syndromes

lar parenchymal amyloid deposition (amyloidoma) (Fig. 75-1*A*) most often occur as isolated phenomena, whereas diffuse interstitial deposition is more often seen in systemic amyloidosis.

Nature of Amyloid

Amyloid was originally identified in tissues by routine histologic examination as a homogenous eosinophilic hyaline material (Fig. 75-1*B* and *C)*. Amyloid binds the dye Congo red, producing orange-red staining by conventional light microscopy. When Congo-red-stained amyloid is examined with crossed polarized lenses, it shows birefringence, staining either apple-green or yellow, depending on orientation of the polarizing lenses to the crystalline axis. Electron microscopic examination of amyloid reveals a dominant (95 percent) fibrillar component with distinctive periodicity, associated with a lesser (5 percent) pentagonal

donut-shaped glyprotein component, physically and chemically identical in all forms of amyloid, is derived from a soluble plasma protein, *soluble amyloid protein* (SAP). X-ray diffraction stuies of amyloid show the fibrils to be arrayed in a beta-pleated sheet configuration. This ac-

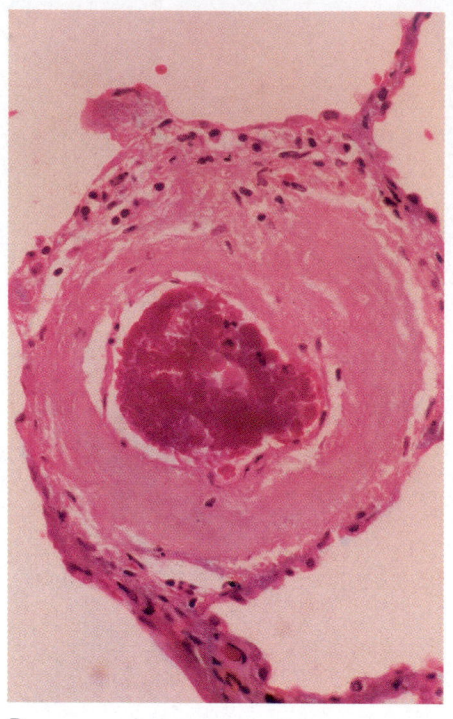

B

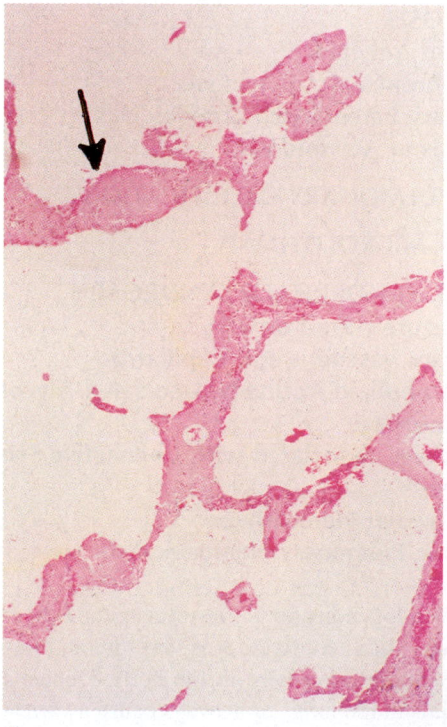

C

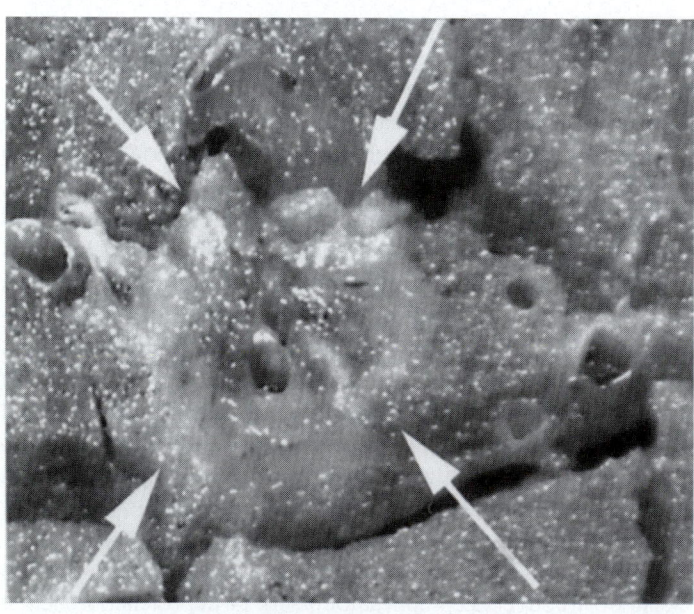

A

FIGURE 75-1   Amyloid deposition. *A*. Amyloidoma. Cut surface of lung with white arrows indicating a dense, wax like lesion that is characteristic of nodular amyloid. Incidental finding at autopsy. *(Courtesy of Leslie A. Litzky, M.D., Department of Pathology and Laboratory Medicine, Hospital of the University of Pennsylvania, Philadelphia, Pennsylvania.) B.* The typical amorphous appearance of amyloid is seen deposited within the wall of a pulmonary venule. Green birefringence on polarized light examination after staining with Congo red will confirm the amyloid nature of the deposit. H&E, ×700. *C*. Amorphous amyloid in the alveolar interstitial space. Arrow indicates a thickened alveolar septum. H&E, ×420.

counts for the ordered binding of Congo red dye which, in turn, causes birefringence.

The diverse protein fibrils in different types of amyloid are derived from soluble precursors, and the resulting deposits are both insoluble and resistant to proteolytic digestion under physiological conditions. Despite the common morphologic features of all types of amyloid, to date 15 different chemical types of amyloid protein have been identified. Systemic and most localized deposits of amyloid are derived from one of three precursor proteins, namely immunoglobulin light chains, amyloid-associated (AA) protein, or transthyretin, previously known as prealbumin. Less common sources of amyloid include β_2-microglobulin in chronic renal failure patients on dialysis, β-protein amyloid in the cerebral senile plaques of Alzheimer's disease, procalcitonin in medullary carcinoma of the thyroid, atrial naturetic factor in isolated cardiac atrial amyloid, and islet cell amyloid polypeptide in the pancreatic islets of patients with type II diabetes. Isolated tracheobronchial and nodular pulmonary parenchymal amyloid deposition are most often immunoglobulin-light-chain-derived, whereas diffuse interstitial pulmonary deposition, usually in the context of systemic amyloidosis, may be derived from immunoglobulin light chains, AA protein, or transthyretin.

Amyloidosis of immunoglobulin light chain origin, *AL amyloid,* is the most common type seen in systemic amyloidosis and the most frequent to cause symptomatic lung disease. AL amyloid usually occurs in association with plasma cell disorders (dyscrasias) which produce a monoclonal immunoglobulin or immunoglobulin fragment (monoclonal gammopathy). The monoclonal immunoglobulins or fragments are produced by a clone of neoplastic plasma cells which, in turn, are derived from B lymphocytes. The neoplastic clone may be clinically manifest as multiple myeloma or may be subclinical (formerly known as *primary amyloidosis*), causing bone marrow plasmacytosis or less commonly a localized monoclonal plasma cell proliferation, as is thought to be the case with localized tracheobronchial amyloid deposition. Most often the source protein is a lambda light chain, either intact or the amino terminal fragment.

AA amyloidosis is a far less common cause of symptomatic amyloidosis of the respiratory tract.[30] The AA protein is derived from an acute-phase reactant found in normal plasma known as *serum amyloid associated* (SAA) *protein* and produced by the liver. Chronic increase in serum acute-phase reactants is an important precondition for the deposition of AA amyloid. AA amyloidosis (previously referred to as *secondary amyloidosis*) was formerly more common in patients with chronic infections (e.g., tuberculosis, leprosy, and chronic osteomyelitis) but is now seen more commonly with noninfectious chronic inflammatory diseases (e.g., rheumatoid arthritis, familial Mediterranean fever, Crohn's disease, and heroin abuse with "skin popping").[4]

Amyloid derived from plasma transthyretin (*senile amyloidosis*) is not uncommon but only infrequently produces clinical disease.[29] This most often takes the form of restrictive cardiomyopathy due to cardiac deposition, and dyspnea due to diffuse interstitial pulmonary deposition is quite rare.

Tracheobronchial Amyloidosis

Amyloid deposition in the tracheobronchial tree can produce either plaques or tumoral masses.[17] The more common presentation as plaques is diffuse, multifocal, and represents submucosal deposition of amyloid. Less commonly, deposition of amyloid in the tracheobronchial tree produces a solitary mass which mimics an endobronchial neoplasm. Tracheobronchial amyloid deposition is most often of light-chain derivation and a localized phenomenon, suggesting that this represents a localized abnormal immune response of bronchial-associated lymphoid tissue (BALT) rather than a systemic immune response.

Diffuse involvement of the airways is apt to be symptomatic, producing cough, stridor, or hemoptysis. In contrast, localized mass lesions are more likely to produce evidence of localized bronchial obstruction (i.e., atelectasis or air trapping), with or without hemoptysis.

Both types of lesions can be readily identified by bronchoscopic examination. However, as is the case with amyloid deposition at all sites, there is a risk of hemorrhage. Although localized tumoral masses may be treated by excision, more diffuse involvement may be treated by laser ablation.[35]

Pulmonary Parenchymal Amyloidosis

Involvement of the pulmonary parenchyma by amyloidosis can be localized in the form of one or multiple macroscopic nodules that mimic neoplasm, or it may produce diffuse interstitial deposition.[23,30,34]

Nodular parenchymal amyloidosis, like tracheobronchial amyloidosis, most often represents a localized abnormal immune response of bronchial-associated lymphoid tissue (Fig. 75-1A). As a rule, solitary amyloid nodules (*amyloidomas*) are incidental radiographic findings in asymptomatic individuals. When multiple, such nodules may be associated with cough, dyspnea, or hemoptysis. These nodules have no distinctive features, although occasionally, they may show radiographic evidence of calcification or cavitation. Usually, the diagnosis of an amyloid nodule is made after surgical resection. Occasionally, the diagnosis has been made by transbronchial biopsy or percutaneous fine-needle aspiration. However, surgical excision of one or more nodules seems prudent, since, on rare occasion, amyloid deposition occurs within a pulmonary neoplasm (e.g., a primary neoplasm such as atypical carcinoid or a metastatic neoplasm such as medullary carcinoma from the thyroid).

Histologically, the amyloid deposit is often associated with an intense inflammatory reaction consisting of plasma cells, macrophages, and multinucleated giant cells. Only occasional chemical analyses are available, and these have revealed that most nodular deposits are of light-chain derivation, although rare cases of amyloid-associated (AA) amyloid have been reported. Interestingly, when the accompanying plasma cells have been analyzed for clonality, they are more often polyclonal than monoclonal. In such cases, the inflammatory cells may therefore be a local reaction to the presence of amyloid, rather than the source of the amyloid precursor light chains.

Widespread, *diffuse interstitial amyloidosis* of the pulmonary parenchyma may produce either a reticulonodular or miliary pattern on the chest radiograph. Such pulmonary involvement occurs most often in patients with systemic amyloidosis, derived from either immunoglobulin light-chain or amyloid-associated protein. Pulmonary interstitial amyloid deposition is rarely sufficiently severe to produce clinical manifestations but, uncommonly, it may produce progressive dyspnea, hemoptysis, or restrictive pulmonary function tests. The deposition of amyloid in the lungs is microscopic and may involve the alveolar septal interstitium, the walls of small blood vessels, or both (Fig. 75-1*B* and *C*). Transbronchial biopsy with Congo red staining is diagnostic, again bearing in mind the potential risk of biopsy-induced hemorrhage.

Diagnosis of Amyloidosis

Diagnosis of amyloidosis requires tissue examination and Congo red staining.[24,37] Whereas the initial recognition of different types of amyloid required chemical extraction of amyloid from tissues followed by amino acid sequencing, immunohistochemistry provides a ready means of classifying most biopsy specimens. Antibodies against immunoglobulin light chains, amyloid-associated protein, and transthyretin can be used immunohistochemically to classify most patients.

One instance has been reported of diffuse interstitial deposition of amyloid associated with ectopic pulmonary uptake of technetium 99m methylene diphosphonate on bone scan. The amyloid was light-chain derived. On biopsy, the deposition of amyloid was associated with ossification and calcification. The technetium binding may therefore have related to ossification rather than direct binding to amyloid.

DIFFUSE PULMONARY CALCIFICATION

Calcification of the pulmonary parenchyma can occur by a variety of mechanisms.[31] *Dystrophic calcification* refers to the deposition of calcium salts, most often crystalline hydroxyapatite, in dead tissue such as within the healing granulomas of tuberculosis. This type of calcification is usually localized; its distinctive radiographic features are sometimes helpful diagnostically (see Chapter 162).

Metastatic calcification refers to the deposition of calcium salts, usually amorphous, in normal tissues (Fig. 75-2). This latter type of calcification occurs in association with some de-

rangement of calcium metabolism, such as primary hyperparathyroidism, secondary hyperparathyroidism of chronic renal failure, hypervitaminosis D, the milk alkali syndrome, sarcoidosis, or increased bone turnover due to multiple myeloma or metastatic carcinoma.

Although metastatic calcification can occur in almost any tissue of the body, it occurs most often in the lungs, kidneys, and the stomach (tissues with more alkaline pH), and the walls of blood vessels. Metastatic calcification in the lungs usually affects the interstitium of the alveolar septa and the walls of bronchioles and pulmonary vessels, sometimes localizing on elastic fibers.

Clinical manifestations of diffuse pulmonary calcification are unusual, occurring most often in patients who are in chronic renal failure, particularly in those on chronic hemodialysis.[5]

Radiographically, metastatic calcification usually takes the form of a diffuse interstitial infiltrate, sometimes with fine nodularity. Less often, confluent patchy consolidation mimicking pneumonia may be seen.[21] Although the calcific nature of the infiltrate is often apparent on routine chest radiograph, CT scan is more sensitive both in detecting the interstitial deposits and in revealing their calcific nature.[12,25] Moreover, CT scan may also demonstrate calcification of chest wall blood vessels, circumstantially implicating calcification as the cause of pulmonary parenchymal abnormalities. Recognition of the calcific nature of the infiltrate is furthered by scanning with technetium 99m.[9]

Only rarely do the patients manifest dyspnea, arterial hypoxemia, and the pulmonary function tests of restrictive pulmonary disease. Unexplained dyspnea in a patient with chronic renal failure or hypercalcemia in the presence of a normal chest radiograph should lead to consideration of high-resolution computerized tomography or technetium scanning.

The mechanism responsible for diffuse pulmonary calcification is unknown. Although high levels of parathyroid hormone or a marked increase in the calcium-phosphate solubility product occur in some patients, diffuse calcification can occur in the absence of either. Ultrastructural observations of minimal, presumably early, lesions show selective deposition of calcium on elastic fibers, suggesting that they may serve as the initial nidus. In contrast to their apparent role in alveolar microlithiasis, extracellular matrix vesicles do not appear to be involved.

ALVEOLAR MICROLITHIASIS

This rare disorder usually presents as an abnormal chest radiograph from an asymptomatic patient (Fig. 75-3*A* and *B*). The chest radiograph is diagnostic, showing a sandlike micronodulation throughout the lung fields. This is caused by the presence of innumerable minute calcified spherules filling the alveolar spaces. The calcification is usually sufficiently dense as to constitute the signature of the disease on the routine radiograph. In some patients, concentration of the spherules in subpleural, paraseptal, and peribronchiolar alveoli can produce linear strands of calcification parallel to or perpendicular to the pleural surface, readily apparent on high-resolution computed tomography. The spherules also bind technetium 99m, which can be a diagnostic adjunct. Although not usually required, bronchoalveolar lavage or biopsy can confirm the diagnosis. Biopsy shows calcified

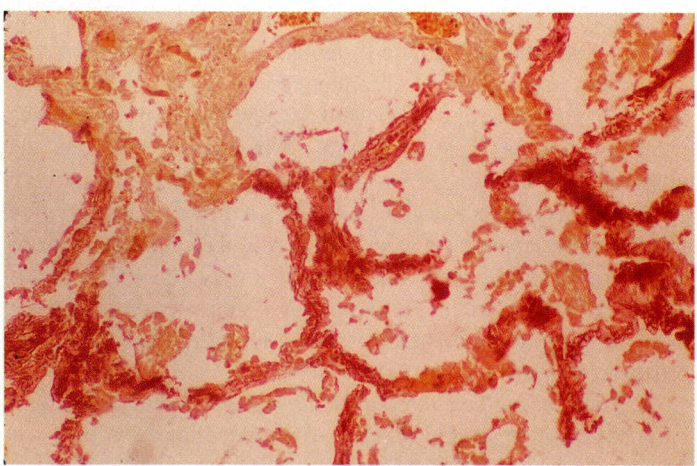

FIGURE 75-2 Metastatic calcification of alveolar septa in a renal dialysis patient. Photomicrograph shows calcium forming a dark red precipitate within the alveolar septa. Alizarin red, ×280.

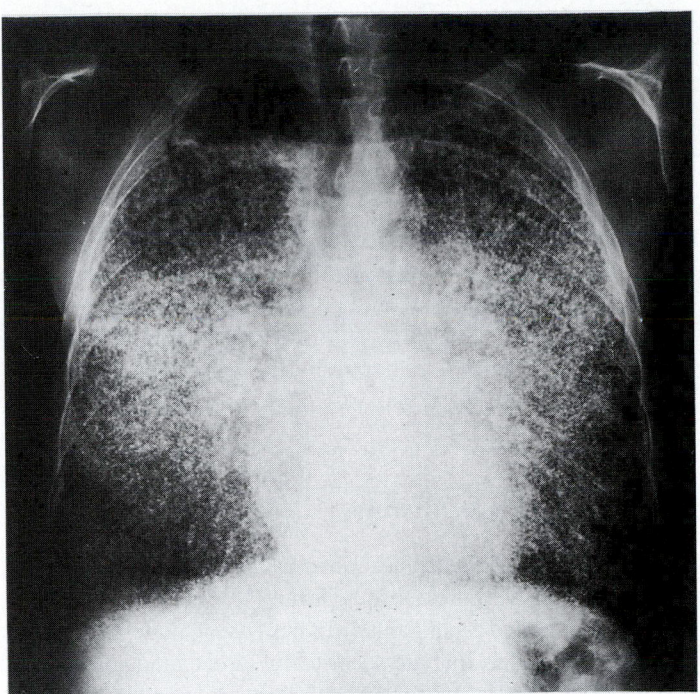

A

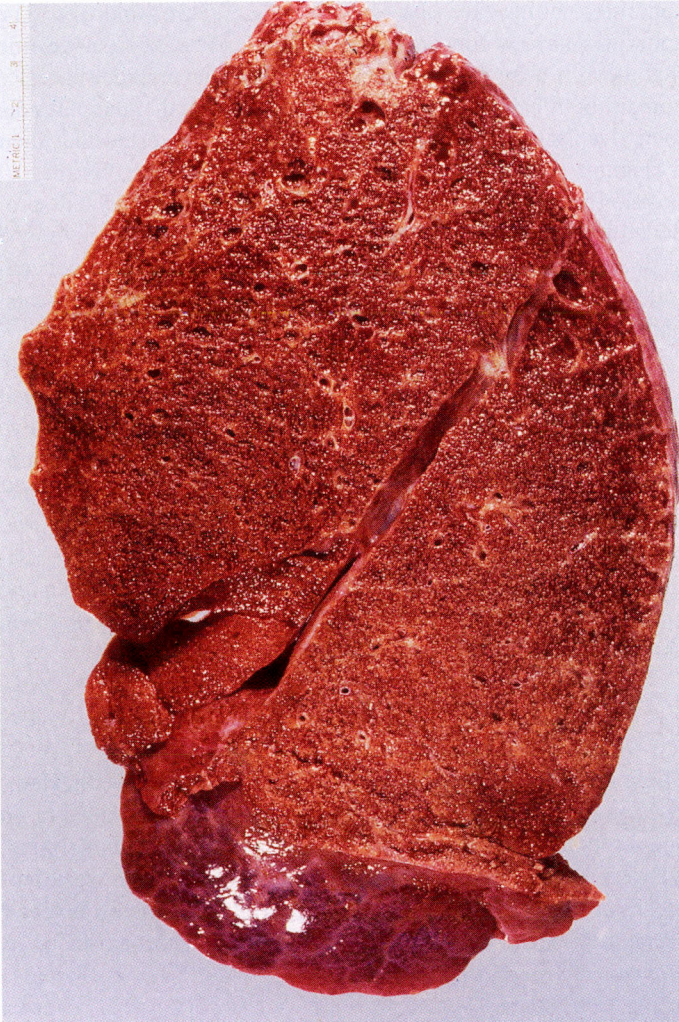

C

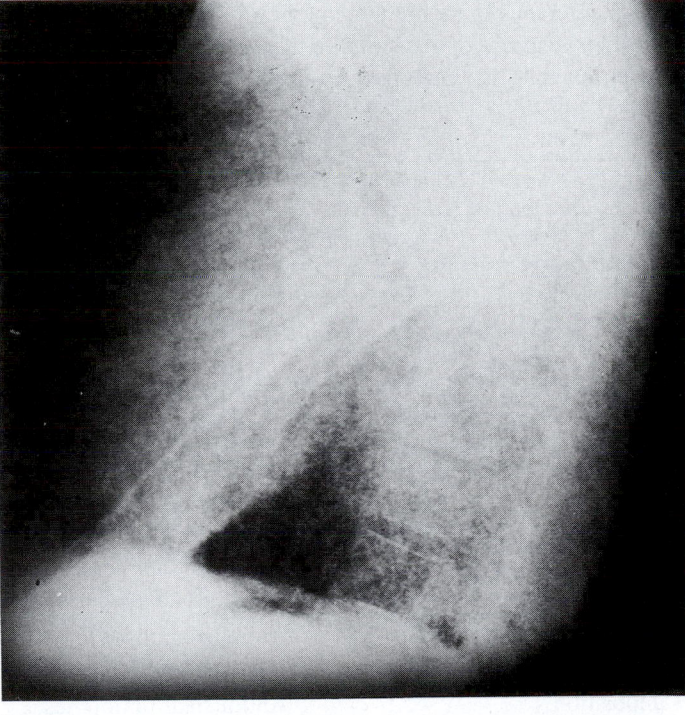

B

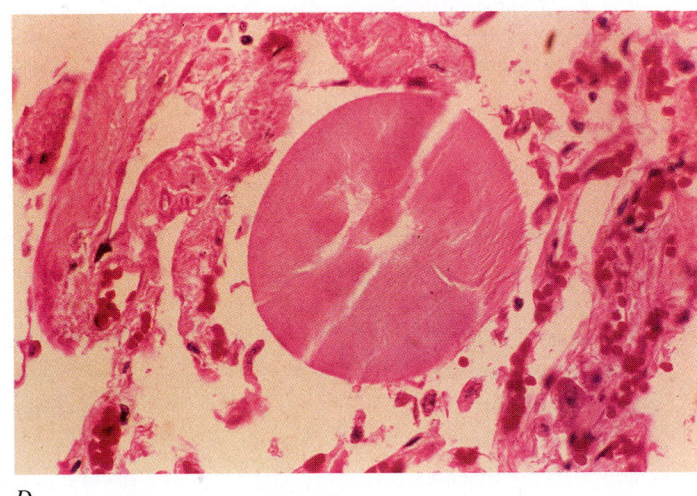

D

FIGURE 75-3   Alveolar microlithiasis in a 46-year-old man admitted for nonpulmonary problems. History included slight dyspnea on exertion and previous episodes of "pneumonia" during 1947, 1950, and 1952. Clinical examination revealed severe restrictive lung disease, pulmonary hypertension, and cor pulmonale. Diagnosis confirmed by lung biopsy. *A* and *B*. Posterior-anterior and lateral chest radiographs demonstrate innumerable, tiny calcified nodules throughout both lung fields. Thin, lucent lines on each side represent normal pleura visualized between the calcified pulmonary parenchyma and the chest wall. Emphysematous blebs in the apices displace the calcifications. *C*. Cut surface of explanted lung from a patient undergoing lung transplantation for primary alveolar microlithiasis. Note the fine nodularity which correlated with the chest radiographs. *(Courtesy of Leslie A. Litzky, M.D., Department of Pathology and Laboratory Medicine, Hospital of the University of Pennsylvania, Philadelphia, Pennsylvania.) D.* Photomicrograph demonstrating a typical calcospherite in an alveolar space. H&E, ×1120.

spherules filling alveolar spaces (Fig. 75-3C and D). The spherules have a concentric lamellated appearance, suggesting that they grow by the addition of successive layers; the spherules contain both calcium and phosphorus. Although the microliths are intra-alveolar, one ultrastructural study has suggested that their formation is initiated in the pulmonary interstitium by the deposition in a collagenous matrix of hydroxyapatite crystals produced by extracellular matrix vesicles. These membrane-bound vesicles are derived from mesenchymal cells and can concentrate calcium ions and liberate phosphate from membrane phospholipids.[2,3]

Although usually asymptomatic at the time of presentation, alveolar microlithiasis, on rare occasion, can produce functional abnormalities. When it does, the findings are those of restrictive pulmonary disease or exercise-induced pulmonary hypertension.[10] In general, no therapy, including bronchoalveolar lavage, has proved effective, although one case report indicates improved oxygenation using nasal continuous positive airway pressure ventilation.[18] Lung transplantation has also been performed in a few patients.[33] The etiology of alveolar microlithiasis is unknown, but some cases appear to be familial.

ALVEOLAR HEMORRHAGE SYNDROMES

These syndromes cause blood to accumulate in the alveoli. Hemorrhage originating proximal to alveoli (e.g., a nose bleed or an endobronchial neoplasm) can fill alveolar spaces with blood, whereas diffuse alveolar hemorrhage is usually the result of bleeding from damaged alveolar septa. The damage to alveolar septa may be identified as an immunologic mechanism or as resulting from exposure to a toxic agent, or the cause may be unknown (Table 75-2).

Pulmonary hemorrhage may occur as an isolated phenomenon or in association with extrapulmonary disease.[1,26,27] Pulmonary involvement may manifest as diffuse alveolar infiltrates on chest radiograph, hemoptysis, or anemia. Immunologic mechanisms include direct antibody mediated injury (e.g., Goodpasture's syndrome), indirect injury by immune complex deposition (e.g., systemic lupus erythematosus), neutrophil activation by antineutrophil cytoplasmic antibodies (e.g., Wegener's granulomatosis) or in association with antiphospholipid antibodies.[7,13,15,19] Associated extrapulmonary disease may include glomerulonephritis, systemic vasculitis, or a connective tissue disease.

Goodpasture's Syndrome

This entity was originally described as an association of alveolar hemorrhage with glomerulonephritis. It was later determined that pulmonary and renal damage in many such patients was mediated by antibodies that are specifically directed against a component of glomerular and other capillary basement membranes, most often the α-3 chain of type IV (basement membrane) collagen. The anti-basement membrane antibodies cause pulmonary hemorrhage only in genetically predisposed individuals, after some injury such as cigarette smoke, viral respiratory infection, or hydrocarbon vapor inhalation exposes alveolar capillary basement membranes to the immune system.[6,16,19,22] Although there are other causes of concomitant alveolar hemorrhage and glomerulonephritis, Goodpasture's syndrome is generally re-

TABLE 75-2

Alveolar Hemorrhage

Syndrome	Mechanism	Serum Marker
Goodpasture's syndrome	Anti-basement-membrane mediated injury to capillaries	Anti-basement membrane antibodies
Pulmonary vasculitis		
Polyarteritis nodosa	Immune-complex-mediated injury	Circulating immune complexes
Wegener's granulomatosis	Pauci-immune* vasculitis involving larger vessels and/or capillaries	c-ANCA† antibodies against proteinase 3
Alveolar capillaritis ± glomerulonephritis	Pauci-immune* capillaritis	p-ANCA† antibodies against myeloperoxidase
Antiphospholipid syndrome	Pauci-immune* capillaritis	Antiphospholipid antibodies
Connective tissue diseases (e.g., systemic lupus erythematosis)	Immune complex deposition, antiphospholipid antibodies or unknown	Antinuclear antibodies, antiphospholipid antibodies
Trimellitic anhydride toxicity	Direct toxic injury	None
Idiopathic pulmonary hemosiderosis	Unknown	None

*Pauci-immune vasculitis denotes absent immunoglobulin or complement deposition on immunofluorescence microscopy
†ANCA denotes anti-neutrophile cytoplasmic antibody

served for disease mediated by anti-glomerular basement membrane antibodies (anti-GBM antibodies) (see Chapter 69).

Goodpasture's syndrome can present with a broad spectrum of clinical findings.[8,26] The "classic" patient presents with massive hemoptysis, dyspnea, diffuse alveolar infiltrates on chest radiograph (Fig. 75-4A and B), and overt glomerulonephritis, often with acute renal failure. However, some patients present with only hemoptysis and subsequently develop overt renal disease months or even years later. On occasion, patients present with acute glomerulonephritis due to anti-GBM antibodies and either develop pulmonary hemorrhage subsequently or never develop pulmonary hemorrhage. Without pulmonary hemorrhage, the entity should not be called "Goodpasture's syndrome."

The histologic findings on lung biopsy in Goodpasture's syndrome are not diagnostic. Routine light-microscopy reveals intra-alveolar hemorrhage, usually associated with intra-alveolar hemosiderin-laden macrophages (Fig. 75-4C). There is no evidence of vasculitis, capillaritis, interstitial or intra-alveolar inflammation, or necrosis. Nonspecific reparative proliferation of the alveolar lining cells may be present. Only occasionally will immunofluorescence microscopy show diagnostic linear deposits of immunoglobulin and/or complement along alveolar capillary walls (Fig. 75-4D). In contrast, kidney biopsy in Goodpasture's syndrome is usually diagnostic: Whereas conventional light microscopy shows nonspecific focal or diffuse glomerulonephritis—which may be crescentic and which may be necrotizing—immunofluorescence microscopy shows linear deposition of immunoglobulin (usually IgG, or rarely IgM or IgA) and frequently shows complement deposition as well.

Even without biopsy, the diagnosis of Goodpasture's syndrome can be made by detecting anti-GBM antibody in the patient's serum. This is most reliably detected by enzyme-linked immunoabsorbent assay (ELISA) or radioimmunoassay (RIA). If these studies are not immediately available, indirect immunofluorescence (using the patient's serum as the primary antibody and normal human or animal kidney as the substrate) provides a less sensitive but rapid and specific assay.

When pulmonary hemorrhage due to Goodpasture's syndrome is life threatening, plasmapheresis for rapid lowering of circulating levels of anti-GBM antibody and administration of intravenous corticosteroids and cyclophosphamide to suppress antibody synthesis can be lifesaving. This therapy has largely replaced emergency nephrectomy. If the patient is not in advanced renal failure at the time of diagnosis, chronic immunosuppression with a combination of corticosteroids and cyclophosphamide can prevent progressive renal damage. If irreversible renal failure has already occurred, the patient can eventually be successfully transplanted once anti-GMB antibodies have disappeared from the serum. Elimination of the antibodies usually can be achieved by immunosuppression alone; in some instances, pretransplant nephrectomy may be required.

Pulmonary Vasculitis and Capillaritis

Fewer than half of the patients with alveolar hemorrhage and associated glomerulonephritis manifest anti-GBM antibodies.[15,27] Most of those without anti-GBM antibodies have evidence of either localized or systemic vasculitis or a connective tissue disease. A rare instance may be due to exposure to a toxic agent (e.g., trimellitic anhydride).[22]

Pulmonary hemorrhage may occur as a consequence of vascular injury within the lung parenchyma, often in association with well-defined systemic vasculitis syndromes (e.g., periarteritis nodosa, Churg-Strauss allergic granulomatosis, Wegener's granulomatosis, Henoch-Schönlein purpura, essential mixed cryoglobulinemia, Behcet's disease) or necrotizing systemic vasculitis that does not fit into any of the well-defined syndromes.[1,8,28]

Pulmonary vascular injury leading to hemorrhage may involve vasculitis of larger vessels (e.g., periarteritis nodosa and Wegener's granulomatosis) or alveolar capillaries (e.g., Wegener's granulomatosis, antineutrophile cytoplasmic antibody-associated alveolar hemorrhage, and systemic lupus erythematosus).[13] Some instances of large-vessel vasculitis and capillaritis are mediated by immune complex deposition with or without complement activation (e.g., periarteritis nodosa and systemic lupus erythematosus). The antigen of the immune complex is not of pulmonary origin (e.g., hepatitis B surface antigen or double-stranded DNA), and the lung is an "innocent bystander." This contrasts with Goodpasture's syndrome, where alveolar capillary basement membrane collagen serves as the antigen.

An increasing number of patients have been found to have alveolar capillaritis without deposition of either immune complexes or anti-GBM antibodies ("pauci-immune capillaritis").[27,28] These have been associated with the development of autoantibodies directed against cytoplasmic components of neutrophils (and monocytes), the antineutrophil cytoplasmic antibodies (ANCAs). Detection of ANCAs entails the use of indirect immunofluorescence and heterologous antibodies against human immunoglobulin to detect autoantibodies bound to neutrophils of affected patients. Ethanol fixation of the neutrophils prior to antibody staining produces one of two patterns when autoantibodies are present: (1) a finely granular centrally accentuated cytoplasmic localization (c-ANCA), (2) a perinuclear localization (p-ANCA).

The usual targets of these antibodies have been identified as proteinase 3 for c-ANCA, and myeloperoxidase for p-ANCA. Both antigens are found in the primary azurophilic granules of neutrophils. When ethanol is used as the fixative, the cellular granules are disrupted: The positively charged myeloperoxidase molecules then migrate toward the negatively charged nucleus to produce the perinuclear pattern, and the neutral proteinase 3 molecules remain dispersed in the cytoplasm to produce the cytoplasmic pattern.

The c-ANCA pattern has been found to be almost uniquely associated with Wegener's granulomatosis. The presence of c-ANCA is near diagnostic of Wegener's granulomatosis. The titer of c-ANCA correlates with disease activity and may, therefore, be used to monitor adequacy of therapy.[13,28]

Alveolar capillaritis associated with p-Anca may be the most common pauci-immune alveolar hemorrhage syndrome. Alveolar hemorrhage may be isolated or more often occur in association with necrotizing glomerulonephritis. Less commonly affected patients may have evidence of widespread systemic vasculitis in the form of periarteritis nodosa. These patients are managed in the same way as patients with Goodpasture's syndrome (i.e., pri-

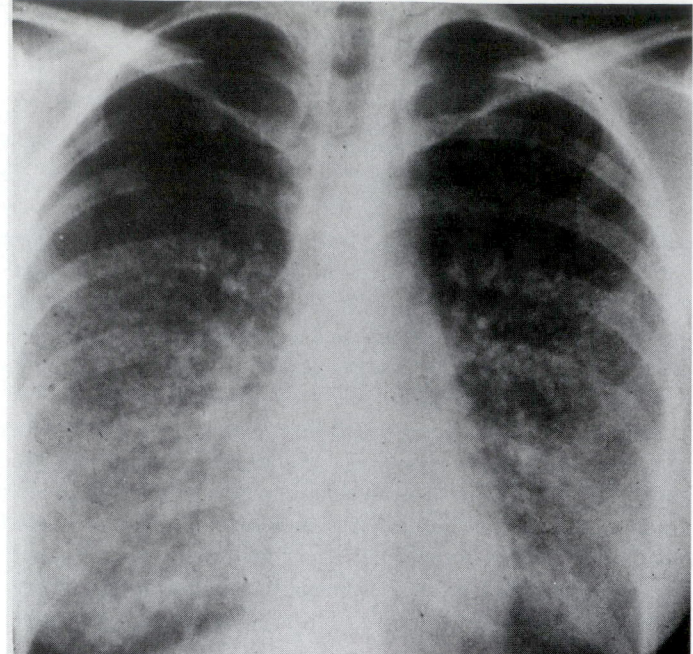

A

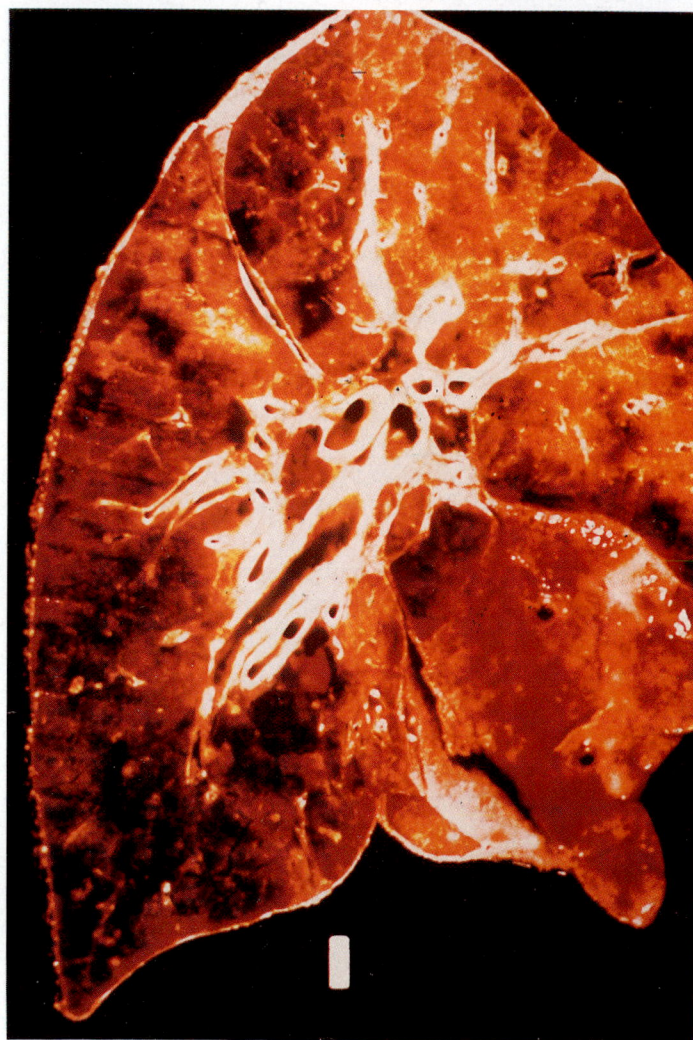

B

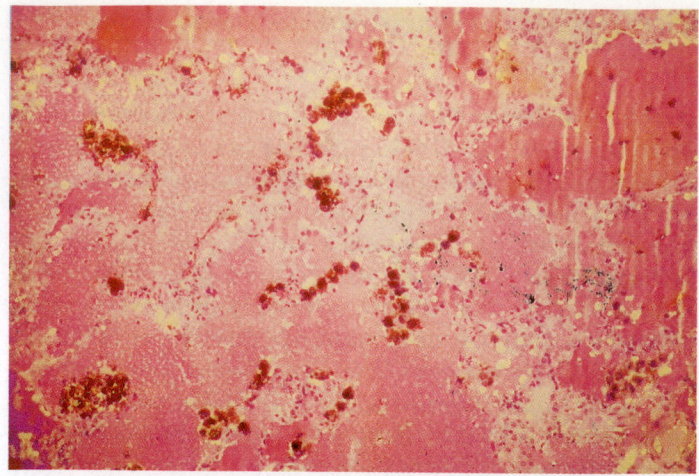

C

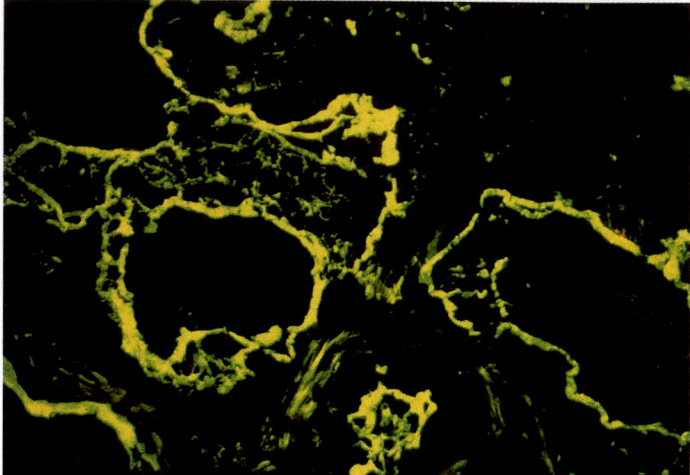

D

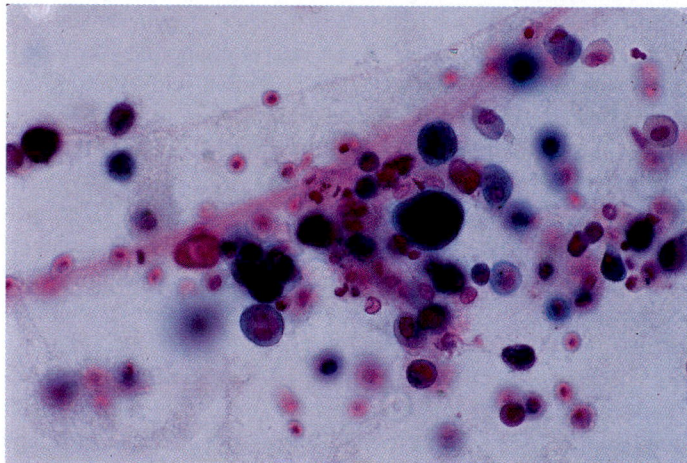

E

FIGURE 75-4 Goodpasture's syndrome. *A.* Chest radiograph showing bilateral alveolar infiltrates, predominantly in the middle and lower lung fields. *B.* Autopsy specimen showing cut surface of lung with massive alveolar hemorrhage. *(Courtesy of Dr. Richard Garnett, Reid Memorial Hospital, Richmond, Indiana.)* *C.* Photomicrograph of intact alveoli, containing both red blood cells and hemosiderin–laden macrophages. H&E, ×45. *D.* Immunofluorescent demonstration of immunoglobulin lining alveolar surfaces in a uniform distribution. Fluoresceinated anti–IgG ×113. *E.* Smear of bronchoalveolar lavage demonstrating hemosiderin laden macrophages. Prussian blue stain. Original magnification ×132. *(Courtesy of Dr. David Lyon, Iankenau Hospital, Wynnewood, Pennsylvania.)*

marily with immunosuppressive therapy with corticosteroids and cyclophosphamide), sometimes augmented by plasmapheresis. Of interest in some patients with p-ANCA-associated alveolar hemorrhage is the presence of anti-basement-membrane antibodies in the serum. These antibodies are directed against basement antigens other than those seen in Goodpasture's syndrome and are thought to be a secondary phenomenon, rather than of pathogenic significance.

Antiphospholipid Antibody-Associated Alveolar Hemorrhage

Patients with serum antibodies directed against membrane phospholipid (antiphospholipid syndrome or APS) display hypercoagulability of their blood.[7,15,19] Clinically, this manifests as peripheral arterial and venous thrombosis, fetal wastage in pregnant women, and thrombocytopenia. Pulmonary involvement can include pulmonary thromboembolism, pulmonary hypertension, or rarely diffuse alveolar hemorrhage. The latter produces fever, dyspnea, and diffuse pulmonary infiltrates on chest radiograph. Alveolar hemorrhage in the APS has been associated with alveolar capillaritis with or without immune complex deposition and with microvascular thrombosis in the lungs.

Antiphospholipid antibodies were first detected in patients with systemic lupus erythematosus (SLE) and were formerly known as the lupus anticoagulant because they prolong some laboratory test of clotting.[38] APS can occur in the absence of SLE. How often these antibodies play a role in pulmonary hemorrhage due to SLE is unknown, as there are other possible mechanisms in that syndrome (see below). In patients with isolated APS and alveolar hemorrhage, corticosteroid treatment, sometimes supplemented by cyclophosphamide, can result in a favorable outcome.

Hemorrhage Associated with Connective Tissue Disease

Diffuse alveolar hemorrhage also occurs as a rare complication of certain connective tissue disease syndromes, most often systemic lupus erythematosus but also rheumatoid arthritis, progressive systemic sclerosis, and mixed connective tissue disease.[21,32,36] Particularly in SLE, other causes of alveolar hemorrhage must be considered, including infection, uremia, and coagulopathy. When such causes have been eliminated, alveolar hemorrhage is sometimes found to be associated with capillaritis, with interstitial pneumonitis, or with immunofluorescent or ultrastructural evidence of immune complex deposition in alveolar septa. However, none of these disorders is consistently associated with pulmonary hemorrhage in SLE. Early diagnosis and treatment with corticosteroids and cytotoxic drugs is associated with favorable outcome, although relapse is not uncommon.

Toxic Alveolar Hemorrhage

At least one agent, trimellitic anhydride, has been associated with the development of alveolar hemorrhage unrelated to the development of either anti-glomerular-basement-membrane antibody or immune-complex-mediated cell injury.[22] Workers exposed to

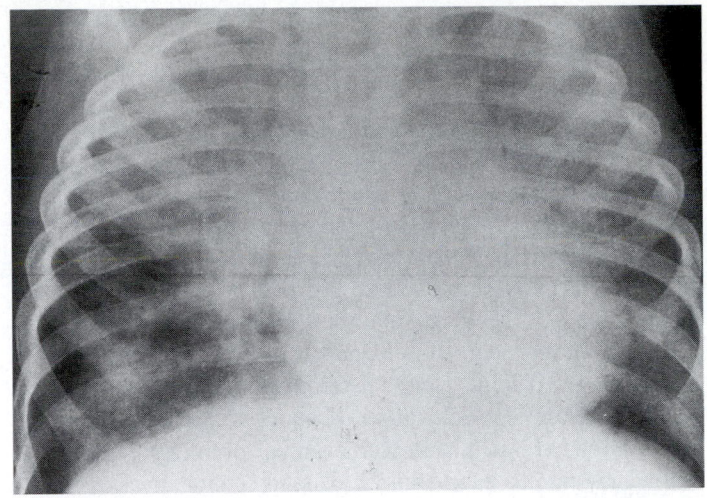

A

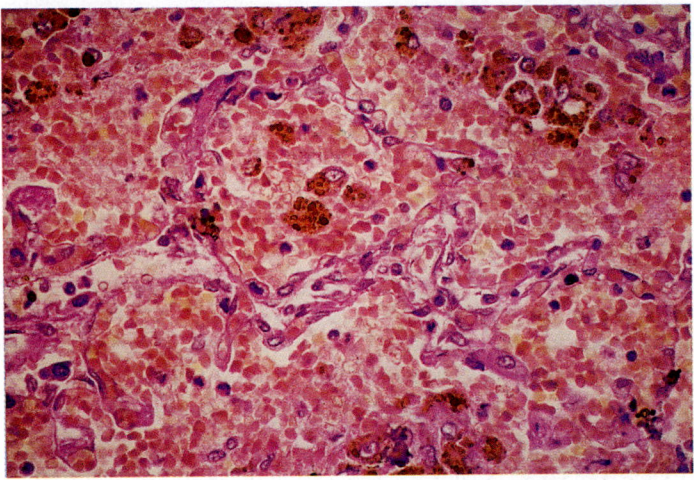

B

FIGURE 75-5   Idiopathic pulmonary hemosiderosis in a 21-month-old child with anemia soon after birth. Iron stain of the sputum showed hemosiderin-laden macrophages. *A.* Chest radiograph showing extensive, bilateral, almost punctate densities throughout both lung fields, most prominent in the perihilar regions where an alveolar filling pattern appears. *B.* Photomicrograph of lung at autopsy, showing intact alveoli containing degenerating red blood cells and hemosiderin-laden macrophages. Immunofluorescence studies for immunoglobulin and complement deposition were negative. H&E, ×131. *(Courtesy of Department of Pathology, St. Christopher's Hospital for Children, Philadelphia, Pennsylvania.)*

dust or fumes containing trimellitic anhydride (a component of certain plastics, paints, and epoxy resins) may develop the acute onset of dyspnea, hemoptysis, fever, pulmonary infiltrates, and anemia due to alveolar hemorrhage. Pathologic study confirms alveolar hemorrhage without damage to basement membranes or deposits of immune complexes; there is no evidence of renal disease. Patients recover with only supportive therapy after exposure to the causative agent ceases.

Trimellitic anhydride acts as a hapten, provoking antibodies which bind to human serum albumin or red blood cells conjugated with this agent. These antibodies are not associated with alveolar hemorrhage but instead are found in workers with acute rhinitis or asthma related to trimellitic anhydride. The mechanism of alveolar hemorrhage is unknown.

Idiopathic Pulmonary Hemosiderosis

When all the above diseases and syndromes have been excluded as likely possibilities, there still remains a small group of patients who develop recurrent diffuse alveolar hemorrhage in the absence of extrapulmonary disease and with no evidence of an immune etiology.[36] These patients are considered to have idiopathic pulmonary hemosiderosis, a diagnosis of exclusion (Fig. 75-5A). Clinically, the patients form a heterogeneous group with respect to the onset and course of disease, which range from fulminant and fatal, to chronic relapse with eventual chronic pulmonary insufficiency due to interstitial fibrosis, to spontaneous remission with little or no residual deficit. The disease usually affects children and young adults.

Pathologic examination reveals nonspecific alveolar hemorrhage without evidence of inflammation, vasculitis, or immune complex deposition (Fig. 75-5B). Only a few observations on ultrastructure are available. These include focal disruption, smudging, or lamination of alveolar capillary basement membranes.

The pathogenesis of this condition remains unknown, and there are no associated antibodies or other serum markers in the idiopathic cases. However, the clinical and morphologic similarity to some cases of alveolar hemorrhage of known immune pathogenesis, the occasional responsiveness to immunosuppressive therapy, the occasional association with celiac sprue—a presumably immunologic disease of the small intestine—and frequent association with a nonspecific elevation of serum IgA all point to an as yet unelucidated immune pathogenesis. Rarely, children with hypersensitivity to cow's milk (Heiner's syndrome) can present with diffuse alveolar hemorrhage.

If the diagnosis proves to be idiopathic pulmonary hemosiderosis, high-dose corticosteroid therapy with or without cyclophosphamide and plasmapheresis is useful in controlling acute bleeding, but the long-term effectiveness of these measures in preventing recurrence or progression of this disease is unknown.[14]

REFERENCES

1. Albelda SM, Gefter WB, Epstein DM, Miller WT: Diffuse pulmonary hemorrhage: a review and classification. *Radiology* 154:289–297, 1985.
2. Bab I, Rosenmann E, Ne'eman Z, Sela J: The occurrence of extracellular matrix vesicles in pulmonary alveolar microlithiasis. *Virch Arch (Pathol Anat)* 391:357–361, 1981.
3. Barnard NJ, Crocker PR, Blainey AD, et al: Pulmonary alveolar microlithiasis. A new analytical approach. *Histopathology* 11:639–645, 1987.
4. Beer TW, Edwards CW: Pulmonary nodules due to reactive systemic amyloidosis (AA) in Crohn's disease. *Thorax* 48(12):1287–1288, 1993.
5. Bestetti-Bosisio M, Cotelli F, Schiaffino E, et al: Lung calcification in long-term dialysed patients: a light and electron microscopic study. *Histopathology* 8:69–79, 1984.
6. Bombassei GJ, Kaplan AA: The association between hydrocarbon exposure and anti-glomerular basement membrane antibody–mediated disease (Goodpasture's syndrome). *Am J Indus Med* 21:141–153, 1992.
7. Bosch X, López-Soto A, Mirapeix E, et al: Antineutrophil cytoplasmic autoantibody-associated alveolar capillaritis in patients presenting with pulmonary hemorrhage. *Arch Pathol Lab Med* 118(5):517–522, 1994.
8. Boyce NW, Holdsworth SR: Pulmonary manifestations of the clinical syndrome of acute glomerulonephritis and lung hemorrhage. *Am J Kidney Dis* 8:31–36, 1986.
9. Brodeur FJ Jr, Kazerooni EA: Metastatic pulmonary calcification mimicking air-space disease. Technetium-99m-MDP SPECT imaging. *Chest* 106(2):620–622, 1994.
10. Brown J, Walfredo L, Felton C: Hemodynamic and pulmonary studies in pulmonary alveolar microlithiasis. *Am J Med* 77:176–178, 1984.
11. Chen KTK: Amyloidosis presenting in the respiratory tract. *Pathol Ann* 24 (Part 1):253–273, 1989.
12. Cluzel P, Grenier P, Bernadac P, et al: Pulmonary alveolar microlithiasis: CT findings. *J Comput Assist Tomogr* 15(6):938–942, 1991.
13. Colby TV: Diffuse pulmonary hemorrhage in Wegener's granulomatosis. *Semin Respir Med* 10:136–140, 1989.
14. Colombo JL, Stolz SM: Treatment of life threatening primary pulmonary hemosiderosis with cyclophosphamide. *Chest* 102:959–960, 1992.
15. Crausman RS, Achenbach GA, Pluss WT, et al: Pulmonary capillaritis and alveolar hemorrhage associated with the antiphospholipid antibody syndrome. *J Rheumatol* 22(3):554–556, 1995.
16. Donaghy M, Rees AJ: Cigarette smoking and lung haemorrhage in glomerulonephritis caused by autoantibodies to glomerular basement membrane. *Lancet* 2:1390–1392, 1983.
17. Felix MA, Levy H, Feldman C, Abramowitz JA: Endobronchial appearance of tracheobronchial amyloidosis. A case report and suggested classification. *S Afr Med J* 75(5):241–242, 1989.
18. Freiberg DB, Young IH, Laks L, et al: Improvement in gas exchange with nasal continuous positive airway pressure in pulmonary alveolar microlithiasis. *Am Rev Respir Dis* 145:1215–1216, 1992.
19. Gertner E, Lie JT: Pulmonary capillaritis, alveolar hemorrhage, and recurrent microvascular thrombosis in primary antiphospholipid syndrome. *J Rheumatol* 20(7):1224–1228, 1993.
20. Hartman TE, Müller NL, Primack SL, et al: Metastatic pulmonary calcification in patients with hypercalcemia: findings on chest radiographs and CT scans. *Am J Roentgenol* 162(4):799–802, 1994.
21. Haupt HM, Moore GW, Hutchins GM: The lung in systemic lupus erythematosus. *Am J Med* 71:791–797, 1981.
22. Herbert FA, Orford R: Pulmonary hemorrhage and edema due to inhalation of resins containing trimellitic anhydride. *Chest* 76:546–551, 1979.
23. Hui AN, Koss MN, Hochholzer L, Wehunt WD: Amyloidosis presenting in the lower respiratory tract. Clinicopathologic, radiologic, immunohistochemical, and histochemical studies on 48 cases. *Arch Pathol Lab Med* 110:212–218, 1986.
24. Husby G. Amyloidosis. *Semin Arthritis Rheum* 22:67–82, 1992.
25. Johkoh T, Ikezoe J, Nagareda T, et al: Metastatic pulmonary calcification: early detection by high-resolution CT. *J Comput Assist Tomogr* 17(3):471–473, 1993.
26. Kelly PT, Haponik EF: Goodpasture's syndrome: molecular and clinical advances. *Medicine* (Baltimore) 73(4):171–185, 1994.
27. Leatherman JW, Davies SF, Hoidal JR: Alveolar hemorrhage syndromes: diffuse microvascular lung hemorrhage in immune and idiopathic disorders. *Medicine* 63:343–361, 1984.

28. Mark EJ, Ramirez JF: Pulmonary capillaritis and hemorrhage in patients with systemic vasculitis. *Arch Pathol Lab Med* 109:413–418, 1985.

29. Pitkanen P, Westermark P, Cornwell GG: Senile systemic amyloidosis. *Am J Pathol* 117:391–399, 1984.

30. Planes C, Kleinknecht D, Brauner M, et al: Diffuse interstitial lung disease due to AA amyloidosis. *Thorax* 42(4):323–324, 1992.

31. Prakash UBS, Barham SS, Rosenow EC, et al: Pulmonary alveolar microlithiasis. *Mayo Clinic Proc* 58:290–300, 1983.

32. Schwab EP, Schumacher HR Jr, Freundlich B, Callegari PE: Pulmonary alveolar hemorrhage in systemic lupus erythematosus. *Semin Arthritis Rheum* 23(1):8–15, 1993.

33. Stamatis G, Zerkowski H–R, Doetsch N, et al: Sequential bilateral lung transplantation for pulmonary alveolar microlithiasis. *Ann Thorac Surg* 56:972–975, 1993.

34. Thompson PJ, Citron KM: Amyloid and the lower respiratory tract. *Thorax* 38:84–87, 1983.

35. Thompson PJ, Ryan G, Laurence BH: Laser photoradiation for tracheobronchial amyloid. *Aust N Z J Med* 16:229–230, 1986.

36. Travis WD, Colby TV, Lombard C, Carpenter HA: A clinicopathologic study of 34 cases of diffuse pulmonary hemorrhage with lung biopsy confirmation. *Am J Surg Pathol* 14:1112–1125, 1990.

37. Utz JP, Swensen SJ, Gertz MA: Pulmonary amyloidosis. The Mayo Clinic Experience from 1980 to 1993. *Ann Int Med* 124:407–413, 1996.

38. Wieslander J: How are anti–neutrophil cytoplasmic autoantibodies detected? *Am J Kidney Dis* 18:154–158, 1991.

39. Zwas ST, Shpilberg O, Huszar M, Rozenman J: Isolated ectopic lung uptake of technetium 99m methylene diphosphonate on bone scintigraphy in primary amyloidosis. *Eur J Nucl Med* 17(5):282–285, 1990.

CHAPTER 76

PULMONARY HISTIOCYTOSIS X

Talmadge E. King, Jr. / Robert S. Crausman

Primary pulmonary histiocytosis X is also called eosinophilic granuloma of the lung and pulmonary Langerhans cell granulomatosis.[20] Like Letterer-Siwe disease and Hand-Schüller-Christian disease, it is characterized by abnormal organ infiltration by Langerhans cells. Langerhans cells are highly differentiated cells in the monocyte-macrophage line that are also found in the dermis of the skin, the reticuloendothelial system, the pleura, and the lung. These related disorders have been grouped under the classification of histiocytosis X.[30] However, the three disorders are clinically distinct.

Letterer-Siwe disease is an acute, often fulminant disease of children less than 2 years of age that is characterized by widespread infiltration of the reticuloendothelial system, bones, and lungs. Hand-Schüller-Christian disease is a more indolent disorder of children and young adults that also typically affects the bones and the lungs. Diabetes insipidus, exophthalmos, and osteolytic skull lesions form the classic clinical triad associated with this disorder. There is some overlap of these diseases; some children present with isolated pulmonary manifestations, and some adults demonstrate more malignant-appearing, disseminated disease.

Primary pulmonary histiocytosis X is an uncommon, smoking-related, interstitial lung disease that primarily affects young adults. Less frequently, solitary osteolytic bone lesions are also seen. Rarely, multifocal or widely disseminated disease more closely approximating the pediatric histiocytoses is described. Advanced disease may mimic idiopathic pulmonary fibrosis; however, it generally follows a more benign and protracted course. Although there is some similarity to other diffuse interstitial lung diseases, primary pulmonary histiocytosis X, as a specific disease entity, is distinct in its clinical, radiologic, and pathologic manifestations.

EPIDEMIOLOGY

The true incidence and prevalence of pulmonary histiocytosis X are unknown. It is likely that some cases are misdiagnosed as idiopathic pulmonary fibrosis. Despite this, pulmonary histiocytosis X is clearly an uncommon, if not rare, disease. No occupational or geographic predisposition has been reported. Among 28 patients seen by our group, we found higher than expected connections to farming (21 percent), woodworking (25 percent), and domestic exposure to animals (77 percent) (unpublished observation of E. Barrett, C. Rose, and T. E. King, Jr.). Of note, nearly all affected persons report a prior smoking history. Thus, tobacco smoke is thought to be an etiologic factor. Other diffuse parenchymal lung diseases associated with cigarette smoking are respiratory bronchiolitis-associated interstitial lung disease and desquamative interstitial pneumonitis.

Most patients present to medical attention in young adulthood (20 to 40 years of age). Pulmonary histiocytosis X can, however, present in any age group. The older literature suggested a male preponderance; however, the recent literature suggests an equal sex distribution, with increasing presentations in middle age. In general, women tend to present at an older age than do men. If the demographics of pulmonary histiocytosis X have truly changed, as the literature would suggest, this may reflect the changing smoking habits of women in our society. Racial factors may also be important in disease pathogenesis. Caucasians are affected much more commonly than people of either African or Asian descent, in whom this disease is very rare.

Pulmonary histiocytosis X has reportedly been associated with a number of malignancies and may be a premalignant condition.[31,38,44] Sadoun and colleagues[38] reported bronchogenic carcinoma in 5 of 95 patients with pulmonary histiocytosis X. Tomashefsi and coworkers[44] found that 10 of 21 patients developed either malignant (n = 9) or nonmalignant tumors—3 lung cancer, 5 extrapulmonary carcinomas, 2 lymphomas, 1 pulmonary carcinoid tumor, and 1 mediastinal ganglioneuroma. Two patients developed two different malignant tumors. Six tumors preceded, three followed, and three occurred concomitantly with the diagnosis of pulmonary histiocytosis X. Lymphoma, both Hodgkin's and non-Hodgkin's, has been reported in association with pulmonary histiocytosis X.[11] The carcinogenic effects of cigarette smoke are probably etiologic for some of these tumors; thus, the relative effects of tobacco in pulmonary histiocytosis X are difficult to discern.

NATURAL HISTORY AND CLINICAL PRESENTATION

Patients with pulmonary histiocytosis X present to medical attention in a variety of ways: as an incidental diagnosis that is suggested by a screening chest radiogram, after pneumothorax, or with respiratory or constitutional symptoms.[6] When symptomatic, patients most often have a nonproductive cough (56 to 70 percent) and, in decreasing order of frequency, dyspnea (40 percent; 87 percent of our patients had breathlessness with exertion on close questioning), chest pain (10 to 21 percent), fatigue (~30 percent), weight loss (20 to 30 percent), and fever (15 percent).[6,12,32] A history of rhinitis has been elicited in 50 percent of the patients with pulmonary histiocytosis X in our clinic population (unpublished observation of E. Barrett, C. Rose, and T. E. King, Jr.).

Pleuritic pain and acute dyspnea with a spontaneous pneumothorax can be a recurrent problem in as many as 25 percent of patients.[40] Pleural thickening or effusion is rarely seen in the absence of a history of pneumothorax.[19] Hemoptysis (13 percent) is occasionally reported,[12,26] and it should prompt consideration of superimposed infection (e.g., *Aspergillus*) or tumor.

Cystic bone lesions are present in 4 to 20 percent of patients with pulmonary histiocytosis X, and they may produce localized pain or a pathologic bone fracture. The exact numbers of patients with bone lesions are not known because complete bone surveys are not routinely performed. Skeletal involvement can be the sole symptomatic manifestation of pulmonary histiocytosis X, or it may precede the more typical pulmonary manifestations. The radiographic pattern is not diagnostic. In most instances, the lesions are solitary and affect the flat bones.

Central nervous system involvement with diabetes insipidus (approximately 15 percent of patients) is also seen with pulmonary histiocytosis X and is thought to portend a worse prognosis.

The physical examination is usually unremarkable. Crackles are not commonly found on chest examination.[15] Digital clubbing is uncommon.[32] Secondary pulmonary hypertension can occur and is probably underappreciated. Manifestations of cor pulmonale are seen in advanced stages. Routine laboratory studies are usually unrevealing, and the peripheral eosinophil count is normal.

RADIOLOGY

Chest Radiograph

The radiographic appearance of pulmonary histiocytosis X can be very characteristic, if not diagnostic. The combination of ill-

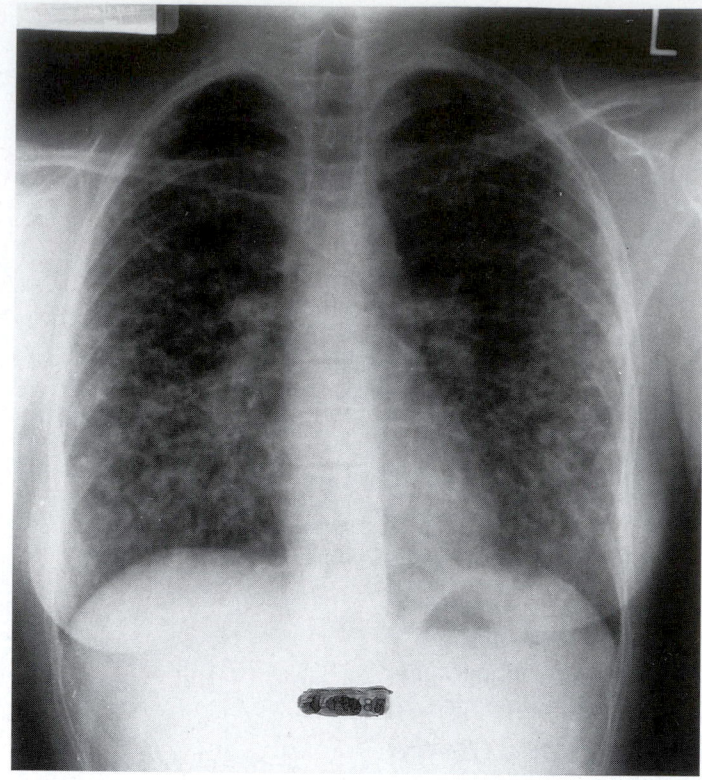

FIGURE 76-1   Pulmonary histiocytosis X in a 22-year-old woman. Chest radiograph demonstrates the classic features of profuse ill-defined nodules, reticulonodular opacities, cysts, costophrenic angle sparing, and preservation of lung volumes.

defined or stellate nodules (2 to 10 mm in size), reticulonodular infiltrates, upper-zone cysts or honeycombing, preservation of lung volume, and costophrenic angle sparing are believed to be highly specific for this disorder.[3,27,28] Typically, the reticulonodular opacities are seen in the middle to upper zone, which parallels the pathology (Fig. 76-1). The total lung volume is most often normal, although both hyperinflation and reduced volume have been described.[12,39] In addition to pulmonary histiocytosis X, lymphangioleiomyomatosis, tuberous sclerosis, chronic hypersensitivity pneumonitis, stage III sarcoidosis, constrictive bronchiolitis, and any interstitial lung disease in a subject with emphysema are interstitial lung diseases that can manifest with increased lung volume.

Small cysts and nodules are the radiographic hallmark of pulmonary histiocytosis X,[27,28] (Fig. 76-2) and occasionally miliary disease is seen. Hilar or mediastinal adenopathy in pulmonary histiocytosis X is rare and should prompt consideration of malignancy as a secondary diagnosis. Pleural thickening is most often due to treated pneumothorax, as pleural involvement by the primary disease process is uncommon. Bone lesions can occur in any bone, including the ribs. On rare occasions, patients come to medical attention with a solitary pulmonary nodule that proves to be pulmonary histiocytosis X on biopsy.[43]

Computed Tomography

The combination of multiple cysts and nodules with a middle-to upper-zone predominance with interstitial thickening in a

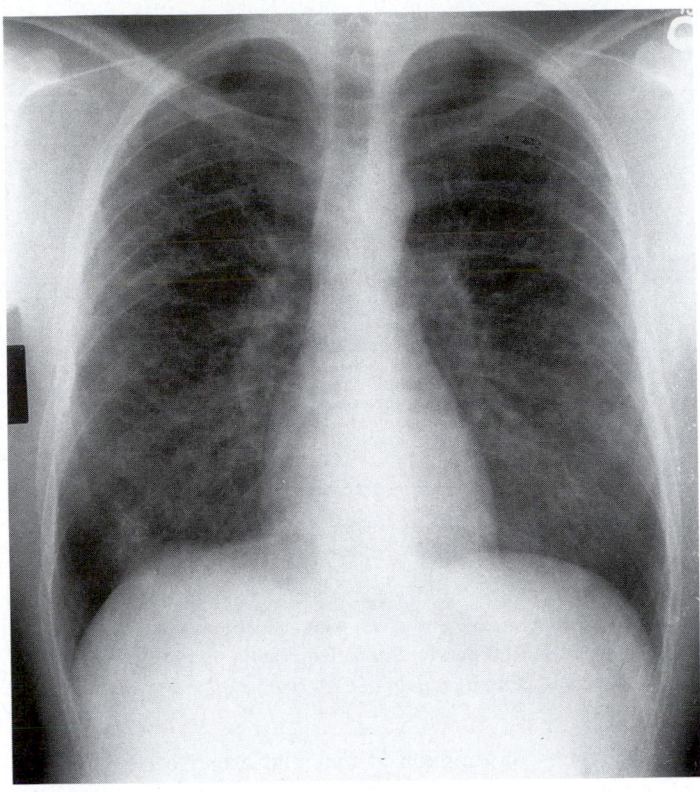

A

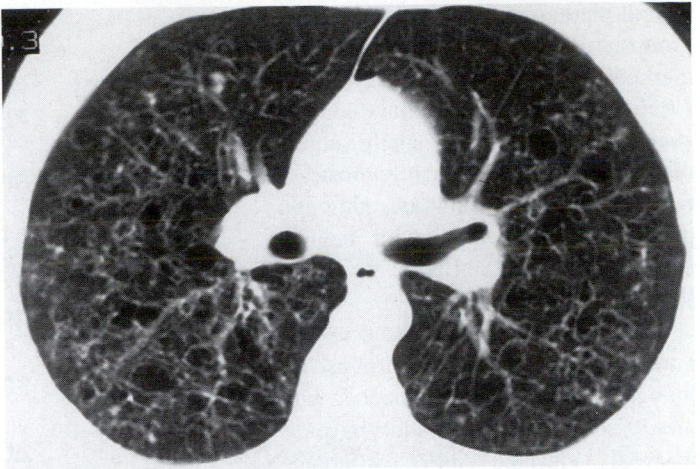

B

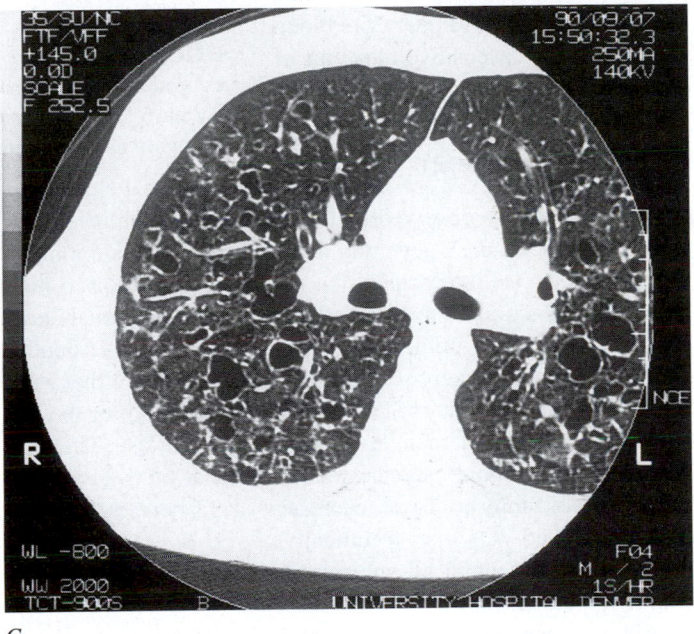

C

young smoker is so characteristic as to be diagnostic of pulmonary histiocytosis X (Fig. 76-2B).[27] The nodules can be well or poorly defined. Occasionally they can be large and bizarrely shaped (Fig. 76-2C). Honeycombing can be seen in advanced disease.

Serial chest CT scanning often suggests a sequence of progression from nodular to cavitating to cystic lesions over time. The degree of cyst formation is often underappreciated with routine chest radiography. Thus, this progression may explain a number of "spontaneous remissions"[47] in the literature reported before the routine use of thin-section CT scanning.

Magnetic Resonance Imaging

The role of MRI in pulmonary histiocytosis X is limited to the evaluation of bony and CNS lesions.

PHYSIOLOGICAL TESTING

Pulmonary Function

Pulmonary function testing of subjects with pulmonary histiocytosis X can potentially demonstrate all possible patterns of function abnormality—normal, obstructive, restrictive, or mixed.[6,9,12,17,21] In general, total lung capacity is well preserved, with nearly normal airflow. The diffusing capacity is most often disproportionately reduced.[12] This pattern of pulmonary function abnormality suggests pulmonary vascular involvement by the disease process. Airflow limitation occurs in a minority of patients and can sometimes be associated with reactive airways, with significant improvement after bronchodilator administration.[12,39] When pres-

FIGURE 76-2 Pulmonary histiocytosis X in a 33-year-old man. *A.* Chest radiograph reveals reticulonodular opacities in midlung zones, cysts, costophrenic angle sparing, and preservation of lung volumes. *B.* Conventional CT scan helps confirm the presence of bilateral reticulonodular opacities and cysts. *C.* High-resolution CT with thin section shows more clearly that the reticulonodular or emphysematous changes on chest radiography are actually cysts. In this instance, few nodules are present. The cysts vary markedly in size and may be larger than 10 mm. The cysts are bizarre in shape, and many are closely related to pulmonary arteries, often mimicking bronchiectasis.

ent, reactive airways disease may reflect coexisting chronic obstructive pulmonary disease (COPD). Classic asthma manifestations are unusual in pulmonary histiocytosis X.

We recently reviewed our experience with 23 patients with pulmonary histiocytosis X and found two major subgroups.[12] The first demonstrated normal total lung capacity, with normal or near-normal airflow. This group had a normal elastic recoil with pulmonary mechanics testing. The second group demonstrated predominantly restrictive disease, with reduced total lung volume and an increased elastic recoil. In both groups, the diffusing capacity was markedly reduced. Those in the restrictive group tended to have longer-standing disease. Only a single subject demonstrated predominantly obstructive pulmonary dysfunction, although obstructive physiology with airflow limitation and hyperinflation is well described in the literature.[6,17]

The mean AaP_{O_2} difference was normal at rest in both subgroups, although a subset of five subjects with more severe disease did have a markedly elevated AaP_{O_2} difference and required supplemental oxygen. The resting pH and Pa_{CO_2} were most often normal. Thus, the resting arterial blood gas was a very insensitive indicator of disease.

Exercise Physiology

Clinically, we have observed that patients with established pulmonary histiocytosis X generally demonstrate a limitation in activity and exercise intolerance that is out of proportion to their pulmonary function abnormalities. In our cross-sectional study of 23 subjects with pulmonary histiocytosis X,[12] we found a markedly decreased exercise capacity as measured by either work achieved (54 ± 4 mean ± SEM percent of predicted) or oxygen utilization ($\dot{V}O_2$, 44 percent ± 3) at maximal exercise. The oxygen pulse at maximal exercise was reduced at 56 ± 3 percent. The anaerobic threshold was decreased at 33 percent ± 1 percent of expected $\dot{V}O_2$ max; specifically, it was ≤40 percent in all subjects in whom it was measured. The maximal ventilatory response ($\dot{V}Emax$, 83 ± 5 percent) was excessive for the maximal level of work. The maximal ventilatory response was not limiting, and the $\dot{V}E$ was well below predicted ventilatory ceilings. Gas exchange abnormalities were reflected by increasing AaP_{O_2} differences with increasing exercise.

Alveolar dead space to tidal volume ratio (V_D/V_T), a parameter thought to reflect pulmonary vascular function, was either abnormally elevated or failed to decrease in most patients (Fig. 76-3). This abnormality suggested either pathologic or functional involvement of the pulmonary vasculature by the disease process.

Two linear regression models derived from pulmonary function indices predicted 73 percent ($r^2 = 0.73$) and 75 percent ($r^2 = 0.75$) of the variability in maximal achieved workload and pre-

dicted oxygen consumption at maximal exercise (% $\dot{V}O_2$ max ex), respectively. The following equation was derived for the maximal achieved workload:

$$\text{maximal achieved workload} = 0.884 - (0.0088 * V_D/V_T \text{ baseline}) - (0.002 * RV) + (0.0044 * DL_{CO}).$$

Here the partial r^2 was V_D/V_T baseline ($r^2 = 0.40$, $p = 0.0007$), RV (0.19, 0.001), and DL_{CO} (0.15, 0.004). Figure 76-4 shows the regression model for the predicted oxygen consumption at maximal exercise.

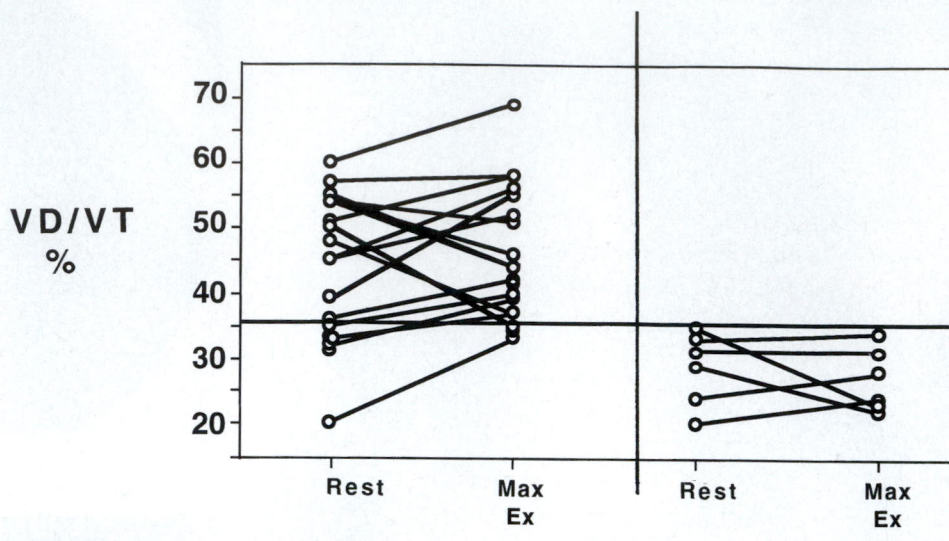

FIGURE 76-3   Dead space to tidal volume ratio (VD/VT%) at rest and maximal exercise in (max ex) patients with pulmonary histiocytosis X (n = 23). Seventeen patients demonstrated either an abnormal VD/VT at rest or response to exercise (left panel). Six patients had a normal VD/VT at rest and normal response to exercise (right panel). *(Based on data of Crausman et al,[12] with permission.)*

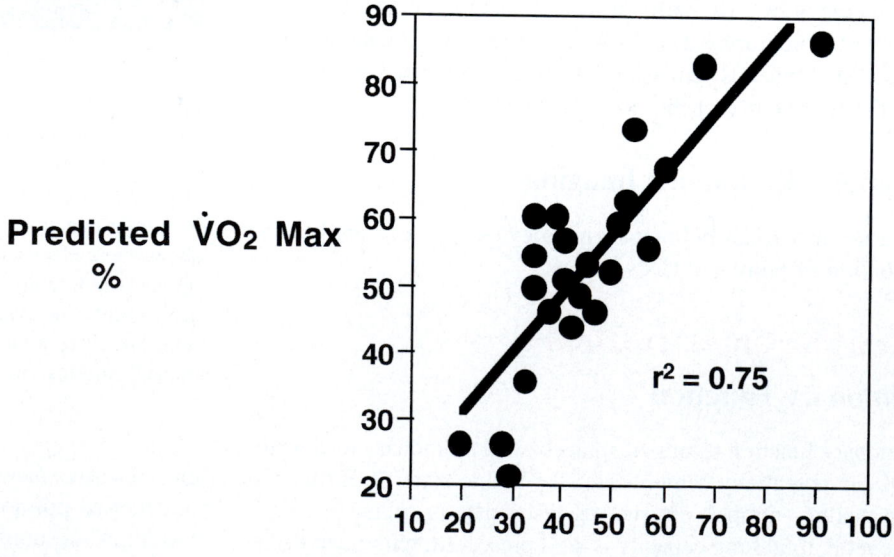

FIGURE 76-4   Correlation between predicted oxygen consumption at maximal exercise ($\dot{V}O_2$ max) and predicted $\dot{V}O_2$ max from the linear regression model: $\dot{V}O_2$ max = 0.062 – (0.0074 * baseline VD/VT) – (0.0014 * RV) + (0.0017 * baseline P(Aa)O_2) + (0.0011 * DL$_{CO}$); $r^2 = 0.75$. *(Based on data of Crausman et al,[12] with permission.)*

Our analysis of the composite results concluded that exercise intolerance in subjects with pulmonary histiocytosis X was due to a combination of mechanical factors and pulmonary vascular involvement by pulmonary histiocytosis X.[12]

HISTOPATHOLOGY

The pathologic cell type of pulmonary histiocytosis X is the Langerhans cell, which is a differentiated cell of the monocyte-macrophage line (Fig. 76-5). Langerhans' cells are normally found in the dermis, the reticuloendothelial system, the lung, and the pleura. They are distinguished by a pale-staining cytoplasm and large nucleus and nucleoli. Electron microscopy can demonstrate the classic pentalaminar cytoplasmic inclusion or Birbeck granule (X-body) (Fig. 76-6). Although this cell can be found in association with cigarette smoking in otherwise healthy persons and with other pulmonary pathologies (e.g., idiopathic pulmonary fibrosis) or in normal lung, its presence is characteristic of pulmonary histiocytosis X.[8,42] In pulmonary histiocytosis X, the Langerhans cells are characteristically found in clusters and significantly outnumber those seen in other lung diseases. Absolute quantitative guidelines for diagnosis of pulmonary histiocytosis X have not been established.

Early inflammatory lesions are centered around the smaller bronchioles and usually contain a mixture of eosinophils, lymphocytes, and neutrophils.[5,6] Pulmonary histiocytosis X is not a granulomatous disorder. Further, lesions are often devoid of eosinophils. Thus, the older term, *eosinophilic granuloma,* is a misnomer. These lesions often affect pulmonary arterioles and venules, and thus the disorder can be described as having a bronchovascular distribution. This vascular involvement has frequently been described; but it has only recently been assessed quantitatively, by Travis and coworkers.[45] They noted evidence of vascular involvement in 80 percent of biopsy specimens. Pseudodesquamative interstitial pneumonia (characterized by the accumulation of alveolar macrophages in the alveolar parenchyma between pulmonary Langerhans cell lesions) and respiratory (smoker's) bronchiolitis (with pigmented macrophages filling the lumen of bronchioles and the surrounding alveolar spaces) were

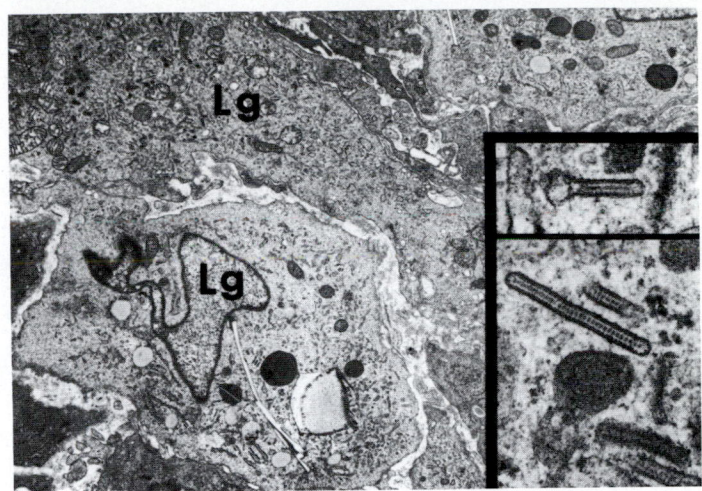

FIGURE 76-6   Electron micrograph of Langerhans cell (Lg) of the lung. Typical X bodies (Birbeck granules) are seen in the two inserts.

also frequently found on lung biopsy.[45] In addition, this group described the frequent presence of intraluminal fibrosis (86 percent of specimens), characterized by mural incorporation, alveolar obliteration, and intraluminal buds. It was mild in extent in 59 percent of specimens, moderate in 20 percent, and marked in 9 percent.[45] These findings support the hypothesis that intraluminal fibrosis serves as a mechanism for alveolar collapse, with progression to interstitial fibrosis and lung remodeling.[18]

Interstitial fibrosis and small cyst formation with a middle- to upper-zone predominance occur with advancing disease. This middle- to upper-zone predominance differs from that of idiopathic pulmonary fibrosis, which generally has a lower zone predominance. More advanced lesions extend widely into the parenchyma of the lung surrounding the bronchovascular structures and produce the so-called stellate lesions that are characteristic of this disorder.[5,17,45]

Older lesions are relatively acellular and produce a diffuse interstitial pathology that can be difficult to distinguish from other forms of end-stage pulmonary fibrosis, with extensive areas of fibrosis and honeycombing accompanying the cystic lesions. The mechanism for cyst formation is unknown. It may be a consequence of central necrosis of older stellate lesions. Alternatively, the cysts may occur as a result of secondary inflammatory foci in relatively avascular areas distal to more advanced bronchovascular lesions. Finally, these cysts may form in part because of more proximal airway obstruction by the stellate lesions.

PATHOGENESIS

The pathogenesis of pulmonary histiocytosis X is unknown. However, the nearly universal association with cigarette smoking strongly implies causation. One hypothesis of disease pathogenesis, the bombesin hypothesis, contends that increased bombesin-like peptide production plays a central role (Fig. 76-7).[2] Bombesin is a neuropeptide produced by neuroendocrine cells, which are increased in the lungs of smokers.[1] Bombesin-like peptides are chemotactic for monocytes, are mitogenic for epithelial cells and fibroblasts, and stimulate cytokine secretion.[2] Thus, there are several attractive features that support the hy-

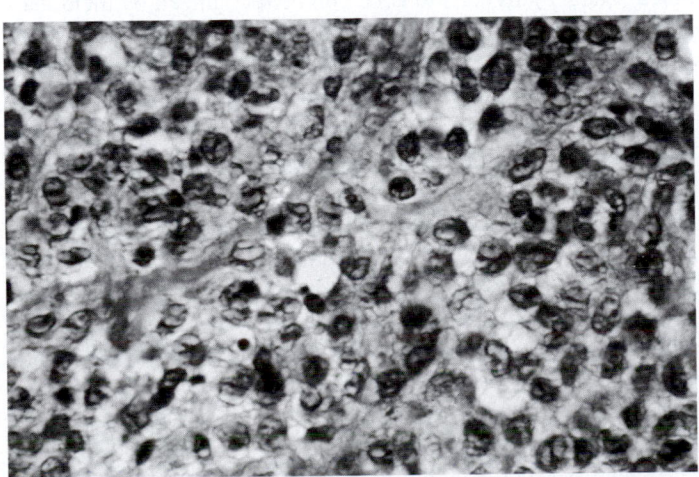

FIGURE 76-5   Lung tissue in primary pulmonary histiocytosis X. The histiocytosis X cells (Langerhans cell) are typical. A characteristic longitudinal groove is seen along the center of some cells. (×96.)

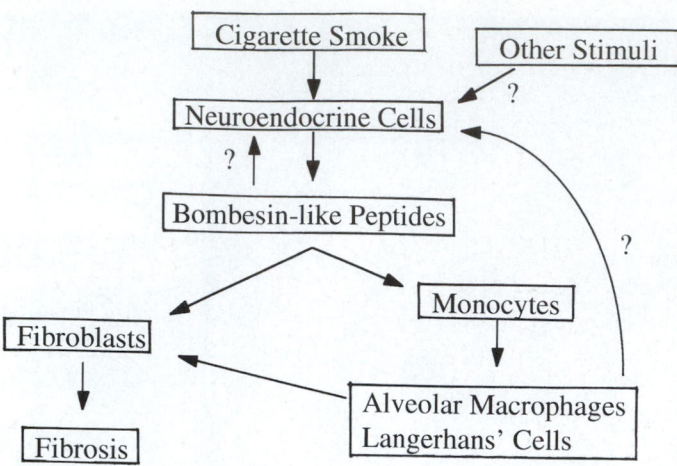

FIGURE 76-7 Hypothetical pathogenetic scheme showing how cigarette smoke–induced neuroendocrine cell hyperplasia may contribute to airway infiltration by mononuclear phagocytes and fibrosis in pulmonary histiocytosis X. In most smokers, the degree of neuroendocrine cell hyperplasia demonstrated in pulmonary histiocytosis X does not occur. Presumably, patients with pulmonary histiocytosis X either are innately more susceptible to cigarette smoke or are exposed to other stimuli which interact synergistically to induce neuroendocrine cell hyperplasia. *(Based on data of Aguayo et al,[2] with permission)*

pothesis that these peptides contribute to the inflammation and fibrosis observed in pulmonary histiocytosis X. Tobacco glycoprotein and other regulatory glycopeptides (e.g., granulocyte-macrophage colony-stimulating factor) have been touted as being potentially important in the pathogenesis of this disease.[49]

Recently, attention has been focused on the processes that may regulate white blood cell traffic in this disorder. These studies suggest that the pathogenesis of pulmonary histiocytosis X entails alterations of the expression of the adhesion molecules that regulate white blood cell/endothelial cell interactions. One important adhesion molecule for neutrophils that is expressed by endothelial cells is intercellular adhesion molecule-1 (ICAM-1). ICAM-1 expression by Langerhans cells from biopsy specimens of subjects with Langerhans cell histiocytosis has been demonstrated. It is interesting to note that the expression of other leukocyte adhesion molecules, such as the β_1 and β_2 integrins, has also been noted.[14,37] The significance of these findings and their relevance to pulmonary histiocytosis X remain to be elucidated.

Alternatively, a viral infection has been suggested as the underlying cause of generalized Langerhans cell histiocytosis.[33,34] There are, however, no convincing data to suggest a role for viral infection as a cause of pulmonary histiocytosis X.

Abnormalities in immune function, with a nonspecific increase in IgG in bronchoalveolar lavage (BAL) fluid,[36] circulating and tissue-bound immune complexes,[25] and abnormalities in T-cell function, have all been observed in association with pulmonary histiocytosis X and may be important in the pathophysiology of this disorder.[40] It is also possible, however, that these findings all represent nonspecific consequences of a generalized activation of immune effector cells.

Although it is not a monoclonal disorder, the clinical similarities between pulmonary histiocytosis X and Langerhans cell histiocytosis and the frequent association with lymphoma do suggest a relationship with malignancy. At present, it is reasonable to think that pulmonary histiocytosis X may be a premalignant condition.

DIAGNOSTIC EVALUATION

The history and physical examination are the first steps in the diagnostic evaluation of a patient suspected of having pulmonary histiocytosis X. Unfortunately, the signs and symptoms of pulmonary histiocytosis X are generally nonspecific and often point to other, more common pulmonary diagnoses. For example, wheezing, cough, and dyspnea in a 50-year-old patient with a prominent smoking history are much more commonly due to COPD than to pulmonary histiocytosis X. However, when present, the history of recurrent pneumothorax, diabetes insipidus, or bone pain can be helpful. A smoking history is a consistent but not essential historical feature, since pulmonary histiocytosis X can occur without antecedent smoking exposure.

Most evaluations for pulmonary histiocytosis X are prompted after an abnormal chest radiograph is obtained. As previously noted, the chest CT, if classic, can be diagnostic, and it should therefore be obtained in all who are suspected of having this disease. We recommend high-resolution chest CT as a prebiopsy step in the evaluation of any patient with diffuse interstitial lung disease suspected of having pulmonary histiocytosis X. A sufficiently characteristic chest CT in association with the appropriate history is believed by many to obviate tissue confirmation. It should be noted that most often chest CT scans in pulmonary histiocytosis X are not classic and can, thus, be confused with those in pulmonary lymphangioleiomyomatosis, tuberous sclerosis, hypersensitivity pneumonitis, sarcoidosis, or idiopathic pulmonary fibrosis. In these instances, further diagnostic evaluation is warranted.

BAL can be of diagnostic value in cases of suspected histiocytosis X.[13] The total number of cells recovered is usually increased (as expected in smokers), and a modest increase in the concentration of neutrophils and eosinophils is frequently noted. In active disease the total number of lymphocytes recovered may also be increased, and a decreased CD4:CD8 ratio has been noted. Langerhans cells in BAL can be recognized by their characteristic staining for S-100 protein or peanut agglutination antigen.[35,48] These cells are also OKT-6 (CD-1) positive, are identified by a specific monoclonal antibody (MT-1) that is currently available,[23] and contain characteristic Birbeck or pentalaminar bodies on electron microscopic evaluation (Fig. 76-6).[7,16] Quantitative criteria for the definitive diagnosis of histiocytosis X based on BAL Langerhans cell numbers have not been conclusively established. A BAL cell differential with more than 5 percent Langerhans cells does, however, strongly suggest the diagnosis.[4,13,40] Lower proportions of Langerhans cells can be seen with other illnesses (current smokers, patients with other interstitial lung disorders or bronchoalveolar carcinoma) and even in normal subjects. Thus, the mere presence of Langerhans cells is of little diagnostic value.

When tissue confirmation is sought, transbronchial biopsy can be sufficient to make the diagnosis.[22] Sampling error and insufficient tissue may account for the substantial number of false-negative or nondiagnostic biopsies. Open or, more recently, video-guided thoracoscopic lung biopsy is generally definitive and can now be done with a minimum of operative risk. Tissue immunostaining with the monoclonal antibody CD-1 (OKT-6) distinguishes Langerhans cells from other histiocytes and can be a useful adjunct in difficult cases.[41] It can be performed on routinely fixed tissue and is less expensive than electron microscopy.

In cases of progressive disease with extensive fibrosis, the number of Langerhans cells present in either tissue specimens or BAL fluid decreases dramatically. Diagnosis at this stage can be difficult regardless of the laboratory methods used. In most cases, the combination of transbronchial lung biopsy and BAL, supplemented with the identification of CD-1–positive cells in tissue and BAL fluid, is highly likely to result in the correct diagnosis.[24]

TREATMENT AND PROGNOSIS

The natural history of pulmonary histiocytosis X is extraordinarily variable, with some patients experiencing spontaneous remission of symptoms and others progressing to end-stage fibrotic lung disease (Table 76-1). Most subjects demonstrate gradual progression with continued cigarette smoking and disease regression with smoking cessation.[47] It is therefore important to stress smoking cessation with these patients (Fig. 76-8). The condition of patients with radiographic sparing of the costophrenic angle is more likely to remain stable or improve than that of patients with costophrenic angle involvement.[28]

Corticosteroids have not been shown to be of any value in the treatment of histiocytosis X. Cytotoxic therapy, which may be of value in the treatment of disseminated disease,[29,46] has not been shown to produce benefit in patients with histiocytosis X. Radiotherapy for symptomatic bone lesions can be palliative. Radiation is not useful in the treatment of the pulmonary manifestations. Lung transplantation has been successfully accomplished in a number of centers. It is a viable option for appropriate patients with end-stage disease.

Gene, monoclonal antibody, and cytokine-based therapies are potential approaches that will likely be of value in the future. Given the vascular impairment seen with this disease and the occasional reports of pulmonary hypertension, it is also tempting to think about vasodilator therapy for symptomatic patients. These approaches remain, however, untried speculations.

TABLE 76-1

Clinical Course of Pulmonary Histiocytosis X

Reference	N	Years of Follow-Up	% Improved	% Stable	% Deteriorated	% Deaths
Basset et al.[6]	67	1–3	13	40	21	25
Friedman et al.[17]	60	Not stated	55*	37	7	2
Colby and Lombard[10]	31	Not stated		74†	19	6
Lacronique et al.[28]	37	1–12‡		65	35	

*Forty patients had essentially no symptoms of residual disease at least 6 months after diagnosis; 13 of these had persistent radiographic abnormalities.
†Stable or with partial or complete resolution.
‡Twenty-six of 37 were followed for >3 years; mean = 5.4 years.
SOURCE: Data from Marcy and Reynolds, 1985.

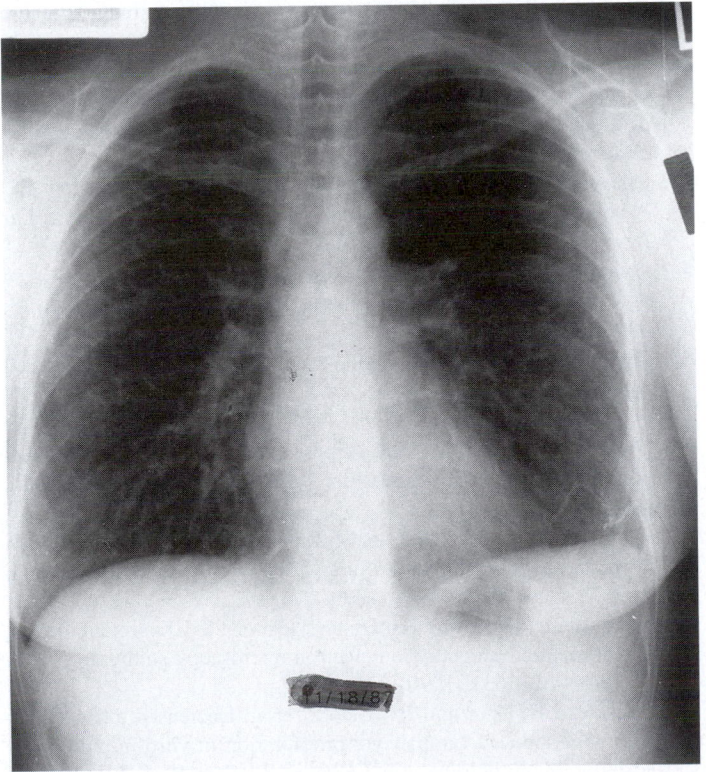

FIGURE 76-8 Follow-up chest radiograph in a 22-year-old woman taken 4 months after the initial film shown in Fig. 76-1. After an open lung biopsy performed on the left hemithorax, she was told to stop smoking and treated with prednisone. The chest radiograph shows marked clearing of the ill-defined nodules and preservation of lung volumes.

REFERENCES

1. Aguayo SM, Kane MA, King TE Jr, et al: Increased levels of bombesin-like peptides in the lower respiratory tract of asymptomatic cigarette smokers. *J Clin Invest* 84:1105–1113, 1989.
2. Aguayo SM, King TE Jr, Waldron JA Jr, et al: Increased pulmonary neuroendocrine cells with bombesin-like immunoreactivity in adult patients with eosinophilic granuloma. *J Clin Invest* 86:838–844, 1990.
3. Aguayo SM, Schwarz MI, Mortenson RL: The role of the chest radiograph in the evaluation of disease severity and clinical course in eosinophilic granuloma. *Am Rev Respir Dis* 141:A61, 1990.
4. Auerswald U, Barth J, Magnussen H: Value of CD-1–positive cells in bronchoalveolar lavage fluid for the diagnosis of pulmonary histiocytosis X. *Lung* 169:305–309, 1991.
5. Auld D: Pathology of eosinophilic granuloma of the lung. *Arch Pathol* 63:113–131, 1959.
6. Basset F, Corrin B, Spencer H, et al: Pulmonary histiocytosis X. *Am Rev Respir Dis* 118:811–820, 1978.
7. Basset F, Soler P, Jaurand MC, Bignon J: Ultrastructural examination of bronchoalveolar lavage for diagnosis of pulmonary histiocytosis X: Preliminary report of 4 cases. *Thorax* 32:303–306, 1977.

8. Casolaro MA, Bernaudin J-F, Saltini C, et al: Accumulation of Langerhans' cells on the epithelial surface of the lower respiratory tract in normal subjects in association with cigarette smoking. *Am Rev Respir Dis* 137:406–411, 1988.

9. Chusid EL: Pulmonary eosinophilic granuloma: Aspects of pulmonary function. *Mt Sinai J Med* 33:116, 1961.

10. Colby TV, Lombard C: Histiocytosis X in the lung. *Hum Pathol* 14:847–856, 1983.

11. Coli A, Bigotti G, Ferrone S: Histiocytosis X arising in Hodgkin's disease: Immunophenotypic characterization with a panel of monoclonal antibodies. *Virchows Arch [A]* 418:369–373, 1991.

12. Crausman RS, Jennings CA, Tuder R, et al: Pulmonary histiocytosis X: Pulmonary function and exercise pathophysiology. *Am J Respir Crit Care Med* 153:426–435, 1996.

13. Danel C, Israel-Biet D, Costabel U, et al: The clinical role of BAL in rare pulmonary diseases. *Eur Respir Rev* 2:83–88, 1991.

14. de Graaf JH, Tamminga RY, Kamps WA, Timens W: Langerhans' cell histiocytosis: Expression of leukocyte cellular adhesion molecules suggests abnormal homing and differentiation. *Am J Pathol* 144:466–472, 1994.

15. Epler GR, Carrington CB, Gaensler EA: Crackles (rales) in the interstitial pulmonary diseases. *Chest* 73:333–339, 1978.

16. Fartasch M, Vigneswaran N, Diepgen TL, Hornstein OP: Immunohistochemical and ultrastructural study of histiocytosis X and non-X histiocytoses. *J Am Acad Dermatol* 23:885–892, 1990.

17. Friedman PJ, Liebow AA, Sokoloff J: Eosinophilic granuloma of lung. *Medicine* 60:385–396, 1981.

18. Fukuda Y, Basset F, Soler P, et al: Intraluminal fibrosis and elastic fiber degradation lead to lung remodeling in pulmonary Langerhans cell granulomatosis (histiocytosis X). *Am J Pathol* 137:415–424, 1990.

19. Guardia J, Pedreira J-D, Esteban R, et al: Early pleural effusion in histiocytosis X. *Arch Intern Med* 139:934–936, 1979.

20. Hance AJ, Cadranel J, Soler P, Basset F: Pulmonary and extrapulmonary Langerhans' cell granulomatosis (histiocytosis X). *Semin Respir Med* 9:349–368, 1988.

21. Hoffman L, Cohn JE, Guenster EA: Respiratory abnormalities in eosinophilic granuloma of the lung: Long-term study of 5 cases. *New Engl J Med* 267:377–389, 1961.

22. Housini I, Tomashefski JF Jr, Cohen A, et al: Transbronchial biopsy in patients with pulmonary eosinophilic granuloma: Comparison with findings on open lung biopsy. *Arch Pathol Lab Med* 118:523–530, 1994.

23. Kahn HJ, Thorner PS: Monoclonal antibody MT1: A marker for Langerhans cell histiocytosis. *Pediatr Pathol* 10:375–384, 1990.

24. King TE Jr: Bronchoscopy in interstitial lung disease, in Feinsilver SH, Fein AM (eds), *Textbook of Bronchoscopy.* Baltimore, Williams & Wilkins, 1995, pp 185–220.

25. King TE Jr, Schwarz MI, Dreisin RE, et al: Circulating immune complexes in pulmonary eosinophilic granuloma. *Ann Intern Med* 91:397–399, 1979.

26. Knight RK: Hemoptysis in eosinophilic granuloma of the lung. *Br J Dis Chest* 73:181–186, 1979.

27. Kulwiec EL, Lynch DA, Aguayo SM, et al: Imaging of pulmonary histiocytosis X. *Radiographics* 12:515–526, 1992.

28. Lacronique J, Roth C, Battesti JP, et al: Chest radiological features of pulmonary histiocytosis X: A report based on 50 adult cases. *Thorax* 37:104–109, 1982.

29. Ladisch S, Gadner H: Treatment of Langerhans cell histiocytosis—Evolution and current approaches. *Br J Cancer* (suppl 23):S41–46, 1994.

30. Lichtenstein L: Histiocytosis X: Intergration of eosinophilic granuloma of bone, "Letterer-Siwe disease" and "Hand-Schüller-Christian disease" as related manifestations of a single nosologic entity. *Arch Pathol* 56:84–102, 1953.

31. Lombard CM, Medeiros LJ, Colby TV: Pulmonary histiocytosis X and carcinoma. *Arch Pathol Lab Med* 111:339–341, 1987.

32. Marcy TW, Reynolds HY: Pulmonary histiocytosis X. *Lung* 163:129–150, 1985.

33. McClain K, Weiss RA: Viruses and Langerhans cell histiocytosis: Is there a link? *Br J Cancer* (suppl 23):S34–36, 1994.

34. Mierau GW, Wills EJ, Steele PO: Ultrastructural studies in Langerhans cell histiocytosis: A search for evidence of viral etiology. *Pediatr Pathol* 14:895–904, 1994.

35. Ornvold K, Ralfkiaer E, Carstensen H: Immunohistochemical study of the abnormal cells in Langerhans cell histiocytosis (histiocytosis X). *Virchows Arch [A]* 416:403–410, 1990.

36. Rowden G: The Langerhans' cells. *Crit Rev Immunol* 3:95–180, 1981.

37. Ruco LP, Stoppacciaro A, Vitolo D, et al: Expression of adhesion molecules in Langerhans' cell histiocytosis. *Histopathology* 23:29–37, 1993.

38. Sadoun D, Vaylet F, Valeyre D, et al: Bronchogenic carcinoma in patients with pulmonary histiocytosis X. *Chest* 101:1610–1613, 1992.

39. Schonfeld N, Frank W, Wenig S, et al: Clinical and radiologic features, lung function and therapeutic results in pulmonary histiocytosis X. *Respiration* 60:38–44, 1993.

40. Schwarz MI: Primary and unclassified interstitial lung diseases, in Schwarz MI, King TE Jr (eds), *Interstitial Lung Disease,* 2d ed. St Louis, Mosby–Year Book, 1993, pp 426–429.

41. Soler P, Chollet S, Jacque C, et al: Immunocytochemical characterization of pulmonary histiocytosis X cells in lung biopsies. *Am J Pathol* 118:439–451, 1985.

42. Soler P, Moreau A, Basset F, Hance AJ: Cigarette smoking–induced changes in the number and differentiated state of pulmonary dendritic cells/Langerhans cells. *Am Rev Respir Dis* 139:1112–1117, 1989.

43. ten Velde GP, Thunnissen FB, van Engelshoven JM, Wouters EF: A solitary pulmonary nodule due to eosinophilic granuloma. *Eur Respir J* 7:1539–1540, 1994.

44. Tomashefski JF, Khiyami A, Kleinerman J: Neoplasms associated with pulmonary eosinophilic granuloma. *Arch Pathol Lab Med* 115:499–506, 1991.

45. Travis WD, Borok Z, Roum JH, et al: Pulmonary Langerhans cell granulomatosis (histiocytosis X): A clinicopathologic study of 48 cases. *Am J Surg Pathol* 17:971–986, 1993.

46. Tsele E, Thomas DM, Chu AC: Treatment of adult Langerhans cell histiocytosis with etoposide. *J Am Acad Dermatol* 27:61–64, 1992.

47. von Essen S, West W, Sitorius M, Rennard SI: Complete resolution of roentgenographic changes in a patient with pulmonary histiocytosis X. *Chest* 98:765–767, 1990.

48. Ye F, Huang SW, Dong HJ: Histiocytosis X: S-100 protein, peanut agglutinin, and transmission electron microscopy study. *Am J Clin Pathol* 94:627–631, 1990.

49. Youkeles LH, Grizzanti JN, Liao Z, et al: Decreased tobacco-glycoprotein–induced lymphocyte proliferation in vitro in pulmonary eosinophilic granuloma. *Am J Respir Crit Care Med* 151:145–150, 1995.

CHAPTER 77

PULMONARY LYMPHANGIOLEIOMYOMATOSIS

Talmadge E. King, Jr. / Robert S. Crausman

LYMPHANGIOLEIOMYOMATOSIS

Pulmonary lymphangioleiomyomatosis is a rare, idiopathic, diffuse, progressive interstitial lung disease that afflicts young women of childbearing age. Pathologically it is characterized by pulmonary interstitial smooth muscle proliferation and cyst formation that mimics pulmonary emphysema.[11,14–16,23,43] It has been variously called myomatosis, angiomyomatosis hyperplasia, lymphangiomatous malformation, diffuse pulmonary leiomyomatosis, and muscular hyperplasia of the lung.

Although pulmonary lymphangioleiomyomatosis is commonly included with the diffuse interstitial lung disease, lymphangioleiomyomatosis has more in common clinically, radiographically, and physiologically with pulmonary emphysema than with either idiopathic pulmonary fibrosis (IPF) or sarcoidosis. Like emphysema, lymphangioleiomyomatosis generally manifests with clinically significant airflow limitation and is often misdiagnosed as asthma or chronic obstructive pulmonary disease (COPD).[4,15,43] Many subjects are evaluated for alpha-1-antitrypsin deficiency. However, lymphangioleiomyomatosis is an interstitial lung disease and should rightly be included with pulmonary histiocytosis X and (stage IV) cystic sarcoidosis as part of a subgroup of cystic interstitial lung diseases. Tuberous sclerosis can be associated with a pathologically indistinguishable pulmonary condition.[10,17,42]

Epidemiology

The incidence and prevalence of pulmonary lymphangioleiomyomatosis is unknown. In the Denver Interstitial Lung Disease Center (supported by a Specialized Center of Research grant from the National Heart, Lung, and Blood Institute) only 16 cases were identified over a 10-year period.[15] This represented fewer than 1 percent of the cases of diffuse parenchymal lung disease seen during this period in the five teaching hospitals of the University of Colorado Health Sciences Center.

This rare disease presents almost exclusively in premenopausal women.[11,14,43] Most patients (70 percent) are age 20 to 40 years at the time of onset of symptoms or diagnosis.[2,8,9,11,12,14,16,19,28,38,46] Only 5 percent of cases are older than age 50 at presentation. The few reported cases occurring in postmenopausal women have most often been associated with estrogen replacement therapy,[1,23,39] although a few exceptions have been noted. Caucasians, and less commonly Asians, are afflicted much more commonly than other racial groups.

Clinical Presentation

Women with lymphangioleiomyomatosis present to medical attention in a variety of ways. Most often, the subjective complaint of dyspnea prompts medical evaluation. Early in the course subjects are frequently misdiagnosed as having asthma. The disease, however, is thought to be inexorably progressive, and patients are ultimately either correctly diagnosed or reclassified as having pulmonary emphysema.

At diagnosis, nearly all subjects complain of dyspnea[14,15,38,43] (Table 77-1). Spontaneous pneumothorax is common and will occur in 50 percent of cases. It is often recurrent, can be bilateral,[6] and may necessitate pleurodesis for more definitive therapy. Barotrauma and cyst rupture can still occur after pleurodesis. This can manifest as pneumomediastinum, pneumoretroperitoneum, pneumoretropharynx, and subcutaneous emphysema. Treatment of these complications following pleurodesis is primarily observant, since they are only rarely associated with significant morbidity (i.e., tension pneumomediastinum or pneumopericardium, which require surgical decompression). Chylothorax, due to obstruction of the thoracic duct or rupture of the lymphatics in the pleura or mediastinum by proliferating smooth-muscle cells, is characteristic of this disorder but is present in only a minority of subjects at diagnosis. Chyle can be recognized by its milky white appearance, high triglyceride level—usually greater than 110 mg/dL—and the presence of chylomicrons. Chyle can be difficult to treat and is typically associated with nutritional wasting and some degree of immunocompromise.[48]

TABLE 77-1

Age and Clinical Manifestations of Patients with Pulmonary Lymphangioleiomyomatosis at Presentation or During Follow-up

Reference	N	Mean Age at Onset (Range)	Cough (%)	Dyspnea (%)	Chest Pain (%)	Hemoptysis (%)	Pneumothorax (%)	Chylothorax (%)	Chylous Ascites (%)
Silverstein (37)	32	39 (18–69)	9*	91*	18*	28	38	78	31
Corrin (14)	28	33 (17–47)	64	86	7	36	43	39	7
Taylor (43)	32	33 Range Not Reported	41	94	34	44	81	28	6
Kitaichi (22)	46	32 (20–63)	54	83	30	24	39	11	4
Crausman (15)	16	32 (26–39)	56	100	—	13	69	—	—
TOTALS	154		47	89	22	30	51	32	10

*n = 22
Wheezing was noted in only 5 of 113. Chyluria was noted in only 3 of 154. Chylopysis was noted in 2 of 154.

Chyloperitoneum (chylous ascites) occurs in approximately 10 percent of cases, more rarely, chyluria (due to abnormal connections between dilated retroperitoneal lymphatics and the renal collecting system), and chylopericardium are also reported. Renal angioleiomyomata, a characteristic pathologic finding in tuberous sclerosis, are also common in lymphangioleiomyomatosis (as many as 50 percent of subjects).[7] They may grow to enormous size prior to clinical detection but only uncommonly affect renal function. Hemoptysis of mild to moderate severity is a well-described manifestation and may be life-threatening.

The physical examination can be unrevealing or may demonstrate end-expiratory rales (22 percent), hyperinflation, decreased or absent breath sounds, ascites and intraabdominal or adnexal masses. Clubbing is uncommon (≤ 5 percent).[23]

Pathology

In lymphangioleiomyomatosis, the primary pathology, proliferation of atypical smooth muscle, occurs around the bronchovascular structures. This abnormal proliferation is not, however, limited to the bronchovascular sheath but also progresses through the pulmonary interstitium. In addition, another unique pathologic feature of lymphangioleiomyomatosis is the occurrence of diffuse, cystic dilatation of the terminal airspaces[4,11,23] (Fig. 77-1). Some degree of hemosiderosis is common[23] and is thought to be a consequence of low-volume hemorrhage due to the rupture of dilated and tortuous venules.

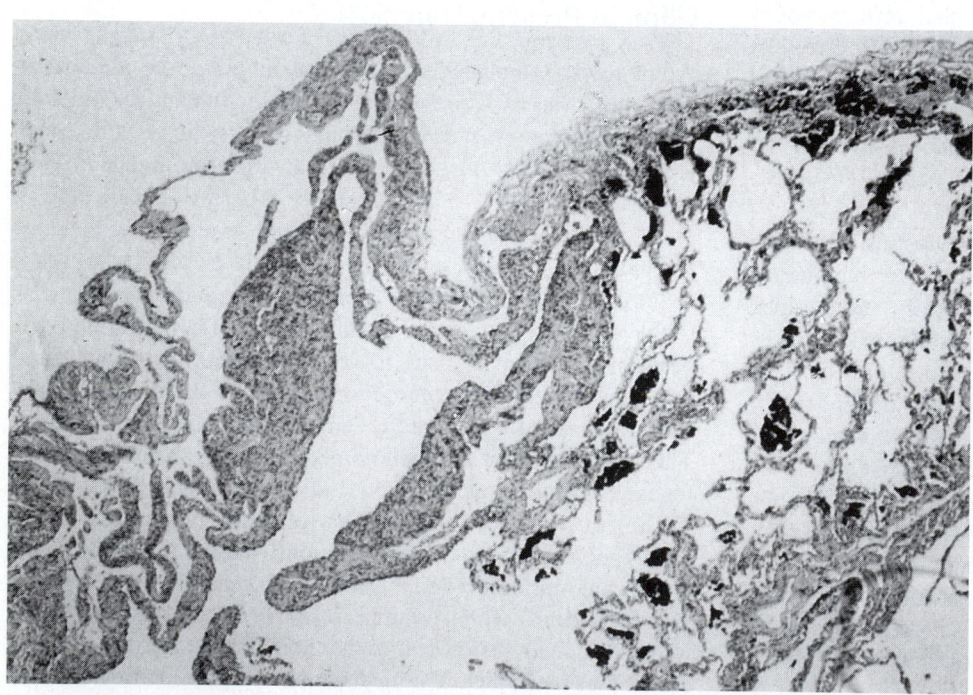

A

FIGURE 77-1 Histopathology of lymphangioleiomyomatosis. *A.* Smooth muscle is irregularly distributed throughout the pulmonary parenchyma. The muscle bundles are often found near blood vessels but extend into the alveolar walls. Intraalveolar collections of macrophages and lymphocytes are also present (right side of figure). *B.* Higher-power view reveals the abnormal smooth-muscle proliferation. The cells appear shorter and more immature than normal smooth muscle. Mitotic figures are rarely encountered.

The atypical proliferating cells resemble vascular smooth-muscle cells but are often somewhat shortened and pleomorphic (Fig. 77-1*B*). The origin of the atypical cells is assumed to be a myosite, but this is controversial. These cells are polyclonal in nature.

Grossly and microscopically the normal architecture is distorted by multiple small cysts ranging from 0.1 cm to several centimeters in diameter (Fig. 77-2). The interstitium is thickened with evidence of smooth-muscle-like proliferation around and within the pulmonary lymphatics, venules, and airways.[11,14] The lymphatic and venous vessels can also be quite tortuous and dilated. Hilar, mediastinal, and retroperitoneal lymph nodes are often involved and enlarged. The thoracic duct is frequently thickened and dilated. Extrapulmonary involvement with renal, retroperitoneal, intraabdominal and pelvic angioleiomyomata commonly occurs.[27,45,49]

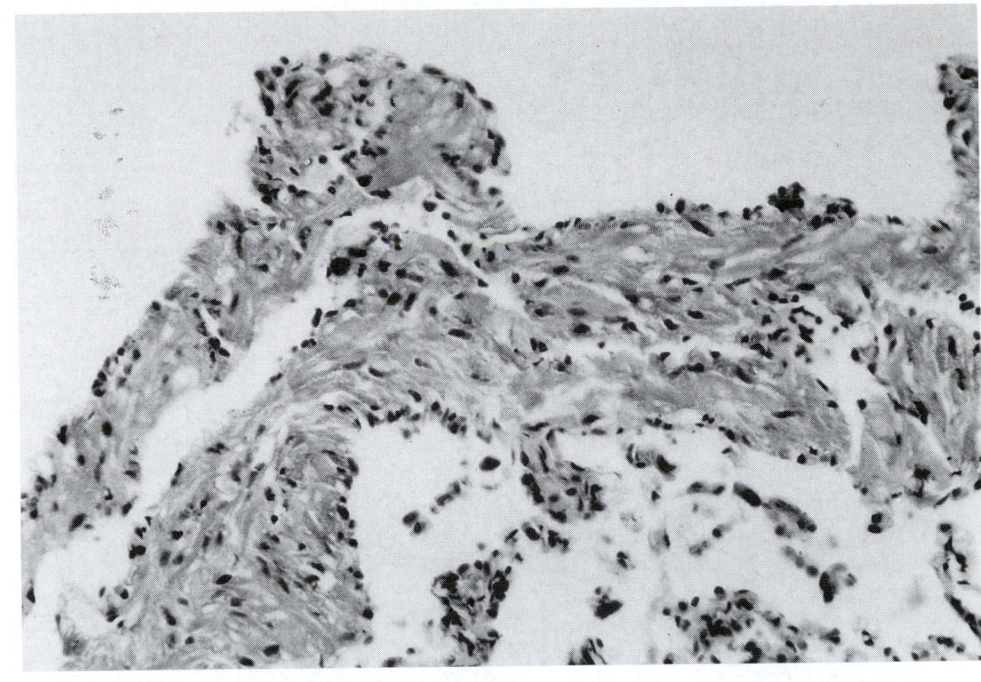

B

FIGURE 77-1   *(Cont.)*

Pathogenesis

Lymphangioleiomyomatosis is primarily a disease of smooth-muscle-like cell proliferation throughout the interstitium of the lungs and within and around the lymphatics of the body. It is unknown whether the proliferation results from an abnormality of the proliferating cells or if the abnormally proliferating cells are simply responding to abnormal stimulation from circulating mediators.

It is very likely that estrogen plays a central role in disease progression. The disease does not present prior to menarche and only rarely after menopause. The few occurences that have been reported in postmenopausal women have most often been in association with hormonal supplementation. The disease is known to accelerate during pregnancy and to abate after oophorectomy. In those with pulmonary disease as part of tuberous sclerosis there is a marked female preponderance.[17] Further, estrogen and progesterone receptors have been demonstrated in biopsy tissue.[5,31]

The mechanism by which interstitial smooth-muscle proliferation causes cyst formation and emphysemalike disease is unknown. The mechanism is thought to result from compression of the conducting airways by the proliferating smooth muscle in the interstitium, but this is controversial.[11,14] Others have postulated that smooth-muscle proliferation within the airways creates a "ball-valve" obstruction which leads to distention of the terminal airspaces. It has also been suggested that elastic fiber degradation related to an imbalance of the elastase/alpha-1-antitrypsin system is a major mechanism leading to the emphysemalike changes.[19] Some combination of these mechanisms probably best explains the pathogenesis.[11,14,40,43]

Pulmonary Physiology

Pulmonary function testing may be very helpful in providing a clue to the diagnosis of lymphangioleiomyomatosis. Lymphangioleiomyomatosis is one of the few interstitial lung diseases which presents with reticulonodular opacities on chest radiograph, increased lung volumes, and an "obstructive" or "mixed" pattern on pulmonary function testing.[9,15,23,43] Lymphangioleiomyomatosis patients are often hyperinflated with an increased total lung volume (TLC) and increased thoracic gas volume (Vtg). Increased gas trapping as evident by an increase in residual volume (RV) and RV/TLC ratio is commonly present even when TLC and Vtg are relatively normal. Often there is evidence of airflow limitation with decreased forced expiratory volume (FEV_1) and vital capacity, FEV_1/FVC. Pulmonary mechanics studies show that mean elastic recoil is reduced and that upstream resistance (R_{us}) is increased.[9,15] Both a loss of elastic recoil and an increase in lung resistance contribute to the observed airflow limitation.

Gas exchange is often abnormal with a markedly reduced diffusing capacity, DL_{CO}, being a characteristic feature. The alveolar-arterial oxygen difference is also increased. There is a diminished exercise performance with a reduced oxygen consumption and low anaerobic threshold in most patients.[15] Exercise causes an abnormal and excessive ventilatory response with high respiratory rate, excessive minute ventilation, and reduced breathing reserve.[15] The baseline or exercise dead space to tidal volume (V_D/V_T) is frequently abnormal[15] (Fig. 77-3). Thus, the primary determinants of this exercise limitation are related to airflow limitation and mechanical factors (i.e., decreased breathing reserve, work of breathing) (Fig. 77-4). However, pulmonary vascular involvement also exerts a significant physiologic effect upon exercise performance, probably because the accompanying increase in physiologic dead space can produce excessive ventilatory requirements that drive $\dot{V}_E$ beyond the ventilatory ceiling. It is this interdependence between airflow limitation (producing a reduced ventilatory ceiling) and pulmonary vascular dysfunction/destruction that leads to severe impairment in exercise performance in many patients with pulmonary lymphangioleiomyomatosis.[15]

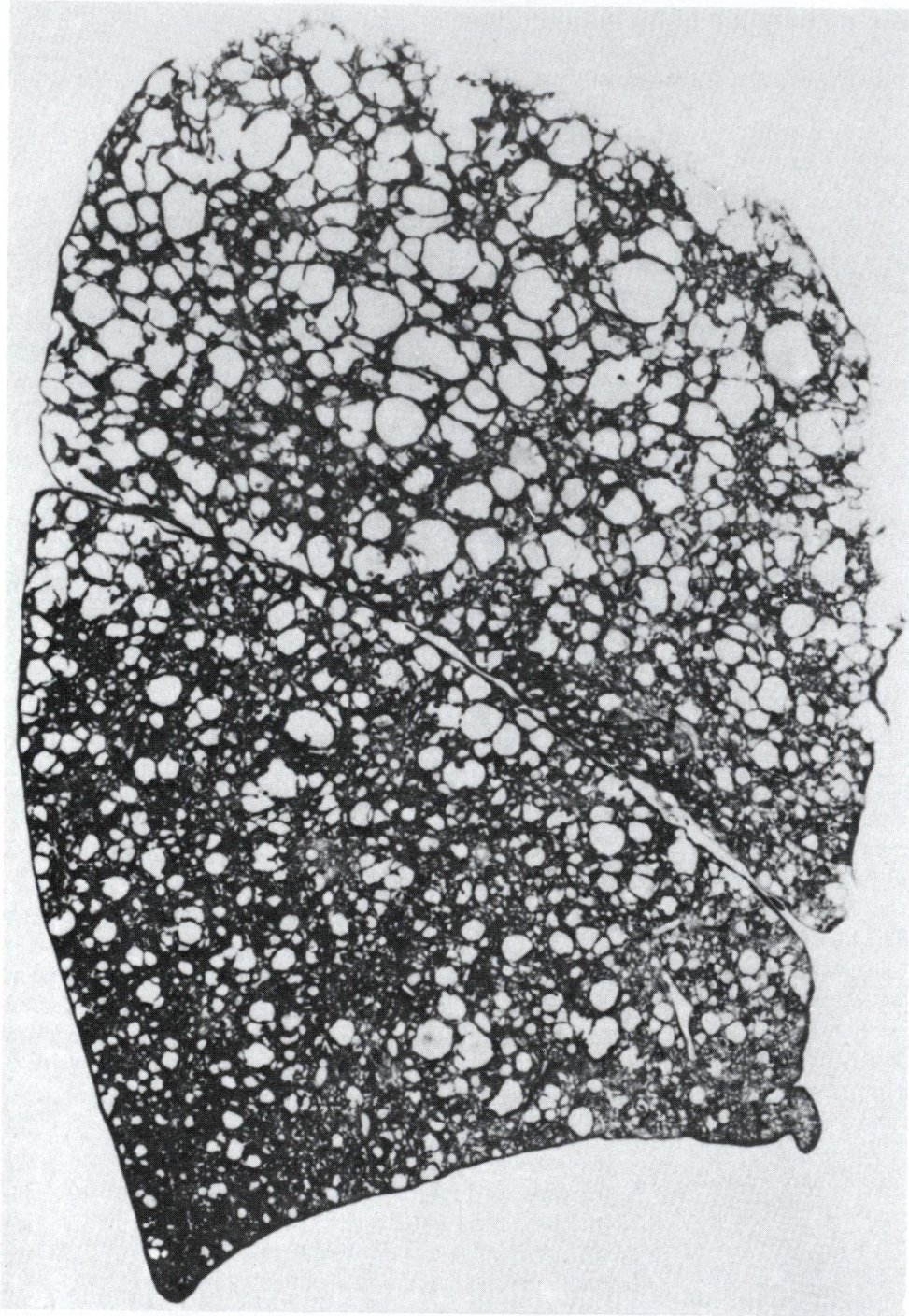

FIGURE 77-2 Pulmonary lymphangioleiomyomatosis causes thin-walled emphysematous spaces leading to the distinctive type of honeycombing. *(From Cornog JL, Enterline HT.[13])*

Radiology

CHEST RADIOGRAPH

The chest radiograph findings in lymphangioleiomyomatosis are variable,[3,11,16,23] ranging from normal early in the course of the disease to severely emphysematouslike changes in advanced disease. Pneumothorax can be an early feature, and chylous pleural effusion can develop at any time during the course (Fig. 77-5). Initial reports of lymphangioleiomyomatosis described a pseudoreticular or nodular pattern of irregular opacities. These opacities result from the compression of smooth-muscle-rich interstitial tissue by more dilated cystic airspaces. Lymphatic obstruction with the development of Kerley B septal lines also contribute to the pattern. Cross-sectional studies show 33 to 62 percent of individuals to have hyperinflation with cystic dilatation of the airspaces, producing relatively radiolucent lung fields.[23,43]

CHEST COMPUTED TOMOGRAPHY

The chest CT is very useful for demonstrating the cystic nature of this disease.[25,29] The high-resolution, thin-section CT scanning is much more sensitive than routine chest radiography.[25,29] Further, the findings of diffuse, homogenous, small (less than 1 cm diameter) thin-walled cysts can be pathopneumonic in an appropriate clinical context[16,29,33,44] (Fig. 77-6). Bilateral lung cysts (100 percent) and ground glass opacities (59 percent) were the most common CT findings in 38 women in the Kyoto study.[23] Nodular opacities 5 percent were uncommonly present, and linear densities were not seen.

There is a close correlation between the extent of the cystic parenchymal replacement in subjects with lymphangioleiomyomatosis (as measured by quantitative high-resolution chest CT) and disease severity (as determined by spirometry, diffusing capacity, lung volume or exercise performance).[16] Thus, chest CT may be of both diagnostic and prognostic importance.

Diagnosis

Lymphangioleiomyomatosis can be readily diagnosed by its characteristic histologic findings on open lung or thoracoscopic biopsy. Often, transbronchial lung biopsy can yield an adequate sample for pathologic evaluation especially when immunohistochemical stains specific for smooth-muscle components; actin or desmin[26] and more recently HMB-45[8,12,21] have been employed to improve diagnostic sensitivity and specificity.

In general, the diagnosis should be strongly suspected in any young woman who presents with emphysema, recurrent pneumothorax, or a chylous pleural effusion. High-resolution chest CT can often confirm the diagnosis and tissue confirmation may not always be necessary, although given the devastating nature of this disorder it is usually recommended. The differential di-

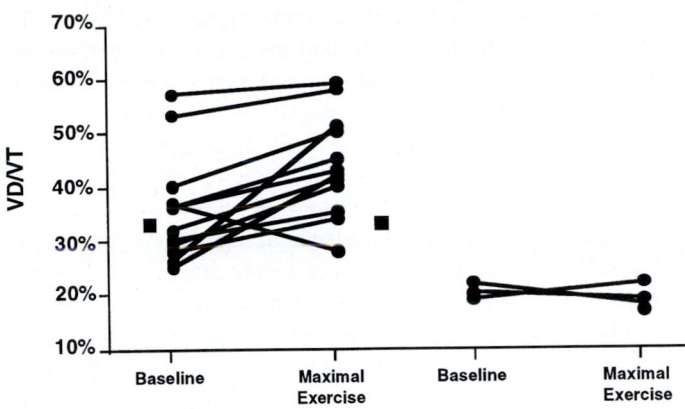

FIGURE 77-3 Pulmonary lymphangioleiomyotosis. Dead space to tidal volume ratio- percent (V_{DS}/V_T) at rest and maximal exercise in patients with LAM (n = 15). *Left panel.* Twelve patients demonstrated an abnormal V_{DS}/V_T either at rest or in response to exercise. *Right panel.* The three subjects with a normal V_{DS}/V_T at rest and normal response to exercise are shown. *(Adapted from Crausman RS, Jennings CJ, Mortenson RL, et al.[15])*

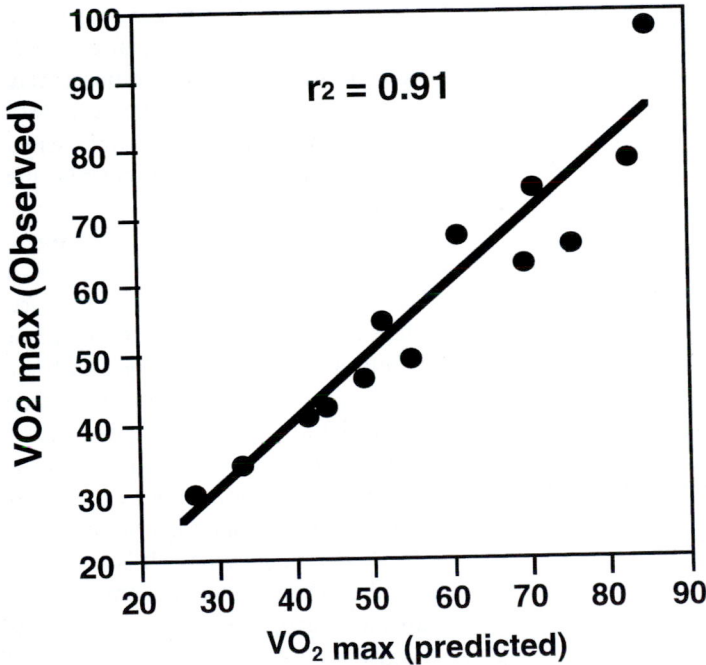

FIGURE 77-4 Linear stepwise regression model derived to determine the variability in exercise capacity. Correlation between percent predicted oxygen consumpton achieved by the patients at maximal exercise ($V_{O_2}max$) and $V_{O_2}max$ predicted from the linear regression equation $V_{O_2}max = 0.40 - (0.0081*baseline\ V_{DS}/V_T) + (0.0070*SGaw)$, $r^2 = 0.91$. Both resting V_{DS}/V_T and SGaw are independent variables in this regression model. For this model, SGaw alone was able to predict 76 percent of the variability, and the addition of baseline V_{DS}/V_T predicted an additional 15 percent of the variability. None of the other airflow or gas exchange variables added significantly to this model's ability to predict maximal achieved oxygen consumption. The stepwise regression procedure determined that the best model for maximal achieved workload should include SGaw and baseline V_{DS}/V_T: Maximal achieved workload = $0.37 - (0.0081*baseline\ V_{DS}/V_T) + (0.0096*SGaw)$. This model was able to predict 76 percent of the variability in maximal achieved workload. *(From Crausman RS, Jennings CJ, Mortenson RL, et al.[15])*

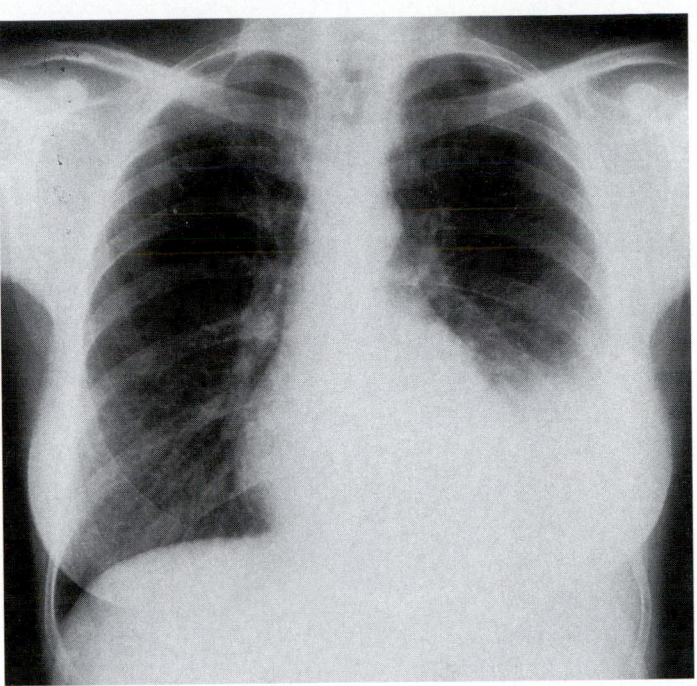

FIGURE 77-5 Posteroanterior radiograph of the chest showing minimal increase in markings in the lower lung zones. A chylothorax is present on the left.

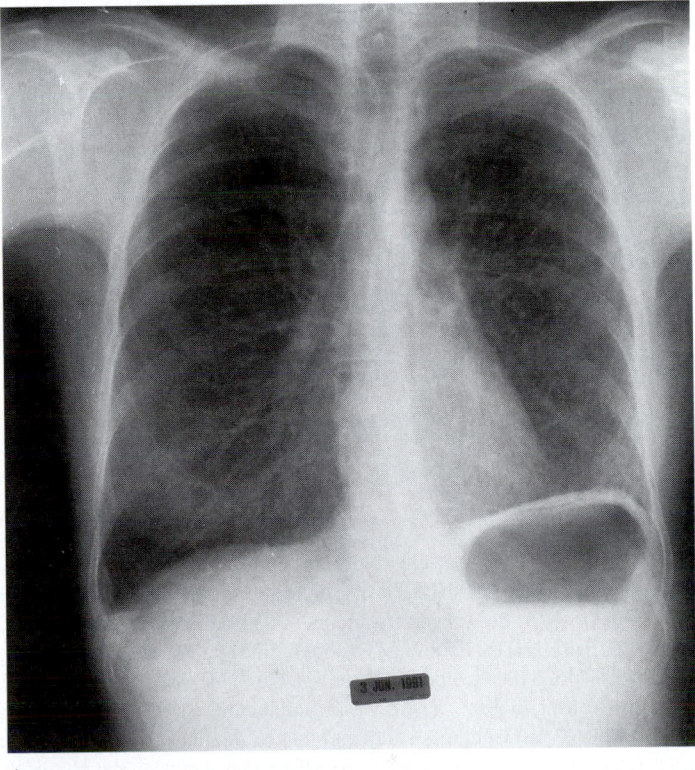

A

FIGURE 77-6 Same patient as in Fig. 77-5, 32 months later. *A.* The current posteroanterior radiograph of the chest shows increased lung volume and difficult-to-see cystic changes in the all lung zones. The pleural changes on the left are secondary to the prior effusion and to an open lung biopsy. *B.* The high-resolution CT scan demonstrates multiple thin-walled cystic airspaces.

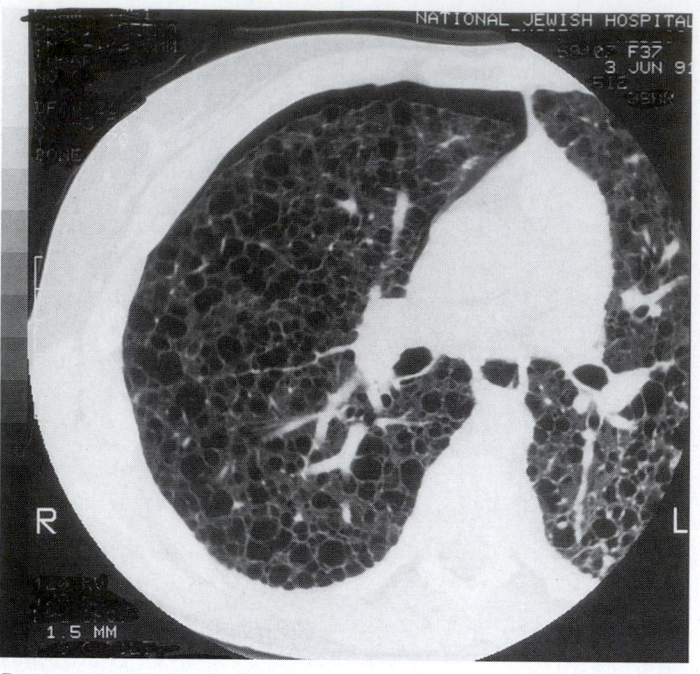

B

FIGURE 77-6   *(Cont.)*

agnosis would also include: emphysema, alpha-1-antitrypsin deficiency, asthma, chronic extrinsic allergic alveolitis, pulmonary histiocytosis X, cystic sarcoidosis, and panacinar emphysema due to intravenous drug use.

Prognosis

The natural history of this disorder is thought to be progressive with a median survival of 8 to 10 years from diagnosis. The prognosis for women with lymphangioleiomyomatosis is variable but generally poor, with about 22 to 62 percent[23,43] succumbing to progressive respiratory failure after 8.5 years from diagnosis (Fig. 77-7). Uncommonly, long-term survival 20 years after diagnosis has been reported.[35] In the two most recent large case series,[23,43] there was an apparent improvement in survival. The reasons for this improved survival are unknown, i.e., bias inherent in the methods, hormonal interventions, better supportive treatments, or a change in the natural history of the disease. Our recent study suggests that the diagnosis is being made at a much earlier stage of the disease.[15] None of our patients were diagnosed after age 40 years. These data also suggest that the rate of progression is quite variable and can occur many years after diagnosis and after menopause.[43] Sudden onset of rapid deterioration is rare later in the course of the disease.[43] Pregnancy and the use of supplemental estrogen are known to accelerate the disease process.[36]

Pulmonary function and histologic pattern of disease have been shown to be predictive of poor survival.[23] An elevated total lung capacity (percent predicted TLC) and reduced FEV_1/FVC ratio were associated with poor survival 2 to 5 years after initial examination. Further, a predominantly cystic pattern of histopathology predicted a worse prognosis than a predominantly muscular pattern. It is unknown whether these patterns represent two distinct histopathologies or different stages in disease evolution.

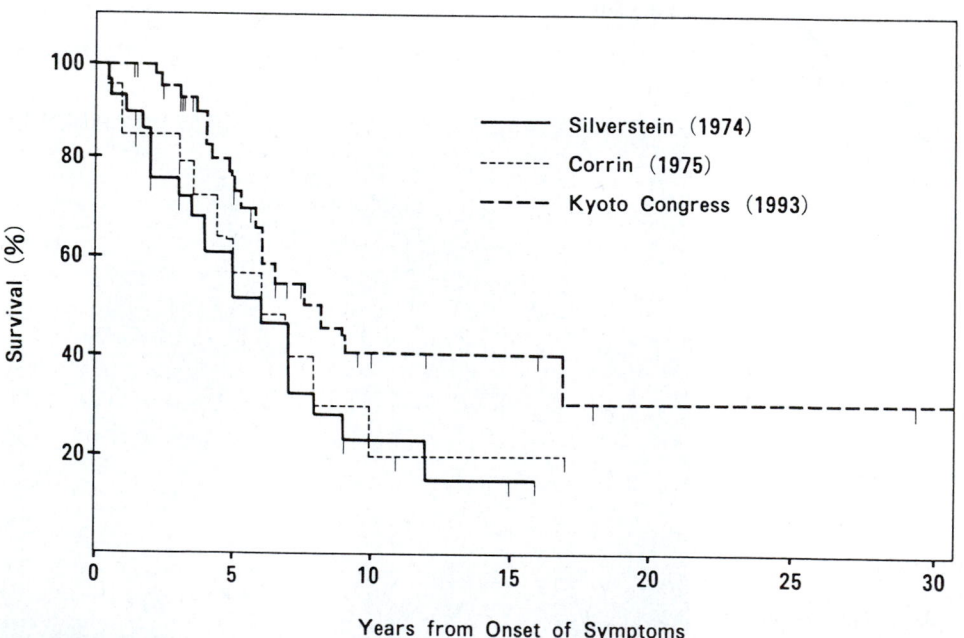

Years from Onset of Symptoms

FIGURE 77-7   Kaplan-Meier plots of actuarial survival of patients with pulmonary lymphangioleiomyomatosis from the onset of symptoms. Three separate reports were analyzed: Silverstein and coworkers in 1974 described the outcome in 31 patients (solid line)[38]; Corrin and coworkers in 1975 described survival in 23 patients (dotted line)[14]; Kitaichi and colleagues in 1995 described the survival of 46 Asian women reported at the 1993 Kyoto Pulmonary Lymphangioleiomyomatosis Congress (dashed line).[23] There was a statistically significant difference between the plot of the patients in the Kyoto Congress study and that of the patients summarized by Silverstein and coworkers (p ≤ 0.01). There were no remarkable differences between the plot of the patients in the Kyoto Congress study and that of the patients reported by Corrin and coworkers or between the plots of the patients summarized by Silverstein and coworkers and those reported by Corrin and coworkers. Interestingly, in a study by Taylor and colleagues[43] the survival appeared to be much better among 32 patients (data not shown). In the Taylor study 78 percent of the patients were alive at the time of writing of the manuscript, with average intervals of 8.5 years since onset of disease in the entire group and 10 years in the group of survivors. In fact, in the Taylor study all deaths occurred within 5 years of the onset of the disease. *(From Kitaichi M, Nishimura K, Itoh H, Izumi T.[23])*

Treatment

Treatment regimens have thus far been unsatisfactory. There is no role for either corticosteroids or cytotoxic agents and there have been few advances since the early recognition that female hormones likely play an etiologic role in the pathogenesis. Oophorectomy, progesterone (10 mg/day), and more recently tamoxifen (20 mg/day) and luteinizing hormone-releasing hormone (LHRH) analogs[34] have been employed with some anecdotal support. Alpha-interferon has also been tried,[24] but in our experience has not been of any benefit primarily because side effects limit use. Only oophorectomy and treatment with progestational agents appear to provide reliable benefit. A recent metanalysis[18] summarized the results of 30 treated cases. Of patients treated early in the course of disease prior to widespread tissue destruction, 5 of 7 with oophorectomy stabilized or improved; 2 of 2 with both oophorectomy and treatment with progesterone stabilized or improved by objective criteria; only 4 of 8 treated with progesterone alone demonstrated stabilization or improvement. Thus, combination therapy with oophorectomy and either progesterone and/or tamoxifen should be considered. Chemical oophorectomy with LHRH analogs may replace surgical oophorectomy as the primary treatment of this disorder, although data are currently lacking.

To date, only lung transplantation offers any hope for cure and should be considered as definitive therapy for any failing patient. Approximately 50 percent of patients with lymphangioleiomyotosis are alive at 3 years following transplant. Unfortunately, reports of recurrent disease in transplanted lungs raise concern regarding even this therapy.[30]

TUBEROUS SCLEROSIS

Tuberous sclerosis (Bourneville's disease) is a rare (varies from 1 per 27,000 to 1 per 100,000 population) autosomal dominant disorder, but up to 68 percent of cases may be new mutations.[41] It affects men or women equally. Mental retardation, seizures, and facial angiofibroma (adenoma sebacium) form the classic clinical triad. The features are variable, however, and some affected individuals can have normal intelligence. Skin lesions are a prominent feature of tuberous sclerosis and are usually present in childhood. These lesions are characterized by hypopigmented spots on the trunk followed by adenoma sebaceum (wartlike lesions distributed in a butterfly pattern over the face and cheeks).

In less than 1 percent of cases, tuberous sclerosis can be associated with pulmonary manifestations that are indistinguishable from those of lymphangioleiomyomatosis (Table 77-2). The onset is generally in the fourth decade of life and rarely before age 20 years. Some have referred to lymphangioleiomyomatosis as a *forme fruste* of tuberous sclerosis.[22,47] The complete triad of tuberous sclerosis is not commonly present in those who develop pulmonary involvement.[47] When pulmonary involvement is present there is a marked female predominance. Dwyer and colleagues[17] reported that in 29 of 34 cases in their series the patients were female. Most patients present with dyspnea. Some have the onset heralded by a spontaneous pneumothorax. Pneumothorax occurs in approximately one-third of patients. Hemoptysis and chest pain are other important features. The radiographic appearance is similar to that of pulmonary lymphangioleiomyomatosis described above.[25] Chylothorax is a rare

TABLE 77-2

Features of Tuberous Sclerosis with and without Involvement of the Lungs

	Without Pulmonary Involvement	*With Pulmonary Involvement*
Age at onset, years	< 20	30 to 35
Sex incidence	1:1	1:5
Family heredity	Yes	Yes
Presenting symptom	Central nervous system disorder	Dyspnea or spontaneous pneumothorax
Mental retardation	Frequent (~60 percent)	Uncommon (~40 percent)
Seizures	Frequent (70–90 percent)	Uncommon (~20 percent)
Facial angiofibroma	Frequent	Frequent
Pneumothorax	Not known (rare)	Frequent
Chylothorax	Not known (rare)	Rare
Angiomyolipoma	Frequent	Frequent

SOURCE: Hauck RW, Konig G, Permanetter W, et al.[20]

complication.[47] The primary histologic lesion is a hamartoma. Similar lesions occur in the brain and can calcify. A micronodular hyperplasia of type II pneumocytes has recently been described.[32] Renal lesions, angioleiomyomata, also occur with high frequency. Other associations include: cardiac rhabdomyoma, sclerotic bone, and periungual fibromas.

There is a decrease in survival for patients with tuberous sclerosis compared to the general population.[37] Renal disease and brain tumors are the most common cause of death.[37] Pulmonary involvement in tuberous sclerosis carries a poor prognosis.[17] Progressive disease is common, and death occurs secondary to respiratory insufficiency within 5 years of the onset of symptoms. Long-term survivors have been described and may occur more frequently today because of improved management of the potential complications, especially cor pulmonale and pneumothorax. No effective treatment has been found. However, because of similarities to lymphangioleiomyomatosis, treatment with progesterone and/or oophorectomy in women is recommended.

REFERENCES

1. Baldi S, Papotti M, Valente ML, et al: Pulmonary lymphangioleiomyomatosis in postmenopausal women: report of two cases and review of the literature. *Eur Respir J* 7:1013–1016, 1994.
2. Banner AS, Carrington CB, Emory WB, et al: Efficacy of oophorectomy in lymphangioleiomyomatosis and benign metastasizing leiomyoma. *New Engl J Med* 305:204–209, 1981.
3. Berger JL: X–ray diagnosis of pulmonary lymphangioleiomyomatosis. *J Tenn Med Assoc* 73:657–658, 1980.
4. Berger JL, Shaff MI: Pulmonary lymphangioleiomyomatosis. *J Comput Assist Tomogr* 5:565–567, 1981.
5. Berger U, Khaghani A, Pomerance A, et al: Pulmonary lymphangioleiomyomatosis and steroid receptors. An immunocytochemical study. *Am J Clin Pathol* 93:609–614, 1990.
6. Berkman N, Bloom A, Cohen P, et al: Bilateral spontaneous pneumothorax as the presenting feature in lymphangioleiomyomatosis. *Respir Med* 89:381–383, 1995.

7. Bernstein SM, Newell JD, Adamczyk D, et al: How common are renal angiomyolipomas in patients with pulmonary lymphangioleiomyomatosis? *Am J Respir Crit Care Med* 152:2138–2143, 1995.

8. Bonetti F, Chiodera PL, Pea M, et al: Transbronchial biopsy in lymphangiomyomatosis of the lung. HMB45 for diagnosis. *Am J Surg Pathol* 17:1092–1102, 1993.

9. Burger CD, Hyatt RE, Staats BA: Pulmonary mechanics in lymphangioleiomyomatosis. *Am Rev Respir Dis* 143:1030–1033, 1991.

10. Capron F, Ameille J, Leclerc P, et al: Pulmonary lymphangioleiomyomatosis and Bourneville's tuberous sclerosis with pulmonary involvement: the same disease? *Cancer* 52:851–855, 1983.

11. Carrington CB, Cugell DW, Gaensler EA, et al: Lymphangioleiomyomatosis. Physiologic-pathologic-radiologic correlations. *Am Rev Respir Dis* 116:977–995, 1977.

12. Chan JKC, Tsang WYW, Pau MY, et al: Lymphangiomyomatosis and angiomyolipoma: closely related entities characterized by hamartomatous proliferation of HMB-45-positive smooth muscle. *Histopathology* 22:445–455, 1993.

13. Cornog JL Jr., Enterline HT: Lymphangiomyoma, a benign lesion of chyliferous lymphatics synonymous with lymphangiopericytoma. *Cancer* 19:1909–1930, 1966.

14. Corrin B, Liebow AA, Friedman PJ: Pulmonary lymphangioleiomyomatosis: a review. *Am J Pathol* 79:348–382, 1975.

15. Crausman RS, Jennings CJ, Mortenson RL, et al: Lymphangioleiomyomatosis: the relative importance of airways and vascular involvement to diminished exercise capacity. *Am J Resp Crit Care Med* in press, 1996.

16. Crausman RS, Lynch DA, Mortenson RL, et al: Quantitative CT predicts the severity of physiologic dysfunction in patients with lymphangioleiomyomatosis. *Chest* 109:131–137, 1996.

17. Dwyer J, Hickie J, Garvan J: Pulmonary tuberous sclerosis. Report of three patients and a review of the literature. *Q J Med* 40:115–125, 1971.

18. Eliasson AH, Phillips YY, Tenholder MF: Treatment of lymphangioleiomyomatosis. A meta-analysis. *Chest* 96:1352–1355, 1989.

19. Fukuda Y, Kawamoto M, Yamamoto A, et al: Role of elastic fiber degradation in emphysema-like lesions of pulmonary lymphangiomyomatosis. *Hum Pathol* 21:1252–1261, 1990.

20. Hauck RW, Konig G, Permanetter W, et al: Tuberous sclerosis with pulmonary involvement. *Respiration* 57:289–292, 1990.

21. Hoon V, Thung SN, Kaneko M, Unger PD: HMB-45 reactivity in renal angiomyolipoma and lymphangioleiomyomatosis. *Arch Pathol Lab Med* 118:732–734, 1994.

22. Jozwiak S: Pulmonary lymphangioleiomyomatosis: a "forme fruste" of tuberous sclerosis? [letter; comment]. *AJR* 155:419, 1990.

23. Kitaichi M, Nishimura K, Itoh H, Izumi T: Pulmonary lymphangioleiomyomatosis: a report of 46 patients including a clinicopathologic study of prognostic factors. *Am J Respir Crit Care Med* 151:527–533, 1995.

24. Klein M, Krieger O, Ruckser R, et al: Treatment of lymphangioleiomyomatosis by ovariectomy, interferon alpha 2b and tamoxifen—a case report. *Arch Gynecol Obstet* 252:99–102, 1992.

25. Lenoir S, Grenier P, Brauner MW, et al: Pulmonary lymphangiomyomatosis and tuberous sclerosis: Comparison of radiographic and thin-section CT findings. *Radiology* 175:329–334, 1990.

26. Matthews TJ, Hornall D, Sheppard MN: Comparison of the use of antibodies to alpha smooth muscle actin and desmin in pulmonary lymphangioleiomyomatosis. *J Clin Pathol* 46:479–480, 1993.

27. McIntosh GS, Dutoit SH, Chronos NV, Kaisary AV: Multiple unilateral renal angiomyolipomas with regional lymphangioleiomyomatosis. *J Urol* 142:1305–1307, 1989.

28. Miller WT, Cornog JL Jr., Sullivan MA: Lymphangiomyomatosis: A clinical-roentgenologic-pathologic syndrome. *Am J Roentgenol Radium Ther Nucl Med* 3:565–672, 1971.

29. Muller NL, Chiles C, Kullnig P: Pulmonary lymphangiomyomatosis: Correlation of CT with radiographic and functional findings. *Radiology* 175:335–339, 1990.

30. Nine JS, Yousem SA, Paradis IL, et al: Lymphangioleiomyomatosis: recurrence after lung transplantation. *J Heart Lung Transplant* 13:714–719, 1994.

31. Ohori NP, Yousem SA, Sonmez-Alpan E, Colby TV: Estrogen and progesterone receptors in lymphangioleiomyomatosis, epithelioid hemangioendothelioma, and sclerosing hemangioma of the lung. *Am J Clin Pathol* 96:529–535, 1991.

32. Popper HH, Juettner-Smolle FM, Pongratz MG: Micronodular hyperplasia of type II pneumocytes—a new lung lesion associated with tuberous sclerosis. *Histopathology* 18:347–354, 1991.

33. Rappaport DC, Weisbrod GL, Herman SJ, Chamberlain DW: Pulmonary lymphangioleiomyomatosis: high-resolution CT findings in four cases. *AJR* 152:961–964, 1989.

34. Rossi GA, Balbi B, Oddera S, et al: Response to treatment with an analog of the luteinizing-hormone-releasing hormone in a patient with pulmonary lymphangioleiomyomatosis. *Am Rev Respir Dis* 143:174–176, 1991.

35. Sawicka EH, Morris AJ: A report of two long-surviving cases of pulmonary lymphangioleiomyomatosis and the response to progesterone therapy. *Br J Dis Chest* 79:400–406, 1985.

36. Shen A, Iseman MD, Waldron JA, King TE: Exacerbation of pulmonary lymphangioleiomyomatosis by exogenous estrogens. *Chest* 91:782–785, 1987.

37. Shepherd CW, Gomez MR, Lie JT, Crowson CS: Causes of death in patients with tuberous sclerosis. *Mayo Clin Proc* 66:792–796, 1991.

38. Silverstein EF, Ellis K, Wolffe M, Jaretzki A: Pulmonary lymphangiomyomatosis. *AJR* 120:832–850, 1974.

39. Sinclair W, Wright JL, Churg A: Lymphangioleiomyomatosis presenting in a postmenopausal woman. *Thorax* 40:475–476, 1985.

40. Sobonya R, Stuart Q, Fleishman J: Pulmonary lymphangioleiomyomatosis: quantitative analysis of lesions producing airflow limitation. *Hum Pathol* 16:1122–1128, 1985.

41. Stefansson K: Tuberous sclerosis. *Mayo Clin Proc* 66:868–872, 1991.

42. Stovin P, Lum C, Flower D, et al: The lungs in lymphangiomyomatosis and in tuberous sclerosis. *Thorax* 30:497–509, 1975.

43. Taylor JR, Ryu J, Colby TV, Raffin TA: Lymphangioleiomyomatosis. Clinical course in 32 patients. *New Engl J Med* 323:1254–1260, 1990.

44. Templeton PA, McLoud TC, Muller NL, et al: Pulmonary lymphangiomyomatosis: CT and pathologic findings. *J Comput Assist Tomogr* 13:54–57, 1989.

45. Torres VE, Bjornsson J, King BF, et al: Extrapulmonary lymphangioleiomyomatosis and lymphangiomatous cysts in tuberous sclerosis complex. *Mayo Clin Proc* 70:641–648, 1995.

46. Urban T, Kuttenn F, Gompel A, et al: Pulmonary lymphangiomyomatosis: follow-up and long-term outcome with antiestrogen therapy; a report of eight cases. *Chest* 102:472–476, 1992.

47. Valensi QJ: Pulmonary lymphangiomyoma, a probable *forme frust* of tuberous sclerosis. *Am Rev Respir Dis* 108:1411–1415, 1973.

48. Valentine VG, Raffin TA: The management of chylothorax. *Chest* 102:586–591, 1992.

49. Woodring JH, Howard RN 2nd, Johnson MV: Massive low-attenuation mediastinal, retroperitoneal, and pelvic lymphadenopathy on CT from lymphangioleiomyomatosis. Case report. *Clin Imaging* 18:7–11, 1994.

CHAPTER 78

THE LUNGS IN PATIENTS WITH INBORN ERRORS OF METABOLISM

Masazumi Adachi

NIEMANN-PICK DISEASE

GAUCHER'S DISEASE

G_{M1} GANGLIOSIDOSIS

SULFATIDE LIPIDOSIS (METACHROMATIC
LEUKODYSTROPHY)

GALACTOSYLCERAMIDE LIPIDOSIS (GLOBOID CELL
LEUKODYSTROPHY—KRABBE'S DISEASE)

GLYCOSPHINGOLIPID LIPIDOSIS (FABRY'S DISEASE)

MUCOPOLYSACCHARIDOSIS

GLYCOGEN STORAGE DISEASE

DISORDERS OF AMINO ACID METABOLISM

CYSTINE STORAGE DISEASE (LIGNAC-FANCONI
DISEASE)

A variety of diseases can be collectively referred to as being *inborn errors of metabolism.* As a result of increasingly sophisticated and complex biochemical and genetic approaches, our knowledge of these disorders has recently expanded greatly. Although many viscera and the central nervous system have been extensively studied in these disorders, comparatively little attention has been paid to the lungs. Most characterizations note that the "stored" material is sometimes deposited in the interalveolar septa or alveoli, that these pathologic changes occasionally lead to pulmonary hypertension and severe pulmonary arteriosclerosis, and that, in some instances, characteristic alterations in the lungs can be demonstrated on radiographic examination. The manifestations of these diseases are diverse. The pulmonary manifestations of selected metabolic disorders are reviewed below.

NIEMANN-PICK DISEASE

Niemann-Pick disease (NPD) is characterized by the excessive accumulation of sphingomyelin (types A and B) and unesterified cholesterol (type C) in the cells of reticuloendothelial and parenchymal tissues of the viscera and/or the brain. The classification of NPD is based on the nature of the primary molecular defect. Types A, B, and C have distinct abnormalities.[10,12] All types are autosomal recessive disorders. Reticular or reticulonodular chest radiographic abnormalities occur in the lungs of most patients afflicted with this disease.

CLINICAL FEATURES

Type A NPD is an acute disorder that affects infants and involves viscera and the nervous system. Almost one-half of affected infants are of Jewish extraction. The onset is insidious, and the children manifest difficulties in feeding and fail to thrive during the early months. The infants show progressive psychomotor deterioration and hepatosplenomegaly. The chest radiograph (Fig. 78-1) shows diffuse reticular infiltration. The infants generally die within the second year of life.

Type B is a chronic infantile form without neurologic involvement. It is less common than types A and C. These infants often have hepatosplenomegaly and lymphadenopathy, which may develop as early as those with type A. However, most patients are in good health until late infancy. The children show increased susceptibility to pneumonia due to diffuse reticular infiltration by the lipids. They die during the juvenile stage.

Type C NPD shows heterogeneous clinical manifestations. It involves viscera and the central nervous system. The initial symptoms usually occur after the first or second year and occasionally after the sixth year of life. Psychomotor deterioration is progressive. Hepatosplenomegaly is less striking than in the previous two types. These patients occasionally survive to adolescence, most often dying between the fifth and fifteenth years of life.

GENETICS

The locus of the genes for types A and B NPD has been identified to be chromosome 11p15.1 to p15.4.[12] The molecular genetics have been derived from three cDNA (designated types 1, 2, and 3),[33] and a total of 12 mutations have been identified as causing the type A and type B disorders.[38] Nine were single base substitutions, and three were small deletions.[38] Type 1 cDNA expressed catalytically active enzyme,[39] and types 2 and 3 cDNA did not express catalytically active enzymes.[38] In type C, the lesion has been mapped to chromosome 18p at genomic marker D18S40.[10]

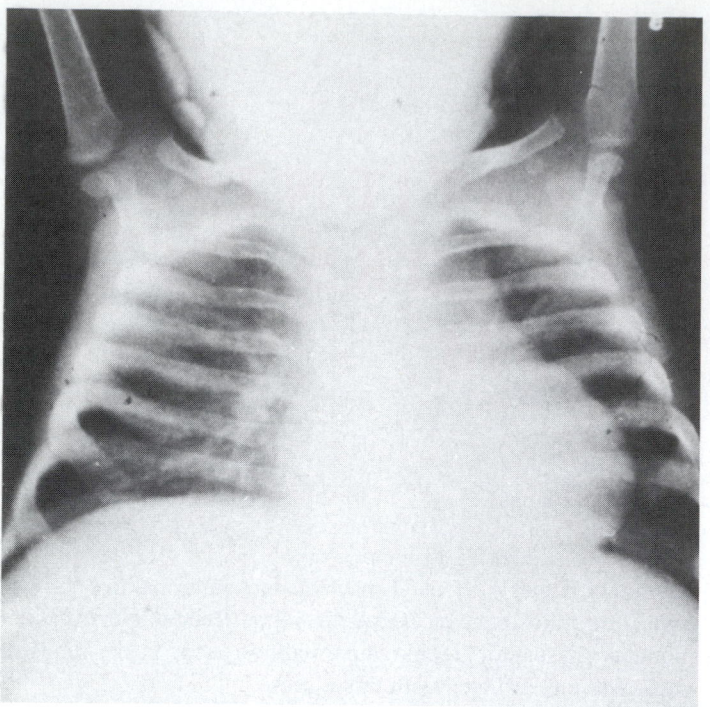

FIGURE 78-1 Chest radiograph of a patient with Niemann-Pick disease (type A) showing bilateral diffuse reticular infiltration.

system. Although the foamy cells are characteristic of this disease, they are not diagnostic without histochemical proof of sphingomyelin (types A and B) or cholesterol (type C).[1] Because the cytoplasmic vacuoles seen in routine sections represent a partly soluble material that has been dissolved during the histologic preparation, frozen sections are often required for this biochemical analysis.

ULTRASTRUCTURE

The foamy cells seen in the tissues of patients with NPD are filled with round to oval cytoplasmic bodies that range from 0.5 to 5 mm in diameter. These bodies are membrane-bound and contain loosely arranged membranous structures in types A and B NPD (Fig. 78-4). Electron-lucent vacuoles that are frequently accompanied by electron-dense membranes are seen in type C NPD. Histochemical preparations for lysosomal enzymes reveal reaction granules in the cytoplasmic inclusion bodies indicating that they are the residua of a cellular effort to eliminate the accumulated lipid material.

BIOCHEMICAL FEATURES

An increase in the sphingomyelin content of the viscera and/or brain from 2 to 30 times normal is the basis for the diagnosis of

PATHOLOGIC FEATURES

The lungs, particularly in type A, are frequently increased in weight, and their cut surfaces show yellow mottling. The liver is markedly enlarged and reaches 2 to 3 times its expected weight. Cut surfaces are diffusely yellow, although the original architecture is usually preserved. The weight of the spleen is often 5 to 6 times normal, and sections show a yellow color with peculiar salmon-pink spots representing malpighian bodies. The lymph nodes are also enlarged. The brains of the patients with types A and C NPD are uniformly reduced in size. On section, the cortex is atrophic, and the gray matter is deep, but the white matter is relatively preserved.

HISTOLOGY

Although some patients have no respiratory disturbances, foamy cells are usually contained in the pulmonary septa and alveoli of most affected individuals (Fig. 78-2). These cells measure 15 to 90 mm in diameter and contain a single nucleus and cytoplasm with numerous fine vacuoles (Fig. 78-3). Similar foamy cells are observed in other visceral organs and the nervous

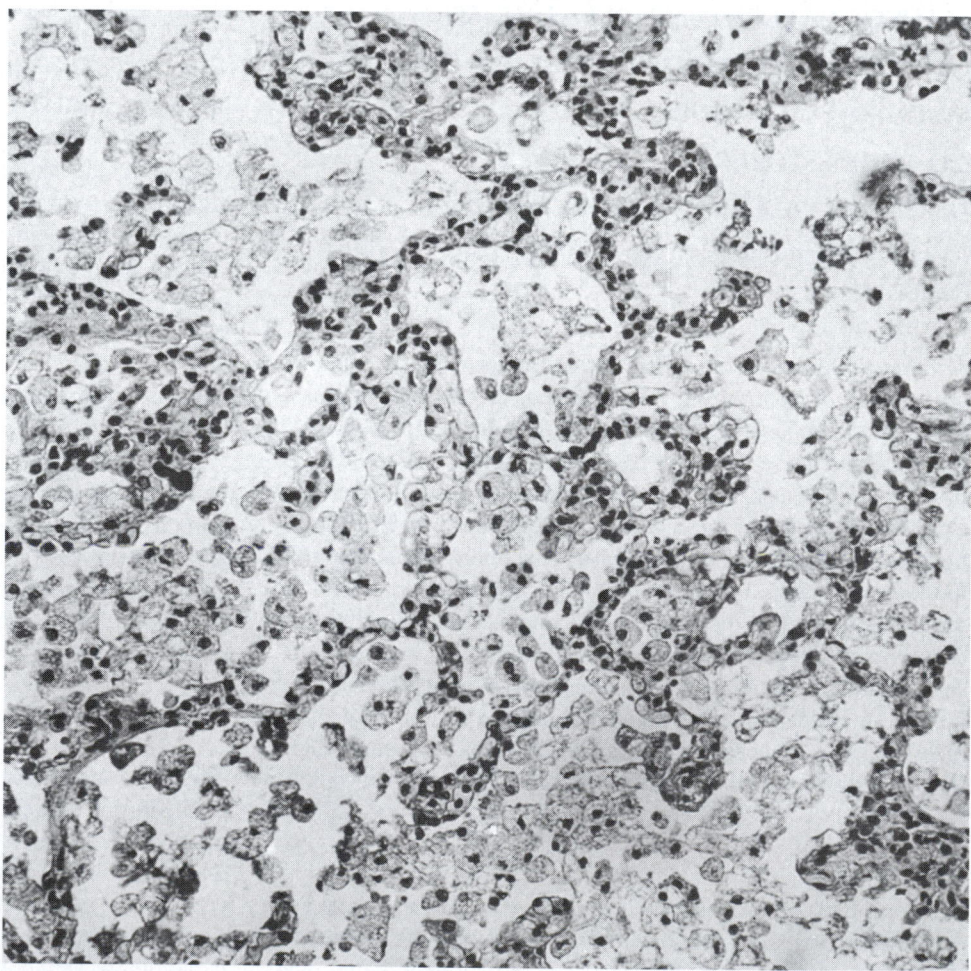

FIGURE 78-2 Sections from lung of a patient with Niemann-Pick disease (type A) exhibiting foamy cells in the alveoli. H&E, ×200.

types A and B NPD. The esterified cholesterol content of the viscera is increased in type C. A deficiency of sphingomyelinase is the primary defect in types A and B,[14] whereas impaired cholesterol esterification is observed in type C.[32]

DIAGNOSIS

Once suspicion of the disease is aroused, types A and B NPD can be diagnosed with biochemical assays of sphingomyelinase in fresh blood samples and frozen tissue. The diagnosis of type C NPD requires analysis of cellular cholesterol esterification and the demonstration of filipin-cholesterol staining in cultured fibroblasts during LDL uptake.[12] Enzyme analysis is not reliable for heterozygote studies, and molecular genetic identification is required. The peripheral smear, bone marrow, and/or lymph nodes or liver should be examined for foamy cells by special histochemical preparations.[1]

GAUCHER'S DISEASE

Gaucher's disease is a hereditary disorder which is transmitted as an autosomal recessive trait. It is characterized by the accumulation of glucosyl ceramide in various organs associated with a deficiency of β-glucosidase.

CLINICAL FEATURES

Three types of this disorder are usually recognized. Type 1, the "adult form," is most common and usually occurs in Ashkenazi Jews. It is a chronic disorder that may start comparatively soon after birth and usually lasts into childhood. It differs from the other types in its lack of neurologic manifestations. Type 2 is the acute form. It occurs in infants and is characterized by progressive neurologic deterioration. The incidence in Jewish families is less than in type 1. Type 3 is the subacute variety. It occurs in juveniles and presents with a more protracted course of neurologic deterioration than the type 2 disorder.

Some patients with the adult form (type 1) die early in life of thrombocytopenia, severe anemia, and pulmonary infections. Hepatosplenomegaly and Gaucher cells in the bone marrow are regular features. The concentration of

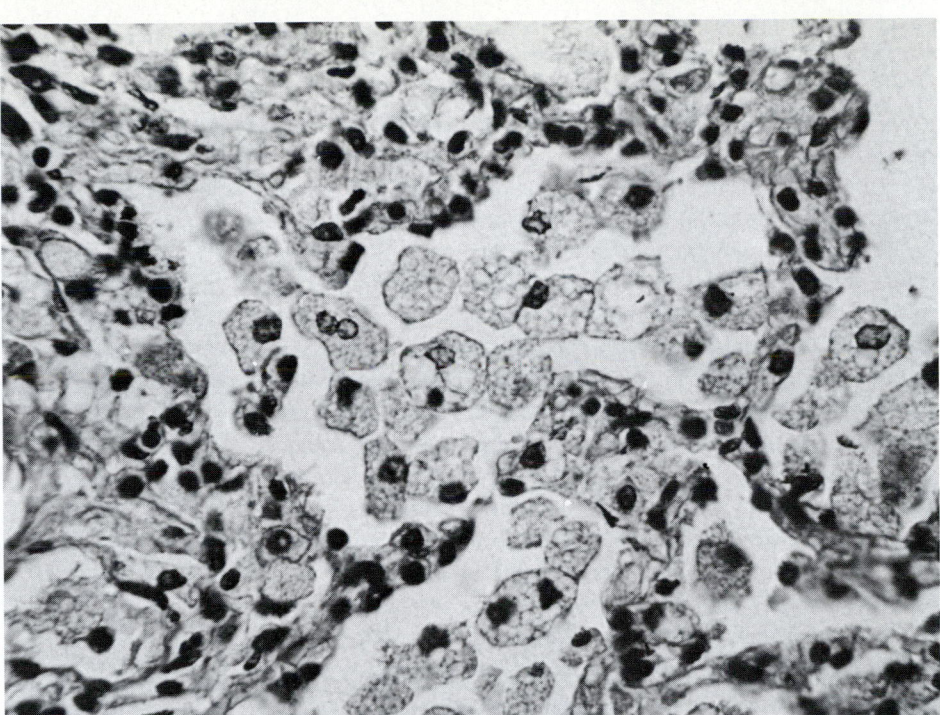

FIGURE 78-3 Under higher magnification, the foamy cells from a patient with Niemann-Pick disease (type A) contain one or two nuclei and numerous fine vacuoles. H&E, ×640.

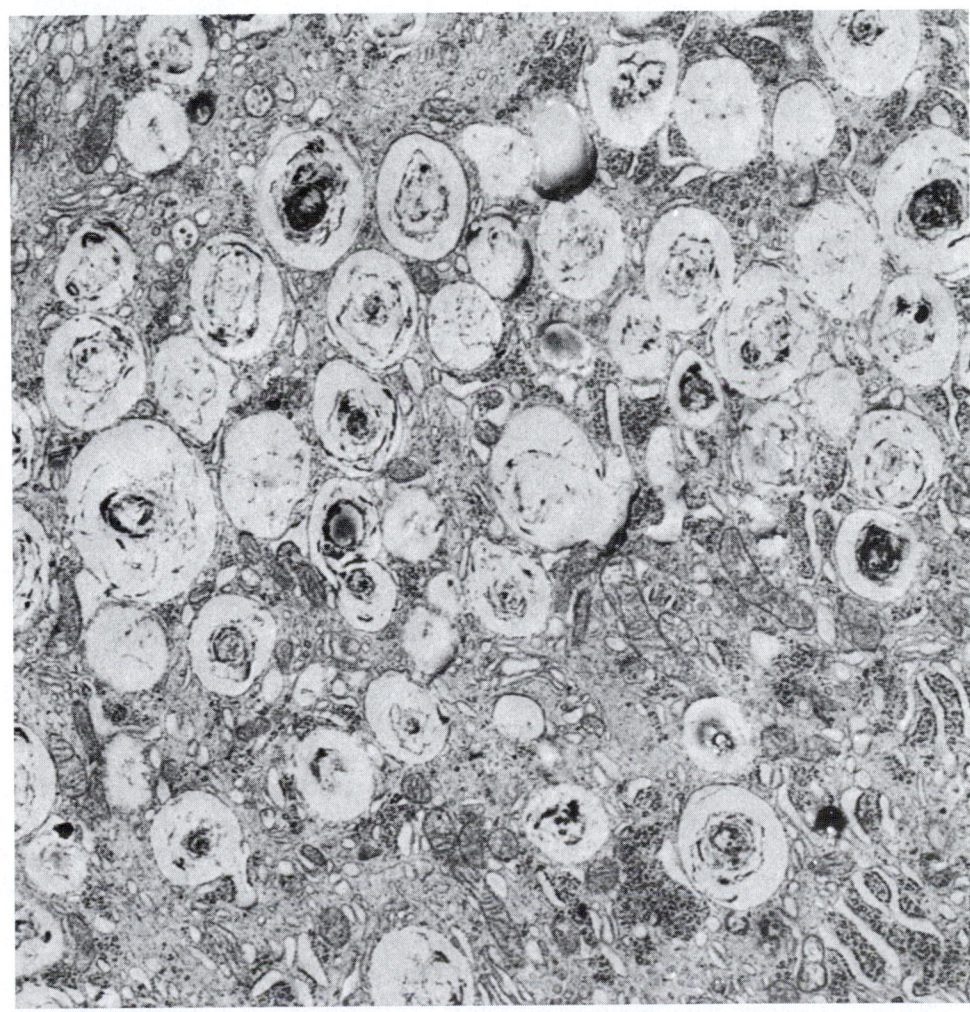

FIGURE 78-4 Electron micrograph of a portion of a foamy cell from a patient with Niemann-Pick disease containing cytoplasmic inclusion bodies which are membrane-bound and contain loosely arranged membranous structures. ×7200.

acid phosphatase in serum is also markedly increased. Pulmonary hypertension and severe pulmonary arteriosclerosis occur in some patients.[37] The reticular pattern of pulmonary infiltration that is characteristic of NPD is rare. Repeated episodes of bone pain are common, and fractures after minor trauma sometimes lead to permanent deformity. Osteolytic changes are frequently seen on radiologic examination.

In type 2, the children develop normally until the age of 3 to 6 months. Thereafter, hepatospenomegaly and lymphadenopathy become prominent, and Gaucher cells are found in the bone marrow. High levels of serum acid phosphatase are sometimes noted as early as 3 months of age. Progressive psychomotor deterioration then sets in, and the patients die within 2 years.

The type 3 disorder presents with a more protracted course of neurologic alterations. Patients with the type 3 variant also show splenomegaly and slowly progressive hepatomegaly. The children often display pulmonary infiltration on radiologic examination. However, the typical reticular pattern is rarely seen. Osteolytic lesions are frequent. About one-half of the patients with this variant have been reported from four interrelated families from the province of Norrbotten in northern Sweden. The mode of inheritance is also consistent with an autosomal recessive trait. E rosette forming peripheral lymphocytes are defective in Gaucher's disease. This abnormality is caused by serum factors, one of which involves ferritin which has been found to be elevated in these patients. This ferritin dysregulation may play a role in the high incidence of cancer in Gaucher patients.[5]

GENETICS

The gene coding acid β-glucosidase is located on chromosome 1 at q21.[40] The gene for the enzyme is approximately 7 kb in length and contains 11 exons. A variety of mutations of this gene have been found to cause Gaucher's disease including missense mutations, frameshift mutations, a splicing mutation, deletions, gene fusions with a pseudogene, and gene conversions.[6] The most common mutation in the Ashkenazic Jewish population is at nucleotide 1226, where an A-to-G alteration causes an amino acid substitution in acid β-glucosidase.[6]

PATHOLOGIC FEATURES

The spleen, liver, and lymph nodes of patients with this disease are markedly enlarged. Gaucher cells are the histologic hallmark of the disease (Fig. 78-5). They are round or polygonal in shape, measure 20 to 80 μm in diameter, and contain fibrils of varying sizes in their cytoplasm which gives the appearance of striation. Histochemically, they show a characteristic reaction staining pink to red with the modified periodic acid Schiff stain for cerebroside.[1] These cells are primarily derived from the reticuloendothelial system. An unusual cardiac and renal involvement with pulmonary hypertension in a 25-year-old black woman who had Gaucher's disease since 1 year of age has also been reported.[41]

Although pulmonary infiltrates are typically seen on chest radiograph evaluations, these infiltrates have not been extensively described in the literature.[37] Severe involvement of the lungs in the adult disorder has been described in three patients with symptoms since infancy followed by juvenile onset dyspnea. Their

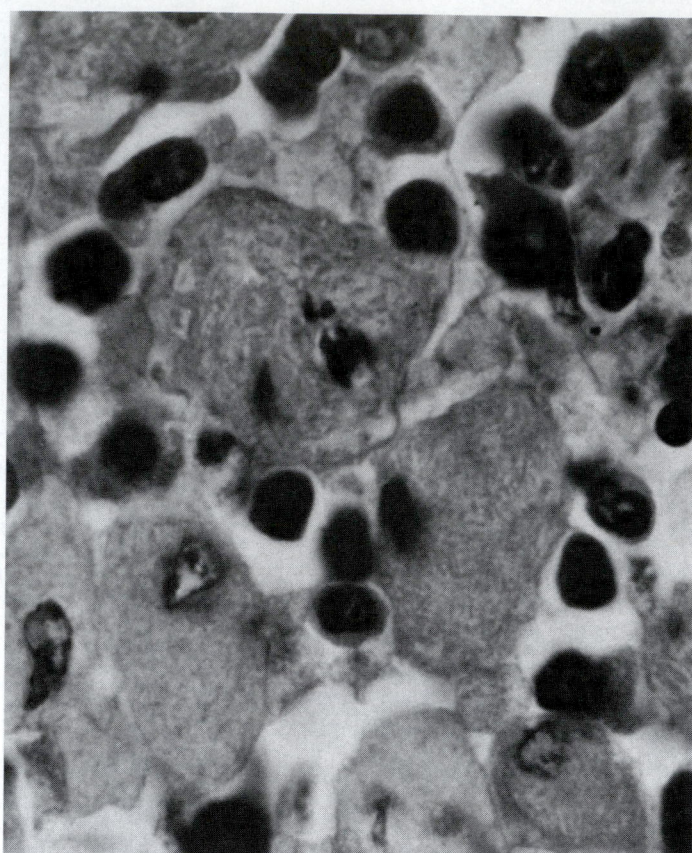

FIGURE 78-5   Gaucher cells from an infant with Gaucher's disease. They contain numerous fibrils and appear striated. H&E, ×1090.

lungs were heavy, and the cut surfaces disclosed diffuse interstitial infiltrates. Gaucher cells were found in the alveolar septa. They were located perivascularly and obliterated air exchange as they filled up the alveoli.[37] Glomoid lesions in pulmonary arterioles with dilatation of postglomoid vessels form angiomatoids typical of grade A3 hypertensive pulmonary vascular disease (Fig. 78-6), and numerous marrow emboli of various ages containing Gaucher cells have also been reported.

Malignant tumors are associated with Gaucher's disease, having been found in one series in 35 out of 275 patients.[23] The associated malignancies are myeloma, Hodgkin's disease, acute myelogenous leukemia, lymphatic leukemia, carcinoma of the lung, breast, kidney, liver, colon, pancreas, skin, mouth, larynx, prostate, and brain.

ULTRASTRUCTURE

The Gaucher cells contain cytoplasmic inclusion bodies which are pleomorphic structures surrounded by a single limiting membrane. These inclusions, called "Gaucher bodies," contain tubular structures measuring 120 to 250 Å in diameter (Fig. 78-7), each of which consists of 10 to 12 fibrils in a characteristic arrangement. The inclusion bodies are derived from the cisternae of the endoplasmic reticulum. Acid phosphatase preparations disclose reaction granules within the Gaucher bodies which indicate the lysosomal character of the inclusion material.

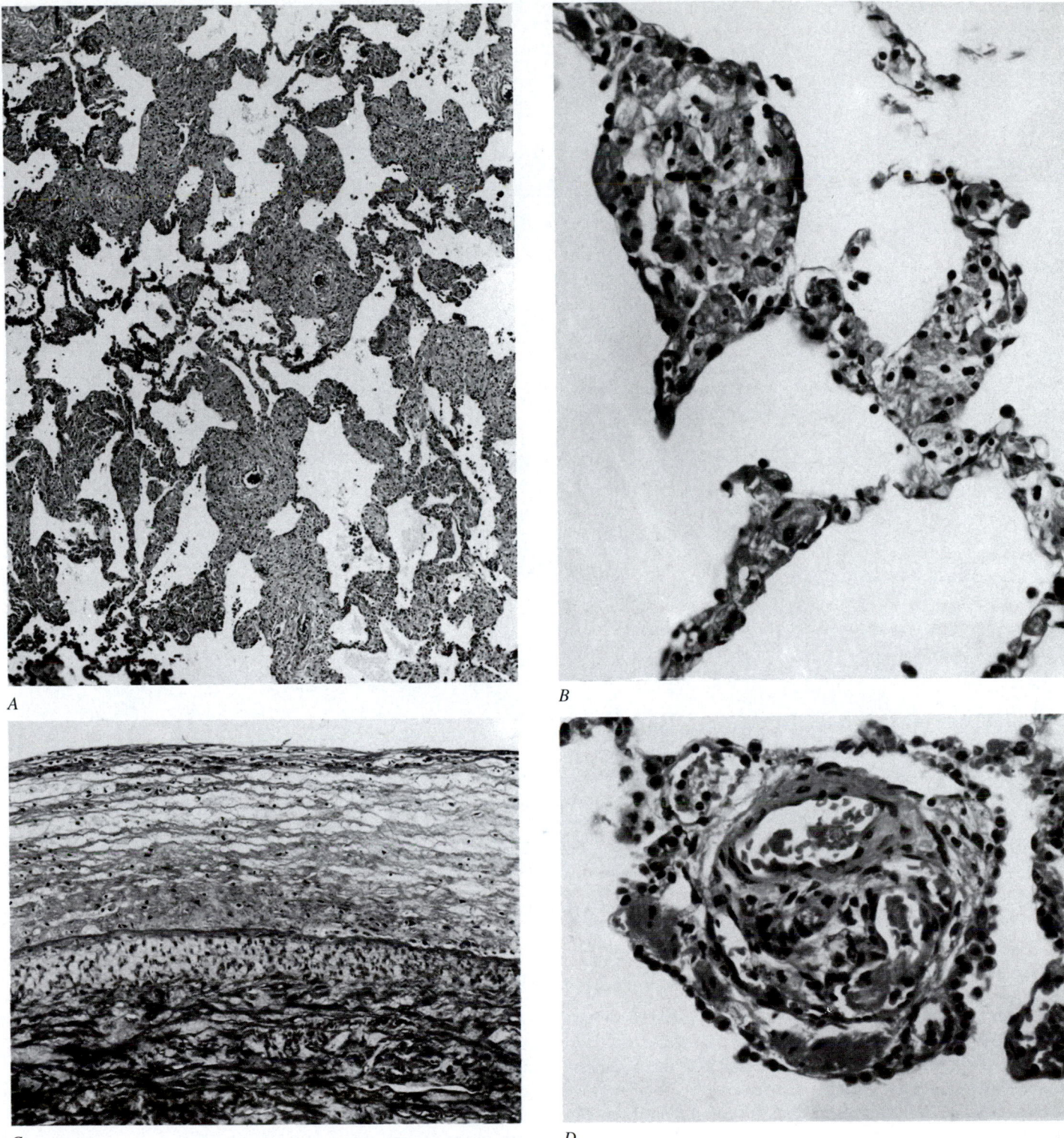

FIGURE 78-6 *A* and *B*. Low- and high-power photomicrographs of pulmonary parenchymal infiltration by Gaucher cells. The vascular bed appears to be absent in much of the tissue and what remains shows distension of capillaries with blood. *C*. Atherosclerotic lesion from the main pulmonary artery. *D*. Glomoid lesion in a pulmonary arteriole with dilatation of postglomoid vessels forming an angiomatoid, typical of grade A3 hypertensive pulmonary vascular disease. *(Courtesy of Dr. GM Hutchins, Am J Med 65:356, 1978.)*

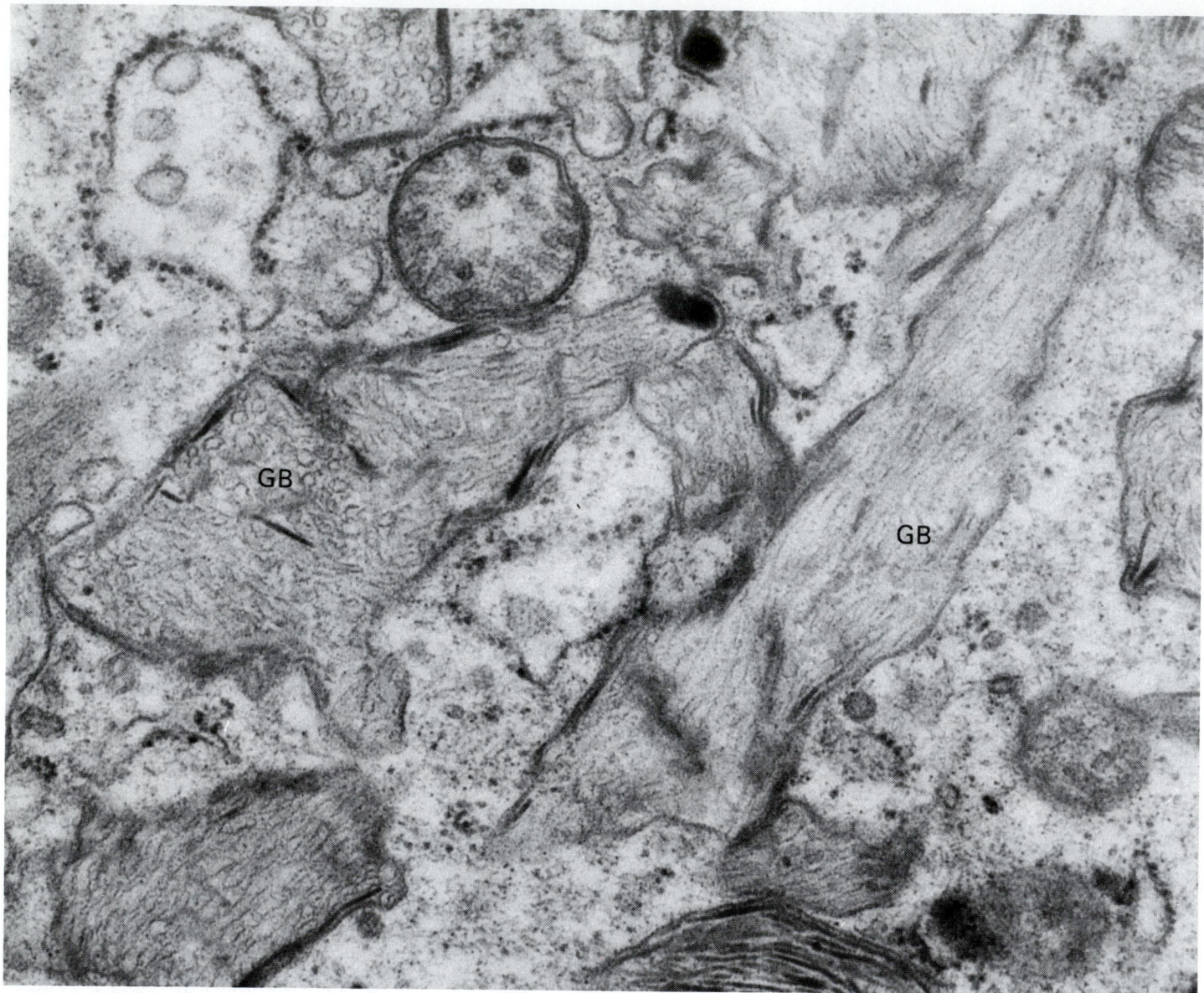

FIGURE 78-7   Electron micrograph of a portion of a Gaucher cell showing pleomorphic Gaucher bodies (GB) which contain tubular structures. ×43,000.

BIOCHEMICAL FEATURES

The organs of patients with the three types of Gaucher's disease almost always have a marked increase in the concentration of glucose-1-ceramide, occasionally exceeding 100 times normal. The enzyme defect in Gaucher's disease is a deficiency of β-glucosidase which catalyzes the cleavage of glucose from glycosyl ceramide.[9]

THERAPY

Bone marrow transplantation has been utilized in severe Gaucher's disease. It was successful in restoring β-glucosidase in mononuclear white blood cells and plasma with complete engraftment of the enzymatically normal donor cells. However, Gaucher cells persisted in the bone marrow. This 8-year-old patient with type 3 Gaucher's disease died of sepsis 13 months after bone marrow transplantation.[34]

DIAGNOSIS

All suspected cases should have a careful radiologic survey of the lungs and bones, identification of Gaucher cells in smears from the bone marrow, and assays of β-glucosidase in leukocytes, or cultured fibroblasts. Should liver biopsy or splenectomy be undertaken, enough fresh frozen tissue (1.0 g) should be preserved for determination of the levels of glycosyl ceramide and β-glucosidase activity. Portions of these tissues should be studied histologically and by electron microscopically. For heterozygote studies, molecular genetic identification is required.

G_{M1} GANGLIOSIDOSIS

Three types of G_{M1} gangliosidosis have been recognized. Type 1 is an infantile form with generalized gangliosidosis, accompanied by bone involvement and psychomotor retardation. Early in the disease, the lungs are unremarkable. Later, bronchopneumonia is common, and the patients usually die of bronchopneumonia before the age of 2 years. Radiologically, abnormalities similar to Hurler's disease are observed after 6 months. Foamy cells are demonstrable in smears of bone marrow. The type 2 disorder is a late infantile, juvenile form with milder bone abnormalities and progressive motor and mental deterioration. The average life span of children with this variant varies from 3 to 10 years. Visceral histiocytosis is less common, but neuronal lipidosis occurs more often than in type 1. The type 3 disorder is an adult, chronic form with juvenile onset of progressive cerebellar dysarthria and slow but progressive motor and intellectual impairment. Long term survival is characteristic of this variant.

GENETICS

The β-galactosidase gene has been mapped to chromosome 3p21-3q21.[27] The cDNA coding for this enzyme has been cloned, and the genomic organization of the gene has been determined. Molecular genetic analysis has demonstrated heterogeneous genetic mutations in infantile G_{M1} gangliosidosis.[47]

PATHOLOGIC AND ULTRASTRUCTURAL FEATURES

Grossly, the liver, spleen, and kidneys of patients with this disease are usually increased in size and weight, but their lungs generally appear normal. The most striking histologic finding is the presence of foamy histiocytes in many visceral organs. In the lungs, these cells are observed in the alveoli and septa. The material in their cytoplasmic vacuoles consists of complex proteolipid compounds.[1] These cells also contain membrane-bound inclusions which consist of moderately electron dense material mixed with fine granules (Fig. 78-8).

BIOCHEMICAL FEATURES

A deficiency of G_{M1}-galactosidase is the underlying basis of this disorder. The deficiency causes ganglioside G_{M1} to accumulate in the different organs.[30] The deficiency of β-galactosidase apparently also interferes with the degradation of mucopolysaccharides.

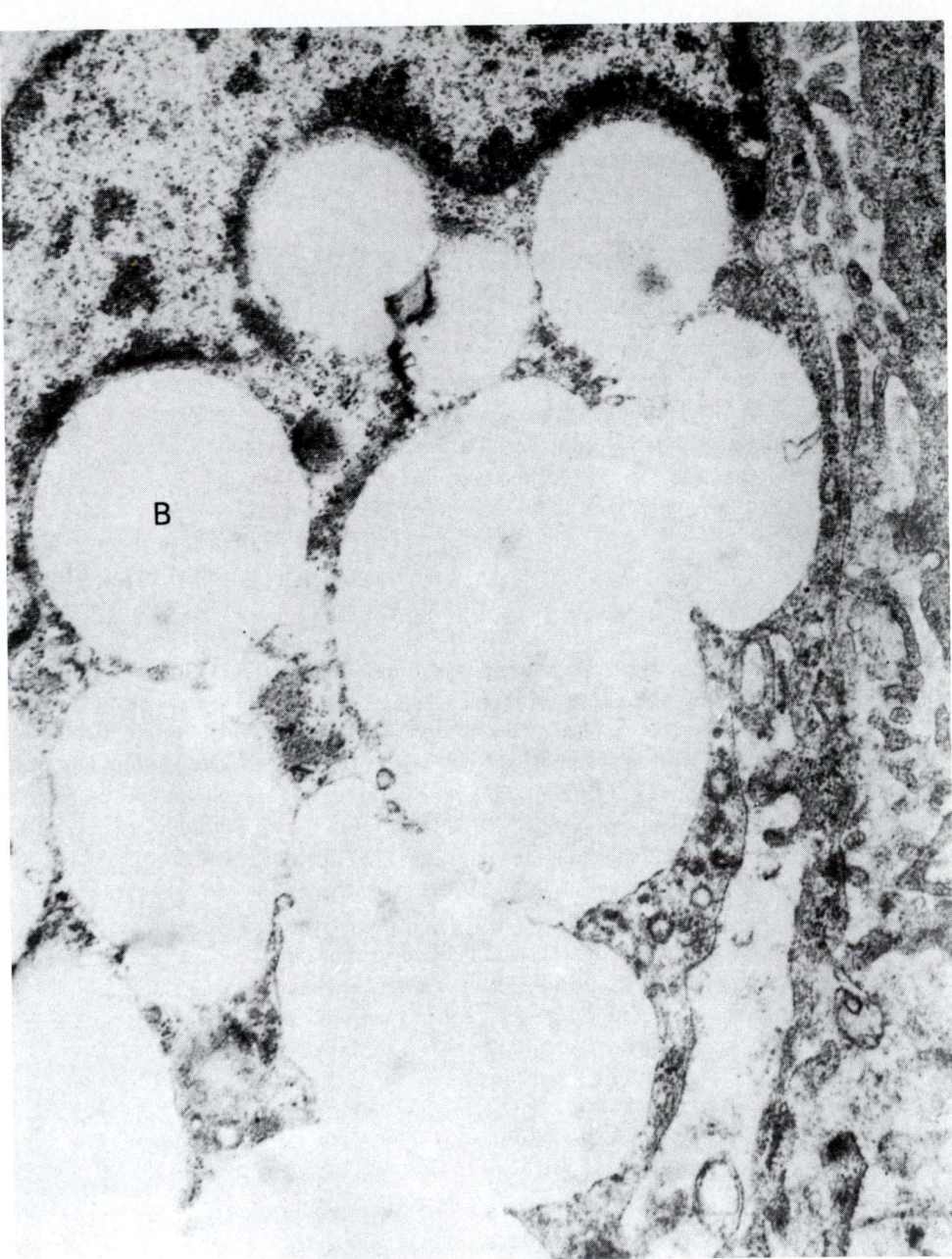

FIGURE 78-8 Electron micrograph of a portion of a foamy cell from a patient with G_{M1} gangliosidosis showing cytoplasmic membrane-bound inclusion bodies (B) which contain electron-lucent material mixed with fine granules. $\times 15,000$.

DIAGNOSIS

The disease can be confirmed by analysis of β-galactosidase activity in leukocytes, urine, and skin. Ultrastructural studies of rectal mucosal biopsies can also be useful.[47] Since enzyme studies are unreliable for heterozygotes, gene analysis is required for carrier detection.

SULFATIDE LIPIDOSIS (METACHROMATIC LEUKODYSTROPHY)

Five categories of sulfatide lipidosis have been identified. It is classified as congenital, late infantile, early juvenile, late juvenile, and adult based on the age of onset of clinical manifestations. In addition, two other types have been identified: multiple sulfate deficiency (MSD) and cerebroside 4-6 sulfatase activator deficiency.[19] The clinical manifestations of these disorders largely reflect the striking changes in the white matter of the brain that occur during the course of the disease. MSD, however, begins with respiratory difficulty in early infancy followed by progressive psychomotor deterioration.[26]

GENETICS

The arylsulfatase A gene is located on chromosome 22 at q13.[15] The mutations underlying the disorder have been identified in 60 to 70 percent of the arylsulfatase A gene.[19] Therefore, carrier studies using genetic analysis are not feasible. The cerebroside sulfatase activator gene is located on chromosome 10 at q21-q22.[17] Its mutations in patients with this disorder are incompletely understood.

PATHOLOGIC AND BIOCHEMICAL FEATURES

Grossly, the visceral organs from patients with sulfatide lipidosis are unremarkable. In contrast, microscopic changes characterized by metachromatic cytoplasmic inclusion bodies are widespread, commonly affecting the lungs. These metachromatic granules are within histiocytes in the interalveolar septa but not in the alveolar spaces or in the vascular walls of the septa. Ultrastructural examination indicates that the cytoplasmic inclusion bodies are composed primarily of lamellar structures and irregular whorls.

Patients afflicted with this disease show a marked increase in the concentration of cerebroside sulftides in their brain and viscera. This abnormality is secondary to the reduced activity of arylsulfatase A and to a lesser degree arylsulfatase B in this disorder.[2,25] Arylsulfatase C is affected only in MSD.

DIAGNOSIS

The most important diagnostic procedure for this disorder is the quantification of arylsulfatase A activity levels in the leukocytes or cultured skin fibroblasts from patients who are suspected to have the disorder. Analysis for sulfatase A in the urine is rapid and simpler but less reliable. Heterozygotes can be identified by leukocyte and fibroblast assays for arylsulfatase A and cerebroside sulfatase.[19]

GALACTOSYLCERAMIDE LIPIDOSIS (GLOBOID-CELL LEUKODYSTROPHY— KRABBE'S DISEASE)

CLINICAL FEATURES

Three clinical forms of galactosylceramide lipidosis (GL) have been described based on the age of the patient at disease onset. In most patients the disease occurs in early infancy, exhibiting its first clinical symptoms at 3 to 6 months of age. The disease is characterized by progressive psychomotor deterioration that generally culminates in death within 2 years. The late infancy form is rare and manifests as mental deterioration, pyramidal signs, and visual impairment in children 2 to 6 years old. The

duration of this variant is aproximately 1 to 5 years. In the adult form, the main clinical manifestation is visual impairment that starts between the ages of 10 and 35 years. Patients with this disease variant also exhibit slowly progressive motor deterioration and usually survive 2 to 10 years from presentation.

GENETICS

GL is transmitted as an autosomal recessive trait. The galactosylceramidase gene has been mapped to chromosome 14.[50] The cDNA or the gene coding for the enzyme has not been cloned and the mutations underlying the disorder have not been characterized.

PATHOLOGIC AND BIOCHEMICAL FEATURES

In this disorder gross pathologic changes are generally confined to the brain. The white matter of all lobes of the brain are extensively affected whereas the cortices and deep gray matter are relatively preserved. Although the visceral organs appear normal, giant cells, similar to the globoid cells in the nervous system, also occur in the lungs, lymph nodes, spleen, and bone marrow. The globoid cells, which are derived from histiocytes, are characterized by large round cell bodies, several peripherally placed nuclei which are 20 to 50 μm in diameter, and fine cytoplasmic granules (Fig. 78-9). Similar lesions have been found in a vari-

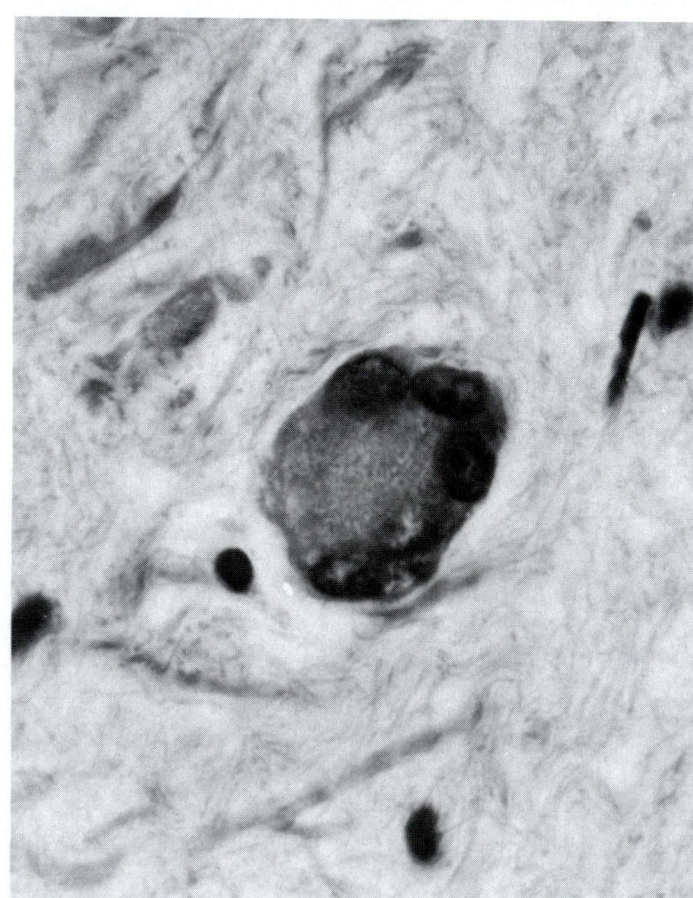

FIGURE 78-9   The globoid cell from a child with Krabbe's disease is characterized by large, round cell bodies containing several peripherally placed nuclei and many cytoplasmic fine granules. H&E, ×1100.

ety of animal models of this disease in sheep, dogs, and the twitcher mouse.[44]

The primary defect in this disorder involves the enzyme galactocerebroside β-galactosidase.[45] This leads to a marked increase in the galactosylceramide concentrations in the white matter of the brain and subsequent cerebral dysfunction.

DIAGNOSIS

In infants suspected of having GL serum, leukocytes or cultured fibroblasts should be studied to quantitate the activity of galactocerebroside β-galactosidase.

GLYCOSPHINGOLIPID LIPIDOSIS (FABRY'S DISEASE)

Glycosphingolipid lipidosis (GSL) is the only sphingolipidosis that is transmitted by the gene on the X chromosome that controls the hydrolytic enzyme, α-galactosidase A. The clinical picture results from the progressive accumulation of globotriaosyl (ceramide) in most visceral organs as well as the brain.

CLINICAL FEATURES

The clinical manifestations of this disease most often occur in men but can be seen in isolated cases of heterozygote women.[35] GSL presents in childhood or adolescence with two types of symptoms: severe pain and telangiectasis. The pain is often in the form of a lightning or burning sensation in the fingers or toes that extends to the palms and soles, respectively. Attacks of abdominal or flank pain simulate those of appendicitis or renal colic. The telangiectasis are symmetrical, involve the superficial layers of the skin, do not bleach on pressure, and are progressive. The oral mucosa, conjunctivae, hips, back, thighs, buttocks, penis, and scrotum are most commonly involved. The area between the umbilicus and the knees is involved less often but can be severely affected. Some patients with this disease develop pulmonary alterations. These alterations range from obstructive disease of the airways to diffuse interstitial abnormalities.[48] Pulmonary function tests in older patients may reveal significant airflow obstruction, a reduced diffusing capacity, and a reduction in the V_{max25} values.[36] Pulmonary complications are a frequent cause of death in this disorder.

GENETICS

The gene that is responsible for this disease has been localized to chromosome Xq22.[7] The α-galactosidase A cDNA and genomic sequences have been isolated, characterized, and used to analyze the mutations causing this disease. Partial gene rearrangements, splice-junction defects, and point mutations have been identified.[12]

PATHOLOGIC FEATURES

When compared to appropriate controls, the lungs from patients with GSL are increased in weight and have cut surfaces that are often congested and edematous. Multiple vacuoles are also ap-

preciated in the alveolar epithelium, airway, and vascular smooth-muscle cells and capillary endothelial cells. Ultrastructural examination shows that both the capillary endothelium and the alveolar type II cells contain laminated inclusions with a periodicity of 50 to 60 Å. This pattern contrasts with the variable periodicity of the lamellar bodies that the type II cells contain in the normal lung. The cytoplasmic inclusion bodies in the ciliated epithelial cells and goblet cells stain darkly with toluidine blue. Ultrastructurally, these inclusion bodies are limited by a single membrane and contain electron dense lamellae arranged in either a parallel or concentric fashion. Alveolar macrophages are devoid of these inclusions.[36]

BIOCHEMICAL FEATURES AND DIAGNOSIS

The primary enzyme defect in this disorder is the absence of α-galactosidase A activity.[8] Affected males can be identified by demonstrating an increase in globotriaosylceramid and by assaying hydrolase activity in serum, leukocytes, tears, and cultured skin fibroblasts.

MUCOPOLYSACCHARIDOSIS

The term *mucopolysaccharidosis* (MPS) refers to a group of genetic diseases manifested by abnormal tissue deposition of acid mucopolysaccharide (glycosaminoglycans). Seven major forms of the disease have been recognized: Hurler syndrome (MPS I), Scheie syndrome (MPS I S, formerly V), Hunter syndrome (MPS II), Sanfillipo syndrome (MPS III), Morquio syndrome (MPS IV), Maroteaux-Lamy syndrome (MPS VI), and Sly syndrome (MPS VII). The most severely affected patients (except for those with type I S) commonly have respiratory involvement, particularly obstructive disease of the airways.

GENETICS

The MPS are transmitted in an autosomal recessive pattern, except for MPS II, which is X-linked. The MPS I gene has been assigned to chromosome 22 at 4p16.3, the MPS II locus to Xq27-28, the gene of the very rare MPS III D (Sanfillipo D) to 12q14, the MPS IV A (Morquio A) gene to 16q24, the MPS VI gene to 5q13-q14, and the MPS VII gene to 7q21-q22.[28]

PATHOLOGIC FEATURES

The visceral organs from patients with MPS can be grossly abnormal. The exact pattern of involvement varies, however, with the type of disease that is manifested. Interestingly, in these patients, the lungs are rarely visibly abnormal. In type I, MPS histologic alterations are seen in almost all organs, including the lungs. The characteristic feature is the presence of an abnormal deposited material in cells that are variously called clear cells, gargoyle cells, Hurler's cells, or balloon cells. They are large, oval or polygonal, measure 20 μm in diameter, and contain pale central nuclei. Frozen sections exhibit metachromatic material that stains with toluidine blue and gives a positive reaction in alcian blue preparations. They also characteristically contain round or oval inclusion bodies that are membrane-bound and display an electron-lucent or low electron-dense material, occasionally mixed with fine granules or lamellae. The histologic changes in types II and III MPS are similar to those of type I. The histologic findings in the other types are less well documented.

BIOCHEMICAL FEATURES

Patients with types I and I S MPS have a deficiency of α-L-iduronidase[4] and increased urinary excretion of dermatan sulfate and heparin sulfate. The deficiency in type II MPS involves iduronate sulfatase.[3] Dermatan sulfate and heparin sulfate are also excreted in abnormally large quantities in the urine of patients with this disorder. Although about 80 percent of the extracted mucopolysaccharide is dermatan sulfate in type I, in type II that portion is about 55 percent. In type III MPS, lesions have been found in the four enzymatic steps involved in the excretion and accumulation of heparin sulfate. The abnormalities are in heparin N-sulfatase in type III A,[20] N-acetyl-α-D glucosaminidase in type III B,[29] acetyl CoA: α-glucosaminide-N-acetyltransferase in type III C,[22] and N-acetyl-α-D-glucosaminide-6-sulfatase in type III D.[21] The enzymatic defects in type IV MPS involve galactosamine-6-sulfate sulfatase in type IV A and β-galactosidase in type IV B. As a result these patients have increased levels of urinary keratan sulfate. Type VI MPS is the result of a deficiency of arylsulfatase B activity,[24] which results in increased urinary excretion of dermatan sulfate, whereas in type VII MPS is the result of the defective degradation of dermatan sulfate and heparin sulfate due to a deficiency of β-glucuronidase.

DIAGNOSIS

The excretion of urinary mucopolysaccharides is markedly increased in many of these disorders. Although metachromatic material can be demonstrated in polymorphonuclear leukocytes and lymphocytes, the diagnosis can only be established by measuring urine mucopolysaccharides with precise identification of the substance excreted. The characteristic enzyme defect of each disorder should also be studied in leukocytes, serum, or fibroblasts from the patient being evaluated.

GLYCOGEN STORAGE DISEASE

Among the major groups of glycogen storage disorders (GSD), Pompe's disease (GSD, type II) frequently shows cardiorespiratory disturbances. Hypotonia, which often develops by 2 months of age, is the cardinal feature of this disorder. The heart is markedly enlarged, and heart failure is common. Most patients die within the first year of life. However, a few survive up to 15 years.

GENETICS

The disease is transmitted as an autosomal recessive trait. It is felt to result from the dysfunction of the structural gene for acid α-glucosidase which is located at chromosome 17 q23.[42]

PATHOLOGIC AND BIOCHEMICAL FEATURES

The lungs and brains of patients with GSD are grossly normal. In contrast, the heart is usually markedly enlarged and increased

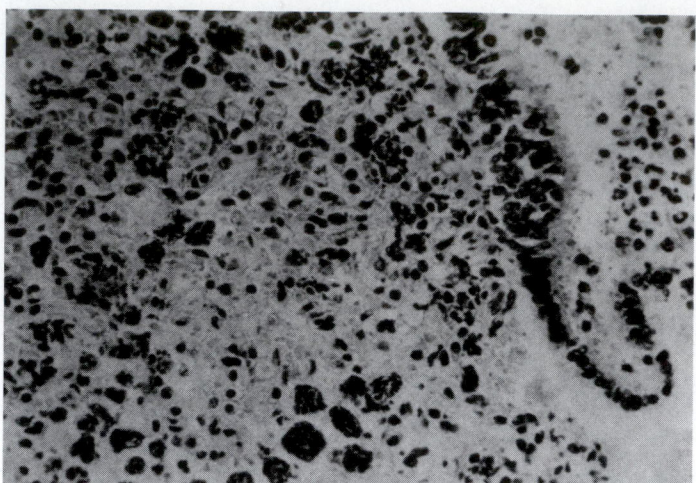

FIGURE 78-10   Intraalveolar and interstitial macrophage laden with glycogen granules (black granules). Best's glycogen stain. (*Courtesy of Dr. H. Spencer.*[43])

in weight. About one-fifth of the patients show thickening of the endocardium similar to that seen in endocardial fibroelastosis. Hepatomegaly is also frequently appreciated. Histologically, GSD is characterized by the massive accumulation of glycogen granules in the cytoplasm of the parenchymal cells of most organs, including the lungs. Foamy alveolar macrophages are also noted which are filled with glycogenlike material (Fig. 78-10). Glycogen is also present in smaller amounts in cartilage cells and mucosal and bronchial epithelial cells.[43] Ultrastructurally, the cytoplasmic inclusion bodies are membrane-bound and contain electron-dense glycogen granules. The massive accumulation of tissue glycogen in this disorder is due to a deficiency in acid maltase (acid α-glucosidase) activity.[18]

DIAGNOSIS

The diagnosis of GSD can be established by demonstrating the increased tissue glycogen concentrations and deficiency of α-glucosidase activity. Studies of urine, muscle tissue, and cultured fibroblasts are helpful in this regard.

DISORDERS OF AMINO ACID METABOLISM

Among the various types of amino acid metabolic disorders, only maple syrup urine disease (MSUD) (leucinosis, branched-chain ketonuria) is occasionally associated with bouts of respiratory embarrassment for which there is no infectious explanation. In affected infants, respiratory distress develops within the first week of life. The infants often become apneic and require respiratory assistance. Severe psychomotor deterioration and episodes of seizures occur during the course of the disease, and the children usually die from intercurrent infections within the first year. However, with the help of a synthetic diet, some patients have survived for as long as 13 years.

Despite severe clinical symptoms in early life, at autopsy only the brain shows specific changes. Grossly, it exhibits microcephaly and microgyria. Histologically it shows a deficiency in myelin sheaths, presumably a result of reduced synthesis of proteolipids.

GENETICS AND BIOCHEMICAL FEATURES

MSUD is an autosomal recessive disorder that is felt to result from abnormalities in the genes of the branched chain α-ketoacid dehydrogenase complex (E1-E3). These genes are on different chromosomes: E1α to chromosome 19q13.1-q13.2, E1β to 6p21-p22, E2 to 1p31, and E3 to 7q31-q32.[11] The mutations in these enzymes cause a deficiency of branched-chain-α-ketoacid dehydrogenase resulting in increased levels of urinary amino acids (leucine, isoleucine, and valine) and plasma branched-chain ketoacids.[11]

DIAGNOSIS

Patients with this disease classically have a maple-syrup-like odor of their urine which can be detected within the first weeks of life. Although the odor is clinically the most distinctive sign of this disease, the diagnosis should be verified by studies of the amino acids and ketoacids in blood and urine. The diagnosis is confirmed by enzymatic studies of leukocytes or cultured skin fibroblasts and lymphoblasts.

CYSTINE STORAGE DISEASE (LIGNAC-FANCONI DISEASE)

This disorder causes widespread pathologic changes in many organs. It is inherited as a simple Mendelian recessive and manifests in children as severe rickets or dwarfism with marked photophobia, amino aciduria, and death from infection or renal dysfunction.

The disease affects the bones, kidneys, lymph nodes, spleen, liver, and lungs. The deposits provoke no cellular reaction and do not alter pulmonary function. The deposits may be mistaken for calcium with Von Kossa's stain if they contain traces of cystine. The cystine is water soluble, and thus sections are best fixed in absolute alcohol. In tissue sections, the crystals are birefringent and form clumps of radiating needlelike crystals when treated with concentrated sulphuric acid and phosphotungstic acid. The crystals in the lungs are mainly distributed within the peribronchial and periarterial reticuloendothelial cells in the alveolar septa (Fig. 78-11).[43]

CONCLUSIONS

Enzyme replacement therapy for these storage diseases is not totally successful at present. However, the birth of children afflicted with inborn errors of metabolism can be prevented by prenatal diagnosis through amniocenteses and analysis of enzyme activity of cultured amniotic cells. Advice for genetic counseling, therefore, seems to be one of the important functions of the physician in those instances where parents are homozygotes or carriers and may produce a baby afflicted with one of these disorders.

REFERENCES

1. Adachi M, Volk BW: Methodology: Histochemistry, in Volk BW, Schneck L (eds), *The Gangliosidoses.* New York, Plenum, 1975, pp 249–264.

2. Austin J, Armstrong D, Shearer L: Metachromatic form of diffuse sclerosis: V. The nature and significance of low sulfatase activity: a controlled study of brain, liver and kidney in four patients with metachromatic leukodystrophy. *Arch Neurol* 13:593–614, 1965.

3. Bach G, Eisenberg F Jr, Cantz M, Neufeld EF: The defect in Hunter syndrome: deficiency of sulfoiduronate sulfatase. *Proc Nat Acad Sci USA* 70:2134–2138, 1973.

4. Bach G, Friedman R, Weissmann B, Neufeld EF: The defect in the Hunter and Scheie syndromes: deficiency of α-L-iduronidase. *Proc Nat Sci USA* 69:2048–2051, 1972.

5. Bassan R, Montanelli A, Barbui T: Interaction between a serum factor and T lymphocytes in Gaucher disease. *Am J Haemat* 18:381–384, 1985.

6. Beutler E, Grabowski GA: Gaucher disease, in Scriver CR, Beaudet AL, Sly WS, Valle D (eds), *The Metabolic and Molecular Bases of Inherited Diseases,* 7th ed, vol 2. New York, McGraw-Hill, 1995, pp 2641–2670.

7. Bishop DF, Calhoun DH, Bernstein HS, et al: Molecular cloning and nucleotide sequencing of a cDNA encording human α-galactosidase A. *Am J Hum Genet* 37:A144, 1985.

8. Brady RO, Gal AE, Bradley RM, et al: Enzyme effect in Fabry's disease: ceramide trihexosidase deficiency. *New Engl J Med* 276:1163–1167, 1967.

9. Brady RO, Kanfer JN, Shapiro D: Metabolism of glucocerebroside: II. Evidence of an enzyme deficiency in Gaucher's disease. *Biochem Biophys Res Commun* 18:211–225, 1965.

10. Carstea ED, Polymeropoulos MH, Parker CC, et al: Linkage of Niemann-Pick disease type C to human chromosome 18. *Proc Natl Acad Sci USA* 90:2002–2004, 1993.

11. Chaung DT, Shih VE: Disorders of branched chain amino acid and keto acid metabolism, in Scriver CR, Beaudet AL, Sly WS, Valle D (eds), *The Metabolic and Molecular Bases of Inherited Diseases,* 7th ed, vol 1. New York, McGraw-Hill, 1995, pp 1239–1277.

12. Da Veiga Pereira L, Desnick RJ, Adler D, et al: Regional assignment of the human acid sphingomyelinase gene (SMPDI) by PCR analysis of somatic cell hybrids and in situ hybridization to 11p15.1–p15.4. *Genomics* 9:229–234, 1991.

13. Desnick RJ, Ioannou YA, Eng CM: α-galactosidase A deficiency: Fabry disease, in Scriver CR, Beaudet CR, Sly WS, Valle D (eds), *The Metabolic and Molecular Bases of Inherited Diseases,* 7th ed, vol 2. New York, McGraw-Hill, 1995, pp 2741–2784.

14. Gal AE, Brady RO, Barranger JA, Pentchev PG: The diagnosis of type A and B Niemann-Pick disease and detection of carriers using leukocytes and a chromogenic analogue of sphingomyelin. *Clin Chim Acta* 104:129–132, 1980.

15. Gustavson K-H, Arancibia W, Eriksson U, Svennerholm L: Deleted ring chromosomes 22 in a mentally retarded boy. *Clin Genet* 29:337–341, 1986.

16. Hirschhorn R: Glycogen storage type II: acid α-glucosidase (acid maltase) deficiency, in Scriver CR, Beaudet AL, Sly WS, Valle D (eds), *The Metabolic and Molecular Bases of Inherited Diseases,* 7th ed, vol 2. New York, McGraw-Hill, 1995, pp 2443–2464.

17. Holtshmidt H, Sandhoff K, Fürst W, et al: The organization of the gene for the human cerebroside sulfate activator protein. *FEBS Lett* 280:267, 1991.

18. Huijing F, van Creveld S, Losekoot G: Diagnosis of generalized glycogen storage disease (Pompe's disease). *J Pediatr* 63:984–987, 1963.

19. Kolodny EH, Fluharty AL: Metachromatic leukodystrophy and multiple sulfatase deficiency: sulfatide lipidosis. In Scriver CR, Beaudet AL, Sly WS, Valle D (eds), *The Metabolic and Molecular Bases of Inherited Diseases,* 7th ed, vol 2. New York, McGraw-Hill, 1995, pp 2693–2739.

20. Kreese H, Neufeld EF: The Sanfillippo A corrective factor: purification and mode of action. *J Biol Chem* 247:2164–2170, 1972.

21. Kreese H, Paschke E, Von Figura K, et al: Sanfillipo disease type D: deficiency of N-acetylglucosamine-6-sulfatase required for heparan sulfate degradation. *Proc Nat Acad Sci USA* 77:6822–6826, 1980.

22. Kreese H, Von Figura K, Klein U: New biochemical subtype of the Sanfillipo syndrome: characterization of the storage material in cultured fibroblasts of Sanfillipo C patients. *Eur J Biochem* 92:333–339, 1978.

23. Lee RE: The pathology of Gaucher disease. *Prog Clin Biol Res* 95:177–217, 1982.

24. Matalon R, Arbogast B, Justice P, et al: Morqiuio's syndrome: deficiency of a chondroitin sulfate N-acetylhexosamine sulfate sulfatase. *Biochem Biophys Res Comm* 61:759–765, 1974.

25. Mehl E, Jatzkewitz H: Evidence for the genetic block in metachromatic leukodystrophy. *Biochem Biophys Res Commun* 19:407–411, 1965.

26. Murphy JV, Wolfe HJ, Balazs ER, Moser HW: A patient with deficiency of arysulfatases A,B,C, and steroid sulfatase associated with storage of sulfatide, cholesterol sulfate and glycosaminoglycans, in Bernsohn J, Grossman HJ (eds), *Lipid Storage Disease.* New York, Academic Press, 1971, pp 67–110.

27. Naylor SL, Elliott RW, Brown JA, Shows TB: Mapping of aminoacylase-1 and β-galactosidase-A to homologous regions of human chromosome 3 and mouse chromosome 9 suggests location of additional genes. *Am J Hum Genet* 34:235–244, 1982.

28. Neufeld EF, Muenzer J: The mucopolysaccharidoses, in Scriber CR, Beaudet AL, Sly WS, Valle D (eds), *The Metabolic and Molecular Bases of Inherited Diseases,* 7th ed, vol 2. New York, McGraw-Hill, 1995, pp 2465–2494.

29. O'Brien JS: Sanfilippo syndrome: profound deficiency of α-acetylglucosaminidase activity in organs and skin fibroblasts from type B patients. *Proc Nat Acad Sci USA* 69:1720–1723, 1970.

30. Okada S, O'Brien JS: Generalized gangliosidosis: beta-galactosidase deficiency. *Science* 160:1002–1004, 1968.

31. Patrick AD: A deficiency of glycocerebrosidase in Gaucher's disease. *Biochem J* 97:17c, 1965.

32. Pentchev PG, Comly ME, Kruth HS, et al: The cholesterol storage disorder of the mutant BALB/c mouse. A primary genetic lesion closely linked to defective esterification of exogenously derived cholesterol and its relationship to human type C Niemann-Pick disease. *J Biol Chem* 261:2772–2777, 1986.

33. Quintern L, Schuchman EH, Levran O, et al: Isolation of cDNA clones encoding human acid sphingomyelinase. Occurrence of alternatively spliced transcripts. *EMBO J* 8:2469–2473, 1989.

34. Rappeport JM, Ginns EI: Bone marrow transplantation in severe Gaucher's disease. *New Engl J Med* 311:84–88, 1984.

35. Rodriguez FH, Hoffman EO, Ordinario AT, Baliga M: Fabry's disease in a heterozygous woman. *Arch Path Lab Med* 109:89–91, 1985.

36. Rosenberg DM, Ferrans VJ, Fulmer JD, et al: Chronic airflow obsruction in Fabry's disease. *Am J Med* 68:898–904, 1980.

37. Schneider EL, Epstein CJ, Kaback MJ, Brandes D: Severe pulmonary involvement in Gaucher's disease. *Am J Med* 63:475–480, 1977.

38. Scuchman EH, Desnick RJ: Niemann-Pick disease types A and B: acid sphingomyelinase deficiencies, in Scriver CR, Beaudet AL, Sly WS, Valle D (eds), *The Metabolic and Molecular Bases of Inherited Diseases,* 7th ed, vol 2. New York, McGraw-Hill, 1995, pp 2601–2624

39. Schuchman EH, Suchi M, Takahashi T, et al: Human acid sphingomyelinase. Isolation, nucleotide sequence and expression of the full-length and alternatively spliced RNAs. *J Biol Chem* 266:8531–8539, 1991.

40. Shafit-Zagardo B, Devine EA, Smith M, et al: Assignment of the gene for acid beta-glucosidase to human chromosome 1. *Am J Hum Genet* 33:564–575, 1981.

41. Smith RRL, Hutchins GM, Sack GH, Ridolfi RL: Unusual cardiac, renal and pulmonary involvement in Gaucher's disease: interstitial glucocerebroside accumulation, pulmonary hypertension and fatal bone marrow embolization. *Am J Med* 65:352–360, 1978.

42. Solomon E, Swallow D, Burgess S, Evans L: Assignment of the human acid alpha-glucosidase gene to chromosome 17 using somatic cell hybrids. *Ann Hum Genet* 42:273–281, 1979.

43. Spencer H: *Pathology of the Lung.* Oxford, Pergamon Press, 1985, pp 753–754.

44. Suzuki K, Suzuku K: The twitcher mouse (a model of human globoid cell leukodystrophy (Krabbe's disease). *Am J Path* 111:394–397, 1983.

45. Suzuki K, Suzuki Y: Globoid cells leukodystrophy (Krabbe's disease) deficiency of galactocerebroside β-galactosidase. *Proc Natl Acad Sci USA* 66:302–309, 1970.

46. Suzuki K, Suzuki Y, Suzuki K: Galactosylceramide lipidosis: globoid-cell leukodystrophy (Krabbe disease), in Scriver CR, Beaudet AL, Sly WS, Valle D (eds), *The Metabolic and Molecular Bases of Inherited Diseases,* 7th ed, vol 2. New York, McGraw-Hill, 1995, pp 2671–2692.

47. Suzuki Y, Sakuraba H, Oshima A: β-galactosidase deficiency (β-galactosidosis): G_{M1} gangliosidosis and Morquio B disease, in Scriber CR, Beaudet AL, Sly WS, Valle D (eds), *The Metabolic and Molecular Bases of Inherited Diseases,* 7th ed, vol 2. New York, McGraw-Hill, 1995, pp 2785–2823.

48. Wise D, Wallace HJ, Jellinek EH: Angiokeratoma corporis diffusum: a clinical study of eight affected families. *Q J Med* 31:177–206, 1962.

49. Yamano T, Shimada M, Okada S, et al: Ultrastructural study of biopsy specimens of rectal mucosa. *Arch Path Lab Med* 106:673–677, 1982.

50. Zlotogora J, Charkraborty S, Knowleton RG, Wenger DA: Krabbe disease locus mapped to chromosome 14 by genetic linkage. *Am J Hum Genet* 47:37–44, 1990.

PART EIGHT

ALVEOLAR DISEASES

CHAPTER 79

ALVEOLAR HEMORRHAGE SYNDROMES

Joseph P. Lynch III / James W. Leatherman

Alveolar hemorrhage is a potentially catastrophic complication of myriad immune and nonimmune disorders. Clinical features are broad, but hemoptysis, infiltrates on chest radiographs, hypoxemia, and progressive respiratory insufficiency are common to diverse etiologies. Nonimmune causes of alveolar hemorrhage include endobronchial tumors, arteriovenous malformations or aneurysms, ulcerative tracheobronchitis, hemorrhagic pneumonia, bronchiectasis, congestive heart failure, uremia, thrombocytopenia or coagulopathy, pulmonary veno-occlusive disease, and massive pulmonary embolism. These nonimmune causes need to be excluded in patients with severe alveolar hemorrhage. Depending upon the clinical scenario, coagulation profiles and ancillary tests (e.g., echocardiogram, pulmonary arteriography, fiberoptic bronchoscopy) may be required to establish a specific diagnosis. In addition, other causes of diffuse parenchymal infiltrates (but without severe alveolar hemorrhage) share features in common with alveolar hemorrhage syndromes (e.g., bronchiolitis obliterans organizing pneumonia, hypersensitivity pneumonitis, pulmonary alveolar proteinosis, and diverse interstitial or alveolar lung disorders). A discussion of these disorders is beyond the scope of this chapter, which focuses primarily on immune-mediated causes of alveolar hemorrhage.

AUTOIMMUNE CAUSES OF ALVEOLAR HEMORRHAGE: DIFFERENTIAL DIAGNOSIS

Autoimmune alveolar hemorrhage results from diffuse injury to the pulmonary microvasculature (termed *capillaritis* or *endotheliitis*)[16,20,30,31,40,44,52] (Table 79-1). Systemic necrotizing vasculitides (principally microscopic polyangiitis and Wegener's granulomatosis) account for the majority of cases of autoimmune alveolar hemorrhage.[16,20,30,31,40] Other causes of autoimmune alveolar hemorrhage include antiglomerular basement membrane antibody disease, collagen vascular disorders (principally systemic lupus erythematosus), exogenous agents (e.g., trimellitic anhydride, isocyanates), or drugs (e.g., D-penicillamine). In many of these disorders, rapidly progressive glomerulonephritis (RPGN) is present concomitantly.[11,30,31] In most patients with autoimmune alveolar hemorrhage and glomerulonephritis, anti-GBM antibody and immune complexes are lacking.[11,30] The term *pauci-immune glomerulonephritis* has been used to refer to this group of patients, who encompass a heterogenous group of disorders (discussed in detail below).[11,30] Idiopathic pulmonary hemosiderosis, a rare cause of recurrent alveolar hemorrhage with no renal or extrapulmonary component, occurs primarily in children and remains a diagnosis of exclusion.[5,49]

Differentiation of these diverse syndromes can usually be accomplished by serological studies and by kidney biopsy.[30] In such cases, lung biopsy is not required.[30] Glomerulonephritis can be demonstrated in the great majority of patients with alveolar hemorrhage complicating Wegener's granulomatosis or microscopic polyangiitis. By contrast, the kidneys may be spared in alveolar hemorrhage associated with collagen vascular disease, bone marrow transplant recipients, or immunocompromised patients.[1,7,35–38] Urinalysis (to look for microscopic hematuria, red cell casts, and proteinuria) and measurement of renal function should always be done in the diagnostic evaluation of alveolar hemorrhage. Findings consistent with glomerulonephritis warrant a prompt and aggressive evaluation, to include percutaneous needle biopsy of the kidney.

CLINICAL FEATURES OF AUTOIMMUNE ALVEOLAR HEMORRHAGE

Irrespective of etiology, the clinical, radiographic, and histopathologic features of alveolar hemorrhage may be similar.

Classical findings are hemoptysis, diffuse alveolar infiltrates, hypoxemia, renal failure, and iron-deficiency anemia.[30,31,40] However, the clinical spectrum is wide, and many of these features may be subtle or absent. In this context, the diagnosis of alveolar hemorrhage may be difficult, as signs and symptoms overlap with diverse etiologies of diffuse alveolar infiltrates. Prompt diagnosis and institution of therapy is vital to avert early mortality from alveolar hemorrhage and late sequelae from end-stage renal failure. Chest radiographs typically reveal bilateral alveolar infiltrates, often with a bat-wing appearance.[40] However, focal, and even unilateral, patterns indistinguishable from pneumonia may occur. Following cessation of bleeding, infiltrates markedly improve or normalize within 24 to 72 h (Fig. 79-1).[30,40] A presumptive diagnosis of alveolar hemorrhage can often be made by a combination of clinical and serological findings and bronchoalveolar lavage (BAL) fluid.[7,25,26,30] Grossly bloody BAL fluid, large numbers of hemosiderin-laden macrophages, and the absence of purulent secretions or ancillary evidence for infection strongly support alveolar hemorrhage as a cause of pul-

monary infiltrates. Ancillary studies including serologies, renal function tests, and urinalysis may support the diagnosis.[26,30,45]

TABLE 79-1

Etiology of Autoimmune Diffuse Alveolar Hemorrhage

Anti-basement membrane antibody disease (Goodpasture's syndrome)

Anti-neutrophil cytoplasmic antibody (ANCA) mediated vasculitis (e.g., Wegener's granulomatosis, microscopic polyangiitis, Churg-Strauss syndrome, pauci-immune glomerulonephritis)

Idiopathic rapidly progressive glomerulonephritis

Collagen vascular disease (e.g., systemic lupus erythematosus)

Immunocompromised status (e.g., bone marrow transplant, AIDS)

Exogenous agents or drugs (e.g., trimellitic anhydride, isocyanates, D-penicillamine, cocaine)

Idiopathic pulmonary hemosiderosis (pathogenesis unknown)

DIAGNOSIS

The Role of Lung Biopsy

The role of lung biopsy in the diagnosis of alveolar hemorrhage and the determination of its etiology is controversial. We believe

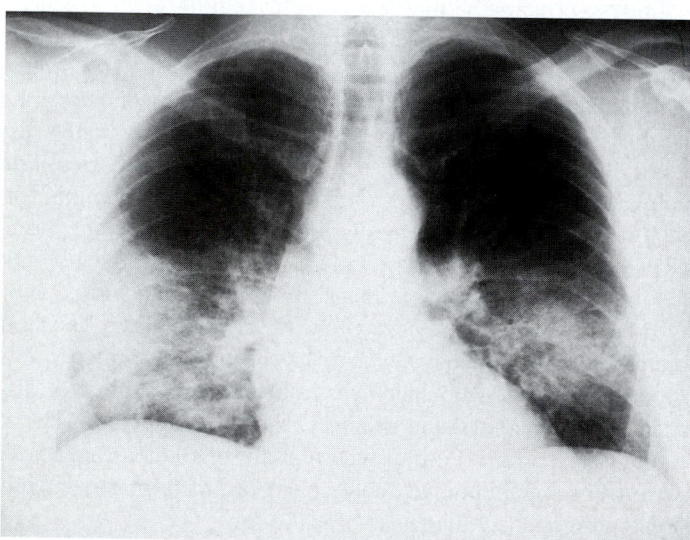

A

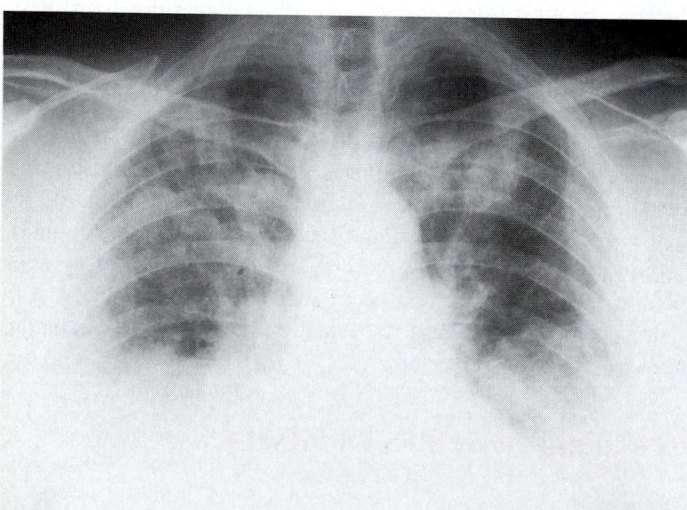

B

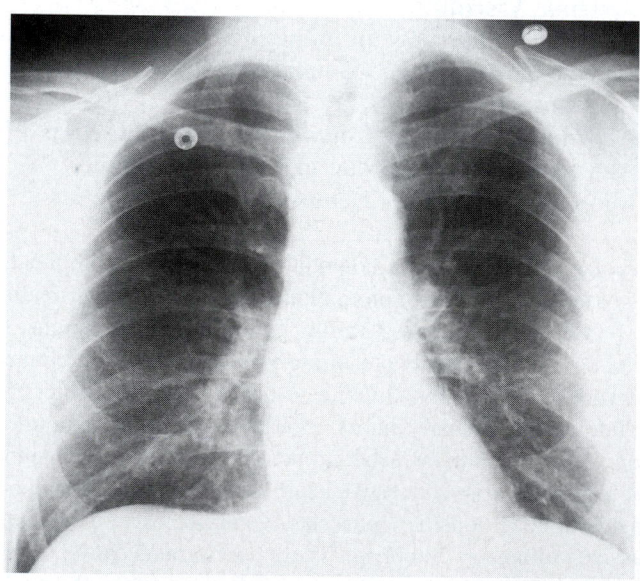

C

FIGURE 79-1 *A.* Idiopathic rapidly progressive glomerulonephritis. PA chest radiograph from a 52-year-old male with rapidly progressive glomerulonephritis, hemoptysis, and bilateral alveolar infiltrates, consistent with alveolar hemorrhage. Bronchoalveolar lavage demonstrated blood-tinged fluid and numerous hemosiderin-laden macrophages. *B.* Idiopathic rapidly progressive glomerulonephritis. PA chest radiograph from the same patient 18 months later with diffuse bilateral alveolar infiltrates representing recurrent massive alveolar hemorrhage. He was treated with pulse methylprednisolone 1 gm daily for 3 days, followed by a gradual corticosteroid taper. *C.* PA chest radiograph from the same patient 3 weeks later demonstrating complete resolution of the alveolar infiltrates.

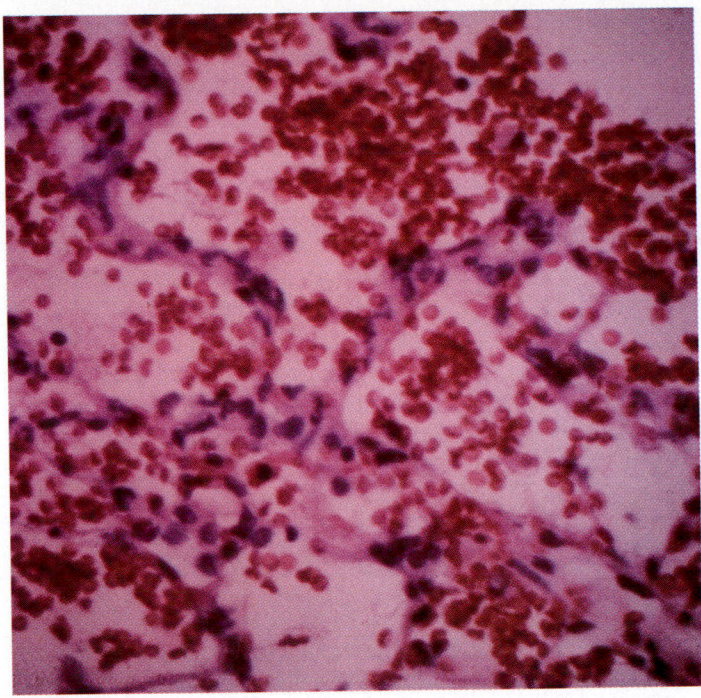

FIGURE 79-2 Postmortem lung biopsy demonstrates large numbers of red blood cells within alveolar spaces in a patient with alveolar hemorrhage due to Wegener's granulomatosis. There is no gross evidence for necrosis or granulomas. The alveolar architecture and septae are well preserved. These histopathologic features are nonspecific. (Hematoxylin-eosin.) *(From Gravelyn TR, Lynch III JP: Alveolar hemorrhage syndromes, IM—Internal Medicine for the Specialist, 1987; (8)1:63–83, copyright Medical Economics Company.)*

the risks of open or thoracoscopic lung biopsy are excessive in patients with severe alveolar hemorrhage and respiratory failure. Postoperative complications such as infection and air leaks may be exacerbated by the corticosteroid or immunosuppressive agents used to treat many of these immune-mediated alveolar hemorrhage syndromes. Further, histologic features are usually nonspecific.[30,37,52] Predominant findings are extensive intraalveolar hemorrhage and necrotizing pulmonary capillaritis (endotheliitis)[33,37,52] (Fig. 79-2). Capillaritis is characterized by neutrophilic infiltration of capillaries, fragmented neutrophils (leukocytoclasis), and necrosis of the capillary walls[33,52] (Fig. 79-3). Loss of the integrity of the alveolar-capillary basement membrane results in leakage of red blood cells and neutrophils into the alveolar space.[52] Hemosiderin-laden macrophages (siderophages) accumulate within the alveolar spaces and interstitium; their presence is a clue to prior episodes of alveolar hemorrhage (Fig. 79-4).[1,25,52]

Capillaritis was initially described as a marker of systemic vasculitis, but may also be observed in myriad disorders associated with alveolar hemorrhage (e.g., systemic lupus erythematosus, collagen vascular disorders, anti-glomerular basement membrane antibody disease, bone marrow transplant recipients, and drug-induced alveolar hemorrhage).[1,14,37,46,52] An associated venulitis and arteriolitis may sometimes be present, but larger vessels are spared.[52] Capillaritis is subtle and often overshadowed by diffuse hemorrhage filling the alveolar spaces.[16,30,52]

Pulmonary capillaritis can be diagnosed by transbronchial biopsy, but this diagnosis is made with greater confidence when a larger biopsy specimen is obtained by video-assisted thoracoscopy or limited thoracotomy.[30,52] Additional pathologic features may be seen in patients with underlying granulomatous vasculitis (e.g., granulomas, necrosis, or eosinophils).[52] Nongranulomatous inflammation in airways and lung interstitium, interstitial fibrosis, diffuse alveolar damage, fibrinous pleuritis, and bronchiolitis obliterans organizing pneumonia have also been described in alveolar hemorrhage associated with anti-neutrophil cytoplasmic antibody (ANCA) syndromes.[52] Histologic findings of alveolar hemorrhage and capillaritis, although distinctive, are nonspecific. Immunofluorescent stains (of lung or kidney) or serologic markers (e.g., anti-GBM antibody or ANCA) are required to differentiate the various causes of autoimmune alveolar hemorrhage (see Table 79-2). Linear deposits of immunoglobulin G (IgG) along alveolar septa is pathognomonic for anti-GBM disease.[24,27,33] A granular, or "lumpy-bumpy" pattern of immune complex deposits may be seen in systemic lupus erythematosis, systemic necrotizing vasculitis, or immune complex-mediated idiopathic rapidly progressive glomerulonephri-

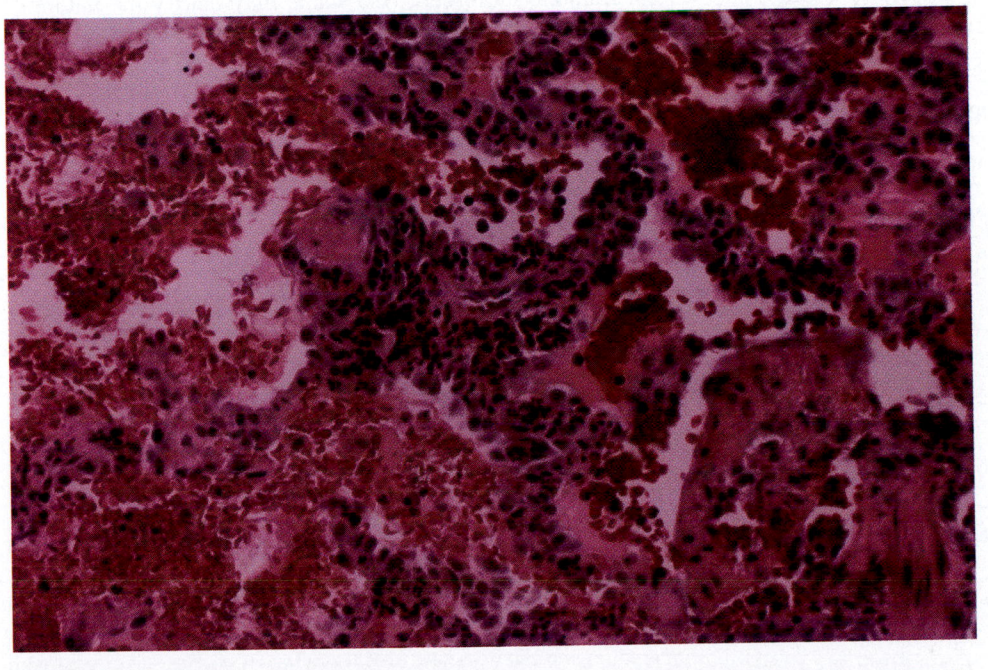

FIGURE 79-3 Pulmonary capillaritis. Intense inflammatory infiltrate involving pulmonary capillaries with intraalveolar hemorrhage (Hematoxylin-cosin). *(Courtesy of Thomas Colby, M.D. From Leatherman,[30] with permission.)*

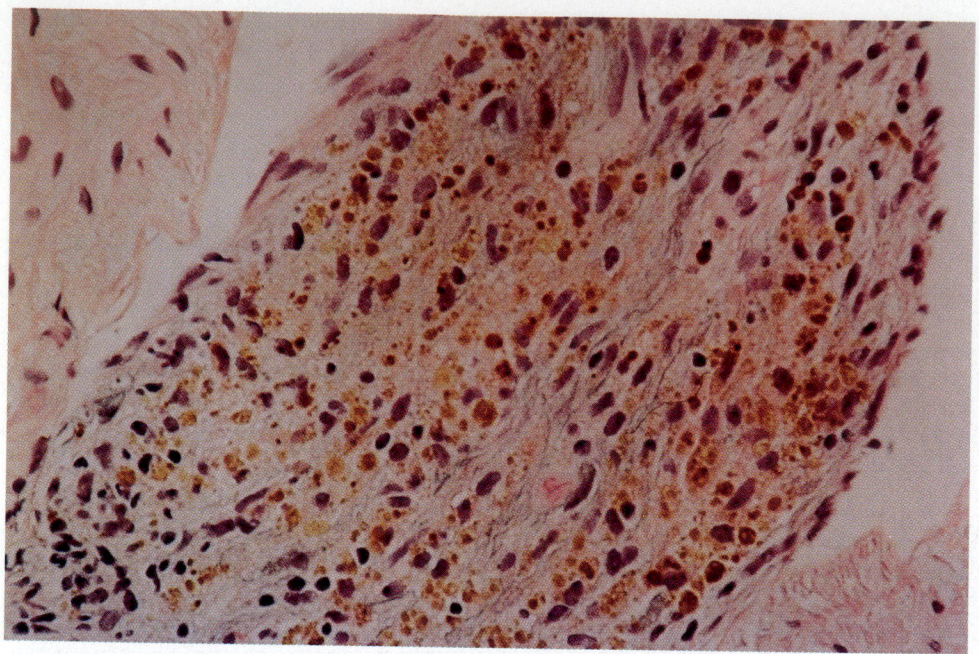

FIGURE 79-4 Hemosiderin-laden macrophages (siderophages) are prominent in the alveolar interstitium in a patient with recurrent alveolar hemorrhage. (Hematoxylin-eosin). *(Courtesy of Joseph Fantone, M.D.)*

with BAL is usually adequate to exclude infectious etiologies and support the diagnosis of alveolar hemorrhage. Bloody or serosanguinous BAL fluid (consistent with active or recent bleeding) or hemosiderin-laden macrophages (a clue to prior episodes of alveolar hemorrhage) may be sufficient to justify initiation of therapy provided clinical and serological features are consistent.[7,25,30,52] Thoracoscopic lung biopsy may be useful in noncritically ill patients with suspected alveolar hemorrhage when ancillary studies, kidney biopsy, and BAL are nondiagnostic.

The Role of Percutaneous Kidney Biopsy

Necrotizing glomerulonephritis is a cardinal (albeit nonspecific) feature of most immune-mediated alveolar hemorrhage syndromes. The histological spectrum is varied, ranging from mild mesangial thickening to severe crescentic glomerulonephritis.[27,30,44] Vasculitis of renal arterioles is rarely found, even in granulomatous vasculitides. Because of the strong association of autoimmune alveolar hemorrhage and glomerulonephritis, percutaneous kidney biopsy should be performed in any patient with suspected alveolar hemorrhage who has abnormalities on urinalysis or renal function tests. Conventional hematoxylin-eosin stains are nonspecific, but the demonstration of glomerular inflammation with necrosis and crescents supports the diagnosis of an immune-mediated etiology (Fig. 79-5). Immunofluorescent (IF) stains may clarify the nature of

tis.[11,13,37,45] In patients with ANCA-associated capillaritis, immune complexes are usually lacking (hence the term *pauci-immune*).[30] When immune alveolar hemorrhage is suspected, a portion of the lung biopsy can be frozen for immunofluorescent (IF) stains, but IF stains of lung tissue are logistically difficult, and nonspecific background staining may lead to misinterpretation. When glomerulonephritis is pres-ent concomitantly, kidney IF stains are more sensitive and reliable.[24,27,30]

Despite the greater accuracy of surgical lung biopsy in evaluating alveolar hemorrhage, we believe fiberoptic bronchoscopy

TABLE 79-2

Autoimmune Diffuse Alveolar Hemorrhage: Pathology and Serology

	Lung Pathology		Renal Pathology		
	Histopathology	*Immunofluorescence*	*Histopathology*	*Immunofluorescence*	*Serology*
ABMA disease (Goodpasture's syndrome)	±Capillaritis	Linear	Variable	Linear	ABMA (± p-ANCA)
Wegener's granulomatosis	Capillaritis (± granulomatous)	Negative	Segmental necrosis, crescents	Pauci-immune	ANCA (c-ANCA>>>p-ANCA)
Microscopic polyangitis	Capillaritis	Negative	Segmental necrosis, crescents	Pauci-immune	ANCA (p-ANCA or c-ANCA)
Systemic lupus erythematosus	Capillaritis	Granular	Variable	Granular	ANA
Idiopathic pulmonary hemosiderosis	±Capillaritis	Negative	Normal	—	Negative

ABMA = anti-basement membrane antibody; ANA = antinuclear antibody; ANCA = anti-neutrophil cytoplasmic antibody; p-ANCA = perinuclear anti-neutrophil cytoplasmic antibody; c-ANCA = cytoplasmic anti-neutrophil cytoplasmic antibody.

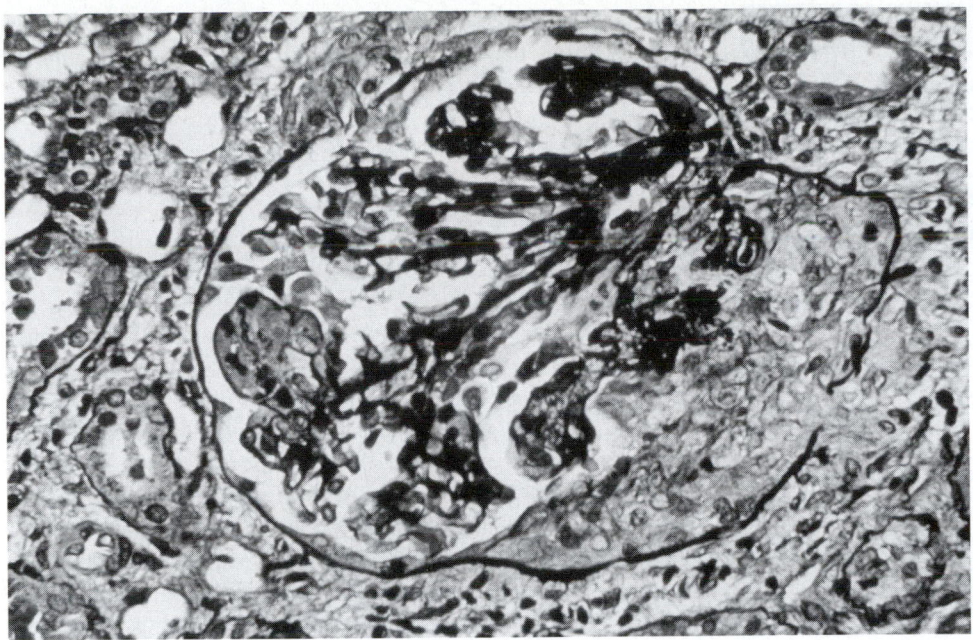

FIGURE 79-5   Segmental necrotizing and crescentic glomerulonephritis due to vasculitis (Hematoxylin-eosin). *(Courtesy of John Crosson, M.D. From Leatherman,[30] with permission.)*

the underlying disorder. Bright linear IF staining along glomerular basement membranes is pathognomonic for anti-GBM disease[24,27,33] (Fig. 79-6). A lumpy-bumpy IF pattern, consistent with deposits of immune complexes, is found in collagen vascular disorders and in idiopathic immune complex-mediated glomerulonephritis.[11,37,52] Negative IF stains are characteristic

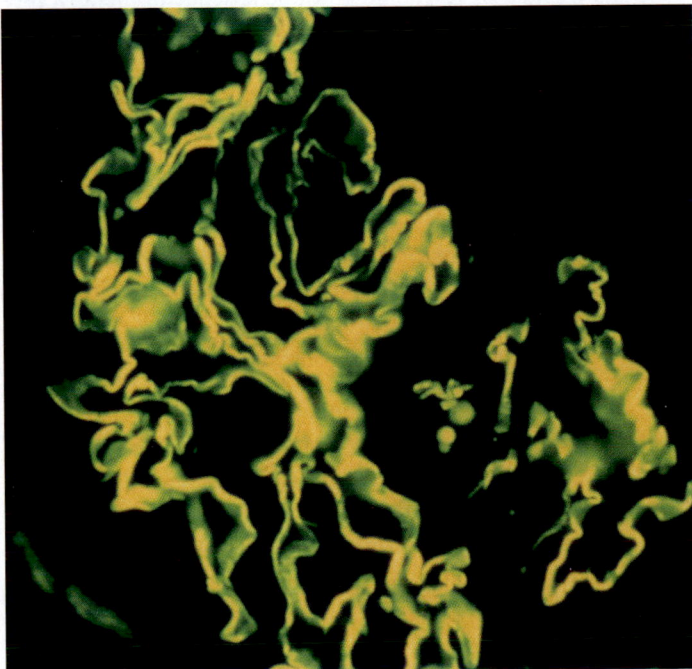

FIGURE 79-6   Linear immunofluorescent staining along glomeruli due to deposition of anti-basement membrane (anti-GBM) antibody. *(Courtesy of John Crosson, M.D. From Leatherman,[30] with permission.)*

of the pauci-immune glomerulonephritis of necrotizing vasculitis.[30,37] Serologies are critically important in defining the underlying disorder responsible for alveolar hemorrhage (particularly ANCA, anti-GBM antibody, and antinuclear antibodies).[26,27,30,38] Recognizing the different pathogenetic mechanisms of these alveolar hemorrhage syndromes is important, as the prognosis and treatment strategies differ.

THERAPY OF IMMUNE-MEDIATED ALVEOLAR HEMORRHAGE

Because of the rarity of the immune-mediated pulmonary-renal syndromes, controlled, randomized trials evaluating therapy are lacking. Corticosteroids are considered part of standard therapy for all the immune-mediated alveolar hemorrhage syndromes (to be discussed in detail later in this chapter). For systemic necrotizing vasculitis, cyclophosphamide (or occasionally other immunosuppressive agents) are combined with cortico-steroids.[4,15,19] The role of cytotoxic agents in other immune-mediated alveolar hemorrhage syndromes needs to be individualized. For severe, fulminant autoimmune alveolar hemorrhage, high-dose intravenous ("pulse") methylprednisolone (1 gm daily for 3 days) is advised (irrespective of underlying etiology),[30] even while pursuing a diagnostic workup. Delaying pulse therapy in a critically ill patient for even a few hours may be catastrophic. Rapid resolution of bleeding can occur, often within 24 to 72 h of initiation of therapy (Fig. 79-7). Following the 3-day pulse, corticosteroids (dose of methylpredisolone 60 to 120 mg per day or equivalent) should be continued for a few days, until control of the bleeding and extrapulmonary manifestations has been achieved. The subsequent dose and rate of corticosteroid taper need to be individualized, based upon clinical, radio-graphic, and serologic response. Cyclophosphamide or other immunosuppressive agents should be withheld until a specific diagnosis mandating treatment with these agents has been substantiated. The specific therapeutic regimen is dictated by the underlying disorder (discussed in detail below). Plasmapheresis is a central component of therapy for anti-GBM disease[24,27] but has no routine role for other disorders. However, anecdotal successes have been cited with plasmapheresis in patients with alveolar hemorrhage complicating SLE or systemic necrotizing vasculitis refractory to corticosteroids or immunosuppressive agents.[4,8,15,38] Plasmapheresis can be considered in patients with severe or progressive alveolar hemorrhage refractory to medical therapy. Measures to ensure adequate oxygenation are also essential. Mechanical ventilatory support, often with positive end-expiratory pressure, may be necessary in fulminant cases of alveolar hemorrhage, to prevent death due to refractory hypoxemia. Transfusion of red blood cells may be required to maintain an

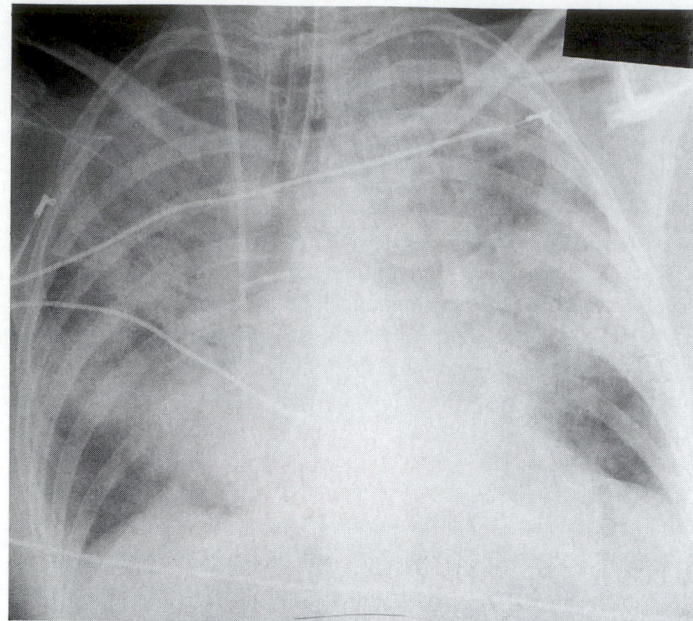

A

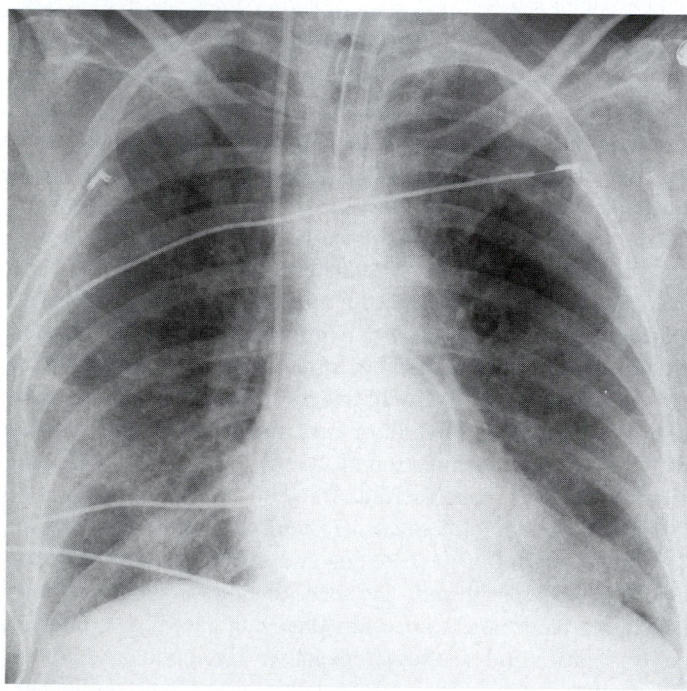

B

FIGURE 79-7 *A.* Alveolar hemorrhage due to microscopic polyarteritis (MPA). PA chest radiograph demonstrating massive alveolar infiltrates involving all lobes. Because of the severity of respiratory failure (requiring 16 cm H_2O of PEEP to achieve acceptable oxygenation), no lung biopsy was performed. Urinalysis demonstrated numerous red cells and occasional red cell casts. Serum creatinine was 1.4 mg%. Pulse methylprednisolone 1 gm daily × 3 days was initiated, and renal biopsy was scheduled for the following morning. *B.* Alveolar hemorrhage due to microscopic polyarteritis (MPA). PA chest radiograph from the same patient 12 h following initiation of pulse methylprednisolone. Marked improvement in alveolar infiltrates is evident. Renal biopsy demonstrated glomerulonephritis and a necrotizing vasculitis involving renal arterioles; no granulomas were present. Cyclophosphamide (2 mg/kg per day) was instituted, and corticosteroids were continued. Within 5 days, the infiltrates had cleared completely and serum creatinine was 0.6 mg%.·

acceptable hemocrit (>25 percent) and adequate blood pressure. In the sections that follow, we will discuss each of the autoimmune alveolar hemorrhage syndromes individually.

SPECIFIC SYNDROMES

Goodpasture's Syndrome

CLINICAL FEATURES

Anti-glomerular basement membrane (anti-GBM) disease (Goodpasture's syndrome), the prototype of pulmonary-renal syndromes, accounts for 18 to 32 percent of immune-mediated alveolar hemorrhage.[20,30] Classically, anti-GBM disease manifests as alveolar hemorrhage and rapidly progressive glomerulonephritis (RPGN).[27] Anti-GBM disease typically affects individuals between age 20 and 45 years, with a distinct male predominance.[24,27] The incidence has been estimated as 0.3 cases per 100,000 population per year.[27] The etiology is not known, but exposure to inhaled hydrocarbons and antecedent viral illnesses, particularly influenza, have been cited as risk factors.[27] The demonstration of anti-GBM antibodies in tissue (typically kidney) or in serum is the cornerstone of the diagnosis.[24,27]

The clinical expression of anti-GBM disease is highly variable. Most patients present with progressive dyspnea, widespread alveolar infiltrates, and hypoxemia; hemoptysis occurs in 80 to 94 percent.[24,27,30] A cardinal feature of Goodpasture's syndrome is the presence of glomerulonephritis. Microscopic hematuria, red cell casts, or proteinuria are almost always present.[24,27,30] Gross hematuria occurs in up to 41 percent of patients. Azotemia is noted in 55 to 71 percent of patients at presentation.[24,27,30] Fatigue and weakness are common. In the absence of therapy, progressive renal insufficiency ensues, often resulting in end-stage renal failure within days to weeks of the onset of symptoms.[24,27,30] Oliguria, severe renal failure, or >50 percent crescents on renal biopsy are associated with a poor prognosis and low rate of recovery of renal function.[24,27,30] The course may be fulminant, with severe renal failure and explosive, life-threatening alveolar hemorrhage. In up to one-third of patients with anti-GBM disease, glomerulonephritis occurs without alveolar hemorrhage; alveolar hemorrhage alone is exceptionally rare.[24,27,30] Chest radiographs typically reveal dense bilateral alveolar infiltrates, often with air-bronchograms.[24,27,30,40] With cessation of bleeding, infiltrates may resolve within 24 to 36 h. Pleural effusions are rare and suggest an alternative diagnosis. Pulmonary function tests are rarely helpful in the acute setting of alveolar hemorrhage. Increases in the diffusing capacity for carbon monoxide (DLCO) occur, due to uptake of carbon monoxide by extravasated alveolar blood.[27] Bloody or serosanguinous BAL fluid suggests alveolar hemorrhage but is nonspecific. Anemia is present in more than 90 percent of cases and may be profound.[24,27,30] Serum iron and ferritin levels are usually decreased, reflecting diminished iron stores.[27] Factors associated with a higher incidence of alveolar hemorrhage include cigarette smoking, exposure to high concentrations of oxygen, upper respiratory tract infections, and increased hydrostatic (pulmonary capillary) pressures.[27]

Serologic assays for anti-GBM antibody are invaluable in confirming the diagnosis and monitoring the adequacy of therapy. Radioimmunoassays or enzyme-linked immunosorbent assays (ELISA) for anti-GBM antibody are highly sensitive (>95 percent) and specific (>97 percent) but are performed in only a few laboratories.[24,27,30] Results are usually not available for several days. Since delay in institution of therapy may preclude a favorable outcome, percutaneous renal biopsy is usually performed while awaiting the results of serum assays. Although the height of serum anti-GBM antibody titer does not correlate with severity of disease, changes in titer over time may be a guide to efficacy of therapy. Rises in titer presage relapse; titers fall as the disease remits.[24,27,30] Treatment can be tapered and discontinued after the antibody has disappeared from the circulation.[24,27,30] Patients with circulating anti-GBM antibodies and ANCA have been described.[9,27,55] Other serologic studies are negative or nondiagnostic.

HISTOPATHOLOGY

Percutaneous kidney biopsy is the preferred invasive procedure to substantiate the diagnosis of anti-GBM disease. Light microscopy demonstrates nonspecific features of a proliferative or necrotizing glomerulonephritis, often with cellular crescents.[24,27] Over time, the crescents may fibrose, and frank glomerulosclerosis, interstitial fibrosis, and tubular atrophy may be observed.[24,27] Although these microscopic features are nonspecific, IF stains are the cornerstone of the diagnosis. Bright linear deposits of immunoglobulin G (IgG) and complement (C3) along glomerular basement membranes are pathognomonic of anti-GBM disease (Fig. 79-6).[27] All four subclasses of IgG are represented, but IgG1 predominates.[27] Rare cases of linear deposits of IgM or IgA have been described.[9,27] Lung biopsies are rarely necessary, as the histologic features on renal biopsy are usually adequate to establish the diagnosis. When lung biopsy has been done, extensive hemorrhage predominates, with accumulation of hemosiderin-laden macrophages within the alveolar spaces.[33] Foci of neutrophilic "capillaritis," hyaline membranes, and diffuse alveolar damage may also be found. Interstitial or intraalveolar inflammation is minimal or absent.[33] Extensive necrosis or large-vessel vasculitis are not a feature. Similar histopathologic features may be seen with a wide gamut of immune-mediated alveolar hemorrhage syndromes. Immunofluorescent stains of lung tissue may be diagnostic, provided a clear linear pattern of immunofluoresence is present. However, IF stains are technically difficult in lung tissue, and autofluorescence may obscure the linear IgG deposits.[30]

PATHOGENESIS

Antibodies are directed against the $\alpha 3$ chain of type IV collagen, an antigen highly expressed in both alveolar and glomerular basement membranes.[27] The pathogenesis of anti-GBM disease remains speculative, but both genetic and environmental factors may play a role. Patients with anti-GBM disease preferentially express certain immunoglobulin Gm allotypes and links between anti-GBM disease and the HLA DR2 histocompatability antigen have been noted.[27] Anecdotal cases of anti-GBM disease have been described in siblings, first cousins, and identical twins, suggesting that a genetic susceptibility may exist.[27] Exposure to cigarette smoke, hydrocarbon-containing solvents, hard metal dust, influenza A2 virus, chlorine gas, and D-penicillamine have been associated with anti-GBM disease.[27,32,34] These exogenous factors may injure the basement membrane, resulting in increased capillary permeability, exposing the Goodpasture antigen ($\alpha 3$ chain) which is then recognized as foreign, eliciting a T-helper cell response. Immunoglobulin synthesis and deposits of IgG along the alveolar and glomerular capillary basement membranes then ensue. Anti-idiotypic (blocking) antibodies and activated T-suppressor (CD8+) cells may modulate the process, but this remains speculative.[27]

TREATMENT

Before the availability of the current therapy and renal dialysis, mortality exceeded 90 percent, with a mean survival of less than 4 months. Currently, with the combination of plasmaphesis, corticosteroids, and cyclophosphamide, mortality has been reduced to less than 20 percent.[24,27,30] Since its introduction as a therapeutic option for anti-GBM disease in the mid-1970s, plasmapheresis was quickly adopted worldwide and has been incorporated in all clinical trials. Because of the rarity of anti-GBM syndrome, only one randomized trial has compared immunosuppressive therapy with the combination of immunosuppressive therapy plus plasma exchange.[24] In that study, plasmapheresis together with immunosuppressive therapy was associated with more rapid disappearance of anti-GBM antibody and improved renal function than treatment with immunosuppressive agents alone.[24] Six of nine patients treated with immunosuppressive agents alone required chronic dialysis compared to two of eight in the plasmapheresis group. Recurrent pulmonary hemorrhage developed in four patients in each group during therapy.

The optimal extent and duration of plasma exchanges have not been defined. Most investigators advocate plasma exchange daily or every other day for 2 to 3 weeks, until the clinical course has improved and serum anti-GBM antibodies are nondetectable.[27] However, less frequent exchanges (i.e., every 3 days) for 30 days may be adequate.[24,27] Immunosuppressive therapy is required to inhibit antibody production and rebound hypersynthesis which may occur following discontinuation of plasma exchange.[27] Either cyclophosphamide (2 mg/kg per day) or azathioprine (2 mg/kg per day), combined with prednisone (1 mg/kg per day) have been used. Most investigators favor oral cyclophosphamide over azathioprine, but studies comparing these agents have not been performed. Treatment of acute, life-threatening alveolar hemorrhage in Goodpasture's syndrome is similar to other autoimmune disorders. Pulse methylprednisolone (1 gm daily for 3 days) is given, followed by a gradual corticosteroid taper. Cyclophosphamide can be initiated once the diagnosis of anti-GBM disease is substantiated by serologies or a pattern of linear immunofluorescence in tissue. This dose of cyclophosphamide is maintained for the duration of therapy, unless complications such as leukopenia necessitate dose reduction. The corticosteroid dose is gradually tapered over the next several weeks. Immunosuppressive or cytotoxic therapy may be discontinued within 3 to 6 months provided a sustained remission has been achieved and anti-GBM antibodies have disappeared.[24,27]

With few exceptions, circulating antibodies clear within 8 weeks, irrespective of the initial titer. Early relapse (within the first 2 months) may occur when circulating antibodies are still present.[27] This typically manifests as alveolar hemorrhage. Risk factors for relapse include infection, volume overload, and cigarette smoking.[27] Late recurrence, associated with renewed antibody synthesis following a remission, has only rarely been documented.[27] In summary, aggressive therapy with plasmapheresis, corticosteroids, and immunosuppressive agents has dramatically improved prognosis. With this approach, 5-year survival exceeds 80 percent, and fewer than 30 percent of patients require chronic dialysis.[24,27] Early recognition and treatment of this syndrome are critical, as the prognosis for recovery of renal function depends upon the initial extent of injury. Recovery of renal function can be expected in patients with minor functional impairment. By contrast, patients manifesting initial serum creatinine >4 mg/dl, oliguria, or greater than 50 percent crescents on renal biopsy rarely recover and usually progress to end-stage renal failure requiring chronic dialysis.[24,27,44] Renal transplantation has been successful in patients with irreversible renal failure, provided serum anti-GBM antibodies are undetectable.[24,30]

Systemic Vasculitis

Diffuse alveolar hemorrhage is a well-recognized complication of microscopic polyangiitis (MPA) and Wegener's granulomatosis but rarely complicates Churg-Strauss syndrome, Behçet's syndrome, mixed cryoglobulinemia, and other systemic necrotizing vasculitides.[15,16,44] Classic polyarteritis nodosa rarely involves the lung.[12,23] Necrotizing small-vessel vasculitis accounts for the majority of autoimmune alveolar hemorrhage syndromes.[16,30,31] Rapidly progressive glomerulonephritis (RPGN) is usually present in each of these alveolar hemorrhage syndromes, but the disease is sometimes limited to the kidneys or lungs. Circulating antibodies directed against components of neutrophils and monocytes (ANCA) have been detected in most patients with these "pulmonary renal syndromes," suggesting a common pathogenesis and mechanism of lung injury in these diverse vasculitic disorders.[11,13]

ANCA-ASSOCIATED VASCULITIDES

Goodpasture's syndrome (anti-GBM disease) was the first of the pulmonary renal syndromes to be immunologically characterized. Subsequent studies documented immune complexes in serum or renal tissue in subsets of patients with pulmonary renal syndromes, particularly systemic lupus erythematosus, Wegener's granulomatosis, and immune complex-mediated glomerulonephritis.[11,16,30] However, more than two-thirds of patients with pulmonary renal syndromes are not mediated by either anti-GBM antibody or immune complexes.[30] As mentioned, the term *pauci-immune glomerulonephritis* has been applied to this group of patients. Some patients with pauci-immune glomerulonephritis and alveolar hemorrhage have clinicopathologic features of Wegener's granulomatosis. Others exhibit a multisystemic small-vessel vasculitis but lack granulomatous inflammation of the respiratory tract. Historically, these patients were considered to have microscopic polyarteritis nodosa.[16] Currently, the term *microscopic polyangiitis* (MPA) is preferred.[23,30]

Some patients have acute alveolar hemorrhage and pauci-immune RPGN but lack evidence for vasculitis elsewhere. The term *idiopathic RPGN* has been used to refer to these patients.[11,30] The availability of serum assays for ANCAs has profoundly influenced the classification of immune alveolar hemorrhage and glomerulonephritis. Most patients with pauci-immune alveolar hemorrhage and glomerulonephritis have circulating ANCA.[11,13,26,45] ANCA-positive patients formerly given a diagnosis of idiopathic RPGN and alveolar hemorrhage are now considered to have microscopic polyangiitis (MPA).[23] The spectrum of ANCA-associated diseases is not limited to patients with pulmonary renal syndromes but includes individuals with microscopic polyangitiis limited to the lung (i.e., manifesting as alveolar hemorrhage) or kidney (i.e., necrotizing glomerulonephritis). To avoid further confusion, brief definitions of the major ANCA-associated vasculitides will be outlined below.

Wegener's Granulomatosis

Wegener's granulomatosis (WG), the most common of the pulmonary vasculitides, typically involves the upper respiratory tract (e.g., sinuses, ears, nasopharynx, oropharynx, trachea), lower respiratory tract (bronchi and lung), and kidney, with varying degrees of disseminated vasculitis[19] (see Chapter 86). Alveolar hemorrhage is a rare complication of WG, reflecting diffuse injury to the lung microvasculature (i.e., capillaritis)[16,19,30] (Fig. 79-8). In this context, rapidly progressive glomerulonephritis is present in more than 90 percent of patients.[16,30,31] The salient histopathologic features of Wegener's granulomatosis include small-vessel vasculitis (involving capillaries, arterioles, venules), geographic necrosis, hemorrhagic infarcts, a mixed inflammatory cellular infiltrate, and a granulomatous component.[19] Circulating antibodies directed against cytoplasmic components of neutrophils (c-ANCA) have been detected in more than 90 percent of patients with active generalized WG and in 40 to 70 percent with active regional WG.[13,26,28,42] Oral cyclophosphamide (2 mg/kg per day) and prednisone is the treatment of choice for WG.[19] With this regimen, remissions are achieved in 70 to 93 percent of patients, with early mortality rates of less than 15 percent.[4,19] Methotrexate may be used in patients with limited disease or those experiencing signficant toxicity from cyclophosphamide.[48] Success has been reported with trimethoprim/sulfamethoxazole, but its role is controversial.[19,48,51]

Churg-Strauss Syndrome (Allergic Angiitis and Granulomatosis)

Churg-Strauss syndrome (CSS), also termed *allergic angiitis and granulomatosis,* is a rare small-vessel vasculitis associated with a prominent allergic component, asthma, and eosinophils in blood or involved tissues[15,29,30] (see Chapter 86). The annual incidence has been estimated at 2.4 cases per million.[54] Pulmonary involvement, primarily asthma, is present in virtually all cases. Focal infiltrates are present on chest radiographs in 30 to 70 percent of cases.[29] Diffuse alveolar hemorrhage is a rare complication.[29,30] Circulating ANCA (either p-ANCA or c-ANCA) have been detected in most patients with CSS.[13,15,23,26] As with other ANCA-associated vasculitides, small vessels (capillaries, venules, and arterioles) are involved.[23,29] Granulomas, eosinophils, and pallisading histiocytes in extravascular tissues are hall-

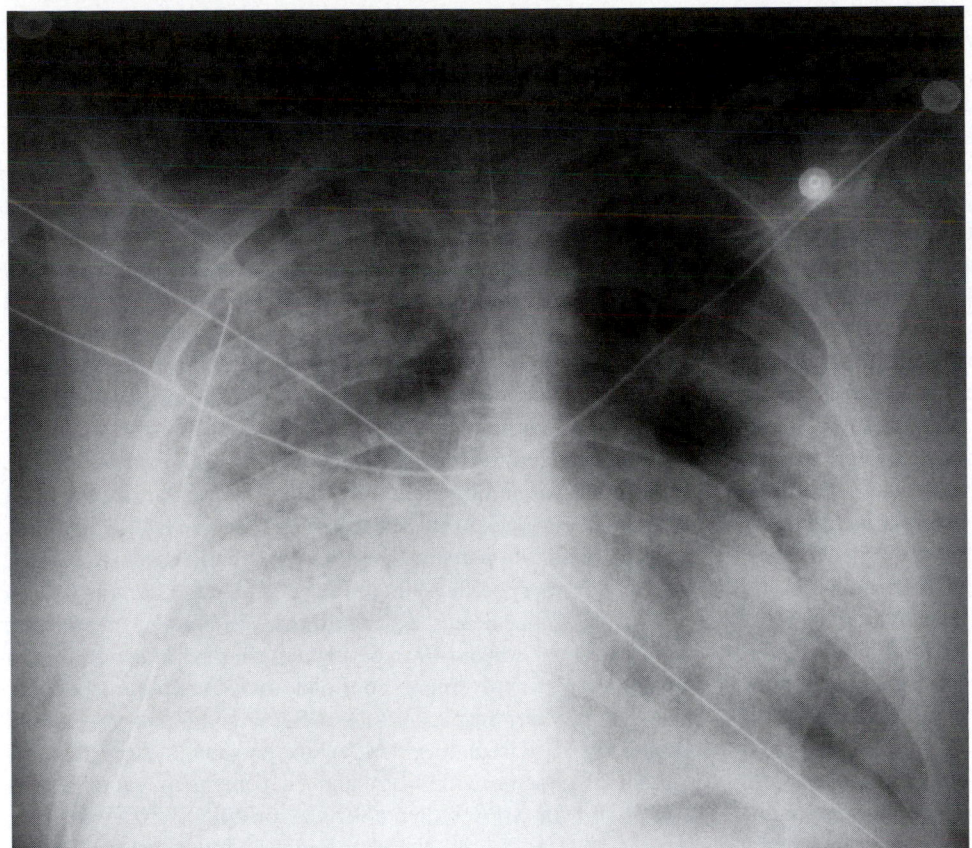

FIGURE 79-8   Wegener's granulomatosis. PA chest radiograph demonstrated bilateral alveolar infiltrates in a 13-year-old female with hemoptysis and respiratory failure. A right chest tube is in place from an open lung biopsy performed 2 days earlier. Open lung biopsy demonstrated capillaritis and massive alveolar hemorrhage. Pulse methylprednisolone, followed by oral cyclophosphamide and prednisone, was associated with a complete remission.

Microscopic Polyangiitis (MPA)

Microscopic polyangiitis (formerly termed *microscopic polyarteritis* or *polyangiitis overlap syndrome*) typically presents with glomerulonephritis and pulmonary capillaritis manifesting as alveolar hemorrhage.[16,23,44] Clinical and serological features of MPA overlap with WG and Churg Strauss syndrome.[4,15,23] Microscopic polyangiitis (MPA) is rare, with an estimated prevalence of 2.4 cases per million.[54] As its name implies, MPA involves small vessels (arterioles, venules, or capillaries); extension to larger vessels occurs in a minority of cases.[23] Small vessels are always spared in classic polyarteritis nodosa (PAN).[15,23] In contrast to Wegener's granulomatosis or Churg-Strauss syndrome, neither granulomas nor eosinophils are prominent in MPA.[23] Circulating ANCA are present in 50 to 90 percent of patients with MPA, suggesting a relationship with other ANCA-associated vasculitides.[13,15,26,45] By contrast, circulating ANCA are present in fewer than 20 percent of patients with classic (macroscopic) polyarteritis nodosa (PAN).[15,23] A necrotizing, crescentic pauci-immune glomerulonephritis is nearly invariably present in MPA but is rare in classical PAN.[4,15,23] Alveolar hemorrhage, which is rarely observed in classical PAN, occurs in 30 to 50 percent of patients with MPA and is often the dominant and most life-threatening manifestation.[16,23,44]

Prednisone, cyclophosphamide, and plasmapheresis, alone or in combination, have been used to treat MPA.[4,12,15,44] Response rates and long-term survival have generally been similar with the various regimens.[15] Most investigators use oral cyclophosphamide (2 mg/kg per day) plus prednisone (1 mg/kg per day, with gradual taper), similar to the regimen used for WG.[4,19] With this approach, favorable responses are achieved in more than 80 percent of patients; 10-year survival exceeds 70 percent.[4,15]

ANCA-ASSOCIATED PULMONARY RENAL SYNDROMES: CLINICAL FEATURES

The clinical and radiologic manifestations of ANCA-associated alveolar hemorrhage are similar to other immune causes. Acute necrotizing glomerulonephritis is nearly always present, but the renal lesion is nonspecific.[11,13] Distinguishing the specific underlying disorder may be difficult. The pathologic lesions in ANCA-associated diseases share characteristic features, regardless of the organ affected. The three key histopathologic findings are a segmental (focal) distribution of vascular injury, infiltration with neutrophils, and fibrinoid necrosis.[23,52] The latter results from lysis of

marks of the disorder.[23,29] Pronounced granulomatous and eosinophilic components distinguish CSS from other vasculitides.[4,15,23] In the classic form of CSS, vasculitis develops after a several-year history of atopy or asthma.[29] The erythrocyte sedimentation rate (ESR), C-reactive protein, and blood eosinophil count are elevated in more than 80 percent of patients during the acute phase of vasculitis or exacerbations.[29] The diagnosis of CSS can be made, even when histologic features are less than definitive, provided the clinical and laboratory features are characteristic.[29]

Because of the rarity of CSS, data on therapy are limited. A variety of treatment regimens employing corticosteroids, immunosuppressive or cytotoxic agents, and plasmapheresis (alone or in combination) have been tried and generally have been equally efficacious.[4,12,15] Corticosteroids achieve remissions in more than 80 percent of patients with CSS and are first-line therapy for mild to moderate cases of CSS.[29] Oral or pulse cyclophosphamide should be added for severe or multisystemic disease or corticosteroid-recalcitrant cases or when unfavorable prognostic factors are present (such as central nervous system or gastrointestinal involvement, cardiomyopathy, severe renal insufficiency, or proteinuria > 1 gm per day).[4,12,15] Plasmapheresis should be considered only in patients failing or experiencing adverse effects from combined therapy.[4,15]

the vascular wall, allowing plasma coagulation factors to enter the interstitium and come into contact with thrombogenic substances, generating fibrin. Neutrophils that infiltrate vessel walls undergo disruption and karyorrhexis, leading to the typical leukocytoclastic pattern of injury in capillaries and venules.[23,52] ANCA-associated vascular injury is accompanied by few, if any, immune deposits (pauci-immune).[23,30] The salient lesion of renal vasculitis is a segmental necrotizing glomerulonephritis, usually accompanied by extracapillary proliferation of Bowmans capsule (crescents)[11,30] (Fig. 79-5). Depending on the duration and extent of renal injury, varying degrees of glomerular fibrosis and sclerosis may be seen. Vasculitis affecting the kidney often involves only the glomerular capillaries; macroscopic arteritis is seldom apparent.[11,19,30] When the lung is involved, the histopathology is nonspecific, demonstrating only capillaritis and intraalveolar hemorrhage.[52] Immune deposits are absent.

Clinical features of ANCA-associated alveolar hemorrhage syndromes overlap. Striking elevations in the erythrocytic sedimentation rate and C-reactive protein may be observed in all the syndromes, particularly when disseminated vasculitis is present.[11,15,16,19,23,29] Anemia and leukocytosis are common. Marked eosinophilia is characteristic of Churg-Strauss syndrome but is not a feature of MPA or WG.[15,23] Extrapulmonary and extrarenal manifestations suggesting small-vessel vasculitis (e.g., palpable purpura, leukocytoclastic vasculitis, mononeuritis multiplex, arthralgias or arthritis, ocular disease, sinusitis) may direct biopsies at these sites. Histologic features of granulomatous vasculitis are consistent with WG or CSS whereas granulomas are lacking in MPA.[23] Radiographic features may discriminate granulomatous vasculitides from MPA. In WG (and less commonly in CSS), focal nodular or cavitary mass lesions may be seen.[19,23,29] These are not found in MPA.[23,44] The diagnosis of CSS can usually be readily established by a pronounced eosinophilic component in the blood or in extravascular sites.[15,23,29] However, discriminating WG from MPA may be difficult or impossible as small-vessel vasculitis is common to both disorders. By definition, WG is associated with concomitant granulomatous inflammation, typically, but not invariably involving the upper and lower respiratory tracts.[19,23] The latter may lead to the highly distinctive features attributed to WG including sinusitis, otitis media, nasal or laryngeotracheal ulcerations, subglottic stenosis, and cavitary pulmonary nodules.

CHARACTERISTICS OF ANTI-NEUTROPHIL CYTOPLASMIC ANTIBODIES (ANCA)

The identification of circulating antibodies directed against cytoplasmic components of neutrophils and monocytes (i.e., ANCA) represented a ma-

jor advance in the classification and understanding of vasculitis.[13,26,42,45] Using ethanol-fixed granulocytes incubated with patient serum, two distinct patterns of ANCA are identified by IF techniques: cytoplasmic (c-ANCA) and perinuclear (p-ANCA)[11,13,26,42,45] (Fig. 79-9). The p-ANCA pattern is an artifact of fixation causing movement of the target antigens to a perinuclear location.[13] These differing IF patterns reflect distinct antigenic specificities.

In both radioimmunoassays and enzyme-linked immunoassays (ELISA), the antibody responsible for c-ANCA is directed against proteinase 3 (PR-3).[13] The p-ANCA pattern is usually due to an antibody to myeloperoxidase (MPO).[11,13] MPO-ANCA is usually associated with small-vessel vasculitis, but multiple p-ANCA antibodies directed against a variety of antigens (e.g., cathepsin G, lactoferrin, and elastin) may be seen in nonvasculitic inflammatory disorders including collagen vascular diseases and inflammatory bowel or liver disease.[13] Therefore, while c-ANCA is more than 90 percent specific for small-vessel vasculitis, p-ANCA is nonspecific.[11] In untreated WG, circulating c-ANCA (PR3-ANCA) are detected in more than 70 percent of patients; the incidence is lower (40 to 65 percent) in patients with limited disease (e.g., involvement confined to the upper respiratory tract).[26,42] By contrast, p-ANCA (MPO-ANCA) is rarely found in WG.[11,26,42] Circulating ANCA are present in more than 90 percent of patients with MPA and 70 percent of patients with CSS.[11,13,23] In MPA either c-ANCA or MPO-ANCA may be present, but MPO is slightly more common.[11,13,23] Serum ANCA, typically p-ANCA, has been detected in more than 50 percent of patients with pauci-immune glomerulonephritis.[11,13,15,23,26,42,45] Circulating ANCA have been found in fewer than 20 percent of patients with classical polyarteritis nodosa

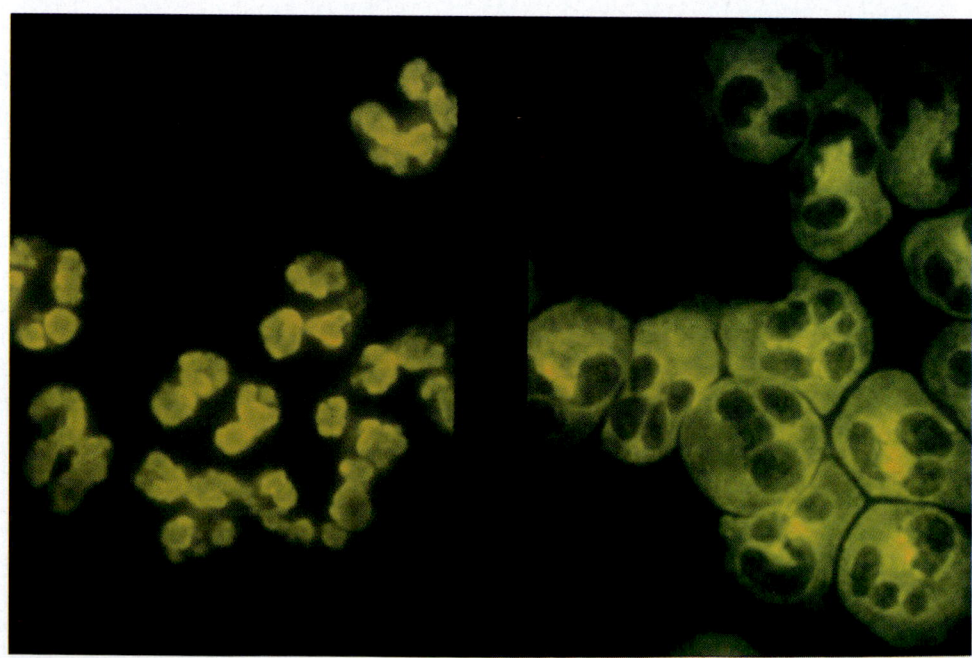

FIGURE 79-9   Indirect immunofluorescent stains demonstrating two distinct types of antineutrophil antibodies. On the left panel, note the perinuclear pattern of immunofluorescence characteristic of p-ANCA (myeloperoxidase epitope). On the right panel, a coarse granular pattern of immunofluorescence within the cytoplasm is evident, characteristic of c-ANCA (proteinase-3 epitope).

(PAN).[15,23] When present, antibodies have shown MPO antigenic specificity.[15,23] Individual patients almost never have both c-ANCA and p-ANCA. Most ANCAs are of the IgG class. However, IgM ANCAs associated with severe alveolar hemorrhage have been described, either concomitant with IgG-ANCA or in the absence of IgG-ANCA.[9,30] It is unknown how often patients with ANCA-negative vasculitis would be ANCA-positive if reagents that detected IgM antibodies were used.

The antigenic specificities of ANCA (i.e., PR3 or MPO) may provide clues to the nature of the underlying disorder and may assist in categorizing the type of disease, but overlap exists. Biopsies are important to differentiate the nature of the underlying vasculitic disorder. For example, patients with c-ANCA and small-vessel vasculitis may be misclassified as MPA if clinically inapparent areas of granulomatous inflammation are overlooked. For clinical purposes, distinguishing Wegener's granulomatosis from MPA is not critical, because therapy and management are similar. Circulating p-ANCA (MPO) or c-ANCA (PR3) are present in more than 70 percent of patients with pauci-immune necrotizing glomerulonephritis (renal vasculitis).[11,13,26,45] ANCA-negative patients usually have disease limited to the kidney. Nearly all patients with concomitant alveolar hemorrhage have circulating ANCA.[11,13] Indeed, a negative ANCA provides very strong evidence against vasculitis as the cause of alveolar hemorrhage and glomerulonephritis. When applied to patients with RPGN, a positive ANCA almost invariably predicts pauci-immune necrotizing glomerulonephritis. In the setting of clinical, laboratory and radiologic features that are highly suggestive of alveolar hemorrhage and RPGN, a positive c-ANCA or MPO-ANCA, together with a negative anti-GBM and ANA assay, is virtually diagnostic of systemic vasculitis (e.g., WG or MPA). Similarly, a positive ANCA (usually MPO-ANCA) is sufficient to diagnose lung-limited MPA, provided the clinical presentation is typical of alveolar hemorrhage and nonimmune causes of lung hemorrhage have been excluded.[13,26] Most patients previously diagnosed as having idiopathic pulmonary hemosiderosis likely had lung-limited MPA or ANCA-associated pulmonary capillaritis.

Problems with using serum ANCA to diagnose vasculitis arise when the clinical presentation is ambiguous. The low incidence of vasculitis in the general population dictates that the positive predictive value of ANCA will be low when applied indiscriminately. Routine assay of serum ANCA in patients with nonspecific respiratory complaints yields a high rate of false positive results.[30] Given the risks of immunosuppressive therapy, misinterpretation of ANCA may lead to devastating consequences. Accordingly, results of serum ANCA assays must be interpreted in light of the entire clinical picture.

Anti-GBM disease and vasculitis have traditionally been viewed as distinct clinicopathologic entities. However, recent studies have found that up to 30 percent of patients with anti-GBM disease (as evidenced by anti-GBM antibody in serum and linear deposits of IgG in kidney biopsy) also have serum MPO-ANCA.[27,30,55] The coexistence of ANCA and anti-GBM antibodies is almost certainly not a chance occurrence, given the rarity of both antibodies in the general population. It is possible that ANCA initiates vascular injury, and anti-GBM antibody then forms in response to the damaged basement membrane. The prognosis for recovery of renal function is better among patients with both anti-GBM antibody and ANCA compared to patients with anti-GBM alone.[27,55]

The role of ANCA in the pathogenesis of vasculitis is uncertain, but these antibodies probably mediate vascular damage. Sera from patients with either c-ANCA or MPO-ANCA induce neutrophils to undergo a respiratory burst with release of reactive oxygen species and proteolytic enzymes.[26] Cytokine-primed neutrophils are stimulated by ANCA to damage human endothelial cells in vitro.[26] These observations, together with correlations of ANCA titer with clinical disease in humans (although imperfect)[28,42] suggest that ANCAs are not innocent markers of vasculitis but play crucial roles in mediating vessel injury.

THERAPY

Therapy of alveolar hemorrhage due to ANCA-associated syndromes depends on the underlying disorder and the extent and severity of symptoms. However, irrespective of etiology, the most immediate concern in patients with severe immune alveolar hemorrhage is to control intrapulmonary bleeding, which may be fatal. Besides general supportive measures, high-dose "pulse" methylprednisolone (followed by a tapering regimen of corticosteroids) should be given. The presence of renal involvement or progression of alveolar hemorrhage on corticosteroids is an indication for adding cyclophosphamide (with or without empiric plasma exchange). Plasma exchange has been used, with anecdotal successes, as therapy for ANCA-associated systemic vasculitis. Because ANCA may play a pivotal role in mediating tissue injury, plasmapheresis may be beneficial in selected patients.

A controlled trial randomized patients with focal necrotizing glomerulonephritis (without anti-GBM antibodies) to either immunosuppression alone (prednisolone, cyclophosphamide, or azathioprine) or immunosuppression *plus* plasma exchange.[41] Fifty-two consecutive patients were stratified according to severity of renal function at the time of entry into the study. In the plasmapheresis group, plasma exchange was performed at least five times within the first week and as needed thereafter. A mean of 9 plasma exchanges was performed. Patients not already on dialysis responded equally well to both regimens (>90 percent improvement). However, among patients with severe renal failure requiring dialysis at the time of entry into the study, plasmapheresis conferred significant benefit. Short-term improvement in renal function was noted in 10 of 11 patients in the plasmapheresis group, compared to only 3 of 8 responses in the control group (immunosuppressive therapy only). This study suggests that combining plasmapheresis and immunosuppression may have a role in selected patients with acute alveolar hemorrhage and severe glomerulonephritis requiring dialysis. When plasma exchange is used to treat ANCA-associated alveolar hemorrhage, it may be preferable to use an apparatus that efficiently removes both IgM and IgG, because of the reported association of IgM-ANCA and alveolar hemorrhage.[9] Protein A immunoadsorption has also been used to treat patients with alveolar hemorrhage and glomerulonephritis, in hopes of removing pathogenic antibodies without producing the side effects of plasma exchange.[10] Additional strategies for patients resistant to conventional therapies include high-dose, intermittent intravenous immunoglobulin G (IVIG).[22,53] The mechanism of action is uncertain but may involve binding of ANCA idiotype by anti-idiotype antibodies in the intravenous IgG preparation.

The role of serial ANCA determinations in following patients with vasculitis is controversial.[26,28,42] We do not base therapeutic decisions on the ANCA titer alone. However, a rising titer should alert the clinician to the possibility of disease exacerbation and clinical follow-up should be intensified. Serial ANCA titers may help differentiate disease relapse from nonimmune causes of pulmonary infiltrates. However, ANCA titers do not obviate the need to aggressively evaluate patients with vasculitis presenting with a new pulmonary process while receiving immunosuppressive therapy.

SYSTEMIC LUPUS ERYTHEMATOSUS

Alveolar hemorrhage is a potentially catastrophic complication of systemic lupus erythematosus (SLE), with mortality rates as high as 50 percent.[37,38] Approximately 10 percent of cases of immune-mediated alveolar hemorrhage have been attributed to SLE.[16,30,31] Alveolar hemorrhage complicating SLE is usually accompanied by other manifestations of active SLE.[37,38] Circulating antinuclear antibody (ANA) is present in more than 99 percent of patients. Alveolar hemorrhage is rarely the sole or presenting feature of SLE.[38] Clinical and radiographic features of alveolar hemorrhage complicating SLE are similar to other alveolar hemorrhage syndromes. However, in SLE-associated alveolar hemorrhage, glomerulonephritis is usually lacking. Diffuse, bilateral alveolar infiltrates, dyspnea, hypoxemia, and hemoptysis are characteristic (Fig. 79-10). With minor episodes, hemoptysis or hypoxemia may be lacking, obscuring the diagnosis. The diffuse pulmonary infiltrates must be differentiated from other pulmonary complications of SLE including lupus pneumonitis,

opportunistic infections, congestive heart failure, uremia, or pulmonary embolism.[38]

Lung biopsy may be needed to exclude alternative diagnoses and corroborate the diagnosis of alveolar hemorrhage.[30,37] However, the risk of lung biopsy may be substantial in critically ill patients with fulminant alveolar hemorrhage and respiratory failure. In addition, as with other immune alveolar hemorrhage syndromes, histopathologic features of alveolar hemorrhage complicating SLE are nonspecific. The dominant feature is intraalveolar hemorrhage and capillaritis, without macroscopic necrosis.[37,52] The small-vessel necrotizing vasculitis rarely extends to arterioles and small muscular arteries in addition to capillaries.[37] Granular deposits of IgG or C3 (consistent with immune complexes) have been found in up to 50 percent of cases of alveolar hemorrhage complicating SLE.[37,38] As noted earlier, because of its potential morbidity, we rarely advise open or thoracoscopic lung biopsy to diagnose alveolar hemorrhage. Provided clinical features are consistent, the diagnosis of alveolar hemorrhage can often be established by fiberoptic bronchoscopy with BAL and transbronchial lung biopsies. Transbronchial biopsies may demonstrate foci of capillaritis with intraalveolar hemorrhage, but due to sampling error, these features may be missed. However, the presence of gross blood in the airways or serosanguinous BAL fluid, large numbers of hemosiderin-laden macrophages, absence of purulent sputum, and lack of infectious organisms by appropriate stains strongly support the diagnosis of autoimmune alveolar hemorrhage[30,38] and justify institution of therapy. Transbronchial lung biopsies may be deferred in acutely ill patients with severe alveolar hemorrhage and respiratory failure. In this context, BAL alone is adequate, primarily to exclude local or infectious causes of bleeding.

Due to the rarity of this syndrome, prospective, controlled trials evaluating therapy have not been performed. As with other causes of immune alveolar hemorrhage, we recommend high-dose intravenous pulse methylprednisolone (1 gm daily for 3 days) for severe alveolar hemorrhage.[31] The dose may be tapered to 60 to 120 mg of methylprednisolone or equivalent by the fourth day, with a gradual taper thereafter. For mild cases, high-dose prednisone (1 mg/kg per day) may be adequate as initial therapy. Symptoms, serial chest radiographs, complete blood counts, and anti-DNA titers reflect efficacy of therapy and guide the rate of taper of corticosteroid. Immunosuppressive or cytotoxic agents may be considered for alveolar hemorrhage refractory to corticosteroids, but data are limited. Plasmapheresis (usually combined with corticosteroids or immunosuppressive agents) has been associated with anecdotal successes for acute flares of SLE or alveolar hemorrhage.[8,38] In one study, plasmapheresis was associated with prompt resolution of life-threatening alveolar hemorrhage in three patients with SLE, two of whom had failed treatment with cyclophosphamide and high-dose corticosteroids.[8] Despite these anecdotal successes, additional studies are required to define the role of plasmapheresis. In randomized, controlled trials, plasmapheresis plus prednisone and cyclophosphamide were no more effective than prednisone and cyclophosphamide alone for severe lupus nephritis.[38] Plasmapheresis is expensive, logistically cumbersome, and should be reserved for patients with severe alveolar hemorrhage refractory to corticosteroids and/or cytotoxic agents.

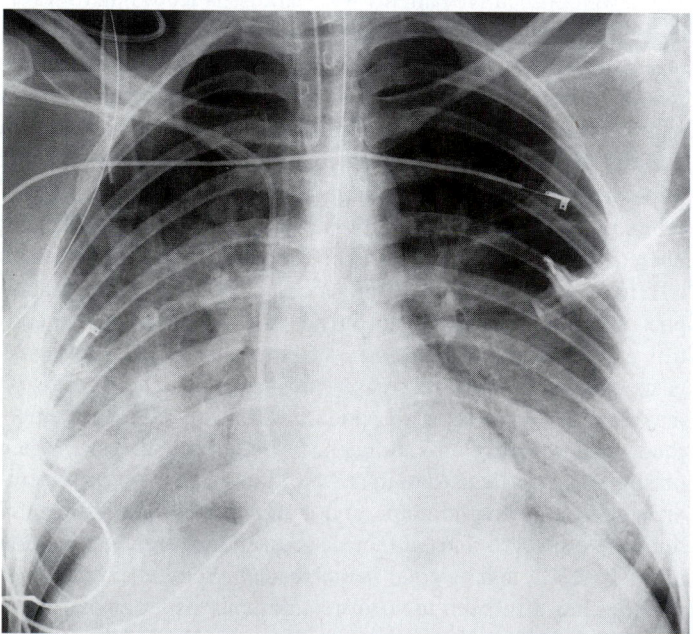

FIGURE 79-10 Systemic lupus erythematosus (SLE). PA chest radiograph reveals extensive bilateral alveolar infiltrates in a 22-year-old female with SLE, hemoptysis, and anemia.

OTHER COLLAGEN VASCULAR DISORDERS

Anecdotal reports of alveolar hemorrhage, with or without capillaritis, have been described in association with rheumatoid arthritis, scleroderma, mixed connective tissue disease, antiphospholipid antibody syndrome, Henoch-Scholein syndrome, and Behçet's disease.[30,46,52] A recent report described two patients with acute polymyositis and severe progressive respiratory failure due to pulmonary capillaritis.[46] Although neither patient had hemoptysis, lung biopsies revealed typical features of alveolar hemorrhage and capillaritis. Dramatic remissions were achieved in both cases with prednisone and cyclophosphamide. Pulmonary capillaritis, recurrent microvascular thrombosis, and alveolar hemorrhage may occur in patients with antiphospholipid antibody syndrome (including patients without apparent thromboemboli).[14] The clinical spectrum ranges from minimal hemoptysis to life-threatening respiratory failure. Only sporadic cases of alveolar hemorrhage complicating other connective vascular disorders have been published. In addition to capillaritis and alveolar hemorrhage, additional histopathologic features on lung biopsies include vasculitis of small and medium muscular pulmonary arteries, diffuse alveolar damage, and bronchiolitis obliterans organizing pneumonia (BOOP).[46,52] In view of the rarity of alveolar hemorrhage complicating these diverse collagen vascular disorders, data regarding therapy are limited. High-dose (pulse) intravenous methylprednisolone is advised as initial treatment. In patients with fulminant or corticosteroid-recalcitrant disease, cyclophosphamide, alone or combined with plasmapheresis, should be added.

Alveolar Hemorrhage in Immunocompromised Hosts

Alveolar hemorrhage may occur in immunocompromised patients. Alveolar hemorrhage may reflect injury to pulmonary endothelial or epithelial cells, (secondary to chemotherapy or radiation toxicity), thrombocytopenia (secondary to bone marrow toxicity), pulmonary edema, pulmonary malignancies, and diverse infectious and nonspecific interstitial pneumonias.[1,7,18,25,35,36,47] The incidence of alveolar hemorrhage in severely immunocompromised hosts with hematologic malignancies or bone marrow transplants has varied from 11 to 64 percent.[1,7,18,25,35,36,47] The variable frequency in large part is due to differing diagnostic criteria for the diagnosis of alveolar hemorrhage. Subclinical alveolar hemorrhage (as evidenced by increased numbers of hemosiderin-laden macrophages in BAL) occurs in up to one-third of immunocompromised hosts with pulmonary infiltrates.[1,7,25] In one retrospective study of 228 immunocompromised patients with suspected pneumonia who underwent BAL, 36 percent of BAL fluids exhibited greater than 20 percent of alveolar macrophages containing hemosiderin, a marker of prior alveolar hemorrhage.[7] The incidence of alveolar hemorrhage was more frequent in cardiac transplant recipients (75 percent) compared to other groups (33 percent). Risk factors for alveolar hemorrhage include thrombocytopenia, coagulopathy, renal failure, alveolar proteinosis, and a smoking history greater than 10 pack years.[7] Surprisingly, alveolar hemorrhage was no more frequent among patients requiring mechanical ventilatory support. Thirty-eight episodes of alveolar hemorrhage (44 percent) were associated with an infectious pneumonia. In 23 percent of the alveolar hemorrhage group and 8 percent of all BALs, alveolar hemorrhage was the *sole* identified cause of pulmonary infiltrates. In contrast to earlier reports, the mortality rate was no higher in patients with alveolar hemorrhage compared to patients without alveolar hemorrhage (approximately 15 percent at 15 days).[7] In summary, subclinical alveolar hemorrhage is common in immunocompromised patients, may have limited prognostic significance, and may reflect pulmonary endothelial or epithelial injury from diverse causes. Other specific causes of alveolar hemorrhage include bronchopulmonary Kaposi's sarcoma and diverse infections (e.g., invasive fungi—particularly *Aspergillus spp*, viruses, *Mycobacteria*, *Legionellae*, and bacteria).[7,18,25] Cardiac or renal failure or platelet dysfunction may precipitate alveolar hemorrhage in patients with underlying injury to the capillary endothelium or alveolar epithelium.[7]

Alveolar Hemorrhage Complicating Bone Marrow Transplantation

Diffuse alveolar hemorrhage occurs in 3 to 31 percent of autologous or allogeneic bone marrow transplant (BMT) recipients receiving pre-BMT conditioning with high-dose chemotherapy or radiation therapy.[1,7,35,36,47] Opportunistic infections or thrombocytopenia account for some cases of alveolar hemorrhage, but a distinct syndrome of alveolar hemorrhage in this population unrelated to infection is well accepted. Risk factors for alveolar hemorrhage which have been cited include age over 40 years, underlying solid tumors, severe oral mucositis, renal failure, airway injury prior to institution of chemotherapy, increased proportions of airway (bronchial) neutrophils and eosinophils, and leukocyte recovery.[35,47] Diffuse alveolar hemorrhage usually develops within 10 to 50 days after BMT, but case reports of alveolar hemorrhage developing immediately following autologous bone marrow transfusion suggest that components within the transfusion (e.g., DMSO) may mediate acute lung injury in some cases.[35,36,47] Chest radiographs typically demonstrate bilateral infiltrates, primarily involving the perihilar, middle, and lower lung zones.[56] In one study of alveolar hemorrhage complicating BMT, the *initial* radiographic pattern was interstitial in 27 patients and alveolar in 10.[56] Chest radiographs were normal in two patients. Over time, diffuse alveolar infiltrates involving all lobes developed in 30 patients, associated with a confluent alveolar pattern in 26.[56] Serosanguinous or frankly bloody BAL fluid, with negative stains for infectious organisms, support the diagnosis of alveolar hemorrhage.[1] However, BAL fluid may be normal even in the face of severe alveolar hemorrhage.[1] The clinical course is variable, but acute, fatal respiratory failure may develop. Mortality rates in patients requiring mechanical ventilatory support typically exceed 50 percent.[35,47,56] Secondary infections are serious and potentially lethal. Coexisting pulmonary processes, most commonly diffuse alveolar damage or infections, were noted in 10 of 11 BMT recipients with alveolar hemorrhage in a recent necropsy series.[1]

Multiple mechanisms may mediate alveolar hemorrhage in this patient population. Diffuse injury to the pulmonary microvasculature, secondary to chemotherapy or radiation therapy, coupled with a heightened inflammatory response in the airways, appear to be operative.[35,47] Bleeding may be amplified by a precipitating factor such as coagulopathy, pulmonary edema, graft-versus-host disease, or infections.[1] Diffuse alveolar damage, a pathologic hallmark seen in toxic lung injury from chemotherapy, radiation therapy, or viral infections, is frequently observed in lung biopsies or necropsies in bone marrow recipients with alveolar hemorrhage.[1,35,47] An association between microangiopathy and alveolar hemorrhage in patients receiving BMT for hematologic malignancies has also been cited.[50] Neutrophils and other inflammatory cells may play important roles in the pathogenesis of alveolar hemorrhage. The onset of alveolar hemorrhage frequently coincides with marrow recovery and reappearance of neutrophils within the circulation or BAL fluid.[35,47] Influx of neutrophils may promote the lung injury by release of oxygen radicals, proteases, and other phlogistic mediators.[36,47]

Although randomized controlled studies have not been performed, a retrospective analysis of 65 episodes of alveolar hemorrhage in marrow transplant recipients noted improved survival in patients receiving high-dose corticosteroids (generally 125 to 250 mg of methylprednisolone every 6 h for the first 4 to 5 days) compared to low-dose corticosteroids (<30 mg per day methylprednisolone or equivalent) or supportive therapy.[35] Respiratory failure developed after the diagnosis of alveolar hemorrhage in 12 of 22 nonintubated patients in the high-dose group compared with 9 of 10 nonintubated patients in the other two groups. Eleven of 12 patients in the supportive therapy group and 9 of 10 patients in the low-dose steroid group died before hospital discharge. By contrast, 29 of 43 patients in the high-dose group died before discharge, a statistically significant increase in survival compared to the other two groups. The incidence of infection was no higher in patients receiving corticosteroids. These findings suggest that aggressive therapy with intravenous methylprednisone 125 to 250 mg every 6 h for 3 to 5 days, followed by oral prednisone, is reasonable.[35] Unfortunately, alveolar hem-orrhage or bloody BAL fluid may be seen in infectious causes of pneumonia (particularly due to CMV or *Aspergillus spp*), and high-dose corticosteroids could be disastrous under these circumstances. Infectious etiologies must be rigorously excluded. Among patients who respond favorably to corticosteroids, the dose can be gradually tapered over 2 to 6 weeks. A more prolonged course is appropriate for patients with graft-versus-host disease or other complications requiring long-term corticosteroid therapy.

Alveolar Hemorrhage Complicating HIV Infection

Diffuse alveolar hemorrhage can complicate human immunodeficiency virus (HIV) infection. The incidence and clinical significance of alveolar hemorrhage is not clear, as additional pulmonary processes (e.g., opportunistic infections, Kaposi's sarcoma) are usually present.[7,18] Subclinical episodes of alveolar hemorrhage are common, as recent studies in HIV-infected patients with pulmonary infiltrates have detected >20 percent hemosiderin-laden macrophages in BAL fluid in 15 to 44 percent of cases.[7,18,21] Pulmonary capillaritis has been cited in oc-

casional patients, most of whom had concomitant opportunistic infections.[18] Cytomegalovirus (CMV) pneumonitis was recently implicated as a cause of alveolar hemorrhage in five patients with acquired immune deficiency syndrome (AIDS).[18] Concomitant features included CMV viremia, multivisceral involvement, and microangiopathic intravascular hemolysis.[18] Four of five met criteria for CMV pneumonitis, with hypoxemia, diffuse pulmonary infiltrates, and lung biopsies demonstrating interstitial inflammation and viral inclusions. CMV exhibits tropism for endothelial cells, and virally infected giant cells within pulmonary endothelial cells were prominent. Schistocytes in peripheral blood likely reflected CMV vascular injury or thrombotic microangiopathy. Antiviral therapy (e.g., ganciclovir) was effective in four of five patients. Undoubtedly, opportunistic pathogens or endobronchial Kaposi's sarcoma account for the majority of cases of alveolar hemorrhage in HIV-infected individuals.[7,18,21] The incidence and appropriate therapy of alveolar hemorrhage of unknown etiology in the setting of AIDS needs to be defined in prospective studies.

Alveolar Hemorrhage due to Exogenous Agents

Certain exogenous agents or drugs (e.g., trimellitic anhydride, isocyanates, D-penicillamine, lymphangiography dye, cocaine, warfarin, prophylthiouracil) are rare causes of alveolar hemorrhage.[30,31] Glomerulonephritis has occurred in alveolar hemorrhage associated with D-penicillamine but not with the other agents.[34] Few lung biopsies have been performed in these cases of alveolar hemorrhage. Histologic findings are nonspecific. Alveolar hemorrhage dominates without immune deposits.[3,17,34,39]

Trimellitic anhydride, a chemical used in manufacturing plastics and epoxy resins, may elicit pulmonary hemorrhage and anemia. In 1979, Herbert and Oxford described seven young men (ages 18 to 21) who developed severe dyspnea, hemoptysis, anemia, and constitutional symptoms following inhalation of trimellitic anhydride (TMA) in poorly ventilated spaces.[17] All affected individuals had close contact with the powder or fumes of an epoxy resin containing TMA. All seven were hypoxemic and anemic. Bilateral pulmonary infiltrates were noted on chest radio-graphs in five. None had renal involvement. Lung biopsies revealed intraalveolar hemorrhage, hemosiderin-laden macro-phages, and nonspecific lung injury; immunofluorescent stains were negative. Six of seven received supportive therapy; one received a brief course of corticosteroids and azathioprine. All recovered within a few days following removal from the offending environment. An immune mechanism is likely, as circulating IgG antibodies against trimellitic protein have been found in some patients with alveolar hemorrhage, suggesting trimellitic anhydride acts as a hapten.[57] Trimellitic anhydride may cause asthma, rhinitis, and hemolytic anemia mediated by IgE antibodies directed against trimellitic protein.[57] Animal models of TMA-induced lung disease have also been developed.[39,57] Induction of serum antibodies against epitopes of TMA produced acute lung injury in guinea pigs, mediated by at least two types of humoral antibodies. It is also possible that TMA may exert a direct toxic effect on alveolar endothelium.

This syndrome is exceptionally rare, as only sporadic cases have been described.

In 1990, Patterson and colleagues described severe alveolar hemorrhage progressing to respiratory failure in a spray painter.[39] Microscopic hematuria was noted, but red cell casts were not detected, and renal biopsy was not performed. Open lung biopsy demonstrated extensive alveolar hemorrhage and siderophages. Immunofluorescent stains for IgG and complement were negative. Prompt recovery ensued following therapy with high-dose corticosteroids. An immune mechanism was supported by several findings: Isocyanates were present in spray paint; isocyanates react with proteins to produce an isocyanate protein conjugate; high levels of IgE and IgG antibodies against diisocyanates were detected in the patient's serum; reexposure to paint sprayed on hot metal reproduced the illness.[39] Thus, exposure to TMA or isocyanates, and possibly other chemicals, can elicit hemorrhagic pneumonitis, likely mediated by circulating antibodies (IgG or IgE) and immune complexes.[39,57]

Sporadic reports of alveolar hemorrhage and glomerulonephritis have been associated with the use of D-penicillamine, a chelating agent used to treat rheumatoid arthritis, Wilson's disease, and diverse autoimmune disorders. In seven cases, the daily dose of penicillamine was high (>1 gm), and the duration of therapy was longer than 10 months.[30,34] Serum anti-GBM antibodies were negative. Immunofluorescent stains were negative in the few lung biopsies performed.[34] Four of seven patients died.[30,34] Two patients treated with combined immunosuppression and plasmapheresis recovered completely.

Mild alveolar hemorrhage occurs in approximately 1 in 3000 patients receiving lymphangiogram dye.[31] The mechanism is not clear. A latency period of 2 to 10 days precedes the onset of dyspnea, pulmonary infiltrates, or hemoptysis. This syndrome is usually mild and self-limited, but at least one fatality has been cited.[31] Extrapulmonary involvement does not occur.

Smoking, snorting, or intravenous "crack" cocaine has been associated with hemoptysis and varying degrees of alveolar hem-orrhage, including rare fatalities. Histopathologic features of cocaine-induced alveolar hemorrhage are nonspecific. The frequency of clinically significant alveolar hemorrhage associated with inhaled or intravenous use of cocaine abuse has not been established. Bailey and colleagues recently reviewed 52 necropsies from cocaine abusers, most of whom died of accidental causes or acute cocaine overdose.[3] Histopathologic aberrations in lung tissue included acute hemorrhage (58 percent), chronic hemorrhage (40 percent), interstitial pneumonitis/fibrosis (38 percent), congestion (88 percent), and intraalveolar edema (77 percent).[3] The incidence of each of these histopathologic features was increased compared to necropsies from age-matched controls who did not abuse cocaine. Thus, alveolar hemorrhage may be common in cocaine abusers, and chronic use could lead to interstitial fibrosis. The mechanism of alveolar hemorrhage is not clear but may relate to direct toxic injury from cocaine or its contaminants, vasospasm, or a combination of both mechanisms.

When drug or hapten-induced alveolar hemorrhage is suspected, immediate avoidance of the implicated agent or drug is essential. For acute or severe cases, a brief course of high-dose

corticosteroids is warranted. Plasmapheresis or cytotoxic agents may be considered for fulminant cases refractory to corticosteroids, but data supporting their use are lacking.

Idiopathic Pulmonary Hemosiderosis

Idiopathic pulmonary hemosiderosis (IPH) is an exceptionally rare cause of alveolar hemorrhage that occurs primarily in infants and children.[5,49] Many children with IPH have a history of milk or gluten sensitivity.[4,49] A subset of adults with celiac sprue manifest IPH, which may respond to elimination of gluten from the diet.[56] Clinical features of IPH are similar to immune causes of alveolar hemorrhage, but extrapulmonary or renal involvement is lacking. Serum or tissue antibodies (including ANCA, immune complexes, anti-GBM antibody) are also absent. A diagnosis of IPH can be made *only* when other specific causes of DAH have been *reliably* excluded. The largest series of IPH, published in 1962, included 112 patients but antedated the availability of anti-GBM antibody or ANCA.[49] Antibodies to lung or kidney were assayed in only six patients. In recent years, with the advent of immunologic and serologic assays, the diagnosis of IPH has rarely been substantiated. It now seems likely that most cases formerly diagnosed as IPH in adults had ANCA-associated vasculitis, microscopic polyangiitis, or underlying collagen vascular disorders.

The clinical course of IPH is variable, but recurrent episodes of alveolar hemorrhage over several years are characteristic. Spontaneous remissions without long-term sequelae have been cited in up to 25 percent of cases.[5,49] One-third to one-half of patients die within 3 years of onset, usually from severe alveolar hemorrhage.[5,49] Sequelae of recurrent episodes of alveolar hemorrhage include pulmonary fibrosis, progressive respiratory

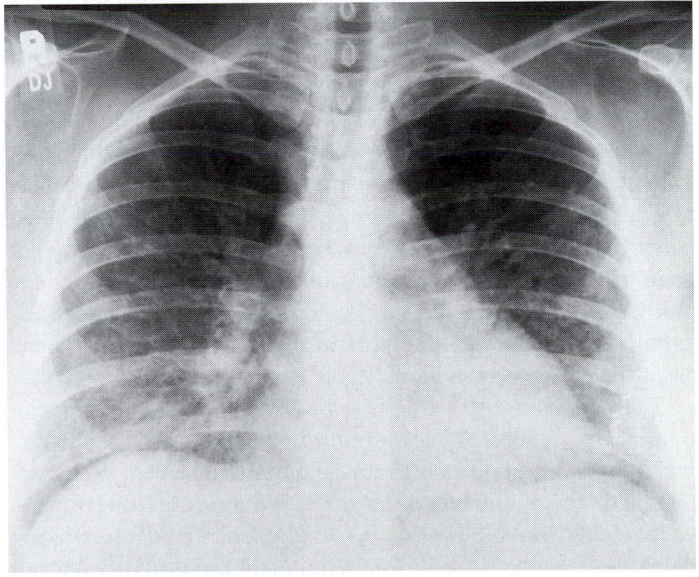

FIGURE 79-11 Idiopathic pulmonary hemosiderosis (IPH). PA chest radiograph demonstrates bilateral reticulonodular infiltrates in a 28-year-old female with idiopathic pulmonary hemosiderosis confirmed 10 years earlier by open lung biopsy. (Note the surgical staples in the left lower lobe from a prior open lung biopsy.)

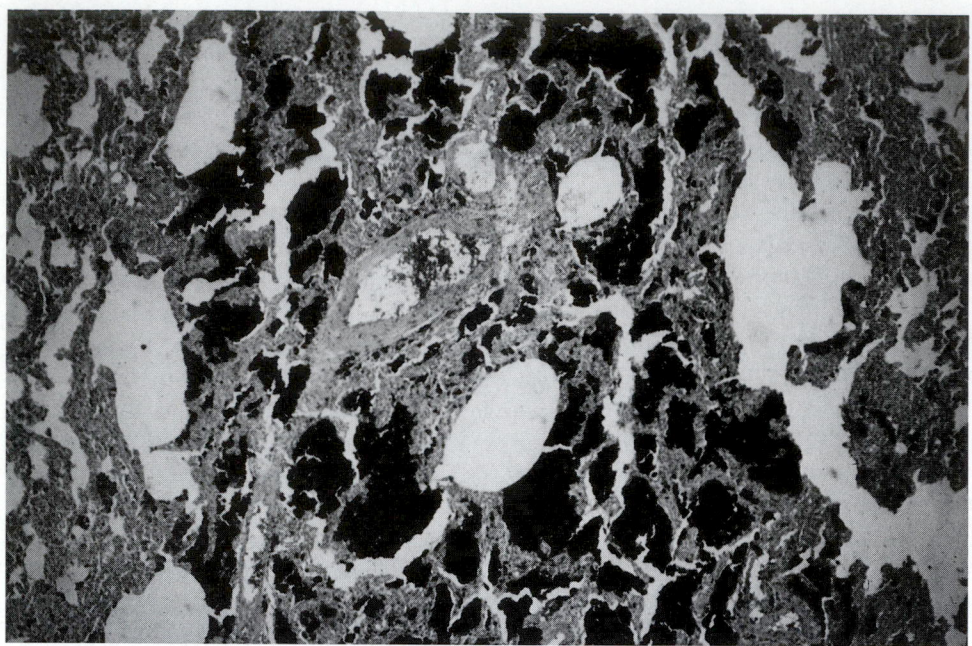

FIGURE 79-12 Idiopathic pulmonary hemosiderosis (IPH). Photomicrograph demonstrating extensive deposits of hemosiderin within alveolar interstitium (Prussian blue stain).

done. Corticosteroids are considered the mainstay of therapy,[5,49] but an epidemiologic survey of 30 children with IPH concluded that corticosteroids did not alter the long-term course or prognosis.[5] Because IPH is life-threatening, most physicians treat acute episodes with daily corticosteroids and taper to the lowest dose which appears to control the disease. Long-term (and possibly indefinite) therapy may be required to prevent recurrences. To minimize side effects, alternate dose corticosteroids should be considered after the acute hemorrhage has resolved. Anecdotal responses have been cited with azathioprine, cyclophosphamide, and plasmapheresis in patients failing corticosteroids.[6] The role of these therapeutic modalities is not clear, particularly given the heightened risk of neoplasia associated with the long-term use of cyclophosphamide. Immunosuppressive or cytotoxic agents should be reserved for patients with corticosteroid-recalcitrant disease or those experiencing serious adverse effects from corticosteroids.

failure, and cor pulmonale.[5,49] During acute episodes, chest radiographs demonstrate bilateral alveolar infiltrates.[2] Following cessation of bleeding, chest radiographs may normalize within 1 to 2 weeks. Reticulonodular infiltrates may be observed as the process is resolving or with recurrent episodes (Fig. 79-11). Computed CT reveals areas of ground glass opacification, representing foci of alveolar hemorrhage.[2] Thickening of interlobular septae and honeycombing may be observed in a subset of patients who progress to pulmonary fibrosis.[2] Hemoptysis may be absent, particularly in young children who may be unable to expectorate blood.[5,49] Iron-deficiency anemia is characteristic and can be profound.[5,49] Iron deficiency may persist despite normal total body iron stores, because hemosiderin within alveolar macrophages is not available to developing erythrocytes. Siderophages may be found in sputum, BAL fluid, or tracheal or gastric aspirates in patients with recent episodes of alveolar hemorrhage. Lung biopsies may reveal fresh areas of alveolar hemorrhage or patchy interstitial fibrosis and aggregates of hemosiderin-laden macrophages from prior episodes of alveolar hemorrhage (Fig. 79-12). Capillaritis has been described in some cases, but macroscopic vasculitis is not found.

The pathogenesis of IPH is not known. In children, associations between IPH and cow's milk hypersensitivity, celiac disease, IgA monoclonal gammopathy, autoimmune hemolytic anemia, and autoimmune thryotoxicosis have been suggested, but a pathogenetic link has not been substantiated.[5,49,57] Resolution of pulmonary symptoms following elimination of mild products or gluten from diet supports a role for exogenous factors in the pathogenesis in at least some cases.[57] No genetic basis has been found, but clusters within families have been described.[49]

In view of the rarity of IPH, optimal therapy is not clear. Controlled studies evaluating therapeutic regimens have not been

REFERENCES

1. Agusti C, Ramirez J, Picardo C, et al: Diffuse alveolar hemorrhage in allogeneic bone marrow transplantation. A postmortem study. *Am J Respir Crit Care Med* 151:1006–1110, 1995.
2. Akyar S, Ozbek SS: Computed tomography findings in idiopathic pulmonary hemosiderosis. *Respiration* 60:63–64, 1993.
3. Bailey ME, Fraire AE, Greenberg SD, et al: Pulmonary histopathology in cocaine abusers. *Hum Pathol* 25:203–207, 1994.
4. Calabrese LH, Hoffman GS, Guillevin L: Therapy of resistant systemic necrotizing vasculitis. Polyarteritis, Churg-Strauss syndrome, Wegener's granulomatosis, and hypersensitivity vasculitis group disorders. *Rheum Dis Clin North Am* 21:41–57, 1995.
5. Chryssanthopoulos C, Cassimos C, Panagiotidou C: Prognostic criteria in idiopathic pulmonary hemosiderosis in children. *Eur J Pediat* 140:123–125, 1983.
6. Columbo JL, Stolz SM: Treatment of life-threatening primary pulmonary hemosiderosis with cyclophosphamide. *Chest* 102:959–960, 1992.
7. De Lassence A, Fleury-Feith J, Escudier E, et al: Alveolar hemorrhage: Diagnostic criteria and results in 194 immunocompromised hosts. *Am J Respir Crit Care Med* 151:157–163, 1995.
8. Erickson RW, Franklin WA, Emlen W: Treatment of hemorrhagic lupus pneumonitis with plasmapheresis. *Semin Arthritis Rheum* 24:114–123, 1994.
9. Esnault VLM, Soleimani B, Keogan MT, et al: Association of IgM with IgG ANCA in patients presenting with pulmonary hemorrhage. *Kidney Int* 41:1304–1310, 1992.
10. Esnault VLM, Testa A, Jayne DRW, et al: Influence of immunoadsorption on the removal of immunoglobulin G autoantibodies in crescentic glomerulonephritis. *Nephron* 65:180–184, 1995.

11. Falk RJ, Hogan S, Carey TS, et al: Clinical course of antineutrophil cytoplasmic autoantibody-associated glomerulonephritis and systemic vasculitis. *Ann Intern Med* 113:656–663, 1990.

12. Fortin PR, Larson MG, Watters AK, et al: Prognostic factors in systemic necrotizing vasculitis of the polyarteritis nodosa group—a review of 45 cases. *J Rheumatol* 22:78–84, 1995.

13. Gaudin PB, Askin FB, Falk RJ, Jennette JC: The pathologic spectrum of pulmonary lesions in patients with anti-neutrophil cytoplasmic autoantibodies specific for anti-proteinase 3 and anti-myeloperoxidase. *Am J Clin Pathol* 104:7–16, 1995.

14. Gertner E, Lie JT: Pulmonary capillaritis, alveolar hemorrhage, and recurrent microvascular thrombosis in primary antiphospholipid syndrome. *J Rheumatol* 20:1224–1228, 1993.

15. Guillevin L, Lhote F, Gayraud M, et al: Prognostic factors in polyarteritis nodosa and Churg-Strauss syndrome. *Medicine* (Baltimore) 75:17–28, 1996.

16. Haworth SJ, Savage CO, Carr D, et al: Pulmonary hemorrhage complicating Wegener's granulomatosis and microscopic polyarteritis. *Br Med J* 290:1175–1178, 1985.

17. Herbert FA, Orford R: Pulmonary hemorrhage and edema due to inhalation of resins containing tri-mellitic anhydride. *Chest* 76:546–551, 1979.

18. Herry I, Cadranel J, Antoine M, et al: Cytomegalovirus-induced alveolar hemorrhage in patients with AIDS: A new clinical entity? *Clin Infect Dis* 22:616–620, 1996.

19. Hoffman GS, Kerr GS, Leavitt RY, et al: Wegener's granulomatosis: an analysis of 158 patients. *Ann Intern Med* 116:488–498, 1992.

20. Holdsworth S, Boyce N, Thomson NM, Atkins RC: The clinical spectrum of acute glomerulonephritis and lung haemorrhage (Goodpasture's syndrome). *Q J Med* 216:75–86, 1985.

21. Hughes-Davies L, Kocjan G, Spittle MF, Miller RF: Occult alveolar haemorrhage in bronchopulmonary Kaposi's sarcoma. *J Clin Pathol* 45:536–537, 1992.

22. Jayne DRW, Davies MJ, Fow CJV, et al: Treatment of systemic vasculitis with pooled intravenous immunoglobulin. *Lancet* 337:1137–1139, 1991.

23. Jennette JC, Falk RJ, Andrassy K, et al: Nomenclature of systemic vasculitides. *Arthritis Rheum* 37:187–192, 1994.

24. Johnson JP, Moore J, Austin AA, et al: Therapy of anti-glomerular basement membrane antibody disease: analysis of prognostic significance of clinical, pathologic, and treatment factors. *Medicine* (Baltimore) 64:219–227, 1985.

25. Kahn FW, Jones JM, England DM: Diagnosis of pulmonary hemorrhage in the immunocompromised host. *Am Rev Respir Dis* 136:155–160, 1987.

26. Kallenberg CGM, Brouwer E, Weening JJ, Cohen-Tervaert JW: Antineutrophil cytoplasmic antibodies: Current diagnostic and pathophysiological potential. *Kidney Int* 46:1–15, 1994.

27. Kelly PT, Haponik EF: Goodpasture's syndrome: molecular and clinical advances. *Medicine* (Baltimore) 73:171–185, 1994.

28. Kerr G, Fleisher TA, Hallahan CW, et al: Limited prognostic value of changes in anti-neutrophil cytoplasmic antibody titer in patients with Wegener's granulomatosis. *Arthritis Rheum* 36:365–371, 1993.

29. Lanham JG, Elkon KB, Pusey CD, et al: Systemic vasculitis with asthma and eosinophilia: a clinical approach to the Churg-Strauss Syndrome. *Medicine* (Baltimore) 63:65–81, 1984.

30. Leatherman J: Autoimmune diffuse alveolar hemorrhage. *Clin Pulm Med* 1:356–364, 1994.

31. Leatherman JW, Davies SF, Hoidal JR: Alveolar hemorrhage syndromes. Diffuse microvascular lung hemorrhage in immune and idiopathic disorders. *Medicine* (Baltimore) 63:343–361, 1984.

32. Lechleither P, Defregger M, Lhotta K, et al: Goodpasture's syndrome: unusual presentation after exposure to hard metal dust. *Chest* 103:956–957, 1993.

33. Lombard CM, Colby TV, Elliott CG: Surgical pathology of the lung in anti-basement membrane antibody-associated Goodpasture's syndrome. *Hum Pathol* 20:445–451, 1989.

34. Louie S, Gamble C, Cross C: Penicillamine associated pulmonary hemorrhage. *J Rheumatol* 13:963–966, 1986.

35. Metcalf JP, Rennard SI, Reed EC, et al: Corticosteroids as adjunctive therapy for diffuse alveolar hemorrhage associated with bone marrow transplantation. *Am J Med* 96:327–334, 1994.

36. Mulder POM, Meinesz A, DeVries EGE, Mulder NH: Diffuse alveolar hemorrhage in autologous bone marrow transplant recipients. *Am J Med* 90:278–280, 1991.

37. Myers JL, Katzenstein AA: Microangiitis in lupus-induced pulmonary hemorrhage. *Am J Clin Pathol* 85:552–556, 1985.

38. Orens J, Martinez FJ, Lynch JP III: Pulmonary manifestations of systemic lupus erythematosus. *Rheum Dis Clin North Am* 20:159–193, 1994.

39. Patterson R, Nugent KM, Harris KE, Eberle ME: Immunologic hemorrhagic pneumonia caused by isocyanates. *Am Rev Respir Dis* 141:226–230, 1990.

40. Primack SL, Miller RR, Muller NL: Diffuse pulmonary hemorrhage: Clinical, pathologic, and imaging features. *Am J Roentgenol* 164:295–300, 1995.

41. Pusey CD, Rees AJ, Evans DJ, et al: Plasma exchange in focal necrotizing glomerulonephritis without anti-GBM antibodies. *Kidney Int* 40:757–763, 1991.

42. Rao JK, Weinberger M, Oddone EZ, et al: The role of antineutrophil cytoplasmic antibody (c-ANCA) testing in the diagnosis of Wegener's granulomatosis. A literature review and meta-analysis. *Ann Intern Med* 123:925–932, 1995.

43. Reznik VM, Griswold WR, Lemire JM, Mendoza SA: Pulmonary hemorrhage in children with glomerulonephritis. *Pediatr Nephrol* 9:83–86, 1995.

44. Savage COS, Winearls CG, Evans DJ, et al: Microscopic polyarteritis: Presentation, pathology, and prognosis. *Q J Med* 56:467–483, 1985.

45. Saxena R, Bygren P, Arvaston B, Wieslander J: Circulating autoantibodies as serological markers in the differential diagnosis of pulmonary renal syndrome. *J Int Med* 238:143–152, 1995.

46. Schwarz MI, Sutarik JM, Nick JA, et al: Pulmonary capillaritis and diffuse alveolar hemorrhage: A primary manifestation of polymyositis. *Am J Resp Crit Care Med* 151:2037–2040, 1995.

47. Sisson JH, Thompson AB, Anderson JR, et al: Airway inflammation predicts diffuse alveolar hemorrhage during bone marrow transplantation in patients with Hodgkin's disease. *Am Rev Respir Dis* 146:439–443, 1992.

48. Sneller MC, Hoffman GS, Talar-Williams C, et al: An analysis of forty-two Wegener's granulomatosis patients treated with methotrexate and prednisone. *Arthritis Rheum* 38:608–613, 1995.

49. Soergel KH, Sommers SC: Idiopathic pulmonary hemosiderosis and related syndromes. *Am J Med* 32:499–511, 1962.

50. Srivastava A, Gottlieb D, Bradstock KF: Diffuse alveolar hemorrhage associated with microangiopathy after allogeneic bone marrow transplantation. *Bone Marrow Transplant* 15:863–867, 1995.

51. Stegeman CA, Cohen Tervaert JV, de Jong PE, et al: Trimethoprim-sulfamethoxazole (co-trimoxazole) for the prevention of relapses of Wegener's granulomatosis. *New Engl J Med* 335:16–20, 1996.

52. Travis WD, Colby TV, Lombard C, et al: A clinicopathologic study of 34 cases of diffuse pulmonary hemorrhage with lung biopsy confirmation. *Am J Surg Pathol* 14:1112–1125, 1990.

53. Tuso P, Moudgil A, Hay J, et al: Treatment of antineutrophil cyto-plasmic antibody-positive systemic vasculitis and glomerulo-nephritis with pooled intravenous gammaglobulin. *Am J Kidney Dis* 20:504–508, 1992.

54. Watts RA, Carruthers DM, Scott DG: Epidemiology of systemic vasculitis: changing incidence or definition? *Semin Arthritis Rheum* 25:28–34, 1995.

55. Weber MFA, Andrassy K, Pullig O, et al: Antineutrophil-cytoplas-mic antibodies and antiglomerular basement membrane antibodies in Goodpasture's syndrome and in Wegener's granulomatosis. *J Am Soc Nephrol* 2:1227–1234, 1992.

56. Witte RJ, Gurney JW, Robbins RA, et al: Diffuse pulmonary hem-orrhage after bone marrow transplantation: Radiographic findings in 39 patients. *Am J Roentgenol* 157:461–464, 1991.

57. Wright PH, Menzies IS, Pouder RE, Keeling PWN: Adult idiopathic pulmonary hemosiderosis and celiac disease. *Q J Med* 50:95–102, 1981.

58. Zeiss CR, Wolkonsky P, Chacon R, et al: Syndromes in workers ex-posed to trimellitic anhydride. *Ann Intern Med* 98:8–12, 1983.

MECHANISMS OF ASPIRATION DISORDERS

Keith M. Robinson / Richard D. Zorowitz

Aspiration involves a spectrum of clinical situations, from laryngeal penetration to frank pulmonary aspiration. Aspiration presumes that the airways and lungs become soiled with nongaseous materials including consistencies that are solid or liquid, caustic or bland, infected or sterile. Pulmonary aspiration can involve segmental or lobar areas of the lung, can be associated with either focal or diffuse inflammatory reactions, and can evolve to include systemic effects such as bacteremia, sepsis, end-organ consequences of hypoxia, and death.[10,17,29,43] *Aspiration pneumonitis* implies the presence of an inflammatory response to aspirated material not associated with infection, whereas *aspiration pneumonia* implies the presence of infection with pneumonitis.[10]

Aspiration may be categorized by several different schema. For instance, aspiration may be described in terms of the degree of the event.[43] *Microaspiration* reflects the entry of subclinical amounts of bacterial and nonbacterial matter into the tracheobronchial tree but may predispose a patient to a more serious event. *Macroaspiration* involving the entry of nonendogenous materials into the lung from oropharyngeal or gastrointestinal sources represents the more serious clinical situation.

Aspiration also may be described as a function of oropharyngeal, esophageal, and gastrointestinal disorders with neuromuscular or mechanical (obstructive) etiologies. Further, medical or surgical interventions meant to treat conditions related or unrelated to swallowing or ventilation unintentionally may cause aspiration and should be considered separately from organic conditions. With an understanding of the normal anatomy and physiology of the larynx, pharynx, esophagus, stomach, and in-

testine, the clinician may better identify the mechanisms of aspiration and the preventable strategies which minimize aspiration and its complications.

NORMAL ANATOMY AND PHYSIOLOGY OF THE AERODIGESTIVE PASSAGE

Aspiration occurs when the integrity of the neuromuscular system used for swallowing becomes altered or impaired anatomically or physiologically (Figs. 80-1 and 80-2). Deglutition is a neurogenically controlled phenomenon requiring intricate cognitive and motor control, integration of sensory information, and multiple levels of central and peripheral reflexic control. Normal deglutition consists of four phases: (1) *oral preparatory;* (2) *oral;* (3) *pharyngeal;* and (4) *esophageal.* A list of the muscles, their innervations and functions, and the phases in which they are associated is found in Table 80-1.

During the *oral preparatory* phase (Fig. 80-3A), food is manipulated in the mouth and masticated if necessary. Mastication involves a repeated cyclical pattern of rotary lateral movement of the labial and mandibular musculature. Some food normally falls into the pharynx during this phase but does not enter the respiratory tree.[32] Once broken down into particles, food is collected into a bolus and held anterolaterally by the tongue against the palate.

During the *oral* phase (Fig. 80-3B), the tongue volitionally propels food posteriorly until the pharyngeal swallow is triggered in the area of the anterior faucial arches, located in the posterior aspect of the mouth. A labial seal is maintained to prevent food or liquid from leaking from the mouth. Tension of the buccal musculature prevents food from falling into the lateral sulci between the mandible and the cheek. The tongue elevates sequentially in an anterior-posterior direction and propels the bolus into the pharynx.[33] The oral phase lasts approximately 1 s and is mediated through cranial nerves VII and XII.

During the *pharyngeal* phase (Fig. 80-3C), the pharyngeal swallow is triggered and moves the bolus through the pharynx. Except for breath holding, the pharyngeal phase of swallowing is the only time during which the larynx is protected directly against aspiration. The pharyngeal swallow is triggered when the bolus passes the anterior faucial arches so that posterior movement of the bolus is not interrupted.[22,30] The soft palate (velum) is elevated and retracted, and the velopharyngeal port is com-

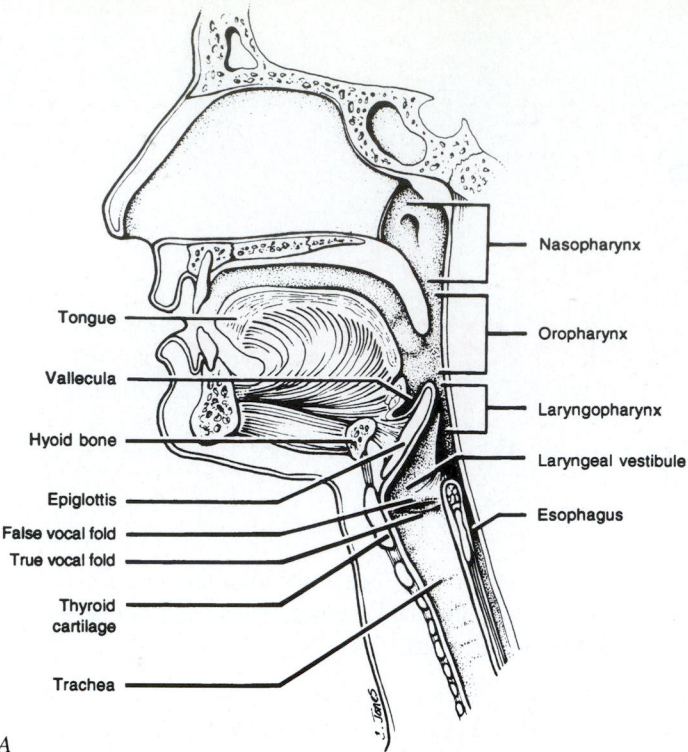

A

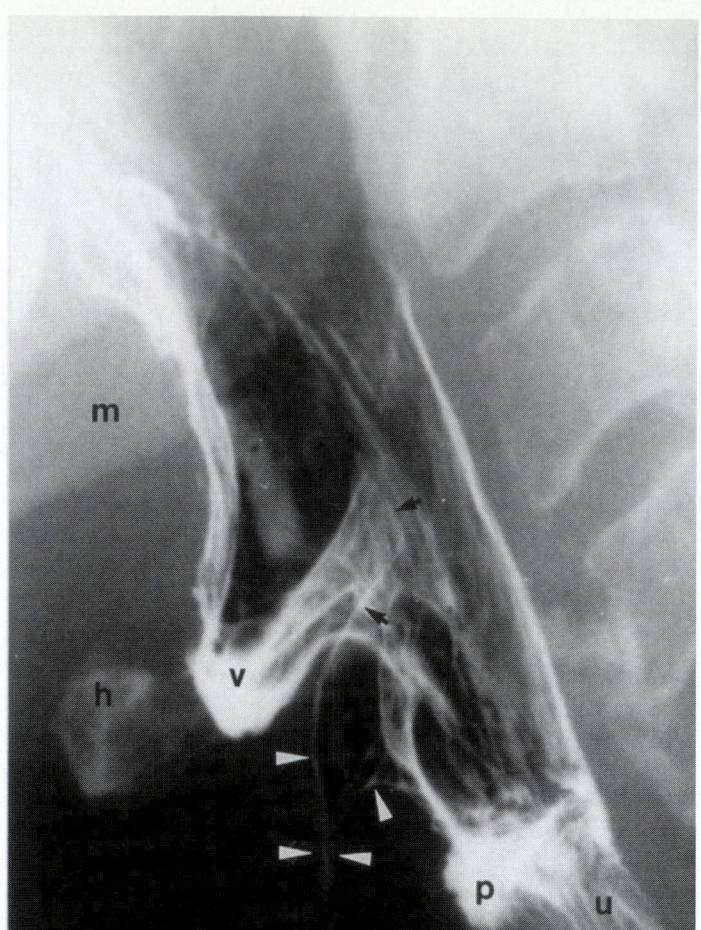

B

FIGURE 80-1 Lateral view of pharynx. *A.* Schematic view. *B.* Radiographic view. This view focuses on structures below the level of the mandible (m). The epiglottis (black arrows) tilts downward during a normal swallow but is not necessary for protection of the airway. It separates the valleculae (v) from the laryngeal vestibule (white arrows) and is tilted upward during the resting state. The valleculae and piriform sinuses (p) are sites for residue which may be aspirated when pharyngeal weakness is present. The upper esophageal sphincter (u) is actively contracted, and the hyoid bone (h) is in its resting position.

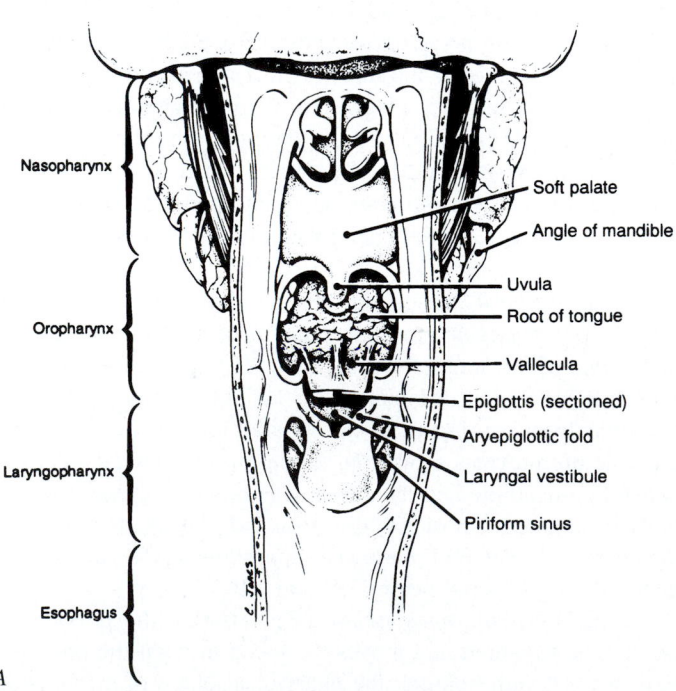

A

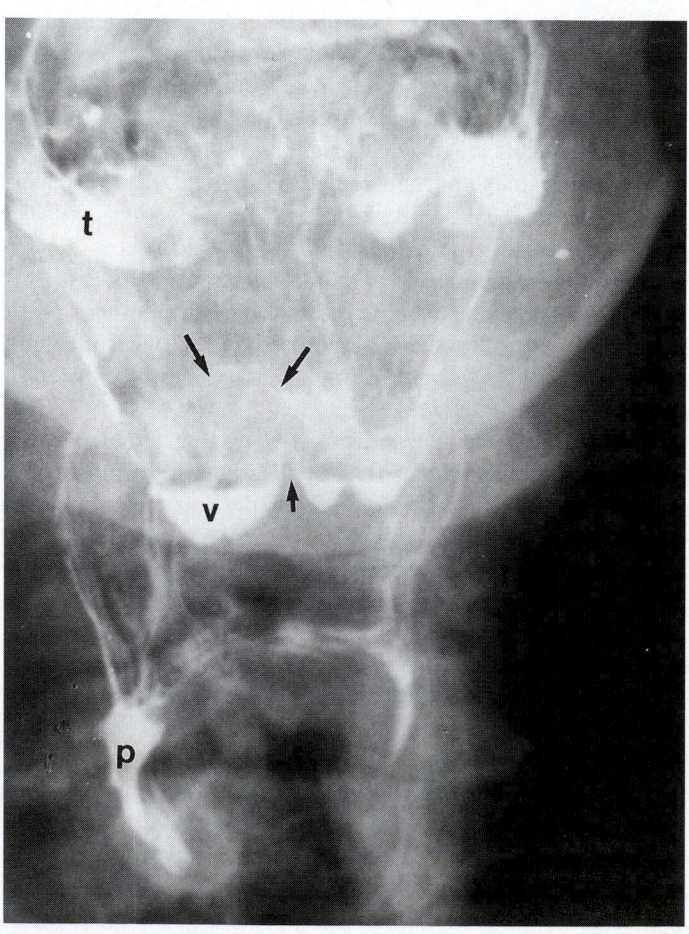

B

FIGURE 80-2 Anteroposterior view of pharynx. *A.* Schematic view. *B.* Radiographic view. The tonsillar pillars (t) are visualized in this view. The median glossoepiglottic fold (small arrow) delineates the two cup–shaped valleculae (v). The epiglottis (large arrows) appears as an inverted U. The piriform sinuses (p) lay along the anterior wall of the mid-hypopharynx.

TABLE 80-1

Muscles Involved in Swallowing

Muscle	Nerve	Stage	Action
Temporalis	V	OP	Elevates, retracts mandible
Masseter	V	OP	Elevates mandible
Pterygoideus medialis	V	OP	Elevates, protracts mandible
Pterygoideus lateralis	V	OP	Depresses, protracts mandible; moves mandible laterally
Obicularis oris	VII	OP,O	Opens, closes, protracts lips
Zygomaticus major	VII	OP,O	Elevates mouth angle upward, backward
Levator labii superioris	VII	OP,O	Elevates upper lip, mouth angle
Depressor labii inferioris	VII	OP,O	Depresses lower lip
Levator anguli oris	VII	OP,O	Elevates mouth angle
Depressor anguli oris	VII	OP,O	Depresses mouth angle
Mentalis	VII	OP,O	Elevates, protracts lower lip
Risorius	VII	OP,O	Retracts mouth angle
Buccinator	VII	OP,O	Flattens, retracts cheek, mouth angle
Hyoglossus	XII	OP,P	Depresses tongue
Genioglossus	XII	OP,P	Depresses, protrudes tongue
Musculus uvulae	IX,X,XI	O	Elevates uvula
Palatoglossus	IX,X,XI	O	Elevates posterior tongue; narrows fauces
Levator veli palatini	IX,X,XI	P	Elevates soft palate
Tensor veli palatini	V	P	Stretches soft palate
Mylohyoideus	V	P	Elevates tongue base, mouth floor, hyoid bone; depresses mandible
Digastricus	V	P	Elevates hyoid bone, tongue base
Geniohyoideus	XII,C1	P	Elevates hyoid bone, tongue
Stylohyoideus	VII	P	Elevates hyoid, tongue base
Thyrohyoideus	XII,C1	P	Depresses larynx, hyoid bone Elevates thyroid cartilage
Styloglossus	XII	P	Elevates, retracts tongue
Palatopharyngeus	IX,X,XI	P	Narrows oropharynx; elevates pharynx
Stylopharyngeus	IX	P	Elevates, dilates pharynx
Salpingopharyngeus	IX,X,XI	P	Elevates nasopharynx
Aryepiglotticus	IX,X	P	Tilts epiglottis downward
Cricoarytenoideus lateralis	IX,X	P	Closes glottis, approximates vocal folds
Thyreoarytenoideus	IX,X	P	Closes glottis, shortens vocal folds
Constrictor pharyngeus superioris	IX,X,XI	P	Compresses pharynx
Constrictor pharyngeus intermedius	IX,X,XI	P	Compresses pharynx
Constrictor pharyngeus inferioris	X,XI	P	Compresses pharynx
Cricopharyngeus	X	P	Closes upper esophageal sphincter

OP = oral preparatory stage; O = oral stage; P = pharyngeal stage.

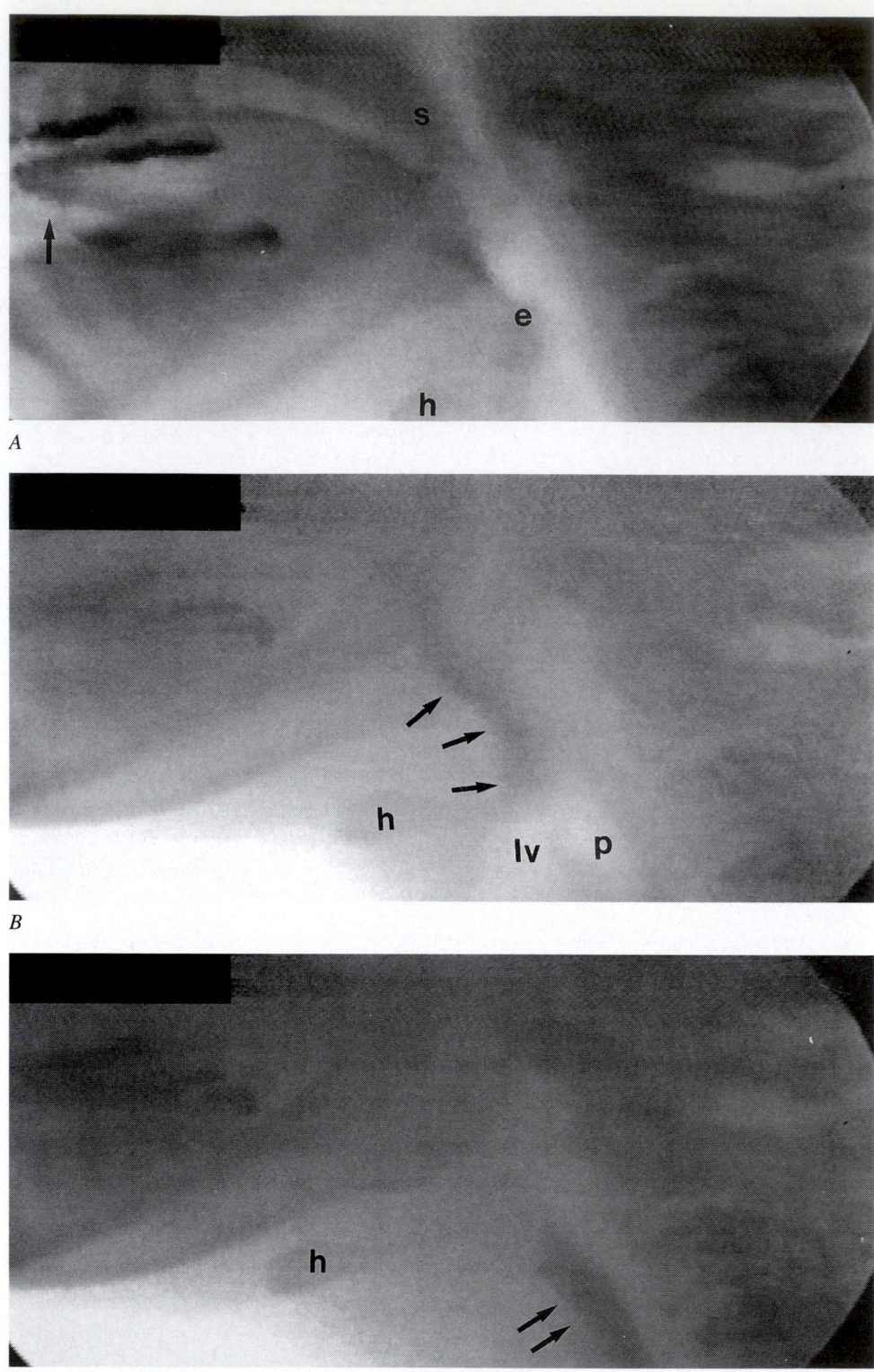

FIGURE 80-3 Phases of deglutition. *A.* Oral preparatory phase. The barium bolus (solid arrow) is masticated using a repeated cyclical pattern of rotary lateral movement of the labial and mandibular musculature. The soft palate (s) is not elevated to allow breathing. The hyoid bone (h) is positioned well below the mandible, and the epiglottis (e) is tilted upward. *B.* Oral phase. The bolus (arrows) has been pushed into the pharynx by elevation and posterior propulsion of the tongue. The soft palate contacts with the posterior pharyngeal wall to obliterate the velopharyngeal port and prevent nasal regurgitation. The hyoid bone (h) is still in its resting position, and the laryngeal vestibule (lv) and hypopharynx (p) are still visible. *C.* Pharyngeal phase. The pharyngeal constrictor muscles shorten and elevate the pharynx while the base of the tongue pushes the bolus toward the esophagus. The nasal passages are still sealed. The hyoid bone (h) is in its most superior and anterior position, correlating with closure of the larynx and the true vocal, false vocal, and ariepiglottic folds. The laryngeal vestibule is closed and cannot be visualized. The upper esophageal sphincter has relaxed, thus allowing the bolus (arrows) to pass into the esophagus.

pletely closed to prevent material from entering the nasal cavity. The true vocal folds, false vocal folds, and aryepiglottic folds close to prevent material from entering the trachea. The larynx and hyoid bone elevate and move forward, relaxing the cricopharyngeus muscle, also known as the upper esophageal sphincter (UES).[20] The tongue pushes the bolus posteriorly and downward through the pharynx, which shortens through elevation of the hypopharynx.[39] Pharyngeal contraction causes a stripping action which minimizes pharyngeal residue.[26] Sensory receptors of the faucial arches, tonsils, soft palate, tongue base, and posterior pharyngeal wall transmits messages centrally through cranial nerve VII[6] and through the superior laryngeal nerve via the tractus solitarius.[35] Motor impulses are mediated through cranial nerves IX and X.[21] The pharyngeal phase lasts approximately 1 s during liquid swallows but may be longer in normal adults for solid consistencies.

The tracheobronchial tree normally provides protection against foreign matter by a medullary reflex arc, mediated through the vagus nerve, which produces a cough. The larynx and carina are especially sensitive to irritation, and the terminal bronchioles and alveoli are very sensitive to corrosive chemical stimuli, such as chlorine. Activation of the reflex results in a deep breath; closure of the epiglottis and vocal folds; forceful contraction of the abdominal and internal intercostal muscles; opening of the epiglottis and vocal folds; and a strong compression of the lungs resulting in air velocities as high as 75 to 100 miles per hour. The generated cough usually extracts any foreign matter present in the respiratory tree.

During the *esophageal* phase, the bolus moves from the pharynx to the stomach. When the bolus reaches the gastroesophageal junction, the lower esophageal sphincter (LES) relaxes, allowing the bolus to enter the stomach. The esophagus consists of striated muscle in the upper third and smooth muscle in the lower two-thirds. The esophagus is innervated throughout its length by two nerve networks: *myenteric* (Auerbach's) and *submucosal* (Meissner's). The myenteric plexus serves as a relay between smooth muscle and the vagus nerve, but its function with respect to striated muscle is unclear. The submucosal plexus primarily controls gastrointestinal secretion and local blood flow.

Active movement within the esophagus occurs by peristalsis. For peristalsis to be effective, contractions must be orderly and sequential from the superior end of the esophagus caudally to the gastroesophageal sphincter. Adequate saliva must be present to propel the bolus toward the stomach. Different types of contractions assist with bolus propulsion. *Primary peristalsis,* which is initiated by a pharyngeal swallow, is the chief mechanism to carry a bolus through the esophagus. Primary peristalsis also produces a stripping wave to empty refluxed gastric contents back into the stomach. If the bolus does not empty into the stomach by primary peristalsis, esophageal distention activates *secondary peristalsis,* which is mediated intrinsically by the myenteric plexus and does not require vagal input. Secondary peristalsis also assists in transport of bicarbonate-containing saliva produced in the mouth to the distal esophagus, where it neutralizes any remaining gastric acid refluxed into the esophagus. In pathologic conditions, nonperistaltic contractions known as *tertiary contractions* may occur and are nonfunctional in the transport process. High-amplitude tertiary contractions causing esophageal spasm usually are perceived as one form of noncardiac chest pain.

The esophagus contains a number of protective mechanisms against reflux and aspiration. First, the tonic contractions of the UES and LES act as physical barriers against gastric contents during the resting state. Pressures in the UES range up to 250 to 350 mmHg in the anteroposterior direction and 80 to 120 mmHg in the lateral direction.[47] In the LES, pressures up to 10 to 30 mmHg relative to intragastric pressure have been recorded and prevent movement between the positive pressure of the abdomen and the negative pressure of the chest. Second, a small portion of the distal esophagus adjacent to the LES is located in the abdomen. Positive intraabdominal pressure tends to keep the stomach and lower esophagus collapsed thereby preventing the transit of boluses into the intrathoracic esophagus. Third, the esophagus enters into the stomach at an acute angle (angle of His) which acts as a one-way valve. The angle decreases when deep inspiration causes descent of the diaphragm and gastric fundus. Even so, the right crus of the diaphragm usually contracts at the same time, preventing reflux by occluding the esophageal lumen.

In addition to afferent and efferent paths, the neural organization of swallowing consists of two centers. One is thought to be located in two regions of the pontine reticular formation:[21] i.e., (1) dorsal, including the nucleus of the solitary tract and adjacent reticular formation, and (2) ventral, corresponding to the lateral reticular formation above the nucleus ambiguus. The dorsal portion appears to initiate and organize the swallowing motor sequence. The ventral portion distributes the motor impulses to the various motor neurons involved with swallowing. In animals, stimulation of the solitary tract or its nucleus in the cat,[35] rat,[27] or sheep[16] can elicit a swallow.

A second swallowing center has been described just anterior to the orbital gyrus in the occipital lobe.[12,22] In animals, single-pulse stimulation of this cortical center causes rhythmic activation of the ipsilateral nucleus of the solitary tract, resulting in a rapid decrease of the frequency of deglutition. Each cortical center is thought to receive information from its contralateral cortical center and oropharyngeal and laryngeal receptors. The center's purpose is not well understood but may be important for repeated swallowing[12] or initiation of the motor sequence of deglutition.[21]

Swallowing is integrated with ventilation so that a bolus inadvertently does not enter the lower respiratory tract. Swallowing usually interrupts the expiratory phase of ventilation, and the completion of expiration occurs at the conclusion of the swallow.[38] If a swallow is initiated during the inspiratory phase of ventilation, inspiration is terminated, and a short expiration usually follows the completion of the swallow. Tidal volume may increase in the breaths following the swallow.[50]

Vomiting, which is diametrically opposed to swallowing, normally should not result in aspiration because of protective mechanisms observed during this reflex. Vomiting can be stimulated from several sources (Table 80-2). Stimuli reach the vomiting center, located bilaterally in the medulla near the tractus solitarius at the level of the dorsal motor nucleus of the vagus nerve. Activation of the vomiting reflex results in a deep breath; elevation of the hyoid bone and larynx with UES opening; glottic and velopharyngeal port closure; simultaneous contraction of the diaphragm and abdominal wall musculature to increase intra-

TABLE 80-2

Afferent Input Involved in Vomiting

Symptom	Source
GI tract irritation and overdistention	Vagal, sympathetic afferents
Drugs (e.g. narcotics, digoxin)	Chemoreceptor trigger zone
Vestibular stimuli	Labyrinth, vestibular nuclei, cerebellum, chemoreceptor trigger zone
Psychic stimuli (visual, auditory)	Cerebral, unknown origin

gastric pressure; and LES relaxation resulting in explusion of gastric contents through the esophagus.

NEUROMUSCULAR MECHANISMS

Dysfunction of the central nervous system, lower sensorimotor neurons, neuromuscular junction, or muscle cells may result in aspiration. Neuromuscular disorders may cause sensory impairment or motor weakness or incoordination which hinders or circumvents the normal protective mechanisms of the gastroesophageal and tracheobronchial systems. Conditions affecting cognitive function may significantly impair intellectual controls which allow swallowing mechanisms to guide boluses safely toward the stomach. Etiologies of aspiration by neuromuscular mechanisms may be divided into two types: (1) dysphagia and (2) gastroesophageal reflux.

Dysphagia

Dysphagia, or swallowing difficulty, refers to symptoms manifested by a disease state but is not itself a disease. However, dysphagia is a convenient way to categorize certain neuromuscular disorders causing aspiration, since aspiration is a serious and prominent manifestation of swallowing problems. Swallowing difficulties resulting in aspiration occur in a variety of neuromuscular disorders (Table 80-3). Many of these conditions result in abnormalities affecting more than one phase of swallowing.

One framework for understanding swallowing and dysphagia involves *adaptation, compensation,* and *decompensation* of deglutition.[3] Normal swallowing involves continuous adaptation of motor function in response to the ongoing conditions during each swallow such as bolus size and consistency, head and neck position, and changes in pharyngeal diameter at different phases of respiration and phonation. When swallowing is impaired, compensation can be observed as a supranormal, protective or reserve ability to prevent aspiration. Compensation involves a variety of voluntary strategies such as chewing food more thoroughly or limiting bolus size, as well as involuntary processes such as contraction of the superior constrictor muscles to close the velopharyngeal opening in the setting of palatal deficiency or kinking of the soft palate in apposition to weak or atrophied

TABLE 80-3

Examples of Neuromuscular Conditions Causing Aspiration

Upper motor neuron
  Stroke
  Traumatic brain injury
  Parkinsonism
  Multiple sclerosis
  Huntington's disease
  Alzheimer's disease
  Neurosyphilis
  Encephalitis
  Meningitis
  Spinocerebellar degeneration
  Olivopontocerebellar atrophy
  Progressive supranuclear palsy
Lower motor neuron
  Poliomyelitis
  Amyotrophic lateral sclerosis (ALS)
  Guillian-Barré syndrome
  Polyneuritis
Neuromuscular junction
  Myaesthenia gravis
  Botulism
  Eaton-Lambert syndrome
Muscle
  Polymyositis
  Dermatomyositis
  Muscular dystrophies—Duchenne (DMD), limb-girdle (LGMD), myotonic (MD), facioscapulohumeral (FSHMD)
  Spinal muscular atrophy (SMA)
  Scleroderma and collagen vascular diseases
  Achalasia
  Metabolic myopathy

tongue to prevent premature leakage and laryngeal penetration. When compensatory strategies fail, decompensation or failure of the swallowing apparatus results. Decompensation occurs both from singular or multiple compromises in adaptational and compensatory mechanisms, including global suppression of the swallowing mechanism by fatigue or impairment of consciousness. Symptoms which are consistent with dysphagia and possible clinical indicators of aspiration are summarized in Table 80-4.

Mechanisms of aspiration due to dysphagia usually are classified temporally with respect to the onset of the pharyngeal swallow.[33] Aspiration *before* the swallow is related to abnormalities in the oral or pharyngeal phases (Fig 80-4). Weak or abnormal tongue movements may cause premature spillage of the bolus into the pharynx. A lesion of the nucleus ambiguus or the brainstem or cortical swallowing centers may result in delay or absence of the onset of the pharyngeal swallow. In either case, the

TABLE 80-4

Symptoms of Dysphagia

Dry mouth
Drooling
Nasal regurgitation
Vomiting
Difficulty clearing phlegm
Postnasal drip
Globus (obstruction)
Odynophagia (pain in throat, chest, or stomach)
Exhaustion after eating or drinking
Dysphonia with or without "wet" voice
Dyspnea
Coughing or choking while eating or drinking
Mouth odor
Heartburn
Chest pain
Weight loss

pharynx is unprepared to transport the bolus safely into the esophagus. The bolus may enter the unprotected trachea, progressing into the bronchial tree if no protective cough is elicited.

Aspiration *during* the swallow usually reflects dysfunction of the laryngeal and pharyngeal musculature (Fig 80-5). Reduced elevation of the larynx and pharynx results from impaired hyoid bone elevation or thyrohyoid or palatopharngeal dysfunction and

may cause defective closure of the laryngeal vestibule. Vocal cord paresis or paralysis may produce an incompetent laryngotracheal port through which food or liquid boluses may pass.

Aspiration *after* the swallow can represent problems in the pharyngeal and esophageal phases of deglutition (Fig 80-6). Weakness of the pharyngeal constrictor muscles may produce residue of the bolus in the valleculae or piriform sinuses, which subsequently spills into the laryngeal vestibule and trachea. The UES may fail to open due to impaired relaxation or distensibility, hypertrophy or hyperplasia, or fibrosis (Fig 80-7). The obstruction may cause filling of the hypopharynx and overflow into the airway.

Similarly, the LES may remain contracted due to defective innervation of the smooth muscle of the esophagus and LES resulting in achalasia (Fig. 80-8). The primary etiology of achalasia usually is idiopathic, but secondary causes may include gastric carcinoma extending to the esophagus, lymphoma, Chagas's disease, irradiation, and certain medications and toxins. Patients with achalasia may experience dysphagia, chest pain, and regurgitation, but pulmonary aspiration may occur due to overflow of saliva and ingested food lodged in the esophagus.

Cerebral lesions can interrupt voluntary control of the preparatory and oral phases. Cortical lesions involving the precentral gyrus may produce contralateral impairment in facial, lip, and tongue motor control and contralateral compromise in pharyngeal peristalsis.[53] A patient with impairments in cognitive function such as concentration or selective attention may not fully masticate food boluses. Oral apraxia seen in stroke or Alzheimer's dementia may result in nonpurposeful sequencing of food by the tongue, lips, and teeth.[19] The bradyphrenia and bradykinesis of Parkinson's disease may challenge attentional vigilance during eating and slow pharyngeal transit.[4,19] In all these cases, boluses may spill prematurely into an open airway due to abnormal or absent lingual control.

Brain-stem lesions may result in compromised sensation of the mouth, tongue, and cheek, delay or absence of the pharyngeal reflex, reduced laryngeal elevation and vocal cord adduction with incomplete glottic closure, and poor cricopharyngeal relaxation.[53] In stroke, for example, a delay or absence of the pharyngeal swallow may cause a bolus to enter an unprotected airway even when the oral stage is normal. Pharyngeal weakness allows accumulation of residue in the valleculae and piriform sinuses which may spill into the larynx after the swallow. In Parkinson's disease, failure of pharyngeal peristalsis by contraction of the pharyngeal constrictors against an unrelaxed cricopharyngeus results in trapping a food bolus in a high-pressure

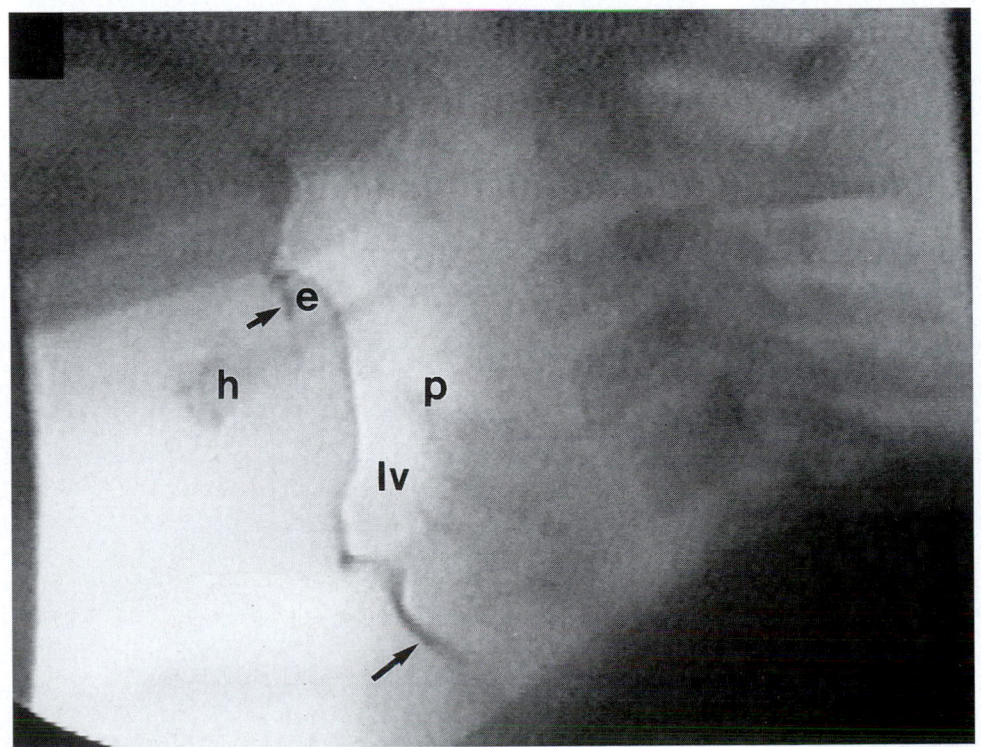

FIGURE 80-4   Aspiration before the swallow. Because of poor lingual control, a liquid bolus has spilled into the vallecula (small arrow), through the laryngeal vestibule (lv), and into the trachea (large arrow). The hyoid bone (h) and epiglottis (e) remain in their resting positions, and the laryngeal vestibule (lv) remains open. The hypopharynx (p) ends at the contracted upper esophageal sphincter.

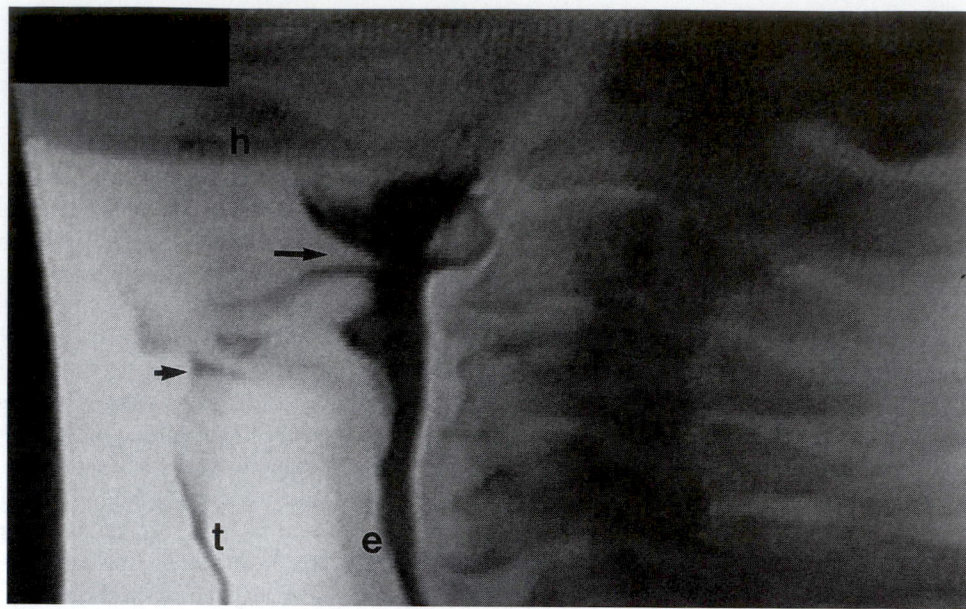

FIGURE 80-5   Aspiration during the swallow. Because of pharyngeal weakness represented in part by partial deflection of the epiglottis (long arrow), a portion of a liquid bolus enters the largyngeal vestibule and passes through the true vocal folds (short arrow) into the trachea (t), while the remainder successfully passes into the esophagus (e). Note that the hyoid bone (h) is in its most elevated position.

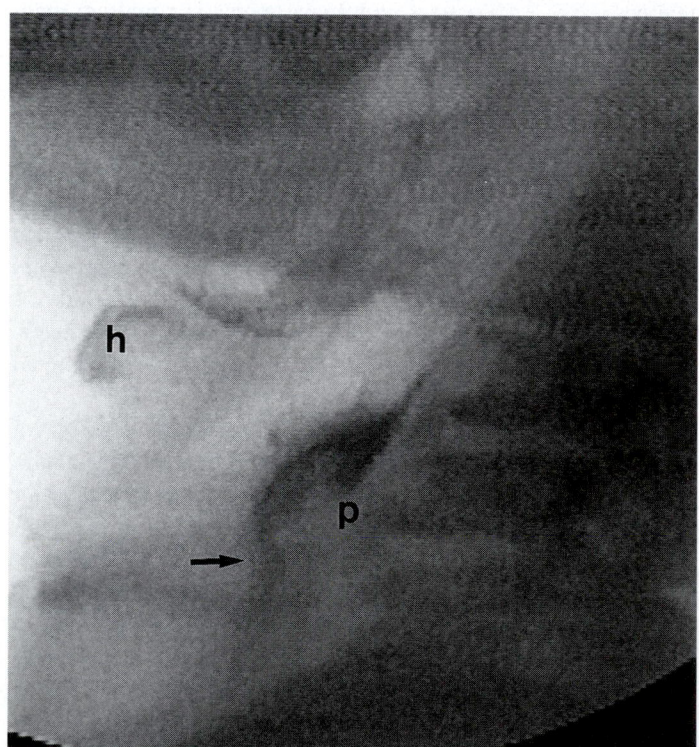

FIGURE 80-6   Aspiration after the swallow. A portion of a liquid bolus pools in the piriform sinuses (p) as a result of pharyngeal weakness. Eventually it spills over the ariepiglottic fold into the trachea (arrow). Note that the hyoid bone (h) is in its resting position.

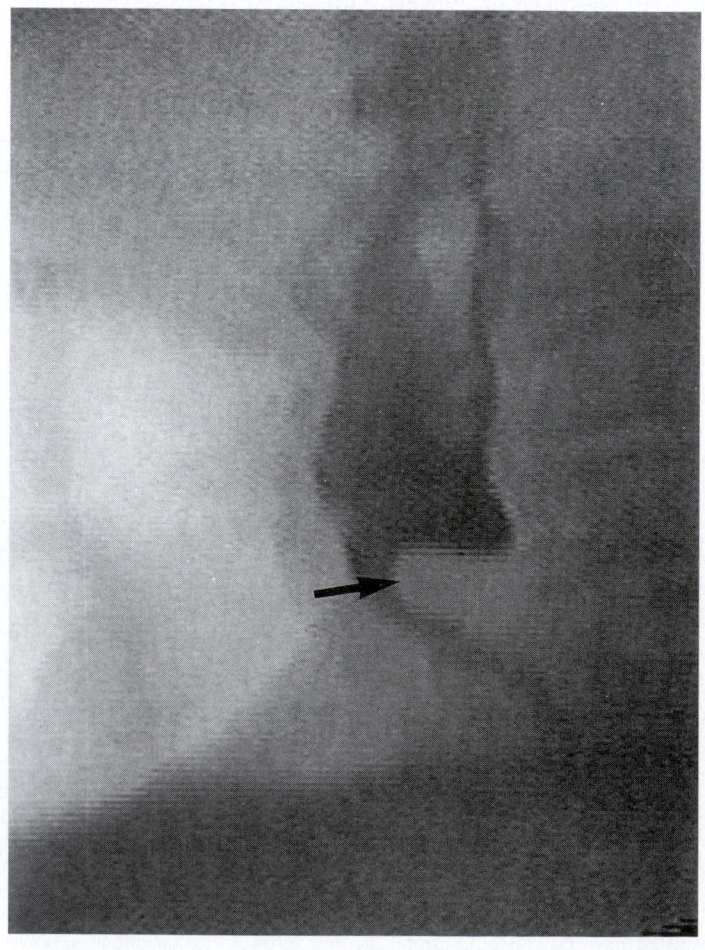

FIGURE 80-7   Cricopharyngeal dysfunction. The upper esophageal sphincter does not completely relax resulting in a "bar" (arrow) that may divert much of this liquid bolus from the esophagus into the airway.

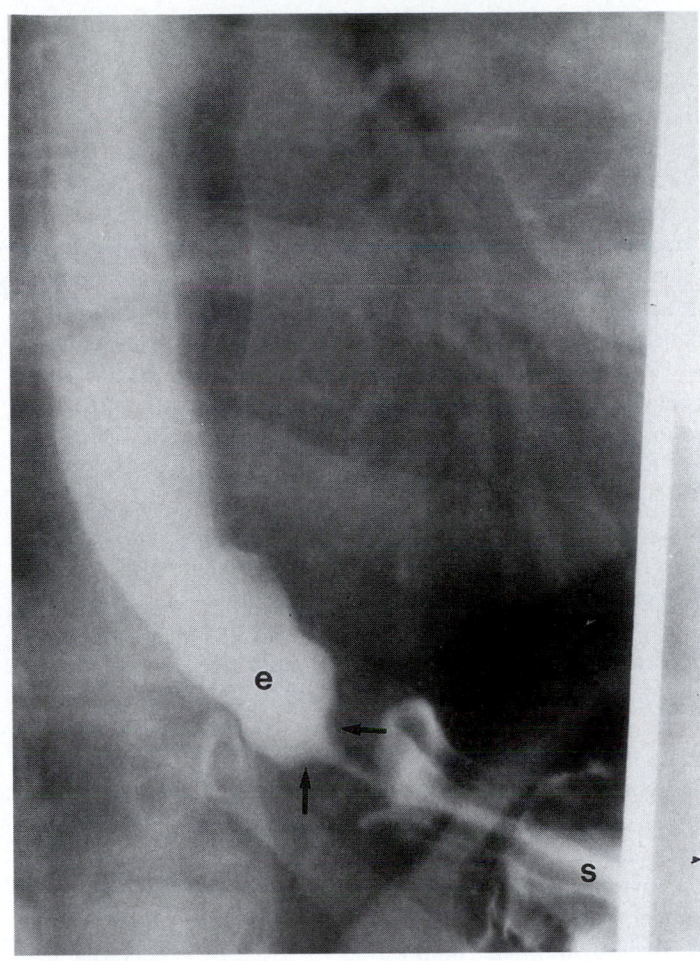

FIGURE 80-8   Achalasia. The esophagus has a characteristic "bird beak" appearance (arrows) where the gastroesophageal junction (g) does not relax and allow passage of boluses. Residue may fill the esophagus and overflow into the airway (e = esophagus; s = stomach).

segment of the lower pharynx ultimately hurling the bolus back toward the pharyngeal and nasopharyngeal opening.[3] During vomiting, weakness or incoordination of the pharyngeal musculature may decrease protection of the larynx allowing vomitus to enter the tracheobronchial tree.

Much investigation of the predictors of aspiration has been directed toward cerebrovascular diseases or stroke. Dysphagia is reported to occur in at least 50 percent of stroke survivors.[5,18,24] Of those, aspiration is reported to occur in up to 75 percent.[18,31] "Silent" aspiration, or aspiration without reflexic cough, is demonstrable in about one-third to one-half of patients.[18] Lesion site or bilaterality are not predictive of dysphagia, aspiration, or their related symptoms.[2] The absence of the gag reflex is neither predictive nor protective of dysphagia and aspiration.[42] The presence of "wet," dysphonic vocalizations may indicate aspiration risk, but its absence does not rule out this possibility.[18] Thinner liquids, such as water, have a higher risk of being aspirated because they are more difficult to manipulate during the oral phase and present less afferent sensory stimulation to trigger the pharyngeal and esophageal reflexes. The single best predictor of aspiration is the presence of an involuntary cough during or for 1 minute after being challenged to drink and swallow 3 ounces of water without interruption.[15]

A voluntary cough, however, does not necessarily indicate an effectively protective cough reflex. The absence of voluntary cough, however, should preclude further oral intake until further investigation.[42] Bedside examination by clinicians may miss up to 40 percent of aspirations seen radiographically.[33] During videofluorographic examination of dysphagic stroke survivors, slow or delayed initiation of the pharyngeal swallow and pharyngeal constrictor weakness were the best predictors of aspiration.[18,24] Penetration of more than 10 percent of a bolus beyond the true vocal folds during videofluorographic evaluation is associated with increased risk of aspiration pneumonia,[15] but findings of residue in the valleculae and piriform sinuses are not associated with aspiration pneumonia.[24]

Stroke survivors with bilateral cranial nerve dysfunction are at the greatest risk of aspiration. Of the 40 percent of dysphagic stroke survivors who aspirate silently,[33] these patients may express fewer subjective complaints and have a weaker cough.[17] Dysphonia is the most common symptom associated with aspiration.[18]

The relative risk of pneumonia in stroke survivors who aspirate radiographically is almost seven times greater than stroke survivors who do not aspirate.[15] The risk of aspiration pneumonia is about five-and-one-half times greater in patients with silent aspiration when compared to nonaspirating stroke survivors. Aspiration pneumonia in stroke survivors occurs about three-and-one-half times more commonly from aspirating liquids than from aspirating solids.

Data have been collected on the incidence of aspiration in other diagnoses. In nonambulatory patients with Parkinsonism, aspiration occurs in up to 46 percent and is seen more commonly with liquid swallows than with solids or semisolids.[51] In multiple sclerosis, bronchopneumonia is a leading direct cause of death, and clinically unsuspected aspiration associated with dysphagia has been correlated with a significantly higher risk of pneumonia.[8] After resection of basal skull tumors, 75 percent of patients aspirated during videofluorographic swallowing studies.[23]

Gastroesophageal Reflux Disease (GERD)

GERD typically presents with symptoms of heartburn and regurgitation and less typically with anginalike chest pain. Tracheopulmonary manifestations of reflux include chronic hoarseness (*reflux laryngitis*) associated with inflammation of the posterior larynx and vocal cords, nocturnal episodes of nonallergic asthma, chronic cough, or sustained hiccups.

For GERD to cause aspiration, gastric secretions and/or bacteria must traverse the LES, esophagus, and UES (Fig. 80-9). Gastric secretions normally have a pH of approximately 0.8 when produced by parietal cells of the stomach. Chemical burns of the airways and lung parenchyma may result when gastric juices are less than a pH of 3.0.[56] Mild desquamation of the parenchyma with delayed regeneration may occur when food particles are greater than a pH of 3.0.[55] Conditions such as Zollinger-Ellison syndrome worsen the risk of GERD due to the propensity for hyperacidity.

Increases in gastric pH create an environment more conducive to supporting bacterial colonization in the stomach. With administration of histamine-2 (H_2) antagonists, antacids, or continuous enteral feedings, bacteria typically found in the duode-

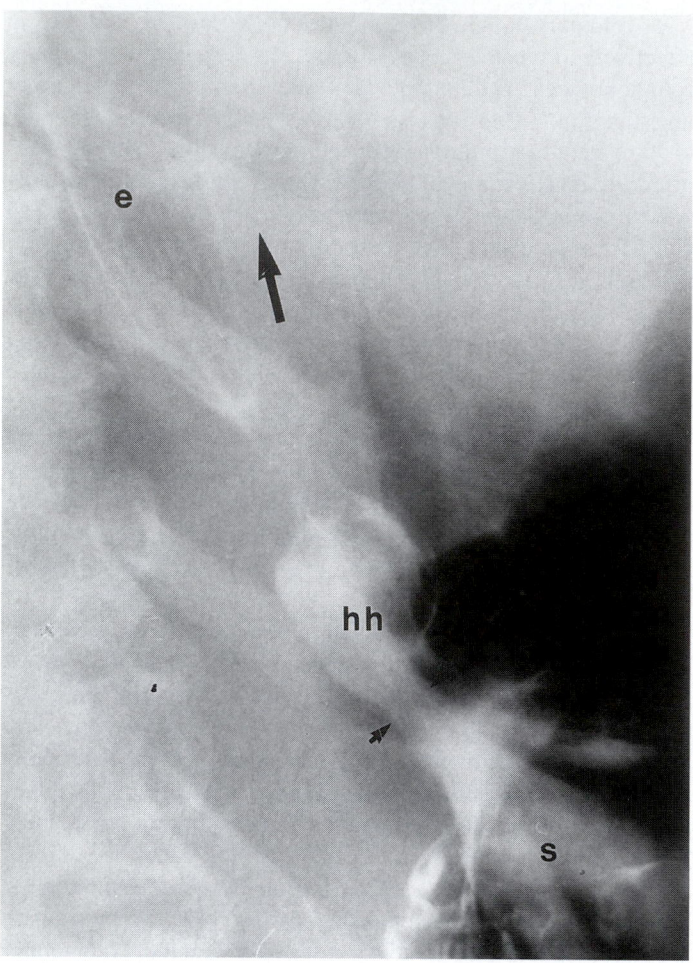

FIGURE 80-9 Gastroesophageal reflux. Incompetence in the LES (small arrows) permits liquid barium to reflux from the stomach (s) to the esophagus (e). A hiatal hernia (hh) commonly may be associated with gastroesophageal reflux.

num (e.g., *Escherichia coli, Streptococcus faecalis, Proteus mirabilis, Pseudomonas maltophilia*) may reflux into and colonize within the stomach independent of oropharyngeal flora.[52] Tracheobronchial contamination then may ensue when GERD occurs. Also, duodenal contents combined with reduced or absent acid secretion may reflux after gastrectomy or in the presence of pyloric dysfunction, resulting in alkaline reflux esophagitis and chronic aspiration.

LES incompetence is most commonly due to transient or chronic reductions in LES tone. The intraabdominal length of the esophagus correlates negatively with the degree of gastroesophageal reflux. Conditions and agents which decrease LES pressure are found in Table 80-5.

The association between hiatal hernia and GERD remains controversial. Hiatal hernias may be found in a large percentage of people, many of whom may be asymptomatic. However, current information suggests that gastric acid may become trapped in the hernial sac, making it more available to reflux into the esophagus when the LES relaxes. A recent study demonstrates that patients with large hiatal hernias tend to have lower LES pressures susceptible to reflux by abrupt increases in intraabdominal pressure.[49]

Esophageal motility must be dysfunctional for gastric secretions to ascend to the UES. However, the primary mechanism that links primary peristaltic dysfunction with reflux is unknown. In patients who aspirate due to GERD, peristalsis usually is not organized but is characterized by tertiary contractions. The amplitude of peristalsis is significantly decreased throughout the esophagus in GERD, while the amplitude of peristalsis is reduced only in the lower esophagus in patients with esophagitis.[41] Absent or incomplete peristaltic contractions result in little or no volume clearance from the involved segments.[25] The degree of peristaltic dysfunction is correlated with the amount of reflux.

The UES represents the final obstacle to aspiration of gastric contents. In patients with aspiration associated with GERD, the resting pressure of the UES is lower than that of normal patients or those with gastroesophageal reflux alone.[41] The primary mechanism for the onset of UES hypotonia is unknown. In addition, UES tone is virtually absent during sleep, during which time reflux does not cause any reflex increase in UES pressure. Without preventive measures such as raising the head of the bed to increase the influence of gravitational forces, gastric secretions have easy access into the respiratory tree.

MECHANICAL MECHANISMS

There are numerous mechanical etiologies of dysphagia, including inflammatory (e.g., Ludwig's angina, retropharyngeal infections), anatomic (e.g., Zenker's diverticulum), traumatic, and cancer-related, but few actually lead to aspiration. Mechanical problems may divert the path of a bolus from the esophagus into the trachea; they may compress nerves resulting in abnormal sensory input or motor function which can cause aspiration. Treatment of these conditions may alleviate or exacerbate symptoms of aspiration.

Ludwig's angina is a submandibular space infection caused by abscesses, caries, or postextraction dental infection.[40] The floor of the mouth becomes erythematous, edematous, and indurated, and the tongue is displaced. The suprahyoid region of the neck becomes swollen and stiff. Asphyxia, aspiration pneumonia, and lung abscess may be potential complications and require intravenous antibiotics. The submandibular abscess may require surgical incision and drainage.

Retropharyngeal infections occur in the space between the posterior pharyngeal wall and the spine. They may be caused acutely by abscesses from the lateral pharyngeal wall or complications from neck trauma, or chronically by complications of osteomyelitis of the cervical spine. Epiglottitis, mediastinitis, meningitis, spontaneous rupture of the larynx with aspiration and asphyxiation, bronchial erosion, pyopneumothorax, and purulent pericarditis may complicate the course of the infection. Antibiotic therapy and surgical drainage may be required to alleviate the condition.

Zenker's diverticulum is an abnormal muscular outpouching that occurs in the cervical esophagus (Fig. 80-10). This outpouching may be located in the midline or laterally and inferior to the cricopharyngeus muscle insertion on the cricoid cartilage (Killian-Mamieson type). The etiology of Zenker's diverticulum is unknown but may be associated with esophageal diseases such as varices, carcinoma, hiatal hernia, and achalasia. These dis-

TABLE 80-5

Examples of Agents and Conditions Causing Decreased LES Pressure

Medications	Hormones and Peptides	Foods	Medical Conditions	Surgical Conditions
Anticholinergics	Calcitonin gene-related peptide	Carminatives (spearmint, peppermint)	Amyloidosis	Lower esophageal sphincter myotomy (Heller)
Barbiturates	Cholecystokinin	Chocolate	Diabetes mellitus	Lower esophageal sphincter resection
Calcium channel blockers	Estrogen	Ethanol	Hypothyroid	
Caffeine	Glucagon	Fat	Pregnancy	
Diazepam	Neuropeptide Y		Scleroderma	
Dopamine	Progesterone		Transient lower esophageal sphincter relaxation	
Meperidine	Somatostatin			
Prostaglandins E_1 and E_2	Secretin			
Theophylline	Vasoactive intestinal polypeptide			

eases occur more commonly in men in their sixth or seventh decade. Symptoms include coughing, choking, or wheezing. Aspiration occurs most often at night, but aspiration pneumonitis occurs in fewer than 10 percent of patients.[54]

Traumatic alteration of the pharyngeal mucosa may lead to aspiration. Blunt trauma due to motor vehicle accidents, gunshot or knife wounds, or falls from significant heights can transform oropharyngeal anatomy or cause nerve damage which results in aspiration. Fistulae allow food to travel directly between the esophagus and the trachea.

Finally, primary tumors and their sequelae may cause aspiration. Tumors of the tongue or floor of the mouth may limit movements of the mandible and tongue resulting in premature spillage of a bolus into an open airway. Pharyngeal or esophageal tumors

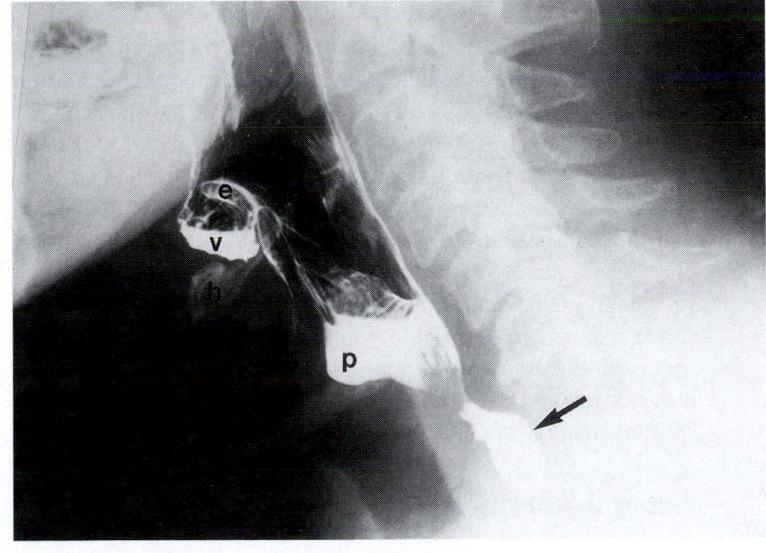

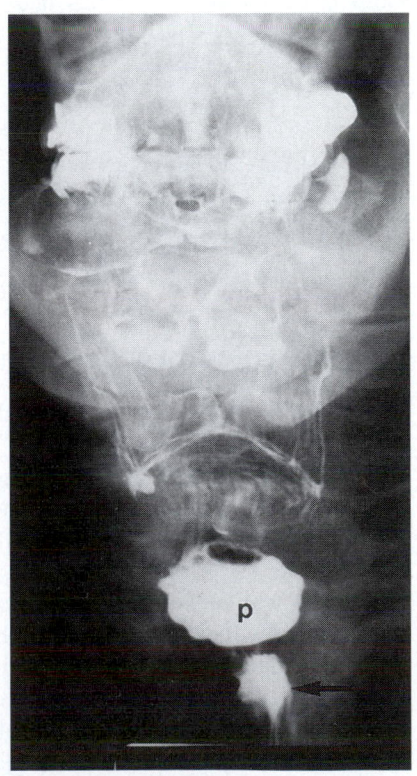

FIGURE 80-10   Zenker's diverticulum. This abnormality is located in the midline just inferior to the upper esophageal sphincter in the cervical esophagus (arrows). Residue may reflux into the pharynx and may be aspirated. *A*. Lateral view. *B*. Anteroposterior view (v = vallecula; e = epiglottis; p = piriform sinus).

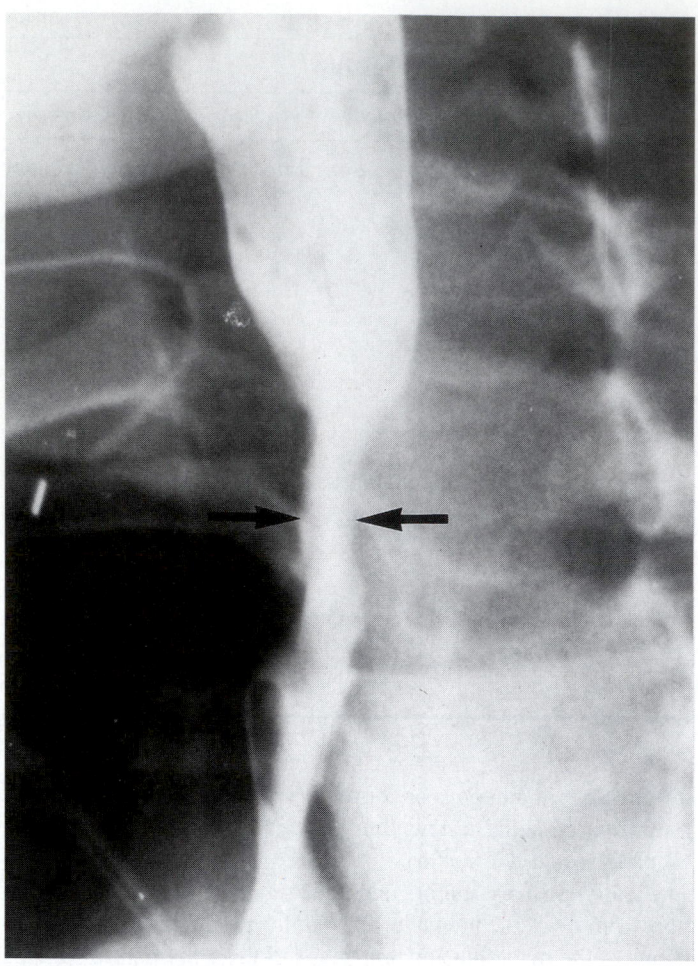

FIGURE 80-11 Esophageal carcinoma. This adenocarcinoma of the esophagus has a characteristic "apple core" appearance. Boluses may lodge in the esophagus or reflux into the pharynx with subsequent aspiration.

may obstruct the alimentary canal, cause backflow into the hypopharynx, and result in spillage of a bolus into the airway (Fig. 80-11).

IATROGENIC MECHANISMS

Nonoral Enteral Feeding

Aspiration not only is an indication for but also is a complication of enteral nutritional support.[28,44] Nasoenteric, gastrostomy, and jejunostomy tubes all have been implicated as a cause of aspiration. The mechanical interruption of the pharynx, gastroesophageal junction, and pylorus of the stomach is presumed to augment any underlying predisposing factors.

Patients with neurogenic dysphagia receiving enteral nutrition by nonoral feeding methods have a higher incidence of aspiration pneumonia than those with dysphagia of mechanical origin. Further, the use of the nasoenteric route for enteral feeding is associated with higher rates of aspiration pneumonia and higher mortality from aspiration pneumonia than gastrostomy or jejunostomy. However, tube size, distal tube location, and feeding

schedules (continuous or intermittent) have not been shown to influence the recurrence of aspiration.[7,11,48]

The use of gastrostomy versus jejunostomy with respect to aspiration risk remains controversial. One review of complications associated with gastrostomy and jejunostomy feedings in patients with neurogenic dysphagia reported no significant difference in aspiration risk.[29] However, another study suggested that patients with clinical or videofluorographic evidence of gastroesophageal reflux, aspiration, gastric atony, and/or gastric outlet obstruction may have a reduced risk of aspiration when jejunostomy tube feedings are used. When these contraindications for the use of a gastrostomy tube are present, the feeding tube should be placed distal to the gastroesophageal and pyloric sphincters, increasing protection against aspiration.[14]

Nosocomial pneumonia may be related to enteral nutrition.[44] Gastrostomy feedings may alkalinize the gastric environment, facilitating bacterial overgrowth (see above discussion of gastroesophageal reflux disease). The use of jejunostomy feedings may result in less alkalinization of the gastric environment but may still result in lowering bacterial colony counts even when reflux and aspiration are present.[36] The usefulness of acidifying enteral formulae to prevent bacterial colonization is being explored but has not yet been firmly established.[13] Monitoring of tracheal secretions in critically ill hospitalized patients requiring tube feeding, especially when mechanically ventilated, using techniques such as methylene blue dye detection and glucose monitoring (glucose-positive indicating reflux and aspiration,) may be useful. However, commonsense interventions, such as keeping these patients in at least a 30-degree semirecumbent position during and up to 1 to 2 hours after enteral feeding, may be more important in preventing aspiration.[34,45,46]

Tracheal Intubation and Tracheostomy

Mechanical interruption of the larynx with a tracheostomy or endotracheal tube is associated with increased risk of aspiration in patients receiving both oral and enteral feedings. For example, in one study, 71.4 percent of the aspirations observed in patients receiving enteral feedings occurred in patients who had artificial airways.[11] A tracheostomy or endotracheal tube will interfere with both laryngeal elevation and laryngeal closure during the pharyngeal phase of swallowing. Further, the cough reflex may be compromised such that there is insufficient subglottic pressure generated by a reflexic cough when laryngeal penetration occurs. Inflation of the tracheostomy cuff is thought to limit, however incompletely, laryngeal and upper airway entry of nongaseous materials.[9,37]

General Anesthesia

The use of general anesthesia for surgical procedures globally depresses consciousness as well as adaptational and compensatory mechanisms that are thought to protect from aspiration. The risk of aspiration is even higher when emergent surgical intervention allows inadequate time for gastric emptying of recently ingested food. Further, when the surgical procedure involves manipulation of the stomach or bowels, the possibility of regurgitation of gastric contents is high.[10] Some investigators have explored the use of artificial airways that aim to prevent the aspiration of regurgitated gastric materials during surgical procedures. These artificial airways provide an esophageal seal that prevents passage of more solid gastric materials yet allows drainage of distal esophageal fluid. The efficacy of these types of airways is not yet established.[1]

Head and Neck Cancer Treatments

Treatments for head and neck cancer may exacerbate swallowing problems which increase the incidence of aspiration. Resections of the retromolar trigone, base of the tongue, and floor of the mouth cause aspiration due to loss of bolus control and premature spillage of the bolus into the pharynx. Resections of the tonsils and superior or lateral pharynx may interfere with bolus transport because of altered sensation or decreased propulsion usually supplied by the pharyngeal constrictor muscles. Resection of the submental muscles impairs the laryngeal elevation and forward movement required to protect the larynx from foreign bodies. Hemilaryngectomy decreases the contact between the base of the tongue and the excised larynx, thus raising the risk of aspiration. Supraglottic laryngectomy, which includes resection of the aryepiglottic folds and one or both of the superior laryngeal nerves, can cause persistent aspiration when the arytenoid cartilage, piriform sinuses, and tongue base are removed. Tracheoesophageal puncture for placement of a prosthetic valve to facilitate voice after laryngectomy can be a site for liquid or secretions to leak into the trachea, both through the fistula and through the prosthesis. Even irradiation of resected tissues may result in tissue necrosis and fibrosis which can limit a significant amount of protective laryngeal movement.

REFERENCES

1. Akhtar TM: Oesophageal vent-laryngeal mask to prevent aspiration of gastric contents. *Br J Anaesth* 72:52–54, 1994.
2. Alberts MJ, Horner J, Gray L, Brazer SR: Aspiration after stroke: lesion analysis by brain MRI. *Dysphagia* 7:170–173, 1992.
3. Buchholz D, Bosma JF, Donner MW: Adaptation, compensation, and decompensation of the pharyngeal swallow. *Gastrointest Radiol* 10:235–239, 1985.
4. Bushmann M, Dobmeyer SM, Leeker L, Perlmutter JS: Swallowing abnormalities and their response to treatment in Parkinson's disease. *Neurology* 39:1309–1314, 1989.
5. DePippo KL, Holas MA, Reding MJ: The Burke dysphagia screening test: validation of its use in patients with stroke. *Arch Phys Med Rehabil* 75:1284–1286, 1994.
6. Donner MW: Swallowing mechanism and neuromuscular disorders. *Sem Roentgenol* 9(4):273–282, 1974.
7. Dotson RG, Robinson RG, Pingleton SK: Gastroesophageal reflux with nasogastric tubes: effect of nasogastric tube size. *Am J Respir Crit Care Med* 149:1659–1662, 1994.
8. Ekberg O, Hildersfors H: Defective closure of the laryngeal vestibule: frequency of pulmonary complications. *AJR* 145:1245–1249, 1985.
9. Elpern EH, Scott MG, Petro L, Ries MH: Pulmonary aspiration in mechanically ventilated patients with tracheostomies. *Chest* 105(2):563–566, 1994.
10. Epstein PE: Aspiration diseases of the lungs, in Fishman AP (ed), *Pulmonary Diseases and Disorders,* 2d ed. New York, McGraw-Hill, 1988, pp 877–890.
11. Flynn KT, Norton LC, Fisher RL: Enteral tube feeding: indications, practices and outcomes. *Image: J Nurs Scholarship* 19:16–19, 1987.
12. Hellemans J, Pelemans W, Vantrappen G: Pharyngoesophageal swallowing disorders and the pharyngoesophageal sphincter. *Med Clin N Am* 65(6):1149–1171, 1981.
13. Heyland D, Bradley C, Mandell LA: Effect of acidified enteral feedings on gastric colonization in the critically ill patient. *Crit Care Med* 20(10):1388–1394, 1992.
14. Hicks ME, Surratt RS, Picus D, et al: Fluoroscopically guided precutaneous gastrostomy and gastroenterostomy: analysis of 158 consecutive cases. *AJR* 154:725–728, 1990.
15. Holas MA, DePippo KL, Reding MJ: Aspiration and relative risk of medical complications following stroke. *Arch Neurol* 51:1051–1053, 1994.
16. Holstege G, Graveland G, Bijker-Biemond C, Schuddeboom I: Location of motoneurons innervating soft palate, pharynx, and upper esophagus. Anatomical evidence for a possible swallowing center in the pontine reticular formation. *Brain Behav Evol* 23:47–62, 1983.
17. Horner J, Massey EW: Silent aspiration following stroke. *Neurology* 38:317–319, 1988.
18. Horner J, Massey EW, Riski JE, et al: Aspiration following stroke: clinical correlates and outcome. *Neurology* 38:1359–1362, 1988.
19. Horner J, Alberts MJ, Dawson DV, Cook GM: Swallowing in Alzheimer's disease. *Alzheimer Dis Assoc Disord* 8(3):177–189, 1994.
20. Jacob P, Kahrilas PJ, Logemann JA, et al: Upper esophageal sphincter opening and modulation during swallowing. *Gastroenterology* 97(6):1469–1478, 1989.
21. Jean A: Brainstem organization of the swallowing network. *Brain Behav Evol* 25:109–116, 1984.
22. Jean A, Car A: Inputs to the swallowing medullary neurons from the peripheral afferent fibers and the swallowing cortical area. *Brain Res* 178:567–572, 1979.
23. Jennings KS, Siroky D, Jackson CG: Swallowing problems after excision of tumors of the skull base: diagnosis and management in 12 patients. *Dysphagia* 7(1):40–44, 1992.
24. Johnson ER, McKenzie SW, Sievers A: Aspiration pneumonia in stroke. *Arch Phys Med Rehabil* 74:973–976, 1993.
25. Kahrilas PJ, Dodds WJ, Hogan WJ: Effect of peristaltic dysfunction on esophageal volume clearance. *Gastroenterology* 94(1):73–80, 1988.
26. Kahrilas PJ, Logemann JA, Lin S, Ergun GA: Pharyngeal clearance during swallowing: a combined manometric and videofluoroscopic study. *Gastroenterology* 103(1):128–136, 1992.
27. Kessler JP, Jean A: Identification of the medullary swallowing regions in the rat. *Exp Brain Res* 57:256–263, 1985.
28. Kohn CL, Keithley JK: Enteral nutrition: potential complications and patient monitoring. *Nurs Clin North Am* 23:339–342, 1989.
29. Lazarus BA, Murphy JB, Culpepper L: Aspiration associated with long-term gastric versus jejunal feeding: a critical analysis of the literature. *Arch Phys Med Rehabil* 71:46–53, 1990.
30. Lederman M: The 17th Knox lecture, delivered 21 June 1974. The oncology of breathing and swallowing. *Clin Radiol* 28:1–14, 1977.
31. Linden P, Siebens AA: Dysphagia: predicting laryngeal penetration. *Arch Phys Med Rehabil* 64:281–284, 1983.
32. Linden P, Tippett D, Johnston J, et al: Bolus position at swallow onset in normal adults: preliminary observations. *Dysphagia* 4:146–150, 1989.
33. Logemann JA: *Evaluation and Treatment of Swallowing Disorders.* Austin, TX, Pro Ed, 1983.
34. Merrill JR: PEG/PEJ and the incidence of aspiration. *Am J Surg* 166:441–442, 1993.

35. Miller AJ: Characteristics of the swallowing reflex induced by peripheral nerve and brain stem stimulation. *Exp Neurol* 34:210–222, 1972.

36. Montecalvo MA, Steger KA, Farber HW, et al: Nutritional outcome and pneumonia in critical care patients randomized to gastric versus jejunal tube feedings. *Crit Care Med* 20(10):1377–1387, 1992.

37. Muz J, Mathog RH, Miller PR, et al: Detection and quantification of laryngotracheopulmonary aspiration with scintigraphy. *Laryngoscope* 97:1180–1185, 1989.

38. Nishino T, Yonezawa T, Honda Y: Effects of swallowing the pattern of continuous respiration in human adults. *Am Rev Respir Dis* 132:1219–1222, 1985.

39. Palmer JB, DuChane AS: Rehabilitation of swallowing disorders due to stroke. *Phys Med Rehabil Clin N Am* 2(3):529–546, 1991.

40. Patterson HC, Kelly LH, Strome RR: Ludwig's angina: an update. *Laryngoscope* 92:370–378, 1982.

41. Patti MG, Debas HT, Pellegrini CA: Esophageal manometry and 24-hour pH monitoring in the diagnosis of pulmonary aspiration secondary to gastroesophageal reflux. *Am J Surg* 163:401–406, 1992.

42. Pennington GR, Krutsch JA: Swallowing disorders: assessment and rehabilitation. *Br J Hosp Med* 44:17–20, 1990.

43. Pennza PT: Aspiration pneumonia, necrotizing pneumonia, and lung abscess. *Emerg Med Clin North Am* 7:279–307, 1989.

44. Pingleton SK: Enteral nutrition as a risk factor for nosocomial pneumonia. *Eur J Clin Microbiol Inf Dis* 8:51–55, 1989.

45. Pingleton SK: Aspiration of enteral feeding in mechanically ventilated patients: how do we monitor? *Crit Care Med* 22(10):1524–1525, 1994.

46. Potts RG, Zaroukian MH, Guerror PA, Baker CD: Comparison of blue dye visualization and glucose oxidase test strip methods for detecting pulmonary aspiration of enteral feedings in intubated adults. *Chest* 103(1):117–121, 1993.

47. Sears VW, Castell JA, Castell DO. Radial and longitudinal asymmetry of human pharyngeal pressures during swallowing. *Gastroenterology* 101:1559–1563, 1991.

48. Sitzmann JV: Nutritional support of the dysphagic patient: methods, risks and complications of therapy. *J Parent Ent Nutr* 14:60–63, 1990.

49. Sloan S, Rademaker AW, Kahrilas PJ: Determinants of gastroesophageal junction incompetence: hiatal hernia, lower esophageal sphincter, or both? *Ann Intern Med* 117:977–982, 1992.

50. Smith J, Wolkove N, Colacone A, Kreisman H: Coordination of eating, drinking, and breathing in adults. *Chest* 96:578–582, 1989.

51. Stroudley J, Walsh M: Radiological assessment of dysphagia in Parkinson's disease. *Br J Radiol* 64(766):890–893, 1991.

52. Tryba M: The gastropulmonary route of infection—fact or fiction? *Am J Med* 91(suppl 2A):135S–146S, 1991.

53. Veis SL, Logemann JA: Swallowing disorders in persons with cerebrovascular accident. *Arch Phys Med Rehabil* 66:372–375, 1985.

54. Welsh GF, Payne WS: The present status of one-stage pharyngoesophageal diverticulectomy. *Surg Clin North Am* 53:953–958, 1973.

55. Wynne JW, Ramphal R, Hood CI: Tracheal mucosal damage after aspiration—a scanning electron microscope study. *Am Rev Respir Dis* 124:728–732, 1981.

56. Wynne JW, DeMarco FJ, Hood CI: Physiological effects of corticosteroids in foodstuff aspiration. *Arch Surg* 116:46–49, 1981.

CHAPTER 81

PULMONARY ALVEOLAR PROTEINOSIS

Anders Persson

PATHOGENESIS

PATHOLOGY

CLINICAL FEATURES

DIAGNOSIS

THERAPY

PROGNOSIS

Pulmonary alveolar proteinosis (PAP) is a remarkable disease of the lungs resulting from the accumulation in the alveoli of a periodic acid–Schiff (PAS)–positive proteinaceous material, rich in phospholipids (Fig. 81-1). Primary PAP is a rare disorder of unknown etiology first reported by Rosen et al. in 1958.[33] Congenital PAP is a similarly rare disorder affecting neonates, in which a subset of the infants have been shown to be deficient in surfactant-associated protein B (SP-B).[8]

Secondary PAP is a similar accumulation of lipoproteinaceous material in the distal airspaces observed with increased frequency in association with a limited set of diverse pathological processes, implying the existence of causal relationships. Acute silicoproteinosis, first recognized by Beuchner and Ansari in 1969,[4] is observed as a response to inhaled silica, and comparable illnesses can be seen on exposure to aluminum dust, titanium dioxide, and other inorganic dusts.[17] There is an increased incidence of secondary PAP in hematologic malignancies and a further correlation with myeloid disorders,[5] suggesting a relationship between PAP and immune dysfunction. An increased frequency of PAP is observed in patients with lysinuric protein intolerance, demonstrating an association between these two rare diseases.[30] In acquired immunodeficiency syndrome (AIDS), varying degrees of accumulation of the lipoproteinaceous materials in association with *Pneumocystis carinii* are recognized.[26,34]

Analysis of the lipoproteinaceous materials accumulating in the airspaces demonstrates that they represent an abnormal accumulation of the normal constituents of surfactant.[2,7,16] In contrast, the accumulation of lipids seen in drug-induced pulmonary lipidoses[17] or the intraalveolar accumulation of proteins arising from paraproteinemias[23] is not a consequence of aberrant metabolism of surfactant and is considered to be distinct from PAP.

PATHOGENESIS

Surfactant is a mixture of lipids and "surfactant-associated proteins" (SP-A, SP-B, SP-C, SP-D), which serves to reduce surface tension and thereby maintain the patency of the distal airspaces (see Chapter 7). The homeostatic mechanisms affecting the quantity and quality of surfactant in the distal airspaces involve the regulation of the synthesis and secretion of surfactant by type II epithelial cells and the clearance of lipids and surfactant-associated proteins from the airspace.[41] A significant proportion of surfactant is recycled by the type II epithelial cell (Fig. 81-2). Surfactant is in part catabolized by macrophages and may also be partially cleared by the mucociliary elevator with subsequent reabsorption in the gastrointestinal tract.

The net rate of synthesis and secretion of surfactant is affected by hypertrophy and hyperplasia of the population of type II cells as well as by modulation of the rate-limiting enzymes responsible for the synthesis of the phospholipids. In the animal model of silicoproteinosis, there is hyperplasia of the type II alveolar epithelial cells and a subset of the cells is markedly hypertrophied, thereby increasing the net synthesis of surfactant and surfactant-associated proteins.[24] However, hyperplasia and hypertrophy of the type II alveolar cells is seen as a reparative process following various types of lung injuries and does not universally result in alveolar lipoproteinosis.

The parameters that regulate the uptake and catabolism of the lipids and surfactant-associated proteins by type II alveolar epithelial cells are not yet understood. Pulmonary alveolar proteinosis is observed with increased frequency in patients with lysinuric protein intolerance, a multisystem disease arising from a defective cationic amino acid transport protein.[30] In a congenital form of PAP, neonates with surfactant-associated protein B (SP-B) deficiency display respiratory insufficiency at birth and an accumulation of surfactantlike material in the distal airspaces.[29] Whether SP-B is directly required for surfactant uptake or participates in other functions of the alveolar type II cell, this organic solvent-soluble protein is clearly an essential participant in surfactant homeostasis.

Pulmonary alveolar proteinosis has been postulated to have a relationship to impaired macrophage maturation or function because of its increased frequency in association with hemato-

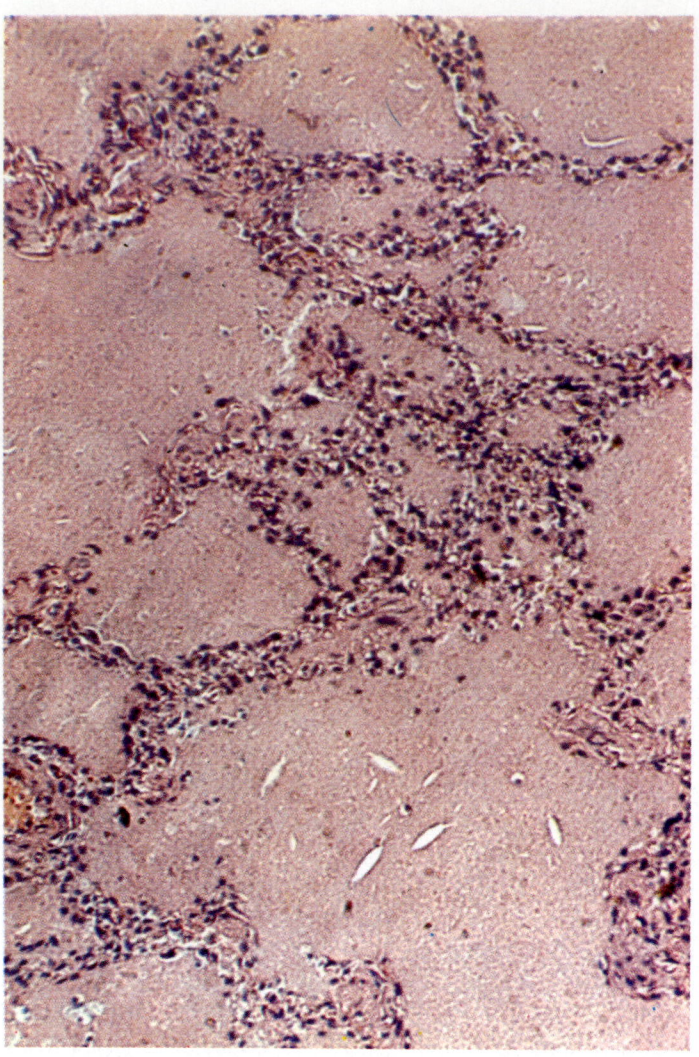

FIGURE 81-1   Light microscopy showing airspaces filled with slightly granular PAS-positive material. *(Courtesy of Dr. W. D. Claypool.)*

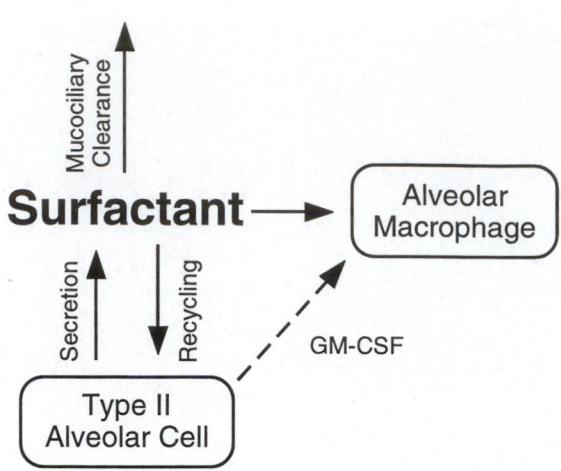

FIGURE 81-2   Pathways of secretion or clearance of surfactant. Solid lines represent identified pathways for surfactant components. The dashed line represents an identified regulatory pathway (GM-CSF–dependent) that may play a role in both surfactant homeostasis and host defense.

logic malignancies and the unusual spectrum of organisms associated with PAP.[1] Targeted deletion of the gene encoding granulocyte-macrophage colony-stimulating factor (GM-CSF) from the mouse genome yielded animals with progressive accumulation of surfactant-like material in the distal airspaces with normal numbers of macrophages and normal synthesis of surfactant-associated proteins.[9,37] Targeted deletion of GM-CSF followed by SP-C promoter-driven expression of the GM-CSF gene in lung epithelial cells reversed the development of alveolar proteinosis in these mice.[18] Targeted deletion of the GM-CSF receptor also resulted in alveolar proteinosis as part of the phenotype.[28] While lung epithelial cells are known to secrete GM-CSF, the alveolar macrophage may be the relevant site of action. Granulocyte-macrophage colony-stimulating factor has been shown to enhance the effectiveness of alveolar macrophages against *Mycobacterium avium intracellulare* complex,[3] and may also facilitate the catabolism of surfactant by macrophages. Mice with severe combined B- and T-cell immunodeficiency (SCID) in a gnotobiotic environment manifest PAP only subsequent to mucosal colonization with *Candida albicans* without evidence of candidal infection of the lungs, sug-

gesting that lymphocyte-macrophage interactions play a role in the pathogenesis of PAP.[39] A case report of combined psoriasis, Fanconi's anemia, and alveolar proteinosis suggests that a common etiology may be a defect in activation of monocyte-macrophage functions.[38] Moreover, PAP is reported in association with malignancies, most commonly with myeloid disorders; upon successful treatment of the underlying malignancy, the PAP has gone into remission.[5]

The deleterious effects of silica and other inorganic dusts on the alveolar macrophage is thought to play a role in the genesis of secondary PAP. The alveolar macrophage from patients with primary PAP is impaired in its functions, and the function of the alveolar macrophage, as reflected by its motility, is improved after whole lung lavage.[13] The clinical remissions of primary PAP observed following whole lung lavage may be a consequence of bringing the amounts of surfactant down to levels that do not overwhelm macrophage function, allowing the normal clearance mechanisms to resume. Either the alveolar macrophage is impaired by the accumulation of surfactant, or impairment of the macrophage results in PAP. In either case, impaired macrophage function may account for the increased incidence of nocardial, fungal, and mycobacterial infections in association with PAP.

Drug-induced pulmonary lipidoses typically involve other organ systems, and the pathological findings are distinct from PAP.[17] Cationic amphiphiles such as chlorphentermine and amiodarone give rise to a pulmonary phospholipidosis by the inhibition of phospholipases, resulting in the net accumulation of phospholipids. They are distinguished from PAP by the absence of increased quantities of the granular PAS-positive proteinaceous debris and surfactant-associated proteins.

PATHOLOGY

On light microscopic examination of the pulmonary parenchyma, the alveoli are filled with a granular PAS base-

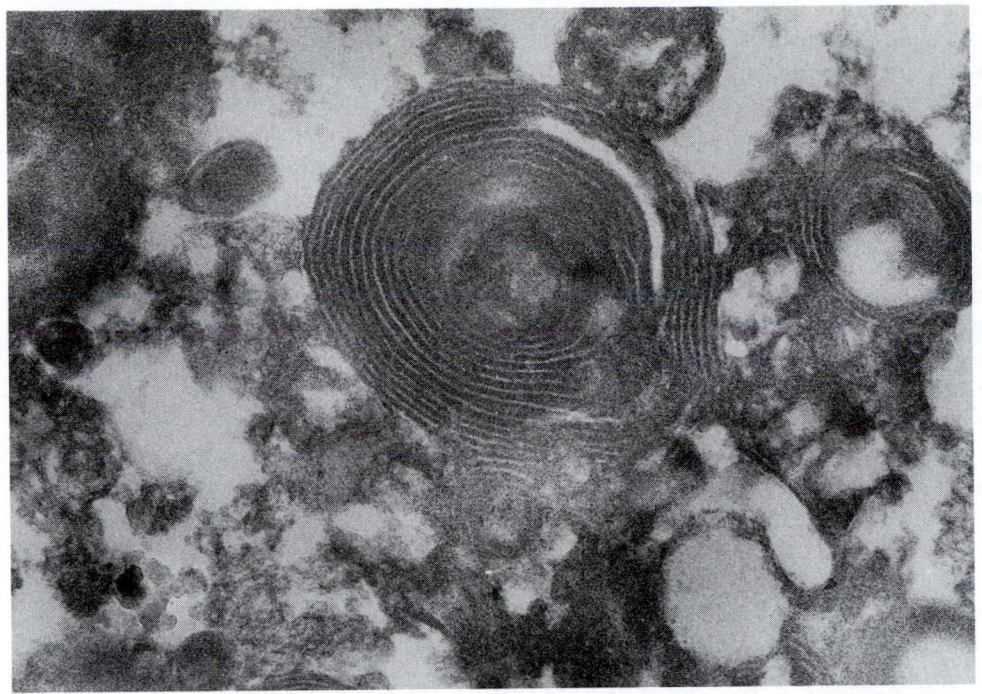

FIGURE 81-3 Electron micrograph of material removed by bronchoalveolar lavage. Tightly packed membranes are arranged concentrically, as in the lamellar bodies of type II cells (×65,000). *(Courtesy of Dr. M. Altose.)*

amounts of sediment obtained on lung lavage yields primarily phospholipids but also shows large quantities of the surfactant-associated proteins. Electron microscopic examination of the material shows multilamellated structures and membranous vesicles as well as granular debris and organic solvent-soluble crystals (Fig. 81-3). The macrophages contain increased quantities of these multilamellated structures.

CLINICAL FEATURES

Primary PAP, a rare disorder with an estimated prevalence of 1 per 100,000, has a fourfold higher incidence in men and occurs predominantly between the ages of 20 and 50.[31] Patients describe a gradual onset of dyspnea with a slowly progressive course, occasionally presenting with cyanosis. There is commonly an accompanying dry cough and rarely hemoptysis, while even less frequently there is pleuritic chest pain, intermittent low-grade fevers, and weight loss.

reactive and diastase-resistant eosinophilic material. The classic pathological description of PAP does not include the interstitial changes and fibrosis that may develop in the course of this disease. Immunohistochemical examination by light microscopy of the material filling the alveoli for surfactant-associated protein A (SP-A) shows uniform staining, while staining of the biopsies from secondary PAP show heterogeneous or focal staining for SP-A.[36] Biochemical analysis of the large

On lung auscultation there are fine end-inspiratory crackles. Rarely, there is evidence of pulmonary hypertension and cor pulmonale. Clubbing is sometimes observed; it may regress if the PAP undergoes remission.

Chest radiographs commonly show bilateral perihilar airspace disease in a "batwing" distribution, sparing the

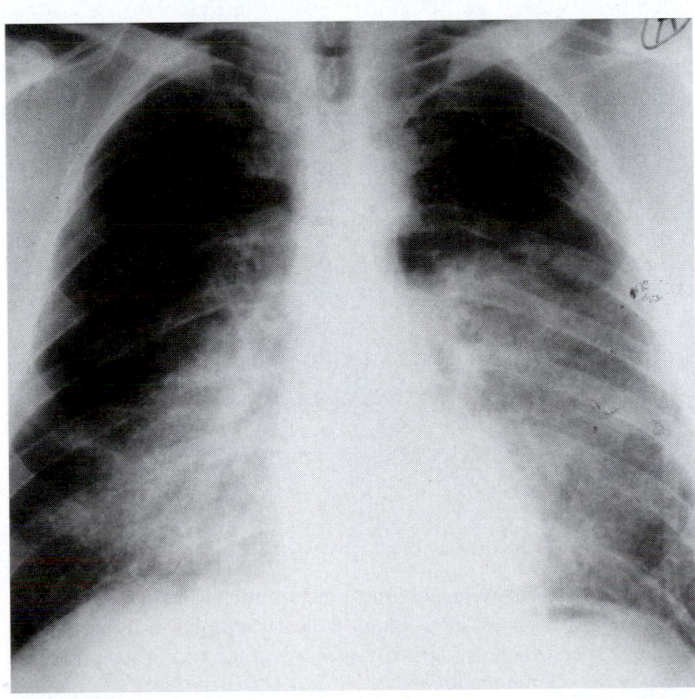

A

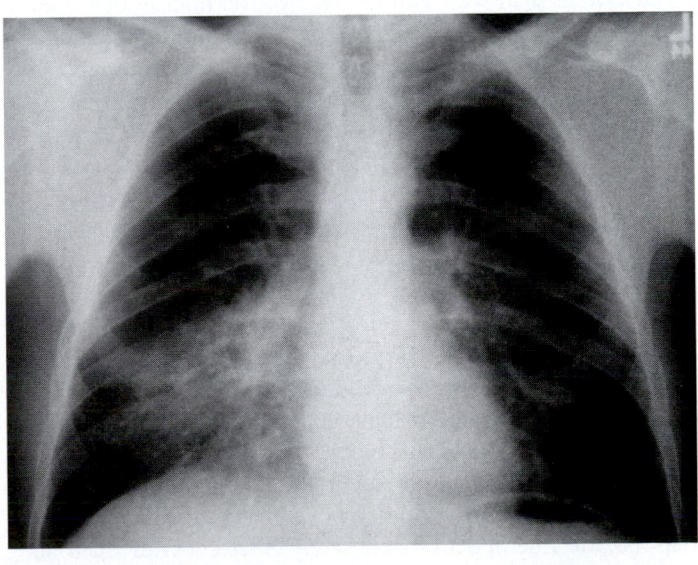

B

FIGURE 81-4 The initial radiograph *(A)* of a 35-year-old with primary PAP shows characteristic symmetrical airspace consolidation; the radiograph immediately after left whole lung lavage *(B)* shows the effectiveness of the lavage. *(Courtesy of Dr. M. Kollef.)*

costophrenic angles (Fig. 81-4), and sometimes simulating the pattern of acute pulmonary edema. On computed tomography (CT) of the chest, a patchy airspace consolidation is commonly seen, and increased interlobular markings are also observed.[25] The differential diagnosis of the CT findings are edema, aspiration, *P. carinii* pneumonia, and sarcoidosis,[15] but the differentiation of PAP from interstitial lung diseases on the basis of CT findings is not certain.[27]

Pulmonary function tests commonly reveal normal expiratory flows and lung volumes or a symmetrical reduction in total lung capacity (TLC), residual volume (RV), and vital capacity (VC). Usually there is a diminished diffusing capacity and arterial hypoxemia with an increased A-a gradient for oxygen. An elevated serum lactate dehydrogenase is sometimes found.[14]

Most of the observed infections are thought to be a consequence rather than a cause of PAP. Fungal pathogens and *Nocardia* have been isolated with increased frequency from the lung lavages and biopsy specimens of patients with PAP. Mycobacterial infections are also observed with increased frequency, most commonly *M. avium intracellulare* complex.[40] A case report of PAP associated with growth of γ-streptococcus that underwent remission with antibiotic treatment,[12] and the association of PAP-like material with *P. carinii* in patients with AIDS suggests that a causal relationship may be present in rare instances.

Differential diagnoses entertained prior to obtaining a pathological specimen reflect a lack of specific clinical and radiographic findings. Common diagnoses include cardiogenic pulmonary edema, granulomatous diseases such as sarcoidosis, atypical pneumonia, and the spectrum of interstitial lung diseases.[10]

DIAGNOSIS

Lung biopsy is almost always necessary for diagnosis. Assay of SP-A in the expectorated sputum may show a 400-fold increase in measureable SP-A.[22] Similarly, electron microscopic examination of expectorated sputum may reveal the multilamellated structures readily identified on bronchoalveolar lavage[6] (Fig. 81-3). However, most patients with PAP do not expectorate significant amounts of material suitable for study, and the rarity of the disease does not warrant the application of these tests. Transbronchial biopsies of affected lung segments frequently yield sufficient tissue to establish the diagnosis of PAP, and when coupled with the findings in the bronchoalveolar lavage, they permit a high degree of confidence in the diagnosis and provide sufficient material to search for infectious agents.[35] Bronchoalveolar lavage will yield a milky or grossly opaque lavagate containing few lipid-laden macrophages and large amounts of eosinophilic PAS-positive extracellular material.[20] More commonly, the diagnoses entertained prior to biopsy suggest to the clinician that a larger biopsy specimen is required to distinguish the possibilities, or the degree of arterial hypoxemia significantly increases the risk of fiberoptic bronchoscopy, therefore an open lung biopsy is obtained. The increased incidence of nocardial, fungal, and mycobacterial infection as well as the association with *P. carinii* suggest that culture and careful examination of the biopsy and lavage for infectious agents should be performed.

THERAPY

Therapeutic decisions in PAP depend on the progression of the illness, the extent of physiological impairment, the presence of coexisting infections, and concurrent illnesses. The natural history of PAP is variable, with numerous reports of spontaneous remission.[21] In the setting of secondary PAP, if the underlying illness is a treatable malignancy, immune deficiency, or infection, treatment of the underlying causes should be effected unless lung function is markedly compromised.

Historically, treatments of primary PAP have included the use of aerosolized proteinases, aerosolized mucolytics, and systemic steroids, but these have been abandoned because of their inefficacy. Currently, the only treatment recognized to be effective is mechanical removal of the proteins and lipids by alveolar lavage. The effectiveness of the procedure is dependent on the volume of lung lavaged; therefore an entire lung is lavaged at one time. Whole lung lavage for the treatment of PAP, first implemented by Ramirez in 1967,[32] is performed with a double-lumen endotracheal tube to allow ventilation of one lung while the other is being lavaged. The ability to tolerate the procedure is dependent on the ability to achieve adequate gas exchange with a single lung. When the patient's impairment is severe, segmental lavage can be performed through the flexible fibreoptic bronchoscope or cardiopulmonary bypass;[11] or hyperbaric oxygen[19] may be employed to permit adequate delivery of oxygen during the lavage of a single lung.

Whole lung lavage is performed under general anesthesia after placement and verification of positioning of a double-lumen endotracheal tube. The lung to be lavaged is briefly ventilated with 100% oxygen and then allowed to become atelectatic. The endotracheal tube should be secure and its position monitored,

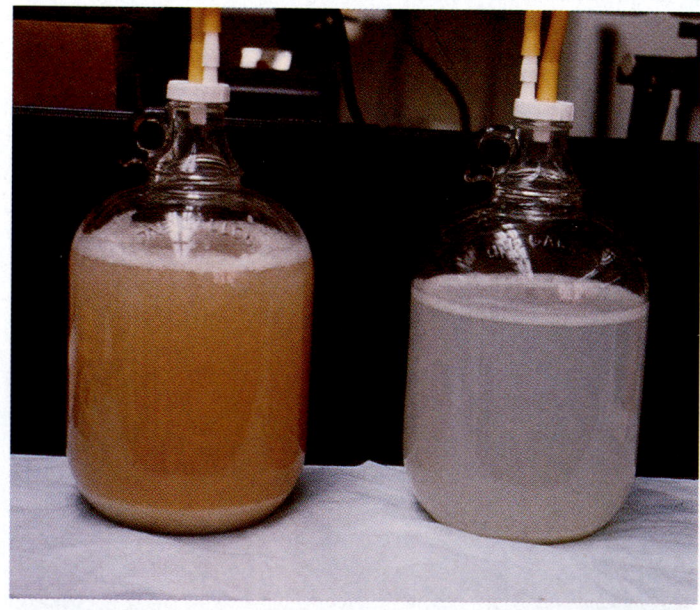

FIGURE 81-5   The lavagate from a therapeutic lavage shows the characteristic turbid appearance, which is nearly opaque in the beginning *(left bottle)* and shows progressive clearing at the end of the procedure *(right bottle)* *(From the author.)*

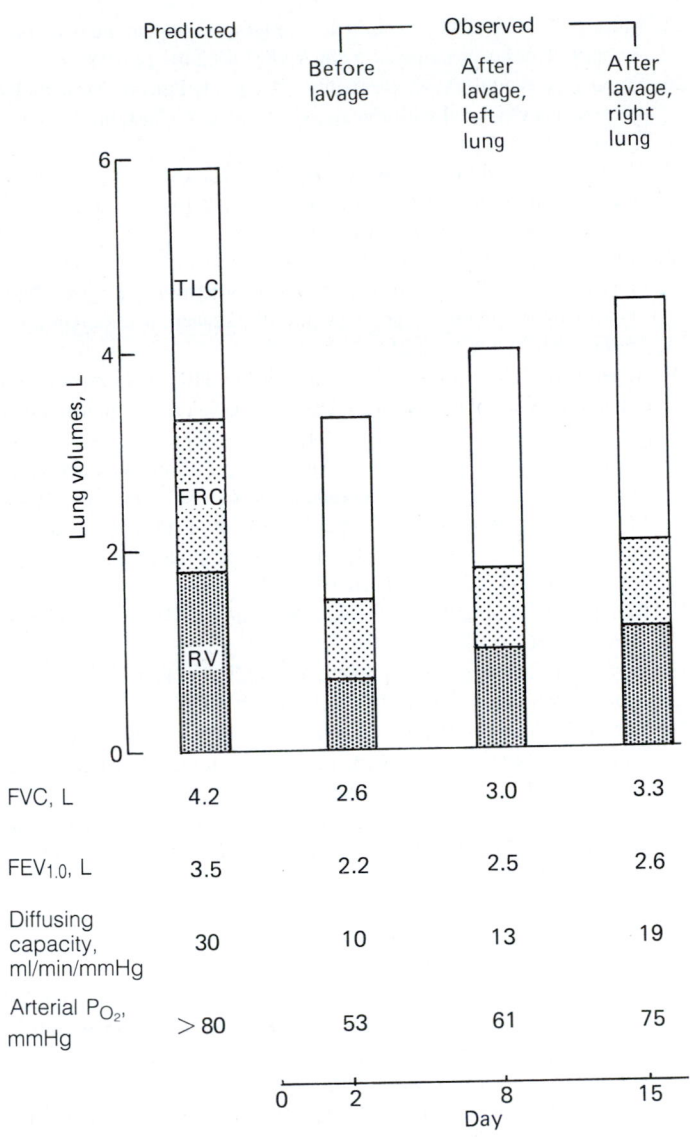

	Predicted	Before lavage	After lavage, left lung	After lavage, right lung
FVC, L	4.2	2.6	3.0	3.3
FEV$_{1.0}$, L	3.5	2.2	2.5	2.6
Diffusing capacity, ml/min/mmHg	30	10	13	19
Arterial P$_{O_2}$, mmHg	> 80	53	61	75

FIGURE 81-6 Pulmonary function tests before and after bronchopulmonary lavage. After lavage, improvement occurs in all lung volumes, diffusing capacity, and arterial P$_{O_2}$. *(Courtesy of Dr. M. Altose.)*

because the hydrostatic pressures achieved during lavage may shift the position of the tube. The team doing the procedure should account for the 37°C saline instilled and recovered and monitor for leakage of lavage fluid into the contralateral lung, the ipsilateral pleural space, or the oropharynx. As warm saline is instilled, the mediastinum shifts toward the opposite side and arterial oxygen tension rises as the shunting of pulmonary arterial blood through the lavaged lung diminishes with increased intraalveolar pressure. Conversely, as the lavaged lung is emptied, the venous blood shunted through the lavaged lung increases and arterial oxygen tension falls. The saline is instilled with a hydrostatic pressure of 30 to 40 cm through large-bore tubing, and flow is stopped for hypotension, leakage or when the rate of flow is significantly decreased. When performed during the first two-thirds of the lavage influx and during the efflux, manual percussion greatly enhances clearance of the proteinaceous materials from the lungs. With each cycle of lavage, the amount of sed-

iment in the lavagate diminishes (Fig. 81-5). On completion of the procedure, ventilation is separately restored to the lavaged lung and the lung is suctioned free of recoverable fluid. A chest radiograph is obtained to exclude a hydropneumothorax and typically shows a diffuse infiltrate in the lavaged lung. Of the total lavage typically comprising 15 to 20 cycles of 1 to 1.5 L, approximately 0.5 to 1 L are not recovered from the lung. Over the course of 2 to 3 days, the retained fluid is absorbed and gas exchange improves, radiographic improvement is also observed (Fig. 81-4). Whole lung lavage can then be performed on the contralateral lung. Patients frequently experience marked improvement in their symptoms soon after lavage, which matches the improvements in lung volumes and gas exchange (Fig. 81-6).

PROGNOSIS

Some patients with primary PAP undergo spontaneous remission. The response to whole lung lavage can be quite dramatic, and some patients appear to have subsequent complete remission. Most patients require repeated lavages to maintain adequate gas exchange, and a significant number have accompanying fibrosis, which worsens the prognosis. Therapy for the congenital PAP associated with SP-B deficiency is currently limited to lung transplantation.

The prognosis of secondary PAP is related to the cause. While whole lung lavage may improve PAP from silica exposure, the long-term prognosis is poor, due to pulmonary fibrosis. The prognosis of PAP associated with malignancy is coupled with the successful treatment of the underlying malignancy. Likewise, PAP in association with immunosuppressed states may be secondary to an infectious agent such as *P. carinii*, and the prognosis is linked to the successful treatment of the pathogen.

REFERENCES

1. Bedrossian CWM, Luna MA, Conklin RH, Miller WC: Alveolar proteinosis as a consequence of immunosuppression. *Hum Pathol* 11:527–535, 1980.
2. Bell DY, Hook GER: Pulmonary alveolar proteinosis: Analysis of airway and alveolar proteins. *Am Rev Respir Dis* 119:979–990, 1979.
3. Bermudez LEM, Young LS: Recombinant granulocyte-macrophage colony-stimulating factor activates human macrophages to inhibit growth or kill *Mycobacterium avium* complex. *J Leuk Biol* 48:67–73, 1990.
4. Buechner HA, Ansari A: Acute silico-proteinosis. *Dis Chest* 55:274–284, 1969.
5. Cordonnier C, Fleury-Feith J, Escudier E, et al: Secondary alveolar proteinosis is a reversible cause of respiratory failure in leukemic patients. *Am J Respir Crit Care Med* 149:788–794, 1994.
6. Costello JF, Moriarty DC, Branthwaite MA, et al: Diagnosis and management of alveolar proteinosis: The role of electron microscopy. *Thorax* 30:121–132, 1975.
7. Crouch E, Persson A, Chang D: Accumulation of surfactant protein D in human pulmonary alveolar proteinosis. *Am J Pathol* 142:241–248, 1993.

8. deMello DE, Nogee LM, Heyman S, et al: Molecular and phenotypic variability in the congenital alveolar proteinosis syndrome associated with inherited surfactant protein B deficiency. *J Pediatr* 125:43–50, 1994.

9. Dranoff G, Crawford AD, Sadelain M, et al: Involvement of granulocyte-macrophage colony stimulating factor in pulmonary hemostasis. *Science* 264:713–716, 1994.

10. duBois RM, McAllister WAC, Branthwaite MA: Alveolar proteinosis: Diagnosis and treatment over a 10-year period. *Thorax* 38:360–363, 1983.

11. Freedman AP, Pelias A, Johnston RF, et al: Alveolar proteinosis lung lavage using partial cardiopulmonary bypass. *Thorax* 36:543–545, 1981.

12. Gumpert BC, Nowacki MR, Amundson DE: Pulmonary alveolar proteinosis: Remission after antibiotic treatment. *West J Med* 161:66–68, 1994.

13. Hoffman RM, Dauber JH, Rogers RM: Improvement in alveolar macrophage migration after therapeutic whole lung lavage in pulmonary alveolar proteinosis. *Am Rev Respir Dis* 139:1030–1032, 1989.

14. Hoffman RM, Rogers RM: Serum and lavage lactate dehydrogenase isoenzymes in pulmonary alveolar proteinosis. *Am Rev Respir Dis* 143:42–46, 1991.

15. Hommeyer SH, Godwin JD, Takasugi JE: Computed tomography of air-space disease. *Radiol Clin North Am* 29:1065–1084, 1991.

16. Honda Y, Kataoka K, Hayashi H, et al: Alterations of acidic phospholipids in bronchoalveolar lavage fluids of patients with pulmonary alveolar proteinosis. *Clin Chim Acta* 181:11–18, 1989.

17. Hook GER: Alveolar proteinosis and phospholipidoses of the lungs. *Toxicol Pathol* 19:483–513, 1991.

18. Huffman JA, Hull WM, Dranoff G, et al: Pulmonary epithelial cell expression of GM-CSF corrects the alveolar proteinosis in GM-CSF deficient mice. *J Clin Invest* 97:649–655, 1996.

19. Jansen HM, Zuurmond WWA, Roos CM, et al: Whole lung lavage under hyperbaric oxygen conditions for alveolar proteinosis with respiratory failure. *Chest* 91:829–832, 1987.

20. Martin RJ, Coalson JJ, Rogers RM, et al: Pulmonary alveolar proteinosis: The diagnosis by segmental lavage. *Am Rev Respir Dis* 121:819–825, 1980.

21. Martinez-Lopez MA, Gomez-Cerezo G, Villasante C, et al: Pulmonary alveolar proteinosis: Prolonged spontaneous remission in two patients. *Eur Respir J* 4:377–379, 1991.

22. Masuda T, Shimura S, Sasaki H, Takishima T: Surfactant apoprotein-A concentration in sputum for diagnosis of pulmonary alveolar proteinosis. *Lancet* 337:4229–4238, 1991.

23. Meijer WG, van Marwijk Kooy M, Ladde BE: A patient with multiple myeloma and respiratory insufficiency due to accumulation of paraprotein in the alveolar space. *Br J Haematol* 87:663–665, 1994.

24. Miller BE, Hook GER: Hypertrophy and hyperplasia of alveolar type II cells in response to silica and other pulmonary toxicants. *Environ Health Perspect* 85:15–23, 1990.

25. Murch CR, Carr DH: Computed tomography appearances of pulmonary alveolar proteinosis. *Clin Radiol* 40:240–243, 1989.

26. Nhieu JTV, Vojtek A-M, Bernaudin J-F, et al: Pulmonary alveolar proteinosis associated with *Pneumocystis carinii*. *Chest* 98:801–805, 1990.

27. Nishimura K, Izumi T, Kitaichi M, et al: The diagnostic accuracy of high-resolution computed tomography in diffuse infiltrative lung diseases. *Chest* 104:1149–1155, 1993.

28. Nishinakamura R, Nakayama N, Hirabayashi Y, et al: Mice deficient for the Il-3/GM-CSF/IL-5 βc receptor exhibit lung pathology and impaired immune response, while βIL3 receptor-deficient mice are normal. *Immunity* 2:211–222, 1995.

29. Nogee LM, deMello DE, Dehner LP, Colten HR: Brief report: Deficiency of pulmonary surfactant protein B in congenital alveolar proteinosis. *New Engl J Med* 328:406–410, 1993.

30. Parto K, Svedstrom E, Majurin M-L, et al: Pulmonary manifestations in lysinuric protein intolerance. *Chest* 104:1176–1182, 1993.

31. Prakash UBS, Barham SS, Carpenter HA, et al: Pulmonary alveolar phospholipoproteinosis: Experience with 34 cases and a review. *Mayo Clin Proc* 62:499–518, 1987.

32. Ramirez R: Pulmonary alveolar proteinosis. *Arch Intern Med* 119:147–156, 1967.

33. Rosen SH, Castleman B, Liebow AA, et al: Pulmonary alveolar proteinosis. *New Engl J Med* 258:1123–1142, 1958.

34. Ruben FL, Talamo TS: Secondary pulmonary alveolar proteinosis occurring in two patients with acquired immune deficiency syndrome. *Am J Med* 80:1187–1190, 1986.

35. Rubinstein I, Mullen JBM, Hoffstein V: Morphologic diagnosis of idiopathic pulmonary alveolar lipoproteinosis—Revisited. *Arch Int Med* 148:813–816, 1988.

36. Singh G, Katyal SL, Bedrossian CWM, Rogers RM: Pulmonary alveolar proteinosis: Staining for surfactant apoproteinosis and in conditions simulating it. *Chest* 83:82–86, 1983.

37. Stanley E, Lieschke GJ, Grail D, et al: Granulocyte/macrophage colony-stimulating factor–deficient mice show no major perturbation of hematopoiesis but develop a characteristic pulmonary pathology. *Proc Natl Acad Sci USA* 91:5592–5596, 1994.

38. Steens RD, Summers QA, Tarala RA: Pulmonary alveolar proteinosis in association with Fanconi's anemia and psoriasis. *Chest* 102:637–638, 1992.

39. Warner T, Balish E: Pulmonary alveolar proteinosis: A spontaneous and inducible disease in immunodeficient germ-free mice. *Am J Pathol* 146:1017–1024, 1995.

40. Witty LA, Tapson VF, Piantadosi CA: Isolation of mycobacteria in patients with pulmonary alveolar proteinosis. *Medicine* 73:103–109, 1994.

41. Wright JR, Dobbs LG: Regulation of pulmonary surfactant secretion and clearance. *Annu Rev Physiol* 53:395–414, 1991.

PART NINE

DISORDERS OF THE PULMONARY CIRCULATION

THE PULMONARY CIRCULATION

Alfred P. Fishman

The normal pulmonary circulation is a low-resistance, highly compliant vascular bed interposed between the two ventricles, lodged within the lungs and thorax. Its initial tone is low. Because of the way in which it is incorporated into the substance of the lung (Fig. 82-1), it can be greatly influenced by changes in airway and pleural pressures, on the one hand, and by the performance of the two ventricles, on the other.[12]

Normally, pulmonary vascular tone is exceedingly low. Also, because the pulmonary vessels are thin-walled and intimately related to the air-containing elements of the lungs, modest changes in external forces can exert rather large hemodynamic effects. Moreover, the pulmonary circulation is poorly equipped for self-regulation. Consequently, it is important to monitor and control perivascular pressures when observations are intended to distinguish between active and passive changes in vascular calibers.

Passive influences can be quite subtle. For example, during each heartbeat, part of the ejectate from the right ventricle is retained with the pulmonary arterial tree, distending its walls, while the remainder flows through the pulmonary microvasculation toward the left side of the heart. How this stroke output is partitioned between the quantity retained and the quantity passing through to the pulmonary capillaries depends on a variety of influences: the intrinsic properties of the pulmonary arterial tree, the pressure drop along the length of the pulmonary arterial tree, the transmural pressures, and the resistance to outflow at the distal end of the arterial tree. A change in breathing pattern or cardiac performance—as may occur during a shift from rest to exercise—can passively affect the partition between the stored and pass-through components of the stroke volume as well as modify the peripheral transmission of the pressure and flow pulses.

Until about 30 years ago, the predominant interest in the pulmonary circulation was on hemodynamics and gas exchange. Since then the focus has widened to include the nonrespiratory and water-exchanging functions of the lungs. Some of the nonrespiratory functions of the pulmonary circulation (e.g., the sieving of particulate matter) are simply mechanical; others are metabolic and endocrine, essential not only for the integrity of pulmonary structure and function (e.g., the generation of surfactant) but also as components of the neurohumoral and metabolic machinery of the body (e.g., the renin-angiotensin system) (Fig. 82-2).

The pulmonary circulation is not the sole blood supply to the lungs: systemic arterial branches (the "bronchial circulation") ensure the vitality of the conducting airways of the lungs and of the structures that support the gas-exchanging apparatus. Ordinarily this blood supply is exceedingly small; however, it is

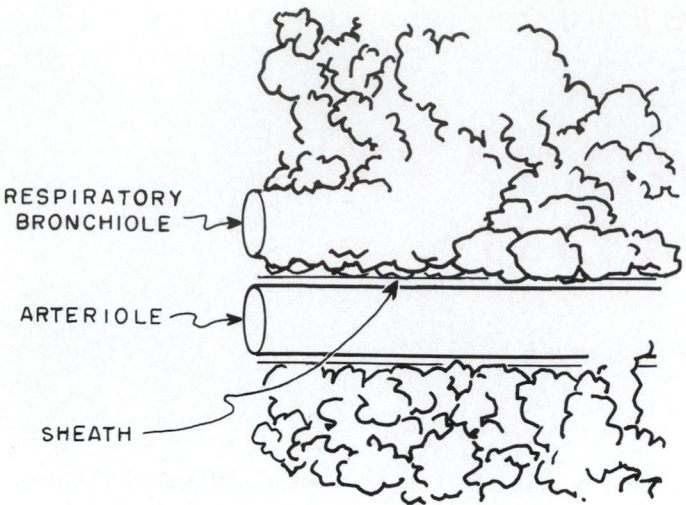

FIGURE 82-1 Incorporation of pulmonary arteriole into pulmonary parenchyma. The fascial sheath enables the vessel to slide in different directions within the lung tissue.

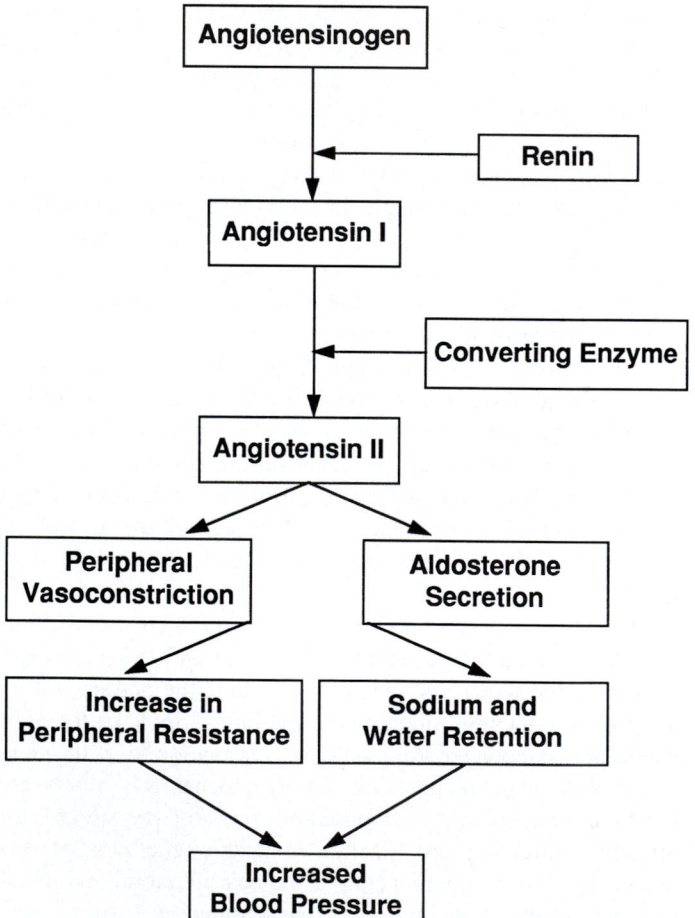

FIGURE 82-2 Renin-angiotensin system. The lungs play a central role in control of systemic blood pressure because of the converting enzyme on the luminal aspect of pulmonary capillary endothelium. Strategic disposition of the enzyme and huge expanse of pulmonary capillary endothelium enable rapid and efficient conversion of angiotensin I to angiotensin II as blood courses through the lungs.

capable of remarkable proliferation when the pulmonary blood is compromised or when the lungs are the seat of certain chronic inflammatory processes.

Finally, both the structure and function of the pulmonary vessels can vary greatly, not only between species (Fig. 82-3) but sometimes also within species. For example, the pulmonary resistance vessels (small arteries and veins) of native human residents at high altitude are more muscular than those of sea-level natives, apparently an adaptation to chronic hypoxia. Also, the pulmonary arterial pressor response to acute hypoxia can vary greatly from species to species. The fetus has thicker-walled media in its arteries and arterioles than does the adult, and these vessels respond more vigorously to vasomotor stimuli in the fetus than in the adult.

In this chapter, unless otherwise stipulated, the designation *normal pulmonary circulation* signifies the pulmonary circulation in the normal adult dweller at sea level (Table 82-1).

PULMONARY HEMODYNAMICS

In clinical practice, thinking about the regulation of the pulmonary circulation centers around the concept of pulmonary vascular resistance (the hindrance offered by a vascular bed to the flow of blood through it). The hindrance changes during vasoconstriction or vasodilation. In the pulmonary circulation, the small pulmonary muscular arteries and arterioles are the only vessels that seem capable of appreciable vasomotor activity. Consequently, these precapillary vessels are generally referred to as *resistance vessels* and pictured as the principal sites of pulmonary vasomotor activity. Other contractile elements, such as perivascular contractile cells, are sometimes invoked to explain active changes in pulmonary vascular resistance, but as a rule, their effects are meager compared to the vasomotor activity of the small muscular arteries and arterioles.

Pulmonary Vascular Resistance

Different approaches have been used to detect changes in pulmonary vascular resistance. However, clinicians rely heavily on calculations of pulmonary vascular resistance based on the following formula:

$$R = \frac{\overline{P}_{PA} - \overline{P}_{LA}}{\overline{Q}_T}$$

where

R = pulmonary vascular resistance, either in R units or dynes $\cdot$ sec^{-1} $\cdot$ cm^5

$\overline{P}_{PA} - \overline{P}_{PV}$ = drop in mean pressure between the pulmonary artery and left atrium, mm Hg (pulmonary wedge pressure, $\overline{P}_{PW}$, is generally substituted for $\overline{P}_{LA}$)

$\overline{Q}_T$ = mean pulmonary blood flow, ml/s

The formula and units above express pulmonary vascular resistance in R (resistance) units. For the normal pulmonary circulation, the value for R is about 0.1 mm Hg $\cdot$ L^{-1} $\cdot$ min^{-1}. Some prefer to express pulmonary vascular resistance in dynes $\cdot$ sec^{-1} $\cdot$ cm^5. To do so, the numerator of the equation is multiplied by 1332. The normal value is then around 100.

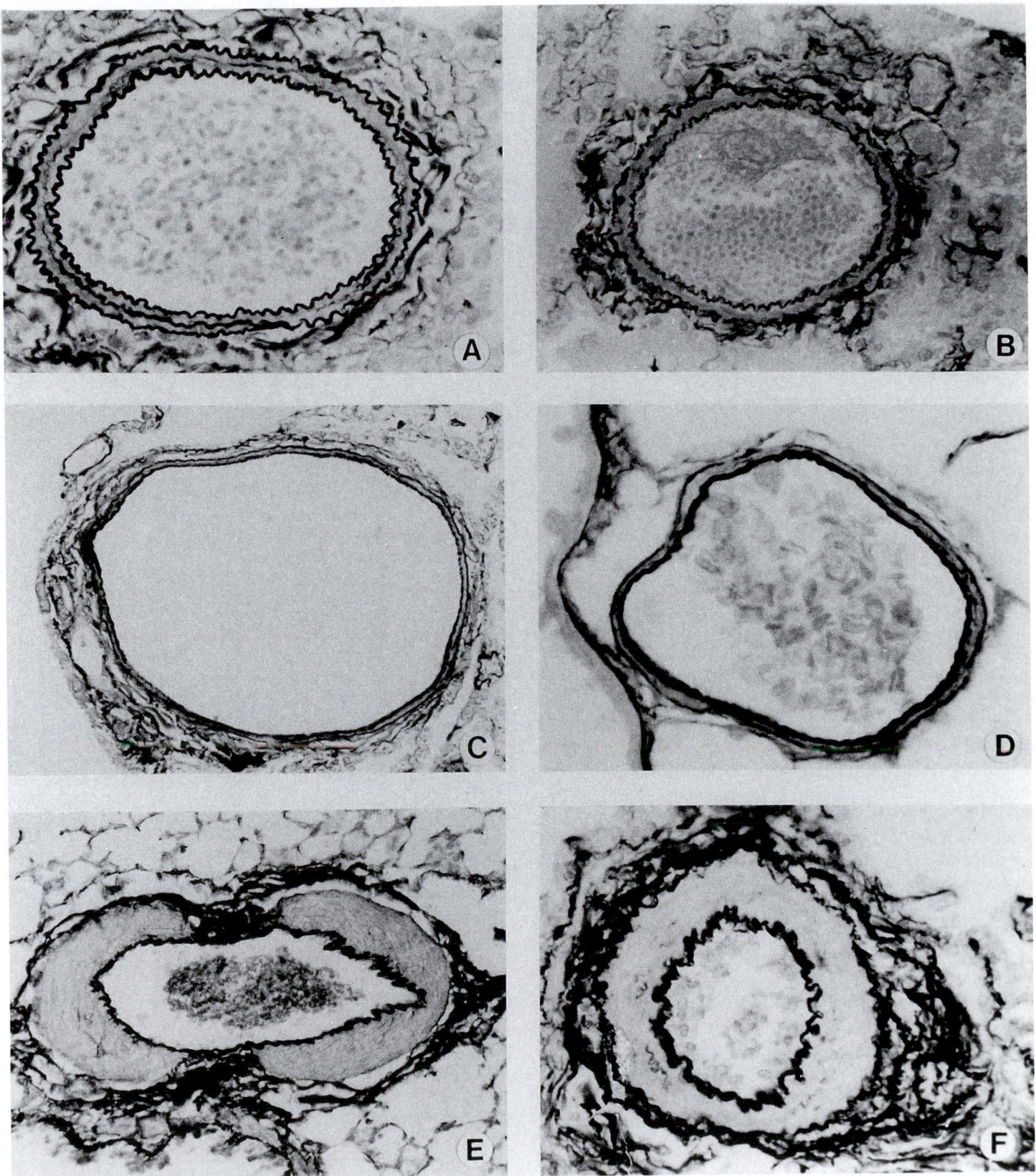

FIGURE 82-3 Muscular pulmonary arteries (resistance vessels) in pulmonary circulation of various animal species. *A.* Dog, ×500. *B.* Cat, ×500. *C.* Human, ×200. *D.* Rat, ×800. *A–D.* Tunica media is relatively thin. *E.* Guinea pig, ×200. *F.* Cow, ×500. Elastic–van Gieson stain. *(Micrographs courtesy of J. M. Kay.)*

TABLE 82-1

Representative Hemodynamic Values for Normal Adult Males at Rest and During Moderate Exercise		
	Rest	*Exercise*
Cardiac output (L/min)	6	16
Heart rate (beats/min)	80	130
Right atrial pressure (mm Hg)	4–6	6–8
Pulmonary artery pressures (mm Hg)		
Systolic	20–25	30–35
Diastolic	10–12	11–14
Mean	14–18	20–25
Pulmonary wedge pressure (mm Hg)	6–9	10–12
Systemic arterial pressure (mm Hg)	120/180	150/95
Mean	90–100	110–120
Pulmonary vascular resistance (units)	0.70–0.95	0.60–0.90

All too often, for the sake of expediency in clinical studies, the pulmonary arterial pressure, per se, is substituted for the pressure difference in the numerator. This omission of the outflow pressure $\overline{P}_{LA}$ is then indicated by referring to the value calculated for resistance as the "total pulmonary vascular resistance." Although this usage may be a practical expedient, the value calculated in this way is bereft of either physiological or physical meaning.

A change in calculated pulmonary vascular resistance (PVR) is generally used to infer that a change has occurred in the calibers of resistance vessels (i.e., in the muscular pulmonary arteries and arterioles). The next step is to judge whether the change is active or passive. This distinction can be difficult if both pulmonary vascular pressures and flows undergo large changes between control and test periods (e.g., in the transition from rest to exercise). In normal persons, in whom pulmonary arterial pressures undergo relatively small changes during exercise despite a doubling of cardiac output (Fig. 82-4), it seems reasonable to interpret a drop in resistance as reflecting pulmonary vasodilation as long as both rest and exercise studies are conducted while the patient is supine. If a shift is made during exercise to an upright position, however, the drop in resistance may reflect recruitment of new vessels in the uppermost parts of the lungs rather than dilation of vessels already open.

In the pulmonary circulation of native residents at high altitude, the muscular media of the small pulmonary arteries and arterioles are thicker and precapillary smooth muscle extends further distally. Because of these anatomic features, pulmonary vascular resistance is ordinarily higher in native residents at altitude than in native residents at sea level.

ALTERNATIVE APPROACHES TO PVR

Physiologists advocate comparisons of the slopes and intercepts of pressure-flow curves, before and after a test stimulus, as a reliable approach (Fig. 82-5). Unfortunately, these curves are usually difficult to obtain in humans because of passive changes that accompany interventions (e.g., before and during assisted ventilation).

A more sophisticated approach to the hindrance of blood flow through a vascular bed is the determination of vascular impedance. Instead of using mean pressures and flows, as in the traditional calculation of pulmonary vascular resistance, vascular impedance takes pulsability into account (Fig. 82-6). This use of pulsatile pressure and flows provides opportunity to gain information about the geometry and viscoelastic properties of the vessels, their dimensions, the sites of wave reflections, the occurrence of pulmonary vasomotor activity, and the relationship between the mechanical performance and energy expenditure of the right ventricle, on the one hand, and the pulmonary circulation, on the other.[38]

PASSIVE MODIFIERS OF PVR

Testing for *active* changes in pulmonary vascular caliber is always haunted by the prospect of overlooking passive changes. Among these, three warrant special mention:

1. An increase in pulmonary arterial or pulmonary venous pressure automatically causes resistance to fall, either by open-

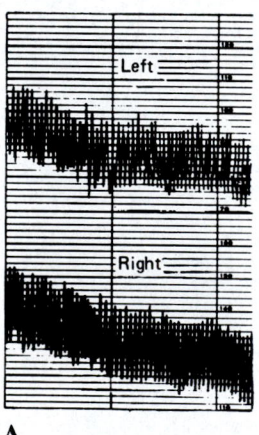 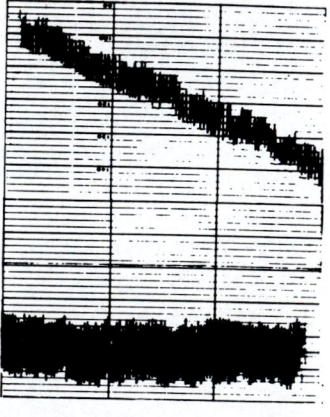

A   B

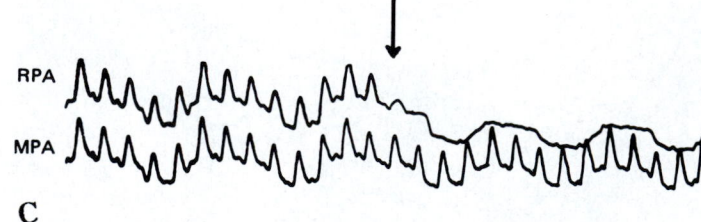

C

FIGURE 82-4   Effect of doubling blood flow through one lung on pulmonary arterial pressure in the main pulmonary artery (MPA). Bronchospirometric tracings of oxygen uptake before (*A*) and after (*B*) occlusion of the right pulmonary artery in a human subject. Oxygen uptake by the right lung ceases. *C*. Pulmonary arterial pressure. Inflation of the balloon (arrow) causes little change in pressure in the main pulmonary artery even though pulmonary blood flow has doubled.

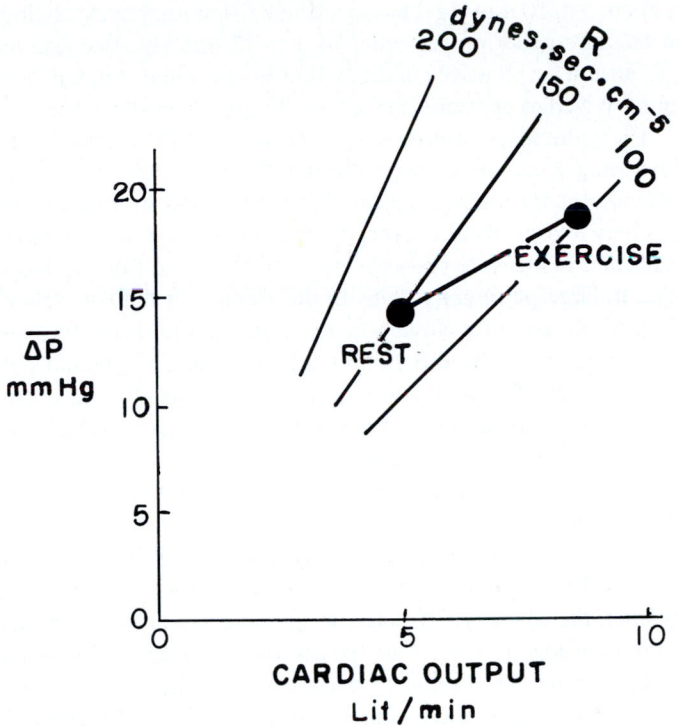

FIGURE 82-5 Pulmonary vascular resistance at rest and during exercise. Background is family of pulmonary vascular resistance curves as isopleths. During exercise, resistance decreases as cardiac output and the difference between pulmonary arterial and left atrial pressures ($\Delta \bar{p}$) increases.

ing segments of the pulmonary microcirculation that were previously closed (recruitment) or by distending resistance vessels that are already open.

2. Lung volumes passively affect pulmonary vascular resistance: calculated pulmonary vascular resistance due to passive influences is lowest at end-expiration and increases as lung volumes move in either direction. This topic is considered in detail in the subsequent section, "The Pulmonary Arterial Microcirculation in Gas Exchange."

3. If alveolar pressure in the portion of the pulmonary vascular bed under consideration exceeds left atrial pressure, conventional calculation of pulmonary vascular resistance as

$$R = \frac{\overline{P}_{PA} - \overline{P}_{PW}}{\dot{\overline{Q}}_T}$$

is meaningless, since alveolar, rather than left atrial, pressure becomes the outflow pressure. This topic is considered later in terms of the zones of the lungs. Here it will suffice to indicate that in the upright lung, resistance to blood flow decreases automatically from top to bottom as, under the influence of gravity, dependent vessels open wider the distention of open *vessels,* and vessels previously closed are forced open ("recruited").

Pulmonary Vascular Pressures

During each respiratory cycle, all intrathoracic vessels are affected to some extent by the swings in pleural pressure. Whether

blood pressure in the pulmonary circulation is referred to atmospheric or to pleural pressure depends on the use to which the results are to be put. For the calculation of pulmonary vascular resistance, mean blood pressures referred to atmosphere are used. In using left atrial pressure as the outflow pressure, care must be taken to ensure that left atrial pressure exceeds alveolar pressure—i.e., that zone 3 conditions prevail (see below).

In contrast to referring pressures to atmosphere, as in the calculation of vascular resistance, the pressures that determine the caliber of vessels (i.e., the transmural pressures) are referred to the intrathoracic pressures that surround them: for the alveolar capillaries, this pressure is calculated as the difference between the luminal pressure in the pulmonary capillaries and the alveolar pressure; for the other pulmonary vessels, the transmural pressure is determined as the difference between luminal and pleural pressure. In practice, esophageal pressure is generally substituted for pleural pressure, and pleural pressure is taken to be equivalent to perivascular pressure.

The pressure drop along the length of the pulmonary vascular tree is compared with that of the systemic circulation in Fig. 82-7. Since pulmonary capillary pressures cannot be measured directly, they are generally estimated to be intermediate between the mean

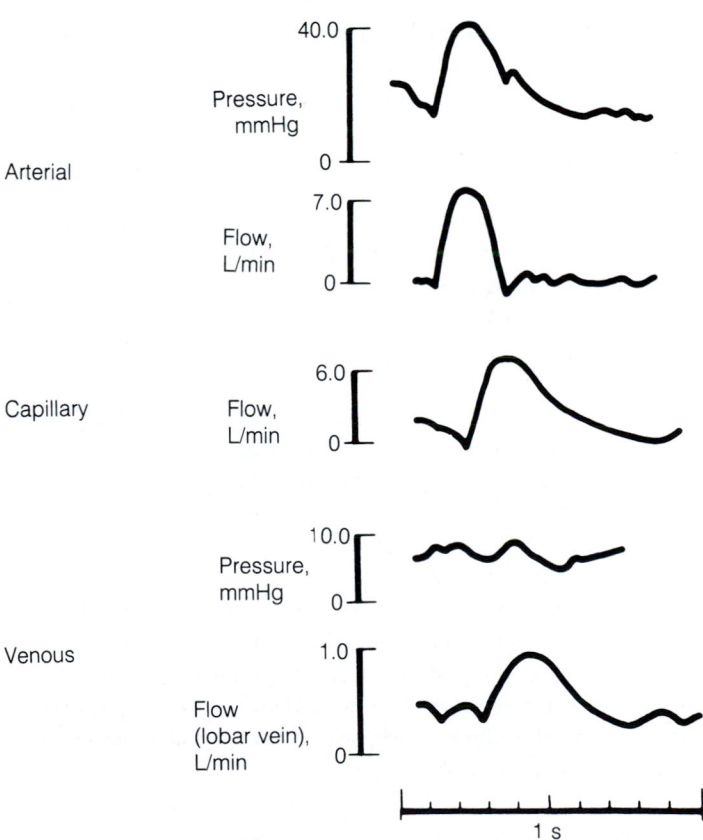

FIGURE 82-6 Transformation of pulsatile pressures and flows in consecutive segments of the pulmonary circulation. Pressure contours between the pulmonary artery and vein undergo considerable transformation, so the pulmonary venous pressure resembles closely the left atrial pressure. In contrast, flow surges ahead under the impulse of the right ventricle, retaining its pulsatile contour in the pulmonary veins. (*Based on data of Fishman,[12] with permission.*)

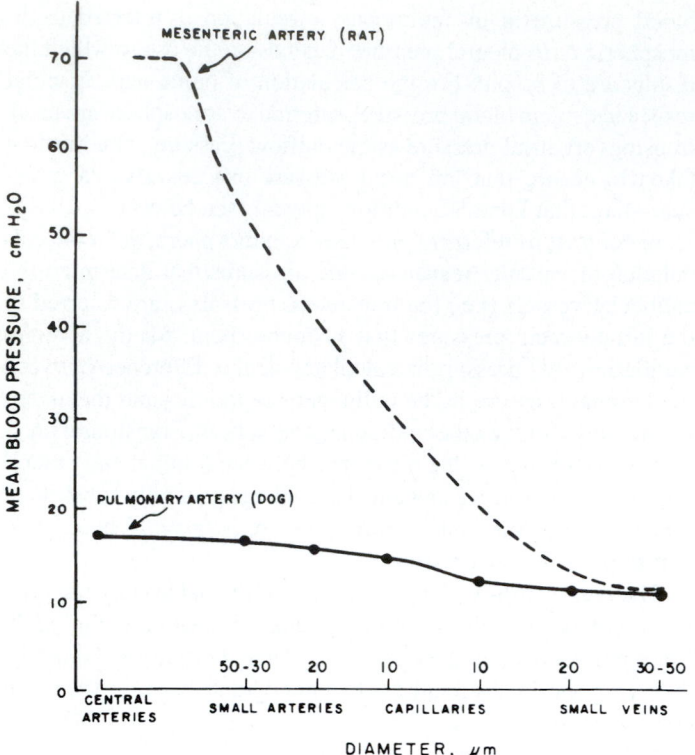

FIGURE 82-7 Pressure drop across the systemic (mesenteric) and pulmonary circulations. The decrements in pressures in the two vascular beds are strikingly different. Measurements were made by direct puncture of arterial and venous segments of the subpleural microcirculation. *(Based on data of Bhattacharya et al,[3] with permission.)*

pulmonary arterial and pulmonary wedge pressures. Pulmonary capillary flow can be recorded with a body plethysmograph and the nitrous oxide method.

PULMONARY ARTERIAL PRESSURES

Ordinarily, the mean pulmonary arterial pressure averages about 10 to 12 mm Hg (on the order of one-eighth of that in the systemic circulation). During systole, pulmonary arterial pressure increases abruptly from diastolic values of 5 to 10 mm Hg to 20 to 30 mm Hg. Aging is associated with a slight increase in pulmonary arterial pressures.

The contour of the pulmonary arterial pressure resembles that recorded at the root of the aorta. Full-bodied pulmonary arterial curves are more apt to be recorded in pulmonary hypertensive states than when pressures are normotensive. Moreover, extrinsic mechanical influences deform contours when pulmonary arterial pressures are low.

LEFT ATRIAL AND PULMONARY WEDGE PRESSURES

The drop in mean pressure between the pulmonary artery and left atrium is small—about 10 mm Hg (about one-eighth of the pressure drop across the systemic circulation) (Fig. 82-7). Micropuncture of subpleural vessels suggests that most of the drop occurs in the pulmonary capillaries.

In intact, unanesthetized humans, the mean left atrial pressure

is about 5 to 10 mm Hg. During a single respiratory cycle, swings in pressure occur on the order of 3 to 12 mm Hg. Because the left atrium is relatively inaccessible in the intact human, pulmonary wedge pressures are generally used as a substitute.

The pulmonary arterial wedge pressure (Pw) is recorded by advancing a cardiac catheter through the right side of the heart and pulmonary arterial tree until it is impacted in a small precapillary vessel. By this procedure, a stagnant column of blood is created to measure pressure at its junction with flowing blood (i.e., in large pulmonary veins in the vicinity of the left atrium) (Fig. 82-8). An alternative practical approach to estimating left atrial pressure is the inflation of a balloon in a segmental pulmonary artery for the recording of pressures distal to an occlusive balloon. The tracing obtained in this way resembles that of the pulmonary arterial wedge pressure.

Various criteria have been advanced to guarantee that a value obtained for Pw is a reliable measure of mean left atrial pressure: Pw less than mean pulmonary arterial and diastolic pressures, fully oxygenated blood withdrawn from the impacted catheter, the characteristic snap of the catheter as it is withdrawn from the wedge position, and the distinctive configuration of the wedge tracing. Unfortunately, even when all criteria are met, the Pw may fail to provide a measure of mean left atrial pressure if the catheter fails to be wedged properly or if the tip is wedged

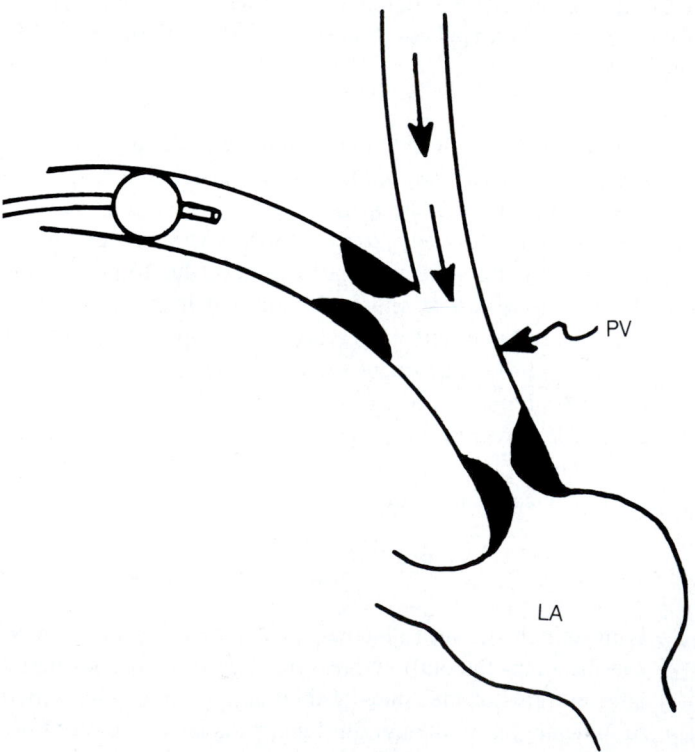

FIGURE 82-8 Meaning of pressure determined distal to an occlusive balloon. After the balloon is inflated, the pressure recorded is that which exists at the conjunction of flowing streams *(two arrows)* and the static pool beyond the occlusive balloon. Narrowing of pulmonary venule (PV) distal to the occlusive balloon, as by venoconstriction, does not affect the use of the postballoon pressure (or pulmonary wedge pressure) as a measure of left atrial pressure until obstruction ensues that closes the channel to the left atrium. *(From Marini: Respiratory Medicine and Intensive Care. Baltimore, Williams & Wilkins, 1981.)*

in an area where alveolar pressure exceeds pulmonary venous pressure (see subsequent section "Zones of the Lungs"), if pulmonary arterial vessels between the catheter tip and the left atrium are occluded, or if the airways or the parenchyma of the intervening lung is sufficiently abnormal to generate abnormal perivascular pressures (e.g., by fibrosis or obstructive airways disease).

In brief, when used critically, the pulmonary arterial wedge pressure, or the balloon-occlusion pressure, usually provides a reliable measure of the mean left atrial pressure. However, because of the possibility that pulmonary venous constriction in various disease states may cause pulmonary capillary pressure to exceed left atrial pressure, it is not used as a measure of pulmonary capillary pressure.

Cardiac Output (Pulmonary Blood Flow) and Oxygen Delivery

Averaged over several respiratory cycles, the outputs of the two ventricles are approximately the same; although the output of the

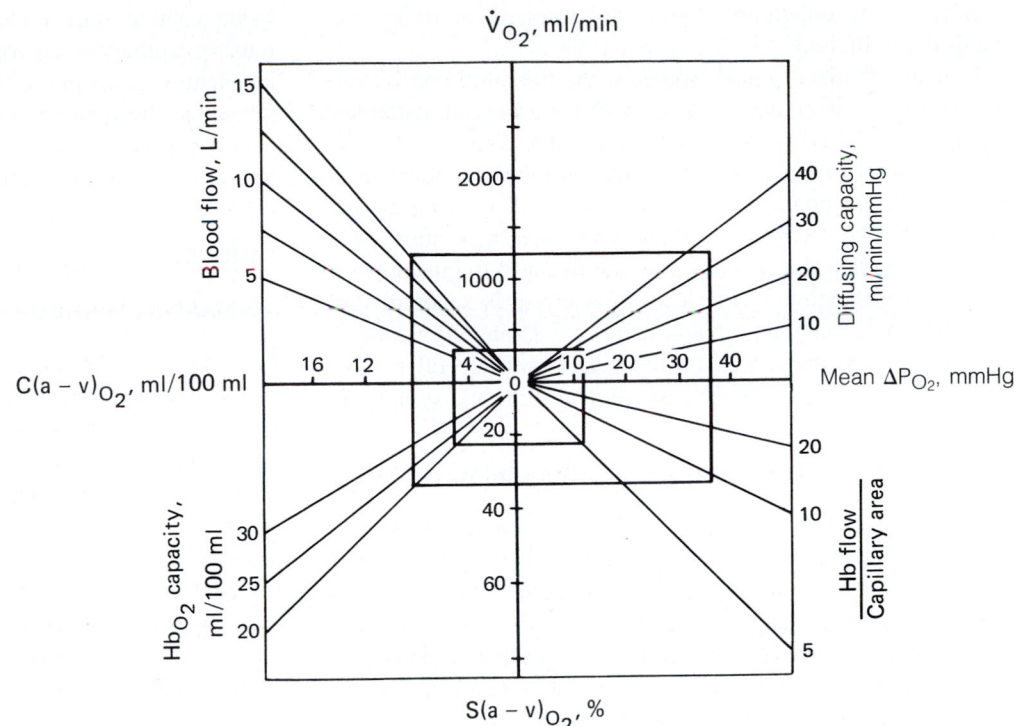

FIGURE 82-9 The Morgan-Murray diagram showing the interplay of the respiration and circulation in satisfying the O_2 requirement at rest and during exercise. At rest *(inner rectangle),* the oxygen uptake $\dot{V}_{O_2}$ is provided by a cardiac output of about 5 L/min and corresponding values for O_2 transport by the blood and diffusing capacity. The increase in O_2 uptake $(\dot{V}_{O_2})$ during exercise *(outer rectangle)* is met by an increase in blood flow, O_2 transport in the blood, and the diffusing capacity of the lungs (EX). A similar diagram can be drawn for O_2 delivery to the tissues.

left ventricle is slightly greater than that of the right ventricle because of the admixture of bronchial venous to pulmonary venous blood, this "anatomic venous admixture" is about 1 to 2 percent of the total left ventricular output. As noted above (Fig. 82-4), doubling of the cardiac output can be accommodated in the capacious pulmonary vascular bed with virtually no increase in mean pulmonary arterial pressure.

In humans, the cardiac output is generally determined by some application of the indicator dilution or Fick principle. For either, reliable determinations require a steady state; the time required to achieve a steady state is generally shorter for the indicator dilution techniques. Also, in practice, indicator dilution techniques are easier to apply. As a result, indicator dilution techniques are quite popular. However, the indicator dilution technique is not as reliable as the Fick technique unless carefully done, and it is apt to be misleading when cardiac output is low (as in heart failure). Other techniques for determining the cardiac output, such as those designed to determine pulmonary capillary blood flow, are neither easy to perform nor reliable.

In order to compare values obtained from subjects of different dimensions, cardiac output is generally expressed in terms of body surface area (i.e., as cardiac index). In normal adults lying quietly at rest, supine and in the postprandial state, the cardiac index averages about 3.12 L/min/m² (SD ± 14).

The primary mission of the coordinated interplay of the respiration, circulation, and blood is to deliver oxygen to tissues and organs in accord with their metabolic needs (Fig. 82-9) and

to carry off the carbon dioxide that they generate in the course of metabolism. In the steady state, cardiac output is matched to metabolic rate: cardiac output (blood flow) increases by 600 to 800 ml per min per 10-ml increase in oxygen uptake ($\Delta \dot{V}_{O_2}$). During heart failure, when blood flow fails to increase normally, the oxygen uptake is sustained by circulatory and ventilatory adjustments in the parameters shown in this figure.

Oxygen delivery is defined as the product of cardiac output and the arterial O_2 content ($\dot{Q}T \times Ca_{O_2}$). An increase in O_2 requirement by the tissues (as during exercise) is ordinarily met by increasing the cardiac output, widening the arteriovenous O_2 difference, or both. In contrast to the roughly linear relation between oxygen uptake and cardiac output during exercise, the relation between oxygen uptake and the arteriovenous oxygen difference is hyperbolic. The relative contribution of an increase in cardiac output and a widening of the arteriovenous oxygen difference to satisfying the tissue requirements for oxygen depends on how the increase in metabolism is induced (by exercise, increase in body temperature, hormones, or drugs).

The "oxygen delivery" to the tissues is equal to the product of the cardiac output and the arterial O_2 content ($\dot{Q}T \times Ca_{O_2}$). Polycythemia enhances O_2 delivery by increasing the O_2 carrying capacity of the blood; but if the increase becomes excessive, complications induced by an increase in red cell mass tend to nullify the advantages of polycythemia for gas exchange. In states of low cardiac output or arterial hypoxemia, O_2 delivery can be enhanced by increasing the oxygen content of arterial blood (e.g., by breathing O_2-enriched inspired air or by mechanical ventilation).

In unanesthetized human subjects, the treadmill and bicycle ergometer are the conventional devices for achieving calibrated and reproducible levels of exercise. The hemodynamic effects of anxiety, caused by lack of familiarity with the procedure, may dominate the response, not only at rest but also during moderate exercise. For this reason, values of $\dot{V}_{O_2}$ at rest are often lower *after* exercise than *before* (i.e., after the threat of the unknown is gone). Quantification of the level of exercise is accomplished either by determining oxygen uptake or by assessing the workload. Tachycardia and the respiratory exchange ratio are often more reliable indices of anxiety than are clinical signs and symptoms.

INTRAPULMONARY DISTRIBUTION OF THE CARDIAC OUTPUT

Matching the blood flow ($\dot{Q}$) to alveolar ventilation ($\dot{V}_A$) is a prime prerequisite for efficiency in gas exchange. A powerful stimulus for rearrangement of local pulmonary blood flow is acute alveolar hypoxia (as might be caused by a local inflammatory process). The classic demonstration of the vasoconstrictor property of acute hypoxia is considered in detail in a subsequent section ("Pulmonary Vasomotor Control").

Pulmonary Blood Volume

In normal humans, the pulmonary blood volume is about 10 percent of the total circulating blood volume. As a rule, it is measured by a variant of the indicator dilution principle. In the hypothetical human male adult weighing 70 kg, this value is approximately 400 to 500 ml. This volume is of interest on several pathophysiological accounts: (1) as a determinant of the mechanical behavior of the lungs, (2) as a reservoir that provides the preload for the left ventricle, (3) as a supply of hemoglobin for alveolar-capillary gas exchange, (4) as a source of water and macromolecules that engage in alveolar-capillary exchange, (5) as a potential mechanism for increasing pulmonary capillary pressures and promoting pulmonary edema, and (6) as a potential mechanism for evoking dyspnea.

Changes in pulmonary blood volume are at the expense of the air volumes. Thus, the vital capacity decreases in acute pulmonary congestion. The pulmonary blood volume varies with body position: it increases when the subject lies down and decreases when he or she stands; it is readily enlarged by intravenous infusions, by immersing the body in water, by inflation of an antigravity suit, by negative-pressure breathing, and by displacement of blood from the systemic circulation (as during systemic vasoconstriction). Conversely, the pulmonary blood volume decreases when the subject stands on his or her head, after a large venesection (one that decreases cardiac output), during positive-pressure breathing or the Valsalva maneuver, and during systemic vasodilatation.

In normal subjects, the pulmonary blood volume appears to be subdivided equally among the pulmonary arteries, capillaries, and veins. In the hypothetical 70-kg man, the pulmonary capillary blood volume can only be estimated: values range from 100 to 200 ml, depending on the method. Upon sitting up, the pulmonary capillary blood volume shares in the overall decrease in pulmonary

blood volume; during exercise, as cardiac output goes up, pulmonary capillary blood volume also increases. More of the increase in volume is accomplished by recruiting new capillaries from the reserve than by dilating open vessels. As capillary blood volume enlarges as a result of recruitment and dilation, the endothelial surface area gas and fluid exchanges enlarge correspondingly.

Induced Changes in Pulmonary Hemodynamics

MECHANICAL VENTILATION

From the hemodynamic point of view, the best-analyzed types of mechanical ventilation are *positive-pressure ventilation* and *positive end-expiratory* ventilation.[43] In the former, airway pressures increase during inflation, returning promptly to atmospheric during expiration; in the latter, raised airway pressure is sustained throughout the breathing cycle. Terminology used in clinical practice generally focuses on the positive end-expiratory pressure (PEEP), and the designation generally refers to *continuous* positive pressure ventilation rather than solely to positive *end-expiratory* pressure (Chapter 176).

In normal humans, the imposition of PEEP at a level of 5 cm H_2O has several hemodynamic consequences: stroke volume, cardiac output, and central blood volume decrease while heart rate is unaffected. Pulmonary arterial pressures (referred to atmospheric pressures) increase, and the increase in alveolar pressure causes pulmonary wedge pressures to exceed left atrial pressures. At higher levels of PEEP, these hemodynamic effects are exaggerated. Stiffening of the lungs by pulmonary edema requires higher levels of PEEP to produce the same effects (e.g., 15 to 40 cm H_2O instead of 5 cm H_2O). At these levels, however, the risk of barotrauma to the lungs also increases markedly.

The cardiac output falls when normal lungs are subjected to PEEP, but how this decrease is effected remains enigmatic. At least three mechanisms have been proposed: the traditional one implicates a decrease in venous return (preload) to the *right* ventricle. The second entails a decrease in *left* ventricular preload and impairment of both right and left ventricular performance. The third attributes a negative inotropic effect to PEEP mediated by way of cardiovascular inhibitory mechanisms in the brain and the local release of prostaglandins. Clearly, the use of PEEP triggers an intricate resetting of regulatory mechanisms that seems to involve mechanical, reflex, and local humoral mechanisms. Which mechanism dominates at any given time may well depend on the experimental and clinical setting.

EXERCISE

The changes in pulmonary vascular pressures, flows, and resistances brought about by light exercise are indicated in Table 82-1. Despite the respiratory swings and the shifts in midposition of the lung during exercise that complicate accurate measurement of pressures, the hemodynamics are quite consistent: at the start of the exercise, the pulmonary arterial mean pressure (referred to atmosphere) increases abruptly by 3 to 5 mm Hg. As exercise continues, a plateau is reached, generally at 1 to 2 mm Hg less than peak values; the increase in systolic pressure is greater than the increase in diastolic pressure. Because of the increase in pulsatility and in mean pulmonary arterial pressure, perfusion of the apices improves.

Direct determinations of left atrial pressure during exercise in intact humans or dogs have not been reported. The pulmonary wedge pressure is generally little affected by mild exercise, but intensification of the exercise tends to increase it. The concept of pulmonary capillary "stress failure" has been advanced as a limiting factor for maximal exercise (see Chapter 85).[49]

PULMONARY VASOMOTOR CONTROL

In the normal pulmonary circulation at sea level, vascular tone is low (i.e., the pulmonary vascular bed is virtually fully dilated) (Fig. 82-10). It is considerably higher in the native resident at high altitude, in whom comparable increments in pulmonary blood flow elicit larger increments in pulmonary arterial pressures.

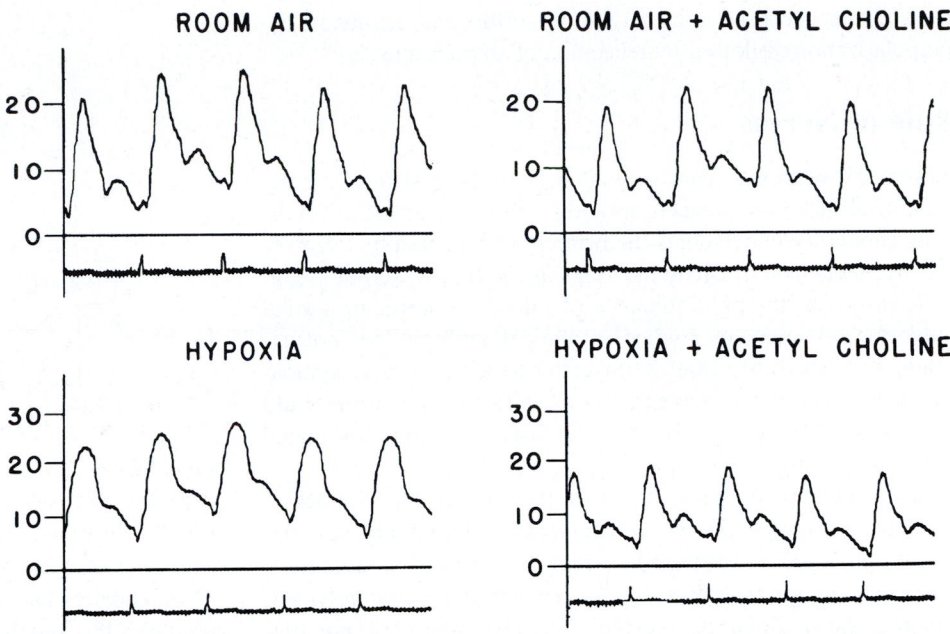

FIGURE 82-10   Effect of initial tone on vasodilator responsiveness. Administration of acetylcholine while the subject is breathing room air *(upper panels)* elicits no vasodilator response because of the low initial tone. During hypoxia, when tone is increased by vasoconstriction, administration of acetylcholine causes a considerable drop in pulmonary arterial pressures. *(From Fritts et al: J Clin Invest 37:99–110, 1958.)*

Initial Tone

The low initial tone in the pulmonary circulation at sea level is attributed to a balance in favor of vasodilation due to substances released by pulmonary vascular endothelium (Fig. 82-11). The predominant mediators in this balance are the vasodilator substances prostacyclin and nitric oxide, on the one hand, and en-

dothelin-1, on the other. The vasodilators are released promptly in response to shear stresses, whereas endothelin-1 is released slowly and is active in more prolonged control of vascular tone.

Ion channels feature prominently in setting pulmonary vascular tone. Paramount among these are several different K^+ channels that are present on vascular smooth muscle: ATP-sensitive, Ca^{2+}-activated, and nonspecific, voltage-gated K^+ channels. Activation of

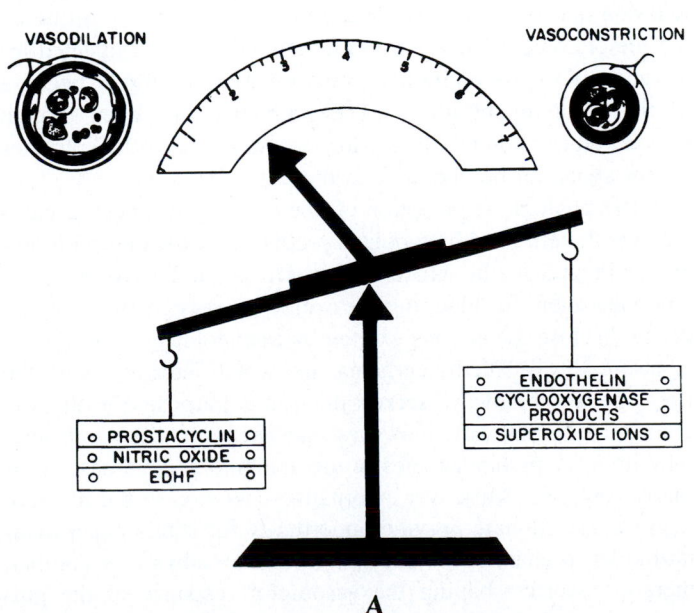

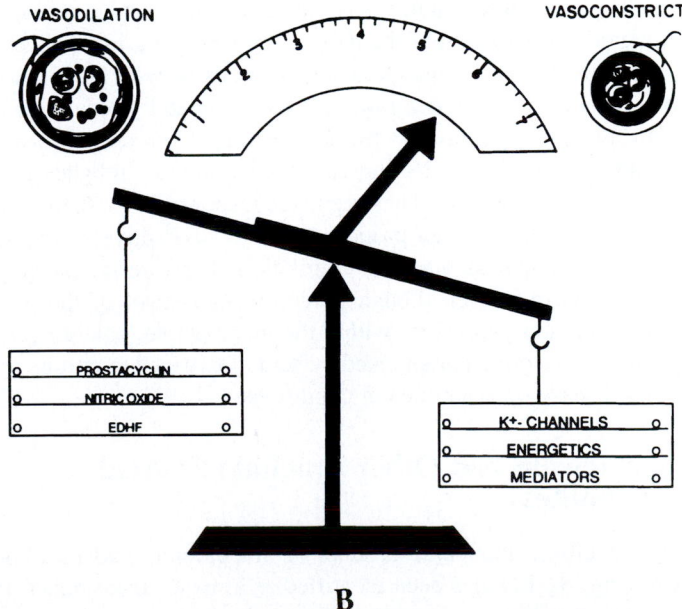

FIGURE 82-11   The balance between vasodilator and vasoconstrictor mediators. *A.* Under normal conditions, breathing ambient air at sea level, the balance favors vasodilation. *B.* During hypoxia, the balance is tilted to vasoconstriction.

these channels causes an increase in K^+ efflux and membrane hyperpolarization, followed by relaxation of smooth muscle.[20]

Role of Nerves

Vasomotor responses can be elicited from the isolated lung devoid of all nervous connections and perfused by artificial fluids. This capability underscores the primary role played by vasomotor mechanisms intrinsic to the lungs in effecting vasomotor control. However, the predominance of intrinsic control in normal subjects or in patients studied in clinical settings does not exclude the possibility that extrinsic influences, such as sympathetic nerves, can contribute important elements of control should the occasion arise (e.g., the "fight or flight reaction" associated with a terrifying experience).[40]

The sympathetic innervation to the pulmonary circulation includes α- and β-adrenergic receptors on pulmonary vascular smooth muscle.[8] α-Adrenergic receptors appear to predominate. The α-adrenergic receptors (e.g., norepinephrine) are constrictor, whereas the β-adrenergic receptors (e.g., isoproterenol) are dilator. In the normal resting adult at sea level, adrenergic activity is modest and α-adrenergic influences predominate. Cholinergic activity does not appear to be implicated at any time in the control of the pulmonary circulation.

Nervous connections from without the lungs can mediate certain reflex effects on the pulmonary circulation. A systemic *depressor reflex* is evoked by an abrupt, large increase in pulmonary arterial or venous pressure and elicits modest bradycardia and *systemic* hypotension; sectioning the vagi abolishes this reflex. The outputs of the two ventricles are automatically adjusted by reflex mechanisms that avoid flooding of the lungs. Stimulation of systemic baro- and chemoreceptors elicits reflex changes in pulmonary vascular tone.

Reflex pathways also exist within the lungs. For example, the juxtacapillary reflex ("J" reflex) is elicited by deformation of the terminal airways (as by edema) to evoke tachypnea, bronchoconstriction, and reluctance to exercise. The Bainbridge reflex is triggered by distention of the pulmonary venoatrial junction and elicits reflex tachycardia. Occasionally, persons with pulmonary hypertension (as do deteriorating experimental preparations) show swings in pulmonary arterial pressure "vasomotor waves" reminiscent of Traube-Hering and Mayer waves. Imbalance in central vasomotor control has been held responsible for their genesis. Finally, it has been proposed that CO_2-sensitive receptors within the lungs can augment ventilation. These reflex patterns demonstrate that even though predominant control of the pulmonary circulation resides within the lungs per se, potential exists for activating a complicated system of extrinsic controls, by either disease or experimental conditions.

Prostacyclin and Other Arachidonic Acid Metabolites

Prostacyclin, a metabolic product or arachidonic acid metabolism (Fig. 82-12), has been identified as a major determinant of initial tone in the pulmonary circulation. Arachidonic acid is metabolized via two major enzymatic pathways: cyclooxygenase and lipoxygenase. The cyclooxygenase pathway gives rise to the

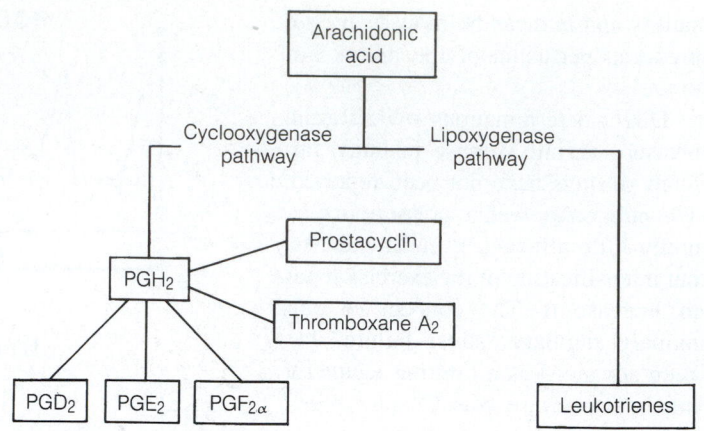

FIGURE 82-12 The arachidonic acid cascade illustrating the two pathways and a few metabolic products capable of pulmonary vasomotor activity. (*Based on data of Fishman,[12] with permission.*)

prostaglandins and thromboxane A_2. The lipoxygenase pathway produces the leukotrienes and 5-, 12-, and 15-hydroxyeicosatetraenoic acids. A separate series of reactions involves a cytochrome P-450 pathway, which produces oxygenated metabolites of arachidonic acid.

Arachidonic acid (eicosanoic acid), a 20-carbon polyunsaturated fatty acid, is the precursor of the prostaglandins (Fig. 82-12). It is released from tissue by deacylation of cellular phospholipids. Upon release, it is metabolized by either the cyclooxygenase or lipoxygenase enzyme systems. Because the arachidonic acid metabolites released from membrane lipids are organ and cell specific, and because experimental conditions strongly influence the metabolism of arachidonic acid, either the cyclooxygenase or lipoxygenase pathway may predominate. Administered arachidonic acid need not have the same metabolic consequences as that generated endogenously. Nor are physiological and pharmacologic doses and patterns of release apt to be identical. Therefore, it is difficult to predict which pathway will dominate or how experimental circumstances are influencing the biologic effects. As a rule, arachidonic acid injected intravenously elicits pulmonary vasoconstriction largely because of the predominant effect of thromboxane A_2, even though prostacyclin, a potent vasodilator, is also released; leukotrienes do not appear to be operative in this circumstance.

Pharmacologic interruption of one pathway has been used to uncover the effect of metabolites produced by the other. For example, indomethacin, which inhibits prostaglandin synthetase, is a popular agent for blocking the cyclooxygenase pathway in order to disclose the actions exerted by metabolites of the lipoxygenase pathway. Diethylcarbamazine, which interferes with the lipoxygenase pathway, serves the same purpose for the cyclooxygenase pathway. However, specificity of these and other inhibitors for particular sites in the arachidonic acid cascade is rarely complete. Moreover, alternative pathways in the metabolism of arachidonate provide opportunity for subtle experimental quirks to channel the cascade into one pathway or another, thereby covertly shaping the vasomotor response of the pulmonary circulation, not only to prostaglandins (exogenous as well as endogenous) but also to inapparent neurohumoral influences and to biologically active molecules. Finally, considerable species variation exists in the intensity of the vasomotor response to particular products of arachidonic acid metabolism.

Considerable diversity of biologic effects exists among the prostaglandins: (1) certain metabolic products of the cyclooxygenase pathway are pulmonary vasoconstrictors (e.g., $PGF_{2\alpha}$, PGE_2, thromboxane A_2), whereas others are pulmonary vasodilators (e.g., PGE_1, PGI_2); PGE_2, which constricts the adult pulmonary vascular bed, dilates the neonatal pulmonary vascular bed; (2) leukotrienes, generated by the lipoxygenase pathway, include potent pulmonary vasoconstrictors; and (3) suspicion is high that the prostaglandins act as intermediaries in pulmonary vasomotor responses to other agents, such as the kallidins, histamine, and isoproterenol.

Prostacyclin (PGI_2) is both a potent pulmonary (and systemic) vasodilator and an antithrombogenic agent. It is formed in pulmonary vascular endothelium (Fig. 82-13) by the action of prostacyclin synthetase on the prostaglandin endoperoxide PGH_2. Shear stress of the endothelium and bradykinin seem to be powerful stimuli for the release of prostacyclin from endothelium.

Thromboxane A_2 is a potent pulmonary vasoconstrictor and a powerful stimulus for platelet aggregation. Prostacyclin antagonizes the effects of thromboxane A_2. An imbalance has been found between the excretion of thromboxane and of prostacyclin metabolites in pulmonary hypertension.[5]

Nitric Oxide

Although the original view of endothelium as a passive lining of blood vessels had long been appreciated to be an oversimplification, particularly with respect to the exchange of water and biologic molecules, full understanding of its biologic role began with the demonstration in isolated aortic preparations that the vasodilation elicited by acetylcholine required the presence of an intact endothelial layer (Fig. 82-14).[14,29] Subsequently, endothelium-derived relaxing factor (EDRF) was pinpointed as the mediator, followed by the identification of nitric oxide as EDRF.

In 1995, largely in recognition of its ubiquitous biologic role as an intercellular messenger in signal transduction in a wide variety of mammalian cells, nitric oxide (NO) was elevated from its lowly status as a gaseous air pollutant to the vaunted position of "molecule of the year"—an endogenous, ubiquitous regulator of a wide range of physiological processes. Although NO is a highly reactive molecule, in minute (physiological) quantities it is safe, transmitting signals and serving diverse biologic functions, such as the regulation of blood pressure. It is short-lived because of its interactions with oxygen. NO also reacts with superoxide radical (O_2^-) and with ferrous hemoproteins, such as guanylate cyclase and hemoglobin. Because of its chemical properties, NO is less specific and less controllable than almost any other transmitter or hormone. Cigarette smoke contains up to 1000 ppm of NO. Silo filler's disease, an interstitial pneumonitis, is caused by exposure to high levels of NO and NO_2.

Nitric oxide is synthesized in endothelial cells from one of the guanidium nitrogens L-arginine by the enzyme nitric oxide synthase (NOS) (Fig. 82-15).[47] Two major forms of NOS enzymes produce NO: constitutive isoforms, in endothelium and neurons, release small quantities of NO, in bursts, to signal ad-

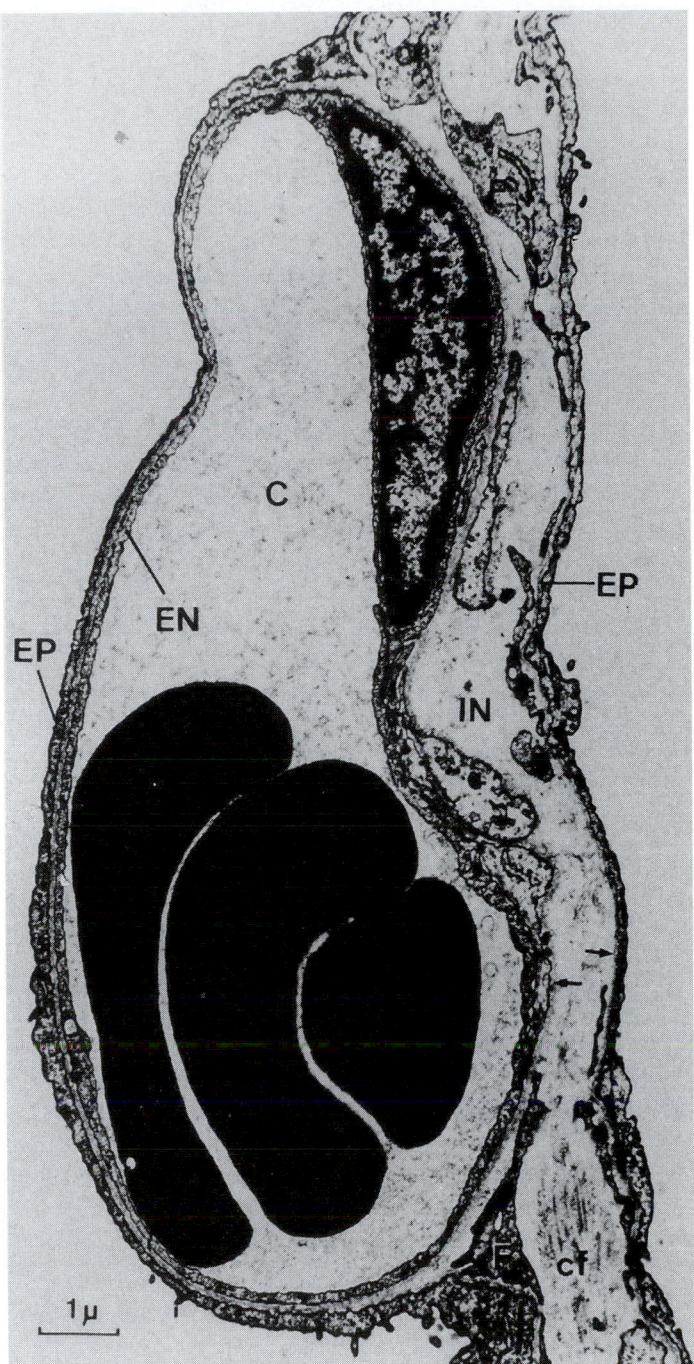

FIGURE 82-13   Cross section of alveolar capillary from human lung lined by endothelium (EN). Endothelial nucleus is striking. Alveolar-capillary barrier is organized into thick (*right*) and thin (*left*) portions. Thick side includes considerable interstitial space (IN), containing connective-tissue elements (e.g., fibers [cf]). In contrast, interstitial space on thin side is obliterated by fusion of basement membranes, which forms a minimal air-blood barrier. C = capillary containing three red corpuscles in its lumen; EP = alveolar epithelium; F = fibroblast. (*Courtesy of E. Weibel.*)

jacent cells; and inducible isoforms, in macrophages, release large amounts of NO continuously and serve to eliminate bacteria and parasites. NOS are a family of complex cytochrome P_{450}-like hemoproteins. NO synthase can be inhibited by methylene blue and by L-N-monomethylarginine, an L-arginine analog.

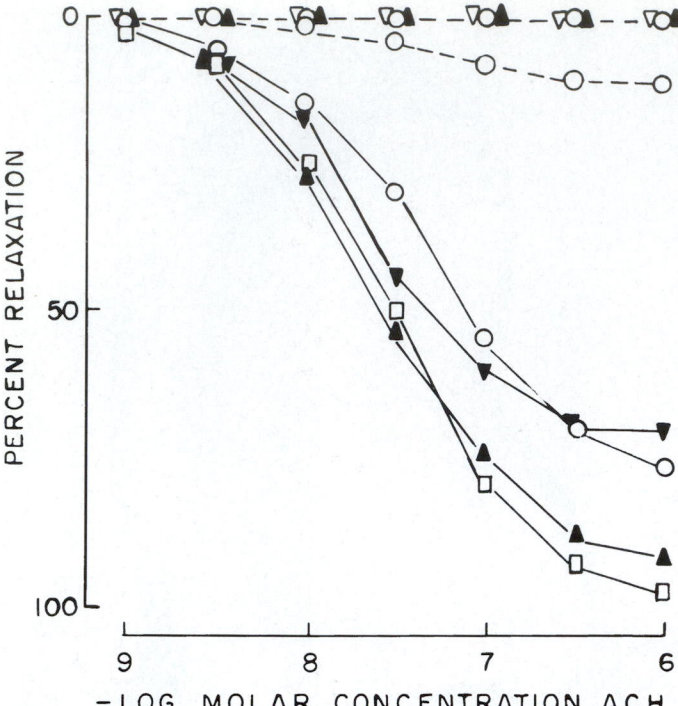

FIGURE 82-14 Influence of endothelium on responses of different vessels to acetylcholine (ACH). Increasing concentrations of acetylcholine were applied to rings of femoral, saphenous, splenic, and pulmonary arteries *(circles)* that had previously been contracted with norepinephrine. Vessels in which endothelium was intact *(solid curves)* responded with increasing vasodilation. In vessels without endothelium *(dashed curves),* virtually no vasodilation occurred. *(From De Mey and Vanhoutte: Circ Res 51:439–447, 1982.)*

Among its biologic functions is the regulation of pulmonary vascular tone.[6,7] Its release is triggered by both physical factors, such as endothelial shear stress, and biochemical influences, such as bradykinin, histamine, and catecholamines. The NO produced by pulmonary endothelial cells is transported by the hemoglobin in the red blood cells to systemic arterioles, where it causes muscle relaxation. The cysteine residue of hemoglobin is active in the transport of NO to the peripheral blood vessels. The NO conveyed to the periphery enters the vascular smooth muscle cell by diffusion to activate adenylate cyclase, leading to an increase in cyclic GMP, which, in turn, causes muscle relaxation (vascular dilation) (Fig. 82-16).

Inhaled nitric oxide is currently being investigated as a therapeutic pulmonary vasodilator.[25,31,34] It is administered by airway and is rapidly removed by hemoglobin in blood. Because it is administered by inhalation, it has opportunity en route to interact with the wide variety of cells that comprise the epithelial lining, autonomic neurons, smooth muscle, and interstitium.

Endothelins

Endothelins (ET-1, ET-2, and ET-3) are a family of short (21 amino acids) peptides produced by endothelial cells.[24] Of the three, ET-1 is the only one produced by endothelial cells. It is a powerful vasoconstrictor and stimulant of cell growth. ET-1 is produced, on physiological demand, from a larger precursor molecule (ECE), which is being intensively investigated for its potential as an avenue for inhibiting endothelin formation in various disease states. Three ET receptors (ETA, ETB, and ETC) have been cloned. ETA receptors on vascular smooth muscle are responsible for vasoconstriction and growth promotion; ETB receptors on endothelium are related to release of prostacyclin or nitric oxide. Binding of endothelin-1 to ETA receptors initiates a cascade leading to vasoconstriction by way of phospholipase C and resulting in an increase in intracellular calcium ion concentration. Binding of endothelins to ETB receptors stimulates vasodilation.[10]

In addition to its direct effects on vascular tone, ET-1 has a wide range of biologic actions, including constriction of extravascular smooth muscle, mitogenesis, and release of other mediators, such as prostacyclin, nitric oxide, and atrial natriuretic peptide. The lungs remove large amounts of endothelin from circulating blood. Within the lungs, ETs are present in the parenchyma and pulmonary vessels. They are powerful bronchoconstrictors. Release of endothelins is stimulated by such receptor-mediated stimuli as epinephrine, angiotensin II, arginine vasopressin, thrombin, transforming growth factor–β, and interleukin-1 and also by hypoxia.[2] The endothelin–receptor antagonist bosentan prevents and reverses pulmonary hypertension in rats.[4] Because of the diversity of their effects and widespread distribution in the body, the role of the endothelins is being explored in a wide variety of diseases, such as hypertension, arteriosclerosis, Raynaud's disease, ulcerative colitis, and renal failure.[39]

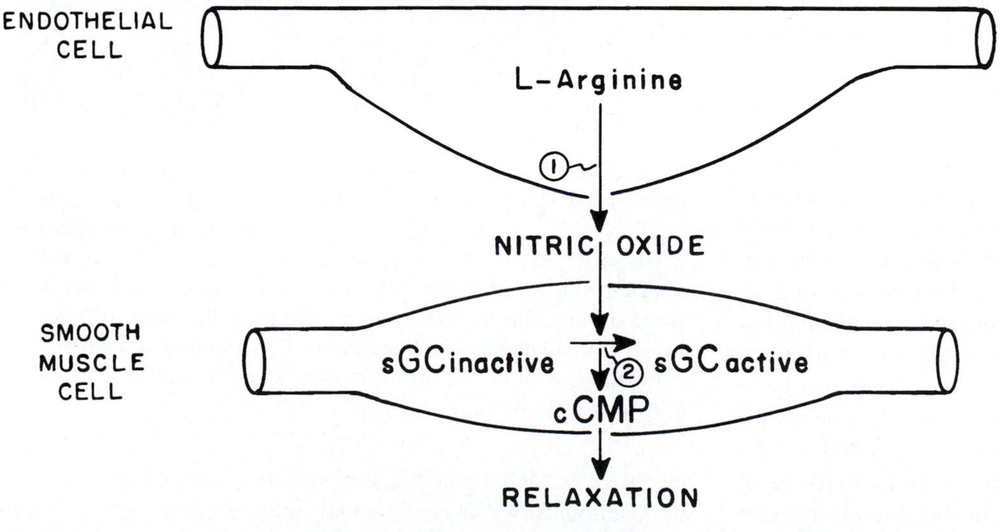

FIGURE 82-15 Synthesis of nitric oxide by vascular endothelium. *1.* The enzyme nitric oxide synthase (NOS) synthesizes nitric oxide from L-arginine. *2.* NO diffuses to the smooth muscle cell, where it activates the enzyme guanylate cyclase via cyclic GMP to smooth-muscle relation.

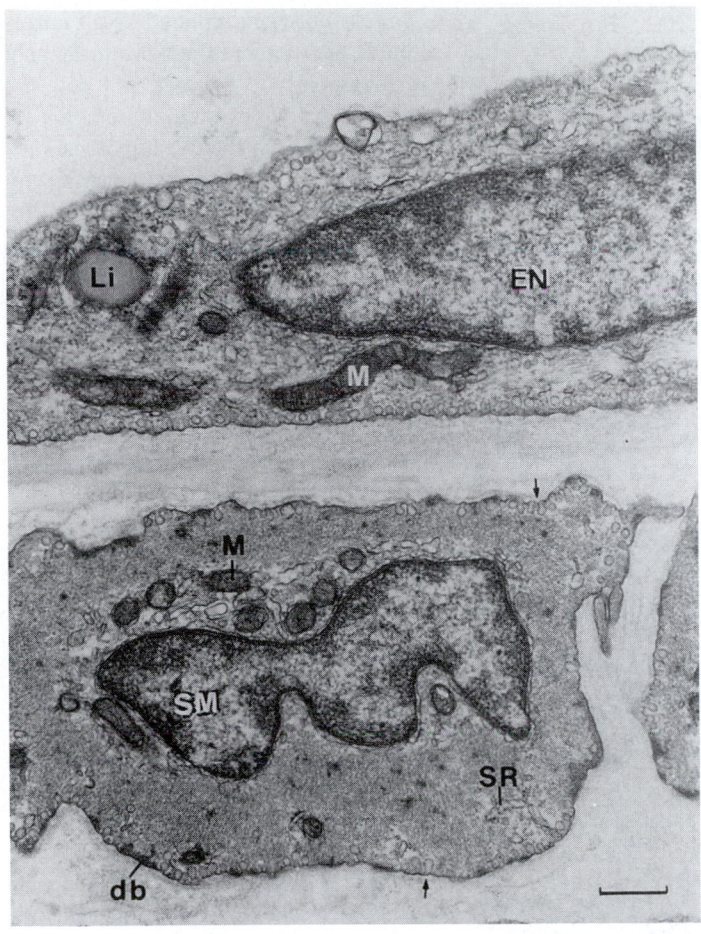

FIGURE 82-16   Electron micrograph of small muscular pulmonary artery from human lung showing endothelium (EN) and single layer of smooth muscle (SM). Thick endothelial cytoplasm and wealth of organelles (*inset*) comprising mitochondria (M), endoplasmic reticulum (ER), lipid droplet (Li), specific granules (asterisks), microtubules (mt), and many vesicles (*arrows*). Cross-sectioned smooth-muscle cells show central nucleus, mitochondria, sarcoplasmic reticulum (SR), membrane-bounded caveolae (*arrows*), filamentous matter with dense bodies (db), and cell-to-cell contacts (circle). cf = collagen fibrils; el = elastic fibers; bars, 0.5 μm. (*Courtesy of E. Weibel.*)

Respiratory Gases and pH

ACUTE HYPOXIA

The classic demonstration of the pressor effect of acute hypoxia on the pulmonary circulation was made by Euler and Liljestrand on the open-chest cat (Fig. 82-17).[9] In the ensuing half-century, acute hypoxia has proved to be a pulmonary vasoconstrictor in virtually all species indigenous to sea level. Euler and Liljestrand not only documented the role of alveolar hypoxia in eliciting the pulmonary pressor response but also appreciated that local hypoxia (as by disease) might automatically redirect blood flow to better-ventilated parts of the lung by eliciting local vasoconstriction.[19] Finally, they anticipated recent studies on the effect of shear on release of endothelial mediators by identifying as a subject for research the response of pulmonary vessels to large increases in pulmonary blood flow.[11]

In human subjects, acute hypoxia causes an increase in pulmonary arterial pressure, does not affect left atrial pressure, and usually produces little increase in cardiac output. The pressor response starts within seconds, generally reaching its peak by 3 min, and attenuates gradually as hypoxia continues.[22] Severe acidosis augments the hypoxic pressor response. The site of pulmonary vasoconstriction in response to acute hypoxia is predominantly at the precapillary level, involving the small muscular arteries and arterioles (Fig. 82-18).

Acute hypoxic vasoconstriction can be relieved by a variety of bronchodilators and vasodilators, such as inhalation anesthetics. Endothelial-derived vasodilators appear to be particularly effective. For example, prostacyclin administered intravenously can blunt or abolish the hypoxic pressor response. Similarly, inhalation of nitric oxide inhibits hypoxic vasoconstriction, whereas inhibitors of nitric oxide synthase augment the hypoxic pressor response by blocking the endogenous synthesis of nitric oxide.

The mechanisms of the hypoxic-pressor response have been investigated for years along two dominant lines: the first postulates a direct effect of hypoxia on the smooth-muscle cells of vascular media; the second proposes the release of a chemical

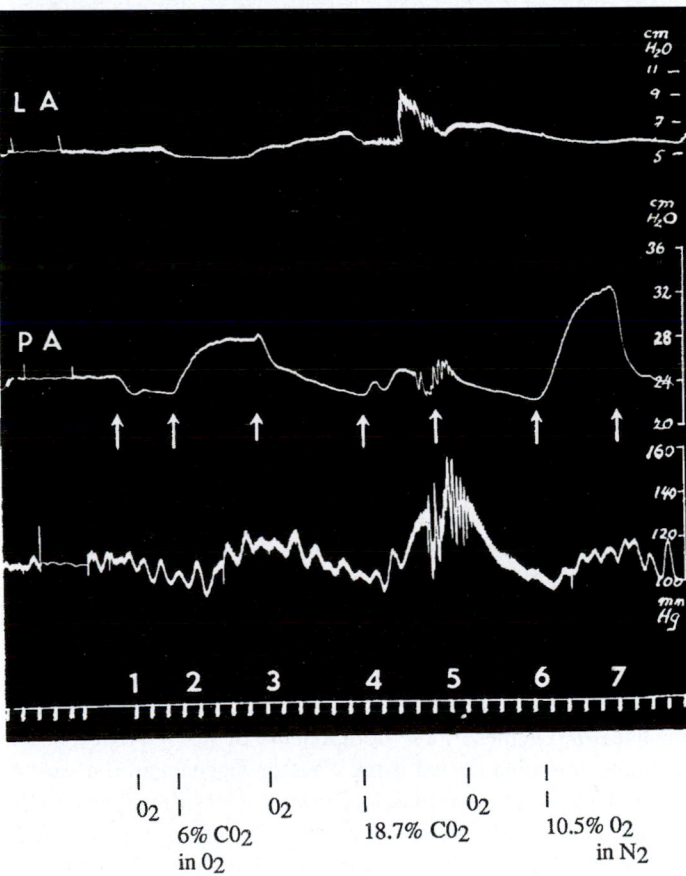

FIGURE 82-17   The classic recordings by Euler and Liljestrand showing the effects of acute hypoxia on the pulmonary arterial (PA) and left atrial (LA) pressures in the open chest cast (labels added). At the far right, breathing 10.5 percent O_2 caused a considerable rise in pulmonary arterial pressure without a corresponding increase in left atrial pressure. (Labels added at bottom of figure.) (*Based on data of Euler and Liljestrand,[9] with permission.*)

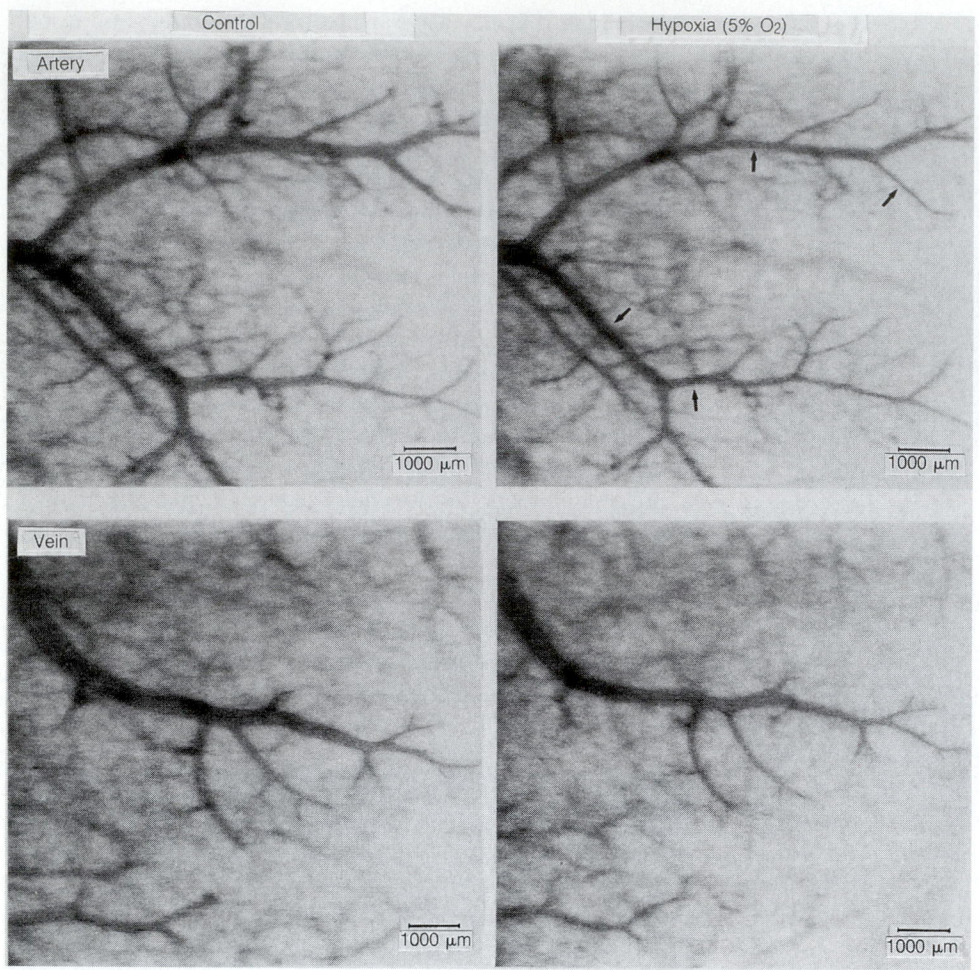

FIGURE 82-18   Direct visualization of the vasoconstrictor effect of acute hypoxia. During breathing of 5 percent O$_2$ in N$_2$, the pulmonary precapillary vessels are attenuated by vasoconstriction, whereas the pulmonary veins undergo no appreciable change. *(Courtesy of Dr. I. Ninomiya, National Cardiovascular Research Institute, Osaka, Japan.)*

and closed when reduced.[1] Still unsettled is the type(s) of potassium channel that responds to hypoxia and how the ionic exchanges through these channels are gated. One attractive hypothesis being tested is that hypoxia is sensed by a hemoprotein in the membrane of the smooth-muscle cell—which, in turn, activates the responsive potassium channel(s).[16]

CHRONIC HYPOXIA

With few exceptions, such as the yak (a native resident at high altitude), chronic hypoxic pulmonary hypertension is a feature of life at high altitude.[18] The exceptions are due to genetic influences that are manifested by variability in the hypoxic pressor response among species and even among strains. Chronic hypoxia elicits anatomic changes in the small pulmonary arteries and arterioles, which have been designated pulmonary vascular remodeling. These fibrocellular changes are characterized by proliferation of the smooth muscle in the vessel walls, causing thickening and peripheral extension of smooth muscle in the media of small muscular arteries and arterioles. Concomitantly, elastin and collagen are synthesized and deposited in the extracellular matrix and adventitia. The end result is an increase in resistance to blood flow and a decrease in distensibility of the pulmonary resistance vessels. The stimuli for remodeling include not only hypoxia but also mechanical forces, such as increase in blood flow, which expose endothelial cells to increased shear stress and activate platelets to release promotors of smooth-muscle cell proliferation. Various genes are expressed in the process of hypoxic-induced vascular remodeling, some attributable to the hypoxia per se and others evoked by the vasoconstrictor response. Agents that block hypoxic pulmonary vasoconstriction also block the development of chronic hypoxic pulmonary hypertension and the remodeling response.[19,30] In essence, a variety of influences, including mechanical factors, growth factors, and mediators, appear to be active in pulmonary vascular remodeling.[42,51] With respect to both acute and chronic hypoxia, one tantalizing enigma is the reason why hypoxia causes pulmonary vessels to constrict and systemic vessels to dilate.

mediator within the lungs during acute hypoxia (e.g., endothelin-1 by pulmonary vascular endothelium). Although both continue to have their proponents, the cumulative evidence favors the view that the hypoxic pressor effect is exerted directly on pulmonary vascular smooth muscle.[4,26,37] Moreover, the many vasoactive substances that have been investigated as possible mediators of this effect (i.e., the postulated "indirect" effect) are actually modulators rather than mediators.[11,50]

The direct effect has been explored along three lines: the sensing mechanism, the transduction mechanism, and the effector mechanism. Of these three components of the hypoxic pressor response, the most settled is the effector mechanism (i.e., an increase in cytosolic calcium concentration).[36] For insights into the sensing and transducing mechanisms, investigators have turned to the type 1 cell of the carotid body that, like the pulmonary myocyte, is stimulated by hypoxia.[23] In both types of cells, hypoxia has been found to inhibit an outward potassium current, thereby causing membrane depolarization and entry of calcium into the cells by way of voltage-dependent calcium channels.[20,33,46] Also in both types of cells, changes in the redox status of the oxygen-sensitive potassium channel or channels may control current flow, so that the channel is open when oxidized

Considerable data about the pulmonary circulation at altitude have been gathered at Morococha, Peru (an altitude of 4540 m), where an ambient PO$_2$ of about 80 mm Hg is associated in adults with a mean pulmonary arterial pressure of about 28 mm Hg (about twice the average value of 12 mm Hg in sea-level residents [Lima], even though cardiac output and

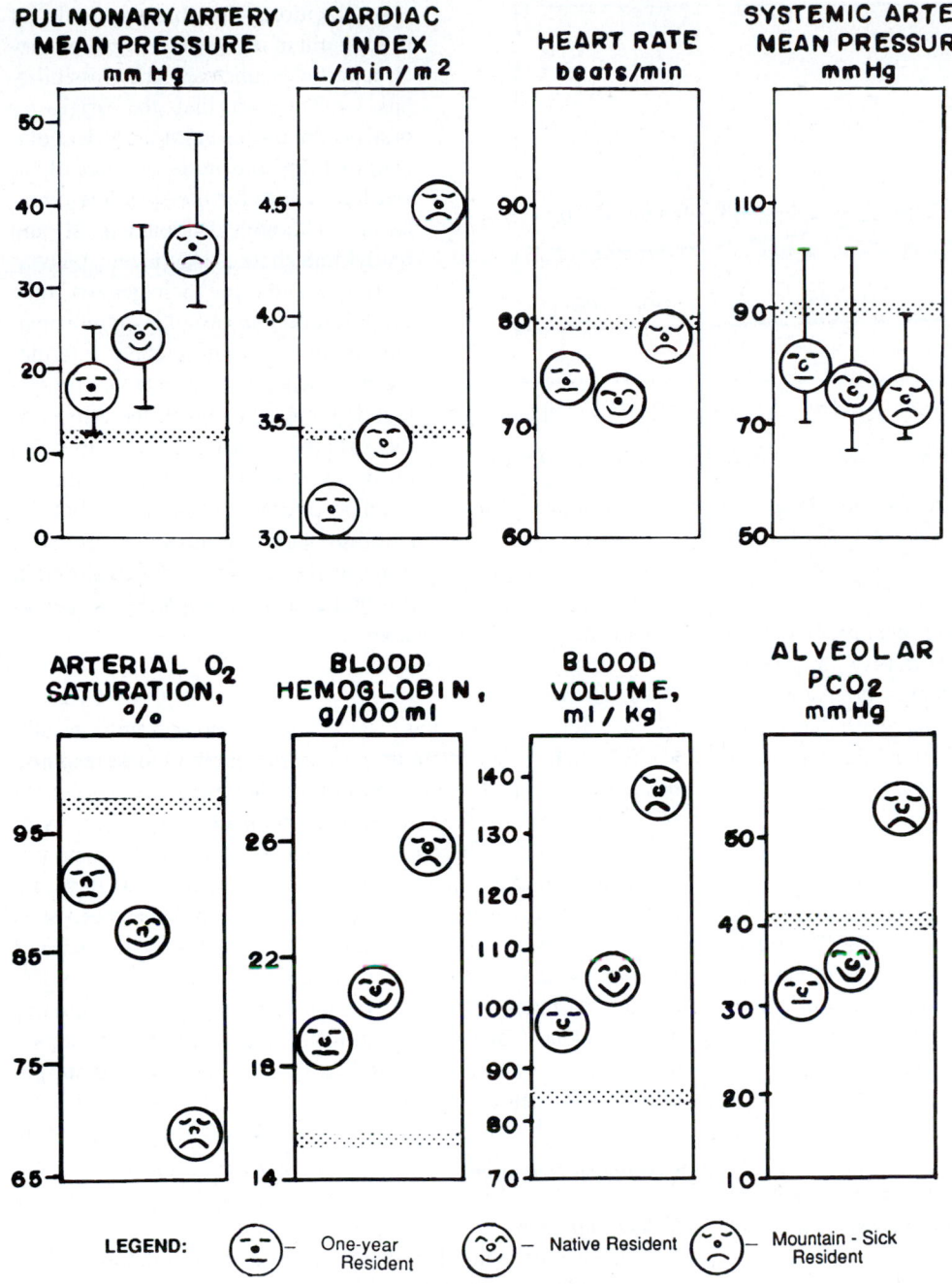

FIGURE 82-19   Schematic representations of respiratory and circulatory measurements in humans at altitude (14,900 feet). The three circles within each rectangle illustrate normal values for the 1-year resident (*left circles*), the native resident (*middle circles*), and the native mountain-sick resident (*right circles*). The facial expressions are intended to indicate the degree of acclimatization.

When native residents of high altitudes take up residence at sea level, pulmonary arterial pressure and pulmonary vascular resistance decrease somewhat, although not to normal (Fig. 82-20). Pulmonary vascular resistance remains high because of anatomic changes in the pulmonary arterial tree elicited by the chronic hypoxia (i.e., by hypertrophy and hyperplasia of the small muscular arteries and arterioles, accompanied by extension of muscle peripherally into precapillary vessels that are ordinarily nonmuscular). In the face of this restructuring of precapillary vessels, the pulmonary capillaries and veins remain unchanged. Polycythemia, because it increases blood viscosity, contributes to the pulmonary hypertension associated with chronic hypoxia.

At sea level, the anatomic lesions of hypoxic pulmonary hypertension gradually revert toward normal. Nonetheless, 2 years after moving sea level, the native high-altitude dweller still shows an inordinate increase in pulmonary arterial pressure, in response to a modest increase in pulmonary blood flow, presumably a consequence of persistent muscularization of the small pulmonary arteries.

Children born at altitude undergo more gradual involution of pulmonary arterial pressures than do those born at sea level. Therefore, up to the age of 5 years, children raised at altitude have uniformly higher pulmonary arterial pressures (around 58/32, 44 mmHg) than do older children at altitude (41/18, 28 mm Hg).

pulmonary wedge pressures are the same) (Fig. 82-19). During moderate exercise, mean pulmonary arterial pressure increases considerably: quadrupling the oxygen uptake intensifies arterial hypoxemia and doubles both the cardiac output (from 3.65 to 7.49 L/min/m²) and the pulmonary arterial pressure (from 41/15, 29 mm Hg, to 77/40, 60 mm Hg).[18] In persons suffering from chronic mountain sickness, in which severe arterial hypoxemia and hypercapnia are secondary to alveolar hypoventilation, pulmonary arterial pressures are much higher. Genetic factors seem to influence human susceptibility to pulmonary hypertension at altitude.

ACUTE HYPERCAPNIA

Although Euler and Liljestrand found an increase in pulmonary arterial pressure during CO_2 breathing, it has since been shown that there is little response to inspired CO_2 if pH is maintained at near-normal levels (they did not measure pH). For example, enrichment of inspired air with tolerable concentration of CO_2 (5 to 7 percent) has little effect on the human pulmonary circulation, presumably because the increase in ventilation minimizes change in blood pH. However, if the ventilatory response is lim-

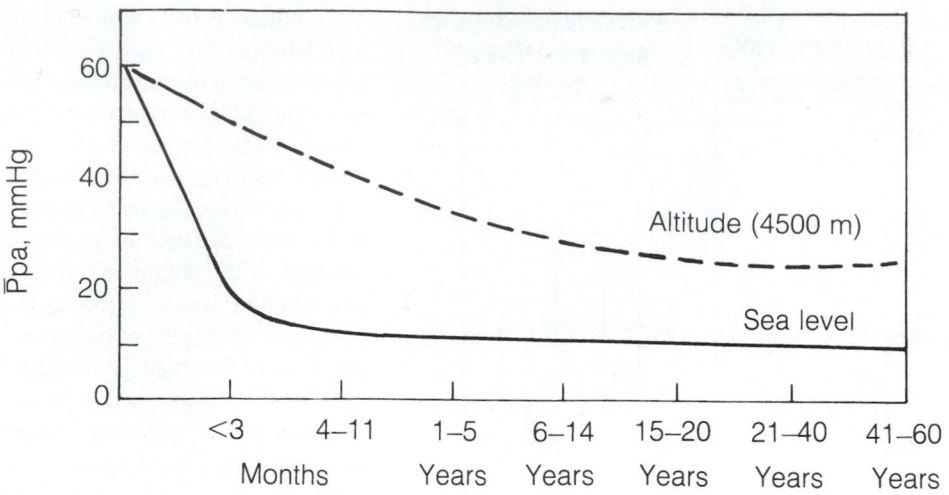

FIGURE 82-20   Return of pulmonary artery pressures to normal after prolonged residence at sea level.

ited (e.g., during anesthesia), a distinct pressor response is evoked as arterial blood becomes acidotic (i.e., as pH falls to 7.2 or less). The combination of moderate to severe acidosis—no matter how induced—and acute hypoxia elicits a greater response than either alone (i.e., the pressor response to acute hypoxia and acute hypercapnia combined is synergistic).

BLOOD PH

Just as severe acidosis elicits pulmonary vasoconstriction, so does severe alkalosis cause pulmonary vasodilatation. The interplay between hypoxia and acidosis is believed to be of considerable importance in areas of alveolar hypoventilation in which the combination of local acidosis and hypoxia promotes the diversion of blood flow to better ventilated parts of the lungs.

Other Vasoactive Substances

A variety of endogenous and exogenous substances have been used to alter the tone of the pulmonary blood vessels, generally the small pulmonary arteries and arterioles.

VASODILATORS

Acetylcholine
As noted above, acetylcholine is a powerful pulmonary vasodilator when pulmonary vascular tone is high (Fig. 82-10). Observations on the role of endothelium in determining the responses of different vessels to acetylcholine marked the beginning of current interest in EDRF and to the identification of nitric oxide as an agent that mimicked the EDRF effects.

Bradykinin
This pulmonary vasodilator is a member of a family of vasoactive polypeptides. It is inactivated by the same converting enzyme(s) in the lungs that convert(s) angiotensin I to II. Although it is consistently a powerful systemic vasodilator, it is not as predictable as a pulmonary vasodilator, usually evoking pulmonary

vasodilatation. The biologic role of bradykinin in regulating the pulmonary circulation is unclear. The possibility has been raised that the origin of bradykinin in the pulmonary vascular endothelium constitutes a source of vasodilator agent for the systemic circulation. Although angiotensin II and bradykinin share a dependency on converting enzyme for their genesis, they act differently on vascular smooth muscle: angiotensin acts without intermediaries, whereas vasoactive prostaglandins are involved in the effects of the kallidins. Indeed, at least in some of the species, the variability in the vasoactive effects of bradykinin and the kallidins has been attributed to variations in the extent to which different prostaglandins are engaged as mediators of the vasodilator response.

Isoproterenol
In the normal pulmonary circulation, isoproterenol usually evokes a barely detectable drop in pressure; the modest response has been attributed to low initial tone due either to the paucity of β-adrenergic receptors or to the low level of their activity in the normal state. The vasodilator response is much more impressive in animal preparations in which initial tone is high and in some patients with pulmonary hypertension. It has been suggested that the pulmonary vasodilator effect of isoproterenol when pulmonary vascular tone is high depends not only on pulmonary vascular adrenergic receptors but also on vasodilator prostaglandins. One complicating feature in the use of isoproterenol as a pulmonary vasodilator is its powerful inotropic effect on the heart.

VASOCONSTRICTORS

Catecholamines
Norepinephrine and phenylephrine, potent stimulators of the α-adrenergic system in the pulmonary circulation, consistently elicit pulmonary vasoconstriction. Epinephrine, which possesses α- and β-adrenergic effects, not only evokes less vasoconstriction on a weight-for-weight basis but can also, depending on the preparation, cause vasodilatation.

Angiotensin II
Angiotensin II, an octapeptide formed in the lungs by the action of converting enzyme from angiotensin I and decapeptide (Fig. 82-2), generally but not invariably elicits pulmonary vasoconstriction. Small doses (0.03 μg/kg/min, administered intravenously) suffice to increase pulmonary arterial pressure without discernible effect on the systemic circulation.

Histamine
Histamine (in doses of 10^{-5} g, given intravenously over a 2-min period) elicits more variable responses. Although species differ-

ence and the type of experimental preparation seem to influence the outcome, as a rule, histamine (like hypoxia) appears to be a powerful pulmonary vasoconstrictor and systemic vasodilator. At one time, it was suspected that histamine was an important local mediator in the regulation of the pulmonary circulation. However, this belief appears to have been discounted.

Discrepant effects of histamine on the pulmonary circulation can be rationalized in terms of H_1 and H_2 receptors and their blocking agents: chlorpheniramine to block H_1 receptors selectively, metiamide to block H_2 receptors. The use of these agents suggests that pulmonary vasoconstriction is mediated by H_1 receptors and vasodilatation by H_2 receptors.

Serotonin

Serotonin (in doses on the order of 10^{-5} g given intravenously over a few minutes) is another vasoconstrictive amine that occurs in the mast cells of some species but not others. It is synthesized in the enterochromaffin cells of the gut from dietary tryptophan. The serotonin released by these cells is largely removed by the liver, the excess being almost completely removed by the endothelial cells of the pulmonary circulation (Fig. 82-21). Any serotonin that escapes the metabolic machinery of the liver and lungs is stored as dense granules in circulating platelets. In addition to direct effects on vessels, airways, and platelets, serotonin enhances vasoconstriction and platelet aggregation pro-

duced by other vasoactive agents, such as norepinephrine and angiotensin II.

Two separate binding sites have been identified for serotonin: S_1 receptor binding sites that are labeled by serotonin and S_2 receptor binding sites that are labeled by serotonin antagonists (e.g., spiperone and ketanserin). The physiological and pharmacologic effects of serotonin (vasomotor activity, bronchoconstriction platelet aggregation) appear to be related to the binding of serotonin to the S_2 receptor; no such effects have been attributed to binding to the S_1 receptor.

The distinction between S_1 receptors and S_2 receptors holds great promise for reexamining the role of serotonin in the bronchoconstriction and pulmonary vasoconstriction evoked by pulmonary embolism. In contrast to histamine, which seems to affect both pulmonary arterial and venous components, serotonin seems to constrict predominantly the precapillary vessels.[3]

THE PULMONARY ARTERIAL MICROCIRCULATION IN GAS EXCHANGE

The pulmonary circulation is designed to operate in concert with alveolar ventilation for the sake of gas exchange. Certain aspects of this interplay warrant special mention: (1) the lungs receive the entire cardiac output; (2) the pulmonary blood flow is about the same as the alveolar ventilation; and (3) although the respiratory and circulatory processes are phasic, the rates are entirely different (i.e., about 15 breaths and 80 heartbeats per minute at rest). Therefore, matching of air and blood for optimal arterialization of mixed venous blood requires delicate tuning of operations that are not in phase, either at rest or during exercise; no vasomotor nerves or neurohumoral substances are at hand to make the speedy and fine adjustments of alveolar blood flow to alveolar ventilation.[44]

Matching of air and blood for optimal gas exchange requires about 300 million alveoli that bear myriad capillary segments in their walls. The interposition of pulmonary capillaries between contiguous alveoli provides an enormous surface area for gas exchange, about 100 m² at rest, which increases further during exercise. The volume of blood in the capillaries at any one instance is approximately 100 to 200 ml, and red blood cells pass from one end of the gas-exchanging network to the other in about 0.75 s.

Four aspects of the distribution of the pulmonary circulation have attracted special attention with re-

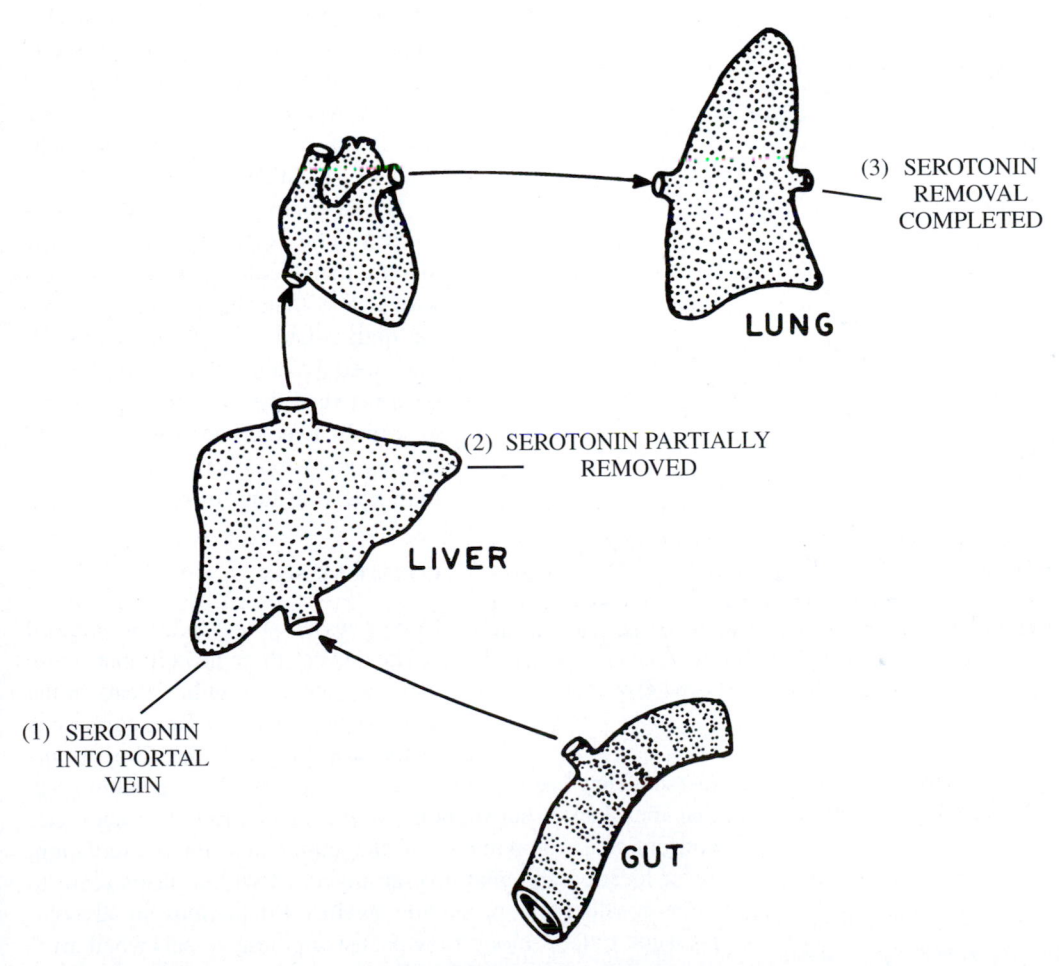

(3) SEROTONIN REMOVAL COMPLETED

LUNG

(2) SEROTONIN PARTIALLY REMOVED

LIVER

(1) SEROTONIN INTO PORTAL VEIN

GUT

FIGURE 82-21 Handling of serotonin by the gut-liver-lung axis. During a single passage, serotonin is partly removed by the liver. Removal is completed by the lungs.

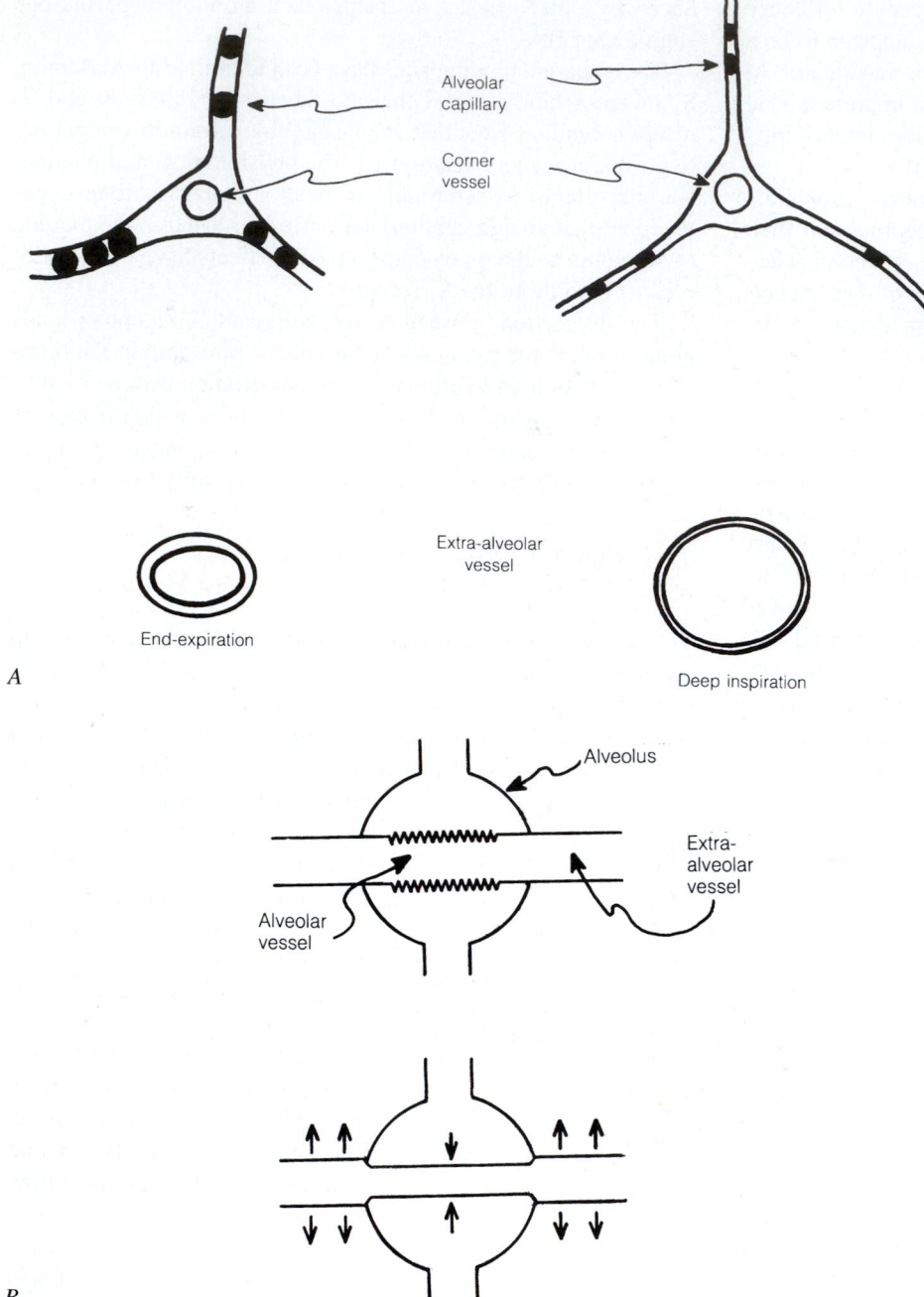

FIGURE 82-22 Schematic representation of the effects of a deep breath on the relative calibers of alveolar capillaries, "corner vessels," and extra-alveolar vessels. *Top:* At end-expiration, the alveolar capillaries (containing red cells) are wide-bored. The relative sizes of corner vessels and of extra-alveolar vessels are also shown. Deep inspiration narrows the alveolar vessels and widens extra-alveolar vessels, leaving inner vessels virtually unchanged in caliber. *Bottom:* The same phenomenon is shown for alveolar and extra-alveolar vessels. *A* represents end-expiration and *B* end-inspiration.

ALVEOLAR VESSELS

Alveolar vessels are capillaries that are contained within the walls that separate adjacent alveoli. They are surround by interstitium that varies in thickness and in the nature and content of cells, collagen, and elastic fibers. The appearance of the alveolar capillaries depends heavily on the route of fixation. Thus, fixation via the airways—which removes the surfactant lining—causes the capillaries to bulge into the alveoli, whereas fixation by perfusion—so that the lung remains air-filled—eliminates these deformations, widens capillaries unnaturally, and does away with alveolar pleats and folds. As the lung expands, alveolar walls unfold, and the connective-tissue elements surrounding them are rearranged. The calibers of the alveolar capillaries depend on the level of lung inflation, and they undergo compression (without change in wall thickness) when alveolar pressures increase. It is clear from the above that impressions of alveolar morphology are meaningful only when full account is taken not only of the route of fixation but also of the way in which the lung was handled during fixation.

As the lungs expand, largely because of the surfactant lining of the alveoli, the alveolar pericapillary pressure is less than the alveolar pressure but higher than the pressure surrounding extra-alveolar vessels. This difference between the interstitial pressures to which alveolar and extra-alveolar vessels are exposed is exaggerated at high levels of lung inflation.

CORNER VESSELS

Corner vessels (Fig. 82-22) are located at sites where three alveoli abut; there they are contained within pleats in the alveolar walls beneath sharp curvatures in the overlying alveolar film of surfactant. They are neither extra-alveolar vessels (see below)—in that they lack a surrounding sleeve of connective tissue—nor conventional components of the pulmonary microcirculation. Their location and anatomic arrangement within pleats seem to offer considerable protection against fluctuations in alveolar pressure. Indeed, blood flow persists in these vessels when alveolar pressure exceeds pulmonary arterial pressure by 10 cm H_2O. Originally pictured as arteriovenous anastomoses, they are now viewed as preferential channels through which blood flow con-

spect to gas exchange: (1) gas-exchanging vessels, (2) effects of gravity, (3) interplay among pressures influencing vascular calibers, and (4) effects of inflation.[17]

Structure and Function

Depending on the perivascular pressures to which they are exposed, three types of intrapulmonary vessels have been distinguished: alveolar, corner, and extra-alveolar (Fig. 82-22).[15,45]

tinues in the face of wide swings in
alveolar pressure.

EXTRA-ALVEOLAR VESSELS

Extra-alveolar vessels are, by definition, small vessels that are not affected
by changes in alveolar pressure but do
enlarge during lung inflation (Fig. 82-
22). The definition is far more precise
for physiologists than for anatomists,
since the designation *extra-alveolar
vessel* appears to include diverse components of the pulmonary microcirculation—notably veins, venules, arteries,
and precapillaries.

Despite the morphologic diversity, the
key to the physiological behavior of the
extra-alveolar vessels appears to be the
connective-tissue sheath that they share. Surrounding the extra-
alveolar vessels is an interstitial space that is bounded by extensions of the fascial sheaths that envelop the trachea and esophagus.
Within the perivascular interstitial space lies loose areolar tissue,
collagenous fibers, and lymph vessels that drain lymph from the
lung parenchyma; in pulmonary edema, excess fluid (and protein)
accumulates within this space. The sheaths extend farther peripherally along the pulmonary arteries than the bronchi; for pulmonary
arteries, and probably for pulmonary veins, the perivascular sheaths
continue peripherally to vessels on the order of 100 μm in diameter.
Dilatation of extra-alveolar vessels during inflation is a consequence
of a drop in the surrounding interstitial pressure.

The degree to which extra-alveolar vessels widen during inflation depends on their initial calibers, which, in turn, vary with
lung volume. During deflation to levels below functional residual capacity (FRC), small arteries and veins tend to close, possibly because of inherent vascular tone abetted by alveolar
hypoxia in the poorly expanded regions. At this time, the site of
maximum resistance to blood flow shifts proximally in the arterial tree.

EFFECTS OF GRAVITY

A variety of techniques have been used
to test the influence of gravity on the
topographic distribution of blood delivered to the lungs. Among these have
been the intravenous injection of a
polysoluble gas (e.g., xenon), the inhalation of a very soluble gas (e.g.,
carbon dioxide), and the intravenous
injection of microaggregated albumin,
followed by radiographic determination of the distribution of radioactivity. Although interpretation of the results of these different methods is
often complicated by individual peculiarities of the techniques, coupled
with the different types of information
that they provide, the results do sug-

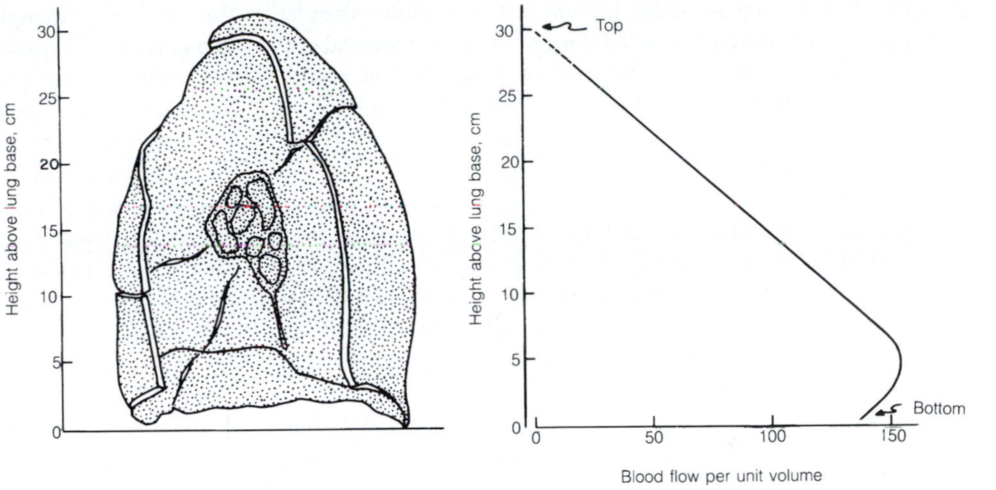

FIGURE 82-23   Blood flow in the upright lung as a function of vertical height. *(Based on data of
Glazier et al,[17] with permission.)*

gest that in the upright lungs, blood flow decreases steadily from
the bottom to the top (Fig. 82-23), that gravity is the compelling
force, and that there is an interplay among pulmonary arterial,
alveolar, and pulmonary venous pressures. As a consequence of
these influences, in a relaxed, seated subject—particularly one
with an elongated thorax—the apices are apt to be poorly perfused, especially in states of pulmonary hypotension or increased
alveolar pressure.

INTERPLAY AMONG PRESSURES INFLUENCING VASCULAR
CALIBERS

In 1960, Banister and Torrance, in West,[48] demonstrated that the
level of alveolar pressure could influence pressure-flow relationships in the pulmonary circulation and drew an analogy between the behavior of the pulmonary arterial, pulmonary venous,
and alveolar pressures and that of a Starling resistor (Fig. 82-
24). The crucial point of their demonstration was that when alveolar pressure (chamber pressure) exceeded venous (downstream)

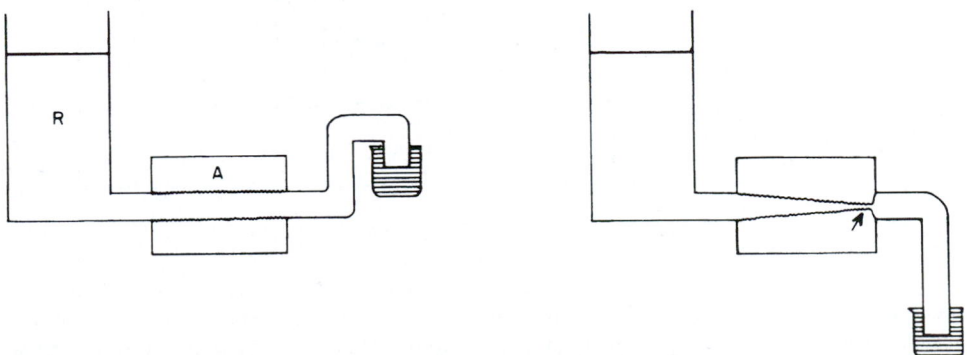

FIGURE 82-24   Principle of a Starling resistor. Thin-walled collapsible tube traverses a closed
chamber (*A*) in which pressure can be varied at will. Fluid flows from reservoir (*R*) into collecting
vessel (striped area), traversing collapsible tube en route. When outflow pressure exceeds chamber
pressure (*left*), flow is determined by difference between inflow and outflow pressure. However,
when chamber pressure exceeds outflow pressure, so that collapsible tube closes (*arrow*), flow is
determined by difference between inflow and chamber pressure. *(From West and Dollery: J Appl
Physiol 20:175, 1965.)*

pressure, the driving pressure became arterial minus alveolar pressure and not arterial minus venous pressure. Permutt and colleagues compared this behavior to that of a waterfall, where height does not influence the flow of water over its brink.[32]

ZONES OF THE LUNGS

Recognition of the effects of alveolar pressure on pressure-flow relationships in the pulmonary circulation, coupled with the formulation of the behavior of pulmonary microvessels in terms of the Starling resistor, paved the way for a model of the topographic distribution of blood flow in the lungs under the influence of gravity. As a result, it is now common to use "zones" of blood flow in the lungs as operative shorthand for specifying the interplay of pulmonary arterial, alveolar, and pulmonary venous pressures (Fig. 82-25).[48]

In the normal, upright lung (estimated height of 25 cm at FRC), about 15 cm is above the left atrium and about 10 cm is below. Assuming that the mean pulmonary arterial pressure measured at the level of the left atrium is around 15 cm H_2O and that left atrial pressure is about 7 cm H_2O, the top few centimeters of the lung will be hypoperfused during most of the cardiac cycle, except for flushes of blood during the peak ejection phase of systole. This zone has been designated as zone 1. In the next-lower zone (zone 2), blood flow increases regularly with distance down the lung. Below zone 2 is another zone of increasing blood flow, zone 3. Finally, a zone 4 may exist near the base; in this zone, blood flow decreases instead of increases.

Zone 1

In the vertical lung, blood flow in zone 1, where alveolar pressure exceeds arterial pressure ($PA > Ppa$), is minimal (Fig. 82-25).

In this zone, although most alveolar capillaries appear to be attenuated or collapsed, extra-alveolar vessels in the alveolar corners often remain open, once again emphasizing that the extra-alveolar vessels are exposed to different forces than are the alveolar vessels. As noted previously, persistence of blood flow through parts of zone 1 presumably occurs via (corner) vessels.

The apices of upright lungs would be deprived of pulmonary blood flow were it not for the pulsatility of pulmonary arterial blood flow; a flush of blood during systole perfuses the apices even though mean pulmonary arterial pressure is too low to sustain blood flow to the apices.

Zone 2

In zone 2, pulmonary arterial pressure exceeds alveolar pressure, which, in turn, exceeds pulmonary venous pressure ($Ppa > PA > Ppv$) (Fig. 82-25). In this constellation of pressures, blood flow is no longer determined by the usual pressure drop across the pulmonary circulation. Instead, the outflow pressure is alveolar pressure and the driving force is the pulmonary arterial-alveolar pressure difference. This hemodynamic situation, in which flow is independent of downstream pressure, has been likened to a "vascular waterfall."

Under the influence of gravity, the pulmonary arterial pressure increases by about 1 cm H_2O per centimeter of distance down the lung, whereas alveolar pressure remains unchanged; the driving pressure and, therefore, the blood flow increase down the zone. Changing relationships between alveolar and luminal pressures then shift outflow pressures from alveolar to pulmonary venous and then back. Flow through the capillaries of zone 2 is pictured as intermittent, as through "sluice gates" that open when pulmonary venous pressures exceed alveolar pressures and close when alveolar pressures exceed pulmonary venous pressures.

Zone 3

It is only in this zone that conventional calculations of pulmonary vascular resistance are valid: since pulmonary venous pressure is greater than alveolar pressure ($Ppa > Ppv > PA$), blood flow is determined by the arteriovenous difference in pressure (since both exceed alveolar pressure) (Fig. 82-25). Resistance to blood flow in zone 3 is less than in zone 2. The driving pressure here remains fixed down to the bottom of the lung because the effect of gravity causes arterial and venous pressures to decrease equally per centimeter of distance as the lung base is approached. Despite the constant driving pressure, flow increases toward the bottom of the lung as resistance decreases. In contrast to zone 2, where the increase in blood flow from top to bottom of the zone is predominantly due to recruitment of vessels that were previously closed in zone 3 a comparable increase in blood flow is effected largely by distention of patient microvessels (i.e., capillaries).

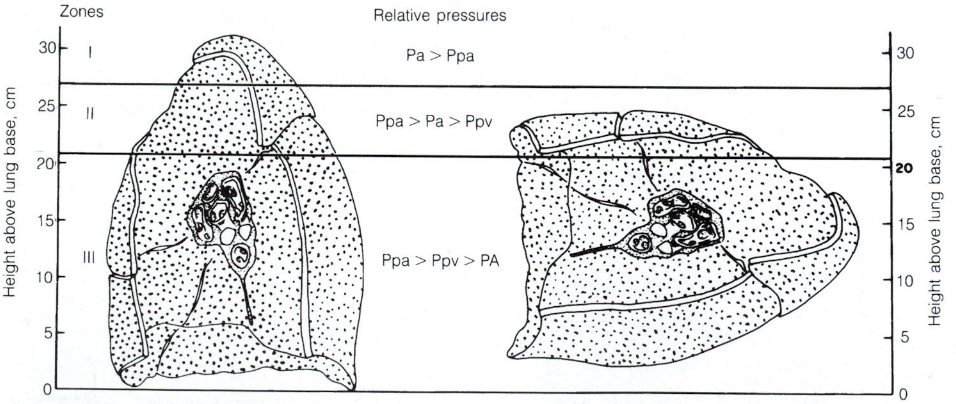

FIGURE 82-25   Zones of the lung. Topographic distribution of pulmonary blood flow according to relationship among pulmonary arterial pressure (Ppa), pulmonary venous pressure (Ppv), and alveolar pressure (PA). Because of effect of surface tension, PA is more accurately pericapillary pressure. Zone 1 (apex): PA > Ppa > Ppv. There is no flow (except through corner vessels) because collapsible vessels close when pericapillary pressure exceeds the pressure inside the vessels. Vessels that close are capillaries and other alveolar vessels up to ~30 μm in diameter. Zone 2: Ppa > PA > Ppv. Driving pressure is Ppa–PA. This difference increases down lung, and so does flow. Zone 3: Ppa > Ppv > PA. Driving pressure is Ppa–Ppv. Although Ppa–Ppv does not change down lung, Ppa and Ppv continue to increase from top to bottom. Flow down zone 3 is less than in zone 2. Zone 4 (appears at residual volume): This region of decreased flow appears during forced exhalation and has been attributed to either an increase in interstitial pressure at lung bases or closure of small airways at low lung volumes as the increase in PA creates either zone 1 or zone 2 conditions. *(From West and Dollery: J Appl Physiol 20:175, 1965.)*

Zone 4

The upright lung includes in its most dependent part, where vascular pressures are highest, an area of decreased blood flow (Fig. 82-23). The zone of reduced flow (zone 4) disappears on deep inflation. This paradox of high vascular pressures and low blood flow is not explicable in terms of the three-zone model, in which pulmonary arterial and pulmonary venous pressures are related to alveolar pressures in predicting distribution of blood flow. The mechanism is believed to reside in the extra-alveolar rather than in the alveolar vessels. Indeed, at residual volume, owing to the increase in perivascular pressure and mechanical distortion of extra-alveolar vessels, the distribution of blood flow throughout the lung is attributable to extra-alveolar vessels.

It is worth emphasizing that zones are a functional rather than an anatomic concept; instead of being fixed topographically, they vary in vertical height according to shifts in the relationships between pulmonary arterial, pulmonary venous, and alveolar pressures. For example, positive-pressure breathing enlarges zone 2 at the expense of zone 3, and zone 1 at the expense of zone 2. Awareness of the functional nature of these relationships affects the interpretation of changes in calculated pulmonary vascular resistance; for vessels in zone 2, because alveolar pressure rather than pulmonary venous pressure is the outlet pressure, the conventional calculation of pulmonary vascular resistance is meaningless; oppositely, for vessels in zone 3, the calculation is meaningful because pulmonary venous pressure rather than alveolar pressure determines the quantity of blood flow.

A change in body position reorients the zones of the lungs. For example, the supine position places more of the lung in zone 3 and virtually eliminates zone 1 (Fig. 82-25).

pended in a sea of air and not embedded in tissue. Indeed, it has now been amply shown that pulmonary vascular calibers do increase appreciably as transmural pressures are raised. But it has also become evident that the relationship between vascular calibers and transmural pressure is far from simple. Moreover, there is no consensus about the extent to which the alveolar capillary bed is distensible.

How recruitment is affected remains unsettled. When blood flow is minimal (as in zone 1), only few capillaries are open; these are predominantly "corner vessels" lodged within septal pleats. As transmural pressures increase, the extent of the open capillary bed enlarges, primarily by recruitment in zone 2 and by dilatation in zone 3. Some believe that as pulmonary arterial pressure increases, critical opening pressures of different arterioles are successively overcome to open new arteriolar domains to blood flow. Others favor the view that capillaries control their own destinies—i.e., that capillaries per se, rather than arterioles, are responsible for opening new portions of the capillary bed, and that both distensibility and recruitment occur at the capillary level.

Despite lingering doubts about the mechanisms at work in the operation of recruitment and distensibility under different conditions, a few generalizations can be made: (1) pulmonary capillaries are more distensible than systemic capillaries, presumably owing to the lack of supporting connective tissue in the lung; (2) both recruitment and distensibility are more affected by changes in pulmonary arterial than in pulmonary venous pressure; and (3) recruitment is the predominant mechanism for enlarging the capillary bed in the apices of the lungs in response to pulsatile flow, whereas recruitment and distensibility probably both contribute—although to different degrees, depending on the circumstances—in the more dependent parts of the lungs.

Effects of Inflation

It was pointed out above ("Pulmonary Vascular Resistance") that at either very high or low levels of lung inflation—no matter how accomplished—pulmonary vascular resistance increases. Inflation of the collapsed, isolated lung with *negative pressure* first *decreases* resistance and then *increases* resistance as high levels of inflation are reached. These observations can be reconciled by attributing the *high resistance* at high levels of inflation (alveolar pressure held constant) to narrowing of alveolar capillaries and the *high resistance* during lung collapse to closure, narrowing, and kinking of alveolar capillaries and extra-alveolar vessels.
Distention and Recruitment   The extent of the alveolar capillary network is quite variable, and the number, size, and shape of the open capillaries depend on the method of fixation for histologic examination as well as on the experimental circumstances. But some uncertainty still persists about the relative roles played by recruitment (opening of new capillaries) or distention (increase in the caliber of patient capillaries) in enlarging the capillary network.

Not very long ago, pulmonary capillary distention was discounted, largely on the basis of extrapolation from the behavior of systemic capillaries. However, attempts to draw analogy between the distensibility of systemic and pulmonary capillaries appear predestined to fail because pulmonary capillaries are sus-

THE BRONCHIAL CIRCULATION

Although popular usage has firmly entrenched the designation *bronchial,* the term is inadequate on two accounts: (1) the systemic blood supply to the lungs originates not only from bronchial arteries but also from the aorta and other intrathoracic arteries, and (2) the systemic arterial blood is delivered not only to the walls of the bronchi but also to the adventitia or large vessels and structures of the lungs.[27]

In the normal lung, the bronchial circulation has the features of a nutrient circulation: it is modest in size (1 to 2 percent of the cardiac output), carries arterialized blood, and is distributed primarily to the airways, blood vessels, and supporting structures of the lungs up to the respiratory bronchioles. Beyond this point, the pulmonary circulation takes over as the nutrient circulation. One likely function of the bronchial circulation is to air-condition the inspired air. For example, the disposition and architecture of the submucosal bronchial venous plexus seem to constitute an anatomic arrangement that could properly adjust the temperature and water content of air passing to and fro in the airways. The nutrient function also comes into play in lung transplantation, where survival of the graft depends critically on an adequate blood supply.

Venous return from the bronchial circulation is via either bronchial or pulmonary veins. From the hilar structures and large bronchi, bronchial venous blood is returned to the right atrium via systemic veins; from more peripheral airways and the substance of the lung, bronchial venous blood is returned to the left atrium by two routes: via bronchopulmonary capillary anastomoses and by "bronchopulmonary veins" that connect bronchial capillaries to small pulmonary veins. The direction taken by bronchial venous outflow is determined by the relative pressures at the outlet of the two systems. For example, an increase in left atrial pressure detours bronchial venous drainage toward the right, rather than the left, atrium. In some animals, functioning communications exist not only between the bronchial and pulmonary capillary circulations but also between the bronchial arteries and other systemic arteries.

Certain features of the bronchial circulation merit special attention: (1) although difficult to demonstrate and of doubtful functional significance, microscopic anastomoses between bronchial and pulmonary arteries do appear to exist at the precapillary level in the normal lung; (2) the bronchial arteries proliferate remarkably in certain types of lung disease, liver disease, and congenital heart disease, often in association with clubbing of the digits; (3) the mechanisms responsible for the proliferation of the bronchial circulation are unclear, but certain influences, such as cortisone, retard its expansion, whereas growth hormone stimulates it; (4) the bronchial veins in the submucosa of the airways form a large plexus that runs the entire length of the tracheobronchial tree, sending off communicating branches to a corresponding venous plexus on the other side of the tracheal muscle; (5) the bronchial venules respond to certain vasoactive agents, notably histamine and bradykinin, as do other systemic venules; and (6) the bronchial venous circulation is involved in the pathogenesis of experimental pulmonary edema produced in the dog and sheep by histamine, endotoxin, and bradykinin.

The Bronchial Circulation in Disease

In the normal lung, the minute bronchial circulation operates covertly. But if the pulmonary circulation to an area is compromised or lost—as by ligation or an embolus—the bronchial circulation proliferates far beyond local metabolic need for viability and function (Fig. 82-26). The stimulus for proliferation is unclear. Expansion of the bronchial arterial circulation is clinically marked in two major categories of disease: (1) those producing severe curtailment of pulmonary atresia and (2) a chronic inflammatory bronchopulmonary process, such as bronchiectasis, old inflammatory cavities, chronic lung abscess, and lung cancer. Because clubbing of the digits, occasionally accompanied by hypertrophic osteoarthropathy, is also common in these disorders, question is often raised about the relationship between clubbing of the digits and expansion of the collateral circulation to the lungs. In contrast to the disorders of the lungs associated with bronchial arterial blood is chronic mitral stenosis, in which hemoptysis usually originates from bronchial veins underlying the tracheobronchial mucosa.

An expanded bronchial arterial circulation can also constitute a hemodynamic burden (a left-to-right shunt). But rarely, as in widespread bronchiectasis, do the connections between the

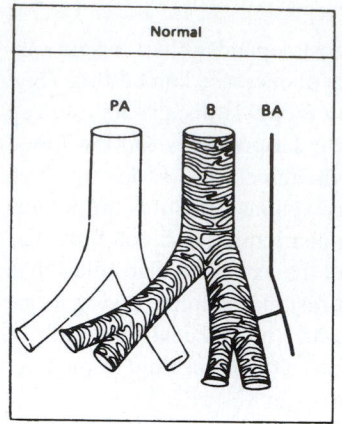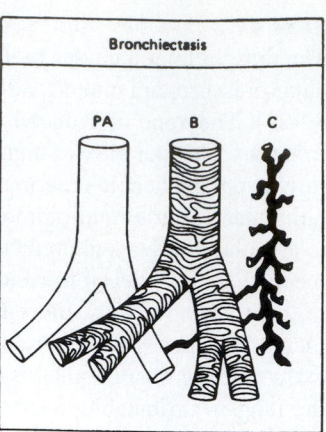

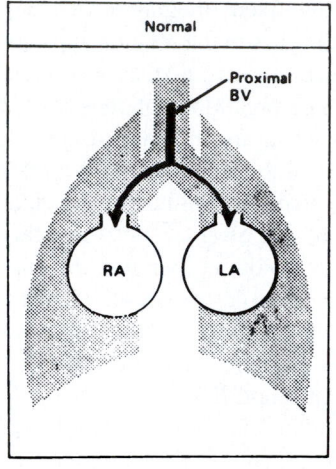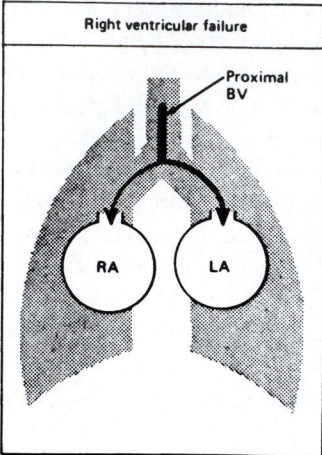

FIGURE 82-26   Schematic representations of bronchial circulation in bronchiectasis and right ventricular failure. *Top:* Bronchial arteries (BA). In chronic suppurative diseases of the lungs, bronchial arteries undergo considerable proliferation. *Bottom:* Bronchial veins (BV). Proximal bronchial veins drain into either right atrium (RA) or left atrium (LA), depending on pressure levels in these two cardiac chambers. Normally most bronchial venous outflow from the lungs enters right atrium (*thicker curved arrow*). However, in right ventricular failure, bronchial venous drainage to left atrium increases.

bronchial and pulmonary arteries enlarge sufficiently to cause cardiac embarrassment. If a wedged pulmonary arterial catheter lodges in the vicinity of bronchopulmonary arterial anastomoses, the pulmonary wedge pressure is apt to be misleading.

As noted above, bronchial venous blood that drains into the left atrium contributes to anatomic venous admixture. Another source of anatomic venous admixture occurs in some patients with cirrhosis of the liver, in whom abnormal anatomic connections allow the passage of portal venous blood into the pulmonary venous system. In an occasional patient with hepatic cirrhosis, the portal-pulmonary blood flow becomes quite extensive (about 5 to 15 percent of the cardiac output). Occasionally, these anastomotic channels enlarge sufficiently to be demonstrable during life with use of indicators or angiography. More often, the quantity of blood shunted from the portal to pulmonary venous system is too small to be measured reliably.

Since primary carcinoma of the lungs often receives much of its blood supply from systemic arteries, particularly if the neoplasm obstructs blood flow to the pulmonary artery, attempts have been made to deliver chemotherapeutic agents to the cancerous site via a bronchial artery. This approach has proved ineffective. Also, in patients in whom life-threatening hemoptysis complicates a carcinoma of the lungs, particulate matter has been injected as bronchial arterial emboli in the hope of occluding the feeder bronchial artery. Unfortunately, selective embolization is, at best, only transiently effective.

THE FETAL AND NEONATAL PULMONARY CIRCULATIONS

Before birth, the lungs play no role in gas exchange; this function is served by the placenta. For the sake of their nutrition and role as a metabolic organ, the lungs are provided with a modest blood flow, and most of the blood returning to the right side of the heart is directed toward the systemic circulation via the foramen ovale and ductus arteriosus. As a result of this diversion, the lungs before birth receive about 10 to 15 percent of the right ventricular output. After birth, as the lungs assume gas-exchanging functions and fetal connections close, the entire output of the right ventricle perfuses the lungs.[35]

In the fetus approaching term, pulmonary arterial and aortic pressure levels are virtually identical; during gestation, blood pressures in both circuits increase in parallel, while pulmonary blood flow increases dramatically. At the same time, pulmonary vascular resistance decreases progressively as the number of minute vessels increases.

Near term, the small muscular arteries, which constitute the "resistance" vessels, are well endowed with smooth muscle. After birth, the media of the small muscular arteries regress rapidly. However, prolonging hypoxia, as by exposing the newborn to a continued decrease in inspired P_{O_2} for 2 weeks, not only retards the normal involution of pulmonary vascular smooth muscle but also leads to the development of new muscle in peripheral precapillary vessels that would otherwise be expected to be devoid of muscle.

Regulation of the Fetal Pulmonary Circulation

Compared to the adult pulmonary circulation, the fetal circulation affords much more vascular resistance, a higher initial tone, and, as has been noted above, a greater vascular reactivity; reactivity increases with gestational age. Also, in contrast to the adult pulmonary circulation, the fetal pulmonary circulation manifests a considerable reactive hyperemia.

The three categories of endothelial-derived substances (prostaglandins, endothelins, and nitric oxide) play an important role in regulating fetal and transitional pulmonary vascular tone.[52] Disturbances in their interplay may culminate in persistent pulmonary hypertension of the newborn. It seems likely, however, that other mediators as well as abnormal developmental changes, entailing growth of vascular smooth muscle and the extracellular matrix, are involved in failure of normal involution after birth of the fetal circulation.

Postnatal Pulmonary Vasodilation

Ventilation of the lungs with air causes a marked drop in pulmonary vascular resistance. Two factors are concerned: predominant is the increase in P_{O_2}; a much lesser role is played by physical expansion of the lungs. The mechanism by which relief of hypoxia exerts its vasodilator effect in the fetus is not settled.

However, the prostaglandins seem to be well established. This prospect stems from two types of observations: (1) distention of the lungs of adult animals results in the release of prostaglandins, particularly those of the E series; and (2) indomethacin blunts the continued drop in pulmonary vascular resistance that would be expected to continue for 10 to 20 min after the initial fall. Moreover, in the fetus, prostaglandin synthetase inhibitors enhance the pulmonary pressor response to acute hypoxia. The role of other vasodilators (e.g., nitric oxide) remains to be defined.[52]

Attention has been called repeatedly in this section to the marked reactivity of the fetal pulmonary circulation. The purposes served by the marked pulmonary vasoreactivity are not certain. But since the increase in fetal pulmonary vascular resistance does direct the bulk of the pulmonary arterial inflow to the placenta, brain, and myocardium, the capability for marked pulmonary vasodilatation may be importantly involved in the circulatory rearrangements after birth.

Fetal hypoxia, no matter how induced, elicits intense pulmonary vasoconstriction. The magnitude of the response increases as gestation advances, consistent with the idea that pulmonary vascular smooth muscle grows increasingly responsive to hypoxia as gestation advances. In contrast to that in the adult, the sympathetic nervous system contributes significantly to initial tone and to the pressor response to acute hypoxia. As in the adult, acidosis elicits pulmonary vasoconstriction and greatly enhances the pulmonary pressor response to acute hypoxia; the more severe the acidosis, the greater the pressor and enhancing effects.

The Ductus Arteriosus

Despite its embryologic origin (as the distal segment of the left sixth aortic arch) and its location as a bridge between the pulmonary artery and the descending aorta, the ductus arteriosus leads a vasomotor life of its own, independent of the two circu-

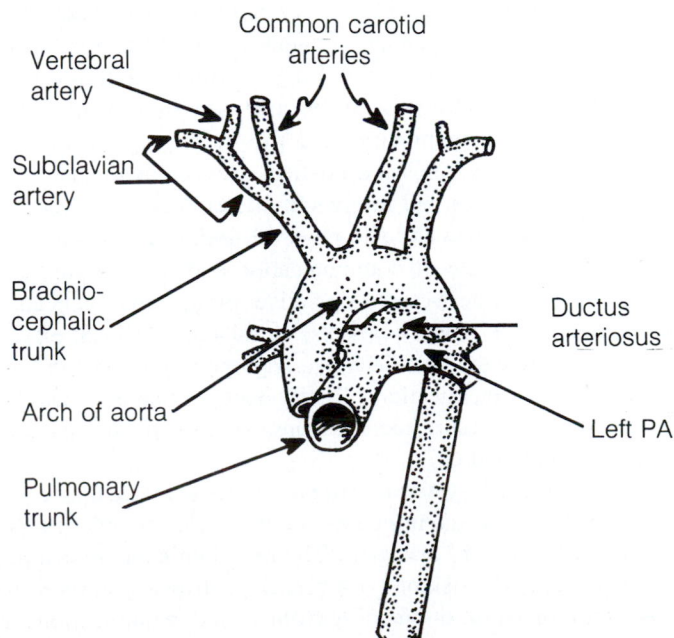

FIGURE 82-27 Relationship between ductus arteriosus and systemic vessels and the aorta. Acute hypoxia constricts pulmonary arteries but dilates the ductus arteriosus and systemic arteries.

lations that it bridges (Fig. 82-27). For example, immediately after birth (i.e., at the switch from the hypoxic environment in utero to the air-filled, oxygen-rich environment of independent neonatal life), the ductus arteriosus contracts vigorously to the point of self-obliteration of its lumen; at the same time, the pulmonary circulation vasodilates.

Closure of the ductus arteriosus immediately after birth depends heavily on prostaglandins in its walls. Conversely, premature closure of the ductus arteriosus (i.e., before birth), as may be caused by transplacental passage of indomethacin taken by the mother, may either cause fetal pulmonary arterial hypertension or interfere with the morphologic development of the pulmonary vascular bed. The vasomotor responses of the ductus arteriosus to prostaglandins and to inhibitors of the cyclooxygenase pathway have been turned to clinical advantage: on the one hand, PGE_2 or PGE_1 has been used to maintain patency of the ductus arteriosus in newborns and in patients with congenital heart disease, who need continued communication between the pulmonary and systemic circulations; on the other hand, indomethacin, an inhibitor of the prostaglandin synthetase element of the cyclooxygenase pathway, has been used to promote closure of a persistent ductus arteriosus in premature infants.

ABNORMAL PULMONARY VASCULAR COMMUNICATIONS

Systemic Artery–Pulmonary Vascular Communications

Communications between a systemic artery and the pulmonary circulation may be acquired or congenital.[41]

ACQUIRED COMMUNICATIONS

Acquired systemic artery–pulmonary communications are much more common than congenital communications. Most are traumatic or iatrogenic and hemodynamically constitute a left-to-right shunt between an intrathoracic systemic artery (coronary, intercostal, or internal mammary) and the pulmonary circulation. Because of the large pressure gradient, flow through such connections can be large, but rarely sufficient to cause left ventricular failure. The characteristic physical finding is a continuous murmur over the site of communication and radiographic evidence either of the vessels operative in the communication (e.g., enlarged pulmonary vessels) or of adjacent local effects (e.g., pleural thickening). Selective angiography reveals the nature of these communications. Rarely does cardiac overload due to left ventricular failure become manifest. Instead, most patients remain asymptomatic.

Other acquired systemic artery–pulmonary vascular communications may complicate intrathoracic neoplasms or chronic inflammatory disorders. Their predominant clinical importance lies in the risk of brisk bleeding. Bronchiectasis is the most common cause of bleeding from such communications. If extensive, bronchial artery–pulmonary arterial inflow may replace pulmonary arterial blood in perfusing an affected lobe or an entire lung.

BRONCHOPULMONARY SEQUESTRATION

Bronchopulmonary sequestration refers to a part of the parenchyma of the lung that has either incomplete or no connection with the airways and is supplied by an aberrant artery from the aorta or one of its branches. Sequestrations are further categorized as either intra- or extralobar: *intralobar* sequestrations have the same pleural covering with the adjacent lung, whereas *extralobar* sequestrations have their own pleural lining (i.e., separate from that of adjacent lung tissue).

Embryology

Bronchopulmonary sequestrations are held to be developmental abnormalities of the embryonic foregut.[80–83] In this respect, they resemble bronchogenic cysts. Sequestration is believed to begin in an accessory lung bud that originates distal to the normal lung bud. Whether the sequestration will be intralobar or extralobar appears to depend on the stage of embryologic development at which this anomaly occurs: if the accessory bud forms before the pleura is formed, the bud remains within the pleura and results in an intralobar sequestration; if it forms after the pleura has formed, it causes an extralobar sequestration that is covered by its own pleura.[84] Both types of sequestrations, but particularly extralobar sequestrations, are often associated with other congenital anomalies of the foregut.

Clinical Manifestations

Bronchopulmonary sequestration is suspected in a patient with recurrent infiltrates about a single chronically affected area containing cystic spaces in a basilar segment of a lower lobe. A clue to the diagnosis may be provided by the presence of a continuous bruit over the chest or axilla on the afflicted side due to shunting of blood from systemic artery to pulmonary vein in the intralobar sequestration.

CONGENITAL PULMONARY ARTERIOVENOUS COMMUNICATIONS

Congenital pulmonary arteriovenous communications between the pulmonary arteries and veins can occur as lesions confined to the lungs or as part of the entity *hereditary hemorrhagic telangiectasia* (Rendu-Osler-Weber disease). In hereditary hemorrhagic telangiestasia, about 15 percent of affected family members have pulmonary arteriovenous fistulas, although about 50 percent of patients with pulmonary arteriovenous fistulas have evidence of other mucocutaneous telangiectases or a family history of hereditary hemorrhagic telangiectasis.

Pulmonary arteriovenous fistulas are local lesions that do not disturb the adjacent pulmonary tissue (i.e., there is no associated atelectasis, bronchiectasis or pneumonia). Generally, the pulmonary artery supplies all the afferent blood, although occasionally, when it occurs in association with hereditary hemorrhagic telangiectasia, some of the afferent supply may be from a bronchial artery or from other systemic arteries. The lesions are multiple in one-third of the cases and are most frequently found in the lower lobes adjacent to the visceral pleura, although they can also be deep in the parenchyma.

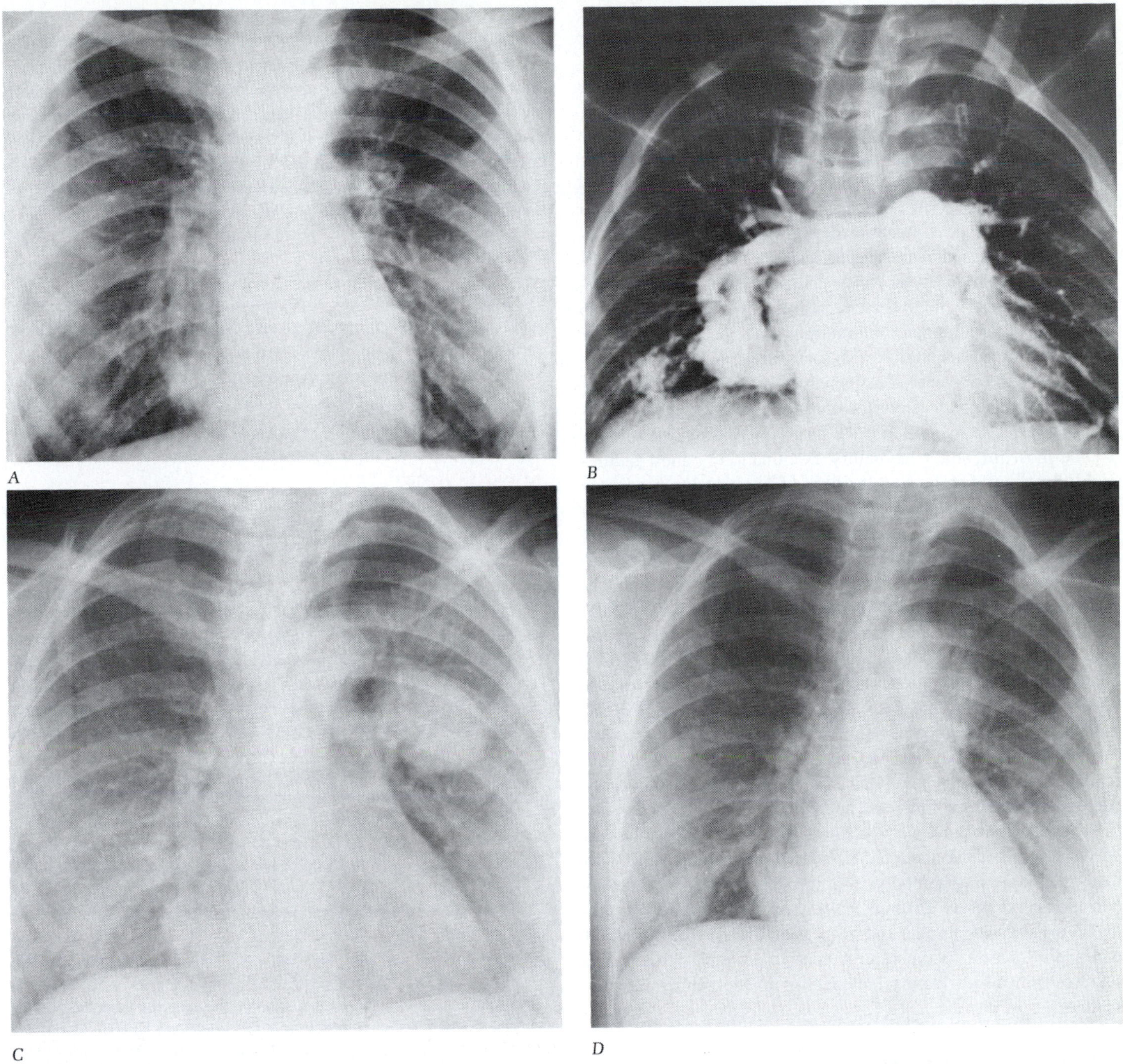

FIGURE 82-28 Pulmonary arteriovenous fistulas in a pregnant 24-year-old woman with hereditary hemorrhagic telangiectasia. *A.* Before pregnancy. Small, nodular densities are seen at both bases and in the left hilus. The shunt was estimated to be 49 percent of the cardiac output. *B.* Arteriogram before pregnancy, demonstrating arteriovenous fistulas of both lower lobes. *C.* Seven months pregnant, the patient was admitted to the hospital with hemoptysis and left hemothorax. The enlargement of the arteriovenous fistulas is striking. The pregnancy was terminated. *D.* Two weeks after termination of pregnancy. The nodular densities have decreased in size. *(Courtesy of M. Rossman.)*

Grossly, the lesions appear as thin-walled aneurysmal sacs connecting the artery and the vein. Thrombotic masses may be present within the aneurysmal sac. Microscopically, the sac walls contain various amounts of muscle, fibrous tissues, and occasionally small amounts of calcium.

The pulmonary arteriovenous fistulas act as bypass routes, allowing mixed venous blood to escape arterialization in the lungs. Despite the hypoxic stimulus, pulmonary hypertension has not occurred; however, the chronic arterial hypoxemia does evoke erythrocytosis and polycythemia.

Clinical Manifestations

Most patients with pulmonary arteriovenous fistulas are asymptomatic and come to medical attention because of an abnormality found on routine radiography. About half of the patients complain of dyspnea. Epistaxis is present in 50 percent of patients, usually in association with hereditary hemorrhagic telangiectasia. These patients may also have GI bleeding, strokes, brain abscesses, or seizures. Most cases are diagnosed in the third or fourth decade of life.

On physical examination, patients with dyspnea usually are cyanotic and clubbed. One-third of all patients will have mucocutaneous telangiectases. A characteristic feature of pulmonary arteriovenous fistula is an extracardiac murmur or bruit. Because pulmonary blood flow increases during inspiration, the intensity of the murmur also increases during inspiration and decreases during expiration. Similarly, the Valsalva maneuver, by transiently decreasing pulmonary blood flow, decreases flow through the fistula and decreases or eliminates the murmur. As expected, the Müller maneuver (forced inspiration with a closed glottis after full expiration) does the opposite (i.e., increases the murmur). Occasionally, for unexplained reasons, the murmur may be atypical and either increase with expiration or be heard only during diastole.

The most important laboratory examination is chest radiography. A solitary fistula takes the form of a coin lesion or a bunch of grapes in the peripheral lung fields (Fig. 82-27). Fewer than 5 percent of pulmonary arteriovenous fistulas contain calcium demonstrable by radiography. Usually, feeding and draining vessels connect the lesion to the hilus. Tomography is useful in demonstrating the continuity of the hilar vessels and the fistula. Fluoroscopy usually demonstrates the pulsating nature of the mass. Angiography is not usually needed to make the diagnosis, but it can be used to demonstrate the vascular nature of the lesion and to determine the exact number of fistulas present. Patients with a significant shunt will have a secondary polycythemia, although if there has been significant bleeding, some patients may actually be anemic. The arterial P_{O_2} is invariably decreased and does not increase appreciably with 100 percent O_2.

Local complications of pulmonary arteriovenous fistulas are due to rupture of the aneurysmal sacs, with bleeding either into the bronchi, causing hemoptysis, or into the pleura, where it produces a hemothorax. Thrombosis within the pulmonary arteriovenous fistula is common and is occasionally the cause of bland and septic emboli to the central nervous system. Strokes and seizures may result from telangiectases in the central nervous system.

Differential Diagnosis

The radiographic shadows may simulate bronchiectasis, tuberculosis, or other granulomatous disease, solitary pulmonary nodules, or metastatic carcinoma. The murmur or bruit must be differentiated from valvular or congenital heart disease. The cause of the cyanosis may erroneously be attributed to congenital heart disease. The normal white blood count, platelets, and spleen help to identify the polycythemia as secondary to hypoxia and not to polycythemia vera.

Treatment

The only available treatment for pulmonary arteriovenous fistulas is excision. Because of the vascular nature of the lesion, wedge resection and lobectomy have been the procedures of choice. Since adjacent lung parenchyma is normal, an attempt is made to preserve as much lung as possible. However, because as many as one-third of the patients have multiple fistulas, recurrence is possible after surgery. Therefore, in all patients with cyanosis and polycythemia, hemoptysis, or rapidly increasing lesions for whom surgery is considered, preoperative pulmonary arteriogram is necessary so that all the fistulas can be identified. Generally, all symptoms due to the pulmonary arteriovenous fistulas are reversed if surgery is successful.

Prognosis

Because the anomaly is uncommon, the natural history is not well understood. Whereas some pulmonary lesions enlarge rapidly, others remain stable or enlarge slightly over a period of years. Serious complications are just as likely to be pulmonary (hemoptysis or hemothorax in about 10 percent) as neurologic (about 10 percent).

REFERENCES

1. Archer SL, Nelson DP, Weir EK: Simultaneous measurements of O_2 radicals and pulmonary vascular reactivity in rat lung. *J Appl Physiol* 67:1903–1911, 1989.
2. Barman SA, Pauly JR: Mechanism of action of endothelin-1 in the canine pulmonary circulation. *J Appl Physiol* 79:2014–2020, 1995.
3. Bhattacharya J, Nanjo S, Staub NC: Micropuncture measurement of lung microvascular pressure during 5-HT infusion. *J Appl Physiol* 52:634–637, 1982.
4. Chen S-J, Chen Y-F, Meng QC, et al: Endothelin–receptor antagonist bosentan prevents and reverses pulmonary hypertension in rats. *J Appl Physiol* 79:2122–2131, 1995.
5. Christman BW, McPherson CD, Newman JH, et al: An imbalance between the excretion of thromboxane and prostacyclin metabolites in pulmonary hypertension. *New Engl J Med* 237:70–75, 1992.
6. Cremona G, Xuan ATD, Higenbottam TW: Endothelium-derived relaxing factor and the pulmonary circulation. *Lung* 169:185–202, 1991.
7. Dinh-Xuan AT: Endothelial modulation of pulmonary vascular tone. *Eur Respir J* 5:757–762, 1992.
8. Downing SE, Lee JC: Nervous control of the pulmonary circulation. *Annu Rev Physiol* 42:199–210, 1980.
9. Euler US von, Liljestrand G: Observations on the pulmonary arterial blood pressure in the cat. *Acta Physiol Scand* 12:301–320, 1946.
10. Filep JG: Endothelin peptides: Biological actions and pathophysiological significance in the lung. *Life Sci* 52:119–133, 1993.
11. Fishman AP: Hypoxia on the pulmonary circulation: How and where it acts. *Circ Res* 38:221–231, 1976.
12. Fishman AP: Pulmonary circulation, in Fishman AP, Fisher AB (eds), *Handbook of Physiology*, sec 3: *The Respiratory System*, vol 1: *Circulation and Nonrespiratory Functions*. Bethesda, Maryland, American Physiological Society, 1985, pp 93–166.
13. Furchgott RF: Role of endothelium in responses of vascular smooth muscle. *Circ Res* 53:557–573, 1983.
14. Furchgott RF, Zawadzki JV: The obligatory role of endothelial cells in the relaxation of arterial smooth muscle by acetylcholine. *Nature* 288:373–376, 1980.
15. Gil J: Organization of microcirculation in the lung. *Annu Rev Physiol* 42:177–186, 1980.
16. Gilles-Gonzalez MA, Ditta GS, Helinski DR: A haemoprotein with kinase activity encoded by the oxygen sensor of *Rhizobium meliloti*. *Nature* 350:170–172, 1991.

17. Glazier JB, Hughes JMB, Maloney JE, West JB: Measurements of capillary dimensions and blood volume in rapidly frozen lungs. *J Appl Physiol* 26:65–76, 1969.

18. Grover RF, Weil JV, Reeves JT: Cardiovascular adaptation to exercise at high altitude. *Exerc Sport Sci Rev* 14:269–302, 1986.

19. Hampl V, Archer SL, Nelson DP, Weir EK: Chronic EDRF inhibition and hypoxia: Effects on pulmonary circulation and systemic blood circulation. *J Appl Physiol* 75:1748–1757, 1993.

20. Hasunuma K, Rodman DM, McMurtry IF: Effects of K^+ channel blockers on vascular tone in the perfused rat lung. *Am Rev Respir Dis* 144:884–887, 1991.

21. Jensen KS, Micco AJ, Czartolomna J, et al: Rapid onset of hypoxic vasoconstriction in isolated lungs. *J Appl Physiol* 72:2018–2023, 1992.

22. Jia L, Bonaventura C, Bonaventura J, Stamler JS: S-Nitrosohaemoglobin: A dynamic activity of blood involved in vascular control. *Nature* 380:221–226, 1996.

23. Lopez-Barneo J, Benot AR, Urena J: Oxygen sensing and the electrophysiology of arterial chemoreceptor cells. *NIPS* 8:191–196, 1993.

24. Luscher TF, Wenzel RR: Endothelin and endothelin antagonists: pharmacology and clinical implications. *Agents Actions Suppl* 45:237–253, 1995.

25. Lynn RJ: Inhaled nitric oxide therapy. *Mayo Clin Proc* 70:247–255, 1995.

26. Madden JA, Vadula M, Kurup VP: Effects of hypoxia and other vasoactive agents on pulmonary and cerebral artery smooth muscle cells. *Am J Physiol* 263:L384–L393, 1992.

27. Magno MG, Fishman AP: Origin, distribution, and blood flow of bronchial circulation in anesthetized sheep. *J Appl Physiol* 53:272–279, 1982.

28. Marshall BE, Hanson CW, Frasch F, Marshall C: Role of hypoxic pulmonary vasoconstriction in pulmonary gas exchange and blood flow distribution. *Intensive Care Med* 20:291–297, 379–389, 1994.

29. Nagao T, Vanhoutte PM: Endothelium-derived hyperpolarizing factor and endothelium-dependent relaxations. *Am J Respir Cell Mol Biol* 8:1–16, 1993.

30. Ono S, Westcott JY, Voelkel NF: PAF antagonists inhibit pulmonary vascular remodeling induced by hypobaric hypoxia in rats. *J Appl Physiol* 73:1084–1092, 1992.

31. Pepke-Zaba J, Higenbottam TW, Dinh-Xuan AT, et al: Inhaled nitric oxide as a cause of selective pulmonary vasodilation in pulmonary hypertension. *Lancet* 338:1173–1174, 1991.

32. Permutt S, Bromberger-Barnea B, Bane HN: Alveolar pressure, pulmonary venous pressure and the vascular waterfall. *Med Thorac* 19:239–260, 1962.

33. Post JM, Hume JR, Archer SL, Weir EK: Direct role for potassium channel inhibition in hypoxic pulmonary vasoconstriction. *Am J Physiol* 262:C882–C890, 1992.

34. Roos CM, Frank DU, Chun X, et al: Chronic inhaled nitric oxide: Effects on pulmonary vascular endothelial function and pathology in rats. *J Appl Physiol* 80:252–260, 1991.

35. Rudolph AM: Fetal and neonatal pulmonary circulation. *Annu Rev Physiol* 41:383–395, 1979.

36. Salvaterra CG, Goldman WF: Acute hypoxia increases cytosolic calcium in cultured pulmonary arterial myocytes. *Am J Physiol* 264:L323–L328, 1993.

37. Shirai M, Sada K, Ninomiya I: Effects of regional alveolar hypoxia and hypercapnia on microcirculation in small pulmonary vessels in cats. *J Appl Physiol* 61:440–448, 1986.

38. Skalak RF, Wiener F, Morkin E, Fishman AP: The energy distribution in the pulmonary circulation: II. Experiments. *Phys Med Biol* 11:437–449, 1966.

39. Stewart DJ: Endothelin in cardiopulmonary disease: factor paracrine vs neurohumoral. *Eur Heart J* 14(Suppl I):48–54, 1993.

40. Szidon JP, Fishman AP: Autonomic control of the pulmonary circulation, in Fishman AP, Hecht H (eds), *Pulmonary Circulation and Interstitial Space*. Chicago, University of Chicago Press, 1969, pp 239–268.

41. Terry P: Pulmonary arteriovenous malformation. *New Engl J Med* 308: 1197–1200, 1983.

42. Tozzi CA, Poiani GJ, Harangozo AM, et al: Pressure-induced connective tissue synthesis in pulmonary artery segments is dependent on intact endothelium. *J Clin Invest* 84:1005–1012, 1989.

43. Versprille A: Basic mechanisms and clinical consequences of cyclic changes in pulmonary blood flow and blood volume during mechanical ventilation. *Eur J Anaesthesiol* 11:15–23, 1994.

44. Wagner WW, Weir EK: *The Pulmonary Circulation and Gas Exchange*. Armonk, NY, Futura Publishing, 1994, pp 1–424.

45. Weibel EW: Lung cell biology, in Fishman AP (ed), *Handbook of Physiology,* sec 3: *The Respiratory System,* vol 1: *Circulation and Nonrespiratory Functions*. Bethesda, MD, American Physiological Society 1985, pp 47–91.

46. Weir EK, Archer SL: The mechanism of acute hypoxic pulmonary vasoconstriction: The tale of two channels. *FASEB J* 9:183–189, 1995.

47. Weir EK, Archer SL, Reeves JT: *Nitric Oxide and Radicals in the Pulmonary Vasculature*. Armonk, NY, Futura Publishing, 1996.

48. West JB: Regional differences in the lung. New York, Academic, 1977, pp 85–165.

49. West JB, Mathieu-Costello O: Stress failure of pulmonary capillaries as a limiting factor for maximal exercise. *Eur J Appl Physiol* 70:99–108, 1995.

50. Yamaguchi K, Asano K, Takasugi T, et al: Modulation of hypoxic pulmonary vasoconstriction by antioxidant enzymes in red blood cells. *Am J Resp Crit Care Med* 153:211–217, 1996.

51. Zhao L, Crawley DE, Hughes JMB, et al: Endothelium-derived relaxing factor activity in rat lung during hypoxic pulmonary vascular remodeling. *J Appl Physiol* 74:1061–1065, 1993.

52. Ziegler JW, Ivy DD, Kinsella JP, Abman SH: The role of nitric oxide, endothelin, and prostaglandins in the transition of the pulmonary circulation. *Clin Perinatol* 22:387–403, 1995.

CHAPTER 83

PULMONARY HYPERTENSION AND COR PULMONALE

Alfred P. Fishman

GENERAL ASPECTS

Definitions

PULMONARY HYPERTENSION

At sea level, pulmonary arterial pressure greater than 20 mm Hg represents pulmonary hypertension. By this criterion, native residents at high altitude are pulmonary hypertensive. For example, at an altitude of about 15,000 ft, mean pulmonary arterial pressures up to 25 mm Hg are regular occurrences.[21] Although the higher pressures are normal at altitude, at sea level such pressures generally imply anatomic curtailment of the pulmonary vascular tree, some hemodynamic abnormality, or a vasoconstrictive influence.

The major importance of high pulmonary arterial pressure is that it increases the work of the right ventricle. In the face of abrupt increments in mean pulmonary arterial pressure of up to 50 mg (e.g., after a large pulmonary embolus), the normal right ventricle can sustain its output. However, larger pressures usually cause either the right ventricle to fail or a life-threatening arrhythmia to occur. The right ventricle can cope with much higher afterloads if they are applied gradually so that the right ventricle can undergo hypertrophy.

A variety of vascular lesions lead to pulmonary hypertension (Fig. 83-1). Some, like those caused by chronic hypoxia, entail thickening of small muscular arteries and peripheral extensions of vascular smooth muscle. Others, such as thrombotic disease, are characterized by eccentric intimal thickening due to organization of clot. A third category is the plexiform lesion, which, in at least some instances, represents healed necrotizing arteritis. These lesions are considered in greater detail with respect to particular diseases.

COR PULMONALE

The term *cor pulmonale* denotes right ventricular enlargement (hypertrophy and/or dilatation) secondary to abnormal lungs, chest bellows, or control of breathing (Fig. 83-2). It has been commonly used as a synonym for pulmonary heart disease. Cor pulmonale may be acute or chronic. The most common cause of acute cor pulmonale is massive embolization of the lungs. In a patient with severe chronic bronchitis and emphysema—i.e., chronic obstructive pulmonary disease (COPD)—it is not uncommon for an acute respiratory infection to precipitate an episode of acute cor pulmonale along with a bout of acute respiratory insufficiency. In chronic cor pulmonale, hypertrophy generally predominates; in acute cor pulmonale, dilatation is the rule.

Pathogenesis of Pulmonary Hypertension

The pathogenetic mechanisms leading to pulmonary hypertension are summarized in Table 83-1. For clinical expediency, these mechanisms are generally sorted into six categories (Table 83-2): (1) *passive*, due to obstruction to pulmonary venous outflow (e.g., fibrosing mediastinitis, mitral stenosis, or left heart failure); (2) *hyperkinetic*, due to abnormally high pulmonary blood

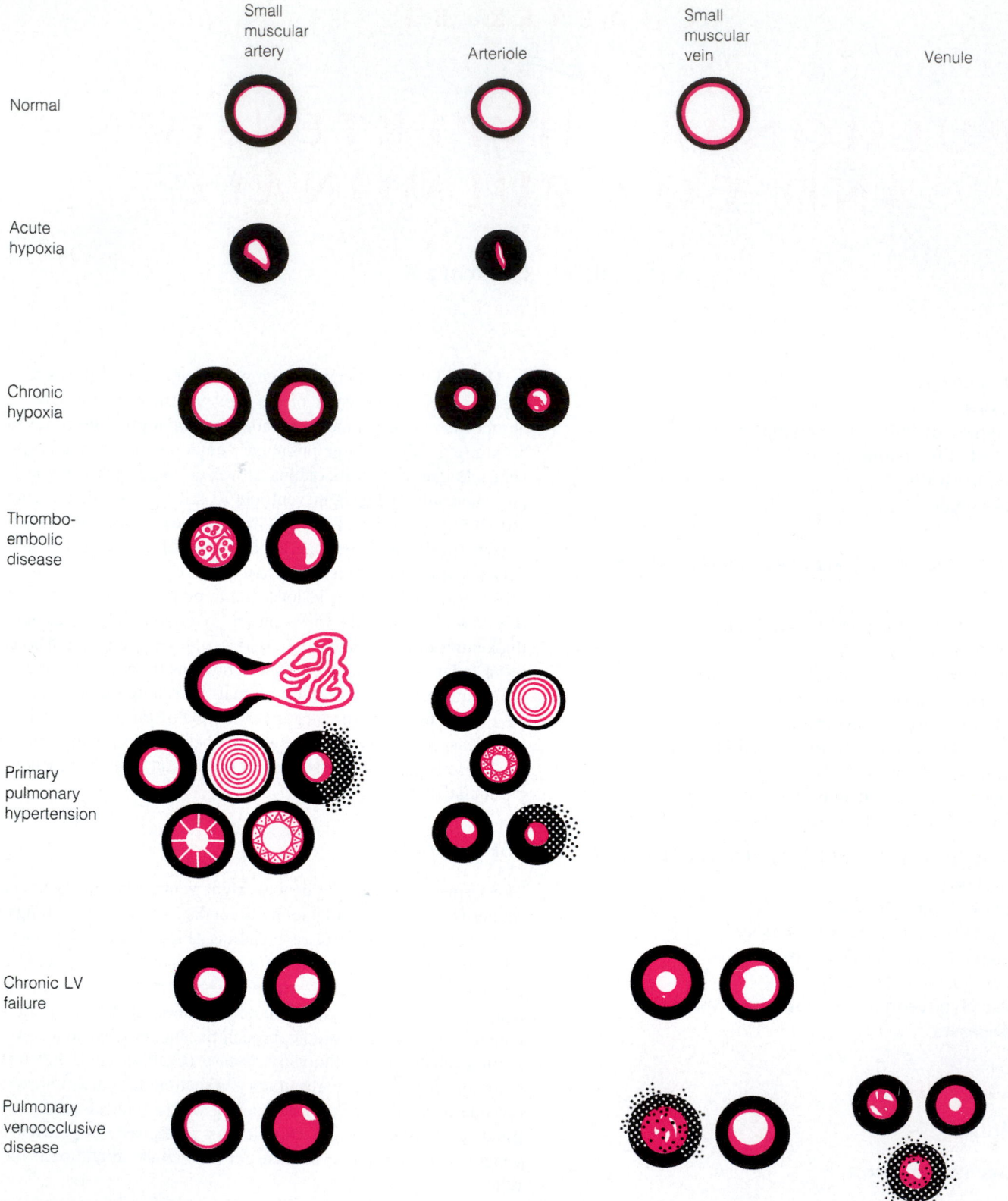

FIGURE 83-1   Diversity of pulmonary vascular lesions in primary pulmonary hypertension and other pulmonary hypertensive disorders.

flow (e.g., left-to-right shunts); (3) *obstructive,* due to pulmonary thromboembolic disease; (4) *obliterative,* due to curtailment of the pulmonary vascular bed by parenchymal disease; (5) *vasoconstrictive,* due to hypoxic vasoconstriction; and (6) *idiopathic* (i.e., without discernible cause). Over time, distinctions between categories tend to become blurred (e.g., thromboembolism complicating obliterative vascular disease). Also, by the time pulmonary hypertension becomes manifest clinically, the pulmonary arterial tree has undergone considerable anatomic alteration in extent and distensibility, thereby limiting its capability of ab-

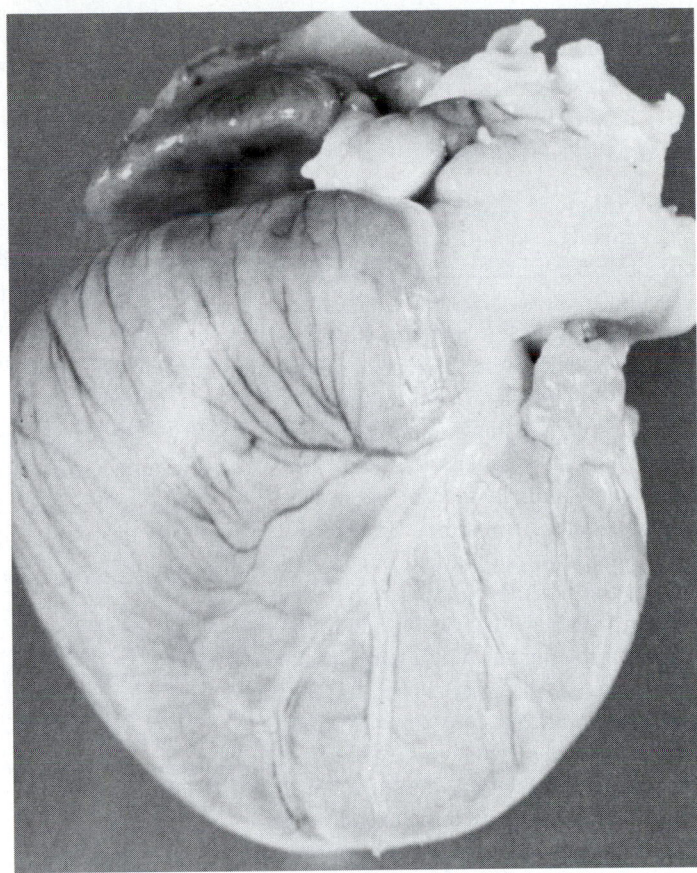

A

B

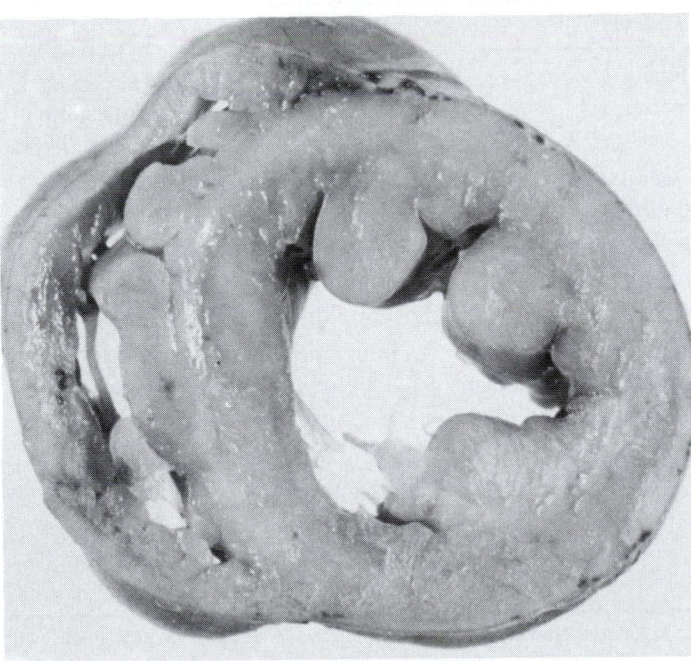

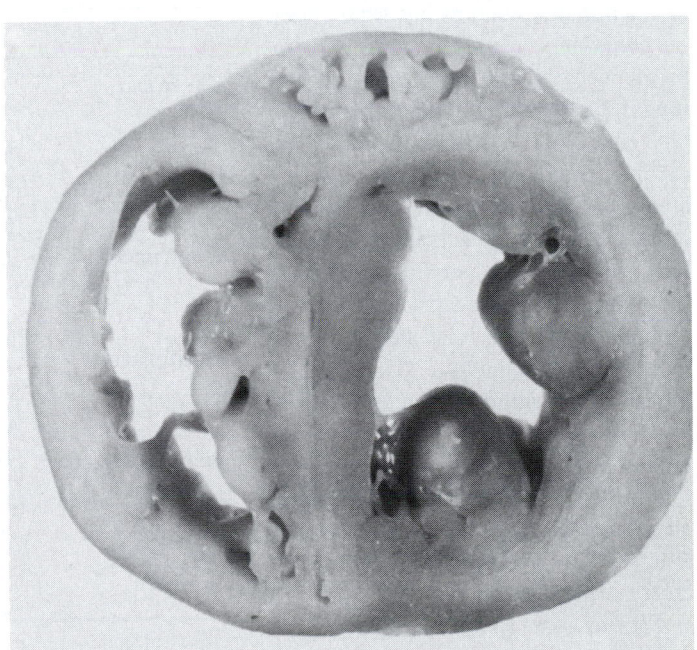

C

D

FIGURE 83-2 Cor pulmonale in experimental pulmonary arterial hypertension in the dog. *A.* Normal heart. *B.* Chronic cor pulmonale secondary to severe pulmonary arterial hypertension. *C.* Cross section of normal heart to show thin wall of the right ventricular cavity. *D.* Cross section of heart with chronic cor pulmonale to show hypertrophy of the right ventricular myocardium and enlargement of the right ventricular cavity. *(Courtesy of Dr. B. Atkinson.)*

sorbing increments in pulmonary blood flow without inordinate increments in pulmonary arterial pressure.

ANATOMIC ALTERATIONS

One common sequel to the various mechanisms outlined above is anatomic curtailment of the pulmonary vascular tree (i.e., thickening of vascular walls, partial or complete obliteration of vascular lumens, peripheral extensions of vascular smooth muscle) (Fig. 83-1).[28] In this situation, modest increments in pulmonary blood flow can elicit inordinate increments in pulmonary vascular pressures (Fig. 83-3). This situation is in marked contrast to that of the normal pulmonary circulation, in which an acute reduction in the extent of the normal pulmonary vascular bed rarely suffices, per se, to raise pulmonary arterial pressures to pulmonary hypertensive levels. In the dog, more than two-thirds of the lungs must be ablated before pulmonary arterial pressures approach hypertensive levels. As indicated in the previous chapter, occlusion of one major pulmonary artery in human beings has little effect on pulmonary arterial pressures. Even in the person with rarefaction of the lungs due to chronic pulmonary emphysema (i.e., unassociated with chronic bronchitis), the striking decrease in the number of minute vessels in the emphysematous areas rarely suffices to elicit pulmonary hypertension. In contrast, widespread occlusion of the pulmonary vascular bed by pulmonary thromboembolic disease commonly causes pulmonary hypertension by obliterating large segments of the pulmonary arterial tree and increasing resistance to blood flow in partly occluded vessels. An increase in vascular tone (e.g., by hypoxia) may further increase resistance.[24]

Perivascular anatomic changes in the pulmonary parenchyma often encroach on the small pulmonary vessels to entrap them in the fibrotic process. In some diseases, such as progressive systemic sclerosis, the parenchymal disease, reflected in interstitial fibrosis, and the pulmonary vascular disease, which leads to widespread occlusion and obstruction of the small muscular arteries, can evolve independently. In the CREST syndrome (calcinosis, Raynaud's phenomenon, esophageal dysfunction, sclerodactyly, and telangiec-

tasis), a variant of scleroderma, pulmonary hypertension sometimes stems solely from obstructive vascular disease of the small muscular arteries, unaccompanied by pulmonary fibrosis. In other connective-tissue disorders, such as lupus erythematosus, combinations of interstitial and intrinsic vascular abnormalities contribute to pulmonary hypertension.

TABLE 83-1

Pathogenetic Mechanisms for Pulmonary Arterial Hypertension and Cor Pulmonale

Mechanisms	Examples
Primary	
Anatomic decrease in cross-sectional area (vessel destruction, encroachment on lumen by hypertherapy) of the pulmonary resistance vessels	(Interstitial fibrosis and granuloma)
Vasoconstriction of pulmonary resistance vessels	Hypoxia and acidosis
Contributory	
Large increments in pulmonary blood flow	Exercise
Increased pressures on the left side of the heart and pulmonary veins	Left ventricular failure or pulmonary veno-occlusive disease
Increased viscosity of the blood	Secondary polycythemia of chronic hypoxia
Unproved	
Compression of pulmonary resistance vessels by raised alveolar pressures in their vicinity	Asthmatic bronchitis

TABLE 83-2

Categories of Pulmonary Hypertension*

	Mechanism	Examples
Passive	Pulmonary venous hypertension	Mitral stenosis, left atrial myxoma, fibrosing mediastinitis pulmonary veno-occlusive disease
Hyperkinetic	Increased pulmonary blood flow*	Left-to-right intracardiac shunts
Obstructive	Thromboembolic pulmonary vascular disease	Widespread pulmonary thrombosis of minute vessels, multiple pulmonary emboli
Obliterative	Inflammatory and/or proliferative pulmonary vascular disease	Interstitial lung disease, primary pulmonary hypertension, schistosomiasis
Venoconstrictive	Hypoxia	Chronic bronchitis and emphysema (COPD)
Idiopathic	Unknown	Dietary pulmonary hypertension, portal-pulmonary hypertension, HIV infection

*Most categories overlap to some extent. For example, increased pulmonary blood flow is usually coupled with anatomic changes in the resistance vessels to produce pulmonary hypertension.

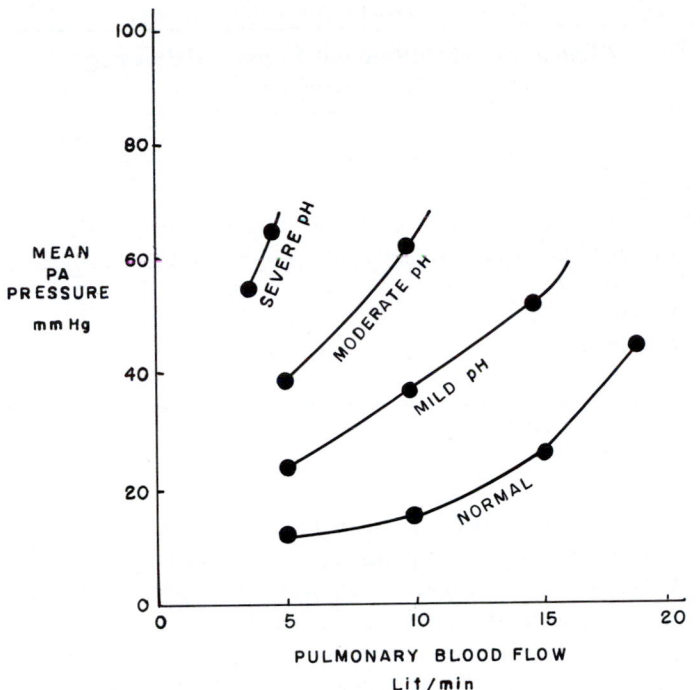

FIGURE 83-3 Schematic pulmonary arterial blood pressure–flow curves for the normal and pulmonary hypertensive circulations. At high levels of pulmonary hypertension, small increments in pulmonary blood flow elicit inordinate increments in pressure.

VASOCONSTRICTIVE MECHANISMS: HYPOXIA, HYPERCAPNIA, ACIDOSIS

Pulmonary vasoconstriction can play a critical role in the pathogenesis of pulmonary hypertension. As indicated in the previous chapter, hypoxia is, by far, the most effective vasoconstrictor encountered clinically; acidosis is next, but is much less powerful.[15,16] Both exert their effects directly on the pulmonary vessels. Although these "powerful" vasoconstrictors generally elicit only modest increments in pulmonary arterial pressure in the normal pulmonary circulation, acute hypoxia can elicit striking pulmonary pressor effects in the fetus and newborn and in persons with pulmonary hypertension who have reactive pulmonary vessels. In chronic hypoxia, sustained vasoconstriction elicits structural changes within a matter of weeks: the media of the small pulmonary arteries and arterioles thicken (Fig. 83-4), and the muscle in the walls of the arterioles extends peripherally into minute vessels that are normally devoid of muscle.[9] Acute hypercapnia has no pressor effect, per se, on the pulmonary circulation. However, it can contribute to pulmonary hypertension by virtue of the acidosis that it produces.

Clinical Manifestations

Because of its large capacity and considerable distensibility, pulmonary vascular disease must be extensive before chronic pulmonary hypertension ensues.[15] Pulmonary hypertension is generally asymptomatic until severe. Not infrequently, suspicion of pulmonary hypertension is raised by the presence of a known

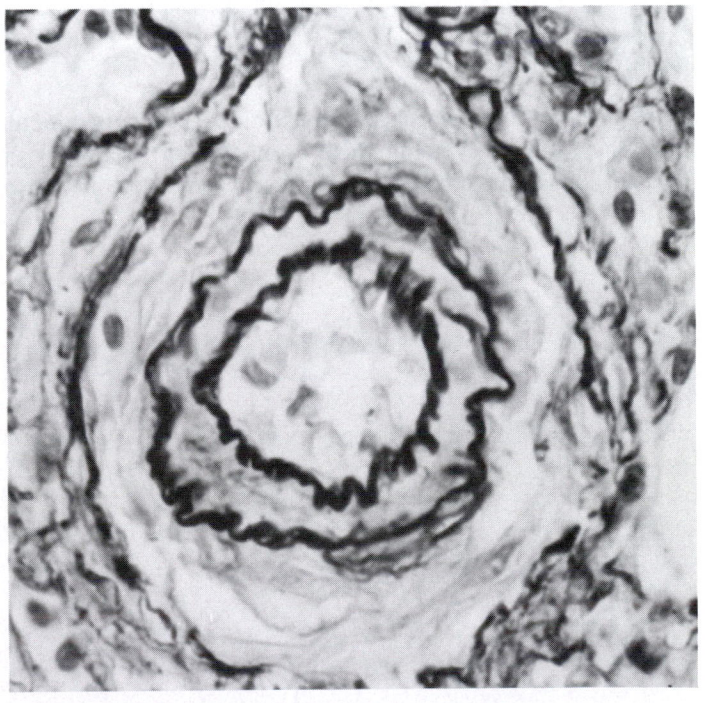

A

B

FIGURE 83-4 Normal and thickened pulmonary resistance vessels. *A.* Pulmonary arteriole showing thin muscular media, double elastic lamina, and widely patent lumen (40 μm). Aldehyde-fuchsin-elastic, ×560. *B.* Pulmonary arteriole from pulmonary hypertensive dog showing marked thickening of the media, decrease in lumen size, and perivascular fibrosis (40 μm). Aldehyde-fuchsin-elastic, ×560. (*Courtesy of Dr. B. Atkinson.*)

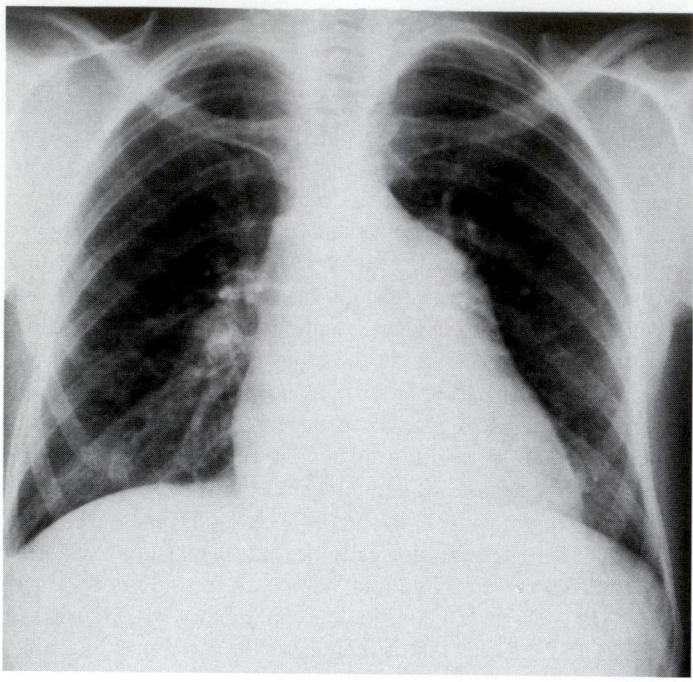

FIGURE 83-5   Multiple pulmonary emboli. The prominent central pulmonary arteries in conjunction with the marked pruning of the peripheral tree reflect the marked pulmonary arterial hypertension.

cause (e.g., mitral stenosis) or by serendipitous discovery of right ventricular enlargement (e.g., by an abnormal electrocardiogram or chest radiograph) (Figs. 83-5 and 83-6). If the right ventricle fails, the typical manifestations appear (systemic venous congestion, tender hepatomegaly, peripheral edema, and ascites).

SYMPTOMS

Symptoms due to pulmonary hypertension are generally difficult to dissociate from symptoms due to underlying pulmonary or cardiac disease. In primary pulmonary hypertension, in which

TABLE 83-3

Clinical Manifestations of Primary Pulmonary Hypertension

Symptom	*Frequency**
Dyspnea	60-90
Fatigue	19
Chest pain	7
Near syncope	5
Syncope	8
Leg edema	3
Palpitations	5

*In percent of patients.

the lesions are confined to the pulmonary arterial tree, the first symptoms attributable to pulmonary hypertension generally occur during exertion, usually in the form of dyspnea and less often as chest pain, dizziness, or syncope. Dyspnea on exertion is by far the most common presenting manifestation of pulmonary hypertension (Table 83-3). Often, because of the lack of other signs or symptoms, it is attributed to deconditioning or anxiety. The mechanism responsible for the dyspnea of pulmonary hypertension is unclear. Anginalike chest pain is common in patients with severe pulmonary hypertension. It is attributed to right ventricular overload and myocardial ischemia.

Syncope, or light-headedness on exertion, is less common but more ominous. It occurs in patients with severe pulmonary hypertension and a fixed low cardiac output. The cause is inadequate cerebral blood flow due to failure to increase the cardiac output along with redistribution of systemic blood flow toward the exercising muscles. Syncope may also occur at rest in association with the onset of bradycardia, presumably vagal in origin. Hoarseness, due to paralysis of the left recurrent laryngeal nerve, may result from trapping of the nerve between the aorta and the dilated left pulmonary artery.

Hemoptysis occurs most often in pulmonary hypertension secondary to pulmonary venous congestion. In mitral stenosis it is generally attributed to bleeding from bronchial veins. Occasionally, hemoptysis occurs in other forms of pulmonary hypertension and may originate in alveolar capillaries, precapillaries, and elsewhere in the pulmonary arterial tree once it has been rendered arteriosclerotic by prolonged severe pulmonary hypertension.

PHYSICAL EXAMINATION

In mild to moderate pulmonary hypertension, physical examination is apt to be unrevealing unless suspicion has been aroused that pulmonary hypertension may be present: right ventricular enlargement is notoriously difficult to

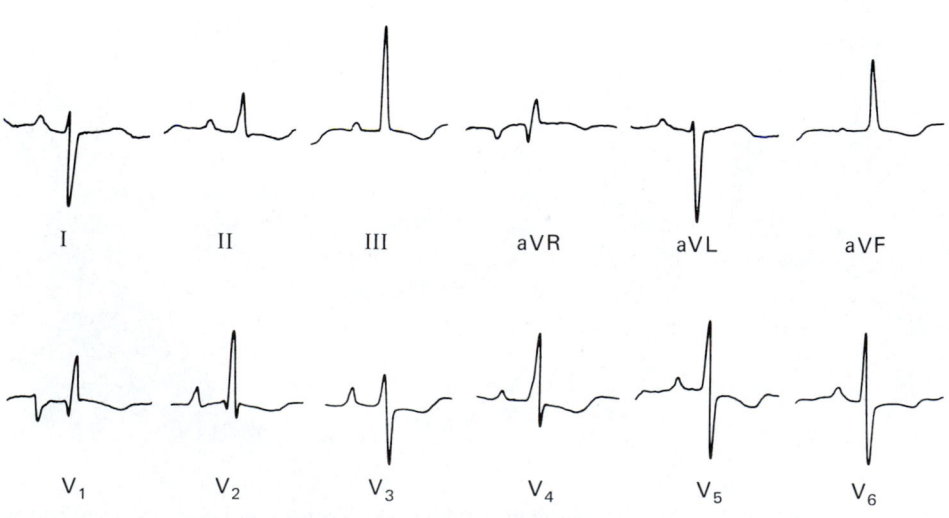

FIGURE 83-6   Twenty-six-year-old woman in whom the first evidence of primary pulmonary hypertension was by electrocardiography. The record shows marked right axis deviation and dominant R waves over the right precordium consistent with right ventricular hypertrophy.

detect on physical exam; prominent closure of the pulmonary valve is apt to be overlooked or discounted, especially in younger people; tricuspid insufficiency or a right ventricular gallop is often delayed until pulmonary hypertension is severe and has led to heart failure.

Once the disease is suspected, the physical exam can offer important clues. When symptoms first become manifest, a large *a* wave generally can be detected in the jugular venous pulse. Auscultation discloses splitting of the second heart sound with accentuation of the pulmonic component. A sharp systolic ejection click over the region of the pulmonary artery is usually heard.

An important sign of cor pulmonale is a right-sided (ventricular), diastolic (S_3) gallop. In timing, it coincides with the third heart sound; it is accentuated by inspiration. Less helpful is the right atrial gallop (S_4), which occurs immediately before the first heart sound and represents an accentuation of the normal atrial sound; it suggests an increase in the filling pressure of the right side of the heart.

As pulmonary hypertension persists, enlargement of the right ventricle (cor pulmonale) becomes evident as a palpable cardiac impulse near the left sternal border and in the hypogastrium. The onset of right ventricular failure is often marked by anorexia and discomfort in the right upper quadrant due to hepatic engorgement.

In time, tricuspid insufficiency develops. It is manifested by a holosystolic murmur, best heard in the fourth interspace to the left of the sternum; the murmur characteristically increases in intensity during inspiration (as do the third and fourth heart sounds). A prominent *v* wave appears in the jugular pulse, and distended neck veins pulsate with each heartbeat; the liver often also shows expansive pulsations that are synchronous with the heartbeat. Hydrothorax and ascites are uncommon, even after right ventricular failure has progressed to the stage of hepatomegaly and pedal edema.

Arrhythmias are not uncommon in cor pulmonale. Common precipitating mechanisms are anxiety and excessive use of bronchodilators. Occasionally, a bout of respiratory failure triggers an episode of atrial tachycardia, nodal rhythm, or a wandering pacemaker; atrial flutter or fibrillation is uncommon. Stimuli that provoke intense adrenergic discharge increase the prospect of adverse effects from therapeutic agents, such as digitalis. As a rule, arrhythmias in cor pulmonale are transient. However, they may be life-threatening if they occur in the presence of disturbances in acid-base balance, arterial hypoxemia, and heightened sympathetic activity. The occurrence of such a life-threatening arrhythmia, usually ventricular fibrillation, is most likely during a bout of acute respiratory failure, with its accompanying disturbances in gas exchange and electrolyte imbalances. Respiratory alkalosis, induced by mechanical hyperventilation and accompanied by hypokalemia, can also be a precipitating mechanism.

Diagnostic Studies

Not infrequently, recognition of the existence of pulmonary hypertension begins with the discovery of right ventricular enlargement on the electrocardiogram or undue prominence of the central pulmonary arteries on the chest radiograph. Echocardiography can help to rule out anatomic abnormalities, such as acquired or congenital mitral valve disease or left atrial myxoma. It can provide evidence of pulmonary hypertension by disclosing flattening of the interventricular septum and right ventricular dilation or hypertrophy. In sustained severe pulmonary hypertension, tricuspid insufficiency is commonly seen.

Cor Pulmonale

GENERAL FEATURES

The common denominator shared by diverse causes listed in Table 83-1 is pulmonary hypertension that stems from a primary disorder of the lungs or respiratory apparatus. Although the anatomic lesions underlying pulmonary hypertension may not be reversible, it is worthy of emphasis that acute hypoxia can generally be alleviated or relieved, thereby decreasing a major vasoconstrictive component of the pulmonary hypertension.

INCIDENCE AND PREVALENCE

The incidence of cor pulmonale varies from country to country, between urban and rural areas, and with exposure to air pollutants. In the United States, cor pulmonale averages about 6 to 7 percent of all types of adult heart disease, and COPD is the most common cause. In Delhi, India, where a large segment of the population lives under conditions of severe air pollution, the incidence has been estimated to be about 16 percent. In Sheffield, England, where air pollution is rife, cor pulmonale constitutes 30 to 40 percent of clinical heart failure. In general, in areas where smoking is widespread, air pollution severe, and chronic bronchitis and emphysema prevalent, the incidence of cor pulmonale is high. Men are more often affected than women because of their greater exposure to air pollutants.

Not all patients with COPD develop cor pulmonale. Many manage (e.g., by pursed-lip breathing —"pink puffers") to maintain arterial oxygenation at near-normal levels, thereby avoiding pulmonary hypertension. In general, the more deranged the ventilation-perfusion balance, the more likely are abnormal blood gases, pulmonary hypertension, and cor pulmonale to develop. Diffuse interstitial lung disease is a less common cause of cor pulmonale and right ventricular failure.

Most pulmonary disorders affect too little of the lungs, or are too circumscribed in their effects on alveolar-capillary gas exchange, to elicit pulmonary hypertension and cor pulmonale. Tuberculosis, although extensive, is rarely the cause of cor pulmonale, unless both lungs are extensively affected by destruction and conglomerate fibrosis or surgical intervention has deranged the functioning of the chest bellows.

Alveolar hypoventilation, secondary to sleep apnea syndromes, is not uncommonly accompanied by pulmonary hypertension and chronic cor pulmonale.

HEMODYNAMIC FEATURES

The normal right ventricle is a thin-walled, distensible muscular pump that accommodates considerable variations in systemic venous return without large changes in filling pressures. In response to chronic pressure overload imposed by the pulmonary hypertension, the right ventricle enlarges, primarily by hypertrophy. This hypertrophy involves mainly the free wall of the right ventricle. In time, if the pressure load continues, the right ventricle will fail. The advent of heart failure is indicated hemodynamically by failure of the cardiac output to increase normally during exercise even though right ventricular end-diastolic pressures (filling pressures) reach abnormally high levels (Fig. 83-7). Salt and water retention, expansion of the plasma volume, and systemic venous congestion follow right ventricular failure; the interstitial water content of the lungs also increases. The mechanisms responsible for the salt and water retention in right ventricular failure are still indefinite.

Recovery reverses the water and electrolyte disturbances. Relief of pulmonary hypertension diminishes the load on the right ventricle, its filling pressures return to normal, and the cardiac output once again responds appropriately to the level of exercise. Support of the heart by cardiotonic agents is much less effective than relief of the afterload (i.e., pulmonary hypertension) in restoring adequate cardiac performance.

The left atrial pressure is normal in cor pulmonale except when circulating blood volume is increased or if cor pulmonale is complicated by left ventricular failure (see below). Experimental observations have raised the prospect that hypertrophy and failure of the right ventricle can lead to disorders in left ventricular performance. One hypothesis has been that hypertrophy of the septal wall of the right ventricle could be etiologically related. However, there is no firm clinical support for this notion.

Indeed, clinical evidence is against this view. For example, at high altitude, where mild to modest pulmonary hypertension is a regular feature of daily life, cardiomegaly is generally confined to the right ventricle. The rare exception is the patient with chronic mountain sickness in whom arterial hypoxemia becomes so severe that it not only elicits severe pulmonary hypertension but also compromises O_2 delivery to the myocardium of both ventricles.

The more usual cause of left ventricular failure in cor pulmonale is independent disease of the left ventricle (Fig. 83-8). In elderly people, it is usually reasonable to implicate the coincidence of independent arteriosclerotic disease of the coronary arteries. In the young patient with cor pulmonale and myocardial impairment (e.g., sarcoidosis), the inclination is to attribute the left ventricular dysfunction to granulomatous impairment of the myocardium. On the other hand, there is little doubt that a damaged or overloaded left ventricle from any cause is not apt to perform well in a patient with persistent hypoxemia and acidosis, particularly if these derangements are severe.

CLINICAL FEATURES

Before the right ventricle fails, preoccupation with the underlying pulmonary disease may divert attention from the presence of pulmonary hypertension and right ventricular enlargement. Each pathogenetic sequence that culminates in cor pulmonale leaves its own imprint on the clinical manifestations. For example, obstructive disease of the airways is usually associated with hyperinflation of the lungs, which shifts the position of the heart and makes heart sounds less audible. Interstitial disorders of the lungs consistently evoke tachypnea.

TREATMENT: GENERAL ASPECTS

Since cor pulmonale is a consequence of pulmonary hypertension, management centers around decreasing the workload of the right ventricle by decreasing pulmonary arterial pressure. In a particular patient, the approach depends on the cause and the underlying pulmonary disorder. Unfortunately, little lasting relief can be expected when anatomic lesions, such as healed multiple pulmonary emboli, are the basis for the pulmonary hypertension. Much more amenable to therapy are pulmonary disorders in which a reversible element can be identified. The most common reversible disorders are those in which ventilation-perfusion imbalances have been acutely increased by an upper respiratory infection (e.g., in the patient with chronic bronchitis and emphysema). Even multiple pulmonary emboli or primary pulmonary hypertension, conditions in which anatomic occlusion of the pulmonary arterial tree is the predominant mechanism, may have a reversible component contributing to pulmonary hypertension.

Of cardinal importance is the prompt achievement of a tolerable level of arterial oxygenation at rest, during exercise, and during sleep, and the institution, when applicable, of adequate treatment for infection. Relief of acute hypercapnia is also critical, but care must be taken to lower arterial P_{CO_2} gradually. Until the hypertrophied right ventricle fails, cor pulmonale requires no cardiotonic program. But once the right ventricle does fail, the usual cardiotonic measures are in order. Among these mea-

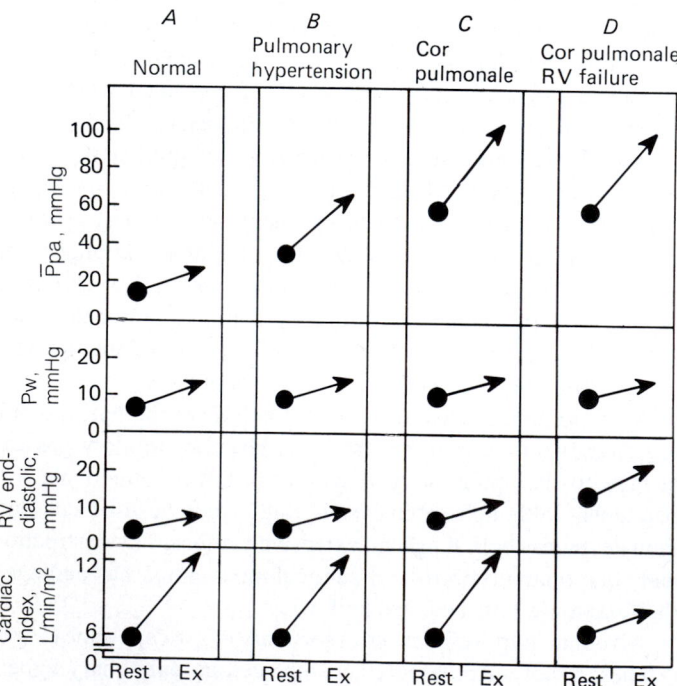

FIGURE 83-7 Schematic representation of evolution of chronic cor pulmonale. Hemodynamic studies at rest and during exercise in a normal subject (*A*). The stage of pulmonary arterial hypertension (*B*) is succeeded by cor pulmonale (*C*), in which the right ventricle performs normally despite pulmonary arterial hypertension but is known to be enlarged because of radiographic and electrocardiographic findings. Once right ventricular failure supervenes (*D*), cardiac output fails to increase normally during exercise, despite an increase of right ventricular filling pressure (end-diastolic) to abnormally high levels.

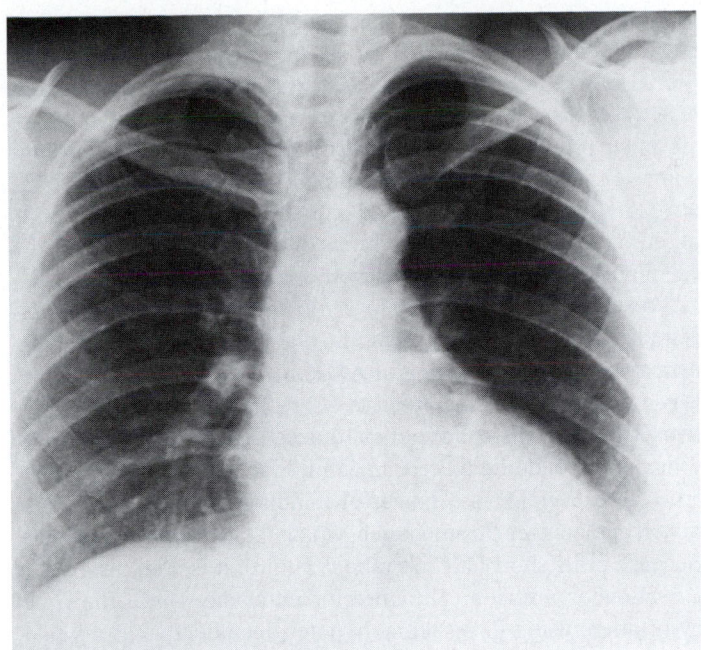

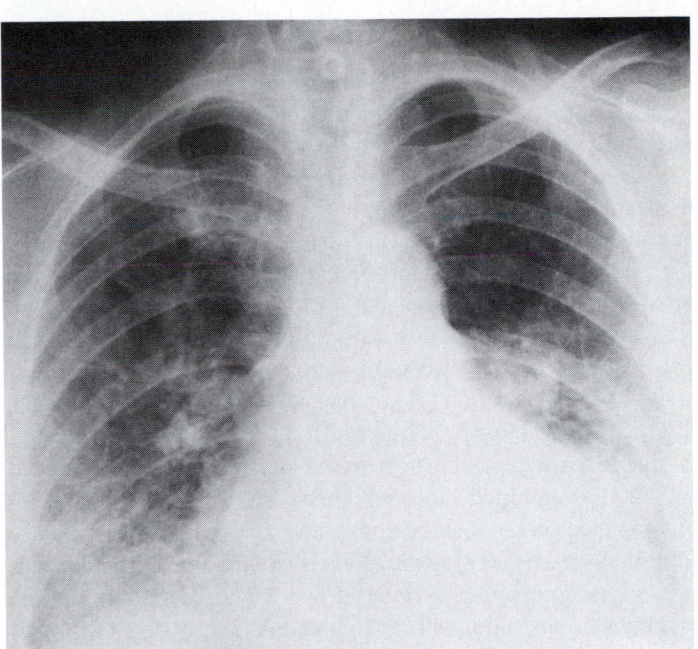

A

B

FIGURE 83-8 Cor pulmonale, right ventricular failure, and pulmonary edema. *A.* In 1956, enlarged heart, cause unknown. The lungs appear normal. *B.* In 1976, increased cardiomegaly is associated with idiopathic interstitial fibrosis (lung biopsy in 1970) and pulmonary edema. *C.* Four days later. Edema has cleared, leaving evidence of interstitial fibrosis.

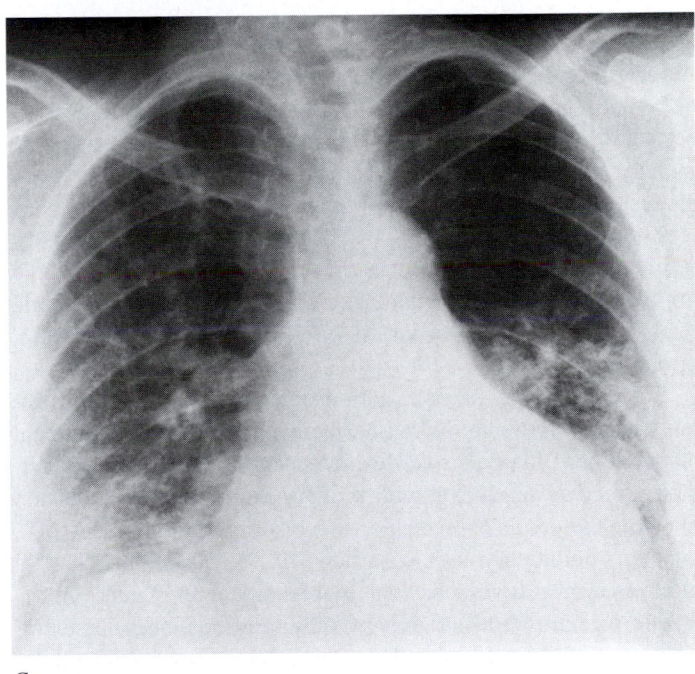

C

sures, bed rest stands out as a strategy by which increments in pulmonary arterial pressure that accompany the activities of daily life can be minimized.

DIURETICS

Diuretics can be helpful in managing cor pulmonale in heart failure, but they must be used cautiously. The lungs share in excess water accumulation of the body; this excess fluid in the lungs further compromises pulmonary gas exchange and may heighten pulmonary vascular resistance. It has now been amply demonstrated that diuretics can improve alveolar ventilation and arterial oxygenation in cor pulmonale. But the use of diuretics engenders hemodynamic side effects that may be troublesome: volume depletion, diminished venous return to the right side of the heart, and a decrease in cardiac output. Another potential complication of powerful diuretics is the production of a hypokalemic metabolic alkalosis, which diminishes the effectiveness of the CO_2 stimulus on the respiratory centers and lessens the ventilatory drive. Also, renal excretion of bicarbonate is compromised when diuretics deplete potassium and chloride. For these reasons, careful monitoring of serum electrolytes—particularly bicarbonate, chloride, and potassium ions—is mandatory once a program of salt depletion, including salt restriction and diuretics, is begun.

OXYGEN THERAPY

The use of supplemental oxygen in obstructive airway disease is employed to relieve hypoxic pulmonary vasoconstriction, to im-

prove the cardiac output, to lessen sympathetic vasoconstriction, and to alleviate tissue hypoxia. Thus, treatment of pulmonary hypertension is part of an overall program to manage severe obstructive airways disease. Two separate trials, that of the Medical Research Council and that of the National Heart, Lung, and Blood Institute (Nocturnal Oxygen Therapy Trial), have shown that intellectual function and survival are improved in chronically hypoxemic patients (arterial P_{O_2} under 55 mm Hg) who are polycythemic (hematocrit greater than 55 percent) and edematous and show P pulmonale on the electrocardiogram. To be effective, however, oxygen must be administered for at least 18 h per day—including at night, when arterial hypoxemia and respiratory acidosis intensify inordinately.

DIGITALIS

This agent is used by some clinicians to support the failing right ventricle; others shy away from this agent even when right-sided heart failure is blatant. They do so on several accounts: (1) the inotropic effect of digitalis on right ventricular performance is modest; (2) if ventricular output increases into the restricted vascular bed, pulmonary arterial pressure will increase further; and (3) patients with cor pulmonale and right ventricular failure are often hypoxemic and somewhat acidotic, thereby predisposed to arrhythmia. Even small doses of digitalis may serve as the trigger. Digitalis seems to benefit patients with demonstrable left ventricular dysfunction. Heart rate is a poor guide to digitalis dosage because hypoxemia, as well as heart failure, evokes tachycardia. Also predisposing to arrhythmia are hypokalemia induced by diuretics and medications given to relieve bronchospasm, including isoproterenol and theophylline. In essence, the safest use of digitalis for its cardiotonic effect is when right ventricular failure is unaccompanied by arterial hypoxemia, acid-base upsets, and the administration of bronchodilators (i.e., in disorders other than obstructive airway disease).

PULMONARY VASODILATORS

A variety of agents have been tried in both secondary and primary pulmonary hypertension. By far the largest experience has been with primary pulmonary hypertension. In secondary pulmonary hypertension, although overall success rates have been modest, occasional instances of dramatic improvement have been reported. Most disappointing has been the use of pulmonary vasodilators in severe COPD: in these patients, no demonstrable improvements in hemodynamics or survival were demonstrable after 1 year's administration of nifedipine (10 mg, by mouth, three times daily).

Calcium channel blockers administered by mouth are the drugs most widely used and the most effective in the chronic treatment of pulmonary hypertensive disorders. These agents are particularly effective in patients with primary pulmonary hypertension in whom there is an appreciable vasoconstrictive component (e.g., hypoxic pulmonary vasoconstriction). The calcium channel blockers diminish vascular tone by preventing an increase in cytosolic calcium concentration by inhibiting the influx of extracellular calcium and the release of calcium from intracellular stores. The two calcium channel blockers that have gained widespread acceptance as pulmonary vasodilators are nifedipine and diltiazem.[2] Less experience has been gained to date with amlodipine, in which potent vasodilator properties seem not to be associated with significant negative inotropic effects.

Experience with primary pulmonary hypertension has established that relatively high doses of calcium channel blockers may be required to effect a significant increase in cardiac output, a decrement in pulmonary vascular resistance, and a decrement in pulmonary arterial pressure. In some instances, the required daily doses of nifedipine and diltiazem have exceeded 200 mg and 700 mg, respectively. The proper dosage can be established by acute testing either with increasing dosages of the calcium channel blockers at hourly intervals or with short-acting vasodilators such as prostacyclin or adenosine. Responders have benefited from improved quality of life and prolonged survival. However, only about one-quarter of patients satisfy the criterion of a significant decrease in pulmonary arterial pressure and pulmonary vascular resistance. The nonresponders not only fail to benefit but also are more prone to adverse side effects, including systemic hypotension, a decrease in cardiac output because of a negative inotropic effect, arrhythmias, and salt and water retention resulting in peripheral edema (which has to be distinguished from the edema of right ventricular failure).

Prostacyclin (also referred to as Flolan, epoprostenol, or PGI_2) is a powerful vasodilator (systemic and pulmonary) and acts by increasing the concentration of AMP in vascular smooth muscle. It is a product of the metabolism of arachidonic acid, which derives from the phospholipid of the cell membrane. Its major source is the endothelial cell. In addition to its vasodilatory properties, prostacyclin is a powerful inhibitor of platelet aggregation; it antagonizes thromboxane, which is generated by platelets. Because of its short half-life (about 3 min), it is administered as a continuous infusion. The dose for intravenous infusion is set by titration, using its systemic hypotensive effective as a guideline to maximum tolerable dosage. Chronic administration is accompanied by an increasing need for higher dosages. This agent is considered in detail subsequently with respect to its use in primary pulmonary hypertension.[4,20,37,40]

Nitric oxide is considered in the previous chapter. The demonstration that nitric oxide is the endothelial-derived relaxing factor has led to trials of inhaled nitric oxide in pulmonary hypertension.[44] Of paramount importance in this regard is its advantage over other vasodilators (with the possible exception of acetylcholine, which induces the release of nitric oxide) of selectively vasodilating pulmonary vessels, thereby reducing pulmonary hypertension, without significantly lowering systemic arterial blood pressure. Currently, inhaled nitric oxide is being tested in a wide array of pulmonary hypertensive states, ranging from the adult respiratory distress syndrome to acquired and congenital heart disease and postoperative surgical management.[26] Limitations to chronic therapy have been imposed by the need for the inhalant route, but apparatus is currently being designed to overcome this limitation.

Nitric oxide is virtually without effect on the normal pulmonary circulation, but it can reduce pulmonary arterial pressures in pulmonary hypertension if increased tone is contributing to the high pulmonary arterial pressures (e.g., in chronic hypoxia and in the fetal circulation). Endothelial-derived nitric oxide is increased in pulmonary vasoconstrictive states apparently serving to blunt the increase. Inhibition of the release of endothelial-derived nitric oxide potentiates the pulmonary pressor response to vasoconstrictive agents (e.g., acute hypoxia).[48]

The list of putative pulmonary vasodilators that have been tried over the years is quite long. Recently, because prostacyclin is costly and not easy to administer, other agents have been put to the test, including other vasodilator derivatives of arachidonic acid metabolism, acetylcholine, and adenosine. Experience with each of these has been much more limited than with prostacyclin or, more recently, with nitric oxide. Some agents, such as captopril, an inhibitor of the angiotensin-converting enzyme, have demonstrated side effects that preclude their use in the treatment of pulmonary hypertension.

ANCILLARY MEASURES

Carbonic anhydrase inhibitors (e.g., acetazolamide) were once first-line therapy for treating patients with chronic hypercapnia. The rationale was to promote diuresis and loss of bicarbonate by the kidney. However, untoward effects, presumably the result of adding metabolic acidosis to the preexisting respiratory acidosis, have led many physicians to abandon the use of acetazolamide as a primary diuretic agent. At present, it is used circumspectly to correct the alkalemia induced by excessive diuresis, volume contraction, and hypochloremia.

Phlebotomy also used to be standard treatment for the polycythemia of chronic hypoxia as the hematocrits went above 55 to 60 percent. However, even though repeated small phlebotomies often result in symptomatic improvement and increased exercise tolerance, it proved difficult to show objective improvement in gas exchange, pulmonary mechanics, or pulmonary arterial pressure after "safe" phlebotomies (i.e., of 250 ml or so); larger phlebotomies were avoided because they occasionally resulted in minor strokes and episodes of hypotension. However, restoring hematocrits gradually (i.e., by repeated 250-ml phlebotomies at intervals of several days or weekly) did decrease pulmonary arterial pressure as hematocrits approached normal levels (i.e., about 50 percent); lower hematocrits offer no further advantage. Therefore, small phlebotomies still have a role when secondary polycythemia becomes severe.

Prognosis

No prospective studies are available concerning the prognosis of chronic cor pulmonale. Observations in the 1950s suggested that once the right ventricle fails and systemic venous congestion ensues, life expectancy is less than 4 years. But the ability to tide these patients over episodes of acute respiratory failure associated with infections and heart failure has improved enormously in the past 5 years. In our own experience, 5 to 10-year survival after the first appearance of peripheral edema is not unusual.

The prognosis for a particular patient with cor pulmonale is inextricably linked to that of the underlying pulmonary disease or disorder. In essence, the circulatory disorders are potentially reversible if the initiating mechanisms can be brought under control. In patients in whom cor pulmonale is a complication of gradual obliteration of small pulmonary arteries by intrinsic disease (emboli) or of interstitial fibrosis, there is little hope for improvement, since the anatomic changes are apt to be fixed, and arterial hypoxemia is rarely striking until it is preterminal. The outlook for longevity is much better in patients with chronic bronchitis and emphysema in whom blood gases can be maintained at near-normal levels.

CLASSIFICATION OF PULMONARY HYPERTENSIVE DISEASES

Most pulmonary hypertensive diseases are due to identifiable causes (Table 83-1). In some instances, however, the cause remains obscure despite the most exhaustive diagnostic workup. Consequently, pulmonary hypertensive diseases are categorized as secondary (due to a known cause) or primary (cause undetermined). In this chapter, primary pulmonary hypertension, a rare disease, is considered at the outset because its manifestations are not clouded by cardiac or pulmonary signs and symptoms attributable to the causes of secondary pulmonary hypertension.

UNEXPLAINED (PRIMARY) PULMONARY HYPERTENSIVE DISEASES

The so-called *primary,* or unexplained, group includes not only diverse pulmonary hypertensive diseases of unknown origin, but also some that occur in segments of the pulmonary vascular tree other than the small muscular arteries and arterioles (i.e., pulmonary capillary or veins).[18]

Primary Pulmonary (Arterial) Hypertension

This section deals with *primary (arterial) pulmonary hypertension* (PPH) that originates as an unexplained disease of the small pulmonary muscular arteries and arterioles. Subsequent sections deal with other categories of unexplained primary pulmonary hypertension—namely, pulmonary veno-occlusive disease and pulmonary capillary hemoangiomatosis.[11]

ETIOLOGY OF PPH

The designation *primary* is intended to convey that the cause of the pulmonary hypertension is unknown. Early in the evolution of the understanding of pulmonary hypertension, certain histologic lesions (e.g., plexiform lesions) became the hallmark of the disease at autopsy. More recently, the histologic lesions proved to be nonspecific. Indeed, in some instances, identical lesions have been found in patients who had recognizable causes of pulmonary hypertension, ranging from Eisenmenger's syndrome to the ingestion of toxic substances (e.g., fenformine). Moreover, members of families who have died of PPH have underscored that the histologic lesions in the pulmonary arteries are not pathognomonic of a single entity that can be categorized as primary pulmonary hypertension. It seems inevitable that in the years ahead, as in the case of pulmonary hypertension caused by identifiable diet and drugs (Table 83-4), an increasing number of instances currently designated as primary will prove to be secondary to some identifiable cause.[39,47]

The common denominator linking the diverse causes of PPH (Fig. 83-9) is believed to be injury to the endothelium of the small muscular arteries and arterioles. Endothelial injury causes obstruction to blood flow not only as a direct local response to injury but also because of concomitant thrombosis and vasoconstriction. Once started, this mechanism tends to be self-perpetuating.

One major obstacle to the identification of the cause of PPH in a particular patient is the long interval between the time of the original insult that initiated the pulmonary vascular occlusive disease and the time at which clinical signs and symptoms appear. Indeed, in some patients, the pulmonary hypertension may be lifelong (i.e., due to unrelieved pulmonary vasoconstriction from birth), due to the persistence of the fetal circulation, or due to amniotic fluid emboli. In others, the pulmonary hy-

TABLE 83-4

Classification of Pulmonary Hypertensive Disease

Disease Category	Example
PRIMARY PULMONARY HYPERTENSION	
Unexplained—pulmonary precapillary	Portal-pulmonary hypertension, dietary pulmonary hypertension, familial primary pulmonary hypertension
Unexplained—pulmonary venous	Pulmonary veno-occlusive disease
Unexplained—pulmonary capillary	Pulmonary capillary hemangiomatosis
SECONDARY PULMONARY HYPERTENSION	
Cardiac disease	
Congenital	Atrial septal defect, Eisenmenger's syndrome
Acquired disease of the left side of heart	Mitral stenosis, left ventricular failure
Respiratory disease	
Intrinsic disease of lung parenchyma or airways	Chronic obstructive pulmonary disease (COPD), interstitial lung disease
Abnormal control of breathing	Postencephalitis syndrome
Abnormal chest bellows	Kyphoscoliosis
Pulmonary vascular diseases	Scleroderma
Systemic diseases affecting lungs	Connective-tissue diseases
Thromboembolic diseases	
Thrombi	Widespread thrombosis of small pulmonary arteries, emboli from systemic veins
Tumor	Lymphangitic carcinoma
Foreign bodies	Talc, schistosomal eggs
Diet and drugs	
Anorexic drugs	Aminorex, fenfluramine
Rapeseed oil	Toxic oil syndrome
Tryptophan	Eosinophilia-myalgia syndrome
Miscellaneous	Inhaled crack, chemotherapeutic agents
Infections	
Viral	HIV infection

pertension can be traced to a few months or years of ingesting pharmacologic and anorectic agents.[6,23] In some instances, PPH has been shown to be a heritable disorder, whereas in others susceptibility to the disease appears to be inherited.

PATHOPHYSIOLOGY

In most patients, in whom the cause is entirely enigmatic, the vascular disease progresses inexorably, albeit at different rates. As a rule, the course has been briefer in young women (i.e., 1 to 2 years between diagnosis and death) than in older men and women. When a toxic substance can be implicated, as was the case in an epidemic in Europe of so-called PPH attributable to the ingestion of the anorectic agent aminorex, removal of the agent from over-the-counter sales arrested the disease. A replay of the aminorex experience can be expected as newer anorectic agents with similar pharmacologic properties appear on the market. The "toxic oil syndrome" in Spain is another relevant epidemic.

As expected from the predominant involvement of pulmonary precapillary vessels, despite marked pulmonary arterial hypertension, pulmonary arterial wedge pressure is normal, and the cardiac output is normal or slightly reduced. In severe pulmonary hypertension, right ventricular end-diastolic pressure and mean right atrial pressure become abnormally high: the conspicuous *a* wave in the right atrium is a reflection of the forceful atrial contraction necessary to fill the hypertrophied right ventricle. As the long-standing overload on the right side of the heart continues, right ventricular failure finally develops.

CLINICAL FEATURES

The first clue may be an abnormal chest radiograph or an electrocardiograph indicative of right ventricular hypertrophy (Figs. 83-5 and 83-6). Initial complaints, particularly easy fatigability and chest discomfort, are often dismissed as neurotic. Direct determination of pulmonary circulatory pressures by cardiac catheterization remains the "gold standard" for establishing the diagnosis. Echocardiography can strongly suggest the diagnosis but has its greatest value in averting numerous cardiac catheterizations: once the baseline echocardiogram has been established at the time of the cardiac catheterization, echocardiography can be extremely useful as a noninvasive approach to monitoring the evolution of the disease and in assessing the response to therapeutic interventions.

When the disease is advanced, dyspnea, particularly during exercise, is common. Many patients are tachypneic and complain of nondescript chest pain as well as breathlessness. Other common symptoms are weakness, fatigue, and syncope; the last is often an ominous manifestation but occasionally disappears spontaneously even though the disease progresses. In time, right-sided heart failure evolves. On occasion, an enlarged pulmonary

```
                          ENDOTHELIAL INJURY

                  Smooth Muscle
                  Growth Factors;
                  Cytokines

INTERACTIONS WITH         HYPERTROPHY OF VASCULAR          PULMONARY
BLOOD CONSTITUENTS          SMOOTH MUSCLE               VASOCONSTRICTION
                       PILING UP OF ENDOTHELIUM

IN-SITU THROMBOSIS
AND RECANALIZATION
                         OBSTRUCTION TO PULMONARY
                              BLOOD FLOW;
                           DECREASE IN AREA OF
                          PULMONARY VASCULAR BED

                           SELF-PERPETUATING
                                 PPH
```

FIGURE 83-9   Proposed pathogenesis of primary pulmonary hypertension. The process begins with injury to endothelium, which sets into motion an interplay that culminates in obliterative pulmonary vascular disease that affects predominantly the small muscular pulmonary arteries.

artery causes hoarseness because of compression of the left recurrent laryngeal nerve.

Systemic arterial hypoxemia, if present, is mild. Late in the disease, many patients develop peripheral cyanosis secondary to reduced cardiac output and peripheral vasoconstriction; central cyanosis also occurs preterminally in some patients because of right-to-left shunting through a patent foramen ovale.

Patients with severe pulmonary hypertension seem prone to sudden death. Thus, death has occurred unexpectedly during normal activities, cardiac catheterization, and surgical procedures, and after the administration of barbiturates or anesthetic agents. In a few instances, bradycardia leading to cardiac arrest has preceded sudden death.

On physical exam, there is no evidence of primary pulmonary or cardiac disease. Otherwise, the cardiac examination is consistent with right ventricular overload, secondary to pulmonary hypertension of any cause.

Early in the evolution of the disease, the chest radiograph appears normal. In time, the central pulmonary arteries become increasingly prominent as the peripheral vessels become attenuated, and the cardiac silhouette enlarges (Fig. 83-10). The electrocardiogram almost invariably shows some evidence of right ventricular overload, usually in conjunction with right atrial impairment (Fig. 83-6). Arrhythmias are uncommon until late in the course of the disease, when they may contribute to syncopal episodes (Fig. 83-11).

In 1981, the National Institutes of Health (NIH) established a nationwide registry to collect and analyze data on PPH. By the

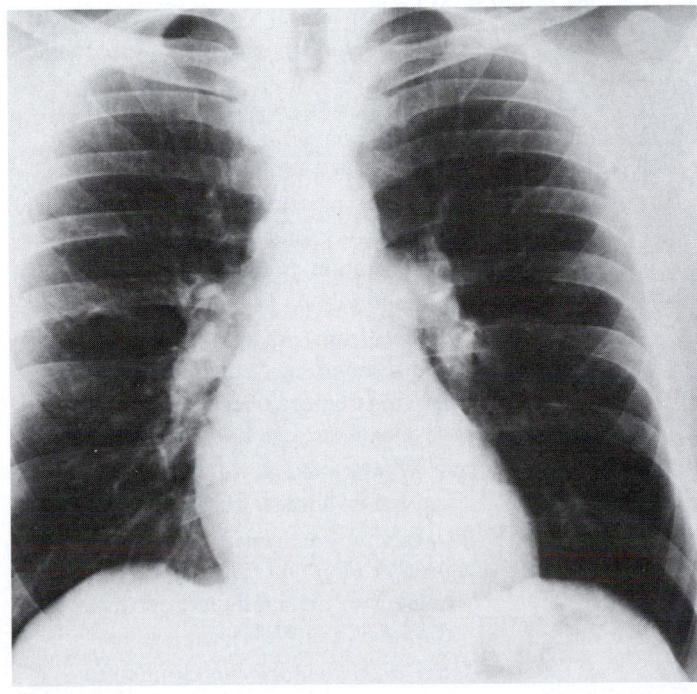

A

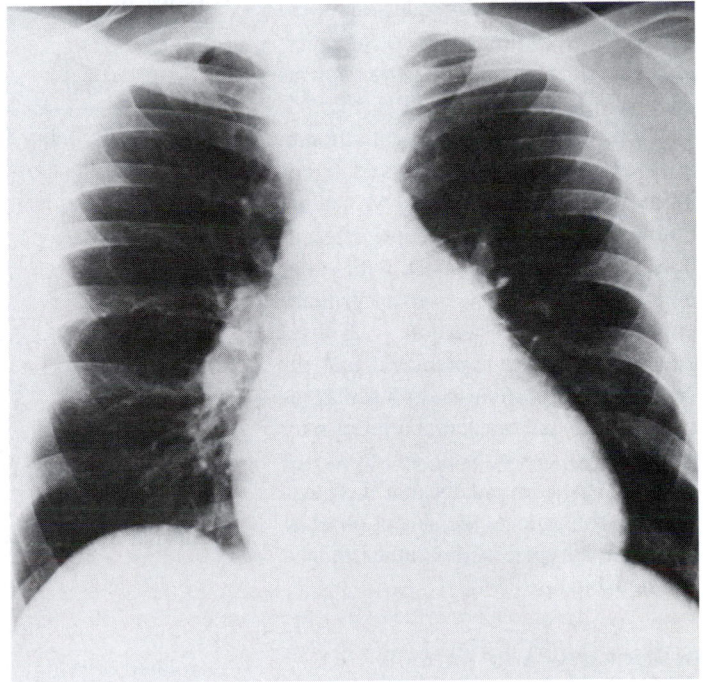

B

FIGURE 83-10   Radiographic changes in primary pulmonary hypertension. *A.* Spontaneous enlargement of the cardiac silhouette in a 30-year-old man in the 14 months between chest radiographs associated with increasing dyspnea. *B.* Decrease in the cardiac silhouette in response to chronic pulmonary vasodilator therapy.

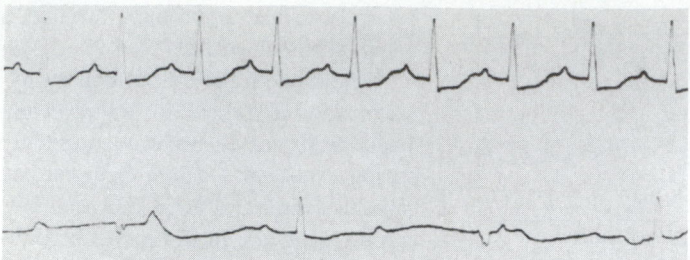

FIGURE 83-12   Vascular lesions at open lung biopsy in patients referred with clinical diagnosis of primary pulmonary hypertension. In
three patients (*A, B, G*) no cause was identified histologically; in the
other five, causes were identified. *A.* Unexplained pulmonary hypertension. Plexiform lesion. *B.* Unexplained pulmonary hypertension.
Small muscular artery. *C.* Pericapillary fibrosis. *D.* Scleroderma. *E.* Systemic lupus erythematosus. *F.* Multiple pulmonary emboli. *G.* Cirrhosis of liver (portal hypertension) and unexplained pulmonary hypertension. *H.* Schistosomiasis. *(A to E courtesy of Dr. G. G. Pietra.)* ➤

FIGURE 83-11   Primary pulmonary hypertension. Bradycardia and
prolongation of atrioventricular conduction progressed to atrioventricular dissociation while patient was on bedpan. Associated with syncope.

close of the registry in 1987, data were available on approximately 200 patients. Criteria for entry of a patient into the national registry included normal pulmonary function tests (except
for a moderate reduction in diffusing capacity), right-sided cardiac catheterization to exclude congenital or acquired heart disease, perfusion scans, angiography if the scans were inconclusive for pulmonary emboli, and serologic testing to rule out
collagen vascular disease. Included in the registry were certain
associated diseases, such as hepatic cirrhosis, because the reason for the association was unclear and because of the suspicion
that the association might provide a clue to etiology.

PATHOLOGY

A variety of lesions have been found in the small muscular (50
to 500 μm in diameter) arteries and arterioles of the lungs of patients who died of PPH (Fig. 83-12). As
noted above, one uncommon but distinctive lesion of the small muscular arteries, the "plexiform lesion," led
pathologists to favor the designation
plexogenic pulmonary hypertension as
the anatomic hallmark of PPH (Fig. 83-
13).[50] Instead of being pathognomonic,
however, this lesion is also found in pulmonary hypertension of known causes
(Table 83-5). Also, at autopsy, thrombotic lesions often coexist with other
obliterative vascular lesions of primary
pulmonary hypertension. Consequently, it is now appreciated that diverse types of intimal and muscular lesions of the small muscular arteries may
give rise to the clinical syndrome of
PPH, and it seems likely that the plexiform lesion reflects the abrupt onset of
pulmonary hypertension rather than a
distinctive cause.[35]

DEMOGRAPHY AND NATURAL
HISTORY

Primary pulmonary (arterial) hypertension is a rare disease. Although the onset may be at any age, symptomatic dis-

ease usually becomes manifest between 30 and 36 years. In childhood, both sexes are equally affected; after puberty, females predominate.

FAMILIAL INCIDENCE

Heritable diseases can be responsible for either primary (unexplained) or secondary pulmonary hypertension. The two primary
diseases are primary pulmonary (arterial) hypertension and familial pulmonary veno-occlusive disease (see below). The secondary diseases include procoagulation disorders, α_1-antipro-
teinase deficiency, cystic fibrosis, and familial idiopathic fibrosis.

Familial primary pulmonary hypertension is rare. Of the 200
patients in the NIH registry, the disease was familial in 12. The
familial type has the same clinical features as PPH in general,
raising the possibility that some instances of sporadic primary
pulmonary hypertension may be familial. The disease is autosomal dominant, it occurs at an earlier age in successive generations (genetic anticipation), and its genetic basis is entirely un-

TABLE 83-5

Types of Histopathologic Lesions in Familial Primary Pulmonary Hypertension

Histopathologic Classification	Characteristic Histopathologic Features
Primary pulmonary arteriopathy with:	
Plexiform lesions, with or without thrombotic lesions	*Plexiform lesions;* medial hypertrophy, eccentric or concentric-laminar intimal proliferation and fibrosis, fibrinoid degeneration-arteritis, dilatation lesions, and thrombotic lesions
Thrombotic lesions	*Thrombi* (fresh, organizing or organized, and recanalized—collander lesions), varying degrees of medial hypertrophy; *no* plexiform lesions
Isolated medial hypertrophy	*Medial hypertrophy; no* appreciable intimal or luminal obstructive lesions
Intimal and medial hypertrophy	*Eccentric or concentric-laminar proliferation and fibrosis;* varying degrees of medial hypertrophy; *no* thrombotic or plexiform lesions
Isolated arteritis	*Active or healed arteritis,* limited to pulmonary arteries; varying degrees of medial hypertrophy, intimal fibrosis, and thrombotic lesions; *no* plexiform lesions

SOURCE: Pietra.[35]

FIGURE 83-12

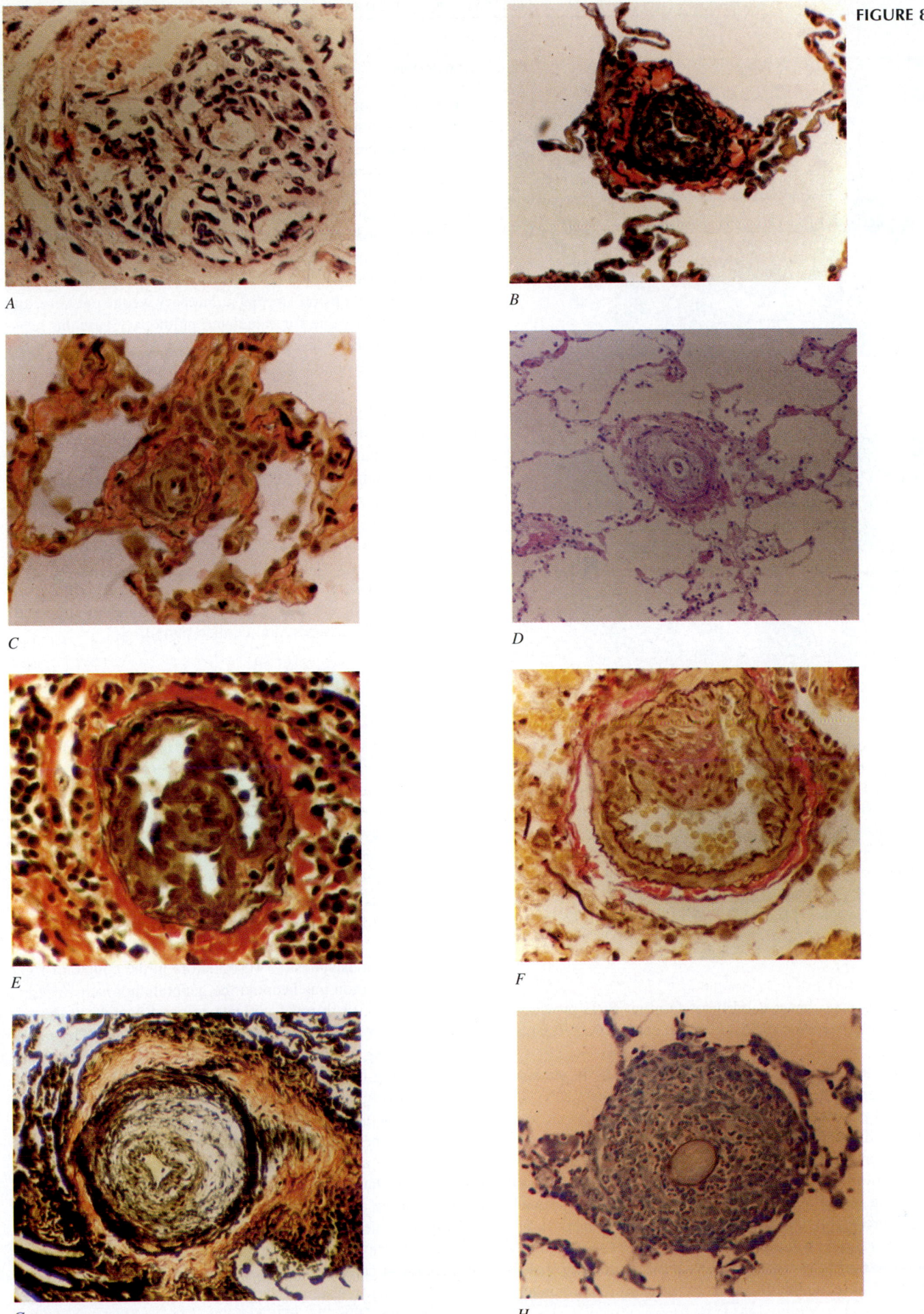

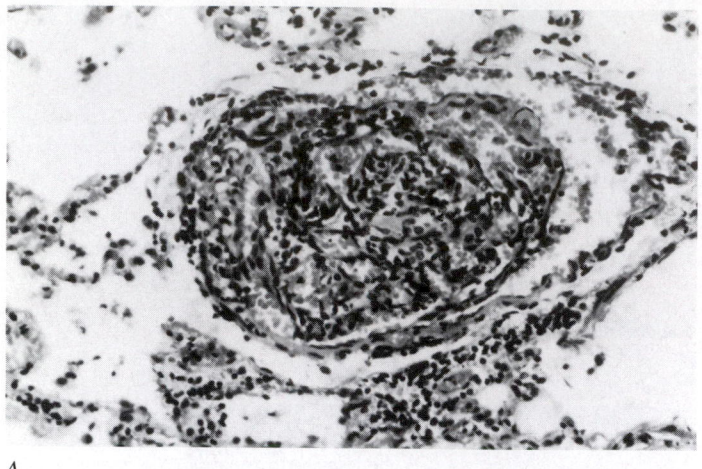

A

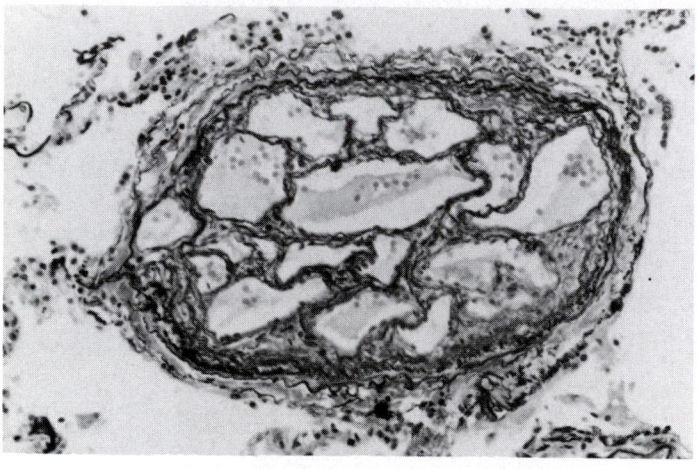

B

FIGURE 83-13   Contrast between plexiform and thromboembolic occlusions. *A.* Plexiform lesions in a muscular pulmonary artery in a 56-year-old woman with primary pulmonary hypertension. There is an active proliferation of intimal cells with capillarylike channels in between. The branch is dilated. To the left is focal destruction of the arterial wall, which contains some lymphocytes and polymorphs. H&E, ×140. *B.* Muscular pulmonary artery in a 63-year-old man with thromboembolic pulmonary hypertension. Many vessels were obstructed by intravascular fibrous septa as remnants of recanalized emboli. Elastic–van Gieson stain, ×140. *(Courtesy of Dr. C. A. Wagenvoort.)*

known. Awareness of the possibility of familial PPH provides opportunity for earlier diagnostic and treatment in affected families.[11,25,30]

Among the important insights provided by autopsy studies were the marked heterogeneity of lesions, the coexistence of thrombotic and plexiform lesions, and the paucity of plexiform lesions. These findings are inconsistent with the World Health Organization consensus statement of 1975, which distinguished between the lesions of PPH and thromboembolic PPH on the basis of plexiform lesions, on the one hand, and eccentric intimal hyperplasia/fibrosis, on the other. Because of the coexistence of these different lesions in families with PPH, there seems to be little reason to continue to regard the plexiform lesion as the hallmark of PPH or to retain the diagnosis of plexogenic pulmonary arteriopathy.

DIAGNOSIS

The diagnosis of PPH is a diagnosis by default. An approach to diagnosis is presented schematically in Table 83-6. Clinical manifestations appear only after the pulmonary vascular disease is moderately severe or severe, and a time delay of 2 years usually ensues before the first symptoms of dyspnea and fatigue and the diagnosis by cardiac catheterization.

The clinical diagnosis is generally made on three grounds: (1) clinical electrocardiographic and radiographic evidence of pulmonary hypertension; (2) right heart catheterization that reveals pulmonary hypertension, normal pulmonary wedge pressure, and abnormally high value for calculated pulmonary vascular resistance; and (3) no evidence for a known cause of pulmonary hypertension in the heart, lungs, control of breathing, or elsewhere in the body.

The paucity of numbers of patients with the disease and the likelihood that diverse causes and pathogenetic mechanisms can produce the same clinical syndrome have complicated descriptions of its natural history. For a while, certain prototypes were regarded as the norm: young women with Raynaud's syndrome, with acute onset of dyspnea and fatigue, and death within 2 years. Now it is appreciated that even though there is such a subset, longevity is not unusual and that the disease may affect all ages, both sexes, and different ethnic groups. Among the predictors of length of survival are the levels of right atrial pressure, pulmonary arterial pressures, and cardiac output.

TREATMENT

For symptomatic relief of breathlessness, supplemental oxygen is almost always part of the therapeutic armamentarium because virtually any change from the awake state at rest may precipitate or aggravate arterial hypoxemia, which, in turn, elicits pulmonary vasoconstriction. Although supplemental oxygen may relieve arterial hypoxemia during exercise or sleep, it may have little effect in patients in whom patency of the foramen ovale allows right-to-left shunting. With the onset of right ventricular failure, the usual cardiotonic regimen is used.

The major focus of therapy has been on vasodilator therapy in the attempt to relieve the pulmonary hypertension.[4,37,38,40,41] Testing for responsiveness to vasodilators in the course of right heart catheterization has become the general approach.[19,32,33,44] However, only one-third of patients respond acutely to the administration of vasodilators. The vasodilators that have been used for acute testing are illustrated in Fig. 83-14. The current mainstay for testing is prostacyclin, which can only be administered intravenously. Inhaled nitric oxide is currently being tested as an alternative, displacing adenosine and prostaglandin E$_1$. Testing for responsiveness also includes trial of calcium channel blockers (nifedipine and diltiazem), since these agents are available for oral use, have few side effects in tolerable dosages, and dosages can be adjusted for optimal benefit.[4,20,38,41]

Responsiveness to a vasodilator agent administered acutely is assessed in terms of a decrease in pulmonary arterial pressure, an increase in cardiac output, and a decrease in calculated pulmonary vascular resistance with little effect on systemic arterial blood pressure (Fig. 83-15). The usual favorable response has

TABLE 83-6

Approach to Patient with Unexplained Pulmonary Hypertension

Initial Appraisal	Goals
History and physical examination	Detect presence of pulmonary hypertension and cor pulmonale
Chest radiograph	
Electrocardiogram	Distinguish between secondary and unexplained pulmonary hypertension
Minimally Invasive Diagnostic Procedures	
Pulmonary function tests	Exclude intrinsic lung disease
Arterial blood gases	Exclude alveolar hypoventilation
Echocardiogram	Chamber size, tricuspid insufficiency, estimate PA pressure, exclude intracardiac shunts*
Blood serologies	Exclude connective tissue diseases
Lung scan	Exclude thromboembolic disease
Invasive (More Definitive) Diagnostic Procedures	
Cardiac catheterization	Gold standard; direct determination of pulmonary hemodynamics; exclude cardiac disease test for vasoresponsiveness
Angiography	Exclude thromboembolic disease
Lung Biopsy	Exclude subtle interstitial lung disease and/or vasculitis

*Also useful in following subsequent course of pulmonary hypertension after cardiac catheterization.

been an increase in cardiac output without change in pulmonary arterial pressure or pulmonary wedge pressure, resulting in a decrease in calculated pulmonary vascular resistance. Along with the increase in cardiac output, there is an improved sense of well-being and exercise tolerance increases. Unfortunately, because of the sustained pulmonary arterial pressures on the rapid heart rate, the work of the right ventricle remains high and improvement is apt to be short-lived.[8]

About 50 percent of patients who undergo vasodilator therapy stabilize or improve on oral agents. The greatest success has been with the calcium channel blockers, notably nifedipine and diltiazem. These agents are given in the maximum tolerated dosage, an amount determined by trial to the point of toxicity for each patient.[38] Those who respond to the calcium channel blockers with a decrease in pulmonary arterial pressure and an increase in cardiac output improve clinically, and their survival is prolonged.

The use of anticoagulants has become a regular feature in the management of primary pulmonary hypertension, since it seems to prolong life. This practice is particularly warranted in patients with a fixed low cardiac output because of slowing of the circulation and the predisposition to thrombosis in the abnormal pulmonary vascular tree. The low cardiac output also increases the possibility of stasis in the systemic venous circulation and of a major thromboembolic event. The usual risks of anticoagulation apply. Warfarin is the drug of choice, and dosage is monitored at an international normalized ratio of 2.0 to 3.0

For the two-thirds who are not responders during acute testing, continuous infusions of prostacyclin have been administered intravenously. For this purpose, an implanted central venous catheter is coupled with a portable infusion pump. Some nonresponders have shown considerable hemodynamic and clinical improvement in response to prolonged therapy. However, complications have arisen from self-administration of the drug and from difficulties with equipment. Some patients have used this technique to advantage for months and, in a few instances, for years. Others have used it as a bridge to lung or heart-lung transplantation.[22,41,45]

Single- or double-lung transplantation is currently being performed as a last resort. Although hemodynamic improvement after surgery can be dramatic, primary pulmonary hypertension poses considerable surgical risk, and the incidence of opportunistic infections postoperatively is high. In addition, rejection phenomena—notably bronchiolitis obliterans—occurs in up to 50 percent of patients within 2 to 3 years after transplantation. One pressing problem is the long waiting periods for suitable lungs for transplantation, so that many patients deteriorate considerably by the time they reach the operating table or die while waiting.

Dietary Pulmonary Hypertension

There is no longer any question that substances taken by mouth can selectively damage the pulmonary circulation. Three instances have been particularly well studied: crotalaria pulmonary hypertension in animals and aminorex and "toxic oil" in humans. Looming on the horizon is a third epidemic in humans due to the ingestion of appetite-suppressing drugs (see below). Although its cause is known, dietary pulmonary hypertension is generally listed as "primary" largely because the clinical course and pulmonary vascular lesions at autopsy in humans are indistinguishable from those of unexplained pulmonary hypertension. However, since dietary pulmonary hypertension suggests a distinct, and possibly identifiable, pathogenetic mechanism, it is considered here separately.[14]

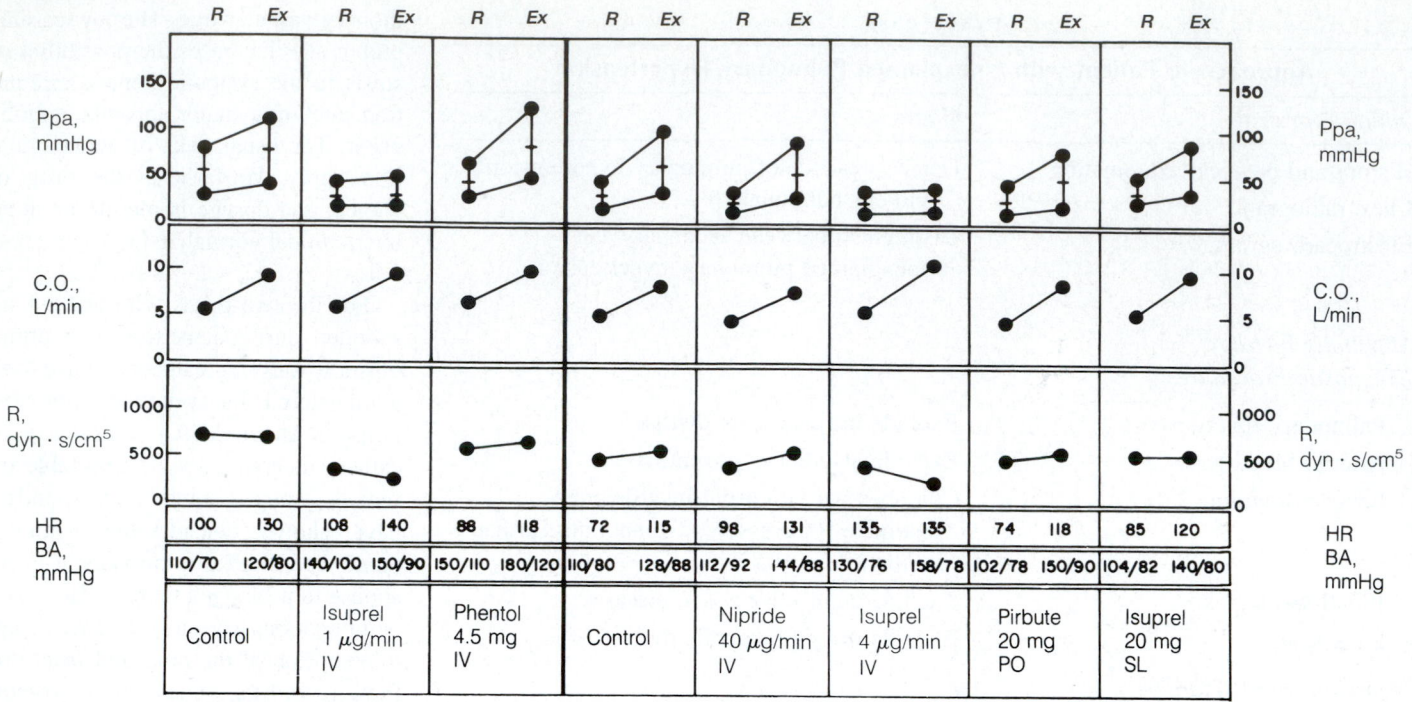

FIGURE 83-14   Repeat vasodilator studies over a 4-month interval. Patient took no medication between trials. Each column contains determinations at rest (R) and during exercise (Ex). *Left three columns* (May 5, 1981): During the control period, as cardiac output increased during exercise, the level of pulmonary arterial pressure (systolic, diastolic, and mean) also increased. Isoproterenol (Isuprel), administered intravenously, was associated with an unchanged pattern of change in cardiac output, but at lower pulmonary arterial pressures. Pulmonary wedge pressures (not shown) remained normal and unchanged. Calculated resistance fell. Phentolamine did not elicit a vasodilator response. *Right five columns* (September 25, 1981): The vasodilator response to isoproterenol, given intravenously, was unchanged. A less impressive response occurred after sodium nitroprusside (Nipride). Oral pirbute and sublingual isoproterenol (*last two columns*) did not elicit a pulmonary vasodilator response. C.O. = cardiac output; R = pulmonary vascular resistance; HR = heart rate; BA = brachial artery; IV = intravenous; PO = per os; SL = sublingual.

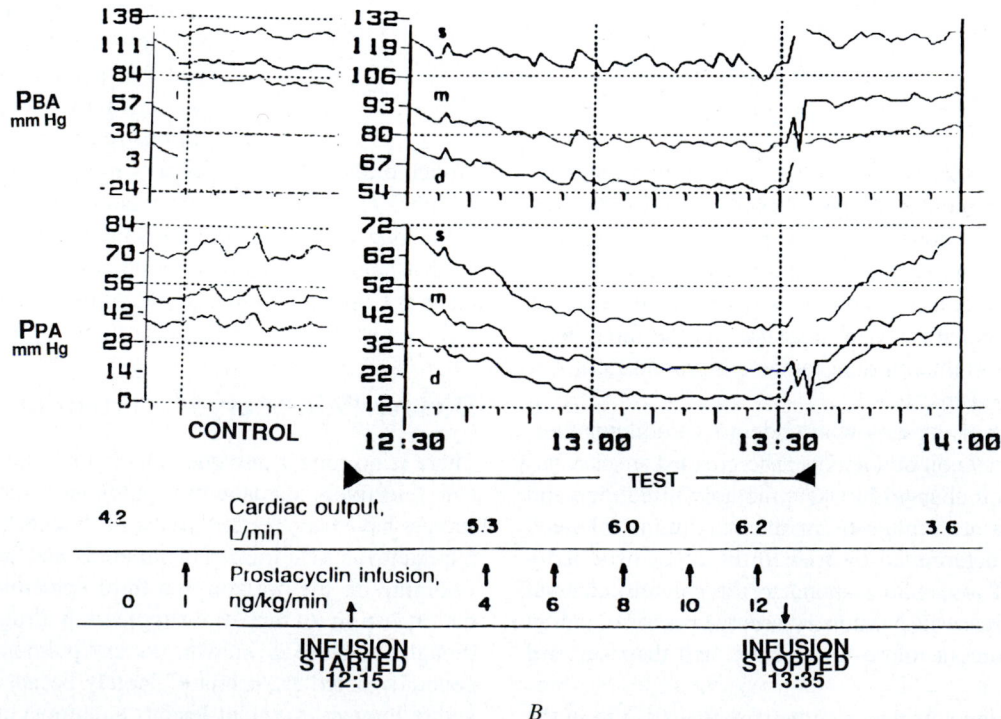

A   *B*

FIGURE 83-15   Prostacyclin infusion in primary pulmonary hypertension illustrating vasodilation in a "responder." The infusion was started at 12:15. Within 15 min (12:30), the pulmonary arterial pressure (Ppa) had begun a dramatic decline despite an increase in cardiac output. The decrease in pulmonary vascular resistance lasted as long as the infusion was continued (until 13:35). After the infusion was stopped (13:35), the Ppa increased rapidly to preinfusion levels and the cardiac output dropped. The changes in systemic arterial pressure (Psa) were much less striking. (*Courtesy of Dr. H. Palevsky.*)

CROTALARIA PULMONARY HYPERTENSION

Crotalaria is a genus of annual shrubs that was introduced into southern states from the tropics and subtropics to restore the soil between crops. Unfortunately, *Crotalaria* is poisonous to humans and animals because of the pyrrolizidine alkaloids that it contains. The major offending pyrrolizidine alkaloid in *C. spectabilis* is monocrotaline. Other species of the shrub, such as *C. fulva*, contain their own distinctive alkaloids (e.g., fulvine). Ingestion of *Crotalaria* by domestic animals (and humans) leads to incapacitating damage of the liver, lungs, and central nervous system. In the West Indies, where poisoning by *C. spectabilis* is endemic in the native population, hepatotoxicity predominates. However, the rat and the nonhuman primate (*Macaca*) manifest primarily the sequelae of pulmonary arterial hypertension (right heart failure and death).

The pyrrolizidine alkaloid monocrotaline does not act directly on the pulmonary circulation of the rat. Instead, monocrotaline apparently has to be converted by the liver to dehydromonocrotaline as a prerequisite for pulmonary vascular toxicity. At autopsy, the pulmonary vascular lesions resemble those produced by severe, long-standing mitral stenosis in humans: medial hypertrophy, necrotizing arteriolitis, and proliferation of mast cells. Moreover, the lesions appear to be morphologically distinct from those of primary pulmonary hypertension, since neither plexiform lesions nor intimal fibrosis is a regular feature.

These experiments have demonstrated conclusively that substances taken by mouth can cause obliterative vascular lesions in the pulmonary circulation.

AMINOREX PULMONARY HYPERTENSION

Between 1966 and 1968, an epidemic of pulmonary hypertension erupted in Switzerland, Austria, and Germany: in these countries, the incidence of pulmonary hypertension increased 20-fold. The epidemic followed the introduction in these countries of an appetite depressant agent, aminorex (2-amino-5-phenyl-2-oxazoline), in November 1965. Aminorex resembles epinephrine and amphetamine in chemical structure; both of these agents release endogenous stores of catecholamines. Aminorex was banned in 1968, and the epidemic subsided. After the drug became unavailable, in many patients the disease continued inexorably to cor pulmonale and death. In some, the level of pulmonary hypertension decreased or stabilized at a tolerable level; in others, it seemed to reverse completely. In contrast to the pulmonary vascular lesions produced by pyrrolizidine alkaloids in the rat, the pathology in humans was typical of PPH, including the plexiform lesions and intimal fibrosis; the liver was spared. Attempts to produce pulmonary hypertension by administering aminorex to experimental animals were consistently unsuccessful.

This outbreak had several important epidemiologic implications: (1) a medication taken by mouth could damage pulmonary arteries and arterioles; (2) since only few of the multitudes who used the agent developed pulmonary hypertension, the possibility was raised of genetic susceptibility (e.g., in some individuals and upon exposure to high altitudes); (3) other anorectic medications that resemble the catecholamines and amphetamines in structure might have similar effects in predisposed individuals (recent experience with phenformin, an anorectic agent that resembles the amphetamines in structure, supports the idea of genetic susceptibility); and (4) pulmonary hypertension can be reversible, particularly when detected early in its course and before pressures reached systemic levels.

TOXIC OIL SYNDROME

Another episode is the story of dietary pulmonary hypertension that unfolded with the occurrence of the "toxic oil syndrome." In May and June 1981, adulterated rapeseed oil, a bootleg pseudo-olive oil sold door to door in Spain, caused an extraordinary epidemic of noncardiogenic pulmonary edema.[14] Twenty thousand persons were affected, and about 375 died. About 2000 experienced sequelae. As a consequence of close surveillance, three stages of the disease have been identified: early (first 6 months), intermediate (6 months to 2 years), and chronic (persisting to date since 1981). From the outset, it was clear that the damage was widespread (affecting lungs, liver, skin, nervous system, immune system, muscle, and fat) and that endothelial injury everywhere features prominently in the pathogenesis of the clinical syndromes.

Early

During the first 3 to 4 months after ingestion of the toxic oil, the lungs were the seat of noncardiogenic pulmonary edema; pleural effusions were also common. Eosinophilia was striking and consistent. Most patients recovered (without pulmonary fibrosis) in 6 months or less. Pulmonary hypertension did occur but reversed spontaneously.

Intermediate

After the first 6 months, thromboembolic phenomena affecting gut, spleen, and other viscera, including lungs, supervened. Weight loss and peripheral neuromuscular dystrophies were common. In patients who had pulmonary hypertension, the blood pressure often seemed to revert toward normal.

Chronic

In this phase (particularly 4 and 5 years after the oil was ingested), pulmonary hypertension and cor pulmonale become increasingly evident. The vascular lesions in the lungs are characterized by intimal fibrosis and proliferation in precapillary vessels in association with organized pulmonary thromboemboli. Plexiform lesions have also been seen. However, neither necrotizing arteritis nor pulmonary fibrosis has been observed.

Unfortunately, the chemical ingredients in the toxic oil responsible for the syndrome remain enigmatic and are unlikely to be uncovered, since the bootleggers provided no recipe for the adulterated cooking oil as they went out of business, and reliable samples are now difficult to come by. Nonetheless, the outbreak showed that ingested material—often in small quantities—could cause widespread endothelial injury that afflicted the lungs. It also underscored the spontaneous reversibility of the pulmonary hypertension (as well as the ineffectiveness of vasodilators tried at different stages in the disease). Most unusual is the sharing of thromboembolism and intimal damage in pathogenesis, a coincidence that is strikingly different from the finding of occasional clots in the pulmonary circulation at autopsy in patients with primary pulmonary hypertension.

Portal-Pulmonary Hypertension

The coincidence of unexplained pulmonary in persons with portal hypertension, generally due to hepatic cirrhosis, has reinforced the idea that malfunction of the liver may allow toxic materials to damage the pulmonary endothelium. Although the logic resembles that applied to dietary pulmonary hypertension, the toxic oil syndrome, aminorex and fenformine pulmonary hypertension, and experimental *Crotalaria* ingestion by animals, direct extrapolation is not possible because not all of the vascular lesions resulting from these various methods are consistent with, or characteristic of, primary pulmonary hypertension. Also, the relatively few instances of portal-pulmonary hypertension, despite the high incidence of hepatic cirrhosis, again suggests that some predisposition, possibly genetic, is operative. Unfortunately, these patients seem to respond poorly to pulmonary vasodilators, and lung transplantation is not an option because of the hepatic cirrhosis.

Pulmonary Hypertension due to Other Appetite-Suppressant Drugs

After the aminorex epidemic, a variety of appetite-suppressant medications were used with little heed to the possibility that these agents might cause pulmonary hypertension. Then, in the early 1990s, Brenot et al called attention to the coincidence in Europe of pulmonary hypertension and the use of fenfluramine derivatives for weight reduction.[6] In 1996, Abenheim et al sounded the alarm that an epidemic might be in the making, especially since the Food and Drug Administration in the United States had approved the use of dexfenfluramine, a major fenfluramine derivative, for the long-term treatment of obesity even though experience with long-term use was extremely sparse.[1] In obese individuals who use anorexic agents for more than 3 months, the risk of pulmonary hypertension was estimated to be more than 30 times the risk in nonusers.

Approval of dexfenfluramine by the FDA was followed by a tremendous increase in sales of dexfenfluramines and other anorectic agents. Isolated reports of pulmonary hypertension following the use of anorexic agents have begun to trickle in, and a registry has been set up to gather information, in a standard way, about the use of anorectic agents and the occurrence of pulmonary hypertension.

At present, a few precautions seem noteworthy: (1) although aminorex and the fenfluramines differ in their pharmacologic characteristics, the pulmonary vascular lesions in the patients who die of pulmonary hypertension with a history of taking either drug are identical; (2) the longer the anorectic agent is used, the more likely is pulmonary hypertension to occur; (3) as in the case of primary pulmonary hypertension in general, early pulmonary hypertension is difficult to diagnose and mortality is high once the disease is established; and (4) pulmonary hypertension in users of anorectic agents is apt to be related to genetic susceptibility.

Pulmonary Veno-Occlusive Disease

In considering pulmonary veno-occlusive disease, it must be borne in mind that pulmonary venous hypertension, especially if

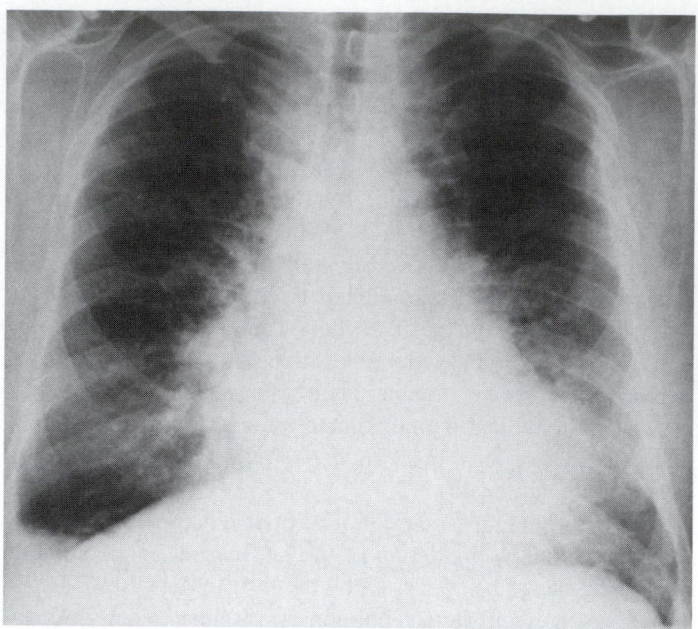

FIGURE 83-16 Pulmonary veno-occlusive disease. Posteroanterior chest radiograph demonstrates pulmonary venous engorgement and edema. Diagnosis established by cardiac catheterization, angiography, and lung biopsy.

severe and protracted (as in chronic mitral valvular disease, left ventricular failure, or mediastinal fibrosis), inevitably elicits pulmonary arterial hypertension. The increment in arterial pressure is not simply passive (i.e., a consequence of back pressure), since it is disproportionately high, suggesting either sustained reflex pulmonary precapillary vasoconstriction or anatomic changes in the precapillary vessels, or both (i.e., possibly reflex at the outset and then anatomic as the pulmonary arterial hypertension continues). That much of the arterial hypertension is anatomic is indicated by the frequent concurrence of medial hypertrophy and fibrosis of the pulmonary muscular arteries, on the one hand, and of intimal fibrosis, on the other. At the same time, the small pulmonary veins become arterialized, with an increase in thickness of the media, often in conjunction with intimal fibrosis.[35,50]

This is a rare disease, a few more than 100 patients having been reported to date. It affects children and adults, the age range varying from 11 days to 76 years; males are affected somewhat more than females. Most reported cases have been diagnosed at autopsy. The cause of this disorder is unknown. Indeed, as in the case of PPH, the possibility of diverse causes is strong.

The pathology is also variable. As a rule, pulmonary veins and venules are predominantly affected by a combination of an inflammatory and thrombotic process; many veins and venules are partly to fully obstructed by intimal fibrosis. The precapillary vessels generally show similar, but less severe, lesions. The intervening capillary bed, with its huge endothelial surface, is spared. Although in situ thrombosis has been suggested as the initiating mechanism of the disorder in the venules, this mechanism is still speculative.

CLINICAL FEATURES

The signs and symptoms are usually the same as those of primary (arterial) pulmonary hypertension. However, certain discrepancies may bring the diagnosis of pulmonary veno-occlusive disease to mind: chest radiography (Fig. 83-16) fails to reveal the expected striking disproportion between the central pulmonary arteries and peripheral pruning of the pulmonary vasculature, sometimes even showing evidences of chronic pulmonary congestion and edema; and the electrocardiogram sometimes fails to show convincing evidence of right ventricular overload. The pulmonary arterial wedge pressure is not helpful because, for unexplained reasons, it is usually normal.

Pulmonary Capillary Hemangiomatosis

Pulmonary capillary hemangiomatosis is a third category of unexplained pulmonary hypertension. The clinical syndrome is exceedingly rare and can mimic that of primary pulmonary hypertension. The diagnosis is made at autopsy.[35]

SECONDARY PULMONARY HYPERTENSIVE DISEASES

This category includes pulmonary hypertension of identifiable causes. The predominant causes are cardiac and pulmonary diseases. The cardiac diseases, such as mitral stenosis, generally elicit pulmonary arterial hypertension by increasing pulmonary venous pressure. Precapillary vasoconstriction, presumably a reflex phenomenon, augments the degree of pulmonary hypertension. Another mechanism is operative in congenital cardiac defects that are associated with an inordinate increase in pulmonary blood flow (e.g., atrial septal defect). The large flow induces anatomic changes in the pulmonary resistance vessels, which, coupled with the large flow, elicit sustained pulmonary hypertension.[10] A third mechanism exerts its effects by way of a high end-diastolic pressure in the left ventricle. This mechanism is operative in left ventricular failure. The pulmonary hypertension is a consequence of parenchymal fibrosis secondary to interstitial edema, trapping of the resistance vessels in the perivascular fibrosis, and reflex arterial vasoconstriction elicited by the pulmonary venous hypertension.

Raised pulmonary venous pressures can also result from obstruction of the large pulmonary veins en route to the left atrium. The underlying cause may be fibrosing mediastinitis (e.g., due to histoplasmosis), neoplastic invasion of lymph nodes (e.g., metastatic carcinoma of the breast), lymphoma (e.g., Hodgkin's disease), or lymphadenitis (e.g., due to sarcoidosis). These types of pulmonary venous occlusion are secondary in contrast to so-called *pulmonary veno-occlusive disease,* whose cause is idiopathic, and the lesions are suggestive of an intraluminal inflammatory process that affects not only the pulmonary veins and venules but, to a lesser extent, the small pulmonary arteries and arterioles.

Cardiac Lung

In chronic pulmonary hypertension due to heart disease, the muscular pulmonary arteries undergo changes that depend on the severity and chronicity of the pulmonary hypertension. These changes may determine the response to medical treatment, the benefit and risk of surgery, and the ultimate outcome. Early in the evolution of the pulmonary hypertension, the changes reflect, in large measure, the initiating mechanism—e.g., predominantly intimal changes in a large left-to-right shunt in contrast to predominantly medial changes in lesions that expose the vessels to systemic arterial pressures (e.g., Eisenmenger's disease). In unremitting chronic pulmonary hypertension, however, such distinctions tend to blur and are often complicated by secondary effects, such as in-site thrombosis, perivascular fibrosis, and decrease in parenchymal elasticity.

In general, chronic pulmonary hypertension may be sustained by two mechanisms: vasoconstrictive, attributable to intrapulmonary reflexes and/or heightened sympathetic activity; and structural changes in the vessels or in their immediate vicinity, which may or may not reverse if pulmonary arterial pressures can be lowered therapeutically. The possibility of vasoconstriction has been the basis for trials of pulmonary vasodilators. The possibility of reversible, albeit gradual, structural changes has been supported by instances of striking relief of pulmonary hypertension 1 to 2 years after surgical treatment of mitral stenosis and long-term improvement in pulmonary arterial pressures in patients with dietary pulmonary hypertension after cessation of the drug.

The considerable impact of cardiac disease on pulmonary performance can be illustrated by the changes induced by chronic congestive heart failure. Because of the stiff lungs and concomitant increase in the work of breathing, ventilation at rest is increased, leading to a mismatch with the low pulmonary blood flow as cardiac output decreases. These patterns account for the near-normal oxygenation of systemic arterial blood at rest in congestive heart failure; sleep disturbances and exercise predispose to arterial hypoxemia. Dependent edema and fibrosis redistribute blood flow to the upper lobes, accounting for a distinctive pattern on the chest radiograph. Pulmonary engorgement and the enlarged heart decrease the total lung capacity and the vital capacity. The FEV_1 and FVC are decreased, but the RV/TLC tends to increase. The diffusing capacity is low not only because of the decrease in air-containing alveolar volume but also because of abnormalities in the alveolar-capillary barrier due to chronic edema and interstitial fibrosis. Exercise limitation in heart failure is attributed to impaired O_2 delivery to peripheral tissues because of the low cardiac output. Enrichment of inspired air with supplemental oxygen improves exercise tolerance. The decrease in pulmonary blood flow predisposes to local thrombosis in the pulmonary vascular bed.

In the management of pulmonary hypertension secondary to congestive heart failure, a cardiotonic regimen that features the use of diuretics and an inhibitor of the angiotensin-converting enzyme (ACE) plays a pivotal role. The role of digitalis is debatable. In general, pulmonary vasodilators (other than ACE inhibitors) have not been shown to be effective in maintenance therapy.[36] Indeed, prostacyclin has promoted morbidity and mortality, and in some patients, acetylcholine infusion elicited pulmonary vasoconstriction instead of vasodilatation. Antagonists of endothelin-1 receptors are being tested.[51]

Thromboembolic Disease

Thromboembolic disease can result in chronic pulmonary hypertension in three major ways: (1) thrombotic occlusion of small pulmonary arteries and arterioles, (2) thromboembolic occlusion

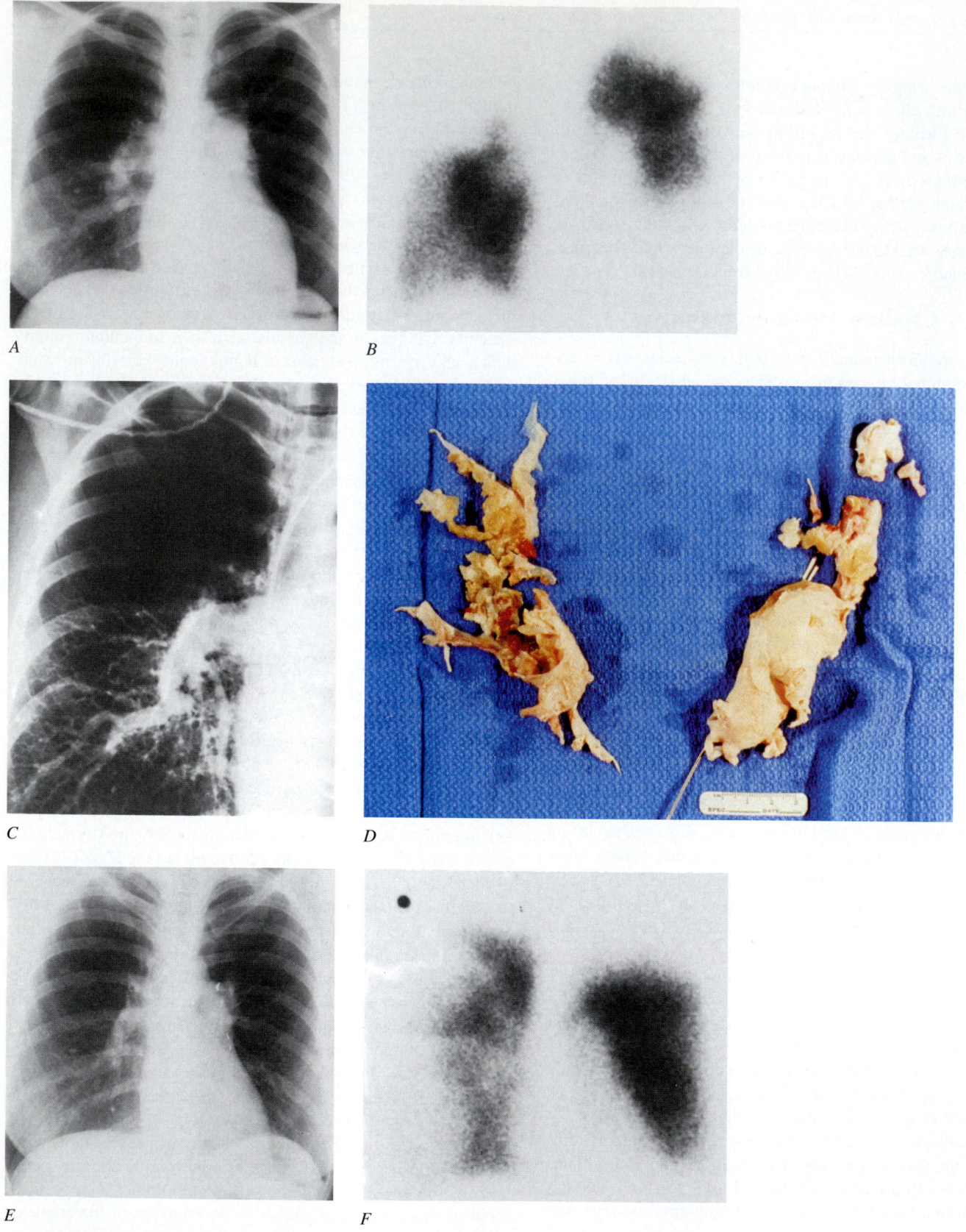

FIGURE 83-17 Chronic pulmonary thromboembolism, before and after surgery, in a 35-year-old woman suspected of having had episodes of pulmonary emboli between 1977 and 1979. Progressive pulmonary hypertension, cor pulmonale, and right ventricular failure. *A.* Preoperative chest radiograph. Pulmonary arterial pressure = 96/78 mm Hg; pulmonary wedge pressure = 4 mm Hg; cardiac output = 3.1 L/min. The chest radiograph reveals hyperlucency and diminished vasculature in the right upper and left lower lobes. Also, cardiomegaly with prominent central pulmonary arteries. *B.* Preoperative perfusion scan. Confirms chest radiograph above. *C.* Preoperative angiogram of right upper lobe showing absence of blood flow. *D.* Organized clot removed by Dr. L. H. Edmunds from the right upper and left lower pulmonary arteries at surgery. *E.* Postoperative (1 year later) chest radiograph. The chest radiograph is virtually normal. Pulmonary arterial pressure = 42/20 mm Hg; cardiac output = 5.0 L/min. *F.* Postoperative perfusion scan. Blood is now perfusing the right upper and left lower lobes. *G.* Postoperative angiogram of right upper lobe. Larger vessels that were previously unfilled (see *C*) now extend to right upper lobe. *(Courtesy of Dr. H. Palevsky.)* ▶

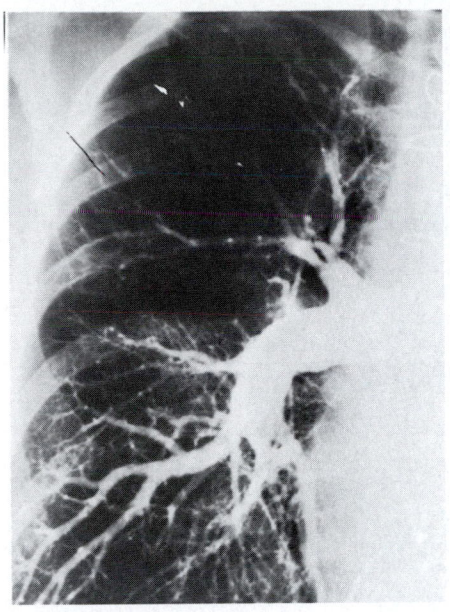

G

FIGURE 83-17   *(Cont.)*

of lobar and segmental pulmonary arteries, and (3) thromboembolic occlusion of large pulmonary arteries (see Chapter 84).

CHRONIC THROMBOTIC OCCLUSION OF SMALL PULMONARY ARTERIES AND ARTERIOLES

Once attributed to one or more showers of small pulmonary emboli, this disorder is currently regarded as widespread thrombosis of the microvessels of the pulmonary arterial tree due to widespread endothelial injury or malfunction.[16] The clinical manifestations and course of this disorder are identical to those of primary pulmonary hypertension. Treatment requires the long-term administration of anticoagulants, such as warfarin and antiplatelet agents.

CHRONIC THROMBOEMBOLIC OCCLUSION OF INTERMEDIATE AND PERIPHERAL PULMONARY ARTERIES

Pulmonary emboli, for which the source is inapparent during life, may be difficult to detect clinically until severe pulmonary hypertension dominates the scene. The typical patient presents with progressive dyspnea that is first attributed to "being out of shape" and is later appreciated as a sign of ill health. Breathlessness on mild exertion is incapacitating; on occasion, the breathlessness is associated with precordial pain. Clinical appraisal indicates the presence of pulmonary hypertension and right ventricular enlargement without evidence of left ventricular, valvular, or pulmonary disease. Perfusion scans may be diagnostic. On occasion, angiography may be needed to clinch the diagnosis.

Treatment

The prophylaxis and treatment of thromboembolic episodes that are clinically evident are described elsewhere (see Chapter 84).

CHRONIC THROMBOEMBOLISM OF MAJOR PULMONARY ARTERIES

The syndrome is a consequence of obstruction of major pulmonary arteries by large emboli that were generally unrecognized and have been progressively incorporated into the arterial walls as organized, occluding pulmonary lesions.

This syndrome is important to recognize, since it lends itself to surgical intervention (Fig. 83-17).[7,13] The diagnosis relies heavily on ventilation-perfusion scanning, which demonstrates perfusion defects that are segmental or larger. Angiography then demonstrates the number and extent of such lesions, which are underestimated by the perfusion scan. Magnetic resonance imaging and fiberoptic angioscopy are being tested for their value in preoperative assessment of the extent and patterns of the lesions. The surgical process of thromboendarterectomy is difficult, with a mortality in experienced hands of up to 15 percent. Long-term improvement is usually dramatic after successful operations, but pulmonary edema of the affected part of the lung may be a serious complication in the postoperative period. Postoperatively, patients require lifelong anticoagulation, and a filter is placed in the inferior vena cava to minimize the chance of recurrence.

Chronic Obstructive Airway Disease

The designation of chronic obstructive *airway* disease includes COPD as well as other obstructive diseases of the airways, such as cystic fibrosis (Fig. 83-18). Although chronic bronchitis and emphysema usually coexist, it is the chronic bronchitis, because of the ventilation-perfusion abnormalities that it produces, that is primarily responsible for the abnormal blood gases that lead to pulmonary hypertension. In these obstructive airway diseases, the onset of arterial hypoxemia coincides with increases in pulmonary arterial pressure to hypertensive levels; as ventilatory insufficiency progresses, respiratory acidosis contributes another stimulus to pulmonary vasoconstriction.[53] The degree of arterial hypoxemia and the level of pulmonary arterial pressure have proved to be reliable prognostic indices. Levels of arterial P_{O_2} less than 55 to 50 mm Hg signify that pulmonary hypertension is present.

ETIOLOGY

In dealing with COPD, one time-honored clinical approach has been the distinction between the "pink puffer" (predominantly emphysema) and the "blue bloater" (predominantly chronic bronchitis) (Fig. 83-19). The pink puffer spends a lifetime breathing through pursed lips—an automatic mechanism for achieving positive-pressure ventilation, which, in turn, maintains arterial P_{CO_2} at near-normal levels. In this group, pulmonary arterial pressures remain at near-normal levels unless some complication, such as a spontaneous pneumothorax or pneumonia, precipitates a bout of severe arterial hypoxemia. In contrast, the blue bloater is continuously on a downhill course of progressive arterial hypoxemia and hypercapnia, which lead to increasing pulmonary hypertension. It is difficult to explain the onset of cor pulmonale in the blue bloater because work of the right ventricle is not greatly increased even when arterial hypoxemia is quite marked (e.g., P_{O_2} of about 35

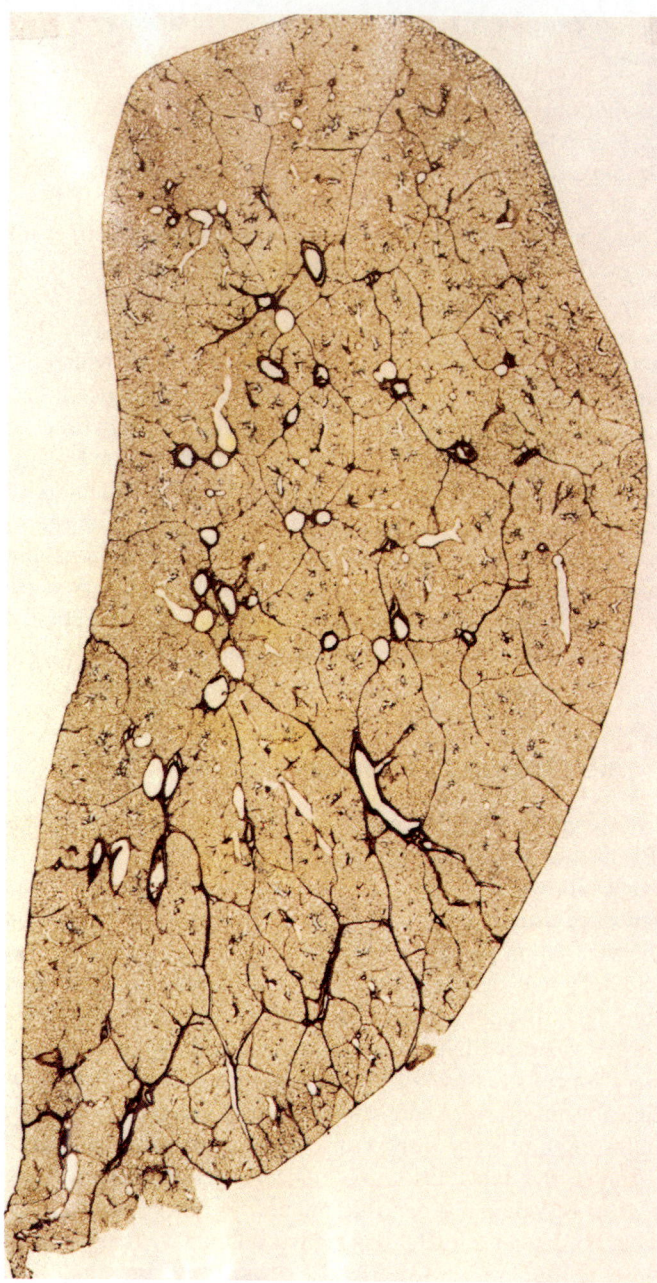

A

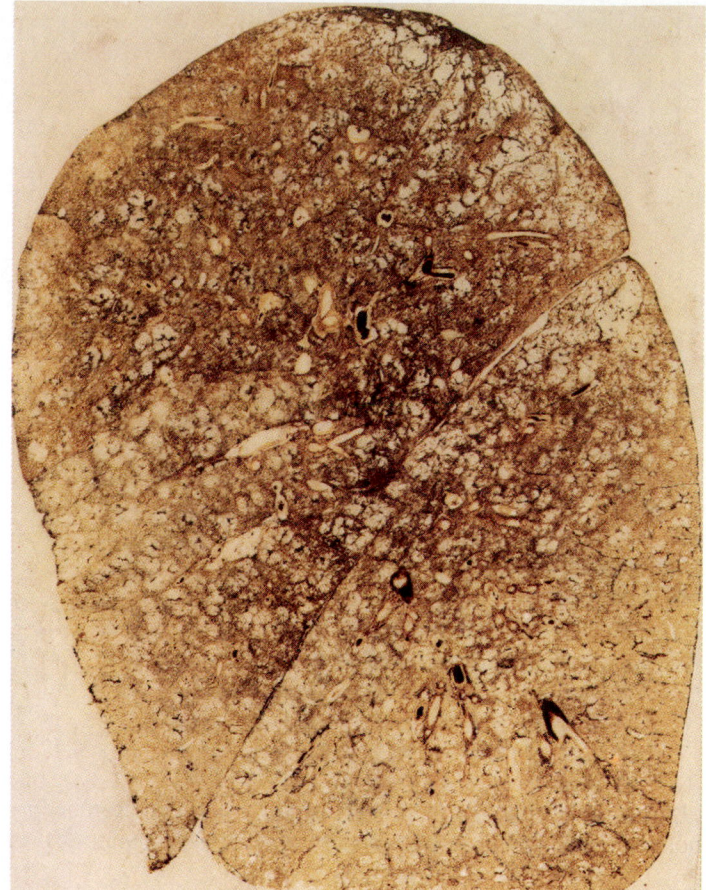

B

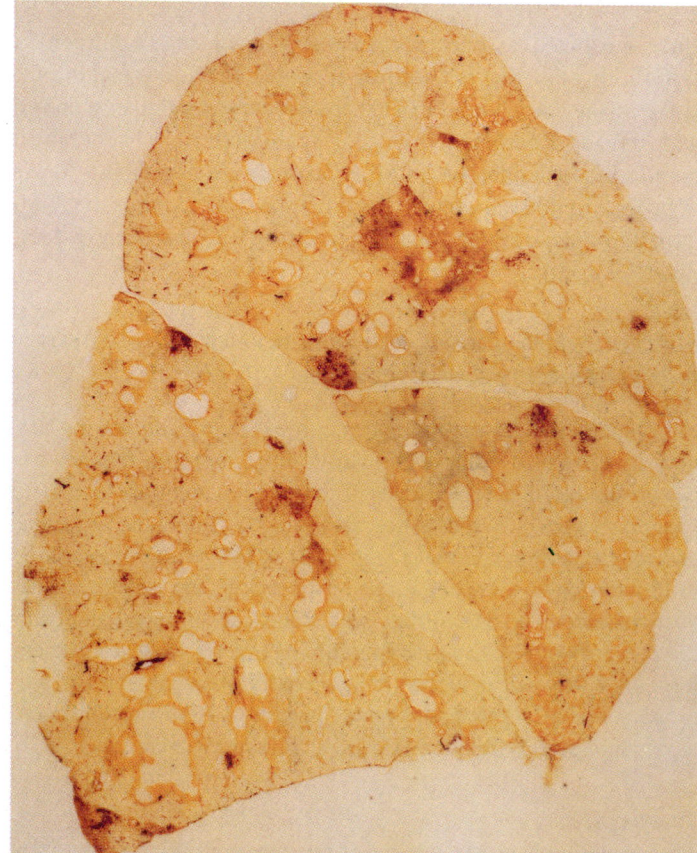

C

FIGURE 83-18   Gough (sagittal) sections. Lung architecture in normal lung and in obstructive airway disease. *A.* Normal lung. Between large airways and vessels, the parenchyma is intact. *B.* Centrilobular emphysema. *C.* Cystic fibrosis. The large airways are dilated and bronchiectatic, whereas the gas-exchanging surface is well preserved. *(Courtesy of Dr. S. Moolten.)*

mm Hg) and accompanied by respiratory acidosis (e.g., P_{CO_2} of about 50 mm Hg). At these levels, mean pulmonary arterial pressure is generally only about 30 mm Hg, and the cardiac output is only moderately increased. Undoubtedly, the blood gas abnormalities increase during sleep and the activities of daily life. Nonetheless, the levels of pulmonary arterial pressure that have been recorded are generally tolerated without difficulty in native residents at high altitude, raising the question of what factors other

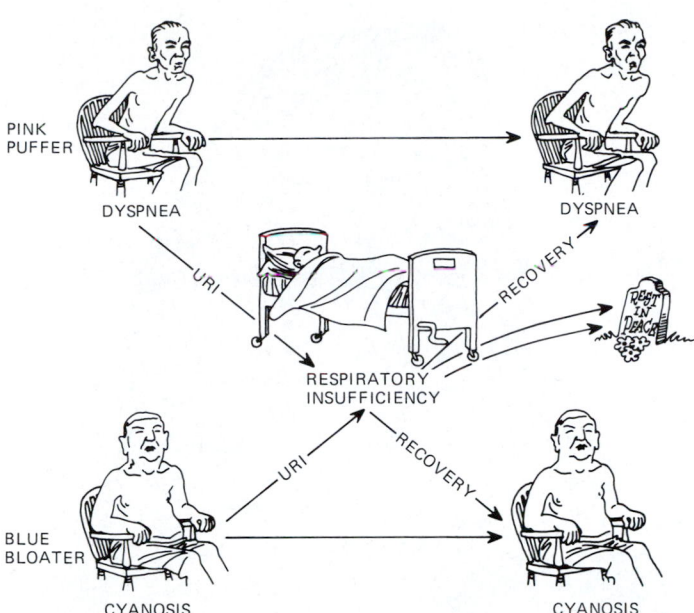

FIGURE 83-19   The pink puffer and the blue bloater. Natural histories. The pink puffer leads a breathless existence that is interrupted by bouts of acute respiratory insufficiency (*center*), from which he or she may recover completely (*upper right*) or go on to a stage of persistent cyanosis and respiratory acidosis (*lower right*). In contrast, the blue bloater generally leads a briefer existence, with more frequent bouts of acute respiratory insufficiency, from which he or she is less apt to recover completely. During the stage of acute respiratory insufficiency, the pink puffer and blue bloater are usually indistinguishable.

than pulmonary hemodynamic abnormalities are at work on the road to right ventricular failure and peripheral edema.[29]

Cystic fibrosis is another common cause of obstructive airways disease that results in pulmonary hypertension (Fig. 83-18C). Here, too, the root cause is persistent alveolar and arterial hypoxia resulting from ventilation-perfusion abnormalities.

Cor pulmonale is uncommon in uncomplicated silicosis, anthrosilicosis, or tuberculosis. On the other hand, it is not uncommon when silicosis, anthrosilicosis, or long-standing fibrotic tuberculosis is complicated by extensive, conglomerate, massive fibrosis, distorted adjacent parenchyma, shrunken lobes, and bronchitis (Fig. 83-20). The likelihood of cor pulmonale is increased further by chronic pleurisy, fibrothorax, or excisional surgery. In such cases, a combination of anatomic restriction of the vascular bed and disturbances in gas exchange is implicated in the pathogenesis of the pulmonary hypertension. The disturbances in gas exchange brought about by an acute respiratory infection are usually the most reversible element of this disorder.

CLINICAL FEATURES

In chronic bronchitis and emphysema, cor pulmonale and right ventricular failure are encountered in three different settings: in the pink puffer during an acute respiratory infection, in the blue bloater who is chronically refractory to all cardiotonic and pulmonary measures, and in the blue bloater during an acute respiratory infection. Not infrequently, in all three categories a bout of florid right ventricular failure is triggered by an acute respiratory infection. But even during a bout of respiratory failure, when blood gases are severely abnormal, rarely is the level of pulmonary hypertension severe enough to account for right ventricular failure.

During a bout of respiratory failure, the clinical pictures of the pink puffer and the blue bloater are often indistinguishable. As the infection subsides, however, it usually becomes clear whether a patient is predominantly emphysematous or bronchitic (Fig. 83-19).

Hyperinflation of the lungs in patients with chronic cor pulmonale secondary to chronic bronchitis and emphysema often obscures enlargement of the right ventricle. Nonetheless, many characteristic features of right ventricular enlargement can be uncovered if looked for carefully: a rhythmic lift of the sternum with each heartbeat, remote but accentuated pulmonary component of the second heart sound, cardiac pulsations in the epigastrium. Right ventricular failure often occurs in a setting of striking cyanosis, unexplained drowsiness or inappropriate behavior, distended neck veins, warm hands, suffused conjunctivae, hepatomegaly, and edema of the extremities. The gallops (S_3 and S_4) of right ventricular failure are generally present, and the murmur of tricuspid insufficiency can usually be elicited if the patient's sensorium is not too blunted to respond to the command, "Take a deep breath." Not only is the liver generally displaced downward by the low diaphragm, it is also enlarged and tender to gentle pressure over the right upper part of the abdomen. Once suspicion is raised that ventilation-perfusion abnormalities are the cause of the clinical picture, an arterial blood sample will confirm that the P_{O_2} is low (less than 40 to 50 mm Hg), the P_{CO_2} is high (more than 50 mm Hg), and respiratory acidosis is present. These blood gas values are rare in left ventricular disorders unless the patient is in frank pulmonary edema.

Radiography is of greater value in suggesting or confirming enlargement of the right ventricle in a patient with chronic bronchitis and emphysema than in proving it. The chest radiograph depends on the state of the underlying pulmonary disorder and on the degree of pulmonary hypertension and right ventricular failure. Most characteristic is the combination of "dirty lungs," prominent pulmonary arterial trunks at the hili, and a pruned peripheral arterial tree. Serial radiographs are generally more useful in detecting cardiomegaly than is a single examination (Fig. 83-21).

Electrocardiographic evidence of right ventricular enlargement is often blurred in patients with bronchitis and emphysema because of rotation and displacement of the heart, widened distances between electrodes and the cardiac surface, and the predominance of dilatation over hypertrophy in the cardiac enlargement. P pulmonale is more a reflection of the effects of hypertension on the right ventricle. If a distinctive pattern of right ventricular enlargement does occur, the degree of cardiomegaly must be severe. Because of these limitations, it is not surprising that the standard criteria for right ventricular enlargement have been satisfied in only one-third of patients with chronic bronchitis and emphysema who have been shown to have right ventricular hypertrophy at autopsy.

The electrocardiographic criteria for right ventricular enlargement in patients with obstructive disease of the airways are summarized elsewhere in this book. One of the most reliable in-

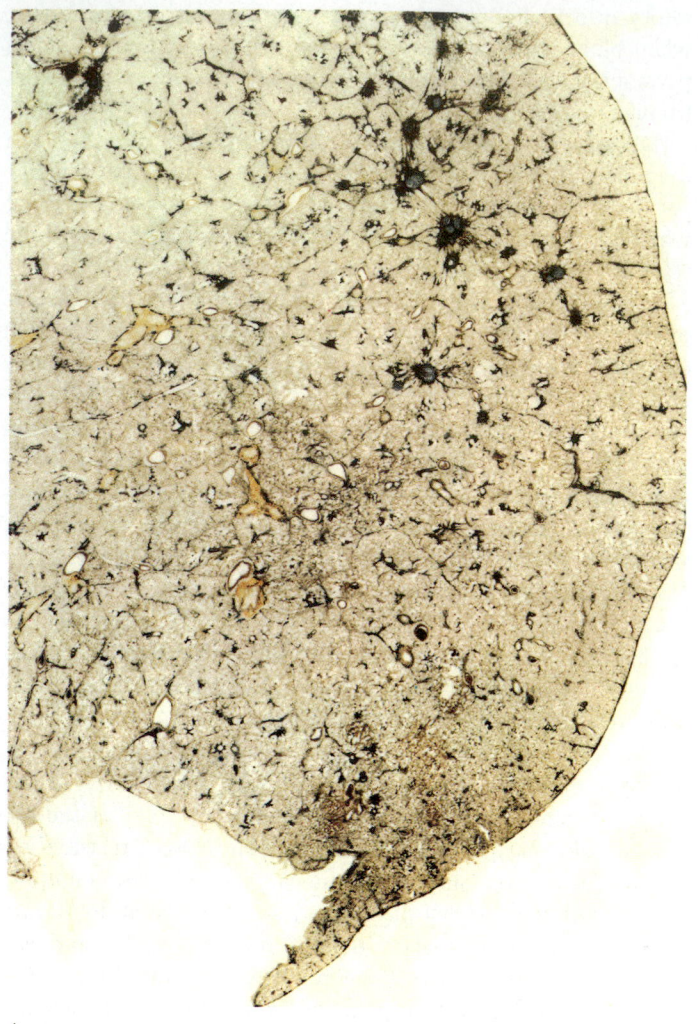

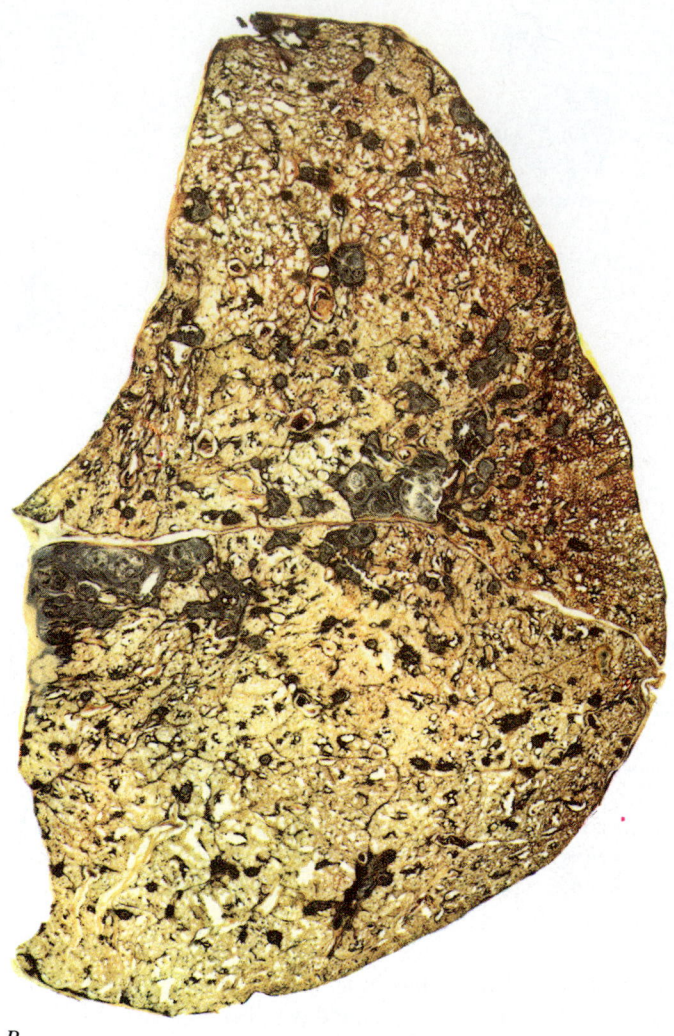

A

B

FIGURE 83-20   Gough (sagittal) sections. *A.* Coalminer's pneumoconiosis. Except for the coal macules (black starts, *upper right*), the architecture is virtually normal. *B.* Anthracosilicotic nodules, predominantly in vicinity of fissure. Background lung shows centrilobular emphysema. *C.* Progressive massive fibrosis. Cor pulmonale is uncommon in *A* unless parenchymal changes are associated with chronic bronchitis (which cannot be seen on these sections). However, cor pulmonale is not uncommon in *B* and *C,* which often derange blood-gas composition severely. *(Courtesy of J. C. Wagner, Cardiff.)* ▶

dexes of right ventricular enlargement in these patients has proved to be variability of successive electrocardiograms that accompanies changing degrees of arterial hypoxemia. As the arterial P_{O_2} drops to distinctly subnormal levels (e.g., below 60 to 70 mm Hg during waking hours), T waves tend to become inverted, biphasic, or flat in the right precordial levels (V_1 to V_3), the mean electrical axis of the QRS shifts 30° or more to the right of the patient's usual axis, ST segments become depressed in leads II, III, and aVF, and right bundle branch block (incomplete or complete) often appears. These changes tend to reverse as arterial oxygenation improves.

TREATMENT

In the patient with obstructive airway disease, as in the patient with *general alveolar hypoventilation* (despite normal lungs), the center of attention is the blood gases: relief of arterial hypoxemia and hypercapnia (acidosis) relieves the pulmonary hypertension. As noted above, a key question is whether the pulmonary hypertension, per se, warrants intervention.[29]

Pulmonary hypertension usually requires no special treatment: pulmonary arterial pressures decrease as a result of management of the obstructive airway disease: antibiotics to clear an acute upper respiratory infection, bronchodilators (notably, but not exclusively, theophylline, which not only relaxes muscle tone in the airways but also enhances cardiac and diaphragmatic contractility, increases mucociliary clearance, and exerts a diuretic effect), and supplemental oxygen as necessary. The 5-year survival rate is generally estimated to be about 50 percent; the lower the pulmonary arterial pressure, the better the prognosis.

The first episodes of right ventricular failure generally respond to a cardiotonic regimen that includes long-term oxygen therapy, diuretics, and digitalis. Each component of this regimen entails some uncertainty. Thus, although long-term oxygen therapy has been shown to improve survival, this benefit is not attributable to improvement in pulmonary hemodynamics.[31,46] As far as diuretics are concerned, chloride-losing agents run the risk of promoting hypercapnia, predisposing to respiratory depression, and aggravating ventilatory insufficiency. The use of digi-

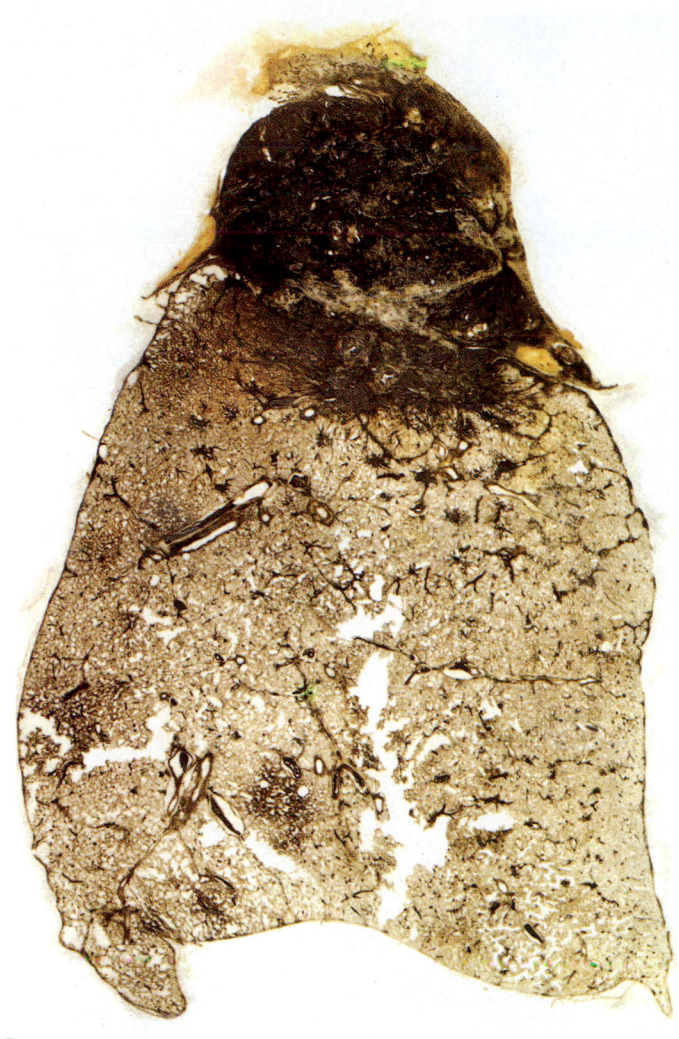

C

FIGURE 83-20   *(Cont.)*

talis must also be undertaken with caution because of the threat of digitalis-associated cardiac arrhythmias during hypoxia.

Right ventricular failure generally responds to clearance of the precipitating mechanism (e.g., an upper respiratory infection). As ventilatory failure increases, however, the margin for recovery from heart failure narrows. Nonetheless, many patients who experience one or more bouts of heart failure per year have survived for 5 to 10 years after the first episode.

Although the considerations above question the need to address pulmonary hypertension in patients with COPD, pulmonary vasodilators have been tried in individual studies. Among the agents tested have been calcium channel blockers and prostacyclin.

Calcium channel blockers have been administered to patients with chronic obstructive (hypoxemic) pulmonary hypertension without improving survival or the quality of life. Indeed, the ventilatory insufficiency seems to have a greater impact on the quality of life than the cardiac failure. Any benefits from the use of calcium channel blockers also seem to diminish with time. No pulmonary vasodilator has proved to be as effective as oxygen in chronic obstructive (hypoxemia) pulmonary disease with respect to either survival or exercise tolerance.

Prostacyclin has had only limited trials in secondary pulmonary hypertension, including COPD.[22] Its use in COPD has not become popular for both practical and theoretical reasons: although its vasodilator effect on pulmonary vessels that are vasoconstricted due to hypoxia increases the cardiac output and the mixed venous O_2 content by decreasing pulmonary vascular resistance, it runs the countervailing risk of aggravating ventilation-perfusion abnormalities; in the few studies to date, the increase in cardiac output resulting from pulmonary vasodilation has left pulmonary arterial pressure virtually unchanged, so the work of the right ventricle has not decreased.

Overall, the sporadic trials of vasodilators in chronic obstructive (hypoxemic) pulmonary disease have shown little benefit: as a rule, pulmonary hemodynamics have shown little improvement, while gas exchange has been further compromised. Also, undesirable systemic side effects have been common. At present, if a pulmonary vasodilator seems to be in order—and this is questionable—there is no more effective pulmonary vasodilator in chronic obstructive (hypoxemic) pulmonary disease than oxygen.[49]

Pulmonary Interstitial Diseases

ETIOLOGY

A wide variety of pathologic processes can evoke pulmonary interstitial fibrosis (Fig. 83-22). The most familiar causes are sarcoidosis, asbestosis, and radiation pneumonitis. Lymphangitic spread of carcinoma within the lungs can produce the same effect (Fig. 83-22). In these disorders, progressive fibrosis and infiltration not only thicken and distort the pulmonary interstitium, replacing the normal mucopolysaccharide matrix with cells and scar tissue, but also entrap the pulmonary blood vessels and obliterate segments of the pulmonary vascular bed. As a result, some segments of the pulmonary vascular bed are amputated, others are encased in scar, and the overall distensibility of the pulmonary parenchyma is diminished. In some disorders, such as silicosis, distortion of the lung due to the pulling of scar tissue on normal and less affected lung intensifies the derangements in the pulmonary parenchyma (Fig. 83-23). Other interstitial processes affect the small airways by encasing them in scar tissue. Disorders such as sarcoidosis affect not only the parenchyma of the lung but also the walls of the airways.

Connective-tissue diseases, particularly systemic lupus erythematosus, progressive systemic sclerosis (scleroderma), and its variant forms, are also common causes. As a rule, these disorders may cause vascular disease without interstitial inflammation and fibrosis.

The common denominator is a pattern of restrictive lung disease that originally focused disproportionately on impairment to diffusion because of thickened alveolar-capillary membranes; hence the designation *alveolar-capillary block*. But since then, disturbances in ventilation-perfusion relationships have been appreciated as dominant features, particularly in the later stages of the disease.

PATHOPHYSIOLOGY

The lungs are stiff (poorly compliant) because of the diffuse interstitial disease, which limits distensibility and increases pulmonary vascular resistance by obliterating small pulmonary ar-

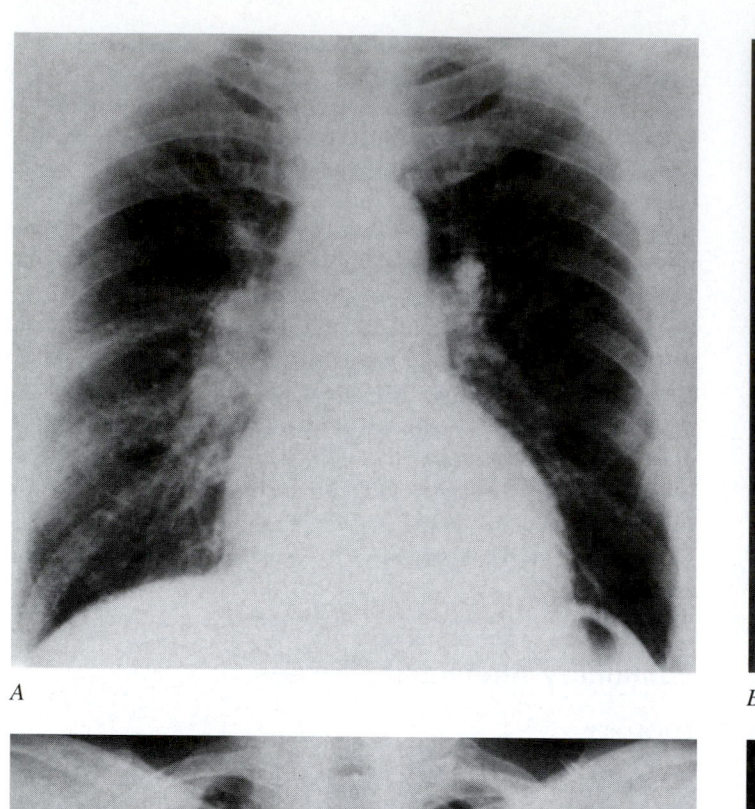

A

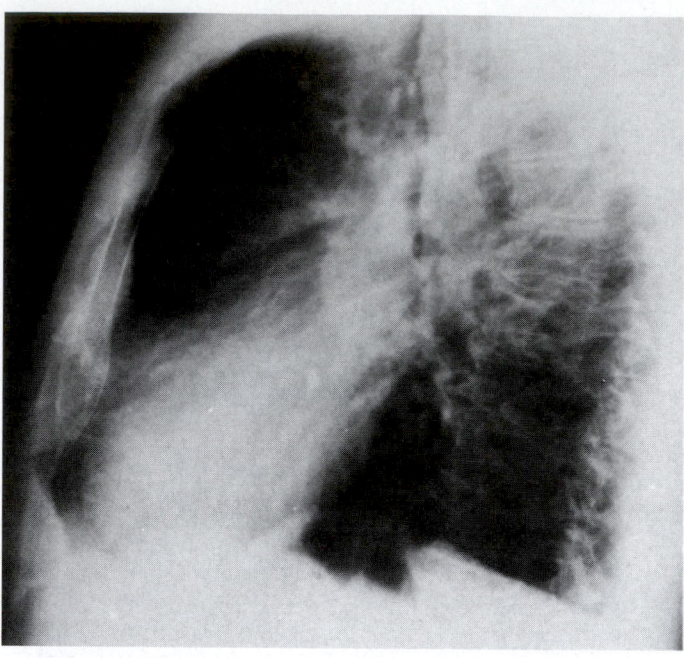

B

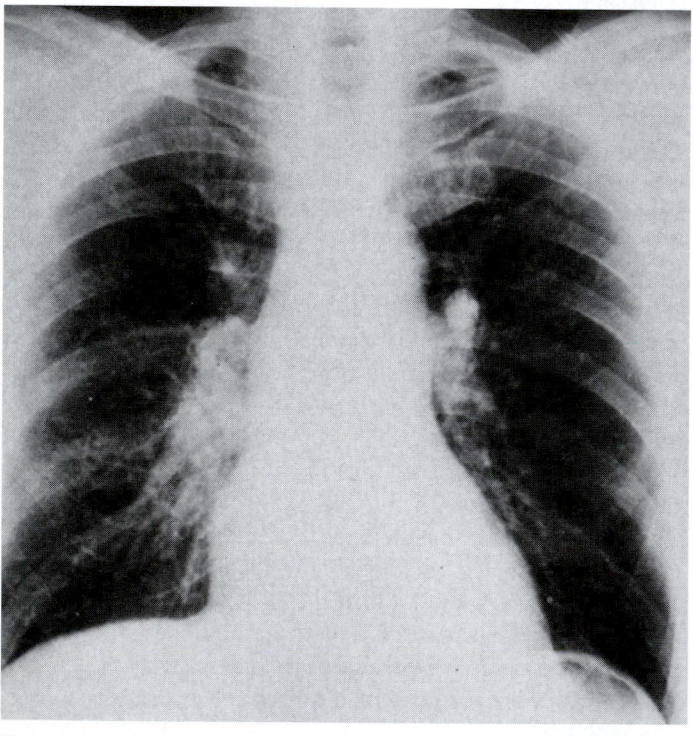

C

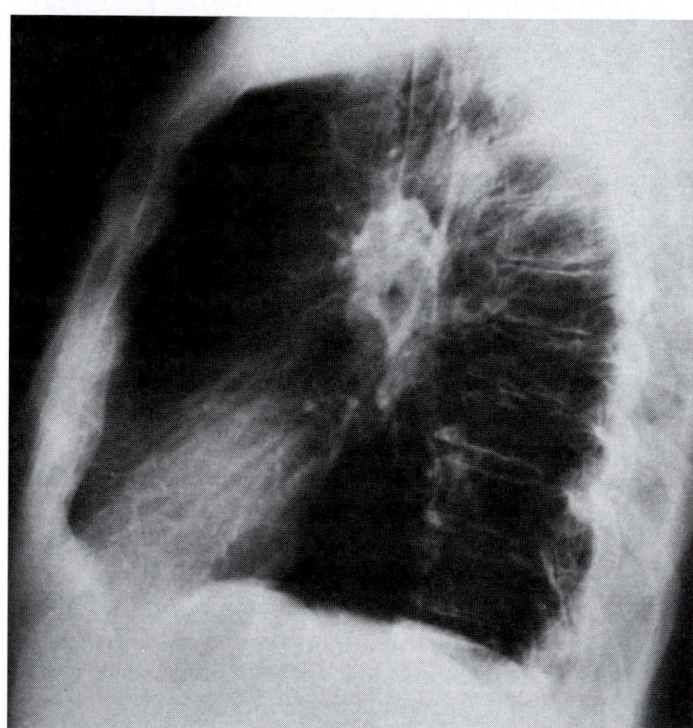

D

FIGURE 83-21 Chronic bronchitis and emphysema. *A* and *B*. Posteroanterior and lateral views during episode of right ventricular failure. *C* and *D*. Posteroanterior and lateral views 3 weeks later, after recovery.

teries and arterioles; their elastic recoil is correspondingly low. In some diseases, such as that due to asbestos, thickening of the pleura can be another factor in reducing pulmonary compliance. O_2 consumption becomes abnormally high, largely because of an increase in the work of breathing.

As the disease progresses, lung volumes undergo gradual, concentric reduction. As an adaptation that minimizes the elastic work of breathing, the minute and alveolar ventilation is high, breathing is rapid and shallow, and the arterial P_{O_2} is near nor-

mal. At this stage, exercise often elicits a precipitous drop in arterial P_{O_2}. When the interstitial process has advanced sufficiently to cast shadows on the chest radiograph (Fig. 83-24), the arterial P_{CO_2} either remains slightly low or begins to increase toward normal, largely as the result of ventilation-perfusion abnormalities (see below). The diffusing capacity decreases progressively as the interstitial fibrosis progresses; even though the value may fall within normal limits at rest, it generally fails to increase normally during graded exercise.

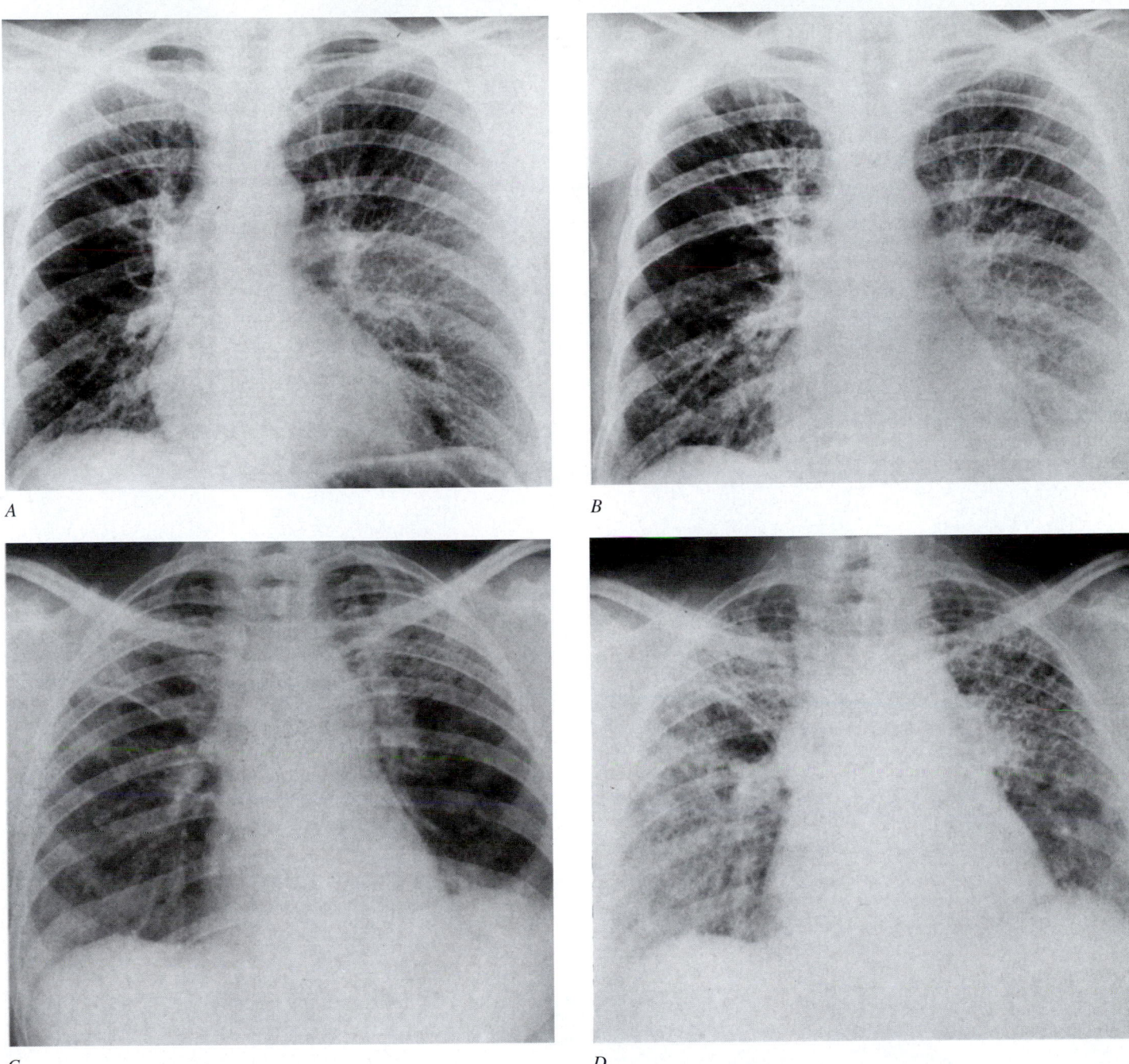

A

B

C

D

FIGURE 83-22 Diffuse interstitial disease. *A* and *B*. Lymphangitic spread of carcinoma of the breast in a 50-year-old woman. In the 2 years between the chest radiographs, dyspnea and tachypnea had progressed. The pulmonary function tests showed severe impairment of diffusion; the electrocardiogram indicated right ventricular enlargement (cor pul- monale). *C* and *D*. Sarcoidosis in a 50-year-old man. In the 2 years be- tween the chest radiographs, pulmonary fibrosis had progressed strik- ingly. At autopsy, pulmonary fibrosis was marked; bronchi were widely dilated, and emphysematous areas were juxtaposed to areas of dense fi- brosis. Cor pulmonale was confirmed.

FIGURE 83-23 Diffuse interstitial disease. Silicosis. *A*. Simple sili- cosis. Right upper lobe. Fine nodularity is evidence of early widespread disease. Hilar adenopathy is also present. *B*. Simple silicosis. The sili- cotic nodules are larger and more profuse. *C*. Progressive massive fi- brosis and emphysema complicating silicosis. A large shadow is seen in the right upper lobe (arrows). In addition, the upper lobes are slightly contracted, whereas the lower lobes are unusually radiolucent. *D*. Same patient as in *C*. Pneumothorax on the right complicates massive fibro- sis. *E*. Progressive massive fibrosis and emphysema complicating sili- cosis. Large bullae are widespread. *F*. Cor pulmonale secondary to pro- gressive massive fibrosis. *[A to D after Dauber JH: Silicosis, in Fishman AP (ed), Update: Pulmonary Diseases and Disorders. New York, Mc- Graw-Hill, 1982, pp 149–166; E and F courtesy of Dr. S. Moolten.]* ▶

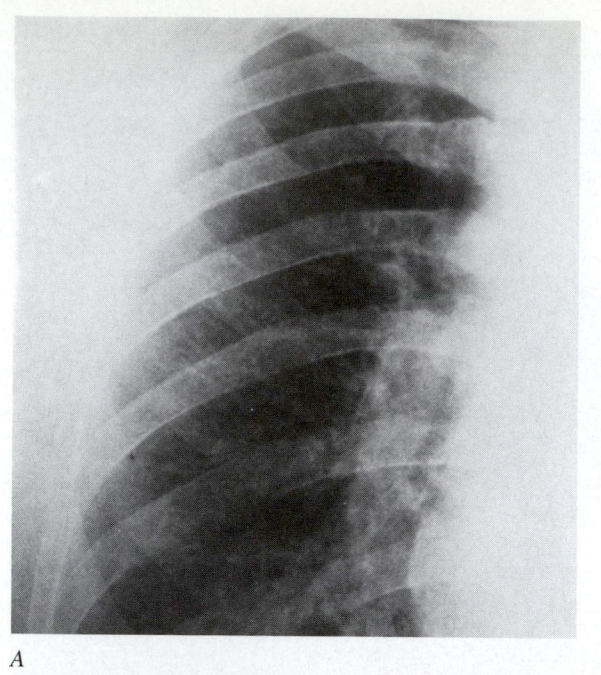

A

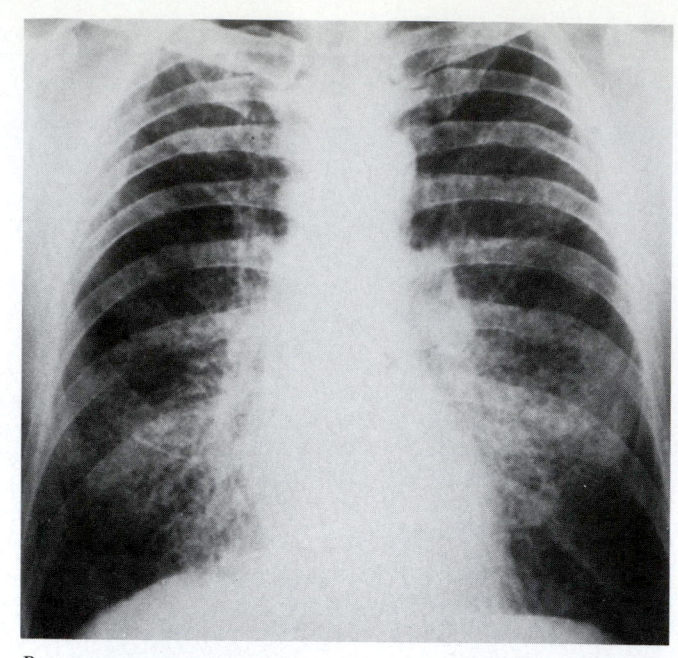

B

FIGURE 83-23

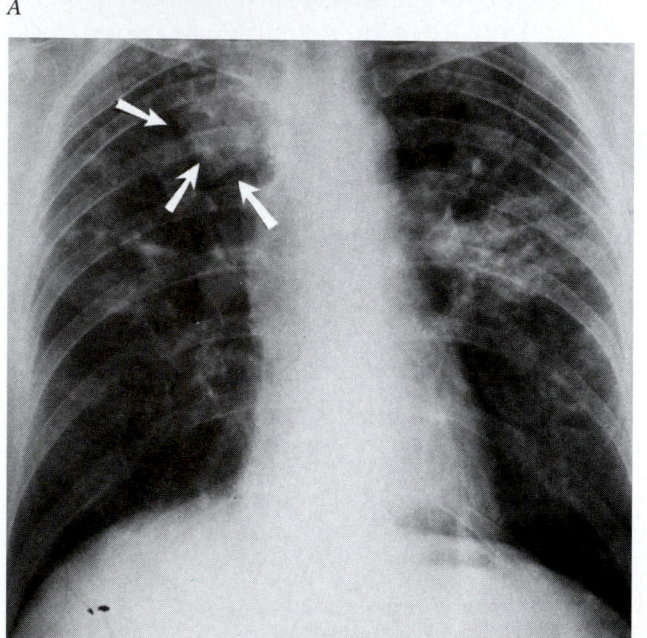

C

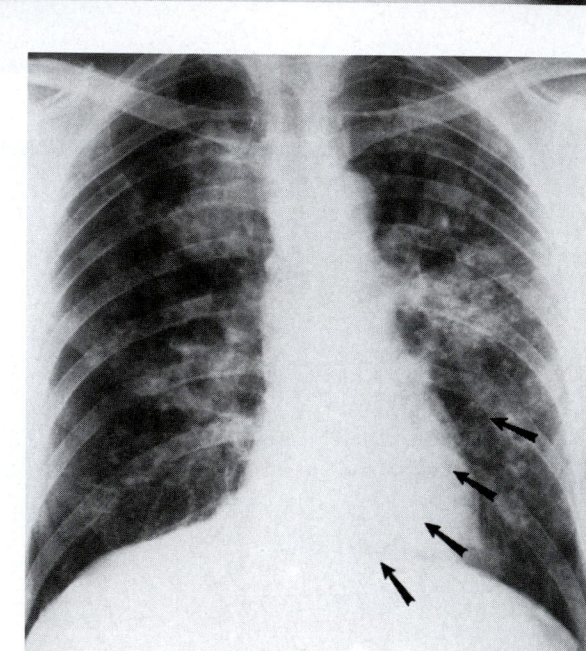

D

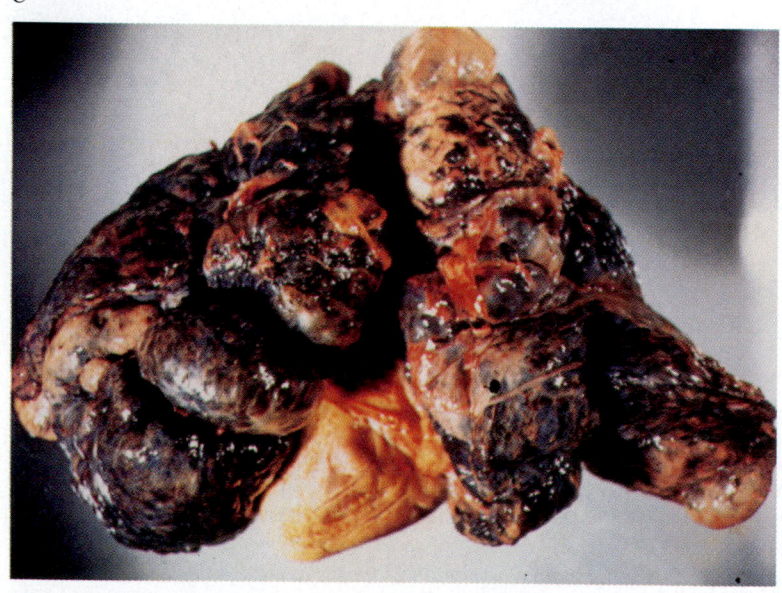

E

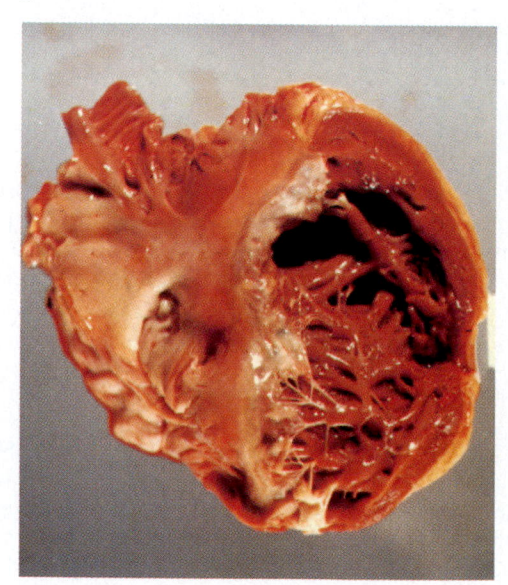

F

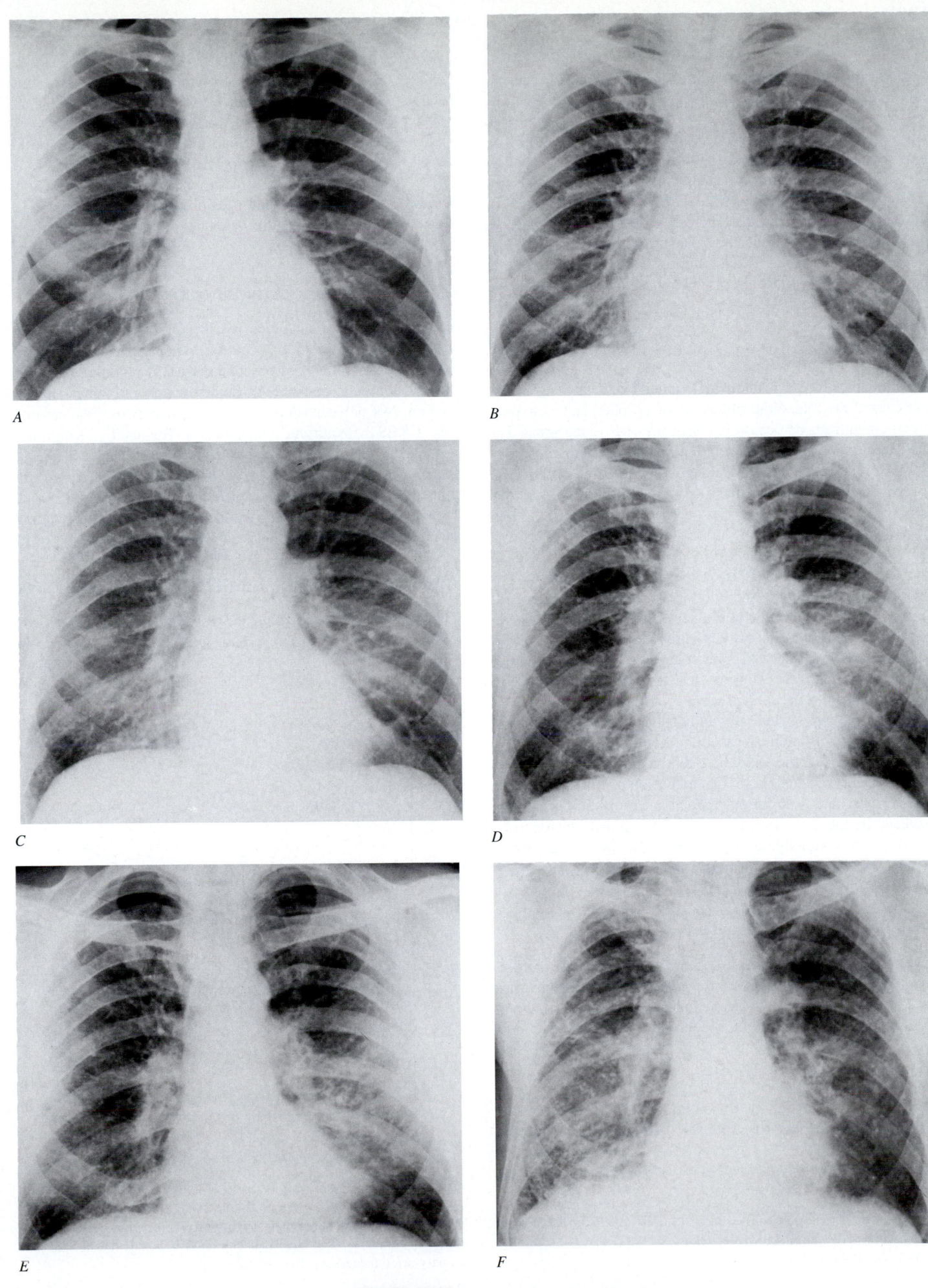

FIGURE 83-24

Derangements in alveolar ventilation and blood flow at a microscopic level are present early in interstitial disease, but in time, progressive disease exaggerates the imbalances sufficiently to cause arterial hypoxemia at rest. As long as the arterial hypoxemia remains mild, pulmonary hypertension is generally modest at rest, increasing during exercise (Fig. 83-25). But as the disease progresses and arterial hypoxemia intensifies, the level of pulmonary hypertension also increases, and cor pulmonale begins to evolve. Arterial eucapnia or hypocapnia is gradually succeeded by hypercapnia. Right ventricular failure occurs late in the course of the disease, in association with severe hypoxemia and respiratory acidosis.

CLINICAL FEATURES

The clinical picture is generally dominated by the disease process that caused the interstitial disease until dyspnea and tachypnea become manifest; on occasion, cough may be troublesome. The chest radiograph and high-resolution computed tomography disclose a diffuse reticular or reticulonodular interstitial pattern (Fig. 83-26) that reflects interstitial fibrosis or infiltration, or both.

TREATMENT

The focus of management is on the underlying lung disease, and success in relieving the pulmonary hypertension depends on the extent to which the pulmonary interstitial disease is reversible. Corticosteroids are generally the first line of attack for the interstitial process. As a rule, they are more effective for cellular than for fibrotic lesions. Immunosuppressive agents are usually the second wave of therapeutic agents. Supplemental oxygen is generally a mainstay of therapy to relieve breathlessness. Pulmonary vasodilators have not had extensive trials. In principle, they may be effective in the early stages of pulmonary hypertension to the extent that vasoconstriction plays a part and ventilation-perfusion abnormalities are not marked. In the late stages, when ventilation-perfusion relationships are seriously deranged, objections to the use of pulmonary vasodilators are the same as the preferences for their use in COPD.

Collagen Vascular Diseases

Suspicion is high that at least some instances of PPH are secondary to systemic connective-tissue disorders. Among those that have been implicated are systemic lupus erythematosus and progressive systemic sclerosis (scleroderma).

SYSTEMIC LUPUS ERYTHEMATOSUS

The lungs as well as the pleura are commonly impaired in systemic lupus erythematosus. Although attention has previously focused on the larger arteries in lupus erythematosus, it has been noted that pulmonary hypertension and cor pulmonale are not uncommon in this disease. As in PPH, females predominate, and many manifest Raynaud's phenomenon. Many of the patients also have positive antinuclear antibodies in the circulation. At autopsy, instead of a vasculitis, the vascular lesions resemble those of PPH. One possible explanation of these lesions is the hypercoagulable state due to lupus anticoagulant in the blood.[3]

PROGRESSIVE SYSTEMIC SCLEROSIS (SCLERODERMA)

In progressive systemic sclerosis, the incidence of pulmonary vascular disease is high; on occasion, the only manifestation may be obliterative pulmonary vascular disease, with pulmonary vascular lesions that resemble those of primary pulmonary hypertension. Not only in scleroderma but also in two of its variants, the CREST syndrome (calcinosis, Raynaud's syndrome, esophageal dysfunction, sclerodactyly, and telangiectasis) and the overlap syndromes (mixed connective-tissue diseases), the clinical picture can be indistinguishable from that of primary pulmonary hypertension unless the extrapulmonary manifestations of these diseases are manifest.[42,43]

Alveolar Hypoventilation Despite Normal Lungs

This topic is considered fully elsewhere in this book. Here it will suffice to consider aspects germane to pulmonary hypertension.

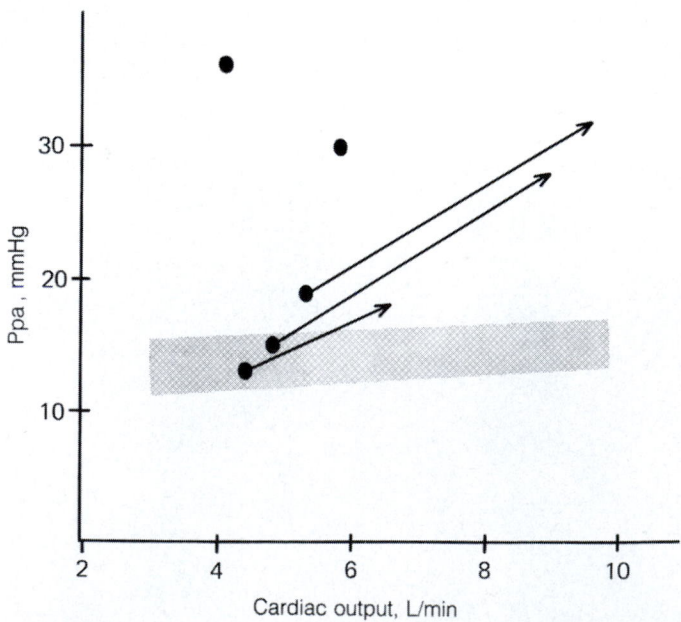

FIGURE 83-25 Pulmonary asbestosis. Hemodynamic observations in five patients. Two of the five had pulmonary hypertension at rest; the other three became pulmonary hypertensive during exercise. ● = at rest; → = exercise. The shaded background indicates the normal pulmonary arterial pressure–flow relationship.

◀ **FIGURE 83-24** Pulmonary asbestosis. Consecutive changes over 18 years. The patient had worked in an asbestos plant for 3 years before the first radiograph shown was taken. *A*. 1937. *B*. 1940. *C*. 1944. *D*. 1947. *E*. 1949. *F*. 1955.

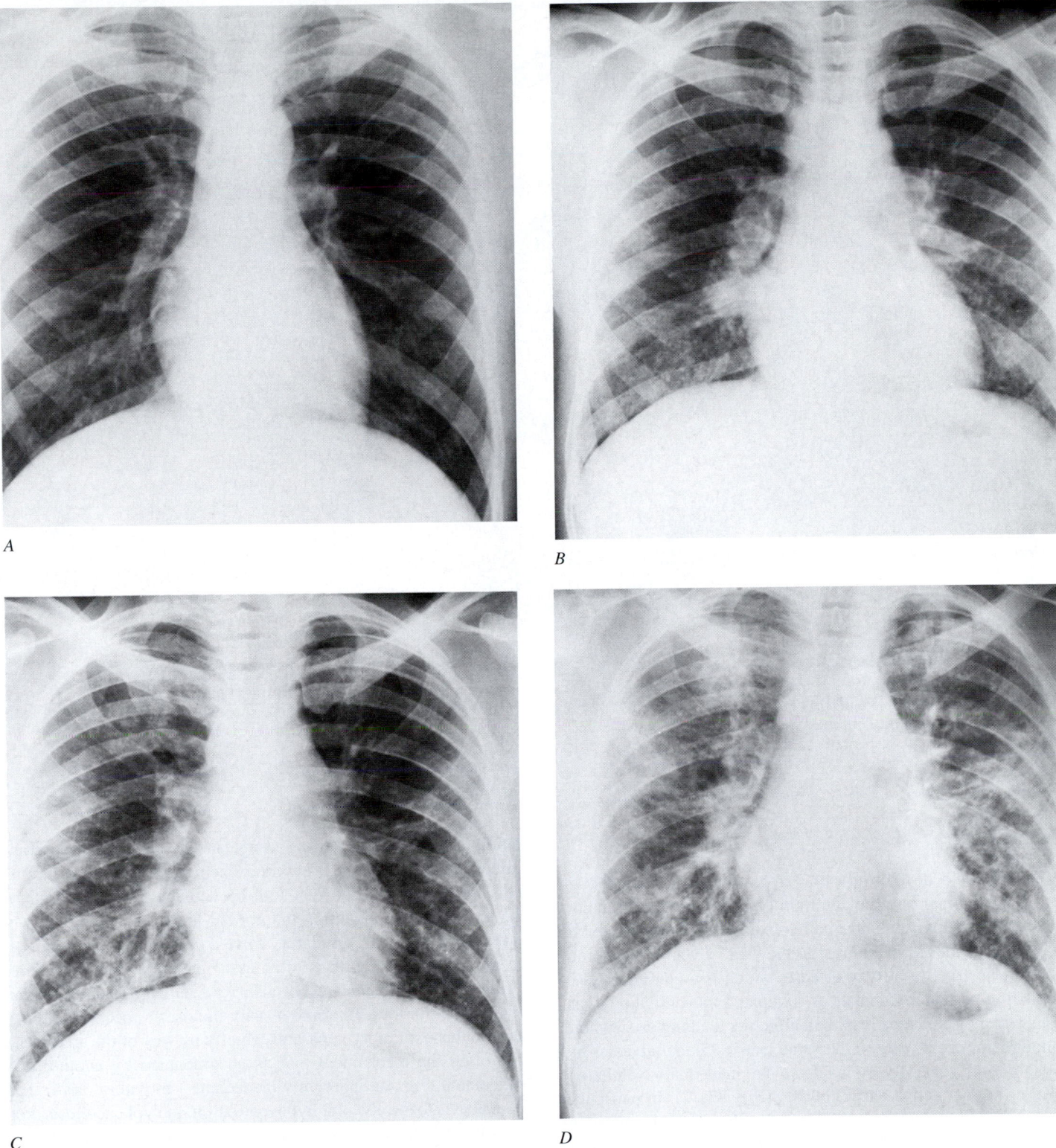

A

B

C

D

FIGURE 83-26   Sarcoidosis. Consecutive stages in evolution of diffuse pulmonary fibrosis, which, in time, became associated with ventilation-perfusion abnormalities and cor pulmonale.

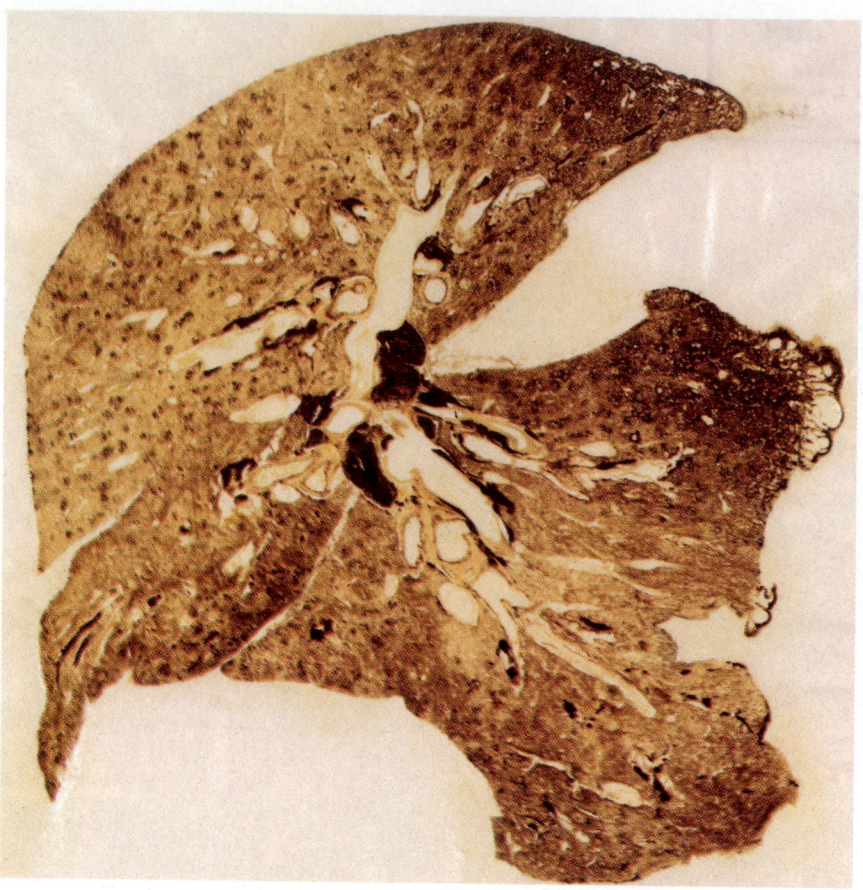

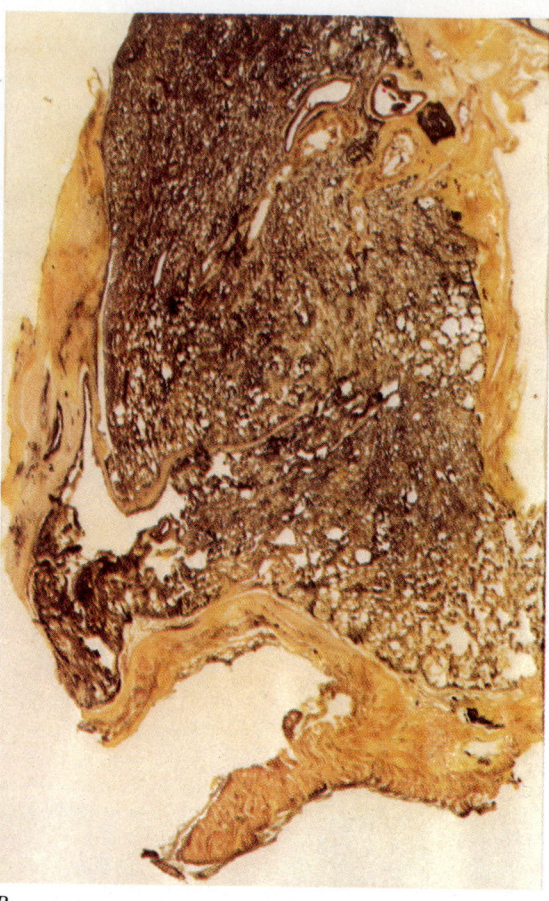

A

B

FIGURE 83-27 Gough (sagittal) sections. *A.* Alveolar hypoventilation secondary to abnormalities in chest wall and pleura. Kyphoscoliosis. *(Courtesy of Dr. J. Gough, Cardiff.) B.* Asbestosis. Encasement of lung by thickened pleura. *(Courtesy of Dr. S. Moolten.)*

ETIOLOGY

In patients who develop alveolar hypoventilation even though their lungs are normal, the common pathogenetic denominators are alveolar hypoxia and arterial hypoxemia, often reinforced by respiratory acidosis. In contrast to the "net" alveolar hypoventilation of obstructive airway disease, which is a consequence of ventilation-perfusion imbalances, alveolar hypoventilation in patients with normal lungs is global, affecting the lung everywhere, although not necessarily to the same extent. Global alveolar hypoventilation generally stems from an inadequate ventilatory drive or an ineffective chest bellows (Fig. 83-27). In particular, a variety of disorders, ranging from the sleep apnea syndromes or a "dead" respiratory center to paralysis of respiratory muscles in the Guillain-Barré syndrome, kyphoscoliosis, and morbid obesity, can be responsible.[5]

PATHOPHYSIOLOGY

The diverse causes share hypoxia and respiratory acidosis as the common pathogenetic mechanism for pulmonary hypertension. However, the routes to hypoxia and acidosis depend somewhat on the cause. In the sleep apnea syndromes, alveolar hypoventi-

lation initially occurs during sleep, and as CO_2 retention continues into waking hours, daytime sleepiness supervenes. In the chronic hypoventilation that follows damage to the respiratory center (as by encephalitis), the normal lungs and chest wall do not receive adequate ventilatory drive. Postpoliomyelitis damage to the respiratory center is often associated not only with paralyzed respiratory muscles but also with damaged nerves to the intercostal muscles. Extreme obesity imposes a mechanical burden on the respiratory apparatus, chiefly by way of the abdomen, but often the mechanical load is accompanied by another derangement (e.g., an inherently inadequate ventilatory drive) that contributes to the alveolar hypoventilation. In kyphoscoliosis, not only is the lung compressed and distorted but the mechanical operation of the chest bellows is compromised and the elastic properties of the lungs and chest wall are abnormal, albeit to different degrees.

Although the routes to hypoxia are different, once the arterial P_{O_2} falls below 40 to 50 mm Hg, the pulmonary arterial walls of the patients undergo the same changes as those that occur spontaneously in native dwellers at high altitude: pulmonary arteries and arterioles manifest muscular hypertrophy, and a self-perpetuating mechanism is instituted for pulmonary hypertension (Fig. 83-28).

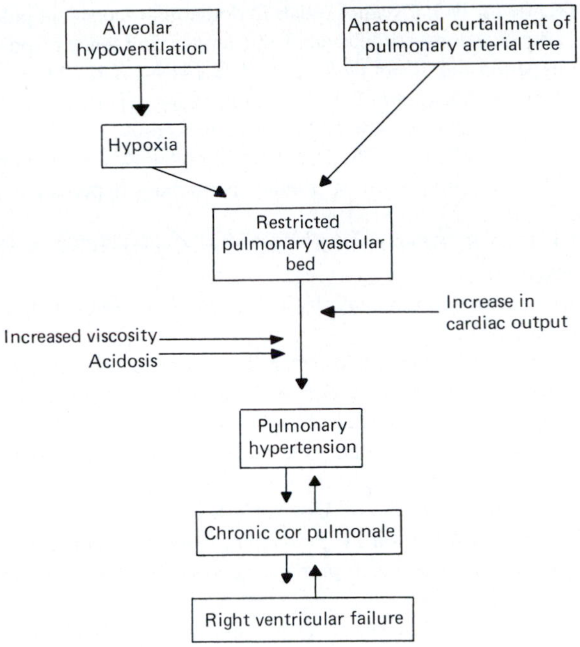

FIGURE 83-28 Evolution of pulmonary hypertension and cor pulmonale in kyphoscoliosis.

CLINICAL FEATURES

These are dominated by the consequences of alveolar hypoxia and hypercapnia and modified by the initiating factors (e.g., kyphoscoliosis). Early in the disorder, when arterial hypoxemia and hypercapnia at rest are minimal, cyanosis may appear during exercise—the result of an inappropriate ventilatory response to increased metabolic demand. During sleep, arterial hypoxemia and hypercapnia intensify, but the blood gases return to near-normal levels during the waking hours. Even at this stage, an upper respiratory infection sometimes topples the subject into acute respiratory failure. On occasion, the first signal of alveolar hypoventilation is right ventricular failure. At that time, cerebral signs of hypercapnia are absent because respiratory acidosis has developed gradually and the kidneys have had time to retain enough bicarbonate.

TREATMENT

Depending on the cause, attention is directed toward relieving arterial hypoxemia and hypercapnia at rest, during sleep, and during exercise (see Chapter 17). If blood gases can be restored to near-normal levels, pulmonary hypertension can be relieved. In the sleep apnea syndromes, mechanical assistance to breathing during sleep using continuous positive-airway pressure has proved effective. For those with obstructive sleep apnea, tracheostomy may be necessary. Treatment of patients with inadequate respiratory musculature is considered elsewhere in this book. Oxygen supplementation must be used with extreme caution because of the threat of increasing hypercapnia.

Viral Diseases

One pathogenetic mechanism that has been repeatedly suggested for primary pulmonary hypertension is some sort of viral infection. The vascular lesions associated with primary pulmonary hypertension have been found at autopsy in several patients with HIV infection.[27,34] This again raises the possibility that some instances of primary pulmonary hypertension may originate in an undetected viral infection that has come and gone long before manifestations of pulmonary hypertension become manifest.

REFERENCES

1. Abenhaum L, Moride Y, Brenot F, et al: Appetite-suppressant drugs and the risk of primary pulmonary hypertension. *New Engl J Med* 335:609–616, 1996.
2. Agostoni P, Doria E, Galli C, et al: Nifedipine reduces pulmonary pressure and vascular tone during short-term but not long-term treatment of pulmonary hypertension in patients with chronic obstructive pulmonary disease. *Am Rev Respir Dis* 139:120–125, 1989.
3. Asherson RA, Cervera R: Review: Antiphospholipid antibodies and the lung. *J Rheumatol* 22:62–66, 1995.
4. Barst RJ, Rubin LJ, McGoon MD, et al: Survival in primary pulmonary hypertension with long-term continuous intravenous prostacyclin. *Ann Intern Med* 121:409–415, 1994.
5. Bergofsky EH, Turino GM, Fishman AP: Cardiorespiratory failure in kyphoscoliosis. *Medicine* 38:263–317, 1959.
6. Brenot F, Herve P, Petitpretz P, et al: Primary pulmonary hypertension and fenfluramine use. *Br Heart J* 70:537–541, 1993.
7. Chitwood WR, Sabiston DC, Wechsler AS: Surgical treatment of unresolved pulmonary embolism. *Clin Chest Med* 5:507–536, 1984.
8. Cremona G, Higenbottam T: Role of prostacyclin in the treatment of primary pulmonary hypertension. *Am J Cardiol* 75:67A–71A, 1995.
9. de Meer K, Heymans HS, Zijlstra WG: Physical adaptation of children to life at high altitude. *Eur J Pediatr* 154:263–272, 1995.
10. Edwards EW: The pathology of secondary pulmonary hypertension, in Fishman AP (ed), *The Pulmonary Circulation: Normal and Abnormal.* Philadelphia, University of Pennsylvania Press, 1990, pp 329–342.
11. Elliott G, Alexander G, Leppert M, et al: Coancestry in apparently sporadic primary pulmonary hypertension. *Chest* 108:973–977, 1995.
12. Eltorky MA, Headley AS, Winer-Muram H, et al: Pulmonary capillary hemangiomatosis: a clinicopathologic review. *Ann Thorac Surg* 57:772–776, 1994.
13. Fedullo PF, Auger WR, Channick RN, et al: Chronic thromboembolic pulmonary hypertension. *Clin Chest Med* 16:353–374, 1995.
14. Fishman AP: Dietary pulmonary hypertension. *Circ Res* 35:657–660, 1974.
15. Fishman AP: Pulmonary circulation, in Fishman AP, Fisher A (eds), *The Handbook of Physiology,* sec 3: *The Respiratory System,* vol I: *Circulation and Nonrespiratory Functions.* Bethesda, American Physiological Society, 1985, pp 93–165.
16. Fishman AP (ed): *The Pulmonary Circulation: Normal and Abnormal.* Philadelphia, University of Pennsylvania Press, 1990, pp 1–522.
17. Fishman AP: Pulmonary thromboembolism: Pathophysiology and clinical features, in Fishman AP (ed), *Pulmonary Diseases and Disorders.* New York, McGraw-Hill, 1980, pp 809–926.
18. Fishman AP, Pietra GG: Primary pulmonary hypertension. *Annu Rev ed* 31:421–431, 1980.

19. Galie N, Ussia G, Passarelli P, et al: Role of pharmacologic tests in the treatment of primary pulmonary hypertension. *Am J Cardiol* 75:55A–62A, 1995.

20. Higenbottam TW, Spiegelhalter D, Scott PJ, et al: Prostacyclin (epoprostenol) and heart-lung transplantation as treatments for severe pulmonary hypertension. *Br Heart J* 70:366–370, 1993.

21. Hurtado A: Chronic mountain sickness. *JAMA* 120:1278–1282, 1942.

22. Jones DK, Higenbottam TW, Wallwork J: Pulmonary vasodilation with prostacyclin in primary and secondary forms of pulmonary hypertension. *Chest* 96:784–789, 1989.

23. Kilbourne EM, Rigau-Perez JG, Heath CW Jr, et al: Clinical epidemiology of toxic-oil syndrome: Manifestations of a new illness. *New Engl J Med* 309:1408–1414, 1983.

24. Kinsella JP, Abman SH: Recent developments in the pathophysiology and treatment of persistent pulmonary hypertension of the newborn. *J Pediatr* 126:853–864, 1995.

25. Loyd JE, Butler MG, Foroud TM, et al: Genetic anticipation and abnormal gender ratio at birth in familial primary pulmonary hypertension. *Am J Respir Crit Care Med* 152:93–97, 1995.

26. Lunn RJ: Inhaled nitric oxide therapy. *Mayo Clin Proc* 70:247–255, 1995.

27. Mani S, Smith GJ: HIV and pulmonary hypertension: A review. *South Med J* 87:357–362, 1994.

28. Mecham RP, Whitehouse LA, Wrenn DS, et al: Smooth muscle–mediated connective tissue remodeling in pulmonary hypertension. *Science* 237:423–426, 1987.

29. Naeji R: Should pulmonary hypertension be treated in chronic obstructive pulmonary disease?, in Weir EK, Archer SL, Reeves JT (eds), *The Diagnosis and Treatment of Pulmonary Hypertension.* New York, Futura Publishing, 1992, pp 209–239.

30. Newman JH, Loyd JE: Familial pulmonary hypertension, in Fishman AP (ed), *The Pulmonary Circulation: Normal and Abnormal.* Philadelphia, University of Pennsylvania Press, 1990, pp 301–314.

31. Nocturnal Oxygen Therapy Trial Group: Continuous or nocturnal oxygen therapy in hypoxemic chronic obstructive lung disease. *Ann Intern Med* 93:391–398, 1980.

32. Nootens M, Schrader B, Kaufmann E, et al: Comparative acute effects of adenosine and prostacyclin in primary pulmonary hypertension. *Chest* 107:54–57, 1995.

33. Palevsky HI, Long W, Crow J, Fishman AP: Prostacyclin and acetylcholine as screening agents for acute pulmonary vasodilator responsiveness in primary pulmonary hypertension. *Circulation* 82:2018–2026, 1990.

34. Petitpretz P, Brenot F, Azarian R, et al: Pulmonary hypertension in patients with human immunodeficiency virus infection: Comparison with primary pulmonary hypertension. *Circulation* 89:2722–2727, 1994.

35. Pietra GG: The histopathology of primary pulmonary hypertension, in: Fishman AP (ed), *The Pulmonary Circulation: Normal and Abnormal.* Philadelphia, University of Pennsylvania Press, 1990, pp 459–472.

36. Porter TR, Taylor DO, Cycan A, et al: Endothelium-dependent pulmonary artery responses in chronic heart failure: Influence of pulmonary hypertension. *J Am Coll Cardiol* 22:1418–1424, 1993.

37. Rich S: Medical treatment of primary pulmonary hypertension: A bridge to transplantation? *Am J Cardiol* 75:63A–66A, 1995.

38. Rich S, Kaufmann E, Levy PS: The effect of high doses of calcium channel blockers on survival in primary pulmonary hypertension. *New Engl J Med* 327:76–81, 1992.

39. Rubin LJ, Rich S: *Primary and Pulmonary Hypertension.* New York, Dekker 1997.

40. Rubin LJ: Primary pulmonary hypertension. *New Engl J Med* 336:111–117, 1997.

41. Rubin LJ, Mendoza J, Hood M, et al: Treatment of primary pulmonary hypertension with continuous intravenous prostacyclin (epoprostenol). *Ann Intern Med* 112:485–491, 1991.

42. Salerni R, Rodnan GP, Leon DF, Shaver JA: Pulmonary hypertension in the CREST syndrome variant of progressive systemic sclerosis (scleroderma). *Ann Intern Med* 86:394–399, 1977.

43. Shuck JW, Oetgen WJ, Tesar JT: Pulmonary vascular response during Raynaud's phenomenon in progressive systemic sclerosis. *Am J Med* 78:221–227, 1985.

44. Sitbon O, Brenot F, Denjean A, et al: Inhaled nitric oxide as a screening vasodilator agent in primary pulmonary hypertension: A dose-response study and comparison with prostacyclin. *Am J Respir Crit Care Med* 151:384–389, 1995.

45. Theodore J, Jamieson SW, Burke CM, et al: Physiologic aspects of human heart-lung transplantation. *Chest* 86:349–357, 1984.

46. Timms RM, Khaja FU, Williams GW: The nocturnal oxygen therapy trial: Hemodynamic response to oxygen therapy in chronic obstructive pulmonary disease. *Ann Intern Med* 102:29–36, 1985.

47. Trell E: Benign, idiopathic pulmonary hypertension. *Acta Med Scand* 193:137–143, 1973.

48. Tuder RM, Flook BE, Voelkel NF: Increased gene expression for VEGF and the VEGF receptors KDR/Flk and Flt in lungs exposed to acute or to chronic hypoxia: Modulation of gene expression by nitric oxide. *J Clin Invest* 95:1798–1807, 1995.

49. Tuxen DV, Powles AC, Mathur PN, et al: Detrimental effects of hydralazine in patients with chronic airflow obstruction and pulmonary hypertension. *Am Rev Respir Dis* 129:388–395, 1984.

50. Wagenvoort CA, Wagenvoort N: *Pathology of Pulmonary Hypertension.* New York, Wiley, 1977.

51. Wei C-M, Lerman A, Rodeheffer RJ, et al: Endothelin in human congestive heart failure. *Circulation* 89:1580–1586, 1994.

52. Weiss JR, Pietra GG, Scharf SM: Primary pulmonary hypertension and the human immunodeficiency virus: Report of two cases and a review of the literature. *Arch Intern Med* 155:2350–2354, 1995.

53. Weitzenblum E, Apprill M, Oswald M, et al: Pulmonary hemodynamics in patients with chronic obstructive pulmonary disease before and during an episode of peripheral edema. *Chest* 105:1377–1382, 1994.

CHAPTER 84

PULMONARY THROMBOEMBOLIC DISEASE

Harold I. Palevsky / Mark A. Kelley / Alfred P. Fishman

The designation *pulmonary thromboembolism* refers to the migration of a clot (or clots) from systemic veins to the pulmonary vascular bed. The term has ominous overtones, since there may be significant morbidity and mortality not only from clots already lodged in the lungs but also because of venous clots still to be released.

It has been estimated that, each year, more than 500,000 people in the United States are affected by pulmonary thromboembolism (Fig. 84-1). In two-thirds of these people, the pulmonary emboli are undiagnosed during life and cause a mortality of at least 30 percent. When pulmonary emboli are correctly diagnosed and treated, the mortality falls to substantially less than 10 percent.[5] That some patients die suddenly and that the disease is not diagnosed until autopsy underscores the pressing need for preventing the formation of thrombi in peripheral veins, for early detection of thrombi that do form, for early and zealous management of peripheral thrombi to avoid embolization to the lungs, for preventing recurrent embolic events, and for promoting the resolution of pulmonary emboli.

SOURCES OF EMBOLI

Most pulmonary emboli (more than 90 percent) come from deep veins in the legs.[44] A clot that is destined to become an embolus generally begins behind a valve in the deep veins of the calf. It then propagates centrally from the sural vein, up the popliteal and femoral veins, and sometimes to the iliac veins. Propagation is faster than is adherence to the venous endothelium, resulting in a free-floating advancing edge that dangles precariously in the venous lumen (Fig. 84-2).

An uncommon but important source of pulmonary emboli, especially in women, is the pelvic veins. Pelvic thrombi may be bland or septic. Usually the pelvic origin of the emboli is suggested by recent pelvic inflammatory disease, recent parturition, recent gynecologic surgery, or clinical signs of pelvic pathology. In men, pelvic vein thrombi may accompany prostatic disease or occur after prostate surgery. Bland emboli evoke few systemic disturbances unless they cause pulmonary infarction. In contrast, septic emboli are usually associated with a history of recent pelvic infection (e.g., septic abortion) and are accompanied by unmistakable evidence of septicemia and multiple pulmonary consolidations that often go on to cavitate.

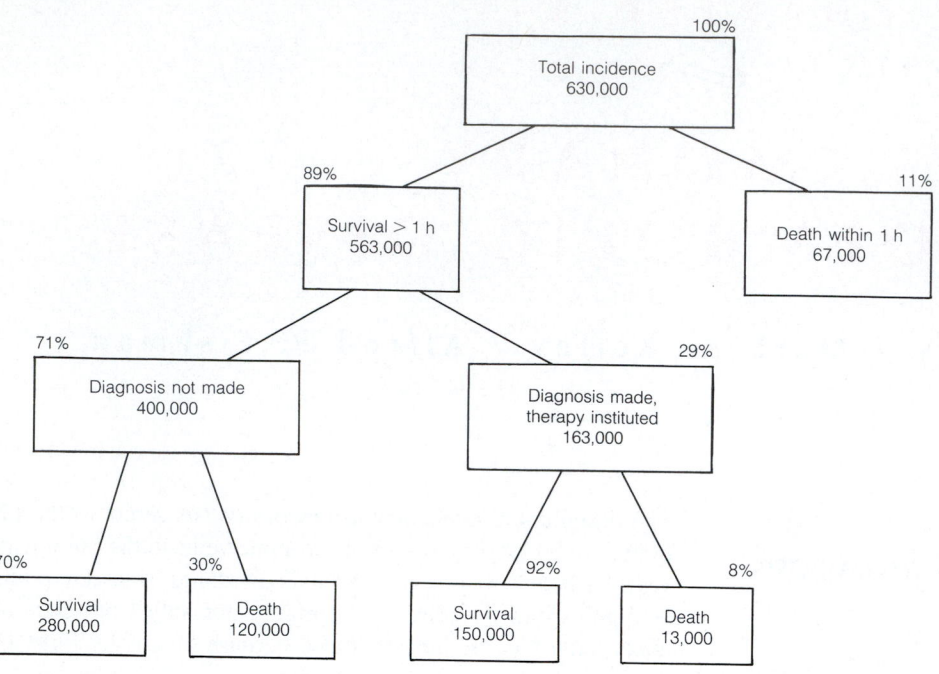

FIGURE 84-1 Estimated incidence and survival statistics for pulmonary embolism in the United States. *(From Dalen and Alpert: Prog Cardiovasc Dis 17:259–270, 1975.)*

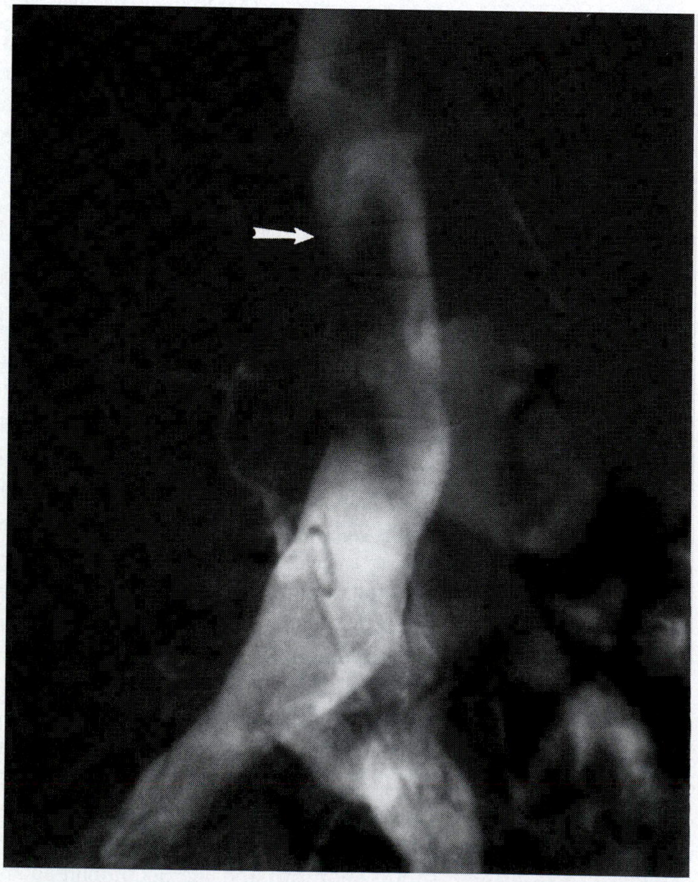

Blood clot is not the only material that ends up as pulmonary emboli. Any particulate matter that gains entry to the venous side of the circulation may lodge in the lungs. Fragments of tissue, parasites, fibers, liquid droplets, and gases find their way into the veins either by injection or as a consequence of trauma; the particles may be sterile or septic. Drug abusers often embolize the lungs with talc and cotton fibers in the course of an intravenous injection. Not only do these particles occlude vessels but they also excite inflammation (e.g., a granulomatous vasculitis) in the walls.

Amniotic fluid embolism is a rare but catastrophic complication of pregnancy.[7] Amniotic fluid gains access to the uterine venous circulation either as a result of vigorous uterine contraction after rupture of the membranes or through tears or surgical incisions in the myometrium or endocervix.

Air embolism can cause a third distinctive clinical picture. The accidental introduction of air into the venous circulation occasionally occurs in the course of intravenous injections, hemodialysis, placement of central venous lines, or induction of an artificial pneumothorax or pneumoperitoneum or after chest injury. The syndromes elicited by fat, amniotic fluid, and air emboli are considered later in this chapter.

FACTORS PREDISPOSING TO VENOUS THROMBOSIS

Over 100 years ago, Virchow identified venous stasis, hypercoagulability, and injury to the venous walls as the factors promoting venous thrombosis (Table 84-1).

Stasis

Venous thrombosis often follows an episode of venous stasis. Even though stasis is clearly important, however, it is generally regarded to be a contributory or precipitating factor rather than a primary initiating mechanism. In favor of this view is the fact that blood trapped in a vein between two ligatures remains fluid for hours. Moreover, venous thrombosis occurs without preceding stasis in women ingesting oral contraceptives, in persons with paroxysmal nocturnal hemoglobinuria, and in familial disorders such as dysfibrinogenemias, antithrombin III deficiency, and homocystinuria.

Stasis predisposes to thrombosis by allowing local accumulation of activated coagulation factors and delaying systemic (hepatic) clearance. The sinuses behind the valves in the deep veins are particularly prone to the effects of low blood flow and stasis.

Elderly patients are particularly prone to venous stasis because of limited mobility, cramped postures imposed by disease, prolonged bed rest during illness, slowing of the circulation by

FIGURE 84-2 Inferior vena caval thrombosis with nonadherent proximal end (arrow). *(Courtesy of Dr. Z. Haskal.)*

TABLE 84-1

Virchow's Triad: Clinical States Predisposing to Venous Thrombosis

Stasis	Immobility
	Bed rest
	Anesthesia
	Congestive heart failure/cor pulmonale
	Prior venous thrombosis
Hypercoagulability	Malignancy
	Anticardiolipin antibody
	Nephrotic syndrome
	Essential thrombocytosis
	Estrogen therapy
	Heparin-induced thrombocytopenia
	Inflammatory bowel disease
	Paroxysmal nocturnal hemoglobinuria
	Disseminated intravascular coagulation
	Protein C and S deficiencies
	Antithrombin III deficiency
Vessel wall injury	Trauma
	Surgery

congestive heart failure, and deep vein varicosities. Even normal persons who sit for a long while with knees flexed, as in a long trip by automobile or airplane, occasionally develop a pulmonary embolus when they disembark.

Postoperative patients, especially those who have undergone extensive and prolonged operations on the abdomen and pelvis, are particularly prone to deep vein thrombosis and pulmonary embolism.[61] Anesthesia, which promotes venous dilation and stasis, coupled with postoperative bed rest, predisposes to the antecedent venous clotting. Embolization is so common in this group of people that much of the available information concerning prophylactic anticoagulation is derived from patients who have undergone surgery.[9] Mechanical devices that generate or augment calf muscle contraction, thereby maintaining venous flow and preventing blood pooling and stasis, are often used postoperatively as an alternative to anticoagulants (see below).

Hypercoagulability

Although hypercoagulable states might be expected to predispose to venous thrombosis, evidence of hypercoagulability in association with thromboembolism is generally difficult to obtain. Nonetheless, in certain clinical disorders, biochemical disorders do predispose to thrombosis.[24] These disorders fall into two broad categories: those that predispose to venous thrombosis and those in which endogenous fibrinolytic mechanisms fail to limit the size of the hemostatic plug.

Among conditions that predispose to venous thrombosis are the hormonal changes of pregnancy and of estrogen usage, which increase procoagulant factor levels (factors XII, V, VIII, fibrinogen), thereby and simultaneously reducing plasma protease inhibitors (antithrombin III, C1 esterase inhibitor) and tipping the balance toward thrombosis. The coagulation system is also acti-

vated by certain malignancies: the tumor cells and their products acting as procoagulants, which activate factor X.

Among the conditions that predispose to thrombosis by decreasing circulating fibrinolytic activity are congenital deficiencies of antithrombin III, protein C, protein S, or plasminogen, congenital resistance to activated protein C (factor V Leiden), hyperhomocystinemia, and increased levels of antiphospholipid antibodies. Each of these has been associated with initial and recurrent deep vein thrombosis and pulmonary embolism. In some of these states (e.g., antithrombin III, protein C, and protein S deficiencies), the frequency of venous thromboembolism during a lifetime is greater than 50 percent.[15]

Endothelial Injury

Endothelial injury predisposes to clotting. Normally, the endothelial lining of blood vessels forms a barrier between cells and proteins in the blood, on the one hand, and the subendothelial connective tissues, on the other. Exposure of blood to the subendothelial basement membrane activates contact-phase coagulation proteins, which, in turn, activate the coagulation cascade. In addition, vascular injury that exposes the subendothelial connective tissues causes activation of platelets, followed by adhesion and aggregation.

Special types of widespread endothelial injury have recently been uncovered. Among these are hyperhomocystinemia and autoimmune injury (e.g., systemic lupus erythematosus). In some patients with systemic lupus erythematosus, as well as a variety of other disorders, a lupuslike anticoagulant (anticardiolipin antibody or antiphospholipid antibody) appears in the blood. Contrary to expectations about anticoagulants, this anticoagulant predisposes to thrombosis. Three mechanisms have been proposed: (1) inhibition of prostacyclin synthesis by endothelium; (2) inhibition of plasminogen activator, thereby decreasing the potential for thrombolysis; and (3) promotion of platelet aggregation due to interaction of the antiphospholipid antibody with the phospholipid in the platelet membranes.

Clot formation is also enhanced by an excessive number of circulating platelets (e.g., essential thrombocytosis) or by damaged platelets (e.g., paroxysmal nocturnal hemoglobinuria or heparin-induced thrombocytopenia). Disseminated intravascular coagulation leads to thrombosis by activating the clotting cascade. The familiar association between malignancy (particularly the mucin-secreting adenocarcinoma) and venous thrombosis has been attributed to low-grade disseminated intravascular coagulation.

THE VESSEL WALL

Injury to the venous wall, as in a hip fracture, may initiate and perpetuate venous thrombosis. The injury produces patchy endothelial damage, which promotes thrombosis by impairing normal antithrombotic mechanisms and by exciting prothrombotic mechanisms. Chemotactic substances, such as fragments of complement (C'3a and C'5a), plasminogen activator, and kallikrein, are released. Exposure of the underlying collagen activates factor XII and prompts the formation of plasmin, the principal fibrinolytic enzyme. The mechanisms of hemostasis, coagulation, and fibrinolysis are complex: they interact and are simultaneously activated after injury. Release of kinins increases vascular permeability so that plasma proteins leak into the collagen matrix and activate Hageman factor. Substances released from tissue damage elsewhere also contribute to coagulation in this setting of vascular injury and stasis. This interplay sets the stage for a propagating thrombus.

Since hours usually pass between the time of fracture and orthopedic intervention, a clot is generally present in deep local veins by the time the patient comes to surgical repair. The problem then is to prevent its extension and release as an embolus to the lungs. The elapsed time between injury and intervention is important with respect to proper anticoagulant therapy.

The same sequence of events is triggered by most elective surgery that entails mobilization or manipulation of vessels. The activation of procoagulant factors as part of the process of wound repair, coupled with the venous stasis and blood pooling promoted by anesthetic agents and immobility, is responsible for thromboembolism as a common and dreaded sequel to surgical procedures. Minimizing manipulation of vascular structures and prophylactic measures to prevent stasis and activation of the systemic clotting cascade—ideally initiated before the surgical procedure—are essential for preventing formation and propagation of thrombus.

PHYSIOLOGICAL CONSEQUENCES

The effects of pulmonary emboli range from imperceptible to disastrous. The physiological and clinical impact depends on three major factors: (1) the extent to which the pulmonary vascular bed is obliterated, the sizes of the affected vessels, and the nature of the emboli; (2) the preexisting cardiopulmonary status of the patient; and (3) secondary effects that follow lodging of the emboli in the lungs—i.e., the local release of neurohumoral substances, such as serotonin and histamine, the occurrence of arterial hypoxemia, which stimulates systemic chemoreceptors, and reflex stimulation of the respiration and circulation.[43]

Respiratory

The hallmark of embolization of the lungs is rapid, shallow breathing (tachypnea) that causes an increase in minute ventilation, which is invariably associated with an increase invariably in dead-space ventilation and usually in alveolar ventilation. Intrapulmonary reflexes, involving the vagus nerves, set the ventilatory pattern. Of the three receptor mechanisms in the lungs (stretch, irritant, and juxtacapillary), only the last two have been shown to play a role in the reflex stimulation of the ventilation by pulmonary emboli.

Occlusion of terminal pulmonary arteries by emboli is accompanied by constriction of the terminal bronchioles. Two mechanisms are held responsible: (1) the release of vasoconstrictive substances from platelet aggregates within the clot and, possibly, from mast cells in the affected lung and (2) hypocapnia secondary to the increase in alveolar ventilation.

Circulatory

Several factors shape the hemodynamic consequences of acute pulmonary emboli. Emboli that are small and few usually cause no hemodynamic upset as long as the preexistent pulmonary vascular bed is normal. Conversely, large emboli to major pulmonary arteries, or a large shower of small emboli, often evoke systemic hypotension, bradycardia, pulmonary hypertension, and a decrease in cardiac output. In persons without cardiopulmonary disease, large increments in pulmonary arterial pressure occur only when more than one-half of the pulmonary vasculature has been compromised by clot (Fig. 84-3). A much smaller burden of clot suffices to evoke pulmonary hypertension with underlying cardiopulmonary disease in patients in whom pulmonary vascular resistance is abnormally high before embolization.

Although the extent to which the pulmonary vascular bed is occluded is of major importance, the pathogenesis of the pulmonary hypertension in pulmonary thromboembolism involves more than mechanical amputation of segments of the pulmonary arterial tree and heightened resistance to blood flow. That other influences are operative is suggested by several observations: the difficulty of generating severe and lasting pulmonary hypertension experimentally by occluding major pulmonary arteries; the frequent disparity between the small size of an acute embolus and the transient, inordinate increase in pulmonary arterial pressure, suggesting reflex vasoconstriction; the consistent but unexplained increase in lung water that occasionally results in frank pulmonary edema, particularly in patients with underlying disease of the left ventricle (Fig. 84-4); and, in contrast to the well-tolerated consequences of cross-clamping pulmonary arteries in the course of a lobectomy or a pneumonectomy, a pulmonary

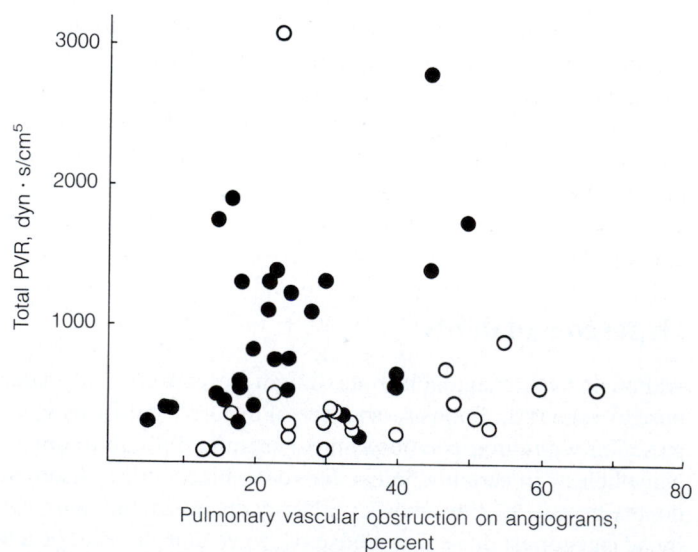

FIGURE 84-3 Hemodynamic consequences of pulmonary embolism and the underlying state of the pulmonary vasculature. Patients in whom the pulmonary vasculature was previously normal (open circles) develop little increase in pulmonary vascular resistance (PVR) until the clot burden exceeds 50 percent. In those with antecedent cardiopulmonary disease (solid circles), the pulmonary vascular resistance increases appreciably with only modest clot burden. (*From Sharma, McIntyre, Sharma, Sasahara: Clin Chest Med 5:421–437, 1984.*)

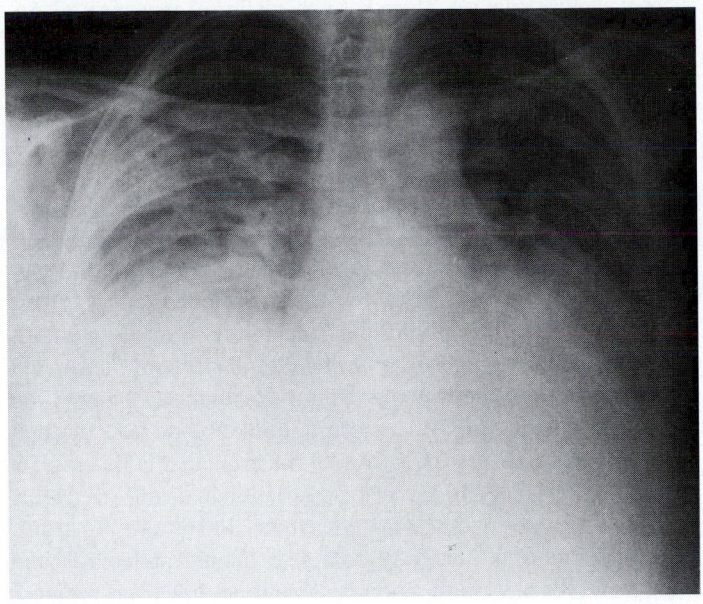

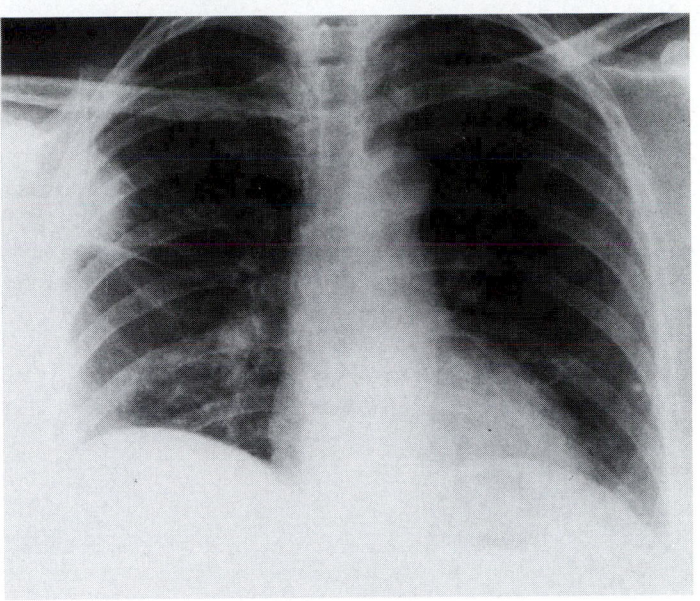

A

FIGURE 84-4   Bilateral pulmonary edema in a 50-year-old patient with pulmonary embolism. *A.* Upon admission, there was overt pul-

B

monary edema. *B.* Ten days later, chest has cleared except for shadow in right upper lobe, which resolved slowly.

embolus that obstructs a lobar pulmonary artery or a main pulmonary artery can be life-threatening.

These discrepancies have prompted a search for additional factors, particularly reflex vasoconstriction and the release of neurohumoral substances. Other evidence supports the idea of a prominent role for humoral mediators in determining the consequences of pulmonary emboli: in experimental models, cyproheptadine (a nonselective serotonin antagonist) and ketanserin (a selective serotonin antagonist) can block many of the hemodynamic and airway responses to pulmonary embolism (e.g., bronchoconstriction, occasionally manifested by localized wheezing) that sometimes occur after pulmonary embolization.[26]

Mediators other than serotonin are released after pulmonary embolization both from the formed elements of the blood (particularly platelets) and from the pulmonary vascular endothelium. These are vasoactive substances that could play a role in determining the clinical consequences of pulmonary emboli. Among the putative vasoconstrictor substances that can be released from the formed elements of the blood are arachidonic acid metabolites, peptidoleukotrienes, platelet-activating factor, and platelet-derived growth factor; the dilators that can be released from the endothelium are a prostacyclin (PGI_2) and endothelium-derived releasing factor (i.e., nitric oxide).[43] In addition to these mediators, neurohumoral reflexes triggered by receptors in the pulmonary vasculature, particularly at bifurcations, may participate in pulmonary vascular response to emboli. The contributions of these substances and reflexes to changes in vascular tone and to the clinical syndrome of pulmonary embolism are still speculative. Whether the increase in pulmonary extravascular water is due to capillary hyperperfusion, to hypertension in the unoccluded parts of the pulmonary circulation, or to damage of endothelium by substances released in the clotting process is currently being investigated.

Pulmonary emboli exert different effects in the normal than in the abnormal lung. Some emboli cause pulmonary infarction.

Although it is not clear why infarction occurs, the consensus is that infarction does not occur unless oxygenation is also compromised locally, either by airway disease or by insufficient bronchial collateral circulation. Chronic congestive heart failure predisposes to infarction, possibly by impeding bronchial venous return to the atria.

Ventilation-Circulation Imbalances

Focal areas of edema and atelectasis often develop in the vicinity of occluded pulmonary arteries. Loss of alveolar surfactant contributes to these changes by promoting alveolar collapse and fluid accumulation. Arterial hypoxemia occurs because of continued blood flow through these hypoventilated, edematous areas of the lung in the vicinity of the occluded pulmonary artery. Because the arterial hypoxemia is only slightly relieved by the breathing of pure O_2, it is designated *anatomic venous admixture.* Venous admixture is sometimes intensified by a low cardiac output (e.g., in massive pulmonary embolism); mixed venous P_{O_2} is then abnormally low. On rare occasions, pulmonary hypertension causes sufficient increase in right atrial pressure to open the foramen ovale and contribute to anatomic venous admixture.

Because of the upsets between alveolar ventilation and alveolar blood flow, there are certain characteristic features of extensive emboli to the lungs: increase in dead-space ventilation, alveolar ventilation, and venous admixture; systemic arterial hypoxemia and hypocapnia; and widening of the alveolar-arterial difference in P_{O_2} ($P_A\text{-}Pa_{O_2}$). Attempts to use the increase in physiological dead space as a measure of the extent of the pulmonary vascular bed that has been amputated by pulmonary emboli have proved unreliable. One plausible explanation for the inadequacy of this measurement is the occurrence of bronchoconstriction in the areas deprived of circulation, thereby partly adjusting the alveolar ventilation to the diminished circulation.

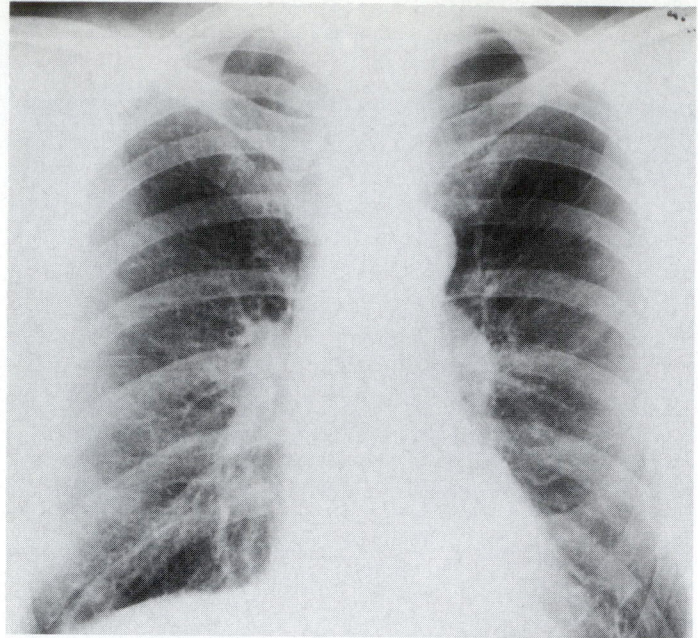

A

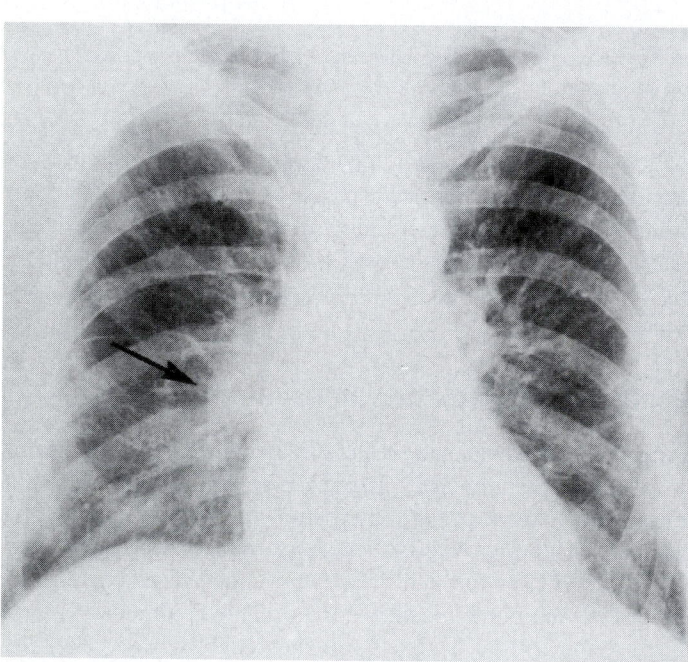

B

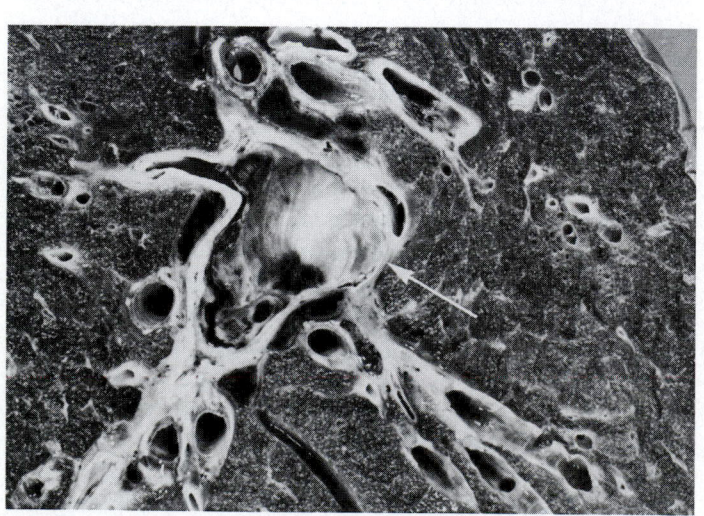

C

FIGURE 84-5 *(left)* Organization of massive thrombus. *A.* In 1967, before embolization of right pulmonary artery. *B.* In 1972, large organized thrombus in right pulmonary artery (arrow). Death followed attempt at surgical removal. Thrombus was confirmed at autopsy. *C.* Another patient. Organized thrombus is seen at autopsy (arrow). Patient died of unrelated cause. *(Courtesy of Dr. G.G. Pietra.)*

NATURAL HISTORY OF CLOTS IN THE LUNGS

Clots that reach the lungs are dealt with in two general ways: fibrinolysis and organization (Fig. 84-5). In addition, large clots in a major pulmonary artery are often disintegrated by the mechanical pounding produced by each cardiac ejection. Overwhelming of the fibrinolytic mechanisms by massive or multiple emboli favors persistence of the clots and their subsequent incorporation into the vascular lining. Resolution of infarction (Fig. 84-6) is accomplished by resumption of blood flow through the occluded vessel, by expansion of the bronchial collateral circulation, or by increasing alveolar ventilation in the affected area. Usually, all three mechanisms contribute. Resolution of a pulmonary embolus is generally complete if only atelectasis and edema are present. If infarction has occurred, however, progressive shrinkage and scarring of the affected area usually follow. In most circumstances, the resultant loss of functional lung has little clinical consequence.

Clinical Manifestations of Deep Venous Thrombosis

Because thrombi so often originate in the deep veins of the legs, particularly those of the calf, careful examination of the legs is indispensable in the search for a source of pulmonary emboli. The characteristic signs are swelling of the leg (most often unilateral), duskiness, pain to deep pressure over the gastrocnemius muscle or to dorsiflexion of the foot (Homan's sign), and palpable deep thrombi. Sometimes the superficial veins are dilated as part of the expansion of the collateral venous circulation. Occasionally, the swollen calf is associated with a tender cord in the femoral triangle. Unfortunately, in at least one-half of patients in whom the legs are the source of deep vein thrombi, the legs appear normal on clinical examination. Conversely, clinical examination that suggests the presence of a clot often proves to be erroneous.

Clinical Manifestations of Pulmonary Emboli

For convenience, four categories of clinical manifestations can be identified. Three of the four categories are acute and run their course in a matter of days: (1) massive occlusion of the pulmonary arterial tree, often by a large embolus that lodges in the central pulmonary arterial tree and arrests blood flow through a

FIGURE 84-6 *(right)* Resolution of a pulmonary infarct. A 48-year-old woman with known adenocarcinoma of the ovary for 2 years was admitted with a swollen leg. *A.* Posteroanterior and lateral views 19 days after admission. The shadow of the pulmonary infarct blends with that of the left pleural effusion and diaphragm. *B.* Twenty-five days after admission. A discrete nodular shadow, about 4 cm in diameter, is seen on the PA view. A lateral body section shows the elliptical appearance of the infarcted area. *C.* Five months after admission. The evidence of pulmonary infarction is gone. *(Courtesy of Dr. S. Eisman.)*

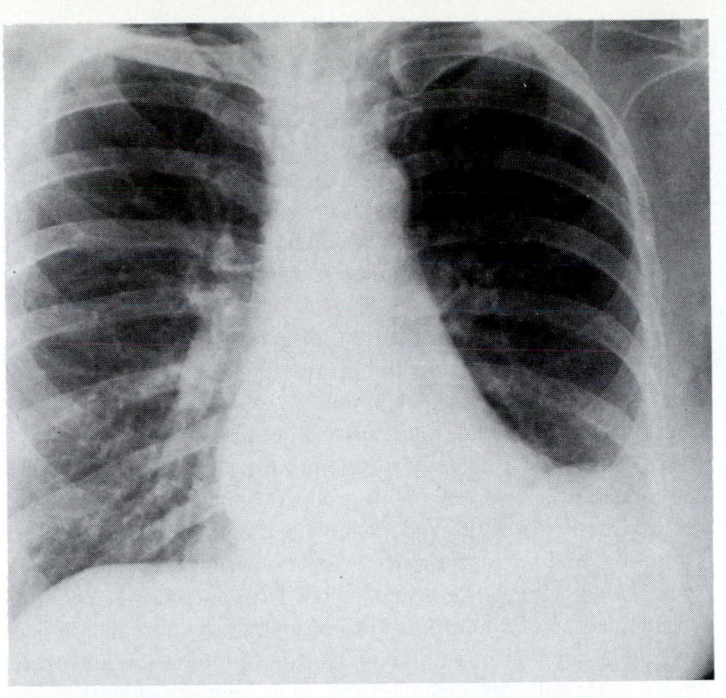
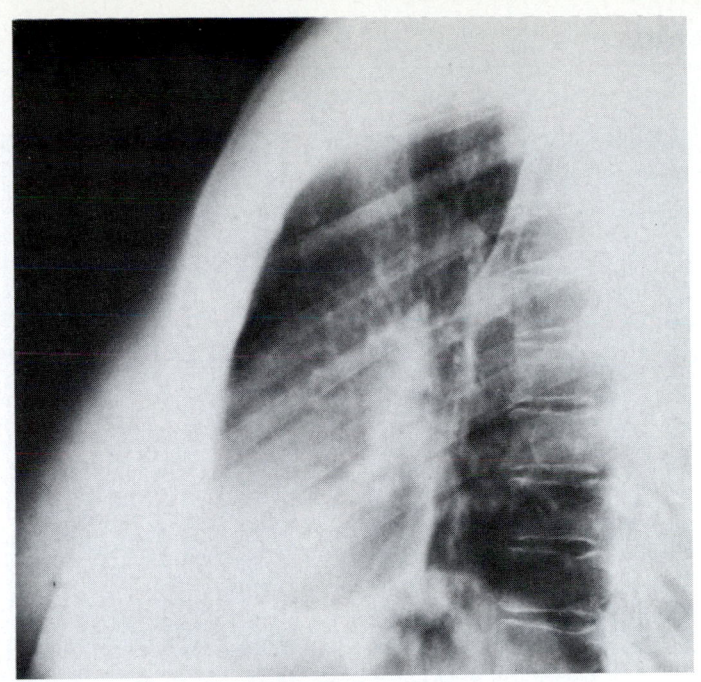

A

FIGURE   84-6

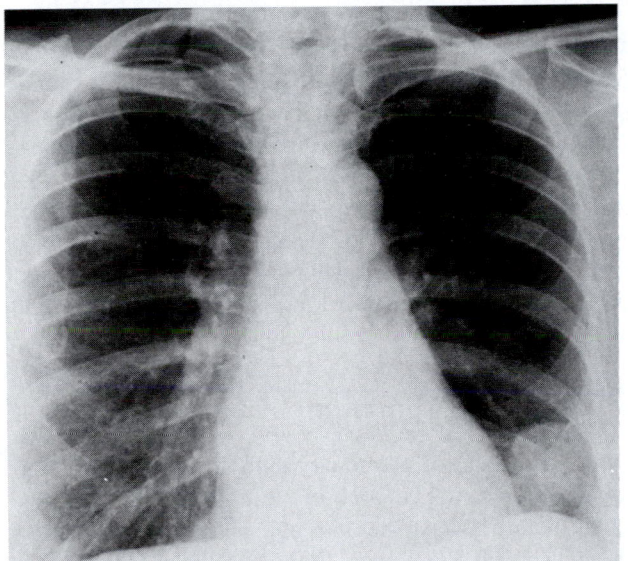
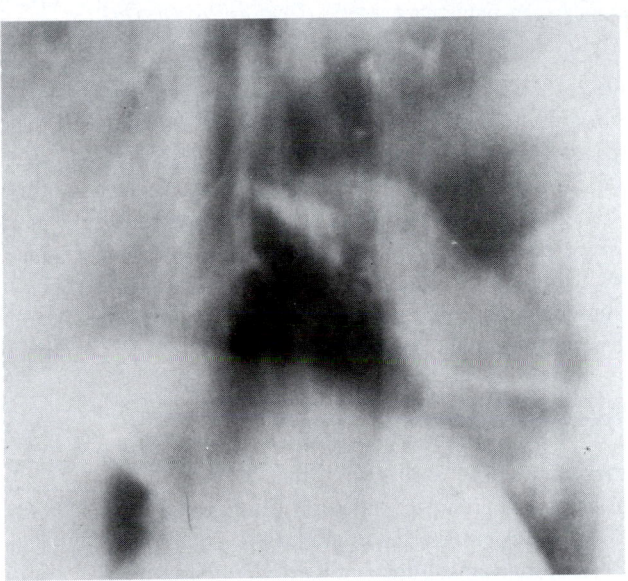

B

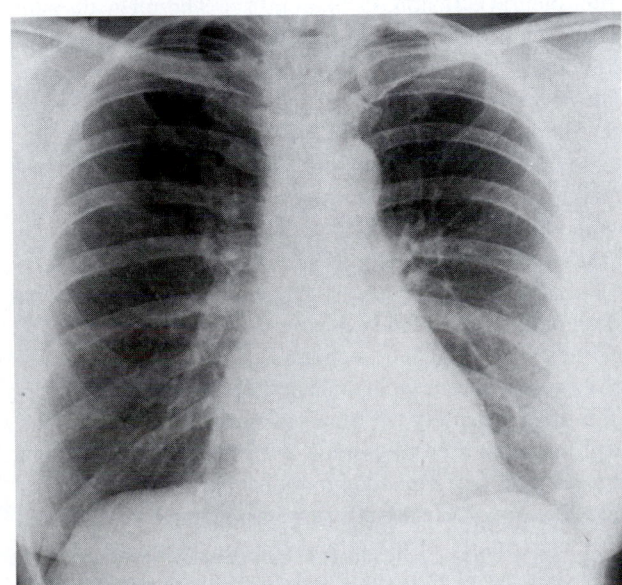
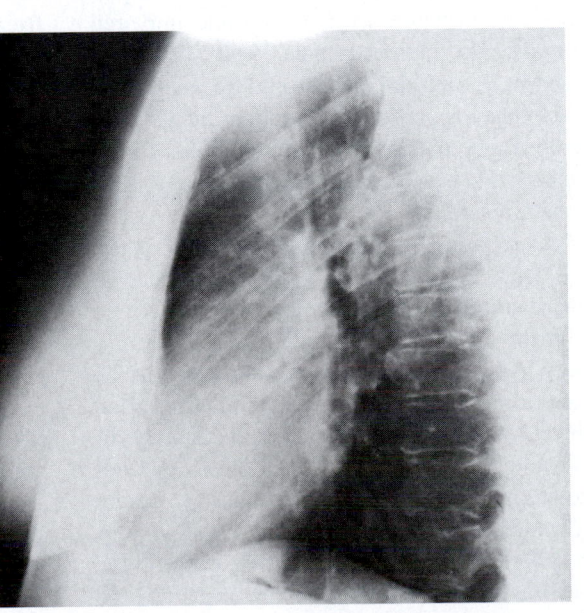

C

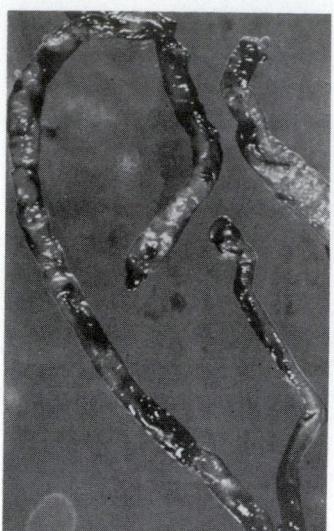 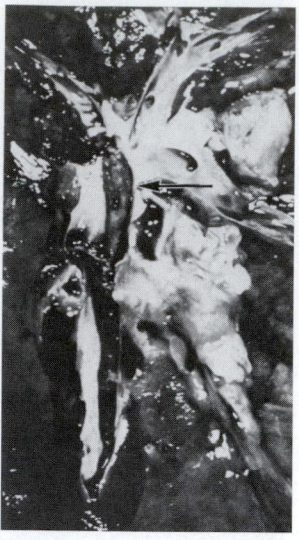

A   *B*

FIGURE 84-7 Thromboembolism. *A.* Massive venous thrombus. *B.* Venous thrombus lodged in pulmonary artery. *(Courtesy of Dr. G.G. Pietra.)*

substantial portion of the pulmonary vascular bed; (2) embolism associated with infarction, an uncommon but distinctive clinical disorder; and (3) embolism without pulmonary infarction, the most common type, in which the degree of vascular obstruction is considerably less than in massive central occlusion. The fourth category, unresolved pulmonary emboli, designates a syndrome that is elicited by a single or repeated embolization of the lungs, often clinically unrecognized, that over months to years results in severe progressive pulmonary hypertension.

Acute Massive Occlusion

The extent of the pulmonary vascular tree that is occluded by large emboli varies from patient to patient.[36] Traditionally, the idea of massive occlusion implies that enough of the pulmonary circulation has been compromised for circulatory collapse to ensue (Fig. 84-7). Fortunately, this group is small. The clinical picture is that of shock—i.e., systemic hypotension and impaired perfusion of vital organs. The patient is pale, weak, listless to the point of apathy, sweaty, nauseated, and oliguric; mentation is often impaired. Tachypnea is particularly striking; tachycardia is a regular feature. Autopsy discloses a large embolus in the vicinity of the bifurcation and evidence that blood flow to at least two lobar arteries was arrested.

Certain clinical signs are associated with this classic, albeit uncommon, emergency. Thus, evidence of pulmonary hypertension can be striking because so much of the pulmonary vascular tree has been occluded by the embolus and the patient is often predisposed to pulmonary hypertension by either underlying cardiac or pulmonary disorder or previous emboli. As a result of the burst of pulmonary hypertension, the pulmonary artery is acutely dilated, producing a visible or palpable impulse in the second left interspace along the sternal border. The sound made by closure of the pulmonary valve is accentuated, sometimes to the point of being palpable. The pulmonary component of the second heart sound often becomes louder than the aortic component, and the second heart sound is narrowly split. Should right ventricular fail-

ure supervene, a right ventricular S_3 gallop or a summation gallop and the murmur of tricuspid insufficiency are often heard along the left lower border of the sternum. Both the clinical manifestations and the electrocardiographic patterns (Fig. 84-8) described above are rarely documented because of the desperate nature of the situation.

Much more common than the disastrous massive occlusion described above are large emboli that compromise the circulation but are not immediately lethal. Many occlude only one lobar artery; some seem to be massive at the outset but then fragment and relocate distally to compromise less and less of the pulmonary vascular tree. In this group, dyspnea, tachypnea, chest pain (usually pleuritic), and anxiety are common features. Fever, sweating, and hemoptysis occur less consistently. Systemic hypotension is a consistent feature but is often mild. Depending on the degree of compromise of the pulmonary circulation and the underlying disorder, the signs and symptoms range from those of massive occlusion to those of pulmonary infarction and peripheral emboli. These are considered subsequently.

On rare occasions, the chest radiograph following massive occlusion of the central pulmonary arteries reveals dilatation and engorgement of the unaffected pulmonary arterial tree, diminished vascularity and increased radiolucency on the affected side, and dilatation of the heart (right ventricle and atrium). Sometimes, the affected vessel does show an abrupt "cutoff" that marks the end of the clot; occasionally, the edge of the embolus is visible. If the thrombus lodges centrally, it may be imaged by transthoracic or transesophageal echocardiography.[10] Angiography is much more definitive in clarifying the nature and extent of the catastrophic event (Fig. 84-9).

Acute Pulmonary Infarction

Only about 10 percent of pulmonary emboli elicit clinical and radiographic evidence of "infarction" (Fig 84-10). In many instances, this picture is due to hemorrhagic pulmonary edema and not to tissue necrosis. Pulmonary "infarction" is generally manifested by acute onset of pleural pain, breathlessness, pleural friction rub, pleural effusion, or hemoptysis. The pleuritic pain is often sharp and localized to the ribs but, depending on the location of the infarct, may be referred to the shoulder or abdomen. As a result of the pain, mobility of one hemithorax may be diminished. Although the acuity of onset and the severity of the pain can simulate those of myocardial ischemia, its pleuritic nature and failure to respond to nitroglycerin usually suffice to establish its identity.

Characteristically, pulmonary infarcts (with or without tissue necrosis) are juxtaposed to pleural surfaces (Fig 84-11). On the chest radiograph, fresh infarcts are usually nonspecific in appearance, often simulating a bronchopneumonia. In time, the affected area evolves into a wedge-shaped opacity at the periphery of the lung. Usually it requires several days for the nondescript infarcted area to assume a distinctive radiographic appearance (Fig. 84-6). Often the infarct is obscured by a pleural effusion, so that only after the effusion has been removed or resorbed does the identity of the infarct become evident.

The nature of the pleural fluid that accompanies pulmonary infarction is considered elsewhere (see Chapter 89). After

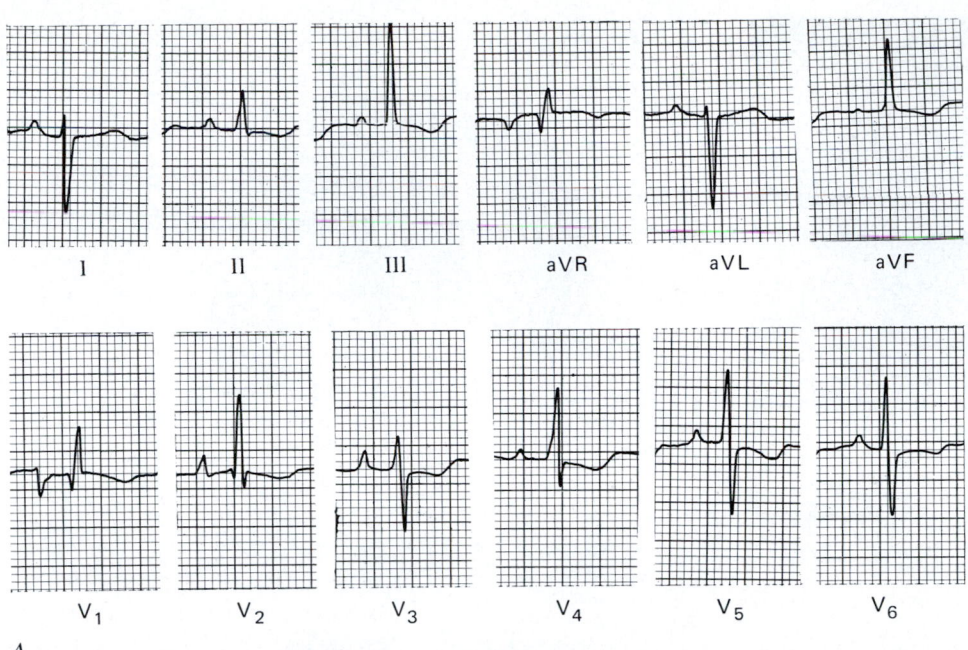

FIGURE 84-8 Massive pulmonary embolism. *A.* Electrocardiogram from a 26-year-old woman who experienced a massive pulmonary embolism. Sinus tachycardia. An RS pattern is seen in lead I and a tall R in lead III, accompanied by T-wave inversion in lead III and leads V_1 to V_6. The precordial transition zone is shifted to the left. The QRS pattern suggests incomplete bundle branch block. At autopsy, fresh massive emboli as well as evidence of old emboli were found in the main pulmonary arteries. *B.* Magnetic resonance image (MRI) of a 66-year-old woman with massive pulmonary embolism that totally occluded the left pulmonary artery. This vessel (PA) projects a gray image associated with little or no blood flow. This contrasts with the black image projected by the lumen of the aorta (Ao), where blood flow is rapid.

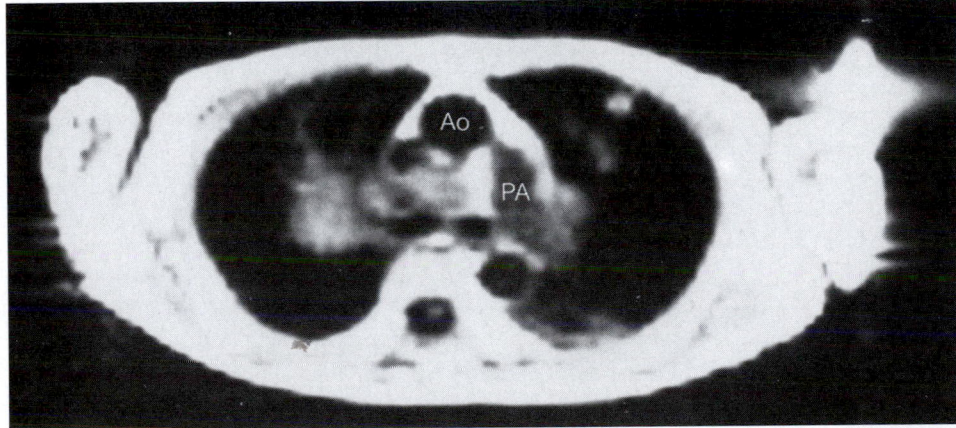

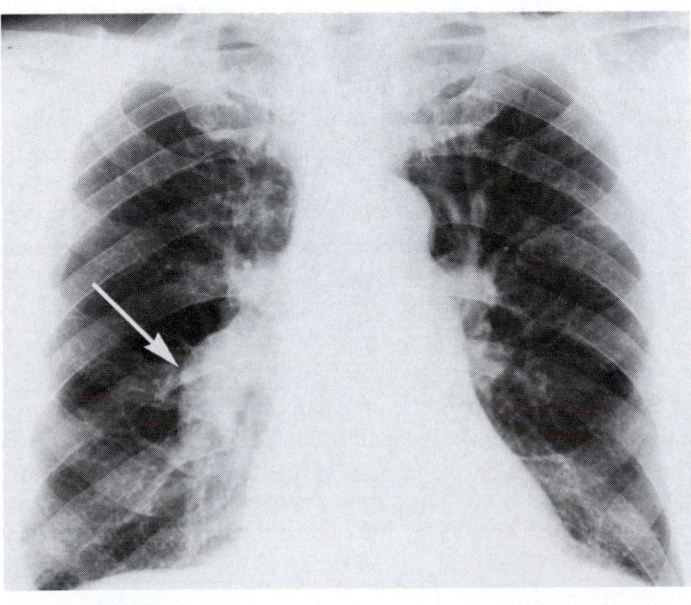
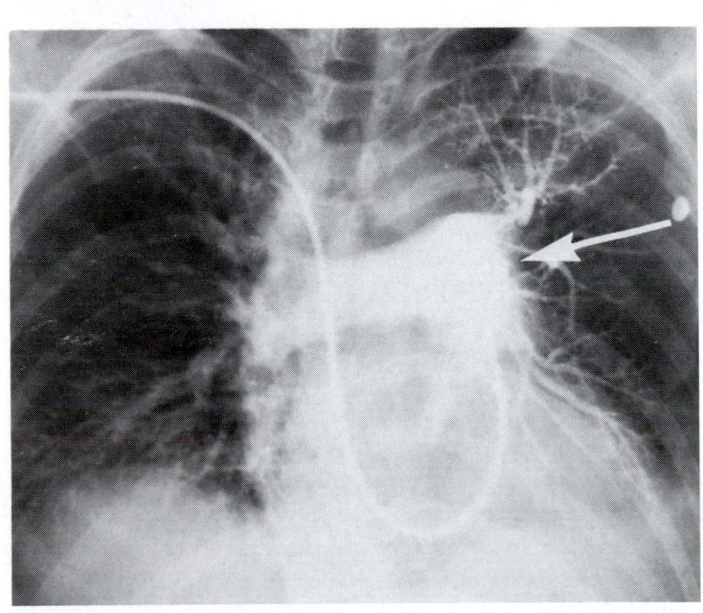

FIGURE 84-9 Massive pulmonary embolism. *A.* Chest radiograph of massive pulmonary embolism. Portable radiograph showing abrupt cut-off of the right pulmonary artery (arrow) and ipsilateral hypovascularity. *B.* Angiogram (another patient). Arrow indicates abrupt cutoff.

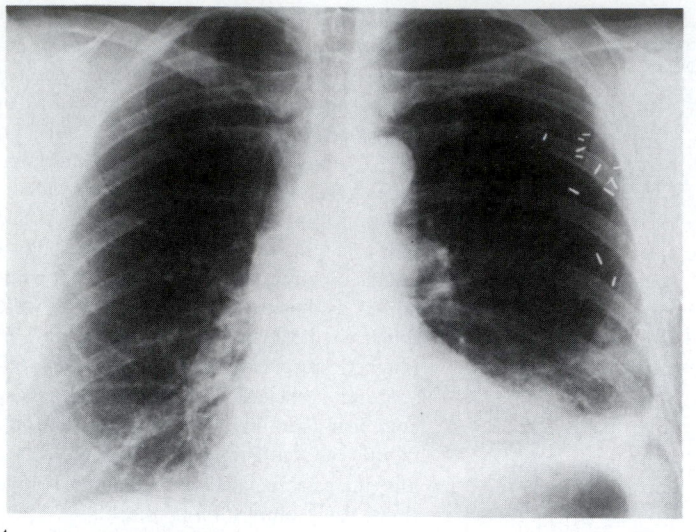

A

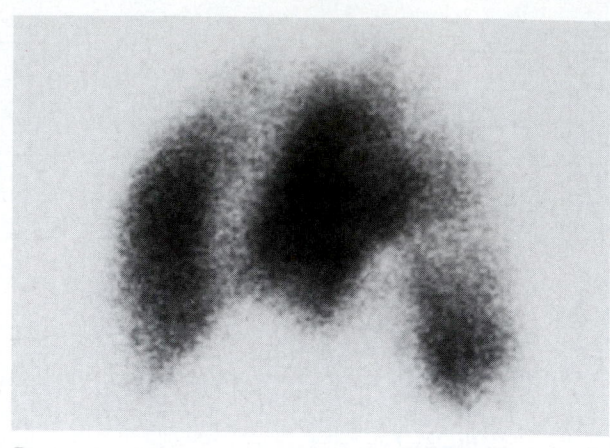

D

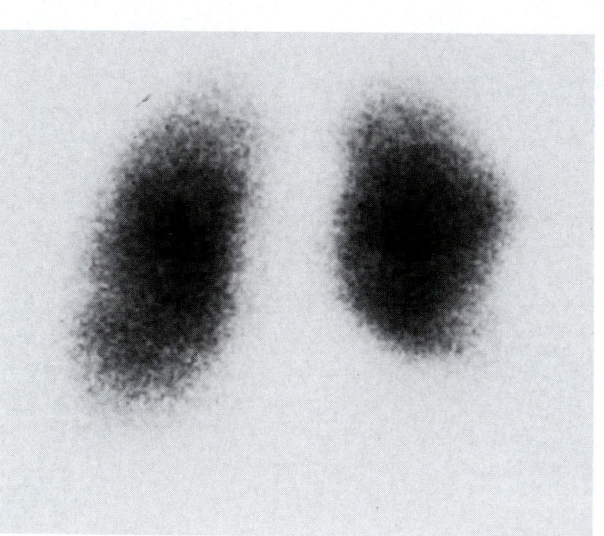

B

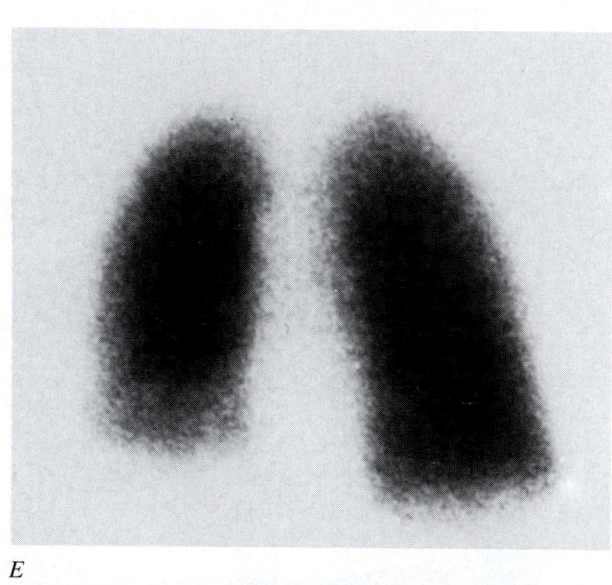

E

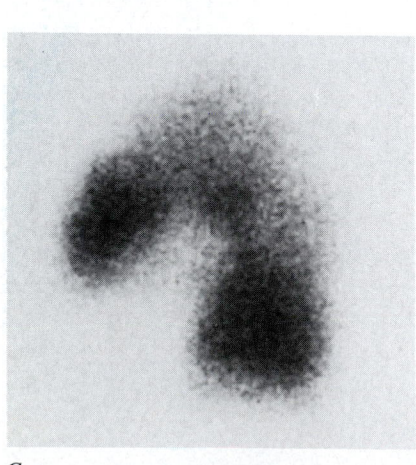

C

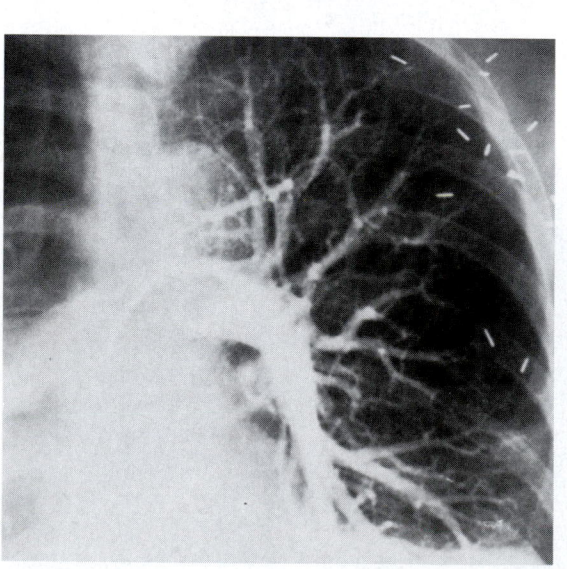

F

FIGURE 84-10   Pulmonary emboli and infarction in a 66-year-old woman who had a recent left radical mastectomy and complained of left pleuritic pain. *A.* Posteroanterior radiograph shows pleural effusion, atelectasis, and pulmonary infiltrate in the left lower lobe. *B, C,* and *D.* Perfusion lung scan. A wedge-shaped defect is present in the left lower lobe on the anterior (*B*), left lateral (*C*), and left anterior oblique (*D*) projections. *E.* Ventilation lung scan (posterior view). Ventilation is decreased at the left base in the area of the abnormality on the chest radiograph. *F.* Selective pulmonary arteriogram. Areas of multiple pulmonary emboli are present in the left lower lobe.

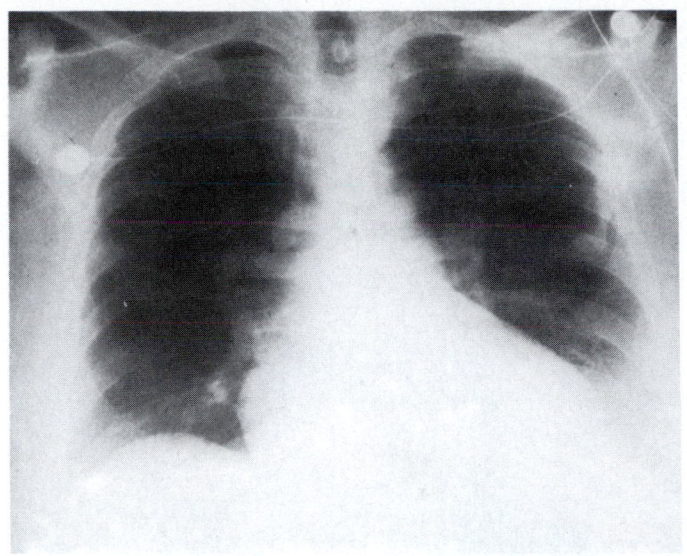

A

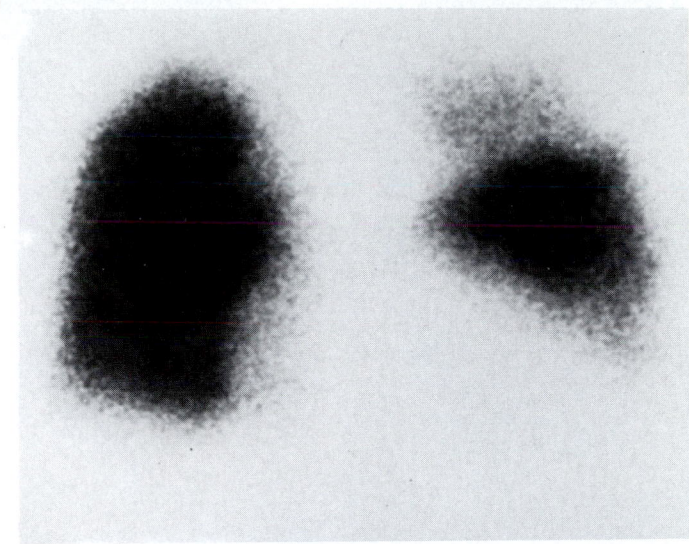

B

FIGURE 84-11 Fatal pulmonary emboli secondary to deep vein thrombosis. *A.* Portable chest radiograph shows mild cardiomegaly and hazy infiltrate at left base. *B.* Perfusion lung scan (anterior projection) shows defect in area of infiltrate and another wedge-shaped defect in left upper lung zone, where chest radiograph showed nothing. *C.* At autopsy, there were multiple pleural-based pulmonary infarcts.

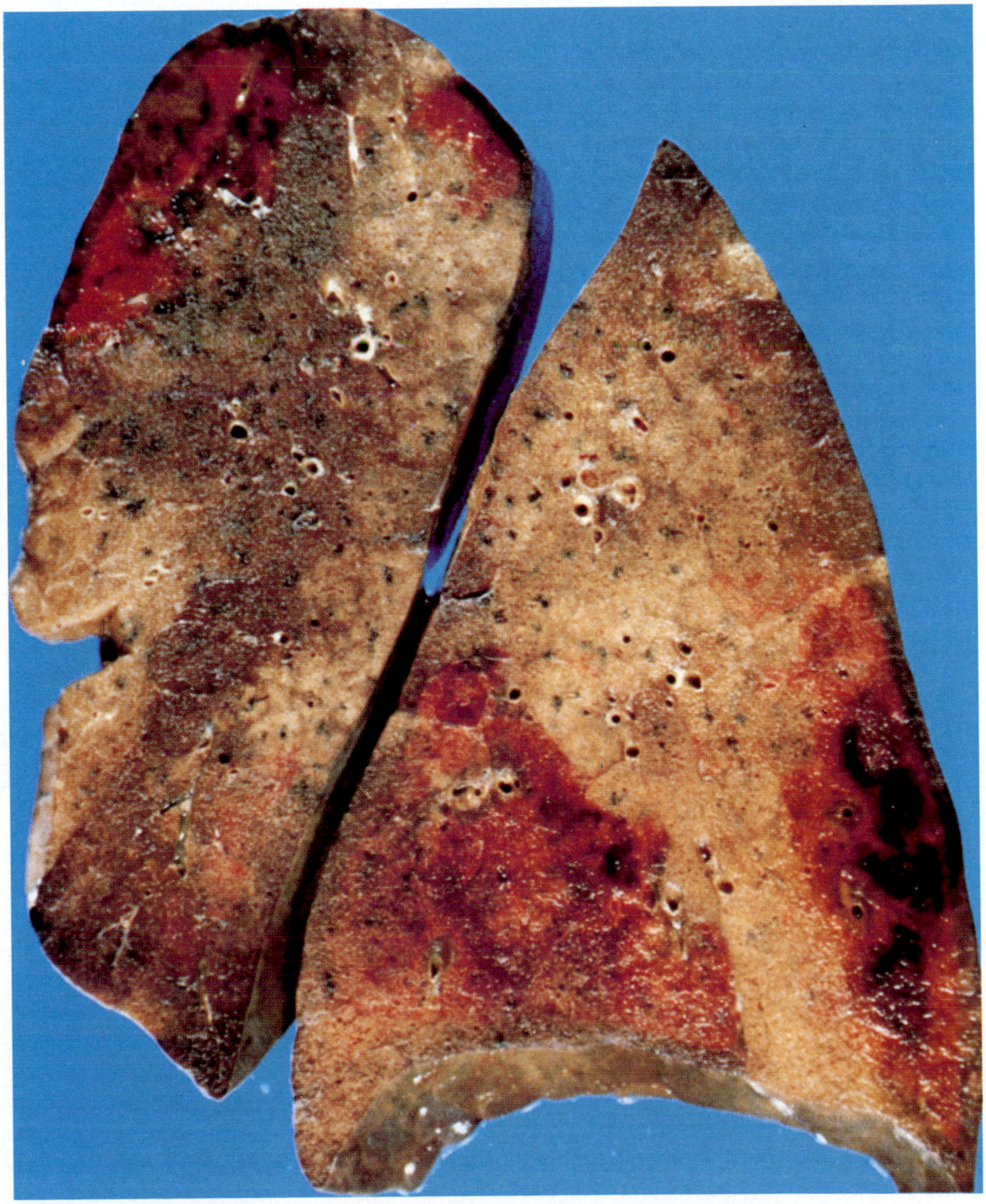

several days, a pulmonary infarct in a costophrenic angle may closely resemble either pleural thickening or free fluid, but often its border is convex toward the hilus (Hampton's hump) rather than concave (Fig. 84-12).

Pulmonary Embolism Without Infarction

Submassive embolization without infarction is the most common and difficult of the thromboembolic syndromes to evaluate (Fig. 84-13). Emboli that do not cause infarction lack the diagnostic specificity of pulmonary infarction (group II) or of massive embolization (group I) (Fig. 84-14). Instead, the hallmarks of this syndrome are meager: unexplained tachypnea, dyspnea, and tachycardia. The more extensive the embolization, the more apt is breathlessness to be severe and persistent; often this unexplained dyspnea is associated with anxiety and substernal oppression. Tachypnea

C

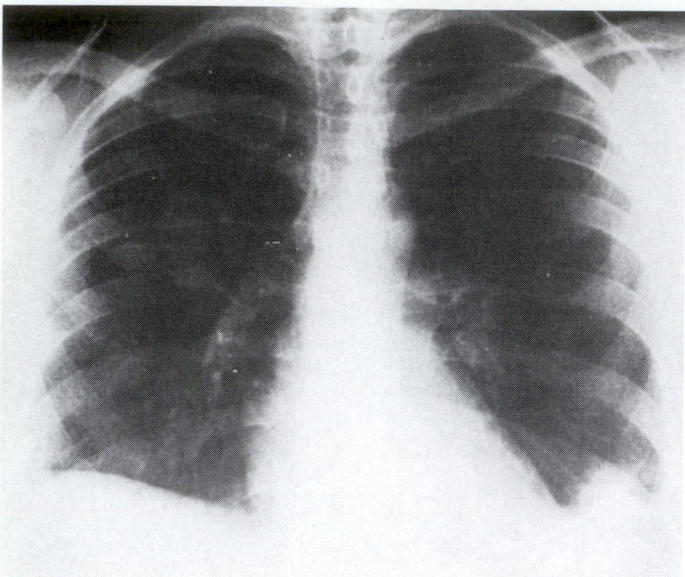

FIGURE 84-12   Hampton hump. A pulmonary infarct presenting as a pleural-based, wedge-shaped parenchymal lesion.

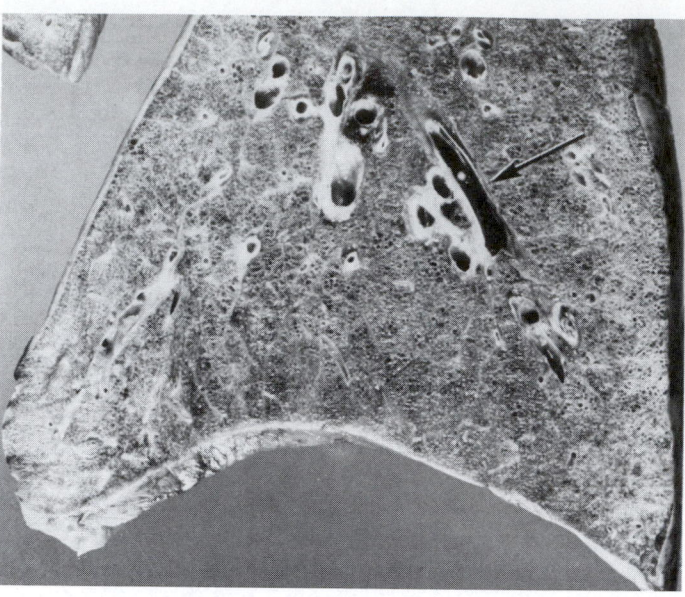

FIGURE 84-13   Pulmonary embolus in a medium-sized vessel without infarction. *(Courtesy of Dr. G.G. Pietra.)*

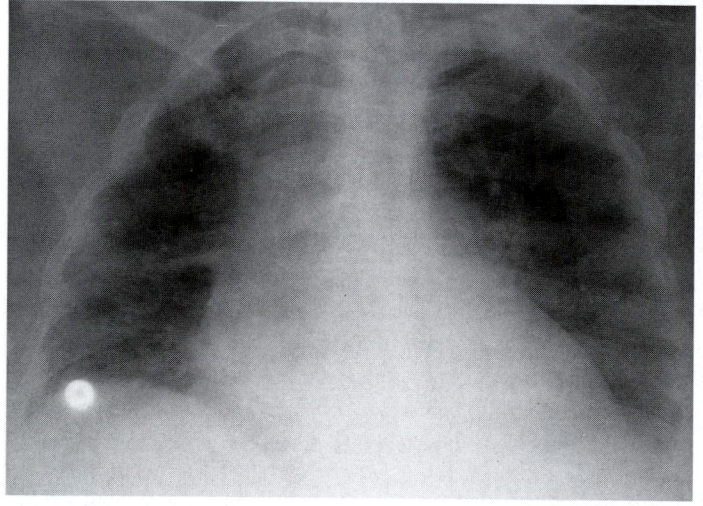

A

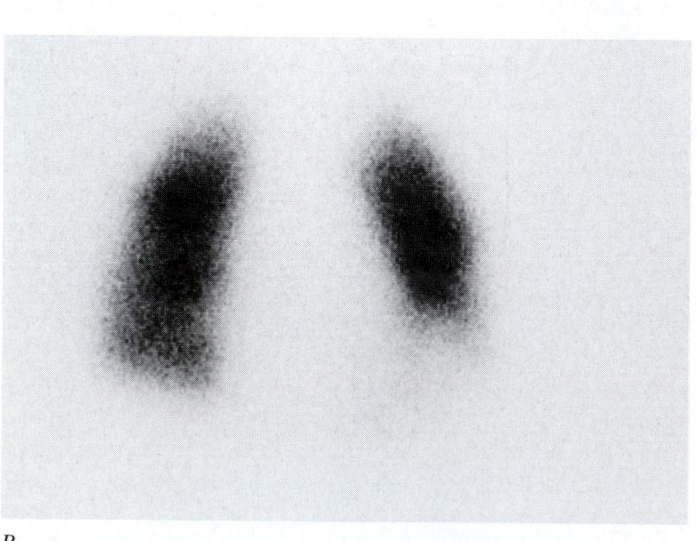

B

C

FIGURE 84-14   Pulmonary embolism without infarction in a 77-year-old woman with the acute onset of dyspnea and tachypnea. *A.* Antero-posterior radiograph (portable technique) shows cardiomegaly without parenchymal infiltrate. *B.* Perfusion lung scan, anterior view, demonstrates a perfusion defect in the left lower lobe. *C.* Angiogram of left lung shows segmental pulmonary artery with filling defect (arrow) and absence of distal filling diagnostic of acute pulmonary embolism. *(Courtesy of Dr. Z. Haskal.)*

and tachycardia persist during sleep. Syncope is not infrequent, usually occurring in association with a large central clot. Recurrent episodes of breathlessness in persons predisposed to venous thrombosis should automatically alert the physician not only to the prospect of pulmonary embolization but also to the possibility of sudden death. Occasionally, especially if right atrial pressures are high (e.g., secondary to pulmonary hypertension), a pulmonary embolus traverses a patent foramen ovale to enter the systemic circulation and produce "paradoxical embolization" of a systemic organ (e.g., the brain or kidney).

The physical examination is rarely helpful except with tachypnea and tachycardia. Pleuritic pain sometimes occurs even though there is no radiographic evidence of pulmonary infarction; it is intensified by deep breathing or by pressure on the overlying ribs. A few rales are occasionally identified in the area of embolism, often in association with a decrease in breath sounds; a local wheeze sometimes occurs.

The chest radiograph is often normal and is rarely diagnostic. One hemidiaphragm is occasionally elevated, presumably as a consequence of ipsilateral reduction in lung volume; platelike areas of atelectasis appear at the lung bases as linear streaks that parallel the diaphragm (Fleischner's lines); or large parts of the lung are avascular (Westermark's sign). Taken separately, these radiographic criteria are rarely diagnostic, but in a candidate for pulmonary embolization, a high diaphragm on one side accompanied by Fleischner's lines, an area of distinct hypovascularity, a nondescript area of pulmonary consolidation, or a small pleural effusion lends support to the impression that embolization has occurred. This impression can be reinforced by lung scans, but angiography may be needed to clinch the diagnosis.

Multiple Pulmonary Emboli (and/or Thrombi)

The category of multiple pulmonary emboli has traditionally included two different kinds of patients. The first subset consists of those who have had documented episodes of systemic venous thrombosis or pulmonary emboli over the years. The repeated emboli gradually give rise to pulmonary hypertension, and the patients may die suddenly or in cor pulmonale and heart failure.[13]

The second subset consists of patients who were formerly categorized as having the *syndrome of multiple pulmonary emboli*. These patients, without prior history of thrombosis or emboli, gradually become incapacitated, usually over a period of months to years, from insidious breathlessness, nondescript episodes of precordial pain, and mounting anxiety. By biopsy or at autopsy, they prove to have widespread occlusive disease due to thrombi or emboli in the minute arteries and arterioles of the lungs.[12] Because of the widespread distribution of these lesions throughout the pulmonary precapillary microcirculation, the relative uniformity of their appearance, and the possibility that they represent local thrombi (due to local malfunction of pulmonary vascular endothelium rather than minute emboli), some clinicians and pathologists now refer to this entity as *pulmonary microthromboembolic disease*. The clinical manifestations and course of the latter disease often mimic those of primary pulmonary hypertension (PPH): progressive breathlessness, right ventricular enlargement (cor pulmonale), and even right ventricular failure without discernible cause (Fig. 84-15),

and most clinicians and pathologists regard this entity to be a histologic subclassification of PPH.

The cause of the widespread pulmonary occlusive disease in this group is generally obscure: the patients lack a clear-cut history of peripheral thromboses or overt emboli, and it is not easy to identify a cause for the localization of the thrombotic process to the precapillary microcirculation of the lungs. Consequently, it is now generally accepted that the likelihood of widespread endothelial damage that predisposes to local pulmonary thrombosis is more tenable than is the idea of a shower of covert organized minute emboli.

The syndrome of multiple pulmonary emboli (or pulmonary microthromboembolic disease) generally terminates in a state of chronic pulmonary hypertension.[13] The latter is considered elsewhere in this book (see Chapter 83). Here it is pertinent to note that more than half of patients with the clinical diagnosis of PPH show widespread thrombotic occlusion of pulmonary arterioles and small muscular arteries at biopsy or autopsy.[12] In some patients, the organized and fresh clots appear to be complications of a slowed circulation. In most instances, however, pulmonary microthrombi appear to have been implicated in the pathogenesis of the clinically unexplained pulmonary hypertension.

Unresolved Pulmonary Embolism

Although virtually all patients who survive large, proximal pulmonary emboli undergo clinical, hemodynamic, and angiographic resolution of the clot, pulmonary emboli occasionally fail to resolve, leaving large segments of the pulmonary arterial tree occluded by organized clot (Fig. 84-5). Prerequisite for making the diagnosis is a high index of suspicion. In a few instances, a large clot organized in a major pulmonary arterial branch has been mistaken for a carcinoma of the lung. A surprising number of these patients give no history of embolic episode. Symptomatically, the main complaint is of progressive dyspnea, initially exertional but gradually requiring less and less activity to bring on. Except for the accentuated P_2 of pulmonary hypertension, the physical findings are not helpful. Arterial hypoxemia generally coexists with the pulmonary hypertension. The electrocardiogram is apt to show right ventricular hypertrophy when cor pulmonale supervenes. The chest radiograph often reveals dilated central pulmonary arteries, sometimes with peripheral pruning over affected parts of the lungs; there may be regions of hypervascularity. Lung scans are most frequently of the high-probability pattern, and angiography demonstrates the nature of the obliterative vascular process. In most patients, the pulmonary hypertension is a harbinger of cor pulmonale.

In recent years, the condition of unresolved pulmonary embolism has proved to be treatable surgically by removal of the organized occlusive clot(s). The surgical procedure consists of thromboendarterectomy rather than embolectomy.[13] Immediately after the occluded vessel is reopened, and for a few days thereafter, the patient is apt to experience "reperfusion" pulmonary edema that is localized to the vascular bed that has been reopened. Thereafter, improvement is often dramatic, clearly arresting the previous downhill course. However, it should be noted that thromboendarterectomy is technically difficult and that even in the most experienced hands, the mortality rate to date is around 10 to 15 percent.

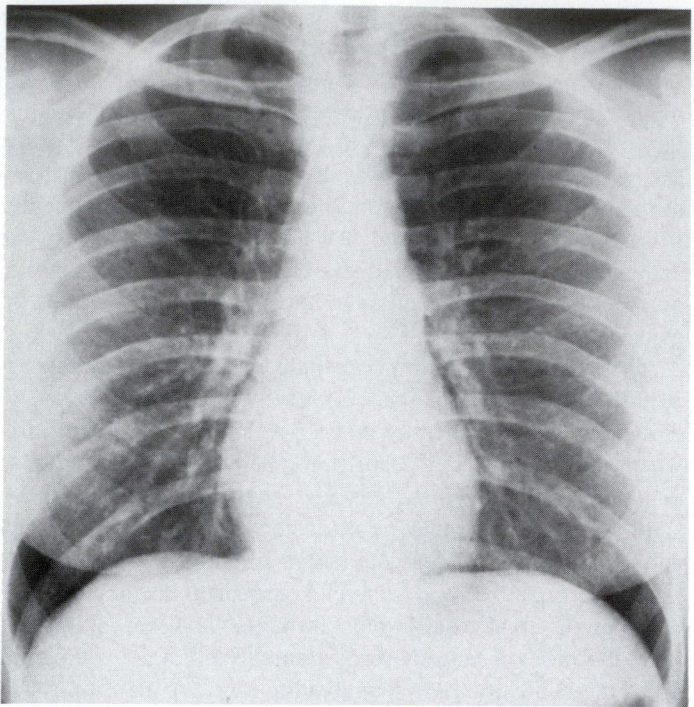

A

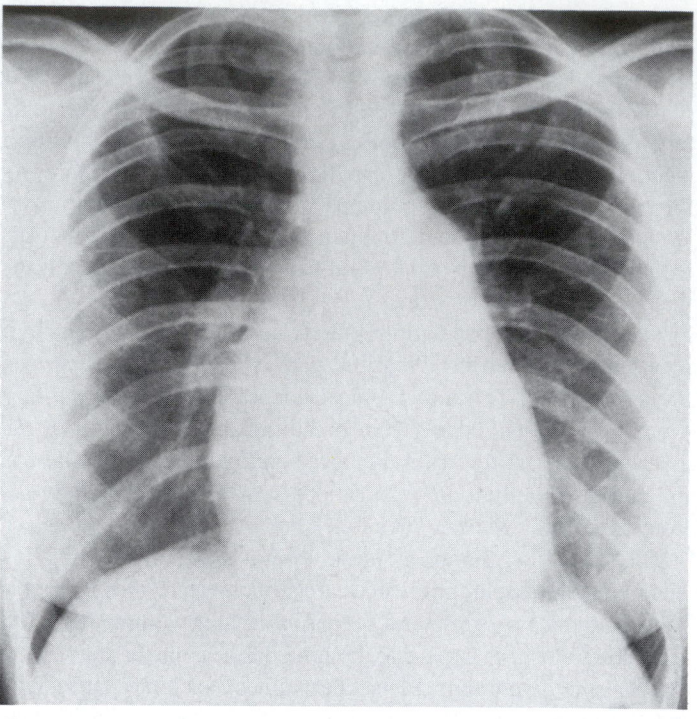

C

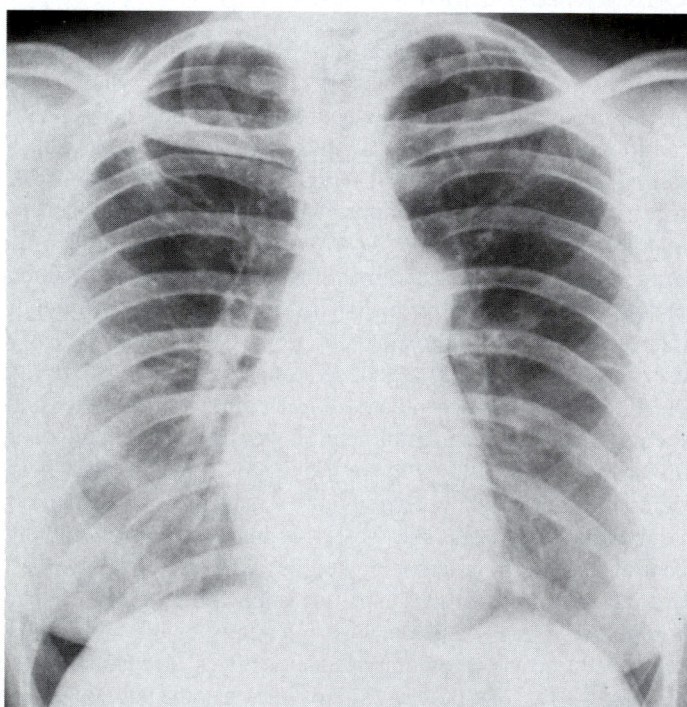

B

FIGURE 84-15   Recurrent pulmonary emboli in a 33-year-old woman who died with a clinical diagnosis of "primary pulmonary hypertension." At autopsy, there was widespread occlusion of small pulmonary arteries by organized clot that had undergone variable degrees of recanalization. *A*. On admission for hemoptysis. Cardiac silhouette is within normal limits. *B*. One year later there was cardiac enlargement with prominent central pulmonary artery. *C*. Two years after admission and shortly before death, there were cardiomegaly, prominent central pulmonary arteries, and bilateral attenuation of vascular markings.

or emboli. This threat emanates from a clot that is propagating beyond its restraints in a peripheral deep vein.

Diagnostic measures are currently directed at pulmonary embolism or thrombus in a systemic deep vein.

Pulmonary Embolism

Most important for the diagnosis of pulmonary embolism is the identification of the person who is predisposed to systemic venous thrombosis. The existence of a predisposing mechanism, particularly venous stasis, in a patient with sudden onset of unexplained breathlessness is of utmost diagnostic importance. Other common important predisposing factors are a carcinoma (especially mucin-secreting adenocarcinoma), the use of oral contraceptives, prolonged bed rest, recent surgery, trauma, congestive heart failure, and preexisting thromboembolic disease. Unfortunately, proving that embolization has occurred can be difficult: as a rule, clinical appraisal, chest radiograph, and conventional laboratory tests neither prove nor disprove that pulmonary embolization has occurred.[46] Pulmonary angiography is the most reliable of the tests currently available, although progress is being made in the use of computed tomography (CT) or magnetic resonance imaging (MRI) to examine the pulmonary vascular bed for thromboemboli.

DIAGNOSTIC MEASURES

It has been noted above that, except for massive pulmonary emboli that threaten life because of circulatory collapse, the clot in the lungs is usually of little therapeutic concern. In time, even an area of "infarcted" lung will clear spontaneously. Much more important is the threat of a recurrent embolus to a pulmonary vascular bed that has been compromised by a previous embolus

CLINICAL SIGNS AND SYMPTOMS

In pulmonary embolism, the diagnostic yield from signs and symptoms is notoriously poor. Tachypnea, pleuritic pain, and hemoptysis are nonspecific (Table 84-2). Similarly, a pleural rub, an exaggerated pulmonic component of the second heart sound, and overt phlebitis occur in other clinical disorders.

The mainstay for the diagnosis of pulmonary embolism is a high degree of clinical suspicion. The so-called classic syndrome of acute shortness of breath, pleuritic chest pain, and acute heart failure is rarely seen. More typical is an aggravation of antecedent dyspnea, the onset of unexplained chest pain or arrhythmia, or the onset of fever.

LABORATORY DATA

The white blood cell count and serial determinations of enzyme concentrations in serum have proved to be of little value in the diagnosis of pulmonary embolism. The white blood cell count is generally normal or slightly increased; at other times, it is quite high. Similarly, the triad of an increase in the concentration of lactic dehydrogenase and bilirubin in the serum coupled with a normal concentration of transaminase, once believed to be suggestive of pulmonary embolism, has proved to be nonspecific.

The determination of the concentrations of fibrin degradation products (D-dimer) in serum, although attractive in principle, suffers from a lack of uniformity in reagents and standards. Moreover, false-positive results have been encountered in such diverse conditions as surgery, trauma, renal disease, and systemic lupus erythematosus. Some investigators have proposed that a negative D-dimer blood test can be used to rule out significant ongoing thrombosis. Until more reliable and specific techniques are developed, however, studies of this kind have little clinical role.[45]

ELECTROCARDIOGRAM

The most common electrocardiographic findings in pulmonary embolism are nonspecific ST-T-wave changes. Except in massive embolization, the pattern of right ventricular strain with an $S_1Q_3T_3$ pattern is unusual. Atrial arrhythmias are common in pulmonary embolism but may also be seen in a variety of other disorders. Thus, the electrocardiogram is nonspecific in the diagnosis of pulmonary embolism, and its major value may be in identifying other clinical disorders (e.g., acute myocardial infarction and pericarditis) that may be confused with pulmonary embolism.

ARTERIAL BLOOD GASES

The diagnostic value of arterial blood gases in pulmonary embolism is supportive at best. As a rule, both the arterial P_{O_2} and

TABLE 84-2

Incidence of Signs and Symptoms of Pulmonary Embolism

	Massive PE* (%)	Submassive PE* (%)	PE Without Preexisting Cardiac or Pulmonary Disease† (%)
Dyspnea	85	82	73
Pleuritic chest pain	64	85	66
Cough	53	52	37
Hemoptysis	23	40	13
Tachypnea	95 (>16 breaths/min)	87 (>16 breaths/min)	70 (>20 breaths/min)
Tachycardia (>100 beats/min)	48	38	30
Increased pulmonic component of second heart sound	58	45	23
Rales	57	60	51
Phlebitis	36	26	11

*SOURCE: Data from NIH-sponsored urokinase and streptokinase clinical trials (*Am J Med* 62:355–360, 1977).
†SOURCE: Data from NIH-sponsored PIOPED study (*Chest* 100:598–603, 1991).

P_{CO_2} are somewhat low. Although arterial blood gases are abnormal in the great majority of patients with pulmonary embolism, similar changes are often seen in conditions that enter into the differential diagnosis of pulmonary embolism. Also, in about 10 to 15 percent of patients with pulmonary embolism, arterial blood gases and alveolar-arterial differences in P_{O_2} are normal. Usually, these patients are young, with a normal pulmonary circulation before embolization and with a modest burden of clot after embolization. Thus, in the diagnosis of pulmonary embolism, arterial blood gases can be weighed only in the balance. Normal arterial blood gases do not exclude the possibility of even major pulmonary emboli. However, the finding of unexplained hypoxemia should raise the possibility of pulmonary embolism; if another explanation is not readily apparent, a ventilation-perfusion lung scan should be obtained.

CHEST RADIOGRAPHY

It is uncommon for the chest radiograph in pulmonary embolism to be normal. More typically, the chest radiograph shows an infiltrate, effusion, or atelectasis, or a combination of the three. Similar findings occur in pneumonia, pleuritis, and congestive heart failure. The classic finding of a peripheral wedge-shaped infarct (Hampton's hump) (Fig. 84-12) is uncommon, whereas Westermark's sign, another "classic" sign, characterized by hypoperfusion of one lung secondary to massive pulmonary embolism, is rare.

Ventilation-Perfusion Lung Scan

The fundamental premise underlying the use of ventilation-perfusion lung scans for the diagnosis of pulmonary embolism is that in most pulmonary diseases or disorders other than pulmonary emboli, the ventilation defect that accompanies a perfusion defect is at least as large as the perfusion defect. In contrast, pulmonary emboli elicit perfusion defects that are unaccompanied by ventilation defects. Interpretation of ventilation-perfusion scans is based on the presence and size of perfusion defects and the correspondence of ventilation and perfusion defects. Scans are classified on these grounds into four categories: normal, high probability, intermediate (or indeterminate) probability, and low probability of pulmonary embolism (Table 84-3).

NORMAL PERFUSION SCANS

Perfusion lung scans, per se (i.e., without accompanying ventilation scans), are sensitive but not specific tests for detection of

---

TABLE 84-3

Criteria for the Interpretation of Ventilation-Perfusion Lung Scans

Normal*
  No perfusion defects
  Perfusion outlines that correspond exactly to the contour of the lungs as seen on the chest radiograph (chest radiograph and/or ventilation scan may be abnormal)

High probability
  ≥2 large (>75 percent of a segment) segmental perfusion defects either without any abnormalities on the chest radiograph or with abnormalities that are considerably larger than corresponding defects in the ventilation scan or the chest radiograph
  ≥2 moderate (≥25 percent and ≤75 percent of a segment) segmental perfusion defects without corresponding defects in the ventilation scan or the chest radiograph plus 1 large mismatched segmental defect
  ≥4 moderate segmental perfusion defects without corresponding defects in the ventilation scan or the chest radiograph

Intermediate probability (indeterminate)
  Not falling into low- or high-probability categories
  Difficult to categorize as low or high probability

Low probability
  Single moderate mismatched segmental perfusion defect in association with normal chest radiograph
  Small (<25 percent of a segment) segmental perfusion defects in association with a normal chest radiograph
  Any perfusion defects involving no more than four segments in one lung and no more than three segments in one region of either lung with *matching* defects on the ventilation scan that are either equal or larger in size
  Nonsegmental perfusion defects (e.g., blunting of the costophrenic angle by a pleural effusion; cardiomegaly; enlarged aorta, hilum, and/or mediastinum; or elevated hemidiaphragm)

---

*Ventilation scan is not necessary to determine if perfusion scan is normal; all other interpretations are based on a comparison of the perfusion and ventilation scans.
SOURCE: Modified after PIOPED criteria (*JAMA* 263:2753–2759, 1990).

---

pulmonary emboli. They are sensitive in that the finding of a normal lung scan excludes even modest-sized (clinically significant) pulmonary emboli. Thus, follow-up study of 515 subjects in whom lung scans had been interpreted as normal (and who had therefore not been anticoagulated) disclosed only one who subsequently had evidence of pulmonary embolism.[35]

ABNORMAL PERFUSION SCANS

Lung scans are not specific for the diagnosis of pulmonary embolism. In persons with abnormal perfusion scans, comparison with ventilation scans improves the accuracy of lung scans for detecting pulmonary embolism (Table 84-3). This holds true even for patients with underlying cardiac or pulmonary disease.[63] Recent efforts, using ventilation-perfusion scans, have focused more on identifying "clinically significant" (larger) pulmonary emboli and on identifying patients at risk for recurrent embolic events (see below) than on identifying all emboli.

HIGH-PROBABILITY LUNG SCANS

The largest perfusion defects—those involving at least 75 percent of a segment—particularly when multiple and not matched by ventilation defects, are likely to represent more significant embolic events. Scans of this type are classified as showing *high probability for pulmonary embolism.* However, the Prospective Investigation of Pulmonary Embolism Diagnosis (PIOPED) study, sponsored by the National Institutes of Health (NIH), found high-probability lung scans to be relatively insensitive: they occurred in only 41 percent of the patients in whom the presence of pulmonary emboli was documented by pulmonary angiography (Table 84-4).[47] Despite this lack of sensitivity, the high-probability scan was accurate: 88 percent of the patients with high-probability lung scans had pulmonary emboli—i.e., positive predictive value of a high-probability scan was 88 percent. However, the predictive value of the high-probability lung scan fell to 74 percent in patients who had a history of pulmonary embolism, presumably because of residual perfusion defects due to the previous pulmonary emboli. One way to overcome this limitation in patients who have had large pulmonary emboli is to obtain follow-up lung scans after they complete their course of anticoagulation: these follow-up scans disclose whether complete resolution of scan defects has taken place and establish a new (not normal) baseline for comparison with lung scans made at some later date should suspicion subsequently arise of recurrent pulmonary embolism.

NON–HIGH-PROBABILITY LUNG SCANS

Intermediate and low probability lung scans are often considered together in dealing with patients suspected of pulmonary emboli, on four accounts. The first is that perfusion defects in both of these categories are smaller and far fewer than in high-probability scans (Table 84-3). In the PIOPED study, most of the emboli that were documented angiographically fell into this category of lung scans: 42 percent of the patients with proven emboli had intermediate-probability lung scans, and 16 percent had low-probability scans (Table 84-4).

Second, distinguishing between intermediate- and low-probability scans is often difficult. In the PIOPED study, concordance

TABLE 84-4

Utility of Lung Scan Interpretations as Determined from Pulmonary Angiography in PIOPED Study

Lung Scan Interpretation	Sensitivity (%)	Specificity (%)	Positive Predictive Value (%)
High probability	41	97	88
Intermediate probability	82	52	33
Low probability	98	10	16

SOURCE: Data from PIOPED study (*JAMA* 263:2753–2759, 1990).

of interpretation among readers of lung scans was only 70 to 75 percent for these categories. Third, the rationale for subsequent diagnostic evaluations and treatment is similar. Finally, in patients suspected of having pulmonary emboli, intermediate- and low-probability scans are not diagnostic.

With respect to management, it has been suggested that in clinically stable patients with intermediate- or low-probability lung scans, anticoagulation does not need to be instituted except to prevent recurrent emboli.[33] The group about which this suggestion was made had the following characteristics: the lung scans were interpreted as "abnormal" but not high probability, the patients had adequate cardiopulmonary reserve, and their lower extremities showed no evidence of deep vein thrombosis by impedance plethysmography. In an outcome study of 371 patients suspected of having had pulmonary emboli who were not anticoagulated, late evidence of deep vein thrombi pulmonary or emboli was found in only 2.7 percent. In a confirmatory study of 1564 patients suspected of pulmonary emboli, 627 fit the profile described above.[34] During long-term follow-up, only 12 patients (1.9 percent; 95 percent confidence limits 0.8 percent to 3.0 percent) demonstrated venous thromboembolism. The implication of these studies is that patients with abnormal but not high-probability lung scans and adequate cardiopulmonary reserve had experienced, at most, modest emboli, which they had tolerated well. Moreover, such patients do not seem to require anticoagulation, since without deep vein thrombosis, they are not at risk for subsequent embolic events.

CORRELATING LUNG SCAN INTERPRETATION WITH CLINICAL ASSESSMENT

The PIOPED study also undertook to correlate the clinical impression of the likelihood of pulmonary embolism with the interpretation of the lung scan.[47] When interpretation of the lung scan and clinical assessment were concordant (both high probability and low probability), diagnostic accuracy was greater than that of the lung scan alone (Table 84-5). In contrast, when interpretation of the lung scan and clinical assessment were discordant, the predictive value of the lung scan was decreased. In as many as two-thirds of patients suspected of pulmonary embolism, the combination of the lung scan and clinical assessment failed to diagnose or exclude pulmonary embolism (Table 81-4). This inability leaves several options for diagnosis and treatment: pulmonary angiography or newer imaging methods for pulmonary emboli or some diagnostic measure (e.g., impedance plethysmography, duplex ultrasound, magnetic resonance venography, or contrast venography) to detect a potential source of emboli in the lower extremities.[31]

Pulmonary Angiography

The pulmonary angiogram continues to be the most accurate diagnostic study for evaluating pulmonary embolism (Fig. 84-16). Two angiographic findings in large vessels are characteristic of pulmonary embolism[22]: a filling defect and a cutoff of the radiopaque stream (Fig. 84-14). Of the two, the filling defect is the more common and reliable. Although angiography in experienced hands has a very low morbidity and mortality, it does entail right heart catheterization and the intravenous injection of contrast material, both of which entail some risk. Nonetheless, in general, angiography poses a minor threat to life when compared with the hazards of pulmonary embolization.

When properly done, using magnification and selective injections and views, pulmonary angiography can detect clots as

TABLE 84-5

Prevalence of Pulmonary Embolism in PIOPED: Value of Correlating Lung Scan Interpretation with Clinical Assessment

		Clinical Assessment		
		High Clinical Suspicion of PE	Intermediate Clinical Suspicion of PE	Low Clinical Suspicion of PE
Lung scan interpretation	High probability of PE	96% (28/29)	88% (70/80)	56% (5/9)
	Intermediate probability of PE	66% (27/41)	28% (66/236)	16% (11/68)
	Low probability of PE	40% (6/15)	16% (30/191)	4% (4/90)

NOTE: PE = pulmonary embolism.
SOURCE: Data modified after *JAMA* 263:2753–2759, 1990.

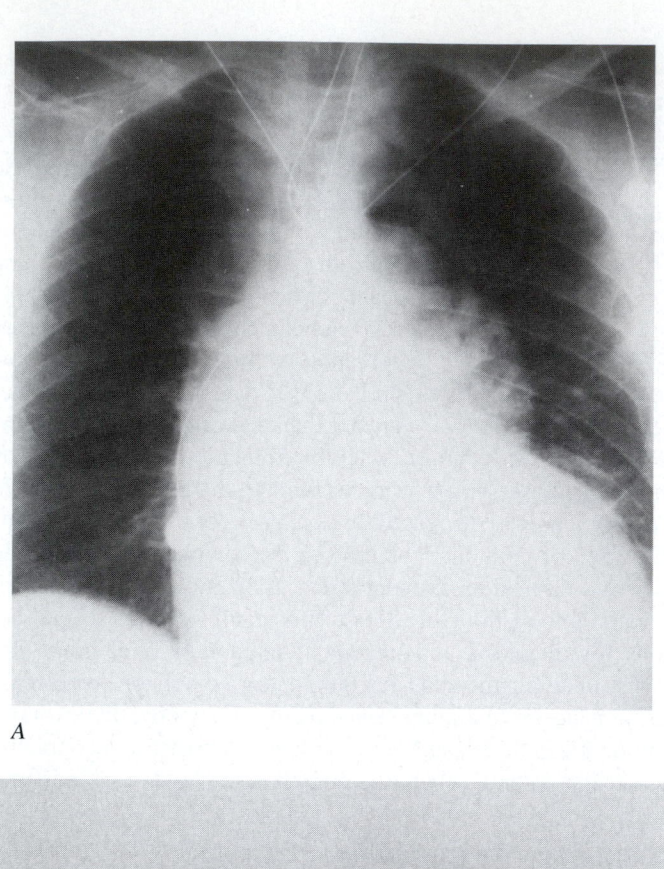

A

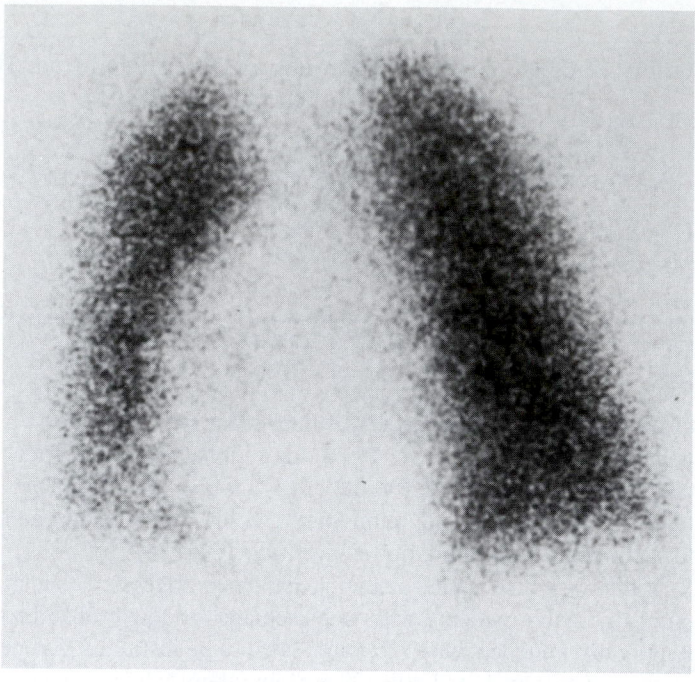

C

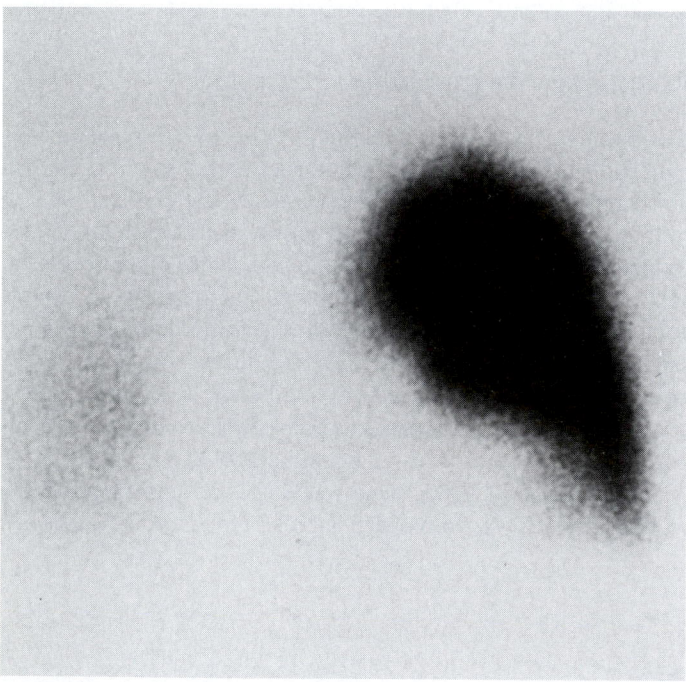

B

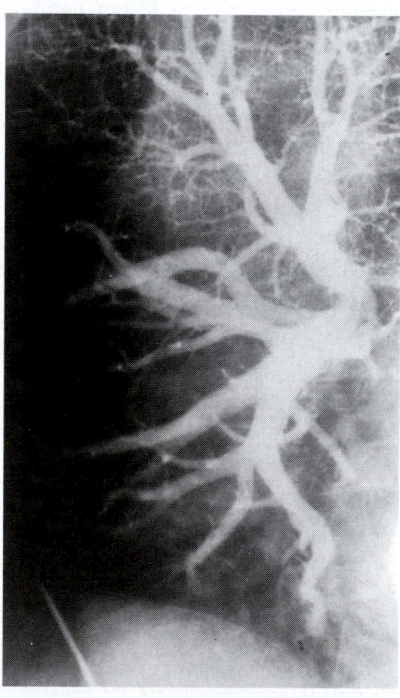

D

FIGURE 84-16   Compression of pulmonary artery simulating massive pulmonary embolism in a 72-year-old man with a history of thoracic aortic aneurysm who presented with sudden onset of dyspnea. *A*. Chest radiograph shows cardiomegaly and enlarged thoracic aorta. Lung markings are decreased in the right lung. *B*. In perfusion lung scan (anterior view), perfusion to the entire right lung is markedly decreased. *C*. Ventilation scan shows no abnormalities attributable to emboli. *D*. Pulmonary arteriogram shows no emboli but extrinsic compression of the right pulmonary artery by the enlarged thoracic aorta.

small as 0.5 mm. With rare exceptions, a normal angiogram excludes the diagnosis of embolism in all but the minute vessels of the lungs. Another exception is incomplete occlusion that allows flow to continue through small pulmonary vessels.

The major flaws of pulmonary angiography are its invasiveness, expense, technical complexity, and limited availability. To reduce these disadvantages, digital subtraction angiography has been developed whereby a bolus of contrast material is injected into a large peripheral vein, and the resultant radiographic image of the pulmonary circulation is enhanced through special computed techniques. Unfortunately, this method has not proved to be as sensitive as pulmonary angiography. Consequently, in most medical centers, its application to the diagnosis of pulmonary embolism has been curtailed.

Another invasive technique that avoids the use of intravenous contrast agents is intravascular ultrasound. Currently investigational, this technique may have more of a role in defining the lesions of unresolved emboli along the walls of central pulmonary arteries than it will in the diagnosis of acute pulmonary embolism.[48]

Other Diagnostic Techniques

COMPUTED TOMOGRAPHY

Recent advances in CT scan technology—helical (spiral) CT and electron-beam CT—have improved visualization of the pulmonary arterial tree to at least the level of segmental arteries (Figure 84-17).[14] Both techniques rapidly acquire images (thoracic scanning time less than 30 min), so that opacification of the pulmonary vasculature following bolus administration of intravenous contrast is at its maximum during scan time. CT provides direct visualization of central pulmonary arterial clots, including nonocclusive thrombi.[17] Unlike ventilation-perfusion scanning, the imaging of the chest by CT has the potential of indicating diagnoses other than pulmonary embolism. However, in contrast to the high sensitivity and low specificity of radionucleotide lung scanning for clot detection, CT is limited by its low sensitivity for the detection of segmental and smaller clots. The clinical significance of the low sensitivity for smaller, peripheral emboli is uncertain. It may well be that this low sensitivity can be offset by combining CT studies with noninvasive studies for deep vein thrombosis.

Published reports on spiral CT angiographic studies have indicated that spiral CT has a sensitivity of 95.5 percent (range, 64 to 100 percent) and a specificity of 97.6 percent (range, 89 to 100 percent) for the detection of pulmonary embolism. Cost-effectiveness analysis has suggested that if sensitivity is greater than 85 percent, an algorithm based on spiral CT evaluation of the lungs and ultrasound evaluation of the legs is more cost-effective than algorithms that include radionucleotide lung scanning and conventional contrast angiography.[57] This suggestion clearly needs to be validated by a large-scale prospective outcome–based trial.

MAGNETIC RESONANCE IMAGING

MRI is also rapidly evolving as a noninvasive method of visualizing pulmonary artery clots (Fig. 84-18). As compared to CT, MRI does not require the use of iodinated intravenous contrast agents. Moreover, pulmonary vascular MRI for pulmonary

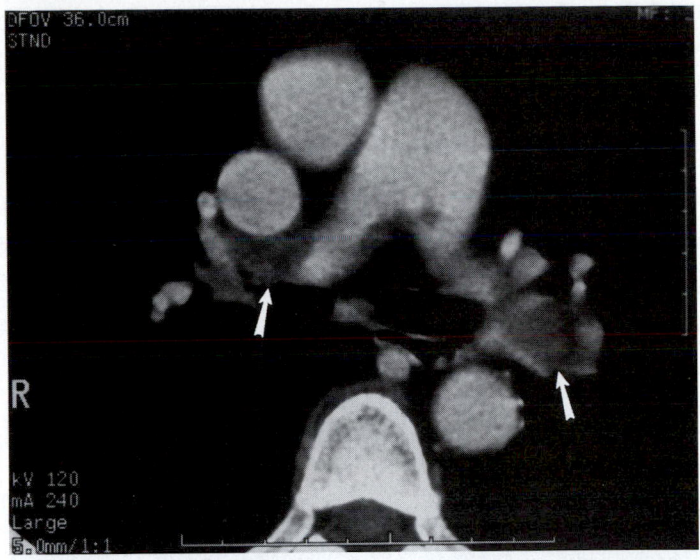

A

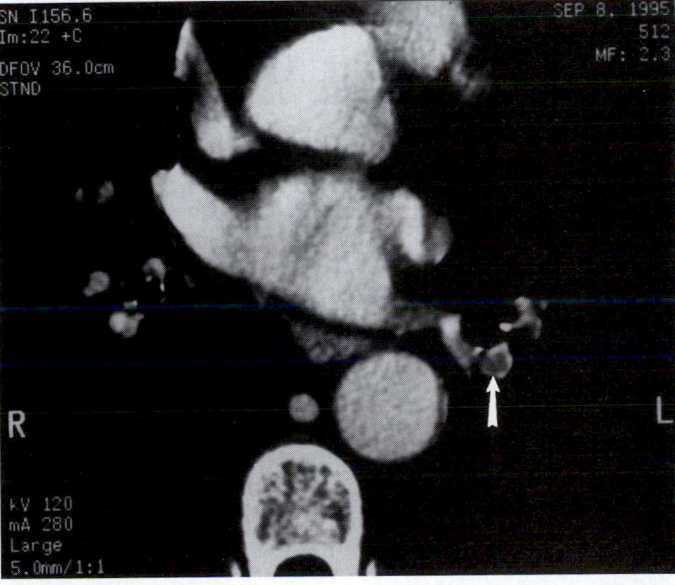

B

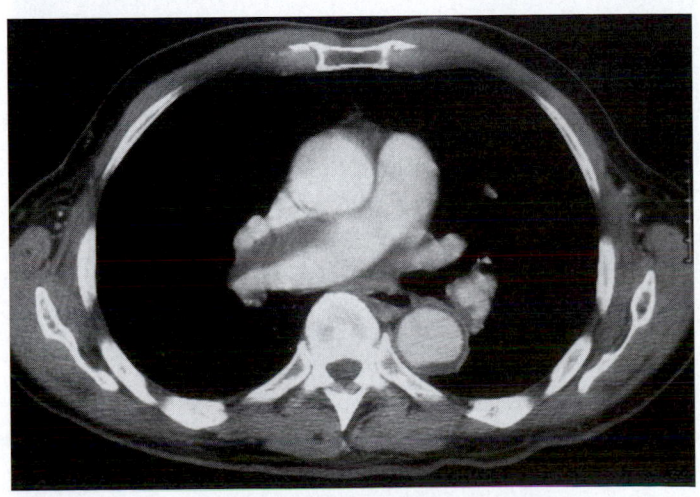

FIGURE 84-17   Helical (spiral) CT scanning. *A.* Magnification view of contrast-enhanced helical (spiral) CT scan of thorax demonstrating massive acute pulmonary thromboemboli in right main pulmonary artery just proximal to its bifurcation and in left descending pulmonary artery. *B.* In a different patient, magnification view of contrast-enhanced helical CT of the thorax demonstrating acute thromboemboli in left-lower-lobe segmental pulmonary arteries. *C.* In a different patient, contrast-enhanced helical CT demonstrating organized mural thrombus along the anterior wall of the proximal right pulmonary artery. (*Courtesy of Dr. W.B. Gefter.*)

C

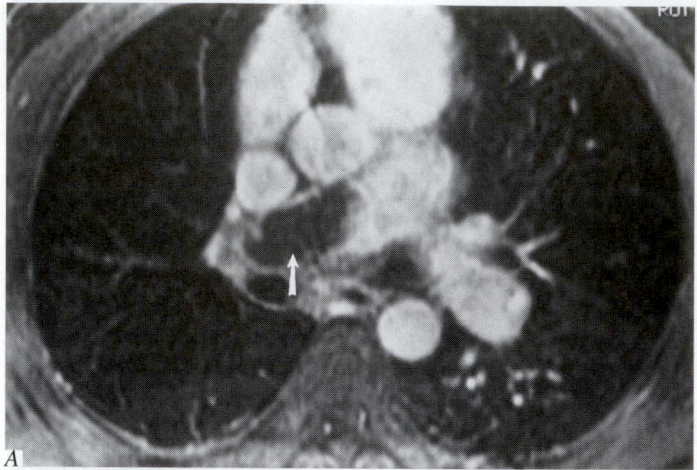

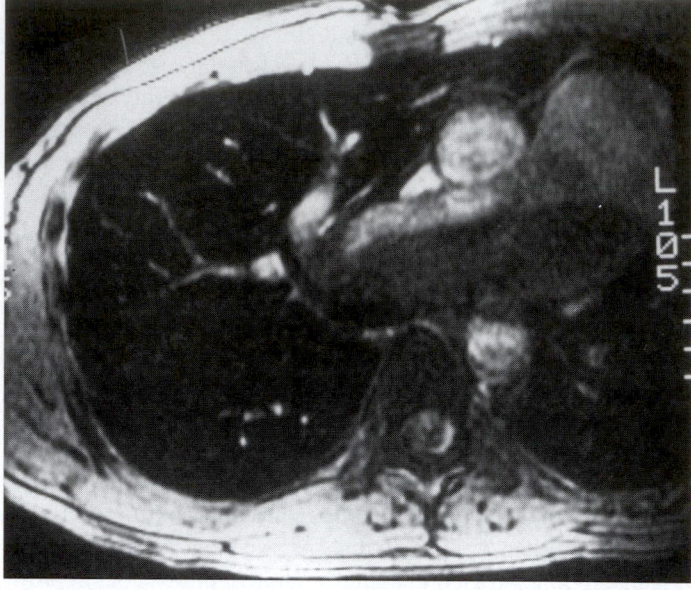

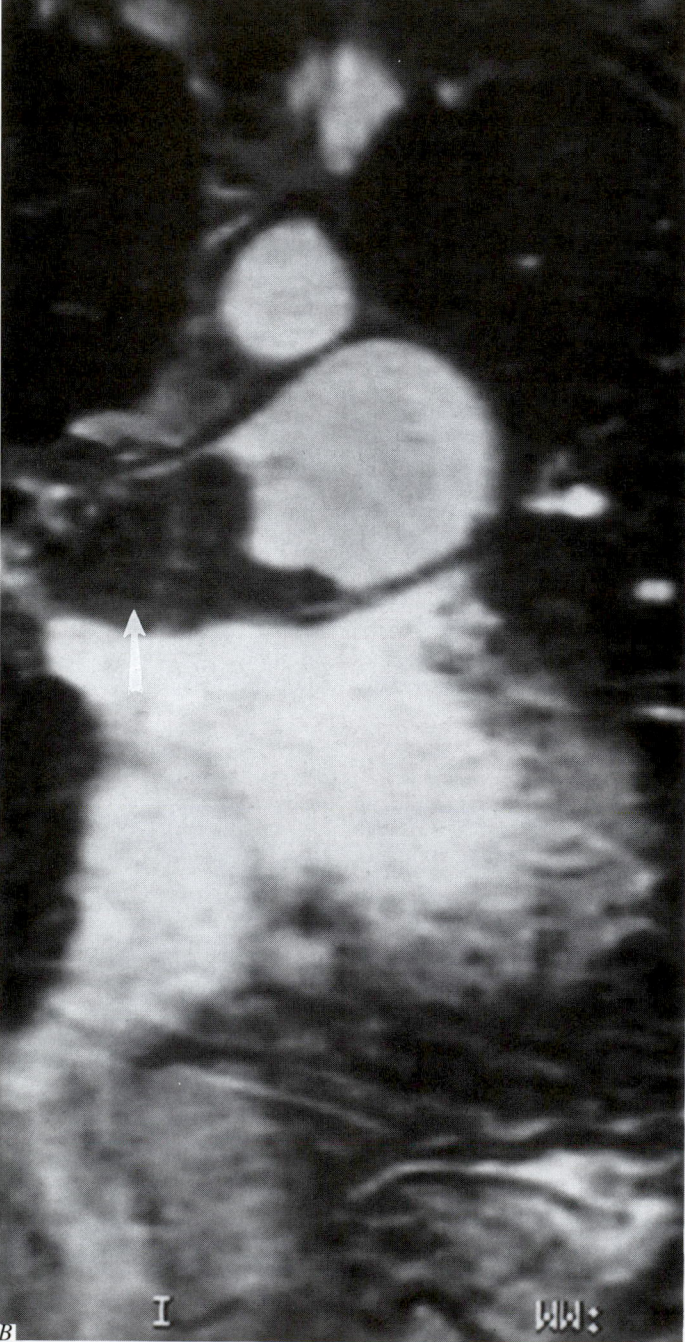

FIGURE 84-18 Axial (*A*) and coronal (*B*) gadolinium-enhanced 3-D time-of-flight gradient echo technique demonstrating large thromboembolus in right main pulmonary artery. *C*. MR image obtained with a fast 2-D time-of-flight gradient-echo sequence in a different patient demonstrating large organized mural thrombus along the posterior wall of the right main pulmonary artery. This patient underwent thromboendarterectomy based solely on the MR findings. (*Courtesy of Dr. W.B. Gefter.*)

emboli may easily be combined with MR venography for evaluation of the pelvic veins and the deep veins of the legs.

The sensitivity of MRI for the detection of pulmonary embolism varies with the size and location of the clot; diagnostic accuracy is good only for segmental or larger clots. As in the case of CT scanning, the inability of this technique to detect small, peripheral emboli may be of minor clinical importance if evaluation for deep vein thrombosis can be easily accomplished. At present, the accuracy of spiral CT scanning appears to be somewhat better than that of MRI.[14] However, the role of MRI in diagnosing thromboembolic disease holds great promise because of technical advances that are shortening image acquisition times (thereby decreasing the image degradation that occurs as a consequence of cardiac and respiratory motion) and enhancing vascular signal intensity.

DEEP VENOUS THROMBOSIS

About two-thirds of venous thrombi are silent and escape clinical detection. Conversely, only about half of the patients who have signs and symptoms attributed to venous thrombosis prove to have the disease.[61] Accurate diagnosis is essential before the start of anticoagulant therapy, since the agents have a morbidity and mortality of their own. Pulmonary emboli usually originate as clots in the deep veins of the lower extremities that propagate proximally to femoral and popliteal veins before migrating to the lungs.[44] As many as one-half of patients with proximal deep vein thrombosis will have had pulmonary emboli that are clinically unsuspected.[27] Therefore, one reasonable approach to establishing the diagnosis of pulmonary embolism is to seek evidence of clot in peripheral veins, bearing in mind that clots in the calves are less likely to be the source of major emboli than those in the thighs and pelvis. Although the search for deep vein thrombosis often does succeed in revealing a venous clot, in nearly one-third of patients with angiographically proven pulmonary embolism, the venogram is normal. Therefore, it must be kept in mind that a normal peripheral venogram does not exclude the diagnosis of pulmonary embolism.[29]

The frequency of fatal thromboembolism underscores the need to find and deal with sources before embolic material is released. However, the wide array of diagnostic measures is generally nonspecific, costly, and troublesome, often forcing the physician to choose between phlebography, radioisotopes, blood tests, plethysmography, ultrasound, and MRI.

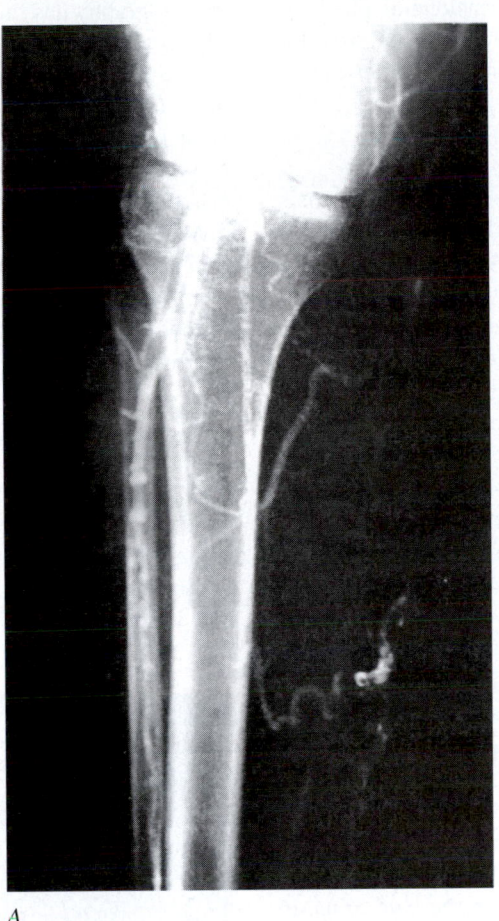 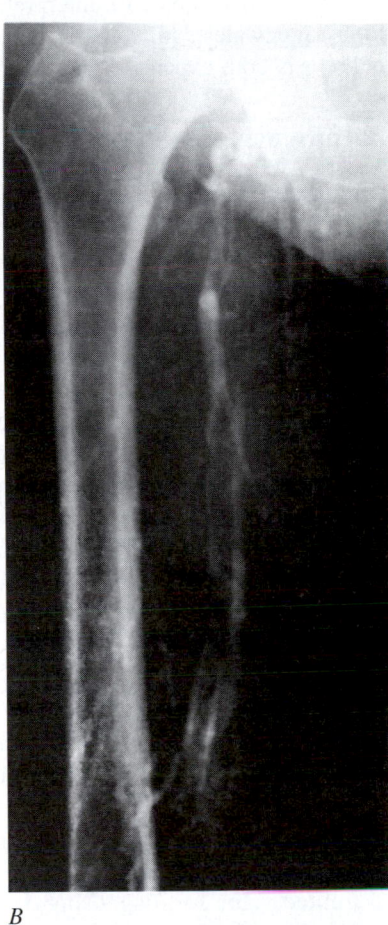

A   *B*

ASCENDING CONTRAST VENOGRAPHY (PHLEBOGRAPHY)

The "gold standard" for the diagnosis of venous thrombosis in the lower extremities is contrast venography (Fig. 84-19). However, this is an invasive procedure that exposes the patient to radiation and to the risks of hemodynamic up-

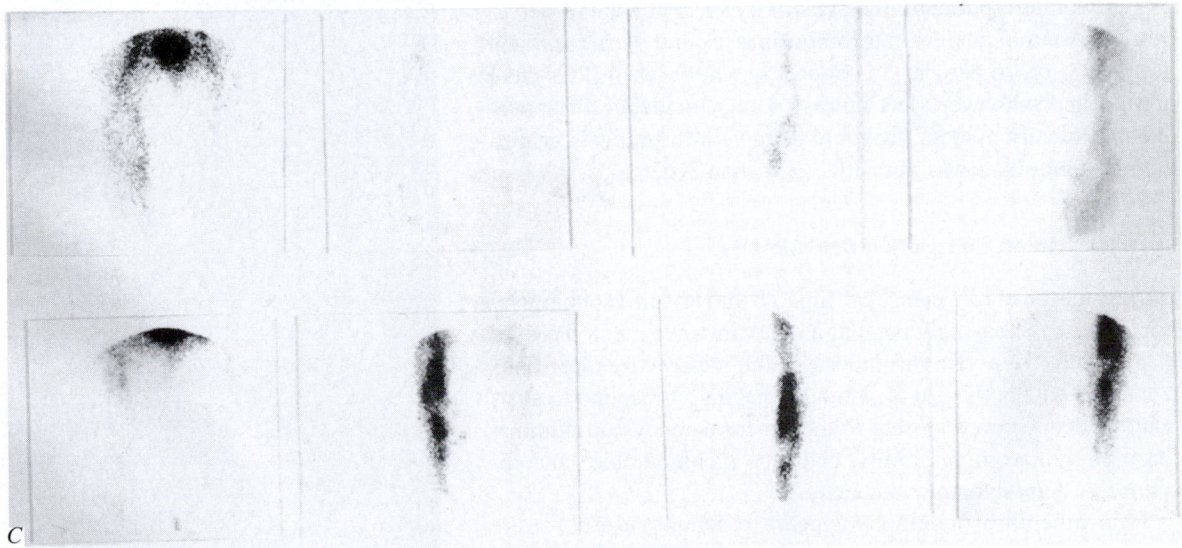

C

FIGURE 84-19 *A.* Venogram, right leg, single view of the popliteal fossae and calf, shows poor filling of all but a single anterior tibial branch. An acute thrombus is seen in the saphenous vein as well as a suggestion of clot, probably in a sural vein. The deep venous system is not opacified, probably because of acute deep venous thrombosis. *B.* Venogram, right leg, single view of the proximal thigh, shows extensive deep vein thrombus and collaterals (suggestive of a chronic process), as well as acute thrombus in the superficial femoral vein. *C.* Antifibrin images. The images in the top row were obtained within 2 h of completion of the venogram shown in *A* and *B;* the images on the bottom row were obtained 24 h later. In each row, the two images on the left are posterior views and the two images on the right are anterior view. They show extensive uptake in the calf, popliteal, and thigh veins, confirming (and matching) the venographic diagnosis of extensive thrombosis. The fact that the patient was not anticoagulated while being imaged with radiolabeled antibody may explain the intense incorporation of the antibody into the clots on the 24-h images. *(Based on data of Alavi et al,[1] with permission.)*

sets and reactions to the injection of large amounts of contrast media. Moreover, in up to 10 to 20 percent of patients, the result may be inadequate for interpretation. Occasionally, phlebography aggravates a phlebitis or precipitates local thrombosis. Finally, it is both expensive and unsuitable for repeated testing.

Noninvasive Methods

Over the past few years, the armamentarium for the diagnosis of deep vein thrombosis has increased considerably, particularly with respect to noninvasive techniques.[18] Although these have proved useful, they have not yet replaced contrast venography as the gold standard. Among these new techniques are impedance plethysmography, real-time (B-mode) ultrasonography, radiolabeled antibody imaging, and magnetic resonance venography. The first two of these are accurate only for clots at or proximal to the popliteal fossae. This does not limit their clinical utility, as those proximal veins are the source of most clinically significant emboli. Radiolabeled antibody imaging and magnetic resonance venography can evaluate the entire venous system for thrombus; this is a potential advantage favoring further development of these techniques.

IMPEDANCE PLETHYSMOGRAPHY

Of the noninvasive techniques available for the diagnosis of deep vein thrombosis, impedance plethysmography (IPG) is the oldest and the best validated. The method is excellent for detection of proximal deep vein thrombosis but is not useful for the detection of thrombus in calf veins. Although serial IPG is of limited value for diagnosing thrombosis in the calf veins, it is useful in detecting proximal propagation of calf vein thrombi. In symptomatic patients, the sensitivity of IPG for the detection of proximal deep vein thrombosis is around 95 percent and its specificity, 96 percent. In patients in whom serial IPGs were normal and who were left untreated, the incidence of subsequent clinically evident proximal deep vein thrombosis or pulmonary embolism was very low (less than 3 percent).[28]

REAL-TIME (B-MODE) ULTRASONOGRAPHY

During the past 15 years, real-time (B-mode) ultrasonography has become increasingly popular as a noninvasive method for the diagnosis of deep vein thrombosis in the lower extremity.[2] This technique entails the use of B-mode imaging ultrasound to evaluate the deep venous system of the leg for patency, intraluminal thrombi, vein compressibility, evidence of blood flow, and response to hemodynamic maneuvers.

Real-time ultrasonography appears to be most useful for the diagnosis of femoral or popliteal deep vein thrombosis; it is neither accurate nor reliable for thrombi in the calf or iliac veins. Unfortunately, the diagnostic yield from this method is operator dependent. Therefore, it is unclear whether the favorable sensitivities and specificities reported from some medical centers are achievable in conventional practice. In most published reports, the sensitivity and specificity of the method for detecting proximal deep vein thrombosis have varied from 78 to 100 percent. For the femoral and popliteal veins, the reported sensitivities range from 88 to 100 percent. However, sensitivities as low as 54 percent have also been reported. Real-time ultrasonography has the potential advantage of being able to identify nonthrombotic causes of leg swelling (e.g., Baker's cyst).

Although this technique does appear promising in most patients for the noninvasive diagnosis of proximal deep vein thrombosis of the lower extremities, real-time ultrasonography is not recommended as the sole study on which to base therapeutic decisions. A cost-effectiveness analysis has suggested that as an individual study, duplex ultrasonography is less cost-effective than IPG in evaluating symptomatic patients suspected of having deep vein thrombosis. Combining an initial duplex study with serial follow-up IPG is recommended as the most cost-effective noninvasive strategy.[30]

MAGNETIC RESONANCE VENOGRAPHY

Magnetic resonance (MR) venography is highly accurate for the diagnosis of deep vein thrombosis, the sensitivity and specificity being comparable to those of ascending contrast venography.[14] Unlike ultrasonography, the technique is not operator dependent. MR venography does not require venous access or the injection

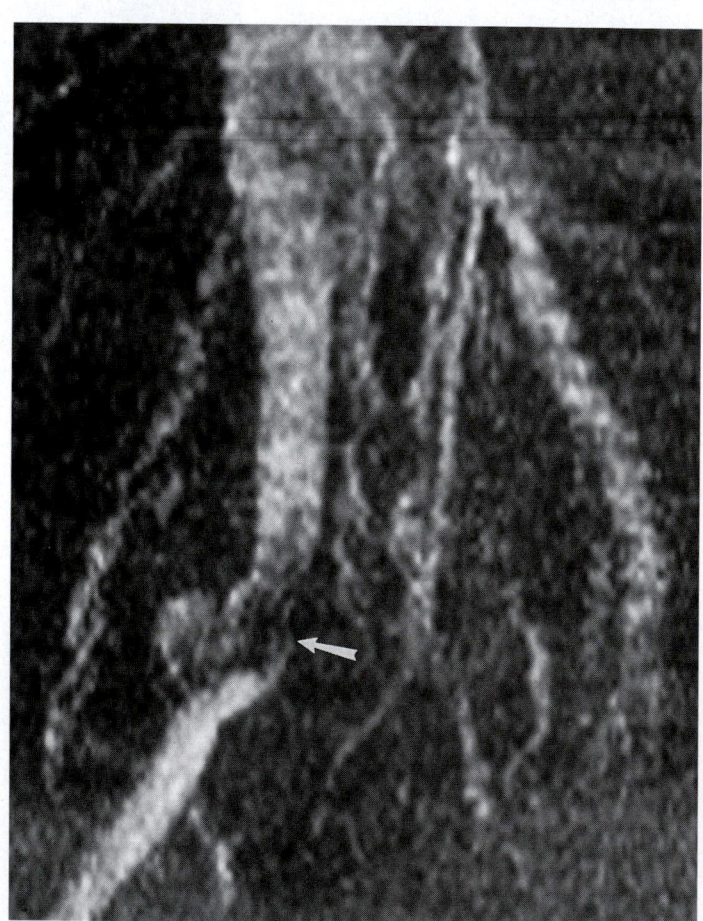

FIGURE 84-20 Gradient-recalled echo MRI of lower inferior vena cava and iliac veins in a 26-year woman with 3 weeks of progressive left leg pain and swelling. Oblique image demonstrates thrombus in the right common iliac vein (arrow) and complete absence of visualization of the left iliac system due to extensive thrombosis. Collateral vessels are visualized.

of contrast agents. MR venography is more sensitive than ultrasonography for lower-extremity deep vein thrombosis, since this technique can adequately image inferior vena cava pelvic veins, the common femoral vein, and the superficial femoral vein in the adductor canal; these areas are difficult to visualize with ultrasonography (Fig. 84-20). MR venography of the pelvis and lower extremities offers an optimal noninvasive method for evaluating and quantifying deep vein thrombosis. It also has potential use in the noninvasive algorithm described below, particularly when coupled with MR angiography of the pulmonary vascular bed.

RADIOLABELED-ANTIBODY IMAGING

The recent development of monoclonal antibodies specific for activated components of the thrombotic process has provided another noninvasive approach to the diagnosis of venous thrombosis. Although a number of different antibodies are being developed, those directed against the NH_2-terminal region of fibrin and against glycoprotein IIb/IIIa complex on platelets have been most intensively studied.

In initial clinical trials, these antibodies, tagged with radiolabel, have demonstrated excellent (greater than 90 percent) sensitivity in detecting thrombosis in both the thigh and calf, particularly in patients not receiving anticoagulants (Fig. 84-19).[1] Such tagged antibodies bind to the entire length of the thrombus and are easily detected by scanning with a gamma camera. Therefore, this technique holds promise of estimating the total extent of clot in the lower extremities instead of providing only positive or negative results for deep vein thrombosis. Initial clinical trials have demonstrated that these antibodies can be safely administered by a peripheral venous injection. However, since they are foreign proteins, most often murine in origin, there is a potential for sensitization. Although initial results have been encouraging, additional clinical trials, large-scale and prospective, are necessary before the use of these antibodies can be endorsed for routine clinical practice.

agnosis and accurate assessment of the extent of the thromboembolic disease.

Basis for the Approach

Certain key observations underlie the approach to management.

1. The vast majority (more than 90 percent) of pulmonary emboli originate as deep vein thrombosis of the lower extremities.
2. Recurrent emboli are associated with proximal deep vein thrombosis, whereas recurrent emboli are rare if there is no proximal deep vein thrombosis.
3. A high-probability lung scan, especially when clinical suspicion of thromboembolism is high and the patient has no history of thromboembolic disease, reliably establishes the presence of pulmonary emboli.
4. A "normal" perfusion scan or a low probability ventilation-perfusion scan is reliable for excluding pulmonary emboli when clinical suspicion of thromboembolism is low.
5. Noninvasive evaluation of the lower extremities (particularly by IPG), especially when repeated, can reliably establish or exclude the diagnosis of proximal deep vein thrombosis.
6. In patients in whom lung scans are not of high probability (Table 84-1) and in whom noninvasive evaluations (e.g., by IPG) of the lower extremities for deep vein thrombosis are negative, especially on successive testing, the prognosis is favorable, even if they are not anticoagulated.

Practicalities of the Approach

Patients who are clinically stable are screened with ventilation-perfusion lung scans and IPG (Fig. 84-21). If both studies yield negative results, other causes of the patients' symptoms are likely. If the lung scan is interpreted as *high probability*, and this interpretation is in keeping with clinical impression, or if the IPG is

APPROACH TO DIAGNOSIS

Integration of the advances and insights noted above has led to a practical approach that emphasizes, on one hand, the important role played by peripheral venous thrombosis in pulmonary embolism and, on the other, the assessment, noninvasively, of the amount of the clot, both in the legs and in the lungs.[37] The approach presupposes stability of the respiration and circulation and is applicable to current conventional therapeutic techniques (e.g., the use of heparin as an anticoagulant). If thrombolytic therapy is being considered, however, the use of invasive diagnostic tests has to be weighed more seriously than usual, since thrombolytic therapy entails hazards that call for considerable confidence in the diagnosis.

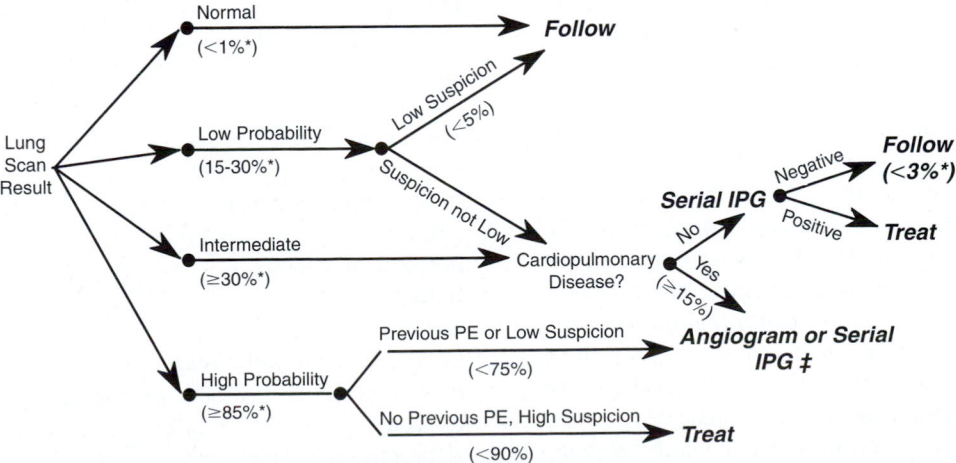

FIGURE 84-21   Approach to management of pulmonary thromboembolism. The likelihood of pulmonary embolism is indicated in parentheses.
*Strongly supported by clinical studies.
†Suggested by clinical studies, needs confirmation.
‡A serially negative impedance plethysmography result may not be sufficient to rule out thromboembolism.   *(Based on data of Kelley MA et al,[37] with permission.)*

positive, the patient should be treated for venous thromboembolic disease. If the lung scan is *non–high probability* (but not normal) and the patient is clinically stable, the decision to treat is often based on the results of IPG: if IPG is negative, particularly on repeated testing, the risk of recurrent thromboembolism is small and treatment for thrombotic disease need not be instituted. Thus, most clinically stable patients can be evaluated noninvasively for the presence of thromboembolic disease. Pulmonary angiography and venography are reserved for the unstable patient or the patient in whom the risks of anticoagulation or thrombolytic therapy are so high that certainty in diagnosis is necessary.

This algorithm has been validated in the outcome studies described above.[33,34] It has been suggested that this approach would decrease the number of pulmonary angiograms needed for the evaluation of patients suspected of pulmonary embolism by approximately 60 percent.[54] Whether newer, less invasive diagnostic methods (e.g., real-time ultrasonography, CT or MR imaging, and monoclonal antibody imaging) can be substituted for invasive procedures is uncertain.

TREATMENT

The treatment of venous thromboembolism can be categorized according to the goal of therapy: (1) prevention of the development of thrombus (i.e., prophylaxis); (2) prevention of clot propagation or recurrence (i.e., anticoagulation); (3) direct treatment of major thromboembolism in unstable patients (i.e., thrombolysis or embolectomy); or (4) removing unresolved thromboembolic material after it has been organized (i.e., thromboendarterectomy).

Prophylaxis

Prophylaxis should be utilized in many common medical conditions and after most surgical procedures lasting longer than 30 minutes (Table 84-6).

Mechanical means for prophylaxis are directed primarily toward limiting venous stasis. Elevating the foot of the bed, encouraging performance of leg exercises, frequent position changes, and gradient elastic stockings are advocated but have never been validated. Intermittent external pneumatic compression of the calf and sometimes the thigh has been shown in selected patients to be as effective as pharmacologic therapy in preventing thrombosis.[32] In some patients—e.g., those with gynecologic malignancy—the combination of pneumatic compression and low-dose heparin administered subcutaneously has been more effective in prophylaxis than has either method alone.

Heparin is the designation for a group of sulfated mucopolysaccharides that exert an antithrombotic effect only when a naturally occurring α_2-globulin inhibitor, antithrombin III, is present. Heparin markedly accelerates the irreversible inhibition of factors IXa, Xa, and thrombin.[6] Less heparin is needed to prevent than to treat a thrombotic process. Because biologic amplification occurs in the coagulation cascade, the amount of heparin needed to inhibit coagulation factors is 1000 times less than that needed to inactivate thrombin.[6]

The recommended dose of heparin for prevention of thromboembolic complications is 5000 units, administered subcutaneously. This therapy is begun 2 h before surgery and is administered thereafter every 8 to 12 h until the patient is either fully ambulatory or discharged. Although this regimen is effective as a prophylactic measure, it is not effective in treating an established thrombotic process.[9]

Standard heparin preparations are effective in preventing the propagation of venous clot. These preparations are polydispersed and composed of heparins that vary considerably in molecular size. Unfortunately, the use of polydispersed heparin is often associated with bleeding complications and with platelet-related side effects (e.g., thrombocytopenia). Recently, low-molecular-weight heparin fractions have been prepared from standard heparin. Low-molecular-weight heparin fractions appear to be as effective as unfractionated heparin in preventing venous thrombosis but cause less bleeding because of a lesser inhibitory effect on platelet function.[55]

Determination of antifactor Xa activity, rather than the activated partial thromboplastin time (aPTT), is used to guide low-molecular-weight heparin therapy because the anticoagulant properties of the low-molecular-weight heparins reside in the an-

---

TABLE 84-6

Common Surgical Procedures and Medical Conditions Predisposing to Deep Venous Thrombosis and Pulmonary Embolism

Surgical procedures
  General surgery in patients > 40 years
  Orthopedic surgery of the lower extremities
  Urologic surgery
  Gynecology and obstetrics
  Neurosurgery
  Trauma*
Medical conditions†
  Low cardiac output states
  Prior thromboembolism
  Obesity
  Polycythemia vera
  Immobilization
  Stroke
  Inflammatory bowel disease
  Paroxysmal nocturnal hemoglobinuria
  Cancer
  Nephrotic syndrome
  Estrogen therapy
  Sepsis
  Lupus anticoagulant

*Especially fractured hip in the elderly and acute injury of the head and spinal cord.
†Other than inherited deficiencies of inhibitors or regulators of coagulation or fibrinolysis.
SOURCE: Based on Consensus Development Conference, National Institutes of Health, March 1986.

tifactor Xa activity. For the low-molecular-weight heparin fractions, an inverse relationship exists between anticoagulant activity (as measured by antifactor Xa) and molecular size.

Anticoagulation

HEPARIN

In most patients, anticoagulation with an intravenous infusion of heparin should be initiated upon suspicion of pulmonary embolism.[25] This therapy should be maintained while diagnostic studies are under way and should not be discontinued until either the evaluation for venous thromboembolism is completed (and negative) or alternative therapies are started.

The dose of heparin that is required depends on the rate of at which the patient metabolizes heparin (a rate that is quite variable) and on the patient's coagulant activity. This requirement accounts for the common finding of large heparin requirements ("heparin resistance") early in pulmonary embolism. In the past, patients were often underdosed with heparin, and substantial delays occurred before adequate prolongation of the aPTT was achieved. This led to the introduction of weight-based dosing nomograms for heparin.[49] The heparin infusion is continued until the patient is adequately anticoagulated with warfarin (see below) or is switched to adjusted-dose subcutaneous heparin therapy for maintenance therapy.[25] Close monitoring of the aPTT, with appropriate adjustments of the heparin infusion, is necessary during the infusion. If bleeding should occur, the heparin infusion is discontinued; if bleeding is severe, heparin can be rapidly neutralized by administration of protamine.

WARFARIN

The time-honored maintenance therapy for deep venous thrombosis and pulmonary embolism has been warfarin, administered orally, with the prothrombin time (PT) used to monitor dosage. Originally, the target PT was one and a half times to twice the control value. However, this regimen was associated with an increasing frequency of bleeding complications. The cause of the increase proved to be a decrease in the sensitivity of the thromboplastin used as test reagent for determining the PT; this unsuspected decrease in sensitivity of the test reagent led, in turn, to the use of higher doses of warfarin to achieve the same prolongation of the PT. In order to control for the variation in the thromboplastins, the PT is now reported both as a time in seconds and as an International Normalized Ratio (INR). The therapeutic range for warfarin therapy of venous thromboembolism is an INR of 2.0 to 3.0.[15]

The antithrombotic action of the vitamin K antagonists that function as oral anticoagulants is not fully effective for about 5 days—the time required for all of the vitamin K–dependent coagulant factors (II, VII, IX, X) to fall to levels that bring the INR to the therapeutic range. Therefore, heparin is continued for 3 to 5 days after warfarin is begun, to allow time for the oral anticoagulant to take effect. The INR should be in the therapeutic range for 2 consecutive days before the heparin infusion is discontinued.

How long warfarin therapy should be continued remains controversial; longer therapy is required for patients who have ongoing risks of thrombosis. The standard treatment is for 3 to 6 months.

Warfarin interacts with many agents. Therefore, consideration of the possibility of enhancement or inhibition of anticoagulation by other medications must be made before warfarin or concurrent medication is started.

The effects of warfarin can be reversed with fresh frozen plasma or vitamin K. The fresh frozen plasma acts more rapidly but is shorter-lived. Vitamin K use may complicate efforts to re-anticoagulate a patient.

LOW-MOLECULAR-WEIGHT HEPARINS

Several low-molecular-weight heparin preparations are currently available. They differ in size distribution and in how they are fractionated.[62] However, all formulations have longer half-lives than unfractionated heparin, and their dose response is more predictable. They also have a lower rate of inducing immune thrombocytopenia.[59] These properties have made possible the intermittent subcutaneous administration of the low-molecular-weight heparins without need for routine laboratory monitoring.[55]

Initial randomized trials of low-molecular-weight heparins versus unfractionated heparin in the initial management of deep vein thrombosis have suggested that low-molecular-weight heparin is at least as effective, with less recurrence of thrombosis and less bleeding.[39,53] Other trials have indicated that outpatient treatment of the person with proximal deep vein thrombosis with subcutaneous low-molecular-weight heparin is as safe and effective as inpatient treatment with intravenous unfractionated heparin.[41] The implications of this finding with respect to the cost of health care and the quality of life are considerable.

At present, even though the low-molecular-weight heparin preparations do appear to be effective and less apt to cause bleeding complications than do the standard heparin preparations, further investigation is necessary before these preparations can replace conventional heparin in routine clinical practice.

OTHER AGENTS UNDER INVESTIGATION

Natural and recombinant hirudins and synthetic thrombin inhibitors are being studied for the prophylaxis and treatment of venous thrombophlebitis. In animal models, both the incidence of venous thrombosis and the size of thrombi have been decreased with the use of these substances. The recombinant hirudins prolong both the aPTT and the bleeding time less than does an equivalent antithrombotic dose of heparin. Although these preliminary results are encouraging, the role of these agents in the management of venous thromboembolism remains to be defined.

Thrombolytic Therapy

Perhaps the most controversial aspect of the management of deep vein thrombosis and pulmonary embolism is the role of thrombolytic therapy. Because of the advent of new thrombolytic agents and the interest in clot dissolution prompted by advances in coronary thrombolysis, the use and role of the

TABLE 84-7

Thrombolytic Therapy for Venous Thromboembolism

Agent	Plasma Clearance ($t_{1/2}$), min	Relative Fibrin Binding	Loading Dose	Hourly Dose	Recommended Duration
Streptokinase (SK)	18–25	Minimal	250,000 IU over 30 min	100,000 IU/h	PE: 24 h DVT: 48–72 h
Urokinase (UK)	13–20	Low	4400 IU/kg over 10 min	4400 IU/kg/h	PE: 12 h DVT: not approved
Tissue-type plasminogen activator (t-PA)	2–6	Moderate	None	50 mg/h	PE: 2 h DVT: not approved

NOTE: PE = pulmonary embolism; DVT = deep vein thrombosis; IU = international units.

agents in treating venous thromboembolic disease continue to be assessed.

Currently, three thrombolytic agents approved by the Food and Drug Administration are available for the treatment of pulmonary embolism: streptokinase, urokinase, and recombinant tissue-type plasminogen activator (Table 84-7).

Streptokinase and urokinase are exogenous systemic activators of the thrombolytic system. Streptokinase is derived from β-hemolytic streptococci, while urokinase is purified from human urine or from human kidney cells in culture. Through different mechanisms, these agents convert circulating plasminogen to plasmin. Streptokinase must first bind to circulating plasminogen before becoming an enzyme capable of cleaving additional plasminogen; urokinase is itself a plasminogen activator. Doses of streptokinase and urokinase sufficient to cause fibrinolysis of thrombi also generate circulating free plasmin that overwhelms and depletes α_2-antiplasmin and other plasma inhibitors. As a result, systemic hemostasis is impaired because of degradation of circulating fibrinogen and other coagulation proteins and because of an increase in fibrin degradation products. Although these exogenous agents dissolve clots, they also anticoagulate the patient, systemically engendering the risk of hemorrhage—particularly from previous sites of injury and invasion, such as arterial puncture. Streptokinase is antigenic, and it requires a loading dose to overcome neutralizing antibodies resulting from prior streptococcal infections.

The Urokinase Pulmonary Embolism Trials, conducted by the National Institutes of Health in the early 1970s, clearly demonstrated that the major advantage of thrombolytic therapy is more rapid clearance of clot from pulmonary arteries.[56] In 1980, the demonstration of a more normal $D_{L_{CO}}$ in patients treated with thrombolytic therapy than in those treated with heparin led to the suggestion that the pulmonary microcirculation is better preserved after thrombolytic therapy than after standard heparin anticoagulation. More recent follow-up of the same patients found that those treated with thrombolytic agents had lower mean pulmonary arterial pressures and pulmonary vascular resistance at rest and during exercise than did patients treated with heparin.[52] The hemodynamic differences were modest, however, and their practical implications are unclear.

In contrast to streptokinase and urokinase, which induce a systemic thrombolytic state in order to dissolve a local clot, tissue-type plasminogen activator affords the prospect of lysing clots by forming the active protease plasmin primarily within the clot.

Fibrinolysis occurs spontaneously when an endogenous serum protease—i.e., blood- or tissue-type plasminogen activator (t-PA)—binds (with high affinity) to a fibrin clot; fibrin-bound plasminogen is then activated to plasmin, which dissolves the clot. In *physiological* amounts, t-PA does not bind to circulating plasminogen. Therefore, it does not produce circulating plasmin, which would induce systemic fibrinolysis or fibrinogenolysis. Nor are circulating inhibitors of plasmin, particularly α_2-antiplasmin, depleted by the clot selective action of t-PA. Indeed, it seems as though the plasmin that is generated locally by t-PA is protected from the circulating α_2-antiplasmin by the thrombus and its environment. In principle, t-PA, because of its intense affinity for fibrin, should have its lytic effects restricted to fibrin in thrombi. At pharmacologic doses, however, some degree of systemic fibrinolysis is the rule.

Proper dosage of t-PA is a critical element in avoidance complications. The administration of 0.50 to 0.75 mg/kg body weight intravenously generally evokes only slight systemic fibrinolysis and degradation of fibrinogen. Initially, t-PA was isolated from uterine tissue; later it was isolated from a cultured line of human melanoma cells. More recently, cloning and expression of the t-PA gene in *Escherichia coli* using recombinant DNA technology have made available large quantities of t-PA for clinical trials.

It is generally accepted that thrombolytic agents should be used in treating life-threatening pulmonary emboli, particularly if the emboli cause hemodynamic instability or respiratory compromise (Fig. 84-22).[16] Less certain is the role of thrombolytic therapy in dealing with submassive pulmonary emboli or large thrombi in proximal deep veins. It has been suggested that patients with large pulmonary emboli who demonstrate right heart dilatation on echocardiography should be treated with thrombolytic agents even in the absence of significant cardiopulmonary compromise.[10] This approach is currently under investigation.

Studies have looked at a variety of dosing protocols and routes of administration for thrombolytic therapy. For full therapeutic doses (Table 84-7), there is no difference in the rate of clot resolution or improvement in hemodynamic parameters when peripheral intravenous infusion of drug has been

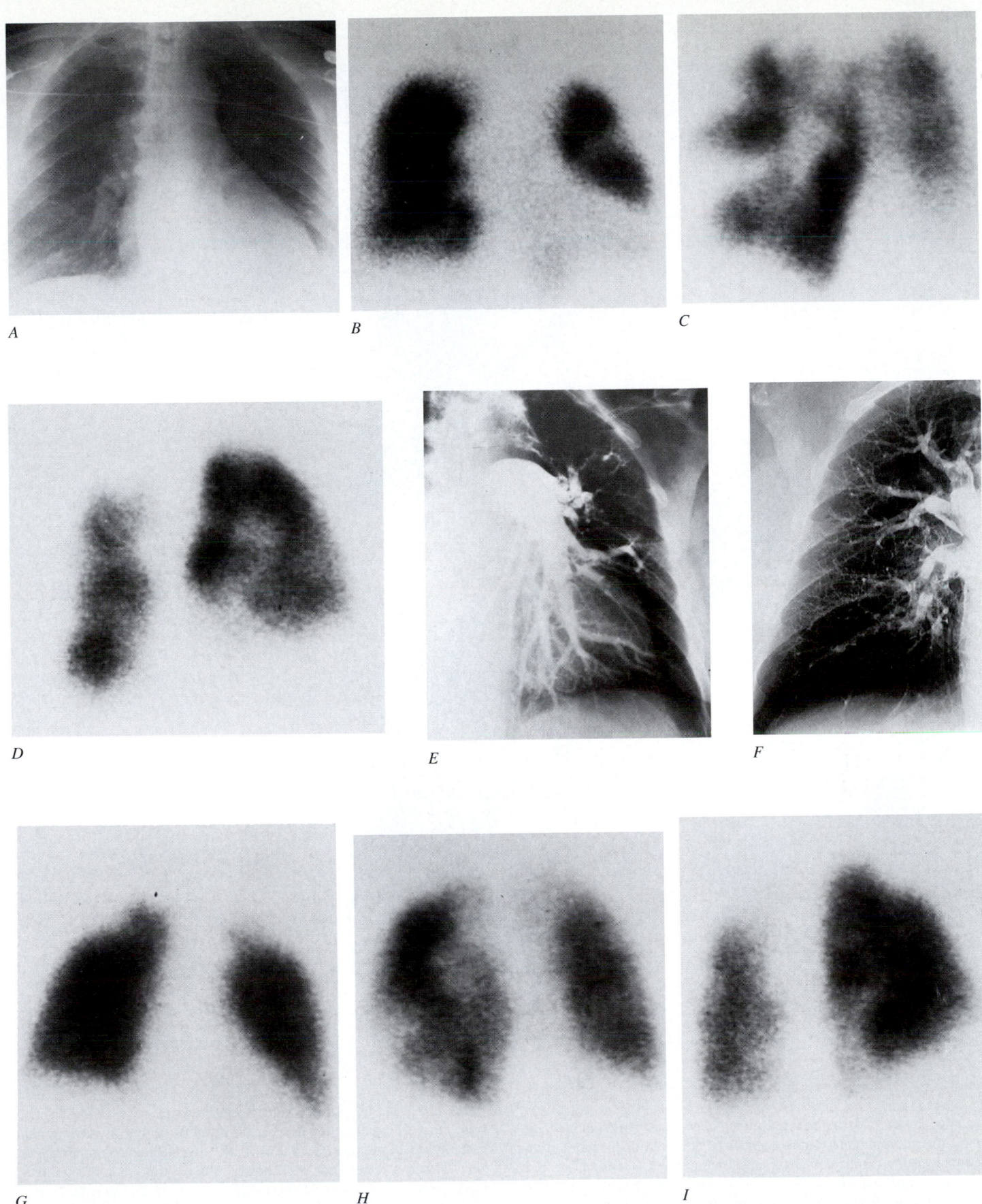

FIGURE 84-22 Streptokinase infusion for large pulmonary emboli in a 72-year-old woman with bilateral ankle fractures and sudden onset of severe dyspnea. *A.* Portable chest radiograph shows slight cardiomegaly and clear lung fields. *B, C,* and *D.* Perfusion scan shows multiple defects in both lungs, well shown in anterior (*B*), left posterior oblique (*C*), and right posterior oblique (*D*) views. Most defects are in the left lung. Ventilation scan (not shown) was normal. *E* and *F.* Pulmonary arteriogram. Multiple emboli are lodged at branching sites of left (*E*) and right (*F*) pulmonary arteries. *G, H,* and *I.* Four days after a 24-h infusion of streptokinase, the perfusion scan shows considerable improvement. Only small defects remain in the anterior (*G*), left posterior oblique (*H*), and right posterior oblique (*I*) projections.

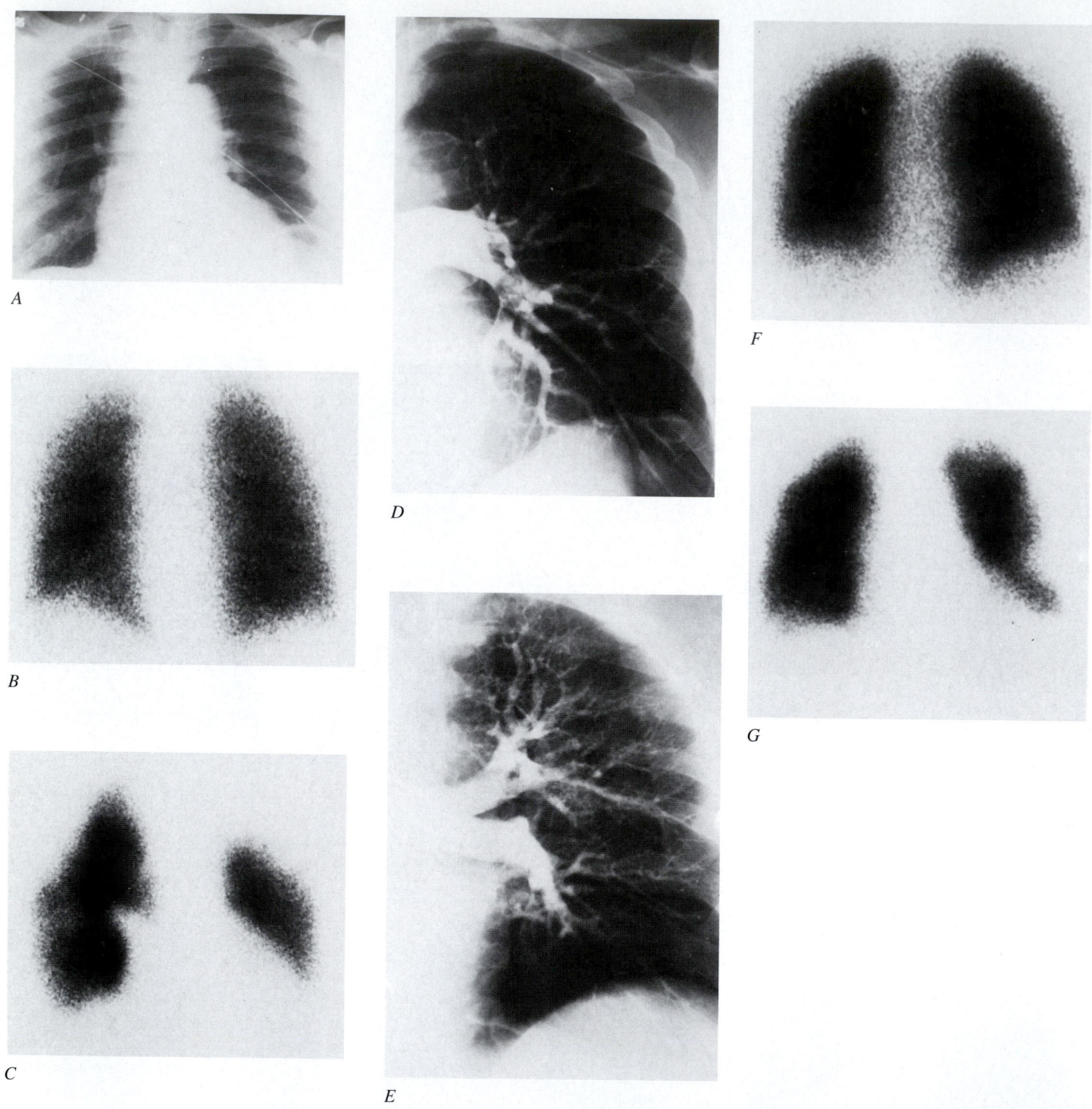

FIGURE 84-23   Tissue-type plasminogen activator (t-PA) in the treatment of acute pulmonary embolism. A 67-year-old man who had undergone an uncomplicated inguinal herniograph 2 weeks before presentation experienced sudden onset of moderate dyspnea and mild left-sided pleuritic chest pain on day of admission. *A*. Portable chest radiograph. *B* and *C*. Equilibrium phase of the initial ventilation lung scan (*B*) and anterior view of the initial perfusion lung scan (*C*). Ventilation-perfusion scan was interpreted as showing high probability for pulmonary embolism. The patient was heparinized before pulmonary angiography. Large pulmonary emboli occlude multiple lobar and segmental arteries of the left lung. Clot was also demonstrated in the right lung. The patient received an infusion of 40 mg of recombinant tissue-type plasminogen activator (rt-PA) over 40 min via a peripheral vein. This is a lesser dose and shorter infusion time than the standard FDA-approved t-PA dose of 100 mg infused over 2 h (Table 84-7). Pulmonary angiography was repeated 90 min after the start of the t-PA infusion. *E*. Post–t-PA pulmonary angiogram shows considerable resolution of the pulmonary emboli. *F* and *G*. Two days after the t-PA infusion, in the equilibrium phase of the follow-up ventilation lung scan (*F*), the anterior view of the follow-up perfusion lung scan (*G*) shows considerable improvement in the perfusion to both lungs.

compared with direct intrapulmonary installation.[58] Direct intrapulmonary infusion may allow for successful clot lysis with lower doses of the thrombolytic agent, thereby reducing the occurrence of systemic bleeding complications. This approach and intermittent bolus administration of the thrombolytic agent, as opposed to continuous intravenous infusion, are currently being studied.

Thrombolytic therapy has also been advocated for the treatment of proximal thrombi in the deep veins of the legs. Thrombolytic therapy results in more rapid and complete clearance of clot from the deep veins, and in better preservation of the venous valves, and seems to evoke fewer long-term complications (venous stasis and ulceration) than does heparin therapy.

However, enthusiasm for the use of thrombolytic therapy in venous thromboembolic disease is tempered by several practical considerations: (1) there have been only few long-term trials that compared thrombolytic therapy and conventional treatment with heparin; (2) thrombolytic therapy carries a greater risk of bleeding than does heparin therapy;[40] (3) the optimal dosage and regimen for thrombolytic therapy, either in pulmonary embolism or in deep vein thrombosis, have not yet been identified (Fig. 84-23); and (4) after a course of thrombolytic therapy, standard anticoagulation with intravenous heparin, followed by either oral warfarin or maintenance subcutaneous heparin, is necessary to prevent recurrent thromboemboli.

Interventional Radiologic Techniques

Rapid restoration of blood flow to the obstructed pulmonary vascular segments is important in patients with major pulmonary emboli. Techniques of mechanical clot disruption with various catheter devices have been described; they can disperse the clot to more distal locations within the pulmonary arterial tree,[4,50] reducing the obstruction of the pulmonary vasculature. Also, when combined with local thrombolytic therapy, the mechanical disruption may facilitate faster clot resolution. Techniques of clot extraction, including transvenous catheter embolectomy, have also been developed.[21] It should be noted that clot extraction techniques should not be employed in patients with an open a foramen ovale because of the potential for systemic embolization during the withdrawal of the catheter and thrombus through the right heart.

Surgical Management

A surgical approach to massive pulmonary embolism was proposed by Trendelenburg in 1908 and first successfully performed by Kirschner in 1924. Survival results were quite poor until the advent of cardiopulmonary bypass. Recent series had reported mortality for pulmonary embolectomy of 30 to 44 percent. Comparisons (nonrandomized) of surgical embolectomy with thrombolytic therapy appear to favor the surgical approach.[23] While the data are far from conclusive, it is clear that surgical embolectomy can serve as an alternative to thrombolytic therapy, especially in patients who have contraindications to thrombolysis or whose condition is too unstable to allow for a trial of medical therapy.[19,42]

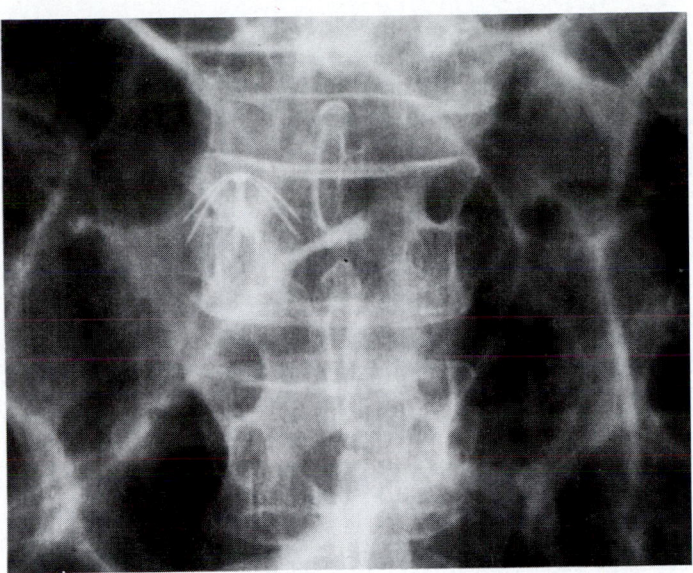

FIGURE 84-24   Umbrella for repeated thromboemboli in a 57-year-old woman with recurrent pulmonary emboli secondary to deep venous thrombosis in the extremities. An umbrella was placed in the inferior vena cava below the renal arteries.

Interruption of the inferior vena cava (IVC) to prevent recurrent pulmonary embolism was initially performed by ligation, plication, or clipping. These procedures have high morbidity and mortality, and they have been abandoned since the development of filter devices. IVC filters can be placed surgically or percutaneously (Fig. 84-24). Currently available filter devices are all quite effective; after placement of the filter, the incidence of pulmonary embolism is 1.9 to 2.4 percent.[3,20] Rarely do the filters occlude. They do not preclude subsequent MR imaging in field strengths of 1.5 Tesla, although some devices do create image artifacts.

PROGNOSIS

In acute pulmonary embolism, once therapeutic measures are taken to prevent further formation of thrombi (anticoagulation) or to deny thrombi in the legs access to the lungs (e.g., interruption or blockade of the IVC), death from embolism is uncommon.[5] Exceptions do occur, even after effective anticoagulation with heparin, particularly if associated disorders persist that predispose to recurrent thrombosis. Also, in some patients who have undergone interruption of the inferior vena cava by placement of a filter, emboli recur, presumably either by way of collateral venous channels or from a thrombus caught in, and propagating through, the IVC filter.

In massive emboli, as clots resolve by fragmentation, dislocation, and fibrinolysis, or are organized and contracted in situ, cardiac output improves, pulmonary artery pressures fall, and right ventricular pressures return to normal. Usually, pulmonary hemodynamics return to original levels in 2 to 8 weeks.

During 1-year follow-up of the patients proven to have pulmonary embolism in the PIOPED study, 23.8 percent of them died. However, only 2.5 percent of the total patient population died of pulmonary embolism (10.5 percent of all deaths), mainly in the setting of clinically suspected recurrent embolic events. Most of the deaths in the study population were attributable to cancer (24.7 percent), sepsis (22.1 percent), or cardiac disease (6.8 percent).[5]

Most surgical patients who are treated at the time of the first embolus recover completely. Chronically ill medical patients are more inclined to recurrence because the underlying disorder that predisposed to thrombosis persists. Exceedingly few patients who are treated go on to develop chronic cor pulmonale. Instead, chronic cor pulmonale is generally a sequela of unrecognized and untreated pulmonary emboli, underscoring the importance of recognizing pulmonary emboli and dealing with them promptly and effectively.

OTHER VARIETIES OF EMBOLIC DISEASE

Fat Emboli

The term *fat embolism* refers to a clinical syndrome of neurologic and respiratory abnormalities that occurs within 12 to 24 h after skeletal trauma, particularly if the injury entails multiple fractures. This syndrome occurs in about 5 percent of patients who have experienced severe and multiple orthopedic injuries: the patient develops fever, unexplained respiratory distress, mental confusion, and often a petechial rash over the body. This syndrome may be mild or progress to respiratory failure and coma. The lungs are the seat of noncardiac pulmonary edema, considerable intrapulmonary shunting, and a low compliance similar to that seen in the adult respiratory distress syndrome. The neurologic findings sometimes progress to stupor and coma without focal neurologic defects. At autopsy, fat deposits are found in many organs, particularly in the pulmonary arteries and the cerebral circulation.

Despite its name, the pathogenesis of fat embolism has not been proved to be the embolization of fat throughout the venous circulation. One suggested explanation is that fractures of the long bones disrupt intramedullary adipose tissue, which then extrudes into the venous circulation. A preferred alternative is that the trauma induces intravascular biochemical changes that cause circulating chylomicrons to aggregate into fat droplets, which, in turn, lodge in the terminal vasculature of various organs. Although there is evidence to support both alternatives, neither has been proved.

PATHOPHYSIOLOGY

The understanding of the end-organ damage caused by fat embolism is incomplete. In the lungs, deposition of the fatty aggregates in the small muscle arteries and arterioles can increase pulmonary artery pressures sufficiently to evoke cor pulmonale. A capillary leak syndrome occurs in fat embolism, presumably due to lysis of the fatty aggregates by lung lipases to form free fatty acids. Thrombocytopenia and the resultant petechiae occur in the fat embolism syndrome, possibly secondary to platelet aggregation by the circulating fat.

CLINICAL FEATURES

The diagnosis of fat embolism syndrome should be considered in any patient who, after severe trauma or orthopedic surgery, develops respiratory distress, mental confusion, or petechiae within 3 days of injury. The rash is usually found in the upper part of the body, including axillae, chest, flanks, conjunctivae, and, at other times, the soft palate. Fever and tachycardia are common. Occasionally, fat can be seen in the retinal vessels.

The hematologic picture is nonspecific. Although increased levels of serum lipase and lipiduria are common in the fat embolism syndrome, these abnormalities are nondiagnostic, since they may occur after any trauma. The chest radiograph is generally normal in the early stages of disease, but it may soon demonstrate the picture of noncardiac pulmonary edema. The arterial blood gases are often abnormal (low P_{O_2}, low P_{CO_2}) despite a normal chest radiograph.

DIAGNOSIS

No single clinical feature or laboratory test establishes the diagnosis of the fat embolism syndrome.[38] However, certain diagnostic hints are useful. The fat embolism syndrome rarely occurs beyond the third day after bony trauma. Arterial hypoxemia, although nonspecific, occurs almost invariably in the fat embolism syndrome. Petechial rash, described above, strongly suggests the disorder. Although high concentrations of lipase in serum are not diagnostic, they may be useful as confirmatory evidence.

TREATMENT

Treatment of the fat embolism syndrome is largely supportive, directed at ensuring proper hydration, managing respiratory manifestations, and dealing with the underlying trauma. None of these measures has any bearing on preventing fat embolism. However, in a prospective study, corticosteroids, given to high-risk patients within 12 h after skeletal trauma, proved effective in reducing the incidence of the fat embolism syndrome.[57] Anecdotal reports also suggest that corticosteroids may be beneficial even after the fat embolism syndrome has developed.

Prevention of the fat embolism syndrome may be possible during orthopedic surgery, particularly involving the hip. One approach is by venting of the intramedullary canal during the insertion of a hip arthroplasty prosthesis.

Air Embolism

Air embolism is a potentially life-threatening disorder in which a large bolus of air that is introduced into the venous circulation travels to the pulmonary circulation. When severe, air embolism can result in total pulmonary arterial obstruction, circulatory collapse, and sudden death.[11] Occasionally, air makes its way into the systemic circulation through either the lungs or a patent foramen ovale, causing infarction in a systemic end-organ, particularly in the central nervous system.

Air embolism may complicate a variety of clinical conditions, including chest injury, instrumentation of central veins, surgery, and hemodialysis. Both the volume and the rate of air introduction are important in producing acute circulatory collapse: a smaller volume injected rapidly into circulation as a bolus may cause as much damage as a larger volume that is introduced slowly. In some patients, the air embolism syndrome is accompanied by noncardiac pulmonary edema and disseminated intravascular coagulation.

The diagnosis of air embolism should be suspected whenever air is accidentally introduced into the venous circulation, particularly when the patient suddenly experiences circulatory collapse. Immediate efforts at resuscitation are directed toward minimizing the volume of the air in the pulmonary circulation: the patient is immediately turned on his or her left side and placed in a head-down (Trendelenburg) position so that the air bubble will remain within the right heart. A central venous or right heart catheter may prove useful in aspirating air from the right side of the circulation. If these efforts and immediate resuscitation prove fruitless, direct open cardiac massage may be successful in restoring the circulation.

More problematic is the continued presence of small air bubbles within the venous and arterial circulations after air embolization. To dissolve these bubbles, the patient is placed immediately on 100 percent oxygen and, if possible, moved to a hyperbaric facility (see Chapter 64). Under hyperbaric conditions, the bubble size can be rapidly reduced. To be most effective, hyperbaric therapy should be instituted promptly.

Amniotic Fluid Embolism

Amniotic fluid embolism is a catastrophic although infrequent complication of labor and delivery. It is characterized by the sudden onset of respiratory distress, cyanosis, central nervous system irritability and seizures, and cardiovascular collapse. Maternal mortality ranges from 60 to 80 percent, with fetal mortality of 40 to 60 percent.[7]

The syndrome is a consequence of amniotic fluid and its cellular components entering the circulation and embolizing to the lungs. The pathophysiology is not a consequence of obstructing the pulmonary vascular bed but, rather, the activation of leukotrienes, prostaglandins, and other vasoactive substances. Endothelin appears to be released, and coagulation cascades activated. The clinical picture resembles anaphylaxis or septic shock more than it does venous thrombosis.

Until recently, the hemodynamic compromise was attributed to the acute development of pulmonary hypertension and right heart failure. Hemodynamic measurements made early in the syndrome now suggest that cardiac function is compromised: decreased left ventricular function and increased left ventricular end-diastolic pressure result in the pulmonary edema and elevated pulmonary arterial pressures.

Treatment is supportive; mechanical ventilation with positive end-expiratory pressure is often required. Based on the suggestion of left heart dysfunction, it is now recommended that diuresis and inotropic support be used in preference to vasodilators. Disseminated intravascular coagulation and bleeding are usually of only short duration, and are managed by transfusion of blood components (e.g., fresh frozen plasma, platelets, and red blood cells).

Sickle Cell Disease

Sickle cell disease affects the lungs by causing local thrombosis and occasionally by embolization of bone marrow elements.

Small pulmonary arteries, arterioles, and capillaries are generally affected. Thrombosis in the pulmonary circulation is part of the general proclivity of red blood cells containing S hemoglobin to sickle under appropriate circumstances, particularly hypoxia; stagnation and clotting follow sickling. In some instances, the thrombus organizes, the vascular lumen is obliterated, and perivascular fibrosis ensues in the adjacent lung; in others, the thrombus recanalizes. Occasionally, infarction occurs.

PATHOPHYSIOLOGY

Of the factors that predispose in thrombosis in the lungs in sickle cell disease, the most important is the low P_{O_2} of mixed venous blood. Not only is the mixed venous P_{O_2} inordinately low but also the O_2 dissociation curve is shifted to the right, thereby handicapping O_2 uptake in the lungs.

Any pulmonary disease that causes alveolar hypoventilation or hypoxemia of blood in the lungs of persons with sickle cell disease favors sickling and thrombosis. Since patients with sickle cell disease are prone to intercurrent pulmonary infections, particularly pneumonia and tuberculosis, they are predisposed to local areas of alveolar hypoventilation and hypoxia. Patients with severe sickle cell anemia and large fractions of hemoglobin S in their red blood cells are particularly susceptible to intense sickling and thrombosis anywhere, including the lungs. However, vulnerability is not restricted to states of hemoglobin S. In some heterozygous sickle states—e.g., hemoglobin SC, S-thalassemia, and hemoglobin SA—enough hemoglobin S is present to cause extensive thrombosis and infarction during an episode of severe hypoxemia, during acidosis, or during septicemia associated with fever and leukocytosis.

CLINICAL FEATURES

The clinical picture of pulmonary infarction in patients with sickle cell disease can mimic or coexist with bronchopneumonia.[60] The latter may promote local hypoxia, which leads to in situ pulmonary thrombosis. An episode often begins with poorly defined or pleuritic chest pain, fever, and sputum that is blood streaked but fails to disclose any specific bacterial cause. A fleeting episode of breathlessness is usually overlooked. Cyanosis is rare because of the severe anemia. The subsequent course is characterized by an unconvincing response to antibiotics and slow clearing; often a linear scar in the lungs remains as a residue of the infarction. Suspicion of infarction should be high in any black person with hemoglobin S and in white people of Greek or Italian descent with S-thalassemia.

Sometimes, occlusive disease is sufficiently extensive to cause pulmonary hypertension and cor pulmonale.[8] For this sequence to evolve, many severe episodes of sickling are required. The cor pulmonale that results is unusual because of its association with a high cardiac output (due to the anemia) and with the intrinsic myocardial damage that generally complicates sickle cell disease.

MANAGEMENT

Management of the patient with pulmonary thrombosis and infarction in sickle cell disease relies heavily on experience with the disease. Few specific measures can be advocated other than conventional supportive treatment. Distinguishing between in situ thrombosis and thromboembolism can be difficult clinically and even with invasive procedures such as angiography, although in situ thrombosis tends to be in small, distal vessels. Moreover, because radiographic contrast materials may promote sickling, they have to be used cautiously. To complicate matters, some patients with sickle cell disease are also at increased risk of thromboemboli because of predisposing factors, such as bed rest, congestive heart failure, and dehydration.

Anticoagulants are generally not used in sickle cell disease, since there are no data to substantiate their effectiveness in treating in situ thrombosis.

REFERENCES

1. Alavi A, Palevsky HI, Gupta N, et al: Radiolabeled antifibrin antibody in the detection of venous thrombosis: Preliminary results. *Radiology* 175:79–85, 1990.

2. Becker DM, Philbrick JT, Abbitt PL: Real-time ultrasonography for the diagnosis of lower extremity deep venous thrombosis: The wave of the future? *Arch Intern Med* 149:1731–1740, 1989.

3. Becker DM, Philbrick JT, Selby JB: Inferior vena cava filters: Indications, safety, effectiveness. *Arch Intern Med* 152:1985–1994, 1992.

4. Brady AJB, Crake T, Oakley CM: Percutaneous catheter fragmentation and distal dispersion of proximal pulmonary embolus. *Lancet* 338:1186–1189, 1991.

5. Carson JL, Kelley MA, Duff A, et al: The clinical course of pulmonary embolism. *New Engl J Med* 326:1240–1245, 1992.

6. Cines DB: Heparin: Do we understand its antithrombotic activity? *Chest* 89:420–426, 1986.

7. Clark SC, Hankins GD, Dudley DA, et al: Amniotic fluid embolism: Analysis of the national registry. *Am J Obstet Gynecol* 172:1158–1167, 1995.

8. Collins FS, Orringer EP: Pulmonary hypertension and cor pulmonale in the sickle cell hemoglobinopathies. *Am J Med* 73:814–821, 1982.

9. Collins R, Scrimgeour A, Yusuf S, Peto R: Reduction in fatal pulmonary embolism and venous thrombosis by perioperative administration of subcutaneous heparin: Overview of results of randomized trials in general, orthopedic, and urologic surgery. *New Engl J Med* 318:1162–1173, 1988.

10. Come PC: Echocardiographic evaluation of pulmonary embolism and its response to therapeutic interventions. *Chest* 101(Suppl): 151S–162S, 1992.

11. Dudney TM, Elliott CG: Pulmonary embolism from amniotic fluid, fat and air. *Prog Cardiovasc Dis* 36:447–474, 1994.

12. Edwards WD: Pulmonary hypertension and related vascular disorders, in Stehbens WE, Lie JT (eds), *Vascular Pathology,* London, Chapman and Hall, 1995, pp 585–621.

13. Fedullo PF, Auger WR, Channick RN, et al: Chronic thromboembolic pulmonary hypertension. *Clin Chest Med* 16:353–374, 1995.

14. Gefter WB, Hatabu H, Holland GA, et al: Pulmonary thromboembolism: Recent developments in diagnosis with CT and MRI imaging. *Radiology* 197:561–574, 1995.

15. Ginsberg JS: Management of venous thromboembolism. *New Engl J Med* 335:1816–1828, 1996.

16. Goldhaber SZ: Recent advances in the diagnosis and lytic therapy of pulmonary embolism. *Chest* 99(Suppl):173S–179S, 1991.

17. Goodman LR, Curtin JJ, Mewissen MW, et al: Detection of pulmonary embolism in patients with unresolved clinical and scintigraphic diagnosis: Helical CT versus angiography. *Am J Radiol* 164:1369–1374, 1995.

18. Grant BJ: Noninvasive tests for acute venous thromboembolism. *Am J Respir Crit Care Med* 149:1044–1047, 1994.

19. Gray HH, Morgan JM, Paneth M, Miller GAH: Pulmonary embolectomy: Its place in the management of pulmonary embolism. *Lancet* 1:1441–1445, 1988.

20. Greenfield L: Caval interruption procedures, in Rutherford RB (ed), *Vascular Surgery.* Philadelphia, Saunders, 1995, pp 1815–1824.

21. Greenfield LJ, Proctor MD, Williams DM, Wakefiled TW: Long-term experience with transvenous catheter embolectomy. *J Vasc Surg* 18:450–453, 1993.

22. Greenspan RH: Pulmonary angiography and the diagnosis of pulmonary embolism. *Prog Cardiovasc Dis* 37:93–105, 1994.

23. Gulba DC, Schmid C, Borst HG, et al: Medical compared with surgical treatment for massive pulmonary embolism. *Lancet* 343:576–577, 1994.

24. Hirsh J, Prins MH, Samama M: Approach to the thrombophilic patient for hemostasis and thrombosis: Basic principles and clinical practice, in Coleman RW, Hirsh J, Marder VJ, Salzman EW (eds), *Hemostasis and Thrombosis: Basic Principles and Clinical Practice,* 3d ed. Philadelphia, Lippincott, 1995, pp 1543–1561.

25. Hommes DW, Bura A, Mazzolai L, et al: Subcutaneous heparin compared with continuous intravenous heparin administration in the initial treatment of deep vein thrombosis: A meta-analysis. *Ann Intern Med* 116:279–284, 1992.

26. Huet Y, Brun-Buisson C, Lemaire F, et al: Cardiopulmonary effects of ketanserin infusion in human pulmonary embolism. *Am Rev Respir Dis* 135:114–117, 1987.

27. Huisman MV, Buller HR, Ten Cate JW, et al: Unexpected high prevalence of silent pulmonary embolism in patients with deep venous thrombosis. *Chest* 95:498–502, 1989.

28. Huisman MV, Buller HR, Ten Cate JW, Vreeken J: Serial impedance plethysmography for suspected deep venous thrombosis in outpatients. *New Engl J Med* 314:823–828, 1986.

29. Hull RD, Hirsh J, Carter CJ, et al: Pulmonary angiography, ventilation lung scanning and venography for clinically suspected pulmonary embolism with abnormal perfusion lung scan. *Ann Intern Med* 98:891–899, 1983.

30. Hull RD, Feldstein W, Pineo GF, Raskob GE: Cost-effectiveness of diagnosis of deep vein thrombosis in symptomatic patients. *Thromb Haemost* 74:189–196, 1995.

31. Hull RD, Feldstein W, Stein PD, Pineo GF: Cost-effectiveness of pulmonary embolism diagnosis. *Arch Intern Med* 156:68–72, 1996.

32. Hull RD, Pineo GF: Intermittent pneumatic compression for the prevention of venous thromboembolism. *Chest* 109:6–9, 1996.

33. Hull RD, Raskob GE, Coates G, et al: A new noninvasive management strategy for patients with suspected pulmonary embolism. *Arch Intern Med* 149:2549–2555, 1989.

34. Hull RD, Raskob GE, Ginsberg JS, et al: A noninvasive strategy for the treatment of patients with suspected pulmonary embolism. *Arch Intern Med* 154:289–297, 1994.

35. Hull RD, Raskob GE, Panju AA: Clinical validity of a normal perfusion lung scan in patients with suspected pulmonary embolism. *Chest* 97:23–26, 1990.

36. Kelley MA, Abbuhl S. Massive pulmonary embolism. *Clin Chest Med* 15:547–560, 1994.

37. Kelley MA, Carson JL, Palevsky HI, Schwartz JS: Diagnosing pulmonary embolism: New facts and strategies. *Ann Intern Med* 114:300–306, 1991.

38. King MB, Harmon KR: Unusual forms of pulmonary embolism. *Clin Chest Med* 15:561–580, 1994.

39. Leizorovicz A, Simonneau G, Decousus H, Boissel JP: Comparison of efficacy and safety of low molecular weight heparins and unfractionated heparin in initial treatment of deep venous thrombosis: a meta-analysis. *Br Med J* 309:299–304, 1994.

40. Levine MN: Thrombolytic therapy for venous thromboembolism: Complications and contraindications. *Clin Chest Med* 16:321–328, 1995.

41. Levine M, Gent M, Hirsh J, et al: A comparison of low-molecular weight heparin administered primarily at home with unfractionated heparin administered in the hospital for proximal deep-vein thrombosis. *New Engl J Med* 334:677–681, 1996.

42. Lund O, Nielsen TT, Ronne K, Schifter S: Pulmonary embolism: Long-term follow-up after treatment with full-dose heparin, streptokinase or embolectomy. *Acta Med Scand* 221:61–71, 1987.

43. Malik AB, Johnson A: Role of humoral mediators in the pulmonary vascular response to the pulmonary embolism, in Weir E, Reeves JT (eds), *Pulmonary Vascular Physiology and Pathophysiology*. New York, Dekker, 1989, pp 445–468.

44. Moser KM: Venous thromboembolism: State of the art. *Am Rev Respir Dis* 141:235–249, 1990.

45. Moser KM: Diagnosing pulmonary embolism: D-dimer needs rigorous evaluation. *Br Med J* 309:1525–1526, 1994.

46. Palevsky HI: The problems of the clinical and laboratory diagnosis of pulmonary embolism. *Semin Nucl Med* 21:276–280, 1991.

47. The PIOPED Investigators: Value of the ventilation/perfusion scan in acute pulmonary embolism: Results of the Prospective Investigation of Pulmonary Embolism Diagnosis (PIOPED). *JAMA* 263:2753–2759, 1990.

48. Porter TR, Mohanty PK, Pandian NG: Intravascular ultrasound imaging of pulmonary arteries: Methodology, clinical applications and future potential. *Chest* 106:1551–1557, 1994.

49. Raschke RA, Reilly BM, Guidry JR, et al: The weight-based heparin dosing nomogram compared with a "standard care" nomogram: A randomized controlled trial. *Ann Intern Med* 119:874–881, 1993.

50. Schmidt-Rode T, Gunther RW: New device for percutaneous fragmentation of pulmonary emboli. *Radiology* 180:135–137, 1991.

51. Schonfeld SA, Ploysongsang Y, Dilisio R, et al: Fat embolism prophylaxis with corticosteroids: A prospective study in high-risk patients. *Ann Intern Med* 99:438–443, 1983.

52. Sharma GVRK, Folland ED, McIntyre KM, Sasahara AA: Long-term hemodynamics of thrombolytic therapy in pulmonary embolic disease (abstract). *J Am Coll Cardiol* 15:65A, 1990.

53. Siragnsa S, Cosmi B, Piuovella F, et al: Low-molecular-weight heparins and unfractionated heparin in the treatment of patients with acute venous thromboembolism: Results of a meta-analysis. *Am J Med* 100:269–277, 1996.

54. Stein PD, Hull RD, Pineo GF: Strategy that includes serial noninvasive leg tests for diagnosis of thromboembolic disease in patient with suspected acute pulmonary embolism based on date from PIOPED. *Arch Intern Med* 155:2101–2104, 1995.

55. Tapson VF, Hull RD: Management of venous thromboembolic disease. The impact of low-molecular weight heparin. *Clin Chest Med* 16:251–294, 1995.

56. Urokinase-streptokinase embolism trial: Phase 2 results. *JAMA* 229:1601–1613, 1974.

57. Van Erkel AR, Van Rossum AB, Bloem JL, et al: Spiral CT angiography for suspect pulmonary embolism: A cost-effectiveness analysis. *Radiology* 201:29–36, 1996.

58. Verstraete M, Miller GAH, Bounamedaux H: Intravenous and intrapulmonary recombinant tissue-type plasminogen activator in the treatment of acute massive pulmonary embolism. *Circulation* 77:353–360, 1988.

59. Warkentin TE, Levine MN, Hirsh J, et al: Heparin-induced thrombocytopenia in patients treated with low-molecular-weight heparin or unfractionated heparin. *New Engl J Med* 332:1330–1335, 1995.

60. Weil JV, Castro O, Malik AB, et al: NHLBI Workshop Summary—Pathogenesis of lung disease in sickle cell hemoglobinopathies. *Am Rev Respir Dis* 148:249–256, 1993.

61. Weinmann EE, Salzman EW: Deep-vein thrombosis. *New Engl J Med* 331:1630–1641, 1994.

62. Wolf H: Low-molecular-weight heparin. *Med Clin North Am* 78:733–743, 1994.

63. Worsley DF, Alavi A, Palevsky HI, Kundel HC: Comparison of diagnostic performance with ventilation-perfusion lung imaging in different patient populations. *Radiology* 199:481–483, 1996.

PULMONARY EDEMA

Daniel P. Schuster

Pulmonary edema is quite simply an abnormal accumulation of extravascular water in the lungs. The normal extravascular water content of the lungs is less than 500 ml. While an accumulation greater than this amount is abnormal by definition, symptoms and physiological dysfunction do not usually develop until the extravascular water content exceeds normal levels by at least 75 to 100 percent. This physiological reserve is made possible by the interstitium, a reservoir that accommodates modest increases in extravascular water (as might develop, say, with exercise) with little derangement in gas exchange or lung mechanics. With greater accumulations of extravascular water resulting in alveolar edema, clinically important effects invariably develop. Thus, one way to classify pulmonary edema is by its location (i.e., as either *interstitial* or *alveolar* edema.)

Pulmonary edema can also be classified according to its cause: *cardiogenic, noncardiogenic, high-pressure, increased permeability,* etc. In this chapter, pulmonary edema will generally be classified as due to an increased hydrostatic pressure gradient across the capillary wall, an increased vascular permeability of the capillary endothelium, or some combination of the two.

When pulmonary edema *is* due to increased vascular permeability, some form of acute lung injury is always responsible. This form of pulmonary edema is typically associated with the acute respiratory distress syndrome (ARDS).[41] Hydrostatic forms of pulmonary edema are usually associated with "heart failure" or "volume overload." While these clinical distinctions are useful for planning further evaluations and treatment, they may not always characterize the pathogenesis of pulmonary edema accurately because, in general, clinicians determine only whether or not hydrostatic pressures are elevated. When these pressures are not in fact elevated, it is assumed that the pathogenesis of pulmonary edema must be due to increased permeability. However, increased hydrostatic pressures *and* increased vascular permeability probably coexist in the pathogenesis of many specific syndromes of pulmonary edema.

DIAGNOSIS

Presentation

Pulmonary edema is usually first suspected when crackles (rales) are heard during the auscultation of a patient with the acute onset of tachypnea and respiratory distress. The crackles are invariably heard at the lung bases; depending on severity, they may be heard in less dependent regions as well. The crackles are produced during each breath by the sudden opening ("popping") of lung units subtended by small airways that have been closed by edema or secretions, with air suddenly bubbling through the liquid. As pulmonary edema worsens, fluid enters larger airways, causing gurgles (rhonchi) to be heard. On the other hand, chest auscultation may be surprisingly normal when pulmonary edema is due to lung injury. Rhonchi are also less common in syndromes of pulmonary edema associated with lung injury than heart failure, despite comparable or even more extensive accumulations of extravascular water. This observation may be the result of differences in how alveolar edema develops in the two conditions.

Despite alveolar filling in pulmonary edema, signs of parenchymal consolidation are unusual, regardless of underlying cause. In patients with airway hyperresponsiveness, wheezing is common, sometimes even with relatively trivial amounts of interstitial edema.

Disturbances in gas exchange depend on the amount of pulmonary edema, the presence or absence of bronchospasm, the effectiveness of hypoxic vasoconstriction in restoring ventilation-perfusion matching, and the presence or absence of any underlying lung disease. With severe pulmonary edema, cyanosis is common. In the absence of underlying lung disease, most patients will be hypocapneic, despite the disturbance in ventilation-perfusion matching. In fact, in the absence of chronic lung disease, *hypercapnea* usually indicates life-threatening respiratory muscle fatigue, premonitory of a respiratory arrest.

If the cause of pulmonary edema is heart failure, the patient may report symptoms associated with cardiac causes (e.g., chest pain, palpitations, a history of orthopnea or paroxysmal nocturnal dyspnea). Signs of myocardial or valvular dysfunction, or signs of coexistent right ventricular hypertension (e.g., *peripheral* edema) may also be present, along with a third or fourth heart sound. If reduced breath sounds are heard at either base during the chest examination along with dullness to percussion, a pleural effusion is probably present; this finding is much more common with cardiogenic than with noncardiogenic causes of pulmonary edema. Pleural friction rubs, however, are not expected in either case.

If pulmonary edema is noncardiogenic, respiratory symptoms other than dyspnea are uncommon. When present, they suggest alternative or associated disorders (e.g., pneumonia, chronic lung disease). On the other hand, dyspnea and tachypnea in ARDS often precede the full development of the characteristic opacities (infiltrates) that develop on the chest radiograph. This disparity may be due to superimposed abnormalities in airway resistance (although clinically obvious bronchospasm in ARDS is unusual), interstitial edema per se (by stimulating so-called interstitial juxtacapillary J receptors), or the poor correlation of the chest radiograph with the actual content of extravascular lung water. Invariably, however, radiographic alveolar infiltrates do then develop over the next several hours.

In all cases of clinically significant pulmonary edema, the most dramatic and consistent aspects of the physical examination include tachypnea, tachycardia, increased work of breathing (intercostal muscle retraction and use of other accessory muscles of respiration during inspiratory effort), and occasionally cyanosis. Systemic hypertension is extremely common (in the absence of shock); in patients with underlying chronic hypertension, blood pressure can become so elevated that a diagnosis of malignant hypertension is mistakenly entertained, sometimes leading to overvigorous antihypertensive treatment and the subsequent development of frank hypotension. Sometimes wheezing is the most prominent auscultatory finding, leading to confusion with an acute asthma attack. Agitation can be striking when pulmonary edema is severe. Hypotension and signs of shock (diaphoresis, cool extremities, ashen color, cyanotic lips and digits) indicate an associated condition, such as myocardial infarction, sepsis, or massive trauma. Likewise, fever should not be present unless infection is the underlying problem.

Diagnostic Tests

CHEST RADIOGRAPHY

The chest radiograph often provides enormously important information about the severity as well as the underlying cause of pulmonary edema. The radiographic appearance of pulmonary edema includes a combination of linear and less well-defined densities, which may eventually coalesce to form an alveolar pattern. In addition, specific causes (e.g., heart failure, volume overload, uremia, and ARDS) are associated with characteristic spatial and temporal patterns of infiltrate.

If pulmonary edema is mild, the radiograph may show only a bilateral perihilar haze with linear opacities extending from the hilum, suggesting interstitial edema. As alveolar filling develops, the linear opacities coalesce radiographically. With further progression, more of the lung parenchyma becomes involved radiographically, occasionally progressing to near-total white-out of both lung fields (Fig 85-1).

Sometimes the radiographic patterns of ARDS and those of heart failure can be readily distinguished from one another. In ARDS the densities tend to be peripheral as well as central, and less gravitationally oriented (from apex to base in the semirecumbent or supine position) than in typical heart failure. Also in ARDS, in the absence of coexisting heart disease or of intravascular volume overload, other radiographic signs of congestive failure (cardiomegaly, perfusion redistribution, increased width of the vascular pedicle, peribronchial cuffing, peripheral septal lines, and pleural effusions) are absent. These differences between the chest radiographic pattern of heart failure and noncardiogenic causes (Figs. 85-1 and 85-2) are most obvious when pulmonary edema is relatively mild and heart failure is relatively chronic. As pulmonary edema becomes more acute and more severe, the radiographic difference between cardiogenic and noncardiogenic causes becomes obscure. By the time mechanical ventilatory support becomes necessary, ascribing a specific origin to the radiographic pattern is often impossible.[52]

Many technical factors influence the radiographic appearance of pulmonary edema, especially rapid shallow breathing and the effects of therapy. Aggressive intravenous fluid administration for shock or hypotension may exacerbate pulmonary edema, whereas diuretics may limit or reduce it. Mechanical ventilation, especially with positive end-expiratory pressure (PEEP) or other modes that significantly increase mean airway pressure (e.g., inverse ratio ventilation) may reduce regional lung density by increasing lung inflation, giving the appearance of radiographic improvement despite continued significant abnormalities in gas exchange. When high airway pressures during mechanical ventilatory support are required for effective ventilation, radiographic signs of barotrauma may quickly become evident (e.g., subcutaneous and mediastinal emphysema, pneumothorax).

Computed tomography (CT) has been used to evaluate the ventral-dorsal distribution of pulmonary infiltrates in supine and prone patients with ARDS.[12,52] In supine patients, the radiographic infiltrates, while always bilateral and diffuse, are usually greater in the more dorsal than ventral lung regions (Fig. 85-1). Since some of these infiltrates resolve when patients are repositioned into the prone position, atelectasis is probably an important reason for such regional inhomogeneity. However, even though ventral-dorsal gradients in lung density (i.e., edema and/or inflation) may be present, injury itself (measured as an increase in vascular permeability) is more evenly distributed (Fig. 85-3).

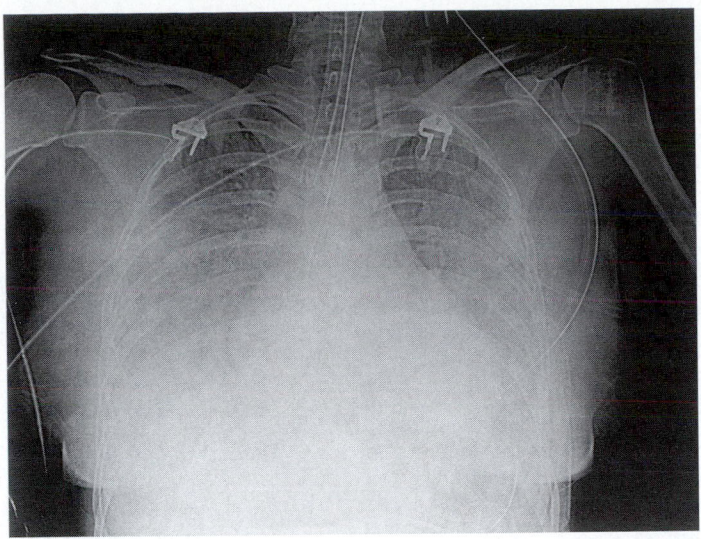

A

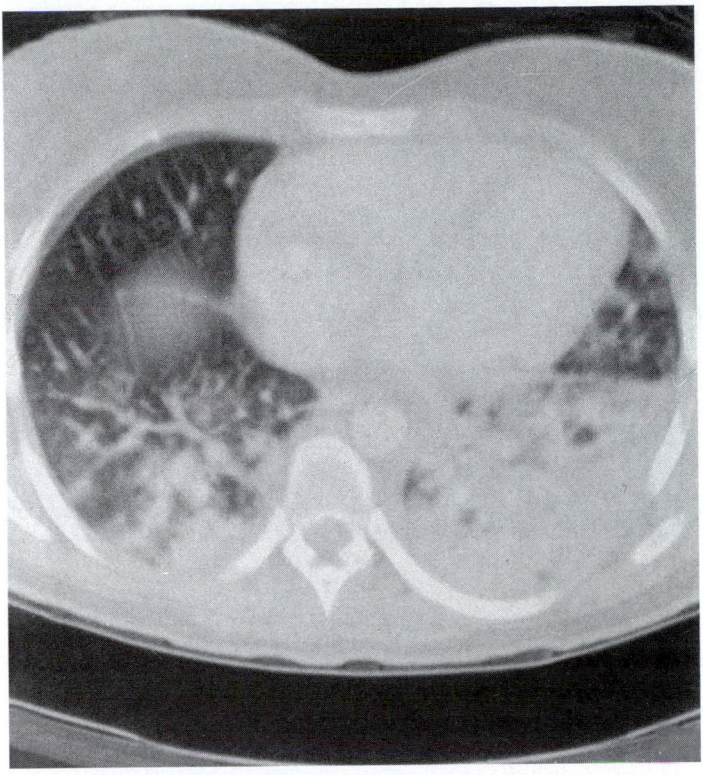

B

FIGURE 85-1 *A:* Portable chest radiograph showing classic diffuse bilateral alveolar infiltrates of a patient with early ARDS. Note the involvement of all lung fields. *B and C:* Two computed tomography scan slices from the same patient. Note that the infiltrates are predominantly in the lower lobes.

Gas Exchange

Measurements of gas exchange, although absolutely vital to management, are not very valuable diagnostically. At first, arterial blood studies usually show a respiratory alkalosis, with varying degrees of hypoxemia. Finger pulse oximetry will show arterial desaturation in proportion to the extent of arterial hypoxemia. If the hypoxemia is relatively resistant to supplemental oxygen administration, the cause may be either intra- or extrapulmonary (e.g., intracardiac) shunting.

Hemodynamic Monitoring

Pulmonary artery catheterization is commonly used as a means of evaluating the cause of pulmonary edema and to guide management. This subject is considered in greater detail in Chapter 82. Although pulmonary edema, high cardiac output, and low ventricular filling pressures are *characteristic* of ARDS, partly treated intravascular volume overload and so-called flash pulmonary edema (in which left ventricular filling pressures are presumably elevated during a period of coronary ischemia but then resolve before pulmonary artery catheterization is actually performed) are examples of clinical problems that can cause confusion with the expected hemodynamics of ARDS. Likewise, although increased cardiac filling pressures are characteristic of heart failure or volume overload, the measured pressures themselves may be elevated artificially (e.g., by increased intrathoracic pressures during mechanical ventilatory support) or as a result of therapy (e.g., volume administration for hypotension). Finally, pulmonary *capillary* pressures may be high even if cardiac filling pressures (i.e., the "wedge" or left atrial pressure) are normal.

Lung Water

Quantifying the *amount* of pulmonary edema might make it possible to detect the onset of pulmonary edema at an early stage,

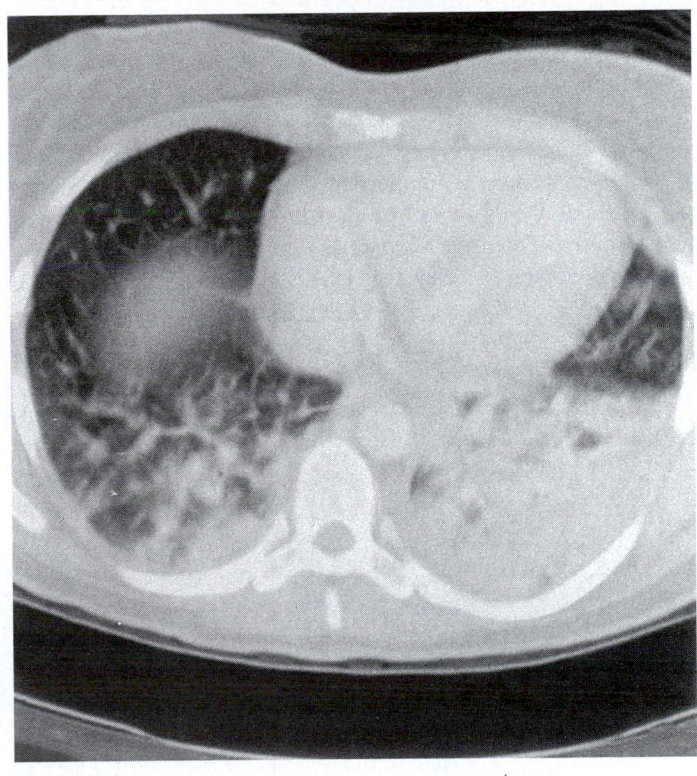

C

to assess its severity, or to predict outcome associated with the development of pulmonary edema. Accordingly, a great deal of effort has been expended over many years to develop clinically appropriate techniques to quantify the amount of extravascular lung water (EVLW) (Table 85-1). These methods range from

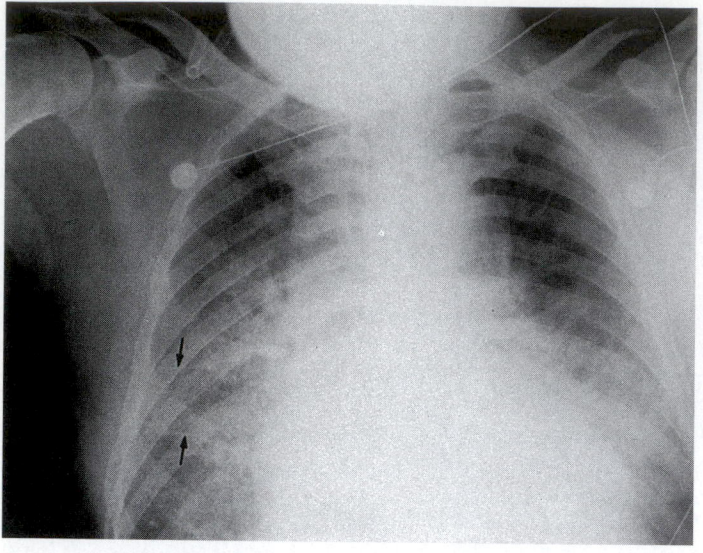

A

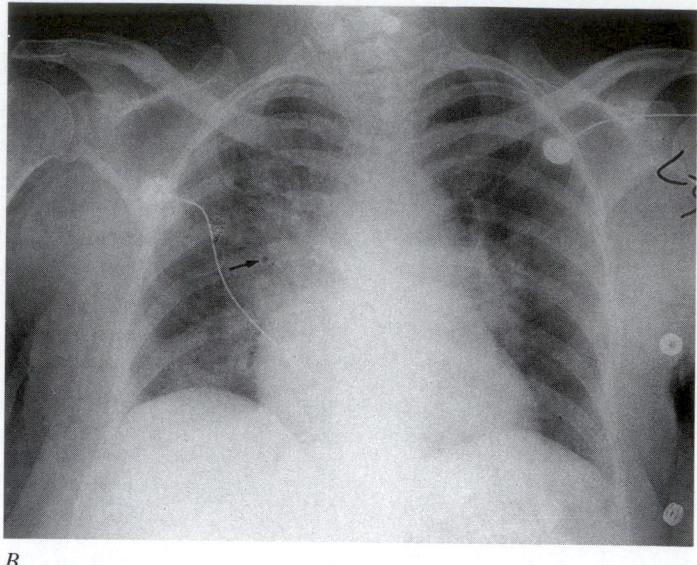

B

FIGURE 85-2 *Left:* Portable chest radiograph of a patient with congestive heart failure. Note the large heart and the presence of Kerley's lines, indicating interstitial septal thickening with fluid (*arrows*). *Right:* Portable chest radiograph of a patient with uremic pulmonary edema. This patient had a BUN of 180 but was clinically volume depleted. The patient was treated with intravenous fluids and hemodialysis with clearing of the infiltrates. Note the presence of a peribronchial cuff of fluid (*arrow*).

semiquantitative assessments of the chest radiograph[52] to invasive catheter-based techniques that depend on the dilution of injected indicators[46] to sophisticated and expensive technologies of nuclear magnetic resonance and positron emission tomographic imaging.[7,40]

Using indicator-dilution methods (the most commonly employed quantitative technique clinically), normal values for EVLW have been determined in human subjects without pulmonary edema and in patients with pulmonary edema associated with both normal and elevated wedge pressures (Fig. 85-4).[27,42,43] Despite the relative ease with which EVLW can be obtained by the indicator-dilution as well as the other techniques, these methods overall have not been widely incorporated into clinical practice, primarily because diagnostic and therapeutic decisions do not depend on the results obtained.

Lung Injury

Since lung injury is so important to the pathogenesis of certain forms of pulmonary edema, a comparable effort has also been spent on developing clinically appropriate ways of quantifying the breakdown in endothelial barrier function that is the *sine qua non* of lung injury. Once again, a range of techniques have been developed, from scoring systems that include measures of gas exchange and chest radiographic involvement to a variety of techniques that can measure a change in vascular or epithelial permeability to protein or other solutes. The latter tests include simple sampling of edema fluid for its protein concentration (predictably low in heart failure but elevated with lung injury) to various radioactive tracer techniques that themselves range greatly in complexity.[8,18,31,34,35]

In general, these methods have shown that vascular permeability to protein may increase by 10-fold or more during pulmonary edema associated with lung injury, while permeability remains relatively unaffected in patients with heart failure.[1,41] However, changes in vascular permeability have not been shown to correlate with outcome from pulmonary edema, and treatment decisions are not dependent on documenting whether or not per-

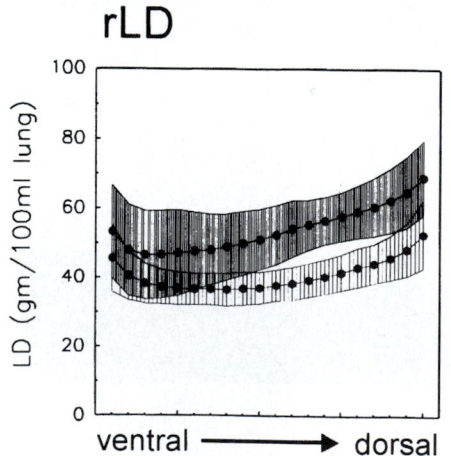

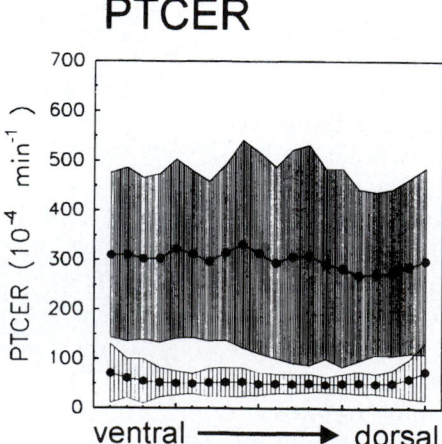

FIGURE 85-3 *Left:* Mean regional lung density (rLD) in normal subjects (*light shading*) and in ARDS patients (*darker shading*) as measured by positron tomography in the supine position. Note the increase in density, especially in the ARDS patients, in the more dorsal lung regions. *Right:* Pulmonary transcapillary escape rate (PTCER), an index of vascular permeability, in the same patients. Unlike lung density, no ventral-dorsal gradient exists for the group as a whole or in individual subjects. (*From Sandiford et al: Am J Respir Crit Care Med 151:737–742, 1995.*)

TABLE 85-1

Clinically Appropriate Methods to Quantify Extravascular Lung Water

Method	Bedside?	Expense	Quantitation	Comments*
CXR	✓	+	Poor	Evaluates density, not EVLW per se; regional inflation artifacts
CT	−	++	Excellent	Same as for CXR
NMR	−	++++	Fair	Poor sensitivity at low (i.e., normal) values; otherwise, same as for CXR
PET	−	++++	Excellent	Measures true EVLW; regional inflation artifacts
ID	✓	+−++	Good-excellent	Measures true EVLW; regional perfusion artifacts

*See text for details about each method; none of the methods can determine whether an increase in EVLW represents noncellular pulmonary edema or cellular water from an inflammatory infiltrate.
Abbreviations: CT = computed tomography; CXR = chest x-radiography; ID = indicator-dilution methods; NMR = nuclear magnetic resonance imaging; PET = positron emission tomography.

meability is abnormal. Accordingly, as with techniques for quantifying lung water, methods for quantifying lung injury per se are still primarily tools for research.

PATHOGENESIS

Normal Fluid Homeostasis

PATHWAYS FOR FLUID EXCHANGE

The principal function of the lungs, of course, is effective and efficient gas exchange. Toward this end, virtually the entire cardiac output flows through the lungs, spreading across an incredibly thin capillary network that reduces the diffusion distance for gas exchange to a minimum.

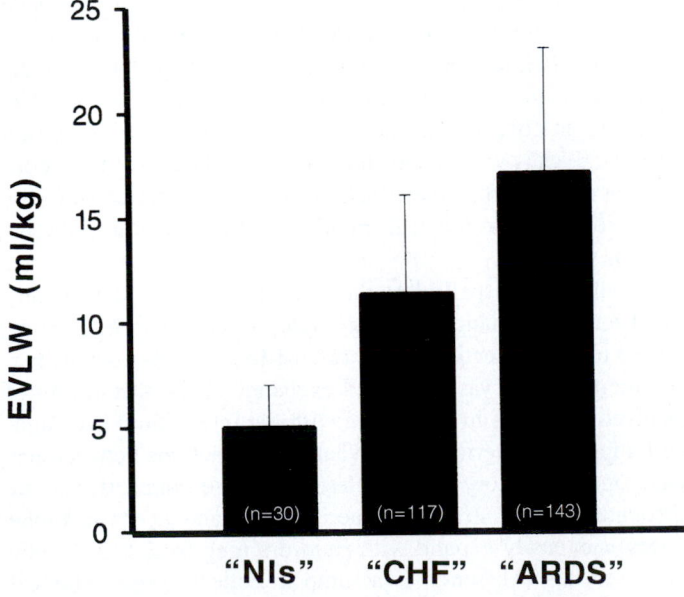

FIGURE 85-4   Average (mean ± SD) amounts of extravascular lung water (EVLW) in patients requiring pulmonary artery catheterization without pulmonary edema (NIs), in patients with pulmonary edema and an elevated pulmonary wedge pressure (congestive heart failure, or CHF), and in patients with pulmonary edema and a wedge pressure under 18 mm Hg (adult respiratory distress syndrome, or ARDS). *(Data combined from references 27, 42, and 43.)*

If gas exchange were the only function of the lungs, the ideal capillary system would limit diffusion across the endothelium to the respiratory gases and would exclude liquid or macromolecular transport altogether. However, the ability to mount a coordinated inflammatory response against both microbial and nonmicrobial invasion is one of many other functions that the lungs must perform. To initiate this response, the endothelium must allow the efflux of inflammatory cells, as well as chemotactic and other regulatory molecules, into the interstitial and alveolar spaces in a controlled manner. Not surprisingly, then, the pulmonary capillary endothelium is permeable (to varying degrees) to water and a wide range of solutes, including macromolecules like albumin and other proteins.

There is a cost, however, to this "leakiness" across the capillary wall. The semipermeable nature of the endothelial barrier and the enormous surface of the capillary bed make the lungs quite vulnerable to minor disturbances in normal physiology. Left uncorrected, these disturbances would quickly lead to excessive fluid leakage from the vascular spaces into alveoli and subsequently to significant disturbances in gas exchange. Instead, the pulmonary lymphatics constitute a drainage system that returns the normal amounts of extravasated fluid to the intravascular blood pool. Under normal conditions in humans, about 10 to 20 ml/h of pulmonary lymph are probably generated each day.[48]

These lymphatic vessels are not present within the alveolar walls. Instead, the first lymphatics are nonmuscular structures that begin at the junctions between respiratory and terminal bronchioles (Fig. 85-5). From there, lymph is directed toward larger muscular lymphatic vessels, which pump the lymph through one-way valves, ensuring the unidirectional flow of lymph toward the hilum under normal conditions. These lymphatics join to form collecting lymphatic vessels, which, in turn, empty into one of the many lymph nodes of the mediastinum, hilum, or lung parenchyma. Finally, lymph exits from these nodes, ultimately returning to the systemic venous system. Since the smooth muscle of the lymphatic pump can overcome most conditions that cause central venous hypertension, interruption of lymphatic drainage does not by itself predispose the lungs to developing pulmonary edema.

Most transvascular fluid exchange in the lungs occurs in vessels less than 200 μ in size (including small arterioles and venules, as well as capillaries), for the simple reason that the vast

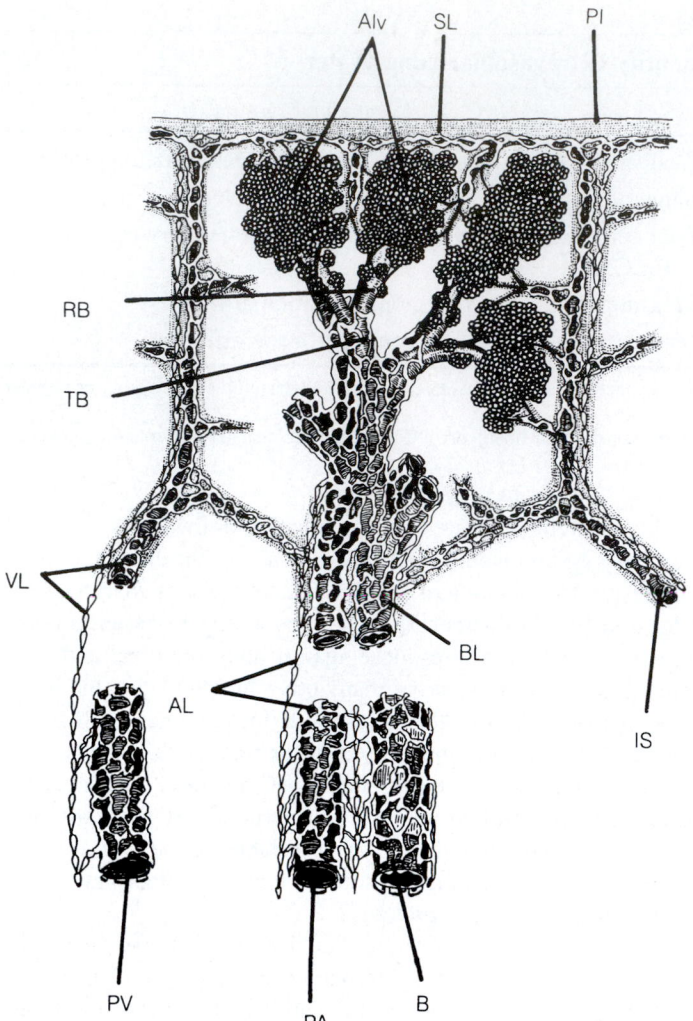

FIGURE 85-5   Distribution of lymphatics in the lung. Note that the lymphatics do not penetrate to the level of the respiratory bronchioles or alveoli. *Abbreviations:* AL = lymphatics and collecting lymphatics related to the pulmonary artery; Alv = alveolar region; B = bronchus; BL = lymphatics related to the bronchus; IS = interlobular septa; PA = pulmonary artery; Pl = pulmonary pleura; PV = pulmonary vein; RB = respiratory bronchiole; SL = septal lymphatics; TB = terminal bronchiole; VL = venous lymphatics.

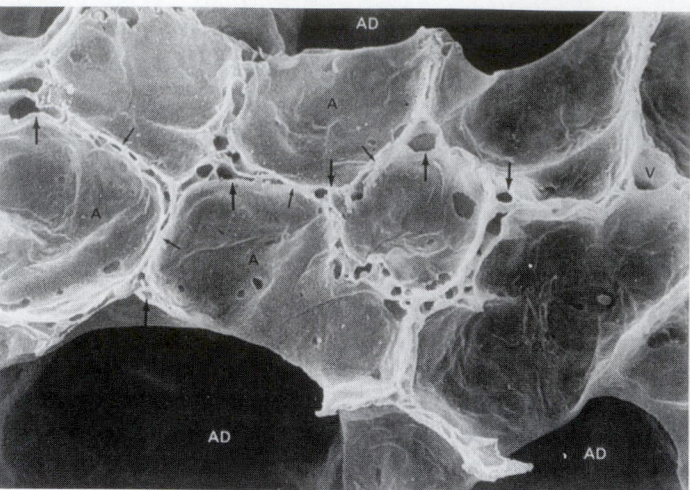

FIGURE 85-6   Demonstration of alveolar and extra-alveolar vessels in a scanning electron micrograph of rabbit lung inflated by air to 80 percent of total lung capacity. The tissue was fixed by vascular perfusion. Bold arrows point to corner vessels; fine arrows point to capillaries in the plane of the septum. *Abbreviations:* A = alveolus; AD = alveolar duct; V = small pre- or postcapillary vessel (×522). Because the lung is hyperinflated, the alveolar vessels are flattened, while the extra-alveolar vessels are widely patent. *(Micrograph courtesy of Dr. Weibel.)*

majority of the endothelial surface resides in vessels of this caliber. Because of uncertainty about the relative contribution of capillary and noncapillary vessels to overall pulmonary transvascular fluid exchange, the term *microvascular* is sometimes used instead of *capillary* when pulmonary fluid balance is discussed.

Another distinction of note is that not all the pulmonary capillaries are "intra-alveolar." (An "intra-alveolar" capillary is one in which its transmural pressure can be influenced directly by alveolar [airway] pressures.) In animal preparations, a substantial portion (perhaps as much as 50 percent) of the normal transvascular fluid exchange can occur from vessels which are "extraalveolar." These vessels, located in so-called alveolar corners at the junction of several alveoli (Fig. 85-6) can leak fluid even when nearby intra-alveolar capillaries are collapsed by increased

airway pressures (as might occur with PEEP during mechanical ventilation).

Even though other vessels of the pulmonary circulation can contribute to water flux in the lungs, it is the alveolar septal capillary that ensures that fluid exchange can occur without compromising gas transfer. This vessel has a unique geometry, being eccentrically placed within the alveolar septum (Fig. 85-7) so that one side is "thin" and the other is "thick." The thin side is composed simply of the apposed basement membranes of the alveolar epithelium and the capillary endothelium; at times the basement membranes actually appear fused to one another. The thick side, in contrast, has an interposed interstitium composed of proteoglycans with a collagen backbone. The interstitial contents has gel-like characteristics; ordinarily, free water with dissolved solutes is excluded from all but a tiny fraction of the interstitial volume.

The thin side, usually less than 0.5 μ in width, seems ideally suited for gas exchange; the thick side, in turn (with its interstitium of loose connective tissue, often 1 to 2 μ wide), seems better suited for transvascular fluid exchange. This interstitium of the alveolar wall is in continuity with the interstitium surrounding lymphatics, arterioles, and venules at junctions between terminal and respiratory bronchioles. The loose connective tissue surrounding these structures (perivascular and peribronchiolar spaces) can easily expand with fluid draining from the alveolar septa, serving in essence as a sump to collect lymph. This expansion of the interstitium and perivascular spaces with fluid yields the appearance of septal lines and peribronchiolar "cuffing" on the chest radiograph of patients with mild (interstitial) pulmonary edema.

The pulmonary capillaries, like those in skeletal muscle and myocardium (among other tissues), are lined by a continuous endothelium with an uninterrupted basement membrane. Capillar-

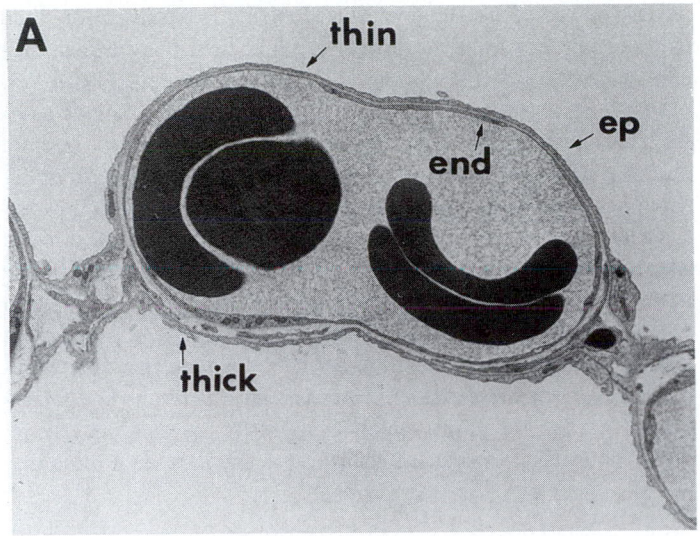

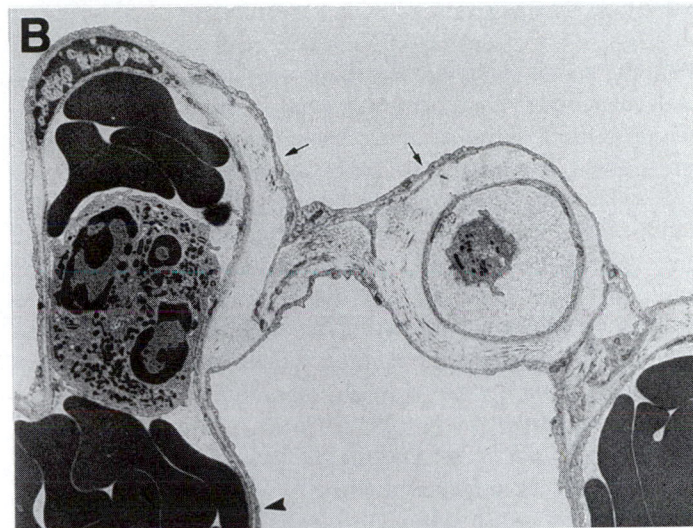

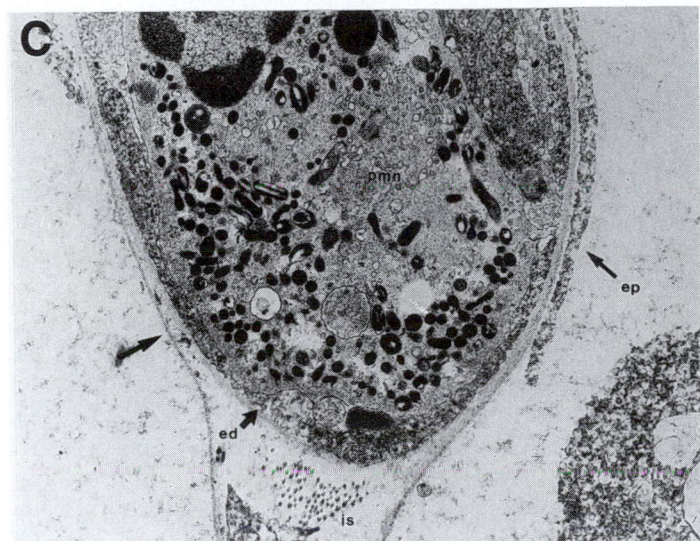

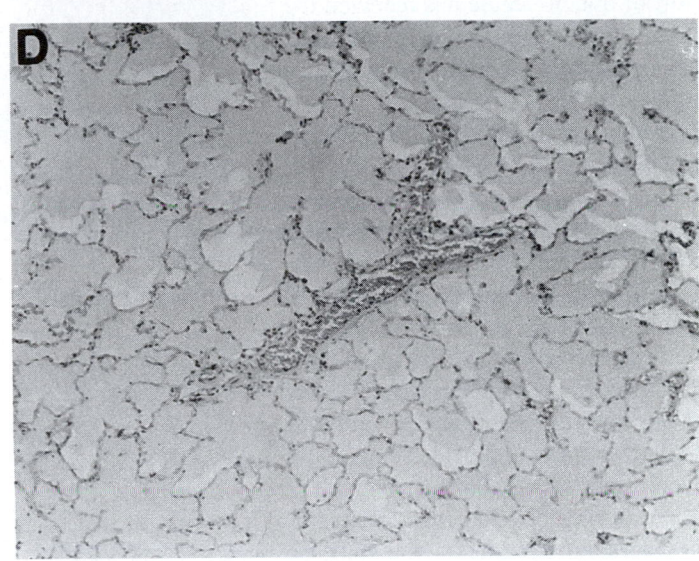

FIGURE 85-7   Micrographs of normal and injured canine lung. *A.* a normal septal pulmonary capillary demonstrating the "thin" and "thick" interfaces with the alveolar epithelium (ep). end = endothelium (×3000). *B.* Marked interstitial edema (*arrows*) with preserved endothelial and epithelial cell surfaces. Note the interstitium of the capillary at the center of the figure is widened circumferentially, whereas in other areas, the thin portion of the barrier is preserved (*arrowhead*) (×3000). *C.* Extensive endothelial and epithelial damage, with denudement of basement membrane (*arrow*) (×10,000). *D.* Alveolar flooding (×100). (*From Velazquez et al: J Appl Physiol 70:2206–2216, 1991.*)

ies in organs with higher rates of fluid exchange (e.g., kidney and small intestine) or in organs such as liver, spleen, and bone marrow are lined by fenestrated or a discontinuous endothelium (sinusoids). Although the continuous endothelium of capillaries like those in the lungs seems best suited to function as a barrier to liquid and solute flux, the barrier does allow the passage of some fluid and solute (e.g., protein).

The precise pathway for the flow of water across the endothelial barrier is still uncertain. The prevailing view is that water flows between cells, through interendothelial junctions that are freely permeable to water but not to larger molecules (see next section). Recently, however, a family of membrane water channel proteins, known as aquaporins, have been identified in many water-permeable tissues such as renal tubules, systemic capillary endothelium, and various tissues of the eye and salivary gland. Two specific members of this family (aquaporin-1 and -5) have been detected in the lung tissue of some species. Aquaporin-1 (channel-integrating protein) has been localized to the alveolar epithelium; the cellular source of aquaporin-5 has not yet been identified.[32] Thus, it is not yet known whether this water channel protein is important in regulating *transvascular* water flow in the lung.

The alveolar epithelium, unlike the capillary endothelium, appears to be virtually impermeable to water or solutes, acting as a final important barrier to fluid accumulation within the airspaces. The exact nature of this imperviousness to alveolar filling is not clear. It may be a function of the epithelial intercellular junctions themselves (see next section). It may also be the result of *fewer* intercellular junctions between alveolar epithelia than capillary endothelia.

PATHWAYS FOR PROTEIN FLUX

With the use of electron microscopy and techniques of cell and molecular biology, a complex picture is emerging about how solutes move from solution in plasma to the lymph of the interstitial space. The transport of each solute from vascular space to interstitial space actually entails a series of interactions with the endothelial cell membrane, instead of the simple movement of inert substances through a porous membrane, as has been the traditional view. Thus, the size, shape, and charge of each molecule, the endothelial surface charge and the structure of intercellular junctions, and the binding characteristics of the solute to membrane surface proteins affect the transport of each solute across the capillary wall.

Since albumin is so important to fluid balance in the lung (because of its effects on oncotic pressure), the transendothelial transport of this molecule has received the greatest attention. However, the same processes that pertain to albumin transport are also relevant to the transport of other important macromolecules.

Since the concentration of protein in lymph (and, therefore, presumably the interstitial spaces) is approximately three-quarters that of plasma, protein clearly leaks from the intravascular compartment to lymph. But exactly where this leak occurs along the microvasculature continues to be a subject of debate. There is evidence that endothelial permeability is not uniform along the length of the microvasculature; protein leak may be greatest at postalveolar (venular) rather than capillary sites.[44] It is also possible that the sites of maximal water and of maximal protein leak are not the same. And in the injured lung, the major sites for water and protein leak may each be quite different than in the normal lung.

A macromolecule like albumin can cross the endothelial barrier in two ways: it can go *through* cells (transcellular transport) or *between* cells (paracellular transport) (Figs. 85-8 and 85-9). Transcellular transport probably occurs via membrane vesicles and/or transcellular channels. The vesicles are spherical portions of pinched-off membrane that can trap albumin after it binds to a membrane receptor, or can carry it off in solution within the vesicle (Fig. 85-9). The vesicle then moves across the cell, eventually releasing its contents into the interstitium.

The nature of transendothelial channels is not as clear; they may simply represent the fusion of more than one vesicle, creating a direct, albeit temporary, path across the cell (Fig. 85-8). Transport via either the vesicular or transcellular channel pathways is independent of changes in either hydrostatic or oncotic pressure gradients across the endothelium. They therefore represent a nondiffusive path for solute flux.

Paracellular transport, on the other hand, takes place through junctions between endothelial cells (Fig. 85-8).[44] These cells make contact with one another at discrete points ("tight junctions"). Molecules with a radius of about 7 nm (70 Å) or less [e.g., albumin with a radius of about 3.6 nm (36 Å)] can move through these junctions. However, these points of contact are many and irregularly placed through the entire length of the cleft between endothelial cells.[6] Thus, each molecule must traverse the cleft via a route that

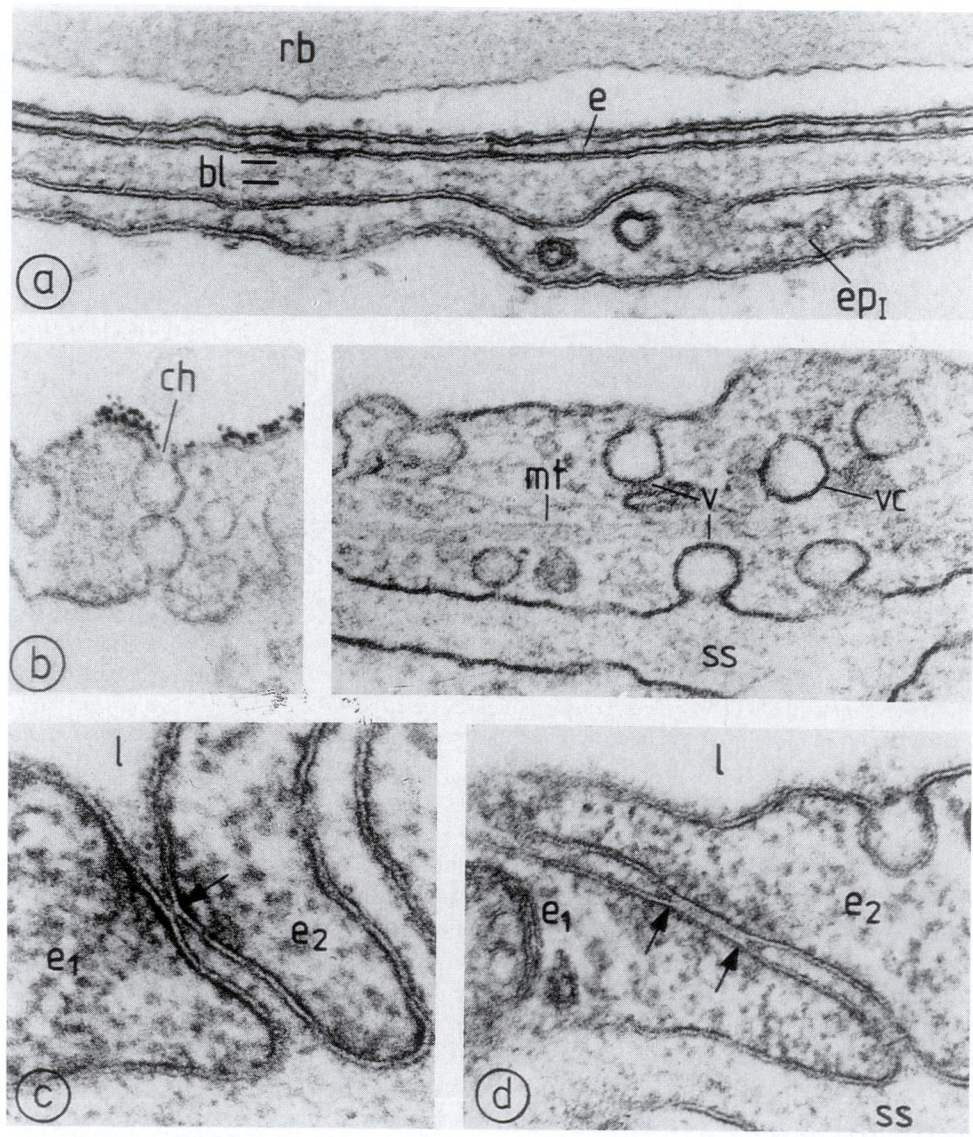

FIGURE 85-8   Electron micrographs of capillary endothelium, showing potential routes for macromolecular flux across the endothelial barrier. *A* and *B:* Vesicles (v) are present in some portions of the endothelium (e) and are absent in others (*A*). Rarely, the vesicles can be found to join, forming transendothelial channels (ch, on left side of panel *B*). Also shown is cationized ferritin on the endothelial lumenal surface. *C* and *D:* Some molecules can also move through tight junctions between endothelial cells (e$_1$, e$_2$). *Abbreviations:* l = lumen; ss = subendothelial space. *A*, ×130,000; *B*, left side, ×83,000; *B*, right side: 100,000; *C*, ×160,000; *D*, ×113,000. (*From Simionescu,*[44] *with permission.*)

is more like a maze than a simple discrete path (Fig. 85-10). The structure of the junctions between noncapillary cells active in lung fluid balance (extraalveolar vessels, alveolar epithelia) is more complex (Fig. 85-11). Furthermore, the tight junctions themselves may be organized differently between cells at various levels (arteriolar, capillary, venular, epithelial), and are probably dynamic structures that actually assemble and disassemble in response to numerous stimuli.

The molecular composition of these junctions is just now beginning to be elucidated.[24,36] Proteins such as zona occludens–1 (ZO-1) in particular have been associated with tight junctions, while cadherins, catenins, and vinculin are associated with other structures in the junction complex, depending on cell type. These various proteins form complexes that link to actin filaments in the cell's cytoskeleton. Intracellular changes in Ca^{++}, induced by a variety of agents, may lead to changes in the distribution of these actin filaments, reversibly altering the conformation of the junction and causing gaps to form between the endothelial cells and permeability to increase (Fig. 85-12).

Endothelial cells also make focal contacts with the extracellular matrix via integrin proteins, such as vitronectin or fibronectin. These adhesion sites may also affect paracellular solute transport, since antibodies or other peptides that interfere with integrin-mediated adhesion increase fluid and macromolecular transport across endothelial cell monolayers in cell culture.[24] Under normal conditions, the paracellular route is probably more important than are the transcellular pathways for protein transport,[49] although this view is not universally held.[49]

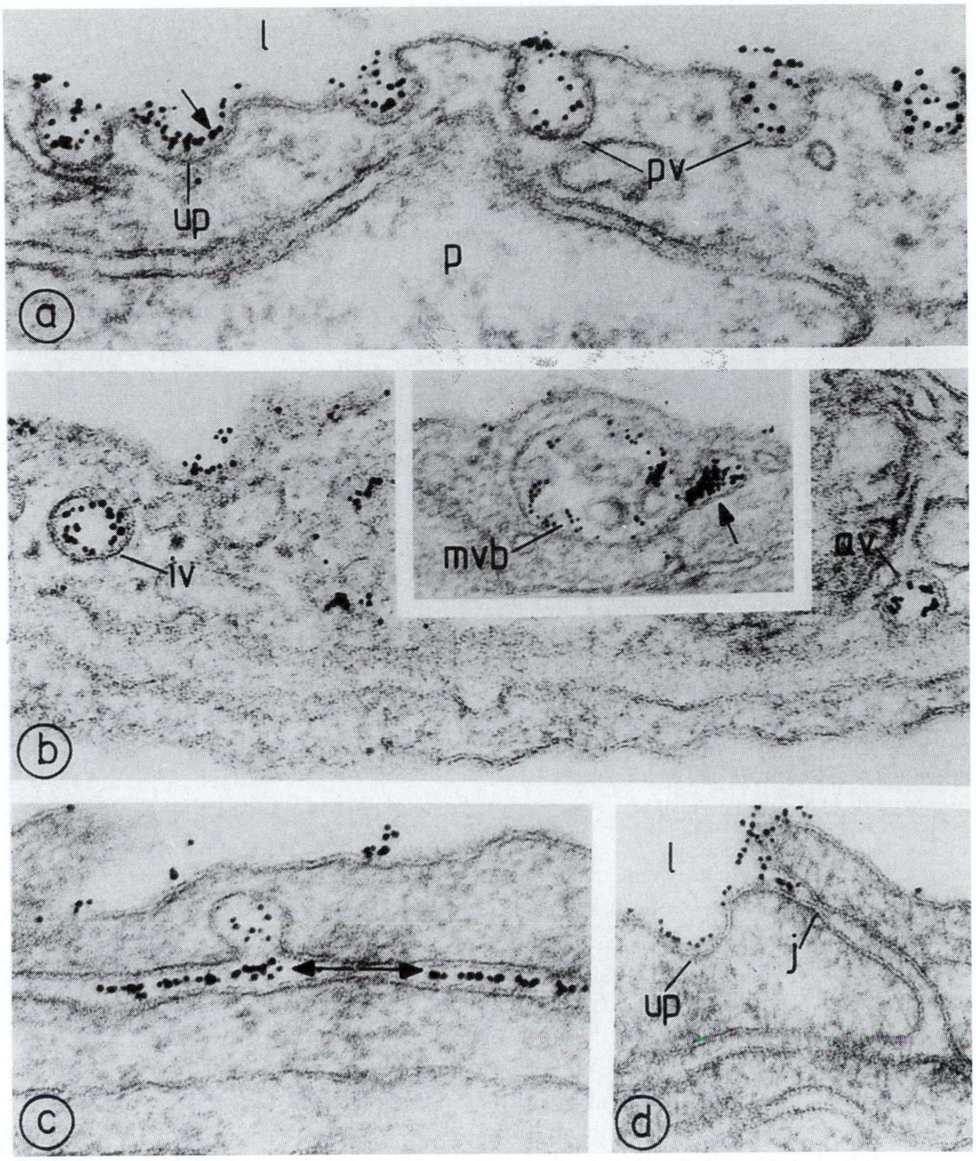

FIGURE 85-9 Transendothelial vesicular transport of albumin tagged to gold particles. *A.* Particles first bind to uncoated pits (up) and plasmalemmal vesicles (pv) ($\times 129,000$). *B.* A few minutes later, they appear internalized (iv); others are open to the abluminal front (av) or are discharging particles into a multivesicular body (mvb) (inset) ($\times 110,000$; inset $\times 81,000$). *C.* Particles are discharged into the subendothelial space (arrows) ($\times 129,000$). *D.* a tight junction restricts the passage of particles between cells ($\times 110,000$). *(From Simionescu,[44] with permission.)*

PHYSIOLOGY OF WATER FLUX

Our current thinking about the pathogenesis of pulmonary edema is strongly conditioned by Starling's classic hypothesis concerning the control of transcapillary fluid movement, now a hundred years old.[33] Simply stated, Starling showed that oncotic forces generated by plasma proteins balanced the hydrostatic pressure that otherwise would drive fluid out of capillaries. In the ensuing decades, his hypothesis has been refined, expanded, and quantified mathematically in many forms.[33] When applied to the lungs and modified to account for the total surface area over which filtration might occur, the hypothesis can be written as an equation:

$$J_v = (L_p * S)\,([P_c - P_i] - \sigma\,[\Pi_c - \Pi_i]) \qquad (1)$$

where

J_v = volume flux of water (ml/min)

S = surface area (cm^2)

L_p = the hydraulic conductivity for water ($cm \cdot min^{-1}$ mm Hg^{-1})

P_c and P_i = the hydrostatic pressure within the capillary and interstitial spaces respectively (mm Hg)

σ = the reflection coefficient for protein (no units)

π_c and π_i = the oncotic pressure within the capillary and interstitial spaces (mm Hg)

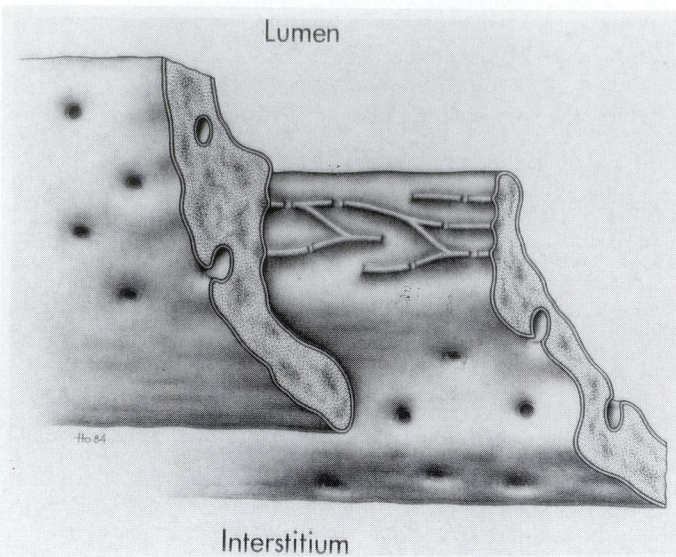

FIGURE 85-10   Diagram illustrating how tight junctions are organized between endothelial cells. The cells are separated, exposing the lateral surface of one endothelial cell. The punctate junctions observed in serial sections actually form lines of contact when reconstructed in three dimensions. Hydrophilic substances (water, electrolytes, small proteins) move between and through the lines of contact via discrete interruptions in the lines. *(From Bundgaard,[6] with permission.)*

The term L_p*S is equivalent to another term often used in mathematical expressions of Starling forces—namely, the filtration coefficient for the conductance of water (K_{fc}) (in ml · min^{-1} · mm Hg^{-1} · 100g^{-1}). Although it is difficult to separately measure S and L_p, expressing K_{fc} this way emphasizes the importance of S on overall fluid balance in the lungs. The term L_p describes the ease with which water traverses the endothelial barrier in response to a step change in hydrostatic pressure. Activity (e.g., exercise) or therapeutic maneuvers (e.g., vasodilators) that increase S (the surface area available for fluid exchange) would, if unopposed, increase EVLW.

If one adds *lymph flow* as a term summarizing the mechanisms responsible for returning fluid to the vascular compartment, the equation could be written as

$$EVLW = (K_{fc})\,([P_c - P_i] - \sigma\,[\Pi_c - \Pi_i]) - lymph\ flow \quad (2)$$

This modification emphasizes that ultimately the amount of pulmonary edema in the lungs represents a balance between the forces responsible for *production* versus those responsible for *resolution*. The fact that lymph is generated at all indicates that the Starling equation (equation 1) is not "balanced"; normally the hydrostatic pressure gradient is slightly greater than the oncotic pressure gradient, and fluid normally moves from the vascular to extravascular space to produce lymph at a slow rate.

The reflection coefficient σ is a mathematical expression for vascular permeability to protein. When a semipermeable membrane is completely impermeable to the proteins responsible for producing oncotic pressure, σ has a value of 1.0; if the membrane provides no resistance to protein diffusion, σ has a value of zero. Technically, there can be different σ's for each type of protein, and σ in equations 1 and 2 represents a weighted aver-

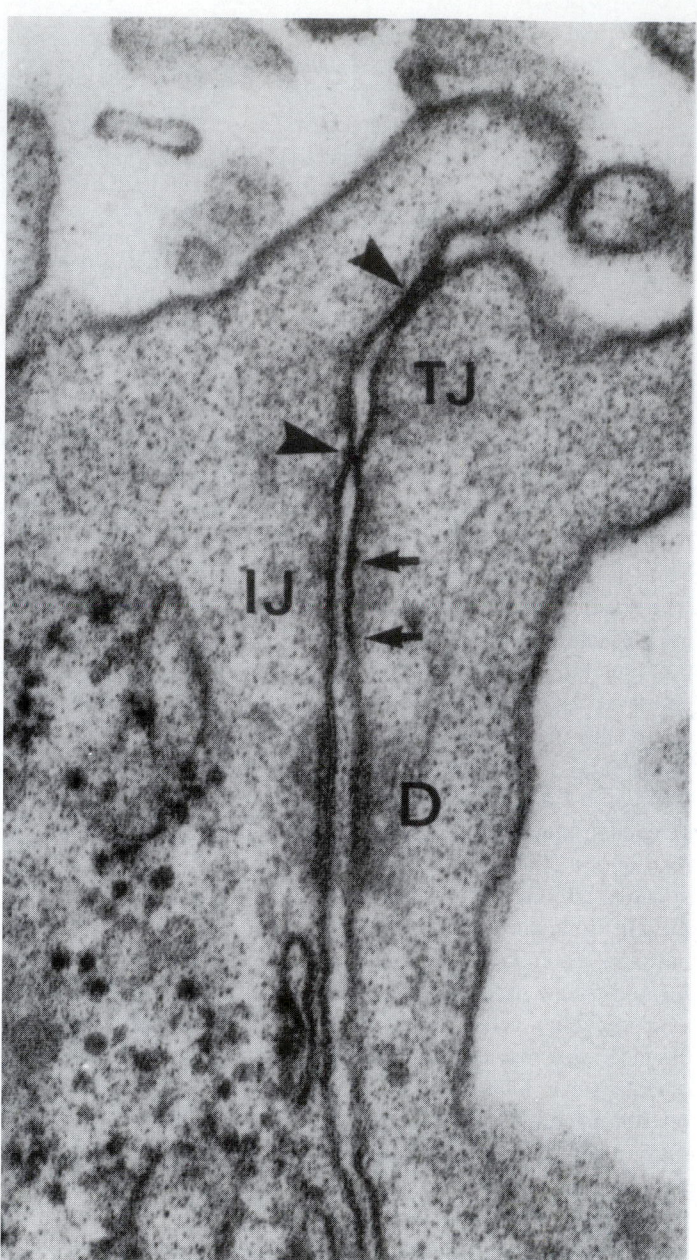

FIGURE 85-11   Junctional complex between two rat airway epithelial cells. Tight junctions (TJ), also known as the zona occludens, are indicated by arrowheads. At the intermediate junction (IJ) between the two arrows, also known as the zona adherens, the interendothelial space is narrowed but open. A desmosome (D) is also shown (×96,000). *(From Schneeberger and Lynch,[36] with permission.)*

age of them all. In effect, σ expresses how changes in vascular permeability modify the impact of an oncotic pressure gradient on EVLW accumulation. In the lungs, the fact that protein is present in lymph is consistent with a σ for the endothelium that is less than 1.0. Estimates for σ depend greatly on the technique used; estimates for albumin usually range between 0.5 and 0.8; estimates for total protein are slightly higher. For the alveolar epithelium, σ is very close to 1.0, essentially expressing mathematically that the alveolar epithelia are virtually impermeable to solutes and fluids.

Although the value of σ less than 1.0 indicates that the en-

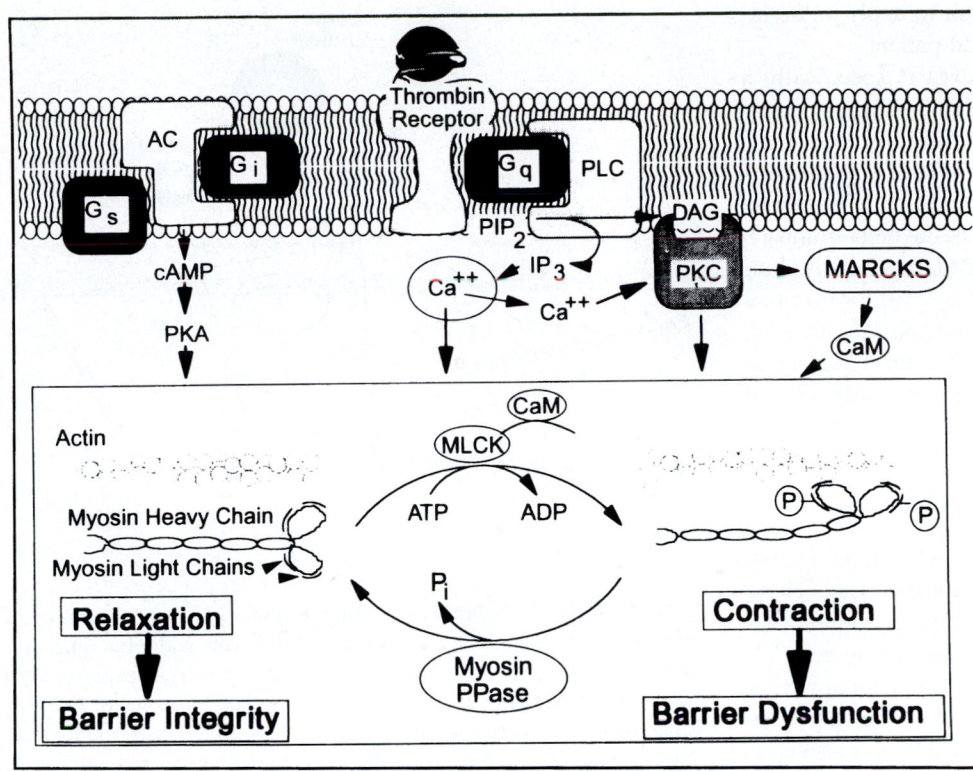

FIGURE 85-12   A proposed model for agonist-induced increases in permeability across the endothelial barrier. In this example, thrombin occupies its receptor, eliciting phospholipase C–mediated increases in cytosolic Ca^{++} and protein kinase C (PKC) activity. The Ca^{++} binds to the binding protein calmodulin (CaM), which, possibly with the participation of the MARCKS protein, in turn activates myosin light-chain kinase (MLCK). By analogy with events that take place in smooth-muscle cells, MLCK phosphorylation may promote cross-bridge formation and cycling between actin and myosin, leading to contraction, gap formation between endothelial cells, and an increase in paracellular protein transport (increased "permeability"). MLCK dephosphorylation by myosin-specific phosphatases (PPase) leads to actin-myosin dissociation, relaxation, and restoration of barrier function to normal. G_i, G_s, and G_q are membrane associated G-proteins; *Abbreviations:* DAG = diacylglycerol; IP_3 = inositol-1,4,5-triphosphate; PIP_2 = phosphatidylinositol-4,5-bisphosphate;   PKA = phosphokinase A. *(From Garcia et al: J Invest Med 43:117, 1995, with permission.)*

nant column of blood caused by balloon occlusion meets flowing blood. Typically, this point is in the large pulmonary veins near the left atrium. If postcapillary venous resistance is minimal and the capillary bed is at the same hydrostatic level as the left atrium, the two pressures are basically equivalent. When left atrial pressure is normal but pulmonary venous resistance is increased, the pulmonary microvascular pressure will be increased but the wedge pressure will be normal. Ordinarily, about 40 percent of the total pulmonary vascular resistance is estimated to be postcapillary (as opposed to the systemic circulation, in which less than 20 percent of the vascular resistance is venous). In many clinical circumstances associated with pulmonary edema, especially those associated with acute lung injury, pulmonary venous vasoconstriction is probably significant. Consequently, pulmonary capillary pressures may frequently be higher than assumed from wedge pressure measurements.

P_c can be estimated accurately, even clinically, by modifying the usual method of reading the WP tracing, as demonstrated in Figure 85-13.[13] The method is based on the observation that the relative magnitude of pulmonary arterial versus pulmonary venous resistance will determine the shape of the pressure decay from pulmonary arterial to wedge pressure. However, even

dothelial barrier is permeable to protein, it is not this fact per se that determines the interstitial oncotic pressure, π_i. At equilibrium, the values for π_c and π_i should be equal, regardless of the value for σ. Rather, it is the total flux of fluid and protein into the interstitium relative to its removal by lymph that determines the ultimate concentration of protein (and thus π_i) in the interstitium. Most estimates of the value for π_i are about 60 to 80 percent of those for π_c.

Neither P_c nor P_i is uniform throughout the lung.[49] Both vary as a result of gravity and the lung's mechanical properties. P_c, however, seems to increase at a greater rate than P_i in lung regions below the left atrium. As a result, the hydrostatic gradient (P_c–P_i) steadily increases below the left atrium, which helps explain why pulmonary edema tends to develop first in the most gravity-dependent portions of the lung.

This is also a useful place to point out that P_c is *not* equivalent to the pulmonary artery occlusion pressure (often called the *wedge pressure*.[49] The wedge pressure, obtained by pulmonary artery catheter balloon occlusion of a segmental pulmonary artery, is a measure of the pressure at the junction where the stag-

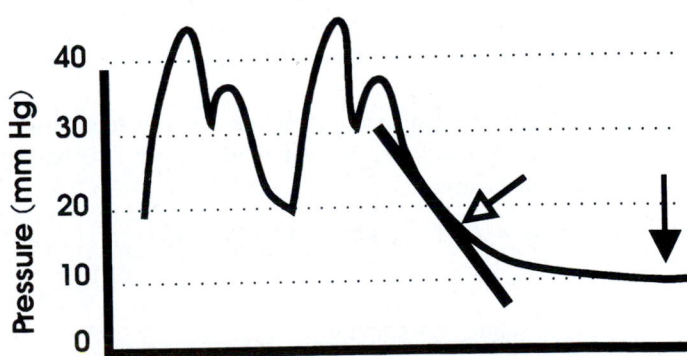

FIGURE 85-13   Diagram illustrating a method for determining the pulmonary capillary pressure, P_c, from a typical pulmonary artery pressure tracing after inflation and balloon occlusion of the pulmonary artery catheter. A straight line is drawn through the rapidly declining portion of the wedge pressure tracing. The inflection point (*open-headed arrow*) corresponds to P_c. In this illustration, the pulmonary artery diastolic pressure is 20 mm Hg, P_c is about 18 mm Hg, and the wedge pressure is only 10 mm Hg.

this relatively simple method can be difficult to apply in the intubated, tachypneic, mechanically ventilated patient.

The Starling equation (equation 1, above) is specifically a model for the development of *interstitial* edema. A similar equation could be written for the movement of fluid from the interstitial to alveolar space—but it is not very useful. Unlike equation 1, linear changes in variables like P_i—which, all other factors being equal, should help drive fluid into the alveolar compartment—actually have little if any effect, primarily because values for L_p are extremely low and σ approaches 1.0 for the alveolar epithelial barrier. Rather, when alveolar edema does develop, the alveolar epithelium seems to suddenly transform, becoming freely permeable to fluid and solutes (a process often termed *alveolar flooding;* see next section).

PHYSIOLOGY OF PROTEIN LEAK

Mathematical models have also been developed for *solute* flux across the endothelium, distinct from those for *fluid* flux. These models usually focus on the transvascular flux of albumin because of its importance in determining oncotic pressure.[34,48,49]

The passive transport of solute across the endothelial barrier can occur two ways: by convection (bulk flow, dependent on pressure gradients) and by diffusion (dependent on concentration gradients). By definition, permeability is the diffusion-dependent process. The capillary endothelial membrane is freely *permeable* to water and small solutes (fewer than a few thousand kDa), but the flux of larger solutes is restricted to varying degrees, depending on size, charge, shape, etc. Thus, the membrane is semipermeable.

A useful model has been to think of the endothelial barrier as full of holes (pores) of specific size. These pores confer size selectivity to the membrane: molecules of a certain size (smaller than a given pore) can cross the membrane, whereas molecules larger than the largest pore cannot (Fig. 85-14). The challenge experimentally has been to quantify the number and size of such pores, and to identify their anatomic equivalents. Since the alveolar epithelium is virtually impenetrable to either water or solutes, a similar model does not work for this barrier. When plasma proteins do appear in the alveolar space, size selectivity for proteins of different size, even at the endothelial level, seems to have been lost.

Like fluid flux, the movement of solute across a semipermeable membrane (in this case, the endothelium) can also be described mathematically:

$$J_S = J_v (1 - \sigma) \, C_{\overline{S}} + PS \, (C_c - C_i) \qquad (3)$$

where

J_S = solute flux (mg/min)
P = permeability (cm/sec)
$C_{\overline{S}}$ = the average molar concentration of solute within the membrane,
$C_c - C_i$ = the solute concentration gradient between the capillary and interstitium (mg/ml)

This equation provides terms for both the convective and diffusive movement of solute (first half of the right side and second half of the right side of equation 3, respectively). The terms

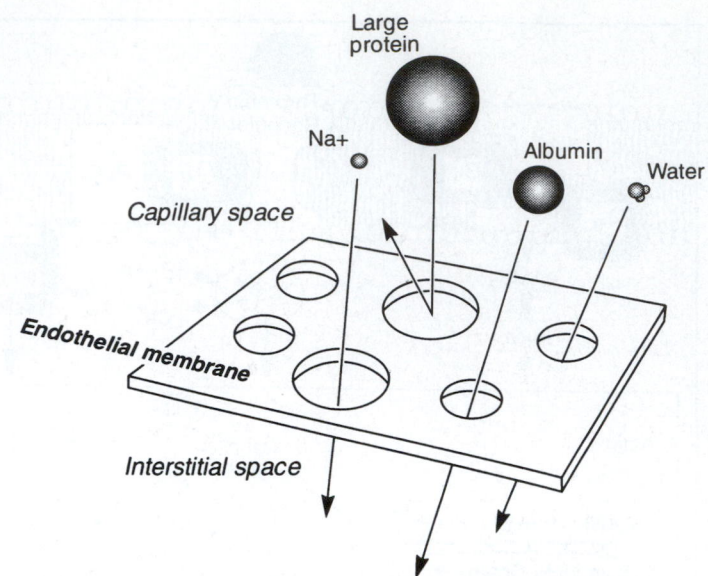

FIGURE 85-14   Diagram illustrating the concept of size selectivity of the endothelial membrane, modeled with a small- and large-pore system. Water and electrolytes can easily traverse the membrane via both pores. Small proteins, like albumin, are only slightly smaller than the small pores, and so access through this system, which is much more numerous than the large pores ($\sim$200:1), is restricted to varying degrees, depending on the level of vascular tissue (arterial, capillary, venular). Large proteins are excluded from traversing the endothelial barrier, even through the large-pore system. (*Modified from Prichard et al: Pulmonary oedema, in Weatherall et al [eds], Oxford Textbook of Medicine, 2d ed.* Oxford, Oxford University Press, 1987.)

"J_v," "S," and "σ" are the same terms used in the Starling equation (equation #1) to describe the volume flow of water (solvent drag) and the surface area of the endothelial membrane. Clearly, then, protein and water fluxes across the endothelial barrier are interdependent processes; changes in permeability affect water flux, and changes in water flux affect solute flux. Accordingly, to fully describe barrier integrity mathematically, L_p, σ, and P (i.e., "permeability") should each be estimated.

A model with pores of two sizes is all that is necessary to produce an excellent fit to experimentally derived lymph and protein flux data.[34,35] The smaller pore is now usually estimated at about 40 to 80 Å in radius; there is less certainty about the large pore, but most estimates range between 100 and 500 Å. The interendothelial cell junction (Fig. 85-8) seems to be a reasonable anatomic correlate of the small pore, since labeled tracers under 70 Å can move through this structure. (Albumin has a radius of 37Å.) The identity of the larger pore is less certain; it may correspond to transendothelial channels formed by the fusion of multiple membrane vesicles (Fig. 85-8); if so, it is not surprising that estimates of large pore size are more variable. The ratio of small to large pores seems to be about 200:1; accordingly, more than 80 percent of the hydraulic conductance appears to take place through the small-pore system.[49]

The "pore" model is obviously a simplified version of reality, and other schemes have been proposed, resulting in so-called pore equivalents. As noted previously (Fig. 85-10),[6] there is in fact no straight route between the vascular and interstitial space through which molecules may pass unencumbered. Nevertheless, even such complex structures as the intercellular junctions can be described mathematically, using the new branch of mathematics known as fractal geometry.[26]

Development of Pulmonary Edema

The Starling equation is a useful paradigm for determining which forces or, more commonly, which *combination* of forces initiate the development of pulmonary edema: increases in "S" or L_p (i.e., K_{fc}), P_c, and π_i should all increase EVLW, assuming that other factors remain unchanged. Likewise, decreases in P_i, σ, π_c and lymph flow should have a similar effect. Clinical examples of these disturbances are listed in Table 85-2. There are no known instances of pulmonary edema in which an increase in π_i is the primary cause. Also, there are no known instances in which changes in vascular permeability affect L_p independently of σ.

Once a disturbance in the Starling forces of equation 1 leads to increased fluid filtration across the endothelial barrier, the sequence of events that ultimately result in the accumulation of excess EVLW are similar regardless of cause. First, as filtration increases, lymph flow is concomitantly augmented. When the capacity of the lymph system is exceeded, fluid accumulates in the loose connective tissue of the bronchovascular sheath, in effect continuously draining the interstitium of the alveolar and/or extra-alveolar capillaries and other microvessels (Fig. 85-15). Once the capacity of the bronchovascular sheath is reached, the alveolar septal interstitium swells (Fig. 85-7). Finally, alveolar flooding develops (Fig. 85-7).

Until recently, most evidence seemed to indicate that when the capacity of the interstitium was finally overwhelmed, fluid entered individual alveoli in an "all-or-none" fashion; i.e., each alveolus was either filled or empty, a process called *alveolar flooding* (Fig. 85-16).[4,48] The events responsible for "flooding,"

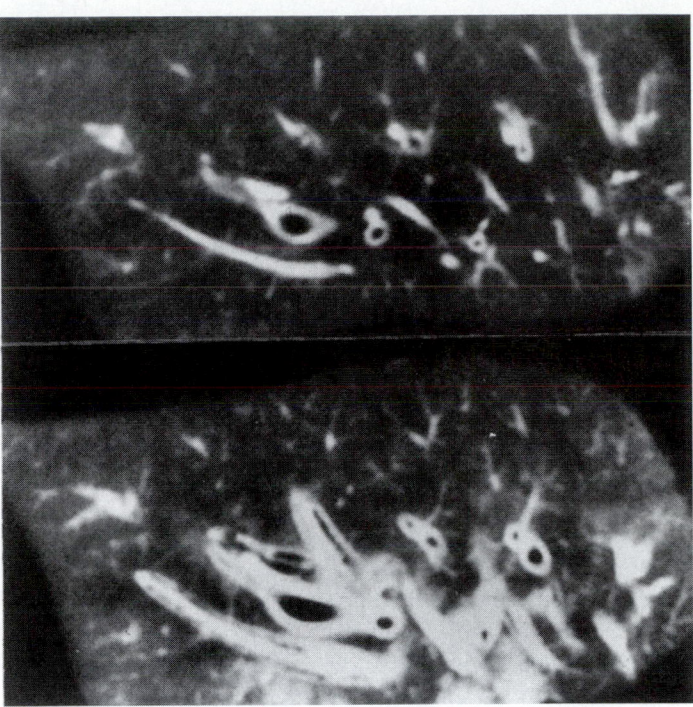

FIGURE 85-15 Computed tomographic scans of a normal dog lobe without edema *(upper figure)* and after an increase in edema of about 150 percent *(lower figure)*. Note the development of vascular engorgement and central peribronchovascular edema, peribronchial cuffing, and hilar edema. *(From Forster et al,[11] with permission.)*

however, are poorly defined. It is possible that the permeability of the epithelium in individual alveolar units changes abruptly (σ near 1.0 changing to a value much closer to 0). Alternatively, the epithelial barrier might first be breached "upstream" from the alveolus, near the terminal bronchiole, with retrograde filling of individual alveoli.[48] Epithelial cell necrosis and complete

TABLE 85-2

Disturbances in Variables of the Starling Equation (Equation 1) Associated with Pulmonary Edema

Variable	Change	Clinical Examples
L_p	↑	ARDS
σ	↓	ARDS
P_c	↑	CHF, volume overload, pulmonary venous hypertension (any cause), HAPE, NPE
P_i	↓	Upper-airway obstruction, reexpansion pulmonary edema
π_c	↓	Severe hypoalbuminemia
π_i	↑	None known

Abbreviations: ARDS = acute respiratory distress syndrome; CHF = congestive heart failure; HAPE = high-altitude pulmonary edema; L_p = hydraulic conductivity for water; NPE = neurogenic pulmonary edema; P_c and P_i = capillary and interstitial hydrostatic pressures respectively; π_c and π_i = capillary and interstitial oncotic pressures respectively; σ = reflection coefficient for protein. The associations listed in the table are probably important in the pathogenesis of the associated clinical disorder, but in many cases more than one variable is abnormal (see discussion in "Overview of Specific Syndromes").

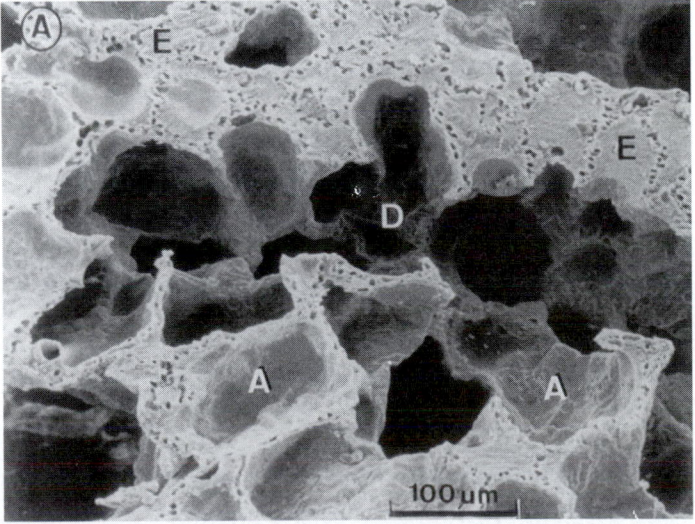

FIGURE 85-16 Scanning electron micrograph from a rabbit lung after the development of pulmonary edema. Note that some alveoli are air-filled (A) and others are flooded with edema (E), even though they are served by the same alveolar duct (D). *(From Bachofen et al,[4] with permission.)*

loss of epithelial barrier integrity, a prominent finding in ARDS and in many models of lung injury (Fig. 85-7), is another possible mechanism. In all likelihood, any of these different mechanisms may be important, depending on the cause and severity of the underlying process. For instance, the more frequent occurrence of rhonchi in pulmonary edema associated with severe heart failure than in ARDS may imply that in patients with cardiogenic pulmonary edema, excess fluid first enters the airspaces at the level of the terminal bronchiole.

The Starling equation, which should apply equally to all lung units regardless of anatomic location, does not adequately explain the markedly heterogeneous development of alveolar edema in any given lung region (Fig. 85-17).[4] Even the notion that alveolar edema develops in an all-or-none fashion as alveolar flooding has recently come under attack (Fig. 85-17).[4] Thus, although the Starling equation is a useful model for the *initiating* events that lead to interstitial edema, the full expression of pulmonary edema as *alveolar* edema is a more complicated and so far inadequately described process.

One particular property of the Starling equation has important clinical implications: as L_p *increases,* or σ or π_c *decreases,* fluid flux across the endothelial barrier becomes *more* sensitive to increases in P_c. Stated differently, as the forces that *oppose* fluid transudation are lost (e.g., the oncotic pressure gradient, membrane permeability), fluid flux becomes increasingly dependent on changes in capillary hydrostatic pressure. This feature forms the basis for the decades-old controversy surrounding fluid management in pulmonary edema (see "Therapy," below).

Another important observation is that increases in P_c do not cause proportionate increases in EVLW (Fig. 85-18).[48] Indeed, P_c can increase over a reasonably broad physiological range without causing pulmonary edema at all. A set of "safety factors" (actually compensatory changes in the other variables of equation 1 as P_c changes) are responsible for this physiological reserve.[48,49] For instance, as P_c increases, the flux of relatively protein-free fluid into the interstitial compartment increases. As a result, pressure within the interstitial compartment (P_i) also increases, interstitial oncotic pressure decreases (because of dilu-

tion), and lymph flow increases. Indeed, lymph flow can increase 10-fold or more.[48,49] With lung injury, however, the overall safety factor is reduced, primarily because as σ decreases, the oncotic pressure gradient ($\pi_c - \pi_i$) is also reduced, and the benefit of diluting interstitial oncotic proteins is lost. Accordingly, EVLW will increase at a lower P_c and at a faster rate than when the endothelial barrier is normal (Fig. 85-18).

MECHANISMS OF INCREASED "PERMEABILITY"

Any condition that reduces the selectivity of the endothelium to solutes of different sizes (quantified as σ in equation 1) will increase both the hydraulic conductivity to water (L_p in equation 1) as well as protein permeability (P in equation 3). Since changes in these biophysical parameters always occur together during acute lung injury, it is necessary to focus only on the mechanisms that increase permeability per se.

The morphologic basis for endothelial injury (unlike epithelial injury) has been difficult to identify in many instances of pulmonary edema associated with lung injury, which might suggest that functional (and potentially reversible) changes in the endothelial barrier are responsible for the increases in vascular permeability that accompany lung injury. Observations of in vitro cell culture systems, in which a variety of chemical and mechanical stimuli cause endothelial cells to contract and gaps to form between cells with reversible increases in permeability across the endothelial cell monolayer,[24] support this conclusion.

The ability of endothelial cells to contract in vitro, thereby increasing permeability, is probably due to Ca++–induced changes in the distribution of actin filaments, which alter the conformation of intercellular junctions. Ca++ is liberated from intracellular stores by both membrane receptor-dependent and receptor-independent processes (Fig. 85-12).[24] The release of Ca++ intracellularly starts with the binding of some agonist to its membrane receptor, inducing a G-protein–mediated increase in phospholipase C activity and hydrolysis of phosphoinositol diphosphate to diacylglycerol and inositol triphosphate. In turn, the liberated cytosolic calcium, in combination with diacylglycerol, activates phosphokinase C (PKC). By phosphorylating (and

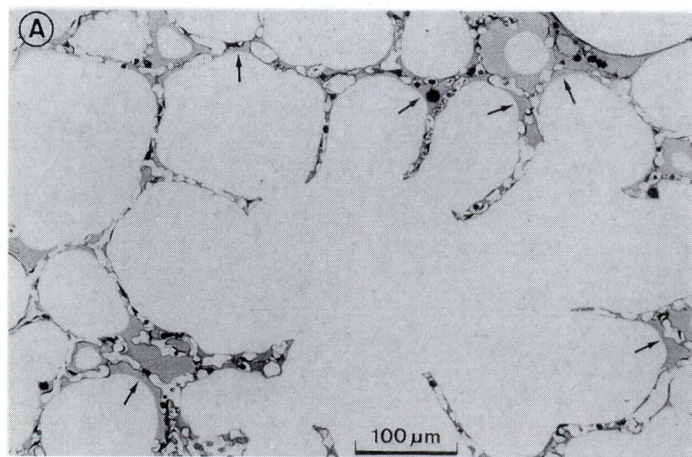

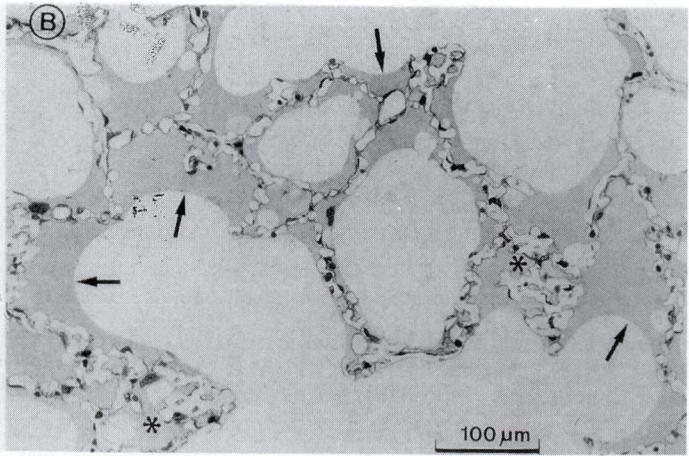

FIGURE 85-17 Electron micrographs of a rabbit lung after the development of pulmonary edema, showing that alveolar filling is not always "all-or-none." *A.* With small amounts of fluid, edema collects at the alveolar corners (*arrows*). *B.* With larger amounts of fluid, menisci form (*arrows*). Asterisks denote irregular septal arrangement in fluid pools. (*From Bachofen et al,*[4] *with permission.*)

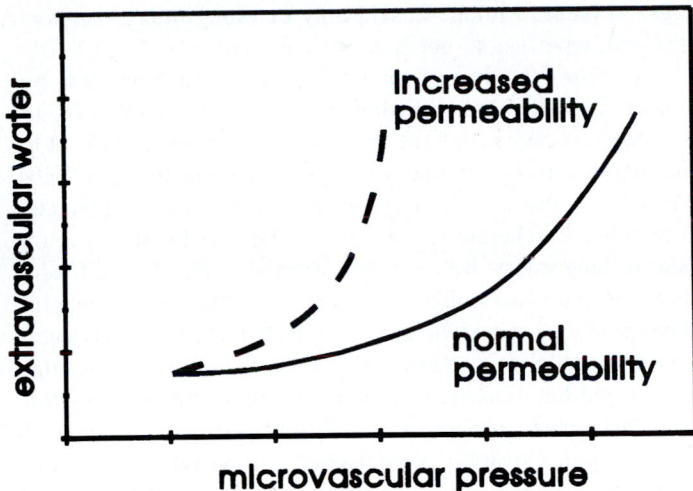

FIGURE 85-18 Diagram illustrating the relationship between extravascular lung water (EVLW) accumulation and microvascular or capillary pressure (P_c). When permeability is normal (as estimated with the filtration coefficient, K_{fc}, and the reflection coefficient, σ), EVLW remains relatively constant until hydrostatic pressure exceeds a critical level (about 18 to 23 mm Hg in a normal lung). This physiological reserve is due to changes in the other variables of the modified Starling equation [Eq. (1) in text]. When permeability is abnormal, EVLW accumulation occurs earlier and at a faster rate. *Abbreviations:* P_i = interstitial hydrostatic pressure; π_c and π_i = capillary and interstitial oncotic pressures, respectively.

thereby activating) a number of other actin-binding proteins (talin, vinculin, etc.), activated PKC, among other mechanisms, can mediate a change in cell shape, thereby increasing permeability at either cell-cell junctions or at cell-matrix focal contacts. PKC can also be activated independently of membrane receptor interactions (e.g., by various eicosanoids and oxygen radicals) that presumably initiate the same sequence of intracellular events (see "Oxidant Stress," below). The extent to which these in vitro observations relate to in vivo phenomena is still unclear.[2]

The development of epithelial cell damage seems to be an important difference distinguishing the pulmonary edema associated with increases in P_c (e.g., congestive heart failure) from that associated with increased permeability (ARDS).[29] For any given amount of excess EVLW, more of it will be alveolar edema when associated with lung injury and epithelial cell damage than when the development of pulmonary edema is driven by increases in hydrostatic pressure alone. The main consequence of this difference, of course, is that gas exchange will be worse (see "Gas Exchange," below). This difference may also be one reason for the generally poor correlation between EVLW and gas exchange; it is not only the *amount* of EVLW but also its *location* (alveolar or interstitial) that affects the efficiency and effectiveness of oxygenation and CO_2 elimination.

OXIDANT STRESS

Various oxidants can damage cell membranes directly by lipid peroxidation and also increase vascular permeability via PKC-

dependent mechanisms. Reactive oxygen species, such as the superoxide anion, hydrogen peroxide, and the hydroxyl radical, are probably most relevant to the pathogenesis of pulmonary edema. Superoxide and hydrogen peroxide are not per se very toxic. However, both participate in the formation of the hydroxyl radical, as well as lipid peroxides and hypohalous acids, all of which are extremely toxic to cell membranes. Whether nitric oxide, alone or in combination with superoxide anion, participates in producing membrane damage is still uncertain.[22] Although the toxic effects of these reactive oxygen species can be attenuated by treatment with oxygen radical scavengers (such as superoxide dismutase and catalase) in experimental settings, the therapeutic value of using oxygen radical scavengers to treat clinical forms of increased permeability pulmonary edema (such as ARDS) is unknown.

The various reactive oxygen species are generated principally from three sources: the breathing of oxygen-enriched inhaled gas, the influx of inflammatory cells (via NADPH-oxidase– and myeloperoxidase-dependent pathways), and after reperfusion of previously ischemic tissue. Enriched oxygen–air mixtures are much more likely to exacerbate than to initiate the injury that leads to pulmonary edema (O_2 toxicity). The other two mechanisms are more likely to be important as initiating events. The mechanisms by which inflammation can cause lung injury are considered in detail in Chapters 165 and 166.

Ischemia-reperfusion injury is a well-established mechanism of injury in several tissues (primarily heart and intestine). How ischemia and reperfusion cause *lung* injury is still unclear. While prolonged tissue ischemia itself is undoubtedly injurious, the events that specifically follow reperfusion are thought to be important for the full expression of ischemia-reperfusion injury (Fig. 85-19). According to one widely held hypothesis, xanthine and hypoxanthine are formed during anaerobic metabolism after adenosine triphosphate and other high-energy phosphates are depleted during ischemia. Concomitantly, cellular membrane dysfunction during ischemia increases calcium ion flux into cells, causing the activation

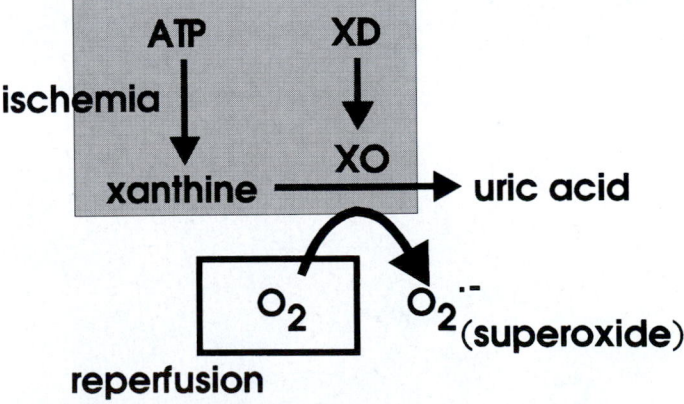

FIGURE 85-19 Diagram illustrating one scenario for the generation of reactive oxygen species (superoxide), which can then lead to additional production of other more toxic molecules. With ischemia (shaded box), ATP is metabolized to xanthine and hypoxanthine, while xanthine dehydrogenase (XD) is converted to xanthine oxidase (XO). With reintroduction of O_2 into the microenvironment during reperfusion (*unshaded box*), O_2 drives the catalysis of xanthine to uric acid in the presence of XO, liberating in the process superoxide anion.

of proteases that stimulate the conversion of xanthine dehydrogenase to xanthine oxidase. Upon reperfusion and the reintroduction of molecular oxygen into the microenvironment, the xanthine oxidase catalyzes xanthine to uric acid.[30] Reactive oxygen metabolites are produced as metabolic by-products; if they are produced in excess, cell damage will result.

According to this hypothesis, tissue hypoxia is a *sine qua non* for the development of ischemia-reperfusion injury. While this prerequisite is easily met in organs such as heart and intestine, it is quite difficult to produce total ischemia in lung tissue; it is even more difficult to render lung tissue severely hypoxic, since the lungs have several sources of oxygen: the pulmonary circulation, the bronchial circulation, and the alveolar gas. Even the reflux of blood into the lungs during left atrial contraction may be enough to support lung tissue integrity.[17] The length of ischemic time and the completeness of tissue hypoxia are important variables in determining whether and to what extent lung tissue damage develops. Mechanical influences, such as atelectasis, may also be at work.[16] The normal low metabolic rate of the lungs, coupled with the relatively little change that develops in the oxygen consumption of lung tissue during exercise or other increases in ventilatory demands, has made it difficult to show that ischemia-reperfusion injury per se is an important mechanism for the development of lung injury in clinically relevant settings. At present, it can be said only that lung injury is *associated* with reperfusion, not *caused* by it.

Sometimes the lungs can be injured as an "innocent bystander" if ischemia-reperfusion injury develops in other organs or tissues. Examples include the pulmonary edema that develops after reperfusion of previously ischemic intestinal tissue or limbs. It is unlikely that reactive oxygen species themselves, generated in peripheral ischemic tissue, are responsible for the development of lung injury, because their reactivity and short diffusion distances make this unlikely. However, circulating xanthine oxidase, produced at peripheral sites of ischemic tissue, may cause lung endothelial injury, especially since the oxygen concentrations in the lung microenvironment are high. Another possibility is that ischemia-reperfusion injury in peripheral tissue leads to neutrophil activation accompanied by the release of proinflammatory and vasoactive mediators into the circulation, which then injure more distant tissues like the lungs.

Stretched Pores and Capillary Stress Failure

It has been known for decades that the vascular permeability of pulmonary capillaries will eventually increase if capillary pressures rise to high enough levels. This phenomenon is often attributed to "stretching" of the interendothelial pores (Fig. 85-20). Capillaries can even rupture under extreme mechanical stress—

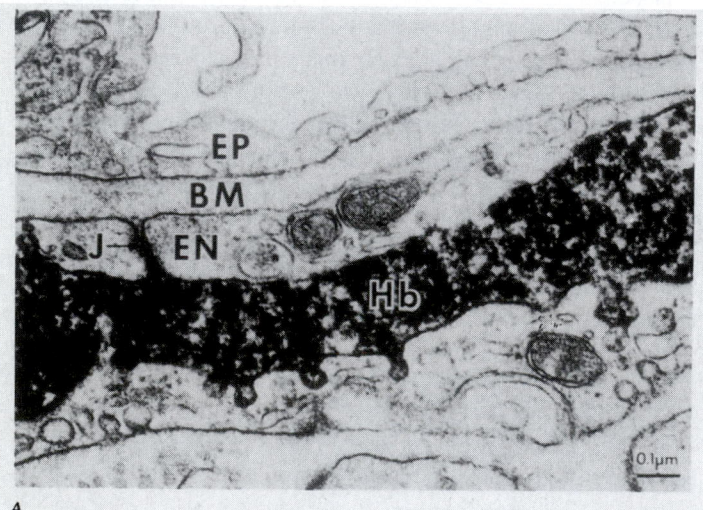

A

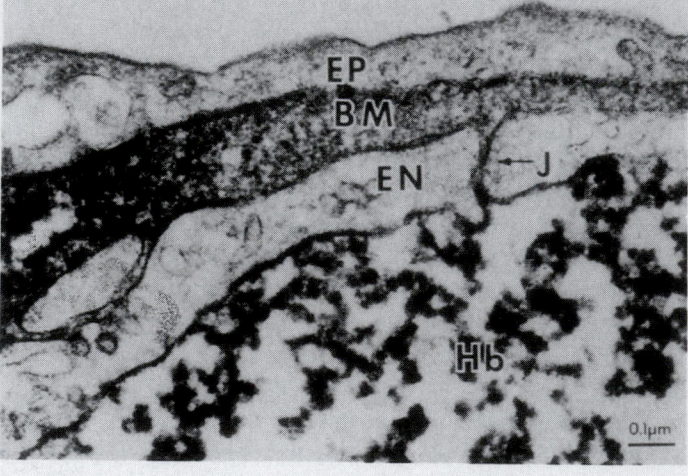

B

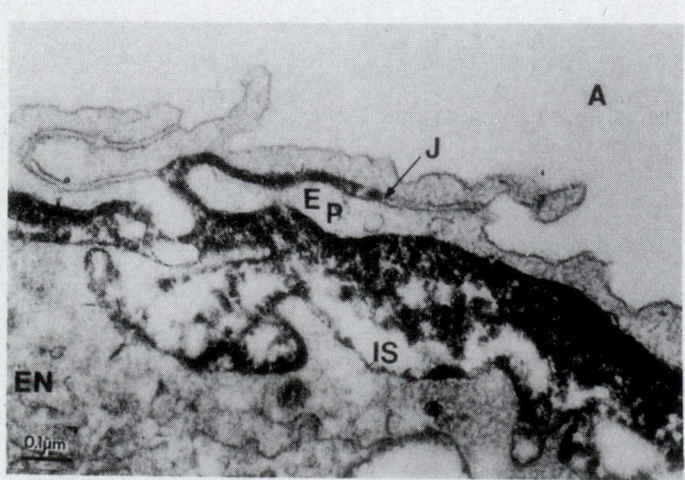

C

FIGURE 85-20 Ultrastructural demonstration of stretched pores in dog lung tissue. *A.* With normal perfusion pressures, electron dense hemoglobin (Hb) (about the same size as albumin) is confined to the capillary lumen and is unable to traverse the junction (J) between endothelial (EN) cells. *B.* With pulmonary capillary hypertension (50 mm Hg), the hemoglobin extends through the junction into the basement membrane (BM). *C.* With continued perfusion under high pressure, the hemoglobin extends from the interstitial space (IS) up to but not through the tight junction between epithelial cells, still leaving the alveolar space (A) free of tracer.

for instance, induced by capillary hydrostatic pressures of 50 mm Hg or more. Since these vascular pressures are so high, this mechanism of injury has usually been discounted as an important cause of clinical pulmonary edema. However, pressures of this magnitude, albeit transient, have been documented clinically.[51] Lung hyperinflation, as might occur with some modes of mechanical ventilation, could exacerbate the effects of high capillary pressures by further increasing capillary wall tensions. Likewise, inflammation ("remodeling") might weaken the normal capillary wall. As a result of these factors, the development of capillary "stress failure" may be more common than was previously thought.[51]

The thinness of the capillary wall, although essential for efficient gas exchange, is probably a key factor for the high wall tensions that presumably develop in capillaries during hydrostatic stress, making them more vulnerable to rupture.[51] With increases in transmural pressure (for example, from any cause of pulmonary venous hypertension) or with increases in the radius of curvature (expanded blood volume or hyperinflation of extra-alveolar capillaries during mechanical ventilation), or some combination of the two, wall stress may reach levels that exceed the tensile strength of the capillary wall. The result would be "stress failure" and capillary rupture (Fig. 85-21).

Type IV collagen within the basement membrane is the most likely molecule responsible for the tensile strength of the capillary wall.[51] However, stress failure apparently develops more easily in some animals (rabbits) than others (dogs, horses),[10,51] possibly because of differences in the capillary dimensions of radius and wall thickness, or possibly because of differences in the composition of the basement membrane. In any case, at some point the molecular structure of the basement membrane is not able to withstand the increase in hydrostatic stress and rupture occurs. This mechanism could be responsible for the hemorrhagic pulmonary edema that develops in some cases of congestive heart failure (especially those that are acute in onset), high-altitude pulmonary edema, or neurogenic pulmonary edema (see relevant sections, below). If the basement membrane is weakened, perhaps by proteases released during inflammation (as might occur in ARDS), stress failure may occur at lower than expected levels of hydrostatic pressure. On the other hand, with chronic elevations of pulmonary venous pressure (mitral steno-

sis or pulmonary vascular occlusive disease), structural remodeling with basement membrane thickening may develop and help to protect the capillary. Not surprisingly, then, in patients with mitral stenosis, pulmonary edema is relatively uncommon, despite very high pulmonary capillary pressures.

PATHOPHYSIOLOGY

Gas Exchange

Pulmonary edema causes hypoxemia by interfering with the normal regional matching of ventilation to perfusion. With continued perfusion of atelectatic and fluid-filled alveoli, the matching can be so disturbed that regions of lung effectively act as a right-to-left intrapulmonary shunt.

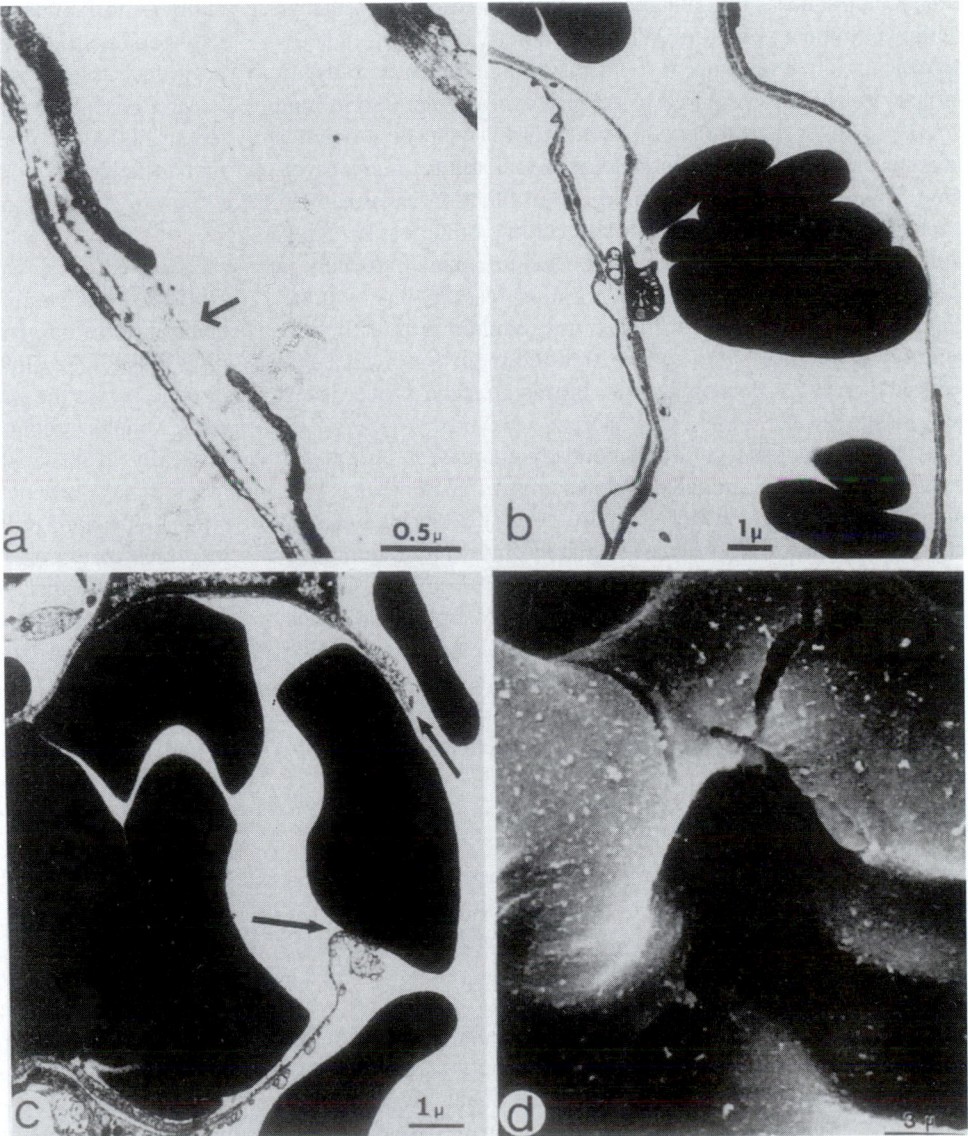

FIGURE 85-21   Electron micrographs of rabbit lung showing stress failure in pulmonary capillaries. *A.* Capillary endothelium is disrupted (*arrow*), but the alveolar epithelium and the two basement membranes are still continuous. *B.* Alveolar epithelial layer (*right*) and capillary endothelial layer (*left*) are disrupted. *C.* Disruption of all layers of the capillary wall, with a red cell appearing to pass through the opening. *D.* Scanning electron micrograph showing breaks in the alveolar epithelium. (*From West and Mathieu-Costello,[51] with permission.*)

In normal persons, intrapulmonary shunt is limited to a small fraction of the total cardiac output. In pulmonary edema, hypoxic pulmonary vasoconstriction can reduce the amount of shunt by limiting perfusion to poorly ventilated lung. In some instances, however (e.g., some cases of sepsis), hypoxic vasoconstriction may be ineffective or absent. In severe cases of pulmonary edema, shunt may approach 25 to 50 percent of the cardiac output. Since blood flowing through a shunt is not exposed to alveolar gas, supplemental oxygen per se is of little value, accounting for the "refractory" nature of hypoxemia in such cases. Instead, airway pressure therapy, supplied during mechanical ventilatory support, is necessary to restore ventilation to some of the nonventilated lung units.

Lung Mechanics

Lung compliance is the change in lung volume for a given change in transpulmonary pressure. When pulmonary edema is clinically significant, the lungs appear to be stiffer; i.e., a greater transpulmonary pressure is required to achieve a given increase in lung volume. However, to reflect the actual intrinsic elastic properties of lung tissue, compliance should be calculated for a given volume of *aeratable* lung (measured as the functional residual capacity). With pulmonary edema, the volume of aeratable lung is reduced. Any associated dysfunction in surfactant, as occurs in ARDS, will exacerbate this decrease in resting lung volume. Thus, most of the need for higher transpulmonary pressures in pulmonary edema can be attributed to the reduction in aeratable lung and not to a decrease in the intrinsic elastic properties of lung tissue per se.

Airway resistance is often modestly increased during pulmonary edema. Occasionally, perhaps most often in patients with underlying bronchial hyperreactivity, airway resistance can increase to the point where wheezing is the most prominent physical finding. In most cases, however, the increase in airway resistance is not of great clinical importance. Which biochemical, humoral, or neural factors are responsible for increased airway resistance in pulmonary edema is not clear. Regardless of the initiating mechanism, β-sympathomimetics and resolution of the pulmonary edema itself are effective treatments.

Work of Breathing

Since changes in mechanical properties increase the airway pressure necessary to achieve a given tidal volume, the work of breathing (measured as the pressure-volume product during spontaneous breaths) is increased in pulmonary edema. This effect is multiplied by the effect of tachypnea. Although the work of breathing in normal subjects comprises only a small proportion of the body's overall oxygen consumption, the work of breathing in severe pulmonary edema (without the benefit of mechanical ventilatory support) may be responsible for 25 to 50 percent of the body's total oxygen consumption. To supply the energy necessary to sustain this level of work, a greater fraction than normal of the cardiac output may have to be diverted from other vital organ systems to the respiratory muscles. For this reason, one of the chief benefits of mechanical ventilatory support during severe pulmonary edema is to reduce the patient's work of breathing so that blood flow can be redirected to other vital organs.

Pulmonary Hemodynamics

The net effect of pulmonary edema on gas exchange is not simply a function of its effect on alveolar ventilation but also of its effect on the regional pattern of blood flow distribution and the matching of regional blood flow to ventilation. Numerous studies have shown that in association with the development of mild to moderate pulmonary hypertension, blood flow is distributed away from areas of alveolar edema, improving ventilation-perfusion matching.[38] Possible acute mechanisms include hypoxic vasoconstriction, vasoconstriction from other mediators, and mechanical forces (vascular compression by edema or atelectasis). Subacutely, in situ thrombosis and vascular obliteration, especially in inflammatory types of pulmonary edema like ARDS, may become important. It appears that patients with ARDS who do in fact de-recruit severely affected capillary beds have a better prognosis than those who do not,[18] suggesting that perfusion redistribution may affect more than just gas exchange in pulmonary edema.

RESOLUTION

Far less is known about the resolution of pulmonary edema than about its development. In principle, *interstitial* edema could simply resolve if the filtrate returned to the pulmonary vascular space directly across the vascular wall or via the lymphatics to the systemic venous circulation. Although lymph flow can increase dramatically in response to increased hydrostatic pressure experimentally, the extent to which lymphatic function increases in clinical forms of pulmonary edema is not known. Furthermore, increases in lymph flow per se seem to play little role in the *clearance* of either alveolar or interstitial edema.[25]

The paths by which *alveolar* edema is cleared also are not known with certainty. Experimentally, under conditions of unchanged Starling forces, fluid instilled directly into the airspaces is cleared predominantly into the pulmonary blood volume.[25] Lymphatic function does not increase, and clearance is unaffected by changes in pulmonary blood flow. However, these observations are not necessarily relevant to clinical forms of pulmonary edema, especially when the development of pulmonary edema is the result of anatomic abnormalities in the alveolocapillary wall.

Pulmonary edema can also be cleared into the pleural space. This may be one reason for the development of pleural effusions after the onset of pulmonary edema. However, the pathways by which fluid moves from the alveolar or interstitial spaces into the pleural space are not known.

While the *pathways* for resolution are not well defined, it does seem clear that the movement of edema out of alveoli is an active, energy-requiring process, at least in lungs with an intact alveolar epithelial barrier. Fluid is reabsorbed from the airspace at a faster rate than protein, leaving the protein concentration of the remaining alveolar fluid to rise progressively. As a result, further clearance takes place against an increasing oncotic pressure gradient. Experimentally, terbutaline, a β-receptor agonist, can increase the rate of liquid clearance, independent of any effect on pulmonary blood or lymph flow, while amiloride (which blocks sodium transport channels in epithelial cells) largely blocks both normal and terbutaline-stimulated clearance.[25] A model of the process is illustrated in Figure 85-22. As sodium is reabsorbed, water follows passively, possibly through newly identified aquaporin water channels (see "Pathways for Fluid Exchange," above).[32]

How alveolar clearance of edema is affected when pulmonary capillary pressures remain elevated by left ventricular dysfunction, when lymphatic clearance is affected by right ventricular failure, or when the alveolar epithelium is injured is not known. Despite lung injury, however, some patients show increasing protein concentrations over time in fluid sampled from the alveolar space. This finding has been interpreted as evidence for continued active transport even in humans with lung injury.[25] This observation could mean that the alveolar barrier can be restored quickly, allowing virtually normal edema clearance, even in injured lungs. Alternatively, the pathways for edema development and for reabsorption could be different; alveolar edema might develop primarily at sites near the terminal airways,[48] leaving the *alveolar* epithelium sufficiently intact to preserve the normal process of edema clearance. In one relatively small study, the prognosis of patients in whom protein concentrations increased was better than in those in whom protein concentrations remained unchanged, suggesting that prognosis could be related to the ability to clear pulmonary edema quickly.[25]

Even less is known about the pathways or mechanisms for *protein* clearance from the alveolar space. Proteins may simply diffuse back into the interstitium, especially if the alveolar epithelium is relatively uninjured. However, in ARDS, when the protein concentration is high enough that hyaline membranes develop (in part representing a precipitate of alveolar protein and other cellular debris), macrophage digestion is probably an important mechanism of resolution.

OVERVIEW OF SPECIFIC SYNDROMES

Table 85-3 lists the most common forms of pulmonary edema and their associated causes or conditions.

Pulmonary Edema Associated with High Transmural Vascular Pressures

CARDIAC DYSFUNCTION

This type of pulmonary edema (congestive heart failure) is perhaps the only one that can present in both acute and chronic forms, a fact not often taken into account when the different types of pulmonary edema are compared. Common precipitating events for acute congestive heart failure include a lack of compliance with diet or drugs in patients with a history of heart failure or hypertension, inadequately or inappropriately treated heart failure, myocardial ischemia, myocardial infarction, uncontrolled

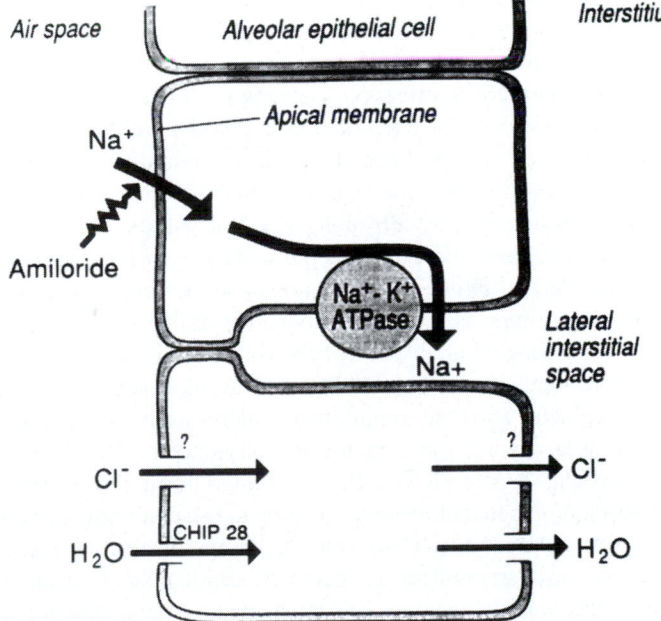

FIGURE 85-22 Diagram illustrating mechanisms for alveolar fluid clearance. Sodium (Na^+) is taken up by amiloride-sensitive channels on the apical surface of the type II alveolar epithelial cell and then actively pumped into the interstitial space by the Na-K-ATPase pumps on the basolateral surface of the cell. Chloride ($Cl-$) probably follows by an incompletely characterized transcellular pathway, which maintains electrical neutrality. Water probably follows via specific water channels, known as aquaporins, including the channellike intrinsic protein, CHIP 28. (*From Matthay et al,[75] with permission.*)

TABLE 85-3
Syndromes of Pulmonary Edema

Associated with high transmural vascular pressures
  Cardiac dysfunction, acute or chronic (see Table 85-4)
  High-altitude pulmonary edema
  Neurogenic pulmonary edema
  After upper-airway obstruction
  After pneumonectomy
Associated with infection
  ARDS (see Chapters 165 and 166)
Associated with reperfusion
  Reexpansion pulmonary edema
  Reimplantation response
  After pulmonary thromboendarterectomy
Associated with aspiration or inhalation of foreign material
  Gastric aspiration
  Smoke or toxic gas inhalation
  O_2 toxicity
  Drowning
Miscellaneous
  ARDS associated with uremia, multiple blood transfusions, pulmonary contusion, fat emboli, drug overdose, pancreatitis, post–coronary bypass

systemic hypertension, various causes of diastolic dysfunction, and both brady- and tachyarrhythmias (Table 85-4).

The severity of symptoms depends greatly on the acuity of presentation. With a more chronic and milder development of pulmonary edema, the patient might report orthopnea, paroxysmal nocturnal dyspnea, and dyspnea on exertion rather than at rest. It is in this type of pulmonary edema that the chest radiograph (typically characterized by cardiac enlargement, pleural effusions, vascular redistribution, vascular engorgement at the hilum, Kerley's lines and a distribution of edema that can include an "interstitial" pattern, a "butterfly" or a "bat-wing" pattern) is most readily distinguished from the acute forms of pulmonary edema (Figs. 85-2 and 85-3).[14]

Although left ventricular dysfunction, with concomitant increases in left ventricular filling and pulmonary capillary pressures, is usually considered to be the principal driving force behind the development of pulmonary edema in this setting, activation of the sympathetic nervous system could significantly reduce systemic venous capacity, effectively redistributing blood from the peripheral to the central blood volume. The net effect would also be an increase in pulmonary capillary pressures. Reversing this effect could explain why venodilator therapy can dramatically resolve symptoms in congestive heart failure without causing a deterioration in systolic function.

Occasionally, pulmonary edema seems to develop in patients with myocardial infarction despite normal wedge pressures.[3] Similar observations have been made in some animal studies in which acute coronary ligation causes pulmonary edema, even in the absence of elevated left atrial filling pressures. Since this experimental effect can be blocked, apparently by pretreatment with indomethacin, it is possible that a potent pulmonary venoconstrictor like thromboxane could at times participate in the pulmonary edema associated with myocardial infarction.

Management of cardiogenic pulmonary edema includes O_2 and mechanical ventilatory support when necessary, morphine (which probably reduces the sympathetically induced increases in afterload and/or increases in central venous blood volume), diuretics, nitroglycerin (especially with myocardial ischemia) or nitroprusside (especially if blood pressure is markedly elevated), control of arrhythmias, inhaled bronchodilators and possibly aminophylline if wheezing is present, dobutamine or dopamine if systolic function or blood pressure needs additional support, and a thorough and expeditious search for a precipitating cause, especially those due to structural cardiac disease like valve or papillary muscle dysfunction or acute coronary thrombosis amenable to thrombolytic or angioplasty therapy.

TABLE 85-4

Common Causes of Congestive Heart Failure

Lack of compliance with diet or drugs for CHF or HTN
Inadequately or inappropriately treated CHF
Myocardial ischemia or infarction
Uncontrolled systemic hypertension
Nonhypertensive causes of diastolic dysfunction
Brady- and tachyarrhythmias
Acute or chronic aortic or mitral valve dysfunction

Abbreviations: CHF = congestive heart failure; HTN = hypertension.

HIGH-ALTITUDE PULMONARY EDEMA

High-altitude pulmonary edema (HAPE) is part of the spectrum of disorders collectively known as *high-altitude illness,* the other major syndromes being acute mountain sickness and cerebral edema.[37] The classic syndrome generally develops in a younger person who rapidly ascends to altitudes above 2500 to 5000 m and then exercises relatively strenuously before acclimatization. HAPE can develop in older persons as well, however, with relatively little exertion above normal activity. Symptoms (first cough, chest pain, and shortness of breath, followed rapidly by respiratory distress, shock, and death if untreated) usually develop within the first few days of exposure. Coexisting symptoms of cerebral edema (headache, confusion, dizziness) are common. Physical signs are nonspecific and consistent with pulmonary edema and cerebral edema. The most common radiographic pattern is diffuse, patchy, bilateral alveolar infiltrates, although a predilection for infiltrates in the right midlung field has been noted by some observers.

The pathogenesis of HAPE is unclear, partly because it is difficult to study (for obvious reasons) and partly because the underlying basis for the development of pulmonary edema appears to be multifactorial.[37] Alveolar hypoxia (from a reduced FiO_2 at altitude as well as the development of alveolar infiltrates), a reduced hypoxic ventilatory response (which would exacerbate alveolar hypoxia), increased fluid retention (common in unacclimatized subjects at altitude), and increased cardiac output (from hypoxemia and excessive exercise, a common clinical correlate) are all factors that would increase both pulmonary vascular resistance and pulmonary blood flow at the same time. These factors would tend to produce pulmonary edema via increased capillary hydrostatic pressures.

Pulmonary artery pressures exceeding 40 mm Hg have been documented in the few cases of HAPE in which pulmonary artery catheterization was performed, while the pulmonary artery occlusion pressure was almost always normal. However, as discussed previously (see "Physiology of Water Flux," above), this finding does not rule out high pulmonary *capillary* pressures, just high *left atrial* pressures. In support of the concept that overperfusion is important to the pathogenesis of this syndrome, subjects with congenital absence of the right pulmonary artery may be more likely to develop HAPE at lower altitudes.[37]

Despite the apparent importance of increased hydrostatic pressures as a driving force in the development of HAPE, bronchoalveolar lavage (BAL) fluid obtained from these patients shows a *high* concentration of protein, consistent with increased vascular permeability. Postmortem findings of alveolar hyaline membranes also confirm an increased capillary leak of protein from the vascular space. The mechanism responsible for the breach in endothelial barrier integrity is not known, but could be stress failure of the alveolar capillaries (see "Stretched Pores and Capillary Stress Failure," above), developing as a result of high pulmonary vascular pressures and hyperperfusion.[51] In some studies, however, inflammatory mediators, especially of the leukotriene series, have been found in high concentrations in BAL fluid, raising the possibility that inflammation could also play a role in the development of increased permeability in this syndrome.

In HAPE, the radiographic infiltrates, though diffuse, are often irregularly distributed throughout the lung fields. This patchy distribution has been confirmed in postmortem studies. An uneven distribution of vasoconstriction and perfusion has usually been invoked as the most convincing explanation, although an underlying mechanism for such a regional difference has never been demonstrated. Alternatively, capillary stress failure, by its very nature, occurs inhomogeneously, and may be a more likely explanation.

Vascular thrombi and fibrin clots are also a common finding at postmortem, giving rise to the hypothesis that microembolization is part of the pathogenesis of HAPE. These findings may be evidence of previous endothelial injury. Again, capillary stress failure provides a mechanism, though unproven, for why such in situ thrombosis would develop.

The concept that increased pulmonary capillary pressures are central to the pathogenesis of HAPE is also supported by remarkable and salutary responses to treatment based on reducing pulmonary pressures. Rapid descent to lower altitudes can have a dramatic effect; sometimes oxygen alone can be used successfully (presumably reducing pulmonary vasoconstriction). Likewise, acetazolamide (a diuretic and ventilatory stimulant) can be useful. Finally, although experience is limited, nifedipine has been used successfully to both treat and prevent HAPE.

NEUROGENIC PULMONARY EDEMA

This relatively rare form of pulmonary edema has many clinical features that are similar to those of HAPE. The distinguishing feature is that in most cases dyspnea, hypoxemia, and radiographic pulmonary infiltrates all develop within a few hours of a well-defined neurologic insult. The most common inciting event is a grand-mal seizure. Some patients develop pulmonary edema with virtually every new attack. However, neurogenic pulmonary edema has also been reported in association with almost all severe forms of neurologic events (head trauma, stroke, intracranial hemorrhage, etc.).

Generally, the radiographic pattern is that of a bilateral, alveolar filling process. Otherwise, the chest radiographic pattern is nonspecific. Given that this form of pulmonary edema usually develops in someone with an impaired level of consciousness, aspiration pneumonitis is often entertained as an alternative diagnosis. Relatively rapid clearing of the infiltrates (in a few days) can be seen with either clinical entity, and so does not help distinguish either as a potential cause.

The problem of aspiration as a potential cause in some cases is made even more difficult because a "delayed" form of neurogenic pulmonary edema has been reported.[45] Except for the slower development of dyspnea, hypoxemia, and radiographic infiltrates, there is little else to distinguish this form from the more acute pattern. Clearly, as additional time elapses, distinguishing this presentation from aspiration or nosocomial infection becomes more difficult.

The pathogenesis of neurogenic pulmonary edema has not been established; it seems to be similar to that hypothesized for HAPE. In experimental animal models, pulmonary venous hypertension is prominent. Clinically, severe (albeit transient) systemic hypertension with left ventricular failure (and elevated pulmonary artery occlusion pressures) has been documented. Simultaneously, systemic venous tone also increases, displacing the peripheral venous blood volume centrally into the lungs. The net effect of these changes is that pulmonary blood volume increases at exactly the same time as pulmonary venous resistance, resulting in a marked elevation of pulmonary capillary pressures. Massive activation of the autonomic nervous system at the time of the neurologic crisis presumably mediates these changes in vascular tone. Both a direct stimulation of pulmonary vessels by the sympathetic nervous system and vasoconstriction in response to systemic catecholamine release are probably involved.

As in HAPE, the protein content of the pulmonary edema fluid in patients and experimental animals with neurogenic pulmonary edema is often relatively high, implying that vascular permeability must be altered in this syndrome. If so, the mechanism remains unclear; again, capillary stress failure, as with HAPE, would be an obvious way to link the observations of markedly increased vascular pressures and proteinaceous edema fluid together.[51] The delayed form of neurogenic pulmonary edema, however, would argue against increased vascular pressures as the only, or even the principal, mechanism underlying the increase in pulmonary vascular permeability, and raise the possibility that the CNS can affect lung vascular permeability directly by other mechanisms.

The sites within the central nervous system that are critical to the development of neurogenic pulmonary edema are not fully established, but certain themes seem to be important. For one, while an intact cervical spine seems to be essential for the development of neurogenic pulmonary edema (in experimental models, cervical transection prevents the development of neurogenic pulmonary edema), spinal pathology itself is rarely if ever associated with the development of this syndrome. Thus, the cervical spine appears to mediate a supraspinal event.

Virtually every form of acute intracerebral pathology has been associated with the development of neurogenic pulmonary edema. Since the most common neurologic events (grand-mal seizures, subarachnoid hemorrhage, head trauma) are associated with increased intracranial pressures, intracranial hypertension is generally considered to be another key etiologic feature. How intracranial hypertension leads to neurogenic pulmonary edema is not known, however, and certainly intracranial hypertension often occurs without the development of pulmonary edema.

Various vasomotor centers of the medulla (so-called areas A_1 and A_5, the nuclei of the solitary tract and the area postrema) have fibers that project onto preganglionic centers in the cervical spinal cord that can increase output along the sympathetic trunk. Some of these areas also have connections to the hypothalamus. Both hypothalamic lesions and stimulation of these medullary areas experimentally can produce neurogenic pulmonary edema.[45] Thus, one possible scenario is that an acute neurologic crisis, accompanied by a marked increase in intracranial pressure, stimulates the hypothalamus and/or vasomotor centers of the medulla, which in turn initiate a massive autonomic discharge mediated by preganglionic centers within the cervical spine.

The potential importance of the medulla in the pathogenesis of neurogenic pulmonary edema is supported by animal experiments in which the instillation of opiates near the respiratory center produced pulmonary edema with a high protein content, providing a mechanism for how the central nervous system could affect the integrity of the pulmonary endothelial barrier directly. Such studies also suggest a possible pathogenesis for pulmonary edema that is associated with narcotic overdose—a syndrome whose clinical features, course, and prognosis are similar to those of other causes of neurogenic pulmonary edema.

The treatment of neurogenic pulmonary edema is supportive and does not differ in any important way from that of the usual patient with ARDS, although special attention must be paid toward therapeutic maneuvers that can increase intracranial pressures (e.g., PEEP). In general, the prognosis is usually good; often, it is more a function of the underlying neurologic problem than the development of pulmonary edema per se.

PULMONARY EDEMA AFTER UPPER-AIRWAY OBSTRUCTION

This form of pulmonary edema can occur sporadically and unexpectedly in circumstances characterized by temporary upper-airway obstruction (near-hanging, strangulation, epiglottitis, thyroid goiter, upper-airway tumor, acromegaly, mediastinal tumor, foreign-body aspiration, or difficult insertion of an endotracheal or tracheostomy tube, among others).[20] In the absence of other complicating conditions, the pulmonary edema usually responds readily to routine supportive measures.

In pulmonary edema associated with upper-airway obstruction, the high transmural capillary pressures are generated by very negative intrapleural pressures that develop when vigorous breathing is attempted to overcome the airway obstruction. The negative pleural pressures, when transmitted to the interstitial space, increase the capillary transmural pressure. Increased autonomic tone, as a reaction to extreme respiratory distress or in response to laryngeal stimulation during intubation, may also cause pulmonary venous vasoconstriction, further increasing the pulmonary capillary transmural hydrostatic pressures. Hypoxic vasoconstriction, especially if unevenly distributed throughout the pulmonary vasculature, could increase the hydrostatic pressures of some capillary beds even further.

In this syndrome of pulmonary edema too, the edema fluid has a relatively high protein concentration, suggesting increased pulmonary vascular permeability. The mechanism for the increase in permeability is uncertain. One possibility is increased transmural vascular pressure complicated by hyperinflation from auto-PEEP, with capillary stress failure and rupture.

PULMONARY EDEMA AFTER LUNG RESECTION

Occasionally, some patients develop pulmonary edema within a few hours of pneumonectomy.[50] Cardiac output is usually normal or high, and cardiac filling pressures are also normal. The pulmonary edema fluid itself has a high protein concentration, most consistent with increased vascular permeability. More direct measures of vascular permeability, however, have not been reported. The course is usually benign. Thus, in the absence of alternative explanations, this clinical picture is most consistent with increased permeability pulmonary edema with (or secondary to) high pulmonary capillary pressures.

Pulmonary Edema Associated with Reperfusion

There are at least three types of pulmonary edema that develop after perfusion has been restored to a previously ischemic lung: reexpansion of previously collapsed lung, reimplantation of a transplanted lung, and pulmonary thromboendarterectomy for chronic pulmonary emboli. Pulmonary edema developing after reperfusion of previously ischemic nonpulmonary tissue may be an example of a similar phenomenon.

REEXPANSION PULMONARY EDEMA

Pulmonary edema can develop, usually ipsilaterally, after a previously atelectatic lung is reexpanded by either large-volume thoracentesis (if associated with a large pleural effusion) or by negative-pressure suction via tube thoracostomy.[19] Typically, symptoms and signs consistent with pulmonary edema develop within minutes to hours of the time the lung is reexpanded.

One possible mechanism for pulmonary edema in these settings is that large negative intrapleural pressures, developed during reexpansion, would decrease interstitial pressures, thereby increasing the hydrostatic gradient for transvascular fluid flow. The result should be a form of hydrostatic pulmonary edema with low protein concentrations.

However, large swings in intrapleural pressures are not necessary for this syndrome to develop, since pulmonary edema can also develop with simple (although relatively rapid) gravity drainage of a large pleural effusion. Furthermore, the protein concentration of the edema fluid in this type of pulmonary edema is often high, suggesting increased vascular permeability. Since the atelectatic lung is usually airless with reduced blood flow, it is probably relatively ischemic. With reexpansion, blood flow and reoxygenation would return abruptly (and indeed, one of the requirements for this syndrome seems to be rapid reexpansion). These are precisely the requirements for the development of ischemia-reperfusion injury (Fig. 85-19). However, as there are no specific markers or inhibitors of ischemia-reperfusion injury, the importance of this mechanism clinically is still unknown. Other mechanisms may be at work. For instance, the lack of mechanical movement by ventilation in the atelectatic lung, in addition to ischemia, may be important.[16]

The treatment of reexpansion pulmonary edema is supportive. The prognosis is not good; mortality has been reported to be as high as 20 percent, possibly because the syndrome often develops in patients with other chronic debilitating disease.

REIMPLANTATION RESPONSE AFTER LUNG ALLOGRAFT TRANSPLANTATION

Virtually all patients develop new pulmonary infiltrates in a lung allograft within the first 48 h after lung transplantation ("reimplantation response").[47] The severity of the response usually reaches a maximum by the fourth postoperative day, clearing rapidly thereafter. Pulmonary vascular permeability is moderately abnormal, not reaching the severity seen in ARDS.[41] The differential diagnosis includes rejection (unusual at such an early time), infection (especially sepsis if both lungs are affected), mucous plugging, or cardiogenic pulmonary edema. The diagnosis of reimplantation injury is supported when the radiographic and gas exchange abnormalities resolve without specific therapy.

Etiologically, reimplantation pulmonary edema may be another example of ischemia-reperfusion injury, or it may be the result of other factors, including surgical trauma and preservation technique.

PULMONARY EDEMA AFTER PULMONARY THROMBOENDARTERECTOMY

This syndrome also develops within the first few postoperative days.[23] The severity of injury is highly variable and unpredictable, but is worsened by relative hyperperfusion of the newly endarterectomized lung ("pulmonary steal"). The edema is limited to the portions of lung that are newly perfused. Denudation of the endothelium with endarterectomy, hyperperfusion, chronic ischemia, and oxidant injury initiated by reperfusion are all possible mechanisms for the development of pulmonary edema in this setting.

Pulmonary Edema Associated with Aspiration or Inhalation of Foreign Material

These cases include the pulmonary aspiration of gastric acid, fresh- and saltwater drowning, and toxic gas and smoke inhalation. Aspiration of foreign material into the airways can cause a number of different clinical syndromes, primarily drowning, mechanical airway obstruction, bronchoconstriction with wheezing, and pulmonary edema. Gas or smoke inhalation is usually characterized by either bronchoconstriction or pulmonary edema, if anything. With both aspiration and toxic inhalations, nosocomial pneumonia may develop eventually, especially in cases that require mechanical ventilatory support or do not resolve quickly. A more complete discussion of these syndromes is found in Chapter 80.

GASTRIC ACID ASPIRATION

The classic animal model of gastric acid aspiration is to instill 2 to 4 ml/kg of concentrated HCl (pH 1.5 to 2.5) directly into the airways, producing a highly lethal model of pulmonary edema.[5] However, aspiration of gastric material at a higher pH is not necessarily clinically benign. Airway obstruction, atelectasis, and pneumonia can all develop, depending on the volume and nature (particulate, infected) of the material aspirated. For this reason, new radiographic chest infiltrates may not simply represent pulmonary edema from chemical pneumonitis.

Aspiration of gastric juice with a pH under 3.0 causes a chemical burn to the airway epithelium, leading to cell death and a local inflammatory reaction characterized by airway edema, bronchoconstriction, and airway closure with atelectasis. Rarely is bronchorrhea itself severe enough to spill over into the distal airways. In some patients, the volume of aspirated material may be sufficiently large or the inflammatory reaction sufficiently severe that the process extends into the lung parenchyma, involving distal airways and alveolar units. At this point, the syndrome may be indistinguishable from any other presentation of ARDS.

Gastric aspiration is often listed as one of the "direct" causes of lung injury. This designation may be misleading because by the time alveolar edema is recognized clinically, intense inflammation is the rule. Thus, acid aspiration can undoubtedly initiate injury, but its full expression may still require an inflammatory host response. In this sense, it is like other causes of ARDS.

Management of pulmonary edema due to gastric acid aspiration is similar to that for any other cause of ARDS. Although some experimental data support the early use of high-dose corticosteroids (presumably suppressing the inflammatory reaction), clinical evidence is lacking, and generally most pulmonologists or intensivists do not use steroids in the early management phase of aspiration-induced pulmonary edema.

The use of prophylactic antibiotics is also controversial. Most pulmonologists and intensivists would avoid using them solely for new pulmonary infiltrates developing within 4 to 24 h of a witnessed aspiration, since infectious pneumonia would be unlikely at this time. However, when the circumstances are less clear, as is often the case, antibiotics are often included in the therapeutic regimen, at least initially, especially if the patient is critically ill.

Since particulates are often present in gastric material, early bronchoscopy, especially in the already intubated patient, can easily be justified to rule out airway obstruction as a complicating factor.

SMOKE AND TOXIC GAS INHALATION

The pathobiology of smoke inhalation is complex, dependent on injury caused by heat, toxins in the gas phase, particulates in the smoke, the total exposure, and the host inflammatory response.[9] Accordingly, there are many different clinical presentations, discussed in greater detail in Chapters 45 and 109.

As with gastric acid aspiration, the pathogenesis of pulmonary edema associated with smoke inhalation is thought to begin with a chemical burn to the upper and lower airways—i.e., diffuse epithelial cell necrosis. The mechanism of injury and cell death is uncertain, but oxidant and lipid peroxidant injuries are likely possibilities. Although distal airway and even parenchymal involvement may be more common after smoke inhalation than after gastric acid aspiration, it is still an unusual event, most commonly associated with massive inhalations. Accordingly, pulmonary edema per se is an unusual early manifestation of smoke inhalation. The development of pulmonary edema in burned patients, *unlike* its development after gastric acid aspiration, may also be exacerbated by the prodigious amounts of fluid administered to the burned patient, and the frequent development of a systemic inflammatory response syndrome with or without frank systemic infection (sepsis). Otherwise, pathogenesis, pathophysiology, and management are similar to those of other causes of ARDS.

DROWNING

Clearance of aspirated fresh water can be very rapid from otherwise normal alveolar units.[28] Surfactant dysfunction may occur with fluid-filled alveoli, resulting in atelectasis. As the fresh water is cleared, serum solutes are diluted and the blood can become hypotonic.

With near-drowning in seawater, water is drawn into the alveoli because seawater is hypertonic relative to plasma. The result is hypovolemia and worsening of the pulmonary edema. The high tonicity, then, impedes clearance.

Miscellaneous

A good example of the difficulty that can be encountered in trying to discern the underlying mechanism of pulmonary edema from clinical characteristics alone is the syndrome of pulmonary edema associated with uremia ("uremic lung"). The classic radiographic description is that of a "butterfly" or "batwing" appearance (i.e., fluffy perihilar haze and infiltrates) (Fig. 85-2). This appearance is consistent with volume overload—a cardinal manifestation of uremia—or cardiac failure, a frequent problem in elderly patients with renal failure.

In some cases, more diffuse and peripheral infiltrates have been seen. When pulmonary edema in these patients has been sampled, the protein concentration has been high, suggesting increased vascular permeability. The mechanism of increased permeability in uremia is unknown; it is possible that high concentrations of some as yet unidentified renally excreted metabolite can affect endothelial integrity. In any case, this entity is very uncommon now that hemodialysis is routinely available.

Despite our advances in understanding, there are still numerous individual cases of pulmonary edema for which the pathogenesis is still obscure, some of which are listed in Table 85-3.

THERAPY

General Measures

The treatment of pulmonary edema is remarkably the same, regardless of cause. However, the *effectiveness* of treatment depends very much on the underlying cause, and whether or not specific treatment for the underlying cause is available and useful. Management primarily entails supportive measures aimed at maintaining cellular and physiological functions (e.g., gas exchange, organ perfusion, aerobic metabolism) while the underlying cause is studied and treated if possible. The supportive measures include oxygen with mechanical ventilatory and airway pressure support if necessary, fluid restriction and/or diuretics when possible, cardiovascular support with hemodynamic monitoring if appropriate, antibiotics for associated infection if present, and nutritional supplementation if mechanical ventilatory support is prolonged (Table 85-5). In the remainder of this section on treatment, some themes relevant to the management of any patient with pulmonary edema are noted. More detailed discussion can be found in chapters reviewing specific clinical syndromes accompanied by pulmonary edema.

Nonpharmacologic Therapies

FLUID MANAGEMENT

As implied by the relationships shown between EVLW and pulmonary capillary pressures shown in Figure 85-18, efforts to reduce pulmonary capillary pressures should have a salutary effect

TABLE 85-5
Therapeutic Principles

Oxygen ± mechanical ventilation ± PEEP/CPAP
Fluid restriction/diuretics (when possible)
Cardiovascular support ± hemodynamic monitoring
Antibiotics for associated infection
Nutritional supplementation for prolonged illness
Expeditious search for an underlying and treatable cause

on the development of pulmonary edema, even when vascular permeability is abnormal. Furthermore, even in ARDS, when the pathogenesis of pulmonary edema is not attributed to pulmonary capillary hypertension, elevated pulmonary capillary pressures may still be a factor, from fluid overload in the management of shock, pulmonary venous vasoconstriction, or concomitant cardiac failure.

Fluid restriction and, when possible, the use of diuretics are commonly employed to reduce pulmonary capillary pressures. Several clinical studies of ARDS indicate that pulmonary function and outcome are better in patients who lose body weight or in whom the wedge pressure falls as a result of diuresis or fluid restriction.[27,39] The strategy of early diuresis/fluid restriction has not been associated with a higher incidence of complications, such as renal failure or hemodynamic compromise, as long as close monitoring ensures adequate organ perfusion.[27]

A long-standing argument has been whether colloid or crystalloid infusions should be used in the fluid management of patients with pulmonary edema, especially patients with ARDS. The argument in favor would suggest that according to equation 1 (see "Physiology of Water Flux," above), increasing plasma oncotic pressure will lead to a reduced transvascular flux of fluid.

There are several arguments against the use of colloid, however. First, colloid infusions are volume expanders as well as oncotic agents. Therefore, they will increase capillary hydrostatic pressures at the same time that they increase oncotic pressures. These effects, obviously, offset one another. Indeed, from equation 1, it can be seen that equivalent increases in hydrostatic pressure and oncotic pressure favor transudation, since the reflection coefficient is less than 1. Second, the oncotic effects of exogenous colloid are transient. Especially in the setting of increased vascular permeability, leakage of colloid at an accelerated pace would be expected, and it could be argued that excess colloid in the pulmonary extravascular space might actually worsen pulmonary edema. Third, the resolution of alveolar edema does not follow the same paths as the development of interstitial edema. Therefore, increasing intravascular colloid concentrations should have little effect on the resolution of alveolar edema. Finally, no clinical studies have shown that the resolution of pulmonary edema is improved by the use of intravenous colloid.

Of course, colloid infusions are very effective blood volume substitutes; therefore they may have a role, although limited, in the acute resuscitation of a hemodynamically unstable patient who also has pulmonary edema. They have no role, however, in the fluid management of pulmonary edema per se. Indeed, as already noted, most studies suggest that outcome in pulmonary edema is improved if fluids can be restricted and diuresis achieved.[27,39]

MECHANICAL VENTILATION

While mechanical ventilation is often initiated during pulmonary edema to improve gas exchange or to reduce the work of breathing, evidence continues to accumulate that another therapeutic goal of mechanical ventilation should be to recruit as many functional lung units as possible, to maintain their patency throughout the respiratory cycle, and to avoid alveolar overdistention.[21]

It is not yet known whether such an approach will affect outcome favorably, but if so, an important clinical marker will be to keep the alveolar plateau pressure below the maximum alveolar distending pressure (in a normal lung, about 35 cm H_2O), reducing the risk of unnecessary hyperinflation.

PEEP is commonly used to increase mean airway pressure, with the twin goals of recruiting previously nonventilated lung and maintaining patency of these units once recruited. From this point of view, the overall effect of PEEP should be a beneficial improvement in gas exchange. However, the overall effects of PEEP are complex (see Chapter 176). With respect to effects on pulmonary edema formation, PEEP tends to *decrease* the hydrostatic pressure gradient for fluid flux in alveolar vessels but *increase* it in extra-alveolar vessels. As a result, PEEP usually has no overall effect on edema formation. However, to the extent that edema may be distributed away from the alveolar compartment, a beneficial effect on gas exchange, in addition to that obtained by opening airways to previously nonventilated lung units, is possible.

Sometimes adequate oxygenation at acceptable levels of F_iO_2 and airway pressure cannot be achieved with the routine use of PEEP. In these cases, additional measures are necessary. Various alternatives are possible, including so-called controlled hypoventilation with permissive hypercapnia, ventilation in the prone position, inverse ratio ventilation, and extracorporeal respiratory support.[21] In the future, tracheal gas insufflation, the intravenous gas exchange catheter, and perfluorocarbon-associated gas exchange (i.e., partial liquid ventilation) may become additional supportive measures. These various topics are discussed in greater detail in other chapters.

Pharmacologic Therapies

The principal pharmacologic therapy for pulmonary edema is oxygen with or without the use of diuretics, as discussed previously. For pulmonary edema specifically due to increased hydrostatic pressures, additional measures to reduce pulmonary capillary pressures will usually be useful, including nitrates, narcotics for pain (specifically associated with myocardial infarction), and nifedipine (or other rapidly acting parenteral agents) for systemic or pulmonary hypertension (especially HAPE). Additional measures to support systolic cardiac function (inotropic agents and/or mechanical assist devices) may be needed for cardiogenic forms of pulmonary edema, in addition to a concerted and timely search for surgically correctable myocardial or valvular causes of pulmonary capillary hypertension.

The pharmacologic treatment for ARDS is discussed in Chapter 166.

REFERENCES

1. Abernathy VJ, Pou NA, Wilson TL, Roselli RJ: Noninvasive measurements of albumin flux into lung interstitium with increased microvascular pressure. *Am J Physiol* 38:H288–H296, 1995.
2. Albelda SM, Sampson PM, Haselton FR, et al: Permeability characterics of cultured endothelial cell monolayers. *J Appl Physiol* 64:308–322, 1988.
3. Altschule MD: Acute pulmonary edema without demonstrable left ventricular failure after myocardial infarction. *Chest* 89:292–293, 1986.
4. Bachofen H, Schurch S, Michel RP, Weibel ER: Experimental hydrostatic pulmonary edema in rabbit lungs. Morphology. *Am Rev Respir Dis* 147:989–996, 1993.
5. Britto J, Demling RH: Aspiration lung injury. *New Horizons* 1:435–439, 1993.
6. Bundgaard M: The three-dimensional organization of tight junctions in a capillary endothelium revealed by serial-section electron microscopy. *J Ultrastruc Res* 88:1–17, 1984.
7. Cutillo AG, Morris AH, Ailion DC, Durney CH: Clinical implications of nuclear magnetic resonance lung research. *Chest* 96:643–652, 1989.
8. Dawson CA, Roerig DL, Linehan JH: Evaluation of endothelial injury in the human lung. *Clin Chest Med* 10:13–24, 1989.
9. Demling RH: Smoke inhalation injury. *New Horizons* 1:422–434, 1993.
10. Ehrhart IC, Hofman WF: Pressure-dependent increase in lung vascular permeability to water but not protein. *J Appl Physiol* 72:211–218, 1992.
11. Forster BB, Muller NL, Mayo JR, et al: High-resolution computed tomography of experimental hydrostatic pulmonary edema. *Chest* 101:1434–1437, 1992.
12. Gattinoni L, Pesenti A, Torresin A, et al: Adult respiratory distress syndrome profiles by computed tomography. *J Thorac Imag* 1:25–30, 1986.
13. Gilbert E, Hakim TS: Derivation of pulmonary capillary pressure from arterial occlusion in intact conditions. *Crit Care Med* 22:986–993, 1994.
14. Gropper MA, Wiener-Kronish JP, Hashimoto S: Acute cardiogenic pulmonary edema. *Clin Chest Med* 15:501–515, 1994.
15. Hainis KD, Sznajder JI, Schraufnagel DE: Lung lymphatics cast from the airspace. *Am J Physiol* 267 (2 Pt 1):L199–205, 1994.
16. Hamvas A, Park CK, Palazzo R, et al: Modifying pulmonary ischemia-reperfusion injury by altering ventilatory strategies during ischemia. *J Appl Physiol* 73:2112–2119, 1992.
17. Hamvas A, Schuster DP: Bronchial and reverse pulmonary venous blood flow protect the lung from ischemia-reperfusion injury. *J Appl Physiol* 77:731–736, 1994.
18. Harris TR, Bernard GR, Brigham KL, et al: Lung microvascular transport properties measured by multiple indicator dilution methods in patients with adult respiratory distress syndrome: A comparison between patients reversing respiratory failure and those failing to reverse. *Am Rev Respir Dis* 141:272–280, 1990.
19. Jackson RM, Veal CF: Re-expansion, re-oxygenation, and rethinking. *Am J Med Sci* 298:44–50, 1989.
20. Kollef MH, Pluss J: Noncardiogenic pulmonary edema following upper airway obstruction: 7 cases and a review of the literature. *Medicine (Baltimore)* 70:91–98, 1991.
21. Kollef MH, Schuster DP: The acute respiratory distress syndrome. *New Engl J Med* 332:27–37, 1995.
22. Kubes P: Nitric oxide affects microvascular permeability in the intact and inflamed vasculature. *Microcirculation* 2:235–244, 1995.

23. Levinson RM, Shure D, Moser KM: Reperfusion pulmonary edema after pulmonary artery thromboendarterectomy. *Am Rev Respir Dis* 134:1241–1245, 1986.

24. Lum H, Malik AB: Regulation of vascular endothelial barrier function. *Am J Physiol* 267:L223–L241, 1994.

25. Matthay MA, Folkesson HG, Campagna A, Kheradmand F: Alveolar epithelial barrier and acute lung injury. *New Horizons* 1:613–622, 1993.

26. McNamee JE: Fractal perspectives in pulmonary physiology. *J Appl Physiol* 71:1–8, 1991.

27. Mitchell JP, Schuller D, Calandrino FS, Schuster DP: Improved outcome based on fluid management in critically ill patients requiring pulmonary artery catheterization. *Am Rev Respir Dis* 145:990–998, 1992.

28. Modell JH: Drowning. *New Engl J Med* 328:253–256, 1994.

29. Montaner JSG, Tsang J, Evans KG, et al: Alveolar epithelial damage: A critical difference between high pressure and oleic acid–induced low pressure pulmonary edema. *J Clin Invest* 77:1786–1796, 1986.

30. Moriwaki Y, Yamamoto T, Suda M, et al: Purification and immunohistochemical tissue localization of human xanthine oxidase. *Biochim Biophys Acta* 1164:327–330, 1993.

31. Peterson BT: Permeability: Theory vs. practice in lung research. *Am J Physiol* 262:L243–L256, 1992.

32. Raina S, Preston GM, Guggino WB, Agre P: Molecular cloning and characterization of an aquaporin cDNA from salivary, lacrimal, and respiratory tissues. *J Biol Chem* 270:1908–1912, 1995.

33. Renkin EM: Cellular aspects of transvascular exchange: A 40-year perspective. *Microcirculation* 1:157–167, 1994.

34. Roselli RJ, Harris TR: Lung fluid and macromolecular transport, in Chang HK, Paiva M (eds), *Respiratory Physiology: An Analytical Approach, Lung Biology in Health and Disease*. New York, Dekker, 1989, pp 633–735.

35. Roselli RJ, Riddle WR: Analysis of noninvasive macromolecular transport measurements in the lung. *J Appl Physiol* 67:2343–2350, 1989.

36. Schneeberger EE, Lynch RD: Structure, function, and regulation of cellular tight junctions. *Am J Physiol* 262:L647–L661, 1992.

37. Schoene RB: Pulmonary edema at high altitude: Review, pathophysiology, and update. *Clin Chest Med* 6:491–507, 1985.

38. Schuster DP: ARDS: Clinical lessons from the oleic acid model of acute lung injury. *Am J Respir Crit Care Med* 149:245–260, 1994.

39. Schuster DP: The case for and against fluid restriction and occlusion pressure reduction in adult respiratory distress syndrome. *New Horizons* 1:478–488, 1993.

40. Schuster DP: Positron emission tomography: Theory and its application to the study of lung disease. *Am Rev Respir Dis* 139:818–840, 1989.

41. Schuster DP: What is acute lung injury? What is ARDS? *Chest* 107:1721–1726, 1995.

42. Sibbald WJ, Short AK, Warshawski FJ, et al: Thermal dye measurements of extravascular lung water in critically ill patients: Intravascular Starling forces and extravascular lung water in the adult respiratory distress syndrome. *Chest* 87:585–592, 1985.

43. Sibbald WJ, Warshawski FJ, Short AK, et al: Clinical studies of measuring extravascular lung water by the thermal dye technique in critically ill patients. *Chest* 83:725–731, 1983.

44. Simionescu M. Lung endothelium: Structure-function correlates, in Crystal RB, West JB (eds), *The Lung: Scientific Foundations*. New York, Raven Press, 1991, pp 301–312.

45. Simon RP: Neurogenic pulmonary edema. *Neurol Clin* 11:309–323, 1993.

46. Sivak ED, Wiedemann HP: Clinical measurement of extravascular lung water. *Crit Care Clin* 2:511–526, 1986.

47. Sleiman C, Mal H, Fournier M, et al: Pulmonary reimplantation response in single-lung transplantation. *Eur Respir J* 8:5–9, 1995.

48. Staub NC: The pathogenesis of pulmonary edema. *Prog Cardiovasc Dis* 23:53–80, 1980.

49. Taylor AE, Barnard JW, Barman SA, Adkins WK: Fluid balance, in Crystal RG, West JB (eds), *The Lung: Scientific Foundations*. New York, Raven Press, 1991, 1147–1161.

50. Turnage WS, Lunn JJ: Postpneumonectomy pulmonary edema: A retrospective analysis of associated variables. *Chest* 103:1646–1650, 1993.

51. West JB, Mathieu-Costello O: Vulnerability of pulmonary capillaries in heart disease. *Circulation* 92:622–631, 1995.

52. Wheeler AP, Carroll FE, Bernard GR: Radiographic issues in adult respiratory distress syndrome. *New Horizons* 1:471–477, 1993.

CHAPTER 86

PULMONARY VASCULITIS

Richard A. DeRemee

DEFINITIONS AND SCOPE

Pulmonary vasculitis is the term applied to inflammation affecting the pulmonary circulation. Pulmonary vasculitis may be a localized phenomenon, but usually it is part of a systemic process. The extrapulmonary manifestations may be more dramatic and consequential than those produced by the pulmonary involvement. Classification of pulmonary vasculitides remains a challenge because diseases such as these of unknown cause cannot be firmly and finally characterized until their etiologic agent or mode of pathogenesis is clarified. Behçet's disease and Takayasu's arteritis are examples of pulmonary vasculitides that rely heavily on clinical criteria for diagnosis and in which there is much blurring and overlap with other syndromes, so that their legitimacy as distinct clinicopathologic entities is doubtful. As new information develops, ideas about pulmonary vasculitides change. The concept of Wegener's granulomatosis is particularly notable, having changed vastly since Wegener's original description, largely due to discovery of the antineutrophil cytoplasmic autoantibody (ANCA).

The main entities to be discussed in this chapter are Wegener's granulomatosis, allergic granulomatosis and angiitis, otherwise referred to as the Churg-Strauss syndrome, and microscopic polyangiitis. Although some dispute may arise between authorities concerning the inclusion of diffuse alveolar hemorrhage syndromes in pulmonary vasculitis, the discussion includes these entities because most patients with alveolar hemorrhage have capillaritis. Behçet's disease and Takayasu's arteritis are given less emphasis even though they have major components in the lung. The discussion concludes with necrotizing sarcoid granulomatosis (NSG) because inflammatory lesions affecting blood vessels occur in this condition. However, unlike the other entities to be discussed, there is neither diffuse alveolar hemorrhage nor significant necrosis and destruction of pulmonary architecture.

Pulmonary vasculitis is relatively rare in the United States, and thus meaningful data regarding incidence and prevalence are difficult to derive. At the Mayo Clinic over a 30-year period, beginning in 1965, approximately 500 new patients were diagnosed with Wegener's granulomatosis and approximately 80 patients were seen with the diagnosis of Churg-Strauss syndrome. These are the two most frequently encountered pulmonary vasculitides. It is even more difficult to obtain data concerning alveolar hemorrhage syndromes because of the multiplicity of causes. Usually some form of systemic vasculitis with concomitant glomerulonephritis is responsible.

At one time, lymphomatoid granulomatosis and bronchocentric granulomatosis were included among the pulmonary vasculitides. However, lymphomatoid granulomatosis is a premalignant or frankly malignant lesion thought to arise from T lymphocytes, and bronchocentric granulomatosis is primarily granulomatous inflammation of airways with only minor vasculitis incidental to the airway inflammation.

COLLAGEN VASCULAR DISEASES WITH MINOR PULMONARY VASCULAR COMPONENTS

Collagen vascular diseases commonly have pulmonary involvement (see Chapter 73). Polyarteritis nodosa was once thought to involve the lung commonly. However, review of reports suggests that most cases, particularly those having peripheral eosinophilia and asthma, would now be classified as the Churg-Strauss syndrome. Polyarteritis nodosa may involve muscular arteries serving the bronchial tree but not the pulmonary artery. Therefore, polyarteritis nodosa does not present with pulmonary symptoms or chest radiographic abnormalities. Other collagen vascular diseases such as systemic lupus erythematosus, rheumatoid arthritis, dermatomyositis, and polymyositis may have an element of vasculitis admixed with interstitial lung disease. The chief clinical manifestation of pulmonary vasculitis in collagen vascular diseases is diffuse alveolar hemorrhage, particularly associated with systemic lupus erythematosus.

DISCOVERY OF ANTINEUTROPHIL CYTOPLASMIC AUTOANTIBODY (ANCA)

Davies and coworkers first described the antineutrophil cytoplasmic autoantibody in association with renal disease in the early 1980s.[12] Subsequently, van derWoude and colleagues showed a close association of antineutrophil cytoplasmic autoantibody with Wegener's granulomatosis.[48] When alcohol-fixed neutrophils are used as substrates for indirect immunofluorescence, two main patterns are recognized. The cytoplasmic or cANCA (Fig. 86-1) displays a coarsely granular cytoplasmic pattern with central accentuation. In contrast, the perinuclear or pANCA (Fig. 86-2) displays a tight rim of immunofluorescence around the nucleus which bears resemblance to an antinuclear antibody and must be differentiated from it. The chief cytoplasmic target antigen for the cANCA pattern is proteinase 3, a serine proteinase in azurophil granules. Myeloperoxidase is the chief target for the pANCA. Other antigens associated with the pANCA pattern have included lactoferrin, neutrophil elastase, and cathepsin G. The three main pulmonary vasculitides associated with antineutrophil cytoplasmic autoantibody are Wegener's granulomatosis, Churg-Strauss syndrome, and microscopic polyangiitis. All these entities involve small-vessel vasculitis, but there is no evidence of the involvement of immune complexes as observed in systemic lupus erythematosus (SLE) or linear immune depositions as seen in Goodpasture's syndrome.

Evidence is mounting to incriminate ANCA directly in the pathogenesis of Wegener's granulomatosis, Churg-Strauss syndrome, and microscopic polyangiitis. In vitro, neutrophils primed

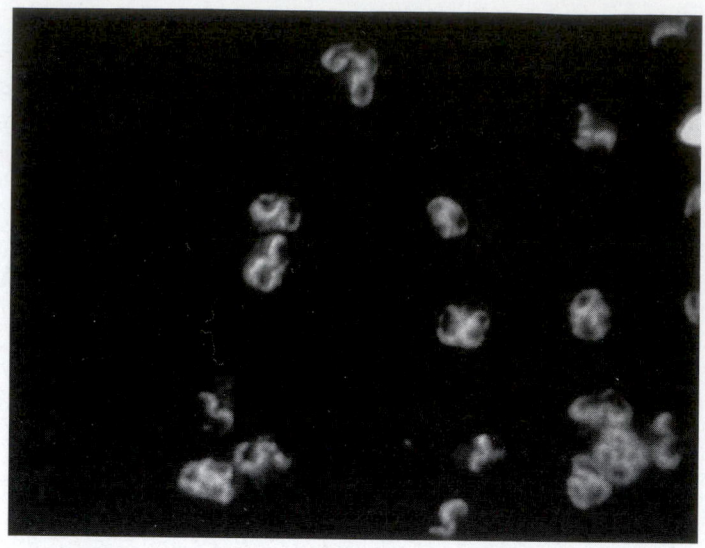

FIGURE 86-2   The antineutrophil cytoplasmic autoantibody with perinuclear pattern, pANCA.

with tumor necrosis factor and other cytokines, when engaged by ANCA to the target antigen exposed on the surface of the cell, discharge their cytoplasmic enzymes, as well as toxic oxygen radicals, and damage tissue, to which they adhere, particularly vascular endothelium.[24] Also, it appears that adhesion molecules are instrumental in fixing the primed neutrophils to the sites where damage occurs. Given the granulomatous nature of some of the lesions, it is likely that T cells have an important role in the pathogenesis.

pANCA is typically associated with primary vasculitic syndromes. Microscopic polyarteritis is chiefly associated with the finding of pANCA. In a review of 2381 patients screened at Mayo Clinic for antineutrophil cytoplasmic autoantibody, there were 42 positive results for pANCA,[17] and 84 positive for cANCA. Of those with pANCA, only 13 or 31 percent had respiratory tract involvement, in contrast to Wegener's granulomatosis, in which the respiratory tract is almost always involved. The predominant clinical syndrome associated with pANCA was nephritis with alveolar hemorrhage.

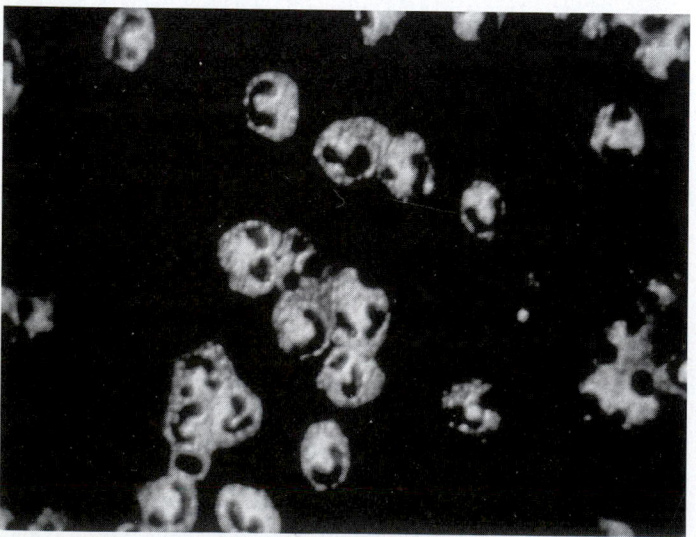

FIGURE 86-1   The antineutrophil cytoplasmic autoantibody with cytoplasmic pattern, cANCA.

TABLE 86-1

Systemic Vasculitides

Large-vessel vasculitis
 Giant cell (temporal) arteritis
 Takayasu arteritis
Medium-vessel vasculitis
 Polyarteritis nodosa
 Kawasaki disease
 Small-vessel vasculitis
 *Wegener's granulomatosis
 *Churg-Strauss syndrome
 *Microscopic polyangiitis
 Henoch-Schönlein purpura
 Essential Cryoglobulinemia vasculitis
 Cutaneous leukocytoclastic angiitis

*ANCA-associated.
SOURCE: Adapted from Jennette et al,[29a] with permission.

Early studies suggested that the titer of antineutrophil cytoplasmic autoantibody closely followed the clinical course. In many cases this is true. But, as evidence has been gathered, it has become apparent that there can be dissociation of the ANCA titer with the clinical course, particularly with the cANCA in Wegener's granulomatosis. Nonetheless, a patient under clinical control manifesting a rising ANCA titer should be observed closely for evidence of recrudescence.

In 1994, an international consensus conference published a revised nomenclature of the systemic vasculitides (Table 86-1). Those entities having a major pulmonary manifestation, namely Wegener's granulomatosis, Churg-Strauss syndrome, and microscopic polyangiitis, have many common pathologic features and are associated with antineutrophil cytoplasmic autoantibody. Accordingly, ANCA can be used as a criterion in approaching the classification of pulmonary vasculitides.

In the discussion to follow, Wegener's granulomatosis, Churg-Strauss syndrome, and microscopic polyangiitis are grouped together under the category of antineutrophil cytoplasmic autoantibody-associated pulmonary vasculitis. Although there are common features among these three entities, there are also substantial differences that allow a relatively clear separation. Disease associated with cANCA is overwhelmingly Wegener's granulomatosis, which is characterized by prominent granulomatous features, as well as vasculitis. Syndromes associated with pANCA have less prominent or absent granulomatous features, and pure, small-vessel vasculitis dominates. In addition, there is a greater diversity of clinical expression of pANCA disease compared to the more uniform manifestations of Wegener's granulomatosis. An exception to this association of the type of antineutrophil cytoplasmic autoantibody with the type of pathology is the Churg-Strauss syndrome, which has prominent granulomatous features but has most often been associated with pANCA rather than cANCA. Whether the distinction between these clinicopathologic subtleties has any rationale in terms of etiology and pathogenesis is yet to be determined.

ANCA-ASSOCIATED VASCULITIDES

Wegener's Granulomatosis

In 1936 and 1939, Friedrich Wegener published his classic papers concerning a new disease that was to be differentiated from the traditional concept of periarteritis nodosa.[51,52] His original three patients experienced a short course to death from renal failure or sepsis. Because there was granulomatous inflammation involving the upper and lower respiratory tracts associated with systemic vasculitis and focal necrotizing glomerulitis, Wegener initially called this disease "rhinogenic granulomatosis," but he later used the

term "pneumogenic granulomatosis." In his view, involvement of both the upper and lower respiratory tracts was the chief manifestations. In 1954 Godman and Churg[22] set down the following criteria for this condition: (1) necrotizing granulomatous inflammation of the upper and/or lower respiratory tracts; (2) generalized focal necrotizing vasculitis involving both arteries and veins; and (3) focal necrotizing glomerulitis. These three criteria became known as the "Wegener's triad."

To the present day, some physicians insist on all three criteria to make the diagnosis of Wegener's granulomatosis. However, about 30 years ago, it was recognized that some patients presented with typical symptoms and histologic findings in the upper or lower respiratory tracts yet failed to have systemic vasculitis or glomerulonephritis. These individuals responded to treatment applied to fully expressed Wegener's granulomatosis, and occasionally they evolved into the complete syndrome. This experience resulted in the formulation of the ELK classification system wherein E stands for the ears, nose and throat or upper respiratory tract, L the lung, and K the kidney (Fig. 86-3).[13] This conception suggested that within the Wegener's granulomatosis spectrum are patients who may have involvement at any of the ELK sites singularly or in combinations. This broadened concept allowed the identification of patients with hitherto unclassifiable disease and provided for the application of treatment traditionally used in the classic ELK disease. Because focal necrotizing glomerulitis was not specific for Wegener's, isolated involvement of the kidney was not considered a part of the Wegener's spectrum until the advent of the antineutrophil cytoplasmic autoantibody test. Because cANCA has high specificity for Wegener's granulomatosis, isolated glomerulonephritis in association with cANCA may be included within the Wegener's spectrum, as may isolated involvement of any major site.[39]

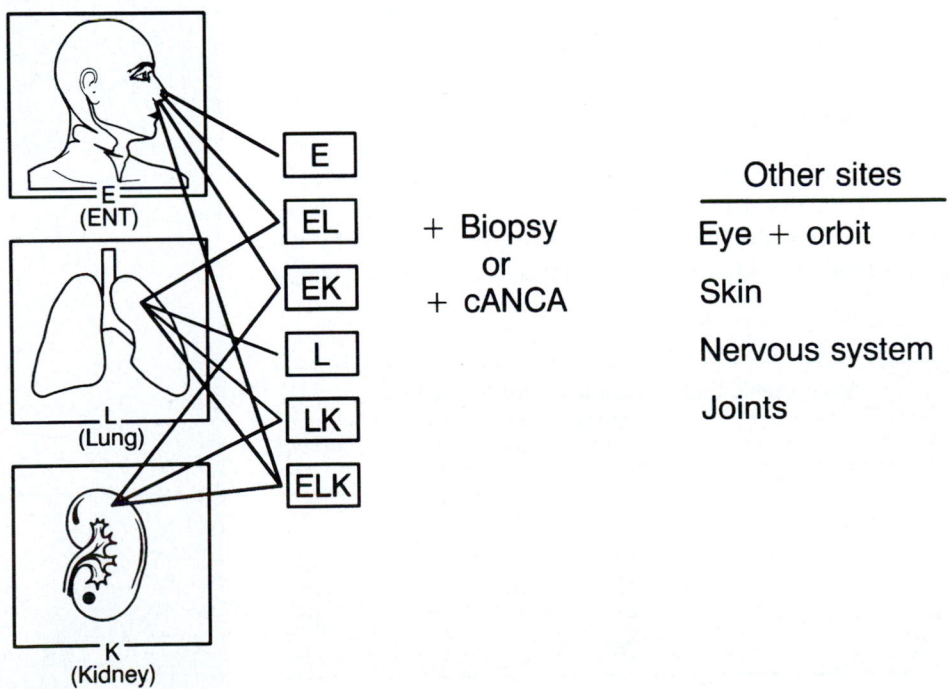

FIGURE 86-3 The ELK classification augmented by cANCA. (*Reproduced by permission from Sarcoidosis and Other Granulomatous Disorders. New York, Marcel Dekker, 1994, vol 73, p 659.*)

Wegener emphasized the vasculitic aspect over the granulomatous character of the disease bearing his name, but in fact the earliest lesion of the condition has since been shown to be a focus of injury and necrosis evolving into a necrotizing palisading granuloma without the participation of vessels.[20] The continuum from granuloma to vasculitis may be important when considering the possible etiology and pathogenesis.

The ELK concept is an extension of observations of "limited" or slowly progressive forms of Wegener's granulomatosis in which the kidney is not involved and there is no evidence of systemic vasculitis. This so-called limited Wegener's denotes the absence of kidney disease and has a more favorable prognosis.[4] The evolution of Wegener's has also been noted in cases of indolent lesions involving the skin and mucous membranes, particularly in the upper respiratory tract that, in retrospect, developed over many years into the fully expressed Wegener's triad.[21]

The ELK concept combines and extends these observations into an up-to-date system. In addition to the major sites E, L, and K, there may be other significant sites of involvement including the eye and orbit, the skin, central and peripheral nervous systems, and the joints. Under the ELK system, any typical manifestation in E, L, or K supported by typical histopathology or a positive cANCA test qualifies for the diagnosis of Wegener's granulomatosis. The American College of Rheumatology has established the following criteria for the diagnosis of Wegener's granulomatosis: (1) a urinary sediment containing red blood cell casts or more than five red blood cells per high-power field; (2) abnormal findings on the chest radiograph (i.e., nodules, cavities, or fixed infiltrates); (3) oral ulcers or nasal discharge; and (4) granulomatous inflammation on biopsy.[32] Note that all cases upon which these criteria were based had demonstrated vasculitis. Thus, cases in the granulomatous phase without vasculitis would be misclassified by adhering to this system. Thus, Wegener's granulomatosis has evolved conceptually with clinical experience and the discovery of new data, particularly related to ANCA.

CLINICAL MANIFESTATIONS

Table 86-2 presents the ELK distribution of 323 patients seen at Mayo Clinic, 174 men and 149 women. No geographic, occupational, or heritable factors were noted. As suggested by the earlier discussion, a wide range of clinical expression and tempo

TABLE 86-2

Wegener's Granulomatosis by ELK Class

Class	Number	Percent
E	38	12
L	34	11
EL	65	20
EK	53	16
LK	55	17
ELK	78	24
	323	100

NOTE: 323 patients (174 men, 149 women, mean age 51.9, age range 12 to 78).

was noted. Some patients experienced chronic nasal obstruction and epistaxis over a number of years that may have been accompanied by gradual deformity or "saddling" of the nose. Others were found in the intensive care unit in respiratory and renal failure with extensive necrotizing lesions of the skin and mononeuritis multiplex. Between these extremes was a wide variety of presentations chiefly defined by the primary anatomic sites of involvement.

Ear, Nose and Throat (E)

E was involved in 72 percent of patients in the Mayo Clinic series (Table 86-2). E includes the nose, paranasal sinus, eustachian tubes, middle ear, the eighth cranial nerve, larynx, trachea, and mastoids. The most common symptom was nasal obstruction with the finding of nasal crusting. A serosanguineous discharge was a frequent accompanying sign. Patients often complained of deep, central facial pain. A "saddling" deformity of the nose was the result of dissolution of the nasal cartilage (Fig. 86-4) which occasionally revealed a central perforation. Chronic otitis media was a frequent finding. Less often encountered was chronic mastoiditis and cholesteatoma formation. Conductive hearing loss was the result of inflammation of the middle ear, but vasculitis involving the cochlea could lead to an additional component of sensory neural loss as well. Ulceration of the vomer was a particularly reliable sign of Wegener's granulomatosis.[36] Subglottic stenosis is most frequently associated with other upper airway involvement but can be seen as an isolated finding associated

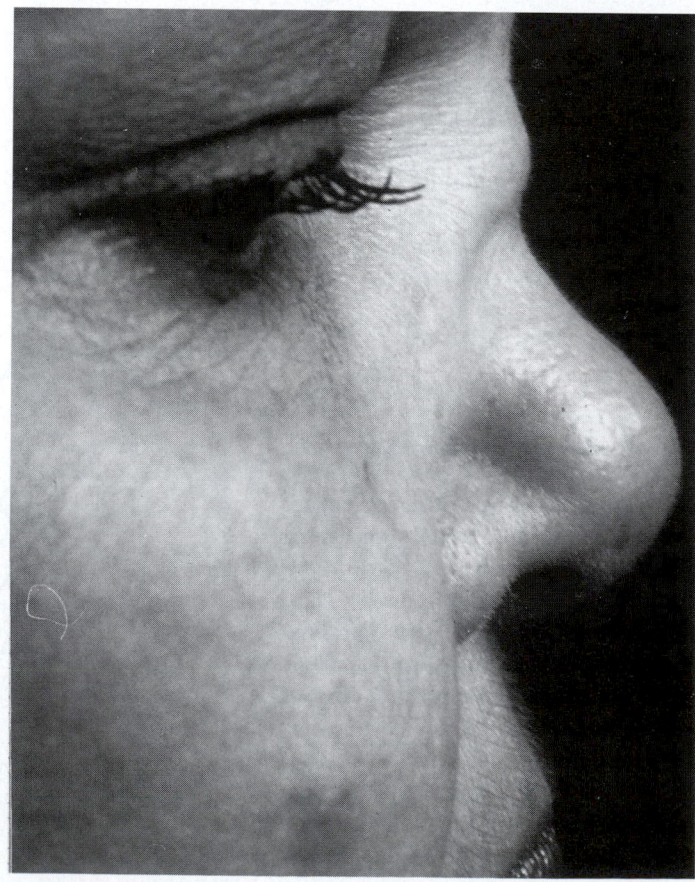

FIGURE 86-4 Saddle nose deformity of Wegener's granulomatosis.

with cANCA. Patients with subglottic stenosis may be mistaken for having asthma because of stridor. A flow volume loop showing flattening of both the inspiratory and expiratory limbs is helpful in directing attention to this lesion. Inflammatory and cicatricial lesions may also involve the trachea and major bronchi and occasionally lead to complete obliteration of a segmental bronchus resulting in atelectasis or recurrent obstructive pneumonia. Rarely, patients may present with an exuberant inflammation of the gums variously described as "mulberry or strawberry" gums which, on biopsy, will yield a typical necrotizing granuloma (Fig. 86-5). Inflammatory lesions of the pinna of the ear may simulate relapsing polychondritis.

Lung (L)

The lung was involved in 72 percent of 323 patients seen at the Mayo Clinic. In 11 percent, the lung was involved alone without apparent disease in the other major organ sites. Patients with lung involvement may be asymptomatic, or they may present with cough and occasionally with hemoptysis. Patients having diffuse alveolar hemorrhage (Fig. 86-6) invariably have severe dyspnea and may develop respiratory failure requiring ventilatory support. As mentioned earlier, inflammatory, cicatricial lesions involving the bronchial tree may result in atelectasis or recurrent obstructive pneumonias. The classic radiographic finding is multiple bilateral pulmonary nodules of varying size and definition which are cavitated in about 50 percent of patients (Figs. 86-7, 86-8). Significant pleural lesions are rare. Accompanying the nodular lesions may be an interstitial or varying degrees of nonspecific infiltrates. CT scanning of the chest can aid in clearer definition of the lesions and disclose cavitation not readily seen on standard chest radiographs (Fig. 86-9). Scanning also may disclose otherwise inapparent pleural lesions. However, it is doubtful that CT adds helpful information to the plain chest radiograph.

Kidney (K)

In the Mayo Clinic series the kidney was involved in 57 percent of cases. The lesion is disclosed by abnormal findings such as proteinuria and urinary red blood cell casts. Kidney involvement is asymptomatic. Clearance studies or the serum creatinine may or may not be altered in very early disease but will change commensurate with the degree of kidney pathology. Some authorities maintain that the kidney is always affected and that normal

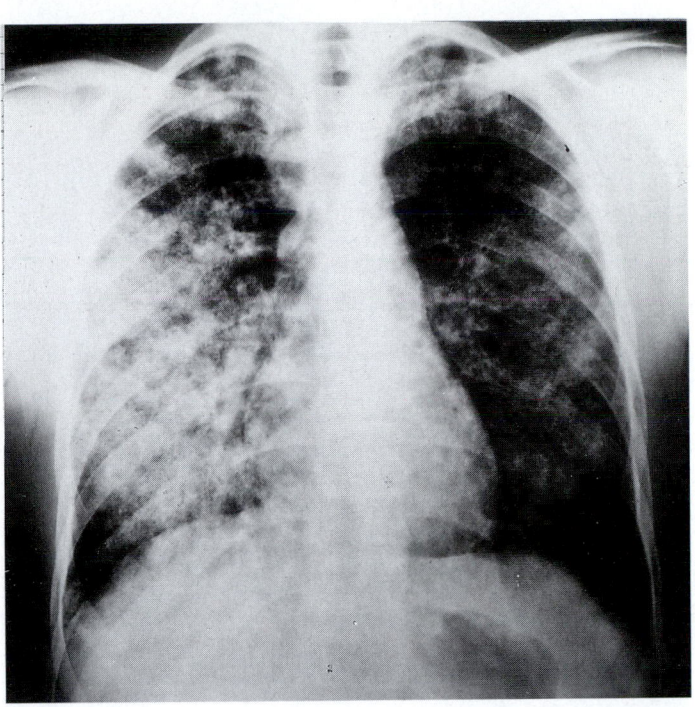

FIGURE 86-6 Chest radiograph of a patient with Wegener's granulomatosis displaying an alveolar filling pattern indicative of diffuse alveolar hemorrhage.

urinalysis, serum creatinine, and creatinine clearance studies are misleading. They would suggest that a renal biopsy be carried out in every patient. However, from a practical standpoint noninvasive renal studies are sufficient to make decisions regarding the extent of renal involvement and the treatment to be selected.

Nervous System

Neurologic involvement occurs in about one-third of patients,[38] without relationship to age or gender. Most of these patients have

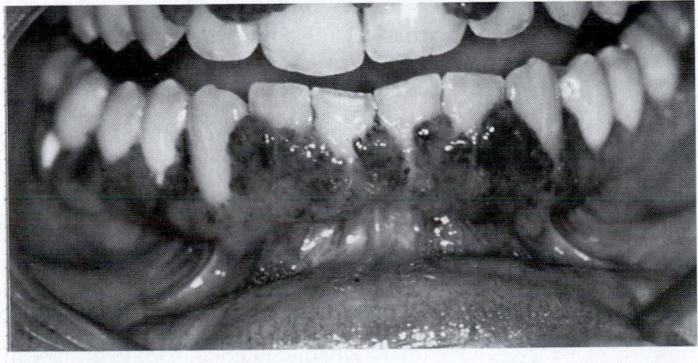

FIGURE 86-5 Strawberry or mulberry gums in a patient with Wegener's granulomatosis.

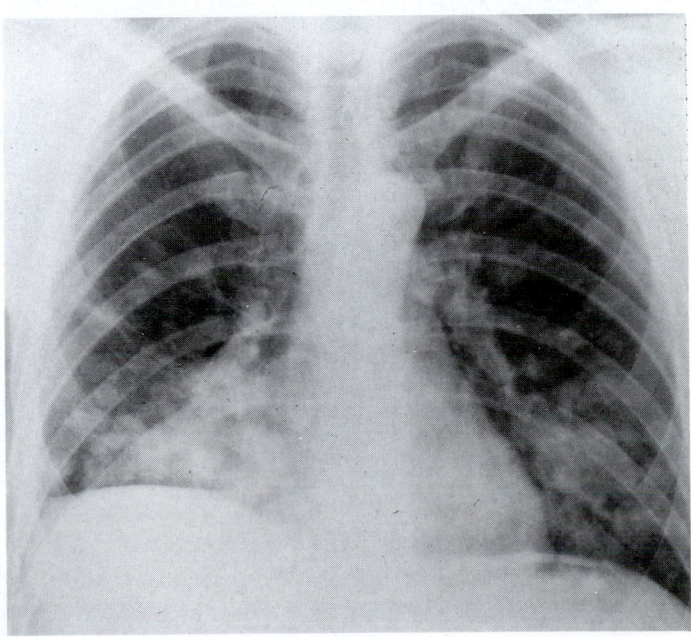

FIGURE 86-7 Chest radiograph of a patient with Wegener's granulomatosis displaying multiple nodules with and without cavitation.

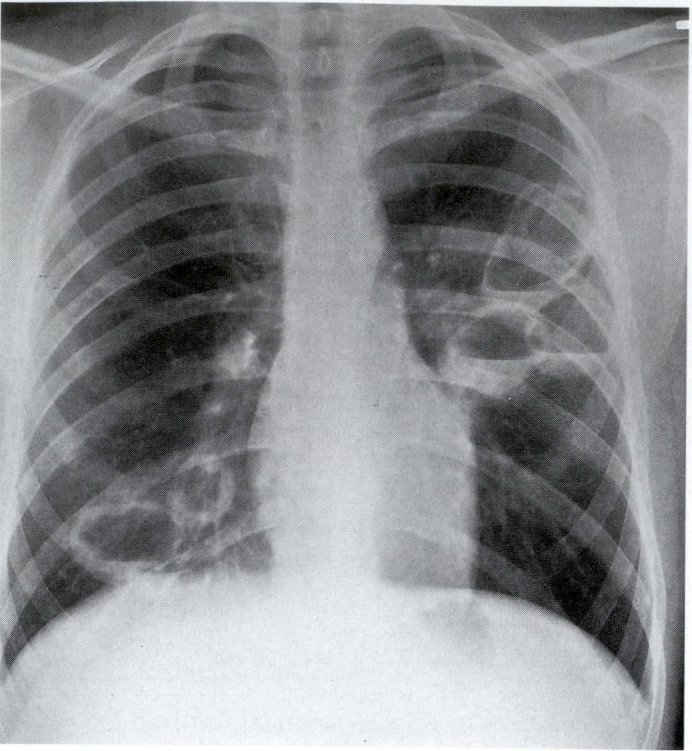

FIGURE 86-8 Chest radiograph of a patient with Wegener's granulomatosis showing multiple large cavities, some with air fluid levels.

peripheral neuropathy, typically in the pattern of mononeuritis multiplex. Occasionally, neurologic features are the presenting symptoms, a finding strongly associated with kidney involvement. Cranial neuropathy occurs, most often affecting the second, sixth, and seventh nerves (Fig. 86-10).

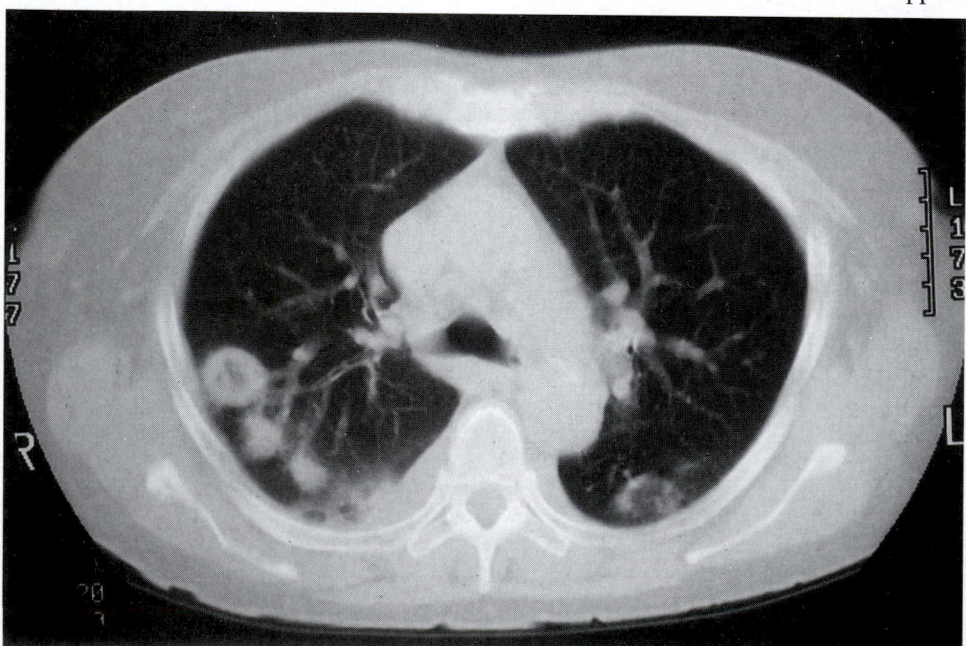

FIGURE 86-9 CT scan of a patient with Wegener's granulomatosis showing multiple nodules, some with cavitation. There are also small bilateral pleural effusions.

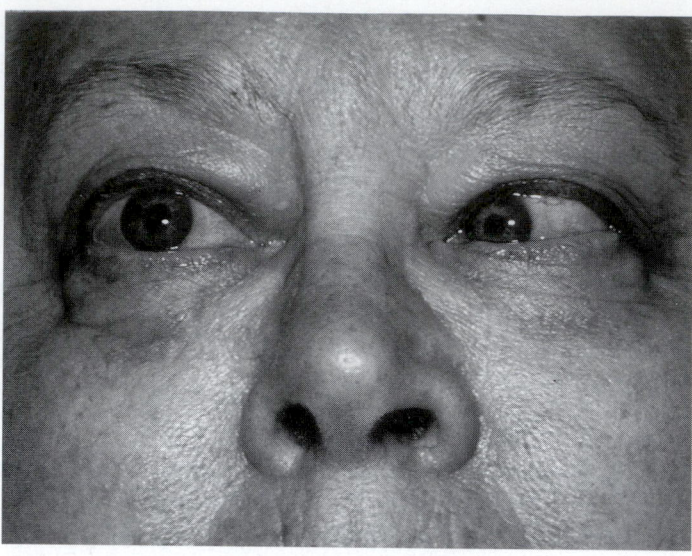

FIGURE 86-10 External ophthalmoplegia of the left eye due to orbital involvement with Wegener's granulomatosis.

Skin

In a series of 244 patients, 34 (14 percent) had skin involvement.[10] Most commonly the pathologic pattern was that of leukocytoclastic vasculitis. Other patterns included extravascular granuloma and pyoderma gangrenosum (Fig. 86-11). The clinical features included palpable purpura, necrotizing ulcerations, papules, nodules, petechiae, superficial erosions, bullae, and erythema, palpable purpura being the most frequent finding. The lower extremities were the most common site for these lesions. The upper extremities were next in order of frequency, with the elbows being a particular place to search for lesions which usually present as nodules that are extravascular granulomas on biopsy. The presence of skin lesions often heralded kidney involvement. It appears that skin involvement is a highly reliable sign of systemic vasculitis.

Eye and Orbit

Eye or orbit complications are common, occurring in 29 percent in one series of 140 patients.[2] A "red eye" may be the introductory symptom and the finding ultimately leading to the diagnosis of Wegener's granulomatosis. If it is painful, the diagnosis of scleritis is most likely, but redness may also be due to conjunctivitis, episcleritis, or corneal ulceration. Intraocular involvement, such as uveitis, retinal vasculitis, and optic neuropathy may be found. The eye may be proptotic due to inflammatory orbital mass or orbital cellulitis. A secondary ocular sign, epiphora, is due to obstruction of the nasolacrimal duct. Obstruction may make the duct subject to infection with frank ulceration into the overlying skin. Involvement of the orbit is to be dif-

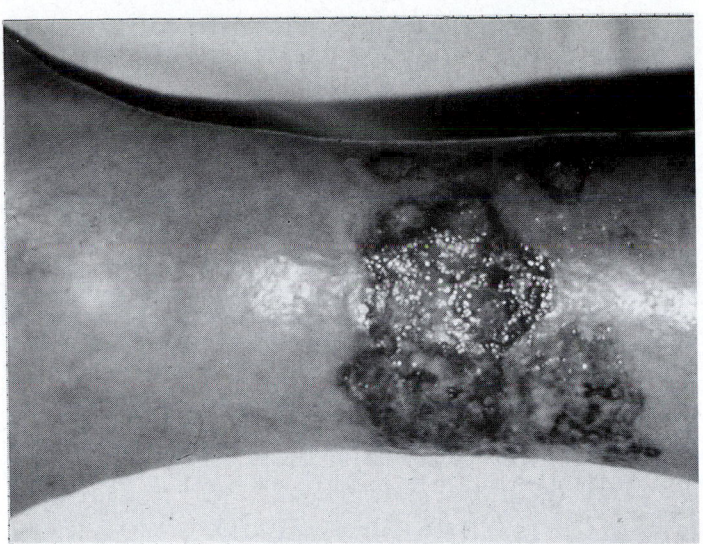

FIGURE 86-11   Pyoderma gangrenosum of the leg in a patient with Wegener's granulomatosis.

ferentiated from Graves' disease, lymphoma, orbital pseudotumor (which may be a manifestation of Wegener's granulomatosis), and even primary or metastatic carcinomas. At times, biopsy of the orbit may be required to confirm Wegener's granulomatosis. MRI or CT scan of the head are appropriately performed when orbital pathology is suspected. Lesions of the eye, particularly scleritis, may persist and progress to a meltdown of the sclera requiring scleral grafting for salvage of the eye even when the disease has been brought under control at other sites. Ocular and orbital pathology may occasionally require enucleation.

Joints

There are no reliable statistics concerning the incidence of joint symptoms and findings in Wegener's granulomatosis, but signs of arthritis are frequent. Frank arthritis of mono- or polyarticular form may be symmetric or asymmetric and is usually migratory. Arthralgias may be the patient's chief complaint. Joint symptoms and findings often correlate with the activity of the disease. Confusion with rheumatoid arthritis might arise, but the arthritis associated with Wegener's granulomatosis is nondeforming and does not become chronic. The onset of frank arthritis may be explosive, developing over a matter of hours, a circumstance in which there is usually a severe clinical course with kidney involvement.

Other Sites

Involvement of the salivary glands has been reported; in these cases, the involvement was the initial manifestation of the disease.[46,49] The prostate is rarely affected, usually presenting with symptoms of prostatitis. Digital rectal examination may reveal a firm nodule

raising the differential diagnosis of carcinoma of the prostate. Acute urinary obstruction due to prostatic involvement may require transurethral prostatectomy or prolonged catheterization awaiting relief from conventional systemic chemotherapy. Other urogenital manifestations have included orchitis, pseudotumor of the bladder, and ulceration of the penis. Perforation of the intestinal tract may result from ischemia secondary to vasculitis.

PATHOLOGY

There are no pathognomonic pathologic features of Wegener's granulomatosis, although the pathology may be highly suggestive. As mentioned above, the necrotizing granuloma dominates the pathologic finding, especially when confined to the upper and/or lower respiratory tracts. Vasculitis is not a prerequisite for the diagnosis of Wegener's granulomatosis. The clinician and pathologist must review the pathologic material jointly, because in the final analysis Wegener's granulomatosis is a clinico-pathologic entity.[16] Infection, particularly due to fungi or acid-fast bacilli, must be excluded.

The characteristic histologic feature is geographic basophilic necrosis with palisaded histiocytes (Fig. 86-12). The earliest lesion is a microabscess beginning as clusters of polymorphonuclear leukocytes that are remote from large foci of necrosis. Giant cells are an important feature. The vasculitis, which involves both small arteries and veins and capillaries, may have granulomatous features with giant cells (Fig. 86-13) or simply be composed of mononuclear cells. Alveolar hemorrhage is found in association with inflammation of the alveolar capillaries, so-called capillaritis (Fig. 86-14). This lesion is not specific for Wegener's and must be supported by typical histopathology elsewhere or the presence of cANCA.

Where the clinical findings are typical or consistent, and there is a positive cANCA, pathologic proof may not be necessary to establish the diagnosis. Biopsies of the upper respiratory tract, including the nose and paranasal sinuses, may show only non-specific inflammation without granuloma or vasculitis. In this case, proof must be sought elsewhere. A transbronchial lung

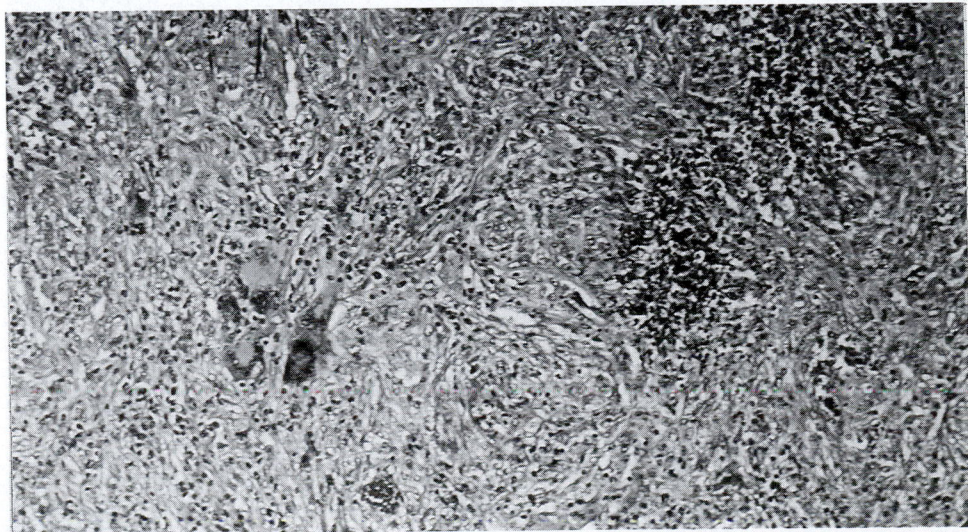

FIGURE 86-12   Geographic basophilic necrosis with palisading histiocytes and giant cells from a lung nodule in a patient with Wegener's granulomatosis.

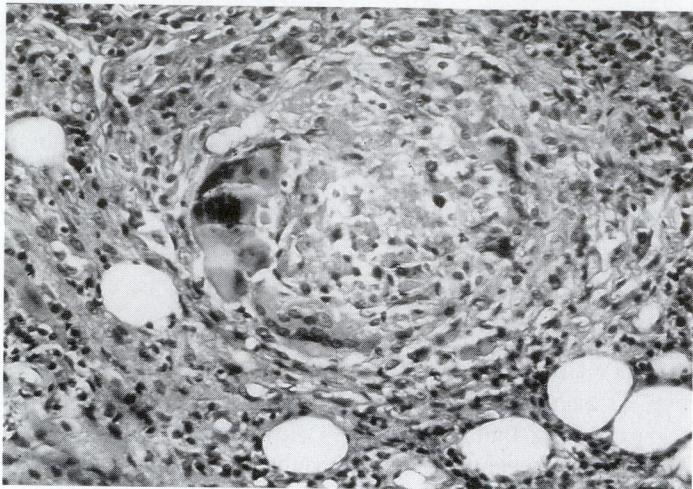

FIGURE 86-13   Granulomatous vasculitis with giant cells in a lung biopsy of a patient with Wegener's granulomatosis.

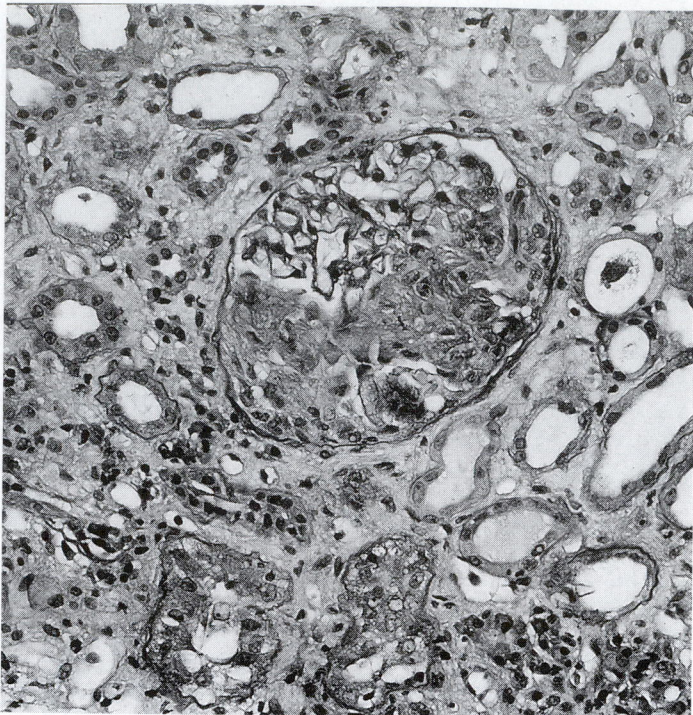

FIGURE 86-15   Focal necrotizing glomerulitis of Wegener's granulomatosis.

biopsy may occasionally support the diagnosis. Thoracoscopic or open lung biopsy may be required if evidence elsewhere is not supportive. The chief finding in the kidney is focal necrotizing glomerulitis (Fig. 86-15) that takes the pattern of rapidly progressive, crescentic glomerulonephritis (Fig. 86-16). Accordingly, the renal pathology is shared with many other conditions including microscopic polyarteritis, Churg-Strauss syndrome, Henoch-Schönlein purpura, systemic lupus erythematosus, Goodpasture's syndrome, and subacute bacterial endocarditis. Granulomatous inflammation may occasionally be seen in the glomerulous and intrarenal arteries. In the skin, the three main pathologic findings are necrotizing vasculitis or leukocytoclastic vasculitis, necrotizing granuloma, and granulomatous vasculitis.

RADIOGRAPHY

The conventional chest radiograph is usually sufficient to disclose significant involvement of the lung. As noted above, the chief manifestation is multiple pulmonary nodules of variable size and definition of which half will be cavitated. The CT scan may give sharper definition of the lesions, but the information revealed is probably not of critical significance. Involvement of the orbit and paranasal sinuses is best detected by either CT scan or MRI (Fig. 86-17). When subglottic stenosis is suspected, plain tomograms of the trachea will often give clear definition of the lesion.

LABORATORY STUDIES

Relatively few simple laboratory tests are helpful in the evaluation of a patient with Wegener's granulomatosis. Anemia is present in up to 50 percent of the patients. It is usually mild except for those having diffuse alveolar hemorrhage, who may present with hemoglobin concentration in the range of 6

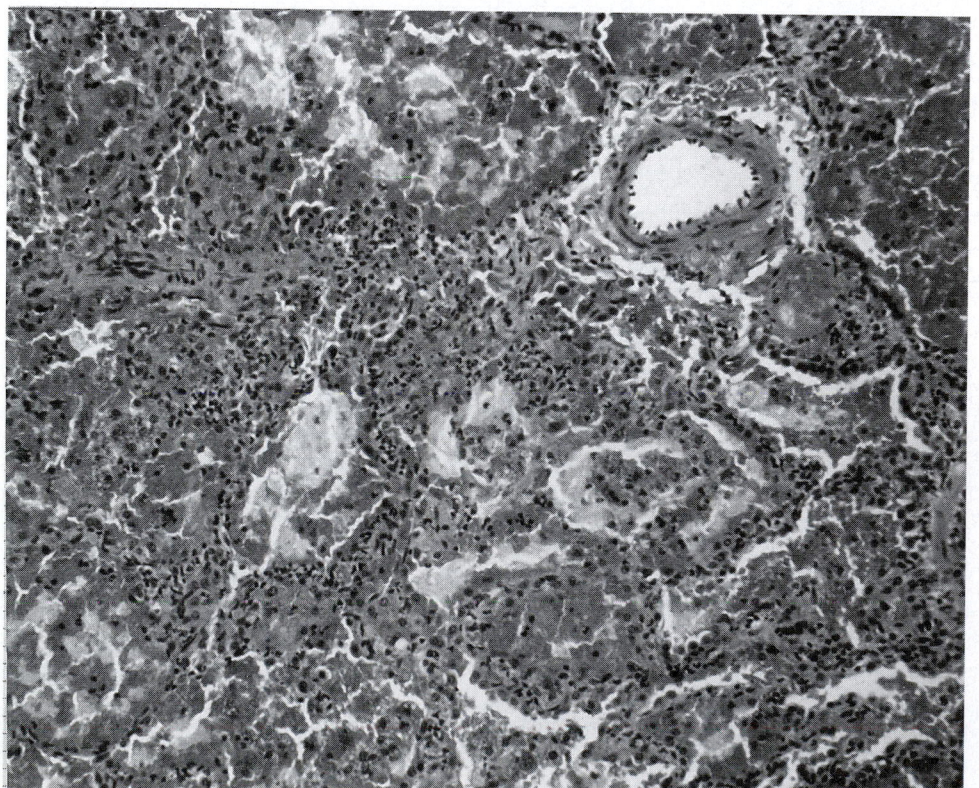

FIGURE 86-14   Alveolar capillaritis causing pulmonary hemorrhage in Wegener's granulomatosis.

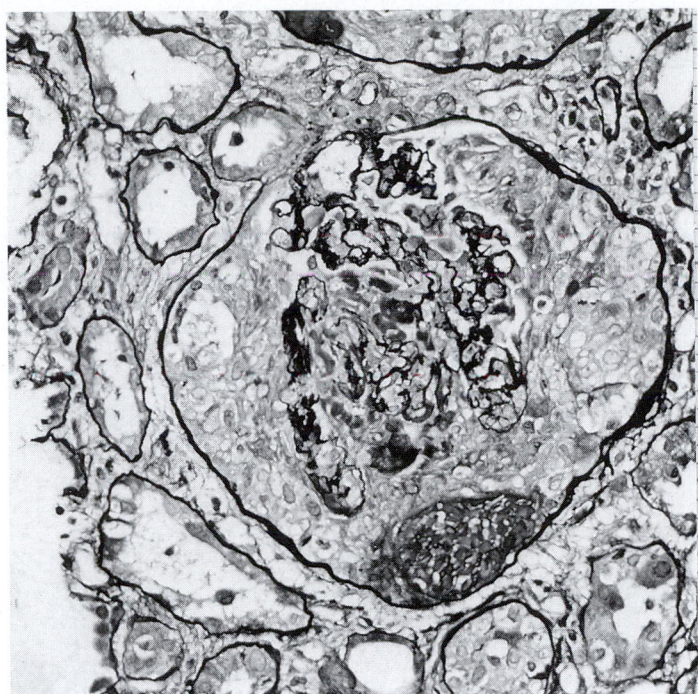

FIGURE 86-16 Rapidly progressive crescentic glomerulonephritis in Wegener's granulomatosis.

to 8 gm/dl. The concentration of iron in the serum may be low, suggestive of iron loss. The peripheral blood smear may show schistocytes and burr cells with a regenerative or hemolytic pattern. Leukocytosis is rarely above 18,000 per cubic mm and is neutrophilic. In contrast to the patients with Churg-Strauss syndrome who manifest a striking eosinophilia, patients with Wegener's granulomatosis rarely show a significant increase in the eosinophil count. The rheumatoid factor may be positive in up to 50 percent of cases and seems to correlate with the extent of the disease. The erythrocyte sedimentation rate may be normal or very elevated if the patient is in a high ELK class. The sedi-

mentation rate is valuable in following the activity of the disease, particularly during treatment. Indicators of kidney disease are most important, particularly the routine urinalysis, serum creatinine, and creatinine clearance. Classic findings on urinalysis are proteinuria with red blood cell casts.

As noted earlier, the presence of cANCA is closely associated with the diagnosis of Wegener's granulomatosis. On occasion, the presence of pANCA has been reported in patients with Wegener's granulomatosis, primarily in patients in whom typical manifestations are limited to the upper or lower respiratory tracts.

Table 86-3 lists signs and symptoms that should prompt consideration of Wegener's granulomatosis and, hence, the ordering of an antineutrophil cytoplasmic autoantibody test. Although clearly valuable in diagnosis, the relation of the ANCA titer to disease activity remains unsettled. Some early data suggested that the titer is helpful in assessing activity and clinical course,[39] but subsequent experience has weakened confidence in this concept. In a large study of patients from the Mayo Clinic and the Unversity of Kiel, Germany, specificity of cANCA for Wegener's granulomatosis was found to exceed 90 percent.[39] When the disease was confined to the upper and/or lower respiratory tracts, without systemic vasculitis, the sensitivity was 67 percent in active disease, dropping to 32 percent during remission. cANCA was positive in many cases considered completely inactive. In patients who had evidence of systemic vasculitis, the sensitivity was 96 percent and dropped to 41 percent when patients entered remission.

CLINICAL COURSE, TREATMENT, AND PROGNOSIS

For over 20 years, the treatment of choice for Wegener's granulomatosis has been cyclophosphamide and prednisone, particularly for those patients with evidence of systemic vasculitis. More recently, trimethoprim/sulfamethoxazole (T/S) has found increasing favor in the treatment of early, predominately granulomatous, disease in the absence of systemic vasculitis.[15] Patients having disease confined to E, L, or EL are started on a double strength T/S tablet twice a day. Significant improvement may occur as early as 10 to 14 days but may require up to 8 weeks.[14] If no improvement is seen after 8 weeks, prednisone is added in doses of 40 to 60 mg on alternate days. If this fails, then conventional treatment with cyclophosphamide at a dose of 2 mg/kg orally can be given. Patients who present in classes EK, LK, or ELK, are started on prednisone 60 to 80 mg daily orally; in 7 to 10 days, when the patient has improved, cyclphosphamide is added at a dosage of 2 mg/kg orally. Once control has been established, the dosage of prednisone is gradually tapered and cyclophosphamide is maintained for one year after the last evidence of stability.

In severely ill patients with rapidly progressive glomerulonephritis and/or alveolar hemorrhage, glucocorticoids are administered intravenously (e.g., a bolus of methylprednisolone 0.5 to 1 g), for three consecutive days followed by prednisone given orally. The use of cyclophosphamide administered intravenously at intervals of 3 to 4 weeks is controversial. In the severely ill patient, gamma globulin given intravenously has shown promising results but cannot as yet be considered to be a proven ther-

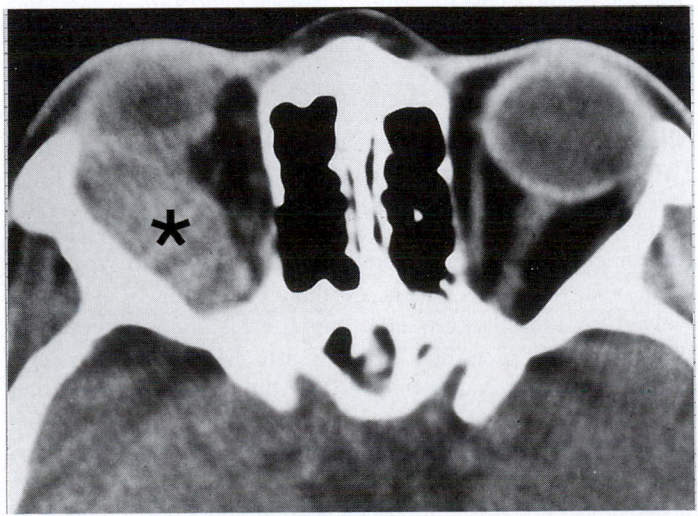

FIGURE 86-17 CT scan of the orbits in a patient with Wegener's granulomatosis showing a mass* in the right orbit causing external ophthalmoplegia.

TABLE 86-3

Findings and Symptoms of Wegener's Granulomatosis

Upper Respiratory Tract—E	Lower Respiratory Tract—L	Kidney—K	Miscellaneous
Nasal obstruction	Chest radiograph— multiple nodules (some cavitated), diffuse alveolar filling pattern	Glomerulonephritis	Necrotizing skin lesions
Epistaxis		Kidney insufficiency or failure	Mononeuritis multiplex
Nasal septum perforation			Nondeforming polyarthritis
Chronic sinusitis	Hemoptysis		Necrotizing vasculitis of arteries and veins in any organ
Chronic otitis media	Dyspnea		
Saddle nose deformity			
Mastoiditis			
Cholesteatoma			
Subglottic stenosis-stridor			
Proptosis			
Red eye—conjunctivitis, scleritis			
Uveitis			
Retinal and optic nerve vasculitis			
Nasolacrimal duct obstruction—epiphora			
Enlarged salivary glands			

apy. In patients who do not tolerate cyclophosphamide, other cytotoxic drugs such as azathioprine, chlorambucil, nitrogen mustard, or methotrexate have been used.

In a series of 151 patients treated at at Mayo Clinic with conventional regimens, the mortality was 28 percent.[18] Survival was 90 percent at 1 year, 87 percent at 2 years, and 76 percent at 5 years. These results contrast with the death rate of 80 percent in the first year that was reported early in the glucocorticoid era.[50] Although involvement of the lungs was more important than involvement of the kidneys in determining overall survivorship, renal involvement was the most important determinant of survival during the first year. Pulmonary involvement was reflected in a high incidence of opportunistic lung infections, a consequence of immunosuppressive treatment. Thus, excessive immunosuppressive therapy can be as dangerous as the underlying disease. For this reason, as already noted, treatment should be based on the extent and tempo of disease. In this context, trimethoprim/sulfamethoxazole is a valuable adjunct in the treatment of early disease and effective in the prevention of relapse following conventional treatment.[47]

When inflammatory insults have left behind fibrotic damage to the nose, subglottic areas, trachea, or bronchi, surgical intervention should be considered. Such intervention, however, is best performed when the underlying disease has been arrested. If not, repairs to the nasal cartilage or the subglottic stenosis may break down and fail.

The saddle nose deformity can be repaired, usually for cosmetic purposes. In our experience, laser treatment to subglottic stenosis is only of temporary benefit; resection of the stenotic area with reanastomosis is the definitive procedure. Obstruction of nasolacrimal ducts can be corrected by surgical means; the

same applies to suppurative dacryocystitis. Patients with severe scleritis leading to "meltdown" may be treated successfully with scleral grafts. Recurrent middle ear infections due to dysfunction of the eustachian tube can be ameliorated by introducing ventilating tubes through the tympanic membrane.

Perhaps the most difficult lesions to correct or modify are those involving ciccatricial stenosis of the major bronchi. Endoscopic techniques, including dilatation and/or the placement of silastic stents are a promising mode of treatment.[11]

Patients with renal failure should be considered for transplantation. In the few patients followed by this author who have been transplanted, the underlying Wegener's granulomatosis has gone into complete remission, probably due to concomitant antirejection treatment.

Allergic Granulomatosis and Angiitis— The Churg-Strauss Syndrome

There are many historical parallels between the Churg-Strauss syndrome and Wegener's granulomatosis. Similar to Wegener's granulomatosis, the concept of the Churg-Strauss syndrome evolved from the background of periarteritis nodosa. Reports in 1939 and 1941 identified cases of asthma and allergies as a unique subset of periarteritis nodosa,[42] but it was the publication of Churg and Strauss in 1951 that clearly delineated the clinical and pathologic features defining a new entity separate from periarteritis nodosa.[7] The new syndrome included the features of severe asthma, fever, and hypereosinophilia, with evidence of systemic vasculitis. The term *allergic granulomatosis and angiitis* was given, but since that time Churg-Strauss syndrome has become the popular designation. In retrospect, nearly one-third of individuals whose disease might have been classified as periarteritis nodosa at one time probably had Churg-Strauss syndrome.[43]

As with Wegener's granulomatosis, Churg-Strauss syndrome has been broadened in concept. All the classic clinical and pathologic criteria for the Churg-Strauss syndrome need not be present in order to invoke the diagnosis.[31] The classic pathologic findings of necrotizing vasculitis, tissue eosinophilia, and extravascular granuloma are not universally present or pathognomonic. The concept of "limited forms"[34] has been applied to cases in which one of the primary diagnostic criteria is missing, and the term *formes frustes*[6] has been applied to patients whose disease has been modified by glucocorticoid treatment of the asthmatic component. However, certain essentials are required to maintain the integrity of the concept of Churg-Strauss syndrome. The eosinophil is the sine qua non, either in the peripheral blood or in tissue. There are two stages with regard to the eosinophil, the first being eosinophilic infiltration of various organs and the second development of vasculitis, tissue necrosis, and granuloma formation. An allergic diathesis is the important clinical counterpart.

CLINICAL MANIFESTATIONS

Respiratory Tract

The typical of symptoms of asthma, namely episodic cough, wheezing, and dyspnea, are the cardinal manifestations. Pulmonary function testing will show airway obstruction relieved by inhalation of bronchodilators. Whereas in Wegener's granulomatosis the chest radiograph typically manifests multiple pulmonary nodules with or without cavitation, in the Churg-Strauss syndrome, the chest radiograph is less distinctive and more variable (Fig. 86-18). There may be fleeting, patchy infiltrates suggesting Löffler's syndrome, or there may be extensive alveolar infiltrates consistent with a pattern of eosinophilic pneumonia. Pure interstitial patterns may be seen infrequently. Multiple poorly circumscribed nodules may occur in Churg-Strauss syndrome, but they are usually smaller and do not cavitate. The Churg-Strauss syndrome may be complicated by diffuse alveolar hemorrhage accompanied by a diffuse bilateral alveolar filling pattern. In one study of 30 patients, only 8 had abnormal chest radiograph[5] in sharp contrast to Wegener's granulomatosis in which an abnormal chest radiograph is typical.

The nose and paranasal sinuses are frequently involved,[41] producing nasal obstruction and rhinorrhea. Nasal polyps and/or crusting are common findings. Nasal perforation occurs occasionally. Abnormal sinus radiographs are seen in approximately one-half of patients. There is a high incidence of allergic rhinitis,[31] so much so that it can be considered a major criterion in making the diagnosis.

Nervous System

Neurologic manifestations are a dominant feature of Churg-Strauss syndrome, occuring in nearly two-thirds of patients.[45] Peripheral neuropathy, especially mononeuritis multiplex, is typical, but distal symmetric polyneuropathy is also common. Less common problems include cerebral infarction, radiculopathy, ischemic optic neuropathy, and bilateral trigeminal neuropathy.

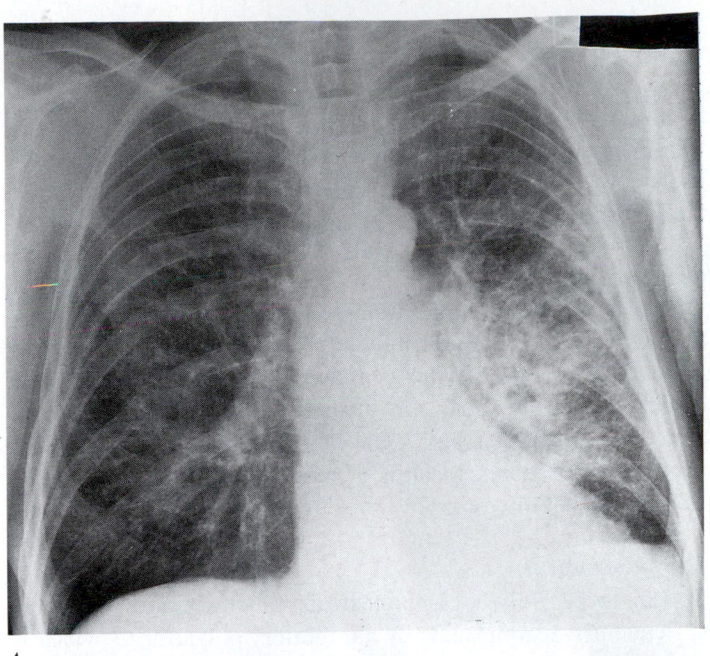

A

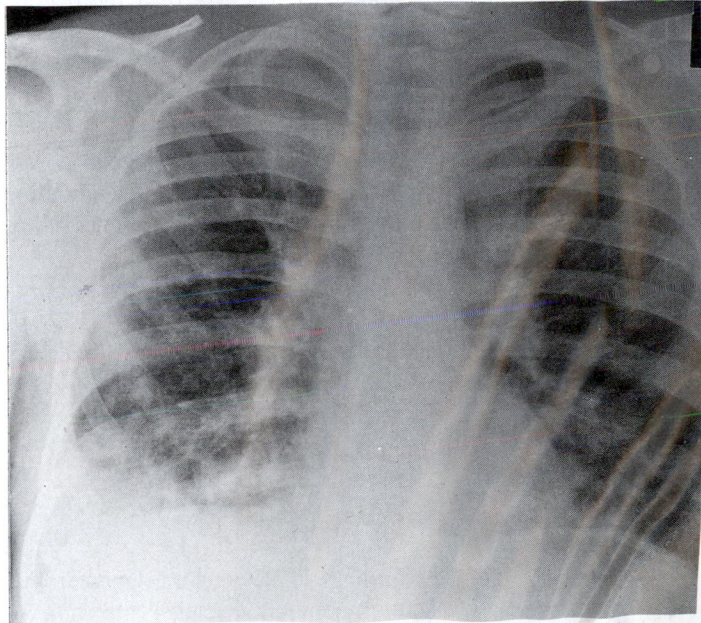

B

FIGURE 86-18 Chest radiographs of patients with Churg-Strauss syndrome: *A.* Nonspecific gnomonic infiltrates. *B.* Multiple vague, patchy infiltrates. *(Reproduced by permission from Mayo Clin Proc 5?, 1977.)*

Asthma usually antedates the onset ... quela.
by several years. Although ... volvement occasionally ... ent, neurologic findings are those reimprove or stabilize with ... thirds of patients, most frefindings and symptoms ... nodules that affect mainly the ... ds, and legs.[5] Other lesions are

Skin

Next in ...
lated t ...
quentl ...
exten ...

petechiae or nonthrombocytopenic purpura, as well as cutaneous infarcts.

Kidney

Significant renal dysfunction is uncommon in Churg-Strauss syndrome, a finding that sharply separates it from Wegener's granulomatosis.

Cardiovascular

Of 15 fatal cases of Churg-Strauss syndrome in one series, 3 patients died of myocardial infarction and 2 of congestive heart failure.[5] A review of Churg-Strauss syndrome found that the cause of fatal outcomes was cardiac failure in 47 percent and pericarditis in 32 percent.[31] The cardiac disease is generally attributed to coronary vasculitis or eosinophilic endocarditis with subsequent endomyocardial fibrosis.

Musculoskeletal

Similar to Wegener's granulomatosis, Churg-Strauss syndrome is frequently accompanied by a migratory polyarthritis which is not erosive or destructive. The chief sites are the ankles, wrists, and knees. Activity of the arthritis tends to reflect the overall activity of the underlying disease. Diffuse myalgias are common, probably due to myositis.

Gastrointestinal

The gastrointestinal tract may be affected, causing small bowel perforations, peritonitis, appendicitis, or mucosal ulceration all due to eosinophilic infiltration and/or vasculitis. Cholecystitis without stones has also been reported.

Genitourinary

Occasional patients have had allergic granuloma involving the prostate and lower urinary tract, which may lead to obstructive uropathy. Although rare, these findings emphasize the need for a thorough physical examination.

PATHOLOGY

The chief histopathologic findings in Churg-Strauss syndrome are necrotizing extravascular granuloma, called the *Churg-Strauss granuloma* or *allergic granuloma*, necrotizing vasculitis of small arteries and veins, prominent eosinophilia of vessels and perivascular tissues with accompanying lymphocytes, plasma cells, and some histiocytes, and fibrinoid necrosis of vessel walls. The allergic or Churg-Strauss granuloma is indicative of systemic disease and is also seen in Wegener's granulomatosis, systemic lupus erythematosus, rheumatoid arthritis, or bacterial endocarditis, and associated with lymphoproliferative diseases. When the Wegener's is hemorrhaged, the pathology is similar to that of other vasculitides, namely focal necrotizing glomerulonephritis. Diffuse alveolar Churg-Strauss hemorrhage, a feature of other systemic are subtle differences in the pathology of jor feature of Wegener's granulomatosis, there of Wegener's granulomatosis tissues is a major feature ... a minor feature ... Wegener's granu-

lomatosis has a coagulative or liquifactive appearance but tends to be more fibrinoid in Churg-Strauss syndrome.

CLINICAL COURSE, TREATMENT, AND PROGNOSIS

Survival has been reported to be 90 percent at 1 year, 76 percent at 3 years, and 62 percent at 5 years in patients treated primarily with glucocorticoids.[5] A short interval between the onset of asthma and the first signs of vasculitis portends an aggressive process. In one series, the mean duration of asthma prior to the onset of vasculitis was 8 years, but only 3.1 years for the 15 patients who died.[5] As indicated earlier, involvement of the heart is a major factor in mortality.

No prospective studies defined appropriate treatment, but glucocorticoids appear to be the mainstay of therapy, since the cytotoxic agents have less effectiveness in the Churg-Strauss syndrome than they do in Wegener's granulomatosis. Treatment with glucocorticoids may last for many years and indeed be lifelong. To lower the risk of side effects, efforts should be made to establish an alternate-day regimen. In fulminating cases, glucocorticoid therapy begins with intravenous administration, as described for Wegener's granulomatosis, followed by oral maintenance dosage of 60 to 80 mg of prednisone daily. The course of the disease can be monitored by observing manifestations in the skin, nervous system, or other anatomic sites. The eosinophil count and sedimentation rate are valuable laboratory parameters. In cases where the ANCA test is positive, it is usually pANCA with a myeloperoxidase target. The titer is helpful in assessing the direction of the clinical course. In the infrequent situation in which the kidney is involved with glomerulonephritis, serial urinalyses and determinations of serum creatinine and renal clearance are essential. Neurologic deficits may persist even after the underlying inflammatory disease has been suppressed.

Microscopic Polyangiitis

Whereas Wegener's granulomatosis and Churg-Strauss syndrome are relatively distinct clinical entities, microscopic polyangiitis is vague. It could be argued that microscopic polyangiitis does not have the clinical consistency to be regarded a distinct clinicopathologic syndrome. It could also be argued that microscopic polyangiitis is best viewed as a pathologic entity having overlap with a number of more clearly recognized syndromes. There may even be dispute concerning the precise definition of microscopic polyangiitis, but what is agreed on is that there is inflammation of small vessels, including venules, arterioles, and capillaries, and that the inflammation is probably not mediated by immune complex deposition. Some authors have suggested that glomerulonephritis, either segmental necrotizing or crescentic, is required for the diagnosis. However, the Chapel Hill Consensus Conference concluded that although glomerulonephritis is often seen, it is not necessary for the diagnosis (Table 86-1). At one time microscopic polyangiitis was called *microscopic polyarteritis nodosa*, but unlike polyarteritis nodosa, which is restricted to involvement of medium-size and small arteries and does not involve small vessels, microscopic polyangiitis usually affects only small vessels.[25] Other terms for microscopic polyangiitis have been used such as *hypersensitivity vasculitis of Zeek* and *cuta-*

neous leukocytoclastic angiitis for patients who have only skin involvement. It is evident that as with other vasculitic entities, microscopic polyangiitis was originally mixed in with polyarteritis nodosa.

Microscopic polyangiitis shares histopathologic findings with Wegener's granulomatosis and Churg-Strauss syndrome and is antineutrophil cytoplasmic autoantibody positive in many cases. It is usually associated with pANCA with a myeloperoxidase target, but can also be associated with cANCA, in which situations there is an argument for considering it a form of Wegener's granulomatosis.

CLINICAL MANIFESTATIONS

In a series of 34 patients reported in the pre-cANCA era, one-third reported prodromal symptoms suggestive of a respiratory illness. Others reported arthralgias, myalgias, all reminiscent of a systemic inflammatory disease.[44] The chief pulmonary manifestation was alveolar hemorrhage, occurring in 10 patients. Five patients had either pleuritic pain or effusion, and 2 manifested pulmonary edema. Although the upper respiratory tract or ears, nose, and throat were frequently involved, no clear-cut manifestations such as ones associated with Wegener's granulomatosis were described. Mouth ulcers were reported in 7 patients. Other significant involvement included the skin, nervous system, gastrointestinal system, the eye, gastrointestinal tract, and the heart. Serological abnormalities of rheumatoid factor, antinuclear antibodies, and immune complexes were common.

CLINICAL COURSE, TREATMENT AND PROGNOSIS

In the patients described above who were given varying regimens of prednisolone, azathioprine, cyclophosphamide, or plasma exchange, the survival rate was 70 percent at 1 year and 65 percent at 5 years.[44] Pulmonary hemorrhage, which developed in nearly one-third, was the most formidable complication.

Diffuse Alveolar Hemorrhage Syndromes

The clinical hallmarks of diffuse alveolar hemorrhage syndromes are a widespread alveolar infiltrate on chest radiography, anemia with the hemoglobin often reduced to 6 to 8 gm/dl, and red cells having microcytic hypochromic indices, occurring in a patient who is usually breathless. (This topic is considered further in Chapter 79). Hemoptysis may or may not be present. Similarly, there may or may not be associated glomerulonephritis.

For many years following the description of fatal alveolar hemorrhage and proliferative glomerulonephritis in young men by Goodpasture[23] it was conventional to label all cases manifesting alveolar hemorrhage and glomerulonephritis as "Goodpasture's syndrome." However, discovery of antiglomerular basement membrane antibodies (anti-GBM) enabled separation of one group of patients with alveolar hemorrhage from others. A second diagnostic group was later identified with discovery that, in rare instances, diffuse alveolar hemorrhage can be associated with systemic lupus erythematosus. With the advent of antineutrophil cytoplasmic autoantibody, a third serologically distinctive group of diseases emerged that is frequently associated with

diffuse alveolar hemorrhage with or without glomerulonephritis. A fourth group of patients who manifest hemoptysis and recurrent alveolar hemorrhage resulting in pulmonary hemosiderosis, but without evidence of glomerulonephritis, has been described and their disease called *idiopathic pulmonary hemosiderosis*. However, this constellation of findings, usually involving young males in whom there is no evidence of other underlying recognized disorder, was reported primarily before the discoveries of anti-GBM (Fig. 86-19), antinuclear antibody, or antineutrophil cytoplasmic autoantibody. It now seems quite likely that idopathic pulmonary hemosiderosis represents a "wastebasket" category that will shrink or even disappear with application of currently available serologic testing.

Although serologic investigations have dissected this group of patients into at least three disease entities, namely anti-GBM disease, systemic lupus erythematosus, and ANCA-associated vasculitis, it is important to note that the causes of these conditions remain unknown. However, their delineation represents a significant advance in understanding of some of the potential mechanisms underlying their development.

GOODPASTURE'S SYNDROME

As indicated above, the term *Goodpasture's syndrome* was used for every case of alveolar hemorrhage with nephritis until the role of the anti-GBM antibody in pathogenesis was conclusively demonstrated. At present Goodpasture's syndrome is applied to cases mediated by anti-GBM antibodies. Alveolar hemorrhage with anti-GBM antibodies but without nephritis is unusual, and, in many cases, nephritis eventually develops. Subsequent studies have shown that the disease is mediated by antibodies that react with NC1 domain of α3 chains in type IV collagen found primarily in basement membranes in the lung and kidney.[26] Why these autoantibodies are formed is unknown. The mortality rate of Goodpasture's syndrome is approximately 50 percent. Indo-

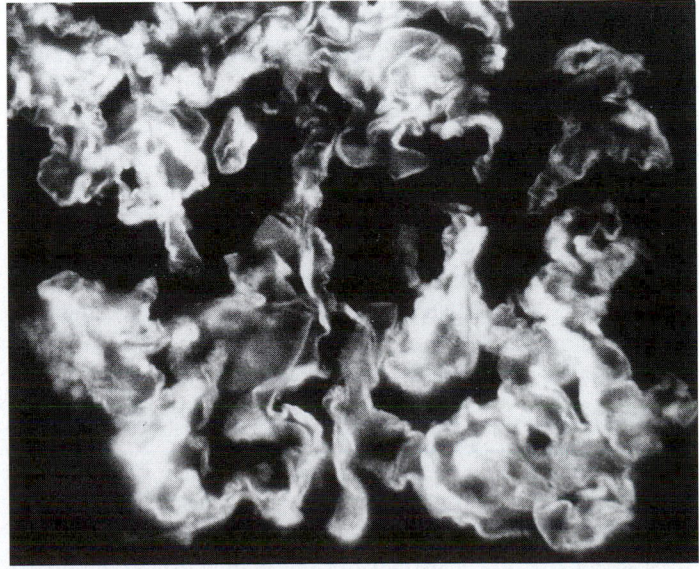

FIGURE 86-19   Kidney biopsy of a patient with Goodpasture's syndrome showing linear immunofluorescence of the glomerular basement membrane due to fixation of IgG anti-GBM antibodies.

lent remitting clinical courses have been described but are decidedly uncommon. The mainstays of treatment are glucocorticoids, cytotoxic agents, particularly cyclophosphamide and azathioprine. Plasmapheresis has been demonstrated to be beneficial in many cases. Up to one-third of patients may have a positive pANCA.

ANCA ASSOCIATED PULMONARY VASCULITIDES

Diffuse alveolar hemorrhage has been chiefly associated with Wegener's granulomatosis and microscopic polyarteritis. Rare cases have been reported with the Churg-Strauss syndrome. The presenting clinical findings are identical to those of other cause. Pathologically there is no evidence of immunoglobulin deposition, as seen in Goodpasture's syndrome or systemic lupus erythematosus. Treatment is similar to that employed for systemic vasculitis with the exception that plamapheresis has not yet been established as a first line treatment although it is reported to be effective in some cases. There is an approximate 50 percent mortality rate.

SYSTEMIC LUPUS ERYTHEMATOSUS (SLE)

There are a number of pleuropulmonary manifestations of SLE that include lupus pneumonitis, lymphocytic interstitial pneumonia, pulmonary embolism associated with lupus anticoagulant, pulmonary hypertension, lupus pruritis, and weakness of the diaphragm (see Chapter 73). The most significant and devastating manifestation is diffuse alveolar hemorrhage, which is, fortunately, rare. Immunofluorescent studies of the lung have revealed evidence of immune complex deposition of a lumpy, bumpy character in the alveolar walls (Fig. 86-20). The antinuclear antibody is invariably positive and there is frequently hypocomplementemia and evidence of nephritis. The frequency of ANCA positivity in SLE-associated alveolar hemorrhage is not known, although some crossover of positive ANA's with pANCA has been described in patients with glomerulonephritis.[3] In one series of 57 patients with systemic lupus erythematosus, there was no one with antineutrophil cytoplasmic autoantibody.[39]

MISCELLANEOUS CAUSES

Rare causes of diffuse alveolar hemorrhage include D-penicillamine, trimelitic anhydride, oxyphenbutazone (thrombocytopenia), mixed cryoglobulinemia, lymphangiography, subacute bacterial endocarditis, tumor related vasculitis, invasive fungal infection, thrombocytopenia, leukemia, Behçet's syndrome, bone marrow transplantation, and Henoch-Schöenlein purpura.

GENERAL CONSIDERATIONS

Identification of an alveolar hemorrhage syndrome constitutes a medical emergency. Often, the patient will be in respiratory distress to a degree requiring assisted ventilation. To aid in making a diagnosis, serologic tests should be ordered immediately for anti-GBM antibody, antinuclear antibody, and ANCA. Where any of these is positive it could be argued that no further diagnostic

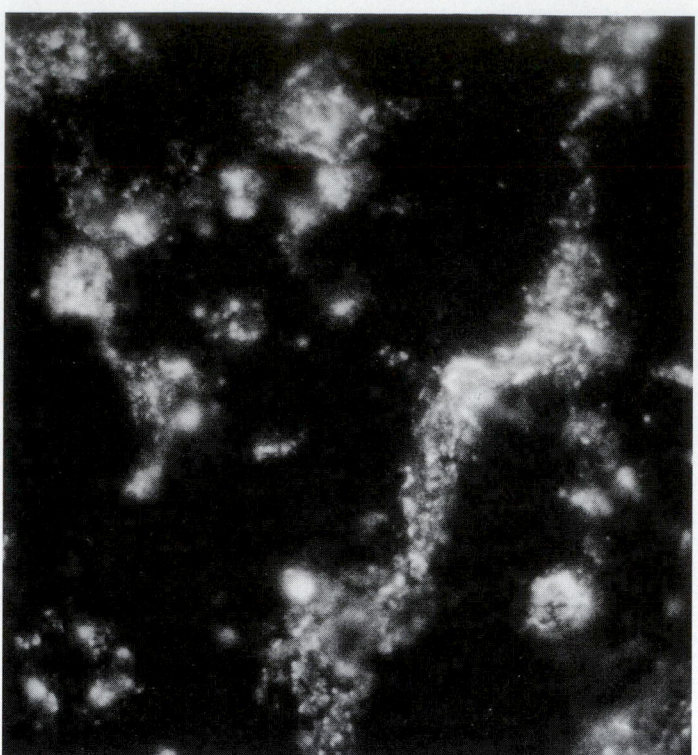

FIGURE 86-20 Lung biopsy of a patient with lupus erythematosus and alveolar hemorrhage showing so-called lumpy, bumpy deposition of immune complexes as demonstrated by immunofluorescence.

work-up is necessary. Anti-GBM antibody is positive in approximately 90 percent of cases of Goodpasture's syndrome. When these serologic studies are negative, kidney or lung biopsy is indicated for pathologic analysis, including immunofluorescence. One might argue that since the treatment is similar among the three major entities there is no necessity to demonstrate a specific serologic association, but plasmapheresis is one therapy in which knowing the specific diagnosis is important. This therapy is effective in Goodpasture's syndrome but is as yet unproven in other alveolar hemorrhage syndromes. There will undoubtedly remain those patients whose disease cannot be classified beyond diffuse alveolar hemorrhage and, if lacking nephritis, will fall into the vague category of idiopathic pulmonary hemosiderosis. However, in all cases, irrespective of cause, there is the common pathology of capillaritis of the alveoli and focal necrotizing glomerulitis or rapidly progressive crescentic glomerulonephritis.

PULMONARY VASCULITIDES NOT ASSOCIATED WITH ANCA

Behçet's Disease

In 1937, a Turkish dermatologist, Behçet, published a report of three patients who had a unique syndrome characterized by oral aphthous ulcerations, genital ulcers, and uveitis.[1] He hypothesized a viral etiology. Subsequently, the term *Behçet's disease* was attached. Similar to Wegener's granulomatosis, Behçet's has been enlarged in scope and concept to be included in the systemic vasculitides. In 1990, an international study group for Behçet's disease set forth specific diagnostic criteria.[29] The sine qua non is aphthous ulcers in addition to two or more of the following: genital ulceration, eye lesions such as anterior/posterior uveitis, hypopyon or retinal vasculitis, skin lesions such as pustules, nodules, erythema nodosum, or dermatographism. The pathergic skin test, present in 85 percent of patients, is a reaction (nodule or pustule) elicited by sterile needle penetration of the skin. Involvement has also been recorded in the lungs, which will be described at greater length. Other organ involvement has included the kidneys, joints, central nervous system, gastrointestinal tract, cardiovascular system, the epididymis, and muscles. Joint involvement is characterized by a nondestructive arthritis.

Although worldwide in distribution, most large series have been reported from the shores of the Mediterranean, particularly Turkey and Greece, as well as the Middle East and Japan. In these areas, men are more frequently affected than women in ratios of up to 3:1. In series reported from Great Britain and the United States, the sex ratio was more balanced.[40] It is most frequently diagnosed between ages 20 to 40 years.

Pathologically there is a nonspecific vasculitis with infiltration of the vessel walls with lymphocytes, plasma cells, and polymorphonuclear leukocytes that is seen with immune complex deposition and complement fixation. These changes lead to occlusion of the vasa vasorum with consequent transmural necrosis and fibrosis. The vasculitis affects veins, venules, capillaries, and arterioles, as well as large vessels. No laboratory blood tests are helpful in making a diagnosis.

Involvement of the respiratory tract has been variously reported in 1 to 5 percent of patients. One of the most significant lesions is aneurysm of the pulmonary arteries with potential erosion into the bronchial tree with consequent exsanguination. The mortality rate has been reported at approximately 50 percent with such involvement. These aneurysms may be either bilateral or unilateral and tend to affect predominately young males. The Hugh-Stovin syndrome involves thrombosis of the pulmonary artery with aneurysm formation, as well as thrombosis of the vena cava. Some authorities feel this is a form of Behçet's disease. When pulmonary artery aneurysm is suspected, either CT scan with contrast, or pulmonary arteriography, is advised. Resection of the aneurysms is indicated and can be lifesaving. Medical treatment for Behçet's disease includes glucocorticoids and a cytotoxic agent such as chlorambucil, azathioprine, or cyclophosphamide. Colchicine in doses up to 1.5 mg/d has been advocated for arthralgias and erythema nodosum.

Takayasu's Arteritis

Takayasu's arteritis affects large vessels, particularly the aorta and its main branches. The pulmonary artery is involved in up to 50 percent of cases. As the radial pulses may often be obtunded or absent, the condition has been referred to otherwise as the "pulseless disease." Pulmonary hypertension may result from the pulmonary vasculitis. Although exceedingly rare, this condition should be considered in all cases of unexplained pulmonary hypertension.

Takayasu's arteritis is rare in the United States. In a 12-year period from 1971 to 1983, only 32 patients were seen with this diagnosis at Mayo Clinic.[27] The disease appears more common in Asians or those of North African descent. Women are predominately affected in ratios as high as 1:25, as reported in a Japanese series. The usual onset is between ages 20 and 30. Some claim the diagnosis should be questioned if it is made over the age of 40.

Approximately half of the patients will present with constitutional symptoms such as fever, malaise, and weight loss. Depending on the severity and location of the obliterative lesions, patients may complain of arm or leg claudication. The diagnosis of arteriosclerotic lesions is raised, but the age of these patients tends to reduce this possibility. The diagnosis of Takayasu's arteritis is made on the basis of clinical suspicion supported by characteristic angiographic findings particularly involving the aorta. Lesions demonstrated by angiography include occlusions, stenosis, irregularity of lumens, ectasia, and aneurysmal formation. Documentation of histopathology is rare in life unless surgery is performed to correct aneurysms, to bypass occlusions, or remedy aortic regurgitation. The lesions are characterized by granulomatous and sclerosing arteritis that is indistinguishable from giant cell (temporal) arteritis.

Glucocorticoids with or without a cytotoxic agent such as cyclophosphamide are the primary forms of therapy, but there are no studies to suggest that this treatment has any remedial value for pulmonary hypertension.

The chief causes of death relate to the complications of the occlusive vascular lesions, including systemic or pulmonary

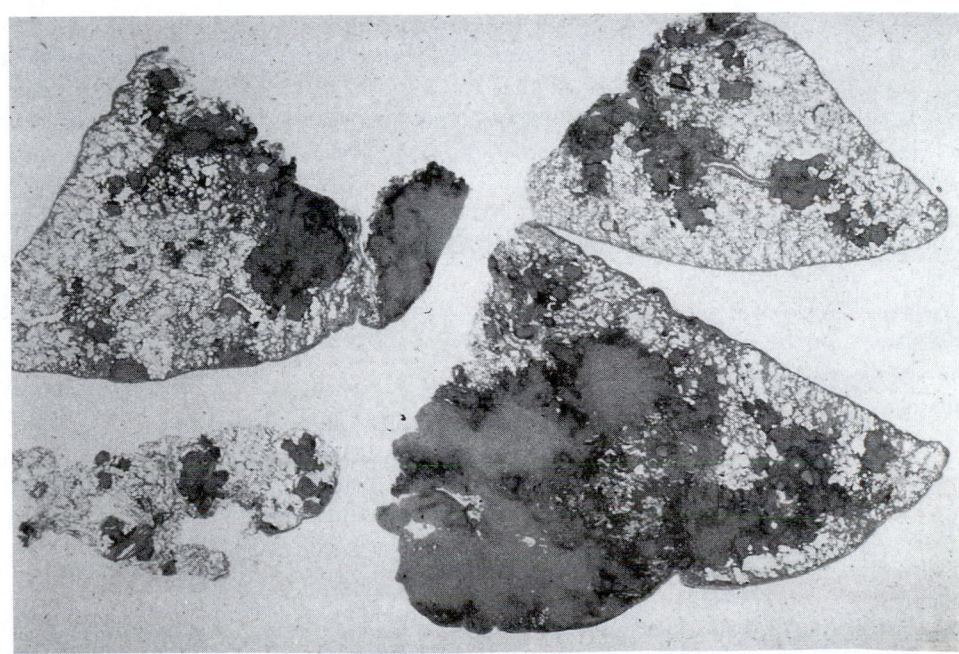

FIGURE 86-21   Low-power photomicrograph of lung revealing coalescing necrotizing granulomas in a patient with necrotizing sarcoid granulomatosis.

hypertension and its ultimate consequences, and aortic valve regurgitation.

Sarcoidosis and Necrotizing Sarcoid Granulomatosis

Involvement of pulmonary blood vessels is a common feature of the pathology of sarcoidosis, but rarely are these manifestations apparent clinically. Pulmonary hypertension may be seen in end-stage sarcoidosis when the pulmonary parenchyma has been destroyed by fibrosis. Diffuse alveolar hemorrhage is not a consequence of sarcoidosis. Pathologically, involvement of the venous system predominates over the arterial system, and rarely sarcoidosis has simulated veno-occlusive disease. About one-third of lung biopsies reveal involvement of both arteries and veins, but only a few cases have been confined to the pulmonary arteries. Lesser involvement of the arterial system may explain the minimal clinical effect. The granulomas may be seen in the adventitia, the media, and the intima, leading to destruction of the elastic tissue and smooth muscle in the vessel walls. However, the endothelium remains intact, and there is no evidence of thrombosis. These features may explain the modest symptomatology.

The lesions of necrotizing sarcoid granulomatosis bear resemblance to those seen in sarcoidosis except for the prominent necrosis and destructive vasculitis. The granulomas may become confluent and are reflected in the appearance (Fig. 86-21) of multiple nodular lesions on the chest radiograph. They are usually multiple and bilateral, but hilar adenopathy commonly seen in stage I sarcoidosis does not occur. In addition, there are no other features of classic sarcoidosis, such as skin involvement or uveitis, and the pathology appears to be confined to the thorax. What is most surprising, considering the extent of the disease apparent on the chest radiograph and the nature of the pathology, is that most of the patients are asymptomatic, which is typical of sarcoidosis generally. Pathologically, veins and arteries are affected by a destructive process that involves the elastic muscular layers of arteries and veins, but again neither thrombosis nor aneurysm formation are seen. Similar to sarcoidosis, the prognosis is good with frequent spontaneous remissions, and a good response is achieved with glucocorticoids. Remember that only a few cases of necrotizing sarcoid granulomatosis have been reported and that the term was coined to cover the ambiguity of whether the lesions represented necrotizing angiitis with a sarcoid reaction or sarcoidosis with necrosis of the granulomas of the blood vessels.

SUMMARY AND GENERAL CONCLUSIONS

Pulmonary vasculitis is rare. When should one suspect pulmonary vasculitis? Cough, hemoptysis, shortness of [breath], and wheezing should immedi[ately] prick one's attention, especially [when the]se symptoms are accompanied

TABLE 86-4

Symptoms and Findings in Churg-Strauss Syndrome

Wheezing, dyspnea (asthma)
Peripheral blood eosinophilia
Allergic rhinitis
Necrotizing skin lesions
Mononeuritis multiplex

by weight loss and fever. Usually, pulmonary symptoms will lead to chest radiography which may reveal almost pathognomonic findings in Wegener's granulomatosis if there are multiple nodules some of which may be cavitary, or an alveolar hemorrhage syndrome if there is a diffuse alveolar filling pattern. Because most cases of pulmonary vasculitis are part of a systemic process, involvement of other organ systems is likely to be present. Accordingly, glomerulonephritis, neurologic signs, particularly mononeuritis multiplex, or changes in the skin may be present. Table 86-3 lists the signs and symptoms that are particularly associated with Wegener's granulomatosis. Table 86-4 lists the main features that suggest the diagnosis of Churg-Strauss syndrome. Regarding this diagnosis, the clinician should not be lulled into complacency by the common disease, asthma, and not look for other manifestations of systemic vasculitis, particularly in the skin and nervous system which are the chief extrapulmonary sites of this syndrome. Microscopic polyangiitis crosses over in many cases with Wegener's granulomatosis and Churg-Strauss syndrome (Table 86-5). It is to be emphasized that these three syndromes are closely associated with ANCA.

Laboratory

Few laboratory tests are necessary to make the diagnosis of pulmonary vasculitis and to monitor the clinical course. A white blood cell count with differential looking for eosinophilia, an erythrocyte sedimentation rate which may give clues to the activity of the process, an ANCA, ANA, and anti-GBM antibody would be the panel of blood tests. A routine urinalysis is a fundamental parameter, with a serum creatinine and creatinine clear-

TABLE 86-5

Comparative Features of Wegener's Granulomatosis (WG), Churg-Strauss Syndrome (CSS), and Microscopic Polyangiitis (MPA)

Feature	WG	CSS	MPA
Asthma	0	++++	0
Eosinophilia (blood, tissue)	+/−	++++	0
History of allergy	0	++++	0
Upper respiratory tract	+++	++	+
Lower respiratroy tract	+++	+++	+
Glomerulonephritis	++	+	++++
Skin lesions	++	+++	++
Mononeuritis multiplex	++	+++	+
Eye lesions	++	0	+
Joint symptoms	++	++	++
Cardiac disease	+/−	++	+/−

ance. Red blood cell casts and proteinuria are the hallmarks of glomerulonephritis.

Radiography

Usually the plain chest radiograph will suffice as the radiographic study. For lesions such as an aneurysm of the pulmonary artery, suspected in the context of Behçet's disease, a chest CT scan with contrast or pulmonary angiography are indicated. When the diagnosis of Takayasu's arteritis is entertained, arteriography, particularly of the aorta, is diagnostic in most cases in the appropriate clinical context. With involvement of the upper respiratory tract, particularly involving the nose and paranasal sinuses, CT scanning of the sinuses and orbits is important. When subglottic stenosis is suspected, tomograms of the trachea may give an accurate definition of the lesion.

Pulmonary Function Tests

Pulmonary function testing has a limited role in pulmonary vasculitis. Where subglottic stenosis is suspected, a flow volume loop will show flattening of both the inspiratory and expiratory limbs consistent with an extrathoracic fixed obstruction. Repeat measurements may be valuable in measuring change with treatment. Diffuse alveolar hemorrhage will cause an increase in the carbon monoxide diffusing capacity, but as a practical matter such measurements are rarely indicated except in a research situation.

Treatment

Having made the diagnosis of pulmonary vasculitis and/or alveolar hemorrhage, one may question the necessity of precision concerning the name given to the particular syndrome or attempting to define its cause, since treatment involves a glucocorticoid with or without a cytotoxic agent for all the entities. There are, however, nuances of clinical course and applications of various modalities that make it worthwhile to make as specific a diagnosis as possible. For instance, in the case of a patient with Wegener's granulomatosis involving the upper and/or lower respiratory tract without systemic vasculitis, trimethoprim/sulfamethoxazole alone may achieve a good response without subjecting the patient to the hazards of systemic glucocorticoids or cytotoxic agents. In the Churg-Strauss syndrome, glucocorticoids are the chief agent, with cytotoxic agents playing a secondary role. Because the patient with Churg-Strauss syndrome may require virtually lifelong treatment, efforts should be made to reduce the long-term side effects of glucocorticoids by developing alternate-day regimens if they are tolerated by the patient. High doses of glucocorticoids are often prescribed, such as 1 mg/kg of prednisone, without a proven rationale. It is essential to appreciate that although the vasculitides conjure a sense of cataclysm and doom, they do not necessarily require toxic regimens.

However, pulmonary vasculitides may produce medical and surgical emergencies. Alveolar hemorrhage syndromes can cause respiratory failure. Apart from the usual regimens of corticosteroids and cytotoxic agents, plasmapheresis has a role in the treatment of Goodpasture's syndrome. In Behçet's disease a pulmonary artery aneurysm may rupture into a bronchus with the potential for exsanguination. Alertness to this possibility may lead to lifesaving surgical intervention. In Takayasu's arteritis various surgical remedies may be necessary, such as the repair of an incompetent aortic valve, the resection of an aortic aneurysm, or the dilatation of a stenosed renal artery.

REFERENCES

1. Behçet H: Über rezidivierende aphthose, durch ein Virus verursachte Geschwure am Mund, am Auge und an den Genitalien. *Derm Wochenschr* 36:1152–1157, 1937.
2. Bullen CL, Liesegang TJ, McDonald TJ, DeRemee RA: Ocular complications of Wegener's granulomatosis. *Ophthalmology* 90:279–290, 1983.
3. Bygren P, Rasmussen N, Isaksson B, Wieslander J: Anti-neutrophil cytoplasm antibodies, anti-GMB antibodies and anti-ds DNA antibodies in glomerulonephritis. *Eur J Clin Invest* 22:783–792, 1992.
4. Carrington CB, Leibow AA: Limited forms of angiitis and granulomatosis of Wegener's type. *Am J Med* 41:497–527, 1966.
5. Chumbley LC, Harrison EG, Jr, DeRemee RA: Allergic granulomatosis and angiitis (Churg-Strauss syndrome) report and analysis of 30 cases. *Mayo Clin Proc* 52:477–484, 1977.
6. Chur A, Brallas M, Cronin SR, Churg J: Formes Frustes of Churg-Strauss syndrome. *Chest* 108:320–323, 1995.
7. Churg J, Strauss L: Allergic granulomatosis, allergic angiitis, and periarteritis nodosa. *Am J Pathol* 27:277–301, 1951.
8. Cohen Tervaert JW, Huitema MG, Hené RJ, et al: Prevention of relapses in Wegener's granulomatosis by treatment based on antineutrophil cytoplasmic antibody titre. *Lancet* 336:709–711, 1990.
9. Crotty CP, DeRemee RA, Winkelmann RK: Cutaneous clinicopathologic correlation of allergic granulomatosis. *J Am Acad Dermatol* 5:571–581, 1981.
10. Daoud MS, Gibson LE, DeRemee RA, et al: Cutaneous Wegener's granulomatosis: clinical, histopathologic, and immunopathologic features of thirty patients. *J Am Acad Dermatol* 31:605–612, 1994.
11. Daum TE, Specks U, Colby TV, et al: Trachobronchial involvement in Wegener's granulomatosis. *Am J Respir Crit Care Med* 151:522–526, 1995.
12. Davies DJ, Moran JE, Niall JF, Ryan GB: Segmental necrotizing glomerulonephritis with antineutrophil antibody: possible arbovirus aetiology? *Br Med J (Clin Res)* 285:606, 1982.
13. DeRemee RA: The nosology of Wegener's granulomatosis utilizing the ELK format augmented by c-ANCA. *Adv Exp Med Biol* 336:209–215, 1993.
14. DeRemee RA: The treatment of Wegener's granulomatosis. *Clin Exp Immunol* 101(suppl 1):23–26, 1995.
15. DeRemee RA, McDonald TJ, Weiland LH: Observations on treatment with antimicrobial agents. *Mayo Clin Proc* 60:27–32, 1985.
16. DeRemee RA, Colby TV: Wegener's granulomatosis, in Thurlbeck WM, Churg AM (eds), *Pathology of the Lung.* New York, Thieme, 1995, pp 401–423.
17. DeRemee RA, Homburger HA, Specks U: Lesions of the respiratory tract associated with the finding of anti-neutrophil cytoplasmic autoantibody with a perinuclear staining pattern. *Mayo Clin Proc* 69:819–824, 1994.
18. DeRemee RA, McDonald TJ, Weiland LH: Aspekte zur Therapie und Verlaufsbeobachtungen der Wegenerschen Granulomatose. *Med Welt* 38:470–473, 1987.

19. DeRemee RA: The treatment of Wegener's granulomatosis with trimethoprim/sulfamethoxazole: illusion or vision? *Arthritis Rheum* 31:1068–1072, 1988.

20. Fienberg R: A morphologic and immunohistoogic study of the evolution of the necrotizing palisading granuloma of pathergic (Wegener's) granulomatosis. *Semin Respir Med* 10:126–132, 1989.

21. Fienberg R: The protracted superficial phenomenon in pathergic (Wegener's) granulomatosis. *Hum Pathol* 12:458–467, 1981.

22. Godman GC, Churg J: Wegener's granulomatosis. Pathology and review of the literature. *Arch Pathol Lab Med* 58:533–553, 1954.

23. Goodpasture EW: The significance of certain pulmonary lesions in relation to the etiology of influenza. *Am J Med Sci* 158:863–870, 1919.

24. Gross WL, Csernok E, Helmchen U: Antineutrophil cytoplasmic autoantibodies, autoantigens, and systemic vasculitis. *APMIS* 103: 81–97, 1995.

25. Guillevin, Lhote F: Polyarteritis nodosa and microscopic polyangiitis. *Clin Exp Immunol* 101(suppl 1):22–23, 1995.

26. Gunwar S, Bejarano PA, Kalluri R, et al: Alveolar basement membrane: molecular properties of the noncollagenous domain (Hexamer) of collagen IV and its reactivity with Goodpasture autoantibodies. *Am J Respir Cell Mol Biol* 5:107–112, 1991.

27. Hall S, Barr W, Lie JT, et al: Takayasu arteritis: a study of 32 North American patients. *Medicine* 64:89–99, 1985.

28. Harkavy J: Vascular allergy pathogenesis of bronchial asthma with recurrent pulmonary infiltrations and eosinophilic polyserositis. *Arch Intern Med* 67:709–734, 1941.

29. International Study Group for Behçet's Disease: Criteria for diagnosis of Behçet's disease. *Lancet* 335:1078–80, 1990.

29a. Jennette JC, Falk RJ, Andrassy K, et al: Nomenclature of systemic vasculitides: The proposal of an interntional consensus conference. *Arthritis Rheum* 37:187–192, 1994.

30. Koffler D, Sandson J, Carr R, Kunkel HG: Immunologic studies concerning the pulmonary lesions in Goodpasture's syndrome. *Am J Pathol* 54:293–306, 1969.

31. Lanham JG, Elkon KB, Pusey CD, Hughes GR: Systemic vasculitis with asthma and eosinophilia: a clinical approach to the Churg-Strauss Syndrome. *Medicine* 63:65–81, 1984.

32. Leavitt RY, Fauci AS, Block DA, et al.: The American College of Rheumatology 1990 criteria for the classification of Wegener's granulomatosis. *Arthritis Rheum* 33:1101–1107, 1990.

33. Lerner RA, Glassock RJ, Dixon FJ: The role of anti-glomerular basement membrane antibody in the pathogenesis of human glomerulonephritis. *J Exp Med* 126:989–1004, 1967.

34. Lie JT: Limited forms of Churg-Strauss syndrome. *Pathol Annual* 28:199–220, 1993.

35. Liebow AA: Pulmonary angiitis and granulomatosis. *Am Rev Resp Dis* 108:1–18, 1973.

36. McDonald TJ, DeRemee RA, Kern EB, et al: Nasal manifestations of Wegener's granulomatosis. *Laryngoscope* 84:2101–2112, 1974.

37. Moriwaki R, Numano F: Takayasu arteritis: follow-up studies for 20 years. *Heart Vessels Suppl* 7:138–145, 1992.

38. Nishino H, Rubino FA, DeRemee RA, et al: Neurologic involvement in Wegener's granulomatosis. *Ann Neurol* 33:4–9, 1993.

39. Nölle B, Specks U, Lüdemann J, et al: Anticytoplasmic autoantibodies: their immunodiagnostic value in Wegener granulomatosis. *Ann Intern Med* 111:28–40, 1989.

40. O'Duffy JD: Vasculitis in Behçet's disease. *Rheum Dis Clin N Amer* 16:423–431, 1990.

41. Olsen KD, Neel HB III, DeRemee RA, Weiland LH: Nasal manifestations of allergic granulomatosis and angiitis (Churg-Strauss syndrome). *Otolaryngol Head Neck Surg* 88:85–89, 1980.

42. Rackemann FM, Greene JE: Periarteritis nodosa and asthma. *Assoc Am Physicians* 54:112–118, 1939.

43. Rose GA, Spencer H: Polyarteritis nodosa. *Q J Med* 26:43–81, 1957.

44. Savage COS, Winearls CG, Evans DJ, et al: Microscopic polyarteritis: presentation, pathology, and prognosis. *Q J Med* 56:467–483, 1985.

45. Sehgal M, Swanson JW, DeRemee RA, Colby TV: Neurologic manifestations of Churg-Strauss syndrome. *Mayo Clin Proc* 70:337–341, 1995.

46. Specks U, Colby TV, Olsen KD, DeRemee RA: Salivary gland involvement in Wegener's granulomatosis. *Arch Otolaryngol Head Neck Surg* 117:218–223, 1991.

47. Stegeman CA, Cohen Tervaert JW, de Jong PE, Kallenberg CGM: Trimethoprim-sulfamethoxazole (co-trimoxazole) for the prevention of relapses of Wegener's granulomatosis. *New Engl J Med* 335: 16–20, 1996.

48. Van der Woude, FJ, Rasmussen N, Lobatto S, et al: Autoantibodies against neutrophils and monocytes: tool for diagnosis and marker of disease activity in Wegener's granulomatosis. *Lancet* 1:425–429, 1985.

49. Vanhauwaert BG, Roskams TA, Vanneste SB, Knockaert DC: Salivary gland involvement as initial presentation of Wegener's disease. *Postgrad Med J* 69:643–645, 1993.

50. Walton EW: Giant cell granuloma of the respiratory tract (Wegener's granulomatosis). *Br Med J* 2:265–270, 1958.

51. Wegener F: Über generalisierte, septische Gefässerkrankungen. *Verhandl Deutsch Ges Pathol.* 29:202–210, 1936.

52. Wegener F: Über eine eigenartige rhinogene Granulomatose mit besonderer Beteiligung des Arteriensystems und der Nieren. *Beitr Pathol* 102:36–68, 1939.

CHAPTER 87

PULMONARY ARTERIOVENOUS MALFORMATIONS

Daniel M. Goodenberger

Pulmonary arteriovenous malformations (PAVMs) were first described relatively recently in medical history; Churton reported the autopsy findings in a young boy with cyanosis in 1897.[7] PAVMs were first diagnosed during life in 1939.[53] As in many later cases, clubbing and polycythemia were present in a 40-year-old man. Based on the correlation of physical with postmortem findings, the triad of cyanosis, clubbing, and polycythemia was identified with PAVM in 1932.[43] Hereditary hemorrhagic telangiectasia (HHT) was first connected to pulmonary arteriovenous malformation in 1938.[47] As described below, HHT is often intimately related to PAVMs—a fact that prompts the following discussion of the history of HHT.

   Hereditary epistaxis was first described in 1865.[3] This report was not generally recognized; nor were subsequent descriptions of telangiectasia, hereditary transmission, and epistaxis by Legg in 1876, or a similar kindred reported by Chiari in 1887. The first widely recognized connection of epistaxis to telangiectasia was made by Rendu in 1896.[46] Osler added three cases, and rec-

ognized familial occurrence in 1901.[36] Weber elucidated the familial nature and lack of coagulation abnormality, and thus earned his eponymic association.[57] By precedence of description, this eponym should be Rendu-Osler-Weber even though Osler-Weber-Rendu is the common usage. Hanes was responsible for naming the syndrome hereditary hemorrhagic telangiectasia, in 1909.

PATHOPHYSIOLOGY

Structure

By far the most common form of PAVM has a pulmonary arterial supply and pulmonary venous drainage.[1] In one series, 60 of 63 PAVMs had a pulmonary arterial blood supply.[10] Approximately 80 percent of PAVMs have a single feeding and a single draining vessel; the remaining 20 percent are complex, with two or more of each.[59] PAVMs appear to develop between precapillary arterioles and venules, with intervening epithelial dysplasia.[34] After development, they are clusters of dilated, tortuous vessels with both arterial and venous elements with no intervening capillary beds.[37]

Number

In one series, more than one-third of the patients had two or more PAVMs.[10] In general, multiple PAVMs correlate with HHT; in the experience of our clinic, most patients with HHT have more than one PAVM.

Size

PAVMs may vary from malformations too small to be seen by radiography or angiography[7,21,58] to those greater than 5 cm in diameter.[19]

Location

Up to 65 percent of PAVMs are located in the lower lobes[58]—a phenomenon that may be due to the increased pulmonary blood

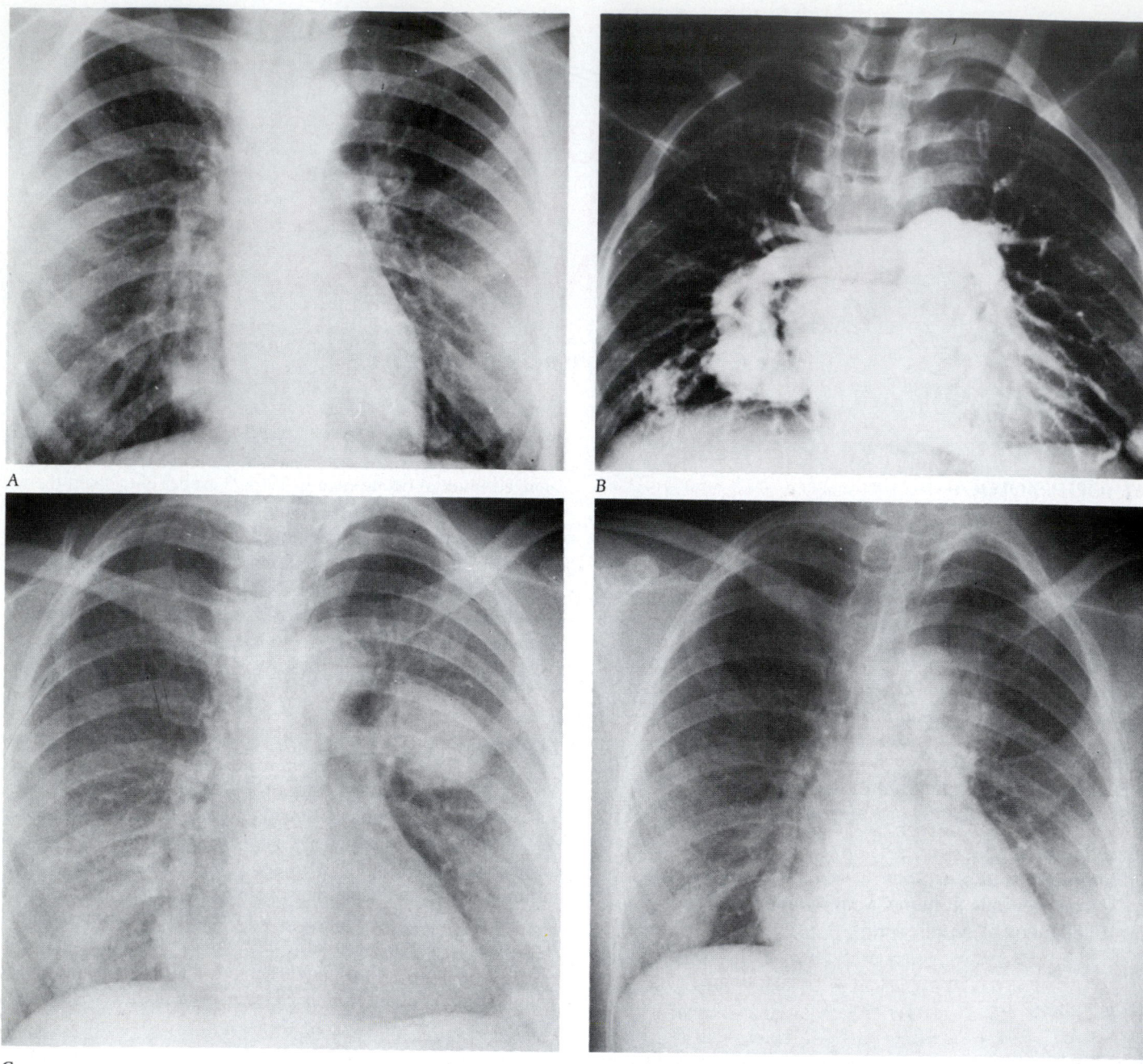

FIGURE 87-1 Pulmonary arteriovenous fistulas in a pregnant 24-year-old woman with hereditary hemorrhagic telangiectasia. *A.* Before pregnancy. Small nodular densities are seen at both bases and in the left hilus. The shunt was estimated to be 49 percent of the cardiac output. *B.* Arteriogram before pregnancy demonstrates arteriovenous fistulas of both lower lobes. *C.* Seven months pregnant, the patient was admitted to the hospital with hemoptysis and left hemothorax. The enlargement of the arteriovenous fistulas is striking. The pregnancy was terminated. *D.* Two weeks after termination of pregnancy, the nodular densities have decreased in size. *(Courtesy of Dr. M. Rossman.)*

flow and pressure, and subsequent "stretch" due to hydrodynamic forces. This location is probably the cause of the often associated orthodeoxia (desaturation in an upright position) and platypnea (dyspnea in an upright position). These symptoms may also occur with cirrhosis, which evidences the pulmonary vascular abnormalities described below. Location may also ac-

count for an increase in right-to-left shunt, which occurs at total lung capacity.[28] PAVMs have been observed to increase in size during pregnancy (Fig. 87-1); this supports the blood flow hypothesis, due to the increased blood volume and hyperdynamic state of pregnancy, although endocrine factors may also have an influence.[6]

Causes and Disease Associations

Early observers thought that all PAVMs were due to HHT.[59] The estimates of frequency of PAVMs due to HHT have varied substantially, from 36 to 100 percent.[4,6,10,19,58]

Estimates of the percentage of patients with HHT who have associated PAVMs also vary from the frequently quoted 15 percent[6] to 20 percent,[44] to 24 percent,[34] and to more than 50 percent.[18] As noted above, the proportion of PAVMs that are multiple has been reported to be approximately one-third;[44] multiple PAVMs are highly associated with HHT.[6] Of note is that the homozygous form of HHT may result in an explosive growth of mucocutaneous telangiectasias and death, with diffuse PAVMs seen in infancy.[26]

Other Associations

Cirrhosis may result in diffuse small arteriovenous connections.[21] Nearly all such patients have cutaneous spider angiomas. The right-to-left shunt is probably due not to true PAVMs but, rather, to vasodilation of pleural vessels, which resemble the cutaneous spiders, and increased numbers of peripheral small arteriolar branches with precapillary arteriole-to-venous connections in the peripheral respiratory lobule. As many as 15 percent may have positive contrast echocardiography indicative of intrapulmonary shunt; many of these patients have shunt eliminated by liver transplantation. A PAVM of significant size, known as a Rasmussen aneurysm, may also develop as a result of tuberculosis.[31] Metastatic thyroid carcinoma, a highly vascular tumor, may mimic pulmonary arteriovenous fistula.[38]

GENETICS

The genetic basis, if any, of isolated PAVMs remains unknown. HHT is an autosomal dominant disease. Its frequency is reported to be 1 to 2 per 100,000 people. Phenotypic variation is extreme, ranging from asymptomatic to severely symptomatic, and from cases with no or few mucocutaneous lesions to those with diffuse cutaneous telangiectasias. For many patients, the disease remains undiagnosed by their primary care physicians, suggesting that disease frequency may be greater than reported, and that some patients with "isolated" PAVMs may actually have HHT.

A gene for HHT was first localized to chromosome 9, region q^{33-34} (9 q^{33-34}).[25,35,49] An early candidate protein was the α_1 chain of type 5 collagen, but this was later shown not to be causative.[20] Further investigation revealed the protein product to be endoglin, the TGF-β receptor.[32] The same work showed the disease to be genetically heterogeneous, with several mutations in the responsible gene. It rapidly became clear that there were other chromosomal mutations resulting in the same syndrome, and the endoglin mutation disease was designated HHT-I; it was noted to be associated more often with PAVMs than were those with non-9q[3] mutations.[33,39] Thus far, a second mutation at 3p22 appears to code for the TGF-β_2 receptor, while a third mutation at 12q has a gene product as yet unknown. The latter abnormality appears not to be associated with PAVMs.[56] It remains to be explored what, if any, genetic abnormalities occur in persons with

isolated PAVMs. The author's opinion is that many such persons will prove to have a poorly expressed phenotype of one of the first two HHT genotypes.

CLINICAL PRESENTATION

The occurrence and frequency of symptoms related to PAVMs depend on how the patients are found—that is, whether they present with manifestations of disease or whether they are discovered as a result of screening.[18] The asymptomatic state is most common when screening is the method of detection, with an incidence ranging from 93 percent,[52] to 55 percent,[6] to 26 percent.[11] The age at onset is usually in the third or fourth decade.[37] The mean age at detection in various series is remarkably constant at 38 to 39 years.[6,11,16] In one series, the patients ranged in age from 5 to 76, with a mean of 36; 26 percent presented at an age less than 21 years.[58] PAVMs are, however, uncommon in childhood; only 4 percent of affected persons are under 10.[18,51] Pulmonary symptoms include dyspnea on exertion, with a frequency ranging from 32 to 71 percent.[10,11,58] Platypnea and orthodeoxia also may occur. Hemoptysis ranges in frequency from 10 to 15 percent.[10,58] Extrapulmonary symptoms include chest pain in 6 percent[12] and epistaxis (largely seen in HHT), ranging from 32 to 85 percent.[11,37] The mean age at onset of epistaxis in HHT is 12 years, with 54 percent of patients presenting by age 10. Severity of epistaxis ranges from mild to severe, with up to 45 episodes per month.[2] Headache is also remarkably common in HHT patients, occurring in 43 percent.[58] Transient ischemic attack occurs in 57 percent of patients with PAVM, and symptomatic cerebrovascular accident in 18 percent.[58]

Physical signs due to the PAVM itself are relatively uncommon. As many as 25 percent of patients may exhibit no findings at all.[10] Hypoxemia is secondary to the right-to-left shunt, with resulting cyanosis and secondary polycythemia. This tends to occur in advanced disease, and is uncommon in our experience. The frequency has been reported to range from less than 10 percent to as much as 50 percent.[4,10] The frequency of clubbing ranges from less than 10 to 20 percent;[4,10] clubbing is nearly always associated with cyanosis. Clubbing may resolve after the PAVM is removed[16] or occluded. A pulmonary bruit, which is often described, is also variable; its frequency, probably influenced by selection bias, ranges from less than 10 percent to 43 percent.[4,10,11]

Telangiectasia has been reported in up to 66 percent of patients with PAVM, depending on the frequency of HHT.[41] These small red vascular blemishes occur most frequently on the face, followed in descending order by the lips, nares, tongue, ears, hands, chest, and feet. They often increase in size and number with age, and cutaneous telangiectasias are seldom identifiable until the second or third decade.[37] We have been struck by the frequency with which classic tongue and lip telangiectasias have been passed off as nonspecific blemishes by primary care physicians.

Laboratory results are nonspecific. A complete blood count may show polycythemia, although in patients with HHT, this tendency may be overcome by iron deficiency anemia. The severely affected person may have arterial hypoxemia at rest; those less severely affected may have orthodeoxia documented by supine and upright arterial blood gases.[60] Arterial blood gases, determined on blood samples drawn while the patient is breathing room air, followed by 100 percent oxygen, may reveal a significant right-to-left shunt.[18]

CLINICAL DIAGNOSIS

Early in the history of this disorder, the diagnosis was made only when it was advanced, when polycythemia and clubbing were present,[53] or after death.[47] Currently, making the diagnosis requires clinical suspicion in the appropriate clinical setting. Diagnosis is approached differently in the two most common situations.

Evaluation of a Radiographic Abnormality

Earlier techniques for determining that a pulmonary nodule detected as an incidental finding was a pulmonary arteriovenous malformation were principally radiographic. Fluoroscopy might reveal the nodule to be pulsatile; a Müller maneuver might cause the lesion to decrease in size, and a Valsalva maneuver might cause it to increase in size. Laminography typically revealed the lesion to be a grapelike cluster, with visible feeding and draining vessels.

A newer kind of chest tomography, the CT scan with contrast enhancement, may show the typical lesion with feeding and draining veins (Fig. 87-2),[47] but vascular tumors may cause false-positive results. A perfusion lung scan may detect a right-to-left shunt. Ordinarily, 95 percent of the technetium-labeled macroaggregated albumin, with an average diameter of approximately 35 μ, is trapped in the pulmonary capillaries. When there is an intracardiac or intrapulmonary shunt, unusually large amounts may pass through the lung and travel to the brain and kidneys, resulting in excess radioactivity in those areas. However, this method cannot differentiate intracardiac from intrapulmonary shunt.

Echocardiography, using indocyanine green as a contrast material, was found to be effective in the diagnosis of intrapulmonary shunt, with delayed appearance of the contrast material in the side of the heart.[50] This was rapidly [follo]ved by the use of agitated saline as

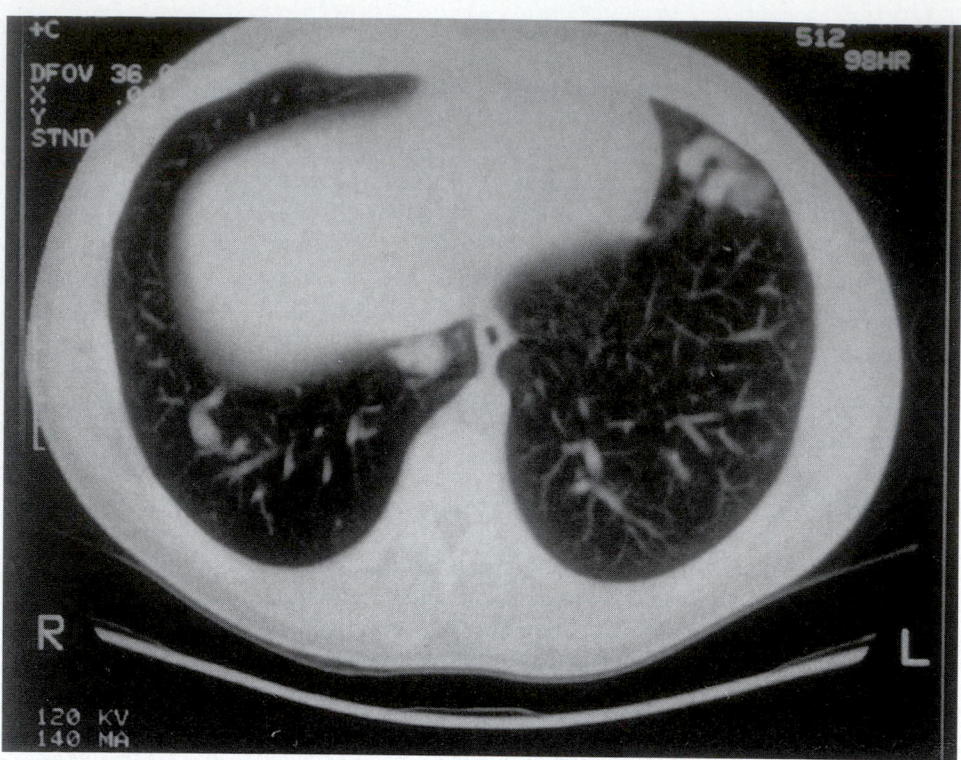

FIGURE 87-2   Characteristic CT image appearance of PAVM in left hemithorax. Portions of two PAVMs are seen in right hemithorax.

contrast (Fig. 87-3).[24] The intrapulmonary nature of the shunt can be determined by the delay, averaging four to five cardiac cycles, of left heart contrast appearance; when the echo is performed

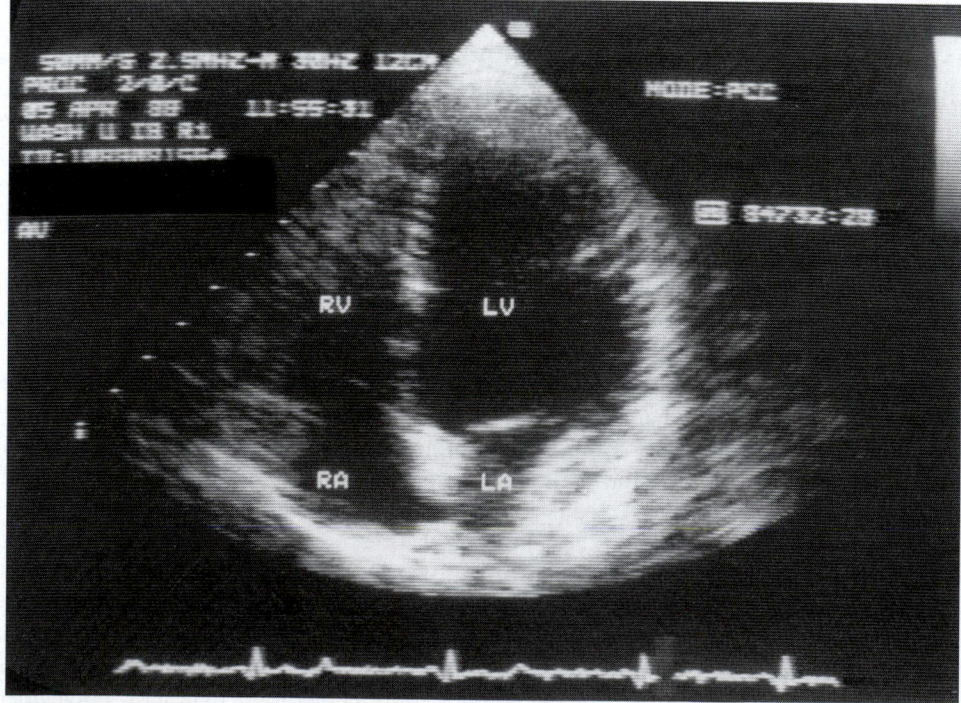

A

FIGURE 87-3   Echocardiographic images using saline contrast: *A.* Before contrast. *B.* Right-sided chamber opacification. *C.* Delayed high-degree left-sided chamber opacification indicative of large intrapulmonary shunt.

transesophageally, the region of a radiographically undetectable PAVM may be inferred by the appearance of contrast in one or another pulmonary vein. If contrast echocardiography is negative, no further workup is indicated for PAVM, and an alternative cause of the pulmonary nodule should be sought. If the contrast echocardiogram is positive, the definitive test is pulmonary angiography. Angiography is 100 percent sensitive, with correct application of the appropriate views, for vessels of 2 mm or more.

Screening of Probands or Relatives

The reported sensitivity of chest radiographs varies widely, depending on whether they are used for screening or in patients with symptomatic disease. Rates of abnormality on the chest radiograph range from 41[52] to 100 percent.[10] Chest radiography does not detect PAVMs less than 20 mm in size (Fig. 87-4), and it may miss larger PAVMs when they are located in radiographically inopportune places, such as the costophrenic sulci, the retrocardiac region, or the proximal hila (Fig. 87-5).[19]

The sensitivity and specificity of chest CT are unknown, although this modality appears to be more sensitive than are chest radiographs.[60] Arterial blood gases, determined on samples drawn while the patient is supine and upright, have been advocated for screening.[60] However, this technique has not proved useful. Arterial blood gases to detect the presence of shunt using room air and 100 percent oxygen have been neither sufficiently sensitive nor sufficiently specific.[18] Gradient-echo MRI shows promise, but it can mistake tumors for PAVMs.[12]

In our clinic, the best screening method has proved to be one that accurately detects right-to-left shunt. Ventilation-perfusion lung scanning has the drawback that it is expensive and time-consuming, requires radiation, and does not separate intracardiac from intrapulmonary shunt. Contrast echocardiography, on the other hand, appears to be 100 percent sensitive and 100 percent specific at levels greater than or equal to trace positive in the previously unembolized patient.[18] The amount of shunt can be roughly quantitated and correlated with AVM size.[4] If it is positive, angiography should be recommended, as levels of shunt greater than trace have never resulted in a false-positive study in our experience. After successful embolization of all visible PAVMs (see "Treatment," below), the contrast echo can remain faintly positive, presumably because of tiny, radiographically invisible AV connections. However, if a contrast echocardiogram remains significantly positive after embolization, we recommend repeat angiography, as we have occasionally found previously undiagnosed AVMs. In all likelihood, the appearance of undiagnosed PAVMs after a very short interval results from the expansion of

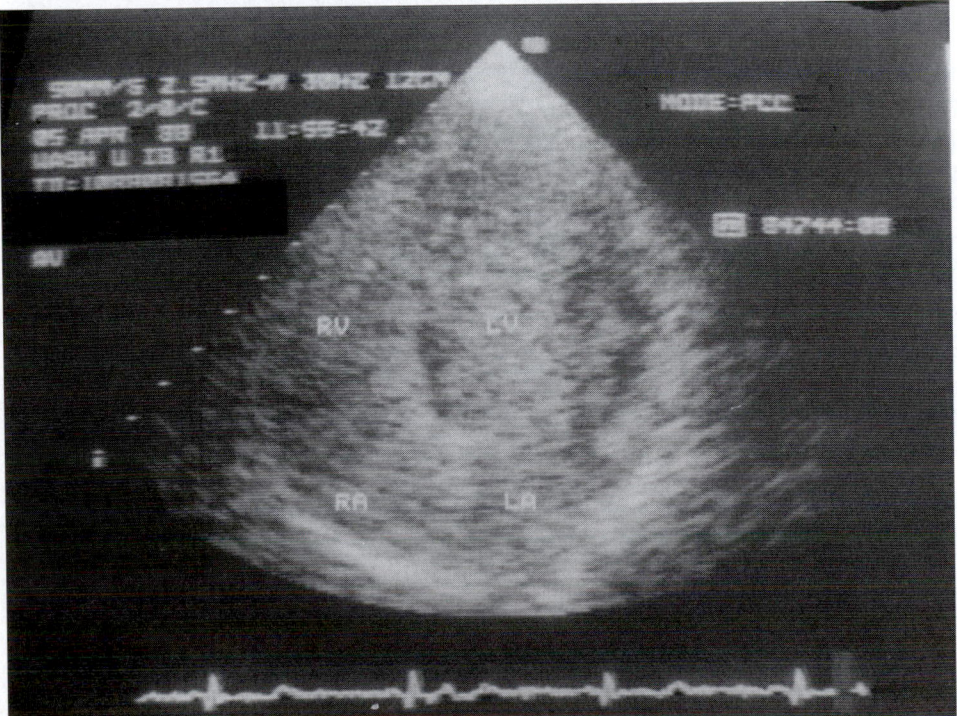

B

C

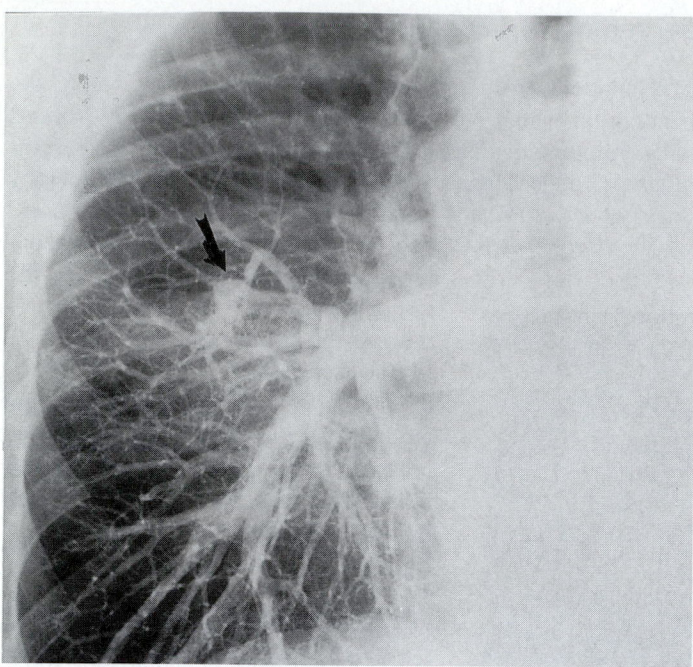

FIGURE 87-4　Example of PAVM not seen on standard chest radiography. Right pulmonary angiogram showing small PAVM (arrow).

small AVMs following the occlusion of larger, lower-resistance PAVMs.

COMPLICATIONS

Pulmonary Complications

Significant hemoptysis occurs in fewer than 10 percent of patients. It may be massive and life threatening. Bronchial telangiectasias may be the cause,[6] but we have found that massive hemoptysis is due to PAVMs.

Hemothorax occurs in approximately 9 percent of patients.[58] Pregnancy may cause PAVMs to enlarge, and has been associated with hemothorax on several occasions.[14,30] Hemothorax may also occur without any other predisposing factors, presumably caused by rupture of large subpleural PAVMs into the pleural space.[9]

Pulmonary hypertension is rare.[55]

Central Nervous System Complications

The pulmonary capillary vascular bed appears to be an important filter for otherwise asymptomatic small emboli, and may also have a significant role in cleansing the bloodstream during transient bacteremias. Most neurologic complications, which occur in 8 to 12 percent of patients with HHT, are complications of PAVMs. In one series, 60 percent were due to PAVM, including abscess, paradoxical embolus, and hypoxemia. Of the remaining neurologic complications, 28 percent were due to cerebral AVMs, 8 percent to spinal AVMs, and 3 percent to portal-systemic encephalopathy.[37,48] Transient ischemic attacks occur in approximately 37 percent of patients with PAVMs.[58] Spinal AVMs occur in up to 5 percent of patients[58] and tend

to run in families.[29] PAVMs can cause symptomatic cerebrovascular accidents (Fig. 87-6); the frequency of this complication ranges from 6 to 18 percent.[10,58] Unfortunately, paradoxical embolization to the brain may be the first manifestation of an occult pulmonary venous malformation.

Brain abscess occurs in 3 to 5 percent of patients with PAVMs.[13] Up to 1 percent of HHT patients may have brain abscesses (1000 times the incidence in the general population). In one series, 5 of 31 patients had recurrent abscess.[40] Up to 8 percent of brain abscesses may be due to PAVMs.[15] Unfortunately, brain abscess may also be the first symptom of an occult PAVM (Fig. 87-7), and many years may elapse before diagnosis of PAVM (Fig. 87-8).

Miscellaneous Complications

The other complications associated with PAVMs are those connected with HHT. Epistaxis is the most common bleeding manifestation. It occurs in up to 85 percent of patients, with 10 per-

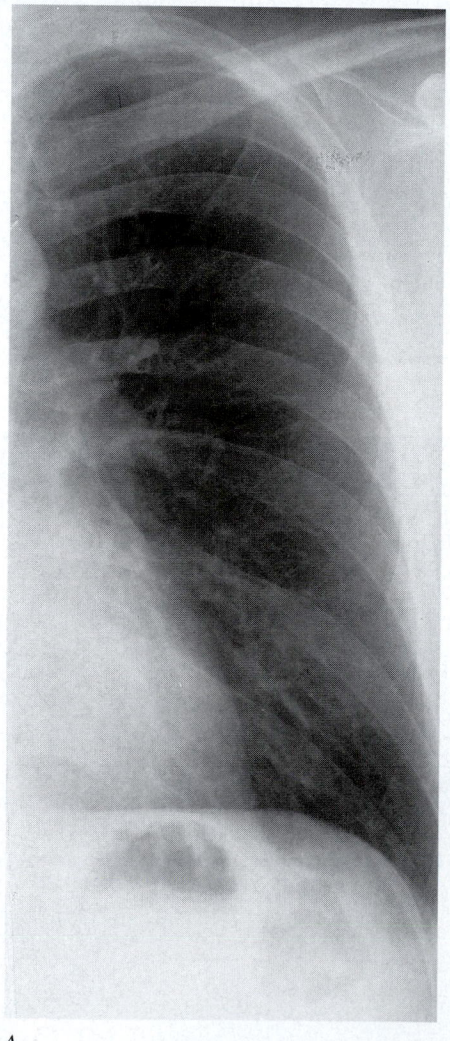

A

FIGURE 87-5　Example of patient with PAVMs that were not seen on standard radiography but were detected by echocardiographic screening: *A.* Before embolization. *B.* Angiogram. *C.* After embolization, showing both coil and balloon emboli.

cent having little or no bleeding and approximately 30 percent each suffering from mild, moderate, or heavy bleeding. GI bleeding, which tends to occur later in life, occurs in 10 to 15 percent of patients. Genitourinary and intracerebral bleeding occurs in less than 10 percent each.[37] AVMs may also occur in the liver; when severe, they are embedded in noncirrhotic fibrous nodules (telangiectasia-associated hepatic fibrosis).[8] On rare occasions, this may result in liver failure.

TREATMENT

Early treatment of PAVMs consisted of thoracotomy and resection. The first successful surgical approach was pneumonectomy, reported in 1942.[23] This treatment resulted in the disappearance of polycythemia. As thoracic surgery improved, the extent of surgery diminished; by 1959, local excision was the procedure of choice.[6] Surgical removal of a PAVM inevitably results in loss of viable lung tissue, a problem for patients with multiple PAVMs; the record is probably held by a patient who underwent

staged bilateral thoracotomies with removal of 23 PAVMs, with substantial symptomatic improvement.[5] Although surgical mortality can be as low as 0,[6] the general anesthesia, morbidity of thoracotomy, and loss of viable lung tissue made a new approach desirable.

Embolization of PAVMs has proved to be an excellent alternative. This procedure was first performed using homemade coils. The procedure was refined and perfected at Johns Hopkins by Terry, White, and colleagues.[54] The original procedure utilized silicone balloons unless the feeding vessel was larger than 9 mm in diameter, in which case embolization coils with thrombogenic Dacron tails were used (Fig. 87-9A).[58] After the silicone breast implant controversy, the balloons became unavailable. All embolizations are now performed with coils of various sizes (Figs. 87-9B and 87-9C). Results have been very good, and embolization therapy is now the procedure of choice, with an apparent mortality of 0, few or no serious complications, no loss of pulmonary parenchyma, and no exposure to anesthesia or thoracotomy.

FIGURE 87-5   *(Cont.)*

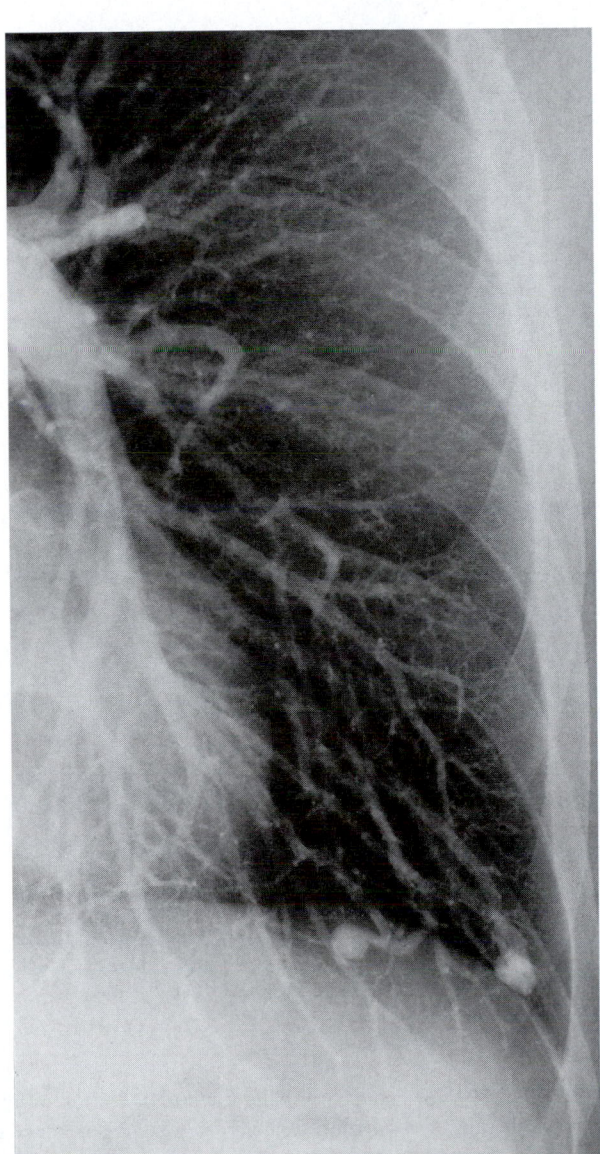

B

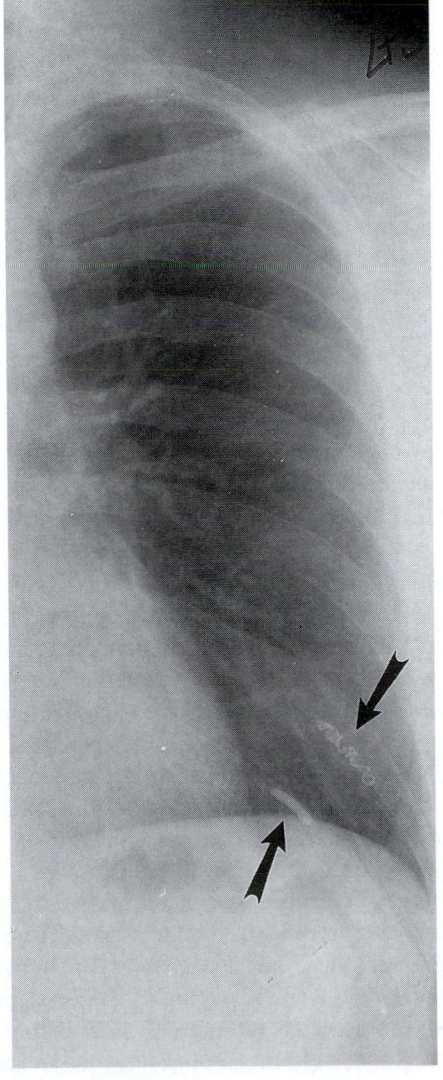

C

standard American Heart Association endocarditis guidelines for antibiotic prophylaxis before embolotherapy seem reasonable. Because of the frequent observation of small persistent left-to-right shunt demonstrated by echocardiography even after successful embolotherapy, antibiotic prophylaxis is recommended for dental and other surgical procedures.

Serious complications of embolotherapy are rare. Air embolism is one potential problem, occurring in less than 5 percent in one series (manifested as perioral paresthesias or angina without permanent effect).[58] Paradoxical embolization has been reported, but with no disastrous symptoms to date. Because of the potential for systemic air and particulate embolism, all intravenous tubing is equipped with micropore filters and embolization precautions are taken. The most common postembolization symptom is pleurisy, reported at rates of 10 percent,[58] 20 percent,[54] and more than 50 percent.[17] The onset may be delayed for up to 9 days, and severity may range from mild pain to a level of discomfort requiring hospitalization. These episodes are sometimes accompanied by large pleural effusions. The effusions and resulting hypoxemia always resolve within several weeks.

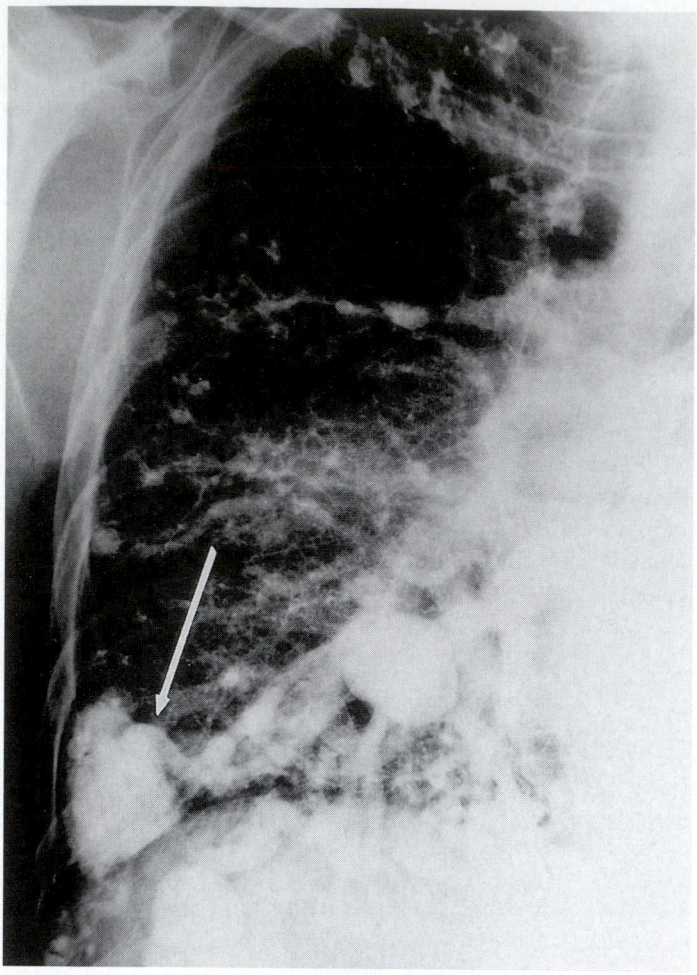

FIGURE 87-6 Right-sided pulmonary angiogram showing multiple PAVMs in a middle-aged man with clubbing, polycythemia, and CT evidence of several prior strokes.

There are some limitations. The feeding vessel must be 2 to 3 mm in diameter or larger. It is technically feasible to embolize most PAVMs, but occasionally this is not possible. In personal experiences involving more than 35 patients with more than 100 PAVMs, only one large central PAVM could not be embolized because of a very short (2 mm), large-diameter (12 mm) feeding vessel and drainage emptying almost immediately into the left atrium. Because systemic embolization would have been nearly inevitable, this patient required thoracotomy and local resection.

Recanalization of the embolized vessel may occur.[45] In general, successful embolization of most or all visible PAVMs results in abatement of hypoxemia and its complications, but approximately 6 percent of patients have diffuse small PAVMs not amenable to embolization. Occlusion of all large PAVMs appears to eliminate the risk of embolic stroke. There is only one report of postembolization stroke, in a patient with multiple residual unoccluded PAVMs. Complex PAVMs must have all feeding vessels embolized for success. Embolotherapy may reduce the risk of brain abscess, but abscess may recur even after successful therapy.[22] Although no data regarding efficacy exist,

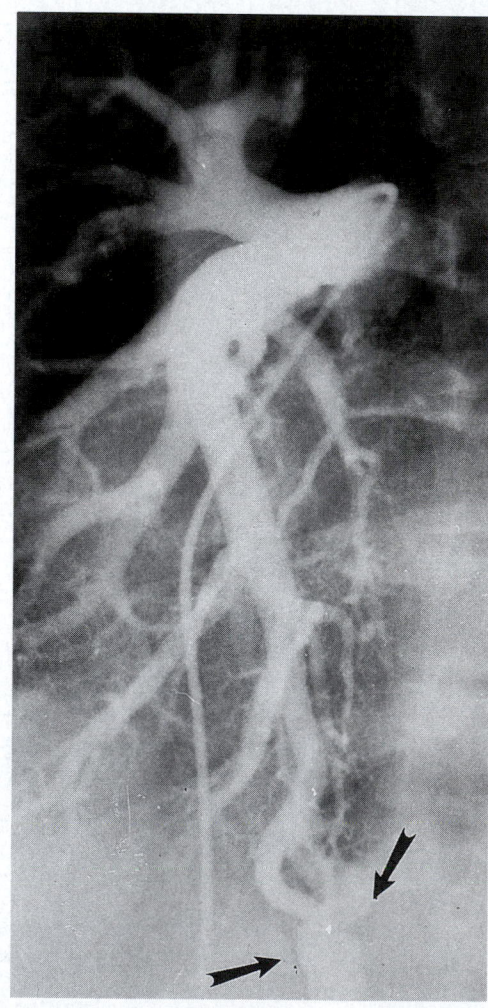

FIGURE 87-7 PAVM detected in patient with HHT after initial presentation with brain abscess: The pulmonary angiogram and lateral chest radiographs were read as normal on several examinations. Right pulmonary angiogram with inferomedial PAVM (arrows).

PROGNOSIS

Early reports suggested a high mortality for patients who did not undergo treatment. Examination of family trees in older reports impresses one with the frequency of death from meningitis, brain abscess, and stroke. Some of this apparently high mortality may be due to selection bias. More recent studies suggest that the prognosis may be more benign, and complications may be nonexistent when PAVMs are discovered by screening.[52] In one series, mortality was approximately 10 percent. Two-thirds of deaths were due to cerebrovascular accident, and all of these patients were cyanotic and polycythemic.[10]

Central nervous system complications may be the most important. Perhaps related to this, single PAVMs less than 2 cm in size appear to have few symptoms or complications.[10]

The issue of enlargement or progression of a PAVM, as well as development of PAVMs de novo after successful therapy, remains unclear, owing to the insensitivity of chest radiographs. Progression of PAVMs appears more likely in those with multiple PAVMs;[52] the rate of progression was 10 percent in one series, predominantly in patients with HHT.[10] Nodules may go from invisible to visible on chest radiographs over 2 years.[27] In part, this is no doubt due to the size-detection threshold noted above. The "doubling time" for individual PAVMs has been estimated to be 20 years. In our clinic, based on repeated angiography over periods of up to 8 years, no new PAVMs have developed in patients who were successfully embolized.

In summary, patients with PAVM can be successfully treated, with resolution of essentially all symptoms and substantial re-

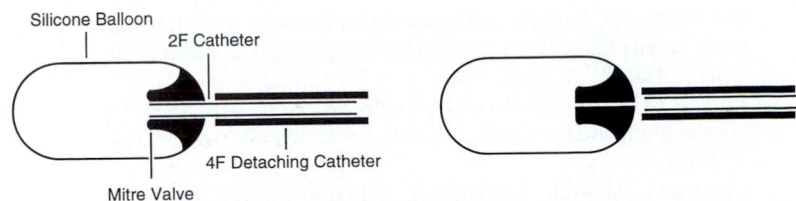

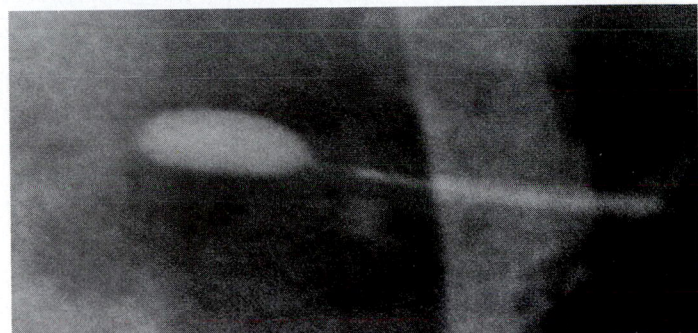

B

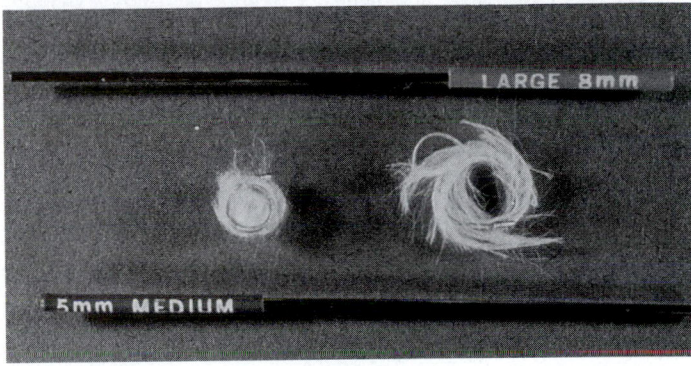

C

FIGURE 87-9 Embolotherapy devices: *A.* Detachable balloon mechanism from catheter. *B.* Fluoroscopic image of balloon in vivo. *C.* Embolization coils of two sizes.

duction in risk of complications. Embolotherapy is the treatment of choice for most patients. The relatives of patients with PAVMs or HHT should be screened with contrast echocardiography to prevent central nervous system complications as the first manifestation of disease.

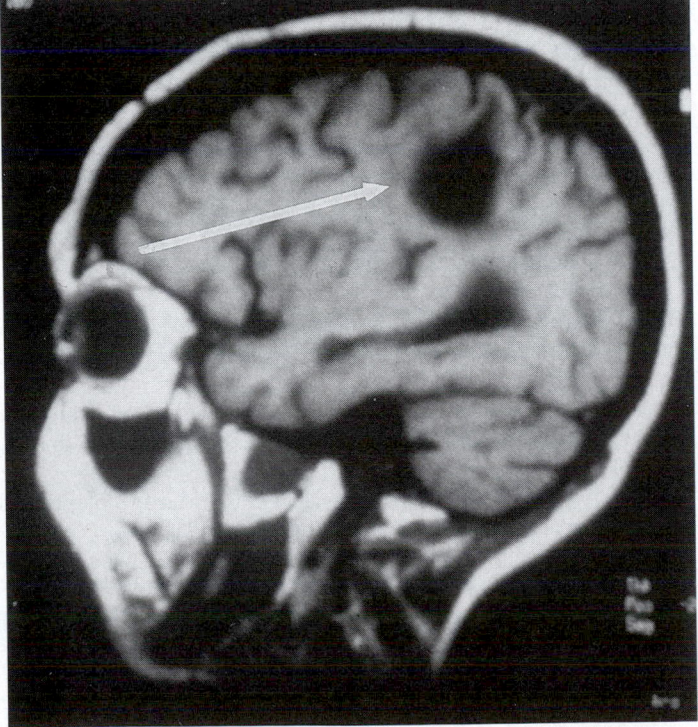

FIGURE 87-8 MRI showing brain abscess residua in patient whose brain abscess preceded diagnosis of pulmonary arteriovenous fistula by 17 years.

REFERENCES

1. Anabtawi IN, Ellison RG, Ellison LT: Pulmonary arteriovenous aneurysms and fistulas: Anatomical variations, embryology, and classification. *Ann Thorac Surg* 1:277–285, 1965.
2. Assar OS, Friedman CM, White RI: The natural history of epistaxis in hereditary hemorrhagic telangiectasia. *Laryngoscope* 101:977–980, 1991.
3. Babbington BG: Hereditary epistaxis. *Lancet* 2:362–363, 1865.
4. Barzilai B, Waggoner A, Spessert C, et al: Two-dimensional contrast echocardiography in the detection and follow-up of congenital pulmonary arteriovenous malformations. *Am J Cardiol* 68:1507–1510, 1991.
5. Brown SE, Wright PW, Renner JW, Riker JB: Staged bilateral tho-

racotomies for multiple pulmonary arteriovenous malformations complicating hereditary hemorrhagic telangiectasia. *J Thorac Cardiovasc Surg* 83:285–289, 1982.

6. Burke CM, Safai C, Nelson DP, Raffin TA: Pulmonary arteriovenous malformations: A critical update. *Am Rev Respir Dis* 134:334–339, 1986.

7. Churton T: Multiple aneurysm of pulmonary artery. *Br Med J* 1:1223, 1897.

8. Cooney T, Sweeney EC, Coll R, Greally M: "Pseudocirrhosis" in hereditary hemorrhagic telangiectasia. *J Clin Pathol* 30:1134–1141, 1977.

9. Dalton ML, Goodwin FC, Bronwell AW, Rutledge R: Intrapleural rupture of pulmonary arteriovenous aneurysm: Report of a case. *Dis Chest* 52:97–100, 1967.

10. Dines DE, Arms RA, Bernatz PE, Gomes MR: Pulmonary arteriovenous fistulas. *Mayo Clin Proc* 49:460–465, 1974.

11. Dines DE, Seward JB, Bernatz PE: Pulmonary arteriovenous fistulas. *Mayo Clin Proc* 58:176–181, 1983.

12. Dinsmore BJ, Gefter WB, Hatabu H, Kressel HY: Pulmonary arteriovenous malformations: Diagnosis by gradient refocused MR imaging. *J Comput Assist Tomogr* 14:918–923, 1990.

13. Dyer NH: Cerebral abscess in hereditary hemorrhagic telangiectasia: Report of two cases in a family. *J Neurol Neurosurg Psychiatry* 30:563–567, 1967.

14. Gammon RB, Miksa AK, Keller FS: Osler-Weber-Rendu disease and pulmonary arteriovenous fistulas: Deterioration and embolotherapy during pregnancy. *Chest* 98:1522–1524, 1990.

15. Gelfand MS, Stephens DS, Howell EI, et al: Brain abscess: Association with pulmonary arteriovenous fistula and hereditary hemorrhagic telangiectasia: Report of three cases. *Am J Med* 85:718–720, 1988.

16. Gomes MR, Bernatz PE, Dines DE: Pulmonary arteriovenous fistulas. *Ann Thorac Surg* 7:582–593, 1969.

17. Goodenberger D, Barzilai B, Picus D: Incidence and timing of pleuritic chest pain after therapeutic pulmonary embolization (abstract). *Chest* 103:159S, 1993.

18. Goodenberger D, Barzilai B, Waggoner A, et al: Frequency of intrapulmonary shunt in relatives of patients with Osler-Weber-Rendu and pulmonary arteriovenous malformation (abstract). *Chest* 98:59S, 1990.

19. Goodenberger D, Spessert C, Waggoner A, et al: Size and location of occult pulmonary arteriovenous malformations (PAVM's) in individuals with Osler-Weber-Rendu (OWR) (abstract). *Am Rev Respir Dis* 143:A663, 1991.

20. Greenspan DS, Northrup H, Au KS, et al: COL5A1: Fine genetic mapping and exclusion as candidate gene in families with nail-patella syndrome, tuberous sclerosis, hereditary hemorrhagic telangiectasia, and Ehlers-Danlos syndrome type II. *Genomics* 25:737–739, 1995.

21. Hales MR: Multiple small arteriovenous fistulae of the lungs. *Am J Pathol* 32:927–943, 1956.

22. Hartnell GG, Jackson JE, Allison DJ: Coil embolization of pulmonary arteriovenous malformations. *Cardiovasc Intervent Radiol* 13:347–350, 1990.

23. Hepburn J, Dauphinee JA: Successful removal of hemangioma of the lung followed by the disappearance of polycythemia. *Am J Med Sci* 204:681–685, 1942.

24. Hernandez A, Strauss AW, McKnight R, Hartmann AF: Diagnosis of pulmonary arteriovenous fistula by contrast echocardiography. *J Pediatr* 93:258–261, 1978.

25. Heutink P, Haitjema T, Breedveld GJ, et al: Linkage of hereditary haemorrhagic telangiectasia to chromosome 9q34 and evidence for locus heterogeneity. *J Med Genet* 31:933–936, 1994.

26. Higgins CB, Wexler L: Clinical and angiographic features of pulmonary arteriovenous fistulas in children. *Radiology* 119:171–175, 1976.

27. Hoffman R, Rabens R: Evolving pulmonary nodules: Multiple pulmonary arteriovenous fistulas. *Am J Roentgenol Radium Ther Nucl Med* 120:861–864, 1974.

28. Huseby JS, Culver BH, Butler J: Pulmonary arteriovenous fistulas: Increase in shunt at high lung volume. *Am Rev Respir Dis* 115:229–232, 1977.

29. Jessurun GA, Kamphuis DJ, van der Zande FH, Nossent JC: Cerebral arteriovenous malformations in the Netherlands Antilles: High prevalence of hereditary hemorrhagic telangiectasia-related single and multiple cerebral arteriovenous malformations. *Clin Neurol Neurosurg* 95:193–198, 1993.

30. LaRoche CM, Wells F, Shneerson J: Massive hemothorax due to enlarging arteriovenous fistula in pregnancy. *Chest* 101:1452–1454, 1992.

31. Lundell M, Finck E: Arteriovenous fistulas originating from Rasmussen aneurysms. *Am J Roentgenol* 140:687–688, 1983.

32. McAllister KA, Grogg KM, Johnson DW, et al: Endoglin, a TGF-beta binding protein of endothelial cells, is the gene for hereditary haemorrhagic telangiectasia type 1. *Nat Genet* 8:345–351, 1994.

33. McAllister KA, Lennon F, Bowles-Biesecker B, et al: Genetic heterogeneity in hereditary haemorrhagic telangiectasia: Possible correlation with clinical phenotype. *J Med Genet* 31:927–932, 1994.

34. McCue CM, Hartenberg M, Nance WE: Pulmonary arteriovenous malformations related to Rendu-Osler-Weber syndrome. *Am J Med Genet* 19:19–27, 1984.

35. McDonald MT, Papenberg KA, Ghosh S, et al: A disease locus for hereditary haemorrhagic telangiectasia maps to chromosome 9q33-34. *Nat Genet* 6:197–204, 1994.

36. Osler W: On a family form of recurring epistaxis, associated with multiple telangiectases of the skin and mucous membranes. *Bull Johns Hopkins Hosp* 12:333–337, 1901.

37. Peery WH: Clinical spectrum of hereditary hemorrhagic telangiectasia (Osler-Weber-Rendu disease). *Am J Med* 82:989–997, 1987.

38. Pierce JA, Reagan WP, Kimball RW: Unusual cases of pulmonary arteriovenous fistulas, with a note on thyroid carcinoma as a cause. *New Engl J Med* 260:901–907, 1959.

39. Porteous ME, Curtis A, Williams O, et al: Genetic heterogeneity in hereditary hemorrhagic telangiectasia. *J Med Genet* 31:925–926, 1994.

40. Press OW, Ramsey PG: Central nervous system infections associated with hereditary hemorrhagic telangiectasia. *Am J Med* 77:86–92, 1984.

41. Przybojewski JZ, Maritz F: Pulmonary arteriovenous fistulas: A case presentation and review of the literature. *S Afr Med J* 57:366–373, 1980.

42. Rankin S, Faling LJ, Pugatch RD: CT diagnosis of pulmonary arteriovenous malformation. *J Comput Assist Tomogr* 6:746–749, 1982.

43. Reading B: Case of congenital telangiectasia of lung, complicated by brain abscess. *Tex St J Med* 28:462–464, 1932.

44. Reilly PJ, Nostrant TT: Clinical manifestations of hereditary hemorrhagic telangiectasia. *Am J Gastroenterol* 79:363–367, 1984.

45. Remy-Jardin M, Wattinne L, Remy J: Transcatheter occlusion of pulmonary arterial circulation and collateral supply: Failures, incidents, and complications. *Radiology* 180:699–705, 1991.

46. Rendu M: Épistaxis répétées chez un sujet porteur de petits angiomes cutanés et muqueux. *Bull Mém Soc Méd Hôp Par* 13:731–733, 1896.

47. Rodes CB: Cavernous hemangiomas of the lung with secondary polycythemia. *JAMA* 110:1914–1915, 1938.

48. Roman G, Fisher M, Perl DP, Poser CM: Neurological manifestations of hereditary hemorrhagic telangiectasia (Rendu-Osler-Weber disease): Report of two cases and review of the literature. *Ann Neurol* 4:130–144, 1978.

49. Shovlin CL, Hughes JM, Tuddenham EG, et al: A gene for hereditary haemorrhagic telangiectasia maps to chromosome 9q3. *Nat Genet* 6:205–209, 1994.

50. Shub C, Tajik AJ, Seward JB, Dines DE: Detecting intrapulmonary right-to-left shunt with contrast echocardiography: Observations in a patient with diffuse pulmonary arteriovenous fistulas. *Mayo Clin Proc* 51:81–84, 1976.

51. Shumacker HB, Waldhausen JA: Pulmonary arteriovenous fistulas in children. *Ann Surg* 158:713–720, 1963.

52. Sluiter-Eringa H, Orie NGM, Sluiter HJ: Pulmonary arteriovenous fistula: Diagnosis and prognosis in noncomplainant patients. *Am Rev Respir Dis* 100:177–188, 1969.

53. Smith HL, Horton BT: Arteriovenous fistula of the lung associated with polycythemia vera: Report of a case in which the diagnosis was made clinically. *Am Heart J* 18:589–592, 1939.

54. Terry PB, White RI, Barth KH, et al: Pulmonary arteriovenous malformations: Physiologic observations and results of therapeutic balloon embolization. *New Engl J Med* 308:1197–1200, 1983.

55. Trell E, Johansson BW, Linell F, Ripa J: Familial pulmonary hypertension and multiple abnormalities of large systemic arteries in Osler's disease. *Am J Med* 53:50–63, 1972.

56. Vincent P, Plauchu H, Hazan J, et al: A third locus for hereditary hemorrhagic telangiectasia maps to chromosome 12q. *Hum Molec Genet* 4:945–949, 1995.

57. Weber FP: Multiple hereditary developmental angiomata (telangiectases) of the skin and mucous membranes associated with recurring hemorrhages. *Lancet* 2:160–162, 1907.

58. White RI Jr, Lynch-Nyhana A, Terry P, et al: Pulmonary arteriovenous malformations: Techniques and long-term outcome of embolotherapy. *Radiology* 169:663–669, 1988.

59. White RI Jr, Mitchell SE, Barth KH, et al: Angioarchitecture of pulmonary arteriovenous malformations: An important consideration before embolotherapy. *Am J Roentgenol* 140:681–686, 1983.

60. White RI Jr: Pulmonary arteriovenous malformations: How do we diagnose them and why is it important to do so? *Radiology* 182:633–635, 1992.

PART TEN

DISORDERS OF THE PLEURAL SPACE

CHAPTER 88

PLEURAL FLUID DYNAMICS AND EFFUSIONS

Gary T. Kinasewitz

In the course of embryologic development, the pleural membranes are formed from mesenchyme to line the space that will separate the lungs from the mediastinum, diaphragm, and chest wall. In principle, the pleural space is designed to behave like brake linings in an automobile, smoothing the movements of the lungs within the thorax during breathing; another function for the pleural space seems to be as a mechanism for coupling the lungs to the chest wall. Neither of these functions appears to be indispensable, however, since obliteration of the pleural space in humans by pleurectomy has no appreciable effect on pulmonary function. Nor do the lungs of the elephant, in which the pleural space is replaced by vascular connective tissue, seem to operate at a disadvantage.

But even though obliteration of the pleural space seems to be of little physiological consequence, the linings are subject to disease and disorders. For example, encasement of the lungs in a thick peel instead of the normal pleural lining can seriously impair pulmonary function. Fluid may accumulate in the pleural space in response to disease of the pleural membranes per se or as a manifestation of a systemic illness affecting many organs. In the latter instance, examination of the pleural fluid can provide a clue to the origin of the underlying disorder. Excess fluid within the pleural space may have serious clinical consequences, and appropriate treatment can produce dramatic symptomatic relief.

ANATOMY OF THE PLEURA

The visceral pleura envelops the entire surface of the lungs: the parietal pleura covers the inner surface of the chest wall, mediastinum, and diaphragm; the visceral pleura invests the lungs everywhere except at the hilum, where the bronchi, pulmonary vessels, and nerves enter the lung substance.[45] Below the merger of visceral and parietal pleura at the hilum, pleural reflections from the dorsal and ventral surface of the lungs usually extend to the diaphragm as a double layer of mesothelial tissue, the pulmonary ligament (Fig. 88-1). In humans, the two pleural cavities are completely separate.

The normal parietal and visceral pleural linings are smooth, glistening, semitransparent membranes. Beneath the single layer of mesothelium that covers the surface is a band of connective tissue containing abundant collagen and elastin. Mesothelial cells vary considerably in size and shape, from flat to columnar. Numerous mitochondria, rough endoplasmic reticulum, and Golgi apparatus are prominent features of cuboidal and columnar cells, suggesting that they are active both in the transport of substances across the pleural surfaces and in ensuring the structure and functions of the pleural space.[46] Microvilli, enmeshed in a matrix of glycoproteins, project from the mesothelial cells, thereby serving as a lubricant and as a device to increase the pleural surface area available for fluid transport.

Although the parietal and visceral membranes are similar in external appearance, important anatomic differences are found beneath the surfaces: beneath the parietal surface, the arrangement of the connective tissue layer is straightforward; in contrast, the submesothelial connective tissue layer of the visceral pleura gives rise to septa that permeate the lungs, creating subdivisions that enhance gas exchange while lending support to the pulmonary parenchyma. Pain fibers are present in the connective-tissue layer of the parietal pleura but not the visceral pleura. These fibers have different origins, depending on the part of the thorax that they innervate: the costal pleura and the peripheral rim of diaphragmatic pleura are innervated by the intercostal

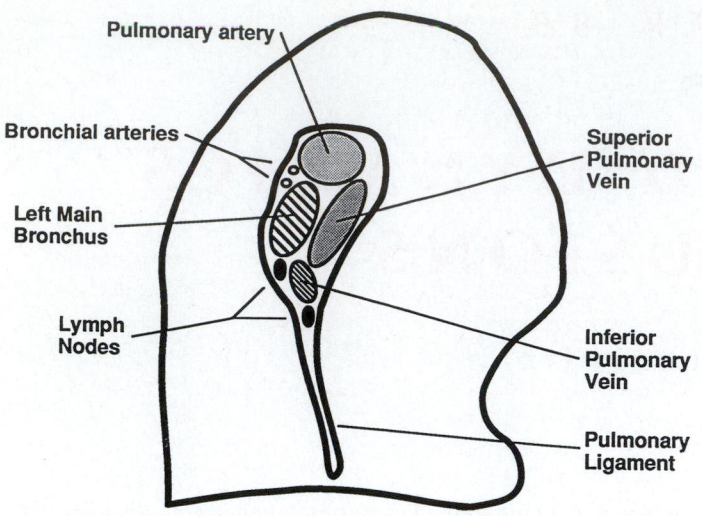

FIGURE 88-1 Diagrammatic illustration of the medial surface of the left lung. The visceral pleura invests the hilar structures and forms the pulmonary ligament. *(From Boggs and Kinasewitz,[4] with permission.)*

nerves; painful stimuli in these regions are sensed in the adjacent chest wall. The central parts of the diaphragm are innervated by the phrenic nerve; stimuli in these areas elicit pain in the ipsilateral shoulder.

The visceral and parietal pleura also differ with respect to blood supply: the parietal pleura is supplied by branches of systemic arteries, the supply depending on the location: the costal, diaphragmatic, and mediastinal aspects receive blood predominantly from systemic arteries in their respective vicinities; branches from these arteries subdivide to form a capillary network beneath the mesothelium of the costal and mediastinal pleura. In contrast, the blood supply to the visceral pleura has a dual origin and is more variable: depending on the species, the blood supply from either the bronchial or pulmonary circulation may predominate. In animals in which the visceral pleura is thin (e.g., the dog), the capillary supply to the visceral pleura is derived almost exclusively from the pulmonary artery tree. In contrast, in humans and in other species in which the visceral pleura is thick, the principal blood supply of the visceral pleura arises from the bronchial circulation. However, irrespective of whether they originate from the bronchial or pulmonary arterial system, the capillaries of the visceral pleura drain into the pulmonary veins.

The lymphatic drainage of the two surfaces differs considerably. The parietal lymphatic system is the major route by which lymph leaves the pleural space. Its mesothelial surface is permeated by pores (stomas) that connect via lacunae to a lymphatic network in the adjacent submesothelial layer.[46] The lymphatics in different regions of the pleural space drain to different nodes: from the costal surface to parasternal and paravertebral nodes; from the mediastinal surface to the tracheobronchial nodes. In contrast to the parietal pleura, the visceral pleura is devoid of lacunae and stomas and the underlying lymphatic vessels appear to drain the pulmonary parenchyma rather than the pleural space.

PHYSIOLOGY OF THE PLEURA

Pleural Liquid Pressures

Elsewhere in this book (see Chapter 12), where pleural pressures have been considered with respect to lung inflation and ventilation, attention focused on "pleural surface pressures." Pleural surface pressure increases by approximately 0.5 cm of water per centimeter of vertical distance from the apex to the base of the lung.[1] Since the hydrostatic pressure in a continuous column of pleural liquid should increase by 1 cm of water for each centimeter of vertical distance, pleural surface pressure appears to be less negative than pleural liquid pressure. To explain this discrepancy, it has been suggested that pleural surface pressure (P_{pl}) is the sum of a negative pleural liquid pressure (P_{liq}) and a positive pleural contact pressure (P_{con}), which develops at points of contact between the visceral and parietal pleura. At any given region of the pleural surface,

$$P_{pl} = P_{liq} + P_{con}$$

Pleural liquid pressure varies as a hydrostatic column, but since there are more points of contact at the top of the lung, the vertical gradient in pleural surface pressure is less than unity.

This explanation for the vertical product in pleural pressure was questioned when measurements of pleural space thickness suggested that the pleural fluid covers the lung as a continuous layer without points of contact. Even in the absence of contact between the visceral and parietal pleura, the observed vertical gradient in pleural pressure may be explained by the viscous flow of a continuous column of fluid through the pleural cavity. Pleural surface pressure and pleural liquid pressure are identical; as fluid flows through the pleural cavity, a portion of the hydrostatic pressure gradient is dissipated in overcoming the resistance to viscous flow.[23] Fluid is filtered through the parietal membrane and flows toward the dependent regions of the pleural cavity, where it is removed by the pleural lymphatics. At any given level within the pleural space, this may be expressed as:

$$P_{pl} = P_{hyd} - (Q \cdot R_v)$$

where P_{hyd} is the hydrostatic pressure gradient (1 cm H_2O/cm vertical distance), Q is the flow of pleural fluid, and R_v is the viscous resistance to flow. When fluid accumulates, the pleural space widens and R_v (which is inversely related to the cube of pleural liquid thickness) falls rapidly; the gradient in pleural pressure approaches the hydrostatic pressure gradient. This mechanism would also explain the horizontal gradients in pleural pressure that have been observed. At the same vertical height, pleural pressure is more negative at the mediastinal than at the costal surface of the lung.[34] The pleural pressure gradient is determined by the lymphatic pumping mechanism; i.e., the pressure needed to produce flow reduces the hydrostatic pressure gradient to less than unity.[33] Alternatively, the buoyancy of the air-filled lung may cause it to rise within the chest and squeeze fluid toward the lower portions of the thoracic cavity, thereby producing a downward flow and the observed pleural pressure gradients.[13]

Currently, the best estimates of pleural surface pressures in humans appear to be made by using an esophageal balloon. Qualitatively, the results are in accord with experimental observations using catheters, micropipettes, and Starling resistors; they indicate that in the normal vertical human lung, a gradient of pleural surface pressure exists from the top to the bottom of the lungs and that this gradient is about 0.2 to 0.5 cm of water per centimeter of vertical height.

Formation of Pleural Fluid

Normally, the composition of the thin layer of fluid between the parietal and visceral pleura is that of an ultrafiltrate of plasma (Table 88-1). The two linings act like semipermeable membranes, so the concentrations of small molecules, such as glucose, are similar in pleural fluid and plasma, whereas the concentrations of macromolecules (e.g., albumin) are considerably lower in pleural fluid than in plasma.

Although the volume of fluid normally present in the pleural space is small (of the order of 5 to 15 ml), the rate of turnover of pleural fluid in humans is rapid and may exceed 1 L per day. Because the rates of fluid entry and efflux are about equal, the volume of pleural fluid remains virtually constant. This equilibrium is accounted for primarily by the forces employed in Starling's equation for "transcapillary" exchange (in reality, "trans-microcirculatory" exchange). According to this equation, net filtration or reabsorption of water (and its solutes) across a semipermeable membrane is determined by balances between the hydrostatic and oncotic pressures on the two sides of the membrane; for the pleural surfaces, which are covered by porous mesothelium, the principal barrier to pleural fluid filtration and reabsorption is the endothelium of the pleural capillaries.[22] Excess water and protein in the pleural space resulting from a dysequilibrium in the Starling forces is left to the pulmonary lymphatics.

For the pleura, Starling's equation can be written as follows:

$$F = k[(P_{cap} - P_{pl}) - \sigma(\pi_{cap} - \pi_{pl})]$$

where

F = the rate of fluid movement,
P and π = the hydrostatic and oncotic pressures respectively
k = the filtration coefficient

σ = the osmotic reflection coefficient for protein, similar to that of muscle capillaries (equals about 0.9)
cap = the capillary
pl = the pleural space.

The normal hydrostatic pressure within the capillaries of the parietal pleura (Fig. 88-2) is probably similar to that in other systemic capillaries (i.e., mean pressure about 25 mmHg); intrapleural pressure is slightly subatmospheric, averaging about −3 mmHg. The resulting hydrostatic pressure difference favors fluid filtration. Opposing this hydrostatic force is the oncotic pressure difference due to the higher concentration of protein in plasma than in pleural fluid. The osmotic force promoting the reabsorption of pleural fluid can be calculated as the product of the osmotic reflection coefficient for protein and the difference between the oncotic pressure of plasma and of pleural fluid: 0.9 (28−5) = 21 mmHg. Because the hydrostatic pressure gradient in parietal pleural capillaries consistently exceeds the oncotic pressure gradient, fluid filters uninterruptedly into the pleural cavity (Fig. 88-1).

In the visceral capillaries, the balance between hydrostatic and oncotic pressures is opposite: even though oncotic pressures are the same as in parietal capillaries, the hydrostatic pressures in the visceral pleural capillaries are lower and are closer to those in the pulmonary capillaries (i.e., about 10 mmHg). Therefore, the balance of hydrostatic and oncotic pressures promotes the reabsorption of fluid across the visceral pleural surfaces. The mesothelium also plays a role in the reabsorption of pleural fluid. Both sodium and chloride are actively transported out of the pleural fluid via a Na^+/H^+ and Cl^-/HCO_3^- double exchange on the serosal surface and a Na^+/K^+ pump on the interstitial side of the mesothelium.[49] As a result of the balance of Starling forces

TABLE 88-1	
Normal Composition of Pleural Fluid*	
Volume	0.1–0.2 ml/kg
Cells/mm³	1000–5000
% mesothelial cells	3–70%
% monocytes	30–75%
% lymphocytes	2–30%
% granulocytes	10%
Protein	1–2 g/dl
% albumin	50–70%
Glucose	≈ plasma level
LDH	<50% plasma level
pH	≥ plasma

*Data from humans and animals.

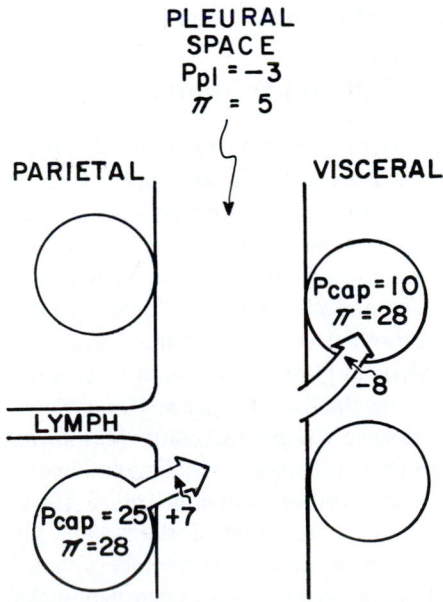

FIGURE 88-2   Distribution of hydrostatic (P) and oncotic (π) pressures across the parietal and visceral pleura. The numbers in the open arrows indicate the net magnitude of the pressure differences that promote filtration and reabsorption across the parietal and visceral pleura, respectively.

across the pleural membranes and the solute-coupled fluid re-sorption by the mesothelium, the volume of fluid within the pleural space tends to be kept at a minimum.

The lymphatics in the parietal pleura provide both a safeguard against excess fluid and a mechanism for recovering proteins from the pleural space and returning them to the circulating plasma. The protein concentration in the capillaries of the parietal and visceral pleura exceeds that of pleural fluid, so a small quantity of protein continually diffuses into the pleural fluid. If there were no mechanism for removing protein from the pleural space, the oncotic gradient opposing the filtration of fluid would dissipate and fluid would accumulate. The pleural lymphatics remove sufficient protein from the pleural cavity to maintain the difference between plasma and pleural fluid protein concentrations, and thereby the volume of pleural fluid, relatively constant.[5] Excess fluid in the pleural space increases lymph flow considerably. Conversely, lymphatic obstruction (see Chapter 90) causes pleural fluid to accumulate.

Excess fluid can accumulate in the pleural space (pleural effusions) as a result either of imbalances in the Starling forces or of structural abnormalities in the vascular and mesothelial linings, impaired lymphatic drainage, or abnormal sites of entry—for instance, congenital defects in the diaphragm in a patient with ascites (Fig. 88-3). An increase in capillary hydrostatic pressure, as in congestive heart failure, or a decrease in plasma oncotic pressure, as in hypoproteinemia, increases the rate of filtration across the parietal pleura and/or decreases the rate of fluid reabsorption across the visceral pleura. A decrease in negative pressure within the pleural space, as occurs in atelectasis, also promotes fluid accumulation in the pleural space. An increase in the permeability of the pleural capillaries, as in pleural inflammation, increases the entry of both fluid and protein into the pleural space. Impairment in lymphatic drainage of the pleural space, as in metastatic neoplastic disease, causes an increase in the protein concentration and in the volume of pleural fluid.

Reactions of Pleura to Injury

The pleural surfaces, lined by mesothelial cells, are subject to injury by substances and cells brought to them via the bloodstream or lymphatics or inadvertently introduced from without, as by penetrating wounds. Injury, often subtle or even covert, may elicit responses ranging from inflammatory to neoplastic (Fig. 88-4). The mesothelium of the peritoneal cavity responds, as does the mesothelium of the pleural spaces.

The mesothelium plays a key role in maintaining the integrity of the pleural membranes. It regulates local blood flow by producing thromboxane and prostacyclin.[43] Mesothelial cell production of plasminogen activators, including urokinase and t-PA, prevents the formation of intrapleural thrombi.[36] The mesothelium is a major source of the hyaluronic acid and other glycosaminoglycans found in pleural fluid. Inflammatory stimuli such as interleukin-1 and tumor necrosis factor elicit mesothelial cell production of interleukin-8 and other chemokines, and induce mesothelial cell expression of leukocyte adhesion molecules such as ICAM-1.[2,11,21] These stimuli induce mesothelial cell tissue factor expression and the secretion of plasminogen activator inhibitors, leading to fibrin deposition on the pleural surface and the development of loculations within the pleural cavity.[19]

The mesothelium also plays an important role in determining whether the normal architecture is restored after pleural injury.[18] Mesothelial cells proliferate and migrate over denuded areas of the membrane to cover the pleural surface. A cytokine-mediated increase in glycosaminoglycan production facilitates repair of the pleura by binding TGF-β or other growth factors and increasing the secretion of both collagen and elastin to rebuild the submesothelial connective tissue layer.[16,39] In addition, mesothelial cell matrix metalloproteinases such as collagenase contribute to the remodeling of the connective-tissue matrix.[29]

Injury caused by immune inflammatory responses is strongly influenced by the nature of the inciting mechanism: cellular or humoral. Thus type I disorders (anaphylactic response initiated by IgE and culminating in the release of mediators) and type II disorders (antibodies against tissue antigens of the host) are rarely implicated in the pathogenesis of immune pleural reactions. In contrast, type III reactions (caused by deposition of circulating immune complexes) and type IV reactions (entailing recognition of foreign antigens by T cells and damage caused by the release of soluble mediators, such as lymphokines) are not infrequent.[7] The traditional examples of pleural disease caused by type III reactions (involving humoral immune mechanisms) are rheumatoid arthritis and lupus erythematosus; postulated, but much less certain, is the role of humoral immune complexes in Wegener's granulomatosis. Also uncertain is the relationship between Dressler's post–myocardial infarction syndrome and type III reactions in producing the postulated autoimmune response. For the type IV reactions (involving cell-mediated immune mechanisms) the prototype is pleural effusion in primary tuberculosis, a delayed hypersensitivity reaction that follows interaction between *M. tuberculosis* and sensitized lymphocytes in the pleural walls and intervening space.[27]

DIAGNOSTIC APPROACH

Clinical Appraisal

The hallmarks of pleural disease are pain, ipsilateral restriction of chest wall motion, breathlessness, fever, and an abnormal chest radiograph. As a rule, inspiratory chest pain caused by pleural inflammation is the most characteristic symptom; typically, it diminishes in intensity as fluid accumulates and separates the pleural surfaces. Fever and tenderness of the chest wall on the affected side often accompany pleural inflammation. A pleural friction rub is often audible before the pleuritis has elicited an appreciable effusion. The rub has a squeaking quality, is loudest on inspiration, but often is also audible during expiration. Sometimes it is confused with a low-pitched, nonmusical wheeze (rhonchus) produced by secretions partly blocking a large airway. Although both can produce vibrations that are palpable on the chest wall, the wheeze that is caused by obstructing secretions is generally eliminated by a cough, whereas the pleural friction rub remains unaffected.

A pleural effusion is difficult to detect on physical examination until more than 300 ml of fluid has accumulated. At that time, chest wall motion lags on the affected side (Hoover's sign), the percussion note over the fluid is flat, both tactile and vocal fremitus are absent, and breath sounds are diminished or inaudible. Above the effusion, compression of lung decreases the gas content per unit volume, to produce the physical findings of consolidation. Thus, bronchial breath sounds, increased transmission of whispered and spoken voice, and *e*-to-*a*(*ā*) changes (egophony) are common physical signs of a large pleural effusion.

The physical findings of a massive pleural effusion (Fig. 88-5) and of atelectasis of an entire lung are identical, with one ex-

ception: both produce dullness to percussion, absent transmission of the spoken and whispered voice, and absent breath sounds; but the pleural effusion increases the size of the affected hemithorax. Therefore, with massive effusion, the trachea is deviated away from the diseased side—in contrast to atelectasis, which causes it to deviate in the direction of the diseased side. This distinction is clinically important, since one disorder is treated by thoracentesis and bronchoscopy is done for the other.

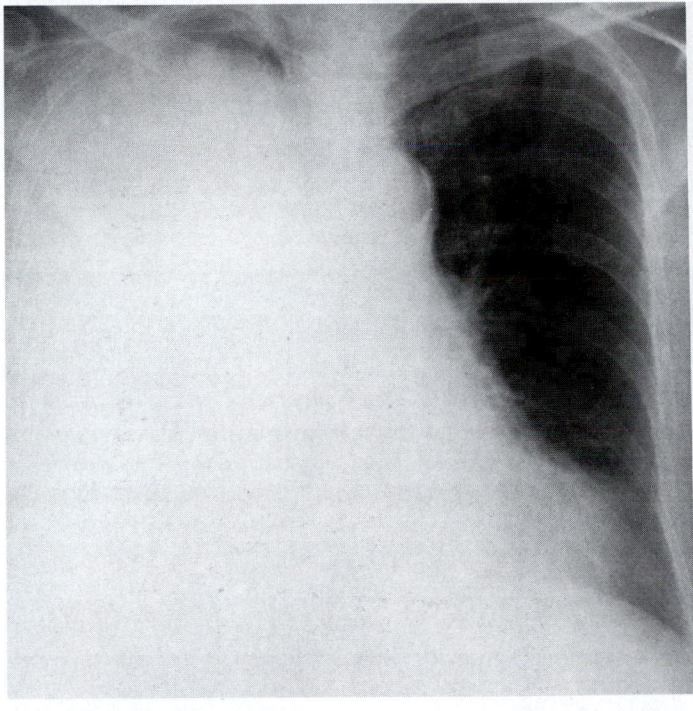

A

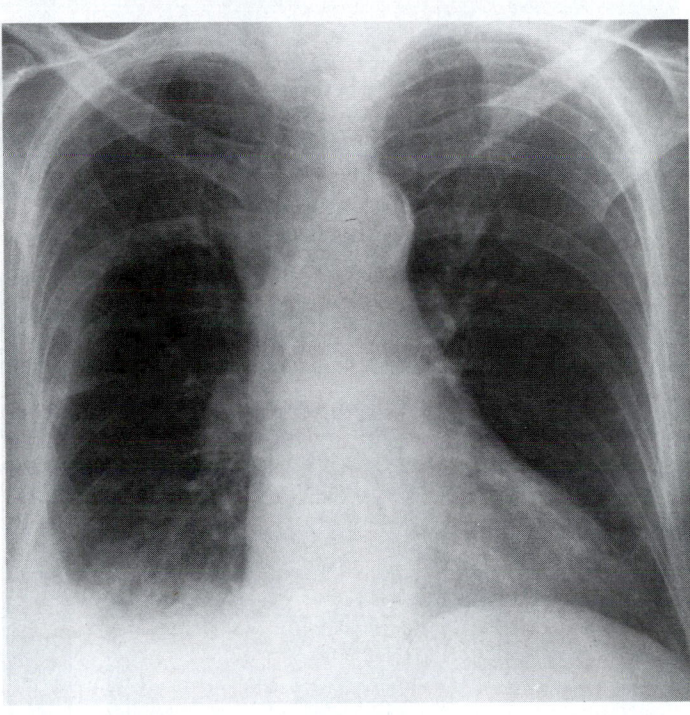

B

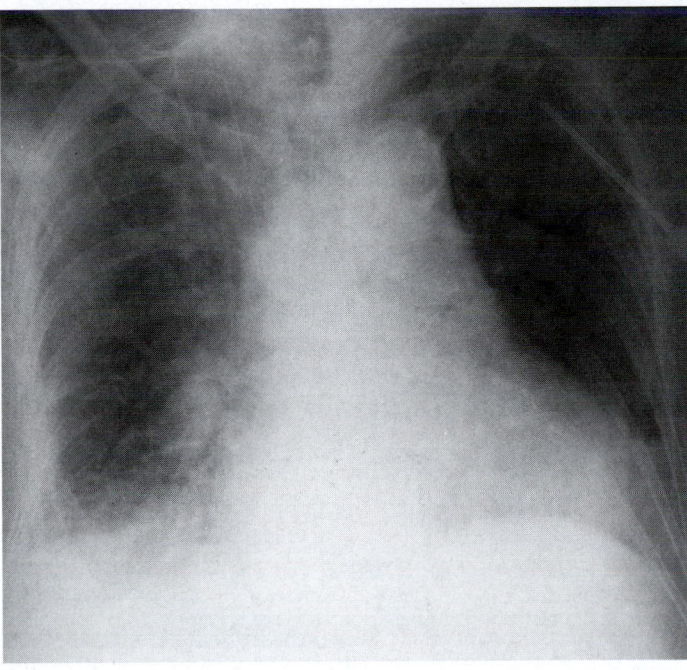

C

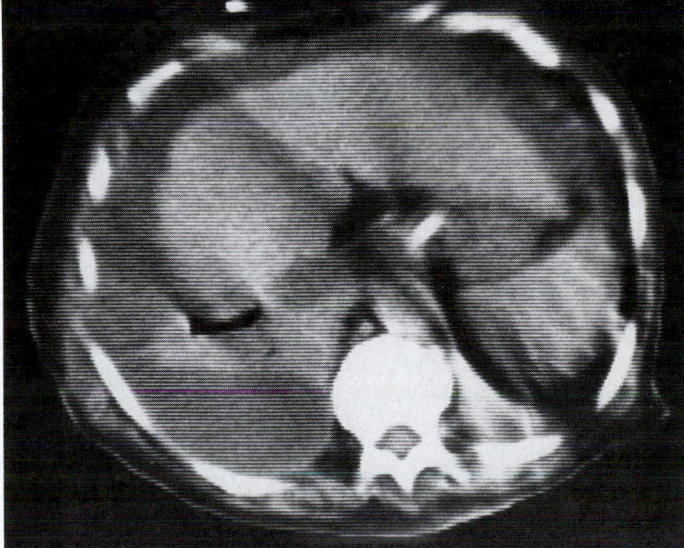

D

FIGURE 88-3   Cirrhosis of the liver, ascites, and pleural effusion in a 72-year-old woman. Autopsy disclosed congenital defects in the right hemidiaphragm. *A.* August 20. Massive pleural effusion on the right. *B.* August 26. After aspiration of pleural effusion. *C.* September 12 (supine). After repeated aspiration and placement of LeVeen shunt. *D.* September 12. CT scan showing ascites and small liver.

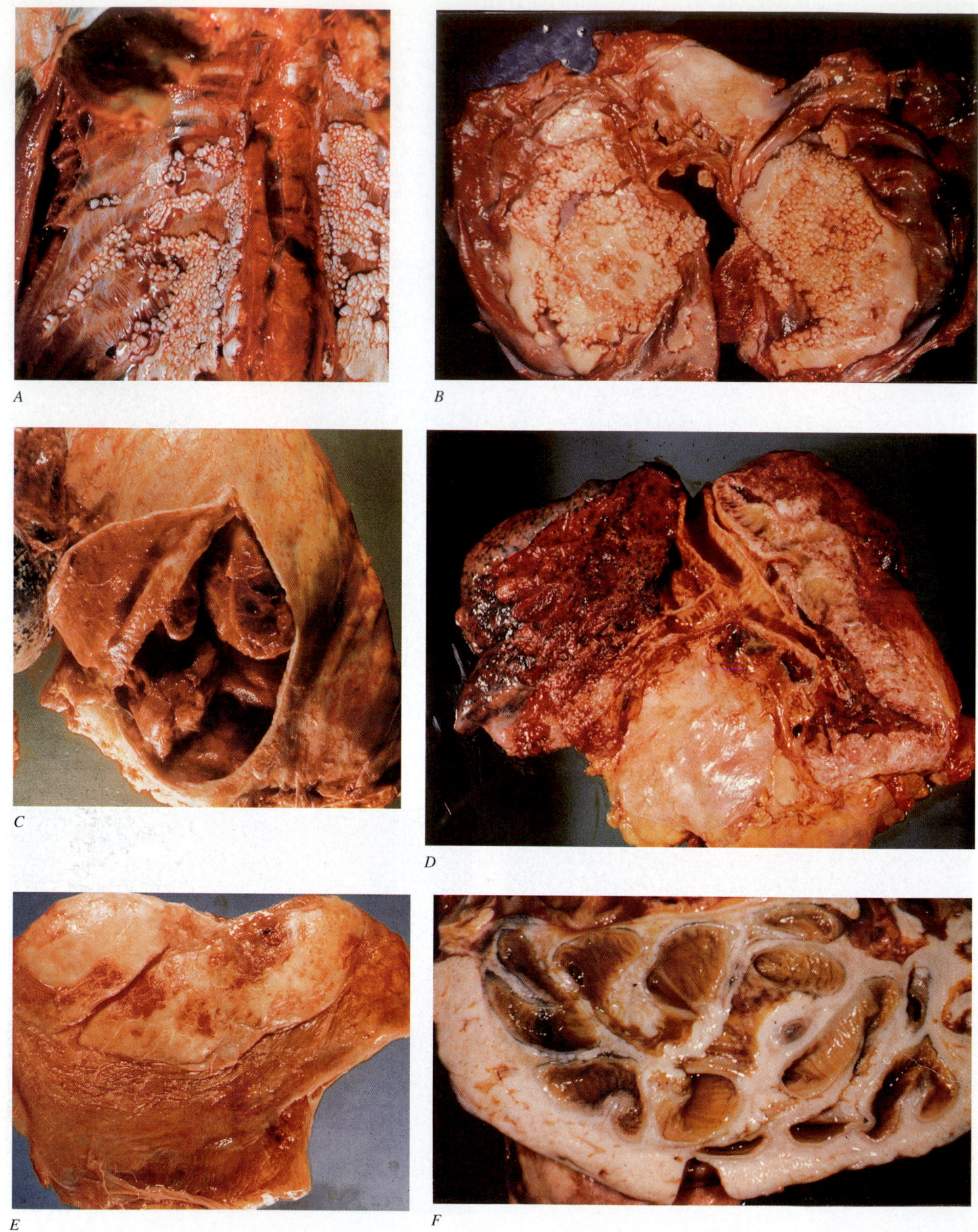

FIGURE 88-4 Examples of mesothelial responses to prolonged injury by asbestos. *A*. Mesothelioma of parietal pleura. *B*. Mesothelioma of thoracic surface of diaphragm. *C*. Window in mesothelioma encasing lung. *D*. Mesothelioma invading lung, pericardium, and heart. *E*. Large plaque on thoracic surface of diaphragm. *F*. Mesothelioma of peritoneal cavity. *(Courtesy of Dr. Sylvan Moolten.)*

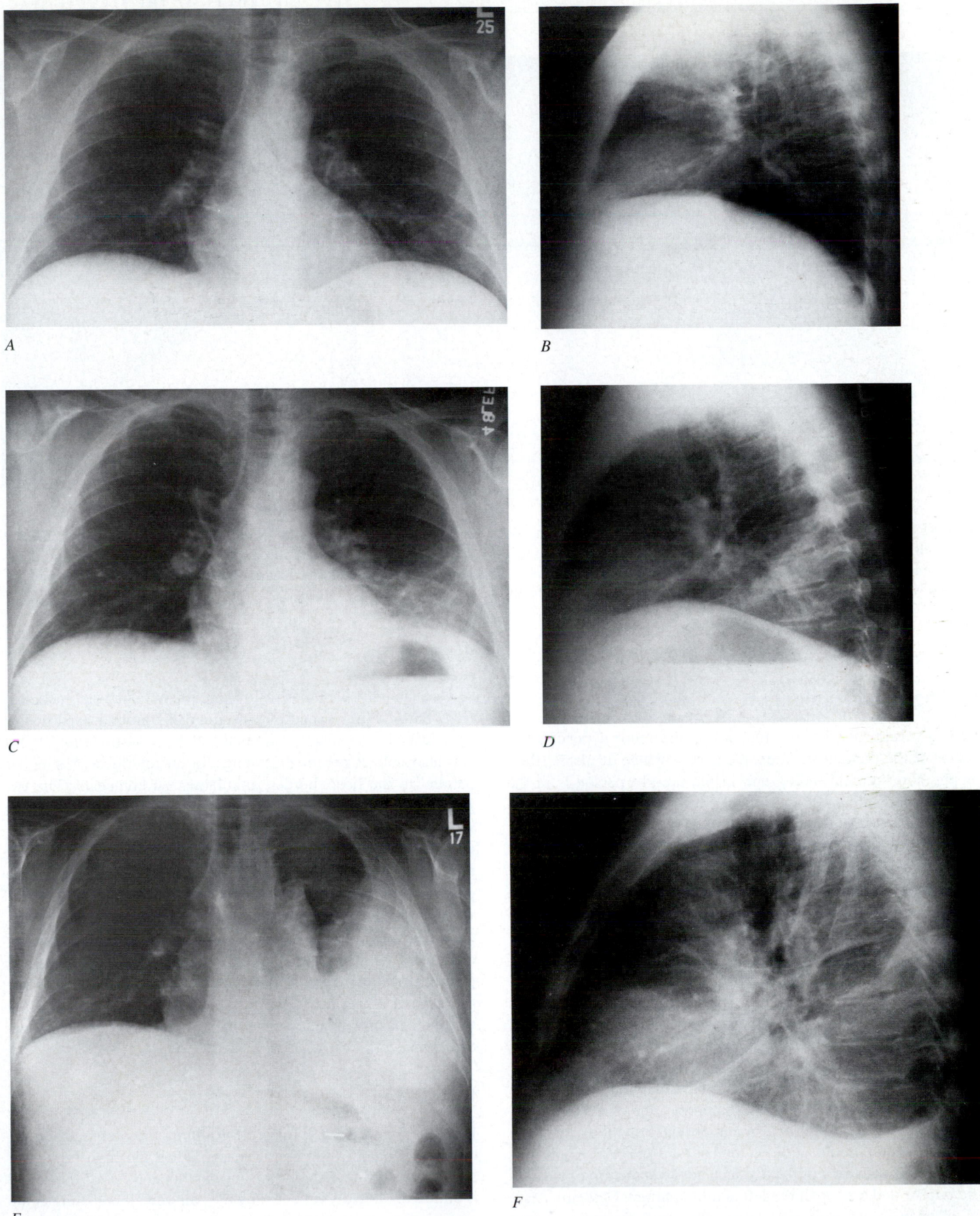

A

B

C

D

E

F

FIGURE 88-5 Evolution of massive effusion in a 35-year-old man with pancreatitis, pancreatic pseudotumor, and ascites. Posteroanterior and lateral radiographs. *A, B.* Before pleural effusion. Normal. *C, D.* Two weeks later. Left pleural effusion and patchy density, probably rep- resenting atelectasis, of left lower lobe. *E, F.* One month after *A* and *B.* Massive left pleural effusion. *G, H.* Three months after *A* and *B,* after multiple thoracenteses. Pleural thickening and pockets of fluid.

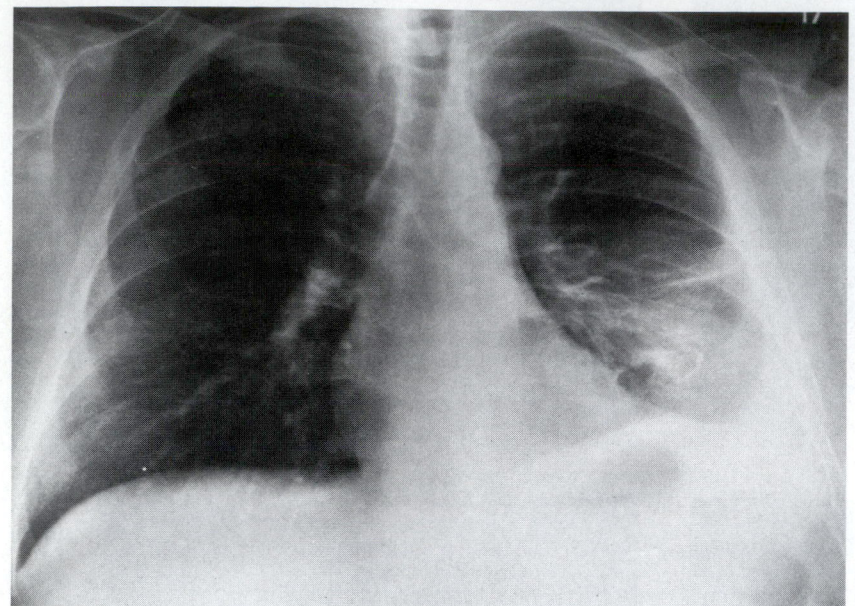

G

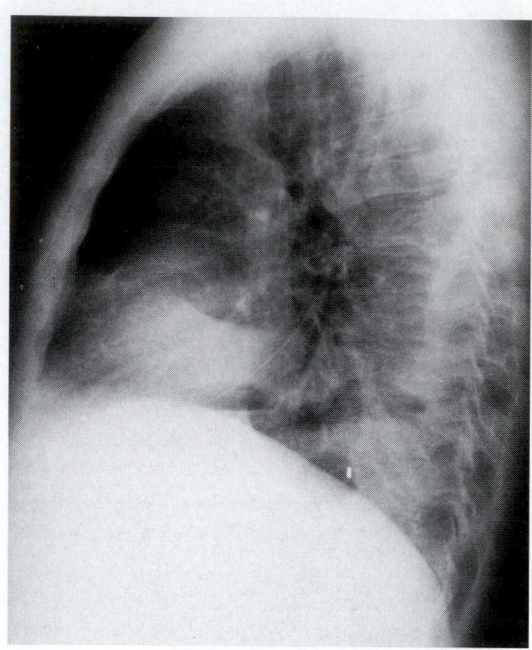

H

FIGURE 88-5 (*cont.*)   Evolution of massive effusion in a 35-year-old man with pancreatitis, pancreatic pseudotumor, and ascites. Posteroanterior and lateral radiographs. *A, B.* Before pleural effusion. Normal. *C, D.* Two weeks later. Left pleural effusion and patchy density, probably representing atelectasis, of left lower lobe. *E, F.* One month after *A* and *B.* Massive left pleural effusion. *G, H.* Three months after *A* and *B,* after multiple thoracenteses. Pleural thickening and pockets of fluid.

Radiographic Evaluation

Because fluid initially accumulates in the more dependent recesses of the thoracic cavities, the first evidence of pleural fluid on the conventional radiograph in the upright person is in the costophrenic sulcus: on the lateral chest radiograph, as little as 200 ml can be detected as blunting of the costophrenic angle (Fig. 88-6); larger effusions (about 500 to 600 ml) are necessary to produce appreciable blunting of the costophrenic angle on the PA radiograph. Even less than 200 ml can be recognized on a lateral decubitus radiograph. On occasion, computed tomography may disclose an effusion that is undetectable by conventional radiography.

The localization of pleural fluid is determined by gravity and the availability of a free pleural space. One common deviation from the usual radiographic appearance of pleural fluid is caused by the accumulation of fluid between diaphragm and the inferior surface of the lung (Fig. 88-7). This intrapulmonary effusion is suspected when one or both hemidiaphragms appear to be elevated for no good reason. Sometimes, the clue to the presence of an intrapulmonic effusion is provided by blunting of the posterior costophrenic angle on the lateral chest radiograph. Another hint is widening of the distance between the top of the gastric bubble and the top of the left hemidiaphragm ($>$2 cm). Also, an effusion on the right side causes the minor fissure to appear closer to the diaphragm than usual. Radiographs taken in the lateral decubitus position often settle the issue by demonstrating the movement of free intrapulmonary fluid from the top of the diaphragm to the dependent chest wall.

Occasionally, pleural effusions are found in unusual locations (Fig. 88-8). Fluid sometimes accumulates around a particular lobe (usually the lower), simulating lobar consolidation. Fluid can also collect paramediastinally, in an interlobar fissure, or parallel to the heart border, simulating cardiomegaly. The explanation generally offered for these anomalous accumulations is localized obliteration of the pleural space either by congenital anomalies or, more often, by inflammatory conditions that force fluid to accumulate in the remaining unaffected part of the pleural space.

As indicated above, the massive pleural effusion often shifts the mediastinum to the opposite side (Fig. 88-5). But should an obstructing endobronchial lesion produce both atelectasis and pleural effusion, the mediastinum is apt to remain in place. Massive pleural effusion without mediastinal shift suggests fixation of the mediastinum and is most often produced by bronchogenic carcinoma.

Ultrasound

Ultrasound is often helpful in determining the presence and location of fluid in the pleural space. When the high-frequency sound wave is directed into the normal thoracic cavity, the sound is almost completely reflected by the "air-containing" lung at the surface. But when pleural fluid is present, an echo-free space that changes shape with respiration can be visualized between the chest wall and the aerated lung. The technique is simple and inexpensive and can be performed at the bedside. It can be extremely helpful in guiding the aspiration of a loculated effusion.

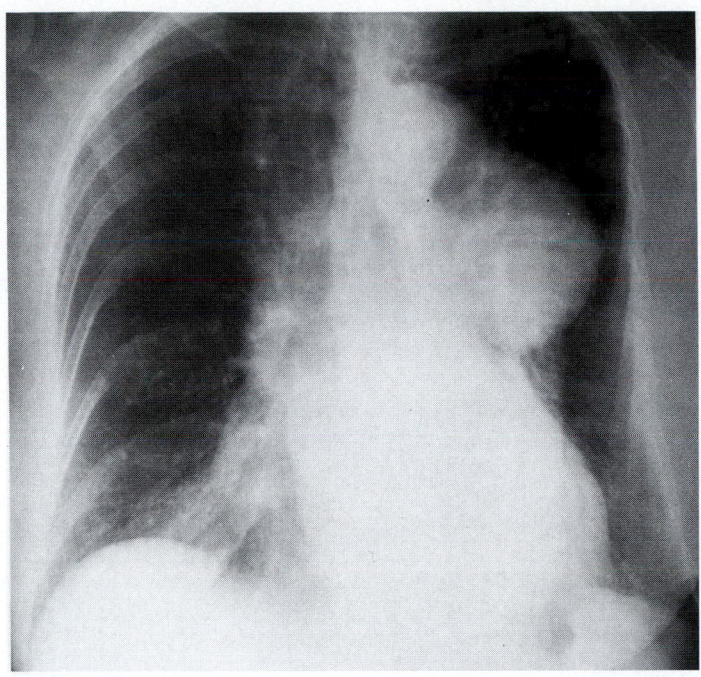

A

FIGURE 88-6 Leaking thoracic aneurysm. *A.* Posteroanterior view. Aneurysm of descending thoracic aorta is clearly visible. No evidence of pleural fluid. *B.* Lateral view. Blunting of costophrenic angle by blood leaking from aneurysm. *C.* CT scan. The large aneurysm and fluid are clearly visible. *(Courtesy of Dr. David Epstein.)*

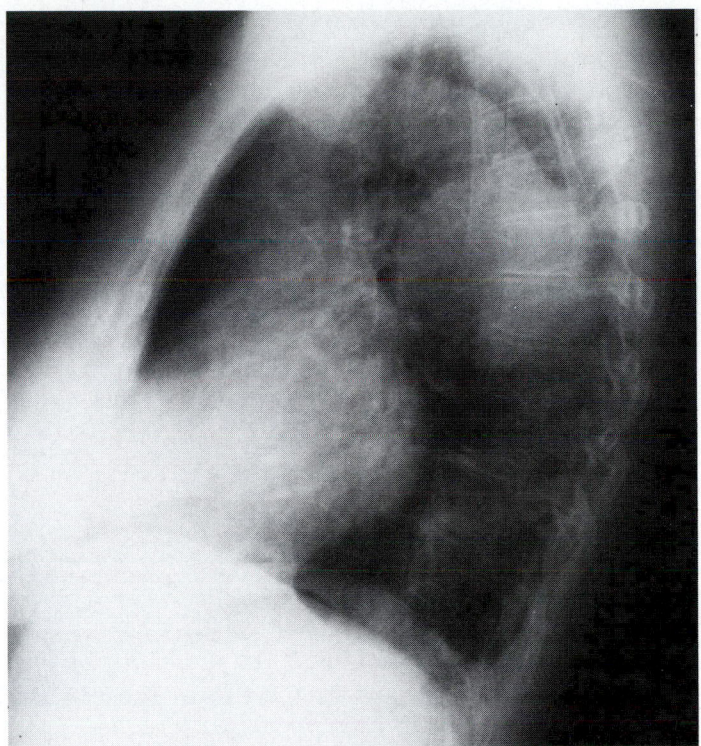

B

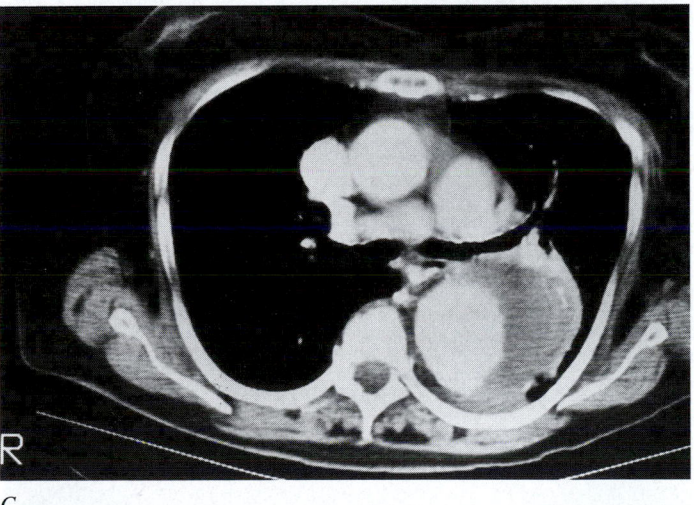

C

Computed Tomography

Computed tomography (CT) can provide useful information in the study of pleural effusions; it permits a view of the underlying parenchyma, which may be obscured by the pleural disease. Occasionally it can be diagnostic—for instance, in distinguishing a peripheral pleural plaque from a pulmonary nodule. It is extremely sensitive in identifying the pleural thickening and calcifications due to asbestos exposure. CT of the pleural space is particularly helpful in distinguishing between a peripheral lung abscess and a loculated empyema: CT of a lung abscess reveals an irregular cavity wall that usually abuts the pleura at an acute angle without displacing the pulmonary vessels and bronchi; in contrast, CT in the case of empyema reveals that the cavity wall is uniform in thickness and that the angle formed at the chest wall is obtuse (Fig. 88-9). If the empyema is very large, the underlying lung may be displaced. While magnetic resonance imaging has become a useful imaging technique for a number of conditions, it provides little useful information about the pleura beyond that available from CT.

Thoracentesis

Thoracentesis is done either to elucidate the cause of an effusion or to relieve dyspnea caused by the effusion. The procedure is technically simple and relatively safe, but it should not be performed in a patient with a bleeding tendency unless the underlying coagulopathy has been corrected by the administration of platelets and/or plasma components. In general, 50 to 100 ml of fluid provides sufficient material for diagnostic studies, whereas a larger quantity is removed during a therapeutic thoracentesis.

Thoracentesis is readily performed at the bedside with the patient sitting upright in a comfortable position, the arms and head supported by an adjustable table. The upper border of a moderate effusion is easily identified at the bedside by the loss of tactile and vocal fremitus and the presence of a flat percussion note. The thoracentesis should be performed in the interspace below this level. While the needle is usually inserted 5 to 10 cm lateral to the spine, the site chosen for its insertion should be free of local disease, to prevent contamination of the pleural space. Effusions that are less than 10 mm thick on decubitus radiographs and those that are loculated should be localized by fluoroscopy or ultrasound before thoracentesis is attempted. The procedure can be performed in the radiology suite, or the ultrasound can

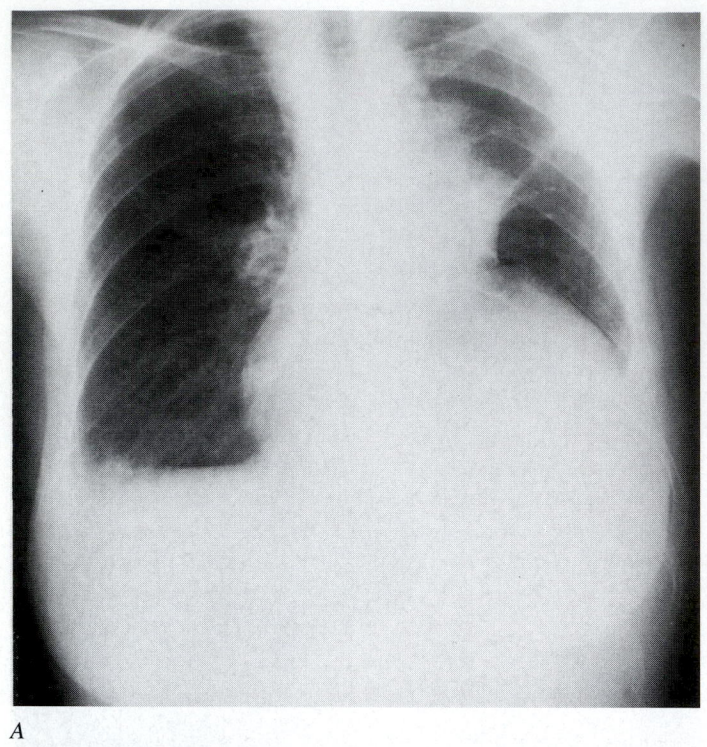

A

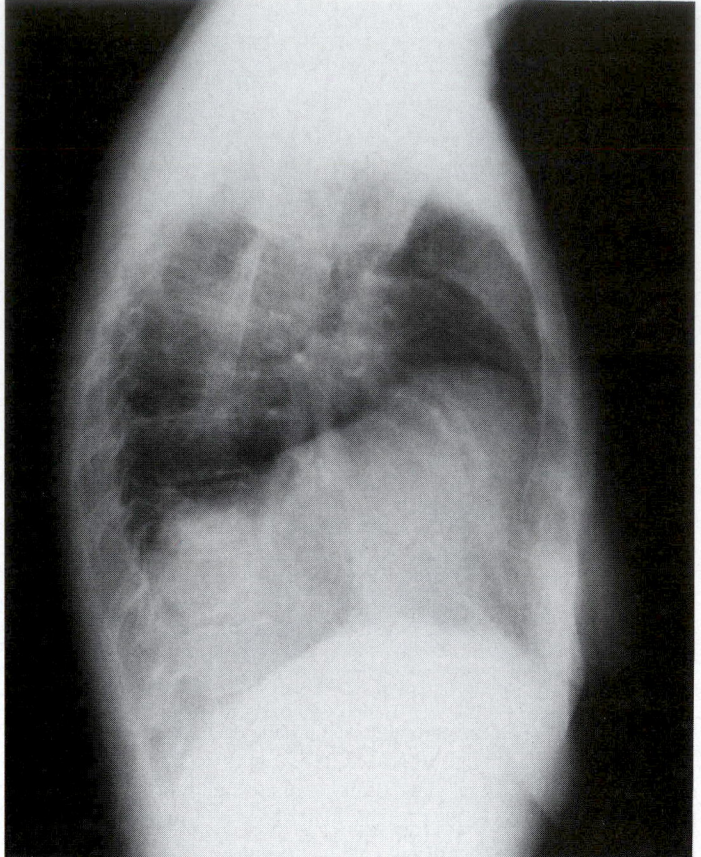

B

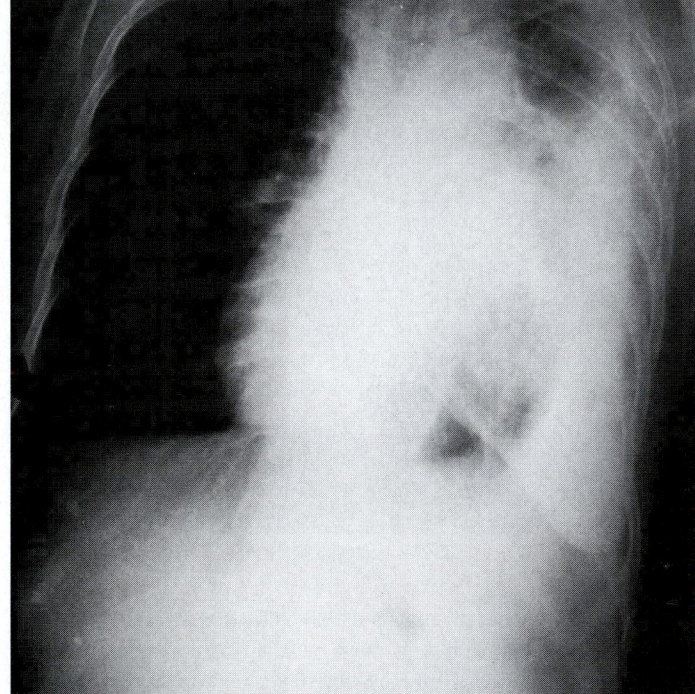

C

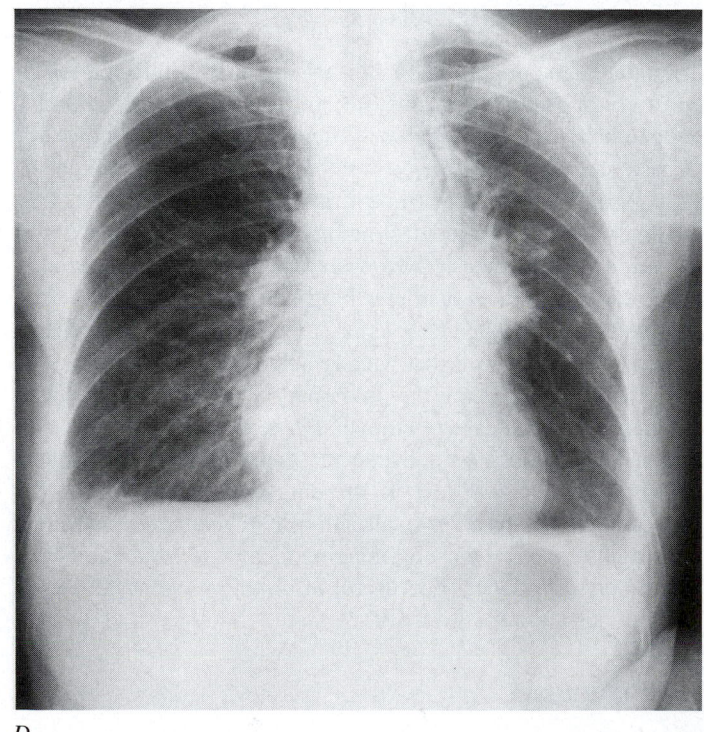

D

FIGURE 88-7   Subpulmonic effusion. Bronchogenic carcinoma in the left lower lobe with mediastinal and pleural metastases in a 65-year-old woman. *A.* Elevation of left diaphragm suggesting subpulmonic effusion. The right costophrenic angle is blunted. *B.* Lateral view of the subpulmonic effusion. *C.* Left lateral decubitus film demonstrating the presence of free pleural fluid. *D.* Radiograph immediately after thoracentesis, showing a small residual effusion and hydropneumothorax.

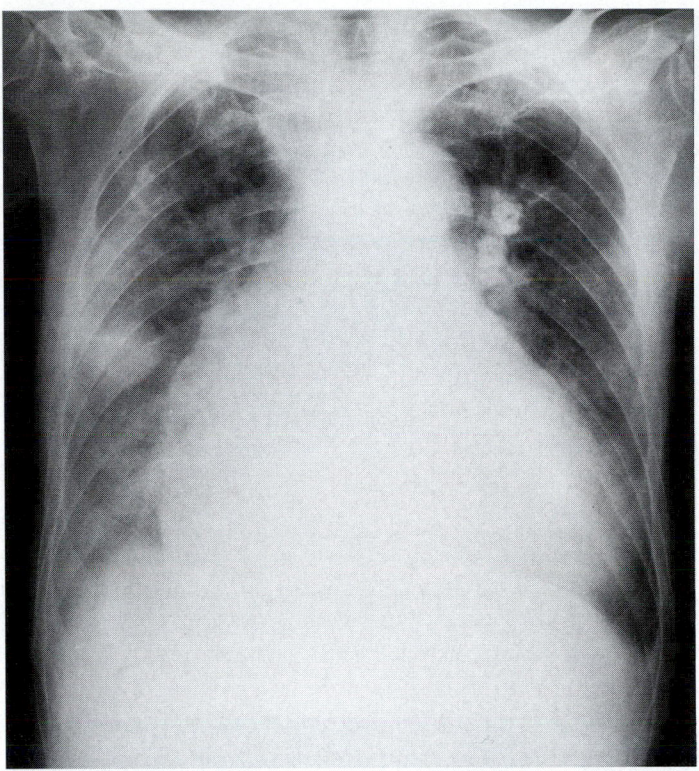

A

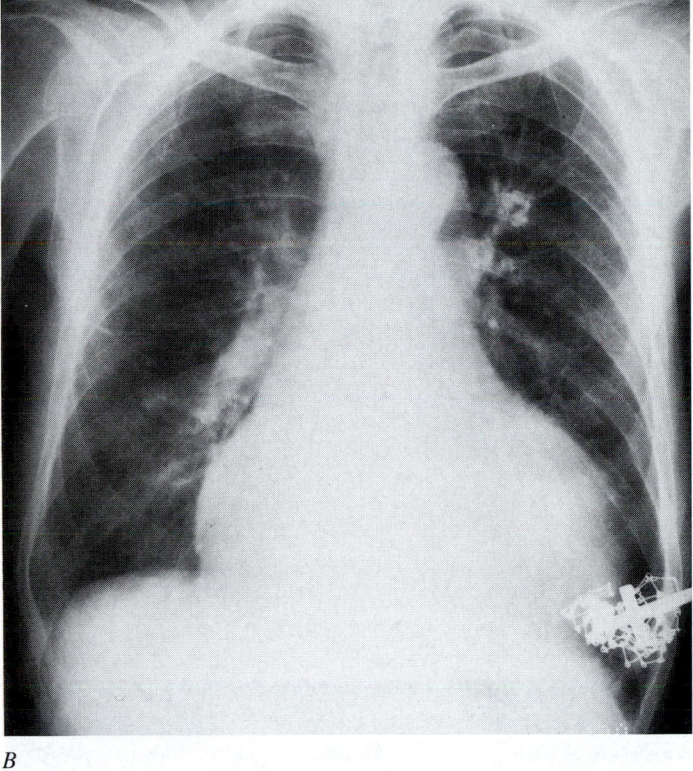

B

C

FIGURE 88-8   Vanishing tumor. Congestive heart failure in a 75-year-old man. *A.* Cardiac enlargement, bilateral pleural effusions, and widening of the superior mediastinum due to venous distention. A masslike lesion is superimposed on the minor septum. *B.* Eight days later after diuresis and loss of weight of 10 lb. The superior mediastinum has narrowed, and the pleural effusion and masslike density have disappeared. The "vanishing tumor" represented loculated pleural fluid. *C.* Thirty-four days after *B.* Changes secondary to left ventricular failure are apparent, and the vanishing tumor has reappeared.

tercostal vessels and nerves lie immediately beneath the ribs. To minimize the danger of injury to these structures, a 20 gauge or larger needle is introduced immediately above the superior aspect of the lower rib and advanced with continuous gentle suction until the parietal membrane is penetrated and fluid is obtained. If air is aspirated, the needle has been advanced too far and the underlying lung has been punctured. The risk of pneumothorax is small if the needle is immediately withdrawn, and the procedure usually can be successfully repeated in an interspace below the initial site. Whenever the effusion is small and the thoracentesis is performed at or below the level of the 10th intercostal space, the needle must be advanced cautiously to avoid penetration of the diaphragm and laceration of the spleen or liver. Most patients will experience pain referred to the ipsilateral shoulder if the diaphragm is injured. In some people, however, this complication is not considered until the operator fully inserts the needle and aspirates blood rather than pleural fluid. Whenever this complication is suspected, the needle should be immediately withdrawn and the patient closely observed for signs of bleeding.

be brought to the bedside, so that proper positioning of the needle can be verified.

The skin is cleansed with iodophor or a similar antiseptic solution, and the underlying tissues, including the periosteum of the rib, are infiltrated with local anesthetic (Fig. 88-10). The in-

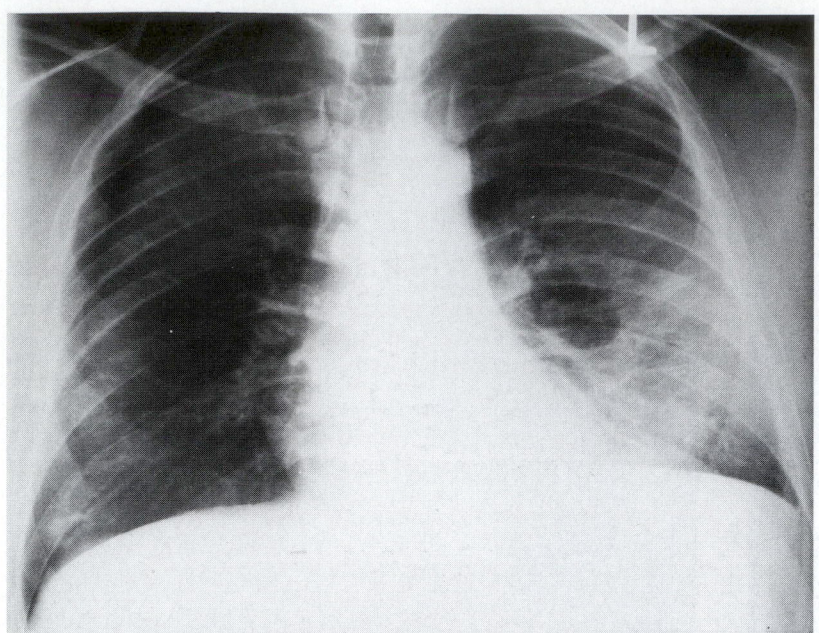

A

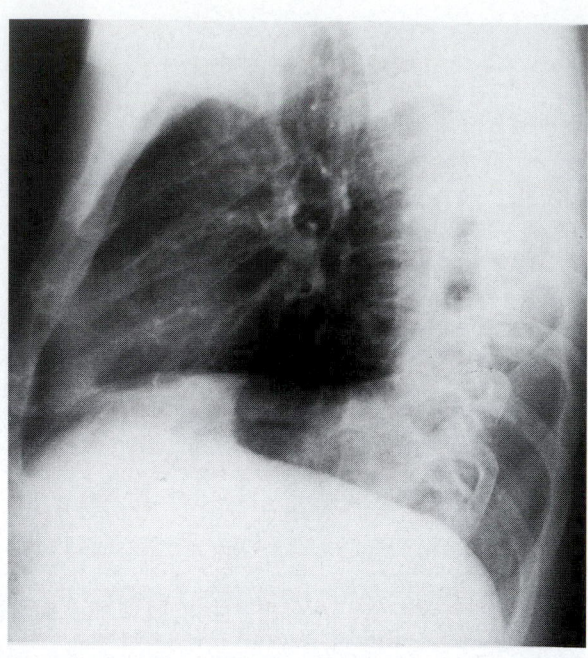

B

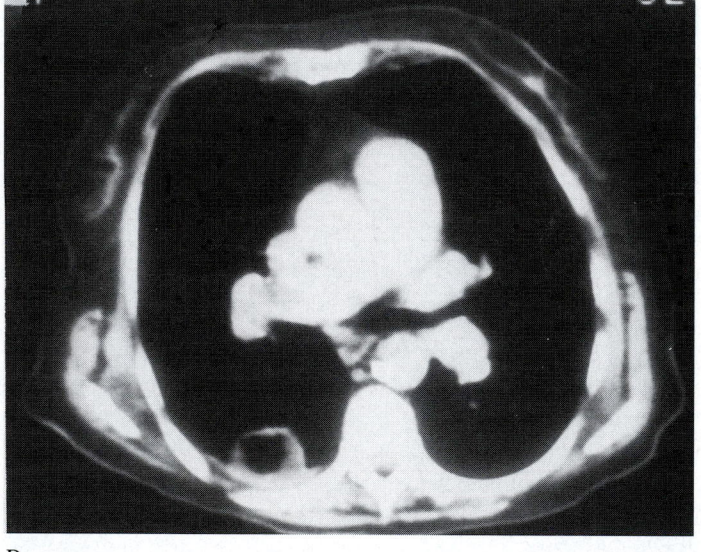

C

D

FIGURE 88-9 Empyema or abscess? Patient with an acute febrile illness. *A*. A density with air in its center is in the left lower lung field. *B*. Lateral film shows that the density is adjacent to the posterior chest wall. *C*. Computed tomography reveals a left pleural density with a smooth border; its margin makes an obtuse angle with the chest wall, characteristic of empyema. *D*. Another patient for comparison. An irregular cavity wall and acute pleural interface in a patient with an abscess in the right lower lobe.

Large effusions often cause dyspnea that can be relieved by therapeutic thoracentesis. In addition to compressing the underlying lung, a large effusion expands the chest wall in the affected hemithorax. Removal of a modest amount of fluid usually alleviates the respiratory discomfort, generally before any improvement in arterial P_{O_2} or in the lung volumes is observed. The relief of symptoms is attributable, in part, to the decrease in the distention of the thoracic cage after thoracentesis, which enables the inspiratory muscles to operate on a more advantageous portion of their length-tension curve.[8] Whether specific receptors are also involved is unknown.

The potential risk of lacerating the visceral pleura and underlying lung increases when the visceral and parietal surfaces are opposed by the withdrawal of a large volume of fluid during

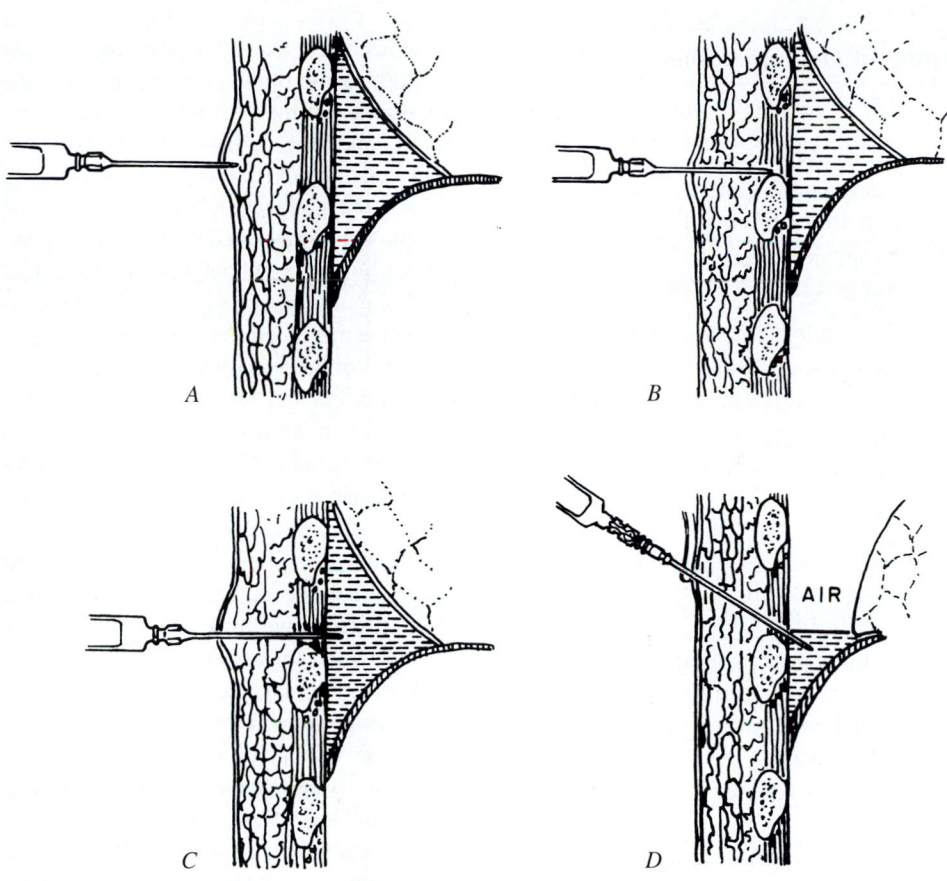

FIGURE 88-10 Thoracentesis. *A*. The skin is anesthetized with a local anesthetic. *B*. The deeper structures, including the periosteum of the rib, are infiltrated with anesthetic. *C*. The needle enters the pleural space, and fluid is aspirated for diagnostic purposes. *D*. A polyethylene catheter is introduced through the needle and directed inferiorly for performance of a therapeutic thoracentesis.

permeability has increased. The increase in capillary permeability is thought to be due to the generation of free radicals when flow is restored to the collapsed lung, creating a reperfusion injury.[20] The abrupt restoration of a strongly negative intrapleural pressure is also thought to play a role in the pathogenesis of the injury.[28] To avoid this complication, an effusion should be drained slowly and the thoracentesis discontinued if the patient develops cough, dyspnea, or pain in the chest. As a rule, no more than 1 L of fluid should be removed at any one thoracentesis.

Pleural Fluid Analysis

Normal pleural fluid resembles water in appearance and clarity and is odorless. It contains about 1000 cells per milliliter, most of which are mesothelial cells and the others, monocytes and lymphocytes. Its chemical composition is summarized in Table 88-1. Abnormalities in these features, supplemented by others, usually succeed in establishing or confirming the cause of the effusion. Although a large battery of tests may be performed, gross and microscopic examination of the fluid and determinations of the concentration of total proteins and lactic dehydrogenase (LDH) usually suffice to establish whether the effusion is a transudate; if so, additional studies are unlikely to yield useful information. The results of these initial tests are usually available from a central laboratory in hours. A portion of the fluid can be refrigerated, and if the effusion is an exudate, additional chemical assays and bacteriologic and cytologic studies can then be obtained (Table 88-2).

GROSS FEATURES

Transudates are generally clear, with only a slightly yellow tint (Fig. 88-11). The more protein and cells, the deeper the color and the more turbid the fluid; exudates that contain large numbers of cells, such as those associated with pneumonia, are usually cloudy; empyema fluid is opaque and viscous. An effusion that is rich in cholesterol has a characteristic satinlike sheen; chylous effusions are milky white.

MICROSCOPIC APPEARANCE

Important information regarding the etiology of an effusion can be obtained from the examination of its cellular composition. Only 5000 to 6000 red blood cells per cubic millimeter—equivalent to adding 1 ml of blood to 1 L of water—suffice to impart a red tint to pleural fluid. This concentration of red blood cells corre-

a therapeutic thoracentesis. To minimize this danger, once the thoracentesis needle enters the pleural space and fluid is aspirated (Fig. 88-10), a plastic catheter can be introduced through the needle and directed inferiorly into the dependent region of the pleural cavity. The metal thoracentesis needle is then withdrawn and its tip shielded with a guard to prevent laceration of the catheter and chest wall. Large quantities of fluid can then be safely aspirated through the plastic catheter.

Complications of thoracentesis include pneumothorax, hemothorax, reexpansion pulmonary edema, and, rarely, air embolism. Leakage of air into the pleural space through the needle is the most common cause of pneumothorax associated with thoracentesis. In a few instances, pneumothorax follows laceration of the visceral pleura. Although the leak usually seals itself quickly, closure may be hastened by having the patient lie on the affected side to decrease the regional alveolar volume and the pressure gradient between the alveoli and the pleural space. If the pneumothorax is large or causes breathlessness, aspiration or even placement of a chest tube is indicated. Hemothorax usually follows trauma to the intercostal vessels; much less often, the cause is an abnormal clotting mechanism.

Pulmonary edema occasionally follows *rapid* reexpansion of the lung. The edema is typically unilateral and the edema fluid has a high protein content, indicating that pulmonary capillary

TABLE 88-2

Useful Tests in the Evaluation of Pleural Effusion

Test	Abnormal Value	Frequently Associated Condition
Red blood cells, per mm³	>100,000	Malignancy, trauma, pulmonary embolism
White blood cells, per mm³	>10,000	Pyogenic infection
neutrophils, %	>50	Acute pleuritis
lymphocytes, %	>90	Tuberculosis, malignancy
eosinophilia, %	>10	Asbestos effusion, pneumothorax, resolving infection
mesothelial cells	absent	Tuberculosis
Protein, PF/S*	>0.5	Exudate
LDH, PF/S	>0.6	Exudate
LDH, IU†	>200	Exudate
Glucose, mg/dl	<60	Empyema, TB, malignancy, rheumatoid arthritis
pH	<7.20	Complicated parapneumonic effusion, empyema, esophageal rupture, TB, malignancy, rheumatoid arthritis
Amylase, PF/S	>1	Pancreatitis
Bacteriologic	positive	Cause of infection
Cytology	positive	Diagnostic of malignancy

*PF/S ratio = pleural fluid to serum ratio.
†IU = concentration in International Units.

sponds roughly to a hemoglobin concentration of 0.015 g/dl of pleural fluid. Grossly bloody effusions in which the concentration of red blood cells exceeds 100,000 per cubic millimeter are usually due to trauma, pulmonary infarction, or malignancy. A traumatic tap usually becomes less hemorrhagic as fluid is removed—a feature that is helpful in distinguishing it from a hemorrhagic effusion.

The white blood cell count of most transudates is under 1000 per cubic millimeter. In neoplastic and tuberculous effusions, the white blood cell count generally ranges between 500 and 2500 per cubic millimeter. A white blood cell count greater than 10,000 per cubic millimeter, in which polymorphonuclear leukocytes predominate, is common in pyogenic infections. But noninfectious processes, notably pulmonary infarction or pancreatitis, can also produce a leukocytosis that can be remarkable on occasion: of the order of 30,000 to 50,000 per cubic millimeter.

The concentration of mesothelial cells is sometimes helpful in interpretation. For example, in tuberculous effu-

sions, fewer than 10 mesothelial cells per 1000 white blood cells are the rule; the absence of mesothelial cells in tuberculous pleuritis is attributed to the fibrinous layer that covers the pleural surface. In nontuberculous pleural effusions the number of mesothelial cells is higher, exceeding 5 per 100 white blood cells. Occasionally, on cytologic examination, reactive mesothelial cells closely resemble those of adenocarcinoma.

Differential white cell counts often provide more insight into etiology than do total counts. For example, a great predominance of mature lymphocytes favors the prospect of neoplasm, lymphoma, or tuberculosis. But a similar pattern is encountered in the pleural fluid of patients with pyogenic pleural infections that are responding to treatment. Polymorphonuclear leukocytes predominate in effusions that accompany pneumonia and pancreatitis. The basis for pleural fluid eosinophilia (>10 percent eosinophils) often remains unexplained. A common cause is air or blood in the pleural space. It also occurs in benign asbestos effusions and in resolving pleural infections. Eosinophilia is uncommon in effusions caused by neoplasms or tuberculosis. Therefore, eosinophilia in pleural fluid generally signifies benignity.

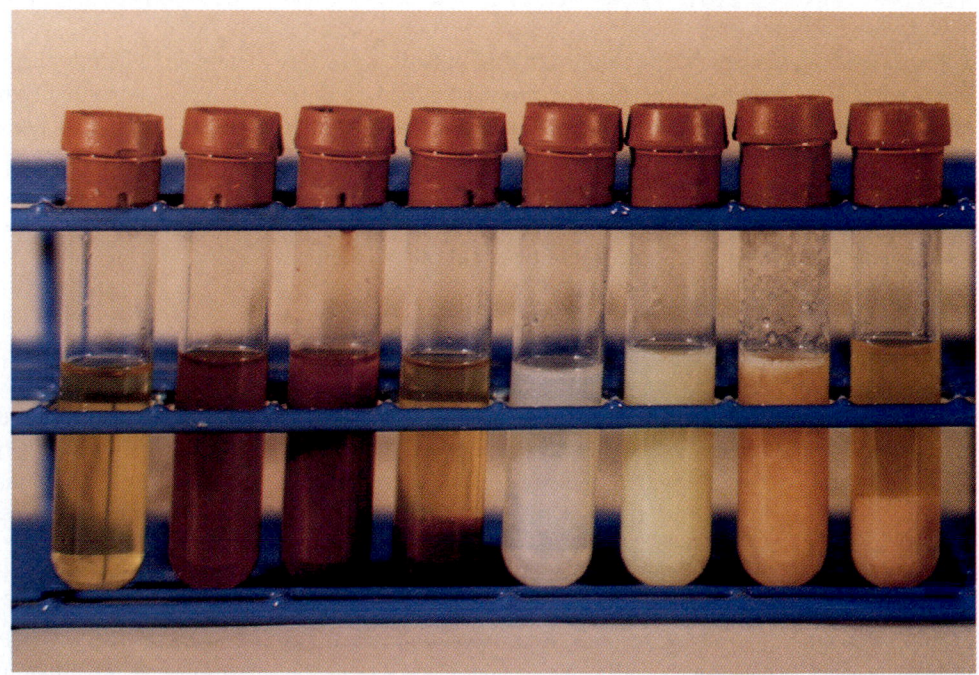

FIGURE 88-11 Appearance of different types of pleural fluid. From left to right is shown a straw-colored transudative effusion, a bloody pleural effusion with 135,000 RBCs per cubic millimeter, a hemothorax, the same hemothorax after centrifugation, a chylothorax, a cholesterol (pseudochylous) effusion, and empyema, and the same empyema after centrifugation. (*From Kinasewitz GT: Pleuritis and pleural effusions, in Bone R: Pulmonary and Critical Care Medicine, Chicago, Mosby–Year Book, 1993, with permission.*)

CHEMICAL ANALYSES

Protein and LDH Measurements   The nature of the effusion is generally designated as either an exudate or a transudate, based on the concentration of protein and LDH in the pleural fluid. For many years, distinction between an exudate and a transudate was based largely on the concentration of total protein: a protein concentration of 3.0 g/dl or more defined an exudate; a transudate contained less than 3.0 g/dl. Better separation of transudates and exudates can be made by comparing the concentrations of total protein and LDH in serum and pleural fluid.[25] Using this approach, pleural fluid is classified as an exudate if it has any one of the following three properties:

1. A ratio of concentration of total protein in pleural fluid to serum >0.5.
2. An absolute value of LDH >200 IU.
3. A ratio of LDH concentrations in pleural fluid to serum >0.6.

Additional tests—including the pleural fluid cholesterol, pleural fluid to serum bilirubin ratio, and pleural fluid to serum albumin gradient—have been used to distinguish transudates from exudates. However, these additional measurements add little to the use of the simple protein and LDH indices.[40]

If the effusion is an exudate, further analysis of the fluid may help determine its origin. However, if none of these three criteria are satisfied, the effusion is a transudate and additional pleural fluid testing is unwarranted.

Glucose   The concentration of glucose in pleural fluid may provide a useful clue to its cause. Proper handling of the sample (use of sodium fluoride) is necessary to avoid artificially low values for glucose concentration due to glycolysis in vitro. In normal subjects, the concentration of glucose in pleural fluid is equal to that in serum. But in bacterial infections of the pleura, rheumatoid disease, tuberculous pleurisy, and malignant effusions, the glucose concentration is usually less than in serum. Only an occasional patient with malignancy or tuberculosis of the pleura will have decreased concentrations of glucose in pleural fluid. In contrast, dramatic and consistent lowering of glucose concentrations (<30 mg/dl) in pleural fluid occurs in most effusions due to rheumatoid pleural disease.

The pH of pleural fluid is sometimes useful in expediting evaluation of an effusion. In handling the sample before analysis, one must take care to avoid artificial changes in pH by collecting the fluid anaerobically and transporting it on ice. As a rule, in effusions in which the concentration of glucose is low and LDH levels are high, the values for pH are low.[10,26] Low values for pleural fluid pH can be expected in empyema, esophageal rupture, hemothorax, rheumatoid pleural disease, and systemic acidosis. A pH of less than 7.20 (or a glucose of less than 40 mg/dl) in a parapneumonic effusion indicates that the effusion is "complicated"—i.e., likely to require chest tube drainage for resolution.[17] Values for pH less than 6.8 are often encountered in empyema or after a communication has been established between the esophagus and the pleural cavity. The mechanism for the low pH depends on the cause. For example, local infection, as in empyema, decreases pH primarily by virtue of lactic acid and CO_2 production by leukocytes. In contrast, pleural fluid pH drops considerably in systemic acidosis, primarily because of its low buffering capacity.

Amylase   The concentration of pancreatic amylase in pleural fluid is abnormally high in effusions secondary to pancreatitis;[30] less consistently, it is increased in patients with malignant effusions produced by primary tumors of the pancreas (Fig. 88-5). High levels of amylase also occur in pleural effusions secondary to esophageal rupture; but in this instance, the amylase is salivary. Occasionally, the concentration of amylase is high in pleural effusions secondary to carcinoma of the lung or other malignancies.

Complement and Antibodies   Complement levels are low in effusions due to rheumatoid disease and systemic lupus erythematosus (SLE). In both disorders, the ratio of complement in pleural fluid to serum is less than 0.4. LE cells are sometimes found in the pleural fluid of patients with SLE, occasionally before they are detected in blood. Also, in patients with active lupus pleuritis, the concentration of antinuclear antibodies in pleural fluid is higher than in the serum.[9] In contrast, the demonstration of rheumatoid factor in pleural fluid is rarely helpful, since levels increase modestly (to about 1:160) in infectious and malignant effusions. Nonetheless, high levels—e.g., >1:640—are uncommon except in rheumatoid pleural effusions.[14]

Other Chemical Tests   A high level of hyaluronic acid in a pleural exudate is highly suggestive of mesothelioma.[37] Although the search for distinctive markers has led to the suggestion that high levels of adenosine deaminase and lysozyme may be helpful in distinguishing tuberculous pleural effusions from malignant pleural effusions, the definite diagnosis of a tuberculous origin still rests on the demonstration of tubercle bacilli—in sputum, pleural fluid, or pleural biopsy.[3] Interleukin-2 receptors are shed from the surface of activated lymphocytes, and elevated levels have been found in tuberculous and rheumatoid effusions.[6]

Lipids   Milky or creamy pleural fluid automatically raises the prospect of chylothorax. The appearance may be deceptive, however, since empyema and pseudochylothorax sometimes look the same, and not all chylothoraces appear milky (Fig. 88-11). The cloudiness in empyema is due to white blood cells. However, in both chylothorax and pseudochylothorax, the milky appearance is due to inordinate quantities of lipids: chylomicrons in a chylothorax and generally lecithin-globulin complexes in pseudochylothorax. Important differences in the behavior of these two kinds of lipids allow a distinction between chylothorax and pseudochylothorax to be made: the addition of ethyl ether clears the fluid in chylothorax but not in pseudochylothorax; triglyceride levels in the pleural fluid are high in chylothorax (>100 mg/dl) but low (<50 mg/dl) in pseudochylothorax.[44] Intermediate values call for lipoprotein electrophoresis to determine if the turbidity is due to chylomicrons.

Cholesterol Pleural Effusion

In certain chronic inflammations of the pleura, notably in tuberculosis or rheumatoid arthritis, the concentration of cholesterol is inordinately high, sometimes exceeding 1000 mg/dl (Fig. 88-12). These levels greatly exceed those generally encountered in chylothorax. The cholesterol is produced by the inflammatory cells in the pleural effusion.[15] Sometimes the fluid is orange; other times it is yellow or green, resembling an empyema. Direct examination of the fluid discloses characteristic rhomboid-shaped crystals. Cholesterol effusions require

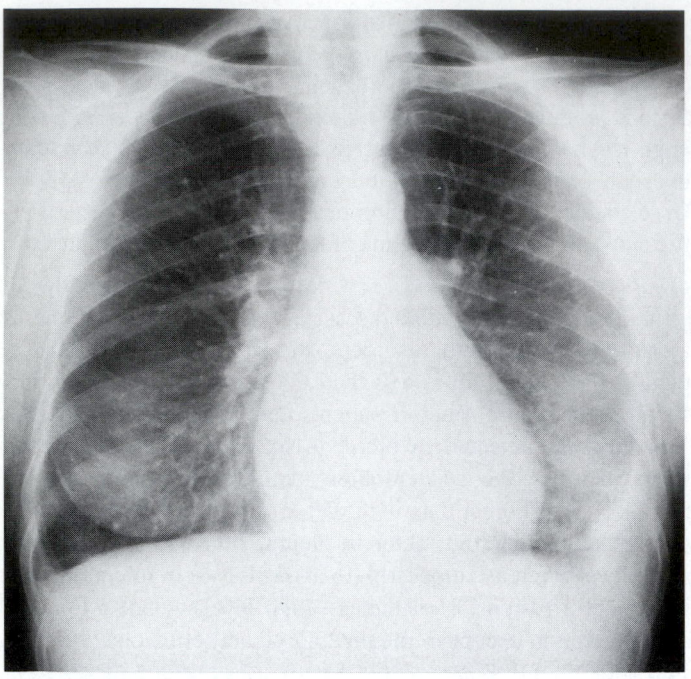

A

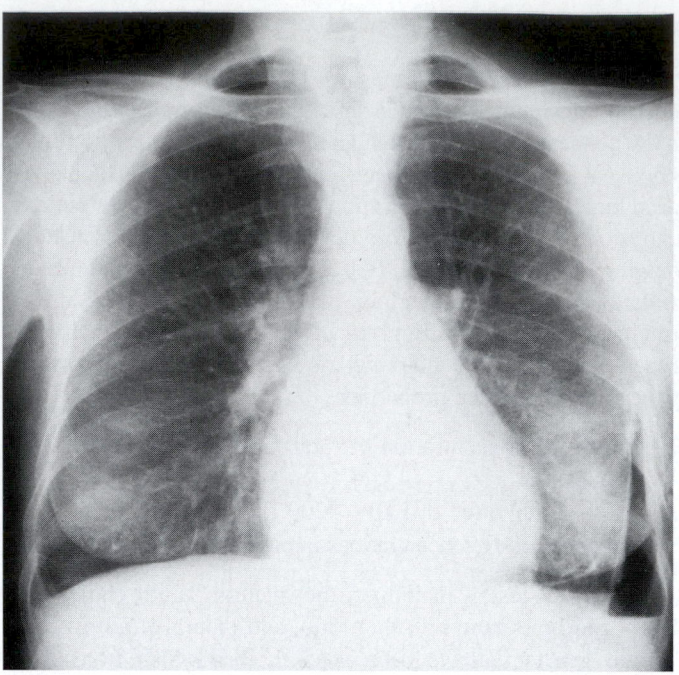

B

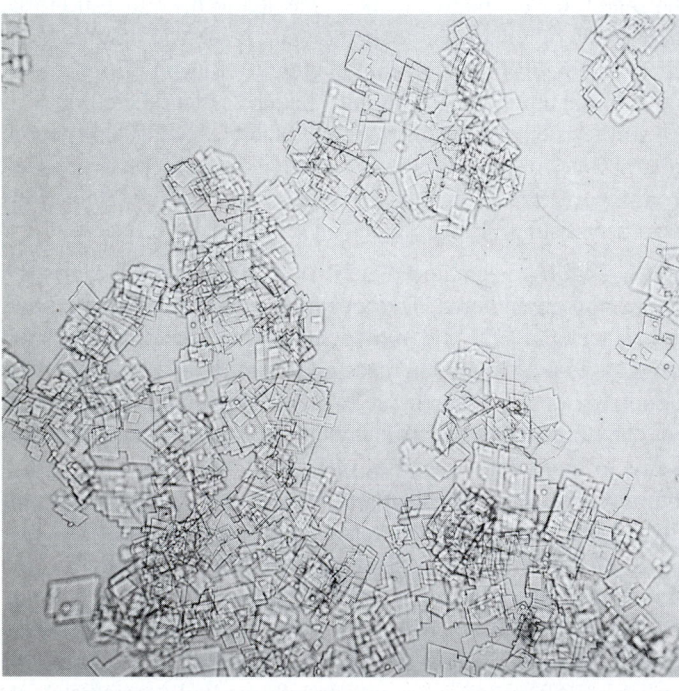

C

FIGURE 88-12   Cholestrol pleural effusion. *A*. Pleural density at left base in a 40-year-old woman with severe rheumatoid arthritis. A chest radiograph 9 years earlier showed "pleural thickening" at the left base. *B*. A pleural pocket is seen at the left base after removal of 80 ml of a turbid orange fluid. Microscopic examination showed cholesterol crystals. Chemical analysis of the orange fluid showed total protein: 6.0 g/dl; glucose: absence (by a qualitative test); total lipid: 5700 mg/dl; cholesterol: 3400 mg/dl, with 14 percent esters. Corresponding blood values were total serum lipids: 263 mg/dl; serum cholesterol: 125 mg/dl, with 60 percent esters. *C*. Photomicrograph of an unstained preparation of pleural fluid. Rhomboid-shaped cholesterol crystals are seen. (×80.)

tuberculous and fungal effusions: 100 ml provides three times as many positive cultures in tuberculous effusions as does 10 ml.

CYTOLOGIC TESTS

Malignant cells in the pleural fluid indicate tumor invasion of either the parietal or visceral pleura. They have prognostic as well as diagnostic significance: patients with pleural effusions secondary to carcinoma of the lung can be expected to die within 1 year; positive pleural cytology in an effusion accompanying carcinoma of the breast or ovary carries a life expectancy of less than 2 years (see Chapter 90).

Carcinomas of the lung and breast and lymphomas are the most common causes of malignant pleural effusions. Malignant cells are found in more than two-thirds of pleural effusions due to carcinoma of the lung or to carcinoma of the breast but in only about one-sixth of patients with lymphoma.

Venous or lymphatic obstruction in the mediastinum causes pleural effusion in the absence of the pleural invasion by neoplasm; in these instances, the fluid does not contain malignant cells.

PLEURAL BIOPSY

When the initial clinical impression suggests a malignant or tuberculous effusion or if pleural fluid analysis fails to establish

no treatment: they are not drained because the collapsed, underlying lung cannot expand.

BACTERIOLOGIC TESTS

In infectious pleuritis, Gram's stain and culture of the pleural fluid are of paramount importance. Recovery of an organism from culture (aerobic or anaerobic) of pleural fluid clinches the cause of the infection.

Acid-fast smears and cultures are routine in evaluating effusions of unknown origin. Concentration of large volumes of fluid before culture increases the prospects for positive cultures in

the cause of an exudative effusion, pleural biopsy is indicated. Closed-needle biopsy of the parietal pleura can be performed at the time of thoracentesis and may provide histologic proof of malignancy or granulomatous pleuritis, even when pleural fluid analysis is not diagnostic.

The technique is similar to that for a thoracentesis except that a special biopsy needle, usually an Abrams' or a Cope's needle, is used to obtain both fluid and the pleural specimen. These are large, blunt-tipped needles with a special hook near the tip to grasp the parietal pleura (Fig. 88-13). The hook is built into the Abrams' needle, whereas a central trocar containing the hook must be introduced through the outer cannula of a Cope's needle. Adequate tissue specimens are obtained with either biopsy needle, so the particular type used depends on the preference of the operator.

The effusion is localized and the site cleansed and anesthetized as previously described for a thoracentesis. A small skin incision is made with a pointed scalpel blade, and the biopsy needle is advanced into the pleural space. Once the pleural space is entered and the fluid is obtained, the biopsy hook is exposed and withdrawn until resistance is felt as the parietal pleura is encountered (Fig. 88-13). The inner cutting edge in the Abrams' needle or the outer cutting cannula of the Cope's needle is then advanced to shear the parietal tissue, and the sample is removed. To minimize the risk of injury to the intercostal vessels and nerves, samples of pleura should be obtained only from the lateral, medial, and inferior margins of the site where the needle punctures the parietal membrane. Parietal pleura, which appears as white to gray tissue attached to the underlying skeletal muscle, should be submitted for histologic examination and mycobacterial and fungal culture.

Pleural biopsy is complementary to cytologic examination of the pleural fluid; when the two tests are performed together, the initial diagnostic attempt will be positive in approximately two-

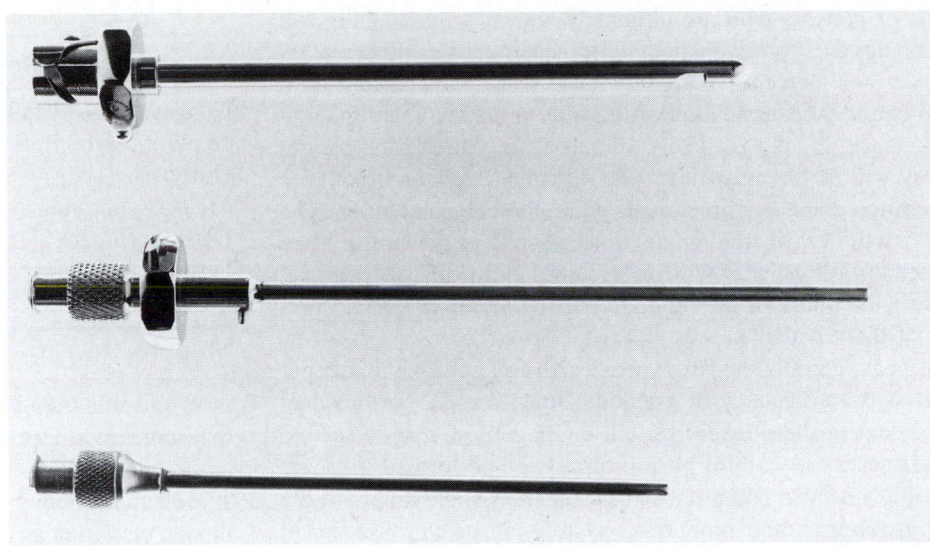

A

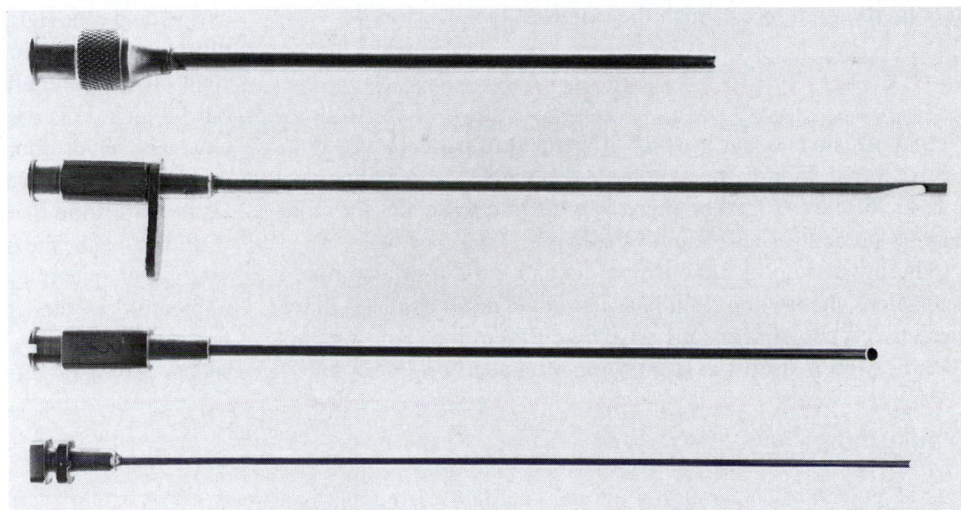

B

FIGURE 88-13   Pleural biopsy needles and technique. *A.* Abrams' needle consists of (1) an outer trocar with a hook, (2) an inner cutting cannula, and (3) a central stylet. *B.* Cope's needle consists of (1) an outer cutting cannula, which is introduced into the pleural space with (2) an inner hollow-beveled trocar, and (3) a central stylet in place. The inner elements are removed, and (4) the blunt-tipped hollow hooked biopsy trocar is introduced to obtain tissue. *C.* Essential steps in a pleural biopsy illustrated using an Abrams' needle: (1) fluid is aspirated to confirm the position of the needle in the pleural space, (2) the needle is withdrawn until the parietal pleura is engaged, and (3) the cutting trocar is advanced to shear the pleura so that the sample can be removed. *(Based on data of Light,[25] with permission.)*

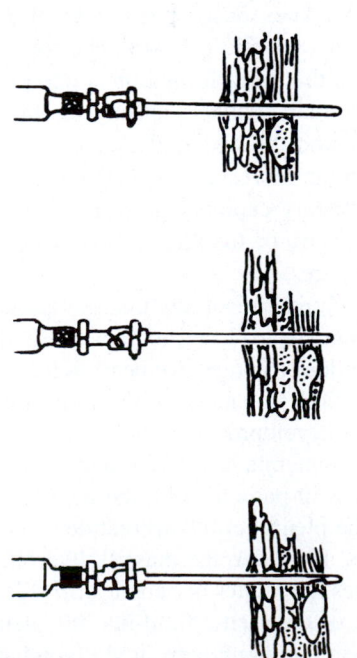

C

thirds of patients who are ultimately shown to have malignant pleural disease.[24,38] Even though the incidence of positive pleural biopsies—40 percent—is slightly lower than the 50 percent yield from cytologic examination of the fluid in patients with pleural malignancy, in approximately 20 percent of patients the pleural biopsy will be the only diagnostic specimen.[42] Pleural biopsy is more often diagnostic in patients with tuberculous pleuritis. The biopsy will demonstrate granulomas or grow organisms in 70 to 80 percent of patients with tuberculous effusions. In contrast, smear and culture of the fluid are positive in fewer than 25 percent of these patients.

Repeat pleural biopsy will increase the diagnostic yield in patients with malignancy or granulomatous disease.[24] More than 90 percent of these disorders will be diagnosed when a second and, if necessary, a third pleural biopsy are performed. In some patients, however, comprehensive evaluation, including multiple pleural biopsies and bronchoscopy to evaluate any associated parenchymal abnormality, fails to reveal the cause of the underlying disorder. Thoracoscopy and visually directed pleural biopsy may be required to establish the origin of the effusion.[31]

TYPES OF PLEURAL EFFUSIONS

Pleural effusions occur in 25 to 50 percent of patients with congestive heart failure, pneumonia, malignancy, and pulmonary embolic disease. Together, these four disorders account for more than 90 percent of all pleural effusions.

The initial step in establishing the cause of an effusion is to determine whether the fluid is a transudate or an exudate. Since these two types of effusions arise by different mechanisms, this classification is useful in identifying the underlying disorder.

Transudates

Pleural fluid formed through a normal capillary membrane is a transudate that is characterized by little protein or other large molecules. Transudates occur when normal relationships between capillary hydrostatic pressure and colloid osmotic pressure are upset, so that fluid formation at one pleural surface exceeds the fluid reabsorptive capacity at the other. Clinical disorders that favor the accumulation of a transudate in the pleural space are an increase in systemic capillary pressure, an increase in pulmonary capillary pressure, a decrease in the colloid osmotic pressure of the plasma, and a marked decrease in intrapleural pressure.

Some of the clinical disorders that are associated with transudates (hydrothorax) are listed in Table 88-3. The overwhelming majority are due to congestive heart failure. The presence of transudative effusions in patients with cardiac disease is best correlated with the development of pulmonary venous hypertension.[48] Hypoalbuminemia also leads to the development of transudative effusions in patients with the nephrotic syndrome and contributes to the pleural effusions that develop in patients with hepatic cirrhosis. However, the massive hydrothorax that sometimes complicates the ascites of hepatic cirrhosis presumably occurs by passage of the ascitic fluid into the pleural space either through defects in the diaphragm or via lymphatics; usually the hydrothorax associated with ascites is on the right.[4] A similar

TABLE 88-3
Causes of Transudative Effusions
Congestive heart failure*
Nephrotic syndrome
Cirrhosis
Meig's syndrome
Hydronephrosis
Peritoneal dialysis
Ex vacuo

*Responsible for >90%

mechanism is thought to be responsible for the pleural effusion that sometimes occurs in the course of hydronephrosis: urine dissects cephalad in the retroperitoneal space and enters the pleural space either directly or via the diaphragmatic lymphatics.[32] Although classified as a transudate because of its low protein content, the effusion has a high creatinine level and is actually a urothorax. In Meigs' syndrome, hydrothorax is associated with ascites and a benign ovarian tumor (fibroma, thecoma, or granulosa cell tumor); in most instances, the effusion is also on the right. The classic effusion in Meig's syndrome is a transudate, but the effusions associated with some ovarian tumors may be exudates. Hydrothorax occasionally occurs during peritoneal dialysis; the chemical composition of the effusion is then similar to that of the dialysate.[41]

Pleural adhesions sometimes prevent the reexpansion of a lung after pneumothorax. The continued absorption of intrapleural gas then produces markedly subatmospheric pleural pressures that favor the formation and accumulation of a transudate (ex vacuo effusion).

TABLE 88-4
Causes of Exudative Effusions
Very common
Parapneumonic
Malignancy
Pulmonary embolism
Common
Abdominal disease
Tuberculous
Traumatic
Collagen vascular
(particularly rheumatoid and SLE)
Unusual
Drug-induced
(e.g., nitrofurantoin)
Asbestos
Dressler's syndrome
Chylothorax
Uremia
Radiation therapy
Sarcoidosis
Yellow-nail syndrome
Ovarian hyperstimulation syndrome

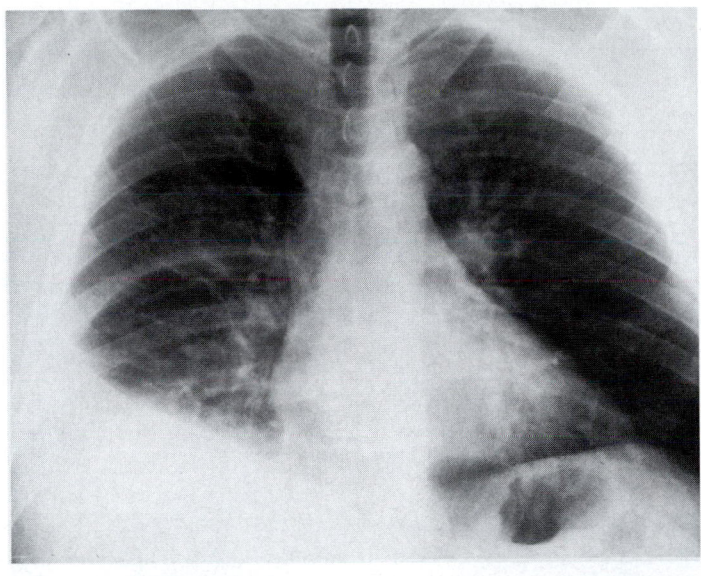

A

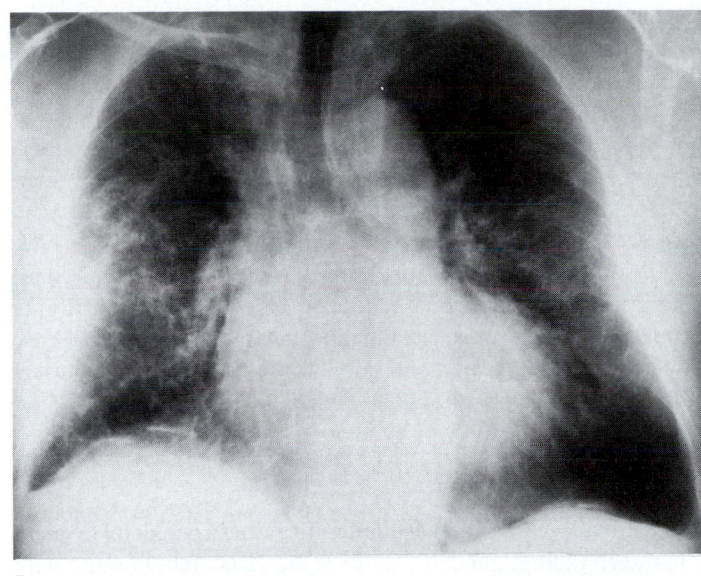

B

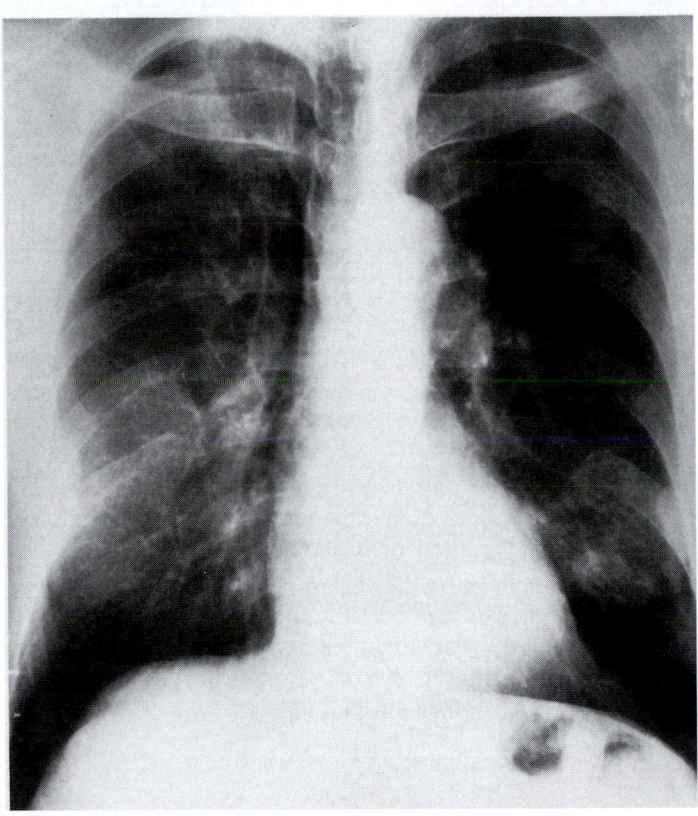

C

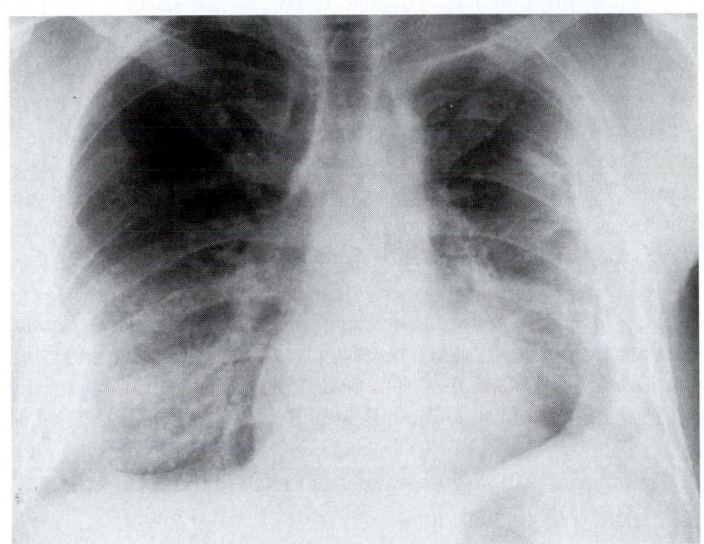

D

FIGURE 88-14   Responses of pleura to asbestos. *A.* Pleural effusion in railroad worker with 6-year history of asbestos exposure. *B.* Calcified pleural plaques. *C.* Bilateral pleural plaques. *D.* Bilateral diffuse pleural thickening. *(Courtesy of Dr. David Murphy.)*

Exudates

An exudate refers to pleural fluid that is formed through abnormally permeable capillary walls and contains higher concentrations of protein than do transudates. The characteristics of an exudative effusion are given in Table 88-2. The altered membrane permeability is usually produced by inflammatory changes in the pleura caused by infection, pulmonary infarction, or neoplasm. As indicated previously, protein is removed from the pleural fluid predominantly by the lymphatics. Therefore, diseases that impair lymphatic drainage of proteins from the pleura (e.g., tuber-

culous pleurisy) increase the protein concentration of the pleural fluid, thereby producing an exudate.

The major causes of exudative pleural effusions are pneumonia, pulmonary neoplasm, and pulmonary embolism (Table 88-4). The incidence of these three disorders is high, and because they frequently produce effusions, together they account for over 80 percent of all exudates.[25]

A variety of gastrointestinal diseases and infradiaphragmatic disorders are also associated with exudative pleural effusions: esophageal perforation, subphrenic abscess, intrahepatic abscess, and abdominal surgery. Pleural effusions also occur at three different phases of pancreatic disease: acute, chronic, and ascitic.[30] In each instance, the fluid is an exudate in which the concentration of amylase in pleural fluid exceeds that in serum. However, the mechanisms differ: transdiaphragmatic lymphatics seem to constitute the predominant route in the acute stage, sinus tracts when there are pancreatic pseudocysts (Fig. 88-5), and congenital foramina when pancreatitis is associated with ascites and pleural effusion.

Most of the other exudative effusions are due to a small number of relatively common conditions. However, occasionally an exudate represents an unusual manifestation of a common disease or a typical manifestation of a rare disorder. Together, the unusual causes of effusion account for less than 5 percent of all exudates.

THICKENED PLEURA

The normal pleura is paper-thin and ordinarily invisible except when seen radiographically on the slant, as is often the case with respect to interlobar fissures that run obliquely. However, organization of protein-rich exudates in the process of healing or of a hemothorax sometimes results in "thickened pleura" that may have clinical consequences.

Exudates that are particularly rich in fibrin often resolve by organization, weaving the visceral and parietal pleural surfaces into a densely fibrous and poorly expansible mat. Not infrequently, pockets containing organisms remain; some of them smolder for a long time, only to undergo recrudescence months to years after the original empyema. If the thickened pleura is sufficiently extensive, the fibrothorax interferes with gas exchange, often to the extent of causing arterial hypoxemia due to "venous admixture"; the "shunt" is usually relieved by decortication.[35] If the underlying lung is affected in the fibrotic process, decortication is seriously handicapped by the lack of a cleavage plane.

Hemothorax is the accumulation of shed blood within the thorax. Usually it is a complication of thoracic trauma; occasionally it is a consequence of a spontaneously bleeding intrathoracic great vessel or an intrapulmonary small vessel, as during spontaneous pneumothorax.[12] Movement of the lungs and heart tends to defibrinate blood in the pleural space, keeping it fluid, unless bleeding is massive or blood is contaminated by products that leak from the abdominal cavity (e.g., bile) or enter from the outside (e.g., bacteria) as a result of trauma.[47] If the blood does clot, it undergoes organization to form "peels" on the visceral and parietal surfaces. Persistent, organized clot encases the lung, as in chronic empyema, often impairing gas exchange in the same way. Decortication focuses primarily on removing the peel from the visceral pleural to free the lung and diaphragm. Blood left in the pleural cavity for more than 4 to 6 weeks often leaves behind a lung damaged by extensive fibrosis; before the fourth week, the peel is usually too fragile to be easily removed.

Among the other common causes of pleural thickening are asbestos and talc (Fig. 88-14). Both are fibrous silicates; indeed, commercial talc is often contaminated with asbestos. Both cause thickening, adhesions, and plaques. The lesions are considered in Chapter 59. A few decades ago, when pneumothorax was a popular form of therapy for tuberculosis, an occasional residuum of pneumothorax treatment was pleural obliteration and fibro-

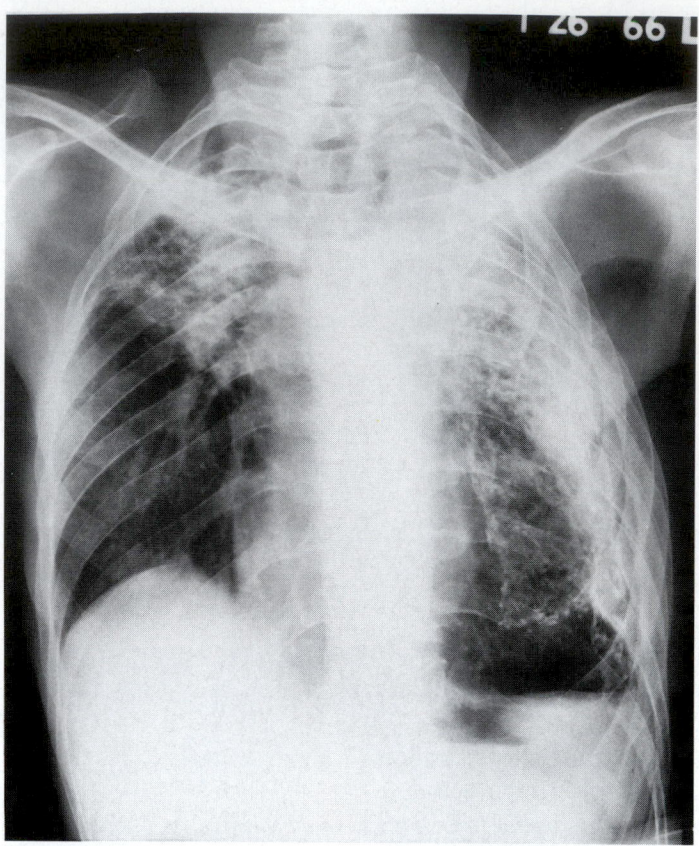

FIGURE 88-15   Fibrothorax with extensive pleural calcification on the left side secondary to therapeutic pneumothorax and empyema in a patient with long-standing tuberculosis. Residual tuberculous disease is present in the right upper lobe.

thorax that resulted in permanent pulmonary collapse (Fig. 88-15). When severe, this complication can cause overdistention of the opposite lung and torsion of the heart and great vessels, requiring thoracoplasty for relief. Fortunately, this complication, now rare, serves as a reminder that persistent pneumothorax is a lingering hazard; pleural obliteration by organization is the desirable end-point after pneumothorax as long as the healing process does not culminate in fibrothorax.

REFERENCES

1. Agostoni E: Mechanics of the pleural space, in Fishman AP (ed), *Handbook of Physiology: The Respiratory System.* Bethesda, MD American Physiological Society, 1986, pp 531–559.
2. Antony VB, Hott JW, Kunkel SL, et al: Pleural mesothelial cell expression of C-C (monocyte chemotactic peptide) and C-X-C (interleukin-8) chemokines. *Am J Respir Cell Mol Biol* 12:581–588, 1995.
3. Banales JL, Pineda PR, Fitzgerald JM, et al: Adenosine deaminase in the diagnosis of tuberculous pleural effusions: A report of 218 patients and review of the literature. *Chest* 99:355–357, 1991.
4. Boggs DS, Kinasewitz GT: Review: Pathophysiology of the pleural space. *Am J Med Sci* 309:53–59, 1995.
5. Broaddus VC, Wiener-Kronish JP, Berthiaume Y, Staub NC: Removal of pleural liquid and protein by lymphatics in awake sheep. *J Appl Physiol* 64:384–390, 1988.

6. Chiang C-S, Chiang C-D, Lin J-W, et al: Neopterin, soluble inter-leukin-2 receptor and adenosine deaminase levels in pleural effusions. *Respiration* 61:150–154, 1994.

7. Daniele RP: The pleura in local and systemic immune disorders, in Chrétien J, Bignon J, Hirsch A (eds), *The Pleura in Health and Disease.* New York, Dekker, 1985, pp 369–383.

8. Estenne M, Yernault JC, De Troyer A: Mechanism of relief of dyspnea after thoracocentesis in patients with large pleural effusions. *Am J Med* 74:813–819, 1983.

9. Good JT, King TE, Antony VB, Sahn SA: Lupus pleuritis: Clinical features and pleural fluid characteristics with special reference to pleural fluid antinuclear antibodies. *Chest* 84:714–718, 1983.

10. Good JT, Taryle DA, Maulitz RM, et al: The diagnostic value of pleural fluid pH. *Chest* 78:55–59, 1980.

11. Goodman RB, Wood RG, Martin TR, et al: Cytokine-stimulated human mesothelial cells produce chemotactic activity for neutrophils including NAP-I/IL-8. *J Immunol* 148:457–465, 1992.

12. Griffith GL, Todd EP, McMillin RD, et al: Acute traumatic hemothorax. *Ann Thorac Surg* 26:204–207, 1978.

13. Grotberg JB, Glucksberg MR: A buoyancy-driven squeeze-film model of intrapleural fluid dynamics: Basic concepts. *J Appl Physiol* 77:1555–1561, 1994.

14. Halla JT, Schrohenloher RE, Volanakis JE: Immune complexes and other laboratory features of pleural effusions. *Ann Intern Med* 92:748–752, 1980.

15. Hamm H, Brohan U, Bohmer R, Missmahl HP: Cholesterol in pleural effusions: A diagnostic aid. *Chest* 92:296–302, 1987.

16. Harvey W, Amlot PL: Collagen production by human mesothelial cells *in vitro. J Pathol* 139:337–347, 1983.

17. Heffner JE, Brown LK, Barbieri C, DeLeo JM: Pleural fluid chemical analysis in parapneumonic effusions: A meta-analysis. *Am J Respir Crit Care Med* 151:1700–1708, 1995.

18. Hott JW, Sparks JA, Godbey SW, Antony VB: Mesothelial cell response to pleural injury: Thrombin-induced proliferation and chemotaxis of rat pleural mesothelial cells. *Am J Respir Cell Mol Biol* 6:421–425, 1992.

19. Idell S, Zwieb C, Kumar A, et al: Pathways of fibrin turnover of human pleural mesothelial cells in vitro. *Am J Respir Cell Mol Biol* 7:414–426, 1992.

20. Jackson RM, Veal CF, Alexander CB, et al: Re-expansion pulmonary edema. *Am Rev Respir Dis* 137:1165–1171, 1988.

21. Jonjic N, Peri G, Bernasconi S, et al: Expression of adhesion molecules and chemotactic cytokines in cultured human mesothelial cells. *J Exp Med* 176:1165–1174, 1992.

22. Kinasewitz GT, Groome LJ, Marshall RP, Diana JN: Permeability of the canine visceral pleura. *J Appl Physiol* 55:121–130, 1983.

23. Lai-Fook SJ: Mechanics of the pleural space: fundamental concepts. *Lung* 165:249–267, 1987.

24. Leslie WK, Kinasewitz GT: Clinical characteristics of the patient with nonspecific pleuritis. *Chest* 94:603–608, 1988.

25. Light RW: *Pleural Diseases.* Philadelphia, Lea & Febiger, 1995.

26. Light RW, MacGregor MI, Ball WC, Luchsinger PC: Diagnostic significance of pleural fluid pH and P_{CO_2}. *Chest* 64:591–596, 1973.

27. Lorgat F, Keraan MM, Lukey PT, Ress SR: Evidence for in vivo generation of cytotoxic T cells. *Am Rev Respir Dis* 145:418–423, 1992.

28. Mahfood S, Hix WR, Aaron BL, et al: Reexpansion pulmonary edema. *Ann Thorac Surg* 45:340–345, 1988.

29. Marshall BC, Santana A, Xu Q-P, et al: Metalloproteinases and tissue inhibitor of metalloproteinases in mesothelial cells. *J Clin Invest* 91:1792–1799, 1993.

30. McKenna JM, Chandrasekhar AJ, Skorton D, et al: The pleuropulmonary complications of pancreatitis. *Chest* 71:197–204, 1977.

31. Menzies R, Charbonneau M: Thoracoscopy for the diagnosis of pleural disease. *Ann Intern Med* 114:271–276, 1991.

32. Miller KS, Wooten S, Sahn SA: Urinothorax: A cause of low pH transudative pleural effusion. *Am J Med* 85:448–449, 1988.

33. Miserocchi G, Negrini D, Pistolesi M, et al: Intrapleural liquid flow down a gravity-dependent hydraulic pressure gradient. *J Appl Physiol* 64:577–584, 1988.

34. Miserocchi G, Pistolesi M, Miniati M, et al: Pleural liquid pressure gradients and intrapleural distribution of injected bolus. *J Appl Physiol* 56:526–532, 1984.

35. Morton JR, Bousky SF, Guinn GA: Physiological evaluation of results of pulmonary decortication. *Ann Thorac Surg* 9:321–326, 1970.

36. Nicholson LJ, Clark JMF, Pittilo RM, et al: The mesothelial cell as a non-thrombogenic surface. *Thromb Haemost* 52:102–104, 1984.

37. Pettersson T, Froseth B, Riska H, Klockars M: Concentration of hyaluronic acid in pleural fluid as a diagnostic aid for malignant mesothelioma. *Chest* 94:1037–1039, 1988.

38. Poe RH, Israel RH, Utell MJ, et al: Sensitivity, specificity, and predictive values of closed pleural biopsy. *Arch Intern Med* 144:325–328, 1984.

39. Rennard SI, Jaurand MC, Bignon J: Role of pleural mesothelial cells in the production of the submesothelial connective tissue matrix of lung. *Am Rev Respir Dis* 130:267–274, 1984.

40. Romero S, Candela A, Martin C, et al: Evaluation of different criteria for the separation of pleural transudates from exudates. *Chest* 104:399–404, 1993.

41. Rudnick MR, Coyle JF, Beck LH, McCurdy DK: Acute massive hydrothorax complicating peritoneal dialysis, report of 2 cases and a review of the literature. *Clin Nephrol* 12:38–44, 1979.

42. Salyer WR, Eggleston JC, Erozan YS: Efficacy of pleural needle biopsy and pleural fluid cytopathology in the diagnosis of malignant neoplasm involving the pleura. *Chest* 67:536–539, 1975.

43. Satoh K, Prescott SM: Culture of mesothelial cells from bovine pericardium and characterization of their arachidonate metabolism. *Biochim Biophys Acta* 930:283–296, 1987.

44. Staats BA, Ellefson RD, Budahn LL: The lipoprotein profile of chylous and nonchylous pleural effusions. *Mayo Clin Proc* 55:700–704, 1980.

45. Von Hayek H: *The Human Lung.* New York, Hafner, 1960, pp 227–233.

46. Wang NS: Mesothelial cells in situ, in Chrétien J, Bignon J, Hirsch A (eds), *The Pleura in Health and Disease.* New York, Dekker, 1985, pp 23–38.

47. Weil PH, Margolis IB: Systematic approach to traumatic hemothorax. *Am J Surg* 142:692–694, 1981.

48. Wiener-Kronish JP, Matthay MA, Callen PW, et al: Relationship of pleural effusions to pulmonary hemodynamics in patients with congestive heart failure. *Am Rev Respir Dis* 132:1253–1256, 1985.

49. Zocchi L, Agostoni E, Cremaschi D: Electrolyte transport across the pleura of rabbits. *Respir Physiol* 86:125–138, 1991.

CHAPTER 89

NONMALIGNANT PLEURAL EFFUSIONS

Richard H. Winterbauer

There are many causes of pleural effusion, and correct diagnosis remains a major challenge to clinicians (Table 89-1). The first step should be sampling the pleural fluid and determining whether it is a transudate or exudate. An exudative pleural effusion results from disease of the pleural surface, while a transudative pleural effusion results from an imbalance of Starling's forces resulting in movement of fluid into the pleural space, i.e., congestive heart failure, cirrhosis with ascites and the nephrotic syndrome (see Chapter 88). The diagnostic focus for exudative effusions is to recognize the responsible intrapleural disease, whereas transudates call for recognition of the systemic disease. Transudative pleural effusions have the following characteristics: (1) the pleural total fluid protein divided by the serum total protein is less than 0.5; (2) the pleural fluid lactic dehydrogenase (LDH) divided by the serum LDH is less than 0.6; and (3) the absolute level of LDH in the pleural fluid is less than two-thirds of the upper normal limit for serum.[38] Exudative pleural effusions do not meet at least one of the above three criteria.

In recent years, other laboratory tests have been proposed to differentiate transudative from exudative pleural effusions. A pleural fluid total cholesterol less than 55 mgm/dl or pleural fluid/serum cholesterol ratio less than 0.3 has been used to identify transudates.[48,61] A serum–pleural effusion albumin gradient (serum albumin level minus pleural effusion albumin level) greater than or equal to 1.2 gm/dl is found in transudates, and exudates have a gradient less than 1.2 g/dl.[55] The ratio of the pleural fluid to total serum bilirubin has also been used with a ratio less than 0.6 for transudates and greater than or equal to 0.6 for exudates.[41] None of these measurements, however, has been shown to be superior to the protein and LDH criteria.[6,54]

In patients likely to have a transudative pleural effusion, the most cost-effective use of the laboratory is to measure the pleural fluid protein and LDH levels initially. If these show that the patient has a transudative pleural effusion, no further laboratory tests on the pleural fluid are indicated. If the patient has an exudative pleural effusion, then the remaining pleural fluid should have these additional tests requested: white blood cell count and differential; glucose; amylase; cytologic examination; and cultures for aerobic and anaerobic bacteria, mycobacteria, and fungi.

Pleural fluid chemical analysis and cell populations are important directives of the diagnostic sequence, although they rarely produce a specific diagnosis.[33,35] For example, a pleural fluid cell population with a high percentage of small lymphocytes suggests that the patient has pleural tuberculosis or pleural malignancy and serves as an indication for a needle or thoracoscopic biopsy of the pleura.[64] Most patients who have more than 10 per-

TABLE 89-1
Differential Diagnosis of Nonmalignant Pleural Effusions

Transudative Pleural Effusions	*Exudative Pleural Effusions*
Congestive heart failure	Infectious diseases
Cirrhosis	Bacterial infections
Peritoneal dialysis	Tuberculosis
Nephrotic syndrome	Fungal infections
Superior vena cava obstruction	Viral infections
Myxedema	Parasitic infections
Pulmonary thromboemboli	Pulmonary thromboembolization
	Gastrointestinal disease
	Pancreatitis
	Esophageal perforation
	Intraabdominal abscesses
	Collagen vascular diseases
	Rheumatoid arthritis
	Lupus erythematosus
	Churg–Strauss syndrome
	Drug-induced pleural disease
	Nitrofurantoin
	Dantrolene
	Methysergide
	Bromocriptine
	Interleukin-2
	Procarbazine
	Amiodarone
	Asbestos exposure
	Chylothorax
	Hemothorax
	Postsurgical
	Abdominal surgery
	Coronary artery bypass
	Sarcoidosis
	Post-cardiac-injury (Dressler's) syndrome
	Uremic pleuritis
	Yellow nail syndrome

*Modified from Light.[33]

cent eosinophils in their pleural fluid have had either blood or air in their pleural spaces; if this is not the case, one should consider a drug reaction, paragonimiasis, or the Churg-Strauss syndrome.[29,33] A pleural fluid glucose below 60 mg/dl narrows the diagnostic possibilities to seven: parapneumonic effusion, malignant effusion, tuberculous effusion, rheumatoid effusion, hemothorax, paragonimiasis, or the Churg-Strauss syndrome.[33] An elevated pleural amylase limits the diagnostic possibilities to three: esophageal rupture, pancreatic disease, or malignant pleural effusion.[33] With esophageal rupture and malignant pleural effusion, the amylase present in the pleural fluid is a salivary type.[24] Depending on the patient, other tests are sometimes useful in determining the cause of a pleural effusion. For example, if a chylothorax is suspected, one should measure the level of triglycerides in the pleural fluid, and measurement of the adenosine deaminase (ADA) is useful in establishing the diagnosis of tuberculous pleuritis.[1]

IMAGING TECHNIQUES IN THE DIAGNOSIS AND MANAGEMENT OF PLEURAL EFFUSIONS

The appearance of pleural fluid on plain chest radiographs may be confusing at times.[51,56] Large amounts of subpulmonic fluid may simulate an elevated diaphragm or subphrenic abscess, and free fluid within the fissure mimics a parenchymal mass. Fluid along the mediastinum may be interpreted as representing a mediastinal mass. These various possibilities frequently can be sorted by the use of computerized tomography (CT) scan of the thorax (Figs. 89-1, 89-2). CT is of great value in distinguishing between parenchymal and pleural disease and is frequently used to separate subpleural lung abscess from an air-containing intrapleural infection. A bolus injection of intravenous contrast medium can sometimes result in significant enhancement of unaerated lung parenchyma and aid in the differentiation.

Recent years have seen an increase in the use of sonography in the management of pleural effusions.[65] Chest sonography has long been used to guide aspiration of small or loculated effusions. Sonography has also been used to find chest wall tumors and provide guidance for biopsy of an area of focal pleural involvement. More recently, criteria have been developed for high-frequency real time sonography recognition of exudates.[65] Exudative pleural effusions typically show complex septated, complex nonseptated, or homogeneously echogenic patterns. Sonographic findings of a thickened pleura and associated parenchymal lesions in the lung are also indicative of an exudate. Homogeneous echogenic effusions are usually hemorraghic or empyema. Transudates are most frequently anechoic, but an anechoic effusion may be either a transudate or an exudate. Sonographic demonstration of an extensively loculated pleural collection usually indicates a poor chance of resolution with thoracentesis or chest tube placement and points to the possible need for more aggressive pleural space drainage procedures.

PARAPNEUMONIC EFFUSIONS AND/OR EMPYEMA

The most common cause of an exudative pleural effusion is pneumonia. Forty percent of the more than 1 million patients in the United States who have bacterial pneumonia each year will have

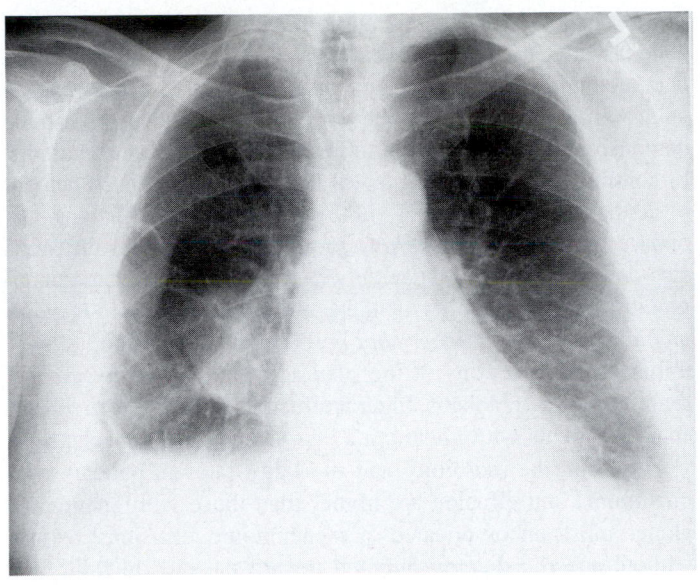

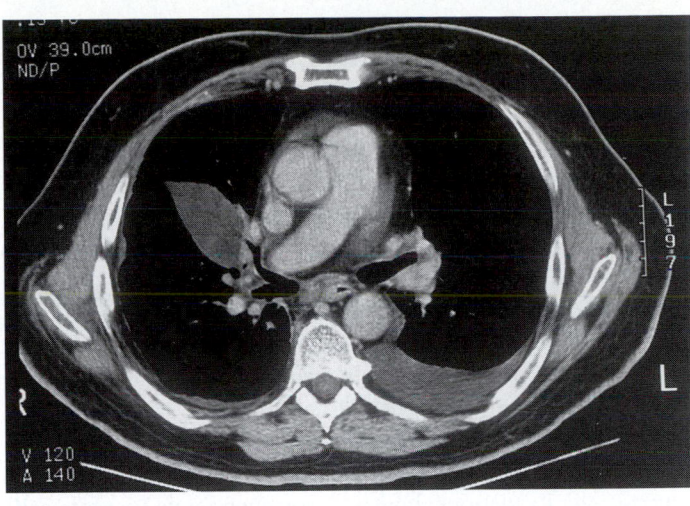

B

A

FIGURE 89-1 *A.* Chest radiograph of a 71-year-old man with insulin-dependent diabetes mellitus and coronary artery disease. Nine years previously, the patient had had a right upper lobectomy for bronchogenic carcinoma. He presents with sudden onset of severe shortness of breath and a PA chest radiograph which shows a right mid-lung mass and multilobulated pleural collection. *B.* Thoracic CT scan revealed the right mid-lung mass to be a loculated pleural fluid collection and the presence of a left-sided pleural effusion. Thoracentesis demonstrated the pleural fluid to be a transudate. With diuresis, the chest radiograph showed complete clearing of the abnormalities. The asymmetric distribution of fluid in the right pleural space was due to the patient's previous thoracotomy and pleural adhesions.

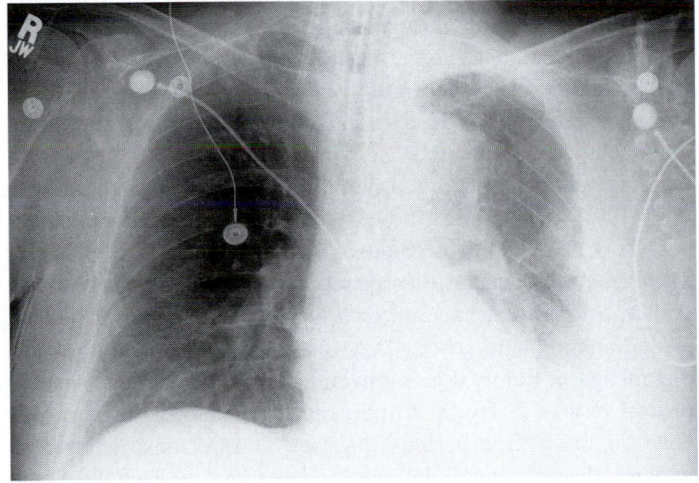

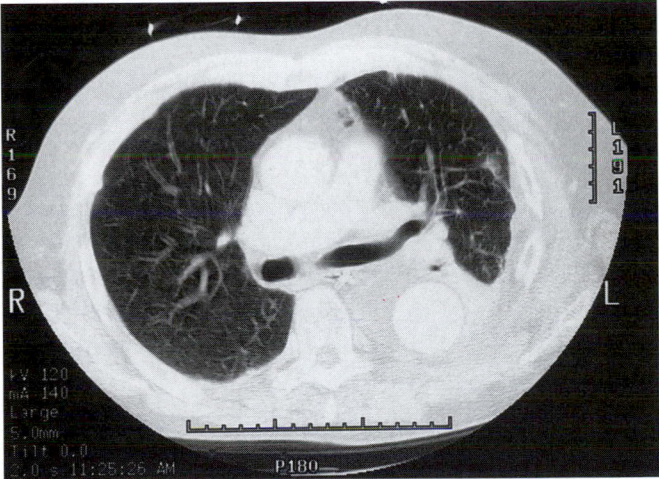

A

B

FIGURE 89-2 *A.* Supine postoperative chest radiograph of 70-year-old man with a chronic dissecting aneurysm of the thoracic aortic repaired by resection and placement of a graft. The radiograph demonstrated diffuse opacification of the left lung compatible with a pleural effusion layering posteriorly. *B.* A CT scan of the chest showed the opacification to be clot surrounding the graft and extending to the left lateral chest wall. No pleural fluid was identified.

a pleural effusion.[34,37] The possibility of a parapneumonic effusion should be considered each time a patient with an acute pneumonia is evaluated. Most parapneumonic effusions are small, but if the depth of the effusion is greater than 10 mm on the decubitus chest radiograph, a diagnostic thoracentesis should be strongly considered.

Pleural effusions secondary to pneumonia arise from an inflammatory process contiguous to the visceral pleura.[34] The effusion derives from fluid entering the lung interstices, transversing the visceral pleura, and accumulating when the rate of accrual exceeds the capacity of the parietal pleural lymphatics to remove fluid. The fluid initially has a low white blood cell count, low concentration of lactic dehydrogenase (LDH), normal concentration of glucose, pH greater than 7.3, and no demonstrable bacteria. This is an "uncomplicated parapneumonic effusion." If appropriate antibiotic therapy for the pulmonary infection is initiated at this stage, the effusion usually does not progress, pleural drainage is frequently unnecessary, and the pleural process reverses with antibiotic therapy. However, if the infection in the pulmonary parenchyma is unchecked, the infectious agent invades the pleural space to create an empyema. Once bacterial infection has involved the pleural space, the effusion rapidly increases in size with an increase in the number of polymorphonuclear leukocytes and fall in pleural fluid pH and glucose.[57] At this point, fibrin frequently is deposited in the pleural space forming semipermeable barriers that envelop or loculate the infected area and lead to regional variation in the composition of pleural fluid (Fig. 89-3). In the region of bacterial proliferation, white blood cells are actively phagocytosing bacteria, and the resultant oxidative burst results in increased production of CO_2 with lowering of the pH and increased consumption of glucose. Neighboring compartments equilibrate glucose and CO_2 across the semipermeable loculations producing a low pH and glucose; the loculations, however, are impervious to white cells and bacteria (Fig. 89-3). Sampling the infected space demonstrates pus and/or bacteria and establishes a diagnosis of empyema thoracis. Fluid from neighboring loculations demonstrates a low pH and low glucose but no bacteria. The latter identifies a complicated parapneumonia effusion and strongly suggests adjacent pleural infection and the possible need for pleural space drainage.[18,21]

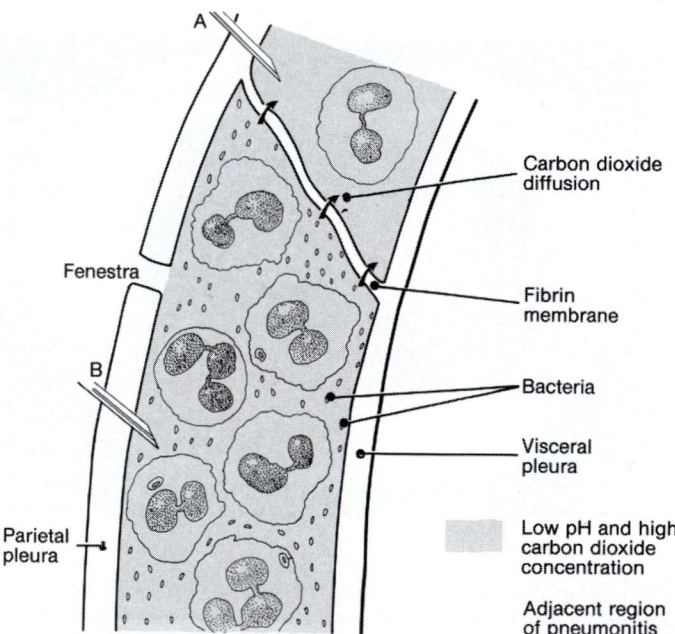

FIGURE 89-3 Compartmentalization of pleural fluid in empyema resulting from inflammation and the formation of semipermeable fibrin membranes. In compartment B of the schematic, bacteria and polymorphonuclear leukocytes abound; pleural fluid sampled from this area will be culture-positive and have an elevated white cell count, low pH, and decreased glucose level. The fibrin membrane prevents migration of bacteria and polymorphonuclear leukocytes to the adjacent compartment A. However, the semipermeable membrane permits diffusion of carbon dioxide from compartment B to compartment A, and glucose diffusion from A to B. Thus, fluid taken from compartment A, although sterile and with a low polymorphonuclear leukocyte count, will have a low pH and glucose, indicating the presence of neighboring infection.

The incidence of parapneumonic effusions and empyema depends, in part, on the infecting organism.[34] For example, a parapneumonic effusion occurs in 50 percent of *Streptococcus pneumoniae* infections of the lung, but the organism can be demonstrated in pleural fluid in fewer than 5 percent of patients. In contrast, culture of the pleural fluid is positive in 20 percent of adults and 80 percent of children with pleural effusions secondary to *Staphylococcus aureus* infections. Pleural effusions also develop in 40 to 50 percent of gram-negative aerobic pneumonias, and the majority of these are culture-positive. *Pseudomonas* species and *Escherichia coli* account for more than two-thirds of all infections of the pleural space caused by aerobic gram-negative organisms. Pleural effusions occur in 30 to 50 percent of patients with pneumonia due to *Legionella* species.

Although the morbidity and mortality rates in patients with pneumonia and effusion are higher than those with pneumonia alone, most uncomplicated parapneumonic effusions resolve without specific therapy directed toward the pleural fluid. Ten percent or less ultimately require pleural drainage for resolution.

An uncomplicated parapneumonic effusion that enlarges in the face of antibiotic therapy, particularly if it causes respiratory discomfort, requires drainage. In some instances, thoracentesis will suffice; however, most patients require a large-diameter (26 to 30 French) chest tube for adequate drainage. The tube should be positioned in the dependent portion of the effusion and connected to an underwater seal drainage system. If the patient fails to improve clinically and radiographically within 48 h, ultrasonic examination of the pleural space is performed to detect undrained loculated fluid; if a pocket is identified, additional chest tubes should be inserted. Decortication and/or open drainage are rarely needed in the management of an uncomplicated parapneumonic effusion.

Direct extension of a pulmonary parenchymal infection into the pleural space causes more than half the cases of empyema; postsurgical infection accounts for an additional 20 percent.[34] Empyema also occurs after penetrating or blunt trauma to the thorax. Sometimes, bacteria from abdominal infection, such as a subdiaphragmatic abscess, cross the diaphragm and enter the pleural space. Rarely does empyema complicate thoracentesis or pleural biopsy. Sixty to 70 percent of patients with empyema have an underlying serious disease. Chronic obstructive pulmonary disease and pulmonary neoplasm are each found in approximately one-third of patients with empyema. Other associated illnesses include alcoholism, diabetes, esophageal disease, and disorders of the central nervous system that lead to aspiration of oropharyngeal contents.

The symptoms of empyema are usually nonspecific. Eighty percent of patients have dyspnea and fever, and 70 percent complain of cough or chest pain.[34] However, some patients with empyema present with only constitutional complaints, such as weight loss, fatigue, and malaise. Evidence of fluid in the pleural space is the principal radiographic finding; most empyema patients also have a recognizable parenchymal infiltrate.

The bacteriology of empyema has changed considerably in the past 50 years.[3,62] Prior to the availability of antibiotics, *S. pneumoniae* and *Streptococcus pyogenes* accounted for most pleural infections. After the use of penicillin became widespread

Labels for Figure 89-3: A · Carbon dioxide diffusion · Fenestra · Fibrin membrane · B · Bacteria · Visceral pleura · Parietal pleura · Low pH and high carbon dioxide concentration · Adjacent region of pneumonitis

in the 1940s, *S. aureus* succeeded *S. pneumoniae* and *S. pyogenes* as the major cause of empyema.[62] Since the advent of β-lactamase-resistant semisynthetic penicillins in the early 1960s, the incidence of staphylococcal empyema has decreased, and infections due to anaerobic bacteria and aerobic gram-negative rods have increased markedly.[3]

Anaerobic organisms are now isolated from up to 75 percent of patients with empyema; about one-half of the isolates consist of only anaerobic organisms and the other one-half of mixed anaerobic and aerobic organisms.[3] Approximately 75 percent of patients with empyema have multiple infecting organisms, averaging three bacterial species per patient.[3] Anaerobic bacteria in the pleural space may originate in the mouth or from a subphrenic source via transdiaphragmatic spread or, less commonly, reach the pleura via the bloodstream. Carious teeth or advanced periodontal disease should alert the clinician to the possibility of anaerobic infection. In children with empyema, the coagulase-positive staphylococcus remains the predominant causative organism; anaerobic organisms are rare in patients younger than 18 years. Despite careful sampling and meticulous culturing, pleural fluids are culture-negative in up to 20 percent of patients with empyema.

The mortality from empyema is formidable, ranging from 11 to 50 percent, depending on the patient population.[33] Contributing to a poor prognosis in patients with empyema are underlying pulmonary disease, especially neoplasm, persistent systemic symptoms, gram-negative bacterial infection, and advanced age.

A good outcome demands prompt recognition, appropriate antibiotic therapy, and adequate pleural drainage. Apart from reducing the risk of sepsis, early antibiotic therapy also decreases the degree of residual pleural fibrosis. The initial choice of antibiotics depends on the results of the Gram stain of pleural fluid and sputum. Antibiotics should be modified when the results of the cultures become available and the in vitro sensitivity patterns of the infecting bacteria are determined. In most patients in whom empyema is suspected, empiric antibiotic therapy is started immediately, i.e., without waiting 24 to 48 h to learn the results from culture. Until proved otherwise, anaerobic involvement is presumed, and an antibiotic that is effective against this group of organisms is started. For patients with empyema thoracis from community-acquired infection, the second-generation cephalosporins, cefotetan or cefoxitin, provide coverage against most aerobic gram-positive cocci, anaerobic bacteria including bacteroides species, and some gram-negative rods (*Hemophilus* species, *Klebsiella* species, *E. coli* and *Enterobacter* species). In the absence of a positive gram stain, erythromycin 2 g daily should be added to cover *Legionella* species and *Chlamydia pneumoniae*. For nosocomial infections, broader coverage is recommended, such as imipenem plus gentamicin. Initially, the antibiotics are administered parenterally. However, should the infection prove to be caused by highly susceptible organisms, oral antibiotics are often substituted after the empyema is adequately drained and signs of sepsis resolved. The duration of antibiotic therapy depends on the individual response. As a rule, antibiotics are continued until (1) the patient is afebrile and the white blood cell count is normal, (2) the tube thoracostomy drainage yields less than 50 ml of fluid daily, and (3) the radiograph shows con-

siderable clearing. Typically, 3 to 6 weeks of antibiotic therapy is required to achieve these results.

Prompt external drainage of infected pleural fluid collections is a mainstay of treatment (Fig. 89-4). However, the optimal method of establishing external drainage remains controversial. Therapeutic options include (1) thoracentesis, (2) non-image-guided chest tube placement, (3) image-guided catheter drainage, (4) thoracotomy with debridement and directed chest tube placement, (5) thoracotomy with pleural decortication, and (6) video-assisted thoracoscopic pleural surgery.

Drainage of pleural collections is indicated in all patients with empyema thoracis. The criteria for drainage of a complicated parapneumonic effusion have been more difficult to establish.[49] Efforts to identify pleural fluid pH, glucose and LDH values that mandate pleural fluid drainage have been unsuccessful. Although pleural fluid pH less than 7.2, glucose less than 40 mg/dl and LDH greater than 1000 IU/l indicate a patient with increased risk for needing pleural drainage, the decision must be individualized. Some patients meeting these criteria may be cured with antibiotics, but most will require pleural drainage for successful resolution of their illness.[5]

Percutaneous drainage is most effective in patients with a short duration of symptoms, free-flowing or unilocular parapneumonic effusions, absence of a thick pleural peel on sonography or CT scans, and fluid that can be aspirated easily by needle. Chest tube placement with or without image guidance is usually the initial procedure. Sonography or CT can accurately guide drainage catheter placement, with sonography the procedure of choice.[28] Catheters ranging from 24 to 30 Fr in outer diameter may be placed under imaging guidance. Radiologically guided pleural drainage procedures have success rates that are slightly increased over that of non-image-guided chest tube drainage.

Once the patient's condition has improved, a decision has to be made about when to remove the chest tube. Criteria for tube removal are: (1) system signs of infection are controlled—usually after 7 to 10 days of therapy; (2) less than 50 ml of fluid is being drained per day; (3) the lung has expanded as fully as possible; and (4) if a bronchopleural fistula was present, it has sealed. Should the volume of unfilled pleural space as determined by contrast agents injected through the chest tube exceed 100 ml, reexpansion of the lung should be attempted before removing the chest tube. To do so sometimes requires the placement of an additional chest tube.

Successful percutaneous tube drainage of an empyema or complicated parapneumonic effusion should see clinical and radiologic improvement in 48 h. If the patient fails to improve, the drainage is either inadequate or, much less commonly, antibiotic selection is incorrect. In patients with inadequate drainage, the choices are: (1) percutaneous insertion of additional chest tubes; (2) intrapleural injection of a fibrinolytic agent; or (3) thoracotomy with digital lysis of adhesions, operative placement of chest tubes with or without decortication.

In 20 to 30 percent of patients with thoracic empyema, antibiotics and drainage with percutaneous chest tubes fail to control the infection. In these patients, thoracotomy with digital lysis of adhesions and operative placement of chest tubes should be strongly considered. Procrastination in moving to thoracot-

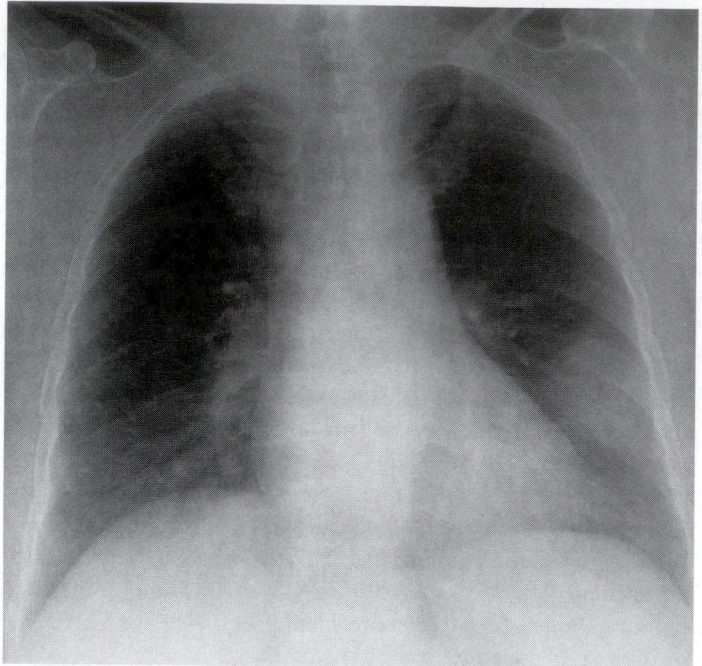

A

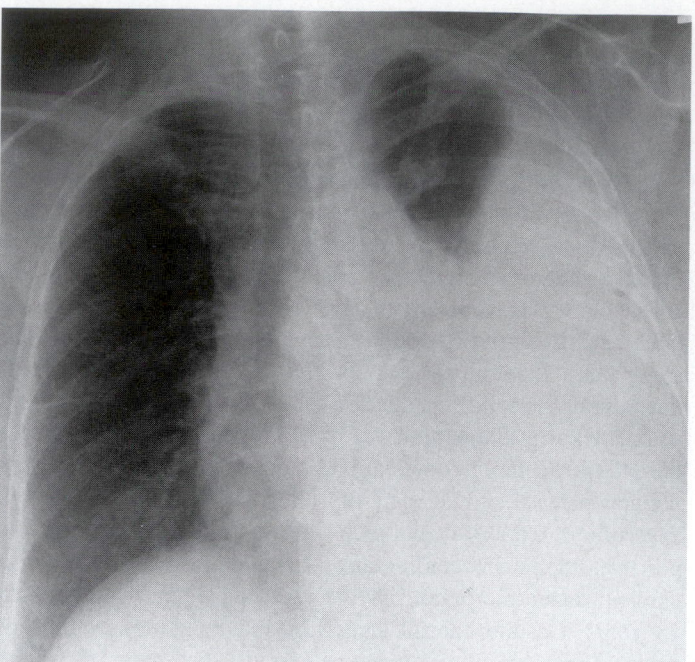

B

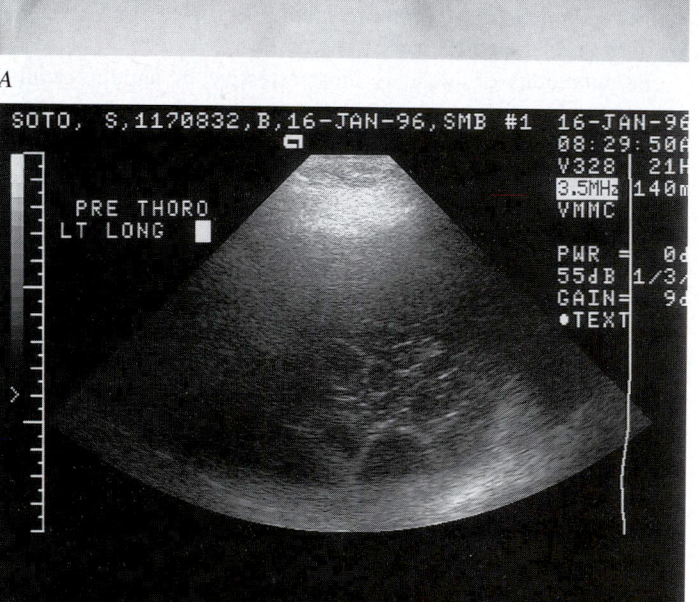

C

D

FIGURE 89-4 *A.* Chest radiograph of a 63-year-old woman with left lower lobe pneumonitis. *B.* The patient developed a large left-sided pleural effusion despite five days of oral antibiotic therapy. *C.* Sono- graphic study of the pleural space showed marked septation throughout the fluid collection. *D.* Adequate drainage was established with thora- cotomy, digital lysis of adhesions, and operative placement of a chest tube.

omy is a common error. Thoracotomy frequently returns the patient to good health most quickly. Decortication is used only for control of pleural infection. It is not used in patients in whom the infection is controlled, but the pleura remains persistently thickened; this type of thickening usually resolves spontaneously over several months (Fig. 89-5).

Experience is growing that demonstrates that intrapleural streptokinase or urokinase can dissolve fibrin membranes and facilitate drainage of the pleural space.[19,50] Either 250,000 units of streptokinase or 100,000 units of urokinase diluted in 100 ml

of normal saline solution can be injected directly through a chest tube into the pleural space. The chest tube is then clamped for 4 h. This form of therapy can be repeated daily up to 14 days, depending on the rapidity of improvement. Successful response is indicated by an increase in the amount of chest tube drainage, radiographic improvement, and decrease in the systemic signs of infection.

Adequate pleural drainage is particularly crucial in an empyema that is accompanied by a bronchopleural fistula. Undrained pleural fluid can spill through the fistula into the lung

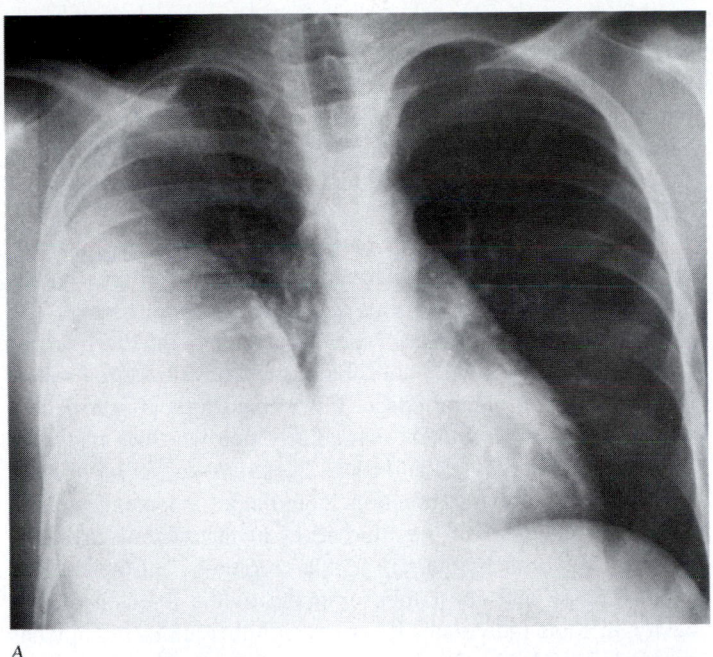

A

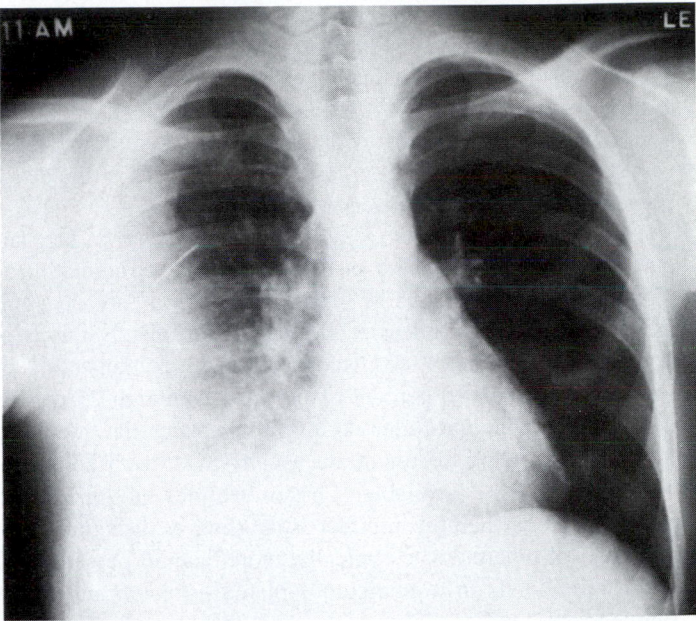

B

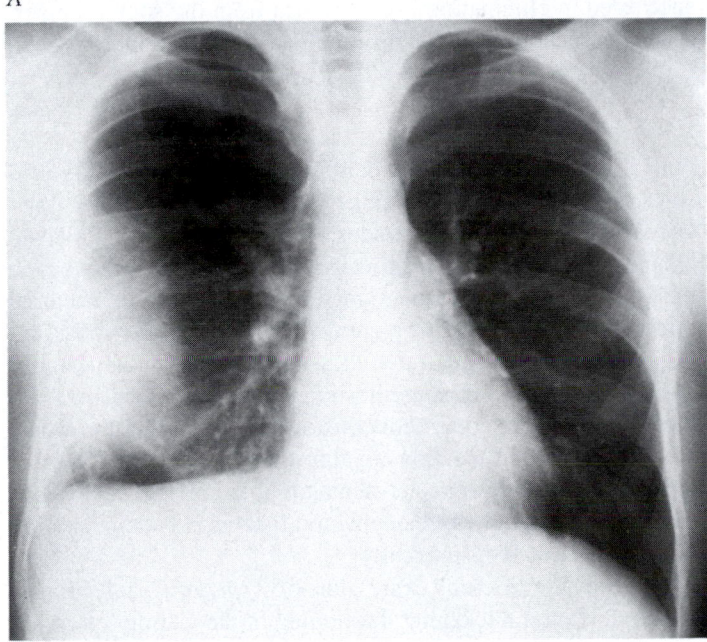

C

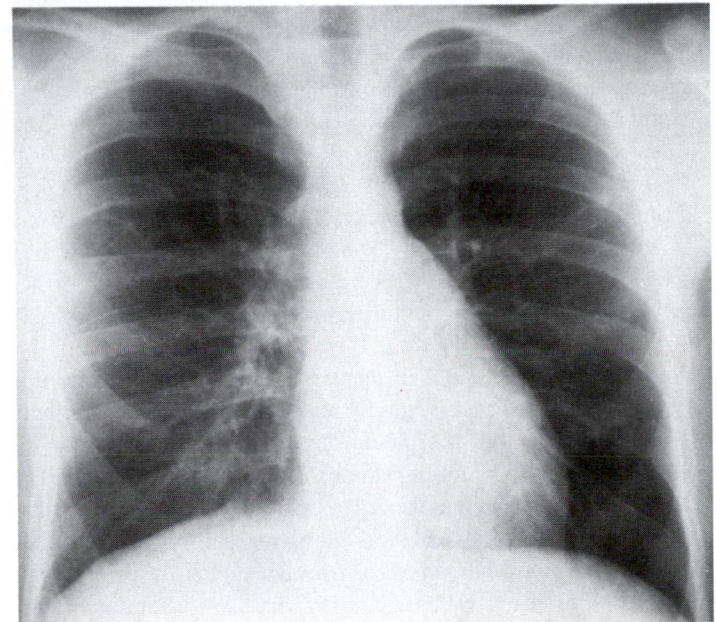

D

FIGURE 89-5 The course of pneumococcal empyema in a 16-year-old immunocompetent patient. *A.* When first seen, the patient has a large volume of loculated pleural fluid with distinct anterior and posterior margins and a meniscus high up on the lateral chest wall forming an obtuse angle between the pleural density and the adjacent parenchyma.

B. Five days after tube thoracostomy the volume of pleural fluid is reduced by over 50 percent. *C.* One month after chest tube removal the patient remains free of symptoms of infection, but significant loculated pleural density remains. *D.* Three months later the pleural abnormality has totally resolved, and the chest radiograph is normal.

and cause a diffuse pneumonitis. A bronchopleural fistula is suspected when the chest radiographs show pleural air-fluid levels and when a patient raises more sputum than anticipated, especially when the production of sputum is position-dependent.

TUBERCULOUS PLEURAL EFFUSIONS

In the United States, tuberculosis is responsible for approximately 2 percent of all pleural effusions.[14] Although usually considered a chronic illness, one-third of patients with tuberculous

pleuritis have an acute illness of less than 1 week duration, and two-thirds seek medical attention within 1 month of the time of onset of symptoms.[32] Nonproductive cough, pleuritic chest pain, and fever occur in most patients; however, as many as 15 percent of patients may be afebrile. Patients with chronic infection frequently present with weight loss, malaise, and dyspnea.

Tuberculous effusions are usually unilateral and moderate in size. In approximately one-third of patients with tuberculous pleural effusions, coexisting parenchymal disease is evident radiographically. If there is no radiographic evidence of parenchymal disease, the infection usually signifies primary tuberculosis. In 65 percent of patients with tuberculous pleuritis in whom the effusion resolves spontaneously, symptomatic parenchymal disease will occur within 12 months.[53] In 30 percent of patients with tuberculous pleural effusion, the *initial* tuberculin skin test is negative. However, a repeat test, within 8 weeks of the development of symptoms, is invariably positive.

A tuberculous effusion is usually serous, may be serosanguineous, but almost never is frankly bloody. Examination of pleural fluid is diagnostic of tuberculosis only if mycobacteria are demonstrated by smear or culture. Unfortunately this is an uncommon occurrence as mycobacteria are demonstrable on smear in less than 10 percent of patients. Although 25 percent of tuberculous pleural fluids do reveal mycobacteria on culture, decisions regarding treatment are usually made well before the culture results are available. Certain features of tuberculous pleural fluid are helpful in either supporting or discounting the diagnosis of tuberculosis. Typically, more than 50 percent of all white blood cells in a tuberculous pleural effusion are mature lymphocytes, and a differential count that reveals more than 80 percent mature lymphocytes strongly suggests either tuberculosis or malignancy. The eosinophil count rarely exceeds 10 percent in tuberculous pleural fluid. Mesothelial cells are rare; indeed, more than 5 percent mesothelial cells in the differential count argues strongly against a tuberculous etiology. A pleural effusion ADA greater than 70 IU/l has shown a sensitivity of 98 percent and specificity of 96 percent for the diagnosis of pleural tuberculosis.[1] Increased ADA levels have also been found in patients with malignancy or empyema, and histologic or bacteriologic confirmation of tuberculosis remains a necessity. The total protein content of the tuberculous effusion tends to be quite high; values above 5 g/dl suggest a tuberculous effusion. The concentration of glucose in pleural fluid is usually greater than 60 mg/dl; the pH varies widely and is of little diagnostic help.

Needle biopsy of the pleura demonstrates granuloma in approximately 80 percent of patients.[30] Pleural tuberculosis is the only nonneoplastic pleural exudate *readily* diagnosed by a pleural biopsy. Culture of the pleural biopsy is helpful as well since *Mycobacterium tuberculosis* can be isolated from over 85 percent of biopsies.[30] Although other diseases, including fungal infection, sarcoidosis, and rheumatoid arthritis, may produce granulomatous pleuritis, more than 95 percent of patients with demonstrable pleural granuloma have tuberculosis.[34]

Even though pleural biopsy and pleural fluid examination fail to substantiate the diagnosis of tuberculosis, empiric antituberculous therapy is appropriate in certain patients. A positive tuberculin skin test in a patient less than 40 years old, in combination with a pleural fluid analysis that is compatible with tuberculosis, is an indication for empiric antituberculous therapy. In contrast, the patient with a suspected tuberculous pleural effusion who is more than 40 years old and who has risk factors for bronchogenic carcinoma should be subjected to thoracoscopy or open pleural biopsy rather than to empiric therapy. The absence of granulomatous inflammation in the open pleural biopsy of a tuberculin-positive patient virtually excludes the diagnosis of tuberculosis and obviates the need for antituberculous therapy.

With antituberculous therapy, the average patient becomes afebrile within 2 weeks; occasionally, fever persists for as long

as 2 months. Radiographic clearing usually occurs in 6 to 12 weeks. Tuberculous effusions may be accompanied by pleural thickening, but the thickening usually undergoes striking resolution in response to antituberculous therapy.[2] Fibrothorax is rare. Therefore, consideration of decortication for pleural thickening should be delayed until the patient has had at least 6 months of antituberculous therapy.

Tuberculosis in the form of pleural disease sometimes becomes manifest in a patient in whom long-dormant tuberculous disease reactivates and forms a bronchopleural fistula. The patient then usually produces sputum and develops fever, sometimes in conjunction with chest pain; most have bacterial superinfections of the pleural space. Empyema thoracis in a patient with previous tuberculosis, particularly one who has never received chemotherapy, should rouse the strong suspicion of reactivation of tuberculous infection. The diagnosis is suggested by the development of an air-fluid level in the pleural cavity. A tuberculous bronchopleural fistula requires antituberculous chemotherapy and chest tube drainage of the infected pleural cavity. In some individuals in whom antituberculous therapy has succeeded in eliminating mycobacteria from the sputum, a persistent bronchopleural fistula requires decortication for relief.

FUNGAL PLEURAL EFFUSIONS

Fungal diseases account for only 1 percent of all pleural effusions.[34] The most common cause is *Aspergillus* infection (usually *A. fumigatus*) which invades the pleural cavity via a bronchopleural fistula complicating lung resection or reactivation tuberculosis. The signs and symptoms mimic chronic bacterial infection of the pleura. In pleural fluid, clumps of hyphae appear as brown suspended particles, and their gross appearance raises a suspicion of aspergillosis. In patients with pleural aspergillosis, precipitating antibodies in the serum and the wheal and flare cutaneous reaction are almost always positive. Optimal therapy consists of surgical evacuation of the pleural cavity, closure or excision of the bronchopleural fistula, and administration of amphotericin B systemically.

An entirely different expression of *Aspergillus* infection is localized pleural thickening developing in the vicinity of an *Aspergillus* mycetoma. This is considered in detail elsewhere (see Chapter 147). However, it is worth emphasizing that occasionally in patients with chronic cavitary or cystic parenchymal disease the *initial* radiographic feature of *Aspergillus* infection is focal pleural fibrosis followed, months later, by a mycetoma in the abnormal adjacent parenchyma.

Approximately 20 percent of patients with acute *Coccidioides immitis* infection show evidence of pleural disease on the chest radiograph, and 70 percent complain of pleuritic chest pain.[33] Free fluid in the pleural cavity is demonstrable in approximately 7 percent of patients. The patients are almost always febrile, and about one-half have either erythema nodosum or erythema multiforme. In about 50 percent of patients, parenchymal infiltrates accompany the pleural effusion.[33] The effusions are usually unilateral. Examination of the pleural fluid reveals a predominance of lymphocytes on the white cell count, a glucose concentration greater than 60 mg/dl, and, rarely, eosinophilia. Pleural fluid cultures are positive for *C. immitis* in 20 percent of patients; culture of the pleural biopsy specimen has a much higher yield.[33] Complement fixation titers higher than 1:16 are common even when the disease is not disseminated. Most patients with primary coccidioidomycosis and pleural effusion do not require systemic antifungal therapy.

Cryptococcosis is another rare cause of pleural effusion. Pleural cryptococcosis appears to result from extension of a primary subpleural cryptococcal infection into the pleural space. More than half of the patients have serious underlying disease, most often either leukemia, lymphoma, or the acquired immunodeficiency syndrome. The pleural effusion is usually unilateral; cultures are positive for the organism in approximately 50 percent of patients.[33,34] Cryptococcal pleural effusions have high titers of cryptococcal antigen. Patients with serious coexisting disease should receive amphotericin B and 5-fluorocytosine. However, immunocompetent patients may recover without specific therapy.

Histoplasmosis rarely produces pleural effusions, i.e., less than 1 percent of patients with histoplasmosis manifest pleural fluid radiographically. Treatment is unnecessary, since the effusion usually resolves spontaneously in several weeks.

VIRAL PLEURAL EFFUSIONS

Pleural effusions occur in approximately 10 percent of patients with adenovirus infections.[33,34] On rare occasions, pleural effusions also occur with infections due to influenza virus, cytomegalovirus, herpes simplex virus, Epstein-Barr virus, and infectious hepatitis. The true incidence of viral infections causing pleural effusions is unknown. Rarely is a particular viral agent identified, so the diagnosis of viral pleural effusion is almost invariably one of exclusion. Many self-limited effusions probably represent undiagnosed viral infections; these would account for approximately 10 to 15 percent of the total of all effusions. A pleural fluid cell count usually reveals a predominance of mononuclear cells.

PARASITIC INFECTIONS OF THE PLEURAL SPACE

Amebic liver abscess is the most common extraintestinal site of infection by E. histolytica.[33] In turn, pleural pulmonary amebiasis is the most common complication of amebic liver abscess and usually due to the erosion of the abscess through the diaphragm to involve the pleural space or lung parenchyma. Serous or sympathetic pleural effusions and atelectasis are common accompaniments of liver abscesses and do not indicate extension of disease. Patients with pleural pulmonary complications present with cough, pleuritic pain, and dyspnea. Empyema due to rupture of the abscess into the pleural cavity presents with sudden respiratory distress and pain and has a substantial mortality. In some instances, a hepatobronchial fistula forms and has been associated with spontaneous drainage of the hepatic abscess. The diagnosis of amebic abscess is suggested by the discovery of "anchovy paste" or "chocolate sauce" pleural fluid. E. histolytica is usually demonstrable in the pleural collection. Treatment consists of metronidazole 750 mg po TID for 5 to 10 days plus

diloxanide furoate 500 mg 3 times a day for 10 days for intraluminal infection.

Human infection by the lung fluke Paragonimus westermani is widely distributed in Africa, Asia, and South America.[33,34] The cercariae are ingested orally, transit the intestinal wall, and migrate through the peritoneal cavity across the diaphragm into the pleural cavities and then into the lungs, where they ultimately lodge. The clinical manifestations of paragonimiasis are eosinophilia and chest complaints, including a cough productive of brown sputum with intermittent hemoptysis. Up to half of patients will have pleural effusions, and in some they may be quite large. The characteristics of the pleural fluid with paragonimiasis are unique in that the glucose is less than 10 mg/dl, the LDH level is above 1000 IU/l, the pH is below 7.1, and the differential count reveals a high percentage of eosinophils.[34] The diagnosis is established by demonstrating the presence of operculated eggs in sputum or feces. A serum complement fixation test is also available and helpful.

The hydatid cysts of E. granulosus form in the liver in 50 to 70 percent of patients and in the lung of 20 to 30 percent of patients.[33] Pleural disease develops when either a hepatic or parenchymal lung cyst ruptures into the pleural space. The patient develops an acute illness with severe chest pain, dyspnea, and sometimes shock, secondary to severe allergic reactions to parasitic antigens suddenly released. The diagnosis is established by recognition of daughter cysts in the pleural fluid. Optimal treatment is surgical resection to drain the pleural space and removal of the original cyst.

PULMONARY EMBOLI

Pleural effusions occur in 30 to 50 percent of patients with pulmonary emboli.[7] Different mechanisms have been postulated to account for the pathogenesis of pleural effusion in these patients and to account for the fact that about 25 percent of the effusions are transudates and about 75 percent are exudates.[7] This topic is covered in detail in Chapter 84.

PANCREATITIS

Approximately 20 percent of patients with acute pancreatitis develop pleural effusions.[34] Although most of the effusions are unilateral and left-sided, the effusion is sometimes bilateral and occasionally only right-sided. The effusion results from contact of the pleura with enzyme-rich peripancreatic fluid that gains access to the pleural space, most commonly via transdiaphragmatic lymphatics, and less often, through a sinus tract between a pancreatic pseudocyst and the pleural space. Rarely, pancreatic fluid can transverse the aortic and esophageal hiatuses into the mediastinum, where an inflammatory response may evoke a mediastinal pseudocyst.[34]

Usually the symptoms of pancreatitis (abdominal pain, nausea, and vomiting) dominate the clinical picture. At times, however, pleuritic chest pain and dyspnea may be the presenting complaint. The diagnosis is established by demonstrating abnormally high levels of amylase in the pleural fluid. The pleural fluid amylase is invariably higher than the serum amylase in pancreatitis-induced pleural effusions, usually with a ratio of 6:1 or more.

High levels of amylase in pleural fluid are not necessarily diagnostic of pancreatic disease; similar increments also occur after esophageal rupture into the pleura and occasionally with a malignant pleural effusion. About 10 percent of patients with malignant pleural effusions have high levels of amylase in their pleural fluids. However, the degree of increase is only slight to moderate in malignant effusions, and isoenzyme analysis will show the amylase to be salivary in type. The pleural fluid associated with pancreatitis is frequently serosanguineous and sometimes bloody. The concentration of glucose in the pleural fluid is normal, and the white blood cell count may vary from 1000 to 50,000 cells per cubic millimeter; as a rule, polymorphonuclear leukocytes predominate.

Pleural effusions secondary to pancreatitis usually resolve promptly as the pancreatic inflammation subsides. If resolution has not occurred within 2 weeks, the possibility of a pancreatic pseudocyst or abscess is likely. The frequency of pleural effusion increases to 40 to 50 percent with each of these complications. Should a sizeable effusion remain after 2 to 3 weeks of nasogastric suction, no oral intake, suppression of pancreatic secretion with atropine, and repeated thoracenteses, the abdomen should be explored surgically, looking for abscess, pseudocyst, and pancreaticopleural sinus. At the time of operation, a pancreatogram is performed to search for the sinus tract that can be ligated or excised. If no sinus is identified, careful dissection of the retroperitoneum in the region of the aortic and esophageal hiatus is undertaken in search of the tract.

ESOPHAGEAL PERFORATION

Approximately two-thirds of esophageal perforations occur as a complication of esophagoscopy.[26] This is particularly true when the procedure is performed in an attempt to remove a foreign body or to dilate an esophageal stricture. Other potential causes include esophageal carcinoma, gastric intubation, chest trauma, and finally, spontaneous rupture as a complication of vomiting (Boerhaave syndrome).

Perforation of the esophagus introduces oropharyngeal contents into the mediastinum, thereby evoking an acute mediastinitis.[39] The inflammatory reaction, in turn, often ruptures through the mediastinal pleura to produce a pleural effusion that is frequently complicated by a pneumothorax: Pleural effusions occur in approximately 60 percent of patients with esophageal perforation; 25 percent have a pneumothorax. The pleural effusion is usually left-sided but is sometimes right-sided or bilateral. Radiographic findings include widening of the mediastinum and pneumomediastinum. Most of the morbidity from esophageal perforation is due to the infection of the mediastinum and the pleural space by oropharyngeal bacterial flora. Clinical symptoms are dominated by chest pain that is usually quite severe. Hematemesis occurs in about half of the patients. Subcutaneous emphysema as a late manifestation occurs in about 10 percent of patients with esophageal rupture.

Examination of the pleural fluid reveals an exudative reaction: the amylase level is high, the pH is very low (frequently less than 6.0), squamous epithelial cells are present, and rarely, there may be ingested food particles. The amylase that has entered the pleural space through the esophageal defect is salivary rather than pancreatic. The treatment of choice for esophageal rupture is exploration of the mediastinum, primary repair of the esophageal tear, and drainage of the pleural space and mediastinum.[26,42]

INTRAABDOMINAL ABSCESS

A pleural effusion occurs in about 80 percent of patients with a subphrenic abscess.[34] The infection usually follows an intraabdominal surgical procedure; splenectomy and exploratory laparotomy for trauma are the more common antecedents. A surgically related subphrenic abscess usually becomes clinically evident 1 to 3 weeks postoperatively. Other predisposing illnesses include gastric, duodenal, or appendiceal perforation, diverticulitis, cholecystitis, pancreatitis, or trauma.

The pleural fluid is an exudate in which polymorphonuclear leukocytes predominate. The pleural fluid white blood count may be as high as 50,000 per cubic millimeter, but the pH is higher than 7.2, and the glucose concentration exceeds 60 mg/dl. It is uncommon for the pleural fluid to become infected.

The diagnosis of a subphrenic abscess is often first made on the basis of a routine chest or abdominal radiograph. An air-fluid level, below the diaphragm and outside the gastrointestinal tract, is demonstrable in about 70 percent of these patients.[34] Abdominal CT scans and ultrasound studies are very effective in diagnosing subphrenic abscesses. A CT-guided percutaneous aspiration of the subphrenic abscess is frequently helpful in finalizing the diagnosis and in identifying the responsible organisms prior to surgical drainage.

About 20 percent of patients with a hepatic abscess develop a pleural effusion; the effusion is usually, though not invariably, right-sided (Fig. 89-6).[34] Most of the patients manifest fever, abdominal pain, and abnormal liver function tests, especially an increase in the concentration of alkaline phosphatase in the blood. CT scanning of the abdomen is currently the most sensitive means of detection; definitive diagnosis can be made using CT scanning as a guide to percutaneous aspiration.

COLLAGEN VASCULAR DISEASES

Rheumatoid Arthritis

Pleural thickening and effusions are the most common pulmonary manifestations of rheumatoid arthritis.[17,22] They are frequently symptomatic and occur in 8 percent of men and 2 percent of women with rheumatoid arthritis in whom chest radiographs are made serially. Autopsy studies have revealed that 40 to 50 percent of patients with rheumatoid arthritis have histologic evidence of pleural disease.[17]

The onset of rheumatoid pleural disease is usually rapid, i.e., over weeks to 3 months, when symptoms reach their peak. Although in most patients pleural disease develops after the onset of joint symptoms, in about 5 percent the pleural disease precedes the arthritis; in another 15 percent, the onset of the pleural disease is simultaneous with the initial episode of synovitis.[22] The severity of arthritis, in terms of the number of joints involved or destruction on joint radiographs, does not correlate with the presence of pleural disease. However, the incidence of pleural

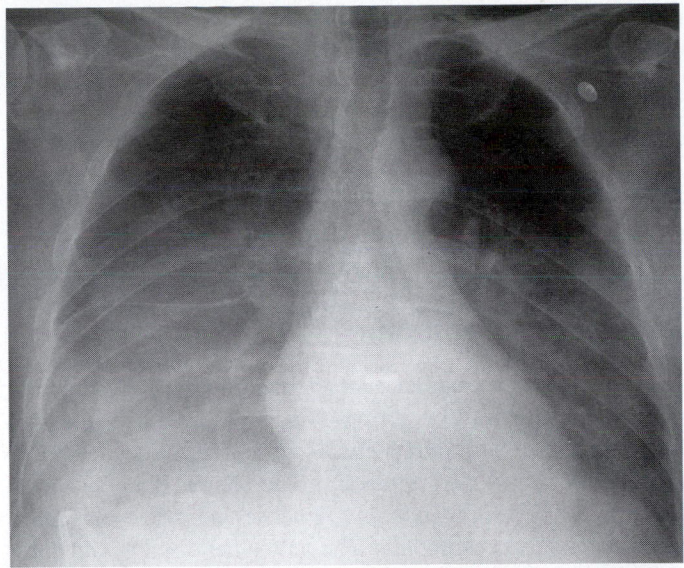

A

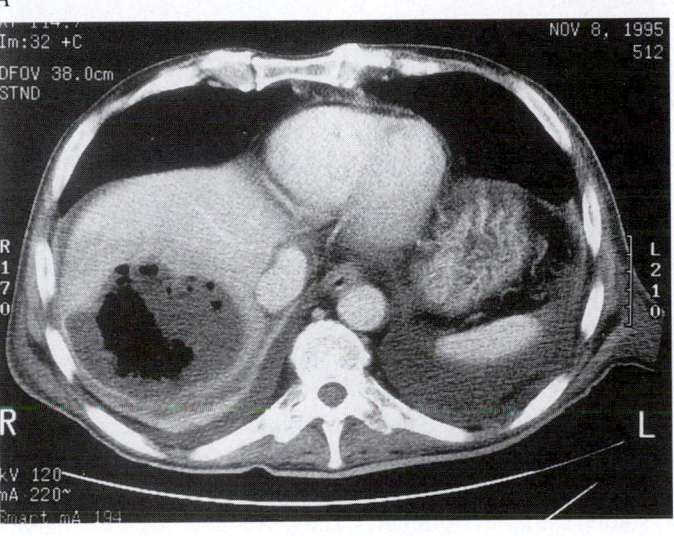

B

FIGURE 89-6 *A*. Chest radiograph of a 62-year-old man with insulin dependent diabetes mellitus and bilateral pleural effusions. *B*. The CT scan revealed a large abscess in the right lobe of the liver complicating chronic pancreatitis. The pleural fluid was an exudate and sterile. Aspirate of the hepatic abscess yielded *Enterococcal* species and *Clostridium* species.

effusions increases in those patients who have high titers of rheumatoid factor and subcutaneous nodules. In some patients, pericardial effusion occurs concurrently. About one-third of patients with rheumatoid pleural effusions have no respiratory symptoms. However, the others notice some combination of pleuritic chest pain, cough, dyspnea, or fever. Sometimes the joint symptoms flare coincident with the onset of the pleural syndrome.

The pleural effusions are usually small in volume but occasionally become large enough to produce respiratory compromise. Eighty percent of patients have a unilateral pleural effusion; in 20 percent, the effusions are bilateral.[22] Both intrapulmonary nodules and diffuse fibrosis sometimes accompany rheumatoid pleural disease. The nodules are often subpleural; at times, they undergo necrosis to produce a pyopneumothorax.

The pleural fluid in rheumatoid arthritis is usually an exudate; the concentration of total protein ranges from 3.5 to 6.0 g/dl and that of lactic dehydrogenase is high.[17] The predominant cell is either the polymorphonuclear leukocyte or, less often, the lymphocyte; a mixture of both cell types is not uncommon. In 80 percent of the patients, the concentration of glucose in the pleural fluid is less than 30 mg. The pH is usually less than 7.2, and the LDH concentration is greater than 700 units. In many patients, the ratio of pleural fluid complement to serum complement is less than 0.4. Pleural biopsy is usually nonspecific but rarely demonstrates pleural rheumatoid nodules that are diagnostic. For the most part, the etiologic diagnosis of the pleural effusion is one of exclusion.

Most patients can be treated with a nonsteroidal anti-inflammatory/analgesic medication such as aspirin, indomethacin, or ibuprofen. Only one-third of patients require systemic corticosteroids for pleural disease. The response to steroids is good, with symptomatic relief and control of pleural fluid volume occurring in more than 75 percent of those treated. The duration of active pleural inflammation is limited in most patients. Fifty percent of patients (both treated and untreated) undergo resolution of the pleural disease within 4 months of onset. Many are left with an asymptomatic, pleural density on chest radiograph. If the patient is asymptomatic and the pleural fluid has not recurred while off therapy for 6 months, the chance of recurrence of the pleural syndrome is small; fewer than 10 percent of patients develop a late recurrence. The postinflammatory pleural residuum is rarely clinically significant, but a few patients show a modest, i.e., 10 percent or less, reduction in vital capacity. An overt fibrothorax that produces symptomatic restrictive ventilatory disease and requires decortication is rare.

However, about 20 percent of the patients develop a chronic, persistent pleural syndrome that tends to flare when therapy is stopped.[22] The therapeutic goal should be symptomatic relief. The frequency of residual pleural fibrosis and restrictive ventilatory defects is higher in this group than in patients who undergo rapid spontaneous remission. There is little evidence to suggest that either nonsteroidal or corticosteroid therapy reduces the degree of long-term respiratory dysfunction. The majority of patients who experience chronic rheumatoid activity undergo remission of the pleural syndrome in 1 to 5 years.

Systemic Lupus Erythematosus (SLE)

Pleural effusions occur in up to 40 percent of patients with SLE (Fig. 89-7).[17,22] Even more have pleuritic chest pain without effusion at some time during the course of their illness. A comparable incidence of pleural effusions has been reported in drug-induced SLE.

In most patients with lupus pleuritis, arthritis or other symptoms precede the pleuritis; however, on occasion, the pleural disease comes first. The pleural effusions are small in volume and bilateral in about 50 percent of the patients; in the remainder, the incidence is about equally divided between the right and left sides.[22] In 20 percent of the patients, the effusions flit from side to side. Chest radiographs often show lesions other than the pleural effusions—parenchymal infiltrates, platelike atelectasis, and cardiomegaly due to either myocardiopathy or pericardial effusion or both.

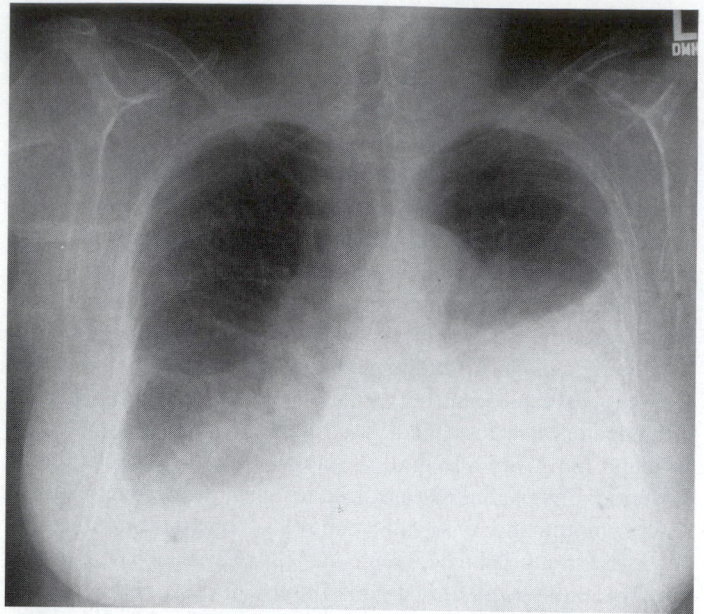

A

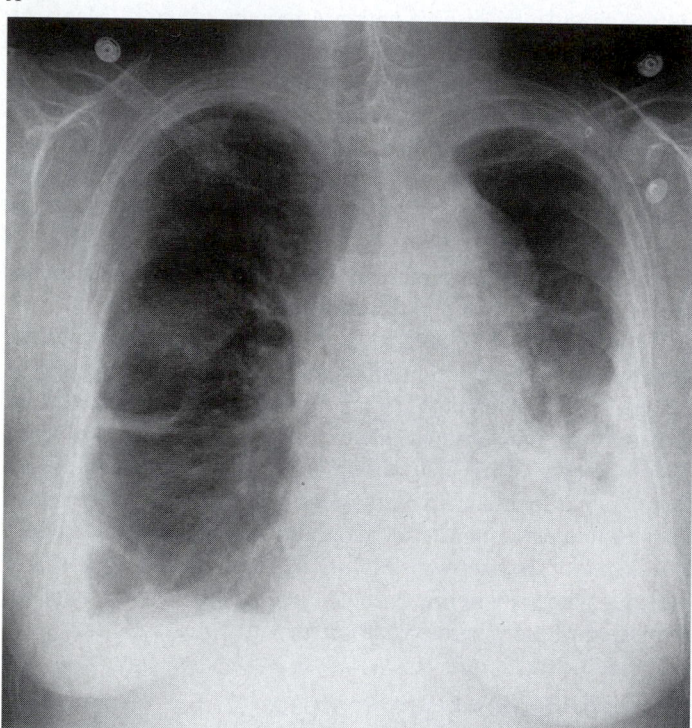

B

FIGURE 89-7   *A.* Chest radiograph of a 60-year-old woman with bilateral pleural effusions from systemic lupus erythematosus. The pleural fluid was an exudate with a pleural fluid to serum C4 ratio of 0.11, pleural fluid ANA titer 1:320, and pleural fluid/serum ANA ratio of 2:1. *B.* The pleural effusions ultimately required pleurodesis for control; talc slurry on the left and surgical parietal pleurectomy on the right.

The pleural fluid is usually clear and yellow; the white cell count reveals a preponderance of polymorphonuclear leukocytes or of lymphocytes.[17] The concentration of complement in the pleural fluid of most patients with lupus pleuritis is subnormal, and the ratio of pleural fluid to serum complement is less than 0.4. In contrast to rheumatoid arthritis, the pH of the SLE effu-

sion is usually higher than 7.20, the concentration of glucose is greater than 60 mg/dl, and the LDH is less than 500 units.[17] A pleural fluid ANA titer greater than or equal to 1:160 and a pleural fluid to serum ANA ratio greater than or equal to 1 is strongly suggestive of lupus pleuritis.[27] The demonstration of LE cells in pleural fluid is diagnostic of lupus pleuritis. The pleural effusion associated with lupus usually responds well to moderate doses of corticosteroids.

Churg-Strauss Syndrome

This syndrome is a disorder characterized by hypereosinophilia and systemic vasculitis occurring in individuals with asthma and allergic rhinitis.[31] Approximately 30 percent of patients with this syndrome have a pleural effusion.[34] The pleural fluid is characterized by a very high LDH, low glucose and pH levels, and a high percentage of eosinophils. The only other disease with comparable findings is paragonimiasis. This syndrome responds well to treatment with corticosteroids.

PLEURAL EFFUSION FROM DRUG REACTIONS

Few pleural effusions are induced by drugs (see Chapters 66 and 67). It is very difficult to make an accurate diagnosis of a drug reaction on clinical grounds. Rechallenge is seldom feasible in clinical practice, and there are no readily available laboratory tests which accurately link the medication to the adverse event. The diagnosis is important, as discontinuation of the drug is frequently followed by a spontaneous reversal of the pleural disease.

Most drug-induced pleural reactions are associated with a parenchymal abnormality. The symptoms sometimes are acute, i.e., chills, fever, cough, and dyspnea develop within hours to days after taking the offending drug. An acute reaction of this type usually develops when prior use has sensitized the patient to the medication. Nitrofurantoin and procarbazine are identified with this pattern of acute illness.[33,34] Acute pleuropulmonary reactions are often accompanied by eosinophilia in both blood and pleural fluid.

If the offending medication is continued, a chronic syndrome developing over weeks to months is apt to occur. Methysergide, dantrolene, and practolol tend to produce a chronic pleural syndrome with effusion and/or fibrosis.[33,34] Pleural disease is occasionally not evident clinically until 2 to 3 years after the initial administration of the drug. The pleural changes are either unilateral or bilateral. After stopping of the medication, the pleural reaction improves in most patients over a period of 6 months; however, some are left with a fibrothorax.

PLEURAL EFFUSION SECONDARY TO ASBESTOS EXPOSURE

Three percent of asbestos workers develop pleural effusions related to their asbestos exposure.[13] There is a direct relationship between the level of asbestos exposure and the development of the pleural effusion. In patients with heavy, moderate, and mild asbestos exposure, the incidence of pleural effusion was 9.2, 3.9, and 0.7 effusions per 10,000 person-years of observation, respectively.[13] The pleural effusion frequently develops within 10 years of the initial exposure, in contrast to the occurrence of pleural plaques and calcification which usually do not occur until more than 10 years after the initial exposure.[13] It is hypothesized that an asbestos fiber is inhaled, passes to the periphery of the lung, ultimately pierces the visceral pleura, and there rubs against and irritates the parietal pleura creating an inflammatory reaction which will lead to effusion and/or plaque.[12] Microscopic examination of the parietal pleura reveals chronic fibrosing pleuritis with varying degrees of inflammation, but asbestos bodies and fibers are conspicuous for their absence in both the pleural plaque and effusion. There is, however, a heavy burden of asbestos fibers and ferruginous bodies in the lymphatic plexus beneath the visceral pleura, and a lung biopsy is necessary to demonstrate the causative agent.

Almost two-thirds of patients with asbestos-related pleural effusions are asymptomatic.[34] Pleuritic chest pain and dyspnea are seen in the other third. Pleural friction rubs are rare. The chest radiograph usually reveals a small or moderate unilateral pleural effusion. In 10 percent of patients, the effusions are bilateral. Approximately 20 percent have associated pleural plaques, fewer than 5 percent have pleural calcification, and fewer than 10 percent develop pulmonary fibrosis. The pleural fluid is either serous or serosanguineous. The total white blood count in the pleural fluid may be as high as 20,000 per cubic millimeter, and either polymorphonuclear leukocytes or mononuclear cells predominate. Pleural fluid eosinophilia is common.

The diagnosis of asbestos pleural effusion is one of exclusion. Patients should be carefully evaluated for mesothelioma or bronchogenic carcinoma. An extensive evaluation, including direct visualization of the pleural space by thoracoscopy, or an open pleural biopsy is necessary to feel confident that all other possibilities have been excluded.

In most patients, asbestos pleural effusion resolves in 1 to 2 years. Approximately 20 percent will progress to massive pleural fibrosis; another 5 percent develop mesotheliomas. In 30 percent of patients, the volume of the effusion waxes and wanes over a long period.

Rounded atelectasis, or folded lung, is an unusual form of asbestos-associated pleural disease that results in a subpleural focus of airless lung.[43] Radiographically such patients present with a subpleural, rounded mass usually at the lung base. Specific for the syndrome is a curvilinear shadow extending from the lower border of the mass toward the hilus, the "comet tail" sign. In most instances, the pleura immediately adjacent to the mass is thickened, often in conjunction with thickening of the lobar fissures. The initial event in the pathogenesis of rounded atelectasis is believed to be thickening of the parietal and visceral pleurae incident to the asbestos exposure; the adjacent pulmonary parenchyma then undergoes atelectasis. Fusion of the parietal and visceral pleurae immobilizes the lung at its periphery, and further atelectasis causes the airless lung to curl, thereby drawing blood vessels and bronchi to the inferior pole of the mass and creating the comet tail. Once radiographically visible, the rounded atelectasis usually does not progress either in size or contour over many years.

CHYLOTHORAX

Most absorbed fat is conveyed to the blood by the thoracic duct in the form of chylomicrons. Fat enters the intestinal lacteal vessels and then travels to the cisterna chyli, a lymphatic structure located on the body of the second lumbar vertebra. From the cisterna chyli, the thoracic duct traverses the esophageal hiatus of the diaphragm to enter the thoracic cavity. The thoracic duct then ascends extrapleurally in the posterior mediastinum along the right side of the anterior surface of the vertebral column in proximity to the esophagus and the pericardium. At the level of the 4th to 6th thoracic vertebra, the duct crosses to the left of the vertebral column and continues cephalad to terminate in the left subclavian vein.

A chylothorax is formed when the thoracic duct is disrupted and chyle enters the pleural space.[15,40] Chyle is a milky, opalescent fluid that contains chylomicrons, triglycerides, and lymphocytes; it is bacteriostatic and nonirritating and has little propensity to form fibrothorax. Fifteen hundred to twenty-five hundred milliliters of chyle normally empty into the venous system daily. The flow of lymph through the thoracic duct can be increased 2 to 10 times the resting level by ingesting fat, whereas ingestion of protein or carbohydrates has little effect on lymph flow. The protein content of chyle is usually above 3 g/dl, and the electrolyte composition is similar to that of serum.

More than 50 percent of chylothoraxes are related to tumor invading the thoracic lymph duct; lymphoma is responsible for 75 percent of the malignancy-associated chylothoraxes.[15,40] Therefore, nontraumatic chylothorax is an indication for a diligent search for malignancy. Trauma is the second leading cause of chylothorax, responsible for 25 percent of cases. Surgery is the most common cause of traumatic chylothorax, especially in operations that mobilize the left subclavian artery. Chylothorax also may be a result of left subclavian lines complicated by clot which obstructs the thoracic duct ostium. Penetrating trauma to the chest, such as gunshot or knife wounds, occasionally sever the thoracic duct, but nonpenetrating trauma can also produce the syndrome. A chylothorax secondary to closed trauma is usually on the right side, and the site of rupture is in the region of the 9th and 10th thoracic vertebra. Falls, motor vehicle accidents, and compressive injuries to the trunk and abdomen are common causes. However, everyday stresses such as coughing, sneezing, vomiting, and lifting heavy objects may produce a chylothorax. Approximately 25 percent of chylothoraxes have no identifiable cause; they are presumed to be secondary to minor trauma. Pulmonary lymphangiomyomatosis, which is a rare interstitial parenchymal disease, has been associated with chylothorax.

The symptoms of chylothorax are almost exclusively related to the volume of fluid in the thoracic cavity. Fever and chest pain are virtually absent. After trauma, the chylothorax usually develops in 2 to 10 days. Lymph collects extrapleurally in the mediastinum after the thoracic duct is disrupted to form a chyloma, a posterior mediastinal mass. In time, the mediastinal pleura ruptures, and chyle enters the pleural space.

A pleural fluid that is white, odorless, and milky in appearance suggests the diagnosis of chylothorax. Effusions of this appearance will be either chylothorax, a pseudochylothorax caused by high lipid levels (cholesterol or lecithin-globulin complexes) in chronic pleural effusions, or an empyema.[58] The first step in differentiation is to centrifuge the fluid. If the supernatant clears, the white color is due to large numbers of white blood cells, and the patient probably has an empyema; the supernatant of a chylous or pseudochylous effusion remains opalescent after centrifugation. Cholesterol crystals are usually easily recognized as rhomboid structures on smears of the sediment. A second way to identify cholesterol is to add 1 to 2 ml of ethyl ether to the pleural fluid, which clears if a high concentration of cholesterol is responsible for the opalescence. Pseudochylothorax accounts for approximately 10 percent of effusions rich in lipids; rheumatoid pleuritis and tuberculosis are the most common underlying diseases for pseudochylothorax.

The best way to establish the diagnosis of chylothorax is to determine the concentrations of the triglyceride in the pleural fluid.[58] Triglyceride concentrations greater than 110 mg/dl usually indicate a chylothorax. Levels below 50 mg/dl virtually exclude a chylothorax. In patients with the intermediate values (between 50 and 110 mg/dl), a lipoprotein analysis of the pleural fluid is performed; the demonstration of chylomicrons by lipoprotein analysis establishes the diagnosis of chylothorax.[58] Remember that not all chylous fluids have a classic milky appearance. Indeed, almost half are either bloody or turbid in appearance. Therefore, determination of the triglyceride content of an exudative fluid of unknown etiology is a must.

Therapeutic efforts should be directed toward correction of the leak rather than simply removing the fluid. The defect in the thoracic duct often closes spontaneously if caused by trauma. In the dyspneic patient, management begins with placement of either a pleuroperitoneal shunt or a chest tube. Efforts are then made to reduce chyle formation; these include placing the patient on constant gastric suction and keeping the patient at bed rest; fluid and nutrition are best supplied by parenteral hyperalimentation. Medium-chain triglycerides have been proposed as a means of providing an oral source of calories to these patients. The rationale is that the medium-chain triglycerides are absorbed into the portal vein directly and thus enter the circulatory system rather than travel through the thoracic duct.

In most instances, the drainage of chyle will slow or stop within the first 7 days following chest tube insertion. Malnutrition and lymphopenia are likely to occur in a patient with chylothorax if large amounts of lymph are drained. If lymph drainage has not stopped spontaneously within 7 days, surgical ligation of the thoracic duct is in order. At the time of surgery, an attempt is made to find the leak in the duct and to ligate on both sides of the leak. In many instances, the leak will not be found, and the thoracic duct is ligated both high and low in the thorax. Tetracycline sclerosis of the pleura is a therapeutic alternative that is reserved for poor-risk patients who are not surgical candidates.

The management of a nontraumatic chylothorax poses a challenge to the clinician to identify the cause of the leak.[60] Lymphoma is a key candidate. Often the patient with lymphoma and chylothorax has no evidence of lymphoma outside the thorax. A CT study of the mediastinum should be done on all such patients. The initial management of the patient with chylothorax suspected of occult intrathoracic lymphoma is as described above: inserting a chest tube, placing the gastrointestinal tract at rest, and preserving the patient's nutritional status by using par-

enteral hyperalimentation. If the CT scan and/or chest radiograph show evidence of intrathoracic tumor, the patient should undergo exploratory thoracotomy. Appropriate biopsies are taken at that time, and the thoracic duct is ligated. In a patient known to have lymphoma or metastatic carcinoma, chylothorax may simply be treated by mediastinal irradiation in anticipation that the leak will stop.

HEMOTHORAX

Hemothorax is the presence of significant amounts of blood in the pleural space (Fig. 89-8). The most common causes are penetrating and nonpenetrating chest trauma.[16,52] Occasionally iatrogenic procedures, such as percutaneous placement of central venous catheters in the subclavian or internal jugular veins, or translumbar aortography, produce a hemothorax.

Hemothorax should be considered to be present when the hematocrit of the pleural fluid is more than half that of the pe-

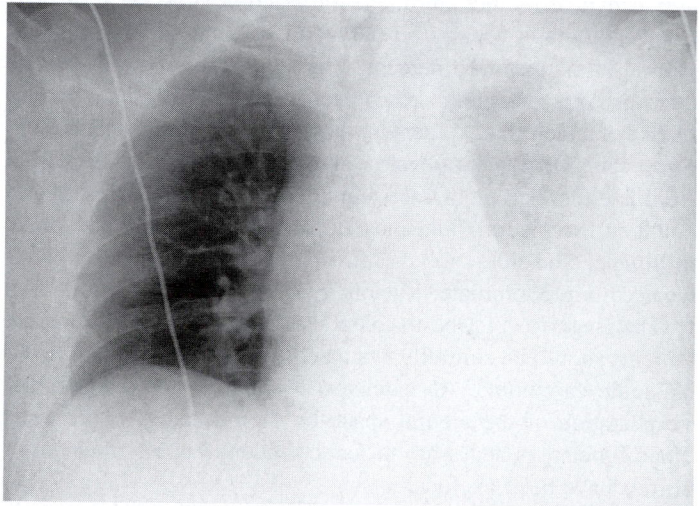

A

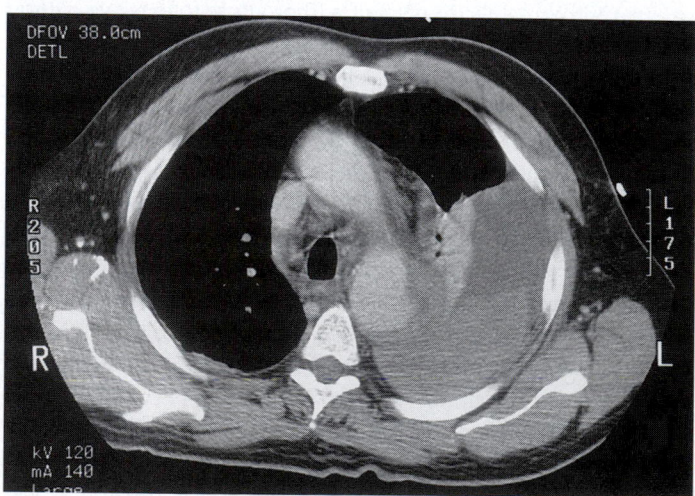

B

FIGURE 89-8 *A.* Admission chest radiograph of a 56-year-old man with a 1-week history of left-sided chest pain showed total opacification of the left hemithorax. Thoracentesis demonstrated a hemothorax. *B.* A CT scan of the thorax showed a dissecting aneurysm of the ascending thoracic aortic with hemorrhage into the left pleural space.

ripheral blood. The diagnosis should be entertained in any individual with thoracic trauma and a pleural effusion on the chest radiograph. A number of bleeding sites may be responsible for the hemothorax, complicating either blunt or penetrating trauma. These sites include pulmonary parenchymal laceration, intercostal vessel laceration, and rupture of pleural adhesions. Much less common is mediastinal injury that causes damage of a major blood vessel or decompression of abdominal hemorrhage through a traumatic diaphragmatic injury. The vast majority of hemothoraxes are due to bleeding from the low-pressure, pulmonary parenchymal vessels; they stop bleeding spontaneously when the hemothorax is evacuated and the pleural surfaces are reapposed.

Chest radiographs in the supine position tend to obscure the diagnosis. Upright radiographs are, therefore, obtained whenever possible. Also, follow-up chest radiographs are taken 24 h after the trauma. In 60 to 80 percent of these patients, an associated pneumothorax is found, after both nonpenetrating and penetrating trauma. The treatment of choice is the immediate insertion of a chest tube. The chest tube is useful to (1) evacuate blood from the pleural space, thereby decreasing the incidence of empyema and/or fibrothorax; (2) stop bleeding from pulmonary parenchyma or pleural lacerations by apposing the pleural surfaces to create a tamponade; and (3) provide a quantitative measure of continued bleeding. Immediate thoracotomy is rarely indicated, since tube thoracostomy controls bleeding in about 85 percent of cases. But cardiac tamponade, continued bleeding, evidence of a major bronchial rupture, or sucking chest wounds require immediate thoracotomy. If bleeding is more than 200 ml/h and shows no signs of slowing over 4 to 6 h, thoracotomy should be seriously considered. Thoracotomy is not indicated for removal of retained blood in patients without active bleeding.[63] The incidence of empyema thoracis is the same in patients undergoing surgical evacuation as in those who are allowed to undergo spontaneous lysis of the pleural clot. Approximately 85 percent of patients with hemothorax and retained blood are left with no pleural abnormalities on follow-up examination.[63]

Empyema occurs in approximately 5 percent of patients with hemothorax. Those with gross contamination of the pleural space at the time of their original injury are most susceptible. Empyema is also more common in patients who are in shock on admission, in those with associated abdominal injuries, and in patients who require prolonged pleural drainage.

An exudative pleural effusion occasionally follows a hemothorax after removal of the chest tubes. This occurs in 15 to 30 percent of patients and is more common in those with residual hemothorax when the tube is removed. When such an effusion does occur, a diagnostic thoracentesis is performed to rule out the possibility of pleural infection. If a pleural infection is not present, the pleural effusion usually clears spontaneously without residual disease. Fewer than 1 percent of patients with hemothorax develop a fibrothorax.

Nontraumatic hemothorax is uncommon. But when it does occur, it usually indicates pleural malignancy. It also occurs during anticoagulant therapy for pulmonary embolus. Other causes include bleeding disorders such as hemophilia or thrombocytopenia, complication of spontaneous pneumothorax, ruptured thoracic aorta, and pancreatic pseudocyst.

POSTSURGICAL PLEURAL EFFUSIONS

Two to 3 days after an upper abdominal surgical procedure, pleural effusions can be identified on the decubitus chest radiograph in up to 70 percent of patients.[10,36,45] The effusions are usually small with only 20 percent measuring more than 10 mm in thickness on the decubitus films. Postoperative pleural effusions are more common in patients undergoing upper abdominal surgical procedures, in patients with postoperative atelectasis, and in those with free abdominal fluid at the time of operation. Large effusions are particularly apt to occur after splenectomy. The effusions resolve spontaneously.

The incidence of pleural effusion following coronary artery bypass surgery is as high as 40 percent.[47] The mechanism is unknown but probably involves trauma to the pleura and pericardium during surgery. Effusions are frequently bilateral or unilateral on the left but rarely unilateral on the right. Proper management is usually observation, and a diagnostic tap is not warranted.

SARCOIDOSIS

Pleural sarcoidosis has typically been identified at thoracotomy or autopsy.[49] Small pleural effusions and pleural thickening from sarcoidosis are rarely extensive enough to produce clinical or physiological consequences and often are not readily apparent on chest radiographs. CT scanning, however, has demonstrated a high incidence of minor pleural abnormalities. Pleural thickening is often seen in association with extensive parenchymal disease. Pleural abnormalities are often located in the lower lung fields and, when apical, should raise a question of *Aspergillus* infection.

A pleural effusion can occur in up to 7 percent of patients with sarcoidosis.[4] One-third of cases are bilateral. Pleural biopsy often reveals multiple noncaseating granuloma.[4,9] Effusions are free-flowing, rarely loculate, and generally small to moderate in size. The fluid is usually an exudate and invariably shows a predominance of lymphocytes. The pleural effusion is rarely associated with acute symptoms such as pleuritic pain, fever, and dyspnea. In some, the effusion may clear spontaneously or with corticosteroid therapy in 1 to 2 months; in others, the effusion can progress to chronic pleural thickening. Because of its relatively rare occurrence, the presence of a pleural effusion in association with pulmonary sarcoidosis should raise a possibility of other causes, including tuberculosis, pneumonia, or heart failure.

POST-CARDIAC-INJURY (DRESSLER'S) SYNDROME

The post-cardiac-injury syndrome consists of fever and pleuropericarditis developing after injury to the pericardium or myocardium.[25] The syndrome has been described following myocardial infarction, cardiac surgery, and blunt chest trauma and occurs in approximately 1 percent of patients with acute myocardial infarction and up to 30 percent of patients undergoing surgical procedures involving the pericardium.[59] Dressler's syndrome is thought to be an immunologic response to damage of the pericardium, and antibodies to cardiac antigens can be demonstrated in many patients.

Affected individuals develop fever, chest pain, pericarditis, pleuritis, and sometimes air space disease after the cardiac injury. Symptoms usually occur in the second or third week following myocardial injury. Almost all patients have a pericardial friction rub, and many have a pericardial effusion. Most patients have a peripheral leukocytosis and an elevated erythrocyte sedimentation rate. The pleural effusion may be either unilateral or bilateral and is usually small.[34] Pericarditis is the dominant clinical feature. The pleural fluid is an exudate with a normal pH and a normal glucose level. Almost a third of patients will have bloody pleural fluid.[34] The pleural fluid cell population will vary from polymorphonuclear predominance to lymphocyte predominance in the more chronic syndromes. The diagnosis is one of exclusion.

UREMIC PLEURITIS

Fibrinous pleuritis is found at autopsy in approximately 20 percent of patients dying of uremia.[34,44] The pleuritis frequently is asymptomatic but sometimes produces pleuritic chest pain, pleural friction rubs, and pleural effusions. The incidence of pleural effusions with uremia is approximately 3 percent; half of the patients are symptomatic. Sometimes, the effusions are quite large and may occupy more than 50 percent of the hemithorax.[34] The fluid is an exudate that is frequently serosanguinous or hemorrhagic. The glucose level is normal, and the differential white blood count reveals a predominance of lymphocytes in most patients. Pleural biopsy results are nonspecific and reveal chronic fibrinous pleuritis. The diagnosis of uremic pleuritis is again one of exclusion in the patient with chronic renal failure. Dialysis is the treatment of choice. With dialysis, the effusion gradually disappears within 4 to 6 weeks in the majority of patients.

YELLOW NAIL SYNDROME

The *yellow nail syndrome* refers to thickening, yellowing, and curvature of all the nails in association with lymph edema; it may be associated with pleural effusions, chronic pulmonary infections, and bronchiectasis.[11,46] The basic abnormality is hypoplasia of the lymphatic vessels. It is conjectured that pleural effusions may develop when a lower respiratory tract infection or pleural inflammation further damages already compromised lymphatic vessels. Pleural effusion occurs in approximately one-third of patients with the yellow nail syndrome.[34] The pleural effusions are bilateral half the time and vary in size from small to massive. The pleural fluid is a clear yellow exudate with normal glucose and predominantly lymphocytes in the pleural fluid differential. No specific treatment is available. Spontaneous remission is very unlikely. If the effusion is large, and produces dyspnea, pleurodesis should be considered.

PLEURAL EFFUSIONS IN PATIENTS WITH AIDS

Pleural effusions occur in up to 27 percent of hospitalized patients with AIDS.[23] A series of 59 AIDS patients with pleural effusions revealed the cause to be infectious in 39 (66 percent), noninfectious in 18 (31 percent), and unknown in 2 (3 percent).[23] Pleural effusions were caused by bacterial pneumonia in 18

(31 percent) patients, *Pneumocystis carinii* pneumonia in 9 (15 percent), *Mycobacterium tuberculosis* in 5 (8 percent), septic embolization in 2 (3 percent), *Nocardia asteroides* in 2 (3 percent), *Cryptococcus neoformans* in 2 (3 percent), and *Mycobacterium avium intracellulare* in 1 (2 percent). Among noninfectious causes (18 patients), hyperalbuminemia was the cause in 11 patients (19 percent), cardiac failure in 3 (5 percent), and atelectasis, Kaposi's sarcoma (KS), uremic pleurisy, and adult respiratory syndrome in 1 (2 percent) each. Patients with AIDS who had pleural effusions had significantly lower serum albumin levels and lower CD4 counts than those without pleural effusions.

In some patients with *Pneumocystis carinii*–associated pleural effusion, the diagnosis can be established by demonstrating the organism in pleural fluid stained with Gomori's methenamine-silver.[20] The pleural fluid is an exudate with pleural fluid glucose and pH normal.[20]

REFERENCES

1. Banales JL, Pineda PR, Fitzgerald JM, et al: Adenosine deaminase in the diagnosis of tuberculous pleural effusions. A report of 218 patients and review of the literature. *Chest* 99:355–357, 1991.
2. Barbas CSV, Cukier A, de Varvalho CRR, et al: The relationship between pleural fluid findings and the development of pleural thickening in patients with pleural tuberculosis. *Chest* 100:1264–1267, 1991.
3. Bartlett JG, Thadepalli H, Gorbach SL, Finegold SM: Bacteriology of empyema. *Lancet* 1:338–340, 1974.
4. Beekman JF, Zimmet SM, Chun BK, et al: Spectrum of pleural involvement in sarcoidosis. *Arch Int Med* 136:323–330, 1976.
5. Berger HA, Morganroth ML: Immediate drainage is not required for all patients with complicated parapneumonic effusions. *Chest* 97:731–735, 1990.
6. Burgess LJ, Maritz FJ, Med M, Taljaard JJF: Comparative analysis of the biochemical parameters used to distinguish between pleural transudates and exudates. *Chest* 107:1604–1609, 1995.
7. Bynum LJ, Wilson JE III: Characteristics of pleural effusions associated with pulmonary embolism. *Arch Intern Med* 136:159–162, 1976.
8. Bynum LJ, Wilson JE III: Radiographic features of pleural effusions in pulmonary embolism. *Am Rev Respir Dis* 117:829–834, 1978.
9. Chusid EL, Siltzbach LE: Sarcoidosis of the pleura. *Ann Int Med* 81:190–194, 1974.
10. Connell TR, Stephens DH, Carlson HC, Brown ML: Upper abdominal abscess: continuing and deadly problem. *Am J Roentgenol* 134:759–765, 1980.
11. Cordasco EM Jr, Beder S, Coltro A, et al: Clinical features of the yellow nail syndrome. *Cleve Clin J Med* 57:472–476, 1990.
12. Craighead JB, Mossman BT: Medical progress. The pathogenesis of asbestos-associated diseases. *New Engl J Med* 306:1446–1455, 1982.
13. Epler GR, McLoud TC, Gaensler EA: Prevalence and incidence of benign asbestos pleural effusion in a working population. *JAMA* 247:617–622, 1982.
14. Epstein DM, Kline LR, Albelda SM, Miller WT: Tuberculous pleural effusions. *Chest* 91:106–109, 1987.
15. Fairfax AJ, McNabb WR, Spiro SG: Chylothorax: a review of 18 cases. *Thorax* 41:880–885, 1986.
16. Griffith GL, Todd EP, McMillin RD, et al: Acute traumatic hemothorax. *Ann Thorac Surg* 26:204–207, 1978.

17. Halla JT, Schronhenloher RE, Volanakis JE: Immune complexes and other laboratory features of pleural effusions. A comparison of rheumatoid arthritis, systemic lupus erythematosus, and other disease. *Ann Intern Med* 92:748–752, 1980.

18. Heffner JE, Brown LK, Barbieri C, DeLeo JM: Pleural fluid chemical analysis in parapneumonic effusions. A meta-analysis. *Am J Respir Crit Care Med* 151:1700–1708, 1995.

19. Henke CA, Leatherman JW: Intrapleurally administered streptokinase in the treatment of acute loculated, nonpurulent parapneumonic effusions. *Am Rev Respir Dis* 145:680–684, 1992.

20. Horowitz ML, Schiff M, Samuels J, et al: Pneumocystis carinii pleural effusion. Pathogenesis and pleural fluid analysis. *Am Rev Respir Dis* 148:232–234, 1993.

21. Houston MC: Pleural fluid pH: diagnostic, therapeutic, and prognostic value. *Am J Surg* 154:333–337, 1987.

22. Hunninghake GW, Fauce AS: Pulmonary involvement in the collagen vascular diseases. *Am Rev Respir Dis* 119:471–503, 1979.

23. Joseph J, Strange C, Sahn SA: Pleural effusions in hospitalized patients with AIDS. *Ann Int Med* 118:856–859, 1993.

24. Joseph J, Viney S, Beck P, et al: A prospective study of amylase-rich pleural effusions with special reference to amylase isoenzyme analysis. *Chest* 102:1455–1459, 1992.

25. Khan AH: The postcardiac injury syndromes. *Clin Cardiol* 15:67–72, 1992.

26. Keszler P, Buzna E: Surgical and conservative management of esophageal perforation. *Chest* 80:158–162, 1981.

27. Khare V, Baethge B, Lang S, et al: Antinuclear antibodies in pleural fluid. *Chest* 106:866–871, 1994.

28. Klein JS, Schultz S, Heffner JE: Interventional radiology of the chest: image-guided percutaneous drainage of pleural effusions, lung abscess and pneumothorax. *Am J Roentgenol* 164:581–588, 1995.

29. Kuhn M, Fitting J, Lewenberger P: Probability of malignancy in pleural fluid eosinophilia. *Chest* 96:992–994, 1989.

30. Kumar S, Seshadri MS, Koshi G, John TJ: Diagnosing tuberculous pleural effusion: Comparative sensitivity of mycobacterial culture and histopathology. *Br Med J* 283:20, 1981.

31. Lanham JG, Elkon KB, Pusey CD, Hughes GR: Systemic vasculitis with asthma and eosinophilia: a clinical approach to the Churg-Strauss syndrome. *Medicine* 63: 65–81, 1984.

32. Levine H, Szanto PB, Cugell DW: Tuberculous pleurisy: An acute illness. *Arch Intern Med* 122:329–332, 1968.

33. Light RW: *Pleural diseases. Disease-a-Month* 28:263–331, 1992.

34. Light RW: *Pleural Diseases*. Baltimore, Williams and Wilkins, 1995.

35. Light RW, Erozan YS, Ball WC Jr: Cells in pleural fluid. Their value in differential diagnosis. *Arch Intern Med* 132:854–860, 1973.

36. Light RW, George RB: Incidence and significance of pleural effusion after abdominal surgery. *Chest* 69:621–626, 1976.

37. Light RW, Girard WM, Jenkinson SG, George RB: Parapneumonic effusions. *Am J Med* 69:507–511, 1980.

38. Light RW, MacGregor MI, Luchinsinger PC, Ball WC Jr: Pleural effusions: the diagnostic separation of transudates and exudates. *Ann Intern Med* 77:507–513, 1972.

39. Maulitz RM, Good JT, Kaplan RL, et al: Pleuropulmonary consequences of esophageal rupture: an experimental model. *Am Rev Respir Dis* 120:363–367, 1979.

40. McFarlane RJ, Holman CW: Chylothorax. *Am Rev Respir Dis* 105:287–291, 1972.

41. Meisel S, Shamiss A, Thaler M, et al: Pleural fluid to serum bilirubin concentration ratio for the separation of transudates from exudates. *Chest* 98:141–144, 1990.

42. Michel L, Grillo HC, Malt RA: Operative and nonoperative management of esophageal perforation. *Ann Surg* 194:57–63, 1981.

43. Mintzer RA, Gore RM, Vogelzang RL, Holz S: Rounded atelectasis and its association with asbestos-induced pleural disease. *Radiology* 139:567–570, 1981.

44. Nidus BD, Matalon R, Cantacuzino D, Eisinger RP: Uremic pleuritis. A clinicopathologic entity. *New Engl J Med* 281:255–256, 1969.

45. Nielsen PH, Jepsen SB, Olsen AD: Postoperative pleural effusion following upper abdominal surgery. *Chest* 96:1133–1135, 1989.

46. Nordkild P, Kromann-Andersen H, Struve-Christensen E: Yellow nail syndrome, the triad of yellow nails, lymphedema, and pleural effusions. *Acta Med Scan* 219:221–227, 1986.

47. Peng M-J, Vargas FS, Cukier A, et al: Postoperative pleural changes after coronary revascularization. *Chest* 10:327–330, 1992.

48. Pfalzer B, Hamm H, Beisiegel U, Ostendorf P: Lipoproteins and apolipoproteins in human pleural effusions. *J Lab Clin Med* 120:483–493, 1992.

49. Poe RH, Marin MG, Israel RH, Kallay MC: Utility of pleural fluid analysis in predicting tube thoracostomy/decortication in parapneumonic effusions. *Chest* 100:963–967, 1991.

50. Pollak JS, Passik CS: Intrapleural urokinase in the treatment of loculated pleural effusions. *Chest* 105:868–873, 1994.

51. Raasch BN, Carsky EW, Lane EJ, et al: Pleural effusion: explanation of some typical appearances. *Am J Roentgenol* 139:899–904, 1982.

52. Rasmussen OV, Brynitz S, Struve-Christensen E: Thoracic injuries. A review of 93 cases. *Scand J Thorac Cardiovasc Surg* 20:71–74, 1986.

53. Roper WH, Waring JJ: Preliminary serofibrinous pleural effusions in military personnel. *Am Rev Respir Dis* 71:616–634, 1955.

54. Romero S, Candela A, Martin C, et al: Evaluation of different criteria for the separation of pleural transudates from exudates. *Chest* 104:399–404, 1993.

55. Roth BJ, O'Meara TF, Cragun WH: The serum-effusion albumen gradient in the evaluation of pleural effusions. *Chest* 98:546–549, 1990.

56. Ruskin JA, Gurney JW, Thorsen MK, Goodman LR: Detection of pleural effusions on supine chest radiographs. *Am J Roentgenol* 148:681–683, 1987.

57. Sahn SA, Taryle DA, Good JT Jr: Experimental empyema. Time course and pathogenesis of pleural fluid acidosis and low pleural fluid glucose. *Am Rev Respir Dis* 120:355–361, 1979.

58. Staats BA, Ellefson RD, Budahn LL, et al: The lipoprotein profile of chylous and nonchylous pleural effusions. *Mayo Clin Proc* 55:700–704, 1980.

59. Stelzner TJ, King TE Jr., Antony VB, Sahn SA: The pleural pulmonary manifestations of the postcardiac injury syndrome. *Chest* 84:383–387, 1983.

60. Strausser JL, Flye MW: Management of nontraumatic chylothorax. *Ann Thoracic Surg* 31:520–526, 1981.

61. Valdes L, Pose A, Suarez J, et al: Cholesterol: a useful parameter for distinguishing between pleural exudates and transudates. *Chest* 99:1097–1102, 1991.

62. Varkey B, Rose HD, Cutty CPK, Politis J: Empyema thoracis during a 10 year period: analysis of 72 cases in comparison to a previous study (1952–1967). *Arch Intern Med* 141:1771–1776, 1981.

63. Wilson JM, Boren CH Jr, Peterson SR, Thomas AN: Traumatic hemothorax: is decortication necessary? *J Thorac Cardiovasc Surg* 77:489–495, 1979.

64. Yam LT: Diagnostic significance of lymphocytes in pleural effusions. *Ann Intern Med* 66:972–982, 1967.

65. Yang P, Luh K, Chang D, et al: The value of sonography in determining the nature of pleural effusion: analysis of 320 cases. *Am J Roentgenol* 159:29–33, 1992.

CHAPTER 90

MALIGNANT PLEURAL EFFUSIONS

Steven A. Sahn

MALIGNANCIES ASSOCIATED WITH PLEURAL EFFUSIONS

PATHOGENESIS

CLINICAL PRESENTATION

CHEST RADIOGRAPHY

PLEURAL FLUID CHARACTERISTICS

DIAGNOSIS

PROGNOSIS

TREATMENT

A malignant pleural effusion is diagnosed by finding exfoliated malignant cells in pleural fluid or by demonstrating these cells in pleural tissue obtained by percutaneous pleural biopsy, thoracoscopy, or thoracotomy or at autopsy. In a number of patients, even though the pleural effusion is caused by the malignancy, neoplastic cells cannot be demonstrated in pleural fluid or pleural tissue and, in fact, probably are not present in these tissues. It makes sense to categorize these pleural effusions associated with malignancy, in which there is no direct pleural involvement with tumor and no other cause for the effusion is found, as paramalignant effusions (Table 90-1).[24] Lymphatic obstruction is the most common cause of a paramalignant effusion and the predominant mechanism for the accumulation of large volumes of fluid in malignancy.[3,21] Other local effects of the tumor causing a paramalignant effusion are bronchial obstruction with either pneumonia or atelectasis and trapped lung. It is important for the clinician to recognize that effusions can result from systemic effects of the tumor and from adverse effects of therapy.

Establishing the diagnosis of a malignant pleural effusion secondary to lung cancer signals incurability. A malignant effusion secondary to a non-lung primary is a manifestation of far advanced disease and is associated with limited survival.[25]

MALIGNANCIES ASSOCIATED WITH PLEURAL EFFUSIONS

Carcinoma of any organ can metastasize to the pleura. However, carcinoma of the lung is the most common malignancy to invade the pleura and produce malignant and paramalignant effusions (Table 90-2).[3,5,12] Carcinoma of the breast is second in incidence

and, in some populations, exceeds lung cancer as a cause of malignant effusions.[28] After lung and breast cancer, the frequency declines markedly, with ovarian and gastric cancer representing 5 percent or less of malignant pleural effusions.[3] Lymphoma accounts for approximately 10 percent of all malignant pleural effusions and is the most common cause of chylothorax. Carcinomas of the lung, breast, ovary, and stomach and lymphomas account for about 80 percent of all malignant pleural effusions. In approximately 7 percent of patients with malignant pleural effusions, the primary site is unknown when the diagnosis of malignant pleural effusion is first established.

A less common cause of malignant pleural effusion, other than metastatic carcinoma, is a primary tumor of the pleura, malignant mesothelioma. The association of asbestos exposure and malignant mesothelioma was documented in the 1960s following an initial report from the Northwestern Cape Province of South Africa[31] and a subsequent study of insulation workers in this country.[29] Owing to the long latency period of 20 to 40 years between exposure and onset of disease and the flurry of shipbuilding activities during World War II, a peak incidence of malignant mesothelioma can be expected to occur in this decade.[11]

PATHOGENESIS

Lymphatics are situated beneath the parietal pleura over the intercostal spaces. As indicated in Chapter 88, an important feature of the parietal pleura is lymphatic stomata, i.e., openings between parietal pleural mesothelial cells. The stomata and their associated lymphatic channels form lymphatic lacunae immediately beneath the mesothelial layer. These lacunae coalesce into collecting lymphatics, which join the intercostal trunk vessels with flow directed mainly toward the mediastinal lymph nodes. The lymphatic system of the parietal pleura plays a major role in the resorption of pleural liquid and proteins; the lymphatics drain to the mediastinum. Interference with the integrity of the lymphatic system anywhere between the parietal pleura and the mediastinal lymph nodes can result in a pleural effusion. Autopsy series have indicated that impaired lymphatic drainage from the pleural space is the predominant mechanism for the accumulation of fluid associated with malignancy: a strong relationship was found between carcinomatous infiltration of the mediastinal lymph nodes and the occurrence of pleural effusion;[3,21] in contrast, no relationship was found between the extent of

TABLE 90-1

Causes of Paramalignant Pleural Effusions

Cause	Comment
Local effects of tumor	
Lymphatic obstruction	Predominant mechanism for pleural fluid accumulation
Bronchial obstruction with pneumonia	Parapneumonic effusion; does not exclude operability in lung cancer
Bronchial obstruction with atelectasis	Transudate; does not exclude operability in lung cancer
Trapped lung	Transudate; due to extensive tumor involvement of visceral pleura
Chylothorax	Disruption of thoracic duct; lymphoma most common cause
Superior vena cava syndrome	Transudate; due to increased systemic venous pressure
Systemic effects of tumor	
Pulmonary embolism	Hypercoagulable state
Hypoalbuminemia	Serum albumin < 1.5 g/dL; associated with anasarca
Complications of therapy	
Radiation therapy	
Early	Pleuritis 6 weeks to 6 months after radiation completed
Late	Fibrosis of mediastinum
	Constrictive pericarditis
	Vena caval obstruction
Chemotherapy	
Methotrexate	Pleuritis or effusion ± blood eosinophilia
Procarbazine	Blood eosinophilia; fever and chills
Cyclophosphamide	Pleuropericarditis
Mitomycin	In association with interstitial disease
Bleomycin	In association with interstitial disease

direct pleural involvement by metastasis and the occurrence of pleural effusion.[21] Further support for this mechanism is provided by the observation that pleural effusions generally do not develop when the pleura is involved by sarcoma because of the characteristic absence of lymphatic metastases.

When pleural metastases occur, tumor cells either "seed" the mesothelial surface or invade the subserous layer: when the

TABLE 90-2

Causes of Malignant Pleural Effusions*

Tumor	n	Percent
Lung	641	36
Breast	449	25
Lymphoma	187	10
Ovary	88	5
Stomach	42	2
Unknown primary	129	7

*N = 1783. Combined data from nine series.

mesothelial surface is involved, abundant tumor cells can be found in pleural fluid; with subserous involvement, a paucity of malignant cells are exfoliated into the pleural space. Tumor involvement of the pleura causes reactive changes in the mesothelium that may lead to mesothelial shedding, mesothelial thickening, and, on occasion, marked pleural fibrosis. Pleural fibrosis, usually observed in the more advanced stage of tumor involvement of the pleura, is at least partially responsible for the low concentrations of glucose and the low pH seen in some malignant pleural effusions and for the failure to achieve pleurodesis after instillation of chemical agents.[9,25]

A bloody, malignant pleural effusion usually results from either direct invasion of blood vessels, occlusion of venules, tumor-induced angiogenesis, or possibly increased capillary permeability due to vasoactive sustances.[21,30] Malignant pleural effusions usually contain a large number of morphologically normal lymphocytes, usually in the 50 to 70 percent range, but less than is seen in tuberculous pleurisy (above 90 percent).[34] Although the reason for the lymphocytosis is not clear, these lymphocytes do seem to be predominantly T lymphocytes that appear to play a role in the local defense against tumor invasion of the pleural cavity. The percentage of mesothelial cells in malignant effusions is variable, ranging from few to a large percentage of the total cells.[30] An abundance of mesothelial cells occurs early in the course of pleural infiltration, before pleural fibrosis and marked infiltration with tumor; in more advanced stages of pleural metastasis, fewer mesothelial cells are generally seen because of pleural fibrosis.

Autopsy data in patients with malignant effusions have provided valuable information about the pathogenesis of pleural metastases.[21] When carcinoma of the lung metastasizes to the pleura, both the visceral and parietal pleural surfaces tend to be involved.[26] The visceral pleural surface is rarely and the parietal pleural surface almost never the sole site of involvement. Parietal pleural involvement in lung cancer probably results from neoplastic spread across the pleural cavity from visceral pleural sites along pleural adhesions that are either preformed or secondary to the malignant process. The pathogenesis of visceral pleural metastasis in lung cancer appears to be through pulmonary artery invasion and embolization. The histologic type of lung cancer does not seem to determine the propensity for pulmonary arterial invasion.[21] Adenocarcinoma of the lung is the most common cell type to involve the pleura because of its peripheral location and spread by contiguity.[3,12] Bilateral pleural metastases in lung cancer are almost always associated with evidence of hepatic involvement and parenchymal invasion of the contralateral lung.

Pleural metastases from primary sites below the diaphragm generally are a manifestation of a tertiary spread from established liver metastases.[21] The data with breast cancer are conflicting: some studies show a high incidence of ipsilateral pleural effusion while others show no such predilection. Probably two mechanisms are operative, chest wall lymphatic invasion resulting in an ipsilateral effusion and hepatic spread with bilateral or contralateral disease.[8]

At diagnosis, pleural effusions are rare in Hodgkin's disease but not infrequent in non-Hodgkin's lymphoma. Pleural effusions can be found in previously untreated patients with non-Hodgkin's lymphoma, even in the absence of detectable intrathoracic lymphadenopathy. However, the pleural effusion is usually not an isolated manifestation of the disease. At autopsy in Hodgkin's disease, lymphomatous infiltration of the lung rather than direct pleural invasion or mediastinal adenopathy has been found in association with the pleural effusion. Lymphomatous invasion of the pleura appears to be an uncommon and late finding in Hodgkin's disease but is seen with increased frequency in non-Hodgkin's lymphoma. As Hodgkin's disease progresses, the incidence of pleural effusion increases and approaches 30 percent. At autopsy, a 30 to 60 percent incidence of pleural effusions and a 7 to 30 percent incidence of pleural nodular infiltrative lesions have been noted.

While pleural effusion in lymphoma can be due to either impaired lymphatic drainage secondary to mediastinal adenopathy, pleural or pulmonary infiltration, or thoracic duct obstruction, impaired lymphatic drainage appears to be the primary mechanism in Hodgkin's disease and direct pleural infiltration the predominant cause in non-Hodgkin's lymphoma.

Malignant mesothelioma (see Chapter 92) is usually a unilateral disease (Fig. 90-1); bilateral tumors are present in < 10 percent of patients.[11] An early manifestation of the tumor is pleural effusion that is reabsorbed or organized and then largely replaced by tumor and fibrosis. At autopsy, the lung is often encased in tumor that involves both visceral and parietal pleural surfaces. The pleural space is often obliterated; the amount of

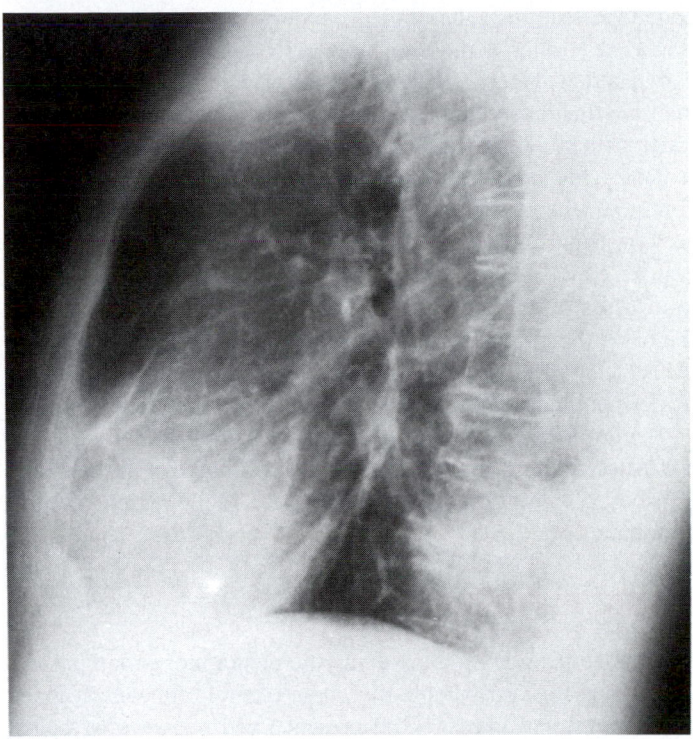

B

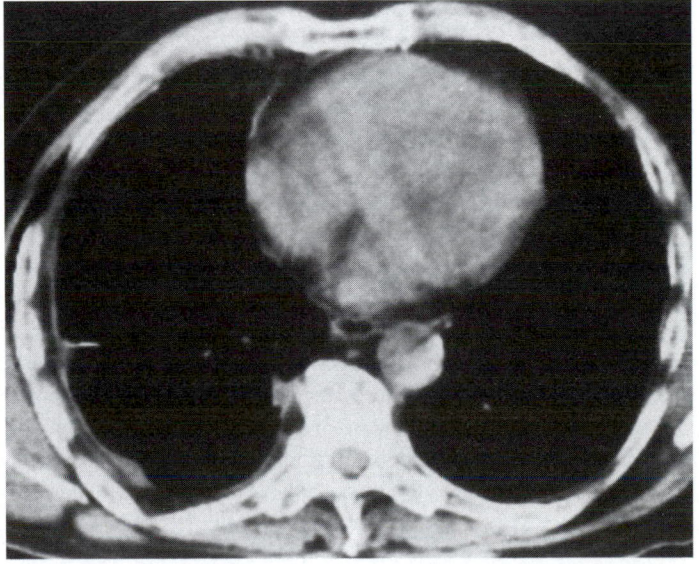

C

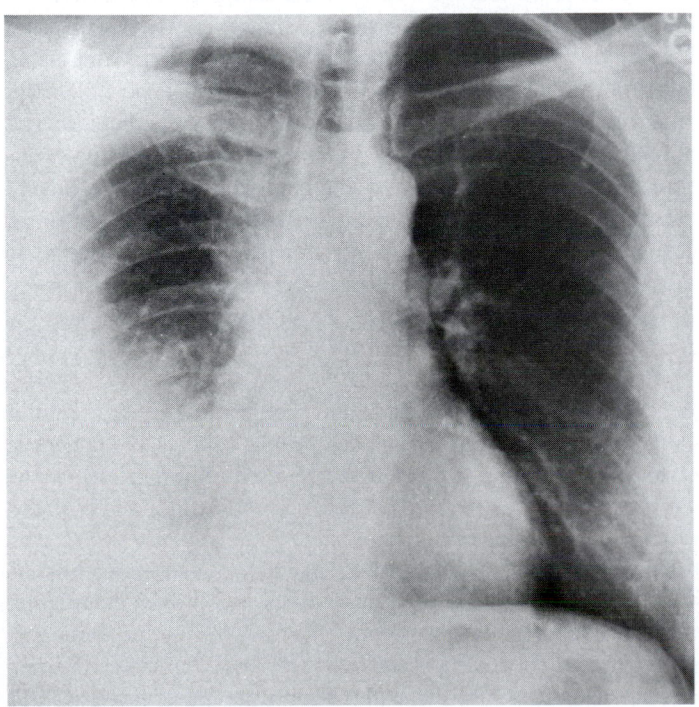

A

FIGURE 90-1 Malignant mesothelioma in a 64-year-old man. *A* and *B*. Diffuse, right-sided involvement. *C*. CT scan shows peripheral disposition of mesothelioma along right pleura. The radiodensity in the right hemithorax is a consequence primarily of pleural tumor with little pleural effusion. Subsequently treated by right extrapleural pneumonectomy. *(Courtesy of Dr. David Murphy.)*

pleural fluid is variable. The tumor seldom penetrates deeply into the lung parenchyma; instead, it extends into interlobar fissures. Hilar lymph nodes are involved by tumor in less than 50 percent of patients. Distant hematogenous metastases are unusual but have been described in liver, bone, adrenals, thyroid, and kidney.

The two distinct histologic types of malignant mesothelioma (epithelial and sarcomatous) generally behave differently.[1] Some patients have mixed tumors with both epithelioid and sarcomatous features. The clinical features of epithelial mesothelioma are similar to those of metastatic carcinoma of the pleura associated with tumor spread by direct extension, i.e., a large pleural effusion and metastases to regional lymph nodes. In contrast, patients with sarcomatous mesotheliomas tend to have features characteristic of sarcomas, i.e., distant metastases are common, whereas there is little or no pleural effusion. These data are consistent with the pathogenesis of pleural effusions in carcinoma of the pleura, i.e., the pleural effusion is due primarily to invasion of the lymphatic system. Moreover, the large bulk of tumor on the pleural surface would be expected to interfere with the removal of pleural fluid by the parietal fluid lymphatics even if the lymphatics were not directly involved with tumor.

Benign asbestos pleural effusions probably develop as a result of the pleural inflammation that occurs during the passage of asbestos fibers across the pleural space to the parietal pleural lymphatics.

CLINICAL PRESENTATION

Patients with carcinoma involving the pleura most often present with symptoms attributable to a large pleural effusion, dyspnea on exertion, and cough.[3] The presence and degree of dyspnea depends on the size of the effusion and the patient's underlying pulmonary function. A moderate to large thoracentesis results in relief of dyspnea in most patients. However, the volume of pleural fluid removed at thoracentesis does not correlate with the change in lung volume. The increase in total lung capacity (TLC) approximates one-third of the volume of fluid removed, while the forced vital capacity (FVC) increases to about a half of the TLC. Indeed, the mechanism of dyspnea caused by a large pleural effusion appears to be multifactorial in origin, probably entailing a decrease in the compliance of the chest wall, a contralateral shift of the mediastinum, and a decrease in ipsilateral lung volume modulated by neurogenic reflexes from the lungs and chest wall. An obstructive pneumonitis, an endobronchial lesion that causes atelectasis, or an infiltrative malignant disease of the pulmonary parenchyma may also contribute to dyspnea and cough.

Since malignant involvement of the pleura signifies far advanced disease, these patients commonly have substantial weight loss and appear chronically ill. Chest pain is often present because of the involvement of the parietal pleura, ribs, or chest wall. However, in one large series of patients with metastatic carcinoma of the pleura, almost 25 percent were "asymptomatic" at the time of presentation.[3] In these patients, the malignant pleural effusion was first suspected on physical examination or diagnosed on routine chest radiograph; in almost 50 percent of patients, the pleural effusion was the first indication of cancer.

The respiratory symptoms of patients with pleural effusion due to lymphoma are indistinguishable in nature and frequency from those due to carcinoma.[33] About 20 percent of patients with lymphoma have no respiratory symptoms when the malignant pleural effusion is diagnosed.

Most patients with carcinoma of the pleura have evidence of a pleural effusion on physical examination when first seen by the physician;[3] physical signs of pleural effusion are to be expected, since the volume of pleural fluid in most malignant effusions is greater than 500 mL. Cachexia and lymphadenopathy are present in about one-third of patients on initial presentation; ipsilateral chest wall tenderness and pleural friction rub are rare.

In contrast to patients with carcinomatous involvement of the pleura, virtually all patients with malignant mesotheliomas are symptomatic when first seen by the physician: in six series of patients encompassing 160 cases of malignant mesothelioma, only one patient was asymptomatic at presentation. Chest pain is the most common presenting symptom and occurs in 60 to 70 percent of patients. Dyspnea and cough are next in frequency and are present in about 25 and 20 percent of patients, respectively.[11]

Pleural effusion due to asbestos exposure is a diagnosis of exclusion. Its frequency of occurrence in exposed workers is estimated to be up to 7 percent.[7] Benign asbestos pleural effusions are the most common manifestation of asbestos-related pleuropulmonary disease in the first 20 years after initial asbestos exposure. Two-thirds of patients with benign asbestos pleural effusion are asymptomatic at presentation, with the effusion diagnosed on a routine chest radiograph. Approximately 20 percent of patients present with pleuritic pain and 10 percent with dyspnea. The effusion generally persists for several months but usually resolves within a year. Recurrent effusions, either on the ipsilateral or contralateral side, occur in approximately 25 percent of patients. Differential diagnosis centers around distinguishing a benign pleural effusion due to asbestos from mesothelioma. Since benign effusions occur sooner after initial exposure than does mesothelioma, i.e., 20 years being the rough dividing line, the pleural effusion in a young asbestos-exposed individual is more likely to represent a benign asbestos-pleurisy than is an effusion that occurs 20 to 40 years after initial exposure. Also, an asymptomatic pleural effusion is more apt to be benign. The absence of other radiographic manifestations of asbestos exposure is not helpful in distinguishing between benign effusion and mesothelioma. Preoccupation with asbestos-related disease occasionally leads to overlooking treatable disorders, such as tuberculous pleurisy or thromboembolic disease.

CHEST RADIOGRAPHY

A pleural effusion ipsilateral to the primary lesion is the rule in carcinoma of the lung.[3] When the primary site of the cancer is elsewhere than the lung, with the possible exception of breast cancer, there seems to be no ipsilateral predilection and bilateral effusions are common.

In three of four patients who present with carcinomatous involvement of the pleura, the pleural effusion is moderate to large, i.e., with volumes ranging from 500 to 2000 mL of fluid. Approximately 10 percent present with effusions of less than 500 mL; another 10 percent present with massive pleural effusions (complete opacification of the hemithorax) (Fig. 90-2). Some 70 per-

If the mediastinum does not shift contralaterally in the face of a large pleural effusion (greater than 1500 mL), malignancy is almost always present and the prognosis is poor. The following diagnoses are then considered: (1) carcinoma of the ipsilateral main-stem bronchus resulting in atelectasis (Fig. 90-4), (2) a fixed mediastinum due to malignant lymph nodes, (3) malignant mesothelioma (the radiodensity represents predominantly tumor with only a small effusion), and (4) extensive tumor infiltration of the ipsilateral lung radiographically mimicking a large effusion. Interstitial infiltrates with effusions (lymphangitic carcinomatosis) and multiple nodules with effusions also suggest a malignant disease.

Depending on the stage of the mesothelioma at the time of presentation, the chest radiograph may show a moderate to large pleural effusion (early) or a lobulated, thickened pleura with extension to the apex of the hemithorax (late).[11] Contralateral mediastinal shift often occurs early, i.e., when the pleural effusion is large; but, as fluid resorbs and is replaced by tumor, the ipsilateral hemithorax shrinks in size and the mediastinal structures either remain in the midline or shift ipsilaterally (Fig. 90-1). Contralateral manifestations of asbestos-induced pleuropulmonary disease, such as pleural plaques with or without calcification and interstitial lung disease, often reinforce the diagnosis. In the more advanced stages of malignant mesothelioma, other radiographic findings are mediastinal widening due to lymph node involvement, an enlarged cardiac silhouette due to pericardial involvement with effusion, and extrapleural lesions such as soft tissue masses or rib destruction.

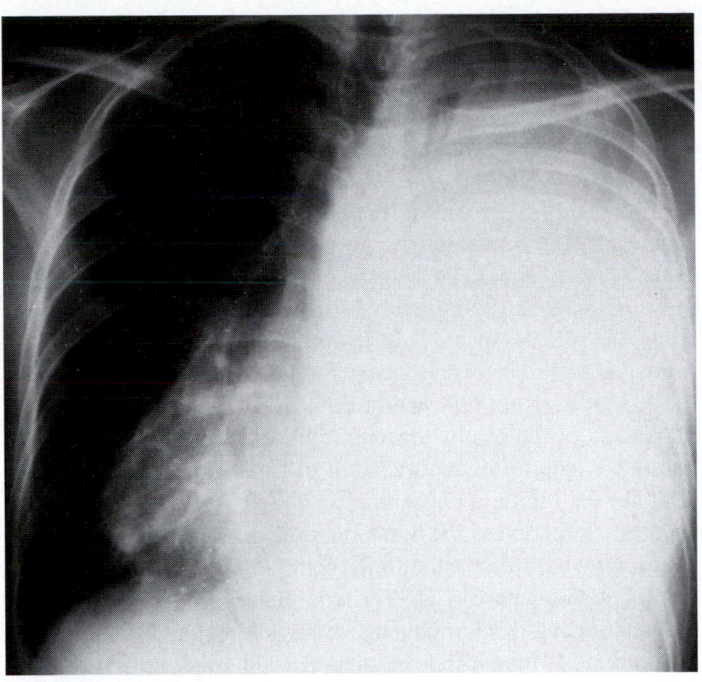

FIGURE 90-2 Carcinoma of the cervix metastatic to the left pleura and mediastinum. The massive pleural effusion is associated with a contralateral shift of the mediastinum.

cent of patients with a massive pleural effusion will have a malignancy.[19]

The finding of bilateral effusions and a normal heart size also suggests a malignant etiology (Fig. 90-3). Approximately 50 percent of patients who present with this radiographic finding have a malignant effusion; however, lupus pleuritis, hypoalbuminemia, constrictive pericarditis, rheumatoid pleurisy, benign asbestos pleural effusion, and cirrhosis must also be considered in the differential diagnosis.

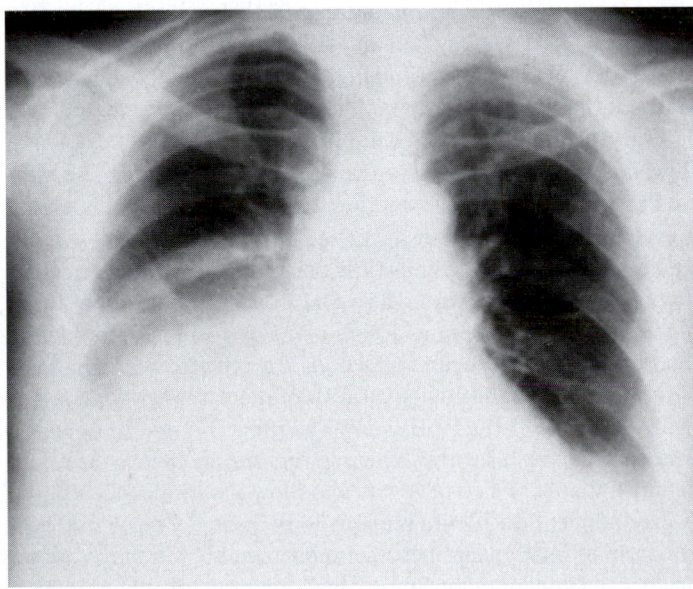

FIGURE 90-3 Carcinoma of the lung involving right lower lobe, with metastasis to right pleura and mediastinal lymph nodes. The pleural effusions are bilateral and the heart size is normal.

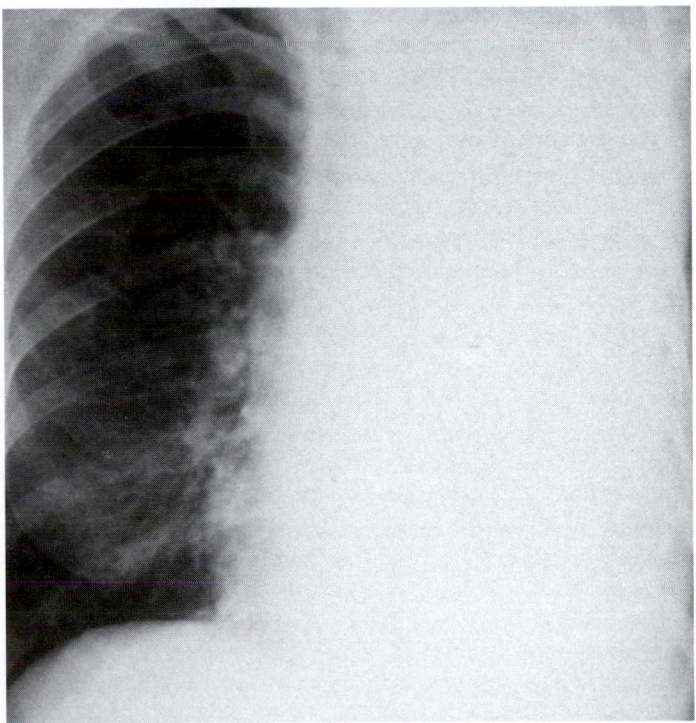

FIGURE 90-4 Carcinoma of the left main-stem bronchus resulting in complete atelectasis of the left lung. The left hemithorax is completely opacified, and the mediastinum has shifted to the side of the bronchial occlusion. The radiographic opacity represents a combination of collapsed lung and pleural fluid.

Benign asbestos pleural effusions are small to moderate (less than 1000 mL) unilateral effusions with evidence of pleural plaques or asbestosis identifiable in less than 20 percent of patients.[7] Calcified pleural plaques are rare, since calcifications require 25 to 40 years from the time of initial asbestos exposure, whereas benign asbestos effusions are the earliest manifestation of asbestos pleuropulmonary disease. Resolution of the effusion usually takes several months. Some patients are left with normal chest radiographs, but most are left with residual abnormalities.[11] These include a blunted costophrenic angle, crow's feet (converging fibrous strands creating a likeness of a bird's foot), rounded atelectasis (in which a portion of the lung periphery has become atelectatic due to pleural adhesions that collapse small bronchi), and diffuse pleural thickening that is sometimes progressive (Fig. 90-5).

PLEURAL FLUID CHARACTERISTICS

Malignant pleural fluid may be serous, serosanguinous, or grossly bloody. The red cell count usually ranges from 30,000 to 50,000 per microliter.[24] The number of nucleated cells in the pleural fluid is modest (1500 to 4000 per microliter) and consists of lymphocytes, macrophages, and mesothelial cells. In about one-half of malignant pleural effusions, lymphocytes predominate (50 to 70 percent of nucleated cells).[34] Malignant cells in pleural fluid are rare in some patients; in others they constitute virtually the complete population.[30] Polymorphonuclear leukocytes usually represent less than 25 percent of the cell population; but, rarely, when pleural inflammation is active, they predominate. Pleural fluid eosinophilia, common in bloody pleural

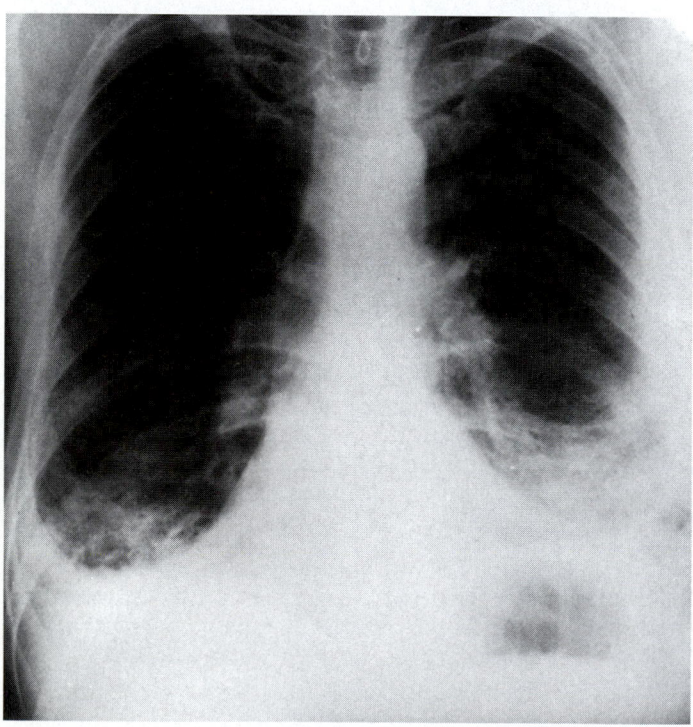

FIGURE 90-5 Bilateral pleural thickening in a 44-year-old man exposed to asbestos for 18 months 20 years ago. Bilateral pleural effusions were succeeded by progressive pleural thickening.

effusions, is inexplicably rare (5 percent) in bloody, malignant effusions.

The pleural fluid in patients who have carcinoma of the pleura is usually an exudate with a protein concentration of about 4 g/dL. However, protein concentrations have been reported in the range of 1.5 to 8.0 g/dL. Often unappreciated is the fact that approximately 5 percent of malignant pleural effusions are transudates.[3,4] These transudates are due either to concomitant congestive heart failure, atelectasis from bronchial obstruction, or the early stages of lymphatic obstruction. Since protein can exit from the pleural space only by parietal pleural lymphatics, a finite period (weeks) is necessary for protein to accumulate (from the 1.5 g/dL of normal pleural liquid) to a level of greater than 50 percent of the serum concentration. Chronic pleural effusions and those with a low pleural fluid pH and glucose tend to have a higher total protein concentration and are virtually never transudates. Sometimes, the ratio of total protein pleural fluid to serum may be low, but the fluid would qualify as an exudate by lactic dehydrogenase (LDH) criteria alone.

In about one-third of patients with malignant pleural effusions at the time of diagnosis, the pleural fluid pH is low (less than 7.30), ranging from 6.95 to 7.29.[25] In these low-pH effusions, the glucose concentration is also low (less than 60 mg/dL, or the ratio of pleural fluid to serum glucose is below 0.5), the lactate concentration is high, the P_{CO_2} is high, and the P_{O_2} is low.[9] On rare occasions, the glucose is as low as 5 mg/dL; but as a rule the concentrations are in the range of 30 to 55 mg/dL.[4]

These low-pH, low-glucose effusions have usually been present for several months and are associated with a large tumor burden and fibrosis of the pleura. The markedly abnormal pleura interferes with glucose transport from blood to pleural fluid; the glucose that does enter is metabolized by normal and malignant pleural cells to form CO_2 and lactate. The abnormal pleural barrier impairs the efflux of these end products of glucose metabolism from the pleural space, resulting in pleural fluid acidosis.[9] About 10 percent of malignant pleural effusions have high amylase concentrations. The finding of a high level of salivary-like isoamylase in a patient without esophageal rupture essentially establishes the diagnosis of malignancy, most likely adenocarcinoma of the lung.

Early in the course of malignant mesothelioma, the pleural fluid may be serous; later, it tends to be hemorrhagic. The effusion associated with malignant mesothelioma is an exudate with a protein concentration in the range of 4 to 5 g/dL and a modest number of nucleated cells (less than 5000 per microliter), predominantly mononuclear. The LDH concentration tends to be higher than in the patient with carcinoma of the pleura; frequently the concentration exceeds 600 IU/L. In 60 percent of patients with malignant mesothelioma, at the time that the diagnosis is made, the pleural fluid pH is low (below 7.30) and the glucose concentration is also low (pleural fluid/serum below 0.5);[10] in contrast, the incidence of low pH and low glucose concentration in carcinoma of the pleura is about 30 percent.[25] The natural progression of malignant mesothelioma resulting in large tumor masses and concomitant fibrosis that obliterate the pleural membrane provides a reasonable explanation for these biochemical findings.[1,11] In some instances of malignant mesothelioma, the viscosity of pleural fluid is greatly increased because of a high concentration of hyaluronic acid. Although a high concentration of hyaluronic acid in pleural fluid does raise the question of malignant mesothelioma as the cause, this test is not specific and only moderately sensitive; thus, it is of no diagnostic value.

The pleural fluid in benign asbestos pleurisy is a sanguineous, lymphocyte-predominate exudate with a variable degree of eosinophilia. During the acute stage there may be a moderate number of polymorphonuclear leukocytes. The pH and glucose are normal (above 7.30 and 60 mg/dL, respectively).

DIAGNOSIS

Malignant pleural effusion can be diagnosed only by demonstrating malignant cells in pleural fluid or pleural tissue. Cytology is a more sensitive test for the diagnosis than percutaneous pleural biopsy, because pleural metastases tend to be focal and the latter is a blind sampling procedure.[12,13,22] The yield on either procedure increases as the disease becomes more advanced. However, the yield from pleural biopsy with proven malignant effusion averages 50 to 60 percent.[12,22] It appears, based on thoracoscopy, that initial pleural metastases begin near the mediastinum and diaphragm; as the disease progresses, tumor spreads cephalad and costally. With improved techniques, the yield from exfoliative cytology now approaches 90 to 95 percent.[12,13,28] If the clinician suspects a malignant effusion, several hundred milliliters of fluid should be removed at the initial diagnostic thoracentesis. This maneuver will not improve the yield on the initial study but, if it is negative, a repeat procedure several days later may provide fluid with fewer degenerative mesothelial cells and freshly exfoliated malignant cells. Percutaneous pleural biopsy should be reserved for the second thoracentesis if the initial pleural fluid cytologic examination is negative. If the second cytologic examination and initial pleural biopsy are negative, a third cytologic examination and second pleural biopsy soon after usually is not diagnostic.

There are several options for the patient with suspected malignancy and negative pleural fluid and pleural tissue examination. These include observation for a few weeks with repeat studies, thoracoscopy,[2,23] or open pleural biopsy. Before proceeding to more invasive procedures, other causes of an exudative pleural effusion must be excluded. Tuberculous pleurisy should always be considered in the patient with a lymphocyte-predominant exudate with or without a positive tuberculin skin test. The yield from pleural biopsy culture and histology, in conjunction with pleural fluid culture, should provide a bacteriologic diagnosis of tuberculous pleurisy in 90 to 95 percent of cases. Even if diagnostic studies are negative, patients with a positive purified protein derivative skin test and a lymphocyte-predominant exudate should be treated for tuberculous pleurisy because of the high risk (70 percent) of developing active pulmonary or extrapulmonary tuberculosis within 5 years if untreated. Bronchoscopy has a low diagnostic yield for an idiopathic pleural effusion without parenchymal lesions on chest radiograph, ipsilateral mediastinal shift, or hemoptysis. The value of computed tomographic examination of the chest in an undiagnosed exudative effusion is unknown and probably not cost effective. If observation is the course undertaken, the clinician would expect a malignant pleural effusion to be stable or to progress and an effusion not due to malignancy to be stable or to regress over time. Failure to identify a malignant pleural effusion for several weeks is rarely a disservice to the patient who has incurable disease. Exceptions are those malignancies that tend to be responsive to therapy, such as breast cancer, prostate cancer, thyroid cancer, small-cell lung carcinoma, germ-cell neoplasms, and lymphomas.

At present, tests on pleural fluids—such as determination of carcinoembryonic antigen, hyaluronic acid, and LDH isoenzymes—have no absolute diagnostic value. Electron microscopic examination of pleural fluid (in contrast to tissue) seems to offer little advantage over routine cytologic examination. Chromosome analysis of pleural fluid may be helpful in the diagnosis of lymphoma, leukemia, and mesothelioma; however, it is expensive and not readily available.[6]

Inflammatory processes involving the pleura may mimic mesothelioma, and patients are often subjected to a battery of tests and consultations before the diagnosis is established. An accurate diagnosis is imperative for proper epidemiologic records, appropriate therapeutic intervention, and litigation. Early in the course of the mesothelioma, establishing a definitive diagnosis may be problematic. Pleural fluid cytology and biopsy may allow the diagnosis of malignancy but usually cannot distinguish between mesothelioma and adenocarcinoma. Sarcomatous type mesothelioma can be confused with rare tumors such as fibrosarcomas or hemangiopericytomas. Thoracoscopic biopsy or open thoracotomy is usually necessary to confirm the diagnosis. Thoracoscopic biopsy has a high diagnostic yield, approaching 100 percent in some series, while the yield for pleural fluid cytology alone is 25 percent and that for combined pleural fluid cytology and closed pleural biopsy is 40 percent.[1] Histochemical and immunochemical studies in conjunction with electron microscopy have improved the accuracy of the diagnosis of malignant mesothelioma.

PROGNOSIS

The diagnosis of a malignant pleural effusion signals a poor prognosis. Patients with carcinoma of the lung, stomach, and ovary tend to have a survival time of only a few months from the time that the malignant effusion is diagnosed; patients with breast cancer may survive longer, several months to years, depending on the response to chemotherapy.[25] Patients with lymphomatous pleural effusions tend to have survival times intermediate between those of breast cancer and other carcinomas.

When pH and glucose concentrations in the malignant pleural effusion are low (7.30 and below 60 mg/dL, respectively), the survival time is less (average 2 months) than in those with a normal pH and glucose (average 10 months).[25] Thus, the pH and glucose in the pleural fluid provide helpful information with respect to a rational plan of palliative treatment.

A pleural effusion in the setting of lung cancer usually excludes operability; however, approximately 5 percent of these patients have a paramalignant effusion or effusion from another cause and may be operable and curable.[5,28] Thus, it is essential to establish the cause of the pleural effusion before deciding that the patient is no longer a candidate for curative surgery.

Survival following the diagnosis of malignant mesothelioma is related to the stage of the disease at the time of presentation.[1] Those patients with only ipsilateral involvement of the pleura and lung survive the longest, whereas those with distant hematogenous metastases have the shortest survival. Chest pain portends a worse prognosis than dyspnea, reflecting a more advanced stage of disease. Overall, the median survival in malignant mesothelioma is about 10 months. The epithelial type has a median survival approximately twice that of the sarcomatous type; long-term survivors of more than 3 years are seen almost exclusively with the epithelial type. As in metastatic carcinoma of the pleura, a low pH effusion in malignant mesothelioma is also predictive of a short survival.

Benign asbestos pleural effusions generally resolve, leaving some residual on the chest radiograph. Although malignant mesothelioma occasionally develops in patients with benign asbestos pleurisy, benign asbestos pleurisy does not appear to be a harbinger of mesothelioma.[7] Obviously, the risk of developing mesothelioma is greater in these asbestos-exposed individuals than in the general population.

TREATMENT

When the pleural effusion has been proved to be malignant or paramalignant and the patient is not a surgical candidate, the type of palliative therapy is weighed, taking into account the patient's general condition, symptoms, and expected survival. Several management options are available (Table 90-3). Asymptomatic patients need not be treated: most will develop progressive pleural effusions that will evoke symptoms and require therapy, but some will reach a steady state of pleural fluid formation and removal and not progress to a symptomatic stage. In the debili-

tated patient in whom a short survival is expected on grounds of general health, extent of disease, and the biochemical characteristics of the pleural fluid, periodic therapeutic thoracentesis as an outpatient is often preferable to hospitalization for tube thoracostomy and intrapleural instillation of a chemical agent.

Pleural abrasion with or without pleurectomy is almost always effective in obliterating the pleural space and controlling a malignant pleural effusion. However, pleurectomy is a major surgical procedure associated with considerable morbidity and some mortality.[20] Accordingly, this procedure is reserved for patients who are in good general condition and who have a reasonably long expected survival or who have failed a sclerosing agent procedure.[16]

In general, systemic chemotherapy is disappointing for the control of malignant pleural effusions. However, some patients with lymphoma, breast cancer, or small-cell carcinoma of the lung manifest a good response to chemotherapy. In patients with carcinoma of the breast, procurement of quantitative data about steroid receptors from a malignant pleural fluid can provide valuable information relating to the potential response to hormonal manipulation.

As a rule, radiation of the hemithorax is contraindicated in malignant pleural effusions from lung cancer, since the adverse effects from radiation pneumonitis outweigh possible benefits of therapy. However, when involvement of mediastinal nodes predominates, radiotherapy may be helpful in patients with lymphoma and lymphomatous chylothorax.

The most cost-effective method of controlling a malignant pleural effusion is chest tube drainage and intrapleural instillation of a chemical agent. A number of antineoplastic and nonantineoplastic chemical agents have been used for pleurodesis with variable success. Currently, the most successful and widely used agents include talc by poudrage or slurry, the tetracyclines (minocycline and doxycycline), *Corynebacterium parvum* (available only in Europe), and bleomycin.[32] Talc by either poudrage or slurry has been shown by numerous investigators to have a success rate of better than 90 percent.[14,27,32] In head-to-head comparisons with tetracycline and bleomycin, talc has been shown to be more effective. Furthermore, talc is readily available, inexpensive, and, when used in the proper doses, has minimal adverse effects.[29] When used as a slurry through a chest tube, talc is less expensive than the tetracycline-like drugs and substantially less expensive than bleomycin.[32] The degree of pain associated with talc has been variously reported from nonexistent to severe. Fever following talc poudrage and slurry is common, occurring from 16 to 69 percent of the time. Fever characteristically occurs 4 to 12 h following talc instillation and may last for 72 h.

Other complications that have been reported with talc include empyema,

TABLE 90-3

Management of Malignant and Paramalignant Pleural Effusions

Option	Comment
Observation	Asymptomatic; most will progress and require therapy
Therapeutic thoracentesis	Prompt relief of dyspnea; recurrence rate variable
Chemotherapy	May be effective in lymphoma, small-cell lung cancer, breast cancer
Radiotherapy	Mediastinal radiation may be effective in lymphoma and with lymphomatous chylothorax
Chest tube drainage only	Usually not effective
Chest tube drainage with talc slurry	Control of effusion in > 90 percent of cases
Thoracoscopy with talc poudrage	Control of effusion in > 90 percent of cases
Pleuroperitoneal shunt	When other options have failed or not indicated; may be useful for chylothorax
Pleural abrasion and pleurectomy	Virtually 100% effective; requires thoracoscopy or thoracotomy

arrhythmia, and respiratory failure including adult respiratory distress syndrome (ARDS) and pneumonitis.[14] It is doubtful that the method of administration (poudrage or slurry) plays a major role in the development of respiratory failure, although the dose may be important, as many reported patients had received 10 or more grams of talc.

Talc that is used for pleurodesis is asbestos-free, but sterility is not required by U.S. Pharmacopeia (USP) standards. Although talc is not packaged sterilely by the manufacturer, limitation on the number of microorganisms is part of USP specifications and total bacterial count cannot exceed 500 per gram. Unsterilized talc contains bacillus species that are generally thought to be nonpathogenic;[15] however, clinically significant disease has been reported primarily in immunocompromised hosts and intravenous drug abusers but also in normal hosts. Sterilization either by prolonged dry heat exposure, ethylene oxide gas, or gamma irradiation is effective.[15]

Before instituting chest tube drainage for intrapleural instillation of a chemical agent, it is necessary to demonstrate that fluid removal improves dyspnea. Determination of the FVC and P_{O_2} during the first 12 h following therapeutic thoracentesis may be misleading. Some patients experience a considerable decrease in P_{O_2} and minimal improvement in pulmonary function despite relief of dyspnea.

Following the initial therapeutic thoracentesis, the recurrence rate and the interval for return of symptoms should be noted. If recurrence is rapid, with return of dyspnea, pleurodesis should be considered. If the expected survival is at least several months, the patient is not debilitated, and the pleural fluid pH is above 7.30, the patient is a good candidate for pleurodesis. However, it is useless to attempt to produce pleurodesis if the lung cannot be expanded fully, as with mainstem bronchial occlusion or trapped lung. Furthermore, demonstrating that pleural fluid pH is below 7.30 not only suggests a short survival time but also predicts a poor response to chemical pleurodesis.[25,27] A large tumor bulk involving the pleural surfaces, seen with low-pH, low-glucose pleural effusions, is associated with diminished effectiveness of the chemical agent.

The technique used for intrapleural instillation of a chemical agent is critical for a good result. The pleural space must be drained as completely as possible so that the instilled agent is not diluted and the pleural surfaces remain in close contact during the time of the initial inflammatory insult. This is accomplished best by tube thoracostomy. If the patient has a large or massive effusion, the fluid should be drained slowly over the first several hours; the chest tube should be clamped intermittently to lessen the likelihood of unilateral pulmonary edema. The position of the chest tube should be checked by chest radiography and the patient positioned to provide optimal drainage. When the chest radiograph demonstrates that the effusion is absent or minimal and the lung is fully expanded (usually by 24 h following chest tube insertion), 5 g of talc in a slurry should be instilled into the pleural space. Following instillation, the tube should be clamped for 1 h. Recent evidence using radiolabeled tetracycline has demonstrated rapid and complete dispersion into the pleural space without patient repositioning.[18] The chest tube can be removed when drainage is below 150 mL/day, usually within 24 to 48 h. If a large volume of drainage persists,

a repeat dose of talc should be instilled. With the properly selected candidate and rigorously applied technique, the malignant effusion is controlled with talc poudrage or slurry in over 90 percent of cases.[14]

A further option available for the patient with intractable symptomatic malignant effusions who cannot undergo pleurodesis is a pleuroperitoneal shunt.[17] These shunts have been found to be safe and effective. The shunt may be particularly beneficial in refractory chylothorax, as it allows recirculation of chyle. Few complications have been associated with the shunt's placement and it can be inserted in patients who are poor surgical candidates. With experienced operators, palliation is obtained in 80 to 90 percent of properly selected patients. The major problem has been shunt failure, which is most commonly due to clotting of the catheter. It is unknown whether patients who have experienced shunt occlusion are at greater risk for occlusion after a new shunt is placed.

In general there is a nihilistic attitude regarding the management of patients with malignant mesothelioma because of the tumor's poor response to chemotherapy and radiation therapy. Early in the course of mesothelioma, the large unilateral pleural effusion causes substantial dyspnea. Talc pleurodesis may be successful in some patients; however, in others, such as patients with a pH below 7.30, the procedure tends not to be successful because of the tumor burden in the pleural space. Parietal pleurectomy tends to be more successful than talc pleurodesis in reducing the recurrence rate of pleural effusion.

REFERENCES

1. Antman KH: Natural history and epidemiology of malignant mesothelioma. *Chest* 103:373S–376S, 1993.
2. Boutin C, Viallat JR, Cargnino P, Farisse P: Thoracoscopy in malignant pleural effusions. *Am Rev Respir Dis* 124:588–592, 1981.
3. Chernow B, Sahn SA: Carcinomatous involvement of the pleura: An analysis of 96 patients. *Am J Med* 63:695–702, 1977.
4. Clarkson B: Relationship between cell type, glucose concentration, and response to treatment in neoplastic effusions. *Cancer* 17:914–928, 1964.
5. Decker DA, Dines DE, Payne WS, et al: The significance of a cytologically negative pleural effusion in bronchogenic carcinoma. *Chest* 74:640–642, 1978.
6. Dewald G, Dines DE, Weiland LH, Gordon H: Usefulness of chromosome examination in the diagnosis of malignant pleural effusions. *New Engl J Med* 295:1494–1500, 1976.
7. Epler GR, McCloud TC, Gaensler EA: Prevalence and incidence of benign asbestos pleural effusion in a working population. *JAMA* 247:617–622, 1982.
8. Fentiman IS, Millis R, Sexton S, Hayward JL: Pleural effusion in breast cancer: A review of 105 cases. *Cancer* 47:2087–2092, 1981.
9. Good JT Jr, Taryle DA, Sahn SA: The pathogenesis of low glucose, low pH malignant effusions. *Am Rev Respir Dis* 131:737–741, 1985.
10. Gottehrer A, Taryle DA, Reed CE, Sahn SA: Pleural fluid analysis in malignant mesothelioma: prognostic implications. *Chest* 100:1003–1006, 1991.
11. Hillerdal G: Malignant mesothelioma in 1982: Review of 4,710 published cases. *Br J Dis Chest* 77:321–343, 1983.
12. Hsu C: Cytologic detection of malignancy in pleural effusion: A review of 5,255 samples from 3,811 patients. *Diagn Cytopathol* 3:8–12, 1987.

13. Johnson WW: The malignant pleural effusion: A review of cytopathologic diagnoses of 584 specimens from 472 consecutive patients. *Cancer* 56:905–909, 1985.

14. Kennedy L, Sahn SA: Talc pleurodesis for the treatment of pneumothorax and pleural effusion. *Chest* 106:1215–1222, 1994.

15. Kennedy L, Vaughan LM, Steed LL, Sahn SA: Sterilization of talc for pleurodesis: Available techniques, efficacy, and cost analysis. *Chest* 107:1032–1034, 1995.

16. Levine MN, Young JE, Ryan ED, Newhouse MT: Pleural effusion in breast cancer: Thoracoscopy for hormone receptor determination. *Cancer* 57:324–327, 1986.

17. Little AG, Ferguson MK, Golomb HM, et al: Pleuroperitoneal shunting for malignant pleural effusions. *Cancer* 58:2740–2743, 1986.

18. Lorch DG, Gordon L, Wooten S, et al: The effect of patient positioning on the distribution of tetracycline in the pleural space during pleurodesis. *Chest* 93:527–529, 1988.

19. Maher GG, Berger HW: Massive pleural effusion: Malignant and nonmalignant causes in 46 patients. *Am Rev Respir Dis* 105:458–460, 1972.

20. Martini N, Bains MS, Beattie EJ Jr: Indications for pleurectomy in malignant effusion. *Cancer* 35:734–738, 1975.

21. Meyer PC: Metastatic carcinoma of the pleura. *Thorax* 21:437–443, 1966.

22. Prakash UBS, Reinman HM: Comparison of needle biopsy with cytologic analysis for the evaluation of pleural effusion: Analysis of 414 cases. *Mayo Clin Proc* 60:158–164, 1985.

23. Rusch VW, Mountain C: Thoracoscopy under regional anesthesia for the diagnosis and management of pleural disease. *Am J Surg* 154:274–278, 1987.

24. Sahn SA: Malignant pleural effusions. *Semin Respir Med* 9:43–53, 1987.

25. Sahn SA, Good JT Jr: Pleural fluid pH in malignant effusions: Diagnostic, prognostic, and therapeutic implications. *Ann Intern Med* 108:345–349, 1988.

26. Sahn SA: Pleural effusion in lung cancer. *Clin Chest Med* 14:189–200, 1993.

27. Sanchez-Armengol A, Rodriguez-Panadero F: Survival and talc pleurodesis in metastatic pleural carcinoma—Revisited. *Chest* 104:1482–1485, 1993.

28. Sears D, Hajdu SI: The cytologic diagnosis of malignant neoplasms in pleural and peritoneal effusions. *Acta Cytol* 31:85–97, 1987.

29. Selikoff IJ, Churg J, Hammond EC: Relation between exposure to asbestos and mesothelioma. *New Engl J Med* 272:560–565,1965.

30. Spriggs AI, Boddington MM: *The Cytology of Effusions,* 2d ed. London, Heinemann, 1968.

31. Wagner JC, Sleggs CA, Marchand P: Diffuse pleural mesothelioma and asbestos exposure in North Western Cape Province. *Br J Industr Med* 17:260–271, 1960.

32. Walker-Renard PB, Vaughan LM, Sahn SA: Chemical pleurodesis for the treatment of malignant pleural effusions. *Ann Intern Med* 120:56–64, 1994.

33. Weick JK, Kiely JM, Harrison EG Jr, et al: Pleural effusion in lymphoma. *Cancer* 31:848–853, 1973.

34. Yam LT: Diagnostic significance of lymphocytes in pleural effusions. *Ann Intern Med* 66:972–982, 1967.

CHAPTER 91

PNEUMOTHORAX

Jay I. Peters / Edward Y. Sako

A pneumothorax is defined as the accumulation of air in the pleural space with secondary lung collapse. Pneumothoraces can be divided into *spontaneous pneumothorax*, which occurs without trauma or obvious cause, and *traumatic pneumothorax,* which occurs as a result of direct trauma to the chest. Spontaneous pneumothorax is subclassified as either a *primary spontaneous* or *secondary spontaneous pneumothorax.* Primary spontaneous pneumothorax occurs in healthy persons and secondary spontaneous pneumothorax in persons with diseases that affect the lung. Traumatic pneumothorax occurs as the result of blunt or penetrating trauma disrupting the lung, bronchus, or the esophagus. A subcategory of traumatic pneumothorax is *iatrogenic pneumothorax,* which occurs as a consequence of diagnostic or therapeutic maneuvers.

PATHOPHYSIOLOGY

The pressure within the pleural space is negative with respect to the alveolar pressure during the entire respiratory cycle. This negative pressure results from the inherent tendency for the lung to collapse (elastic recoil) and of the chest wall to expand. The negative intrapleural pressure is not uniform throughout the pleural space; a gradient of 0.25 cm of water per centimeter of vertical distance can be measured between the apex and the base of the lung. At the apex, the pressure is more negative than at the base, and this pressure difference tends to favor a greater distention of the alveoli located in this region.

When a communication develops between an alveolus and the pleural space, air will move from the alveolus into the pleural space until there is equalization of pressure or until the communication is sealed. The same happens with a communication between the chest wall and the pleural cavity. Although the mechanism responsible for spontaneous pneumothorax is not clear, experimental overdistention of normal lungs results in rupture of subpleural alveoli.[37] Air can dissect along the bronchovascular sheath medially to produce pneumomediastinum, which may be accompanied by subcutaneous emphysema or pneumothorax (Fig. 91-1), or it can dissect to the peripheral portion of the lung.[26] Peripheral dissection of air may result in an air-containing space within or immediately below the visceral pleura. Pathologic studies of resected lung from patients with spontaneous pneumothorax usually show one or both of these types of air-spaces, a bleb or a bulla. A bulla is lined partly by a thickened fibrotic pleura and partly by fibrous tissue within the lung itself, whereas a bleb is situated entirely within the pleura. A pneumothorax occurs when these peripheral bullae or blebs become distended and rupture into the pleural space.

The main physiological consequences of a pneumothorax are a decrease in the vital capacity of the lung and a decrease in Pa_{O_2}. Total lung capacity, functional residual capacity, and diffusing capacity are also reduced, though less than vital capacity. Air in the pleural space eliminates the gravitational gradients of pleural pressure and regional lung volume so that regional ventilation is uniform. The reduction in arterial Pa_{O_2} appears to be caused by low ventilation-perfusion ($\dot{V}_A/\dot{Q}$) ratios, anatomic shunts, and, occasionally, alveolar hypoventilation. Anthonisen reported that lungs demonstrate airway closure at low lung volumes and suggested that airway closure is the main cause of $\dot{V}_A/\dot{Q}$ imbalance in patients with pneumothorax.[5] If perfusion to the collapsed lung is preserved, there is an increase in pulmonary shunt and substantial hypoxemia. If perfusion to the collapsed lung is reduced by hypoxic vasoconstriction, hypoxemia may be minimal. Pneumothoraces occupying less than 25 percent of the hemithorax are not usually associated with increased shunts.[27] Under normal circumstances, despite the degree of pneumotho-

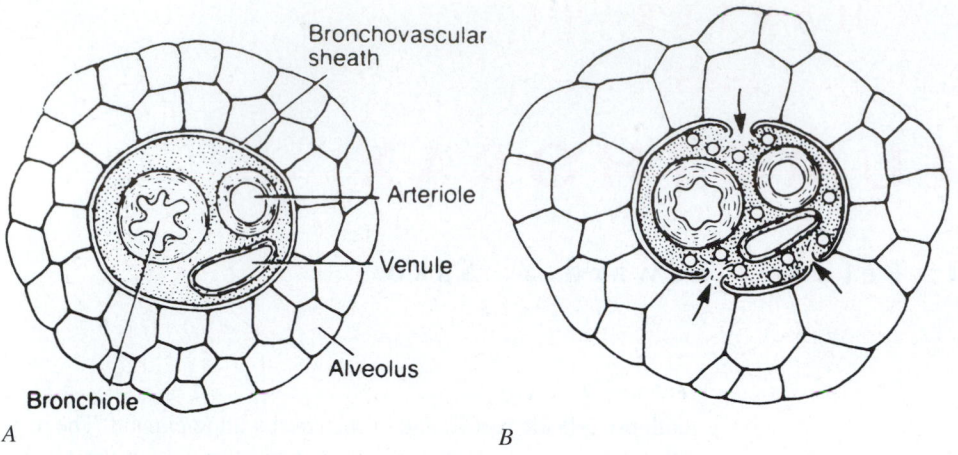

FIGURE 91-1   Proposed mechanism of alveolar rupture in spontaneous pneumothorax. *A.* Normal structures. *B.* Overdistention of marginal alveoli. Pressure in the adjacent bronchovascular sheath remains lower than in the overdistended alveoli. This pressure gradient may lead to rupture of the alveoli with dissection of air towards the pleura or mediastinum. (*From Maunder: Arch Intern Med 144:1449, 1984.*)

rax, hypoxemia tends to abate within 24 h, presumably because of redistribution of pulmonary blood flow.

In the healthy person, the decrease in vital capacity and Pa_{O_2} is well tolerated. In patients with compromised pulmonary function before the pneumothorax, the decrease in vital capacity may lead to alveolar hypoventilation and respiratory acidosis. When air is evacuated from the pleural space, the Pa_{O_2} usually improves. In animal studies, the Pa_{O_2} returns to baseline immediately after reexpansion of the lung. In humans, normalization of the Pa_{O_2} takes longer and may occur over hours to several days. The delay in improvement may be related to the duration of the pneumothorax.

REABSORPTION OF PLEURAL GASES

Gas reabsorption from the pleural space is achieved by simple diffusion from the pleural space into the venous blood. The rate of gas reabsorption depends on four variables: (1) the pressure gradient for the gases between the pleural space in relation to the venous blood, (2) the diffusion properties for the gases present in the pleural space, (3) the area of contact between the pleural gas and the pleura, and (4) the permeability of the pleural surface. (A thickened, fibrotic pleura will absorb less than normal pleura.)

The solubility and diffusion properties of different gases vary considerably, and the speed of reabsorption will depend on the type of gas. Oxygen will be absorbed 62 times faster than nitrogen, the slowest gas to be reabsorbed. Carbon dioxide will be absorbed 23 times faster than oxygen, and carbon dioxide and water vapor will equilibrate almost instantaneously. If a patient develops a pneumothorax while receiving 100 percent oxygen, the pleural gas will be composed mostly of oxygen and contain no nitrogen. The pneumothorax will reabsorb much faster for two reasons: the pneumothorax will be filled with the more soluble oxygen, and the pressure gradient between the pneumothorax and the venous blood will be larger, because 100 percent

oxygen will wash out nitrogen from the alveoli and, eventually, the venous blood.

Under normal circumstances, the total gas pressure in the pneumothorax is within a few millimeters of mercury of that of the atmosphere, or 760 mmHg. Tissue gas tensions are close to those of systemic venous blood: typically $pCO_2 = 46$ mmHg, $pO_2 = 40$ mmHg, $pH_2O = 47$ mmHg, and $pN_2 = 569$ mmHg, giving a total pressure of 702 mmHg. This positive-pressure gradient between the pneumothorax and the venous blood constitutes the driving force responsible for gas reabsorption from a pneumothorax.

If the gas in the pneumothorax equilibrates with tissue in terms of pO_2 and pCO_2, the pN_2 must be about 627 mmHg (atmospheric pressure less the sum of pO_2, pCO_2, and pH_2O), and N_2 is reabsorbed. This reabsorption decreases the volume of the pneumothorax, but decreases its total pressure only slightly, so that pO_2 and pCO_2 increase. As they equilibrate with tissue, pN_2 again rises and is reabsorbed in a continuing cycle (Fig. 91-2).[39] The time required to absorb all gases in a pneumothorax is quite variable.

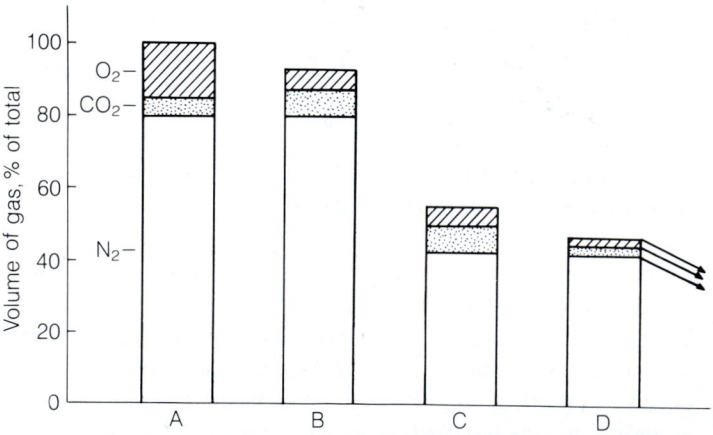

FIGURE 91-2   Hypothetical representation of the resorption of a spontaneous pneumothorax. *A.* Closed pleural space after leak has stopped. The alveolar gas in the space contains 15 percent O_2, 5% CO_2, and 80% N_2. *B.* CO_2 and O_2 have quickly equilibrated with the surrounding tissues; the amount of N_2 in the pneumothorax is unchanged. The pneumothorax is already decreased by about 10 percent. *C.* The number of N_2 molecules is unchanged, but the total volume of the pneumothorax has decreased (see *B*). Therefore, the outward diffusion of N_2 increases because pN_2 in the pleural space is greater than pN_2 in the tissues. As N_2 diffuses out, the total volume of gas in the pleural space decreases and concentrations of O_2 and CO_2 increase. As a result, O_2 and CO_2 diffuse out of the pleural space. *D.* The high N_2 concentration promotes the exit of N_2 from the pleural space and continues the cycle by which the pneumothorax grows smaller. (*From Farhi: JAMA 188:986, 1964.*)

It has been estimated that between 1 and 6 percent of a pneumothorax is absorbed in 24 h.[31]

SYNDROMES

Primary Spontaneous Pneumothorax

Primary spontaneous pneumothorax occurs most commonly in men in the third and fourth decades of life. Probably the most accurate estimate on the incidence of primary spontaneous pneumothorax comes from a population-based study of the residents of Olmsted County, Minnesota, where complete medical records are maintained and patients are served by a single medical community. Between 1950 and 1974, 141 cases of spontaneous pneumothorax (77 primary, 64 secondary) occurred among the county's population.[42] The age-adjusted incidence of primary spontaneous pneumothorax was 7.4/100,000/year for males and 1.2/100,000/year for females. The male-to-female predominance for primary spontaneous pneumothorax ranges from 6-to-1 to 3-to-1. A familial tendency has been noted, and the HLA haplotype A_2B_{40}[52] or the α_1-antitrypsin phenotypes M_1M_2 have been implicated as risk factors. Women more often have a family history of pneumothorax and develop their first spontaneous pneumothorax 2 to 5 years earlier than men.

Tobacco smoking increases the risk of spontaneous pneumothorax. The quantity of cigarettes per day and the length of exposure are dominant risk factors. The relative risk of spontaneous pneumothorax is more than 20 times higher in men who smoke one-half pack per day and 100 times higher in men who smoke one pack per day than in nonsmokers. One review of 402 patients with spontaneous primary pneumothorax reported that 92 percent of the patients were smokers or ex-smokers.[27] Another study showed that patients who had stopped smoking more than one year before their first spontaneous pneumothorax had no recurrence during a follow-up of 5.2 years.[35]

Patients with primary spontaneous pneumothorax tend to be taller and thinner than control populations. Military recruits who developed spontaneous pneumothorax were, on the average, 2 in taller and 25 lb lighter than the typical military recruit.[44] In the series of Melton and colleagues, primary spontaneous pneumothorax increased with height and reached an incidence of 200 per 100,000 person-years for subjects at least 76 in tall.[42] Pleural pressure is most negative at the apices, and the degree of negativity relates to the height of the lungs. The alveoli of taller persons are subjected to greater mean distending pressures. Over a long period, this phenomenon could lead to the formation of subpleural blebs in a taller population genetically predisposed to bleb formation. Data suggest that some cases of spontaneous pneumothorax are inherited through an autosomal-dominant gene with variable penetrance while others appear to be due to an X-linked recessive gene.[1]

The cause of primary spontaneous pneumothorax is most often the rupture of subpleural blebs or bullae on the apical portion of the upper lobes. The pathogenesis of these subpleural blebs or bullae is unknown. They have been attributed to intrinsic abnormality of connective tissue (e.g., Marfan's syndrome), to inflammation of the bronchioles, or to overdistension of alveoli with poor collateral ventilation.

Blebs are demonstrated on chest radiographs in only 20 percent of cases, although their visualization may be facilitated radiographically in expiration or at the time of maximal pulmonary collapse. Computed tomography often reveals small blebs or bullae that are not visualized on plain radiographs. At the time of thoracotomy, subpleural blebs or bullae are identified in 85 to 100 percent of cases.[22]

The rate of recurrence after a primary spontaneous pneumothorax is approximately 25 percent (range: 23 to 52 percent) and usually occurs within 2 years of the first episode. The rate of recurrence may increase with each successive pneumothorax. Gobbel and coworkers found the risk of recurrence increased to more than 60 percent after the second pneumothorax and to 83 percent after the third.[22] Although there is no predilection for the right or left hemithorax with the initial episode, more than 75 percent of recurrences occur on the same side as the first pneumothorax. Despite the documentation that pleural blebs occur bilaterally in many patients with primary spontaneous pneumothorax, the risk of contralateral pneumothorax is only 5 to 10 percent.

Secondary Pneumothorax

Secondary spontaneous pneumothorax is more serious than primary spontaneous pneumothorax because, by definition, the patient already has underlying lung disease. The incidence of secondary spontaneous pneumothorax is similar to that of primary spontaneous pneumothorax. In Olmsted County, Minnesota, the incidence of secondary spontaneous pneumothorax was 6.3/100,000/year for males and 2.0/100,000/year for females.[42] On average, patients with secondary spontaneous pneumothorax are 15 to 20 years older than patients with primary spontaneous pneumothorax.

Many different pulmonary diseases have been associated with spontaneous pneumothorax, but chronic obstructive pulmonary disease (COPD) is the most common cause of secondary spontaneous pneumothorax. The Veterans Administration Cooperative Study on Pneumothorax noted that pneumothorax tended to occur in patients with moderately severe COPD, with a quarter of the participants having an FEV_1 below 1 L and a mean FEV_1/FVC ratio of 57 percent.[33] Persistent bronchopleural fistula was also noted to be common in patients with obstructive lung disease, and 35 percent of patients had an air leak for more than 5 days. Although the mortality for recurrent pneumothorax was only 1.5 percent in the VA Cooperative Study, previous studies with secondary pneumothorax in patients with COPD have a combined mortality of 16 percent.

The incidence of spontaneous pneumothorax in patients with cystic fibrosis is high. One study found that spontaneous pneumothorax occurred in 12.5 percent of 144 patients with cystic fibrosis over 10 years of age.[36] Pneumothorax in patients with cystic fibrosis tended to occur in older patients with severe pulmonary disease. Pneumothorax is an ominous complication of cystic fibrosis, and the recurrence rate of spontaneous pneumothorax treated with tube thoracostomy alone approaches 50 percent.[10] In one study, the median survival after the first spontaneous pneumothorax was only 29.9 months.[53]

Many other diseases may be associated with spontaneous pneumothorax. The following list gives some idea of the broad spectrum of diseases associated with spontaneous secondary pneumothorax, but it is by no means complete: asthma, sarcoidosis, tuberculosis, idiopathic pulmonary fibrosis, eosinophilic granuloma, lymphangioleiomyomatosis, acute bacterial pneumonia (especially staphylococcosis), *Pneumocystis carinii* pneumonia, lung abscess, radiation therapy, pulmonary carcinoma, pulmonary metastasis (especially sarcomas), pulmonary infarction, idiopathic pulmonary hemorrhage, pulmonary alveolar proteinosis, coccidioidomycosis, tuberous sclerosis, von Recklinghausen's disease, Wegener's granulomatosis, and complications of chemotherapy in the treatment of malignancy.

Traumatic Pneumothorax

Trauma is the most common cause of pneumothorax. Between 1950 and 1974, there were 318 cases of pneumothorax in Olmsted County, Minnesota. Trauma was responsible for 177 of these cases (56 percent), of which 102 were iatrogenic.[42] Iatrogenic cases have increased over the past 20 years because of increased use of invasive diagnostic procedures such as percutaneous lung aspiration, transbronchial biopsy, and insertion of central venous and pulmonary artery catheters.

Iatrogenic pneumothorax most commonly occurs as a complication of procedures. The leading cause of iatrogenic pneumothorax is transthoracic needle aspiration.[18] Pneumothorax occurs in about 30 percent of patients undergoing this procedure, and 10 percent of patients require tube thoracostomy. The risk of pneumothorax in transthoracic needle aspiration increases in patients with COPD or if the lesion is deep in the lung. The risk of pneumothorax with central venous catheterization has been reported between 3 to 6 percent.[13] Subclavian catheterization carries a significantly higher risk than internal jugular catheterization. Pneumothorax may also occur with thoracentesis, transbronchial biopsy, Wang needle aspiration, liver biopsy, intercostal nerve block, mediastinoscopy, and tracheostomy. Pneumothorax may not be evident immediately after the procedure, but most cases develop within the first 24 h. Another cause of pneumothorax that is frequently overlooked is chest tube malfunction. Common causes of chest tube malfunction include inadequate securing of the chest tube to the drainage system, failing to fill the U-manometer in the waterseal chamber, failing to refill the water in the suction control chamber, and permitting intermittent disconnection of the system during diagnostic or therapeutic studies.

Mechanical ventilation is a frequent, potentially lethal cause of iatrogenic pneumothorax. The overall incidence of pneumothorax during mechanical ventilation is about 5 percent, but it may be as high as 35 percent in patients with an inflammatory disease such as aspiration pneumonia.[16] The incidence of pneumothorax is also increased during mechanical ventilation if patients have chronic pulmonary disease, receive positive end-expiratory pressure, or have right main-stem intubation.[16] Clinically, the patients become tachypneic and may fight the ventilator. Peak inspiratory pressure often rises suddenly from a coexisting fall in lung compliance. Resulting barotrauma leads to a pneumothorax that may rapidly progress to a tension pneumothorax. Radiographs of critically ill patients are frequently obtained only in the supine position. In a study by Tocino and colleagues, supine and semierect radiographs were obtained in 88 critically ill patients with 112 cases of pneumothorax.[54] The radiologist initially failed to detect the pneumothorax in 30 percent of the cases. Any increased lucency in a supine film should be evaluated by erect or decubitus views to detect the presence of a pneumothorax. If erect or decubitus films cannot be obtained, CT scans of the chest may be necessary.

Noniatrogenic traumatic pneumothorax can result from either penetrating or nonpenetrating chest injury. Penetrating chest trauma produces a pneumothorax by allowing air to enter the pleural cavity directly through the chest wall. In addition, if the visceral pleura is penetrated, air may leak from the tracheobronchial tree. If the continuity of the chest wall is disrupted, an open pneumothorax is produced. If the opening in the chest wall is larger than the diameter of the trachea (1.2 to 1.5 cm in an adult), air movement occurs through the pathway of least resistance, and air is preferentially inspired into the thoracic cavity through the open chest wound. Any open chest wound must be occluded to assure adequate ventilation of the patient.

Pneumothorax is also a frequent finding in patients with blunt trauma to the chest. The visceral pleura may be lacerated secondary to a rib fracture or dislocation; however, in almost one-half of patients with pneumothorax secondary to blunt trauma, there are no associated rib fractures. This is especially common with blunt trauma to the chest secondary to blast injuries and high-altitude falls into water. In such incidents, the abrupt increase in the pressure gradient between the alveolus and the adjacent bronchovesicular sheath causes disruption of the alveolar membrane. Dissection of air through the interstitial space results in either pneumothorax or pneumomediastinum.

Occasionally, patients with traumatic pneumothorax have coexisting injuries of the tracheobronchial tree or of the esophagus. In a patient with a traumatic pneumothorax, fiberoptic bronchoscopy should be performed in the presence of hemoptysis or a persistent air leak. Eighty percent of injuries to the tracheobronchial tree are within 2.5 cm of the carina, most commonly on the right side at the membranous-cartilaginous interface. The main lobar bronchi and the cervical trachea are the next most common sites of injury.

Traumatic rupture of the esophagus usually produces a hydropneumothorax. Therefore, if a patient with a traumatic pneumothorax also has a pleural effusion, the possibility of esophageal rupture should be entertained. Almost all patients with perforation of the thoracic esophagus also have dysphagia and pneumomediastinum. An elevated pleural fluid amylase concentration is a reliable screening procedure for esophageal rupture. Once the diagnosis is suspected, contrast radiographic studies of the esophagus should be performed as soon as possible. Untreated, esophageal rupture results in mediastinitis and septic shock; therefore, a high index of suspicion is essential in making an early diagnosis.

Catamenial Pneumothorax

Catamenial pneumothorax is a pneumothorax that occurs in conjunction with menstruation and is usually recurrent. Catamenial pneumothorax is a rare disorder, and fewer than 100 cases of catamenial pneumothorax and one case of catamenial pneumomediastinum have been reported in the literature in English. However, these numbers probably underestimate the frequency of this disorder. Catamenial pneumothorax represents 3 to 6 percent of spontaneous pneumothorax in women.[12]

Most women affected by catamenial pneumothorax are in the third to fourth decade of life. The diagnosis of this syndrome is based on recurrent pneumothorax occurring within 48 to 72 h of the onset of menses. The majority (90 to 95 percent) of catamenial pneumothoraces affect the right hemithorax, but isolated left-side or bilateral pneumothoraces have been reported.

The pathogenesis of catamenial pneumothorax is not definitely known. Twenty to 40 percent of women with catamenial pneumothorax have documented pelvic endometriosis. One theory suggests pleural and/or diaphragmatic endometrial implants as being responsible for this disorder;[41] however, only one-third of women have implants at the time of thoracotomy. Theories also include peritoneal air entering the thoracic cavity through diaphragmatic defects during menstruation, intrapulmonary implants causing bronchiolar obstruction, and the production of prostaglandin $F_{2\alpha}$ by endometrial tissue resulting in bronchiolar and vascular constriction.[34]

Catamenial pneumothorax is usually treated by the administration of oral contraceptives to suppress ovulation. Danazol, a weak androgen, suppresses ovulation and has been used in a few cases. Hysterectomy with bilateral oophorectomy will induce surgical menopause and thus prevent pneumothorax. Since many patients are at childbearing age, thoracotomy with pleural abrasion or pleurectomy have been performed to prevent recurrent pneumothorax.

Pneumothorax in Acquired Immunodeficiency Syndrome

Since the early 1980s, there have been an increasing number of reports describing the association between pneumothorax or pneumomediastinum and the acquired immunodeficiency syndrome (AIDS). About 2 to 5 percent of patients with AIDS experience pneumothorax unrelated to trauma or a pulmonary procedure. Patients receiving inhaled pentamidine prophylaxis and those with a history of *Pneumocystis carinii* pneumonia (PCP) are at greatest risk. Although pneumothorax may occur as a late sequela of PCP, 95 percent of patients have active PCP at the time of presentation.[50] Therefore, PCP treatment is recommended in any patient with AIDS who presents with a spontaneous pneumothorax.

The large number of pneumothoraces seen in patients with AIDS is thought to be secondary to the high incidence of subpleural cystic disease seen in AIDS patients with PCP. These lesions occur most frequently at the apices of the lungs and consist of necrotic alveoli filled with PCP organisms, macrophages, eosinophilic exudate, and fibrous material. Histologic examination of patients who have recovered from PCP demonstrates both subpleural blebs and bullae as well as pneumatoceles. Because of the necrotizing nature of the pneumonia, spontaneous pneumothorax is notoriously difficult to treat. Persistent air leaks often require tube thoracostomy for 3 to 4 weeks, and up to one-quarter of patients require surgical intervention.

The incidence of bilateral cystic disease in these patients is extremely high, and the incidence of contralateral pneumothorax was about 50 percent in one study.[50] Therefore, if surgical intervention is planned, some authors recommend preoperative CT scans of the chest and median sternotomy in patients with significant bilateral disease. Others recommend early thoracoscopic therapy in good surgical candidates to avoid prolonged hospitalization.

Pneumothorax in patients with AIDS can also occur with pyogenic infections, Kaposi's sarcoma, cytomegalovirus, and mycobacterial disease. With the rise of AIDS, the frequency of pulmonary tuberculosis has increased within the general population. Between 1 and 3 percent of all patients hospitalized for pulmonary tuberculosis will have a pneumothorax, which often requires prolonged periods of chest drainage. In cases of tuberculosis, surgery should not be considered until the patient has received antituberculous therapy for at least 6 weeks.

CLINICAL FEATURES

The main symptoms with the development of a pneumothorax are chest pain and dyspnea, which occur in 95 percent of patients. The pain is usually acute, localized to the side of the pneumothorax, and typically pleuritic. Cough, hemoptysis, orthopnea, and Horner's syndrome are uncommon manifestations of a pneumothorax.[27,32] A small percentage of patients are asymptomatic or complain only of generalized malaise.

Spontaneous pneumothorax usually occurs at rest, and fewer than 10 percent of them occur during strenuous exercise. In primary spontaneous pneumothorax, both the dyspnea and chest pain may subsequently abate over the first 24 h. This may explain why nearly half of patients have symptoms for 2 days before seeking medical attention and why 18 percent wait for more than a week.[27] Most patients with secondary spontaneous pneumothorax have more-severe symptoms, and dyspnea frequently seems out of proportion to the size of the pneumothorax.

Small pneumothoraces (less than 20 percent) are usually not detectable on physical exam. In patients with obstructive lung disease, even larger pneumothoraces may be difficult to detect. On physical exam, vital signs are usually normal, with the exception of moderate tachycardia. Examination of the chest may reveal the affected side to be larger and move less during respiration. Tactile fremitus is absent, the percussion note is hyperresonant, and breath sounds are absent or reduced on the side with the pneumothorax. Hamman's sign may be detected. This sign, also heard with pneumomediastinum, has been described as crunching or clicking noises synchronous with the heartbeat but influenced by respiration and body position. Severe tachycardia, with a heart rate above 140 beats a minute, hypotension, cyanosis, or tracheal deviation, suggests the possibility of a tension pneumothorax.

Arterial blood gases often show hypoxemia and perhaps hypocarbia from hyperventilation. Hypoxemia is usually mild in primary spontaneous pneumothorax when less than 25 percent of the lung is affected. When more than 25 percent of the lung is involved, pulmonary shunts occur more frequently and hypoxemia may be severe. In patients with secondary spontaneous pneumothorax, pulmonary reserve is already diminished and life-threatening hypoxemia and hypercarbia may be present. In a study by Dines et al., the mean Pa_{O_2} was 48 mmHg and the mean pCO_2 was 58 mmHg when patients with emphysema presented with a spontaneous pneumothorax.[19]

Patients with a left pneumothorax may show changes suggesting an anterolateral myocardial infarction. A rightward shift of the frontal QRS axis and clockwise rotation of the heart result in a diminution of precordial R-wave voltage, a decrease in the QRS amplitude, and precordial T-wave inversion.[59] These electrocardiographic features differ from a transmural myocardial infarction because of the absence of ST-segment elevation or significant Q waves. An anterior subendocardial infarction may present with T-wave inversion but without the rightward shift in the frontal axis. The electrocardiographic changes with a left pneumothorax may normalize when the patient is in the upright or right lateral decubitus position.

RADIOGRAPHIC APPEARANCE

The diagnosis of a pneumothorax is established by demonstrating the outer margin of the visceral pleura (and lung) separated from the parietal pleura (and chest wall) by a lucent gas space devoid of pulmonary vessels (Fig. 91-3). The pleural line may be difficult to detect with a small pneumothorax unless high-quality PA and lateral chest films are obtained and viewed under a bright light. In erect patients, pleural gas collects over the apex, and the space between the lung and chest wall is most notable there. In the supine position, gas migrates along the broad ventral surface of the lung, making detection on a frontal radiograph difficult. In the supine position, the juxtacardiac area, the lateral chest wall, and the subpulmonic region are the best areas to search for evidence of pneumothorax. When a suspected pneumothorax is not definitely seen on an inspiratory film, an expiratory film may be helpful. At end-expiration, the constant volume of the pneumothorax gas is accentuated by the reduction in the size of the hemithorax. Therefore, the pneumothorax is more easily recognized. Similar accentuation can be obtained with lateral decubitus studies of the appropriate side.

It is very important to differentiate the pleural line of a pneumothorax from that of a skinfold, clothing, tubing, or chest wall artifact. Careful inspection of the film may show that the artifact extends beyond the thorax, or that lung markings are visible beyond the apparent pleural line. In the absence of underlying lung disease, the pleural line of a pneumothorax usually parallels the shape of the chest wall. Artifactual densities generally do not parallel the course of the chest wall over their entire length. Avascular bullae or thin-walled cysts can be mistaken for a pneumothorax. The pleural line caused by a pneumothorax is usually bowed at its center toward the lateral chest wall. As opposed to a pneumothorax, the inner margins of bullae or cysts are, in general, concave rather than convex and do not exactly conform to the contour of the costophrenic sulcus. A pneumothorax with a pleural adhesion may also simulate bullae or lung cysts. A synechia tends to form a straight line connecting the lung to the

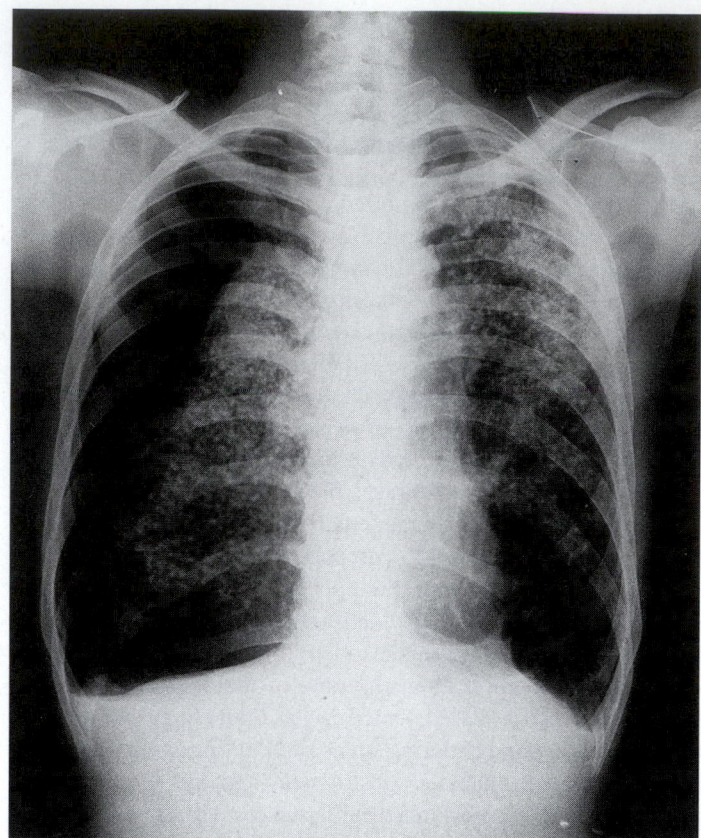

FIGURE 91-3 Patient with nodular silicosis and a spontaneous secondary pneumothorax. The visceral pleural line is clearly seen with the absence of vascular workings beyond the pleural line. There are cicatricial bullae in both bases.

parietal pleura; bullae or cysts have rounded edges. Such features are not 100 percent specific, and the use of tomography (standard or computed) may be required to differentiate a loculated pneumothorax from a cyst or bulla. Pleural effusions occur coincident with pneumothorax in 20 to 25 percent of cases. Hemopneumothorax occurs in 2 to 3 percent of cases of spontaneous pneumothorax. Bleeding is believed to represent rupture or tearing of vascular adhesions between the visceral and parietal pleura as the lung collapses.

Quantification of the size of a pneumothorax is helpful; unfortunately, however, the methods for quantifying lack uniformity and are by no means precise. Light suggested the measurement of the average diameters of the collapsed lung and of the affected hemithorax, with the cubing of these diameters to estimate the percentage of collapsed lung.[32] For example, if the diameter of the collapsed lung is 6 cm and the diameter of the hemithorax is 10 cm, the collapsed lung is estimated by the formula $100 - 6^3/10^3$. Thus, the estimated size of the pneumothorax is 78 percent.[32] Rhea and coworkers proposed the use of a nomogram to calculate the size of the pneumothorax.[47] With this method, the average intrapleural distance is calculated by measuring the interpleural distance at the apex and at the midpoints of both the upper and lower lungs. These three values are then averaged, and the number is reported on a nomogram, which gives an estimated size of the pneumothorax. An example of these calculations is shown in Fig. 91-4.

The most common radiographic manifestations of tension pneumothorax are mediastinal shift, diaphragmatic depression, and rib cage expansion (Fig. 91-5). Any significant degree of displacement of the mediastinum from the midline position on maximum inspiration, or any depression of the diaphragm, should be taken as evidence of tension. The degree of lung collapse is an unreliable sign for or against collapse, since underlying lung disease may prevent collapse even in the presence of tension.

CT scans of the chest are being used with increasing frequency in patients with pneumothorax. CT scans may be necessary to diagnose pneumothorax in critically ill patients when upright or decubitus films are not possible. CT scans may prove helpful in predicting the rate of recurrence in patients with spontaneous pneumothorax. One study demonstrated that patients who have larger or more numerous blebs on thoracic CT scans are more likely to have recurrence.[60]

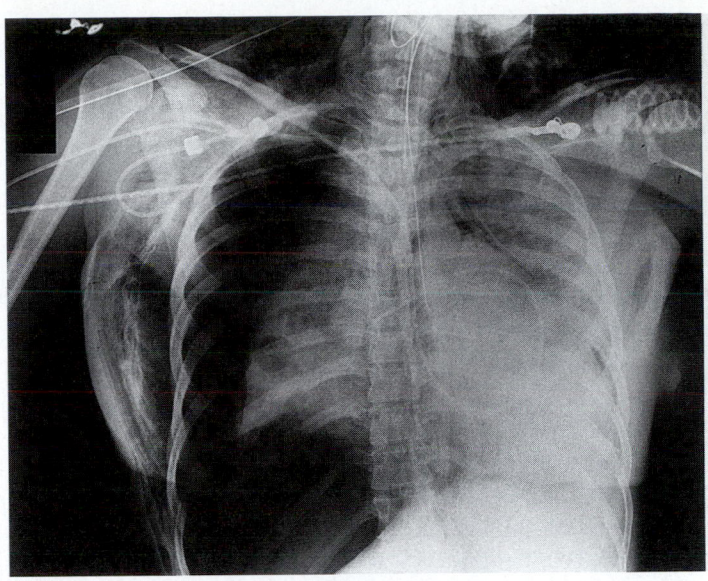

FIGURE 91-5   Right tension pneumothorax in a young patient with staphylococcal endocarditis and septic emboli. There is marked depression of the right hemidiaphragm, shift of the mediastinum, and subcutaneous emphysema. *Note:* The pulmonary artery catheter, endotracheal tube, and nasogastric tube (midchest) are all displaced to the left.

THERAPY

The basic tenets of therapy for pneumothorax are to evacuate the space, achieve closure of the leak, and either assess the risk of recurrence or ensure some means of reducing this risk. A variety of treatment methods and adjuncts exist. The choice is dependent on many factors, including the clinical status of the patient, the cause of the pneumothorax, evidence for concomitant lung disease, prior history of pneumothorax, risk of recurrence, and, finally, the experience and preferred techniques of the physicians caring for the patient.[30] Major categories of treatment methods are listed below, followed by suggested guidelines for their application.

Observation

Simple observation of the patient with a pneumothorax requires evidence that the air leak is sealed (i.e., that there is no further progression of the pneumothorax). This form of management is generally reserved for asymptomatic patients with a small (<20 percent) unilateral pneumothorax.

A suggested protocol is the performance of serial chest radiographs over the initial 24 h to assess for further progression of the pneumothorax. Some have suggested that this approach could be performed safely on an outpatient basis with close observation and limited patient activity. This form of management is risky because complications may occur rapidly, with potential morbidity. In one study of observation, a 5 percent mortality was reported owing to the development of tension pneumothorax from an unrecognized pleural leak.[45] Inpatient monitoring during the initial phase of therapy also allows the use of adjunct measures such as supplemental oxygen, which increases the rate of absorption of pleural gas. Depending on the circumstances and level of patient compliance, continued follow-up may be done on an outpatient basis.

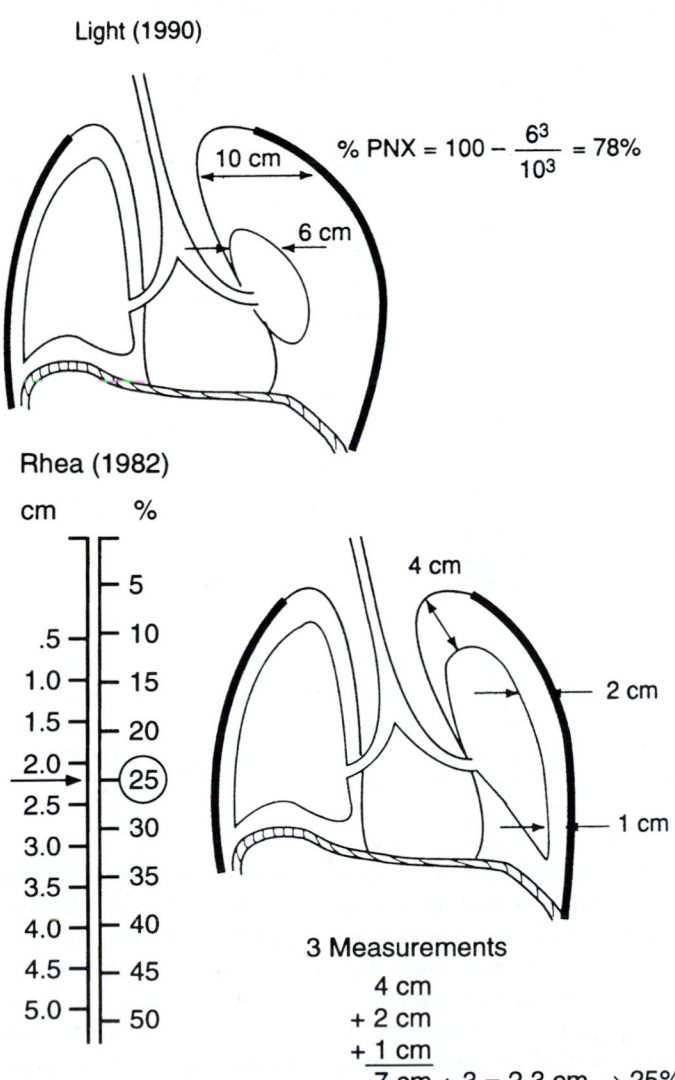

$$\% \text{ PNX} = 100 - \frac{6^3}{10^3} = 78\%$$

Light (1990)

10 cm

6 cm

Rhea (1982)

cm   %

5

.5   10

1.0   15

1.5   20

2.0   25

2.5   30

3.0

3.5   35

4.0   40

4.5   45

5.0   50

4 cm

2 cm

1 cm

3 Measurements

4 cm
+ 2 cm
+ 1 cm
7 cm ÷ 3 = 2.3 cm → 25%

FIGURE 91-4   Estimation of the size of the pneumothorax according to the method described by Light[32] and Rhea et al.[47] [*From Beauchchamp, in Pearson (ed), Textbook of Thoracic Surgery, 1995, 1043.*]

Aspiration

Aspiration of a pneumothorax has been advocated by some, with varied levels of success.[25] In a randomized study of needle aspiration versus tube thoracostomy, there was a higher immediate recurrence rate with the needle aspiration, although approximately 66 percent of patients had resolution of their pneumothorax. The recurrence rates at 3 months were similar to those for patients treated initially with tube thoracostomy. While the initial recurrence was somewhat high, it was suggested that needle aspiration may be considered as a first line of therapy, with initial close follow-up.[4] Review of five separate studies in the literature suggests that aspiration is successful in 65 percent of patients with primary spontaneous pneumothorax but in only about 35 percent of patients with secondary spontaneous pneumothorax.[1,6,7,25,28]

The procedure consists of insertion of a No. 16 or 18 French plastic catheter under local anesthesia using sterile technique. The recommended point of insertion is the second anterior intercostal space in the midclavicular line. The catheter is connected to a three-way stopcock and a large-volume syringe. Aspiration is performed until no further gas can be withdrawn. Follow-up chest radiographs are performed, with aspiration repeated once within 24 h if the first attempt is unsuccessful. If large volumes are aspirated without resolution or the second attempt is unsuccessful, a tube thoracostomy should be performed.

LONG-TERM ASPIRATION

This entails the placement of an indwelling catheter into the pleural space for continual removal of the interpleural gas. The classic method is the use of standard tube thoracostomy. For uncomplicated pneumothorax without evidence of significant amounts of fluid or blood, one may use tubes ranging in size from No. 16 to 24 French to minimize the discomfort of a larger tube in the intercostal space.

The tube is then connected to a pleural drainage system. Commercial systems commonly employ variations on the three-chamber system (Fig. 91-6). The three-chamber system consists of a fluid collection chamber attached to a water-seal chamber to allow egress of gas from the pleural space, but in a one-way fashion. The final connection is to a manometer bottle, which regulates the degree of suction being applied to the system. In most

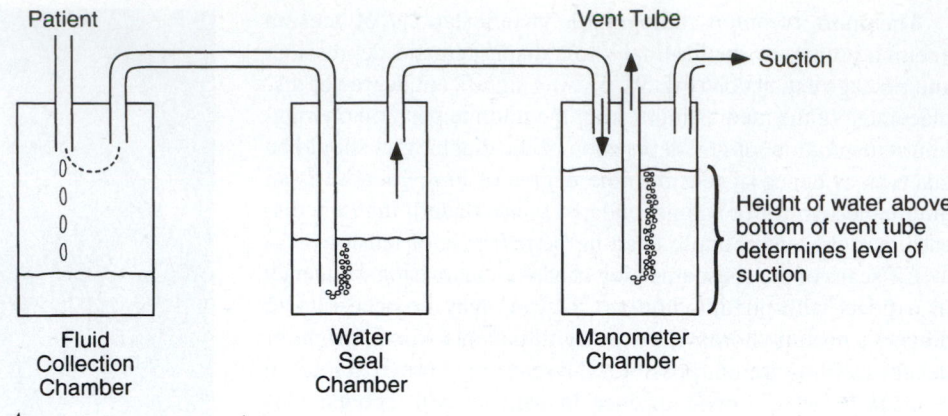

A

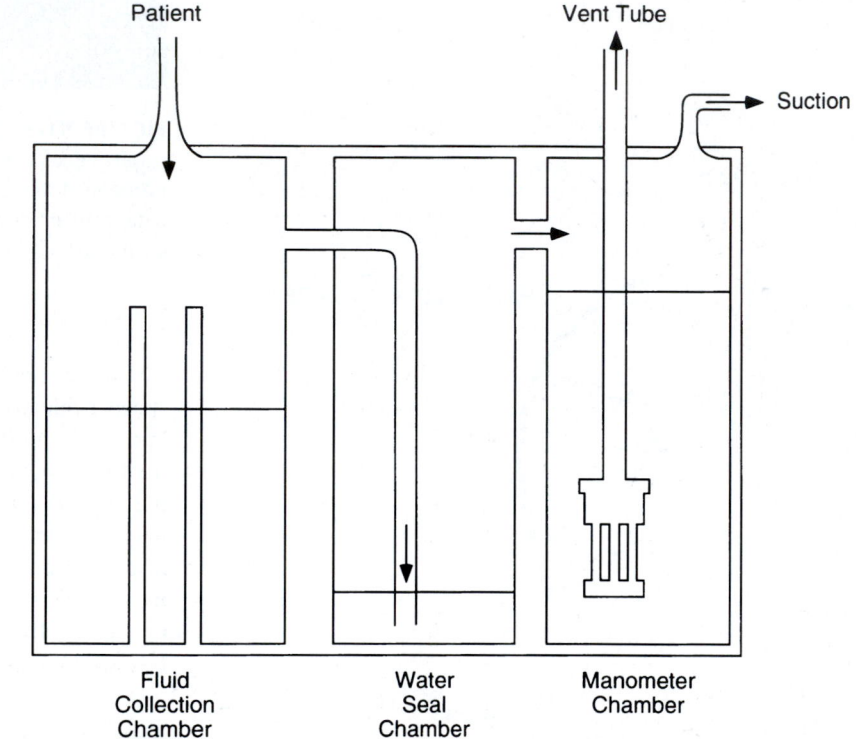

B

FIGURE 91-6   Three-bottle chest tube drainage system (*A*). The system consists of a collection bottle, a water-seal bottle, and a suction-control bottle. The collection bottle allows sterile drainage from the pleural spaces. The water-seal bottle acts as a one-way valve in the absence of suction, and the suction bottle allows for the regulation of negative pressure applied to the pleural space. Commercially available, compartmentalized plastic drainage system (*B*).

cases, after placement of tube thoracostomy, suction is applied for the initial 24 h. If an air leak exists, as evidenced by continual or intermittent egress of gas through the water seal chamber, suction is maintained. Once there is no evidence of an active air leak, the tube may be placed to an underwater seal. After an additional period of observation of 12 to 24 h, the chest tube may be removed if the pneumothorax does not recur.[43] Tube thoracostomy alone will result in closure of an air leak in most cases by complete evacuation of the pleural space and apposition of the visceral and parietal pleura. Persistence of an air leak for more than 72 h generally presages a leak that will not close by this regimen and should prompt consideration of more aggressive therapy, usually surgical with or without some form of pleurodesis.[23]

In order to have a less traumatic method of placement of an indwelling tube, as well as to minimize the discomfort from a large-bore tube in the intercostal space, a variety of smaller catheters have been suggested for use as an interpleural drain.[46] The method of placement is similar to needle aspiration, although the indwelling catheter is left in place and attached to pleural drainage system as described above. Potential problems with smaller catheters relate to a greater propensity for blockage of the tube. Also, the smaller size makes them more prone to kinking, clotting from blood or fluid, and sealing around the tube by the lung, resulting in a loculated pneumothorax. In cases in which the pneumothorax is associated with significant amounts of blood or fluid, tube thoracostomy using a larger-bore chest tube (26 to 32 French) is recommended.

A variation on the use of pleural drainage systems has been the substitution of a one-way valve to permit greater mobility by the patient.[9] The most common is the Heimlich flutter valve, which may have some application in cases in which long-term indwelling catheterization is required but surgical therapy is declined or not possible. This valve is not widely recommended, however, owing to a potential for problems with blockage, which may not be immediately recognized on an outpatient basis.

Pleurodesis

Pleurodesis is an adjunct to the other forms of therapy. The goal is to achieve pleural symphysis, or adhesion of the visceral and parietal pleura to obliterate the pleural space. Sealing the visceral and parietal pleura together will prevent future air leaks and prohibit the lung from "falling away" from the chest wall. The basic mechanism entails chemical or physical irritation of the pleural surface to promote an inflammatory response and subsequent adhesion formation.

Chemical pleurodesis may be used in combination with tube thoracostomy or surgical therapy. A number of pleural irritants have been suggested, including quinacrine, silver nitrate, bleomycin, autologous blood, tetracycline, and talc. Tetracycline and talc have been the most effective and popular.

Experimental studies of tetracycline revealed it to be the only agent capable of sufficient pleural fibrosis formation when compared to hydrochloric acid, quinacrine, nitrogen mustard, bleomycin, or sodium hydroxide.[48] A clinical, prospective trial of tetracycline pleurodesis showed a significant reduction in the recurrence rate of pneumothorax, from 41 to 25 percent.[33] Tetracycline pleurodesis did not appear to have any long-term adverse effect on the pulmonary function or the chest radiograph. Tetracycline, however, is no longer commercially available. Minocycline and doxyclycline have recently been suggested as replacements for tetracycline, but long-term efficacy is not known.[8]

Talc has also been shown to be a very effective sclerosing agent when applied as a slurry or when insufflated in dry form over the visceral pleural surface. In an experimental study, talc was noted to be as efficacious as mechanical abrasion.[11] The intermediate effect of tetracycline was also noted in the study. Tetracycline pleurodesis may be more effective than a chest tube alone, but it resulted in minimal pleural fibrosis. This confirms anecdotal evidence that the degree of pleural symphysis with tetracycline is less than that with talc or mechanical abrasion. In a meta-analysis, talc achieved a "success rate" of 91 percent.[29]

As an adjunct to tube thoracostomy, the chemical of choice is suspended in fluid and instilled through the tube. The tube is clamped for 6 to 8 h, then placed back to either suction or water seal. Periodically changing patient position during this period is believed to effect more even distribution of the irritant. Typical doses are 0.5 to 1.0 gm of doxycycline in 50 to 100 ml normal saline, 600 mg of minocycline in 50 to 100 ml of normal saline, and 2 to 10 gm of talc in 100 to 200 ml of normal saline. General requirements for the performance of chemical pleurodesis via the tube are that pleural fluid output be less than 150 to 200 ml a day and that there be no air leak. Success is largely dependent on apposition of the visceral and parietal pleura during the period of inflammation while the tube is clamped. Excessive pleural fluid will dilute the sclerosing agent, and an air leak will allow the lung to separate from the chest wall. Pleurodesis in the face of an air leak has been tried,[2,38] but in our experience it has rarely been successful.

As an adjunct to surgical therapy, the most commonly described material is talc. Sterile, asbestos-free talc is insufflated during thoracoscopy or thoracotomy to coat the visceral pleural surface. Typically, 2 to 10 gm is used.[15,29]

Mechanical pleurodesis is performed as part of a surgical procedure. It may consist of simple abrasion of the parietal pleural surface or may entail stripping of the parietal pleura (pleurectomy). The second method has a greater potential for complications, including injury to an intercostal neurovascular bundle or excessive bleeding from the large raw surface area. Also considered in this category is the use of an Nd:YAG laser or an argon beam coagulator, which essentially cauterizes the pleural surface.[55] Experimental studies have not borne out their effectiveness.[11]

The performance of pleurodesis is somewhat controversial, owing to the degree of pleural symphysis that can be obtained with these methods. Either talc or mechanical pleurodesis, especially pleurectomy, results in rather significant adhesion formation. There are concerns that future surgical procedures, such as pulmonary resection, open lung biopsy, and lung transplantation, may be hampered by this degree of pleural symphysis. The application of pleurodesis thus depends on an assessment of the risk of recurrent pneumothorax and the potential morbidity to the patient should a recurrence occur versus the potential for later operative procedures in the thorax. One suggested compromise is limitation of the pleurodesis to the apical area, as this is the most common location for air leaks to occur. Later thoracic procedures may be done, albeit with more difficulty, by entrance inferior to the area of pleurodesis and subsequent adhesion lysis apically. Localized pleurodesis is not possible when it is performed as an adjunct to tube thoracostomy. A second potential compromise is the use of tetracycline analogs such as minocycline or doxycycline. Experimental studies and anecdotal reports indicate that with the use of tetracycline, the degree of pleural symphysis and density of adhesions are not as great as with talc or mechanical pleurodesis.[3,11]

Operative Therapy

Operative treatment is generally thought to be the most effective in assuring expansion of the lung, with complete evacuation of the pleural space, and providing for the best means of reducing the risk of recurrence. In addition, it provides a means of potentially identifying an air leak and closing it. However, increased patient discomfort, risks of general anesthesia, and greater costs of the procedures, combined with moderate success of the less invasive methods, result in restricted application of surgery for pneumothorax.

Operative therapy is indicated in cases in which the above-mentioned techniques have failed, with a persistence or recurrence of the pneumothorax, or in cases of initial presentation of patients with factors suggesting increased risk of later recurrence. This risk of recurrence also includes an assessment of the potential morbidity to the patient should another pneumothorax occur.

Longitudinal studies have indicated that after tube thoracostomy treatment of a spontaneous pneumothorax, the recurrence rate is approximately 30 percent. Among patients in whom the disease recurs once, the subsequent recurrence rate continues to increase.[20] Evidence suggests that a more definitive procedure—namely surgery—is indicated with the first recurrence. In patients with underlying lung disease, such a large bulla is also believed to have an increased risk of recurrence, and in most cases, surgery is indicated for the initial episode. Patients who have high-risk lifestyles, such as pilots or scuba divers, or patients who may not have ready access to medical care may possess a relative indication for surgical treatment of a first occurrence of spontaneous pneumothorax because of the risk to the patient should a pneumothorax occur. Patients who present with bilateral or tension pneumothorax may also fall in this category of morbidity assessment.

Patients with a pneumothorax from any cause who have a persistent air leak despite chronic aspiration therapy should also be considered for operative therapy. An air leak that fails to close after 72 h of suction has a very low chance of closing spontaneously. This is the recommended time for surgical referral.[23] Finally, patients in whom the previous forms of therapy result in incomplete reexpansion of the lung should be considered for surgery. This situation may reflect loculation of the pneumothorax or trapping of the lung by a fibrotic "peel," which will require surgery to be released.

Thoracoscopy　Thoracoscopy, though a relatively old procedure, has enjoyed a resurgence in recent years, owing to the advent of video assistance (video-assisted thoracoscopic surgery, or VATS), a greater emphasis on "minimally invasive surgery," and increasing patient acceptance because of less discomfort and decreased length of hospital stay. The decreased morbidity is the result of the ability to examine the pleural space and manipulate the lung without significant muscle division or rib spreading.[15]

In most cases, the technique requires general anesthesia with double-lumen endotracheal ventilation. Up to three separate ports are placed in the intercostal spaces to effect installation of the camera as well as manipulating devices. The entire lung can be inspected and a search for the air leak carried out. Generally speaking, the apical area is the location, and this area can then be closed with the use of a stapler. In patients with concomitant lung disease, particularly COPD, the staple line can be reinforced with the aid of bovine pericardium to minimize persistence of air leaks.[14] The pleural surface can then be abraded or talc insufflated, as mentioned above, to achieve some degree of pleural adhesion following reexpansion of the lung. Long-term follow-up of recurrence rates has shown results similar to those for open thoracotomy.

The less invasive nature of this method compared to open thoracotomy has prompted earlier and more frequent surgical referral. While the risks associated with general anesthesia remain, overall costs are generally less than thoracotomy owing to a decreased postoperative period.

Open Thoracotomy　Classically, thoracotomy was believed to be the ultimate and most effective form of therapy for pneumothorax. Recurrence rates are generally less than 2 percent.[17] Thoracotomy allows examination of the lung for the site of an air leak, enables lysis of previous adhesions that may lead to a loculated pneumothorax, and enables the release of a fibrotic peel that occasionally forms, leading to incomplete reexpansion of the lung. Drawbacks include the potential risks associated with general anesthesia, increased costs, and the significant amount of patient discomfort. Discomfort is generally most severe with a standard lateral or posterolateral thoracotomy with muscle division and rib spreading.

In an effort to minimize the level of discomfort, variations have been developed, including the use of smaller incisions, so-called muscle-sparing thoracotomies, and the axillary thoracotomy. Lung examination and air leak closure and possible pleurodesis or pleurectomy can then still be performed.[17]

While thoracoscopy has supplanted thoracotomy as the surgical treatment of pneumothorax in many institutions, open thoracotomy remains a valuable option in the treatment of complicated cases.

Suggested Guidelines for Therapy

Based on the relative efficacy of the various forms of therapy (Table 91-1), combined with relative risks for the major categories of pneumothorax, the following guidelines are suggested:

PRIMARY PNEUMOTHORAX

Patients with a first-time primary spontaneous pneumothorax who are asymptomatic and whose pneumothorax is thought to be less than 20 percent may be treated with observation and sometimes adjunct measures, including the use of supplemental oxygen. Patients with primary spontaneous pneumothorax who are symptomatic or whose pneumothorax is greater than 20 percent should undergo an attempt at catheter aspiration. Subsequent small- or large-tube thoracostomy is indicated for failure of simple aspiration.

Patients who undergo successful tube thoracostomy with complete lung reexpansion and absence of an air leak may be considered for further chemical pleurodesis, with doxycycline as the suggested agent. This will reduce the risk of recurrence, but it should not completely obviate the ability to perform later surgical procedures. Patients with tube thoracostomies that have persistent air leaks for more than 72 h should be referred for surgical therapy.

Because of the progressive increase in risk of recurrence, patients with their first recurrence of a primary pneumothorax should be referred for surgical therapy, preferably thoracoscopy with stapling of the air leak and pleural abrasion. Indications for surgery in primary pneumothorax are listed in Table 91-2.

TABLE 91-1

Recurrence of Primary Spontaneous Pneumothorax After Various Therapies

Therapy	Recurrence (%)
Observation	30–40
Aspiration	25–40
Chest tube drainage	25–30
Pleurodesis (tetracycline)	20–25
Pleurodesis (talc)	7–15
Surgery	0.6–2

SECONDARY PNEUMOTHORAX

In general, therapy for secondary pneumothorax should be more aggressive because of the higher rate of recurrence due to the underlying lung pathology. Specific conditions with pneumothorax as a common occurrence are as listed below.

COPD   Most cases of pneumothorax in patients with COPD should be treated with some form of long-term aspiration, typically tube thoracostomy. If the pneumothorax was relatively well tolerated by the patient, chemical pleurodesis with doxycycline should be performed if there is complete reexpansion and absence of an air leak. If the COPD is believed to be severe, the pneumothorax episode was poorly tolerated, or an air leak persists longer than 72 h, more-aggressive therapy should be considered.[57] Recommended therapy would be thoracoscopy with talc insufflation or mechanical pleurodesis. Patients with severe COPD are unlikely to tolerate any form of surgical pulmonary resection. Therefore, this approach provides a better means of achieving lower risk of recurrence.

Cystic Fibrosis   In a retrospective review of patients with cystic fibrosis and pneumothorax, the entire spectrum of therapeutic options were utilized as clinically indicated.[53] Patients undergoing surgical therapy did better and had fewer episodes of recurrence and complications. Therefore, this is the primary recommendation for this subgroup of patients. Because of the growing application of lung transplantation to patients with cystic fibrosis, localized pleurodesis is recommended as an adjunct to surgical closure of the air leak.

AIDS   For most AIDS patients presenting with a pneumothorax, tube thoracostomy is the primary mode of initial treatment. Because of the high primary and secondary treatment failure rates, patients who have no air leak with complete lung reexpansion should undergo talc slurry pleurodesis. For patients with a persistent air leak who are felt to be poor surgical risks because of severe debilitation, a Heimlich valve may be utilized. For patients who are deemed good risks for surgery, thoracoscopy with talc insufflation is recommended.[58]

Other Conditions   While there are insufficient data to make firm recommendations for the following situations, some suggestions are offered. Patients having pneumothorax secondary to iatrogenic causes may be treated with observation or aspiration according to the guidelines previously listed. Patients who have a pneumothorax secondary to trauma should have large-bore tube thoracostomy, because there is a high association with hemothorax and the margin of safety may be decreased owing to other injury. Patients who experience a pneumothorax while on positive-pressure ventilation should have tube thoracostomy placement to avoid progression to a tension pneumothorax. Patients who present with bilateral pneumothoraces or a tension pneumothorax, but who are not on positive-pressure ventilation, should have placement of tube thoracostomy. Further therapy with regard to chemical pleurodesis versus surgery is dependent on underlying lung pathology.

COMPLICATIONS

Tension Pneumothorax

A tension pneumothorax is present when the intrapleural pressure is greater than atmospheric throughout expiration and often during inspiration as well. The term *expiratory tension pneumothorax* has been proposed to highlight the fact that in a spontaneously breathing person, pleural pressure must be negative in relation to atmospheric pressure during part of the respiratory cycle for air to enter the pleural space. The mechanism responsible for tension pneumothorax is the disruption of the visceral or parietal pleura in such a manner that a one-way valve develops. During inspiration, the respiratory muscles contract and create negative intrapleural pressure, allowing for air movement into the pleural space. Then, during expiration, when the expiratory muscles relax, the pleural pressure becomes positive and the one-way valve prevents the egress of air from the pleural space. As a tension pneumothorax progresses, the pleural pressure remains positive during a greater portion of the inspiratory cycle.

Tension pneumothorax can occur after a spontaneous pneumothorax but is more common after a traumatic pneumothorax or with mechanical ventilation. A tension pneumothorax may develop because of improper connection of a one-way flutter valve to the chest tube. The clinical picture associated with the development of a tension pneumothorax is striking. Patients appear acutely ill, with labored breathing, tachypnea, marked

TABLE 91-2

Indications for Surgery in Primary Spontaneous Pneumothorax

First episode
  Prolonged air leak
  Incomplete reexpansion of lung
  Associated single large bulla
  Occupational hazard (flight personnel, divers)
  Absence of medical facility in isolated areas
  Tension pneumothorax*
  Hemopneumothorax*
  Bilateral pneumothorax*

Second Episode
  Ipsilateral recurrence
  Contralateral recurrence after first pneumothorax*

*Relative indication.

tachycardia, profuse diaphoresis, and cyanosis. On physical examination, patients often exhibit distended neck veins, tracheal deviations to the side opposite the pneumothorax, subcutaneous emphysema, and hypotension. Patients receiving mechanical ventilation often develop a sudden increase in their peak and plateau pressures, with an associated decrease in the oxygen saturation.

Tension pneumothorax should be suspected in any patient with a pneumothorax whose condition deteriorates acutely, or in any patient with cardiopulmonary collapse after a procedure known to cause a pneumothorax. One should also suspect a tension pneumothorax in any patient undergoing cardiopulmonary resuscitation who is difficult to ventilate or develops electromechanical dissociation.

The decompensation of the cardiopulmonary status in patients with tension pneumothorax is usually attributed to diminished venous return and low cardiac output. Animal studies demonstrate that cardiac output is maintained by the tachycardia and the increase in negative intrathoracic pressure during inspiration.[24] Deterioration has been shown to be related to severe hypoxemia, probably because of increased shunting and $\dot{V}_A/\dot{Q}$ mismatch in the compressed lung. Preterminally, animals develop CO_2 retention and respiratory acidosis. The importance of negative intrathoracic pressure swings in maintaining cardiac output was demonstrated by the precipitous fall in cardiac output when mechanical ventilation was initiated.[24]

When the diagnosis of a tension pneumothorax is considered, the patient should be given a high concentration of oxygen to alleviate the extreme hypoxemia seen with this syndrome. Radiographic documentation may not be possible in an emergency situation. A large-bore needle should be inserted into the second anterior intercostal space. Optimally, the needle should be connected to a syringe partly filled with sterile saline. Air bubbling outward through the fluid confirms the diagnosis. The needle or its plastic outer sheath should be left in place, and the patient should be prepared for immediate tube thoracostomy.

Bronchopleural Fistula

Most air leaks seal within 24 to 48 h. Only 3 to 5 percent of patients with pneumothorax have a persisting air leak.[51] If an air leak persists for more than 48 h, continuous suction for 8 to 10 days results in only minimal increase in pulmonary healing.[49] Placement of a second chest tube may help, but surgery should be considered after 3 to 4 days of tube drainage.[23]

Patients with cystic fibrosis or COPD are at increased risk for the development of persistent bronchopleural fistula. For those who are not candidates for thoracotomy, the fistula may be localized by bronchoscopic balloon catheter occlusion and subsequently injected with a variety of substances to promote sealing of the air leak. Fibrin glue, liquid bioadhesive (isobutyl 2-cyanocrylate), sterile gelatin sponge, and even lead shot have been used for this purpose.[2] Autologous "blood patch" pleurodesis has also been accomplished, using 50 to 100 ml of the patient's blood and injecting it into the chest tube. In our experience, however, these patients almost all come to thoracoscopic surgery because these procedures usually fail, and the air leak persists for more than 7 to 10 days.

Reexpansion Pulmonary Edema

Unilateral pulmonary edema may occur when the lung is rapidly reexpanded, whether the cause of the collapse is pleural effusion or a pneumothorax. Occasionally, reexpansion pulmonary edema becomes bilateral and necessitates intubation and mechanical ventilation. Animal models demonstrate that reexpansion pulmonary edema occurs when a pneumothorax has been present for 3 days or more and the lung has been expanded with more than –20 cm H_2O pleural pressure. Reexpansion pulmonary edema appears to be due to increased permeability of the pulmonary capillaries that are damaged by mechanical stress during reexpansion of the lung. Reperfusion injury due to free radicals may also be responsible for increased capillary permeability.

Typically, a persistent cough or tightness of the chest develops immediately after chest tube insertion, and the patient develops hypoxemia and, occasionally, hypotension. Symptoms usually progress for 24 to 48 h. If the patient survives the first 48 h, recovery is usually complete. In 1988, Mahfood and colleagues[40] reviewed the literature of reexpansion pulmonary edema and found only 53 cases, but 11 (21 percent) were fatal. When thoracostomy is performed for a spontaneous pneumothorax of unknown duration, the tube should be connected to underwater-seal drainage rather than to negative pressure. If the lung fails to fully expand after 12 to 24 h, negative pressure can be applied to the pleural space.

REFERENCES

1. Abolnik IZ, Lossos IS, Zlotogora J, Braver R: On the inheritance of spontaneous pneumothorax. *Am J Med* 40:155–158, 1991.
2. Almassi GH, Haasler GB: Chemical pleurodesis in the presence of persistent air leak. *Ann Thorac Surg* 47:786–787, 1989.
3. Almind M, Lange P, Viskum K: Spontaneous pneumothorax: Comparison of simple drainage, talc pleurodesis, and tetracycline pleurodesis. *Thorax* 44:627–630, 1989.
4. Andrivet P, Kamael D, Teboul JL, et al: Spontaneous pneumothorax: Comparison of thoracic drainage vs. immediate or delayed needle aspiration. *Chest* 108:335–339, 1995.
5. Anthonisen NR: Regional lung function in spontaneous pneumothorax. *Am Rev Respir Dis* 115:873–876, 1977.
6. Archer GJ, Hamilton AA, Upadhyay R, et al: Results of simple aspiration of pneumothoraces. *Br J Dis Chest* 79:177–182, 1985.
7. Belvelacqua FA, Aranda C: Management of spontaneous pneumothorax with small lumen catheter manual aspiration. *Chest* 81:693–694, 1985.
8. Berger R: Pleurodesis for spontaneous pneumothorax: Will the procedure of choice please stand up? (editorial). *Chest* 106:992–994, 1994.
9. Bernstein A, Waqaruddin M, Shah M: Management of spontaneous pneumothorax using a Heimlich flutter valve. *Thorax* 28:386–389, 1973.
10. Boat TF, Di Sant'Agnese PA, Warwick WJ, Handwerger SA: Pneumothorax in cystic fibrosis. *JAMA* 209:1498–1504, 1969.
11. Bresticker MA, Oba J, LoCicero III J, Greene R: Optimal pleurodesis: A comparison study. *Ann Thorac Surg* 55:364–367, 1993.
12. Carter EJ, Ettenshon DB: Catamenial pneumothorax. *Chest* 98:713–716, 1990.
13. Conces DJ, Holden RW: Aberrant locations and complications in initial placement of subclavian vein catheters. *Arch Surg* 119:293–295, 1984.

14. Cooper JD: Technique to reduce air leaks after resection of emphysematous lung. *Ann Thorac Surg* 57:1038–1039, 1994.

15. Daniel TM, Tribble CG, Rogers BM: Thoracoscopy and talc poudrage for pneumothoraces and effusions. *Ann Thorac Surg* 50:186–189, 1990.

16. DeLatorre FJ, Tomasa A, Klamburg J, et al: Incidence of pneumothorax and pneumomediastinum in patients with aspiration pneumonia requiring ventilatory support. *Chest* 72:141–144, 1977.

17. Deslauriers J, Beaulieu M, Despres JP, et al: Transaxillary pleurectomy for treatment of spontaneous pneumothorax. *Ann Thorac Surg* 30:569–574, 1980.

18. Despars JA, Sassoon CS, Light RW: Incidence and significance of iatrogenic pneumothorax. *Chest* 98:138S, 1990.

19. Dines DE, Clagett OT, Payne WS: Spontaneous pneumothorax in emphysema. *Mayo Clin Proc* 45:481–487, 1970.

20. Gaensler EA: Parietal pleurectomy for recurrent spontaneous pneumothorax. *Surg Gynecol Obstet* 102:293–308, 1956.

21. Gammon RB, Shin MS, Buchalter SE: Pulmonary barotrauma in mechanical ventilation. *Chest* 102:568–572, 1992.

22. Gobbel WG Jr, Rhea WG Jr, Nelson IA, Daniel RA Jr: Spontaneous pneumothorax. *J Thorac Cardiovasc Surg* 46:331–345, 1963.

23. Granke K, Fischer CR, Gago O, et al: The efficacy and timing of operative intervention for spontaneous pneumothorax. *Ann Thorac Surg* 42:540–542, 1986.

24. Gustman P, Yerger L, Wanner A: Immediate cardiovascular effects of tension pneumothorax. *Am Rev Respir Dis* 127:171–174, 1983.

25. Hamilton AAD, Archer GJ: Treatment of pneumothorax by single aspiration. *Thorax* 38:934–936, 1983.

26. Jantz MA, Pierson DJ: Pneumothorax and barotrauma. *Clin Chest Med* 15:75–91, 1994.

27. Jenkinson SG: Pneumothorax. *Clin Chest Med* 6:153–161, 1985.

28. Jones JS: A place for aspiration in the treatment of spontaneous pneumothorax. *Thorax* 40:66–67, 1985.

29. Kennedy L, Sahn SA: Talc pleurodesis for the treatment of pneumothorax and pleural effusion. *Chest* 106:1215–1222, 1994.

30. Kirby TJ, Ginsberg RJ: Management of the pneumothorax and barotrauma. *Clin Chest Med* 13:97–112, 1992.

31. Kircher LT Jr, Swartzel RC: Spontaneous pneumothorax and its treatment. *JAMA* 155:24–29, 1967.

32. Light RW: *Pleural Diseases,* 3d ed. Philadelphia, Lea & Febiger, 1990, pp 237–262.

33. Light RW, O'Hara VS, Moritz TE, et al, for the Department of Veterans Affairs Cooperative Study Group on Spontaneous Pneumothorax: Intrapleural tetracycline for the prevention of recurrent spontaneous pneumothorax: Results of a Department of Veterans Affairs cooperative study. *JAMA* 264:2224–2230, 1990.

34. Lillington GA, Mitchell SP, Wood GA: Catamenial pneumothorax. *JAMA* 219:1328–1332, 1972.

35. Lippert HL, Lung O, Bleguard S, Larsen HV: Independent risk factors for cumulative recurrence rate after first spontaneous pneumothorax. *Eur Respir J* 4:324–331, 1991.

36. Luck SR, Raffensperger JG, Sullivan HJ, Gibson LE: Management of pneumothorax in children with chronic pulmonary disease. *J Thorac Cardiovasc Surg* 74:834–839, 1977.

37. Macklin MT, Macklin CC: Malignant interstitial emphysema of the lungs and mediastinum as an important occult complication in many respiratory diseases and other conditions: An interpretation of clinical literature in light of laboratory experiment. *Medicine* 23:281–351, 1944.

38. Macoviak JA, Stephenson LW, Ochs R, Edmunds LH Jr: Tetracycline pleurodesis during active pulmonary-pleural air leak for prevention of recurrent pneumothorax. *Chest* 81:78–81, 1982.

39. Magnussen H, Perry SF, Willmer H, Piiper J: Transpleural diffusion of inert gases in excised lung lobes of the dog. *Respir Physiol* 20:1–15, 1974.

40. Mahfood S, Hix WR, Aaron BL, Blaes P, Watson DC: Reexpansion pulmonary edema. *Ann Thorac Surg* 45:340–345, 1988.

41. Maurer ER, Schaal JA, Mendez FL: Chronic recurrent spontaneous pneumothorax due to endometriosis of the diaphragm. *JAMA* 168:2013–2014, 1958.

42. Melton LJ, Hepper NG, Offord KP: Incidence of spontaneous pneumothorax in Olmsted County, Minnesota: 1950 to 1974. *Am Rev Respir Dis* 120:1379–1382, 1979.

43. Miller KS, Sahn SA: Chest tubes: Indications, techniques, management and complications. *Chest* 91:258–264, 1987.

44. O'Hara VS: Spontaneous pneumothorax. *Milit Med* 143:32–35, 1978.

45. O'Rourke JP, Yee ES: Civilian spontaneous pneumothorax: Treatment options and long-term results. *Chest* 96:1302–1306, 1989.

46. Peters J, Kubitschek KR: Clinical evaluation of percutaneous pneumothorax catheter. *Chest* 86:714–717, 1984.

47. Rhea JT, DeLuca SA, Greene RE: Determining the size of pneumothorax in the upright patient. *Radiology* 144:733–736, 1982.

48. Sahn SA, Good JT Jr: The effect of common sclerosing agents on the rabbit pleural space. *Am Rev Respir Dis* 124:65–67, 1981.

49. Schoenenberger RA, Haefeli WE, Weiss P, Ritz RF: Timing of invasive procedures in therapy for primary and secondary spontaneous pneumothorax. *Arch Surg* 126:764–766, 1991.

50. Sepkowitz KA, Telzak EE, Gold JW, et al: Pneumothorax in patients with AIDS. *Ann Intern Med* 114:455–459, 1991.

51. Seremetis MG: The management of spontaneous pneumothorax. *Chest* 57:68–68, 1970.

52. Sharpe IK, Ahmad M, Braun W: Familial spontaneous pneumothorax and HLA antigens. *Chest* 78:264–268, 1980.

53. Spector ML, Stern RC: Pneumothorax in cystic fibrosis: A 26-year experience. *Ann Thorac Surg* 47:204–207, 1989.

54. Tocino IM, Miller MH, Fairfar WR: Distribution of pneumothorax in the supine and semierect critically ill adult. *AJR Am J Roentgenol* 144:901–905, 1985.

55. Torre M, Belloni P: Nd:YAG laster pleurodesis through thoracscopy: New curative therapy in spontaneous pneumothorax. *Ann Thoracic Surg* 47:887–889, 1989.

56. Vallee P, Sullivan M, Richardson H, et al: Sequential treatment of a simple pneumothorax. *Ann Emerg Med* 5:45–47, 1988.

57. Videm V, Pillgram-Larsen J, Ellingsen O, et al: Spontaneous pneumothorax in chronic obstructive pulmonary disease: Complications, treatment and recurrences. *Eur J Respir Dis* 71:365–371, 1987.

58. Wait MA, Dal Nogare AR: Treatment of AIDS-related spontaneous pneumothorax. *Chest* 106:693–696, 1994.

59. Walston A, Brewer DL, Kitchens CS, Krook JE: The electrocardiographic manifestations of spontaneous left pneumothorax. *Ann Intern Med* 80:375–379, 1974.

60. Warner BW, Bailey WW, Shipley RT: Value of computed tomography of the lung in the management of primary spontaneous pneumothorax. *Am J Surg* 162:39–42, 1991.

CHAPTER 92

MALIGNANT MESOTHELIOMA AND OTHER PRIMARY PLEURAL TUMORS

Steven M. Albelda / Daniel H. Sterman / Leslie A. Litzky

The pleura is a membranous structure covering the entire surface of the lung and lining the inside of the chest cavity. It is composed of a thin mesothelial layer with underlying fibroblasts and varying amounts of collagenous fibrous tissue with interdigitating capillaries and venules. The most common tumors of the pleura are metastatic neoplasms, predominantly of lung, breast, or colonic origin. Tumors arising primarily from the pleura are rare but still constitute a variety of benign and malignant lesions from several different cells of origin, some of which have yet to be identified.

MALIGNANT MESOTHELIOMA

The most common primary malignant tumor of the pleura is malignant mesothelioma, an insidious neoplasm with a dismal prognosis arising from the mesothelial surfaces of the pleural and peritoneal cavities as well as from the tunica vaginalis and pericardium. Eighty percent of all cases of mesothelioma are pleural in origin.

Epidemiology

The incidence of mesothelioma in the United States is estimated to be 2200 cases per year, with reported rates increasing by as much as 50 percent in the past decade.[5,35] Incidence is also increasing worldwide, particularly in Great Britain, where 2700 to 3000 deaths are expected annually by the year 2020.[34] After that time, mesothelioma rates are expected to drop in England and other developed countries because of recent legislation aimed at reducing asbestos exposure in the workplace and the general environment. In contrast, mesothelioma incidence rates are predicted to escalate indefinitely in the third world because of poor regulation of asbestos mining and widespread industrial and household utilization of asbestos.[5]

Etiology

ASBESTOS EXPOSURE

The predominant cause of malignant mesothelioma in humans is now clearly established as inhalational exposure to asbestos. Approximately 70 percent of cases of pleural mesothelioma are associated with documented asbestos exposure. In ancient Greece, the philosopher Pliny first associated asbestos exposure and lung disease with the observation that slaves working in asbestos mines were less healthy than other slaves. It was not until 1960, with the publication by Wagner and colleagues of a series of 33 mesothelioma cases occurring in a crocidolite mining community in South Africa, that the etiologic connection between asbestos and mesothelioma was established. Wagner's study was soon followed by several other accounts of mesothelioma afflicting asbestos workers at locations around the world.[5]

Although the lifetime risk of developing mesothelioma among asbestos workers is thought to be as high as 8 to 13 percent, there is no direct correlation of pleural disease incidence to the amount or duration of asbestos exposure. This is not true for peritoneal mesothelioma, however, as it has been shown to occur more commonly in patients with heavy asbestos exposure. The absence of a definite dose-response relationship between asbestos and pleural mesothelioma is of significant concern because as many as 8 million persons living in the United States have been occupationally exposed to asbestos over the past 50 years. Also, many well-documented cases of mesothelioma occur after very brief or low-level exposures to asbestos (i.e., spouses of asbestos workers exposed by washing clothes).[5,35]

Asbestos is not a specific molecule but the commercial name for a group of hydrated magnesium silicate fibrous minerals divided into two major types: the serpentines and the amphiboles. Serpentine chrysotile fibers are curly and pliable, whereas the amphiboles (crocidolite, amosite, tremolite, anthophyllite, actinolite) are long and needlelike. The carcinogenicity of certain types of asbestos is thought to be due primarily to physical properties of the fibers rather than their chemical composition. Fibers with a high length-to-width ratio, such as crocidolite, are considered more carcinogenic. Amosite has an intermediate risk, chrysotile the lowest. Ninety percent of the asbestos currently used in the United States is obtained from Canada.[5] It is unclear whether the cases of mesothelioma attributed to chrysotile exposure are caused by the chrysotile itself or by contaminating tremolite. In addition, other fibrous materials, such as fiber glass, milled to the same size standards, may carry a similar cancer risk.

MOLECULAR PATHOGENESIS

The long latency period from asbestos exposure to the development of mesothelioma is approximately 30 to 40 years, suggesting the necessity of multiple genetic alterations for eventual malignant transformation of the mesothelium. Despite extensive investigatory effort, the exact mechanisms of asbestos carcinogenesis have not yet been fully elucidated. In rodent model systems, asbestos fibers act like tumor promoters in combination with a carcinogen, eliciting proliferation of mesothelial cells. Asbestos fibers can also interact with the mitotic spindle to cause missegregation of chromosomes and aneuploidy. In rat pleural mesothelial cells, asbestos fibers and erionite have been shown to induce the protooncogenes c-fos and c-jun in a prolonged and dose-responsive manner.[25,33] Several growth factors, putatively secreted by mesothelial/mesothelioma cells in an autocrine fashion, have been implicated in various stages of mesothelioma tumorigenesis. Platelet-derived growth factors A and B (PDGF A and B), insulinlike growth factors I and II (IGF I and II), basic fibroblast growth factor (bFGF), and transforming growth factor-β1,2, and 3 (TGF β1,2, and 3) constitute a complex mixture of autocrine and paracrine stimuli for mesothelioma cell proliferation as well as initiation of tumor angiogenesis.[18]

Analysis of explanted human mesotheliomas and cultured human mesothelioma cell lines has revealed a number of cytogenetic aberrations that may predispose to the development of the malignant phenotype. Partial or total loss of chromosomes 1, 3, and 4, deletions of 9p, and monosomy of chromosome 22 are

the most common abnormalities seen.[27,47,50] For mesotheliomas, 9p deletions have been associated with the loss of function of the p16^{INK4} cdk inhibitor, a putative tumor suppresser gene, engendering unchecked cdk4-mediated phosphorylation of the retinoblastoma 1 (Rb1) gene product and leading to loss of regulation of cell division.[19,22,27,50] Monosomy 22, the most frequent numerical cytogenetic abnormality in mesothelioma, has recently been correlated with mutations in the neurofibromatosis 2 (NF2) tumor suppresser gene—mutations more commonly associated with acoustic neuromas, schwannomas, and meningiomas.[7,22] The ubiquitous presence of the Wilms' tumor suppresser gene (WT1) in human mesotheliomas raises the possibility that alterations in this gene or binding of the WT1 gene product to the p53 tumor suppresser may predispose to mesothelial cell carcinogenesis.[10] In addition, several researchers have noted the presence of SV40-like sequences in human mesotheliomas, including the SV40 large T antigen (Tag). As Tag is capable of binding to and inactivating functional p53 in vitro, inhibiting its tumor suppresser capabilities, Tag expression in human mesotheliomas is potentially related to the development of the malignant phenotype.[14]

GENETIC PREDISPOSITION

Hirvonen et al recently described an increased incidence of mesothelioma among asbestos-exposed individuals in Finland found to be lacking the glutathione-S-transferase M1 (GSTM1) gene and carrying the "slow-acetylator" type of the N-acetyltransferase 2 (NAT-2) gene.[21] The GSTM1 gene is important in the detoxification of several carcinogens, including polycyclic aromatic hydrocarbons; NAT-2 is associated with the biotransformation of aromatic amines.

OTHER ETIOLOGIC FACTORS

The development of malignant pleural mesothelioma has also been associated in rare cases with other etiologic factors, including therapeutic irradiation, intrapleural thorium dioxide (Thorotrast), and inhalation of other fibrous silicates such as erionite. Epidemiologic studies of a region in central Anatolia (Turkey) with an abnormally high incidence of pleural mesothelioma (22 per 10,000 individuals over 25 years old) implicated routine household use of a locally ubiquitous silicate, zeolite, as a potential etiologic agent.[3]

Pathology

GROSS PATHOLOGY

Malignant mesothelioma's gross appearance is that of firm, grayish tumor coalescing on the visceral and parietal pleural surfaces into discrete plaques and nodules. The lung can be completely covered with a thick rind of tumor that can reach diameters of 5 cm or more with only minimal penetration of the underlying lung parenchyma. Adjacent structures are involved at an early stage, with invasion of the chest wall, pericardium, diaphragm, and interlobar fissures (Fig. 92-1A and B). Seventy percent of patients will have mediastinal lymph node involvement at au-

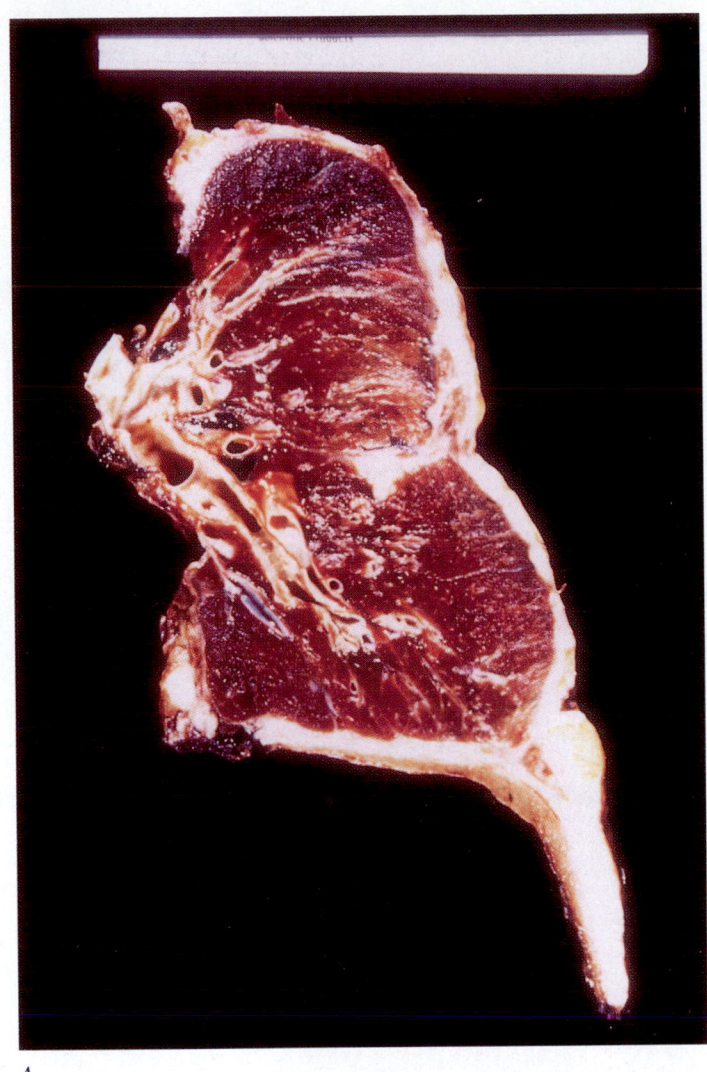

A

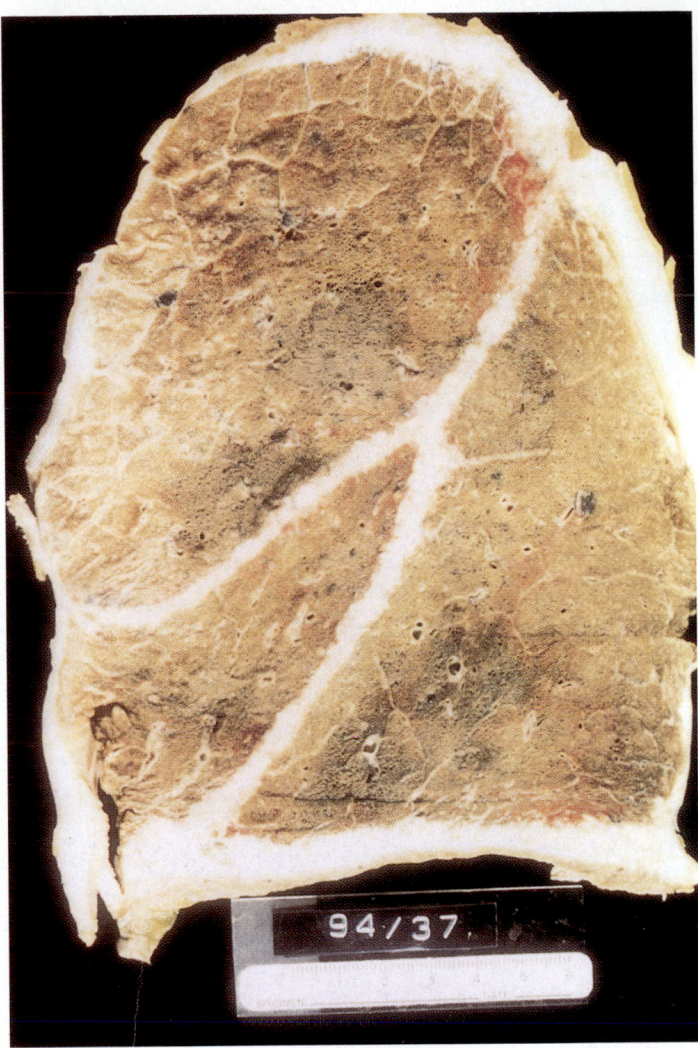

B

FIGURE 92-1   *A.* Transverse section of an extrapleural pneumonectomy surgical specimen with the entire right lung, parietal and visceral pleurae, portions of pericardium, and the majority of the right hemidiaphragm. Note the thick rind of tumor along the pleural surface encasing the lung and invading the diaphragm. *B.* Postmortem mesothelioma specimen with overnight formalin inflation and fixation. The right lung pictured is covered by a thick, whitish rind of tumor involving the entire pleural surface, which has also infiltrated and demarcated the interlobar fissures.

topsy. Hematogenous metastases are more common than previously thought, particularly in liver, lung, bone, and adrenal glands.

HISTOLOGY

Malignant mesothelioma is typically classified into three histologic subtypes—epithelial, sarcomatoid, and biphasic (Fig. 92-2). This categorization is somewhat of an oversimplification in that the larger the tissue sample, the more frequent the histologic variation. Nonetheless, the classification scheme has general diagnostic and prognostic utility. The epithelial variant (Fig. 92-2*A*) is the most common, making up 50 to 60 percent of all mesotheliomas. Typical histologies of this subtype include tubulopapillary, glandular, and solid epithelioid patterns. Sarcomatoid mesotheliomas (Fig. 92-2*B*) are composed of malignant spindled cells, which may mimic malignant mesenchymal tumors such as fibrosarcoma or leiomyosarcomas. Biphasic, or mixed, mesotheliomas (Fig. 92-2*C*) have epithelioid and sarcomatoid features,

but multiple tissue sections may be needed to demonstrate both components.

Epithelial mesotheliomas differ from those with sarcomatoid histology in clinical course and presentation. The former behave similarly to metastatic carcinomas to the pleura in that they present with large pleural effusions and metastases to regional lymph nodes, while the latter are more similar to pleural sarcomas in presenting with bulky tumor masses, minimal pleural fluid, and blood-borne metastases.[5]

HISTOCHEMISTRY

Due to ease and low cost, histochemical stains for the presence of intracytoplasmic mucin are still favored as a means of differentiating adenocarcinomas from epithelial mesotheliomas. Mucicarmine and periodic acid–Schiff (PAS) with diastase are the two most frequently used histochemical stains in excluding the diagnosis of adenocarcinoma. The use of histochemical staining

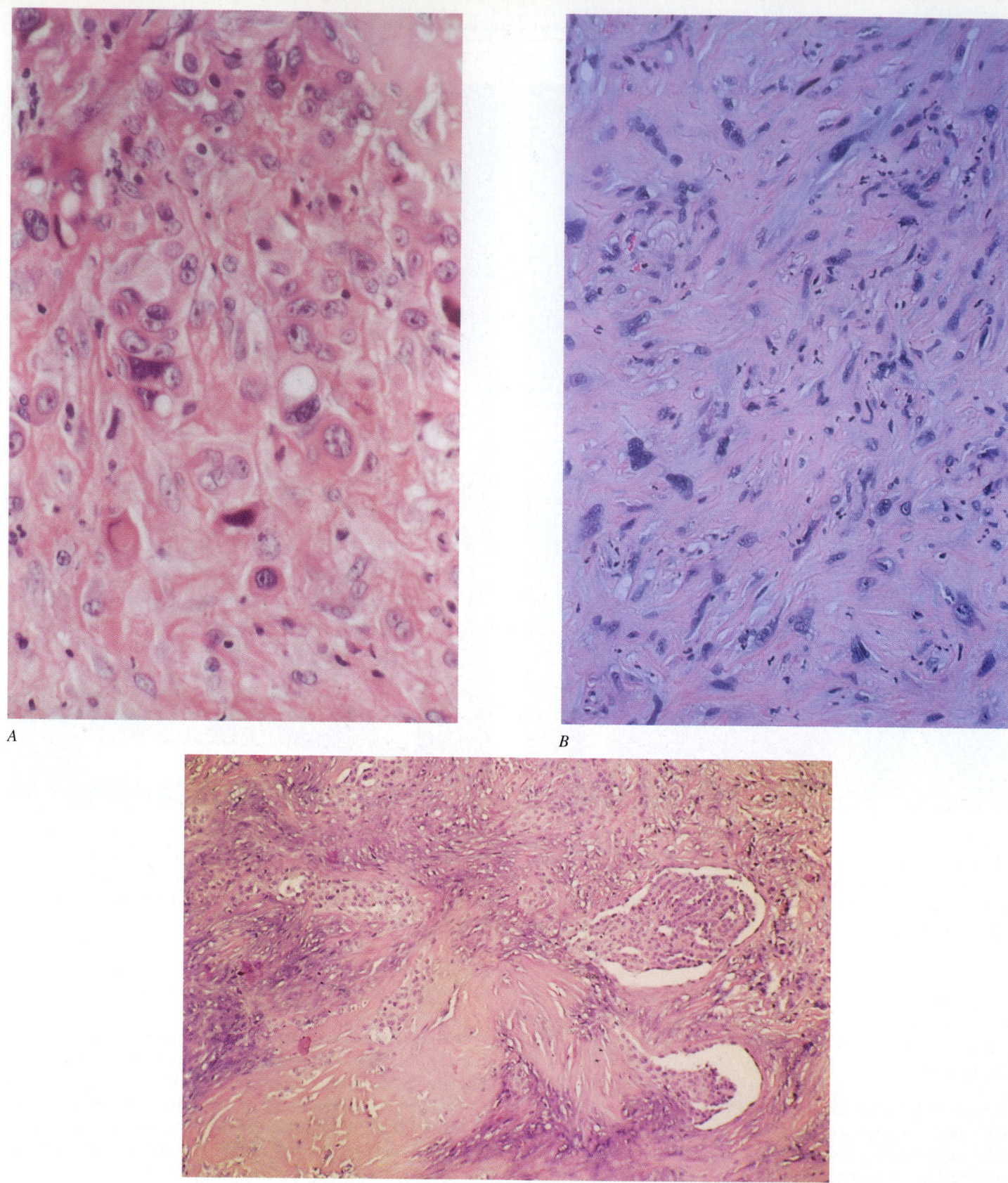

FIGURE 92-2 *A.* Photomicrograph of an epithelial malignant meso-thelioma. These sheets of pleomorphic cells are epithelial in appearance, with eosinophilic cytoplasm and fairly well defined cell borders. Note the cytoplasmic vacuoles, which can lead to confusion with a signet ring type of adenocarcinoma. By electron microscopy, these vacuoles can be shown to contain crystallized hyaluronic acid (H&E, ×400). *B.* Pho-tomicrograph of a sarcomatoid malignant mesothelioma. This tumor has a malignant mesenchymal appearance with bizarre spindled cells and a growth pattern resembling that of a sarcoma. These cells demonstrated strong cytokeratin positivity on immunohistochemical staining, distin-guishing this tumor from a sarcoma (H&E, ×400). *C.* Photomicrograph of a biphasic malignant mesothelioma. This tumor demonstrates several areas of epithelioid histology with a papillary growth pattern seen against a background of spindled and more poorly differentiated ep-ithelioid cells (H&E, ×200).

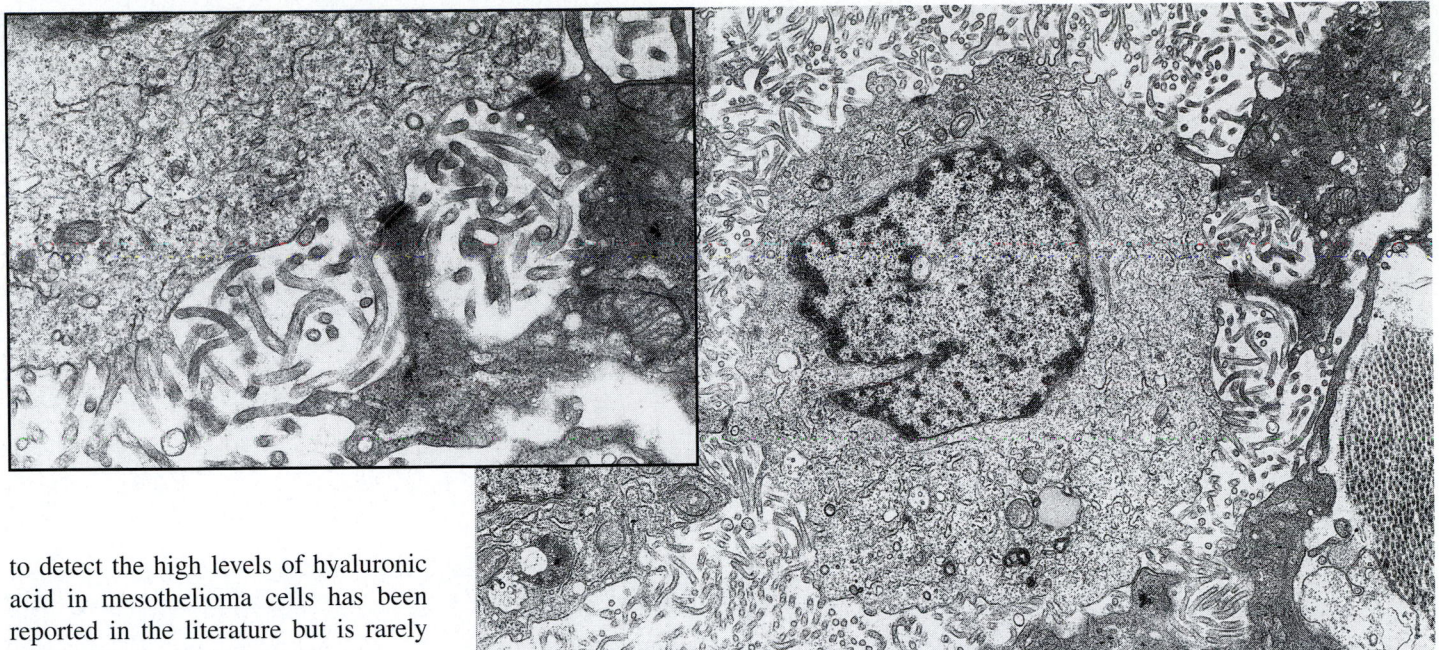

FIGURE 92-3   Electron micrograph of a human mesothelioma cell showing abundant microvilli arising from the cell surface and prominent desmosomes (×10,500; inset, ×30,000). *(Courtesy of Dr. Giuseppe G. Pietra, Department of Pathology and Laboratory Medicine, University of Pennsylvania Medical Center, Philadelphia, Pennsylvania.)*

to detect the high levels of hyaluronic acid in mesothelioma cells has been reported in the literature but is rarely relied upon in clinical practice.

ELECTRON MICROSCOPY

Ultrastructural analysis has traditionally been considered the gold standard for the diagnosis of malignant mesothelioma. Well-differentiated epithelial mesotheliomas have characteristically long, thin, "bushy" microvilli over much of the free cell surface, in addition to prominent desmosomes and numerous tonofilaments (Fig. 92-3). By contrast, the microvilli of adenocarcinomas tend to be short and more sparse, with a concentration on the apical cell surface. It has been reported that a villous length/diameter ratio of 15 or more favors a diagnosis of mesothelioma.[51] The sarcomatoid variant also contains cytokeratin and vimentin filaments, with some intracellular attachments and rare microvilli. Electron microscopic studies may be inconclusive in poorly differentiated tumors of both subtypes.

IMMUNOHISTOCHEMISTRY

Because it can be somewhat difficult to differentiate the epithelioid form of mesothelioma from metastatic adenocarcinoma and the sarcomatous form from true mesenchymal tumors, a number of immunohistologic approaches have been employed.[12,29,43,52,53] The most commonly used approach to diagnosis has been one of "diagnosis by exclusion." Tumors are usually first stained with a panel of antibodies that positively identify adenocarcinoma cells. As a rule, mesotheliomas do not stain with antibodies directed against carcinoembryonic antigen (CEA), Leu-M1, and B72.3 (a high-molecular-weight mucinlike epithelial tumor antigen) that are typically positive in most adenocarcinomas. Taken together, these three antibodies have a fairly high specificity and sensitivity for the differential diagnosis of epithelial mesothelioma versus pulmonary adenocarcinoma. This approach may not, however, reliably exclude metastatic adenocarcinomas from other primary sites such as the kidney, ovary, and prostate. An-

tibodies to cytokeratin and epithelial membrane antigen (EMA) will stain both mesotheliomas and adenocarcinomas and are therefore not helpful.

Sarcomatoid mesothelial cells characteristically coexpress vimentin and cytokeratin. Vimentin immunoreactivity is present in sarcomatoid mesotheliomas, soft tissue sarcomas, and a sufficient number of epithelial tumors to be of little utility in this differential diagnosis. Although soft tissue sarcomas may be focally positive for cytokeratin, strong cytokeratin positivity favors a diagnosis of sarcomatoid mesothelioma or spindle-cell carcinoma. Desmin positivity is characteristic of some types of soft tissue sarcomas but can also be found in malignant mesotheliomas.[23]

It has been much more difficult to obtain antibodies that reliably and specifically identify mesothelioma, especially in paraffin-fixed sections. A number of antibodies have been shown to be useful in small studies, including: antithrombomodulin, anti-*N*-cadherin, monoclonal antibody (mAb) K1, mAb ME1, mAb MOC-31, mAb HBME-1 (epithelial mesotheliomas), and a polyclonal antibody—AMAD-2 (reviewed in Ref. 43). One recently described marker that may prove to be particularly valuable in the diagnosis of mesothelioma is the Wilms' tumor 1 (WT1) gene product.[2] WT1 is a tumor suppresser gene that is primarily restricted to mesenchymally derived tissue and therefore appears to be selectively expressed in tumors of mesodermal origin, such as mesothelioma. Northern analysis and immunostaining of multiple frozen tumors for WT1 message or protein product revealed selective expression in mesotheliomas (Fig. 92-4*A* and *B*) with little or no positivity in non-small-cell lung carcinomas and in adenocarcinomas of varying origins (Fig. 92-4*C* and *D*).

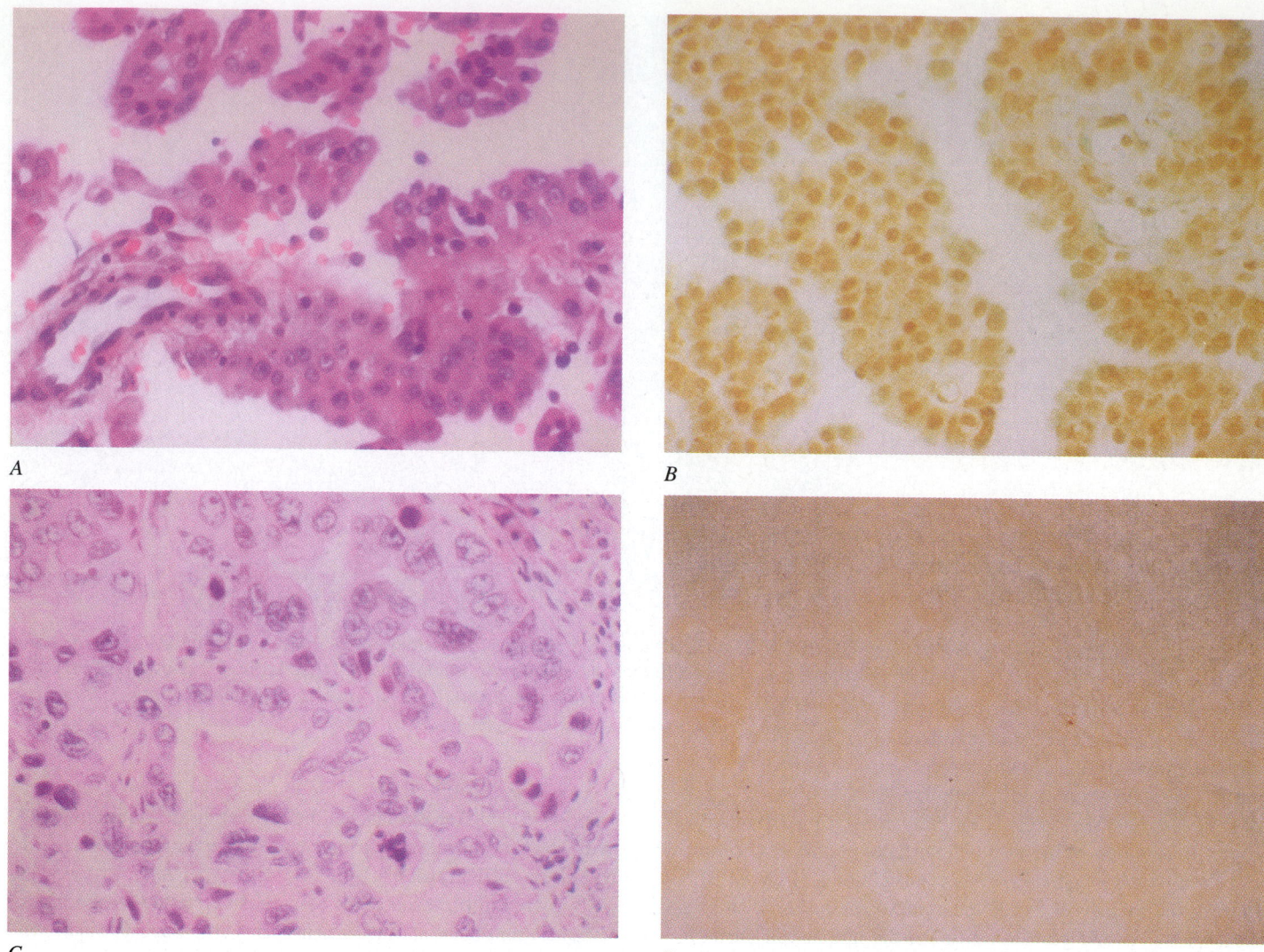

FIGURE 92-4 *A.* Photomicrograph of an epithelial mesothelioma (H&E, ×400). *B.* Photomicrograph of epithelial mesothelioma demonstrating positive nuclear staining with an antibody to the Wilms' tumor 1 (WT1) gene product (×400). *C.* Photomicrograph of an adenocarcinoma metastatic to the pleura (H&E, ×400). *D.* Photomicrograph of pleural adenocarcinoma stained with an anti-WT1 antibody (×400). Only minimal background staining is present.

Clinical Presentation

Malignant pleural mesothelioma most commonly presents in the fifth to seventh decades of life. Most patients diagnosed with mesothelioma earlier in life have a history of childhood asbestos exposure. The most frequent presenting symptoms of pleural mesothelioma are nonpleuritic chest pain (60 to 70 percent of patients), dyspnea (25 percent), and cough (20 percent). Some patients are asymptomatic at diagnosis, with unilateral pleural effusions found incidentally on routine chest radiographs. Mesothelioma is typically a unilateral disease—only 10 percent of patients with mesothelioma have bilateral involvement. In more advanced stages of disease, physical findings may include unilateral dullness to percussion throughout the hemithorax, palpable chest wall masses, and scoliosis toward the side of the malignancy.[3,5,35]

Radiographic Presentation

The most common initial radiographic manifestation of pleural mesothelioma is a large unilateral pleural effusion with contralateral mediastinal shift (Fig. 92-5A). Sixty percent of patients will have right-sided lesions; only 5 to 10 percent have bilateral disease. Occasionally, mesothelioma can present as a pleural mass or with diffuse pleural thickening with involvement of the interlobar fissures in the absence of pleural effusion. Only 20 percent of patients with pleural mesothelioma will have radiographic signs of asbestosis (i.e., bibasilar interstitial fibrosis), although many will have evidence of pleural plaques and/or calcifications. In later stages of disease, ipsilateral mediastinal shift is seen secondary to encompassment of the lung by a thick rind of tumor and resultant significant unilateral loss of lung volume. Patients with advanced mesothelioma may also have radio-

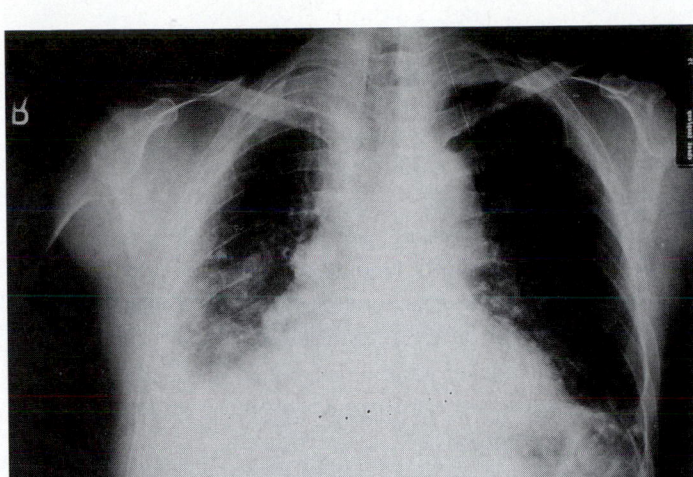

A

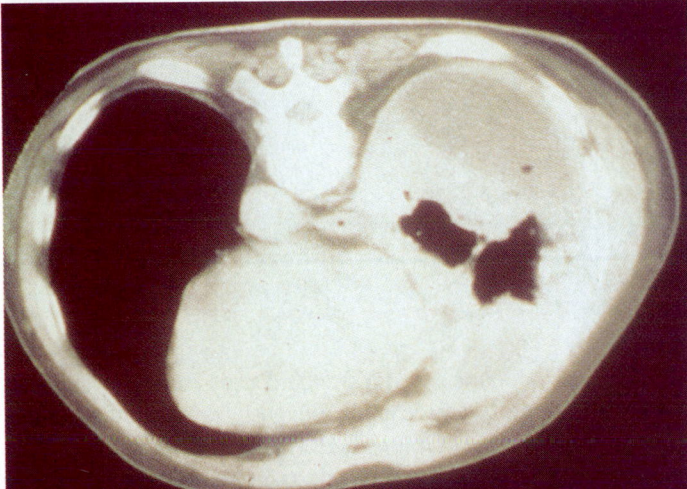

B

FIGURE 92-5 *A.* Posteroanterior chest radiograph in a patient with malignant pleural mesothelioma demonstrating significant right-sided pleural effusion and diffuse pleural thickening associated with marked volume loss of the right hemithorax. No definite calcified pleural plaques are seen. *B.* Computed axial tomographic image from a patient with pleural mesothelioma, illustrating complete encasement of the ipsilateral lung with a thick rind of tumor, neoplastic invasion of the interlobar fissures, small residual pleural effusion, and marked unilateral volume loss.

graphic findings of mediastinal widening due to direct tumor invasion or lymph node involvement, enlargement of the cardiac margins secondary to pericardial invasion with effusion, and evidence of rib destruction or soft tissue masses extending from the chest wall. Chest computed tomography (CT) is important in detecting invasion of chest wall, ribs, and mediastinal structures (Fig. 92-5*B*). Coronal magnetic resonance imaging (MRI) is helpful in discerning the extent of disease, particularly extension of pleural mesothelioma through the diaphragm into the peritoneal cavity.[30]

Laboratory Studies

Although there are no specific serum biomarkers for malignant mesothelioma, evaluation of pleural fluid may be beneficial. Effusions associated with mesothelioma are strongly exudative, with elevated protein concentrations in the range of 4 to 5 g/dL and a lymphocytic predominance. Pleural fluid lactate dehydrogenase (LDH) concentrations often exceed those of patients with carcinomatous pleural effusions, with levels greater than 600 IU/L. In patients with advanced disease and extensive involvement of visceral and parietal pleura, pleural fluid pH and glucose are commonly low.[40] In addition, the pleural effusion associated with mesothelioma is characteristically highly viscous, presumably because of elevated concentrations of hyaluronic acid. An increased pleural fluid hyaluronidase level is suggestive but not diagnostic of mesothelioma.[5] The cytokine profile of pleural effusions related to mesothelioma is somewhat unique in that high concentrations of interleukin-6 (IL-6) are found with relatively low levels of IL-1β and tumor necrosis factor-α. These elevated intrapleural levels of IL-6 in patients with malignant mesothelioma are postulated to induce systemic manifestations such as fever, cachexia, and thrombocytosis.[31] Pulmonary function testing typically demonstrates a restrictive pattern resulting from pleural effusions, tumor encasement of the lung, or chest wall involvement.

Diagnosis

The differential diagnosis of malignant pleural mesothelioma includes both benign and malignant processes. Inflammatory reactions such as chronic, organized empyema can mimic the dense pleural thickening and large, viscous pleural effusions characteristic of mesothelioma. As discussed above, epithelial mesotheliomas can be extremely difficult to distinguish grossly and histologically from metastatic adenocarcinoma to the pleura from any number of primary sources, including lung, breast, stomach, kidney, ovary, and prostate. Sarcomas such as fibrosarcoma and malignant fibrous histiocytoma can present in similar fashion and infiltrate like sarcomatous mesotheliomas. The mixed-cellular type of mesothelioma can bear a significant histologic resemblance to sarcomatoid carcinomas and synovial sarcoma.[3]

Accurate diagnosis of malignant mesothelioma is important in the event of subsequent litigation, for proper epidemiologic records, and for appropriate therapeutic intervention. Thoracentesis or closed pleural biopsy can often establish the diagnosis of pleural malignancy but may not provide enough diagnostic material to confirm the presence of mesothelioma. Cytologic evaluation of pleural fluid is helpful for detecting the presence of malignancy but has difficulty in distinguishing epithelioid mesothelioma from adenocarcinoma and the sarcomatoid type from fibrosarcomas or hemangiopericytomas. Immunohistochemical markers and monoclonal antibodies may aid in differentiating mesothelioma from adenocarcinoma on cytology specimens. In addition, certain cytopathological features of cells obtained from pleural fluid have been found to correlate well with the presence of mesothelioma, including papillary aggregates, multinucleation with atypia, cell-to-cell apposition, nuclear pleomorphism, and macronucleoli.[44]

Surgical intervention, via video-assisted thoracoscopic biopsy or open thoracotomy, is often necessary to firmly establish the diagnosis. Boutin and colleagues from Marseille prospectively evaluated thoracoscopy for the diagnosis of malignant pleural mesothelioma in 188 consecutive patients from 1973 to 1990 and found that thoracoscopic biopsy was diagnostic in 98 percent of cases, compared with only 26 percent for thoracentesis alone, and 39 percent for fluid cytology and closed pleural biopsy. These procedures were performed under local anesthesia in an endoscopy suite with minimal morbidity or complications.[9]

Concurrent bronchoscopy may be important in distinguishing between mesothelioma and metastatic adenocarcinoma of the lung, as endobronchial lesions are rarely seen in mesothelioma. In addition, mediastinoscopy plays an increasingly important role in the diagnosis and staging of mesothelioma, as recent studies have documented the significant negative prognostic implications of mediastinal nodal invasion in this disease.[45] Approximately 10 percent of patients who undergo a diagnostic procedure for mesothelioma will seed the biopsy site with tumor cells, later developing chest wall recurrences. This complication can potentially be prevented by prophylactic radiation therapy to the surgical incision or thoracentesis sites.[3,10]

Staging

The staging of malignant mesothelioma has proven to be more controversial than that of many other tumors. The most commonly used schema was devised by Butchart in 1976[13] (Table 92-1). Although useful, its ability to predict survival is weakened by lack of inclusion of lymph node involvement and chest wall invasion.

For this reason, the Union Internationale Contre le Cancer (UICC) in 1990 first proposed a staging system based upon the

TABLE 92-1

Butchart Staging System

Stage I	Tumor confined within the "capsule" of the parietal pleura
Stage II	Tumor invading chest wall or involving mediastinal structures
Stage III	Tumor penetrating diaphragm to involve peritoneum; involvement of opposite pleura; lymph node involvement outside the chest
Stage IV	Distant blood-borne metastases

TABLE 92-2

International Mesothelioma Interest Group (IMIG) Staging System

T1	T1a: Tumor limited to ipsilateral parietal pleura
	T1b: Tumor involving ipsilateral parietal pleura, with scattered foci of tumor on visceral pleural surface
T2	Tumor involving all ipsilateral pleural surfaces with diaphragmatic invasion or extension into underlying pulmonary parenchyma
T3	Involvement of the endothoracic fascia; mediastinal fat; solitary, resectable chest wall focus; or nontransmural pericardial invasion
T4	Diffuse extension into chest wall, peritoneum, spine, mediastinal organs, contralateral pleura, internal surface of pericardium or myocardium
N0	No regional lymph nodes metastases
N1	Metastases in the ipsilateral bronchopulmonary or hilar lymph nodes
N2	Metastases in the subcarinal or ipsilateral mediastinal lymph nodes
N3	Metastases in the contralateral mediastinal or internal mammary lymph nodes or any supraclavicular node metastasis

STAGING:

Stage I	Ia: T1aN0M0
	Ib: T1bN0M0
Stage II	T2N0M0
Stage III	Any T3M0, any N1M0, any N2M0
Stage IV	Any T4, any N3, any M1

TNM (tumor/node/metastasis) standard used for many other tumors. More recently, Rusch and colleagues from the International Mesothelioma Interest Group (IMIG) proposed an updated staging system based upon tumor descriptors, providing precise anatomic definitions of the local extent of the primary tumor. This staging system (Table 92-2) was designed to provide the framework for proper analysis of prospective clinical trials of new treatment modalities.[38]

Clinical Course and Complications

Mesothelioma exerts its morbidity and mortality via inexorable local invasion. Patients typically develop shortness of breath and chest pain as tumor and fibrosis gradually obliterate the pleural space and replace any pleural fluid. As the tumor spreads, it covers both visceral and parietal pleural surfaces, encasing the ipsilateral lung with a thick, fibrous peel that extends into interlobar fissures and occasionally into lung parenchyma. Deoxygenated blood is shunted through the trapped lung, leading to significant dyspnea and hypoxemia that is often refractory to supplemental oxygen. Dyspnea also results from abnormal chest wall mechanics secondary to tumor invasion into ribs as well as intercostal nerves and muscles. Local invasion of crucial thoracic structures can result in dysphagia, hoarseness, cord compression, brachial plexopathy, Horner's syndrome, and superior vena cava syndrome. Hilar and mediastinal lymph node involvement occurs in less than 50 percent of patients but is a harbinger of poor prognosis. Distant metastatic disease, by hematogenous spread, is unusual in mesothelioma but may present in liver, bone, brain, adrenals, thyroid, and kidney. Metastatic disease is typically an end-stage manifestation of malignant mesothelioma.[3,5,35]

Mortality

Median survival of patients with mesothelioma is between 6 and 18 months and is not significantly affected by currently available standard therapeutic interventions. Patients die from local extension and respiratory failure; tumor extension below the diaphragm may result in death from small bowel obstruction. Patients may also die from arrhythmias, heart failure, or stroke caused by tumor invasion of the heart or pericardium.[3,5,35]

Paraneoplastic Syndromes

Disseminated intravascular coagulation, migratory thrombophlebitis, thrombocytosis, Coombs-positive hemolytic anemia, hypoglycemia, and hypercalcemia associated with secretion of a parathyroid hormone–like peptide have all been described in the setting of mesothelioma.[3]

Prognostic Factors

At the time of presentation with mesothelioma, poor prognosis is indicated by thrombocytosis, fever of unknown origin, sarcomatous or mixed histology, age above 65 years, and poor performance status. A better prognosis is associated with epithelial histology, stage I disease, age under 55, performance status of 0 to 1, absence of chest pain, and the presence of symptoms for more than 6 months prior to establishment of diagnosis.[25,33] Epithelial mesotheliomas have been reported to have a significantly improved prognosis as compared with the sarcomatoid and biphasic forms.[3] In a study performed at the University of Lund in Sweden, patients with purely epithelial mesotheliomas survived significantly longer than those whose tumors had a sarcomatoid component (674 versus 471 days). Patients with tubulopapillary mesotheliomas, a subtype of the epithelial form, had the longest mean survival (775 days), prompting the investigators to conclude that the tubulopapillary form should be reclassified as "low-grade mesotheliomas."[26]

CURRENT APPROACHES TO TREATMENT OF MESOTHELIOMA

For many years, a nihilistic attitude has existed among many physicians and surgeons caring for patients with malignant mesothelioma because of the tumor's characteristically poor response to multiple forms of therapy. Much of this pessimism has been justified, but emerging therapies may offer hope for improved palliation, prolonged survival, and even possible cure of patients with mesothelioma.

Chemotherapy

Despite multiple single-agent and combination chemotherapy trials in patients with mesothelioma over the past two decades, there is currently little indication for primary use of this modality. Response rates to single-agent chemotherapy have been dismal, ranging from 0 to 20 percent. Doxorubicin has the highest single-agent response rate; methotrexate and cisplatin have demonstrated little efficacy. Combination therapy with mitomycin and cisplatin showed significant activity in animal models but only 25 percent total response rates in clinical trials.[5,33] A recent study of intensive combination chemotherapy with cyclophosphamide, doxorubicin, and cisplatin performed at the M. D. Anderson Cancer Center in Houston reported only 7 partial responses out of 23 patients (30 percent), with a median survival time after initiation of therapy of only 14 months.[41]

Radiation Therapy

Mesothelioma is actually more responsive to radiation than non-small-cell lung cancer; however, "curative" radiotherapy with an attempt to treat the entire involved pleural surface is technically difficult and associated with a high risk of radiation pneumonitis, myelitis, hepatitis, and myocarditis. There have been anecdotal reports of long-term survivals following high-dose external-beam irradiation and even intrapleural administration of radioactive isotopes, but most studies have shown no significant effect upon overall survival in patients with mesothelioma. Radiation therapy may play a palliative role in mesothelioma for the prevention of chest wall recurrences after thoracoscopy/thoracotomy and in improving local control after pleurectomy or extrapleural pneumonectomy.[1,5,10]

Surgical Approaches to Treatment of Mesothelioma

Although potentially associated with significant morbidity, surgical treatment of mesothelioma has been useful in palliating the major symptoms of the disease; in selected cases, it has led to some improvement in patient survival.[45] With the increased use of thoracoscopy, more patients with mesothelioma are being diagnosed at earlier stages, at which point they may be candidates for more aggressive attempts at surgical "cure."

PLEURODESIS

By far the most common and bothersome symptom of patients with mesothelioma is persistent dyspnea from large unilateral pleural effusions. A reasonable approach to palliation of this disabling dyspnea is complete drainage of the pleural effusion via tube thoracostomy or video thoracoscopy and then introduction of an irritative agent into the pleural space by injection or insufflation. The goal is to produce an inflammatory reaction of the parietal and visceral pleural surfaces, resulting in obliteration of the pleural space (i.e., pleurodesis) and thus precluding significant reaccumulation of pleural fluid. Multiple compounds have been used in the past to achieve pleural symphysis, including tetracycline, minocycline, quinacrine, and bleomycin. At present, the most widely used compound for pleurodesis is sterile talc, either as a powder or slurry (see Chap. 90). Unfortunately, chemical pleurodesis is often unsuccessful in patients with mesothelioma because of bulky tumor covering the pleural cavity and preventing apposition of inflamed pleural surfaces.

PLEUROPERITONEAL SHUNT

Pleuroperitoneal shunting is an alternative approach to relieving the unrelenting dyspnea resulting from the rapid reaccumulation of pleural fluid in patients with a hemithorax diffusely involved with mesothelioma.[48] This procedure involves insertion of a catheter into the pleural space, which is tunneled subcutaneously into the peritoneal cavity. A manual pump and one-way valve are interposed, allowing the patient to control the drainage of pleural fluid from the affected hemithorax. One theoretical problem, which has been borne out by anecdotal reports, is the rapid spread of mesothelioma to the abdomen, with subsequent development of bowel obstruction.[36]

PLEURECTOMY

Parietal pleurectomy—open surgical stripping of the pleura and pericardium from the apex of the lung to the diaphragm—is more successful than talc pleurodesis in reducing the recurrence of pleural effusion in mesothelioma. Pleurectomy alone has not been shown to prolong survival; however, there are reports that the combination of parietal pleurectomy with postoperative intrapleural therapy and/or external beam irradiation resulted in a median survival of 22.5 months and a 2-year survival rate of 41 percent in a select group of 27 patients, predominantly with the epithelial subtype.[1,39,45]

EXTRAPLEURAL PNEUMONECTOMY

Extrapleural pneumonectomy (EPP) is a much more radical surgical procedure involving the complete removal of the ipsilateral lung along with the parietal and visceral pleura, pericardium with portions of the phrenic nerve, and the majority of the hemidiaphragm (Fig. 92-1A). Used alone, EPP is an excellent means of palliating the profound dyspnea and orthopnea associated with the significant ventilation/perfusion mismatch resulting from lung encasement by tumor.[45,46]

Without adjuvant therapy, however, EPP has not been shown to significantly prolong survival in patients with mesothelioma. Investigators have combined EPP with sequential postoperative chemotherapy (doxorubicin, cyclophosphamide, and cisplatin for four to six cycles) and up to 5500 cGy adjuvant radiotherapy to the postoperative hemithorax. Other groups have used intracavitary chemotherapy, postoperative irradiation, and postresectional intracavitary photodynamic therapy. In these contexts, EPP is designed as a cytoreductive and not a curative procedure.[45,46]

It should be noted that EPP is associated with significant morbidity and an operative mortality that ranges from 5 to 35 percent, depending on the experience of the center and the preoperative condition of the patient. Patient recruitment must therefore be highly selective, with candidates for this multimodal approach undergoing extensive preoperative evaluation, including chest MRI with sagittal views to assess mediastinal and diaphragmatic involvement, full pulmonary function testing with quantitative ventilation-perfusion scanning for patients with borderline FEV_1, and echocardiography to evaluate mediastinal invasion and ventricular function (crucial before treatment with anthracycline chemotherapy). Using this combined-modality

schema, at least one group has demonstrated improved short- and long-term survival in patients with mesothelioma; median overall survival was 16 months, but this improved to 24 months for those with the epithelial subtype. Patients in this study who had epithelial mesothelioma and no mediastinal lymph node involvement at resection had a remarkable 5-year survival rate of 45 percent.[45]

Treatment of Nonpleural Forms of Mesothelioma

Patients recently diagnosed with peritoneal mesothelioma appear to have an improved prognosis relative to the pleural form. This may reflect the technical ease of delivery of intraperitoneal chemotherapy as well as the capacity for multiple resections/debulking of peritoneal masses. One-third of 25 patients with peritoneal mesothelioma in a Dana-Farber phase II series remain disease-free at 2 to 3 years after treatment. There is no effective therapy for mesothelioma of the pericardium or tunica vaginalis; these neoplasms share the dismal prognosis of the pleural form of the disease.[5]

NEW THERAPEUTIC APPROACHES

Despite the small but significant improvement in survival achieved with intensive multimodality therapy for mesothelioma, it is obvious that less morbid, more effective interventions are needed. Many investigators over the past two decades have attempted to treat this disease primarily by direct instillation of chemotherapeutic and other compounds into the pleural space, but with minimal success.[24,39,46] Based upon reports that mesothelioma patients with greater amounts of intratumoral lymphocytic infiltration had improved median survival rates, several groups have looked at immunotherapy as an alternative means of achieving better tumor response rates.[28,37]

Immunotherapy

The use of compounds to stimulate an antitumor immune response against pleural malignancy stemmed from the observation that patients who developed empyemas postthoracotomy for primary lung carcinoma had improved survival rates. Subsequently, intrapleural bacille Calmette-Guérin (BCG) was studied as a surgical adjuvant, but no significant benefit was seen. Several systemic immunotherapies have been administered to patients with mesothelioma, including interleukin-2 (IL-2) and interferon-gamma (IFN-γ), both of which demonstrated limited efficacy and significant side effects. Subcutaneous IFN-α-2a was found to have some efficacy, one complete response, and three partial responses out of 25 patients studied and was well tolerated clinically.[6,15,20,37] One recent European phase I–II study of intrapleural IL-2 administered by continuous infusion via an intrapleural catheter revealed a 19 percent partial response rate with marked dose-related toxicity, primarily the development of ipsilateral empyemas.[20] Of note were the high ratios of intrapleural/systemic IL-2 levels approaching 1,000:1, particularly in the highest doses.

Boutin's group in Marseilles, France, has pioneered the intrapleural administration of immunostimulants to treat mesothelioma, and has demonstrated significant responses with both intrapleural IL-2 and IFN-γ.[8,11] Most impressive were the results of intrapleural IFN-γ in patients with early-stage mesothelioma (Butchart stage I and II). A total of 89 patients were treated over 46 months with an overall response rate of 20 percent. Eight patients had histologically confirmed complete responses and nine had partial responses with greater than 50 percent reduction in tumor volume. Overall, patients with stage I disease had a response rate of 45 percent. The effectiveness of IFN-γ against mesothelioma was thought to be mediated in part by direct inhibitory effects upon mesothelioma cell growth as well as by decreased intrapleural IL-6 production, with resultant activation of tumor-directed macrophages and cytotoxic T-lymphocytes.[31] Other investigators have focused their attention on the use of colony-stimulating factors such as granulocyte colony-stimulating factor (G-CSF) to initiate an antitumor immune response.

Gene Therapy

In the absence of other effective, nontoxic therapies for malignant mesothelioma, several groups of investigators have looked to the newly evolving technologies of gene therapy for new treatment modalities. One approach has been intrapleural delivery of replication-deficient recombinant adenovirus (rAd) that has been genetically engineered to contain the herpes simplex virus thymidine kinase gene (HSV*tk*).[32] It is hoped that administration of AdHSV*tk* into the pleural cavity of patients with mesothelioma will transduce the tumor cells, enabling them to express viral *tk,* and conferring upon them sensitivity to the normally nontoxic antiviral drug ganciclovir (GCV). Viral *tk,* unlike mammalian kinases, can catalyze the rate-limiting step of the production of GCV-triphosphate, a strong cellular toxin that inhibits function of DNA polymerase. By virtue of the "bystander effect" in which GCV-triphosphate and possibly other toxic metabolites pass through gap junctions between transduced and nontransduced tumor cells, established mesothelioma tumors have been successfully eradicated in several animal models. This approach is now in a phase I clinical trial.[16,42]

Other gene therapy approaches to the treatment of mesothelioma under investigation include a vaccinia virus–IL-2 construct for direct intratumoral injection and a recombinant adenovirus containing the wild-type p53 gene, which is purported to transduce mesothelioma cells, causing overexpression of wild-type p53 and inducing apoptosis.

OTHER PRIMARY PLEURAL NEOPLASMS

Solitary, benign fibrous tumors of the pleura, previously referred to as "benign mesotheliomas," are approximately one-third as common as malignant mesothelioma and are thought to arise from a different cell of origin. Whereas mesotheliomas derive from altered mesothelial cells, benign fibrous tumors appear to come from submesothelial fibrous tissue. Although the peak age range of affected patients is similar (40 to 70 years), benign fibrous tumors can affect patients of all ages, including children

as young as 5 years old. In addition, there is no significant association of benign fibrous tumors of the pleura with asbestos exposure or other environmental agents.[17]

Clinical Presentation

Patients with solitary fibrous tumors of the pleura are usually asymptomatic and are diagnosed incidentally at routine chest radiography, but they can present with nonpleuritic chest pain, dyspnea, cough, or pleural effusion. A large proportion (up to 40 percent) of patients present with symptomatic hypoglycemia, thought to be secondary to elaboration of insulinlike growth factors. Clubbing of fingers and toes is common, as are diffuse arthralgias, but the incidence of pulmonary hypertrophic osteoarthropathy is controversial.[17]

Radiography

Benign fibrous tumors typically present radiographically as large, rounded, well-circumscribed pleura-based masses, but occasionally they can appear to be intraparenchymal. Some of these masses can be very large (over 15 cm in diameter) and can cause clinically significant compression of the lung. About 17 percent will present with an ipsilateral pleural effusion. Asbestos-related pleural plaques are rare.[17]

Gross Pathology

Solitary fibrous tumors of the pleura typically arise from a pedicle off of the visceral pleural surface but rarely invade the visceral pleura itself (Fig. 92-6*A*). They are usually well-circumscribed, firm, encapsulated, occasionally lobulated masses that vary in size from 1 cm in diameter to more than 30 cm. When sectioned, the cut surface may reveal a whorled appearance, with associated areas of hemorrhage and/or necrosis.[17]

Microscopic Pathology

Histologically, benign fibrous tumors have what has been described as a "patternless pattern" (Fig. 92-6*B*). Sections often show fascicles of interlacing spindlelike cells interspersed between areas of variably dense collagenous material. Cuboidal mesothelial cells may be trapped within these collagenous collections. These mesothelial cells have elongated nuclei, small nucleoli, and infrequent mitotic figures. Multiple vascular channels run between the spindle cells, varying in size from capillaries to small arteries. Immunoperoxidase staining of solitary fibrous tumors is generally nonreactive with all antibodies except vimentin, but recent reports have shown consistent positive staining with an antibody directed against CD34[49] (Fig. 92-6*C*). Anti-CD34 has been found to stain endothelium positively, as well as some vascular and smooth muscle tumors. Negative staining for a panel of other markers, such as cytokeratin, helps to distinguish solitary fibrous tumors from a host of benign and malignant pleural neoplasms.[49] Electron microscopy of the spindle cells does not demonstrate the prominent microvilli and tonofilaments seen in malignant mesothelioma.

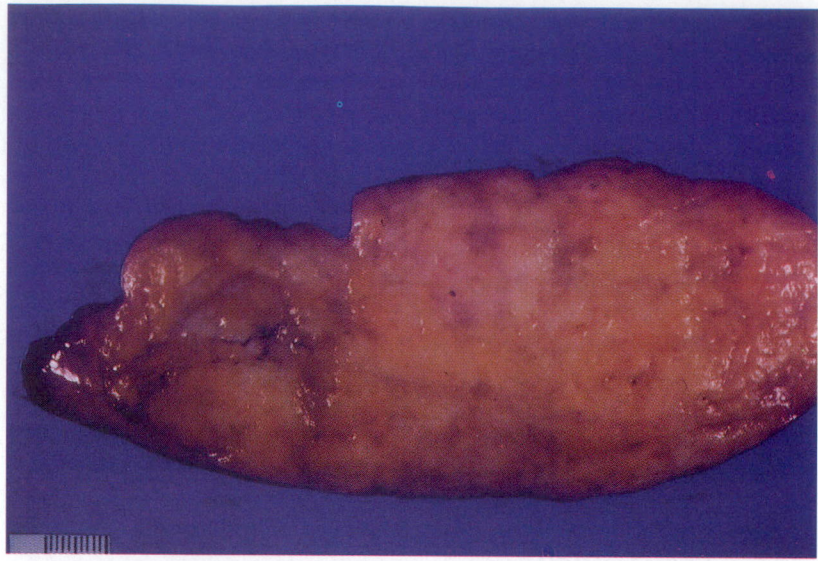

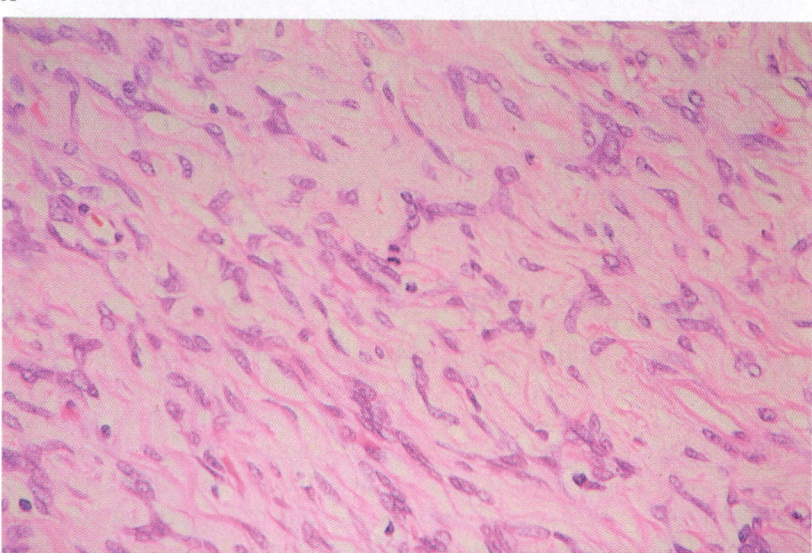

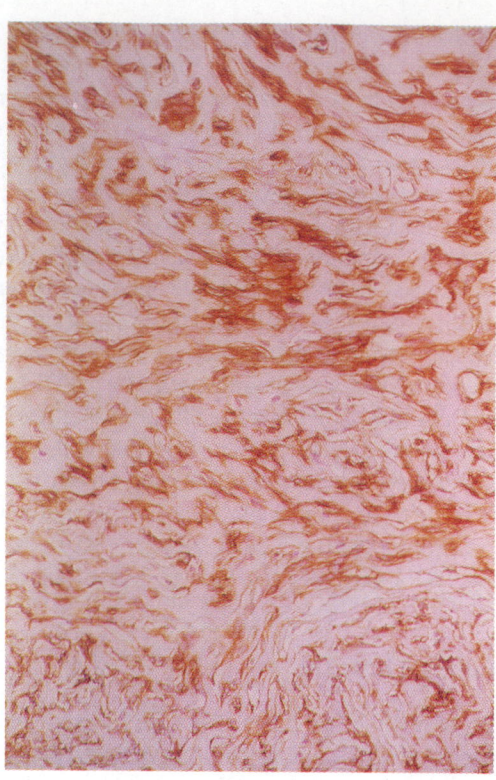

FIGURE 92-6 *A.* Gross photograph of a surgically resected, solitary, benign pleural fibrous tumor. Note the well-circumscribed nature of this firm, slightly lobulated mass with its smooth-cut surface and punctate areas of hemorrhage and necrosis. (Courtesy of Dr. Matt van de Rijn, Department of Pathology and Laboratory Medicine, University of Pennsylvania Medical Center, Philadelphia, Pennsylvania.) *B.* Photomicrograph of a typical solitary fibrous tumor demonstrating the "patternless-pattern" (H&E, ×400). (Courtesy of Dr. Matt van de Rijn.) *C.* Photomicrograph of a section of solitary fibrous tumor stained with an antibody directed against CD-34, a cell surface marker found commonly on endothelial cells and some smooth muscle and vascular tumors (×400). Positive staining for CD-34 helps distinguish these lesions from mesotheliomas and other pleural neoplasms. *(Courtesy of Dr. Matt van de Rijn.)*

Treatment

Surgical resection of solitary, benign fibrous tumors of the pleura is curative with little risk of recurrence. There is typically a discrete separation between the tumor and underlying compressed lung, so pulmonary resection is usually unnecessary. Some tumors may require a limited chest wall resection. A small percentage of patients will develop recurrences several decades after surgical resection and may die from extensive local disease.[17] Some of these recurrent, localized fibrous tumors of the pleura demonstrate more aggressive histologic features but are often successfully cured by surgical excision, in particular the pedunculated lesions.

Other Primary Pleural Tumors

A wide variety of benign and malignant neoplasms arising from multiple cell types of the pleural lining have been described, including soft tissue sarcomas (liposarcoma, leiomyosarcoma, fibrosarcoma, synovial sarcoma), granulocytic sarcomas, malignant and benign fibrous histiocytomas, fibromyxomas, and spindle-cell carcinoma. Each of these lesions can be differentiated from benign fibrous tumors by a characteristic immunohistochemical pattern.[49] Pleural endometriomas are nonneoplastic ectopic foci of endometrial tissue that may wax and wane with the menstrual cycle and can precipitate recurrent pneumothoraxes (catamenial pneumothorax).

REFERENCES

1. Aisner J: Current approach to malignant mesothelioma of the pleura. *Chest* 107:332S–344S, 1995.

2. Amin KM, Litzky LA, Smythe WR, et al: Wilms' tumor 1 susceptibility (WT1) gene products are selectively expressed in malignant mesothelioma. *Am J Pathol* 146:344–356, 1995.

3. Antman KH, Pass HI, Li FP, et al: Benign and malignant mesothelioma, in DeVita VT Jr, Hellman S, Rosenberg SA (eds): *Cancer: Principles and Practice of Oncology,* 4th ed. Philadelphia, Lippincott, 1993, pp 1489–1508.

4. Antman KH: Malignant mesothelioma: Prognostic variables in a registry of 180 patients, the Dana-Farber Cancer Institute and Brigham and Women's Hospital experience over two decades, 1965–1985. *J Clin Oncol* 6:147–153, 1988.

5. Antman KH: Natural history and epidemiology of malignant mesothelioma. *Chest* 103:373S–376S, 1993.

6. Astoul P, Viallat JR, Laurent JC, et al: Intrapleural recombinant IL-2 in passive immunotherapy for malignant pleural effusion. *Chest* 103:209–213, 1993.

7. Bianchi AB, Mitsunaga SI, Cheng JQ, et al: High frequency of inactivating mutations in the neurofibromatosis type 2 gene (NF2) in primary malignant mesotheliomas. *Proc Natl Acad Sci USA* 92:10854–10858, 1995.

8. Boutin C, Nussbaum E, Monnet I, et al: Intrapleural treatment with recombinant gamma-interferon in early stage malignant mesothelioma. *Cancer* 74:2460–2467, 1994.

9. Boutin C, Rey F, Gouvernet J, et al: Thoracoscopy in pleural malignant mesothelioma: A prospective study of 188 consecutive patients. *Cancer* 72:389–403, 1993.

10. Boutin C, Rey F, Viallat JR: Prevention of malignant seeding after invasive diagnostic procedures in patients with pleural mesothelioma. *Chest* 108:754–758, 1995.

11. Boutin C, Viallat JR, Van Zandwijk N, et al: Activity of intrapleural recombinant gamma-interferon in malignant mesothelioma. *Cancer* 67:2033–2037, 1991.

12. Brown RW, Clark GM, Tandon AK, Allred DC: Multiple-marker immunohistochemical phenotypes distinguishing malignant pleural mesothelioma from pulmonary adenocarcinoma. *Hum Pathol* 24:347–354, 1993.

13. Butchart EG, Ashcroft T, Barnsley WC, Holden MP: Pleuropneumonectomy in the management of diffuse malignant mesothelioma of the pleura: Experience with 29 patients. *Thorax* 31:15–24, 1976.

14. Carbone M, Pass HI, Rizzo P, et al: Simian virus 40-like DNA sequences in human pleural mesothelioma. *Oncogene* 9:1781–1790, 1994.

15. Christmas TI, Manning LS, Garlepp MJ, et al: Effect of interferon-α2a on malignant mesothelioma. *J Interferon Res* 13:9–12, 1993.

16. Elshami A, Kucharczuk J, Zhang H, et al: Treatment of pleural mesothelioma in an immunocompetent rat model utilizing adenoviral transfer of the HSV-thymidine kinase gene. *Hum Gene Ther* 7:141–148, 1996.

17. England DM, Hochholzer L, McCarthy MJ: Localized benign and malignant fibrous tumors of the pleura: A clinicopathologic review of 223 cases. *Am J Surg Pathol* 13:640–658, 1989.

18. Fitzpatrick DR, Peroni DJ, Bielefeldt-Ohmann H: The role of growth factors and cytokines in the tumorigenesis and immunobiology of malignant mesothelioma. *Am J Respir Cell Mol Biol* 12:455–460, 1995.

19. Gerwin BI: Asbestos and the mesothelial cell: A molecular trail to mitogenic stimuli and supressor gene suspects. *Am J Respir Cell Mol Biol* 11:507–508, 1994.

20. Goey SH, Eggermont AMM, Punt CJA, et al: Intrapleural administration of interleukin 2 in pleural mesothelioma: a phase I-II study. *Br J Cancer* 72:1283–1288, 1995.

21. Hirvonen A, Pelin K, Tammilehto L, et al: Inherited GSTM1 and NAT2 defects as concurrent risk modifiers in asbestos-related human malignant mesothelioma. *Cancer Res* 55:2981–2983, 1995.

22. Huncharek M: Genetic factors in the aetiology of malignant mesothelioma. *Eur J Cancer* 31A:1741–1747, 1995.

23. Hurlimann J: Desmin and neural marker expression in mesothelial cells and mesotheliomas. *Hum Pathol* 25:753–757, 1994.

24. Ike O, Shimuzu V, Hitomi S, et al: Treatment of malignant pleural effusions with doxorubicin hydrochloride-containing ply (L-lactic acid) microspheres. *Chest* 99:911–915, 1991.

25. Janssen YM, Heintz NH, Marsh JP, et al: Induction of c-fos and c-jun proto-oncogenes in target cells of the lung and pleura by carcinogenic fibers. *Am J Respir Cell Mol Biol* 11:522–530, 1994.

26. Johansson L, Lindén CJ: Aspects of histopathological subtype as a prognostic factor in 85 pleural mesotheliomas. *Chest* 109:109–114, 1996.

27. Knudson A: Asbestos and mesothelioma: Genetic lessons from a tragedy. *Proc Natl Acad Sci USA* 92:10819–10820, 1995.

28. Leigh RA, Webster I: Lymphocytic infiltration of pleural mesothelioma and its significance for suvival. *S Afr Med J* 61:1007–1009, 1982.

29. McCaughey WTE, Colby TV, Battifora H, et al: Diagnosis of diffuse malignant mesothelioma: Experience of a US/Canadian mesothelioma panel. *Mod Pathol* 4:342–353, 1991.

30. Miller WT Jr, Gefter WB, Miller WT Sr: Asbestos-related chest diseases: Plain radiographic findings. *Semin Roentgenol* 27:102–120, 1992.

31. Monti G, Jaurand MC, Monnet I, et al: Intrapleural production of interleukin 6 during mesothelioma and its modulation by gamma-interferon treatment. *Cancer Res* 54:4419–4423, 1994.

32. Moolten FL, Wells JM: Curability of tumors bearing herpes thymidine kinase genes transferred by retroviral vectors. *J Natl Cancer Inst* 82:297–300, 1990.

33. Mossman BT: Carcinogenesis and related cell and tissue responses to asbestos: A review. *Ann Occup Hyg* 38:617–624, 1994.

34. Peto J, Hodgson JT, Matthews FE, Jones JR: Continuing increase in mesothelioma mortality in Britain. *Lancet* 345:535–539, 1995.

35. Pisani RJ, Colby TV, Williams DE: Malignant mesothelioma of the pleura. *Mayo Clin Proc* 63:1234–1244, 1988.

36. Prior AJ, Ball AB: Intestinal obstruction complicating malignant mesothelioma of the pleura. *Respir Med* 87:147–148, 1993.

37. Robinson BWS, Manning LS, Bowman RV, et al: The scientific basis for the immunotherapy of human malignant mesothelioma. *Eur Respir Rev* 3:195–198, 1993.

38. Rusch VW: A proposed new international TNM staging system for malignant pleural mesothelioma. *Chest* 108:1122–1128, 1995.

39. Rusch VW: Pleurectomy/decortication and adjuvant therapy for malignant mesothelioma. *Chest* 103:382S–384S, 1993.

40. Sahn S, Good JT Jr: Pleural fluid pH in malignant effusions: diagnostic, prognostic, and therapeutic implications. *Ann Intern Med* 108:345–349, 1988.

41. Shin DM, Fossella FV, Umsowasdi T, et al: Prospective study of combination chemotherapy with cyclophosphamide, doxorubicin, and cisplatin for unresectable or metastatic malignant pleural mesothelioma. *Cancer* 76:2230–2236, 1995.

42. Smythe WR, Hwang HC, Amin KM, et al: Treatment of experimental human mesothelioma using adenovirus transfer of the herpes simplex-thymidine kinase gene. *Ann Surg* 222:78–86, 1995.

43. Soler AP, Knudsen KA, Jaurand MC, et al: The differential expression of N cadherin and E-cadherin distinguishes pleural mesotheliomas from lung adenocarcinomas. *Hum Pathol* 26:1363–1469, 1995.

44. Stevens MW, Leong AS, Fazzalari NL, et al: Cytopathology of malignant mesothelioma: A stepwise logistic regression analysis. *Diagn Cytopathol* 9:334–341, 1992.

45. Sugarbaker DJ, Jaklitsch MT, Liptay MJ: Mesothelioma and radical multimodality therapy: Who benefits? *Chest* 107(Suppl):345S–350S, 1995.

46. Sugarbaker DJ: Extrapleural pneumonectomy, chemotherapy and radiotherapy in the treatment of diffuse malignant pleural mesothelioma. *J Thorac Cardiovasc Surg* 102:10–15, 1991.

47. Taguchi T, Jhanwar SC, Seigfied JM, et al: Recurrent deletions of specific chromosomal sites in 1p, 3p, 6q, and 9p in human malignant mesothelioma. *Cancer Res* 53:4349–4355, 1993.

48. Tsang V, Fernando HC, Goldstraw P: Pleuroperitoneal shunt for recurrent malignant pleural effusions. *Thorax* 45:369–372, 1990.

49. van de Rijn M, Lombard CM, Rouse RV: Expression of CD34 by solitary fibrous tumors of the pleura, mediastinum, and lung. *Am J Surg Pathol* 18:814–820, 1994.

50. Walker C, Everitt J, Barrett JC: Possible cellular and molecular mechanisms for asbestos carcinogenicity. *Am J Ind Med* 2:253–273, 1992.

51. Warhol MJ, Hickey WF, Corson JM: Malignant mesothelioma: Ultrastructural distinction from adenocarcinoma. *Am J Surg Pathol* 6:307, 1982.

52. Wick MR, Loy T, Mills SE, et al: Malignant epithelioid pleural mesothelioma versus peripheral pulmonary adenocarcinoma: A histochemical, ultrastructural and immunohistologic study of 103 cases. *Hum Pathol* 21:759–766, 1990.

53. Zeng L, Fleury-Feith J, Monnet I, et al: Immunocytochemical characterization of cell lines from human malignant mesothelioma. *Hum Pathol* 25:227–234, 1994.

APPENDIXES

APPENDIX A

RESPIRATORY QUESTIONNAIRE

Name _____ Social Security no. _____ Date _____

Plant _____ Sex _____ Date of birth _____ Age _____

Questionnaire administered by _____

I. Occupational history: Please list entire work history, starting with present job and going back to first job. (Use extra sheet if necessary.)

Industry (or company) and location	From	To	Specific job

	Yes	No	Number of years
A. Have you ever worked in a dusty job?			
1. In a mine?			
2. In a quarry?			
3. In a foundry?			
4. In a pottery?			
5. In a cotton, flax, or hemp mill?			
6. With asbestos?			
7. In a brick plant?			
8. As a sandblaster?			
9. In the manufacture of glass, ceramics, or abrasives?			
10. In other dusty jobs? Specify_____			
B. Have your ever worked with chemicals?			
1. Solvents? Specify_____			
2. Acids? Specify_____			
3. Lead?			
4. Plastics? Specify_____			
5. TDI?			

	Yes	No

II. Previous illnesses

A. Have you ever had any of the following problems?

1. Asthma? . . . .

2. Emphysema? . . . .

3. Chronic bronchitis? . . . .

4. Pneumonia? . . . .

5. Tuberculosis? . . . .

6. Pleurisy? . . . .

7. Heart trouble of any type? . . . .

B. Have you ever had surgery on your chest or lungs? . . . .

    If yes, specify. _____

    _____

C. Chest x-rays

    Last one (date) _____

    Ever abnormal? . . . .

D. Tuberculosis skin test

    Last one (date) _____

    Positive? . . . .

III. Symptoms

A. Cough

1. Do you usually cough first thing in the morning? . . . .

2. Do you usually cough at other times during the day or night? . . . .

Skip 3 to 6 if answer to 1 and 2 is "no." Answer if "yes."

3. Do you cough on most days for as much as 3 months of the year? . . . .

4. For how many years have you had this cough?

    Less than 2 years _____

    2 to 5 years _____

    5 years or more _____

5. Do you cough more on any particular day of the week? . . . .

    If yes, which day? _____

6. Do you cough during any particular season of the year? . . . .

    If yes, which season? _____

B. Sputum

1. Do you usually bring up phlegm, sputum, or mucus from your chest first thing in the morning? . . . .

2. Do you usually bring up phlegm, sputum, or mucus from your chest at other times of the day or night? . . . .

Skip 3 and 4 if answer to 1 and 2 is "no." Answer if "yes."

3. Do you bring up phlegm, sputum, or mucus from your chest on most days for as much as 3 months of the year? . . . .

4. For how many years have you raised phlegm, sputum, or mucus from your chest?

    Less than 2 years _____

    2 to 5 years _____

    5 years or more _____

C. Wheezing

1. Does your breathing ever sound wheezy? . . . .

2. Have you ever had attacks of shortness of breath with wheezing? . . . .

3. Have you ever had a feeling of tightness in your chest? . . . .

Skip 4 to 6 if answer to 1, 2, and 3 is "no." Answer if "yes."

4. At what age did wheezing first occur? _____

5. How frequently does wheezing occur?

    Daily _____

    Nightly _____

    A few times per week _____

	Yes	No

A few times per month _____

A few times per year _____

6. Is it worse on any particular day of the week?

What day? _____

D. Breathlessness

1. Do you get short of breath when walking on level ground? . . . .

2. Do you get short of breath while walking up stairs? . . . .

3. How many flights of stairs can you climb up without stopping?

1 to 2? _____

2 to 3? _____

More than 3? _____

E. Hemoptysis

1. Have you ever coughed up blood from your chest? If yes, when
was the last time this happened? _____ . . . .

IV. Smoking

A. Smoking (currently)

1. Do you now smoke regularly (cigarettes, pipe, cigars)? . . . .

Skip 2 to 6 if answer
to 1 is "no." Answer if
"yes."

2. How old were you when you started smoking?

_____

3. For how many years have you smoked regularly?

_____

4. How many cigarettes do you now smoke each day?

_____

5. How much pipe tobacco do you now smoke each week?

_____

6. How many cigars do you now smoke each day?

_____

B. Smoking (formerly)

1. Have you ever smoked regularly? . . . .

Skip 2 to 7 if answer
to 1 is "no." Answer if
"yes."

2. How old were you when you started smoking regularly?

_____

3. For how many years did you smoke regularly?

_____

4. When did you quit smoking?

Month _____

Year _____

5. How many cigarettes did you usually smoke per day?

_____

6. How much pipe tobacco did you usually smoke per week?

_____

7. How many cigars did you usually smoke per day?

_____

V. Additional comments

NORMAL VALUES

TYPICAL VALUES FOR A 20-YEAR-OLD SEATED MAN*

Ventilation (BTPS)

Tidal volume, L	0.6
Frequency, breaths/min	12
Minute volume, L/min	7.2
Respiratory dead space, ml	150
Alveolar ventilation, L/min	5.4

Lung Volumes and Capacities (BTPS)

Inspiratory capacity (IC), L	3.0
Expiratory reserve volume (ERV), L	1.9
Vital capacity (VC), L	4.9
Residual volume (RV), L	1.4
Functional residual capacity (FRC), L	3.2
Total lung capacity (TLC), L	6.3
Residual volume/total lung capacity $\times 100$ (RV/TLC,%)	22

Mechanics of Breathing

Forced vital capacity (FVC), L	4.9
Forced expiratory volume, first second (FEV_1), L	4.0
Maximum voluntary ventilation (MVV), L/min	170
Forced expiratory volume in 1 s/forced vital capacity $\times 100\%$ (FEV_1/FVC,%)	83
Forced expiratory volume in 3 s/forced vital capacity $\times 100\%$ (FEV_3/FVC,%)	97
Forced expiratory flow during middle half of FVC (FEF_{25-75}), L/s	4.7
Forced inspiratory flow at the middle of FIVC (FIF_{50}), L/s	5.0
Static compliance of the lungs (Cst, L), L/cm H_2O	0.2
Compliance of lungs and thoracic cage, L/cm H_2O	0.1
Airway resistance at FRC (Raw), cm H_2O/L/s	1.5
Pulmonary resistance at FRC, cm H_2O/L/s	2.0
Airway conductance at FRC (Gaw), L/s/cm H_2O	0.66
Specific conductance (Gaw/V_L)	0.22
Work of quiet breathing, (kg · m)/min	0.5
Maximum work of breathing, (kg · m)/breath	10
Maximum inspiratory pressure, mmHg	−75
Maximum expiratory pressure, mmHg	120

Distribution of Inspired Gas

Single-breath N_2 test (ΔN_2 from 750 to 1250 ml in expired gas), % N_2	<1.5
Alveolar N_2 after 7 min of breathing O_2, % N_2	<2.5
Closing volume (CV), ml	400
CV/VC $\times 100\%$	8
Closing capacity (CC), ml	1900

CC/TLC $\times 100\%$	30
Slope of phase III in single-breath N_2 test, % N_2/L	<2

Gas Exchange

O_2 consumption at rest (STPD), ml/min	240
CO_2 output at rest (STPD), ml/min	192
Respiratory exchange ratio (R), CO_2 output/O_2 uptake	0.8

ALVEOLAR GAS

$P_{A_{O_2}}$, mmHg	105
$P_{A_{CO_2}}$, mmHg	40

ARTERIAL BLOOD

Pa_{O_2}, mmHg	95
Sa_{O_2}, %	98
pH	7.41
Pa_{CO_2}, mmHg	40
Pa_{O_2}, while breathing 100% O_2, mmHg	640

Alveolar Ventilation

Alveolar ventilation, L/min	4.2
Physiological dead space/tidal volume $\times 100$ (V_D/V_T, %)	<30
Alveolar-arterial P_{O_2}, P(A-a)$_{O_2}$, mmHg	<10

Diffusing Capacity

Diffusing capacity at rest for CO, single-breath ($DL_{CO_{sb}}$), ml CO/min/mmHg	29
Diffusing capacity per unit alveolar volume (DL/VA)	4.8

Control of Ventilation

Ventilatory response to hypercapnia, L/min/per Δ Pa_{CO_2} mmHg	>0.5
Ventilatory response to hypoxia, L/min per ΔS_{O_2} (%)	>0.2
Arterial blood P_{O_2} during moderate exercise, mmHg	95

Pulmonary Hemodynamics

Pulmonary blood flow (cardiac output), L/min	5.4
Pulmonary artery pressure, systolic/diastolic, mmHg	25/8
Pulmonary capillary blood volume, ml	100
Pulmonary "capillary" blood pressure (wedge), mmHg	<10

*Height = 165 cm; weight = 64 kg; body surface area = 1.7 m².

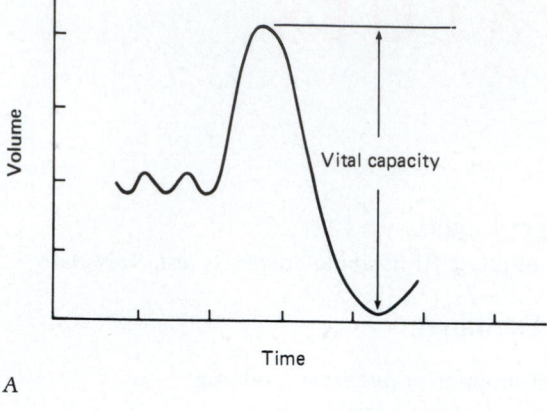

A

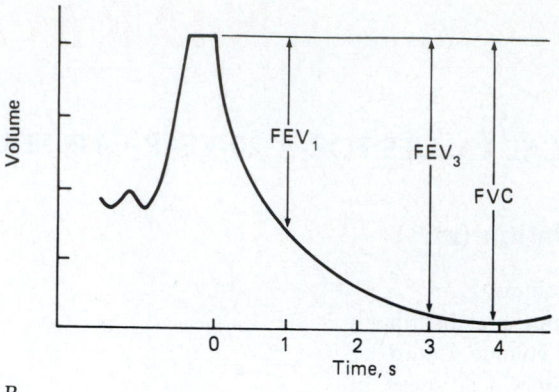

B

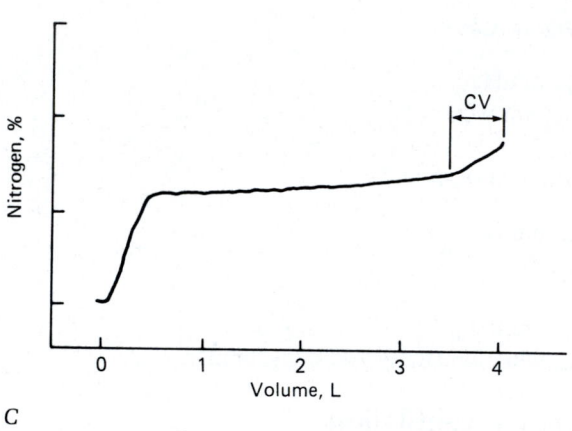

C

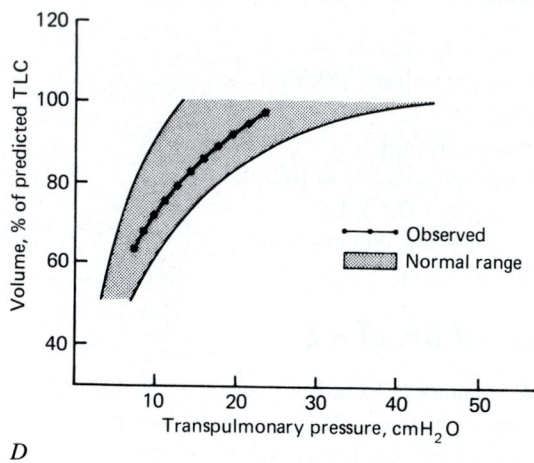

D

Figure B-1. Representative tracings and graphs commonly used in assessing pulmonary function. *A*. Lung volumes (vital capacity). *B*. Mechanics of breathing (forced expiratory volumes). *C*. Distribution of inspired gas (closing volumes). *D*. Mechanics of breathing (compliance of lungs).

APPENDIX C

TERMS AND SYMBOLS IN RESPIRATORY PHYSIOLOGY

GENERAL SYMBOLS

P
: Partial pressure in blood or gas.
  P_{O_2} = partial pressure of O_2

$\overline{X}$
: A bar over the symbol indicates a mean value.
  $\overline{P}$ = mean pressure, as distinct from instantaneous pressure

$\dot{X}$
: A time derivative (rate) is indicated by a dot above the symbol.
  $\dot{V}_{O_2}$ = O_2 consumption per minute
  $\dot{V}_{CO_2}$ = CO_2 production per minute

% X
: Percent sign preceding a symbol indicates percentage of the predicted normal value.

X/Y%
: Percent sign following a symbol indicates a ratio function with the ratio expressed as a percentage. Both components of the ratio must be designated.
  FEV_1/FVC, % = 100 × FEV_1/FVC

X_A, Xa
: A small capital letter or a lower-case letter on the same line following a primary symbol is a qualifier to further define the primary symbol. Alternatively, subscript letters may be used.
  $X_A = X_A$, $Xa = X_a$

$P_{E_{CO_2}}$
: Additional qualifiers of the primary symbol may be identified as shown.

GAS PHASE SYMBOLS

PRIMARY SYMBOLS

V
: Volume of gas.

$\dot{V}$
: Flow of gas.

F
: Fractional concentration of a gas.

Qualifying Symbols

I
: Inspired.
  V_I = inspired volume

E
: Expired.
  V_E = expired volume

A
: Alveolar.
  V_A = alveolar volume
  $\dot{V}_A$ = alveolar ventilation per minute

T
: Tidal.
  V_T = tidal volume

D
: Dead space.
  V_D = volume of dead space
  $\dot{V}_D$ = dead-space ventilation per minute

B
: Barometric.
  P_B = barometric pressure

STPD
: Standard conditions: temperature 0°C, pressure 760 mmHg, and dry (0 mmHg water vapor).

BTPS
: Body conditions: body temperature and ambient pressure, saturated with water vapor at these conditions.

ATPD
: Ambient temperature and pressure, dry.

ATPS
: Ambient temperature and pressure, saturated with water vapor at these conditions.

an	Anatomic.
p	Physiological.
f	Respiratory frequency, per minute.
max	Maximum.
t	Time.

BLOOD PHASE SYMBOLS

Primary Symbols

Q	Volume of blood.
$\dot{Q}$	Blood flow.
	$\dot{Q}$ = cardiac output, L/min
C	Concentration in the blood phase.
	C_{N_2} = concentration of N_2 in blood, ml of N_2 per 100 ml of blood
S	Saturation in the blood phase.
	S_{O_2} = saturation of hemoglobin with O_2, percent

Qualifying Symbols

a	Arterial.
	Ca_{O_2} = concentration of O_2 in arterial blood, ml of O_2 per 100 ml of blood
c	Capillary.
	Cc_{O_2} = concentration of O_2 in capillary blood, ml of O_2 per 100 ml of blood
c′	Pulmonary end-capillary.
	Pc'_{CO_2} = partial pressure of CO_2 in end-capillary blood, mmHg
v	Venous.
	Cv_{O_2} = concentration of O_2 in venous blood, ml of O_2 per 100 ml of blood
$\bar{v}$	Mixed venous.
	$C\bar{v}_{O_2}$ = concentration of O_2 in mixed venous blood, ml of O_2 per 100 ml of blood

VENTILATION AND LUNG MECHANICS TESTS AND SYMBOLS

Static Lung Volumes*

PRIMARY COMPARTMENTS

RV	Residual volume. Volume of air remaining in the lungs after maximum expiration.
CV	Closing volume. Volume of air expired from the onset of airways closure to residual volume. May be expressed as a fraction of VC: CV/VC,%.
ERV	Expiratory reserve volume. Maximum volume of air expired from the resting end-expiratory level.
V_T	Tidal volume. Volume of air inspired or expired with each breath during quiet breathing. When tidal volume is used in gas-exchange formulations, this symbol is used. When indicating a subdivision of lung volumes, the symbol TV may be used.
IRV	Inspiratory reserve volume. Maximum volume of air inspired from the end-tidal inspiratory level.

Lung Capacities†

IC	Inspiratory capacity. The sum of IRV and TV.
IVC	Inspiratory vital capacity. Maximum volume of air inspired from the point of maximum expiration.
VC	Vital capacity. Maximum volume of air expired from the point of maximum inspiration.
FRC	Functional residual capacity. Sum of RV and ERV. FRC is the volume of air remaining in the lungs at the resting end-expiratory position.
TLC	Total lung capacity. Volume of air in the lungs after maximum inspiration. Also, the sum of all volume compartments of the lungs.
RV/TLC,%	Residual volume to total lung capacity ratio, expressed as a percentage.
CC	Closing capacity. Closing volume plus residual volume, may be expressed as a ratio of TLC: CC/TLC,%.

*Expressed at BTPS.
†Combinations of volumes for practical purposes.

Forced Respiratory Maneuvers During Spirometry*

FVC	Forced vital capacity. The maximum volume of air forcibly expired from total lung capacity.
FIVC	Forced inspiratory vital capacity. Maximum volume of air forcibly inspired starting from residual volume.
FEV_t	Timed forced expiratory volume. Volume of air expired in a specified time in the course of the forced vital capacity maneuver.
	FEV_1 = volume of air expired during the first second of the FVC
FEV_t/FVC, %	Ratio of time forced expiratory volume to forced vital capacity, expressed as a percentage.
FEF_x	Forced expiratory flow, related to some portion of the FVC curve. Modifiers refer to the amount of the FVC that has been expired at the time of measurement.
$FEF_{200\text{-}1200}$	Forced expiratory flow between 200 and 1200 ml of the FVC (formerly called the maximum expiratory flow rate).
$FEF_{25\text{-}75}$	Forced expiratory flow during middle half of the FVC (formerly called the maximum midexpiratory flow rate).
PEF	Peak expiratory flow. Highest value for expiratory flow.
$\dot{V}max_x$	Maximum flow when x percent of the FVC has been expired.
	$\dot{V}max_{75}$ = flow (instantaneous) when 75 percent of the FVC has been expired
FIF_x	Forced inspiratory flow. As in the case of the FEF, appropriate modifiers designate the volume at which flow is being measured. Unless otherwise specified, the volume qualifiers indicate the volume inspired from RV at the point of measurement.
	$FIF_{25\text{-}75}$ = forced inspiratory flow during the middle half of the FIVC
$I\dot{V}max_x$	Maximum inspiratory flow (instantaneous) when x percent of the FIVC has been inspired.
MVV	Maximum voluntary ventilation. Volume of air exhaled during maximum breathing efforts within a specified time period. Formerly called maximum breathing capacity. If breathing frequency is set by the examiner, it is indicated by the qualifier.
	MVV_{60} = MVV at a breathing frequency of 60 per minute

Measurements Related to Ventilation

$\dot{V}_E$	Expired volume per minute (BTPS).
$\dot{V}_I$	Inspired volume per minute (BTPS).
$\dot{V}_{CO_2}$	Carbon dioxide production per minute (STPD).
$\dot{V}_{O_2}$	Oxygen consumption per minute (STPD).
R	Respiratory exchange ratio, the ratio of CO_2 output to O_2 intake in the lungs.
$\dot{V}_A$	Alveolar ventilation per minute (BTPS).
$\dot{V}_D$	Ventilation per minute of the physiological dead space (BTPS) defined by the equation

$$\dot{V}_D = \dot{V}_E \frac{Pa_{CO_2} - P_{E_{CO_2}}}{Pa_{CO_2} - P_{I_{CO_2}}}$$

V_D	Volume of the physiological dead space, calculated as $\dot{V}_D/f$.
$\dot{V}_{D_{an}}$	Ventilation per minute of the anatomic dead space, that portion of the conducting airway in which no significant gas exchange occurs (BTPS).
$V_{D_{an}}$	Volume of the anatomic dead space (BTPS).

Mechanics of Breathing†

PRESSURE TERMS

Paw	Pressure at any point along the airways.
Pao	Pressure at the airway opening.
Ppl	Pleural pressure.
P_A	Alveolar pressure.
Pbs	Pressure at the body surface.
Pes	Esophageal pressure: used to estimate Ppl.
P_A–Pbs	Transthoracic pressure.
P_A–Ppl	Transpulmonary pressure.
Ppl–Pbs	Pressure difference across the chest wall.
Paw–Ppl	Transbronchial pressure, estimated as difference between airway and pleural pressures.

*All values at BTPS.
†All pressures expressed relative to ambient pressure unless otherwise specified.

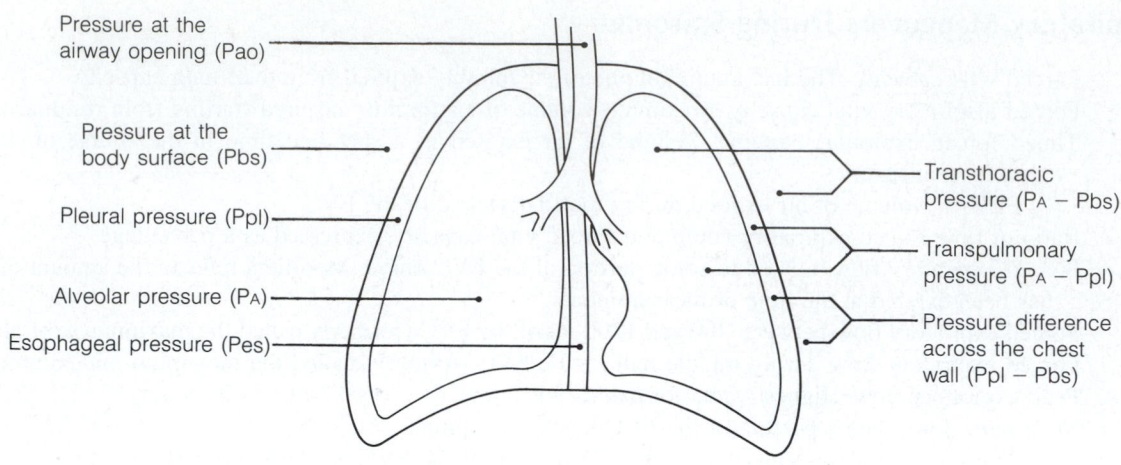

FLOW-PRESSURE RELATIONSHIPS*

R	General symbol for frictional resistance, defined as the ratio of pressure difference to flow.
Raw	Airway resistance, calculated from pressure difference between airway opening (Pao) and alveoli (PA) divided by the airflow, cm H_2O/L/s.
RL	Total pulmonary resistance, measured by relating flow-dependent transpulmonary pressure to airflow at the mouth.
Rti	Tissue resistance (viscous resistance of lung tissue), calculated as difference between RL and Raw.
Rus	Resistance of the airways on the upstream (alveolar) side of the point in the airways where intraluminal pressure equals Ppl, i.e., equal pressure point. Measured during a forced expiration.
Rds	Resistance of the airways on the downstream (mouth) side of the point in the airways where intraluminal pressure equals Ppl, i.e., equal pressure point. Measured during a forced expiration.
Gaw	Airway conductance, reciprocal of Raw.
Gaw/VL	Specific conductance, airway conductance, expressed per liter of lung volume at which Gaw is measured.
$\dot{W}$	Rate of work or power. Expressed either in kpm/min or J/s (watt).

VOLUME-PRESSURE RELATIONSHIPS

C	General symbol for compliance of the lungs, chest wall, or total respiratory system. Volume change per unit change in applied pressure. For the lungs, the applied pressure is the pressure difference across the lungs, or transpulmonary pressure, Pao–Ppl; for the chest wall, the applied pressure is the transthoracic pressure, Ppl–Pbs; for the entire respiratory system, the applied pressure is Pao–Pbs.
Cdyn	Dynamic compliance. Value for compliance determined at time of zero gas flow at the mouth during uninterrupted breathing. The respiratory frequency appears as a qualifier. $Cdyn_{40}$ = dynamic compliance at a respiratory frequency of 40 per minute
Cst	Static compliance, value for compliance determined on the basis of measurements made during a period of zero airflow.
C/VL	Specific compliance. Compliance divided by the lung volume at which it is determined, usually FRC.
Pst	Static pulmonary pressure at a specified lung volume. Pst_{TLC} = static recoil pressure of the lung measured at TLC (maximum recoil pressure)
W	Mechanical work of breathing.

DIFFUSING CAPACITY TESTS AND SYMBOLS

DL_x, D_x	Diffusing capacity of the lung expressed as volume (STPD) of gas (x) uptake per minute per unit alveolar-capillary pressure difference for the gas used. A modifier can be used to designate the technique:
	      $DL_{CO/sb}$ = single-breath CO diffusing capacity
	      $DL_{CO/ss}$ = steady-state CO diffusing capacity

DM	Diffusing capacity of the alveolar-capillary membrane (STPD).

*Unless otherwise specified, all resistance measurements assumed to be made at FRC.

θ Reaction rate coefficient for red blood cells. Determined as the volume of gas (STPD) that will combine per minute with 1 unit volume of blood per unit of gas tension. If the specific gas is not stated, θ is assumed to refer to CO and is a function of existing O_2 tension.

Vc   Capillary blood volume. This should be Qc for consistency with other symbols, but Vc is entrenched in the literature. In the equation that follows for 1/DL, Vc represents the effective pulmonary capillary blood volume, i.e., capillary blood volume in intimate association with alveolar gas.

1/DL   Total resistance to diffusion, including resistance to diffusion of test gas across the alveolar-capillary membrane, through plasma in the capillary, and across the red blood cell membrane (1/DM), the resistance to diffusion with the red cell arising from the chemical reaction of the test gas and hemoglobin (1/θVc), according to the formulation

$$\frac{1}{D_L} = \frac{1}{D_M} + \frac{1}{\theta V_c}$$

DL/VA   Diffusing capacity per unit of alveolar volume. DL is expressed STPD, and VA is expressed in liters, BTPS.

BLOOD GAS SYMBOLS

Symbols for these values are readily composed by combining general symbols. Some examples include the following.

Pa_{CO_2} Arterial CO_2 tension, mmHg.

Sa_{O_2} Arterial O_2 saturation, percent.

Cc'_{O_2} Oxygen content of pulmonary end-capillary blood, ml of O_2 per 100 ml of blood.

$PA_{O_2} - Pa_{O_2}$
$P(A\text{-}a)_{O_2}$ Alveolar-arterial difference in the partial pressure of O_2, mmHg.

$Ca_{O_2} - C\overline{v}_{O_2}$ O_2 content difference between arterial and mixed venous blood (arteriovenous O_2 difference), ml of O_2 per 100 ml of blood.

PULMONARY SHUNT SYMBOLS

$\dot{Q}s$ Flow of blood via shunts. This is usually determined as percent of cardiac output ($\dot{Q}$) while breathing 100% O_2, according to the equation

$$\frac{\dot{Q}s}{\dot{Q}} = \frac{Cc' - Ca}{Cc' - C\overline{v}},$$

where

$$\frac{\dot{Q}s}{\dot{Q}} = \text{"anatomic" venous admixture}$$

and

$Cc'_{O_2} = O_2$ content of end-capillary blood
$Ca_{O_2} = O_2$ content of arterial blood
$C\overline{v}_{O_2} = O_2$ content of mixed venous blood

INDEX

Index

Page numbers followed by *f* indicate figures; page numbers followed by *t* indicate tables.

ISBN 0-07-911167-X

ISBN 0-07-021179-5